How to use this book

This book provides information about prescription and over-the-counter medicines. It is written in everyday language, making it a valuable reference guide for consumers.

On this page, you'll find general information about how to use this book. An illustration showing how the listings of closely related medicines are organized appears on the back of this page.

About the entries

The drug entries are arranged alphabetically like an encyclopedia. ***If you already know what entry the drug belongs to,*** you can turn directly to it.

If you know only the drug's generic or brand name, the best way to find your information is to use the index at the back of this book. It will tell you what entry includes that drug and the page number it starts on.

For more information

For general guidelines about medicines, see *To the Reader* (page v), which also discusses this book's content and USP in depth. In addition to the entries, this book has a glossary with over 400 medical terms plus the following supplemental appendixes:

- ***Appendix 1*** *Combination Chemotherapy,*
- ***Appendix 2*** *Additional Monographs,*
- ***Appendix 3*** *Additional Products and Uses,*
- ***Appendix 4*** *Pictograms,*
- ***Appendix 5*** *Categories of Use,*
- ***Appendix 6*** *The Medicine Chart,*
- ***Appendix 7*** *Pregnancy Precaution Listing,*
- ***Appendix 8*** *Breast-feeding Precaution Listing, and*
- ***Appendix 9*** *Athletes Precautions.*

See illustration on the back of this page.

Sample entry

Title section: lists the drug's commonly used brand names in both the United States and Canada.

Precautions: tells you what to avoid or be careful of when using the drug and when medical supervision is required.

Proper use of this medicine: tells how to store and use the drug, including information such as what to do if you miss a dose.

Additional information: gives details about other uses that are not shown in the product labeling.

included in product labeling, clofibrate is used in certa patients with the following medical condition:
• Certain types of diabetes insipidus (water diabetes)

Other than the above information, there is no additional information relating to proper use, precautions, or side effects for this use.

Annual revision: 07/26/91

CLOMIPHENE Systemic

Some commonly used brand names are:

In the U.S.
Clomid — Serophene
Milophene

In Canada
Clomi — Serophene

Another com ly used name is clomifene.

Description

Clomip (KLOE-mi-feen) is used as a fertili medicine i ome women who are unable to become pre nant.

Clomiphene probably works by changing the hormo balance of the body. In women, this causes ovulation occur and prepares the body for pregnancy.

Clomiphene may also be used for other conditions both females and males as determined by your doctor.

The following information applies only to female p tients taking clomiphene. Check with your doctor if y are a male and have any questions about the use of cl miphene.

Clomiphene is available only with your doctor's pr scription, in the following dosage form:

Oral
• Tablets (U.S. and Canada)

It is very important that you read and understand t following information. If any of it causes you special co cern, do not decide against using this medicine witho first checking with your doctor. Also, **if you have a questions** or if you want more information about this me icine or your medical problem, **ask your doctor, nurse, rmacist.**

Before Using This Medicine

eciding to use a medicine, the risks of taking t icine must be weighed against the good it will d his is a decision you and your doctor will make. F clomiphene, the following should be considered:

Allergies—Tell your doctor if you have ever had any unusual or allergic reaction to clomiphene. Also tell your doctor and pharmacist if you are allergic to any other substances, such as foods, preservatives, or dyes.

Pregnancy—There is a chance that clomiphene may cause birth defects if it is taken after you become pregnant. **Stop taking this medicine and tell your doctor immediately if you think you have become pregnant** while still taking clomiphene.

If you become pregnant as a result of using this medicine, there is a chance of a multiple birth (for example, twins, triplets) occurring.

Other medical problems—The presence of other medical problems may affect the use of clomiphene. Make sure you tell your doctor if you have any other medical problems, especially:
• Cyst on ovary—Clomiphene may cause the cyst to increase in size
• Endometriosis—Inducing ovulation (including using clomiphene) may worsen endometriosis because the body estrogen level is increased; estrogen can cause growth of endometriosis implants
• Fibroid tumors of the uterus—Clomiphene may cause fibroid tumors to increase in size
• Inflamed veins due to blood clots
• Liver disease (or history of)
• Mental depression
• Unusual vaginal bleeding—Some irregular vaginal bleeding is a sign that the lining of the uterus is growing too much or is a sign of cancer of the uterus lining; these problems must be ruled out before clomiphene is used because clomiphene can make these conditions worse

Other medicines—Although certain medicines should not be used together at all, in other cases two different medicines may be used together even if an interaction might occur. In these cases, your doctor may want to change the dose, or other precautions may be necessary. When you are taking clomiphene, it is especially important that your doctor and pharmacist know if you are taking any other prescription or nonprescription (over-the-counter [OTC]) medicine.

Before you begin using any new medicine (prescription or nonprescription) or if you develop any new medical problem while you are using this medicine, check with your ctor, nurse, or pharmacist.

Proper Use of This Medicine

ke this medicine only as directed by your doctor. If are to begin on Day 5, count the first day of your menstrual period as Day 1. Beginning on Day 5, take the correct dose every day for as many days as your doctor

ordered. To help you to remember to take your dose of medicine, take it at the same time every day.

If you miss a dose of this medicine, take it as soon as possible. If you do not remember until it is time for the next dose, take both doses together; then go back to your regular dosing schedule. If you miss more than one dose, check with your doctor.

To store this medicine:
• Keep out of the reach of children.
• Store away from heat and direct light.
• Do not store in the bathroom, near the kitchen sink, or in other damp places. Heat or moisture may cause the medicine to break down.
• Do not keep outdated medicine or medicine no longer needed. Be sure that any discarded medicine is out of the reach of children.

Precautions While Using This Medicine

It is very important that your doctor check your progress at regular visits to make sure this medicine is working and to check for unwanted effects.

At certain times in your menstrual cycle, your doctor may want you to use an ovulation prediction test kit. **Follow your doctor's instructions carefully.** Ovulation is controlled by luteinizing hormone (LH). LH is present in the blood and urine in very small amounts during most of the menstrual cycle but rises suddenly for a short time in the middle of the menstrual cycle. This sharp rise, the LH surge, usually causes ovulation within about 30 hours. A woman is most likely to become pregnant if she has intercourse within the 24 hours after detecting the LH surge. Ovulation prediction test kits are used to test for this large amount of LH in the urine. This method is better for predicting ovulation than measuring daily basal body temperature. It is important that intercourse take place at the correct time to give you the best chance of becoming pregnant.

There is a chance that clomiphene may cause birth defects if it is taken after you become pregnant. **Stop taking this medicine and tell your doctor immediately if you think you have become pregnant** while still taking clomiphene.

This medicine may cause blurred vision, difficulty in reading, or other changes in vision. It may also cause some people to become dizzy or lightheaded. **Make sure you know how you react to this medicine before you drive, use machines, or do anything else that could be dangerous if you are not clear-headed or able to see well.** If these reactions are especially bothersome, check with your doc-

Side Effects of This Medicine

ong with its needed effects, a medicine may cause ne unwanted effects. Although not all of these side effects may occur, if they do occur they may need medical attention.

When this medicine is used for a short time at low doses, serious side effects usually are rare. **However, check with your doctor immediately** if any of the following side effects occur:

More common
Bloating
Stomach or pelvic pain

Less common or rare
Shortness of breath (sudden)

Check with your doctor as soon as possible if any of the following side effects occur:

Less common or rare
Blurred vision
Decreased or double vision or other vision problems
Sensitivity of eyes to light
Yellow eyes or skin

Other side effects may occur that usually do not need medical attention. These side effects may go away during treatment as your body adjusts to the medicine. However, check with your doctor if any of the following side effects continue or are bothersome:

More common
Hot flashes

Less common or rare
Breast discomfort
Dizziness or lightheadedness
Headache
Heavy menstrual periods or bleeding between periods
Mental depression
Nausea or vomiting
Nervousness
Restlessness or trouble in sleeping
Tiredness

Other side effects not listed above may also occur in som patients. If you notice any other effects, check with you ctor.

Additional Information

medicine has been approved for marketing for a c in use, experience may show that it is also useful for other medical problems. Although not specifically included in product labeling, clomiphene is used in certain patients with the following medical conditions:
• Male infertility caused by low production of sperm
• Certain problems of the male sexual organs caused by pituitary or hypothalamus gland problems (diagnosis)

For males taking this medicine for treatment of infertility caused by low sperm production:
• To decide on the best treatment for your medical problem, your doctor should be told:
—if you have ever had any unusual or allergic reaction to clomiphene.
—if you have either of the following medical problems:
Liver disease
Mental depression

Before using this medicine: explains what you and your health care professional should consider in advance, such as allergies and special diet restrictions.

Side effects: lists both common and rare side effects of the drug and whether they require medical attention.

Description: tells how to pronounce the drug's name, what the drug is used for, what dosage forms are available, and if a doctor must prescribe the drug.

Turn to the last page for the new "Fast-finder" subject guide.

COMPLETE DRUG REFERENCE

1994 Edition

United States Pharmacopeia

Consumer Reports Books
A Division of Consumers Union

Yonkers, New York

Library of Congress Catalog Card Number: 81-640842
ISBN: 0-89043-677-0

First printing, November 1993

Manufactured in the United States of America

Published simultaneously by USPC, Inc., under the title *USP DI, Volume II (Advice for the Patient)*, Fourteenth Edition, 1994. Previous editions of this book appeared under the title *United States Pharmacopeia Drug Information for the Consumer*.

Complete Drug Reference, 1994 Edition, is a Consumer Reports Book published by Consumers Union, the nonprofit organization that publishes *Consumer Reports*, the monthly magazine of test reports, product Ratings, and buying guidance. Established in 1936, Consumers Union is chartered under the Not-For-Profit Corporation Law of the State of New York.

The purposes of Consumers Union, as stated in its charter, are to provide consumers with information and counsel on consumer goods and services, to give information on all matters relating to the expenditure of the family income, and to initiate and to cooperate with individual and group efforts seeking to create and maintain decent living standards.

Consumers Union derives its income solely from the sale of *Consumer Reports* and other publications. In addition, expenses of occasional public service efforts may be met, in part, by nonrestrictive, noncommercial contributions, grants, and fees. Consumers Union accepts no advertising or product samples and is not beholden in any way to any commercial interest. Its Ratings and reports are solely for the use of the readers of its publications. Neither the Ratings nor the reports nor any Consumers Union publications, including this book, may be used in advertising or for any commercial purpose. Consumers Union will take all steps open to it to prevent such uses of its material, its name, or the name of *Consumer Reports*.

NOTICE AND WARNING

Concerning U. S. Patent or Trademark Rights

The inclusion in *Complete Drug Reference* of entry on any drug in respect to which patent or trademark rights may exist shall not be deemed, and is not intended as, a grant of, or authority to exercise, any right or privilege protected by such patent or trademark. All such rights and privileges are vested in the patent or trademark owner, and no other person may exercise the same without express permission, authority, or license secured from such patent or trademark owner.

The listing of selected brand names is intended only for ease of reference. The inclusion of a brand name does not mean the USPC or Consumers Union has any particular knowledge that the brand listed has properties different from other brands of the same drug, nor should it be interpreted as an endorsement by the USPC or by Consumers Union. Similarly, the fact that a particular brand has not been included does not indicate that the product has been judged to be unsatisfactory or unacceptable.

For permission to copy or utilize portions of this text, address inquiries to the Secretary of the USPC Board of Trustees, 12601 Twinbrook Parkway, Rockville, Maryland 20852.

Turn to the last page for the new "Fast-finder" subject guide.

Contents

Complete Drug Reference

Foreword to the Consumer Reports Books Edition

For 174 years, the United States Pharmacopeia has set official standards of strength, quality, purity, packaging, and labeling for medical products in the United States. And for 58 years Consumers Union, through its magazine *Consumer Reports*, has served as this country's foremost source for authoritative, reliable, and unbiased product testing and buying guidance. It thus seems only natural that these two organizations, both dedicated to the consumer's well-being, should join forces to publish a layman's guide to prescription and over-the-counter drugs.

At one time or another, most of us find it necessary to use some type of medical drug. In fact, many people feel that medical treatment is only effective when it includes drug therapy. It's not surprising, then, that in 1993 it is estimated that Americans will spend $60.7 billion on prescription drugs, and another $11.4 billion on nonprescription drugs. Moreover, studies show that up to 50 percent of all prescriptions are taken incorrectly, and as many as 70 percent of all patients receive little or no counseling about drug usage, including, interactions with food or other drugs, and possible side effects. It is apparent that there is a grave need for a straightforward, objective guide to drugs that cautions and informs the consumer about the role of prescription drugs as a routine part of medical care.

Complete Drug Reference lists almost every medicine, prescription and nonprescription, available in the United States and Canada. It provides consumers with up-to-date information about drug usage and potential side effects. Organized alphabetically by generic or family name, each entry includes different dosage forms and common brand names—over 9,000 different brand and generic entries in all. It is well indexed according to both generic and brand names, making it easy to look up any medication. Most important, unlike other drug information books available to the consumer, notably the *Physicians' Desk Reference,* the information presented in this guide is not controlled by drug manufacturers or anyone connected with the drug industry. Rather, *Complete Drug Reference* is a consensus book put together by many experts—physicians, pharmacists, pharmacologists, dentists, nurses, chemists, microbiologists, and other individuals particularly qualified to judge drugs—and is supported by 33 advisory panels representing differing medical specialties, health professionals, and consumers. The guide is reviewed by so many experts that it is constantly in revision, with the result that it may contain the latest precautions and side effects of a particular drug before the information is readily available elsewhere.

We believe that the therapeutic use of drugs deserves much closer scrutiny by physicians, pharmacists, and patients than is usually the case. Even the exacting approval process undertaken by the Food and Drug Administration (FDA) cannot possibly guarantee that all drugs on the market are totally safe and effective. Post-marketing surveillance by physicians and patients should therefore be an integral part of drug usage. It is also important that patients report the side effects of drugs to their physicians and that the physicians relay that information to the FDA, if only so that future editions of *Complete Drug Reference* may reflect that new knowledge and experience.

The material contained in this book is presented in a direct, factual manner with a refreshing absence of editorial opinion or biased discussions about the relative merits of one drug over another. Each profile of a specific drug lists indications, proper usage, precautions, and side effects. The language is easily understood and targeted specifically to the patient. *Complete Drug Reference* is the most comprehensive drug information book available to the public, and we are proud to present it to our readers.

To The Reader

When purchasing a medicine, whether over-the-counter (nonprescription) or with a doctor's prescription, you may have questions about its usefulness to you, the best way to take it, possible side effects, and precautions to take to avoid complications. For instance, some medicines should be taken with meals, others between meals. Some may make you drowsy while others may tend to keep you awake. Alcoholic or other beverages, other medicines, certain foods, or smoking may affect the way your medicine works. As for side effects, some are merely bothersome and may go away while others may require medical attention.

Complete Drug Reference contains information which may provide general answers to some of your questions as well as suggestions for the correct use of your medicine. *It is important to remember, however, that the human body is very complex and medicines may act differently on different people—and even in the same person at different times. If you want additional information about your medicine or its possible side effects, ask your doctor, nurse, or pharmacist. They are there to help you.*

How to Use This Book:

Complete Drug Reference contains a section of general information about the correct use of any medicine, as well as individual discussions of a wide variety of commonly and not so commonly used medicines. *You should read both the general information and the information specific to the medicine you are taking.* See page xxv for this general information.

Each medicine has a generic name that all manufacturers who make that medicine must use. Some manufacturers also create a brand name to put on the label and to use in advertising. *Look in the index* for the generic name or the brand name of the medicine about which you have questions. We have put the generic names and common brand names in the same index, so you do not have to know whether the name you have is a generic name or a brand name. However, it is a good idea for you to learn both the generic and the brand names of the medicines you are using and even to write them down and keep them for future use.

Although the informational monographs generally appear in alphabetical order by generic name, there are numerous occasions when closely related medicines are grouped under a family name. Therefore, the surest way to find the page number of the information about each medicine is to *look in the index first*.

The information for each medicine is presented according to the area of the body which is affected. As a general rule, information for one type of use will not be the same as for other types of use. Thus, if you take tetracycline capsules by mouth for their systemic effect in treating an infection, the information will not be the same as for tetracycline ointment, which is applied directly to the skin for its topical effects. And both of these will be different from the information for tetracyclines used in the eye. The common divisions used in this publication are:

- *BUCCAL*—For general effects throughout the body when a medicine is placed in the cheek pocket and slowly absorbed.
- *DENTAL*—For local effects when applied to the teeth or gums.
- *INHALATION*—For local, and in some cases systemic, effects when inhaled into the lungs.
- *INTRA-AMNIOTIC*—For local effects when a medicine is injected into the sac that contains the fetus and amniotic fluid.
- *INTRACAVERNOSAL*—For local effects in the penis when a medicine is given by injection.
- *LINGUAL*—For general effects throughout the body when a medicine is absorbed through the lining of the mouth.
- *MUCOSAL*—For local effects when applied directly to mucous membranes (for example, the inside of the mouth).
- *NASAL*—For local effects when used in the nose.
- *OPHTHALMIC*—For local effects when applied directly to the eyes.
- *ORAL-LOCAL*—For local effects in the gastrointestinal tract when taken by mouth (i.e., not absorbed into the body).

- *OTIC*—For local effects when used in the ear.
- *PARENTERAL-LOCAL*—For local effects in a specific area of the body when given by injection.
- *RECTAL*—For local, and in some cases systemic, effects when used in the rectum.
- *SUBLINGUAL*—For general effects throughout the body when a medicine is placed under the tongue and slowly absorbed.
- *SYSTEMIC*—For general effects throughout the body; applies to most medicines when taken by mouth or given by injection.
- *TOPICAL*—For local effects when applied directly to the skin.
- *VAGINAL*—For local, and in some cases systemic, effects when used in the vagina.

Notice:

The information about the drugs contained herein is general in nature and is intended to be used in consultation with your health care providers. It is not intended to replace specific instructions or directions or warnings given to you by your physician or other prescriber or accompanying a particular product. The information is selective and it is not claimed that it includes all known precautions, contraindications, effects, or interactions possibly related to the use of a drug. The information may differ from that contained in the product labeling which is required by law. The information is not sufficient to make an evaluation as to the risks and benefits of taking a particular drug in a particular case and is not medical advice for individual problems and should not alone be relied upon for these purposes. Since the inclusion or exclusion of particular information about a drug is judgmental in nature and since opinion as to drug usage may differ, you may wish to consult additional sources. Should you desire additional information or if you have any questions as to how this information may relate to you in particular, ask your doctor, nurse, pharmacist, or other health care provider.

Since new drugs are constantly being marketed and since previously unreported side effects, newly recognized precautions, or other new information for any given drug may come to light at any time, continuously updated drug information sources should be consulted as necessary.

There are many brands of drugs on the market. The listing of selected brand names is intended only for ease of reference. The inclusion of a brand name does not mean the USPC or Consumers Union has any particular knowledge that the brand listed has properties different from other brands of the same drug, nor should it be interpreted as an endorsement by the USPC or Consumers Union. Similarly, the fact that a brand name has not been included does not indicate that that particular brand has been judged to be unsatisfactory or unacceptable.

If any of the information in this book causes you special concern, do not decide against taking any medicine prescribed for you without first checking with your doctor.

About USPC:

The information in this volume is prepared by the United States Pharmacopeial Convention, Inc. (USPC), the organization that sets the official standards of strength, quality, purity, packaging, and labeling for medical products used in the United States.

The United States Pharmacopeial Convention is an independent, not-for-profit corporation composed of delegates from the accredited colleges of medicine and pharmacy in the U.S.; state medical and pharmaceutical associations; many national associations concerned with medicines, such as the American Medical Association, the American Nurses Association, the American Dental Association, the National Association of Retail Druggists, and the American Pharmaceutical Association; and various departments of the federal government, including the Food and Drug Administration. In addition, four members of the Convention have been appointed by the Board of Trustees specifically to represent the public. USPC was established 174 years ago, and is the only national body that represents the professions of both pharmacy and medicine.

The first convention came into being on January 1, 1820, and within the year published the first national drug formulary of the United States. The *U.S. Pharmacopeia* of 1820 contained 217 drug names, divided into two groups according to the level of general acceptance and usage.

When Congress passed the first major drug safety law in 1906, the standards recognized by that statute were those set forth in the *United States Pharmacopeia* and in the *National Formulary*. Today, the *USP* and *NF* continue to be the official U.S. compendia for standards for drugs and for the inactive ingredients in drug dosage forms. The *United States Pharmacopeia* is the world's oldest regularly revised national pharmacopeia and is generally accepted as being the most influential.

The work of the USPC is carried out by the Committee of Revision. This committee of experts is elected by the Convention and currently consists of 114 outstanding physicians, pharmacists, dentists, nurses, chemists, microbiologists, and other individuals particularly qualified to judge the merits of drugs and the standards and information that should apply to them. Committee members serve without pay and are assisted by numerous advisory panels, other outside reviewers, and USPC staff.

The United States Pharmacopeial Convention 1990–1995

Officers

MARK NOVITCH, M.D.
President
Kalamazoo, MI

DONALD R. BENNETT, M.D., PH.D.
Vice-President
Chicago, IL

JOHN T. FAY, JR., PH.D.
Treasurer
San Clemente, CA

ARTHUR HULL HAYES, JR., M.D.
Past President
New Rochelle, NY

JEROME A. HALPERIN
Secretary
Rockville, MD

[1]At large.
[2]Representing pharmacy.
[3]Public member.
[4]Representing medicine.
[5]12601 Twinbrook Parkway, Rockville, MD 20852.
[6]Deceased.

General Committee of Revision

JEROME A. HALPERIN[5], *Executive Director, USPC, Chairman*

LEE T. GRADY, PH.D.[5], *Director, Drug Standards Division*

KEITH W. JOHNSON[5], *Director, Drug Information Division*

LOYD V. ALLEN, JR., PH.D.
Oklahoma City, OK

JERRY R. ALLISON, PH.D.
New Brunswick, NY

THOMAS J. AMBROSIO, PH.D.
Somerville, NJ

GREGORY E. AMIDON, PH.D.
Kalamazoo, MI

NORMAN W. ATWATER, PH.D.
Hopewell, NJ

HENRY L. AVALLONE, B.SC.
North Brunswick, NJ

LEONARD C. BAILEY, PH.D.
Piscataway, NJ

JOHN A. BELIS, M.D.
Hershey, PA

LESLIE Z. BENET, PH.D.
San Francisco, CA

JUDY P. BOEHLERT, PH.D.
Nutley, NJ

JAMES C. BOYLAN, PH.D.
Abbott Park, IL

LYNN R. BRADY, PH.D.[6]
(1990–1992)
Seattle, WA

R. EDWARD BRANSON, PH.D.
Beltsville, MD

WILLIAM H. BRINER, CAPT., B.S.
Durham, NC

STEPHEN R. BYRN, PH.D.
West Lafayette, IN

PETER R. BYRON, PH.D.
Richmond, VA

HERBERT S. CARLIN, D.SC.
Chappaqua, NY

DENNIS L. CASEY, PH.D.
Raritan, NJ

LESTER CHAFETZ, PH.D.
Kansas City, MO

VIRGINIA C. CHAMBERLAIN, PH.D.
Rockville, MD

WEI-WEI, CHANG, PH.D.
(1992–)
Morris Plains, NJ

MARY BETH CHENAULT, B.S.
Harrisonburg, VA

ZAK T. CHOWHAN, PH.D.
Palo Alto, CA

SEBASTIAN G. CIANCIO, D.D.S.
Buffalo, NY

MURRAY S. COOPER, PH.D.
Islamorada, FL

LLOYD E. DAVIS, PH.D., D.V.M.
Urbana, IL

LEON ELLENBOGEN, PH.D.
Clifton, NJ
R. MICHAEL ENZINGER, PH.D.
(1990–1992)
Kalamazoo, MI
CLYDE R. ERSKINE, B.S., M.B.A.
Newtown Square, PA
EDWARD A. FITZGERALD, PH.D.
Bethesda, MD
EVERETT FLANIGAN, PH.D.
Kankakee, IL
KLAUS G. FLOREY, PH.D.
Princeton, NJ
THOMAS S. FOSTER, PHARM.D.
Lexington, KY
JOSEPH F. GALLELLI, PH.D.
Bethesda, MD
ROBERT L. GARNICK, PH.D.
So. San Francisco, CA
DOUGLAS D. GLOVER, M.D., R.PH.
Morgantown, WV
ALAN M. GOLDBERG, PH.D.
Baltimore, MD
BURTON J. GOLDSTEIN, M.D.
Miami, FL
DENNIS K. J. GORECKI, PH.D.
Saskatoon, Saskatchewan, Canada
MICHAEL J. GROVES, PH.D.
Lake Forest, IL
ROBERT M. GUTHRIE, M.D.
Columbus, OH
SAMIR A. HANNA, PH.D.
Lawrenceville, NJ
STANLEY L. HEM, PH.D.
West Lafayette, IN
JOY HOCHSTADT, PH.D.
New York, NY
DAVID W. HUGHES, PH.D.
Nepean, Ontario, Canada
NORMAN C. JAMIESON, PH.D.
St. Louis, MO
RICHARD D. JOHNSON, PHARM.D., PH.D.
Kansas City, MO
JUDITH K. JONES, M.D., PH.D.
Arlington, VA
STANLEY A. KAPLAN, PH.D.
Baltimore, MD
HERBERT E. KAUFMAN, M.D.
New Orleans, LA
DONALD KAYE, M.D.
Philadelphia, PA
PAUL E. KENNEDY, PH.D.
West Conshohocken, PA
JAY S. KEYSTONE, M.D.
Toronto, Ontario, Canada
ROSALYN C. KING, PHARM.D., M.P.H.
Silver Spring, MD
GORDON L. KLEIN, M.D.
Galveston, TX
JOSEPH E. KNAPP, PH.D.
Pittsburgh, PA
JOHN B. LANDIS, PH.D.
(1990–1992)
Kalamazoo, MI
THOMAS P. LAYLOFF, PH.D.
St. Louis, MO
LEWIS J. LEESON, PH.D.
Summit, NJ
JOHN W. LEVCHUK, PH.D.
Rockville, MD
ROBERT D. LINDEMAN, M.D.
Albuquerque, NM
CHARLES H. LOCHMULLER, PH.D.
Durham, NC
EDWARD G. LOVERING, PH.D.
Ottawa, Ontario, Canada
CATHERINE M. MACLEOD, M.D.
Chicago, IL
CAROL S. MARCUS, PH.D., M.D.
Torrance, CA
THOMAS MEDWICK, PH.D.
Piscataway, NJ
ROBERT F. MORRISSEY, PH.D.
New Brunswick, NJ
TERRY E. MUNSON, B.S.
Fairfax, VA
HAROLD S. NELSON, M.D.
Denver, CO
WENDEL L. NELSON, PH.D.
Seattle, WA
MARIA I. NEW, M.D.
New York, NY
SHARON C. NORTHUP, PH.D.
Round Lake, IL
JEFFERY L. OTTO, PH.D.
(1992–)
Broomfield, CO
GARNET E. PECK, PH.D.
West Lafayette, IN
ROBERT V. PETERSEN, PH.D.
Salt Lake City, UT
ROSEMARY C. POLOMANO, R.N., M.S.N.
Philadelphia, PA
THOMAS P. REINDERS, PHARM.D.
Richmond, VA
CHRISTOPHER T. RHODES, PH.D.
West Kingston, RI
JOSEPH R. ROBINSON, PH.D.
Madison, WI
LARY A. ROBINSON, M.D.
Omaha, NE
DAVID B. ROLL, PH.D.
Salt Lake City, UT
THEODORE J. ROSEMAN, PH.D.
Round Lake, IL
SANFORD H. ROTH, M.D.
Phoenix, AZ
LEONARD P. RYBAK, M.D.
Springfield, IL
RONALD J. SAWCHUK, PH.D.
Minneapolis, MN
GORDON D. SCHIFF, M.D.
Chicago, IL
ANDREW J. SCHMITZ, JR., M.S.[6]
(1990–1992)
Huntington, NY
RALPH F. SHANGRAW, PH.D.
Baltimore, MD
ALBERT L. SHEFFER, M.D.
Boston, MA
ELI SHEFTER, PH.D.
San Diego, CA
ERIC B. SHEININ, PH.D.
Rockville, MD
ROBERT L. SIEGLE, M.D.
San Antonio, TX
EDWARD B. SILBERSTEIN, M.D.
Cincinnati, OH
JOSEPH E. SINSHEIMER, PH.D.
Ann Arbor, MI
MARILYN DIX SMITH, PH.D.
Dayton, NJ
BURTON E. SOBEL, M.D.
St. Louis, MO
E. JOHN STABA, PH.D.
Minneapolis, MN
ROBERT S. STERN, M.D.
Boston, MA

JAMES T. STEWART, PH.D.
Athens, GA
HENRY S. I. TAN, PH.D.
Cincinnati, OH
THEODORE G. TONG, PHARM.D.
Tucson, AZ
SALVATORE J. TURCO, PHARM.D.
Philadelphia, PA
CLARENCE T. UEDA, PHARM.D., PH.D.
Omaha, NE
ELIZABETH B. VADAS, PH.D.
Pointe Claire-Dorval, Quebec, Canada
HUIB J. M. VAN DE DONK, PH.D.
Bilthoven, The Netherlands
STANLEY VAN DEN NOORT, M.D.
Irvine, CA
VINCENT S. VENTURELLA, PH.D.
Murray Hill, NJ
ROBERT E. VESTAL, M.D.
Boise, ID
JAMES A. VISCONTI, PH.D.
Columbus, OH
EDWARD W. VOSS, JR., PH.D.
Urbana, IL
PHILIP D. WALSON, M.D.
Columbus, OH
PAUL F. WHITE, PH.D., M.D.
Dallas, TX
ROBERT G. WOLFANGEL, PH.D.
St. Louis, MO
MANFRED E. WOLFF, PH.D.
San Diego, CA
WESLEY E. WORKMAN, PH.D.
(1992–)
St. Louis, MO
LINDA R. WUHL, PH.D.
(1993–)
Thousand Oaks, CA
JOHN W. YARBRO, M.D., PH.D.
Springfield, IL
GEORGE ZOGRAFI, PH.D.
Madison, WI

Executive Committee of Revision (1992–1993)
JEROME A. HALPERIN, *Chairman*
NORMAN W. ATWATER, PH.D.
CLYDE R. ERSKINE (March 1, 1993–June 30, 1993)
BURTON J. GOLDSTEIN, M.D.
ROBERT V. PETERSEN, PH.D.
ANDREW J. SCHMITZ, JR.[6] (July 1, 1992–November 21, 1992)

ROBERT S. STERN, M.D.
PAUL F. WHITE, M.D.

Drug Information Division Executive Committee
HERBERT S. CARLIN, D.SC., *Chairman*
JAMES C. BOYLAN, PH.D.
SEBASTIAN G. CIANCIO, D.D.S.
LLOYD E. DAVIS, D.V.M., PH.D.
JAY S. KEYSTONE, M.D.
ROBERT D. LINDEMAN, M.D.
MARIA I. NEW, M.D.
ROSEMARY C. POLOMANO, R.N., M.S.N.
THOMAS P. REINDERS, PHARM.D.
GORDON D. SCHIFF, M.D.
ALBERT L. SHEFFER, M.D.
THEODORE G. TONG, PHARM.D.
ROBERT E. VESTAL, M.D.
JOHN W. YARBRO, M.D., PH.D.

Drug Standards Division Executive Committee
KLAUS G. FLOREY, PH.D., *Chairman*
JERRY R. ALLISON, PH.D.
JUDY P. BOEHLERT, PH.D.
CAPT. WILLIAM H. BRINER, B.S.
LESTER CHAFETZ, PH.D.
ZAK T. CHOWHAN, PH.D.
MURRAY S. COOPER, PH.D.
JOSEPH F. GALLELLI, PH.D.
ROBERT L. GARNICK, PH.D. (1992–)
DAVID W. HUGHES, PH.D.
JOHN B. LANDIS, PH.D. (1990–1992)
LEWIS J. LEESON, PH.D.
THOMAS MEDWICK, PH.D.
ROBERT F. MORRISSEY, PH.D.
SHARON C. NORTHUP, PH.D.
RALPH F. SHANGRAW, PH.D.
JAMES T. STEWART, PH.D.

Drug Nomenclature Committee
HERBERT S. CARLIN, D.SC., *Chairman*
WILLIAM M. HELLER, PH.D., *Consultant/Advisor*
LESTER CHAFETZ, PH.D.
LLOYD E. DAVIS, D.V.M., PH.D.
EVERETT FLANIGAN, PH.D. (1992–)
DOUGLAS D. GLOVER, M.D.
DAVID W. HUGHES, PH.D.
RICHARD D. JOHNSON, PHARM.D., PH.D.
JOHN B. LANDIS, PH.D. (1990–1992)
ROSEMARY C. POLOMANO, R.N., M.S.N.
THOMAS P. REINDERS, PHARM.D.
ERIC B. SHEININ, PH.D.
PHILIP D. WALSON, M.D.

Drug Information Division Advisory Panels 1990–1995

Members who serve as Chairs are listed first.

The information presented in this text represents an ongoing review of the drugs contained herein and represents a consensus of various viewpoints expressed. The individuals listed below have served on the USP Advisory Panels for the 1990–1995 revision period and have contributed to the development of the 1993 USP DI data base. Such listing does not imply that these individuals have reviewed all of the material in this text or that they individually agree with all statements contained herein.

Anesthesiology
Paul F. White, Ph.D., M.D., *Chair*, Dallas, TX; David R. Bevan, M.B., FFARCS, MRCP, Vancouver, British Columbia; Eugene Y. Cheng, M.D., Milwaukee, WI; Charles J. Coté, M.D., Chicago, IL; Roy Cronnelly, M.D., Ph.D., Somerset, CA; Robert Feinstein, M.D., St. Louis, MO; Peter S.A. Glass, M.D., Durham, NC; Michael B. Howie, M.D., Columbus, OH; Beverly A. Krause, C.R.N.A., M.S., St. Louis, MO; Carl Lynch III, M.D., Ph.D., Charlottesville, VA; Carl Rosow, M.D., Ph.D., Boston, MA; Peter S. Sebel, M.B., Ph.D., Atlanta, GA; Walter L. Way, M.D., San Francisco, CA; Matthew B. Weinger, M.D., San Diego, CA; Richard Weiskopf, M.D., San Francisco, CA; David H. Wong, Pharm.D., M.D., Long Beach, CA

Cardiovascular and Renal Drugs
Burton E. Sobel, M.D., *Chair*, St. Louis, MO; William P. Baker, M.D., Ph.D., Bethesda, MD; Nils U. Bang, M.D., Indianapolis, IN; Emmanuel L. Bravo, M.D., Cleveland, OH; Mary Jo Burgess, M.D., Salt Lake City, UT; James H. Chesebro, M.D., Boston, MA; Peter Corr, Ph.D., St. Louis, MO; Dwain L. Eckberg, M.D., Richmond, VA; Ruth Eshleman, Ph.D., W. Kingston, RI; William H. Frishman, M.D., Bronx, NY; Edward D. Frohlich, M.D., New Orleans, LA; Martha Hill, Ph.D., R.N., Baltimore, MD; Norman M. Kaplan, M.D., Dallas, TX; Michael Lesch, M.D., Detroit, MI; Manuel Martinez-Maldonado, M.D., Decatur, GA; Patrick A. McKee, M.D., Oklahoma City, OK; Dan M. Roden, M.D., Nashville, TN; Michael R. Rosen, M.D., New York, NY; Jane Schultz, R.N., B.S.N., Rochester, MN; Robert L. Talbert, Pharm.D., San Antonio, TX; Raymond L. Woosley, M.D., Ph.D., Washington, DC

Clinical Immunology/Allergy/Rheumatology
Albert L. Sheffer, M.D., *Chair*, Boston, MA; John A. Anderson, M.D., Detroit, MI; Emil Bardana, Jr., M.D., Portland, OR; John Baum, M.D., Rochester, NY; Debra Danoff, M.D., Montreal, Quebec; Daniel G. de Jesus, M.D., Ph.D., Vanier, Ontario; Elliott F. Ellis, M.D., Jacksonville, FL; Patricia A. Fraser, M.D., Boston, MA; Frederick E. Hargreave, M.D., Hamilton, Ontario; Evelyn V. Hess, M.D., Cincinnati, OH; Jean M. Jackson, M.D., Boston, MA; Stephen R. Kaplan, M.D., Buffalo, NY; Sandra M. Koehler, Milwaukee, WI; Richard A. Moscicki, M.D., Newton, MA; Shirley Murphy, M.D., Albuquerque, NM; Gary S. Rachelefsky, M.D., Los Angeles, CA; Robert E. Reisman, M.D., Buffalo, NY; Robert L. Rubin, Ph.D., La Jolla, CA; Daniel J. Stechschulte, M.D., Kansas City, KS; Virginia S. Taggert, Bethesda, MD; Joseph A. Tami, Pharm.D., San Antonio, TX; John H. Toogood, M.D., London, Ontario; Martin D. Valentine, M.D., Baltimore, MD; Michael Weinblatt, M.D., Boston, MA; Dennis Michael Williams, Pharm.D., Chapel Hill, NC; Stewart Wong, Ph.D., Brookfield, CT

Clinical Toxicology/Substance Abuse
Theodore G. Tong, Pharm.D., *Chair*, Tucson, AZ; John Ambre, M.D., Ph.D., Chicago, IL; Usoa E. Busto, Pharm.D., Toronto, Ontario; Darryl Inaba, Pharm.D., San Francisco, CA; Edward P. Krenzelok, Pharm.D., Pittsburgh, PA; Michael Montagne, Ph.D., Boston, MA; Sven A. Normann, Pharm.D., Tampa, FL; Gary M. Oderda, Pharm.D., Salt Lake City, UT; Paul Pentel, M.D., Minneapolis, MN; Rose Ann Soloway, R.N., Washington, DC; Daniel A. Spyker, M.D., Ph.D., Rockville, MD; Anthony R. Temple, M.D., Ft. Washington, PA; Anthony Tommasello, Pharm.D., Baltimore, MD; Joseph C. Veltri, Pharm.D., Salt Lake City, UT; William A. Watson, Pharm.D., Kansas City, MO

Consumer Interest/Health Education
Gordon D. Schiff, M.D., *Chair*, Chicago, IL; Michael J. Ackerman, Ph.D., Bethesda, MD; Barbara Aranda-Naranjo, R.N., San Antonio, TX; Frank J. Ascione, Pharm.D., Ph.D., Ann Arbor, MI; Judith I. Brown, Silver Spring, MD; Jose Camacho, Austin, TX; Margaret A. Charters, Ph.D., Syracuse, NY; Jennifer Cross, San Francisco, CA; William G. Harless, Ph.D., Bethesda, MD; Louis H. Kompare, Lake Buena Vista, FL; Margo Kroshus, R.N., B.S.N., Rochester, MN; Marilyn Lister, Wakefield, Quebec; Margaret Lueders, Seattle, WA; Frederick S. Mayer, R.Ph., M.P.H., Sausalito, CA; Nancy Milio, Ph.D., Chapel Hill, NC; Irving Rubin, Port Washington, NY; T. Donald Rucker, Ph.D., River Forest, IL; Stephen B. Soumerai, Sc.D., Boston, MA; Carol A. Vetter, Rockville, MD

Critical Care Medicine
Catherine M. MacLeod, M.D., *Chair*, Chicago, IL; William Banner, Jr., M.D., Salt Lake City, UT; Philip S. Barie, M.D., New York, NY; Thomas P. Bleck, M.D., Charlottesville, VA; Roger C. Bone, M.D., Chicago, IL; Susan S. Fish, Pharm.D., Boston, MA; Edgar R. Gonzalez, Pharm.D., Richmond, VA; Robert Gottesman, Rockville, MD; Michael Halperin, M.D., Denver, CO; John W. Hoyt, M.D., Pittsburgh, PA; Sheldon A. Magder, M.D., Montreal, Quebec; Henry Masur, M.D., Bethesda, MD; Joseph E. Parrillo, M.D., Chicago, IL; Sharon Peters, M.D., St. John's, Newfoundland; Domenic A. Sica, M.D., Richmond, VA; Martin G. Tweeddale, M.B., Ph.D., Vancouver, British Columbia

Dentistry
Sebastian G. Ciancio, D.D.S., *Chair*, Buffalo, NY; Donald F. Adams, D.D.S., Portland, OR; Karen A. Baker, M.S. Pharm., Iowa City, IA; Stephen A. Cooper, D.M.D., Ph.D., Philadelphia, PA; Frederick A. Curro, D.M.D., Ph.D., Jersey City,

NJ; Paul J. Desjardins, D.M.D., Ph.D., Newark, NJ; Tommy W. Gage, D.D.S., Ph.D., Dallas, TX; Stephen F. Goodman, D.D.S., New York, NY; Daniel A. Haas, D.D.S., Ph.D., Toronto, Ontario; Richard E. Hall, D.D.S., Ph.D., Buffalo, NY; Lireka P. Joseph, Dr.P.H., Rockville, MD; Janice Lieberman, Fort Lee, NJ; Laurie Lisowski, Buffalo, NY; Clarence L. Trummel, D.D.S., Ph.D., Farmington, CT; Joel M. Weaver, II, D.D.S., Ph.D., Columbus, OH; Clifford W. Whall, Jr., Ph.D., Chicago, IL; Raymond P. White, Jr., D.D.S., Ph.D., Chapel Hill, NC; Ray C. Williams, D.M.D., Boston, MA

Dermatology
Robert S. Stern, M.D., *Chair*, Boston, MA; Beatrice B. Abrams, Ph.D., Somerville, NJ; Richard D. Baughman, M.D., Hanover, NH; Michael Bigby, M.D., Boston, MA; Janice T. Chussil, R.N., M.S.N., Portland, OR; Stuart Maddin, M.D., Vancouver, British Columbia; Milton Orkin, M.D., Minneapolis, MN; Neil H. Shear, M.D., Toronto, Ontario; Edgar Benton Smith, M.D., Galveston, TX; Dennis P. West, M.S. Pharm., Lincolnshire, IL; Gail M. Zimmerman, Portland, OR

Diagnostic Agents—Nonradioactive
Robert L. Siegle, M.D., *Chair*, San Antonio, TX; Kaizer Aziz, Ph.D., Rockville, MD; Robert C. Brasch, M.D., San Francisco, CA; Nicholas Harry Malakis, M.D., Bethesda, MD; Robert F. Mattrey, M.D., San Diego, CA; James A. Nelson, M.D., Seattle, WA; Jovitas Skucas, M.D., Rochester, NY; Gerald L. Wolf, Ph.D., M.D., Charlestown, MA

Drug Information Science
James A. Visconti, Ph.D., *Chair*, Columbus, OH; Marie A. Abate, Pharm.D., Morgantown, WV; Ann B. Amerson, Pharm.D., Lexington, KY; Philip O. Anderson, Pharm.D., San Diego, CA; Danial E. Baker, Pharm.D., Spokane, WA; C. David Butler, Pharm.D., M.B.A., Oak Brook, IL; Linda L. Hart, Pharm.D., San Francisco, CA; Edward J. Huth, M.D., Philadelphia, PA; John M. Kessler, Pharm.D., Chapel Hill, NC; R. David Lauper, Pharm.D., Emeryville, CA; Domingo R. Martinez, Pharm.D., Birmingham, AL; William F. McGhan, Pharm.D., Ph.D., Philadelphia, PA; John K. Murdoch, B.Sc.Phm., Toronto, Ontario; Kurt A. Proctor, Ph.D., Alexandria, VA; Arnauld F. Scafidi, M.D., M.P.H., Rockville, MD; John A. Scarlett, M.D., Austin, TX; Gary H. Smith, Pharm.D., Tucson, AZ; Dennis F. Thompson, Pharm.D., Oklahoma City, OK; William G. Troutman, Pharm.D., Albuquerque, NM; Lee A. Wanke, M.S., Houston, TX

Drug Utilization Review
Judith K. Jones, M.D., Ph.D., *Chair*, Arlington, VA; John F. Beary, III., M.D., Washington, DC; James L. Blackburn, Pharm.D., Saskatoon, Saskatchewan; Richard S. Blum, M.D., East Hills, NY; Amy Cooper-Outlaw, Pharm.D., Stone Mountain, GA; Joseph W. Cranston, Jr., Ph.D., Chicago, IL; W. Gary Erwin, Pharm.D., Philadelphia, PA; Jere E. Goyan, Ph.D., Northvale, NJ; Duane M. Kirking, Ph.D., Ann Arbor, MI; Karen E. Koch, Pharm.D., Tupelo, MS; Aida A. LeRoy, Pharm.D., Arlington, VA; Jerome Levine, M.D., Baltimore, MD; Richard W. Lindsay, M.D., Charlottesville, VA; Deborah M. Nadzam, R.N., Ph.D., Oakbrook Terrace, IL; William Z. Potter, M.D., Ph.D., Bethesda, MD; Louise R. Rodriquez, M.S., Washington, DC; Stephen P. Spielberg, M.D., Ph.D., West Point, PA; Suzan M. Streichenwein, M.D., Houston, TX; Brian L. Strom, M.D., Philadelphia, PA; Michael Weintraub, M.D., Rockville, MD; Antonio Carlos Zanini, M.D., Ph.D., Sao Paulo, Brazil

Endocrinology
Maria I. New, M.D., *Chair*, New York, NY; Ronald D. Brown, M.D., Oklahoma City, OK; R. Keith Campbell, Pharm.D., Pullman, WA; David S. Cooper, M.D., Baltimore, MD; Betty J. Dong, Pharm.D., San Francisco, CA; Andrea Dunaif, M.D., New York, NY; Anke A. Ehrhardt, Ph.D., New York, NY; Nadir R. Farid, M.D., Riyadh, Saudi Arabia; John G. Haddad, Jr., M.D., Philadelphia, PA; Michael M. Kaplan, M.D., Southfield, MI; Harold E. Lebovitz, M.D., Brooklyn, NY; Marvin E. Levin, M.D., Chesterfield, MO; Marvin M. Lipman, M.D., Scarsdale, NY; Barbara Lippe, M.D., Los Angeles, CA; Barbara J. Maschak-Carey, R.N., M.S.N., Philadelphia, PA; James C. Melby, M.D., Boston, MA; Walter J. Meyer, III., M.D., Galveston, TX; Rita Nemchik, R.N., M.S., C.D.E., Florence, NJ; Daniel A. Notterman, M.D., New York, NY; Ron Gershon Rosenfeld, M.D., Stanford, CA; Paul Saenger, M.D., Bronx, NY; Leonard Wartofsky, M.D., Washington, DC

Family Practice
Robert M. Guthrie, M.D., *Chair*, Columbus, OH; Jack A. Brose, D.O., Athens, OH; Jannet M. Carmichael, Pharm.D., Reno, NV; Jacqueline A. Chadwick, M.D., Scottsdale, AZ; Mark E. Clasen, M.D., Ph.D., Dayton, OH; Lloyd P. Haskell, M.D., West Borough, MA; Luis A. Izquierdo-Mora, M.D., Rio Piedras, PR; Edward L. Langston, M.D., Houston, TX; Charles D. Ponte, Pharm.D., Morgantown, WV; Jack M. Rosenberg, Pharm.D., Ph.D., Brooklyn, NY; John F. Sangster, M.D., London, Ontario; Theodore L. Yarboro, Sr., M.D., M.P.H., Sharon, PA

Gastroenterology
Gordon L. Klein, M.D., *Chair*, Galveston, TX; Karl E. Anderson, M.D., Galveston, TX; William Balistreri, M.D., Cincinnati, OH; Paul Bass, Ph.D., Madison, WI; Rosemary R. Berardi, Pharm.D., Ann Arbor, MI; Raymond F. Burk, M.D., Nashville, TN; George D. Ferry, M.D., Houston, TX; Thomas Q. Garvey, III, M.D., Potomac, MD; Donald J. Glotzer, M.D., Boston, MA; Flavio Habal, M.D., Toronto, Ontario; Paul E. Hyman, M.D., Torrance, CA; Bernard Mehl, D.P.S., New York, NY; William J. Snape, Jr., M.D., Torrance, CA; Ronald D. Soltis, M.D., Minneapolis, MN; C. Noel Williams, M.D., Halifax, Nova Scotia; Hyman J. Zimmerman, M.D., Washington, DC

Geriatrics
Robert E. Vestal, M.D., *Chair*, Boise, ID; Darrell R. Abernethy, M.D., Providence, RI; William B. Abrams, M.D., West Point, PA; Jerry Avorn, M.D., Boston, MA; Robert A. Blouin, Pharm.D., Lexington, KY; S. George Carruthers, M.D., Halifax, Nova Scotia; Lynn E. Chaitovitz, Rockville, MD; Terry Fulmer, R.N., Ph.D., New York, NY; Philip P. Gerbino, Pharm.D., Philadelphia, PA; Pearl S. German, Sc.D., Baltimore, MD; David J. Greenblatt, M.D., Boston, MA; Martin D. Higbee, Pharm.D., Tucson, AZ; Brian B. Hoffman, M.D., Palo Alto, CA; J. Edward Jackson, M.D., San Diego, CA; Peter P. Lamy, Ph.D., Baltimore, MD; Joseph V. Levy, Ph.D., San Francisco, CA; Paul A. Mitenko, M.D., FRCPC, Nanaimo, British Columbia; John E. Morley, M.B., B.Ch., St. Louis, MO; Jay Roberts, Ph.D., Philadelphia, PA; Louis J. Rubenstein, R.Ph., Alexandria, VA; Janice B. Schwartz, M.D., San Francisco, CA; Alexander M.M. Shepherd, M.D., San Antonio, TX; William Simonson, Pharm.D., Portland, OR; Daniel S. Sitar, Ph.D., Winnipeg, Manitoba; Mary K. Walker, R.N., Ph.D., Lexington, KY; Alastair J. J. Wood, M.D., Nashville, TN

Hematologic and Neoplastic Disease

John W. Yarbro, M.D., Ph.D., *Chair*, Springfield, IL; Joseph S. Bailes, M.D., McAllen, TX; Laurence H. Baker, D.O., Detroit, MI; Barbara D. Blumberg, Dallas, TX; Helene G. Brown, B.S., Los Angeles, CA; Nora L. Burnham, Pharm.D., Princeton, NJ; William J. Dana, Pharm.D., Houston, TX; Connie Henke-Yarbro, R.N., B.S.N., Springfield, IL; William H. Hryniuk, M.D., San Diego, CA; B. J. Kennedy, M.D., Minneapolis, MN; Barnett Kramer, M.D., Rockville, MD; Brigid G. Leventhal, M.D., Baltimore, MD; Michael J. Mastrangelo, M.D., Philadelphia, PA; David S. Rosenthal, M.D., Cambridge, MA; Richard L. Schilsky, M.D., Chicago, IL; Rowena N. Schwartz, Pharm.D., Pittsburgh, PA; Roy L. Silverstein, M.D., New York, NY; Samuel G. Taylor, IV, M.D., Chicago, IL; Raymond B. Weiss, M.D., Washington, DC

Infectious Disease Therapy

Donald Kaye, M.D., *Chair*, Philadelphia, PA; Robert Austrian, M.D., Philadelphia, PA; C. Glenn Cobbs, M.D., Birmingham, AL; Joseph W. Cranston, Jr., Ph.D., Chicago, IL; John J. Dennehy, M.D., Danville, PA; Courtney V. Fletcher, Pharm. D., Minneapolis, MN; Earl H. Freimer, M.D., Toledo, OH; Marc LeBel, Pharm.D., Quebec, Quebec; John D. Nelson, M.D., Dallas, TX; Lindsay E. Nicolle, M.D., Winnipeg, Manitoba; Alvin Novick, M.D., New Haven, CT; Charles G. Prober, M.D., Stanford, CA; Douglas D. Richman, M.D., San Diego, CA; Spotswood L. Spruance, M.D., Salt Lake City, UT; Roy T. Steigbigel, M.D., Stony Brook, NY; Paul F. Wehrle, M.D., San Clemente, CA

International Health

Rosalyn C. King, Pharm.D., M.P.H., *Chair*, Silver Spring, MD; Fernando Antezana, Ph.D., Geneva, Switzerland; Walter M. Batts, Rockville, MD; Eugenie Brown, Pharm.D., Kingston, Jamaica; Alan Cheung, Pharm.D., M.P.H., Washington, DC; Mary Couper, M.D., Geneva, Switzerland; Gabriel Daniel, Washington, DC; S. Albert Edwards, Pharm.D., Lincolnshire, IL; Enrique Fefer, Ph.D., Washington, DC; Peter H. M. Fontilus, Curacao, Netherlands Antilles; Marcellus Grace, Ph.D., New Orleans, LA; George B. Griffenhagen, Washington, DC; Gan Ee Kiang, Penang, Malaysia; Thomas Langston, Silver Spring, MD; Thomas Lapnet-Moustapha, Yaounde, Cameroon; David Lee, B.A., M.D., Panama City, Panama; Aissatov Lo, Ka-Olack, Senegal; Stuart M. MacLeod, M.D., Hamilton, Ontario; Russell E. Morgan, Jr., Dr.P.H., Chevy Chase, MD; David Ofori-Adjei, M.D., Accra, Ghana; S. Ofosu-Amaah, M.D., New York, NY; James Rankin, Arlington, VA; Olikoye Ransome-Kuti, M.D., Lagos, Nigeria; Budiono Santoso, M.D., Ph.D., Yogyakarta, Indonesia; Carmen Selva, Ph.D., Madrid, Spain; Valentin Vinogradov, Moscow, Russia; Fela Viso-Gurovich, Mexico City, Mexico; William B. Walsh, M.D., Chevy Chase, MD; Lawrence C. Weaver, Ph.D., Minneapolis, MN; Albert I. Wertheimer, Ph.D., Philadelphia, PA

Neurology

Stanley van den Noort, M.D., *Chair*, Irvine, CA; William T. Beaver, M.D., Washington, DC; Elizabeth U. Blalock, M.D., Anaheim, CA; James C. Cloyd, Pharm.D., Minneapolis, MN; David M. Dawson, M.D., West Roxbury, MA; Kevin Farrell, M.D., Vancouver, British Columbia; Kathleen M. Foley, M.D., New York, NY; Anthony E. Lang, M.D., Toronto, Ontario; Ira T. Lott, M.D., Orange, CA; James R. Nelson, M.D., La Jolla, CA; J. Kiffin Penry, M.D., Winston-Salem, NC; Neil H. Raskin, M.D., San Francisco, CA; Alfred J. Spiro, M.D., Bronx, NY; M. DiAnn Turek, R.N., Lansing, MI

Nursing Practice

Rosemary C. Polomano, R.N., M.S.N., *Chair*, Philadelpia, PA; Mecca S. Cranley, R.N., Ph.D., Buffalo, NY; Jan M. Ellerhorst-Ryan, R.N., M.S.N., Cincinnati, OH; Linda Felver, Ph.D., R.N., Sedro Woolley, WA; Hector Hugo Gonzalez, R.N., Ph.D., San Antonio, TX; Mary Harper, R.N., Ph.D., Rockville, MD; Ada K. Jacox, R.N., Ph.D., Baltimore, MD; Patricia Kummeth, R.N., M.S., Rochester, MN; Ida M. Martinson, R.N., Ph.D., San Francisco, CA; Carol P. Patton, R.N., Ph.D., J.D., Detroit, MI; Ginette A. Pepper, R.N., Ph.D., Englewood, CO; Geraldine A. Peterson, R.N., M.A., Potomac, MD; Linda C. Pugh, R.N., Ph.D., York, PA; Sharon S. Rising, R.N., C.N.M., Cheshire, CT; Marjorie Ann Spiro, R.N., B.S., C.S.N., Scarsdale, NY

Nutrition and Electrolytes

Robert D. Lindeman, M.D., *Chair*, Albuquerque, NM; Hans Fisher, Ph.D., New Brunswick, NJ; Walter H. Glinsmann, M.D., Washington, DC; Helen Andrews Guthrie, M.S., Ph.D., State College, PA; Steven B. Heymsfield, M.D., New York, NY; K. N. Jeejeebhoy, M.D., Toronto, Ontario; Leslie M. Klevay, M.D., Grand Forks, ND; Bonnie Liebman, M.S., Washington, DC; Sudesh K. Mahajan, M.D., Grosse Point Woods, MI; Craig J. McClain, M.D., Lexington, KY; Jay M. Mirtallo, M.S., Columbus, OH; Sohrab Mobarhan, M.D., Maywood, IL; Robert M. Russell, M.D., Boston, MA; Harold H. Sandstead, M.D., Galveston, TX; William J. Stone, M.D., Nashville, TN; Carlos A. Vaamonde, M.D., Miami, FL; Stanley Wallach, M.D., New York, NY

Obstetrics and Gynecology

Douglas D. Glover, M.D., *Chair*, Morgantown, WV; Rudi Ansbacher, M.D., Ann Arbor, MI; Florence Comite, M.D., New Haven, CT; James W. Daly, M.D., Columbia, MO; Marilynn C. Frederiksen, M.D., Chicago, IL; Charles B. Hammond, M.D., Durham, NC; Barbara A. Hayes, M.A., New Rochelle, NY; Art Jacknowitz, Pharm.D., Morgantown, WV; William J. Ledger, M.D., New York, NY; Andre-Marie Leroux, M.D., Vanier, Ontario; William A. Nahhas, M.D., Dayton, OH; Warren N. Otterson, M.D., Shreveport, LA; Samuel A. Pasquale, M.D., New Brunswick, NJ; Johanna Perlmutter, M.D., Boston, MA; Robert W. Rebar, M.D., Cincinnati, OH; Richard H. Reindollar, M.D., Boston, MA; G. Millard Simmons, M.D., Morgantown, WV; J. Benjamin Younger, M.D., Birmingham, AL

Ophthalmology

Herbert E. Kaufman, M.D., *Chair*, New Orleans, LA; Steven R. Abel, Pharm.D., Indianapolis, IN; Jules Baum, M.D., Boston, MA; Lee R. Duffner, M.D., Miami, FL; David L. Epstein, M.D., Durham, NC; Allan J. Flach, Pharm.D., M.D., San Francisco, CA; Vincent H. L. Lee, Ph.D., Los Angeles, CA; Steven M. Podos, M.D., New York, NY; Kirk R. Wilhelmus, M.D., Houston, TX; Thom J. Zimmerman, M.D., Ph.D., Louisville, KY

Otorhinolaryngology

Leonard P. Rybak, M.D., *Chair*, Springfield, IL; Robert E. Brummett, Ph.D., Portland, OR; Robert A. Dobie, M.D., San Antonio, TX; Linda J. Gardiner, M.D., Fort Myers, FL; David Hilding, M.D., Price, UT; David B. Hom, M.D., Minneapolis, MN; Helen F. Krause, M.D., Pittsburgh, PA; Richard L. Mabry, M.D., Dallas, TX; Lawrence J. Marentette, M.D., Minneapolis, MN; Robert A. Mickel, M.D., Ph.D., West Los Angeles, CA; Randal A. Otto, M.D., San Antonio, TX; Richard W. Waguespack, M.D., Birmingham, AL; William R. Wilson, M.D., Washington, DC

Parasitic Disease

Jay S. Keystone, M.D., *Chair*, Toronto, Ontario; Michele Barry, M.D., New Haven, CT; Frank J. Bia, M.D., M.P.H., Guilford, CT; David Botero, M.D., Medellin, Colombia; David D. Freedman, M.D., Birmingham, AL; Elaine C. Jong, M.D., Seattle, WA; Dennis D. Juranek, M.D., Atlanta, GA; Donald J. Krogstad, M.D., New Orleans, LA; Douglas W. MacPherson, M.D., Hamilton, Ontario; Edward K. Markell, M.D., San Francisco, CA; Theodore Nash, M.D., Bethesda, MD; Murray Wittner, M.D., Bronx, NY

Pediatrics

Philip D. Walson, M.D., *Chair*, Columbus, OH; Jacob V. Aranda, M.D., Ph.D., Montreal, Quebec; Cheston M. Berlin, Jr., M.D., Hershey, PA; Nancy Jo Braden, M.D., Phoenix, AZ; Patricia J. Bush, Ph.D., Washington, DC; Marion J. Finkel, M.D., East Hanover, NJ; George S. Goldstein, M.D., Elmsford, NY; Ralph E. Kauffman, M.D., Detroit, MI; Gideon Koren, M.D., Toronto, Ontario; Joan M. Korth-Bradley, Pharm.D., Ph.D., Philadelphia, PA; Richard Leff, Pharm.D., Kansas City, KS; Carolyn Lund, R.N., M.S., San Francisco, CA; Wayne Snodgrass, M.D., Galveston, TX; Celia A. Viets, M.D., Ottawa, Canada; John T. Wilson, M.D., Shreveport, LA; Sumner J. Yaffe, M.D., Bethesda, MD; Karin E. Zenk, Pharm.D., Irvine, CA

Pharmacy Practice

Thomas P. Reinders, Pharm.D., *Chair*, Richmond, VA; Olya Duzey, M.S., Big Rapids, MI; Yves Gariepy, B.Sc.Pharm., Quebec, Quebec; Ned Heltzer, M.S., New Castle, DE; Lester S. Hosto, B.S., Little Rock, AR; Martin J. Jinks, Pharm.D., Pullman, WA; Frederick Klein, B.S., Montvale, NJ; Calvin H. Knowlton, Ph.D., Lumberton, NJ; Patricia A. Kramer, B.S., Bismarck, ND; Dennis McCallum, Pharm.D., Rochester, MN; Shirley P. McKee, B.S., Houston, TX; William A. McLean, Pharm.D., Ottawa, Ontario; Gladys Montañez, B.S., Santurce, PR; Donald L. Moore, B.S., Kokomo, IN; John E. Ogden, M.S., Washington, DC; Henry A. Palmer, Ph.D., Storrs, CT; Lorie G. Rice, B.A., M.P.H., San Francisco, CA; Mike R. Sather, M.S., Albuquerque, NM; Albert Sebok, B.S., Twinsburg, OH; William E. Smith, Pharm.D., M.P.H., Auburn University, AL; Susan East Torrico, B.S., Orlando, FL; J. Richard Wuest, Pharm.D., Cincinnati, OH; Glenn Y. Yokoyama, Pharm.D., Pasadena, CA

Psychiatric Disease

Burton J. Goldstein, M.D., *Chair*, Miami Beach, FL; Magda Campbell, M.D., New York, NY; Alex A. Cardoni, M.S. Pharm., Hartford, CT; James L. Claghorn, M.D., Houston, TX; N. Michael Davis, M.S., Miami, FL; Larry Ereshefsky, Pharm.D., San Antonio, TX; W. Edwin Fann, M.D., Houston, TX; Alan J. Gelenberg, M.D., Tucson, AZ; Tracy R. Gordy, M.D., Austin, TX; Paul Grof, M.D., Ottawa, Ontario; Russell T. Joffe, M.D., Toronto, Ontario; Harriet P. Lefley, Ph.D., Miami, FL; Nathan Rawls, Pharm.D., Memphis, TN; Jarrett W. Richardson, III, M.D., Rochester, MN; Ruth Robinson, Saskatoon, Saskatchewan; Matthew V. Rudorfer, M.D., Rockville, MD; Karen A. Theesen, Pharm.D., Omaha, NE

Pulmonary Disease

Harold S. Nelson, M.D., *Chair*, Denver, CO; Richard C. Ahrens, M.D., Iowa City, IA; Eugene R. Bleecker, M.D., Baltimore, MD; William W. Busse, M.D., Madison, WI; Christopher Fanta, M.D., Boston, MA; Mary K. Garcia, R.N., Missouri City, TX; Nicholas Gross, M.D., Hines, IL; Leslie Hendeles, Pharm.D., Gainesville, FL; Elliot Israel, M.D., Boston, MA; Susan Janson-Bjerklie, R.N., Ph.D., San Francisco, CA; John W. Jenne, M.D., Hines, IL; H. William Kelly, Pharm.D., Albuquerque, NM; James P. Kemp, M.D., San Diego, CA; Henry Levison, M.D., Toronto, Ontario; Gail Shapiro, M.D., Seattle, WA; Stanley J. Szefler, M.D., Denver, CO

Radiopharmaceuticals

Carol S. Marcus, Ph.D., M.D., *Chair*, Torrance, CA; Capt. William H. Briner, B.S., Durham, NC; Ronald J. Callahan, Ph.D., Boston, MA; Janet F. Eary, M.D., Seattle, WA; Joanna S. Fowler, Ph.D., Upton, NY; David L. Gilday, M.D., Toronto, Ontario; David A. Goodwin, M.D., Palo Alto, CA; David L. Laven, N.Ph., C.R.Ph., FASCP, Bay Pines, FL; Andrea H. McGuire, M.D., Des Moines, IA; Peter Paras, Ph.D., Rockville, MD; Barry A. Siegel, M.D., St. Louis, MO; Edward B. Silberstein, M.D., Cincinnati, OH; Dennis P. Swanson, M.S., Pittsburgh, PA; Mathew L. Thakur, Ph.D., Philadelphia, PA; Henry N. Wellman, M.D., Indianapolis, IN

Surgical Drugs and Devices

Lary A. Robinson, M.D., *Chair*, Omaha, NE; Gregory Alexander, M.D., Rockville, MD; Norman D. Anderson, M.D., Baltimore, MD; Alan R. Dimick, M.D., Birmingham, AL; Jack Hirsh, M.D., Hamilton, Ontario; Manucher J. Javid, M.D., Madison, WI; Henry J. Mann, Pharm.D., Minneapolis, MN; Kurt M. W. Niemann, M.D., Birmingham, AL; Robert P. Rapp, Pharm.D., Lexington, KY; Ronald Rubin, M.D., Boston, MA

Urology

John A. Belis, M.D., *Chair*, Hershey, PA; Culley C. Carson, M.D., Chapel Hill, NC; Richard A. Cohen, M.D., Red Bank, NJ; B. J. Reid Czarapata, R.N., Washington, DC; Jean B. de Kernion, M.D., Los Angeles, CA; Warren Heston, Ph.D., New York, NY; Mark V. Jarowenko, M.D., Hershey, PA; Mary Lee, Pharm.D., Chicago, IL; Marguerite C. Lippert, M.D., Charlottesville, VA; Penelope A. Longhurst, Ph.D., Philadelphia, PA; Tom F. Lue, M.D., San Francisco, CA; Michael G. Mawhinney, Ph.D., Morgantown, WV; Martin G. McLoughlin, M.D., Vancouver, British Columbia; Randall G. Rowland, M.D., Ph.D., Indianapolis, IN; J. Patrick Spirnak, M.D., Cleveland, OH; William F. Tarry, M.D., Morgantown, WV; Keith N. Van Arsdalen, M.D., Philadelphia, PA

Veterinary Medicine

Lloyd E. Davis, D.V.M., Ph.D., *Chair*, Urbana, IL; Arthur L. Aronson, D.V.M., Ph.D., Raleigh, NC; Gordon W. Brumbaugh, D.V.M., Ph.D., College Station, TX; Gordon L. Coppoc, D.V.M., Ph.D., West Lafayette, IN; Sidney A. Ewing, D.V.M., Ph.D., Stillwater, OK; Stuart D. Forney, M.S., Fort Collins, CO; William G. Huber, D.V.M., Ph.D., Sun City West, AZ; William L. Jenkins, D.V.M., Baton Rouge, LA; Vernon Corey Langston, D.V.M., Ph.D., Mississippi State, MS; Mark G. Papich, D.V.M., Raleigh, NC; John W. Paul, D.V.M., Somerville, NJ; Thomas E. Powers, D.V.M., Ph.D., Columbus, OH; Charles R. Short, D.V.M., Ph.D., Baton Rouge, LA; Richard H. Teske, D.V.M., Ph.D., Rockville, MD; Jeffrey R. Wilcke, D.V.M., M.S., Blacksburg, VA

Drug Information Division Additional Contributors

The information presented in this text represents an ongoing review of the drugs contained herein and represents a consensus of various viewpoints expressed. In addition to the individuals listed below, many schools, associations, pharmaceutical companies, and governmental agencies have provided comment or otherwise contributed to the development of the 1994 USP DI data base. Such listing does not imply that these individuals have reviewed all of the material in this text or that they individually agree with all statements contained herein.

Donald I. Abrams, M.D., San Francisco, CA
Herbert L. Abrams, M.D., Stanford, CA
Jonathan Abrams, M.D., Albuquerque, NM
Martin Alda, M.D., Ottawa, Ontario, Canada
Bruce D. Anderson, Pharm.D., Tampa, FL
Susan G. Arbuck, M.D., Bethesda, MD
G. Richard Arthur, Ph.D., Boston, MA
Louis V. Avioli, M.D., St. Louis, MO
Patsy Barnett, Pharm.D., Bay Pines, FL
Joseph M. Baron, M.D., Chicago, IL
LuAnne Barron, Birmingham, AL
Robert W. Beightol, Pharm.D., Roanoke, VA
William Bell, M.D., Baltimore, MD
John M. Bennett, M.D., Chicago, IL
Patricia Bennett, B.S.Pharm., Cincinnati, OH
Charles B. Berde, M.D., Ph.D., Boston, MA
Michael A. Bettmann, M.D., Boston, MA
Jerry G. Blaivas, M.D., New York, NY
M. Donald Blaufox, M.D., Bronx, NY
Henry G. Bone, III, M.D., Detroit, MI
Wayne E. Bradley, Richmond, VA
Michael Brady, M.D., Columbus, OH
Robert E. Braun, D.D.S., Buffalo, NY
Myron Brazin, M.D., Denville, NJ
Orval Brown, M.D., Dallas, TX
Wesley G. Byerly, Pharm.D., Winston-Salem, NC
James E. Caldwell, M.D., San Francisco, CA
Karim A. Calis, Pharm.D., Rockville, MD
Michael Camilleri, M.D., Rochester, MN
Bruce A. Chabner, M.D., Bethesda, MD
Cyril R. Clarke, Ph.D., Stillwater, OK
Katie Clarke, RN, Lincolnshire, IL
Arthur Cocco, M.D., Baltimore, MD
Dr. R.E. Coleman, Sheffield, England
James W. Cooper, Ph.D., Athens, GA
Clinton N. Corder, Ph.D., M.D., Oklahoma City, OK
Carolyn R. Corn, M.D., Oklahoma City, OK
Deborah Cotton, M.D., Boston, MA
Fred F. Cowan, Ph.D., Portland, OR
Thomas D. DeCillis, North Port, FL
Carel P. de Haseth, Ph.D., Netherland Antilles (Caribbean)
Margo A. Denke, M.D., Dallas, TX
Virgil C. Dias, Pharm.D., Kansas City, MO
Barry D. Dickinson, Ph.D., Chicago, IL
Dr. Cosmo DiFazio, Charlottesville, VA
Ananias C. Diokno, M.D., Royal Oak, MI
Gerald D. Dodd, M.D., Houston, TX
James E. Doherty, M.D., Little Rock, AR
Ross Donehover, M.D., Baltimore, MD
Sue Duran, R.Ph., MS, Auburn University, AL
Suzanne Eastman, B.S., R.Ph., Cincinnati, OH
Timothy J. Eberlein, M.D., Cambridge, MA
Avi I. Einzig, M.D., Bronx, NY
Charles N. Ellis, M.D., Ann Arbor, MI
William Fant, Cincinnati, OH
Dave Ferguson, M.D., Bethesda, MD
Anne Gilbert Feuer, B.S., Cincinnati, OH
Suzanne Fields, Pharm.D., San Antonio, TX
Robert A. Figlin, M.D., Los Angeles, CA
Alex Finkbeiner, M.D., Little Rock, AR
Richard I. Fisher, M.D., Maywood, IL
Maria Font, Vicenza, Italy
Tammy Fox, B.S., R.Ph., Cincinnati, OH
Dr. Ruth Francis-Floyd, Gainesville, FL
Carl J. Friedman, M.D., Philadelphia, PA
Jose P.B. Gallardo, R.Ph., Iowa City, IA
Abhimanyu Garg, M.D., Dallas, TX
Edward Genton, M.D., New Orleans, LA
Anne A. Gershon, M.D., New York, NY
Michael J. Glade, Ph.D., Chicago, IL
Wallace A. Gleason, M.D., Houston, TX
Charles J. Glueck, M.D., Cincinnati, OH
Micheline Andel Goldwire, Brooklyn, NY
K. Lance Gould, M.D., Houston, TX
MAJ. John D. Grabenstein, MS, Fort Sam Houston, TX
Martin D. Green, M.D., Rockville, MD
Robert Greenberg, M.D., Hanover, NH
Scott M. Grundy, M.D., Ph.D., Dallas, TX
Carl Grunfeld, M.D., San Francisco, CA
David R. P. Guay, Pharm.D., St. Paul, MN
Renato Gusmao, Washington, DC
Angela M. Hadbavny, M.S., Pharm.D., Pittsburgh, PA
Nortin M. Hadler, M.D., Chapel Hill, NC
William M. Hadley, Ph.D., Albuquerque, NM
Richard E. Harris, M.D., Cincinnati, OH
Steven T. Harris, M.D., San Francisco, CA
Edward A. Hartshorn, Ph.D., League City, TX
Peggy E. Hayes, Pharm.D., East Hanover, NJ
Duncan H. Haynes, Ph.D., Miami, FL
Alfred D. Heggie, M.D., Cleveland, OH
Bryan N. Henderson, II, D.D.S., Dallas, TX
Melvin B. Heyman, M.D., San Francisco, CA
M. Ho, M.D., Pittsburgh, PA
Vincent C. Ho, M.D., Vancouver, British Columbia, Canada
M.E. Hoar, Springfield, MA
Robert Hodgeman, B.S., R.Ph., Cincinnati, OH
Frankie Ann Holmes, M.D., Houston, TX
David C. Hooper, M.D., Boston, MA

Colin W. Howden, M.D., Columbia, SC
Walter T. Hughes, M.D., Memphis, TN
John Iazzetta, Pharm.D., Toronto, Ontario, Canada
Rodney D. Ice, Ph.D., Atlanta, GA
D. Roger Illingworth, Portland, OR
Ann L. Janer, M.S., Auburn, AL
Bela Janszky, New York, NY
Janet P. Jaramilla, Pharm.D., Chicago, IL
V. Craig Jordan, Ph.D., Madison, WI
Dr. S. Joy, Rochester, NY
Hugh F. Kabat, Ph.D., Albuquerque, NM
Alan Kanada, Pharm.D., Denver, CO
Selna Kaplan, M.D., Ph.D., San Francisco, CA
Mary Carman Kasparek, Vanier, Ont., Canada
John J. Kavanagh, M.D., Houston, TX
Ronald Kleinman, M.D., Boston, MA
Sandra Knowles, B.Pharm., Toronto, Ontario, Canada
John Koepke, Pharm.D., Columbus, OH
Barbara A. Konkle, M.D., Philadelphia, PA
Joseph Kostick, Rochester MN
Donald P. Kotler, M.D., New Rochelle, NY
Joseph A. Kovacs, M.D., Bethesda, MD
Daryl E. Krepps, B.S.P., Ottawa, Ont. Canada
G. T. Krishnamurthy, M.D., Portland, OR
Dr. Debbie Kuapp, West Lafayette, IN
Lee Kudrow, M.D., Encino, CA
Paul B. Kuehn, Ph.D., Woodinville, WA
Robert Kuhn, Pharm.D., Lexington, KY
Thomas L. Kurt, M.D., Dallas, TX
Cathy Kwaitkowski, B.S., R.Ph., Cincinnati, OH
John R. LaMontagne, Bethesda, MD
Carol Lang, MS, RD, Washington, DC
Victor Lanzotti, M.D., Springfield, IL
Belle Lee, Pharm.D., San Francisco, CA
Cathy E. Lennon, R.N., Boston, MA
Joseph Levy, M.D., New York, NY
Christopher D. Lind, M.D., Nashville, TN
Timothy O. Lipman, M.D., Washington, DC
Scott M. Lippman, M.D., Houston, TX
Don Long, M.D., Baltimore, MD
Margaret H. Macgillivray, M.D., Buffalo, NY
Howard I. Maibach, M.D., San Francisco, CA
Frank Marcus, M.D., Tucson, AZ
Joseph E. Margarone, D.D.S., Buffalo, NY
Maurie Markman, M.D., Cleveland, OH
J. Jeffrey Marshall, M.D., Decatur, GA
Micheline Mathews-Roth, M.D., Boston, MA
Alice Lorraine McAfee, Pharm.D., San Pedro, CA
Norman L. McElroy, San Jose, CA
Ross E. McKinney, M.D., Durham, NC
Anne McNulty, M.D., Waterbury, CT
Janie Menchaca-Wilson, Ph.D., R.N., San Antonio, TX
Edgar L. Milford, M.D., Ann Arbor, MI
Craig S. Miller, D.D.S., Lexington, KY
Donald Miller, Pharm.D., Fargo, ND
Ronald D. Miller, M.D., San Francisco, CA
Joel S. Mindel, M.D., Ph.D., New York, NY
Bernard L. Mirkin, M.D., Chicago, IL
Linda Miwa, Pharm.D., Arlington, VA
Mary E. Mortensen, M.D., Columbus, OH
Mardi K. Mountford,, Atlanta, GA
Robyn Mueller, B.S., R.Ph., Cumberland, RI
Martha D. Mullett, M.D., Morgantown, WV
Serpil Nebioglu, M.D., Tandogan-Ankara, Turkey
David Nierenberg, M.D., Honover, NH
Cheryl Nunn-Thompson, Pharm.D., Chicago, IL
Robert P. Nussenblatt, M.D., Bethesda, MD
Dr. Patience Obih, New Orleans, LA
Linda K. Ohri, Pharm.D., Omaha, NE
Karen S. Oles, Pharm.D., Winston-Salem, NC
Susan Orenstein, M.D., Pittsburgh, PA
James R. Oster, M.D., Miami, FL
Judith M. Ozbun, R.Ph., M.S., Fargo, ND
Robert H. Palmer, M.D., King of Prussia, PA
David C. Pang, Ph.D., Chicago, IL
Michael F. Para, M.D., Columbus, OH
Carmen Alerany Pardo, Barcelona, Spain
Satyapal R. Pareddy, B.Pharm., Brooklyn, NY
Hee-Myung Park, M.D., Indianapolis, IN
Robert C. Park, M.D., Washington, DC
David R. Parkinson, M.D., Bethesda, MD
Albert Patterson, Hines, IL
Bruce Peterson, M.D., Minneapolis, MN
Neil A. Petry, M.S., Ann Arbor, MI
Philip A. Pizzo, M.D., Bethesda, MD
Therese Poirier, Pharm.D., Pittsburgh, PA
James Ponto, R.Ph., Iowa City, IA
Carol M. Proudfit, Ph.D., Chicago, IL
Norbert P. Rapoza, Ph.D., Chicago, IL
B. Redman, D.O., Detroit, MI
Alfred J. Remillard, Pharm.D., Saskatoon, Saskatchewan, Canada
Ann Richards, Pharm.D., San Antonio, TX
Cara Rieseaman, Pharm.D., San Antonio, TX
Daniel C. Robinson, Pharm.D., Los Angeles, CA
Leslie Rocher, M.D., Royal Oak, MI
Hector M. Rodriguez, Mexico D.F., Mexico
John Rodman, M.D., New York, NY
Wolfgang Rosch, M.D., Frankfurt, German
Maura K. Roush, M.D., San Antonio, TX
Erick K. Rowinsky, M.D., Baltimore, MD
Frederick Ruben, M.D., Pittsburgh, PA
Jean A. Rumsfield, Pharm.D., Lincolnshire, IL
Mary Russell, R.D., Durham, NC
Michael S. Saag, M.D., Birmingham, AL
Frank Sacks, M.D., Boston, MA
Eugene L. Saenger, M.D., Cincinnati, OH
Evelyn Salerno, Pharm.D., Hialeah, FL
Jay P. Sanford, M.D., Dallas, TX
Subbiah Sangiah, Ph.D., Stillwater, OK
Gisele A. Sarosy, M.D., Bethesda, MD
John J. Savarese, M.D., Boston, MA
Sheila Kelly Scarim, Pharm.D., Indianapolis, IN
Anthony J. Schaeffer, Chicago, IL
Alan F. Schatzberg, M.D., Stanford, CA
Renslow Scherer, M.D., Chicago, IL
Gerald Schiffman, M.D., Brooklyn, NY
Steven M. Schnittman, M.D., Rockville, MD
Gustav Schonfeld, M.D., St. Louis, MO
Tim Schroeder, M.D., Cincinnati, OH
Jerome Seidenfeld, Ph.D., Chicago, IL
Charles F. Seifert, Pharm.D., Oklahoma City, OK
Sandra L. Sessoms, M.D., Houston, TX
Allen Shaughnessy, Pharm.D., Harrisburg, PA
Yvonne M. Shevchuk, Pharm.D., Saskatoon, Saskatchewan, Canada
Mitchell Shub, M.D., Phoenix, AZ
Frederick P. Siegal, M.D., New Hyde Park, NY
Gary G. Sladek, M.D., Bethesda, MD
Howard R. Sloan, M.D., Bronx, NY
Geralynn B. Smith, M.S., Detroit, MI
John R. Smith, M.S., Ph.D., Portland, OR
Steven J. Smith, Ph.D., Chicago, IL
Elliott M. Sogol, Ph.D., Research Triangle Park, NC

Harry Spiera, M.D., New York, NY
E. Spierings, M.D., Chesnut Hill, MA
Alexander S.D. Spiers, M.D., Albany, NY
John J. Stern, M.D., Philadelphia, PA
David Stuhr, Denver, CO
Alan Sugar, M.D., Boston, MA
Jay Sullivan, M.D., Memphis, TN
Linda Gore Sutherland, Pharm.D., Laramie, WY
Mario Sznol, M.D., Bethesda, MD
M. E. Teresi, Iowa City, IA
Daniel Thibaud, M.D., Switzerland
James C. Thompson, M.D., Galveston, TX
Michael G. Tierney, M.Sc., Ottawa, Ontario, Canada
Kenneth J. Tomecki, M.D., Cleveland, OH
William Treem, M.D., Hartford, CT
Jayme Trott, Pharm.D., San Antonio, TX
Theodore F. Tsai, M.D., Bethesda, MD
Nanette Turcaso, Pharm.D., Salt Lake City, UT
Nicholas Vogelzang, M.D., Chicago, IL
Mann Vohra, PLD, Halifax, Nova Scotia, Canada
Paul A. Volberding, M.D., San Francisco, CA
Charles Wabner, M.D., Springfield, IL
Andrea Wall, B.S., R.Ph., Cincinnati, OH
Carla Wallace, Pharm.D., Lexington, KY
William Warner, Ph.D., New York, NY
Elizabeth Warren-Bolton, Washington, DC
Gary Wasserman, DO, Kansas City, MO
Evelyn E. Watson, Oak Ridge, TN
Michael Weber, M.D., Irvine, CA
Dr. K. Weeraewiya, Geneva, Switzerland
R. S. Weinstein, M.D., Augusta, GA
Rochelle Weiss, Ph.D., Lincolnshire, IL
Thom Welch, M.D., Cincinnati, OH
T. Wellems, M.D., Bethesda, MD
Timothy E. Welty, Pharm.D., Bismarck, ND
John White, Pharm.D., Spokane, WA
Richard J. Whitley, M.D., Birmingham, AL
Catherine Wilfert, M.D., Durham, NC
Robert F. Wilkens, M.D., Seattle, WA
Robert G. Wolfangel, Ph.D., St. Louis, MO
M. Michael Wolfe, M.D., Boston, MA
Paul D. Woolf, M.D., Rochester, NY
Donna Wowhuter, R.N., Rochester, MN
Corinne Zara Yahni, Barcelona, Spain
Katherine E. Yutzy, Goshen, IN
John M. Zajecka, M.D., Chicago, IL
Mark Zetin, M.D., Orange, CA
Frederic J. Zucchero, M.A., R.Ph., St. Louis, MO

Headquarters Staff

DRUG INFORMATION DIVISION

Director: Keith W. Johnson

Assistant Director: Georgie M. Cathey

Administrative Staff: Jaime A. Ramirez *(Administrative Assistant),* Albert Crucillo, Mayra L. Rios

Senior Drug Information Specialists: Nancy Lee Dashiell, Esther H. Klein *(Supervisor),* Angela Méndez Mayo *(Spanish Publications Coordinator)*

Drug Information Specialists: Joyce Carpenter, Ann Corken, Debra A. Edwards, Robin Isham-Schermerhorn, Jymeann King, Doris Lee *(Supervisor),* Denise Seldon

Veterinary Drug Information Specialist: Amy Neal

Coordinator, Patient Counseling and Education Programs: Stacy M. Hartranft

Computer Applications Specialist: David Gillikin

Publications Development Staff: Diana M. Blais *(Supervisor)*, Anne M. Lawrence *(Associate)*, Dorothy Raymond *(Assistant)*, Darcy Schwartz *(Assistant)*

Library Services: Florence A. Hogan *(Coordinator)*, Terri Rikhy *(Assistant),* Madeleine Welsch

Research Assistants: Marie Kotomori, Annamarie J. Sibik

Consultants: Sandra Lee Boyer, David W. Hughes, S. Ramakrishnan Iyer, Wanda Janicki, Marcelo Vernengo

Scholar in Residence: Duane M. Kirking, University of Michigan

Student Interns/Externs: Carmelina Battista, Albany College of Pharmacy; Nilam Dhanani, University of Pittsburgh; Sharon Gelmini, West Virginia University; Bill Kutney, University of North Carolina, Chapel Hill; Jeann Lee, University of Illinois, Chicago; Mark Sanders, University of Arkansas

Visiting Scholars: O. O. Omoyele, Lagos, Nigeria; Omowunmi Osibo, Lagos, Nigeria

USPC ADMINISTRATIVE STAFF

Executive Director: Jerome A. Halperin

Associate Executive Director: Joseph G. Valentino

Assistant Executive Director for Professional and Public Affairs: Jacqueline L. Eng

Director, Finance: Abe Brauner

Director, Operations: J. Robert Strang

Director, Personnel: Arlene Bloom

Fulfillment/Facilities Manager: Drew J. Lutz

DRUG STANDARDS DIVISION

Director: Lee T. Grady

Assistant Directors: Charles H. Barnstein *(Revision)*, Barbara B. Hubert, *(Scientific Administration)*, Robert H. King *(Technical Services)*

Senior Scientists: Roger Dabbah, V. Srinivasan, William W. Wright

Scientists: Frank P. Barletta, Vivian A. Gray, W. Larry Paul

Senior Scientific Associate: Susan W. Brobst

Scientific Associate: Todd L. Cecil

Technical Editors: Ann K. Ferguson, Melissa M. Smith

Supervisor of Administration: Anju K. Malhotra

Support Staff: Glenna Etherton, Theresa H. Lee, Cecilia Luna, Maureen Rawson, Margaret Traynor, Ernestene Williams

Drug Research and Testing Laboratory: Richard F. Lindauer *(Director)*

Hazard Communications: James J. Lenahan, Linda Shear

Consultants: J. Joseph Belson, Zorach R. Glaser, Aubrey S. Outschoorn

MARKETING

Director: Joan Blitman

Senior Product Manager: Mitchell A. Lapides *(Electronic Applications)*

Marketing Associates: Jennifer C. Glenn, Dana L. McCullah

Marketing Representative: Susan M. Williams *(Electronic Applications)*

Marketing Assistant: Susan D. Harmon

PUBLICATION SERVICES

Director: Patricia H. Morgenstern

Managing Editors: A. V. Precup *(USP DI)*, Sandra Boynton *(USP-NF)*

Editorial Associates: *USP DI*—Ellen R. Loeb *(Senior Editorial Associate)*, Carol M. Griffin, Carol N. Hankin, Harriet S. Nathanson, Ellen D. Smith, Barbara A. Visco; *USP-NF*—Jesusa D. Cordova *(Senior Editorial Associate)*, Ellen Elovitz, John Pahle, Margaret Kay Walshaw

USAN Staff: Carolyn A. Fleeger *(Editor)*, Gerilynne Seigneur

Typesetting Systems Coordinator: Jean E. Dale

Typesetting Staff: Susan L. Entwistle *(Supervisor)*, Donna Alie, Deborah R. Connelly, Lauren Taylor Davis, M. T. Samahon, Micheline Tranquille

Graphics: Gail M. Oring *(Manager)*, Cristy Gonzalez, Tia C. Morfessis, Mary P. Regan, Greg Varhola

Word Processing: Barbara A. Bowman *(Supervisor)*, Frances Rampp, Susan Schartman, Jane Shulman

Also Contributing: Jennifer Nathanson, Proofreader; Deborah James, Typesetter; and Terri A. DeIuliis, Graphics.

PRACTITIONER REPORTING PROGRAMS

Assistant Executive Director for Practitioner Reporting Programs: Diane D. Cousins

Staff: Robin A. Baldwin, Shawn C. Becker, Jean Canada, Alice C. Curtis, Ilze Mohseni, Joanne Pease, Susmita Samanta, Anne Paula Thompson, Mary Susan Zmuda

Members of the USPC and the Institutions and Organizations Represented as of August 1, 1992

Officers and Board of Trustees

President: Mark Novitch, M.D.
Vice President: Donald R. Bennett, M.D.
Treasurer: John T. Fay, Jr., Ph.D.
Trustees Representing Medical Sciences: Edwin D. Bransome, Jr., M.D.; J. Richard Crout, M.D.
Trustees Representing Pharmaceutical Sciences: Jordan L. Cohen, Ph.D.; James T. Doluisio, Ph.D.
Trustee Representing the Public: Grace Powers Monaco, J.D.
Trustees at Large: John V. Bergen, Ph.D., Joseph A. Mollica, Ph.D.
Past President: Arthur Hull Hayes, Jr., M.D.

United States Government Services

Department of the Army: Col. William O. Hiner, Jr.
Food and Drug Administration: Carl C. Peck, M.D.
National Institute of Standards and Technology: Stanley D. Rasberry
Navy Surgeon General's Office/Bureau of Medicine and Surgery: Captain R. Whiten
Office of the Surgeon General, U.S. Air Force: Col. John M. Hammond
United States Public Health Service: Richard M. Church
U.S. Office of Consumer Affairs: Howard Seltzer
Department of Veterans Affairs: John Ogden
Health Care Financing Administration: Robert E. Wren

National Organizations

American Association of Pharmaceutical Scientists: Ralph F. Shangraw, Ph.D.
American Chemical Society: Norman C. Jamieson, Ph.D.
American Dental Association: Clifford W. Whall, Ph.D.
American Hospital Association: William R. Reid
American Medical Association: Joseph W. Cranston, Jr., Ph.D.
American Nurses Association: Linda Cronenwett, Ph.D., R.N., F.A.A.N.
American Pharmaceutical Association: Arthur H. Kibbe, Ph.D.
American Society for Clinical Pharmacology & Therapeutics: William J. Mroczek, M.D.
American Society of Consultant Pharmacists: Milton S. Moskowitz
American Society of Hospital Pharmacists: Stephanie Y. Crawford, Ph.D.
American Society for Pharmacology and Experimental Therapeutics: Kenneth L. Dretchen
American Society for Quality Control: Anthony M. Carfagno
American Veterinary Medical Association: Lloyd Davis, D.V.M., Ph.D.
Association of Food and Drug Officials: David R. Work, J.D.
Association of Official Analytical Chemists: Thomas Layloff, Jr.
Chemical Manufacturers Association: Andrew J. Schmitz, Jr.
Cosmetic, Toiletry & Fragrance Association, Inc.: G.N. McEwen, Jr., Ph.D., J.D.
Drug Information Association: Elizabeth B. D'Angelo, Ph.D.
Generic Pharmaceutical Industry Association: William F. Haddad
Health Industry Manufacturers Association: Dee Simons
National Association of Boards of Pharmacy: Carmen Catizone
National Association of Chain Drug Stores, Inc.: Saul Schneider
National Wholesale Druggists' Association: Bruce R. Siecker, R. Ph., Ph.D.
Nonprescription Drug Manufacturers Association: R. William Soller, Ph.D.
Parenteral Drug Association, Inc.: Peter E. Manni, Ph.D.
Pharmaceutical Manufacturers Association: Maurice Q. Bectel

Other Organizations and Institutions

Alabama

Auburn University, School of Pharmacy: Kenneth N. Barker, Ph.D.
Samford University School of Pharmacy: H. Anthony McBride, Ph.D.
University of Alabama School of Medicine: Robert B. Diasio, M.D.
University of South Alabama, College of Medicine: Samuel J. Strada, Ph.D.
Medical Association of the State of Alabama: Paul A. Palmisano, M.D.
Alabama Pharmaceutical Association: Mitchel C. Rothholz

Alaska

Alaska Pharmaceutical Association: Jackie Warren, R.Ph.

Arizona

University of Arizona, College of Medicine: John D. Palmer, Ph.D., M.D.

University of Arizona, College of Pharmacy: Michael Mayersohn, Ph.D.

Arizona Pharmacy Association: Edward Armstrong

Arkansas

University of Arkansas for Medical Sciences, College of Pharmacy: Kenneth G. Nelson, Ph.D.

Arkansas Pharmacists Association: Norman Canterbury, P.D.

California

Loma Linda University Medical Center: Ralph Cutler, M.D.

Stanford University School of Medicine: Brian B. Hoffman, M.D.

University of California, Davis, School of Medicine: Larry Stark, Ph.D.

University of California, San Diego, School of Medicine: Harold J. Simon, M.D., Ph.D.

University of California, San Francisco, School of Medicine: Walter L. Way, M.D.

University of Southern California, School of Medicine: Wayne R. Bidlack, Ph.D.

University of California, San Francisco, School of Pharmacy: Richard H. Guy, Ph.D.

University of Southern California, School of Pharmacy: Robert T. Koda, Pharm.D., Ph.D.

University of the Pacific, School of Pharmacy: Alice Jean Matuszak, Ph.D.

California Pharmacists Association: Robert P. Marshall, Pharm.D.

Colorado

University of Colorado School of Pharmacy: Merrick Lee Shively, Ph.D.

Colorado Pharmacal Association: Thomas G. Arthur, R.Ph.

Connecticut

University of Connecticut, School of Medicine: Paul F. Davern

University of Connecticut, School of Pharmacy: Karl A. Nieforth, Ph.D.

Connecticut Pharmaceutical Association: Henry A. Palmer, Ph.D.

Delaware

Delaware Pharmaceutical Society: Charles J. O'Connor

Medical Society of Delaware: John M. Levinson, M.D.

District of Columbia

George Washington University: Janet Elgert-Madison, Pharm.D.

Georgetown University, School of Medicine: Arthur Raines, Ph.D.

Howard University, College of Medicine: Sonya K. Sobrian, Ph.D.

Howard University, College of Pharmacy & Pharmacal Sciences: Wendell T. Hill, Jr., Pharm.D.

Florida

Southeastern College of Pharmacy: William D. Hardigan, Ph.D.

University of Florida, College of Medicine: Thomas F. Muther, Ph.D.

University of Florida, College of Pharmacy: Michael A. Schwartz, Ph.D.

University of South Florida, College of Medicine: Joseph J. Krzanowski, Jr., Ph.D.

Florida Pharmacy Association: "Red" Camp

Georgia

Medical College of Georgia, School of Medicine: David W. Hawkins, Pharm.D.

Mercer University School of Medicine: W. Douglas Skelton, M.D.

Mercer University, Southern School of Pharmacy: Hewitt W. Matthews, Ph.D.

Morehouse School of Medicine: Ralph W. Trottier, Jr., Ph.D., J.D.

University of Georgia, College of Pharmacy: Stuart Feldman, Ph.D.

Medical Association of Georgia: E.D. Bransome, Jr., M.D.

Georgia Pharmaceutical Association, Inc.: Larry R. Braden

Idaho

Idaho State University, College of Pharmacy: Eugene I. Isaacson, Ph.D.

Idaho State Pharmaceutical Association: Doris Denney

Illinois

Chicago Medical School/University of Health Sciences: Velayudhan Nair, Ph.D., D.Sc.

Loyola University of Chicago Stritch School of Medicine: Erwin Coyne, Ph.D.

Northwestern University Medical School: Marilynn C. Frederiksen, M.D.

Rush Medical College of Rush University: Paul G. Pierpaoli, M.S.

Southern Illinois University, School of Medicine: Lionard Rybak, M.D., Ph.D.

University of Chicago, Pritzker School of Medicine: Patrick T. Horn, M.D., Ph.D.

University of Illinois, College of Medicine: Marten M. Kernis, Ph.D.

Chicago College of Pharmacy: David J. Slatkin, Ph.D.

Illinois Pharmacists Association: Ronald W. Gottrich

Illinois State Medical Society: Vincent A. Costanzo, Jr., M.D.

Indiana

Butler University, College of Pharmacy: Wagar H. Bhatti, Ph.D.

Purdue University, School of Pharmacy and Pharmacal Sciences: Garnet E. Peck, Ph.D.

Indiana State Medical Association: Edward Langston, M.D.

Iowa

Drake University, College of Pharmacy: Sidney L. Finn, Ph.D.

University of Iowa, College of Medicine: John E. Kasik, M.D., Ph.D.

University of Iowa, College of Pharmacy: Robert A. Wiley, Ph.D.

Iowa Pharmacists Association: Steve C. Firman, R.Ph.

Kansas

University of Kansas, School of Pharmacy: Siegfried Lindenbaum, Ph.D.

Kansas Pharmacists Association: Robert R. Williams

Kentucky

University of Kentucky, College of Medicine: John M. Carney, Ph.D.

University of Kentucky, College of Pharmacy: Patrick P. DeLuca, Ph.D.

University of Louisville, School of Medicine: Peter P. Rowell, Ph.D.

Kentucky Medical Association: Ellsworth C. Seeley, M.D.

Kentucky Pharmacists Association: Chester L. Parker, Pharm.D.

Louisiana

Louisiana State University School of Medicine in New Orleans: Paul L. Kirkendol, Ph.D.

Northeast Louisiana University, School of Pharmacy: William M. Bourn, Ph.D.

Tulane University, School of Medicine: Floyd R. Domer, Ph.D.

Xavier University of Louisiana: Barry A. Bleidt, Ph.D., R.Ph.

Louisiana State Medical Society: Henry W. Jolly, Jr., M.D.

Louisiana Pharmacists Association: Patricia M. Williford

Maryland

Johns Hopkins University, School of Medicine: E. Robert Feroli, Jr., Pharm.D.

University of Maryland, School of Medicine: Edson X. Albuquerque, M.D., Ph.D.

Uniformed Services University of the Health Sciences, F. Edward Hebert School of Medicine: Louis R. Cantilena, Jr., M.D., Ph.D.

University of Maryland, School of Pharmacy: Larry L. Augsburger, Ph.D.

Medical and Chirurgical Faculty of the State of Maryland: Frederick Wilhelm, M.D.

Maryland Pharmacists Association: Nicholas C. Lykos, P.D.

Massachusetts

Harvard Medical School: Peter Goldman, M.D.

Massachusetts College of Pharmacy and Allied Health Sciences: David A. Williams, Ph.D.

Northeastern University, College of Pharmacy and Allied Health Professions: John L. Neumeyer, Ph.D.

Tufts University, School of Medicine: John Mazzullo, M.D.

University of Massachusetts Medical School: Brian Johnson, M.D.

Massachusetts Medical Society: Errol Green, M.D.

Michigan

Ferris State College, School of Pharmacy: Gerald W.A. Slywka, Ph.D.

Michigan State University, College of Human Medicine: John Penner, M.D.

University of Michigan, College of Pharmacy: Ara G. Paul, Ph.D.

University of Michigan Medical Center: Jeoffrey K. Stross, M.D.

Wayne State University, School of Medicine: Ralph E. Kauffman, M.D.

Wayne State University, College of Pharmacy and Allied Health Professions: Janardan B. Nagwekar, Ph.D.

Michigan Pharmacists Association: Patrick L. McKercher, Ph.D.

Minnesota

Mayo Medical School: James J. Lipsky, M.D.

University of Minnesota, College of Pharmacy: E. John Staba, Ph.D.

University of Minnesota Medical School, Minneapolis: Jack W. Miller, Ph.D.

Minnesota Medical Association: Harold Seim, M.D.

Minnesota State Pharmaceutical Association: Arnold D. Delger

Mississippi

University of Mississippi, School of Medicine: James L. Achord, M.D.

University of Mississippi, School of Pharmacy: Robert W. Cleary, Ph.D.

Mississippi State Medical Association: Charles L. Mathews

Mississippi Pharmacists Association: Mike Kelly

Missouri

St. Louis College of Pharmacy: John W. Zuzack, Ph.D.

St. Louis University, School of Medicine: Alvin H. Gold, Ph.D.

University of Missouri, Columbia, School of Medicine: John W. Yarbro, M.D.

University of Missouri-Kansas City, School of Medicine: Paul Cuddy, Pharm.D.

University of Missouri, Kansas City, School of Pharmacy: Lester Chafetz, Ph.D.

Washington University, School of Medicine: H. Mitchell Perry, Jr., M.D.

Missouri Pharmaceutical Association: George L. Oestreich

Montana

The University of Montana, School of Pharmacy & Allied Health Sciences: David S. Forbes, Ph.D.

Nebraska

Creighton University, School of Medicine: Michael C. Makoid, Ph.D.

Creighton University School of Pharmacy and Allied Health Professions: Kenneth R. Keefner, Ph.D.

University of Nebraska, College of Medicine: Manuchair Ebadi, Ph.D.

University of Nebraska, College of Pharmacy: Clarence T. Ueda, Pharm.D., Ph.D.

Nebraska Pharmacists Association: Rex C. Higley, R.Ph.

Nevada

Nevada Pharmacists Association: Steven P. Bradford

New Hampshire

Dartmouth Medical School: James J. Kresel, Ph.D.

New Hampshire Pharmaceutical Association: William J. Lancaster, P.D.

New Jersey

University of Medicine and Dentistry of New Jersey, New Jersey Medical School: Sheldon B. Gertner, Ph.D.

Rutgers, The State University of New Jersey, College of Pharmacy: John L. Colaizzi, Ph.D.

Medical Society of New Jersey: Joseph N. Micale, M.D.

New Jersey Pharmaceutical Association: Stephen J. Csubak, Ph.D.

New Mexico

University of New Mexico, College of Pharmacy: William M. Hadley, Ph.D.

New Mexico Pharmaceutical Association: Hugh Kabat, Ph.D.

New York

Albert Einstein College of Medicine of Yeshiva University: Walter G. Levine, Ph.D.

City University of New York, Mt. Sinai School of Medicine: Joel S. Mindel

Columbia Univ. College of Physicians and Surgeons: Michael R. Rosen, M.D.

Cornell University Medical College: Lorraine J. Gudas, Ph.D.

Long Island University, Arnold and Marie Schwartz College of Pharmacy and Health Sciences: Jack M. Rosenberg, Ph.D.

New York Medical College: Mario A. Inchiosa, Jr., Ph.D.

New York University School of Medicine: Norman Altzuler, Ph.D.

State University of New York, Buffalo, School of Medicine: Robert J. McIsaac, Ph.D.

State University of New York, Buffalo, School of Pharmacy: Robert M. Cooper

State University of New York, Health Science Center, Syracuse: Oliver M. Brown, Ph.D.

St. John's University, College of Pharmacy and Allied Health Professions: Albert A. Belmonte, Ph.D.

Union University, Albany College of Pharmacy: David W. Newton, Ph.D.

University of Rochester, School of Medicine and Dentistry: Michael Weintraub, M.D.

Medical Society of the State of New York: Richard S. Blum, M.D.

Pharmaceutical Society of the State of New York: Bruce Moden

North Carolina

Bowman Gray School of Medicine, Wake Forest University: Jack W. Strandhoy, Ph.D.

Campbell University, School of Pharmacy: Antoine Al-Achi, Ph.D.

Duke University Medical Center: William J. Murray, M.D., Ph.D.

East Carolina University, School of Medicine: A-R. A. Abdel-Rahman, Ph.D.

University of North Carolina, Chapel Hill, School of Medicine: George Hatfield, Ph.D.

University of North Carolina, Chapel Hill, School of Pharmacy: Richard J. Kowalsky, Pharm.D.

North Carolina Pharmaceutical Association: George H. Cocolas, Ph.D.

North Carolina Medical Society: T. Reginald Harris, M.D.

North Dakota

University of North Dakota, School of Medicine: David W. Hein, Ph.D.

North Dakota State University, College of Pharmacy: William M. Henderson, Ph.D.

North Dakota Medical Association: Vernon E. Wagner

North Dakota Pharmaceutical Association: William H. Shelver, Ph.D.

Ohio

Case Western Reserve University, School of Medicine: Kenneth A. Scott, Ph.D.

Medical College of Ohio at Toledo: R. Douglas Wilkerson, Ph.D.

Northeastern Ohio University, College of Medicine: Ralph E. Berggren, M.D.

Ohio Northern University, College of Pharmacy: Joseph Theodore, Ph.D.

Ohio State University, College of Medicine: Robert Guthrie, M.D.

Ohio State University, College of Pharmacy: Michael C. Gerald, Ph.D.

University of Cincinnati, College of Medicine: Leonard T. Sigell, Ph.D.

University of Cincinnati, College of Pharmacy: Henry S.I. Tan, Ph.D.

University of Toledo, College of Pharmacy: Norman F. Billups, Ph.D.

Wright State University, School of Medicine: John O. Lindower, M.D., Ph.D.

Ohio State Medical Association: Janet K. Bixel, M.D.

Ohio State Pharmaceutical Association: J. Richard Wuest

Oklahoma

University of Oklahoma College of Medicine: Ronald D. Brown, M.D.

Southwestern Oklahoma State University, School of Pharmacy: W. Steven Pray, Ph.D.

University of Oklahoma, College of Pharmacy: Loyd V. Allen, Jr., Ph.D.

Oklahoma State Medical Association: Clinton Nicholas Corder, M.D., Ph.D.

Oklahoma Pharmaceutical Association: Carl D. Lyons

Oregon

Oregon Health Sciences University, School of Medicine: Hall Downes, M.D., Ph.D.

Oregon State University, College of Pharmacy: Randall L. Vanderveen, Ph.D.

Pennsylvania

Duquesne University, School of Pharmacy: Lawrence H. Block, Ph.D.

Hahnemann University, School of Medicine: Vincent J. Zarro, M.D.

Medical College of Pennsylvania: Athole G. McNeil Jacobi, M.D.

Pennsylvania State University, College of Medicine: John D. Connor, Ph.D.

Philadelphia College of Pharmacy and Science: Alfonso R. Gennaro, Ph.D.

Temple University, School of Medicine: Ronald J. Tallarida, Ph.D.
Temple University, School of Pharmacy: Murray Tuckerman, Ph.D.
University of Pennsylvania, School of Medicine: Marilyn E. Hess, Ph.D.
University of Pittsburgh, School of Pharmacy: Terrence L. Schwinghammer, Pharm.D.
Pennsylvania Medical Society: Benjamin Calesnick, M.D.
Pennsylvania Pharmaceutical Association: Joseph A. Mosso R.Ph.

Puerto Rico
Universidad Central del Caribe, School of Medicine: Jesús Santos-Martínez, Ph.D.
University of Puerto Rico, College of Pharmacy: Benjamin P. de Gracia, Ph.D.
University of Puerto Rico, School of Medicine: Walmor C. De Mello, M.D., Ph.D.

Rhode Island
Brown University Program in Medicine: Darrell R. Abernethy, M.D., Ph.D.
University of Rhode Island, College of Pharmacy: Thomas E. Needham, Ph.D.

South Carolina
Medical University of South Carolina, College of Medicine: Herman B. Daniell, Ph.D.
Medical University of South Carolina, College of Pharmacy: Paul J. Niebergall, Ph.D.
University of South Carolina, College of Pharmacy: Robert L. Beamer, Ph.D.

South Dakota
South Dakota State University, College of Pharmacy: Gary S. Chappell, Ph.D.
South Dakota State Medical Association: Robert D. Johnson
South Dakota Pharmaceutical Association: James Powers

Tennessee
East Tennessee State University, Quillen College of Medicine: Ernest A. Daigneault, Ph.D.
Meharry Medical College, School of Medicine: Dolores C. Shockley, Ph.D.
University of Tennessee, College of Medicine: Murray Heimberg, M.D., Ph.D.
University of Tennessee, College of Pharmacy: Dick R. Gourley, Pharm.D.
Vanderbilt University, School of Medicine: David H. Robertson, M.D.
Tennessee Pharmacists Association: Roger L. Davis, Pharm.D.

Texas
Texas A & M University, College of Medicine: Marsha A. Raebel, Pharm.D.
Texas Southern University, College of Pharmacy and Health Sciences: Victor Padron, Ph.D.
University of Houston, College of Pharmacy: Mustafa Lokhandwala, Ph.D.
University of Texas, Austin, College of Pharmacy: James T. Doluisio, Ph.D.
University of Texas, Medical Branch at Galveston: George T. Bryan, M.D.
University of Texas Medical School, Houston: Jacques E. Chelly, M.D., Ph.D.
University of Texas Medical School, San Antonio: Alexander M.M. Shepherd, M.D., Ph.D.
Texas Medical Association: Robert H. Barr, M.D.
Texas Pharmaceutical Association: Shirley McKee, R.Ph.

Utah
University of Utah, College of Pharmacy: David B. Roll, Ph.D.
Utah Pharmaceutical Association: Robert V. Peterson, Ph.D.
Utah Medical Association: David A. Hilding, M.D.

Vermont
University of Vermont, College of Medicine: John J. McCormack, Ph.D.
Vermont Pharmacists Association: James S. Craddock

Virginia
Medical College of Hampton Roads: William J. Cooke, Ph.D.
Medical College of Virginia/Virginia Commonwealth University, School of Pharmacy: William H. Barr, Pharm.D., Ph.D.
University of Virginia, School of Medicine: Peyton E. Weary, M.D.
The Medical Society of Virginia: Richard W. Lindsay, M.D.
Virginia Pharmaceutical Association: Daniel A. Herbert

Washington
Washington State University, College of Pharmacy: Martin J. Jinks, Pharm.D.
Washington State Pharmacists Association: Danial E. Baker

West Virginia
Marshall University, School of Medicine: John L. Szarek, Ph.D.
West Virginia University, School of Medicine: Douglas D. Glover, M.D.
West Virginia University Medical Center, School of Pharmacy: Arthur I. Jacknowitz, Pharm.D.

Wisconsin
Medical College of Wisconsin: Garrett J. Gross, Ph.D.
University of Wisconsin, Madison, School of Pharmacy: Chester A. Bond, Pharm.D.
University of Wisconsin Medical School, Madison: Joseph M. Benforado, M.D.
State Medical Society of Wisconsin: Thomas L. Adams, CAE
Wisconsin Pharmacists Association: Dennis Dziczkowski, R.Ph.

Wyoming
University of Wyoming, School of Pharmacy: Kenneth F. Nelson, Ph.D.
Wyoming Medical Society: R. W. Johnson, Jr.
Wyoming Pharmaceutical Association: Linda G. Sutherland

Members-at-Large

Norman W. Atwater, Ph.D., Hopewell, NJ
Cheston M. Berlin, Jr., M.D., The Milton S. Hershey Medical Ctr.
Fred S. Brinkley, Jr., Texas State Board of Pharmacy
Herbert S. Carlin, D.Sc., Chappaqua, NY
Jordan Cohen, Ph.D., College of Pharmacy, University of Kentucky
John L. Cova, Ph.D., Health Insurance Assoc. of America
Enrique Fefer, Ph.D., Pan American Health Organization
Leroy Fevang, Canadian Pharmaceutical Association
Klaus G. Florey, Ph.D., Squibb Institute for Medical Research
Lester Hosto, Ph.D., Arkansas State Board of Pharmacy
Jay S. Keystone, M.D., Tropical Disease Unit, Toronto General Hospital
Calvin M. Kunin, M.D., Ohio State University
Marvin Lipman, M.D., Scarsdale, NY
Joseph A. Mollica, Ph.D., DuPont Merck Pharmaceuticals
Stuart L. Nightingale, M.D., Food and Drug Administration
Daniel A. Nona, Ph.D., The American Council on Pharmaceutical Education
Mark Novitch, M.D., The Upjohn Company
Charles A. Pergola, SmithKline Beecham Consumer Brands
Donald O. Schiffman, Ph.D., Genealogy Unlimited
Carl E. Trinca, Ph.D., American Association of Colleges of Pharmacy

Members-at-Large (representing other countries that provide legal status to *USP* or *NF*)

Prof. T. D. Arias, Estafeta Universitaria, Panama, Republica De Panama
Keith Bailey, M.A., D.Phil., Canadian Bureau of Drug Research
Quintin L. Kintanar, M.D., Ph.D., National Science & Technology Authority, Bicutan, Taguig, Philippines
Marcelo Jorge Vernego, Ph.D., Pan American Health Organization - Rio de Janeiro, Brasil

Members-at-Large (Public)

Clement Bezold, Ph.D., Alternative Futures Association
Alexander Grant, Food and Drug Administration
Grace Powers Monaco, J.D., Washington, DC
Paul G. Rogers, National Council on Patient Information and Education
Frances M. West, J.D., Wilmington, DE

Ex-Officio Members

Joseph M. Benforado, M.D., Madison, WI
Joseph P. Buckley, Ph.D., Houston, TX
Estelle G. Cohen, M.A., Baltimore, MD
Leo E. Hollister, M.D., Houston, TX
Paul F. Parker, Lexington, KY

Committee Chairmen

Credentials Committee: Peyton E. Weary, M.D.
Nominating Committee for the General Committee of Revision: Walter L. Way, M.D.
Nominating Committee for Officers and Trustees: Joseph M. Benforado, M.D.
Resolutions Committee: J. Richard Crout, M.D.
General Committee of Revision: Jerome A. Halperin
Constitution and Bylaws Committee: John V. Bergen, Ph.D.

Honorary Members

George F. Archambault, Pharm.D., J.D., Bethesda, MD
William J. Kinnard, Jr., Ph.D., Baltimore, MD
Lloyd C. Miller, Ph.D., Escondido, CA
John H. Moyer, M.D., D.Sc., Palmyra, PA
John A. Owen, Jr., M.D., Charlottesville, VA
Harry C. Shirkey, M.D., Cincinnati, OH
Linwood F. Tice, D.Sc., Philadelphia, PA

General Information About Use of Medicines

Information about the proper use of medicines is of two types. One type is drug specific and applies to a certain medicine or group of medicines only. The other type is general in nature and applies to the use of any medicine.

The information that follows is general in nature. For your own safety, health, and well-being, however, it is important that you learn about the proper use of your specific medicines as well. You can get this information from your health care provider, or find it in the individual listings of this book.

Before Using Your Medicine

Before you use any medicine, your health care provider should be told:

—if you have ever had an allergic or unusual reaction to any medicine, food, or other substance, such as yellow dye or sulfites.

—if you are on a low-salt, low-sugar, or any other special diet. Most medicines contain more than their active ingredient, and many liquid medicines contain alcohol.

—*if you are pregnant or if you plan to become pregnant*. Certain medicines may cause birth defects or other problems in the unborn child. For other medicines, safe use during pregnancy has not been established. *The use of any medicine during pregnancy must be carefully considered* and should be discussed with a health care professional.

—*if you are breast-feeding*. Some medicines may pass into the breast milk and cause unwanted effects in the baby.

—*if you are now taking or have taken any medicines or dietary supplements in the recent past*. Do not forget over-the-counter (nonprescription) medicines such as pain relievers, laxatives, and antacids or dietary supplements.

—*if you have any medical problems* other than the one(s) for which your medicine was prescribed.

—*if you have difficulty remembering things or reading labels.*

Storage of Your Medicine

It is important to store your medicines properly. Guidelines for proper storage include:

- *Keep out of the reach of children* and in the original container.
- Store away from heat and direct light.
- Do not store capsules or tablets in the bathroom, near the kitchen sink, or in other damp places. Heat or moisture may cause the medicine to break down. Also, do not leave the cotton plug in a medicine container that has been opened since it may draw moisture into the container.
- Keep liquid medicines from freezing.
- Do not store medicines in the refrigerator unless directed to do so.
- Do not leave your medicines in an automobile for long periods of time.
- Do not keep outdated medicine or medicine no longer needed. Be sure that any discarded medicine is out of the reach of children.

Proper Use of Your Medicine

Take medicine only as directed, at the right time, and for the full length of time prescribed by your health care provider. If you are using an over-the-counter (nonprescription) medicine, follow the directions on the label, unless otherwise directed by your health care provider. If you feel that your medicine is not working for you, check with your health care provider.

Unless your pharmacist has packaged different medicines together in a "bubble-pack," different medicines should never be mixed in one container. It is best to keep your medicines tightly capped in their original containers when not in use. Do not remove the label since directions for use and other special information appear on it.

To avoid mistakes, do not take medicine in the dark. Always read the label before taking, noting especially the expiration date, if any, of the contents.

For oral (by mouth) medicines:

- In general, it is best to take oral medicines with a full glass of water. However, follow your health care provider's directions. Some medicines should be taken with food while others should be taken on an empty stomach.
- When taking most long-acting forms of a medicine, each dose should be swallowed whole. Do not break, crush, or chew before swallowing unless you have been specifically told that it is allright to do so.
- If you are taking liquid medicines, you might consider using a specially marked measuring spoon or other device to measure each dose accurately. Ask your pharmacist about these devices. The average household teaspoon may not hold the right amount of liquid.

- Oral medicine may come in a number of different dosage forms such as tablets, capsules, and liquids. If you have trouble swallowing the dosage form prescribed for you, check with your health care provider. There may be another dosage form that would be better for you.
- Child-resistant caps on medicines for oral use have greatly decreased the number of accidental poisonings and are required by law. However, if you find it hard to open such caps, you may ask your pharmacist for a regular, easier-to-open cap. He or she is authorized by law to furnish you with a regular cap if you request it. You must make this request, however, each time you get a prescription filled.

For skin patches:

- Apply the patch to a clean, dry skin area with little or no hair and free of scars, cuts, or irritation. Remove the previous patch before applying a new one.
- Apply a new patch if the first one becomes loose or falls off.
- Apply each dose to a different area of skin to prevent skin irritation or other problems.
- Do not try to trim or cut the adhesive patch to adjust the dosage. Check with your health care provider if you think the medicine is not working as it should.

For inhalers:

- Medicines that come in inhalers usually come with patient directions. *Read the directions carefully before using the medicine.* If you do not understand the directions, or if you are not sure how to use the inhaler, check with your health care provider.
- Since different types of inhalers may not be used the same way, it is very important to carefully follow the directions given to you.

For ophthalmic (eye) drops:

- To prevent contamination, do not let the eye drop applicator tip touch any surface (including the eye) and keep the container tightly closed.
- How to apply: First, wash hands. Tilt your head back and, with the index finger, pull the lower eyelid away from the eye to form a pouch. Drop the medicine into the pouch and gently close your eyes. Do not blink. Keep your eyes closed for 1 or 2 minutes.
- If your medicine is for glaucoma or inflammation of the eye: With the middle finger of the same hand, apply pressure to the inside corner of the eye (and continue to apply pressure for 1 or 2 minutes after the medicine has been placed in the eye). This will help prevent the medicine from being absorbed into the body and causing side effects.
- After applying the eye drops, wash your hands to remove any medicine that may be on them.
- The bottle may not be full; this is to provide proper drop control.

For ophthalmic (eye) ointments:

- To prevent contamination of the eye ointment, do not let the applicator tip touch any surface (including the eye). After using, wipe the tip of the ointment tube with a clean tissue and keep the tube tightly closed.
- How to apply: First, wash your hands. Pull the lower eyelid away from the eye to form a pouch. Squeeze a thin strip of ointment into the pouch. A 1-cm (approximately ⅓-inch) strip of ointment is usually enough unless otherwise directed. Gently close your eyes and keep them closed for 1 or 2 minutes.
- After applying the eye ointment, wash your hands to remove any medicine that may be on them.

For nasal (nose) drops:

- How to use: Blow your nose gently, without squeezing. Tilt your head back while standing or sitting up, or lie down on your back on a bed and hang your head over the side. Place the drops into each nostril and keep your head tilted back for a few minutes to allow the medicine to spread throughout the nose.
- Rinse the dropper with hot water and dry with a clean tissue. Replace the cap right after use. To avoid the spread of infection, do not use the container for more than one person.

For nasal (nose) spray:

- How to use: Blow your nose gently, without squeezing. With your head upright, spray the medicine into each nostril. Sniff briskly while squeezing the bottle quickly and firmly.
- Rinse the tip of the spray bottle with hot water, taking care not to suck water into the bottle, and dry with a clean tissue. Replace the cap right after cleaning. To avoid the spread of infection, do not use the container for more than one person.

For otic (ear) drops:

- To prevent contamination of the ear drops, do not touch the applicator tip to any surface (including the ear).
- How to apply: First, wash your hands. Lie down or tilt your head so that the ear into which the medicine is to be placed faces up. For adults, gently pull the ear lobe up and back to straighten the ear canal. (For children, gently pull the ear lobe down and back to straighten the ear canal). Drop the medicine into the ear canal. Keep the ear facing up for several minutes to allow the medicine to run to the bottom of the ear canal. A sterile cotton plug may be gently inserted into the ear opening to prevent the medicine from leaking out.
- The bottle may not be full; this is to provide proper drop control.
- Do not rinse the dropper after use. Wipe the tip of the dropper with a clean tissue and keep the container tightly closed.

For rectal suppositories:

- How to insert suppository: First, wash your hands. Remove the foil wrapper and moisten the suppository with water. Lie down on your side and push the suppository well up into the rectum with your finger. If the suppository is too soft to insert because of storage in a warm place, chill the suppository in the refrigerator for 30 minutes or run cold water over it before removing the foil wrapper.
- Wash your hands after you have inserted the suppository.

For rectal cream or ointment:

- Bathe and dry the rectal area. Apply a small amount of cream or ointment and rub it in gently.
- If your health care provider wants you to insert the medicine into the rectum: First, attach the plastic applicator tip onto the opened tube. Insert the applicator tip into the rectum and gently squeeze the tube to deliver the cream. Remove the applicator tip from the tube and wash with hot, soapy water. Replace the cap of the tube after use.
- Wash your hands after you have inserted the medicine.

For vaginal medicines:

- How to insert the medicine. First, wash your hands. Use the special applicator. Follow any special directions that are provided by the manufacturer. However, if you are pregnant, check with your health care provider before using the applicator to insert the medicine.
- Lie on your back with your knees drawn up. Using the applicator, insert the medicine into the vagina as far as you can without using force or causing discomfort. Release the medicine by pushing on the plunger. Wait several minutes before getting up.
- Wash the applicator and your hands with soap and warm water.

Precautions While Using Your Medicine

Never give your medicine to anyone else. It has been prescribed for your personal medical problem and may not be the correct treatment for or may even be harmful to another person.

Many medicines should not be taken with other medicines or with alcoholic beverages. Follow your health care provider's directions to help avoid problems.

Before having any kind of surgery (including dental surgery) or emergency treatment, tell the physician or dentist about any medicine you are taking.

If you think you have taken an overdose of any medicine or if a child has taken a medicine by accident: Call your poison control center or your health care provider at once. Keep those telephone numbers handy. Also, keep a bottle of Ipecac Syrup safely stored in your home in case you are told to cause vomiting. Read the directions on the label of Ipecac Syrup before using.

Side Effects of Your Medicine

Along with its intended effects, a medicine may cause some unwanted effects. Some of these side effects may need medical attention, while others may not. It is important for you to know what side effects may occur and what you should do if you notice signs of them. Ask your health care provider about the possible side effects of the medicines you are taking. If you notice any unusual reactions or side effects that you were not told about, check with your health care provider.

Additional Information

It is a good idea for you to learn both the generic and brand names of your medicine and even to write them down and keep them for future use.

Many prescriptions may not be refilled unless your pharmacist has first checked with your health care provider. *To save time, do not wait until you have run out of medicine before requesting a refill.* This is especially important if you must take your medicine every day.

When traveling:

- Carry your medicine with you rather than putting it in your checked luggage. Checked luggage may get lost or misplaced or may be stored in very cold or very hot areas.
- Make sure a source of medicine is available where you are traveling to or take a large enough supply to last during your visit. It is also a good idea to take a copy of your written prescription with you in case you need it.

If you want more information about your medicines, ask your health care provider. *Do not be embarrassed to ask questions* about any medicine you are taking. To help you remember, it may be helpful to write down any questions and bring them with you on your next visit to your health care provider.

Avoiding Medicine Mishaps

Tips Against Tampering

Over-the-counter (OTC) or nonprescription medicines are now packaged so that you can more easily notice signs of tampering. A tamper-resistant package is now required either to be unique so that it cannot be copied with materials that are easy to find, or to have a barrier or indicator (that has an identifying characteristic, such as a pattern, picture, or logo) that will be easily noticed if it is broken. For two-piece, unsealed, hard gelatin capsules, two tamper-resistant features are required. Improved packaging also includes the use of special wrappers, seals, or caps on the outer and/or inner containers, or sealing each dose in its own pouch. Even with such packaging, however, no system is completely safe. It is important that you do your part by checking for signs of tampering whenever you buy and use a medicine.

The following information may help you detect possible signs of tampering. For some products, these tips will be helpful only if you already know how the product usually looks.

Protecting yourself

General common sense suggestions include the following:

- When buying a drug product, *consider* the dosage form (for example, capsules, tablets, syrup), the type of packaging, and the tamper-resistant features. Ask yourself: Would it be easy for someone to tamper with this product? Will I be able to determine whether or not this product has been tampered with?
- *Look very carefully* at the outer packaging of the drug product before you buy it. After you buy it, also check the inner packaging as soon as possible.
- If the medicine has a protective packaging feature, it should be described in the labeling. This description is required to be placed so that it will not be affected if the feature is broken or missing. If the feature is broken or missing, *do not buy* the product. If you have already purchased the product, return it to the store. Always be sure to tell someone in charge about any problems.
- *Do not take* medicines that show even the slightest signs of tampering or don't seem quite right.
- Never take medicines in the dark or in poor lighting. *Read* the label and check each dose of medicine before you take it.

What to look for

Packaging

- Are there breaks, cracks, or holes in the outer or inner wrapping or protective cover or seal?
- Does the outer or inner covering appear to have been disturbed, unwrapped, or replaced?
- Does a plastic or other shrink band (tight-fitting wrap) around the top of the bottle appear distorted or stretched, as though it had been rolled down and then put back into place? Is the band missing? Has the band been slit and retaped?
- Is the bottom of the container intact?
- Does the container appear to be too full or not full enough?
- Is the cap on tight?
- Are there bits of paper or glue stuck on the rim of the container that make it seem the container once had a bottle seal?
- Is the cotton plug or filler in the bottle torn, sticky, or stained, or does it appear to have been taken out and put back?
- Do eye drops have a protective seal? All eye drops must be sealed when they are made, in order to keep them germ-free. Do not use if there is any sign of a broken or removed seal.
- Check the bottom as well as the top of a tube. Is the tube properly sealed? Metal tubes crimped up from the bottom like a tube of toothpaste should be firmly sealed.
- Are the expiration date, lot number, and other information the same on both the container and its outer wrapping or box?

Liquids

- Is the medicine the usual color? Thickness?
- Is a normally clear liquid cloudy or colored?
- Are there particles (small pieces) in the bottom of the bottle or floating in the solution? For some liquids, called suspensions, floating particles are normal.
- Does the medicine have a strange or different odor (for example, bleach, acid, gasoline-like, or other pungent or sharp odor) or taste?

Tablets

- Do the tablets look different than they usually do? Do they have unusual spots or markings? If they normally are shiny and smooth, are some dull or rough? Is there anything unusual about the color?
- Are the tablets all the same size and thickness?
- If there is printing on the tablets, do they all have the same imprint? Is the imprint missing from any?
- Do the tablets have a strange or different odor or taste?
- Are any of the tablets broken?

Capsules

• Do the capsules look different than they usually do? Are any cracked or dented? Are they all the same size and color?

• Do they have their normal shiny appearance or are some dull or have fingerprints on them as though they have been handled?

• Are the capsules all the same length?

• Does the filling in all the capsules look the same? Is it stuck together?

• If there is printing on the capsules, do they all have the same imprint? Is the imprint missing from any? Do the imprints all line up the same way?

• Do the capsules have an unexpected or unusual odor or taste?

Tubes and jars (ointments, creams, pastes, etc.)

• Does the product or container look different than usual?

• Are ointments and creams smooth and non-gritty? Have they separated?

Be a wise consumer. Look for signs of tampering before you buy a medicine and again each time you take a dose. Also, pay attention to the daily news in order to learn about any reported tampering.

It is important to understand that a change in the appearance or condition of a product may not mean that the package has been tampered with. The manufacturer may have changed the color of a medicine or its packaging. Also, the product may be breaking down with age or it may have had rough or unusual handling in shipping. In addition, some minor product variations may be normal.

Whenever you suspect that something is unusual about a medicine or its packaging, take it to your pharmacist. He or she is familiar with most products and their packaging. If there are serious concerns or problems, your pharmacist should report it to the USP Drug Product Problem Reporting Program (USP DPPR) at 1-800-638-6725, or other appropriate authorities.

Accidental Poisoning

Over 1 million children 5 years of age and younger were accidentally poisoned in 1992. Of these, over 100,000 required hospital emergency room treatment, according to information provided by the American Association of Poison Control Centers. In 1992, 29 children 5 years of age and younger died as a result of poisoning.

Adults also may be accidentally poisoned, most often through carelessness or lack of information. For example, the sleepy adult who takes a medicine in the dark and winds up getting the wrong one, or the adult who decides to take the medicine prescribed for a friend to treat "the same symptoms."

Drug poisoning from an accidental overdose is 1 of the 3 types of accidental poisoning that contributes to these figures. The other 2 are household chemical poisoning from accidental ingestion or contact, and vapor poisoning—for example, carbon monoxide, usually from a car.

Children are ready victims

The natural curiosity of children makes them ready victims of poisoning. Children explore everywhere and investigate their environment. What they find frequently goes into their mouths. They do not understand danger and possibly cannot read warning labels.

Accidental poisoning from medicine is especially dangerous in small children because the strength of most medicines that may be ingested is often based on their use in adults. Even a small quantity of an adult dose can sometimes poison a child.

Preventing poisoning from medicines

• Store medicines out of the sight and reach of children, preferably in a locked cabinet—not in the bathroom medicine cabinet or in a food cabinet.

• Use child-resistant closures on pain relievers and other potentially harmful products whether you have children living with you or only as occasional visitors. Adults who have difficulty opening child-resistant closures may request traditional, easy-to-open packaging for their medicines. Always store medicines in a secure place.

• Always replace lids and return medicines to their storage place after use, even if you will be using them again soon.

• If you are called to the telephone or to answer the door while you are taking medicine, take the container with you or put the medicine out of the reach of small children. Children act quickly—usually when no one is watching.

• Date medicines when purchased and clean out your medicines periodically. Discard prescription medicines that are past their expiration or "beyond use" date. As medicines grow old, the chemicals in them may change. In general, medicines that do not have an expiration date should not be kept for more than 1 year. Carefully discard any medicines so that children cannot get them. Rinse containers well before discarding in the trash.

• Take only those medicines prescribed for you and give medicines only to those for whom prescribed. A medicine that worked well for one person may harm another.

• It is best to keep all medicines in their original containers with their labels intact. The label contains valuable information for taking the medicine properly. Also, in case of accidental poisoning, it is important to know the ingredients in a drug product and any emergency instructions from the manufacturer. While prescription medicines usually do not list ingredients, information on the label makes it possible for your pharmacist to identify the contents.

• Ask your pharmacist to include on the label the number of tablets or capsules that he or she put in the container. In case of poisoning, it may be important to know roughly how many tablets or capsules were taken.

• Do not trust your memory—read the label before using the medicine, and take it as directed.

• If a medicine container has no label or the label has been defaced so that you are not absolutely sure what it says, do not use it.

• Turn on a light when taking or giving medicines at night or in a dark room.

• Label medicine containers with poison symbols, especially if you have children, individuals with poor vision, or other persons in your home who cannot read well.

• Teach children that medicine is not candy by calling each medicine by its proper name.

• Do not take medicines in front of children. They may wish to imitate you.

• Communicate these safety rules to any babysitters you have and remember them if you babysit or are visiting a house with children. Children are naturally curious and can get into a pocketbook, briefcase, or overnight bag that contains medicines.

What to do if a poisoning happens

Remember:

• There may be no immediate, significant symptoms or warning signs, particularly in a child.

• Nothing you can give will work equally well in all cases of poisoning. In fact, one "antidote" may counteract the effects of another.

• Many poisons act quickly, leaving little time for treatment.

Therefore:

• Do not wait to see what effect the poison will have or if symptoms of overdose develop. If you think someone has swallowed medicine or a household product, immediately call a Poison Control Center (listed in the white pages of your telephone book under "Poison Control" or inside the front cover with other emergency numbers), health care provider, hospital, or rescue squad. These numbers should be posted beside every telephone in the house, as should those of your pharmacist, the police, the fire department, and ambulance services. (Some poison control centers have TTY capability for the deaf. Check with your local center if you or someone in your family requires this service.)

• Have the container with you when you call so you can read the label on the product for ingredients.

• Describe what, when, and how much was taken and the age and condition of the person poisoned—for example, if the person is vomiting, choking, drowsy, shows a change in color or temperature of skin, is conscious or unconscious, or is convulsing.

• *Do not induce vomiting* unless instructed by medical personnel. *Do not induce vomiting or force liquids* into a person who is convulsing, unconscious, or very drowsy.

• Stay calm and in control of the situation.

Keep a bottle of Ipecac Syrup stored in a secure place in your home for emergency use. It is available at pharmacies in 1 ounce bottles without prescription. Ipecac Syrup is often recommended to induce vomiting in cases of poisoning.

Activated Charcoal also is sometimes recommended in certain types of poisoning and you may wish to add a supply to your emergency medicines. It is available without a prescription. Before using this medicine for poisoning, however, call for medical advice. There are a number of types of poisoning for which this substance should *not* be used. When you are directed to use it, be aware that Activated Charcoal acts by adsorbing (holding) the poison so that it can be eliminated from the body before it is absorbed into the bloodstream. Therefore, any other medicine taken within two hours of the Activated Charcoal may similarly be tied up and not taken up by the body. Also, if you are told to use both Ipecac Syrup and Activated Charcoal to treat poisoning, do not take the Activated Charcoal until *after* you have taken the Ipecac Syrup to cause vomiting and the vomiting has stopped. This will usually take about 30 minutes.

A first aid book that describes emergency treatment of poisoning, or a chart of emergency measures to take that can be posted in some central place in your home, can be useful if medical help is not readily available in your area. If you must rely on these sources of information, however, familiarize yourself fully with the various procedures listed so that in an emergency you will not waste time trying to match the poison with treatment.

Getting the Most Out of Your Medicines

Most consumers are concerned with getting the best value for their money. However, there are many who ignore this consideration when it comes to medicines. These are the people—up to 50% of all drug consumers in the United States according to some research studies—who do not follow drug use directions accurately.

To get the most out of your medicines, there are certain things that you must do. Although your health care providers will be working with you, you also have a responsibility for your own health.

Communicating With Your Health Care Provider

The exchange of information is central to good medical care. Your health care provider needs to know about you, your medical history, and your current complaints. In turn, you need to know about the recommendations your health care provider is making and what the alternative treatments might be. You will have to ask questions—and answer some too. Communication is a two-way street.

Giving information

To make an intelligent diagnosis and prescription for care, your health care provider needs to know about your past and present medical history, including all the illnesses you have ever had; current symptoms; the drugs you are taking; any allergies or sensitivities to foods, medicines, or other things; your smoking, drinking, and exercise habits; vaccinations; operations; accidents requiring hospitalization; illnesses that run in your family; the cause of death of your closest relatives; and other relevant information.

Many health care providers have a standard "medical history" form they will ask you to fill out when they see you for the first time, or they may ask the questions and write down the answers for you. If you will be visiting a health care provider for the first time, prepare yourself before you go by thinking about the questions that might be asked and jotting down the answers—including dates—so that you will not forget an important item. Once your "medical history" is in the health care provider's files, subsequent visits will take less time.

You will, however, have to supply each health care provider you see—every time you see one—with complete information about what happened since your last visit. It is important that your records are updated so the health care provider can make sound recommendations for your continued treatment, or treatment of any new problems.

It will simplify things if you develop a "medical history" file for yourself at home and keep one for each family member for whom you are responsible. Setting up the file will take time. However, once it is established, you need only to keep it up-to-date and remember to take it with you when you see a health care provider. This will be easier than having to repeat the information time after time and running the risk of confusing or forgetting details.

It is also a good idea to carry in your wallet a card that summarizes your chronic medical conditions, the medicines you are taking, and your allergies and drug sensitivities. You should keep this card as up-to-date as possible. Many pharmacists provide these cards as a service.

"Medical history" checklist

A "medical history" checklist covers the following information:

- All the serious illnesses you have ever had and the approximate dates.
- Your current symptoms, if any.
- **All** the medicines and dietary supplements you are taking or have taken in the recent past, including prescription and nonprescription medicines (pain relievers, antacids, laxatives, and cold medicines, etc.) and home remedies. This is especially important if you are seeing more than one health care provider; if you are having surgery, including dental or emergency treatment; or if you obtain your medicines from more than one source.
- **Any** allergies or sensitivities to medicines, foods, or other substances.
- Your smoking, drinking, and exercise habits.
- Any recent changes in your lifestyle or personal habits. New job? Retired? Change of residence? Death in family? Married? Divorced? Other?
- Any special diet you are on—low-sugar, low-sodium, or a diet to lose or gain weight.
- If you are pregnant, plan to become pregnant, or if you are breast-feeding an infant.
- All the vaccinations and vaccination boosters you have had, with dates if possible.
- Any operations you have had, including dental and those performed on an outpatient basis, and any accidents that have required hospitalization.
- Illnesses that run in your family.
- Cause of death of closest relatives.

Remember, be sure to tell your health care provider at each visit if there have been any changes since your last visit.

Getting information

You need to understand what you are being directed to do so that you can follow the instructions. A number of medical problems can be handled without the use of drugs. Some of these lend themselves to a standard list of instructions that your health care provider may have had printed up for your use. If the instructions are not provided in written form, you may want to write them down or ask the health care provider to write them down for you.

If you do not have time to jot down everything while you are still with your health care provider, sit down in the waiting room before you leave and write down the information while it is still fresh in your mind and you can still ask questions. If you have been given a prescription, ask for written information about the drug. Your pharmacist can also answer questions when you have your prescription filled.

For your health care provider to be able to serve you well, you must communicate all that you know about your present health condition at every visit. In order to benefit from the advice for which you have paid—and you have paid not only in dollars, but in terms of time, taxes, insurance, and transportation costs—your health care provider must communicate full instructions for your care. Then it is up to you to carry out those instructions precisely. If there is a failure in any part of this system, you will pay an even higher price—physically and financially—for your health care.

What you need to know about your medicines

There are a number of things that you should know about each medicine you are taking. These include:

- The medicine's generic and brand name.
- How it will help you and the expected results. How it makes you feel. How long it takes to begin working.
- How much to take at one time.
- How often to take the medicine.
- How long it will be necessary to take the medicine.
- When to take it. Before, during, after meals? At bedtime? At any other special times?
- How to take it. With water? With fruit juice? How much?
- What to do about a missed dose.
- Foods, drinks, or other medicines not to be taken while taking a medicine.
- Restrictions on activities while taking a medicine. May I drive a car or operate other motor vehicles?
- Side effects to be expected. What to do if they appear. How to minimize the side effects. How soon will they go away?
- When to seek help if there are problems.
- How long to wait before reporting no change in symptoms.
- How to store the medicine. Should the unused portion be saved for future use?
- The expiration date.
- The cost of the medicine.
- How to have your prescription refilled, if necessary.

Other issues or important information about your medicine that you may want to consider include the following:

- Ask your health care provider about the ingredients in the prescription and over-the-counter (OTC) medicines you are taking and whether there may be a conflict with other medicines you are taking. Your health care provider can help you avoid dangerous combinations or drug products that contain ingredients to which you are allergic or sensitive.
- Ask your health care provider for help in developing a system for taking your medicines properly, particularly if you are taking a number of them on a daily basis. (When you are a patient in a hospital, ask for instruction in managing your medicines on your own before you are discharged.) Do not hesitate or be embarrassed to ask questions or ask for help.
- If you are over 60 years of age, ask your health care provider if the dose of the medicine prescribed is right for you. Some medicines may have to be given in lower doses to certain older individuals.
- If you are taking several different medicines, ask your health care provider if all of them are necessary for you. You should take only those medicines that you need.
- Medicines should be kept in the container they came in. However, if this is not possible when you are at work or away from home, ask your pharmacist to provide or recommend a suitable container or a more convenient package to transport your medicines safely. Tablets can be broken or chipped or can deteriorate in "pill boxes," which can make the dosage somewhat smaller than prescribed. Medicines that are similar in appearance can be confused if they are in the same container and you could take the wrong medicine in the wrong amount. In rare cases, some medicines can interact with the metal of these boxes, causing harmful effects. Medicines like nitroglycerin can evaporate, altering the quantity you may receive in any given tablet.
- Some people have trouble taking tablets or capsules. Your health care provider will know if another dosage form is available, or if tablets can be crushed or capsule contents dissolved and taken in a liquid. If this is an ongoing problem, ask your prescriber to write the prescription for the dosage form you can take most comfortably.
- Child-resistant caps are required by law on most prescription medicines for oral use to protect children from accidental poisoning. These containers are designed so that children will have difficulty opening them. Since many adults also find these containers hard to open, the law allows consumers to request traditional, easy-to-open packaging for their drugs. If you do not use child-resistant packaging, however, make sure that your medicines are stored where small children cannot see or reach them. If you use child-resistant containers, ask your pharmacist to show you how to open them.

Consumer education is one of the most important responsibilities of your health care provider. To supplement what you learn during your visit to your health care provider, ask if there is any written information about your medicines that you can take home with you. Your health care provider may also have available various reference books or computerized drug information that you can consult for details about precautions, side effects, and proper use of your medicines.

Your Health Care Team

Your health care team will be made up of several different health care providers. Each of these individuals will play an important part in the overall provision of your health care. It is important that you understand the roles of each of these providers and what you should be able to expect from each of them.

Your dentist

In addition to providing care and maintenance of your mouth, teeth, and gums, your dentist is also an essential member of your overall health care team since your oral health and general health often affect one another.

In providing dental treatment, your dentist should base his or her decisions upon an extensive knowledge of your current condition and past medical and dental history. Because the dentist is a prescriber of medications, it is very important that he or she is aware of your **full** medical and dental history. A complete medical and dental history should include the information that is listed in the "Medical history checklist" section above. Even if you do not consider this information important, you should inform your dentist as fully as possible.

In the treatment of any dental/oral problem your dentist should make every effort to inform you as fully as possible about the nature of the problem. He or she should explain why this problem has occurred, the advantages and disadvantages of available treatments (including no treatment), and what types of preventive measures can be employed to avoid future problems. These measures may include periodic visits to the dentist, and a general awareness of the manner in which dental and overall health may affect one another. In any type of treatment, your dentist should always allow you to ask questions, and should be willing to answer them to your satisfaction.

In selecting a dentist, it is important to keep in mind the role of the dentist as a member of the health care team, and the extent of the information that he or she should be asking for and providing. There are also several practical issues that you should consider, such as:

- Is the dentist a specialist or general practitioner?
- What are the office hours?
- Is the dentist or his/her associates available after office hours by phone? In emergencies, will you be able to contact a dentist?
- What is the office policy on cancellations?
- What types of payment are accepted at the office?
- What is the office policy on x-ray procedures?
- What infection control procedures (for instance, wearing masks and gloves, sterilizing instruments, etc.) does the office use?
- Is the dentist willing to work with other medical and/or dental specialists that you may be seeing?

Your dentist should be an integral part of your health care team. In treating problems and providing general maintenance of your oral health, your dentist should base decisions upon a full dental and medical history. He or she should also be willing to answer any questions that you have regarding your oral health, any medications prescribed, and preventive measures to avoid future problems.

Your nurse

Depending upon the setting, type of therapy being administered, and state regulations, the role of the nurse in your health care team may vary. Registered nurses practice in diverse health care settings, such as hospitals, out-patient clinics or physicians' offices, schools, workplaces, homes, and long-term care facilities like nursing homes and retirement centers. Some nurses, including certified nurse practitioners and midwives, hold a master's degree in nursing and may assume the role of primary health care provider in practice by themselves or in joint practices with physicians. In most states, nurse practitioners may prescribe medications. Clinical nurse specialists also have a master's degree in nursing and specialize in a particular area of health care. In some hospitals, long-term care facilities, and out-patient care settings, licensed practical nurses (LPNs) have certain responsibilities in administering medication to patients. LPNs usually work under the supervision of a RN or physician. Nursing aides assist RNs and LPNs with different kinds of patient care activities. In most places where people receive health care, RNs may be the primary source of information for drug therapies and other medical treatments. It is important that you be aware of the roles and responsibilities of the nurses participating in your health care.

Professional nurses participate with other health professionals, such as physicians and pharmacists, to ensure that your drug therapy is safe and effective and to monitor any effects (both desired and negative) from the medication. You may be admitted to the hospital so that nurses can administer medications and monitor your response to therapy. In hospitals or long-term care facilities, nurses are responsible for administering your medications in their proper dosage form and dose, and at correct time intervals, as well as monitoring your response to these medications. At home or in out-patient settings, nurses should ensure that you have the proper information and support of others, if needed, to get the medication and take it as prescribed. When nurses administer medication, they should explain why you are receiving this medication, how it works, any possible side effects, special precautions or actions that you must take while using the medication, and any potential interactions with other medications.

If you experience any side effects or symptoms from a medication, you should always tell your health care provider. It is important that these reactions be detected before they become serious or permanent. You can seek advice about possible ways to minimize these side effects from your nurse. Your health care provider should also be made aware of any additional medical problems or conditions (such as pregnancy) that you may have, since these can also affect the safety and effectiveness of a medication.

You should view the professional nurse as someone who can help to clarify drug information. In most health care settings, nurses are accessible and can answer your questions or direct you to others who can assist you. Professional nurses are skilled in the process of patient teaching. To make sure that patients learn important information about their health problem and its treatment, RNs often use a combination of teaching methods, such as verbal instruction, written materials, demonstration, and audiovisual instructions. Above all, professional nurses should teach at a time and level that are appropriate for you. RNs can also help you design a medication schedule that fits your lifestyle and may be less likely to cause unwanted side effects.

Your pharmacist

Your pharmacist is an important member of your health care team. In addition to performing traditional services, such as dispensing medications, your pharmacist can help you understand your medications and how to take them safely and effectively. By keeping accurate and up-to-date records and monitoring your use of medications, your pharmacist can help to protect you from improper drug therapy, unwanted side effects, and dangerous drug interactions. You should expect your pharmacist to provide these services.

To provide you with the best possible care, your pharmacist should be informed about your current condition and medication history. Your personal medication history should include the information that is listed in the "Medical history checklist" section above. Your pharmacist should also be aware of any special packaging needs that you may have (such as child-resistant or easy-to-open containers). Your pharmacist should keep accurate and up-to-date records that contain this information. If you visit a new pharmacy that does not have access to your medication records, it is important that you inform that pharmacist as fully as possible about your medical history or provide him or her with a copy of your medication records from your previous pharmacy. In general, in order to get the most out of your pharmacy services, it is best to get all of your medications (including OTCs) from the same pharmacy.

Your pharmacist should be a knowledgeable and approachable source of information about your medications. Some of the information that your pharmacist should explain to you about your medications is listed in the "What you need to know about your medicines" section above. Ideally, this information should also be provided in written form, so that you may refer to it later if you have any questions or problems. The pharmacist should always be willing to answer any questions that you have regarding your medications, and should also be willing to contact your physician or other health care professionals (dentist, nurses, etc.) on your behalf if necessary.

Your pharmacist can also help you with information on the costs of your medicines. Many medicines are available from more than one company. They may have equal effects, but may have different costs. Your insurance company, HMO, or other third-party payment group may reimburse you for only some of these medications or only for part of their costs. Your pharmacist will be able to tell you which of these medications are covered by your payment plan or cost less.

In selecting a pharmacist, it is important that you understand the role of the pharmacist as a member of your health care team and the extent of information that he or she should be asking for and providing. Because pharmacies can offer different types of services and have different policies regarding patient information, some of the issues that you should consider in selecting a pharmacist also relate to the pharmacy where that person practices. There are several issues regarding the pharmacist and pharmacy that you should consider, such as:

- What other professional services, such as written information that you can take home or home delivery, does the pharmacy offer?
- Are you able to talk to your pharmacist without other people hearing you?
- Can the pharmacist be reached easily by phone? Is a pharmacist available twenty-four hours (including weekends and holidays) by phone?
- What types of payment are accepted in the pharmacy?
- Does the pharmacy accept your HMO or third-party payment plan?
- Does the pharmacy offer any specialized services, such as diabetes education?

You should select your pharmacist and pharmacy as carefully as you select your physician, and stay with the same pharmacy so that all of your medication records are in the same place. This will help to ensure that your records are accurate and up-to-date and will allow you to develop a beneficial relationship with your pharmacist.

Your physician

One of the most important health care decisions that you will make is your choice of a personal physician. The physician is central to your health care team, and is responsible for helping you maintain your overall health. In addition to detecting and treating ailments or adverse conditions, your physician and his or her coworkers should also serve as primary sources of health care information. Because the physician plays such an important role in your overall health care, it is important that you understand the full range of the physician's role as health care and information provider.

In providing any type of treatment or counseling, your physician should base his or her decisions upon an extensive knowledge of your current condition and past medical history. A complete medical history should include the information that is listed in the "Medical history checklist" section above. Your physician should keep accurate and comprehensive medical records containing this information. Because your treatment (and your health) is dependent upon a full disclosure of your medical history, as well as any factors that may currently be affecting your health (i.e., stress, smoking, drug use, etc.), it is important that you inform your physician as fully as possible, even if you might not consider this information important.

It is important that you inform your personal physician of any other physicians (such as specialists or subspecialists), dentists, or other health care providers that you are seeing. You should also inform your physician as to which pharmacy you use or intend to use, so that he or she may contact the pharmacist if necessary.

In treating any health problem, your physician should make every effort to help you understand completely the nature of the problem and its treatment. He or she should take the time to explain the problem, why it may have occurred, and what preventive measures (if any) can be taken to avoid it in the future. Your physician should explain fully the reasons for any prescribed treatment. He or she should also be willing to discuss alternative therapies, especially if you are uncomfortable with the one that has been prescribed. Your physician should always be willing to answer all of your questions to your satisfaction.

In selecting a physician, you should look for one who will provide a full range and depth of services. Asking for a full medical history and providing complete information about your treatment and medications are some of these services. There are several other issues that you may want to consider. Does your physician:

- Consult peers with specialty training for difficult problems?
- Inquire about your general health as well as specific problems?
- Have a good working relationship with your pharmacist? With the nurses and staff at his/her office?
- Periodically have you bring in bottles or labels from all of the medications (prescription and nonprescription) that you are taking or have at home?
- Periodically check the status of your vaccinations?
- Refer to an affiliated testing facility?

You may also want to consider your physician's medical credentials. Your local medical society should be able to provide specific facts about your physician's training, experience, and membership in professional societies.

One of the most important issues in contemporary health care is that of cost and payment. Your physician should be sensitive to the costs of your treatment and the manner in which you intend to pay for this and related medications. If you belong to an HMO or third-party payment plan, be sure that your physician is aware of your involvement in the plan. You should also be aware of the different types of payment that are accepted at the physician's office.

In prescribing medications, your physician should take into account the manner in which you intend to pay for your drugs, and should be aware of any specific concerns regarding the costs of your treatment and medication. He or she should also explain why brand or generic drugs may be preferable in certain situations.

In selecting a physician, there are also several practical issues and matters of convenience that you should consider, such as:

- Is the office convenient to your home or work?
- What are the office hours?
- Is your physician or his/her associates or partners available (twenty-four hours) by phone? In emergencies, will you be able to contact a physician?
- Are you able to arrange appointments to fit your schedule? What is the office policy on cancellations?
- Is the physician well regarded in the community? Does he or she have a reputation for listening to patients and answering questions?
- Does the physician have admitting privileges at a hospital of your preference?
- Does he/she participate in your health plan?

In addition to the considerations already mentioned, your physician should be sensitive to the special concerns of treating the elderly. Older patients can present disease processes differently from younger adults, can react differently to certain drugs and dosages, and may have preexisting conditions that require special treatments to be prescribed.

There are also several special issues to consider in your selection of a pediatrician or family physician. If your child is not old enough to understand all instructions and information, it is important that your child's physician explain to you any information pertaining to the nature of a problem and all instructions for medications. When your child is of school age, the physician should speak directly to the child as well, asking and answering questions, and providing information about cause and prevention of medical problems and the use of medications. He or she should choose a dosage form and dose that is appropriate for your child's age and explain what to do if your child has certain symptoms, such as fever, vomiting, etc. (including the amount and type of medicine to give and when to call him or her for advice).

Your physician should be a primary source of information about your health and any medications that you are taking. In providing treatment for medical problems or conditions, the physician should base decisions upon a full medical history and be willing to answer any questions that you have regarding your health, treatment, and medications.

Managing Your Medicines

To get the full benefit and reduce risks in taking your prescribed medicines, it is important to take the right medicine and dose at correct time intervals for the length of time prescribed. Bad effects can result from taking too much or too little of a medicine, or taking it too often or not often enough.

Establishing a system

Whether you are taking one or several medicines, develop a system for taking them. It can be just as difficult to remember whether you took your once-a-day high blood pressure medicine as it can be to keep track of a number of medicines that need to be taken several times a day. Many medicines also have special instructions that can further complicate proper use.

Establish a way of knowing whether you took your medicines and took them properly, then make that a part of your daily routine. If you take only 1 or 2 medicines a day, you may only need to take them at the same time that you perform some other regular task, such as brushing your teeth or getting dressed. For most people, a check-off record can also be a handy way of managing multiple medicines. Keep your medicine record with a pencil or pen in a handy, visible place next to where you take your medicines. Check off each dose as you take it. If you skip a dose, for whatever reason, make a note about what happened and what you did on the back of the record or the bottom of the sheet.

Try to take your medicines on time, but a half hour early or late usually is not going to upset things drastically. If you are more than several hours late and are getting close to your next scheduled dose, however, check with your health care provider if you did not receive instructions for what to do about a missed dose. You may also find this information in the entries included in this book.

Also be sure to note any unwanted effects or anything unusual that happens to you that may be connected with your medicines, or if a medicine does not do what you expect. Remember that some medicines take a while before they start having a noticeable effect.

If you keep a check-off record faithfully, you will know for sure whether or not you took your medicine. You will also have a complete record for your health care providers to review when you visit any one of them again. This information can help them determine if the medicine is working properly or causing unwanted side effects, or whether adjustments should be made in your medicines and/or doses.

If your medicines or the instructions for taking them are changed, correct your record or make a new one. Keep the old record until you are sure you or your health care providers no longer need that information.

You might want to color code your medicine containers to help you tell them apart. If you are having trouble reading labels or if you are color-blind, codes that can be recognized by touch (rubber bands, a cotton ball, or a piece of emery board, for instance) can be attached to the container. If you code your medicines, be sure these identifications are included on any medicine record you use. If necessary, ask your pharmacist to type medicine labels in large letters for easier reading.

A check-off list is not the only method to record medicine use. If this system does not work for you, ask your health care provider to help you develop an alternative. Be sure he or she knows all the medicines prescribed for you and any nonprescription medicines you take regularly, the hours you usually eat your meals, and any special diet you are following.

Informed management

Your medicines have been prescribed for you and your condition. You should ask your health care provider what benefits to expect, what side effects may occur, and when to report any side effects. If your symptoms go away, do not decide on your own that you are well and stop taking your medicine. If you stop too soon, the symptoms may come back. Finish all of the medicine if you have been told to do so by your health care provider. However, if you develop diarrhea or other unpleasant side effects, do not continue with the medicine just because you were told to finish it. Call your health care provider and report these effects. A change in dose or in the kind of medicine you are taking may be necessary.

When you are given a prescription for a medicine, ask the person who wrote it to explain it to you. For example, does "four times a day" mean one in the morning, one at noon, one in the evening, and one at bedtime; or does it mean every six hours around the clock? When a prescription says "take as needed," ask how close together the doses can be taken and what the maximum number of doses you can take in one day should be. Does "take with liquids" mean with water, milk, or something else? Are there some liquids that should avoided? What does "take with food" mean? At every meal time (some people must eat six meals a day), or with a snack? Do not trust your memory—have the instructions written down. To follow the instructions for taking your medicines, you must understand exactly what the prescriber wants you to do in order to "take as directed."

When the pharmacist dispenses your medicine, you have another opportunity to clarify information received or to ask other questions. Before you leave, check the label on your medicine to be sure it matches the prescription and your understanding of what you are to do. If it does not, ask more questions.

The key to getting the most from your prescribed treatments is following instructions accurately and intelligently. If you have questions or doubts about the prescribed treatment, do not decide not to take the medicine or otherwise fail to follow the prescribed regimen. Discuss your questions and doubts with your health care provider.

The time and effort put into setting up a system to manage your medicines and establish a routine for taking them will pay off by relieving anxiety and helping you get the most from your prescribed treatment.

Taking Your Medicine

To take medicines safely and get the greatest benefit from them, it is important to establish regular habits so that you are less likely to make mistakes.

Before taking any medicine, read the label and any accompanying information. If you would like more information, you can consult books to learn the purpose, side effects, and other information about the medicine. If you have unanswered questions, check with your health care provider.

The label on the container of a prescription medicine should bear your first and last name; the name of the prescriber; the pharmacy address and telephone number; the prescription number so it can be located for refills or in case of emergency; the date of dispensing; and directions for use. Some states or provinces may have additional requirements. If the name of the drug product is not on the label, ask the pharmacist to include the brand (if any) and generic names. An expiration date may also appear. All of this information is important in identifying your medicines and using them properly. In general, the labels on the containers should never be removed and all medicines should be kept in their original containers.

Some tips for taking medicines safely and accurately include the following:

- Read the label of each medicine container three times:
  - —before you remove it from its storage place,
  - —before you take the lid off the container to remove the dose, and
  - —before you replace the container in its storage place.
- Never take medicines in the dark even if you believe you know exactly where to find them.
- Use standard measuring devices to take your medicines (the household teaspoon, cup, and glass vary widely in the amount they hold). Ask your pharmacist for help with measuring.
- Set bottles and boxes of medicines on a clear area, well back from the edge of the surface to prevent containers and/or caps from being knocked to the floor.
- When pouring liquid medicines, pick up the container with the label against the palm of your hand to protect it from being stained by dripping medicine.
- Wipe off the top and neck of bottles of liquid medicines to keep labels from being obscured, and to make it less likely that the lid will stick.
- Shake all liquid suspensions of drug products before pouring so that ingredients are mixed thoroughly.
- If you are to take medicine with water, take a full, 8 ounce glassful, not just enough to get it down. Too little liquid with some medicines can prevent the medicine from working like it should or can cause throat irritation if the medicine does not get completely to the stomach.
- Replace the lid on one container before opening another to avoid accidental confusion of lids, labels, and medicines.
- When you are called to the door or telephone or are otherwise interrupted while taking your medicine, take the container with you or put the medicine up out of the reach of small children. It only takes a second for them to take an overdose. When you return, check the label of the medicine to be sure you have the right one before taking it.
- Do not crush tablets or open capsules to take the powder or granules with food or beverages unless you have checked with your health care provider and know that this will not affect the way that the medicine works. If you have difficulty swallowing a tablet or capsule, check with your health care provider about the availability of a different dosage form.
- Follow any diet instructions or other treatment measures prescribed by your health care provider.
- If at any point you realize you have taken the wrong medicine or the wrong amount, call your health care provider immediately. In an emergency, call your local emergency number.

When you have finished taking your medicines, mark it down immediately on your medication calendar to avoid "double dosing." Also, make notes of any unusual changes in your body: change in weight, color or amount of urine, perspiration, or sputum; your pulse, temperature, or any other items you may have been instructed to observe for your condition or your medicine.

When your medicines are being managed by someone else, for example, when you are a patient in a hospital or nursing home, question what is happening to you and communicate what you know about your previous drug therapy—or any other treatments. If you know you always take 1, not 2, of a certain tablet, say so and ask that your record be checked before you take the medicine. If you are there for pain in your back and they are putting drops in your eyes, speak up. If you know you took that medicine an hour ago, tell the nurse. Your concerns may be unfounded—your health care provider may have forgotten to tell you about a change in your therapy, and different brands of the same drug may not look alike. Then again, you might be right.

Many hospitals and nursing homes now offer counseling in medicine management as part of their discharge planning for patients. If you or a family member is getting ready to come home, ask your health care provider if you can be part of such instruction since you will have to manage the medicines at home.

The "Expiration Date" on Medicine Labels

To assure that a drug product meets applicable standards of identity, strength, quality, and purity at the time of use, an "expiration date" is added by the manufacturer to the label of most prescription and nonprescription drug products.

The expiration date on a drug product is valid only as long as the product is stored in the original, unopened container under the storage conditions specified by the manufacturer. Among other things, drugs can be affected by humidity, temperature, light, and even air. A medicine taken after the expiration date may have changed in potency or may have formed harmful material as it deteriorates (for example, as sometimes happens with tetracyclines). In other instances, for injectables, eye drops, or other sterile products, contamination with germs may have occurred. The safest rule is not to use any medicine beyond the expiration date.

Preventing deterioration

A drug begins to deteriorate the minute it is made. This rate of deterioration is factored in by the manufacturer in calculating the expiration date. Keeping the drug product in the container supplied by the pharmacist helps slow down deterioration. Storing the drug in the prescribed manner—for example, in a light-resistant container or in a cool, dry place (not the bathroom medicine cabinet)—also helps. The need for medicines to be kept in their pharmacist-dispensed containers and to be stored properly to minimize deterioration cannot be overstressed.

Patients sometimes ask their health care providers to prescribe a large quantity of a particular medicine they are taking in order to "economize." This may be a false economy; especially if, as a result of the medicine's deterioration, the illness is not properly treated, or the medicine causes an unexpected reaction. Therefore, your health care provider may recommend against this practice.

Sometimes deterioration can be recognized by physical changes in the drug, such as a change in odor or appearance. For example, aspirin tablets develop a vinegar odor when they break down. These changes are not true of all drugs, however, and the absence of physical changes should not be assumed to mean no deterioration has occurred.

Some liquid medicines mixed at the pharmacy will have a "beyond use" date on the label. This expiration date is calculated from the date of preparation in the pharmacy. This is a definite date, after which you should discard any of the medicine that remains.

If your prescription medicines do not bear an "expiration" or "beyond use" date, your dispensing pharmacist is the best person to advise you about how long they can be safely utilized.

About the Medicines You Are Taking

New Drugs—From Idea to Marketplace

To be sold legitimately in the United States, new drugs must pass through a rigorous system of approval specified in the Food, Drug, and Cosmetic Act and supervised by the Food and Drug Administration (FDA). Except for certain drugs subject to other regulatory provisions, no new drug for human use may be marketed in this country unless FDA has approved a "New Drug Application" (NDA) for it.

The idea

The creation of a new drug usually starts with an idea. Most likely that idea results from the study of a disease or group of symptoms, or may come from observations of clinical research. This may involve many years of study, or the idea may occur from an accidental discovery in a research laboratory or may be a coincidental discovery, as happened with penicillin.

Idea development takes place most often in the laboratory of a pharmaceutical company, but may also happen in laboratories at research institutions like the National Institutes of Health, at medical centers and universities, or in the laboratory of a chemical company.

Animal testing

The idea for a new drug is first tested on animals to help determine how toxic the substance may be. Most drugs interfere in some way with normal body functions. These animal studies are designed to discover the degree of that interference and the extent of the toxic effects.

After successful animal testing, perhaps over several years, the sponsors of the new drug apply to the FDA for an Investigational New Drug (IND) application—approval to test in humans. As part of their request, the sponsoring manufacturer must submit the information about the drug that was found as a result of the animal studies plus a detailed outline of the proposed human testing and information about the researchers to be involved in the human trials.

Human testing

Drug testing in humans usually consists of three consecutive phases. "Informed consent" must be secured from all volunteers participating in this testing.

Phase I testing is most often done on young, healthy adults. This testing is done on a relatively small number of subjects, generally between 20 and 80. Its purpose is to learn more about the biochemistry of the drug, how it acts on the body, and how the body reacts to it. The procedure differs for some drugs, however. For example, Phase I testing of drugs used to treat cancer involves actual patients with the disease from the beginning of testing.

During Phase II, small controlled clinical studies designed to test the effectiveness and relative safety of the drug are done on closely monitored patients who have the disease for which the drug is being tested. Their numbers seldom go beyond 100 to 200 patients. Some volunteers for Phase II testing who have severely complicating conditions may be excluded.

A "control" group of people of comparable physical and disease types is used to do double-blind, controlled experiments for most drugs. These are conducted by medical investigators thoroughly familiar with the disease and this type of research. In a double-blind experiment, the patient, the health care provider, and other personnel do not know or are "blind" as to whether the patient is receiving the drug being tested, another active drug, or no medicine at all (a placebo or "sugar pill"). This helps eliminate bias and assures the accuracy of results. The findings of these tests are statistically analyzed to determine whether they are "significant" or due to chance alone.

Phase III consists of larger studies. This testing is performed after effectiveness of the drug has been established initially and is intended to gather additional evidence of effectiveness for specific uses of the drug. These studies also help discover adverse drug reactions that may occur with the drug. Phase III studies involve a few hundred to several thousand patients who have the disease the drug is intended to treat.

Patients with additional diseases or those receiving other therapy may be included in later Phase II and Phase III studies, since they would be expected to be representative of certain segments of the population who will be receiving the drug following approval for marketing.

Final approval

When a sponsor believes the investigational studies on a drug have shown it to be safe and effective in treating specific conditions, a New Drug Application (NDA) is submitted to FDA, accompanied by all the documentation from the company's research. This includes everything they know about the medicine as well as the complete records of all the animal and human testing. This documentation can run to many thousands of pages.

The application, together with its documentation, must then be reviewed by FDA physicians, pharmacologists, chemists, statisticians, and other professionals experienced in evaluating new drugs. Proposed information for the physician and pharmacist that is to be placed on the label of the medicine and in its package insert is screened for accuracy, completeness, and conformity to FDA-approved wording.

The regulations call for the FDA to review an NDA within 180 days. This period may be extended and, in fact, takes an average of 2 to 3 years. When all research phases are considered, the actual time it takes from idea to marketplace may be 8 to 10 years or even longer. However, for drugs representing major therapeutic advances, FDA may "fast-track" the approval process to try to get those drugs to patients who need them as soon as possible.

After approval

After a drug is marketed, the manufacturer must inform the FDA of any unexpected side effects or toxicity that comes to its attention. Consumers and health care professionals have an important role in helping to identify any previously unreported effects. New information may be added to the drug's labeling or the FDA can withdraw approval for marketing at any time if new evidence indicates the drug presents an "imminent hazard."

Generic drugs

After a new drug is approved for marketing, a patent will generally protect the financial interests of the drug's developer for a number of years after approval. The traditional protection period is for 17 years but in reality the period is much less because of the extended period of time needed to gain approval before marketing can begin. Recognizing that a considerable part of a drug's patent life may be tied up in the approval process, Congress in 1984 passed a law providing patent extension for drugs whose commercial sale may have been unduly delayed because of the approval process.

Any manufacturer can apply for permission to produce and market a drug after the patent for the drug has expired. Following a procedure called an Abbreviated New Drug Application (ANDA), the applicant must show that its product is bioequivalent to the originator's product. Although the extensive clinical testing the originator had to complete during the drug's development does not have to be repeated, comparative testing between the products in question must be done to ensure that the products will indeed be therapeutically equivalent.

Drug Names

Every drug must have a nonproprietary name; that is, a name that is available for each manufacturer of it to use. These names are commonly called generic names.

Although FDA requires that the generic name of a drug product be placed on its labeling, manufacturers often coin brand (trade) names to use in promotion of their particular product. In general, brand names are shorter, catchier, and easier to use than the corresponding generic name. The brand name manufacturer will then emphasize its proprietary product name (i.e., one that cannot be used by anyone else) in its advertising and other promotions. In many instances, the consumer may not recognize that a drug being sold under one particular brand name is indeed available under other brand names or by generic

A

name. Ask your pharmacist if you have any questions about the names of your medicines.

Drug Quality

After an NDA or an ANDA has been approved, the manufacturer of that product must then meet all requirements relating to production, including current Good Manufacturing Practice regulations of the Food and Drug Administration (FDA) and any applicable standards relating to strength, quality, purity, packaging, and labeling that are established by the *United States Pharmacopeia* (USP).

It should be obvious that the mere placing of a brand name on the label does not in itself assure the quality of the product inside the container. Rather, the quality of a product depends on the manufacturer's ability to create a good mix of inactive ingredients into which to put the active ingredient to make the final dosage form (for example, tablet, capsule, syrup, or suppository) *and* to do so consistently from batch to batch.

Routine product testing by the manufacturer is required by the Good Manufacturing Practice regulations of the FDA (the FDA itself does not routinely test all products, except in cases where there is a suspicion that something might be wrong). In addition to governmental standards, drug products must meet public standards of strength, quality, and purity that are published in the USP. In order to market their products, all manufacturers in the United States must meet USP-established standards unless they specifically choose not to meet the standards for a particular product, in which case that product's label must state that it is "not USP" (this occurs very rarely).

Differences in Drug Products

Although standards to ensure strength, quality, purity, and bioequivalence exist for drug products, the standards allow for variations in certain factors that may produce other differences from product to product. These product variations may be important or of concern to some patients since not all patients are "equivalent." For example, the size, shape, and coating may vary and, therefore, be harder or easier for some patients to swallow; an oral liquid will taste good to some patients and taste awful to others; one manufacturer may use lactose as an inactive ingredient in its product while a therapeutically equivalent product may use some other inactive ingredient; one product may contain sugar or alcohol while another product may not.

In deciding to use one therapeutically equivalent product over another, consumers should keep the following in mind:

- Consider convenience factors that may be important in relation to the use of a drug product (for example, ease of taking a particular dosage form).
- Don't overlook the convenience of the package. The package must protect the drug in accordance with USP requirements, but packages can be quite different in their ease of carrying, storing, opening, and measuring.
- If you have a known allergy or any type of dietary restriction, you need to be aware of the pharmaceutic or "inactive" ingredients that may be present in medicines you have to take. These inactive ingredients may vary from product to product.
- Price is always a consideration. The selection of the specific product to be dispensed may be the most significant factor in the price of a prescription. Talk to the pharmacist about it. Depending on state laws and regulations, the consumer may need to talk to the physician first about changing brands, as the pharmacist may have no alternative but to dispense the specific product the physician originally prescribed.

Aside from differences in the drug product, there are many other factors that you often cannot control that may influence the effectiveness of a medicine. For example, your diet, body chemistry, medical conditions, or other drugs you are taking may affect how much of a dose of a particular medicine gets into the body.

For a majority of the drugs you might take, slight differences in the amount of drug made available to the body will not make any therapeutic difference. For other drugs, the precise amount that gets into the body is more critical. For example, some heart medicines or medicines for epilepsy may create problems for the patient if the dose delivered to the body varies for some reason.

For those drugs that fall in the critical category, it is probably a good idea to stay on the specific product you started on, with any changes being made only if the prescribing health care provider is aware of the change. Your health care provider can help you with questions about these medicines. Also, if you are on such a medicine and you feel that a certain batch is more potent or does not work as well as previous batches, check with your health care provider.

ACETAMINOPHEN Systemic

This information applies to the following medicines:

Acetaminophen (a-seat-a-MIN-oh-fen)
Acetaminophen and Caffeine (kaf-EEN)

Some commonly used brand names are:

For Acetaminophen

In the U.S.

Aceta Elixir
Aceta Tablets
Acetaminophen Uniserts
Actamin
Actamin Extra
Aminofen
Aminofen Max
Anacin-3 Children's Elixir
Anacin-3 Children's Tablets
Anacin-3, Infants'
Anacin-3 Maximum Strength Caplets
Anacin-3 Maximum Strength Tablets
Anacin-3 Regular Strength Tablets
Apacet Capsules
Apacet Elixir
Apacet Extra Strength Caplets
Apacet Extra Strength Tablets
Apacet, Infants'
Apacet Regular Strength Tablets
Arthritis Pain Formula Aspirin Free
Banesin
Dapa
Dapa X-S
Datril Extra-Strength
Dolanex
Dorcol Children's Fever and Pain Reducer
Feverall, Children's
Feverall Junior Strength
Feverall Sprinkle Caps, Children's
Feverall Sprinkle Caps Junior Strength
Genapap Children's Elixir
Genapap Children's Tablets
Genapap Extra Strength Caplets
Genapap Extra Strength Tablets
Genapap, Infants'
Genapap Regular Strength Tablets
Genebs Extra Strength Caplets
Genebs Regular Strength Tablets
Genebs X-Tra
Halenol Elixir
Halenol Extra Strength Caplets
Halenol Extra Strength Tablets
Halenol Regular Strength Tablets
Liquiprin Children's Elixir
Liquiprin Infants' Drops
Meda Cap
Myapap Elixir
Myapap, Infants'
Neopap
Oraphen-PD
Panadol, Children's
Panadol, Infants'
Panadol Junior Strength Caplets
Panadol Maximum Strength Caplets
Panadol Maximum Strength Tablets
Panex
Panex-500
Phenaphen Caplets
Redutemp
Ridenol Caplets
Snaplets-FR
St. Joseph Aspirin-Free Fever Reducer for Children
Suppap-120
Suppap-325
Suppap-650
Tapanol Extra Strength Caplets
Tapanol Extra Strength Tablets
Tempra
Tempra D.S.
Tempra, Infants'
Tempra Syrup
Tenol
Tylenol Children's Elixir
Tylenol Children's Tablets
Tylenol Extra-Strength Adult Liquid Pain Reliever
Tylenol Extra Strength Caplets
Tylenol Extra Strength Gelcaps
Tylenol Extra Strength Tablets
Tylenol, Infants'
Tylenol Junior Strength Caplets
Tylenol Junior Strength Tablets
Tylenol Regular Strength Caplets
Tylenol Regular Strength Tablets
Ty-Pap
Ty-Pap, Infants'
Ty-Pap Syrup
Ty-Tab Caplets
Ty-Tab Capsules
Ty-Tab, Children's
Ty-Tab Tablets
Valadol Liquid
Valadol Tablets
Valorin
Valorin Extra

Generic name product may also be available.

In Canada

Abenol
Anacin-3
Anacin-3 Extra Strength
Apo-Acetaminophen
Atasol Caplets
Atasol Drops
Atasol Elixir
Atasol Forte Caplets
Atasol Forte Tablets
Atasol Tablets
Exdol
Exdol Strong
Panadol
Panadol Extra Strength
Robigesic
Rounox
Tempra Caplets
Tempra Chewable Tablets
Tempra Drops
Tempra Syrup
Tylenol Caplets
Tylenol Chewable Tablets
Tylenol Drops
Tylenol Gelcaps
Tylenol Elixir
Tylenol Junior Strength Caplets
Tylenol Tablets

Generic name product may also be available.

Other commonly used names are APAP and paracetamol.

For Acetaminophen and Caffeine

In the U.S.

Actamin Super
Aspirin-Free Excedrin Caplets
Summit

In Canada

Excedrin Caplets
Excedrin Extra Strength Caplets

Description

Acetaminophen is used to relieve pain and reduce fever. Unlike aspirin, it does not relieve the redness, stiffness, or swelling caused by rheumatoid arthritis. However, it may relieve the pain caused by mild forms of arthritis.

This medicine is available without a prescription; however, your medical doctor or dentist may have special instructions on the proper dose of acetaminophen for your medical condition.

Acetaminophen is available in the following dosage forms:

Oral

Acetaminophen

- Capsules (U.S. and Canada)
- Oral granules (in packets) (U.S.)
- Oral liquid (drops) for babies (U.S. and Canada)
- Oral liquid for children (U.S. and Canada)
- Oral liquid for adults (U.S.)
- Oral powders (in capsules) (U.S.)
- Oral suspension (drops) for babies (U.S.)
- Tablets (U.S. and Canada)
- Chewable tablets (U.S. and Canada)

Acetaminophen and Caffeine
- Capsules (U.S.)
- Tablets (U.S. and Canada)

Rectal

Acetaminophen
- Suppositories (U.S. and Canada)

It is very important that you read and understand the following information. If any of it causes you special concern, check with your doctor or pharmacist. Also, *if you have any questions* or if you want more information about this medicine or your medical problem, *ask your doctor, nurse, or pharmacist.*

Before Using This Medicine

If you are taking this medicine without a prescription, carefully read and follow any precautions on the label. For acetaminophen, the following should be considered:

Allergies—Tell your doctor if you have ever had any unusual or allergic reaction to acetaminophen or to aspirin. Also tell your doctor and pharmacist if you are allergic to any other substances, such as foods, preservatives, or dyes.

Pregnancy—Although studies have not been done in pregnant women, acetaminophen has not been reported to cause birth defects or other problems.

Breast-feeding—Although acetaminophen passes into the breast milk in small amounts, it has not been reported to cause problems in nursing babies.

Children—This medicine has been tested in children and has not been shown to cause different side effects or problems than it does in adults. However, some children's products containing acetaminophen also contain aspartame, which may be dangerous if it is given to children with phenylketonuria.

Older adults—Acetaminophen has been tested and has not been shown to cause different side effects or problems in older people than it does in younger adults.

Other medicines—Although certain medicines should not be used together at all, in other cases two different medicines may be used together even if an interaction might occur. In these cases, your doctor may want to change the dose, or other precautions may be necessary. Tell your doctor and pharmacist if you are taking any other prescription or nonprescription (over-the-counter [OTC]) medicine.

Other medical problems—The presence of other medical problems may affect the use of acetaminophen. Make sure you tell your doctor if you have any other medical problems, especially:
- Alcohol abuse or
- Kidney disease (severe) or
- Hepatitis or other liver disease—The chance of serious side effects may be increased
- Phenylketonuria—Some brands of acetaminophen contain aspartame, which can make your condition worse

Before you begin using any new medicine (prescription or nonprescription) or if you develop any new medical problem while you are using this medicine, check with your doctor, nurse, or pharmacist.

Proper Use of This Medicine

Unless otherwise directed by your physician or dentist:
- *Do not take more of this medicine than is recommended on the package label.* If too much is taken, liver damage may occur.
- *Children up to 12 years of age should not take this medicine more than 5 times a day.*

To use *acetaminophen oral granules* (e.g., Snaplets-FR):
- Just before the medicine is to be taken, open the number of packets needed for one dose. Mix the granules inside of the packets with a small amount of soft food, such as applesauce, ice cream, or jam. Eat the acetaminophen granules along with the food.

To use *acetaminophen oral powders* (e.g., Feverall Sprinkle Caps [Children's or Junior Strength]):
- These capsules are not intended to be swallowed whole. Instead, just before the medicine is to be taken, open the number of capsules needed for one dose. Empty the powder from each capsule into 1 teaspoonful of water or other liquid. Drink the medicine along with the liquid. You may drink more liquid after taking the medicine. You may also mix the powder with a small amount of soft food, such as applesauce, ice cream, or jam. Eat the acetaminophen powder along with the food, right away.

For patients using *acetaminophen suppositories:*
- If the suppository is too soft to insert, chill it in the refrigerator for 30 minutes or run cold water over it before removing the foil wrapper.
- To insert the suppository:

  —First remove the foil wrapper and moisten the suppository with cold water. Lie down on your side and use your finger to push the suppository well up into the rectum.

Storage—To store this medicine:
- Keep out of the reach of children.
- Store away from heat and direct light.
- Do not store acetaminophen tablets (including caplets and gelcaps), capsules, or granules in the bathroom, near the kitchen sink, or in other damp places. Heat or moisture may cause the medicine to break down.
- Keep the liquid and suppository forms of this medicine from freezing.

- Do not keep outdated medicine or medicine no longer needed. Be sure that any discarded medicine is out of the reach of children.

Precautions While Using This Medicine

If you will be taking this medicine for a long time, especially in high doses (more than eight 325-mg or five 500-mg doses a day), your doctor should check your progress at regular visits.

Check with your medical doctor or dentist:

- if you are taking this medicine to relieve pain, including arthritis pain, and the pain lasts for more than 10 days for adults or 5 days for children or if the pain gets worse, if new symptoms occur, or if the painful area is red or swollen. These could be signs of a serious condition that needs medical or dental treatment.
- if you are taking this medicine to bring down a fever, and the fever lasts for more than 3 days or returns, if the fever gets worse, if new symptoms occur, or if redness or swelling is present. These could be signs of a serious condition that needs treatment.
- if you are taking this medicine for a sore throat, and the sore throat is very painful, lasts for more than 2 days, or occurs together with or is followed by fever, headache, skin rash, nausea, or vomiting.

Check the labels of all over-the-counter (OTC), nonprescription, and prescription medicines you now take. If any contain acetaminophen be especially careful, since taking them while taking this medicine may lead to overdose. If you have any questions about this, check with your medical doctor, dentist, or pharmacist.

If you will be taking more than an occasional 1 or 2 doses of acetaminophen, *do not drink alcoholic beverages.* To do so may increase the chance of liver damage, especially if you drink large amounts of alcoholic beverages regularly, if you take more acetaminophen than is recommended on the package label, or if you take it regularly for a long time.

Taking certain other medicines together with acetaminophen may increase the chance of unwanted effects. The risk will depend on how much of each medicine you take every day, and on how long you take the medicines together. If your medical doctor or dentist directs you to take these medicines together on a regular basis, follow his or her directions carefully. However, *do not take any of the following medicines together with acetaminophen for more than a few days, unless your doctor has directed you to do so and is following your progress:*

Aspirin or other salicylates
Diclofenac (e.g., Voltaren)
Diflunisal (e.g., Dolobid)
Fenoprofen (e.g., Nalfon)
Floctafenine (e.g., Idarac)
Flurbiprofen, oral (e.g., Ansaid)
Ibuprofen (e.g., Motrin)
Indomethacin (e.g., Indocin)
Ketoprofen (e.g., Orudis)
Ketorolac (e.g., Toradol)
Meclofenamate (e.g., Meclomen)
Mefenamic acid (e.g., Ponstel)
Naproxen (e.g., Naprosyn)
Phenylbutazone (e.g., Butazolidin)
Piroxicam (e.g., Feldene)
Sulindac (e.g., Clinoril)
Tiaprofenic acid (e.g., Surgam)
Tolmetin (e.g., Tolectin)

Acetaminophen may interfere with the results of some medical tests. Before you have any medical tests, tell the doctor in charge if you have taken acetaminophen within the past 3 or 4 days. If possible, it is best to check with the doctor first, to find out whether this medicine may be taken during the 3 or 4 days before the test.

For *diabetic patients:*

- Acetaminophen may cause false results with some blood glucose (sugar) tests. If you notice any change in your test results, or if you have any questions about this possible problem, check with your doctor, nurse, or pharmacist. This is especially important if your diabetes is not well-controlled.

For patients taking one of the products that contain *caffeine* in addition to acetaminophen:

- Caffeine may interfere with the results of a test that uses dipyridamole (e.g., Persantine) to help find out how well your blood is flowing through certain blood vessels. Therefore, you should not have any caffeine for at least 4 hours before the test.

If you think that you or anyone else may have taken an overdose of acetaminophen, get emergency help at once, even if there are no signs of poisoning. Signs of severe poisoning may not appear for 2 to 4 days after the overdose is taken, but treatment to prevent liver damage or death must be started as soon as possible. Treatment started more than 24 hours after the overdose is taken may not be effective.

Side Effects of This Medicine

Along with its needed effects, a medicine may cause some unwanted effects. Although not all of these side effects may occur, if they do occur they may need medical attention.

Check with your doctor immediately if any of the following side effects occur:

Rare

Yellow eyes or skin

Symptoms of overdose

Diarrhea; increased sweating; loss of appetite; nausea or vomiting; stomach cramps or pain; swelling, pain, or tenderness in the upper abdomen or stomach area

Also, check with your doctor as soon as possible if any of the following side effects occur:

Rare

Bloody or black, tarry stools; bloody or cloudy urine; pain in lower back and/or side (severe and/or sharp); pinpoint red spots on skin; skin rash, hives, or itching; sudden decrease in amount of urine; unexplained sore throat and fever; unusual bleeding or bruising; unusual tiredness or weakness

Other side effects not listed above may also occur in some patients. If you notice any other effects, check with your doctor.

Annual revision: 07/09/91

ACETAMINOPHEN, CALCIUM CARBONATE, POTASSIUM AND SODIUM BICARBONATES, AND CITRIC ACID Systemic

A commonly used brand name in the U.S. is Alka-Seltzer Advanced Formula.

Description

Acetaminophen, calcium carbonate, potassium and sodium bicarbonate, and citric acid (a-seat-a-MIN-oh-fen, KAL-see-um KAR-boe-nate, poe-TAS-ee-um and SOE-dee-um bi-KAR-boe-nates, and SI-trik AS-id) combination is used to relieve pain occurring together with heartburn, sour stomach, or acid indigestion. The acetaminophen in this combination medicine is the pain reliever. The calcium carbonate and potassium and sodium bicarbonates in this combination medicine are antacids. They neutralize stomach acid by combining with it to form a new substance that is not an acid.

There is another medicine with a similar brand name, i.e., Alka-Seltzer Effervescent Pain Reliever and Antacid. Alka-Seltzer Effervescent Pain Reliever and Antacid contains aspirin rather than acetaminophen, and also has a lot more sodium than Alka-Seltzer Advanced Formula. *Be sure that you are getting the right product.*

This medicine is available without a prescription; however, your doctor may have special instructions on the proper dose for your medical condition.

Acetaminophen, calcium carbonate, potassium and sodium bicarbonates, and citric acid combination is available in the following dosage form:

Oral

- Effervescent tablets (U.S.)

It is very important that you read and understand the following information. If any of it causes you special concern, check with your doctor or pharmacist. Also, *if you have any questions* or if you want more information about this medicine or your medical problem, *ask your doctor, nurse, or pharmacist.*

Before Using This Medicine

If you are taking this medicine without a prescription, carefully read and follow any precautions on the label. For acetaminophen, calcium carbonate, potassium and sodium bicarbonates, and citric acid combination, the following should be considered:

Allergies—Tell your doctor if you have ever had any unusual or allergic reaction to acetaminophen or aspirin, or to any medicine that contains calcium, potassium, or sodium bicarbonate. Also tell your doctor and pharmacist if you are allergic to any other substances, such as foods, preservatives, or dyes.

Diet—Make certain your doctor and pharmacist know if you are on any special diet, such as a low-sodium or low-sugar diet. This medicine contains about 140 mg of sodium in each tablet.

Pregnancy—Although acetaminophen, potassium and sodium bicarbonates, and citric acid have not been reported to cause birth defects or other problems in humans, studies on birth defects have not been done in humans. However, you should not take more than an occasional 1 or 2 doses of this medicine if you tend to retain (keep) body water, because the sodium in it can cause you to retain body water. This can result in swelling and weight gain.

Breast-feeding—Acetaminophen and calcium (from the calcium carbonate) pass into the breast milk in small amounts. However, they have not been reported to cause problems in nursing babies.

Children—Acetaminophen has been tested in children and, in effective doses, has not been shown to cause different side effects or problems than it does in adults. However, antacids should not be given to young children (under 6 years of age) unless ordered by their doctor. Small children with stomach problems usually cannot describe their symptoms very well. They should be checked by a doctor, because they may have a condition that needs other treatment.

Older adults—Acetaminophen has been tested and has not been shown to cause different side effects or problems in older people than it does in younger adults. However, the sodium and potassium in this combination medicine can be harmful to some elderly people, especially if large amounts of the medicine are taken regularly.

Other medicines—Although certain medicines should not be used together at all, in other cases two different medicines may be used together even if an interaction might occur. In these cases, your doctor may want to change the dose, or other precautions may be necessary. When you are taking this combination medicine, it is especially important that your doctor and pharmacist know if you are taking any of the following:

- Alcohol—The chance of liver damage may be increased
- Digitalis glycosides (heart medicine)—The chance of unwanted effects may be increased
- Etidronate (e.g., Didronel) or
- Ketoconazole (e.g., Nizoral) or
- Methenamine (e.g., Mandelamine) or
- Tetracyclines (medicine for infection), taken by mouth—Antacids can keep these medicines from working properly
- Mecamylamine (e.g., Inversine)—Antacids can increase the risk of unwanted effects by causing mecamylamine to stay in your body longer than usual

Other medical problems—The presence of other medical problems may affect the use of this combination medicine. Make sure you tell your doctor if you have any other medical problems, especially:

- Alcohol abuse or
- Hepatitis or other liver disease—The chance of serious side effects, including liver damage, may be increased
- Appendicitis (symptoms of, such as stomach or lower abdominal pain, cramping, bloating, soreness, nausea, or vomiting)—Antacids can make your condition worse; also, people who may have appendicitis need medical attention and should not try to treat themselves
- Constipation (severe and continuing) or
- Hemorrhoids or
- Intestinal blockage—Calcium carbonate can make these conditions worse
- Dehydration (loss of body fluid because of sweating, diarrhea, vomiting)—Higher blood levels of the potassium in this combination medicine and an increased chance of serious side effects may occur
- Edema (swelling of face, fingers, feet, or lower legs caused by too much water in the body) or
- Heart disease or
- High blood pressure or
- Toxemia of pregnancy—Sodium can make these conditions worse
- Familial periodic paralysis—Potassium may make one form of this condition worse
- Kidney disease or
- Sarcoidosis or
- Underactive parathyroid gland—The chance of unwanted effects may be increased
- Phenylketonuria—This combination medicine also contains phenylalanine (from aspartame), which can make your condition worse; the amount of phenylalanine in each tablet is 4.2 mg

Proper Use of This Medicine

Unless otherwise directed by your doctor, do not take more of this medicine than is recommended on the package label. If too much is taken, liver damage or other serious side effects may occur.

To use this medicine:

- This medicine must be taken in the form of a liquid that is made from the tablets. Do not swallow the tablets or any pieces of the tablets.
- To make the liquid, place the number of tablets needed for one dose (1 or 2 tablets) into a glass. Then add ½ glass (4 ounces) of cool water.
- Check to be sure that the tablets have disappeared completely. This shows that all of the medicine is in the liquid. Then drink all of the liquid. You may drink the liquid while it is still fizzing or after the fizzing stops.
- Add a little more water to the glass and drink that, to make sure that you are taking all of the medicine.

Missed dose—If your doctor has directed you to take this medicine according to a regular schedule and you miss a dose, take it as soon as you remember. However, if it is almost time for your next dose, skip the missed dose and go back to your regular dosing schedule. Do not double doses.

Storage—To store this medicine:

- Keep out of the reach of children.
- Store away from heat and direct light.
- Do not store this medicine in the bathroom, near the kitchen sink, or in other damp places. Heat or moisture may cause the medicine to break down.
- Do not keep outdated medicine or medicine no longer needed. Be sure that any discarded medicine is out of the reach of children.

Precautions While Using This Medicine

If you will be taking this medicine for a long time (more than 10 days in a row), your doctor should check your progress at regular visits.

Check with your doctor if your pain and/or upset stomach last for more than 10 days or if they get worse, if new symptoms occur, or if the painful area is red or swollen. These could be signs of a serious condition that needs medical treatment.

The antacids in this combination medicine can keep other medicines from working properly if the 2 medicines are taken too close together. *Always take this medicine:*

- *At least 3 hours before or after taking ketoconazole (e.g., Nizoral).*
- *At least 3 or 4 hours before or after taking a tetracycline antibiotic by mouth.*
- *At least 1 or 2 hours before or after taking any other medicine by mouth.*

Check the labels of all over-the-counter (OTC), nonprescription, and prescription medicines you now take. If any contain acetaminophen, calcium, sodium, or potassium be especially careful, since taking them while taking this medicine could cause an overdose. If you have any questions about this, check with your doctor or pharmacist.

Taking certain other medicines together with acetaminophen may increase the chance of unwanted effects. The risk will depend on how much of each medicine you take every day, and on how long you take the medicines together. If your medical doctor or dentist directs you to take these medicines together on a regular basis, follow his or her directions carefully. However, *do not take any of the following medicines together with acetaminophen for more than a few days, unless your doctor has directed you to do so and is following your progress:*

Aspirin or other salicylates
Diclofenac (e.g., Voltaren)
Diflunisal (e.g., Dolobid)
Fenoprofen (e.g., Nalfon)
Floctafenine (e.g., Idarac)
Flurbiprofen, oral (e.g., Ansaid)
Ibuprofen (e.g., Motrin)
Indomethacin (e.g., Indocin)
Ketoprofen (e.g., Orudis)
Ketorolac (e.g., Toradol)
Meclofenamate (e.g., Meclomen)
Mefenamic acid (e.g., Ponstel)
Naproxen (e.g., Naprosyn)
Phenylbutazone (e.g., Butazolidin)
Piroxicam (e.g., Feldene)
Sulindac (e.g., Clinoril)
Tiaprofenic acid (e.g., Surgam)
Tolmetin (e.g., Tolectin)

If you will be taking more than an occasional 1 or 2 doses of this medicine:

- *Do not drink alcoholic beverages.* Drinking alcoholic beverages while you are taking acetaminophen may increase the chance of liver damage, especially if you drink large amounts of alcoholic beverages regularly, if you take more acetaminophen than is recommended on the package label, or if you take it regularly for a long time.
- *Do not also drink a lot of milk or eat a lot of milk products.* To do so may increase the chance of side effects.
- To prevent side effects caused by too much sodium in the body, you may need to limit the amount of sodium in the foods you eat. Some foods that contain large amounts of sodium are canned soup, canned vegetables, pickles, ketchup, green and ripe (black) olives, relish, frankfurters and other sausage-type meats, soy sauce, and carbonated beverages. If you have any questions about this, check with your doctor, nurse, or pharmacist.

This medicine may interfere with the results of some medical tests. Before you have any medical tests, tell the doctor in charge if you have taken this medicine within the past 3 or 4 days. If possible, it is best to check with the doctor first, to find out whether this medicine may be taken during the 3 or 4 days before the test.

For diabetic patients:

- This medicine may cause false results with some blood glucose (sugar) tests. If you notice any change in your test results, or if you have any questions about this possible problem, check with your doctor, nurse, or pharmacist. This is especially important if your diabetes is not well-controlled.

If you think that you or anyone else may have taken an overdose of this medicine, get emergency help at once, even if there are no signs of poisoning. Signs of severe poisoning may not appear for 2 to 4 days after the overdose is taken, but treatment to prevent liver damage or death must be started as soon as possible. Treatment started more than 24 hours after the overdose is taken may not be effective.

Side Effects of This Medicine

Along with its needed effects, a medicine may cause some unwanted effects. Although the following side effects occur very rarely when 1 or 2 doses of this combination medicine is taken occasionally, they may be more likely to occur if:

- too much medicine is taken.
- the medicine is taken several times a day.
- the medicine is taken for more than a few days in a row.

Check with your doctor immediately if any of the following side effects occur:

Rare

Yellow eyes or skin

Symptoms of overdose

Confusion; diarrhea; increased sweating; irregular or slow heartbeat; loss of appetite; nausea or vomiting; numbness or tingling in hands, feet, or lips; shortness of breath or difficult breathing; stomach cramps or pain; swelling, pain, or tenderness in the upper abdomen or stomach area; unexplained anxiety; weakness or heaviness of legs

Also, check with your doctor as soon as possible if any of the following side effects occur:

Rare

Cloudy urine, frequent urge to urinate, or sudden decrease in the amount of urine; constipation (severe and continuing); difficult, burning, or painful urination; headache (continuing); increased blood pressure; mood or mental changes; muscle pain or twitching; nervousness or restlessness; pain in lower back, abdomen (stomach), and/or side; skin rash, hives, or itching; slow breathing; swelling of face, fingers, ankles, feet, or lower legs; unexplained sore throat and fever; unpleasant taste; unusual bleeding or bruising; unusual tiredness or weakness; weight gain (unusual)

Other side effects may occur that usually do not need medical attention. These side effects may go away during treatment as your body adjusts to the medicine. However, check with your doctor if any of the following side effects continue or are bothersome:

Less common

Constipation (mild); increased thirst

Other side effects not listed above may also occur in some patients. If you notice any other effects, check with your doctor.

Annual revision: 07/09/91

ACETAMINOPHEN AND SALICYLATES Systemic†

This information applies to the following medicines:

- Acetaminophen and Aspirin (a-seat-a-MIN-oh-fen and AS-pir-in)
- Acetaminophen, Aspirin, and Caffeine (kaf-EEN)
- Acetaminophen, Aspirin, and Caffeine, Buffered
- Acetaminophen, Aspirin, Salicylamide (sal-i-SILL-a-mide), and Caffeine
- Acetaminophen, Aspirin, and Salicylamide, Buffered
- Acetaminophen and Salicylamide
- Acetaminophen, Salicylamide, and Caffeine

Some commonly used brand names are:

For Acetaminophen and Aspirin

In the U.S.

Gemnisyn

For Acetaminophen, Aspirin, and Caffeine

In the U.S.

Duradyne
Excedrin Extra-Strength Caplets
Excedrin Extra-Strength Tablets
Goody's Extra Strength Tablets
Goody's Headache Powders

Note: In Canada, Excedrin contains acetaminophen and caffeine, but no aspirin.

For Acetaminophen, Aspirin, and Caffeine, Buffered

In the U.S.

Buffets II
Gelpirin
Supac
Vanquish Caplets

For Acetaminophen, Aspirin, Salicylamide, and Caffeine

In the U.S.

Saleto
Tri-Pain Caplets

For Acetaminophen, Aspirin, and Salicylamide, Buffered

In the U.S.

Presalin

For Acetaminophen and Salicylamide

In the U.S.

Duoprin

For Acetaminophen, Salicylamide, and Caffeine

In the U.S.

Rid-A-Pain Compound
S-A-C

†Not commercially available in Canada.

Description

Acetaminophen and salicylate combination medicines relieve pain and reduce fever. They may be used to relieve occasional pain caused by mild inflammation or arthritis (rheumatism). However, neither acetaminophen nor salicylamide is as effective as aspirin for treating chronic or severe pain, or other symptoms, caused by inflammation or arthritis. Some of these combination medicines do not contain any aspirin. Even those that do contain aspirin may not contain enough to be effective in treating these conditions.

A few reports have suggested that acetaminophen and salicylates may work together to cause kidney damage or cancer of the kidney or urinary bladder. This may occur if large amounts of both medicines are taken together for a very long time. However, taking usual amounts of these combination medicines for a short time has not been shown to cause these unwanted effects. Also, these effects are not likely to occur with either acetaminophen or a salicylate used alone, even if large amounts have been taken for a long time. Therefore, for long-term use, it may be best to use either acetaminophen or a salicylate, but not both, unless you are under a doctor's care.

Before giving any of these combination medicines to a child, check the package label very carefully. Some of these medicines are too strong for use in children. If you are not certain whether a specific product can be given to a child, or if you have any questions about the amount to give, check with your doctor, nurse, or pharmacist.

These medicines are available without a prescription. However, your doctor may have special instructions on the proper dose of these medicines for your medical condition.

These medicines are available in the following dosage forms:

Oral

Acetaminophen and Aspirin
- Tablets (U.S.)

Acetaminophen, Aspirin, and Caffeine
- Oral powders (U.S.)
- Tablets (U.S.)

Acetaminophen, Aspirin, and Caffeine, Buffered
- Tablets (U.S.)

Acetaminophen, Aspirin, Salicylamide, and Caffeine
- Tablets (U.S.)

Acetaminophen, Aspirin, and Salicylamide, Buffered
- Tablets (U.S.)

Acetaminophen and Salicylamide
- Capsules (U.S.)

Acetaminophen, Salicylamide, and Caffeine
- Capsules (U.S.)
- Tablets (U.S.)

It is very important that you read and understand the following information. If any of it causes you special concern, check with your doctor or pharmacist. Also, *if you have any questions* or if you want more information about this medicine or your medical problem, *ask your doctor, nurse, or pharmacist.*

Before Using This Medicine

If you are taking this medicine without a prescription, carefully read and follow any precautions on the label. For acetaminophen and salicylate combinations, the following should be considered:

Allergies—Tell your doctor if you have ever had any unusual or allergic reaction to acetaminophen, aspirin or other salicylates including methyl salicylate (oil of wintergreen), or to any of the following medicines:

Diclofenac (e.g., Voltaren)
Diflunisal (e.g., Dolobid)
Fenoprofen (e.g., Nalfon)
Floctafenine (e.g., Idarac)
Flurbiprofen, oral (e.g., Ansaid)
Ibuprofen (e.g., Motrin)
Indomethacin (e.g., Indocin)
Ketoprofen (e.g., Orudis)
Ketorolac (e.g., Toradol)
Meclofenamate (e.g., Meclomen)
Mefenamic acid (e.g., Ponstel)
Naproxen (e.g., Naprosyn)
Oxyphenbutazone (e.g., Tandearil)
Phenylbutazone (e.g., Butazolidin)
Piroxicam (e.g., Feldene)
Sulindac (e.g., Clinoril)
Suprofen (e.g., Suprol)
Tiaprofenic acid (e.g., Surgam)
Tolmetin (e.g., Tolectin)
Zomepirac (e.g., Zomax)

Also tell your doctor and pharmacist if you are allergic to any other substances, such as foods, preservatives, or dyes.

Pregnancy—
- *For Acetaminophen*: Studies on birth defects have not been done in humans. However, acetaminophen has not been reported to cause birth defects or other problems.
- *For Aspirin*: Studies in humans have not shown that aspirin causes birth defects. However, aspirin has been shown to cause birth defects in animals.

  Do not take aspirin during the last 3 months of pregnancy unless it has been ordered by your doctor. Some reports have suggested that too much use of aspirin late in pregnancy may cause a decrease in the newborn's weight and possible death of the fetus or newborn infant. However, the mothers in these reports had been taking much larger amounts of aspirin than are usually recommended. Studies of mothers taking aspirin in the doses that are usually recommended did not show these unwanted effects. However, there is a chance that regular use of aspirin late in pregnancy may cause unwanted effects on the heart or blood flow in the fetus or newborn infant.

  Use of aspirin during the last 2 weeks of pregnancy may cause bleeding problems in the fetus before or during delivery, or in the newborn infant. Also, too much use of aspirin during the last 3 months of pregnancy may increase the length of pregnancy, prolong labor, cause other problems during delivery, or cause severe bleeding in the mother before, during, or after delivery.
- *For Salicylamide*: Studies on birth defects have not been done in humans.
- *For Caffeine*: Studies in humans have not shown that caffeine causes birth defects. However, use of large amounts of caffeine by the mother during pregnancy may cause problems with the heart rhythm of the fetus and may affect the growth of the fetus. Studies in animals have shown that caffeine causes birth defects when given in very large doses (amounts equal to the amount of caffeine in 12 to 24 cups of coffee a day).

Breast-feeding—
- *For Acetaminophen and for Aspirin:* Although acetaminophen and aspirin have not been reported to cause problems in nursing babies, these medicines pass into the breast milk.
- *For Caffeine:* Caffeine (contained in some of these combination medicines) passes into the breast milk in small amounts. Taking caffeine in the amounts present in these medicines has not been reported to cause problems in nusing babies. However, studies have shown that babies may appear jittery and have trouble in sleeping when their mothers drink large

amounts of caffeine-containing beverages. Therefore, breast-feeding mothers who use these medicines should probably limit the amount of caffeine they take in from other medicines or from beverages.

Children—

- *For Acetaminophen*: Acetaminophen has been tested in children and, in effective doses, has not been shown to cause different side effects or problems than it does in adults.
- *For Aspirin and for Salicylamide*: *Do not give a medicine containing aspirin or salicylamide to a child with symptoms of a virus infection, especially flu or chickenpox, without first discussing its use with your child's doctor*. This is very important because aspirin may cause a serious illness called Reye's syndrome in children with fever caused by a virus infection, especially flu or chickenpox. Children who do not have a virus infection may also be more sensitive to the effects of aspirin, especially if they have a fever or have lost large amounts of body fluid because of vomiting, diarrhea, or sweating. This may increase the chance of side effects during treatment.
- *For Caffeine*: There is no specific information comparing use of caffeine in children up to 12 years of age with use in other age groups. However, caffeine is not expected to cause different side effects or problems in children than it does in adults.

Teenagers—*Teenagers with fever or other symptoms of a virus infection, especially flu or chickenpox, should check with a doctor before taking this medicine*. The aspirin in this combination medicine may cause a serious illness called Reye's syndrome in teenagers with fever caused by a virus infection, especially flu or chickenpox.

Older adults—Elderly people may be more likely than younger adults to develop serious kidney problems if they take large amounts of these combination medicines for a long time. Therefore, it is best that elderly people not take this medicine for more than 5 days in a row unless they are under a doctor's care.

- *For Acetaminophen*: Acetaminophen has been tested and, in effective doses, has not been shown to cause different side effects or problems in older people than it does in younger adults.
- *For Aspirin*: People 60 years of age and older are especially sensitive to the effects of aspirin. This may increase the chance of side effects during treatment.
- *For Caffeine*: Many medicines have not been studied specifically in older people. Therefore, it may not be known whether they work exactly the same way they do in younger adults or if they cause different side effects or problems in older people. There is no specific information comparing use of caffeine in the elderly with use in other age groups.

Other medicines—Although certain medicines should not be used together at all, in other cases two different medicines may be used together even if an interaction might occur. In these cases, your doctor may want to change the dose, or other precautions may be necessary. When you are taking an acetaminophen and salicylate combination, it is especially important that your doctor and pharmacist know if you are taking any of the following:

- Anticoagulants (blood thinners) or
- Carbenicillin by injection (e.g., Geopen) or
- Cefamandole (e.g., Mandol) or
- Cefoperazone (e.g., Cefobid) or
- Cefotetan (e.g., Cefotan) or
- Dipyridamole (e.g., Persantine) or
- Divalproex (e.g., Depakote) or
- Heparin or
- Inflammation or pain medicine, except narcotics, or
- Moxalactam (e.g., Moxam) or
- Pentoxifylline (e.g., Trental) or
- Plicamycin (e.g., Mithracin) or
- Ticarcillin (e.g., Ticar) or
- Valproic acid (e.g., Depakene)—Taking these medicines together with aspirin (present in some of these combination medicines) may increase the chance of serious bleeding
- Antidiabetics, oral (diabetes medicine you take by mouth)—Aspirin (present in some of these combination medicines) may increase the effects of the antidiabetic medicine; a change in dose may be needed if aspirin is taken regularly
- Ketoconazole (e.g., Nizoral) or
- Tetracyclines (medicine for infection), taken by mouth—Antacids (present in buffered forms of these combination medicines) can keep the ketoconazole or tetracycline from working properly if taken too close to them
- Methotrexate (e.g., Mexate)—Taking aspirin (present in some of these combination medicines) together with methotrexate may increase the chance of serious side effects
- Probenecid (e.g., Benemid)—Aspirin (present in some of these combination medicines) can keep probenecid from working properly when it is used to treat gout
- Sulfinpyrazone (e.g., Anturane)—Aspirin (present in some of these combination medicines) can keep sulfinpyrazone from working properly when it is used to treat gout; also, taking aspirin together with sulfinpyrazone may increase the chance of bleeding
- Urinary alkalizers (medicine that makes the urine less acid, such as acetazolamide [e.g., Diamox], calcium- and/or magnesium-containing antacids, dichlorphenamide [e.g., Daranide], methazolamide [e.g., Neptazane], potassium or sodium citrate and/or citric acid, sodium bicarbonate [baking soda])—These medicines may make aspirin (present in some of these combination medicines) less effective by causing it to be removed from the body more quickly

Other medical problems—The presence of other medical problems may affect the use of acetaminophen and salicylate combinations. Make sure you tell your doctor if you have any other medical problems, especially:

- Alcohol abuse or
- Asthma, allergies, and nasal polyps (history of) or

- Hepatitis or other liver disease or
- Kidney disease—The chance of serious side effects may be increased
- Anemia or
- Stomach ulcer or other stomach problems—Aspirin (present in some of these combination medicines) may make these conditions worse
- Gout—Aspirin (present in some of these combination medicines) can make this condition worse and can also lessen the effects of some medicines used to treat gout
- Heart disease—Caffeine (present in some of these combination medicines) can make your condition worse
- Hemophilia or other bleeding problems—Aspirin (present in some of these combination medicines) increases the chance of serious bleeding

Before you begin using any new medicine (prescription or nonprescription) or if you develop any new medical problem while you are using this medicine, check with your doctor, nurse, or pharmacist.

Proper Use of This Medicine

Take this medicine with food or a full glass (8 ounces) of water to lessen the chance of stomach upset.

Unless otherwise directed by your doctor:

- *Do not take more of this medicine than directed on the package label.* Taking too much acetaminophen may cause liver damage or lead to other medical problems because of an overdose. Also, taking too much aspirin can cause stomach problems or lead to other medical problems because of an overdose.
- *Children up to 12 years of age should not take this medicine more often than 5 times a day.*

Check with your doctor before taking one of these combination medicines to treat severe or chronic inflammation or arthritis (rheumatism). These combination medicines may not relieve the severe pain, redness, swelling, or stiffness caused by these conditions unless very large amounts are taken for a long time. *It is best not to take acetaminophen and salicylate combination medicines in large amounts for a long time* unless you are under a doctor's care.

If a combination medicine containing aspirin has a strong vinegar-like odor, do not use it. This odor means the medicine is breaking down. If you have any questions about this, check with your pharmacist.

Storage—To store this medicine:

- Keep out of the reach of children. Overdose of the salicylates in these combination medicines is very dangerous in young children.
- Store away from heat and direct light.
- Do not store tablets (including caplets), capsules, or powders in the bathroom, near the kitchen sink, or in other damp places. Heat or moisture may cause the medicine to break down.
- Do not keep outdated medicine or medicine no longer needed. Be sure that any discarded medicine is out of the reach of children.

Precautions While Using This Medicine

If you will be taking this medicine for a long time, or in high doses, *your doctor should check your progress at regular visits.* This is especially important for elderly people, who may be more likely than younger adults to develop serious kidney problems if they take large amounts of this medicine for a long time.

Check with your doctor:

- If you are taking this medicine to relieve pain and the pain lasts for more than 10 days (5 days for children), if the pain gets worse, if new symptoms occur, or if the painful area is red or swollen. These could be signs of a serious condition that needs treatment.
- If you are taking this medicine to bring down a fever, and the fever lasts for more than 3 days or returns, if your fever gets worse, if new symptoms occur, or if redness or swelling is present. These could be signs of a serious condition that needs treatment.
- If you are taking this medicine for a sore throat, and the sore throat is very painful, lasts for more than 2 days, or occurs together with or is followed by fever, headache, skin rash, nausea, or vomiting.

Do not take any of the combination medicines containing aspirin for 5 days before any surgery, including dental surgery, unless otherwise directed by your medical doctor or dentist. Taking aspirin during this time may cause bleeding problems.

Check the label of all over-the-counter (OTC), nonprescription, and prescription medicines you now take. If any contain acetaminophen or aspirin or other salicylates, including bismuth subsalicylate (e.g., Pepto-Bismol), be especially careful. Also, be careful if you regularly apply a shampoo or other medicine containing salicylic acid to your skin or scalp. Taking or using any of these medicines together with this combination medicine may lead to overdose. If you have any questions about this, check with your doctor or pharmacist.

If you will be taking more than an occasional 1 or 2 doses of this medicine, *do not drink alcoholic beverages.* Stomach problems may be more likely to occur if you drink alcoholic beverages while you are taking aspirin. Also, liver damage may be more likely to occur if you drink large amounts of alcoholic beverages while you are taking acetaminophen.

Taking certain other medicines together with acetaminophen and salicylates may increase the chance of unwanted effects. The risk will depend on how much of each medicine you take every day, and on how long you take the medicines together. If your medical doctor or dentist directs you to take these medicines together on a regular basis, follow his or her directions carefully. However, *do not take any of the following medicines together with any of these combination medicines for more than a few days, unless your doctor has directed you to do so and is following your progress:*

Diclofenac (e.g., Voltaren)
Diflunisal (e.g., Dolobid)
Fenoprofen (e.g., Nalfon)
Floctafenine (e.g., Idarac)
Flurbiprofen, oral (e.g., Ansaid)
Ibuprofen (e.g., Motrin)
Indomethacin (e.g., Indocin)
Ketoprofen (e.g., Orudis)
Ketorolac (e.g., Toradol)
Meclofenamate (e.g., Meclomen)
Mefenamic acid (e.g., Ponstel)
Naproxen (e.g., Naprosyn)
Phenylbutazone (e.g., Butazolidin)
Piroxicam (e.g., Feldene)
Sulindac (e.g., Clinoril)
Tiaprofenic acid (e.g., Surgam)
Tolmetin (e.g., Tolectin)

The antacid present in buffered forms of these combination medicines can keep other medicines from working properly. To prevent this problem, *always take this medicine:*

- *At least 3 hours before or after taking ketoconazole (e.g., Nizoral).*
- *At least 3 or 4 hours before or after taking a tetracycline antibiotic by mouth.*
- *At least 1 or 2 hours before or after taking any other medicine by mouth.*

If you are taking a laxative containing cellulose, do not take it within 2 hours of taking this medicine. Taking them close together may make this medicine less effective by preventing the salicylate in it from being absorbed by your body.

Acetaminophen and salicylate combinations may interfere with the results of some medical tests. Before you have any medical tests, tell the doctor in charge if you have taken any of these combination medicines within the past 3 or 4 days. If possible, it is best to check with the doctor first, to find out whether the medicine may be taken during the 3 or 4 days before the test.

For diabetic patients:

- Acetaminophen and salicylate combinations may cause false results with some blood and urine glucose (sugar) tests. If you notice any change in your test results, or if you have any questions about this possible problem, check with your doctor, nurse, or pharmacist. This is especially important if your diabetes is not well-controlled.

For patients taking one of the products that contain *caffeine:*

- Caffeine may interfere with the results of a test that uses dipyridamole (e.g., Persantine) to help find out how well your blood is flowing through certain blood vessels. Therefore, you should not have any caffeine for at least 4 hours before the test.

If you think that you or anyone else may have taken an overdose of this medicine, get emergency help at once. Taking an overdose of a salicylate may cause unconsciousness or death. The first symptom of an aspirin overdose may be ringing or buzzing in the ears. Other signs include convulsions (seizures), hearing loss, confusion, severe drowsiness or tiredness, severe excitement or nervousness, and unusually fast or deep breathing. Signs of severe acetaminophen overdose may not appear until 2 to 4 days after the overdose is taken, but treatment to prevent liver damage or death must be started within 24 hours or less after the overdose is taken.

Side Effects of This Medicine

Along with its needed effects, a medicine may cause some unwanted effects. Although not all of these side effects may occur, if they do occur they may need medical attention.

Check with your doctor immediately if any of the following side effects occur:

Less common or rare

Difficulty in swallowing; dizziness, lightheadedness, or feeling faint (severe); flushing, redness, or other change in skin color; shortness of breath, troubled breathing, tightness in chest, or wheezing; sudden decrease in amount of urine; swelling of eyelids, face, or lips

Signs and symptoms of overdose

Agitation, anxiety, excitement, irritability, nervousness, or restlessness; any loss of hearing; bloody urine; confusion or delirium; convulsions (seizures); diarrhea (severe or continuing); dizziness or lightheadedness; drowsiness (severe); fast or deep breathing; fast or irregular heartbeat (for medicines containing caffeine); frequent urination (for medicines containing caffeine); hallucinations (seeing, hearing, or feeling things that are not there); headache (severe or continuing); increased sensitivity to touch or pain (for medicines containing caffeine); increased sweating; loss of appetite; muscle trembling or twitching (for medicines containing caffeine); nausea or vomiting (continuing, sometimes with blood); ringing or buzzing in ears (continuing); seeing flashes of "zig-zag" lights (for medicines containing caffeine); stomach cramps or pain (severe or continuing); swelling, pain, or tenderness in the upper abdomen or stomach area; trouble in sleeping (for medicines containing caffeine); uncontrollable flapping movements of the hands, especially in elderly patients; unexplained fever; unusual thirst; vision problems

Signs of overdose in children

Changes in behavior; drowsiness or tiredness (severe); fast or deep breathing

Also, check with your doctor as soon as possible if any of the following side effects occur:

Less common or rare

Bloody or black, tarry stools; cloudy urine; pain in lower back and/or side (severe and/or sharp); skin rash, hives, or itching; swelling of face, fingers, feet, or lower legs; unexplained sore throat and fever; unusual bleeding or bruising; unusual tiredness or weakness; vomiting of blood or material that looks like coffee grounds; weight gain; yellow eyes or skin

Other side effects may occur that usually do not need medical attention. These side effects may go away during treatment as your body adjusts to the medicine. However, check with your doctor if any of the following side effects continue or are bothersome:

More common

Heartburn or indigestion (for medicines containing aspirin); nausea, vomiting, or stomach pain (for medicines containing aspirin)

Less common

Drowsiness (for medicines containing salicylamide); trouble in sleeping, nervousness, or jitters (for medicines containing caffeine)

Some side effects may occur after you have stopped taking these combination medicines, especially if you have taken large amounts of them for a long time. *Check with your doctor immediately* if any of these side effects occur after you have stopped taking this medicine:

Rare

Bloody or cloudy urine; decreased urination; swelling of face, fingers, feet, or lower legs; weight gain

Other side effects not listed above may also occur in some patients. If you notice any other effects, check with your doctor.

Annual revision: 04/30/93

ACETAMINOPHEN, SALICYLATES, AND CODEINE Systemic†

This information applies to the following medicines:

Acetaminophen, Aspirin, Salicylamide (sal-i-SILL-a-mide), Codeine, and Caffeine (kaf-EEN)

A commonly used brand name in the U.S. is Rid-A-Pain with Codeine.

†Not commercially available in Canada.

Description

Acetaminophen (a-seat-a-MIN-oh-fen), aspirin (AS-pir-in), salicylamide (sal-i-SILL-a-mide), codeine (KOE-deen), and caffeine (kaf-EEN) combination is used to relieve pain. Aspirin and salicylamide belong to the group of medicines called salicylates. Codeine belongs to the group of medicines called narcotic analgesics (nar-KOT-ik an-al-JEE-zicks). A narcotic analgesic, acetaminophen, and a salicylate used together may provide better pain relief than any of these medicines used alone. In some cases, relief of pain may come with lower doses of each medicine.

Narcotic analgesics act in the central nervous system (CNS) to relieve pain. Many of their side effects are also caused by actions in the CNS. When narcotics are used for a long time, your body may get used to them so that larger amounts are needed to relieve pain. This is called tolerance to the medicine. Also, when narcotics are used for a long time or in large doses, they may become habit-forming (causing mental or physical dependence). Physical dependence may lead to withdrawal symptoms when you stop taking the medicine.

Acetaminophen and salicylates do not become habit-forming when taken for a long time or in large doses, but they may cause other unwanted effects if too much is taken.

This medicine is available without a prescription, in the following dosage form:

Oral

Acetaminophen, Aspirin, Salicylamide, Codeine, and Caffeine

- Tablets (U.S.)

It is very important that you read and understand the following information. If any of it causes you special concern, check with your doctor or pharmacist. Also, *if you have any questions* or if you want more information about this medicine or your medical problem, *ask your doctor, nurse, or pharmacist.*

Before Using This Medicine

In deciding to use a medicine, the risks of taking the medicine must be weighed against the good it will do. This is a decision you and your doctor will make. For acetaminophen, salicylate, and codeine combination, the following should be considered:

Allergies—Tell your doctor if you have ever had any unusual or allergic reaction to acetaminophen, aspirin or other salicylates including methyl salicylate (oil of wintergreen), codeine, or any of the following medicines:

Diclofenac (e.g., Voltaren)
Diflunisal (e.g., Dolobid)
Fenoprofen (e.g., Nalfon)
Floctafenine (e.g., Idarac)
Flurbiprofen, oral (e.g., Ansaid)
Ibuprofen (e.g., Motrin)
Indomethacin (e.g., Indocin)
Ketoprofen (e.g., Orudis)
Ketorolac (e.g., Toradol)
Meclofenamate (e.g., Meclomen)
Mefenamic acid (e.g., Ponstel)
Naproxen (e.g., Naprosyn)
Oxyphenbutazone (e.g., Tandearil)
Phenylbutazone (e.g., Butazolidin)
Piroxicam (e.g., Feldene)
Sulindac (e.g., Clinoril)
Suprofen (e.g., Suprol)
Tiaprofenic acid (e.g., Surgam)
Tolmetin (e.g., Tolectin)
Zomepirac (e.g., Zomax)

Also tell your doctor and pharmacist if you are allergic to any other substances, such as foods, preservatives, or dyes.

Pregnancy—

- *For acetaminophen*: Acetaminophen has not been reported to cause birth defects or other problems in humans. However, studies on birth defects with acetaminophen have not been done in humans.
- *For aspirin*: Studies in humans have not shown that aspirin causes birth defects. However, it has caused birth defects in animal studies.

  Do not take aspirin during the last 3 months of pregnancy unless it has been ordered by your doctor. Some reports have suggested that too much use of aspirin late in pregnancy may cause a decrease in the newborn's weight and possible death of the fetus or newborn infant. However, the mothers in these reports had been taking much larger amounts of aspirin than are usually recommended. Studies of mothers taking aspirin in the doses that are usually recommended did not show these effects. However, regular use of aspirin late in pregnancy may cause unwanted effects on the heart or blood flow in the fetus or in the newborn infant. Also, use of aspirin during the last 2 weeks of pregnancy may cause bleeding problems in the fetus before or during delivery or in the newborn infant.

  Too much use of aspirin during the last 3 months of pregnancy may increase the length of pregnancy, prolong labor, cause other problems during delivery, or cause severe bleeding in the mother before, during, or after delivery.
- *For codeine*: Although studies on birth defects with codeine have not been done in humans, codeine has not been reported to cause birth defects in humans. Animal studies have not shown that codeine causes birth defects, but it slowed development of bones and caused a decrease in successful pregnancies.

  Too much use of a narcotic during pregnancy may cause the fetus to become dependent on the medicine. This may lead to withdrawal side effects in the newborn baby. Also, codeine may cause breathing problems in the newborn baby if taken just before or during delivery.
- *For caffeine*: Studies in humans have not shown that caffeine (contained in some of these combination medicines) causes birth defects. However, studies in animals have shown that caffeine causes birth defects when given in very large doses (amounts equal to those present in 12 to 24 cups of coffee a day).

Breast-feeding—These combination medicines have not been reported to cause problems in nursing babies. However, acetaminophen, aspirin, caffeine, and codeine pass into the breast milk.

Children and teenagers—*Do not give a medicine containing aspirin or other salicylates to a child or a teenager with symptoms of a virus infection, especially flu or chickenpox, without first discussing its use with your child's doctor.* This is very important because aspirin may cause a serious illness called Reye's syndrome in children with fever caused by a virus infection, especially flu or chickenpox. Children who do not have a virus infection may also be more sensitive to the effects of aspirin, especially if they have a fever or have lost large amounts of body fluid because of vomiting, diarrhea, or sweating. This may increase the chance of side effects during treatment.

The codeine in this combination medicine may cause breathing problems, especially in children younger than 2 years of age. These children are usually more sensitive than adults to the effects of codeine. Also, unusual excitement or restlessness may be more likely to occur in children receiving codeine.

Older adults—Elderly people are especially sensitive to the effects of aspirin and codeine. This may increase the chance of side effects, especially breathing problems caused by codeine, during treatment.

Other medicines—Although certain medicines should not be used together at all, in other cases two different medicines may be used together even if an interaction might occur. In these cases, your doctor may want to change the dose, or other precautions may be necessary. When you are taking an acetaminophen, salicylate, and codeine combination, it is especially important that your doctor and pharmacist know if you are taking any of the following:

- Anticoagulants (blood thinners) or
- Carbenicillin by injection (e.g., Geopen) or
- Cefamandole (e.g., Mandol) or
- Cefoperazone (e.g., Cefobid) or
- Cefotetan (e.g., Cefotan) or
- Dipyridamole (e.g., Persantine) or

- Divalproex (e.g., Depakote) or
- Heparin or
- Medicine for inflammation or pain, except narcotics, or
- Moxalactam (e.g., Moxam) or
- Pentoxifylline (e.g., Trental) or
- Plicamycin (e.g., Mithracin) or
- Ticarcillin (e.g., Ticar) or
- Valproic acid (e.g., Depakene)—Taking these medicines together with aspirin may increase the chance of bleeding
- Antidepressants, tricyclic (amitriptyline [e.g., Elavil], amoxapine [e.g., Asendin], clomipramine [e.g., Anafranil], desipramine [e.g., Pertofrane], doxepin [e.g., Sinequan], imipramine [e.g., Tofranil], nortriptyline [e.g., Aventyl], protriptyline [e.g., Vivactil], trimipramine [e.g., Surmontil]) or
- Central nervous system (CNS) depressants—Taking these medicines together with codeine may increase the chance of serious side effects
- Antidiabetics, oral (diabetes medicine you take by mouth)—Aspirin may increase the effects of the antidiabetic medicine; a change in the dose of the antidiabetic medicine may be needed if aspirin is taken regularly
- Methotrexate (e.g., Mexate)—Taking aspirin together with methotrexate may increase the chance of serious side effects
- Naltrexone (e.g., Trexan)—Naltrexone keeps codeine from working to relieve pain; people taking naltrexone should take pain relievers that do not contain a narcotic
- Probenecid (e.g., Benemid)—Aspirin can keep probenecid from working properly for treating gout
- Sulfinpyrazone (e.g., Anturane)—Aspirin can keep sulfinpyrazone from working properly for treating gout; also, taking aspirin together with sulfinpyrazone may increase the chance of bleeding
- Urinary alkalizers (medicine that makes the urine less acid, such as acetazolamide [e.g., Diamox], dichlorphenamide [e.g., Daranide], methazolamide [e.g., Neptazane], potassium or sodium citrate and/or citric acid)—These medicines may make aspirin less effective by causing it to be removed from the body more quickly

Other medical problems—The presence of other medical problems may affect the use of acetaminophen, salicylate, and codeine combinations. Make sure you tell your doctor if you have any other medical problems, especially:

- Alcohol and/or other drug abuse (or history of) or
- Asthma, allergies, and nasal polyps (history of) or
- Brain disease or head injury or
- Colitis or
- Convulsions (seizures) (history of) or
- Emotional problems or mental illness or
- Emphysema, asthma, or chronic lung disease or
- Hepatitis or other liver disease or
- Kidney disease or
- Underactive thyroid—The chance of serious side effects may be increased
- Anemia or
- Stomach ulcer or other stomach problems—Aspirin may make these conditions worse
- Enlarged prostate or problems with urination or
- Gallbladder disease or gallstones—Codeine may add to some of the effects of these medical problems
- Gout—Aspirin can make this condition worse and can also lessen the effects of some medicines used to treat gout
- Heart disease—Caffeine can make your condition worse
- Hemophilia or other bleeding problems or
- Vitamin K deficiency—Aspirin increases the chance of serious bleeding

Before you begin using any new medicine (prescription or nonprescription) or if you develop any new medical problem while you are using this medicine, check with your doctor, nurse, or pharmacist.

Proper Use of This Medicine

Take this medicine only as directed by your medical doctor or dentist. Do not take more of it, do not take it more often, and do not take it for a longer time than your medical doctor or dentist ordered. This is especially important for children and the elderly, who are usually more sensitive than other people to the effects of the aspirin and the codeine in this medicine. If too much codeine is taken, it may become habit-forming (causing mental or physical dependence) or lead to medical problems because of an overdose. Also, taking too much acetaminophen or aspirin may increase the chance of other unwanted effects, including stomach problems or kidney or liver damage, or lead to medical problems because of an overdose.

If you think that this medicine is not working properly after you have been taking it for a few weeks, *do not increase the dose.* Instead, check with your medical doctor or dentist.

Take this medicine with food and a full glass (8 ounces) of water to lessen stomach irritation. Also, do not lie down for about 15 or 30 minutes after swallowing the medicine. This helps to prevent irritation that may lead to trouble in swallowing.

Do not take this medicine if it has a strong vinegar-like odor. This odor means the aspirin in it is breaking down. If you have any questions about this, check with your doctor or pharmacist.

Missed dose—If your doctor has ordered you to take this medicine according to a regular schedule and you miss a dose, take it as soon as you remember. However, if it is almost time for your next dose, skip the missed dose and go back to your regular dosing schedule. *Do not double doses.*

Storage—To store this medicine:

- Keep out of the reach of children. Overdose is very dangerous in young children.
- Store away from heat and direct light.
- Do not store this medicine in the bathroom, near the kitchen sink, or in other damp places. Heat or moisture may cause the medicine to break down.

- Do not keep outdated medicine or medicine no longer needed. Be sure that any discarded medicine is out of the reach of children.

Precautions While Using This Medicine

If you will be taking this medicine for a long time (for example, for several months at a time) or in large amounts, your doctor should check your progress at regular visits.

Check the labels of all nonprescription (over-the-counter [OTC]) and prescription medicines you now take. If any contain a narcotic, acetaminophen, aspirin, or other salicylates, including diflunisal, be especially careful, since taking them while taking this medicine may lead to overdose. If you have any questions about this, check with your doctor or pharmacist.

Too much use of certain other medicines together with the acetaminophen or aspirin contained in this combination medicine may increase the chance of unwanted effects. The risk will depend on how much of each medicine you take every day, and on how long you take the medicines together. If your doctor directs you to take these medicines together on a regular basis, follow his or her directions carefully. However, do not take any of the following medicines together with this combination medicine for more than a few days, unless your doctor has directed you to do so and is following your progress:

Diclofenac (e.g., Voltaren)
Diflunisal (e.g., Dolobid)
Fenoprofen (e.g., Nalfon)
Floctafenine (e.g., Idarac)
Flurbiprofen, oral (e.g., Ansaid)
Ibuprofen (e.g., Motrin)
Indomethacin (e.g., Indocin)
Ketoprofen (e.g., Orudis)
Ketorolac (e.g., Toradol)
Meclofenamate (e.g., Meclomen)
Mefenamic acid (e.g., Ponstel)
Naproxen (e.g., Naprosyn)
Phenylbutazone (e.g., Butazolidin)
Piroxicam (e.g., Feldene)
Sulindac (e.g., Clinoril)
Tiaprofenic acid (e.g., Surgam)
Tolmetin (e.g., Tolectin)

The codeine in this medicine will add to the effects of alcohol and other CNS depressants (medicines that slow down the nervous system, possibly causing drowsiness). Some examples of CNS depressants are antihistamines or medicine for hay fever, other allergies, or colds; sedatives, tranquilizers, or sleeping medicine; other prescription pain medicine or narcotics; barbiturates; medicine for seizures; muscle relaxants; or anesthetics, including some dental anesthetics. Also, liver problems may be more likely to occur if you drink large amounts of alcoholic beverages while taking acetaminophen. In addition, stomach problems may be more likely to occur if you drink alcoholic beverages while you are taking aspirin. *Do not drink alcoholic beverages, and check with your doctor before taking any of the medicines listed above, while you are using this medicine.*

This medicine may cause some people to become drowsy, dizzy, or lightheaded, or to feel a false sense of well-being. *Make sure you know how you react to this medicine before you drive, use machines, or do anything else that could be dangerous if you are dizzy or are not alert and clearheaded.*

Dizziness, lightheadedness, or fainting may occur, especially when you get up suddenly from a lying or sitting position. Getting up slowly may help lessen this problem. If you do feel dizzy, lightheaded, or faint, lying down for a while may help.

Nausea or vomiting may occur, especially after the first couple of doses. This effect may go away if you lie down for a while. However, if nausea or vomiting continues, check with your doctor.

Before having any kind of surgery, dental work, or emergency treatment, tell the medical doctor or dentist in charge that you are taking this medicine.

Do not take this medicine for 5 days before any surgery, including dental surgery, unless otherwise directed by your medical doctor or dentist. Taking aspirin during this time may cause bleeding problems.

If you are taking a laxative containing cellulose, take this medicine at least 2 hours before or after you take the laxative. Taking these medicines too close together may lessen the effects of the aspirin in this combination medicine.

Codeine may cause dryness of the mouth. For temporary relief, use sugarless candy or gum, melt bits of ice in your mouth, or use a saliva substitute. However, if your mouth continues to feel dry for more than 2 weeks, check with your dentist. Continuing dryness of the mouth may increase the chance of dental disease, including tooth decay, gum disease, and fungus infections.

For diabetic patients:

- This combination medicine may cause false results with some blood and urine glucose (sugar) tests. If you notice any change in your test results, or if you have any questions about this possible problem, check with your doctor, nurse, or pharmacist. This is especially important if your diabetes is not well-controlled.

This combination medicine may interfere with the results of some medical tests. Before you have any medical tests, tell the doctor in charge if you have taken any of these combination medicines within the past 3 or 4 days. If possible, it is best to check with the doctor first, to find out whether the medicine may be taken during the 3 or 4 days before the test.

The caffeine in this combination medicine may interfere with the results of a test that uses dipyridamole (e.g., Persantine) to help find out how well your blood is flowing through certain blood vessels. Therefore, you should avoid caffeine for at least 4 hours before the test.

If you have been taking this medicine regularly for several weeks or more, *do not suddenly stop taking it without first checking with your doctor.* Depending on which of these medicines you have been taking, and the amount you have been taking every day, your doctor may want you to reduce gradually the amount you are taking before stopping completely, in order to lessen the chance of withdrawal side effects.

If you think you or someone else may have taken an overdose of this medicine, get emergency help at once. Taking an overdose of this medicine or taking alcohol or CNS depressants with this medicine may lead to unconsciousness or death. Signs of overdose of this medicine include convulsions (seizures); hearing loss or ringing or buzzing in the ear; severe confusion, excitement, nervousness, or restlessness; severe dizziness or drowsiness; shortness of breath or troubled breathing; and severe weakness.

Side Effects of This Medicine

Along with its needed effects, a medicine may cause some unwanted effects. Although not all of these side effects may occur, if they do occur they may need medical attention.

Get emergency help immediately if any of the following symptoms of overdose occur:

Any loss of hearing; bloody urine; cold, clammy skin; confusion (severe); convulsions (seizures); diarrhea (severe or continuing); dizziness or lightheadedness (severe); drowsiness (severe); excitement, nervousness, or restlessness (severe); hallucinations (seeing, hearing, or feeling things that are not there); headache (severe or continuing); hive-like swellings (large) on face, eyelids, mouth, lips, and/or tongue; increased sweating; low blood pressure; nausea or vomiting (severe or continuing); pinpoint pupils of eyes; ringing or buzzing in the ears (continuing); shortness of breath or troubled breathing; slow heartbeat; stomach cramps or pain (severe or continuing); swelling, pain, or tenderness in the upper abdomen or stomach area; thirst (continuing); uncontrollable flapping movements of the hands, especially in elderly patients; unexplained fever; vision problems; weakness (severe)

Also, check with your doctor as soon as possible if any of the following side effects occur:

More common

Nausea or vomiting; stomach pain

Less common or rare

Bloody or black, tarry stools; cloudy urine; confusion; difficult, painful, or decreased urination; difficulty in swallowing; fast or pounding heartbeat; irregular breathing; mental depression; pain in lower back and/or side (severe and/or sharp); pinpoint red spots on skin; redness or flushing of face or other change in skin color; skin rash, hives, or itching; sore throat and fever; swelling of face, fingers, feet, or lower legs; trembling or uncontrolled muscle movements; unusual bleeding or bruising; unusual excitement or restlessness, especially in children; unusual tiredness or weakness; vomiting of blood or material that looks like coffee grounds; weight gain; wheezing or tightness in chest; yellow eyes or skin

Other side effects may occur that usually do not need medical attention. These side effects may go away during treatment as your body adjusts to the medicine. However, check with your doctor if any of the following side effects continue or are bothersome:

More common

Constipation (especially with long-term use); drowsiness; heartburn or indigestion

Less common or rare

Dizziness, lightheadedness, or feeling faint; dryness of mouth; false sense of well-being; general feeling of discomfort or illness; headache; loss of appetite; trouble in sleeping; unusual nervousness or restlessness

After you stop using this medicine, your body may need time to adjust. The length of time this takes depends on which of these medicines you were taking, the amount of medicine you were taking, and how long you took it. During this time check with your doctor if you notice any of the following side effects:

Body aches; diarrhea; fever, runny nose, or sneezing; gooseflesh; increased sweating; increased yawning; loss of appetite; nausea or vomiting; nervousness, restlessness, or irritability; shivering or trembling; stomach cramps; trouble in sleeping; unusually large pupils of eyes; weakness

Other side effects not listed above may also occur in some patients. If you notice any other effects, check with your doctor.

Annual revision: 09/14/91
Interim revision: 04/23/93

ACETAMINOPHEN, SODIUM BICARBONATE, AND CITRIC ACID Systemic†

A commonly used brand name in the U.S. is Bromo-Seltzer‡.

†Not commercially available in Canada.

‡The Bromo-Seltzer available in Canada is different from that available in the U.S. The Canadian product contains sodium bicarbonate and citric acid, but no acetaminophen. It is used as an antacid.

Description

Acetaminophen, sodium bicarbonate, and citric acid (a-seat-a-MIN-oh-fen, SOE-dee-um bi-KAR-boe-nate, and SI-trik AS-id) combination is used to relieve pain occurring together with heartburn, sour stomach, or acid indigestion. The acetaminophen in this combination medicine is the pain reliever. The sodium bicarbonate in this medicine is an antacid. It neutralizes stomach acid by combining with it to form a new substance that is not an acid.

This medicine is available without a prescription; however, your doctor may have special instructions on the proper dose for your medical condition.

Acetaminophen, sodium bicarbonate, and citric acid combination is available in the following dosage form:

Oral

- Effervescent granules (U.S.)

It is very important that you read and understand the following information. If any of it causes you special concern, check with your doctor or pharmacist. Also, *if you have any questions* or if you want more information about this medicine or your medical problem, *ask your doctor, nurse, or pharmacist.*

Before Using This Medicine

If you are taking this medicine without a prescription, carefully read and follow any precautions on the label. For acetaminophen, sodium bicarbonate, and citric acid combination, the following should be considered:

Allergies—Tell your doctor if you have ever had any unusual or allergic reaction to acetaminophen or aspirin, or to sodium bicarbonate. Also tell your doctor and pharmacist if you are allergic to any other substances, such as foods, preservatives, or dyes.

Diet—Make certain your doctor and pharmacist know if you are on a low-sodium, low-sugar, or any other special diet. This medicine contains a large amount of sodium (more than 750 mg for each 325 mg of acetaminophen).

Pregnancy—Although studies on birth defects have not been done in humans, the ingredients in this combination medicine have not been reported to cause birth defects in humans. However, you should avoid this medicine if you tend to retain (keep) body water because the sodium in it can cause you to retain body water. This can result in swelling and weight gain.

Breast-feeding—Acetaminophen passes into the breast milk in small amounts. However, acetaminophen, sodium bicarbonate, and citric acid have not been reported to cause problems in nursing babies.

Children—Acetaminophen has been tested in children and has not been shown to cause different side effects or problems than it does in adults. However, sodium bicarbonate should not be given to young children (under 6 years of age) unless ordered by their doctor. Small children with stomach problems usually cannot describe their symptoms very well. They should be checked by a doctor, because they may have a condition that needs other treatment.

Older adults—Acetaminophen has been tested and has not been shown to cause different side effects or problems in older people than it does in younger adults. However, the large amount of sodium in this combination medicine can be harmful to some elderly people. Therefore, it is best that older people not use this medicine for more than 5 days in a row, unless otherwise directed by their doctor.

Other medicines—Although certain medicines should not be used together at all, in other cases two different medicines may be used together even if an interaction might occur. In these cases, your doctor may want to change the dose, or other precautions may be necessary. When you are taking this combination medicine, it is especially important that your doctor and pharmacist know if you are taking any of the following:

- Alcohol—The chance of liver damage may be increased
- Ketoconazole (e.g., Nizoral) or
- Methenamine (e.g., Mandelamine) or
- Tetracyclines (medicine for infection), taken by mouth—Sodium bicarbonate can keep these medicines from working properly
- Mecamylamine (e.g., Inversine)—Sodium bicarbonate can increase the risk of unwanted effects by causing mecamylamine to stay in your body longer than usual

Other medical problems—The presence of other medical problems may affect the use of acetaminophen, sodium bicarbonate, and citric acid combination. Make sure you tell your doctor if you have any other medical problems, especially:

- Alcohol abuse or
- Hepatitis or other liver disease—The chance of serious side effects, including liver damage, may be increased
- Appendicitis (symptoms of, such as stomach or lower abdominal pain, cramping, bloating, soreness, nausea, or vomiting)—Sodium bicarbonate can make your condition

worse; also, people who may have appendicitis need medical attention and should not try to treat themselves

- Edema (swelling of face, fingers, feet, or lower legs caused by too much water in the body) or
- Heart disease or
- High blood pressure or
- Toxemia of pregnancy—The sodium in this combination medicine can make these conditions worse
- Kidney disease—The chance of serious side effects may be increased

Proper Use of This Medicine

Unless otherwise directed by your doctor, do not take more of this medicine than is recommended on the package label. If too much is taken, liver damage or other serious side effects may occur.

To use this medicine:

- This medicine must be taken in the form of a liquid that is made from the effervescent granules. Do not swallow the granules themselves.
- To make the liquid, pour the amount of effervescent granules directed on the package into a glass. Then add ½ glass (4 ounces) of cool water.
- Drink all of the liquid. You may drink the liquid while it is still fizzing or after the fizzing stops.
- Add a little more water to the glass and drink that, to make sure that you get the full amount of the medicine.

Missed dose—If your doctor has directed you to take this medicine according to a regular schedule and you miss a dose, take it as soon as you remember. However, if it is almost time for your next dose, skip the missed dose and go back to your regular dosing schedule. Do not double doses.

Storage—To store this medicine:

- Keep out of the reach of children.
- Store away from heat and direct light.
- Do not store this medicine in the bathroom, near the kitchen sink, or in other damp places. Heat or moisture may cause the medicine to break down.
- Do not keep outdated medicine or medicine no longer needed. Be sure that any discarded medicine is out of the reach of children.

Precautions While Using This Medicine

If you will be taking this medicine for a long time (more than 10 days in a row), your doctor should check your progress at regular visits.

Check with your doctor if your pain and/or upset stomach last for more than 10 days or if they get worse, if new symptoms occur, or if the painful area is red or swollen. These could be signs of a serious condition that needs medical treatment.

The sodium bicarbonate in this combination medicine can keep other medicines from working properly if the 2 medicines are taken too close together. *Always take this medicine:*

- *At least 3 hours before or after taking ketoconazole (e.g., Nizoral).*
- *At least 3 or 4 hours before or after taking a tetracycline antibiotic by mouth.*
- *At least 1 or 2 hours before or after taking any other medicine by mouth.*

Check the labels of all nonprescription (over-the-counter [OTC]) and prescription medicines you now take. If any contain acetaminophen or sodium be especially careful, since taking them while taking this medicine could cause an overdose. If you have any questions about this, check with your doctor or pharmacist.

Taking certain other medicines together with acetaminophen may increase the chance of unwanted effects. The risk will depend on how much of each medicine you take every day, and on how long you take the medicines together. If your medical doctor or dentist directs you to take these medicines together on a regular basis, follow his or her directions carefully. However, *do not take any of the following medicines together with acetaminophen for more than a few days, unless your doctor has directed you to do so and is following your progress:*

Aspirin or other salicylates
Diclofenac (e.g., Voltaren)
Diflunisal (e.g., Dolobid)
Fenoprofen (e.g., Nalfon)
Floctafenine (e.g., Idarac)
Flurbiprofen, oral (e.g., Ansaid)
Ibuprofen (e.g., Motrin)
Indomethacin (e.g., Indocin)
Ketoprofen (e.g., Orudis)
Ketorolac (e.g., Toradol)
Meclofenamate (e.g., Meclomen)
Mefenamic acid (e.g., Ponstel)
Naproxen (e.g., Naprosyn)
Phenylbutazone (e.g., Butazolidin)
Piroxicam (e.g., Feldene)
Sulindac (e.g., Clinoril)
Tiaprofenic acid (e.g., Surgam)
Tolmetin (e.g., Tolectin)

If you will be taking more than an occasional 1 or 2 doses of this medicine:

- *Do not drink alcoholic beverages.* Drinking alcoholic beverages while you are taking acetaminophen may increase the chance of liver damage, especially if you drink large amounts of alcoholic beverages regularly, if you take more acetaminophen than is recommended on the package label, or if you take it regularly for a long time.

- *Do not also drink a lot of milk or eat a lot of milk products.* To do so may increase the chance of side effects.
- To prevent side effects caused by too much sodium in the body, you may need to limit the amount of sodium in the foods you eat. Some foods that contain large amounts of sodium are canned soup, canned vegetables, pickles, ketchup, green and ripe (black) olives, relish, frankfurters and other sausage-type meats, soy sauce, and carbonated beverages. If you have any questions about this, check with your doctor, nurse, or pharmacist.

Acetaminophen may interfere with the results of some medical tests. Before you have any medical tests, tell the doctor in charge if you have taken acetaminophen within the past 3 or 4 days. If possible, it is best to check with the doctor first, to find out whether this medicine may be taken during the 3 or 4 days before the test.

For diabetic patients:

- Acetaminophen may cause false results with some blood glucose (sugar) tests. If you notice any change in your test results, or if you have any questions about this possible problem, check with your doctor, nurse, or pharmacist. This is especially important if your diabetes is not well-controlled.

If you think that you or anyone else may have taken an overdose of this medicine, get emergency help at once, even if there are no signs of poisoning. Signs of severe acetaminophen poisoning may not appear for 2 to 4 days after the overdose is taken, but treatment to prevent liver damage or death must be started as soon as possible. Treatment started more than 24 hours after the overdose is taken may not be effective.

Side Effects of This Medicine

Along with its needed effects, a medicine may cause some unwanted effects. Although the following side effects occur very rarely when 1 or 2 doses of this combination medicine is taken occasionally, they may be more likely to occur if:

- too much medicine is taken.
- the medicine is taken several times a day.
- the medicine is taken for more than a few days in a row.

Check with your doctor immediately if any of the following side effects occur:

Rare

Yellow eyes or skin

Symptoms of overdose

Diarrhea; increased sweating; loss of appetite; nausea or vomiting; stomach cramps or pain; swelling, pain, or tenderness in the upper abdomen or stomach area

Also, check with your doctor as soon as possible if any of the following side effects occur:

Less common or rare

Abdominal or stomach pain; cloudy urine, frequent urge to urinate, or sudden decrease in amount of urine; headache (continuing); increased blood pressure; mood or mental changes; muscle pain or twitching; nervousness or restlessness; pain (severe and/or sharp) in lower back and/or side; skin rash, hives, or itching; slow breathing; swelling of face, fingers, ankles, feet, or lower legs; unexplained sore throat and fever; unpleasant taste; unusual bleeding or bruising; unusual tiredness or weakness; weight gain

Other side effects may occur that usually do not need medical attention. These side effects may go away during treatment as your body adjusts to the medicine. However, check with your doctor if any of the following side effects continue or are bothersome:

Less common

Increased thirst

Other side effects not listed above may also occur in some patients. If you notice any other effects, check with your doctor.

Annual revision: 07/09/91

ACETOHYDROXAMIC ACID Systemic†

A commonly used brand name in the U.S. is Lithostat.

†Not commercially available in Canada.

Description

Acetohydroxamic acid (a-SEE-toe-hye-drox-AM-ik AS-id) is used to keep kidney stones from forming and to stop the growth of existing stones. Such stone build-up is often caused by certain bacterial infections. The bacteria produce an enzyme that makes the urine too alkaline. Under such conditions, kidney stones tend to form and, once formed, to grow in size. Acetohydroxamic acid stops the enzyme action and so reduces the chance for stones to form. This medicine is not used to dissolve existing stones and is not used in place of surgery.

It is sometimes used to make antibiotics or similar medicines work better when treating kidney or urinary tract infections.

Acetohydroxamic acid is available only with your doctor's prescription, in the following dosage form:

Oral

- Tablets (U.S.)

It is very important that you read and understand the following information. If any of it causes you special concern, check with your doctor. Also, *if you have any questions* or if you want more information about this medicine or your medical problem, *ask your doctor, nurse, or pharmacist.*

Before Using This Medicine

In deciding to use a medicine, the risks of taking the medicine must be weighed against the good it will do. This is a decision you and your doctor will make. For acetohydroxamic acid, the following should be considered:

Allergies—Tell your doctor if you have ever had any unusual or allergic reaction to acetohydroxamic acid. Also tell your doctor and pharmacist if you are allergic to any other substances, such as foods, preservatives, or dyes.

Pregnancy—Acetohydroxamic acid should not be used during pregnancy since it has been shown to cause serious birth defects in animals. Effective methods of contraception (birth control) must be used during treatment with this medicine to prevent a pregnancy that could result in birth defects. Be sure you have discussed this with your doctor.

Breast-feeding—It is not known whether acetohydroxamic acid passes into the breast milk. Although no problems have been reported in nursing babies, its use in breast-feeding mothers is not recommended.

Children—Although there is no specific information comparing use of acetohydroxamic acid in children with use in other age groups, it is not expected to cause different side effects or problems in children than it does in adults.

Older adults—Many medicines have not been studied specifically in older people. Therefore, it may not be known whether they work exactly the same way they do in younger adults or if they cause different side effects or problems in older people. There is no specific information comparing use of acetohydroxamic acid in the elderly with use in other age groups.

Other medicines—Although certain medicines should not be used together at all, in many cases two different medicines may be used together even if an interaction might occur. In these cases, your doctor may want to change the dose, or other precautions may be necessary. When you are taking acetohydroxamic acid it is especially important that your doctor and pharmacist know if you are taking the following:

- Iron supplements or any other medicine containing iron, taken by mouth—Use with acetohydroxamic acid may decrease effects of both medicines; iron supplements by injection may be needed

Other medical problems—The presence of other medical problems may affect the use of acetohydroxamic acid. Make sure you tell your doctor if you have any other medical problems, especially:

- Anemia or other blood disorders or
- Blood clots (history of) or
- Phlebitis (vein inflammation)—If you have one of these conditions, use of acetohydroxamic acid increases the risk of problems occurring
- Other kidney disorders—Higher blood levels of acetohydroxamic acid may result and a change in your dose may be needed

Before you begin using any new medicine (prescription or nonprescription) or if you develop any new medical problem while you are using this medicine, check with your doctor, nurse, or pharmacist.

Proper Use of This Medicine

Acetohydroxamic acid works best when taken on an empty stomach. Take the medicine 1 hour before or 2 hours after meals if possible.

Take this medicine exactly as ordered by your doctor. This is especially important because it is used along with antibiotics or other medicine to clear up the infection.

Do not miss any doses. Skipped doses may delay treatment progress and your recovery. When too many doses are missed, stone formation and growth may start again. Remember that this medicine is intended to prevent kidney stones and the surgery that is sometimes required to remove them.

Missed dose—If you do miss a dose of acetohydroxamic acid, take it as soon as possible. Then go back to your regular dosing schedule. Do not double doses.

Storage—To store this medicine:

- Keep out of the reach of children.
- Store away from heat and direct light.
- Do not store in the bathroom, near the kitchen sink, or in other damp places. Heat or moisture may cause the medicine to break down.
- Do not keep outdated medicine or medicine no longer needed. Be sure that any discarded medicine is out of the reach of children.

Precautions While Using This Medicine

Your doctor should check your progress at regular visits to make sure that this medicine is working properly and does not cause unwanted effects.

Do not take any form of iron by mouth while you are taking acetohydroxamic acid. Taking the 2 medicines together will keep both medicines from working properly.

Do not drink alcoholic beverages while you are taking acetohydroxamic acid. To do so may cause a rash to appear on the arms and face about 30 to 45 minutes after you drink the alcohol. Also, the skin may become flushed and feel warm and tingling. This reaction lasts about 30 minutes and can be very strong in some patients.

If you suspect you may have become pregnant during treatment with acetohydroxamic acid, stop taking the medicine immediately and check with your doctor.

Side Effects of This Medicine

Along with its needed effects, a medicine may cause some unwanted effects. The following side effects may be caused by blood clots. If they occur, they need immediate medical attention. *Stop taking this medicine and get emergency help immediately* if any of the following side effects occur:

More common

Headache (severe or sudden); loss of coordination (sudden); pains in chest, groin, or legs (especially in calves of legs); shortness of breath (sudden); slurred speech (sudden); vision changes (sudden)

Other side effects may occur that require medical attention. Check with your doctor as soon as possible if any of the following side effects occur:

More common

Anxiety, confusion, or mental depression; loss of appetite; nausea or vomiting; nervousness, shakiness, or tremors; unusual tiredness or weakness

Other side effects may occur that usually do not need medical attention. These side effects may go away during treatment as your body adjusts to the medicine. However, check with your doctor if any of the following side effects continue or are bothersome:

More common

General feeling of discomfort or illness; headache (mild)

Less common

Hair loss; skin rash (non-itching) on arms and face

Other side effects not listed above may also occur in some patients. If you notice any other effects, check with your doctor at once.

Annual revision: 12/11/92

ACETYLCYSTEINE Inhalation

Some commonly used brand names are:

In the U.S.

Mucomyst
Mucosil
Generic name product may also be available.

In Canada

Airbron
Mucomyst

Description

Acetylcysteine (a-se-teel-SIS-teen) belongs to the group of medicines called mucolytics (medicines that destroy or dissolve mucus). It is usually given by inhalation but may be given in other ways in a hospital.

Acetylcysteine is used to help make breathing easier in conditions such as bronchitis, emphysema, tuberculosis, and other lung diseases. It may also be used in patients with a tracheostomy. Acetylcysteine liquefies (thins) or dissolves mucus so that it may be coughed up. Sometimes the mucus may have to be removed by suction.

This medicine is available only with your doctor's prescription, in the following dosage form:

Inhalation

- Solution (U.S. and Canada)

It is very important that you read and understand the following information. If any of it causes you special concern, check with your doctor. Also, *if you have any questions* or if you want more information about this medicine or your medical problem, *ask your doctor, nurse, or pharmacist.*

Before Using This Medicine

In deciding to use a medicine, the risks of taking the medicine must be weighed against the good it will do. This is a decision you and your doctor will make. For acetylcysteine, the following should be considered:

Allergies—Tell your doctor if you have ever had any unusual or allergic reaction to acetylcysteine. Also tell your doctor and pharmacist if you are allergic to any other substances, such as foods, preservatives, or dyes.

Pregnancy—Acetylcysteine has not been studied in pregnant women. However, acetylcysteine has not been shown to cause birth defects or other problems in animal studies when given in doses larger than the recommended human dose.

Breast-feeding—It is not known whether acetylcysteine passes into the breast milk. However, this medicine has not been reported to cause problems in nursing babies.

Children—Although there is no specific information comparing use of acetylcysteine in children with use in other age groups, this medicine is not expected to cause different side effects or problems in children than it does in adults.

Older adults—Many medicines have not been studied specifically in older people. Therefore, it may not be known whether they work exactly the same way they do in younger adults or if they cause different side effects or problems in older people. There is no specific information comparing use of acetylcysteine in the elderly with use in other age groups.

Other medical problems—The presence of other medical problems may affect the use of acetylcysteine. Make sure you tell your doctor if you have any other medical problems, especially:

- Asthma or
- Other lung disease—Acetylcysteine may make the condition worse

Before you begin using any new medicine (prescription or nonprescription) or if you develop any new medical problem while you are using this medicine, check with your doctor, nurse, or pharmacist.

Proper Use of This Medicine

Use acetylcysteine only as directed. Do not use more of it and do not use it more often than your doctor ordered. To do so may increase the chance of side effects.

If you are using this medicine at home, make sure you understand exactly how to use it. If you have any questions about this, check with your doctor.

After using acetylcysteine, try to cough up the loosened or thinned mucus. If this does not work, it may have to be suctioned out. This will prevent too much mucus from accumulating in the lungs. If you have any questions about this, check with your doctor.

Missed dose—If you miss a dose of this medicine, use it as soon as possible. Then use any remaining doses for that day at regularly spaced intervals.

Storage—To store this medicine:

- Keep out of the reach of children.
- Before the container is opened, store it away from heat and direct light.
- After the container is opened, store it in the refrigerator. However, keep the medicine from freezing.
- Do not keep outdated medicine or medicine no longer needed. Be sure that any discarded medicine is out of the reach of children.

Precautions While Using This Medicine

If your condition does not improve or if it becomes worse, check with your doctor.

Side Effects of This Medicine

Along with its needed effects, a medicine may cause some unwanted effects. Although not all of these side effects may occur, if they do occur they may need medical attention.

Check with your doctor as soon as possible if any of the following side effects occur:

Less common

Spitting up blood; wheezing, tightness in chest, or difficulty in breathing (especially in asthma patients)

Rare

Skin rash or other irritation

Other side effects may occur that usually do not need medical attention. These side effects may go away during treatment as your body adjusts to the medicine. However, check with your doctor if any of the following side effects continue or are bothersome:

Less common

Clammy skin; fever; increase in amount of mucus in lungs; irritation or soreness of mouth, throat, or lungs; nausea or vomiting; runny nose

For patients using a face mask for inhalation of acetylcysteine:

- The mask may leave a stickiness on your face. This can be removed with water.

When you use acetylcysteine, you may notice that the medicine has an unpleasant odor at first. However, this smell will go away soon after you use the medicine.

Other side effects not listed above may also occur in some patients. If you notice any other effects, check with your doctor.

Annual revision: 05/28/91

ACYCLOVIR Systemic

A commonly used brand name in the U.S. and Canada is Zovirax. Other commonly used names are aciclovir and acycloguanosine.

Description

Acyclovir (ay-SYE-kloe-veer) belongs to the family of medicines called antivirals, which are used to treat infections caused by viruses. Usually these medicines work for only one kind or group of virus infections.

Acyclovir is used to treat the symptoms of herpes virus infections of the genitals (sex organs), the skin, the brain, and mucous membranes. Although acyclovir will not cure herpes, it does help relieve the pain and discomfort and helps the sores (if any) heal faster. Acyclovir is also used to treat chickenpox.

Acyclovir may also be used for other virus infections as determined by your doctor. However, it does not work in treating certain viruses, such as the common cold.

Acyclovir is available only with your doctor's prescription, in the following dosage forms:

Oral

- Capsules (U.S.)
- Oral suspension (U.S.)
- Tablets (Canada)

Parenteral

- Injection (U.S. and Canada)

It is very important that you read and understand the following information. If any of it causes you special concern, check with your doctor. Also, *if you have any questions* or if you want more information about this medicine or your medical problem, *ask your doctor, nurse, or pharmacist.*

Before Using This Medicine

In deciding to use a medicine, the risks of taking the medicine must be weighed against the good it will do. This is a decision you and your doctor will make. For acyclovir, the following should be considered:

Allergies—Tell your doctor if you have ever had any unusual or allergic reaction to acyclovir or ganciclovir. Also tell your doctor and pharmacist if you are allergic to any other substances, such as foods, sulfites or other preservatives, or dyes.

Pregnancy—Acyclovir has been used in pregnant women and has not been reported to cause birth defects or other problems. However, studies have not been done in humans. Studies in rabbits have shown that acyclovir given by injection may keep the fetus from becoming attached to the lining of the uterus (womb). However, acyclovir has not been shown to cause birth defects or other problems in mice given many times the usual human dose, or in rats or rabbits given several times the usual human dose.

Breast-feeding—Acyclovir passes into the breast milk. However, it has not been reported to cause problems in nursing babies.

Children—A limited number of studies have been done using oral acyclovir in children, and it has not caused different effects or problems in children than it does in adults.

Older adults—Acyclovir has been used in the elderly and has not been shown to cause different side effects or problems in older people than it does in younger adults.

Other medicines—Although certain medicines should not be used together at all, in many cases two different medicines may be used together even if an interaction might occur. In these cases, changes in dose or other precautions may be necessary. If you are receiving acyclovir by injection it is especially important that your doctor and pharmacist know if you are taking any of the following:

- Carmustine (e.g., BiCNU) or
- Cisplatin (e.g., Platinol) or
- Combination pain medicine containing acetaminophen and aspirin (e.g., Excedrin) or other salicylates or
- Cyclosporine (e.g., Sandimmune) or
- Deferoxamine (e.g., Desferal) (with long-term use) or
- Gold salts (medicine for arthritis) or
- Inflammation or pain medicine, except narcotics, or
- Lithium (e.g., Lithane) or
- Other medicine for infection or
- Penicillamine (e.g., Cuprimine) or
- Plicamycin (e.g., Mithracin) or
- Streptozocin (e.g., Zanosar)—Concurrent use of these medicines with acyclovir by injection may increase the chance for side effects, especially when kidney disease is present

Other medical problems—The presence of other medical problems may affect the use of acyclovir. Make sure you tell your doctor if you are receiving acyclovir by injection and have any of the following medical problems, especially:

- Kidney disease—Kidney disease may increase blood levels of acyclovir, increasing the chance of side effects
- Nerve disease—Acyclovir by injection may increase the chance for nervous system side effects

Before you begin using any new medicine (prescription or nonprescription) or if you develop any new medical problem while you are using this medicine, check with your doctor, nurse, or pharmacist.

Proper Use of This Medicine

Patient information about the treatment of herpes is available with this medicine. Read it carefully before using this medicine.

Acyclovir is best used as soon as possible after the symptoms of herpes infection (for example, pain, burning, blisters) begin to appear.

Acyclovir capsules, tablets, and oral suspension may be taken with meals.

If you are taking acyclovir for the *treatment of chickenpox*, it is best to start taking acyclovir as soon as possible after the first sign of the chickenpox rash, usually within one day.

If you are using *acyclovir oral suspension*, use a specially marked measuring spoon or other device to measure each dose accurately. The average household teaspoon may not hold the right amount of liquid.

Do not use after the expiration date on the label. The medicine may not work properly. Check with your pharmacist if you have any questions about this.

To help clear up your herpes infection, *keep taking acyclovir for the full time of treatment,* even if your symptoms begin to clear up after a few days. *Do not miss any doses.* However, *do not use this medicine more often or for a longer time than your doctor ordered.*

Dosing—The dose of acyclovir will be different for different patients. *Follow your doctor's orders or the directions on the label.* The following information includes only the average doses of acyclovir. Your dose may be different if you have kidney disease. *If your dose is different, do not change it* unless your doctor tells you to do so.

- The number of capsules or tablets or teaspoonfuls of suspension that you take depends on the strength of the medicine. Also, *the number of doses you take each day, the time allowed between doses, and the length of time you take the medicine depend on the medical problem for which you are taking acyclovir.*
- For *oral* dosage forms (capsules, oral suspension, or tablets):
  —Adults and children 12 years of age and older: 200 to 800 milligrams two to five times a day for up to ten days.
  —Children 2 to 12 years of age: Treatment of chickenpox, up to 800 milligrams per dose (dose is based on body weight) four times a day for five days.
  —Children up to 2 years of age: Dose must be determined by the doctor.
- For *injection* dosage form:
  —Adults and children 12 years of age and older: Dose is based on body weight (5 to 10 milligrams of acyclovir per kilogram [2.3 to 4.6 milligrams per pound] of body weight). It is given slowly into a vein over at least a one-hour period and repeated every eight hours for up to ten days.
  —Children up to 12 years of age: Dose is based on body weight or body size. It is given slowly into a vein over at least a one-hour period and repeated every eight hours for up to ten days.

Missed dose—If you do miss a dose of this medicine, take it as soon as possible. However, if it is almost time for your next dose, skip the missed dose and go back to your regular dosing schedule. Do not double doses.

Storage—To store this medicine:
- Keep out of the reach of children.
- Store away from heat and direct light.
- Do not store the capsule or tablet form of this medicine in the bathroom, near the kitchen sink, or in other damp places. Heat or moisture may cause the medicine to break down.
- Do not keep outdated medicine or medicine no longer needed. Be sure that any discarded medicine is out of the reach of children.

Precautions While Using This Medicine

Women with genital herpes may be more likely to get cancer of the cervix (mouth of the womb). Therefore, it is very important that Pap tests be taken at least once a year to check for cancer. Cervical cancer can be cured if found and treated early.

If your symptoms do not improve within a few days, or if they become worse, check with your doctor.

The areas affected by herpes should be kept as clean and dry as possible. Also, wear loose-fitting clothing to avoid irritating the sores (blisters).

It is important to remember that acyclovir will not keep you from spreading herpes to others.

Herpes infection of the genitals can be caught from or spread to your partner during any sexual activity. Even though you may get herpes if your partner has no symptoms, the infection is more likely to be spread if sores are present. This is true until the sores are completely healed and the scabs have fallen off. *Therefore, it is best to avoid any sexual activity if either you or your sexual partner has any symptoms of herpes.* The use of a latex condom ("rubber") may help prevent the spread of herpes. However, spermicidal (sperm-killing) jelly or a diaphragm will probably not help.

Side Effects of This Medicine

Along with its needed effects, a medicine may cause some unwanted effects. Although not all of these side effects may occur, if they do occur they may need medical attention.

Check with your doctor immediately if any of the following side effects occur:

For acyclovir injection only

More common

Pain, swelling, or redness at place of injection

Less common (more common with rapid injection)

Abdominal or stomach pain; decreased frequency of urination or amount of urine; increased thirst; loss of appetite; nausea or vomiting; unusual tiredness or weakness

Rare

Confusion; convulsions (seizures); hallucinations (seeing, hearing, or feeling things that are not there); trembling

Other side effects may occur that usually do not need medical attention. These side effects may go away during treatment as your body adjusts to the medicine. However, check with your doctor if any of the following side effects continue or are bothersome:

For oral acyclovir only

Less common (especially seen with long-term use or high doses)

Diarrhea; headache; lightheadedness; nausea or vomiting

Other side effects not listed above may also occur in some patients. If you notice any other effects, check with your doctor.

Additional Information

Once a medicine has been approved for marketing for a certain use, experience may show that it is also useful for other medical problems. Although not specifically included in product labeling, acyclovir by injection is used in certain patients with the following medical conditions:

- Disseminated neonatal herpes simplex (widespread infection in the newborn)
- Herpes simplex (prevention of)

Other than the above information, there is no additional information relating to proper use, precautions, or side effects for these uses.

Annual revision: 06/17/92

ACYCLOVIR Topical

A commonly used brand name in the U.S. and Canada is Zovirax. Other commonly used names are aciclovir and acycloguanosine.

Description

Acyclovir (ay-SYE-kloe-veer) belongs to the family of medicines called antivirals. Antivirals are used to treat infections caused by viruses. Usually they work for only one kind or group of virus infections.

Topical acyclovir is used to treat the symptoms of herpes simplex virus infections of the skin, mucous membranes, and genitals (sex organs). Although topical acyclovir will not cure herpes simplex, it may help relieve the pain and discomfort and may help the sores (if any) heal faster. Topical acyclovir may also be used for other conditions as determined by your doctor.

Acyclovir is available only with your doctor's prescription, in the following dosage form:

Topical

- Ointment (U.S. and Canada)

It is very important that you read and understand the following information. If any of it causes you special concern, check with your doctor. Also, *if you have any questions* or if you want more information about this medicine or your medical problem, *ask your doctor, nurse, or pharmacist.*

Before Using This Medicine

In deciding to use a medicine, the risks of using the medicine must be weighed against the good it will do. This is a decision you and your doctor will make. For acyclovir, the following should be considered:

Allergies—Tell your doctor if you have ever had any unusual or allergic reaction to acyclovir. Also tell your doctor and pharmacist if you are allergic to any other substances, such as preservatives or dyes.

Pregnancy—Topical acyclovir has not been studied in pregnant women. However, this medication has not been shown to cause birth defects or other problems in animal studies using mice, rats, or rabbits.

Breast-feeding—It is not known whether topical acyclovir passes into the breast milk. However, acyclovir ointment has not been reported to cause problems in nursing babies, even though small amounts of topical acyclovir are absorbed through the mother's skin and mucous membranes.

Children—Although there is no specific information comparing the use of topical acyclovir in children with use in other age groups, this medicine is not expected to cause different side effects or problems in children than it does in adults.

Older adults—Many medicines have not been studied specifically in older people. Therefore, it may not be known whether they work exactly the same way they do in younger adults. Although there is no specific information comparing the use of topical acyclovir in the elderly with use in other age groups, this medicine is not expected to cause different side effects or problems in older people than it does in younger adults.

Other medicines—Although certain medicines should not be used together at all, in other cases two different medicines may be used together even if an interaction might occur. In these cases, your doctor may want to change the dose, or other precautions may be necessary. Tell your doctor and pharmacist if you are using any other topical prescription or nonprescription (over-the-counter [OTC]) medicine that is to be applied to the same area of the skin.

Before you begin using any new medicine (prescription or nonprescription) or if you develop any new medical problem while you are using this medicine, check with your doctor, nurse, or pharmacist.

Proper Use of This Medicine

Acyclovir may come with patient information about herpes simplex infections. Read this information carefully. If you have any questions, check with your doctor, nurse, or pharmacist.

Do not use this medicine in the eyes.

Acyclovir is best used as soon as possible after the symptoms of herpes infection (for example, pain, burning, or blisters) begin to appear.

Use a finger cot or rubber glove when applying this medicine. This will help keep you from spreading the infection to other areas of your body. Apply enough medicine to completely cover all the sores (blisters). A 1.25-cm (approximately ½-inch) strip of ointment applied to each area of the affected skin measuring 5 × 5 cm (approximately 2 × 2 inches) is usually enough, unless otherwise directed by your doctor.

To help clear up your herpes infection, *continue using acyclovir for the full time of treatment,* even if your symptoms begin to clear up after a few days. *Do not miss any doses.* However, *do not use this medicine more often or for a longer time than your doctor ordered.*

Missed dose—If you do miss a dose of this medicine, apply it as soon as possible. However, if it is almost time for your next dose, skip the missed dose and go back to your regular dosing schedule.

Storage—To store this medicine:

- Keep out of the reach of children.
- Store away from heat and direct light.
- Keep the medicine from freezing.
- Do not keep outdated medicine or medicine no longer needed. Be sure that any discarded medicine is out of the reach of children.

Precautions While Using This Medicine

Women with genital herpes may be more likely to get cancer of the cervix (mouth of the womb). Therefore, it is very important that Pap tests be taken at least once a year to check for cancer. Cervical cancer can be cured if found and treated early.

If your symptoms do not improve within 1 week, or if they become worse, check with your doctor.

The areas affected by herpes should be kept as clean and dry as possible. Also, wear loose-fitting clothing to avoid irritating the sores (blisters).

Herpes infection of the genitals can be caught from or spread to your partner during any sexual activity. Although you may get herpes even though your sexual partner has no symptoms, the infection is more likely to be spread if sores are present. This is true until the sores are completely healed and the scabs have fallen off. The use of a condom (prophylactic) may help prevent the spread of herpes. However, spermicidal (sperm-killing) jelly or a diaphragm will not help prevent the spread of herpes. *Therefore, it is best to avoid any sexual activity if either you or your partner has any symptoms of herpes. It is also important to remember that acyclovir will not keep you from spreading herpes to others.*

Side Effects of This Medicine

Along with its needed effects, a medicine may cause some unwanted effects. The following side effects may go away during treatment as your body adjusts to the medicine. However, check with your doctor if any of these effects continue or are bothersome:

More common

Mild pain, burning, or stinging

Less common

Itching

Rare

Skin rash

Other side effects not listed above may also occur in some patients. If you notice any other effects, check with your doctor.

Annual revision: 01/15/92

ALCOHOL AND ACETONE Topical†

Some commonly used brand names in the U.S. are Seba-Nil Liquid Cleanser, Tyrosum Liquid, and Tyrosum Packets.

†Not commercially available in Canada.

Description

Alcohol and acetone (AL-koe-hol and A-se-tone) combination is used to clean oily or greasy skin associated with acne or other oily skin conditions.

This medicine is available without a prescription; however, your doctor may have special instructions on the proper use of this medicine for your medical condition.

Alcohol and acetone combination is available in the following dosage forms:

Topical

- Detergent lotion (U.S.)
- Pledgets (U.S.)

It is very important that you read and understand the following information. If any of it causes you special concern, check with your doctor or pharmacist. Also, *if you have any questions* or if you want more information about this medicine or your medical problem, *ask your doctor, nurse, or pharmacist.*

Before Using This Medicine

If you are using this medicine without a prescription, carefully read and follow any precautions on the label. For alcohol and acetone combination, the following should be considered:

Allergies—Tell your doctor if you have ever had any unusual or allergic reaction to alcohol or acetone. Also tell your doctor and pharmacist if you are allergic to any other substances, such as preservatives or dyes.

Pregnancy—Topical alcohol and acetone combination has not been shown to cause birth defects or other problems in humans.

Breast-feeding—Topical alcohol and acetone combination has not been reported to cause problems in nursing babies.

Children—This medicine should not be used on children up to 8 years of age. In older children, although there is no specific information comparing use of alcohol and acetone with use in other age groups, this medicine is not expected to cause different side effects or problems in older children than it does in adults.

Older adults—Many medicines have not been tested in older people. Therefore, it may not be known whether they work exactly the same way they do in younger adults. Although there is no specific information comparing use of alcohol and acetone in the elderly with use in other age groups, this medicine is not expected to cause different side effects or problems in older people than it does in younger adults.

Other medicines—Although certain medicines should not be used together at all, in other cases two different medicines may be used together even if an interaction might occur. In these cases, your doctor may want to change the dose, or other precautions may be necessary. Tell your doctor and pharmacist if you are using any other topical prescription or nonprescription (over-the-counter [OTC]) medicine that is to be applied to the same area of the skin.

Other medical problems—The presence of other medical problems may affect the use of alcohol and acetone combination. Make sure you tell your doctor if you have any other medical problems, especially:

- Burns or wounds—Alcohol and acetone combination may cause severe irritation if applied to burns or wounds

Before you begin using any new medicine (prescription or nonprescription) or if you develop any new medical problem while you are using this medicine, check with your doctor, nurse, or pharmacist.

Proper Use of This Medicine

Keep this medicine away from the eyes, the inside of the nose, and the lips.

This medicine is flammable. Do not use near heat, near open flame, or while smoking.

To use the *lotion form* of this medicine:

- Put a small amount of this medicine on a gauze pad or cotton ball and apply by wiping or rubbing over the face and other affected areas to remove dirt and surface oil.

To use the *pledget form* of this medicine:

- Apply by wiping or rubbing over the face and other affected areas to remove dirt and surface oil.

After applying this medicine, do not rinse the affected areas with water, since this will remove the medicine.

Missed dose—If you are using this medicine on a regular schedule and you miss a dose, apply it as soon as possible. Then go back to your regular dosing schedule.

Storage—To store this medicine:

- Keep out of the reach of children.
- Store away from heat and direct light.
- Keep the lotion form of this medicine from freezing.

- Do not keep outdated medicine or medicine no longer needed. Be sure that any discarded medicine is out of the reach of children.

Precautions While Using This Medicine

When using alcohol and acetone combination, do not use any of the following preparations on the same affected area, unless otherwise directed by your doctor:

Abrasive soaps or cleaners
Any other topical acne preparation or preparation containing a peeling agent (for example, benzoyl peroxide, resorcinol, salicylic acid, sulfur, or tretinoin [vitamin A acid])
Cosmetics or soaps that dry the skin
Medicated cosmetics
Other alcohol-containing preparations
Other topical medicine for the skin

To use any of the above preparations on the same affected area as this medicine may cause severe irritation of the skin

Side Effects of This Medicine

Along with its needed effects, a medicine may cause some unwanted effects. Although not all of these side effects may occur, if they do occur they may need medical attention.

Check with your doctor as soon as possible if any of the following side effects occur:

Irritation, pain, redness, or swelling of skin; skin infection

Other side effects may occur that usually do not need medical attention. These side effects may go away during treatment as your body adjusts to the medicine. However, check with your doctor or pharmacist if the following side effect continues or is bothersome:

Burning or stinging of skin

Other side effects may also occur in some patients. If you notice any other effects, check with your doctor or pharmacist.

Annual revision: 01/15/92

ALCOHOL AND SULFUR Topical

Some commonly used brand names are:

In the U.S.
Liquimat Creamy Beige
Liquimat Dark
Liquimat Light
Liquimat Medium
Liquimat Natural Beige
Transact
Xerac

In Canada
Postacne

Description

Alcohol and sulfur (AL-koe-hol and SUL-fur) combination is used in the treatment of acne and oily skin. Some of the products are tinted a flesh color and can be used as a makeup or cover-up.

This medicine is available without a doctor's prescription; however, your doctor may have special instructions on the proper use of this medicine for your medical condition.

Alcohol and sulfur combination is available in the following dosage forms:

Topical
- Gel (U.S.)
- Lotion (U.S. and Canada)

It is very important that you read and understand the following information. If any of it causes you special concern, check with your doctor or pharmacist. Also, *if you have any questions* or if you want more information about this medicine or your medical problem, *ask your doctor, nurse, or pharmacist.*

Before Using This Medicine

If you are using this medicine without a prescription, carefully read and follow any precautions on the label. For alcohol and sulfur combination, the following should be considered:

Allergies—Tell your doctor if you have ever had any unusual or allergic reaction to alcohol or sulfur. Also tell your doctor and pharmacist if you are allergic to any other substances, such as preservatives or dyes.

Pregnancy—Topical alcohol and sulfur combination has not been shown to cause birth defects or other problems in humans.

Breast-feeding—Topical alcohol and sulfur combination has not been reported to cause problems in nursing babies.

Children—This medicine should not be used for children up to 8 years of age. In older children, although there is no specific information comparing use of alcohol and sulfur with use in other age groups, this medicine is not expected to cause different side effects or problems than it does in adults.

Older adults—Many medicines have not been studied specifically in older people. Therefore, it may not be known whether they work exactly the same way they do in younger adults. Although there is no specific information comparing use of alcohol and sulfur in the elderly with use in other age groups, this medicine is not expected to cause different side effects or problems in older people than it does in younger adults.

Other medicines—Although certain medicines should not be used together at all, in other cases two different medicines may be used together even if an interaction might occur. In these cases, your doctor may want to change the dose, or other precautions may be necessary. Tell your doctor and pharmacist if you are using any other topical prescription or nonprescription (over-the-counter [OTC]) medicine that is to be applied to the same area of the skin.

Before you begin using any new medicine (prescription or nonprescription) or if you develop any new medical problem while you are using this medicine, check with your doctor, nurse, or pharmacist.

Proper Use of This Medicine

Before using this medicine, wash or cleanse the affected areas thoroughly and gently pat dry. Then apply a small amount of this medicine to the affected areas and rub in gently.

Keep this medicine away from the eyes, the inside of the nose, and the lips. If you accidentally get some in your eyes, flush them thoroughly with water.

This medicine is flammable. Do not use near heat, near open flame, or while smoking.

Use this medicine only as directed. Do not use it more often than recommended on the label, unless otherwise directed by your doctor.

Missed dose—If you miss a dose of this medicine, apply it as soon as possible. Then go back to your regular dosing schedule.

Storage—To store this medicine:
- Keep out of the reach of children.
- Store away from heat and direct light.
- Keep the medicine from freezing.
- Do not keep outdated medicine or medicine no longer needed. Be sure that any discarded medicine is out of the reach of children.

Precautions While Using This Medicine

When using alcohol and sulfur combination, do not use any of the following preparations on the same affected area, unless otherwise directed by your doctor.

Abrasive soaps or cleansers
Any other topical acne preparation or preparation containing a peeling agent (for example, benzoyl peroxide, resorcinol, salicylic acid, or tretinoin [vitamin A acid])
Cosmetics or soaps that dry the skin
Medicated cosmetics
Other alcohol-containing preparations
Other topical medicine for the skin

To use any of the above preparations on the same affected area as this medicine may cause severe irritation of the skin.

Do not use any topical mercury-containing preparation, such as ammoniated mercury ointment, on the same affected area as this medicine. To do so may cause a foul odor, may be irritating to the skin, and may stain the skin black. If you have any questions about this, check with your doctor or pharmacist.

Side Effects of This Medicine

Along with its needed effects, a medicine may cause some unwanted effects. Although not all of these side effects may occur, if they do occur they may need medical attention.

Check with your doctor as soon as possible if the following side effect occurs:

Skin irritation not present before use of this medicine

Other side effects may occur that usually do not need medical attention. These side effects may go away during treatment as your body adjusts to the medicine. However, check with your doctor or pharmacist if any of the following side effects continue or are bothersome:

Burning or stinging of skin; dryness or peeling of skin (may occur after a few days)

Other side effects not listed above may also occur in some patients. If you notice any other effects, check with your doctor or pharmacist.

Annual revision: 01/15/92

ALGLUCERASE Systemic

A commonly used brand name in the U.S. and Canada is Ceredase.

Description

Alglucerase (al-GLOO-ser-ace) is used to treat Gaucher's disease caused by the lack of a certain enzyme, glucocerebrosidase, in the body. This enzyme is necessary for your body to use fats.

Alglucerase is made from human placenta tissue that is collected after a baby is born. Before it is used, the tissue is tested for hepatitis and human immunodeficiency virus (HIV). This is similar to the testing that a blood bank does on donated blood before it is given to anyone else.

Alglucerase is available with your doctor's prescription, in the following dosage form:

Parenteral

- Injection (U.S. and Canada)

It is very important that you read and understand the following information. If any of it causes you special concern, check with your doctor. Also, *if you have any questions* or if you want more information about this medicine or your medical problem, *ask your doctor, nurse, or pharmacist.*

Before Receiving This Medicine

In deciding to use a medicine, the risks of receiving the medicine must be weighed against the good it will do. This is a decision you and your doctor will make. For alglucerase, the following should be considered:

Allergies—Tell your doctor if you have ever had any unusual or allergic reaction to alglucerase. Also tell your doctor and pharmacist if you are allergic to any other substances, such as foods, preservatives, or dyes.

Pregnancy—Studies have not been done in either humans or animals.

Breast-feeding—It is not known whether alglucerase passes into human breast milk.

Children—This medicine has been tested in a limited number of children. In effective doses, the medicine has not been shown to cause different side effects or problems than it does in adults.

Older adults—Many medicines have not been studied specifically in older people. Therefore, it may not be known whether they work exactly the same way they do in younger adults or if they cause different side effects or problems in older people. There is no specific information comparing use of alglucerase in the elderly with use in other age groups.

Other medicines—Although certain medicines should not be used together at all, in other cases two different medicines may be used together even if an interaction might occur. In these cases, your doctor may want to change the dose, or other precautions may be necessary. Tell your doctor and pharmacist if you are taking any other prescription or nonprescription (over-the-counter [OTC]) medicines.

Before you begin using any new medicine (prescription or nonprescription) or if you develop any new medical problem while you are using this medicine, check with your doctor, nurse, or pharmacist.

Proper Use of This Medicine

This medicine will not cure Gaucher's disease but it does help control it. Therefore, you must continue to receive it if you expect to keep your condition under control. You may have to receive alglucerase for the rest of your life. If Gaucher's disease is not treated, it can cause serious blood, liver, skeletal, or spleen problems.

Dosing—The dose of alglucerase will be different for different patients. The dose is based on body weight and will be determined by your doctor. *Follow your doctor's orders.*

Precautions While Receiving This Medicine

It is important that your doctor check your progress while you are receiving alglucerase to make sure that the dosage is correct for you.

Side Effects of This Medicine

Since alglucerase is made from human tissue, it is possible that diseases caused by viruses could be passed on. Examples of such diseases are hepatitis and HIV infection. These problems have not been reported to date, however, and are unlikely since the tissue is tested before being used. If you have questions or concerns about this, check with your doctor.

Along with its needed effects, a medicine may cause some unwanted effects. The following side effects may go away during treatment as your body adjusts to the medicine.

However, check with your doctor if any of these effects continue or are bothersome:

Less common

Abdominal discomfort; chills; fever; nausea and vomiting; swelling at place of injection

Other side effects not listed above may also occur in some patients. If you notice any other effects, check with your doctor.

Annual revision: 01/18/93

ALLOPURINOL Systemic

Some commonly used brand names are:

In the U.S.

Lopurin
Zyloprim

Generic name product may also be available.

In Canada

Alloprin
Apo-Allopurinol
Novopurol
Purinol
Zyloprim

Description

Allopurinol (al-oh-PURE-i-nole) is used to treat chronic gout (gouty arthritis). This condition is caused by too much uric acid in the blood.

This medicine works by causing less uric acid to be produced by the body. Allopurinol will not relieve a gout attack that has already started. Also, it does not cure gout, but it will help prevent gout attacks. However, it works only after you have been taking it regularly for a few months. Allopurinol will help prevent gout attacks only as long as you continue to take it.

Allopurinol is also used to prevent or treat other medical problems that may occur if too much uric acid is present in the body. These include certain kinds of kidney stones or other kidney problems.

Allopurinol is available only with your doctor's prescription in the following dosage form:

Oral

- Tablets (U.S. and Canada)

It is very important that you read and understand the following information. If any of it causes you special concern, check with your doctor. Also, *if you have any questions* or if you want more information about this medicine or your medical problem, *ask your doctor, nurse, or pharmacist.*

Before Using This Medicine

In deciding to use a medicine, the risks of taking the medicine must be weighed against the good it will do. This is a decision you and your doctor will make. For allopurinol, the following should be considered:

Allergies—Tell your doctor if you have ever had any unusual or allergic reaction to allopurinol. Also tell your doctor and pharmacist if you are allergic to any other substances, such as foods, preservatives, or dyes.

Pregnancy—Although studies on birth defects have not been done in humans, allopurinol has not been reported to cause problems in humans. In one study in mice, large amounts of allopurinol caused birth defects and other unwanted effects. However, allopurinol did not cause birth defects or other problems in rats or rabbits given doses up to 20 times the amount usually given to humans.

Breast-feeding—Allopurinol passes into the breast milk. However, this medicine has not been reported to cause problems in nursing babies.

Children—This medicine has been tested in children and, in effective doses, has not been shown to cause different side effects or problems than it does in adults.

Older adults—Many medicines have not been studied specifically in older people. Therefore, it may not be known whether they work exactly the same way they do in younger adults or if they cause different side effects or problems in older people. There is no specific information comparing use of allopurinol in the elderly with use in other age groups.

Other medicines—Although certain medicines should not be used together at all, in other cases two different medicines may be used together even if an interaction might occur. In these cases, your doctor may want to change the dose, or other precautions may be necessary. When you are taking allopurinol, it is especially important that your doctor and pharmacist know if you are taking any of the following:

- Anticoagulants (blood thinners)—Allopurinol may increase the chance of bleeding; changes in the dose of the anticoagulant may be needed, depending on blood test results
- Azathioprine (e.g., Imuran) or
- Mercaptopurine (e.g., Purinethol)—Allopurinol may cause higher blood levels of azathioprine or mercaptopurine, leading to an increased chance of serious side effects

Other medical problems—The presence of other medical problems may affect the use of allopurinol. Make sure

you tell your doctor if you have any other medical problems, especially:

- Diabetes mellitus (sugar diabetes) or
- High blood pressure or
- Kidney disease—There is an increased risk of severe allergic reactions or other serious effects; a change in the dose of allopurinol may be needed

Proper Use of This Medicine

If this medicine upsets your stomach, it may be taken after meals. If stomach upset (indigestion, nausea, vomiting, diarrhea, or stomach pain) continues, check with your doctor.

In order for this medicine to help you, it must be taken regularly as ordered by your doctor.

To help prevent kidney stones while taking allopurinol, adults should drink at least 10 to 12 full glasses (8 ounces each) of fluids each day unless otherwise directed by their doctor. Check with the doctor about the amount of fluids that children should drink each day while receiving this medicine. Also, your doctor may want you to take another medicine to make your urine less acid. It is important that you follow your doctor's instructions very carefully.

For patients taking allopurinol for *gout:*

- After you begin to take allopurinol, gout attacks may continue to occur for a while. However, if you take this medicine regularly as directed by your doctor, the attacks will gradually become less frequent and less painful. After you have been taking allopurinol regularly for several months, they may stop completely.
- Allopurinol is used to help prevent gout attacks. It will not relieve an attack that has already started. *Even if you take another medicine for gout attacks, continue to take this medicine also.*

Missed dose—If you miss a dose of this medicine, take it as soon as possible. However, if it is almost time for your next dose, skip the missed dose and go back to your regular dosing schedule. Do not double doses.

Storage—To store this medicine:

- Keep out of the reach of children.
- Store away from heat and direct light.
- Do not store this medicine in the bathroom, near the kitchen sink, or in other damp places. Heat or moisture may cause the medicine to break down.
- Do not keep outdated medicine or medicine no longer needed. Be sure that any discarded medicine is out of the reach of children.

Before you begin using any new medicine (prescription or nonprescription) or if you develop any new medical problem while you are using this medicine, check with your doctor, nurse, or pharmacist.

Precautions While Using This Medicine

Your doctor should check your progress at regular visits. A blood test may be needed to make sure that this medicine is working properly and is not causing unwanted effects.

Drinking too much alcohol may increase the amount of uric acid in the blood and lessen the effects of allopurinol. Therefore, people with gout and other people with too much uric acid in the body should be careful to limit the amount of alcohol they drink.

Taking too much vitamin C may make the urine more acidic and increase the possibility of kidney stones forming while you are taking allopurinol. Therefore, check with your doctor before you take vitamin C while taking this medicine.

Check with your doctor immediately:

- *if you notice a skin rash, hives, or itching while you are taking allopurinol.*
- *if chills, fever, joint pain, muscle aches or pains, sore throat, or nausea or vomiting occur, especially if they occur together with or shortly after a skin rash.*

Very rarely, these effects may be the first signs of a serious reaction to the medicine.

Allopurinol may cause some people to become drowsy or less alert than they are normally. *Make sure you know how you react to this medicine before you drive, use machines, or do anything else that could be dangerous if you are not alert.*

Side Effects of This Medicine

Along with its needed effects, a medicine may cause some unwanted effects. Although not all of these side effects may occur, if they do occur they may need medical attention.

Stop taking this medicine and check with your doctor immediately if any of the following side effects occur:

More common

Skin rash or sores, hives, or itching

Rare

Black, tarry stools; bleeding sores on lips; blood in urine or stools; chills, fever, muscle aches or pains, nausea, or vomiting—especially if occurring with or shortly after a skin rash; difficult or painful urination; pinpoint red spots on skin; redness, tenderness, burning, or peeling of skin; red and/or irritated eyes; red, thickened, or scaly skin; shortness of breath, troubled breathing, tightness in chest, or wheezing; sores, ulcers, or white spots in mouth or on lips; sore throat and fever; sudden decrease in amount of urine; swelling in upper abdominal (stomach) area; swelling of face, fingers, feet, or lower legs; unusual bleeding or bruising; unusual weakness; weight gain (rapid); yellow eyes or skin

Also, check with your doctor as soon as possible if any of the following side effects occur:

Rare

Loosening of fingernails; numbness, tingling, pain, or weakness in hands or feet; pain in lower back or side; unexplained nosebleeds

Other side effects may occur that usually do not need medical attention. These side effects may go away during treatment as your body adjusts to the medicine. However, check with your doctor if any of the following side effects continue or are bothersome:

Less common or rare

Diarrhea; drowsiness; headache occurring without other side effects; indigestion; nausea or vomiting occurring without a skin rash or other side effects; stomach pain occurring without other side effects; unusual hair loss

Other side effects not listed above may also occur in some patients. If you notice any other effects, check with your doctor.

Annual revision: 08/28/91

ALPHA$_1$-PROTEINASE INHIBITOR, HUMAN Systemic

A commonly used brand name in the U.S. and Canada is Prolastin. Another commonly used name is alpha$_1$-antitrypsin.

Description

Alpha$_1$-proteinase (AL-fa wun PRO-teen-ayce) inhibitor (alpha$_1$-PI) is used to treat emphysema caused by the lack of a certain protein, alpha$_1$-antitrypsin, in the body. This medicine replaces the protein when the body does not produce enough by itself.

Alpha$_1$-PI is prepared from human blood obtained from many donors. Each donor's blood is tested for human immunodeficiency virus (HIV) and hepatitis B virus before it is used to prepare this medicine. Also, alpha$_1$-PI is treated with heat to further reduce the risk of transmission of virus infections. However, no procedure has been found to be totally effective in removing viruses from blood products.

There have not been any reports of hepatitis developing in any patients receiving alpha$_1$-PI. However, as a precaution, before you receive this medicine, you should be immunized against hepatitis B with hepatitis B vaccine. This will help prevent infection by any hepatitis virus that may have been in the blood used to prepare alpha$_1$-PI. In some cases, there may not be enough time for the immunization to take effect before the alpha$_1$-PI needs to be given. Therefore, you may be given hepatitis B immune globulin at the same time that you receive the hepatitis B vaccine.

Alpha$_1$-PI is given once a week. Your doctor may want you to receive this medicine on a regular basis for a long time. However, at the present time, it is not known what the effects of this medicine are when it is used regularly to treat emphysema caused by lack of alpha$_1$-antitrypsin. Be sure you have discussed this with your doctor.

Alpha$_1$-PI is administered only by or under the immediate supervision of your doctor. It is available in the following dosage form:

Parenteral

- Injection (U.S. and Canada)

It is very important that you read and understand the following information. If any of it causes you special concern, check with your doctor. Also, *if you have any questions* or if you want more information about this medicine or your medical problem, *ask your doctor, nurse, or pharmacist.*

Before Receiving This Medicine

In deciding to use a medicine, the risks of taking the medicine must be weighed against the good it will do. This is a decision you and your doctor will make. For alpha$_1$-proteinase inhibitor, the following should be considered:

Allergies—Tell your doctor if you have ever had any unusual or allergic reaction to alpha$_1$-proteinase inhibitor. Also tell your doctor and pharmacist if you are allergic to any other substances, such as foods, preservatives, or dyes.

Pregnancy—Studies on effects in pregnancy have not been done in either humans or animals.

Breast-feeding—This medicine has not been reported to cause problems in nursing babies.

Children—Studies on this medicine have been done only in adult patients and there is no specific information about its use in children. Therefore, be sure to discuss with your doctor the use of this medicine in children.

Older adults—Many medicines have not been tested in older people. Therefore, it may not be known whether they work exactly the same way they do in younger adults or if they cause different side effects or problems in older people. There is no specific information about the use of alpha$_1$-proteinase inhibitor in the elderly.

Other medicines—Although certain medicines should not be used together at all, in other cases two different medicines may be used together even if an interaction might occur. In these cases, your doctor may want to change the dose, or other precautions may be necessary. When you are taking alpha$_1$-proteinase inhibitor, it is especially important that your doctor and pharmacist know if you are taking other prescription or nonprescription (over-the-counter [OTC]) medicine.

Before you begin using any new medicine (prescription or nonprescription) or if you develop any new medical problem while you are using this medicine, check with your doctor, nurse, or pharmacist.

Proper Use of This Medicine

In order for alpha$_1$-proteinase inhibitor (alpha$_1$-PI) to work properly, it is important that you receive this medicine once a week on a regular schedule. If you have any questions about this, check with your doctor.

Side Effects of This Medicine

Along with its needed effects, a medicine may cause some unwanted effects. The following side effects usually do not require medical attention. However, check with your doctor if any of these effects continue or are bothersome:

Less common or rare

Chills and fever; dizziness or lightheadedness; fever up to 102 °F (38.9 °C)

Note: Chills and fever may occur several hours after you receive this medicine but are usually mild and only temporary. Also, fever up to 102 °F (38.9 °C) may occur up to 12 hours after you receive this medicine and will disappear within about 24 hours.

Other side effects not listed above may also occur in some patients. If you notice any other effects, check with your doctor.

Annual revision: 4/17/91

ALPROSTADIL Intracavernosal

Some commonly used brand names are:

In the U.S.
Prostin VR Pediatric

In Canada
Prostin VR

Other commonly used names are PGE_1 and prostaglandin E_1.

Description

Alprostadil (al-PROSS-ta-dil) belongs to the group of medicines called vasodilators. Vasodilators cause blood vessels to expand, thereby increasing blood flow. Alprostadil is used to produce erections in some impotent men. When alprostadil is injected into the penis (intracavernosal), it increases blood flow to the penis, which results in an erection.

Alprostadil injection should not be used as a sexual aid by men who are not impotent. If the medicine is not used properly, permanent damage to the penis and loss of the ability to have erections could result.

Alprostadil is available only with your doctor's prescription, in the following dosage form:

Parenteral

- Injection (U.S. and Canada)

It is very important that you read and understand the following information. If any of it causes you special concern, check with your doctor. Also, *if you have any questions* or if you want more information about this medicine or your medical problem, *ask your doctor, nurse, or pharmacist.*

Before Using This Medicine

In deciding to use a medicine, the risks of taking the medicine must be weighed against the good it will do. This is a decision you and your doctor will make. For alprostadil, the following should be considered:

Allergies—Tell your doctor if you have ever had any unusual or allergic reaction to alprostadil. Also tell your doctor and pharmacist if you are allergic to any other substances, such as foods, preservatives, or dyes.

Older adults—Many medicines have not been studied specifically in older people. Therefore, it may not be known whether they work exactly the same way they do in younger adults or it they cause different side effects or problems in older people. There is no specific information comparing the use of alprostadil in the elderly with use in other age groups.

Other medicines—Although certain medicines should not be used together at all, in other cases two different medicines may be used together even if an interaction might occur. In these cases, your doctor may want to change the dose, or other precautions may be necessary. Tell your doctor and pharmacist if you are taking any other prescription or nonprescription (over-the-counter [OTC]) medicine.

Other medical problems—The presence of other medical problems may affect the use of alprostadil. Make sure you tell your doctor if you have any other medical problems, especially:

- Bleeding problems or
- Liver disease—These conditions increase the risk of bleeding at the place of injection
- Priapism (history of) or
- Sickle cell disease—Patients with these conditions have an increased risk of priapism (erection lasting longer than 4 hours) while using alprostadil

Proper Use of This Medicine

To give *alprostadil injection*:

- Cleanse the injection site with alcohol. Using a sterile needle, *inject the medicine slowly and directly into the base of the penis as instructed by your doctor. Alprostadil should not be injected just under the skin.* The injection is usually not painful. If the injection is very painful or you notice bruising or swelling at the place of injection, that means you have been injecting the medicine under the skin. Stop, withdraw the needle, and reposition it properly before continuing with the injection.
- After you have completed the injection, put pressure on the place of injection to prevent bruising. Then massage your penis as instructed by your doctor. This helps the medicine spread to all parts of the penis, so that the medicine will work better.

This medicine usually begins to work in about 5 to 10 minutes. You should attempt intercourse within 10 to 30 minutes after injecting the medicine.

Do not use the same injection site each time you use alprostadil. Rather, rotate injection sites with each use, to prevent skin problems.

Storage—To store this medicine:

- Keep out of the reach of children.
- Refrigerate. Keep the medicine from freezing.

Precautions While Using This Medicine

Use alprostadil injection exactly as directed by your doctor. Do not use more of it and do not use it more often than ordered. If too much is used, the erection lasts too long and does not reverse when it should. This condition is called priapism, and it can be very dangerous. If the erection is not reversed, the blood supply to the penis may be cut off and permanent damage may occur.

Contact your doctor immediately if the erection lasts for longer than 4 hours or if it becomes painful. This may be a sign of priapism and must be treated right away to prevent permanent damage.

If you notice bleeding at the site when you inject alprostadil, put pressure on the spot until the bleeding stops. If it doesn't stop, check with your doctor.

Side Effects of This Medicine

Along with its needed effects, a medicine may cause some unwanted effects. Although not all of these side effects may occur, if they do occur they may need medical attention.

Check with your doctor immediately if the following side effect occurs:

Rare

Erection continuing for more than 4 hours

Other side effects may occur that usually do not need medical attention. These side effects may go away during treatment as your body adjusts to the medicine. However, check with your doctor if any of the following side effects continue or are bothersome:

More common

Pain at place of injection; pain during erection (burning or aching)

Rare

Bruising or bleeding at place of injection; swelling at place of injection

Other side effects not listed above may also occur in some patients. If you notice any other effects, check with your doctor.

Annual revision: 04/08/92

ALTRETAMINE Systemic

Some commonly used brand names are:

In the U.S.
Hexalen

In Canada
Hexastat

Another commonly used name is hexamethylmelamine.

Description

Altretamine (al-TRET-a-meen) belongs to the group of medicines called antineoplastics. It is used to treat cancer of the ovaries.

Altretamine interferes with the growth of cancer cells, which are eventually destroyed. Since the growth of normal body cells may also be affected by altretamine, other effects will also occur. Some of these may be serious and must be reported to your doctor. Other effects may not be serious but may cause concern. Some effects may not occur for months or years after the medicine is used.

Before you begin treatment with altretamine, you and your doctor should talk about the good this medicine will do as well as the risks of using it.

Altretamine is available only with your doctor's prescription in the following dosage form:

Oral

- Capsules (U.S. and Canada)

It is very important that you read and understand the following information. If any of it causes you special concern, check with your doctor. Also, *if you have any questions* or if you want more information about this medicine or your medical problem, *ask your doctor, nurse, or pharmacist.*

Before Using This Medicine

In deciding to use a medicine, the risks of taking the medicine must be weighed against the good it will do. This is a decision you and your doctor will make. For altretamine, the following should be considered:

Allergies—Tell your doctor if you have ever had any unusual or allergic reaction to altretamine.

Pregnancy—There is a chance that this medicine may cause birth defects if either the male or female is taking it at the time of conception or if it is taken during pregnancy. In addition, many cancer medicines may cause sterility which could be permanent. Although sterility has not been reported with this medicine, it does occur in animals and the possibility should be kept in mind.

Be sure that you have discussed this with your doctor before taking this medicine. It is best to use some kind of birth control while you are taking altretamine. Tell your doctor right away if you think you have become pregnant while taking altretamine.

Breast-feeding—Because altretamine may cause serious side effects, breast-feeding is generally not recommended while you are taking it.

Children—There is no specific information comparing use of altretamine in children with use in other age groups.

Older adults—Many medicines have not been studied specifically in older people. Therefore, it may not be known whether they work exactly the same way they do in younger adults. Although there is no specific information comparing use of altretamine in the elderly with use in other age groups, this medicine is not expected to cause different side effects or problems in older people than it does in younger adults.

Other medicines—Although certain medicines should not be used together at all, in other cases two different medicines may be used together even if an interaction might occur. In these cases, your doctor may want to change the dose, or other precautions may be necessary. When you are taking altretamine, it is especially important that your doctor and pharmacist know if you are taking any of the following:

- Amphotericin B by injection (e.g., Fungizone) or
- Antithyroid agents (medicine for overactive thyroid) or
- Azathioprine (e.g., Imuran) or
- Chloramphenicol (e.g., Chloromycetin) or
- Colchicine or
- Flucytosine (e.g., Ancobon) or
- Ganciclovir (e.g., Cytovene) or
- Interferon (e.g., Intron A, Roferon-A) or
- Plicamycin (e.g., Mithracin) or
- Zidovudine (e.g., AZT, Retrovir) or
- If you have ever been treated with x-rays or cancer medicines—Altretamine may increase the effects of these medicines or radiation therapy on the blood
- Monoamine oxidase (MAO) inhibitors (furazolidone [e.g., Furoxone], isocarboxazid [e.g., Marplan], phenelzine [e.g., Nardil], procarbazine [e.g., Matulane], selegiline [e.g., Eldepryl], tranylcypromine [e.g., Parnate])—Taking altretamine while you are taking MAO inhibitors may cause a severe drop in blood pressure

Other medical problems—The presence of other medical problems may affect the use of altretamine. Make sure you tell your doctor if you have any other medical problems, especially:

- Chickenpox (including recent exposure) or
- Herpes zoster (shingles)—Risk of severe disease affecting other parts of the body
- Nervous system problems—May be worsened by altretamine
- Infection—Altretamine may decrease your body's ability to fight infection

- Kidney disease—Effects may be increased because of slower removal of altretamine from the body
- Liver disease—Effects may be changed because altretamine is activated and cleared from the body by the liver

Before you begin using any new medicine (prescription or nonprescription) or if you develop any new medical problem while you are using this medicine, check with your doctor, nurse, or pharmacist.

Proper Use of This Medicine

This medicine often causes nausea and vomiting. However, it is very important that you continue to receive the medicine even if you begin to feel ill. Taking this medicine after meals will lessen stomach upset. Ask your doctor, nurse, or pharmacist for other ways to lessen these effects.

Missed dose—If you miss a dose of this medicine, take it as soon as possible. However, if it is almost time for your next dose, skip the missed dose and go back to your regular dosing schedule. Do not double doses.

Storage—To store this medicine:

- Keep out of the reach of children.
- Store away from heat and direct light.
- Do not store in the bathroom, near the kitchen sink, or in other damp places. Heat or moisture may cause the medicine to break down.
- Do not keep outdated medicine or medicine no longer needed. Be sure that any discarded medicine is out of the reach of children.

Precautions While Using This Medicine

It is very important that your doctor check your progress at regular visits to make sure that this medicine is working properly and to check for unwanted effects.

While you are being treated with altretamine, and after you stop treatment with it, *do not have any immunizations (vaccinations) without your doctor's approval.* Altretamine may lower your body's resistance and there is a chance you might get the infection the immunization is meant to prevent. In addition, other persons living in your household should not take oral polio vaccine since there is a chance they could pass the polio virus on to you. Also, avoid persons who have taken oral polio vaccine. Do not get close to them and do not stay in the same room with them for very long. If you cannot take these precautions, you should consider wearing a protective face mask that covers the nose and mouth.

Altretamine can temporarily lower the number of white blood cells in your blood, increasing the chance of getting an infection. It can also lower the number of platelets, which are necessary for proper blood clotting. If this occurs, there are certain precautions you can take, especially when your blood count is low, to reduce the risk of infection or bleeding:

- If you can, avoid people with infections. *Check with your doctor immediately* if you think you are getting an infection or if you get a fever or chills, cough or hoarseness, lower back or side pain, or painful or difficult urination.
- *Check with your doctor immediately* if you notice any unusual bleeding or bruising; black, tarry stools; blood in urine or stools; or pinpoint red spots on your skin.
- Be careful when using a regular toothbrush, dental floss, or toothpick. Your medical doctor, dentist, or nurse may recommend other ways to clean your teeth and gums. Check with your medical doctor before having any dental work done.
- Do not touch your eyes or the inside of your nose unless you have just washed your hands and have not touched anything else in the meantime.
- Be careful not to cut yourself when you are using sharp objects such as a safety razor or fingernail or toenail cutters.
- Avoid contact sports or other situations where bruising or injury could occur.

Side Effects of This Medicine

Along with their needed effects, medicines like altretamine can sometimes cause unwanted effects such as blood problems and other side effects. These and others are described below. Also, because of the way these medicines act on the body, there is a chance that they might cause other unwanted effects that may not occur until months or years after the medicine is used. These delayed effects may include certain types of cancer, such as leukemia. Discuss these possible effects with your doctor.

Although not all of these side effects may occur, if they do occur they may need medical attention.

Check with your doctor or nurse immediately if any of the following side effects occur:

Less common or rare

Black, tarry stools; blood in urine or stools; cough or hoarseness; fever or chills; lower back or side pain; painful or difficult urination; pinpoint red spots on skin; unusual bleeding or bruising; unusual tiredness

Check with your doctor as soon as possible if any of the following side effects occur:

More common

Anxiety; clumsiness; confusion; dizziness; mental depression; numbness in arms or legs; weakness

Rare

Convulsions (seizures); skin rash or itching

Other side effects may occur that usually do not need medical attention. These side effects may go away during treatment as your body adjusts to the medicine. Also, your doctor or nurse may be able to tell you about ways to prevent or reduce some of these side effects. Check with your doctor if any of the following side effects continue or are bothersome or if you have any questions about them:

More common

Nausea and vomiting

Less common

Diarrhea; loss of appetite; stomach cramps

Other side effects not listed above may also occur in some patients. If you notice any other effects, check with your doctor.

Annual revision: 07/23/92

AMANTADINE Systemic

Some commonly used brand names are:

In the U.S.

Symadine
Symmetrel

Generic name product may also be available.

In Canada

Symmetrel

Description

Amantadine (a-MAN-ta-deen) is an antiviral. It is used to prevent or treat certain influenza (flu) infections (type A). It may be given alone or along with flu shots. Amantadine will not work for colds, other types of flu, or other virus infections.

Amantadine also is an antidyskinetic. It is used to treat Parkinson's disease, sometimes called paralysis agitans or shaking palsy. It may be given alone or with other medicines for Parkinson's disease. By improving muscle control and reducing stiffness, this medicine allows more normal movements of the body as the disease symptoms are reduced. Amantadine is also used to treat stiffness and shaking caused by certain medicines used to treat nervous, mental, and emotional conditions.

Amantadine may be used for other conditions as determined by your doctor.

Amantadine is available only with your doctor's prescription, in the following dosage forms:

Oral

- Capsules (U.S. and Canada)
- Syrup (U.S. and Canada)

It is very important that you read and understand the following information. If any of it causes you special concern, check with your doctor. Also, *if you have any questions* or if you want more information about this medicine or your medical problem, *ask your doctor, nurse, or pharmacist.*

Before Using This Medicine

In deciding to use a medicine, the risks of taking the medicine must be weighed against the good it will do. This is a decision you and your doctor will make. For amantadine, the following should be considered:

Allergies—Tell your doctor if you have ever had any unusual or allergic reaction to amantadine. Also tell your doctor and pharmacist if you are allergic to any other substances, such as foods, preservatives, or dyes.

Pregnancy—Studies have not been done in humans. However, studies in some animals have shown that amantadine is harmful to the fetus and causes birth defects.

Breast-feeding—Amantadine passes into breast milk. However, the effects of amantadine in newborn babies and infants are not known.

Children—This medicine has been tested in children over one year of age and has not been shown to cause different side effects or problems in these children than it does in adults. There is no specific information comparing the use of amantadine in children under one year of age with use in other age groups.

Older adults—Elderly people are especially sensitive to the effects of amantadine. Confusion, difficult urination, blurred vision, constipation, and dry mouth, nose, and throat may be especially likely to occur.

Other medicines—Although certain medicines should not be used together at all, in other cases two different medicines may be used together even if an interaction might occur. In these cases, your doctor may want to change the dose, or other precautions may be necessary. When you are taking amantadine, it is especially important that your doctor and pharmacist know if you are taking any of the following:

- Amphetamines or
- Appetite suppressants (diet pills), except fenfluramine (e.g., Pondimin), or

- Caffeine (e.g., NoDoz) or
- Chlophedianol (e.g., Ulone) or
- Cocaine or
- Medicine for asthma or other breathing problems or
- Medicine for colds, sinus problems, or hay fever or other allergies (including nose drops or sprays) or
- Methylphenidate (e.g., Ritalin) or
- Nabilone (e.g., Cesamet) or
- Pemoline (e.g., Cylert)—The use of amantadine with these medicines may increase the chance of unwanted effects such as nervousness, irritability, trouble in sleeping, and possibly seizures or irregular heartbeat
- Anticholinergics (medicine for abdominal or stomach spasms or cramps)—The use of amantadine with these medicines may increase the chance of unwanted effects such as blurred vision, dryness of the mouth, confusion, hallucinations, and nightmares

Other medical problems—The presence of other medical problems may affect the use of amantadine. Make sure you tell your doctor if you have any other medical problems, especially:

- Eczema (recurring)—Amantadine may cause or worsen eczema
- Epilepsy or other seizures (history of)—Amantadine may increase the frequency of convulsions (seizures) in patients with a seizure disorder
- Heart disease or other circulation problems or
- Swelling of feet and ankles—Amantadine may increase the chance of swelling of the feet and ankles, and may worsen heart disease or circulation problems
- Kidney disease—Amantadine is removed from the body by the kidneys; patients with kidney disease will need to receive a lower dose of amantadine
- Mental or emotional illness—Higher doses of amantadine may cause confusion, hallucinations, and nightmares

Before you begin using any new medicine (prescription or nonprescription) or if you develop any new medical problem while you are using this medicine, check with your doctor, nurse, or pharmacist.

Proper Use of This Medicine

For patients *taking amantadine to prevent or treat flu infections:*

- Talk to your doctor about the possibility of getting a flu shot if you have not had one yet.
- This medicine is *best taken before exposure, or as soon as possible after exposure,* to people who have the flu.
- To help keep yourself from getting the flu, *keep taking this medicine for the full time of treatment.* Or if you already have the flu, continue taking this medicine for the full time of treatment even if you begin to feel better after a few days. This will help to clear up your infection completely. If you stop taking this medicine too soon, your symptoms may return. This medicine should be taken for at least 2 days after all your flu symptoms have disappeared.
- This medicine works best when there is a constant amount in the blood. *To help keep the amount constant, do not miss any doses. Also, it is best to take the doses at evenly spaced times day and night.* For example, if you are to take 2 doses a day, the doses should be spaced about 12 hours apart. If this interferes with your sleep or other daily activities, or if you need help in planning the best times to take your medicine, check with your doctor, nurse, or pharmacist.
- If you are using the oral liquid form of amantadine, use a specially marked measuring spoon or other device to measure each dose accurately. The average household teaspoon may not hold the right amount of liquid.

For patients *taking amantadine for Parkinson's disease or movement problems* caused by certain medicines used to treat nervous, mental, and emotional conditions:

- *Take this medicine exactly as directed by your doctor.* Do not miss any doses and do not take more medicine than your doctor ordered.
- Improvement in the symptoms of Parkinson's disease usually occurs in about 2 days. However, in some patients this medicine must be taken for up to 2 weeks before full benefit is seen.

Dosing—The dose of amantadine will be different for different patients. *Follow your doctor's orders or the directions on the label.* The following information includes only the average doses of amantadine. Your dose may be different if you have kidney disease. *If your dose is different, do not change it* unless your doctor tells you to do so.

- The number of capsules or teaspoonfuls of suspension that you take depends on the strength of the medicine. Also, *the number of doses you take each day, the time allowed between doses, and the length of time you take the medicine depend on the medical problem for which you are taking amantadine.*
- For the *treatment or prevention of flu*:
  —Older adults: 100 milligrams once a day.
  —Adults and children 12 years of age and older: 200 milligrams once a day, or 100 milligrams two times a day.
  —Children 9 to 12 years of age: 100 milligrams two times a day.
  —Children 1 to 9 years of age: Dose is based on body weight and must be determined by the doctor.
- For the *treatment of Parkinson's disease or movement problems*:
  —Older adults: 100 milligrams once a day to start. The dose may be increased slowly over time, if needed.
  —Adults: 100 milligrams one or two times a day.
  —Children: Dose has not been determined.

Missed dose—If you miss a dose of this medicine, take it as soon as possible. This will help to keep a constant amount of medicine in the blood. However, if it is almost time for your next dose, skip the missed dose and go back to your regular dosing schedule. Do not double doses.

Storage—To store this medicine:

- Keep out of the reach of children.
- Store away from heat and direct light.
- Do not store the capsule form of this medicine in the bathroom, near the kitchen sink, or in other damp places. Heat or moisture may cause the medicine to break down.
- Keep the oral liquid form of this medicine from freezing.
- Do not keep outdated medicine or medicine no longer needed. Be sure that any discarded medicine is out of the reach of children.

Precautions While Using This Medicine

Drinking alcoholic beverages while taking this medicine may cause increased side effects such as circulation problems, dizziness, lightheadedness, fainting, or confusion. Therefore, *do not drink alcoholic beverages while you are taking this medicine.*

This medicine may cause some people to become dizzy, confused, or lightheaded, or to have blurred vision or trouble concentrating. *Make sure you know how you react to this medicine before you drive, use machines, or do anything else that could be dangerous if you are dizzy or are not alert or able to see well.* If these reactions are especially bothersome, check with your doctor.

Getting up suddenly from a lying or sitting position may also be a problem because of the dizziness, lightheadedness, or fainting that may be caused by this medicine. Getting up slowly may help. If this problem continues or gets worse, check with your doctor.

Amantadine may cause dryness of the mouth, nose, and throat. For temporary relief of mouth dryness, use sugarless candy or gum, melt bits of ice in your mouth, or use a saliva substitute. However, if your mouth continues to feel dry for more than 2 weeks, check with your doctor or dentist. Continuing dryness of the mouth may increase the chance of dental disease, including tooth decay, gum disease, and fungus infections.

This medicine may cause purplish red, net-like, blotchy spots on the skin. This problem occurs more often in females and usually occurs on the legs and/or feet after this medicine has been taken regularly for a month or more. Although the blotchy spots may remain as long as you are taking this medicine, they usually go away gradually within 2 to 12 weeks after you stop taking the medicine. If you have any questions about this, check with your doctor.

For patients *taking amantadine to prevent or treat flu infections:*

- If your symptoms do not improve within a few days, or if they become worse, check with your doctor.

For patients *taking amantadine for Parkinson's disease or movement problems* caused by certain medicines used to treat nervous, mental, and emotional conditions:

- *Patients with Parkinson's disease must be careful not to overdo physical activities as their condition improves and body movements become easier* since injuries resulting from falls may occur. Such activities must be gradually increased to give your body time to adjust to changing balance, circulation, and coordination.
- Some patients may notice that this medicine gradually loses its effect while they are taking it regularly for a few months. If you notice this, check with your doctor. Your doctor may want to adjust the dose or stop the medicine for a while and then restart it to restore its effect.
- *Do not suddenly stop taking this medicine without first checking with your doctor* since your Parkinson's disease may get worse very quickly. Your doctor may want you to reduce your dose gradually before stopping the medicine completely.

Side Effects of This Medicine

Along with its needed effects, a medicine may cause some unwanted effects. Although not all of these side effects may occur, if they do occur they may need medical attention.

Check with your doctor immediately if any of the following side effects occur:

Less common

Blurred vision; confusion (especially in elderly patients); difficult urination (especially in elderly patients); fainting; hallucinations (seeing, hearing, or feeling things that are not there)

Rare

Convulsions (seizures); decreased vision or any change in vision; difficulty in coordination; irritation and swelling of the eye; mental depression; skin rash; swelling of feet or lower legs; unexplained shortness of breath

Other side effects may occur that usually do not need medical attention. These side effects may go away during treatment as your body adjusts to the medicine. However, check with your doctor if any of the following side effects continue or are bothersome:

More common

Difficulty concentrating; dizziness or lightheadedness; headache; irritability; loss of appetite; nausea; nervousness; purplish red, net-like, blotchy spots on skin; trouble in sleeping or nightmares

Less common or rare

Constipation; dryness of the mouth, nose, and throat; vomiting

Other side effects not listed above may also occur in some patients. If you notice any other effects, check with your doctor.

Additional Information

Once a medicine has been approved for marketing for a certain use, experience may show that it is also useful for other medical problems. Although this use is not included in product labeling, amantadine is used in certain patients with the following medical condition:

- Unusual tiredness or weakness associated with multiple sclerosis

Other than the above information, there is no additional information relating to proper use, precautions, or side effects for this use.

Annual revision: 02/23/93

AMINOBENZOATE POTASSIUM Systemic

Some commonly used brand names in the U.S. and Canada are Potaba, Potaba Envules, and Potaba Powder.

Other commonly used names are KPAB, potassium aminobenzoate, and potassium para-aminobenzoate.

Description

Aminobenzoate potassium (a-mee-noe-BEN-zoe-ate poe-TAS-ee-um) is used to treat fibrosis, a condition in which the skin and underlying tissues tighten and become less flexible. This condition occurs in such diseases as dermatomyositis, morphea, Peyronie's disease, scleroderma, and linear scleroderma.

Aminobenzoate potassium is also used to treat a certain type of inflammation (nonsuppurative inflammation) that occurs in such diseases as dermatomyositis, pemphigus, and Peyronie's disease.

This medicine is available only with your doctor's prescription in the following dosage forms:

Oral

- Capsules (U.S. and Canada)
- Oral Solution (U.S. and Canada)
- Powder for Oral Solution (U.S. and Canada)
- Tablets (U.S. and Canada)

It is very important that you read and understand the following information. If any of it causes you special concern, check with your doctor or pharmacist. Also, *if you have any questions* or if you want more information about this medicine or your medical problem, *ask your doctor, nurse, or pharmacist.*

Before Using This Medicine

In deciding to use a medicine, the risks of taking the medicine must be weighed against the good it will do. This is a decision you and your doctor will make. For aminobenzoate potassium, the following should be considered:

Allergies—Tell your doctor if you have ever had any unusual or allergic reaction to aminobenzoate potassium or aminobenzoic acid (PABA). Also tell your doctor and pharmacist if you are allergic to any other substances, such as foods, preservatives, or dyes.

Diet—Make certain your doctor and pharmacist know if you are on any special diet, such as a low-sodium or low-sugar diet.

Pregnancy—Studies on effects in pregnancy have not been done in either humans or animals.

Breast-feeding—Aminobenzoate potassium has not been reported to cause problems in nursing babies.

Children—Although there is no specific information comparing use of this medicine in children with use in other age groups, it is not expected to cause different side effects or problems in children than it does in adults.

Older adults—Elderly people may be more sensitive to certain symptoms of the low blood sugar side effect. These symptoms include confusion, difficulty in concentration, and headache. In addition, these symptoms may be harder to detect in elderly persons than in younger adults. This may increase the chance of problems during treatment with this medicine.

Other medicines—Although certain medicines should not be used together at all, in other cases two different medicines may be used together even if an interaction might occur. In these cases, your doctor may want to change the dose, or other precautions may be necessary. When you are taking aminobenzoate potassium, it is especially important that your doctor and pharmacist know if you are taking any of the following:

- Aminosalicylates or
- Sulfonamides (sulfa medicine)—Aminobenzoate potassium may decrease the effects of these medicines

Other medical problems—The presence of other medical problems may affect the use of aminobenzoate potassium. Make sure you tell your doctor if you have any other medical problems, especially:

- Diabetes mellitus (sugar diabetes) or
- Hypoglycemia (low blood sugar)—The risk of the medicine causing hypoglycemia (low blood sugar) may be increased
- Kidney disease—Aminobenzoate potassium is excreted by the kidneys, and higher blood levels of the medicine may result if kidney disease is present

Before you begin using any new medicine (prescription or nonprescription) or if you develop any new medical problem while you are using this medicine, check with your doctor, nurse, or pharmacist.

Proper Use of This Medicine

Take this medicine with meals or snacks to lessen the possibility of stomach upset. If stomach upset continues, check with your doctor.

For patients taking the *capsule or tablet form* of aminobenzoate potassium:

- Take each dose with a full glass (8 ounces) of water or milk to lessen the possibility of stomach upset.
- Patients using the tablets should dissolve them in water before taking. This also will help lessen the possibility of stomach upset.

For patients using the *powder form* of this medicine:

- This medicine should never be taken in its dry form. Instead, always mix it with water or citrus juice, as directed.
- To mask the taste of aminobenzoate potassium, you may dissolve the powder in citrus drinks instead of in water. However, if you do dissolve the powder in water, drinking a citrus juice or a carbonated beverage immediately after each dose of medicine will also help mask the taste.
- The flavor of this medicine is improved if the solution is chilled before you take it.
- For patients using the *two-gram individual packets of powder*:
  —Dissolve one packet (2 grams) of aminobenzoate potassium in a full glass (8 ounces) of water or citrus juice.
  —Stir well to dissolve powder.
- For patients using the *bulk powder form* of this medicine:
  —Use a specially marked measuring spoon or other device to measure out the correct amount of medicine. Your doctor or pharmacist can help you with this.
  —To make a 10-percent solution of this medicine:
    - Choose a container that is resistant to light, such as an amber glass container, a metal container, or a plastic container that you cannot see through. Make sure the container is large enough to measure one liter (approximately one quart).
    - Place 100 grams (approximately 3 ounces) of aminobenzoate potassium powder in the container.
    - Add enough water or citrus juice to make one liter (approximately one quart) of solution and stir well.
    - Store the solution in a container that is resistant to light, such as an amber glass container, a metal container, or a plastic container that you cannot see through.
    - Keep the solution refrigerated. Stir well before pouring each dose. Discard the unused portion after one week.

For this medicine to be effective, it must be taken every day as ordered by your doctor. It may take 3 or more months before you begin to see an improvement in your condition.

Missed dose—If you miss a dose of this medicine, take it as soon as possible. However, if it is within 2 hours of your next dose, skip the missed dose and go back to your regular dosing schedule. Do not double doses.

Storage—To store this medicine:

- Keep out of the reach of children.
- Store away from heat and direct light.
- Do not store the medicine in the bathroom, near the kitchen sink, or in other damp places. Heat or moisture may cause the medicine to break down.
- Store the liquid form of this medicine in the refrigerator. However, keep the medicine from freezing. Store the liquid form of this medicine in a container that is resistant to light, such as an amber glass container, a metal container, or a plastic container that you cannot see through.
- Discard the unused portion of the liquid form of this medicine after one week.
- Do not keep outdated medicine or medicine no longer needed. Be sure that any discarded medicine is out of the reach of children.

Precautions While Using This Medicine

While you are taking this medicine, it is important that your doctor check your progress at regular visits.

Check with your doctor right away if you cannot eat normally while taking this medicine because of nausea, loss of appetite, or for any other reason. Taking this medicine when you have not been eating normally for several days may cause low blood sugar (hypoglycemia).

If symptoms of low blood sugar (hypoglycemia) appear, stop taking this medicine, eat or drink something containing sugar, and check with your doctor right away. Good sources of sugar are table sugar mixed in water, sugar cubes, orange juice, corn syrup, or honey. One popular source of sugar is a glassful of orange juice containing 2 or 3 teaspoonfuls of table sugar.

- *Tell someone ahead of time to take you to your doctor or to a hospital right away if you begin to feel that you may pass out. If you do pass out, emergency help should be gotten at once.*
- Even if you correct the symptoms of low blood sugar by eating or drinking something with sugar, it is very important to call your doctor right away. The effects this medicine has on low blood sugar may last for a few days, and the symptoms may return often during this period of time.

Side Effects of This Medicine

Along with its needed effects, a medicine may cause some unwanted effects. Although not all of these side effects may occur, if they do occur they may need medical attention.

Check with your doctor as soon as possible if any of the following side effects occur:

Less common or rare

Chills; fever; skin rash; sore throat

Symptoms of low blood sugar

Anxiety; chills; cold sweats; confusion; cool pale skin; difficulty in concentration; drowsiness; excessive hunger; fast heartbeat; headache; nervousness; shakiness; unsteady walk; unusual tiredness or weakness

Other side effects may occur that usually do not need medical attention. These side effects may go away during treatment as your body adjusts to the medicine. However, check with your doctor if either of the following side effects continues or is bothersome:

More common

Loss of appetite; nausea

Other side effects not listed above may also occur in some patients. If you notice any other effects, check with your doctor.

Annual revision: 11/21/91

AMINOGLUTETHIMIDE Systemic

A commonly used brand name in the U.S. and Canada is Cytadren.

Description

Aminoglutethimide (a-mee-noe-gloo-TETH-i-mide) acts on a part of the body called the adrenal cortex. It affects production of steroids and also has some other effects. Aminoglutethimide is used to treat some kinds of tumors that affect the adrenal cortex. Also, it is sometimes used when the adrenal cortex is overactive without being cancerous.

In addition, aminoglutethimide is sometimes used to treat certain other conditions as determined by your doctor.

Aminoglutethimide is available only with your doctor's prescription, in the following dosage form:

Oral

- Tablets (U.S. and Canada)

It is very important that you read and understand the following information. If any of it causes you special concern, check with your doctor. Also, *if you have any questions* or if you want more information about this medicine or your medical problem, *ask your doctor, nurse, or pharmacist.*

Before Using This Medicine

In deciding to use a medicine, the risks of taking the medicine must be weighed against the good it will do. This is a decision you and your doctor will make. For aminoglutethimide, the following should be considered:

Allergies—Tell your doctor if you have ever had any unusual or allergic reaction to glutethimide or aminoglutethimide. Also tell your doctor and pharmacist if you are allergic to any other substances, such as foods, preservatives, or dyes.

Pregnancy—Aminoglutethimide has been shown to cause birth defects in humans and animals. However, this medicine may be needed in serious diseases or in other situations that threaten the mother's life. Be sure you have discussed this with your doctor before taking this medicine.

Breast-feeding—It is not known whether aminoglutethimide passes into breast milk. However, this medicine has not been reported to cause problems in nursing babies.

Children—There is no specific information comparing use of aminoglutethimide in children with use in other age groups. However, there is a chance that aminoglutethimide could cause premature growth and sexual development in males or development of male features in females.

Older adults—Lack of energy is more likely to occur in the elderly, who are usually more sensitive to the effects of aminoglutethimide.

Other medicines—Although certain medicines should not be used together at all, in other cases two different medicines may be used together even if an interaction might occur. In these cases, your doctor may want to change the dose, or other precautions may be necessary. When you are taking aminoglutethimide it is especially important that your doctor and pharmacist know if you are taking any of the following:

- Dexamethasone (e.g., Decadron)—Aminoglutethimide increases the rate at which dexamethasone is removed from the body

Other medical problems—The presence of other medical problems may affect the use of aminoglutethimide. Make sure you tell your doctor if you have any other medical problems, especially:

- Chickenpox (including recent exposure) or
- Herpes zoster (shingles)—Risk of severe disease affecting other parts of the body
- Infection—May affect the adrenal cortex. If a steroid supplement is being used, a change in dose may be needed
- Kidney disease or
- Liver disease—Effects of aminoglutethimide may be increased because of slower removal from the body
- Underactive thyroid—Aminoglutethimide can cause underactive thyroid

Before you begin using any new medicine (prescription or nonprescription) or if you develop any new medical problem while you are using this medicine, check with your doctor, nurse, or pharmacist.

Proper Use of This Medicine

Take this medicine only as directed by your doctor. Do not take more or less of it, and do not take it more often than your doctor ordered.

This medicine sometimes causes nausea and vomiting. This effect usually goes away or lessens after you have taken the medicine for a while. It is very important that you continue to use this medicine even if you begin to feel ill. Ask your doctor, nurse, or pharmacist for ways to lessen these effects. *Do not stop taking this medicine without first checking with your doctor.*

If you vomit shortly after taking a dose of aminoglutethimide, check with your doctor. You will be told whether to take the dose again or to wait until the next scheduled dose.

Missed dose—If you miss a dose of this medicine and remember within 2 to 4 hours of the missed dose, take it as soon as possible. Then go back to your regular dosing schedule. However, if it is almost time for your next dose, skip the missed dose and go back to your regular dosing schedule. Do not double doses.

Storage—To store this medicine:

- Keep out of the reach of children.
- Store away from heat and direct light.
- Do not store in the bathroom, near the kitchen sink, or in other damp places. Heat or moisture may cause the medicine to break down.
- Do not keep outdated medicine or medicine no longer needed. Be sure that any discarded medicine is out of the reach of children.

Precautions While Using This Medicine

It is very important that your doctor check your progress at regular visits to make sure that the medicine is working properly and does not cause unwanted effects.

Your doctor may want you to carry a medical identification card or wear a bracelet stating that you are taking this medicine.

Before you have any kind of surgery (including dental surgery) or emergency treatment, tell the medical doctor or dentist in charge that you are taking this medicine. Because this medicine affects the adrenal gland, extra steroids may be needed.

Check with your doctor right away if you get an injury, infection, or illness of any kind. This medicine may weaken your body's defenses against infection or inflammation.

This medicine may cause some people to become dizzy, drowsy, or less alert than they are normally. *Make sure you know how you react to this medicine before you drive, use machines, or do anything else that could be dangerous if you are dizzy or are not alert.*

Side Effects of This Medicine

Along with its needed effects, a medicine may cause some unwanted effects. Some side effects will have signs or symptoms that you can see or feel. Your doctor may watch for others by doing certain tests. Some of the unwanted effects that may be caused by aminoglutethimide are listed below. Although not all of these side effects may occur, if they do occur they may need medical attention.

Check with your doctor immediately if any of the following side effects occur:

Rare

Black, tarry stools; blood in urine or stools; cough or hoarseness; fever or chills; lower back or side pain; painful or difficult urination; pinpoint red spots on skin; unusual bleeding or bruising; yellow eyes or skin

Check with your doctor as soon as possible if the following side effects occur:

Less common

Darkening of skin; mental depression

Rare

Neck tenderness or swelling

This medicine may also cause the following side effects that your doctor will watch for:

More common

Low red blood cell count; low white blood cell count

Other side effects may occur that usually do not need medical attention. These side effects may go away during treatment as your body adjusts to the medicine. However, check with your doctor or nurse if any of the following side effects continue or are bothersome:

More common

Clumsiness; dizziness or lightheadedness (especially when getting up from a lying or sitting position); drowsiness; lack of energy; loss of appetite; measles-like skin rash or itching on face and/or palms of hands; nausea; uncontrolled eye movements

Less common or rare

Deepening of voice in females; headache; increased hair growth in females; irregular menstrual periods; mental depression; muscle pain; vomiting

Other side effects not listed above may also occur in some patients. If you notice any other effects, check with your doctor.

Additional Information

Once a medicine has been approved for marketing for a certain use, experience may show that it is also useful for other medical problems. Although these uses are not included in product labeling, aminoglutethimide is used in certain patients with the following medical conditions:

- Breast cancer
- Prostate cancer

Other than the above information, there is no additional information relating to proper use, precautions, or side effects for these uses.

Annual revision: 04/09/93

AMINOGLYCOSIDES Systemic

This information applies to the following medicines:

Amikacin (am-i-KAY-sin)
Gentamicin (jen-ta-MYE-sin)
Kanamycin (kan-a-MYE-sin)
Neomycin (nee-oh-MYE-sin)
Netilmicin (ne-til-MYE-sin)
Streptomycin (strep-toe-MYE-sin)
Tobramycin (toe-bra-MYE-sin)

Some commonly used brand names are:

For Amikacin

In the U.S.

Amikin

Generic name product may also be available.

In Canada

Amikin

For Gentamicin

In the U.S.

Garamycin
Jenamicin
G-Mycin

Generic name product may also be available.

In Canada

Cidomycin
Garamycin

For Kanamycin†

In the U.S.

Kantrex

Generic name product may also be available.

For Neomycin†

In the U.S.

Generic name product may be available.

For Netilmicin

In the U.S.

Netromycin

In Canada

Netromycin

For Streptomycin

In the U.S.

Generic name product may be available.

In Canada

Generic name product may be available.

For Tobramycin

In the U.S.

Nebcin

Generic name product may also be available.

In Canada

Nebcin

†Not commercially available in Canada.

Description

Aminoglycosides (a-mee-noe-GLYE-koe-sides) are used to treat serious bacterial infections. They work by killing bacteria or preventing their growth.

Aminoglycosides are given by injection to treat serious bacterial infections in many different parts of the body. In addition, some aminoglycosides may be given by irrigation (applying a solution of the medicine to the skin or mucous membranes or washing out a body cavity) or by inhalation into the lungs. Streptomycin may also be given for tuberculosis (TB). These medicines may be given with 1 or more other medicines for bacterial infections, or they may be given alone. Aminoglycosides may also be used for other conditions as determined by your doctor. However, aminoglycosides will not work for colds, flu, or other virus infections.

Aminoglycosides given by injection are usually used for serious bacterial infections for which other medicines may not work. However, aminoglycosides may also cause some serious side effects, including damage to your hearing, sense of balance, and kidneys. These side effects may be more likely to occur in elderly patients and newborn infants. *You and your doctor should talk about the good these medicines may do as well as the risks of receiving them.*

Aminoglycosides are to be administered only by or under the immediate supervision of your doctor. They are available in the following dosage forms:

Inhalation

Amikacin
- Inhalation solution (U.S.)

Gentamicin
- Inhalation solution (U.S.)

Kanamycin
- Inhalation solution (U.S.)

Tobramycin
- Inhalation solution (U.S.)

Irrigation

Kanamycin
- Irrigation solution (U.S.)

Parenteral

Amikacin
- Injection (U.S. and Canada)

Gentamicin
- Injection (U.S. and Canada)

Kanamycin
- Injection (U.S.)

Neomycin
- Injection (U.S.)

Netilmicin
- Injection (U.S. and Canada)

Streptomycin
- Injection (U.S. and Canada)

Tobramycin
- Injection (U.S. and Canada)

It is very important that you read and understand the following information. If any of it causes you special concern, check with your doctor. Also, *if you have any questions* or if you want more information about this medicine or your medical problem, *ask your doctor, nurse, or pharmacist.*

Before Receiving This Medicine

In deciding to use a medicine, the risks of taking the medicine must be weighed against the good it will do. This is a decision you and your doctor will make. For aminoglycosides, the following should be considered:

Allergies—Tell your doctor if you have ever had any unusual or allergic reaction to any of the aminoglycosides. Also tell your doctor and pharmacist if you are allergic to any other substances, such as foods, sulfites, or other preservatives.

Pregnancy—Studies on most of the aminoglycosides have not been done in pregnant women. Some reports have shown that aminoglycosides, especially streptomycin and tobramycin, may cause damage to the infant's hearing, sense of balance, and kidneys if the mother was receiving the medicine during pregnancy. However, this medicine may be needed in serious diseases or other situations that threaten the mother's life. Be sure you have discussed this with your doctor.

Breast-feeding—Aminoglycosides pass into breast milk in small amounts. However, they are not absorbed very much when taken by mouth. To date, aminoglycosides have not been reported to cause problems in nursing babies.

Children—Children are especially sensitive to the effects of aminoglycosides. Damage to hearing, sense of balance, and kidneys is more likely to occur in premature infants and neonates.

Older adults—Elderly people are especially sensitive to the effects of aminoglycosides. Serious side effects, such as damage to hearing, sense of balance, and kidneys may occur in elderly patients.

Other medicines—Although certain medicines should not be used together at all, in other cases two different medicines may be used together even if an interaction might occur. In these cases, your doctor may want to change the dose, or other precautions may be necessary. When you are receiving aminoglycosides it is especially important that your doctor and pharmacist know if you are taking any of the following:

- Aminoglycosides, used on the skin or mucous membranes and by injection at the same time; or more than one aminoglycoside at a time or
- Anti-infectives by mouth or by injection (medicine for infection) or
- Capreomycin (e.g., Capastat) or
- Carmustine (e.g., BiCNU) or
- Chloroquine (e.g., Aralen) or
- Cisplatin (e.g., Platinol) or
- Combination pain medicine containing acetaminophen and aspirin (e.g., Excedrin) or other salicylates (with large amounts taken regularly) or
- Cyclosporine (e.g., Sandimmune) or
- Deferoxamine (e.g., Desferal) (with long-term use) or

- Gold salts (medicine for arthritis) or
- Hydroxychloroquine (e.g., Plaquenil) or
- Inflammation or pain medicine, except narcotics, or
- Lithium (e.g., Lithane) or
- Methotrexate (e.g., Mexate) or
- Penicillamine (e.g., Cuprimine) or
- Plicamycin (e.g., Mithracin) or
- Quinine (e.g., Quinamm) or
- Streptozocin (e.g., Zanosar) or
- Tiopronin (e.g., Thiola)—Use of any of these medicines with aminoglycosides may increase the chance of hearing, balance, or kidney side effects

Other medical problems—The presence of other medical problems may affect the use of the aminoglycosides. Make sure you tell your doctor if you have any other medical problems, especially:

- Kidney disease—Patients with kidney disease may have increased aminoglycoside blood levels and increased chance of side effects
- Loss of hearing and/or balance (eighth-cranial-nerve disease)—High aminoglycoside blood levels may cause hearing loss or balance disturbances
- Myasthenia gravis or
- Parkinson's disease—Aminoglycosides may cause muscular problems, resulting in further muscle weakness

Before you begin using any new medicine (prescription or nonprescription) or if you develop any new medical problem while you are using this medicine, check with your doctor, nurse, or pharmacist.

Proper Use of This Medicine

To help clear up your infection completely, *aminoglycosides must be given for the full time of treatment,* even if you begin to feel better after a few days. Also, this medicine works best when there is a certain amount in the blood or urine. To help keep the correct level, aminoglycosides must be given on a regular schedule.

Dosing—The dose of aminoglycosides will be different for different patients. *Follow your doctor's orders or the directions on the label.* The following information includes only the average doses of aminoglycosides. Your dose may be different if you have kidney disease. *If your dose is different, do not change it* unless your doctor tells you to do so.

The dose of most aminoglycosides is based on body weight and must be determined by your doctor. The medicine is injected into a muscle or vein. Depending on the aminoglycoside prescribed, doses are given at different times and for different lengths of time. These times are as follows:

- *For amikacin*

  —Adults and children: The dose is given every eight or twelve hours for seven to ten days.

  —Newborn babies: The dose is given every twelve hours for seven to ten days.

  —Premature babies: The dose is given every eighteen to twenty-four hours for seven to ten days.
- *For gentamicin*

  —Adults and children: The dose is given every eight hours for seven to ten days or more.

  —Infants: The dose is given every eight to sixteen hours for seven to ten days or more.

  —Premature and full-term newborn babies: The dose is given every twelve to twenty-four hours for seven to ten days or more.
- *For kanamicin*

  —Adults and children: The dose is given every eight or twelve hours for seven to ten days.
- *For netilmicin*

  —Adults and children: The dose is given every eight or twelve hours for seven to fourteen days.
- *For tobramycin*

  —Adults and adolescents: The dose is given every six to eight hours for seven to ten days or more.

  —Older infants and children: The dose is given every six to sixteen hours.

  —Premature and full-term newborn babies: The dose is given every twelve to twenty-four hours.
- *For streptomycin*—The dose of streptomycin is often not based on body weight and the amount given depends on the disease being treated.

  —*Treatment of tuberculosis (TB):*

  • Adults and adolescents: 1 gram injected into a muscle once a day. This will be reduced to two or three times a week, if possible. This medicine must be given with other medicines for tuberculosis (TB).

  • Children: Dose is based on body weight and must be determined by your doctor. This dose is injected into a muscle once a day. This medicine must be given with other medicines for tuberculosis (TB).

  —*Treatment of bacterial infections:*

  • Adults and adolescents: 250 milligrams to 1 gram of streptomycin is injected into a muscle every six to twelve hours.

  • Children: Dose is based on body weight and must be determined by your doctor. This dose is injected into a muscle every six to twelve hours.

Side Effects of This Medicine

Along with its needed effects, a medicine may cause some unwanted effects. Although not all of these side effects may occur, if they do occur they may need medical attention.

Check with your doctor or nurse immediately if any of the following side effects occur:

More common

Any loss of hearing; clumsiness or unsteadiness; dizziness; greatly increased or decreased frequency of urination or amount of urine; increased thirst; loss of appetite; nausea or vomiting; numbness, tingling, or burning of face or mouth (streptomycin only); muscle twitching, or convulsions (seizures); ringing or buzzing or a feeling of fullness in the ears

Less common

Any loss of vision (streptomycin only); skin rash, itching, redness, or swelling

Rare

Difficulty in breathing; drowsiness; weakness

In addition, leg cramps, skin rash, fever, and convulsions (seizures) may occur when gentamicin is given by injection into the muscle or a vein, and into the spinal fluid.

For up to several weeks after you stop receiving this medicine, it may still cause some side effects that need medical attention. Check with your doctor if you notice any of the following side effects or if they get worse:

Any loss of hearing; clumsiness or unsteadiness; dizziness; greatly increased or decreased frequency of urination or amount of urine; increased thirst; loss of appetite; nausea or vomiting; ringing or buzzing or a feeling of fullness in the ears

Other side effects not listed above may also occur in some patients. If you notice any other effects, check with your doctor.

Annual revision: 02/23/93

AMINOSALICYLATE SODIUM Systemic

Some commonly used brand names are:

In the U.S.

Tubasal

In Canada

Nemasol Sodium

Another commonly used name is PAS.

Description

Aminosalicylate sodium (a-mee-noe-sal-I-si-late soe-dee-um) belongs to the family of medicines called anti-infectives. It is used along with one or more other medicines, to help the body overcome tuberculosis (TB). It will not work for colds, flu, or other virus infections.

Aminosalicylate sodium is available only with your doctor's prescription, in the following dosage form:

Oral

- Tablets (U.S. and Canada)

It is very important that you read and understand the following information. If any of it causes you special concern, check with your doctor. Also, *if you have any questions* or if you want more information about this medicine or your medical problem, *ask your doctor, nurse, or pharmacist.*

Before Using This Medicine

In deciding to use a medicine, the risks of taking the medicine must be weighed against the good it will do. This is a decision you and your doctor will make. For aminosalicylate sodium, the following should be considered:

Allergies—Tell your doctor if you have ever had any unusual or allergic reaction to aminosalicylate sodium, aspirin or other salicylates, including methyl salicylate (oil of wintergreen), or to other related medicines such as sulfonamides (sulfa medicine). Also tell your doctor and pharmacist if you are allergic to any other substances, such as foods, preservatives, or dyes.

Pregnancy—In one study where aminosalicylates were taken with other medicines for tuberculosis, there was an increase in birth defects. However, other studies have not shown aminosalicylates to cause birth defects.

Breast-feeding—Aminosalicylate sodium passes into the breast milk. However, this medicine has not been reported to cause problems in nursing babies.

Children—There is no specific information comparing use of aminosalicylate sodium in children with use in other age groups.

Older adults—Many medicines have not been studied specifically in older people. Therefore, it may not be known whether they work exactly the same way they do in younger adults or if they cause different side effects or problems in older people. There is no specific information comparing use of aminosalicylate sodium in the elderly with use in other age groups.

Other medicines—Although certain medicines should not be used together at all, in other cases two different medicines may be used together even if an interaction might occur. In these cases, your doctor may want to change the dose, or other precautions may be necessary. When

you are taking aminosalicylate sodium, it is especially important that your doctor and pharmacist know if you are taking any of the following:

- Aminobenzoates (e.g., Potaba)—Use of aminosalicylate sodium with aminobenzoates may decrease the effectiveness of aminosalicylate sodium

Other medical problems—The presence of other medical problems may affect the use of aminosalicylate sodium. Make sure you tell your doctor if you have any other medical problems, especially:

- Glucose-6-phosphate dehydrogenase (G6PD) deficiency—Aminosalicylate sodium may cause or worsen this blood problem
- Heart disease or other circulation problems—The sodium in aminosalicylate sodium may cause or worsen heart or circulation problems
- Kidney disease (severe)—Patients with kidney disease may have an increase in side effects
- Liver disease (severe)—Patients with severe liver disease may have an increase in side effects
- Stomach ulcer—Aminosalicylate sodium may cause stomach irritation

Before you begin using any new medicine (prescription or nonprescription) or if you develop any new medical problem while you are using this medicine, check with your doctor, nurse, or pharmacist.

Proper Use of This Medicine

Aminosalicylate sodium may be taken with or after meals or with an antacid if it upsets your stomach.

To help clear up your tuberculosis (TB) completely, *it is important that you keep taking this medicine for the full time of treatment* even if you begin to feel better after a few weeks. Since TB may take a long time to clear up, you may have to take the medicine every day for as long as 1 to 2 years or more. If you stop taking this medicine too soon, your symptoms may return.

This medicine works best when there is a constant amount in the blood. *To help keep the amount constant, do not miss any doses. Also, it is best to take the doses at evenly spaced times day and night.* For example, if you are to take 3 doses a day, doses should be spaced about 8 hours apart. If this interferes with your sleep or other daily activities, or if you need help in planning the best times to take your medicine, check with your doctor, nurse, or pharmacist.

Dosing—The dose of aminosalicylate sodium will be different for different patients. *Follow your doctor's orders or the directions on the label.* The following information includes only the average doses of aminosalicylate sodium. This medicine comes in tablets as aminosalicylate sodium (the salt form), but your doctor bases the dose on the amount of aminosalicylate acid (the acid form of the medicine) in the tablet. *If your dose is different, do not change it* unless your doctor tells you to do so.

- For the *tablet* dosage form:
  —Adults and children 12 years of age and older: 3.3 to 4 grams (aminosalicylate acid) every eight hours, or 5 to 6 grams (aminosalicylate acid) every twelve hours. This medicine must be taken with other medicines used to treat tuberculosis (TB).
  —Younger children: The dose is based on body weight and must be determined by the doctor. Depending on the size of the dose, the medicine may be given every six or eight hours. this medicine must be taken with other medicines used to treat tuberculosis (TB).

Missed dose—If you miss a dose of this medicine, take it as soon as possible. This will help to keep a constant amount of medicine in the blood. However, if it is almost time for your next dose, skip the missed dose and go back to your regular dosing schedule. Do not double doses.

Storage—To store this medicine:

- Keep out of the reach of children.
- Store away from heat and direct light.
- Do not store in the bathroom, near the kitchen sink, or in other damp places. Heat or moisture may cause the medicine to break down.
- Do not keep outdated medicine or medicine no longer needed. Be sure that any discarded medicine is out of the reach of children.

Precautions While Using This Medicine

If your symptoms do not improve within 2 to 3 weeks, or if they become worse, check with your doctor.

Do not take aminosalicylate sodium within 6 hours of taking rifampin. Taking the 2 medicines too close together may keep rifampin from working properly.

For diabetic patients:

- *This medicine may cause false test results with some urine sugar tests.* Check with your doctor before changing your diet or the dosage of your diabetes medicine.

Side Effects of This Medicine

Along with its needed effects, a medicine may cause some unwanted effects. Although not all of these side effects may occur, if they do occur they may need medical attention.

Check with your doctor immediately if any of the following side effects occur:

More common

Fever; joint pains; skin rash or itching; unusual tiredness or weakness

Less common

Abdominal pain (severe); backache; headache; lower back pain; pain or burning while urinating; paleness of skin; sore throat; yellow eyes or skin

Check with your doctor as soon as possible if any of the following side effects occur:

Less common—with long-term, high-dose therapy

Changes in menstrual periods; decreased sexual ability in males; dry, puffy skin; swelling of front part of neck; weight gain (unusual)

Other side effects may occur that usually do not need medical attention. These side effects may go away during treatment as your body adjusts to the medicine. However, check with your doctor if any of the following side effects continue or are bothersome:

More common

Diarrhea; loss of appetite; nausea and vomiting; stomach pain (mild)

Other side effects not listed above may also occur in some patients. If you notice any other effects, check with your doctor.

Annual revision: 02/23/93

AMIODARONE Systemic

A commonly used brand name in the U.S. and Canada is Cordarone.

Description

Amiodarone (am-ee-OH-da-rone) belongs to the group of medicines known as antiarrhythmics. It is used to correct irregular heartbeats to a normal rhythm.

Amiodarone produces its helpful effects by slowing nerve impulses in the heart and acting directly on the heart tissues.

This medicine is available only with your doctor's prescription, in the following dosage form:

Oral

- Tablets (U.S. and Canada)

It is very important that you read and understand the following information. If any of it causes you special concern, check with your doctor. Also, *if you have any questions* or if you want more information about this medicine or your medical problem, *ask your doctor, nurse, or pharmacist.*

Before Using This Medicine

In deciding to use a medicine, the risks of taking the medicine must be weighed against the good it will do. This is a decision you and your doctor will make. For amiodarone, the following should be considered:

Allergies—Tell your doctor if you have ever had any unusual or allergic reaction to amiodarone. Also tell your doctor and pharmacist if you are allergic to any other substances, such as foods, preservatives, or dyes.

Pregnancy—Amiodarone has been shown to cause thyroid problems in babies whose mothers took amiodarone when pregnant. In addition, there is concern that amiodarone could cause slow heartbeat in the newborn. However, this medicine may be needed in serious situations that threaten the mother's life. Be sure you have discussed this with your doctor before taking this medicine.

Breast-feeding—Although amiodarone passes into breast milk, it has not been shown to cause problems in nursing babies. However, amiodarone has been shown to cause growth problems in rats. It may be necessary for you to stop breast-feeding during treatment. Be sure you have discussed the risks and benefits of the medicine with your doctor.

Children—Amiodarone can cause serious side effects in any patient. Therefore, it is especially important that you discuss with the child's doctor the good that this medicine may do as well as the risks of using it.

Older adults—Elderly patients may be more likely to get thyroid problems with this medicine. Also, difficulty in walking and numbness, tingling, trembling, or weakness in hands or feet are more likely to occur in the elderly.

Other medicines—Although certain medicines should not be used together at all, in other cases two different medicines may be used together even if an interaction might occur. In these cases, your doctor may want to change the dose, or other precautions may be necessary. When you are taking amiodarone, it is especially important that your doctor and pharmacist know if you are taking any of the following:

- Anticoagulants (blood thinners) or
- Other heart medicine or
- Phenytoin (e.g., Dilantin)—Effects may be increased

Other medical problems—The presence of other medical problems may affect the use of amiodarone. Make sure

you tell your doctor if you have any other medical problems, especially:

- Liver disease—Effects may be increased because of slower removal from the body
- Thyroid problems—Risk of overactive or underactive thyroid is increased

Before you begin using any new medicine (prescription or nonprescription) or if you develop any new medical problem while you are using this medicine, check with your doctor, nurse, or pharmacist.

Proper Use of This Medicine

Take amiodarone exactly as directed by your doctor even though you may feel well. Do not take more medicine than ordered and do not miss any doses.

Dosing—The dose of amiodarone will be different for different patients. *Follow your doctor's orders or the directions on the label.* The following information includes only the average doses of amiodarone. *If your dose is different, do not change it* unless your doctor tells you to do so:

- For *oral* dosage form (tablets):
  - For treatment of *ventricular arrhythmias:*
    - Adults—At first, 800 to 1600 milligrams (mg) per day taken in divided doses. Then, 600 to 800 mg per day for one month. Then, 400 mg per day.
    - Children—Dose is based on body weight and must be determined by your doctor. The dose for the first ten days is usually 10 mg per kilogram (4.55 mg per pound) of body weight per day. Then, the dose is decreased to 5 mg per kilogram (2.27 mg per pound) of body weight per day. After several weeks, the dose is then decreased to 2.5 mg per kilogram (1.14 mg per pound) of body weight per day.

Missed dose—If you do miss a dose of this medicine, do not take the missed dose at all and do not double the next one. Instead, go back to your regular dosing schedule. If you miss two or more doses in a row, check with your doctor.

Storage—To store this medicine:

- Keep out of the reach of children.
- Store away from heat and direct light.
- Do not store in the bathroom, near the kitchen sink, or in other damp places. Heat or moisture may cause the medicine to break down.
- Do not keep outdated medicine or medicine no longer needed. Be sure that any discarded medicine is out of the reach of children.

Precautions While Using This Medicine

It is important that your doctor check your progress at regular visits to make sure the medicine is working properly. This will allow for changes to be made in the amount of medicine you are taking, if necessary.

Your doctor may want you to carry a medical identification card or bracelet stating that you are taking this medicine.

Before having any kind of surgery (including dental surgery) or emergency treatment, tell the medical doctor or dentist in charge that you are taking this medicine.

Amiodarone increases the sensitivity of your skin to sunlight; too much exposure could cause a serious burn. Your skin may continue to be sensitive to sunlight for several months after treatment with this medicine is stopped. A burn can occur even through window glass or thin cotton clothing. If you must go out in the sunlight, *cover your skin and wear a wide-brimmed hat. A special sun-blocking cream should also be used;* it must contain zinc or titanium oxide because other sunscreens will not work. *In case of a severe burn, check with your doctor.*

After you have taken this medicine for a long time, it may cause a blue-gray color to appear on your skin, especially in areas exposed to the sun, such as your face, neck, and arms. This color will usually fade after treatment with amiodarone has ended, although it may take several months. However, check with your doctor if this effect occurs.

Side Effects of This Medicine

Along with its needed effects, a medicine may cause some unwanted effects. Although not all of these side effects may occur, if they do occur they may need medical attention. Also, some side effects may not appear until several weeks or months, or even years, after you start taking amiodarone.

Check with your doctor immediately if any of the following side effects occur:

More common

Cough; painful breathing; shortness of breath

Check with your doctor as soon as possible if any of the following side effects occur:

More common

Fever (slight); numbness or tingling in fingers or toes; sensitivity of skin to sunlight; trembling or shaking of hands; trouble in walking; unusual and uncontrolled movements of the body; weakness of arms or legs

Less common

Blue-gray coloring of skin on face, neck, and arms; blurred vision or blue-green halos seen around objects; coldness; dry eyes; dry, puffy skin; fast or irregular heartbeat; nervousness; pain and swelling in scrotum; sensitivity of eyes to light; sensitivity to heat; slow heartbeat; sweating; swelling of feet or lower legs; trouble in sleeping; unusual tiredness; weight gain or loss

Rare

Skin rash; yellow eyes or skin

Other side effects may occur that usually do not need medical attention. These side effects may go away during treatment as your body adjusts to the medicine. However, check with your doctor if any of the following side effects continue or are bothersome:

More common

Constipation; headache; loss of appetite; nausea and vomiting

Less common

Bitter or metallic taste; decreased sexual ability in males; decrease in sexual interest; dizziness; flushing of face

After you stop using this medicine, your body may need time to adjust. The length of time this takes depends on the amount of medicine you were using and how long you used it. During this period of time check with your doctor if you notice any of the following side effects:

Cough; fever (slight); painful breathing; shortness of breath

Other side effects not listed above may also occur in some patients. If you notice any other effects, check with your doctor.

Annual revision: 04/13/93

AMMONIATED MERCURY Topical

Description

Ammoniated mercury (a-MOE-nee-ay-ted MER-kyoo-ree) is used to treat psoriasis, minor skin infections, and other skin disorders.

Some strengths of this medicine are available only with your doctor's prescription. Others are available without a prescription; however, your doctor may have special instructions on the proper use of this medicine for your medical condition.

Ammoniated mercury is available in the following dosage form:

Topical

- Ointment (U.S.)

It is very important that you read and understand the following information. If any of it causes you special concern, check with your doctor or pharmacist. Also, *if you have any questions* or if you want more information about this medicine or your medical problem, *ask your doctor, nurse, or pharmacist.*

Before Using This Medicine

If you are using this medicine without a prescription, carefully read and follow any precautions on the label. For ammoniated mercury, the following should be considered:

Allergies—Tell your doctor if you have ever had any unusual or allergic reaction to ammoniated mercury. Also tell your doctor and pharmacist if you are allergic to any other substances, such as preservatives or dyes.

Pregnancy—Studies on effects in pregnancy have not been done in either humans or animals. However, ammoniated mercury is absorbed through the skin.

Breast-feeding—This medicine is absorbed through the skin. It is not known whether it passes into the breast milk. However, ammoniated mercury has not been reported to cause problems in nursing babies.

Children—Use is not recommended, since children are especially sensitive to the effects of ammoniated mercury. This may increase the chance of side effects during treatment.

Older adults—Many medicines have not been studied specifically in older people. Therefore, it may not be known whether they work exactly the same way they do in younger adults or if they cause different side effects or problems in older people. There is no specific information comparing use of ammoniated mercury in the elderly with use in other age groups.

Other medicines—Although certain medicines should not be used together at all, in other cases two different medicines may be used together even if an interaction might occur. In these cases, your doctor may want to change the dose, or other precautions may be necessary. Tell your doctor and pharmacist if you are using any other prescription or nonprescription (over-the-counter [OTC]) medicine.

Other medical problems—The presence of other medical problems may affect the use of ammoniated mercury.

Make sure you tell your doctor if you have any other medical problems, especially:

- Deep or open wounds or
- Serious burns—Use of ammoniated mercury on these areas may cause mercury poisoning

Before you begin using any new medicine (prescription or nonprescription) or if you develop any new medical problem while you are using this medicine, check with your doctor, nurse, or pharmacist.

Proper Use of This Medicine

It is very important that you use this medicine only as directed. Do not use more of it and do not use it more often than recommended on the label, unless otherwise directed by your doctor. To do so may increase the chance of absorption through the skin and the risk of mercury poisoning.

Do not use this medicine on deep or open wounds or serious burns. To do so may cause mercury poisoning.

Keep this medicine away from the eyes.

Apply enough ointment to cover the affected area, and rub in gently.

Missed dose—If you miss a dose of this medicine, apply it as soon as possible. However, if it is almost time for your next dose, skip the missed dose and go back to your regular dosing schedule.

Storage—To store this medicine:

- Keep out of the reach of children.
- Store away from heat and direct light.
- Keep the medicine from freezing.
- Do not keep outdated medicine or medicine no longer needed. Be sure that any discarded medicine is out of the reach of children.

Precautions While Using This Medicine

Do not use any topical iodine-containing preparations (for example, iodine solution, iodine tincture, or povidone-iodine) *on the same affected area as this medicine.* To do so may increase the possibility of side effects. If you have any questions about this, check with your doctor or pharmacist.

Do not use any sulfur-containing preparations on the same affected area as this medicine. To do so may cause a foul odor, may irritate the skin, and may stain the skin black. If you have any questions about this, check with your doctor or pharmacist.

Side Effects of This Medicine

Along with its needed effects, a medicine may cause some unwanted effects. Although not all of these side effects may occur, if they do occur they may need medical attention.

Check with your doctor as soon as possible if any of the following side effects occur:

Skin infection or irritation not present before use of this medicine

Symptoms of mercury poisoning

Cloudy urine; dizziness; headache (continuing or severe); irritation, soreness, or swelling of gums; nausea; skin rash or unusual redness of skin

Other side effects not listed above may also occur in some patients. If you notice any other effects, check with your doctor or pharmacist.

Annual revision: 11/21/91

AMPHETAMINES Systemic

This information applies to the following medicines:

Amphetamine (am-FET-a-meen)
Amphetamine and Dextroamphetamine Resin Complex
Dextroamphetamine (dex-troe-am-FET-a-meen)
Methamphetamine (meth-am-FET-a-meen)

Some commonly used brand names are:

For Amphetamine†

In the U.S.

Generic name product is available.

Another commonly used name is amfetamine.

For Amphetamine and Dextroamphetamine Resin Complex†

In the U.S.

Biphetamine 12½
Biphetamine 20

For Dextroamphetamine

In the U.S.

Dexedrine
Dexedrine Spansule
Oxydess II
Spancap No.1

Generic name product may also be available.

In Canada

Dexedrine
Dexedrine Spansule

Another commonly used name is dexamfetamine.

For Methamphetamine†

In the U.S.

Desoxyn
Desoxyn Gradumet

Another commonly used name is metamfetamine.

†Not commercially available in Canada.

Description

Amphetamines (am-FET-a-meens) belong to the group of medicines called central nervous system (CNS) stimulants. They are used to treat children with attention-deficit hyperactivity disorder (ADHD). Amphetamines increase attention and decrease restlessness in children who are overactive, unable to concentrate for very long or are easily distracted, and have unstable emotions. These medicines are used as part of a total treatment program that also includes social, educational, and psychological treatment.

Amphetamine and dextroamphetamine are also used in the treatment of narcolepsy (uncontrollable desire for sleep or sudden attacks of deep sleep).

Amphetamines should not be used for weight loss or weight control or to combat unusual tiredness or weakness or replace rest. When used for these purposes, they may be dangerous to your health.

These medicines are available only with a doctor's prescription. Prescriptions cannot be refilled. A new prescription must be obtained from your doctor each time you or your child needs this medicine.

Amphetamines are available in the following dosage forms:

Oral

- Amphetamine
  - Tablets (U.S.)
- Amphetamine and Dextroamphetamine Resin Complex
  - Capsules (U.S.)
- Dextroamphetamine
  - Extended-release capsules (U.S. and Canada)
  - Tablets (U.S. and Canada)
- Methamphetamine
  - Tablets (U.S.)
  - Extended-release tablets (U.S.)

It is very important that you read and understand the following information. If any of it causes you special concern, check with your doctor. Also, *if you have any questions* or if you want more information about this medicine or your medical problem, *ask your doctor, nurse, or pharmacist.*

Before Using This Medicine

In deciding to use a medicine, the risks of taking the medicine must be weighed against the good it will do. This is a decision you and your doctor will make. For amphetamines, the following should be considered:

Allergies—Tell your doctor if you have ever had any unusual or allergic reaction to amphetamine, dextroamphetamine, ephedrine, epinephrine, isoproterenol, metaproterenol, methamphetamine, norepinephrine, phenylephrine, phenylpropanolamine, pseudoephedrine, or terbutaline. Also tell your doctor and pharmacist if you are allergic to any other substances, such as foods, preservatives, or dyes.

Pregnancy—Studies have not been done in humans. However, animal studies have shown that amphetamines may increase the chance of birth defects if taken during the early months of pregnancy.

In addition, overuse of amphetamines during pregnancy may increase the chances of a premature delivery and of having a baby with a low birth weight. Also, the baby may become dependent on amphetamines and experience withdrawal effects such as agitation and drowsiness.

Breast-feeding—Amphetamines pass into breast milk. Although this medicine has not been reported to cause problems in nursing babies, it is best not to breast-feed while you are taking an amphetamine. Be sure you have discussed this with your doctor.

Children—When amphetamines are used for long periods of time in children, they may cause unwanted effects on behavior and growth. Before these medicines are given to a child, you should discuss their use with your child's doctor.

Older adults—Many medicines have not been studied specifically in older people. Therefore, it may not be known whether they work exactly the same way they do in younger adults or if they cause different side effects or problems in older people. There is no specific information comparing use of amphetamines in the elderly with use in other age groups.

Other medicines—Although certain medicines should not be used together at all, in many cases 2 different medicines may be used together even if an interaction might occur. In these cases, changes in dose or other precautions may be necessary. When you are taking amphetamines it is especially important that your doctor and pharmacist know if you are taking any of the following:

- Amantadine (e.g., Symmetrel) or
- Caffeine (e.g., NoDoz) or
- Chlophedianol (e.g., Ulone) or
- Methylphenidate (e.g., Ritalin) or
- Nabilone (e.g., Cesamet) or
- Pemoline (e.g., Cylert)—Use of these medicines may increase the CNS stimulation effects of amphetamines and cause unwanted effects such as nervousness, irritability, trouble in sleeping, and possibly convulsions (seizures)
- Appetite suppressants (diet pills), except fenfluramine (e.g., Pondimin), or
- Medicine for asthma or other breathing problems or
- Medicine for colds, sinus problems, or hay fever or other allergies (including nose drops or sprays)—Use of these medicines may increase the CNS stimulation effects of amphetamines and cause unwanted effects such as nervousness, irritability, trouble in sleeping, and possibly convulsions (seizures), as well as unwanted effects on the heart and blood vessels

- Beta-blockers (acebutolol [e.g., Sectral], atenolol [e.g., Tenormin], carteolol [e.g., Cartrol], labetalol [e.g., Normodyne], metoprolol [e.g., Lopressor], nadolol [e.g., Corgard], oxprenolol [e.g., Trasicor], penbutolol [e.g., Levatol], pindolol [e.g., Visken], propranolol [e.g., Inderal], sotalol [e.g., Sotacor], timolol [e.g., Blocadren])—Use of amphetamines with beta-blockers may increase the chance of high blood pressure and heart problems
- Cocaine—Use by persons taking amphetamines may cause a severe increase in blood pressure and other unwanted effects, including nervousness, irritability, trouble in sleeping, and possible convulsions (seizures)
- Digitalis glycosides (heart medicine)—Amphetamines may cause additive effects, resulting in irregular heartbeat
- Meperidine—Use of meperidine by persons taking amphetamines is not recommended because the chance of serious side effects (such as high fever, convulsions, and coma) may be increased
- Monoamine oxidase (MAO) inhibitors (furazolidone [e.g., Furoxone], isocarboxazid [e.g., Marplan], phenelzine [e.g., Nardil], procarbazine [e.g., Matulane], selegiline [e.g., Eldepryl], tranylcypromine [e.g., Parnate])—Taking amphetamines while you are taking or within 2 weeks of taking monoamine oxidase (MAO) inhibitors may increase the chance of serious side effects such as sudden and severe high blood pressure or fever
- Thyroid hormones—The effects of either these medicines or amphetamines may be increased; unwanted effects may occur in patients with heart or blood vessel disease
- Tricyclic antidepressants (amitriptyline [e.g., Elavil], amoxapine [e.g., Asendin], clomipramine [e.g., Anafranil], desipramine [e.g., Pertofrane], doxepin [e.g., Sinequan], imipramine [e.g., Tofranil], nortriptyline [e.g., Aventyl], protriptyline [e.g., Vivactil], trimipramine [e.g., Surmontil])—Although tricyclic antidepressants may be used with amphetamines to help make them work better, using the 2 medicines together may increase the chance of fast or irregular heartbeat, severe high blood pressure, or high fever

Other medical problems—The presence of other medical problems may affect the use of amphetamines.Make sure you tell your doctor if you have any other medical problems, especially:

- Anxiety or tension (severe) or
- Drug abuse or dependence, (history of) or
- Glaucoma or
- Heart or blood vessel disease or
- High blood pressure or
- Mental illness (severe), especially in children, or
- Overactive thyroid or
- Tourette's syndrome (history of) or other tics—Amphetamines may make the condition worse

Before you begin using any new medicine (prescription or nonprescription) or if you develop any new medical problem while you are using this medicine, check with your doctor, nurse, or pharmacist.

Proper Use of This Medicine

For patients taking *the short-acting form* of this medicine:

- Take the last dose for each day at least 6 hours before bedtime to help prevent trouble in sleeping.

For patients taking *the long-acting form* of this medicine:

- Take the daily dose about 10 to 14 hours before bedtime to help prevent trouble in sleeping.
- These capsules or tablets should be swallowed whole. Do not break, crush, or chew them before swallowing.

Take this medicine only as directed by your doctor. Do not take more or less of it, do not take it more often, and do not take it for a longer time than your doctor ordered. If too much is taken, it may become habit-forming (causing mental or physical dependence).

If you think this medicine is not working properly after you have taken it for several weeks, *do not increase the dose.* Instead, check with your doctor.

Missed dose—If you miss a dose of this medicine and your dosing schedule is:

- One dose a day—Take the missed dose as soon as possible, but not later than stated above, to prevent trouble in sleeping. However, if you do not remember the missed dose until the next day, skip it and go back to your regular dosing schedule. Do not double doses.
- Two or three doses a day—If you remember within an hour or so of the missed dose, take the dose right away. However, if you do not remember until later, skip it and go back to your regular dosing schedule. Do not double doses.

Storage—To store this medicine:

- Keep out of the reach of children.
- Store away from heat and direct light.
- Do not store the capsule or tablet form of this medicine in the bathroom, near the kitchen sink, or in other damp places. Heat or moisture may cause the medicine to break down.
- Keep the liquid form of this medicine from freezing.
- Do not keep outdated medicine or medicine no longer needed. Be sure that any discarded medicine is out of the reach of children.

Precautions While Using This Medicine

Your doctor should check your progress at regular visits to make sure that this medicine does not cause unwanted effects.

If you will be taking this medicine in large doses for a long time, *do not stop taking it without first checking with your doctor.* Your doctor may want you to reduce gradually the amount you are taking before stopping completely.

This medicine may cause some people to feel a false sense of well-being or to become dizzy, lightheaded, or less alert than they are normally. *Make sure you know how you react to this medicine before you drive, use machines, or do anything else that could be dangerous if you are dizzy or are not alert.*

Before you have any medical tests, tell the medical doctor in charge that you are taking this medicine. The results of the metyrapone test may be affected by this medicine.

If you have been using this medicine for a long time and you think you may have become mentally or physically dependent on it, check with your doctor. Some signs of dependence on amphetamines are:

- A strong desire or need to continue taking the medicine.
- A need to increase the dose to receive the effects of the medicine.
- Withdrawal effects (for example, mental depression, nausea or vomiting, stomach cramps or pain, trembling, unusual tiredness or weakness) occurring after the medicine is stopped.

Side Effects of This Medicine

Along with its needed effects, a medicine may cause some unwanted effects. Although not all of these side effects may occur, if they do occur they may need medical attention.

Check with your doctor as soon as possible if any of the following side effects occur:

More common

Irregular heartbeat

Rare

Chest pain; fever, unusually high; skin rash or hives; uncontrolled movements of head, neck, arms, and legs

With long-term use or high doses

Difficulty in breathing; dizziness or feeling faint; increased blood pressure; mood or mental changes; pounding heartbeat; unusual tiredness or weakness

Other side effects may occur that usually do not need medical attention. These side effects may go away during treatment as your body adjusts to the medicine. However, check with your doctor if any of the following side effects continue or are bothersome:

More common

False sense of well-being; irritability; nervousness; restlessness; trouble in sleeping

Note: After these stimulant effects have worn off, drowsiness, trembling, unusual tiredness or weakness, or mental depression may occur.

Less common

Blurred vision; changes in sexual desire or decreased sexual ability; constipation; diarrhea; dizziness or lightheadedness; dryness of mouth or unpleasant taste; fast or pounding heartbeat; headache; increased sweating; loss of appetite; nausea or vomiting; stomach cramps or pain; weight loss

After you stop using this medicine, your body may need time to adjust. The length of time this takes depends on the amount of medicine you were using and how long you used it. During this period of time check with your doctor if you notice any of the following side effects:

Mental depression; nausea or vomiting; stomach cramps or pain; trembling; unusual tiredness or weakness

Other side effects not listed above may also occur in some patients. If you notice any other effects check with your doctor.

Annual revision: 06/21/91

AMPHOTERICIN B Systemic

A commonly used brand name in the U.S. and Canada is Fungizone Intravenous.

Generic name product may also be available in the U.S.

Description

Amphotericin (am-foe-TER-i-sin) B is an antifungal. It is used to help the body overcome serious fungus infections. It may also be used for other problems as determined by your doctor.

Amphotericin B is available only with your doctor's prescription. It is available in the following dosage form:

Parenteral

- Injection (U.S. and Canada)

It is very important that you read and understand the following information. If any of it causes you special concern, check with your doctor. Also, *if you have any questions* or if you want more information about this medicine or your medical problem, *ask your doctor, nurse, or pharmacist.*

Before Receiving This Medicine

In deciding to use a medicine, the risks of taking the medicine must be weighed against the good it will do. This is a decision you and your doctor will make. For amphotericin B, the following should be considered:

Allergies—Tell your doctor if you have ever had any unusual or allergic reaction to amphotericin B. Also tell your doctor and pharmacist if you are allergic to any other substances, such as foods, preservatives, or dyes.

Pregnancy—Amphotericin B has not been reported to cause birth defects or other problems in humans.

Breast-feeding—Amphotericin B has not been reported to cause problems in nursing babies.

Children—Although there is no specific information comparing use of amphotericin B in children with use in other age groups, this medicine is not expected to cause different side effects or problems in children than it does in adults.

Older adults—Many medicines have not been studied specifically in older people. Therefore, it may not be known whether they work exactly the same way they do in younger adults or if they cause different side effects or problems in older people. There is no specific information comparing use of amphotericin B in the elderly with use in other age groups.

Other medicines—Although certain medicines should not be used together at all, in other cases two different medicines may be used together even if an interaction might occur. In these cases, your doctor may want to change the dose, or other precautions may be necessary. When you are taking amphotericin B, it is especially important that your doctor and pharmacist know if you are taking any of the following:

- Antineoplastics (cancer medicine) or
- Antithyroid agents (medicine for overactive thyroid) or
- Azathioprine (e.g., Imuran) or
- Chloramphenicol (e.g., Chloromycetin) or
- Colchicine or
- Cyclophosphamide (e.g., Cytoxan) or
- Flucytosine (e.g., Ancobon) or
- Ganciclovir (e.g., Cytovene) or
- Interferon (e.g., Intron A, Roferon-A) or
- Mercaptopurine (e.g., Purinethol) or
- Zidovudine (e.g., AZT, Retrovir) or
- X-ray treatment—Use of amphotericin B with any of these medicines or x-ray treatment may increase the chance of side effects affecting the blood
- Bumetanide (e.g., Bumex) or
- Carmustine (e.g., BiCNU) or
- Cisplatin (e.g., Platinol) or
- Combination pain medicine containing acetaminophen and aspirin (e.g., Excedrin) or other salicylates (with large amounts taken regularly) or
- Cyclosporine (e.g., Sandimmune) or
- Deferoxamine (e.g., Desferal) (with long-term use) or
- Ethacrynic acid (e.g., Edecrin) or
- Furosemide (e.g., Lasix) or
- Gold salts (medicine for arthritis) or
- Indapamide (e.g., Lozol) or
- Inflammation or pain medicine, except narcotics, or
- Lithium (e.g., Lithane) or
- Other medicine for infection or
- Plicamycin (e.g., Mithracin) or
- Streptozocin (e.g., Zanosar) or
- Tiopronin (e.g., Thiola) or
- Thiazide diuretics (water pills)—Using these medicines with amphotericin B may increase the risk of side effects affecting the kidneys
- Corticosteroids (cortisone-like medicine) or
- Corticotropin (ACTH)—Use of amphotericin B with these medicines may cause changes in the blood that may increase the chance for heart problems
- Digitalis glycosides (heart medicine)—Use of amphotericin B with digitalis medicines (such as digoxin) may cause changes in the blood that may increase the chance of heart problems
- Methotrexate (e.g., Mexate) or
- Penicillamine (e.g., Cuprimine)—Using these medicines with amphotericin B may increase the risk of side effects affecting the blood and the kidneys

Other medical problems—The presence of other medical problems may affect the use of amphotericin B. Make sure you tell your doctor if you have any other medical problems, especially:

- Kidney disease—Amphotericin B may cause side effects affecting the kidneys

Before you begin using any new medicine (prescription or nonprescription) or if you develop any new medical problem while you are using this medicine, check with your doctor, nurse, or pharmacist.

Proper Use of This Medicine

Dosing—The dose of amphotericin B will be different for different patients. The following information includes only the average doses of amphotericin B. Your dose may be different if you have kidney disease.

- For the *injection* dosage form:
  - —Adults and children: A small test dose is usually given first to see how you react to the medicine. The dose is then slowly increased, depending on what your infection is and how well you tolerate the medicine. The dose must be determined by your doctor.

Side Effects of This Medicine

Along with its needed effects, a medicine may cause some unwanted effects. Although not all of these side effects may occur, if they do occur they may need medical attention.

Check with your doctor or nurse immediately if any of the following side effects occur:

More common

With intravenous injection

Fever and chills; headache; increased or decreased urination; irregular heartbeat; muscle cramps or pain; nausea; pain at the place of injection; unusual tiredness or weakness; vomiting

Less common or rare
With intravenous injection
Blurred or double vision; convulsions (seizures); numbness, tingling, pain, or weakness in hands or feet; shortness of breath, troubled breathing, wheezing, or tightness in chest; skin rash or itching; sore throat and fever; unusual bleeding or bruising
With spinal injection
Blurred vision or any change in vision; difficult urination; numbness, tingling, pain, or weakness

Other side effects may occur that usually do not need medical attention. These side effects may go away during treatment as your body adjusts to the medicine. However, check with your doctor if any of the following side effects continue or are bothersome:

More common
With intravenous injection
Diarrhea; headache; indigestion; loss of appetite; nausea or vomiting; stomach pain
Less common
With spinal injection
Back, leg, or neck pain; dizziness or lightheadedness; headache; nausea or vomiting

Other side effects not listed above may also occur in some patients. If you notice any other effects, check with your doctor.

Annual revision: 02/23/93

AMPHOTERICIN B Topical†

A commonly used brand name in the U.S. is Fungizone.

†Not commercially available in Canada.

Description

Amphotericin (am-foe-TER-i-sin) B belongs to the family of medicines called antifungals. Amphotericin B topical preparations are used to treat fungus infections.

Amphotericin B is available only with your doctor's prescription, in the following dosage forms:

Topical
- Cream (U.S.)
- Lotion (U.S.)
- Ointment (U.S.)

It is very important that you read and understand the following information. If any of it causes you special concern, check with your doctor. Also, *if you have any questions* or if you want more information about this medicine or your medical problem, *ask your doctor, nurse, or pharmacist.*

Before Using This Medicine

In deciding to use a medicine, the risks of using the medicine must be weighed against the good it will do. This is a decision you and your doctor will make. For amphotericin B, the following should be considered:

Allergies—Tell your doctor if you have ever had any unusual or allergic reaction to amphotericin B. Also tell your doctor and pharmacist if you are allergic to any other substances, such as preservatives or dyes.

Pregnancy—Amphotericin B topical preparations have not been shown to cause birth defects or other problems in humans.

Breast-feeding—Amphotericin B topical preparations have not been reported to cause problems in nursing babies.

Children—Although there is no specific information comparing use of amphotericin B topical preparations in children with use in other age groups, this medicine is not expected to cause different side effects or problems in children than it does in adults.

Older adults—Many medicines have not been studied specifically in older people. Therefore, it may not be known whether they work exactly the same way they do in younger adults. Although there is no specific information comparing use of topical amphotericin B preparations in the elderly with use in other age groups, these preparations are not expected to cause different side effects or problems in older people than they do in younger adults.

Other medicines—Although certain medicines should not be used together at all, in other cases two different medicines may be used together even if an interaction might occur. In these cases, your doctor may want to change the dose, or other precautions may be necessary. Tell your doctor and pharmacist if you are using any other topical prescription or nonprescription (over-the-counter [OTC]) medicine that is to be applied to the same area of the skin.

Before you begin using any new medicine (prescription or nonprescription) or if you develop any new medical problem while you are using this medicine, check with your doctor, nurse, or pharmacist.

Proper Use of This Medicine

Apply enough amphotericin B to cover the affected areas, and rub in gently.

Do not apply an occlusive dressing (airtight covering such as kitchen plastic wrap) over this medicine since it may cause irritation of the skin. If you have any questions about this, check with your doctor.

To help clear up your infection completely, *it is very important that you keep using this medicine for the full time of treatment,* even if your symptoms begin to clear up after a few days. Since fungus infections may be very slow to clear up, you may have to continue using this medicine every day for several months or longer. If you stop using this medicine too soon, your symptoms may return. *Do not miss any doses.*

Missed dose—If you do miss a dose of this medicine, apply it as soon as possible. Then go back to your regular dosing schedule.

Storage—To store this medicine:

- Keep out of the reach of children.
- Store away from heat and direct light.
- Keep the medicine from freezing.
- Do not keep outdated medicine or medicine no longer needed. Be sure that any discarded medicine is out of the reach of children.

Precautions While Using This Medicine

If your skin problem does not improve within 1 to 2 weeks, or if it becomes worse, check with your doctor.

When amphotericin B is rubbed into the affected skin areas, it may stain the skin slightly, especially if it is applied to areas on or around the nails. It may also stain the nails.

For patients using the *cream or lotion form* of this medicine:

- If either of these forms stain your clothing, the stain may be removed by hand-washing the clothing with soap and warm water.

For patients using the *ointment form* of this medicine:

- If this form stains your clothing, the stain may be removed with a standard cleaning fluid.

Side Effects of This Medicine

Along with its needed effects, a medicine may cause some unwanted effects. Although not all of these side effects may occur, if they do occur they may need medical attention.

Check with your doctor as soon as possible if any of the following side effects occur:

Less common

Burning, itching, redness, or other sign of irritation not present before use of this medicine

Rare

Skin rash

Other side effects may occur that usually do not need medical attention. These side effects may go away during treatment as your body adjusts to the medicine. However, check with your doctor if the following side effect continues or is bothersome:

Less common—for cream only

Dryness of skin

Other side effects not listed above may also occur in some patients. If you notice any other effects, check with your doctor.

Annual revision: 11/21/91

AMYL NITRITE Systemic

Generic name product available in the U.S. and Canada.

Description

Amyl nitrite (AM-il NYE-trite) is related to the nitrate medicines and is used by inhalation to relieve the pain of angina attacks. It works by relaxing blood vessels and increasing the supply of blood and oxygen to the heart while reducing its work load.

Amyl nitrite may also be used for other conditions as determined by your doctor.

This medicine comes in a glass capsule covered by a protective cloth. The cloth covering allows you to crush the glass capsule between your fingers without cutting yourself.

On the street, this medicine and others like it are sometimes called "poppers." They have been used by some people to cause a "high" or to improve sex. Use in this way is not recommended. Amyl nitrite can cause serious harmful effects if too much is inhaled.

Amyl nitrite is available only with your doctor's prescription, in the following dosage form:

Inhalation

- Glass capsules (U.S. and Canada)

It is very important that you read and understand the following information. If any of it causes you special concern, check with your doctor. Also, *if you have any questions* or if you want more information about this medicine or your medical problem, *ask your doctor, nurse, or pharmacist.*

Before Using This Medicine

In deciding to use a medicine, the risks of taking the medicine must be weighed against the good it will do. This is a decision you and your doctor will make. For amyl nitrite, the following should be considered:

Allergies—Tell your doctor if you have ever had any unusual or allergic reaction to amyl nitrite or nitrates. Also tell your doctor and pharmacist if you are allergic to any other substances, such as foods or dyes.

Pregnancy—Studies on effects in pregnancy have not been done in either humans or animals. However, use of amyl nitrite is not recommended during pregnancy because it could cause serious problems in the unborn baby.

Breast-feeding—It is not known whether amyl nitrite passes into breast milk. However, use of amyl nitrite is not recommended during breast-feeding, because it may cause unwanted effects in nursing babies.

Children—Studies on this medicine have been done only in adult patients and there is no specific information comparing use of amyl nitrite in children with use in other age groups.

Older adults—Dizziness or lightheadedness may be more likely to occur in the elderly, who are usually more sensitive to the effects of amyl nitrite.

Other medicines—Although certain medicines should not be used together at all, in other cases two different medicines may be used together even if an interaction might occur. In these cases, your doctor may want to change the dose, or other precautions may be necessary. When you are taking amyl nitrite, it is especially important that your doctor and pharmacist know if you are taking any of the following:

- Amantadine (e.g., Symmetrel) or
- Antidepressants (medicine for depression) or
- Antihypertensives (high blood pressure medicine) or
- Antipsychotics (medicine for mental illness) or
- Bromocriptine (e.g., Parlodel) or
- Diuretics (water pills) or
- Levodopa (e.g., Dopar) or
- Medicine for heart disease or
- Nabilone (e.g., Cesamet)—in high doses or
- Narcotic pain medicine or
- Nimodipine (e.g., Nimotop) or
- Pentamidine (e.g., Pentam) or
- Pimozide (e.g., Orap) or
- Promethazine (e.g., Phenergan) or
- Trimeprazine (e.g., Temaril)—May increase dizziness or lightheadedness when getting up from a lying or sitting position

It is also important that your doctor and pharmacist know if you are using any of the following medicines in the eye:

- Levobunolol (e.g., Betagan) or
- Metipranolol (e.g., Optipranolol) or
- Timolol (e.g., Timoptic)—May increase dizziness or lightheadedness when getting up from a lying or sitting position

Other medical problems—The presence of other medical problems may affect the use of amyl nitrite. Make sure you tell your doctor if you have any other medical problems, especially:

- Anemia (severe)
- Glaucoma—Amyl nitrite may make this condition worse
- Overactive thyroid
- Recent stroke, heart attack, or head injury

Before you begin using any new medicine (prescription or nonprescription) or if you develop any new medical problem while you are using this medicine, check with your doctor, nurse, or pharmacist.

Proper Use of This Medicine

To use amyl nitrite:

- *When you begin to feel an attack of angina starting (chest pains or a tightness or squeezing in the chest), sit down. Then crush the cloth-covered glass capsule containing amyl nitrite between your finger and thumb. Pass it back and forth close to your nose and inhale the vapor several (1 to 6) times.* Since you may become dizzy, lightheaded, or faint soon after using amyl nitrite, it is best to sit or lie down rather than stand while the medicine is working. If you become dizzy or faint while sitting, take several deep breaths of air and either bend forward with your head between your knees or lie down with your feet elevated.
- Remain calm and you should feel better in a few minutes.

Use this medicine exactly as directed by your doctor, and do not use more than your doctor ordered. Using too much amyl nitrite may cause a dangerous overdose. If the medicine does not seem to be working as well after you have used it for a while, check with your doctor. *Do not increase the dose on your own.*

Dosing—*Follow your doctor's orders or the directions on the label.* The following information includes only the average doses of amyl nitrite:

- For *inhalation* dosage form:
  —Adults: 0.18 or 0.3 milliliter (1 ampul) taken by inhaling the vapor of amyl nitrite through the nose. Dose may be repeated within 1 to 5 minutes if pain is not relieved. *If you still have chest pain after a total of 2 doses in a 10-minute period, contact your doctor or have someone take you to a hospital emergency room without delay.*

Storage—To store this medicine:

- Keep out of the reach of children.
- Store away from heat and direct light.
- Do not store in the bathroom or in the kitchen. Heat may cause the medicine to break down.
- Do not keep outdated medicine or medicine no longer needed. Be sure that any discarded medicine is out of the reach of children.

Precautions While Using This Medicine

Amyl nitrite is extremely flammable. Keep it away from heat or any open flame, especially when crushing the capsule. Amyl nitrite can catch fire very easily and cause serious burns.

Dizziness or lightheadedness may occur, especially when you get up from a lying or sitting position. Getting up slowly may help, but if the problem continues or gets worse, check with your doctor.

Drinking alcohol while you are taking this medicine may make the dizziness or lightheadedness worse and may cause a serious drop in blood pressure. Check with your doctor before drinking alcoholic beverages.

After using a dose of amyl nitrite, you may get a mild headache that lasts for a short time. This is a common side effect and is no cause for alarm. However, if this effect continues, or if the headaches are severe, check with your doctor.

Side Effects of This Medicine

Along with its needed effects, a medicine may cause some unwanted effects. Although not all of these side effects may occur, if they do occur they may need medical attention.

Check with your doctor as soon as possible if any of the following side effects occur:

Rare

Skin rash; unusual tiredness or weakness

Signs and symptoms of overdose

Bluish-colored lips, fingernails, or palms of hands; dizziness (extreme) or fainting; feeling of extreme pressure in head; shortness of breath; unusual tiredness or weakness; weak and fast heartbeat

Other side effects may occur that usually do not need medical attention. These side effects may go away during treatment as your body adjusts to the medicine. However, check with your doctor if any of the following side effects continue or are bothersome:

More common

Dizziness or lightheadedness, especially when getting up from a lying or sitting position; fast pulse; flushing of face and neck; headache (mild); nausea or vomiting; restlessness

Other side effects not listed above may also occur in some patients. If you notice any other effects, check with your doctor.

Annual revision: 04/12/93

ANABOLIC STEROIDS Systemic

This information applies to the following medicines:

Nandrolone (NAN-droe-lone)
Oxandrolone (ox-AN-droe-lone)
Oxymetholone (ox-i-METH-oh-lone)
Stanozolol (stan-OH-zoe-lole)

Some commonly used brand names are:

For Nandrolone

In the U.S.

Anabolin
Anabolin LA-100
Androlone
Androlone 50
Androlone D
Deca-Durabolin
Durabolin
Hybolin Decanoate
Hybolin-Improved
Kabolin
Nandrobolic
Nandrobolic L.A.
Neo-Durabolic

Generic name product may also be available.

In Canada

Deca-Durabolin
Durabolin

For Oxandrolone†‡

In the U.S.

Anavar

For Oxymetholone

In the U.S.

Anadrol

In Canada

Anapolon 50

For Stanozolol
In the U.S.
Winstrol
In Canada
Winstrol

†Not commercially available in Canada.
‡Product is no longer being manufactured but may still be in circulation.

Description

This medicine belongs to the group of medicines known as anabolic (an-a-BOL-ik) steroids. They are related to testosterone, a male sex hormone. Anabolic steroids help to rebuild tissues that have become weak because of serious injury or illness. A diet high in proteins and calories is necessary with anabolic steroid treatment.

Anabolic steroids are used for several reasons:

- to help patients gain weight after a severe illness, injury, or continuing infection. They also are used when patients fail to gain or maintain normal weight because of unexplained medical reasons.
- to treat certain types of anemia.
- to treat certain kinds of breast cancer in some women.
- to treat hereditary angioedema, which causes swelling of the face, arms, legs, throat, windpipe, bowels, or sexual organs.

Anabolic steroids may also be used for other conditions as determined by your doctor.

Anabolic steroids are available only with your doctor's prescription, in the following dosage forms:

Oral
Oxandrolone
- Tablets (U.S.)

Oxymetholone
- Tablets (U.S. and Canada)

Stanozolol
- Tablets (U.S. and Canada)

Parenteral
Nandrolone
- Injection (U.S. and Canada)

It is very important that you read and understand the following information. If any of it causes you special concern, check with your doctor. Also, *if you have any questions* or if you want more information about this medicine or your medical problem, *ask your doctor, nurse, or pharmacist.*

Before Using This Medicine

In deciding to use a medicine, the risks of taking the medicine must be weighed against the good it will do. This is a decision you and your doctor will make. For anabolic steroids, the following should be considered:

Allergies—Tell your doctor if you have ever had any unusual or allergic reaction to anabolic steroids or androgens (male sex hormones). Also tell your doctor and pharmacist if you are allergic to any other substances, such as foods, preservatives, or dyes.

Pregnancy—Anabolic steroids are not recommended during pregnancy. They may cause the development of male features in the female fetus and premature growth and development of male features in the male fetus. Be sure you have discussed this with your doctor.

Breast-feeding—It is not known whether anabolic steroids can cause problems in nursing babies. There is very little experience with their use in mothers who are breast-feeding.

Children—Anabolic steroids may cause children to stop growing. In addition, they may make male children develop too fast sexually and may cause male-like changes in female children.

Older adults—When elderly male patients are treated with anabolic steroids, they may have an increased risk of enlarged prostate or cancer of the prostate.

Other medicines—Although certain medicines should not be used together at all, in other cases two different medicines may be used together even if an interaction might occur. In these cases, your doctor may want to change the dose, or other precautions may be necessary. When you are taking anabolic steroids, it is especially important that your doctor and pharmacist know if you are taking any of the following:

- Acetaminophen (e.g., Tylenol) (with long-term, high-dose use) or
- Amiodarone (e.g., Cordarone) or
- Androgens (male hormones) or
- Anti-infectives by mouth or by injection (medicine for infection) or
- Antithyroid agents (medicine for overactive thyroid) or
- Carbamazepine (e.g., Tegretol) or
- Carmustine (e.g., BiCNU) or
- Chloroquine (e.g., Aralen) or
- Dantrolene (e.g., Dantrium) or
- Daunorubicin (e.g., Cerubidine) or
- Disulfiram (e.g., Antabuse) or
- Divalproex (e.g., Depakote) or
- Estrogens (female hormones) or
- Etretinate (e.g., Tegison) or
- Gold salts (medicine for arthritis) or
- Hydroxychloroquine (e.g., Plaquenil) or
- Mercaptopurine (e.g., Purinethol) or
- Methotrexate (e.g., Mexate) or
- Methyldopa (e.g., Aldomet) or
- Naltrexone (e.g., Trexan) (with long-term, high-dose use) or
- Oral contraceptives (birth control pills) containing estrogen or
- Phenothiazines (acetophenazine [e.g., Tindal], chlorpromazine [e.g., Thorazine], fluphenazine [e.g., Prolixin], mesoridazine [e.g., Serentil], perphenazine [e.g., Trilafon], prochlorperazine [e.g., Compazine], promazine [e.g., Sparine], promethazine [e.g., Phenergan], thioridazine

[e.g., Mellaril], trifluoperazine [e.g., Stelazine], triflupromazine [e.g., Vesprin], trimeprazine [e.g., Temaril]) or
- Phenytoin (e.g., Dilantin) or
- Plicamycin (e.g., Mithracin) or
- Valproic acid (e.g., Depakene)—Taking anabolic steroids with any of these medicines may increase the chances of liver damage. Your doctor may want you to have extra blood tests to check for this if you must take both medicines
- Anticoagulants, oral (blood thinners you take by mouth)—Anabolic steroids can increase the effect of these medicines and possibly cause excessive bleeding

Other medical problems—The presence of other medical problems may affect the use of anabolic steroids. Make sure you tell your doctor if you have any other medical problems, especially:
- Breast cancer (in males and some females)
- Diabetes mellitus (sugar diabetes)—Anabolic steroids can decrease blood sugar levels
- Enlarged prostate or
- Prostate cancer—Anabolic steroids may make these conditions worse by causing more enlargement of the prostate or more growth of a tumor
- Heart or blood vessel disease—Anabolic steroids can worsen these conditions by increasing blood cholesterol levels
- Kidney disease
- Liver disease
- Too much calcium in the blood (or history of) (in females)—Anabolic steroids may worsen this condition by raising the amount of calcium in the blood even more

Proper Use of This Medicine

Take this medicine only as directed. Do not take more of it and do not take it more often than your doctor ordered. To do so may increase the chance of side effects.

In order for this medicine to work properly, it is important that you follow a diet high in proteins and calories. If you have any questions about this, check with your doctor, nurse, or pharmacist.

Missed dose—If you miss a dose of this medicine and your dosing schedule is:
- One dose a day—Take the missed dose as soon as possible. However, if you do not remember it until the next day, skip the missed dose and go back to your regular dosing schedule. Do not double doses.
- More than one dose a day—Take the missed dose as soon as possible. However, if it is almost time for your next dose, skip the missed dose and go back to your regular dosing schedule. Do not double doses.

If you have any questions about this, check with your doctor.

Storage—To store this medicine:
- Keep out of the reach of children.
- Store away from heat and direct light.
- Do not store the tablet form of this medicine in the bathroom, near the kitchen sink, or in other damp places. Heat or moisture may cause the medicine to break down.
- Keep the liquid form of this medicine from freezing.
- Do not keep outdated medicine or medicine no longer needed. Be sure that any discarded medicine is out of the reach of children.

Precautions While Using This Medicine

Your doctor should check your progress at regular visits to make sure that this medicine does not cause unwanted effects.

For diabetic patients:
- This medicine may affect blood sugar levels. If you notice a change in the results of your blood or urine sugar tests or if you have any questions, check with your doctor.

Side Effects of This Medicine

Tumors of the liver, liver cancer, or peliosis hepatis, a form of liver disease, have occurred during long-term, high-dose therapy with anabolic steroids. Although these effects are rare, they can be very serious and may cause death. Discuss these possible effects with your doctor.

Along with its needed effects, a medicine may cause some unwanted effects. Although not all of these side effects may occur, if they do occur they may need medical attention.

Check with your doctor immediately if any of the following side effects occur:

For both females and males

Less common

Yellow eyes or skin

Rare (with long-term use)

Black, tarry, or light-colored stools; dark-colored urine; purple- or red-colored spots on body or inside the mouth or nose; sore throat and/or fever; vomiting of blood

Also, check with your doctor as soon as possible if any of the following side effects occur:

For both females and males

Less common

Bone pain; nausea or vomiting; sore tongue; swelling of feet or lower legs; unusual bleeding; unusual weight gain

Rare (with long-term use)

Abdominal or stomach pain; feeling of discomfort (continuing); headache (continuing); hives; loss of appetite (continuing); unexplained weight loss; unpleasant breath odor (continuing)

For females only

More common

Acne or oily skin; enlarging clitoris; hoarseness or deepening of voice; irregular menstrual periods; unnatural hair growth; unusual hair loss

Less common

Mental depression; unusual tiredness

For young males (boys) only

More common

Acne; enlarging penis; increased frequency of erections; unnatural hair growth

Less common

Unexplained darkening of skin

For sexually mature males only

More common

Enlargement of breasts or breast soreness; frequent or continuing erections; frequent urge to urinate

For elderly males only

Less common

Difficult or frequent urination

Other side effects may occur that usually do not need medical attention. These side effects may go away during treatment as your body adjusts to the medicine. However, check with your doctor if any of the following side effects continue or are bothersome:

For both females and males

Less common

Chills; diarrhea; feeling of abdominal or stomach fullness; muscle cramps; trouble in sleeping; unusual decrease or increase in sexual desire

For males only

More common

Acne

Less common

Decreased sexual ability

Other side effects not listed above may also occur in some patients. If you notice any other effects, check with your doctor.

Additional Information

Once a medicine has been approved for marketing for a certain use, experience may show that it is also useful for other medical problems. Although these uses are not included in product labeling, anabolic steroids may be used in certain patients with the following medical conditions:

- Certain blood clotting diseases
- Growth failure
- Turner's syndrome

Other than the above information, there is no additional information relating to proper use, precautions, or side effects for these uses.

Annual revision: 06/20/92

ANDROGENS Systemic

This information applies to the following medicines:

Fluoxymesterone (floo-ox-i-MES-te-rone)
Methyltestosterone (meth-ill-tess-TOSS-te-rone)
Testosterone (tess-TOSS-te-rone)

Some commonly used brand names are:

For Fluoxymesterone

In the U.S.

Android-F
Halotestin
Generic name product may also be available.

In Canada

Halotestin

For Methyltestosterone

In the U.S.

Android-5
Android-10
Android-25
Oreton
Testred
Virilon
Generic name product may also be available.

In Canada

Metandren

For Testosterone

In the U.S.

Andro 100
Andro-Cyp 100
Andro-Cyp 200
Andro L.A. 200
Andronaq-50
Andronaq-LA
Andronate 100
Andronate 200
Andropository 100
Andryl 200
Delatest
Delatestryl
depAndro 100
depAndro 200
Depotest
Depo-Testosterone
Duratest-100
Duratest-200
Durathate-200
Everone
Histerone-50
Histerone-100
T-Cypionate
Testa-C
Testamone 100
Testaqua
Testex
Testoject-50
Testoject-LA
Testone L.A. 100
Testone L.A. 200
Testred Cypionate 200
Testrin P.A.
Virilon IM
Generic name product may also be available.

In Canada

Delatestryl
Depo-Testosterone Cypionate
Malogen
Malogex

Description

Androgens (AN-droe-jens) are male hormones. Some androgens are naturally produced in the body and are necessary for the normal sexual development of males.

Androgens are used for several reasons, such as:

- to replace the hormone when the body is unable to produce enough on its own.
- to stimulate the beginning of puberty in certain boys who are late starting puberty naturally.
- to treat certain types of breast cancer in females.

In addition, some of these medicines may be used for other conditions as determined by your doctor.

Androgens are available only with your doctor's prescription, in the following dosage forms:

Oral

Fluoxymesterone
- Tablets (U.S. and Canada)

Methyltestosterone
- Capsules (U.S.)
- Buccal tablets (U.S. and Canada)
- Oral tablets (U.S. and Canada)

Parenteral

Testosterone
- Injection (U.S. and Canada)

Topical

Testosterone
- Ointment

It is very important that you read and understand the following information. If any of it causes you special concern, check with your doctor. Also, *if you have any questions* or if you want more information about this medicine or your medical problem, *ask your doctor, nurse, or pharmacist.*

Before Using This Medicine

In deciding to use a medicine, the risks of taking the medicine must be weighed against the good it will do. This is a decision you and your doctor will make. For androgens, the following should be considered:

Allergies—Tell your doctor if you have ever had any unusual or allergic reaction to androgens or anabolic steroids. Also tell your doctor and pharmacist if you are allergic to any other substances, such as foods, preservatives, or dyes.

Pregnancy—Androgens are not recommended during pregnancy. They have been shown to cause the development of male features in female babies and premature (too early) development of male features in male babies in humans.

Breast-feeding—Use is not recommended in nursing mothers, since androgens may pass into the breast milk and may cause unwanted effects in the nursing baby, such as premature (too early) sexual development in males and development of male features in female babies.

Children—Androgens may cause children to stop growing. In addition, androgens may make male children develop too fast sexually and may cause male-like changes in female children.

Older adults—When elderly male patients are treated with androgens, they may have an increased risk of enlarged prostate or growth of cancer of the prostate. For this reason, a prostate examination and a blood test to check for prostate cancer is often done before androgens are prescribed for men over the age of 50 years. These examinations may be repeated during treatment.

Other medicines—Although certain medicines should not be used together at all, in other cases two different medicines may be used together even if an interaction might occur. In these cases, your doctor may want to change the dose, or other precautions may be necessary. When you are taking androgens, it is especially important that your doctor and pharmacist know if you are taking any of the following:

- Acetaminophen (e.g., Tylenol) (with long-term, high-dose use) or
- Amiodarone (e.g., Cordarone) or
- Anabolic steroids (nandrolone [e.g., Anabolin], oxandrolone [e.g., Anavar], oxymetholone [e.g., Anadrol], stanozolol [e.g., Winstrol]) or
- Anti-infectives by mouth or by injection (medicine for infection) or
- Antithyroid agents (medicine for overactive thyroid) or
- Carbamazepine (e.g., Tegretol) or
- Carmustine (e.g., BiCNU) or
- Chloroquine (e.g., Aralen) or
- Dantrolene (e.g., Dantrium) or
- Daunorubicin (e.g., Cerubidine) or
- Disulfiram (e.g., Antabuse) or
- Divalproex (e.g., Depakote) or
- Estrogens (female hormones) or
- Etretinate (e.g., Tegison) or
- Gold salts (medicine for arthritis) or
- Hydroxychloroquine (e.g., Plaquenil) or
- Mercaptopurine (e.g., Purinethol) or
- Methotrexate (e.g., Mexate) or
- Methyldopa (e.g., Aldomet) or
- Naltrexone (e.g., Trexan) (with long-term, high-dose use) or
- Oral contraceptives (birth control pills) containing estrogen or
- Phenothiazines (acetophenazine [e.g., Tindal], chlorpromazine [e.g., Thorazine], fluphenazine [e.g., Prolixin], mesoridazine [e.g., Serentil], perphenazine [e.g., Trilafon], prochlorperazine [e.g., Compazine], promazine [e.g., Sparine], promethazine [e.g., Phenergan], thioridazine [e.g., Mellaril], trifluoperazine [e.g., Stelazine], triflupromazine [e.g., Vesprin], trimeprazine [e.g., Temaril]) or
- Phenytoin (e.g., Dilantin) or
- Plicamycin (e.g., Mithracin) or

- Valproic acid (e.g., Depakene)—All of these medicines and androgens can cause liver damage. Your doctor may want you to have extra blood tests that tell about your liver, while you are taking any of these medicines with an androgen.
- Anticoagulants (blood thinners)—Androgens can increase the effect of these medicines and possibly cause excessive bleeding

Other medical problems—The presence of other medical problems may affect the use of androgens. Make sure you tell your doctor if you have any other medical problems, especially:

- Breast cancer (in males) or
- Prostate cancer—Androgens can cause growth of these tumors
- Diabetes mellitus (sugar diabetes)—Androgens can increase blood sugar levels. Careful monitoring of blood glucose should be done
- Edema (swelling of face, hands, feet, or lower legs) or
- Kidney disease or
- Liver disease—These conditions can be worsened by the fluid retention (keeping too much body water) that can be caused by androgens. Also, liver disease can prevent the body from getting the medicine out of the bloodstream as fast as it normally would. This could increase the chance of side effects
- Enlarged prostate—Androgens can cause further enlargement of the prostate
- Heart or blood vessel disease—Androgens can make these conditions worse because androgens may increase blood cholesterol levels. Also, androgens can cause fluid retention (keeping too much body water), which also can worsen heart or blood vessel disease

Before you begin using any new medicine (prescription or nonprescription) or if you develop any new medical problem while you are using this medicine, check with your doctor, nurse, or pharmacist.

Proper Use of This Medicine

For patients taking *fluoxymesterone* or the *capsule or regular tablet form of methyltestosterone*:

- Take this medicine with food to lessen possible stomach upset, unless otherwise directed by your doctor.

For patients using the *buccal tablet form of methyltestosterone:*

- *This medicine should not be swallowed whole.* It is meant to be absorbed through the lining of the mouth. Place the tablet in the upper or lower pouch between your gum and the side of your cheek. Let the tablet slowly dissolve there. Do not eat, drink, chew, or smoke while the tablet is dissolving. It is important that you brush your teeth or thoroughly rinse out your mouth after the tablet has completely dissolved and you can no longer taste it. This will help prevent tooth decay and cavities from the sugar in the tablet, as well as mouth irritation or soreness.

Take this medicine only as directed. Do not take more of it and do not take it more often than your doctor ordered. To do so may increase the chance of side effects.

Missed dose—If you miss a dose of this medicine and your dosing schedule is:

- One dose a day—Take the missed dose as soon as possible. However, if you do not remember it until the next day, skip the missed dose and go back to your regular dosing schedule. Do not double doses.
- More than one dose a day—Take the missed dose as soon as possible. However, if it is almost time for your next dose, skip the missed dose and go back to your regular dosing schedule. Do not double doses.

If you have any questions about this, check with your doctor.

Storage—To store this medicine:

- Keep out of the reach of children.
- Store away from heat and direct light.
- Do not store in the bathroom, near the kitchen sink, or in other damp places. Heat or moisture may cause the medicine to break down.
- Keep the injection form of this medicine from freezing.
- Do not keep outdated medicine or medicine no longer needed. Be sure that any discarded medicine is out of the reach of children.

Precautions While Using This Medicine

Your doctor should check your progress at regular visits to make sure this medicine does not cause unwanted effects.

For *diabetic patients*:

- This medicine may affect blood sugar levels. If you notice a change in the results of your blood or urine sugar tests or if you have any questions, check with your doctor.

Side Effects of This Medicine

Discuss these possible effects with your doctor:

- Tumors of the liver, liver cancer, or peliosis hepatis (a form of liver disease), have occurred during long-term, high-dose therapy with androgens. Although these effects are rare, they can be very serious and may cause death.
- When androgens are used in women, especially in high doses, male-like changes may occur, such as hoarseness or deepening of the voice, unnatural hair growth, or unusual hair loss. Most of these changes will go away if the medicine is stopped as soon as the changes are noticed. However, some changes,

such as voice changes or enlarged clitoris, may not go away.

- When androgens are used in high doses in males, they interfere with the production of sperm. This effect is usually temporary and only happens during the time you are taking the medicine. However, discuss this possible effect with your doctor if you are planning on having children.

Along with its needed effects, a medicine may cause some unwanted effects. Although not all of these side effects appear very often, when they do occur they may require medical attention.

Check with your doctor immediately if any of the following side effects occur:

For both females and males

Less common

Itching of skin; yellow eyes or skin

Rare (with long-term use and/or high doses)

Black, tarry, or light-colored stools; dark-colored urine; purple- or red-colored spots on body or inside the mouth or nose; sore throat or fever; vomiting of blood

Also, check with your doctor as soon as possible if any of the following side effects occur:

For both females and males

Less common

Changes in skin color; confusion; constipation; dizziness; flushing or redness of skin; headache (frequent or continuing); increased thirst; increase in urination; mental depression; nausea or vomiting; swelling of feet or lower legs; unusual bleeding; unusual tiredness; weight gain (rapid)

Rare (with long-term use and/or high doses)

Abdominal or stomach pain (continuing); feeling of discomfort (continuing); hives; loss of appetite (continuing); pain, tenderness, or swelling in the upper abdominal or stomach area; unpleasant breath odor (continuing)

For females only

More common

Acne or oily skin; decreased breast size; enlarged clitoris; hoarseness or deepening of voice; irregular menstrual periods; male type of baldness; unnatural and excessive hair growth

For males only

More common

Breast soreness; enlargement of breasts; frequent or continuing erections; frequent urge to urinate

Less common

Chills; difficult urination; pain in scrotum or groin

For prepubertal boys only

Less common

Acne; early growth of pubic hair; enlargement of penis; increased frequency of erections

Other side effects may occur that usually do not need medical attention. These side effects may go away during treatment as your body adjusts to the medicine. However, check with your doctor if any of the following side effects continue or are bothersome:

For both females and males

Less common

Acne (mild); diarrhea; increase in pubic hair growth; infection, redness, pain, or other irritation at the place of injection (for patients receiving testosterone by injection); irritation or soreness of mouth or unusual watering of mouth (for patients taking buccal tablet form of methyltestosterone); stomach pain; trouble in sleeping; unusual decrease or increase in sexual desire

For males only

Less common

Decrease in testicle size; impotence

Other side effects not listed above may also occur in some patients. If you notice any other effects, check with your doctor.

Additional Information

Once a medicine has been approved for marketing for a certain use, experience may show that it is also useful for other medical problems. Although these uses are not included in product labeling, androgens are used in certain patients with the following medical conditions:

- Anemias (some types of blood diseases)
- Delayed growth spurt
- Development of male features in transsexuals
- Microphallus (under-development of the penis)
- Lichen sclerosus (a skin problem of the vulva)

Other than the above information, there is no additional information relating to proper use, precautions, or side effects for these uses.

Annual revision: 06/30/92

ANDROGENS AND ESTROGENS Systemic

This information applies to the following medicines:

Diethylstilbestrol (dye-eth-il-stil-BESS-trole) and Methyltestosterone (meth-il-tes-TOSS-ter-one)
Estrogens, Conjugated (ESS-troe-jenz, CON-ju-gate-ed), and Methyltestosterone
Estrogens, Esterified (ess-TAIR-i-fyed), and Methyltestosterone
Fluoxymesterone (floo-ox-e-MESS-ter-own) and Ethinyl Estradiol (ETH-in-il ess-tra-DYE-ole)
Testosterone (tess-TOSS-ter-own) and Estradiol

Some commonly used brand names are:

For Diethylstilbestrol and Methyltestosterone
In the U.S.
Tylosterone

Another commonly used name for diethylstilbestrol is DES.

For Estrogens, Conjugated, and Methyltestosterone
In the U.S.
Premarin with Methyltestosterone
In Canada
Premarin with Methyltestosterone

For Estrogens, Esterified, and Methyltestosterone
In the U.S.
Estratest
Estratest H.S.

For Fluoxymesterone and Ethinyl Estradiol
In the U.S.
Halodrin

For Testosterone and Estradiol
In the U.S.

Andrest 90-4	Duo-Gen L.A.
Andro-Estro 90-4	Dura-Dumone 90/4
Androgyn L.A.	Duratestin
De-Comberol	Menoject-L.A.
Deladumone	OB
Delatestadiol	Teev
depAndrogyn	Tes Est Cyp
Depo-Testadiol	Test-Estro Cypionate
Depotestogen	Valertest No. 1
Duo-Cyp	Valertest No. 2

Generic name product may also be available.

In Canada

Climacteron	Neo-Pause
Duogex L.A.	

Description

Androgens (AN-droe-jens) and estrogens (ESS-troe-jens) are hormones. Estrogens are produced by the body in greater amounts in females. They are necessary for normal sexual development of the female and for regulation of the menstrual cycle during the childbearing years. Androgens are produced by the body in greater amounts in males. However, androgens are also present in females in small amounts.

The ovaries and adrenal glands begin to produce less of these hormones after menopause. This combination product is prescribed to make up for this lower production of hormones. This may relieve signs of menopause, such as hot flashes and unusual sweating, chills, faintness, or dizziness.

Androgens and estrogens may also be used for other conditions as determined by your doctor.

There is no medical evidence to support the belief that the use of estrogens (contained in this combination medicine) will keep the patient feeling young, keep the skin soft, or delay the appearance of wrinkles. Nor has it been proven that the use of estrogens during the menopause will relieve emotional and nervous symptoms, unless these symptoms are caused by other menopausal symptoms, such as hot flashes.

A paper called "Information for the Patient" should be given to you with your prescription. Read this carefully. Also, before you use an androgen and estrogen product, you and your doctor should discuss the good that it will do as well as the risks of using it.

This medicine is available only with your doctor's prescription, in the following dosage forms:

Oral

Diethylstilbestrol and Methyltestosterone
- Tablets (U.S.)

Estrogens, Conjugated, and Methyltestosterone
- Tablets (U.S. and Canada)

Estrogens, Esterified, and Methyltestosterone
- Tablets (U.S.)

Fluoxymesterone and Ethinyl Estradiol
- Tablets (U.S.)

Parenteral

Testosterone and Estradiol
- Injection (U.S. and Canada)

It is very important that you read and understand the following information. If any of it causes you special concern, check with your doctor. Also, *if you have any questions* or if you want more information about this medicine or your medical problem, *ask your doctor, nurse, or pharmacist.*

Before Using This Medicine

In deciding to use a medicine, the risks of taking the medicine must be weighed against the good it will do. This is a decision you and your doctor will make. For androgen and estrogen combination products, the following should be considered:

Allergies—Tell your doctor if you have ever had any unusual or allergic reaction to androgens, anabolic steroids, or estrogens. Also tell your doctor and pharmacist if you are allergic to any other substances, such as foods, preservatives, or dyes.

Pregnancy—Estrogens (contained in this combination medicine) are not recommended for use during pregnancy, since some estrogens have been shown to cause serious birth defects in humans. Some daughters of women who took diethylstilbestrol (DES) during pregnancy have developed reproductive (genital) tract problems and, rarely, cancer of the vagina and/or uterine cervix when they reached childbearing age. Some sons of women who took DES during pregnancy have developed urinary-genital tract problems.

Androgens (contained in this combination medicine) should not be used during pregnancy because they may cause male-like changes in a female baby.

Breast-feeding—Use of this medicine is not recommended in nursing mothers. Estrogens pass into the breast milk and their possible effect on the baby is not known. It is not known if androgens pass into breast milk. However, androgens may cause unwanted effects in nursing babies such as too early sexual development in males or male-like changes in females.

Older adults—This medicine has been tested and has not been shown to cause different side effects or problems in older women than it does in younger females.

Other medicines—Although certain medicines should not be used together at all, in other cases two different medicines may be used together even if an interaction might occur. In these cases, your doctor may want to change the dose, or other precautions may be necessary. When you are taking an androgen and estrogen combination product, it is especially important that your doctor and pharmacist know if you are taking any of the following:

- Acetaminophen (e.g., Tylenol) (with long-term, high-dose use) or
- Amiodarone (e.g., Cordarone) or
- Anabolic steroids (nandrolone [e.g., Anabolin], oxandrolone [e.g., Anavar], oxymetholone [e.g., Anadrol], stanozolol [e.g., Winstrol]) or
- Anti-infectives by mouth or by injection (medicine for infection) or
- Antithyroid agents (medicine for overactive thyroid) or
- Carbamazepine (e.g., Tegretol) or
- Carmustine (e.g., BiCNU) or
- Chloroquine (e.g., Aralen) or
- Dantrolene (e.g., Dantrium) or
- Daunorubicin (e.g., Cerubidine) or
- Disulfiram (e.g., Antabuse) or
- Divalproex (e.g., Depakote) or
- Etretinate (e.g., Tegison) or
- Gold salts (medicine for arthritis) or
- Hydroxychloroquine (e.g., Plaquenil) or
- Mercaptopurine (e.g., Purinethol) or
- Methotrexate (e.g., Mexate) or
- Methyldopa (e.g., Aldomet) or
- Naltrexone (e.g., Trexan) (with long-term, high-dose use) or
- Phenothiazines (acetophenazine [e.g., Tindal], chlorpromazine [e.g., Thorazine], fluphenazine [e.g., Prolixin], mesoridazine [e.g., Serentil], perphenazine [e.g., Trilafon], prochlorperazine [e.g., Compazine], promazine [e.g., Sparine], promethazine [e.g., Phenergan], thioridazine [e.g., Mellaril], trifluoperazine [e.g., Stelazine], triflupromazine [e.g., Vesprin], trimeprazine [e.g., Temaril]) or
- Phenytoin (e.g., Dilantin) or
- Plicamycin (e.g., Mithracin) or
- Valproic acid (e.g., Depakene)—Androgens, estrogens, and all of these medicines can cause liver damage. Your doctor may want you to have extra blood tests that tell about your liver, while you are taking any of these medicines with an androgen and estrogen combination product
- Anticoagulants (blood thinners)—Androgens can cause an increased effect of blood thinners, which could lead to uncontrolled or excessive bleeding
- Cyclosporine (e.g., Sandimmune)—Estrogens can increase the chances of toxic effects to the kidney or liver from cyclosporine because estrogens can interfere with the body's ability to get the cyclosporine out of the bloodstream as it normally would

Other medical problems—The presence of other medical problems may affect the use of androgen and estrogen combination products. Make sure you tell your doctor if you have any other medical problems, especially:

- Blood clots (or history of during previous estrogen therapy)—Estrogens may worsen blood clots or cause new clots to form
- Breast cancer (active or suspected)—Estrogens may cause growth of the tumor
- Changes in vaginal bleeding of unknown causes—Some irregular vaginal bleeding is a sign that the lining of the uterus is growing too much or is a sign of cancer of the uterus lining; estrogens may make these conditions worse
- Diabetes mellitus (sugar diabetes)—Androgens can decrease blood sugar levels
- Edema (swelling of feet or lower legs caused by retaining [keeping] too much body water) or
- Heart or circulation disease or
- Kidney disease or
- Liver disease—Androgens can worsen these conditions because androgens cause the body to retain extra fluid (keep too much body water). Also, heart or circulation disease can be worsened by androgens because androgens may increase blood cholesterol levels
- Endometriosis—Estrogens may worsen endometriosis by causing growth of endometriosis implants
- Fibroid tumors of the uterus—Estrogens may cause fibroid tumors to increase in size
- Gallbladder disease or gallstones (or history of)—There is no clear evidence as to whether estrogens increase the risk of gallbladder disease or gallstones
- Jaundice (or history of during pregnancy)—Estrogens use may worsen or cause jaundice in these patients
- Liver disease—Toxic drug effects may occur in patients with liver disease because the body is not able to get this medicine out of the bloodstream as it normally would
- Porphyria—Estrogens can worsen porphyria

Before you begin using any new medicine (prescription or nonprescription) or if you develop any new medical problem while you are using this medicine, check with your doctor, nurse, or pharmacist.

Proper Use of This Medicine

For patients taking any of the androgen and estrogen products by mouth:

- *Take this medicine only as directed by your doctor. Do not take more of it and do not take it for a longer time than your doctor ordered.* Try to take the medicine at the same time each day to reduce the possibility of side effects and to allow it to work better.
- Nausea may occur during the first few weeks after you start taking estrogens. This effect usually disappears with continued use. If the nausea is bothersome, it can usually be prevented or reduced by taking each dose with food or immediately after food.

Missed dose—If you miss a dose of this medicine and your dosing schedule is:

- One dose a day—Take the missed dose as soon as possible. However, if you do not remember it until the next day, skip the missed dose and go back to your regular dosing schedule. Do not double doses.
- More than one dose a day—Take the missed dose as soon as possible. However, if it is almost time for your next dose, skip the missed dose and go back to your regular dosing schedule. Do not double doses.

If you have any questions about this, check with your doctor.

Storage—To store this medicine:

- Keep out of the reach of children.
- Store away from heat and direct light.
- Do not store in the bathroom medicine cabinet because the heat or moisture may cause the medicine to break down.
- Keep the injectable form of this medicine from freezing.
- Do not keep outdated medicine or medicine no longer needed. Be sure that any discarded medicine is out of the reach of children.

Precautions While Using This Medicine

It is very important that your doctor check your progress at regular visits to make sure this medicine does not cause unwanted effects. These visits will usually be every 6 to 12 months, but many doctors require them more often.

It is not yet known whether the use of estrogen increases the risk of breast cancer in women. Therefore, it is very important that you regularly check your breasts for any unusual lumps or discharge. You should also have a mammogram (x-ray picture of the breasts) done if your doctor recommends it.

In some patients using estrogens, tenderness, swelling, or bleeding of the gums may occur. Brushing and flossing your teeth carefully and regularly and massaging your gums may help prevent this. See your dentist regularly to have your teeth cleaned. Check with your medical doctor or dentist if you have any questions about how to take care of your teeth and gums, or if you notice any tenderness, swelling, or bleeding of your gums.

For diabetic patients:

- This medicine may affect blood sugar levels. If you notice a change in the results of your blood or urine sugar tests or if you have any questions, check with your doctor.

If you think that you may have become pregnant, check with your doctor immediately. Continued use of this medicine during pregnancy may cause birth defects or future health problems in the child.

In studies with oral contraceptives (birth control pills) containing estrogens, cigarette smoking during the use of estrogens was shown to cause an increased risk of serious side effects affecting the heart or blood circulation, such as dangerous blood clots, heart attack, or stroke. The risk increased as the amount of smoking and the age of the smoker increased. Women aged 35 and over were at greatest risk when they smoked while using oral contraceptives containing estrogens. It is not known if this risk exists with the use of androgens and estrogens for symptoms of menopause. However, smoking may make estrogens less effective.

Do not give this medicine to anyone else. Your doctor has prescribed it specifically for you after studying your health record and the results of your physical examination. Androgens and estrogens may be dangerous for some people because of differences in their health and body chemistry.

Side Effects of This Medicine

Discuss these possible effects with your doctor:

- Tumors of the liver, liver cancer, and peliosis hepatis (a form of liver disease) have occurred during long-term, high-dose therapy with androgens. Although these effects are rare, they can be very serious and may cause death.
- When androgens are used in women, especially in high doses, male-like changes may occur, such as hoarseness or deepening of the voice, unnatural hair growth, or unusual hair loss. Most of these changes will go away if the medicine is stopped as soon as the changes are noticed. However, some changes, such as voice changes, may not go away.
- The prolonged use of estrogens has been reported to increase the risk of endometrial cancer (cancer of the uterus lining) in women after menopause. The

risk seems to increase as the dose and the length of use increase. When estrogens are used in low doses for less than one year, there is less risk. The risk is also reduced if a progestin (another female hormone) is added to, or replaces part of, your estrogen dose. If the uterus has been removed by surgery (total hysterectomy), there is no risk of endometrial cancer.

- It is not yet known whether the use of estrogens increases the risk of breast cancer in women. Although some large studies show an increased risk, most studies and information gathered to date do not support this idea.

Along with its needed effects, a medicine may cause some unwanted effects. Although not all of these side effects may occur, if they do occur they may need medical attention.

Check with your doctor immediately if any of the following side effects occur:

Less common

Yellow eyes or skin

Rare

Uncontrolled jerky muscle movements; vomiting of blood (with long-term use or high doses)

Also, check with your doctor as soon as possible if any of the following side effects occur:

More common

Acne or oily skin (severe); breast pain or tenderness; changes in vaginal bleeding (spotting, breakthrough bleeding, prolonged or heavier bleeding, or complete stoppage of bleeding); enlarged clitoris; enlargement or decrease in size of breasts; hoarseness or deepening of voice; swelling of feet or lower legs; unnatural hair growth; unusual hair loss; weight gain (rapid)

Less common or rare

Confusion; dizziness; flushing or redness of skin; headaches (frequent or continuing); hives (especially at place of injection); shortness of breath (unexplained); skin rash, hives, or itching; unusual bleeding; unusual tiredness or drowsiness

With long-term use or high doses

Black, tarry, or light-colored stools; dark-colored urine; general feeling of discomfort or illness (continuing); hives (frequent or continuing); loss of appetite (continuing); lump in, or discharge from breast; nausea (severe); pain, swelling, or tenderness in stomach or upper abdomen (continuing); purple- or red-colored spots on body or inside the mouth or nose; sore throat or fever (continuing); unpleasant breath odor (continuing); vomiting (severe)

Other side effects may occur that usually do not need medical attention. These side effects may go away during treatment as your body adjusts to the medicine. However, check with your doctor if any of the following side effects continue or are bothersome:

More common

Bloating of abdomen or stomach; cramps of abdomen or stomach; loss of appetite (temporary); nausea (mild); stomach pain (mild); unusual increase in sexual desire; vomiting (mild)

Less common

Constipation; diarrhea (mild); dizziness (mild); headaches (mild); infection, redness, pain, or other irritation at place of injection; migraine headaches; problems in wearing contact lenses; trouble in sleeping

Also, many women who are taking a progestin (another type of female hormone) with this medicine will begin to have monthly vaginal bleeding again, similar to menstrual periods. This effect will continue for as long as this medicine is used. However, monthly bleeding will not occur in women who have had the uterus removed by surgery (total hysterectomy).

Other side effects not listed above may also occur in some patients. If you notice any other effects, check with your doctor.

Annual revision: 06/30/92

ANESTHETICS Dental

This information applies to the following medicines:

Benzocaine (BEN-zoe-kane)
Butacaine (BYOO-ta-kane)
Dyclonine (DYE-kloe-neen)
Lidocaine (LYE-doe-kane)
Tetracaine (TET-ra-kane)

Some commonly used brand names are:

For Benzocaine

In the U.S.

Americaine
Anbesol Maximum Strength
Baby Anbesol
Baby Orajel
Baby Orajel Nighttime Formula

Benzodent	Orabase-B
Children's Chloraseptic	Orabase-O
Chloraseptic Cool Mint Flavor	Orajel
Hurricaine	Rid-A-Pain
Maximum Strength Orajel	Spec-T
	T-Caine
	Tyrobenz

In Canada

Baby Anbesol	Sabex Teething Syrup
Dentocaine	

Another commonly used name is ethyl aminobenzoate.

For Butacaine

In the U.S.

Butyn

For Dyclonine

In the U.S.

Children's Sucrets	Sucrets Wild Cherry Regular Strength
Sucrets Maximum Strength	

For Lidocaine

In the U.S.

Xylocaine	Xylocaine Viscous

Generic name product may also be available.

In Canada

Xylocaine	Xylocaine Viscous

Another commonly used name is lignocaine.

For Tetracaine*

In Canada

Supracaine

*Dental use product not commercially available in the U.S.

Description

Dental anesthetics (an-ess-THET-iks) are used in the mouth to relieve pain or irritation caused by many conditions. Examples include toothache, teething, and sores in the mouth. Also, some of these medicines are used to relieve pain or irritation caused by dentures or other dental appliances, including braces. However, if you have an infection or a lot of large sores in your mouth, check with your medical doctor or dentist before using a dental anesthetic because other kinds of treatment may be needed. Also, the chance of side effects is increased.

One form of lidocaine is also used to relieve pain caused by certain throat conditions. Some forms of benzocaine and dyclonine are also used to relieve sore throat pain.

Some of these medicines are available only with your medical doctor's or dentist's prescription. Others are available without a prescription; however, your medical doctor or dentist may have special instructions on the proper use and dose for your medical problem.

These medicines are available in the following dosage forms:

Dental

Benzocaine
- Aerosol solution (U.S.)
- Jelly for adults (U.S.)
- Jelly for children (U.S. and Canada)
- Dental paste (U.S.)
- Lozenges for adults (U.S.)
- Lozenges for children (U.S.)

Butacaine
- Dental ointment (U.S.)

Dyclonine
- Lozenges (U.S.)
- Solution (U.S.)

Lidocaine
- Aerosol solution (U.S. and Canada)
- Ointment (U.S. and Canada)
- Solution (U.S. and Canada)

Tetracaine
- Aerosol solution (Canada)

It is very important that you read and understand the following information. If any of it causes you special concern, check with your doctor. Also, *if you have any questions* or if you want more information about this medicine or your medical problem, *ask your doctor, nurse, or pharmacist.*

Before Using This Medicine

If you are taking this medicine without a prescription, carefully read and follow any precautions on the label. For dental anesthetics, the following should be considered:

Allergies—Tell your doctor if you have ever had any unusual or allergic reaction to a local anesthetic, especially one that was applied to any part of the body as a liquid, cream, ointment, or spray. Also tell your doctor and pharmacist if you are allergic to any other substances, such as foods, preservatives, or dyes.

Pregnancy—Dental anesthetics have not been reported to cause birth defects or other problems in humans.

Breast-feeding—Dental anesthetics have not been reported to cause problems in nursing babies.

Children—Children may be especially sensitive to the effects of lidocaine. This may increase the chance of serious side effects during treatment. Also, benzocaine may be absorbed into the bodies of young children and cause unwanted effects. Before benzocaine is used for children under 2 years of age, you should discuss its use with your medical doctor or dentist. Nonprescription (over-the-counter [OTC]) children's products containing local anesthetics are not likely to cause problems in children older than 2 years of age. However, be careful not to give adult-strength products to children, and do not use more medicine than directed on the package label, unless otherwise directed by a medical doctor or a dentist.

Older adults—Elderly people are especially sensitive to the effects of many local anesthetics. This may increase the chance of side effects during treatment, especially with lidocaine. Nonprescription (over-the-counter [OTC]) products containing local anesthetics are not likely to cause problems. However, be careful not to use more medicine than directed on the package label, unless otherwise directed by a medical doctor or a dentist.

Other medicines—Although certain medicines should not be used together at all, in other cases two different medicines may be used together even if an interaction might occur. In these cases, your doctor may want to change the dose, or other precautions may be necessary. Before you use a dental anesthetic, check with your medical doctor, dentist, or pharmacist if you are taking any other prescription or nonprescription (over-the-counter [OTC]) medicine.

Before you begin using any new medicine (prescription or nonprescription) or if you develop any new medical problem while you are using this medicine, check with your doctor, nurse, or pharmacist.

Proper Use of This Medicine

For safe and effective use of this medicine:

- Follow your medical doctor's or dentist's instructions if this medicine was prescribed.
- Follow the manufacturer's package directions if you are treating yourself.
- *Do not use more of this medicine, do not use it more often, and do not use it for a longer time than directed.* To do so may increase the chance of absorption into the body and the chance of side effects. This is particularly important for young children and elderly patients, especially with lidocaine.

For patients using *the viscous (very thick) liquid form of lidocaine* (e.g., Xylocaine Viscous):

- This medicine may cause serious side effects, especially in young children, if too much of it is swallowed. Be certain that you understand exactly how you are to use this medicine, and whether or not you are to swallow it. Also, *be very careful to measure the exact amount of medicine that you are to use.*
- If you are using this medicine for a problem in the mouth, you may apply it to the sore places with a cotton-tipped applicator. Or, you may swish the measured amount of medicine around in your mouth until you are certain that it has reached all of the sore places. *Do not swallow the medicine unless your medical doctor or dentist has told you to do so.*
- If you are using this medicine for a problem in the throat, gargle with the measured amount of medicine as directed by your doctor. *Do not swallow the medicine unless your doctor has told you to do so.*
- If you are using this medicine for a young child, be sure that you understand exactly how this medicine should be used. Follow the medical doctor's or dentist's orders very carefully.

For patients using *aerosol or spray forms of a dental anesthetic*:

- Be very careful not to inhale (breathe in) the medicine, and do not spray the back of your mouth or throat with it, unless your medical doctor or dentist orders you to do so. This helps to prevent unwanted effects.

For patients using *throat lozenge forms of benzocaine or dyclonine:*

- These lozenges should be dissolved slowly in the mouth. Do not bite or chew them.

To use *benzocaine dental paste* (e.g., Orabase-B):

- Do not rub or try to spread the medicine with your finger while you are applying it, because the medicine will become crumbly and gritty. Use a cotton-tipped applicator to dab small amounts of the medicine onto the sore places.

To use the *mouthwash or gargle form of dyclonine* (e.g., Sucrets Maximum Strength):

- This medicine may be swished around in the mouth or gargled, without being swallowed. It may also be sprayed into the mouth, then swallowed. While spraying, be careful not to inhale (breathe in) the medicine. If you will be swallowing the medicine, be very careful not to use more of it than directed by your medical doctor or dentist or recommended on the package label.

Dental anesthetics should be used only for conditions being treated by your medical doctor or dentist or for problems listed in the package directions. *Do not use any of them for other problems without first checking with your medical doctor or dentist.* These medicines should not be used if certain kinds of infections are present.

Missed dose—If your medical doctor or dentist has directed you to use this medicine on a regular schedule, and you miss a dose, use it as soon as possible. However, if it is almost time for your next dose, skip the missed dose and go back to your regular dosing schedule. Do not double doses.

Storage—To store this medicine:

- Keep out of the reach of children.
- Store away from heat and direct light.
- Do not store throat lozenge forms of benzocaine or dyclonine in the bathroom, near the kitchen sink, or in other damp places. Heat or moisture may cause the medicine to break down.
- Keep the medicine from freezing.
- Do not puncture, break, or burn aerosol containers, even when they are empty.
- Do not keep outdated medicine or medicine no longer needed. Be sure that any discarded medicine is out of the reach of children.

Precautions While Using This Medicine

Check with your medical doctor or dentist:

- if you are using this medicine to relieve a sore throat, and the sore throat lasts for more than two days, or if it gets worse or returns.
- if you are using this medicine for any condition other than a sore throat, and your condition does not improve after you have been using this medicine regularly for a few days, or if it becomes worse.
- if you notice any redness, irritation, or sores that were not present before you started using this medicine.

False test results may occur if benzocaine, butacaine, or lidocaine is present in your body when a certain laboratory test is done. This test uses a medicine called bentiromide (e.g., Chymex) to show how well your pancreas is working. You should not use any products containing benzocaine, butacaine, or lidocaine for about 72 hours (3 days) before this test is done.

If you are using this medicine in the back of the mouth, or in the throat, *do not eat or drink anything for one hour after using it.* When this medicine is applied to these areas, it may interfere with swallowing and cause choking.

Do not chew gum or food while your mouth or throat feels numb after you use this medicine. To do so may cause an injury. You may accidentally bite your tongue or the inside of your cheeks.

If you are using this medicine to relieve a toothache, remember that it should not be used for a long time. It is meant to relieve toothache pain temporarily, until the problem causing the toothache can be corrected. *Call your dentist as soon as possible to arrange for treatment.*

Side Effects of This Medicine

Along with its needed effects, a medicine may cause some unwanted effects. Although not all of these side effects may occur, if they do occur they may need medical attention.

Stop using this medicine and check with your medical doctor or dentist immediately if any of the following side effects occur:

Less common or rare

Swellings on skin or in mouth or throat

Signs and symptoms of too much medicine being absorbed by the body

Blurred or double vision; convulsions (seizures); dizziness; drowsiness; increased sweating; ringing or buzzing in the ears; shivering or trembling; slow or irregular heartbeat; unusual anxiety, excitement, nervousness, or restlessness; unusual paleness

Also, check with your medical doctor or dentist as soon as possible if any of the following side effects occur:

Less common or rare

Burning, stinging, swelling, or tenderness not present before treatment; skin rash, redness, itching, or hives in or around the mouth

Other side effects not listed above may also occur in some patients. If you notice any other effects, check with your medical doctor or dentist.

Annual revision: June 1990

ANESTHETICS Ophthalmic

This information applies to the following medicines:

Proparacaine (proe-PARE-a-kane)
Tetracaine (TET-ra-kane)

Some commonly used brand names are:

For Proparacaine

In the U.S.

Ak-Taine
Alcaine
I-Paracaine
Kainair
Ocu-Caine
Ophthaine
Ophthetic
Spectro-Caine

Generic name product may also be available.

In Canada

Ak-Taine
Alcaine
Ophthaine
Ophthetic

Another commonly used name is proxymetacaine.

For Tetracaine

In the U.S.

Pontocaine

Generic name product may also be available.

In Canada

Pontocaine

Generic name product may also be available.

Description

Proparacaine and tetracaine are local anesthetics that are used in the eye to cause numbness or loss of feeling. They are used before certain procedures such as measuring of eye pressure, removing foreign objects or sutures (stitches) from the eye, and performing certain eye examinations.

These medicines are to be administered only by or under the immediate supervision of your doctor. They are available in the following dosage forms:

Ophthalmic

Proparacaine
- Ophthalmic solution (U.S. and Canada)

Tetracaine
- Ophthalmic ointment (U.S.)
- Ophthalmic solution (U.S. and Canada)

It is very important that you read and understand the following information. If any of it causes you special concern, check with your doctor. Also, *if you have any questions* or if you want more information about this medicine or your medical problem, *ask your doctor, nurse, or pharmacist.*

Before Receiving This Medicine

In deciding to use a medicine, the risks of using the medicine must be weighed against the good it will do. This is a decision you and your doctor will make. For local anesthetics used in the eye, the following should be considered:

Allergies—Tell your doctor if you have ever had any unusual or allergic reaction after use of a local anesthetic in the eye. Such a reaction may include severe itching, pain, redness, or swelling of the eye or eyelid, or severe and continuing watering of the eyes.

Also, tell your doctor if you have ever had any unusual or allergic reaction to tetracaine or other local anesthetics, such as benzocaine, butacaine, butamben, chloroprocaine, procaine, or propoxycaine, when given by injection or applied to the skin.

In addition, tell your doctor if you have ever had an allergic reaction to aminobenzoic acid (also called para-aminobenzoic acid [PABA]), or if you are allergic to any other substances, such as foods, preservatives, or dyes.

Pregnancy—Although studies on effects in pregnancy have not been done in either humans or animals, proparacaine and tetracaine have not been reported to cause birth defects or other problems in humans.

Breast-feeding—Proparacaine and tetracaine have not been reported to cause problems in nursing babies.

Children—Although there is no specific information comparing use of ophthalmic anesthetics in children with use in other age groups, these medicines are not expected to cause different side effects or problems in children than they do in adults.

Older adults—Many medicines have not been studied specifically in older people. Therefore, it may not be known whether they work exactly the same way they do in younger adults. Although there is no specific information comparing use of ophthalmic anesthetics in the elderly with use in other age groups, these medicines are not expected to cause different side effects or problems in older people than they do in younger adults.

Other medicines—Although certain medicines should not be used together at all, in other cases two different medicines may be used together even if an interaction might occur. In these cases, your doctor may want to change the dose, or other precautions may be necessary. Before receiving a local anesthetic in the eye, tell your doctor if you are taking any other prescription or nonprescription (over-the-counter [OTC]) medicine.

Other medical problems—The presence of other medical problems may affect the use of local anesthetics in the eye. Make sure you tell your doctor if you have any other medical problems, especially:
- Allergies or
- Heart disease or
- Overactive thyroid—The risk of unwanted effects may be increased

Precautions After Receiving This Medicine

After a local anesthetic is applied to the eye, *do not rub or wipe the eye until the anesthetic has worn off or feeling in the eye returns.* To do so may cause injury or damage to the eye. The effects of these medicines usually last for about 20 minutes. However, if more than one dose is applied, the effects may last longer.

If you get one of these medicines on your fingers, it may cause a rash with dryness and cracking of the skin. If you touch your eye after this medicine has been applied, wash your hands as soon as possible.

Side Effects of This Medicine

Along with its needed effects, a medicine may cause some unwanted effects. Although not all of these side effects may occur, if they do occur they may need medical attention.

Tell your doctor immediately if any of the following side effects occur shortly after this medicine has been applied:

Symptoms of too much medicine being absorbed into the body—very rare

Dizziness or drowsiness; increased sweating; irregular heartbeat; muscle twitching or trembling; nausea or vomiting; shortness of breath or troubled breathing; unusual excitement, nervousness, or restlessness; unusual tiredness or weakness

Other side effects may occur that usually do not need medical attention. Mild stinging or eye irritation may occur as soon as tetracaine is applied or up to several hours after proparacaine is applied. Although these side effects usually are not serious, *check with your doctor as soon as possible if any of the following side effects are severe,* because you may be having an allergic reaction to the medicine. Also, check with your doctor if any of these effects continue or are bothersome:

Less common

Burning, stinging, redness, or other irritation of eye

Rare

Itching, pain, redness, or swelling of the eye or eyelid; watering of eyes

Other side effects not listed above may also occur in some patients. If you notice any other effects, check with your doctor.

Annual revision: 09/14/91

ANESTHETICS Parenteral-Local

This information applies to the following medicines:

- Bupivacaine (byoo-PIV-a-kane)
- Chloroprocaine (klor-oh-PROE-kane)
- Etidocaine (e-TI-doe-kane)
- Etidocaine and Epinephrine (ep-i-NEF-rin)
- Lidocaine (LYE-doe-kane)
- Mepivacaine (me-PIV-a-kane)
- Mepivacaine and Levonordefrin (lee-voe-nor-DEF-rin)
- Prilocaine (PRIL-oh-kane)
- Prilocaine and Epinephrine
- Procaine (PROE-kane)
- Propoxycaine and Procaine (proe-POX-i-kane)
- Tetracaine (TET-ra-kane)

Some commonly used brand names are:

For Bupivacaine

In the U.S.

Marcaine
Marcaine Spinal
Sensorcaine
Sensorcaine-MPF
Sensorcaine-MPF Spinal

Generic name product may also be available.

In Canada

Marcaine

For Chloroprocaine

In the U.S.

Nesacaine
Nesacaine-MPF

Generic name product may also be available.

In Canada

Nesacaine-CE

For Etidocaine

In the U.S.

Duranest
Duranest-MPF

For Lidocaine

In the U.S.

Dalcaine
Dilocaine
L-Caine
Lidoject-1
Lidoject-2
Nervocaine
Octocaine
Xylocaine
Xylocaine-MPF
Xylocaine-MPF with Glucose

Generic name product may also be available.

In Canada

Octocaine-50
Octocaine-100
Xylocaine
Xylocaine with Glucose
Xylocaine Test Dose

Generic name product may also be available.

Another commonly used name is lignocaine.

For Mepivacaine

In the U.S.

Carbocaine
Carbocaine with Neo-Cobefrin
Isocaine
Polocaine
Polocaine-MPF

Generic name product may also be available.

In Canada

Carbocaine
Isocaine 2%
Isocaine 3%
Polocaine

For Prilocaine

In the U.S.

Citanest Forte
Citanest Plain

In Canada

Citanest Forte
Citanest Plain

Generic name product may also be available.

For Procaine

In the U.S.

Novocain

Generic name product may also be available.

In Canada

Novocain

For Propoxycaine and Procaine

In the U.S.

Ravocaine and Novocain with Levophed
Ravocaine and Novocain with Neo-Cobefrin

For Tetracaine

In the U.S.

Pontocaine

In Canada

Pontocaine

Description

Parenteral-local anesthetics (an-ess-THET-iks) are given by injection to cause loss of feeling before and during surgery, dental procedures (including dental surgery), or labor and delivery. These medicines do not cause loss of consciousness.

These medicines are given only by or under the immediate supervision of a medical doctor or dentist, or by a specially trained nurse, in the doctor's office or in a hospital.

These medicines are available in the following dosage forms:

Parenteral

Bupivacaine
- Injection (U.S. and Canada)

Chloroprocaine
- Injection (U.S. and Canada)

Etidocaine
- Injection (U.S.)

Lidocaine
- Injection (U.S. and Canada)

Mepivacaine
- Injection (U.S. and Canada)

Prilocaine
- Injection (U.S. and Canada)

Procaine
- Injection (U.S. and Canada)

Propoxycaine and Procaine
- Injection (U.S.)

Tetracaine
- Injection (U.S. and Canada)

Before Receiving This Medicine

In deciding to use a medicine, the risks of using the medicine must be weighed against the good it will do. This is a decision you and your medical doctor, dentist, or nurse will make. For local anesthetics, the following should be considered:

Allergies—Tell your medical doctor, dentist, or nurse if you have ever had any unusual or allergic reaction to a local anesthetic or to epinephrine (e.g., Adrenalin). Also tell your medical doctor, dentist, nurse, or pharmacist if you are allergic to any other substances, such as sulfites or other preservatives, especially aminobenzoic acid (also called para-aminobenzoic acid [PABA]).

Pregnancy—Local anesthetics have not been reported to cause birth defects in humans.

Use of a local anesthetic during labor and delivery may rarely cause unwanted effects. These medicines may increase the length of labor by making it more difficult for the mother to bear down (push). They may also cause unwanted effects in the fetus or newborn baby, especially if certain medical problems are present at the time of delivery. Before receiving a local anesthetic for labor and delivery, you should discuss with your doctor the good that this medicine will do as well as the risks of receiving it.

Breast-feeding—It is not known whether local anesthetics pass into the breast milk. However, these medicines have not been reported to cause problems in nursing babies.

Children—Children may be especially sensitive to the effects of parenteral-local anesthetics. This may increase the chance of side effects.

Older adults—Elderly people are especially sensitive to the effects of parenteral-local anesthetics. This may increase the chance of side effects.

Other medicines—Although certain medicines should not be used together at all, in other cases two different medicines may be used together even if an interaction might occur. In these cases, your medical doctor, dentist, or nurse may want to change the dose, or other precautions may be necessary. It is very important that you tell the person in charge if you are taking:

- Any other medicine, prescription or nonprescription (over-the-counter [OTC]), or
- "Street" drugs, such as amphetamines ("uppers"), barbiturates ("downers"), cocaine (including "crack"), marijuana, phencyclidine (PCP, "angel dust"), and heroin or other narcotics—Serious side effects may occur if anyone gives you a local anesthetic without knowing that you have taken another medicine

Other medical problems—The presence of other medical problems may affect the use of local anesthetics. Make sure you tell your medical doctor, dentist, or nurse if you have *any* other medical problems, especially:

- Malignant hyperthermia (very high fever, fast and irregular heartbeat, muscle spasms or tightness, and breathing problems occurring during, or soon after, use of an anesthetic) (history of, in yourself or in any close relative)—The chance of an attack of malignant hyperthermia is increased. Some anesthetics are more likely than others to cause this unwanted effect. Your medical doctor, dentist, or nurse will want to avoid using them

Precautions After Receiving This Medicine

For patients going home before the numbness or loss of feeling caused by a local anesthetic wears off:

- During the time that the injected area feels numb, serious injury can occur without your knowing about it. Be especially careful to avoid injury until the anesthetic wears off or feeling returns to the area.
- If you have received a local anesthetic injection in your mouth, do not chew gum or food while your mouth feels numb. You may injure yourself by biting your tongue or the inside of your cheeks.

Side Effects of This Medicine

Along with its needed effects, a medicine may cause some unwanted effects. Although not all of these side effects may occur, if they do occur they may need medical attention. While you are in the hospital or your medical doctor's or dentist's office, your medical doctor, dentist, or nurse will carefully follow the effects of any medicine you have received. However, some effects may not be noticed until later.

Check with your doctor immediately if any of the following side effects occur:

Less common or rare

Skin rash, hives, or itching

Also, check with your dentist if you have received a local anesthetic for dental work, and the feeling of numbness or tingling in your lips and mouth does not go away within a few hours, or if you have difficulty in opening your mouth.

Other side effects not listed above may also occur in some patients. If you notice any other effects, check with your medical doctor or dentist.

Annual revision: 01/30/92

ANESTHETICS Rectal

This information applies to the following medicines:

Benzocaine (BEN-zoe-kane)
Dibucaine (DYE-byoo-kane)
Pramoxine (pra-MOX-een)
Tetracaine (TET-ra-kane)

Some commonly used brand names are:

For Benzocaine

Americaine Hemorrhoidal

Another commonly used name is ethyl aminobenzoate.

For Dibucaine

Nupercainal

Generic name product may also be available.

Another commonly used name is cinchocaine.

For Pramoxine

Fleet Relief
ProctoFoam/non-steroid
Tronolane
Tronothane

Another commonly used name is pramocaine.

For Tetracaine

Pontocaine Cream

For Tetracaine and Menthol

Pontocaine Ointment

Description

Rectal anesthetics (an-ess-THET-iks) are used to relieve the pain and itching of hemorrhoids (piles) and other rectal disorders. However, if you have hemorrhoids that bleed, especially after a bowel movement, check with your doctor before using this medicine. Bleeding may mean that you have a condition that needs other treatment.

These medicines are available without a prescription; however, your doctor may have special instructions on the proper use and dose for your medical problem.

These medicines are available in the following dosage forms:

Rectal

Benzocaine
- Ointment (U.S.)

Dibucaine
- Ointment (U.S. and Canada)

Pramoxine
- Aerosol foam (U.S.)
- Cream (U.S. and Canada)
- Ointment (U.S.)
- Suppositories (U.S.)

Tetracaine
- Cream (U.S.)

Tetracaine and Menthol
- Ointment (U.S.)

It is very important that you read and understand the following information. If any of it causes you special concern, check with your doctor. Also, *if you have any questions* or if you want more information about this medicine or your medical problem, *ask your doctor, nurse, or pharmacist.*

Before Using This Medicine

If you are taking this medicine without a prescription, carefully read and follow any precautions on the label. For rectal anesthetics, the following should be considered:

Allergies—Tell your doctor if you have ever had any unusual or allergic reaction to a local anesthetic, especially one that was applied to any part of the body as a liquid, cream, ointment, or spray. Also tell your doctor and pharmacist if you are allergic to any other substances, such as foods, preservatives, or dyes.

Pregnancy—Rectal anesthetics have not been reported to cause birth defects or other problems in humans.

Breast-feeding—Rectal anesthetics have not been reported to cause problems in nursing babies.

Children—Children may be especially sensitive to the effects of local anesthetics. This may increase the chance of side effects during treatment.

Older adults—Elderly people are especially sensitive to the effects of local anesthetics. This may increase the chance of side effects during treatment.

Other medicines—Although certain medicines should not be used together at all, in other cases two different medicines may be used together even if an interaction might occur. In these cases, your doctor may want to change the dose, or other precautions may be necessary. Before you use a rectal anesthetic, check with your doctor or pharmacist if you are taking any other prescription or nonprescription (over-the-counter [OTC]) medicine.

Other medical problems—The presence of other medical problems may affect the use of rectal anesthetics. Make sure you tell your doctor if you have any other medical problems, especially:

- Infection at or near place of treatment or
- Large sores, broken skin, or severe injury at or near place of treatment—The chance of unwanted effects may be increased

Before you begin using any new medicine (prescription or nonprescription) or if you develop any new medical problem while you are using this medicine, check with your doctor, nurse, or pharmacist.

Proper Use of This Medicine

For safe and effective use of this medicine:

- Follow your doctor's instructions if this medicine was prescribed.
- Follow the manufacturer's package directions if you are treating yourself.
- *Do not use more of this medicine, do not use it more often, and do not use it for a longer time than directed.* To do so may increase the chance of absorption into the body and the chance of unwanted effects.

To use the *rectal ointment or cream:*

- This medicine usually comes with patient directions. Read them carefully before using this medicine.
- This medicine may be applied with a "finger cot" or the applicator that comes in the package.
- If you use the applicator, wash it carefully after each use.
- If you are using the product that comes in pre-filled applicators, each applicator is meant to be used only once. Throw the applicator away after using it.

To use *pramoxine aerosol rectal foam* (e.g., Proctofoam/non-steroid):

- This medicine usually comes with patient directions. Read them carefully before using this medicine.
- This medicine is used with a special applicator. Do not insert any part of the aerosol container into the rectum.
- Take the applicator apart and wash it carefully after each use.

To use *suppositories:*

- If the suppository is too soft to insert, chill it in the refrigerator for 30 minutes or run cold water over it before removing the foil wrapper.
- To insert the suppository: First remove the foil wrapper and moisten the suppository with cold water. Lie down on your side and use your finger to push the suppository well up into the rectum.

This medicine should be used only for conditions being treated by your doctor or for problems listed on the package label. *Do not use it for other problems without first checking with your doctor.* This medicine should not be used if certain kinds of infections are present.

Missed dose—If your doctor has directed you to use this medicine on a regular schedule and you miss a dose, use it as soon as possible. However, if it is almost time for your next dose, skip the missed dose and go back to your regular dosing schedule.

Storage—To store this medicine:

- Keep out of the reach of children.
- Store away from heat and direct light.
- Keep the medicine from freezing.
- Do not puncture, break, or burn the pramoxine aerosol foam container, even after it is empty.
- Do not keep outdated medicine or medicine no longer needed. Be sure that any discarded medicine is out of the reach of children.

Precautions While Using This Medicine

Check with your doctor:

- If your condition does not improve after you have been using this medicine regularly for a few days, or if it becomes worse.
- If you notice any rash, redness, or irritation that was not present before you started using this medicine.

False test results may occur if benzocaine or tetracaine is present in your body when a certain laboratory test is done. This test uses a medicine called bentiromide (e.g., Chymex) to show how well your pancreas is working. You should not use any products containing benzocaine or tetracaine for about 72 hours (3 days) before this test is done.

Side Effects of This Medicine

Along with its needed effects, a medicine may cause some unwanted effects. Although not all of these side effects may occur, if they do occur they may need medical attention.

Stop using this medicine and check with your doctor immediately if any of the following side effects occur:

Signs and symptoms of too much medicine being absorbed by the body

Blurred or double vision; convulsions (seizures); dizziness; drowsiness; increased sweating; ringing or buzzing in ears; shivering or trembling; slow or irregular heartbeat; unusual anxiety, excitement, nervousness, or restlessness; unusual paleness

Also, check with your doctor as soon as possible if any of the following side effects occur:

Less common

Burning, stinging, swelling, or tenderness not present before treatment; skin rash, redness, itching, or hives at or near place of application

Other side effects not listed above may also occur in some patients. If you notice any other effects, check with your doctor.

Annual revision: June 1990

ANESTHETICS Topical

This information applies to the following medicines:

Benzocaine (BEN-zoe-kane)
Benzocaine and Menthol (MEN-thol)
Butamben (byoo-TAM-ben)
Dibucaine (DYE-byoo-kane)
Lidocaine (LYE-doe-kane)
Pramoxine (pra-MOX-een)
Pramoxine and Menthol
Tetracaine (TET-ra-kane)
Tetracaine and Menthol

Some commonly used brand names are:

For Benzocaine
In the U.S
Americaine
Benzocol
Generic name product may also be available.

Another commonly used name is ethyl aminobenzoate.

For Benzocaine and Menthol
In the U.S.
Dermoplast
In Canada
Dermoplast

For Butamben
In the U.S.
Butesin Picrate

Another commonly used name is butyl aminobenzoate.

For Dibucaine
In the U.S.
Nupercainal Cream
Nupercainal Ointment
Generic name product may also be available.
In Canada
Nupercainal Ointment

Another commonly used name is cinchocaine.

For Lidocaine
In the U.S.
Xylocaine
Generic name product may also be available.
In Canada
Xylocaine

Another commonly used name is lignocaine.

For Pramoxine
In the U.S.
Prax
Tronothane
In Canada
Tronothane

Another commonly used name is pramocaine.

For Pramoxine and Menthol
In the U.S.
Pramegel
In Canada
Pramegel

For Tetracaine
In the U.S.
Pontocaine Cream

For Tetracaine and Menthol
In the U.S.
Pontocaine Ointment

Description

This medicine belongs to a group of medicines known as topical local anesthetics (an-ess-THET-iks). Topical anesthetics are used to relieve the pain, itching, and redness of minor skin disorders. These include sunburn or other minor burns, insect bites or stings, poison ivy, poison oak, poison sumac, and minor cuts and scratches.

Topical anesthetics deaden the nerve endings in the skin. They do not cause unconsciousness as general anesthetics used for surgery do.

Most topical anesthetics are available without a prescription; however, your doctor may have special instructions on the proper use and dose for your medical problem.

These medicines are available in the following dosage forms:

Topical

Benzocaine
- Cream (U.S.)
- Ointment (U.S.)
- Topical aerosol solution (U.S.)

Benzocaine and Menthol
- Lotion (U.S.)
- Topical aerosol solution (U.S. and Canada)

Butamben
- Ointment (U.S.)

Dibucaine
- Cream (U.S.)
- Ointment (U.S. and Canada)

Lidocaine
- Ointment (U.S. and Canada)

Pramoxine
- Cream (U.S. and Canada)
- Lotion (U.S.)

Pramoxine and Menthol
- Gel (U.S. and Canada)

Tetracaine
- Cream (U.S.)

Tetracaine and Menthol
- Ointment (U.S.)

It is very important that you read and understand the following information. If any of it causes you special concern, check with your doctor or pharmacist. Also, *if you have any questions* or if you want more information about this medicine or your medical problem, *ask your doctor, nurse, or pharmacist.*

Before Using This Medicine

If you are using this medicine without a prescription, carefully read and follow any precautions on the label. For topical anesthetics, the following should be considered:

Allergies—Tell your doctor if you have ever had any unusual or allergic reaction to a local anesthetic, especially when applied to the skin or other areas of the body. Also tell your doctor and pharmacist if you are allergic to any other substances, such as foods, preservatives, or dyes, especially aminobenzoic acid (also called para-aminobenzoic acid [PABA]), to parabens (preservatives in many foods and medicines), or to paraphenylenediamine (a hair dye).

Pregnancy—Although studies on effects in pregnancy have not been done in humans, topical anesthetics have not been reported to cause problems in humans. Lidocaine has not been shown to cause birth defects or other problems in animal studies. Other topical anesthetics have not been studied in animals.

Breast-feeding—Topical anesthetics have not been reported to cause problems in nursing babies.

Children—Benzocaine may be absorbed through the skin of young children and cause unwanted effects. Before benzocaine is used for children under 2 years of age, you should discuss its use with your child's doctor. There is no specific information comparing use of other topical anesthetics in children with use in other age groups.

Older adults—Many medicines have not been studied specifically in older people. Therefore, it may not be known whether they work exactly the same way they do in younger adults or if they cause different side effects or problems in older people. There is no specific information comparing use of topical anesthetics in the elderly with use in other age groups.

Other medicines—Although certain medicines should not be used together at all, in other cases two different medicines may be used together even if an interaction might occur. In these cases, your doctor may want to change the dose, or other precautions may be necessary. Tell your doctor or pharmacist if you are taking any other prescription or nonprescription (over-the-counter [OTC]) medicine.

Other medical problems—The presence of other medical problems may affect the use of topical anesthetics. Before using a topical anesthetic, check with your doctor or pharmacist if you have any other medical problems, especially:
- Infection at or near the place of application or
- Large sores, broken skin, or severe injury at the area of application—The chance of side effects may be increased

Before you begin using any new medicine (prescription or nonprescription) or if you develop any new medical problem while you are using this medicine, check with your doctor, nurse, or pharmacist.

Proper Use of This Medicine

For safe and effective use of this medicine:
- Follow your doctor's instructions if this medicine was prescribed.
- Follow the manufacturer's package directions if you are treating yourself.
- Unless otherwise directed by your doctor, *do not use this medicine on large areas, especially if the skin is broken or scraped. Also, do not use it more often than directed on the package label, or for more than a few days at a time.* To do so may increase the chance of absorption through the skin and the chance of unwanted effects. This is especially important when benzocaine is used for children younger than 2 years of age.

This medicine should be used only for problems being treated by your doctor or conditions listed in the package directions. *Check with your doctor before using it for other problems, especially if you think that an infection may be present.* This medicine should not be used to treat certain kinds of skin infections or serious problems, such as severe burns.

Read the package label very carefully to see if the product contains any alcohol. Alcohol is flammable and can catch on fire. *Do not use any product containing alcohol near a fire or open flame, or while smoking. Also, do not smoke after applying one of these products until it has completely dried.*

If you are using this medicine on your face, *be very careful not to get it in your eyes.* If you are using an aerosol or spray form of this medicine, spray it on your hand or an applicator (for example, a sterile gauze pad or a cotton swab) before applying it to your face.

For patients using *butamben:*

- Butamben may stain clothing. To avoid this, do not touch your clothing while applying the medicine. Also, cover the treated area with a loose bandage after applying butamben, to protect your clothes.

Missed dose—If your doctor has ordered you to use this medicine according to a regular schedule and you miss a dose, use it as soon as possible. However, if it is almost time for your next dose, skip the missed dose and use your next dose at the regularly scheduled time.

Storage—To store this medicine:

- Keep out of the reach of children.
- Store away from heat and direct light.
- Keep the medicine from freezing.
- Do not puncture, break, or burn aerosol containers, even when they are empty.
- Do not keep outdated medicine or medicine no longer needed. Be sure that any discarded medicine is out of the reach of children.

Precautions While Using This Medicine

Stop using this medicine and check with your doctor:

- *If your condition does not improve within a few days, or if it gets worse.*
- *If the area you are treating becomes infected.*
- *If you notice a skin rash, burning, stinging, swelling, or any other sign of irritation that was not present when you began using this medicine.*
- *If you swallow any of the medicine.*

Side Effects of This Medicine

Along with its needed effects, a medicine may cause some unwanted effects. Although not all of these side effects may occur, if they do occur they may need medical attention.

Check with your doctor immediately if any of the following side effects occur:

Less common

Swellings on skin, mouth, or throat (large)

Symptoms of too much medicine being absorbed by the body—very rare

Blurred or double vision; convulsions (seizures); dizziness; drowsiness; increased sweating; ringing or buzzing in the ears; shivering or trembling; slow or irregular heartbeat; unusual anxiety, excitement, nervousness, or restlessness; unusual paleness

Also, check with your doctor as soon as possible if any of the following side effects occur:

Burning, stinging, or tenderness not present before treatment; skin rash, redness, itching, or hives

Other side effects not listed above may also occur in some patients. If you notice any other effects, check with your doctor.

Annual revision: 09/14/91

ANESTHETICS, GENERAL Systemic

This information applies to the following medicines:

Enflurane (EN-floo-rane)
Etomidate (e-TOM-i-date)
Halothane (HA-loe-thane)
Isoflurane (eye-soe-FLURE-ane)
Ketamine (KEET-a-meen)
Methohexital (meth-oh-HEX-i-tal)
Methoxyflurane (meth-ox-ee-FLOO-rane)
Nitrous (NYE-trus) Oxide
Propofol (PROE-po-fole)
Thiamylal (thye-AM-i-lal)
Thiopental (thye-oh-PEN-tal)

Some commonly used brand names are:

For Enflurane

In the U.S.

Ēthrane

Generic name product may also be available.

In Canada

Ēthrane

For Etomidate†

In the U.S.

Amidate

For Halothane

In the U.S.

Fluothane

Generic name product may also be available.

In Canada

Fluothane Somnothane

For Isoflurane

In the U.S.

Forane

In Canada
Forane

For Ketamine
In the U.S.
Ketalar

In Canada
Ketalar

For Methohexital
In the U.S.
Brevital

In Canada
Brietal

Another commonly used name is methohexitone.

For Methoxyflurane
In the U.S.
Penthrane

For Nitrous Oxide
In the U.S.
Generic name product available.

In Canada
Generic name product available.

For Propofol
In the U.S.
Diprivan

In Canada
Diprivan

For Thiamylal
In the U.S.
Surital

In Canada
Surital

For Thiopental
In the U.S.
Pentothal
Generic name product may also be available.

In Canada
Pentothal

Another commonly used name is thiopentone.

---

†Not commercially available in Canada.

Description

General anesthetics (an-ess-THET-iks) are normally used to produce loss of consciousness before and during surgery. However, for obstetrics (labor and delivery) or certain minor procedures, an anesthetic may be given in small amounts to relieve anxiety or pain without causing unconsciousness. Also, some of the anesthetics may be used for certain procedures in a medical doctor's or dentist's office.

Some barbiturate (bar-BI-tyoo-rate) anesthetics (thiamylal and thiopental) are also sometimes used to control convulsions (seizures) caused by certain medicines or seizure disorders. Thiopental may be used to reduce pressure on the brain in certain conditions. Barbiturate anesthetics may also be used for other conditions as determined by your doctor.

General anesthetics are usually given by inhalation or by injection into a vein. However, certain barbiturate anesthetics may be given rectally to help produce sleep before surgery or certain procedures. Although most general anesthetics can be used by themselves in producing loss of consciousness, some are often used together. This allows for more effective anesthesia in certain patients.

General anesthetics are given only by or under the immediate supervision of a medical doctor or dentist trained to use them. If you will be receiving a general anesthetic during surgery, your doctor or anesthesiologist will give you the medicine and closely follow your progress.

General anesthetics are available in the following dosage forms:

Inhalation

Enflurane
- Inhalation (U.S. and Canada)

Halothane
- Inhalation (U.S. and Canada)

Isoflurane
- Inhalation (U.S. and Canada)

Methoxyflurane
- Inhalation (U.S.)

Nitrous oxide
- Inhalation (U.S. and Canada)

Parenteral

Etomidate
- Injection (U.S.)

Ketamine
- Injection (U.S. and Canada)

Methohexital
- Injection (U.S. and Canada)

Propofol
- Injection (U.S. and Canada)

Thiamylal
- Injection (U.S. and Canada)

Thiopental
- Injection (U.S. and Canada)

Rectal

Methohexital
- Rectal solution (U.S. and Canada)

Thiamylal
- Rectal solution (U.S and Canada)

Thiopental
- Rectal solution (U.S. and Canada)
- Rectal suspension (U.S.)

It is very important that you read and understand the following information. If any of it causes you special concern, check with your doctor. Also, *if you have any questions* or if you want more information about this medicine or your medical problem, *ask your doctor, nurse, or pharmacist.*

Before Receiving This Medicine

In deciding to use a medicine, the risks of taking the medicine must be weighed against the good it will do. This is a decision you and your doctor will make. For general anesthetics, the following should be considered:

Allergies—Tell your doctor if you have ever had any unusual or allergic reaction to barbiturates or general anesthetics. Also tell your doctor and pharmacist if you are allergic to any other substances, such as foods, preservatives, or dyes.

Pregnancy—

- *For barbiturate anesthetics (methohexital, thiamylal, and thiopental)*—Methohexital has not been studied in pregnant women. However, it has not been shown to cause birth defects or other problems in animal studies. Studies on effects in pregnancy with thiamylal and thiopental have not been done in either humans or animals. However, use of barbiturate anesthetics during pregnancy may affect the nervous system in the fetus.
- *For etomidate*—Etomidate has not been studied in pregnant women. Although studies in animals have not shown etomidate to cause birth defects, it has been shown to cause other unwanted effects in the animal fetus when given in doses usually many times the human dose.
- *For inhalation anesthetics (enflurane, halothane, isoflurane, methoxyflurane, and nitrous oxide)*—Enflurane, halothane, isoflurane, methoxyflurane, and nitrous oxide have not been studied in pregnant women. However, studies in animals have shown that inhalation anesthetics may cause birth defects or other harm to the fetus.

  When used as an anesthetic for an abortion, enflurane, halothane, or isoflurane may cause increased bleeding.

  When used in small doses to relieve pain during labor and delivery, halothane may slow delivery and increase bleeding in the mother after the baby is born. These effects do not occur with small doses of enflurane, isoflurane, or methoxyflurane. However, they may occur with large doses of these anesthetics.
- *For ketamine*—Ketamine has not been studied in pregnant women. Studies in animals have not shown that ketamine causes birth defects, but it caused damage to certain tissues when given in large amounts for a long period of time.
- *For propofol*—Propofol has not been studied in pregnant women. Although studies in animals have not shown propofol to cause birth defects, it has been shown to cause deaths in nursing mothers and their offspring when given in doses usually many times the human dose.

General anesthetics may cause unwanted effects, such as drowsiness, in the newborn baby if large amounts are given to the mother during labor and delivery.

Breast-feeding—Barbiturate anesthetics (methohexital, thiamylal, and thiopental), halothane, and propofol pass into the breast milk. However, general anesthetics have not been reported to cause problems in nursing babies.

Children—Anesthetics given by inhalation and ketamine have been tested in children and have not been shown to cause different side effects or problems in children than they do in adults.

Although there is no specific information comparing use of barbiturate anesthetics (methohexital, thiamylal, and thiopental), etomidate, or propofol in children with use in other age groups, these medicines are not expected to cause different side effects or problems in children than they do in adults.

Older adults—Elderly people are especially sensitive to the effects of the barbiturate anesthetics (methohexital, thiamylal, and thiopental), etomidate, propofol, and anesthetics given by inhalation. This may increase the chance of side effects.

Ketamine has not been shown to cause different side effects or problems in older people than it does in younger adults.

Other medicines—Although certain medicines should not be used together at all, in other cases 2 different medicines may be used together even if an interaction might occur. In these cases, your doctor may want to change the dose, or other precautions may be necessary. When you are receiving general anesthetics, it is especially important that your doctor and pharmacist know if you are taking any of the following:

- "Street" drugs, such as amphetamines ("uppers"), barbiturates ("downers"), cocaine, marijuana, phencyclidine (PCP or "angel dust"), and heroin or other narcotics—Serious, possibly fatal, side effects may occur if your medical doctor or dentist gives you an anesthetic without knowing that you have taken another medicine

Other medical problems—The presence of other medical problems may affect the use of general anesthetics. Make sure you tell your doctor if you have any other medical problems, especially:

- Malignant hyperthermia, during or shortly after receiving an anesthetic (history of, or family history of). Signs of malignant hyperthermia include very high fever, fast and irregular heartbeat, muscle spasms or tightness, and breathing problems—This side effect may occur again

Before you begin using any new medicine (prescription or nonprescription) or if you develop any new medical problem while you are receiving this medicine, check with your doctor, nurse, or pharmacist.

Precautions After Receiving This Medicine

For patients going home within 24 hours after receiving a general anesthetic:

- General anesthetics may cause some people to feel drowsy, tired, or weak for up to a few days after they have been given. They may also cause problems with coordination and one's ability to think. Therefore, for at least 24 hours (or longer if necessary) *after receiving a general anesthetic, do not drive, use machines, or do anything else that could be dangerous if you are not alert.*

- Unless otherwise directed by your medical doctor or dentist, *do not drink alcoholic beverages or take other CNS depressants (medicines that slow down the nervous system, possibly causing drowsiness) for about 24 hours after you have received a general anesthetic.* To do so may add to the effects of the anesthetic. Some examples of CNS depressants are antihistamines or medicine for hay fever, other allergies, or colds; other sedatives, tranquilizers, or sleeping medicine; prescription pain medicine or narcotics; other barbiturates; medicine for seizures; and muscle relaxants.

Side Effects of This Medicine

Along with its needed effects, a medicine may cause some unwanted effects. Although not all of these side effects may occur, if they do occur they may need medical attention. While you are receiving a general anesthetic, your doctor will closely follow its effects. However, some effects may not be noticed until later.

Check with your doctor as soon as possible if any of the following side effects occur within 2 weeks after you have received an anesthetic:

Rare

Abdominal or stomach pain; back or leg pain; black or bloody vomit; fever; headache (severe); increase or decrease in amount of urine; loss of appetite; nausea (severe); pale skin; unusual tiredness or weakness; weakness of wrist and fingers; weight loss (unusual); yellow eyes or skin

Other side effects may occur that usually do not need medical attention. The following side effects may go away as the effects of the anesthetic wear off. However, check with your doctor if any of the following side effects continue or are bothersome:

More common

Shivering or trembling

Less common

Blurred or double vision or other vision problems; dizziness, lightheadedness, or feeling faint; drowsiness; headache; mood or mental changes; nausea (mild) or vomiting; nightmares or unusual dreams

Other side effects not listed above may also occur in some patients. If you notice any other effects, check with your doctor.

Additional Information

Once a medicine has been approved for marketing for a certain use, experience may show that it is also useful for other medical problems. Although these uses are not included in product labeling, thiopental is used in certain patients with the following medical conditions:

- Hypoxia, cerebral (shortage of oxygen supplied to the brain) or
- Ischemia, cerebral (shortage of blood supplied to the brain)

Other than the above information, there is no additional information relating to proper use, precautions, or side effects for these uses.

Annual revision: 07/22/91

ANGIOTENSIN-CONVERTING ENZYME (ACE) INHIBITORS Systemic

This information applies to the following medicines:

Benazepril (ben-AY-ze-pril)
Captopril (KAP-toe-pril)
Enalapril (e-NAL-a-pril)
Enalaprilat (e-NAL-a-pril-at)
Fosinopril (foe-SIN-oh-pril)
Lisinopril (lyse-IN-oh-pril)
Quinapril (KWIN-a-pril)
Ramipril (ra-MI-pril)

Some commonly used brand names are:

For Benazepril†
In the U.S.
Lotensin

For Captopril
In the U.S.
Capoten
In Canada
Capoten

For Enalapril
In the U.S.
Vasotec
In Canada
Vasotec

For Enalaprilat
In the U.S.
Vasotec
In Canada
Vasotec

For Fosinopril†
In the U.S.
Monopril

For Lisinopril
In the U.S.
Prinivil
Zestril
In Canada
Prinivil
Zestril

For Quinapril†
In the U.S.
Accupril

For Ramipril†
In the U.S.
Altace

†Not commercially available in Canada.

Description

ACE inhibitors belong to the class of medicines called high blood pressure medicines (antihypertensives). They are used to treat high blood pressure (hypertension).

High blood pressure adds to the workload of the heart and arteries. If it continues for a long time, the heart and arteries may not function properly. This can damage the blood vessels of the brain, heart, and kidneys, resulting in a stroke, heart failure, or kidney failure. High blood pressure may also increase the risk of heart attacks. These problems may be less likely to occur if blood pressure is controlled.

Some of these medicines are also used to treat congestive heart failure.

These medicines may also be used for other conditions as determined by your doctor.

The exact way that these medicines work is not known. They block an enzyme in the body that is necessary to produce a substance that causes blood vessels to tighten. As a result, they relax blood vessels. This lowers blood pressure and increases the supply of blood and oxygen to the heart.

These medicines are available only with your doctor's prescription, in the following dosage forms:

Oral

Benazepril
- Tablets (U.S.)

Captopril
- Tablets (U.S. and Canada)

Enalapril
- Tablets (U.S. and Canada)

Fosinopril
- Tablets (U.S.)

Lisinopril
- Tablets (U.S. and Canada)

Quinapril
- Tablets (U.S.)

Ramipril
- Capsules (U.S.)

Parenteral

Enalaprilat
- Injection (U.S. and Canada)

It is very important that you read and understand the following information. If any of it causes you special concern, check with your doctor. Also, *if you have any questions* or if you want more information about this medicine or your medical problem, *ask your doctor, nurse, or pharmacist.*

Before Using This Medicine

In deciding to use a medicine, the risks of taking the medicine must be weighed against the good it will do. This is a decision you and your doctor will make. For the angiotensin-converting enzyme (ACE) inhibitors, the following should be considered:

Allergies—Tell your doctor if you have ever had any unusual or allergic reaction to benazepril, captopril, enalapril, fosinopril, lisinopril, quinapril, or ramipril. Also tell your doctor and pharmacist if you are allergic to any other substances, such as foods, preservatives, or dyes.

Pregnancy—Use of angiotensin-converting enzyme (ACE) inhibitors during pregnancy, especially in the second and third trimesters (after the first three months) can cause low blood pressure, severe kidney failure, too much potassium, or even death in the newborn. *Therefore, it is important that you check with your doctor immediately if you think that you may be pregnant.* Be sure that you have discussed this with your doctor before taking this medicine. In addition, if you are taking:

- *Benazepril*—Benazepril has not been shown to cause birth defects in animals when given in doses more than 3 times the highest recommended human dose.
- *Captopril*—Studies in rabbits and rats at doses up to 400 times the recommended human dose have shown that captopril causes an increase in deaths of the fetus and newborn. Also, captopril has caused deformed skulls in the offspring of rabbits given doses 2 to 70 times the recommended human dose.
- *Enalapril*—Studies in rats at doses many times the recommended human dose have shown that use of enalapril causes the fetus to be smaller than normal. Studies in rabbits have shown that enalapril causes an increase in fetal death. Enalapril has not been shown to cause birth defects in rats or rabbits.
- *Fosinopril*—Studies in rats have shown that fosinopril causes the fetus to be smaller than normal. Studies in rabbits have shown that fosinopril causes fetal death, probably due to extremely low blood pressure. In rats, birth defects such as skeletal and facial deformities were seen. However, it is not clear that the deformities were related to fosinopril. Birth defects were not seen in rabbits.

- *Lisinopril*—Studies in mice and rats at doses many times the recommended human dose have shown that use of lisinopril causes a decrease in successful pregnancies, a decrease in the weight of infants, and an increase in infant deaths. It has also caused a decrease in successful pregnancies and abnormal bone growth in rabbits. Lisinopril has not been shown to cause birth defects in mice, rats, or rabbits.
- *Quinapril*—Studies in rats have shown that quinapril causes lower birth weights and changes in kidney structure of the fetus. However, birth defects were not seen in rabbits given quinapril.
- *Ramipril*—Studies in animals have shown that ramipril causes lower birth weights.

Breast-feeding—
- *Benazepril, captopril, and fosinopril*—These medicines pass into breast milk.
- *Enalapril, lisinopril, quinapril, or ramipril*—It is not known whether these medicines pass into breast milk. However, these medicines have not been reported to cause problems in nursing babies.

Children—Children may be especially sensitive to the blood pressure–lowering effect of ACE inhibitors. This may increase the chance of side effects or other problems during treatment. Therefore, it is especially important that you discuss with the child's doctor the good that this medicine may do as well as the risks of using it.

Older adults—This medicine has been tested in a limited number of patients 65 years of age or older and has not been shown to cause different side effects or problems in older people than it does in younger adults.

Other medicines—Although certain medicines should not be used together at all, in other cases two different medicines may be used together even if an interaction might occur. In these cases, your doctor may want to change the dose, or other precautions may be necessary. When you are taking or receiving ACE inhibitors it is especially important that your doctor and pharmacist know if you are taking any of the following:
- Diuretics (water pills)—Effects on blood pressure may be increased. In addition, some diuretics make the increase in potassium in the blood caused by ACE inhibitors even greater
- Potassium-containing medicines or supplements or
- Salt substitutes or
- Low-salt milk—Use of these substances with ACE inhibitors may result in an unusually high potassium level in the blood, which can lead to heart rhythm and other problems

Other medical problems—The presence of other medical problems may affect the use of the ACE inhibitors. Make sure you tell your doctor if you have any other medical problems, especially:
- Diabetes mellitus (sugar diabetes)—Increased risk of potassium levels in the body becoming too high
- Heart or blood vessel disease or
- Heart attack or stroke (recent)—Lowering blood pressure may make problems resulting from these conditions worse
- Kidney disease or
- Liver disease—Effects may be increased because of slower removal from the body
- Kidney transplant—Increased risk of kidney disease caused by ACE inhibitors
- Systemic lupus erythematosus (SLE)—Increased risk of blood problems caused by ACE inhibitors
- Previous reaction to any ACE inhibitor involving hoarseness; swelling of face, mouth, hands, or feet; or sudden trouble in breathing—Reaction is more likely to occur again

Before you begin using any new medicine (prescription or nonprescription) or if you develop any new medical problem while you are using this medicine, check with your doctor, nurse, or pharmacist.

Proper Use of This Medicine

To help you remember to take your medicine, try to get into the habit of taking it at the same time each day.

For patients taking *captopril:*
- This medicine is best taken on an empty stomach 1 hour before meals, unless you are otherwise directed by your doctor.

For patients taking this medicine *for high blood pressure:*
- In addition to the use of the medicine your doctor has prescribed, treatment for your high blood pressure may include weight control and care in the types of foods you eat, especially foods high in sodium. Your doctor will tell you which of these are most important for you. You should check with your doctor before changing your diet.
- Many patients who have high blood pressure will not notice any signs of the problem. In fact, many may feel normal. It is very important that you *take your medicine exactly as directed* and that you keep your appointments with your doctor even if you feel well.
- Remember that this medicine will not cure your high blood pressure but it does help control it. Therefore, you must continue to take it as directed if you expect to lower your blood pressure and keep it down. *You may have to take high blood pressure medicine for the rest of your life.* If high blood pressure is not treated, it can cause serious problems such as heart failure, blood vessel disease, stroke, or kidney disease.

Missed dose—If you miss a dose of this medicine, take it as soon as possible. However, if it is almost time for your next dose, skip the missed dose and go back to your regular dosing schedule. Do not double doses.

Storage—To store this medicine:
- Keep out of the reach of children.
- Store away from heat and direct light.
- Do not store in the bathroom, near the kitchen sink, or in other damp places. Heat or moisture may cause the medicine to break down.
- Do not keep outdated medicine or medicine no longer needed. Be sure that any discarded medicine is out of the reach of children.

Precautions While Using This Medicine

It is important that your doctor check your progress at regular visits to make sure that this medicine is working properly and to check for unwanted effects.

For patients taking this medicine *for high blood pressure:*
- *Do not take other medicines unless they have been discussed with your doctor.* This especially includes over-the-counter (nonprescription) medicines for appetite control, asthma, colds, cough, hay fever, or sinus problems, since they may tend to increase your blood pressure.

Dizziness or lightheadedness may occur after the first dose of this medicine, especially if you have been taking a diuretic (water pill). Make sure you know how you react to this medicine before you drive, use machines, or do anything else that could be dangerous if you are dizzy.

Check with your doctor right away if you become sick while taking this medicine, especially with severe or continuing nausea and vomiting or diarrhea. These conditions may cause you to lose too much water and lead to low blood pressure.

Dizziness, lightheadedness, or fainting may also occur if you exercise or if the weather is hot. Heavy sweating can cause loss of too much water and low blood pressure. Use extra care during exercise or hot weather.

Avoid alcoholic beverages until you have discussed their use with your doctor. Alcohol may make the low blood pressure effect worse and/or increase the possibility of dizziness or fainting.

Before having any kind of surgery (including dental surgery) or emergency treatment, tell the medical doctor or dentist in charge that you are taking this medicine.

For patients taking *captopril or fosinopril:*
- Before you have any medical tests, tell the doctor in charge that you are taking this medicine. The results of some tests may be affected by this medicine.

Side Effects of This Medicine

Along with its needed effects, a medicine may cause some unwanted effects. Although not all of these side effects may occur, if they do occur they may need medical attention.

Check with your doctor immediately if any of the following side effects occur:

Rare

Fever and chills; hoarseness; swelling of face, mouth, hands, or feet; trouble in swallowing or breathing (sudden)

Check with your doctor as soon as possible if any of the following side effects occur:

Less common

Dizziness, lightheadedness, or fainting; skin rash, with or without itching, fever, or joint pain

Rare

Abdominal pain, abdominal distention, fever, nausea, or vomiting; chest pain

Signs and symptoms of too much potassium in the body

Confusion; irregular heartbeat; nervousness; numbness or tingling in hands, feet, or lips; shortness of breath or difficulty breathing; weakness or heaviness of legs

Other side effects may occur that usually do not need medical attention. These side effects may go away during treatment as your body adjusts to the medicine. However, check with your doctor if any of the following side effects continue or are bothersome:

More common

Cough (dry, continuing)

Less common

Diarrhea; headache; loss of taste; nausea; unusual tiredness

Other side effects not listed above may also occur in some patients. If you notice any other effects, check with your doctor.

Additional Information

Once a medicine has been approved for marketing for a certain use, experience may show that it is also useful for other medical problems. Although these uses are not included in product labeling, ACE inhibitors are used in certain patients with the following medical conditions:
- Hypertension in scleroderma (high blood pressure in patients with hardening and thickening of the skin)
- Renal crisis in scleroderma (kidney problems in patients with hardening and thickening of the skin)

Other than the above information, there is no additional information relating to proper use, precautions, or side effects for these uses.

Annual revision: 07/12/92

ANGIOTENSIN-CONVERTING ENZYME (ACE) INHIBITORS AND HYDROCHLOROTHIAZIDE Systemic†

This information applies to the following medicines:

Captopril (KAP-toe-pril) and Hydrochlorothiazide (hye-droe-klor-oh-THYE-a-zide)
Enalapril (e-NAL-a-pril) and Hydrochlorothiazide
Lisinopril (lyse-IN-oh-pril) and Hydrochlorothiazide

Some commonly used brand names in the U.S. are:

For Captopril and Hydrochlorothiazide†
Capozide

For Enalapril and Hydrochlorothiazide†
Vaseretic

For Lisinopril and Hydrochlorothiazide†
Prinzide
Zestoretic

†Not commercially available in Canada.

Description

This combination belongs to the class of medicines called high blood pressure medicines (antihypertensives). It is used to treat high blood pressure (hypertension).

High blood pressure adds to the workload of the heart and arteries. If it continues for a long time, the heart and arteries may not function properly. This can damage the blood vessels of the brain, heart, and kidneys, resulting in a stroke, heart failure, or kidney failure. High blood pressure may also increase the risk of heart attacks. These problems may be less likely to occur if blood pressure is controlled.

The exact way in which captopril, enalapril, and lisinopril work is not known. They block an enzyme in the body that is necessary to produce a substance that causes blood vessels to tighten. As a result, they relax blood vessels. This lowers blood pressure and increases the supply of blood and oxygen to the heart. Hydrochlorothiazide helps reduce the amount of salt and water in the body by acting on the kidneys to increase the flow of urine; this also helps to lower blood pressure.

This combination may also be used for other conditions as determined by your doctor.

This medicine is available only with doctor's prescription, in the following dosage forms:

Oral

Captopril and Hydrochlorothiazide
- Tablets (U.S.)

Enalapril and Hydrochlorothiazide
- Tablets (U.S.)

Lisinopril and Hydrochorothiazide
- Tablets (U.S.)

It is very important that you read and understand the following information. If any of it causes you special concern, check with your doctor. Also, *if you have any questions* or if you want more information about this medicine or your medical problem, *ask your doctor, nurse, or pharmacist.*

Before Using This Medicine

In deciding to use a medicine, the risks of taking the medicine must be weighed against the good it will do. This is a decision you and your doctor will make. For the angiotensin-converting enzyme (ACE) inhibitors and hydrochlorothiazide, the following should be considered:

Allergies—Tell your doctor if you have ever had any unusual or allergic reaction to enalapril, captopril, lisinopril, sulfonamides (sulfa drugs), bumetanide, furosemide, acetazolamide, dichlorphenamide, or methazolamide or to hydrochlorothiazide or any of the other thiazide diuretics (water pills). Also tell your doctor and pharmacist if you are allergic to any other substances, such as foods, sulfites or other preservatives, or dyes.

Pregnancy—Studies with this combination medicine have not been done in pregnant women. However, use of any of the ACE inhibitors (captopril, enalapril, lisinopril) during pregnancy, especially in the second and third trimesters (after the first three months) can cause low blood pressure, kidney failure, too much potassium, or even death in newborns. *Therefore, it is important that you check with your doctor immediately if you think that you may be pregnant.* Be sure that you have discussed this with your doctor before taking this medicine. In addition, if your medicine contains:

- *Captopril*—Studies in rabbits and rats at doses up to 400 times the recommended human dose have shown that captopril causes an increase in death of the fetus and newborn. Also, captopril has caused deformed skulls in the offspring of rabbits given doses 2 to 70 times the recommended human dose.
- *Enalapril*—Studies in rats at doses many times the recommended human dose have shown that use of enalapril causes the fetus to be smaller than normal. Studies in rabbits have shown that enalapril causes an increase in fetal death. Enalapril has not been shown to cause birth defects in rats or rabbits.
- *Lisinopril*—Studies in mice and rats at doses many times the recommended human dose have shown that use of lisinopril causes a decrease in successful pregnancies, a decrease in the weight of infants, and an increase in infant deaths. It has also caused a decrease in successful pregnancies and abnormal bone growth in rabbits. Lisinopril has not been shown to cause birth defects in mice, rats, or rabbits.
- *Hydrochlorothiazide*—Hydrochlorothiazide has not been shown to cause birth defects or other problems

in animal studies. However, when hydrochlorothiazide is used during pregnancy, it may cause side effects including jaundice, blood problems, and low potassium in the newborn baby.

Breast-feeding—
- *Captopril*—Passes into breast milk. However, this medicine has not been reported to cause problems in nursing babies.
- *Enalapril or lisinopril*—It is not known whether enalapril or lisinopril passes into breast milk. However, these medicines have not been reported to cause problems in nursing babies.
- *Hydrochlorothiazide*—Passes into breast milk. However, this medicine has not been reported to cause problems in nursing babies.

Children—Children may be especially sensitive to the blood pressure–lowering effect of ACE inhibitors. This may increase the chance of side effects or other problems during treatment. Extra caution may be necessary when using hydrochlorothiazide in infants with jaundice because it can make this condition worse. Therefore, it is especially important that you discuss with the child's doctor the good that this medicine may do as well as the risks of using it.

Older adults—Dizziness or lightheadedness and symptoms of too much potassium loss may be more likely to occur in the elderly, who may be more sensitive to the effects of this medicine.

Other medicines—Although certain medicines should not be used together at all, in other cases two different medicines may be used together even if an interaction might occur. In these cases, your doctor may want to change the dose, or other precautions may be necessary. When taking ACE inhibitors and hydrochlorothiazide it is especially important that your doctor and pharmacist know if you are taking any of the following:
- Cholestyramine or
- Colestipol—Use with thiazide diuretics may prevent the diuretic from working properly; the diuretic should be taken at least 1 hour before or 4 hours after cholestyramine or colestipol
- Digitalis glycosides (heart medicine)—If potassium levels in the body are decreased, symptoms of digitalis toxicity may occur
- Diuretics (water pills)—Effects on blood pressure may be increased
- Lithium (e.g., Lithane)—Risk of lithium overdose, even at low doses, may be increased
- Potassium-containing medicines or supplements or
- Salt substitutes or
- Low-salt milk—Use of these substances with ACE inhibitors may result in an unusually high potassium level in the blood, which can lead to heart rhythm and other problems

Other medical problems—The presence of other medical problems may affect the use of the ACE inhibitors. Make sure you tell your doctor if you have any other medical problems, especially:
- Diabetes mellitus (sugar diabetes)—Increased risk of potassium levels in the body becoming too high
- Gout (or history of)—Hydrochlorothiazide may increase the amount of uric acid in the body, which can lead to gout
- Heart or blood vessel disease or
- Heart attack or stroke (recent)—Lowering blood pressure may make problems resulting from these conditions worse
- Kidney disease or
- Liver disease—Effects may be increased because of slower removal from the body
- Kidney transplant—Increased risk of kidney disease caused by ACE inhibitors
- Pancreatitis (inflammation of the pancreas)—Hydrochlorothiazide can make this condition worse
- Systemic lupus erythematosus (SLE) (or history of)—Hydrochlorothiazide may worsen the condition, and there is an increased risk of blood problems caused by ACE inhibitors
- Previous reaction to captopril, enalapril, or lisinopril involving hoarseness; swelling of face, mouth, hands, or feet; or sudden trouble in breathing—Reaction is more likely to occur again

Before you begin using any new medicine (prescription or nonprescription) or if you develop any new medical problem while you are using this medicine, check with your doctor, nurse, or pharmacist.

Proper Use of This Medicine

To help you remember to take your medicine, try to get into the habit of taking it at the same time each day.

For patients taking *captopril and hydrochlorothiazide:*
- This medicine is best taken on an empty stomach 1 hour before meals, unless you are otherwise directed by your doctor.

For patients taking this medicine *for high blood pressure:*
- In addition to the use of the medicine your doctor has prescribed, treatment for your high blood pressure may include weight control and care in the types of foods you eat, especially foods high in sodium. Your doctor will tell you which of these are most important for you. You should check with your doctor before changing your diet.
- Many patients who have high blood pressure will not notice any signs of the problem. In fact, many may feel normal. It is very important that you *take your medicine exactly as directed* and that you keep your appointments with your doctor even if you feel well.
- Remember that this medicine will not cure your high blood pressure but it does help control it. Therefore, you must continue to take it as directed if you expect to lower your blood pressure and keep it down. *You may have to take high blood pressure medicine for*

the rest of your life. If high blood pressure is not treated, it can cause serious problems such as heart failure, blood vessel disease, stroke, or kidney disease.

This medicine may cause you to have an unusual feeling of tiredness when you begin to take it. You may also notice an increase in the amount of urine or in your frequency of urination. After you have taken the medicine for a while, these effects should lessen. In general, to keep the increase in urine from affecting your sleep:

- If you are to take a single dose a day, take it in the morning after breakfast.
- If you are to take more than one dose a day, take the last dose no later than 6 p.m., unless otherwise directed by your doctor.

However, it is best to plan your dose or doses according to a schedule that will least affect your personal activities and sleep. Ask your doctor, nurse, or pharmacist to help you plan the best time to take this medicine.

Missed dose—If you miss a dose of this medicine, take it as soon as possible. However, if it is almost time for your next dose, skip the missed dose and go back to your regular dosing schedule. Do not double doses.

Storage—To store this medicine:

- Keep out of the reach of children.
- Store away from heat and direct light.
- Do not store in the bathroom, near the kitchen sink, or in other damp places. Heat or moisture may cause the medicine to break down.
- Do not keep outdated medicine or medicine no longer needed. Be sure that any discarded medicine is out of the reach of children.

Precautions While Using This Medicine

It is important that your doctor check your progress at regular visits to make sure that this medicine is working properly and to check for unwanted effects.

Dizziness or lightheadedness may occur, especially after the first dose of this medicine. Make sure you know how you react to the medicine before you drive, use machines, or do anything else that could be dangerous if you are dizzy.

Check with your doctor right away if you become sick while taking this medicine, especially with severe or continuing nausea and vomiting or diarrhea. These conditions may cause you to lose too much water and lead to low blood pressure.

Dizziness, lightheadedness, or fainting may also occur if you exercise or if the weather is hot. Heavy sweating can cause loss of too much water and low blood pressure. Use extra care during exercise or hot weather.

Avoid alcoholic beverages until you have discussed their use with your doctor. Alcohol may make the low blood pressure effect worse and/or increase the possibility of dizziness or fainting.

Before having any kind of surgery (including dental surgery) or emergency treatment, tell the medical doctor or dentist in charge that you are taking this medicine.

For patients taking *captopril and hydrochlorothiazide:*

- Before you have any medical tests, tell the doctor in charge that you are taking this medicine. The results of some tests may be affected by this medicine.

For patients taking this medicine *for high blood pressure:*

- *Do not take other medicines unless they have been discussed with your doctor.* This especially includes over-the-counter (nonprescription) medicines for appetite control, asthma, colds, cough, hay fever, or sinus problems, since they may tend to increase your blood pressure.

For *diabetic patients:*

- Hydrochlorothiazide (contained in this combination medicine) may raise blood sugar levels. While you are taking this medicine, be especially careful in testing for sugar in your urine.

Hydrochlorothiazide (contained in this combination medicine) may cause your skin to be more sensitive to sunlight than it is normally. Exposure to sunlight, even for brief periods of time, may cause a skin rash, itching, redness or other discoloration of the skin, or a severe sunburn. When you first begin taking this medicine:

- Stay out of direct sunlight, especially between the hours of 10:00 a.m. and 3:00 p.m., if possible.
- Wear protective clothing, including a hat. Also, wear sunglasses.
- Apply a sun block product that has a skin protection factor (SPF) of at least 15. Some patients may require a product with a higher SPF number, especially if they have a fair complexion. If you have any questions about this, check with your doctor or pharmacist.
- Apply a sun block lipstick that has an SPF of at least 15 to protect your lips.
- Do not use a sunlamp or tanning bed or booth.

If you have a severe reaction from the sun, check with your doctor.

Before you have any medical tests, tell the doctor in charge that you are taking this medicine. The results of some tests may be affected by this medicine.

Side Effects of This Medicine

Along with its needed effects, a medicine may cause some unwanted effects. Although not all of these side effects may occur, if they do occur they may need medical attention.

Check with your doctor immediately if any of the following side effects occur:

Rare

Fever and chills; hoarseness; swelling of face, mouth, hands, or feet; trouble in swallowing or breathing (sudden)

Check with your doctor as soon as possible if any of the following side effects occur:

Less common

Dizziness, lightheadedness, or fainting; skin rash, with or without itching, fever, or joint pain

Rare

Chest pain; joint pain; lower back or side pain; stomach pain (severe) with nausea and vomiting; unusual bleeding or bruising; yellow eyes or skin

Signs and symptoms of too much or too little potassium in the body

Dryness of mouth; increased thirst; irregular heartbeats; mood or mental changes; muscle cramps or pain; numbness or tingling in hands, feet, or lips; weakness or heaviness of legs; weak pulse

Other side effects may occur that usually do not need medical attention. These side effects may go away during treatment as your body adjusts to the medicine. However, check with your doctor if any of the following side effects continue or are bothersome:

More common

Cough (dry, continuing)

Less common

Diarrhea; headache; increased sensitivity of skin to sunlight (skin rash, itching, redness or other discoloration or skin or severe sunburn after exposure to sunlight); loss of appetite; loss of taste; stomach upset; unusual tiredness

Other side effects not listed above may also occur in some patients. If you notice any other effects, check with your doctor.

Additional Information

Once a medicine has been approved for marketing for a certain use, experience may show that it is also useful for other medical problems. Although this use is not included in product labeling, ACE inhibitors and hydrochlorothiazide are used in certain patients with the following medical condition:

- Congestive heart failure

Other than the above information, there is no additional information relating to proper use, precautions, or side effects for this use.

Annual revision: 07/28/92

ANISTREPLASE Systemic†

A commonly used brand name in the U.S. is Eminase.

Other commonly used names are anisoylated plasminogen-streptokinase activator complex and APSAC.

†Not commercially available in Canada.

Description

Anistreplase (an-EYE-strep-lase) is a long-acting form of streptokinase, which belongs to the group of medicines called thrombolytic agents. These medicines are used to break up (lyse) or dissolve blood clots that have formed in certain blood vessels. Clots in blood vessels that carry blood to the heart may cause a heart attack. Anistreplase is used to break up clots that are causing a heart attack. This increases the flow of blood to the heart and lessens the chance of serious heart damage.

Anistreplase may cause bleeding in some people, because it can also break up blood clots that are needed to stop bleeding after a cut or other injury.

Anistreplase is given only by or under the direct supervision of a doctor. It is available in the following dosage form:

Parenteral

- Injection (U.S.)

Precautions After Receiving This Medicine

Anistreplase can cause bleeding that usually is not serious. However, serious bleeding may occur in some people. *To help prevent serious bleeding, follow any instructions given by your doctor or nurse very carefully. Also, move around as little as possible, and do not get out of bed on your own, unless your doctor or nurse tells you it is all right to do so.*

Side Effects of This Medicine

Along with its needed effects, a medicine may cause some unwanted effects. Although not all of these side effects may occur, if they do occur they may need medical attention. After you have received anistreplase, your doctor or nurse will closely follow its effects. However, *tell your doctor or nurse immediately if you notice any of the following side effects:*

More common

Bleeding or oozing from cuts or around the place of injection

Less common or rare

Bruising; chills and/or shivering; fast or irregular breathing; skin rash, hives, and/or itching; shortness of breath, troubled breathing, tightness in chest, and/or wheezing

Signs of bleeding inside the body

Abdominal or stomach pain or swelling; back pain or backaches; constipation; coughing up blood; dizziness; headaches (severe or continuing); joint pain, stiffness, or swelling; muscle pain or stiffness (severe or continuing); nosebleeds; unexpected or unusually heavy bleeding from vagina; vomiting of blood or material that looks like coffee grounds

Some side effects may occur a few weeks after you have received anistreplase. During this time, check with your doctor as soon as possible if you notice any of the following side effects:

Rare

Bloody or cloudy urine; fever, chills and/or shivering; muscle aches; pinpoint red spots on skin; stomach upset; swelling of ankles

Other side effects not listed above may also occur in some patients. If you notice any other effects, check with your doctor.

Annual revision: June 1990

ANTACIDS Oral

Some commonly used brand names are:

In the U.S.

Advanced Formula Di-Gel[11]
Alamag[1]
Algenic Alka[4]
Algicon[4]
Alka-Mints[9]
Alkets[13]
Almacone[3]
Almacone II[3]
Alma-Mag Improved[3]
Alma-Mag #4 Improved[3]
AlternaGEL[8]
Alu-Cap[8]
Aludrox[3]
Alu-Tab[8]
Amitone[9]
Amphojel[8]
AntaGel[3]
AntaGel-II[3]
Basaljel[7]
Bisodol[10 19]
Calcilac[9]
Calglycine[9]
Camalox[2]
Chooz[9]
Creamalin[1]
Dialume[8]
Dicarbosil[9]
Di-Gel[3 25]
Equilet[9]
Foamicon[5]
Gas-is-gon[6]
Gaviscon[4 5]
Gaviscon-2[5]
Gaviscon Extra Strength Relief Formula[4]
Gelamal[1]
Gelusil[3]
Gelusil-II[3]
Genalac[9]
Genaton[5]
Glycate[9]
Kudrox Double Strength[1]
Losotron Plus[18]
Lowsium[17]
Lowsium Plus[18]
Maalox[1]
Maalox Extra Strength[1]
Maalox Plus, Extra Strength[3]
Maalox TC[1]
Maalox Whip[1]
Magnagel[4]
Magnatril[22]
Mag-Ox 400[21]
Mallamint[9]
Maox[21]
Marblen[12]
Mi-Acid[3]
Mintox[1]
Mintox Plus[3]
Mygel[3]
Mygel II[3]
Mylanta[3]
Mylanta-II[3]
Nephrox[8]
Noralac[12]
Phillips' Milk of Magnesia[20]
Riopan[17]
Riopan Plus[18]
Riopan Plus 2[18]
Rolaids[16]
Rolaids Calcium Rich[9]
Rolaids Sodium Free[10]
Rulox[1]
Rulox No. 1[1]
Rulox No. 2[1]
Simaal Gel[3]
Simaal 2 Gel[3]
Spastosed[12]
Tempo[23]
Titracid[9]
Titralac[9]
Titralac Extra Strength[9]
Titralac Plus[14]
Triconsil[6]
Tums[9]
Tums E-X[9]
Tums Liquid Extra Strength[9]
Tums Liquid Extra Strength with Simethicone[14]
Uro-Mag[21]
WinGel[1]

In Canada

Algicon[4]
Alu-Tab[8]
Amphojel[8]
Amphojel 500[1]
Amphojel Plus[3 24]
Antiflux[17]
Basaljel[8]
Diovol[1]
Diovol Ex[1]
Diovol Plus[3 24]
Gaviscon[5 8]
Gelusil[1]
Gelusil Extra Strength[1]
Maalox[1]
Maalox Plus[3]
Maalox TC[1]
Mylanta-2[3]
Mylanta-2 Extra Strength[3]
Mylanta-2 Plain[1]
Neutralca-S[1]
Phillips' Milk of Magnesia[20]
Riopan[17]
Riopan Extra Strength[17]
Riopan Plus[18]
Riopan Plus Extra Strength[18]
Robalate[15]
Univol[1]

Note: For quick reference the following antacids are numbered to match the corresponding brand names.

This information applies to the following medicines:
1. Alumina (a-LOO-mi-na) and Magnesia (mag-NEE-zha)
2. Alumina, Magnesia, and Calcium Carbonate (KAL-see-um KAR-boe-nate)
3. Alumina, Magnesia, and Simethicone (si-METH-i-kone)
4. Alumina and Magnesium Carbonate (mag-NEE-zhum)
5. Alumina and Magnesium Trisilicate (trye-SILL-i-kate)
6. Alumina, Magnesium Trisilicate, and Sodium Bicarbonate (SOE-dee-um)
7. Aluminum Carbonate (a-LOO-mi-num), Basic
8. Aluminum Hydroxide (hye-DROX-ide)*†
9. Calcium Carbonate*
10. Calcium Carbonate and Magnesia
11. Calcium Carbonate, Magnesia, and Simethicone
12. Calcium and Magnesium Carbonates
13. Calcium and Magnesium Carbonates and Magnesium Oxide (mag-NEE-zhum OX-ide)
14. Calcium Carbonate and Simethicone
15. Dihydroxyaluminum Aminoacetate (dye-hye-DROX-ee-a-LOO-mi-num a-mee-noe-ASS-e-tate)
16. Dihydroxyaluminum Sodium Carbonate
17. Magaldrate (MAG-al-drate)*
18. Magaldrate and Simethicone
19. Magnesium Carbonate and Sodium Bicarbonate
20. Magnesium Hydroxide*†
21. Magnesium Oxide
22. Magnesium Trisilicate, Alumina, and Magnesia
23. Simethicone, Alumina, Calcium Carbonate, and Magnesia
24. Simethicone, Alumina, Magnesium Carbonate, and Magnesia

*Generic name product may also be available in U.S.
†Generic name product available in Canada.

Description

Antacids are taken by mouth to relieve heartburn, sour stomach, or acid indigestion. They work by neutralizing excess stomach acid. Some antacid combinations also contain simethicone, which may relieve the symptoms of excess gas. Antacids alone or in combination with simethicone may also be used to treat the symptoms of stomach or duodenal ulcers.

With larger doses than those used for the antacid effect, magnesium hydroxide (magnesia) and magnesium oxide antacids produce a laxative effect. The information that follows applies only to their use as an antacid.

Some antacids, like aluminum carbonate and aluminum hydroxide, may be prescribed with a low-phosphate diet to treat hyperphosphatemia (too much phosphate in the blood). Aluminum carbonate and aluminum hydroxide may also be used with a low-phosphate diet to prevent the formation of some kinds of kidney stones. Aluminum hydroxide may also be used for other conditions as determined by your doctor.

These medicines are available without a prescription. However, your doctor may have special instructions on the proper use and dose of these medicines for your medical problem. They are available in the following dosage forms:

Oral

Alumina and Magnesia
- Oral suspension (U.S. and Canada)
- Tablets (Canada)
- Chewable tablets (U.S. and Canada)

Alumina, Magnesia, and Calcium Carbonate
- Oral suspension (U.S.)
- Chewable tablets (U.S.)

Alumina, Magnesia, and Simethicone
- Oral suspension (U.S. and Canada)
- Chewable tablets (U.S. and Canada)

Alumina and Magnesium Carbonate
- Oral suspension (U.S. and Canada)
- Chewable tablets (U.S. and Canada)

Alumina and Magnesium Trisilicate
- Chewable tablets (U.S. and Canada)

Alumina, Magnesium Trisilicate, and Sodium Bicarbonate
- Chewable tablets (U.S.)

Aluminum Carbonate, Basic
- Capsules (U.S.)
- Gel (U.S.)
- Tablets (U.S.)

Aluminum Hydroxide
- Capsules (U.S. and Canada)
- Gel (U.S. and Canada)
- Tablets (U.S. and Canada)

Calcium Carbonate
- Chewing gum (U.S.)
- Oral suspension (U.S.)
- Tablets (U.S.)
- Chewable tablets (U.S.)

Calcium Carbonate and Magnesia
- Chewable tablets (U.S.)

Calcium Carbonate, Magnesia, and Simethicone
- Tablets (U.S.)

Calcium and Magnesium Carbonates
- Oral suspension (U.S.)
- Tablets (U.S.)
- Chewable tablets (U.S.)

Calcium and Magnesium Carbonates and Magnesium Oxide
- Tablets (U.S.)

Calcium Carbonate and Simethicone
- Oral suspension (U.S.)
- Chewable tablets (U.S.)

Dihydroxyaluminum Aminoacetate
- Tablets (Canada)

Dihydroxyaluminum Sodium Carbonate
- Chewable tablets (U.S.)

Magaldrate
- Oral suspension (U.S. and Canada)
- Tablets (U.S.)
- Chewable tablets (U.S. and Canada)

Magaldrate and Simethicone
- Oral suspension (U.S. and Canada)
- Chewable tablets (U.S. and Canada)

Magnesium Carbonate and Sodium Bicarbonate
- For oral suspension (U.S.)

Magnesium Hydroxide
- Milk of magnesia (U.S. and Canada)
- Tablets (U.S. and Canada)
- Chewable Tablets (U.S. and Canada)

Magnesium Oxide
- Capsules (U.S.)
- Tablets (U.S.)

Magnesium Trisilicate, Alumina, and Magnesia
- Oral suspension (U.S.)
- Chewable tablets (U.S.)

Simethicone, Alumina, Calcium Carbonate, and Magnesia
- Chewable tablets (U.S.)

Simethicone, Alumina, Magnesium Carbonate, and Magnesia
- Chewable tablets (U.S. and Canada)

It is very important that you read and understand the following information. If any of it causes you special concern, check with your doctor or pharmacist. Also, *if you have any questions* or if you want more information about this medicine or your medical problem, *ask your doctor, nurse, or pharmacist.*

Before Using This Medicine

If you are taking this medicine without a prescription, carefully read and follow any precautions on the label. For antacids, the following should be considered:

Allergies—Tell your doctor or pharmacist if you have ever had any unusual or allergic reaction to aluminum-, calcium-, magnesium-, simethicone-, or sodium bicarbonate–containing medicines. Also tell your doctor and pharmacist if you are allergic to any other substances, such as foods, preservatives, or dyes.

Diet—Make certain your doctor and pharmacist know if you are on a low-sodium diet. Some antacids contain large amounts of sodium.

Pregnancy—Studies have not been done in either humans or animals. However, there have been reports of antacids causing side effects in babies whose mothers took antacids for a long time, especially in high doses during pregnancy. Also, sodium-containing medicines should be avoided if you tend to retain (keep) body water.

Breast-feeding—These medicines have not been reported to cause problems in nursing babies.

Children—Antacids should not be given to young children (under 6 years of age) unless ordered by their doctor. Since children cannot usually describe their symptoms very well, a doctor should first check the child. The child may have a condition that needs other treatment. If so, antacids will not help and may even cause unwanted effects or make the condition worse. In addition, aluminum- or magnesium-containing medicines may cause serious side effects when given to premature or very young children, especially those who have kidney disease or who are dehydrated.

Older adults—Aluminum-containing antacids should not be used by elderly persons with bone problems or with Alzheimer's disease. The aluminum may cause their condition to get worse.

Other medicines—Although certain medicines should not be used together at all, in other cases two different medicines may be used together even if an interaction might occur. In these cases, your doctor may want to change the dose, or other precautions may be necessary. When you are taking antacids, it is especially important that your doctor and pharmacist know if you are taking any of the following:

- Cellulose sodium phosphate (e.g., Calcibind)—Calcium-containing antacids may decrease the effects of cellulose sodium phosphate; use with magnesium-containing antacids may prevent either medicine from working properly; antacids should not be taken within 1 hour of cellulose sodium phosphate
- Isoniazid taken by mouth (e.g., INH)—Aluminum-containing antacids may decrease the effects of isoniazid; isoniazid should be taken at least 1 hour before or after the antacid
- Ketoconazole (e.g., Nizoral) or
- Methenamine (e.g., Mandelamine)—Antacids may decrease the effects of ketoconazole or methenamine; these medicines should be taken 3 hours before the antacid
- Mecamylamine (e.g., Inversine)—Antacids may increase the effects and possibly the side effects of mecamylamine
- Sodium polystyrene sulfonate resin (SPSR) (e.g., Kayexalate)—This medicine may decrease the effects of antacids
- Tetracyclines (medicine for infection) taken by mouth—Use with antacids may decrease the effects of both medicines; antacids should not be taken within 3 to 4 hours of tetracyclines

Other medical problems—The presence of other medical problems may affect the use of antacids. Make sure you tell your doctor if you have any other medical problems, especially:

- Alzheimer's disease (for aluminum-containing antacids only) or
- Appendicitis (or signs of) or
- Bone fractures or
- Colitis or
- Constipation (severe and continuing) or
- Hemorrhoids or
- Inflamed bowel or
- Intestinal blockage or
- Intestinal or rectal bleeding—Antacids may make these conditions worse
- Colostomy or
- Ileostomy—Use of antacids may cause the body to retain (keep) water and electrolytes such as sodium and/or potassium
- Diarrhea (continuing)—Aluminum-containing antacids may cause the body to lose too much phosphorus; magnesium-containing antacids may make diarrhea worse
- Edema (swelling of feet or lower legs) or
- Heart disease or
- Liver disease or
- Toxemia of pregnancy—Use of sodium-containing antacids may cause the body to retain (keep) water
- Kidney disease—Antacids may cause higher blood levels of aluminum, calcium, or magnesium, which may increase the risk of serious side effects
- Sarcoidosis—Use of calcium-containing antacids may cause kidney problems or too much calcium in the blood

- Underactive parathyroid glands—Use with calcium-containing antacids may cause too much calcium in the blood

Before you begin using any new medicine (prescription or nonprescription) or if you develop any new medical problem while you are using this medicine, check with your doctor, nurse, or pharmacist.

Proper Use of This Medicine

For safe and effective use of this medicine:

- Follow your doctor's instructions if this medicine was prescribed.
- Follow the manufacturer's package directions if you are treating yourself.

For patients taking the *chewable tablet form* of this medicine:

- Chew the tablets well before swallowing. This is to allow the medicine to work faster and be more effective.

For patients taking this medicine for a *stomach or duodenal ulcer:*

- Take it exactly as directed and for the full time of treatment as ordered by your doctor, to obtain maximum relief of your symptoms.
- Take it 1 and 3 hours after meals and at bedtime for best results, unless otherwise directed by your doctor.

For patients taking *aluminum carbonate* or *aluminum hydroxide* to *prevent kidney stones:*

- Drink plenty of fluids for best results, unless otherwise directed by your doctor.

For patients taking *aluminum carbonate* or *aluminum hydroxide* for *hyperphosphatemia* (too much phosphate in the blood):

- Your doctor may want you to follow a low-phosphate diet. If you have any questions about this, check with your doctor.

Missed dose—If your doctor has told you to take this medicine on a regular schedule and you miss a dose, take it as soon as possible. However, if it is almost time for your next dose, skip the missed dose and go back to your regular dosing schedule. Do not double doses.

Storage—To store this medicine:

- Keep out of the reach of children.
- Store away from heat and direct light.
- Do not store the capsule, tablet, or powder form of this medicine in the bathroom, near the kitchen sink, or in other damp places. Heat or moisture may cause the medicine to break down.
- Keep the liquid form of this medicine from freezing.
- Do not keep outdated medicine or medicine no longer needed. Be sure that any discarded medicine is out of the reach of children.

Precautions While Using This Medicine

If this medicine has been ordered by your doctor and you will be taking it in large doses, or for a long time, your doctor should check your progress at regular visits. This is to make sure the medicine does not cause unwanted effects.

Some tests may be affected by this medicine. Tell the doctor in charge that you are taking this medicine before you have any tests to determine how much acid your stomach produces.

Do not take this medicine:

- *if you have any signs of appendicitis or inflamed bowel* (such as stomach or lower abdominal pain, cramping, bloating, soreness, nausea, or vomiting). Instead, check with your doctor as soon as possible.
- *within 1 to 2 hours or more of taking other medicine by mouth.* To do so may keep the other medicine from working properly.

For patients on a *sodium-restricted diet:*

- Some antacids (especially sodium bicarbonate–containing ones) contain a large amount of sodium. If you have any questions about this, check with your doctor or pharmacist.

For patients taking this medicine as an *antacid:*

- *Do not take it for more than 2 weeks unless otherwise directed by your doctor.* Antacids should be used only for occasional relief.
- If your stomach problem is not helped by the antacid or if it keeps coming back, check with your doctor.
- Using magnesium- or sodium bicarbonate–containing antacids too often, or in high doses, may produce a laxative effect. This happens fairly often and depends on the individual's sensitivity to the medicine.

For patients taking *aluminum-containing antacids* (including magaldrate):

- Before you have any test in which a radiopharmaceutical will be used, tell the doctor in charge that you are taking this medicine. The results of the test may be affected by aluminum-containing antacids.

For patients taking *calcium-* or *sodium bicarbonate–containing antacids:*

- *Do not take the antacid with large amounts of milk or milk products.* To do so may increase the chance of side effects.

Side Effects of This Medicine

Along with its needed effects, a medicine may cause some unwanted effects. Although the following side effects occur very rarely when this medicine is taken as recommended, they may be more likely to occur if:

- too much medicine is taken.
- it is taken in large doses.
- it is taken for a long time.
- it is taken by patients with kidney disease.

Check with your doctor as soon as possible if any of the following side effects (which may be signs of overdose) occur:

For aluminum-containing antacids (including magaldrate)

Bone pain; constipation (severe and continuing); feeling of discomfort (continuing); loss of appetite (continuing); mood or mental changes; muscle weakness; swelling of wrists or ankles; weight loss (unusual)

For calcium-containing antacids

Constipation (severe and continuing); difficult or painful urination; frequent urge to urinate; headache (continuing); loss of appetite (continuing); mood or mental changes; muscle pain or twitching; nausea or vomiting; nervousness or restlessness; slow breathing; unpleasant taste; unusual tiredness or weakness

For magnesium-containing antacids (including magaldrate)

Difficult or painful urination (with magnesium trisilicate); dizziness or lightheadedness; irregular heartbeat; mood or mental changes; unusual tiredness or weakness

For sodium bicarbonate–containing antacids

Frequent urge to urinate; headache (continuing); loss of appetite (continuing); mood or mental changes; muscle pain or twitching; nausea or vomiting; nervousness or restlessness; slow breathing; swelling of feet or lower legs; unpleasant taste; unusual tiredness or weakness

Other side effects may occur that usually do not need medical attention. These side effects may go away during treatment as your body adjusts to the medicine. However, check with your doctor if any of the following side effects continue or are bothersome:

More common

Chalky taste

Less common

Constipation (mild); diarrhea or laxative effect; increased thirst; speckling or whitish discoloration of stools; stomach cramps

Other side effects not listed above may also occur in some patients. If you notice any other effects, check with your doctor.

Annual revision: 04/06/92

ANTHRALIN Topical

Some commonly used brand names are:

In the U.S.

Anthra-Derm
Drithocreme
Drithocreme HP
Dritho-Scalp
Lasan
Lasan 0.1
Lasan 0.2
Lasan 0.4
Lasan HP-1

In Canada

Anthraforte 1
Anthraforte 2
Anthraforte 3
Anthranol 0.1
Anthranol 0.2
Anthranol 0.4
Anthrascalp

Another commonly used name is dithranol.

Description

Anthralin (AN-thra-lin) is used to treat psoriasis. It may also be used to treat other skin conditions as determined by your doctor.

In the U.S., this medicine is available only with your doctor's prescription. In Canada, this medicine should be used only on the advice of your doctor.

This medicine is available in the following dosage forms:

Topical

- Cream (U.S. and Canada)
- Ointment (U.S. and Canada)

It is very important that you read and understand the following information. If any of it causes you special concern, check with your doctor. Also, *if you have any questions* or if you want more information about this medicine or your medical problem, *ask your doctor, nurse, or pharmacist.*

Before Using This Medicine

In deciding to use a medicine, the risks of using the medicine must be weighed against the good it will do. This is a decision you and your doctor will make. For anthralin, the following should be considered:

Allergies—Tell your doctor if you have ever had any unusual or allergic reaction to anthralin. Also tell your doctor and pharmacist if you are allergic to any other substances, such as preservatives or dyes.

Pregnancy—Anthralin may be absorbed through the skin. However, studies on effects in pregnancy have not been done in either humans or animals.

Breast-feeding—Anthralin may be absorbed through the mother's skin. It is not known whether anthralin passes into the breast milk. However, this medicine has not been reported to cause problems in nursing babies.

Children—Studies on this medicine have been done only in adult patients, and there is no specific information comparing use of anthralin in children with use in other age groups.

Older adults—Many medicines have not been studied specifically in older people. Therefore, it may not be known whether they work exactly the same way they do in younger adults or if they cause different side effects or problems in older people. There is no specific information comparing use of anthralin in the elderly with use in other age groups.

Other medicines—Although certain medicines should not be used together at all, in other cases two different medicines may be used together even if an interaction might occur. In these cases, your doctor may want to change the dose, or other precautions may be necessary. Tell your doctor and pharmacist if you are using any other prescription or nonprescription (over-the-counter [OTC]) medicine.

Other medical problems—The presence of other medical problems may affect the use of anthralin. Make sure you tell your doctor if you have any other medical problems, especially:

- Skin diseases or problems (other)—Anthralin may make the condition worse

Before you begin using any new medicine (prescription or nonprescription) or if you develop any new medical problem while you are using this medicine, check with your doctor, nurse, or pharmacist.

Proper Use of This Medicine

Keep this medicine away from the eyes and other mucous membranes, such as the mouth and the inside of the nose.

Do not apply this medicine to blistered, raw, or oozing areas of the skin or scalp.

Do not use this medicine on your face or sex organs or in the folds and creases of your skin. If you have any questions about this, check with your doctor.

Use this medicine only as directed. Do not use more of it, do not use it more often, and do not use it for a longer time than your doctor ordered. To do so may increase the chance of side effects.

Anthralin may be used in different ways. In some cases, it is applied at night and allowed to remain on the affected areas overnight, then washed off the next morning or before the next application. In other cases, it may be applied and allowed to remain on the affected areas for a short period of time (usually 10 to 30 minutes), then washed off. (This is called short contact treatment.) Make sure you understand exactly how you are to use this medicine. If you have any questions about this, check with your doctor.

Anthralin may cause irritation of normal skin. If it does, petrolatum may be applied to the skin or scalp around the affected areas for protection.

Apply a thin layer of anthralin to only the affected area of the skin or scalp and rub in gently.

Immediately after applying this medicine, wash your hands to remove any medicine that may be on them.

For patients using *anthralin for short contact* (usually 10 to 30 minutes) treatment:

- After applying anthralin, allow the medicine to remain on the affected area for 10 to 30 minutes or as directed by your doctor. Then remove the medicine by bathing, if the anthralin was applied to the skin, or by shampooing, if it was applied to the scalp.

For patients using the *cream form* of anthralin for overnight treatment:

- If anthralin cream is applied to the skin, any medicine remaining on the affected areas the next morning should be removed by bathing.
- If anthralin cream is applied to the scalp, shampoo to remove the scales and any medicine remaining on the affected areas from the previous application. Dry the hair and, after parting, rub the cream into the affected areas. Check with your doctor to see when the cream should be removed.

For patients using the *ointment form* of anthralin for overnight treatment:

- If anthralin ointment is applied to the skin at night, any ointment remaining on the affected areas the next morning should be removed with warm liquid petrolatum followed by bathing.
- If anthralin ointment is applied to the scalp at night, use a shampoo the next morning to clean the scalp.

Missed dose—If you miss a dose of this medicine, apply it as soon as possible. However, if it is almost time for your next dose, skip the missed dose and go back to your regular dosing schedule. Do not double doses.

Storage—To store this medicine:

- Keep out of the reach of children.
- Store away from heat and direct light.
- Keep the medicine from freezing.
- Do not keep outdated medicine or medicine no longer needed. Be sure that any discarded medicine is out of the reach of children.

Precautions While Using This Medicine

Anthralin may stain the skin, hair, fingernails, clothing, bed linens, or bathtub or shower:

- Avoid getting the medicine on your clothing or on bed linens. Protective dressings may be used, unless you have been otherwise directed by your doctor.
- The stain on the skin or hair will wear off in several weeks after you stop using this medicine.
- To prevent staining of your hands, you may wear plastic gloves when you apply this medicine.
- If the medicine is applied to the scalp at night, check with your doctor to see if you may wear a plastic cap to prevent staining of the pillow.
- To remove any medicine on the surface of the bathtub or shower, wash it with hot water immediately after bathing or showering. Then use a household cleanser to remove any remaining deposit of the medicine on the bathtub or shower.

Side Effects of This Medicine

Anthralin has been shown to cause tumors (some cancerous) in animals. However, there have been no reports of anthralin causing tumors in humans.

Along with its needed effects, a medicine may cause some unwanted effects. Although not all of these side effects may occur, if they do occur they may need medical attention.

Check with your doctor as soon as possible if any of the following side effects occur:

More common

Redness or other skin irritation not present before use of this medicine

Rare

Skin rash

Other side effects not listed above may also occur in some patients. If you notice any other effects, check with your doctor.

Additional Information

Once a medicine has been approved for marketing for a certain use, experience may show that it is also useful for other medical problems. Although this use is not included in product labeling, anthralin is used in certain patients with the following medical condition:

- Alopecia areata (a certain type of baldness)

Other than the above information, there is no additional information relating to proper use, precautions, or side effects for this use.

Annual revision: 01/15/92

ANTICHOLINERGICS/ANTISPASMODICS Systemic

This information applies to the following medicines:

Anisotropine (an-iss-oh-TROE-peen)
Atropine (A-troe-peen)
Belladonna (bell-a-DON-a)
Clidinium (kli-DI-nee-um)
Dicyclomine (dye-SYE-kloe-meen)
Glycopyrrolate (glye-koe-PYE-roe-late)
Homatropine (hoe-MA-troe-peen)
Hyoscyamine (hye-oh-SYE-a-meen)
Isopropamide (eye-soe-PROE-pa-mide)
Mepenzolate (me-PEN-zoe-late)
Methantheline (meth-AN-tha-leen)
Methscopolamine (meth-skoe-POL-a-meen)
Oxyphencyclimine (ox-i-fen-SYE-kli-meen)
Pirenzepine (peer-EN-ze-peen)
Propantheline (proe-PAN-the-leen)
Scopolamine (scoe-POL-a-meen)
Tridihexethyl (trye-dye-hex-ETH-il)

Some commonly used brand names are:

For Anisotropine†
In the U.S.
Valpin 50

Generic name product may also be available.

Another commonly used name is octatropine.

For Atropine
In the U.S.
Generic name product available.
In Canada
Generic name product available.

For Belladonna†
In the U.S.
Generic name product available.

For Clidinium†
In the U.S.
Quarzan

For Dicyclomine
In the U.S.
Antispas
A-Spas
Bentyl
Di-Spaz
Neoquess
Or-Tyl
Spasmoject

Generic name product may also be available.

In Canada
Bentylol
Formulex
Lomine
Spasmoban

Another commonly used name is dicycloverine.

For Glycopyrrolate
In the U.S.
Robinul
Robinul Forte
Generic name product may also be available.
In Canada
Robinul
Robinul Forte
Another commonly used name is glycopyrronium bromide.

For Homatropine†
In the U.S.
Homapin

For Hyoscyamine
In the U.S.
Anaspaz
Cystospaz
Cystospaz-M
Gastrosed
Levsin
Levsinex Timecaps
Levsin S/L
Neoquess
In Canada
Levsin

For Isopropamide†
In the U.S.
Darbid

For Mepenzolate†
In the U.S.
Cantil

For Methantheline†
In the U.S.
Banthine
Another commonly used name is methanthelinium.

For Methscopolamine†
In the U.S.
Pamine
Another commonly used name for methscopolamine is hyoscine methobromide.

For Oxyphencyclimine†
In the U.S.
Daricon

For Pirenzepine*
In Canada
Gastrozepin

For Propantheline
In the U.S.
Norpanth
Pro-Banthine
Generic name product may also be available.
In Canada
Pro-Banthine
Propanthel

For Scopolamine
In the U.S.
Transderm-Scōp
Generic name product may also be available.
In Canada
Buscopan
Transderm-V
Another commonly used name for scopolamine is hyoscine hydrobromide.

For Tridihexethyl†
In the U.S.
Pathilon

*Not commercially available in the U.S.
†Not commercially available in Canada.

Description

The anticholinergics/antispasmodics are a group of medicines that include the natural belladonna alkaloids (atropine, belladonna, hyoscyamine, and scopolamine) and related products.

The anticholinergics/antispasmodics are used to relieve cramps or spasms of the stomach, intestines, and bladder. Some are used together with antacids or other medicine in the treatment of peptic ulcer. Others are used to prevent nausea, vomiting, and motion sickness.

Anticholinergics/antispasmodics are also used in certain surgical and emergency procedures. In surgery, some are given by injection before anesthesia to help relax you and to decrease secretions, such as saliva. During anesthesia and surgery, atropine, glycopyrrolate, hyoscyamine, and scopolamine are used to help keep the heartbeat normal. Atropine is also given by injection to help relax the stomach and intestines for certain types of examinations. Some anticholinergics are also used to treat poisoning caused by medicines such as neostigmine and physostigmine, certain types of mushrooms, and poisoning by "nerve" gases or organic phosphorous pesticides (for example, demeton [Systox], diazinon, malathion, parathion, and ronnel [Trolene]). Also, anticholinergics can be used for painful menstruation, runny nose, and to prevent urination during sleep.

These medicines may also be used for other conditions as determined by your doctor.

The anticholinergics/antispasmodics are available only with your doctor's prescription in the following dosage forms:

Oral

Anisotropine
- Tablets (U.S.)

Atropine
- Tablets (U.S.)
- Soluble tablets (U.S.)

Belladonna
- Tincture (U.S.)

Clidinium
- Capsules (U.S.)

Dicyclomine
- Capsules (U.S. and Canada)
- Syrup (U.S. and Canada)
- Tablets (U.S. and Canada)
- Extended-release Tablets (Canada)

Glycopyrrolate
- Tablets (U.S. and Canada)

Homatropine
- Tablets (U.S.)

Hyoscyamine
- Extended-release capsules (U.S.)
- Elixir (U.S.)
- Oral solution (U.S. and Canada)
- Tablets (U.S.)

Isopropamide
- Tablets (U.S.)

Mepenzolate
- Tablets (U.S.)

Methantheline
- Tablets (U.S.)

Methscopolamine
- Tablets (U.S.)

Oxyphencyclimine
- Tablets (U.S.)

Pirenzepine
- Tablets (Canada)

Propantheline
- Tablets (U.S. and Canada)

Scopolamine
- Tablets (Canada)

Tridihexethyl
- Tablets (U.S.)

Parenteral

Atropine
- Injection (U.S. and Canada)

Dicyclomine
- Injection (U.S. and Canada)

Glycopyrrolate
- Injection (U.S. and Canada)

Hyoscyamine
- Injection (U.S. and Canada)

Scopolamine
- Injection (U.S. and Canada)

Rectal

Scopolamine
- Suppositories (Canada)

Transdermal

Scopolamine
- Transdermal disk (U.S. and Canada)

It is very important that you read and understand the following information. If any of it causes you special concern, check with your doctor. Also, *if you have any questions* or if you want more information about this medicine or your medical problem, *ask your doctor, nurse, or pharmacist.*

Before Using This Medicine

In deciding to use a medicine, the risks of taking the medicine must be weighed against the good it will do. This is a decision you and your doctor will make. For anticholinergics/antispasmodics the following should be considered:

Allergies—Tell your doctor if you have ever had any unusual or allergic reaction to any of the natural belladonna alkaloids (atropine, belladonna, hyoscyamine, and scopolamine), iodine or iodides, or any related products. Also, tell your doctor and pharmacist if you are allergic to any other substances, such as foods, preservatives, or dyes.

Pregnancy—If you are pregnant or if you may become pregnant, make sure your doctor knows if your medicine contains any of the following:

- *Atropine*—Atropine has not been shown to cause birth defects or other problems in animals. However, when injected into humans during pregnancy, atropine has been reported to increase the heartbeat of the fetus.
- *Belladonna*—Studies on effects in pregnancy have not been done in either humans or animals.
- *Clidinium*—Clidinium has not been studied in pregnant women. However, clidinium has not been shown to cause birth defects or other problems in animal studies.
- *Dicyclomine*—Dicyclomine has been associated with a few cases of human birth defects but dicyclomine has not been confirmed as the cause.
- *Glycopyrrolate*—Glycopyrrolate has not been studied in pregnant women. However, glycopyrrolate did not cause birth defects in animal studies, but did decrease the chance of becoming pregnant and in the newborn's chance of surviving after weaning.
- *Hyoscyamine*—Studies on effects in pregnancy have not been done in either humans or animals. However, when injected into humans during pregnancy, hyoscyamine has been reported to increase the heartbeat of the fetus.
- *Isopropamide*—Studies on effects in pregnancy have not been done in either humans or animals.
- *Mepenzolate*—Mepenzolate has not been studied in pregnant women. However, studies in animals have not shown that mepenzolate causes birth defects or other problems.
- *Propantheline*—Studies on effects in pregnancy have not been done in either humans or animals.
- *Scopolamine*—Studies on effects in pregnancy have not been done in either humans or animals.

Breast-feeding—Although these medicines may pass into the breast milk, they have not been reported to cause problems in nursing babies. However, the flow of breast milk may be reduced in some patients. The use of dicyclomine in nursing mothers has been reported to cause breathing problems in infants.

Children—Unusual excitement, nervousness, restlessness, or irritability and unusual warmth, dryness, and flushing of skin are more likely to occur in children, who are usually more sensitive to the effects of anticholinergics. Also, when anticholinergics are given to children during hot weather, a rapid increase in body temperature may occur. In infants and children, especially those with spastic paralysis or brain damage, this medicine may be more likely to cause severe side effects. Shortness of breath or difficulty in breathing has occurred in children taking dicyclomine.

Older adults—Confusion or memory loss; constipation; difficult urination; drowsiness; dryness of mouth, nose, throat, or skin; and unusual excitement, nervousness, restlessness, or irritability may be more likely to occur in the elderly, who are usually more sensitive than younger adults to the effects of anticholinergics. Also, eye pain may occur, which may be a sign of glaucoma.

Other medicines—Although certain medicines should not be used together at all, in other cases two different medicines may be used together even if an interaction might occur. In these cases, your doctor may want to change the dose, or other precautions may be necessary. When you are taking anticholinergics/antispasmodics, it is especially important that your doctor and pharmacist know if you are taking any of the following:

- Antacids or
- Diarrhea medicine containing kaolin or attapulgite or
- Ketoconazole (e.g., Nizoral)—Using these medicines with an anticholinergic may lessen the effects of the anticholinergic
- Central nervous system (CNS) depressants (medicines that cause drowsiness)—Taking scopolamine with CNS depressants may increase the effects of either medicine
- Other anticholinergics (medicine for abdominal or stomach spasms or cramps) or
- Tricyclic antidepressants (amitriptyline [e.g., Elavil], amoxapine [e.g., Asendin], clomipramine [e.g., Anafranil], desipramine [e.g., Pertofrane], doxepin [e.g., Sinequan], imipramine [e.g., Tofranil], nortriptyline [e.g., Aventyl], protriptyline [e.g., Vivactil], trimipramine [e.g., Surmontil])—Taking anticholinergics with tricyclic antidepressants or other anticholinergics may cause an increase the effects of the anticholinergic
- Potassium chloride (e.g., Kay Ciel)—Using this medicine with an anticholinergic may make gastrointestinal problems caused by potassium worse

Other medical problems—The presence of other medical problems may affect the use of anticholinergics/antispasmodics. Make sure you tell your doctor if you have any other medical problems, especially:

- Bleeding problems (severe)—These medicines may increase heart rate, which would make bleeding problems worse
- Brain damage (in children)—May increase the CNS effects of this medicine
- Colitis (severe) or
- Dryness of mouth (severe and continuing) or
- Enlarged prostate or
- Fever or
- Glaucoma or
- Heart disease or
- Hernia (hiatal) or
- High blood pressure (hypertension) or
- Intestinal blockage or other intestinal problems or
- Lung disease (chronic) or
- Myasthenia gravis or
- Toxemia of pregnancy or
- Urinary tract blockage or difficult urination—These medicines may make these conditions worse
- Down's syndrome (mongolism)—These medicines may cause an increase in pupil dilation and heart rate
- Kidney disease or
- Liver disease—Higher blood levels may occur and cause an increase in side effects
- Overactive thyroid—These medicines may further increase heart rate
- Spastic paralysis (in children)—This condition may increase the effects of the anticholinergic

Before you begin using any new medicine (prescription or nonprescription) or if you develop any new medical problem while you are using this medicine, check with your doctor, nurse, or pharmacist.

Proper Use of This Medicine

Take this medicine only as directed. Do not take more of it, do not take it more often, and do not take it for a longer time than your doctor ordered. To do so may increase the chance of side effects.

Missed dose—If you miss a dose of this medicine, take it as soon as possible. However, if it is almost time for your next dose, skip the missed dose and go back to your regular dosing schedule. Do not double doses.

For patients *taking any of these medicines by mouth:*

- Take this medicine 30 minutes to 1 hour before meals unless otherwise directed by your doctor.

To use the *rectal suppository* form of *scopolamine:*

- If the suppository is too soft to insert, chill it in the refrigerator for 30 minutes or run cold water over it before removing the foil wrapper.
- To insert the suppository: First remove the foil wrapper and moisten the suppository with cold water. Lie down on your side and use your finger to push the suppository well up into the rectum.

To use the *transdermal disk* form of *scopolamine:*

- This medicine usually comes with patient directions. Read them carefully before using this medicine.
- Wash and dry your hands thoroughly before and after handling.
- Apply the disk to the hairless area of skin behind the ear. Do not place over any cuts or irritations.

Storage—To store this medicine:

- Keep out of the reach of children. Overdose is especially dangerous in young children.
- Store away from heat and direct light.
- Do not store the capsule or tablet form of this medicine in the bathroom, near the kitchen sink, or in other damp places. Heat or moisture may cause the medicine to break down.
- Keep the liquid form of this medicine tightly closed and keep it from freezing. Do not refrigerate the syrup form of this medicine.
- Do not keep outdated medicine or medicine no longer needed. Be sure that any discarded medicine is out of the reach of children.

Precautions While Using This Medicine

If you think you or someone else may have taken an overdose, get emergency help at once. Taking an overdose of any of the belladonna alkaloids or taking scopolamine with alcohol or other CNS depressants may lead to unconsciousness and possibly death. Some signs of overdose are clumsiness or unsteadiness; dizziness; severe drowsiness; fever; hallucinations (seeing, hearing, or feeling things that are not there); confusion; shortness of breath or troubled breathing; slurred speech; unusual excitement, nervousness, restlessness, or irritability; fast heartbeat; and unusual warmth, dryness, and flushing of skin.

These medicines may make you sweat less, causing your body temperature to increase. *Use extra care not to become overheated during exercise or hot weather while you are taking this medicine,* since overheating may result in heat stroke. Also hot baths or saunas may make you dizzy or faint while you are taking this medicine.

Check with your doctor before you stop using this medicine. Your doctor may want you to reduce gradually the amount you are using before stopping completely. Stopping this medicine may cause withdrawal side effects such as vomiting, sweating, and dizziness.

Anticholinergics may cause some people to have blurred vision. *Make sure your vision is clear before you drive or do anything else that could be dangerous if you are not able to see well.* These medicines may also cause your eyes to become more sensitive to light than they are normally. Wearing sunglasses may help lessen the discomfort from bright light.

These medicines, especially in high doses, may cause some people to become dizzy or drowsy. *Make sure you know how you react to this medicine before you drive, use machines, or do anything else that could be dangerous if you are dizzy or are not alert.*

Dizziness, lightheadedness, or fainting may occur, especially when you get up from a lying or sitting position. Getting up slowly may help lessen this problem.

These medicines may cause dryness of the mouth, nose, and throat. For temporary relief of mouth dryness, use sugarless candy or gum, melt bits of ice in your mouth, or use a saliva substitute. However, if your mouth continues to feel dry for more than 2 weeks, check with your medical doctor or dentist. Continuing dryness of the mouth may increase the chance of dental disease, including tooth decay, gum disease, and fungus infections.

For patients taking *isopropamide:*

- Make sure your doctor knows if you are planning to have any future thyroid tests. The results of the thyroid test may be affected by the iodine in this medicine.

For patients taking *scopolamine:*

- This medicine will add to the effects of alcohol and other CNS depressants (medicines that slow down the nervous system, possibly causing drowsiness). Some examples of CNS depressants are antihistamines or medicine for hay fever, other allergies, or colds; sedatives, tranquilizers, or sleeping medicine; prescription pain medicine or narcotics; barbiturates; medicine for seizures; muscle relaxants; or anesthetics, including some dental anesthetics. *Check with your doctor before taking any of the above while you are using this medicine.*

For patients *taking any of these medicines by mouth:*

- Do not take this medicine within 2 or 3 hours of taking antacids or medicine for diarrhea. Taking antacids or antidiarrhea medicines and this medicine too close together may prevent this medicine from working properly.

Side Effects of This Medicine

Along with its needed effects, a medicine may cause some unwanted effects. Although not all of these side effects may occur, if they do occur they may need medical attention.

Check with your doctor as soon as possible if any of the following side effects occur:

Rare

Confusion (especially in the elderly); dizziness, lightheadedness (continuing), or fainting; eye pain; skin rash or hives

Symptoms of overdose

Blurred vision (continuing) or changes in near vision; clumsiness or unsteadiness; confusion; convulsions (seizures); difficulty in breathing, muscle weakness (severe), or tiredness (severe); dizziness; drowsiness (severe); dryness of mouth, nose, or throat (severe); fast heartbeat; fever; hallucinations (seeing, hearing, or feeling things that are not there); slurred speech; unusual excitement, nervousness, restlessness, or irritability; unusual warmth, dryness, and flushing of skin

Other side effects may occur that usually do not need medical attention. These side effects may go away during treatment as your body adjusts to the medicine. However, check with your doctor if any of the following side effects continue or are bothersome:

More common

Constipation (less common with hyoscyamine); decreased sweating; dryness of mouth, nose, throat, or skin

Less common or rare

Bloated feeling; blurred vision; decreased flow of breast milk; difficult urination; difficulty in swallowing; drowsiness (more common with high doses of any of these medicines and with usual doses of scopolamine when given by mouth or by injection); false sense of well-being (for scopolamine only); headache; increased sensitivity of eyes to light; lightheadedness (with injection); loss of memory; nausea or vomiting; redness or other signs of irritation at place of injection; trouble in sleeping (for scopolamine only); unusual tiredness or weakness

For patients using *scopolamine:*

- After you stop using scopolamine, your body may need time to adjust. The length of time this takes depends on the amount of scopolamine you were using and how long you used it. During this period of time check with your doctor if you notice any of the following side effects:

  Anxiety; irritability; nightmares; trouble in sleeping

For patients using the *transdermal disk* of *scopolamine:*

- While using the disk or even after removing it, your eyes may become more sensitive to light than usual. You may also notice the pupil in one eye is larger than the other. Check with your doctor if this side effect continues or is bothersome.

Other side effects not listed above may also occur in some patients. If you notice any other effects, check with your doctor.

Additional Information

Once a medicine has been approved for marketing for a certain use, experience may show that it is also useful for other medical problems. Although these uses are not included in product labeling, anticholinergics/antispasmodics are used in certain patients with the following medical conditions:

- Diarrhea
- Excessive watering of mouth

Other than the above information, there is no additional information relating to proper use, precautions, or side effects for these uses.

Annual revision: 01/29/92

ANTICOAGULANTS Systemic

This information applies to the following medicines:

Anisindione (an-iss-in-DYE-one)
Dicumarol (dye-KOO-ma-role)
Warfarin (WAR-far-in)

This information does *not* apply to heparin.

Some commonly used brand names are:

For Anisindione
In the U.S.
Miradon

For Dicumarol
In the U.S.
Generic name product available.

Another commonly used name is dicoumarol.

For Warfarin
In the U.S.
Coumadin
Panwarfin
Sofarin
Generic name product may also be available.

In Canada
Coumadin
Warfilone

Description

Anticoagulants decrease the clotting ability of the blood and therefore help to prevent harmful clots from forming in the blood vessels. These medicines are sometimes called blood thinners, although they do not actually thin the blood. They also will not dissolve clots that already have formed, but they may prevent the clots from becoming larger and causing more serious problems. They are often used as treatment for certain blood vessel, heart, and lung conditions.

In order for an anticoagulant to help you without causing serious bleeding, it must be used properly and all of the precautions concerning its use must be followed exactly. Be sure that you have discussed the use of this medicine with your doctor. It is very important that you understand all of your doctor's orders and that you are willing and able to follow them exactly.

Anticoagulants are available only with your doctor's prescription, in the following dosage forms:

Oral

Anisindione
- Tablets (U.S.)

Dicumarol
- Tablets (U.S.)

Warfarin
- Tablets (U.S. and Canada)

Parenteral

Warfarin
- Injection (U.S.)

It is very important that you read and understand the following information. If any of it causes you special concern, check with your doctor. Also, *if you have any questions* or if you want more information about this medicine or your medical problem, *ask your doctor, nurse, or pharmacist.*

Before Using This Medicine

In deciding to use a medicine, the risks of taking the medicine must be weighed against the good it will do. This is a decision you and your doctor will make. For anticoagulants, the following should be considered:

Allergies—Tell your doctor if you have ever had any unusual or allergic reaction to an anticoagulant. Also tell your doctor and pharmacist if you are allergic to any other substances, such as foods, preservatives, or dyes.

Pregnancy—Anticoagulants may cause birth defects. They may also cause other problems affecting the physical or mental growth of the fetus or newborn baby. In addition, use of this medicine during the last 6 months of pregnancy may increase the chance of severe, possibly fatal, bleeding in the fetus. If taken during the last few weeks of pregnancy, anticoagulants may cause severe bleeding in both the fetus and the mother before or during delivery and in the newborn infant.

Do not begin taking this medicine during pregnancy, and do not become pregnant while taking it, unless you have first discussed the possible effects of this medicine with your doctor. Also, if you suspect that you may be pregnant and you are already taking an anticoagulant, check with your doctor at once. Your doctor may suggest that you take a different anticoagulant that is less likely to harm the fetus or the newborn infant during all or part of your pregnancy. Anticoagulants may also cause severe bleeding in the mother if taken soon after the baby is born.

Breast-feeding—Warfarin is not likely to cause problems in nursing babies. Other anticoagulants may pass into the breast milk. A blood test can be done to see if unwanted effects are occurring in the nursing baby. If necessary, another medicine that will overcome any unwanted effects of the anticoagulant can be given to the baby.

Children—Very young babies may be especially sensitive to the effects of anticoagulants. This may increase the chance of bleeding during treatment.

Older adults—Elderly people are especially sensitive to the effects of anticoagulants. This may increase the chance of bleeding during treatment.

Other medicines—Although certain medicines should not be used together at all, in other cases two different medicines may be used together even if an interaction might occur. In these cases, your doctor may want to change the dose, or other precautions may be necessary. *Many different medicines can affect the way anticoagulants work in your body.* Therefore, it is very important that your doctor and pharmacist know if you are taking *any* other prescription or nonprescription (over-the-counter [OTC]) medicine, even aspirin, laxatives, vitamins, or antacids.

Other medical problems—The presence of other medical problems may affect the use of anticoagulants. Make sure you tell your doctor if you have *any* other medical problems, or if you are now being treated by any other medical doctor or dentist. Many medical problems and treatments will affect the way your body responds to this medicine.

Also, it is important that you tell your doctor if you have recently had any of the following conditions or medical procedures:

- Childbirth or
- Falls or blows to the body or head or
- Fever lasting more than a couple of days or
- Heavy or unusual menstrual bleeding or
- Insertion of intrauterine device (IUD) or
- Medical or dental surgery or
- Severe or continuing diarrhea or
- Spinal anesthesia or
- X-ray (radiation) treatment—The risk of serious bleeding may be increased

Before you begin using any new medicine (prescription or nonprescription) or if you develop any new medical problem while you are using this medicine, check with your doctor, nurse, or pharmacist.

Proper Use of This Medicine

Take this medicine only as directed by your doctor. Do not take more or less of it, do not take it more often, and do not take it for a longer time than your doctor ordered. This is especially important for elderly patients, who are especially sensitive to the effects of anticoagulants.

Your doctor should check your progress at regular visits. A blood test must be taken regularly to see how fast your blood is clotting. This will help your doctor decide on the proper amount of anticoagulant you should be taking each day.

Missed dose—If you miss a dose of this medicine, take it as soon as possible. Then go back to your regular dosing schedule. If you do not remember until the next day, do not take the missed dose at all and do not double the next one. *Doubling the dose may cause bleeding.* Instead, go back to your regular dosing schedule. It is recommended that you keep a record of each dose as you take it to avoid mistakes. Also, be sure to give your doctor a record of any doses you miss. If you have any questions about this, check with your doctor.

Storage—To store this medicine:

- Keep out of the reach of children.
- Store away from heat and direct light.
- Do not store this medicine in the bathroom, near the kitchen sink, or in other damp places. Heat or moisture may cause the medicine to break down.
- Do not keep outdated medicine or medicine no longer needed. Be sure that any discarded medicine is out of the reach of children.

Precautions While Using This Medicine

Tell all medical doctors, dentists, and pharmacists you go to that you are taking this medicine.

Check with your doctor, nurse, or pharmacist before you start or stop taking any other medicine. This includes any nonprescription (over-the-counter [OTC]) medicine, even aspirin or acetaminophen. Many medicines change the way this medicine affects your body. You may not be able to take the other medicine, or the dose of your anticoagulant may need to be changed.

It is important that you carry identification stating that you are using this medicine. If you have any questions about what kind of identification to carry, check with your doctor, nurse, or pharmacist.

While you are taking this medicine, it is very important that you avoid sports and activities that may cause you to be injured. Report to your doctor any falls, blows to the body or head, or other injuries, since serious internal bleeding may occur without your knowing about it.

Be careful to avoid cutting yourself. This includes taking special care in brushing your teeth and in shaving. Use a soft toothbrush and floss gently. Also, it is best to use an electric shaver rather than a blade.

Drinking too much alcohol may change the way this anticoagulant affects your body. You should not drink regularly on a daily basis or take more than 1 or 2 drinks at any time. If you have any questions about this, check with your doctor.

The foods that you eat may also affect the way this medicine affects your body. Eat a normal, balanced diet while you are taking this medicine. Do not go on a reducing diet, make other changes in your eating habits, start taking vitamins, or begin using other nutrition supplements unless you have first checked with your doctor, nurse, or pharmacist. Also, check with your doctor if you are unable to eat for several days or if you have continuing stomach upset, diarrhea, or fever. These precautions are important because the effects of the anticoagulant depend on the amount of vitamin K in your body. Therefore, it is best to have the same amount of vitamin K in your body every day. Some multiple vitamins and some nutrition supplements contain vitamin K. Vitamin K is also present in meats, dairy products (such as milk, cheese, and yogurt), and green, leafy vegetables (such as broccoli, cabbage, collard greens, kale, lettuce, and spinach). It is especially important that you do not make large changes in the amounts of these foods that you eat every day while you are taking an anticoagulant.

After you stop taking this medicine, your body will need time to recover before your blood clotting ability returns to normal. Your pharmacist or doctor can tell you how long this will take depending on which anticoagulant you were taking. Use the same caution during this period of time as you did while you were taking the anticoagulant.

Side Effects of This Medicine

Along with its needed effects, a medicine may cause some unwanted effects. Although not all of these side effects may occur, if they do occur they may need medical attention.

Check with your doctor immediately if any of the following side effects occur:

Less common or rare

Blue or purple color of toes and pain in toes; cloudy or dark urine; difficult or painful urination; sores, ulcers, or white spots in mouth or throat; sore throat and fever or chills; sudden decrease in amount of urine; swelling of face, feet, or lower legs; unusual tiredness or weakness; unusual weight gain; yellow eyes or skin

Since many things can affect the way your body reacts to this medicine, you should always watch for signs of unusual bleeding. Unusual bleeding may mean that your body is getting more medicine than it needs. *Check with your doctor immediately if any of the following signs of overdose occur:*

Bleeding from gums when brushing teeth; unexplained bruising or purplish areas on skin; unexplained nosebleeds; unusually heavy bleeding or oozing from cuts or wounds; unusually heavy or unexpected menstrual bleeding

Signs and symptoms of bleeding inside the body

Abdominal or stomach pain or swelling; back pain or backaches; blood in urine; bloody or black tarry stools; constipation; coughing up blood; dizziness; headache (severe or continuing); joint pain, stiffness, or swelling; vomiting blood or material that looks like coffee grounds

Also, check with your doctor as soon as possible if any of the following side effects occur:

Less common or rare

Diarrhea (more common with dicumarol); nausea or vomiting; skin rash, hives, or itching; stomach cramps or pain

For patients taking *anisindione* (e.g., Miradon):

- Depending on your diet, this medicine may cause your urine to turn orange. Since it may be hard to tell the difference between blood in the urine and this normal color change, check with your doctor if you notice any color change in your urine.

Other side effects may occur that usually do not need medical attention. These side effects may go away during treatment as your body adjusts to the medicine. However, check with your doctor if any of the following side effects continue or are bothersome:

More common
Bloated feeling or gas (with dicumarol)

Less common
Blurred vision or other vision problems (with anisindione); loss of appetite; unusual hair loss

Other side effects not listed above may also occur in some patients. If you notice any other effects, check with your doctor.

Annual revision: June 1990

ANTICONVULSANTS, DIONE Systemic†

This information applies to the following medicines:
Paramethadione (par-a-meth-a-DYE-one)
Trimethadione (trye-meth-a-DYE-one)

Some commonly used brand names are:

For Paramethadione†
In the U.S.
Paradione

For Trimethadione†
In the U.S.
Tridione
Tridione Dulcets

†Not commercially available in Canada.

Description

Dione anticonvulsants are used to control certain types of seizures in the treatment of epilepsy. These medicines act on the central nervous system (CNS) to reduce the number of seizures.

This medicine is available only with your doctor's prescription in the following dosage forms:

Oral
Paramethadione
- Capsules (U.S.)

Trimethadione
- Capsules (U.S.)
- Oral solution (U.S.)
- Tablets (U.S.)

It is very important that you read and understand the following information. If any of it causes you special concern, check with your doctor. Also, *if you have any questions* or if you want more information about this medicine or your medical problem, *ask your doctor, nurse, or pharmacist.*

Before Using This Medicine

In deciding to use a medicine, the risks of taking the medicine must be weighed against the good it will do. This is a decision you and your doctor will make. For dione anticonvulsants, the following should be considered:

Allergies—Tell your doctor if you have ever had any unusual or allergic reaction to anticonvulsant medicines. Also tell your doctor and pharmacist if you are allergic to any other substances, such as foods, preservatives, or dyes.

Pregnancy—There have been reports of increased birth defects when dione anticonvulsants were used during pregnancy. The use of an effective method of birth control is recommended during treatment with dione anticonvulsants. Be sure you have discussed this with your doctor before taking this medicine. Dione anticonvulsants may also cause a bleeding problem in the mother during delivery and in the newborn. Doctors can help prevent this by giving vitamin K to the mother during delivery, and to the baby immediately after birth.

Breast-feeding—It is not known whether this medicine passes into breast milk.

Children—Although there is no specific information comparing use of dione anticonvulsants in children with use in other age groups, these medicines are not expected to cause different side effects or problems in children than they do in adults.

Older adults—Many medicines have not been studied specifically in older people. Therefore, it may not be known whether they work exactly the same way they do in younger adults. Although there is no specific information comparing use of dione anticonvulsants in the elderly with use in other age groups, these medicines are not expected to cause different side effects or problems in older people than they do in younger adults.

Other medicines—Although certain medicines should not be used together at all, in other cases 2 different medicines may be used together even if an interaction might occur. In these cases, your doctor may want to change the dose, or other precautions may be necessary. When you are taking dione anticonvulsants, it is especially important that your doctor and pharmacist know if you are taking any of the following:

- Central nervous system (CNS) depressants (medicine that causes drowsiness) or
- Tricyclic antidepressants (medicine for depression)—Using these medicines together may increase the CNS depressant effects

Other medical problems—The presence of other medical problems may affect the use of the dione anticonvulsants. Make sure you tell your doctor if you have any other medical problems, especially:

- Blood disease (severe) or
- Diseases of the eye or optic nerve or
- Kidney disease (severe) or
- Liver disease (severe)—Dione anticonvulsants may make the condition worse
- Porphyria—Trimethadione may make the condition worse

Before you begin using any new medicine (prescription or nonprescription) or if you develop any new medical problem while you are using this medicine, check with your doctor, nurse, or pharmacist.

Proper Use of This Medicine

For patients taking *paramethadione capsules:*

- Swallow the capsules whole. Do not crush, chew, or break them before swallowing.

For patients taking *trimethadione tablets:*

- The tablets may be chewed or crushed and dissolved in a small amount of water before they are swallowed.

If this medicine upsets your stomach, take it with a small amount of food or milk unless otherwise directed by your doctor.

This medicine must be taken every day in regularly spaced doses as ordered by your doctor.

Dosing—The dose of dione anticonvulsants will be different for different patients. *Follow your doctor's orders or the directions on the label.* The following information includes only the average doses of paramethadione and trimethadione. *If your dose is different, do not change it* unless your doctor tells you to do so.

For paramethadione

- For *oral* dosage forms (capsules):
  —Adults and adolescents: To start, 300 milligrams three or four times a day. Your doctor may increase your dose by 300 milligrams every week until seizures are controlled or side effects appear.
  —Children 6 years of age and over: 300 milligrams three times a day.
  —Children 2 to 6 years of age: 200 milligrams three times a day.
  —Children up to 2 years of age: 100 milligrams three times a day.

For trimethadione

- For *oral* dosage forms (capsules, solution, tablets):
  —Adults and adolescents: To start, 300 milligrams three or four times a day. Your doctor may increase your dose by 300 milligrams every week until seizures are controlled or side effects appear.
  —Children 6 years of age and over: 300 milligrams three or four times a day.
  —Children 2 to 6 years of age: 200 milligrams three times a day.
  —Children up to 2 years of age: 100 milligrams three times a day.

Missed dose—If you miss a dose of this medicine, take it as soon as possible. However, if it is almost time for your next dose, skip the missed dose and go back to your regular dosing schedule. If only one dose is missed, it may be taken at bedtime.

Storage—To store this medicine:

- Keep out of the reach of children.
- Store away from heat and direct light.
- Do not store the capsule or tablet form of this medicine in the bathroom, near the kitchen sink, or in other damp places. Heat or moisture may cause the medicine to break down.
- Keep the liquid form of this medicine from freezing.
- Do not keep outdated medicine or medicine no longer needed. Be sure that any discarded medicine is out of the reach of children.

Precautions While Using This Medicine

It is very important that your doctor check your progress at regular visits, especially during the first few months of treatment with this medicine.

If you have been taking this medicine regularly, do not stop taking it without first checking with your doctor. Your doctor may want you to reduce gradually the amount you are taking before stopping completely. Stopping this medicine suddenly may cause seizures.

This medicine may cause your eyes to become more sensitive to bright light than they are normally, making it difficult for you to see well. Wearing sunglasses and avoiding too much exposure to bright light may help lessen the discomfort. You may also have difficulty seeing in light that changes in brightness. If you notice this effect, be especially careful when driving at night.

This medicine will add to the effects of alcohol and other CNS depressants (medicines that slow down the nervous system, possibly causing drowsiness). Some examples of CNS depressants are antihistamines or medicine for hay fever, other allergies, or colds; sedatives, tranquilizers, or sleeping medicine; prescription pain medicine or narcotics; barbiturates; medicine for seizures; muscle relaxants; or anesthetics, including some dental anesthetics. *Check with your doctor before taking any of the above while you are using this medicine.*

This medicine may cause some people to become drowsy or less alert than they are normally. *Make sure you know how you react to this medicine before you drive, use machines, or do anything else that could be dangerous if you are not alert.* After you have taken this medicine for a while, this effect may not be so bothersome.

Before having any kind of surgery, dental treatment, or emergency treatment, tell the medical doctor or dentist in charge that you are taking this medicine. Taking dione anticonvulsants together with medicines that are used during surgery or dental or emergency treatments may increase the CNS depressant effects.

Be sure to tell your doctor as soon as possible if you have a sore throat, fever, or general feeling of tiredness, or if you notice any unusual bleeding or bruising, such as reddish or purplish spots on the skin, or recurring nosebleeds or bleeding gums.

Check with your doctor as soon as possible if you suspect you have become pregnant.

Side Effects of This Medicine

Along with its needed effects, a medicine may cause some unwanted effects. Although not all of these side effects may occur, if they do occur they may need medical attention.

Check with your doctor as soon as possible if any of the following side effects occur:

More common

Changes in vision, such as glare or snowy image, caused by bright light, or double vision

Rare

Confusion; convulsions (seizures); dark or cloudy urine; dizziness; fever; loss of appetite or weight; muscle weakness (severe), especially drooping eyelids, difficulty in chewing, swallowing, talking, or breathing, and unusual tiredness; nausea or vomiting; pain in abdomen or joints; skin rash or itching; sore throat and fever; swelling of face, hands, legs, and feet; swollen glands; unusual bleeding or bruising, such as recurring nosebleeds, bleeding gums, or vaginal bleeding, or red or purple spots on skin; unusual tiredness or weakness; yellow eyes or skin

Symptoms of overdose

Clumsiness or unsteadiness; dizziness (severe); drowsiness (severe); nausea (severe)

Other side effects may occur that usually do not need medical attention. These side effects may go away during treatment as your body adjusts to the medicine. However, check with your doctor if any of the following side effects continue or are bothersome:

More common

Dizziness; drowsiness; headache; increased sensitivity of eyes to light; irritability

Less common

Behavior or mood changes; blood pressure changes; hair loss; hiccups; stomach pain or upset; tingling, burning, or prickly sensations; trouble in sleeping

Other side effects not listed above may also occur in some patients. If you notice any other effects, check with your doctor.

Annual revision: 01/29/93

ANTICONVULSANTS, HYDANTOIN Systemic

This information applies to the following medicines:

Ethotoin (ETH-oh-toyn)
Mephenytoin (me-FEN-i-toyn)
Phenytoin (FEN-i-toyn)

Some commonly used brand names are:

For Ethotoin†
In the U.S.
Peganone

For Mephenytoin
In the U.S.
Mesantoin
In Canada
Mesantoin

For Phenytoin
In the U.S.
Dilantin
Dilantin-125
Dilantin Infatabs
Dilantin Kapseals
Dilantin-30 Pediatric
Diphenylan
Phenytex

Generic name product may also be available.

In Canada
Dilantin
Dilantin-30
Dilantin-125
Dilantin Infatabs

Another commonly used name is diphenylhydantoin.

†Not commercially available in Canada.

Description

Hydantoin anticonvulsants (hye-DAN-toyn an-tye-kon-VUL-sants) are used most often to control certain convulsions or seizures in the treatment of epilepsy. Phenytoin may also be used for other conditions as determined by your doctor.

In seizure disorders, these medicines act on the central nervous system (CNS) to reduce the number and severity of seizures. Hydantoin anticonvulsants may also produce some unwanted effects. These depend on the patient's individual condition, the amount of medicine taken, and how long it has been taken. It is important that you know what the side effects are and when to call your doctor if they occur.

Hydantoin anticonvulsants are available only with your doctor's prescription, in the following dosage forms:

Oral

Ethotoin
- Tablets (U.S.)

Mephenytoin
- Tablets (U.S. and Canada)

Phenytoin
- Extended capsules (U.S. and Canada)
- Prompt capsules (U.S.)
- Oral suspension (U.S. and Canada)
- Chewable tablets (U.S. and Canada)

Parenteral

Phenytoin
- Injection (U.S. and Canada)

It is very important that you read and understand the following information. If any of it causes you special concern, check with your doctor. Also, *if you have any questions* or if you want more information about this medicine or your medical problem, *ask your doctor, nurse, or pharmacist.*

Before Using This Medicine

In deciding to use a medicine, the risks of taking the medicine must be weighed against the good it will do. This is a decision you and your doctor will make. For hydantoin anticonvulsants, the following should be considered:

Allergies—Tell your doctor if you have ever had any unusual or allergic reaction to any hydantoin anticonvulsant medicine. Also tell your doctor and pharmacist if you are allergic to any other substance, such as foods, preservatives, or dyes.

Pregnancy—Although most mothers who take medicine for seizure control deliver normal babies, there have been reports of increased birth defects when these medicines were used during pregnancy. It is not definitely known if any of these medicines are the cause of such problems.

Also, pregnancy may cause a change in the way hydantoin anticonvulsants are absorbed in your body. You may have more seizures, even though you are taking your medicine regularly. Your doctor may need to increase the anticonvulsant dose during your pregnancy.

In addition, when taken during pregnancy, this medicine may cause a bleeding problem in the mother during delivery and in the newborn. This may be prevented by giving vitamin K to the mother during delivery, and to the baby immediately after birth.

Breast-feeding—Ethotoin and phenytoin pass into the breast milk in small amounts. It is not known whether mephenytoin passes into breast milk. Be sure you have discussed the risks and benefits of the medicine with your doctor.

Children—Some side effects, especially bleeding, tender, or enlarged gums and enlarged facial features, are more likely to occur in children and young adults. Also, unusual and excessive hair growth may occur, which is more noticeable in young girls. In addition, some children may not do as well in school after using high doses of this medicine for a long time.

Older adults—Some medicines may affect older patients differently than they do younger patients. Overdose is more likely to occur in elderly patients and in patients with liver disease.

Other medicines—Although certain medicines should not be used together at all, in other cases 2 different medicines may be used together even if an interaction might occur. In these cases, your doctor may want to change the dose, or other precautions may be necessary. When you are taking or receiving hydantoin anticonvulsants, it is especially important that your doctor and pharmacist know if you are taking any of the following:

- Alcohol or
- Central nervous system (CNS) depressants (medicine that causes drowsiness)—Long-term use of alcohol may decrease the blood levels of hydantoin anticonvulsants, resulting in decreased effects; use of hydantoin anticonvulsants in cases where a large amount of alcohol is consumed may increase the blood levels of the hydantoin, resulting in an increased risk of side effects

- Aminophylline (e.g., Somophyllin) or
- Caffeine (e.g., NoDoz) or
- Oxtriphylline (e.g., Choledyl) or
- Theophylline (e.g., Somophyllin-T)—Hydantoin anticonvulsants may make these medicines less effective

- Amiodarone (e.g., Cordarone)—Use with phenytoin and possibly with other hydantoin anticonvulsants may increase blood levels of the hydantoin, resulting in an increase in serious side effects

- Antacids or
- Medicine containing calcium—Use of antacids or calcium supplements may decrease the absorption of phenytoin; doses of antacids and phenytoin or calcium supplements and phenytoin should be taken 2 to 3 hours apart

- Anticoagulants (blood thinners) or
- Chloramphenicol (e.g., Chloromycetin) or
- Cimetidine (e.g., Tagamet) or
- Disulfiram (e.g., Antabuse) (medicine for alcoholism) or
- Isoniazid (INH) (e.g., Nydrazid) or
- Phenylbutazone (e.g., Butazolidin) or
- Sulfonamides (sulfa drugs)—Blood levels of hydantoin anticonvulsants may be increased, increasing the risk of serious side effects; hydantoin anticonvulsants may increase the effects of the anticoagulants at first, but with continued use may decrease the effects of these medicines

- Corticosteroids (cortisone-like medicines) or
- Estrogens (female hormones) or
- Oral contraceptives (birth-control pills) containing estrogens—Hydantoin anticonvulsants may decrease the effects of these medicines; use of hydantoin anticonvulsants

with oral, estrogen-containing contraceptives may result in breakthrough bleeding and contraceptive failure; the amount of estrogen in the oral contraceptive may need to be increased to stop the bleeding and decrease the risk of pregnancy

- Diazoxide (e.g., Proglycem)—Use with hydantoin anticonvulsants may decrease the effects of both medicines; therefore, these medicines should not be taken together
- Fluconazole (e.g., Diflucan)—Blood levels of phenytoin may be increased, increasing the chance of side effects
- Lidocaine—Risk of slow heartbeat may be increased. Other effects of lidocaine may be decreased because hydantoin anticonvulsants may cause it to be removed from the body more quickly
- Methadone (e.g., Dolophine, Methadose)—Long-term use of phenytoin may bring on withdrawal symptoms in patients being treated for drug dependence
- Phenacemide (e.g., Phenurone)—Use with hydantoin anticonvulsants may increase the risk of serious side effects
- Rifampin (e.g., Rifadin)—Use with phenytoin may decrease the effects of phenytoin; your doctor may need to adjust your dosage
- Streptozocin (e.g., Zanosar)—Phenytoin may decrease the effects of streptozocin; therefore, these medicines should not be used together
- Sucralfate (e.g., Carafate)—Use of sucralfate may decrease the absorption of hydantoin anticonvulsants
- Valproic acid (e.g., Depakene, Depakote)—Use with phenytoin, and possibly other hydantoin anticonvulsants, may increase seizure frequency and increase the risk of serious liver side effects, especially in infants

Other medical problems—The presence of other medical problems may affect the use of hydantoin anticonvulsants. Make sure you tell your doctor if you have any other medical problems, especially:

- Alcohol abuse—Blood levels of phenytoin may be decreased, decreasing its effects
- Blood disease—Risk of serious infections rarely may be increased by hydantoin anticonvulsants
- Diabetes mellitus (sugar diabetes) or
- Porphyria or
- Systemic lupus erythematosus—Hydantoin anticonvulsants may make the condition worse
- Fever above 101 °F for longer than 24 hours—Blood levels of hydantoin anticonvulsants may be decreased, decreasing the medicine's effects
- Heart disease—Administration of phenytoin by injection may change the rhythm of the heart
- Kidney disease or
- Liver disease—Blood levels of hydantoin anticonvulsants may be increased, leading to an increase in serious side effects
- Thyroid disease—Blood levels of thyroid hormones may be decreased

Before you begin using any new medicine (prescription or nonprescription) or if you develop any new medical problem while you are using this medicine, check with your doctor, nurse, or pharmacist.

Proper Use of This Medicine

For patients taking the *liquid form* of this medicine:

- Shake the bottle well before using.
- Use a specially marked measuring spoon, a plastic syringe, or a small measuring cup to measure each dose accurately. The average household teaspoon may not hold the right amount of liquid.

For patients taking the *chewable tablet form* of this medicine:

- Tablets may be chewed or crushed before they are swallowed, or may be swallowed whole.

For patients taking the *capsule form* of this medicine:

- Swallow the capsule whole.

If this medicine upsets your stomach, take it with food, unless otherwise directed by your doctor. The medicine should always be taken at the same time in relation to meals to make sure that it is absorbed in the same way.

To control your medical problem, *take this medicine every day* exactly as ordered by your doctor. Do not take more or less of it than your doctor ordered. To help you remember to take the medicine at the correct times, try to get into the habit of taking it at the same time each day.

Dosing—The dose of hydantoin anticonvulsants will be different for different patients. *Follow your doctor's orders or the directions on the label.* The following information includes only the average doses of ethotoin, mephenytoin, and phenytoin. *If your dose is different, do not change it* unless your doctor tells you to do so.

- The number of capsules or tablets or teaspoonfuls of suspension that you take depends on the strength of the medicine. Also, *the number of doses you take each day, the time allowed between doses, and the length of time you take the medicine depend on the medical problem for which you are using an hydantoin anticonvulsant.*

For ethotoin

- For *oral* dosage form (tablets):

  —Adults and adolescents: To start, 125 to 250 milligrams four to six times a day. Your doctor may increase your dose gradually over several days if needed. However, the dose is usually not more than 3000 milligrams a day.

  —Children: To start, up to 750 milligrams a day, based on the age and weight of the child. The doctor may increase the dose gradually if needed.

For mephenytoin

- For *oral* dosage form (tablets):

  —Adults and adolescents: To start, 50 to 100 milligrams once a day. Your doctor may increase your dose by 50 to 100 milligrams a day at weekly intervals if needed. However, the dose is usually not more than 1200 milligrams a day.

—Children: To start, 25 to 50 milligrams once a day. The doctor may increase the dose by 25 to 50 milligrams a day at weekly intervals if needed. However, the dose is usually not more than 400 milligrams a day.

For phenytoin

- For *oral* dosage forms (capsules, chewable tablets, or suspension):
  —Adults and adolescents: To start, 100 to 125 milligrams three times a day. Your doctor may adjust your dose at intervals of seven to ten days if needed.
  —Children: Dose is based on body weight or body surface area. The usual dose is 5 milligrams of phenytoin per kilogram (2.3 milligrams per pound) of body weight to start. The doctor may adjust the dose if needed.
  —Older adults: Dose is based on body weight. The usual dose is 3 milligrams per kilogram (1.4 milligrams per pound) of body weight. The doctor may need to adjust the dose based on your response to the medicine.
- For *injection* dosage form:
  —Adults and children: Dose is based on illness being treated, and body weight or body surface area of the patient. The medicine is usually injected into a vein.

Missed dose—*If you miss a dose of this medicine* and your dosing schedule is:

- One dose a day—Take the missed dose as soon as possible. However, if you do not remember the missed dose until the next day, skip it and go back to your regular dosing schedule. Do not double doses.
- More than one dose a day—Take the missed dose as soon as possible. However, if it is within 4 hours of your next dose, skip the missed dose and go back to your regular dosing schedule. Do not double doses.

If you miss doses for 2 or more days in a row, check with your doctor.

Storage—To store this medicine:

- Keep out of the reach of children.
- Store away from heat and direct light.
- Do not store in the bathroom, near the kitchen sink, or in other damp places. Heat or moisture may cause the medicine to break down.
- Keep the liquid form of this medicine from freezing. Do not refrigerate.
- Do not keep outdated medicine or medicine no longer needed. Be sure any discarded medicine is out of the reach of children.

Precautions While Using This Medicine

Your doctor should check your progress at regular visits, especially during the first few months of treatment with this medicine. During this time the amount of medicine you are taking may have to be changed often to meet your individual needs.

Do not start or stop taking any other medicine without your doctor's advice. Other medicines may affect the way this medicine works.

This medicine will add to the effects of alcohol and other CNS depressants (medicines that slow down the nervous system, possibly causing drowsiness). Some examples of CNS depressants are antihistamines or medicine for hay fever, other allergies, or colds; sedatives, tranquilizers, or sleeping medicine; prescription pain medicine or narcotics; barbiturates; other medicine for seizures; muscle relaxants; or anesthetics, including some dental anesthetics. *Check with your doctor before taking any of the above while you are using this medicine.*

Do not take this medicine within 2 to 3 hours of taking antacids or medicine for diarrhea. Taking these medicines too close to taking hydantoin anticonvulsants may make the hydantoins less effective.

Do not change brands or dosage forms of phenytoin without first checking with your doctor. Different products may not work the same way. If you refill your medicine and it looks different, check with your pharmacist.

If you have been taking this medicine regularly for several weeks or more, do not suddenly stop taking it. Your doctor may want you to reduce gradually the amount you are taking before stopping completely.

Your doctor may want you to carry a medical identification card or bracelet stating that you are taking this medicine.

For diabetic patients:

- This medicine may affect blood sugar levels. If you notice a change in the results of your blood or urine sugar tests or if you have any questions, check with your doctor.

Before you have any medical tests, tell the doctor in charge that you are taking this medicine. The results of some tests (including the dexamethasone, metyrapone, or Schilling tests, and certain thyroid function tests) may be affected by this medicine.

Before having any kind of surgery, dental treatment, or emergency treatment, tell the medical doctor or dentist in charge that you are taking this medicine. Taking hydantoin anticonvulsants together with medicines that are used during surgery or dental or emergency treatments may cause increased side effects.

This medicine may cause some people to become dizzy, lightheaded, drowsy, or less alert than they are normally. After you have taken this medicine for a while, this effect may not be so bothersome. However, *make sure you know how you react to this medicine before you drive, use machines, or do anything else that could be dangerous if you are dizzy or are not alert.*

Oral contraceptives (birth control pills) containing estrogen may not work properly if you take them while you are taking hydantoin anticonvulsants. Unplanned pregnancies may occur. You should use a different or additional means of birth control while you are taking hydantoin anticonvulsants. If you have any questions about this, check with your doctor or pharmacist.

For patients taking *phenytoin* or *mephenytoin*:

- In some patients (usually younger patients), tenderness, swelling, or bleeding of the gums (gingival hyperplasia) may appear soon after phenytoin or mephenytoin treatment is started. To help prevent this, brush and floss your teeth carefully and regularly and massage your gums. Also, *see your dentist every 3 months to have your teeth cleaned. If you have any questions about how to take care of your teeth and gums, or if you notice any tenderness, swelling, or bleeding of your gums, check with your doctor or dentist.*

Side Effects of This Medicine

Along with its needed effects, a medicine may cause some unwanted effects. Although not all of these side effects may occur, if they do occur they may need medical attention.

Check with your doctor as soon as possible if any of the following side effects or signs of overdose occur:

More common

Bleeding, tender, or enlarged gums (rare with ethotoin); clumsiness or unsteadiness; confusion; continuous, uncontrolled back-and-forth and/or rolling eye movements—may be sign of overdose; enlarged glands in neck or underarms; fever; increase in seizures; mood or mental changes; muscle weakness or pain; skin rash or itching; slurred speech or stuttering—may be sign of overdose; sore throat; trembling—may be sign of overdose; unusual excitement, nervousness, or irritability

Rare

Bone malformations; burning pain at place of injection; chest discomfort; chills and fever; dark urine; dizziness; frequent breaking of bones; headache; joint pain; learning difficulties—in children taking high doses for a long time; light gray–colored stools; loss of appetite; nausea or vomiting; pain of penis on erection; restlessness or agitation; slowed growth; stomach pain (severe); troubled or quick, shallow breathing; uncontrolled jerking or twisting movements of hands, arms, or legs; uncontrolled movements of lips, tongue, or cheeks; unusual bleeding (such as nosebleeds) or bruising; unusual tiredness or weakness; weight loss (unusual); yellow eyes or skin

Rare (with long-term use of phenytoin)

Numbness, tingling, or pain in hands or feet

Symptoms of overdose

Blurred or double vision; clumsiness or unsteadiness (severe); confusion (severe); dizziness or drowsiness (severe); staggering walk

Other side effects may occur that usually do not need medical attention. These side effects may go away during treatment as your body adjusts to the medicine. However, check with your doctor if any of the following side effects continue or are bothersome:

More common

Constipation; dizziness (mild); drowsiness (mild)

Less common

Diarrhea (with ethotoin); enlargement of jaw; muscle twitching; swelling of breasts—in males; thickening of lips; trouble in sleeping; unusual and excessive hair growth on body and face (more common with phenytoin); widening of nose tip

Other side effects not listed above may also occur in some patients. If you notice any other effects, check with your doctor.

Additional Information

Once a medicine has been approved for marketing for a certain use, experience may show that it is also useful for other medical problems. Although these uses are not included in product labeling, phenytoin is used in certain patients with the following medical conditions:

- Cardiac arrythmias caused by digitalis medicine (changes in your heart rhythm)
- Episodic dyscontrol (certain behavior disorders)
- Myotonia congenita or
- Myotonic muscular dystrophy or
- Neuromyotonia (certain muscle disorders)
- Paroxysmal choreoathetosis (certain movement disorders)
- Tricyclic antidepressant poisoning
- Trigeminal neuralgia (tic douloureux)

Other than the above information, there is no additional information relating to proper use, precautions, or side effects for these uses.

Annual revision: 03/09/93

ANTICONVULSANTS, SUCCINIMIDE Systemic

This information applies to the following medicines:

Ethosuximide (eth-oh-SUX-i-mide)
Methsuximide (meth-SUX-i-mide)
Phensuximide (fen-SUX-i-mide)

Some commonly used brand names are:

For Ethosuximide
In the U.S.
Zarontin
In Canada
Zarontin

For Methsuximide
In the U.S.
Celontin
In Canada
Celontin

Another commonly used name is mesuximide.

For Phensuximide†
In the U.S.
Milontin

†Not commercially available in Canada.

Description

Succinimide anticonvulsants are used to control certain seizures in the treatment of epilepsy. These medicines act on the central nervous system (CNS) to reduce the number and severity of seizures.

This medicine is available only with your doctor's prescription, in the following dosage forms:

Oral

Ethosuximide
- Capsules (U.S. and Canada)
- Syrup (U.S. and Canada)

Methsuximide
- Capsules (U.S. and Canada)

Phensuximide
- Capsules (U.S.)

It is very important that you read and understand the following information. If any of it causes you special concern, check with your doctor. Also, *if you have any questions* or if you want more information about this medicine or your medical problem, *ask your doctor, nurse, or pharmacist.*

Before Using This Medicine

In deciding to use a medicine, the risks of taking the medicine must be weighed against the good it will do. This is a decision you and your doctor will make. For succinimide anticonvulsants, the following should be considered:

Allergies—Tell your doctor if you have ever had any unusual or allergic reaction to anticonvulsant medicines. Also tell your doctor and pharmacist if you are allergic to any other substances, such as foods, preservatives, or dyes.

Pregnancy—Although succinimide anticonvulsants have not been shown to cause problems in humans, there have been unproven reports of increased birth defects associated with the use of other anticonvulsant medicines.

Breast-feeding—Ethosuximide passes into breast milk. It is not known whether methsuximide or phensuximide passes into breast milk. However, these medicines have not been reported to cause problems in nursing babies.

Children—Succinimide anticonvulsants are not expected to cause different side effects or problems in children than they do in adults.

Older adults—Many medicines have not been studied specifically in older people. Therefore, it may not be known whether they work exactly the same way they do in younger adults. Although there is no specific information comparing use of succinimide anticonvulsants in the elderly to use in other age groups, they are not expected to cause different side effects or problems in older people than they do in younger adults.

Other medicines—Although certain medicines should not be used together at all, in other cases two different medicines may be used together even if an interaction might occur. In these cases, your doctor may want to change the dose, or other precautions may be necessary. When you are taking succinimide anticonvulsants, it is especially important that your doctor and pharmacist know if you are taking any of the following:

- Central nervous system (CNS) depressants (medicines that cause drowsiness)—Using these medicines together may increase the CNS depressant effects
- Haloperidol (e.g., Haldol)—A change in the pattern and/or the frequency of seizures may occur; the dose of either medicine may need to be changed

Other medical problems—The presence of other medical problems may affect the use of succinimide anticonvulsants. Make sure you tell your doctor if you have any other medical problems, especially:

- Blood disease or
- Intermittent porphyria or
- Kidney disease (severe) or
- Liver disease—Succinimide anticonvulsants may make the condition worse

Before you begin using any new medicine (prescription or nonprescription) or if you develop any new medical problem while you are using this medicine, check with your doctor, nurse, or pharmacist.

Proper Use of This Medicine

This medicine must be taken every day in regularly spaced doses as ordered by your doctor. Do not take more or less of it than your doctor ordered.

If this medicine upsets your stomach, take it with food or milk unless otherwise directed by your doctor.

Missed dose—If you miss a dose of this medicine, take it as soon as possible. However, if it is within 4 hours of your next dose, skip the missed dose and go back to your regular dosing schedule. Do not double doses.

Storage—To store this medicine:

- Keep out of the reach of children.
- Store away from heat and direct light.
- Do not store the capsule form of this medicine in the bathroom, near the kitchen sink, or in other damp places. Heat or moisture may cause the medicine to break down.
- Keep the liquid form of this medicine from freezing. Do not refrigerate.
- Do not keep outdated medicine or medicine that is no longer needed. Be sure any discarded medicine is out of the reach of children.

Precautions While Using This Medicine

Your doctor should check your progress at regular visits, especially during the first few months of treatment with this medicine. During this time the amount of medicine you are taking may have to be changed often to meet your individual needs.

If you have been taking a succinimide anticonvulsant regularly, do not stop taking it without first checking with your doctor. Your doctor may want you to reduce gradually the amount you are taking before stopping completely. Stopping this medicine suddenly may cause seizures.

Do not start or stop taking any other medicine without your doctor's advice. Other medicines may affect the way this medicine works.

This medicine will add to the effects of alcohol and other CNS depressants (medicines that slow down the nervous system, possibly causing drowsiness). Some examples of CNS depressants are antihistamines or medicine for hay fever, other allergies, or colds; sedatives, tranquilizers, or sleeping medicine; prescription pain medicine or narcotics; barbiturates; medicine for seizures; muscle relaxants; or anesthetics, including some dental anesthetics. *Check with your doctor before taking any of the above while you are using this medicine.*

This medicine may cause some people to become drowsy or less alert than they are normally. *Make sure you know how you react to this medicine before you drive, use machines, or do anything else that could be dangerous if you are not alert.* After you have taken this medicine for a while, this effect may lessen.

Before having any kind of surgery, dental treatment, or emergency treatment, tell the medical doctor or dentist in charge that you are taking this medicine. Taking succinimide anticonvulsants together with medicines that are used during surgery or dental or emergency treatments may increase the CNS depressant effects.

Your doctor may want you to carry a medical identification card or bracelet stating that you are taking this medicine.

For patients taking *methsuximide*:

- Do not use capsules that are not full or in which the contents have melted, because they may not work properly.

Side Effects of This Medicine

Along with its needed effects, a medicine may cause some unwanted effects. Although not all of these side effects may occur, if they do occur they may need medical attention.

Check with your doctor as soon as possible if any of the following side effects occur:

More common

Muscle pain; skin rash and itching; swollen glands; sore throat and fever

Less common

Aggressiveness; difficulty in concentration; mental depression; nightmares

Rare

Chills; increased chance of certain types of seizures; mood or mental changes; nosebleeds or other unusual bleeding or bruising; shortness of breath; sores, ulcers, or white spots on lips or in mouth; unusual tiredness or weakness; wheezing, tightness in chest, or troubled breathing

Symptoms of overdose

Drowsiness (severe); nausea and vomiting (severe); troubled breathing

Other side effects may occur that usually do not need medical attention. These side effects may go away during treatment as your body adjusts to the medicine. However, check with your doctor if any of the following side effects continue or are bothersome:

More common

Clumsiness or unsteadiness; dizziness; drowsiness; headache; hiccups; loss of appetite; nausea and vomiting; stomach cramps

Less common
Irritability

Phensuximide may cause the urine to turn pink, red, or red-brown. This is harmless and is to be expected while you are taking this medicine.

Other side effects not listed above may also occur in some patients. If you notice any other effects, check with your doctor.

Annual revision: 10/21/92

ANTIDEPRESSANTS, MONOAMINE OXIDASE (MAO) INHIBITOR Systemic

This information applies to the following medicines:

Isocarboxazid (eye-soe-kar-BOX-a-zid)
Phenelzine (FEN-el-zeen)
Tranylcypromine (tran-ill-SIP-roe-meen)

Note: This information does *not* apply to furazolidone, procarbazine, or selegiline.

Some commonly used brand names are:

For Isocarboxazid
In the U.S.
Marplan
In Canada
Marplan

For Phenelzine
In the U.S.
Nardil
In Canada
Nardil

For Tranylcypromine
In the U.S.
Parnate
In Canada
Parnate

Description

Monoamine oxidase (MAO) inhibitors are taken by mouth to relieve certain types of mental depression. They work by blocking the action of a chemical substance known as monoamine oxidase (MAO) in the nervous system.

Although these medicines are very effective for certain patients, they may also cause some unwanted reactions if not taken in the right way. It is very important to avoid certain foods, beverages, and medicines while you are being treated with an MAO inhibitor. Your doctor, nurse, or pharmacist will help you obtain a list to carry in your wallet or purse as a reminder of which products you should avoid.

MAO inhibitors are available only with your doctor's prescription, in the following dosage forms:

Oral
Isocarboxazid
- Tablets (U.S. and Canada)

Phenelzine
- Tablets (U.S. and Canada)

Tranylcypromine
- Tablets (U.S. and Canada)

It is very important that you read and understand the following information. If any of it causes you special concern, check with your doctor. Also, *if you have any questions* or if you want more information about this medicine or your medical problem, *ask your doctor, nurse, or pharmacist.*

Before Using This Medicine

In deciding to use a medicine, the risks of taking the medicine must be weighed against the good it will do. This is a decision you and your doctor will make. For monoamine oxidase (MAO) inhibitors, the following should be considered:

Allergies—Tell your doctor if you have ever had any unusual or allergic reaction to any MAO inhibitor. Also tell your doctor and pharmacist if you are allergic to any other substances, such as foods, preservatives, or dyes.

Diet—Dangerous reactions such as sudden high blood pressure may result when MAO inhibitors are taken with certain foods or drinks. The following foods should be avoided:

- Foods that have a high tyramine content (most common in foods that are aged or fermented to increase their flavor), such as cheeses; fava or broad bean pods; yeast or meat extracts; smoked or pickled meat, poultry or fish; fermented sausage (bologna, pepperoni, salami, summer sausage) or other fermented meat; sauerkraut; or any overripe fruit. If a list of these foods and beverages is not given to you, ask your doctor, nurse, or pharmacist to provide one.
- Alcoholic beverages or alcohol-free or reduced-alcohol beer and wine.
- Large amounts of caffeine-containing food or beverages such as coffee, tea, cola, or chocolate.

Pregnancy—Tranylcypromine (and probably isocarboxazid and phenelzine) crosses the placenta. A limited study in humans showed an increased risk of birth defects when these medicines were taken during the first trimester. In animal studies, MAO inhibitors caused a slowing of growth and increased excitability in the newborn when very large doses were given to the mother during pregnancy.

Breast-feeding—Tranylcypromine passes into the breast milk; it is not known whether isocarboxazid or phenelzine passes into breast milk. Problems in nursing babies have not been reported.

Children—Studies on these medicines have been done only in adult patients and there is no specific information comparing use of MAO inhibitors in children with use in other age groups. However, animal studies have shown that these medicines may slow growth in the young. Therefore, be sure to discuss with your doctor the use of these medicines in children.

Older adults—Dizziness or lightheadedness may be especially likely to occur in elderly patients, who are usually more sensitive than younger adults to these effects of MAO inhibitors.

Other medicines—Although certain medicines should not be used together at all, in other cases 2 different medicines may be used together even if an interaction might occur. In these cases, your doctor may want to change the dose, or other precautions may be necessary. When you are taking MAO inhibitors, it is especially important that your doctor and pharmacist know if you are taking any of the following:

- Amphetamines or
- Antihypertensives (high blood pressure medicine) or
- Appetite suppressants (diet pills) or
- Cyclobenzaprine (e.g., Flexeril) or
- Fluoxetine (e.g., Prozac) or
- Levodopa (e.g., Dopar, Larodopa) or
- Maprotiline (e.g., Ludiomil) or
- Medicine for asthma or other breathing problems or
- Medicines for colds, sinus problems, or hay fever or other allergies (including nose drops or sprays) or
- Meperidine (e.g., Demerol) or
- Methylphenidate (e.g., Ritalin) or
- Monoamine oxidase (MAO) inhibitors, other, including furazolidone (e.g., Furoxone), procarbazine (e.g., Matulane), or selegiline (e.g., Eldepryl), or
- Tricyclic antidepressants (amitriptyline [e.g., Elavil], amoxapine [e.g., Asendin], clomipramine [e.g., Anafranil], desipramine [e.g., Pertofrane], doxepin [e.g., Sinequan], imipramine [e.g., Tofranil], nortriptyline [e.g., Aventyl], protriptyline [e.g., Vivactil], trimipramine [e.g., Surmontil])—Using these medicines while you are taking or within 2 weeks of taking MAO inhibitors may cause serious side effects such as sudden highly elevated body temperature, extremely high blood pressure, severe convulsions, and death; however, sometimes certain of these medicines may be used together under close supervision by your doctor
- Antidiabetics, oral (diabetes medicine you take by mouth) or
- Insulin—MAO inhibitors may change the amount of antidiabetic medicine you need to take
- Buspirone (e.g., BuSpar)—Use with MAO inhibitors may cause high blood pressure
- Carbamazepine (e.g., Tegretol)—Use with MAO inhibitors may increase seizures
- Central nervous system (CNS) depressants (medicines that cause drowsiness)—Using these medicines with MAO inhibitors may increase the CNS and other depressant effects
- Cocaine—Cocaine use by persons taking MAO inhibitors, including furazolidone and procarbazine, may cause a severe increase in blood pressure
- Dextromethorphan—Use with MAO inhibitors may cause excitement, high blood pressure, and fever
- Trazodone or
- Tryptophan used as a food supplement or a sleep aid—Use of these medicines by persons taking MAO inhibitors, including furazolidone and procarbazine, may cause mental confusion, excitement, shivering, trouble in breathing, or fever

Other medical problems—The presence of other medical problems may affect the use of MAO inhibitors. Make sure you tell your doctor if you have any other medical problems, especially:

- Alcohol abuse—Drinking alcohol while you are taking an MAO inhibitor may cause serious side effects
- Angina (chest pain) or
- Headaches (severe or frequent)—These conditions may interfere with warning signs of other more serious side effects
- Asthma or bronchitis—Some medicines used to treat these conditions may cause serious side effects when used while you are taking an MAO inhibitor
- Diabetes mellitus (sugar diabetes)—These medicines may change the amount of insulin or oral antidiabetic medication that you need
- Epilepsy—Seizures may occur more often
- Heart or blood vessel disease or
- Liver disease or
- Mental illness (or history of) or
- Parkinson's disease or
- Recent heart attack or stroke—MAO inhibitors may make the condition worse
- High blood pressure—Condition may be affected by these medicines
- Kidney disease—Higher blood levels of MAO inhibitors may occur, which increases the chance of side effects
- Overactive thyroid or
- Pheochromocytoma (PCC)—Serious side effects may occur

Proper Use of This Medicine

Sometimes this medicine must be taken for several weeks before you begin to feel better. Your doctor should check your progress at regular visits, especially during the first few months of treatment, to make sure that this medicine is working properly and to check for unwanted effects.

Take this medicine only as directed by your doctor. Do not take more of it, do not take it more often, and do not take it for a longer time than your doctor ordered.

Missed dose—If you miss a dose of this medicine, take it as soon as possible. However, if it is within 2 hours of your next dose, skip the missed dose and go back to your regular dosing schedule. Do not double doses.

Storage—To store this medicine:

- Keep out of the reach of children.
- Store away from heat and direct light.
- Do not store in the bathroom, near the kitchen sink, or in other damp places. Heat or moisture may cause the medicine to break down.
- Do not keep outdated medicine or medicine no longer needed. Be sure that any discarded medicine is out of the reach of children.

Precautions While Using This Medicine

When taken with certain foods, drinks, or other medicines, MAO inhibitors can cause very dangerous reactions such as sudden high blood pressure (also called hypertensive crisis). To avoid such reactions, *obey the following rules of caution:*

- Do not eat foods that have a high tyramine content (most common in foods that are aged or fermented to increase their flavor), such as cheeses; fava or broad bean pods; yeast or meat extracts; smoked or pickled meat, poultry, or fish; fermented sausage (bologna, pepperoni, salami, and summer sausage) or other fermented meat; sauerkraut; or any overripe fruit. If a list of these foods is not given to you, ask your doctor, nurse, or pharmacist to provide one.
- Do not drink alcoholic beverages or alcohol-free or reduced-alcohol beer and wine.
- Do not eat or drink large amounts of caffeine-containing food or beverages such as coffee, tea, cola, or chocolate.
- Do not take any other medicine unless approved or prescribed by your doctor. This especially includes over-the-counter (OTC) or nonprescription medicine, such as that for colds (including nose drops or sprays), cough, asthma, hay fever, and appetite control; "keep awake" products; or products that make you sleepy.

This medicine will add to the effects of alcohol and other CNS depressants (medicines that slow down the nervous system, possibly causing drowsiness). Some examples of CNS depressants are antihistamines or medicine for hay fever, other allergies, or colds; sedatives, tranquilizers, or sleeping medicine; prescription pain medicine or narcotics; barbiturates; medicine for seizures; muscle relaxants; or anesthetics, including some dental anesthetics. *Check with your doctor before taking any of the above while you are using this medicine.*

Check with your doctor or hospital emergency room immediately if severe headache, stiff neck, chest pains, fast heartbeat, or nausea and vomiting occur while you are taking this medicine. These may be symptoms of a serious side effect that should have a doctor's attention.

Do not stop taking this medicine without first checking with your doctor. Your doctor may want you to reduce gradually the amount you are using before stopping completely.

Dizziness, lightheadedness, or fainting may occur, especially when you get up from a lying or sitting position. *Getting up slowly may help.* When you get up from lying down, sit on the edge of the bed with your feet dangling for 1 or 2 minutes. Then stand up slowly. If the problem continues or gets worse, check with your doctor.

This medicine may cause blurred vision or make some people drowsy or less alert than they are normally. *Make sure you know how you react to this medicine before you drive, use machines, or do anything else that could be dangerous if you are unable to see well or are not alert.*

Before having any kind of surgery, dental treatment, or emergency treatment, tell the medical doctor or dentist in charge that you are using this medicine or have used it within the past 2 weeks.

Your doctor may want you to carry an identification card stating that you are using this medicine.

For patients with *angina* (chest pain):

- This medicine may cause you to have an unusual feeling of good health and energy. However, *do not suddenly increase the amount of exercise you get without discussing it with your doctor.* Too much activity could bring on an attack of angina.

For *diabetic* patients:

- This medicine may affect blood sugar levels. While you are using this medicine, be especially careful in testing for sugar in your blood or urine. If you have any questions about this, check with your doctor.

After you stop using this medicine, you must continue to obey the rules of caution for at least 2 weeks concerning food, drink, and other medicine, since these things may continue to react with MAO inhibitors.

Side Effects of This Medicine

Along with its needed effects, a medicine may cause some unwanted effects. Although not all of these side effects may occur, if they do occur they may need medical attention.

Stop taking this medicine and get emergency help immediately if any of the following side effects occur:

Symptoms of unusually high blood pressure (hypertensive crisis)

Chest pain (severe); enlarged pupils; fast or slow heartbeat; headache (severe); increased sensitivity of eyes to light; increased sweating (possibly with fever or cold, clammy skin); nausea and vomiting; stiff or sore neck

Check with your doctor as soon as possible if any of the following side effects occur:

More common

Dizziness or lightheadedness (severe), especially when getting up from a lying or sitting position

Less common

Diarrhea; fast or pounding heartbeat; swelling of feet or lower legs; unusual excitement or nervousness

Rare

Dark urine; fever; skin rash; slurred speech; sore throat; staggering walk; yellow eyes or skin

Symptoms of overdose

Anxiety (severe); confusion; convulsions (seizures); cool, clammy skin; dizziness (severe); drowsiness (severe); fast and irregular pulse; fever; hallucinations (seeing, hearing, or feeling things that are not there); headache (severe); high or low blood pressure; muscle stiffness; sweating; troubled breathing; trouble in sleeping (severe); unusual irritability

Other side effects may occur that usually do not need medical attention. These side effects may go away during treatment as your body adjusts to the medicine. However, check with your doctor if any of the following side effects continue or are bothersome:

More common

Blurred vision; decreased amount of urine; decreased sexual ability; dizziness or lightheadedness (mild), especially when getting up from a lying or sitting position; drowsiness; headache (mild); increased appetite (especially for sweets) or weight gain; increased sweating; muscle twitching during sleep; restlessness; shakiness or trembling; tiredness and weakness; trouble in sleeping; weakness

Less common or rare

Chills; constipation; decreased appetite; dryness of mouth

Other side effects not listed above may also occur in some patients. If you notice any other effects, check with your doctor.

Additional Information

Once a medicine has been approved for marketing for a certain use, experience may show that it is also useful for other medical problems. Although these uses are not included in product labeling, phenelzine and tranylcypromine are used in certain patients with the following medical conditions:

- Headache
- Panic disorder

Other than the above information, there is no additional information relating to proper use, precautions, or side effects for this use.

Annual revision: 06/15/92

ANTIDEPRESSANTS, TRICYCLIC Systemic

This information applies to the following medicines:

Amitriptyline (a-mee-TRIP-ti-leen)
Amoxapine (a-MOX-a-peen)
Clomipramine (cloe-MIP-ra-meen)
Desipramine (dess-IP-ra-meen)
Doxepin (DOX-e-pin)
Imipramine (im-IP-ra-meen)
Nortriptyline (nor-TRIP-ti-leen)
Protriptyline (proe-TRIP-ti-leen)
Trimipramine (trye-MIP-ra-meen)

Some commonly used brand names are:

For Amitriptyline

In the U.S.

Elavil
Endep
Emitrip
Enovil

Generic name product may also be available.

In Canada

Apo-Amitriptyline
Novotriptyn
Elavil
PMS Amitriptyline
Levate

Generic name product may also be available.

For Amoxapine

In the U.S.

Asendin

Generic name product may also be available.

In Canada

Asendin

For Clomipramine

In the U.S.

Anafranil

In Canada

Anafranil

For Desipramine

In the U.S.

Norpramin

Generic name product may also be available.

In Canada

Norpramin
Pertofrane

Generic name product may also be available.

For Doxepin

In the U.S.

Sinequan

Generic name product may also be available.

In Canada

Novo-Doxepin
Triadapin
Sinequan

For Imipramine
In the U.S.
Janimine
Norfranil
Tipramine
Tofranil
Tofranil-PM
Generic name product may also be available.
In Canada
Apo-Imipramine
Impril
Novopramine
PMS Imipramine
Tofranil
Generic name product may also be available.

For Nortriptyline
In the U.S.
Aventyl
Pamelor
Generic name product may also be available.
In Canada
Aventyl

For Protriptyline
In the U.S.
Vivactil
In Canada
Triptil

For Trimipramine
In the U.S.
Surmontil
Generic name product may also be available.
In Canada
Apo-Trimip
Novo-Tripramine
Rhotrimine
Surmontil

Description

Tricyclic antidepressants ("mood elevators") are used to relieve mental depression.

One form of this medicine (imipramine) is also used to treat enuresis (bedwetting) in children. Another form (clomipramine) is used to treat obsessive-compulsive disorders. Tricyclic antidepressants may be used for other conditions as determined by your doctor.

These medicines are available only with your doctor's prescription, in the following dosage forms:

Oral

Amitriptyline
- Syrup (Canada)
- Tablets (U.S. and Canada)

Amoxapine
- Tablets (U.S. and Canada)

Clomipramine
- Capsules (U.S.)
- Tablets (Canada)

Desipramine
- Tablets (U.S. and Canada)

Doxepin
- Capsules (U.S. and Canada)
- Oral solution (U.S.)

Imipramine
- Capsules (U.S.)
- Tablets (U.S. and Canada)

Nortriptyline
- Capsules (U.S. and Canada)
- Oral solution (U.S.)

Protriptyline
- Tablets (U.S. and Canada)

Trimipramine
- Capsules (U.S. and Canada)
- Tablets (Canada)

Parenteral

Amitriptyline
- Injection (U.S.)

Imipramine
- Injection (U.S.)

It is very important that you read and understand the following information. If any of it causes you special concern, check with your doctor. Also, *if you have any questions* or if you want more information about this medicine or your medical problem, *ask your doctor, nurse, or pharmacist.*

Before Using This Medicine

In deciding to use a medicine, the risks of taking the medicine must be weighed against the good it will do. This is a decision you and your doctor will make. For tricyclic antidepressants, the following should be considered:

Allergies—Tell your doctor if you have ever had any unusual or allergic reaction to any tricyclic antidepressant or to carbamazepine, maprotiline, or trazodone. Also tell your doctor and pharmacist if you are allergic to any other substances, such as foods, preservatives, or dyes.

Pregnancy—Studies have not been done in pregnant women. However, there have been reports of newborns suffering from muscle spasms and heart, breathing, and urinary problems when their mothers had taken tricyclic antidepressants immediately before delivery. Also, studies in animals have shown that some tricyclic antidepressants may cause unwanted effects in the fetus.

Breast-feeding—Tricyclic antidepressants pass into the breast milk. Doxepin has been reported to cause drowsiness in the nursing baby.

Children—Children are especially sensitive to the effects of this medicine. This may increase the chance of side effects during treatment. However, side effects in children taking this medicine for bedwetting usually disappear upon continued use. The most common of these are nervousness, sleeping problems, tiredness, and mild stomach upset. If these side effects continue or are bothersome, check with your doctor.

Older adults—Drowsiness, dizziness, confusion, vision problems, dryness of mouth, constipation, and problems in urinating are more likely to occur in elderly patients, who are usually more sensitive than younger adults to the effects of tricyclic antidepressants.

Other medicines—Although certain medicines should not be used together at all, in other cases 2 different medicines may be used together even if an interaction might occur. In these cases, your doctor may want to change the dose, or other precautions may be necessary. When you are taking a tricyclic antidepressant, it is especially important that your doctor and pharmacist know if you are taking any of the following:

- Antipsychotics (medicine for mental illness) or
- Clonidine (e.g., Catapres)—Using these medicines with tricyclic antidepressants may increase the CNS depressant effects and increase the chance of serious side effects
- Antithyroid agents (medicine for overactive thyroid) or
- Cimetidine (e.g., Tagamet)—Using these medicines with tricyclic antidepressants may increase the chance of serious side effects
- Amphetamines or
- Appetite suppressants (diet pills) or
- Ephedrine or
- Epinephrine (e.g., Adrenalin) or
- Isoproterenol (e.g., Isuprel) or
- Medicine for asthma or other breathing problems or
- Medicine for colds, sinus problems, or hay fever or other allergies or
- Phenylephrine (e.g., Neo-Synephrine)—Using these medicines with tricyclic antidepressants may increase the risk of serious effects on the heart
- Central nervous system (CNS) depressants—Using these medicines with tricyclic antidepressants may increase the CNS depressant effects
- Guanadrel (e.g., Hylorel) or
- Guanethidine (e.g., Ismelin)—Tricyclic antidepressants may keep these medicines from working as well
- Methyldopa (e.g., Aldomet) or
- Metoclopramide (e.g., Reglan) or
- Metyrosine (e.g., Demser) or
- Pemoline (e.g., Cylert) or
- Pimozide (e.g., Orap) or
- Promethazine (e.g., Phenergan) or
- Rauwolfia alkaloids (alseroxylon [e.g., Rauwiloid], deserpidine [e.g., Harmonyl], rauwolfia serpentina [e.g., Raudixin], reserpine [e.g., Serpasil]) or
- Trimeprazine (e.g., Temaril)—Tricyclic antidepressants may cause certain side effects to be more severe and occur more often
- Metrizamide—The risk of seizures may be increased
- Monoamine oxidase (MAO) inhibitors (furazolidone [e.g., Furoxone], isocarboxazid [e.g., Marplan], phenelzine [e.g., Nardil], procarbazine [e.g., Matulane], selegiline [e.g., Eldepryl], tranylcypromine [e.g., Parnate])—Taking tricyclic antidepressants while you are taking or within 2 weeks of taking monoamine oxidase (MAO) inhibitors may cause sudden highly elevated body temperature, extremely high blood pressure, severe convulsions, and death; however, sometimes certain of these medicines may be used together under close supervision by your doctor

Other medical problems—The presence of other medical problems may affect the use of tricyclic antidepressants. Make sure you tell your doctor if you have any other medical problems, especially:

- Alcohol abuse (or history of)—Drinking alcohol may cause increased CNS depressant effects
- Asthma or
- Bipolar disorder (manic-depressive illness) or
- Blood disorders or
- Convulsions (seizures) or
- Difficult urination or
- Enlarged prostate or
- Glaucoma or increased eye pressure or
- Heart disease or
- High blood pressure (hypertension) or
- Schizophrenia—Tricyclic antidepressants may make the condition worse
- Kidney disease or
- Liver disease—Higher blood levels of tricyclic antidepressants may result, increasing the chance of side effects
- Overactive thyroid or
- Stomach or intestinal problems—Tricyclic antidepressants may cause an increased chance of serious side effects

Before you begin using any new medicine (prescription or nonprescription) or if you develop any new medical problem while you are using this medicine, check with your doctor, nurse, or pharmacist.

Proper Use of This Medicine

To lessen stomach upset, take this medicine with food, even for a daily bedtime dose, unless your doctor has told you to take it on an empty stomach.

Take this medicine only as directed by your doctor, to benefit your condition as much as possible. Do not take more of it, do not take it more often, and do not take it for a longer time than your doctor ordered.

Sometimes this medicine must be taken for several weeks before you begin to feel better. Your doctor should check your progress at regular visits.

To use *doxepin oral solution:*

- This medicine is to be taken by mouth even though it comes in a dropper bottle. The amount you should take should be measured with the dropper provided with your prescription and diluted just before you take each dose. Dilute each dose with about one-half glass (4 ounces) of water, milk, citrus fruit juice, tomato juice, or prune juice. Do not mix this medicine with grape juice or carbonated beverages since these may decrease the medicine's effectiveness.
- Doxepin oral solution must be mixed immediately before you take it. Do not prepare it ahead of time.

Missed dose—If you miss a dose of this medicine and your dosing schedule is:

- One dose a day at bedtime—Do not take the missed dose in the morning since it may cause disturbing side effects during waking hours. Instead, check with your doctor.

- More than one dose a day—Take the missed dose as soon as possible. However, if it is almost time for your next dose, skip the missed dose, and go back to your regular dosing schedule. Do not double doses.

If you have any questions about this, check with your doctor.

Storage—To store this medicine:

- Keep out of the reach of children. Overdose of this medicine is very dangerous in young children.
- Store away from heat and direct light.
- Do not store the tablet or capsule form of this medicine in the bathroom, near the kitchen sink, or in other damp places. Heat or moisture may cause the medicine to break down.
- Keep the liquid form of this medicine from freezing.
- Do not keep outdated medicine or medicine no longer needed. Be sure that any discarded medicine is out of the reach of children.

Precautions While Using This Medicine

It is very important that your doctor check your progress at regular visits to allow dosage adjustments and to help reduce side effects.

This medicine will add to the effects of alcohol and other CNS depressants (medicines that slow down the nervous system, possibly causing drowsiness). Some examples of CNS depressants are antihistamines or medicine for hay fever, other allergies, or colds; sedatives, tranquilizers, or sleeping medicine; prescription pain medicine or narcotics; barbiturates; medicine for seizures; muscle relaxants; or anesthetics, including some dental anesthetics. *Check with your medical doctor or dentist before taking any of the above while you are taking this medicine.*

This medicine may cause some people to become drowsy. *If this occurs, do not drive, use machines, or do anything else that could be dangerous if you are not alert.*

Dizziness, lightheadedness, or fainting may occur, especially when you get up from a lying or sitting position. Getting up slowly may help. If this problem continues or gets worse, check with your doctor.

This medicine may cause dryness of the mouth. For temporary relief, use sugarless gum or candy, melt bits of ice in your mouth, or use a saliva substitute. However, if your mouth continues to feel dry for more than 2 weeks, check with your medical doctor or dentist. Continuing dryness of the mouth may increase the chance of dental disease, including tooth decay, gum disease, and fungus infections.

Tricyclic antidepressants may cause your skin to be more sensitive to sunlight than it is normally. Exposure to sunlight, even for brief periods of time, may cause a skin rash, itching, redness or other discoloration of the skin, or a severe sunburn. When you begin taking this medicine:

- Stay out of direct sunlight, especially between the hours of 10:00 a.m. and 3:00 p.m., if possible.
- Wear protective clothing, including a hat. Also, wear sunglasses.
- Apply a sun block product that has a skin protection factor (SPF) of at least 15. Some patients may require a product with a higher SPF number, especially if they have a fair complexion. If you have any questions about this, check with your doctor or pharmacist.
- Apply a sun block lipstick that has an SPF of at least 15 to protect your lips.
- Do not use a sunlamp or tanning bed or booth.

If you have a severe reaction from the sun, check with your doctor.

Before you have any medical tests, tell the medical doctor in charge that you are taking this medicine. The results of the metyrapone test may be affected by this medicine.

Before having any kind of surgery, dental treatment, or emergency treatment, tell the medical doctor or dentist in charge that you are using this medicine.

For diabetic patients:

- This medicine may affect blood sugar levels. If you notice a change in the results of your blood or urine sugar tests or if you have any questions, check with your doctor.

Do not stop taking this medicine without first checking with your doctor. Your doctor may want you to reduce gradually the amount you are using before stopping completely. This may help prevent a possible worsening of your condition and reduce the possibility of withdrawal symptoms such as headache, nausea, and/or an overall feeling of discomfort.

The effects of this medicine may last for 3 to 7 days after you have stopped taking it. Therefore, all the precautions stated here must be observed during this time.

For patients taking protriptyline:

- If taken late in the day, protriptyline may interfere with nighttime sleep.

Side Effects of This Medicine

Along with its needed effects, a medicine may cause some unwanted effects. Although not all of these side effects may occur, if they do occur they may need medical attention.

Stop taking this medicine and get emergency help immediately if any of the following side effects occur:

Reported for amoxapine only—rare

Convulsions (seizures); difficult or fast breathing; fever with increased sweating; high or low (irregular) blood pressure; loss of bladder control; muscle stiffness (severe); pale skin; unusual tiredness or weakness

Check with your doctor as soon as possible if any of the following side effects occur:

Less common

Blurred vision; confusion or delirium; constipation (especially in the elderly); decreased sexual ability (more common with amoxapine and clomipramine); difficulty in speaking or swallowing; eye pain; fainting; fast or irregular heartbeat (pounding, racing, skipping); hallucinations; loss of balance control; mask-like face; nervousness or restlessness; problems in urinating; shakiness or trembling; shuffling walk; slowed movements; stiffness of arms and legs

Reported for amoxapine only (in addition to the above)—less common

Lip smacking or puckering; puffing of cheeks; rapid or worm-like movements of tongue; uncontrolled chewing movements; uncontrolled movements of hands, arms, or legs

Rare

Anxiety; breast enlargement in both males and females; hair loss; inappropriate secretion of milk—in females; increased sensitivity to sunlight; irritability; muscle twitching; red or brownish spots on skin; ringing, buzzing, or other unexplained sounds in the ears; seizures (more common with clomipramine); skin rash and itching; sore throat and fever; swelling of face and tongue; swelling of testicles (more common with amoxapine); trouble with teeth or gums (more common with clomipramine); weakness; yellow eyes or skin

Symptoms of acute overdose

Confusion; convulsions (seizures); disturbed concentration; drowsiness (severe); enlarged pupils; fast, slow, or irregular heartbeat; fever; hallucinations (seeing, hearing, or feeling things that are not there); restlessness and agitation; shortness of breath or troubled breathing; unusual tiredness or weakness (severe); vomiting

Other side effects may occur that usually do not need medical attention. These side effects may go away during treatment as your body adjusts to the medicine. However, check with your doctor if any of the following side effects continue or are bothersome:

More common

Dizziness; drowsiness; dryness of mouth; headache; increased appetite (may include craving for sweets); nausea; tiredness or weakness (mild); unpleasant taste; weight gain

Less common

Diarrhea; heartburn; increased sweating; trouble in sleeping (more common with protriptyline, especially when taken late in the day); vomiting

Certain side effects of this medicine may occur after you have stopped taking it. Check with your doctor if you notice any of the following effects:

Headache; irritability; nausea, vomiting, or diarrhea; restlessness; trouble in sleeping, with vivid dreams; unusual excitement

Reported for amoxapine only (in addition to the above)

Lip smacking or puckering; puffing of cheeks; rapid or worm-like movements of the tongue; uncontrolled chewing movements; uncontrolled movements of arms or legs

Other side effects not listed above also may occur in some patients. If you notice any other effects, check with your doctor.

Additional Information

Once a medicine has been approved for marketing for a certain use, experience may show that it is also useful for other medical problems. Although these uses are not included in product labeling, tricyclic antidepressants are used in certain patients with the following medical conditions:

- Attention deficit hyperactivity disorder (hyperactivity in children) (desipramine, imipramine, and protriptyline)
- Bulimia (uncontrolled eating, followed by vomiting) (amitriptyline, clomipramine, desipramine, and imipramine)
- Cocaine withdrawal (desipramine and imipramine)
- Headache prevention (for certain types of frequent or continuing headaches) (most tricyclic antidepressants)
- Itching with hives due to cold temperature exposure (doxepin)
- Narcolepsy (extreme tendency to fall asleep suddenly) (clomipramine, desipramine, imipramine, and protriptyline)
- Neurogenic pain (a type of continuing pain) (amitriptyline, clomipramine, desipramine, doxepin, imipramine, nortriptyline, and trimipramine)
- Panic disorder (clomipramine, desipramine, doxepin, nortriptyline, and trimipramine)
- Stomach ulcer (amitriptyline, doxepin, and trimipramine)
- Urinary incontinence (imipramine)

Other than the above information, there is no additional information relating to proper use, precautions, or side effects for these uses.

Annual revision: 05/22/92
Interim revision(s): 06/1/92; 03/01/93

ANTIDIABETICS, ORAL Systemic

This information applies to the following medicines:

Acetohexamide (a-set-oh-HEX-a-mide)
Chlorpropamide (klor-PROE-pa-mide)
Glipizide (GLIP-i-zide)
Glyburide (GLYE-byoo-ride)
Tolazamide (tole-AZ-a-mide)
Tolbutamide (tole-BYOO-ta-mide)

Some commonly used brand names are:

For Acetohexamide

In the U.S.
Dymelor
Generic name product may also be available.

In Canada
Dimelor
Generic name product may also be available.

For Chlorpropamide

In the U.S.
Diabinese
Glucamide
Generic name product may also be available.

In Canada
Apo-Chlorpropamide
Novopropamide
Diabinese
Generic name product may also be available.

For Glipizide

In the U.S.
Glucotrol

For Glyburide

In the U.S.
DiaBeta
Micronase

In Canada
DiaBeta
Euglucon
Another commonly used name is glibenclamide.

For Tolazamide

In the U.S.
Tolamide
Tolinase
Generic name product may also be available.

For Tolbutamide

In the U.S.
Oramide
Orinase
Generic name product may also be available.

In Canada
Apo-Tolbutamide
Novobutamide
Mobenol
Orinase
Generic name product may also be available.

Description

Oral antidiabetics (diabetes medicine you take by mouth) may help reduce the amount of sugar in the blood by causing your pancreas gland to make more insulin. They are used to treat certain types of diabetes mellitus (sugar diabetes).

Oral antidiabetics can usually be used only by adults who develop diabetes after 30 years of age and who do not require insulin shots (or who usually do not require more than 20 Units of insulin a day) to control their condition. This type of diabetic patient is said to have non–insulin-dependent diabetes mellitus (or NIDDM), sometimes known as maturity-onset or Type II diabetes. Oral antidiabetics do not help diabetic patients who have insulin-dependent diabetes mellitus (or IDDM), sometimes known as juvenile-onset or Type I diabetes.

Chlorpropamide may also be used for other conditions as determined by your doctor.

Oral antidiabetic medicines do not help diabetic patients who are insulin-dependent (type I). However, non–insulin-dependent (type II) diabetic patients who are taking oral antidiabetics may have to temporarily switch to insulin if they:

- develop diabetic coma or ketoacidosis.
- have a severe injury or burn.
- develop a severe infection.
- are to have major surgery.
- are pregnant.

Before you begin treatment with this medicine, you and your doctor should talk about the good the medicine will do as well as the risks of using it. You should also find out about other possible ways to treat your diabetes such as by diet alone or by diet plus insulin.

Oral antidiabetics are available only with your doctor's prescription, in the following dosage forms:

Oral

Acetohexamide
- Tablets (U.S. and Canada)

Chlorpropamide
- Tablets (U.S. and Canada)

Glipizide
- Tablets (U.S.)

Glyburide
- Tablets (U.S. and Canada)

Tolazamide
- Tablets (U.S.)

Tolbutamide
- Tablets (U.S. and Canada)

It is very important that you read and understand the following information. If any of it causes you special concern, check with your doctor. Also, *if you have any questions* or if you want more information about this medicine or your medical problem, *ask your doctor, nurse, or pharmacist.*

Before Using This Medicine

In deciding to use a medicine, the risks of taking the medicine must be weighed against the good it will do. This is a decision you and your doctor will make. For oral antidiabetic medicines, the following should be considered:

Allergies—Tell your doctor if you have ever had any unusual or allergic reaction to oral antidiabetic medicines, or to sulfonamide-type (sulfa) medications, including thiazide diuretics (a certain type of water pill). Also tell your doctor and pharmacist if you are allergic to any other substances, such as foods, preservatives, or dyes.

Diet—If you have non–insulin-dependent (type II) diabetes, your doctor may try to control your condition by prescribing a personal meal plan for you before prescribing medicine. Such a diet is low in refined carbohydrates (foods such as sugar and candy used for quick energy) and fat. The daily number of calories in this meal plan should be adjusted by a dietitian to help you reach and maintain a proper body weight. Oral antidiabetics are less effective if you are greatly overweight. It may be very important for you to follow a planned weight reduction diet. In addition, meals and snacks are arranged to meet the energy needs of your body at different times of the day.

Many people with type II diabetes are able to control their diabetes by carefully following their prescribed meal and exercise plan. Oral antidiabetics are prescribed only when additional help is needed.

Pregnancy—Oral antidiabetics should not be used during pregnancy. Insulin may be needed to keep blood sugar levels as close to normal as possible. Poor control of blood sugar levels may cause birth defects or death of the fetus. In addition, use of oral antidiabetics during pregnancy may cause the newborn baby to have low blood sugar levels. This may last for several days following birth.

Breast-feeding—Chlorpropamide passes into the breast milk and its use is not recommended because it could cause low blood sugar in the baby. Although it is not known if the other oral antidiabetics pass into breast milk and these medicines have not been shown to cause problems in humans, the chance always exists.

Children—There is little information about the use of oral antidiabetic agents in children. Type II diabetes is unusual in this age group.

Older adults—The elderly may be more sensitive than younger adults to the effects of oral antidiabetics. Also, elderly patients who take chlorpropamide are more likely to retain (keep) too much body water.

Other medicines—Although certain medicines should not be used together at all, in other cases two different medicines may be used together even if an interaction might occur. In these cases, your doctor may want to change the dose, or other precautions may be necessary. *Do not take any other medicine, unless prescribed or approved by your doctor*. When you are taking oral antidiabetic drugs, it is especially important that your doctor and pharmacist know if you are taking any of the following:

- Anticoagulants (blood thinners)—The effect of either the blood thinner or the antidiabetic medicine may be increased or decreased if the 2 medicines are used together
- Appetite control medicines or
- Asthma medicines or
- Cough or cold medicines or
- Hay fever or allergy medicines—Many medicines (including nonprescription [over-the-counter]) products can affect the control of your blood glucose (sugar)
- Aspirin or other salicylates or
- Chloramphenicol (e.g., Chloromycetin) or
- Guanethidine (e.g., Ismelin) or
- Sulfonamides (sulfa medicine)—These medicines may increase the chances of low blood sugar
- Beta-blockers (acebutolol [e.g., Sectral], atenolol [e.g., Tenormin], carteolol [e.g., Cartrol], labetalol [e.g., Normodyne], metoprolol [e.g., Lopressor], nadolol [e.g., Corgard], oxprenolol [e.g., Trasicor], penbutolol [e.g., Levatol], pindolol [e.g., Visken], propranolol [e.g., Inderal], sotalol [e.g., Sotacor], timolol [e.g., Blocadren])—Beta-blockers may increase the risk of high or low blood sugar occurring. They can also block symptoms of low blood sugar (such as fast heartbeat or high blood pressure). Because of this, a diabetic patient might not know that he or she had low blood sugar and might not immediately take the proper steps to raise the blood sugar level. Beta-blockers can also cause low blood sugar to last longer
- Monoamine oxidase (MAO) inhibitors (furazolidone [e.g., Furoxone], isocarboxazid [e.g., Marplan], pargyline [e.g., Eutonyl], phenelzine [e.g., Nardil], procarbazine [e.g., Matulane], or tranylcypromine [e.g., Parnate])—Taking oral antidiabetic medicines while you are taking (or within 2 weeks of taking) monoamine oxidase (MAO) inhibitors may increase the chances of low blood sugar occurring

Other medical problems—The presence of other medical problems may affect the use of the oral antidiabetic medicines. Make sure you tell your doctor if you have any other medical problems, especially:

- Heart disease—Chlorpropamide causes some patients to retain (keep) more body water than usual. Heart disease may worsened by this extra body water
- Infection (severe)—Insulin may be needed temporarily to control diabetes in patients with severe infection because changes in blood sugar may occur rapidly and without much warning
- Kidney disease or
- Liver disease—Low blood sugar may be more likely to occur because the kidney or liver is not able to get the medicine out of the blood stream as it normally would. Also, people with kidney disease who take chlorpropamide are more likely to retain (keep) too much body water
- Thyroid disease
- Underactive adrenal glands (untreated) or
- Underactive pituitary gland (untreated)—Patients with these conditions may be more likely to develop low blood sugar (hypoglycemia) while taking oral antidiabetic medicines

Before you begin using any new medicine (prescription or nonprescription) or if you develop any new medical problem while you are using this medicine, check with your doctor, nurse, or pharmacist.

Proper Use of This Medicine

Follow carefully your special meal plan, since this is the most important part of controlling your diabetes and is necessary if the medicine is to work properly.

Take your oral antidiabetics only as directed by your doctor. Do not take more or less of it than your doctor ordered, and take it at the same time each day. This will help to control your blood sugar levels.

Missed dose—If you miss a dose of this medicine, take it as soon as possible. However, if it is almost time for your next dose, skip the missed dose and go back to your regular dosing schedule. Do not double doses.

Storage—To store this medicine:
- Keep out of the reach of children.
- Store away from heat and direct light.
- Do not store in the bathroom, near the kitchen sink, or in other damp places. Heat or moisture may cause the medicine to break down.
- Do not keep outdated medicine or medicine no longer needed. Be sure that any discarded medicine is out of the reach of children.

Precautions While Using This Medicine

Your doctor will want to check your progress at regular visits, especially during the first few weeks that you take this medicine.

Test for sugar in your blood or urine as directed by your doctor. This is important in making sure your diabetes is being controlled and provides an early warning when it is not.

Do not take any other medicine, unless prescribed or approved by your doctor. This especially includes nonprescription (over-the-counter [OTC]) medicine such as that for colds, cough, asthma, hay fever, or appetite control.

Avoid drinking alcoholic beverages until you have discussed their use with your doctor. Some patients who drink alcohol while taking this medicine may suffer stomach pain, nausea, vomiting, dizziness, pounding headache, sweating, or flushing (redness of face and skin). In addition, alcohol may produce hypoglycemia (low blood sugar).

Oral antidiabetic medicines may cause your skin to be more sensitive to sunlight than it is normally. Exposure to sunlight, even for brief periods of time, may cause a skin rash, itching, redness or other discoloration of the skin, or a severe sunburn.

When you begin taking this medicine:
- Stay out of direct sunlight, especially between the hours of 10:00 a.m. and 3:00 p.m., if possible.
- Wear protective clothing, including a hat. Also, wear sunglasses.
- Apply a sun block product that has a skin protection factor (SPF) of at least 15. Some patients may require a product with a higher SPF number, especially if they have a fair complexion. If you have any questions about this, check with your doctor or pharmacist.
- Apply a sun block lipstick that has an SPF of at least 15 to protect your lips.
- Do not use a sunlamp or tanning bed or booth.

If you have a severe reaction from the sun, check with your doctor.

Eat or drink something containing sugar and check with your doctor right away if mild symptoms of low blood sugar (hypoglycemia) appear. Good sources of sugar are glucose tablets or gel or fruit juice, corn syrup, honey, non-diet soft drinks, or sugar cubes or table sugar (dissolved in water). It is a good idea also to check your blood sugar to confirm that it is low.

- *If severe symptoms such as convulsions (seizures) or unconsciousness occur, diabetics should not eat or drink anything.* There is a chance that they could choke from not swallowing correctly. Emergency medical help should be obtained immediately.
- *Symptoms of low blood sugar (hypoglycemia) are:*
  Abdominal or stomach pain (mild)
  Anxious feeling
  Chills (continuing)
  Cold sweats
  Confusion
  Convulsions (seizures)
  Cool pale skin
  Difficulty in concentration
  Drowsiness
  Excessive hunger
  Fast heartbeat
  Headache (continuing)
  Nausea or vomiting (continuing)
  Nervousness
  Shakiness
  Unconsciousness
  Unsteady walk
  Unusual tiredness or weakness
  Vision changes
- Different people may have different symptoms of hypoglycemia. It is important that you learn your own signs of low blood sugar so that you can treat it quickly.
- *These symptoms may occur if you:*
  —delay or miss a scheduled meal or snack.
  —exercise much more than usual.

—cannot eat because of nausea and vomiting.

—drink a significant amount of alcohol.

- *Tell someone to take you to your doctor or to a hospital right away if the symptoms do not improve after eating or drinking a sweet food.*
- Even if you correct these symptoms by eating sugar, it is very important to call your doctor or hospital emergency service right away, since the blood sugar–lowering effects of this medicine may last for days and the symptoms may return often during this time.

Before having any kind of surgery, dental treatment, or emergency treatment, tell the medical doctor or dentist in charge that you are taking this medicine.

You should wear a medical I.D. bracelet or chain at all times. In addition, you should carry an identification card that says you have diabetes and that lists your medications.

Side Effects of This Medicine

The use of oral antidiabetics has been reported to increase the risk of death from heart and blood vessel disease. A report based on a study by the University Group Diabetes Program (UGDP) compared the use of one of the oral medicines (tolbutamide) to the use of diet alone or diet plus insulin. Although only tolbutamide was studied, other oral antidiabetics may cause a similar effect since all these medicines are related chemically and in the way they work.

Along with their needed effects, oral antidiabetics may cause some unwanted effects. Although not all of these side effects may occur, if they do occur they may need medical attention.

Check with your doctor as soon as possible if any of the following side effects occur:

Rare

Chest pain; chills; coughing up blood; dark urine; fever; general feeling of illness; increased sweating; itching of the skin; light-colored stools; increased amounts of sputum (phlegm); shortness of breath; sore throat; unusual bleeding or bruising; unusual tiredness or weakness (continuing and unexplained); yellow eyes or skin

Symptoms of overdose (hypoglycemia)

Abdominal or stomach pain (mild); anxious feeling; chills (continuing); cold sweats; confusion; convulsions (seizures); cool, pale skin; difficulty in concentration; drowsiness; excessive hunger; fast heartbeat; headache (continuing); nausea or vomiting (continuing); nervousness; shakiness; unconsciousness; unsteady walk; unusual tiredness or weakness; vision changes

Other side effects may occur that usually do not need medical attention. These side effects may go away during treatment as your body adjusts to the medicine. However, check with your doctor if any of the following side effects continue or are bothersome:

More common

Changes in taste (for tolbutamide); constipation; diarrhea; dizziness; drowsiness (mild); headache; heartburn; increased or decreased appetite; nausea; vomiting; stomach pain, fullness, or discomfort

Less common or rare

Hives; increased sensitivity of skin to sun; skin redness, itching, or rash

For patients taking chlorpropamide:

- Some patients who take chlorpropamide may retain (keep) more body water than usual. Check with your doctor as soon as possible if any of the following signs occur:

  Breathing difficulty; shortness of breath

Other side effects not listed above may also occur in some patients. If you notice any other effects, check with your doctor.

Additional Information

Once a medicine has been approved for marketing for a certain use, experience may show that it is also useful for other medical problems. Although this use is not included in product labeling, chlorpropamide is used in certain patients with the following medical condition:

- Diabetes insipidus (water diabetes)

If you are taking this medicine for water diabetes, the advice listed above that relates to diet and urine testing for patients with *sugar* diabetes *does not apply to you.* However, the advice about hypoglycemia (low blood sugar) does apply to you. Call your doctor right away if you feel any of the symptoms described.

Annual revision: July 1990

ANTIDYSKINETICS Systemic

This information applies to the following medicines:

Benztropine (BENZ-troe-peen)
Biperiden (bye-PER-i-den)
Ethopropazine (eth-oh-PROE-pa-zeen)
Procyclidine (proe-SYE-kli-deen)
Trihexyphenidyl (trye-hex-ee-FEN-i-dill)

Note: This information does *not* apply to Amantadine, Carbidopa and Levodopa, Diphenhydramine, Haloperidol, and Levodopa.

Some commonly used brand names are:

For Benztropine

In the U.S.
Cogentin
Generic name product may also be available.

In Canada
Apo-Benztropine
Cogentin
PMS Benztropine
Generic name product may also be available.

Another commonly used name is benzatropine.

For Biperiden

In the U.S.
Akineton

In Canada
Akineton

For Ethopropazine

In the U.S.
Parsidol

In Canada
Parsitan

Another commonly used name is profenamine.

For Procyclidine

In the U.S.
Kemadrin

In Canada
Kemadrin
PMS Procyclidine
Procyclid

For Trihexyphenidyl

In the U.S.
Artane
Artane Sequels
Trihexane
Trihexy
Generic name product may also be available.

In Canada
Apo-Trihex
Artane
Artane Sequels
PMS Trihexyphenidyl

Description

Antidyskinetics are used to treat Parkinson's disease, sometimes referred to as "shaking palsy." By improving muscle control and reducing stiffness, this medicine allows more normal movements of the body as the disease symptoms are reduced. It is also used to control severe reactions to certain medicines such as reserpine (e.g., Serpasil) (medicine to control high blood pressure) or phenothiazines, chlorprothixene (e.g., Taractan), thiothixene (e.g., Navane), loxapine (e.g., Loxitane), and haloperidol (e.g., Haldol) (medicines for nervous, mental, and emotional conditions).

Antidyskinetics may also be used for other conditions as determined by your doctor.

These medicines are available only with your doctor's prescription in the following dosage forms:

Oral

Benztropine
- Tablets (U.S. and Canada)

Biperiden
- Tablets (U.S. and Canada)

Ethopropazine
- Tablets (U.S. and Canada)

Procyclidine
- Elixir (Canada)
- Tablets (U.S. and Canada)

Trihexyphenidyl
- Extended-release capsules (U.S. and Canada)
- Elixir (U.S. and Canada)
- Tablets (U.S. and Canada)

Parenteral

Benztropine
- Injection (U.S. and Canada)

Biperiden
- Injection (U.S.)

It is very important that you read and understand the following information. If any of it causes you special concern, check with your doctor. Also, *if you have any questions* or if you want more information about this medicine or your medical problem, *ask your doctor, nurse, or pharmacist.*

Before Using This Medicine

In deciding to use a medicine, the risks of taking the medicine must be weighed against the good it will do. This is a decision you and your doctor will make. For antidyskinetics, the following should be considered:

Allergies—Tell your doctor if you have ever had any unusual or allergic reaction to antidyskinetics. Also tell your doctor and pharmacist if you are allergic to any other substances, such as foods, preservatives, or dyes.

Pregnancy—Studies on effects in pregnancy have not been done in either humans or animals. However, antidyskinetics have not been shown to cause problems in humans.

Breast-feeding—It is not known if antidyskinetics pass into breast milk. Although most medicines pass into breast milk in small amounts, many of them may be used safely while breast-feeding. Mothers who are taking these medicines and who wish to breast-feed should discuss this with their doctor.

Since antidyskinetics tend to decrease the secretions of the body, it is possible that the flow of breast milk may be reduced in some patients.

Children—Children may be especially sensitive to the effects of antidyskinetics. This may increase the chance of side effects during treatment.

Older adults—Agitation, confusion, disorientation, hallucinations, memory loss, and mental changes are more likely to occur in elderly patients, who are usually more sensitive to the effects of antidyskinetics.

Other medicines—Although certain medicines should not be used together at all, in other cases 2 different medicines may be used together even if an interaction might occur. In these cases, your doctor may want to change the dose, or other precautions may be necessary. When you are taking an antidyskinetic, it is especially important that your doctor and pharmacist know if you are taking any of the following:

- Anticholinergics (medicine for abdominal or stomach spasms or cramps) or
- Central nervous system (CNS) depressants (medicine that causes drowsiness) or
- Tricyclic antidepressants (medicine for depression)—Using these medicines together with antidyskinetics may result in additive effects, increasing the chance of unwanted effects

Other medical problems—The presence of other medical problems may affect the use of antidyskinetics. Make sure you tell your doctor if you have any other medical problems, especially:

- Difficult urination or
- Enlarged prostate or
- Glaucoma or
- Heart or blood vessel disease or
- High blood pressure or
- Intestinal blockage or
- Myasthenia gravis or
- Uncontrolled movements of hands, mouth, or tongue—Antidyskinetics may make the condition worse
- Kidney disease or
- Liver disease—Higher blood levels of the antidyskinetics may result, increasing the chance of side effects

Before you begin using any new medicine (prescription or nonprescription) or if you develop any new medical problem while you are using this medicine, check with your doctor, nurse, or pharmacist.

Proper Use of This Medicine

Take this medicine only as directed by your doctor. Do not take more of it, do not take it more often, and do not take it for a longer period of time than your doctor ordered. To do so may increase the chance of side effects.

To lessen stomach upset, take this medicine with meals or immediately after meals, unless otherwise directed by your doctor.

Dosing—The dose of antidyskinetics will be different for different patients. *Follow your doctor's orders or the directions on the label.* The following information includes only the average doses of benztropine, biperiden, ethopropazine, procyclidine, and trihexyphenidyl. *If your dose is different, do not change it* unless your doctor tells you to do so.

The number of capsules, tablets, or teaspoonfuls of elixir that you take depends on the strength of the medicine. Also, *the number of doses you take each day, the time allowed between doses, and the length of time you take the medicine depend on the medical problem for which you are taking antidyskinetics.*

For benztropine

- For *oral* dosage forms (tablets):
  - —For Parkinson's disease or certain severe side effects caused by some other medicines:
    - Adults—To start, 0.5 to 4 milligrams (mg) a day, depending on your condition. Your doctor will adjust your dose as needed; however, the dose is usually not more than 6 mg a day.
    - Children—Use and dose must be determined by your doctor.
- For *injection* dosage form:
  - —For Parkinson's disease or certain severe side effects caused by some other medicines:
    - Adults—1 to 4 mg a day, depending on your condition. Your doctor will adjust your dose as needed; however, the dose is usually not more than 6 mg a day.
    - Children—Use and dose must be determined by your doctor.

For biperiden

- For *oral* dosage forms (tablets):
  - —For Parkinson's disease or certain severe side effects caused by some other medicines:
    - Adults—2 mg up to four times a day. Your doctor will adjust your dose, depending on your condition; however, the dose is usually not more than 16 mg a day.
    - Children—Use and dose must be determined by your doctor.
- For *injection* dosage form:
  - —For Parkinson's disease or certain severe side effects caused by some other medicines:
    - Adults—2 mg, injected into a muscle or vein. The dose may be repeated if needed; however, the dose is usually not given more than four times a day.
    - Children—Use and dose is based on body weight and must be determined by your doctor.

For ethopropazine

- For *oral* dosage forms (tablets):
  - —For Parkinson's disease or certain severe side effects caused by some other medicines:
    - Adults—50 mg one or two times a day. Your doctor will adjust your dose as needed; however, the dose is usually not more than 600 mg a day.

- Children—Use and dose must be determined by your doctor.

For procyclidine

- For *oral* dosage forms (elixir or tablets):
  - —For Parkinson's disease or certain severe side effects caused by some other medicines:
    - Adults—To start, 2.5 mg three times a day after meals. Your doctor may need to adjust your dose, depending on your condition.
    - Children—Use and dose must be determined by your doctor.

For trihexyphenidyl

- For *extended-release oral* dosage forms (extended-release capsules):
  - —For Parkinson's disease or certain severe side effects caused by some other medicines:
    - Adults—5 mg after breakfast. Your doctor may add another 5 mg dose to be taken twelve hours later, depending on your condition.
    - Children: Use and dose must be determined by your doctor.
- For other *oral* dosage forms (elixir or tablets):
  - —For Parkinson's disease or certain severe side effects caused by some other medicines:
    - Adults—To start, 1 to 2 mg a day. Your doctor may adjust your dose as needed; however, the dose is usually not more than 15 mg a day.
    - Children—Use and dose must be determined by your doctor.

Missed dose—If you miss a dose of this medicine, take it as soon as possible. However, if it is within 2 hours of your next dose, skip the missed dose and go back to your regular dosing schedule. Do not double doses.

Storage—To store this medicine:

- Keep out of the reach of children.
- Store away from heat and direct light.
- Do not store the capsule or tablet form of this medicine in the bathroom, near the kitchen sink, or in other damp places. Heat or moisture may cause the medicine to break down.
- Keep the liquid form of this medicine from freezing.
- Do not keep outdated medicine or medicine no longer needed. Be sure that any discarded medicine is out of the reach of children.

Precautions While Using This Medicine

Your doctor should check your progress at regular visits, especially for the first few months you take this medicine. This will allow your dosage to be changed as necessary to meet your needs.

Your doctor may want you to have your eyes examined by an ophthalmologist (eye doctor) before and also sometime later during treatment.

Do not stop taking this medicine without first checking with your doctor. Your doctor may want you to reduce gradually the amount you are taking before stopping completely, to prevent side effects or the worsening of your condition.

This medicine will add to the effects of alcohol and other CNS depressants (medicines that slow down the nervous system, possibly causing drowsiness). Some examples of CNS depressants are antihistamines or medicine for hay fever, other allergies, or colds; sedatives, tranquilizers, or sleeping medicine; prescription pain medicine or narcotics; barbiturates; medicine for seizures; muscle relaxants; or anesthetics, including some dental anesthetics. *Check with your doctor before taking any of the above while you are using this medicine.*

Do not take this medicine within 1 hour of taking medicine for diarrhea. Taking these medicines too close together will make this medicine less effective.

If you think you or anyone else has taken an overdose of this medicine, get emergency help at once. Taking an overdose of this medicine may lead to unconsciousness. Some signs of an overdose are clumsiness or unsteadiness; seizures; severe drowsiness; severe dryness of mouth, nose and throat; fast heartbeat; hallucinations (seeing, hearing, or feeling things that are not there); mood or mental changes; shortness of breath or troubled breathing; trouble in sleeping; and unusual warmth, dryness, and flushing of skin.

This medicine may cause your eyes to become more sensitive to light than they are normally. Wearing sunglasses and avoiding too much exposure to bright light may help lessen the discomfort.

This medicine may cause some people to have blurred vision or to become drowsy, dizzy, or less alert than they are normally. *Make sure you know how you react to this medicine before you drive, use machines, or do anything else that could be dangerous if you are dizzy or are not alert or able to see well.*

Dizziness, lightheadedness, or fainting may occur, especially when you get up from lying or sitting. Getting up slowly may help. If the problem continues or gets worse, check with your doctor.

This medicine may make you sweat less, causing your body temperature to increase. *Use extra care to avoid becoming overheated during exercise or hot weather while you are taking this medicine, since overheating may result in heat stroke.* Also, hot baths or saunas may make you feel dizzy or faint while you are taking this medicine.

This medicine may cause dryness of the mouth. For temporary relief, use sugarless candy or gum, melt bits of ice in your mouth, or use a saliva substitute. However, if your mouth continues to feel dry for more than 2 weeks, check with your medical doctor or dentist. Continuing dryness of the mouth may increase the chance of dental disease, including tooth decay, gum disease, and fungus infections.

Side Effects of This Medicine

Along with its needed effects, a medicine may cause some unwanted effects. Although not all of these side effects may occur, if they do occur they may need medical attention.

Check with your doctor as soon as possible if any of the following side effects occur:

Rare

Confusion (more common in the elderly or with high doses); eye pain; skin rash

Symptoms of overdose

Clumsiness or unsteadiness; drowsiness (severe); dryness of mouth, nose, or throat (severe); fast heartbeat; hallucinations (seeing, hearing, or feeling things that are not there); mood or mental changes; seizures; shortness of breath or troubled breathing; trouble in sleeping; warmth, dryness, and flushing of skin

Other side effects may occur that usually do not need medical attention. These side effects may go away during treatment as your body adjusts to the medicine. However, check with your doctor if any of the following side effects continue or are bothersome:

More common

Blurred vision; constipation; decreased sweating; difficult or painful urination (especially in older men); drowsiness; dryness of mouth, nose, or throat; increased sensitivity of eyes to light; nausea or vomiting

Less common or rare

Dizziness or lightheadedness when getting up from a lying or sitting position; false sense of well-being (especially in the elderly or with high doses); headache; loss of memory (especially in the elderly); muscle cramps; nervousness; numbness or weakness in hands or feet; soreness of mouth and tongue; stomach upset or pain; unusual excitement (more common with large doses of trihexyphenidyl)

After you stop using this medicine, your body may need time to adjust. The length of time this takes depends on the amount of medicine you were using and how long you used it. During this period of time check with your doctor if you notice any of the following side effects:

Anxiety; difficulty in speaking or swallowing; dizziness or lightheadedness when getting up from a lying or sitting position; fast heartbeat; loss of balance control; mask-like face; muscle spasms, especially of face, neck, and back; restlessness or desire to keep moving; shuffling walk; stiffness of arms or legs; trembling and shaking of hands and fingers; trouble in sleeping; twisting movements of body

Other side effects not listed above may also occur in some patients. If you notice any other effects, check with your doctor.

Annual revision: 05/11/93

ANTIFIBRINOLYTIC AGENTS Systemic

This information applies to the following medicines:

Aminocaproic Acid (a-mee-noe-ka-PROE-ik ASS-id)
Tranexamic Acid (tran-ex-AM-ik ASS-id)

Some commonly used brand names are:

For Aminocaproic Acid

In the U.S.

Amicar
Generic name product may also be available.

In Canada

Amicar

For Tranexamic Acid

In the U.S.

Cyklokapron

In Canada

Cyklokapron

Description

Antifibrinolytic agents are used to treat serious bleeding, especially when the bleeding occurs after dental surgery or certain other kinds of surgery. These medicines are also sometimes given before an operation to prevent serious bleeding in patients with hemophilia or other medical problems that increase the chance of serious bleeding.

Antifibrinolytic agents may also be used for other conditions as determined by your doctor.

Antifibrinolytic agents are available only with your doctor's prescription, in the following dosage forms:

Oral

Aminocaproic acid
- Syrup (U.S. and Canada)
- Tablets (U.S. and Canada)

Tranexamic acid
- Tablets (U.S. and Canada)

Parenteral

Aminocaproic acid
- Injection (U.S. and Canada)

Tranexamic acid
- Injection (U.S. and Canada)

It is very important that you read and understand the following information. If any of it causes you special concern, check with your doctor. Also, *if you have any questions* or if you want more information about this medicine or your medical problem, *ask your doctor, nurse, or pharmacist.*

Before Using This Medicine

In deciding to use a medicine, the risks of taking the medicine must be weighed against the good it will do. This is a decision you and your doctor will make. For antifibrinolytic agents, the following should be considered:

Allergies—Tell your doctor if you have ever had any unusual or allergic reaction to aminocaproic acid or tranexamic acid. Also tell your doctor and pharmacist if you are allergic to any other substances, such as foods, preservatives, or dyes.

Pregnancy—Studies on birth defects have not been done in humans. However, these medicines have been given to pregnant women with no known birth defects or other problems occurring.

In animal studies, aminocaproic acid has caused birth defects and other unwanted effects.

Tranexamic acid has not been shown to cause birth defects or other problems in animal studies.

Breast-feeding—These medicines have not been reported to cause problems in nursing babies. However, small amounts of tranexamic acid pass into the breast milk.

Children—Although there is no specific information comparing the use of aminocaproic acid or tranexamic acid in children with use in other age groups, these medicines are not expected to cause different side effects or problems in children than they do in adults.

Older adults—
- *For aminocaproic acid*: Although there is no specific information comparing use of aminocaproic acid in the elderly with use in other age groups, it is not expected to cause different side effects or problems in older people than it does in younger adults.
- *For tranexamic acid*: Tranexamic acid has been tested and has not been shown to cause different side effects or problems in older people than it does in younger adults.

Other medicines—Although certain medicines should not be used together at all, in other cases two different medicines may be used together even if an interaction might occur. In these cases, your doctor may want to change the dose, or other precautions may be necessary. Tell your doctor and pharmacist if you are taking any other prescription or nonprescription (over-the-counter [OTC]) medicine.

Other medical problems—The presence of other medical problems may affect the use of antifibrinolytic agents. Make sure you tell your doctor if you have any other medical problems, especially:
- Blood clots or a history of medical problems caused by blood clots or
- Color vision problems or
- Heart disease or
- Kidney disease or
- Liver disease—The chance of side effects may be increased

Before you begin using any new medicine (prescription or nonprescription) or if you develop any new medical problem while you are using this medicine, check with your doctor, nurse, or pharmacist.

Proper Use of This Medicine

Take this medicine only as directed by your doctor. Do not take more or less of it, do not take it more often, and do not take it for a longer time than your doctor ordered. To do so may increase the chance of unwanted effects.

Missed dose—
- *For aminocaproic acid* (e.g., Amicar): If you miss a dose, take it as soon as possible. However, if you do not remember until it is almost time for your next dose, double the next dose. Then go back to your regular dosing schedule.
- *For tranexamic acid* (e.g., Cyklokapron): If you miss a dose, take it as soon as possible. Then take any remaining doses for the day at regularly spaced times. Do not double doses. If you have any questions about this, check with your doctor.

Storage—To store this medicine:
- Keep out of the reach of children.
- Store away from heat and direct light.
- Do not store the tablet form of this medicine in the bathroom, near the kitchen sink, or in other damp places. Heat or moisture may cause the medicine to break down.
- Do not keep outdated medicine or medicine no longer needed. Be sure that any discarded medicine is out of the reach of children.

Precautions While Using This Medicine

If you will be taking tranexamic acid for longer than several days, your doctor may want you to have your eyes checked regularly by an ophthalmologist (eye doctor).

This will allow your doctor to check for unwanted effects that may be caused by this medicine.

Side Effects of This Medicine

Along with its needed effects, a medicine may cause some unwanted effects. Although not all of these side effects may occur, if they do occur they may need medical attention.

The same effect that makes aminocaproic acid or tranexamic acid help prevent or stop bleeding also makes it possible for them to cause blood clots that could be dangerous. Check with your doctor immediately if any of the following possible signs and symptoms of blood clots occur:

Rare

Headache (severe and sudden); loss of coordination (sudden); pains in chest, groin, or legs, especially the calves; shortness of breath (sudden); slurred speech (sudden); vision changes (sudden); weakness or numbness in arm or leg

Also, check with your doctor as soon as possible if any of the following side effects occur:

Less common or rare

For aminocaproic acid

Dizziness; headache; muscle pain or weakness (severe and continuing); red or bloodshot eyes; ringing or buzzing in ears; skin rash; slow or irregular heartbeat—with the injection only; stomach cramps or pain; stuffy nose; sudden decrease in amount of urine; swelling of face, feet, or lower legs; unusual tiredness or weakness; weight gain (rapid)

For tranexamic acid

Blurred vision or other changes in vision; dizziness or lightheadedness; unusual tiredness or weakness

Other side effects may occur that usually do not need medical attention. These side effects may go away during treatment as your body adjusts to the medicine. However, check with your doctor if any of the following side effects continue or are bothersome:

For aminocaproic acid or tranexamic acid

Diarrhea; nausea or vomiting; unusual menstrual discomfort

Other side effects not listed above may also occur in some patients. If you notice any other effects, check with your doctor.

Annual revision: 09/12/91

ANTIFUNGALS, AZOLE Vaginal

This information applies to the following medicines:

Butoconazole (byoo-toe-KOE-na-zole)
Clotrimazole (kloe-TRIM-a-zole)
Econazole (e-KONE-a-zole)
Miconazole (mi-KON-a-zole)
Terconazole (ter-KONE-a-zole)
Tioconazole (tye-oh-KONE-a-zole)

Some commonly used brand names are:

For Butoconazole

In the U.S.

Femstat

In Canada

Femstat

For Clotrimazole

In the U.S.

Gyne-Lotrimin
Mycelex-G

In Canada

Canesten
Canesten 1
Canesten 3
Canesten 10%
Myclo

For Econazole*

In Canada

Ecostatin

For Miconazole

In the U.S.

Monistat 3
Monistat 7

In Canada

Monistat
Monistat 3
Monistat 5
Monistat 7

For Terconazole

In the U.S.

Terazol 3
Terazol 7

In Canada

Terazol 3
Terazol 7

For Tioconazole

In the U.S.

Vagistat

In Canada

Gyno-Trosyd

*Not commercially available in the U.S.

Description

Vaginal azoles (A-zoles) are used to treat fungus (yeast) infections of the vagina.

Most vaginal azoles are available only with your doctor's prescription, in the following dosage forms:

Vaginal

Butoconazole

- Cream (U.S. and Canada)
- Suppositories (Canada)

Clotrimazole
- Cream (U.S. and Canada)
- Tablets (U.S. and Canada)

Econazole
- Suppositories (Canada)

Miconazole
- Cream (U.S. and Canada)
- Suppositories (U.S. and Canada)
- Tampons (Canada)

Terconazole
- Cream (U.S. and Canada)
- Suppositories (U.S. and Canada)

Tioconazole
- Ointment (U.S. and Canada)
- Suppositories (Canada)

It is very important that you read and understand the following information. If any of it causes you special concern, check with your doctor. Also, *if you have any questions* or if you want more information about this medicine or your medical problem, *ask your doctor, nurse, or pharmacist.*

Before Using This Medicine

In deciding to use a medicine, the risks of using the medicine must be weighed against the good it will do. This is a decision you and your doctor will make. For vaginal azoles, the following should be considered:

Allergies—Tell your doctor if you have ever had any unusual or allergic reaction to any of the azoles. Also tell your doctor and pharmacist if you are allergic to any other substances, such as foods, preservatives, or dyes.

Pregnancy—Studies have not been done in humans during the first trimester of pregnancy. Vaginal azoles have not been shown to cause birth defects or other problems in humans when used during the second and third trimesters.

Breast-feeding—It is not known whether vaginal azoles pass into the breast milk. However, these medicines have not been shown to cause problems in nursing babies.

Children—Studies on these medicines have been done only in adult patients, and there is no specific information comparing use of vaginal azoles in children with use in other age groups.

Older adults—Many medicines have not been studied specifically in older people. Therefore, it may not be known whether they work exactly the same way they do in younger adults. Although there is no specific information comparing use of vaginal azoles in the elderly with use in other age groups, they are not expected to cause different side effects or problems in older people than they do in younger adults.

Other medicines—Although certain medicines should not be used together at all, in other cases two different medicines may be used together even if an interaction might occur. In these cases, your doctor may want to change the dose, or other precautions may be necessary. Tell your doctor and pharmacist if you are using any other vaginal prescription or nonprescription (over-the-counter [OTC]) medicine.

Before you begin using any new medicine (prescription or nonprescription) or if you develop any new medical problem while you are using this medicine, check with your doctor, nurse, or pharmacist.

Proper Use of This Medicine

Vaginal azoles usually come with patient directions. Read them carefully before using this medicine.

Use this medicine at bedtime, unless otherwise directed by your doctor. The vaginal tampon form of miconazole should be left in the vagina overnight and removed the next morning.

This medicine is usually inserted into the vagina with an applicator. However, if you are pregnant, check with your doctor before using the applicator.

To help clear up your infection completely, *it is very important that you keep using this medicine for the full time of treatment,* even if your symptoms begin to clear up after a few days. If you stop using this medicine too soon, your symptoms may return. *Do not miss any doses.* Also, *do not stop using this medicine if your menstrual period starts during the time of treatment.*

Missed dose—If you do miss a dose of this medicine, insert it as soon as possible. However, if it is almost time for your next dose, skip the missed dose and go back to your regular dosing schedule.

Storage—To store this medicine:
- Keep out of the reach of children.
- Store away from heat and direct light.
- Do not store the vaginal suppository or vaginal tablet form of this medicine in the bathroom, near the kitchen sink, or in other damp places. Heat or moisture may cause the medicine to break down.
- Keep the vaginal cream, ointment, and suppository forms of this medicine from freezing.
- Do not keep outdated medicine or medicine no longer needed. Be sure that any discarded medicine is out of the reach of children.

Precautions While Using This Medicine

If your symptoms do not improve within a few days, or if they become worse, check with your doctor.

Vaginal medicines usually will come out of the vagina during treatment. To keep the medicine from getting on your clothing, wear a minipad or sanitary napkin. The use of nonmedicated tampons (like those used for menstrual periods) is not recommended since they may soak up the medicine.

To help clear up your infection completely and to help make sure it does not return, good health habits are also required.

- Wear cotton panties (or panties or pantyhose with cotton crotches) instead of synthetic (for example, nylon or rayon) panties.
- Wear only clean panties.

If you have any questions about this, check with your doctor, nurse, or pharmacist.

Many vaginal infections are spread by having sex. A male sexual partner may carry the fungus on or in his penis. While you are using this medicine, it may be a good idea for your partner to wear a condom during sex to avoid re-infection. Also, it may be necessary for your partner to be treated. *Do not stop using this medicine if you have sex during treatment.*

Certain brands of vaginal azoles contain oils in the cream bases the medicine is put in. Oils can weaken latex rubber condoms, diaphragms, or cervical caps. This increases the chances of a condom breaking during sexual intercourse. The rubber in cervical caps or diaphragms may break down faster and wear out sooner. Check with your doctor, nurse, or pharmacist to make sure the vaginal azole product you are using can be used with latex rubber birth control devices.

Some women may want to use a douche before the next dose. Some doctors will allow the use of a vinegar and water douche or other douche. However, others do not allow any douching. If you do use a douche, *do not overfill the vagina.* To do so may push the douche up into the uterus and possibly cause inflammation or infection. Also, *do not douche if you are pregnant since this may harm the fetus.* If you have any questions about this, check with your doctor, nurse, or pharmacist.

Side Effects of This Medicine

Along with its needed effects, a medicine may cause some unwanted effects. Although not all of these side effects may occur, if they do occur they may need medical attention.

Check with your doctor as soon as possible if any of the following side effects occur:

Less common

Vaginal burning, itching, discharge, or other irritation not present before use of this medicine

Rare

Skin rash or hives

Other side effects may occur that usually do not need medical attention. These side effects may go away during treatment as your body adjusts to the medicine. However, check with your doctor if any of the following side effects continue or are bothersome:

Less common or rare

Abdominal or stomach cramps or pain; burning or irritation of penis of sexual partner; headache

Other side effects not listed above may also occur in some patients. If you notice any other effects, check with your doctor.

Annual revision: 04/21/92
Interim revision: 07/23/92

ANTIGLAUCOMA AGENTS, CHOLINERGIC, LONG-ACTING Ophthalmic

This information applies to the following medicines:

Demecarium (dem-e-KARE-ee-um)
Echothiophate (ek-oh-THYE-oh-fate)
Isoflurophate (eye-soe-FLURE-oh-fate)

Some commonly used brand names are:

For Demecarium
In the U.S.
Humorsol

For Echothiophate
In the U.S.
Phospholine Iodide
In Canada
Phospholine Iodide

Another commonly used name is ecothiopate.

For Isoflurophate
In the U.S.
Floropryl

Other commonly used names are DFP, difluorophate, and dyflos.

Description

Demecarium, echothiophate, and isoflurophate are used in the eye to treat certain types of glaucoma and other eye conditions. They may also be used in the diagnosis of certain eye conditions.

These medicines are available only with your doctor's prescription, in the following dosage forms:

Ophthalmic

Demecarium
- Ophthalmic solution (eye drops) (U.S.)

Echothiophate
- Ophthalmic solution (eye drops) (U.S. and Canada)

Isoflurophate
- Ophthalmic ointment (eye ointment) (U.S.)

It is very important that you read and understand the following information. If any of it causes you special concern, check with your doctor. Also, *if you have any questions* or if you want more information about this medicine or your medical problem, *ask your doctor, nurse, or pharmacist.*

Before Using This Medicine

In deciding to use a medicine, the risks of taking the medicine must be weighed against the good it will do. This is a decision you and your doctor will make. For demecarium, echothiophate, or isoflurophate, the following should be considered:

Allergies—Tell your doctor if you have ever had any unusual or allergic reaction to demecarium, echothiophate, or isoflurophate. Also tell your doctor and pharmacist if you are allergic to any other substances, such as preservatives.

Pregnancy—Because of the toxicity of these medicines in general, demecarium, echothiophate, and isoflurophate are not recommended during pregnancy.

Breast-feeding—Demecarium, echothiophate, and isoflurophate may be absorbed into the body. These medicines are not recommended during breast-feeding, because they may cause unwanted effects in nursing babies. It may be necessary for you to use another medicine or to stop breast-feeding during treatment. Be sure you have discussed the risks and benefits of the medicine with your doctor.

Children—Demecarium, echothiophate, or isoflurophate can cause serious side effects in any patient. When this medicine is used for a long time, eye cysts may occur. These eye cysts occur more often in children than in adults. Therefore, it is especially important that you discuss with the child's doctor the good that this medicine may do as well as the risks of using it.

Older adults—Many medicines have not been tested in older people. Therefore, it may not be known whether they work exactly the same way they do in younger adults or if they cause different side effects or problems in older people. There is no specific information about the use of these medicines in the elderly. However, demecarium, echothiophate, or isoflurophate can cause serious side effects in any patient.

Other medicines—Although certain medicines should not be used together at all, in other cases two different medicines may be used together even if an interaction might occur. In these cases, your doctor may want to change the dose, or other precautions may be necessary. When you are taking demecarium, echothiophate, or isoflurophate, it is especially important that your doctor and pharmacist know if you are taking any of the following:

- Amantadine (e.g., Symmetrel) or
- Anticholinergics (medicine to help reduce stomach acid and for abdominal or stomach spasms or cramps) or
- Antidepressants (medicine for depression) or
- Antidyskinetics (medicine for Parkinson's disease or other conditions affecting control of muscles) or
- Antihistamines or
- Antimyasthenics (ambenonium [e.g., Mytelase], neostigmine [e.g., Prostigmin], pyridostigmine [e.g., Mestinon]) or
- Antipsychotics (medicine for mental illness) or
- Buclizine (e.g., Bucladin) or
- Carbamazepine (e.g., Tegretol) or
- Cyclizine (e.g., Marezine) or
- Cyclobenzaprine (e.g., Flexeril) or
- Disopyramide (e.g., Norpace) or
- Flavoxate (e.g., Urispas) or
- Ipratropium (e.g., Atrovent) or
- Meclizine (e.g., Antivert) or
- Methylphenidate (e.g., Ritalin) or
- Orphenadrine (e.g., Norflex) or
- Oxybutynin (e.g., Ditropen) or
- Procainamide (e.g., Pronestyl) or
- Promethazine (e.g., Phenergan) or
- Quinidine (e.g., Quinidex) or
- Trimeprazine (e.g., Temaril)—May increase the possibility of side effects or toxic effects; use of these medicines with demecarium, echothiophate, or isoflurophate is not recommended except under close supervision by your doctor
- Malathion (topical) (e.g., Prioderm)—May increase the possibility of side effects or toxic effects, especially if large amounts of malathion are used

Pesticides or insecticides—Make sure you tell your doctor if you have been exposed recently to pesticides or insecticides.

Other medical problems—The presence of other medical problems may affect the use of demecarium, echothiophate, or isoflurophate. Make sure you tell your doctor if you have any other medical problems, especially:

- Asthma or
- Epilepsy or
- Heart disease or
- High blood pressure or
- Myasthenia gravis or
- Overactive thyroid or
- Parkinsonism or
- Stomach ulcer or other stomach problems or
- Urinary tract blockage—If this medicine is absorbed into the body, it may make the condition worse
- Down's syndrome (mongolism)—Medicine may cause these children to become hyperactive
- Eye disease or problems (other)—May increase absorption of this medicine into the body or may make the condition worse

Before you begin using any new medicine (prescription or nonprescription) or if you develop any new medical

problem while you are using this medicine, check with your doctor, nurse, or pharmacist.

Proper Use of This Medicine

To use the *ophthalmic solution (eye drops) form* of this medicine:

- First, wash your hands. With the middle finger, apply pressure to the inside corner of the eye (and continue to apply pressure for 1 or 2 minutes after the medicine has been placed in the eye). Tilt the head back and with the index finger of the same hand, pull the lower eyelid away from the eye to form a pouch. Drop the medicine into the pouch and gently close the eyes. Do not blink. Keep the eyes closed for 1 or 2 minutes to allow the medicine to be absorbed.
- Remove any excess solution around the eye with a clean tissue, being careful not to touch the eye.
- Immediately after using the eye drops, wash your hands to remove any medicine that may be on them.
- To keep the medicine as germ-free as possible, do not touch the applicator tip to any surface (including the eye). Also, keep the container tightly closed.

To use the *ophthalmic ointment (eye ointment) form* of this medicine:

- First, wash your hands. Then pull the lower eyelid away from the eye to form a pouch. Squeeze a thin strip of ointment into the pouch. A ½-cm (approximately ¼-inch) strip of ointment is usually enough unless otherwise directed by your doctor. Gently close the eyes and keep them closed for 1 or 2 minutes to allow the medicine to be absorbed.
- Immediately after using the eye ointment, wash your hands to remove any medicine that may be on them.
- Since isoflurophate loses its effectiveness when exposed to moisture, do not wash the tip of the ointment tube or allow it to touch any moist surface (including the eye).
- To keep the medicine as germ-free as possible, do not touch the applicator tip to any surface (including the eye). After using this eye ointment, wipe the tip of the ointment tube with a clean tissue and keep the tube tightly closed.
- Since an eye ointment usually causes blurred vision for a short time after you apply it, ask your doctor if the dose (or one of the doses if you use more than 1 dose a day) can be applied at bedtime.

It is very important that you use this medicine only as directed. Do not use more of it and do not use it more often than your doctor ordered. To do so may increase the chance of too much medicine being absorbed into the body and the chance of side effects.

Missed dose—If you miss a dose of this medicine and your dosing schedule is:

- One dose every other day—Apply the missed dose as soon as possible if you remember it on the day it should be applied. However, if you do not remember the missed dose until the next day, apply it at that time. Then skip a day and start your dosing schedule again. Do not double doses.
- One dose a day—Apply the missed dose as soon as possible. However, if you do not remember the missed dose until the next day, skip the missed dose and go back to your regular dosing schedule. Do not double doses.
- More than one dose a day—Apply the missed dose as soon as possible. However, if it is almost time for your next dose, skip the missed dose and go back to your regular dosing schedule. Do not double doses.

If your dosing schedule is different from all of the above and you miss a dose of this medicine, or if you have any questions about this, check with your doctor.

Storage—To store this medicine:

- Keep out of the reach of children. Overdose of demecarium, echothiophate, or isoflurophate is very dangerous in young children.
- Store away from heat and direct light.
- Keep this medicine from freezing.
- Do not keep outdated medicine or medicine no longer needed. Be sure that any discarded medicine is out of the reach of children.

Precautions While Using This Medicine

If you are using this medicine for glaucoma, your doctor should check your eye pressure at regular visits to make sure the medicine is working.

If you will be using this medicine for a long time, your doctor should examine your eyes at regular visits to make sure this medicine does not cause unwanted effects.

Before you have any kind of surgery (including eye surgery), dental treatment, or emergency treatment, tell the medical doctor or dentist in charge and the anesthesiologist or anesthetist (the person who puts you to sleep) that you are using this medicine or have used it within the past month.

Avoid breathing in even small amounts of carbamate- or organophosphate-type insecticides or pesticides (for example, carbaryl [Sevin], demeton [Systox], diazinon, malathion, parathion, ronnel [Trolene], or TEPP). They may add to the effects of this medicine. Farmers, gardeners, residents of communities undergoing insecticide or pesticide spraying or dusting, workers in plants manufacturing such products, or other persons exposed to such poisons should protect themselves by wearing a mask over the nose and mouth, changing clothes frequently, and washing hands often.

Make sure your vision is clear before you drive, use machines, or do anything else that could be dangerous if you are not able to see well. This is because:

- After you apply this medicine to your eyes, your pupils may become unusually small. This may cause you to see less well at night or in dim light.
- After you begin using this medicine, your vision may be blurred or there may be a change in your near or distant vision.
- The eye ointment form of this medicine usually causes blurred vision for a short time after you apply it.

Side Effects of This Medicine

Along with its needed effects, a medicine may cause some unwanted effects. Although not all of these side effects may occur, if they do occur they may need medical attention.

Check with your doctor immediately if any of the following side effects occur:

Rare

Veil or curtain appearing across part of vision

Symptoms of too much medicine being absorbed into the body

Increased sweating; loss of bladder control; muscle weakness; nausea, vomiting, diarrhea, or stomach cramps or pain; shortness of breath, tightness in chest, or wheezing; slow or irregular heartbeat; unusual tiredness or weakness; watering of mouth

Note: The most common of these symptoms, especially in children, are nausea, vomiting, diarrhea, and stomach cramps or pain. Too much medicine being absorbed is rare with the eye ointment form of this medicine.

Other side effects may occur that usually do not need medical attention. These side effects may go away during treatment as your body adjusts to the medicine. However, check with your doctor if any of the following side effects continue or are bothersome:

Blurred vision or change in near or distant vision; burning, redness, stinging, or other eye irritation; difficulty in seeing at night or in dim light; eye pain; headache or browache; twitching of eyelids; watering of eyes

Other side effects not listed above may also occur in some patients. If you notice any other effects, check with your doctor.

Annual revision: 09/13/91

ANTIHISTAMINES Systemic

This information applies to the following medicines:

Astemizole (a-STEM-mi-zole)
Azatadine (a-ZA-ta-deen)
Bromodiphenhydramine (broe-moe-dye-fen-HYE-dra-meen)
Brompheniramine (brome-fen-EER-a-meen)
Carbinoxamine (kar-bi-NOX-a-meen)
Cetirizine (se-TI-ra-zeen)
Chlorpheniramine (klor-fen-EER-a-meen)
Clemastine (KLEM-as-teen)
Cyproheptadine (si-proe-HEP-ta-deen)
Dexchlorpheniramine (dex-klor-fen-EER-a-meen)
Dimenhydrinate (dye-men-HYE-dri-nate)
Diphenhydramine (dye-fen-HYE-dra-meen)
Diphenylpyraline (dye-fen-il-PEER-a-leen)
Doxylamine (dox-ILL-a-meen)
Hydroxyzine (hye-DROX-i-zeen)
Loratadine (lor-AT-a-deen)
Phenindamine (fen-IN-da-meen)
Pyrilamine (peer-ILL-a-meen)
Terfenadine (ter-FEN-a-deen)
Tripelennamine (tri-pel-ENN-a-meen)
Triprolidine (trye-PROE-li-deen)

Some commonly used brand names are:

For Astemizole
In the U.S.
Hismanal
In Canada
Hismanal

For Azatadine
In the U.S.
Optimine
In Canada
Optimine

For Bromodiphenhydramine
Another commonly used name for bromodiphenhydramine is bromazine. Bromodiphenhydramine is not available by itself in the U.S. and Canada. However, it is available in cough/cold combination products.

For Brompheniramine
In the U.S.
Bromphen
Chlorphed
Codimal-A
Conjec-B
Cophene-B
Dehist
Diamine T.D.
Dimetane
Dimetane Extentabs
Histaject Modified
Nasahist B
ND-Stat Revised
Oraminic II
Veltane
Generic name product may also be available.
In Canada
Dimetane
Dimetane Extentabs

For Carbinoxamine
Carbinoxamine is not available by itself in the U.S. and Canada. However, it is available in cough/cold combination products.

For Cetirizine*
In Canada
Reactine

For Chlorpheniramine
In the U.S.
Aller-Chlor
Chlo-Amine
Chlor-100
Chlorate
Chlor-Niramine
Chlor-Pro
Chlor-Pro 10
Chlorspan-12
Chlortab-4
Chlortab-8
Chlor-Trimeton
Chlor-Trimeton Repetabs
Genallerate
PediaCare Allergy Formula
Pfeiffer's Allergy
Phenetron
Phenetron Lanacaps
Telachlor
Teldrin
Trymegen

Generic name product may also be available.

In Canada
Chlor-Tripolon
Novopheniram

Another commonly used name is chlorphenamine.

For Clemastine
In the U.S.
Tavist
Tavist-1

In Canada
Tavist

For Cyproheptadine
In the U.S.
Periactin

Generic name product may also be available.

In Canada
Periactin

For Dexchlorpheniramine
In the U.S.
Dexchlor
Poladex T.D.
Polaramine
Polaramine Repetabs

Generic name product may also be available.

In Canada
Polaramine
Polaramine Repetabs

For Dimenhydrinate
In the U.S.
Calm X
Dimetabs
Dinate
Dommanate
Dramamine
Dramamine Chewable
Dramamine Liquid
Dramanate
Dramocen
Dramoject
Dymenate
Hydrate
Marmine
Nico-Vert
Tega-Vert
Triptone Caplets
Vertab

Generic name product may also be available.

In Canada
Apo-Dimenhydrinate
Gravol
Gravol L/A
Nauseatol
Novodimenate
PMS-Dimenhydrinate
Travamine

Generic name product may also be available.

For Diphenhydramine
In the U.S.
AllerMax Caplets
Aller-med
Banophen
Banophen Caplets
Beldin
Belix
Bena-D 10
Bena-D 50
Benadryl
Benadryl 25
Benadryl Kapseals
Benahist 10
Benahist 50
Ben-Allergin-50
Benoject-10
Benoject-50
Benylin Cough
Bydramine Cough
Compoz
Diphenacen-50
Diphenadryl
Diphen Cough
Diphenhist
Diphenhist Captabs
Dormarex 2
Fynex
Genahist
Gen-D-phen
Hydramine
Hydramine Cough
Hydramyn
Hydril
Hyrexin-50
Nervine Nighttime Sleep-Aid
Nidryl
Noradryl
Nordryl
Nordryl Cough
Nytol Maximum Strength
Nytol with DPH
Phendry
Phendry Children's Allergy Medicine
Sleep-Eze 3
Sominex Formula 2
Tusstat
Twilite Caplets
Uni-Bent Cough
Wehdryl-10
Wehdryl-50

Generic name product may also be available.

In Canada
Allerdryl
Benadryl
Insomnal

Generic name product may also be available.

For Diphenylpyraline
Diphenylpyraline is not available by itself in the U.S. and Canada. However, it is available in cough/cold combination products.

For Doxylamine
In the U.S.
Unisom Nighttime Sleep Aid
In Canada
Doxylamine is not available by itself in Canada. However, it is available in cough/cold combination products.

For Hydroxyzine
In the U.S.
Anxanil
Atarax
E-Vista
Hydroxacen
Hyzine-50
Quiess
Vistaject-25
Vistaject-50
Vistaril
Vistazine 50

Generic name product may also be available.

In Canada
Apo-Hydroxyzine
Atarax
Multipax
Novohydroxyzin

Generic name product may also be available.

For Loratadine
In the U.S.
Claritin
In Canada
Claritin

For Phenindamine†
In the U.S.
Nolahist

For Pyrilamine†
In the U.S.
Nisaval

Generic name product may also be available.

Another commonly used name is mepyramine.

For Terfenadine

In the U.S.

Seldane

In Canada

Seldane — Seldane Caplets

For Tripelennamine

In the U.S.

PBZ — Pelamine

PBZ-SR

Generic name product may also be available.

In Canada

Pyribenzamine

For Triprolidine

In the U.S.

Actidil — Myidil

Alleract

Generic name product may also be available.

In Canada

Triprolidine is not available by itself in Canada. However, it is available in cough/cold combination products.

---

*Not commercially available in the U.S.

†Not commercially available in Canada.

Description

Antihistamines are used to relieve or prevent the symptoms of hay fever and other types of allergy. They work by preventing the effects of a substance called histamine, which is produced by the body.

Some of the antihistamines are also used to prevent motion sickness, nausea, vomiting, and dizziness. In patients with Parkinson's disease, diphenhydramine may be used to decrease stiffness and tremors. Also, the syrup form of diphenhydramine is used to relieve the cough due to colds or hay fever. In addition, since antihistamines may cause drowsiness as a side effect, some of them may be used to help people go to sleep.

Hydroxyzine is used in the treatment of nervous and emotional conditions to help control anxiety. It can also be used to help control anxiety and produce sleep before surgery.

Antihistamines may also be used for other conditions as determined by your doctor.

Some antihistamine preparations are available only with your doctor's prescription. Others are available without a prescription. However, your doctor may have special instructions on the proper dose of the medicine for your medical condition.

These medicines are available in the following dosage forms:

Oral

Astemizole
- Oral suspension (Canada)
- Tablets (U.S. and Canada)

Azatadine
- Tablets (U.S. and Canada)

Brompheniramine
- Elixir (U.S. and Canada)
- Tablets (U.S. and Canada)
- Extended-release tablets (U.S. and Canada)

Cetirizine
- Tablets (Canada)

Chlorpheniramine
- Extended-release capsules (U.S.)
- Syrup (U.S. and Canada)
- Tablets (U.S. and Canada)
- Chewable tablets (U.S.)
- Extended-release tablets (U.S. and Canada)

Clemastine
- Syrup (U.S. and Canada)
- Tablets (U.S. and Canada)

Cyproheptadine
- Syrup (U.S. and Canada)
- Tablets (U.S. and Canada)

Dexchlorpheniramine
- Syrup (U.S. and Canada)
- Tablets (U.S. and Canada)
- Extended-release tablets (U.S. and Canada)

Dimenhydrinate
- Capsules (U.S.)
- Extended-release capsules (Canada)
- Elixir (Canada)
- Syrup (U.S.)
- Tablets (U.S. and Canada)
- Chewable tablets (U.S.)

Diphenhydramine
- Capsules (U.S. and Canada)
- Elixir (U.S. and Canada)
- Syrup (U.S.)
- Tablets (U.S.)

Doxylamine
- Tablets (U.S.)

Hydroxyzine
- Capsules (U.S. and Canada)
- Oral suspension (U.S.)
- Syrup (U.S. and Canada)
- Tablets (U.S.)

Loratadine
- Tablets (U.S. and Canada)

Phenindamine
- Tablets (U.S.)

Pyrilamine
- Tablets (U.S.)

Terfenadine
- Oral suspension (Canada)
- Tablets (U.S. and Canada)

Tripelennamine
- Elixir (U.S.)
- Tablets (U.S. and Canada)
- Extended-release tablets (U.S.)

Triprolidine
- Syrup (U.S.)
- Tablets (U.S.)

Parenteral

Brompheniramine
- Injection (U.S.)

Chlorpheniramine
- Injection (U.S. and Canada)

Dimenhydrinate
- Injection (U.S. and Canada)

Diphenhydramine
- Injection (U.S. and Canada)

Hydroxyzine
- Injection (U.S. and Canada)

Rectal

Dimenhydrinate
- Suppositories (Canada)

It is very important that you read and understand the following information. If any of it causes you special concern, check with your doctor or pharmacist. Also, *if you have any questions* or if you want more information about this medicine or your medical problem, *ask your doctor, nurse, or pharmacist.*

Before Using This Medicine

In deciding to use a medicine, the risks of taking the medicine must be weighed against the good it will do. This is a decision you and your doctor will make. For antihistamines, the following should be considered:

Allergies—Tell your doctor if you have ever had any unusual or allergic reaction to antihistamines. Also tell your doctor and pharmacist if you are allergic to any other substances, such as foods, preservatives, or dyes.

Diet—Make certain your doctor and pharmacist know if you are on a low-sodium, low-sugar, or any other special diet. Most medicines contain more than their active ingredient, and many liquid medicines contain alcohol.

Pregnancy—Most antihistamines have not been studied in pregnant women. Although these antihistamines have not been shown to cause problems in humans, studies in animals have shown that some other antihistamines, such as meclizine (e.g., Antivert) and cyclizine (e.g., Marezine), may cause birth defects.

Also, studies in animals have shown that terfenadine, when given in doses several times the human dose, lowers the birth weight and increases the risk of death of the offspring.

Hydroxyzine is not recommended for use in the first months of pregnancy since it has been shown to cause birth defects in animal studies when given in doses up to many times the usual human dose. Be sure you have discussed this with your doctor.

Breast-feeding—Small amounts of antihistamines pass into the breast milk. Use is not recommended since babies are more susceptible to the side effects of antihistamines, such as unusual excitement or irritability. Also, since these medicines tend to decrease the secretions of the body, it is possible that the flow of breast milk may be reduced in some patients. It is not known yet whether astemizole, loratadine, and terfenadine cause these same side effects.

Children—Serious side effects, such as convulsions (seizures), are more likely to occur in younger patients and would be of greater risk to infants than to older children or adults. In general, children are more sensitive to the effects of antihistamines. Also, nightmares or unusual excitement, nervousness, restlessness, or irritability may be more likely to occur in children.

Older adults—Elderly patients are usually more sensitive to the effects of antihistamines. Confusion; difficult or painful urination; dizziness; drowsiness; feeling faint; or dryness of mouth, nose, or throat may be more likely to occur in elderly patients. Also, nightmares or unusual excitement, nervousness, restlessness, or irritability may be more likely to occur in elderly patients.

Other medicines—Although certain medicines should not be used together at all, in other cases different medicines may be used together even if an interaction might occur. In these cases, your doctor may want to change the dose, or other precautions may be necessary. When you are taking antihistamines it is especially important that your doctor and pharmacist know if you are taking any of the following:

- Anticholinergics (medicine for abdominal or stomach spasms or cramps)—Side effects, such as dryness of mouth, of antihistamines or anticholinergics may be more likely to occur
- Central nervous system (CNS) depressants—Effects, such as drowsiness, of CNS depressants or antihistamines may be worsened; also, taking maprotiline or tricyclic antidepressants may cause some side effects of either of these medicines, such as dryness of mouth, to become more severe
- Erythromycin (e.g., E-Mycin) or
- Itraconazole (e.g., Sporanox) or
- Ketoconazole (e.g., Nizoral)—Use of these medicines with astemizole and terfenadine may cause heart problems, such as an irregular heartbeat; these medicines should not be used together
- Monoamine oxidase (MAO) inhibitors (furazolidone [e.g., Furoxone], isocarboxazid [e.g., Marplan], phenelzine [e.g., Nardil], procarbazine [e.g., Matulane], tranylcypromine [e.g., Parnate])—If you are now taking, or have taken within the past 2 weeks, any of the MAO inhibitors, the side effects of the antihistamines may become more severe; these medicines should not be used together

Other medical problems—The presence of other medical problems may affect the use of antihistamines. Make sure you tell your doctor if you have any other medical problems, especially:

- Enlarged prostate or
- Urinary tract blockage or difficult urination—Antihistamines may make urinary problems worse
- Glaucoma—These medicines may cause a slight increase in inner eye pressure that may make the condition worse
- Liver disease—Higher blood levels of astemizole or terfenadine may result, which may increase the chance of heart problems

Before you begin using any new medicine (prescription or nonprescription) or if you develop any new medical problem while you are using this medicine, check with your doctor, nurse, or pharmacist.

Proper Use of This Medicine

Antihistamines are used to relieve or prevent the symptoms of your medical problem. Take them only as directed. Do not take more of them and do not take them more often than recommended on the label, unless otherwise directed by your doctor. To do so may increase the chance of side effects.

Missed dose—If you are taking this medicine regularly and you miss a dose, take it as soon as possible. However, if it is almost time for your next dose, skip the missed dose and go back to your regular dosing schedule. Do not double doses.

For patients *taking this medicine by mouth:*

- Antihistamines can be taken with food or a glass of water or milk to lessen stomach irritation if necessary.
- If you are taking the extended-release tablet form of this medicine, swallow the tablets whole. Do not break, crush, or chew before swallowing.

For patients taking *dimenhydrinate or diphenhydramine for motion sickness:*

- Take this medicine at least 30 minutes or, even better, 1 to 2 hours before you begin to travel.

For patients using the *suppository form of this medicine:*

- To insert suppository: First remove the foil wrapper and moisten the suppository with cold water. Lie down on side and use your finger to push the suppository well up into the rectum. If the suppository is too soft to insert, chill the suppository in the refrigerator for 30 minutes or run cold water over it, before removing the foil wrapper.

For patients using the *injection form of this medicine:*

- If you will be giving yourself the injections, make sure you understand exactly how to give them. If you have any questions about this, check with your doctor, nurse, or pharmacist.

Storage—To store this medicine:

- Keep out of the reach of children, since overdose may be very dangerous in children.
- Store away from heat and direct light.
- Do not store the capsule or tablet form of this medicine in the bathroom medicine cabinet, near the kitchen sink, or in other damp places. Heat or moisture may cause the medicine to break down.
- Keep the liquid form of this medicine from freezing.
- Do not keep outdated medicine or medicine no longer needed. Be sure that any discarded medicine is out of the reach of children.

Precautions While Using This Medicine

Before you have any skin tests for allergies, tell the doctor in charge that you are taking this medicine. The results of the test may be affected by this medicine.

When taking antihistamines on a regular basis, make sure your doctor knows if you are taking large amounts of aspirin at the same time (as in arthritis or rheumatism). Effects of too much aspirin, such as ringing in the ears, may be covered up by the antihistamine.

Antihistamines will add to the effects of alcohol and other CNS depressants (medicines that slow down the nervous system, possibly causing drowsiness). Some examples of CNS depressants are sedatives, tranquilizers, or sleeping medicine; prescription pain medicine or narcotics; barbiturates; medicine for seizures; muscle relaxants; or anesthetics, including some dental anesthetics. *Check with your doctor before taking any of the above while you are using this medicine.*

This medicine may cause some people to become drowsy or less alert than they are normally. Even if taken at bedtime, it may cause some people to feel drowsy or less alert on arising. Some antihistamines are more likely to cause drowsiness than others (astemizole, loratadine, and terfenadine, for example, rarely produce this effect). *Make sure you know how you react to the antihistamine you are taking before you drive, use machines, or do anything else that could be dangerous if you are not alert.*

Antihistamines may cause dryness of the mouth, nose, and throat. Some antihistamines are more likely to cause dryness of the mouth than others (astemizole, loratadine, and terfenadine, for example, rarely produce this effect). For temporary relief of mouth dryness, use sugarless candy or gum, melt bits of ice in your mouth, or use a saliva substitute. However, if your mouth continues to feel dry for more than 2 weeks, check with your medical doctor or dentist. Continuing dryness of the mouth may increase the chance of dental disease, including tooth decay, gum disease, and fungus infections.

For patients using *dimenhydrinate, diphenhydramine, or hydroxyzine:*

- This medicine controls nausea and vomiting. For this reason, it may cover up the signs of overdose caused by other medicines or the symptoms of appendicitis. This will make it difficult for your doctor to diagnose these conditions. Make sure your doctor knows that you are taking this medicine if you have other symptoms of appendicitis such as stomach or lower abdominal pain, cramping, or soreness. Also, if you think you may have taken an overdose of any medicine, tell your doctor that you are taking this medicine.

For patients using *diphenhydramine or doxylamine as a sleeping aid:*

- If you are already taking a sedative or tranquilizer, do not take this medicine without consulting your doctor first.

Side Effects of This Medicine

Along with its needed effects, a medicine may cause some unwanted effects. Although not all of these side effects may occur, if they do occur they may need medical attention.

Check with your doctor immediately if the following side effect occurs:

Less common or rare—with high doses of astemizole or terfenadine only

Fast or irregular heartbeat

Also, check with your doctor as soon as possible if any of the following side effects occur:

Less common or rare

Sore throat and fever; unusual bleeding or bruising; unusual tiredness or weakness

Symptoms of overdose

Clumsiness or unsteadiness; convulsions (seizures); drowsiness (severe); dryness of mouth, nose, or throat (severe); feeling faint; flushing or redness of face; hallucinations (seeing, hearing, or feeling things that are not there); shortness of breath or troubled breathing; trouble in sleeping

Other side effects may occur that usually do not need medical attention. These side effects may go away during treatment as your body adjusts to the medicine. However, check with your doctor or pharmacist if any of the following side effects continue or are bothersome:

More common—rare with astemizole, loratadine, and terfenadine; less common with cetirizine

Drowsiness; thickening of mucus

Less common or rare

Blurred vision or any change in vision; confusion; difficult or painful urination; dizziness; dryness of mouth, nose, or throat; fast heartbeat; increased sensitivity of skin to sun; increased sweating; loss of appetite (increased appetite with astemizole and cyproheptadine); nightmares; ringing or buzzing in ears; skin rash; stomach upset or stomach pain (more common with pyrilamine and tripelennamine); unusual excitement, nervousness, restlessness, or irritability; weight gain (with astemizole and cyproheptadine only)

Other side effects not listed above may also occur in some patients. If you notice any other effects, check with your doctor or pharmacist.

Additional Information

Once a medicine has been approved for marketing for a certain use, experience may show that it is also useful for other medical problems. Although this use is not included in product labeling, astemizole, cetirizine, loratadine, and terfenadine are used in certain patients with asthma.

Other than the above information, there is no additional information relating to proper use, precautions, or side effects for this use.

Annual revision: 08/21/91
Interim revision(s): 11/08/91; 09/22/92; 04/21/93

ANTIHISTAMINES AND DECONGESTANTS Systemic

Some commonly used brand names are:

In the U.S.—

Actacin[25]
Actagen[25]
Actifed[25]
Actifed 12-Hour[25]
Alamine[11]
Alersule[9]
Allent[6]
Allerest[11]
Allerest 12 Hour[11]
Allerest 12 Hour Caplets[11]
Allerfrin[25]
Allergy Formula Sinutab [18]
Allergy Relief Medicine[11]
Allerphed[25]
Amaril D[13]
Amaril D Spantab[13]
Anamine[14]
Anamine T.D.[14]
Aprodrine[25]
A.R.M. Maximum Strength Caplets[11]
Atrohist Sprinkle[5]
Benadryl Decongestant[19]
Benylin Decongestant[19]
Brexin L.A.[14]
Bromatap[4]
Bromatapp[4]
Bromfed[6]
Bromfed-PD[6]
Bromophen T.D.[3]
Brompheril[18]
Carbiset[7]
Carbodec[7]
Carbodec TR[7]
Cardec-S[7]
Cenafed Plus[25]
Chlorafed[14]
Chlorafed H.S. Timecelles[14]
Chlorafed Timecelles[14]
Chlor-Rest[11]
Chlor-Trimeton Decongestant[14]
Chlor-Trimeton Decongestant Repetabs[14]
Codimal-L.A.[14]
Coltab Children's[9]
Comhist[12]

Comhist LA[12]
Condrin-LA[11]
Conex D.A.[11]
Contac 12-Hour[11]
Contac Maximum Strength 12-Hour Caplets[11]
Cophene No.2[14]
Co-Pyronil 2[14]
Dallergy-D[9 14]
Dallergy Jr.[6]
Decohist[9]
Deconamine[14]
Deconamine SR[14]
Decongestabs[13]
Dehist[11]
Demazin[11]
Demazin Repetabs[11]
Dexaphen SA[18]
Dexophed[18]
Dihistine[9]
Dimaphen S.A.[3]
Dimetane Decongestant[2]
Dimetane Decongestant Caplets[2]
Dimetapp[4]
Dimetapp Extentabs[4]
Disobrom[18]
Disophrol[18]
Disophrol Chronotabs[18]
Dorcol Children's Cold Formula[14]
Drixoral[6 18]
Drize[11]
Duralex[14]
Dura-Tap PD[14]
Dura-Vent/A[11]
Endafed[6]
Fedahist[14]
Fedahist Decongestant[14]
Fedahist Gyrocaps[14]
Fedahist Timecaps[14]
Genac[25]
Genamin[11]
Genatap[4]
Gencold[11]
Histabid Duracaps[11]
Histalet[14]
Histalet Forte[16]
Histamic[13]
Histatab Plus[9]
Histatan[15]
Hista-Vadrin[10]
Histor-D[9]
12-Hour Cold[11]
Isoclor[14]
Isoclor Timesules[14]
Klerist-D[14]
Kronofed-A Jr. Kronocaps[14]
Kronofed-A Kronocaps[14]
Myfed[25]
Myfedrine Plus[14]
Myhistine[9]
Myminic[11]
Myphetapp[4]
Naldecon[13]
Naldecon Pediatric Drops[13]
Naldecon Pediatric Syrup[13]
Naldelate[13]
Naldelate Pediatric Syrup [13]
Nalgest[13]
Napril[14]
Nasahist[10]
ND Clear T.D.[14]
New-Decongest[13]
New-Decongest Pediatric Syrup[13]
Nolamine[8]
Norafed[25]
Noraminic[11]
Normatane[3]
Novafed A[14]
Novahistine[9]
Oragest S.R.[11]
Oraminic Spancaps[11]
Ornade Spansules[11]
Panadyl[23]
PediaCare Cold Formula[14]
Phenergan-D[23]
Phenergan VC[22]
Phentox Compound[13]
Pherazine VC[22]
Poly-Histine-D[20]
Poly-Histine-D Ped[20]
Prometh VC Plain[22]
Promethazine VC[22]
Pseudo-Chlor[14]
Pseudo-gest Plus[14]
Resaid S.R.[11]
Resporal TR[18]
Rhinolar-EX[11]
Rhinolar-EX 12[11]
Rinade B.I.D.[14]
Rondec[7]
Rondec Drops[7]
Rondec-TR[7]
R-Tannate[15]
Ru-Tuss[9]
Ru-Tuss II[11]
Ryna[14]
Rynatan[15]
Seldane-D[24]
Sinucon Pediatric Drops[13]
Snaplets-D[11]
Sudafed Plus[14]
Tamine S.R.[3]
Tavist-D[17]
T-Dry[14]
T-Dry Junior[14]
Triaminic-12[11]
Triaminic Allergy[11]
Triaminic Chewables[11]
Triaminic Cold[11]
Triaminic Oral Infant Drops[21]
Triaminic TR[21]
Trifed[25]
Trinalin Repetabs[1]
Trind[11]
Tri-Nefrin Extra Strength[11]
Triofed[25]
Triotann[15]
Tri-Phen-Chlor[13]
Tri-Phen-Chlor T.D.[13]
Triphenyl[11]
Triphenyl T.D.[21]
Tripodrine[25]
Triposed[25]
Tussanil Plain[9]
Vasominic T.D.[13]
Veltap[3]

In Canada—

Actifed[25]
Benylin Cold[14]
Chlor-Tripolon Decongestant[11 14]
Chlor-Tripolon Decongestant Extra Strength[14]
Chlor-Tripolon Decongestant Repetabs[14]
Corsym[11]
Dimetapp[3]
Dimetapp Extentabs[3]
Dimetapp Oral Infant Drops[3]
Drixoral[18]
Drixtab[18]
Novahistex[14]
Ornade[11]
Ornade-A.F.[11]
Ornade Spansules[11]
Triaminic[11 21]
Triaminic Oral Infant Drops[21]
Trinalin Repetabs[1]

Note: For quick reference the following antihistamine and decongestant combinations are numbered to match the corresponding brand names.

This information applies to the following medicines:

1. Azatadine (a-ZA-ta-deen) and Pseudoephedrine (soo-doe-e-FED-rin)
2. Brompheniramine (brome-fen-EER-a-meen) and Phenylephrine (fen-ill-EF-rin)
3. Brompheniramine, Phenylephrine, and Phenylpropanolamine (fen-ill-proe-pa-NOLE-a-meen)
4. Brompheniramine and Phenylpropanolamine
5. Brompheniramine, Phenyltoloxamine (fen-ill-toe-LOX-a-meen), and Phenylephrine
6. Brompheniramine and Pseudoephedrine
7. Carbinoxamine (kar-bi-NOX-a-meen) and Pseudoephedrine
8. Chlorpheniramine (klor-fen-EER-a-meen), Phenindamine (fen-IN-da-meen), and Phenylpropanolamine
9. Chlorpheniramine and Phenylephrine
10. Chlorpheniramine, Phenylephrine, and Phenylpropanolamine
11. Chlorpheniramine and Phenylpropanolamine
12. Chlorpheniramine, Phenyltoloxamine, and Phenylephrine
13. Chlorpheniramine, Phenyltoloxamine, Phenylephrine, and Phenylpropanolamine
14. Chlorpheniramine and Pseudoephedrine
15. Chlorpheniramine, Pyrilamine (peer-ILL-a-meen), and Phenylephrine
16. Chlorpheniramine, Pyrilamine, Phenylephrine, and Phenylpropanolamine
17. Clemastine (KLEM-as-teen) and Phenylpropanolamine
18. Dexbrompheniramine (dex-brom-fen-EER-a-meen) and Pseudoephedrine
19. Diphenhydramine (dye-fen-HYE-dra-meen) and Pseudoephedrine
20. Pheniramine (fen-EER-a-meen), Phenyltoloxamine, Pyrilamine, and Phenylpropanolamine
21. Pheniramine, Pyrilamine, and Phenylpropanolamine
22. Promethazine (proe-METH-a-zeen) and Phenylephrine
23. Promethazine and Pseudoephedrine
24. Terfenadine (ter-FEN-a-deen) and Pseudoephedrine
25. Triprolidine (trye-PROE-li-deen) and Pseudoephedrine

Description

Antihistamine and decongestant combinations are used to treat the nasal congestion (stuffy nose), sneezing, and runny nose caused by colds and hay fever.

Antihistamines work by preventing the effects of a substance called histamine, which is produced by the body.

Antihistamines contained in these combinations are: brompheniramine, chlorpheniramine, dexbrompheniramine, diphenhydramine, pheniramine, phenyltoloxamine, pyrilamine, terfenadine, and triprolidine.

The decongestants, such as phenylephrine, phenylpropanolamine (also known as PPA), and pseudoephedrine produce a narrowing of blood vessels. This leads to clearing of nasal congestion, but it may also cause an increase in blood pressure in patients who have high blood pressure.

Some of these combinations are available only with your doctor's prescription. Others are available without a prescription; however, your doctor may have special instructions on the proper dose of the medicine for your medical condition. They are available in the following dosage forms:

Oral

Azatadine and Pseudoephedrine
- Extended-release tablets (U.S. and Canada)

Brompheniramine and Phenylephrine
- Elixir (U.S.)
- Tablets (U.S.)

Brompheniramine, Phenylephrine, and Phenylpropanolamine
- Elixir (U.S. and Canada)
- Oral solution (Canada)
- Tablets (Canada)
- Extended-release tablets (U.S. and Canada)

Brompheniramine and Phenylpropanolamine
- Elixir (U.S.)
- Tablets (U.S.)
- Extended-release tablets (U.S.)

Brompheniramine, Phenyltoloxamine, and Phenylephrine
- Extended-release capsules (U.S.)

Brompheniramine and Pseudoephedrine
- Extended-release capsules (U.S.)
- Syrup (U.S.)
- Tablets (U.S.)

Carbinoxamine and Pseudoephedrine
- Oral solution (U.S.)
- Syrup (U.S.)
- Tablets (U.S.)
- Extended-release tablets (U.S.)

Chlorpheniramine, Phenindamine, and Phenylpropanolamine
- Extended-release tablets (U.S.)

Chlorpheniramine and Phenylephrine
- Extended-release capsules (U.S.)
- Elixir (U.S.)
- Syrup (U.S.)
- Tablets (U.S.)
- Chewable tablets (U.S.)

Chlorpheniramine, Phenylephrine, and Phenylpropanolamine
- Extended-release capsules (U.S.)
- Tablets (U.S.)

Chlorpheniramine and Phenylpropanolamine
- Extended-release capsules (U.S. and Canada)
- Granules (U.S.)
- Oral solution (U.S. and Canada)
- Extended-release oral suspension (Canada)
- Syrup (U.S. and Canada)
- Tablets (U.S.)
- Chewable tablets (U.S.)
- Extended-release tablets (U.S.)

Chlorpheniramine, Phenyltoloxamine, and Phenylephrine
- Extended-release capsules (U.S.)
- Tablets (U.S.)

Chlorpheniramine, Phenyltoloxamine, Phenylephrine, and Phenylpropanolamine
- Extended-release capsules (U.S.)
- Oral solution (U.S.)
- Syrup (U.S.)
- Extended-release tablets (U.S.)

Chlorpheniramine and Pseudoephedrine
- Capsules (U.S. and Canada)
- Extended-release capsules (U.S. and Canada)
- Oral solution (U.S.)
- Syrup (U.S.)
- Tablets (U.S. and Canada)
- Extended-release tablets (U.S. and Canada)

Chlorpheniramine, Pyrilamine, and Phenylephrine
- Oral suspension (U.S.)
- Tablets (U.S.)
- Extended-release tablets (U.S.)

Chlorpheniramine, Pyrilamine, Phenylephrine, and Phenylpropanolamine
- Tablets (U.S.)

Clemastine and Phenylpropanolamine
- Extended-release tablets (U.S.)

Dexbrompheniramine and Pseudoephedrine
- Extended-release capsules (Canada)
- Syrup (Canada)
- Tablets (U.S. and Canada)
- Extended-release tablets (U.S. and Canada)

Diphenhydramine and Pseudoephedrine
- Capsules (U.S.)
- Oral solution (U.S.)
- Tablets (U.S.)

Pheniramine, Phenyltoloxamine, Pyrilamine, and Phenylpropanolamine
- Extended-release capsules (U.S.)
- Elixir (U.S.)

Pheniramine, Pyrilamine, and Phenylpropanolamine
- Oral solution (U.S. and Canada)
- Extended-release tablets (U.S. and Canada)

Promethazine and Phenylephrine
- Syrup (U.S.)

Promethazine and Pseudoephedrine
- Tablets (U.S.)

Terfenadine and Pseudoephedrine
- Extended-release tablets (U.S.)

Triprolidine and Pseudoephedrine
- Capsules (U.S.)
- Extended-release capsules (U.S.)
- Syrup (U.S. and Canada)
- Tablets (U.S. and Canada)

It is very important that you read and understand the following information. If any of it causes you special concern, check with your doctor or pharmacist. Also, *if you have any questions* or if you want more information about this medicine or your medical problem, *ask your doctor, nurse, or pharmacist.*

Before Using This Medicine

If you are taking this medicine without a prescription, carefully read and follow any precautions on the label. For antihistamine and decongestant combinations, the following should be considered:

Allergies—Tell your doctor if you have ever had any unusual or allergic reaction to antihistamines or to amphetamine, dextroamphetamine (e.g., Dexedrine), ephedrine (e.g., Ephed II), epinephrine (e.g., Adrenalin), isoproterenol (e.g., Isuprel), metaproterenol (e.g., Alupent), methamphetamine (e.g., Desoxyn), norepinephrine (e.g., Levophed), phenylephrine (e.g., Neo-Synephrine), pseudoephedrine (e.g., Sudafed), PPA (e.g., Dexatrim), or terbutaline (e.g., Brethine).

Pregnancy—The occasional use of antihistamine and decongestant combinations is not likely to cause problems in the fetus or in the newborn baby. However, when these medicines are used at higher doses and/or for a long time, the chance that problems might occur may increase. For the individual ingredients of these combinations, the following apply:

- *Alcohol*—Some of these combination medicines contain alcohol. Too much use of alcohol during pregnancy may cause birth defects.
- *Antihistamines*—Antihistamines have not been shown to cause problems in humans.
- *Phenylephrine*—Studies on birth defects have not been done in either humans or animals with phenylephrine.
- *Phenylpropanolamine*—Studies on birth defects have not been done in either humans or animals with phenylpropanolamine. However, it seems that women who take phenylpropanolamine in the weeks following delivery are more likely to suffer mental or mood changes.
- *Pseudoephedrine*—Studies on birth defects with pseudoephedrine have not been done in humans. In animal studies pseudoephedrine did not cause birth defects but did cause a decrease in average weight, length, and rate of bone formation in the animal fetus when administered in high doses.
- *Promethazine*—Phenothiazines, such as promethazine (contained in some of these combination medicines [e.g., Phenergan-D]), have been shown to cause jaundice and muscle tremors in a few newborn infants whose mothers received phenothiazines during pregnancy. Also, the newborn baby may have blood clotting problems if promethazine is taken by the mother within 2 weeks before delivery.

Breast-feeding—Small amounts of antihistamines and decongestants pass into the breast milk. Use is not recommended since the chances are greater for this medicine to cause side effects, such as unusual excitement or irritability, in the nursing baby. Also, since antihistamines tend to decrease the secretions of the body, it is possible that the flow of breast milk may be reduced in some patients. It is not known yet whether terfenadine causes these same side effects.

Children—Very young children are usually more sensitive to the effects of this medicine. Increases in blood pressure, nightmares or unusual excitement, nervousness, restlessness, or irritability may be more likely to occur in children. Also, mental changes may be more likely to occur in young children taking combination medicines that contain phenylpropanolamine. *Before giving any of these combination medicines to a child, check the package label very carefully. Some of these medicines are too strong for use in children.* If you are not certain whether a specific product can be given to a child, or if you have any questions about the amount to give, check with your doctor, nurse, or pharmacist.

Older adults—Confusion, difficult and painful urination, dizziness, drowsiness, dryness of mouth, or convulsions (seizures) may be more likely to occur in the elderly, who are usually more sensitive to the effects of this medicine. Also, nightmares or unusual excitement, nervousness, restlessness, or irritability may be more likely to occur in elderly patients.

Other medicines—Although certain medicines should not be used together at all, in other cases different medicines may be used together even if an interaction might occur. In these cases, your doctor may want to change the dose, or other precautions may be necessary. When you are taking antihistamines it is especially important that your doctor and pharmacist know if you are taking any of the following:

- Anticholinergics (medicine for abdominal or stomach spasms or cramps)—Side effects, such as dryness of mouth, of antihistamines or anticholinergics may be more likely to occur
- Central nervous system (CNS) depressants—Effects, such as drowsiness, of CNS depressants or antihistamines may be worsened
- Erythromycin (e.g., E-Mycin) or
- Ketoconazole (e.g., Nizoral)—Use of these medicines with the terfenadine-containing combination may cause heart problems, such as an irregular heartbeat; these medicines should not be used together
- Monoamine oxidase (MAO) inhibitors (furazolidone [e.g., Furoxone], isocarboxazid [e.g., Marplan], phenelzine [e.g., Nardil], procarbazine [e.g., Matulane], selegiline [e.g., Eldepryl], tranylcypromine [e.g., Parnate])—If you are now taking, or have taken within the past 2 weeks, any of the MAO inhibitors, the side effects of the antihistamines may become more severe; these medicines should not be used together
- Rauwolfia alkaloids (alseroxylon [e.g., Rauwiloid], deserpidine [e.g., Harmonyl], rauwolfia serpentina [e.g., Raudixin], reserpine [e.g., Serpasil])—These medicines may increase or decrease the effect of the decongestant

- Tricyclic antidepressants (amitriptyline [e.g., Elavil], amoxapine [e.g., Asendin], clomipramine [e.g., Anafranil], desipramine [e.g., Pertofrane], doxepin [e.g., Sinequan], imipramine [e.g., Tofranil], maprotiline [e.g., Ludiomil], nortriptyline [e.g., Aventyl], protriptyline [e.g., Vivactil], trimipramine [e.g., Surmontil])—Effects, such as drowsiness, of CNS depressants or antihistamines may be worsened; also, taking these medicines together may cause some of their side effects, such as dryness of mouth, to become more severe

Also, if you are taking one of the combinations containing phenylpropanolamine or pseudoephedrine and are also taking:

- Amantadine (e.g., Symmetrel) or
- Amphetamines or
- Appetite suppressants (diet pills), except fenfluramine (e.g., Pondimin) or
- Beta-blockers (acebutolol [e.g., Sectral], atenolol [e.g., Tenormin], carteolol [e.g., Cartrol], labetalol [e.g., Normodyne], metoprolol [e.g., Lopressor], nadolol [e.g., Corgard], oxprenolol [e.g., Trasicor], penbutolol [e.g., Levatol], pindolol [e.g., Visken], propanolol [e.g., Inderal], sotalol [e.g., Sotacor], timolol [e.g., Blocadren]) or
- Caffeine (e.g., NoDoz) or
- Chlophedianol (e.g., Ulo) or
- Medicine for asthma or other breathing problems or
- Medicine for colds, sinus problems, or hay fever or other allergies (including nose drops or sprays) or
- Methylphenidate (e.g., Ritalin) or
- Pemoline (e.g., Cylert)—Using any of these medicines together with an antihistamine and decongestant combination may cause excessive stimulant side effects, such as difficulty in sleeping, heart rate problems, nervousness, and irritability

Other medical problems—The presence of other medical problems may affect the use of antihistamine and decongestant combinations. Make sure you tell your doctor if you have any other medical problems, especially:

- Diabetes mellitus (sugar diabetes)—The decongestant in this medicine may put diabetic patients at a greater risk of having heart or blood vessel disease
- Enlarged prostate or
- Urinary tract blockage or difficult urination—Some of the effects of antihistamines may make urinary problems worse
- Glaucoma—A slight increase in inner eye pressure may occur
- Heart or blood vessel disease or
- High blood pressure—The decongestant in this medicine may cause the blood pressure to increase and may also speed up the heart rate
- Liver disease—Higher blood levels of terfenadine may result, which may increase the chance of heart problems (for terfenadine-containing combination only)
- Overactive thyroid—If the overactive thyroid has caused a fast heart rate, the decongestant in this medicine may cause the heart rate to speed up further

Before you begin using any new medicine (prescription or nonprescription) or if you develop any new medical problem while you are using this medicine, check with your doctor, nurse, or pharmacist.

Proper Use of This Medicine

Take this medicine only as directed. Do not take more of it and do not take it more often than recommended on the label, unless otherwise directed by your doctor. To do so may increase the chance of side effects.

If this medicine irritates your stomach, you may take it with food or a glass of water or milk, to lessen the irritation.

For patients *taking the extended-release capsule or tablet form of this medicine:*

- Swallow it whole.
- Do not crush, break, or chew before swallowing.
- If the capsule is too large to swallow, you may mix the contents of the capsule with applesauce, jelly, honey, or syrup and swallow without chewing.

Missed dose—If you are taking this medicine regularly and you miss a dose, take it as soon as possible. However, if it is almost time for your next dose, skip the missed dose and go back to your regular dosing schedule. Do not double doses.

Storage—To store this medicine:

- Keep out of the reach of children.
- Store away from heat and direct light.
- Do not store in the bathroom, near the kitchen sink, or in other damp places. Heat or moisture may cause the medicine to break down.
- Keep the liquid form of this medicine from freezing.
- Do not keep outdated medicine or medicine no longer needed. Be sure that any discarded medicine is out of the reach of children.

Precautions While Using This Medicine

Before you have any skin tests for allergies, tell the doctor in charge that you are taking this medicine. The results of the test may be affected by the antihistamine in this medicine.

When taking antihistamines (contained in this combination medicine) on a regular basis, make sure your doctor knows if you are taking large amounts of aspirin at the same time (as in arthritis or rheumatism). Effects of too much aspirin, such as ringing in the ears, may be covered up by the antihistamine.

The antihistamine in this medicine will add to the effects of alcohol and other CNS depressants (medicines that slow down the nervous system, possibly causing drowsiness). Some examples of CNS depressants are other antihistamines or medicine for hay fever, other allergies, or colds; sedatives, tranquilizers, or sleeping medicine; prescription pain medicine or narcotics; barbiturates; medicine for seizures; muscle relaxants; or anesthetics, including some dental anesthetics. *Check with your doctor before taking any of the above while you are taking this medicine.*

The antihistamine in this medicine may cause some people to become drowsy, dizzy, or less alert than they are normally. *Some antihistamines are more likely to cause drowsiness than others (terfenadine, for example, rarely produces this effect). Make sure you know how you react before you drive, use machines, or do anything else that could be dangerous if you are dizzy or are not alert.*

The decongestant in this medicine may add to the central nervous system (CNS) stimulant and other effects of phenylpropanolamine (PPA)-containing diet aids. *Do not use medicines for diet or appetite control while taking this medicine unless you have checked with your doctor.*

The decongestant in this medicine may cause some people to be nervous or restless or to have trouble in sleeping. If you have trouble in sleeping, *take the last dose of this medicine for each day a few hours before bedtime.* If you have any questions about this, check with your doctor.

Antihistamines may cause dryness of the mouth, nose, and throat. Some antihistamines are more likely to cause dryness of the mouth than others (terfenadine, for example, rarely produces this effect). For temporary relief, use sugarless candy or gum, melt bits of ice in your mouth, or use a saliva substitute. However, if your mouth continues to feel dry for more than 2 weeks, check with your dentist. Continuing dryness of the mouth may increase the chance of dental disease, including tooth decay, gum disease, and fungus infections.

For patients *using promethazine-containing medicine:*

- This medicine controls nausea and vomiting. For this reason, it may cover up the signs of overdose caused by other medicines or the symptoms of intestinal blockage. This will make it difficult for your doctor to diagnose these conditions. Make sure your doctor knows that you are taking this medicine if you have other symptoms such as stomach or lower abdominal pain, cramping, or soreness. Also, if you think you may have taken an overdose of any medicine, tell your doctor that you are taking this medicine.

Side Effects of This Medicine

Along with its needed effects, a medicine may cause some unwanted effects. Although serious side effects occur rarely when this medicine is taken as recommended, they may be more likely to occur if:

- too much medicine is taken.
- it is taken in large doses.
- it is taken for a long period of time.

Get emergency help immediately if any of the following symptoms of overdose occur:

Clumsiness or unsteadiness; convulsions (seizures); drowsiness (severe); dryness of mouth, nose, or throat (severe); flushing or redness of face; hallucinations (seeing, hearing, or feeling things that are not there); headache (continuing); shortness of breath or troubled breathing; slow, fast, or irregular heartbeat; trouble in sleeping

For promethazine only

Muscle spasms (especially of neck and back); restlessness; shuffling walk; tic-like (jerky) movements of head and face; trembling and shaking of hands

Also, check with your doctor as soon as possible if any of the following side effects occur:

Rare

Mood or mental changes; sore throat and fever; tightness in chest; unusual bleeding or bruising; unusual tiredness or weakness

Other side effects may occur that usually do not need medical attention. These side effects may go away during treatment as your body adjusts to the medicine. However, check with your doctor or pharmacist if any of the following side effects continue or are bothersome:

More common—rare with terfenadine-containing combination

Drowsiness; thickening of the bronchial secretions

Less common—more common with high doses

Blurred vision; confusion; difficult or painful urination; dizziness; dryness of mouth, nose, or throat; headache; loss of appetite; nightmares; pounding heartbeat; ringing or buzzing in ears; skin rash; stomach upset or pain (more common with pyrilamine and tripelennamine); unusual excitement, nervousness, restlessness, or irritability

Other side effects not listed above may also occur in some patients. If you notice any other effects, check with your doctor.

Annual revision: 08/01/92
Interim revision: 09/22/92

ANTIHISTAMINES, DECONGESTANTS, AND ANALGESICS Systemic

This information applies to the following medicines:

Brompheniramine (brom-fen-EER-a-meen), Phenylephrine (fen-ill-ef-rin), Phenylpropanolamine (fen-ill-proe-pa-nole-a-meen), and Acetaminophen (a-seat-a-min-oh-fen)
Brompheniramine, Phenylpropanolamine, and Acetaminophen
Brompheniramine, Phenylpropanolamine, and Aspirin (AS-pir-in)
Chlorpheniramine (klor-fen-EER-a-meen), Phenylephrine, and Acetaminophen†
Chlorpheniramine, Phenylephrine, Acetaminophen, and Caffeine (kaf-EEN)
Chlorpheniramine, Phenylephrine, Acetaminophen, and Salicylamide (sal-i-sill-a-mide)
Chlorpheniramine, Phenylephrine, Acetaminophen, Salicylamide, and Caffeine
Chlorpheniramine, Phenylpropanolamine, and Acetaminophen
Chlorpheniramine, Phenylpropanolamine, Acetaminophen, and Caffeine
Chlorpheniramine, Phenylpropanolamine, and Aspirin
Chlorpheniramine, Phenylpropanolamine, Aspirin, and Caffeine
Chlorpheniramine, Phenyltoloxamine (fen-ill-tole-OX-a-meen), Phenylpropanolamine, and Acetaminophen
Chlorpheniramine, Pseudoephedrine (soo-doe-e-FED-rin), and Acetaminophen
Chlorpheniramine, Pyrilamine (peer-ILL-a-meen), Phenylephrine, and Acetaminophen
Chlorpheniramine, Pyrilamine, Phenylephrine, Phenylpropanolamine, and Acetaminophen
Dexbrompheniramine (dex-brome-fen-EER-a-meen), Pseudoephedrine, and Acetaminophen
Diphenhydramine (dye-fen-HYE-dra-meen), Phenylpropanolamine, and Aspirin
Diphenhydramine, Pseudoephedrine, and Acetaminophen
Pheniramine (fen-EER-a-meen), Phenylephrine, Sodium Salicylate (SOE-dee-um sa-LI-si-late), and Caffeine
Pheniramine, Pyrilamine, Phenylpropanolamine, and Aspirin
Phenyltoloxamine, Phenylpropanolamine, and Acetaminophen
Pyrilamine, Phenylephrine, Aspirin, and Caffeine
Pyrilamine, Phenylpropanolamine, Acetaminophen, and Caffeine
Triprolidine (trye-PROE-li-deen), Pseudoephedrine, and Acetaminophen

Some commonly used brand names are:

For Brompheniramine, Phenylephrine, Phenylpropanolamine, and Acetaminophen*
In Canada
Dimetapp-A
Dimetapp-A Pediatric

For Brompheniramine, Phenylpropanolamine, and Acetaminophen†
In the U.S.
Dimetapp Plus Caplets

For Brompheniramine, Phenylpropanolamine, and Aspirin†
In the U.S.
Alka-Seltzer Plus Maximum Strength Sinus Allergy Medicine

For Chlorpheniramine, Phenylephrine, and Acetaminophen†
In the U.S.
Aclophen
Advanced Formula Dristan
Advanced Formula Dristan Caplets
Histagesic Modified

For Chlorpheniramine, Phenylephrine, Acetaminophen, and Caffeine†
In the U.S.
Dristan-AF
Korigesic
In Canada
Dristan-AF Plus

For Chlorpheniramine, Phenylephrine, Acetaminophen, and Salicylamide†
In the U.S.
Rhinogesic
Salphenyl

For Chlorpheniramine, Phenylephrine, Acetaminophen, Salicylamide, and Caffeine†
In the U.S.
Kolephrin

For Chlorpheniramine, Phenylpropanolamine, and Acetaminophen
In the U.S.
Allerest Headache Strength
Allerest Sinus Pain Formula
Alumadrine
BQ Cold
Chlor-Trimeton Sinus Caplets
Conex Plus
Coricidin 'D' Decongestant
Coricidin Demilets
Coricidin Maximum Strength Sinus Headache
Dapacin Cold
Duadacin
Extreme Cold Formula Caplets
Phenate T.D.
Pyrroxate
Remcol Cold
Sinarest
Sinarest Extra Strength
Sinulin
Triaminicin
Tylenol Cold Medication
4-Way Cold
In Canada
Coricidin 'D' Medilets

For Chlorpheniramine, Phenylpropanolamine, Acetaminophen, and Caffeine†
In the U.S.
Sinapils

For Chlorpheniramine, Phenylpropanolamine, and Aspirin
In the U.S.
Alka-Seltzer Plus Cold
Sine-Off Sinus Medicine
In Canada
Coricidin 'D'

For Chlorpheniramine, Phenylpropanolamine, Aspirin, and Caffeine*
In Canada
Dristan

For Chlorpheniramine, Phenyltoloxamine, Phenylpropanolamine, and Acetaminophen†
In the U.S.
Norel Plus

For Chlorpheniramine, Pseudoephedrine, and Acetaminophen
In the U.S.
Children's Tylenol Cold
Codimal
Comtrex A/S
Comtrex A/S Caplets
Maximum Strength Tylenol Allergy Sinus Caplets
Phenapap Sinus Headache & Congestion
Sine-Off Maximum Strength Allergy/Sinus Formula Caplets
Singlet
Sinutab
Sinutab Maximum Strength
TheraFlu/Flu and Cold Medicine
Thera-Hist
Tricom Caplets
In Canada
Sinutab Extra Strength
Sinutab Regular

For Chlorpheniramine, Pyrilamine, Phenylephrine, and Acetaminophen
In the U.S.
ND-Gesic

For Chlorpheniramine, Pyrilamine, Phenylephrine, Phenylpropanolamine, and Acetaminophen†
In the U.S.
Covangesic

For Dexbrompheniramine, Pseudoephedrine, and Acetaminophen†
In the U.S.
Drixoral Plus

For Diphenhydramine, Phenylpropanolamine, and Aspirin†
In the U.S.
Alka-Seltzer Plus Nighttime Cold

For Diphenhydramine, Pseudoephedrine, and Acetaminophen†
In the U.S.
Benadryl Plus
Benadryl Plus Nighttime Liquid

For Pheniramine, Phenylephrine, Sodium Salicylate, and Caffeine†
In the U.S.
Scot-tussin Original 5-Action Cold Medicine

For Pheniramine, Pyrilamine, Phenylpropanolamine, and Aspirin†
In the U.S.
Fiogesic

For Phenyltoloxamine, Phenylpropanolamine, and Acetaminophen
In the U.S.
Sinubid
In Canada
Sinutab SA

For Pyrilamine, Phenylephrine, Aspirin, and Caffeine*
In Canada
Dristan Formula P

For Pyrilamine, Phenylpropanolamine, Acetaminophen, and Caffeine†
In the U.S.
Histosal

For Triprolidine, Pseudoephedrine, and Acetaminophen
In the U.S.
Actifed Plus
Actifed Plus Caplets
In Canada
Actifed-A

---

*Not commercially available in the U.S.
†Not commercially available in Canada.

Description

Antihistamine, decongestant, and analgesic combinations are taken by mouth to relieve the sneezing, runny nose, sinus and nasal congestion (stuffy nose), fever, headache, and aches and pain, of colds, influenza, and hay fever. These combinations do not contain any ingredient to relieve coughs.

Antihistamines are used to relieve or prevent the symptoms of hay fever and other types of allergy. They may also help relieve some symptoms of the common cold, such as sneezing and runny nose. They work by preventing the effects of a substance called histamine, which is produced by the body. Antihistamines contained in these combinations are: brompheniramine, chlorpheniramine, dexbrompheniramine, diphenydramine, pheniramine, phenyltoloxamine, pyrilamine, and triprolidine.

Decongestants, such as phenylephrine, phenylpropanolamine (also known as PPA), and pseudoephedrine produce a narrowing of blood vessels. This leads to clearing of nasal congestion, but it may also cause an increase in blood pressure in patients who have high blood pressure.

Analgesics, such as acetaminophen and salicylates (e.g., aspirin, salicylamide, sodium salicylate), are used in these combination medicines to help relieve fever, headache, aches, and pain.

Some of these medicines are available without a prescription. However, your doctor may have special instructions on the proper dose of these medicines for your medical condition. They are available in the following dosage forms:

Oral

Brompheniramine, Phenylephrine, Phenylpropanolamine, and Acetaminophen
- Oral solution (Canada)
- Tablets (Canada)

Brompheniramine, Phenylpropanolamine, and Acetaminophen
- Tablets (U.S.)

Brompheniramine, Phenylpropanolamine, and Aspirin
- Effervescent tablets (U.S.)

Chlorpheniramine, Phenylephrine, and Acetaminophen
- Tablets (U.S.)

Chlorpheniramine, Phenylephrine, Acetaminophen, and Caffeine
- Tablets (U.S. and Canada)

Chlorpheniramine, Phenylephrine, Acetaminophen, and Salicylamide
- Capsules (U.S.)
- Tablets (U.S.)

Chlorpheniramine, Phenylephrine, Acetaminophen, Salicylamide, and Caffeine
- Capsules (U.S.)

Chlorpheniramine, Phenylpropanolamine, and Acetaminophen
- Capsules (U.S.)
- Tablets (U.S.)
- Chewable tablets (U.S. and Canada)
- Effervescent tablets (U.S.)
- Extended-release tablets (U.S.)

Chlorpheniramine, Phenylpropanolamine, Acetaminophen, and Caffeine
- Tablets (U.S.)

Chlorpheniramine, Phenylpropanolamine, and Aspirin
- Oral solution (U.S.)
- Tablets (U.S. and Canada)

Chlorpheniramine, Phenylpropanolamine, Aspirin, and Caffeine
- Capsules (Canada)
- Tablets (Canada)

Chlorpheniramine, Phenyltoloxamine, Phenylpropanolamine, and Acetaminophen
- Capsules (U.S.)

Chlorpheniramine, Pseudoephedrine, and Acetaminophen
- Capsules (U.S. and Canada)
- For oral solution (U.S.)
- Oral solution (U.S.)

• Chewable tablets (U.S.)
• Tablets (U.S. and Canada)

Chlorpheniramine, Pyrilamine, Phenylephrine, and Acetaminophen
• Tablets (U.S.)

Chlorpheniramine, Pyrilamine, Phenylephrine, Phenylpropanolamine, and Acetaminophen
• Tablets (U.S.)

Dexbrompheniramine, Pseudoephedrine, and Acetaminophen
• Extended-release tablets (U.S.)

Diphenhydramine, Phenylpropanolamine, and Aspirin
• Oral solution (U.S.)

Diphenhydramine, Pseudoephedrine, and Acetaminophen
• Oral solution (U.S.)
• Tablets (U.S.)

Pheniramine, Phenylephrine, Sodium Salicylate, and Caffeine
• Oral solution (U.S.)

Pheniramine, Pyrilamine, Phenylpropanolamine, and Aspirin
• Tablets (U.S.)

Phenyltoloxamine, Phenylpropanolamine, and Acetaminophen
• Extended-release tablets (U.S. and Canada)

Pyrilamine, Phenylephrine, Aspirin, and Caffeine
• Tablets (Canada)

Pyrilamine, Phenylpropanolamine, Acetaminophen, and Caffeine
• Tablets (U.S.)

Triprolidine, Pseudoephedrine, and Acetaminophen
• Tablets (U.S. and Canada)

It is very important that you read and understand the following information. If any of it causes you special concern, check with your doctor or pharmacist. Also, *if you have any questions* or if you want more information about this medicine or your medical problem, *ask your doctor, nurse, or pharmacist.*

Before Using This Medicine

If you are taking this medicine without a prescription, carefully read and follow any precautions on the label. For antihistamine, decongestant, and analgesic combinations the following should be considered:

Allergies—Tell your doctor if you have ever had any unusual or allergic reaction to any of the ingredients contained in this medicine. If this medicine contains *aspirin* or *another salicylate*, before taking it, check with your doctor if you have ever had any unusual or allergic reaction to any of the following medicines:

Diclofenac (e.g., Voltaren)
Diflunisal (e.g., Dolobid)
Fenoprofen (e.g., Nalfon)
Floctafenine
Flurbiprofen, by mouth (e.g., Ansaid)
Ibuprofen (e.g., Motrin)
Indomethacin (e.g., Indocin)
Ketoprofen (e.g., Orudis)
Meclofenamate (e.g., Meclomen)
Mefenamic acid (e.g., Ponstel)
Methyl salicylate (oil of wintergreen)
Naproxen (e.g., Naprosyn)
Oxyphenbutazone (e.g., Tandearil)
Phenylbutazone (e.g., Butazolidin)
Piroxicam (e.g., Feldene)
Sulindac (e.g., Clinoril)
Suprofen (e.g., Suprol)
Tiaprofenic acid (e.g., Surgam)
Tolmetin (e.g., Tolectin)
Zomepirac (e.g., Zomax).

Also tell your doctor and pharmacist if you are allergic to any other substances, such as foods, preservatives, or dyes.

Pregnancy—The occasional use of antihistamine, decongestant, and analgesic combinations is not likely to cause problems in the fetus or in the newborn baby. However, when these medicines are used at higher doses and/or for a long time, the chance that problems might occur may increase. For the individual ingredients of these combinations, the following apply:

- *Acetaminophen*—Acetaminophen has not been shown to cause birth defects or other problems in humans. However, studies on birth defects have not been done in humans.
- *Alcohol*—Some of these combination medicines contain large amounts of alcohol. Too much use of alcohol during pregnancy may cause birth defects.
- *Antihistamines*—Antihistamines have not been shown to cause problems in humans.
- *Caffeine*—Studies in humans have not shown that caffeine causes birth defects. However, studies in animals have shown that caffeine causes birth defects when given in very large doses (amounts equal to the amount of caffeine contained in 12 to 24 cups of coffee a day).
- *Phenylephrine*—Studies on birth defects have not been done in either humans or animals with phenylephrine.
- *Phenylpropanolamine*—Studies on birth defects have not been done in either humans or animals with phenylpropanolamine. However, it seems that women who take phenylpropanolamine in the weeks following delivery are more likely to suffer mental or mood changes.
- *Pseudoephedrine*—Studies on birth defects with pseudoephedrine have not been done in humans. In animal studies pseudoephedrine did not cause birth defects but did cause a decrease in average weight, length, and rate of bone formation in the animal fetus when administered in high doses.
- *Salicylates (e.g., aspirin)*—Salicylates have not been shown to cause birth defects in humans. Studies on birth defects in humans have been done with aspirin, but not with salicylamide. However, salicylates have been shown to cause birth defects in animals.

Regular use of salicylates late in pregnancy may cause unwanted effects on the heart or blood flow in the fetus or newborn baby. Use of salicylates during the last 2 weeks of pregnancy may cause bleeding problems in the fetus before or during delivery, or in the newborn baby. Also, too much use of salicylates during the last 3 months of pregnancy may increase the length of pregnancy, prolong labor, cause other problems during delivery, or cause severe bleeding in the mother before, during, or after delivery. *Do not take aspirin during the last 3 months of pregnancy unless it has been ordered by your doctor.*

Breast-feeding—If you are breast-feeding the chance that problems might occur depends on the ingredients of the combination. For the individual ingredients of these combinations, the following apply:

- *Acetaminophen*—Acetaminophen passes into the breast milk. However, it has not been shown to cause problems in nursing babies.
- *Alcohol*—Alcohol passes into the breast milk. However, the amount of alcohol in recommended doses of this medicine does not usually cause problems in nursing babies.
- *Antihistamines*—Use is not recommended since the chances are greater for this medicine to cause side effects, such as unusual excitement or irritability, in the nursing baby. Also, since antihistamines tend to decrease the secretions of the body, it is possible that the flow of breast milk may be reduced in some women.
- *Caffeine*—Small amounts of caffeine pass into the breast milk and may build up in the nursing baby. However, the amount of caffeine in recommended doses of this medicine does not usually cause problems in nursing babies.
- *Decongestants (e.g., phenylephrine, phenylpropanolamine, pseudoephedrine)*—Phenylephrine and phenylpropanolamine have not been shown to cause problems in nursing babies. Pseudoephedrine passes into the breast milk and may cause unwanted effects in nursing babies (especially newborn and premature babies) of mothers taking this medicine.
- *Salicylates (e.g., aspirin, salicylamide, sodium salicylate)*—Salicylates pass into the breast milk. Although salicylates have not been reported to cause problems in nursing babies, it is possible that problems may occur if large amounts are taken regularly.

Children—Very young children are usually more sensitive to the effects of this medicine. Increases in blood pressure, nightmares, unusual excitement, nervousness, restlessness, or irritability may be more likely to occur in children. Also, mental changes may be more likely to occur in young children taking these combination medicines.

Before giving any of these combination medicines to a child, check the package label very carefully. Some of these medicines are too strong for use in children. If you are not certain whether a specific product can be given to a child, or if you have any questions about the amount to give, check with your doctor or pharmacist.

Do not give aspirin or other salicylates to a child with a fever or other symptoms of a virus infection, especially flu or chickenpox, without first discussing its use with your child's doctor. This is very important because salicylates may cause a serious illness called Reye's syndrome in children with fever caused by a virus infection, especially flu or chickenpox. Also, children may be more sensitive to the aspirin or other salicylates contained in some of these medicines, especially if they have a fever or have lost large amounts of body fluid because of vomiting, diarrhea, or sweating.

Teenagers—*Do not give aspirin or other salicylates to a teenager with a fever or other symptoms of a virus infection, especially flu or chickenpox, without first discussing its use with your child's doctor.* This is very important because salicylates may cause a serious illness called Reye's syndrome in teenagers with fever caused by a virus infection, especially flu or chickenpox.

Older adults—The elderly are usually more sensitive to the effects of this medicine. Confusion, difficult or painful urination, dizziness, drowsiness, feeling faint, or dryness of mouth, nose, or throat may be more likely to occur in elderly patients. Also, nightmares or unusual excitement, nervousness, restlessness, or irritability may be more likely to occur in the elderly.

Other medicines—Although certain medicines should not be used together at all, in other cases two different medicines may be used together even if an interaction might occur. In these cases, your doctor may want to change the dose, or other precautions may be necessary. When you are taking antihistamine, decongestant, and analgesic combinations it is especially important that your doctor and pharmacist know if you are taking *any* other prescription or nonprescription (over-the-counter [OTC]) medicine, for example, aspirin or other medicine for allergies. Some medicines may change the way this medicine affects your body. Also, the effect of other medicines may be increased or reduced by some of the ingredients in this medicine.

Other medical problems—The presence of other medical problems may affect the use of antihistamine, decongestant, and analgesic combinations. Make sure you tell your doctor if you have any other medical problems, especially:

- Alcohol abuse—Acetaminophen-containing medicines increase the chance of liver damage
- Anemia—Taking a salicylate-containing medicine may make the anemia worse

- Asthma, allergies, and nasal polyps, history of, or
- Asthma attacks—Taking a salicylate-containing medicine may cause an allergic reaction in which breathing becomes difficult; also, although antihistamines open tightened bronchial passages, other effects of the antihistamines may cause secretions to become thick so that during an asthma attack it might be difficult to cough them up
- Diabetes mellitus (sugar diabetes)—The decongestant in this medicine may put the patient with diabetes at a greater risk of having heart or blood vessel disease
- Enlarged prostate or
- Urinary tract blockage or difficult urination—Some of the effects of antihistamines may cause urinary problems to get worse
- Glaucoma—A slight increase in inner eye pressure may occur
- Gout—Aspirin- or sodium salicylate–containing medicine may make the gout worse and reduce the benefit of the medicines used for gout
- Hemophilia or other bleeding problems—Aspirin- or sodium salicylate–containing medicine increase the chance of bleeding
- Hepatitis or other liver disease—There is a greater chance of side effects because the medicine is not broken down and may build up in the body; also, if liver disease is severe there is a greater chance that aspirin-containing medicine may cause bleeding
- Heart or blood vessel disease or
- High blood pressure—The decongestant in this medicine may cause the blood pressure to increase and may also speed up the heart rate; also, caffeine-containing medicine, if taken in large amounts may have a similar effect on the heart
- Kidney disease (severe)—The kidneys may be affected, especially if too much of this medicine is taken for a long time
- Overactive thyroid—If the overactive thyroid has caused a fast heart rate, the decongestant in this medicine may cause the heart rate to speed up further
- Stomach ulcer or other stomach problems—Salicylate-containing medicine may make the ulcer worse or cause bleeding of the stomach

Proper Use of This Medicine

Take this medicine only as directed. Do not take more of it and do not take it more often than recommended on the label, unless otherwise directed by your doctor. To do so may increase the chance of side effects.

If this medicine irritates your stomach, you may take it with food or a glass of water or milk, to lessen the irritation.

For patients taking the extended-release tablet form of this medicine:

- Swallow the tablets whole.
- Do not crush, break, or chew before swallowing.

If a combination medicine containing aspirin has a strong vinegar-like odor, do not use it. This odor means the medicine is breaking down. If you have any questions about this, check with your pharmacist.

Missed dose—If you must take this medicine regularly and you miss a dose, take it as soon as possible. However, if it is almost time for your next dose, skip the missed dose and go back to your regular dosing schedule. Do not double doses.

Storage—To store this medicine:

- Keep this medicine out of the reach of children. Overdose is very dangerous in young children.
- Store away from heat and direct light.
- Do not store the capsule or tablet form of this medicine in the bathroom, near the kitchen sink, or in other damp places. Heat or moisture may cause the medicine to break down.
- Keep the liquid form of this medicine from freezing.
- Do not keep outdated medicine or medicine no longer needed. Be sure that any discarded medicine is out of the reach of children.

Precautions While Using This Medicine

Before you have any skin tests for allergies, tell the doctor in charge that you are taking this medicine. The results of the test may be affected by the antihistamine in this medicine.

Check with your doctor if your symptoms do not improve or become worse, or if you have a high fever.

The antihistamine in this medicine will add to the effects of alcohol and other CNS depressants (medicines that slow down the nervous system, possibly causing drowsiness). Some examples of CNS depressants are other antihistamines or medicine for hay fever, other allergies, or colds; sedatives, tranquilizers, or sleeping medicine; prescription pain medicine or narcotics; barbiturates; medicine for seizures; muscle relaxants; or anesthetics, including some dental anesthetics. *Check with your doctor before taking any of the above while you are taking this medicine.*

Also, stomach problems may be more likely to occur if you drink alcoholic beverages while taking a medicine that contains aspirin. In addition, drinking large amounts of alcoholic beverages while taking a medicine that contains acetaminophen may cause liver damage.

The antihistamine in this medicine may cause some people to become drowsy, dizzy, or less alert than they are normally. *Make sure you know how you react before you drive, use machines, or do anything else that could be dangerous if you are dizzy or are not alert.*

The decongestant in this medicine may cause some people to become nervous or restless or to have trouble in sleeping. If you have trouble in sleeping, *take the last dose of this medicine for each day a few hours before bedtime.* If you have any questions about this, check with your doctor.

Also, this medicine may add to the central nervous system (CNS) stimulant and other effects of phenylpropanolamine (PPA)-containing diet aids. *Do not use medicines for diet or appetite control while taking this medicine unless you have checked with your doctor.*

Before having any kind of surgery (including dental surgery) or emergency treatment, tell the medical doctor or dentist in charge that you are taking this medicine.

Antihistamines may cause dryness of the mouth, nose, and throat. For temporary relief of mouth dryness, use sugarless candy or gum, melt bits of ice in your mouth, or use a saliva substitute. However, if your mouth continues to feel dry for more than 2 weeks, check with your dentist. Continuing dryness of the mouth may increase the chance of dental disease, including tooth decay, gum disease, and fungus infections.

Check the label of all over-the-counter (OTC), nonprescription, and prescription medicines you now take. If any contain acetaminophen or aspirin or other salicylates, including diflunisal or bismuth subsalicylate (e.g., Pepto-Bismol), be especially careful. This combination medicine contains acetaminophen and/or a salicylate. Therefore, taking it while taking any other medicine that contains these drugs may lead to overdose. If you have any questions about this, check with your doctor or pharmacist.

For patients taking *aspirin-containing medicine*:

- Do not take aspirin-containing medicine for 5 days before any surgery, including dental surgery, unless otherwise directed by your medical doctor or dentist. Taking aspirin during this time may cause bleeding problems.

For diabetic patients taking *salicylate-containing medicine,* false urine sugar test results may occur:

- If you take 8 or more 325-mg (5-grain) doses of aspirin every day for several days in a row.
- If you take 8 or more 325-mg (5-grain), or 4 or more 500-mg (10-grain), doses of sodium salicylate a day.

Smaller doses or occasional use usually will not affect urine sugar tests. If you have any questions about this, check with your doctor, nurse, or pharmacist, especially if your diabetes is not well controlled.

Side Effects of This Medicine

Along with its needed effects, a medicine may cause some unwanted effects. Although serious side effects occur rarely when this medicine is taken as recommended, they may be more likely to occur if:

- too much medicine is taken.
- it is taken in large doses.
- it is taken for a long time.

Get emergency help immediately if any of the following symptoms of overdose occur:

For all combinations

Clumsiness or unsteadiness; convulsions (seizures); drowsiness (severe); dryness of mouth, nose, or throat (severe); fast heartbeat; flushing or redness of face; hallucinations (seeing, hearing, or feeling things that are not there); headache (continuing and/or severe); increased sweating; muscle spasms (especially of neck and back); nausea or vomiting (severe or continuing); shortness of breath or troubled breathing; stomach cramps or pain (severe or continuing); trouble in sleeping

For acetaminophen-containing only

Diarrhea; loss of appetite; swelling or tenderness in the upper abdomen or stomach area

Note: Signs of severe acetaminophen overdose may not appear until 2 to 4 days after the overdose is taken, but treatment to prevent liver damage or death must be started within 24 hours or less after the overdose is taken.

For salicylate-containing only

Any loss of hearing; bloody urine; changes in behavior (in children); confusion; diarrhea (severe or continuing); drowsiness or tiredness (severe, especially in children); fast or deep breathing (especially in children); fever; ringing or buzzing in ears (continuing); uncontrollable flapping movements of the hands (especially in elderly patients); unusual thirst; vision problems

Also, check with your doctor as soon as possible if any of the following side effects occur:

More common

Nausea or vomiting; stomach pain (mild)

Less common or rare

Bloody or black tarry stools; changes in urine or problems with urination; skin rash, hives, or itching; sore throat and fever; swelling of face, feet, or lower legs; tightness in chest; unusual bleeding or bruising; unusual tiredness or weakness; vomiting of blood or material that looks like coffee grounds; weight gain (unusual); yellow eyes or skin

Other side effects may occur that usually do not need medical attention. These side effects may go away during treatment as your body adjusts to the medicine. However, check with your doctor if any of the following side effects continue or are bothersome:

More common

Drowsiness; heartburn or indigestion (for salicylate-containing medicines); thickening of mucus

Less common—more common with high doses

Blurred vision; confusion; difficult or painful urination; dizziness; dryness of mouth, nose, or throat; headache; loss of appetite; nightmares; pounding heartbeat; ringing or buzzing in ears; skin rash; stomach upset or stomach pain; unusual excitement, nervousness, restlessness, or irritability

Not all of the side effects listed above have been reported for each of these medicines, but they have been reported for at least one of them. There are some similarities among these combination medicines, so many of the above side effects may occur with any of these medicines.

Other side effects not listed above may also occur in some patients. If you notice any other effects, check with your doctor.

Annual revision: 07/08/91

ANTIHISTAMINES, DECONGESTANTS, AND ANTICHOLINERGICS Systemic†

Some commonly used brand names in the U.S. are:

- Atrohist L.A.[1]
- AH-chew[2]
- D.A. Chewable[2]
- Dallergy[2]
- Dura-Vent/DA[2]
- Extendryl[2]
- Extendryl JR[2]
- Extendryl SR[2]
- Histor-D Timecelles[2]
- OMNIhist L.A.[2]
- Phenahist-TR[3]
- Phenchlor SHA[3]
- Prehist D[2]
- Rhinolar[4]
- Ru-Tuss[3]
- Stahist[3]

Note: For quick reference the following antihistamine, decongestant, and anticholinergic combinations are numbered to match the corresponding brand names.

This information applies to the following medicines:

1. Brompheniramine (brome-fen-EER-a-meen), Phenyltoloxamine (fen-ill-toe-LOX-a-meen), Pseudoephedrine (soo-doe-e-FED-rin), and Atropine (A-troe-peen)†
2. Chlorpheniramine (klor-fen-EER-a-meen), Phenylephrine (fen-ill-EF-rin), and Methscopolamine (meth-skoe-POL-a-meen)†
3. Chlorpheniramine, Phenylephrine, Phenylpropanolamine (fen-ill-proe-pa-NOLE-a-meen), Atropine, Hyoscyamine (hye-oh-SYE-a-meen), and Scopolamine (skoe-POL-a-meen)†
4. Chlorpheniramine, Phenylpropanolamine, and Methscopolamine†

†Not commercially available in Canada.

Description

Antihistamine, decongestant, and anticholinergic combinations are used to treat the nasal congestion (stuffy nose) and runny nose caused by allergies.

Antihistamines work by preventing the effects of a substance called histamine, which is produced by the body. Antihistamines contained in these combinations are brompheniramine, chlorpheniramine, and phenyltoloxamine.

The decongestants in these combinations, phenylephrine, phenylpropanolamine (also known as PPA), and pseudoephedrine, produce a narrowing of blood vessels. This leads to clearing of nasal congestion, but it may also cause an increase in blood pressure in patients who have high blood pressure.

Anticholinergics, such as atropine, hyoscyamine, methscopolamine, and scopolamine may help produce a drying effect in the nose and chest.

These combinations are available only with your doctor's prescription in the following dosage forms:

Oral

Brompheniramine, Phenyltoloxamine, Pseudoephedrine, and Atropine
- Extended-release tablets (U.S.)

Chlorpheniramine, Phenylephrine, and Methscopolamine
- Extended-release capsules (U.S.)
- Syrup (U.S.)
- Tablets (U.S.)
- Chewable tablets (U.S.)
- Extended-release tablets (U.S.)

Chlorpheniramine, Phenylephrine, Phenylpropanolamine, Atropine, Hyoscyamine, and Scopolamine
- Extended-release tablets (U.S.)

Chlorpheniramine, Phenylpropanolamine, and Methscopolamine
- Extended-release capsules (U.S.)

It is very important that you read and understand the following information. If any of it causes you special concern, check with your doctor or pharmacist. Also, *if you have any questions* or if you want more information about this medicine or your medical problem, *ask your doctor, nurse, or pharmacist.*

Before Using This Medicine

In deciding to use a medicine, the risks of taking the medicine must be weighed against the good it will do. This is a decision you and your doctor will make. For antihistamine, decongestant, and anticholinergic combinations, the following should be considered:

Allergies—Tell your doctor if you have ever had any unusual or allergic reaction to antihistamines, anticholinergics, or to amphetamine, dextroamphetamine (e.g., Dexedrine), ephedrine (e.g., Ephed II), epinephrine (e.g.,

Adrenalin), isoproterenol (e.g., Isuprel), metaproterenol (e.g., Alupent), methamphetamine (e.g., Desoxyn), norepinephrine (e.g., Levophed), phenylephrine (e.g., Neo-Synephrine), phenylpropanolamine [PPA] (e.g., Dexatrim), pseudoephedrine (e.g., Sudafed), or terbutaline (e.g., Brethine). Also, tell your doctor and pharmacist if you are allergic to any other substances, such as foods, preservatives, or dyes.

Pregnancy—For the individual ingredients of these combinations, the following apply:

- *Antihistamines*—Antihistamines have not been shown to cause problems in humans.
- *Atropine*—Studies on effects in pregnancy have not been done in humans. Atropine has not been shown to cause birth defects or other problems in animals.
- *Hyoscyamine*—Studies on effects in pregnancy have not been done in either humans or animals.
- *Methscopolamine*—Studies on effects in pregnancy have not been done in either humans or animals.
- *Phenylephrine*—Studies on birth defects have not been done in either humans or animals with phenylephrine.
- *Phenylpropanolamine*—Studies on birth defects have not been done in either humans or animals with phenylpropanolamine. However, it seems that some women who take phenylpropanolamine in the weeks following delivery are more likely to suffer mental or mood changes.
- *Pseudoephedrine*—Studies on birth defects with pseudoephedrine have not been done in humans. In animal studies pseudoephedrine did not cause birth defects but did cause a decrease in average weight, length, and rate of bone formation in the animal fetus when high doses were given.
- *Scopolamine*—Studies on effects in pregnancy have not been done in pregnant women. However, studies in animals at doses many times the human dose have shown that scopolamine causes a small increase in the number of fetal deaths.

Breast-feeding—Small amounts of antihistamines. decongestants, and anticholinergics may pass into the breast milk. Use is not recommended since this medicine may cause side effects, such as unusual excitement or irritability, in the nursing baby. Also, since this medicine tends to decrease the secretions of the body, it is possible that the flow of breast milk may be reduced in some women.

Children—Very young children are usually more sensitive than adults to the effects of this medicine. Increases in blood pressure, nightmares or unusual excitement, nervousness, restlessness, or irritability may be more likely to occur in children. Also, mental changes may be more likely to occur in young children taking combination medicines that contain phenylpropanolamine. Also, when anticholinergics are given to children during hot weather, a rapid increase in body temperature may occur, which may lead to heat stroke. In infants and children, especially those with spastic paralysis or brain damage, this medicine may be especially likely to cause severe side effects.

Older adults—Confusion or memory loss, difficult and painful urination, dizziness, drowsiness, dryness of mouth, or convulsions (seizures) may be more likely to occur in the elderly, who are usually more sensitive than younger adults to the effects of this medicine. Also, nightmares or unusual excitement, nervousness, restlessness, or irritability may be more likely to occur in elderly patients. In addition, eye pain may occur, which may be a sign of glaucoma.

Other medicines—Although certain medicines should not be used together at all, in other cases different medicines may be used together even if an interaction might occur. In these cases, your doctor may want to change the dose, or other precautions may be necessary. When you are taking this medicine it is especially important that your doctor and pharmacist know if you are taking any of the following:

- Amantadine (e.g., Symmetrel) or
- Amphetamines or
- Appetite suppressants (diet pills), except fenfluramine (e.g., Pondimin), or
- Beta-adrenergic blocking agents (acebutolol [e.g., Sectral], atenolol [e.g., Tenormin], betaxolol [e.g., Kerlone], carteolol [e.g., Cartrol], labetalol [e.g., Normodyne], metoprolol [e.g., Lopressor], nadolol [e.g., Corgard], oxprenolol [e.g., Trasicor], penbutolol [e.g., Levatol], pindolol [e.g., Visken], propanolol [e.g., Inderal], sotalol [e.g., Sotacor], timolol [e.g., Blocadren]) or
- Caffeine (e.g., NoDoz) or
- Chlophedianol (e.g., Ulone) or
- Cocaine or
- Digitalis glycosides (heart medicine) or
- Medicine for asthma or other breathing problems or
- Medicine for colds, sinus problems, or hay fever or other allergies (including nose drops or sprays) or
- Methylphenidate (e.g., Ritalin) or
- Nabilone (e.g., Cesamet) or
- Pemoline (e.g., Cylert)—Using any of these medicines together with a decongestant-containing combination may cause excessive stimulant side effects, such as difficulty in sleeping, heart rate problems, nervousness, and irritability
- Central nervous system (CNS) depressants—Using these combinations with CNS depressants may worsen the effects (e.g., drowsiness) of CNS depressants or antihistamines
- Monoamine oxidase (MAO) inhibitors (furazolidone [e.g., Furoxone], isocarboxazid [e.g., Marplan], phenelzine [e.g., Nardil], procarbazine [e.g., Matulane], selegiline [e.g., Eldepryl], tranylcypromine [e.g., Parnate])—If you are now taking, or have taken within the past 2 weeks, any of the MAO inhibitors, the side effects of the antihistamines may become more severe; these medicines should not be used together

- Other anticholinergics (medicine for abdominal or stomach spasms or cramps)—Side effects of antihistamines or anticholinergics, such as dryness of mouth, may be more likely to occur
- Potassium chloride (e.g., Kay Ciel)—Using this medicine with an anticholinergic-containing medicine may make gastrointestinal problems caused by potassium worse
- Rauwolfia alkaloids (alseroxylon [e.g., Rauwiloid], deserpidine [e.g., Harmonyl], rauwolfia serpentina [e.g., Raudixin], reserpine [e.g., Serpasil])—These medicines may increase or decrease the effect of the decongestant in this medicine
- Tricyclic antidepressants (amitriptyline [e.g., Elavil], amoxapine [e.g., Asendin], clomipramine [e.g., Anafranil], desipramine [e.g., Pertofrane], doxepin [e.g., Sinequan], imipramine [e.g., Tofranil], nortriptyline [e.g., Aventyl], protriptyline [e.g., Vivactil], trimipramine [e.g., Surmontil])—Effects, such as drowsiness, may be worsened; also, taking these medicines together may make some of the anticholinergic side effects, such as dryness of mouth, become more severe

Other medical problems—The presence of other medical problems may affect the use of antihistamine, decongestant, and anticholinergic combinations. Make sure you tell your doctor if you have any other medical problems, especially:

- Brain damage in children or
- Down's syndrome or
- Dryness of mouth (severe and continuing) or
- Enlarged prostate or
- Fever or
- Glaucoma or
- Intestinal blockage or other intestinal problems or
- Kidney disease or
- Liver disease or
- Lung disease or
- Mental or emotional problems or
- Myasthenia gravis or
- Urinary tract blockage or difficult urination—These medicines may make these conditions worse
- Diabetes mellitus (sugar diabetes)—The decongestant in this medicine may put diabetic patients at a greater risk of having heart or blood vessel disease
- Heart or blood vessel disease or
- High blood pressure—The decongestant and anticholinergic in this medicine may cause the blood pressure to increase and may also speed up the heart rate
- Overactive thyroid—If the overactive thyroid has caused a fast heart rate, the decongestant and anticholinergic in this medicine may cause the heart rate to speed up further

Before you begin using any new medicine (prescription or nonprescription) or if you develop any new medical problem while you are using this medicine, check with your doctor, nurse, or pharmacist.

Proper Use of This Medicine

Take this medicine only as directed. Do not take more of it and do not take it more often than recommended on the label, unless otherwise directed by your doctor. To do so may increase the chance of side effects.

If this medicine irritates your stomach, you may take it with food or a glass of water or milk, to lessen the irritation.

For patients *taking the extended-release capsule or extended-release tablet form of this medicine:*

- Swallow the capsule or tablet whole.
- Do not crush, break, or chew before swallowing.
- If the capsule is too large to swallow, you may mix the contents of the capsule with applesauce, jelly, honey, or syrup and swallow without chewing.

Dosing—The dose of these combination medicines will be different for different patients. *Follow your doctor's orders or the directions on the label.* The following information includes only the average doses for these combinations. *If your dose is different, do not change it* unless your doctor tells you to do so:

- The number of capsules or tablets or teaspoonfuls of syrup that you take depends on the strength of the medicine. Also, the number of doses you take each day and the time between doses depends on whether you are taking a short-acting or long-acting form of this medicine.
- For *regular (short-acting)* dosage forms (capsules, syrup, or tablets):
  —Adults and children 12 years of age and older: 1 capsule, tablet, or 1 to 2 teaspoonfuls every four to six hours.
  —Children:
    - Up to 6 years of age: Dose must be determined by the doctor.
    - 6 to 12 years of age: 1 chewable tablet or 1 teaspoonful of syrup every four hours.
- For *long-acting* dosage forms (extended-release capsules or tablets):
  —Adults and children 12 years of age and older: 1 capsule or tablet every twelve hours.
  —Children up to 12 years of age: Dose must be determined by the doctor.

Missed dose—If you miss a dose of this medicine, take it as soon as possible. However, if it is almost time for your next dose, skip the missed dose and go back to your regular dosing schedule. Do not double doses.

Storage—To store this medicine:

- Keep out of the reach of children.
- Store away from heat and direct light.
- Do not store in the bathroom, near the kitchen sink, or in other damp places. Heat or moisture may cause the medicine to break down.
- Keep the liquid form of this medicine from freezing.
- Do not keep outdated medicine or medicine no longer needed. Be sure that any discarded medicine is out of the reach of children.

Precautions While Using This Medicine

Check with your doctor if your symptoms do not improve or become worse, or if you have a high fever.

Before you have any skin tests for allergies, tell the doctor in charge that you are taking this medicine. The results of the test may be affected by the antihistamine in this medicine.

These medicines may make you sweat less, causing your body temperature to increase. *Use extra care not to become overheated during exercise or hot weather while you are taking this medicine,* since overheating may result in heat stroke. Also hot baths or saunas may make you dizzy or faint while you are taking this medicine.

The anticholinergic contained in this medicine may cause some people to have blurred vision. *Make sure your vision is clear before you drive or do anything else that could be dangerous if you are not able to see well.* These medicines may also cause your eyes to become more sensitive to light than they are normally. Wearing sunglasses may help lessen the discomfort from bright light.

These medicines may cause some people to become dizzy or drowsy. *Make sure you know how you react to this medicine before you drive, use machines, or do anything else that could be dangerous if you are dizzy or are not alert.*

The decongestant in this medicine may cause some people to be nervous or restless or to have trouble in sleeping. If you have trouble in sleeping, *take the last dose of this medicine for each day a few hours before bedtime.* If you have any questions about this, check with your doctor.

The decongestant in this medicine may add to the central nervous system (CNS) stimulant and other effects of phenylpropanolamine (PPA)-containing diet aids. *Do not use medicines for diet or appetite control while taking this medicine unless you have checked with your doctor.*

Before having any kind of surgery (including dental surgery) or emergency treatment, tell the medical doctor or dentist in charge that you are taking this medicine.

This medicine may cause dryness of the mouth, nose, and throat. For temporary relief, use sugarless candy or gum, melt bits of ice in your mouth, or use a saliva substitute. However, if your mouth continues to feel dry for more than 2 weeks, check with your dentist. Continuing dryness of the mouth may increase the chance of dental disease, including tooth decay, gum disease, and fungus infections.

If you think you or someone else may have taken an overdose, get emergency help at once. Taking an overdose of this medicine or taking this medicine with alcohol or other CNS depressants may lead to unconsciousness and possibly death.

Side Effects of This Medicine

Along with its needed effects, a medicine may cause some unwanted effects. Although not all of these side effects may occur, if they do occur they may need medical attention.

Get emergency help immediately if any of the following symptoms of overdose occur:

Clumsiness or unsteadiness; convulsions (seizures); drowsiness (severe); dryness of mouth, nose, or throat (severe); fast heartbeat; flushing or redness of face; hallucinations (seeing, hearing, or feeling things that are not there); headache (continuing); shortness of breath or troubled breathing; trouble in sleeping

Also, check with your doctor as soon as possible if any of the following side effects occur:

Rare

Mood or mental changes; skin rash, hives, or itching; sore throat and fever; tightness in chest; unusual bleeding or bruising; unusual tiredness or weakness

Other side effects may occur that usually do not need medical attention. These side effects may go away during treatment as your body adjusts to the medicine. However, check with your doctor or pharmacist if any of the following side effects continue or are bothersome:

More common

Drowsiness; thickening of the bronchial secretions

Less common—more common with high doses

Blurred vision; confusion; difficult or painful urination; dizziness; dryness of mouth, nose, or throat; headache; loss of appetite; nightmares; pounding heartbeat; ringing or buzzing in ears; skin rash; unusual excitement, nervousness, restlessness, or irritability

Other side effects not listed above may also occur in some patients. If you notice any other effects, check with your doctor.

Annual revision: 05/03/93

ANTIHISTAMINES, PHENOTHIAZINE-DERIVATIVE Systemic

This information applies to the following medicines:

Methdilazine (meth-DILL-a-zeen)
Promethazine (proe-METH-a-zeen)
Trimeprazine (trye-MEP-ra-zeen)

Some commonly used brand names are:

For Methdilazine†

In the U.S.

Tacaryl

For Promethazine

In the U.S.

Anergan 25	Pro-50
Anergan 50	Prometh-25
Pentazine	Prometh-50
Phenameth	Promethegan
Phenazine 25	Prorex-25
Phenazine 50	Prorex-50
Phencen-50	Prothazine
Phenergan	Prothazine Plain
Phenergan Fortis	V-Gan-25
Phenergan Plain	V-Gan-50
Phenoject-50	

Generic name product may also be available.

In Canada

Histantil	PMS Promethazine
Phenergan	

Generic name product may also be available.

For Trimeprazine

In the U.S.

Temaril

Generic name product may also be available.

Another commonly used name for trimeprazine is alimemazine.

In Canada

Panectyl

†Not commercially available in Canada.

Description

Phenothiazine (FEE-noe-THYE-a-zeen)-derivative antihistamines are used to relieve or prevent the symptoms of hay fever and other types of allergy. They work by preventing the effects of a substance called histamine, which is produced by the body.

Some of these antihistamines are also used to prevent motion sickness, nausea, vomiting, and dizziness. In addition, some of them may be used to help people go to sleep and control their anxiety before or after surgery.

Phenothiazine-derivative antihistamines may also be used for other conditions as determined by your doctor.

In the U.S. these antihistamines are available only with your doctor's prescription. In Canada some are available without a prescription. However, your doctor may have special instructions on the proper dose of the medicine for your medical condition.

These medicines are available in the following dosage forms:

Oral

Methdilazine
- Syrup (U.S.)
- Tablets (U.S.)
- Chewable tablets (U.S.)

Promethazine
- Syrup (U.S. and Canada)
- Tablets (U.S. and Canada)

Trimeprazine
- Extended-release capsules (U.S.)
- Syrup (U.S. and Canada)
- Tablets (U.S. and Canada)

Parenteral

Promethazine
- Injection (U.S. and Canada)

Rectal

Promethazine
- Suppositories (U.S.)

It is very important that you read and understand the following information. If any of it causes you special concern, check with your doctor. Also, *if you have any questions* or if you want more information about this medicine or your medical problem, *ask your doctor, nurse, or pharmacist*.

Before Using This Medicine

In deciding to use a medicine, the risks of taking the medicine must be weighed against the good it will do. This is a decision you and your doctor will make. For phenothiazine-derivative antihistamines, the following should be considered:

Allergies—Tell your doctor if you have ever had any unusual or allergic reaction to these medicines or to phenothiazines. Also tell your doctor and pharmacist if you are allergic to any other substances, such as foods, preservatives, or dyes.

Pregnancy—Methdilazine, promethazine, and trimeprazine have not been studied in pregnant women. In animal studies, promethazine has not been shown to cause birth defects. However, other phenothiazine medicines have been shown to cause jaundice and muscle tremors in a few newborn babies whose mothers received them during pregnancy. Also, the newborn baby may have blood clotting problems if promethazine is taken by the mother within 2 weeks before delivery.

Breast-feeding—Small amounts of antihistamines pass into the breast milk. Use is not recommended since babies are more sensitive to the side effects of antihistamines, such as unusual excitement or irritability. Also, with the use of phenothiazine-derivative antihistamines there is the chance that the nursing baby may be more at risk of having difficulty in breathing while sleeping or of the sudden infant death syndrome (SIDS). However, more studies are needed to confirm this.

In addition, since these medicines tend to decrease the secretions of the body, it is possible that the flow of breast milk may be reduced in some patients.

Children—Serious side effects, such as convulsions (seizures), are more likely to occur in younger patients and would be of greater risk to infants than to older children or adults. In general, children are more sensitive to the effects of antihistamines. Also, nightmares or unusual excitement, nervousness, restlessness, or irritability may be more likely to occur in children. *The use of phenothiazine-derivative antihistamines is not recommended in children who have a history of difficulty in breathing while sleeping, or a family history of sudden infant death syndrome (SIDS).*

Children who show signs of Reye's syndrome should not be given phenothiazine-derivative antihistamines, especially by injection. Seizures or uncontrolled movements that may occur with phenothiazine-derivative antihistamines may be thought to be symptoms of Reye's syndrome.

Adolescents—Adolescents who show signs of Reye's syndrome should not be given phenothiazine-derivative antihistamines, especially by injection. Seizures or uncontrolled movements that may occur with phenothiazine-derivative antihistamines may be thought to be symptoms of Reye's syndrome.

Older adults—Elderly patients are especially sensitive to the effects of antihistamines. Confusion; difficult or painful urination; dizziness; drowsiness; feeling faint; or dryness of mouth, nose, or throat may be more likely to occur in elderly patients. Also, nightmares or unusual excitement, nervousness, restlessness, or irritability may be more likely to occur in elderly patients. In addition, uncontrolled movements may be more likely to occur in elderly patients taking phenothiazine-derivative antihistamines.

Other medicines—Although certain medicines should not be used together at all, in other cases two different medicines may be used together even if an interaction might occur. In these cases, your doctor may want to change the dose, or other precautions may be necessary. When taking phenothiazine-derivative antihistamines, it is especially important that your doctor and pharmacist know if you are taking/receiving any of the following:

- Amoxapine (e.g., Asendin) or
- Antipsychotics (medicine for mental illness) or
- Methyldopa (e.g., Aldomet) or
- Metoclopramide (e.g., Reglan) or
- Metyrosine (e.g., Demser) or
- Pemoline (e.g., Cylert) or
- Pimozide (e.g., Orap) or
- Rauwolfia alkaloids (alseroxylon [e.g., Rauwiloid], deserpidine [e.g., Harmonyl], rauwolfia serpentina [e.g., Raudixin], reserpine [e.g., Serpasil])—Side effects, such as uncontrolled body movements, of these medicines may become more severe and frequent if they are used together with phenothiazine-derivative antihistamines
- Anticholinergics (medicine for abdominal or stomach spasms or cramps)—Side effects of phenothiazine-derivative antihistamines or anticholinergics, such as dryness of mouth, may be more likely to occur
- Antithyroid agents (medicine for overactive thyroid)—Serious side effects may be more likely to occur when antithyroid agents are taken together with phenothiazine-derivative antihistamines
- Central nervous system (CNS) depressants—Effects of CNS depressants or antihistamines, such as drowsiness, may be made more severe; also, taking maprotiline or tricyclic antidepressants may cause some side effects of antihistamines, such as dryness of mouth, to become more severe
- Contrast agent, injected into spinal canal—If you are having an x-ray test of the head, spinal canal, or nervous system for which you are going to receive an injection into the spinal canal, phenothiazine-derivative antihistamines may increase the chance of seizures; stop taking any phenothiazine-derivative antihistamine 48 hours before the test and do not start taking it until 24 hours after the test
- Levodopa—When used together with phenothiazine-derivative antihistamines, the levodopa may not work as it should
- Monoamine oxidase (MAO) inhibitors (furazolidone [e.g., Furoxone], isocarboxazid [e.g., Marplan], phenelzine [e.g., Nardil], procarbazine [e.g., Matulane], tranylcypromine [e.g., Parnate])—If you are now taking or have taken within the past 2 weeks any of the MAO inhibitors, the side effects of the phenothiazine-derivative antihistamines may become more severe; these medicines should not be used together

Other medical problems—The presence of other medical problems may affect the use of antihistamines. Make sure you tell your doctor if you have any other medical problems, especially:

- Asthma attacks—Although antihistamines open bronchial passages that are narrowed due to allergies, they may also cause secretions to become thick so that during an asthma attack it might be difficult to cough them up
- Blood disease or
- Heart or blood vessel disease—These medicines may cause more serious conditions to develop
- Enlarged prostate or
- Urinary tract blockage or difficult urination—Phenothiazine-derivative antihistamines may cause urinary problems to become worse
- Epilepsy or
- Reye's syndrome—Phenothiazine-derivative antihistamines, especially promethazine given by injection, may increase the chance of seizures or uncontrolled movements
- Glaucoma—These medicines may cause a slight increase in inner eye pressure that may worsen the condition
- Jaundice—Phenothiazine-derivative antihistamines may make the condition worse

- Liver disease—Phenothiazine-derivative antihistamines may build up in the body, which may increase the chance of side effects such as muscle spasms

Before you begin using any new medicine (prescription or nonprescription) or if you develop any new medical problem while you are using this medicine, check with your doctor, nurse, or pharmacist.

Proper Use of This Medicine

Antihistamines are used to relieve or prevent the symptoms of your medical problem. Take them only as directed. Do not take more of them and do not take them more often than recommended on the label, unless otherwise directed by your doctor. To do so may increase the chance of side effects.

For patients *taking this medicine by mouth:*

- Antihistamines can be taken with food or a glass of water or milk to lessen stomach irritation if necessary.
- If you are taking the *extended-release capsule* form of this medicine, swallow it whole. Do not break, crush, or chew before swallowing.

For patients taking *promethazine for motion sickness:*

- Take this medicine 30 minutes to 1 hour before you begin to travel.

For patients using the *suppository form of this medicine:*

- To insert suppository: First remove the foil wrapper and moisten the suppository with cold water. Lie down on side and use your finger to push the suppository well up into the rectum. If the suppository is too soft to insert, chill the suppository in the refrigerator for 30 minutes or run cold water over it, before removing the foil wrapper.

For patients using the *injection form of this medicine:*

- If you will be giving yourself the injections, make sure you understand exactly how to give them. If you have any questions about this, check with your doctor, nurse, or pharmacist.

Missed dose—If you are taking this medicine regularly and you miss a dose, take it as soon as possible. However, if it is almost time for your next dose, skip the missed dose and go back to your regular dosing schedule. Do not double doses.

Storage—To store this medicine:

- Keep out of the reach of children, since overdose may be very dangerous in children.
- Store away from heat and direct light.
- Do not store the capsule or tablet form of this medicine in the bathroom medicine cabinet, near the kitchen sink, or in other damp places. Heat or moisture may cause the medicine to break down.
- Keep the liquid form of this medicine from freezing.
- Do not keep outdated medicine or medicine no longer needed. Be sure that any discarded medicine is out of the reach of children.

Precautions While Using This Medicine

Tell the doctor in charge that you are taking this medicine before you have any skin tests for allergies. The results of the test may be affected by this medicine.

When taking phenothiazine-derivative antihistamines on a regular basis, make sure your doctor knows if you are taking large amounts of aspirin at the same time (as in arthritis or rheumatism). Effects of too much aspirin, such as ringing in the ears, may be covered up by the antihistamine.

Phenothiazine-derivative antihistamines will add to the effects of alcohol and other CNS depressants (medicines that slow down the nervous system, possibly causing drowsiness). Some examples of CNS depressants are sedatives, tranquilizers, or sleeping medicine; prescription pain medicine or narcotics; barbiturates; medicine for seizures; muscle relaxants; or anesthetics, including some dental anesthetics. *Check with your doctor before taking any of the above while you are using this medicine.*

This medicine may cause some people to become drowsy or less alert than they are normally. Even if taken at bedtime, it may cause some people to feel drowsy or less alert on arising. *Make sure you know how you react to the phenothiazine-derivative antihistamine you are taking before you drive, use machines, or do anything else that could be dangerous if you are not alert.*

Phenothiazine-derivative antihistamines may cause dryness of the mouth, nose, and throat. For temporary relief of mouth dryness, use sugarless candy or gum, melt bits of ice in your mouth, or use a saliva substitute. However, if your mouth continues to feel dry for more than 2 weeks, check with your medical doctor or dentist. Continuing dryness of the mouth may increase the chance of dental disease, including tooth decay, gum disease, and fungus infections.

This medicine controls nausea and vomiting. For this reason, it may cover up the signs of overdose caused by other medicines or the symptoms of appendicitis. This will make it difficult for your doctor to diagnose these conditions. Make sure your doctor knows that you are taking this medicine if you have other symptoms of appendicitis such as stomach or lower abdominal pain, cramping, or soreness. Also, if you think you may have taken an overdose of any medicine, tell your doctor that you are taking this medicine.

Side Effects of This Medicine

Along with its needed effects, a medicine may cause some unwanted effects. Although not all of these side effects may occur, if they do occur they may need medical attention.

Check with your doctor as soon as possible if any of the following side effects occur:

Less common or rare

Sore throat and fever; unusual bleeding or bruising; unusual tiredness or weakness

Symptoms of overdose

Clumsiness or unsteadiness; convulsions (seizures); drowsiness (severe); dryness of mouth, nose, or throat (severe); feeling faint; flushing or redness of face; hallucinations (seeing, hearing, or feeling things that are not there); muscle spasms (especially of neck and back); restlessness; shortness of breath or troubled breathing; shuffling walk; tic-like (jerky) movements of head and face; trembling and shaking of hands; trouble in sleeping

Other side effects may occur that usually do not need medical attention. These side effects may go away during treatment as your body adjusts to the medicine. However, check with your doctor or pharmacist if any of the following side effects continue or are bothersome:

More common

Drowsiness (less common with methdilazine); thickening of mucus

Less common or rare

Blurred vision or any change in vision; burning or stinging of rectum (with rectal suppository); confusion; difficult or painful urination; dizziness; dryness of mouth, nose, or throat; fast heartbeat; feeling faint; increased sensitivity of skin to sun; increased sweating; loss of appetite; nightmares; ringing or buzzing in ears; skin rash; unusual excitement, nervousness, restlessness, or irritability

Other side effects not listed above may also occur in some patients. If you notice any other effects, check with your doctor or pharmacist.

Annual revision: 07/08/91

ANTI-INFLAMMATORY AGENTS, NONSTEROIDAL Ophthalmic

This information applies to the following medicines:

Diclofenac (dye-KLOE-fen-ak)
Flurbiprofen (flure-BI-proe-fen)
Indomethacin (in-doe-METH-a-sin)
Suprofen (soo-PROE-fen)

Some commonly used brand names are:

For Diclofenac
In the U.S.
Voltaren Ophthalmic
In Canada
Voltaren Ophtha

For Flurbiprofen
In the U.S.
Ocufen
In Canada
Ocufen

For Indomethacin*
In Canada
Indocid

For Suprofen
In the U.S.
Profenal

*Not commercially available in the U.S.

Description

Ophthalmic anti-inflammatory medicines are used in the eye to lessen problems that can occur during or after some kinds of eye surgery. Sometimes, the pupil of the eye gets smaller during an operation. This makes it more difficult for the surgeon to reach some areas of the eye. Some of these medicines are used to help prevent this. Also, some of them are used after eye surgery, to relieve effects such as inflammation or edema (too much fluid in the eye).

These medicines may also be used for other conditions, as determined by your ophthalmologist (eye doctor).

These medicines are available only with your doctor's prescription, in the following dosage forms:

Ophthalmic

Diclofenac
- Ophthalmic solution (U.S. and Canada)

Flurbiprofen
- Ophthalmic solution (U.S. and Canada)

Indomethacin
- Ophthalmic suspension (Canada)

Suprofen
- Ophthalmic solution (U.S.)

It is very important that you read and understand the following information. If any of it causes you special concern, check with your doctor. Also, *if you have any questions* or if you want more information about this medicine or your medical problem, *ask your doctor, nurse, or pharmacist.*

Before Using This Medicine

In deciding to use a medicine, the risks of taking the medicine must be weighed against the good it will do. This is a decision you and your doctor will make. For ophthalmic anti-inflammatory medicines, the following should be considered:

Allergies—Tell your doctor if you have ever had any unusual or allergic reaction to one of the ophthalmic anti-inflammatory medicines or other serious reactions, especially asthma or wheezing, runny nose, or hives, to any of the following medicines:

Aspirin or other salicylates
Diclofenac (e.g., Voltaren)
Diflunisal (e.g., Dolobid)
Etodolac (e.g., Lodine)
Fenoprofen (e.g., Nalfon)
Floctafenine (e.g., Idarac)
Flurbiprofen, oral (e.g., Ansaid)
Ibuprofen (e.g., Motrin)
Indomethacin (e.g., Indocin)
Ketoprofen (e.g., Orudis)
Ketorolac (e.g., Toradol)
Meclofenamate (e.g., Meclomen)
Mefenamic acid (e.g., Ponstel)
Nabumetone (e.g., Relafen)
Naproxen (e.g., Naprosyn)
Oxyphenbutazone (e.g., Tandearil)
Phenylbutazone (e.g., Butazolidin)
Piroxicam (e.g., Feldene)
Sulindac (e.g., Clinoril)
Suprofen (e.g., Suprol)
Tenoxicam (e.g., Mobiflex)
Tiaprofenic acid (e.g., Surgam)
Tolmetin (e.g., Tolectin)
Zomepirac (e.g., Zomax)

Also tell your doctor and pharmacist if you are allergic to any other substances, such as foods, preservatives, or dyes.

Pregnancy—Although studies on birth defects have not been done in pregnant women after use of these medicines in the eye, ophthalmic anti-inflammatory medicines have not been reported to cause birth defects or other problems. Studies have been done in animals receiving anti-inflammatory medicines by mouth in amounts that are much greater than the amounts used in the eye. These medicines did not cause birth defects in these studies. However, they decreased the weight or slowed the growth of the fetus and caused other, more serious, harmful effects on the fetus when they were given in amounts that were large enough to cause harmful effects in the mother. Also, when these medicines were given to animals late in pregnancy, they increased the length of pregnancy or prolonged labor.

Breast-feeding—It is not known whether any of these medicines pass into the breast milk after they are placed in the eye. Diclofenac, indomethacin, and suprofen pass into the breast milk when they are are taken by mouth. It is not known whether flurbiprofen passes into the breast milk when it is taken by mouth. However, these medicines have not been shown to cause problems in nursing babies.

Children—These medicines have been studied only in adults, and there is no specific information about their use in children.

Older adults—These medicines have been tested and have not been shown to cause different side effects or problems in older people than they do in younger adults.

Other medical problems—The presence of other medical problems may affect the use of these medicines. Make sure you tell your doctor if you have any other medical problems, especially:

- Hemophilia or other bleeding problems—The possibility of bleeding may be increased

Proper Use of This Medicine

To use:

- First, wash your hands. With the middle finger, apply pressure to the inside corner of the eye (and continue to apply pressure for 1 or 2 minutes after the medicine has been placed in the eye). Tilt the head back and with the index finger of the same hand, pull the lower eyelid away from the eye to form a pouch. Drop the medicine into the pouch and gently close your eyes. Do not blink. Keep your eyes closed for 1 or 2 minutes to allow the medicine to come into contact with the irritation. If you think you did not get the drop of medicine into your eye properly, use another drop.
- Remove any excess solution around the eye with a clean tissue, being careful not to touch the eye.
- Immediately after using the eye drops, wash your hands to remove any medicine that may be on them.
- To keep the medicine as germ-free as possible, do not touch the applicator tip to any surface (including the eye). Also, always keep the container tightly closed.

Do not use this medicine more often or for a longer time than your doctor ordered. To do so may increase the chance of side effects.

Do not use any leftover medicine for future eye problems without first checking with your doctor. If certain kinds of infection are present, using this medicine may make the infection worse and possibly lead to eye damage.

Dosing—The dose of these medicines will be different for different patients. *Follow your doctor's orders or the directions on the label.* The following information includes only the average doses of these medicines. *If your dose is different, do not change it* unless your doctor tells you to do so.

For diclofenac

- Adults:
  —For use before an eye operation: Your doctor or nurse will probably give you the medicine before your operation.
  —To relieve inflammation or edema in the eye: 1 drop in the eye 3 to 5 times a day.
- Children: To be determined by the doctor.

For flurbiprofen

- Adults:
  —For use before an eye operation: Your doctor or nurse will probably give you the medicine before your operation.
  —To relieve inflammation: 1 drop in the eye every 4 hours.
- Children: To be determined by the doctor.

For indomethacin

- Adults:
  —For use before an eye operation: Your doctor or nurse will probably give you the medicine before your operation.
  —To relieve inflammation or edema in the eye: 1 drop in the eye 4 times a day.
- Children: To be determined by the doctor.

For suprofen

- Adults:
  —For use before an eye operation: Your doctor or nurse will probably give you the medicine before your operation.
  —To relieve inflammation or edema in the eye: To be determined by the doctor.
- Children: To be determined by the doctor.

Missed dose—If you miss a dose of this medicine, apply it as soon as possible. But if it is almost time for your next dose, skip the missed dose and go back to your regular dosing schedule.

Storage—To store this medicine:

- Keep out of the reach of children.
- Store away from heat and direct light.
- Keep the medicine from freezing.
- Do not keep outdated medicine or medicine no longer needed. Be sure that any discarded medicine is out of the reach of children.

Precautions While Using This Medicine

Wearing soft (hydrogel) contact lenses during treatment with diclofenac has caused severe irritation (redness and itching) in some people. Therefore, *do not wear soft contact lenses during the time that you are being treated with diclofenac.*

Side Effects of This Medicine

Along with its needed effects, a medicine may cause some unwanted effects. Check with your doctor as soon as possible if any of the following side effects occur:

Less common or rare

Bleeding in the eye or redness or swelling of the eye or the eyelid (not present before you started using this medicine or becoming worse while you are using this medicine); itching or tearing

Other side effects may occur that usually do not need medical attention. The following side effects usually do not need medical attention. However, check with your doctor if they continue or are bothersome.

More common

Burning or stinging after application

Other side effects not listed above may also occur in some patients. If you notice any other effects, check with your doctor.

Annual revision: 09/08/92

ANTI-INFLAMMATORY ANALGESICS Systemic

This information applies to the following medicines:

Diclofenac (dye-KLOE-fen-ak)
Diflunisal (dye-FLOO-ni-sal)
Fenoprofen (fen-oh-PROE-fen)
Floctafenine (flok-ta-FEN-een)
Flurbiprofen (flure-BI-proe-fen)
Ibuprofen (eye-byoo-PROE-fen)
Indomethacin (in-doe-METH-a-sin)
Ketoprofen (kee-toe-PROE-fen)
Meclofenamate (me-kloe-FEN-am-ate)
Mefenamic (me-fe-NAM-ik) Acid
Naproxen (na-PROX-en)
Phenylbutazone (fen-ill-BYOO-ta-zone)
Piroxicam (peer-OX-i-kam)
Sulindac (sul-IN-dak)
Tiaprofenic (tie-a-pro-FEN-ik) Acid
Tolmetin (TOLE-met-in)

This information does *not* apply to aspirin or other salicylates or to etodolac (e.g., Lodine), ketorolac (e.g., Toradol), Nabumetone (e.g., Relafen), or Oxaprozin (e.g., Daypro).

Some commonly used brand names are:

For Diclofenac

In the U.S.

Voltaren

In Canada

Voltaren
Voltaren SR

For Diflunisal

In the U.S.

Dolobid

In Canada

Dolobid

For Fenoprofen

In the U.S.

Nalfon
Nalfon 200

Generic name product may also be available.

In Canada

Nalfon

For Floctafenine*

In Canada

Idarac

For Flurbiprofen

In the U.S.

Ansaid

In Canada

Ansaid
Froben

Generic name product may also be available.

For Ibuprofen

In the U.S.

Aches-N-Pain
Advil
Advil Caplets
Children's Advil
Dolgesic
Genpril
Genpril Caplets
Haltran
Ibren
Ibumed
Ibuprin
Ibupro-600
Ibuprohm
Ibuprohm Caplets
Ibu-Tab
Ibutex
Ifen
Medipren
Medipren Caplets
Midol 200 Caplets
Motrin
Motrin-IB
Motrin-IB Caplets
Nuprin
Nuprin Caplets
Pamprin-IB
PediaProfen
Profen
Ro-Profen
Rufen
Trendar

Generic name product may also be available.

In Canada

Actiprofen Caplets
Advil
Advil Caplets
Amersol
Apo-Ibuprofen
Medipren
Medipren Caplets
Motrin
Motrin-IB Caplets
Novoprofen
Nuprin

Generic name product may also be available.

For Indomethacin

In the U.S.

Indameth
Indocin
Indocin SR

Generic name product may also be available.

In Canada

Apo-Indomethacin
Indocid
Indocid SR
Novomethacin

Another commonly used name is indometacin.

For Ketoprofen

In the U.S.

Orudis

In Canada

Orudis
Orudis-E
Orudis-SR
Rhodis
Rhodis-E

For Meclofenamate†

In the U.S.

Meclofen
Meclomen

Generic name product may also be available.

For Mefenamic Acid

In the U.S.

Ponstel

Generic name product may also be available.

In Canada

Ponstan

For Naproxen

In the U.S.

Anaprox
Anaprox DS
Naprosyn

In Canada

Anaprox
Apo-Napro-Na
Apo-Naproxen
Naprosyn
Naprosyn-SR
Naxen
Novonaprox
Novonaprox Sodium
Synflex

For Phenylbutazone

In the U.S.

Butatab
Butazolidin
Butazone

Generic name product may also be available.

In Canada

Alka-Butazolidin
Alkabutazone
Alka-Phenylbutazone
Apo-Phenylbutazone
Butazolidin
Intrabutazone
Novobutazone
Phenylone Plus

Generic name product may also be available.

For Piroxicam

In the U.S.

Feldene

In Canada

Apo-Piroxicam
Feldene
Novopirocam

For Sulindac

In the U.S.

Clinoril

Generic name product may also be available.

In Canada

Apo-Sulin
Clinoril
Novo-Sundac

For Tiaprofenic Acid*

In Canada

Surgam

For Tolmetin

In the U.S.

Tolectin 200
Tolectin 600
Tolectin DS

In Canada
Tolectin 200
Tolectin 400
Tolectin 600

*Not commercially available in the U.S.
†Not commercially available in Canada.

Description

Anti-inflammatory analgesics (also called nonsteroidal anti-inflammatory drugs [NSAIDs]) are used to relieve some symptoms caused by arthritis (rheumatism), such as inflammation, swelling, stiffness, and joint pain. However, this medicine does not cure arthritis and will help you only as long as you continue to take it.

Some of these medicines are also used to relieve other kinds of pain or to treat other painful conditions, such as:

- gout attacks;
- bursitis;
- tendinitis;
- sprains, strains, or other injuries; or
- menstrual cramps.

Ibuprofen is also used to reduce fever.

Anti-inflammatory analgesics may also be used to treat other conditions as determined by your doctor.

Any anti-inflammatory analgesic can cause side effects, especially when it is used for a long time or in large doses. Some of the side effects are painful or uncomfortable. Others can be more serious, resulting in the need for medical care and sometimes even death. If you will be taking this medicine for more than one or two months or in large amounts, you should discuss with your doctor the good that it can do as well as the risks of taking it. Also, it is a good idea to ask your doctor about other forms of treatment that might help to reduce the amount of this medicine that you take and/or the length of treatment.

One of the anti-inflammatory analgesics, phenylbutazone, is especially likely to cause very serious side effects. These serious side effects are more likely to occur in patients 40 years of age or older than in younger adults, and the risk becomes greater as the patient's age increases. Before you take phenylbutazone, be sure that you have discussed its use with your doctor. *Also, do not use phenylbutazone to treat any painful condition other than the one for which it was prescribed by your doctor.*

Although ibuprofen may be used instead of aspirin to treat many of the same medical problems, it must not be used by people who are allergic to aspirin.

The 200-mg strength of ibuprofen is available without a prescription. However, your medical doctor or dentist may have special instructions on the proper dose of ibuprofen for your medical condition.

Other anti-inflammatory analgesics and other strengths of ibuprofen are available only with your medical doctor's or dentist's prescription. These medicines are available in the following dosage forms:

Oral

Diclofenac
- Delayed-release tablets (U.S. and Canada)
- Extended-release tablets (Canada)

Diflunisal
- Tablets (U.S. and Canada)

Fenoprofen
- Capsules (U.S. and Canada)
- Tablets (U.S. and Canada)

Floctafenine
- Tablets (Canada)

Flurbiprofen
- Tablets (U.S. and Canada)

Ibuprofen
- Capsules (Canada)
- Oral suspension (U.S.)
- Tablets (U.S. and Canada)

Indomethacin
- Capsules (U.S. and Canada)
- Extended-release capsules (U.S. and Canada)
- Oral suspension (U.S.)

Ketoprofen
- Capsules (U.S. and Canada)
- Delayed-release tablets (Canada)
- Extended-release tablets (Canada)

Meclofenamate
- Capsules (U.S.)

Mefenamic Acid
- Capsules (U.S. and Canada)

Naproxen
- Oral suspension (U.S. and Canada)
- Tablets (U.S. and Canada)
- Extended-release tablets (Canada)

Phenylbutazone
- Capsules (U.S.)
- Tablets (U.S. and Canada)
- Buffered tablets (Canada)
- Delayed-release tablets (Canada)

Piroxicam
- Capsules (U.S. and Canada)

Sulindac
- Tablets (U.S. and Canada)

Tiaprofenic Acid
- Tablets (Canada)

Tolmetin
- Capsules (U.S. and Canada)
- Tablets (U.S. and Canada)

Rectal

Diclofenac
- Suppositories (Canada)

Indomethacin
- Suppositories (U.S. and Canada)

Ketoprofen
- Suppositories (Canada)

Naproxen
- Suppositories (Canada)

Piroxicam
- Suppositories (Canada)

It is very important that you read and understand the following information. If any of it causes you special concern, check with your doctor. Also, *if you have any questions* or if you want more information about this medicine or your medical problem, *ask your doctor, nurse, or pharmacist.*

Before Using This Medicine

In deciding to use a medicine, the risks of taking the medicine must be weighed against the good it will do. This is a decision you and your doctor will make. For the anti-inflammatory analgesics, the following should be considered:

Allergies—Tell your doctor if you have ever had any unusual or allergic reaction to any of the anti-inflammatory analgesics, or to any of the following medicines:

- Aspirin or other salicylates
- Ketorolac (e.g., Toradol)
- Oxyphenbutazone (e.g., Oxalid, Tandearil)
- Suprofen (e.g., Suprol)
- Zomepirac (e.g., Zomax)

Also tell your doctor and pharmacist if you are allergic to any other substances, such as foods, preservatives, or dyes.

Diet—Make certain your doctor and pharmacist know if you are on any special diet, such as a low-sodium or low-sugar diet. Some of these medicines contain sodium or sugar.

Pregnancy—Studies on birth defects with these medicines have not been done in humans. However, there is a chance that these medicines may cause unwanted effects on the heart or blood flow of the fetus or newborn baby if they are taken regularly during the last few months of pregnancy. Also, studies in animals have shown that these medicines, if taken late in pregnancy, may increase the length of pregnancy, prolong labor, or cause other problems during delivery.

Studies in animals have not shown that fenoprofen, floctafenine, flurbiprofen, ibuprofen, ketoprofen, naproxen, phenylbutazone, piroxicam, tiaprofenic acid, or tolmetin causes birth defects. Diflunisal caused birth defects of the spine and ribs in rabbits, but not in mice or rats. Diclofenac and meclofenamate caused unwanted effects on the formation of bones in animals. Indomethacin caused slower development of bones and damage to nerves in animals. In some animal studies, sulindac caused unwanted effects on the development of bones and organs. Studies on birth defects with mefenamic acid have not been done in animals.

Even though most of these medicines did not cause birth defects in animals, many of them did cause other harmful or toxic effects on the fetus, usually when they were given in such large amounts that the pregnant animals became sick.

Breast-feeding—

- *For indomethacin:* Indomethacin passes into the breast milk and has been reported to cause unwanted effects in nursing babies.
- *For phenylbutazone:* Phenylbutazone passes into the breast milk and may cause unwanted effects, such as blood problems, in nursing babies.
- *For meclofenamate:* Use of meclofenamate by nursing mothers is not recommended because in animal studies it caused unwanted effects on the newborn's development.
- *For piroxicam:* Studies in animals have shown that piroxicam may decrease the amount of milk.

Although other anti-inflammatory analgesics have not been reported to cause problems in nursing babies, diclofenac, diflunisal, fenoprofen, mefenamic acid, flurbiprofen, naproxen, piroxicam, and tolmetin pass into the breast milk. It is not known whether floctafenine, ibuprofen, ketoprofen, meclofenamate, sulindac, or tiaprofenic acid passes into human breast milk.

Children—

- *For ibuprofen:* Ibuprofen has been tested in children 6 months of age and older with fevers and in children 12 months of age and older with arthritis. It has not been shown to cause different side effects or problems than it does in adults.
- *For indomethacin and for tolmetin:* Indomethacin and tolmetin have been tested in children 2 years of age and older and have not been shown to cause different side effects or problems than they do in adults.
- *For naproxen:* Studies with naproxen in children 2 years of age and older have shown that skin rash may be more likely to occur.
- *For other anti-inflammatory analgesics:* There is no specific information on the use of other anti-inflammatory analgesics in children.

Most of these medicines, especially indomethacin and phenylbutazone, can cause serious side effects in any patient. Therefore, it is especially important that you discuss with the child's doctor the good that this medicine may do as well as the risks of using it.

Older adults—Certain side effects, such as confusion, swelling of the face, feet, or lower legs, or sudden decrease in the amount of urine, may be especially likely to occur in elderly patients, who are usually more sensitive than younger adults to the effects of anti-inflammatory analgesics. Also, elderly people are more likely than younger adults to get very sick if these medicines cause stomach problems. With phenylbutazone, blood problems may also be more likely to occur in the elderly.

Other medicines—Although certain medicines should not be used together at all, in other cases two different medicines may be used together even if an interaction might occur. In these cases, your doctor may want to change the dose, or other precautions may be necessary. When you are taking an anti-inflammatory analgesic, it is especially important that your doctor and pharmacist know if you are taking any of the following:

- Amphotericin B by injection (e.g., Fungizone) or
- Antineoplastics (cancer medicine) or
- Antithyroid agents (medicine for overactive thyroid) or
- Azathioprine (e.g., Imuran) or
- Chloramphenicol (e.g., Chloromycetin) or
- Colchicine or
- Cyclophosphamide (e.g., Cytoxan) or
- Flucytosine (e.g., Ancobon) or
- Interferon (e.g., Intron A, Roferon-A) or
- Mercaptopurine (e.g., Purinethol) or
- Penicillamine (e.g., Cuprimine)—The chance of serious side effects may be increased, especially with phenylbutazone
- Anticoagulants (blood thinners) or
- Cefamandole (e.g., Mandol) or
- Cefoperazone (e.g., Cefobid) or
- Cefotetan (e.g., Cefotan) or
- Heparin or
- Moxalactam (e.g., Moxam) or
- Plicamycin (e.g., Mithracin)—The chance of bleeding may be increased
- Aspirin—The chance of serious side effects may be increased if aspirin is used together with an anti-inflammatory analgesic on a regular basis
- Digitalis glycosides (heart medicine) or
- Lithium (e.g., Lithane) or
- Methotrexate (e.g., Mexate) or
- Phenytoin (e.g., Dilantin)—Higher blood levels of these medicines and an increased chance of side effects may occur
- Probenecid (e.g., Benemid)—Higher blood levels of the anti-inflammatory analgesic and an increased chance of side effects may occur
- Triamterene (e.g., Dyrenium)—The chance of kidney problems may be increased, especially with indomethacin
- Zidovudine (e.g., AZT, Retrovir)—The chance of serious side effects may be increased, especially with indomethacin or phenylbutazone

Other medical problems—The presence of other medical problems may affect the use of anti-inflammatory analgesics. Make sure you tell your doctor if you have any other medical problems, especially:

- Alcohol abuse or
- Bleeding problems or
- Colitis, stomach ulcer, or other stomach problems or
- Diabetes mellitus (sugar diabetes) or
- Hepatitis or other liver disease or
- Kidney disease or history of or
- Rectal irritation or bleeding, recent, or
- Systemic lupus erythematosus (SLE) or
- Tobacco use (or recent history of)—The chance of side effects may be increased
- Anemia or
- Asthma or
- Epilepsy or
- Fluid retention (swelling of feet or lower legs) or
- Heart disease or
- High blood pressure or
- Mental illness or
- Parkinson's disease or
- Polymyalgia rheumatica or
- Temporal arteritis—Some anti-inflammatory analgesics may make these conditions worse
- Ulcers, sores, or white spots in mouth—Ulcers, sores, or white spots in the mouth sometimes mean that the medicine is causing serious side effects; if these sores or spots are already present before you start taking the medicine, it will be harder for you and your doctor to recognize that these side effects might be occurring

Before you begin using any new medicine (prescription or nonprescription) or if you develop any new medical problem while you are using this medicine, check with your doctor, nurse, or pharmacist.

Proper Use of This Medicine

For patients taking *a capsule, tablet (including caplet), or liquid form* of this medicine:

- To lessen stomach upset, these medicines should be taken with food or an antacid. This is especially important when you are taking indomethacin, mefenamic acid, phenylbutazone, or piroxicam, which should always be taken with food or an antacid. Your doctor may want you to take the first few doses of other anti-inflammatory analgesics 30 minutes before meals or 2 hours after meals. This helps the medicine to work a little faster when you first begin to take it. However, after the first few doses, take the medicine with food or an antacid.
- It is not necessary to take delayed-release (enteric-coated) tablets with food or an antacid, because the enteric coating helps protect your stomach from the irritating effects of the medicine.
- If you will be taking your medicine together with an antacid, one that contains magnesium and aluminum hydroxides (e.g., Maalox) may be the best kind of antacid to use, unless your doctor has directed you to use another antacid. However, do not mix the liquid form of ibuprofen, indomethacin, or naproxen together with an antacid, or any other liquid, before taking it. To do so may cause the medicine to break down. If stomach upset (indigestion, nausea, vomiting, stomach pain, or diarrhea) continues or if you have any questions about how you should be taking this medicine, check with your doctor, nurse, or pharmacist.
- *Take tablet or capsule forms of these medicines with a full glass (8 ounces) of water.* Also, do not lie down for about 15 to 30 minutes after taking the

medicine. This helps to prevent irritation that may lead to trouble in swallowing.

- Some anti-inflammatory analgesic tablets must be swallowed whole, not crushed or broken. These include diclofenac tablets (e.g., Voltaren), diflunisal tablets (e.g., Dolobid), ketoprofen delayed-release (enteric-coated) tablets (e.g., Orudis-E), ketoprofen extended-release tablets (e.g., Orudis-SR), naproxen extended-release tablets (e.g., Naprosyn-SR), phenylbutazone tablets (e.g., Butazolidin), and phenylbutazone delayed-release (enteric-coated) tablets (e.g., Intrabutazone).

For patients using *a suppository form* of this medicine:

- If the suppository is too soft to insert, chill it in the refrigerator for 30 minutes or run cold water over it before removing the foil wrapper.
- To insert the suppository: First remove the foil wrapper and moisten the suppository with cold water. Lie down on your side and use your finger to push the suppository well up into the rectum.
- Indomethacin suppositories should be kept inside the rectum for at least one hour so that all of the medicine can be absorbed by your body. This helps the medicine work better.

For patients taking *200-mg (nonprescription) strength ibuprofen:*

- This medicine comes with a patient information sheet. Read it carefully. If you have any questions about this information, check with your doctor or pharmacist.

For safe and effective use of this medicine, do not take more of it, do not take it more often, and do not take it for a longer time than ordered by your medical doctor or dentist or directed on the 200-mg (nonprescription) strength ibuprofen package label. Taking too much of any of these medicines may increase the chance of unwanted effects, especially in elderly patients.

When used for severe or continuing arthritis, this medicine must be taken regularly as ordered by your doctor in order for it to help you. These medicines usually begin to work within one week, but in severe cases up to two weeks or even longer may pass before you begin to feel better. Also, several weeks may pass before you feel the full effects of the medicine.

For patients taking *mefenamic acid:*

- *Always take mefenamic acid with food or antacids.*
- *Do not take mefenamic acid for more than 7 days at a time* unless otherwise directed by your doctor. To do so may increase the chance of side effects, especially in elderly patients.

For patients taking *phenylbutazone:*

- Phenylbutazone is intended to treat your current medical problem only. *Do not take it for any other aches or pains.* Also, phenylbutazone should be used for the shortest time possible because of the chance of serious side effects, especially in patients who are 40 years of age or older.

Missed dose—If your medical doctor or dentist has ordered you to take this medicine according to a regular schedule, and you miss a dose, take it as soon as you remember. However, if it is almost time for your next dose, skip the missed dose and go back to your regular dosing schedule. (For long-acting medicines or extended-release dosage forms that are only taken once or twice a day, take the missed dose only if you remember within an hour or two after the dose should have been taken. If you do not remember until later, skip the missed dose and go back to your regular dosing schedule.) Do not double doses.

Storage—To store this medicine:

- Keep out of the reach of children.
- Store away from heat and direct light.
- Do not store tablets or capsules in the bathroom, near the kitchen sink, or in other damp places. Heat or moisture may cause the medicine to break down.
- Keep liquid and suppository forms of this medicine from freezing.
- Do not keep outdated medicine or medicine no longer needed. Be sure that any discarded medicine is out of the reach of children.

Precautions While Using This Medicine

If you will be taking this medicine for a long time, as for arthritis (rheumatism), your doctor should check your progress at regular visits. Your doctor may want to do certain tests to find out if unwanted effects are occurring, especially if you are taking phenylbutazone. The tests are very important because serious side effects, including ulcers, bleeding, or blood problems, can occur without any warning.

Stomach problems may be more likely to occur if you drink alcoholic beverages while being treated with this medicine. Also, alcohol may add to the depressant side effects of phenylbutazone. Therefore, *do not regularly drink alcoholic beverages while taking this medicine,* unless otherwise directed by your doctor.

Taking acetaminophen or aspirin or other salicylates together with an anti-inflammatory analgesic may increase the chance of unwanted effects. The risk will depend on how much of each medicine you take every day, and on how long you take the medicines together. If your medical doctor or dentist directs you to take these medicines together on a regular basis, follow his or her directions carefully. However, *do not take acetaminophen or aspirin or other salicylates together with this medicine for more than a few days, unless your doctor has directed you to do so and is following your progress.*

For patients taking *the buffered form of phenylbutazone (e.g., Alka-Butazolidin):*

- If you are also taking a tetracycline antibiotic, *do not take buffered phenylbutazone within 1 to 3 hours of taking the antibiotic.* Buffered phenylbutazone contains antacids that may make the tetracycline less effective in treating your infection by causing less of it to be absorbed into your body.

Before having any kind of surgery (including dental surgery), tell the medical doctor or dentist in charge that you are taking this medicine.

This medicine may cause some people to become confused, drowsy, dizzy, lightheaded, or less alert than they are normally. They may also cause blurred vision or other vision problems in some people. *Make sure you know how you react to this medicine before you drive, use machines, or do anything else that could be dangerous if you are dizzy or are not alert and able to see well.* If these reactions are especially bothersome, check with your doctor.

For patients taking *mefenamic acid:*

- If diarrhea occurs while you are using this medicine, *stop taking it and check with your doctor immediately. Do not take it again without first checking with your doctor,* because severe diarrhea may occur each time you take it.

Some people who take anti-inflammatory analgesics may become more sensitive to sunlight than they are normally. Exposure to sunlight, even for brief periods of time, may cause severe sunburn; skin rash, redness, itching, or discoloration; or vision changes. When you begin taking this medicine:

- Stay out of direct sunlight, especially between the hours of 10:00 a.m. and 3:00 p.m., if possible.
- Wear protective clothing, including a hat and sunglasses.
- Apply a sun block product that has a skin protection factor (SPF) of at least 15. Some patients may require a product with a higher SPF number, especially if they have a fair complexion. If you have any questions about this, check with your doctor or pharmacist.
- Do not use a sunlamp or tanning bed or booth.

If you have a severe reaction from the sun, check with your doctor.

Serious side effects, including ulcers or bleeding, can occur during treatment with this medicine. Sometimes serious side effects can occur without any warning. However, possible warning signs often occur, including severe abdominal or stomach cramps, pain, or burning; black, tarry stools; severe, continuing nausea, heartburn, or indigestion; and/or vomiting of blood or material that looks like coffee grounds. *Stop taking this medicine and check with your doctor immediately if you notice any of these warning signs.*

Check with your doctor immediately if chills, fever, muscle aches or pains, or other influenza-like symptoms occur, especially if they occur shortly before, or together with, a skin rash. Very rarely, these effects may be the first signs of a serious reaction to this medicine.

Anti-inflammatory analgesics may cause a serious type of allergic reaction called anaphylaxis. Although this is rare, it may occur more often in patients who are allergic to aspirin or to any other anti-inflammatory analgesic. *Anaphylaxis requires immediate medical attention.* The most serious signs of this reaction are very fast or irregular breathing, gasping for breath, wheezing, or fainting. Other signs may include changes in color of the skin of the face; very fast but irregular heartbeat or pulse; hive-like swellings on the skin; and puffiness or swellings of the eyelids or around the eyes. If these effects occur, get emergency help at once. Ask someone to drive you to the nearest hospital emergency room. If this is not possible, do not try to drive yourself. Call an ambulance, lie down, cover yourself to keep warm, and prop your feet higher than your head. Stay in that position until help arrives.

For patients taking *ibuprofen* without a prescription:

- Check with your medical doctor or dentist:
  —if your symptoms do not improve or if they get worse.
  —if you are using this medicine to bring down a fever and the fever lasts more than 3 days or returns.
  —if the painful area becomes red or swollen.

Side Effects of This Medicine

Along with its needed effects, a medicine may cause some unwanted effects. Although not all of these side effects may occur, if they do occur they may need medical attention.

Stop taking this medicine and check with your doctor immediately if any of the following side effects occur:

More common—for mefenamic acid only

Diarrhea

More common—for phenylbutazone only

Swelling of face, hands, feet, or lower legs; weight gain (rapid)

Symptoms of phenylbutazone overdose

Bluish color of fingernails, lips, or skin; headache (severe and continuing)

Rare—for all anti-inflammatory analgesics

Abdominal or stomach pain, cramping, or burning (severe); bloody or black tarry stools; chest pain; convulsions (seizures); fainting; hive-like swellings (large) on face, eyelids, mouth, lips, or tongue; nausea, heartburn, and/or indigestion (severe and continuing);

shortness of breath, troubled breathing, wheezing, or tightness in chest or fast or irregular breathing; sore throat, fever, and chills; sudden decrease in amount of urine; unusual bleeding or bruising; vomiting of blood or material that looks like coffee grounds

Also, check with your doctor as soon as possible if any of the following side effects occur:

More common

Bleeding from rectum (with suppositories); headache (severe), especially in the morning (for indomethacin only); skin rash

Less common or rare

Bleeding or crusting sores on lips; bloody or cloudy urine or any problem with urination, such as difficult, burning, or painful urination; frequent urge to urinate; sudden, large increase in the amount of urine; or loss of bladder control; blurred vision or any change in vision; burning feeling in throat, chest, or stomach; confusion, forgetfulness, mental depression, or other mood or mental changes; cough or hoarseness; decreased hearing, any other change in hearing, or ringing or buzzing in ears; eye pain, irritation, dryness, redness, and/or swelling; fever with or without chills; hallucinations (seeing, hearing, or feeling things that are not there); headache (severe), throbbing, or with fever and stiff neck; hives, itching of skin, or any other skin problem, such as redness, tenderness, burning, peeling, thickening, or scaliness; increased blood pressure; irregular heartbeat; loosening or splitting of fingernails; muscle cramps, pain, or weakness; numbness, tingling, pain, or weakness in hands or feet; pain in lower back and/or side (severe); pinpoint red spots on skin; sores, ulcers, or white spots on lips or in mouth; spitting blood; swelling and/or tenderness in upper abdominal or stomach area; swelling of face, feet, or lower legs (if taking phenylbutazone, stop taking it and check with your doctor immediately); swollen and/or painful glands (especially in the neck or throat area); thirst (continuing); unexplained nosebleeds; unexplained runny nose or sneezing; unexplained, unexpected, or unusually heavy vaginal bleeding; unusual tiredness or weakness; weight gain (rapid) (if taking phenylbutazone, stop taking it and check with your doctor immediately); yellow eyes or skin

Other side effects may occur that usually do not need medical attention. These side effects may go away during treatment as your body adjusts to the medicine. However, check with your doctor if any of the following side effects continue or are bothersome:

More common

Abdominal or stomach cramps, pain, or discomfort (mild to moderate); diarrhea (if taking mefenamic acid, stop taking it and check with your doctor immediately); dizziness, drowsiness, or lightheadedness; headache (mild to moderate); heartburn, indigestion, nausea, or vomiting

Less common or rare

Bitter taste or other taste change; bloated feeling, gas, or constipation; decreased appetite or loss of appetite; fast or pounding heartbeat; flushing or hot flushes; general feeling of discomfort or illness; increased sensitivity of skin to sunlight; increased sweating; irritation, dryness, or soreness of mouth; nervousness, irritability, or trembling; rectal irritation (with suppositories); trouble in sleeping; unexplained weight loss; unusual tiredness or weakness without any other symptoms

Although not all of the side effects listed above have been reported for all of these medicines, they have been reported for at least one of them. However, since all anti-inflammatory analgesics are very similar, it is possible that any of the above side effects may occur with any of these medicines.

Some side effects may occur many days or weeks after you have stopped using phenylbutazone. During this time *check with your doctor immediately* if you notice any of the following side effects:

Sore throat and fever; ulcers, sores, or white spots in mouth; unusual bleeding or bruising; unusual tiredness or weakness

Other side effects not listed above may also occur in some patients. If you notice any other effects, check with your doctor.

Annual revision: June 1990

ANTIMYASTHENICS Systemic

This information applies to the following medicines:

Ambenonium (am-be-NOE-nee-um)
Neostigmine (nee-oh-STIG-meen)
Pyridostigmine (peer-id-oh-STIG-meen)

Some commonly used brand names are:

For Ambenonium†
In the U.S.
Mytelase Caplets

For Neostigmine
In the U.S.
Prostigmin

Generic name product may also be available.

In Canada
Prostigmin

For Pyridostigmine
In the U.S.
Mestinon
Mestinon Timespans
Regonol

In Canada
Mestinon
Mestinon-SR
Regonol

†Not commercially available in Canada.

Description

Antimyasthenics are given by mouth or by injection to treat myasthenia gravis. Neostigmine may also be given by injection as a test for myasthenia gravis. Sometimes neostigmine is given by injection to prevent or treat certain urinary tract or intestinal disorders. In addition, neostigmine or pyridostigmine may be given by injection as an antidote to certain types of muscle relaxants used in surgery.

These medicines are available only with your doctor's prescription in the following dosage forms:

Oral

Ambenonium
- Tablets (U.S.)

Neostigmine
- Tablets (U.S. and Canada)

Pyridostigmine
- Syrup (U.S.)
- Tablets (U.S. and Canada)
- Extended-release tablets (U.S. and Canada)

Parenteral

Neostigmine
- Injection (U.S. and Canada)

Pyridostigmine
- Injection (U.S. and Canada)

It is very important that you read and understand the following information. If any of it causes you special concern, check with your doctor. Also, *if you have any questions* or if you want more information about this medicine or your medical problem, *ask your doctor, nurse, or pharmacist.*

Before Using This Medicine

In deciding to use a medicine, the risks of taking the medicine must be weighed against the good it will do. This is a decision you and your doctor will make. For the antimyasthenics, the following should be considered:

Allergies—Tell your doctor if you have ever had any unusual or allergic reaction to ambenonium, bromides, neostigmine, or pyridostigmine. Also tell your doctor and pharmacist if you are allergic to any other substances, such as foods, preservatives, or dyes.

Pregnancy—Antimyasthenics have not been reported to cause birth defects; however, muscle weakness has occurred temporarily in some newborn babies whose mothers took antimyasthenics during pregnancy.

Breast-feeding—Antimyasthenics have not been reported to cause problems in nursing babies.

Children—Although there is no specific information comparing use of antimyasthenics in children with use in other age groups, these medicines are not expected to cause different side effects or problems in children than they do in adults.

Older adults—Many medicines have not been studied specifically in older people. Therefore, it may not be known whether they work exactly the same way they do in younger adults. Although there is not much information comparing use of antimyasthenics in the elderly with use in other age groups, these medicines are not expected to cause different side effects or problems in older people than they do in younger adults.

Other medicines—Although certain medicines should not be used together at all, in other cases 2 different medicines may be used together even if an interaction might occur. In these cases, your doctor may want to change the dose, or other precautions may be necessary. When you are taking an antimyasthenic, it is especially important that your doctor and pharmacist know if you are using any of the following:

- Demecarium (e.g., Humorsol) or
- Echothiophate (e.g., Phospholine Iodide) or
- Isoflurophate (e.g., Floropryl) or
- Malathion (e.g., Prioderm)—Using these medicines with antimyasthenics may result in serious side effects
- Guanadrel (e.g., Hylorel) or
- Guanethidine (e.g., Ismelin) or
- Mecamylamine (e.g., Inversine) or
- Procainamide (e.g., Pronestyl) or
- Trimethaphan (e.g., Arfonad)—The effects of these medicines may interfere with the actions of the antimyasthenics

Other medical problems—The presence of other medical problems may affect the use of the antimyasthenics. Make sure you tell your doctor if you have any other medical problems, especially:

- Intestinal blockage or
- Urinary tract blockage or
- Urinary tract infection—These medicines may make the condition worse

Proper Use of This Medicine

Your doctor may want you to take this medicine with food or milk to help lessen the chance of side effects. If you have any questions about how you should be taking this medicine, check with your doctor.

Take this medicine only as directed. Do not take more of it, do not take it more often, and do not take it for a longer time than your doctor ordered. To do so may increase the chance of side effects.

If you are taking this medicine *for myasthenia gravis*:

- When you first begin taking this medicine, your doctor may want you to keep a daily record of:
  —the time you take each dose.
  —how long you feel better after taking each dose.
  —how long you feel worse.
  —any side effects that occur.

This is to help your doctor decide whether the dose of this medicine should be increased or decreased and how often the medicine should be taken in order for it to be most effective in your condition.

Missed dose—If you miss a dose of this medicine, take it as soon as you remember. However, if it is almost time for your next dose, skip the missed dose and go back to your regular dosing schedule. Do not double doses.

Storage—To store this medicine:

- Keep out of the reach of children.
- Store away from heat and direct light.
- Do not store the tablet form of this medicine in the bathroom, near the kitchen sink, or in other damp places. Heat or moisture may cause the medicine to break down.
- Keep the syrup form of pyridostigmine from freezing.
- Do not keep outdated medicine or medicine no longer needed. Be sure that any discarded medicine is out of the reach of children.

Side Effects of This Medicine

Along with its needed effects, a medicine may cause some unwanted effects. Although not all of these side effects may occur, if they do occur they may need medical attention.

Check with your doctor immediately if any of the following side effects occur:

Symptoms of overdose

Blurred vision; clumsiness or unsteadiness; confusion; convulsions (seizures); diarrhea (severe); increase in bronchial secretions or watering of mouth (excessive); increasing muscle weakness (especially in the arms, neck, shoulders, and tongue); muscle cramps or twitching; nausea or vomiting (severe); shortness of breath, troubled breathing, wheezing, or tightness in chest; slow heartbeat; slurred speech; stomach cramps or pain (severe); unusual irritability, nervousness, restlessness, or fear; unusual tiredness or weakness

Also, check with your doctor as soon as possible if any of the following side effects occur:

Rare

Redness, swelling, or pain at place of injection (for pyridostigmine injection only); skin rash (does not apply to ambenonium)

Other side effects may occur that usually do not need medical attention. These side effects may go away during treatment as your body adjusts to the medicine. However, check with your doctor if any of the following side effects continue or are bothersome:

More common

Diarrhea; increased sweating; increased watering of mouth; nausea or vomiting; stomach cramps or pain

Less common

Frequent urge to urinate; increase in bronchial secretions; unusually small pupils; unusual watering of eyes

Other side effects not listed above may also occur in some patients. If you notice any other effects, check with your doctor.

Annual revision: 09/30/91

ANTIPYRINE AND BENZOCAINE Otic

Some commonly used brand names are:

In the U.S.

- Aurafair
- Auralgan
- Aurodex
- Oto

In Canada

- Auralgan

Description

Antipyrine (an-tee-PYE-reen) and benzocaine (BEN-zoe-kane) combination is used in the ear to help relieve the pain, swelling, and redness of some ear infections. It will not cure the infection itself. This medicine is also used to help remove ear wax.

In the U.S., this medicine is available only with your doctor's prescription. In Canada, this medicine is available without a prescription. However, your doctor may have special instructions on the proper dose for your ear problem. This medicine is available in the following dosage form:

Otic

- Otic solution (U.S. and Canada)

It is very important that you read and understand the following information. If any of it causes you special concern, check with your doctor or pharmacist. Also, *if you have any questions* or if you want more information about this medicine or your medical problem, *ask your doctor, nurse, or pharmacist.*

Before Using This Medicine

In deciding to use a medicine, the risks of using the medicine must be weighed against the good it will do. This is a decision you and your doctor will make. For antipyrine and benzocaine combination, the following should be considered:

Allergies—Tell your doctor if you have ever had any unusual or allergic reaction to antipyrine or benzocaine or other local anesthetics. Also tell your doctor and pharmacist if you are allergic to any other substances, such as foods, preservatives, or dyes.

Pregnancy—Although studies on effects in pregnancy have not been done in either humans or animals, this medicine has not been reported to cause problems in humans.

Breast-feeding—It is not known whether this medicine passes into the breast milk. However, this medicine has not been reported to cause problems in nursing babies.

Children—This medicine has been tested in children and, in effective doses, has not been shown to cause different side effects or problems than it does in adults.

Older adults—Many medicines have not been studied specifically in older people. Therefore, it may not be known whether they work exactly the same way they do in younger adults. Although there is no specific information comparing use of antipyrine and benzocaine in the elderly with use in other age groups, this medicine is not expected to cause different side effects or problems in older people than it does in younger adults.

Other medical problems—The presence of other medical problems may affect the use of antipyrine and benzocaine combination. Make sure you tell your doctor if:

- Your ear is draining—The chance of unwanted effects may be increased

Proper Use of This Medicine

You may warm the ear drops to body temperature (37 °C or 98.6 °F) by holding the bottle in your hand for a few minutes before applying the drops.

To use:

- Lie down or tilt the head so that the affected ear faces up. Gently pull the earlobe up and back for adults (down and back for children) to straighten the ear canal. Drop the medicine into the ear canal. Keep the ear facing up for about 5 minutes to allow the medicine to be absorbed. A sterile cotton plug may be moistened with a few drops of this medicine and gently inserted into the ear opening to prevent the medicine from leaking out.
- To keep the medicine as germ-free as possible, do not touch the dropper to any surface (including the ear).
- *Do not rinse the dropper after use.* Wipe the tip of the dropper with a clean tissue and keep the container tightly closed.

If you are using this medicine to help remove ear wax, the ear should be flushed with warm water after you have used this medicine for 2 or 3 days. Make sure that you know how to do this. If you have any questions about how to flush the ear with water, check with your doctor.

Missed dose—If you miss a dose of this medicine, use it as soon as you remember. However, if it is almost time for your next dose, skip the missed dose and go back to your regular dosing schedule.

Storage—To store this medicine:

- Keep out of the reach of children.
- Store away from heat and direct light.
- Keep the medicine from freezing.
- Do not keep outdated medicine or medicine no longer needed. Be sure that any discarded medicine is out of the reach of children.

Side Effects of This Medicine

Along with its needed effects, a medicine may cause some unwanted effects. Check with your doctor if either effect continues or is bothersome:

Itching or burning in the ear

Other side effects not listed above may also occur in some patients. If you notice any other effects, check with your doctor.

Annual revision: 09/14/91

ANTITHYROID AGENTS Systemic

This information applies to the following medicines:

Methimazole (meth-IM-a-zole)
Propylthiouracil (proe-pill-thye-oh-YOOR-a-sill)

Some commonly used brand names are:

For Methimazole

In the U.S.
Tapazole

In Canada
Tapazole

Another commonly used name for methimazole is thiamazole.

For Propylthiouracil

In the U.S.
Available as generic name product.

In Canada
Propyl-Thyracil

Description

Methimazole and propylthiouracil are used to treat conditions in which the thyroid gland produces too much thyroid hormone.

These medicines work by making it harder for the body to use iodine to make thyroid hormone. They do not block the effects of thyroid hormone that was made by the body before their use was begun.

Methimazole and propylthiouracil are available only with your doctor's prescription, in the following dosage forms:

Oral

Methimazole
- Tablets (U.S. and Canada)

Propylthiouracil
- Tablets (U.S. and Canada)

It is very important that you read and understand the following information. If any of it causes you special concern, check with your doctor. Also, *if you have any questions* or if you want more information about this medicine or your medical problem, *ask your doctor, nurse, or pharmacist.*

Before Using This Medicine

In deciding to use a medicine, the risks of taking the medicine must be weighed against the good it will do. This is a decision you and your doctor will make. For antithyroid agents, the following should be considered:

Allergies—Tell your doctor if you have ever had any unusual or allergic reaction to methimazole or propylthiouracil. Also tell your doctor and pharmacist if you are allergic to any other substances, such as foods, preservatives, or dyes.

Pregnancy—Use of too large a dose during pregnancy may cause problems in the fetus. However, use of the proper dose, with careful monitoring by the doctor, is not likely to cause problems.

Breast-feeding—These medicines pass into breast milk. (Methimazole passes into breast milk more freely and in higher amounts than propylthiouracil.) However, your doctor may allow you to continue to breast-feed, if your dose is low and the infant gets frequent check-ups. If you are taking a large dose, it may be necessary for you to stop breast-feeding during treatment.

Children—This medicine has been used in children and, in effective doses, has not been shown to cause different side effects or problems in children than it does in adults.

Teenagers—This medicine has been used in teenagers and, in effective doses, has not been shown to cause different side effects or problems in teenagers than it does in adults.

Older adults—Elderly people may have an increased chance of certain side effects during treatment. Your doctor may need to take special precautions while you are taking this medicine.

Other medicines—Although certain medicines should not be used together at all, in other cases two different medicines may be used together even if an interaction might occur. In these cases, your doctor may want to change the dose, or other precautions may be necessary. When you are taking antithyroid agents, it is especially important that your doctor and pharmacist know if you are taking any of the following:

- Amiodarone or
- Iodinated glycerol or
- Potassium iodide (e.g., Pima)—The use of these medicines may change the effect of antithyroid agents
- Anticoagulants (blood thinners)—The use of antithyroid agents may affect the way anticoagulants work in your body
- Digitalis glycosides—The use of antithyroid agents may affect the amount of digitalis glycosides in the bloodstream

Other medical problems—The presence of other medical problems may affect the use of antithyroid agents. Make sure you tell your doctor if you have any other medical problems, especially:

- Liver disease—The body may not get this medicine out of the bloodstream at the usual rate, which may increase the chance of side effects

Before you begin using any new medicine (prescription or nonprescription) or if you develop any new medical problem while you are using this medicine, check with your doctor, nurse, or pharmacist.

Proper Use of This Medicine

Use this medicine only as directed by your doctor. Do not use more or less of it and do not use it more often or for a longer time than your doctor ordered. To do so may increase the chance of side effects.

This medicine works best when there is a constant amount in the blood. *To help keep the amount constant, do not miss any doses. Also, if you are taking more than one dose a day, it is best to take the doses at evenly spaced times day and night.* For example, if you are to take 3 doses a day, the doses should be spaced about 8 hours apart. If this interferes with your sleep or other daily activities, or if you need help in planning the best times to take your medicine, check with your doctor, nurse, or pharmacist.

Food in your stomach may change the amount of methimazole that is able to enter the bloodstream. To make sure that you always get the same effects, try to take methimazole at the same time in relation to meals every day. That is, always take it with meals or always take it on an empty stomach.

Missed dose—If you miss a dose of this medicine, take it as soon as possible. If it is almost time for your next dose, take both doses together. Then go back to your regular dosing schedule. If you miss more than one dose or if you have any questions about this, check with your doctor.

Storage—To store this medicine:

- Keep out of the reach of children.
- Store away from heat and direct light.
- Do not store in the bathroom, near the kitchen sink, or in other high-moisture areas. Heat or moisture may cause the medicine to break down.
- Do not keep outdated medicine or medicine no longer needed. Be sure that any discarded medicine is out of the reach of children.

Precautions While Using This Medicine

It is very important that your doctor check your progress at regular visits to make sure that this medicine is working properly and to check for unwanted effects.

It may take several days or weeks for this medicine to work. However, *do not stop taking this medicine without first checking with your doctor.* Some medical problems may require several years of continuous treatment.

Before having any kind of surgery (including dental surgery) or emergency treatment, *tell the medical doctor or dentist in charge that you are taking this medicine.*

Check with your doctor right away if you get an injury, infection, or illness of any kind. Your doctor may want you to stop taking this medicine or change the amount you are taking.

While you are being treated with antithyroid agents, and after you stop treatment with it, *do not have any immunizations (vaccinations) without your doctor's approval.* Antithyroid agents may lower your body's resistance and there is a chance you might get the infection the immunization is meant to prevent. In addition, other persons living in your household should not take or have recently taken oral polio vaccine since there is a chance they could pass the polio virus on to you. Also, avoid other persons who have taken oral polio vaccine. Do not get close to them, and do not stay in the same room with them for very long. If you cannot take these precautions, you should consider wearing a protective face mask that covers the nose and mouth.

Before you have any medical tests, tell the doctor in charge that you are taking this medicine. The results of some tests may be affected by this medicine.

Side Effects of This Medicine

Along with its needed effects, a medicine may cause some unwanted effects. Although not all of these side effects may occur, if they do occur they may need medical attention.

Check with your doctor immediately if any of the following side effects occur:

Less common

Cough; fever or chills (continuing or severe); general feeling of discomfort, illness or weakness; hoarseness; mouth sores; pain, swelling, or redness in joints; throat infection

Rare

Yellow eyes or skin

Check with your doctor as soon as possible if any of the following side effects occur:

More common

Fever (mild and temporary); skin rash or itching

Rare

Backache; black, tarry stools; blood in urine or stools; shortness of breath; increase in bleeding or bruising; increase or decrease in urination; numbness or tingling of fingers, toes, or face; pinpoint red spots on skin; swelling of feet or lower legs; swollen lymph nodes; swollen salivary glands

Symptoms of overdose

Changes in menstrual periods; coldness; constipation; dry, puffy skin; headache; listlessness or sleepiness; muscle aches; swelling in the front of the neck; unusual tiredness or weakness; weight gain (unusual)

Other side effects may occur that usually do not need medical attention. These side effects may go away during treatment as your body adjusts to the medicine. However, check with your doctor if any of the following side effects continue or are bothersome:

Less common

Dizziness; loss of taste (for methimazole); nausea; stomach pain; vomiting

Other side effects not listed above may also occur in some patients. If you notice any other effects, check with your doctor.

Annual revision: 04/21/92

APOMORPHINE Systemic†

Available in the U.S. as generic name product.

†Not commercially available in Canada.

Description

Apomorphine (a-poe-MOR-feen) is used in the emergency treatment of certain types of poisoning and overdose. It is given by injection to cause vomiting of the poison. However, it has generally been replaced by syrup of ipecac for the treatment of poisonings and overdoses.

Ordinarily, apomorphine is not used if strychnine, corrosives such as alkalies (lye) and strong acids, or petroleum products such as kerosene, gasoline, coal oil, fuel oil, paint thinner, or cleaning fluid have been swallowed, since it may cause seizures, additional injury to the throat, or pneumonia. Also, it should not be given to unconscious or very drowsy persons, since the vomited material may enter the lungs and cause pneumonia.

This medicine may also be used for other conditions as determined by your doctor.

Apomorphine is available only on prescription and should be administered only by or under the immediate supervision of a doctor. It is available in the following dosage form:

Parenteral

- Injection (U.S.)

It is very important that you read and understand the following information. If any of it causes you special concern, check with your doctor. Also, *if you have any questions* or if you want more information about this medicine or your medical problem, *ask your doctor, nurse, or pharmacist.*

Before Receiving This Medicine

In deciding to use a medicine, the risks of taking the medicine must be weighed against the good it will do. This is a decision you and your doctor will make. For apomorphine, the following should be considered:

Allergies—Tell your doctor if you have ever had any unusual or allergic reaction to codeine, hydromorphone, levorphanol, morphine, opium alkaloids, oxycodone, or oxymorphone.

Pregnancy—Studies have not been done in either humans or animals.

Breast-feeding—Apomorphine has not been reported to cause problems in nursing babies.

Children—Children are especially sensitive to the effects of apomorphine. This may increase the chance of side effects during treatment.

Older adults—Elderly people are especially sensitive to the effects of apomorphine. This may increase the chance of side effects during treatment.

Other medicines—Although certain medicines should not be used together at all, in other cases two different medicines may be used together even if an interaction might occur. In these cases, your doctor may want to change the dose, or other precautions may be necessary. When you are going to receive apomorphine, it is especially important that your doctor know if you are taking any of the following:

- Antiemetics (medicine for nausea or vomiting)—The antiemetic medicine may decrease the effect of apomorphine; also, CNS depressant effects, such as drowsiness, may be increased

Other medical problems—The presence of other medical problems may affect the use of apomorphine. Make sure you tell your doctor if you have any other medical problems, especially:

- Heart disease
- Nausea and vomiting (predisposition to)
- Seizures (epilepsy)

Proper Use of This Medicine

Immediately after receiving an injection of this medicine, adults should drink a full glass (8 ounces) of water and children should drink ½ to 1 full glass (4 to 8 ounces) of water. This is to help the medicine cause vomiting of the poison.

Side Effects of This Medicine

Along with its needed effects, a medicine may cause some unwanted effects. Although not all of these side effects may occur, if they do occur they may need medical attention.

Check with your doctor or nurse immediately if any of the following side effects occur:

Drowsiness (severe); shortness of breath or troubled breathing; slow heartbeat; vomiting (continuing)

Other side effects may occur that usually do not need medical attention. These side effects may go away during treatment as your body adjusts to the medicine. However, check with your doctor if any of the following side effects continue or are bothersome:

More common

Drowsiness; increased sweating; increased watering of mouth; nausea; unusual tiredness or weakness

Less common or rare

Dizziness or lightheadedness especially when getting up from a lying or sitting position (more common in patients with Parkinson's disease); false sense of well-being; fast heartbeat; fast or irregular breathing; restlessness; trembling

Other side effects not listed above may also occur in some patients. If you notice any other effects, check with your doctor.

Additional Information

Once a medicine has been approved for marketing for a certain use, experience may show that it is also useful for other medical problems. Although this use is not included in product labeling, apomorphine is used in certain patients with Parkinson's disease.

For patients receiving this medicine *as part of the treatment for Parkinson's disease*:

- Drowsiness, dizziness or lightheadedness, especially when getting up from a lying or sitting position, and mild nausea and vomiting may occur. However, these effects do not last long.

There is no additional information relating to proper use, precautions, or side effects for this use.

Annual revision: 09/04/91

APPETITE SUPPRESSANTS Systemic

This information applies to the following medicines:

Benzphetamine (benz-FET-a-meen)
Diethylpropion (dye-eth-il-PROE-pee-on)
Mazindol (MAY-zin-dole)
Phendimetrazine (fen-dye-MET-ra-zeen)
Phentermine (FEN-ter-meen)

Note: This information does *not* apply to Fenfluramine or Phenylpropanolamine.

Some commonly used brand names are:

For Benzphetamine†
In the U.S.
Didrex

Another commonly used name is benzfetamine.

For Diethylpropion
In the U.S.
M-Orexic
Tenuate
Tenuate Dospan
Tepanil
Tepanil Ten-Tab

Generic name product may also be available.

In Canada
Nobesine-75
Tenuate
Tenuate Dospan

Another commonly used name is amfepramone.

For Mazindol
In the U.S.
Mazanor
Sanorex

In Canada
Sanorex

For Phendimetrazine†
In the U.S.
Adipost
Anorex
Appecon
Bacarate
Bontril PDM
Bontril Slow-Release
Dital
Dyrexan-OD
Marlibar A
Melfiat-105 Unicelles
Metra
Neocurb
Obalan
Obe-Del
Obeval
Obezine
Panrexin M
Panrexin MTP
Parzine
Phendiet
Phendiet-105
Phendimet
Phentra
Plegine
Prelu-2
PT 105
Rexigen
Rexigen Forte
Slyn-LL
Statobex
Tega-Nil
Trimcaps
Trimstat
Trimtabs
Wehless
Wehless-105 Timecelles
Weightrol
Wescoid
X-Trozine
X-Trozine LA

Generic name product may also be available.

For Phentermine
In the U.S.
Adipex-P
Dapex-37.5
Fastin
Ionamin
Obe-Mar
Obe-Nix
Obephen
Obermine
Obestin-30
Oby-Trim
Panshape
Phentercot
Phentride
Phentride Caplets
Phentrol
Phentrol 2
Phentrol 4
Phentrol 5
T-Diet
Teramin
Wilpowr
Zantryl

Generic name product may also be available.

In Canada
- Fastin
- Ionamin

†Not commercially available in Canada.

Description

Appetite suppressants are used in the short-term treatment of obesity. For a few weeks, these medicines in combination with dieting, exercise, and changes in eating habits can help obese patients lose weight. However, since their appetite-reducing effect is only temporary, they are useful only for the first few weeks of dieting until new eating habits are established.

These medicines are available only with your doctor's prescription, in the following dosage forms:

Oral

Benzphetamine
- Tablets (U.S.)

Diethylpropion
- Extended-release capsules (Canada)
- Tablets (U.S. and Canada)
- Extended-release tablets (U.S. and Canada)

Mazindol
- Tablets (U.S. and Canada)

Phendimetrazine
- Capsules (U.S.)
- Extended-release capsules (U.S.)
- Tablets (U.S.)
- Extended-release tablets (U.S.)

Phentermine
- Capsules (U.S. and Canada)
- Resin capsules (U.S. and Canada)
- Tablets (U.S.)

It is very important that you read and understand the following information. If any of it causes you special concern, check with your doctor. Also, *if you have any questions* or if you want more information about this medicine or your medical problem, *ask your doctor, nurse, or pharmacist.*

Before Using This Medicine

In deciding to use a medicine, the risks of taking the medicine must be weighed against the good it will do. This is a decision you and your doctor will make. For appetite suppressants, the following should be considered:

Allergies—Tell your doctor if you have ever had any unusual or allergic reaction to this medicine or amphetamine, dextroamphetamine, ephedrine, epinephrine, isoproterenol, metaproterenol, methamphetamine, norepinephrine, phenylephrine, phenylpropanolamine, pseudoephedrine, terbutaline, or other appetite suppressants. Also tell your doctor and pharmacist if you are allergic to any other substances, such as foods, preservatives, or dyes.

Pregnancy—
- *Benzphetamine*—Benzphetamine must not be used during pregnancy because it may harm the fetus. Be sure you have discussed this with your doctor. If you think you may have become pregnant during treatment with benzphetamine, tell your doctor immediately.
- *Diethylpropion*—Diethylpropion has not been reported to cause birth defects or other problems in human and animal studies.
- *Mazindol*—Studies in animals have shown that mazindol increases the chance of rib malformations, and also increases the chance of death in the newborn when given in large doses.
- *Phendimetrazine* and *phentermine*—These medicines have not been shown to cause birth defects or other problems in humans.

Breast-feeding—Diethylpropion and benzphetamine are excreted in breast milk. It is not known if other appetite suppressants are excreted in breast milk. However, problems in nursing babies have not been reported.

Children—Appetite suppressants should not be used by children up to 12 years of age.

Older adults—Many medicines have not been studied specifically in older people. Therefore, it may not be known whether they work exactly the same way they do in younger adults or if they cause different side effects or problems in older people. There is no specific information comparing use of appetite suppressants in the elderly to use in other age groups.

Other medicines—Although certain medicines should not be used together at all, in other cases two different medicines may be used together even if an interaction might occur. In these cases, your doctor may want to change the dose, or other precautions may be necessary. When you are taking appetite suppressants, it is especially important that your doctor and pharmacist know if you are taking any of the following:
- Amantadine (e.g., Symmetrel) or
- Amphetamines or
- Caffeine (e.g., NoDoz) or
- Chlophedianol (e.g., Ulone) or
- Cocaine or
- Medicine for asthma or other breathing problems or
- Medicine for colds, sinus problems, or hay fever or other allergies (including nose drops or sprays) or
- Methylphenidate (e.g., Ritalin) or
- Nabilone (e.g., Cesamet) or
- Other appetite suppressants (diet pills) or
- Pemoline (e.g., Cylert)—Using these medicines with appetite suppressants may increase the CNS stimulant effects
- Monoamine oxidase (MAO) inhibitors (furazolidone [e.g., Furoxone], isocarboxazid [e.g., Marplan], phenelzine [e.g., Nardil], procarbazine [e.g., Matulane], selegiline [e.g., Eldepryl], tranylcypromine [e.g., Parnate])—Taking appetite suppressants while you are taking or within 2 weeks

of taking monoamine oxidase (MAO) inhibitors may cause sudden extremely high blood pressure; at least 14 days should be allowed between stopping treatment with one medicine and starting treatment with the other

Other medical problems—The presence of other medical problems may affect the use of appetite suppressants. Make sure you tell your doctor if you have any other medical problems, especially:

- Alcohol abuse (or history of) or
- Drug abuse or dependence (or history of)—Dependence on appetite suppressants may develop
- Diabetes mellitus (sugar diabetes)—The amount of insulin or oral antidiabetic medicine that you need to take may change
- Epilepsy—Diethylpropion may increase the risk of seizures
- Glaucoma or
- Heart or blood vessel disease or
- High blood pressure or
- Mental illness (severe) or
- Overactive thyroid—Appetite suppressants may make the condition worse
- Kidney disease—Higher blood levels of mazindol may occur, increasing the chance of serious side effects

Before you begin using any new medicine (prescription or nonprescription) or if you develop any new medical problem while you are using this medicine, check with your doctor, nurse, or pharmacist.

Proper Use of This Medicine

For patients taking the *short-acting form* of this medicine:

- Take the last dose for each day about 4 to 6 hours before bedtime to help prevent trouble in sleeping.

For patients taking the *long-acting form* of this medicine:

- Take the daily dose about 10 to 14 hours before bedtime to help prevent trouble in sleeping.
- These capsules or tablets are to be swallowed whole. Do not break, crush, or chew before swallowing.

For patients taking *mazindol*:

- To help prevent trouble in sleeping, if you are taking this medicine in a:

  —*1-mg tablet,* take the last dose for each day about 4 to 6 hours before bedtime.

  —*2-mg tablet,* take the dose once each day about 10 to 14 hours before bedtime.

Take this medicine only as directed by your doctor. Do not take more of it, do not take it more often, and do not take it for a longer time than your doctor ordered. If too much is taken, it may become habit-forming.

If you think this medicine is not working properly after you have taken it for a few weeks, *do not increase the dose.* Instead, check with your doctor.

Storage—To store this medicine:

- Keep out of the reach of children.
- Store away from heat and direct light.
- Do not store in the bathroom, near the kitchen sink, or in other damp places. Heat or moisture may cause the medicine to break down.
- Do not keep outdated medicine or medicine no longer needed. Be sure that any discarded medicine is out of the reach of children.

Precautions While Using This Medicine

Your doctor should check your progress at regular visits to make sure that this medicine does not cause unwanted effects.

This medicine may cause some people to feel a false sense of well-being or to become dizzy, lightheaded, drowsy, or less alert than they are normally. *Make sure you know how you react to this medicine before you drive, use machines, or do anything else that could be dangerous if you are dizzy or are not alert.*

Before having any kind of surgery, dental treatment, or emergency treatment, tell the medical doctor or dentist in charge that you are using this medicine.

If you have been taking this medicine for a long time or in large doses and *you think you may have become mentally or physically dependent on it, check with your doctor.*

- Some signs of dependence on appetite suppressants are:

  —a strong desire or need to continue taking the medicine.

  —a need to increase the dose to receive the effects of the medicine.

  —withdrawal side effects (for example, mental depression, nausea or vomiting, stomach cramps or pain, trembling, unusual tiredness or weakness when you stop taking the medicine).

For *diabetic patients*:

- This medicine may affect blood sugar levels. If you notice a change in the results of your urine or blood sugar test or if you have any questions, check with your doctor.

If you have been taking this medicine in large doses for a long time, *do not stop taking it without first checking with your doctor.* Your doctor may want you to reduce gradually the amount you are taking before stopping completely.

Side Effects of This Medicine

Along with its needed effects, a medicine may cause some unwanted effects. Although not all of these side effects may occur, if they do occur they may need medical attention.

Check with your doctor as soon as possible if any of the following side effects occur:

More common

Increased blood pressure

Less common or rare

Confusion or mental depression; mental illness; skin rash or hives; sore throat and fever; unusual bleeding or bruising

Symptoms of overdose

Abdominal or stomach cramps; diarrhea (severe); fast breathing; fever; hallucinations (seeing, hearing or feeling things that are not there); high or low blood pressure; hostility; irregular heartbeat; nausea or vomiting (severe); panic state; restlessness; tremor

Other side effects may occur that usually do not need medical attention. These side effects may go away during treatment as your body adjusts to the medicine. However, check with your doctor if any of the following side effects continue or are bothersome:

More common

False sense of well-being; irritability; nervousness or restlessness; trouble in sleeping

Note: After these stimulant effects have worn off, drowsiness, trembling, unusual tiredness or weakness, or mental depression may occur.

Less common or rare

Blurred vision; changes in sexual desire or decreased sexual ability; constipation; diarrhea; difficult or painful urination; dizziness or lightheadedness; drowsiness; dryness of mouth; fast or pounding heartbeat; frequent urge to urinate or increased urination; headache; increased sweating; nausea or vomiting; stomach cramps or pain; unpleasant taste

Although not all of the side effects listed above have been reported for all of these medicines, they have been reported for at least one of them. However, since all of the appetite suppressants are very similar, any of the above side effects may occur with any of these medicines.

After you stop using this medicine, your body may need time to adjust. The length of time this takes depends on the amount of medicine you were using and how long you used it. During this time check with your doctor if you notice any of the following side effects:

Mental depression; nausea or vomiting; stomach cramps or pain; trembling; unusual tiredness or weakness

Other side effects not listed above may also occur in some patients. If you notice any other effects, check with your doctor.

Annual revision: 06/25/91

APRACLONIDINE Ophthalmic†

A commonly used brand name in the U.S. is Iopidine.

Other commonly used names are aplonidine and p-aminoclonidine.

†Not commercially available in Canada.

Description

Apraclonidine (a-pra-KLOE-ni-deen) is used just before and after certain types of eye surgery (argon laser trabeculoplasty, argon laser iridotomy, and Nd YAG laser posterior capsulotomy). The medicine is used to control or prevent a rise in pressure within the eye that can occur after this type of surgery.

This medicine is given in the hospital at the time of the surgery in the following dosage form:

Ophthalmic

- Ophthalmic solution (eye drops) (U.S.)

It is very important that you read and understand the following information. If any of it causes you special concern, check with your doctor. Also, *if you have any questions* or if you want more information about this medicine or your medical problem, *ask your doctor, nurse, or pharmacist.*

Before Receiving This Medicine

In deciding to use a medicine, the risks of using the medicine must be weighed against the good it will do. This is a decision you and your doctor will make. For apraclonidine, the following should be considered:

Allergies—Tell your doctor if you have ever had any unusual or allergic reaction to apraclonidine or clonidine. Also tell your doctor and pharmacist if you are allergic to any other substances, such as preservatives.

Pregnancy—Studies on effects in pregnancy have not been done in either humans or animals.

Breast-feeding—It is not known whether apraclonidine passes into the breast milk. However, your doctor may want you to stop breast-feeding during the day of your surgery.

Children—Studies on this medicine have been done only in adult patients, and there is no specific information comparing use of apraclonidine in children with use in other age groups.

Older adults—Many medicines have not been studied specifically in older people. Therefore, it may not be known whether they work exactly the same way they do in younger adults or if they cause different side effects or problems in older people. There is no specific information comparing use of apraclonidine in the elderly with use in other age groups.

Other medicines—Although certain medicines should not be used together at all, in other cases two different medicines may be used together even if an interaction might occur. In these cases, your doctor may want to change the dose, or other precautions may be necessary. Tell your doctor and pharmacist if you are using any other prescription or nonprescription (over-the-counter [OTC]) medicine.

Other medical problems—The presence of other medical problems may affect the use of apraclonidine. Make sure you tell your doctor if you have any other medical problems, especially:

- Heart or blood vessel disease or
- High blood pressure—Apraclonidine may make the condition worse
- Unusual reaction to a medicine that reduces the pressure within the eye—Apraclonidine is a strong reducer of eye pressure
- Vasovagal attack (history of)—The signs and symptoms are paleness, nausea, sweating, slow heartbeat, sudden and severe tiredness or weakness, and possibly fainting, usually brought on by emotional stress caused by fear or pain. Apraclonidine may cause this reaction to happen again

Side Effects of This Medicine

Along with its needed effects, a medicine may cause some unwanted effects. Although not all of these side effects may occur, if they do occur they may need medical attention.

Check with your doctor or nurse as soon as possible if the following side effect occurs:

Less common or rare

Irregular heartbeat

Check with your doctor or nurse if any of the following side effects continue or are bothersome:

More common

Increase in size of pupil of eye; paleness of eye or inner lining of eyelid; raising of upper eyelid

Less common or rare

Redness of eye or inner lining of eyelid; swelling of eyelid; watering of eye

Other side effects not listed above may also occur in some patients. If you notice any other effects, check with your doctor or nurse.

Annual revision: 11/21/91

ASCORBIC ACID (Vitamin C) Systemic

Some commonly used brand names are:

In the U.S.

Ascorbicap
Cebid Timecelles
Cecon
Cee-500
Cemill
Cenolate
Cetane
Cetane 500
Cevalin
Cevi-Bid
Ce-Vi-Sol
Flavorcee
Sunkist

Generic name product may also be available.

In Canada

Apo-C
Ce-Vi-Sol
Kamu Jay
Sunkist

Generic name product may also be available.

Description

Vitamins (VYE-ta-mins) are compounds that you *must* have for growth and health. They are needed in small amounts only and are usually available in the foods that you eat. Ascorbic (a-SKOR-bik) acid, also known as vitamin C, is necessary for healthy bones and teeth as well as the general make-up of the body; it may have other effects as well.

Lack of vitamin C can lead to a condition called scurvy, which causes muscle weakness, swollen and bleeding gums, loss of teeth, and bleeding under the skin, as well as tiredness and depression. Wounds also do not heal easily. Your doctor may treat scurvy by prescribing vitamin C for you.

Patients with the following conditions may be more likely to have a deficiency of ascorbic acid:

- Alcoholism
- Burns
- Cancer
- Diarrhea (prolonged)
- Fever (prolonged)
- Infection (prolonged)
- Intestinal diseases
- Overactive thyroid (hyperthyroidism)

- Stomach ulcer
- Stress (continuing)
- Surgical removal of stomach
- Tuberculosis

Also, the following groups of people may have a deficiency of ascorbic acid:

- Infants receiving unfortified formulas
- Smokers
- Patients using an artificial kidney (on hemodialysis)
- Individuals who do heavy manual labor on a daily basis
- Patients who undergo surgery
- Individuals who are exposed to long periods of cold temperatures

If any of these conditions apply to you, you should take ascorbic acid supplements only on the advice of your doctor after need has been established.

Ascorbic acid may be used for other conditions as determined by your doctor.

Claims that vitamin C is effective for preventing senility and the common cold, and for treating asthma, some mental problems, cancer, hardening of the arteries, allergies, eye ulcers, blood clots, gum disease, and pressure sores have not been proven. Although vitamin C is being used to prevent certain types of cancer, there is not enough information to show that this is effective.

Most strengths of vitamin C are available without a prescription. However, it may be a good idea to check with your doctor before taking vitamin C on your own.

Vitamin C is available in the following dosage forms:

Oral

- Extended-release capsules (U.S. and Canada)
- Oral solution (U.S. and Canada)
- Syrup (U.S.)
- Tablets (U.S. and Canada)
- Chewable tablets (U.S. and Canada)
- Effervescent tablets (U.S.)
- Extended-release tablets (U.S. and Canada)

Parenteral

- Injection (U.S. and Canada)

It is very important that you read and understand the following information. If any of it causes you special concern, check with your doctor or pharmacist. Also, *if you have any questions* or if you want more information about this dietary supplement or your medical problem, *ask your doctor, nurse, pharmacist, or dietitian.*

Importance of Diet

Ascorbic acid supplements should be taken only if you cannot get enough vitamins in your diet; however, some diets may not contain all of the vitamins you need. This may occur with rapid weight loss, unusual diets (such as some reducing diets in which choice of foods is limited), prolonged intravenous feeding, or malnutrition. A balanced diet should provide all the vitamins you normally need.

In order to get enough vitamins and minerals in your diet, it is important that you eat a balanced and varied diet. Follow carefully any diet program your doctor may recommend. For your specific vitamin and/or mineral needs, ask your doctor or dietitian for a list of appropriate foods.

Ascorbic acid is found in various foods, including citrus fruits (oranges, lemons, grapefruit), green vegetables (peppers, broccoli, cabbage), tomatoes, and potatoes. It is best to eat fresh fruits and vegetables whenever possible since they contain the most vitamins. Food processing may destroy some of the vitamins. For example, exposure to air, drying, salting, or cooking (especially in copper pots), mincing of fresh vegetables, or mashing potatoes may reduce the amount of ascorbic acid in foods. Freezing does not usually cause loss of vitamin C unless foods are stored for a very long time.

Vitamins alone will not take the place of a good diet and will not provide energy. Your body also needs other substances found in food such as protein, minerals, carbohydrates, and fat. Vitamins themselves often cannot work without the presence of other foods.

In some cases, it may not be possible for you to get enough food to supply you with the proper vitamins. In other cases, the amount of vitamins you need may be increased above normal. Therefore, a vitamin supplement may be needed.

Experts have developed a list of recommended dietary allowances (RDA) for most of the vitamins. The RDA are not an exact number but a general idea of how much you need. They do not cover amounts needed for problems caused by a serious lack of vitamins.

The RDA for ascorbic acid are:

Infants and children—
- Birth to 6 months of age: 30 milligrams (mg) per day.
- 6 months to 1 year of age: 35 mg per day.
- 1 to 3 years of age: 40 mg per day.
- 4 to 10 years of age: 45 mg per day.

Adolescent and adult males—
- 11 to 14 years of age: 50 mg per day.
- 15 years of age and over: 60 mg per day.

Adolescent and adult females—
- 11 to 14 years of age: 50 mg per day.
- 15 years of age and over: 60 mg per day.

Pregnant females—70 mg per day.

Breast-feeding females—
- First 6 months: 95 mg per day.
- Second 6 months: 90 mg per day.

Smokers—100 mg per day.

Remember:

- The total amount of each vitamin that you get every day includes what you get from the foods that you eat *and* what you may take as a supplement.
- Your total amount should not be greater than the RDA, unless ordered by your doctor. Taking too much ascorbic acid over a period of time may cause harmful effects.

Before Using This Dietary Supplement

In deciding to use a dietary supplement, the risks of taking the dietary supplement must be weighed against the good it will do. This is a decision you and your doctor will make. For ascorbic acid, the following should be considered:

Allergies—Tell your doctor if you have ever had any unusual or allergic reaction to ascorbic acid. Also, tell your doctor and pharmacist if you are allergic to any other substances, such as foods, sulfites or other preservatives, or dyes.

Pregnancy—It is especially important that you are receiving enough vitamins when you become pregnant and that you continue to receive the right amount of vitamins throughout your pregnancy. Healthy fetal growth and development depend on a steady supply of nutrients from mother to fetus.

However, taking too much vitamin C may not be good for the fetus and may cause your baby to need more than the usual amount after birth.

Breast-feeding—It is especially important that you receive the right amounts of vitamins so that your baby will also get the vitamins needed to grow properly. You should also check with your doctor if you are giving your baby an unfortified formula. In that case, the baby must get the vitamins needed some other way. However, taking large amounts of a dietary supplement while breast-feeding may be harmful to the mother and/or baby and should be avoided.

Children—Normal daily requirements vary according to age. It is especially important that children receive enough vitamins in their diet for healthy growth and development. Although there is no specific information about the use of vitamins in children in doses higher than the normal daily requirements, it is not expected to cause different side effects or problems in children than in adults.

Older adults—It is important that older people continue to receive enough vitamins in their diet for good health. Although there is no specific information about the use of vitamins in older people in doses higher than the normal daily requirements, it is not expected to cause different side effects or problems in older people than in younger adults.

Medicines or other dietary supplements—Although certain medicines or dietary supplements should not be used together at all, in other cases they may be used together even if an interaction might occur. In these cases, your doctor may want to change the dose, or other precautions may be necessary. Tell your doctor and pharmacist if you are taking any other dietary supplement or any prescription or nonprescription (over-the-counter [OTC]) medicine.

Other medical problems—The presence of other medical problems may affect the use of ascorbic acid. Make sure you tell your doctor if you have any other medical problems, especially:

- Diabetes mellitus (sugar diabetes)—Very high doses of ascorbic acid may interfere with tests for sugar in the urine
- Glucose-6-phosphate dehydrogenase (G6PD) deficiency—High doses of ascorbic acid may cause hemolytic anemia
- Kidney stones (history of)—High doses of ascorbic acid may increase risk of kidney stones in the urinary tract
- Sickle cell anemia or other blood problems—High doses of ascorbic acid may bring on a crisis

Proper Use of This Dietary Supplement

Do not take more than the recommended daily amount. Vitamin C is not stored in the body. If you take more than you need, the extra will pass into your urine. There is a chance that high doses could cause stones to form in your urinary tract. Very large doses may also interfere with tests for sugar in diabetics and with tests for blood in the stool. Some people believe that taking very large doses of vitamins (called megadoses or megavitamin therapy) is useful for treating certain medical problems. Studies have not proven this. Large doses should be taken only under the direction of your doctor after need has been identified.

For patients taking the *oral liquid form* of ascorbic acid:

- This preparation is to be taken by mouth even though it comes in a dropper bottle.
- This dietary supplement may be dropped directly into the mouth or mixed with cereal, fruit juice, or other food.

Missed dose—If you miss taking a vitamin for one or more days there is no cause for concern, since it takes some time for your body to become seriously low in vitamins. However, if your doctor has recommended that you take this vitamin, try to remember to take it as directed every day.

Storage—To store this dietary supplement:

- Keep out of the reach of children.
- Store away from heat and direct light.

- Do not store in the bathroom, near the kitchen sink, or in other damp places. Heat or moisture may cause the dietary supplement to break down.
- Keep the oral liquid form of this dietary supplement from freezing.
- Do not keep outdated dietary supplements or those no longer needed. Be sure that any discarded dietary supplement is out of the reach of children.

Side Effects of This Dietary Supplement

Along with its needed effects, a dietary supplement may cause some unwanted effects. Although not all of these side effects may occur, if they do occur, they may need medical attention.

Check with your doctor as soon as possible if the following side effect occurs:

Less common or rare—with high doses

Side or lower back pain

Other side effects may occur that usually do not need medical attention. These side effects may go away during treatment as your body adjusts to the dietary supplement. However, check with your doctor or pharmacist as soon as possible if any of the following side effects continue or are bothersome:

Less common or rare—with high doses

Diarrhea; dizziness or faintness (with the injection only); flushing or redness of skin; headache; increase in urination (mild); nausea or vomiting; stomach cramps

Other side effects not listed above may also occur in some patients. If you notice any other effects, check with your doctor or pharmacist.

Additional Information

Once a medicine or dietary supplement has been approved for marketing for a certain use, experience may show that it is also useful for other medical problems. Although these uses are not included in product labeling, ascorbic acid is used in certain patients with the following medical conditions:

- Overdose of iron (to help another drug in decreasing iron levels in the body)
- Methemoglobinemia (a blood disease)

Other than the above information, there is no additional information relating to proper use, precautions, or side effects for these uses.

Annual revision: 04/14/92

ASPARAGINASE Systemic

Some commonly used brand names are:

In the U.S.
Elspar

In Canada
Kidrolase

Another commonly used name is colaspase.

Description

Asparaginase (a-SPARE-a-gin-ase) belongs to the group of medicines known as enzymes. It is used to treat some kinds of cancer.

All cells need a chemical called asparagine to stay alive. Normal cells can make this chemical for themselves, while cancer cells cannot. Asparaginase breaks down asparagine in the body. Since the cancer cells cannot make more asparagine, they die.

Before you begin treatment with asparaginase, you and your doctor should talk about the good this medicine will do as well as the risks of using it.

Asparaginase is to be administered only by or under the supervision of your doctor. It is available in the following dosage form:

Parenteral

- Injection (U.S. and Canada)

It is very important that you read and understand the following information. If any of it causes you special concern, check with your doctor. Also, *if you have any questions* or if you want more information about this medicine or your medical problem, *ask your doctor, nurse, or pharmacist.*

Before Using This Medicine

In deciding to use a medicine, the risks of taking the medicine must be weighed against the good it will do. This is a decision you and your doctor will make. For asparaginase, the following should be considered:

Allergies—Tell your doctor if you have ever had any unusual or allergic reaction to asparaginase.

Pregnancy—Asparaginase has not been studied in pregnant women. However, studies in mice and rats have shown that asparaginase in doses 5 times the usual human dose slows the weight gain of infants and may also increase the risk of birth defects or cause a decrease in successful pregnancies. In addition, doses slightly less than the human dose have caused birth defects in rabbits.

It is best to use some kind of birth control while you are receiving asparaginase. Tell your doctor right away if you think you have become pregnant while receiving asparaginase.

Breast-feeding—It is not known whether asparaginase passes into breast milk. However, because asparaginase may cause serious side effects, breast-feeding is generally not recommended while you are receiving it.

Children—This medicine has been tested in children and has not been shown to cause different side effects or problems than it does in adults. In fact, the side effects of this medicine seem to be less severe in children than in adults.

Older adults—Many medicines have not been studied specifically in older people. Therefore, it may not be known whether they work exactly the same way they do in younger adults or if they cause different side effects or problems in older people. There is no specific information comparing use of asparaginase in the elderly with use in other age groups.

Other medicines—Although certain medicines should not be used together at all, in other cases two different medicines may be used together even if an interaction might occur. In these cases, your doctor may want to change the dose, or other precautions may be necessary. When you are receiving asparaginase it is especially important that your doctor and pharmacist know if you are taking any of the following:

- Probenecid (e.g., Benemid) or
- Sulfinpyrazone (e.g., Anturane)—Asparaginase may raise the concentration of uric acid in the blood. Since these medicines are used to lower uric acid levels, they may not work as well in patients receiving asparaginase
- If you have ever been treated with x-rays or cancer medicines—Asparaginase may increase the total effects of these medications and radiation therapy

Other medical problems—The presence of other medical problems may affect the use of asparaginase. Make sure you tell your doctor if you have any other medical problems, especially:

- Chickenpox (including recent exposure) or
- Herpes zoster (shingles)—Risk of severe disease affecting other parts of the body
- Diabetes mellitus (sugar diabetes)—Asparaginase may increase glucose (sugar) in the blood
- Gout or
- Kidney stones—Asparaginase may increase levels of uric acid in the body, which can cause gout or kidney stones
- Infection—Asparaginase can reduce your body's ability to fight infection
- Liver disease—Asparaginase may worsen the condition
- Pancreatitis (inflammation of the pancreas)—Asparaginase may cause pancreatitis

Before you begin using any new medicine (prescription or nonprescription) or if you develop any new medical problem while you are using this medicine, check with your doctor, nurse, or pharmacist.

Proper Use of This Medicine

This medicine is usually given together with certain other medicines. If you are using a combination of medicines, it is important that you receive each one at the proper time. If you are taking some of these medicines by mouth, ask your doctor, nurse, or pharmacist to help you plan a way to remember to take them at the right times.

While you are using this medicine, your doctor may want you to drink extra fluids so that you will pass more urine. This will help prevent kidney problems and keep your kidneys working well.

This medicine often causes nausea, vomiting, and loss of appetite. However, it is very important that you continue to receive the medicine, even if you begin to feel ill. After several doses, your stomach upset should lessen. Ask your doctor, nurse, or pharmacist for ways to lessen these effects.

Precautions While Using This Medicine

It is very important that your doctor check your progress at regular visits to make sure that this medicine is working properly and to check for unwanted effects.

While you are being treated with asparaginase, and after you stop treatment with it, *do not have any immunizations (vaccinations) without your doctor's approval.* Asparaginase may lower your body's resistance and there is a chance you might get the infection the immunization is meant to prevent. In addition, other persons living in your household should not take oral polio vaccine since there is a chance they could pass the polio virus on to you. Also, avoid persons who have taken oral polio vaccine. Do not get close to them, and do not stay in the same room with them for very long. If you cannot take these precautions, you should consider wearing a protective face mask that covers the nose and mouth.

Before you have any medical tests, tell the medical doctor in charge that you are receiving this medicine. The results of thyroid tests may be affected by this medicine.

Side Effects of This Medicine

Along with its needed effects, a medicine may cause some unwanted effects. Some side effects will have signs or symptoms that you can see or feel. Your doctor may watch for others by doing certain tests. Some of the unwanted effects that may be caused by asparaginase are listed below. Although not all of these effects may occur, if they do occur, they may need medical attention.

Also, because of the way these medicines act on the body, there is a chance that they might cause other unwanted effects that may not occur until months or years after the medicine is used. These delayed effects may include certain types of cancer, such as leukemia. Discuss these possible effects with your doctor.

Check with your doctor or nurse immediately if any of the following side effects occur:

More common

Joint pain; puffy face; skin rash or itching; stomach pain (severe) with nausea and vomiting; trouble in breathing

Rare

Fever or chills; headache (severe); inability to move arm or leg; unusual bleeding or bruising

Check with your doctor or nurse as soon as possible if any of the following side effects occur:

Less common

Confusion; drowsiness; frequent urination; hallucinations (seeing, hearing, or feeling things that are not there); lower back or side pain; mental depression; nervousness; sores in mouth or on lips; swelling of feet or lower legs; unusual thirst; unusual tiredness

Rare

Convulsions (seizures); pain in lower legs

This medicine may also cause the following side effect that your doctor will watch for:

More common

Liver problems

Other side effects may occur that usually do not need medical attention. These side effects may go away during treatment as your body adjusts to the medicine. Also, your doctor or nurse may be able to tell you about ways to prevent or reduce some of these side effects. Check with your doctor or nurse if any of the following side effects continue or are bothersome or if you have any questions about them:

More common

Headache (mild); loss of appetite; nausea or vomiting; stomach cramps; weight loss

After you stop receiving asparaginase, it may still produce some side effects that need attention. During this period of time, *check with your doctor or nurse immediately* if any of the following side effects occur:

Headache (severe); inability to move arm or leg; stomach pain (severe) with nausea and vomiting

Other side effects not listed above may also occur in some patients. If you notice any other effects, check with your doctor or nurse.

Annual revision: 04/09/93

ASPIRIN, SODIUM BICARBONATE, AND CITRIC ACID Systemic

A commonly used brand name in the U.S. and Canada is Alka-Seltzer Effervescent Pain Reliever and Antacid.

Other commonly used names for aspirin are acetylsalicylic acid and ASA. Because Aspirin is a brand name in Canada, ASA is the term that commonly appears on Canadian product labels.

Description

Aspirin, sodium bicarbonate, and citric acid (AS-pir-in, SOE-dee-um bye-KAR-boe-nate, and SI-trik AS-id) combination is used to relieve pain occurring together with heartburn, sour stomach, or acid indigestion.

The aspirin in this combination is the pain reliever. Aspirin belongs to the group of medicines known as salicylates (sa-LISS-ih-lates) and to the group of medicines known as anti-inflammatory analgesics. The sodium bicarbonate in this medicine is an antacid. It neutralizes stomach acid by combining with it to form a new substance that is not an acid.

Aspirin, sodium bicarbonate, and citric acid combination may also be used to lessen the chance of heart attack, stroke, or other problems that may occur when a blood vessel is blocked by blood clots. The aspirin in this medicine helps prevent dangerous blood clots from forming. However, this effect of aspirin may increase the chance of serious bleeding in some people. Therefore, aspirin should be used for this purpose only when your doctor decides, after studying your medical condition and history, that the danger of blood clots is greater than the risk of bleeding. *Do not take aspirin to prevent blood clots or a heart attack unless it has been ordered by your doctor.*

There is another medicine with a similar brand name, i.e., Alka-Seltzer Advanced Formula. Alka-Seltzer Advanced Formula contains acetaminophen rather than aspirin, and will not prevent blood clots from forming or cause bleeding problems. Also, it does not have as much sodium as Alka-Seltzer Effervescent Pain Reliever and Antacid. *Be sure that you are getting the right product.*

This combination medicine is available without a prescription. However, your doctor may have special instructions on the proper dose for your medical condition.

Aspirin, sodium bicarbonate, and citric acid combination is available in the following dosage form:

Oral

- Effervescent tablets (U.S. and Canada)

It is very important that you read and understand the following information. If any of it causes you special concern, check with your doctor or pharmacist. Also, *if you have any questions* or if you want more information about this medicine or your medical problem, *ask your doctor, nurse, or pharmacist.*

Before Using This Medicine

If you are taking this medicine without a prescription, carefully read and follow any precautions on the label. For aspirin, sodium bicarbonate, and citric acid combination, the following should be considered:

Allergies—Tell your doctor if you have ever had any unusual or allergic reaction to aspirin or other salicylates, including methyl salicylate (oil of wintergreen), or to any of the following medicines:

Diclofenac (e.g., Voltaren)
Diflunisal (e.g., Dolobid)
Etodolac (e.g., Lodine)
Fenoprofen (e.g., Nalfon)
Floctafenine (e.g., Idarac)
Flurbiprofen, oral (e.g., Ansaid)
Ibuprofen (e.g., Motrin)
Indomethacin (e.g., Indocin)
Ketoprofen (e.g., Orudis)
Ketorolac (e.g., Toradol)
Meclofenamate (e.g., Meclomen)
Mefenamic acid (e.g., Ponstel)
Naproxen (e.g., Naprosyn)
Oxyphenbutazone (e.g., Tandearil)
Phenylbutazone (e.g., Butazolidin)
Piroxicam (e.g., Feldene)
Sulindac (e.g., Clinoril)
Suprofen (e.g., Suprol)
Tiaprofenic acid (e.g., Surgam)
Tolmetin (e.g., Tolectin)
Zomepirac (e.g., Zomax)

Also tell your doctor and pharmacist if you are allergic to any other substances, such as foods, preservatives, or dyes.

Diet—Make certain your doctor and pharmacist know if you are on any special diet, such as a low-sodium or low-sugar diet. This medicine contains a large amount of sodium (more than 500 mg in each tablet).

Pregnancy—Studies in humans have not shown that aspirin causes birth defects in humans. However, it has been shown to cause birth defects in animal studies.

Do not take aspirin during the last 3 months of pregnancy unless it has been ordered by your doctor. Some reports have suggested that too much use of aspirin late in pregnancy may cause a decrease in the newborn's weight and possible death of the fetus or newborn infant. However, the mothers in these reports had been taking much larger amounts of aspirin than are usually recommended. Studies of mothers taking aspirin in the doses that are usually recommended did not show these unwanted effects. However, there is a chance that regular use of aspirin late in pregnancy may cause unwanted effects on the heart or blood flow in the fetus or in the newborn infant.

Use of aspirin during the last 2 weeks of pregnancy may cause bleeding problems in the fetus before or during delivery or in the newborn infant. Also, too much use of aspirin during the last 3 months of pregnancy may increase the length of pregnancy, prolong labor, cause other problems during delivery, or cause severe bleeding in the mother before, during, or after delivery.

The sodium in this combination medicine can cause you to retain (keep) body water. This may result in swelling and weight gain. Therefore, you should not use this combination medicine if you tend to retain body water.

Breast-feeding—Aspirin passes into the breast milk. However, aspirin (in the amounts used to relieve pain or prevent blood clots), sodium bicarbonate, and citric acid have not been reported to cause problems in nursing babies.

Children—*Do not give any medicine containing aspirin to a child with fever or other symptoms of a virus infection, especially flu or chickenpox, without first discussing its use with your child's doctor.* This is very important because aspirin may cause a serious illness called Reye's syndrome in children with fever caused by a virus infection, especially flu or chickenpox. Children who do not have a virus infection may also be more sensitive to the effects of aspirin, especially if they have a fever or have lost large amounts of body fluid because of vomiting, diarrhea, or sweating. This may increase the chance of side effects during treatment.

Teenagers—*Teenagers with fever or other symptoms of a virus infection, especially flu or chickenpox, should check with a doctor before taking this medicine.* The aspirin in this combination medicine may cause a serious illness called Reye's syndrome in teenagers with fever caused by a virus infection, especially flu or chickenpox.

Older adults—People 60 years of age and older are especially sensitive to the effects of aspirin. This may increase the chance of side effects during treatment. Also, the sodium in this combination medicine can be harmful to some elderly people, especially if large amounts of the medicine are taken regularly. Therefore, it is best that older people not use this medicine for more than 5 days in a row, unless otherwise directed by their doctor.

Other medicines—Although certain medicines should not be used together at all, in other cases two different medicines may be used together even if an interaction might occur. In these cases, your doctor may want to change the dose, or other precautions may be necessary. When you are taking this combination medicine, it is especially important that your doctor and pharmacist know if you are taking any of the following:

- Anticoagulants (blood thinners) or
- Carbenicillin by injection (e.g., Geopen) or
- Cefamandole (e.g., Mandol) or
- Cefoperazone (e.g., Cefobid) or
- Cefotetan (e.g., Cefotan) or
- Dipyridamole (e.g., Persantine) or
- Divalproex (e.g., Depakote) or
- Heparin or
- Moxalactam (e.g., Moxam) or
- Pentoxifylline (e.g., Trental) or
- Plicamycin (e.g., Mithracin) or
- Ticarcillin (e.g., Ticar) or
- Valproic acid (e.g., Depakene)—Use of these medicines together with aspirin may increase the chance of bleeding
- Antidiabetics, oral (diabetes medicine you take by mouth)—Aspirin may increase the effects of these medicines; a change in dose may be needed
- Ketoconazole (e.g., Nizoral) or
- Methenamine (e.g., Mandelamine) or
- Tetracyclines (medicine for infection), taken by mouth—Sodium bicarbonate can keep these medicines from working properly
- Mecamylamine (e.g., Inversine)—Sodium bicarbonate may increase the chance of unwanted effects by causing mecamylamine to stay in your body longer than usual
- Medicine for pain and/or inflammation (except narcotics) or
- Methotrexate (e.g., Mexate)—The chance of serious side effects may be increased
- Probenecid (e.g., Benemid) or
- Sulfinpyrazone (e.g., Anturane)—Aspirin can keep these medicines from working properly when they are used to treat gout

Other medical problems—The presence of other medical problems may affect the use of this combination medicine. Make sure you tell your doctor if you have any other medical problems, especially:

- Anemia or
- Stomach ulcer or other stomach problems—Aspirin can make these conditions worse
- Appendicitis (symptoms of, such as stomach or lower abdominal pain, cramping, bloating, soreness, nausea, or vomiting)—Sodium bicarbonate can make your condition worse; also, people who may have appendicitis need medical attention and should not try to treat themselves
- Asthma, allergies, and nasal polyps (history of) or
- Kidney disease or
- Liver disease—The chance of serious side effects may be increased
- Edema (swelling of face, fingers, feet, or lower legs caused by too much water in the body) or
- Heart disease or
- High blood pressure or
- Toxemia of pregnancy—The sodium in this combination medicine can make these conditions worse
- Gout—Aspirin can make this condition worse and can also lessen the effects of some medicines used to treat gout
- Hemophilia or other bleeding problems—Aspirin increases the chance of serious bleeding

Before you begin using any new medicine (prescription or nonprescription) or if you develop any new medical problem while you are using this medicine, check with your doctor, nurse, or pharmacist.

Proper Use of This Medicine

Unless otherwise directed by your doctor, do not take more of this medicine than is recommended on the package label. If too much is taken, serious side effects may occur.

To use this medicine:

- This medicine must be taken in the form of a liquid that is made from the tablets. Do not swallow the tablets or any pieces of the tablets.
- To make the liquid, place the number of tablets needed for one dose (1 or 2 tablets) into a glass. Then add ½ glass (4 ounces) of cool water.
- Check to be sure that the tablets have disappeared completely. This shows that all of the medicine is in the liquid. Then drink all of the liquid. You may drink the liquid while it is still fizzing or after the fizzing stops.
- Add a little more water to the glass and drink that, to make sure that you get the full amount of the medicine.

Missed dose—If your doctor has ordered you to take this medicine according to a regular schedule and you miss a dose, take it as soon as you remember. However, if it is almost time for your next dose, skip the missed dose and go back to your regular dosing schedule. Do not double doses.

Storage—To store this medicine:

- Keep out of the reach of children. Overdose is very dangerous in young children.
- Store away from heat and direct light.
- Do not store in the bathroom, near the kitchen sink, or in other damp places. Heat or moisture may cause the medicine to break down.
- Do not keep outdated medicine or medicine no longer needed. Be sure that any discarded medicine is out of the reach of children.

Precautions While Using This Medicine

If you will be taking this medicine for a long time (more than 5 days in a row for children or 10 days in a row for adults), your doctor should check your progress at regular visits.

Check with your doctor if your pain and/or upset stomach last for more than 10 days for adults or 5 days for children or if they get worse, if new symptoms occur, or if the painful area is red or swollen. These could be signs of a serious condition that needs medical treatment.

The sodium bicarbonate in this combination medicine can keep other medicines from working properly if the 2 medicines are taken too close together. *Always take this medicine:*

- *At least 3 hours before or after taking ketoconazole (e.g., Nizoral).*
- *At least 3 or 4 hours before or after taking a tetracycline antibiotic by mouth.*
- *At least 1 or 2 hours before or after taking any other medicine by mouth.*

If you are also taking a laxative that contains cellulose, take this combination medicine at least 2 hours before or after you take the laxative. Taking the medicines too close together may lessen the effects of aspirin.

Check the labels of all nonprescription (over-the-counter [OTC]) and prescription medicines you now take. If any contain aspirin or other salicylates, including bismuth subsalicylate (e.g., Pepto-Bismol) or salicylic acid (present in some shampoos or medicines for your skin), or if any contain sodium, be especially careful. Using other salicylate-containing or other sodium-containing products while taking this medicine may lead to overdose. If you have any questions about this, check with your doctor or pharmacist.

Do not take aspirin for 5 days before any surgery, including dental surgery, unless otherwise directed by your medical doctor or dentist. Taking aspirin during this time may cause bleeding problems.

For patients taking this medicine to lessen the chance of a heart attack, stroke, or other problems caused by blood clots:

- *Take only the amount of aspirin ordered by your doctor.* If you need a medicine to relieve pain, a fever, or arthritis, your doctor may not want you to take extra aspirin. It is a good idea to discuss this with your doctor, so that you will know ahead of time what medicine to take.
- *Do not stop taking this medicine for any reason without first checking with the doctor who directed you to take it.*

Taking certain other medicines together with a salicylate may increase the chance of unwanted effects. The risk will depend on how much of each medicine you take every day, and on how long you take the medicines together. If your doctor directs you to take these medicines together on a regular basis, follow his or her directions carefully. However, *do not take any of the following medicines together with a salicylate for more than a few days, unless your doctor has directed you to do so and is following your progress*:

Acetaminophen (e.g., Tylenol)
Diclofenac (e.g., Voltaren)
Diflunisal (e.g., Dolobid)
Etodolac (e.g., Lodine)
Fenoprofen (e.g., Nalfon)
Floctafenine (e.g., Idarac)
Flurbiprofen, oral (e.g., Ansaid)
Ibuprofen (e.g., Motrin)
Indomethacin (e.g., Indocin)
Ketoprofen (e.g., Orudis)
Ketorolac (e.g., Toradol)
Meclofenamate (e.g., Meclomen)
Mefenamic acid (e.g., Ponstel)
Naproxen (e.g., Naprosyn)
Phenylbutazone (e.g., Butazolidin)
Piroxicam (e.g., Feldene)
Sulindac (e.g., Clinoril)
Tiaprofenic acid (e.g., Surgam)
Tolmetin (e.g., Tolectin)

If you will be taking more than an occasional 1 or 2 doses of this medicine:

- *Do not drink alcoholic beverages.* Drinking alcoholic beverages while you are taking aspirin, especially if you take aspirin regularly or in large amounts, may increase the chance of stomach problems.
- *Do not drink a lot of milk or eat a lot of milk products.* To do so may increase the chance of side effects.
- To prevent side effects caused by too much sodium in the body, you may need to limit the amount of sodium in the foods you eat. Some foods that contain large amounts of sodium are canned soup, canned vegetables, pickles, ketchup, green and ripe (black) olives, relish, frankfurters and other sausage-type meats, soy sauce, and carbonated beverages. If you have any questions about this, check with your doctor, nurse, or pharmacist.

Before you have any medical tests, tell the doctor in charge that you are taking this medicine. The results of some tests may be affected by the aspirin in this combination medicine.

For *diabetic patients:*

- Aspirin can cause false urine glucose (sugar) test results if you regularly take 8 or more 324-mg, or 4 or more 500-mg (extra-strength), tablets a day. Smaller amounts or occasional use of aspirin usually will not affect the test results. However, check with your doctor, nurse, or pharmacist if you notice any change in your urine glucose test results. This is especially important if your diabetes is not well-controlled.

If you think that you or anyone else may have taken an overdose, get emergency help at once. Taking an overdose of aspirin may cause unconsciousness or death, especially in young children. Signs of overdose include convulsions (seizures), hearing loss, confusion, ringing or buzzing in the ears, severe drowsiness or tiredness, severe excitement or nervousness, and fast or deep breathing.

Side Effects of This Medicine

Along with its needed effects, a medicine may cause some unwanted effects. Although the following side effects occur very rarely when 1 or 2 doses of this combination medicine is taken occasionally, they may be more likely to occur if:

- too much medicine is taken.
- the medicine is taken several times a day.
- the medicine is taken for more than a few days in a row.

Get emergency help immediately if any of the following side effects occur:

Any loss of hearing; bloody urine; confusion; convulsions (seizures); diarrhea (severe or continuing); difficulty in swallowing; dizziness, lightheadedness, or feeling faint (severe); drowsiness (severe); excitement or nervousness (severe); fast or deep breathing; flushing, redness, or other change in skin color; hallucinations (seeing, hearing, or feeling things that are not there); nausea or vomiting (severe or continuing); shortness of breath, troubled breathing, tightness in chest, or wheezing; stomach pain (severe or continuing); swelling of eyelids, face, or lips; unexplained fever; uncontrollable flapping movements of the hands (especially in elderly patients); vision problems

Symptoms of overdose in children

Changes in behavior; drowsiness or tiredness (severe); fast or deep breathing

Also, check with your doctor as soon as possible if any of the following side effects occur:

Less common or rare

Bloody or black, tarry stools; frequent urge to urinate; headache (severe or continuing); increased blood pressure; loss of appetite (continuing); mood or mental changes; muscle pain or twitching; ringing or buzzing in ears (continuing); skin rash, hives, or itching; slow breathing; swelling of face, fingers, ankles, feet, or lower legs; unpleasant taste; unusual tiredness or weakness; vomiting of blood or material that looks like coffee grounds; weight gain (unusual)

Other side effects may occur that usually do not need medical attention. These side effects may go away during treatment as your body adjusts to the medicine. However, check with your doctor or pharmacist if any of the following side effects continue or are bothersome:

Heartburn or indigestion; increased thirst; nausea or vomiting; stomach pain (mild)

Other side effects not listed above may also occur in some patients. If you notice any other effects, check with your doctor.

Annual revision: 02/24/92

ATOVAQUONE Systemic

A commonly used brand name in the U.S. and Canada is Mepron. Another commonly used name is 566C80.

Description

Atovaquone (a-TOE-va-kwone) is used to treat pneumocystis (noo-moe-SISS-tis) pneumonia (PCP), a very serious kind of pneumonia. This particular kind of pneumonia occurs commonly in patients whose immune systems are not working normally, such as cancer patients, transplant patients, and patients with acquired immune deficiency syndrome (AIDS).

This medicine is available only with your doctor's prescription, in the following dosage form:

Oral

- Tablets (U.S. and Canada)

It is very important that you read and understand the following information. If any of it causes you special concern, check with your doctor. Also, *if you have any questions* or if you want more information about this medicine or your medical problem, *ask your doctor, nurse, or pharmacist.*

Before Receiving This Medicine

In deciding to use a medicine, the risks of taking the medicine must be weighed against the good it will do. This is a decision you and your doctor will make. For atovaquone, the following should be considered:

Allergies—Tell your doctor if you have ever had any unusual or allergic reaction to atovaquone. Also tell your doctor and pharmacist if you are allergic to any other substances, such as foods, preservatives, or dyes.

Pregnancy—Atovaquone has not been studied in pregnant women. However, studies in rabbits have shown an increase in miscarriages and other harmful effects in the mother and fetus. Before taking this medicine, make sure your doctor knows if you are pregnant or if you may become pregnant.

Breast-feeding—It is not known whether atovaquone passes into human breast milk. However, it was found in the milk of rats. Be sure you have discussed the risks and benefits of atovaquone with your doctor.

Children—Atovaquone has been tested in a limited number of children 5 months of age to 13 years old. It is not known if this medicine causes different side effects or problems in children than it does in adults.

Older adults—Many medicines have not been studied specifically in older people. Therefore, it may not be known whether they work exactly the same way they do in younger adults or if they cause different side effects or problems in older people. There is no specific information comparing use of atovaquone in the elderly with use in other age groups.

Other medicines—Although certain medicines should not be used together at all, in other cases two different medicines may be used together even if an interaction might occur. In these cases, your doctor may want to change the dose, or other precautions may be necessary. Tell your doctor and pharmacist if you are taking any other prescription or nonprescription (over-the-counter [OTC]) medicine.

Other medical problems—The presence of other medical problems may affect the use of atovaquone. Make sure you tell your doctor if you have any other medical problems, especially:

- Stomach or intestinal disorders—Atovaquone may not work properly in patients with some kinds of stomach or intestinal problems

Before you begin using any new medicine (prescription or nonprescription) or if you develop any new medical problem while you are using this medicine, check with your doctor, nurse, or pharmacist.

Proper Use of This Medicine

It is important that you take atovaquone with a high fat meal. This will make sure the medicine is fully absorbed into the body.

To help clear up your infection completely, *keep taking your medicine for the full time of treatment,* even if you begin to feel better after a few days. If you stop taking this medicine too soon, your symptoms may return.

Atovaquone works best when there is a constant amount in the blood. *To help keep the amount constant, do not miss any doses.*

Dosing—The dose of atovaquone may be different for different patients. *Follow your doctor's orders or the directions on the label.* The following information includes only the average doses of atovaquone. *If your dose is different, do not change it* unless your doctor tells you to do so.

- For the *oral* dosage form (capsules):
  —For treatment of *Pneumocystis carinii* pneumonia (PCP):
    - Adults—750 milligrams (mg) taken with food three times a day for twenty-one days.
    - Children—Use and dose must be determined by your doctor.

Missed dose—If you miss a dose of this medicine, take it as soon as possible. This will help to keep a constant amount of medicine in the blood. However, if it is almost time for your next dose, skip the missed dose and go back to your regular dosing schedule. Do not double doses.

Storage—To store this medicine:

- Keep out of the reach of children.
- Store away from heat and direct light.
- Do not store in the bathroom, near the kitchen sink, or in other damp places. Heat or moisture may cause the medicine to break down.
- Do not keep outdated medicine or medicine no longer needed. Be sure that any discarded medicine is out of the reach of children.

Precautions While Using This Medicine

If your symptoms do not improve within a few days, or if they become worse, check with your doctor.

Side Effects of This Medicine

Along with its needed effects, a medicine may cause some unwanted effects. Although not all of these side effects may occur, if they do occur they may need medical attention.

Check with your doctor immediately if any of the following side effects occur:

More common

Fever; skin rash

Other side effects may occur that usually do not need medical attention. These side effects may go away during treatment as your body adjusts to the medicine. However, check with your doctor if any of the following side effects continue or are bothersome:

More common

Cough; diarrhea; headache; nausea; trouble in sleeping; vomiting

Other side effects not listed above may also occur in some patients. If you notice any other effects, check with your doctor.

Annual revision: 04/21/93

ATROPINE Ophthalmic

This information applies to the following medicines:

Atropine (A-troe-peen)
Homatropine (hoe-MA-troe-peen)
Scopolamine (skoe-POL-a-meen)

Some commonly used brand names are:

For Atropine

In the U.S.

Atropair
Atropine-Care
Atropine Sulfate S.O.P.
Atropisol
Isopto Atropine
I-Tropine
Ocu-Tropine

Generic name product may also be available.

In Canada

Atropisol
Isopto Atropine
Minims Atropine

Generic name product may also be available.

For Homatropine

In the U.S.

AK-Homatropine
I-Homatrine
Isopto Homatropine
Spectro-Homatropine

Generic name product may also be available.

In Canada

Isopto Homatropine
Minims Homatropine

Generic name product may also be available.

For Scopolamine

In the U.S.

Isopto Hyoscine

Another commonly used name is hyoscine.

Description

Ophthalmic atropine, homatropine, and scopolamine are used to dilate (enlarge) the pupil of the eye. They are used before eye examinations, before and after eye surgery, and to treat certain eye conditions.

These medicines are available only with your doctor's prescription, in the following dosage forms:

Ophthalmic

Atropine
- Ophthalmic ointment (U.S. and Canada)
- Ophthalmic solution (eye drops) (U.S. and Canada)

Homatropine
- Ophthalmic solution (eye drops) (U.S. and Canada)

Scopolamine
- Ophthalmic solution (eye drops) (U.S.)

It is very important that you read and understand the following information. If any of it causes you special concern, check with your doctor. Also, *if you have any questions* or if you want more information about this medicine or your medical problem, *ask your doctor, nurse, or pharmacist.*

Before Using This Medicine

In deciding to use a medicine, the risks of using the medicine must be weighed against the good it will do. This is a decision you and your doctor will make. For ophthalmic atropine, homatropine, and scopolamine, the following should be considered:

Allergies—Tell your doctor if you have ever had any unusual or allergic reaction to atropine, homatropine, or scopolamine. Also tell your doctor and pharmacist if you are allergic to any other substances, such as certain preservatives.

Pregnancy—Studies on effects in pregnancy have not been done in either humans or animals. However, this medicine may be absorbed into the body.

Breast-feeding—This medicine may be absorbed into the body. Atropine passes into the breast milk in very small amounts and may cause side effects, such as fast pulse, fever, or dry skin, in babies of nursing mothers using ophthalmic atropine. Homatropine and scopolamine have not been reported to cause problems in nursing babies.

Children—Infants and young children and children with blond hair or blue eyes may be especially sensitive to the effects of atropine, homatropine, or scopolamine. This may increase the chance of side effects during treatment.

Older adults—Elderly people are especially sensitive to the effects of atropine, homatropine, or scopolamine. This may increase the chance of side effects during treatment.

Other medicines—Although certain medicines should not be used together at all, in other cases two different medicines may be used together even if an interaction might occur. In these cases, your doctor may want to change the dose, or other precautions may be necessary. Tell your doctor and pharmacist if you are using any other prescription or nonprescription (over-the-counter [OTC]) medicine.

Other medical problems—The presence of other medical problems may affect the use of ophthalmic atropine, homatropine, or scopolamine. Make sure you tell your doctor if you have any other medical problems, especially:

- Brain damage (in children) or
- Down's syndrome (mongolism) (in children and adults) or
- Glaucoma or
- Other eye diseases or problems or
- Spastic paralysis (in children)—Use of ophthalmic atropine, homatropine, or scopolamine may make the condition worse

Before you begin using any new medicine (prescription or nonprescription) or if you develop any new medical problem while you are using this medicine, check with your doctor, nurse, or pharmacist.

Proper Use of This Medicine

To use the *eye-drop form* of this medicine:

- First, wash your hands. With the middle finger, apply pressure to the inside corner of the eye (and continue to apply pressure for 2 or 3 minutes after the medicine has been placed in the eye). Tilt the head back and with the index finger of the same hand, pull the lower eyelid away from the eye to form a pouch. Drop the medicine into the pouch and gently close the eyes. Do not blink. Keep the eyes closed for 1 or 2 minutes to allow the medicine to be absorbed.

- Immediately after using the eye drops, wash your hands to remove any medicine that may be on them. If you are using the eye drops for an infant or child, be sure to wash his or her hands immediately afterwards also, and do not let any of the medicine get in his or her mouth. In addition, wipe off any medicine that may have accidentally gotten on the infant or child, including his or her face or eyelids.
- To keep the medicine as germ-free as possible, do not touch the applicator tip to any surface (including the eye). Also, keep the container tightly closed.

To use the *ointment form* of this medicine:

- First, wash your hands. Then pull the lower eyelid away from the eye to form a pouch. Squeeze a thin strip of ointment into the pouch. A ⅓- to ½-cm (approximately ⅛-inch in infants and young children and ¼-inch in older children and adults) strip of ointment is usually enough unless otherwise directed by your doctor. Gently close the eyes and keep them closed for 1 or 2 minutes to allow the medicine to be absorbed.
- Immediately after using the eye ointment, wash your hands to remove any medicine that may be on them. If you are using the eye ointment for an infant or child, be sure to wash his or her hands immediately afterwards also, and do not let any of the medicine get in his or her mouth. In addition, wipe off any medicine that may have accidentally gotten on the infant or child, including his or her face or eyelids.
- To keep the medicine as germ-free as possible, do not touch the applicator tip to any surface (including the eye). After using the eye ointment, wipe the tip of the ointment tube with a clean tissue and keep the tube tightly closed.

Use this medicine only as directed. Do not use more of it and do not use it more often than your doctor ordered. To do so may increase the chance of too much medicine being absorbed into the body and the chance of side effects. *This is especially important when this medicine is used in infants and children, since overdose is very dangerous in infants and children.*

Missed dose—If you miss a dose of this medicine and your dosing schedule is:

- One dose a day—Apply the missed dose as soon as possible. However, if you do not remember the missed dose until the next day, skip the missed dose and go back to your regular dosing schedule. Do not double doses.
- More than one dose a day—Apply the missed dose as soon as possible. However, if it is almost time for your next dose, skip the missed dose and go back to your regular dosing schedule. Do not double doses.

Storage—To store this medicine

- Keep out of the reach of children. Overdose of this medicine is very dangerous for infants and children.
- Store away from heat and direct light.
- Keep this medicine from freezing.
- Do not keep outdated medicine or medicine no longer needed. Be sure that any discarded medicine is out of the reach of children.

Precautions While Using This Medicine

After you apply this medicine to your eyes:

- Your pupils will become unusually large and you will have blurring of vision, especially for close objects. *Make sure your vision is clear before you drive, use machines, or do anything else that could be dangerous if you are not able to see well.*
- Your eyes will become more sensitive to light than they are normally. *Wear sunglasses to protect your eyes from sunlight and other bright lights.*

These effects may continue for several days after you stop using this medicine. However, check with your doctor if they continue longer than:

- 14 days if you are using atropine.
- 3 days if you are using homatropine.
- 7 days if you are using scopolamine.

Side Effects of This Medicine

Along with its needed effects, a medicine may cause some unwanted effects. Although not all of these side effects may occur, if they do occur they may need medical attention.

Check with your doctor immediately if any of the following side effects occur:

Symptoms of too much medicine being absorbed into the body

Clumsiness or unsteadiness; confusion or unusual behavior; dizziness; dryness of skin; fast or irregular heartbeat; fever; flushing or redness of face; hallucinations (seeing, hearing, or feeling things that are not there); skin rash; slurred speech; swollen stomach in infants; thirst or unusual dryness of mouth; unusual drowsiness, tiredness, or weakness

Other side effects may occur that usually do not need medical attention. These side effects may go away during treatment as your body adjusts to the medicine. However,

check with your doctor if any of the following side effects continue or are bothersome:

Blurred vision; eye irritation not present before use of this medicine; increased sensitivity of eyes to light; swelling of the eyelids

Other side effects not listed above may also occur in some patients. If you notice any other effects, check with your doctor.

Annual revision: 11/21/91

ATROPINE, HYOSCYAMINE, METHENAMINE, METHYLENE BLUE, PHENYL SALICYLATE, AND BENZOIC ACID Systemic†

Some commonly used brand names are:

In the U.S.

Atrosept	Urimed
Dolsed	Urinary Antiseptic No. 2
Hexalol	Urised
Prosed/DS	Uriseptic
Trac Tabs 2X	Uritab
UAA	Uritin
Uridon Modified	Uro-Ves

†Not commercially available in Canada.

Description

Atropine (A-troe-peen), hyoscyamine (hye-oh-SYE-a-meen), methenamine (meth-EN-a-meen), methylene (METH-i-leen) blue, phenyl salicylate (FEN-ill sa-LI-si-late), and benzoic acid (ben-ZOE-ik AS-id) combination medicine is an anticholinergic, anti-infective, and analgesic. It is given by mouth to help relieve the discomfort caused by urinary tract infections; however, it will not cure the infection itself. This combination medicine may also be used for other conditions as determined by your doctor.

This medicine is available only with your doctor's prescription in the following dosage form:

Oral

- Tablets (U.S.)

It is very important that you read and understand the following information. If any of it causes you special concern, check with your doctor. Also, *if you have any questions* or if you want more information about this medicine or your medical problem, *ask your doctor, nurse, or pharmacist.*

Before Using This Medicine

In deciding to use a medicine, the risks of taking the medicine must be weighed against the good it will do. This is a decision you and your doctor will make. For this combination medicine, the following should be considered:

Allergies—Tell your doctor if you have ever had any unusual or allergic reaction to any of the belladonna alkaloids such as atropine, hyoscyamine, and scopolamine, or to aspirin or other salicylates. Also tell your doctor and pharmacist if you are allergic to any other substances, such as foods, preservatives, or dyes.

Diet—While you are taking this combination medicine, it is important for your urine to be acidic. To do this, your doctor may recommend that you eat more protein and such foods as cranberries (especially cranberry juice with vitamin C added), plums, or prunes. You should avoid foods that make the urine more alkaline, such as most fruits (especially citrus fruits and juices), milk, and other dairy products.

Pregnancy—Studies have not been done in either humans or animals.

Breast-feeding—Although methenamine and very small amounts of atropine and hyoscyamine (contained in this combination medicine) pass into the breast milk, this medicine has not been reported to cause problems in nursing babies.

Children—Unusual excitement, nervousness, restlessness or irritability, and unusual warmth, dryness, and flushing of skin are more likely to occur in children, who are usually more sensitive to the effects of atropine and hyoscyamine (contained in this combination medicine). Also, when atropine and hyoscyamine are given to children during hot weather, a rapid increase in body temperature may occur. In infants and children, especially those with spastic paralysis or brain damage, this medicine may be more likely to cause severe side effects.

Older adults—Confusion or memory loss, constipation, difficult urination, excitement, agitation, drowsiness, or dryness of mouth may be more likely to occur in elderly patients, who are usually more sensitive than younger adults to the effects of atropine and hyoscyamine. Also, this combination medicine may cause eye pain in patients who have untreated glaucoma.

Other medicines—Although certain medicines should not be used together at all, in other cases two different medicines may be used together even if an interaction might occur. In these cases, your doctor may want to change the dose, or other precautions may be necessary. When you are taking this combination medicine, it is especially important that your doctor and pharmacist know if you are taking any of the following:

- Antacids or
- Diarrhea medicine containing kaolin or attapulgite or
- Thiazide diuretics (water pills) or
- Urinary alkalizers (medicine that makes the urine less acid, such as acetazolamide [e.g., Diamox], calcium- and/or magnesium-containing antacids, dichlorphenamide [e.g., Daranide], methazolamide [e.g., Neptazone], potassium or sodium citrate and/or citric acid, sodium bicarbonate [baking soda])—Use with these medicines may decrease the effects of this combination medicine
- Ketoconazole (e.g., Nizoral)—Use with this combination medicine may reduce the effects of ketoconazole
- Other anticholinergics (medicine for abdominal or stomach spasms or cramps)—Use with these medicines may increase the effects of atropine and hyoscyamine
- Potassium chloride (e.g., Slow K or K-Dur)—May worsen or cause an increase in lesions (sores) of the stomach or intestine
- Sulfonamides (sulfa medicine)—Use with this combination medicine may increase the risk of crystals forming in the urine

Other medical problems—The presence of other medical problems may affect the use of this combination medicine. Make sure you tell your doctor if you have any other medical problems, especially:

- Bleeding problems (severe)—This combination medicine may increase heart rate, which would make bleeding problems worse
- Brain damage (in children)—May increase the central nervous system (CNS) effects of this combination medicine
- Colitis (severe) or
- Dryness of mouth (severe or continuing) or
- Enlarged prostate or
- Fever or
- Glaucoma or
- Heart disease or
- Hernia (hiatal) or
- High blood pressure or
- Intestinal blockage or other intestinal or stomach problems or
- Lung disease or
- Myasthenia gravis or
- Toxemia of pregnancy or
- Urinary tract blockage or difficult urination—This combination medicine may make these conditions worse
- Dehydration or
- Kidney disease or
- Liver disease—Higher levels of medicine may result and increase the risk of side effects
- Overactive thyroid—May increase the heart rate

Before you begin using any new medicine (prescription or nonprescription) or if you develop any new medical problem while you are using this medicine, check with your doctor, nurse, or pharmacist.

Proper Use of This Medicine

Take this medicine only as directed. Do not take more of it, do not take it more often, and do not take it for a longer time than your doctor ordered. To do so may increase the chance of side effects.

Each dose should be taken with a full glass (8 ounces) of water or other liquid (except citrus juices and milk). Drink plenty of water or other liquids every day, unless otherwise directed by your doctor. Drinking enough liquids will help your kidneys work better and lessen your discomfort.

To help clear up your infection completely, *keep taking this medicine for the full time of treatment* even if you begin to feel better after a few days. *Do not miss any doses.*

In order for this medicine to work well, your urine must be acid (pH 5.5 or below). To make sure that your urine is acid:

- Before you start taking this medicine, check your urine with phenaphthazine paper or another test to see if it is acid. If you have any questions about this, check with your doctor or pharmacist.
- You may need to change your diet; however, check with your doctor first if you are on a special diet (for example, for diabetes). To help make your urine more acid you should avoid most fruits (especially citrus fruits and juices), milk and other dairy products, and other foods which make the urine more alkaline. Eating more protein and foods such as cranberries (especially cranberry juice with vitamin C added), plums, or prunes may also help. If your urine is still not acid enough, check with your doctor.

Dosing—The dose of this combination medicine will be different for different patients. *Follow your doctor's orders or the direction on the label.* The following information includes only the average doses of this combination medicine. *If your dose is different, do not change it* unless your doctor tells you to do so.

- For *oral* dosage form (tablets):
  - —For relief of urinary tract symptoms:
    - Adults and children 12 years of age and older—1 to 2 tablets four times a day.
    - Children 6 to 12 years of age—Dose must be determined by the doctor.
    - Children up to 6 years of age—Use is not recommended.

Missed dose—If you miss a dose of this medicine, take it as soon as possible. However, if it is almost time for your next dose, skip the missed dose and go back to your regular dosing schedule. Do not double doses.

Storage—To store this medicine:

- Keep out of the reach of children.
- Store away from heat and direct light.
- Do not store this medicine in the bathroom, near the kitchen sink, or in other damp places. Heat or moisture may cause the medicine to break down.
- Do not keep outdated medicine or medicine no longer needed. Be sure that any discarded medicine is out of the reach of children.

Precautions While Using This Medicine

If your symptoms do not improve within a few days or if they become worse, check with your doctor.

These medicines may make you sweat less, causing your body temperature to increase. *Use extra care not to become overheated during exercise or hot weather while you are taking this medicine,* since overheating may result in heat stroke. Also, hot baths or saunas may make you dizzy or faint while you are taking this medicine.

This medicine may cause some people to have blurred vision. *Make sure you know how you react to this medicine before you drive, use machines, or do anything else that could be dangerous if you are not able to see well. If your vision continues to be blurred, check with your doctor.*

This medicine may cause dryness of the mouth. For temporary relief, use sugarless candy or gum, melt bits of ice in your mouth, or use a saliva substitute. However, if your mouth continues to feel dry for more than 2 weeks, check with your dentist. Continuing dryness of the mouth may increase the chance of dental disease, including tooth decay, gum disease, and fungus infections.

Do not take this medicine within 2 or 3 hours of taking antacids or medicine for diarrhea. Taking antacids or antidiarrhea medicines and this medicine too close together may prevent this medicine from working properly.

Side Effects of This Medicine

Along with its needed effects, a medicine may cause some unwanted effects. Although not all of these side effects may occur, if they do occur they may need medical attention.

Check with your doctor as soon as possible if any of the following side effects occur:

Less common or rare

Blurred vision; eye pain; skin rash or hives

Symptoms of overdose

Blood in urine and/or stools; diarrhea; dizziness; drowsiness (severe); fast heartbeat; flushing or redness of face; headache (severe or continuing); lower back pain; pain or burning while urinating; ringing or buzzing in the ears; shortness of breath or troubled breathing; sweating; unusual tiredness or weakness

Other side effects may occur that usually do not need medical attention. These side effects may go away during treatment as your body adjusts to the medicine. However, check with your doctor if any of the following side effects continue or are bothersome:

Less common

Difficult urination (more common with large doses taken over a prolonged period of time); dryness of mouth, nose, or throat; nausea or vomiting; stomach upset or pain (more common with large doses taken over a prolonged period of time)

This medicine may cause your urine and/or stools to turn blue or blue-green. This is to be expected while you are taking this medicine.

Other side effects not listed above may also occur in some patients. If you notice any other effects, check with your doctor.

Annual revision: 05/11/93

ATTAPULGITE Oral

Some commonly used brand names are:

In the U.S.

- Diar-Aid
- Diasorb
- Kaopectate
- Kaopectate Advanced Formula
- Kaopectate Maximum Strength
- Rheaban
- St. Joseph Antidiarrheal

In Canada

- Fowler's Diarrhea Tablets
- Kaopectate

Description

Attapulgite is taken by mouth to treat diarrhea. Attapulgite is a clay-like powder believed to work by adsorbing the bacteria or germ that may be causing the diarrhea.

This medicine is available without a prescription; however, the product's directions and warnings should be carefully followed. In addition, your doctor may have special instructions on the proper dose or use of attapulgite medicine for your medical condition.

Attapulgite is available in the following dosage forms:

Oral

Attapulgite
- Oral suspension (U.S. and Canada)
- Tablets (U.S. and Canada)
- Chewable tablets (U.S. and Canada)

It is very important that you read and understand the following information. If any of it causes you special concern, check with your doctor or pharmacist. Also, *if you have any questions* or if you want more information about this medicine or your medical problem, *ask your doctor, nurse, or pharmacist.*

Before Using This Medicine

If you are taking this medicine without a prescription, carefully read and follow any precautions on the label. For attapulgite, the following should be considered:

Pregnancy—This medicine is not absorbed into the body and is not likely to cause problems.

Breast-feeding—This medicine is not absorbed into the body and is not likely to cause problems.

Children—The fluid loss caused by diarrhea may result in a severe condition. For this reason, antidiarrheals must not be given to young children (under 3 years of age) without first checking with their doctor. In older children with diarrhea, antidiarrheals may be used, but it is also very important that a sufficient amount of liquids be given to replace the fluid lost by the body. If you have any questions about this, check with your doctor, nurse, or pharmacist.

Older adults—The fluid loss caused by diarrhea may result in a severe condition. For this reason, elderly persons with diarrhea, in addition to using an antidiarrheal, must receive a sufficient amount of liquids to replace the fluid lost by the body. If you have any questions about this, check with your doctor, nurse, or pharmacist.

Other medicines—Although certain medicines should not be used together at all, in other cases two different medicines may be used together even if an interaction might occur. In these cases, your doctor may want to change the dose, or other precautions may be necessary. *If you are taking any other medicine, do not take it within 2 to 3 hours of attapulgite.* Taking the medicines at the same time may prevent the other medicine from being absorbed by your body. If you have any questions about this, check with your doctor, nurse, or pharmacist.

Other medical problems—The presence of other medical problems may affect the use of attapulgite. Make sure you tell your doctor if you have any other medical problems, especially:

- Dysentery—This condition may get worse; a different kind of treatment may be needed

Before you begin using any new medicine (prescription or nonprescription) or if you develop any new medical problem while you are using this medicine, check with your doctor, nurse, or pharmacist.

Proper Use of This Medicine

Take this medicine after each loose bowel movement following the directions in the product package, unless otherwise directed by your doctor.

Importance of diet and fluid intake while treating diarrhea:

- *In addition to using medicine for diarrhea, it is very important that you replace the fluid lost by the body and follow a proper diet.* For the first 24 hours you should drink plenty of clear liquids, such as ginger ale, decaffeinated cola, decaffeinated tea, broth, and gelatin. During the next 24 hours you may eat bland foods, such as cooked cereals, bread, crackers, and applesauce. Fruits, vegetables, fried or spicy foods, bran, candy, and caffeine and alcoholic beverages may make the condition worse.
- If too much fluid has been lost by the body due to the diarrhea a serious condition may develop. Check with your doctor as soon as possible if any of the following signs of too much fluid loss occur:

  Decreased urination
  Dizziness and lightheadedness
  Dryness of mouth
  Increased thirst
  Wrinkled skin

Storage—To store this medicine:
- Keep out of the reach of children.
- Store away from heat and direct light.
- Keep the liquid form of this medicine from freezing.
- Do not keep outdated medicine or medicine no longer needed. Be sure that any discarded medicine is out of the reach of children.

Precautions While Using This Medicine

Check with your doctor if your diarrhea does not stop after 1 or 2 days or if you develop a fever.

Side Effects of This Medicine

Along with its needed effects, a medicine may cause some unwanted effects. No serious side effects have been reported for this medicine. However, constipation may occur in some patients, especially if they take a lot of it. Check with your doctor as soon as possible if constipation continues or is bothersome.

Other side effects not listed above may also occur in some patients. If you notice any other effects, check with your doctor.

Annual revision: 07/31/91

AZATHIOPRINE Systemic

A commonly used brand name in the U.S. and Canada is Imuran.

Description

Azathioprine (ay-za-THYE-oh-preen) belongs to the group of medicines known as immunosuppressive agents. It is used to reduce the body's natural immunity in patients who receive organ transplants. It is also used to treat rheumatoid arthritis. Azathioprine may also be used for other conditions as determined by your doctor.

Azathioprine is a very strong medicine. You and your doctor should talk about the need for this medicine and its risks. Even though azathioprine may cause side effects that could be very serious, remember that it may be required to treat your medical problem.

Azathioprine is available only with your doctor's prescription, in the following dosage forms:

Oral

- Tablets (U.S. and Canada)

Parenteral

- Injection (U.S. and Canada)

It is very important that you read and understand the following information. If any of it causes you special concern, check with your doctor. Also, *if you have any questions* or if you want more information about this medicine or your medical problem, *ask your doctor, nurse, or pharmacist.*

Before Using This Medicine

In deciding to use a medicine, the risks of taking the medicine must be weighed against the good it will do. This is a decision you and your doctor will make. For azathioprine, the following should be considered:

Allergies—Tell your doctor if you have ever had any unusual or allergic reaction to azathioprine. Also tell your doctor and pharmacist if you are allergic to any other substances, such as foods, preservatives, or dyes.

Pregnancy—Use of azathioprine is not recommended during pregnancy. It may cause birth defects if either the male or the female is using it at the time of conception. The use of birth control methods is recommended. If you have any questions about this, check with your doctor.

Breast-feeding—Azathioprine passes into breast milk. Because this medicine may cause serious side effects, breast-feeding is generally not recommended while you are using it.

Children—This medicine has been tested in children and, in effective doses, has not been shown to cause different side effects or problems than it does in adults.

Older adults—Many medicines have not been studied specifically in older people. Therefore, it may not be known whether they work exactly the same way they do in younger adults. Although there is no specific information comparing use of azathioprine in the elderly with use in other age groups, this medicine is not expected to cause different side effects or problems in older people than it does in younger adults.

Other medicines—Although certain medicines should not be used together at all, in other cases two different medicines may be used together even if an interaction might occur. In these cases, your doctor may want to change the dose, or other precautions may be necessary. When taking or receiving azathioprine it is especially important that your doctor and pharmacist know if you are taking any of the following:

- Allopurinol (e.g., Zyloprim)—May interfere with removal of azathioprine from the body; effects of azathioprine (including toxicity) may be increased
- Chlorambucil (e.g., Leukeran) or
- Corticosteroids (cortisone-like medicine) or
- Cyclophosphamide (e.g., Cytoxan) or
- Cyclosporine (e.g., Sandimmune) or
- Mercaptopurine (e.g., Purinethol) or
- Muromonab-CD3 (monoclonal antibody) (e.g., Orthoclone OKT3)—There may be an increased risk of infection and cancer because azathioprine reduces the body's ability to fight them

Other medical problems—The presence of other medical problems may affect the use azathioprine. Make sure you tell your doctor if you have any other medical problems, especially:

- Chickenpox (including recent exposure) or
- Herpes zoster (shingles)—Risk of severe disease affecting other parts of the body

- Gout—Allopurinol (used to treat gout) may increase wanted and unwanted effects of azathioprine
- Infection—Azathioprine decreases your body's ability to fight infection
- Kidney disease or
- Liver disease—Effects of azathioprine may be increased because of slower removal from the body
- Pancreatitis (inflammation of the pancreas)—Azathioprine can cause pancreatitis

Before you begin using any new medicine (prescription or nonprescription) or if you develop any new medical problem while you are using this medicine, check with your doctor, nurse, or pharmacist.

Proper Use of This Medicine

Use this medicine only as directed by your doctor. Do not use more or less of it, and do not use it more often than your doctor ordered. The exact amount of medicine you need has been carefully worked out. Taking too much may increase the chance of side effects, while taking too little may not properly treat your condition.

This medicine is sometimes given together with certain other medicines. If you are using a combination of medicines, make sure that you take each one at the proper time and do not mix them up. Ask your doctor, nurse, or pharmacist to help you plan a way to remember to take your medicines at the right times.

Do not stop taking this medicine without first checking with your doctor.

Azathioprine sometimes causes nausea or vomiting. Taking this medicine after meals or at bedtime may lessen stomach upset. Ask your doctor, nurse, or pharmacist for other ways to lessen these effects.

If you vomit shortly after taking a dose of azathioprine, check with your doctor. You will be told whether to take the dose again or to wait until the next scheduled dose.

Missed dose—If you miss a dose of this medicine and your dosing schedule is:

- One dose a day—Do not take the missed dose at all and do not double the next one. Instead, go back to your regular dosing schedule and check with your doctor.
- More than one dose a day—Take the missed dose as soon as you remember it. If it is time for your next dose, take both doses together, then go back to your regular dosing schedule. If you miss more than one dose, check with your doctor.

Storage—To store this medicine:

- Keep out of the reach of children.
- Store away from heat and direct light.
- Do not store in the bathroom, near the kitchen sink, or in other damp places. Heat or moisture may cause the medicine to break down.
- Do not keep outdated medicine or medicine no longer needed. Be sure that any discarded medicine is out of the reach of children.

Precautions While Using This Medicine

It is very important that your doctor check your progress at regular visits to make sure that this medicine is working properly and to check for unwanted effects.

While you are being treated with azathioprine, and after you stop treatment with it, *do not have any immunizations (vaccinations) without your doctor's approval.* Azathioprine lowers your body's resistance and there is a chance you might get the infection the immunization is meant to prevent. In addition, other persons living in your household should not take oral polio vaccine since there is a chance they could pass the polio virus on to you. Also, avoid persons who have recently taken oral polio vaccine. Do not get close to them, and do not stay in the same room with them for very long. If you cannot take these precautions, you should consider wearing a protective face mask that covers the nose and mouth.

Azathioprine can temporarily lower the number of white blood cells in your blood, increasing the chance of getting an infection. It can also lower the number of platelets, which are necessary for proper blood clotting. If this occurs, there are certain precautions you can take, especially when your blood count is low, to reduce the risk of infection or bleeding:

- If you can, avoid people with infections. *Check with your doctor immediately* if you think you are getting an infection or if you get a fever or chills, cough or hoarseness, lower back or side pain, or painful or difficult urination.
- *Check with your doctor immediately* if you notice any unusual bleeding or bruising; black, tarry stools; blood in urine or stools; or pinpoint red spots on your skin.
- Be careful when using a regular toothbrush, dental floss, or toothpick. Your medical doctor, dentist, or nurse may recommend other ways to clean your teeth and gums. Check with your medical doctor before having any dental work done.
- Do not touch your eyes or the inside of your nose unless you have just washed your hands and have not touched anything else in the meantime.
- Be careful not to cut yourself when you are using sharp objects such as a safety razor or fingernail or toenail cutters.
- Avoid contact sports or other situations where bruising or injury could occur.

Side Effects of This Medicine

Along with its needed effects, a medicine may cause some unwanted effects. Some side effects will have signs or symptoms that you can see or feel. Your doctor will watch for others by doing certain tests.

Also, because of the way these medicines act on the body, there is a chance that they might cause other unwanted effects that may not occur until months or years after the medicine is used. These delayed effects may include certain types of cancer, such as leukemia, lymphoma, or skin cancer. However, the risk of cancer seems to be lower in people taking azathioprine for arthritis. Discuss these possible effects with your doctor.

Check with your doctor immediately if any of the following side effects occur:

More common

Unusual tiredness or weakness

Less common

Cough or hoarseness; fever or chills; lower back or side pain; painful or difficult urination

Rare

Black, tarry stools; blood in urine or stools; fast heartbeat; fever (sudden); muscle or joint pain; nausea, vomiting, and diarrhea (severe); pinpoint red spots on skin; redness or blisters on skin; stomach pain (severe) with nausea and vomiting; unusual bleeding or bruising; unusual feeling of discomfort or illness (sudden)

Check with your doctor as soon as possible if any of the following side effects occur:

Rare

Shortness of breath; sores in mouth and on lips; stomach pain; swelling of feet or lower legs

This medicine may also cause the following side effect that your doctor will watch for:

Less common

Liver problems

For patients taking this medicine *for rheumatoid arthritis:*

- Signs and symptoms of blood problems (black, tarry stools; blood in urine or stools; cough or hoarseness; fever or chills; lower back or side pain; painful or difficult urination; pinpoint red spots on skin; unusual tiredness or weakness; or unusual bleeding or bruising) are less likely to occur in patients taking azathioprine for rheumatoid arthritis than for transplant rejection. This is because lower doses are often used.

Other side effects may occur that usually do not need medical attention. These side effects may go away during treatment as your body adjusts to the medicine. However, check with your doctor if any of the following side effects continue or are bothersome:

More common

Loss of appetite; nausea or vomiting

Less common

Skin rash

After you stop using this medicine, it may still produce some side effects that need attention. During this period of time *check with your doctor immediately* if you notice any of the following:

Black, tarry stools; blood in urine; cough or hoarseness; fever or chills; lower back or side pain; painful or difficult urination; pinpoint red spots on skin; unusual bleeding or bruising

Other side effects not listed above may also occur in some patients. If you notice any other effects, check with your doctor.

Additional Information

Once a medicine has been approved for marketing for a certain use, experience may show that it is also useful for other medical problems. Although these uses are not included in product labeling, azathioprine is used in certain patients with the following medical conditions:

- Bowel disease, inflammatory
- Hepatitis, chronic active
- Cirrhosis, biliary
- Lupus erythematosus, systemic
- Glomerulonephritis
- Nephrotic syndrome
- Myopathy, inflammatory
- Myasthenia gravis
- Dermatomyositis, systemic
- Pemphigoid
- Pemphigus

Other than the above information, there is no additional information relating to proper use, precautions, or side effects for these uses.

Annual revision: 05/06/93

AZITHROMYCIN Systemic†

A commonly used brand name in the U.S. is Zithromax.

†Not commercially available in Canada.

Description

Azithromycin (az-ith-roe-MYE-sin) is used to treat bacterial infections in many different parts of the body. It works by killing bacteria or preventing their growth. However, this medicine will not work for colds, flu, or other virus infections. Azithromycin may be used for other problems as determined by your doctor.

Azithromycin is available only with your doctor's prescription, in the following dosage form:

Oral

- Capsules (U.S.)

It is very important that you read and understand the following information. If any of it causes you special concern, check with your doctor. Also, *if you have any questions* or if you want more information about this medicine or your medical problem, *ask your doctor, nurse, or pharmacist.*

Before Using This Medicine

In deciding to use a medicine, the risks of taking the medicine must be weighed against the good it will do. This is a decision you and your doctor will make. For azithromycin, the following should be considered:

Allergies—Tell your doctor if you have ever had any unusual or allergic reaction to azithromycin or to any related medicines such as erythromycin. Also tell your doctor and pharmacist if you are allergic to any other substances, such as foods, preservatives, or dyes.

Pregnancy—Azithromycin has not been studied in pregnant women. However, azithromycin has not been shown to cause birth defects or other problems in animal studies.

Breast-feeding—It is not known whether azithromycin passes into breast milk.

Children—This medicine has been tested in a limited number of children up to the age of 16. In effective doses, the medicine has not been shown to cause different side effects of problems than it does in adults.

Older adults—This medicine has been tested in a limited number of elderly patients and has not been shown to cause different side effects or problems in older people than it does in younger adults.

Other medicines—Although certain medicines should not be used together at all, in other cases two different medicines may be used together even if an interaction might occur. In these cases, your doctor may want to change the dose, or other precautions may be necessary. When you are taking azithromycin, it is especially important that your doctor and pharmacist know if you are taking any of the following:

- Antacids, aluminum- and magnesium-containing—Antacids may decrease the amount of azithromycin in the blood, which may decrease its effects. To avoid problems, azithromycin should be taken at least one hour before or at least 2 hours after taking antacids

Other medical problems—The presence of other medical problems may affect the use of azithromycin. Make sure you tell your doctor if you have any other medical problems, especially:

- Liver disease—Patients with liver disease may have an increased chance of side effects

Before you begin using any new medicine (prescription or nonprescription) or if you develop any new medical problem while you are using this medicine, check with your doctor, nurse, or pharmacist.

Proper Use of This Medicine

Azithromycin should be taken at least one hour before or at least 2 hours after meals. Taking azithromycin with food may decrease the amount of medicine that gets into your blood and keep the medicine from working properly.

To help clear up your infection completely, *keep taking azithromycin for the full time of treatment,* even if you begin to feel better after a few days. If you stop taking this medicine too soon, your symptoms may return.

Dosing—The dose of azithromycin will be different for different patients. *Follow your doctor's orders or the directions on the label.* The following information includes only the average doses of azithromycin. *If your dose is different, do not change it* unless your doctor tells you to do so.

- For bronchitis, strep throat, pneumonia, and skin infections:

  —Adults and children 16 years of age and older: 500 mg on the day 1, then 250 mg once a day on days 2 through 5.

  —Children up to 16 years of age: To be determined by doctor.
- For chlamydia infections:

  —Adults and children 16 years of age and older: 1000 mg taken once as a single dose.

  —Children up to 16 years of age: To be determined by doctor.

Missed dose—If you miss a dose of this medicine, take it as soon as possible. However, if it is almost time for your next dose, skip the missed dose and go back to your regular dosing schedule. Do not double doses.

Storage—To store this medicine:

- Keep out of the reach of children.
- Store away from heat and direct light.
- Do not store in the bathroom, near the kitchen sink, or in other damp places. Heat or moisture may cause the medicine to break down.
- Do not keep outdated medicine or medicine no longer needed. Be sure that any discarded medicine is out of the reach of children.

Precautions While Using This Medicine

If your symptoms do not improve within a few days, or if they become worse, check with your doctor.

Side Effects of This Medicine

Along with its needed effects, a medicine may cause some unwanted effects. Although not all of these side effects may occur, if they do occur they may need medical attention.

Stop taking this medicine and get emergency help immediately if any of the following side effects occur:

Rare

Difficulty in breathing; skin rash; swelling of face, mouth, neck, hands, and feet

Other side effects may occur that usually do not need medical attention. These side effects may go away during treatment as your body adjusts to the medicine. However, check with your doctor if any of the following side effects continue or are bothersome:

Less common

Diarrhea; nausea; stomach pain or discomfort; vomiting

Rare

Dizziness; headache

Other side effects not listed above may also occur in some patients. If you notice any other effects, check with your doctor.

Additional Information

Once a medicine has been approved for marketing for a certain use, experience may show that it is also useful for other medical problems. Although this use is not included in product labeling, azithromycin is used in certain patients with the following medical condition:

- Mycoplasmal pneumonia

Other than the above information, there is no additional information relating to proper use, precautions, or side effects for this use.

Annual revision: 01/05/93

AZTREONAM Systemic†

A commonly used brand name in the U.S. is Azactam.

†Not commercially available in Canada.

Description

Aztreonam (az-TREE-oh-nam) is an antibiotic that is used to treat infections caused by bacteria. It works by killing bacteria or preventing their growth.

Aztreonam is used to treat bacterial infections in many different parts of the body. It is sometimes given with other antibiotics. This medicine will not work for colds, flu, or other virus infections.

This medicine is available only with your doctor's prescription. It is available in the following dosage form:

Parenteral

- Injection (U.S.)

It is very important that you read and understand the following information. If any of it causes you special concern, check with your doctor. Also, *if you have any questions* or if you want more information about this medicine or your medical problem, *ask your doctor, nurse, or pharmacist.*

Before Receiving This Medicine

In deciding to use a medicine, the risks of taking the medicine must be weighed against the good it will do. This is a decision you and your doctor will make. For aztreonam, the following should be considered:

Allergies—Tell your doctor if you have ever had any unusual or allergic reaction to aztreonam. Also tell your doctor and pharmacist if you are allergic to any other substances, such as foods, preservatives, or dyes.

Pregnancy—Studies have not been done in humans. However, aztreonam has not been shown to cause birth defects

B

or other problems in studies in rabbits and rats given up to 15 times the highest human daily dose.

Breast-feeding—Aztreonam passes into the breast milk in small amounts. However, this medicine is not absorbed when taken by mouth, and problems have not been seen in nursing babies.

Children—This medicine has been tested in a limited number of children up to 12 years of age and has not been shown to cause different side effects or problems in children than it does in adults.

Older adults—Aztreonam has been tested in a limited number of patients 65 years of age or older and has not been shown to cause different side effects or problems in older people than it does in younger adults.

Other medicines—Although certain medicines should not be used together at all, in other cases two different medicines may be used together even if an interaction might occur. In these cases, your doctor may want to change the dose, or other precautions may be necessary. Tell your doctor or pharmacist if you are taking any other prescription or nonprescription (over-the-counter [OTC]) medicine.

Other medical problems—The presence of other medical problems may affect the use of aztreonam. Make sure you tell your doctor if you have any other medical problems, especially:

- Cirrhosis (liver disease)—Patients receiving high doses of aztreonam for a long time, who also have severe liver disease, may have an increased chance of side effects
- Kidney disease—Patients with kidney disease may have an increased chance of side effects

Before you begin using any new medicine (prescription or nonprescription) or if you develop any new medical problem while you are using this medicine, check with your doctor, nurse, or pharmacist.

Proper Use of This Medicine

To help clear up your infection completely, *aztreonam must be given for the full time of treatment,* even if you begin to feel better after a few days. Also, this medicine works best when there is a constant amount in the blood or urine. To help keep the amount constant, aztreonam must be given on a regular schedule.

Dosing—The dose of aztreonam will be different for different patients. *Follow your doctor's orders or the directions on the label.* The following information includes only the average doses of aztreonam. Your dose may be different if you have kidney disease. *If your dose is different, do not change it* unless your doctor tells you to do so.

- For *injection* dosage form:
  - —Adults and children 12 years of age and older: 1 to 2 grams injected slowly into a vein over a twenty- to sixty-minute period. This is repeated every six to twelve hours.
  - —Children up to 12 years of age: Dosage is based on body weight and must be determined by your doctor.

Side Effects of This Medicine

Along with its needed effects, a medicine may cause some unwanted effects. Although not all of these side effects may occur, if they do occur they may need medical attention.

Check with your doctor immediately if any of the following side effects occur:

Less common

Pain, swelling, or redness at place of injection; skin rash, redness, or itching

Other side effects may occur that usually do not need medical attention. These side effects may go away during treatment as your body adjusts to the medicine. However, check with your doctor if any of the following side effects continue or are bothersome:

Less common or rare

Abdominal or stomach cramps; nausea, vomiting, or diarrhea

Other side effects not listed above may also occur in some patients. If you notice any other effects, check with your doctor.

Annual revision: 02/23/93

B

BACILLUS CALMETTE-GUÉRIN (BCG) LIVE Mucosal-Local

Some commonly used brand names are:

In the U.S.

TheraCys

TICE BCG

In Canada

ImmuCyst

Description

Bacillus Calmette-Guérin (BCG) is used as a solution that is run through a tube (instilled through a catheter) into the bladder to treat bladder cancer. The exact way it works against cancer is not known, but it may work by stimulating the body's immune system.

BCG is to be administered only by or under the immediate supervision of your doctor. It is available in the following dosage form:

Mucosal-Local

- Bladder instillation (U.S. and Canada)

It is very important that you read and understand the following information. If any of it causes you special concern, check with your doctor. Also, *if you have any questions* or if you want more information about this medicine or your medical problem, *ask your doctor, nurse, or pharmacist.*

Before Receiving This Medicine

In deciding to use a medicine, the risks of taking the medicine must be weighed against the good it will do. This is a decision you and your doctor will make. For BCG, the following should be considered:

Allergies—Tell your doctor if you have ever had any unusual or allergic reaction to BCG.

Pregnancy—BCG has not been studied in pregnant women or animals. Make sure your doctor knows if you are pregnant or if you may become pregnant before receiving BCG.

Breast-feeding—It is not known whether BCG passes into the breast milk.

Children—There is no specific information comparing use of BCG for treatment of cancer in children with use in other age groups.

Older adults—This medicine has been tested and has not been shown to cause different side effects or problems in older people than it does in younger adults.

Other medicines—Although certain medicines should not be used together at all, in other cases two different medicines may be used together even if an interaction might occur. In these cases, your doctor may want to change the dose, or other precautions may be necessary. When receiving BCG it is especially important that your doctor and pharmacist know if you are taking any of the following:

- Adrenocorticoids (cortisone-like medicine) or
- Amphotericin B by injection (e.g., Fungizone) or
- Antineoplastics (cancer medicine) or
- Antithyroid agents (medicine for overactive thyroid) or
- Azathioprine (e.g., Imuran) or
- Chlorambucil (e.g., Leukeran) or
- Chloramphenicol (e.g., Chloromycetin) or
- Colchicine or
- Cyclophosphamide (e.g., Cytoxan) or
- Cyclosporine (e.g., Sandimmune) or
- Flucytosine (e.g., Ancobon) or
- Interferon (e.g., Intron A, Roferon-A) or
- Mercaptopurine (e.g., Purinethol) or
- Methotrexate (e.g., Mexate) or
- Muromonab-CD3 (e.g., Orthoclone OKT3) or
- Plicamycin (e.g., Mithracin) or
- Zidovudine (e.g., Retrovir)—Because these medicines reduce the body's natural immunity, they may prevent BCG from stimulating the immune system and will cause it to be less effective. In addition, the risk of infection may be increased

Other medical problems—The presence of other medical problems may affect the use of BCG. Make sure you tell your doctor if you have any other medical problems, especially:

- Fever—Infection may be present and could cause problems
- Immunity problems—BCG treatment is less effective and there is a risk of infection
- Urinary tract infection—Infection and irritation of the bladder may occur

Before you begin using any new medicine (prescription or nonprescription) or if you develop any new medical problem while you are using this medicine, check with your doctor, nurse, or pharmacist.

Proper Use of This Medicine

Your doctor will ask you to empty your bladder completely before the solution is instilled into it.

Follow your doctor's instructions carefully about how long to hold the solution in your bladder:

- The solution should be held in your bladder for 2 hours. If you think you cannot hold it, tell your doctor or nurse.
- During the first hour, your doctor may have you lie for 15 minutes each on your stomach, back, and each side.
- When you do empty your bladder, you should be sitting down.

It is important that you drink extra fluids for several hours after each treatment with BCG so that you will pass more urine. Also, empty your bladder frequently. This will help prevent bladder problems.

BCG is a live product. In other words, it contains active bacteria that can cause infection. Some bacteria will be present for several hours in urine that you pass after each treatment with BCG. Any urine that you pass during the first 6 hours after each treatment should be disinfected with an equal amount (usually about 1 cup) of undiluted household bleach. After the bleach is added to the urine, it should be allowed to sit for 15 minutes before it is flushed. If you have any questions about this, check with your doctor.

Precautions While Using This Medicine

While you are being treated with BCG, and for 6 to 12 weeks after you stop treatment with it, avoid contact with people who have tuberculosis. If you think you have been exposed to someone with tuberculosis, tell your doctor.

While you are being treated with BCG and for a few weeks after you stop treatment with it, do not have any immunizations (vaccinations) without your doctor's approval.

Side Effects of This Medicine

Along with its needed effects, a medicine may cause some unwanted effects. Although not all of these side effects may occur, if they do occur they may need medical attention.

Check with your doctor as soon as possible if any of the following side effects occur:

More common

Blood in urine; fever and chills; frequent urge to urinate; increased frequency of urination; joint pain; nausea and vomiting; painful urination (severe or continuing)

Rare

Cough; skin rash

Other side effects may occur that usually do not need medical attention. These side effects may go away during treatment as your body adjusts to the medicine. However, check with your doctor if any of the following side effects continue or are bothersome or if you have any questions about them:

More common

Burning during first urination after treatment

After you stop using this medicine, your body may need time to adjust. The length of time this takes depends on the amount of medicine you were using and how long you used it. During this period of time (up to 6 months after treatment with BCG) check with your doctor if you notice any of the following side effects:

Cough; fever

Other side effects not listed above may also occur in some patients. If you notice any other effects, check with your doctor.

Annual revision: 06/14/91

BACLOFEN Systemic

A commonly used brand name in the U.S. and Canada is Lioresal. Generic name product may also be available in the U.S.

Description

Baclofen (BAK-loe-fen) is used to help relax certain muscles in your body. It relieves the spasms, cramping, and tightness of muscles caused by medical problems such as multiple sclerosis or certain injuries to the spine. Baclofen does not cure these problems, but it may allow other treatment, such as physical therapy, to be more helpful in improving your condition.

Baclofen acts on the central nervous system (CNS) to produce its muscle relaxant effects. Its actions on the CNS may also cause some of the medicine's side effects. Baclofen may also be used to relieve other conditions as determined by your doctor.

This medicine is available only with your doctor's prescription, in the following dosage form:

Oral

- Tablets (U.S. and Canada)

It is very important that you read and understand the following information. If any of it causes you special concern, check with your doctor. Also, *if you have any questions* or if you want more information about this medicine or your medical problem, *ask your doctor, nurse, or pharmacist.*

Before Using This Medicine

In deciding to use a medicine, the risks of taking the medicine must be weighed against the good it will do. This is a decision you and your doctor will make. For baclofen, the following should be considered:

Allergies—Tell your doctor if you have ever had any unusual or allergic reaction to baclofen. Also tell your doctor and pharmacist if you are allergic to any other substances, such as foods, preservatives, or dyes.

Pregnancy—Studies on birth defects with baclofen have not been done in humans. However, studies in animals have shown that baclofen, when given in doses several times the human dose, increases the chance of hernias and incomplete or slow development of bones in the fetus, and of lower birth weight.

Breast-feeding—Baclofen passes into the breast milk. However, this medicine has not been reported to cause problems in nursing babies.

Children—Studies on this medicine have been done only in adult patients, and there is no specific information comparing use of baclofen in children with use in other age groups.

Older adults—Side effects such as hallucinations, confusion or mental depression, other mood or mental changes, and severe drowsiness may be especially likely to occur in elderly patients, who are usually more sensitive than younger adults to the effects of baclofen.

Other medicines—Although certain medicines should not be used together at all, in other cases two different medicines may be used together even if an interaction might occur. In these cases, your doctor may want to change the dose, or other precautions may be necessary. When you are taking baclofen, it is especially important that your doctor and pharmacist know if you are taking any of the following:

- Antidepressants, tricyclic (amitriptyline [e.g., Elavil]), amoxapine [e.g., Asendin], clomipramine [e.g., Anafranil], desipramine [e.g., Pertofrane], doxepin [e.g., Sinequan], imipramine [e.g., Tofranil], nortriptyline [e.g., Aventyl], protriptyline [e.g., Vivactil], trimipramine [e.g., Surmontil]) or
- Central nervous system (CNS) depressants—The chance of side effects may be increased

Other medical problems—The presence of other medical problems may affect the use of baclofen. Make sure you tell your doctor if you have any other medical problems, especially:

- Diabetes mellitus (sugar diabetes)—Baclofen may raise blood sugar levels
- Epilepsy or
- Kidney disease or
- Mental or emotional problems or
- Stroke or other brain disease—The chance of side effects may be increased

Before you begin using any new medicine (prescription or nonprescription) or if you develop any new medical problem while you are using this medicine, check with your doctor, nurse, or pharmacist.

Proper Use of This Medicine

Missed dose—If you miss a dose of this medicine, and you remember within an hour or so of the missed dose, take it as soon as you remember. However, if you do not remember until later, skip the missed dose and go back to your regular dosing schedule. Do not double doses.

Storage—To store this medicine:

- Keep out of the reach of children.
- Store away from heat and direct light.
- Do not store in the bathroom, near the kitchen sink, or in other damp places. Heat or moisture may cause the medicine to break down.
- Do not keep outdated medicine or medicine no longer needed. Be sure that any discarded medicine is out of the reach of children.

Precautions While Using This Medicine

Do not suddenly stop taking this medicine. Unwanted effects may occur if the medicine is stopped suddenly. Check with your doctor for the best way to reduce gradually the amount you are taking before stopping completely.

This medicine will add to the effects of alcohol and other CNS depressants (medicines that slow down the nervous system, possibly causing drowsiness). Some examples of CNS depressants are antihistamines or medicine for hay fever, other allergies, or colds; sedatives, tranquilizers, or sleeping medicine; prescription pain medicine or narcotics; barbiturates; medicine for seizures; other muscle relaxants; or anesthetics, including some dental anesthetics. *Check with your doctor before taking any of the above while you are using baclofen.*

This medicine may cause drowsiness, dizziness, vision problems, or clumsiness or unsteadiness in some people. *Make sure you know how you react to this medicine before you drive, use machines, or do anything else that could be dangerous if you are not alert, well-coordinated, and able to see well.*

For *diabetic patients:*

- This medicine may cause your blood sugar levels to rise. If you notice a change in the results of your blood or urine sugar test or if you have any questions about this, check with your doctor.

Side Effects of This Medicine

Along with its needed effects, a medicine may cause some unwanted effects. Although not all of these side effects may occur, if they do occur they may need medical attention.

Check with your doctor as soon as possible if any of the following side effects occur:

Rare

Bloody or dark urine; chest pain; fainting; hallucinations (seeing or hearing things that are not there); mental depression or other mood changes; ringing or buzzing in the ears; skin rash or itching

Symptoms of overdose

Blurred or double vision; convulsions (seizures); muscle weakness (severe); shortness of breath or unusually slow or troubled breathing; vomiting

Other side effects may occur that usually do not need medical attention. These side effects may go away during treatment as your body adjusts to the medicine. However, check with your doctor if any of the following side effects continue or are bothersome:

More common

Confusion; dizziness or lightheadedness; drowsiness; nausea; unusual weakness, especially muscle weakness

Less common or rare

Abdominal or stomach pain or discomfort; clumsiness, unsteadiness, trembling, or other problems with muscle control; constipation; diarrhea; difficult or painful urination or decrease in amount of urine; false sense of well-being; frequent urge to urinate or uncontrolled urination; headache; loss of appetite; low blood pressure; muscle or joint pain; numbness or tingling in hands or feet; pounding heartbeat; sexual problems in males; slurred speech or other speech problems; stuffy nose; swelling of ankles; trouble in sleeping; unexplained muscle stiffness; unusual excitement; unusual tiredness; weight gain

Some side effects may occur after you have stopped taking this medicine, especially if you stop taking it suddenly. *Check with your doctor immediately* if any of the following effects occur:

Convulsions (seizures); hallucinations (seeing or hearing things that are not there); increase in muscle spasm, cramping, or tightness; mood or mental changes; unusual nervousness or restlessness

Other side effects not listed above may also occur in some patients. If you notice any other effects, check with your doctor.

Additional Information

Once a medicine has been approved for marketing for a certain use, experience may show that it is also useful for other medical problems. Although this use is not included in product labeling, baclofen is used in certain patients with trigeminal neuralgia (severe burning or stabbing pain along the nerves in the face); also called "tic douloureux."

There is no additional information relating to proper use, precautions, or side effects for this use of baclofen.

Annual revision: 07/09/91

BARBITURATES Systemic

This information applies to the following medicines:

Amobarbital (am-oh-BAR-bi-tal)
Aprobarbital (a-proe-BAR-bi-tal)
Butabarbital (byoo-ta-BAR-bi-tal)
Mephobarbital (me-foe-BAR-bi-tal)
Metharbital (meth-AR-bi-tal)
Pentobarbital (pen-toe-BAR-bi-tal)
Phenobarbital (fee-noe-BAR-bi-tal)
Secobarbital (see-koe-BAR-bi-tal)
Secobarbital and Amobarbital (see-koe-BAR-bi-tal and am-oh-BAR-bi-tal)

Some commonly used brand names are:

For Amobarbital

In the U.S.

Amytal

Generic name product may also be available.

In Canada

Amytal

For Aprobarbital†

In the U.S.

Alurate

For Butabarbital

In the U.S.

Butalan
Butisol
Sarisol No. 2

Generic name product may also be available.

In Canada

Butisol

For Mephobarbital

In the U.S.

Mebaral

In Canada

Mebaral

For Metharbital*†

In other countries

Gemonil

For Pentobarbital
In the U.S.
Nembutal
Generic name product may also be available.
In Canada
Nembutal
Nova Rectal
Novopentobarb

For Phenobarbital
In the U.S.
Barbita
Luminal
Solfoton
Generic name product may also be available.
In Canada
Ancalixir
Generic name product may also be available.

For Secobarbital
In the U.S.
Seconal
Generic name product may also be available.
In Canada
Novosecobarb
Seconal

For Secobarbital and Amobarbital
In the U.S.
Tuinal
In Canada
Tuinal

*Not commercially available in the U.S.
†Not commercially available in Canada.

Description

Barbiturates (bar-BI-tyoo-rates) belong to the group of medicines called central nervous system (CNS) depressants (medicines that slow down the nervous system). They act on the brain and CNS to produce effects that may be helpful or harmful. This depends on the individual patient's condition and response and the amount of medicine taken.

Some of the barbiturates may be used before surgery to relieve anxiety or tension. In addition, some of the barbiturates are used as anticonvulsants to help control seizures in certain disorders or diseases, such as epilepsy. Barbiturates may also be used for other conditions as determined by your doctor.

The barbiturates have been used to treat insomnia (sleeplessness); but if they are used regularly (for example, every day) for insomnia, they are usually not effective for longer than 2 weeks. The barbiturates have also been used to relieve nervousness or restlessness during the daytime. However, the barbiturates have generally been replaced by safer medicines for the treatment of insomnia and daytime nervousness or tension.

If too much of a barbiturate is used, it may become habit-forming.

Barbiturates should not be used for anxiety or tension caused by the stress of everyday life.

These medicines are available only with your doctor's prescription, in the following dosage forms:

Oral

Amobarbital
- Capsules (U.S. and Canada)
- Tablets (U.S. and Canada)

Aprobarbital
- Elixir (U.S.)

Butabarbital
- Capsules (U.S.)
- Elixir (U.S.)
- Tablets (U.S. and Canada)

Mephobarbital
- Tablets (U.S. and Canada)

Metharbital
- Tablets (Other countries)

Pentobarbital
- Capsules (U.S. and Canada)
- Elixir (U.S.)

Phenobarbital
- Capsules (U.S.)
- Elixir (U.S. and Canada)
- Tablets (U.S. and Canada)

Secobarbital
- Capsules (U.S. and Canada)

Secobarbital and Amobarbital
- Capsules (U.S. and Canada)

Parenteral

Amobarbital
- Injection (U.S. and Canada)

Pentobarbital
- Injection (U.S. and Canada)

Phenobarbital
- Injection (U.S. and Canada)

Secobarbital
- Injection (U.S.)

Rectal

Pentobarbital
- Suppositories (U.S. and Canada)

It is very important that you read and understand the following information. If any of it causes you special concern, check with your doctor. Also, *if you have any questions* or if you want more information about this medicine or your medical problem, *ask your doctor, nurse, or pharmacist.*

Before Using This Medicine

In deciding to use a medicine, the risks of taking the medicine must be weighed against the good it will do. This is a decision you and your doctor will make. For barbiturates, the following should be considered:

Allergies—Tell your doctor if you have ever had any unusual or allergic reaction to barbiturates. Also tell your doctor and pharmacist if you are allergic to any other substances, such as foods, preservatives, or dyes.

Pregnancy—Barbiturates have been shown to increase the chance of birth defects in humans. However, this medicine may be needed in serious diseases or other situations that threaten the mother's life. Be sure you have discussed this and the following information with your doctor:

- Taking barbiturates regularly during pregnancy may cause bleeding problems in the newborn infant. In addition, taking barbiturates regularly during the last 3 months of pregnancy may cause the baby to become dependent on the medicine. This may lead to withdrawal side effects in the baby after birth.
- One study in humans has suggested that barbiturates taken during pregnancy may increase the chance of brain tumors in the baby.
- Barbiturates taken for anesthesia during labor and delivery may reduce the force and frequency of contractions of the uterus; this may prolong labor and delay delivery.
- Use of barbiturates during labor may cause breathing problems in the newborn infant.

Breast-feeding—Barbiturates pass into the breast milk and may cause drowsiness, slow heartbeat, shortness of breath, or troubled breathing in babies of nursing mothers taking this medicine.

Children—Unusual excitement may be more likely to occur in children, who are usually more sensitive than adults to the effects of barbiturates.

Older adults—Confusion, mental depression, and unusual excitement may be more likely to occur in the elderly, who are usually more sensitive than younger adults to the effects of barbiturates.

Other medicines—Although certain medicines should not be used together at all, in other cases 2 different medicines may be used together even if an interaction might occur. In these cases, your doctor may want to change the dose, or other precautions may be necessary. When you are taking a barbiturate, it is especially important that your doctor and pharmacist know if you are taking any of the following:

- Adrenocorticoids (cortisone-like medicine) or
- Anticoagulants (blood thinners) or
- Carbamazepine or
- Corticotropin (ACTH)—Barbiturates may decrease the effects of these medicines
- Central nervous system (CNS) depressants (medicines that cause drowsiness)—Using these medicines with barbiturates may result in increased CNS depressant effects
- Divalproex sodium or
- Valproic acid—Using these medicines with barbiturates may change the amount of either medicine that you need to take
- Oral contraceptives (birth control pills) containing estrogens—Barbiturates may decrease the effectiveness of these oral contraceptives, and you may need to change to a different type of birth control

Other medical problems—The presence of other medical problems may affect the use of barbiturates. Make sure you tell your doctor if you have any other medical problems, especially:

- Alcohol abuse (or history of) or
- Drug abuse or dependence (or history of)—Dependence on barbiturates may develop
- Anemia (severe) or
- Asthma (history of), emphysema, or other chronic lung disease or
- Diabetes mellitus (sugar diabetes) or
- Hyperactivity (in children) or
- Mental depression or
- Overactive thyroid or
- Porphyria (or history of)—Barbiturates may make the condition worse
- Kidney disease or
- Liver disease—Higher blood levels of barbiturates may result, increasing the chance of side effects
- Pain—Barbiturates may cause unexpected excitement or mask important symptoms of more serious problems
- Underactive adrenal gland—Barbiturates may interfere with the effects of other medicines needed for this condition

Before you begin using any new medicine (prescription or nonprescription) or if you develop any new medical problem while you are using this medicine, check with your doctor, nurse, or pharmacist.

Proper Use of This Medicine

For patients taking the *extended-release capsule or tablet form* of this medicine:

- These capsules or tablets are to be swallowed whole. Do not break, crush, or chew before swallowing.

For patients using the *rectal suppository form* of this medicine:

- To insert the suppository: First remove the foil wrapper and moisten the suppository with cold water. Lie down on your side and use your finger to push the suppository well up into the rectum.
- Wash your hands with soap and water.

Use this medicine only as directed by your doctor. Do not use more of it, do not use it more often, and do not use it for a longer time than your doctor ordered. If too much is used, it may become habit-forming (causing mental or physical dependence).

If you think this medicine is not working properly after you have taken it for a few weeks, *do not increase the dose.* To do so may increase the chance of your becoming dependent on the medicine. Instead, check with your doctor.

If you are taking this medicine for epilepsy, it must be taken every day in regularly spaced doses as ordered by your doctor in order for it to control your seizures. This is necessary to keep a constant amount of medicine in the blood. To help keep the amount constant, do not miss any doses.

Missed dose—If you are taking this medicine regularly (for example, every day as in epilepsy) and you do miss a dose, take it as soon as possible. However, if it is almost time for your next dose, skip the missed dose and go back to your regular dosing schedule. Do not double doses.

Storage—To store this medicine:

- Keep out of the reach of children since overdose is especially dangerous in children.
- Store away from heat and direct light.
- Do not store the capsule or tablet form of this medicine in the bathroom, near the kitchen sink, or in other damp places. Heat or moisture may cause the medicine to break down.
- Keep the liquid form of this medicine from freezing.
- Store the suppository form of this medicine in the refrigerator.
- Do not keep outdated medicine or medicine no longer needed. Be sure that any discarded medicine is out of the reach of children.

Precautions While Using This Medicine

If you will be using this medicine regularly for a long time:

- Your doctor should check your progress at regular visits.
- Do not stop using it without first checking with your doctor. Your doctor may want you to reduce gradually the amount you are using before stopping completely.

This medicine will add to the effects of alcohol and other CNS depressants (medicines that slow down the nervous system, possibly causing drowsiness). Some examples of CNS depressants are antihistamines or medicine for hay fever, other allergies, or colds; sedatives, tranquilizers, or sleeping medicine; prescription pain medicine or narcotics; medicine for seizures; muscle relaxants; or anesthetics, including some dental anesthetics. *Check with your doctor before taking any of the above while you are using this medicine.*

Before you have any medical tests, tell the medical doctor in charge that you are taking this medicine. The results of the metyrapone test may be affected by this medicine.

If you have been using this medicine for a long time and you think that you may have become mentally or physically dependent on it, check with your doctor. Some signs of mental or physical dependence on barbiturates are:

- a strong desire or need to continue taking the medicine.
- a need to increase the dose to receive the effects of the medicine.
- withdrawal side effects (for example, anxiety or restlessness, convulsions [seizures], feeling faint, nausea or vomiting, trembling of hands, trouble in sleeping) occurring after the medicine is stopped.

If you think you or someone else may have taken an overdose of this medicine, get emergency help at once. Taking an overdose of a barbiturate or taking alcohol or other CNS depressants with the barbiturate may lead to unconsciousness and possibly death. Some signs of an overdose are severe drowsiness, severe confusion, severe weakness, shortness of breath or slow or troubled breathing, slurred speech, staggering, and slow heartbeat.

This medicine may cause some people to become dizzy, lightheaded, drowsy, or less alert than they are normally. Even if taken at bedtime, it may cause some people to feel drowsy or less alert on arising. *Make sure you know how you react to this medicine before you drive, use machines, or do anything else that could be dangerous if you are dizzy or are not alert.*

Oral contraceptives (birth control pills) containing estrogen may not work properly if you take them while you are taking barbiturates. Unplanned pregnancies may occur. You should use a different or additional means of birth control while you are taking barbiturates. If you have any questions about this, check with your doctor or pharmacist.

Side Effects of This Medicine

Along with its needed effects, a medicine may cause some unwanted effects. Although not all of these side effects may occur, if they do occur they may need medical attention.

Check with your doctor immediately if any of the following side effects occur:

Rare

Bleeding sores on lips; chest pain; fever; muscle or joint pain; red, thickened, or scaly skin; skin rash or hives; sores, ulcers, or white spots in mouth (painful); sore throat and/or fever; swelling of eyelids, face, or lips; wheezing or tightness in chest

Also, check with your doctor as soon as possible if any of the following side effects occur:

Less common

Confusion; mental depression; unusual excitement

Rare

Hallucinations (seeing, hearing, or feeling things that are not there); unusual bleeding or bruising; unusual tiredness or weakness

With long-term or chronic use

Bone pain, tenderness, or aching; loss of appetite; muscle weakness; weight loss (unusual); yellow eyes or skin

Symptoms of overdose

Confusion (severe); decrease in or loss of reflexes; drowsiness (severe); fever; irritability (continuing); low body temperature; poor judgment; shortness of breath or slow or troubled breathing; slow heartbeat; slurred speech; staggering; trouble in sleeping; unusual movements of the eyes; weakness (severe)

Other side effects may occur that usually do not need medical attention. These side effects may go away during treatment as your body adjusts to the medicine. However, check with your doctor if any of the following side effects continue or are bothersome:

More common

Clumsiness or unsteadiness; dizziness or lightheadedness; drowsiness; "hangover" effect

Less common

Anxiety or nervousness; constipation; feeling faint; headache; irritability; nausea or vomiting; nightmares or trouble in sleeping

For very ill patients:

- Confusion, mental depression, and unusual excitement may be more likely to occur in very ill patients.

After you stop using this medicine, your body may need time to adjust. If you took this medicine in high doses or for a long time, this may take up to about 15 days. During this period of time check with your doctor if any of the following side effects occur (usually occur within 8 to 16 hours after medicine is stopped):

Anxiety or restlessness; convulsions (seizures); dizziness or lightheadedness; feeling faint; hallucinations (seeing, hearing, or feeling things that are not there); muscle twitching; nausea or vomiting; trembling of hands; trouble in sleeping, increased dreaming, or nightmares; vision problems; weakness

Other side effects not listed above may also occur in some patients. If you notice any other effects, check with your doctor.

Additional Information

Once a medicine has been approved for marketing for a certain use, experience may show that it is also useful for other medical problems. Although this use is not included in product labeling, phenobarbital is used in certain patients with the following medical condition:

- Hyperbilirubinemia (high amount of bile pigments in the blood that may lead to jaundice)

Other than the above information, there is no additional information relating to proper use, precautions, or side effects for these uses.

Annual revision: 01/27/92

BARBITURATES, ASPIRIN, AND CODEINE Systemic

This information applies to the following medicines:

Butalbital (byoo-TAL-bi-tal), Aspirin (AS-pir-in), and Codeine (KOE-deen)

Phenobarbital (fee-noe-BAR-bi-tal), Aspirin, and Codeine

Some commonly used brand names are:

For Butalbital, Aspirin, Codeine, and Caffeine

In the U.S.

Ascomp with Codeine No.3
Butalbital Compound with Codeine
Butinal with Codeine No.3
Fiorinal with Codeine No.3
Idenal with Codeine
Isollyl with Codeine

Generic name product may also be available.

In Canada‡

Fiorinal-C ¼
Fiorinal-C ½
Tecnal-C ¼
Tecnal-C ½

For Phenobarbital, Aspirin, and Codeine*

In Canada‡

Phenaphen with Codeine No.2
Phenaphen with Codeine No.3
Phenaphen with Codeine No.4

*Not commercially available in the U.S.

‡In Canada, *Aspirin* is a brand name. Acetylsalicylic acid is the generic name in Canada. ASA, a synonym for acetylsalicylic acid, is the term that commonly appears on Canadian product labels.

Description

Barbiturate (bar-BI-tyoo-rate), aspirin, and codeine combinations are used to relieve headaches and other kinds of pain. These combination medicines may provide better pain relief than either aspirin or codeine used alone. In some cases, relief of pain may come at lower doses of each medicine.

Codeine is a narcotic analgesic (nar-KOT-ik an-al-JEE-zik) that acts in the central nervous system (CNS) to relieve pain. Many of its side effects are also caused by actions in the CNS. Butalbital and phenobarbital belong to the group of medicines called barbiturates. Barbiturates also act in the CNS to produce their effects.

When you use a barbiturate or codeine for a long time, your body may get used to the medicine so that larger amounts are needed to produce the same effects. This is called tolerance to the medicine. Also, barbiturates and codeine may become habit-forming (causing mental or physical dependence) when they are used for a long time or in large doses. Physical dependence may lead to withdrawal symptoms when you stop taking the medicine. In patients who get headaches, the first symptom of withdrawal may be new (rebound) headaches.

The butalbital, aspirin, and codeine combination also contains caffeine (kaf-EEN). Caffeine may help to relieve headaches. However, caffeine can also cause physical dependence when it is used for a long time. This may lead to withdrawal (rebound) headaches when you stop taking it.

Aspirin is not a narcotic and does not cause physical dependence. However, it may cause other unwanted effects if too much is taken.

These combination medicines are available only with your doctor's prescription, in the following dosage forms:

Oral

Butalbital, Aspirin, Codeine, and Caffeine
- Capsules (U.S. and Canada)
- Tablets (U.S.)

Phenobarbital, Aspirin, and Codeine
- Capsules (Canada)

It is very important that you read and understand the following information. If any of it causes you special concern, check with your doctor. Also, *if you have any questions* or if you want more information about this medicine or your medical problem, *ask your doctor, nurse, or pharmacist*.

Before Using This Medicine

In deciding to use a medicine, the risks of taking the medicine must be weighed against the good it will do. This is a decision you and your doctor will make. For barbiturate, aspirin, and codeine combinations, the following should be considered:

Allergies—Tell your doctor if you have ever had any unusual or allergic reaction to aspirin or other salicylates including methyl salicylate (oil of wintergreen); butalbital, phenobarbital, or other barbiturates; caffeine; codeine; or any of the following medicines:

Diclofenac (e.g., Voltaren)
Diflunisal (e.g., Dolobid)
Etodolac (e.g., Lodine)
Fenoprofen (e.g., Nalfon)
Floctafenine (e.g., Idarac)
Flurbiprofen, oral (e.g., Ansaid)
Ibuprofen (e.g., Motrin)
Indomethacin (e.g., Indocin)
Ketoprofen (e.g., Orudis)
Ketorolac (e.g., Toradol)
Meclofenamate (e.g., Meclomen)
Mefenamic acid (e.g., Ponstel)
Nabumetone (e.g., Relafen)
Naproxen (e.g., Naprosyn)
Oxyphenbutazone (e.g., Tandearil)
Phenylbutazone (e.g., Butazolidin)
Piroxicam (e.g., Feldene)
Sulindac (e.g., Clinoril)
Suprofen (e.g., Suprol)
Tenoxicam (e.g., Mobiflex)
Tiaprofenic acid (e.g., Surgam)
Tolmetin (e.g., Tolectin)
Zomepirac (e.g., Zomax)

Also tell your doctor and pharmacist if you are allergic to any other substances, such as foods, preservatives, or dyes.

Pregnancy—
- *For butalbital or phenobarbital:* Barbiturates have been shown to increase the chance of birth defects in humans. Also, one study in humans has suggested that barbiturates taken during pregnancy may increase the chance of brain tumors in the baby. Barbiturates may cause breathing problems in the newborn baby if taken just before or during delivery.
- *For aspirin:* Although studies in humans have not shown that aspirin causes birth defects, aspirin has caused birth defects in animal studies.

  Do not take aspirin during the last 3 months of pregnancy unless it has been ordered by your doctor. Some reports have suggested that use of aspirin late in pregnancy may cause a decrease in the newborn's weight and possible death of the fetus or newborn baby. However, the mothers in these reports had been taking much larger amounts of aspirin than are usually recommended. Studies of mothers taking aspirin in the doses that are usually recommended did not show these unwanted effects.

  There is a chance that regular use of aspirin late in pregnancy may cause unwanted effects on the heart or blood flow in the fetus or in the newborn baby. Also, use of aspirin during the last 2 weeks of pregnancy may cause bleeding problems in the fetus before or during delivery or in the newborn baby. In addition, too much use of aspirin during the last 3 months of pregnancy may increase the length of pregnancy, prolong labor, cause other problems during delivery, or cause severe bleeding in the mother before, during, or after delivery.
- *For codeine:* Although studies on birth defects with codeine have not been done in pregnant women, it has not been reported to cause birth defects. However, it may cause breathing problems in the newborn baby if taken just before or during delivery. Codeine did not cause birth defects in animal studies, but it caused slower development of bones and other harmful effects in the fetus.
- *For caffeine:* Studies in humans have not shown that caffeine causes birth defects. However, use of large amounts of caffeine during pregnancy may cause problems with the heart rhythm and the growth of the fetus. Also, studies in animals have shown that caffeine causes birth defects when given in very large doses (amounts equal to those in 12 to 24 cups of coffee a day).

Breast-feeding—Although this combination medicine has not been reported to cause problems, the chance always exists, especially if the medicine is taken for a long time or in large amounts.

- *For butalbital or phenobarbital:* Barbiturates pass into the breast milk and may cause drowsiness, unusually slow heartbeat, shortness of breath, or troubled breathing in nursing babies.
- *For aspirin:* Aspirin passes into the breast milk. However, taking aspirin in the amount present in these combination medicines has not been reported to cause problems in nursing babies.
- *For codeine:* Codeine passes into the breast milk in small amounts. However, it has not been reported to cause problems in nursing babies.
- *For caffeine:* The caffeine in the butalbital, aspirin, and codeine combination medicine passes into the breast milk in small amounts. Taking caffeine in the amounts present in this combination medicine has not been reported to cause problems in nursing babies. However, studies have shown that nursing babies may appear jittery when their mothers drink large amounts of caffeine-containing beverages. Therefore, breast-feeding mothers who use caffeine-containing medicines should probably limit the amount of caffeine they take in from other medicines or from beverages.

Children—

- *For butalbital or phenobarbital:* Although barbiturates often cause drowsiness, some children become excited after taking them.
- *For aspirin: Do not give a medicine containing aspirin to a child with fever or other symptoms of a virus infection, especially flu or chickenpox, without first discussing its use with your child's doctor.* This is very important because aspirin may cause a serious illness called Reye's syndrome in children with fever caused by a virus infection, especially flu or chickenpox. Children who do not have a virus infection may also be more sensitive to the effects of aspirin, especially if they have a fever or have lost large amounts of body fluid because of vomiting, diarrhea, or sweating. This may increase the chance of side effects during treatment.
- *For caffeine:* There is no specific information comparing use of caffeine in children up to 12 years of age with use in other age groups. However, caffeine is not expected to cause different side effects or problems in children than it does in adults.

Teenagers—*Teenagers with fever or other symptoms of a virus infection, especially flu or chickenpox, should check with a doctor before taking this medicine.* The aspirin in this combination medicine may cause a serious illness called Reye's syndrome in teenagers with fever caused by a virus infection, especially flu or chickenpox.

Older adults—

- *For butalbital or phenobarbital:* Confusion, depression, or excitement may be especially likely to occur in elderly patients, who are usually more sensitive than younger adults to the effects of barbiturates.
- *For aspirin:* Elderly patients are more sensitive than younger adults to the effects of aspirin. This may increase the chance of side effects during treatment.
- *For codeine:* Breathing problems may be especially likely to occur in elderly patients, who are usually more sensitive than younger adults to the effects of codeine.
- *For caffeine:* Many medicines have not been studied specifically in older people.Therefore, it may not be known whether they work exactly the same way they do in younger adults or if they cause different side effects or problems in older people. There is no specific information comparing use of caffeine in the elderly with use in other age groups.

Other medicines—Although certain medicines should not be used together at all, in other cases two different medicines may be used together even if an interaction might occur. In these cases, your doctor may want to change the dose, or other precautions may be necessary. When you are taking this combination medicine, it is especially important that your doctor and pharmacist know if you are taking any of the following:

- Adrenocorticoids (cortisone-like medicines) or
- Carbamazepine or
- Contraceptives, oral (birth control pills) containing estrogens or
- Corticotropin (ACTH)—Barbiturates, especially phenobarbital, may make these medicines less effective
- Antacids, large amounts taken regularly, especially calcium- and/or magnesium-containing antacids or sodium bicarbonate (baking soda), or
- Urinary alkalizers (medicine that makes the urine less acid, such as acetazolamide [e.g., Diamox], dichlorphenamide [e.g., Daranide], methazolamide [e.g., Neptazane], potassium or sodium citrate and/or citric acid)—These medicines may cause aspirin to be removed from the body faster than usual, which may shorten the length of time that aspirin is effective; acetazolamide, dichlorphenamide, and methazolamide may also increase the chance of side effects when taken together with aspirin
- Anticoagulants (blood thinners) or
- Heparin—Use of these medicines together with aspirin may increase the chance of bleeding; also, barbiturates, especially phenobarbital, may decrease the effects of anticoagulants
- Antidepressants, tricyclic (amitriptyline [e.g., Elavil], amoxapine [e.g., Asendin], clomipramine [e.g., Anafranil], desipramine [e.g., Pertofrane], doxepin [e.g., Sinequan], imipramine [e.g., Tofranil], nortriptyline [e.g., Aventyl], protriptyline [e.g., Vivactil], trimipramine [e.g., Surmontil]) or
- Central nervous system (CNS) depressants (medicines that often cause drowsiness)—These medicines may add to

the effects of barbiturates and codeine and increase the chance of drowsiness or other side effects
- Divalproex (e.g., Depakote) or
- Methotrexate (e.g., Mexate) or
- Valproic acid (e.g., Depakene) or
- Vancomycin (e.g., Vancocin)—The chance of serious side effects may be increased
- Naltrexone (e.g., Trexan)—Naltrexone blocks the pain-relieving effect of codeine
- Probenecid (e.g., Benemid) or
- Sulfinpyrazone (e.g., Anturane)—Aspirin can keep these medicines from working properly for treating gout

Other medical problems—The presence of other medical problems may affect the use of butalbital, aspirin, and codeine combination. Make sure you tell your doctor if you have any other medical problems, especially:
- Alcohol abuse (or history of) or
- Drug abuse or dependence (or history of)—Dependence on barbiturates and/or codeine may develop
- Asthma, especially if occurring together with other allergies and nasal polyps (history of), or
- Brain disease or head injury or
- Colitis or
- Convulsions (seizures) (history of) or
- Emphysema or other chronic lung disease or
- Enlarged prostate or problems with urination or
- Gallbladder disease or gallstones or
- Hyperactivity (in children) or
- Kidney disease or
- Liver disease—The chance of serious side effects may be increased
- Diabetes mellitus (sugar diabetes) or
- Mental depression or
- Overactive thyroid or
- Porphyria (or history of)—Barbiturates can make these conditions worse
- Gout—Aspirin can make this condition worse and can also lessen the effects of some medicines used to treat gout
- Heart disease (severe)—The caffeine in the butalbital, aspirin, and codeine combination can make some kinds of heart disease worse
- Hemophilia or other bleeding problems or
- Vitamin K deficiency—Aspirin increases the chance of serious bleeding
- Stomach ulcer, especially with a history of bleeding, or other stomach problems—Aspirin can make your condition worse

Before you begin using any new medicine (prescription or nonprescription) or if you develop any new medical problem while you are using this medicine, check with your doctor, nurse, or pharmacist.

Proper Use of This Medicine

Take this medicine with food or a full glass (8 ounces) of water to lessen stomach irritation.

Do not take this medicine if it has a strong vinegar-like odor. This odor means the aspirin in it is breaking down. If you have any questions about this, check with your doctor or pharmacist.

Take this medicine only as directed by your doctor. Do not take more of it, do not take it more often, and do not take it for a longer time than your doctor ordered. If a barbiturate or codeine is taken regularly (for example, every day), it may become habit-forming (causing mental or physical dependence). Regular use of caffeine can also cause physical dependence. Dependence is especially likely to occur in people who take these medicines to relieve frequent headaches. Also, taking too much of this combination medicine may cause stomach problems or other medical problems.

This medicine will relieve a headache best if you *take it as soon as the headache begins.* If you get warning signs of a migraine, take this medicine as soon as you are sure that the migraine is coming. This may even stop the headache pain from occurring. *Lying down in a quiet, dark room for a while after taking the medicine also helps to relieve headaches.*

People who get a lot of headaches may need to take a different medicine to help prevent headaches. *It is important that you follow your doctor's directions about taking the other medicine, even if your headaches continue to occur.* Headache-preventing medicines may take several weeks to start working. Even after they do start working, your headaches may not go away completely. However, your headaches should occur less often, and they should be less severe and easier to relieve than before. This will reduce the amount of headache relievers that you need. If you do not notice any improvement after several weeks of headache-preventing treatment, check with your doctor.

Missed dose—If your doctor has ordered you to take this medicine according to a regular schedule and you miss a dose, take it as soon as you remember. However, if it is almost time for your next dose, skip the missed dose and go back to your regular dosing schedule. Do not double doses.

Storage—To store this medicine:
- Keep out of the reach of children. Overdose is especially dangerous in young children.
- Store away from heat and direct light.
- Do not store this medicine in the bathroom, near the kitchen sink, or in other damp places. Heat or moisture may cause the medicine to break down.
- Do not keep outdated medicine or medicine no longer needed. Be sure that any discarded medicine is out of the reach of children.

Precautions While Using This Medicine

Check with your doctor:
- If the medicine stops working as well as it did when you first started using it. This may mean that you

are in danger of becoming dependent on the medicine. *Do not try to get better pain relief by increasing the dose.*
- *If you are having headaches more often than you did before you started using this medicine.* This is especially important if a new headache occurs within 1 day after you took your last dose of headache medicine, headaches begin to occur every day, or a headache continues for several days in a row. This may mean that you are dependent on the headache medicine. *Continuing to take this medicine will cause even more headaches later on.* Your doctor can give you advice on how to relieve the headaches.

Check the labels of all nonprescription (over-the-counter [OTC]) and prescription medicines you now take. If any contain a narcotic, a barbiturate, aspirin, or other salicylates including diflunisal, be especially careful, since taking them while taking this medicine may cause an overdose. If you have any questions about this, check with your doctor or pharmacist.

The barbiturate and the codeine in this medicine will add to the effects of alcohol and other CNS depressants (medicines that slow down the nervous system, possibly causing drowsiness). Some examples of CNS depressants are antihistamines or medicine for hay fever, other allergies, or colds; sedatives, tranquilizers, or sleeping medicine; other prescription pain medicine or narcotics; other barbiturates; medicine for seizures; muscle relaxants; or anesthetics, including some dental anesthetics. Also, stomach problems may be more likely to occur if you drink alcoholic beverages while you are taking aspirin. Therefore, *do not drink alcoholic beverages, and check with your doctor before taking any of the medicines listed above, while you are using this medicine.*

This medicine may cause some people to become drowsy, dizzy, or lightheaded, or to feel a false sense of well-being. *Make sure you know how you react to this medicine before you drive, use machines, or do anything else that could be dangerous if you are dizzy or are not alert and clearheaded.*

Dizziness, lightheadedness, or fainting may occur, especially when you get up suddenly from a lying or sitting position. Getting up slowly may help lessen this problem. Lying down for a while may relieve these effects.

Nausea or vomiting may occur, especially after the first couple of doses. This effect may go away if you lie down for a while. However, if nausea or vomiting continues, check with your doctor.

Before having any kind of surgery (including dental surgery) or emergency treatment, tell the medical doctor or dentist in charge that you are taking this medicine. Serious side effects can occur if your medical doctor or dentist gives you certain medicines without knowing that you have taken a barbiturate or codeine.

Do not take this medicine for 5 days before any planned surgery, including dental surgery, unless otherwise directed by your medical doctor or dentist. Taking aspirin during this time may cause bleeding problems.

Before you have any medical tests, tell the person in charge that you are taking this medicine. The caffeine in the butalbital, aspirin, and codeine combination interferes with the results of certain tests that use dipyridamole (e.g., Persantine) to help show how well blood is flowing to your heart. Caffeine should not be taken for 8 to 12 hours before the test. The results of some other tests may also be affected by this medicine.

If you have been taking large amounts of this medicine, or if you have been taking it regularly for several weeks or more, *do not suddenly stop using it without first checking with your doctor.* Your doctor may want you to reduce gradually the amount you are taking before stopping completely, to lessen the chance of withdrawal side effects.

If you think you or anyone else may have taken an overdose of this medicine, get emergency help at once. Taking an overdose of this medicine or taking alcohol or CNS depressants with this medicine may lead to unconsciousness or death. Signs of overdose of this medicine include convulsions (seizures); hearing loss; confusion; ringing or buzzing in the ears; severe excitement, nervousness, or restlessness; severe dizziness; severe drowsiness; unusually slow or troubled breathing; and severe weakness.

Side Effects of This Medicine

Along with its needed effects, a medicine may cause some unwanted effects. Although not all of these side effects may occur, if they do occur they may need medical attention.

The following side effects may mean that a serious allergic reaction is occurring. Check with your doctor or get emergency help immediately if they occur, especially if several of them occur at the same time.

Less common or rare

Bluish discoloration or flushing or redness of skin (occurring together with other effects listed in this section); coughing, shortness of breath, troubled breathing, tightness in chest, or wheezing; difficulty in swallowing; dizziness or feeling faint (severe); hive-like swellings (large) on eyelids, face, lips, or tongue; skin rash, itching, or hives; stuffy nose (occurring together with other effects listed in this section)

Also check with your doctor immediately if any of the following side effects occur, especially if several of them occur together:

Rare

Bleeding or crusting sores on lips; chest pain; fever with or without chills; red, thickened, or scaly skin; sores, ulcers, or white spots in mouth (painful); sore throat (unexplained); tenderness, burning, or peeling of skin

Symptoms of overdose

Anxiety, confusion, excitement, irritability, nervousness, restlessness, or trouble in sleeping (severe, especially with products containing caffeine); cold, clammy skin; convulsions (seizures); diarrhea (severe or continuing); dizziness, lightheadedness, drowsiness, or weakness (severe); frequent urination (for products containing caffeine); hallucinations (seeing, hearing, or feeling things that are not there); increased sensitivity to touch or pain (for products containing caffeine); increased thirst; low blood pressure; muscle trembling or twitching (for products containing caffeine); nausea or vomiting (severe or continuing), sometimes with blood; pinpoint pupils of eyes; ringing or buzzing in ears (continuing) or hearing loss; seeing flashes of "zig-zag" lights (for products containing caffeine); slow, fast, or irregular heartbeat; slow, fast, irregular, or troubled breathing; slurred speech; staggering; stomach pain (severe); uncontrollable flapping movements of the hands (especially in elderly patients); unusual movements of the eyes; vision problems

Also, check with your doctor as soon as possible if any of the following side effects occur:

Less common or rare

Bloody or black, tarry stools; bloody urine; confusion or mental depression; pinpoint red spots on skin; skin rash, hives, or itching (without other signs of an allergic reaction to aspirin listed above); sore throat and fever; stomach pain (severe); swollen or painful glands; trembling or uncontrolled muscle movements; unusual bleeding or bruising; unusual excitement (mild); unusual tiredness or weakness (mild)

Other side effects may occur that usually do not need medical attention. These side effects may go away during treatment as your body adjusts to the medicine. However, check with your doctor if any of the following side effects continue or are bothersome:

More common

Bloated or "gassy" feeling; dizziness, lightheadedness, or drowsiness (mild); heartburn or indigestion; nausea, vomiting, or stomach pain (occurring without other symptoms of overdose)

Other side effects not listed above may also occur in some patients. If you notice any other effects, check with your doctor.

Annual revision: 07/14/92

BARIUM SULFATE Diagnostic

Description

Barium sulfate is a radiopaque agent. Radiopaque agents are drugs used to help diagnose certain medical problems. Since radiopaque agents are opaque to (block) x-rays, the areas of the body in which they are localized will appear white on the x-ray film. This creates the needed distinction, or contrast, between one organ and other tissues. The contrast will help the doctor see any special conditions that may exist in that organ or part of the body.

Barium sulfate is taken by mouth or given rectally by enema. If taken by mouth, it makes the esophagus, stomach, and/or small intestine opaque to the x-rays so that they can be "photographed." If it is given by enema, the colon and/or small intestine can be seen and photographed by x-rays.

Barium sulfate is to be used only by or under the direct supervision of a doctor.

It is very important that you read and understand the following information. If any of it causes you special concern, check with your doctor. Also, *if you have any questions* or if you want more information about this test or your medical problem, *ask your doctor, nurse, or pharmacist.*

Before Having This Test

In deciding to use a diagnostic test, any risks of the test must be weighed against the good it will do. This is a decision you and your doctor will make. Also, test results may be affected by other things. For barium sulfate, the following should be considered:

Allergies—Tell your doctor if you have ever had any unusual or allergic reaction to barium sulfate. Also, tell your doctor if you are allergic to any other substances, such as foods, preservatives, or dyes.

Pregnancy—X-rays of the abdomen are usually not recommended during pregnancy. This is to avoid exposing the fetus to radiation. Be sure you have discussed this with your doctor.

Breast-feeding—Barium sulfate does not pass into the breast milk. This medicine has not been reported to cause problems in nursing babies.

Children—Although there is no specific information comparing use of barium sulfate in children with use in other age groups, this agent is not expected to cause different side effects or problems in children than it does in adults.

Older adults—This contrast agent has been used in older people and has not been shown to cause different side effects or problems in them than it does in younger adults.

Other medical problems—The presence of other medical problems may affect the use of barium sulfate. Make sure you tell your doctor if you have any other medical problems, especially:

- Asthma, hay fever, or other allergies (history of)—If you have a history of these conditions, the risk of having a reaction, such as an allergic reaction to the additives in the barium sulfate preparation, is greater
- Intestinal blockage or perforation—Barium sulfate may make this condition worse

Preparation For This Test

Your doctor may have special instructions for you in preparation for your test. If you have not received such instructions or if you do not understand them, check with your doctor in advance.

For some tests your doctor may tell you not to eat after 8 the evening before the test. You may be allowed to drink small amounts of clear liquids until midnight; however, check first with your doctor. For other tests you may need to eat meals free of fiber and bulk the day before the test. You may also need to use a laxative.

Precautions After Having This Test

Make sure to drink plenty of liquids after the test. Otherwise, barium sulfate may cause severe constipation.

Side Effects of This Medicine

Along with its needed effects, a radiopaque agent may cause some unwanted effects. Although not all of these side effects may occur, if they do occur they may need medical attention.

Check with your doctor immediately if any of the following side effects occur:

Rare

Bloating; severe, continuing constipation; severe cramping; nausea or vomiting; stomach or lower abdominal pain; tightness in chest or troubled breathing; troubled breathing; wheezing

Other side effects may occur that usually do not need medical attention. These side effects may go away as your body adjusts to this agent. However, check with your doctor if any of the following side effects continue or are bothersome:

More common

Constipation or diarrhea; cramping

Other side effects not listed above may also occur in some patients. If you notice any other effects, check with your doctor.

Annual revision: 09/16/92

BELLADONNA ALKALOIDS AND BARBITURATES Systemic

This information applies to the following medicines:

Atropine (A-troe-peen), Hyoscyamine (hye-oh-SYE-a-meen), Scopolamine (skoe-POL-a-meen), and Phenobarbital (fee-noe-BAR-bi-tal)
Atropine and Phenobarbital
Belladonna and Butabarbital (byoo-ta-BAR-bi-tal)
Belladonna and Phenobarbital
Hyoscyamine and Phenobarbital

Some commonly used brand names are:

For Atropine, Hyoscyamine, Scopolamine, and Phenobarbital

In the U.S.

Barbidonna
Barbidonna No. 2
Barophen
Bellalphen
Donnamor
Donnapine
Donnatal
Donnatal Extentabs
Donnatal No. 2
Donphen
Hyosophen
Kinesed
Malatal
Relaxadon
Spaslin
Spasmolin
Spasmophen
Spasquid
Susano

Generic name product may also be available.

In Canada

Donnatal
Donnatal Extentabs

For Atropine and Phenobarbital†

In the U.S.

Antrocol

For Belladonna and Butabarbital†

In the U.S.

Butibel

For Belladonna and Phenobarbital†

In the U.S.

Chardonna-2

For Hyoscyamine and Phenobarbital†

In the U.S.

Levsin-PB
Levsin with Phenobarbital

†Not commercially available in Canada.

Description

Belladonna alkaloids and barbiturates are combination medicines taken to relieve cramping and spasms of the stomach and intestines. They are used also to decrease the amount of acid formed in the stomach.

These medicines are available only with your doctor's prescription in the following dosage forms:

Oral

Atropine, Hyoscyamine, Scopolamine, and Phenobarbital
- Capsules (U.S.)
- Elixir (U.S. and Canada)
- Tablets (U.S. and Canada)
- Chewable tablets (U.S.)
- Extended-release tablets (U.S. and Canada)

Atropine and Phenobarbital
- Capsules (U.S.)
- Elixir (U.S.)
- Tablets (U.S.)

Belladonna and Butabarbital
- Elixir (U.S.)
- Tablets (U.S.)

Belladonna and Phenobarbital
- Tablets (U.S.)

Hyoscyamine and Phenobarbital
- Elixir (U.S.)
- Oral solution (U.S.)
- Tablets (U.S.)

It is very important that you read and understand the following information. If any of it causes you special concern, check with your doctor. Also, *if you have any questions* or if you want more information about this medicine or your medical problem, *ask your doctor, nurse, or pharmacist.*

Before Using This Medicine

In deciding to use a medicine, the risks of taking the medicine must be weighed against the good it will do. This is a decision you and your doctor will make. For belladona alkaloids and barbiturates, the following should be considered:

Allergies—Tell your doctor if you have ever had any unusual or allergic reaction to belladonna alkaloids (atropine, belladonna, hyoscyamine, and scopolamine) or to barbiturates (butabarbital, phenobarbital). Also, tell your doctor and pharmacist if you are allergic to any other substances, such as foods, preservatives, or dyes.

Pregnancy—Belladonna alkaloids have not been shown to cause problems in humans. However, barbiturates (contained in this medicine) have been shown to increase the chance of birth defects in humans. Also, when taken during pregnancy, barbiturates may cause bleeding problems in the newborn baby. Be sure that you have discussed this with your doctor before taking this medicine.

Breast-feeding—Belladonna alkaloids or barbiturates have not been shown to cause problems in nursing babies. However, traces of the belladonna alkaloids and barbiturates pass into the breast milk. Also, because the belladonna alkaloids tend to decrease the secretions of the body, it is possible that the flow of breast milk may be reduced in some patients.

Children—Severe side effects may be more likely to occur in infants and children, especially those with spastic paralysis or brain damage. Unusual excitement, nervousness, restlessness, or irritability and unusual warmth, dryness, and flushing of skin are more likely to occur in children, who are usually more sensitive to the effects of belladonna alkaloids. Also, when belladonna alkaloids are given to children during hot weather, a rapid increase in body temperature may occur. In addition, the barbiturate in this medicine could cause some children to become hyperactive.

Older adults—Confusion or memory loss; constipation; difficult urination; drowsiness; dryness of mouth, nose, throat, or skin; and unusual excitement, nervousness, restlessness, or irritability may be more likely to occur in the elderly, who are usually more sensitive than younger adults to the effects of belladonna alkaloids and barbiturates. Also, eye pain may occur, which may be a sign of glaucoma.

Other medicines—Although certain medicines should not be used together at all, in other cases two different medicines may be used together even if an interaction might occur. In these cases, your doctor may want to change the dose, or other precautions may be necessary. When you are taking belladonna alkaloids and barbiturates, it is especially important that your doctor and pharmacist know if you are taking any of the following:

- Adrenocorticoids (cortisone-like medicine) or
- Corticotropin (ACTH)—Belladonna alkaloids and barbiturates may decrease the response to these medicines
- Antacids or
- Diarrhea medicine containing kaolin or attapulgite—These medications may decrease the response to belladonna alkaloids
- Anticholinergics (medicine for abdominal or stomach spasms or cramps)—Belladonna alkaloids and barbiturates may increase the response to anticholinergics
- Anticoagulants (blood thinners)—Belladonna alkaloids and barbiturates may decrease the effect of this medicine
- Central nervous system (CNS) depressants (medicines that cause drowsiness)—The CNS effects of either medicine could be increased
- Ketoconazole (e.g., Nizoral)—Using ketoconazole with this combination medicine may lessen the effects of ketoconazole and barbiturates
- Monoamine oxidase (MAO) inhibitors (furazolidone [e.g., Furoxone], isocarboxazid [e.g., Marplan], phenelzine [e.g., Nardil], procarbazine [e.g., Matulane], selegiline [Eldepryl]; tranylcypromine [e.g., Parnate])—Taking belladonna alkaloids and barbiturates while you are taking or within 2 weeks of taking monoamine oxidase inhibitors may increase the effects of the barbiturates
- Potassium chloride (e.g., Slow K or K-Dur)—May cause an increase in lesions (sores) of the stomach or intestine

Other medical problems—The presence of other medical problems may affect the use of belladonna alkaloids and barbiturates. Make sure you tell your doctor if you have any other medical problems, especially:

- Asthma, emphysema, or other chronic lung disease or
- Dryness of mouth (severe and continuing) or
- Enlarged prostate or
- Glaucoma or
- Heart disease or
- Hyperactivity (in children) or
- Intestinal blockage or other intestinal problems or
- Urinary tract blockage or difficult urination—Belladonna alkaloids and barbiturates may make these conditions worse
- Brain damage (in children) or
- Spastic paralysis (in children)—These conditions may increase the effects of the medicine
- Down's syndrome (mongolism)—This condition may increase the side effects of the medicine
- Kidney disease or
- Liver disease—Higher levels of the belladonna alkaloid and barbiturate may result, possibly leading to increased side effects

Before you begin using any new medicine (prescription or nonprescription) or if you develop any new medical problem while you are using this medicine, check with your doctor, nurse, or pharmacist.

Proper Use of This Medicine

Take this medicine about ½ to 1 hour before meals, unless otherwise directed by your doctor.

Take this medicine only as directed. Do not take more or less of it, do not take it more often, and do not take it for a longer time than your doctor ordered. To do so may increase the chance of side effects.

Missed dose—If you miss a dose of this medicine, take it as soon as possible. However, if it is almost time for your next dose, skip the missed dose and go back to your regular dosing schedule. Do not double doses.

Storage—To store this medicine:

- Keep this medicine out of the reach of children. Overdose of belladonna alkaloids and barbiturates is especially dangerous in young children.
- Store away from heat and direct light.
- Do not store the capsule or tablet form of this medicine in the bathroom, near the kitchen sink, or in other damp places. Heat or moisture may cause the medicine to break down.
- Keep the liquid form of this medicine from freezing.
- Do not keep outdated medicine or medicine no longer needed. Be sure that any discarded medicine is out of the reach of children.

Precautions While Using This Medicine

This medicine will add to the effects of alcohol and other CNS depressants (medicines that slow down the nervous system, possibly causing drowsiness). Some examples of CNS depressants are antihistamines or medicine for hay fever, other allergies, or colds; sedatives, tranquilizers, or sleeping medicine; prescription pain medicine or narcotics; barbiturates; medicine for seizures; muscle relaxants; or anesthetics, including some dental anesthetics. *Check with your doctor before taking any of the above while you are taking this medicine.*

Do not take this medicine within 1 hour of taking antacids or medicine for diarrhea. Taking them too close together will make the belladonna alkaloids less effective.

Belladonna alkaloids will often make you sweat less, causing your body temperature to increase. *Use extra care not to become overheated during exercise or hot weather while you are taking this medicine,* as overheating could possibly result in heat stroke. This is especially important in children taking belladonna alkaloids.

This medicine may cause your eyes to become more sensitive to light than they are normally. Wearing sunglasses and avoiding too much exposure to bright light may help lessen the discomfort.

This medicine may cause some people to have blurred vision or to become drowsy, dizzy, or less alert than they are normally. *Make sure you know how you react to this medicine before you drive, use machines, or do anything else that could be dangerous if you are not alert or able to see well.*

This medicine may cause dryness of the mouth, nose, and throat. For temporary relief of mouth dryness, use sugarless candy or gum, melt bits of ice in your mouth, or use a saliva substitute. However, if your mouth continues to feel dry for more than 2 weeks, check with your dentist. Continuing dryness of the mouth may increase the chance of dental disease, including tooth decay, gum disease, and fungus infections.

Side Effects of This Medicine

Along with its needed effects, a medicine may cause some unwanted effects. Although not all of these side effects may occur, if they do occur they may need medical attention.

Check with your doctor as soon as possible if any of the following side effects occur:

Rare

Eye pain; skin rash or hives; sore throat and fever; unusual bleeding or bruising; yellow eyes or skin

Symptoms of overdose

Blurred vision (continuing) or changes in near vision; clumsiness or unsteadiness; confusion; convulsions (seizures); dizziness (continuing); drowsiness (severe); dryness of mouth, nose, or throat (severe); fast heartbeat; fever; hallucinations (seeing, hearing, or feeling things that are not there); shortness of breath or troubled breathing; slurred speech; unusual excitement, nervousness, restlessness, or irritability; unusual warmth, dryness, and flushing of skin

Other side effects may occur that usually do not need medical attention. These side effects may go away during treatment as your body adjusts to the medicine. However, check with your doctor if any of the following side effects continue or are bothersome:

More common

Constipation; decreased sweating; dizziness; drowsiness; dryness of mouth, nose, throat, or skin

Less common or rare

Bloated feeling; blurred vision; decreased flow of breast milk; difficult urination; difficulty in swallowing; headache; increased sensitivity of eyes to sunlight; loss of memory; nausea or vomiting; unusual tiredness or weakness

Other side effects not listed above may also occur in some patients. If you notice any other effects, check with your doctor.

Annual revision: 01/13/92

BENTIROMIDE Diagnostic†

A commonly used brand name in the U.S. is Chymex.

†Not commercially available in Canada.

Description

Bentiromide (ben-TEER-oh-mide) is used to help find out if the pancreas is working the way it should. The pancreas helps break down the bentiromide almost the same way it helps to break down food.

After bentiromide is broken down, a part of it appears in the urine. By measuring how much appears in the urine, your doctor can tell how well your pancreas is working.

How the test is done: After you take bentiromide, all of your urine is collected for the next six hours. The total amount is measured and a small sample is saved and examined.

Bentiromide is to be used only under the supervision of a doctor. It is available in the following dosage form:

Oral

- Oral solution (U.S.)

It is very important that you read and understand the following information. If any of it causes you special concern, check with your doctor. Also, *if you have any questions* or if you want more information about this test or your medical problem, *ask your doctor, nurse, or pharmacist.*

Before Having This Test

In deciding to use a diagnostic test, any risks of the test must be weighed against the good it will do. This is a decision you and your doctor will make. Also, test results may be affected by other things. For the test using bentiromide, the following should be considered:

Allergies—Tell your doctor if you have ever had any unusual or allergic reaction to bentiromide. Also tell your doctor if you are allergic to any other substances, such as foods, preservatives, or dyes.

Diet—Eating prunes or cranberries shortly before the bentiromide test period starts will affect test results. Avoid these foods for 3 days before the test.

Pregnancy—Studies with bentiromide have not been done in pregnant women. However, in animal studies bentiromide has not been shown to cause birth defects or other problems.

Breast-feeding—It is not known whether bentiromide passes into the breast milk. However, this medicine has not been reported to cause problems in nursing babies.

Children—Studies on this medicine have been done only in older children and adult patients, and there is no specific information comparing use of bentiromide in children up to 6 years of age with use in other age groups.

Older adults—Many medicines have not been studied specifically in older people. Therefore, it may not be known whether they work exactly the same way they do in younger adults or if they cause different side effects or problems in older people. There is no specific information comparing use of bentiromide in the elderly with use in other age groups.

Other medicines—Although certain medicines should not be used together at all, in other cases two different medicines may be used together even if an interaction might occur. In these cases, your doctor may want to change the dose, or other precautions may be necessary. When you are taking bentiromide it is especially important that your doctor know if you are taking or using any of the following:

- Acetaminophen (e.g., Tylenol) or
- Chloramphenicol (e.g., Chloromycetin) or
- Local anesthetics (e.g., benzocaine and lidocaine) or
- Para-aminobenzoic acid (PABA)-containing preparations (e.g., sunscreens and some multivitamins) or
- Procainamide (e.g., Pronestyl) or
- Sulfonamides (sulfa medicines) or
- Thiazide diuretics (water pills)—Use of these medicines during the test period will affect the test results
- Pancreatic supplements (e.g., pancrelipase)—Use of pancreatic supplements may give false test results

Other medical problems—The presence of other medical problems may affect the results of the test. Make sure you tell your doctor if you have any other medical problems, especially:

- Disease of the stomach and intestines or
- Kidney disease or
- Liver disease (severe)—These medical problems may cause false test results

Before you begin using any new medicine (prescription or nonprescription) or if you develop any new medical problem while you are using this medicine, check with your doctor, nurse, or pharmacist.

Preparation For This Test

Your doctor may ask you to avoid certain medicines or foods for at least 72 hours before this test is done. *Follow your doctor's instructions carefully.* Otherwise, this test may not work and may have to be done again.

Unless otherwise directed by your doctor:

- Do not eat anything after midnight the night before the test. Some foods may affect the results of the test.
- Urinate before taking bentiromide. You should have an empty bladder when you take the test.
- After taking bentiromide, drink a large glass of water (at least 8 ounces). Drink another large glass of water in 2 hours and then 2 more glasses of water in the next 4 hours. This will help increase the amount of urine, which is needed for testing.

Side Effects of This Medicine

Along with its needed effects, a medicine may cause some unwanted effects. Although not all of these side effects may occur, if they do occur they may need medical attention.

Check with your doctor or nurse immediately if either of the following side effects occurs:

Rare

Shortness of breath or troubled breathing

Other side effects may occur that usually do not need medical attention. These side effects should go away as the effects of the medicine wear off. However, check with your doctor if any of the following side effects continue or are bothersome:

More common

Diarrhea; headache

Less common or rare

Gas; nausea and vomiting; weakness

Other side effects not listed above may also occur in some patients. If you notice any other effects, check with your doctor.

Annual revision: 12/02/92

BENZODIAZEPINES Systemic

This information applies to the following medicines:

Alprazolam (al-PRAZ-oh-lam)
Bromazepam (broe-MA-ze-pam)
Chlordiazepoxide (klor-dye-az-e-POX-ide)
Clonazepam (kloe-NA-ze-pam)
Clorazepate (klor-AZ-e-pate)
Diazepam (dye-AZ-e-pam)
Estazolam (ess-TA-zoe-lam)
Flurazepam (flure-AZ-e-pam)
Halazepam (hal-AZ-e-pam)
Ketazolam (kee-TAY--zoe-lam)
Lorazepam (lor-AZ-e-pam)
Nitrazepam (nye-TRA-ze-pam)
Oxazepam (ox-AZ-e-pam)
Prazepam (PRAZ-e-pam)
Quazepam (KWA-ze-pam)
Temazepam (tem-AZ-e-pam)
Triazolam (trye-AY-zoe-lam)

Some commonly used brand names are:

For Alprazolam

In the U.S.

Xanax

In Canada

Apo-Alpraz
Novo-Alprazol
Nu-Alpraz
Xanax

For Bromazepam*

In Canada

Lectopam

For Chlordiazepoxide

In the U.S.

Libritabs — Lipoxide

Librium

Generic name product may also be available.

In Canada

Apo-Chlordiazepoxide — Novopoxide

Librium — Solium

For Clonazepam

In the U.S.

Klonopin

In Canada

Rivotril

For Clorazepate

In the U.S.

Gen-XENE — Tranxene T-Tab

Tranxene-SD

Generic name product may also be available.

In Canada

Apo-Clorazepate — Tranxene

Novoclopate

For Diazepam

In the U.S.

Diazepam Intensol — Valrelease

T-Quil — Vazepam

Valium — Zetran

Generic name product may also be available.

In Canada

Apo-Diazepam — PMS Diazepam

Diazemuls — Valium

Novodipam — Vivol

Generic name product may also be available.

For Estazolam†

In the U.S.

ProSom

For Flurazepam

In the U.S.

Dalmane

Durapam

Generic name product may also be available.

In Canada

Apo-Flurazepam — Novoflupam

Dalmane — Somnol

For Halazepam†

In the U.S.

Paxipam

For Ketazolam*

In Canada

Loftran

For Lorazepam

In the U.S.

Alzapam — Lorazepam Intensol

Ativan

Generic name product may also be available.

In Canada

Apo-Lorazepam — Novolorazem

Ativan — Nu-Loraz

For Nitrazepam*

In Canada

Mogadon

For Oxazepam

In the U.S.

Serax

Generic name product may also be available.

In Canada

Apo-Oxazepam — Serax

Novoxapam — Zapex

For Prazepam†

In the U.S.

Centrax

Generic name product may also be available.

For Quazepam†

In the U.S.

Doral

For Temazepam

In the U.S.

Razepam — Restoril

Generic name product may also be available.

In Canada

Restoril

For Triazolam

In the U.S.

Halcion

In Canada

Apo-Triazo — Novotriolam

Halcion — Nu-Triazo

Generic name product may also be available.

---

*Not commercially available in the U.S.

†Not commercially available in Canada.

Description

Benzodiazepines (ben-zoe-dye-AZ-e-peens) belong to the group of medicines called central nervous system (CNS) depressants (medicines that slow down the nervous system).

Some benzodiazepines are used to relieve nervousness or tension. Others are used in the treatment of insomnia (trouble in sleeping). However, if used regularly (for example, every day) for insomnia, they are usually not effective for more than a few weeks.

One of the benzodiazepines, diazepam, is also used to help relax muscles or relieve muscle spasm. Another benzodiazepine, alprazolam, is also used in the treatment of panic disorder. Clonazepam, clorazepate, and diazepam are also used to treat certain convulsive (seizure) disorders, such as epilepsy. The benzodiazepines may also be used for other conditions as determined by your doctor.

Benzodiazepines should not be used for nervousness or tension caused by the stress of everyday life.

These medicines are available only with your doctor's prescription, in the following dosage forms:

Oral

Alprazolam
- Tablets (U.S. and Canada)

Bromazepam
- Tablets (Canada)

- Chlordiazepoxide
  - Capsules (U.S. and Canada)
  - Tablets (U.S.)
- Clonazepam
  - Tablets (U.S. and Canada)
- Clorazepate
  - Capsules (U.S. and Canada)
  - Tablets (U.S.)
- Diazepam
  - Extended-release capsules (U.S.)
  - Oral solution (U.S.)
  - Tablets (U.S. and Canada)
- Estazolam
  - Tablets (U.S.)
- Flurazepam
  - Capsules (U.S. and Canada)
  - Tablets (Canada)
- Halazepam
  - Tablets (U.S.)
- Ketazolam
  - Capsules (Canada)
- Lorazepam
  - Oral solution (U.S.)
  - Tablets (U.S. and Canada)
  - Sublingual tablets (Canada)
- Nitrazepam
  - Tablets (Canada)
- Oxazepam
  - Capsules (U.S.)
  - Tablets (U.S. and Canada)
- Prazepam
  - Capsules (U.S.)
  - Tablets (U.S.)
- Quazepam
  - Tablets (U.S.)
- Temazepam
  - Capsules (U.S. and Canada)
  - Tablets (U.S.)
- Triazolam
  - Tablets (U.S. and Canada)

Parenteral

- Chlordiazepoxide
  - Injection (U.S. and Canada)
- Diazepam
  - Injection (U.S. and Canada)
- Lorazepam
  - Injection (U.S. and Canada)

Rectal

- Diazepam
  - Rectal solution (U.S. and Canada)

It is very important that you read and understand the following information. If any of it causes you special concern, check with your doctor. Also, *if you have any questions* or if you want more information about this medicine or your medical problem, *ask your doctor, nurse, or pharmacist.*

Before Using This Medicine

In deciding to use a medicine, the risks of taking the medicine must be weighed against the good it will do. This is a decision you and your doctor will make. For benzodiazepines, the following should be considered:

Allergies—Tell your doctor if you have ever had any unusual or allergic reaction to benzodiazepines. Also tell your doctor and pharmacist if you are allergic to any other substances, such as foods, preservatives, or dyes.

Pregnancy—Chlordiazepoxide and diazepam have been reported to increase the chance of birth defects when used during the first 3 months of pregnancy. Although similar problems have not been reported with the other benzodiazepines, the chance always exists since all of the benzodiazepines are related.

Studies in animals have shown that clonazepam, lorazepam, and temazepam cause birth defects or other problems, including death of the animal fetus.

Too much use of benzodiazepines during pregnancy may cause the baby to become dependent on the medicine. This may lead to withdrawal side effects after birth. Also, use of benzodiazepines during pregnancy, especially during the last weeks, may cause drowsiness, slow heartbeat, shortness of breath, or troubled breathing in the newborn infant.

Benzodiazepines given just before or during labor may cause weakness in the newborn infant. When diazepam is given in high doses (especially by injection) within 15 hours before delivery, it may cause breathing problems, muscle weakness, difficulty in feeding, and body temperature problems in the newborn infant.

Breast-feeding—Benzodiazepines may pass into the breast milk and cause drowsiness, slow heartbeat, shortness of breath, or troubled breathing in nursing babies of mothers taking this medicine.

Children—Most of the side effects of these medicines are more likely to occur in children, especially the very young. These patients are usually more sensitive than adults to the effects of benzodiazepines.

When clonazepam is used for long periods of time in children, it may cause unwanted effects on physical and mental growth. These effects may not be noticed until many years later. Before this medicine is given to children for long periods of time, you should discuss its use with your child's doctor.

Older adults—Most of the side effects of these medicines are more likely to occur in the elderly, who are usually more sensitive to the effects of benzodiazepines.

Taking benzodiazepines for trouble in sleeping may cause more daytime drowsiness in elderly patients than in younger adults. In addition, falls and related injuries may be more likely to occur in elderly patients taking benzodiazepines.

Other medicines—Although certain medicines should not be used together at all, in other cases 2 different medicines may be used together even if an interaction might occur. In these cases, your doctor may want to change the dose, or other precautions may be necessary. When you are taking or receiving benzodiazepines it is especially important that your doctor and pharmacist know if you are taking any of the following:

- Central nervous system (CNS) depressants (medicine that causes drowsiness)—The CNS depressant effects of either these medicines or benzodiazepines may be increased; your doctor may want to change the dose of either or both medicines

Other medical problems—The presence of other medical problems may affect the use of benzodiazepines. Make sure you tell your doctor if you have any other medical problems, especially:

- Alcohol abuse (or history of) or
- Drug abuse or dependence (or history of)—Dependence on benzodiazepines may develop
- Brain disease—CNS depression and other side effects of benzodiazepines may be more likely to occur
- Difficulty in swallowing (in children) or
- Emphysema, asthma, bronchitis, or other chronic lung disease or
- Glaucoma or
- Hyperactivity or
- Mental depression or
- Mental illness (severe) or
- Myasthenia gravis or
- Porphyria or
- Sleep apnea (temporarily stopping of breathing during sleep)—Benzodiazepines may make the condition worse
- Epilepsy or history of seizures—Although clonazepam and diazepam are used in treating epilepsy, starting or suddenly stopping treatment with these medicines may increase seizures
- Kidney or liver disease—Higher blood levels of benzodiazepines may result, increasing the chance of side effects

Before you begin using any new medicine (prescription or nonprescription) or if you develop any new medical problem while you are using this medicine, check with your doctor, nurse, or pharmacist.

Proper Use of This Medicine

For patients taking *diazepam extended-release capsules:*

- Swallow capsules whole.
- Do not crush, break, or chew the capsules before swallowing.

For patients taking *lorazepam oral solution:*

- Each dose may be diluted with water, soda or soda-like beverages, or semisolid food, such as applesauce or pudding.

For patients taking *lorazepam sublingual tablets:*

- Do not chew or swallow the tablet. This medicine is meant to be absorbed through the lining of the mouth. Place the tablet under your tongue (sublingual) and let it slowly dissolve there. Do not swallow for at least 2 minutes.

Take this medicine only as directed by your doctor. Do not take more of it, do not take it more often, and do not take it for a longer time than your doctor ordered. If too much is taken, it may become habit-forming (causing mental or physical dependence).

If you think this medicine is not working properly after you have taken it for a few weeks, *do not increase the dose.* Instead, check with your doctor.

For patients taking this medicine *for epilepsy or other seizure disorder:*

- *In order for this medicine to control your seizures, it must be taken every day in regularly spaced doses as ordered by your doctor.* This is necessary to keep a constant amount of the medicine in the blood. To help keep the amount constant, do not miss any doses.

For patients taking this medicine *for insomnia:*

- *Do not take this medicine when your schedule does not permit you to get a full night's sleep (7 to 8 hours).* If you must wake up before this, you may continue to feel drowsy and may experience memory problems, because the effects of the medicine have not had time to wear off.

For patients taking *flurazepam:*

- *When you begin to take this medicine, your sleeping problem will improve somewhat the first night. However, 2 or 3 nights may pass before you receive the full effects of this medicine.*

Missed dose—If you are taking this medicine regularly (for example, every day as for epilepsy) and you miss a dose, take it right away if you remember within an hour or so of the missed dose. However, if you do not remember until later, skip the missed dose and go back to your regular dosing schedule. Do not double doses.

Storage—To store this medicine:

- Keep out of the reach of children. Overdose of benzodiazepines may be especially dangerous in children.
- Store away from heat and direct light.
- Do not store the capsule or tablet form of this medicine in the bathroom, near the kitchen sink, or in other damp places. Heat or moisture may cause the medicine to break down.
- Keep the liquid form of this medicine from freezing.
- Do not keep outdated medicine or medicine no longer needed. Be sure that any discarded medicine is out of the reach of children.

Precautions While Using This Medicine

If you will be *taking this medicine regularly for a long time:*

- Your doctor should check your progress at regular visits to make sure that this medicine does not cause unwanted effects. If you are taking clonazepam, this is also important during the first few months of treatment.
- If you are taking this medicine for nervousness or tension or for panic disorder, check with your doctor at least every 4 months to make sure you need to continue taking this medicine.
- If you are taking estazolam, flurazepam, quazepam, temazepam, or triazolam for insomnia (trouble in sleeping), and you think you need this medicine for more than 7 to 10 days, be sure to discuss it with your doctor. Insomnia that lasts longer than this may be a sign of another medical problem.

If you will be taking this medicine in large doses or for a long time, do not stop taking it without first checking with your doctor. Your doctor may want you to reduce gradually the amount you are taking before stopping completely. Stopping this medicine suddenly may cause withdrawal side effects. Also, if you are taking this medicine for epilepsy or another seizure disorder, stopping this medicine suddenly may cause seizures.

For patients taking this medicine *for epilepsy or another seizure disorder:*

- Your doctor may want you to carry a medical identification card or bracelet stating that you are taking this medicine.

This medicine will add to the effects of alcohol and other CNS depressants (medicines that slow down the nervous system, possibly causing drowsiness). Some examples of CNS depressants are antihistamines or medicine for hay fever, other allergies, or colds; sedatives, tranquilizers, or sleeping medicine; prescription pain medicine or narcotics; barbiturates; medicine for seizures; muscle relaxants; or anesthetics, including some dental anesthetics. This effect may last for a few days after you stop taking this medicine. *Check with your doctor before taking any of the above while you are taking this medicine.*

If you think you or someone else may have taken an overdose of this medicine, get emergency help at once. Taking an overdose of a benzodiazepine or taking alcohol or other CNS depressants with the benzodiazepine may lead to unconsciousness and possibly death. Some signs of an overdose are continuing slurred speech or confusion, severe drowsiness, severe weakness, and staggering.

Before you have any medical tests, tell the medical doctor in charge that you are taking this medicine. The results of the metyrapone test may be affected by chlordiazepoxide.

If you develop any unusual and strange thoughts or behavior while you are taking this medicine, be sure to discuss it with your doctor. Some changes that have occurred in people taking this medicine are like those seen in people who drink alcohol and then act in a manner that is not normal. Other changes may be more unusual and extreme, such as confusion, agitation, and hallucinations (seeing, hearing, or feeling things that are not there).

This medicine may cause some people, especially older persons, to become drowsy, dizzy, lightheaded, clumsy or unsteady, or less alert than they are normally. Even if taken at bedtime, it may cause some people to feel drowsy or less alert on arising. *Make sure you know how you react to this medicine before you drive, use machines, or do anything else that could be dangerous if you are dizzy or are not alert.*

If you have been taking this medicine for insomnia, you may have difficulty sleeping (rebound insomnia) for the first few nights after you stop taking the medicine.

Side Effects of This Medicine

Along with its needed effects, a medicine may cause some unwanted effects. Although not all of these side effects may occur, if they do occur they may need medical attention.

Check with your doctor as soon as possible if any of the following side effects occur:

Less common or rare

Behavior problems, including difficulty in concentrating and outbursts of anger; confusion or mental depression; convulsions (seizures); hallucinations (seeing, hearing, or feeling things that are not there); hypotension (low blood pressure); impaired memory—may be more common with triazolam; muscle weakness; skin rash or itching; sore throat, fever, and chills; trouble in sleeping; ulcers or sores in mouth or throat (continuing); uncontrolled movements of body, including the eyes; unusual bleeding or bruising; unusual excitement, nervousness, or irritability; unusual tiredness or weakness (severe); yellow eyes or skin

Symptoms of overdose

Confusion (continuing); drowsiness (severe); shakiness; slow heartbeat, shortness of breath, or troubled breathing; slow reflexes; slurred speech (continuing); staggering; weakness (severe)

Other side effects may occur that usually do not need medical attention. These side effects may go away during treatment as your body adjusts to the medicine. However, check with your doctor if any of the following side effects continue or are bothersome:

More common

Clumsiness or unsteadiness; dizziness or lightheadedness; drowsiness; slurred speech

Less common or rare

Abdominal or stomach cramps or pain; blurred vision or other changes in vision; changes in sexual drive or performance; constipation; diarrhea; dryness of mouth or increased thirst; false sense of well-being; fast or pounding heartbeat; headache; increased bronchial secretions or watering of mouth; muscle spasm; nausea or vomiting; problems with urination; trembling; unusual tiredness or weakness

Not all of the side effects listed above have been reported for each of these medicines, but they have been reported for at least one of them. All of the benzodiazepines are similar, so any of the above side effects may occur with any of these medicines.

For patients having *chlordiazepoxide, diazepam, or lorazepam injected:*

- Check with your doctor if there is redness, swelling, or pain at the place of injection.

After you stop using this medicine, your body may need time to adjust. If you took this medicine in high doses or for a long time, this may take up to 3 weeks. During this period of time check with your doctor if you notice any of the following side effects:

More common

Irritability; nervousness; trouble in sleeping

Less common

Abdominal or stomach cramps; confusion; fast or pounding heartbeat; increased sense of hearing; increased sensitivity to touch and pain; increased sweating; loss of sense of reality; mental depression; muscle cramps; nausea or vomiting; sensitivity of eyes to light; tingling, burning, or prickly sensations; trembling

Rare

Confusion as to time, place, or person; convulsions (seizures); feelings of suspicion or distrust; hallucinations (seeing, hearing, or feeling things that are not there)

Other side effects not listed above may also occur in some patients. If you notice any other effects, check with your doctor.

Additional Information

Once a medicine has been approved for marketing for a certain use, experience may show that it is also useful for other medical problems. Although these uses are not included in product labeling, some of the benzodiazepines are used in certain patients with the following medical conditions:

- Nausea and vomiting caused by cancer chemotherapy
- Tension headache
- Tremors

Other than the above information, there is no additional information relating to proper use, precautions, or side effects for these uses.

Annual revision: 08/04/92

BENZONATATE Systemic†

A commonly used brand name in the U.S. is Tessalon.

†Not commercially available in Canada.

Description

Benzonatate (ben-ZOE-na-tate) is used to relieve coughs due to colds or influenza (flu). It is sometimes used to relieve the cough that occurs with smoking, asthma, or emphysema. However, in patients with an unusually large amount of mucus or phlegm with the cough, medicines like benzonatate that suppress the cough are generally not recommended.

Benzonatate relieves cough by acting directly on the lungs and the breathing passages. It also acts on the cough center in the brain.

This medicine is available only with your doctor's prescription, in the following dosage form:

Oral

- Capsules (U.S.)

It is very important that you read and understand the following information. If any of it causes you special concern, check with your doctor. Also, *if you have any questions* or if you want more information about this medicine or your medical problem, *ask your doctor, nurse, or pharmacist.*

Before Using this Medicine

In deciding to use a medicine, the risks of taking the medicine must be weighed against the good it will do. This is a decision you and your doctor will make. For benzonatate, the following should be considered:

Allergies—Tell your doctor if you have ever had any unusual or allergic reaction to benzonatate or to tetracaine or other local anesthetics. Also tell your doctor and pharmacist if you are allergic to any other substances, such as foods, preservatives, or dyes.

Pregnancy—Studies on effects in pregnancy have not been done in either humans or animals.

Breast-feeding—It is not known whether benzonatate passes into the breast milk. However, this medicine has not been reported to cause problems in nursing babies.

Children—Children may tend to chew the capsule before swallowing it. This may cause numbness (loss of feeling) in the mouth and throat, and choking may occur.

Older adults—Many medicines have not been studied specifically in older people. Therefore, it may not be known whether they work exactly the same way they do in younger adults or if they cause different side effects or problems in older people. There is no specific information comparing use of benzonatate in the elderly with use in other age groups.

Other medicines—Although certain medicines should not be used together at all, in other cases 2 different medicines may be used together even if an interaction might occur. In these cases, your doctor may want to change the dose, or other precautions may be necessary. When you are taking benzonatate it is especially important that your doctor and pharmacist know if you are taking any of the following:

- Central nervous system (CNS) depressants—The depressant effects of either these medicines or benzonatate may be increased

Before you begin using any new medicine (prescription or nonprescription) or if you develop any new medical problem while you are using this medicine, check with your doctor, nurse, or pharmacist.

Proper Use of This Medicine

Do not chew the capsules before swallowing them. If the benzonatate contained in the capsules comes in contact with the mouth, it may cause the mouth and throat to become numb (loss of feeling) and choking may occur.

Missed dose—If you must take this medicine regularly and you miss a dose, take it as soon as possible. However, if it is almost time for your next dose, skip the missed dose and go back to your regular dosing schedule. Do not double doses.

Storage—To store this medicine:

- Store away from heat and direct light.
- Keep out of the reach of children.
- Do not store this medicine in the bathroom, near the kitchen sink, or in other damp places. Heat or moisture may cause the medicine to break down.
- Do not keep outdated medicine or medicine no longer needed. Be sure that any discarded medicine is out of the reach of children.

Precautions While Using This Medicine

If your cough has not become better after 7 days or if you have a high fever, skin rash, or continuing headache with the cough, check with your doctor. These signs may mean that you have other medical problems.

Side Effects of This Medicine

Along with its needed effects, a medicine may cause some unwanted effects. Although not all of these side effects may occur, if they do occur they may need medical attention.

Check with your doctor as soon as possible if any of the following side effects occur:

Symptoms of overdose

Convulsions (seizures); restlessness; trembling

Other side effects may occur that usually do not need medical attention. These side effects may go away during treatment as your body adjusts to the medicine. However, check with your doctor or pharmacist if any of the following side effects continue or are bothersome:

Less common or rare

Constipation; dizziness (mild); drowsiness (mild); nausea or vomiting; skin rash; stuffy nose

Other side effects not listed above may also occur in some patients. If you notice any other effects, check with your doctor.

Annual revision: 05/15/91

BENZOYL PEROXIDE Topical

Some commonly used brand names are:

In the U.S.

Acne Aid 10 Cream
Acne-5 Lotion
Acne-10 Lotion
Ben-Aqua-2½ Gel
Ben-Aqua-5 Gel
Ben-Aqua-10 Gel
Ben-Aqua-5 Lotion
Ben-Aqua-10 Lotion
Ben-Aqua Masque 5
Benoxyl 5 Lotion
Benoxyl 10 Lotion
Benzac Ac 2½ Gel
Benzac Ac 5 Gel
Benzac Ac 10 Gel
Benzac 5 Gel
Benzac 10 Gel
Benzac W 2½ Gel
Benzac W 5 Gel
Benzac W 10 Gel
Benzac W Wash 5
Benzac W Wash 10
BenzaShave 5 Cream
BenzaShave 10 Cream
Brevoxyl 4 Gel
Clearasil Maximum Strength Medicated Anti-Acne 10 Tinted Cream
Clearasil Maximum Strength Medicated Anti-Acne 10 Vanishing Cream
Clearasil Maximum Strength Medicated Anti-Acne 10 Vanishing Lotion
Clear By Design 2.5 Gel
Cuticura Acne 5 Cream
Del-Aqua-5 Gel
Del-Aqua-10 Gel
Desquam-E 2.5 Gel
Desquam-E 5 Gel
Desquam-E 10 Gel
Desquam-X 10 Bar
Desquam-X 2.5 Gel
Desquam-X 5 Gel
Desquam-X 10 Gel
Desquam-X 5 Wash
Desquam-X 10 Wash
Dry and Clear Double Strength 10 Cream
Dry and Clear 5 Lotion
Dryox 5 Gel
Dryox 10 Gel
Dryox 20 Gel
Dryox Wash 5
Dryox Wash 10
Fostex 10 Bar
Fostex 10 Cream
Fostex 5 Gel
Fostex 10 Gel
Fostex 10 Wash
Loroxide 5.5 Lotion
Neutrogena Acne Mask 5
Noxzema Clear-ups Maximum Strength 10 Lotion
Noxzema Clear-ups On-The-Spot 10 Lotion
Oxy 10 Daily Face Wash
Oxy 5 Tinted Lotion
Oxy 10 Tinted Lotion
Oxy 5 Vanishing Lotion
Oxy 10 Vanishing Lotion
PanOxyl AQ 2½ Gel
PanOxyl AQ 5 Gel
PanOxyl AQ 10 Gel
PanOxyl 5 Bar
PanOxyl 10 Bar
PanOxyl 5 Gel
PanOxyl 10 Gel
Persa-Gel 5
Persa-Gel 10
Persa-Gel W 5
Persa-Gel W 10
pHisoAc BP 10 Cream
Propa P.H. 10 Acne Cover Stick
Propa P.H. 10 Liquid Acne Soap
Stri-Dex Maximum Strength Treatment 10 Cream
Theroxide 5 Lotion
Theroxide 10 Lotion
Theroxide 10 Wash
Topex 10 Lotion
Vanoxide 5 Lotion
Xerac BP 5 Gel
Xerac BP 10 Gel
Zeroxin-5 Gel
Zeroxin-10 Gel

Generic name product may also be available.

In Canada

Acetoxyl 2.5 Gel
Acetoxyl 5 Gel
Acetoxyl 10 Gel
Acetoxyl 20 Gel
Acnomel B.P. 5 Lotion
Benoxyl 5 Lotion
Benoxyl 10 Lotion
Benoxyl 20 Lotion
Benoxyl 5 Wash
Benoxyl 10 Wash
Benzac W 5 Gel
Benzac W 10 Gel
Benzagel 5 Acne Lotion
Benzagel 5 Acne Wash
Benzagel 5 Gel
Benzagel 10 Gel
Clearasil BP Plus 5 Cream
Clearasil BP Plus 5 Lotion
Dermoxyl Aqua 5 Gel
Dermoxyl 2.5 Gel
Dermoxyl 5 Gel
Dermoxyl 10 Gel
Dermoxyl 20 Gel
Desquam-X 5 Bar
Desquam-X 5 Gel
Desquam-X 10 Gel
Desquam-X 5 Wash
Desquam-X 10 Wash
H_2Oxyl 2.5 Gel
H_2Oxyl 5 Gel
H_2Oxyl 10 Gel
H_2Oxyl 20 Gel
Loroxide 5 Lotion with Flesh-Tinted Base
Oxyderm 5 Lotion
Oxyderm 10 Lotion
Oxyderm 20 Lotion
Oxy 5 Vanishing Formula Lotion
PanOxyl 5 Bar
PanOxyl 10 Bar
PanOxyl 5 Gel
PanOxyl 10 Gel
PanOxyl 15 Gel
PanOxyl 20 Gel
Topex 5 Lotion

Description

Benzoyl peroxide (BEN-zoe-ill per-OX-ide) is used to treat acne. It may also be used for other conditions as determined by your doctor.

Some of these preparations are available only with your doctor's prescription. Others are available without a prescription; however, your doctor may have special instructions on the proper use of benzoyl peroxide for your medical condition.

Benzoyl peroxide is available in the following dosage forms:

Topical

- Cleansing bar (U.S. and Canada)
- Cream (U.S. and Canada)
- Gel (U.S. and Canada)
- Lotion (U.S. and Canada)
- Cleansing lotion (U.S. and Canada)
- Facial mask (U.S.)
- Stick (U.S.)

It is very important that you read and understand the following information. If any of it causes you special concern, check with your doctor. Also, *if you have any questions* or if you want more information about this medicine or your medical problem, *ask your doctor, nurse, or pharmacist.*

Before Using This Medicine

If you are using this medicine without a prescription, carefully read and follow any precautions on the label. For benzoyl peroxide, the following should be considered:

Allergies—Tell your doctor if you have ever had any unusual or allergic reaction to benzoyl peroxide. Also tell your doctor and pharmacist if you are allergic to any other substances, such as preservatives or dyes.

Pregnancy—Studies on effects in pregnancy have not been done in either humans or animals. However, benzoyl peroxide may be absorbed through the skin.

Breast-feeding—Benzoyl peroxide may be absorbed through the mother's skin. It is not known whether it passes into the breast milk. However, this medicine has not been reported to cause problems in nursing babies.

Children—For children up to 12 years of age: Studies on this medicine have been done only in adult patients, and there is no specific information comparing use of benzoyl peroxide with use in other age groups. For children 12 years of age and older: Although there is no specific information comparing use of benzoyl peroxide in children with use in other age groups, this medicine is not expected to cause different side effects or problems in children 12 years of age and older than it does in adults.

Older adults—Many medicines have not been studied specifically in older people. Therefore, it may not be known whether they work exactly the same way they do in younger adults. Although there is no specific information comparing use of benzoyl peroxide in the elderly with use in other age groups, this medicine is not expected to cause different side effects or problems in older people than it does in younger adults.

Other medicines—Although certain medicines should not be used together at all, in other cases two different medicines may be used together even if an interaction might occur. In these cases, your doctor may want to change the dose, or other precautions may be necessary. Tell your doctor and pharmacist if you are using any other topical prescription or nonprescription (over-the-counter [OTC]) medicine that is to be applied to the same area of the skin.

Other medical problems—The presence of other medical problems may affect the use of benzoyl peroxide. Make sure you tell your doctor if you have any other medical problems, especially:

- Red or raw skin—Irritation will occur if benzoyl peroxide is used on red or raw skin

Before you begin using any new medicine (prescription or nonprescription) or if you develop any new medical problem while you are using this medicine, check with your doctor, nurse, or pharmacist.

Proper Use of This Medicine

To use the *cream, gel, lotion, or stick form* of benzoyl peroxide:

- Before applying, wash the affected area with nonmedicated soap and water or with a degreasing cleanser and then gently pat dry with a towel.
- Apply enough medicine to cover the affected areas, and rub in gently.

To use the *shave cream form* of benzoyl peroxide:

- Wet the area to be shaved.
- Apply a small amount of the shave cream and gently rub over entire area.
- Shave.
- Rinse the area and pat dry.
- After-shave lotions or other drying face products should not be used, without checking with your doctor first.

To use the *cleansing bar, cleansing lotion, or soap form* of benzoyl peroxide:

- Use to wash the affected areas as directed.

To use the *facial mask form* of benzoyl peroxide:

- Before applying, wash the affected area with a nonmedicated cleanser. Then rinse and pat dry.
- Using a circular motion, apply a thin layer of the mask evenly over the affected area.
- Allow the mask to dry for 15 to 25 minutes.
- Then rinse thoroughly with warm water and pat dry.

Use benzoyl peroxide only as directed. Do not use more of it and do not use it more often than recommended on the label, unless otherwise directed by your doctor.

Keep this medicine away from the eyes, other mucous membranes, such as the mouth, lips, and inside of the nose, and sensitive areas of the neck.

Do not apply benzoyl peroxide to raw or irritated skin.

Missed dose—If you miss a dose of this medicine, apply or use it as soon as possible. Then go back to your regular dosing schedule.

Storage—To store this medicine:

- Keep out of the reach of children.
- Store away from heat and direct light.
- Keep the cream, gel, or liquid form of this medicine from freezing.
- Do not keep outdated medicine or medicine no longer needed. Be sure that any discarded medicine is out of the reach of children.

Precautions While Using This Medicine

If your skin problem has not improved within 4 to 6 weeks, check with your doctor.

If this medicine causes too much redness, peeling, or dryness of your skin, check with your doctor. It may be necessary for you to reduce the number of times a day that you use the medicine and/or use a weaker strength of the medicine.

When using benzoyl peroxide, do not use any of the following preparations on the same affected area as this medicine, unless otherwise directed by your doctor:

Abrasive soaps or cleansers
Alcohol-containing preparations
Any other topical acne preparation or preparation containing a peeling agent (for example, resorcinol, salicylic acid, sulfur, or tretinoin [vitamin A acid])

Cosmetics or soaps that dry the skin
Medicated cosmetics
Other topical medicine for the skin

To use any of the above preparations on the same affected area as benzoyl peroxide may cause severe irritation of the skin.

This medicine may bleach hair or colored fabrics.

Side Effects of This Medicine

Along with its needed effects, a medicine may cause some unwanted effects. Although not all of these side effects may occur, if they do occur they may need medical attention.

Check with your doctor as soon as possible if any of the following side effects occur:

Less common or rare

Painful irritation of skin, including burning, blistering, crusting, itching, severe redness, or swelling; skin rash

Symptoms of overdose

Burning, itching, scaling, redness, or swelling of skin (severe)

Other side effects may occur that usually do not need medical attention. These side effects may go away during treatment as your body adjusts to the medicine. However, check with your doctor or pharmacist if any of the following side effects continue or are bothersome:

Less common

Dryness or peeling of skin (may occur after a few days); feeling of warmth, mild stinging, and redness of skin

Other side effects not listed above may also occur in some patients. If you notice any other effects, check with your doctor or pharmacist.

Additional Information

Once a medicine has been approved for marketing for a certain use, experience may show that it is also useful for other medical problems. Although these uses are not included in product labeling, benzoyl peroxide is used in certain patients with the following medical conditions:

- Decubital ulcer (bed sores)
- Stasis ulcer (a certain type of ulcer)

Other than the above information, there is no additional information relating to proper use, precautions, or side effects for these uses.

Annual revision: 01/15/92

BETA-ADRENERGIC BLOCKING AGENTS Ophthalmic

This information applies to the following medicines:

Betaxolol (be-TAX-oh-lol)
Carteolol (KAR-tee-oh-lole)
Levobunolol (lee-voe-BYOO-noe-lole)
Metipranolol (met-i-PRAN-oh-lol)
Timolol (TYE-moe-lole)

Some commonly used brand names are:

For Betaxolol

In the U.S.

Betoptic
Betoptic S

In Canada

Betoptic

For Carteolol†

In the U.S.

Ocupress

For Levobunolol

In the U.S.

Betagan C Cap B.I.D.
Betagan C Cap Q.D.
Betagan Standard Cap

In Canada

Betagan C Cap B.I.D.
Betagan Standard Cap

For Metipranolol†

In the U.S.

OptiPranolol

For Timolol

In the U.S.

Timoptic
Timoptic in Ocudose

In Canada

Apo-Timop
Gen-Timolol
Timoptic

†Not commercially available in Canada.

Description

Betaxolol, carteolol, levobunolol, metipranolol, and timolol are used to treat certain types of glaucoma. They appear to work by reducing the production of fluid in the eye. This lowers the pressure in the eye.

These medicines are available only with your doctor's prescription, in the following dosage forms:

Ophthalmic

Betaxolol
- Ophthalmic solution (eye drops) (U.S. and Canada)
- Ophthalmic suspension (eye drops) (U.S.)

Carteolol
- Ophthalmic solution (eye drops) (U.S.)

Levobunolol
- Ophthalmic solution (eye drops) (U.S. and Canada)

Metipranolol
- Ophthalmic solution (eye drops) (U.S.)

Timolol
- Ophthalmic solution (eye drops) (U.S. and Canada)

It is very important that you read and understand the following information. If any of it causes you special concern, check with your doctor. Also, *if you have any questions* or if you want more information about this medicine or your medical problem, *ask your doctor, nurse, or pharmacist.*

Before Using This Medicine

In deciding to use a medicine, the risks of taking the medicine must be weighed against the good it will do. This is a decision you and your doctor will make. For ophthalmic beta-adrenergic blocking agents, the following should be considered:

Allergies—Tell your doctor if you have ever had any unusual or allergic reaction to any of the beta-adrenergic blocking agents, either ophthalmic or systemic, such as acebutolol, atenolol, betaxolol, bisoprolol, carteolol, labetalol, levobunolol, metipranolol, metoprolol, nadolol, oxprenolol, penbutolol, pindolol, propranolol, sotalol, or timolol. Also tell your doctor and pharmacist if you are allergic to any other substances, such as sulfites or preservatives.

Pregnancy—Ophthalmic beta-adrenergic blocking agents may be absorbed into the body. These medicines have not been studied in pregnant women. Studies in animals have not shown that betaxolol, levobunolol, metipranolol, or timolol causes birth defects. However, very large doses of carteolol given by mouth to pregnant rats have been shown to cause wavy ribs in rat babies. In addition, some studies in animals have shown that beta-adrenergic blocking agents increase the chance of death in the animal fetus. Before using ophthalmic beta-adrenergic blocking agents, make sure your doctor knows if you are pregnant or if you may become pregnant.

Breast-feeding—Betaxolol and timolol, and maybe other beta-adrenergic blocking agents, when taken by mouth, may pass into the breast milk. Since ophthalmic beta-adrenergic blocking agents may be absorbed into the body, they, too, may pass into the breast milk. However, it is not known whether ophthalmic beta-adrenergic blocking agents pass into the breast milk, and these medicines have not been reported to cause problems in nursing babies.

Children—Infants may be especially sensitive to the effects of ophthalmic beta-adrenergic blocking agents. This may increase the chance of side effects during treatment.

Older adults—Elderly people are especially sensitive to the effects of ophthalmic beta-adrenergic blocking agents. If too much medicine is absorbed into the body, the chance of side effects during treatment may be increased.

Other medicines—Although certain medicines should not be used together at all, in other cases two different medicines may be used together even if an interaction might occur. In these cases, your doctor may want to change the dose, or other precautions may be necessary. Tell your doctor and pharmacist if you are using any other prescription or nonprescription (over-the-counter [OTC]) medicine.

Other medical problems—The presence of other medical problems may affect the use of ophthalmic beta-adrenergic blocking agents. Make sure you tell your doctor if you have any other medical problems, especially:

- Asthma (or history of), chronic bronchitis, emphysema, or other lung disease—Severe breathing problems, including death due to bronchospasm (spasm of the bronchial tubes), have been reported in patients with asthma following use of some ophthalmic beta-adrenergic blocking agents (carteolol, levobunolol, metipranolol, and timolol). Although most often not a problem, the possibility of wheezing or troubled breathing also exists with betaxolol
- Diabetes mellitus (sugar diabetes) or
- Hypoglycemia (low blood sugar)—Ophthalmic beta-adrenergic blocking agents may cover up some signs and symptoms of hypoglycemia (low blood sugar), such as fast heartbeat and trembling, although they do not cover up other signs, such as dizziness or sweating
- Heart or blood vessel disease—Ophthalmic beta-adrenergic blocking agents may decrease heart activity
- Overactive thyroid—Ophthalmic beta-adrenergic blocking agents may cover up certain signs and symptoms of hyperthyroidism (overactive thyroid). Suddenly stopping the use of ophthalmic beta-adrenergic blocking agents may cause a sudden and dangerous increase in thyroid symptoms

Before you begin using any new medicine (prescription or nonprescription) or if you develop any new medical problem while you are using this medicine, check with your doctor, nurse, or pharmacist.

Proper Use of This Medicine

To use:

- First, wash your hands. With the middle finger, apply pressure to the inside corner of the eye (and continue to apply pressure for 1 or 2 minutes after the medicine has been placed in the eye). *This is especially important if the ophthalmic beta-adrenergic blocking agent is used to treat infants and children.* Tilt the head back and with the index finger of the same hand, pull the lower eyelid away from the eye to form a pouch. Drop the medicine into the pouch and gently close the eyes. Do not blink. Keep the eyes closed for 1 or 2 minutes to allow the medicine to be absorbed.
- Immediately after using the eye drops, wash your hands to remove any medicine that may be on them.

- To keep the medicine as germ-free as possible, do not touch the applicator tip to any surface (including the eye). Also, keep the container tightly closed.
- If you are using the medication with the compliance cap (C Cap):

  —Before using the eye drops for the first time, make sure the number 1 or the correct day of the week appears in the window on the cap.

  —Remove the cap and use the eye drops as directed.

  —Replace the cap. Holding the cap between your thumb and forefinger, rotate the bottle until the cap clicks to the next position. This will tell you the time of your next dose.

  —After every dose, rotate the bottle until the cap clicks to the position that tells you the time of your next dose.

Use this medicine only as directed. Do not use more of it and do not use it more often than your doctor ordered. To do so may increase the chance of too much medicine being absorbed into the body and the chance of side effects.

Dosing—The dose of betaxolol, carteolol, levobunolol, metipranolol, or timolol will be different for different patients. *Follow your doctor's orders or the directions on the label.* The following information includes only the average doses. *If your dose is different, do not change it* unless your doctor tells you to do so.

The number of doses of medicine that you use also depends on the strength of the medicine.

For betaxolol, carteolol, or metipranolol
- For *ophthalmic drops* dosage forms:
  —For glaucoma:
  - Adults and older children—Topical, to the conjunctiva, 1 drop two times a day.
  - Infants and younger children—Dose must be determined by the doctor.

For levobunolol or timolol
- For *ophthalmic drops* dosage forms:
  —For glaucoma:
  - Adults and older children—Topical, to the conjunctiva, 1 drop one or two times a day.
  - Infants and younger children—Dose must be determined by the doctor.

Missed dose—If you miss a dose of this medicine and your dosing schedule is:
- One dose a day—Use the missed dose as soon as possible. However, if you do not remember the missed dose until the next day, skip the missed dose and go back to your regular dosing schedule. Do not double doses.
- More than one dose a day—Use the missed dose as soon as possible. However, if it is almost time for your next dose, skip the missed dose and go back to your regular dosing schedule. Do not double doses.

If you have any questions about this, check with your doctor.

Storage—To store this medicine:
- Keep out of the reach of children.
- Store away from heat and direct light.
- Keep this medicine from freezing.
- Do not keep outdated medicine or medicine no longer needed. Be sure that any discarded medicine is out of the reach of children.

Precautions While Using This Medicine

Your doctor should check your eye pressure at regular visits to make certain that your glaucoma is being controlled.

Before you have any kind of surgery, dental treatment, or emergency treatment, tell the medical doctor or dentist in charge that you are using this medicine. Using an ophthalmic beta-adrenergic blocking agent during this time may cause an increased risk of side effects.

For diabetic patients:
- *Ophthalmic beta-adrenergic blocking agents may affect blood sugar levels. They may also cover up some signs of hypoglycemia (low blood sugar),* such as trembling or increase in pulse rate or blood pressure. However, other signs of low blood sugar, such as dizziness or sweating, are not affected. If you notice a change in the results of your blood or urine sugar tests or if you have any questions, check with your doctor.

Some ophthalmic beta-adrenergic blocking agents (betaxolol, carteolol, and metipranolol) may cause your eyes to become more sensitive to light than they are normally. Wearing sunglasses and avoiding too much exposure to bright light may help lessen the discomfort.

Side Effects of This Medicine

Along with its needed effects, a medicine may cause some unwanted effects. Although not all of these side effects may occur, if they do occur they may need medical attention.

Check with your doctor as soon as possible if any of the following side effects occur:

More common

Redness of eyes or inside of eyelids

Less common or rare

Blurred vision or other change in vision; different size pupils of the eyes; discoloration of the eyeball; droopy upper eyelid; eye pain; redness or irritation of the tongue; seeing double; swelling, irritation or inflammation of eye or eyelid (severe)

Symptoms of too much medicine being absorbed into the body

Anxiety or nervousness; burning or prickling feeling on body; change in taste; chest pain; clumsiness or unsteadiness; confusion or mental depression; coughing, wheezing, or troubled breathing; decreased sexual ability; diarrhea; dizziness or feeling faint; drowsiness; hair loss; hallucinations (seeing, hearing, or feeling things that are not there); headache; irregular, slow, or pounding heartbeat; muscle or joint aches or pain; nausea or vomiting; raw or red areas of the skin; runny, stuffy, or bleeding nose; skin rash, hives, or itching; swelling of feet, ankles, or lower legs; trouble in sleeping; unusual tiredness or weakness

Other side effects may occur that usually do not need medical attention. These side effects may go away during treatment as your body adjusts to the medicine. However, check with your doctor if any of the following side effects continue or are bothersome:

More common

Decreased night vision; stinging of eye or other eye irritation (when medicine is applied)

Less common or rare

Browache; crusting of eyelashes; dryness of eye; increased sensitivity of eye to light; redness, itching, stinging, burning, or watering of eye or other eye irritation

Other side effects not listed above may also occur in some patients. If you notice any other effects, check with your doctor.

Annual revision: 05/12/93

BETA-ADRENERGIC BLOCKING AGENTS Systemic

This information applies to the following medicines:

Acebutolol (a-se-BYOO-toe-lole)
Atenolol (a-TEN-oh-lole)
Betaxolol (be-TAX-oh-lol)
Bisoprolol (bis-OH-proe-lol)
Carteolol (KAR-tee-oh-lole)
Labetalol (la-BET-a-lole)
Metoprolol (me-TOE-proe-lole)
Nadolol (NAY-doe-lole)
Oxprenolol (ox-PREN-oh-lole)
Penbutolol (pen-BYOO-toe-lole)
Pindolol (PIN-doe-lole)
Propranolol (proe-PRAN-oh-lole)
Sotalol (SOE-ta-lole)
Timolol (TIM-oh-lole)

Some commonly used brand names are:

For Acebutolol
In the U.S.
Sectral
In Canada
Monitan
Sectral

For Atenolol
In the U.S.
Tenormin
Generic name product may also be available.
In Canada
Apo-Atenolol
Novo-Atenol
Tenormin

For Betaxolol†
In the U.S.
Kerlone

For Bisoprolol†
In the U.S.
Zebeta

For Carteolol†
In the U.S.
Cartrol

For Labetalol
In the U.S.
Normodyne
Trandate
In Canada
Trandate

For Metoprolol
In the U.S.
Lopressor
Toprol-XL
In Canada
Apo-Metoprolol
Apo-Metoprolol (Type L)
Betaloc
Betaloc Durules
Lopresor
Lopresor SR
Novometoprol
Generic name product may also be available.

For Nadolol
In the U.S.
Corgard
In Canada
Corgard
Syn-Nadolol
Generic name product may also be available.

For Oxprenolol*
In Canada
Slow-Trasicor
Trasicor

For Penbutolol†
In the U.S.
Levatol

For Pindolol
In the U.S.
Visken

In Canada
Novo-Pindol
Syn-Pindolol
Visken

For Propranolol
In the U.S.
Inderal
Inderal LA
Generic name product may also be available.
In Canada
Apo-Propranolol
Detensol
Inderal
Inderal LA
Novopranol
pms Propranolol
Generic name product may also be available.

For Sotalol
In the U.S.
Betapace
In Canada
Sotacor

For Timolol
In the U.S.
Blocadren
Generic name product may also be available.
In Canada
Apo-Timol
Blocadren
Novo-Timol

*Not commercially available in the U.S.
†Not commercially available in Canada.

Description

This group of medicines is known as beta-adrenergic blocking agents, beta-blocking agents, or, more commonly, beta-blockers. Beta-blockers are used in the treatment of high blood pressure (hypertension). Some beta-blockers are also used to relieve angina (chest pain) and in heart attack patients to help prevent additional heart attacks. Beta-blockers are also used to correct irregular heartbeat, prevent migraine headaches, and treat tremors. They may also be used for other conditions as determined by your doctor.

Beta-blockers work by affecting the response to some nerve impulses in certain parts of the body. As a result, they decrease the heart's need for blood and oxygen by reducing its workload. They also help the heart to beat more regularly.

Beta-adrenergic blocking agents are available only with your doctor's prescription, in the following dosage forms:

Oral

Acebutolol
- Capsules (U.S.)
- Tablets (Canada)

Atenolol
- Tablets (U.S. and Canada)

Betaxolol
- Tablets (U.S.)

Bisoprolol
- Tablets (U.S.)

Carteolol
- Tablets (U.S.)

Labetalol
- Tablets (U.S. and Canada)

Metoprolol
- Tablets (U.S. and Canada)
- Extended-release tablets (U.S. and Canada)

Nadolol
- Tablets (U.S. and Canada)

Oxprenolol
- Tablets (Canada)
- Extended-release tablets (Canada)

Penbutolol
- Tablets (U.S.)

Pindolol
- Tablets (U.S. and Canada)

Propranolol
- Extended-release capsules (U.S. and Canada)
- Oral solution (U.S.)
- Tablets (U.S. and Canada)

Sotalol
- Tablets (U.S. and Canada)

Timolol
- Tablets (U.S. and Canada)

Parenteral

Atenolol
- Injection (U.S.)

Labetalol
- Injection (U.S. and Canada)

Metoprolol
- Injection (U.S. and Canada)

Propranolol
- Injection (U.S. and Canada)

It is very important that you read and understand the following information. If any of it causes you special concern, check with your doctor. Also, *if you have any questions* or if you want more information about this medicine or your medical problem, *ask your doctor, nurse, or pharmacist.*

Before Using This Medicine

In deciding to use a medicine, the risks of taking the medicine must be weighed against the good it will do. This is a decision you and your doctor will make. For the beta-blockers, the following should be considered:

Allergies—Tell your doctor if you have ever had any unusual or allergic reaction to the beta-blocker medicine prescribed. Also tell your doctor and pharmacist if you are allergic to any other substances, such as foods, preservatives, or dyes.

Pregnancy—Use of some beta-blockers during pregnancy has been associated with low blood sugar, breathing problems, a lower heart rate, and low blood pressure in the newborn infant. Other reports have not shown unwanted effects on the newborn infant. Animal studies have shown some beta-blockers to cause problems in pregnancy when used in doses many times the usual human dose. Before taking any of these medicines, make sure your doctor knows if you are pregnant or if you may become pregnant.

Breast-feeding—It is not known whether bisoprolol, carteolol, or penbutolol passes into breast milk. All other beta-blockers pass into breast milk. Problems such as slow heartbeat, low blood pressure, and trouble in breathing have been reported in nursing babies. Mothers who are taking beta-blockers and who wish to breast-feed should discuss this with their doctor.

Children—Some of these medicines have been used in children and, in effective doses, have not been shown to cause different side effects or problems in children than they do in adults.

Older adults—Some side effects are more likely to occur in the elderly, who are usually more sensitive to the effects of beta-blockers. Also, beta-blockers may reduce tolerance to cold temperatures in elderly patients.

Other medicines—Although certain medicines should not be used together at all, in other cases 2 different medicines may be used together even if an interaction might occur. In these cases, your doctor may want to change the dose, or other precautions may be necessary. When you are taking or receiving a beta-blocker it is especially important that your doctor and pharmacist know if you are taking any of the following:

- Allergen immunotherapy (allergy shots) or
- Allergen extracts for skin testing—Beta-blockers may increase the risk of serious allergic reaction to these medicines
- Aminophylline (e.g., Somophyllin) or
- Caffeine (e.g., NoDoz) or
- Dyphylline (e.g., Lufyllin) or
- Oxtriphylline (e.g., Choledyl) or
- Theophylline (e.g., Somophyllin-T)—The effects of both these medicines and beta-blockers may be blocked; in addition, theophylline levels in the body may be increased, especially in patients who smoke
- Antidiabetics, oral (diabetes medicine you take by mouth) or
- Insulin—There is an increased risk of hyperglycemia (high blood sugar); beta-blockers may cover up certain symptoms of hypoglycemia (low blood sugar) such as increases in pulse rate and blood pressure, and may make the hypoglycemia last longer
- Calcium channel blockers (bepridil [e.g., Bepadin], diltiazem [e.g., Cardizem], felodipine [e.g., Plendil], flunarizine [e.g., Sibelium], isradipine [e.g., DynaCirc], nicardipine [e.g., Cardene], nifedipine [e.g., Procardia], nimodipine [e.g., Nimotop], verapamil [e.g., Calan]) or
- Clonidine (e.g., Catapres) or
- Guanabenz (e.g., Wytensin)—Effects on blood pressure may be increased. In addition, unwanted effects may occur if clonidine, guanabenz, or a beta-blocker is stopped suddenly after use together. Unwanted effects on the heart may occur when beta-blockers are used with calcium channel blockers
- Cocaine—Cocaine may block the effects of beta-blockers; in addition, there is an increased risk of high blood pressure, fast heartbeat, and possibly heart problems if you use cocaine while taking a beta-blocker
- Monoamine oxidase (MAO) inhibitors (furazolidone [e.g., Furoxone], isocarboxazid [e.g., Marplan], phenelzine [e.g., Nardil], procarbazine [e.g., Matulane], selegiline [e.g., Eldepryl], tranylcypromine [e.g., Parnate])—Taking beta-blockers while you are taking or within 2 weeks of taking monoamine oxidase (MAO) inhibitors may cause severe high blood pressure

Other medical problems—The presence of other medical problems may affect the use of the beta blockers. Make sure you tell your doctor if you have any other medical problems, especially:

- Allergy, history of (asthma, eczema, hay fever, hives), or
- Bronchitis or
- Emphysema—Severity and duration of allergic reactions to other substances may be increased; in addition, beta-blockers can increase trouble in breathing
- Bradycardia (unusually slow heartbeat) or
- Heart or blood vessel disease—There is a risk of further decreased heart function; also, if treatment is stopped suddenly, unwanted effects may occur
- Diabetes mellitus (sugar diabetes)—Beta-blockers may cause hyperglycemia (high blood sugar) and circulation problems; in addition, if your diabetes medicine causes your blood sugar to be too low, beta-blockers may cover up some of the symptoms (fast heartbeat), although they will not cover up other symptoms such as dizziness or sweating
- Kidney disease or
- Liver disease—Effects of beta-blockers may be increased because of slower removal from the body
- Mental depression (or history of)—May be increased by beta-blockers
- Myasthenia gravis or
- Psoriasis—Beta-blockers may make these conditions worse
- Overactive thyroid—Stopping beta-blockers suddenly may increase symptoms; beta-blockers may cover up fast heartbeat, which is a sign of overactive thyroid

Before you begin using any new medicine (prescription or nonprescription) or if you develop any new medical problem while you are using this medicine, check with your doctor, nurse, or pharmacist.

Proper Use of This Medicine

For patients taking the *extended-release capsule or tablet* form of this medicine:

- Swallow the capsule or tablet whole.
- Do not crush, break (except metoprolol succinate extended-release tablets, which may be broken in half), or chew before swallowing.

For patients taking the *concentrated oral solution* form of *propranolol:*

- This medicine is to be taken by mouth even though it comes in a dropper bottle. The amount you should take is to be measured only with the specially marked dropper.

- Mix the medicine with some water, juice, or a carbonated drink. After drinking all the liquid containing the medicine, rinse the glass with a little more liquid and drink that also, to make sure you get all the medicine.

  If you prefer, you may mix this medicine with applesauce or pudding instead.
- Mix the medicine immediately before you are going to take it. Throw away any mixed medicine that you do not take immediately. Do not save medicine that has been mixed.

Ask your doctor about checking your pulse rate before and after taking beta-blocking agents. Then, while you are taking this medicine, check your pulse regularly. If it is much slower than your usual rate (or less than 50 beats per minute), check with your doctor. A pulse rate that is too slow may cause circulation problems.

To help you remember to take your medicine, try to get into the habit of taking it at the same time each day.

For patients taking this medicine *for high blood pressure:*

- In addition to the use of the medicine your doctor has prescribed, treatment for your high blood pressure may include weight control and care in the types of foods you eat, especially foods high in sodium. Your doctor will tell you which of these are most important for you. You should check with your doctor before changing your diet.
- Many patients who have high blood pressure will not notice any signs of the problem. In fact, many may feel normal. However, if high blood pressure is not treated, it can cause serious problems such as heart failure, blood vessel disease, stroke, or kidney disease.
- Remember that this medicine will not cure your high blood pressure but it does help control it. It is very important that you *take your medicine exactly as directed*, even if you feel well. You must continue to take it as directed if you expect to lower your blood pressure and keep it down. *You may have to take high blood pressure medicine for the rest of your life.* Also, it is very important to keep your appointments with your doctor, even if you feel well.

Dosing—The dose of beta-blocker will be different for different patients. *Follow your doctor's orders or the directions on the label.* The following information includes only the average doses. *If your dose is different, do not change it* unless your doctor tells you to do so.

The number of capsules or tablets or teaspoonfuls of solution that you take depends on the strength of the medicine. Also, *the number of doses you take each day, the time allowed between doses, and the length of time you take the medicine depend on the medical problem for which you are taking the beta-blocker.*

For acebutolol

- For *oral* dosage forms (capsules and tablets):
  - —For angina (chest pain) or irregular heartbeat:
    - Adults—200 milligrams (mg) two times a day. The dose may be increased up to a total of 1200 mg a day.
    - Children—Dose must be determined by your doctor.
  - —For high blood pressure:
    - Adults—200 to 800 mg a day as a single dose or divided into two daily doses.
    - Children—Dose must be determined by your doctor.

For atenolol

- For *oral* dosage form (tablets):
  - —For angina (chest pain):
    - Adults—50 to 100 mg once a day.
  - —For high blood pressure:
    - Adults—25 to 100 mg once a day.
    - Children—Dose must be determined by your doctor.
  - —For treatment after a heart attack:
    - Adults—50 mg ten minutes after the last intravenous dose, followed by another 50 mg twelve hours later. Then 100 mg once a day or 50 mg two times a day for six to nine days or until discharge from hospital.
- For *injection* dosage form:
  - —For treatment of heart attacks:
    - Adults—5 mg given over 5 minutes. The dose is repeated ten minutes later.

For betaxolol

- For *oral* dosage form (tablets):
  - —For high blood pressure:
    - Adults—10 mg once a day. Your doctor may double your dose after seven to fourteen days.
    - Children—Dose must be determined by your doctor.

For bisoprolol

- For *oral* dosage form (tablets):
  - —For high blood pressure:
    - Adults—5 to 10 mg once a day.
    - Children—Dose must be determined by your doctor.

For carteolol

- For *oral* dosage form (tablets):
  - —For high blood pressure:
    - Adults—2.5 to 10 mg once a day.
    - Children—Dose must be determined by your doctor.

For labetalol

- For *oral* dosage form (tablets):
  —For high blood pressure:
  - Adults—100 to 400 mg two times a day.
  - Children—Dose must be determined by your doctor.
- For *injection* dosage form:
  —For high blood pressure:
  - Adults—20 mg injected slowly over two minutes with additional injections of 40 and 80 mg given every ten minutes if needed, up to a total of 300 mg; may be given instead as an infusion at a rate of 2 mg per minute to a total dose of 50 to 300 mg.
  - Children—Dose must be determined by your doctor.

For metoprolol

- For *regular (short-acting) oral* dosage form (tablets):
  —For high blood pressure or angina (chest pain):
  - Adults—100 to 450 mg a day, taken as a single dose or in divided doses.
  - Children—Dose must be determined by your doctor.

  —For treatment after a heart attack:
  - Adults—50 mg every six hours starting fifteen minutes after last intravenous dose. Then 100 mg two times a day for three months to 1 year.
- For *long-acting oral* dosage forms (extended-release tablets):
  —For high blood pressure or angina (chest pain):
  - Adults—Up to 400 mg once a day.
  - Children—Dose must be determined by your doctor.
- For *injection* dosage form:
  —For treatment of a heart attack:
  - Adults—5 mg every two minutes for three doses.

For nadolol

- For *oral* dosage form (tablets):
  —For angina (chest pain):
  - Adults—40 to 240 mg once a day.

  —For high blood pressure:
  - Adults—40 to 320 mg once a day.
  - Children—Dose must be determined by your doctor.

For oxprenolol

- For *regular (short-acting) oral* dosage form (tablets):
  —For high blood pressure:
  - Adults—20 mg three times a day. Your doctor may increase your dose up to 480 mg a day.
  - Children—Dose must be determined by your doctor.
- For *long-acting oral* dosage form (extended-release tablets):
  —For high blood pressure:
  - Adults—80 to 160 mg once a day.
  - Children—Dose must be determined by your doctor.

For penbutolol

- For *oral* dosage form (tablets):
  —For high blood pressure:
  - Adults—20 mg once a day.
  - Children—Dose must be determined by your doctor.

For pindolol

- For *oral* dosage form (tablets):
  —For high blood pressure:
  - Adults—5 mg two times a day. Your doctor may increase your dose up to 60 mg a day.
  - Children—Dose must be determined by your doctor.

For propranolol

- For *regular (short-acting) oral* dosage forms (tablets and oral solution):
  —For angina (chest pain):
  - Adults—80 to 320 mg a day taken in two, three, or four divided doses.

  —For irregular heartbeat:
  - Adults—10 to 30 mg three or four times a day.
  - Children—500 micrograms (0.5 mg) to 4 mg per kilogram of body weight a day taken in divided doses.

  —For high blood pressure:
  - Adults—40 mg two times a day. Your doctor may increase your dose up to 640 mg a day.
  - Children—500 micrograms (0.5 mg) to 4 mg per kilogram of body weight a day taken in divided doses.

  —For diseased heart muscle (cardiomyopathy):
  - Adults—20 to 40 mg three or four times a day.

  —For treatment after a heart attack:
  - Adults—180 to 240 mg a day taken in divided doses.

  —For treating pheochromocytoma:
  - Adults—30 to 160 mg a day taken in divided doses.

  —For preventing migraine headaches:
  - Adults—20 mg four times a day. Your doctor may increase your dose up to 240 mg a day.

  —For trembling:
  - Adults—40 mg two times a day. Your doctor may increase your dose up to 320 mg a day.

- For *long-acting oral* dosage form (extended-release capsules):
  - —For high blood pressure:
    - Adults—80 to 160 mg once a day. Doses up to 640 mg once a day may be needed in some patients.
  - —For angina (chest pain):
    - Adults—80 to 320 mg once a day.
  - —For preventing migraine headaches:
    - Adults—80 to 240 mg once a day.
- For *injection* dosage form:
  - —For irregular heartbeat:
    - Adults—1 to 3 mg given at a rate not greater than 1 mg per minute. Dose may be repeated after two minutes and again after four hours if needed.
    - Children—10 to 100 micrograms (0.01 to 0.1 mg) per kilogram of body weight given intravenously every six to eight hours.

For sotalol

- For *oral* dosage form (tablets):
  - —For irregular heartbeat:
    - Adults—80 mg two times a day. Your doctor may increase your dose up to 320 mg per day taken in two or three divided doses.
    - Children—Dose must be determined by your doctor.

For timolol

- For *oral* dosage form (tablets):
  - —For high blood pressure:
    - Adults—10 mg two times a day. Your doctor may increase your dose up 60 mg per day taken as a single dose or in divided doses.
    - Children—Dose must be determined by your doctor.
  - —For treatment after a heart attack:
    - Adults—10 mg two times a day.
  - —For preventing migraine headaches:
    - Adults—10 mg two times a day. Your doctor may increase your dose up to 30 mg once a day or in divided doses.

Missed dose—Do not miss any doses. This is especially important when you are taking only one dose per day. Some conditions may become worse if this medicine is not taken regularly.

If you do miss a dose of this medicine, take it as soon as possible. However, if it is within 4 hours of your next dose (8 hours when using atenolol, betaxolol, bisoprolol, carteolol, labetalol, nadolol, penbutolol, sotalol, or extended-release [long-acting] metoprolol, oxprenolol, or propranolol), skip the missed dose and go back to your regular dosing schedule. Do not double doses.

Storage—To store this medicine:

- Keep out of the reach of children.
- Store away from heat and direct light.
- Do not store in the bathroom, near the kitchen sink, or in other damp places. Heat or moisture may cause the medicine to break down.
- Do not keep outdated medicine or medicine no longer needed. Be sure that any discarded medicine is out of the reach of children.

Precautions While Using This Medicine

It is important that your doctor check your progress at regular visits. This is to make sure the medicine is working for you and to allow the dosage to be changed if needed.

Do not stop taking this medicine without first checking with your doctor. Your doctor may want you to reduce gradually the amount you are taking before stopping completely. Some conditions may become worse when the medicine is stopped suddenly, and the danger of heart attack is increased in some patients.

Make sure that you have enough medicine on hand to last through weekends, holidays, or vacations. You may want to carry an extra written prescription in your billfold or purse in case of an emergency. You can then have it filled if you run out of medicine while you are away from home.

Your doctor may want you to carry medical identification stating that you are taking this medicine.

Before having any kind of surgery (including dental surgery) or emergency treatment, tell the medical doctor or dentist in charge that you are taking this medicine.

For *diabetic patients:*

- *This medicine may cause your blood sugar levels to rise.* Also, *this medicine may cover up signs of hypoglycemia (low blood sugar),* such as change in pulse rate.

This medicine may cause some people to become dizzy, drowsy, or lightheaded. *Make sure you know how you react to this medicine before you drive, use machines, or do anything else that could be dangerous if you are dizzy or are not alert.* If the problem continues or gets worse, check with your doctor.

Beta-blockers may make you more sensitive to cold temperatures, especially if you have blood circulation problems. Beta-blockers tend to decrease blood circulation in the skin, fingers, and toes. Dress warmly during cold weather and be careful during prolonged exposure to cold, such as in winter sports.

Chest pain resulting from exercise or physical exertion is usually reduced or prevented by this medicine. This may tempt a patient to be overly active. *Make sure you discuss with your doctor a safe amount of exercise for your medical problem.*

Before you have any medical tests, tell the doctor in charge that you are taking this medicine. The results of some tests may be affected by this medicine.

Before you have any allergy shots, tell the doctor in charge that you are taking a beta-blocker. Beta-blockers may cause you to have a serious reaction to the allergy shot.

For patients with *allergies to foods, medicines, or insect stings:*

- There is a chance that this medicine will cause allergic reactions to be worse and harder to treat. If you have a severe allergic reaction while you are being treated with this medicine, check with a doctor right away so that it can be treated. Be sure to tell the doctor that you are taking a beta-blocker.

For patients taking this medicine *for high blood pressure:*

- *Do not take other medicines unless they have been discussed with your doctor.* This especially includes over-the-counter (nonprescription) medicines for appetite control, asthma, colds, cough, hay fever, or sinus problems since they may tend to increase your blood pressure.

For patients taking *labetalol by mouth:*

- *Dizziness, lightheadedness, or fainting may occur, especially when you get up from a lying or sitting position.* This is more likely to occur when you first start taking labetalol or when the dose is increased. *Getting up slowly may help.* When you get up from lying down, sit on the edge of the bed with your feet dangling for 1 to 2 minutes. Then stand up slowly. If the problem continues or gets worse, check with your doctor.
- The dizziness, lightheadedness, or fainting is also more likely to occur if you drink alcohol, stand for long periods of time, or exercise, or if the weather is hot. *While you are taking this medicine, be careful to limit the amount of alcohol you drink. Also, use extra care during exercise or hot weather or if you must stand for long periods of time.*

For patients receiving *labetalol by injection:*

- It is very important that you lie down flat while receiving labetalol and for up to 3 hours afterward. If you try to get up too soon, you may become dizzy or faint. *Do not try to sit or stand until your doctor or nurse tells you to do so.*

Side Effects of This Medicine

Along with its needed effects, a medicine may cause some unwanted effects. Although not all of these side effects may occur, if they do occur they may need medical attention.

Check with your doctor as soon as possible if any of the following side effects occur:

Less common

Breathing difficulty and/or wheezing; cold hands and feet; mental depression; shortness of breath; slow heartbeat (especially less than 50 beats per minute); swelling of ankles, feet, and/or lower legs

Rare

Back pain or joint pain; chest pain; confusion (especially in elderly); dark urine—for acebutolol, bisoprolol, or labetalol; dizziness or lightheadedness when getting up from a lying or sitting position; fever and sore throat; hallucinations (seeing, hearing, or feeling things that are not there); irregular heartbeat; red, scaling, or crusted skin; skin rash; unusual bleeding and bruising; yellow eyes or skin—for acebutolol, bisoprolol, or labetalol

Signs and symptoms of overdose (in the order in which they may occur)

Slow heartbeat; dizziness (severe) or fainting; fast or irregular heartbeat; difficulty in breathing; bluish-colored fingernails or palms of hands; convulsions (seizures)

Other side effects may occur that usually do not need medical attention. These side effects may go away during treatment as your body adjusts to the medicine. However, check with your doctor if any of the following side effects continue or are bothersome:

More common

Decreased sexual ability; dizziness or lightheadedness; drowsiness (slight); trouble in sleeping; unusual tiredness or weakness

Less common or rare

Anxiety and/or nervousness; changes in taste—for labetalol only; constipation; diarrhea; dry, sore eyes; frequent urination—for acebutolol and carteolol only; itching of skin; nausea or vomiting; nightmares and vivid dreams; numbness and/or tingling of fingers and/or toes; numbness and/or tingling of skin, especially on scalp—for labetalol only; stomach discomfort; stuffy nose

Although not all of the side effects listed above have been reported for all of these medicines, they have been reported for at least one of them. Since all of the beta-adrenergic blocking agents are very similar, any of the above side effects may occur with any of these medicines. However, they may be more or less common with some agents than with others.

After you have been taking a beta-blocker for a while, it may cause unpleasant or even harmful effects if you stop taking it too suddenly. After you stop taking this medicine or while you are gradually reducing the amount you are taking, check with your doctor right away if any of the following occur:

Chest pain; fast or irregular heartbeat; general feeling of discomfort or illness or weakness; headache; shortness of breath (sudden); sweating; trembling

For patients taking *labetalol:*

- You may notice a tingling feeling on your scalp when you first begin to take labetalol. This is to be expected and usually goes away after you have been taking labetalol for a while.

Other side effects not listed above may also occur in some patients. If you notice any other effects, check with your doctor.

Additional Information

Once a medicine has been approved for marketing for a certain use, experience may show that it is also useful for other medical problems. Although these uses are not included in product labeling, some beta-blockers are used in certain patients with the following medical conditions:

- Glaucoma
- Neuroleptic-induced akathisia (restlessness or the need to keep moving caused by some medicines used to treat nervousness or mental and emotional disorders)

Other than the above information, there is no additional information relating to proper use, precautions, or side effects for these uses.

Annual revision: 05/13/93

BETA-ADRENERGIC BLOCKING AGENTS AND THIAZIDE DIURETICS Systemic

This information applies to the following medicines:

Atenolol (a-TEN-oh-lole) and Chlorthalidone (klor-THAL-i-doan)
Labetalol (la-BET-a-lole) and Hydrochlorothiazide (hye-droe-klor-oh-THYE-a-zide)
Metoprolol (me-TOE-proe-lole) and Hydrochlorothiazide
Nadolol (NAY-doe-lole) and Bendroflumethiazide (ben-droe-floo-meth-EYE-a-zide)
Pindolol (PIN-doe-lole) and Hydrochlorothiazide
Propranolol (proe-PRAN-oh-lole) and Hydrochlorothiazide
Timolol (TIM-oh-lole) and Hydrochlorothiazide

Some commonly used brand names are:

For Atenolol and Chlorthalidone
In the U.S. and Canada
Tenoretic

For Labetalol and Hydrochlorothiazide†
In the U.S.
Normozide
Trandate HCT

For Metoprolol and Hydrochlorothiazide†
In the U.S.
Lopressor HCT

For Nadolol and Bendroflumethiazide
In the U.S. and Canada
Corzide

For Pindolol and Hydrochlorothiazide*
In Canada
Viskazide

For Propranolol and Hydrochlorothiazide
In the U.S.
Inderide
Inderide LA
Generic name product may also be available.
In Canada
Inderide

For Timolol and Hydrochlorothiazide
In the U.S. and Canada
Timolide

*Not commercially available in the U.S.
†Not commercially available in Canada.

Description

Beta-blocker and thiazide diuretic combinations belong to the group of medicines known as antihypertensives (high blood pressure medicine). Both ingredients of the combination control high blood pressure, but work in different ways. Beta-blockers (atenolol, labetalol, metoprolol, nadolol, pindolol, propranolol, and timolol) reduce the workload on the heart as well as having other effects. Thiazide diuretics (bendroflumethiazide, chlorthalidone, and hydrochlorothiazide) reduce the amount of fluid pressure in the body by increasing the flow of urine.

High blood pressure adds to the workload of the heart and arteries. If it continues for a long time, the heart and arteries may not function properly. This can damage the blood vessels of the brain, heart, and kidneys, resulting in a stroke, heart failure, or kidney failure. High blood pressure may also increase the risk of heart attacks. These problems may be less likely to occur if blood pressure is controlled.

Beta-blocker and thiazide diuretic combinations are available only with your doctor's prescription, in the following dosage forms:

Oral

Atenolol and chlorthalidone
- Tablets (U.S. and Canada)

Labetalol and hydrochlorothiazide
- Tablets (U.S.)

Metoprolol and hydrochlorothiazide
- Tablets (U.S.)

Nadolol and bendroflumethiazide
- Tablets (U.S. and Canada)

Pindolol and hydrochlorothiazide
- Tablets (Canada)

Propranolol and hydrochlorothiazide
- Extended-release capsules (U.S.)
- Tablets (U.S. and Canada)

Timolol and hydrochlorothiazide
- Tablets (U.S. and Canada)

It is very important that you read and understand the following information. If any of it causes you special concern, check with your doctor. Also, *if you have any questions* or if you want more information about this medicine or your medical problem, *ask your doctor, nurse, or pharmacist.*

Before Using This Medicine

In deciding to use a medicine, the risks of taking the medicine must be weighed against the good it will do. This is a decision you and your doctor will make. For the beta-adrenergic blocking agents (also known as beta-blocking agents or, more commonly, beta-blockers) and thiazide diuretics, the following should be considered:

Allergies—Tell your doctor if you have ever had any unusual or allergic reaction to beta-blockers, sulfonamides (sulfa drugs), bumetanide, furosemide, acetazolamide, dichlorphenamide, methazolamide, or to any of the thiazide diuretics. Also tell your doctor and pharmacist if you are allergic to any other substances, such as foods, preservatives, or dyes.

Pregnancy—Although adequate studies in pregnant women have not been done, use of some beta-blockers during pregnancy has been associated with low blood sugar, breathing problems, a slower heart rate, and low blood pressure in the newborn infant. However, other reports have shown no unwanted effects in the newborn infant. Animal studies have shown some beta-blockers to cause problems in pregnancy when used in doses many times the usual human dose.

Studies with thiazide diuretics have not been done in pregnant women. However, use during pregnancy may cause side effects such as jaundice, blood problems, and low potassium in the newborn infant. Animal studies have not shown thiazide diuretic medicines to cause birth defects even when used in doses several times the usual human dose.

Breast-feeding—Although beta-blockers and thiazide diuretics pass into the breast milk, these medicines have not been reported to cause problems in nursing babies.

Children—Although there is no specific information about the use of this medicine in children, it is not expected to cause different side effects or problems in children than it does in adults.

Older adults—Some side effects, especially dizziness or lightheadedness and signs and symptoms of too much potassium loss, may be more likely to occur in the elderly, who are usually more sensitive to the effects of this medicine. Also, beta-blockers may reduce tolerance to cold temperatures in elderly patients.

Other medicines—Although certain medicines should not be used together at all, in other cases 2 different medicines may be used together even if an interaction might occur. In these cases, your doctor may want to change the dose, or other precautions may be necessary. When taking beta-adrenergic blocking agents, or more commonly, beta-blockers and thiazide diuretics it is especially important that your doctor and pharmacist know if you are taking any of the following:

- Adrenocorticoids (cortisone-like medicines)—May decrease the wanted effects of thiazide diuretics, and may increase unwanted effects such as hypokalemia (low levels of potassium in the body)
- Aminophylline (e.g., Somophyllin) or
- Caffeine (e.g., NoDoz) or
- Dyphylline (e.g., Lufylline) or
- Oxtriphylline (e.g., Choledyl) or
- Theophylline (e.g., Somophyllin-T)—The effects of both these medicines and beta-blockers may be blocked; in addition, theophylline levels in the body may be increased, especially in patients who smoke
- Antidiabetics, oral (diabetes medicine you take by mouth) or
- Insulin—There is an increased risk of hypoglycemia (low blood sugar) or hyperglycemia (high blood sugar); beta-blockers may cover up certain symptoms of hypoglycemia, such as increases in pulse rate and blood pressure, and may make the hypoglycemia last longer
- Clonidine (e.g., Catapres) or
- Diltiazem (e.g., Cardizem) or
- Guanabenz (e.g., Wytensin) or
- Nicardipine (e.g., Cardene) or
- Nifedipine (e.g., Procardia) or
- Nimodipine (e.g., Nimotop) or
- Verapamil (e.g., Calan)—Effects on blood pressure may be increased. In addition, unwanted effects may occur if clonidine, guanabenz, or a beta-blocker are stopped suddenly after use together
- If you use cocaine—Cocaine may block the effects of beta-blockers; in addition, there is an increased risk of high blood pressure, fast heartbeat, and possibly heart problems
- Digitalis glycosides (heart medicine)—Thiazide diuretics can cause hypokalemia (low levels of potassium in the body), which can increase the unwanted effects of digitalis medicines
- Lithium—Thiazide diuretics can increase the effects of lithium, possibly leading to symptoms of overdose
- Methenamine—Thiazide diuretics can make methenamine less effective

- Monoamine oxidase (MAO) inhibitors (furazolidone [e.g., Furoxone], isocarboxazid [e.g., Marplan], pargyline [e.g., Eutonyl], phenelzine [e.g., Nardil], procarbazine [e.g., Matulane], tranylcypromine [e.g., Parnate])—Taking beta-blockers and thiazide diuretics while you are taking or within 2 weeks of taking monoamine oxidase (MAO) inhibitors may cause severe high blood pressure

Other medical problems—The presence of other medical problems may affect the use of the beta-blockers and thiazide diuretics. Make sure you tell your doctor if you have any other medical problems, especially:

- Allergy, history of (asthma, eczema, hay fever, hives), or
- Bronchitis or
- Emphysema—Severity and duration of allergic reactions to other substances may be increased; in addition, beta-blockers can increase trouble in breathing
- Bradycardia (unusually slow heartbeat) or
- Heart or blood vessel disease—There is a risk of further decreased heart function; also, if treatment is stopped suddenly, unwanted effects may occur
- Diabetes mellitus (sugar diabetes)—Beta-blockers may cover up fast heartbeat associated with hypoglycemia (low blood sugar), but not dizziness and sweating; in addition, beta-blockers may cause hypoglycemia and circulation problems, and thiazide diuretics may change the amount of antidiabetic medicine needed
- Kidney disease—Effects of beta-blockers may be increased
- Liver disease—Effects of beta-blockers may be increased; thiazide diuretics may cause unwanted effects
- Mental depression (or history of)—May be increased by beta-blockers
- Overactive thyroid—Sudden withdrawal of beta-blockers may increase symptoms; beta-blockers may cover up fast heartbeat

Before you begin using any new medicine (prescription or nonprescription) or if you develop any new medical problem while you are using this medicine, check with your doctor, nurse, or pharmacist.

Proper Use of This Medicine

Importance of diet:

- When prescribing medicine for your condition, your doctor may also prescribe a personal diet for you. Such a diet may be low in sodium (salt). Most people eat much more sodium than they need. Too much sodium in the diet may increase blood pressure. Some foods that contain large amounts of sodium are canned soup, pickles, ketchup, green and ripe olives, relish, frankfurters, soy sauce, and carbonated beverages. Your doctor may want you to limit the amounts of these and other high-sodium foods in your diet. High blood pressure medicine is usually more effective when such a diet is properly followed.
- Also, it may be very important for you to go on a reducing diet.
- However, check with your doctor before changing your diet.

Many patients who have high blood pressure will not notice any signs of the problem. In fact, many may feel normal. It is very important that you *take your medicine exactly as directed*. Also, keep your appointments with your doctor even if you feel well.

Remember that this medicine will not cure your high blood pressure but it does help control it. Therefore, you must continue to take it as directed if you expect to lower your blood pressure and keep it down. *You may have to take high blood pressure medicine for the rest of your life*. If high blood pressure is not treated, it can cause serious problems such as heart failure, blood vessel disease, stroke, or kidney disease.

For patients taking the *extended-release tablet* form of this medicine:

- Swallow the tablet whole.
- Do not crush, break, or chew before swallowing.

To help you remember to take your medicine, try to get into the habit of taking it at the same time each day.

Ask your doctor about checking your pulse rate before and after taking beta-blocking agents. Then, while you are taking this medicine, check your pulse regularly. If it is much slower than your usual rate (or less than 50 beats per minute), check with your doctor. A pulse rate that is too slow may cause circulation problems.

The thiazide diuretic (e.g., bendroflumethiazide, chlorthalidone, or hydrochlorothiazide) contained in this combination medicine may cause you to have an unusual feeling of tiredness when you begin to take it. You may also notice an increase in the amount of urine or in your frequency of urination. After you take the medicine for a while, these effects should lessen. To keep the increase in urine from affecting your sleep:

- If you are to take a single dose a day, take it in the morning after breakfast.
- If you are to take more than one dose a day, take the last dose no later than 6 p.m., unless otherwise directed by your doctor.

However, it is best to plan your dose or doses according to a schedule that will least affect your personal activities and sleep. Ask your doctor, nurse, or pharmacist to help you plan the best time to take this medicine.

Do not miss any doses. This is especially important when you are taking only one dose per day. Some conditions may become worse when this medicine is not taken regularly.

Missed dose—If you do miss a dose of this medicine, take it as soon as possible. However, if it is within 4 hours of your next dose (8 hours when using atenolol and chlorthalidone, labetalol and hydrochlorothiazide, nadolol and bendroflumethiazide, or extended-release propranolol and hydrochlorothiazide), skip the missed dose and go back to your regular dosing schedule. Do not double doses.

Storage—To store this medicine:

- Keep out of the reach of children.
- Store away from heat and direct light.
- Do not store in the bathroom, near the kitchen sink, or in other damp places. Heat or moisture may cause the medicine to break down.
- Do not keep outdated medicine or medicine no longer needed. Be sure that any discarded medicine is out of the reach of children.

Precautions While Using This Medicine

It is important that your doctor check your progress at regular visits. This is to make sure the medicine is properly controlling your blood pressure and to allow the dosage to be changed if needed.

Do not stop taking this medicine without first checking with your doctor. Your doctor may want you to reduce gradually the amount you are taking before stopping completely. Some conditions may become worse when the medicine is stopped suddenly, and the risk of heart attack is increased in some patients.

Make sure that you have enough medicine on hand to last through weekends, holidays, or vacations. You may want to carry an extra written prescription in your billfold or purse in case of an emergency. You can then have it filled if you run out of medicine while you are away from home.

Your doctor may want you to carry a medical identification card stating that you are taking this medicine.

Do not take other medicines unless they have been discussed with your doctor. This especially includes over-the-counter (nonprescription) medicines for appetite control, asthma, colds, cough, hay fever, or sinus problems since they may tend to increase your blood pressure.

Before having any kind of surgery (including dental surgery) or emergency treatment, tell the medical doctor or dentist in charge that you are taking this medicine.

For *diabetic patients*:

- *This medicine may cause your blood sugar levels to rise or to fall.* Also, *this medicine may cover up signs of hypoglycemia (low blood sugar),* such as change in pulse rate. While you are taking this medicine, be especially careful in testing for sugar in your urine. If you have any questions about this, check with your doctor.

The thiazide diuretic contained in this medicine may cause a loss of potassium from your body.

- To help prevent this, your doctor may want you to:
  —eat or drink foods that have a high potassium content (for example, orange or other citrus fruit juices), or
  —take a potassium supplement, or
  —take another medicine to help prevent the loss of the potassium in the first place.
- It is very important to follow these directions. Also, it is important not to change your diet on your own. This is more important if you are already on a special diet (as for diabetes), or if you are taking a potassium supplement or a medicine to reduce potassium loss. Extra potassium may not be necessary and, in some cases, too much potassium could be harmful.

Check with your doctor if you become sick and have severe or continuing vomiting or diarrhea. These problems may cause you to lose additional water and potassium.

This medicine may cause some people to become dizzy, drowsy, lightheaded, or less alert than they are normally. *Make sure you know how you react to this medicine before you drive, use machines, or do anything else that could be dangerous if you are dizzy or are not alert.* If the problem continues or gets worse, check with your doctor.

The beta-blocker (atenolol, labetalol, metoprolol, nadolol, pindolol, propranolol, or timolol) contained in this medicine may make you more sensitive to cold temperatures, especially if you have blood circulation problems. It tends to decrease blood circulation in the skin, fingers, and toes. Dress warmly during cold weather and be careful during prolonged exposure to cold, such as in winter sports.

This medicine may cause your skin to be more sensitive to sunlight than it is normally. Exposure to sunlight, even for brief periods of time, may cause a skin rash, itching, redness or other discoloration of the skin, or a severe sunburn. When you begin taking this medicine:

- Stay out of direct sunlight, especially between the hours of 10:00 a.m. and 3:00 p.m., if possible.
- Wear protective clothing, including a hat. Also, wear sunglasses.
- Apply a sun block product that has a skin protection factor (SPF) of at least 15. Some patients may require a product with a higher SPF number, especially if they have a fair complexion. If you have any questions about this, check with your doctor or pharmacist.
- Apply a sun block lipstick that has an SPF of at least 15 to protect your lips.
- Do not use a sunlamp or tanning bed or booth.

If you have a severe reaction from the sun, check with your doctor.

Before you have any medical tests, tell the doctor in charge that you are taking this medicine. The results of some tests may be affected by this medicine.

For patients with allergies to foods, medicines, or insect stings:

- There is a chance that this medicine will cause allergic reactions to be worse and harder to treat. If you have a severe allergic reaction while you are being treated with this medicine, check with a doctor right away so that it can be treated.

Side Effects of This Medicine

Along with its needed effects, a medicine may cause some unwanted effects. Although not all of these side effects may occur, if they do occur they may need medical attention.

Check with your doctor as soon as possible if any of the following side effects occur:

Less common

Breathing difficulty and/or wheezing; cold hands and feet; confusion (especially in elderly); hallucinations (seeing, hearing, or feeling things that are not there); irregular heartbeat; mental depression; slow pulse (especially less than 50 beats per minute)

Rare

Chest pain; dark urine; fever and sore throat; joint pain; lower back or side pain; red, scaling, or crusted skin; skin rash or hives; stomach pain (severe) with nausea and vomiting; swelling of ankles, feet, and/or lower legs; unusual bleeding or bruising; yellow eyes or skin

Signs of too much potassium loss

Dryness of mouth; increased thirst; irregular heartbeats; mood or mental changes; muscle cramps or pain; weak pulse

Signs and symptoms of overdose (in the order in which they may occur)

Slow heartbeat; dizziness (severe) or fainting; difficulty in breathing; bluish-colored fingernails or palms of hands; convulsions (seizures)

Other side effects may occur that usually do not need medical attention. These side effects may go away during treatment as your body adjusts to the medicine. However, check with your doctor if any of the following side effects continue or are bothersome:

More common

Decreased sexual ability; dizziness or lightheadedness; drowsiness (slight); trouble in sleeping; unusual tiredness or weakness

Less common

Anxiety or nervousness; changes in taste—for labetalol and hydrochlorothiazide only; constipation; diarrhea; dry, sore eyes; increased sensitivity of skin to sunlight (skin rash, itching, redness or other discoloration of skin, or severe sunburn); itching of skin; loss of appetite; nausea or vomiting; nightmares and vivid dreams; numbness and/or tingling of skin, especially on scalp—for labetalol and hydrochlorothiazide only; numbness or tingling of fingers and toes; stomach discomfort or upset; stuffy nose

Although not all of the above side effects have been reported for all of these medicines, they have been reported for at least one of the beta-adrenergic blockers or thiazide diuretics. Since all of the beta-adrenergic blocking agents are very similar and the thiazide diuretics are also very similar, any of the above side effects may occur with any of these medicines. However, they may be more common with some combinations than with others.

After you have been taking this medicine for a while, it may cause unpleasant or even harmful effects if you stop taking it too suddenly. After you stop taking this medicine or while you are gradually reducing the amount you are taking, check with your doctor right away if any of the following occur:

Chest pain; fast or irregular heartbeat; general feeling of discomfort, illness, or weakness; headache; shortness of breath (sudden); sweating; trembling

Other side effects not listed above may also occur in some patients. If you notice any other effects, check with your doctor.

Annual revision: July 1990

BETA-CAROTENE—For Dietary Supplement (Vitamin) Systemic

A commonly used brand name in the U.S. is Solatene.

Generic name product may also be available in the U.S. and Canada.

Description

Vitamins (VYE-ta-mins) are compounds that you *must* have for growth and health. They are needed in small amounts only and are usually available in the foods that you eat. Beta-carotene (bay-ta-KARE-oh-teen) is converted in the body to vitamin A, which is necessary for normal growth and health and for healthy eyes and skin. In the absence of a dietary source of vitamin A, a lack of beta-carotene may also lead to a deficiency of vitamin

A, which may cause a rare condition called night blindness (problems seeing in the dark). It may also cause dry eyes, eye infections, skin problems, and slowed growth. Your doctor may treat these problems by prescribing beta-carotene or vitamin A for you.

Beta-carotene or vitamin A supplements may be needed in patients with the following conditions:

- Cystic fibrosis
- Diarrhea, continuing
- Illness, long-term
- Injury, serious
- Liver disease
- Malabsorption problems
- Pancreas disease

If any of these conditions apply to you, you should take beta-carotene only on the advice of your doctor after need has been established.

Claims that beta-carotene is effective as a sunscreen have not been proven. Although beta-carotene is being studied for its ability to prevent certain types of cancer, there is not enough information to show that this treatment is effective.

Beta-carotene is available without a prescription. However, it may be a good idea to check with your doctor before taking beta-carotene on your own.

Beta-carotene is available in the following dosage forms:

Oral

- Capsules (U.S. and Canada)
- Tablets (U.S. and Canada)

It is very important that you read and understand the following information. If any of it causes your special concern, check with your doctor or pharmacist. Also, *if you have any questions* or if you want more information about this dietary supplement or your medical problems, *ask your doctor, nurse, pharmacist, or dietitian.*

Importance of Diet

Vitamin supplements should be taken only if you cannot get enough vitamins in your diet; however, some diets may not contain all of the vitamins you need. This may occur with rapid weight loss, unusual diets (such as some reducing diets in which choice of foods is very limited), prolonged intravenous feeding, or malnutrition. A balanced diet should provide all the vitamins you normally need.

In order to get enough vitamins and minerals in your diet, it is important that you eat a balanced and varied diet. Follow carefully any diet program your doctor may recommend. For specific vitamin and/or mineral needs, ask your doctor or dietitian for a list of appropriate foods.

Beta-carotene is found in carrots; dark-green leafy vegetables, such as spinach, green leaf lettuce; tomatoes; sweet potatoes; broccoli; cantaloupe; and winter squash. The body converts beta-carotene into vitamin A. Ordinary cooking does not destroy beta-carotene.

Vitamins alone will not take the place of a good diet and will not provide energy. Your body needs other substances found in food, such as protein, minerals, carbohydrates, and fat. Vitamins themselves often cannot work without the presence of other foods. For example, some fat is needed so that beta-carotene can be absorbed into the body.

In some cases, it may not be possible for you to get enough food to supply you with the proper vitamins. In other cases, the amount of vitamins you need may be increased above normal. Therefore, a vitamin supplement may be needed.

Before Using This Dietary Supplement

If you are taking this dietary supplement without a prescription, carefully read and follow any precautions on the label. For beta-carotene, the following should be considered:

Allergies—Tell your doctor if you have ever had any unusual or allergic reaction to beta-carotene. Also tell your doctor and pharmacist if you are allergic to any other substances, such as foods, preservatives, or dyes.

Pregnancy—It is especially important that you are receiving enough vitamins when you become pregnant and that you continue to receive the right amount of vitamins throughout your pregnancy. The healthy growth and development of the fetus depend on a steady supply of nutrients from the mother.

However, animal studies have shown that extremely large doses of beta-carotene given during pregnancy may cause miscarriages.

Breast-feeding—It is especially important that you receive the right amounts of vitamins so that your baby will also get the vitamins needed to grow properly. However, taking large amounts of a dietary supplement while breast-feeding may be harmful to the mother and/or baby and should be avoided.

Children—Normal daily requirements vary according to age. It is especially important that children receive enough vitamins in their diet for healthy growth and development.

Older adults—It is important that older people continue to receive enough vitamins in their diet for good health.

Medicines or other dietary supplements—Although certain medicines or dietary supplements should not be used together at all, in other cases they may be used together even if an interaction might occur. In these cases, your doctor may want to change the dose, or other precautions may be necessary. Tell your doctor and pharmacist if you are taking any other dietary supplement or any prescription or nonprescription (over-the-counter [OTC]) medicine.

Other medical problems—The presence of other medical problems may affect the use of beta-carotene. Make sure you tell your doctor if you have any other medical problems, especially:

- Kidney disease or
- Liver disease—These conditions may cause high blood levels of beta-carotene, which may increase the chance of side effects

Proper Use of This Dietary Supplement

Beta-carotene is safer than vitamin A (retinol) because vitamin A can be harmful in high doses. If you have high blood levels of vitamin A, then your body will convert less beta-carotene to vitamin A. However, you should take large doses of beta-carotene only under the direction of your doctor after need has been identified.

Missed dose—If you miss taking a vitamin for one or more days there is no cause for concern, since it takes some time for your body to become seriously low in vitamins. However, if your doctor has recommended that you take this vitamin, try to remember to take it as directed every day.

Storage—To store this dietary supplement:

- Keep out of the reach of children.
- Store away from heat and direct light.
- Do not store in the bathroom, near the kitchen sink, or in other damp places. Heat or moisture may cause the dietary supplement to break down.
- Keep the dietary supplement from freezing. Do not refrigerate.
- Do not keep outdated dietary supplements or those no longer needed. Be sure that any discarded dietary supplement is out of the reach of children.

Side Effects of This Dietary Supplement

Along with its needed effects, a dietary supplement may cause some unwanted effects. The following side effects may go away during treatment as your body adjusts to the dietary supplement. However, check with your doctor if any of the following side effects continue or are bothersome:

More common

Yellowing of palms, hand, or soles of feet, and to a lesser extent the face (this may be a sign that your dose of beta-carotene as a nutritional supplement is too high)

Rare

Diarrhea; dizziness; joint pain; unusual bleeding or bruising

Other side effects not listed above may also occur in some patients. If you notice any other effects, check with your doctor.

Annual revision: 11/27/91
Interim revision: 05/11/92

BETA-CAROTENE—For Photosensitivity Systemic

A commonly used brand name in the U.S. is Solatene.

Generic name product may also be available in the U.S. and Canada.

Description

Beta-carotene (bay-ta-KARE-oh-teen) is used to prevent or treat a sun reaction (photosensitivity) in patients with a disease called erythropoietic protoporphyria.

It may also be used to treat other conditions as determined by your doctor. However, beta-carotene has not been shown to be effective as a sunscreen.

Beta-carotene is available without a prescription. However, it may be a good idea to check with your doctor before taking it on your own.

Beta-carotene is available in the following dosage forms:

Oral

- Capsules (U.S. and Canada)
- Tablets (U.S. and Canada)

It is very important that you read and understand the following information. If any of it causes you special concern, check with your doctor or pharmacist. Also, *if you have any questions* or if you want more information about this medicine or your medical problem, *ask your doctor, nurse, or pharmacist.*

Before Using This Medicine

If you are taking this medicine without a prescription, carefully read and follow any precautions on the label. For beta-carotene, the following should be considered:

Allergies—Tell your doctor if you have ever had any unusual or allergic reaction to beta-carotene. Also tell your doctor and pharmacist if you are allergic to any other substances, such as foods, preservatives, or dyes.

Pregnancy—Beta-carotene has not been studied in pregnant women. However, studies in animals have shown that beta-carotene in extremely large doses causes miscarriages. Before taking this medicine, make sure your doctor knows if you are pregnant or if you may become pregnant.

Breast-feeding—Beta-carotene has not been reported to cause problems in nursing babies.

Children—This medicine has been tested in children and, in effective doses, has not been shown to cause different side effects or problems in children than it does in adults.

Older adults—Many medicines have not been studied specifically in older people. Therefore, it may not be known whether they work exactly the same way they do in younger adults. Although there is no specific information comparing use of beta-carotene in the elderly with use in other age groups, it is not expected to cause different side effects or problems in older people than it does in younger adults.

Other medicines—Although certain medicines should not be used together at all, in other cases two different medicines may be used together even if an interaction might occur. In these cases, your doctor may want to change the dose, or other precautions may be necessary. Tell your doctor and pharmacist if you are taking any other prescription or nonprescription (over-the-counter [OTC]) medicine.

Other medical problems—The presence of other medical problems may affect the use of beta-carotene. Make sure you tell your doctor if you have any other medical problems, especially:

- Kidney disease or
- Liver disease—These conditions may cause high blood levels of beta-carotene, which may increase the chance of side effects

Before you begin using any new medicine (prescription or nonprescription) or if you develop any new medical problem while you are using this medicine, check with your doctor, nurse, or pharmacist.

Proper Use of This Medicine

Missed dose—If you miss a dose of this medicine, take it as soon as possible. However, if it is almost time for your next dose, skip the missed dose and go back to your regular dosing schedule. Do not double doses.

Storage—To store this medicine:

- Keep out of the reach of children.
- Store away from heat and direct light.
- Do not store in the bathroom, near the kitchen sink, or in other damp places. Heat or moisture may cause the medicine to break down.
- Keep the medicine from freezing. Do not refrigerate.
- Do not keep outdated medicine or medicine no longer needed. Be sure that any discarded medicine is out of the reach of children.

Side Effects of This Medicine

Along with its needed effects, a medicine may cause some unwanted effects. The following side effects may go away during treatment as your body adjusts to the medicine. However, check with your doctor if any of the following side effects continue or are bothersome:

More common

Yellowing of palms, hands, or soles of feet, and to a lesser extent the face

Rare

Diarrhea; dizziness; joint pain; unusual bleeding or bruising

Other side effects not listed above may also occur in some patients. If you notice any other effects, check with your doctor.

Additional Information

Once a medicine has been approved for marketing for a certain use, experience may show that it is also useful for other medical problems. Although this use is not included in product labeling, beta-carotene is used in certain patients with the following medical condition:

- Polymorphous light eruption (a type of sun reaction)

Other than the above information, there is no additional information relating to proper use, precautions, or side effects for this use.

Annual revision: 11/27/91

BETHANECHOL Systemic

Some commonly used brand names are:

In the U.S.

Duvoid
Urecholine
Urabeth

Generic name product may also be available.

In Canada

Duvoid
Urecholine

Description

Bethanechol (be-THAN-e-kole) is taken to treat certain disorders of the urinary tract or bladder. It helps to cause urination and emptying of the bladder. Bethanechol may also be used for other conditions as determined by your doctor.

Bethanechol is available only with your doctor's prescription in the following dosage forms:

Oral

- Tablets (U.S. and Canada)

Parenteral

- Injection (U.S. and Canada)

It is very important that you read and understand the following information. If any of it causes you special concern, check with your doctor. Also, *if you have any questions* or if you want more information about this medicine or your medical problem, *ask your doctor, nurse, or pharmacist.*

Before Using This Medicine

In deciding to use a medicine, the risks of taking the medicine must be weighed against the good it will do. This is a decision you and your doctor will make. For bethanechol, the following should be considered:

Allergies—Tell your doctor if you have ever had any unusual or allergic reaction to bethanechol. Also tell your doctor and pharmacist if you are allergic to any other substances, such as foods, preservatives, or dyes.

Pregnancy—Studies on effects in pregnancy have not been done in either humans or animals.

Breast-feeding—It is not known whether bethanechol passes into the breast milk.

Children—Although there is no specific information comparing use of bethanechol in children with use in other age groups, this medicine is not expected to cause different side effects or problems in children than it does in adults.

Older adults—Many medicines have not been studied specifically in older people. Therefore, it may not be known whether they work exactly the same way they do in younger adults. Although there is no specific information comparing use of bethanechol in the elderly with use in other age groups, it is not expected to cause different side effects or problems in older people than it does in younger adults.

Other medicines—Although certain medicines should not be used together at all, in other cases two different medicines may be used together even if an interaction might occur. In these cases, your doctor may want to change the dose, or other precautions may be necessary. Tell your doctor and pharmacist if you are taking any other prescription or nonprescription (over-the-counter [OTC]) medicine.

Other medical problems—The presence of other medical problems may affect the use of bethanechol. Make sure you tell your doctor if you have any other medical problems, especially:

- Asthma or
- Epilepsy or
- Heart or blood vessel disease or
- Intestinal blockage or
- Low blood pressure or
- Parkinson's disease or
- Recent bladder or intestinal surgery or
- Stomach ulcer or other stomach problems or
- Urinary tract blockage or difficult urination—Bethanechol may make these conditions worse
- High blood pressure—Bethanechol may cause a rapid fall in blood pressure
- Overactive thyroid—Bethanechol may further increase the chance of heart problems

Before you begin using any new medicine (prescription or nonprescription) or if you develop any new medical problem while you are using this medicine, check with your doctor, nurse, or pharmacist.

Proper Use of This Medicine

Take this medicine on an empty stomach (either 1 hour before or 2 hours after meals) to lessen the possibility of nausea and vomiting, unless otherwise directed by your doctor.

Take this medicine only as directed. Do not take more of it, do not take it more often, and do not take it for a longer time than your doctor ordered. To do so may increase the chance of side effects.

Dosing—The dose of bethanechol will be different for different patients. *Follow your doctor's orders or the directions on the label.*

Missed dose—If you miss a dose of this medicine and you remember within an hour or so of the missed dose, take it right away. However, if you do not remember until 2 or more hours after, skip the missed dose and go back to your regular dosing schedule. Do not double doses.

Storage—To store this medicine:
- Keep out of the reach of children.
- Store away from heat and direct light.
- Do not store the tablet form of this medicine in the bathroom, near the kitchen sink, or in other damp places. Heat or moisture may cause the medicine to break down.
- Do not keep outdated medicine or medicine no longer needed. Be sure that any discarded medicine is out of the reach of children.

Precautions While Using This Medicine

Dizziness, lightheadedness, or fainting may occur, especially when you get up from a lying or sitting position. Getting up slowly may help lessen this problem.

Side Effects of This Medicine

Along with its needed effects, a medicine may cause some unwanted effects. Although not all of these side effects may occur, if they do occur they may need medical attention.

Check with your doctor as soon as possible if any of the following side effects occur:

Rare—more common with the injection

Shortness of breath, wheezing, or tightness in chest

Other side effects may occur that usually do not need medical attention. These side effects may go away during treatment as your body adjusts to the medicine. However, check with your doctor if any of the following side effects continue or are bothersome:

Less common or rare—more common with the injection

Belching; blurred vision or change in near or distance vision; diarrhea; dizziness or lightheadedness; feeling faint; frequent urge to urinate; headache; increased watering of mouth or sweating; nausea or vomiting; redness or flushing of skin or feeling of warmth; seizures; sleeplessness, nervousness, or jitters; stomach discomfort or pain

Other side effects not listed above may also occur in some patients. If you notice any other effects, check with your doctor.

Additional Information

Once a medicine has been approved for marketing for a certain use, experience may show that it is also useful for other medical problems. Although these uses are not included in product labeling, bethanechol is used in certain patients with the following medical conditions:
- Certain stomach problems
- Gastroesophageal reflux (caused by acid in the stomach washing back up into the esophagus)
- Megacolon (an abnormally large or dilated colon)

Other than the above information, there is no additional information relating to proper use, precautions, or side effects for these uses.

Annual revision: 05/12/93

BIOTIN Systemic

A commonly used brand name in the U.S. is Bio-Tn.

Generic name product is available in the U.S. and Canada.

Other commonly used names are vitamin H, coenzyme R, or vitamin Bw.

Description

Vitamins (VYE-ta-mins) are compounds that you must have for growth and health. They are needed in only small amounts and are usually available in the foods that you eat. Biotin (BYE-oh-tin) is necessary for normal metabolism.

A lack of biotin is rare. However, if it occurs it may lead to skin rash, loss of hair, high blood levels of cholesterol, and heart problems.

Patients with the following conditions may be more likely to have a deficiency of biotin:
- Genetic disorder of biotin deficiency
- Seborrheic determatitis in infants
- Surgical removal of the stomach

If any of these conditions apply to you, you should take biotin supplements only on the advice of your doctor after need has been established.

Claims that biotin supplements are effective in the treatment of acne, eczema (a type of skin disorder), or hair loss have not been proven.

Some preparations are available only with your doctor's prescription. Others are available without a prescription;

however, your doctor may have special instructions on the proper use and dose for your condition.

Biotin supplements are available in the following dosage forms:

Oral

- Capsules (U.S.)
- Tablets (U.S. and Canada)

It is very important that you read and understand the following information. If any of it causes you special concern, check with your doctor. Also, *if you have any questions* or if you want more information about this dietary supplement or your medical problem, *ask your doctor, nurse, or dietitian.*

Importance of Diet

Many nutritionists recommend that, if possible, people should get all the biotin they need from foods. Some people may need more biotin than normal. For such people a supplement is important.

In order to get enough vitamins and minerals in your diet, it is important that you eat a balanced and varied diet. Follow carefully any diet program your doctor may recommend. For your specific vitamin and/or mineral needs, ask your doctor or dietitian for a list of appropriate foods.

Biotin is found in various foods, including liver, cauliflower, salmon, carrots, bananas, soy flour, cereals, and yeast. Biotin content of food is reduced by cooking and preserving.

Experts have developed a list of recommended dietary allowances (RDA) for most vitamins and some minerals. The RDA are not an exact number but a general idea of how much you need. They do not cover amounts needed for problems caused by a serious lack of vitamins and minerals. Because lack of biotin is rare, there are no RDA for it. The following intakes are thought to be plenty for most individuals:

Infants and children—
- Birth to 6 months of age: 10 micrograms (mcg) a day.
- 6 months to 1 year of age: 15 mcg a day.
- 1 to 3 years of age: 20 mcg a day.
- 4 to 6 years of age: 25 mcg a day.
- 7 to 10 years of age: 30 mcg a day.

Adolescents and adults—30 to 100 mcg a day.

Before Using This Dietary Supplement

If you are taking this dietary supplement without a prescription, carefully read and follow any precautions on the label. For biotin, the following should be considered:

Pregnancy—It is especially important that you are receiving enough vitamins and minerals when you become pregnant and that you continue to receive the right amount of vitamins and minerals throughout your pregnancy. The healthy growth and development of the fetus depend on a steady supply of nutrients from the mother. However, taking large amounts of a dietary supplement in pregnancy may be harmful to the mother and/or fetus and should be avoided.

Children—It is especially important that children receive enough biotin in their diet for healthy growth and development. Although there is no specific information comparing the use of biotin in children with use in other age groups, this medicine is not expected to cause different side effects or problems in children than in adults.

Older adults—It is important that older people continue to receive enough biotin in their daily diets.

Proper Use of This Dietary Supplement

Some people believe that taking very large doses of a vitamin or mineral (called megadoses) is useful for treating certain medical problems. Studies have not proven this. Large doses should be taken only under the direction of your doctor after need has been identified.

Missed dose—If you miss taking biotin supplements for one or more days there is no cause for concern, since it takes some time for your body to become seriously low in biotin. However, if your doctor has recommended that you take biotin, try to remember to take it as directed every day.

Storage—To store this dietary supplement:

- Keep out of the reach of children.
- Store away from heat and direct light.
- Do not store in the bathroom, near the kitchen sink, or in other damp places. Heat or moisture may cause the dietary supplement to break down.
- Keep the dietary supplement from freezing. Do not refrigerate.
- Do not keep outdated dietary supplements or those no longer needed. Be sure that any discarded dietary supplement is out of the reach of children.

Side Effects of This Dietary Supplement

No side effects have been reported for biotin, However, check with your doctor if you notice any unusual effects while you are taking it.

Annual revision: 09/26/91
Interim revision: 06/02/92

BISMUTH SUBSALICYLATE Oral

A commonly used brand name in the U.S. and Canada is Pepto-Bismol.

Description

Bismuth subsalicylate (BIS-muth sub-sa-LIS-a-late) is used to treat diarrhea. It is also used to relieve the symptoms of an upset stomach, such as heartburn, indigestion, and nausea.

This medicine is available without a prescription; however, your doctor may have special instructions on the proper use and dose for your medical problem. Bismuth subsalicylate is available in the following dosage forms:

Oral
- Oral suspension (U.S. and Canada)
- Chewable tablets (U.S. and Canada)

It is very important that you read and understand the following information. If any of it causes you special concern, check with your doctor or pharmacist. Also, *if you have any questions* or if you want more information about this medicine or your medical problem, *ask your doctor, nurse, or pharmacist.*

Before Using This Medicine

If you are taking this medicine without a prescription, carefully read and follow any precautions on the label. For bismuth subsalicylate, the following should be considered:

Allergies—Tell your doctor if you have ever had any unusual or allergic reaction to bismuth subsalicylate or to other salicylates, such as aspirin, including methyl salicylate (oil of wintergreen), or to any of the following medicines:

- Carprofen (e.g., Rimadyl)
- Diclofenac (e.g., Voltaren)
- Diflunisal (e.g., Dolobid)
- Fenoprofen (e.g., Nalfon)
- Floctafenine (e.g., Idarac)
- Flurbiprofen taken by mouth (e.g., Ansaid)
- Ibuprofen (e.g., Motrin)
- Indomethacin (e.g., Indocin)
- Ketoprofen (e.g., Orudis)
- Ketorolac (e.g., Toradol)
- Meclofenamate (e.g., Meclomen)
- Mefenamic acid (e.g., Ponstel)
- Naproxen (e.g., Naprosyn)
- Oxyphenbutazone (e.g., Tandearil)
- Phenylbutazone (e.g., Butazolidin)
- Piroxicam (e.g., Feldene)
- Sulindac (e.g., Clinoril)
- Suprofen (e.g., Suprol)
- Tiaprofenic acid (e.g., Surgam)
- Tolmetin (e.g., Tolectin)
- Zomepirac (e.g., Zomax)

Also tell your doctor and pharmacist if you are allergic to any other substances, such as certain foods, sulfites or other preservatives, or dyes.

Diet—Make certain your doctor and pharmacist know if you are on any special diet, such as a low-sodium or low-sugar diet.

Pregnancy—The occasional use of bismuth subsalicylate is not likely to cause problems in the fetus or in the newborn baby. However, based on what is known about the use of other salicylates, especially at high doses and for long periods of time, the following information may also apply for bismuth subsalicylate.

Salicylates have not been shown to cause birth defects in humans. However, studies in animals have shown that salicylates may cause birth defects.

There is a chance that regular use of salicylates late in pregnancy may cause unwanted effects on the heart or blood flow in the fetus or in the newborn infant.

Use of salicylates during the last 2 weeks of pregnancy may cause bleeding problems in the fetus before or during delivery or in the newborn infant. Also, too much use of salicylates during the last 3 months of pregnancy may increase the length of pregnancy, prolong labor, cause other problems during delivery, or cause severe bleeding in the mother before, during, or after delivery.

Breast-feeding—Salicylates pass into the breast milk. Although they have not been shown to cause problems in nursing babies, it is possible that problems may occur if large amounts of salicylates are taken regularly.

Children—The fluid loss caused by diarrhea may result in a severe condition. For this reason, medicine for diarrhea must not be given to young children (under 3 years of age) without first checking with their doctor. In older children with diarrhea, medicine for diarrhea may be used, but it is also very important that a sufficient amount of liquids be given to replace the fluid lost by the body. If you have any questions about this, check with your doctor, nurse, or pharmacist.

Also, children are usually more sensitive to the effects of salicylates, especially if they have a fever or have lost large amounts of body fluid because of vomiting, diarrhea, or sweating.

The bismuth in this medicine may cause severe constipation in children.

In addition, do not use this medicine to treat nausea or vomiting in children or teenagers who have or are recovering from the flu or chickenpox. If nausea or vomiting is present, check with the child's doctor because this could be an early sign of Reye's syndrome.

Older adults—The fluid loss caused by diarrhea may result in a severe condition. For this reason, elderly persons with diarrhea should not take this medicine without first checking with their doctor. It is also very important that a sufficient amount of liquids be taken to replace the fluid lost by the body. If you have any questions about this, check with your doctor, nurse, or pharmacist.

Also, the elderly may be more sensitive to the effects of salicylates. This may increase the chance of side effects during treatment. In addition, the bismuth in this medicine may cause severe constipation in the elderly.

Other medicines—Although certain medicines should not be used together at all, in other cases two different medicines may be used together even if an interaction might occur. In these cases, your doctor may want to change the dose, or other precautions may be necessary. When taking bismuth subsalicylate it is especially important that your doctor and pharmacist know if you are taking any of the following:

- Anticoagulants (blood thinners) or
- Heparin—The salicylate in this medicine may increase the chance of bleeding
- Antidiabetics, oral (diabetes medicine you take by mouth)—This medicine may make the levels of sugar in the blood become too low
- Medicine for pain and/or inflammation (except narcotics)—If these medicines contain salicylates, use of bismuth subsalicylate (which also contains salicylate) may lead to increased side effects and overdose
- Probenecid (e.g., Benemid) or
- Sulfinpyrazone (e.g., Anturane)—Bismuth subsalicylate may make these medicines less effective for treating gout
- Tetracyclines by mouth (medicine for infection)—The tablet form of bismuth subsalicylate should be taken at least 1 to 3 hours before or after tetracyclines; otherwise it may decrease the effectiveness of the tetracycline

Other medical problems—The presence of other medical problems may affect the use of bismuth subsalicylate. Make sure you tell your doctor if you have any other medical problems, especially:

- Dysentery—This condition may get worse; a different kind of treatment may be needed
- Gout—The salicylate in this medicine may worsen the gout and make the medicines taken for gout less effective
- Hemophilia or other bleeding problems—The salicylate in this medicine may increase the chance of bleeding
- Kidney disease—There is a greater chance of side effects because the body may be unable to get rid of the bismuth subsalicylate
- Stomach ulcer—Use of this medicine may make the ulcer worse

Before you begin using any new medicine (prescription or nonprescription) or if you develop any new medical problem while you are using this medicine, check with your doctor, nurse, or pharmacist.

Proper Use of This Medicine

For safe and effective use of this medicine:

- Follow your doctor's instructions if this medicine was prescribed.
- Follow the manufacturer's package directions if you are treating yourself.

For patients using this medicine to treat diarrhea:

- *It is very important that the fluid lost by the body be replaced and that a proper diet be followed.* For the first 24 hours you should drink plenty of clear liquids, such as ginger ale, decaffeinated cola, decaffeinated tea, broth, and gelatin. During the next 24 hours you may eat bland foods, such as cooked cereals, bread, crackers, and applesauce. Fruits, vegetables, fried or spicy foods, bran, candy, and caffeine and alcoholic beverages may make the diarrhea worse.
- If too much fluid has been lost by the body due to the diarrhea a serious condition may develop. Check with your doctor as soon as possible if any of the following signs of too much fluid loss occur:

  Decreased urination
  Dizziness and lightheadedness
  Dryness of mouth
  Increased thirst
  Wrinkled skin

Missed dose—If your doctor has ordered you to take this medicine according to a regular schedule and you miss a dose, take it as soon as you remember. However, if it is almost time for your next dose, skip the missed dose and go back to your regular dosing schedule. Do not double doses.

Storage—To store this medicine:

- Keep out of the reach of children. Overdose is very dangerous in young children.
- Store away from heat and direct light.
- Do not store the tablet form of this medicine in the bathroom, near the kitchen sink, or in other damp places. Heat or moisture may cause the medicine to break down.
- Keep the liquid form of this medicine from freezing.
- Do not keep outdated medicine or medicine no longer needed. Be sure that any discarded medicine is out of the reach of children.

Precautions While Using This Medicine

Check the labels of all over-the-counter (OTC), nonprescription, and prescription medicines you now take. If any contain aspirin or other salicylates, be especially careful. Using other salicylate-containing products while taking this medicine may lead to overdose. If you have any questions about this, check with your doctor or pharmacist.

For diabetic patients:

- False urine sugar test results may occur if you are regularly taking large amounts of bismuth subsalicylate or other salicylates.
- Smaller doses or occasional use of bismuth subsalicylate usually will not affect urine sugar tests. However, check with your doctor, nurse, or pharmacist (especially if your diabetes is not well-controlled) if:
  —you are not sure how much salicylate you are taking every day.
  —you notice any change in your urine sugar test results.
  —you have any other questions about this possible problem.

If you think that you or anyone else may have taken an overdose, get emergency help at once. Taking an overdose of this medicine may cause unconsciousness or death. Signs of overdose include convulsions (seizures), hearing loss, confusion, ringing or buzzing in the ears, severe drowsiness or tiredness, severe excitement or nervousness, and fast or deep breathing.

If you are taking this medicine for diarrhea, check with your doctor:

- if your symptoms do not improve within 2 days or if they become worse.
- if you also have a high fever.

Side Effects of This Medicine

Along with its needed effects, a medicine may cause some unwanted effects. Although not all of these side effects may occur, if they do occur they may need medical attention.

When this medicine is used occasionally or for short periods of time at low doses, side effects usually are rare. However, check with your doctor immediately if any of the following side effects occur, since they may indicate that too much medicine is being taken:

Anxiety; any loss of hearing; confusion; constipation (severe); diarrhea (severe or continuing); difficulty in speaking or slurred speech; dizziness or lightheadedness; drowsiness (severe); fast or deep breathing; headache (severe or continuing); increased sweating; increased thirst; mental depression; muscle spasms (especially of face, neck, and back); muscle weakness; nausea or vomiting (severe or continuing); ringing or buzzing in ears (continuing); stomach pain (severe or continuing); trembling; uncontrollable flapping movements of the hands (especially in elderly patients) or other uncontrolled body movements; vision problems

In some patients bismuth subsalicylate may cause dark tongue and/or grayish black stools. This is only temporary and will go away when you stop taking this medicine.

Other side effects not listed above may also occur in some patients. If you notice any other effects, check with your doctor.

Annual revision: 02/03/92

BLEOMYCIN Systemic

A commonly used brand name in the U.S. and Canada is Blenoxane.

Description

Bleomycin (blee-oh-MYE-sin) belongs to the general group of medicines called antineoplastics. It is used to treat some kinds of cancer.

Bleomycin seems to act by interfering with the growth of cancer cells, which are eventually destroyed. Since the growth of normal body cells may also be affected by bleomycin, other effects will also occur. Some of these may be serious and must be reported to your doctor. Other effects, like darkening of skin or hair loss, may not be serious but may cause concern. Some effects may not occur for months or years after the medicine is used.

This medicine may also be used for other conditions, as determined by your doctor.

Before you begin treatment with bleomycin, you and your doctor should talk about the good this medicine will do as well as the risks of using it.

Bleomycin is to be administered only by or under the immediate supervision of your doctor. It is available in the following dosage form:

Parenteral

- Injection (U.S. and Canada)

It is very important that you read and understand the following information. If any of it causes you special concern, check with your doctor. Also, *if you have any questions* or if you want more information about this medicine or your medical problem, *ask your doctor, nurse, or pharmacist.*

Before Using This Medicine

In deciding to use a medicine, the risks of taking the medicine must be weighed against the good it will do. This is a decision you and your doctor will make. For bleomycin, the following should be considered:

Allergies—Tell your doctor if you have ever had any unusual or allergic reaction to bleomycin.

Pregnancy—Studies have not been done in pregnant women. However, there is a chance that this medicine may cause birth defects if either the male or female is receiving it at the time of conception or if it is used during pregnancy. Studies in mice given large doses of bleomycin have shown that it causes birth defects. In addition, many cancer medicines may cause sterility which could be permanent. Although sterility has not been reported with this medicine, the possibility should be kept in mind.

Be sure that you have discussed this with your doctor before receiving this medicine. It is best to use some kind of birth control while you are receiving bleomycin. However, do not use oral contraceptives ("the Pill") since they may interfere with this medicine. Tell your doctor right away if you think you have become pregnant while receiving bleomycin.

Breast-feeding—Because bleomycin may cause serious side effects, breast-feeding is generally not recommended while you are receiving it.

Children—Although there is no specific information about the use of bleomycin in children, it is not expected to cause different side effects or problems in children than it does in adults.

Older adults—Lung problems are more likely to occur in elderly patients (over 70 years of age), who are usually more sensitive to the effects of bleomycin.

Other medical problems—The presence of other medical problems may affect the use of bleomycin. Make sure you tell your doctor if you have any other medical problems, especially:

- Kidney disease—Effects of bleomycin may be increased because of slower removal from the body
- Liver disease—Bleomycin can cause liver problems
- Lung disease—Bleomycin may worsen the condition

Smoking—Tell your doctor if you smoke. The risk of lung problems is increased in people who smoke.

Before you begin using any new medicine (prescription or nonprescription) or if you develop any new medical problem while you are using this medicine, check with your doctor, nurse, or pharmacist.

Proper Use of This Medicine

Bleomycin is sometimes given together with certain other medicines. If you are using a combination of medicines, it is important that you receive each medicine at the proper time. If you are taking some of these medicines by mouth, ask your doctor, nurse, or pharmacist to help you plan a way to take them at the right times.

Bleomycin often causes nausea, vomiting, and loss of appetite. However, it is very important that you continue to receive the medicine, even if you begin to feel ill. Ask your doctor, nurse, or pharmacist for ways to lessen these effects.

Precautions While Using This Medicine

It is very important that your doctor check your progress at regular visits to make sure that this medicine is working properly and to check for unwanted effects.

Before having any kind of surgery (including dental surgery) or emergency treatment, *tell the medical doctor or dentist in charge that you are receiving or have received this medicine.*

Side Effects of This Medicine

Along with their needed effects, medicines like bleomycin can sometimes cause unwanted effects such as loss of hair, lung problems, and other side effects. These and others are described below. Also, because of the way these medicines act on the body, there is a chance that they might cause other unwanted effects that may not occur until months or years after the medicine is used. These delayed effects may include certain types of cancer, such as leukemia. Discuss these possible effects with your doctor.

Although not all of these side effects may occur, if they do occur they may need medical attention.

Check with your doctor or nurse immediately if the following side effects occur:

More common

Fever and chills (occurring within 3 to 6 hours after a dose)

Less common

Confusion; faintness; wheezing

Rare

Chest pain (sudden severe); weakness in arms or legs (sudden)

Check with your doctor or nurse as soon as possible if any of the following side effects occur:

More common

Cough; shortness of breath; sores in mouth and on lips

Other side effects may occur that usually do not need medical attention. These side effects may go away during

treatment as your body adjusts to the medicine. Also, your doctor or nurse may be able to tell you about ways to prevent or reduce some of these side effects. Check with your doctor or nurse if any of the following side effects continue or are bothersome or if you have any questions about them:

More common

Darkening or thickening of skin; dark stripes on skin; itching of skin; skin rash or colored bumps on fingertips, elbows, or palms; skin redness or tenderness; swelling of fingers; vomiting and loss of appetite

Less common

Changes in fingernails or toenails; weight loss

Bleomycin may cause a temporary loss of hair in some people. After treatment has ended, normal hair growth should return, although it may take several months.

Side effects that affect your lungs (for example, cough and shortness of breath) may be more likely to occur if you smoke.

After you stop receiving bleomycin, it may still produce some side effects that need attention. During this period of time, check with your doctor or nurse *immediately* if you notice either of the following:

Cough; shortness of breath

Other side effects not listed above may also occur in some patients. If you notice any other effects, check with your doctor or nurse.

Additional Information

Once a medicine has been approved for marketing for a certain use, experience may show that it is also useful for other medical problems. Although this use is not included in product labeling, bleomycin is used in certain patients with the following medical condition:

- Verruca vulgaris (warts)

For patients being treated with bleomycin for warts:

- Bleomycin is used to treat severe cases of warts when other treatments have not worked.
- Before using bleomycin, tell your doctor if you have problems with circulation. Bleomycin can cause paleness or coldness in fingers treated for warts.
- Bleomycin is injected directly into the wart. Because it is not absorbed into the body, it does not cause loss of hair, lung problems, or other unwanted effects described above. However, it may cause burning or pain at the place of injection. Skin rash or itching, nail loss, and pain or coldness in the finger where bleomycin was injected have also been reported.

Other than the above information, there is no additional information relating to proper use, precautions, or side effects for these uses.

Annual revision: July 1990

BOTULINUM TOXIN TYPE A Parenteral-Local

A commonly used brand name in the U.S. is Oculinum.

Description

Botulinum toxin type A (BOT-yoo-lye-num) is used to treat certain eye conditions, such as:

- Blepharospasm—A condition in which the eyelid will not stay open, because of a spasm of a muscle of the eye.
- Strabismus—A condition in which the eyes do not line up properly.

Botulinum toxin type A is injected into the surrounding muscle or tissue of the eye, but not into the eye itself. Depending on your condition, more than one treatment may be required.

This medicine is to be administered only by, or under the immediate supervision of, your doctor. It is available in the following dosage form:

Parenteral-Local

- Injection (U.S.)

It is very important that you read and understand the following information. If any of it causes you special concern, check with your doctor. Also, *if you have any questions* or if you want more information about this medicine or your medical problem, *ask your doctor, nurse, or pharmacist.*

Before Receiving This Medicine

In deciding to receive a medicine, the risks of receiving the medicine must be weighed against the good it will do. This is a decision you and your doctor will make. For botulinum toxin type A, the following should be considered:

Allergies—Tell your doctor if you have ever had any unusual or allergic reaction to botulinum toxin type A. Also tell your doctor and pharmacist if you are allergic to any other substances.

Pregnancy—Studies on effects in pregnancy have not been done in either humans or animals.

Breast-feeding—It is not known whether botulinum toxin type A passes into the breast milk. However, this medicine has not been reported to cause problems in nursing babies.

Children—Studies on this medicine have been done only in adult patients, and there is no specific information comparing use of botulinum toxin type A in children up to 12 years of age with use in other age groups.

Older adults—Many medicines have not been studied specifically in older people. Therefore, it may not be known whether they work exactly the same way they do in younger adults. Although there is no specific information comparing use of botulinum toxin type A in the elderly with use in other age groups, this medicine is not expected to cause different side effects or problems in older people than it does in younger adults.

Other medicines—Although certain medicines should not be used together at all, in other cases two different medicines may be used together even if an interaction might occur. In these cases, your doctor may want to change the dose, or other precautions may be necessary. Tell your doctor and pharmacist if you are using any other ophthalmic prescription or nonprescription (over-the-counter [OTC]) medicine.

Other medical problems—The presence of other medical problems may affect the use of botulinum toxin type A. Make sure you tell your doctor if you have any other medical problems, especially:

- Heart problems or other medical conditions that may worsen with rapidly increasing activity—Treatment with botulinum toxin type A may give you better vision and the desire to become more active in your daily life; this may put a strain on your heart and body
- Infection with *Clostridium botulinum* toxin (botulism poisoning), history of—Persons with a history of infection with *Clostridium botulinum* toxin (botulism poisoning) may have produced antibodies that may interfere with botulinum toxin type A therapy and make it less effective

Precautions After Receiving This Medicine

After you have received this medicine and your vision is better, you may find that you are a lot more active than you were before. You should increase your activities slowly and carefully to allow your heart and body time to get stronger. Also, before you start any exercise program, check with your doctor.

Side Effects of This Medicine

Along with its needed effects, a medicine may cause some unwanted effects. Although not all of these side effects may occur, if they do occur they may need medical attention.

Check with your doctor as soon as possible if any of the following side effects occur:

More common

Dryness of the eye; inability to close the eyelid completely

Less common or rare

Decreased blinking; irritation of the cornea (colored portion) of the eye; turning outward or inward of the edge of the eyelid

Other side effects may occur that usually do not need medical attention. These side effects may go away as your body adjusts to the medicine. However, check with your doctor if any of the following side effects continue or are bothersome:

More common

Blue or purplish bruise on eyelid; drooping of the upper eyelid; eye pointing upward or downward instead of straight ahead; irritation or watering of the eye; sensitivity of the eye to light

Less common or rare

Difficulty finding the location of objects; double vision; skin rash; swelling of the eyelid skin

Other side effects not listed above may also occur in some patients. If you notice any other effects, check with your doctor.

Additional Information

Once a medicine has been approved for marketing for a certain use, experience may show that it is also useful for other medical problems. Although these uses are not included in product labeling, botulinum toxin type A is used in certain patients with the following medical conditions:

- Spasms of the face
- Spasms of the neck

Annual revision: 01/09/92

BROMOCRIPTINE Systemic

A commonly used brand name in the U.S. and Canada is Parlodel.

Description

Bromocriptine (broe-moe-KRIP-teen) belongs to the group of medicines known as ergot alkaloids. It is used to treat certain menstrual problems or as a fertility medicine in some women who are unable to become pregnant. It is also used to stop milk production in some women who have abnormal milk leakage. Bromocriptine blocks release of a hormone called prolactin from the pituitary gland. Prolactin affects the menstrual cycle and milk production.

Bromocriptine is also used to treat some people who have Parkinson's disease. It works by stimulating certain parts of the brain and nervous system that are involved in this disease.

Bromocriptine is also used to treat acromegaly (overproduction of growth hormone) and pituitary prolactinomas (tumors of the pituitary gland).

Bromocriptine may be used to stop milk production after abortion or after the delivery of a baby in women who should not breast-feed for medical reasons or in women who do not wish to breast-feed. However, some serious side effects have occurred during the use of bromocriptine to stop milk flow after pregnancy or abortion. These side effects have included strokes, seizures (convulsions), and heart attacks. Some deaths have also occurred. You should discuss with your doctor the good that this medicine will do as well as the risks of using it.

Bromocriptine may also be used for other conditions as determined by your doctor.

Bromocriptine is available only with your doctor's prescription, in the following dosage forms:

Oral

- Capsules (U.S. and Canada)
- Tablets (U.S. and Canada)

It is very important that you read and understand the following information. If any of it causes you special concern, check with your doctor. Also, *if you have any questions* or if you want more information about this medicine or your medical problem, *ask your doctor, nurse, or pharmacist.*

Before Using This Medicine

In deciding to use a medicine, the risks of taking the medicine must be weighed against the good it will do. This is a decision you and your doctor will make. For bromocriptine, the following should be considered:

Allergies—Tell your doctor if you have ever had any unusual or allergic reaction to bromocriptine or other ergot medicines such as ergotamine. Also tell your doctor and pharmacist if you are allergic to any other substances, such as foods, preservatives, or dyes.

Pregnancy—Bromocriptine is not generally recommended for use during pregnancy. However, bromocriptine can be used during pregnancy in certain patients who are closely monitored by their doctor.

Breast-feeding—This medicine stops milk from being produced.

Teenagers—This medicine has been tested in teenagers and, in effective doses, has not been shown to cause different side effects or problems than it does in adults.

Older adults—Side effects such as confusion, hallucinations, or uncontrolled body movements may be more likely to occur in older patients.

Other medicines—Although certain medicines should not be used together at all, in other cases two different medicines may be used together even if an interaction might occur. In these cases, your doctor may want to change the dose, or other precautions may be necessary. When you are taking bromocriptine, it is especially important that your doctor and pharmacist know if you are taking any of the following:

- Ergot alkaloids (dihydroergotamine [e.g., D.H.E. 45], ergoloid mesylates [e.g., Hydergine], ergonovine [e.g., Ergotrate], ergotamine [e.g., Gynergen], methylergonovine [e.g., Methergine], methysergide [e.g., Sansert])—Severe cases of high blood pressure have occurred with the use of bromocriptine. This may be made worse with the use of ergot alkaloids
- Estrogens (female hormones) or
- Oral contraceptives (birth control pills) or
- Progestins (hydroxyprogesterone [e.g., Delalutin], medroxyprogesterone [e.g., Provera], megestrol [e.g., Megace], norethindrone [e.g., Norlutin], norethindrone acetate [e.g., Norlutate], norgestrel [e.g., Ovrette], progesterone [e.g., Lipo-Lutin])—These medicines may interfere with the effects of bromocriptine when it is used to treat amenorrhea (abnormal stoppage of menstrual periods) or galactorrhea (milk flow that occurs abnormally, without nursing)

Other medical problems—The presence of other medical problems may affect the use of bromocriptine. Make sure you tell your doctor if you have any other medical problems, especially:

- High blood pressure (history of) or
- Pregnancy-induced high blood pressure (history of)—Rarely, bromocriptine can make the high blood pressure worse

- Liver disease—Toxic effects of bromocriptine may occur in patients with liver disease because the body is not able to get the bromocriptine out of the bloodstream as it normally would
- Mental problems (history of)—Bromocriptine may make certain mental problems worse

Before you begin using any new medicine (prescription or nonprescription) or if you develop any new medical problem while you are using this medicine, check with your doctor, nurse, or pharmacist.

Proper Use of This Medicine

If bromocriptine upsets your stomach, it may be taken with meals or milk. Also, taking the dose at bedtime may help to lessen nausea if it occurs. If stomach upset continues, check with your doctor. Your doctor may recommend that you take the first dose vaginally.

Dosing—The dose of bromocriptine will be different for different patients. *Follow your doctor's orders or the directions on the label.* The following information includes only the average doses of bromocriptine. *If your dose is different, do not change it* unless your doctor tells you to do so.

The number of capsules or tablets that you take depends on the strength of the medicine. Also, *the number of doses you take each day, the time allowed between doses, and the length of time you take the medicine depend on the medical problem for which you are taking bromocriptine.*

- For *oral* dosage forms (capsules and tablets):
  —Adults and teenagers:
    - For acromegaly: 1.25 to 100 milligrams a day.
    - For female infertility: 1.25 to 7.5 milligrams a day, taken one to three times a day.
    - For menstrual cycle irregularity: 1.25 to 7.5 milligrams a day, taken one to three times a day.
    - For Parkinson's disease: 1.25 to 300 milligrams a day.
    - For pituitary tumors: 1.25 to 20 milligrams a day.
    - For unexpected breast milk production: 1.25 to 7.5 milligrams a day, taken one to three times a day.

Missed dose—If you miss a dose of this medicine and remember it within 4 hours, take the missed dose when you remember it. However, if a longer time has passed, skip the missed dose and go back to your regular dosing schedule. Do not double doses.

Storage—To store this medicine:

- Keep out of the reach of children.
- Store away from heat and direct light.
- Do not store in the bathroom, near the kitchen sink, or in other damp places. Heat or moisture may cause the medicine to break down.
- Do not keep outdated medicine or medicine no longer needed. Be sure that any discarded medicine is out of the reach of children.

Precautions While Using This Medicine

It is important that your doctor check your progress at regular visits, to make sure that this medicine is working and to check for unwanted effects.

This medicine may cause some people to become drowsy, dizzy, or less alert than they are normally. *Make sure you know how you react to this medicine before you drive, use machines, or do anything else that could be dangerous if you are dizzy or are not alert.*

Dizziness is more likely to occur after the first dose of bromocriptine. It may be helpful if you get up slowly from a lying or sitting position. Taking the first dose at bedtime or when you are able to lie down may also lessen problems. Your doctor may also recommend that you take the first dose vaginally.

Bromocriptine may cause dryness of the mouth. For temporary relief, use sugarless candy or gum, melt bits of ice in your mouth, or use a saliva substitute. However, if dry mouth continues for more than 2 weeks, check with your medical doctor or dentist. Continuing dryness of the mouth may increase the chance of dental disease, including tooth decay, gum disease, and fungus infections.

It may take several weeks for bromocriptine to work. Do not stop taking this medicine or reduce the amount you are taking without first checking with your doctor.

Drinking alcohol while you are taking bromocriptine may cause you to have a certain reaction. *Avoid alcoholic beverages until you have discussed this with your doctor.* Some of the symptoms you may have if you drink any alcohol while you are taking this medicine are:

Blurred vision
Chest pain
Confusion
Fast or pounding heartbeat
Flushing or redness of face
Nausea
Sweating
Throbbing headache
Vomiting
Weakness (severe)

For females who are able to bear children and who are *taking this medicine for menstrual problems, to stop milk production, for acromegaly, or for pituitary tumors:*

- It is best to use some type of birth control while you are taking bromocriptine. However, do not use oral contraceptives ("the Pill") since they may prevent this medicine from working. If you wish to become pregnant, you and your doctor should decide on the best time for you to stop using birth control. Tell your doctor right away if you think you have become pregnant while taking this medicine. You and your doctor should discuss whether or not you should continue to take bromocriptine during pregnancy.

- *Check with your doctor right away* if you get blurred vision, a sudden headache, or severe nausea and vomiting.

For females *taking bromocriptine for infertility:*

- In general, it is best to use some type of birth control when you start taking bromocriptine. However, do not use oral contraceptives ("the Pill") since they may prevent this medicine from working. When your normal menstrual cycle returns, you and your doctor can decide on the best time for you to stop using birth control. Tell your doctor right away if you think you have become pregnant while taking this medicine. You and your doctor should discuss whether or not you should continue to take bromocriptine during pregnancy.
- *Check with your doctor right away* if you get blurred vision, a sudden headache, or severe nausea and vomiting.

Side Effects of This Medicine

Along with its needed effects, a medicine may cause some unwanted effects. Although not all of these side effects may occur, if they do occur they may need medical attention.

Some serious side effects have occurred during the use of bromocriptine to stop milk flow after pregnancy or abortion. These side effects have included strokes, seizures (convulsions), and heart attacks. Some deaths have also occurred. You should discuss with your doctor the good that this medicine will do as well as the risks of using it.

Check with your doctor immediately if any of the following side effects occur:

Rare

Black, tarry stools; bloody vomit; chest pain (severe); convulsions (seizures); fainting; fast heartbeat; headache (unusual); increased sweating; nausea and vomiting (continuing or severe); nervousness; shortness of breath (unexplained); vision changes (such as blurred vision or temporary blindness); weakness (sudden)

Check with your doctor as soon as possible if any of the following side effects occur:

Less common—reported more often in patients with Parkinson's disease

Confusion; hallucinations (seeing, hearing, or feeling things that are not there); uncontrolled movements of the body, such as the face, tongue, arms, hands, head, and upper body

Rare—reported more often in patients taking large doses

Abdominal or stomach pain (continuing or severe); increased frequency of urination; loss of appetite (continuing); lower back pain; runny nose (continuing); weakness

Other side effects may occur that usually do not need medical attention. These side effects may go away during treatment as your body adjusts to the medicine. However, check with your doctor if any of the following side effects continue or are bothersome:

More common

Dizziness or lightheadedness, especially when getting up from a lying or sitting position; nausea

Less common

Constipation; diarrhea; drowsiness or tiredness; dry mouth; leg cramps at night; loss of appetite; mental depression; stomach pain; stuffy nose; tingling or pain in fingers and toes when exposed to cold; vomiting

Some side effects may be more likely to occur in patients who are taking bromocriptine for Parkinson's disease, acromegaly, or pituitary tumors since they may be taking larger doses.

Other side effects not listed above may also occur in some patients. If you notice any other effects, check with your doctor.

Additional Information

Once a medicine has been approved for marketing for a certain use, experience may show that it is also useful for other medical problems. Although these uses are not included in product labeling, bromocriptine is used in certain patients with the following medical conditions:

- Male infertility caused by excess prolactin (a hormone) in the blood
- Neuroleptic malignant syndrome

Other than the above information, there is no additional information relating to proper use, precautions, or side effects for these uses.

Annual revision: 06/04/93

BRONCHODILATORS, ADRENERGIC Inhalation

This information applies to the following medicines:

- Albuterol (al-BYOO-ter-ole)
- Bitolterol (bye-TOLE-ter-ole)
- Epinephrine (ep-i-NEF-rin)
- Fenoterol (fen-OH-ter-ole)
- Isoetharine (eye-soe-ETH-a-reen)
- Isoproterenol (eye-soe-proe-TER-e-nole)
- Metaproterenol (met-a-proe-TER-e-nole)
- Pirbuterol (peer-BYOO-ter-ole)
- Procaterol (proe-KAY-ter-ole)
- Racepinephrine (race-ep-i-NEF-rin)
- Terbutaline (ter-BYOO-ta-leen)

Some commonly used brand names are:

For Albuterol

In the U.S.

Proventil
Ventolin
Ventolin Rotacaps

Generic name product may also be available.

In Canada

Ventolin
Ventolin Rotacaps

Another commonly used name is salbutamol.

For Bitolterol

In the U.S.

Tornalate

For Epinephrine

In the U.S.

Adrenalin
AsthmaHaler
Bronitin Mist
Bronkaid Mist
Bronkaid Mist Suspension
Medihaler-Epi
Primatene Mist
Primatene Mist Suspension

Generic name product may also be available.

In Canada

Bronkaid Mistometer
Medihaler-Epi

For Fenoterol*

In Canada

Berotec

For Isoetharine

In the U.S.

Arm-a-Med Isoetharine
Bronkometer
Bronkosol
Dey-Dose Isoetharine
Dey-Dose Isoetharine S/F
Dey-Lute Isoetharine
Dey-Lute Isoetharine S/F
Dispos-a-Med Isoetharine

Generic name product may also be available.

For Isoproterenol

In the U.S.

Aerolone
Dey-Dose Isoproterenol
Dispos-a-Med Isoproterenol
Isuprel
Isuprel Mistometer
Medihaler-Iso
Norisodrine Aerotrol
Vapo-Iso

Generic name product may also be available.

In Canada

Isuprel
Isuprel Mistometer
Medihaler-Iso

For Metaproterenol

In the U.S.

Alupent
Arm-a-Med Metaproterenol
Dey-Dose Metaproterenol
Dey-Lute Metaproterenol
Metaprel

Generic name product may also be available.

In Canada

Alupent

For Pirbuterol

In the U.S.

Maxair

For Procaterol*

In Canada

Pro-Air

For Racepinephrine

In the U.S.

AsthmaNefrin
Dey-Dose Racepinephrine
Vaponefrin

In Canada

Vaponefrin

For Terbutaline

In the U.S.

Brethaire

In Canada

Bricanyl

*Not commercially available in the U.S.

Description

Adrenergic bronchodilators are medicines that open up the bronchial tubes (air passages) of the lungs. They are taken by oral inhalation to treat the symptoms of bronchial asthma, chronic bronchitis, emphysema, and other lung diseases. They relieve cough, wheezing, shortness of breath, and troubled breathing by increasing the flow of air through the bronchial tubes.

Some of these medicines are also taken by oral inhalation to prevent bronchospasm (wheezing or difficulty in breathing) caused by exercise. In addition, some of these medicines are taken by oral inhalation to prevent attacks of bronchial asthma and bronchospasm. Also, racepinephrine may be used in the treatment of croup.

All of these medicines, except some epinephrine preparations, are available only with your doctor's prescription. Although some of the epinephrine preparations are available without a prescription, your doctor may have special instructions on the proper dose of epinephrine for your medical condition.

These medicines are available in the following dosage forms:

Inhalation

Albuterol
- Capsules for inhalation (U.S. and Canada)
- Inhalation aerosol (U.S. and Canada)
- Inhalation solution (U.S. and Canada)

Bitolterol
- Inhalation aerosol (U.S.)

Epinephrine
- Inhalation aerosol (U.S. and Canada)
- Inhalation solution (U.S.)

Fenoterol
- Inhalation aerosol (Canada)
- Inhalation solution (Canada)

Isoetharine
- Inhalation aerosol (U.S.)
- Inhalation solution (U.S.)

Isoproterenol
- Inhalation aerosol (U.S. and Canada)
- Inhalation solution (U.S. and Canada)

Metaproterenol
- Inhalation aerosol (U.S. and Canada)
- Inhalation solution (U.S. and Canada)

Pirbuterol
- Inhalation aerosol (U.S.)

Procaterol
- Inhalation aerosol (Canada)

Racepinephrine
- Inhalation solution (U.S. and Canada)

Terbutaline
- Inhalation aerosol (U.S. and Canada)

It is very important that you read and understand the following information. If any of it causes you special concern, check with your doctor. Also, *if you have any questions* or if you want more information about this medicine or your medical problem, *ask your doctor, nurse, or pharmacist.*

Before Using This Medicine

In deciding to use a medicine, the risks of taking the medicine must be weighed against the good it will do. This is a decision you and your doctor will make. For inhalation adrenergic bronchodilators, the following should be considered:

Allergies—Tell your doctor if you have ever had any unusual or allergic reaction to albuterol, bitolterol, epinephrine, fenoterol, isoetharine, isoproterenol, metaproterenol, pirbuterol, procaterol racepinephrine, terbutaline, or other inhalation medicines. Also tell your doctor and pharmacist if you are allergic to any other substances, such as foods, preservatives, or dyes.

Pregnancy—
- *For albuterol, bitolterol, and metaproterenol*: Albuterol, bitolterol, and metaproterenol have not been studied in pregnant women. However, studies in animals have shown that albuterol, bitolterol, and metaproterenol cause birth defects when given in doses many times the usual human inhalation dose.
- *For epinephrine and racepinephrine*: Epinephrine and racepinephrine have not been studied in pregnant women. However, studies in animals have shown that epinephrine causes birth defects when given in doses many times the usual human inhalation dose. Use of epinephrine or racepinephrine during pregnancy may decrease the supply of oxygen to the fetus.
- *For fenoterol*: Fenoterol has not been shown to cause birth defects or other problems in humans.
- *For isoetharine and isoproterenol*: Studies on birth defects with isoetharine or isoproterenol have not been done in either humans or animals.
- *For pirbuterol*: Pirbuterol has not been studied in pregnant women. However, in some animal studies, pirbuterol has been shown to cause miscarriage and death of the animal fetus when given in doses many times the usual human inhalation dose.
- *For procaterol*: Procaterol has not been studied in pregnant women.
- *For terbutaline*: Terbutaline has not been studied in pregnant women. It has not been shown to cause birth defects in animal studies when given in doses many times the human inhalation dose. However, terbutaline may delay labor.

Breast-feeding—
- *For albuterol, bitolterol, fenoterol, isoetharine, isoproterenol, metaproterenol, pirbuterol, and procaterol*: Although it is not known whether albuterol, bitolterol, fenoterol, isoetharine, isoproterenol, metaproterenol, pirbuterol, or procaterol passes into the breast milk, these medicines have not been reported to cause problems in nursing babies.
- *For epinephrine and racepinephrine*: Epinephrine passes into the breast milk. Epinephrine and racepinephrine may cause unwanted side effects in babies of mothers using epinephrine or racepinephrine.
- *For terbutaline*: Although terbutaline passes into the breast milk, it has not been reported to cause problems in nursing babies.

Children—Although there is no specific information about the use of albuterol, bitolterol, fenoterol, isoetharine, isoproterenol, metaproterenol, pirbuterol, procaterol, racepinephrine, or terbutaline in children, these medicines are not expected to cause different side effects or problems in children than they do in adults.

Infants and children may be especially sensitive to the effects of epinephrine. Fainting has occurred after epinephrine was given to children with asthma.

Older adults—Many medicines have not been tested in older people. Therefore, it may not be known whether they work exactly the same way they do in younger adults or if they cause different side effects or problems in older people. There is no specific information about the use of inhalation adrenergic bronchodilators in the elderly.

Other medicines—Although certain medicines should not be used together at all, in other cases two different medicines may be used together even if an interaction might occur. In these cases, your doctor may want to change the dose, or other precautions may be necessary. When you are using inhalation adrenergic bronchodilators, it is especially important that your doctor and pharmacist know if you are taking any of the following:

- Beta-blockers (acebutolol [e.g., Sectral], atenolol [e.g., Tenormin], betaxolol [e.g., Betoptic, Kerlone], carteolol [e.g., Cartrol], labetalol [e.g., Normodyne], levobunolol [e.g., Betagan], metoprolol [e.g., Lopressor], nadolol [e.g., Corgard], oxprenolol [e.g., Trasicor], penbutolol [e.g., Levatol], pindolol [e.g., Visken], propranolol [e.g., Inderal], sotalol [e.g., Sotacor], timolol [e.g., Blocadren, Timoptic])—These medicines may prevent the adrenergic bronchodilators from working properly

- Cocaine or
- Ergoloid mesylates (e.g., Hydergine) or
- Ergotamine (e.g., Gynergen) or
- Maprotiline (e.g., Ludiomil) or
- Tricyclic antidepressants (medicine for depression)—The effects of these medicines on the heart and blood vessels may be increased
- Digitalis glycosides (heart medicine)—The chance of irregular heartbeat may be increased
- Monoamine oxidase (MAO) inhibitors (furazolidone [e.g., Furoxone], isocarboxazid [e.g., Marplan], pargyline [e.g., Eutonyl], phenelzine [e.g., Nardil], procarbazine [e.g., Matulane], tranylcypromine [e.g., Parnate])—Using adrenergic bronchodilators while you are taking or within 2 weeks of taking monoamine oxidase (MAO) inhibitors may increase the effects of MAO inhibitors

Other medical problems—The presence of other medical problems may affect the use of inhalation adrenergic bronchodilators. Make sure you tell your doctor if you have any other medical problems, especially:

- Brain damage
- Convulsions (seizures) (or history of)
- Diabetes mellitus (sugar diabetes)—Adrenergic bronchodilators may make the condition worse; your doctor may need to change the dose of your diabetes medicine
- Heart or blood vessel disease or
- High blood pressure—Adrenergic bronchodilators may make the condition worse
- Mental disease—Epinephrine may make the condition worse
- Overactive thyroid—The chance of side effects may be increased
- Parkinson's disease—Epinephrine may temporarily increase certain symptoms of Parkinson's disease, such as rigidity and tremor

Before you begin using any new medicine (prescription or nonprescription) or if you develop any new medical problem while you are using this medicine, check with your doctor, nurse, or pharmacist.

Proper Use of This Medicine

For patients using *epinephrine, isoetharine, isoproterenol, or racepinephrine*:

- Do not use if the solution turns pinkish to brownish in color or if it becomes cloudy.

Some epinephrine preparations are available without a doctor's prescription. However, *do not use this medicine without a doctor's prescription, unless your medical problem has been diagnosed as asthma by a doctor.*

Some of these preparations may come with patient directions. Read them carefully before using this medicine.

If you are using this medicine in a nebulizer or in a combination nebulizer and respirator, make sure you understand exactly how to use it. If you have any questions about this, check with your doctor or pharmacist.

For patients using the *inhalation aerosol* form of this medicine:

- *Keep spray away from the eyes because it may cause irritation.*
- *Do not take more than 2 inhalations of this medicine at any one time,* unless otherwise directed by your doctor. Allow 1 to 2 minutes after the first inhalation to make certain that a second inhalation is necessary.
- Save your applicator. Refill units of this medicine may be available.

Use this medicine only as directed. Do not use more of it and do not use it more often than recommended on the label, unless otherwise directed by your doctor. To do so may increase the chance of serious side effects. Inhalation aerosol medicines have been reported to cause death when too much of the medicine was used.

Missed dose—If you are using this medicine regularly and you miss a dose, use it as soon as possible. Then use any remaining doses for that day at regularly spaced intervals. Do not double doses.

Storage—To store this medicine:

- Keep out of the reach of children.
- Store away from heat.
- Store the solution form of this medicine away from direct light. Store the inhalation aerosol form of this medicine away from direct sunlight.
- Keep the medicine from freezing.
- Do not puncture, break, or burn the inhalation aerosol container, even if it is empty.
- Do not keep outdated medicine or medicine no longer needed. Be sure that any discarded medicine is out of the reach of children.

Precautions While Using This Medicine

If you still have trouble breathing after using this medicine, or if your condition becomes worse, check with your doctor at once.

For *diabetic patients* using *epinephrine*:

- This medicine may cause your blood sugar levels to rise. If you notice a change in the results of your blood or urine sugar tests or if you have any questions, check with your doctor.

For patients using the aerosol form of this medicine:

- If you are also using the inhalation aerosol form of an adrenocorticoid (cortisone-like medicine, such as beclomethasone, dexamethasone, flunisolide, or triamcinolone) or ipratropium, *use the adrenergic bronchodilator inhalation aerosol first and then wait about 5 minutes before using the adrenocorticoid or ipratropium inhalation aerosol*, unless otherwise directed by your doctor. This will allow the adrenocorticoid or ipratropium inhalation aerosol to better reach the passages of the lungs (bronchioles) after the adrenergic bronchodilator inhalation aerosol opens them.

For patients using *albuterol inhalation aerosol*:

- If you use all of the medicine in one canister (container) in less than 2 weeks, check with your doctor. You may be using too much of the medicine.

Dryness of the mouth and throat may occur after use of this medicine. Rinsing the mouth with water after each dose may help prevent the dryness.

Some of these preparations may contain sulfites as a preservative. Sulfites may cause an allergic reaction in some people. *If you know that you are allergic to sulfites, do not use this medicine until you have carefully read the label or checked with your doctor or pharmacist to make sure the medicine does not contain sulfites.* Signs of an allergic reaction to sulfites include bluish coloration of skin; severe dizziness or feeling faint; continuing flushing or redness of face or skin; increased wheezing or difficulty in breathing; skin rash, hives, or itching; or swelling of face, lips, or eyelids. *If any of these signs occur, check with your doctor immediately.*

Side Effects of This Medicine

In some animal studies, albuterol and terbutaline were shown to increase the chance of benign (not cancerous) tumors. Terbutaline was also shown to increase the chance of ovarian cysts. The doses given were many times the inhalation dose of albuterol and the oral dose of terbutaline given to humans. It is not known if albuterol or terbutaline increases the chance of tumors in humans, or if terbutaline increases the chance of ovarian cysts in humans.

Along with its needed effects, a medicine may cause some unwanted effects. Although not all of these side effects may occur, if they do occur they may need medical attention.

Check with your doctor immediately if any of the following side effects occur:

Bluish coloration of skin; dizziness (severe) or feeling faint; flushing or redness of face or skin (continuing); increased wheezing or difficulty in breathing; skin rash, hives, or itching; swelling of face, lips, or eyelids

Check with your doctor as soon as possible if any of the following side effects occur:

Rare

Chest discomfort or pain; irregular heartbeat; numbness in hands or feet; unusual bruising

With high doses

Hallucinations (seeing, hearing, or feeling things that are not there)

Symptoms of overdose

Chest discomfort or pain (continuing or severe); chills or fever; convulsions (seizures); dizziness or lightheadedness (continuing or severe); fast or slow heartbeat (continuing); headache (continuing or severe); increase or decrease in blood pressure (severe); irregular or pounding heartbeat (continuing or severe); muscle cramps (severe); nausea or vomiting (continuing or severe); shortness of breath or troubled breathing (severe); trembling (severe); unusual anxiety, nervousness, or restlessness; unusually large pupils or blurred vision; unusual paleness and coldness of skin; weakness (severe)

Other side effects may occur that usually do not need medical attention. These side effects may go away during treatment as your body adjusts to the medicine. However, check with your doctor if any of the following side effects continue or are bothersome:

More common

Nervousness or restlessness; trembling

Less common

Coughing or other bronchial irritation; dizziness or lightheadedness; drowsiness; dryness or irritation of mouth or throat; fast or pounding heartbeat; flushing or redness of face or skin; headache; increased sweating; increase in blood pressure; muscle cramps or twitching; nausea or vomiting; trouble in sleeping; unusual paleness; weakness

Not all of the side effects listed above have been reported for each of these medicines, but they have been reported for at least one of them. All of the adrenergic bronchodilators are similar, so any of the above side effects may occur with any of these medicines.

While you are using albuterol, bitolterol, fenoterol, metaproterenol, or terbutaline, you may notice an unusual or unpleasant taste. Also, pirbuterol may cause changes in smell or taste. These effects may be expected and will go away when you stop using the medicine.

Isoproterenol may cause the saliva to turn pinkish to red. This is to be expected while you are using this medicine.

Other side effects not listed above may also occur in some patients. If you notice any other effects, check with your doctor.

Annual revision: July 1990

BRONCHODILATORS, ADRENERGIC Oral/Injection

This information applies to the following medicines:

Albuterol (al-BYOO-ter-ole)
Ephedrine (e-FED-rin)
Epinephrine (ep-i-NEF-rin)
Ethylnorepinephrine (ETH-il-nor-ep-i-NEF-rin)
Fenoterol (fen-OH-ter-ole)
Isoproterenol (eye-soe-proe-TER-e-nole)
Metaproterenol (met-a-proe-TER-e-nole)
Terbutaline (ter-BYOO-ta-leen)

Some commonly used brand names are:

For Albuterol

In the U.S.

Proventil
Ventolin
Proventil Repetabs

Generic name product may also be available.

In Canada

Novosalmol
Ventolin

Another commonly used name is salbutamol.

For Ephedrine

In the U.S.

Ephed II

Generic name product may also be available.

In Canada

Generic name product may be available.

For Epinephrine

In the U.S.

Adrenalin
EpiPen Jr. Auto-Injector
EpiPen Auto-Injector
Sus-Phrine

Generic name product may also be available.

In Canada

Adrenalin
EpiPen Jr. Auto-Injector
EpiPen Auto-Injector

Generic name product may also be available.

For Ethylnorepinephrine

In the U.S.

Bronkephrine

For Fenoterol*

In Canada

Berotec

For Isoproterenol

In the U.S.

Isuprel
Isuprel Glossets

Generic name product may also be available.

In Canada

Isuprel

Generic name product may also be available.

For Metaproterenol

In the U.S.

Alupent
Metaprel

Generic name product may also be available.

In Canada

Alupent

For Terbutaline

In the U.S.

Brethine
Bricanyl

In Canada

Bricanyl

*Not commercially available in the U.S.

Description

Adrenergic bronchodilators are medicines that open up the bronchial tubes (air passages) of the lungs. They are used to treat the symptoms of bronchial asthma, chronic bronchitis, emphysema, and other lung diseases. They relieve cough, wheezing, shortness of breath, and troubled breathing by increasing the flow of air through the bronchial tubes.

Ephedrine may also be used for the relief of nasal congestion in hay fever or other allergies. Ephedrine injection may be used to treat low blood pressure. In addition, ephedrine may be used in the treatment of narcolepsy (uncontrolled desire for sleep or sudden attacks of sleep) and certain types of mental depression.

Epinephrine injection (not including the auto-injector or the sterile suspension) may also be used in certain heart conditions. In addition, epinephrine injection may be used in eye surgery to stop bleeding, reduce congestion, and dilate the pupil. It may also be applied topically to the skin or mucous membranes to stop bleeding.

Epinephrine injection (including the auto-injector but not the sterile suspension) is used in the emergency treatment of allergic reactions to insect stings, medicines, foods, or other substances. It relieves skin rash, hives, and itching; wheezing; and swelling of the lips, eyelids, tongue, and inside of nose.

Isoproterenol injection and tablets may also be used in the treatment of certain heart disorders.

Adrenergic bronchodilators may be used for other conditions as determined by your doctor.

Ephedrine capsules and syrup are available without a prescription. However, your doctor may have special instructions on the proper dose of ephedrine for your medical condition.

All of the other adrenergic bronchodilators are available only with your doctor's prescription.

These medicines are available in the following dosage forms:

Oral

Albuterol
- Oral solution (Canada)
- Syrup (U.S.)
- Tablets (U.S. and Canada)
- Extended-release tablets (U.S.)

Ephedrine
- Capsules (U.S.)
- Syrup (U.S.)

Fenoterol
- Tablets (Canada)

Isoproterenol
- Tablets (U.S. and Canada)

Metaproterenol
- Syrup (U.S. and Canada)
- Tablets (U.S. and Canada)

Terbutaline
- Tablets (U.S. and Canada)

Parenteral

Albuterol
- Injection (Canada)

Ephedrine
- Injection (U.S. and Canada)

Epinephrine
- Injection (U.S. and Canada)

Ethylnorepinephrine
- Injection (U.S.)

Isoproterenol
- Injection (U.S. and Canada)

Terbutaline
- Injection (U.S.)

It is very important that you read and understand the following information. If any of it causes you special concern, check with your doctor. Also, *if you have any questions* or if you want more information about this medicine or your medical problem, *ask your doctor, nurse, or pharmacist.*

Before Using This Medicine

In deciding to use a medicine, the risks of taking the medicine must be weighed against the good it will do. This is a decision you and your doctor will make. For adrenergic bronchodilators taken by mouth or given by injection, the following should be considered:

Allergies—Tell your doctor if you have ever had any unusual or allergic reaction to albuterol, ephedrine, epinephrine, ethylnorepinephrine, fenoterol, isoproterenol, metaproterenol, or terbutaline. Also tell your doctor and pharmacist if you are allergic to any other substances, such as foods, preservatives, or dyes.

Pregnancy—
- *For albuterol*: Albuterol has not been studied in pregnant women. However, studies in animals have shown that albuterol causes birth defects when given in doses many times the usual human dose. In addition, although albuterol has been reported to delay preterm labor when taken by mouth, it has not been shown to stop preterm labor or prevent labor at term.
- *For ephedrine*: Studies on birth defects with ephedrine have not been done in either humans or animals. When ephedrine is used just before or during labor, its effects on the newborn infant or on the growth and development of the child are not known.
- *For epinephrine*: Epinephrine has not been studied in pregnant women. However, studies in animals have shown that epinephrine causes birth defects when given in doses many times the usual human dose. Also, use of epinephrine during pregnancy may decrease the supply of oxygen to the fetus. Epinephrine is not recommended for use during labor since it may delay the second stage of labor. In addition, high doses of epinephrine that decrease contractions of the uterus may result in excessive bleeding when used during labor and delivery.
- *For ethylnorepinephrine and isoproterenol*: Studies on birth defects with ethylnorepinephrine or isoproterenol have not been done in either humans or animals.
- *For fenoterol*: Fenoterol has not been shown to cause birth defects or other problems in humans.
- *For metaproterenol*: Metaproterenol has not been studied in pregnant women. However, studies in animals have shown that metaproterenol causes birth defects when given in doses many times the usual human dose. Also, studies in animals have shown that metaproterenol causes death of the animal fetus when given in doses many times the usual human dose.
- *For terbutaline*: Terbutaline has not been studied in pregnant women. It has not been shown to cause birth defects in animal studies when given in doses many times the usual human dose. However, terbutaline given by injection during pregnancy has been reported to cause an unusually fast heartbeat in the fetus. Although terbutaline is used to delay preterm labor, it may also delay labor at term.

Breast-feeding—
- *For albuterol, fenoterol, isoproterenol, and metaproterenol*: It is not known whether albuterol, fenoterol, isoproterenol, or metaproterenol passes into the breast milk. However, these medicines have not been reported to cause problems in nursing babies.
- *For ephedrine and epinephrine*: Ephedrine and epinephrine pass into the breast milk and may cause unwanted side effects in babies of mothers using ephedrine or epinephrine.
- *For terbutaline*: Although terbutaline passes into the breast milk, it has not been reported to cause problems in nursing babies.

Children—Although there is no specific information about the use of albuterol, ethylnorepinephrine, fenoterol, isoproterenol, metaproterenol, or terbutaline in children, these medicines are not expected to cause different side effects or problems in children than they do in adults.

Infants may be especially sensitive to the effects of ephedrine.

Infants and children may be especially sensitive to the effects of epinephrine. Fainting has occurred after epinephrine was given to children with asthma.

Older adults—Many medicines have not been tested in older people. Therefore, it may not be known whether

they work exactly the same way they do in younger adults or if they cause different side effects or problems in older people. There is no specific information about the use of adrenergic bronchodilators in the elderly.

Other medicines—Although certain medicines should not be used together at all, in other cases two different medicines may be used together even if an interaction might occur. In these cases, your doctor may want to change the dose, or other precautions may be necessary. When you are taking adrenergic bronchodilators, it is especially important that your doctor and pharmacist know if you are taking any of the following:

- Beta-blockers (acebutolol [e.g., Sectral], atenolol [e.g., Tenormin], betaxolol [e.g., Betoptic, Kerlone], carteolol [e.g., Cartrol], labetalol [e.g., Normodyne], levobunolol [e.g., Betagan], metoprolol [e.g., Lopressor], nadolol [e.g., Corgard], oxprenolol [e.g., Trasicor], penbutolol [e.g., Levatol], pindolol [e.g., Visken], propranolol [e.g., Inderal], sotalol [e.g., Sotacor], timolol [e.g., Blocadren, Timoptic])—These medicines may prevent the adrenergic bronchodilators from working properly
- Cocaine or
- Ergoloid mesylates (e.g., Hydergine) or
- Ergotamine (e.g., Gynergen) or
- Maprotiline (e.g., Ludiomil) or
- Tricyclic antidepressants (medicine for depression)—The effects of these medicines on the heart and blood vessels may be increased
- Digitalis glycosides (heart medicine)—The chance of irregular heartbeat may be increased
- Monoamine oxidase (MAO) inhibitors (furazolidone [e.g., Furoxone], isocarboxazid [e.g., Marplan], pargyline [e.g., Eutonyl], phenelzine [e.g., Nardil], procarbazine [e.g., Matulane], tranylcypromine [e.g., Parnate])—Taking adrenergic bronchodilators while you are taking or within 2 weeks of taking monoamine oxidase (MAO) inhibitors may increase the effects of MAO inhibitors

Other medical problems—The presence of other medical problems may affect the use of adrenergic bronchodilators. Make sure you tell your doctor if you have any other medical problems, especially:

- Brain damage
- Convulsions (seizures) (history of)
- Diabetes mellitus (sugar diabetes)—Adrenergic bronchodilators may make the condition worse; your doctor may need to change the dose of your diabetes medicine
- Enlarged prostate—Ephedrine may make the condition worse
- Heart or blood vessel disease or
- High blood pressure—Adrenergic bronchodilators may make the condition worse
- Mental disease—Epinephrine may make the condition worse
- Overactive thyroid—The chance of side effects may be increased
- Parkinson's disease—Epinephrine may temporarily increase certain symptoms of Parkinson's disease, such as rigidity and tremor

Before you begin using any new medicine (prescription or nonprescription) or if you develop any new medical problem while you are using this medicine, check with your doctor, nurse, or pharmacist.

Proper Use of This Medicine

For patients taking *albuterol extended-release tablets:*

- Swallow the tablet whole.
- Do not crush, break, or chew before swallowing.

For patients taking *ephedrine:*

- Ephedrine may cause trouble in sleeping. To help prevent this, *take the last dose of ephedrine for each day a few hours before bedtime.* If you have any questions about this, check with your doctor.

For patients taking *isoproterenol sublingual tablets*:

- Do not chew or swallow the tablet. This medicine is meant to be absorbed through the lining of the mouth. Place the tablet under your tongue (sublingual) and let it slowly dissolve there. Do not swallow until the tablet has dissolved completely.

For patients using the *injection* form of this medicine:

- Do not use the epinephrine solution or suspension if it turns pinkish to brownish in color or if the solution becomes cloudy.
- *Use this medicine only for the conditions for which it was prescribed by your doctor.*
- Keep this medicine ready for use at all times. Also, keep the telephone numbers for your doctor and the nearest hospital emergency room readily available.
- Check the expiration date on the injection regularly. Replace the medicine before that date.
- This medicine is for injection only. If you will be giving yourself the injections, make sure you understand exactly how to give them. If you have any questions about this, check with your doctor.

For patients using *epinephrine injection* for an *allergic reaction emergency*:

- If an allergic reaction as described by your doctor occurs, *use the epinephrine injection immediately.*
- Notify your doctor immediately or go to the nearest hospital emergency room. If you have used the epinephrine injection, be sure to tell your doctor.
- If you have been stung by an insect, remove the insect's stinger with your fingernails, if possible. Be careful not to squeeze, pinch, or push it deeper into the skin. Ice packs or sodium bicarbonate (baking soda) soaks, if available, may then be applied to the area stung.
- If you are using the epinephrine auto-injector (automatic injection device):

  —It is important that you do not remove the safety cap on the auto-injector until you are ready to use it. This prevents accidental activation of the device during storage and handling.

—Epinephrine auto-injector comes with patient directions. Read them carefully before you actually need to use this medicine. Then, when an emergency arises, you will know how to inject the epinephrine.

—To use the epinephrine auto-injector:

- Remove the gray safety cap.
- Place the black tip on the thigh, at a right angle to the leg.
- Press hard into the thigh until the auto-injector functions. Hold in place for several seconds. Then remove the auto-injector and discard.
- Massage the injection area for 10 seconds.

Use this medicine only as directed. Do not use more of it and do not use it more often than your doctor ordered, or more than recommended on the label unless otherwise directed by your doctor. To do so may increase the chance of side effects.

Missed dose—If you are using this medicine regularly and you miss a dose, use it as soon as possible. Then use any remaining doses for that day at regularly spaced intervals. Do not double doses.

Storage—To store this medicine:

- Keep out of the reach of children.
- Store away from heat and direct light.
- Do not store the capsule or tablet form of this medicine in the bathroom, near the kitchen sink, or in other damp places. Heat or moisture may cause the medicine to break down.
- Keep the injection or syrup form of this medicine from freezing.
- Store the suspension form of epinephrine injection in the refrigerator.
- Do not keep outdated medicine or medicine no longer needed. Be sure that any discarded medicine is out of the reach of children.

Precautions While Using This Medicine

If after using this medicine for asthma or other breathing problems you still have trouble breathing, or if your condition becomes worse, check with your doctor at once.

For *diabetic patients* using *epinephrine*:

- This medicine may cause your blood sugar levels to rise. If you notice a change in the results of your blood or urine sugar tests or if you have any questions, check with your doctor.

For patients using *epinephrine injection* (including the auto-injector but not the sterile suspension) or *ethylnorepinephrine injection*:

- Some of the injection preparations may contain sulfites as a preservative. Sulfites may cause an allergic reaction in some people. If you know that you are allergic to sulfites, carefully read the label on the injection or check with your doctor or pharmacist to find out if the injection contains sulfites.
- Although epinephrine injection may contain sulfites, it is still used to treat serious allergic reactions or other emergency conditions because other medicines may not work properly in a life-threatening situation.
- If you have any questions about when or whether you should use an epinephrine injection that contains sulfites, check with your doctor.
- Signs of an allergic reaction to sulfites include bluish coloration of skin; severe dizziness or feeling faint; continuing flushing or redness of face or skin; increased wheezing or difficulty in breathing; skin rash, hives, or itching; or swelling of face, lips, or eyelids. *If any of these signs occur, check with your doctor immediately.*

Side Effects of This Medicine

In some animal studies, albuterol and terbutaline were shown to increase the chance of benign (not cancerous) tumors. Terbutaline was also shown to increase the chance of ovarian cysts. The doses given were many times the oral dose of albuterol or terbutaline given to humans. It is not known if albuterol or terbutaline increases the chance of tumors in humans, or if terbutaline increases the chance of ovarian cysts in humans.

Along with its needed effects, a medicine may cause some unwanted effects. Although not all of these side effects may occur, if they do occur they may need medical attention.

Check with your doctor immediately if any of the following side effects occur:

Bluish coloration of skin; dizziness (severe) or feeling faint; flushing or redness of face or skin (continuing); increased wheezing or difficulty in breathing; skin rash, hives, or itching; swelling of face, lips, or eyelids

Check with your doctor as soon as possible if any of the following side effects occur:

Rare

Chest discomfort or pain; irregular heartbeat

With high doses

Hallucinations (seeing, hearing, or feeling things that are not there); mood or mental changes (reported for ephedrine only)

Symptoms of overdose

Bluish coloration of skin; chest discomfort or pain (continuing or severe); chills or fever; convulsions (seizures); dizziness or lightheadedness (continuing or severe); fast or slow heartbeat (continuing); headache (continuing or severe); increase or decrease in blood pressure (severe); irregular or pounding heartbeat (continuing or severe); muscle cramps (severe); nausea or vomiting (continuing or severe); shortness of breath or troubled breathing (severe); trembling (severe); unusual anxiety, nervousness, or restlessness; unusually large pupils or blurred vision; unusual paleness and coldness of skin; weakness (severe)

Other side effects may occur that usually do not need medical attention. These side effects may go away during treatment as your body adjusts to the medicine. However, check with your doctor if any of the following side effects continue or are bothersome:

More common

Nervousness or restlessness; trembling

Less common

Difficult or painful urination; dizziness or lightheadedness; drowsiness; fast or pounding heartbeat; flushing or redness of face or skin; headache; heartburn; increased sweating; increase in blood pressure; loss of appetite; muscle cramps or twitching; nausea or vomiting; trouble in sleeping; unusual paleness; weakness

Not all of the side effects listed above have been reported for each of these medicines, but they have been reported for at least one of them. All of the adrenergic bronchodilators are similar, so any of the above side effects may occur with any of these medicines.

While you are using albuterol, fenoterol, metaproterenol, or terbutaline, you may notice an unusual or unpleasant taste. This may be expected and will go away when you stop using the medicine.

Isoproterenol sublingual (under-the-tongue) tablets may cause the saliva to turn pinkish to red. This is to be expected while you are using this medicine.

Other side effects not listed above may also occur in some patients. If you notice any other effects, check with your doctor.

Additional Information

Once a medicine has been approved for marketing for a certain use, experience may show that it is also useful for other medical problems. Although these uses are not included in product labeling, some of the adrenergic bronchodilators are used in certain patients with the following medical conditions:

- Premature labor (terbutaline)
- Urticaria (hives) (ephedrine)
- Hemorrhage (bleeding) of gums and teeth (epinephrine)
- Priapism (prolonged abnormal erection of penis) (epinephrine)

Other than the above information, there is no additional information relating to proper use, precautions, or side effects for these uses.

Annual revision: July 1990

BRONCHODILATORS, XANTHINE-DERIVATIVE Systemic

This information applies to the following medicines:

Aminophylline (am-in-OFF-i-lin)
Dyphylline (DYE-fi-lin)
Oxtriphylline (ox-TRYE-fi-lin)
Theophylline (thee-OFF-i-lin)

Some commonly used brand names are:

For Aminophylline

In the U.S.

Aminophyllin
Phyllocontin
Somophyllin
Somophyllin-DF
Truphylline

Generic name product may also be available.

In Canada

Corophyllin
Palaron
Phyllocontin
Phyllocontin-350

Generic name product may also be available.

For Dyphylline

In the U.S.

Dilor
Dilor-400
Dyflex
Dyflex 400
Lufyllin
Lufyllin-400
Neothylline
Thylline

Generic name product may also be available.

In Canada

Protophylline

For Oxtriphylline

In the U.S.

Choledyl
Choledyl Delayed-release
Choledyl SA

Generic name product may also be available.

In Canada

Apo-Oxtriphylline
Choledyl
Choledyl SA
Novotriphyl

For Theophylline

In the U.S.

Accurbron
Aerolate
Aerolate III
Aerolate Jr.
Aerolate Sr.
Aquaphyllin
Asmalix
Bronkodyl
Constant-T
Duraphyl
Elixicon
Elixomin
Elixophyllin
Elixophyllin SR
Lanophyllin
Lixolin
Quibron-T Dividose
Quibron-T/SR Dividose

Respbid	Theoclear L.A.-260 Cenules
Slo-bid Gyrocaps	Theocot
Slo-Phyllin	Theo-Dur
Slo-Phyllin Gyrocaps	Theo-Dur Sprinkle
Solu-Phyllin	Theolair
Somophyllin-CRT	Theolair-SR
Somophyllin-T	Theomar
Sustaire	Theon
Theo-24	Theophylline SR
Theo 250	Theospan-SR
Theobid Duracaps	Theostat 80
Theobid Jr. Duracaps	Theo-Time
Theochron	Theovent Long-Acting
Theoclear-80	T-Phyl
Theoclear L.A.-130 Cenules	Truxophyllin
	Uniphyl

Generic name product may also be available.

In Canada

Elixophyllin	Somophyllin-T
PMS Theophylline	Theochron
Pulmophylline	Theo-Dur
Quibron-T	Theolair
Quibron-T/SR	Theolair-SR
Slo-Bid	Theo-SR
Somophyllin-12	Uniphyl

For Theophylline Sodium Glycinate

In the U.S.

Synophylate

Description

Xanthine-derivative bronchodilators are used to treat and/or prevent the symptoms of bronchial asthma, chronic bronchitis, and emphysema. These medicines relieve cough, wheezing, shortness of breath, and troubled breathing. They work by opening up the bronchial tubes (air passages of the lungs) and increasing the flow of air through them.

Aminophylline and theophylline may also be used for other conditions as determined by your doctor.

The oral liquid, uncoated or chewable tablet, capsule, and rectal enema dosage forms of xanthine-derivative bronchodilators may be used for treatment of the acute attack and for chronic (long-term) treatment. If rectal enemas are used, they should not be used for longer than 48 hours because they may cause rectal irritation. The enteric-coated tablet and extended-release dosage forms are usually used only for chronic treatment. Sometimes, aminophylline rectal suppositories may be used but they generally are not recommended because of possible poor absorption.

These medicines are available only with your doctor's prescription, in the following dosage forms:

Oral

Aminophylline
- Oral solution (U.S. and Canada)
- Tablets (U.S. and Canada)
- Enteric-coated tablets (U.S.)
- Extended-release tablets (U.S. and Canada)

Dyphylline
- Elixir (U.S. and Canada)
- Oral solution (Canada)
- Tablets (U.S. and Canada)

Oxtriphylline
- Oral solution (U.S. and Canada)
- Syrup (U.S. and Canada)
- Tablets (U.S. and Canada)
- Delayed-release tablets (U.S.)
- Extended-release tablets (U.S. and Canada)

Theophylline
- Capsules (U.S. and Canada)
- Extended-release capsules (U.S. and Canada)
- Elixir (U.S. and Canada)
- Oral solution (U.S. and Canada)
- Oral suspension (U.S.)
- Syrup (U.S.)
- Tablets (U.S. and Canada)
- Extended-release tablets (U.S. and Canada)

Theophylline Sodium Glycinate
- Elixir (U.S.)

Parenteral

Aminophylline
- Injection (U.S. and Canada)

Aminophylline and Sodium Chloride
- Injection (U.S.)

Dyphylline
- Injection (U.S.)

Theophylline in Dextrose
- Injection (U.S. and Canada)

Rectal

Aminophylline
- Enema (U.S.)
- Suppositories (U.S. and Canada)

It is very important that you read and understand the following information. If any of it causes you special concern, check with your doctor. Also, *if you have any questions* or if you want more information about this medicine or your medical problem, *ask your doctor, nurse, or pharmacist.*

Before Using This Medicine

In deciding to use a medicine, the risks of taking the medicine must be weighed against the good it will do. This is a decision you and your doctor will make. For xanthine-derivative bronchodilators, the following should be considered:

Allergies—Tell your doctor if you have ever had any unusual or allergic reaction to aminophylline, caffeine, dyphylline, ethylenediamine (contained in aminophylline), oxtriphylline, theobromine, or theophylline. Also tell your doctor and pharmacist if you are allergic to any other substances, such as foods, preservatives, or dyes.

Diet—Make certain your doctor and pharmacist know if you are on any special diet, such as a low-sodium or low-sugar diet or a high-protein, low-carbohydrate or low-protein, high-carbohydrate diet.

Avoid eating or drinking large amounts of caffeine-containing foods or beverages, such as chocolate, cocoa, tea, coffee, and cola drinks, because they may increase the central nervous system (CNS) stimulant effects of the xanthine-derivative bronchodilators.

Also, eating charcoal broiled foods every day while taking aminophylline, oxtriphylline, or theophylline may keep these medicines from working properly.

Pregnancy—Studies on birth defects have not been done in humans. However, some studies in animals have shown that theophylline (including aminophylline and oxtriphylline) causes birth defects when given in doses many times the human dose. Also, use of aminophylline, oxtriphylline, or theophylline during pregnancy may cause unwanted effects such as fast heartbeat, jitteriness, irritability, gagging, vomiting, and breathing problems in the newborn infant. Studies on birth defects with dyphylline have not been done in either humans or animals.

Breast-feeding—Theophylline passes into the breast milk and may cause irritability, fretfulness, or trouble in sleeping in nursing babies of mothers taking aminophylline, oxtriphylline, or theophylline. Although dyphylline passes into the breast milk, it has not been reported to cause problems in nursing babies.

Children—The side effects of xanthine-derivative bronchodilators are more likely to occur in newborn infants, who are usually more sensitive to the effects of these medicines.

Older adults—The side effects of xanthine-derivative bronchodilators are more likely to occur in elderly patients, who are usually more sensitive than younger adults to the effects of these medicines.

Other medicines—Although certain medicines should not be used together at all, in other cases two different medicines may be used together even if an interaction might occur. In these cases, your doctor may want to change the dose, or other precautions may be necessary. When you are taking xanthine-derivative bronchodilators, it is especially important that your doctor and pharmacist know if you are taking any of the following:

- Adrenocorticoids (cortisone-like medicine)—Use of these medicines with aminophylline and sodium chloride injection may result in too much sodium in the blood
- Beta-blockers (acebutolol [e.g., Sectral], atenolol [e.g., Tenormin], betaxolol [e.g., Kerlone], carteolol [e.g., Cartrol], labetalol [e.g., Normodyne], metoprolol [e.g., Lopressor], nadolol [e.g., Corgard], oxprenolol [e.g., Trasicor], penbutolol [e.g., Levatol], pindolol [e.g., Visken], propranolol [e.g., Inderal], sotalol [e.g., Sotacor], timolol [e.g., Blocadren])—Use of these medicines with xanthine-derivative bronchodilators may prevent either the beta-blocker or the bronchodilator from working properly
- Cimetidine (e.g., Tagamet) or
- Ciprofloxacin or
- Erythromycin (e.g., E-Mycin) or
- Nicotine chewing gum (e.g., Nicorette) or
- Norfloxacin or
- Ranitidine (e.g., Zantac) or
- Troleandomycin (e.g., TAO)—These medicines may increase the effects of aminophylline, oxtriphylline, or theophylline
- Phenytoin (e.g., Dilantin)—The effects of phenytoin may be decreased by aminophylline, oxtriphylline, or theophylline
- Smoking tobacco or marijuana—If you smoke or have smoked tobacco or marijuana regularly within the last 2 years, the amount of medicine you need may vary, depending on how much and how recently you have smoked

Other medical problems—The presence of other medical problems may affect the use of xanthine-derivative bronchodilators. Make sure you tell your doctor if you have any other medical problems, especially:

- Alcohol abuse (or history of) or
- Fever or
- Liver disease or
- Respiratory infections, such as influenza (flu)—The effects of aminophylline, oxtriphylline, or theophylline may be increased
- Diarrhea—The absorption of xanthine-derivative bronchodilators, especially the extended-release dosage forms, may be decreased; therefore, the effects of these medicines may be decreased
- Enlarged prostate or
- Heart disease or
- High blood pressure or
- Stomach ulcer (or history of) or other stomach problems—Xanthine-derivative bronchodilators may make the condition worse
- Fibrocystic breast disease—Symptoms of this disease may be increased by xanthine-derivative bronchodilators
- Irritation or infection of the rectum or lower colon—Aminophylline rectal enema may make the condition worse, since rectal use of this medicine may be irritating
- Kidney disease—The effects of dyphylline may be increased
- Overactive thyroid—The effects of aminophylline, oxtriphylline, or theophylline may be decreased

Before you begin using any new medicine (prescription or nonprescription) or if you develop any new medical problem while you are using this medicine, check with your doctor, nurse, or pharmacist.

Proper Use of This Medicine

For patients *taking this medicine by mouth:*

- If you are taking the *capsule, tablet, liquid, or extended-release (not including the once-a-day capsule or tablet) form* of this medicine, *it works best when taken with a glass of water on an empty stomach* (either 30 minutes to 1 hour before meals or 2 hours after meals). That way the medicine will get into the blood sooner. However, in some cases your doctor may want you to take this medicine with meals or right after meals to lessen stomach upset. If you have any questions about how you should be taking this medicine, check with your doctor.

- If you are taking the *once-a-day capsule or tablet form* of this medicine, *some products are to be taken each morning after fasting overnight and at least 1 hour before eating. However, other products are to be taken in the morning or evening with or without food. Be sure you understand exactly how to take the medicine prescribed for you.* Try to take the medicine about the same time each day.
- There are several different forms of xanthine-derivative bronchodilator capsules and tablets. If you are taking:

  —enteric-coated or delayed-release tablets, swallow the tablets whole. Do not crush, break, or chew before swallowing.

  —extended-release capsules, swallow the capsule whole. Do not crush, break, or chew before swallowing.

  —extended-release tablets, swallow the tablets whole. Do not break (unless tablet is scored for breaking), crush, or chew before swallowing.

For patients using the *aminophylline enema:*

- This medicine usually comes with patient directions. Read them carefully before using this medicine.
- If crystals form in the solution, dissolve them by placing the closed container of solution in warm water. If the crystals do not dissolve, do not use the medicine.

Use this medicine only as directed by your doctor. Do not use more of it, do not use it more often, and do not use it for a longer time than your doctor ordered. To do so may increase the chance of serious side effects.

In order for this medicine to help your medical problem, it must be taken every day in regularly spaced doses as ordered by your doctor. This is necessary to keep a constant amount of this medicine in the blood. To help keep the amount constant, do not miss any doses.

Missed dose—If you do miss a dose of this medicine, take it as soon as possible. However, if it is almost time for your next dose, skip the missed dose and go back to your regular dosing schedule. Do not double doses.

Storage—To store this medicine:

- Keep out of the reach of children.
- Store away from heat and direct light.
- Do not store the capsule or tablet form of this medicine in the bathroom, near the kitchen sink, or in other damp places. Heat or moisture may cause the medicine to break down.
- Keep the liquid form of this medicine from freezing.
- Do not keep outdated medicine or medicine no longer needed. Be sure that any discarded medicine is out of the reach of children.

Precautions While Using This Medicine

Your doctor should check your progress at regular visits, especially for the first few weeks after you begin using this medicine. A blood test may be taken to help your doctor decide whether the dose of this medicine should be changed.

Do not change brands or dosage forms of this medicine without first checking with your doctor. Different products may not work the same way. If you refill your medicine and it looks different, check with your pharmacist.

This medicine may add to the central nervous system (CNS) stimulant effects of caffeine-containing foods or beverages such as chocolate, cocoa, tea, coffee, and cola drinks. *Avoid eating or drinking large amounts of these foods or beverages while using this medicine.* If you have any questions about this, check with your doctor.

For patients using *aminophylline, oxtriphylline, or theophylline*:

- Do not eat charcoal-broiled foods every day while using this medicine since these foods may keep the medicine from working properly.
- *Check with your doctor at once if you develop symptoms of influenza (flu) or a fever* since either of these may increase the chance of side effects with this medicine.
- Also, *check with your doctor if diarrhea occurs* because the dose of this medicine may need to be changed.

For patients using the *aminophylline enema*:

- If burning or other irritation of the rectal area occurs after you use this medicine and if it continues or becomes worse, check with your doctor.

Side Effects of This Medicine

Along with its needed effects, a medicine may cause some unwanted effects. Although not all of these side effects may occur, if they do occur they may need medical attention.

Check with your doctor as soon as possible if any of the following side effects occur:

Less common

Heartburn and/or vomiting

Rare

Skin rash or hives (with aminophylline only)

Symptoms of overdose

Bloody or black, tarry stools; confusion or change in behavior; convulsions (seizures); diarrhea; dizziness or lightheadedness; fast breathing; fast, pounding, or irregular heartbeat; flushing or redness of face; headache; increased urination; irritability; loss of appetite;

muscle twitching; nausea (continuing or severe) or vomiting; stomach cramps or pain; trembling; trouble in sleeping; unusual tiredness or weakness; vomiting blood or material that looks like coffee grounds

Other side effects may occur that usually do not need medical attention. These side effects may go away during treatment as your body adjusts to the medicine. However, check with your doctor if any of the following side effects continue or are bothersome:

More common

Nausea; nervousness or restlessness

Less common

Burning or irritation of rectum (for rectal enema only)

Other side effects not listed above may also occur in some patients. If you notice any other effects, check with your doctor.

Additional Information

Once a medicine has been approved for marketing for a certain use, experience may show that it is also useful for other medical problems. Although this use is not included in product labeling, aminophylline and theophylline are used in certain patients with the following medical condition:

- Apnea (breathing problem) in newborns

Other than the above information, there is no additional information relating to proper use, precautions, or side effects for this use.

Annual revision: July 1990

BUPROPION Systemic†

A commonly used brand name in the U.S. is Wellbutrin.
Another commonly used name is amfebutamone.

†Not commercially available in Canada.

Description

Bupropion (byoo-PROE-pee-on) is an antidepressant or "mood elevator." It works in the central nervous system (CNS) to relieve mental depression.

This medicine is available only with your doctor's prescription, in the following dosage form:

Oral

- Tablets (U.S.)

It is very important that you read and understand the following information. If any of it causes you special concern, check with your doctor. Also, *if you have any questions* or if you want more information about this medicine or your medical problem, *ask your doctor, nurse, or pharmacist.*

Before Using This Medicine

In deciding to use a medicine, the risks of taking the medicine must be weighed against the good it will do. This is a decision you and your doctor will make. For bupropion, the following should be considered:

Allergies—Tell your doctor if you have ever had any unusual or allergic reaction to bupropion. Also tell your doctor and pharmacist if you are allergic to any other substances, such as foods, preservatives, or dyes.

Pregnancy—Studies have not been done in pregnant women. However, bupropion has not been reported to cause birth defects or other problems in animal studies.

Breast-feeding—Bupropion passes into breast milk. Because it may cause unwanted effects in nursing babies, use of bupropion is not recommended during breast-feeding.

Children—Studies on this medicine have been done only in adult patients, and there is no specific information comparing use of bupropion in children with use in other age groups.

Older adults—This medicine has been tested in a limited number of patients 60 years of age and older and has not been shown to cause different side effects or problems in older people than it does in younger adults.

Other medicines—Although certain medicines should not be used together at all, in other cases 2 different medicines may be used together even if an interaction might occur. In these cases, your doctor may want to change the dose, or other precautions may be necessary. When you are taking bupropion, it is especially important that your doctor and pharmacist know if you are taking any of the following:

- Alcohol or
- Antipsychotics (medicine for mental illness) or
- Fluoxetine (e.g., Prozac) or
- Lithium (e.g., Lithane) or
- Maprotiline (e.g., Ludiomil) or
- Trazodone (e.g., Desyrel) or
- Tricyclic antidepressants (amitriptyline [e.g., Elavil], amoxapine [e.g., Asendin], clomipramine [e.g., Anafranil], desipramine [e.g., Pertofrane], doxepin [e.g., Sinequan], imipramine [e.g., Tofranil], nortriptyline [e.g.,

Aventyl], protriptyline [e.g., Vivactil], trimipramine [e.g., Surmontil])—Using these medicines with bupropion may increase the risk of seizures
- Monoamine oxidase (MAO) inhibitors (furazolidone [e.g., Furoxone], isocarboxazid [e.g., Marplan], phenelzine [e.g., Nardil], procarbazine [e.g., Matulane], selegiline [e.g., Eldepryl], tranylcypromine [e.g., Parnate])—Taking bupropion while you are taking or within 2 weeks of taking monoamine oxidase (MAO) inhibitors may increase the chance of side effects; at least 14 days should be allowed between stopping treatment with one medicine and starting treatment with the other

Other medical problems—The presence of other medical problems may affect the use of bupropion. Make sure you tell your doctor if you have any other medical problems, especially:

- Anorexia nervosa or
- Brain tumor or
- Bulimia or
- Head injury, history of, or
- Seizure disorder—The risk of seizures may be increased when bupropion is taken by patients with these conditions
- Bipolar disorder (manic-depressive illness) or
- Other nervous, mental, or emotional conditions—Bupropion may make the condition worse
- Heart attack (recent) or heart disease—Bupropion may cause unwanted effects on the heart
- Kidney disease or
- Liver disease—Higher blood levels of bupropion may result, increasing the chance of side effects

Proper Use of This Medicine

Use bupropion only as directed by your doctor. Do not use more of it, do not use it more often, and do not use it for a longer time than your doctor ordered. To do so may increase the chance of side effects.

To lessen stomach upset, this medicine may be taken with food, unless your doctor has told you to take it on an empty stomach.

Usually this medicine must be taken for several weeks before you feel better. Your doctor should check your progress at regular visits.

Missed dose—If you miss a dose of this medicine, take it as soon as possible. However, if it is within 4 hours of your next dose, skip the missed dose and go back to your regular dosing schedule. Do not double doses.

Storage—To store this medicine:

- Keep out of the reach of children.
- Store away from heat and direct light.
- Do not store in the bathroom, near the kitchen sink, or in other damp places. Heat or moisture may cause the medicine to break down.
- Do not keep outdated medicine or medicine no longer needed. Be sure that any discarded medicine is out of the reach of children.

Precautions While Using This Medicine

Your doctor should check your progress at regular visits, especially during the first few months of treatment with this medicine. The amount of bupropion you take may have to be changed often to meet the needs of your condition and to help avoid unwanted effects.

If you have been taking this medicine regularly, do not stop taking it without first checking with your doctor. Your doctor may want you to reduce gradually the amount you are taking before stopping completely. This will help reduce the possibility of side effects.

Drinking of alcoholic beverages should be limited or avoided, if possible, while taking bupropion. This will help prevent unwanted effects.

This medicine may cause some people to feel a false sense of well-being, or to become drowsy, dizzy, or less alert than they are normally. *Make sure you know how you react to this medicine before you drive, use machines, or do anything else that could be dangerous if you are dizzy or are not alert and clearheaded.*

Side Effects of This Medicine

Along with its needed effects, a medicine may cause some unwanted effects. Although not all of these side effects may occur, if they do occur they may need medical attention.

Check with your doctor as soon as possible if any of the following side effects occur:

More common

Agitation or excitement; anxiety; confusion; fast or irregular heartbeat; headache (severe); restlessness; trouble in sleeping

Less common

Hallucinations; skin rash

Rare

Fainting; convulsions (seizures), especially with higher doses

Other side effects may occur that usually do not need medical attention. These side effects may go away during treatment as your body adjusts to the medicine. However, check with your doctor if any of the following side effects continue or are bothersome:

More common

Constipation; decrease in appetite; dizziness; dryness of mouth; increased sweating; nausea or vomiting; tremor; weight loss (unusual)

Less common

Blurred vision; difficulty concentrating; drowsiness; fever or chills; hostility or anger; tiredness; unusual feeling of well-being

Other side effects not listed above may also occur in some patients. If you notice any other effects, check with your doctor.

Annual revision: 07/24/91

BUSERELIN Systemic*

A commonly used brand name in Canada is Suprefact.

*Not commercially available in the U.S.

Description

Buserelin (BYOO-se-rel-in) is used to treat cancer of the prostate gland.

It is similar to a hormone normally released from the hypothalamus gland. When given regularly, buserelin decreases testosterone levels. Reducing the amount of testosterone in the body is one way of treating cancer of the prostate.

Buserelin is available only with your doctor's prescription, in the following dosage forms:

Nasal

- Nasal solution (Canada)

Parenteral

- Injection (Canada)

It is very important that you read and understand the following information. If any of it causes you special concern, check with your doctor. Also, *if you have any questions* or if you want more information about this medicine or your medical problem, *ask your doctor, nurse, or pharmacist.*

Before Using This Medicine

In deciding to use a medicine, the risks of taking the medicine must be weighed against the good it will do. This is a decision you and your doctor will make. For buserelin, the following should be considered:

Allergies—Tell your doctor if you have ever had any unusual or allergic reaction to buserelin.

Fertility—Buserelin causes sterility which may be permanent. If you intend to have children, discuss this with your doctor before receiving this medicine.

Older adults—Many medicines have not been studied specifically in older people. Therefore, it may not be known whether they work exactly the same way they do in younger adults. Although there is no specific information comparing use of buserelin in the elderly to use in other age groups, it has been used mostly in elderly patients and is not expected to cause different side effects or problems in older people than it does in younger adults.

Before you begin using any new medicine (prescription or nonprescription) or if you develop any new medical problem while you are using this medicine, check with your doctor, nurse, or pharmacist.

Proper Use of This Medicine

Buserelin comes with patient directions. Read these instructions carefully.

For patients using the *injection* form of this medicine:

- Use the syringes provided in the kit. Other syringes may not provide the correct dose. These disposable syringes and needles are already sterilized and designed to be used one time only and then discarded. If you have any questions about the use of disposable syringes, check with your doctor, nurse, or pharmacist.
- After use, dispose of the syringes and needles in a safe manner. If a special container is not provided, ask your doctor, nurse, or pharmacist about the best way to dispose of syringes and needles.

For patients using the *nasal solution* form of this medicine:

- Use the nebulizer (spray pump) provided. Directions about how to use it are included. If you have any questions about the use of the nebulizer, check with your doctor, nurse, or pharmacist.

Use this medicine only as directed by your doctor. Do not use more or less of it, and do not use it more often than your doctor ordered. The exact amount of medicine you need has been carefully worked out. Using too much may increase the chance of side effects, while using too little may not improve your condition.

Buserelin sometimes causes unwanted effects such as hot flashes or decreased sexual ability. It may also cause a temporary increase in pain, trouble in urinating, or weakness in your legs when you begin to use it. However, it is very important that you continue to use the medicine, even after you begin to feel better. *Do not stop using this medicine without first checking with your doctor.*

Missed dose—If you miss a dose of this medicine, use it as soon as possible. However, if it is almost time for the next dose, skip the missed dose and go back to your regular dosing schedule. Do not double doses.

Storage—To store this medicine:

- Keep out of the reach of children.
- Store away from heat and direct light.
- Keep the medicine from freezing.
- Do not keep outdated medicine or medicine no longer needed. Dispose of used syringes properly in the container provided. Be sure that any discarded medicine is out of the reach of children.

Precautions While Using This Medicine

It is very important that your doctor check your progress at regular visits to make sure that this medicine is working properly and to check for unwanted effects.

Side Effects of This Medicine

Along with its needed effects, a medicine may cause some unwanted effects. Some side effects will have signs or symptoms that you can see or feel. Your doctor may watch for others by doing certain tests. Some of the unwanted effects that may be caused by buserelin are listed below. Although not all of these side effects may occur, if they do occur they may need medical attention.

The following side effects are symptoms of a flareup of your condition that may occur during the first few days of treatment. After a few days, these symptoms should lessen. However, they may require medical attention. Check with your doctor if any of the following side effects occur or get worse:

Bone pain; numbness or tingling of hands or feet; trouble in urinating; weakness in legs

Other side effects may occur that usually do not need medical attention. These side effects may go away during treatment as your body adjusts to the medicine. However, check with your doctor if any of the following side effects continue or are bothersome:

More common

Decrease in sexual desire; impotence; sudden sweating and feelings of warmth ("hot flashes")

Less common

Burning, itching, redness, or swelling at place of injection; diarrhea; dry or sore nose (with nasal solution); headache (with nasal solution); increased sweating (with nasal solution); loss of appetite; nausea or vomiting; swelling and increased tenderness of breasts; swelling of feet or lower legs

Other side effects not listed above may also occur in some patients. If you notice any other effects, check with your doctor.

Annual revision: 05/05/93

BUSPIRONE Systemic

A commonly used brand name in the U.S. and Canada is BuSpar.

Description

Buspirone (byoo-SPYE-rone) is used to treat certain anxiety disorders or to relieve the symptoms of anxiety. However, buspirone is usually not used for anxiety or tension caused by the stress of everyday life.

It is not known exactly how buspirone works to relieve the symptoms of anxiety.

Buspirone is available only with your doctor's prescription, in the following dosage form:

Oral

- Tablets (U.S. and Canada)

It is very important that you read and understand the following information. If any of it causes you special concern, check with your doctor. Also, *if you have any questions* or if you want more information about this medicine or your medical problem, *ask your doctor, nurse, or pharmacist.*

Before Using This Medicine

In deciding to use a medicine, the risks of taking the medicine must be weighed against the good it will do. This is a decision you and your doctor will make. For buspirone, the following should be considered:

Allergies—Tell your doctor if you have ever had any unusual or allergic reaction to buspirone. Also tell your doctor and pharmacist if you are allergic to any other substances, such as foods, preservatives, or dyes.

Pregnancy—Buspirone has not been studied in pregnant women. However, buspirone has not been shown to cause birth defects or other problems in animal studies.

Breast-feeding—It is not known whether buspirone passes into the breast milk of humans.

Children—Studies on this medicine have been done only in adult patients, and there is no specific information comparing use of buspirone in children up to 18 years of age with use in other age groups.

Older adults—This medicine has been tested and has not been shown to cause different side effects or problems in older people than it does in younger adults.

Other medicines—Although certain medicines should not be used together at all, in other cases 2 different medicines may be used together even if an interaction might occur. In these cases, your doctor may want to change the dose, or other precautions may be necessary. When you are taking buspirone, it is especially important that your doctor and pharmacist know if you are taking any of the following:

- Monoamine oxidase (MAO) inhibitors (furazolidone [e.g., Furoxone], isocarboxazid [e.g., Marplan], phenelzine [e.g., Nardil], procarbazine [e.g., Matulane], selegiline at doses more than 10 mg a day [e.g., Eldepryl], tranylcypromine [e.g., Parnate])—Taking buspirone while you are taking or within 2 weeks of taking monoamine oxidase (MAO) inhibitors may cause high blood pressure

Other medical problems—The presence of other medical problems may affect the use of buspirone. Make sure you tell your doctor if you have any other medical problems, especially:

- Drug abuse or dependence (history of)—There is a possibility that buspirone could become habit-forming, causing mental or physical dependence
- Kidney disease or
- Liver disease—The effects of buspirone may be increased, which may increase the chance of side effects

Before you begin using any new medicine (prescription or nonprescription) or if you develop any new medical problem while you are using this medicine, check with your doctor, nurse, or pharmacist.

Proper Use of This Medicine

Take buspirone only as directed by your doctor. Do not take more of it, do not take it more often, and do not take it for a longer time than your doctor ordered. To do so may increase the chance of unwanted effects.

After you begin taking buspirone, 1 to 2 weeks may pass before you feel the full effects of this medicine.

Dosing—The dose of buspirone will be different for different patients. *Follow your doctor's orders or the directions on the label.* The following information includes only the average doses of buspirone. *If your dose is different, do not change it* unless your doctor tells you to do so.

- The number of tablets that you take depends on the strength of the medicine. Also, *the number of doses you take each day, the time allowed between doses, and the length of time you take the medicine depend on the medical problem for which you are taking buspirone.*
- For *oral* dosage forms (tablets):
  —Adults: To start, 5 milligrams three times a day. Your doctor may increase your dose by 5 milligrams a day every few days if needed. However, the dose is usually not more than 60 milligrams a day.
  —Children up to 18 years of age: Dose must be determined by the doctor.

Missed dose—If you are taking this medicine regularly and you miss a dose, take it as soon as possible. However, if it is almost time for your next dose, skip the missed dose and go back to your regular dosing schedule. Do not double doses.

Storage—To store this medicine:

- Keep out of the reach of children.
- Store away from heat and direct light.
- Do not store in the bathroom, near the kitchen sink, or in other damp places. Heat or moisture may cause the medicine to break down.
- Do not keep outdated medicine or medicine no longer needed. Be sure that any discarded medicine is out of the reach of children.

Precautions While Using This Medicine

If you will be using buspirone regularly for a long time, your doctor should check your progress at regular visits to make sure the medicine does not cause unwanted effects.

Buspirone, when taken with alcohol or other CNS depressants (medicines that slow down the nervous system, possibly causing drowsiness), may increase the chance of drowsiness. Some examples of CNS depressants are antihistamines or medicine for hay fever, other allergies, or colds; sedatives, tranquilizers, or sleeping medicine; prescription pain medicine or narcotics; barbiturates; medicine for seizures; muscle relaxants; or anesthetics, including some dental anesthetics. Check with your doctor before taking any of the above while you are taking this medicine.

Buspirone may cause some people to become dizzy, lightheaded, drowsy, or less alert than they are normally. *Make sure you know how you react to this medicine before you drive, use machines, or do anything else that could be dangerous if you are dizzy or are not alert.*

If you think you or someone else may have taken an overdose of buspirone, get emergency help at once. Some symptoms of an overdose are severe dizziness or drowsiness; severe stomach upset, including nausea or vomiting; or unusually small pupils.

Side Effects of This Medicine

Along with its needed effects, a medicine may cause some unwanted effects. Although not all of these side effects may occur, if they do occur they may need medical attention.

Check with your doctor as soon as possible if any of the following side effects occur:

Rare

Chest pain; confusion or mental depression; fast or pounding heartbeat; muscle weakness; numbness, tingling, pain, or weakness in hands or feet; sore throat or fever; uncontrolled movements of the body

Symptoms of overdose

Dizziness (severe); drowsiness (severe); stomach upset, including nausea or vomiting (severe); unusually small pupils

Other side effects may occur that usually do not need medical attention. These side effects may go away during treatment as your body adjusts to the medicine. However, check with your doctor if any of the following side effects continue or are bothersome:

More common

Dizziness or lightheadedness; headache; nausea; restlessness, nervousness, or unusual excitement

Less common or rare

Blurred vision; decreased concentration; drowsiness (more common with doses of more than 20 mg per day); dryness of mouth; muscle pain, spasms, cramps, or stiffness; ringing in the ears; stomach upset; trouble in sleeping, nightmares, or vivid dreams; unusual tiredness or weakness

Other side effects not listed above may also occur in some patients. If you notice any other effects, check with your doctor.

Annual revision: 03/09/93

BUSULFAN Systemic

A commonly used brand name in the U.S. and Canada is Myleran.

Description

Busulfan (byoo-SUL-fan) belongs to the group of medicines known as alkylating agents. It is used to treat some kinds of cancer.

Busulfan seems to act by interfering with the function of the bone marrow. Since the growth of normal body cells may also be affected by busulfan, other effects will also occur. Some of these may be serious and must be reported to your doctor. Other effects may not be serious but may cause concern. Some effects may not occur for months or years after the medicine is used.

Before you begin treatment with busulfan, you and your doctor should talk about the good this medicine will do as well as the risks of using it.

Busulfan is available only with your doctor's prescription, in the following dosage form:

Oral

- Tablets (U.S. and Canada)

It is very important that you read and understand the following information. If any of it causes you special concern, check with your doctor. Also, *if you have any questions* or if you want more information about this medicine or your medical problem, *ask your doctor, nurse, or pharmacist.*

Before Using This Medicine

In deciding to use a medicine, the risks of taking the medicine must be weighed against the good it will do. This is a decision you and your doctor will make. For busulfan, the following should be considered:

Allergies—Tell your doctor if you have ever had any unusual or allergic reaction to busulfan.

Pregnancy—Although only one case has been reported, there is a chance that this medicine may cause birth defects if either the male or the female is taking it at the time of conception or if it is taken during pregnancy. In addition, many cancer medicines may cause sterility which could be permanent. Sterility may occur with busulfan and the possibility should be kept in mind.

Be sure that you have discussed this with your doctor before taking this medicine. It is best to use some kind of birth control while you are taking busulfan. Tell your doctor right away if you think you have become pregnant while taking busulfan.

Breast-feeding—It is not known whether busulfan passes into breast milk. However, because this medicine may cause serious side effects, breast-feeding is generally not recommended while you are taking it.

Children—Although there is no specific information comparing use of busulfan in children with use in other age groups, this medicine is not expected to cause different side effects or problems in children than it does in adults.

Older adults—Many medicines have not been studied specifically in older people. Therefore, it may not be known whether they work exactly the same way they do in younger adults. Although there is no specific information comparing use of busulfan in the elderly with use in other age groups, this medicine is not expected to cause different side effects or problems in older people than it does in younger adults.

Other medicines—Although certain medicines should not be used together at all, in other cases two different medicines may be used together even if an interaction might occur. In these cases, your doctor may want to change the dose, or other precautions may be necessary. When taking busulfan it is especially important that your doctor and pharmacist know if you are taking any of the following:

- Amphotericin B by injection (e.g., Fungizone) or
- Antithyroid agents (medicine for overactive thyroid) or
- Azathioprine (e.g., Imuran) or
- Chloramphenicol (e.g., Chloromycetin) or
- Colchicine or
- Flucytosine (e.g., Ancobon) or
- Ganciclovir (e.g., Cytovene) or
- Interferon (e.g., Intron A, Roferon-A) or
- Plicamycin (e.g., Mithracin) or
- Zidovudine (e.g., AZT, Retrovir) or
- If you have ever been treated with x-rays or cancer medicines—Busulfan may increase the effects of these medicines or radiation therapy on the blood
- Probenecid (e.g., Benemid) or
- Sulfinpyrazone (e.g., Anturane)—Busulfan may raise the amount of uric acid in the blood. Since these medicines are used to lower uric acid levels, they may not be as effective in patients taking busulfan

Other medical problems—The presence of other medical problems may affect the use of busulfan. Make sure you tell your doctor if you have any other medical problems, especially:

- Chickenpox (including recent exposure) or
- Herpes zoster (shingles)—Risk of severe disease affecting other parts of the body
- Gout (history of) or
- Kidney stones (or history of)—Busulfan may increase levels of uric acid in the body, which can cause gout or kidney stones
- Head injury or
- Convulsions (history of)—Very high doses of busulfan can cause convulsions
- Infection—Busulfan may decrease your body's ability to fight infection

Before you begin using any new medicine (prescription or nonprescription) or if you develop any new medical problem while you are using this medicine, check with your doctor, nurse, or pharmacist.

Proper Use of This Medicine

Take this medicine only as directed by your doctor. Do not take more or less of it, and do not take it more often than your doctor ordered. The exact amount of medicine you need has been carefully worked out. Taking too much may increase the chance of side effects, while taking too little may not improve your condition.

Take each dose at the same time each day to make sure it has the best effect.

While you are taking this medicine, your doctor may want you to drink extra fluids so that you will pass more urine. This will help prevent kidney problems and keep your kidneys working well.

This medicine sometimes causes nausea and vomiting. However, it is very important that you continue to use the medicine, even if you begin to feel ill. *Do not stop taking this medicine without first checking with your doctor.* Ask your doctor, nurse, or pharmacist for ways to lessen these effects.

If you vomit shortly after taking a dose of busulfan, check with your doctor. You will be told whether to take the dose again or to wait until the next scheduled dose.

Missed dose—If you miss a dose of this medicine, skip the missed dose and go back to your regular dosing schedule. Do not double doses.

Storage—To store this medicine:

- Keep out of the reach of children.
- Store away from heat and direct light.
- Do not store in the bathroom, near the kitchen sink, or in other damp places. Heat or moisture may cause the medicine to break down.
- Do not keep outdated medicine or medicine no longer needed. Be sure that any discarded medicine is out of the reach of children.

Precautions While Using This Medicine

It is very important that your doctor check your progress at regular visits to make sure that this medicine is working properly and to check for unwanted effects.

While you are being treated with busulfan, and after you stop treatment with it, *do not have any immunizations (vaccinations) without your doctor's approval.* Busulfan may lower your body's resistance and there is a chance you might get the infection the immunization is meant to prevent. In addition, other persons living in your household should not take oral polio vaccine since there is a chance they could pass the polio virus on to you. Also, avoid persons who have recently taken oral polio vaccine. Do not get close to them, and do not stay in the same room with them for very long. If you cannot take these precautions, you should consider wearing a protective face mask that covers the nose and mouth.

Busulfan can temporarily lower the number of white blood cells in your blood, increasing the chance of getting an infection. It can also lower the number of platelets, which are necessary for proper blood clotting. If this occurs, there are certain precautions you can take, especially when your blood count is low, to reduce the risk of infection or bleeding:

- If you can, avoid people with infections. *Check with your doctor immediately* if you think you are getting an infection or if you get a fever or chills, cough or hoarseness, lower back or side pain, or painful or difficult urination.
- *Check with your doctor immediately* if you notice any unusual bleeding or bruising; black, tarry stools; blood in urine or stools; or pinpoint red spots on your skin.
- Be careful when using a regular toothbrush, dental floss, or toothpick. Your medical doctor, dentist, or nurse may recommend other ways to clean your teeth and gums. Check with your medical doctor before having any dental work done.
- Do not touch your eyes or the inside of your nose unless you have just washed your hands and have not touched anything else in the meantime.
- Be careful not to cut yourself when you are using sharp objects such as a safety razor or fingernail or toenail cutters.
- Avoid contact sports or other situations where bruising or injury could occur.

Before you have any medical tests, tell the medical doctor in charge that you are taking this medicine. The results of some body tissue studies may be affected by this medicine.

Side Effects of This Medicine

Along with their needed effects, medicines like busulfan can sometimes cause unwanted effects such as lung problems, blood problems, and other side effects. These and others are described below. Also, because of the way these medicines act on the body, there is a chance that they might cause other unwanted effects that may not occur until months or years after the medicine is used. These delayed effects may include certain types of cancer, such as leukemia. Discuss these possible effects with your doctor.

Although not all of these side effects may occur, if they do occur they may need medical attention.

Check with your doctor or nurse immediately if any of the following side effects occur:

More common

Black, tarry stools; blood in urine or stools; pinpoint red spots on skin; unusual bleeding or bruising

Less common

Cough or hoarseness; fever or chills; lower back or side pain; painful or difficult urination

Check with your doctor as soon as possible if any of the following side effects occur:

Less common

Joint pain; shortness of breath; sores in mouth and on lips; swelling of feet or lower legs

Rare

Blurred vision

Other side effects may occur that usually do not need medical attention. These side effects may go away during treatment as your body adjusts to the medicine. Also, your doctor or nurse may be able to tell you about ways to prevent or reduce some of these side effects. Check with your doctor or nurse if any of the following side effects continue or are bothersome or if you have any questions about them:

More common

Darkening of skin; missed or irregular menstrual periods

Less common

Confusion; diarrhea; dizziness; loss of appetite; nausea and vomiting; unusual tiredness or weakness; weight loss (sudden)

After you stop taking busulfan, it may still produce some side effects that need attention. During this period of time, check with your doctor if you notice any of the following:

Black, tarry stools; blood in urine or stools; cough or hoarseness; fever or chills; lower back or side pain; painful or difficult urination; pinpoint red spots on skin; shortness of breath; unusual bleeding or bruising

Other side effects not listed above may also occur in some patients. If you notice any other effects, check with your doctor.

Annual revision: 06/12/92

BUTALBITAL AND ACETAMINOPHEN Systemic†

Some commonly used brand names are:

For Butalbital and Acetaminophen†

In the U.S.

Bancap	Phrenilin Forte
Bucet	Sedapap
Conten	Tencon
Phrenilin	Triaprin

Generic name product may also be available.

For Butalbital, Acetaminophen, and Caffeine†

In the U.S.

Amaphen	Fioricet
Anolor-300	Isocet
Anoquan	Isopap
Arcet	Medigesic
Butace	Pacaps
Dolmar	Pharmagesic
Endolor	Repan
Esgic	Tencet
Esgic-Plus	Triad
Ezol	Two-Dyne
Femcet	

Generic name product may also be available.

†Not commercially available in Canada.

Description

Butalbital (byoo-TAL-bi-tal) and acetaminophen (a-seat-a-MIN-oh-fen) combination is a pain reliever and relaxant. It is used to treat tension headaches. Butalbital belongs to the group of medicines called barbiturates (bar-BI-tyoo-rates). Barbiturates act in the central nervous system (CNS) to produce their effects.

When you take butalbital for a long time, your body may get used to it so that larger amounts are needed to produce the same effects. This is called tolerance to the medicine. Also, butalbital may become habit-forming (causing mental or physical dependence) when it is used for a long time or in large doses. Physical dependence may lead to withdrawal side effects when you stop taking the medicine. In patients who get headaches, the first symptom of withdrawal may be new (rebound) headaches.

Some butalbital and acetaminophen combinations also contain caffeine (kaf-EEN). Caffeine may help to relieve headaches. However, caffeine can also cause physical dependence when it is used for a long time. This may lead to withdrawal (rebound) headaches when you stop taking it.

Butalbital and acetaminophen combination may also be used for other kinds of headaches or other kinds of pain as determined by your doctor.

Butalbital and acetaminophen combinations are available only with your doctor's prescription in the following dosage forms:

Oral

Butalbital and Acetaminophen
- Capsules (U.S.)
- Tablets (U.S.)

Butalbital, Acetaminophen, and Caffeine
- Capsules (U.S.)
- Tablets (U.S.)

It is very important that you read and understand the following information. If any of it causes you special concern, check with your doctor. Also, *if you have any questions* or if you want more information about this medicine or your medical problem, *ask your doctor, nurse, or pharmacist.*

Before Using This Medicine

In deciding to use a medicine, the risks of taking the medicine must be weighed against the good it will do. This is a decision you and your doctor will make. For butalbital and acetaminophen combinations, the following should be considered:

Allergies—Tell your doctor if you have ever had any unusual or allergic reaction to butalbital or other barbiturates, or to acetaminophen, aspirin, or caffeine. Also tell your doctor and pharmacist if you are allergic to any other substances, such as foods, preservatives, or dyes.

Pregnancy—
- *For butalbital:* Barbiturates such as butalbital have been shown to increase the chance of birth defects in humans. Also, one study in humans has suggested that barbiturates taken during pregnancy may increase the chance of brain tumors in the baby.

  Butalbital may cause breathing problems in the newborn baby if taken just before or during delivery.
- *For acetaminophen:* Although studies on birth defects with acetaminophen have not been done in pregnant women, it has not been reported to cause birth defects or other problems.
- *For caffeine:* Studies in humans have not shown that caffeine (contained in some of these combination medicines) causes birth defects. However, use of large amounts of caffeine during pregnancy may cause problems with the heart rhythm and the growth of the fetus. Also, studies in animals have shown that caffeine causes birth defects when given in very large doses (amounts equal to those present in 12 to 24 cups of coffee a day).

Breast-feeding—
- *For butalbital:* Barbiturates such as butalbital pass into the breast milk and may cause drowsiness, unusually slow heartbeat, shortness of breath, or troubled breathing in nursing babies.

- *For acetaminophen:* Although acetaminophen has not been shown to cause problems in nursing babies, it passes into the breast milk in small amounts.
- *For caffeine:* Caffeine (present in some butalbital and acetaminophen combinations) passes into the breast milk in small amounts. Taking caffeine in the amounts present in these medicines has not been shown to cause problems in nursing babies. However, studies have shown that nursing babies may appear jittery and have trouble in sleeping when their mothers drink large amounts of caffeine-containing beverages. Therefore, breast-feeding mothers who use caffeine-containing medicines should probably limit the amount of caffeine they take in from other medicines or from beverages.

Children—

- *For butalbital:* Although barbiturates such as butalbital often cause drowsiness, some children become excited after taking them.
- *For acetaminophen:* Acetaminophen has been tested in children and, in effective doses, has not been shown to cause different side effects or problems than it does in adults.
- *For caffeine:* There is no specific information comparing use of caffeine in children up to 12 years of age with use in other age groups. However, caffeine is not expected to cause different side effects or problems in children than it does in adults.

Older adults—

- *For butalbital:* Certain side effects, such as confusion, excitement, or mental depression, may be especially likely to occur in elderly patients, who are usually more sensitive than younger adults to the effects of the butalbital in this combination medicine.
- *For acetaminophen:* Acetaminophen has been tested and has not been shown to cause different side effects or problems in older people than it does in younger adults.
- *For caffeine:* Many medicines have not been studied specifically in older people. Therefore, it may not be known whether they work exactly the same way they do in younger adults or if they cause different side effects or problems in older people. There is no specific information comparing use of caffeine in the elderly with use in other age groups.

Other medicines—Although certain medicines should not be used together at all, in other cases two different medicines may be used together even if an interaction might occur. In these cases, your doctor may want to change the dose, or other precautions may be necessary. When you are taking a butalbital and acetaminophen combination, it is especially important that your doctor and pharmacist know if you are taking any of the following:

- Adrenocorticoids (cortisone-like medicines) or
- Anticoagulants (blood thinners), or
- Carbamazepine (e.g., Tegretol) or
- Contraceptives, oral (birth control pills) containing estrogen, or
- Corticotropin (e.g., ACTH)—Butalbital may make these medicines less effective
- Antidepressants, tricyclic (amitriptyline [e.g., Elavil], amoxapine [e.g., Asendin], clomipramine [e.g., Anafranil], desipramine [e.g., Pertofrane], doxepin [e.g., Sinequan], imipramine [e.g., Tofranil], nortriptyline [e.g., Aventyl], protriptyline [e.g., Vivactil], trimipramine [e.g., Surmontil]) or
- Central nervous system (CNS) depressants (medicines that often cause drowsiness)—These medicines may add to the effects of butalbital and increase the chance of drowsiness or other side effects
- Divalproex (e.g., Depakote) or
- Valproic acid (e.g., Depakene)—The chance of side effects may be increased

Other medical problems—The presence of other medical problems may affect the use of butalbital and acetaminophen combinations. Make sure you tell your doctor if you have any other medical problems, especially:

- Alcohol abuse (or history of) or
- Drug abuse or dependence (or history of)—Dependence on butalbital may develop; also, acetaminophen may cause liver damage in people who abuse alcohol
- Asthma (or history of), emphysema, or other chronic lung disease or
- Hepatitis or other liver disease or
- Hyperactivity (in children) or
- Kidney disease—The chance of serious side effects may be increased
- Diabetes mellitus (sugar diabetes) or
- Mental depression or
- Overactive thyroid or
- Porphyria (or history of)—Butalbital can make these conditions worse
- Heart disease (severe)—The caffeine in some butalbital and acetaminophen combinations can make some kinds of heart disease worse

Before you begin using any new medicine (prescription or nonprescription) or if you develop any new medical problem while you are using this medicine, check with your doctor, nurse, or pharmacist.

Proper Use of This Medicine

Take this medicine only as directed by your doctor. Do not take more of it, do not take it more often, and do not take it for a longer time than your doctor ordered. If butalbital and acetaminophen combination is taken regularly (for example, every day), it may become habit-forming (causing mental or physical dependence). The caffeine in some butalbital and acetaminophen combinations can also increase the chance of dependence. Dependence is especially likely to occur in patients who take these medicines to relieve frequent headaches. Taking too much of this medicine may also lead to liver damage or other medical problems.

This medicine will relieve a headache best if you *take it as soon as the headache begins.* If you get warning signs of a migraine, take this medicine as soon as you are sure that the migraine is coming. This may even stop the headache pain from occurring. *Lying down in a quiet, dark room for a while after taking the medicine also helps to relieve headaches.*

People who get a lot of headaches may need to take a different medicine to help prevent headaches. *It is important that you follow your doctor's directions about taking the other medicine, even if your headaches continue to occur.* Headache-preventing medicines may take several weeks to start working. Even after they do start working, your headaches may not go away completely. However, your headaches should occur less often, and they should be less severe and easier to relieve than before. This will reduce the amount of headache relievers that you need. If you do not notice any improvement after several weeks of headache-preventing treatment, check with your doctor.

Missed dose—If your doctor has ordered you to take this medicine according to a regular schedule and you miss a dose, take it as soon as you remember. However, if it is almost time for your next dose, skip the missed dose and go back to your regular dosing schedule. *Do not double doses.*

Storage—To store this medicine:

- Keep out of the reach of children. Overdose is especially dangerous in young children.
- Store away from heat and direct light.
- Do not store this medicine in the bathroom, near the kitchen sink, or in other damp places. Heat or moisture may cause the medicine to break down.
- Do not keep outdated medicine or medicine no longer needed. Be sure that any discarded medicine is out of the reach of children.

Precautions While Using This Medicine

Check with your doctor:

- If the medicine stops working as well as it did when you first started using it. This may mean that you are in danger of becoming dependent on the medicine. *Do not try to get better pain relief by increasing the dose.*
- *If you are having headaches more often than you did before you started taking this medicine.* This is especially important if a new headache occurs within 1 day after you took your last dose of this medicine, headaches begin to occur every day, or a headache continues for several days in a row. This may mean that you are dependent on the medicine. *Continuing to take this medicine will cause even more headaches later on.* Your doctor can give you advice on how to relieve the headaches.

Check the labels of all nonprescription (over-the-counter [OTC]) or prescription medicines you now take. If any contain a barbiturate or acetaminophen, be especially careful, since taking them while taking this medicine may lead to overdose. If you have any questions about this, check with your doctor or pharmacist.

The butalbital in this medicine will add to the effects of alcohol and other CNS depressants (medicines that slow down the nervous system, possibly causing drowsiness). Some examples of CNS depressants are antihistamines or medicine for hay fever, other allergies, or colds; sedatives, tranquilizers, or sleeping medicine; other prescription pain medicine; narcotics; other barbiturates; medicine for seizures; muscle relaxants; or anesthetics, including some dental anesthetics. Also, drinking large amounts of alcoholic beverages regularly while taking this medicine may increase the chance of liver damage, especially if you take more of this medicine than your doctor ordered or if you take it regularly for a long time. *Therefore, do not drink alcoholic beverages, and check with your doctor before taking any of the medicines listed above, while you are using this medicine.*

This medicine may cause some people to become drowsy, dizzy, or lightheaded. *Make sure you know how you react to this medicine before you drive, use machines, or do anything else that could be dangerous if you are dizzy or are not alert and clearheaded.*

Before you have any medical tests, tell the person in charge that you are taking this medicine. Caffeine (present in some butalbital and acetaminophen combinations) interferes with the results of certain tests that use dipyridamole (e.g., Persantine) to help show how well blood is flowing to your heart. Caffeine should not be taken for 8 to 12 hours before the test. The results of other tests may also be affected by butalbital and acetaminophen combinations.

Before having any kind of surgery (including dental surgery) or emergency treatment, tell the medical doctor or dentist in charge that you are taking this medicine. Serious side effects can occur if your medical doctor or dentist gives you certain medicines without knowing that you have taken butalbital.

If you have been taking large amounts of this medicine, or if you have been taking it regularly for several weeks or more, *do not suddenly stop taking it without first checking with your doctor.* Your doctor may want you to reduce gradually the amount you are taking before stopping completely in order to lessen the chance of withdrawal side effects.

If you think you or anyone else may have taken an overdose of this medicine, get emergency help at once. Taking an overdose of this medicine or taking alcohol or CNS depressants with this medicine may lead to unconsciousness or possibly death. Signs of butalbital overdose include severe drowsiness, confusion, severe weakness, shortness of breath or unusually slow or troubled breathing, slurred speech, staggering, and unusually slow heartbeat. Signs of severe acetaminophen poisoning may not occur until 2 to 4 days after the overdose is taken, but treatment to prevent liver damage or death must be started within 24 hours or less after the overdose is taken.

Side Effects of This Medicine

Along with its needed effects, a medicine may cause some unwanted effects. Although not all of these side effects may occur, if they do occur they may need medical attention.

Check with your doctor immediately if any of the following side effects occur, especially if several of them occur together:

Rare

Bleeding or crusting sores on lips; chest pain; fever with or without chills; hive-like swellings (large) on eyelids, face, lips, and/or tongue; muscle cramps or pain; red, thickened, or scaly skin; shortness of breath, troubled breathing, tightness in chest, or wheezing; skin rash, itching, or hives; sores, ulcers, or white spots in mouth (painful); sore throat

Symptoms of overdose

Anxiety, confusion, excitement, irritability, nervousness, restlessness, or trouble in sleeping (severe, especially with products containing caffeine); convulsions (seizures) (for products containing caffeine); diarrhea, especially if occurring together with increased sweating, loss of appetite, and stomach cramps or pain; dizziness, lightheadedness, drowsiness, or weakness, (severe); frequent urination (for products containing caffeine); hallucinations (seeing, hearing, or feeling things that are not there); increased sensitivity to touch or pain (for products containing caffeine); muscle trembling or twitching (for products containing caffeine); nausea or vomiting, sometimes with blood; ringing or other sounds in ears (for products containing caffeine); seeing flashes of "zig-zag" lights (for products containing caffeine); shortness of breath or unusually slow or troubled breathing; slow, fast, or irregular heartbeat; slurred speech; staggering; swelling, pain, or tenderness in the upper abdomen or stomach area; unusual movements of the eyes

Also, check with your doctor as soon as possible if any of the following side effects occur:

Less common

Confusion (mild); mental depression; unusual excitement (mild)

Rare

Bloody or black, tarry stools; bloody urine; pinpoint red spots on skin; swollen or painful glands; unusual bleeding or bruising; unusual tiredness or weakness (mild)

Other side effects may occur that usually do not need medical attention. These side effects may go away during treatment as your body adjusts to the medicine. However, check with your doctor if any of the following side effects continue or are bothersome:

More common

Bloated or "gassy" feeling; dizziness or lightheadedness (mild); drowsiness (mild); nausea, vomiting, or stomach pain (occurring without other symptoms of overdose)

Other side effects not listed above may also occur in some patients. If you notice any other effects, check with your doctor.

Annual revision: 07/14/92

BUTALBITAL AND ASPIRIN Systemic

Some commonly used brand names are:

For Butalbital and Aspirin†

In the U.S.

Axotal

For Butalbital, Aspirin‡, and Caffeine

In the U.S.

Butalgen
Fiorgen
Fiorinal
Fiormor
Fortabs
Isobutal
Isobutyl
Isolin
Isollyl
Laniroif
Lanorinal
Marnal
Vibutal

Generic name product may also be available.

In Canada

Fiorinal
Tecnal

Other commonly used names for this combination medicine are butalbital-AC and butalbital compound.

†Not commercially available in Canada.

‡In Canada, *Aspirin* is a brand name. Acetylsalicylic acid is the generic name in Canada. ASA, a synonym for acetylsalicylic acid, is the term that commonly appears on Canadian product labels.

Description

Butalbital (byoo-TAL-bi-tal) and aspirin (AS-pir-in) combination is a pain reliever and relaxant. It is used to treat tension headaches. Butalbital belongs to the group of medicines called barbiturates (bar-BI-tyoo-rates). Barbiturates act in the central nervous system (CNS) to produce their effects.

When you use butalbital for a long time, your body may get used to it so that larger amounts are needed to produce the same effects. This is called tolerance to the medicine. Also, butalbital may become habit-forming (causing mental or physical dependence) when it is used for a long time or in large doses. Physical dependence may lead to withdrawal side effects when you stop taking the medicine. In patients who get headaches, the first symptom of withdrawal may be new (rebound) headaches.

Some of these medicines also contain caffeine (kaf-EEN). Caffeine may help to relieve headaches. However, caffeine can also cause physical dependence when it is used for a long time. This may lead to withdrawal (rebound) headaches when you stop taking it.

Butalbital and aspirin combination is sometimes also used for other kinds of headaches or other kinds of pain, as determined by your doctor.

Butalbital and aspirin combination is available only with your doctor's prescription, in the following dosage forms:

Oral

Butalbital and Aspirin
- Tablets (U.S.)

Butalbital, Aspirin, and Caffeine
- Capsules (U.S. and Canada)
- Tablets (U.S. and Canada)

It is very important that you read and understand the following information. If any of it causes you special concern, check with your doctor. Also, *if you have any questions* or if you want more information about this medicine or your medical problem, *ask your doctor, nurse, or pharmacist.*

Before Using This Medicine

In deciding to use a medicine, the risks of taking the medicine must be weighed against the good it will do. This is a decision you and your doctor will make. For butalbital and aspirin combinations, the following should be considered:

Allergies—Tell your doctor if you have ever had any unusual or allergic reaction to butalbital or other barbiturates; aspirin or other salicylates, including methyl salicylate (oil of wintergreen); caffeine; or any of the following medicines:

Diclofenac (e.g., Voltaren)
Diflunisal (e.g., Dolobid)
Etodolac (e.g., Lodine)
Fenoprofen (e.g., Nalfon)
Floctafenine (e.g., Idarac)
Flurbiprofen, oral (e.g., Ansaid)
Ibuprofen (e.g., Motrin)
Indomethacin (e.g., Indocin)
Ketoprofen (e.g., Orudis)
Ketorolac (e.g., Toradol)
Meclofenamate (e.g., Meclomen)
Mefenamic acid (e.g., Ponstel)
Nabumetone (e.g., Relafen)
Naproxen (e.g., Naprosyn)
Oxyphenbutazone (e.g., Tandearil)
Phenylbutazone (e.g., Butazolidin)
Piroxicam (e.g., Feldene)
Sulindac (e.g., Clinoril)
Suprofen (e.g., Suprol)
Tenoxicam (e.g., Mobiflex)
Tiaprofenic acid (e.g., Surgam)
Tolmetin (e.g., Tolectin)
Zomepirac (e.g., Zomax)

Also tell your doctor and pharmacist if you are allergic to any other substances, such as foods, preservatives, or dyes.

Pregnancy—
- *For butalbital:* Barbiturates such as butalbital have been shown to increase the chance of birth defects in humans. Also, one study in humans has suggested that barbiturates taken during pregnancy may increase the chance of brain tumors in the baby. Butalbital may cause breathing problems in the newborn baby if taken just before or during delivery.
- *For aspirin:* Although studies in humans have not shown that aspirin causes birth defects, it has caused birth defects in animal studies.

  Do not take aspirin during the last 3 months of pregnancy unless it has been ordered by your doctor. Some reports have suggested that use of aspirin late in pregnancy may cause a decrease in the newborn's weight and possible death of the fetus or newborn baby. However, the mothers in these reports had been taking much larger amounts of aspirin than are usually recommended. Studies of mothers taking aspirin in the doses that are usually recommended did not show these unwanted effects.

  There is a chance that regular use of aspirin late in pregnancy may cause unwanted effects on the heart or blood flow in the fetus or in the newborn baby. Also, use of aspirin during the last 2 weeks of pregnancy may cause bleeding problems in the fetus before or during delivery or in the newborn baby. In addition, too much use of aspirin during the last 3 months of pregnancy may increase the length of pregnancy, prolong labor, cause other problems during delivery, or cause severe bleeding in the mother before, during, or after delivery.
- *For caffeine:* Studies in humans have not shown that caffeine causes birth defects. However, use of large amounts of caffeine during pregnancy may cause problems with the heart rhythm and the growth of the fetus. Also, studies in animals have shown that caffeine causes birth defects when given in very large

doses (amounts equal to the amount in 12 to 24 cups of coffee a day).

Breast-feeding—Although this combination medicine has not been reported to cause problems, the chance always exists, especially if the medicine is taken for a long time or in large amounts.

- *For butalbital:* Barbiturates such as butalbital pass into the breast milk and may cause drowsiness, unusually slow heartbeat, shortness of breath, or troubled breathing in nursing babies.
- *For aspirin:* Aspirin passes into the breast milk. However, taking aspirin in the amounts present in these combination medicines has not been reported to cause problems in nursing babies.
- *For caffeine:* The caffeine in some of these combination medicines passes into the breast milk in small amounts. Taking caffeine in the amounts present in these medicines has not been reported to cause problems in nursing babies. However, studies have shown that nursing babies may appear jittery and have trouble in sleeping when their mothers drink large amounts of caffeine-containing beverages. Therefore, breast-feeding mothers who use caffeine-containing medicines should probably limit the amount of caffeine they take in from other medicines or from beverages.

Children—

- *For butalbital:* Although barbiturates such as butalbital often cause drowsiness, some children become excited after taking them.
- *For aspirin: Do not give a medicine containing aspirin to a child with fever or other symptoms of a virus infection, especially flu or chickenpox, without first discussing its use with your child's doctor.* This is very important because aspirin may cause a serious illness called Reye's syndrome in children with fever caused by a virus infection, especially flu or chickenpox. Children who do not have a virus infection may also be more sensitive to the effects of aspirin, especially if they have a fever or have lost large amounts of body fluid because of vomiting, diarrhea, or sweating. This may increase the chance of side effects during treatment.
- *For caffeine:* There is no specific information comparing use of caffeine in children up to 12 years of age with use in other age groups. However, caffeine is not expected to cause different side effects or problems in children than it does in adults.

Teenagers—*Teenagers with fever or other symptoms of a virus infection, especially flu or chickenpox, should check with a doctor before taking this medicine.* The aspirin in this combination medicine may cause a serious illness called Reye's syndrome in teenagers with fever caused by a virus infection, especially flu or chickenpox.

Older adults—

- *For butalbital:* Confusion, depression, or excitement may be especially likely to occur in elderly patients, who are usually more sensitive than younger adults to the effects of butalbital.
- *For aspirin:* Elderly patients are more sensitive than younger adults to the effects of aspirin. This may increase the chance of side effects during treatment.
- *For caffeine:* Many medicines have not been studied specifically in older people. Therefore, it may not be known whether they work exactly the same way they do in younger adults or if they cause different side effects or problems in older people. There is no specific information comparing use of caffeine in the elderly with use in other age groups.

Other medicines—Although certain medicines should not be used together at all, in other cases two different medicines may be used together even if an interaction might occur. In these cases, your doctor may want to change the dose, or other precautions may be necessary. When you are taking a butalbital and aspirin combination, it is especially important that your doctor and pharmacist know if you are taking any of the following:

- Adrenocorticoids (cortisone-like medicines) or
- Carbamazepine (e.g., Tegretol) or
- Contraceptives, oral (birth control pills), containing estrogen or
- Corticotropin (e.g., ACTH)—Butalbital may make these medicines less effective
- Antacids, large amounts taken regularly, especially calcium- and/or magnesium-containing antacids or sodium bicarbonate (baking soda), or
- Urinary alkalizers (medicine that makes the urine less acid, such as acetazolamide [e.g., Diamox], dichlorphenamide [e.g., Daranide], methazolamide [e.g., Neptazane], potassium or sodium citrate and/or citric acid)—These medicines may cause aspirin to be removed from the body faster than usual, which may shorten the time that aspirin is effective; acetazolamide, dichlorphenamide, and methazolamide may also increase the chance of side effects when taken together with aspirin
- Anticoagulants (blood thinners) or
- Heparin—Use of these medicines together with aspirin may increase the chance of bleeding; also, butalbital may cause anticoagulants to be less effective
- Antidepressants, tricyclic (amitriptyline [e.g., Elavil], amoxapine [e.g., Asendin], clomipramine [e.g., Anafranil], desipramine [e.g., Pertofrane], doxepin [e.g., Sinequan], imipramine [e.g., Tofranil], nortriptyline [e.g., Aventyl], protriptyline [e.g., Vivactil], trimipramine [e.g., Surmontil]) or
- Central nervous system (CNS) depressants (medicines that often cause drowsiness)—These medicines may add to the effects of butalbital and increase the chance of drowsiness or other side effects
- Divalproex (e.g., Depakote) or
- Methotrexate (e.g., Folex, Mexate) or
- Valproic acid (e.g., Depakene) or
- Vancomycin (e.g., Vancocin)—The chance of serious side effects may be increased

- Probenecid (e.g., Benemid) or
- Sulfinpyrazone (e.g., Anturane)—Aspirin can keep these medicines from working properly for treating gout

Other medical problems—The presence of other medical problems may affect the use of butalbital and aspirin combinations. Make sure you tell your doctor if you have any other medical problems, especially:

- Alcohol abuse (or history of) or
- Drug abuse or dependence (or history of)—Dependence on butalbital may develop
- Asthma, especially if occurring together with other allergies and nasal polyps (or history of), or
- Emphysema or other chronic lung disease or
- Hyperactivity (in children) or
- Kidney disease or
- Liver disease—The chance of serious side effects may be increased
- Diabetes mellitus (sugar diabetes) or
- Mental depression or
- Overactive thyroid or
- Porphyria (or history of)—Butalbital may make these conditions worse
- Gout—Aspirin can make this condition worse and can also lessen the effects of some medicines used to treat gout
- Heart disease (severe)—The caffeine in some of these combination medicines can make some kinds of heart disease worse
- Hemophilia or other bleeding problems or
- Vitamin K deficiency—Aspirin increases the chance of serious bleeding
- Stomach ulcer, especially with a history of bleeding, or other stomach problems—Aspirin can make your condition worse

Before you begin using any new medicine (prescription or nonprescription) or if you develop any new medical problem while you are using this medicine, check with your doctor, nurse, or pharmacist.

Proper Use of This Medicine

Take this medicine with food or a full glass (8 ounces) of water to lessen stomach irritation.

Do not take this medicine if it has a strong vinegar-like odor. This odor means the aspirin in it is breaking down. If you have any questions about this, check with your doctor or pharmacist.

Take this medicine only as directed by your doctor. Do not take more of it, do not take it more often, and do not take it for a longer time than your doctor ordered. If butalbital and aspirin combination is taken regularly (for example, every day), it may become habit-forming (causing mental or physical dependence). The caffeine in some butalbital and aspirin combinations can also increase the chance of dependence. Dependence is especially likely to occur in patients who take this medicine to relieve frequent headaches. Taking too much of this combination medicine can also lead to stomach problems or to other medical problems.

This medicine will relieve a headache best if you *take it as soon as the headache begins.* If you get warning signs of a migraine, take this medicine as soon as you are sure that the migraine is coming. This may even stop the headache pain from occurring. *Lying down in a quiet, dark room for a while after taking the medicine also helps to relieve headaches.*

People who get a lot of headaches may need to take a different medicine to help prevent headaches. *It is important that you follow your doctor's directions about taking the other medicine, even if your headaches continue to occur.* Headache-preventing medicines may take several weeks to start working. Even after they do start working, your headaches may not go away completely. However, your headaches should occur less often, and they should be less severe and easier to relieve than before. This will reduce the amount of headache relievers that you need. If you do not notice any improvement after several weeks of headache-preventing treatment, check with your doctor.

Missed dose—If your doctor has ordered you to take this medicine according to a regular schedule and you miss a dose, take it as soon as you remember. However, if it is almost time for your next dose, skip the missed dose and go back to your regular dosing schedule. Do not double doses.

Storage—To store this medicine:

- Keep out of the reach of children. Overdose is especially dangerous in young children.
- Store away from heat and direct light.
- Do not store this medicine in the bathroom, near the kitchen sink, or in other damp places. Heat or moisture may cause the medicine to break down.
- Do not keep outdated medicine or medicine no longer needed. Be sure that any discarded medicine is out of the reach of children.

Precautions While Using This Medicine

Check with your doctor:

- If the medicine stops working as well as it did when you first started using it. This may mean that you are in danger of becoming dependent on the medicine. *Do not try to get better pain relief by increasing the dose.*
- *If you are having headaches more often than you did before you started using this medicine.* This is especially important if a new headache occurs within 1 day after you took your last dose of headache medicine, headaches begin to occur every day, or a headache continues for several days in a row. This may mean that you are dependent on the headache

medicine. *Continuing to take this medicine will cause even more headaches later on.* Your doctor can give you advice on how to relieve the headaches.

Check the labels of all nonprescription (over-the-counter [OTC]) and prescription medicines you now take. If any contain a barbiturate, aspirin, or other salicylates, including diflunisal, be especially careful, since taking them while taking this medicine may lead to overdose. If you have any questions about this, check with your doctor or pharmacist.

The butalbital in this medicine will add to the effects of alcohol and other CNS depressants (medicines that slow down the nervous system, possibly causing drowsiness). Some examples of CNS depressants are antihistamines or medicine for hay fever, other allergies, or colds; sedatives, tranquilizers, or sleeping medicine; other prescription pain medicine or narcotics; other barbiturates; medicine for seizures; muscle relaxants; or anesthetics, including some dental anesthetics. Also, stomach problems may be more likely to occur if you drink alcoholic beverages while you are taking aspirin. Therefore, *do not drink alcoholic beverages, and check with your doctor before taking any of the medicines listed above, while you are using this medicine.*

This medicine may cause some people to become drowsy, dizzy, or lightheaded. *Make sure you know how you react to this medicine before you drive, use machines, or do anything else that could be dangerous if you are dizzy or are not alert and clearheaded.*

Before having any kind of surgery (including dental surgery) or emergency treatment, tell the medical doctor or dentist in charge that you are taking this medicine. Serious side effects may occur if your medical doctor or dentist gives you certain other medicines without knowing that you have taken butalbital.

Do not take this medicine for 5 days before any planned surgery, including dental surgery, unless otherwise directed by your medical doctor or dentist. Taking aspirin during this time may cause bleeding problems.

Before you have any medical tests, tell the person in charge that you are taking this medicine. Caffeine (present in some butalbital and aspirin combinations) interferes with the results of certain tests that use dipyridamole (e.g., Persantine) to help show how well blood is flowing to your heart. Caffeine should not be taken for 8 to 12 hours before the test. The results of some other tests may also be affected by butalbital and aspirin combinations.

If you have been taking large amounts of this medicine, or if you have been taking it regularly for several weeks or more, *do not suddenly stop using it without first checking with your doctor.* Your doctor may want you to reduce gradually the amount you are taking before stopping completely, to lessen the chance of withdrawal side effects.

If you think you or anyone else may have taken an overdose of this medicine, get emergency help at once. Taking an overdose of this medicine or taking alcohol or CNS depressants with this medicine may lead to unconsciousness or death. Symptoms of overdose of this medicine include convulsions (seizures); hearing loss; confusion; ringing or buzzing in the ears; severe excitement, nervousness, or restlessness; severe dizziness; severe drowsiness; shortness of breath or troubled breathing; and severe weakness.

Side Effects of This Medicine

Along with its needed effects, a medicine may cause some unwanted effects. Although not all of these side effects may occur, if they do occur they may need medical attention.

The following side effects may mean that a serious allergic reaction is occurring. Check with your doctor or get emergency help immediately if they occur, especially if several of them occur at the same time.

Less common or rare

Bluish discoloration or flushing or redness of skin (occurring together with other effects listed in this section); coughing, shortness of breath, troubled breathing, tightness in chest, or wheezing; difficulty in swallowing; dizziness or feeling faint (severe); hive-like swellings (large) on eyelids, face, lips, or tongue; skin rash, itching, or hives; stuffy nose (occurring together with other effects listed in this section)

Also check with your doctor immediately if any of the following side effects occur, especially if several of them occur together:

Rare

Bleeding or crusting sores on lips; chest pain; fever with or without chills; red, thickened, or scaly skin; sores, ulcers, or white spots in mouth (painful); sore throat (unexplained); tenderness, burning, or peeling of skin

Symptoms of overdose

Anxiety, confusion, excitement, irritability, nervousness, restlessness, or trouble in sleeping (severe, especially with products containing caffeine); convulsions (seizures, with products containing caffeine); diarrhea (severe or continuing); dizziness, lightheadedness, drowsiness, or weakness (severe); frequent urination (for products containing caffeine); hallucinations (seeing, hearing, or feeling things that are not there); increased sensitivity to touch or pain (for products containing caffeine); increased thirst; muscle trembling or twitching (for products containing caffeine); nausea or vomiting (severe or continuing), sometimes with blood; ringing or buzzing in ears (continuing) or hearing loss; seeing flashes of "zig-zag" lights (for products containing caffeine); slow, fast, or irregular heartbeat; slow, fast, irregular, or troubled breathing; slurred speech;

staggering; stomach pain (severe); uncontrollable flapping movements of the hands, especially in elderly patients; unusual movements of the eyes; vision problems

Also, check with your doctor as soon as possible if any of the following side effects occur:

Less common or rare

Bloody or black, tarry stools; bloody urine; confusion or mental depression; muscle cramps or pain; pinpoint red spots on skin; swollen or painful glands; unusual bleeding or bruising; unusual excitement (mild)

Other side effects may occur that usually do not need medical attention. These side effects may go away during treatment as your body adjusts to the medicine. However, check with your doctor if any of the following side effects continue or are bothersome:

More common

Bloated or "gassy" feeling; dizziness or lightheadedness (mild); drowsiness (mild); heartburn or indigestion; nausea, vomiting, or stomach pain (occurring without other symptoms of overdose)

Other side effects not listed above may also occur in some patients. If you notice any other effects, check with your doctor.

Annual revision: 07/14/92

CAFFEINE Systemic

C

Some commonly used brand names are:

For Caffeine

In the U.S.

Caffedrine	NoDoz
Caffedrine Caplets	Quick Pep
Dexitac	Vivarin

Generic name product may also be available.

For Citrated Caffeine

In the U.S.

Generic name product may be available.

Description

Caffeine (kaf-FEEN) belongs to the group of medicines called central nervous system (CNS) stimulants. It is used to help restore mental alertness when unusual tiredness or weakness or drowsiness occurs. Caffeine's use as an alertness aid should be only occasional. It is not intended to replace sleep and should not be used routinely for this purpose.

Caffeine is also used in combination with ergotamine or with certain pain relievers, such as aspirin or acetaminophen, for relief of headaches or menstrual tension. When used in this way, caffeine may increase the effectiveness of the other medicines. Caffeine is sometimes used in combination with an antihistamine to overcome the drowsiness caused by the antihistamine.

Caffeine may also be used for other conditions as determined by your doctor.

Caffeine is present in coffee, tea, soft drinks, cocoa, and chocolate.

As a medicine, it is available without a prescription; however, your doctor or pharmacist may have special instructions on its proper use. Caffeine is available in the following dosage forms:

Oral

Caffeine
- Extended-release capsules (U.S.)
- Tablets (U.S.)

Citrated caffeine
- Tablets (U.S.)

It is very important that you read and understand the following information. If any of it causes you special concern, check with your doctor or pharmacist. Also, *if you have any questions* or if you want more information about this medicine or your medical problem, *ask your doctor, nurse, or pharmacist.*

Before Using This Medicine

If you are taking this medicine without a prescription, carefully read and follow any precautions on the label. For caffeine, the following should be considered:

Allergies—Tell your doctor if you have ever had any unusual or allergic reaction to aminophylline, caffeine, dyphylline, oxtriphylline, theobromine (also found in cocoa or chocolate), or theophylline. Also tell your doctor and pharmacist if you are allergic to any other substances, such as foods, preservatives, or dyes.

Pregnancy—Studies in humans have not shown that caffeine causes birth defects. However, studies in animals have shown that caffeine causes birth defects when given in very large doses (amounts equal to 12 to 24 cups of coffee a day) and problems with bone growth when given in smaller doses. In addition, use of large amounts of caffeine by the mother during pregnancy may cause problems with the heart rhythm of the fetus.

Breast-feeding—Caffeine passes into breast milk in small amounts and may build up in the nursing baby. Studies have shown that babies may appear jittery and have trouble in sleeping when their mothers drink large amounts of caffeine-containing beverages.

Children—With the exception of infants, there is no specific information comparing use of caffeine in children with use in other age groups. However, this medicine is not expected to cause different side effects or problems in children than it does in adults.

Older adults—Many medicines have not been studied specifically in older people. Therefore, it may not be known whether they work exactly the same way they do in younger adults or if they cause different side effects or problems in older people. There is no specific information comparing use of caffeine in the elderly with use in other age groups.

Other medicines—Although certain medicines should not be used together at all, in other cases 2 different medicines may be used together even if an interaction might occur. In these cases, your doctor may want to change the dose, or other precautions may be necessary. When you are taking caffeine, it is especially important that your doctor and pharmacist know if you are taking any of the following:

- Amantadine (e.g., Symmetrel) or
- Amphetamines (e.g., Desoxyn, Dexedrine) or
- Appetite suppressants (diet pills), except fenfluramine (e.g., Pondimin), or
- Chlophedianol (e.g., Ulone) or
- Cocaine or
- Medicine for asthma or other breathing problems or
- Medicine for colds, sinus problems, hay fever or other allergies (including nose drops or sprays) or
- Methylphenidate (e.g., Ritalin) or
- Nabilone (e.g., Cesamet) or
- Other medicines or beverages containing caffeine or
- Pemoline (e.g., Cylert)—Using these medicines with caffeine may increase the CNS-stimulant effects, such as nervousness, irritability, or trouble in sleeping, or possibly

convulsions (seizures) or changes in the rhythm of your heart
- Monoamine oxidase (MAO) inhibitors (furazolidone [e.g., Furoxone], isocarboxazid [e.g., Marplan], phenelzine [e.g., Nardil], procarbazine [e.g., Matulane], selegiline [e.g., Eldepryl], tranylcypromine [e.g., Parnate])—Taking large amounts of caffeine while you are taking or within 2 weeks of taking monoamine oxidase (MAO) inhibitors may cause extremely high blood pressure or dangerous changes in the rhythm of your heart; taking small amounts of caffeine may cause mild high blood pressure and fast heartbeat; at least 14 days should be allowed between stopping treatment with an MAO inhibitor and starting treatment with caffeine

Other medical problems—The presence of other medical problems may affect the use of caffeine. Make sure you tell your doctor if you have any other medical problems, especially:
- Agoraphobia (fear of being in open places) or
- Anxiety or
- Heart disease or
- High blood pressure or
- Panic attacks or
- Stomach ulcer or
- Trouble in sleeping—Caffeine may make the condition worse
- Liver disease—Higher blood levels of caffeine may result, increasing the chance of side effects

Proper Use of This Medicine

For patients taking the *extended-release form* of this medicine:
- Swallow the capsule whole.
- Do not break, crush, or chew the capsule before swallowing.

Take caffeine in capsule or tablet form only as directed. Do not take more of it, do not take it more often, and do not take it for a longer time than directed. Taking too much may increase the chance of side effects. It may also become habit-forming.

If you think this medicine is not working properly after you have taken it for a long time, *do not increase the dose.* To do so may increase the chance of side effects.

Storage—To store this medicine:
- Keep out of the reach of children. Young children are especially sensitive to caffeine's side effects.
- Store away from heat and direct light.
- Do not store in the bathroom, near the kitchen sink, or in other damp places. Heat or moisture may cause the medicine to break down.
- Do not keep outdated medicine or medicine no longer needed. Be sure that any discarded medicine is out of the reach of children.

Precautions While Using This Medicine

Capsules or tablets containing caffeine are for occasional use only. They should not be used instead of sleep. If unusual tiredness or weakness or drowsiness continues or returns often, check with your doctor.

The recommended dose of this medicine contains about the same amount of caffeine as a cup of coffee. Do not drink large amounts of caffeine-containing coffee, tea, or soft drinks while you are taking this medicine. Also, do not take large amounts of other medicines that contain caffeine. To do so may cause unwanted effects.

The amount of caffeine in some common foods and beverages is as follows:
- Coffee, brewed—40 to 180 milligrams (mg) per cup.
- Coffee, instant—30 to 120 mg per cup.
- Coffee, decaffeinated—3 to 5 mg per cup.
- Tea, brewed American—20 to 90 mg per cup.
- Tea, brewed imported—25 to 110 mg per cup.
- Tea, instant—28 mg per cup.
- Tea, canned iced—22 to 36 mg per 12 ounces.
- Cola and other soft drinks, caffeine-containing—36 to 90 mg per 12 ounces.
- Cola and other soft drinks, decaffeinated—0 mg per 12 ounces.
- Cocoa—4 mg per cup.
- Chocolate, milk—3 to 6 mg per ounce.
- Chocolate, bittersweet—25 mg per ounce.

Caffeine may cause nervousness or irritability, trouble in sleeping, dizziness, or a fast or pounding heartbeat. If these effects occur, discontinue the use of caffeine-containing beverages or medicines, or large amounts of chocolate-containing products.

To prevent trouble in sleeping, do not take caffeine-containing beverages or medicines too close to bedtime.

Side Effects of This Medicine

Along with its needed effects, a medicine may cause some unwanted effects. Although not all of these side effects may occur, they may be more likely to occur if caffeine is taken in large doses or more often than recommended. If they do occur, they may need medical attention.

Check with your doctor as soon as possible if any of the following side effects occur:

More common

Diarrhea; dizziness; fast heartbeat; nausea (severe); nervousness; severe jitters in newborn babies; tremors; trouble in sleeping; vomiting

Symptoms of overdose

Abdominal or stomach pain; agitation, anxiety, excitement, or restlessness; confusion or delirium; convulsions (seizures)—in acute overdose; fast or irregular heartbeat; fever; frequent urination; headache; increased sensitivity to touch or pain; irritability; muscle trembling or twitching; nausea and vomiting, sometimes with blood; painful, swollen abdomen or vomiting in newborn babies; ringing or other sounds in ears; seeing flashes of "zig-zag" lights; trouble in sleeping; whole-body tremors in newborn babies

Other side effects may occur that usually do not need medical attention. These side effects may go away during treatment as your body adjusts to the medicine. However, check with your doctor if any of the following side effects continue or are bothersome:

More common

Nausea (mild); nervousness or jitters (mild)

After you stop using this medicine, your body may need time to adjust. The length of time this takes depends on the amount of medicine you were using and how long you used it. During this time check with your doctor if you notice any of the following side effects:

More common

Anxiety; dizziness; headache; irritability; muscle tension; nausea; nervousness; stuffy nose; unusual tiredness

Other side effects not listed above may also occur in some patients. If you notice any other effects, check with your doctor.

Additional Information

Once a medicine has been approved for marketing for a certain use, experience may show that it is also useful for other medical problems. Although these uses are not included in product labeling, caffeine is used in certain patients with the following medical conditions:

- Neonatal apnea (breathing problems in newborn babies)
- Postoperative infant apnea (breathing problems after surgery in young babies)
- Psychiatric disorders requiring ECT (electroconvulsive or shock therapy)

Other than the above information, there is no additional information relating to proper use, precautions, or side effects for these uses.

Annual revision: 11/11/91

CALCITONIN Systemic

Some commonly used brand names are:

For Calcitonin-Human†

In the U.S.

Cibacalcin

For Calcitonin-Salmon

In the U.S.

Calcimar

Miacalcin

In Canada

Calcimar

†Not commercially available in Canada.

Description

Calcitonin (kal-si-TOE-nin) is used to treat Paget's disease of bone. It also may be used to prevent continuing bone loss in women with postmenopausal osteoporosis and to treat hypercalcemia (too much calcium in the blood). This medicine may be used to treat other conditions as determined by your doctor.

Calcitonin is available only with your doctor's prescription, in the following dosage forms:

Parenteral

Calcitonin-Human

- Injection (U.S.)

Calcitonin-Salmon

- Injection (U.S. and Canada)

It is very important that you read and understand the following information. If any of it causes you special concern, check with your doctor. Also, *if you have any questions* or if you want more information about this medicine or your medical problem, *ask your doctor, nurse, or pharmacist.*

Before Using This Medicine

In deciding to use a medicine, the risks of taking the medicine must be weighed against the good it will do. This is a decision you and your doctor will make. For calcitonin, the following should be considered:

Allergies—Tell your doctor if you have ever had any unusual or allergic reaction to calcitonin or other proteins. Also tell your doctor and pharmacist if you are allergic to any other substances, such as foods, preservatives, or dyes.

Diet—Make certain your doctor and pharmacist know if your diet includes large amounts of calcium-containing foods and/or vitamin D–containing foods, such as milk or other dairy products. Calcium and vitamin D may cause the calcitonin to be less effective in treating a high blood calcium. Also let your doctor and pharmacist know if you are on any special diet, such as low-sodium or low-sugar diet.

Pregnancy—Calcitonin has not been studied in pregnant women. However, in animal studies, calcitonin has been shown to lower the birth weight of the baby when the mother was given a dose of calcitonin many times the human dose.

Breast-feeding—Calcitonin has not been reported to cause problems in nursing babies. However, studies in animals have shown that calcitonin may decrease the flow of breast milk.

Children—Studies on this medicine have been done only in adult patients, and there is no specific information comparing the use of calcitonin in children with use in other age groups. Therefore, be sure to discuss with your doctor the use of this medicine in children.

Older adults—Many medicines have not been studied specifically in older people. Therefore, it may not be known whether they work exactly the same way they do in younger adults. Although there is no specific information comparing the use of calcitonin in the elderly with use in other age groups, this medicine is not expected to cause different side effects or problems in older people than it does in younger adults. Calcitonin is often used in elderly patients.

Other medicine—Although certain medicines should not be used together at all, in other cases two different medicines may be used together even if an interaction might occur. In these cases, your doctor may want to change the dose, or other precautions may be necessary. When you are using calcitonin, it is especially important that your doctor and pharmacist know if you are using any other prescription or nonprescription (over-the-counter [OTC]) medicine.

Before you begin using any new medicine (prescription or nonprescription) or if you develop any new medical problem while you are using this medicine, check with your doctor, nurse, or pharmacist.

Proper Use of This Medicine

This medicine is for injection only. If you will be giving yourself the injections, make sure you understand exactly how to give them, including how to fill the syringe before injection. If you have any questions about this, check with your doctor.

Use the calcitonin only when the contents of the syringe are clear and colorless. Do not use it if it looks grainy or discolored.

Take this medicine only as directed by your doctor. Do not take more of it and do not take it more often than your doctor ordered.

Missed dose—If you miss a dose of this medicine and your dosing schedule is:

- Two doses a day—If you remember within 2 hours of the missed dose, give it right away. Then go back to your regular dosing schedule. But if you do not remember the missed dose until later, skip it and go back to your regular dosing schedule. Do not double doses.
- One dose a day—Give the missed dose as soon as possible. Then go back to your regular dosing schedule. If you do not remember the missed dose until the next day, skip it and go back to your regular dosing schedule. Do not double doses.
- One dose every other day—Give the missed dose as soon as possible if you remember it on the day it should be given. Then go back to your regular dosing schedule. If you do not remember the missed dose until the next day, give it at that time. Then skip a day and start your dosing schedule again.
- One dose three times a week—Give the missed dose the next day. Then set each injection back a day for the rest of the week. Go back to your regular Monday-Wednesday-Friday schedule the following week. Do not double doses.

If you have any questions about this, check with your doctor.

Storage—To store this medicine:

- Keep out of the reach of children.
- Store away from heat and direct light.
- Store *calcitonin-human* at a temperature below 77 °F. Do not refrigerate. Use prepared solution within 6 hours.
- Store *calcitonin-salmon* in the refrigerator. However, keep it from freezing.
- Do not keep outdated medicine or medicine no longer needed. Be sure that any discarded medicine is out of the reach of children.

Precautions While Using This Medicine

Your doctor should check your progress at regular visits to make sure that this medicine does not cause unwanted effects.

If you are using this medicine for hypercalcemia (too much calcium in the blood), your doctor may want you to follow a low-calcium diet. If you have any questions about this, check with your doctor.

Side Effects of This Medicine

Along with its needed effects, a medicine may cause some unwanted effects. Although not all of these side effects may occur, if they do occur they may need medical attention.

Check with your doctor as soon as possible if either of the following side effects occurs:

Rare

Skin rash or hives

Other side effects may occur that usually do not need medical attention. These side effects may go away during treatment as your body adjusts to the medicine. However, check with your doctor if any of the following side effects continue or are bothersome:

More common

Diarrhea; flushing or redness of face, ears, hands, or feet; loss of appetite; nausea or vomiting; pain, redness, soreness, or swelling at place of injection; stomach pain

Less common

Increased frequency of urination

Rare

Chills; dizziness; headache; pressure in chest; stuffy nose; tenderness or tingling of hands or feet; trouble in breathing; weakness

Other side effects not listed above may also occur in some patients. If you notice any other effects, check with your doctor.

Additional Information

Once a medicine has been approved for marketing for a certain use, experience may show that it is also useful for other medical problems. Although this use is not included in product labeling, calcitonin is used in certain patients with the following medical condition:

- Osteoporosis caused by hormone problems, certain drugs, and other causes

Other than the above information, there is no additional information relating to proper use, precautions, or side effects for these uses.

Annual revision: 05/13/92

CALCIUM CHANNEL BLOCKING AGENTS Systemic

This information applies to the following medicines:

Bepridil (BE-pri-dil)
Diltiazem (dil-TYE-a-zem)
Felodipine (fe-LOE-di-peen)
Flunarizine (floo-NAR-i-zeen)
Isradipine (is-RA-di-peen)
Nicardipine (nye-KAR-de-peen)
Nifedipine (nye-FED-i-peen)
Nimodipine (nye-MOE-di-peen)
Verapamil (ver-AP-a-mil)

Some commonly used brand names are:

For Bepridil†
In the U.S.
Bepadin
Vascor

For Diltiazem
In the U.S.
Cardizem
Cardizem CD
Cardizem SR
In Canada
Apo-Diltiaz
Cardizem
Cardizem SR
Novo-Diltazem
Nu-Diltiaz
Syn-Diltiazem
Generic name product may also be available.

For Felodipine
In the U.S.
Plendil
In Canada
Plendil
Renedil

For Flunarizine*
In Canada
Sibelium

For Isradipine†
In the U.S.
DynaCirc

For Nicardipine
In the U.S.
Cardene
In Canada
Cardene

For Nifedipine
In the U.S.
Adalat
Procardia
Procardia XL
Generic name product may also be available.
In Canada
Adalat
Adalat FT
Adalat P.A.
Apo-Nifed
Novo-Nifedin
Nu-Nifed

For Nimodipine
In the U.S.
Nimotop

In Canada
Nimotop

For Verapamil
In the U.S.
Calan
Calan SR
Isoptin
Isoptin SR
Verelan
Generic name product may also be available.
In Canada
Apo-Verap
Isoptin
Isoptin SR
Novo-Veramil
Nu-Verap
Generic name product may also be available.

*Not commercially available in the U.S.
†Not commercially available in Canada.

Description

Bepridil, diltiazem, felodipine, flunarizine, isradipine, nicardipine, nifedipine, nimodipine, and verapamil belong to the group of medicines called calcium channel blockers.

Calcium channel blocking agents affect the movement of calcium into the cells of the heart and blood vessels. As a result, they relax blood vessels and increase the supply of blood and oxygen to the heart while reducing its workload.

Some of the calcium channel blocking agents are used to relieve and control angina pectoris (chest pain).

Some are also used to treat high blood pressure (hypertension). High blood pressure adds to the workload of the heart and arteries. If it continues for a long time, the heart and arteries may not function properly. This can damage the blood vessels of the brain, heart, and kidneys, resulting in a stroke, heart failure, or kidney failure. High blood pressure may also increase the risk of heart attacks. These problems may be less likely to occur if blood pressure is controlled.

Flunarizine is used to prevent migraine headaches.

Nimodipine is used to prevent and treat problems caused by a burst blood vessel in the head (also known as a ruptured aneurysm or subarachnoid hemorrhage).

Other calcium channel blocking agents may also be used for these and other conditions as determined by your doctor.

These medicines are available only with your doctor's prescription, in the following dosage forms:

Oral

Bepridil
- Tablets (U.S.)

Diltiazem
- Extended-release capsules (U.S. and Canada)
- Tablets (U.S. and Canada)

Felodipine
- Extended-release tablets (U.S. and Canada)

Flunarizine
- Capsules (Canada)

Isradipine
- Capsules (U.S.)

Nicardipine
- Capsules (U.S. and Canada)

Nifedipine
- Capsules (U.S. and Canada)
- Tablets (Canada)
- Extended-release tablets (U.S. and Canada)

Nimodipine
- Capsules (U.S. and Canada)

Verapamil
- Extended-release capsules (U.S.)
- Tablets (U.S. and Canada)
- Extended-release tablets (U.S. and Canada)

Parenteral

Diltiazem
- Injection (U.S.)

Verapamil
- Injection (U.S. and Canada)

It is very important that you read and understand the following information. If any of it causes you special concern, check with your doctor. Also, *if you have any questions* or if you want more information about this medicine or your medical problem, *ask your doctor, nurse, or pharmacist.*

Before Using This Medicine

In deciding to use a medicine, the risks of taking the medicine must be weighed against the good it will do. This is a decision you and your doctor will make. For the calcium channel blocking agents, the following should be considered:

Allergies—Tell your doctor if you have ever had any unusual or allergic reaction to bepridil, diltiazem, felodipine, flunarizine, isradipine, nicardipine, nifedipine, nimodipine, or verapamil. Also tell your doctor and pharmacist if you are allergic to any other substances, such as foods, preservatives, or dyes.

Pregnancy—Calcium channel blockers have not been studied in pregnant women. However, studies in animals have shown that large doses of calcium channel blockers cause birth defects, prolonged pregnancy, poor bone development, and stillbirth.

Breast-feeding—Although bepridil, diltiazem, nifedipine, verapamil, and possibly other calcium channel blockers, pass into breast milk, they have not been reported to cause problems in nursing babies.

Children—Although there is no specific information comparing use of this medicine in children with use in other age groups, it is not expected to cause different side effects or problems in children than it does in adults.

Older adults—Elderly people may be especially sensitive to the effects of calcium channel blockers. This may increase the chance of side effects during treatment.

Other medicines—Although certain medicines should not be used together at all, in other cases two different medicines may be used together even if an interaction might occur. In these cases, your doctor may want to change the dose, or other precautions may be necessary. When taking calcium channel blockers it is especially important that your doctor and pharmacist know if you are taking any of the following:

- Acetazolamide (e.g., Diamox) or
- Amphotericin B by injection (e.g., Fungizone) or
- Corticosteroids (cortisone-like medicine) or
- Dichlorphenamide (e.g., Daranide) or
- Diuretics (water pills) or
- Methazolamide (e.g., Naptazane)—These medicines can cause hypokalemia (low levels of potassium in the body), which can increase the unwanted effects of bepridil
- Beta-blockers (acebutolol [e.g., Sectral], atenolol [e.g., Tenormin], betaxolol [e.g., Kerlone], carteolol [e.g., Cartrol], labetalol [e.g., Normodyne], metoprolol [e.g., Lopressor], nadolol [e.g., Corgard], oxprenolol [e.g., Trasicor], penbutolol [e.g., Levatol], pindolol [e.g., Visken], propranolol [e.g., Inderal], sotalol [e.g., Sotacor], timolol [e.g., Blocadren])—Effects of both may be increased. In addition, unwanted effects may occur if a calcium channel blocker or a beta-blocker is stopped suddenly after use together
- Carbamazepine (e.g., Tegretol) or
- Cyclosporine (e.g., Sandimmune) or
- Procainamide (e.g., Pronestyl) or
- Quinidine (e.g., Quinidex)—Effects of these medicines may be increased if they are used with some calcium channel blockers
- Digitalis glycosides (heart medicine)—Effects of these medicines may be increased if they are used with some calcium channel blockers
- Disopyramide (e.g., Norpace)—Effects of some calcium channel blockers on the heart may be increased

Also, tell your doctor or pharmacist if you are using any of the following medicines in the eye:

- Betaxolol (e.g., Betoptic) or
- Levobunolol (e.g., Betagan) or
- Metipranolol (e.g., OptiPranolol) or
- Timolol (e.g., Timoptic)—Effects on the heart and blood pressure may be increased

Other medical problems—The presence of other medical problems may affect the use of the calcium channel blockers. Make sure you tell your doctor if you have any other medical problems, especially:

- Heart rhythm problems (history of)—Bepridil can cause serious heart rhythm problems
- Kidney disease or
- Liver disease—Effects of the calcium channel blocker may be increased
- Mental depression (history of)—Flunarizine may cause mental depression
- Parkinson's disease or similar problems—Flunarizine can cause parkinsonian-like effects
- Other heart or blood vessel disorders—Calcium channel blockers may make some heart conditions worse

Before you begin using any new medicine (prescription or nonprescription) or if you develop any new medical problem while you are using this medicine, check with your doctor, nurse, or pharmacist.

Proper Use of This Medicine

Take this medicine exactly as directed even if you feel well and do not notice any signs of chest pain. Do not take more of this medicine and do not take it more often than your doctor ordered. Do not miss any doses.

For patients taking *bepridil:*

- If this medicine causes upset stomach, it can be taken with meals or at bedtime.

For patients taking *diltiazem extended-release capsules:*

- Swallow the capsule whole, without crushing or chewing it.
- *Do not change to another brand without checking with your physician.* Different brands have different doses. If you refill your medicine and it looks different, check with your pharmacist.

For patients taking *nifedipine or verapamil extended-release capsules:*

- Swallow the capsule whole, without crushing or chewing it.

For patients taking *regular nifedipine or extended-release felodipine or nifedipine tablets:*

- Swallow the tablet whole, without breaking, crushing, or chewing it.
- If you are taking *Procardia XL*, you may sometimes notice what looks like a tablet in your stool. That is just the empty shell that is left after the medicine has been absorbed into your body.

For patients taking *verapamil extended-release tablets:*

- Swallow the tablet whole, without crushing or chewing it. However, if your doctor tells you to, you may break the tablet in half.
- Take the medicine with food or milk.

For patients taking this medicine *for high blood pressure:*

- In addition to the use of the medicine your doctor has prescribed, appropriate treatment for your high blood pressure may include weight control and care in the types of food you eat, especially foods high in sodium (salt). Your doctor will tell you which factors are most important for you. You should check with your doctor before changing your diet.
- Many patients who have high blood pressure will not notice any signs of the problem. In fact, many may

feel normal. It is very important that you *take your medicine exactly as directed* and that you keep your appointments with your doctor even if you feel well.

- Remember that this medicine will not cure your high blood pressure but it does help control it. Therefore, you must continue to take it as directed if you expect to lower your blood pressure and keep it down. *You may have to take high blood pressure medicine for the rest of your life.* If high blood pressure is not treated, it can cause serious problems such as heart failure, blood vessel disease, stroke, or kidney disease.

Missed dose—If you do miss a dose of this medicine, take it as soon as possible. However, if it is almost time for your next dose, skip the missed dose and go back to your regular dosing schedule. Do not double doses.

Storage—To store this medicine:

- Keep out of the reach of children.
- Store away from heat and direct light.
- Do not store in the bathroom, near the kitchen sink, or in other damp places. Heat or moisture may cause the medicine to break down.
- Do not keep outdated medicine or medicine no longer needed. Be sure that any discarded medicine is out of the reach of children.

Precautions While Using This Medicine

It is important that your doctor check your progress at regular visits. This will allow your doctor to make sure the medicine is working properly and to change the dosage if needed.

If you have been using this medicine regularly for several weeks, do not suddenly stop using it. Stopping suddenly may bring on your previous problem. Check with your doctor for the best way to reduce gradually the amount you are taking before stopping completely.

Chest pain resulting from exercise or physical exertion is usually reduced or prevented by this medicine. This may tempt you to be overly active. *Make sure you discuss with your doctor a safe amount of exercise for your medical problem.*

After taking a dose of this medicine you may get a headache that lasts for a short time. This effect is more common if you are taking felodipine, isradipine, or nifedipine. This should become less noticeable after you have taken this medicine for a while. If this effect continues or if the headaches are severe, check with your doctor.

In some patients, tenderness, swelling, or bleeding of the gums may appear soon after treatment with this medicine is started. Brushing and flossing your teeth carefully and regularly and massaging your gums may help prevent this. *See your dentist regularly to have your teeth cleaned. Check with your medical doctor or dentist if you have any questions about how to take care of your teeth and gums, or if you notice any tenderness, swelling, or bleeding of your gums.*

For patients taking *bepridil, diltiazem,* or *verapamil*:

- *Ask your doctor how to count your pulse rate. Then, while you are taking this medicine, check your pulse regularly.* If it is much slower than your usual rate, or less than 50 beats per minute, check with your doctor. A pulse rate that is too slow may cause circulation problems.

For patients taking *flunarizine:*

- This medicine may cause some people to become drowsy or less alert than they are normally. This is more likely to happen when you begin to take it or when you increase the amount of medicine you are taking. *Make sure you know how you react to this medicine before you drive, use machines, or do anything else that could be dangerous if you are not alert.*

For patients taking this medicine *for high blood pressure:*

- *Do not take other medicines unless they have been discussed with your doctor.* This especially includes over-the-counter (nonprescription) medicines for appetite control, asthma, colds, cough, hay fever, or sinus problems, since they may tend to increase your blood pressure.

Side Effects of This Medicine

Along with its needed effects, a medicine may cause some unwanted effects. Although not all of these side effects may occur, if they do occur they may need medical attention.

Not all of the side effects listed below have been reported for each of these medicines, but they have been reported for at least one of them. Since many of the effects of calcium channel blockers are similar, some of these side effects may occur with any of these medicines. However, they may be more common with some of these medicines than with others.

Check with your doctor as soon as possible if any of the following side effects occur:

Less common

Breathing difficulty, coughing, or wheezing; irregular or fast, pounding heartbeat; skin rash; slow heartbeat (less than 50 beats per minute—bepridil, diltiazem, and verapamil only); swelling of ankles, feet, or lower legs (more common with felodipine and nifedipine)

For flunarizine only—less common

Loss of balance control; mask-like face; mental depression; shuffling walk; stiffness of arms or legs; trembling and shaking of hands and fingers; trouble in speaking or swallowing

Rare

Bleeding, tender, or swollen gums; chest pain (may appear about 30 minutes after medicine is taken); fainting; painful, swollen joints (for nifedipine only); trouble in seeing (for nifedipine only)

For flunarizine and verapamil only—rare

Unusual secretion of milk

Other side effects may occur that usually do not need medical attention. These side effects may go away during treatment as your body adjusts to the medicine. However, check with your doctor if any of the following side effects continue or are bothersome:

More common

Drowsiness (for flunarizine only); increased appetite and/or weight gain (for flunarizine only)

Less common

Constipation; diarrhea; dizziness or lightheadedness (more common with bepridil and nifedipine); dryness of mouth (for flunarizine only); flushing and feeling of warmth (more common with nicardipine and nifedipine); headache (more common with felodipine, isradipine, and nifedipine); nausea (more common with bepridil and nifedipine); unusual tiredness or weakness

Other side effects not listed above may also occur in some patients. If you notice any other effects, check with your doctor.

Additional Information

Once a medicine has been approved for marketing for a certain use, experience may show that it is also useful for other medical problems. Although these uses are not included in product labeling, calcium channel blockers are used in certain patients with the following medical conditions:

- Hypertrophic cardiomyopathy (a heart condition) (verapamil)
- Raynaud's phenomenon (circulation problems) (nicardipine and nifedipine)

Other than the above information, there is no additional information relating to proper use, precautions, or side effects for these uses.

Annual revision: 08/21/92

CALCIUM SUPPLEMENTS Systemic

This information applies to the following medicines:

Calcium Carbonate (KAL-see-um KAR-boh-nate)
Calcium Chloride (KLOR-ide)
Calcium Citrate (SIH-trayt)
Calcium Glubionate (gloo-BY-oh-nate)
Calcium Gluceptate
Calcium Gluceptate and Calcium Gluconate (GLOO-coh-nate)
Calcium Gluconate
Calcium Glycerophosphate (gliss-er-o-FOS-fate) and Calcium Lactate (LAK-tate)
Calcium Lactate
Calcium Lactate-Gluconate and Calcium Carbonate
Dibasic (dy-BAY-sic) Calcium Phosphate (FOS-fate)
Tribasic (try-BAY-sic) Calcium Phosphate

Note: This information does *not* apply to calcium carbonate used as an antacid.

Some commonly used brand names are:

For Calcium Carbonate

In the U.S.

BioCal
Calcarb 600
Calci-Chew
Calciday 667
Calcilac
Calcium 600
Calglycine
Caltrate 600
Chooz
Dicarbosil
Gencalc
Mallamint
Nephro-Calci
Os-Cal 500
Oysco
Oysco 500 Chewable
Oyst-Cal 500
Oyst-Cal 500 Chewable
Oystercal 500
Rolaids Calcium Rich
Super Calcium 1200
Titralac
Tums
Tums E-X

Generic name product may also be available.

In Canada

Apo-Cal
Calcite 500
Calcium 500
Calsan
Caltrate 300
Caltrate 600
Caltrate Chewable
Mega-Cal
Nu-Cal
Os-Cal
Os-Cal Chewable

Generic name product may also be available.

For Calcium Chloride

In the U.S.

Generic name product may be available.

In Canada

Calciject

Generic name product may also be available.

For Calcium Citrate†

In the U.S.

Citracal
Citracal Liquitabs

Generic name product may also be available.

For Calcium Glubionate

In the U.S.

Neo-Calglucon

In Canada

Calcium-Sandoz§

For Calcium Gluceptate and Calcium Gluconate*

In Canada

Calcium Stanley

For Calcium Gluconate
In the U.S.
Kalcinate
Generic name product may also be available.
In Canada
Generic name product may be available.

For Calcium Glycerophosphate and Calcium Lactate†
In the U.S.
Calphosan

For Calcium Lactate
In the U.S.
Generic name product may be available.
In Canada
Generic name product may be available.

For Calcium Lactate-Gluconate and Calcium Carbonate*
In Canada
Calcium-Sandoz Forte
Gramcal

For Dibasic Calcium Phosphate†
In the U.S.
Generic name product may be available.

For Tribasic Calcium Phosphate†
In the U.S.
Posture

*Not commercially available in the U.S.
†Not commercially available in Canada.
§In Canada, calcium glubionate is known as calcium glucono-galacto gluconate.

Description

Calcium supplements are taken by patients who are unable to get enough calcium in their regular diet or who have a need for more calcium. They are used to prevent or treat several conditions that may cause hypocalcemia (not enough calcium in the blood). The body needs calcium to make strong bones. Calcium is also needed for the heart, muscles, and nervous system to work properly.

The bones serve as a storage site for the body's calcium. They are continuously giving up calcium to the bloodstream and then replacing it as the body's need for calcium changes from day to day. When there is not enough calcium in the blood to be used by the heart and other organs, your body will take the needed calcium from the bones. When you eat foods rich in calcium, the calcium will be restored to the bones and the balance between your blood and bones will be maintained.

Pregnant women, nursing mothers, children, and adolescents may need more calcium than they normally get from eating calcium-rich foods. Adult women may take calcium supplements to help prevent a bone disease called osteoporosis. Osteoporosis, which causes thin, porous, easily broken bones, may occur in women after menopause, but may sometimes occur in elderly men also. Osteoporosis in women past menopause is thought to be caused by a reduced amount of ovarian estrogen (a female hormone). However, a diet low in calcium for many years, especially in the younger adult years, may add to the risk of developing it. Other bone diseases in children and adults are also treated with calcium supplements.

These medicines may also be used for other conditions as determined by your doctor.

Some of these preparations are available only with your doctor's prescription. Others are available without a prescription; however, your doctor may have special instructions on the proper use and dose for your medical problem.

Calcium supplements are available in the following dosage forms:

Oral

Calcium Carbonate
- Capsules (U.S. and Canada)
- Oral suspension (U.S.)
- Tablets (U.S. and Canada)
- Chewable tablets (U.S. and Canada)

Calcium Citrate
- Tablets (U.S.)
- Tablets for solution (U.S.)

Calcium Glubionate
- Syrup (U.S. and Canada)

Calcium Gluceptate and Calcium Gluconate
- Oral solution (Canada)

Calcium Gluconate
- Tablets (U.S. and Canada)

Calcium Lactate
- Tablets (U.S. and Canada)

Calcium Lactate-Gluconate and Calcium Carbonate
- Tablets for solution (Canada)

Dibasic Calcium Phosphate
- Tablets (U.S.)

Tribasic Calcium Phosphate
- Tablets (U.S.)

Parenteral

Calcium Chloride
- Injection (U.S. and Canada)

Calcium Glubionate
- Injection (Canada)

Calcium Gluceptate
- Injection (U.S.)

Calcium Gluconate
- Injection (U.S. and Canada)

Calcium Glycerophosphate and Calcium Lactate
- Injection (U.S.)

A calcium "salt" contains calcium along with another substance, such as carbonate or gluconate. Some calcium salts have more calcium (elemental calcium) than others. For example, the amount of calcium in calcium carbonate is greater than that in calcium gluconate. To give you an idea of how different calcium supplements vary in calcium content, the following chart explains how many tablets of each type of supplement will provide 1000 milligrams of elemental calcium. When you look for a calcium supplement, be sure the number of milligrams on the label refers to the amount of elemental calcium, and not to the strength of each tablet.

Calcium supplement	Strength of each tablet (in milligrams)	Amount of elemental calcium per tablet (in milligrams)	Number of tablets to provide 1000 milligrams of calcium
Calcium carbonate	625	250	4
	650	260	4
	750	300	4
	835	334	3
	1250	500	2
	1500	600	2
Calcium citrate	950	200	5
Calcium gluconate	500	45	22
	650	58	17
	1000	90	11
Calcium lactate	325	42	24
	650	84	12
Calcium phosphate, dibasic	500	115	9
Calcium phosphate, tribasic	800	304	4
	1600	608	2

It is very important that you read and understand the following information. If any of it causes you special concern, check with your doctor or pharmacist. Also, *if you have any questions* or if you want more information about this medicine or your medical problems, *ask your doctor, nurse, pharmacist, or dietitian.*

Importance of Diet

Many nutritionists recommend that, if possible, people should get all the calcium they need from foods. However, many people do not get enough calcium from food. For example, people on weight-loss diets may consume too little food to provide enough calcium. Others may not be able to tolerate milk products because their bodies lack an enzyme called lactase, which helps the body digest milk. Still others may need more calcium than normal. For such people, a calcium supplement is important.

In order to get enough vitamins and minerals in your diet, it is important that you eat a balanced and varied diet. Follow carefully any diet program your doctor may recommend. For your specific vitamin and/or mineral needs, ask your doctor or dietitian for a list of appropriate foods.

Experts have developed a list of Recommended Dietary Allowances (RDA) of calcium. The RDA is not an exact number but a general idea of how much you need every day. The RDA do not cover amounts needed for problems caused by a serious lack of calcium.

The RDA for calcium are as follows:

Infants and children—
- Birth to 6 months of age: 400 milligrams (mg) a day.
- 6 months to 1 year of age: 600 mg a day.
- 1 to 10 years of age: 800 mg a day.

Adolescent and adult males—
- 11 to 24 years of age: 1200 mg a day.
- 24 years of age and over: 800 mg a day.

Adolescent and adult females—
- 11 to 24 years of age: 1200 mg a day.
- 24 years of age and over: 800 mg a day.

Pregnant women—1200 mg a day.

Breast-feeding women—1200 mg a day.

Getting the proper amount of calcium in the diet every day and participating in weight-bearing exercise (walking, dancing, bicycling, aerobics, jogging), especially during the early years of life (up to about 35 years of age) is most important in helping to build and maintain bones as dense as possible to prevent the development of osteoporosis in later life.

The following table includes some calcium-rich foods. The calcium content of these foods can supply the daily RDA for calcium if the foods are eaten regularly in sufficient amounts.

Food (amount)	Milligrams of calcium
Nonfat dry milk, reconstituted (1 cup)	375
Lowfat, skim, or whole milk (1 cup)	290 to 300
Yogurt (1 cup)	275 to 400
Sardines with bones (3 ounces)	370
Ricotta cheese, part skim (½ cup)	340
Salmon, canned, with bones (3 ounces)	285
Cheese, Swiss (1 ounce)	272
Cheese, cheddar (1 ounce)	204
Cheese, American (1 ounce)	174
Cottage cheese, lowfat (1 cup)	154
Tofu (4 ounces)	154
Shrimp (1 cup)	147
Ice milk (¾ cup)	132

Vitamin D helps prevent calcium loss from your bones. It is sometimes called "the sunshine vitamin" because it is made in your skin when you are exposed to sunlight. If you get outside in the sunlight every day for 15 to 30 minutes, you should get all the vitamin D you need. However, in northern locations in winter, the sunlight may be too weak to make vitamin D in the skin. Vitamin D may also be obtained from your diet or from multivitamin preparations. Most milk is fortified with vitamin D.

Do not use bonemeal or dolomite as a source of calcium. The Food and Drug Administration has issued warnings that bonemeal and dolomite could be dangerous because these products may contain lead.

Remember:
- The total amount of calcium that you get every day includes what you get from food *and* what you may take as a supplement. Read the labels of processed foods. Many foods now have added calcium.
- This total intake of calcium need not be greater than the recommended amounts, unless ordered by your doctor. In some cases, excessive amounts of calcium may be harmful by causing kidney stones or kidney impairment.

Before Using This Dietary Supplement

If you are taking this dietary supplement without a prescription, carefully read and follow any precautions on the label. For calcium supplements, the following should be considered:

Pregnancy—It is especially important that you are receiving enough calcium when you become pregnant and that you continue to receive the right amount of calcium throughout your pregnancy. The healthy growth and development of the fetus depend on a steady supply of nutrients from the mother. However, taking large amounts of a dietary supplement during pregnancy may be harmful to the mother and/or fetus and should be avoided.

Breast-feeding—It is especially important that you receive the right amount of calcium so that your baby will also get the calcium needed to grow properly. However, taking large amounts of a dietary supplement while breast-feeding may be harmful to the mother and/or baby and should be avoided.

Children—It is especially important that children receive enough calcium in their diet for healthy growth and development. Although there is no specific information about the use of calcium in children in doses higher than the normal daily requirements, it is not expected to cause different side effects or problems in children than in adults. Injectable forms of calcium should not be given to children because of the risk of irritating the injection site.

Older adults—It is important that older people continue to receive enough calcium in their daily diets. However, some older people may need to take extra calcium or larger doses because they do not absorb calcium as well as younger people. Check with your doctor if you have any questions about the amount of calcium you should be taking in each day.

Medicines or other dietary supplements—Although certain medicines or dietary supplements should not be used together at all, in other cases they may be used together even if an interaction might occur. In these cases, your doctor may want to change the dose, or other precautions may be necessary. When you are taking calcium supplements, it is especially important that your doctor and pharmacist know if you are taking any of the following:

- Calcium-containing medicines, other—Taking excess calcium may cause too much calcium in the blood or urine and lead to medical problems
- Cellulose sodium phosphate (e.g., Calcibind)—Use with calcium supplements may decrease the effects of cellulose sodium phosphate
- Digitalis glycosides (heart medicine)—Use with calcium supplements by injection may increase the chance of irregular heartbeat
- Etidronate (e.g., Didronel)—Use with calcium supplements may decrease the effects of etidronate; etidronate should not be taken within 2 hours of calcium supplements
- Gallium nitrate (e.g., Ganite)—Use with calcium supplements may cause gallium nitrate to not work properly
- Magnesium sulfate (for injection)—Use with calcium supplements may cause either medicine to be less effective
- Phenytoin (e.g., Dilantin)—Use with calcium supplements may decrease the effects of both medicines; calcium supplements should not be taken within 1 to 3 hours of phenytoin
- Tetracyclines (medicine for infection) taken by mouth—Use with calcium supplements may decrease the effects of tetracycline; calcium supplements should not be taken within 1 to 3 hours of tetracyclines

Other medical problems—The presence of other medical problems may affect the use of calcium supplements. Make sure you tell your doctor if you have any other medical problems, especially:

- Diarrhea or
- Stomach or intestinal problems—Extra calcium or specific calcium preparations may be necessary in these conditions
- Heart disease—Calcium by injection may increase the chance of irregular heartbeat
- Hypercalcemia or
- Hypercalciuria—Calcium supplements may make these conditions worse
- Hyperparathyroidism or
- Sarcoidosis—Calcium supplements may increase the chance of hypercalcemia (too much calcium in the blood)
- Hypoparathyroidism—Use of calcium phosphate may cause high blood levels of phosphorus which could increase the chance of side effects
- Kidney disease or stones—Too much calcium may increase the chance of kidney stones

Proper Use of This Dietary Supplement

Drink a full glass (8 ounces) of water or juice when taking a calcium supplement. However, if you are taking calcium carbonate as a phosphate binder in kidney dialysis, it is not necessary to drink a glass of water.

This dietary supplement is best taken 1 to 1½ hours after meals, unless otherwise directed by your doctor. However, patients with a condition known as achlorhydria may not absorb calcium supplements on an empty stomach and should take them with meals.

For patients taking *the chewable tablet form* of this dietary supplement:

- Chew the tablets completely before swallowing.

For patients taking *the syrup form* of this dietary supplement:

- Take the syrup before meals. This will allow the dietary supplemernt to work faster.
- Mix in water or fruit juice for infants or children.

Take this dietary supplement only as directed. Do not take more of it and do not take it more often than recommended on the label. To do so may increase the chance of side effects.

Missed dose—If you are taking this dietary supplement on a regular schedule and you miss a dose, take it as soon as possible, then go back to your regular dosing schedule.

Storage—To store this dietary supplement:

- Keep out of the reach of children.
- Store away from heat and direct light.
- Do not store in the bathroom, near the kitchen sink, or in other damp places. Heat or moisture may cause the dietary supplement to break down.
- Keep the liquid form of this dietary supplement from freezing.
- Do not keep outdated dietary supplements or those no longer needed. Be sure that any discarded dietary supplement is out of the reach of children.

Precautions While Using This Dietary Supplement

If this dietary supplement has been ordered for you by your doctor and you will be taking it in large doses or for a long time, your doctor should check your progress at regular visits. This is to make sure the medicine is working properly and does not cause unwanted effects.

Do not take calcium supplements within 1 to 2 hours of taking other medicine by mouth. To do so may keep the other medicine from working properly.

Unless you are otherwise directed by your doctor, to make sure that calcium is used properly by your body:

- *Do not take other medicines or dietary supplements containing large amounts of calcium, phosphates, magnesium, or vitamin D unless your doctor has told you to do so or approved.*
- *Do not take calcium supplements within 1 to 2 hours of eating large amounts of fiber-containing foods, such as bran and whole-grain cereals or breads, especially if you are being treated for hypocalcemia (not enough calcium in your blood).*
- *Do not drink large amounts of alcohol or caffeine-containing beverages (usually more than 8 cups of coffee a day), or use tobacco.*

Recently, some calcium carbonate tablets have been shown to break up too slowly in the stomach to be properly absorbed into the body. If the calcium carbonate tablets you purchase are not specifically labeled as being "USP," check with your pharmacist. He or she may be able to help you determine which tablets are best.

Side Effects of This Dietary Supplement

Along with its needed effects, a dietary supplement may cause some unwanted effects. Although the following side effects occur very rarely when the calcium supplement is taken as recommended, they may be more likely to occur if:

- It is taken in large doses.
- It is taken for a long time.
- It is taken by patients with kidney disease.

Check with your doctor as soon as possible if any of the following side effects occur:

More common (for injection form only)

Dizziness; flushing and/or sensation of warmth or heat; irregular heartbeat; nausea or vomiting; skin redness, rash, pain, or burning at injection site; sweating; tingling sensation

Rare

Drowsiness; difficult or painful urination; nausea or vomiting (continuing); weakness

Early signs of overdose

Constipation (severe); dryness of mouth; headache (continuing); increased thirst; irritability; loss of appetite; mental depression; metallic taste; unusual tiredness or weakness

Late signs of overdose

Confusion; drowsiness (severe); high blood pressure; increased sensitivity of eyes or skin to light; irregular, fast, or slow heartbeat; unusually large amount of urine or increased frequency of urination

Other side effects not listed above may also occur in some patients. If you notice any other effects, check with your doctor.

Additional Information

Once a medicine or dietary supplement has been approved for marketing for a certain use, experience may show that it is also useful for other medical problems. Although this use is not included in product labeling, calcium supplements are used in certain patients with the following medical condition:

- Hyperphosphatemia (too much phosphate in the blood)

Other than the above information, there is no additional information relating to proper use, precautions, or side effects for this use.

Annual revision: 06/10/92

CAPREOMYCIN Systemic

A commonly used brand name in the U.S. and Canada is Capastat.

Description

Capreomycin (kap-ree-oh-MYE-sin) is used to treat tuberculosis (TB). It is given with one or more other medicines for TB.

Capreomycin is available only with your doctor's prescription, in the following dosage form:

Parenteral
- Injection (U.S. and Canada)

It is very important that you read and understand the following information. If any of it causes you special concern, check with your doctor. Also, *if you have any questions* or if you want more information about this medicine or your medical problem, *ask your doctor, nurse, or pharmacist.*

Before Receiving This Medicine

In deciding to use a medicine, the risks of taking the medicine must be weighed against the good it will do. This is a decision you and your doctor will make. For capreomycin, the following should be considered:

Allergies—Tell your doctor if you have ever had any unusual or allergic reaction to capreomycin. Also tell your doctor and pharmacist if you are allergic to any other substances, such as foods, preservatives, or dyes.

Pregnancy—Capreomycin has not been studied in pregnant women. However, studies in rats given several times the human dose have shown that capreomycin may cause "wavy ribs" in the fetus.

Breast-feeding—It is not known whether capreomycin passes into breast milk. However, capreomycin has not been reported to cause problems in nursing babies.

Children—Studies on this medicine have been done only in adult patients, and there is no specific information comparing use of capreomycin in children with use in other age groups.

Older adults—Many medicines have not been studied specifically in older people. Therefore, it may not be known whether they work exactly the same way they do in younger adults or if they cause different side effects or problems in older people. There is no specific information comparing use of capreomycin in the elderly with use in other age groups.

Other medicines—Although certain medicines should not be used together at all, in other cases two different medicines may be used together even if an interaction might occur. In these cases, your doctor may want to change the dose, or other precautions may be necessary. When you are receiving capreomycin, it is especially important that your doctor and pharmacist know if you are taking any of the following:

- Aminoglycosides by injection (amikacin [e.g., Amikin], gentamicin [e.g., Garamycin], kanamycin [e.g., Kantrex], neomycin [e.g., Mycifradin], netilmicin [e.g., Netromycin], streptomycin, tobramycin [e.g., Nebcin]) or
- Anti-infectives by mouth or by injection (medicine for infection) or
- Carmustine (e.g., BiCNU) or
- Chloroquine (e.g., Aralen) or
- Cisplatin (e.g., Platinol) or
- Combination pain medicine containing acetaminophen and aspirin (e.g., Excedrin) or other salicylates (with large amounts taken regularly) or
- Cyclosporine (e.g., Sandimmune) or
- Deferoxamine (e.g., Desferal) (with long-term use) or
- Gold salts (medicine for arthritis) or
- Hydroxychloroquine (e.g., Plaquenil) or
- Inflammation or pain medicines, except narcotics, or
- Lithium (e.g., Lithane) or
- Methotrexate (e.g., Mexate) or
- Penicillamine (e.g., Cuprimine) or
- Plicamycin (e.g., Mithracin) or
- Quinine (e.g., Quinamm) or
- Streptozocin (e.g., Zanosar) or
- Tiopronin (e.g., Thiola)—Use of any of these medicines with capreomycin may increase the chance of hearing, balance, or kidney side effects

Other medical problems—The presence of other medical problems may affect the use of capreomycin. Make sure you tell your doctor if you have any other medical problems, especially:

- Eighth-cranial-nerve disease (loss of hearing and/or balance)—Capreomycin may cause hearing and balance side effects
- Kidney disease—Capreomycin may cause serious side effects affecting the kidneys
- Myasthenia gravis or
- Parkinson's disease—Capreomycin may cause muscular weakness

Before you begin using any new medicine (prescription or nonprescription) or if you develop any new medical problem while you are using this medicine, check with your doctor, nurse, or pharmacist.

Proper Use of This Medicine

Dosing—The dose of capreomycin will be different for different patients. The following information includes only the average doses of capreomycin. Your dose may be different if you have kidney disease.

- For *injection* dosage form:
  - —Adults and adolescents: 1 gram of capreomycin injected into the muscle once a day for 60 to 120 days. After this time, 1 gram of capreomycin is injected into the muscle 2 or 3 times a week. This medicine must be given with other medicines to treat tuberculosis (TB).
  - —Children: Dose has not been determined.

Side Effects of This Medicine

Along with its needed effects, a medicine may cause some unwanted effects. Although not all of these side effects may occur, if they do occur they may need medical attention.

Check with your doctor as soon as possible if any of the following side effects occur:

More common

Greatly increased or decreased frequency of urination or amount of urine; increased thirst; loss of appetite; nausea; vomiting

Less common

Any loss of hearing; clumsiness or unsteadiness; difficulty in breathing; dizziness; drowsiness; fever; irregular heartbeat; itching; muscle cramps or pain; pain, redness, hardness, unusual bleeding, or a sore at the place of injection; ringing or buzzing or a feeling of fullness in the ears; skin rash; swelling; unusual tiredness or weakness

Other side effects not listed above may also occur in some patients. If you notice any other effects, check with your doctor.

Annual revision: 02/23/93

CAPSAICIN Topical

Some commonly used brand names are:

In the U.S.
Zostrix
Zostrix–HP

In Canada
Axsain
Zostrix

Description

Capsaicin (cap-SAY-sin) is used to help relieve a certain type of pain known as neuralgia (new-RAL-ja). Capsaicin is also used to temporarily help relieve the pain from osteoarthritis (OS-te-o-ar-THRI-tis) or rheumatoid arthritis (ROO-ma-toid ar-THRI-tis). This medicine will not cure any of these conditions.

Neuralgia is a pain from the nerves near the surface of your skin. This pain may occur after an infection with herpes zoster (shingles). It may also occur if you have diabetic neuropathy (di-a-BET-ick new-ROP-a-thee). Diabetic neuropathy is a condition that occurs in some persons with diabetes. The condition causes tingling and pain in the feet and toes. Capsaicin will help relieve the pain of diabetic neuropathy, but it will not cure diabetic neuropathy or diabetes.

Capsaicin may also be used for neuralgias caused by other conditions as determined by your doctor.

Capsaicin is available without a prescription; however, your doctor may have special instructions on the proper use of this medicine.

Topical

- Cream (U.S. and Canada)

It is very important that you read and understand the following information. If any of it causes you special concern, check with your doctor or pharmacist. Also, *if you have any questions* or if you want more information about this medicine or your medical problem, *ask your doctor, nurse, or pharmacist.*

Before Using This Medicine

If you are using this medicine without a prescription, carefully read and follow any precautions on the label. For capsaicin, the following should be considered:

Allergies—Tell your doctor if you have ever had any unusual or allergic reaction to capsaicin or to the fruit of capsicum plants (for example, hot peppers). Also tell your doctor and pharmacist if you are allergic to any other substances, such as foods, preservatives, or dyes.

Pregnancy—Capsaicin has not been reported to cause birth defects or other problems in humans.

Breast-feeding—Capsaicin has not been reported to cause problems in nursing babies.

Children—Use is not recommended for infants and children up to 2 years of age, except as directed by your doctor. In children 2 years of age and older, this medicine is not expected to cause different side effects or problems than it does in adults.

Older adults—Many medicines have not been studied specifically in older people. Therefore, it may not be known whether they work exactly the same way they do in younger adults. Although there is no specific information comparing use of capsaicin in the elderly with use in other age groups, this medicine is not expected to cause different side effects or problems in older people than it does in younger adults.

Other medical problems—The presence of other medical problems may affect the use of capsaicin. Make sure you tell your doctor if you have any other medical problems, especially:

- Broken or irritated skin on area to be treated with capsaicin

Before you begin using any new medicine (prescription or nonprescription) or if you develop any new medical problem while you are using this medicine, check with your doctor, nurse, or pharmacist.

Proper Use of This Medicine

If you are using capsaicin for the treatment of neuralgia caused by herpes zoster, do not apply the medicine until the zoster sores have healed.

It is not necessary to wash the areas to be treated before you apply capsaicin, but doing so will not cause harm.

Apply a small amount of cream and use your fingers to rub it well into the affected area so that little or no cream is left on the surface of the skin afterwards.

Wash your hands with soap and water after applying capsaicin to avoid getting the medicine in your eyes or on other sensitive areas of the body. However, if you are using capsaicin for arthritis in your hands, do not wash your hands for at least 30 minutes after applying the cream.

If a bandage is being used on the treated area, it should not be applied tightly.

When you first begin to use capsaicin, a warm, stinging, or burning sensation (feeling) may occur. This sensation is related to the action of capsaicin on the skin, and is to be expected. Although this sensation usually disappears after the first several days of treatment, it may last 2 to 4 weeks or longer. Heat, humidity, clothing, bathing in warm water, or sweating may increase the sensation. However, the sensation usually occurs less often and is less severe the longer you use the medicine. Reducing the number of doses of capsaicin that you use each day will not lessen the sensation, and may lengthen the period of time that you get the sensation. Also, reducing the number of doses you use may reduce the amount of pain relief that you get.

Capsaicin must be used regularly every day as directed if it is to work properly. Even then, it may not relieve your pain right away. The length of time it takes to work depends on the type of pain you have. In persons with arthritis, pain relief usually begins within 1 to 2 weeks. In most persons with neuralgia, relief usually begins within 2 to 4 weeks, although with head and neck neuralgias, relief may take as long as 4 to 6 weeks.

Once capsaicin has begun to relieve pain, you must continue to use it regularly 3 or 4 times a day to keep the pain from returning. If you stop using capsaicin and your pain returns, you can begin using it again.

Dosing—The dose of capsaicin may be different for different patients. *Follow your doctor's orders or the directions on the label.* The following information includes only the average dose of capsaicin. *If your dose is different, do not change it* unless your doctor tells you to do so:

- Apply regularly 3 or 4 times a day and rub in well.

Missed dose—If you miss a dose of this medicine, use it as soon as possible. However, if it is almost time for your next dose, skip the missed dose and go back to your regular dosing schedule. Do not double doses.

Storage—To store this medicine:

- Keep out of the reach of children.
- Store away from heat and direct light.
- Keep the medicine from freezing. Do not refrigerate.
- Do not keep outdated medicine or medicine no longer needed. Be sure that any discarded medicine is out of the reach of children.

Precautions While Using This Medicine

If capsaicin gets into your eyes or on other sensitive areas of the body, it will cause a burning sensation. If capsaicin gets into your eyes, flush your eyes with water. If capsaicin gets on other sensitive areas of your body, wash the areas with warm (not hot) soapy water.

If your condition gets worse, or does not improve after 1 month, stop using this medicine and check with your doctor.

Side Effects of This Medicine

Along with its needed effects, a medicine may cause some unwanted effects. Although not all of these side effects may occur, if they do occur they may need medical attention. Some side effects may occur that usually do not need medical attention. These side effects may go away during treatment as your body adjusts to the medicine.

However, check with your doctor if any of the following side effects continue or are bothersome:

More common

Warm, stinging, or burning feeling at the place of treatment

Other side effects not listed above may also occur in some patients. If you notice any other effects, check with your doctor.

Annual revision: 07/14/92

CARBACHOL Ophthalmic

Some commonly used brand names in the U.S. and Canada are Isopto Carbachol and Miostat.

Another commonly used name is carbamylcholine.

Description

Carbachol (KAR-ba-kole) is used in the eye to treat glaucoma. Sometimes it is also used in eye surgery.

This medicine is available only with your doctor's prescription, in the following dosage forms:

Ophthalmic

- Intraocular solution (U.S. and Canada)
- Ophthalmic solution (U.S. and Canada)

It is very important that you read and understand the following information. If any of it causes you special concern, check with your doctor. Also, *if you have any questions* or if you want more information about this medicine or your medical problem, *ask your doctor, nurse, or pharmacist.*

Before Using This Medicine

In deciding to use a medicine, the risks of taking the medicine must be weighed against the good it will do. This is a decision you and your doctor will make. For carbachol, the following should be considered:

Allergies—Tell your doctor if you have ever had any unusual or allergic reaction to carbachol. Also tell your doctor and pharmacist if you are allergic to any other substances, such as preservatives.

Pregnancy—Carbachol may be absorbed into the body. However, carbachol has not been shown to cause birth defects or other problems in humans.

Breast-feeding—Carbachol may be absorbed into the mother's body. However, carbachol has not been reported to cause problems in nursing babies.

Children—Although there is no specific information comparing use of carbachol in children with use in other age groups, this medicine is not expected to cause different side effects or problems in children than it does in adults.

Older adults—Many medicines have not been studied specifically in older people. Therefore, it may not be known whether they work exactly the same way they do in younger adults. Although there is no specific information comparing use of carbachol in the elderly with use in other age groups, this medicine is not expected to cause different side effects or problems in older people than it does in younger adults.

Other medicines—Although certain medicines should not be used together at all, in other cases two different medicines may be used together even if an interaction might occur. In these cases, your doctor may want to change the dose, or other precautions may be necessary. Tell your doctor and pharmacist if you are using any other prescription or nonprescription (over-the-counter [OTC]) medicine.

Other medical problems—The presence of other medical problems may affect the use of carbachol. Make sure you tell your doctor if you have any other medical problems, especially:

- Asthma or
- Eye problems (other) or
- Heart disease or
- Overactive thyroid or
- Parkinson's disease or
- Stomach ulcer or other stomach problems or
- Urinary tract blockage—Carbachol may make the condition worse

Before you begin using any new medicine (prescription or nonprescription) or if you develop any new medical problem while you are using this medicine, check with your doctor, nurse, or pharmacist.

Proper Use of This Medicine

Use this medicine only as directed. Do not use more of it and do not use it more often than your doctor ordered. To do so may increase the chance of too much medicine being absorbed into the body and the chance of side effects.

To use:

- First, wash your hands. With the middle finger, apply pressure to the inside corner of the eye (and continue to apply pressure for 1 or 2 minutes after the medicine has been placed in the eye). Tilt the head back and with the index finger of the same hand, pull the lower eyelid away from the eye to form a pouch. Drop the medicine into the pouch and gently close the eyes. Do not blink. Keep the eyes closed for 1 or 2 minutes to allow the medicine to be absorbed.
- Immediately after using the eye drops, wash your hands to remove any medicine that may be on them.
- To keep the medicine as germ-free as possible, do not touch the applicator tip to any surface (including the eye). Also, keep the container tightly closed.

Missed dose—If you miss a dose of this medicine, apply it as soon as possible. However, if it is almost time for your next dose, skip the missed dose and go back to your regular dosing schedule. Do not double doses.

Storage—To store this medicine:

- Keep out of the reach of children.
- Store away from heat and direct light.
- Keep the medicine from freezing.
- Do not keep outdated medicine or medicine no longer needed. Be sure that any discarded medicine is out of the reach of children.

Precautions While Using This Medicine

Your doctor should check your eye pressure at regular visits.

After you apply this medicine to your eyes, your pupils may become unusually small. This may cause you to see less well at night or in dim light. *Be especially careful if you drive, use machines, or do anything else at night or in dim light that could be dangerous if you are not able to see well.*

Also, for a short time after you apply this medicine, your vision may be blurred or there may be a change in your near or distant vision. *Make sure your vision is clear before you drive, use machines, or do anything else that could be dangerous if you are not able to see well.*

Side Effects of This Medicine

Along with its needed effects, a medicine may cause some unwanted effects. Although not all of these side effects may occur, if they do occur they may need medical attention.

Check with your doctor as soon as possible if any of the following side effects occur:

Symptoms of too much medicine being absorbed into the body

Diarrhea, stomach cramps or pain, or vomiting; flushing or redness of face; frequent urge to urinate; increased sweating; shortness of breath, wheezing, or tightness in chest; watering of mouth

Other side effects may occur that usually do not need medical attention. These side effects may go away during treatment as your body adjusts to the medicine. However, check with your doctor if any of the following side effects continue or are bothersome:

More common

Blurred vision or change in near or distant vision; eye pain

Less common

Headache; irritation of eyes; twitching of eyelids

Other side effects not listed above may also occur in some patients. If you notice any other effects, check with your doctor.

Annual revision: 11/21/91

CARBAMAZEPINE Systemic

Some commonly used brand names are:

In the U.S.

Epitol
Tegretol

Generic name product may also be available.

In Canada

Apo-Carbamazepine
Mazepine
Novocarbamaz
PMS Carbamazepine
Tegretol
Tegetrol Chewtabs
Tegetrol CR

Description

Carbamazepine (kar-ba-MAZ-e-peen) is used to control some types of seizures in the treatment of epilepsy. It is also used to relieve pain due to trigeminal neuralgia (tic douloureux). It should not be used for other more common aches or pains.

Carbamazepine may also be used for other conditions as determined by your doctor.

This medicine is available only with your doctor's prescription, in the following dosage forms:

Oral
- Suspension (U.S.)
- Tablets (U.S. and Canada)
- Chewable tablets (U.S. and Canada)
- Extended-release tablets (Canada)

It is very important that you read and understand the following information. If any of it causes you special concern, check with your doctor. Also, *if you have any questions* or if you want more information about this medicine or your medical problem, *ask your doctor, nurse, or pharmacist.*

Before Using This Medicine

In deciding to use a medicine, the risks of taking the medicine must be weighed against the good it will do. This is a decision you and your doctor will make. For carbamazepine, the following should be considered:

Allergies—Tell your doctor if you have ever had any unusual or allergic reaction to carbamazepine or to any of the tricyclic antidepressants, such as amitriptyline, amoxapine, clomipramine, desipramine, doxepin, imipramine, nortriptyline, protriptyline, or trimipramine. Also tell your doctor and pharmacist if you are allergic to any other substances, such as foods, preservatives, or dyes.

Pregnancy—Carbamazepine has not been studied in pregnant women. However, there have been reports of babies having low birth weight, small head size, skull and facial defects, underdeveloped fingernails, and delays in growth when their mothers had taken carbamazepine in high doses during pregnancy. In addition, birth defects have been reported in some babies when the mothers took other medicines for epilepsy during pregnancy. Also, studies in animals have shown that carbamazepine causes birth defects when given in large doses. Therefore, the use of carbamazepine during pregnancy should be discussed with your doctor.

Breast-feeding—Carbamazepine passes into the breast milk, and in some cases the baby may receive enough of it to cause unwanted effects. In animal studies, carbamazepine has affected the growth and appearance of the nursing babies.

Children—Behavior changes are more likely to occur in children.

Older adults—Confusion; restlessness and nervousness; irregular, pounding, or unusually slow heartbeat; and chest pain may be especially likely to occur in elderly patients, who are usually more sensitive than younger adults to the effects of carbamazepine.

Other medicines—Although certain medicines should not be used together at all, in other cases two different medicines may be used together even if an interaction might occur. In these cases, your doctor may want to change the dose, or other precautions may be necessary. When you are taking carbamazepine, it is especially important that your doctor and pharmacist know if you are taking any of the following:

- Adrenocorticoids (cortisone-like medicine)—The effects of adrenocorticoids may be decreased
- Anticoagulants (blood thinners)—The effects of anticoagulants may be decreased; monitoring of blood clotting time may be necessary during and after carbamazepine treatment
- Cimetidine (e.g., Tagamet)—Blood levels of carbamazepine may be increased, leading to an increase in serious side effects
- Diltiazem (e.g., Cardizem) or
- Erythromycin (e.g., E-Mycin, Erythrocin, Ilosone) or
- Propoxyphene (e.g., Darvon) or
- Verapamil (e.g., Calan)—Blood levels of carbamazepine may be increased; these medicines should not be used with carbamazepine
- Estrogens (female hormones) or
- Quinidine or
- Oral contraceptives (birth control pills), containing estrogen—The effects of these medicines may be decreased; use of a nonhormonal method of birth control or an oral contraceptive containing only a progestin may be necessary
- Isoniazid (e.g., INH)—The risk of serious side effects may be increased
- Monoamine oxidase (MAO) inhibitors (furazolidone [e.g., Furoxone], isocarboxazid [e.g., Marplan], phenelzine [e.g., Nardil], procarbazine [e.g., Matulane], tranylcypromine [e.g., Parnate])—Taking carbamazepine while you are taking or within 2 weeks of taking monoamine oxidase (MAO) inhibitors may cause sudden high body temperature, extremely high blood pressure, and severe convulsions; at least 14 days should be allowed between stopping treatment with one medicine and starting treatment with the other
- Other anticonvulsants (seizure medicine)—The effects of these medicines may be decreased; in addition, if these medicines and carbamazepine are used together during pregnancy, the risk of birth defects may be increased
- Tricyclic antidepressants (amitriptyline [e.g., Elavil], amoxapine [e.g., Asendin], clomipramine [e.g., Anafranil], desipramine [e.g., Pertofrane], doxepin [e.g., Sinequan], imipramine [e.g., Tofranil], nortriptyline [e.g., Aventyl], protriptyline [e.g., Vivactil], trimipramine [e.g., Surmontil])—Central nervous system depressant effects of carbamazepine may be increased while the anticonvulsant effects of carbamazepine may be decreased; seizures may occur more frequently

Other medical problems—The presence of other medical problems may affect the use of carbamazepine. Make sure you tell your doctor if you have any other medical problems, especially:

- Alcohol abuse (or history of) or
- Anemia or other blood problems or
- Behavioral problems or
- Diabetes mellitus (sugar diabetes) or
- Glaucoma or

- Heart or blood vessel disease or
- Problems with urination—Carbamazepine may make the condition worse
- Kidney disease or
- Liver disease—Higher blood levels of carbamazepine may result, increasing the chance of side effects

Before you begin using any new medicine (prescription or nonprescription) or if you develop any new medical problem while you are using this medicine, check with your doctor, nurse, or pharmacist.

Proper Use of This Medicine

Carbamazepine should be taken with meals to lessen the chance of stomach upset (nausea and vomiting).

It is very important that you take this medicine exactly as directed by your doctor to obtain the best results and lessen the chance of serious side effects. Do not take more of it, do not take it more often, and do not take it for a longer time than your doctor ordered.

If you are taking this medicine for pain relief:

- Carbamazepine is *not* an ordinary pain reliever. It should be used only when a doctor prescribes it for certain kinds of pain. *Do not take carbamazepine for any other aches or pains.*

If you are taking this medicine for epilepsy:

- *Do not suddenly stop taking this medicine without first checking with your doctor.* To keep your seizures under control, it is usually best to gradually reduce the amount of carbamazepine you are taking before stopping completely.

Missed dose—If you miss a dose of this medicine, take it as soon as possible. However, if it is almost time for your next dose, skip the missed dose and go back to your regular dosing schedule. Do not double doses. However, if you miss more than one dose a day, check with your doctor.

Storage—To store this medicine:

- Keep out of the reach of children.
- Store away from heat and direct light.
- *Do not store the tablet forms of carbamazepine in the bathroom, near the kitchen sink, or in other damp places. Heat or moisture may cause the medicine to break down and become less effective.*
- Keep the liquid form of this medicine from freezing.
- Do not keep outdated medicine or medicine no longer needed. Be sure that any discarded medicine is out of the reach of children.

Precautions While Using This Medicine

It is very important that your doctor check your progress at regular visits. Your doctor may want to have certain tests done to see if you are receiving the right amount of medicine or if certain side effects may be occurring without your knowing it. Also, the amount of medicine you are taking may have to be changed often.

This medicine will add to the effects of alcohol and other CNS depressants (medicines that slow down the nervous system, possibly causing drowsiness). Some examples of CNS depressants are antihistamines or medicine for hay fever, other allergies, or colds; sedatives, tranquilizers, or sleeping medicine; prescription pain medicine or narcotics; barbiturates; medicine for seizures; muscle relaxants; or anesthetics, including some dental anesthetics. *Check with your doctor before taking any of the above while you are using this medicine.*

This medicine may cause some people to become drowsy, dizzy, lightheaded, or less alert than they are normally, especially when they are starting treatment or increasing the dose. It may also cause blurred or double vision, weakness, or loss of muscle control in some people. *Make sure you know how you react to this medicine before you drive, use machines, or do anything else that could be dangerous if you are not alert and well-coordinated or able to see well.*

Some people who take carbamazepine may become more sensitive to sunlight than they are normally. Exposure to sunlight, even for brief periods of time, may cause a skin rash, itching, redness or other discoloration of the skin, or a severe sunburn. When you begin taking this medicine:

- Stay out of direct sunlight, especially between the hours of 10:00 a.m. and 3:00 p.m., if possible.
- Wear protective clothing, including a hat. Also, wear sunglasses.
- Apply a sun block product that has a skin protection factor (SPF) of at least 15. Some patients may require a product with a higher SPF number, especially if they have a fair complexion. If you have any questions about this, check with your doctor or pharmacist.
- Apply a sun block lipstick that has an SPF of at least 15 to protect your lips.
- Do not use a sunlamp or tanning bed or booth.

If you have a severe reaction from the sun, check with your doctor.

For diabetic patients:

- Carbamazepine may affect urine sugar levels. While you are using this medicine, be especially careful when testing for sugar in your urine. If you notice a change in the results of your urine sugar tests or have any questions about this, check with your doctor.

Before having any medical tests, tell the medical doctor in charge that you are taking this medicine. The results of some pregnancy tests and the metyrapone test may be affected by this medicine.

Before having any kind of surgery, dental treatment, or emergency treatment, tell the medical doctor or dentist in charge that you are taking this medicine.

Your doctor may want you to carry a medical identification card or bracelet stating that you are taking this medicine.

Side Effects of This Medicine

Along with its needed effects, a medicine may cause some unwanted effects. Although not all of these side effects may occur, if they do occur they may need medical attention.

Check with your doctor immediately if any of the following side effects occur:

Rare

Black, tarry stools; blood in urine or stools; bone or joint pain; cough or hoarseness; darkening of urine; lower back or side pain; nosebleeds or other unusual bleeding or bruising; painful or difficult urination; pain, tenderness, swelling, or bluish color in leg or foot; pale stools; pinpoint red spots on skin; shortness of breath or cough; sores, ulcers, or white spots on lips or in the mouth; sore throat, chills, and fever; swollen or painful glands; unusual tiredness or weakness; wheezing, tightness in chest, or troubled breathing; yellow eyes or skin

Symptoms of overdose

Body spasm in which head and heels are bent backward and body is bowed forward; clumsiness or unsteadiness; convulsions (seizures)—especially in small children; dizziness (severe) or fainting; drowsiness (severe); fast or irregular heartbeat; high or low blood pressure (hypertension or hypotension); irregular, slow, or shallow breathing; large pupils; nausea or vomiting (severe); overactive reflexes followed by underactive reflexes; poor control in body movements (for example, when reaching or stepping); sudden decrease in amount of urine; trembling, twitching, or abnormal body movements

In addition, check with your doctor as soon as possible if any of the following side effects occur:

More common

Blurred vision or double vision; continuous back-and-forth eye movements

Less common

Behavioral changes (especially in children); confusion, agitation, or hostility (especially in the elderly); diarrhea (severe); headache (continuing); increase in seizures; nausea and vomiting (severe); skin rash, hives, or itching; unusual drowsiness

Rare

Chest pain; difficulty in speaking or slurred speech; fainting; frequent urination; irregular, pounding, or unusually slow heartbeat; mental depression with restlessness and nervousness or other mood or other mental changes; numbness, tingling, pain, or weakness in hands and feet; rapid weight gain; rigidity; ringing, buzzing, or other unexplained sounds in the ears; sudden decrease in amount of urine; swelling of face, hands, feet, or lower legs; trembling; uncontrolled body movements; visual hallucinations (seeing things that are not there)

Other side effects may occur that usually do not need medical attention. These side effects may go away during treatment as your body adjusts to the medicine. However, check with your doctor if any of the following side effects continue or are bothersome:

More common

Clumsiness or unsteadiness; dizziness (mild); drowsiness (mild); lightheadedness; nausea or vomiting (mild)

Less common or rare

Aching joints or muscles; constipation; diarrhea; dryness of mouth; headache; increased sensitivity of skin to sunlight (skin rash, itching, redness or other discoloration of skin, or severe sunburn); increased sweating; irritation or soreness of tongue or mouth; loss of appetite; loss of hair; muscle or abdominal cramps; sexual problems in males; stomach pain or discomfort

Other side effects not listed above may also occur in some patients. If you notice any other effects, check with your doctor.

Additional Information

Once a medicine has been approved for marketing for a certain use, experience may show that it is also useful for other medical problems. Although these uses are not included in product labeling, carbamazepine is used in certain patients with the following medical conditions:

- Neurogenic pain (a type of continuing pain)
- Bipolar disorder (manic-depressive illness)
- Central partial diabetes insipidus (water diabetes)
- Alcohol withdrawal
- Psychotic disorders (severe mental illness)

Other than the above information, there is no additional information relating to proper use, precautions, or side effects for these uses.

Annual revision: 04/29/91

CARBOHYDRATES AND ELECTROLYTES Systemic

This information applies to the following medicines:

Dextrose and Electrolytes
Oral Rehydration Salts
Rice Syrup Solids and Electrolytes

Some commonly used brand names are:

For Dextrose and Electrolytes

In the U.S.

Naturalyte
Pedialyte
Rehydralyte
Resol‡

In Canada

Lytren
Pedialyte

For Oral Rehydration Salts*§

In Canada

Gastrolyte
Rapolyte

For Rice Syrup Solids and Electrolytes†

In the U.S.

Ricelyte

Other commonly used names are oral rehydration salts, ORS-bicarbonate, and ORS-citrate.§

*Not commercially available in the U.S.
†Not commercially available in Canada.
‡ Resol is available to hospitals only.
§Distributed by the World Health Organization (WHO).

Description

Carbohydrate and electrolytes combination is used to treat or prevent dehydration (the loss of too much water from the body) that may occur with severe diarrhea, especially in babies and young children. Although this medicine does not immediately stop the diarrhea, it replaces the water and some important salts (electrolytes), such as sodium and potassium, that are lost from the body during diarrhea, and helps prevent more serious problems. Some carbohydrate and electrolytes solutions may also be used after surgery when food intake has been stopped.

This medicine is available without a prescription; however, your doctor may have special instructions on the proper use and dose for you or your child.

Carbohydrate and electrolytes combination is available in the following dosage forms:

Oral

- Solution (U.S. and Canada)
- Powder for oral solution (Canada)

It is very important that you read and understand the following information. If any of it causes you special concern, check with your doctor or pharmacist. Also, *if you have any questions* or if you want more information about this medicine or your medical problem, *ask your doctor, nurse, or pharmacist.*

Before Using This Medicine

If you are taking this medicine without a prescription, carefully read and follow any precautions on the label. For carbohydrate and electrolytes solutions, the following should be considered:

Allergies—Tell your doctor if you have ever had any unusual or allergic reaction to medicines containing potassium, sodium, citrates, rice, or sugar. Also tell your doctor and pharmacist if you are allergic to any other substances, such as foods, preservatives, or dyes.

Pregnancy—Carbohydrate and electrolytes solutions have not been shown to cause birth defects or other problems in humans.

Breast-feeding—This medicine has not been reported to cause problems in nursing babies. Breast-feeding should continue, if possible, during treatment with carbohydrate and electrolytes solution.

Children—This medicine has been tested in children and, in effective doses, appears to be safe and effective in children. This medicine has not been tested in premature infants.

Older adults—This medicine has been tested and has been shown to be well tolerated by older people.

Other medicines—Although certain medicines should not be used together at all, in other cases two different medicines may be used together even if an interaction might occur. In these cases, your doctor may want to change the dose, or other precautions may be necessary. Tell your doctor and pharmacist if you are taking any other prescription or nonprescription (over-the-counter [OTC]) medicine.

Other medical problems—The presence of other medical problems may affect the use of carbohydrate and electrolytes solutions. Make sure you tell your doctor if you have any other medical problems, especially:

- Difficult urination—This condition may prevent the carbohydrate and electrolytes solution from working properly
- Inability to drink or
- Vomiting (severe and continuing)—Treatment by injection may need to be given to patients with these conditions
- Intestinal blockage—Carbohydrate and electrolytes solution may be harmful if given to patients with this condition

Before you begin using any new medicine (prescription or nonprescription) or if you develop any new medical problem while you are using this medicine, check with your doctor, nurse, or pharmacist.

Proper Use of This Medicine

For patients using the *commercial powder form* of this medicine:

- Add 7 ounces of boiled, cooled tap water to the entire contents of one powder packet. Shake or stir the container for 2 or 3 minutes until all the powder is dissolved.

- Do not add more water to the solution after it is mixed.
- Do not boil the solution.
- Make and use a fresh solution each day.

For patients using the *powder form* of this medicine *distributed by the World Health Organization (WHO):*

- Add the entire contents of one powder packet to enough drinking water to make one quart (32 ounces) or liter of solution. Shake the container for 2 or 3 minutes until all the powder is dissolved.
- Do not add more water to the solution after it is mixed.
- Do not boil the solution.
- Make and use a fresh solution each day.

Babies and small children should be given the solution slowly, in small amounts, with a spoon, as often as possible, during the first 24 hours of diarrhea.

Take as directed. Do not take it for a longer time than your doctor has recommended. To do so may increase the chance of side effects.

Storage—To store this medicine:

- Keep out of the reach of children.
- Store away from heat and direct light.
- Do not store the powder packets in the bathroom, near the kitchen sink, or in other damp places. Heat or moisture may cause the medicine to break down.
- Store the liquid in the refrigerator. However, keep the medicine from freezing.
- Make a fresh solution each day. Discard unused solution at the end of each day. Be sure that any discarded medicine is out of the reach of children.

Precautions While Using This Medicine

Eat soft foods, if possible, such as rice cereal, bananas, cooked peas or beans, and potatoes to keep up nutrition until the diarrhea stops and regular food and milk can be taken again. Breast-fed infants should be given breast milk between doses of the solution.

If your diarrhea does not improve in 1 or 2 days, or if it becomes worse, check with your doctor.

Also, *check with your doctor immediately* if your baby or child appears to have severe thirst, doughy skin, sunken eyes, dizziness or lightheadedness, tiredness or weakness, irritability, difficult urination, loss of weight, or convulsions (seizures). These signs may mean that too much water has been lost from the body.

For patients (except nursing babies) using the *powder form* of this medicine:

- Drink plain water whenever thirsty between doses of solution.

For patients taking the *premixed liquid form* of this medicine:

- Do not drink fruit juices or eat foods containing added salt until the diarrhea has stopped.

Side Effects of This Medicine

Along with its needed effects, a medicine may cause some unwanted effects. Although not all of these side effects may occur, if they do occur they may need medical attention.

Check with your doctor as soon as possible if any of the following side effects occur:

Symptoms of too much sodium (salt) in the body

Convulsions (seizures); dizziness; fast heartbeat; high blood pressure; irritability; muscle twitching; restlessness; swelling of feet or lower legs; weakness

Symptoms of too much fluid in the body

Puffy eyelids

Other side effects may occur that usually do not need medical attention. These side effects may go away during treatment as your body adjusts to the medicine. However, check with your doctor if the following side effect continues or is bothersome:

More common

Vomiting (mild)

Other side effects not listed above may also occur in some patients. If you notice any other effects, check with your doctor.

Annual revision: 12/02/92

CARBOL-FUCHSIN Topical

A commonly used brand name in the U.S. is Castel Plus.
Another commonly used name is Castellani Paint.
Generic name product may also be available.

Description

Carbol-fuchsin (kar-bol-FOOK-sin) is used to treat fungus infections, including athlete's foot and ringworm of the nails. It may also be used as a drying agent in skin conditions where there is too much moisture. This medicine may also be used for other infections as determined by your doctor.

Some preparations containing carbol-fuchsin topical solution are available only with your doctor's prescription. Others are available without a prescription; however, your doctor may have special instructions on the use of topical carbol-fuchsin solutions for your medical condition.

Topical carbol-fuchsin is available in the following dosage form:

Topical
- Solution (U.S.)

It is very important that you read and understand the following information. If any of it causes you special concern, check with your doctor or pharmacist. Also, *if you have any questions* or if you want more information about this medicine or your medical problem, *ask your doctor, nurse, or pharmacist.*

Before Using This Medicine

If you are using this medicine without a prescription, carefully read and follow any precautions on the label. For carbol-fuchsin, the following should be considered:

Allergies—Tell your doctor if you have ever had any unusual or allergic reaction to carbol-fuchsin. Also tell your doctor and pharmacist if you are allergic to any other substances, such as preservatives or dyes.

Pregnancy—Studies in humans have not shown that carbol-fuchsin causes birth defects or other problems in humans.

Breast-feeding—Carbol-fuchsin has not been reported to cause problems in nursing babies.

Children—If you are treating an infant or child with eczema, do not use carbol-fushsin more than once a day. Although there is no specific information comparing use of carbol-fuchsin in children treated for other conditions with use in other age groups, this medicine is not expected to cause different side effects or problems in children than it does in adults.

Older adults—Many medicines have not been studied specifically in older people. Therefore, it may not be known whether they work exactly the same way they do in younger adults or if they cause different side effects or problems in older people. There is no specific information comparing use of carbol-fuchsin in the elderly with use in other age groups.

Other medicines—Although certain medicines should not be used together at all, in other cases two different medicines may be used together even if an interaction might occur. In these cases, your doctor may want to change the dose, or other precautions may be necessary. Tell your doctor and pharmacist if you are using any other topical prescription or nonprescription (over-the-counter [OTC]) medicine that is to be applied to the same area of the skin.

Before you begin using any new medicine (prescription or nonprescription) or if you develop any new medical problem while you are using this medicine, check with your doctor, nurse, or pharmacist.

Proper Use of This Medicine

Carbol-fuchsin is a poison if swallowed. Use only on the affected areas as directed. Do not swallow this medicine.

Before applying this medicine, wash the affected areas with soap and water, and dry thoroughly.

Using an applicator or swab, apply this medicine only to the affected areas. Do not apply to large areas of the body, unless otherwise directed by your doctor.

When this medicine is applied to the fingers or toes, do not bandage them.

To help clear up your infection completely, *it is very important that you keep using this medicine for the full time of treatment,* even if your symptoms begin to clear up after a few days. Since fungus infections may be very slow to clear up, you may have to continue using this medicine every day for as long as several months or more. If you stop using this medicine too soon, your symptoms may return. *Do not miss any doses.*

Missed dose—If you do miss a dose of this medicine, apply it as soon as possible. However, if it is almost time for your next dose, skip the missed dose and go back to your regular dosing schedule.

Storage—To store this medicine:
- Keep out of the reach of children.
- Store away from heat and direct light.
- Keep the medicine from freezing.
- Do not keep outdated medicine or medicine no longer needed. Be sure that any discarded medicine is out of the reach of children.

Precautions While Using This Medicine

If your skin problem does not improve within 1 week, or if it becomes worse, check with your doctor.

This medicine will stain skin and clothing. Avoid getting it on your clothes. The stain will slowly wear off from your skin.

Side Effects of This Medicine

Along with its needed effects, a medicine may cause some unwanted effects. Although not all of these side effects may occur, if they do occur they may need medical attention.

Check with your doctor as soon as possible if the following side effect occurs:

Skin irritation not present before use of this medicine

Other side effects may occur that usually do not need medical attention. These side effects may go away during treatment as your body adjusts to the medicine. However, check with your doctor if the following side effect continues or is bothersome:

Mild, temporary stinging

Other side effects not listed above may also occur in some patients. If you notice any other effects, check with your doctor.

Annual revision: 02/10/92

CARBONIC ANHYDRASE INHIBITORS Systemic

This information applies to the following medicines:

Acetazolamide (a-set-a-ZOLE-a-mide)
Dichlorphenamide (dye-klor-FEN-a-mide)
Methazolamide (meth-a-ZOLE-a-mide)

Some commonly used brand names are:

For Acetazolamide

In the U.S.

Ak-Zol
Dazamide
Diamox
Diamox Sequels

Generic name product may also be available.

In Canada

Acetazolam
Apo-Acetazolamide
Diamox
Diamox Sequels

For Dichlorphenamide

In the U.S.

Daranide

Another commonly used name is diclofenamide.

For Methazolamide

In the U.S.

Neptazane

In Canada

Neptazane

Description

Carbonic anhydrase inhibitors are used to treat glaucoma. Acetazolamide is also used as an anticonvulsant to control certain seizures in the treatment of epilepsy. It is also sometimes used to prevent or lessen some effects in mountain climbers who climb to high altitudes, and to treat other conditions as determined by your doctor.

These medicines are available only with your doctor's prescription, in the following dosage forms:

Oral

Acetazolamide
- Extended-release capsules (U.S. and Canada)
- Tablets (U.S. and Canada)

Dichlorphenamide
- Tablets (U.S.)

Methazolamide
- Tablets (U.S. and Canada)

Parenteral

Acetazolamide
- Injection (U.S. and Canada)

It is very important that you read and understand the following information. If any of it causes you special concern, check with your doctor. Also, *if you have any questions* or if you want more information about this medicine or your medical problem, *ask your doctor, nurse, or pharmacist.*

Before Using This Medicine

In deciding to use a medicine, the risks of taking the medicine must be weighed against the good it will do. This is a decision you and your doctor will make. For carbonic anhydrase inhibitors, the following should be considered:

Allergies—Tell your doctor if you have ever had any unusual or allergic reaction to carbonic anhydrase inhibitors, sulfonamides (sulfa drugs), or thiazide diuretics (a type of water pill). Also tell your doctor and pharmacist if you are allergic to any other substances, such as foods, preservatives, or dyes.

Pregnancy—Carbonic anhydrase inhibitors have not been shown to cause birth defects or other problems in humans. However, studies in animals have shown that they cause birth defects when given in very high doses. Before taking this medicine, make sure your doctor knows if you are pregnant or if you may become pregnant.

Breast-feeding—Although carbonic anhydrase inhibitors may pass into the breast milk, they have not been reported to cause problems in nursing babies.

Children—Although there is no specific information about the use of carbonic anhydrase inhibitors in children, they are not expected to cause different side effects or problems in children than they do in adults.

Older adults—Many medicines have not been tested in older people. Therefore, it may not be known whether they work exactly the same way they do in younger adults. Although there is no specific information about the use of carbonic anhydrase inhibitors in the elderly, they are not expected to cause different side effects or problems in older people than they do in younger adults.

Other medicines—Although certain medicines should not be used together at all, in other cases two different medicines may be used together even if an interaction might occur. In these cases, your doctor may want to change the dose, or other precautions may be necessary. When you are using carbonic anhydrase inhibitors, it is especially important that your doctor and pharmacist know if you are using any of the following:

- Amphetamines or
- Mecamylamine (e.g., Inversine) or
- Quinidine (e.g., Quinidex)—Use of carbonic anhydrase inhibitors may increase the chance of side effects
- Methenamine (e.g., Mandelamine)—Use of carbonic anhydrase inhibitors may decrease the effectiveness of methenamine

Other medical problems—The presence of other medical problems may affect the use of carbonic anhydrase inhibitors. Make sure you tell your doctor if you have any other medical problems, especially:

- Diabetes mellitus (sugar diabetes)—Use of carbonic anhydrase inhibitors may increase the patient's blood and urine sugar concentrations
- Emphysema or other chronic lung disease—Use of carbonic anhydrase inhibitors may increase the risk of acidosis (shortness of breath, troubled breathing)
- Gout or
- Low blood levels of potassium or sodium—Use of carbonic anhydrase inhibitors may make the condition worse
- Kidney disease or stones—Higher blood levels of carbonic anhydrase inhibitors may result, which may increase the chance of side effects; also, these medicines may make the condition worse
- Liver disease—Use of carbonic anhydrase inhibitors may increase the risk of electrolyte imbalance and may make the condition worse
- Underactive adrenal gland (Addison's disease)—Use of carbonic anhydrase inhibitors may increase the risk of electrolyte imbalance

Before you begin using any new medicine (prescription or nonprescription) or if you develop any new medical problem while you are using this medicine, check with your doctor, nurse, or pharmacist.

Proper Use of This Medicine

Take this medicine only as directed. Do not take more of it and do not take it more often than your doctor ordered. To do so may increase the chance of side effects without increasing the effectiveness of this medicine.

This medicine may be taken with meals to lessen the chance of stomach upset. However, if stomach upset (nausea or vomiting) continues, check with your doctor.

This medicine may cause an increase in the amount of urine or in your frequency of urination. If you continue to take the medicine every day, these effects should lessen or stop. To keep the increase in urine from affecting your nighttime sleep:

- If you are to take a single dose a day, take it in the morning after breakfast.
- If you are to take more than one dose a day, take the last dose no later than 6 p.m., unless otherwise directed by your doctor.

However, it is best to plan your dose or doses according to a schedule that will least affect your personal activities and sleep. Ask your doctor, nurse, or pharmacist to help you plan the best time to take this medicine.

Missed dose—If you miss a dose of this medicine, take it as soon as possible. However, if it is almost time for your next dose, skip the missed dose and go back to your regular dosing schedule. Do not double doses.

Storage—To store this medicine:

- Keep out of the reach of children.
- Store away from heat and direct light.
- Do not store the capsule or tablet form of this medicine in the bathroom, near the kitchen sink, or in other damp places. Heat or moisture may cause the medicine to break down.
- Do not keep outdated medicine or medicine no longer needed. Be sure that any discarded medicine is out of the reach of children.

Precautions While Using This Medicine

This medicine may cause some people to feel drowsy, dizzy, lightheaded, or more tired than they are normally. *Make sure you know how you react to this medicine before you drive, use machines, or do anything else that could be dangerous if you are not alert.*

It is important that your doctor check your progress at regular visits. Your doctor may want to do certain tests to see if the medicine is working properly or to see if certain side effects may be occurring without your knowing it.

This medicine may cause a loss of potassium from your body. To help prevent this, your doctor may want you to eat or drink foods that have a high potassium content (for example, orange or other citrus fruit juices) or take a potassium supplement. It is very important to follow these directions. Also, it is important not to change your diet on your own. This is more important if you are already on a special diet (as for diabetes) or if you are taking a potassium supplement. Extra potassium may not be necessary and, in some cases, too much potassium could be harmful.

For *diabetic patients:*

- This medicine may raise blood and urine sugar levels. While you are using this medicine, be especially careful in testing for sugar in your blood or urine. If you have any questions about this, check with your doctor.

Your doctor may want you to increase the amount of fluids you drink while you are taking this medicine. This is to prevent kidney stones. However, do not increase the amount of fluids you drink without first checking with your doctor.

For patients taking *acetazolamide as an anticonvulsant*:

- *If you have been taking acetazolamide regularly for several weeks or more, do not suddenly stop taking it.* Your doctor may want you to reduce gradually the amount you are taking before stopping completely.

Side Effects of This Medicine

Along with its needed effects, a medicine may cause some unwanted effects. Although not all of these side effects may occur, if they do occur they may need medical attention.

Check with your doctor immediately if either of the following side effects occurs:

Rare

Shortness of breath or trouble in breathing

Also, check with your doctor as soon as possible if any of the following side effects occur:

More common

Unusual tiredness or weakness

Less common

Blood in urine; difficult urination; mental depression; pain in lower back; pain or burning while urinating; sudden decrease in amount of urine

Rare

Bloody or black, tarry stools; clumsiness or unsteadiness; confusion; convulsions (seizures); darkening of urine; fever; hives, itching of skin, skin rash, or sores; muscle weakness (severe); pale stools; ringing or buzzing in the ears; sore throat; trembling; unusual bruising or bleeding; yellow eyes or skin

Symptoms of too much potassium loss

Dryness of mouth; increased thirst; irregular heartbeats; mood or mental changes; muscle cramps or pain; nausea or vomiting; unusual tiredness or weakness; weak pulse

Also, check with your doctor if you have any changes in your vision (especially problems with seeing faraway objects) when you first begin taking this medicine.

Other side effects may occur that usually do not need medical attention. These side effects may go away during treatment as your body adjusts to the medicine. However, check with your doctor if any of the following side effects continue or are bothersome:

More common

Diarrhea; general feeling of discomfort or illness; increase in frequency of urination or amount of urine (rare with methazolamide); loss of appetite; metallic taste in mouth; nausea or vomiting; numbness, tingling, or burning in hands, fingers, feet, toes, mouth, lips, tongue, or anus; weight loss

Less common or rare

Constipation; dizziness or lightheadedness; drowsiness; feeling of choking or lump in the throat; headache; increased sensitivity of eyes to sunlight; loss of taste and smell; nervousness or irritability

Other side effects not listed above may also occur in some patients. If you notice any other effects, check with your doctor.

Annual revision: June 1990

CARBOPLATIN Systemic

Some commonly used brand names are:

In the U.S.

Paraplatin

In Canada

Paraplatin
Paraplatin-AQ

Description

Carboplatin (KAR-boe-pla-tin) belongs to the group of medicines known as alkylating agents. It is used to treat some kinds of cancer.

Carboplatin interferes with the growth of cancer cells, which are eventually destroyed. Since the growth of normal body cells may also be affected by carboplatin, other effects will also occur. Some of these may be serious and must be reported to your doctor. Other effects may not be serious but may cause concern. Some effects may not occur for months or years after the medicine is used.

Before you begin treatment with carboplatin, you and your doctor should talk about the good this medicine will do as well as the risks of using it.

Carboplatin is to be administered only by or under the immediate supervision of your doctor. It is available in the following dosage form:

Parenteral

- Injection (U.S. and Canada)

It is very important that you read and understand the following information. If any of it causes you special concern, check with your doctor. Also, *if you have any questions* or if you want more information about this medicine or your medical problem, *ask your doctor, nurse, or pharmacist.*

Before Using This Medicine

In deciding to use a medicine, the risks of taking the medicine must be weighed against the good it will do. This is a decision you and your doctor will make. For carboplatin, the following should be considered:

Allergies—Tell your doctor if you have ever had any unusual or allergic reaction to carboplatin, cisplatin, or any other platinum-containing substance.

Pregnancy—There is a chance that this medicine may cause birth defects if either the male or female is taking it at the time of conception or if it is taken during pregnancy. Carboplatin causes toxic or harmful effects and birth defects in rats. In addition, many cancer medicines may cause sterility which could be permanent. Although sterility has not been reported with this medicine, the possibility should be kept in mind.

Be sure that you have discussed these possible effects with your doctor before receiving this medicine. It is best to use some kind of birth control while you are receiving carboplatin. However, do not use oral contraceptives ("the Pill") since they may interfere with this medicine. Tell your doctor right away if you think you have become pregnant while receiving carboplatin. Before receiving carboplatin, make sure your doctor knows if you are pregnant or if you may become pregnant.

Breast-feeding—Because carboplatin may cause serious side effects, breast-feeding is generally not recommended while you are receiving it.

Children—Studies on this medicine have been done only in adult patients and there is no specific information comparing use of carboplatin in children with use in other age groups.

Older adults—Some side effects of carboplatin (especially blood problems or numbness or tingling in fingers or toes) may be more likely to occur in the elderly.

Other medicines—Although certain medicines should not be used together at all, in other cases two different medicines may be used together even if an interaction might occur. In these cases, your doctor may want to change the dose, or other precautions may be necessary. When receiving carboplatin it is especially important that your doctor and pharmacist know if you have every been treated with x-rays or cancer medicines or if you are taking any of the following:

- Amphotericin B by injection (e.g., Fungizone) or
- Antithyroid agents (medicine for overactive thyroid) or
- Azathioprine (e.g., Imuran) or
- Chloramphenicol (e.g., Chloromycetin) or
- Colchicine or
- Flucytosine (e.g., Ancobon) or
- Interferon (e.g., Intron A, Roferon-A) or
- Ganciclovir (e.g., Cytovene)
- Plicamycin (e.g., Mithracin) or
- Zidovudine (e.g., AZT, Retrovir)—Carboplatin may increase the effects of these medicines or radiation on the blood

Other medical problems—The presence of other medical problems may affect the use of carboplatin. Make sure you tell your doctor if you have any other medical problems, especially:

- Chickenpox (including recent exposure) or
- Herpes zoster (shingles)—Risk of severe disease affecting other parts of the body
- Hearing problems—May be worsened by carboplatin
- Infection—reduces immunity to infection
- Kidney disease—Effects may be increased because of slower removal from the body

Before you begin using any new medicine (prescription or nonprescription) or if you develop any new medical problem while you are using this medicine, check with your doctor, nurse, or pharmacist.

Proper Use of This Medicine

This medicine is sometimes given together with certain other medicines. If you are using a combination of medicines, it is important that you receive each one at the proper time. If you are taking some of these medicines by mouth, ask your doctor, nurse, or pharmacist to help you plan a way to take them at the right times.

This medicine usually causes nausea and vomiting that may sometimes be severe. However, it is very important that you continue to receive the medicine, even if you begin to feel ill. Ask your doctor, nurse, or pharmacist for ways to lessen these effects, especially if they are severe.

Precautions While Using This Medicine

It is very important that your doctor check your progress at regular visits to make sure that this medicine is working properly and to check for unwanted effects.

While you are being treated with carboplatin, and after you stop treatment with it, *do not have any immunizations (vaccinations) without your doctor's approval.* Carboplatin may lower your body's resistance and there is a chance you might get the infection the immunization is meant to prevent. In addition, other persons living in your household should not take or should not have recently taken oral polio vaccine since there is a chance they could pass the polio virus on to you. Also, avoid other persons who have taken oral polio vaccine. Do not get close to them, and do not stay in the same room with them for very long. If you cannot take these precautions, you should consider wearing a protective face mask that covers the nose and mouth.

Carboplatin can lower the number of white blood cells in your blood temporarily, increasing the chance of getting an infection. It can also lower the number of platelets, which are necessary for proper blood clotting. If this occurs, there are certain precautions you can take, especially when your blood count is low, to reduce the risk of infection or bleeding:

- If you can, avoid people with infections. *Check with your doctor immediately* if you think you are getting an infection or if you get a fever or chills, cough or hoarseness, lower back or side pain, or painful or difficult urination.
- *Check with your doctor immediately* if you notice any unusual bleeding or bruising; black, tarry stools; blood in urine or stools; or pinpoint red spots on your skin.
- Be careful when using a regular toothbrush, dental floss, or toothpick. Your medical doctor, dentist, or nurse may recommend other ways to clean your teeth and gums. Check with your medical doctor before having any dental work done.
- Do not touch your eyes or the inside of your nose unless you have just washed your hands and have not touched anything else in the meantime.
- Be careful not to cut yourself when you are using sharp objects such as a safety razor or fingernail or toenail cutters.
- Avoid contact sports or other situations where bruising or injury could occur.

Side Effects of This Medicine

Along with their needed effects, medicines like carboplatin can sometimes cause unwanted effects such as blood problems, ear and kidney problems, and other side effects. These and others are described below. Also, because of the way these medicines act on the body, there is a chance that they might cause other unwanted effects that may not occur until months or years after the medicine is used. These delayed effects may include certain types of cancer, such as leukemia. Discuss these possible effects with your doctor.

Although not all of these side effects may occur, if they do occur they may need medical attention.

Check with your doctor or nurse immediately if any of the following side effects occur:

Less common

Black, tarry stools; blood in urine or stools; cough or hoarseness; fever or chills; lower back or side pain; painful or difficult urination; pinpoint red spots on skin; skin rash or itching; unusual bleeding or bruising

Rare

Wheezing

Check with your doctor as soon as possible if any of the following side effects occur:

More common

Pain at place of injection

Less common

Numbness or tingling in fingers or toes

Rare

Blurred vision; ringing in ears; sores in mouth and on lips

Other side effects may occur that usually do not need medical attention. These side effects may go away during treatment as your body adjusts to the medicine. Also, your doctor or nurse may be able to tell you about ways to prevent or reduce some of these side effects. Check with your doctor or nurse if any of the following side effects continue or are bothersome or if you have any questions about them:

More common

Nausea and vomiting; unusual tiredness or weakness

Less common

Constipation or diarrhea; loss of appetite

This medicine may cause a temporary loss of hair in some people. After treatment with carboplatin has ended, normal hair growth should return.

Other side effects not listed above may also occur in some patients. If you notice any other effects, check with your doctor.

Annual revision: 06/03/92

CARBOPROST Systemic

Some commonly used brand names are:

In the U.S.
Hemabate

In Canada
Prostin/15M

Description

Carboprost (KAR-boe-prost) is given by injection to cause abortion. It is an oxytocic, which means it acts by causing the uterus to contract the way it does during labor and also helps the cervix to dilate.

Carboprost may also be used for other purposes as determined by your doctor.

Carboprost is to be administered only by or under the immediate care of your doctor. It is available in the following dosage form:

Parenteral

- Injection (U.S. and Canada)

It is very important that you read and understand the following information. If any of it causes you special concern, check with your doctor. Also, *if you have any questions* or if you want more information about this medicine or your medical problem, *ask your doctor, nurse, or pharmacist.*

Before Receiving This Medicine

In deciding to use a medicine, the risks of taking the medicine must be weighed against the good it will do. This is a decision you and your doctor will make. For carboprost, the following should be considered:

Allergies—Tell your doctor if you have ever had any unusual or allergic reaction to carboprost or other oxytocics (medicines that stimulate the uterus to contract). Also tell your doctor and pharmacist if you are allergic to any other substances, such as foods, preservatives, or dyes.

Other medicines—Although certain medicines should not be used together at all, in other cases two different medicines may be used together even if an interaction might occur. In these cases, your doctor may want to change the dose, or other precautions may be necessary. Tell your doctor if you are taking any prescription or nonprescription (over-the-counter [OTC]) medicine.

Other medical problems—The presence of other medical problems may affect the use of carboprost. Make sure you tell your doctor if you have any other medical problems, especially:

- Adrenal gland disease (history of)—Carboprost stimulates the body to produce steroids
- Anemia—In some patients, abortion with carboprost may result in loss of blood that may require a transfusion
- Asthma (or history of) or
- Lung disease—Carboprost may cause narrowing of the blood vessels in the lungs or narrowing of the lung passages
- Diabetes mellitus (sugar diabetes) (history of)
- Epilepsy (or history of)—Rarely, seizures have occurred with use of carboprost
- Fibroid tumors of the uterus or
- Uterus surgery (history of)—There is an increased risk of rupture of the uterus
- Glaucoma—Rarely, the pressure within the eye has increased during use of carboprost
- Heart or blood vessel disease (or history of) or
- High blood pressure (or history of) or
- Low blood pressure (or history of)—Carboprost may cause changes in heart function or blood pressure changes
- Jaundice (history of)
- Kidney disease (or history of)
- Liver disease (or history of)—The body may not get carboprost out of the bloodstream at the usual rate, which may make the medicine work longer or cause toxic effects

Side Effects of This Medicine

Along with its needed effects, a medicine may cause some unwanted effects. Although not all of these side effects may occur, if they do occur they may need medical attention.

Tell the doctor or nurse immediately if any of the following side effects occur:

Less common or rare

Fast or slow heartbeat; headache (severe and continuing); hives or skin rash; increased pain of the uterus; pale, cool, blotchy skin on arms or legs; pressing or painful feeling in chest; shortness of breath; swelling of face, inside the nose, and eyelids; tightness in chest; trouble in breathing; weak or absent pulse in arms or legs; wheezing

Check with the doctor or nurse as soon as possible if any of the following side effects occur:

Constipation; pain or inflammation at place of injection; tender or mildly bloated abdomen or stomach

Other side effects may occur that usually do not need medical attention. These side effects usually go away after the medicine is stopped. However, let the doctor or nurse know if any of the following side effects continue or are bothersome:

More common

Diarrhea; nausea; vomiting

Less common or rare

Chills or shivering; dizziness; fever (temporary); flushing or redness of face; headache; stomach cramps or pain

This procedure may result in some effects, which occur after the procedure is completed, that need medical attention. Check with your doctor if you notice any of the following:

Chills or shivering (continuing); fever (continuing); foul-smelling vaginal discharge; increase in uterus bleeding; pain in lower abdomen

Other side effects not listed above may also occur in some patients. If you notice any other effects, check with your doctor or nurse.

Annual revision: 10/26/92

CARMUSTINE Systemic

A commonly used brand name in the U.S. and Canada is BiCNU. Another commonly used name is BCNU.

Description

Carmustine (kar-MUS-teen) belongs to the group of medicines known as alkylating agents. It is used to treat some kinds of cancer.

Carmustine interferes with the growth of cancer cells, which are eventually destroyed. Since the growth of normal body cells may also be affected by carmustine, other effects will also occur. Some of these may be serious and must be reported to your doctor. Other effects, like hair loss, may not be serious but may cause concern. Some effects may not occur for months or years after the medicine is used.

Before you begin treatment with carmustine, you and your doctor should talk about the good this medicine will do as well as the risks of using it.

Carmustine is to be administered only by or under the immediate supervision of your doctor. It is available in the following dosage form:

Parenteral

- Injection (U.S. and Canada)

It is very important that you read and understand the following information. If any of it causes you special concern, check with your doctor. Also, *if you have any questions* or if you want more information about this medicine or your medical problem, *ask your doctor, nurse, or pharmacist.*

Before Using This Medicine

In deciding to use a medicine, the risks of taking the medicine must be weighed against the good it will do. This is a decision you and your doctor will make. For carmustine, the following should be considered:

Allergies—Tell your doctor if you have ever had any unusual or allergic reaction to carmustine.

Pregnancy—There is a chance that this medicine may cause birth defects if either the male or female is taking it at the time of conception or if it is taken during pregnancy. Carmustine causes toxic or harmful effects in the fetus of rats and rabbits and causes birth defects in rats at doses about the same as the human dose. In addition, many cancer medicines may cause sterility which could be permanent. Although this has only been reported in animals with this medicine, the possibility should be kept in mind.

Be sure that you have discussed this with your doctor before receiving this medicine. It is best to use some kind of birth control while you are receiving carmustine. Tell your doctor right away if you think you have become pregnant while receiving carmustine.

Breast-feeding—Because carmustine may cause serious side effects, breast-feeding is generally not recommended while you are receiving it.

Children—Although there is no specific information comparing use of carmustine in children with use in other age groups, this medicine is not expected to cause different side effects or problems in children than it does in adults.

Older adults—Many medicines have not been studied specifically in older people. Therefore, it may not be known whether they work exactly the same way they do in younger adults or if they cause different side effects or problems in older people. There is no specific information comparing use of carmustine in the elderly with use in other age groups.

Other medicines—Although certain medicines should not be used together at all, in other cases two different medicines may be used together even if an interaction might occur. In these cases, your doctor may want to change the dose, or other precautions may be necessary. When you are receiving carmustine, it is especially important that your doctor and pharmacist know if you are taking any of the following:

- Amphotericin B by injection (e.g., Fungizone) or
- Antithyroid agents (medicine for overactive thyroid) or
- Azathioprine (e.g., Imuran) or
- Chloramphenicol (e.g., Chloromycetin) or

- Colchicine or
- Flucytosine (e.g., Ancobon) or
- Ganciclovir (e.g., Cytovene) or
- Interferon (e.g., Intron A, Roferon-A) or
- Plicamycin (e.g., Mithramycin) or
- Zidovudine (e.g., AZT, Retrovir) or
- If you have ever been treated with x-rays or cancer medicines—Carmustine may increase the effects of these medicines or radiation therapy on the blood

Other medical problems—The presence of other medical problems may affect the use of carmustine. Make sure you tell your doctor if you have any other medical problems, especially:

- Chickenpox (including recent exposure) or
- Herpes zoster (shingles)—Risk of severe disease affecting other parts of the body
- Infection—Carmustine decreases your body's ability to fight infection
- Kidney disease—Effects of carmustine may be increased because of slower removal from the body
- Liver disease—Carmustine may cause side effects to the liver
- Lung disease—Risk of lung problems caused by carmustine may be increased

Smoking—Increased risk of lung problems

Before you begin using any new medicine (prescription or nonprescription) or if you develop any new medical problem while you are using this medicine, check with your doctor, nurse, or pharmacist.

Proper Use of This Medicine

Carmustine is sometimes given together with certain other medicines. If you are using a combination of medicines, it is important that you receive each one at the proper time. If you are taking some of these medicines by mouth, ask your doctor, nurse, or pharmacist to help you plan a way to take them at the right times.

This medicine often causes nausea and vomiting, which usually last no longer than 4 to 6 hours. It is very important that you continue to receive the medicine, even if you begin to feel ill. Ask your doctor, nurse, or pharmacist for ways to lessen these effects.

Precautions While Using This Medicine

It is very important that your doctor check your progress at regular visits to make sure that this medicine is working properly and to check for unwanted effects.

While you are being treated with carmustine, and after you stop treatment with it, *do not have any immunizations (vaccinations) without your doctor's approval.* Carmustine may lower your body's resistance and there is a chance you might get the infection the immunization is meant to prevent. In addition, other persons living in your household should not take oral polio vaccine since there is a chance they could pass the polio virus on to you. Also, avoid persons who have taken oral polio vaccine. Do not get close to them, and do not stay in the same room with them for very long. If you cannot take these precautions, you should consider wearing a protective face mask that covers the nose and mouth.

Carmustine can temporarily lower the number of white blood cells in your blood, increasing the chance of getting an infection. It can also lower the number of platelets, which are necessary for proper blood clotting. If this occurs, there are certain precautions you can take, especially when your blood count is low, to reduce the risk of infection or bleeding:

- If you can, avoid people with infections. *Check with your doctor immediately* if you think you are getting an infection or if you get a fever or chills, cough or hoarseness, lower back or side pain, or painful or difficult urination.
- *Check with your doctor immediately* if you notice any unusual bleeding or bruising; black, tarry stools; blood in urine or stools; or pinpoint red spots on your skin.
- Be careful when using a regular toothbrush, dental floss, or toothpick. Your medical doctor, dentist, or nurse may recommend other ways to clean your teeth and gums. Check with your medical doctor before having any dental work done.
- Do not touch your eyes or the inside of your nose unless you have just washed your hands and have not touched anything else in the meantime.
- Be careful not to cut yourself when you are using sharp objects such as a safety razor or fingernail or toenail cutters.
- Avoid contact sports or other situations where bruising or injury could occur.

If carmustine accidentally seeps out of the vein into which it is injected, it may damage some tissues and cause scarring. *Tell the doctor or nurse right away if you notice redness, pain, or swelling at the place of injection.*

Side Effects of This Medicine

Along with its needed effects, a medicine may cause some unwanted effects. Some side effects will have signs or symptoms that you can see or feel. Your doctor may watch for others by doing certain tests. Some of the unwanted effects that may be caused by carmustine are listed below. Although not all of these effects may occur, if they do occur, they may need medical attention.

Also, because of the way these medicines act on the body, there is a chance that they might cause other unwanted effects that may not occur until months or years after the medicine is used. These delayed effects may include certain types of cancer, such as leukemia. Discuss these possible effects with your doctor.

Check with your doctor or nurse immediately if any of the following side effects occur:

Less common

Black, tarry stools; blood in urine or stools; cough or hoarseness; fever or chills; lower back or side pain; painful or difficult urination; pain or redness at place of injection; pinpoint red spots on skin; unusual bleeding or bruising

Check with your doctor or nurse as soon as possible if any of the following side effects occur:

More common

Shortness of breath

Less common

Flushing of face; sores in mouth and on lips; unusual tiredness or weakness

Rare

Decrease in urination; swelling of feet or lower legs

This medicine may also cause the following side effects that your doctor will watch for:

More common

Low red blood cell count; low white blood cell count

Rare

Liver problems

Other side effects may occur that usually do not need medical attention. These side effects may go away during treatment as your body adjusts to the medicine. Also, your doctor or nurse may be able to tell you about ways to prevent or reduce some of these side effects. Check with your doctor or nurse if any of the following side effects continue or are bothersome or if you have any questions about them:

More common

Nausea and vomiting (usually lasting no longer than 4 to 6 hours)

Less common

Diarrhea; discoloration of skin along vein of injection; dizziness; loss of appetite; skin rash and itching; trouble in swallowing; trouble in walking

This medicine may cause a temporary loss of hair in some people. After treatment with carmustine has ended, normal hair growth should return.

Side effects that affect your lungs (for example, cough and shortness of breath) may be more likely to occur if you smoke.

After you stop receiving carmustine, it may still produce some side effects that need attention. During this period of time check with your doctor or nurse if you notice any of the following:

Black, tarry stools; blood in urine or stools; cough or hoarseness; fever or chills; lower back or side pain; painful or difficult urination; pinpoint red spots on skin; shortness of breath; unusual bleeding or bruising

Other side effects not listed above may also occur in some patients. If you notice any other effects, check with your doctor or nurse.

Annual revision: 04/09/93

CELLULOSE SODIUM PHOSPHATE Systemic†

A commonly used brand name in the U.S. is Calcibind.

†Not commercially available in Canada.

Description

Cellulose sodium phosphate (SELL-u-lose SO-dee-um FOS-fate) is used to prevent the formation of calcium-containing kidney stones. It is used in patients whose bodies absorb too much calcium from their food.

Cellulose sodium phosphate works by combining with the calcium and some other minerals in food. This prevents the calcium from reaching the kidneys where the stones are formed.

Cellulose sodium phosphate is available only with your doctor's prescription, in the following dosage form:

Oral

- Powder for oral suspension (U.S.)

It is very important that you read and understand the following information. If any of it causes you special concern, check with your doctor. Also, *if you have any questions* or if you want more information about this medicine or your medical problem, *ask your doctor, nurse, or pharmacist.*

Before Using This Medicine

In deciding to use a medicine, the risks of taking the medicine must be weighed against the good it will do. This is a decision you and your doctor will make. For cellulose sodium phosphate, the following should be considered:

Allergies—Tell your doctor if you have ever had any unusual or allergic reaction to cellulose sodium phosphate. Also tell your doctor and pharmacist if you are allergic to any other substances, such as foods, preservatives, or dyes.

Diet—Make certain your doctor and pharmacist know if you are on any special diet, such as a low-sodium or low-sugar diet. Also tell your doctor or pharmacist if your diet contains large amounts of milk or other dairy products, spinach (or other dark green leafy vegetables), chocolate, brewed tea, or rhubarb or if you are taking vitamin C or magnesium supplements.

Pregnancy—Studies have not been done in either humans or animals. However, pregnant women usually need more calcium in their diet, and should not take cellulose sodium phosphate unless it is clearly needed. Be sure you have discussed the risks and benefits with your doctor.

Breast-feeding—It is not known whether cellulose sodium phosphate passes into breast milk. However, this medicine has not been reported to cause problems in nursing babies.

Children—Although there is no specific information comparing use of cellulose sodium phosphate in children with use in any other age group, its use is not recommended in children up to 16 years of age because of the increased need for calcium in growing children.

Older adults—Many medicines have not been studied specifically in older people. Therefore, it may not be known whether they work exactly the same way they do in younger adults or if they cause different side effects or problems in older people. There is no specific information comparing use of cellulose sodium phosphate in the elderly with use in other age groups.

Other medicines—Although certain medicines should not be used together at all, in other cases two different medicines may be used together even if an interaction might occur. In these cases, your doctor may want to change the dose, or other precautions may be necessary. When you are taking cellulose sodium phosphate, it is especially important that your doctor and pharmacist know if you are taking any of the following:

- Calcium supplements, or calcium containing antacids or laxatives—Use may lead to too much calcium in the body, preventing the cellulose sodium phosphate from working properly
- Magnesium supplements, or magnesium containing antacids or laxatives—Cellulose sodium phosphate and magnesium should not be taken within 1 hour of each other

Other medical problems—The presence of other medical problems may affect the use of cellulose sodium phosphate. Make sure you tell your doctor if you have any other medical problems, especially:

- Bone disease—Cellulose sodium phosphate may make the condition worse
- Edema or swelling or
- Heart disease—The high sodium content of cellulose sodium phosphate may cause the body to hold water
- Intestinal problems or
- Parathyroid disease or problems—Cellulose sodium phosphate may increase the risk of bone problems

Before you begin using any new medicine (prescription or nonprescription) or if you develop any new medical problem while you are using this medicine, check with your doctor, nurse, or pharmacist.

Proper Use of This Medicine

Take this medicine mixed in a full glass (8 ounces) of water, soft drink, or fruit juice. After drinking all the liquid containing the medicine, rinse the glass with a little more liquid. Drink that also to make sure you get all the medicine.

It is very important that you take cellulose sodium phosphate with meals. If this medicine is taken an hour or more after a meal, it will not work properly.

Take cellulose sodium phosphate only as directed. Do not take more of it, do not take it more often, and do not take it for a longer time than your doctor ordered. To do so may increase the chance of side effects.

Drink at least a full glass (8 ounces) of water, a soft drink, or fruit juice every hour while you are awake, unless otherwise directed by your doctor. This also will help prevent kidney stones while you are taking cellulose sodium phosphate.

Missed dose—If you miss a dose of this medicine, skip the missed dose and go back to your regular dosing schedule. Do not double doses.

Storage—To store this medicine:

- Keep out of the reach of children.
- Store away from heat and direct light.
- Do not store in the bathroom, near the kitchen sink, or in other damp places. Heat or moisture may cause the medicine to break down.
- Do not keep outdated medicine or medicine no longer needed. Be sure that any discarded medicine is out of the reach of children.

Precautions While Using This Medicine

It is important that your doctor check your progress at regular visits. This is to make sure cellulose sodium phosphate is working properly and does not cause unwanted effects.

If you are taking a magnesium supplement, take it at least one hour before or after you take cellulose sodium phosphate. Otherwise, the magnesium may combine with this medicine and keep it from working properly.

Do not take vitamin C, or eat spinach (or other dark green leafy vegetables), chocolate, brewed tea, or rhubarb while you are taking cellulose sodium phosphate. They may increase the chance of kidney stones.

Do not drink milk or eat milk products (for example, cheese, ice cream, and yogurt) while you are taking this medicine, because dairy products are high in calcium. Drinking milk or eating milk products may keep cellulose sodium phosphate from working properly.

While you are taking cellulose sodium phosphate, do not eat salty foods or use extra salt on foods. To do so may increase the chance of unwanted effects.

For patients on a low-sodium diet:

- This medicine contains sodium. If you have any questions about this, check with your doctor, nurse, or pharmacist.

Side Effects of This Medicine

Along with its needed effects, a medicine may cause some unwanted effects. Although not all of these side effects may occur, if they do occur they may need medical attention.

Check with your doctor as soon as possible if any of the following side effects occur:

With long-term use

Convulsions (seizures); drowsiness; loss of appetite; mood or mental changes; muscle spasms or twitching; nausea or vomiting; trembling; unusual tiredness or weakness

Other side effects may occur that usually do not need medical attention. These side effects may go away during treatment as your body adjusts to the medicine. However, check with your doctor if any of the following side effects continue or are bothersome:

More common

Abdominal or stomach discomfort; loose bowel movements or diarrhea

Other side effects not listed above may also occur in some patients. If you notice any other effects, check with your doctor.

Annual revision: 12/02/92

CEPHALOSPORINS Systemic

This information applies to the following medicines:

Cefaclor (SEF-a-klor)
Cefadroxil (sef-a-DROX-ill)
Cefamandole (sef-a-MAN-dole)
Cefazolin (sef-A-zoe-lin)
Cefixime (sef-IX-eem)
Cefmetazole (sef-MET-a-zole)
Cefonicid (se-FON-i-sid)
Cefoperazone (sef-oh-PER-a-zone)
Ceforanide (se-FOR-a-nide)
Cefotaxime (sef-oh-TAKS-eem)
Cefotetan (sef-oh-TEE-tan)
Cefoxitin (se-FOX-i-tin)
Cefprozil (sef-PROE-zil)
Ceftazidime (sef-TAY-zi-deem)
Ceftizoxime (sef-ti-ZOX-eem)
Ceftriaxone (sef-try-AX-one)
Cefuroxime (se-fyoor-OX-eem)
Cephalexin (sef-a-LEX-in)
Cephalothin (sef-A-loe-thin)
Cephapirin (sef-a-PYE-rin)
Cephradine (SEF-ra-deen)
Moxalactam (MOX-a-lak-tam)

Some commonly used brand names are:

For Cefaclor

In the U.S.
Ceclor

In Canada
Ceclor

For Cefadroxil

In the U.S.
Duricef   Ultracef
Generic name product may also be available.

In Canada
Duricef

For Cefamandole

In the U.S.
Mandol

In Canada
Mandol

For Cefazolin

In the U.S.
Ancef   Zolicef
Kefzol
Generic name product may also be available.

In Canada
Ancef   Kefzol

For Cefixime

In the U.S.
Suprax

In Canada
Suprax

For Cefmetazole†

In the U.S.
Zefazone

For Cefonicid

In the U.S.
Monocid

In Canada
Monocid

For Cefoperazone

In the U.S.
Cefobid

In Canada
Cefobid

For Ceforanide†
In the U.S.
Precef

For Cefotaxime
In the U.S.
Claforan
In Canada
Claforan

For Cefotetan
In the U.S.
Cefotan
In Canada
Cefotan

For Cefoxitin
In the U.S.
Mefoxin
In Canada
Mefoxin

For Cefprozil†
In the U.S.
Cefzil

For Ceftazidime
In the U.S.
Ceptaz
Fortaz
Tazicef
Tazidime
In Canada
Ceptaz
Fortaz

For Ceftizoxime
In the U.S.
Cefizox
In Canada
Cefizox

For Ceftriaxone
In the U.S.
Rocephin
In Canada
Rocephin

For Cefuroxime
In the U.S.
Ceftin
Kefurox
Zinacef
In Canada
Zinacef

For Cephalexin
In the U.S.
Cefanex
C-Lexin
Keflet
Keflex
Keftab
Generic name product may also be available.
In Canada
Apo-Cephalex
Ceporex
Keflex
Novolexin
Nu-Cephalex

For Cephalothin
In the U.S.
Keflin
Generic name product may also be available
In Canada
Ceporacin
Keflin

For Cephapirin
In the U.S.
Cefadyl
Generic name product may also be available.
In Canada
Cefadyl

For Cephradine
In the U.S.
Anspor
Velosef
Generic name product may also be available.
In Canada
Velosef

For Moxalactam†
In the U.S.
Moxam

†Not commercially available in Canada.

Description

Cephalosporins (sef-a-loe-SPOR-ins) are used in the treatment of infections caused by bacteria. They work by killing bacteria or preventing their growth.

Cephalosporins are used to treat infections in many different parts of the body. They are sometimes given with other antibiotics. Some cephalosporins are also given by injection to prevent infections before, during, and after surgery. However, cephalosporins will not work for colds, flu, or other virus infections.

Cephalosporins are available only with your doctor's prescription, in the following dosage forms:

Oral

Cefaclor
- Capsules (U.S. and Canada)
- Oral suspension (U.S. and Canada)

Cefadroxil
- Capsules (U.S. and Canada)
- Oral suspension (U.S. and Canada)
- Tablets (U.S.)

Cefixime
- Oral suspension (U.S. and Canada)
- Tablets (U.S. and Canada)

Cefprozil
- Oral suspension (U.S.)
- Tablets (U.S.)

Cefuroxime
- Tablets (U.S.)

Cephalexin
- Capsules (U.S. and Canada)
- Oral suspension (U.S. and Canada)
- Tablets (U.S. and Canada)

Cephradine
- Capsules (U.S. and Canada)
- Oral suspension (U.S.)

Parenteral

Cefamandole
- Injection (U.S. and Canada)

Cefazolin
- Injection (U.S. and Canada)

Cefmetazole
- Injection (U.S.)

Cefonicid
- Injection (U.S. and Canada)

Cefoperazone
- Injection (U.S. and Canada)

Ceforanide
- Injection (U.S.)

Cefotaxime
- Injection (U.S. and Canada)

Cefotetan
- Injection (U.S. and Canada)

Cefoxitin
- Injection (U.S. and Canada)

Ceftazidime
- Injection (U.S. and Canada)

Ceftizoxime
- Injection (U.S. and Canada)

Ceftriaxone
- Injection (U.S. and Canada)

Cefuroxime
- Injection (U.S. and Canada)

Cephalothin
- Injection (U.S. and Canada)

Cephapirin
- Injection (U.S. and Canada)

Cephradine
- Injection (U.S.)

Moxalactam
- Injection (U.S.)

It is very important that you read and understand the following information. If any of it causes you special concern, check with your doctor. Also, *if you have any questions* or if you want more information about this medicine or your medical problem, *ask your doctor, nurse, or pharmacist.*

Before Using This Medicine

In deciding to use a medicine, the risks of taking the medicine must be weighed against the good it will do. This is a decision you and your doctor will make. For the cephalosporins, the following should be considered:

Allergies—Tell your doctor if you have ever had any unusual or allergic reaction to any of the cephalosporins, penicillins, penicillin-like medicines, or penicillamine. Also tell your doctor and pharmacist if you are allergic to any other substances, such as foods, preservatives, or dyes.

Pregnancy—Studies have not been done in humans. However, most cephalosporins have not been reported to cause birth defects or other problems in animal studies. Studies in rabbits have shown that cefoxitin may increase the risk of miscarriages and cause other problems. Studies in rats and mice have shown that moxalactam causes a decrease in the animal's ability to live after birth. Moxalactam has not been shown to cause birth defects or other problems in rats and mice given up to 20 times the usual human dose.

Breast-feeding—Most cephalosporins pass into human breast milk, usually in small amounts. However, cephalosporins have not been reported to cause problems in nursing babies.

Children—Many cephalosporins have been tested in children and, in effective doses, have not been shown to cause different side effects or problems than they do in adults. However, there are some cephalosporins that have not been tested in children up to 1 year of age.

Older adults—Cephalosporins have been used in the elderly, and they are not expected to cause different side effects or problems in older people than they do in younger adults.

Other medicines—Although certain medicines should not be used together at all, in other cases 2 different medicines may be used together even if an interaction might occur. In these cases, your doctor may want to change the dose, or other precautions may be necessary. When you are taking a cephalosporin, it is especially important that your doctor and pharmacist know if you are taking any of the following:

- Alcohol and alcohol-containing medicine (cefamandole, cefmetazole, cefoperazone, cefotetan, and moxalactam only)—Using alcohol and these cephalosporins together may cause abdominal or stomach cramps, nausea, vomiting, headache, dizziness or lightheadedness, shortness of breath, sweating, or facial flushing; this reaction usually begins within 15 to 30 minutes after alcohol is consumed and usually goes away over several hours
- Anticoagulants (blood thinners) or
- Carbenicillin by injection (e.g., Geopen) or
- Dipyridamole (e.g., Persantine) or
- Divalproex (e.g., Depakote) or
- Heparin (e.g., Panheprin) or
- Pentoxifylline (e.g., Trental) or
- Plicamycin (e.g., Mithracin) or
- Sulfinpyrazone (e.g., Anturane) or
- Ticarcillin (e.g., Ticar) or
- Thrombolytic agents or
- Valproic acid (e.g., Depakene)—Any of these medicines may increase the chance of bleeding, especially when used with cefamandole, cefmetazole, cefoperazone, cefotetan, or moxalactam
- Probenecid (e.g., Benemid) (except cefoperazone, ceforanide, ceftazidime, ceftriaxone, moxalactam)—Probenecid increases the blood level of many cephalosporins. Although probenecid may be given with a cephalosporin by your doctor to purposely increase the blood level to treat some infections, in other cases, this effect may be unwanted and may increase the chance of side effects

Other medical problems—The presence of other medical problems may affect the use of cephalosporins. Make sure you tell your doctor if you have any other medical problems, especially:

- Bleeding problems, history of (cefamandole, cefmetazole, cefoperazone, cefotetan, and moxalactam only)—These medicines may increase the chance of bleeding

- Kidney disease—Some cephalosporins need to be given at a lower dose to people with kidney disease. Also, cephalothin, especially, may increase the chance of kidney damage
- Liver disease (cefoperazone only)—Cefoperazone needs to be given at a lower dose to people with liver and kidney disease
- Phenylketonuria—Cefprozil oral suspension contains phenylalanine
- Stomach or intestinal disease, history of (especially colitis, including colitis caused by antibiotics, or enteritis)—Cephalosporins may cause colitis in some patients

Proper Use of This Medicine

Cephalosporins may be taken on a full or empty stomach. If this medicine upsets your stomach, it may help to take it with food. Cefuroxime axetil tablets should be taken with food to increase absorption of the medicine.

For patients taking the *oral liquid* form of this medicine:

- This medicine is to be taken by mouth even if it comes in a dropper bottle. If this medicine does not come in a dropper bottle, use a specially marked measuring spoon or other device to measure each dose accurately. The average household teaspoon may not hold the right amount of liquid.
- Do not use after the expiration date on the label since the medicine may not work properly after that date. Check with your pharmacist if you have any questions about this.

For patients unable to swallow *cefuroxime axetil tablets* whole:

- Cefuroxime axetil tablets may be crushed and mixed with food (e.g., applesauce, ice cream) or drinks (apple, orange, or grape juice, or chocolate milk) to cover up the strong, lasting, bitter taste.

To help clear up your infection completely, *keep taking this medicine for the full time of treatment,* even if you begin to feel better after a few days. *If you have a "strep" infection, you should keep taking this medicine for at least 10 days. This is especially important in "strep" infections since serious heart or kidney problems could develop later* if your infection is not cleared up completely. Also, if you stop taking this medicine too soon, your symptoms may return.

This medicine works best when there is a constant amount in the blood or urine. *To help keep the amount constant, do not miss any doses. Also, it is best to take the doses at evenly spaced times, day and night.* For example, if you are to take 4 doses a day, the doses should be spaced about 6 hours apart. If this interferes with your sleep or other daily activities, or if you need help in planning the best times to take your medicine, check with your doctor, nurse, or pharmacist.

Missed dose—If you do miss a dose of this medicine, take it as soon as possible. This will help to keep a constant amount of medicine in the blood or urine. However, if it is almost time for your next dose, skip the missed dose and go back to your regular dosing schedule. Do not double doses.

Storage—To store this medicine:

- Keep out of the reach of children.
- Store away from heat and direct light.
- Do not store the capsule or tablet form of this medicine in the bathroom, near the kitchen sink, or in other damp places. Heat or moisture may cause the medicine to break down.
- Store the oral liquid form of most cephalosporins in the refrigerator because heat will cause this medicine to break down. However, keep the medicine from freezing. Follow the directions on the label. Cefixime oral suspension and Ceporex oral suspension do not need to be refrigerated.
- Do not keep outdated medicine or medicine no longer needed. Be sure that any discarded medicine is out of the reach of children.

Precautions While Using This Medicine

If your symptoms do not improve within a few days, or if they become worse, check with your doctor.

For diabetic patients:

- *This medicine may cause false test results with some urine sugar tests.* Check with your doctor before changing your diet or the dosage of your diabetes medicine.

For patients with phenylketonuria (PKU):

- Cefprozil oral suspension contains phenylalanine. Check with your doctor before taking this medicine.

In some patients, cephalosporins may cause diarrhea:

- Severe diarrhea may be a sign of a serious side effect. *Do not take any diarrhea medicine without first checking with your doctor.* Diarrhea medicines may make your diarrhea worse or make it last longer.
- For mild diarrhea, diarrhea medicine containing kaolin or attapulgite (e.g., Kaopectate tablets, Diasorb) may be taken. However, other kinds of diarrhea medicine should not be taken. They may make your diarrhea worse or make it last longer.
- If you have any questions about this or if mild diarrhea continues or gets worse, check with your doctor or pharmacist.

For patients receiving *cefamandole, cefmetazole, cefoperazone, cefotetan, or moxalactam by injection:*

- Drinking alcoholic beverages or taking other alcohol-containing preparations (for example, elixirs, cough syrups, tonics, or injections of alcohol) while receiving these medicines may cause problems. The problems may occur if you consume alcohol even several days after you stop taking the cephalosporin. Drinking alcoholic beverages may result in increased side effects such as abdominal or stomach cramps, nausea, vomiting, headache, fainting, fast or irregular heartbeat, difficult breathing, sweating, or redness of the face or skin. These effects usually start within 15 to 30 minutes after you drink alcohol and may not go away for up to several hours. Therefore, *you should not drink alcoholic beverages or take other alcohol-containing preparations while you are receiving these medicines and for several days after stopping them.*

Side Effects of This Medicine

Along with its needed effects, a medicine may cause some unwanted effects. Although not all of these side effects may occur, if they do occur they may need medical attention.

Check with your doctor immediately if any of the following side effects occur:

Less common or rare

Abdominal or stomach cramps and pain (severe); watery and severe diarrhea, which may also be bloody; fever (these side effects may also occur up to several weeks after you stop taking this medicine); unusual bleeding or bruising (more common for cefamandole, cefmetazole, cefoperazone, cefotetan, and moxalactam)

Rare

Blistering, peeling, or loosening of skin; convulsions (seizures); decrease in urine output; dizziness or lightheadedness; fever; joint pain; loss of appetite; pain, redness, and swelling at place of injection; skin rash, itching, redness, or swelling; trouble in breathing

Other side effects may occur that usually do not need medical attention. These side effects may go away during treatment as your body adjusts to the medicine. However, check with your doctor if any of the following side effects continue or are bothersome:

More common (less common with some cephalosporins)

Diarrhea (mild); nausea and vomiting; sore mouth or tongue; stomach cramps (mild)

Less common or rare

Vaginal itching or discharge

Other side effects not listed above may also occur in some patients. If you notice any other effects, check with your doctor.

Annual revision: 09/13/92

CHARCOAL, ACTIVATED Oral

This information applies to the following medicines:

Activated Charcoal (AK-ti-vay-ted CHAR-kole)
Activated Charcoal and Sorbitol (SOR-bi-tole)

Some commonly used brand names are:

For Activated Charcoal

In the U.S.

Actidose-Aqua
Charcocaps
Insta-Char
Insta-Char Aqueous Suspension
Liqui-Char

Generic name product may also be available.

In Canada

Aqueous Charcodote
Charac-50
Insta-Char Aqueous Suspension
Pediatric Aqueous Charcodote

Generic name product may also be available.

For Activated Charcoal and Sorbitol

In the U.S.

Actidose with Sorbitol
Charcoaid

In Canada

Charac-tol 50
Charcodote
Charcodote TFS
Pediatric Charcodote

Description

Activated charcoal is used in the emergency treatment of certain kinds of poisoning. It helps prevent the poison from being absorbed by the body. Ordinarily, this medicine should not be used in poisoning if corrosive agents such as alkalis (lye) and strong acids, iron, boric acid, lithium, petroleum products (e.g., kerosene, gasoline, coal oil, fuel oil, paint thinner, cleaning fluid), ethyl alcohol, or methyl alcohol have been swallowed, since it will not prevent these poisons from being absorbed into the body.

Some activated charcoal products contain sorbitol. Sorbitol is a sweetener. It also works as a laxative, for the elimination of the poison from the body. *Products that contain sorbitol should be given only under the direct supervision of a doctor because severe diarrhea and vomiting may result.*

Activated charcoal (without sorbitol) may also be used to relieve diarrhea and intestinal gas.

Activated charcoal is available without a doctor's prescription; however, before using this medicine for poisoning, call a poison control center, your doctor, or an emergency room for advice. Also, your doctor may have special instructions on the proper use of this medicine for diarrhea or intestinal gas. Activated charcoal is available in the following dosage forms:

Oral

Activated Charcoal
- Capsules (U.S. and Canada)
- Powder (U.S. and Canada)
- Oral suspension (U.S. and Canada)
- Tablets (U.S.)

Activated Charcoal and Sorbitol
- Oral suspension (U.S. and Canada)

It is very important that you read and understand the following information. If any of it causes you special concern, check with your doctor or pharmacist. Also, *if you have any questions* or if you want more information about this medicine or your medical problem, *ask your doctor, nurse, or pharmacist.*

Before Using This Medicine

In deciding to use a medicine, the risks of taking the medicine must be weighed against the good it will do. This is a decision you and your doctor will make. Before you use activated charcoal *for diarrhea or intestinal gas,* the following should be considered:

Allergies—Tell your doctor if you have ever had any unusual or allergic reaction to activated charcoal. Also tell your doctor and pharmacist if you are allergic to any other substances, such as foods, preservatives, or dyes.

Diet—Make certain your doctor and pharmacist know if you are on a low-sodium, low-sugar, or any other special diet. Most medicines contain more than their active ingredient.

Pregnancy—Activated charcoal has not been reported to cause birth defects or other problems in humans.

Breast-feeding—Activated charcoal has not been reported to cause problems in nursing babies.

Children—In babies and children under 3 years of age, activated charcoal should not be used regularly to relieve diarrhea and gas, since it may affect the child's nutrition. Also, the fluid loss caused by diarrhea may result in a severe condition. For this reason, a medicine for diarrhea must not be given to children without first checking with their doctor. If medicine for diarrhea is used, it is also very important that a sufficient amount of liquids be given to replace the fluid lost by the body. If you have any questions about this, check with your doctor, nurse, or pharmacist.

Older adults—Many medicines have not been studied specifically in older people. Therefore, it may not be known whether they work exactly the same way they do in younger adults. Although there is no specific information comparing the use of activated charcoal in the elderly, this medicine is not expected to cause different side effects or problems in older people than it does in younger adults.

However, the fluid loss caused by diarrhea may result in a severe condition. For this reason, elderly persons with diarrhea, in addition to using a medicine for diarrhea, must receive a sufficient amount of liquids to replace the fluid lost by the body. If you have any questions about this, check with your doctor, nurse, or pharmacist.

Other medicines—Although certain medicines should not be used together at all, in other cases two different medicines may be used together even if an interaction might occur. In these cases, your doctor may want to change the dose, or other precautions may be necessary. Tell your doctor and pharmacist if you are taking any other prescription or nonprescription (over-the-counter [OTC]) medicine.

Other medical problems—The presence of other medical problems may affect the use of activated charcoal to relieve diarrhea. Make sure you tell your doctor if you have any other medical problems, especially:

- Dysentery—This condition may get worse; a different kind of treatment may be needed

Before you begin using any new medicine (prescription or nonprescription) or if you develop any new medical problem while you are using this medicine, check with your doctor, nurse, or pharmacist.

Proper Use of This Medicine

Do not take this medicine mixed with chocolate syrup, ice cream, or sherbet, since it may prevent the medicine from working properly.

For patients taking this medicine *for poisoning*:

- *Before taking this medicine for the treatment of poisoning, call a poison control center, your doctor, or an emergency room for advice.* It is a good idea to have these telephone numbers readily available.
- *It is very important that you shake the liquid form of this medicine well before taking it, some might have settled in the bottom. Be sure to drink all the liquid to get the full dose of activated charcoal.*
- If you have been told to take both this medicine and ipecac syrup to treat the poisoning, *do not take this medicine until after you have taken the ipecac syrup to cause vomiting and the vomiting has stopped. This is usually about 30 minutes.*

For patients taking this medicine *for diarrhea or intestinal gas:*

- *If you are taking any other medicine, do not take it within 2 hours of the activated charcoal.* Taking other medicines together with activated charcoal may prevent the other medicine from being absorbed by your body. If you have any questions about this, check with your doctor, nurse, or pharmacist.

Importance of diet and fluid intake while treating diarrhea:

- *In addition to using medicine for diarrhea, it is very important that you replace the fluid lost by the body and follow a proper diet.* For the first 24 hours you should drink plenty of caffeine-free clear liquids, such as ginger ale, decaffeinated cola, decaffeinated tea, broth, or gelatin. During the next 24 hours you may eat bland foods, such as cooked cereals, bread, crackers, and applesauce. Fruits, vegetables, fried or spicy foods, bran, candy, caffeine, and alcoholic beverages may make the condition worse.
- If too much fluid has been lost by the body due to the diarrhea, a serious condition may develop. Check with your doctor as soon as possible if any of the following signs of too much fluid loss occur:

  Decreased urination
  Dizziness and lightheadedness
  Dryness of mouth
  Increased thirst
  Wrinkled skin

Storage—To store this medicine:

- Keep out of the reach of children.
- Store away from heat and direct light.
- Do not store the capsule, tablet, or powder form of this medicine in the bathroom, near the kitchen sink, or in other damp places. Heat or moisture may cause the medicine to break down.
- Keep the liquid form of this medicine from freezing.
- Do not keep outdated medicine or medicine no longer needed. Be sure that any discarded medicine is out of the reach of children.

Precautions While Using This Medicine

For patients taking this medicine *for diarrhea or intestinal gas:*

- If you are taking this medicine for intestinal gas and your condition has not improved after 7 days, check with your doctor.
- If you are taking this medicine for diarrhea and your condition has not improved after 2 days or if you have fever with the diarrhea, check with your doctor.

Side Effects of This Medicine

Along with its needed effects, a medicine may cause some unwanted effects. Although not all of these side effects may occur, if they do occur they may need medical attention.

Check with your doctor as soon as possible if the following side effect occurs:

Rare

Swelling or pain in stomach

Other side effects may occur that usually do not need medical attention. These side effects may go away during treatment as your body adjusts to the medicine. However, check with your doctor if any of the following side effects continue:

More common (for sorbitol-containing preparations only)

Diarrhea; vomiting

Activated charcoal will cause your stools to turn black. This is to be expected while you are taking this medicine.

There have not been any other side effects reported with this medicine. However, if you notice any other effects, check with your doctor.

Annual revision: 08/16/91

CHENODIOL Systemic†

A commonly used brand name in the U.S. is Chenix.
Another commonly used name is chenodeoxycholic acid.

†Not commercially available in Canada.

Description

Chenodiol (kee-noe-DYE-ole) is used in the treatment of gallstone disease. It is taken by mouth to dissolve the gallstones.

Chenodiol is used in patients who do not need to have their gallbladder removed or in those in whom surgery is best avoided because of other medical problems. However, chenodiol works only in those patients who have a working gallbladder and whose gallstones are made of cholesterol. Chenodiol works best when these stones are small and of the "floating" type.

Chenodiol is available only with your doctor's prescription, in the following dosage form:

Oral

- Tablets (U.S.)

It is very important that you read and understand the following information. If any of it causes you special concern, check with your doctor. Also, *if you have any questions* or if you want more information about this medicine or your medical problem, *ask your doctor, nurse, or pharmacist.*

Before Using This Medicine

In deciding to use a medicine, the risks of taking the medicine must be weighed against the good it will do. This is a decision you and your doctor will make. For chenodiol, the following should be considered:

Allergies—Tell your doctor if you have ever had any unusual or allergic reaction to chenodiol or to other bile acid products.

Diet—If you have gallstones, your doctor may prescribe chenodiol and a personal high-fiber diet for you. Some foods that are high in fiber are whole grain breads and cereals, bran, fruit, and green, leafy vegetables. It has been found that such a diet may help dissolve the stones faster and may keep new stones from forming.

It may also be important for you to go on a reducing diet. However, check with your doctor before going on any diet.

Pregnancy—Chenodiol is not recommended for use during pregnancy. It has been shown to cause liver and kidney problems in animals when given in doses many times the human dose. Be sure you have discussed this with your doctor.

Breast-feeding—It is not known whether chenodiol passes into the breast milk. However, this medicine has not been reported to cause problems in nursing babies.

Children—Studies on this medicine have been done only in adult patients, and there is no specific information comparing use of chenodiol in children with use in other age groups.

Older adults—Many medicines have not been studied specifically in older people. Therefore, it may not be known whether they work exactly the same way they do in younger adults. Although there is no specific information comparing use of chenodiol in the elderly with use in other age groups, this medicine is not expected to cause different side effects or problems in older people than it does in younger adults.

Other medicines—Although certain medicines should not be used together at all, in other cases two different medicines may be used together even if an interaction might occur. In these cases, your doctor may want to change the dose, or other precautions may be necessary. Tell your doctor and pharmacist if you are taking any other prescription or nonprescription (over-the-counter [OTC]) medicine.

Other medical problems—The presence of other medical problems may affect the use of chenodiol. Make sure you tell your doctor if you have any other medical problems, especially:

- Biliary tract problems or
- Blood vessel disease or
- Pancreatitis (inflammation of pancreas)—These conditions may make it necessary to have surgery since treatment with chenodiol would take too long
- Liver disease—Liver disease may become worse with use of chenodiol

Before you begin using any new medicine (prescription or nonprescription) or if you develop any new medical problem while you are using this medicine, check with your doctor, nurse, or pharmacist.

Proper Use of This Medicine

Take chenodiol with food or milk for best results, unless otherwise directed by your doctor.

Take chenodiol for the full time of treatment, even if you begin to feel better. If you stop taking this medicine too soon, the gallstones may not dissolve as fast or may not dissolve at all.

Missed dose—If you miss a dose of this medicine, take it as soon as possible. However, if it is almost time for your next dose, skip the missed dose and go back to your regular dosing schedule. Do not double doses.

Storage—To store this medicine:

- Keep out of the reach of children.
- Store away from heat and direct light.
- Do not store in the bathroom, near the kitchen sink, or in other damp places. Heat or moisture may cause the medicine to break down.
- Do not keep outdated medicine or medicine no longer needed. Be sure that any discarded medicine is out of the reach of children.

Precautions While Using This Medicine

Do not take aluminum-containing antacids (e.g., ALternaGel, Maalox) while taking chenodiol. To do so may keep the chenodiol from working properly.

It is important that your doctor check your progress at regular visits. Laboratory tests will have to be done every few months while you are taking this medicine to make sure that the gallstones are dissolving and your liver is working properly.

Check with your doctor immediately if severe abdominal or stomach pain, especially toward the upper right side, and severe nausea and vomiting occur. These symptoms may mean that you have other medical problems or that your gallstone condition needs your doctor's attention.

Side Effects of This Medicine

Along with its needed effects, a medicine may cause some unwanted effects. Although not all of these side effects may occur, if they do occur they may need medical attention.

Check with your doctor as soon as possible if the following side effect occurs:

Less common or rare

Diarrhea (severe)

Other side effects may occur that usually do not need medical attention. These side effects may go away during treatment as your body adjusts to the medicine. However, check with your doctor if any of the following side effects continue or are bothersome:

More common

Diarrhea (mild)

Less common or rare

Constipation; frequent urge for bowel movement; gas or indigestion (usually disappears within 2 to 4 weeks after the beginning of treatment); loss of appetite; nausea or vomiting; stomach cramps or pain

Other side effects not listed above may also occur in some patients. If you notice any other effects, check with your doctor.

Annual revision: 06/12/91

CHLOPHEDIANOL Systemic*

A commonly used brand name in Canada is Ulone.

*Not commercially available in the U.S.

Description

Chlophedianol (kloe-fe-DYE-a-nole) is used to relieve dry, irritating coughs. This medicine should not be used when there is mucus or phlegm (pronounced flem) with the cough.

Chlophedianol is available without a doctor's prescription; however, your doctor may have special instructions on the proper use of this medicine. It is available in the following dosage form:

Oral

- Syrup (Canada)

It is very important that you read and understand the following information. If any of it causes you special concern, check with your doctor or pharmacist. Also, *if you have any questions* or if you want more information about this medicine or your medical problem, *ask your doctor, nurse, or pharmacist.*

Before Using This Medicine

If you are taking this medicine without a prescription, carefully read and follow any precautions on the label. For chlophedianol, the following should be considered:

Allergies—Tell your doctor if you have ever had any unusual or allergic reaction to chlophedianol. Also tell your doctor and pharmacist if you are allergic to any other substances, such as foods, preservatives, or dyes.

Pregnancy—Studies on effects in pregnancy have not been done in either humans or animals.

Breast-feeding—It is not known whether chlophedianol passes into the breast milk. However, this medicine has not been reported to cause problems in nursing babies.

Children—This medicine has been tested in children 2 years of age or older. In effective doses, the medicine has not been shown to cause different side effects or problems in children then it does in adults.

Older adults—Many medicines have not been studied specifically in older people. Therefore, it may not be known whether they work exactly the same way they do in younger adults or if they cause different side effects or problems in older people. There is no specific information comparing use of chlophedianol in the elderly with use in other age groups.

Other medicines—Although certain medicines should not be used together at all, in other cases two different medicines may be used together even if an interaction might occur. In these cases, your doctor may want to change the dose, or other precautions may be necessary. When you are taking chlophedianol, it is especially important that your doctor and pharmacist know if you are taking any of the following:

- Amantadine (e.g., Symmetrel) or
- Amphetamines or
- Appetite suppressants (diet pills), except fenfluramine (e.g., Pondimin) or
- Caffeine (e.g., NoDoz) or
- Cocaine or
- Medicine for asthma or other breathing problems or
- Medicine for colds, sinus problems, or hay fever or other allergies (including nose drops or sprays) or

• Methylphenidate (e.g., Ritalin) or
• Pemoline (e.g., Cylert)—The stimulant effects of either these medicines or chlophedianol may become greater
• Central nervous system (CNS) depressants (medicine that causes drowsiness)—Effects, such as drowsiness, of CNS depressants or chlophedianol may become greater

Other medical problems—The presence of other medical problems may affect the use of chlophedianol. Make sure you tell your doctor if you have any other medical problems.

Before you begin using any new medicine (prescription or nonprescription) or if you develop any new medical problem while you are using this medicine, check with your doctor, nurse, or pharmacist.

Proper Use of This Medicine

Do not take liquids immediately after taking this medicine. To do so may decrease the soothing effect of the syrup.

Take this medicine only as directed. Do not take more of it and do not take it more often than your doctor ordered. To do so may increase the chance of side effects.

Missed dose—If you are taking this medicine on a regular schedule and you miss a dose, take it as soon as possible. However, if it is almost time for your next dose, skip the missed dose and go back to your regular dosing schedule. Do not double doses.

Storage—To store this medicine:

- Keep out of the reach of children.
- Store away from heat and direct light.
- Keep the syrup from freezing.
- Do not keep outdated medicine or medicine no longer needed. Be sure that any discarded medicine is out of the reach of children.

Precautions While Using This Medicine

If your cough has not improved after 7 days, or if you have a high fever, skin rash, or continuing headache with the cough, check with your doctor. These signs may mean that you have other medical problems.

This medicine will add to the effects of alcohol and other CNS depressants (medicines that slow down the nervous system, possibly causing drowsiness). Some examples of CNS depressants are antihistamines or medicine for hay fever, other allergies, or colds; sedatives, tranquilizers, or sleeping medicine; prescription pain medicine or narcotics; barbiturates; medicine for seizures; muscle relaxants; or anesthetics, including some dental anesthetics. *Check with your doctor before taking any of the above while you are taking this medicine.*

This medicine may also add to the effects of CNS stimulants, such as appetite suppressants and caffeine-containing beverages like tea, coffee, cocoa, and cola drinks. *Avoid drinking large amounts of these beverages while taking this medicine.* If you have any questions about this, check with your doctor.

This medicine may cause some people to become drowsy or less alert than they are normally. *Make sure you know how you react to this medicine before you drive, use machines, or do anything else that could be dangerous if you are not alert.*

Side Effects of This Medicine

Along with its needed effects, a medicine may cause some unwanted effects. Although not all of these side effects may occur, if they do occur they may need medical attention.

Check with your doctor as soon as possible if any of the following side effects occur:

Rare

Hallucinations (seeing, hearing, or feeling things that are not there); nightmares; skin rash or hives; unusual excitement or irritability

With large doses

Blurred vision; drowsiness or dizziness; dryness of the mouth; nausea or vomiting

Other side effects not listed above may also occur in some patients. If you notice any other effects, check with your doctor.

Annual revision: 06/12/91

CHLORAL HYDRATE Systemic

Some commonly used brand names are:

In the U.S.

Aquachloral Supprettes

Generic name product may also be available.

In Canada

Novochlorhydrate

Generic name product may also be available.

Description

Chloral hydrate (KLOR-al HYE-drate) belongs to the group of medicines called sedatives and hypnotics. It is sometimes used before surgery or certain procedures to relieve anxiety or tension or to produce sleep. In addition, chloral hydrate may be used with analgesics (pain medicine) for control of pain following surgery.

Chloral hydrate has been used in the treatment of insomnia (trouble in sleeping) and to help calm or relax patients who are nervous or tense. However, this medicine has generally been replaced by other medicines for the treatment of insomnia and nervousness or tension.

Chloral hydrate comes in different strengths. Serious problems, including deaths, have occurred when children were given the wrong strength. *Make sure your doctor has told your pharmacist how many milligrams (mg), not just the number of capsules, teaspoonfuls, or suppositories, your child should receive.*

This medicine is available only with your doctor's prescription, in the following dosage forms:

Oral

- Capsules (U.S. and Canada)
- Syrup (U.S. and Canada)

Rectal

- Suppositories (U.S.)

It is very important that you read and understand the following information. If any of it causes you special concern, check with your doctor. Also, *if you have any questions* or if you want more information about this medicine or your medical problem, *ask your doctor, nurse, or pharmacist.*

Before Using This Medicine

In deciding to use a medicine, the risks of taking the medicine must be weighed against the good it will do. This is a decision you and your doctor will make. For chloral hydrate, the following should be considered:

Allergies—Tell your doctor if you have ever had any unusual or allergic reaction to chloral hydrate. Also tell your doctor and pharmacist if you are allergic to any other substances, such as foods, preservatives, or dyes.

Pregnancy—Studies on birth defects have not been done in either humans or animals. Too much use of chloral hydrate during pregnancy may cause the baby to become dependent on the medicine. This may lead to withdrawal side effects after birth.

Breast-feeding—Chloral hydrate passes into the breast milk and may cause drowsiness in babies of mothers using this medicine.

Children—This medicine comes in different strengths. Serious problems, including deaths, have occurred when children were given the wrong strength. *Make sure your doctor has told your pharmacist how many milligrams (mg), not just the number of capsules, teaspoonfuls, or suppositories, your child should receive.* With proper use, this medicine is not expected to cause different side effects or problems in children than it does in adults.

Older adults—Many medicines have not been studied specifically in older people. Therefore, it may not be known whether they work exactly the same way they do in younger adults. Although there is no specific information comparing use of chloral hydrate in the elderly with use in other age groups, this medicine is not expected to cause different side effects or problems in older people than it does in younger adults.

Other medicines—Although certain medicines should not be used together at all, in other cases 2 different medicines may be used together even if an interaction might occur. In these cases, your doctor may want to change the dose, or other precautions may be necessary. When taking chloral hydrate it is especially important that your doctor and pharmacist know if you are taking any of the following:

- Anticoagulants (blood thinners)—Chloral hydrate may change the amount of anticoagulant you need to take
- Central nervous system (CNS) depressants (medicine that causes drowsiness) or
- Tricyclic antidepressants (medicine for depression)—Using these medicines together may increase the CNS and other depressant effects

Other medical problems—The presence of other medical problems may affect the use of chloral hydrate. If you are taking this medicine by mouth or using the rectal suppository form of chloral hydrate, make sure you tell your doctor if you have any other medical problems, especially:

- Colitis or
- Proctitis or inflammation of the rectum—Chloral hydrate used rectally may make the condition worse
- Drug abuse or dependence (or history of)—Dependence on chloral hydrate may develop
- Esophagitis or inflammation of the esophagus, or
- Gastritis or inflammation of the stomach, or
- Stomach ulcers—Chloral hydrate taken by mouth may make the condition worse
- Heart disease—Chloral hydrate may make the condition worse
- Kidney disease or
- Liver disease—Higher blood levels of chloral hydrate may occur, increasing the chance of side effects
- Porphyria—Acute attacks may be set off by chloral hydrate

Before you begin using any new medicine (prescription or nonprescription) or if you develop any new medical problem while you are using this medicine, check with your doctor, nurse, or pharmacist.

Proper Use of This Medicine

Use this medicine only as directed by your doctor. Do not use more of it, do not use it more often, and do not use it for a longer time than your doctor ordered. If too much is used, it may become habit-forming.

For patients taking *chloral hydrate capsules:*

- Swallow the capsule whole. Do not chew since the medicine may cause an unpleasant taste.
- Take this medicine with a full glass (8 ounces) of water, fruit juice, or ginger ale to lessen stomach upset.

For patients taking *chloral hydrate syrup:*

- Take each dose of medicine mixed with ½ glass (4 ounces) of water, fruit juice, or ginger ale to improve flavor and lessen stomach upset.

For patients using *chloral hydrate rectal suppositories:*

- If the suppository is too soft to insert, chill it in the refrigerator for 30 minutes or run cold water over it before removing the foil wrapper.
- To insert suppository, first remove the foil wrapper and moisten the suppository with cold water. Lie down on your side and use your finger to push the suppository well up into the rectum.

Dosing—The dose of chloral hydrate will be different for different patients. *Follow your doctor's orders or the directions on the label.* The following information includes only the average doses of chloral hydrate. *If your dose is different, do not change it* unless your doctor tells you to do so.

- This medicine comes in different strengths. *Make sure your doctor has told your pharmacist how many milligrams (mg), not just the number of capsules, teaspoonfuls, or suppositories, your child should receive.*
- The number of capsules or teaspoonfuls of syrup that you take, or suppositories that you use, depends on the strength of the medicine. Also, *the number of doses you take each day, the time allowed between doses, and the length of time you take the medicine depend on the medical problem for which you are taking chloral hydrate.*
- For *oral* dosage forms (capsules or syrup):
  —Adults:
    - For trouble in sleeping or sedation before surgery: 500 to 1000 milligrams taken thirty minutes before bedtime or surgery.
    - For daytime sedation: 250 milligrams taken three times a day after meals.

  —Children:
    - For trouble in sleeping: Dose is based on body weight. The usual dose is 50 milligrams per kilogram [23 milligrams per pound]. The dose is usually not more than 1000 milligrams.
    - For daytime sedation: Dose is based on body weight. The usual dose is 8.3 milligrams per kilogram [3.8 milligrams per pound]. The dose is usually not more than 500 milligrams, taken three times a day after meals.
    - For sedation before an EEG (electroencephalograph) test: Dose is based on body weight. The usual dose is 20 to 25 milligrams per kilogram [9 to 11 milligrams per pound].
- For *rectal* dosage forms (suppositories):
  —Adults:
    - For trouble in sleeping: 500 to 1000 milligrams at bedtime.
    - For daytime sedation: 325 milligrams three times a day.

  —Children:
    - For trouble in sleeping: Dose is based on body weight. The usual dose is 50 milligrams per kilogram [23 milligrams per pound]. The dose is usually not more than 1000 milligrams.
    - For daytime sedation: Dose is based on body weight. The usual dose is 8.3 milligrams per kilogram [3.8 milligrams per pound], given three times a day.

Missed dose—If you miss a dose of this medicine, skip the missed dose and go back to your regular dosing schedule. Do not double doses.

Storage—To store this medicine:

- Keep out of the reach of children. Overdose of chloral hydrate is especially dangerous in children.
- Store away from heat and direct light.
- Do not store the capsule form of this medicine in the bathroom, near the kitchen sink, or in other damp places. Heat or moisture may cause the medicine to break down.
- Keep the syrup form of this medicine from freezing.
- Do not keep outdated medicine or medicine no longer needed. Be sure that any discarded medicine is out of the reach of children.

Precautions While Using This Medicine

If you will be using this medicine regularly for a long time:

- Your doctor should check your progress at regular visits to make sure that this medicine does not cause unwanted effects.
- Do not stop using it without first checking with your doctor. Your doctor may want you to reduce gradually the amount you are using before stopping completely.

This medicine will add to the effects of alcohol and other CNS depressants (medicines that slow down the nervous system, possibly causing drowsiness). Some examples of CNS depressants are antihistamines or medicine for hay fever, other allergies, or colds; sedatives, tranquilizers, or sleeping medicine; prescription pain medicine or narcotics; barbiturates; medicine for seizures; muscle relaxants; or anesthetics, including some dental anesthetics. *Check with your doctor before taking any of the above while you are using this medicine.*

If you think you or someone else may have taken an overdose of this medicine, get emergency help at once. Taking an overdose of chloral hydrate or taking alcohol or other CNS depressants with chloral hydrate may lead to unconsciousness and possibly death. Some signs of an overdose are continuing confusion, difficulty in swallowing, convulsions (seizures), severe drowsiness, severe weakness, shortness of breath or troubled breathing, staggering, and slow or irregular heartbeat.

This medicine may cause some people to become dizzy, lightheaded, drowsy, or less alert than they are normally. Even if taken at bedtime, it may cause some people to feel drowsy or less alert on arising. *Make sure you know how you react to this medicine before you drive, use machines, or do anything else that could be dangerous if you are dizzy or are not alert.*

Side Effects of This Medicine

Along with its needed effects, a medicine may cause some unwanted effects. Although not all of these side effects may occur, if they do occur they may need medical attention.

Check with your doctor as soon as possible if any of the following side effects occur:

Less common

Skin rash or hives

Rare

Confusion; hallucinations (seeing, hearing, or feeling things that are not there); unusual excitement

Symptoms of overdose

Confusion (continuing); convulsions (seizures); difficulty in swallowing; drowsiness (severe); low body temperature; nausea, vomiting, or stomach pain (severe); shortness of breath or troubled breathing; slow or irregular heartbeat; slurred speech; staggering; weakness (severe)

Other side effects may occur that do not need medical attention. These side effects may go away during treatment as your body adjusts to the medicine. However, check with your doctor if any of the following side effects continue or are bothersome:

More common

Nausea; stomach pain; vomiting

Less common

Clumsiness or unsteadiness; diarrhea; dizziness or lightheadedness; drowsiness; "hangover" effect

After you stop using this medicine, your body may need time to adjust. The length of time this takes depends on the amount of medicine you were using and how long you used it. During this period of time, check with your doctor if you notice any of the following side effects:

Confusion; hallucinations (seeing, hearing, or feeling things that are not there); nausea or vomiting; nervousness; restlessness; stomach pain; trembling; unusual excitement

Other side effects not listed above may also occur in some patients. If you notice any other effects, check with your doctor.

Annual revision: 03/09/93
Interim revision: 08/12/93

CHLORAMBUCIL Systemic

A commonly used brand name in the U.S. and Canada is Leukeran.

Description

Chlorambucil (klor-AM-byoo-sill) belongs to the group of medicines called alkylating agents. It is used to treat some kinds of cancer.

Chlorambucil interferes with the growth of cancer cells, which are eventually destroyed. Since the growth of normal body cells may also be affected by chlorambucil, other effects will also occur. Some of these may be serious and must be reported to your doctor. Other effects may not be serious but may cause concern. Some effects may not occur for months or years after the medicine is used.

Before you begin treatment with chlorambucil, you and your doctor should talk about the good this medicine will do as well as the risks of using it.

Chlorambucil may also be used for other conditions as determined by your doctor.

Chlorambucil is available only with your doctor's prescription, in the following dosage form:

Oral

- Tablets (U.S. and Canada)

It is very important that you read and understand the following information. If any of it causes you special concern, check with your doctor. Also, *if you have any questions* or if you want more information about this medicine or your medical problem, *ask your doctor, nurse, or pharmacist.*

Before Using This Medicine

In deciding to use a medicine, the risks of taking the medicine must be weighed against the good it will do.

This is a decision you and your doctor will make. For chlorambucil, the following should be considered:

Allergies—Tell your doctor if you have ever had any unusual or allergic reaction to chlorambucil or other cancer medicines.

Pregnancy—This medicine may cause birth defects if either the male or female is taking it at the time of conception or if it is taken during pregnancy. In addition, many cancer medicines may cause sterility which could be permanent. Sterility has been reported with this medicine and the possibility should be kept in mind.

Be sure that you have discussed this with your doctor before taking this medicine. It is best to use some kind of birth control while you are taking chlorambucil. Tell your doctor right away if you think you have become pregnant while taking chlorambucil.

Breast-feeding—Because chlorambucil may cause serious side effects, breast-feeding is generally not recommended while you are taking it.

Children—In general, this medicine has not been shown to cause different side effects or problems in children than it does in adults. However, some children with nephrotic syndrome (a kidney disease) may be more likely to have convulsions (seizures).

Older adults—Many medicines have not been studied specifically in older people. Therefore, it may not be known whether they work exactly the same way they do in younger adults or if they cause different side effects or problems in older people. There is no specific information comparing use of chlorambucil in the elderly with use in other age groups.

Other medicines—Although certain medicines should not be used together at all, in other cases two different medicines may be used together even if an interaction might occur. In these cases, your doctor may want to change the dose, or other precautions may be necessary. When taking chlorambucil it is especially important that your doctor and pharmacist know if you are taking any of the following:

- Amphotericin B by injection (e.g., Fungizone) or
- Antithyroid agents (medicine for overactive thyroid) or
- Chloramphenicol (e.g., Chloromycetin) or
- Colchicine or
- Flucytosine (e.g., Ancobon) or
- Ganciclovir (e.g., Cytovene) or
- Interferon (e.g., Intron A, Roferon-A) or
- Plicamycin (e.g., Mithracin) or
- Zidovudine (e.g., AZT, Retrovir) or
- If you have ever been treated with x-rays or cancer medicines—Chlorambucil may increase the effects of these medicines or radiation therapy on the blood
- Azathioprine (e.g., Imuran) or
- Corticosteroids (cortisone-like medicine) or
- Cyclophosphamide (e.g., Cytoxan) or
- Cyclosporine (e.g., Sandimmune) or
- Mercaptopurine (e.g., Purinethol) or
- Muromonab-CD3 (monoclonal antibody) (e.g., Orthoclone OKT3)—There may be an increased risk of infection and development of cancer because chlorambucil decreases the body's ability to fight them
- Probenecid (e.g., Benemid) or
- Sulfinpyrazone (e.g., Anturane)—Chlorambucil may increase the amount of uric acid in the blood. Since these medicines are used to lower uric acid levels, they may not work as well in patients taking chlorambucil

Other medical problems—The presence of other medical problems may affect the use of chlorambucil. Make sure you tell your doctor if you have any other medical problems, especially:

- Chickenpox (including recent exposure) or
- Herpes zoster (shingles)—Risk of severe disease affecting other parts of the body
- Convulsions (seizures) (history of) or
- Head injury—Increased risk of seizures
- Gout or
- Kidney stones (history of)—Chlorambucil may increase levels of uric acid in the body, which can cause gout or kidney stones
- Infection—Chlorambucil decreases your body's ability to fight infection

Before you begin using any new medicine (prescription or nonprescription) or if you develop any new medical problem while you are using this medicine, check with your doctor, nurse, or pharmacist.

Proper Use of This Medicine

Take this medicine only as directed by your doctor. Do not take more or less of it, and do not take it more often than your doctor ordered. The exact amount of medicine you need has been carefully worked out. Taking too much may increase the chance of side effects, while taking too little may not improve your condition.

Chlorambucil is sometimes given together with certain other medicines. If you are using a combination of medicines, make sure that you take each one at the proper time and do not mix them. Ask your doctor, nurse, or pharmacist to help you plan a way to remember to take your medicines at the right times.

While you are using chlorambucil, your doctor may want you to drink extra fluids so that you will pass more urine. This will help prevent kidney problems and keep your kidneys working well.

This medicine sometimes causes nausea and vomiting. However, it is very important that you continue to use the medicine, even if you begin to feel ill. *Do not stop using this medicine without first checking with your doctor.* Ask your doctor, nurse, or pharmacist for ways to lessen these effects.

If you vomit shortly after taking a dose of chlorambucil, check with your doctor. You will be told whether to take the dose again or to wait until the next scheduled dose.

Missed dose—If you miss a dose of this medicine and your dosing schedule is:

- One dose a day—Take the missed dose as soon as possible. Then go back to your regular dosing schedule. However, if you do not remember the missed dose until the next day, do not take it at all. Instead, take your regularly scheduled dose. Do not double doses.
- More than one dose a day—Take the missed dose as soon as possible. Then go back to your regular dosing schedule. However, if it is almost time for your next dose, skip the missed dose and go back to your regular dosing schedule. Do not double doses.

Storage—To store this medicine:

- Keep out of the reach of children.
- Store away from heat and direct light.
- Do not store in the bathroom, near the kitchen sink, or in other damp places. Heat or moisture may cause the medicine to break down.
- Do not keep outdated medicine or medicine no longer needed. Be sure that any discarded medicine is out of the reach of children.

Precautions While Using This Medicine

It is very important that your doctor check your progress at regular visits to make sure this medicine is working properly and to check for unwanted effects.

While you are being treated with chlorambucil, and after you stop treatment with it, *do not have any immunizations (vaccinations) without your doctor's approval.* Chlorambucil may lower your body's resistance and there is a chance you might get the infection the immunization is meant to prevent. In addition, other persons living in your household should not take oral polio vaccine since there is a chance they could pass the polio virus on to you. Also, avoid persons who have recently taken oral polio vaccine. Do not get close to them, and do not stay in the same room with them for very long. If you cannot take these precautions, you should consider wearing a protective face mask that covers the nose and mouth.

Chlorambucil can temporarily lower the number of white blood cells in your blood, increasing the chance of getting an infection. It can also lower the number of platelets, which are necessary for proper blood clotting. If this occurs, there are certain precautions you can take, especially when your blood count is low, to reduce the risk of infection or bleeding:

- If you can, avoid people with infections. *Check with your doctor immediately* if you think you are getting an infection or if you get a fever or chills, cough or hoarseness, lower back or side pain, or painful or difficult urination.
- *Check with your doctor immediately* if you notice any unusual bleeding or bruising; black, tarry stools; blood in urine or stools; or pinpoint red spots on your skin.
- Be careful when using a regular toothbrush, dental floss, or toothpick. Your medical doctor, dentist, or nurse may recommend other ways to clean your teeth and gums. Check with your medical doctor before having any dental work done.
- Do not touch your eyes or the inside of your nose unless you have just washed your hands and have not touched anything else in the meantime.
- Be careful not to cut yourself when you are using sharp objects such as a safety razor or fingernail or toenail cutters.
- Avoid contact sports or other situations where bruising or injury could occur.

Side Effects of This Medicine

Along with their needed effects, medicines like chlorambucil can sometimes cause unwanted effects such as blood problems and other side effects. These and others are described below. Also, because of the way these medicines act on the body, there is a chance that they might cause other unwanted effects that may not occur until months or years after the medicine is used. These delayed effects may include certain types of cancer, such as leukemia. Discuss these possible effects with your doctor.

Although not all of these side effects may occur, if they do occur they may need medical attention.

Check with your doctor or nurse immediately if any of the following side effects occur:

Less common

Black, tarry stools; blood in urine or stools; cough or hoarseness; fever or chills; lower back or side pain; painful or difficult urination; pinpoint red spots on skin; sores in mouth and on lips; unusual bleeding or bruising

Check with your doctor as soon as possible if any of the following side effects occur:

Less common

Joint pain; skin rash; swelling of feet or lower legs

Rare

Agitation; confusion; convulsions (seizures); hallucinations (seeing, hearing, or feeling things that are not there); muscle twitching; shortness of breath; tremors; trouble in walking; weakness (severe) or paralysis; yellow eyes or skin

Other side effects may occur that usually do not need medical attention. These side effects may go away during treatment as your body adjusts to the medicine. Also, your doctor or nurse may be able to tell you about ways to prevent or reduce some of these side effects. Check with your doctor or nurse if any of the following side effects continue or are bothersome or if you have any questions about them:

Less common

Changes in menstrual period; itching of skin; nausea and vomiting

After you stop using chlorambucil, it may still produce some side effects that need attention. During this period of time, check with your doctor if you notice any of the following side effects:

Black, tarry stools; blood in urine or stools; cough or hoarseness; fever or chills; lower back or side pain; painful or difficult urination; pinpoint red spots on skin; shortness of breath; unusual bleeding or bruising

Other side effects not listed above may also occur in some patients. If you notice any other effects, check with your doctor.

Additional Information

Once a medicine has been approved for marketing for a certain use, experience may show that it is also useful for other medical problems. Although these uses are not included in product labeling, chlorambucil is used in certain patients with the following medical conditions:

- Polycythemia vera
- Nephrotic syndrome

Other than the above information, there is no additional information relating to proper use, precautions, or side effects for these uses.

Annual revision: 06/11/92

CHLORAMPHENICOL Ophthalmic

Some commonly used brand names are:

In the U.S.

- Ak-Chlor Ophthalmic Ointment
- Ak-Chlor Ophthalmic Solution
- Chloracol Ophthalmic Solution
- Chlorofair Ophthalmic Ointment
- Chlorofair Ophthalmic Solution
- Chloromycetin Ophthalmic Ointment
- Chloromycetin for Ophthalmic Solution
- Chloroptic Ophthalmic Solution
- Chloroptic S.O.P.
- Econochlor Ophthalmic Ointment
- Econochlor Ophthalmic Solution
- I-Chlor Ophthalmic Solution
- Ocu-Chlor Ophthalmic Ointment
- Ocu-Chlor Ophthalmic Solution
- Ophthochlor Ophthalmic Solution
- Spectro-Chlor Ophthalmic Ointment
- Spectro-Chlor Ophthalmic Solution

In Canada

- Ak-Chlor Ophthalmic Solution
- Chloromycetin Ophthalmic Ointment
- Chloromycetin for Ophthalmic Solution
- Chloroptic Ophthalmic Solution
- Chloroptic S.O.P.
- Fenicol Ophthalmic Ointment
- Ophtho-Chloram Ophthalmic Solution
- Pentamycetin Ophthalmic Ointment
- Pentamycetin Ophthalmic Solution
- Sopamycetin Ophthalmic Ointment
- Sopamycetin Ophthalmic Solution

Description

Chloramphenicol (klor-am-FEN-i-kole) belongs to the family of medicines called antibiotics. Chloramphenicol ophthalmic preparations are used to treat infections of the eye. This medicine may be given alone or with other medicines that are taken by mouth for eye infections.

Chloramphenicol is available only with your doctor's prescription, in the following dosage forms:

Ophthalmic

- Ophthalmic ointment (eye ointment) (U.S. and Canada)
- Ophthalmic solution (eye drops) (U.S. and Canada)

It is very important that you read and understand the following information. If any of it causes you special concern, check with your doctor. Also, *if you have any questions* or if you want more information about this medicine or your medical problem, *ask your doctor, nurse, or pharmacist.*

Before Using This Medicine

In deciding to use a medicine, the risks of taking the medicine must be weighed against the good it will do. This is a decision you and your doctor will make. For chloramphenicol, the following should be considered:

Allergies—Tell your doctor if you have ever had any unusual or allergic reaction to chloramphenicol. Also tell your doctor and pharmacist if you are allergic to any other substances, such as preservatives.

Pregnancy—Chloramphenicol ophthalmic preparations have not been shown to cause birth defects or other problems in humans.

Breast-feeding—Chloramphenicol ophthalmic preparations have not been reported to cause problems in nursing babies.

Children—Studies on this medicine have been done only in adult patients, and there is no specific information comparing use of this medicine in children with use in other age groups.

Older adults—Many medicines have not been studied specifically in older people. Therefore, it may not be known whether they work exactly the same way they do in younger adults or if they cause different side effects or problems in older people. There is no specific information comparing use of this medicine in the elderly with use in other age groups.

Other medicines—Although certain medicines should not be used together at all, in other cases two different medicines may be used together even if an interaction might occur. In these cases, your doctor may want to change the dose, or other precautions may be necessary. Tell your doctor and pharmacist if you are using any other prescription or nonprescription (over-the-counter [OTC]) medicine.

Before you begin using any new medicine (prescription or nonprescription) or if you develop any new medical problem while you are using this medicine, check with your doctor, nurse, or pharmacist.

Proper Use of This Medicine

For patients using the *eye drop form* of chloramphenicol:

- Although the bottle may not be full, it contains exactly the amount of medicine your doctor ordered.
- To use:
  —First, wash your hands. Then tilt the head back and pull the lower eyelid away from the eye to form a pouch. Drop the medicine into the pouch and gently close the eyes. Do not blink. Keep the eyes closed for 1 or 2 minutes to allow the medicine to come into contact with the infection.

  —If you think you did not get the drop of medicine into your eye properly, use another drop.

  —To keep the medicine as germ-free as possible, do not touch the applicator tip or dropper to any surface (including the eye). Also, keep the container tightly closed.

To use the *eye ointment form* of chloramphenicol:

- First, wash your hands. Then pull the lower eyelid away from the eye to form a pouch. Squeeze a thin strip of ointment into the pouch. A 1-cm (approximately ⅓-inch) strip of ointment is usually enough unless otherwise directed by your doctor. Gently close the eyes and keep them closed for 1 or 2 minutes to allow the medicine to come into contact with the infection.
- To keep the medicine as germ-free as possible, do not touch the applicator tip to any surface (including the eye). After using chloramphenicol eye ointment, wipe the tip of the ointment tube with a clean tissue and keep the tube tightly closed.

To help clear up your infection completely, *keep using this medicine for the full time of treatment*, even if your symptoms begin to clear up after a few days. If you stop using this medicine too soon, your symptoms may return. *Do not miss any doses.*

Missed dose—If you do miss a dose of this medicine, apply it as soon as possible. However, if it is almost time for your next dose, skip the missed dose and go back to your regular dosing schedule.

Storage—To store this medicine:

- Keep out of the reach of children.
- Store away from heat and direct light.
- Keep the medicine from freezing.
- Do not keep outdated medicine or medicine no longer needed. Be sure that any discarded medicine is out of the reach of children.

Precautions While Using This Medicine

If your symptoms do not improve within a few days, or if they become worse, check with your doctor.

Side Effects of This Medicine

Along with its needed effects, a medicine may cause some unwanted effects. Although not all of these side effects may occur, if they do occur they may need medical attention.

Check with your doctor immediately if any of the following side effects occur:

Rare

Pale skin; sore throat and fever; unusual bleeding or bruising; unusual tiredness or weakness (the above side effects may also occur weeks or months after you stop using this medicine)

Check with your doctor as soon as possible if any of the following side effects occur:

Less common

Burning, itching, redness, skin rash, swelling, or other sign of irritation not present before use of this medicine

Other side effects may occur that usually do not need medical attention. These side effects may go away during treatment as your body adjusts to the medicine. However, check with your doctor if either of the following side effects continues or is bothersome:

Less common

Burning or stinging

After application, eye ointments may be expected to cause your vision to blur for a few minutes.

Other side effects not listed above may also occur in some patients. If you notice any other effects, check with your doctor.

Annual revision: 01/15/92

CHLORAMPHENICOL Otic

Some commonly used brand names are:

In the U.S.

Chloromycetin

Generic name product may also be available.

In Canada

Chloromycetin

Sopamycetin

Description

Chloramphenicol (klor-am-FEN-i-kole) belongs to the family of medicines called antibiotics. Chloramphenicol otic drops are used to treat infections of the ear canal. This medicine may be used alone or with other medicines that are taken by mouth for ear canal infections.

Chloramphenicol is available only with your doctor's prescription, in the following dosage form:

Otic

- Solution (U.S. and Canada)

It is very important that you read and understand the following information. If any of it causes you special concern, check with your doctor. Also, *if you have any questions* or if you want more information about this medicine or your medical problem, *ask your doctor, nurse, or pharmacist.*

Before Using This Medicine

In deciding to use a medicine, the risks of using the medicine must be weighed against the good it will do. This is a decision you and your doctor will make. For chloramphenicol otic, the following should be considered:

Allergies—Tell your doctor if you have ever had any unusual or allergic reaction to chloramphenicol. Also tell your doctor and pharmacist if you are allergic to any other substances, such as preservatives.

Pregnancy—Chloramphenicol otic drops have not been shown to cause birth defects or other problems in humans.

Breast-feeding—Chloramphenicol otic drops have not been reported to cause problems in nursing babies.

Children—Although there is no specific information comparing use of chloramphenicol otic drops in children with use in other age groups, this medicine is not expected to cause different side effects or problems in children than it does in adults.

Older adults—Many medicines have not been studied specifically in older people. Therefore, it may not be known whether they work exactly the same way they do in younger adults or if they cause different side effects or problems in older people. There is no specific information comparing use of this medicine in the elderly with use in other age groups.

Other medicines—Although certain medicines should not be used together at all, in other cases two different medicines may be used together even if an interaction might occur. In these cases, your doctor may want to change the dose, or other precautions may be necessary. Tell your doctor and pharmacist if you are using any other prescription or nonprescription (over-the-counter [OTC]) medicine.

Other medical problems—The presence of other medical problems may affect the use of chloramphenicol ear drops. Make sure you tell your doctor if you have any other medical problems, especially:

- Opening in your ear drum—This medicine may cause unwanted effects if it goes past the ear drum into the middle ear

Before you begin using any new medicine (prescription or nonprescription) or if you develop any new medical problem while you are using this medicine, check with your doctor, nurse, or pharmacist.

Proper Use of This Medicine

To use:

- Lie down or tilt the head so that the infected ear faces up. Gently pull the earlobe up and back for adults (down and back for children) to straighten the ear canal. Drop the medicine into the ear canal. Keep the ear facing up for about 1 or 2 minutes to allow the medicine to come into contact with the infection. A sterile cotton plug may be gently inserted into the ear opening to prevent the medicine from leaking out.

- To keep the medicine as germ-free as possible, do not touch the dropper to any surface (including the ear). Also, keep the container tightly closed.

To help clear up your infection completely, *keep using this medicine for the full time of treatment,* even if your symptoms begin to clear up after a few days. If you stop using this medicine too soon, your symptoms may return. *Do not miss any doses.*

Missed dose—If you do miss a dose of this medicine, apply it as soon as possible. However, if it is almost time for your next dose, skip the missed dose and go back to your regular dosing schedule.

Storage—To store this medicine:
- Keep out of the reach of children.
- Store away from heat and direct light.
- Keep the medicine from freezing.
- Do not keep outdated medicine or medicine no longer needed. Be sure that any discarded medicine is out of the reach of children.

Precautions While Using This Medicine

If your symptoms do not improve within a few days, or if they become worse, check with your doctor.

Side Effects of This Medicine

Along with its needed effects, a medicine may cause some unwanted effects. Although not all of these side effects may occur, if they do occur they may need medical attention.

Check with your doctor immediately if any of the following side effects occur:

Rare

Pale skin; sore throat and fever; unusual bleeding or bruising; unusual tiredness or weakness (the above side effects may also occur weeks or months after you stop using this medicine)

Check with your doctor as soon as possible if any of the following side effects occur:

Less common

Burning, itching, redness, skin rash, swelling, or other sign of irritation not present before use of this medicine

Other side effects not listed above may also occur in some patients. If you notice any other effects, check with your doctor.

Annual revision: 02/10/92

CHLORAMPHENICOL Systemic

Some commonly used brand names are:

In the U.S.
Chloromycetin
Generic name product may also be available.

In Canada
Chloromycetin
Novochlorocap

Description

Chloramphenicol (klor-am-FEN-i-kole) is used in the treatment of infections caused by bacteria. It works by killing bacteria or preventing their growth.

Chloramphenicol is used to treat serious infections in different parts of the body. It is sometimes given with other antibiotics. However, chloramphenicol should not be used for colds, flu, other virus infections, sore throats or other minor infections, or to prevent infections.

Chloramphenicol should only be used for serious infections in which other medicines do not work. This medicine may cause some serious side effects, including blood problems and eye problems. Symptoms of the blood problems include pale skin, sore throat and fever, unusual bleeding or bruising, and unusual tiredness or weakness. *You and your doctor should talk about the good this medicine will do as well as the risks of taking it.*

Chloramphenicol is available only with your doctor's prescription, in the following dosage forms:

Oral
- Capsules (U.S. and Canada)
- Oral suspension (U.S.)

Parenteral
- Injection (U.S. and Canada)

It is very important that you read and understand the following information. If any of it causes you special concern, check with your doctor. Also, *if you have any questions* or if you want more information about this medicine or your medical problem, *ask your doctor, nurse, or pharmacist.*

Before Using This Medicine

In deciding to use a medicine, the risks of taking the medicine must be weighed against the good it will do.

This is a decision you and your doctor will make. For chloramphenicol, the following should be considered:

Allergies—Tell your doctor if you have ever had any unusual or allergic reaction to chloramphenicol. Also tell your doctor and pharmacist if you are allergic to any other substances, such as foods, preservatives, or dyes.

Pregnancy—Chloramphenicol has not been shown to cause birth defects in humans. However, use is not recommended within a week or two of your delivery date. Chloramphenicol may cause gray skin color, low body temperature, bloated stomach, uneven breathing, drowsiness, pale skin, sore throat and fever, unusual bleeding or bruising, unusual tiredness or weakness, or other problems in the infant.

Breast-feeding—Chloramphenicol passes into the breast milk and has been shown to cause unwanted effects, such as pale skin, sore throat and fever, unusual bleeding or bruising, unusual tiredness or weakness, or other problems in nursing babies. It may be necessary for you to take another medicine or to stop breast-feeding during treatment. Be sure you have discussed the risks and benefits of the medicine with your doctor.

Children—Newborn infants are especially sensitive to the side effects of chloramphenicol because they cannot remove the medicine from their body as well as older children and adults.

Older adults—Many medicines have not been studied specifically in older people. Therefore, it may not be known whether they work exactly the same way they do in younger adults or if they cause different side effects or problems in older people. There is no specific information comparing use of chloramphenicol in the elderly with use in other age groups.

Other medicines—Although certain medicines should not be used together at all, in other cases two different medicines may be used together even if an interaction might occur. In these cases, your doctor may want to change the dose, or other precautions may be necessary. When you are taking chloramphenicol, it is especially important that your doctor and pharmacist know if you are taking any of the following:

- Alfentanil or
- Antidiabetics, oral (diabetes medicine you take by mouth) or
- Phenobarbital or
- Warfarin (e.g., Coumadin)—Use of chloramphenicol with these medicines may increase the chance of side effects of these medicines

- Amphotericin B by injection (e.g., Fungizone) or
- Antineoplastics (cancer medicine) or
- Antithyroid agents (medicine for overactive thyroid) or
- Azathioprine (e.g., Imuran) or
- Colchicine or
- Cyclophosphamide (e.g., Cytoxan) or
- Ethotoin (e.g., Peganone) or
- Flucytosine (e.g., Ancobon) or
- Ganciclovir (e.g., Cytovene) or
- Interferon (e.g., Intron A, Roferon-A) or
- Mephenytoin (e.g., Mesantoin) or
- Mercaptopurine (e.g., Purinethol) or
- Methotrexate (e.g., Mexate) or
- Phenytoin (e.g., Dilantin) or
- Plicamycin (e.g., Mithracin) or
- Zidovudine (e.g., AZT, Retrovir) or
- X-ray treatment—Use of chloramphenicol with any of these medicines or with x-ray treatment may increase the risk of blood problems

- Clindamycin (e.g., Cleocin) or
- Erythromycins (medicine for infection) or
- Lincomycin (e.g., Lincocin)—Use of chloramphenicol with any of these medicines may decrease the effectiveness of these medicines

- Phenytoin (e.g., Dilantin)—Use of chloramphenicol with phenytoin may increase the chance of blood problems or increase the side effects of phenytoin

Other medical problems—The presence of other medical problems may affect the use of chloramphenicol. Make sure you tell your doctor if you have any other medical problems, especially:

- Anemia, bleeding, or other blood problems—Chloramphenicol may cause blood problems
- Liver disease—Patients with liver disease may have an increased risk of side effects

Before you begin using any new medicine (prescription or nonprescription) or if you develop any new medical problem while you are using this medicine, check with your doctor, nurse, or pharmacist.

Proper Use of This Medicine

Chloramphenicol is best taken with a full glass (8 ounces) of water on an empty stomach (either 1 hour before or 2 hours after meals), unless otherwise directed by your doctor.

For patients taking the oral liquid form of this medicine:

- Use a specially marked measuring spoon or other device to measure each dose accurately. The average household teaspoon may not hold the right amount of liquid.

To help clear up your infection completely, *keep taking this medicine for the full time of treatment,* even if you begin to feel better after a few days. *Do not miss any doses.*

Missed dose—If you do miss a dose of this medicine, take it as soon as possible. However, if it is almost time for your next dose and your dosing schedule is:

- Two doses a day—Space the missed dose and the next dose 5 to 6 hours apart.
- Three or more doses a day—Space the missed dose and the next dose 2 to 4 hours apart.

Then go back to your regular dosing schedule.

Storage—To store this medicine:

- Keep out of the reach of children.
- Store away from heat and direct light.
- Do not store the capsule form of this medicine in the bathroom, near the kitchen sink, or in other damp places. Heat or moisture may cause the medicine to break down.
- Keep the oral liquid form of this medicine from freezing.
- Do not keep outdated medicine or medicine no longer needed. Be sure that any discarded medicine is out of the reach of children.

Precautions While Using This Medicine

If your symptoms do not improve within a few days, or if they become worse, check with your doctor.

It is very important that your doctor check you at regular visits for any blood problems that may be caused by this medicine.

Chloramphenicol may cause blood problems. These problems may result in a greater chance of infection, slow healing, and bleeding of the gums. Therefore, you should be careful when using regular toothbrushes, dental floss, and toothpicks. Dental work, whenever possible, should be done before you begin taking this medicine or delayed until your blood counts have returned to normal. Check with your medical doctor or dentist if you have any questions about proper oral hygiene (mouth care) during treatment.

For diabetic patients:

- *This medicine may cause false test results with urine sugar tests.* Check with your doctor before changing your diet or the dosage of your diabetes medicine.

Side Effects of This Medicine

Along with its needed effects, a medicine may cause some serious unwanted effects. Although not all of these side effects may occur, if they do occur they may need medical attention.

Stop taking this medicine and get emergency help immediately if any of the following side effects occur:

Rare—in babies only

Bloated stomach; drowsiness; gray skin color; low body temperature; uneven breathing; unresponsiveness

Also, *check with your doctor immediately* if any of the following side effects occur:

Less common

Pale skin; sore throat and fever; unusual bleeding or bruising; unusual tiredness or weakness (the above side effects may also occur up to weeks or months after you stop taking this medicine)

Rare

Confusion, delirium, or headache; eye pain, blurred vision, or loss of vision; numbness, tingling, burning pain, or weakness in the hands or feet; skin rash, fever, or difficulty in breathing

Other side effects may occur that usually do not need medical attention. These side effects may go away during treatment as your body adjusts to the medicine. However, check with your doctor if any of the following side effects continue or are bothersome:

Less common

Diarrhea; nausea or vomiting

Other side effects not listed above may also occur in some patients. If you notice any other effects, check with your doctor.

Annual revision: 05/13/92

CHLORAMPHENICOL Topical

A commonly used brand name in the U.S. and Canada is Chloromycetin.

Description

Chloramphenicol (klor-am-FEN-i-kole) belongs to the family of medicines called antibiotics. Chloramphenicol cream is used to treat infections of the skin. It may be used alone or with other medicines that are taken by mouth for skin infections.

Chloramphenicol is available only with your doctor's prescription, in the following dosage form:

Topical

- Cream (U.S. and Canada)

It is very important that you read and understand the following information. If any of it causes you special concern, check with your doctor. Also, *if you have any questions* or if you want more information about this medicine or your medical problem, *ask your doctor, nurse, or pharmacist.*

Before Using This Medicine

In deciding to use a medicine, the risks of using the medicine must be weighed against the good it will do. This is a decision you and your doctor will make. For chloramphenicol, the following should be considered:

Allergies—Tell your doctor if you have ever had any unusual or allergic reaction to chloramphenicol. Also tell your doctor and pharmacist if you are allergic to any other substances, such as preservatives or dyes.

Pregnancy—Topical chloramphenicol has not been shown to cause birth defects or other problems in humans.

Breast-feeding—Topical chloramphenicol has not been reported to cause problems in nursing babies.

Children—Although there is no specific information comparing use of topical chloramphenicol in children with use in other age groups, this medicine is not expected to cause different side effects or problems in children than it does in adults.

Older adults—Many medicines have not been studied specifically in older people. Therefore, it may not be known whether they work exactly the same way they do in younger adults or if they cause different side effects or problems in older people. There is no specific information comparing use of this medicine in the elderly with use in other age groups.

Other medicines—Although certain medicines should not be used together at all, in other cases two different medicines may be used together even if an interaction might occur. In these cases, your doctor may want to change the dose, or other precautions may be necessary. Tell your doctor and pharmacist if you are using any other prescription or nonprescription (over-the-counter [OTC]) medicine.

Before you begin using any new medicine (prescription or nonprescription) or if you develop any new medical problem while you are using this medicine, check with your doctor, nurse, or pharmacist.

Proper Use of This Medicine

Before applying this medicine, wash the affected area with soap and water, and dry thoroughly.

To help clear up your infection completely, *keep using this medicine for the full time of treatment,* even if your symptoms begin to clear up after a few days. If you stop using this medicine too soon, your symptoms may return. *Do not miss any doses.* However, *do not use this medicine more often or for a longer time than your doctor ordered.*

Missed dose—If you do miss a dose of this medicine, apply it as soon as possible. However, if it is almost time for your next dose, skip the missed dose and go back to your regular dosing schedule.

Storage—To store this medicine:
- Keep out of the reach of children.
- Store away from heat and direct light.
- Keep the medicine from freezing.
- Do not keep outdated medicine or medicine no longer needed. Be sure that any discarded medicine is out of the reach of children.

Precautions While Using This Medicine

If your skin problem does not improve within 1 week, or if it becomes worse, check with your doctor.

Side Effects of This Medicine

Along with its needed effects, a medicine may cause some unwanted effects. Although not all of these side effects may occur, if they do occur they may need medical attention.

Check with your doctor immediately if any of the following side effects occur:

Rare

Pale skin; sore throat and fever; unusual bleeding or bruising; unusual tiredness or weakness (the above side effects may also occur weeks or months after you stop using this medicine)

Check with your doctor as soon as possible if any of the following side effects occur:

More common

Burning, itching, redness, skin rash, swelling, or other sign of irritation not present before use of this medicine

Other side effects not listed above may also occur in some patients. If you notice any other effects, check with your doctor.

Annual revision: 02/10/92

CHLORDIAZEPOXIDE AND AMITRIPTYLINE Systemic†

Some commonly used brand names in the U.S. are Limbitrol and Limbitrol DS.

Generic name product may also be available.

†Not commercially available in Canada.

Description

Chlordiazepoxide (klor-dy-az-e-POX-ide) and amitriptyline (a-mee-TRIP-ti-leen) combination is used to treat mental depression that occurs with anxiety or nervous tension.

This medicine is available only with your doctor's prescription, in the following dosage form:

Oral

- Tablets (U.S.)

It is very important that you read and understand the following information. If any of it causes you special concern, check with your doctor. Also, *if you have any questions* or if you want more information about this medicine or your medical problem, *ask your doctor, nurse, or pharmacist.*

Before Using This Medicine

In deciding to use a medicine, the risks of taking the medicine must be weighed against the good it will do. This is a decision you and your doctor will make. For chlordiazepoxide and amitriptyline combination, the following should be considered:

Allergies—Tell your doctor if you have ever had any unusual or allergic reaction to chlordiazepoxide (e.g., Librium) or other benzodiazepines (such as alprazolam [e.g., Xanax], bromazepam [e.g., Lectopam], clonazepam [e.g., Klonopin], clorazepate [e.g., Tranxene], diazepam [e.g., Valium], estazolam [e.g., ProSom], flurazepam [e.g., Dalmane], halazepam [e.g., Paxipam], ketazolam [e.g., Loftran], lorazepam [e.g., Ativan], midazolam [e.g., Versed], nitrazepam [e.g., Mogadon], oxazepam [e.g., Serax], prazepam [e.g., Centrax], quazepam [e.g., Doral], temazepam [e.g., Restoril], triazolam [e.g., Halcion]) or to amitriptyline (e.g., Elavil) or other tricyclic antidepressants (such as amoxapine [e.g., Asendin], clomipramine [e.g., Anafranil], desipramine [e.g., Pertofrane], doxepin [e.g., Sinequan], imipramine [e.g., Tofranil], nortriptyline [e.g., Aventyl], protriptyline [e.g., Vivactil], trimipramine [e.g., Surmontil]).

Also tell your doctor and pharmacist if you are allergic to any other substances, such as foods, preservatives, or dyes.

Pregnancy—

- *Chlordiazepoxide*: Chlordiazepoxide has been reported to increase the chance of birth defects when used during the first 3 months of pregnancy.

  In addition, overuse of chlordiazepoxide during pregnancy may cause the baby to become dependent on the medicine. This may lead to withdrawal side effects in the baby after birth.

  Use of chlordiazepoxide during pregnancy, especially during the last weeks, may cause drowsiness, slow heartbeat, shortness of breath, or troubled breathing in the newborn baby. Chlordiazepoxide given just before or during labor may cause weakness in the newborn baby.
- *Amitriptyline*: Studies with amitriptyline have not been done in pregnant women. However, studies in animals have shown amitriptyline to cause birth defects when used in doses many times the human dose. Also, there have been reports of newborns suffering from muscle spasms and heart, breathing, and urinary problems when their mothers had taken tricyclic antidepressants (such as amitriptyline) immediately before delivery.

Breast-feeding—Chlordiazepoxide may pass into the breast milk and cause drowsiness, slow heartbeat, shortness of breath, or troubled breathing in babies of mothers taking this medicine. Although amitriptyline has also been found in breast milk, it has not been reported to cause problems in nursing babies.

Children—Children may be especially sensitive to the effects of chlordiazepoxide and amitriptyline combination. This may increase the chance of side effects during treatment.

Older adults—Elderly people are especially sensitive to the effects of chlordiazepoxide and amitriptyline combination. This may increase the chance of side effects during treatment.

Other medicines—Although certain medicines should not be used together at all, in other cases 2 different medicines may be used together even if an interaction might occur. In these cases, your doctor may want to change the dose, or other precautions may be necessary. When you are taking chlordiazepoxide and amitriptyline combination, it is especially important that your doctor and pharmacist know if you are taking any of the following:

- Alcohol or
- Central nervous system (CNS) depressants (medicines that cause drowsiness)—Using these medicines with chlordiazepoxide and amitriptyline combination may increase the CNS depressant effects

- Amphetamines or
- Appetite suppressants (diet pills) or
- Medicine for asthma or other breathing problems or

- Medicine for colds, sinus problems, or hay fever or other allergies (including nose drops or sprays)—Using these medicines with chlordiazepoxide and amitriptyline combination may increase the risk of serious effects on your heart
- Antacids—Taking these medicines with chlordiazepoxide and amitriptyline combination may delay the combination medicine's effects
- Antihypertensives (high blood pressure medicine)—Taking these medicines with chlordiazepoxide and amitriptyline combination may increase the chance of low blood pressure (hypotension)
- Antithyroid agents (medicine for overactive thyroid) or
- Cimetidine (e.g., Tagamet)—Taking these medicines with chlordiazepoxide and amitriptyline combination may increase the chance of serious side effects
- Monoamine oxidase (MAO) inhibitors (furazolidone [e.g., Furoxone], isocarboxazid [e.g., Marplan], phenelzine [e.g., Nardil], procarbazine [e.g., Matulane], selegiline [e.g., Eldepryl], tranylcypromine [e.g., Parnate])—Taking chlordiazepoxide and amitriptyline combination while you are taking or within 2 weeks of taking monoamine oxidase (MAO) inhibitors may cause sudden very high body temperature, extremely high blood pressure, and severe convulsions; however, sometimes certain of these medicines may be used with this combination medicine under close supervision by your doctor

Other medical problems—The presence of other medical problems may affect the use of chlordiazepoxide and amitriptyline combination. Make sure you tell your doctor if you have any other medical problems, especially:

- Alcohol abuse (or history of) or
- Drug abuse or dependence (or history of)—Dependence on this medicine may develop
- Bipolar disorder (manic-depressive illness) or
- Blood problems or
- Difficulty in urinating or
- Emphysema, asthma, bronchitis, or other chronic lung disease or
- Enlarged prostate or
- Glaucoma or increased eye pressure or
- Heart disease or
- Mental illness (severe) or
- Myasthenia gravis or
- Porphyria—Chlordiazepoxide and amitriptyline combination may make the condition worse
- Epilepsy or history of seizures—The risk of seizures may be increased
- Hyperactivity—Chlordiazepoxide and amitriptyline combination may cause unexpected effects
- Kidney disease or
- Liver disease—Higher blood levels of chlordiazepoxide and amitriptyline may occur, increasing the chance of side effects
- Overactive thyroid or
- Stomach or intestinal problems—Use of this combination medicine may result in more serious problems

Before you begin using any new medicine (prescription or nonprescription) or if you develop any new medical problem while you are using this medicine, check with your doctor, nurse, or pharmacist.

Proper Use of This Medicine

To reduce stomach upset, take this medicine immediately after meals or with food unless your doctor has told you to take it on an empty stomach.

Sometimes this medicine must be taken for several weeks before you begin to feel better. Your doctor should check your progress at regular visits.

Take this medicine only as directed by your doctor. Do not take more of it, do not take it more often, and do not take it for a longer period of time than your doctor ordered. If too much is taken, it may increase unwanted effects or become habit-forming (causing mental or physical dependence).

If you think this medicine is not working properly after you have taken it for a few weeks, *do not increase the dose.* Instead, check with your doctor.

Dosing—The dose of chlordiazepoxide and amitriptyline combination will be different for different patients. *Follow your doctor's orders or the directions on the label.* The following information includes only the average doses of chlordiazepoxide and amitriptyline combination. *If your dose is different, do not change it* unless your doctor tells you to do so.

- The number of tablets that you take depends on the strength of the medicine. Also, *the number of doses you take each day, the time allowed between doses, and the length of time you take the medicine depend on the medical problem for which you are taking chlordiazepoxide and amitriptyline combination.*
- For *oral* dosage forms (tablets):
  —Adults and adolescents: To start, 5 milligrams of chlordiazepoxide and 12.5 milligrams of amitriptyline or 10 milligrams of chlordiazepoxide and 25 milligrams of amitriptyline, taken three or four times a day. The doctor may adjust your dose if needed. However, the dose is usually not greater than 10 milligrams of chlordiazepoxide and 25 milligrams of amitriptyline taken six times a day.
  —Children up to 12 years of age: Dose must be determined by the doctor.

Missed dose—If you miss a dose of this medicine, skip the missed dose and go back to your regular dosing schedule. Do not double doses.

Storage—To store this medicine:

- Keep out of the reach of children. Overdose of this medicine is very dangerous in young children.
- Store away from heat and direct light.

- Do not store in the bathroom, near the kitchen sink, or in other damp places. Heat or moisture may cause the medicine to break down.
- Do not keep outdated medicine or medicine no longer needed. Be sure that any discarded medicine is out of the reach of children.

Precautions While Using This Medicine

It is very important that your doctor check your progress at regular visits to allow dose adjustments and help reduce side effects.

Do not stop taking this medicine without first checking with your doctor. Your doctor may want you to reduce gradually the amount you are using before stopping completely. This may help prevent a possible worsening of your condition and reduce the possibility of withdrawal symptoms such as headache, nausea, and/or an overall feeling of discomfort.

This medicine will add to the effects of alcohol and other CNS depressants (medicines that slow down the nervous system, possibly causing drowsiness). Some examples of CNS depressants are antihistamines or medicine for hay fever, other allergies, or colds; sedatives, tranquilizers, or sleeping medicine; prescription pain medicine or narcotics; barbiturates; medicine for seizures; muscle relaxants; or anesthetics, including some dental anesthetics. This effect may last for a few days after you stop taking this medicine. *Check with your doctor before taking any of the above while you are using this medicine.*

For diabetic patients:

- This medicine may affect blood sugar levels. If you notice a change in the results of your blood or urine sugar tests or if you have any questions, check with your doctor.

Before you have any medical tests, tell the medical doctor in charge that you are taking this medicine. The results of the metyrapone test may be affected by this medicine.

Before having any surgery, any dental treatment, or emergency treatment, tell the medical doctor or dentist in charge that you are using this medicine. Taking chlordiazepoxide and amitriptyline combination together with medicines that are used during surgery or dental or emergency treatments may increase the CNS depressant effects.

This medicine may cause some people to become dizzy, lightheaded, drowsy, or less alert than they are normally. Even if taken at bedtime, it may cause some people to feel drowsy or less alert on arising. *Make sure you know how you react to this medicine before you drive, use machines, or do anything else that could be dangerous if you are dizzy or are not alert.*

Dizziness, lightheadedness, or fainting may occur when you get up from a lying or sitting position. Getting up slowly may help. If this problem continues or gets worse, check with your doctor.

Chlordiazepoxide and amitriptyline combination may cause dryness of the mouth. For temporary relief, use sugarless candy or gum, melt bits of ice in your mouth, or use a saliva substitute. However, if your mouth continues to feel dry for more than 2 weeks, check with your medical doctor or dentist. Continuing dryness of the mouth may increase the chance of dental disease, including tooth decay, gum disease, and fungus infections.

Chlordiazepoxide and amitriptyline combination may cause your skin to be more sensitive to sunlight than it is normally. Exposure to sunlight, even for brief periods of time, may cause a skin rash, itching, redness or other discoloration of the skin, or a severe sunburn. When you begin taking this medicine:

- Stay out of direct sunlight, especially between the hours of 10:00 a.m. and 3:00 p.m., if possible.
- Wear protective clothing, including a hat. Also, wear sunglasses.
- Apply a sun block product that has a skin protection factor (SPF) of at least 15. Some patients may require a product with a higher SPF number, especially if they have a fair complexion. If you have any questions about this, check with your doctor or pharmacist.
- Apply a sun block lipstick that has an SPF of at least 15 to protect your lips.
- Do not use a sunlamp or tanning bed or booth.

If you have a severe reaction from the sun, check with your doctor.

Side Effects of This Medicine

Along with its needed effects, a medicine may cause some unwanted effects. Although not all of these side effects may occur, if they do occur they may need medical attention.

Check with your doctor as soon as possible if any of the following side effects occur:

Less common

Blurred vision or other changes in vision; confusion or hallucinations (seeing, hearing, or feeling things that are not there); constipation; difficulty in urinating; eye pain; fainting; irregular heartbeat; mental depression; shakiness; trouble in sleeping; unusual excitement, nervousness, or irritability

Rare

Convulsions (seizures); increased sensitivity to sunlight; skin rash and itching; sore throat and fever; yellow eyes or skin

Symptoms of overdose

Agitation; confusion; convulsions (seizures); dizziness or lightheadedness (severe); drowsiness (severe); enlarged pupils; fast or irregular heartbeat; fever; hallucinations; muscle stiffness or rigidity; vomiting (severe)

Other side effects may occur that usually do not need medical attention. These side effects may go away during treatment as your body adjusts to the medicine. However, check with your doctor if any of the following side effects continue or are bothersome:

More common

Bloating; clumsiness or unsteadiness; dizziness or lightheadedness; drowsiness; dryness of mouth or unpleasant taste; headache; weight gain

Less common

Diarrhea; nausea or vomiting; unusual tiredness or weakness

After you stop using this medicine, your body may need time to adjust. If you took this medicine in high doses or for a long time, this may take up to 2 weeks. *During this time check with your doctor if you notice any of the following side effects:*

Convulsions (seizures); headache; increased sweating; irritability or restlessness; muscle cramps; nausea or vomiting; stomach cramps; trembling; trouble in sleeping, with vivid dreams

Other side effects not listed above may also occur in some patients. If you notice any other effects, check with your doctor.

Annual revision: 03/19/93

CHLORDIAZEPOXIDE AND CLIDINIUM Systemic

Some commonly used brand names are:

In the U.S.

Clindex
Clinoxide
Clipoxide
Librax
Lidox
Lidoxide
Zebrax

Generic name product may also be available.

In Canada

Apo-Chlorax
Corium
Librax

Description

Chlordiazepoxide (klor-dye-az-e-POX-ide) and clidinium (kli-DI-nee-um) is a combination of medicines used to relax the digestive system and to reduce stomach acid. It is used to treat stomach and intestinal problems such as ulcers and colitis.

Chlordiazepoxide belongs to the group of medicines known as benzodiazepines. It is a central nervous system (CNS) depressant (a medicine that slows down the nervous system).

Clidinium belongs to the group of medicines known as anticholinergics. It helps lessen the amount of acid formed in the stomach. Clidinium also helps relieve abdominal or stomach spasms or cramps.

This combination is available only with your doctor's prescription, in the following dosage form:

Oral

- Capsules (U.S. and Canada)

It is very important that you read and understand the following information. If any of it causes you special concern, check with your doctor. Also, *if you have any questions* or if you want more information about this medicine or your medical problem, *ask your doctor, nurse, or pharmacist.*

Before Using This Medicine

In deciding to use a medicine, the risks of taking the medicine must be weighed against the good it will do. This is a decision you and your doctor will make. For chlordiazepoxide and clidinium, the following should be considered:

Allergies—Tell your doctor if you have ever had any unusual or allergic reaction to benzodiazepines such as alprazolam [e.g., Xanax], bromazepam [e.g., Lectopam], chlordiazepoxide [e.g., Librium], clonazepam [e.g., Klonopin], clorazepate [e.g., Tranxene], diazepam [e.g., Valium], flurazepam [e.g., Dalmane], halazepam [e.g., Paxipam], ketazolam [e.g., Loftran], lorazepam [e.g., Ativan], midazolam [e.g., Versed], nitrazepam [e.g., Mogadon], oxazepam [e.g., Serax], prazepam [e.g., Centrax], temazepam [e.g., Restoril], or triazolam [e.g., Halcion], or to clidinium or any of the belladonna alkaloids (atropine, belladonna, hyoscyamine, and scopolamine). Also tell your doctor and pharmacist if you are allergic to any other substances, such as foods, preservatives, or dyes.

Pregnancy—Clidinium (contained in this combination) has not been studied in pregnant women. However, clidinium has not been shown to cause birth defects or other problems in animal studies. Chlordiazepoxide (contained also in this combination) may cause birth defects if taken during the first 3 months of pregnancy. In addition, too much use of this medicine during pregnancy may cause the baby to become dependent on the medicine. This may lead to withdrawal side effects after birth. Make sure your doctor knows if you are pregnant or if you may become pregnant before taking chlordiazepoxide and clidinium.

Breast-feeding—Chlordiazepoxide may pass into the breast milk and cause unwanted effects, such as excessive drowsiness, in nursing babies. Also, because clidinium tends to decrease the secretions of the body, it is possible that the flow of breast milk may be reduced in some patients.

Children—There is no specific information comparing use of chlordiazepoxide and clidinium in children with use in other age groups. However, children are especially sensitive to the effects of chlordiazepoxide and clidinium. Therefore, this may increase the chance of side effects during treatment.

Older adults—Confusion or memory loss; constipation; difficult urination; drowsiness; dryness of mouth, nose, throat, or skin; and unusual excitement or agitation may be more likely to occur in the elderly, who are usually more sensitive than younger adults to the effects of chlordiazepoxide and clidinium.

Other medicines—Although certain medicines should not be used together at all, in other cases 2 different medicines may be used together even if an interaction might occur. In these cases, your doctor may want to change the dose, or other precautions may be necessary. When you are taking chlordiazepoxide and clidinium it is especially important that your doctor and pharmacist know if you are taking any of the following:

- Antacids or
- Diarrhea medicine containing kaolin or attapulgite—These medicines may reduce the blood levels of chlordiazepoxide and clidinium, which may decrease their effects; they should be taken at least 2 to 3 hours before or after the chlordiazepoxide and clidinium combination
- Central nervous system (CNS) depressants (medicines that cause drowsiness) or
- Other anticholinergics (medicines for abdominal or stomach spasms or cramps)—Use with chlordiazepoxide and clidinium may increase the side effects of either medicine
- Ketoconazole (e.g., Nizoral)—Chlordiazepoxide and clidinium may reduce the blood level of ketoconazole, which may decrease its effects; therefore, chlordiazepoxide and clidinium should be taken at least 2 hours after ketoconazole
- Potassium chloride (e.g., Kay Ciel)—Use of chlordiazepoxide and clidinium may worsen or cause sores of the stomach or intestine

Other medical problems—The presence of other medical problems may affect the use of chlordiazepoxide and clidinium. Make sure you tell your doctor if you have any other medical problems, especially:

- Difficult urination or
- Dryness of mouth (severe and continuing) or
- Emphysema, asthma, bronchitis, or other chronic lung disease or
- Enlarged prostate or
- Glaucoma or
- Hiatal hernia or
- High blood pressure (hypertension) or
- Intestinal blockage or
- Mental depression or
- Mental illness (severe) or
- Myasthenia gravis or
- Ulcerative colitis (severe)—Use of chlordiazepoxide and clidinium may make these conditions worse
- Drug abuse or dependence—Taking chlordiazepoxide (contained in this combination) may become habit-forming, causing mental or physical dependence
- Kidney disease or
- Liver disease—Higher blood levels of chlordiazepoxide and clidinium may result, possibly increasing the chance of side effects
- Overactive thyroid—Use of chlordiazepoxide and clidinium may further increase the heart rate

Before you begin using any new medicine (prescription or nonprescription) or if you develop any new medical problem while you are using this medicine, check with your doctor, nurse, or pharmacist.

Proper Use of This Medicine

Take this medicine about ½ to 1 hour before meals unless otherwise directed by your doctor.

Take this medicine only as directed by your doctor. Do not take more of it, do not take it more often, and do not take it for a longer time than your doctor ordered. If too much is taken, it may become habit-forming.

Missed dose—If you miss a dose of this medicine, take it as soon as possible. However, if it is almost time for your next dose, skip the missed dose and go back to your regular dosing schedule. Do not double doses.

Storage—To store this medicine:

- Keep out of the reach of children.
- Store away from heat and direct light.
- Do not store the capsule form of this medicine in the bathroom, near the kitchen sink, or in other damp places. Heat or moisture may cause the medicine to break down.
- Do not keep outdated medicine or medicine no longer needed. Be sure that any discarded medicine is out of the reach of children.

Precautions While Using This Medicine

If you will be taking this medicine regularly for a long time your doctor should check your progress at regular visits.

Do not take this medicine within an hour of taking medicine for diarrhea. Taking them too close together will make this medicine less effective.

This medicine may cause some people to have blurred vision or to become dizzy, lightheaded, drowsy, or less alert than they are normally. *Make sure you know how you react to this medicine before you drive, use machines, or do anything else that could be dangerous if you are dizzy or are not alert or able to see well.*

This medicine will add to the effects of alcohol and other CNS depressants (medicines that slow down the nervous system, possibly causing drowsiness). Some examples of CNS depressants are sedatives, tranquilizers, or sleeping medicine; prescription pain medicine or narcotics; barbiturates; medicine for seizures; muscle relaxants; or anesthetics, including some dental anesthetics. *Check with your doctor before taking any of the above while you are using this medicine and also for a few days after you stop taking it.*

This medicine will often make you sweat less, causing your body temperature to increase. *Use extra care not to become overheated during exercise or hot weather while you are taking this medicine* as this could possibly result in heat stroke. Also, hot baths or saunas may make you feel dizzy or faint while you are taking this medicine.

Your mouth, nose, and throat may feel very dry while you are taking this medicine. For temporary relief of mouth dryness, use sugarless candy or gum, melt bits of ice in your mouth, or use a saliva substitute. However, if your mouth continues to feel dry for more than 2 weeks, check with your dentist. Continuing dryness of the mouth may increase the chance of dental disease, including tooth decay, gum disease, and fungus infections.

Check with your doctor if you develop intestinal problems such as constipation. This is especially important if you are taking other medicine while you are taking chlordiazepoxide and clidinium. If these problems are not corrected, serious complications may result.

If you will be taking this medicine in large doses or for a long time, do not stop taking it without first checking with your doctor. Your doctor may want you to reduce gradually the amount you are taking before stopping completely.

Side Effects of This Medicine

Along with its needed effects, a medicine may cause some unwanted effects. Although not all of these side effects may occur, if they do occur they may need medical attention.

Check with your doctor as soon as possible if any of the following side effects occur:

Less common or rare

Constipation; eye pain; mental depression; skin rash or hives; slow heartbeat, shortness of breath, or troubled breathing; sore throat and fever; trouble in sleeping; unusual excitement, nervousness, or irritability; yellow eyes or skin

Symptoms of overdose

Confusion; difficult urination; drowsiness (severe); dryness of mouth, nose, or throat (severe); fast heartbeat; unusual warmth, dryness, and flushing of skin

Other side effects may occur that usually do not need medical attention. These side effects may go away during treatment as your body adjusts to the medicine. However, check with your doctor if any of the following side effects continue or are bothersome:

More common

Bloated feeling; decreased sweating; dizziness; drowsiness; dryness of mouth; headache

Less common

Blurred vision; decreased sexual ability; loss of memory; nausea; unusual tiredness or weakness

After you stop using this medicine, your body may need time to adjust. The length of time this takes depends on the amount of medicine you were using and how long you used it. During this time check with your doctor if you notice any of the following side effects:

Convulsions (seizures); muscle cramps; nausea or vomiting; stomach cramps; trembling

Other side effects not listed above may also occur in some patients. If you notice any other effects, check with your doctor.

Annual revision: 01/29/92

CHLORHEXIDINE Dental†

A commonly used brand name in the U.S. is Peridex.

†Not commercially available in Canada.

Description

Chlorhexidine (klor-HEX-i-deen) is used to treat gingivitis. It helps to reduce the inflammation (redness) and swelling of your gums and to control gum bleeding.

Gingivitis is caused by the bacteria that grow in the coating (plaque) that forms on your teeth between tooth brushings. Chlorhexidine destroys the bacteria, thereby preventing the gingivitis from occurring. However, chlorhexidine does *not* prevent plaque and tartar from forming; proper tooth brushing and flossing are still necessary and important.

Chlorhexidine is available only with your dentist's or medical doctor's prescription, in the following dosage form:

Dental

- Oral rinse (U.S.)

It is very important that you read and understand the following information. If any of it causes you special concern, check with your doctor. Also, *if you have any questions* or if you want more information about this medicine or your medical problem, *ask your doctor, nurse, or pharmacist.*

Before Using This Medicine

In deciding to use a medicine, the risks of using the medicine must be weighed against the good it will do. This is a decision you and your doctor will make. For chlorhexidine, the following should be considered:

Allergies—Tell your doctor if you have ever had any unusual or allergic reaction to this medicine or to skin disinfectants containing chlorhexidine. Also tell your doctor and pharmacist if you are allergic to any other substances, such as foods, preservatives, or dyes.

Pregnancy—Chlorhexidine has not been studied in pregnant women. However, chlorhexidine has not been shown to cause birth defects or other problems in animal studies.

Breast-feeding—It is not known whether chlorhexidine passes into the breast milk. However, this medicine has not been reported to cause problems in nursing babies.

Children—Studies on this medicine have been done only in adult patients, and there is no specific information comparing use of this medicine in children with use in other age groups.

Older adults—Many medicines have not been studied specifically in older people. Therefore, it may not be known whether they work exactly the same way they do in younger adults or if they cause different side effects or problems in older people. There is no specific information comparing use of this medicine in the elderly with use in other age groups.

Other medicines—Although certain medicines should not be used together at all, in other cases two different medicines may be used together even if an interaction might occur. In these cases, your doctor may want to change the dose, or other precautions may be necessary. Tell your doctor and pharmacist if you are using any other prescription or nonprescription (over-the-counter [OTC]) medicine that is to be used in the mouth.

Other medical problems—The presence of other medical problems may affect the use of chlorhexidine. Make sure you tell your doctor if you have any other medical problems, especially:

- Front-tooth fillings (especially those having rough surfaces)—Chlorhexidine may cause staining that, in some cases, may be impossible to remove and may require replacement of the filling
- Gum problems (other)—Use of chlorhexidine may make the condition worse

Before you begin using any new medicine (prescription or nonprescription) or if you develop any new medical problem while you are using this medicine, check with your doctor, nurse, or pharmacist.

Proper Use of This Medicine

Chlorhexidine oral rinse should be used after you have brushed and flossed your teeth. Rinse the toothpaste completely from your mouth with water before using the oral rinse. Do not eat or drink for several hours after using the oral rinse.

The cap on the original container of chlorhexidine can be used to measure the 15 mL (½ fluid ounce) dose of this medicine. Fill the cap to the "fill line." If you do not receive the dental rinse in its original container, make sure you have a measuring device to measure out the correct dose. Your pharmacist can help you with this.

Swish chlorhexidine around in the mouth for 30 seconds. Then spit out. *Use the medicine full strength.* Do not mix with water before using. *Do not swallow the medicine.*

Missed dose—If you miss a dose of this medicine, use it as soon as possible. However, if it is almost time for your next dose, skip the missed dose and go back to your regular dosing schedule. Do not double doses.

Storage—To store this medicine:

- Keep out of the reach of children.
- Store away from heat and direct light.
- Keep the medicine from freezing.
- Do not keep outdated medicine or medicine that is no longer needed. Be sure any discarded medicine is out of the reach of children.

Precautions While Using This Medicine

Chlorhexidine may have a bitter aftertaste. Do not rinse your mouth with water immediately after using chlorhexidine, since this will increase the bitterness.

Chlorhexidine may change the way foods taste to you. Sometimes this effect may last up to 4 hours after you use the oral rinse. In most cases, this effect will become less noticeable as you continue to use the medicine. When you stop using chlorhexidine, your taste should return to normal.

Chlorhexidine may cause staining and an increase in tartar (calculus) on your teeth. Brushing with a tartar-control toothpaste and flossing your teeth daily may help reduce this tartar build-up and staining. In addition, you should visit your dentist at least every 6 months to have your teeth cleaned and your gums examined.

If you think that a child weighing 22 pounds (10 kg) or less has swallowed more than 4 ounces of the dental rinse, *get emergency help at once.* In addition, if a child of any age drinks the dental rinse, *get emergency help at once if the child has symptoms of alcohol intoxication,* such as slurred speech, sleepiness, or staggering or stumbling walk.

Side Effects of This Medicine

Along with its needed effects, a medicine may cause some unwanted effects. Although not all of these side effects may occur, if they do occur they may need medical attention.

Check with your doctor immediately if any of the following side effects occur:

Nasal congestion; shortness of breath or troubled breathing; skin rash, hives, or itching; swelling of face

Other side effects may occur that usually do not need medical attention. These side effects may go away during treatment as your body adjusts to the medicine. However, check with your dentist or medical doctor if any of the following side effects continue or are bothersome:

More common

Change in taste; increase in tartar (calculus) on teeth; staining of teeth, mouth, tooth fillings, and dentures or other mouth appliances

Less common or rare

Mouth irritation; tongue tip irritation

Other side effects not listed above may also occur in some patients. If you notice any other effects, check with your dentist or medical doctor.

Annual revision: 03/04/92

CHLORMEZANONE Systemic†

A commonly used brand name in the U.S. is Trancopal Caplets.

†Not commercially available in Canada.

Description

Chlormezanone (klor-MEZ-an-own) is used to relieve nervousness or tension. This medication should not be used for nervousness or tension caused by the stress of everyday life.

Chlormezanone is available only with your doctor's prescription, in the following dosage form:

Oral

- Tablets (U.S.)

It is very important that you read and understand the following information. If any of it causes you special concern, check with your doctor. Also, *if you have any questions* or if you want more information about this medicine or your medical problem, *ask your doctor, nurse, or pharmacist.*

Before Using This Medicine

In deciding to use a medicine, the risks of taking the medicine must be weighed against the good it will do. This is a decision you and your doctor will make. For chlormezanone, the following should be considered:

Allergies—Tell your doctor if you have ever had any unusual or allergic reaction to chlormezanone. Also tell your doctor and pharmacist if you are allergic to any other substances, such as foods, preservatives, or dyes.

Pregnancy—Studies on effects in pregnancy have not been done in either humans or animals.

Breast-feeding—Chlormezanone has not been reported to cause problems in nursing babies.

Children—Although there is no specific information comparing use of chlormezanone in children with use in other age groups, this medicine is not expected to cause different side effects or problems in children than it does in adults.

Older adults—Many medicines have not been studied specifically in older people. Therefore, it may not be known whether they work exactly the same way they do in younger adults. Although there is no specific information comparing use of chlormezanone in the elderly with use in other age groups, this medicine is not expected to cause different side effects or problems in older people than it does in younger adults.

Other medicines—Although certain medicines should not be used together at all, in other cases two different medicines may be used together even if an interaction might occur. In these cases, your doctor may want to change the dose, or other precautions may be necessary. When you are taking chlormezanone, it is especially important that your doctor and pharmacist know if you are taking any of the following:

- Central nervous system (CNS) depressants (medicine that causes drowsiness) or
- Tricyclic antidepressants (medicine for depression)—Concurrent use may increase the CNS depressant effects of either these medications or chlormezanone

Other medical problems—The presence of other medical problems may affect the use of chlormezanone. Make sure you tell your doctor if you have any other medical problems, especially:

- Drug abuse or dependence (or history of)—Dependence on chlormezanone may develop
- Kidney disease or
- Liver disease—Higher blood levels of chlormezanone may occur, increasing the chance of side effects

Before you begin using any new medicine (prescription or nonprescription) or if you develop any new medical problem while you are using this medicine, check with your doctor, nurse, or pharmacist.

Proper Use of This Medicine

Take this medicine only as directed by your doctor. Do not take more of it, do not take it more often, and do not take it for a longer time than your doctor ordered. If too much chlormezanone is taken, it may become habit-forming. Also, taking too much of this medicine may increase the chance of side effects.

Dosing—The dose of chlormezanone will be different for different patients. *Follow your doctor's orders or the directions on the label.* The following information includes only the average doses of chlormezanone. *If your dose is different, do not change it* unless your doctor tells you to do so.

- The number of tablets that you take depends on the strength of the medicine. Also, *the number of doses you take each day, the time allowed between doses, and the length of time you take the medicine depend on the medical problem for which you are taking chlormezanone.*
- For *oral* dosage forms (tablets):
  —Adults and adolescents: 100 to 200 milligrams three or four times a day.
  —Children 5 to 12 years of age: 50 to 100 milligrams three or four times a day.
  —Children up to 5 years of age: Dose must be determined by the doctor.

Missed dose—If you miss a dose of this medicine and remember within an hour or so of the missed dose, take it right away. However, if you do not remember until later, skip the missed dose and go back to your regular dosing schedule. Do not double doses.

Storage—To store this medicine:

- Keep out of the reach of children.
- Store away from heat and direct light.
- Do not store in the bathroom, near the kitchen sink, or in other damp places. Heat or moisture may cause the medicine to break down.
- Do not keep outdated medicine or medicine no longer needed. Be sure that any discarded medicine is out of the reach of children.

Precautions While Using This Medicine

If you will be taking chlormezanone regularly for a long time:

- Your doctor should check your progress at regular visits.
- Check with your doctor at least every 4 months to make sure you need to continue taking this medicine.

If you will be taking this medicine in large doses or for a long time, do not stop taking it without first checking with your doctor. Your doctor may want you to reduce gradually the amount you are taking before stopping completely.

Chlormezanone will add to the effects of alcohol and other CNS depressants (medicines that slow down the nervous system, possibly causing drowsiness). Some examples of CNS depressants are antihistamines or medicine for hay fever, other allergies, or colds; sedatives, tranquilizers, or sleeping medicine; prescription pain medicine or narcotics; barbiturates; medicine for seizures; muscle relaxants; or anesthetics, including some dental anesthetics. *Check with your doctor before taking any of the above while you are using this medicine.*

If you think you or someone else may have taken an overdose of this medicine, get emergency help at once. Taking an overdose of chlormezanone or taking alcohol or other CNS depressants with chlormezanone may lead to unconsciousness and possibly death. Some signs of an overdose are severe confusion, severe drowsiness, loss of reflexes, and continuing unusual tiredness or weakness.

This medicine may cause some people to become dizzy, drowsy, or less alert than they are normally. Even if taken at bedtime, it may cause some people to feel drowsy or less alert on arising. *Make sure you know how you react to this medicine before you drive, use machines, or do anything else that could be dangerous if you are dizzy or are not alert.*

Side Effects of This Medicine

Along with its needed effects, a medicine may cause some unwanted effects. Although not all of these side effects may occur, if they do occur they may need medical attention.

Check with your doctor as soon as possible if any of the following side effects occur:

Less common

Confusion; mental depression

Rare

Abdominal or stomach pains; aching muscles and joints; fever and chills; skin rash or itching (severe); swelling of feet or lower legs; yellow eyes or skin; unusual excitement

Signs and/or symptoms of overdose

Confusion (severe); drowsiness (severe); loss of reflexes; unusual tiredness or weakness (continuing)

Other side effects may occur that usually do not need medical attention. These side effects may go away during treatment as your body adjusts to the medicine. However, check with your doctor if any of the following side effects continue or are bothersome:

More common

Drowsiness

Less common

Clumsiness or unsteadiness; difficulty in urination; dizziness; flushing or redness of skin; headache; nausea; trembling; weakness

Other side effects not listed above may also occur in some patients. If you notice any other effects, check with your doctor.

Annual revision: 03/09/93

CHLOROQUINE Systemic

Some commonly used brand names are:

In the U.S.

Aralen

Aralen HCl

Generic name product may also be available.

In Canada

Aralen

Description

Chloroquine (KLOR-oh-kwin) is a medicine used to prevent and treat malaria and to treat some conditions such as liver disease caused by protozoa. It is also used in the treatment of arthritis to help relieve inflammation, swelling, stiffness, and joint pain and to help control the symptoms of lupus erythematosus (lupus; SLE).

This medicine may be given alone or with one or more other medicines. It may also be used for other conditions as determined by your doctor.

Chloroquine is available only with your doctor's prescription, in the following dosage forms:

Oral

- Tablets (U.S. and Canada)

Parenteral

- Injection (U.S.)

It is very important that you read and understand the following information. If any of it causes you special concern, check with your doctor. Also, *if you have any questions* or if you want more information about this medicine or your medical problem, *ask your doctor, nurse, or pharmacist.*

Before Using This Medicine

In deciding to use a medicine, the risks of taking the medicine must be weighed against the good it will do. This is a decision you and your doctor will make. For chloroquine, the following should be considered:

Allergies—Tell your doctor if you have ever had any unusual or allergic reaction to chloroquine or hydroxychloroquine. Also tell your doctor and pharmacist if you are allergic to any other substances, such as foods, preservatives, or dyes.

Pregnancy—Unless you are taking it for malaria or liver disease caused by protozoa, use of this medicine is not recommended during pregnancy. In animal studies, chloroquine has been shown to cause damage to the central nervous system (brain and spinal cord) of the fetus, including damage to hearing, sense of balance, bleeding inside the eyes, and other eye problems. However, when given in low doses (once a week) to prevent malaria, this medicine has not been shown to cause birth defects or other problems in humans.

Breast-feeding—Chloroquine passes into the breast milk. Chloroquine has not been reported to cause problems in nursing babies to date. However, babies and children are especially sensitive to the effects of chloroquine.

Children—Children are especially sensitive to the effects of chloroquine. This may increase the chance of side effects during treatment. Overdose is especially dangerous in children. Taking as little as 1 tablet (300-mg strength) has resulted in the death of a small child.

Older adults—Many medicines have not been studied specifically in older people. Therefore, it may not be known whether they work exactly the same way they do in younger adults or if they cause different side effects or problems in older people. There is no specific information comparing use of chloroquine in the elderly with use in other age groups.

Other medicines—Although certain medicines should not be used together at all, in other cases 2 different medicines may be used together even if an interaction might occur. In these cases, your doctor may want to change the dose, or other precautions may be necessary. Tell your doctor and pharmacist if you are taking any other prescription or nonprescription (over-the-counter [OTC]) medicine.

Other medical problems—The presence of other medical problems may affect the use of chloroquine. Make sure you tell your doctor if you have any other medical problems, especially:

- Blood disease (severe)—Chloroquine may cause blood disorders
- Eye or vision problems—Chloroquine may cause serious eye side effects, especially in high doses
- Glucose-6-phosphate dehydrogenase (G6PD) deficiency—Chloroquine may cause serious blood side effects in patients with this deficiency
- Liver disease—May decrease the removal of chloroquine from the blood, increasing the chance of side effects
- Nerve or brain disease (severe), including convulsions (seizures)—Chloroquine may cause muscle weakness and, in high doses, seizures
- Porphyria—Chloroquine may cause episodes of porphyria to occur more frequently
- Psoriasis—Chloroquine may bring on severe attacks of psoriasis
- Stomach or intestinal disease (severe)—Chloroquine may cause stomach or intestinal irritation

Before you begin using any new medicine (prescription or nonprescription) or if you develop any new medical problem while you are using this medicine, check with your doctor, nurse, or pharmacist.

Proper Use of This Medicine

Take this medicine with meals or milk to lessen possible stomach upset, unless otherwise directed by your doctor.

Keep this medicine out of the reach of children. Children are especially sensitive to the effects of chloroquine and overdose is especially dangerous in children. Taking as little as 1 tablet (300-mg strength) has resulted in the death of a small child.

It is very important that you *take this medicine only as directed.* Do not take more of it, do not take it more often, and do not take it for a longer time than your doctor ordered. To do so may increase the chance of serious side effects.

If you are taking this medicine to help keep you from getting malaria, *keep taking it for the full time of treatment.* If you already have malaria, you should still keep taking this medicine for the full time of treatment even if you begin to feel better after a few days. This will help to clear up your infection completely. If you stop taking this medicine too soon, your symptoms may return.

Chloroquine works best when you take it on a regular schedule. For example, if you are to take it once a week to prevent malaria, it is best to take it on the same day each week. Or if you are to take 2 doses a day, 1 dose may be taken with breakfast and the other with the evening meal. *Make sure that you do not miss any doses.* If you have any questions about this, check with your doctor, nurse, or pharmacist.

For patients taking chloroquine *to prevent malaria:*

- Your doctor may want you to start taking this medicine 1 to 2 weeks before you travel to an area where there is a chance of getting malaria. This will help you to see how you react to the medicine. Also, it will allow time for your doctor to change to another medicine if you have a reaction to this medicine.
- Also, you should keep taking this medicine while you are in the area and for 4 weeks after you leave the area. No medicine will protect you completely from malaria. However, to protect you as completely as possible, *it is important to keep taking this medicine for the full time your doctor ordered.* Also, if fever develops during your travels or within 2 months after you leave the area, *check with your doctor immediately.*

For patients taking chloroquine *for arthritis or lupus:*

- This medicine must be taken regularly as ordered by your doctor in order for it to help you. It may take up to several weeks before you begin to feel better. It may take up to 6 months before you feel the full benefit of this medicine.

Missed dose—If you do miss a dose of this medicine and your dosing schedule is:

- One dose every seven days—Take the missed dose as soon as possible. Then go back to your regular dosing schedule.
- One dose a day—Take the missed dose as soon as possible. But if you do not remember until the next day, skip the missed dose and go back to your regular dosing schedule. Do not double doses.
- More than one dose a day—Take it right away if you remember within an hour or so of the missed dose. But if you do not remember until later, skip the missed dose and go back to your regular dosing schedule. Do not double doses.

If you have any questions about this, check with your doctor.

Storage—To store this medicine:

- Keep out of the reach of children. Overdose of chloroquine is very dangerous in children.
- Store away from heat and direct light.
- Do not store in the bathroom, near the kitchen sink, or in other damp places. Heat or moisture may cause the medicine to break down.
- Do not keep outdated medicine or medicine no longer needed. Be sure that any discarded medicine is out of the reach of children.

Precautions While Using This Medicine

If you will be taking this medicine for a long time, *it is very important that your doctor check you at regular visits* for any blood problems or muscle weakness that may be caused by this medicine. In addition, *check with your doctor immediately if blurred vision, difficulty in reading, or any other change in vision occurs during or after treatment.* Your doctor may want you to have your eyes checked by an ophthalmologist (eye doctor).

If your symptoms do not improve within a few days (or a few weeks or months for arthritis), or if they become worse, check with your doctor.

Chloroquine may cause blurred vision, difficulty in reading, or other change in vision. It may also cause some people to become lightheaded. *Make sure you know how you react to this medicine before you drive, use machines, or do anything else that could be dangerous if you are not able to see well.* If these reactions are especially bothersome, check with your doctor.

Malaria is spread by mosquitoes. If you are living in, or will be traveling to, an area where there is a chance of getting malaria, the following mosquito-control measures will help to prevent infection:

- If possible, sleep under mosquito netting to avoid being bitten by malaria-carrying mosquitoes.
- Wear long-sleeved shirts or blouses and long trousers to protect your arms and legs, especially from dusk through dawn when mosquitoes are out.
- Apply mosquito repellent to uncovered areas of the skin from dusk through dawn when mosquitoes are out.

Side Effects of This Medicine

Along with its needed effects, a medicine may cause some unwanted effects. Although not all of these side effects may occur, if they do occur they may need medical attention. When this medicine is used for short periods of time, side effects usually are rare. However, when it is used for a long time and/or in high doses, side effects are more likely to occur and may be serious.

Check with your doctor immediately if any of the following side effects occur:

Less common

Blurred vision or any other change in vision

Note: The above side effects may also occur or get worse after you stop taking this medicine.

Rare

Convulsions (seizures); fatigue; feeling faint or lightheaded; increased muscle weakness; mood or other mental changes; ringing or buzzing in ears or any loss of hearing; sore throat and fever; unusual bleeding or bruising; weakness

Symptoms of overdose

Drowsiness; headache; increased excitability

Other side effects may occur that usually do not need medical attention. These side effects may go away during treatment as your body adjusts to the medicine. However, check with your doctor if any of the following side effects continue or are bothersome:

More common

Diarrhea; difficulty in seeing to read; headache; itching (more common in black patients); loss of appetite; nausea or vomiting; stomach cramps or pain

Less common

Bleaching of hair or increased hair loss; blue-black discoloration of skin, fingernails, or inside of mouth; skin rash

Other side effects not listed above may also occur in some patients. If you notice any other effects, check with your doctor.

Additional Information

Once a medicine has been approved for marketing for a certain use, experience may show that it is also useful for other medical problems. Although these uses are not included in product labeling, chloroquine is used in certain patients with the following medical conditions:

- Arthritis in children
- High levels of calcium in the blood associated with sarcoidosis
- Various skin disorders

Other than the above information, there is no additional information relating to proper use, precautions, or side effects for these uses.

Annual revision: 07/06/92

CHLOROXINE Topical

A commonly used brand name in the U.S. is Capitrol.

Description

Chloroxine (klor-OX-een) is used in the treatment of dandruff and seborrheic dermatitis of the scalp.

This medicine is available only with your doctor's prescription, in the following dosage form:

Topical
- Lotion shampoo (U.S.)

It is very important that you read and understand the following information. If any of it causes you special concern, check with your doctor. Also, *if you have any questions* or if you want more information about this medicine or your medical problem, *ask your doctor, nurse, or pharmacist.*

Before Using This Medicine

In deciding to use a medicine, the risks of using the medicine must be weighed against the good it will do. This is a decision you and your doctor will make. For chloroxine, the following should be considered:

Allergies—Tell your doctor if you have ever had any unusual or allergic reaction to chloroxine, clioquinol (iodochlorhydroxyquin), iodoquinol (diiodohydroxyquin), or edetate disodium. Also tell your doctor and pharmacist if you are allergic to any other substances, such as preservatives or dyes.

Pregnancy—Studies on effects in pregnancy have not been done in either humans or animals.

Breast-feeding—It is not known whether chloroxine passes into the breast milk. However, this medicine has not been reported to cause problems in nursing babies.

Children—Studies on this medicine have been done only in adult patients, and there is no specific information comparing use of this medicine in children with use in other age groups.

Older adults—Many medicines have not been studied specifically in older people. Therefore, it may not be known whether they work exactly the same way they do in younger adults or if they cause different side effects or problems in older people. There is no specific information comparing use of this medicine in the elderly with use in other age groups.

Other medicines—Although certain medicines should not be used together at all, in other cases two different medicines may be used together even if an interaction might occur. In these cases, your doctor may want to change the dose, or other precautions may be necessary. Tell your doctor and pharmacist if you are using any other topical prescription or nonprescription (over-the-counter [OTC]) medicine that is to be applied to the same area of the skin.

Before you begin using any new medicine (prescription or nonprescription) or if you develop any new medical problem while you are using this medicine, check with your doctor, nurse, or pharmacist.

Proper Use of This Medicine

Do not use this medicine if blistered, raw, or oozing areas are present on your scalp, unless otherwise directed by your doctor.

Keep this medicine away from the eyes. If you should accidentally get some in your eyes, flush them thoroughly with cool water. Check with your doctor if eye irritation continues or is bothersome.

To use:
- Wet the hair and scalp with lukewarm water. Apply enough chloroxine to the scalp to work up a lather, and rub in well. Allow the lather to remain on the scalp for about 3 minutes, then rinse. Apply the medicine again and rinse thoroughly. Use the medicine two times a week or as directed by your doctor.

Storage—To store this medicine:
- Keep out of the reach of children.
- Store away from heat and direct light.
- Keep the medicine from freezing.
- Do not keep outdated medicine or medicine no longer needed. Be sure that any discarded medicine is out of the reach of children.

Precautions While Using This Medicine

This medicine may slightly discolor light-colored hair (for example, bleached, blond, or gray).

Side Effects of This Medicine

Along with its needed effects, a medicine may cause some unwanted effects. Although not all of these side effects may occur, if they do occur they may need medical attention.

Check with your doctor as soon as possible if any of the following side effects occur:

Irritation or burning of scalp not present before use of this medicine; skin rash

Other side effects may occur that usually do not need medical attention. However, check with your doctor if either of the following side effects continues or is bothersome:

Dryness or increased itching of scalp

Other side effects not listed above may also occur in some patients. If you notice any other effects, check with your doctor.

Annual revision: 02/10/92

CHLORZOXAZONE AND ACETAMINOPHEN Systemic*

A commonly used brand name in Canada is Parafon Forte.

Another commonly used name for this combination medicine is chlorzoxazone with APAP.

*Not commercially available in the U.S.

Description

Chlorzoxazone (klor-ZOX-a-zone) and acetaminophen (a-seat-a-MIN-oh-fen) combination medicine is used to help relax certain muscles in your body and relieve the pain and discomfort caused by strains, sprains, or other injuries to your muscles. However, this medicine does not take the place of rest, exercise or physical therapy, or other treatment that your doctor may recommend for your medical problem.

Chlorzoxazone acts in the central nervous system (CNS) to produce its muscle relaxant effects. Its actions in the CNS may also produce some of its side effects.

In Canada, this medicine is available without a prescription.

This medicine is available in the following dosage forms:

Oral

- Tablets (Canada)

It is very important that you read and understand the following information. If any of it causes you special concern, check with your doctor or pharmacist. Also, *if you have any questions* or if you want more information about this medicine or your medical problem, *ask your doctor, nurse, or pharmacist.*

Before Using This Medicine

If you are taking this medicine without a prescription, carefully read and follow any precautions on the label. For chlorzoxazone and acetaminophen combination, the following should be considered:

Allergies—Tell your doctor if you have ever had any unusual or allergic reaction to acetaminophen, chlorzoxazone, or aspirin. Also tell your doctor and pharmacist if you are allergic to any other substances, such as foods, preservatives, or dyes.

Pregnancy—Although studies on birth defects with chlorzoxazone or acetaminophen have not been done in pregnant women, these medicines have not been reported to cause birth defects or other problems.

Breast-feeding—Chlorzoxazone and acetaminophen have not been shown to cause problems in nursing babies. However, acetaminophen passes into the breast milk in small amounts.

Children—Studies on this combination medicine have been done only in adult patients, and there is no specific information about its use in children. However, chlorzoxazone and acetaminophen have been tested separately in children. In effective doses, these medicines have not been shown to cause different side effects or problems in children than they do in adults.

Older adults—Many medicines have not been studied specifically in older people. Therefore, it may not be known whether they work exactly the same way they do in younger adults or if they cause different side effects or problems in older people. There is no specific information comparing the use of chlorzoxazone and acetaminophen combination or of chlorzoxazone alone in the elderly with use in other age groups. However, acetaminophen has been tested and has not been shown to cause different side effects or problems in older people than it does in younger adults.

Other medicines—Although certain medicines should not be used together at all, in other cases two different medicines may be used together even if an interaction might occur. In these cases, your doctor may want to change the dose, or other precautions may be necessary. When you are taking chlorzoxazone and acetaminophen combination, it is especially important that your doctor and pharmacist know if you are taking any of the following:

- Antidepressants, tricyclic (amitriptyline [e.g., Elavil], amoxapine [e.g., Asendin], clomipramine [e.g., Anafranil], desipramine [e.g., Pertofrane], doxepin [e.g., Sinequan], imipramine [e.g., Tofranil], nortriptyline [e.g., Aventyl], protriptyline [e.g., Vivactil], trimipramine [e.g., Surmontil]) or
- Central nervous system (CNS) depressants (medicines that often cause drowsiness)—These medicines may add to the effects of chlorzoxazone and increase the chance of drowsiness or other side effects

Other medical problems—The presence of other medical problems may affect the use of chlorzoxazone and acetaminophen combination. Make sure you tell your doctor if you have any other medical problems, especially:

- Alcohol abuse or
- Allergies (asthma, eczema, hay fever, hives) or
- Hepatitis or other liver disease or
- Kidney disease—The chance of side effects may be increased

Before you begin using any new medicine (prescription or nonprescription) or if you develop any new medical problem while you are using this medicine, check with your doctor, nurse, or pharmacist.

Proper Use of This Medicine

Take this medicine only as directed. Do not take more of it, do not take it more often, and do not take it for a longer time than directed on the package label or by your doctor. To do so may increase the chance of side effects. This medicine may cause liver damage if too much is taken.

Missed dose—If you miss a dose of this medicine, take it as soon as you remember. However, if it is almost time for your next dose, skip the missed dose and go back to your regular dosing schedule. Do not double doses.

Storage—To store this medicine:

- Keep out of the reach of children.
- Store away from heat and direct light.
- Do not store this medicine in the bathroom, near the kitchen sink, or in other damp places. Heat or moisture may cause the medicine to break down.
- Do not keep outdated medicine or medicine no longer needed. Be sure that any discarded medicine is out of the reach of children.

Precautions While Using This Medicine

If you will be taking this medicine for a long time (for example, for several months at a time), your doctor should check your progress at regular visits.

Check the labels of all nonprescription (over-the-counter [OTC]) and prescription medicines you now take. If any contain acetaminophen, be especially careful since taking them while taking this medicine may lead to overdose. If you have any questions about this, check with your doctor, nurse, or pharmacist.

This medicine will add to the effects of alcohol and other CNS depressants (medicines that slow down the nervous system, possibly causing drowsiness). Some examples of CNS depressants are antihistamines or medicine for hay fever, other allergies, or colds; sedatives, tranquilizers, or sleeping medicine; prescription pain medicine or narcotics; barbiturates; medicine for seizures; or anesthetics, including some dental anesthetics. Also, the risk of liver damage from acetaminophen may be greater if you use large amounts of alcoholic beverages with acetaminophen. Therefore, *do not drink alcoholic beverages, and check with your doctor before taking any of the medicines listed above, while you are taking this medicine.*

Taking the acetaminophen in this combination medicine together with certain other medicines may increase the chance of unwanted effects. The risk will depend on how much of each medicine you take every day, and on how long you take the medicines together. If your medical doctor or dentist directs you to take these medicines together on a regular basis, follow his or her directions carefully. However, *do not take any of the following medicines together with chlorzoxazone and acetaminophen combination for more than a few days, unless your doctor has directed you to do so and is following your progress.*

Aspirin or other salicylates
Diclofenac (e.g., Voltaren)
Diflunisal (e.g., Dolobid)
Etodolac (e.g., Lodine)
Fenoprofen (e.g., Nalfon)
Floctafenine (e.g., Idarac)
Flurbiprofen, oral (e.g., Ansaid)
Ibuprofen (e.g., Motrin)
Indomethacin (e.g., Indocin)
Ketoprofen (e.g., Orudis)
Ketorolac (e.g., Toradol)
Meclofenamate (e.g., Meclomen)
Mefenamic acid (e.g., Ponstel)
Naproxen (e.g., Naprosyn)
Phenylbutazone (e.g., Butazolidin)
Piroxicam (e.g., Feldene)
Sulindac (e.g., Clinoril)
Tiaprofenic acid (e.g., Surgam)
Tolmetin (e.g., Tolectin)

This medicine may cause some people to become drowsy, dizzy, or less alert than they are normally. *Make sure you know how you react to this medicine before you drive, use machines, or do anything else that could be dangerous if you are dizzy or are not alert.*

Acetaminophen may interfere with the results of some medical tests. Before you have any medical tests, tell the doctor in charge if you have taken acetaminophen within the past 3 or 4 days. If possible, it is best to check with the doctor first, to find out whether this medicine may be taken during the 3 or 4 days before the test.

For *diabetic patients:*

- Acetaminophen may cause false results with some blood glucose (sugar) tests. If you notice any change in your test results, or if you have any questions about this possible problem, check with your doctor, nurse, or pharmacist. This is especially important if your diabetes is not well-controlled.

If you think that you or anyone else may have taken an overdose of this medicine, get emergency help at once. Signs of overdose of this medicine include fast or irregular breathing and severe muscle weakness. Signs of severe acetaminophen poisoning may not appear for 2 to 4 days after the overdose is taken, but treatment to prevent liver damage or death must be started within 24 hours or less after the overdose is taken.

Side Effects of This Medicine

Along with its needed effects, a medicine may cause some unwanted effects. Although not all of these side effects may occur, if they do occur they may need medical attention.

Check with your doctor immediately if any of the following side effects occur:

Rare

Hive-like swellings (large) on face, eyelids, mouth, lips, or tongue; sudden decrease in amount of urine

Symptoms of overdose

Diarrhea; fast or irregular breathing; increased sweating; loss of appetite; muscle weakness (severe); nausea or vomiting; pain, tenderness, or swelling in upper abdomen or stomach area; stomach cramps or pain

Also, check with your doctor as soon as possible if any of the following side effects occur:

Rare

Bloody or black, tarry stools; bloody or cloudy urine; difficult or painful urination; frequent urge to urinate; pain in lower back and/or side (severe and/or sharp); pinpoint red spots on skin; skin rash, hives, itching, or redness; sore throat and fever; unusual bleeding or bruising; unusual tiredness or weakness; yellow eyes or skin

Other side effects may occur that usually do not need medical attention. These side effects may go away during treatment as your body adjusts to the medicine. However, check with your doctor if any of the following side effects continue or are bothersome:

More common

Dizziness or lightheadedness; drowsiness

Less common

Constipation; headache; heartburn; unusual excitement, nervousness, restlessness, or irritability

This medicine sometimes causes the urine to turn orange or reddish purple. This is not harmful and will go away when you stop taking the medicine. If you have any questions about this, check with your doctor.

Other side effects not listed above may also occur in some patients. If you notice any other effects, check with your doctor.

Annual revision: 06/01/92

CHOLECYSTOGRAPHIC AGENTS, ORAL Diagnostic

This information applies to the following medicines:

Iocetamic Acid (eye-oh-se-TAM-ik)
Iopanoic Acid (eye-oh-pa-NOE-ik)
Ipodate (EYE-poe-date)
Tyropanoate (tye-roe-pa-NOE-ate)

Some commonly used brand names:

For Iocetamic Acid†

In the U.S.
Cholebrine

Other
Colebrin
Colebrina

For Iopanoic Acid

In the U.S.
Telepaque

In Canada
Telepaque

Other
Cistobil
Colegraf
Felombrine
Jopanonsyre
Neocontrast

For Ipodate†

In the U.S.
Bilivist
Oragrafin Calcium
Oragrafin Sodium

Other
Biloptin

Another commonly used name for ipodate sodium is sodium iopodate.

For Tyropanoate

In the U.S.
Bilopaque

In Canada
Bilopaque

Other
Lumopaque

Another commonly used name is sodium tyropanoate.

†Not commercially available in Canada.

Description

Oral cholecystographic (ko-le-sis-to-GRAF-ik) agents are radiopaque agents. Radiopaque agents are drugs used to help diagnose certain medical problems. These agents contain iodine, which absorbs x-rays. Depending on how the radiopaque agent is given, it builds up in certain areas of the body. When radiopaque agents are inside the body they will appear white on the x-ray film. This creates the needed distinction, or contrast, between one organ and other tissues. This will help the doctor see any special conditions that may exist in that organ or part of the body.

The oral cholecystographic agents are taken by mouth before x-ray tests to help check for problems of the gallbladder and the biliary tract. Ipodate may also be used for other conditions as determined by your doctor.

These radiopaque agents are to be given only by or under the direct supervision of a doctor. They are available in the following dosage forms:

Oral

- Iocetamic acid
  - Tablets (U.S.)
- Iopanoic acid
  - Tablets (U.S. and Canada)
- Ipodate
  - Capsules (U.S.)
  - Oral suspension (U.S.)
- Tyropanoate
  - Capsules (U.S. and Canada)

It is very important that you read and understand the following information. If any of it causes you special concern, check with your doctor. Also, *if you have any questions* or if you want more information about this test or your medical problem, *ask your doctor, nurse, or pharmacist.*

Before Having This Test

In deciding to use a diagnostic test, any risks of the test must be weighed against the good it will do. This is a decision you and your doctor will make. Also, test results may be affected by other things. For cholecystographic agents, the following should be considered:

Allergies—Tell your doctor if you have ever had any unusual or allergic reaction to iodine, to products containing iodine (for example, iodine-containing foods, such as seafoods, cabbage, kale, rape [turnip-like vegetable], turnips, or iodized salt), or to other radiopaque agents. Also tell your doctor if you are allergic to any other substance, such as preservatives.

Pregnancy—Studies on effects in pregnancy have not been done in humans with any of these agents. Studies in animals have been done only with iocetamic acid, which has not been shown to cause birth defects or other problems. However, on rare occasions, other radiopaque agents containing iodine have caused hypothyroidism (underactive thyroid) in the baby when given in late pregnancy. Also, x-rays of the abdomen are usually not recommended during pregnancy. This is to avoid exposing the fetus to radiation. Be sure you have discussed this with your doctor.

Breast-feeding—Iocetamic acid, iopanoic acid, and tyropanoate pass into the breast milk, and the other agents may pass into the breast milk also. However, these radiopaque agents have not been reported to cause problems in nursing babies.

Children—Although there is no specific information comparing use of cholecystographic agents in children with use in other age groups, tests using iopanoic acid and ipodate in children have not shown that these agents cause different side effects or problems in children than they do in adults.

Older adults—Many medicines have not been studied specifically in older people. Therefore, it may not be known whether they work exactly the same way they do in younger adults. Although there is no specific information comparing use of cholecystographic agents in the elderly with use in other age groups, these agents are not expected to cause different side effects or problems in older people than they do in younger adults.

Other medicines—Although certain medicines should not be used together at all, in other cases two different medicines may be used together even if an interaction might occur. In these cases, your doctor may want to change the dose, or other precautions may be necessary. Tell your doctor if you are taking any other prescription or nonprescription (over-the-counter [OTC]) medicine.

Other medical problems—The presence of other medical problems may affect the use of cholecystographic agents. Make sure you tell your doctor if you have any other medical problems, especially:

- Asthma, hay fever, or other allergies (history of)—Patients with these conditions have a greater chance of having a reaction, such as an allergic reaction
- Heart disease—Other problems, such as low blood pressure or slow heartbeat, may occur
- Kidney disease or
- Liver disease (severe)—Serious kidney problems may result
- Overactive thyroid—A sudden increase in symptoms, such as fast heartbeat or palpitations, fatigue, nervousness, excessive sweating, and muscle weakness may occur

Preparation For This Test

Dosing—Take this radiopaque agent with water after dinner the evening or evenings before the examination, following the directions of your doctor.

Do not eat or drink anything but water after taking the medicine. Also, avoid smoking or chewing gum.

Your doctor may order a special diet or use of a laxative or enema in preparation for your test, depending on the type of test. If you have not received such instructions or if you do not understand them, check with your doctor in advance.

Precautions After Having This Test

Make sure your doctor knows if you are planning to have any future thyroid tests. The results of the thyroid test may be affected, even weeks or months later, by the iodine in this agent.

Side Effects of This Medicine

Along with its needed effects, a medicine may cause some unwanted effects. Although not all of these side effects may occur, if they do occur they may need medical attention.

Check with your doctor or nurse immediately if any of the following side effects occur:

Rare

Itching; skin rash or hives; swelling of skin; unusual bleeding or bruising (with iopanoic acid only)

Symptoms of overdose

Severe diarrhea; severe nausea and vomiting; problems with urination

Other side effects may occur that usually do not need medical attention. These side effects should go away as the effects of the radiopaque agent wear off. However, check with your doctor if any of the following side effects continue or are bothersome:

More common

Mild diarrhea; mild to moderate nausea and vomiting

Less common

Abdominal or stomach spasms or cramps; severe diarrhea; difficult or painful urination; dizziness; frequent urge to urinate; headache; heartburn; severe or continuing nausea and vomiting

Other side effects not listed above may also occur in some patients. If you notice any other effects, check with your doctor.

Additional Information

Once a medicine has been approved for marketing for a certain use, experience may show that it is also useful for other medical problems. Although not specifically included in product labeling, ipodate is used in certain patients with the following medical condition:

- Graves' disease

In addition to the above information, for patients with Graves' disease taking ipodate:

- Ipodate is used in patients with Graves' disease, who have an overactive thyroid, to reduce the amount of thyroid hormone produced by the thyroid gland.
- *Use this medicine only as directed by your doctor.* Do not take more of it, do not take it more often, and do not take it for a longer period of time than your doctor ordered. To do so may increase the chance of side effects.
- In order for it to work properly, *ipodate must be taken every day, as ordered by your doctor.*
- The information given above in the section *Preparation For This Test* will not apply to you.

Other than the above information, there is no additional information relating to proper use, precautions, or side effects for these uses.

Annual revision: 07/27/92

CHOLESTYRAMINE Oral

Some commonly used brand names are:

In the U.S.

Cholybar
Questran
Questran Light

In Canada

Questran
Questran Light

Description

Cholestyramine (koe-less-TEAR-a-meen) is used to remove substances called bile acids from your body. With some liver problems, there is too much bile acid in your body and this can cause severe itching. Cholestyramine is also used to lower high cholesterol levels in the blood. This may help prevent medical problems caused by cholesterol clogging the blood vessels.

Cholestyramine works by attaching to certain substances in the intestine. Since cholestyramine is not absorbed into the body, these substances also pass out of the body without being absorbed.

Cholestyramine may also be used for other conditions as determined by your doctor.

Cholestyramine is available only with your doctor's prescription, in the following dosage forms:

Oral

- Chewable bar (U.S.)
- Powder (U.S. and Canada)

It is very important that you read and understand the following information. If any of it causes you special concern, check with your doctor. Also, *if you have any questions* or if you want more information about this medicine or your medical problem, *ask your doctor, nurse, or pharmacist.*

Before Using This Medicine

In deciding to use a medicine, the risks of taking the medicine must be weighed against the good it will do. This is a decision you and your doctor will make. For cholestyramine, the following should be considered:

Allergies—Tell your doctor if you have ever had any unusual or allergic reaction to cholestyramine. Also tell your doctor and pharmacist if you are allergic to any other substances, such as foods, preservatives, or dyes.

Pregnancy—Cholestyramine is not absorbed into the body and is not likely to cause problems. However, it may reduce absorption of vitamins into the body. Ask your doctor whether you need to take extra vitamins.

Breast-feeding—Cholestyramine is not absorbed into the body and is not likely to cause problems. However, the reduced absorption of vitamins by the mother may affect the nursing infant.

Children—There is no specific information comparing use of cholestyramine in children with use in other age groups. However, use is not recommended in children under 2 years of age since cholesterol is needed for normal development.

Older adults—Side effects may be more likely to occur in patients over 60 years of age, who are usually more sensitive to the effects of cholestyramine.

Other medicines—Although certain medicines should not be used together at all, in other cases two different medicines may be used together even if an interaction might occur. In these cases, your doctor may want to change the dose, or other precautions may be necessary. When you are taking cholestyramine it is especially important that your doctor and pharmacist know if you are taking any of the following:

- Anticoagulants (blood thinners)—The effects of the anticoagulant may be altered
- Digitalis glycosides (heart medicine) or
- Diuretics (water pills) or
- Penicillin G, taken by mouth or
- Phenylbutazone or
- Propranolol (e.g., Inderal) or
- Tetracyclines, taken by mouth (medicine for infection) or
- Thyroid hormones or
- Vancomycin, taken by mouth—Cholestyramine may prevent these medicines from working properly

Other medical problems—The presence of other medical problems may affect the use of cholestyramine. Make sure you tell your doctor if you have any other medical problems, especially:

- Bleeding problems or
- Constipation or
- Gallstones or
- Heart or blood vessel disease or
- Hemorrhoids or
- Stomach ulcer or other stomach problems or
- Underactive thyroid—Cholestyramine may make these conditions worse
- Kidney disease—There is an increased risk of the developing electrolyte problems
- Phenylketonuria—The sugar-free brand of cholestyramine powder contains aspartame, which can cause problems in people with this condition. It is best if you avoid using this product. Phenylalanine in aspartame, is included in sugar-free preparations, and should be avoided

Before you begin using any new medicine (prescription or nonprescription) or if you develop any new medical problem while you are using this medicine, check with your doctor, nurse, or pharmacist.

Proper Use of This Medicine

Take this medicine exactly as directed by your doctor. Try not to miss any doses and do not take more medicine than your doctor ordered.

For patients taking *the powder form* of this medicine:

- *This medicine should never be taken in its dry form, since it could cause you to choke.* Instead, always mix as follows:

  —Place the medicine in 2 ounces of any beverage and mix thoroughly. Then add an additional 2 to 4 ounces of beverage and again mix thoroughly (it will not dissolve) before drinking. After drinking all the liquid containing the medicine, rinse the glass with a little more liquid and drink that also, to make sure you get all the medicine.

  —You may also mix this medicine with milk in hot or regular breakfast cereals, or in thin soups such as tomato or chicken noodle soup. Or you may add it to some pulpy fruits such as crushed pineapple, pears, peaches, or fruit cocktail.

For patients taking *the chewable bar form* of this medicine:

- Chew each bite well before swallowing.

For patients taking this medicine *for high cholesterol*:

- Importance of diet—Before prescribing medicine for your condition, your doctor will probably try to control your condition by prescribing a personal diet for you. Such a diet may be low in fats, sugars, and/or cholesterol. Many people are able to control their condition by carefully following their doctor's orders for proper diet and exercise. Medicine is prescribed only when additional help is needed. *Follow carefully the special diet your doctor gave you,* since the medicine is effective only when a schedule of diet and exercise is properly followed.

- Also, this medicine is less effective if you are greatly overweight. It may be very important for you to go on a reducing diet. However, check with your doctor before going on any diet.
- Remember that this medicine will not cure your cholesterol problem but it will help control it. Therefore, you must continue to take it as directed if you expect to lower your cholesterol level.

Missed dose—If you miss a dose of this medicine, take it as soon as possible. Then go back to your regular dosing schedule. However, if it is almost time for your next dose, skip the missed dose and go back to your regular dosing schedule. Do not double doses.

Storage—To store this medicine:

- Keep out of the reach of children.
- Store away from heat and direct light.
- Do not store in the bathroom, near the kitchen sink, or in other damp places. Heat or moisture may cause the medicine to break down.
- Do not keep outdated medicine or medicine no longer needed. Be sure that any discarded medicine is out of the reach of children.

Precautions While Using This Medicine

It is very important that your doctor check your progress at regular visits. This will allow your doctor to see if the medicine is working properly and to decide if you should continue to take it.

Do not take any other medicine unless prescribed by your doctor since cholestyramine may change the effect of other medicines.

Do not stop taking this medicine without first checking with your doctor. When you stop taking this medicine, your blood cholesterol levels may increase again. Your doctor may want you to follow a special diet to help prevent this from happening.

Side Effects of This Medicine

In some animal studies, cholestyramine was found to cause tumors. It is not known whether cholestyramine causes tumors in humans.

Along with its needed effects, a medicine may cause some unwanted effects. Although not all of these side effects may occur, if they do occur they may need medical attention.

Check with your doctor immediately if either of the following side effects occurs:

Rare

Black, tarry stools; stomach pain (severe) with nausea and vomiting

Check with your doctor as soon as possible if either of the following side effects occurs:

More common

Constipation

Rare

Loss of weight (sudden)

Other side effects may occur that usually do not need medical attention. These side effects may go away during treatment as your body adjusts to the medicine. However, check with your doctor if any of the following side effects continue or are bothersome:

More common

Heartburn or indigestion; nausea or vomiting; stomach pain

Less common

Belching; bloating; diarrhea; dizziness; headache

Other side effects not listed above may also occur in some patients. If you notice any other effects, check with your doctor.

Additional Information

Once a medicine has been approved for marketing for a certain use, experience may show that it is also useful for other medical problems. Although these uses are not included in product labeling, cholestyramine is used in certain patients with the following medical conditions:

- Digitalis glycoside overdose
- Excess oxalate in the urine

Other than the above information, there is no additional information relating to proper use, precautions, or side effects for these uses.

Annual revision: 08/08/91

CHORIONIC GONADOTROPIN Systemic

Some commonly used brand names are:

In the U.S.

A.P.L. Profasi
Pregnyl

Generic name product may also be available.

In Canada

A.P.L. Profasi HP

Generic name product may also be available.

Another commonly used name is human chorionic gonadotropin (hCG).

Description

Chorionic gonadotropin (kor-ee-ON-ik goe-NAD-oh-troe-pin) is a drug whose actions are almost the same as those of luteinizing (loo-te-in-eye-ZING) hormone (LH), which is produced by the pituitary gland. It is a hormone also normally produced by the placenta in pregnancy. Chorionic gonadotropin has different uses for females and males.

In females, chorionic gonadotropin is used to help conception occur. It is usually given in combination with other drugs such as menotropins and urofollitropin. Many women being treated with these drugs usually have already tried clomiphene alone (e.g., Serophene) and have not been able to conceive yet. Chorionic gonadotropin is also used in *in vitro* fertilization (IVF) programs.

In males, LH and chorionic gonadotropin stimulate the testes to produce male hormones such as testosterone. Testosterone causes the enlargement of the penis and testes and the growth of pubic and underarm hair. It also increases the production of sperm.

Although chorionic gonadotropin has been prescribed to help some patients lose weight, it should *never* be used this way. When used improperly, chorionic gonadotropin can cause serious problems.

Chorionic gonadotropin is to be administered only by or under the immediate supervision of your doctor. It is available in the following dosage form:

Parenteral

- Injection (U.S. and Canada)

It is very important that you read and understand the following information. If any of it causes you special concern, check with your doctor. Also, *if you have any questions* or if you want more information about this medicine or your medical problem, *ask your doctor, nurse, or pharmacist.*

Before Using This Medicine

In deciding to use a medicine, the risks of taking the medicine must be weighed against the good it will do. This is a decision you and your doctor will make. For chorionic gonadotropin, the following should be considered:

Allergies—Tell your doctor if you have ever had any unusual or allergic reaction to chorionic gonadotropin. Also tell your doctor and pharmacist if you are allergic to any other substances, such as foods, preservatives, or dyes.

Pregnancy—If you become pregnant as a result of using this medicine with menotropins (e.g., Pergonal) or urofollitropin (e.g., Metrodin), there is an increased chance of a multiple pregnancy (for example, twins, triplets).

Children—Chorionic gonadotropin, when used for treating cryptorchidism (a birth defect where the testes remain inside the body), has caused the sexual organs of some male children to develop too rapidly.

Other medicines—Although certain medicines should not be used together at all, in other cases two different medicines may be used together even if an interaction might occur. In these cases, your doctor may want to change the dose, or other precautions may be necessary. Tell your doctor and pharmacist if you are taking any prescription or nonprescription (over-the-counter [OTC]) medicine.

Other medical problems—The presence of other medical problems may affect the use of chorionic gonadotropin. Make sure you tell your doctor if you have any other medical problems, especially:

- Cancer of the prostate—Increases in the amount of testosterone in the bloodstream may make this condition worse
- Cyst on ovary or
- Fibroid tumors of the uterus—Chorionic gonadotropin can cause further growth of cysts on the ovary or fibroid tumors of the uterus
- Pituitary gland enlargement or tumor—Chorionic gonadotropin can cause the pituitary gland or a pituitary tumor to increase in size
- Unusual vaginal bleeding—Irregular vaginal bleeding is a sign that the endometrium is growing too much, of endometrial cancer, or of other hormone imbalances; the increases in estrogen production caused by ovulation can aggravate these problems of the endometrium. If other hormone imbalances are present, they should be treated before beginning ovulation induction

Before you begin using any new medicine (prescription or nonprescription) or if you develop any new medical problem while you are using this medicine, check with your doctor, nurse, or pharmacist.

Precautions While Using This Medicine

It is very important that your doctor check your progress at regular visits to make sure that the medicine is working and to check for unwanted effects.

For women *taking this medicine to become pregnant:*

- Record your basal body temperature every day if told to do so by your doctor, so that you will know if you have begun to ovulate. It is important that intercourse take place around the time of ovulation to give you the best chance of becoming pregnant. Your doctor will likely want to monitor the development of the ovarian follicle(s) by measuring the amount of estrogen in your bloodstream and by checking the size of the follicle(s) with ultrasound examinations.

Side Effects of This Medicine

Along with its needed effects, a medicine may cause some other effects. Although not all of these side effects may occur, if they do occur they may need medical attention.

Check with your doctor as soon as possible if any of the following side effects occur:

For females only

More common

Bloating (mild); stomach or pelvic pain

Less common or rare

Abdominal or stomach pain (severe); bloating (moderate to severe); decreased amount of urine; feeling of indigestion; nausea, vomiting, or diarrhea (continuing or severe); pelvic pain (severe); shortness of breath; swelling of feet or lower legs; weight gain (rapid)

For boys only

Less common

Acne; enlargement of penis and testes; growth of pubic hair; increase in height (rapid)

Other side effects may occur that usually do not need medical attention. These side effects may go away during treatment as your body adjusts to the medicine. However, check with your doctor if any of the following side effects continue or are bothersome:

Less common

Enlargement of breasts; headache; irritability; mental depression; pain at place of injection; tiredness

After you stop receiving this medicine, it may continue to cause some side effects which require medical attention. During this period of time check with your doctor if you notice either of the following side effects:

For females only

Less common or rare

Abdominal or stomach pain (severe); bloating (moderate to severe); decreased amount of urine; feeling of indigestion; nausea, vomiting, or diarrhea (continuing or severe); pelvic pain (severe); shortness of breath; weight gain (rapid)

Other side effects not listed above may also occur in some patients. If you notice any other effects, check with your doctor.

Annual revision: 07/26/92

CHROMIC PHOSPHATE P 32 Therapeutic

A commonly used brand name in the U.S. is Phosphocol P 32.

Description

Chromic phosphate (KROME-ik FOS-fate) P 32 is a radiopharmaceutical (ray-dee-oh-far-ma-SOO-ti-kal). Radiopharmaceuticals are agents used to diagnose certain medical problems or treat certain diseases.

Chromic phosphate P 32 is used to treat cancer or related problems. It is put by catheter into the pleura (sac that contains the lungs) or into the peritoneum (sac that contains the liver, stomach, and intestines) to treat the leaking of fluid inside these areas that is caused by cancer. It may also be given by injection to treat cancer in certain organs such as the ovaries and prostate.

Chromic phosphate P 32 is to be given only by or under the direct supervision of a doctor with specialized training in nuclear medicine. It is available in the following dosage form:

Parenteral

- Suspension (U.S.)

It is very important that you read and understand the following information. If any of it causes you special concern, check with your doctor. Also, *if you have any questions* or if you want more information about this medicine or your medical problem, *ask your doctor, nuclear medicine physician and/or technologist, nuclear pharmacist, or nurse.*

Before Using This Medicine

In deciding to use a medicine, the risks of taking the medicine must be weighed against the good it will do. This is a decision you and your doctor will make. For

chromic phosphate P 32, the following should be considered:

Pregnancy—Radiopharmaceuticals are usually not recommended for use during pregnancy to avoid exposing the fetus to radiation. However, some treatment using radiopharmaceuticals may be required even during pregnancy. Be sure you have discussed this with your doctor.

Breast-feeding—Chromic phosphate P 32 passes into the breast milk. If you must receive this radiopharmaceutical, it may be necessary for you to stop breast-feeding during treatment. Be sure you have discussed this with your doctor.

Children—There is no specific information comparing use of chromic phosphate P 32 in children with use in other age groups.

Older adults—Many medicines have not been studied specifically in older people. Therefore, it may not be known whether they work exactly the same way they do in younger adults. Although there is no specific information comparing use of chromic phosphate P 32 in the elderly with use in other age groups, this medicine is not expected to cause different side effects or problems in older people than it does in younger adults.

Before you begin using any new medicine (prescription or nonprescription) or if you develop any new medical problem while you are using this medicine, check with your doctor, nuclear medicine physician and/or technologist, nuclear pharmacist, or nurse.

Preparation for This Treatment

Your doctor may have special instructions for you in preparation for your treatment. If you have not received such instructions or if you do not understand them, check with your doctor in advance.

Side Effects of This Medicine

Along with its needed effects, a medicine may cause some unwanted effects. Although not all of these side effects may occur, if they do occur they may need medical attention.

Check with your doctor or nurse immediately if any of the following side effects occur:

Less common or rare

Abdominal or stomach pain (severe); chest pain; chills and/or fever; dry cough; nausea and vomiting (severe); sore throat and fever; troubled breathing; unusual bleeding or bruising; unusual tiredness or weakness

Other side effects may occur that usually do not need medical attention. These side effects may go away during treatment as your body adjusts to the medicine. However, check with your doctor if any of the following side effects continue or are bothersome:

More common

Abdominal or stomach cramps; diarrhea; feeling of discomfort; loss of appetite; nausea and vomiting; weakness

Other side effects not listed above may also occur in some patients. If you notice any other effects, check with your doctor.

Annual revision: 05/18/92

CHROMIUM SUPPLEMENTS Systemic

This information applies to the following medicines:

Chromic Chloride (KROME-ik KLOR-ide)
Chromium (KROH-mee-um)

For Chromic Chloride

In the U.S.

Generic name product is available.

In Canada

Generic name product is available.

For Chromium

In the U.S.

Generic name product is available.

In Canada

Generic name product is available.

Description

Chromium supplements are used to prevent or treat chromium deficiency.

The body needs chromium for normal growth and health. For patients who are unable to get enough chromium in their regular diet or who have a need for more chromium, chromium supplements may be necessary. They are generally taken by mouth but some patients may have to receive them by injection.

Lack of chromium may lead to nerve problems and may decrease the body's ability to use sugar properly.

There is not enough evidence to show that chromium supplements may improve the way your body uses sugar (glucose tolerance).

Some chromium preparations are available only with your doctor's prescription. Others are available without a prescription; however, your doctor may have special instructions on the proper use and dose for your condition.

Chromium supplements are available in the following dosage forms:

Oral

Chromium
- Tablets (U.S. and Canada)

Parenteral

Chromic Chloride
- Injection (U.S. and Canada)

It is very important that you read and understand the following information. If any of it causes you special concern, check with your doctor or pharmacist. Also, *if you have any questions* or if you want more information about this dietary supplement or your medical problem, *ask your doctor, nurse, pharmacist, or dietitian.*

Importance of Diet

Many nutritionists recommend that, if possible, people should get all the chromium they need from foods. However, some people do not get enough chromium from their diet. For example, people on weight-loss diets may consume too little food to provide enough chromium. Others may need more chromium than normal. For such people, a chromium supplement is important.

In order to get enough vitamins and minerals in your regular diet, it is important that you eat a balanced and varied diet. Follow carefully any diet program your doctor may recommend. For your specific vitamin and/or mineral needs, ask your doctor or dietitian for a list of appropriate foods.

Chromium is found in various foods, including brewer's yeast, calf liver, American cheese, and wheat germ.

Experts have developed a list of recommended dietary allowances (RDA) for most vitamins and some minerals. The RDA are not an exact number but a general idea of how much you need. They do not cover amounts needed for problems caused by serious lack of vitamins and minerals.

Because a lack of chromium is rare, there are no RDA for it. The following intakes are thought to be plenty for most individuals:

Infants and children—
- Birth to 6 months of age: 10–40 micrograms (mcg) per day.
- 6 months to 1 year of age: 20–60 mcg per day.
- 1 to 3 years of age: 20–80 mcg per day.
- 4 to 6 years of age: 30–120 mcg per day.
- 7 to 10 years of age: 50–200 mcg per day.

Adolescents and adults—50–200 mcg per day.

Before Using This Dietary Supplement

If you are taking this dietary supplement without a prescription, carefully read and follow any precautions on the label. For chromium, the following should be considered:

Allergies—Tell your doctor if you have ever had any unusual or allergic reaction to chromium. Also tell your doctor and pharmacist if you are allergic to any other substances, such as foods, preservatives, or dyes.

Pregnancy—It is especially important that you are receiving enough vitamins and minerals when you become pregnant and that you continue to receive the right amount of vitamins and minerals throughout your pregnancy. The healthy growth and development of the fetus depend on a steady supply of nutrients from the mother. However, taking large amounts of a dietary supplement during pregnancy may be harmful to the mother and/or fetus and should be avoided.

Breast-feeding—It is important that you receive the right amounts of vitamins and minerals so that your baby will also get the vitamins and minerals needed to grow properly. However, taking large amounts of a dietary supplement while breast-feeding may be harmful to the mother and/or baby and should be avoided.

Children—It is especially important that children receive enough chromium in their diet for healthy growth and development. Although there is no specific information about the use of chromium in children in doses higher than normal daily requirements, it is not expected to cause different side effects or problems in children than it does in adults.

Older adults—It is important that older people continue to receive enough vitamins in their diet for good health. This medicine has been tested and has not been shown to cause different side effects or problems in older people than it does in younger adults.

Medicines or other dietary supplements—Although certain medicines or dietary supplements should not be used together at all, in other cases they may be used together even if an interaction might occur. In these cases, your doctor may want to change the dose, or other precautions may be necessary. Tell your doctor and pharmacist if you are using any other dietary supplement or any prescription or over-the-counter (OTC) medication.

Other medical problems—The presence of other medical problems may affect the use of chromium. Make sure you tell your doctor if you have any other medical problems, especially:

- Diabetes mellitus (sugar diabetes)—Taking chromium supplements when you have a chromium deficiency may cause a change in the amount of insulin you need

Proper Use of This Dietary Supplement

Some people believe that taking very large doses of a vitamin or mineral (called megadoses) is useful for treating certain medical problems. Studies have not proven this. Large doses should be taken only under the direction of your doctor after need has been identified.

Missed dose—If you miss taking chromium supplements for one or more days there is no cause for concern, since it takes some time for your body to become seriously low in chromium. However, if your doctor has recommended that you take chromium, try to remember to take it as directed every day.

Storage—To store this dietary supplement:

- Keep out of the reach of children.
- Store away from heat and direct light.
- Do not store in the bathroom, near the kitchen sink, or in other damp places. Heat or moisture may cause the dietary supplement to break down.
- Keep the dietary supplement from freezing. Do not refrigerate.
- Do not keep outdated dietary supplements or those no longer needed. Be sure that any discarded dietary supplement is out of the reach of children.

Side Effects of This Dietary Supplement

No side effects have been reported for chromium. However, check with your doctor if you notice any unusual effects while you are taking it.

Annual revision: 03/24/92

CHYMOPAPAIN Parenteral-Local

A commonly used brand name in the U.S. and Canada is Chymodiactin.

Description

Chymopapain (kye-moe-PAP-ane) is injected directly into a herniated ("slipped") disk in the spine to dissolve part of the disk and relieve the pain and other problems caused by the disk pressing on a nerve. Before you receive chymopapain, you will be given an anesthetic (either a general anesthetic to put you to sleep or a local anesthetic).

Very rarely, use of chymopapain may cause serious side effects, including paralysis of the legs or death. Another dangerous side effect of chymopapain injection is a severe allergic reaction called anaphylaxis. This side effect occurs in less than 1% of the patients receiving the medicine, but it occurs more often in women than in men. Before receiving chymopapain, you should discuss its use, and the possibility of anaphylaxis or other serious side effects, with your doctor.

Chymopapain injections are given only in a hospital, usually in an operating room, by your surgeon. This medicine is available in the following dosage form:

Parenteral

- Injection (U.S. and Canada)

It is very important that you read and understand the following information. If any of it causes you special concern, check with your doctor. Also, *if you have any questions* or if you want more information about this medicine or your medical problem, *ask your doctor, nurse, or pharmacist.*

Before Receiving This Medicine

In deciding to use a medicine, the risks of receiving the medicine must be weighed against the good it will do. This is a decision you and your doctor will make. For chymopapain, the following should be considered:

Allergies—Tell your doctor if you have ever had any unusual or allergic reaction to chymopapain, papaya, meat tenderizer, contact lens cleaning solutions, beer, or iodine. Also tell your doctor if you are allergic to any other substances, such as foods, preservatives, or dyes.

Pregnancy—Studies on birth defects or other problems relating to pregnancy have not been done in either humans or animals.

Breast-feeding—Chymopapain has not been reported to cause problems in nursing babies.

Children—Studies on this medicine have been done only in adult patients, and there is no specific information comparing use of chymopapain in children with use in other age groups.

Older adults—Many medicines have not been studied specifically in older people. Therefore, it may not be known whether they work exactly the same way they do in younger adults or if they cause different side effects or problems in older people. There is no specific information comparing use of chymopapain in the elderly with use in other age groups.

Other medicines—Although certain medicines should not be used together at all, in other cases two different medicines may be used together even if an interaction might occur. In these cases, your doctor may want to change the dose, or other precautions may be necessary. Before you receive chymopapain, it is important that your doctor know if you are taking any other prescription or nonprescription (over-the-counter [OTC]) medicine.

Other medical problems—The presence of other medical problems may affect the use of chymopapain. Make sure you tell your doctor if you have ever received an injection of chymopapain, if you have had back surgery, or if you have any other medical problems, especially:

- Allergies or
- Stroke or bleeding in the brain (or if any member of your family has ever had these problems) or
- High blood pressure (hypertension)—The chance of side effects may be increased

Side Effects of This Medicine

Along with its needed effects, a medicine may cause some unwanted effects. Very rarely, use of chymopapain has caused serious side effects, including paralysis of the legs or death. Also, this medicine may cause dangerous allergic reactions, especially in women.

Although not all of the following side effects may occur, if they do occur they may need medical attention. Tell your doctor or nurse if any of the following side effects occur:

Rare

Abdominal or stomach cramps or pain; constipation (severe); decreased or uncontrolled urination; fast or irregular breathing; headache (sudden, severe, and continuing); pain, tenderness, changes of skin color, hot skin, or swelling of leg or foot; runny nose; shortness of breath, troubled breathing, tightness in chest, or wheezing; skin rash, redness, hives, or itching; swelling of abdomen or stomach; uncontrolled bowel movements; vomiting; weakness in legs (severe) or problems with moving legs

Other side effects may occur that usually do not need medical attention. Pain and muscle spasms in the lower back may last for several days after you have received this medicine. Stiffness or soreness in the back may last for several months. Other side effects may go away after a short time. However, check with your doctor if any of the following side effects continue or are bothersome:

More common

Back pain, stiffness, or soreness; muscle spasms in lower back

Less common or rare

Cramps, pain, or mild weakness in legs; dizziness; feeling of burning in lower back; headache; nausea; numbness or tingling in legs or toes

Some side effects may not appear until several days or weeks after you have received chymopapain. Check with your doctor as soon as possible if any of the following side effects occur within one month after you have received this medicine:

Back pain or muscle weakness (sudden and severe); skin rash, hives, or itching

Other side effects not listed above may also occur in some patients. If you notice any other effects, check with your doctor.

Annual revision: 08/28/91

CICLOPIROX Topical

A commonly used brand name in the U.S. and Canada is Loprox.

Description

Ciclopirox (sye-kloe-PEER-ox) is used to treat infections caused by a fungus. It works by killing the fungus or preventing its growth.

Ciclopirox is applied to the skin to treat:

- ringworm of the body (tinea corporis);
- ringworm of the foot (tinea pedis; athlete's foot);
- ringworm of the groin (tinea cruris; jock itch);
- "sun fungus" (tinea versicolor; pityriasis versicolor); and
- certain other fungus infections, such as Candida (Monilia) infections.

Ciclopirox is available only with your doctor's prescription, in the following dosage forms:

Topical

- Cream (U.S. and Canada)
- Lotion (U.S. and Canada)

It is very important that you read and understand the following information. If any of it causes you special concern, check with your doctor. Also, *if you have any questions* or if you want more information about this medicine or your medical problem, *ask your doctor, nurse, or pharmacist.*

Before Using This Medicine

In deciding to use a medicine, the risks of taking the medicine must be weighed against the good it will do.

This is a decision you and your doctor will make. For ciclopirox, the following should be considered:

Allergies—Tell your doctor if you have ever had any unusual or allergic reaction to ciclopirox. Also tell your doctor and pharmacist if you are allergic to any other substances, such as preservatives or dyes.

Pregnancy—Ciclopirox has not been studied in pregnant women. However, this medication has not been shown to cause birth defects or other problems in animal studies.

Breast-feeding—It is not known whether ciclopirox passes into the breast milk. However, this medicine has not been reported to cause problems in nursing babies.

Children—Studies on this medicine have been done only in adult patients, and there is no specific information comparing use of ciclopirox in children under the age of 10 with use in other age groups.

Older adults—Many medicines have not been studied specifically in older people. Therefore, it may not be known whether they work exactly the same way they do in younger adults. Although there is no specific information comparing use of ciclopirox in the elderly with use in other age groups, this medicine is not expected to cause different side effects or problems in older people than it does in younger adults.

Other medicines—Although certain medicines should not be used together at all, in other cases two different medicines may be used together even if an interaction might occur. In these cases, your doctor may want to change the dose, or other precautions may be necessary. Tell your doctor and pharmacist if you are using any other topical prescription or nonprescription (over-the-counter [OTC]) medicine that is to be applied to the same area of the skin.

Before you begin using any new medicine (prescription or nonprescription) or if you develop any new medical problem while you are using this medicine, check with your doctor, nurse, or pharmacist.

Proper Use of This Medicine

Apply enough ciclopirox to cover the affected and surrounding skin areas and rub in gently.

Keep this medicine away from the eyes.

When ciclopirox is used to treat certain types of fungus infections of the skin, an occlusive dressing (airtight covering, such as kitchen plastic wrap) should *not* be applied over the medicine. To do so may irritate the skin. *Do not apply an airtight covering over this medicine unless you have been directed to do so by your doctor.*

To help clear up your infection completely, *it is very important that you keep using ciclopirox for the full time of treatment,* even if your symptoms begin to clear up after a few days. Since fungus infections may be very slow to clear up, you may have to continue using this medicine every day for several weeks or more. If you stop using this medicine too soon, your symptoms may return. *Do not miss any doses.*

Missed dose—If you do miss a dose of this medicine, apply it as soon as possible. However, if it is almost time for your next dose, skip the missed dose and go back to your regular dosing schedule.

Storage—To store this medicine:
- Keep out of the reach of children.
- Store away from heat and direct light.
- Keep the medicine from freezing.
- Do not keep outdated medicine or medicine no longer needed. Be sure that any discarded medicine is out of the reach of children.

Precautions While Using This Medicine

If your skin problem does not improve within 2 to 4 weeks, or if it becomes worse, check with your doctor.

To help clear up your infection completely and to help make sure it does not return, good health habits are also required. The following measures will help reduce chafing and irritation and will also help keep the area cool and dry.

- *For patients using ciclopirox for ringworm of the groin:*
  - —Avoid wearing underwear that is tight-fitting or made from synthetic materials (for example, rayon or nylon). Instead, wear loose-fitting, cotton underwear.
  - —Use a bland, absorbent powder (for example, talcum powder) or an antifungal powder (for example, tolnaftate) on the skin. It is best to use the powder between the times you use ciclopirox.
- *For patients using ciclopirox for ringworm of the foot:*
  - —Carefully dry the feet, especially between the toes, after bathing.
  - —Avoid wearing socks made from wool or synthetic materials (for example, rayon or nylon). Instead, wear clean, cotton socks and change them daily or more often if the feet sweat freely.
  - —Wear sandals or well-ventilated shoes (for example, shoes with holes).
  - —Use a bland, absorbent powder (for example, talcum powder) or an antifungal powder (for example, tolnaftate) between the toes, on the feet, and in socks and shoes freely once or twice a day. It is best to use the powder between the times you use ciclopirox.

If you have any questions about these measures, check with your doctor, nurse, or pharmacist.

Side Effects of This Medicine

Along with its needed effects, a medicine may cause some unwanted effects. Although not all of these side effects may occur, if they do occur they may need medical attention.

Check with your doctor as soon as possible if any of the following side effects occur:

Rare

Burning, itching, redness, swelling, blistering, oozing, or other sign of irritation not present before use of this medicine

Other side effects not listed above may also occur in some patients. If you notice any other effects, check with your doctor.

Annual revision: 11/21/91

CINOXACIN Systemic†

A commonly used brand name in the U.S. is Cinobac.

†Not commercially available in Canada.

Description

Cinoxacin (sin-OX-a-sin) is used to prevent and treat infections of the urinary tract. It will not work for other infections or for colds, flu, or other virus infections.

Cinoxacin is available only with your doctor's prescription, in the following dosage form:

Oral

- Capsules (U.S.)

It is very important that you read and understand the following information. If any of it causes you special concern, check with your doctor. Also, *if you have any questions* or if you want more information about this medicine or your medical problem, *ask your doctor, nurse, or pharmacist.*

Before Using This Medicine

In deciding to use a medicine, the risks of taking the medicine must be weighed against the good it will do. This is a decision you and your doctor will make. For cinoxacin, the following should be considered:

Allergies—Tell your doctor if you have ever had any unusual or allergic reaction to cinoxacin or to any related medicines such as ciprofloxacin (e.g., Cipro), enoxacin (e.g. Penetrex), lomefloxacin (e.g. Maxaquin), nalidixic acid (e.g., NegGram), norfloxacin (e.g., Noroxin), or ofloxacin (e.g., Floxin). Also tell your doctor and pharmacist if you are allergic to any other substances, such as foods, preservatives, or dyes.

Pregnancy—Studies have not been done in humans. However, use is not recommended during pregnancy since cinoxacin has been shown to cause bone development problems in young animals.

Breast-feeding—It is not known whether cinoxacin passes into the breast milk. However, other related medicines do pass into the breast milk. Since cinoxacin has been shown to cause bone development problems in young animals, use is not recommended in nursing mothers.

Children—Since this medicine has been shown to cause bone development problems in young animals, its use is not recommended in children.

Older adults—Many medicines have not been studied specifically in older people. Therefore, it may not be known whether they work exactly the same way they do in younger adults. Although there is no specific information comparing use of cinoxacin in the elderly with use in other age groups, this medicine is not expected to cause different side effects or problems in older people than it does in younger adults.

Other medical problems—The presence of other medical problems may affect the use of cinoxacin. Make sure you tell your doctor if you have any other medical problems, especially:

- Kidney disease—Patients with kidney disease may have an increased risk of side effects

Before you begin using any new medicine (prescription or nonprescription) or if you develop any new medical problem while you are using this medicine, check with your doctor, nurse, or pharmacist.

Proper Use of This Medicine

Cinoxacin may be taken with food, unless you are otherwise directed by your doctor.

Do not give this medicine to infants or children under 12 years of age, unless otherwise directed by your doctor.

It has been shown to cause bone development problems in young animals.

To help clear up your infection completely, *keep taking this medicine for the full time of treatment,* even if you begin to feel better after a few days. If you stop taking this medicine too soon, your symptoms may return.

This medicine works best when there is a constant amount in the urine. *To help keep the amount constant, do not miss any doses. Also, it is best to take the doses at evenly spaced times, day and night.* For example, if you are to take 4 doses a day, the doses should be spaced about 6 hours apart. If this interferes with your sleep or other daily activities, or if you need help in planning the best times to take your medicine, check with your doctor, nurse, or pharmacist.

Dosing—The dose of cinoxacin will be different for different patients. *Follow your doctor's orders or the directions on the label.* The following information includes only the average doses of cinoxacin. Your dose may be different if you have kidney disease. *If your dose is different, do not change it* unless your doctor tells you to do so.

- The number of capsules that you take depends on the strength of the medicine. Also, *the number of doses you take each day, the time allowed between doses, and the length of time you take the medicine depend on the medical problem for which you are taking cinoxacin.*
- For the *prevention* of urinary tract infections:
  —Adults: 250 milligrams (mg) at bedtime for up to five months.
  —Children up to 18 years of age: Use is generally not recommended because it may cause bone development problems.
- For the *treatment* of urinary tract infections:
  —Adults: 250 milligrams (mg) every six hours; or 500 mg every twelve hours for seven to fourteen days.
  —Children up to 18 years of age: Use is generally not recommended because it may cause bone development problems.

Missed dose—If you do miss a dose of this medicine, take it as soon as possible. This will help to keep a constant amount of medicine in the urine. However, if it is almost time for your next dose, skip the missed dose and go back to your regular dosing schedule. Do not double doses.

Storage—To store this medicine:

- Keep out of the reach of children.
- Store away from heat and direct light.
- Do not store in the bathroom, near the kitchen sink, or in other damp places. Heat or moisture may cause the medicine to break down.
- Do not keep outdated medicine or medicine no longer needed. Be sure that any discarded medicine is out of the reach of children.

Precautions While Using This Medicine

If your symptoms do not improve within a few days, or if they become worse, check with your doctor.

This medicine may also cause some people to become dizzy. *Make sure you know how you react to this medicine before you drive, use machines, or do anything else that could be dangerous if you are dizzy.* If this reaction is especially bothersome, check with your doctor.

Side Effects of This Medicine

Along with its needed effects, a medicine may cause some unwanted effects. Although not all of these side effects may occur, if they do occur they may need medical attention.

Check with your doctor as soon as possible if any of the following side effects occur:

More common

Skin rash, itching, redness, or swelling

Less common

Dizziness; headache

Other side effects may occur that usually do not need medical attention. These side effects may go away during treatment as your body adjusts to the medicine. However, check with your doctor if any of the following side effects continue or are bothersome:

Less common

Diarrhea; loss of appetite; nausea; stomach cramps; vomiting

Other side effects not listed above may also occur in some patients. If you notice any other effects, check with your doctor.

Annual revision: 04/15/93

CISPLATIN Systemic

Some commonly used brand names are:

In the U.S.
Platinol
Platinol-AQ

In Canada
Platinol
Platinol-AQ

Generic name product may also be available.

Description

Cisplatin (sis-PLA-tin) belongs to the group of medicines known as alkylating agents. It is used to treat some kinds of cancer.

Cisplatin interferes with the growth of cancer cells, which are eventually destroyed. Since the growth of normal body cells may also be affected by cisplatin, other effects will also occur. Some of these may be serious and must be reported to your doctor. Other effects may not be serious but may cause concern. Some effects may not occur for months or years after the medicine is used.

Before you begin treatment with cisplatin, you and your doctor should talk about the good this medicine will do as well as the risks of using it.

Cisplatin is to be administered only by or under the immediate supervision of your doctor. It is available in the following dosage form:

Parenteral
- Injection (U.S. and Canada)

It is very important that you read and understand the following information. If any of it causes you special concern, check with your doctor. Also, *if you have any questions* or if you want more information about this medicine or your medical problem, *ask your doctor, nurse, or pharmacist.*

Before Using This Medicine

In deciding to use a medicine, the risks of taking the medicine must be weighed against the good it will do. This is a decision you and your doctor will make. For cisplatin, the following should be considered:

Allergies—Tell your doctor if you have ever had any unusual or allergic reaction to cisplatin.

Pregnancy—There is a chance that this medicine may cause birth defects if either the male or female is taking it at the time of conception or if it is taken during pregnancy. Cisplatin causes toxic or harmful effects in the fetus in humans and birth defects in mice. In addition, many cancer medicines may cause sterility which could be permanent. Although sterility has not been reported with this medicine, the possibility should be kept in mind.

Be sure that you have discussed this with your doctor before receiving this medicine. It is best to use some kind of birth control while you are receiving cisplatin. Tell your doctor right away if you think you have become pregnant while receiving cisplatin.

Breast-feeding—Because cisplatin may cause serious side effects, breast-feeding is generally not recommended while you are receiving it.

Children—Hearing problems and loss of balance are more likely to occur in children, who are usually more sensitive to the effects of cisplatin.

Older adults—Many medicines have not been studied specifically in older people. Therefore, it may not be known whether they work exactly the same way they do in younger adults or if they cause different side effects or problems in older people. There is no specific information comparing use of cisplatin in the elderly with use in other age groups.

Other medicines—Although certain medicines should not be used together at all, in other cases two different medicines may be used together even if an interaction might occur. In these cases, your doctor may want to change the dose, or other precautions may be necessary. When receiving cisplatin it is especially important that your doctor and pharmacist know if you are taking any of the following:

- Amphotericin B by injection (e.g., Fungizone) or
- Antithyroid agents (medicine for overactive thyroid) or
- Azathioprine (e.g., Imuran) or
- Chloramphenicol (e.g., Chloromycetin) or
- Colchicine or
- Flucytosine (e.g., Ancobon) or
- Ganciclovir (e.g., Cytovene) or
- Interferon (e.g., Introl A, Roferon-A) or
- Plicamycin (e.g., Mithracin) or
- Zidovudine (e.g., AZT, Retrovir) or
- If you have ever been treated with x-rays or cancer medicines—Cisplatin may increase the effects of these medicines or radiation therapy on the blood
- Anti-infectives by mouth or by injection (medicine for infection) or
- Chloroquine (e.g., Aralen) or
- Combination pain medicine containing acetaminophen and aspirin (e.g., Excedrin) or other salicylates (with large amounts taken regularly) or
- Cyclosporine (e.g., Sandimmune) or
- Deferoxamine (e.g., Desferal) (with long-term use) or
- Gold salts or
- Hydroxychloroquine (e.g., Plaquenil) or
- Inflammation or pain medicine, except narcotics, or
- Lithium (e.g., Lithane) or
- Penicillamine (e.g., Cuprimine) or
- Plicamycin (e.g., Mithracin) or
- Quinine (e.g., Quinamm) or
- Tiopronin (e.g., Thiola)—Risk of ear and kidney problems caused by cisplatin is increased

- Probenecid (e.g., Benemid) or
- Sulfinpyrazone (e.g., Anturane)—Cisplatin may raise the amount of uric acid in the blood. Since these medicines are used to lower uric acid levels, they may not work as well in patients receiving cisplatin

Other medical problems—The presence of other medical problems may affect the use of cisplatin. Make sure you tell your doctor if you have any other medical problems, especially:

- Chickenpox (including recent exposure) or
- Herpes zoster (shingles)—Risk of severe disease affecting other parts of the body
- Gout (history of) or
- Kidney stones (history of)—Cisplatin may increase levels of uric acid in the body, which can cause gout or kidney stones
- Hearing problems—May be worsened by cisplatin
- Infection—Cisplatin decreases your body's ability to fight infection
- Kidney disease—Effects may be increased because of slower removal of cisplatin from the body

Before you begin using any new medicine (prescription or nonprescription) or if you develop any new medical problem while you are using this medicine, check with your doctor, nurse, or pharmacist.

Proper Use of This Medicine

This medicine is sometimes given together with certain other medicines. If you are using a combination of medicines, it is important that you receive each one at the proper time. If you are taking some of these medicines by mouth, ask your doctor, nurse, or pharmacist to help you plan a way to take them at the right times.

While you are receiving this medicine, your doctor may want you to drink extra fluids so that you will pass more urine. This will help prevent kidney problems and keep your kidneys working well.

This medicine usually causes nausea and vomiting that may be severe. However, it is very important that you continue to receive the medicine, even if you begin to feel ill. Ask your doctor, nurse, or pharmacist for ways to lessen these effects, especially if they are severe.

Precautions While Using This Medicine

It is very important that your doctor check your progress at regular visits to make sure that this medicine is working properly and to check for unwanted effects.

While you are being treated with cisplatin, and after you stop treatment with it, *do not have any immunizations (vaccinations) without your doctor's approval.* Cisplatin may lower your body's resistance and there is a chance you might get the infection the immunization is meant to prevent. In addition, other persons living in your household should not take oral polio vaccine since there is a chance they could pass the polio virus on to you. Also, avoid persons who have recently taken oral polio vaccine. Do not get close to them, and do not stay in the same room with them for very long. If you cannot take these precautions, you should consider wearing a protective face mask that covers the nose and mouth.

Cisplatin can temporarily lower the number of white blood cells in your blood, increasing the chance of getting an infection. It can also lower the number of platelets, which are necessary for proper blood clotting. If this occurs, there are certain precautions you can take, especially when your blood count is low, to reduce the risk of infection or bleeding:

- If you can, avoid people with infections. *Check with your doctor immediately* if you think you are getting an infection or if you get a fever or chills, cough or hoarseness, lower back or side pain, or painful or difficult urination.
- *Check with your doctor immediately* if you notice any unusual bleeding or bruising; black, tarry stools; blood in urine or stools; or pinpoint red spots on your skin.
- Be careful when using a regular toothbrush, dental floss, or toothpick. Your medical doctor, dentist, or nurse may recommend other ways to clean your teeth and gums. Check with your medical doctor before having any dental work done.
- Do not touch your eyes or the inside of your nose unless you have just washed your hands and have not touched anything else in the meantime.
- Be careful not to cut yourself when you are using sharp objects such as a safety razor or fingernail or toenail cutters.
- Avoid contact sports or other situations where bruising or injury could occur.

If cisplatin accidentally seeps out of the vein into which it is injected, it may damage some tissues and cause scarring. *Tell the doctor or nurse right away if you notice redness, pain, or swelling at the place of injection.*

Side Effects of This Medicine

Along with their needed effects, medicines like cisplatin can sometimes cause unwanted effects such as blood problems, ear and kidney problems, and other side effects. These and others are described below. Also, because of the way these medicines act on the body, there is a chance that they might cause other unwanted effects that may not occur until months or years after the medicine is used. These delayed effects may include certain types of cancer, such as leukemia. Discuss these possible effects with your doctor.

Although not all of these side effects may occur, if they do occur they may need medical attention.

Check with your doctor or nurse immediately if any of the following side effects occur:

Less common

Black, tarry stools; blood in urine or stools; cough or hoarseness; fever or chills; lower back or side pain; painful or difficult urination; pain or redness at place of injection; pinpoint red spots on skin; unusual bleeding or bruising

Rare

Dizziness or faintness (shortly after a dose); fast heartbeat (shortly after a dose); swelling of face (shortly after a dose); wheezing (shortly after a dose)

Check with your doctor as soon as possible if any of the following side effects occur:

More common

Joint pain; loss of balance; lower back or side pain; ringing in ears; swelling of feet or lower legs; trouble in hearing; unusual tiredness or weakness

Less common

Convulsions (seizures); loss of reflexes; loss of taste; numbness or tingling in fingers or toes; trouble in walking

Rare

Agitation or confusion; blurred vision; change in ability to see colors (especially blue or yellow); sores in mouth and on lips

Other side effects may occur that usually do not need medical attention. These side effects may go away during treatment as your body adjusts to the medicine. Also, your doctor or nurse may be able to tell you about ways to prevent or reduce some of these side effects. Check with your doctor or nurse if any of the following side effects continue or are bothersome or if you have any questions about them:

More common

Nausea and vomiting (severe)

Less common

Loss of appetite

After you stop receiving cisplatin, it may still produce some side effects that need attention. During this period of time check with your doctor if you notice any of the following side effects:

Black, tarry stools; blood in urine or stools; cough or hoarseness; decrease in urination; fever or chills; loss of balance; lower back or side pain; painful or difficult urination; pinpoint red spots on skin; ringing in ears; swelling of feet or lower legs; trouble in hearing; unusual bleeding or bruising

Other side effects not listed above may also occur in some patients. If you notice any other effects, check with your doctor.

Annual revision: 06/03/93

CITRATES Systemic

This information applies to the following medicines:

Potassium Citrate (poe-TASS-ee-um SIH-trayt)
Potassium Citrate and Citric Acid (SIH-trik A-sid)
Potassium Citrate and Sodium (SOE-dee-um) Citrate
Sodium Citrate and Citric Acid
Tricitrates (Try-SIH-trayts)

Some commonly used brand names are:

For Potassium Citrate

In the U.S.

Urocit-K

For Potassium Citrate and Citric Acid

In the U.S.

Polycitra-K
Polycitra-K Crystals

For Potassium Citrate and Sodium Citrate

In the U.S.

Citrolith

For Sodium Citrate and Citric Acid

In the U.S.

Bicitra
Oracit

In Canada

Oracit

Other commonly used names for sodium citrate and citric acid are Albright's solution and modified Shohl's solution.

For Tricitrates

In the U.S.

Polycitra-LC
Polycitra Syrup

Description

Citrates (SIH-trayts) are used to make the urine more alkaline (less acid). This helps prevent certain kinds of kidney stones. Citrates are sometimes used with other medicines to help treat kidney stones that may occur with gout. They are also used to make the blood more alkaline in certain conditions.

Citrates are available only with your doctor's prescription, in the following dosage forms:

Oral

Potassium Citrate

- Tablets (U.S.)

Potassium Citrate and Citric Acid
- Oral solution (U.S.)
- Crystals for oral solution (U.S.)

Potassium Citrate and Sodium Citrate
- Tablets (U.S.)

Sodium Citrate and Citric Acid
- Oral solution (U.S. and Canada)

Tricitrates
- Oral solution (U.S.)

It is very important that you read and understand the following information. If any of it causes you special concern, check with your doctor. Also, *if you have any questions* or if you want more information about this medicine or your medical problem, *ask your doctor, nurse, or pharmacist.*

Before Using This Medicine

In deciding to use a medicine, the risks of taking the medicine must be weighed against the good it will do. This is a decision you and your doctor will make. For citrates, the following should be considered:

Allergies—Tell your doctor if you have ever had any unusual or allergic reaction to potassium citrate or potassium. Also tell your doctor and pharmacist if you are allergic to any other substances, such as foods, preservatives, or dyes.

Pregnancy—Studies on effects in pregnancy have not been done in either humans or animals.

Breast-feeding—Although it is not known whether citrates pass into the breast milk, this medicine has not been reported to cause problems in nursing babies.

Children—Although there is no specific information comparing use of citrates in children with use in other age groups, these medicines are not expected to cause different side effects or problems in children than they do in adults.

Older adults—Many medicines have not been studied specifically in older people. Therefore, it may not be known whether they work exactly the same way they do in younger adults or if they cause different side effects or problems in older people. There is no specific information comparing use of citrates in the elderly with use in other age groups.

Other medicines—Although certain medicines should not be used together at all, in other cases two different medicines may be used together even if an interaction might occur. In these cases, your doctor may want to change the dose, or other precautions may be necessary. When you are taking citrates, it is especially important that your doctor and pharmacist know if you are taking any of the following:

- Amiloride (e.g., Midamor) or
- Benazepril (e.g., Lotensin) or
- Captopril (e.g., Capoten) or
- Digitalis glycosides (heart medicine) or
- Enalapril (e.g., Vasotec) or
- Fosinopril (e.g., Monotril) or
- Heparin (e.g., Panheprin) or
- Lisinopril (e.g., Prinivil; Zestril) or
- Medicines for inflammation or pain (except narcotics) or
- Potassium-containing medicines (other) or
- Quinapril (e.g., Accuprol) or
- Ramipril (e.g., Altase) or
- Salt substitutes, low-salt foods or milk or
- Spironolactone (e.g., Aldactone) or
- Triamterene (e.g., Dyrenium)—Use with potassium-containing citrates may further increase potassium blood levels, possibly leading to serious side effects
- Antacids, especially those containing aluminum or sodium bicarbonate—Use with citrates may increase the risk of kidney stones; also, citrates may increase the amount of aluminum in the blood and cause serious side effects, especially in patients with kidney problems
- Methenamine (e.g., Mandelamine)—Use with citrates may make the methenamine less effective
- Quinidine (e.g., Quinidex)—Use with citrates may cause quinidine to build up in the bloodstream, possibly leading to serious side effects

Other medical problems—The presence of other medical problems may affect the use of citrates. Make sure you tell your doctor if you have any other medical problems, especially:

- Addison's disease (underactive adrenal glands) or
- Diabetes mellitus (sugar diabetes) or
- Kidney disease—The potassium in potassium-containing citrates may worsen or cause heart problems in patients with these conditions
- Diarrhea (chronic)—Treatment with citrates may not be effective; a change in dose of citrate may be needed
- Edema (swelling of the feet or lower legs) or
- High blood pressure or
- Toxemia of pregnancy—The sodium in sodium-containing citrates may cause the body to retain (keep) water
- Heart disease—The sodium in sodium-containing citrates may cause the body to retain (keep) water; the potassium in potassium-containing citrates may make heart disease worse
- Intestinal or esophageal blockage—Potassium citrate tablets may cause irritation of the stomach or intestines
- Stomach ulcer or other stomach problems—Potassium citrate–containing products make make these conditions worse
- Urinary tract infection—Citrates may make conditions worse

Before you begin using any new medicine (prescription or nonprescription) or if you develop any new medical problem while you are using this medicine, check with your doctor, nurse, or pharmacist.

Proper Use of This Medicine

For patients taking the *tablet form of this medicine:*

- Swallow the tablets whole. Do not crush, chew, or suck the tablet.

- Take with a full glass (8 ounces) of water.
- *If you have trouble swallowing the tablets or they seem to stick in your throat, check with your doctor at once.* If this medicine is not completely swallowed and not properly dissolved, it can cause severe irritation.

For patients taking the *liquid form of this medicine:*

- Dilute with a full glass (6 ounces) of water or juice and drink; follow with additional water, if desired.
- Chill, but do *not* freeze, this medicine before taking it, for a better taste.

For patients taking the *crystals form of this medicine:*

- Add the contents of one packet to at least 6 ounces of cool water or juice.
- Stir well to make sure the crystals are completely dissolved.
- Drink all the mixture to be sure you are taking the correct dose. Follow with additional water or juice, if desired.

Take each dose immediately after a meal or within 30 minutes after a meal or bedtime snack. This helps prevent the medicine from causing stomach pain or a laxative effect.

Drink at least a full glass (8 ounces) of water or other liquid (except milk) every hour during the day (about 3 quarts a day), unless otherwise directed by your doctor. This will increase the flow of urine and help prevent kidney stones.

Take this medicine only as directed by your doctor. Do not take more of it, do not take it more often, and do not take it for a longer time than your doctor ordered. *This is especially important if you are also taking a diuretic (water pill) or digitalis medicine for your heart.*

Dosing—The dose of citrates will be different for different patients. *Follow your doctor's orders or the directions on the label.*

Missed dose—If you miss a dose of this medicine, take it as soon as possible if remembered within 2 hours. However, if it is almost time for your next dose, skip the missed dose and go back to your regular dosing schedule. Do not double doses.

Storage—To store this medicine:

- Keep out of the reach of children.
- Store away from heat and direct light.
- Do not store in the bathroom, near the kitchen sink, or in other damp places. Heat or moisture may cause the medicine to break down.
- Keep the liquid form of this medicine from freezing.
- Do not keep outdated medicine or medicine no longer needed. Be sure that any discarded medicine is out of the reach of children.

Precautions While Using This Medicine

It is important that your doctor check your progress at regular visits. This is to make sure the medicine is working properly and to check for unwanted effects.

Do not eat salty foods or use extra table salt on your food while you are taking citrates. This will help prevent kidney stones and unwanted effects.

Check with your doctor before starting any strenuous physical exercise, especially if you are out of condition and are taking any other medication. Exercise and certain medications may increase the amount of potassium in the blood.

For patients taking *potassium citrate–containing medicines:*

- Do not use salt substitutes and low-salt milk unless told to do so by your doctor. They may contain potassium.
- *Check with your doctor at once if you are taking the tablet form and notice black, tarry stools or other signs of stomach or intestinal bleeding.*
- Do not be alarmed if you notice what appears to be a whole tablet in the stool after taking potassium citrate tablets. Your body has received the proper amount of medicine from the tablet and has expelled the tablet shell. However, it is a good idea to check with your doctor also.
- If you are on a potassium-rich or potassium-restricted diet, check with your doctor, nurse, or pharmacist. Potassium citrate–containing medicines contain a large amount of potassium.

For patients taking *sodium citrate–containing medicines:*

- If you are on a sodium-restricted diet, check with your doctor, nurse, or pharmacist. Sodium citrate–containing medicines contain a large amount of sodium.

Side Effects of This Medicine

Along with its needed effects, a medicine may cause some unwanted effects. Although not all of these side effects may occur, if they do occur they may need medical attention.

Stop taking this medicine and check with your doctor immediately if any of the following side effects occur:

Rare

Abdominal or stomach pain or cramping (severe); black, tarry stools; vomiting (severe), sometimes with blood

Also, check with your doctor as soon as possible if any of the following side effects occur:

Confusion; convulsions (seizures); dizziness; high blood pressure; irregular or fast heartbeat; irritability; mood or mental changes; muscle pain or twitching; nervousness or restlessness; numbness or tingling in hands, feet, or lips; shortness of breath, difficult breathing, or slow breathing; swelling of feet or lower legs; unexplained anxiety; unpleasant taste; unusual tiredness or weakness; weakness or heaviness of legs

Other side effects may occur that usually do not need medical attention. These side effects may go away during treatment as your body adjusts to the medicine. However, check with your doctor if any of the following side effects continue or are bothersome:

Less common

Abdominal or stomach soreness or pain (mild); diarrhea or loose bowel movements; nausea or vomiting

Other side effects not listed above may also occur in some patients. If you notice any other effects, check with your doctor.

Annual revision: 01/18/93

CLARITHROMYCIN Systemic†

A commonly used brand name in the U.S. is Biaxin.

†Not commercially available in Canada.

Description

Clarithromycin (kla-RITH-roe-mye-sin) is used to treat bacterial infections in many different parts of the body. It works by killing bacteria or preventing their growth. However, this medicine will not work for colds, flu, or other virus infections. Clarithromycin may be used for other problems as determined by your doctor.

Clarithromycin is available only with your doctor's prescription, in the following dosage form:

Oral

- Tablets (U.S.)

It is very important that you read and understand the following information. If any of it causes you special concern, check with your doctor. Also, *if you have any questions* or if you want more information about this medicine or your medical problem, *ask your doctor, nurse, or pharmacist.*

Before Using This Medicine

In deciding to use a medicine, the risks of taking the medicine must be weighed against the good it will do. This is a decision you and your doctor will make. For clarithromycin, the following should be considered:

Allergies—Tell your doctor if you have ever had any unusual or allergic reaction to clarithromycin or to any related medicines such as erythromycin. Also tell your doctor and pharmacist if you are allergic to any other substances, such as foods, preservatives, or dyes.

Pregnancy—Clarithromycin has not been studied in pregnant women. However, studies in animals have shown that clarithromycin causes birth defects and other problems. Before taking this medicine, make sure your doctor knows if you are pregnant or if you may become pregnant.

Breast-feeding—Clarithromycin passes into breast milk.

Children—Studies on this medicine have not been done in children up to 12 years of age. In effective doses, the medicine has not been shown to cause different side effects or problems in children over the age of 12 than it does in adults.

Older adults—This medicine has been tested in a limited number of elderly patients and has not been shown to cause different side effects or problems in older people than it does in younger adults.

Other medicines—Although certain medicines should not be used together at all, in other cases two different medicines may be used together even if an interaction might occur. In these cases, your doctor may want to change the dose, or other precautions may be necessary. When you are taking clarithromycin, it is especially important that your doctor and pharmacist know if you are taking any of the following:

- Theophylline (e.g., Theodur, Slo-Bid)—Clarithromycin may increase the chance of side effects of theophylline
- Zidovudine (e.g., Retrovir)—Clarithromycin may decrease the amount of zidovudine in the blood

Other medical problems—The presence of other medical problems may affect the use of clarithromycin. Make sure you tell your doctor if you have any other medical problems, especially:

- Kidney disease—Patients with severe kidney disease may have an increased chance of side effects

Before you begin using any new medicine (prescription or nonprescription) or if you develop any new medical problem while you are using this medicine, check with your doctor, nurse, or pharmacist.

Proper Use of This Medicine

Clarithromycin may be taken with meals or on an empty stomach.

To help clear up your infection completely, *keep taking clarithromycin for the full time of treatment,* even if you begin to feel better after a few days. If you stop taking this medicine too soon, your symptoms may return.

Dosing—The dose of clarithromycin will be different for different patients. *Follow your doctor's orders or the directions on the label.* The following information includes only the average doses of clarithromycin. Your dose may be different if you have kidney disease. *If your dose is different, do not change it* unless your doctor tells you to do so:

- Adults and children 12 years of age and older: 250 mg to 500 mg every twelve hours.
- Children up to 12 years of age: To be determined by doctor.

Missed dose—If you miss a dose of this medicine, take it as soon as possible. However, if it is almost time for your next dose, skip the missed dose and go back to your regular dosing schedule. Do not double doses.

Storage—To store this medicine:

- Keep out of the reach of children.
- Store away from heat and direct light.
- Do not store in the bathroom, near the kitchen sink, or in other damp places. Heat or moisture may cause the medicine to break down.
- Do not keep outdated medicine or medicine no longer needed. Be sure that any discarded medicine is out of the reach of children.

Precautions While Using This Medicine

If your symptoms do not improve within a few days, or if they become worse, check with your doctor.

Side Effects of This Medicine

Side effects may occur that usually do not need medical attention. These side effects may go away during treatment as your body adjusts to the medicine. However, check with your doctor if any of the following side effects continue or are bothersome:

Less common

Abnormal taste; diarrhea; headache; nausea; stomach pain or discomfort

Other side effects not listed above may also occur in some patients. If you notice any other effects, check with your doctor.

Additional Information

Once a medicine has been approved for marketing for a certain use, experience may show that it is also useful for other medical problems. Although these uses are not specifically included in product labeling, clarithromycin is used in certain patients with the following medical conditions:

- Legionnaires' disease
- *Mycobacterium avium* complex (MAC)

Other than the above information, there is no additional information relating to proper use, precautions, or side effects for these uses.

Annual revision: 06/16/92

CLINDAMYCIN Systemic

Some commonly used brand names are:

In the U.S.

Cleocin

Cleocin Pediatric

Generic name product may also be available.

In Canada

Dalacin C

Dalacin C Palmitate

Dalacin C Phosphate

Description

Clindamycin is used to treat bacterial infections. It will not work for colds, flu, or other virus infections.

Clindamycin is available only with your doctor's prescription, in the following dosage forms:

Oral

- Capsules (U.S. and Canada)
- Oral solution (U.S. and Canada)

Parenteral

- Injection (U.S. and Canada)

It is very important that you read and understand the following information. If any of it causes you special concern, check with your doctor. Also, *if you have any questions* or if you want more information about this medicine or your medical problem, *ask your doctor, nurse, or pharmacist.*

Before Using This Medicine

In deciding to use a medicine, the risks of taking the medicine must be weighed against the good it will do. This is a decision you and your doctor will make. For clindamycin, the following should be considered:

Allergies—Tell your doctor if you have ever had any unusual or allergic reaction to clindamycin, lincomycin, or doxorubicin. Also tell your doctor and pharmacist if you are allergic to any other substances, such as foods, preservatives, or dyes.

Pregnancy—Clindamycin has not been reported to cause birth defects or other problems in humans.

Breast-feeding—Clindamycin passes into the breast milk. However, clindamycin has not been reported to cause problems in nursing babies.

Children—This medicine has been tested in children and, in effective doses, has not been reported to cause different side effects or problems than it does in adults.

Older adults—Many medicines have not been studied specifically in older people. Therefore, it may not be known whether they work exactly the same way they do in younger adults or if they cause different side effects or problems in older people. There is no specific information comparing use of clindamycin in the elderly with use in other age groups.

Other medicines—Although certain medicines should not be used together at all, in other cases two different medicines may be used together even if an interaction might occur. In these cases, your doctor may want to change the dose, or other precautions may be necessary. When you are taking clindamycin, it is especially important that your doctor and pharmacist know if you are taking any of the following:

- Chloramphenicol (e.g., Chloromycetin) or
- Diarrhea medicine containing kaolin or attapulgite or
- Erythromycins (medicine for infection)—Taking these medicines along with clindamycin may decrease the effects of clindamycin

Other medical problems—The presence of other medical problems may affect the use of clindamycin. Make sure you tell your doctor if you have any other medical problems, especially:

- Kidney disease (severe) or
- Liver disease (severe)—Severe kidney or liver disease may increase blood levels of this medicine, increasing the chance of side effects
- Stomach or intestinal disease, history of (especially colitis, including colitis caused by antibiotics, or enteritis)—Patients with a history of stomach or intestinal disease may have an increased chance of side effects

Before you begin using any new medicine (prescription or nonprescription) or if you develop any new medical problem while you are using this medicine, check with your doctor, nurse, or pharmacist.

Proper Use of This Medicine

For patients taking the *capsule form* of clindamycin:

- *The capsule form of clindamycin should be taken with a full glass (8 ounces) of water or with meals* to prevent irritation of the esophagus (tube between the throat and stomach).

For patients taking the *oral liquid form* of clindamycin:

- Use a specially marked measuring spoon or other device to measure each dose accurately. The average household teaspoon may not hold the right amount of liquid.
- Do not use after the expiration date on the label. The medicine may not work properly after this date. Check with your pharmacist if you have any questions about this.

To help clear up your infection completely, *keep taking this medicine for the full time of treatment,* even if you begin to feel better after a few days. *If you have a "strep" infection, you should keep taking this medicine for at least 10 days. This is especially important in "strep" infections. Serious heart problems could develop later* if your infection is not cleared up completely. Also, if you stop taking this medicine too soon, your symptoms may return.

This medicine works best when there is a constant amount in the blood. *To help keep the amount constant, do not miss any doses. Also, it is best to take each dose at evenly spaced times day and night.* For example, if you are to take 4 doses a day, doses should be spaced about 6 hours apart. If this interferes with your sleep or other daily activities, or if you need help in planning the best times to take your medicine, check with your doctor, nurse, or pharmacist.

Missed dose—If you do miss a dose of this medicine, take it as soon as possible. This will help to keep a constant amount of medicine in the blood. However, if it is almost time for your next dose, skip the missed dose and go back to your regular dosing schedule. Do not double doses.

Storage—To store this medicine:

- Keep out of the reach of children.
- Store away from heat and direct light.
- Do not store the capsule form of this medicine in the bathroom, near the kitchen sink, or in other damp places. Heat or moisture may cause the medicine to break down.
- Do not refrigerate the oral liquid form of clindamycin. If chilled, the liquid may thicken and be difficult to pour. Follow the directions on the label.

- Do not keep outdated medicine or medicine no longer needed. Be sure that any discarded medicine is out of the reach of children.

Precautions While Using This Medicine

It is important that your doctor check your progress at regular visits.

If your symptoms do not improve within a few days, or if they become worse, check with your doctor.

In some patients, clindamycin may cause diarrhea.

- Severe diarrhea may be a sign of a serious side effect. *Do not take any diarrhea medicine without first checking with your doctor.* Diarrhea medicines, such as loperamide (Imodium A-D) or diphenoxylate and atropine (Lomotil), may make your diarrhea worse or make it last longer.
- For mild diarrhea, diarrhea medicine containing attapulgite (e.g., Kaopectate tablets, Diasorb) may be taken. However, attapulgite may keep clindamycin from being absorbed into the body. Therefore, these diarrhea medicines should be taken at least 2 hours before or 3 to 4 hours after you take clindamycin by mouth. Other kinds of diarrhea medicine should not be taken. They may make your diarrhea worse or make it last longer.
- If you have any questions about this or if mild diarrhea continues or gets worse, check with your doctor or pharmacist.

Before having surgery (including dental surgery) with a general anesthetic, tell the medical doctor or dentist in charge that you are taking clindamycin.

Side Effects of This Medicine

Along with its needed effects, a medicine may cause some unwanted effects. Although not all of these side effects may occur, if they do occur they may need medical attention.

Check with your doctor immediately if any of the following side effects occur:

More common

Abdominal or stomach cramps and pain (severe); abdominal tenderness; diarrhea (watery and severe), which may also be bloody; fever
(the above side effects may also occur up to several weeks after you stop taking this medicine)

Less common

Sore throat and fever; skin rash, redness, and itching; unusual bleeding or bruising

Other side effects may occur that usually do not need medical attention. These side effects may go away during treatment as your body adjusts to the medicine. However, check with your doctor if any of the following side effects continue or are bothersome:

More common

Diarrhea (mild); nausea and vomiting; stomach pain

Less common

Itching of rectal, or genital (sex organ) areas

Other side effects not listed above may also occur in some patients. If you notice any other effects, check with your doctor.

Annual revision: 08/12/92

CLINDAMYCIN Topical

Some commonly used brand names are:

In the U.S.

Cleocin T Gel
Cleocin T Lotion
Cleocin T Topical Solution

In Canada

Dalacin T Topical Solution

Description

Clindamycin (klin-da-MYE-sin) belongs to the family of medicines called antibiotics. Topical clindamycin is used to help control acne. It may be used alone or with one or more other medicines that are used on the skin or taken by mouth for acne. Topical clindamycin may also be used for other problems as determined by your doctor.

Clindamycin is available only with your doctor's prescription, in the following dosage forms:

Topical

- Gel (U.S.)
- Solution (U.S. and Canada)
- Suspension (U.S.)

It is very important that you read and understand the following information. If any of it causes you special concern, check with your doctor. Also, ***if you have any questions*** or if you want more information about this medicine or your medical problem, ***ask your doctor, nurse, or pharmacist.***

Before Using This Medicine

In deciding to use a medicine, the risks of using the medicine must be weighed against the good it will do. This is a decision you and your doctor will make. For clindamycin, the following should be considered:

Allergies—Tell your doctor if you have ever had any unusual or allergic reaction to this medicine or any of the other clindamycins (by mouth or by injection) or to lincomycin. Also tell your doctor and pharmacist if you are allergic to any other substances, such as preservatives or dyes.

Pregnancy—Clindamycin has not been studied in pregnant women. However, this medication has not been shown to cause birth defects or other problems in animal studies.

Breast-feeding—Small amounts of clindamycin are absorbed through the skin. However, this medicine has not been reported to cause problems in nursing babies.

Children—Studies on this medicine have been done only in adult patients, and there is no specific information comparing use of this medicine in children up to 12 years of age with use in other age groups.

Older adults—Many medicines have not been studied specifically in older people. Therefore, it may not be known whether they work exactly the same way they do in younger adults. Although there is no specific information comparing use of this medicine in the elderly with use in other age groups, this medicine is not expected to cause different side effects or problems in older people than it does in younger adults.

Other medicines—Although certain medicines should not be used together at all, in other cases two different medicines may be used together even if an interaction might occur. In these cases, your doctor may want to change the dose, or other precautions may be necessary. Tell your doctor and pharmacist if you are using any other prescription or nonprescription (over-the-counter [OTC]) medicine.

Other medical problems—The presence of other medical problems may affect the use of clindamycin. Make sure you tell your doctor if you have any other medical problems, especially:

- History of stomach or intestinal disease (especially colitis, including colitis caused by antibiotics, or enteritis)—These conditions may increase the chance of side effects that affect the stomach and intestines

Before you begin using any new medicine (prescription or nonprescription) or if you develop any new medical problem while you are using this medicine, check with your doctor, nurse, or pharmacist.

Proper Use of This Medicine

Before applying this medicine, thoroughly wash the affected areas with warm water and soap, rinse well, and pat dry.

When applying the medicine, use enough to cover the affected area lightly. *You should apply the medicine to the whole area usually affected by acne, not just to the pimples themselves.* This will help keep new pimples from breaking out.

You should avoid washing the acne-affected areas too often. This may dry your skin and make your acne worse. Washing with a mild, bland soap 2 or 3 times a day should be enough, unless you have oily skin. If you have any questions about this, check with your doctor.

Clindamycin will not cure your acne. However, to help keep your acne under control, *keep using this medicine for the full time of treatment,* even if your symptoms begin to clear up after a few days. You may have to continue using this medicine every day for months or even longer in some cases. If you stop using this medicine too soon, your symptoms may return. *It is important that you do not miss any doses.*

Missed dose—If you do miss a dose of this medicine, apply it as soon as possible. However, if it is almost time for your next dose, skip the missed dose and go back to your regular dosing schedule.

For patients using the *topical solution form* of clindamycin:

- After washing or shaving, it is best to wait 30 minutes before applying this medicine. The alcohol in it may irritate freshly washed or shaved skin.
- This medicine contains alcohol and is flammable. *Do not use near heat, near open flame, or while smoking.*
- To apply this medicine:

  —This medicine comes in a bottle with an applicator tip, which may be used to apply the medicine directly to the skin. Use the applicator with a dabbing motion instead of a rolling motion (not like a roll-on deodorant, for example). Tilt the bottle and press the tip firmly against your skin. If needed, you can make the medicine flow faster from the applicator tip by slightly increasing the pressure against the skin. If the medicine flows too fast, use less pressure. If the applicator tip becomes dry, turn the bottle upside down and press the tip several times to moisten it.

  —Since this medicine contains alcohol, it will sting or burn. In addition, it has an unpleasant taste if it gets on the mouth or lips. Therefore, *do not get this medicine in the eyes, nose, or mouth, or on other mucous membranes.* Spread the medicine away from these areas when applying. If this medicine does get in the eyes, wash them out immediately, but carefully, with large amounts of cool tap water. If your eyes still burn or are painful, check with your doctor.

- It is important that you do not use this medicine more often than your doctor ordered. It may cause your skin to become too dry or irritated.

For patients using the *topical suspension form* of clindamycin:

- *Shake well* before applying.

Storage—To store this medicine:

- Keep out of the reach of children.
- Store away from heat and direct light.
- Keep the medicine from freezing.
- Do not keep outdated medicine or medicine no longer needed. Be sure that any discarded medicine is out of the reach of children.

Precautions While Using This Medicine

If your acne does not improve within about 6 weeks, or if it becomes worse, check with your doctor or pharmacist. However, treatment of acne may take up to 8 to 12 weeks before full improvement is seen.

If your doctor has ordered another medicine to be applied to the skin along with this medicine, it is best to apply them at different times (for example, morning and evening). This may help keep your skin from becoming too irritated. Also, if the medicines are used too close together, they may not work properly.

For patients using the *topical solution form* of clindamycin:

- This medicine may cause the skin to become unusually dry, even with normal use. If this occurs, check with your doctor.

In some patients, clindamycin may cause diarrhea.

- Severe diarrhea may be a sign of a serious side effect. *Do not take any diarrhea medicine without first checking with your doctor.* Diarrhea medicines may make your diarrhea worse or make it last longer.
- For mild diarrhea, only diarrhea medicine containing kaolin (e.g., Kaopectate liquid) or attapulgite (e.g., Kaopectate tablets, Diasorb) may be taken. Other kinds of diarrhea medicine (e.g., Imodium A.D. or Lomotil) should not be taken. They may make your condition worse or make it last longer.
- If you have any questions about this or if mild diarrhea continues or gets worse, check with your doctor or pharmacist.

You may continue to use cosmetics (make-up) while you are using this medicine for acne. However, it is best to use only "water-base" cosmetics. Also, it is best not to use cosmetics too heavily or too often. They may make your acne worse. If you have any questions about this, check with your doctor.

Side Effects of This Medicine

Along with its needed effects, a medicine may cause some unwanted effects. Although not all of these side effects may occur, if they do occur they may need medical attention.

Check with your doctor immediately if any of the following side effects occur:

Rare

Abdominal or stomach cramps, pain, and bloating (severe); diarrhea (watery and severe), which may also be bloody; fever; increased thirst; nausea or vomiting; unusual tiredness or weakness; weight loss (unusual)—these side effects may also occur up to several weeks after you stop using this medicine

Also, check with your doctor as soon as possible if any of the following side effects occur:

Less common

Skin rash, itching, redness, swelling, or other sign of irritation not present before use of this medicine

Other side effects may occur that usually do not need medical attention. These side effects may go away during treatment as your body adjusts to the medicine. However, check with your doctor if any of the following side effects continue or are bothersome:

More common

Dryness, scaliness, or peeling of skin (for the topical solution)

Less common

Abdominal pain; diarrhea (mild); irritation or oiliness of skin; stinging or burning feeling of skin

Other side effects not listed above may also occur in some patients. If you notice any other effects, check with your doctor.

Annual revision: 02/10/92

CLIOQUINOL Topical

A commonly used brand name in the U.S. and Canada is Vioform. Another commonly used name is iodochlorhydroxyquin.

Description

Clioquinol (klye-oh-KWIN-ole) belongs to the family of medicines called anti-infectives. Clioquinol topical preparations are used to treat skin infections.

Clioquinol is available without a prescription; however, your doctor may have special instructions on the proper use of this medicine for your medical problem. It is available in the following dosage forms:

Topical
- Cream (U.S. and Canada)
- Ointment (U.S. and Canada)

It is very important that you read and understand the following information. If any of it causes you special concern, check with your doctor or pharmacist. Also, *if you have any questions* or if you want more information about this medicine or your medical problem, *ask your doctor, nurse, or pharmacist.*

Before Using This Medicine

If you are using this medicine without a prescription, carefully read and follow any precautions on the label. For clioquinol, the following should be considered:

Allergies—Tell your doctor if you have ever had any unusual or allergic reaction to clioquinol, chloroxine (e.g., capitrol), iodine, or iodine-containing preparations. Also tell your doctor and pharmacist if you are allergic to any other substances, such as preservatives or dyes.

Pregnancy—Clioquinol topical preparations have not been shown to cause birth defects or other problems in humans.

Breast-feeding—Clioquinol topical preparations have not been reported to cause problems in nursing babies.

Children—Clioquinol is not recommended in children under 2 years of age. Although there is no specific information comparing use of this medicine in children 2 years of age and over with use in other age groups, this medicine is not expected to cause different side effects or problems in children than it does in adults.

Older adults—Many medicines have not been studied specifically in older people. Therefore, it may not be known whether they work exactly the same way they do in younger adults. Although there is no specific information comparing use of this medicine in the elderly with use in other age groups, this medicine is not expected to cause different side effects or problems in older people than it does in younger adults.

Other medicines—Although certain medicines should not be used together at all, in other cases two different medicines may be used together even if an interaction might occur. In these cases, your doctor may want to change the dose, or other precautions may be necessary. Tell your doctor and pharmacist if you are using any other prescription or nonprescription (over-the-counter [OTC]) medicine.

Before you begin using any new medicine (prescription or nonprescription) or if you develop any new medical problem while you are using this medicine, check with your doctor, nurse, or pharmacist.

Proper Use of This Medicine

Before applying this medicine, wash the affected area with soap and water, and dry thoroughly.

Do not use this medicine in or around the eyes.

To use the *cream form* of this medicine:
- Apply a thin layer of cream to the affected area and rub in gently until the cream disappears.

To use the *ointment form* of this medicine:
- Apply a thin layer of ointment to the affected area and rub in gently.

To help clear up your infection completely, *keep using this medicine for the full time of treatment,* even if your symptoms have disappeared. *Do not miss any doses.*

Missed dose—If you do miss a dose of this medicine, apply it as soon as possible. However, if it is almost time for your next dose, skip the missed dose and go back to your regular dosing schedule.

Storage—To store this medicine:
- Keep out of the reach of children.
- Store away from heat and direct light.
- Keep the medicine from freezing.
- Do not keep outdated medicine or medicine no longer needed. Be sure that any discarded medicine is out of the reach of children.

Precautions While Using This Medicine

If your skin problem does not improve within 1 to 2 weeks, or if it becomes worse, check with your doctor.

This medicine may stain clothing, skin, hair, and nails yellow. Avoid getting this medicine on your clothing since bleaching may not remove the stain.

Before you have any medical tests, tell the doctor in charge that you are using this medicine. The results of some tests may be affected by this medicine.

Side Effects of This Medicine

Along with its needed effects, a medicine may cause some unwanted effects. Although not all of these side effects may occur, if they do occur they may need medical attention.

Check with your doctor immediately if any of the following side effects occur:

Rare

Itching, skin rash, redness, swelling, or other sign of irritation not present before use of this medicine

Other side effects not listed above may also occur in some patients. If you notice any other effects, check with your doctor.

Annual revision: 02/10/92

CLIOQUINOL AND HYDROCORTISONE Topical

Some commonly used brand names are:

In the U.S.

- Vioform-Hydrocortisone Cream
- Vioform-Hydrocortisone Lotion
- Vioform-Hydrocortisone Mild Cream
- Vioform-Hydrocortisone Mild Ointment
- Vioform-Hydrocortisone Ointment

In Canada

- Vioform-Hydrocortisone Cream
- Vioform-Hydrocortisone Mild Cream
- Vioform-Hydrocortisone Ointment

Another commonly used name is iodochlorhyroxyquin and hydrocortisone.

Description

Clioquinol (klye-oh-KWIN-ole) and hydrocortisone (hye-droe-KOR-ti-sone) is a combined anti-infective and cortisone-like medicine. Clioquinol and hydrocortisone topical preparations are used to treat infections of the skin and to help provide relief from the redness, itching, and discomfort of many skin problems.

Clioquinol and hydrocortisone combination is available only with your doctor's prescription, in the following dosage forms:

Topical

- Cream (U.S. and Canada)
- Lotion (U.S.)
- Ointment (U.S. and Canada)

It is very important that you read and understand the following information. If any of it causes you special concern, check with your doctor. Also, *if you have any questions* or if you want more information about this medicine or your medical problem, *ask your doctor, nurse, or pharmacist.*

Before Using This Medicine

In deciding to use a medicine, the risks of taking the medicine must be weighed against the good it will do. This is a decision you and your doctor will make. For clioquinol and hydrocortisone combination, the following should be considered:

Allergies—Tell your doctor if you have ever had any unusual or allergic reaction to clioquinol, hydrocortisone, chloroxine (e.g., Capitrol), iodine, or iodine-containing preparations. Also tell your doctor and pharmacist if you are allergic to any other substances, such as preservatives or dyes.

Pregnancy—Clioquinol and hydrocortisone topical preparations may be absorbed through the mother's skin. This medicine has not been shown to cause birth defects or other problems in humans. However, studies in animals have shown that it causes birth defects. Use of large amounts on the skin or use for a long time is not recommended during pregnancy.

Breast-feeding—Clioquinol and hydrocortisone topical preparations have not been reported to cause problems in nursing babies.

Children—Clioquinol and hydrocortisone combination is not recommended in children up to 2 years of age. Although there is no specific information comparing use of clioquinol and hydrocortisone combination in children over 2 years of age with use in other age groups, this medicine is not expected to cause different side effects or problems in these children than it does in adults.

Older adults—Many medicines have not been studied specifically in older people. Therefore, it may not be known whether they work exactly the same way they do in younger adults. Although there is no specific information comparing use of clioquinol and hydrocortisone combination in the elderly with use in other age groups, this medicine is not expected to cause different side effects or problems in older people than it does in younger adults.

Other medicines—Although certain medicines should not be used together at all, in other cases two different medicines may be used together even if an interaction might

occur. In these cases, your doctor may want to change the dose, or other precautions may be necessary. Tell your doctor and pharmacist if you are using any other prescription or nonprescription (over-the-counter [OTC]) medicine.

Other medical problems—The presence of other medical problems may affect the use of clioquinol and hydrocortisone topical preparations. Make sure you tell your doctor if you have any other medical problems, especially:

- Skin infection (other)—Use of clioquinol and hydrocortisone topical preparations may make the condition worse

Before you begin using any new medicine (prescription or nonprescription) or if you develop any new medical problem while you are using this medicine, check with your doctor, nurse, or pharmacist.

Proper Use of This Medicine

Before applying this medicine, wash the affected area with soap and water, and dry thoroughly.

Do not use this medicine in or around the eyes or on infants and children up to 2 years of age.

To use the *cream form* of this medicine:

- Apply a thin layer of cream to the affected area and rub in gently until cream disappears.

To use the *lotion form* of this medicine:

- Gently squeeze bottle and apply a few drops of lotion to the affected area. Rub in gently until lotion disappears.

To use the *ointment form* of this medicine:

- Apply a thin layer of ointment to the affected area and rub in gently.

Do not bandage or otherwise wrap the area of the skin being treated unless directed to do so by your doctor.

Check with your doctor before using this medicine on any other skin problems. It should not be used on certain kinds of bacterial, virus, or fungus skin infections.

To help clear up your infection completely, *keep using this medicine for the full time of treatment*, even if your symptoms have disappeared. *Do not miss any doses.* However, *do not use this medicine more often or for a longer time than your doctor ordered.* To do so may increase the chance of absorption through the skin and the chance of side effects. In addition, too much use, especially on thin skin areas (for example, face, armpits, groin), may result in thinning of the skin and stretch marks.

Missed dose—If you do miss a dose of this medicine, apply it as soon as possible. However, if it is almost time for your next dose, skip the missed dose and go back to your regular dosing schedule.

Storage—To store this medicine:

- Keep out of the reach of children.
- Store away from heat and direct light.
- Keep the medicine from freezing.
- Do not keep outdated medicine or medicine no longer needed. Be sure that any discarded medicine is out of the reach of children.

Precautions While Using This Medicine

If your skin problem does not improve within 1 to 2 weeks, or if it becomes worse, check with your doctor.

This medicine may be absorbed through the skin, and too much use can affect growth. *Children who must use this medicine should be followed closely by their doctor.*

This medicine may stain clothing, skin, hair, and nails yellow. Avoid getting this medicine on your clothing. Bleaching may not remove the stain.

Side Effects of This Medicine

Along with its needed effects, a medicine may cause some unwanted effects. Although not all of these side effects may occur, if they do occur they may need medical attention.

Check with your doctor immediately if any of the following side effects occur:

Rare

Blistering, burning, itching, peeling, skin rash, redness, swelling, or other sign of irritation not present before use of this medicine

With prolonged use

Thinning of skin with easy bruising

Other side effects not listed above may also occur in some patients. If you notice any other effects, check with your doctor.

Annual revision: 02/10/92

CLOFAZIMINE Systemic†

A commonly used brand name in the U.S. is Lamprene.

†Not commercially available in Canada.

Description

Clofazimine (kloe-FA-zi-meen) is taken to treat leprosy (Hansen's disease). It is sometimes given with other medicines for leprosy. When this medicine is used to treat "flare-ups" of leprosy, it may be given with a cortisone-like medicine. Clofazimine may also be used for other problems as determined by your doctor.

This medicine is available only with your doctor's prescription, in the following dosage form:

Oral

- Capsules (U.S.)

It is very important that you read and understand the following information. If any of it causes you special concern, check with your doctor. Also, *if you have any questions* or if you want more information about this medicine or your medical problem, *ask your doctor, nurse, or pharmacist.*

Before Using This Medicine

In deciding to use a medicine, the risks of taking the medicine must be weighed against the good it will do. This is a decision you and your doctor will make. For clofazimine, the following should be considered:

Allergies—Tell your doctor if you have ever had any unusual or allergic reaction to clofazimine. Also tell your doctor and pharmacist if you are allergic to any other substances, such as foods, preservatives, or dyes.

Pregnancy—Clofazimine has not been studied in pregnant women. Although the skin of babies born to mothers who took clofazimine during pregnancy was deeply discolored, this medicine has not been shown to cause birth defects or other problems in humans. A gradual fading of the discoloration may occur over a period of about a year. Some animal studies have not shown that clofazimine causes birth defects. However, studies in mice have shown that clofazimine may cause slow bone formation of the skull and a decrease in successful pregnancies. Before you take clofazimine, make sure your doctor knows if you are pregnant or if you may become pregnant.

Breast-feeding—Clofazimine passes into the breast milk. Use is not recommended in nursing mothers.

Children—Studies on this medicine have been done only in adult patients, and there is no specific information comparing use of clofazimine in children with use in other age groups.

Older adults—Many medicines have not been studied specifically in older people. Therefore, it may not be known whether they work exactly the same way they do in younger adults or if they cause different side effects or problems in older people. There is no specific information comparing use of clofazimine in the elderly with use in other age groups.

Other medicines—Although certain medicines should not be used together at all, in other cases two different medicines may be used together even if an interaction might occur. In these cases, your doctor may want to change the dose, or other precautions may be necessary. Tell your doctor and pharmacist if you are taking any other prescription or nonprescription (over-the-counter [OTC]) medicine.

Other medical problems—The presence of other medical problems may affect the use of clofazimine. Make sure you tell your doctor if you have any other medical problems, especially:

- Liver disease—Clofazimine may on rare occasion cause hepatitis and liver disease
- Stomach or intestinal problems, history of—Clofazimine often causes some stomach upset, but on rare occasion may cause severe, sharp abdominal pain and burning, which may be a sign of a serious side effect

Before you begin using any new medicine (prescription or nonprescription) or if you develop any new medical problem while you are using this medicine, check with your doctor, nurse, or pharmacist.

Proper Use of This Medicine

Clofazimine should be taken with meals or milk.

To help clear up your leprosy completely, *it is very important that you keep taking clofazimine for the full time of treatment,* even if you begin to feel better after a few months. You may have to take it every day for as long as 2 years to life. If you stop taking this medicine too soon, your symptoms may return.

This medicine works best when there is a constant amount in the blood. *To help keep the amount constant, do not miss any doses. Also, it is best to take each dose at the same time every day.* If you need help in planning the best time to take your medicine, check with your doctor, nurse, or pharmacist.

Dosing—The dose of clofazimine will be different for different patients. *Follow your doctor's orders or the directions on the label.* The following information includes only the average doses of clofazimine. *If your dose is different, do not change it* unless your doctor tells you to do so.

- The number of capsules that you take depends on the strength of the medicine. Also, *the number of doses you take each day, the time allowed between doses, and the length of time you take the medicine depend on the medical problem for which you are taking clofazimine.*
- For the *treatment of leprosy (Hansen's disease)*:
  —Adults and teenagers: 50 to 100 milligrams once a day. This medicine must be taken with other medicines for the treatment of Hansen's disease.
  —Children: Dose must be determined by the doctor.

Missed dose—If you miss a dose of this medicine, take it as soon as possible. However, if it is almost time for your next dose, skip the missed dose and go back to your regular dosing schedule. Do not double doses.

Storage—To store this medicine:

- Keep out of the reach of children.
- Store away from heat and direct light.
- Do not store in the bathroom, near the kitchen sink, or in other damp places. Heat or moisture may cause the medicine to break down.
- Do not keep outdated medicine or medicine no longer needed. Be sure that any discarded medicine is out of the reach of children.

Precautions While Using This Medicine

If your symptoms do not improve within 1 to 3 months, or if they become worse, check with your doctor. It may take up to 6 months before the full benefit of this medicine is seen.

Clofazimine may cause pink or red to brownish-black discoloration of the skin within a few weeks after you start taking it. Because of the skin discoloration, some patients may become depressed. The discoloration will go away when you stop taking this medicine. However, it may take several months or years for the skin to clear up completely. *If skin discoloration causes you to feel very depressed or to have thoughts of suicide, check with your doctor immediately.*

This medicine may cause some people to become dizzy, drowsy, or less alert than they are normally. *Make sure you know how you react to this medicine before you drive, use machines, or do anything else that could be dangerous if you are dizzy or are not alert or able to see well.* If these reactions are especially bothersome, check with your doctor.

Clofazimine may cause your skin to become more sensitive to sunlight than it is normally. Exposure to sunlight, even for brief periods of time, may cause a skin rash, itching, redness, or other discoloration of the skin, or a severe sunburn. When you begin taking this medicine:

- Stay out of direct sunlight, especially between the hours of 10:00 a.m. and 3:00 p.m., if possible.
- Wear protective clothing, including a hat. Also, wear sunglasses.
- Apply a sun block product that has a skin protection factor (SPF) of at least 15. Some patients may require a product with a higher SPF number, especially if they have a fair complexion. If you have any questions about this, check with your doctor or pharmacist.
- Apply a sun block lipstick that has an SPF of at least 15 to protect your lips.
- Do not use a sunlamp or tanning bed or booth.

If you have a severe reaction, check with your doctor.

Clofazimine may also cause dry, rough, or scaly skin. A skin cream, lotion, or oil may help to treat this problem.

Side Effects of This Medicine

Along with its needed effects, a medicine may cause some unwanted effects. Although not all of these side effects may occur, if they do occur they may need medical attention.

Check with your doctor immediately if any of the following side effects occur:

Rare

Bloody or black, tarry stools; colicky or burning abdominal or stomach pain; mental depression; yellow eyes or skin—may be an orange color if already have a pink to brownish-black skin or eye discoloration

Other side effects may occur that usually do not need medical attention. These side effects may go away during treatment as your body adjusts to the medicine. However, check with your doctor if any of the following side effects continue or are bothersome:

More common

Diarrhea; dry, rough, or scaly skin; loss of appetite; nausea or vomiting; pink or red to brownish-black discoloration of skin and eyes; skin rash and itching

Less common or rare

Changes in taste; dryness, burning, itching, or irritation of the eyes; increased sensitivity of skin to sunlight

Clofazimine commonly causes discoloration of the feces, lining of the eyelids, sputum, sweat, tears, and urine. Usually this side effect does not require medical attention, but the discoloration may not go away. However, *clofazimine may also cause bloody or black, tarry stools. This side effect may be a symptom of serious bleeding problems that do require medical attention.*

Other side effects not listed above may also occur in some patients. If you notice any other effects, check with your doctor.

Annual revision: 02/23/93

CLOFIBRATE Systemic

Some commonly used brand names are:

In the U.S.
Abitrate
Atromid-S
Generic name product may also be available.

In Canada
Atromid-S
Claripex
Novofibrate

Description

Clofibrate (kloe-FYE-brate) is used to lower cholesterol and triglyceride (fat-like substances) levels in the blood. This may help prevent medical problems caused by such substances clogging the blood vessels.

Clofibrate may also be used for other conditions as determined by your doctor.

Clofibrate is available only with your doctor's prescription, in the following dosage form:

Oral

- Capsules (U.S. and Canada)

It is very important that you read and understand the following information. If any of it causes you special concern, check with your doctor. Also, *if you have any questions* or if you want more information about this medicine or your medical problem, *ask your doctor, nurse, or pharmacist.*

Before Using This Medicine

In addition to its helpful effects in treating your medical problem, this medicine may have some harmful effects.

You may have read or heard about a study called the World Health Organization (WHO) Study. This study compared the effects in patients who used clofibrate with effects in those who used a placebo (sugar pill). The results of this study suggested that clofibrate might increase the patient's risk of cancer, liver disease, and pancreatitis (inflammation of the pancreas), although it might also decrease the risk of heart attack. It may also increase the risk of gallstones and problems from gallbladder surgery. Other studies have not found all of these effects. Be sure you have discussed this with your doctor before taking this medicine.

In deciding to use a medicine, the risks of taking the medicine must be weighed against the good it will do. This is a decision you and your doctor will make. For clofibrate, the following should be considered:

Allergies—Tell your doctor if you have ever had any unusual or allergic reaction to clofibrate. Also tell your doctor and pharmacist if you are allergic to any other substances, such as foods, preservatives, or dyes.

Diet—Before prescribing medicine for your condition, your doctor will probably try to control your condition by prescribing a personal diet for you. Such a diet may be low in fats, sugars, and/or cholesterol. Many people are able to control their condition by carefully following their doctors' orders for proper diet and exercise. *Medicine is prescribed only when additional help is needed* and is effective only when a schedule of diet and exercise is properly followed.

Also, this medicine is less effective if you are greatly overweight. It may be very important for you to go on a reducing diet. However, check with your doctor before going on any diet.

Make certain your doctor and pharmacist know if you are on a low-sodium, low-sugar, or any other special diet. Most medicines contain more than their active ingredient.

Pregnancy—Use of clofibrate is not recommended during pregnancy. Although studies have not been done in pregnant women, studies in rabbits have shown that the fetus may not be able to break down and get rid of this medicine as well as the mother. Because of this, it is possible that clofibrate may be harmful to the fetus if you take it while you are pregnant or for up to several months before you become pregnant. Be sure that you have discussed this with your doctor before taking this medicine, especially if you plan to become pregnant in the near future.

Breast-feeding—Clofibrate passes into breast milk. This medicine is not recommended during breast-feeding because it may cause unwanted effects in nursing babies.

Children—Studies on this medicine have been done only in adult patients, and there is no specific information comparing use of clofibrate in children with use in other age groups. However, use is not recommended in children under 2 years of age since cholesterol is needed for normal development.

Older adults—Many medicines have not been studied specifically in older people. Therefore, it may not be known whether they work exactly the same way they do in younger adults. Although there is no specific information comparing use of clofibrate in the elderly with use in other age groups, this medicine is not expected to cause different side effects or problems in older people than it does in younger adults.

Other medicines—Although certain medicines should not be used together at all, in other cases two different medicines may be used together even if an interaction might occur. In these cases, your doctor may want to change the dose, or other precautions may be necessary. When you are taking clofibrate, it is especially important that your doctor and pharmacist know if you are taking the following:

- Anticoagulants (blood thinners)—Use with clofibrate may increase the effects of the anticoagulant

Other medical problems—The presence of other medical problems may affect the use of clofibrate. Make sure you tell your doctor if you have any other medical problems, especially:

- Gallstones or
- Stomach or intestinal ulcer—May make these conditions worse
- Heart disease or
- Kidney disease or
- Liver disease—Higher blood levels may result and increase the risk of side effects
- Underactive thyroid—Clofibrate may cause or make muscle disease worse

Before you begin using any new medicine (prescription or nonprescription) or if you develop any new medical problem while you are using this medicine, check with your doctor, nurse, or pharmacist.

Proper Use of This Medicine

Use this medicine only as directed by your doctor. Do not use more or less of it, and do not use it more often or for a longer time than your doctor ordered.

Follow carefully the special diet your doctor gave you. This is the most important part of controlling your condition and is necessary if the medicine is to work properly.

Stomach upset may occur but usually lessens after a few doses. Take this medicine with food or immediately after meals to lessen possible stomach upset.

Missed dose—If you miss a dose of this medicine, take it as soon as possible. However, if it is almost time for your next dose, skip the missed dose and go back to your regular dosing schedule. Do not double doses.

Storage—To store this medicine:

- Keep out of the reach of children.
- Store away from heat and direct light.
- Do not store in the bathroom, near the kitchen sink, or in other damp places. Heat or moisture may cause the medicine to break down.
- Do not keep outdated medicine or medicine no longer needed. Be sure that any discarded medicine is out of the reach of children.

Precautions While Using This Medicine

It is very important that your doctor check your progress at regular visits. This will allow your doctor to see if the medicine is working properly to lower your cholesterol and triglyceride levels and to decide if you should continue to take it.

Do not stop taking this medicine without first checking with your doctor. When you stop taking this medicine, your blood fat levels may increase again. Your doctor may want you to follow a special diet to help prevent that.

Side Effects of This Medicine

Along with its needed effects, a medicine may cause some unwanted effects. Although not all of these side effects may occur, if they do occur they may need medical attention.

Check with your doctor immediately if you think you have taken an overdose or if any of the following side effects occur:

Rare

Chest pain; irregular heartbeat; shortness of breath; stomach pain (severe) with nausea and vomiting

Check with your doctor as soon as possible if any of the following side effects occur:

Rare

Blood in urine; cough or hoarseness; decrease in urination; fever or chills; lower back or side pain; painful or difficult urination; swelling of feet or lower legs

Other side effects may occur that usually do not need medical attention. These side effects may go away during treatment as your body adjusts to the medicine. However, check with your doctor if any of the following side effects continue or are bothersome:

More common

Diarrhea; nausea

Less common or rare

Decreased sexual ability; headache; increased appetite or weight gain (slight); muscle aches or cramps; sores in mouth and on lips; stomach pain, gas, or heartburn; unusual tiredness or weakness; vomiting

Other side effects not listed above may also occur in some patients. If you notice any other effects, check with your doctor.

Additional Information

Once a medicine has been approved for marketing for a certain use, experience may show that it is also useful for other medical problems. Although this use is not included in product labeling, clofibrate is used in certain patients with the following medical condition:

- Certain types of diabetes insipidus (water diabetes)

Other than the above information, there is no additional information relating to proper use, precautions, or side effects for this use.

Annual revision: 11/24/92

CLOMIPHENE Systemic

Some commonly used brand names are:

In the U.S.

Clomid
Milophene
Serophene

In Canada

Clomid
Serophene

Another commonly used name is clomifene.

Description

Clomiphene (KLOE-mi-feen) is used as a fertility medicine in some women who are unable to become pregnant.

Clomiphene probably works by changing the hormone balance of the body. In women, this causes ovulation to occur and prepares the body for pregnancy.

Clomiphene may also be used for other conditions in both females and males as determined by your doctor.

The following information applies only to female patients taking clomiphene. Check with your doctor if you are a male and have any questions about the use of clomiphene.

Clomiphene is available only with your doctor's prescription, in the following dosage form:

Oral

- Tablets (U.S. and Canada)

It is very important that you read and understand the following information. If any of it causes you special concern, check with your doctor. Also, *if you have any questions* or if you want more information about this medicine or your medical problem, *ask your doctor, nurse, or pharmacist.*

Before Using This Medicine

In deciding to use a medicine, the risks of taking the medicine must be weighed against the good it will do. This is a decision you and your doctor will make. For clomiphene, the following should be considered:

Allergies—Tell your doctor if you have ever had any unusual or allergic reaction to clomiphene. Also tell your doctor and pharmacist if you are allergic to any other substances, such as foods, preservatives, or dyes.

Pregnancy—There is a chance that clomiphene may cause birth defects if it is taken after you become pregnant. *Stop taking this medicine and tell your doctor immediately if you think you have become pregnant* while still taking clomiphene.

If you become pregnant as a result of using this medicine, there is a chance of a multiple birth (for example, twins, triplets) occurring.

Other medicines—Although certain medicines should not be used together at all, in other cases two different medicines may be used together even if an interaction might occur. In these cases, your doctor may want to change the dose, or other precautions may be necessary. When you are taking clomiphene, it is especially important that your doctor and pharmacist know if you are taking any other prescription or nonprescription (over-the-counter [OTC]) medicine.

Other medical problems—The presence of other medical problems may affect the use of clomiphene. Make sure you tell your doctor if you have any other medical problems, especially:

- Cyst on ovary—Clomiphene may cause the cyst to increase in size
- Endometriosis—Inducing ovulation (including using clomiphene) may worsen endometriosis because the body estrogen level is increased; estrogen can cause growth of endometriosis implants
- Fibroid tumors of the uterus—Clomiphene may cause fibroid tumors to increase in size
- Inflamed veins due to blood clots
- Liver disease (or history of)
- Mental depression
- Unusual vaginal bleeding—Some irregular vaginal bleeding is a sign that the lining of the uterus is growing too much or is a sign of cancer of the uterus lining; these problems must be ruled out before clomiphene is used because clomiphene can make these conditions worse

Before you begin using any new medicine (prescription or nonprescription) or if you develop any new medical problem while you are using this medicine, check with your doctor, nurse, or pharmacist.

Proper Use of This Medicine

Take this medicine only as directed by your doctor. If you are to begin on Day 5, count the first day of your menstrual period as Day 1. Beginning on Day 5, take the correct dose every day for as many days as your doctor ordered. To help you to remember to take your dose of medicine, take it at the same time every day.

Missed dose—If you miss a dose of this medicine, take it as soon as possible. If you do not remember until it is time for the next dose, take both doses together; then go back to your regular dosing schedule. If you miss more than one dose, check with your doctor.

Storage—To store this medicine:

- Keep out of the reach of children.
- Store away from heat and direct light.
- Do not store in the bathroom, near the kitchen sink, or in other damp places. Heat or moisture may cause the medicine to break down.

- Do not keep outdated medicine or medicine no longer needed. Be sure that any discarded medicine is out of the reach of children.

Precautions While Using This Medicine

It is very important that your doctor check your progress at regular visits to make sure this medicine is working and to check for unwanted effects.

At certain times in your menstrual cycle, your doctor may want you to use an ovulation prediction test kit. *Follow your doctor's instructions carefully.* Ovulation is controlled by luteinizing hormone (LH). LH is present in the blood and urine in very small amounts during most of the menstrual cycle but rises suddenly for a short time in the middle of the menstrual cycle. This sharp rise, the LH surge, usually causes ovulation within about 30 hours. A woman is most likely to become pregnant if she has intercourse within the 24 hours after detecting the LH surge. Ovulation prediction test kits are used to test for this large amount of LH in the urine. This method is better for predicting ovulation than measuring daily basal body temperature. It is important that intercourse take place at the correct time to give you the best chance of becoming pregnant.

There is a chance that clomiphene may cause birth defects if it is taken after you become pregnant. *Stop taking this medicine and tell your doctor immediately if you think you have become pregnant* while still taking clomiphene.

This medicine may cause blurred vision, difficulty in reading, or other changes in vision. It may also cause some people to become dizzy or lightheaded. *Make sure you know how you react to this medicine before you drive, use machines, or do anything else that could be dangerous if you are not clear-headed or able to see well.* If these reactions are especially bothersome, check with your doctor.

Side Effects of This Medicine

Along with its needed effects, a medicine may cause some unwanted effects. Although not all of these side effects may occur, if they do occur they may need medical attention.

When this medicine is used for a short time at low doses, serious side effects usually are rare. *However, check with your doctor immediately* if any of the following side effects occur:

More common

Bloating; stomach or pelvic pain

Less common or rare

Shortness of breath (sudden)

Check with your doctor as soon as possible if any of the following side effects occur:

Less common or rare

Blurred vision; decreased or double vision or other vision problems; sensitivity of eyes to light; yellow eyes or skin

Other side effects may occur that usually do not need medical attention. These side effects may go away during treatment as your body adjusts to the medicine. However, check with your doctor if any of the following side effects continue or are bothersome:

More common

Hot flashes

Less common or rare

Breast discomfort; dizziness or lightheadedness; headache; heavy menstrual periods or bleeding between periods; mental depression; nausea or vomiting; nervousness; restlessness or trouble in sleeping; tiredness

Other side effects not listed above may also occur in some patients. If you notice any other effects, check with your doctor.

Additional Information

Once a medicine has been approved for marketing for a certain use, experience may show that it is also useful for other medical problems. Although these uses are not included in product labeling, clomiphene is used in certain patients with the following medical conditions:

- Male infertility caused by low production of sperm
- Certain problems of the male sexual organs caused by pituitary or hypothalamus gland problems (diagnosis)

For males taking this medicine for treatment of infertility caused by low sperm production:

- To decide on the best treatment for your medical problem, your doctor should be told:
  —if you have ever had any unusual or allergic reaction to clomiphene.
  —if you have either of the following medical problems:
  Liver disease
  Mental depression
- If you miss a dose of this medicine, take it as soon as possible. If you do not remember until it is time for the next dose, take both doses together, then go back to your regular dosing schedule. If you miss more than one dose, check with your doctor.
- It is important that your doctor check your progress at regular visits to find out if clomiphene is working and to check for unwanted effects.

- This medicine may cause vision problems, dizziness, or lightheadedness. *Make sure you know how you react to this medicine before you drive, use machines, or do anything else that could be dangerous if you are dizzy or are not clear-headed or able to see well.*
- Along with its needed effects, a medicine may cause some unwanted effects. Although not all of these side effects may occur, if they do occur they may need medical attention. When this medicine is used for short periods of time at low doses, serious side effects usually are rare. However, check with your doctor if any of the following side effects occur:

  Less common or rare

  Blurred vision; decreased or double vision or other vision problems; sensitivity of eyes to light; yellow eyes or skin

- Other side effects may occur that usually do not need medical attention. These side effects may go away during treatment as your body adjusts to the medicine. However, check with your doctor if any of the following side effects continue or are bothersome:

  Less common or rare

  Breast enlargement; dizziness or lightheadedness; headache; mental depression; nausea or vomiting; nervousness; restlessness; tiredness; trouble in sleeping

Other than the above information, there is no additional information relating to proper use, precautions, or side effects for these uses.

Annual revision: July 1990

CLONIDINE Systemic

Some commonly used brand names are:

In the U.S.
- Catapres
- Catapres-TTS
- Generic name product may also be available.

In Canada
- Catapres
- Dixarit

Description

Clonidine (KLOE-ni-deen) belongs to the general class of medicines called antihypertensives. It is used to treat high blood pressure (hypertension).

High blood pressure adds to the workload of the heart and arteries. If it continues for a long time, the heart and arteries may not function properly. This can damage the blood vessels of the brain, heart, and kidneys, resulting in a stroke, heart failure, or kidney failure. Hypertension may also increase the risk of heart attacks. These problems may be less likely to occur if blood pressure is controlled.

Clonidine works by controlling nerve impulses along certain nerve pathways. As a result, it relaxes blood vessels so that blood passes through them more easily. This helps to lower blood pressure.

Clonidine may also be used for other conditions as determined by your doctor.

Clonidine is available only with your doctor's prescription, in the following dosage forms:

Oral
- Tablets (U.S. and Canada)

Transdermal
- Skin patch (U.S.)

It is very important that you read and understand the following information. If any of it causes you special concern, check with your doctor. Also, *if you have any questions* or if you want more information about this medicine or your medical problem, *ask your doctor, nurse, or pharmacist.*

Before Using This Medicine

In deciding to use a medicine, the risks of taking the medicine must be weighed against the good it will do. This is a decision you and your doctor will make. For clonidine, the following should be considered:

Allergies—Tell your doctor if you have ever had any unusual or allergic reaction to clonidine. Also tell your doctor and pharmacist if you are allergic to any other substance, such as foods, preservatives, or dyes.

Pregnancy—Clonidine has not been studied in pregnant women. However, studies in animals have shown that clonidine causes harmful effects in the fetus, but not birth defects.

Breast-feeding—Although clonidine passes into breast milk, it has not been reported to cause problems in nursing babies.

Children—Children may be more sensitive than adults to clonidine. Clonidine overdose has been reported when children accidentally took this medicine.

Older adults—Dizziness or faintness may be more likely to occur in the elderly, who are more sensitive than younger adults to the effects of clonidine.

Other medicines—Although certain medicines should not be used together at all, in other cases two different medicines may be used together even if an interaction might occur. In these cases, your doctor may want to change the dose, or other precautions may be necessary. When you are taking clonidine, it is especially important that your doctor and pharmacist know if you are taking any of the following:

- Beta-blockers (acebutolol [e.g., Sectral], atenolol [e.g., Tenormin], betaxolol [e.g., Kerlone], carteolol [e.g., Cartrol], labetalol [e.g., Normodyne], metoprolol [e.g., Lopressor], nadolol [e.g., Corgard], oxprenolol [e.g., Trasicor], penbutolol [e.g., Levatol], pindolol [e.g., Visken], propranolol [e.g., Inderal], sotalol [e.g., Sotacor], timolol [e.g., Blocadren])—These medicines may increase the risk of harmful effects when clonidine treatment is stopped suddenly
- Tricyclic antidepressants (amitriptyline [e.g., Elavil], amoxapine [e.g., Asendin], clomipramine [e.g., Anafranil], desipramine [e.g., Pertofrane], doxepin [e.g., Sinequan], imipramine [e.g., Tofranil], nortriptyline [e.g., Aventyl], protriptyline [e.g., Vivactil], trimipramine [e.g., Surmontil])—These medicines may decrease clonidine's effects on blood pressure

Other medical problems—The presence of other medical problems may affect the use of clonidine. Make sure you tell your doctor if you have any other medical problems, especially:

- Heart or blood vessel disease—Clonidine may make these conditions worse
- Irritated or scraped skin (with transdermal system [skin patch] only)—The effects of clonidine may be increased if the skin patch is placed on an area of scraped or irritated skin because more medicine is absorbed into the body
- Kidney disease—Effects of clonidine may be increased because of slower removal of clonidine from the body
- Mental depression (history of) or
- Raynaud's syndrome—Clonidine may make these conditions worse
- Polyarteritis nodosa or
- Scleroderma or
- Systemic lupus erythematosus (SLE)—with transdermal system (skin patch) only—Effects of clonidine may be decreased because absorption of this medicine into the body is blocked

Before you begin using any new medicine (prescription or nonprescription) or if you develop any new medical problem while you are using this medicine, check with your doctor, nurse, or pharmacist.

Proper Use of This Medicine

For patients taking this medicine *for high blood pressure*:

- In addition to the use of the medicine your doctor has prescribed, treatment for your high blood pressure may include weight control and care in the types of foods you eat, especially foods high in sodium. Your doctor will tell you which of these are most important for you. You should check with your doctor before changing your diet.
- Many patients who have high blood pressure will not notice any signs of the problem. In fact, many may feel normal. It is very important that you *take your medicine exactly as directed* and that you keep your appointments with your doctor even if you feel well.
- Remember that this medicine will not cure your high blood pressure but it does help control it. Therefore, you must continue to use it as directed if you expect to lower your blood pressure and keep it down. *You may have to take high blood pressure medicine for the rest of your life.* If high blood pressure is not treated, it can cause serious problems such as heart failure, blood vessel disease, stroke, or kidney disease.

For patients using the *transdermal system (skin patch)*:

- *Use this medicine exactly as directed by your doctor.* It will work only if applied correctly. *This medicine usually comes with patient instructions. Read them carefully before using.*
- Do not try to trim or cut the adhesive patch to adjust the dosage. Check with your doctor if you think the medicine is not working as it should.
- Apply the patch to a clean, dry area of skin on your upper arm or chest. Choose an area with little or no hair and free of scars, cuts, or irritation.
- The system should stay in place even during showering, bathing, or swimming. If the patch becomes loose, cover it with the extra adhesive overlay provided. Apply a new patch if the first one becomes too loose or falls off.
- Each dose is best applied to a different area of skin to prevent skin problems or other irritation.
- After removing a used patch, fold the patch in half with the sticky sides together. Make sure to dispose of it out of the reach of children.

To help you remember to use your medicine, try to get into the habit of using it at regular times. If you are taking the tablets, take them at the same time each day. If you are using the transdermal system (skin patch), try to change it at the same time and day of the week.

Dosing—The dose of clonidine will be different for different patients. *Follow your doctor's orders or the directions on the label.* The following information includes only the average doses of clonidine used for the treatment of high blood pressure. *If your dose is different, do not change it* unless your doctor tells you to do so:

- For *oral* dosage form (tablets):
  - —For high blood pressure:
    - Adults—100 mcg (0.1 mg) two times a day. Your doctor may increase your dose up to 200

mcg (0.2 mg) to 600 mcg (0.6 mg) a day taken in divided doses.

- Children—Use and dose must be determined by your doctor.

- For *transdermal* dosage form (skin patch):
  - —For high blood pressure:
    - Adults—One transdermal dosage system (skin patch) applied once a week.
    - Children—Use and dose must be determined by your doctor.

Missed dose—If you miss a dose of this medicine, take it or use it as soon as possible. Then go back to your regular dosing schedule. *If you miss 2 or more doses of the tablets in a row or if you miss changing the transdermal patch for 3 or more days, check with your doctor right away.* If your body goes without this medicine for too long, your blood pressure may go up to a dangerously high level and some unpleasant effects may occur.

Storage—To store this medicine:

- Keep out of the reach of children.
- Store away from heat and direct light.
- Do not store in the bathroom, near the kitchen sink, or in other damp places. Heat or moisture may cause the medicine to break down.
- Do not keep outdated medicine or medicine no longer needed. Be sure that any discarded medicine is out of the reach of children.

Precautions While Using This Medicine

It is important that your doctor check your progress at regular visits to make sure that this medicine is working properly.

Check with your doctor before you stop using this medicine. Your doctor may want you to reduce gradually the amount you are using before stopping completely.

Make sure that you have enough clonidine on hand to last through weekends, holidays, or vacations. You should not miss any doses. You may want to ask your doctor for another written prescription for clonidine to carry in your wallet or purse. You can then have it filled if you run out of medicine when you are away from home.

For patients taking this medicine *for high blood pressure*:

- *Do not take other medicines unless they have been discussed with your doctor.* This especially includes over-the-counter (nonprescription) medicines for appetite control, asthma, colds, cough, hay fever, or sinus problems, since they may tend to increase your blood pressure.

Clonidine will add to the effects of alcohol and other CNS depressants (medicines that slow down the nervous system, possibly causing drowsiness). Some examples of CNS depressants are antihistamines or medicine for hay fever, other allergies, or colds; sedatives, tranquilizers, or sleeping medicine; prescription pain medicine or narcotics; barbiturates; medicine for seizures; muscle relaxants; or anesthetics, including some dental anesthetics. *Check with your doctor before taking any of the above while you are using this medicine.*

Clonidine may cause some people to become drowsy or less alert than they are normally. This is more likely to happen when you begin to take it or when you increase the amount of medicine you are taking. *Make sure you know how you react to this medicine before you drive, use machines, or do anything else that could be dangerous if you are not alert.*

Before having any kind of surgery (including dental surgery) or emergency treatment, *tell the medical doctor or dentist in charge that you are using this medicine.*

Dizziness, lightheadedness, or fainting may occur after you take this medicine, especially when you get up from a lying or sitting position. Getting up slowly may help, but if the problem continues or gets worse, check with your doctor.

The dizziness, lightheadedness, or fainting is also more likely to occur if you drink alcohol, stand for long periods of time, exercise, or if the weather is hot. While you are taking clonidine, be careful to limit the amount of alcohol you drink. Also, use extra care during exercise or hot weather or if you must stand for a long time.

Clonidine may cause dryness of the mouth. For temporary relief, use sugarless candy or gum, melt bits of ice in your mouth, or use a saliva substitute. However, if your mouth continues to feel dry for more than 2 weeks, check with your medical doctor or dentist. Continuing dryness of the mouth may increase the chance of dental disease, including tooth decay, gum disease, and fungus infections.

Side Effects of This Medicine

Along with its needed effects, a medicine may cause some unwanted effects. Although not all of these side effects may occur, if they do occur they may need medical attention.

Check with your doctor immediately if any of the following side effects occur:

Signs and symptoms of overdose

Difficulty in breathing; dizziness (extreme) or faintness; pinpoint pupils of eyes; slow heartbeat; unusual tiredness or weakness (extreme)

Check with your doctor as soon as possible if any of the following side effects occur:

More common—with transdermal system (skin patch) only

Itching or redness of skin

Less common

Mental depression; swelling of feet and lower legs

Rare

Paleness or cold feeling in fingertips and toes; vivid dreams or nightmares

Other side effects may occur that usually do not need medical attention. These side effects may go away during treatment as your body adjusts to the medicine. However, check with your doctor if any of the following side effects continue or are bothersome:

More common

Constipation; dizziness; drowsiness; dryness of mouth; unusual tiredness or weakness

Less common

Darkening of skin—with transdermal system (skin patch) only; decreased sexual ability; dizziness, lightheadedness, or fainting, especially when getting up from a lying or sitting position; dry, itching, or burning eyes; loss of appetite; nausea or vomiting; nervousness

After you have been using this medicine for a while, it may cause unpleasant or even harmful effects if you stop taking it too suddenly. After you stop taking this medicine, *check with your doctor immediately* if any of the following occur:

Anxiety or tenseness; chest pain; fast or pounding heartbeat; headache; increased salivation; nausea; nervousness; restlessness; shaking or trembling of hands and fingers; stomach cramps; sweating; trouble in sleeping; vomiting

Other side effects not listed above may also occur in some patients. If you notice any other effects, check with your doctor.

Additional Information

Once a medicine has been approved for marketing for a certain use, experience may show that it is also useful for other medical problems. Although this use is not included in product labeling, clonidine is used in certain patients with the following medical conditions:

- Migraine headache
- Symptoms associated with menopause or menstrual discomfort
- Symptoms of withdrawal associated with alcohol, nicotine, or narcotics
- Gilles de la Tourette's syndrome

Other than the above information, there is no additional information relating to proper use, precautions, or side effects for these uses.

Annual revision: 05/17/93

CLONIDINE AND CHLORTHALIDONE Systemic

A commonly used brand name in the U.S. and Canada is Combipres. Generic name product may also be available in the U.S.

Description

Clonidine (KLOE-ni-deen) and chlorthalidone (klor-THAL-i-done) combinations are used in the treatment of high blood pressure (hypertension).

High blood pressure adds to the workload of the heart and arteries. If it continues for a long time, the heart and arteries may not function properly. This can damage the blood vessels of the brain, heart, and kidneys resulting in a stroke, heart failure, or kidney failure. Hypertension may also increase the risk of heart attacks. These problems may be less likely to occur if blood pressure is controlled.

Clonidine works by controlling nerve impulses along certain body nerve pathways. As a result, it relaxes blood vessels so that blood passes through them more easily. The chlorthalidone in this combination is a diuretic (water pill) that helps reduce the amount of water in the body by increasing the flow of urine.

Clonidine and chlorthalidone combination is available only with your doctor's prescription, in the following dosage form:

Oral

- Tablets (U.S. and Canada)

It is very important that you read and understand the following information. If any of it causes you special concern, check with your doctor. Also, *if you have any questions* or if you want more information about this medicine or your medical problem, *ask your doctor, nurse, or pharmacist.*

Before Using This Medicine

In deciding to use a medicine, the risks of taking the medicine must be weighed against the good it will do. This is a decision you and your doctor will make. For clonidine and chlorthalidone, the following should be considered:

Allergies—Tell your doctor if you have ever had any unusual or allergic reaction to clonidine, chlorthalidone, sulfonamides (sulfa drugs), or other thiazide diuretics (water pills). Also tell your doctor and pharmacist if you are allergic to any other substance, such as foods, preservatives, or dyes.

Pregnancy—Studies with clonidine have not been done in humans. Although clonidine has not been shown to cause birth defects in animals, it has been shown to cause toxic or harmful effects in the fetus in animals even at doses of only one-third the maximum human dose. When chlorthalidone is used during pregnancy, it may cause side effects including jaundice, blood problems, and low potassium in the newborn infant. Be sure you have discussed this with your doctor before taking this medicine.

Breast-feeding—Although both clonidine and chlorthalidone pass into breast milk, they have not been reported to cause problems in nursing babies.

Children—There is no specific information about the use of clonidine and chlorthalidone in children.

Older adults—Dizziness or faintness and signs of too much potassium loss may be more likely to occur in the elderly, who are more sensitive to the effects of clonidine and chlorthalidone.

Other medicines—Although certain medicines should not be used together at all, in other cases two different medicines may be used together even if an interaction might occur. In these cases, your doctor may want to change the dose, or other precautions may be necessary. When you are taking clonidine and chlorthalidone, it is especially important that your doctor and pharmacist know if you are taking any of the following:

- Adrenocorticoids (cortisone-like medicines)—Chlorthalidone may decrease some effects and increase others
- Beta-blockers (acebutolol [e.g., Sectral], atenolol [e.g., Tenormin], betaxolol [Kerlone], carteolol [e.g., Cartrol], labetalol [e.g., Normodyne], metoprolol [e.g., Lopressor], nadolol [e.g., Corgard], oxprenolol [e.g., Trasicor], penbutolol [e.g., Levatol], pindolol [e.g., Visken], propranolol [e.g., Inderal], sotalol [e.g., Sotacor], timolol [e.g., Blocadren])—May increase the risk of harmful effects when clonidine treatment is stopped suddenly
- Digitalis glycosides (heart medicine)—Chlorthalidone may cause low potassium in the blood, which can lead to symptoms of digitalis toxicity
- Lithium (e.g., Lithane)—Risk of lithium overdose, even at usual doses, may be increased
- Methenamine (e.g., Mandelamine)—Chlorthalidone may reduce the effects of methenamine
- Tricyclic antidepressants (amitriptyline [e.g., Elavil], amoxapine [e.g., Asendin], clomipramine [e.g., Anafranil], desipramine [e.g., Pertofrane], doxepin [e.g., Sinequan], imipramine [e.g., Tofranil], nortriptyline [e.g., Aventyl], protriptyline [e.g., Vivactil], trimipramine [e.g., Surmontil])—May decrease the effects of clonidine on blood pressure

Other medical problems—The presence of other medical problems may affect the use of clonidine and chlorthalidone. Make sure you tell your doctor if you have any other medical problems, especially:

- Diabetes mellitus (sugar diabetes)—Chlorthalidone may change the amount of diabetes medicine needed
- Gout—Chlorthalidone may increase the amount of uric acid in the blood, which can lead to gout
- Heart or blood vessel disease
- Kidney disease—Effects may be increased because of slower removal of clonidine from the body. If severe, chlorthalidone may not work
- Liver disease—If chlorthalidone causes loss of too much water from the body, liver disease can become much worse
- Lupus erythematosus (history of)—Chlorthalidone may worsen the condition
- Mental depression (history of)
- Pancreatitis (inflammation of the pancreas)
- Raynaud's syndrome

Before you begin using any new medicine (prescription or nonprescription) or if you develop any new medical problem while you are using this medicine, check with your doctor, nurse, or pharmacist.

Proper Use of This Medicine

This medicine may cause you to have an unusual feeling of tiredness when you begin to take it. You may also notice an increase in the amount of urine or in your frequency of urination. After taking the medicine for a while, these effects should lessen. In general, to keep the increase in urine from affecting your sleep:

- If you are to take a single dose a day, take it in the morning after breakfast.
- If you are to take more than one dose a day, take the last dose no later than 6 p.m., unless otherwise directed by your doctor.

However, it is best to plan your dose or doses according to a schedule that will least affect your personal activities and sleep. Ask your doctor, nurse, or pharmacist to help you plan the best time to take this medicine.

Importance of diet:

- When prescribing medicine for your condition, your doctor may also prescribe a personal diet for you. Such a diet may be low in sodium (salt). Most people eat much more sodium than they need and too much sodium in the diet may increase blood pressure. Some foods that contain large amounts of sodium are canned soup, pickles, ketchup, green and ripe olives, relish, frankfurters, soy sauce, and carbonated beverages. Your doctor may want you to limit the amounts of these and other high-sodium foods in your diet. High blood pressure medicine is usually more effective when such a diet is properly followed.
- Also, it may be very important for you to go on a reducing diet. However, check with your doctor before changing your diet.

Many patients who have high blood pressure will not notice any signs of the problem. In fact, many may feel normal. It is very important that you *take your medicine exactly as directed* and that you keep your appointments with your doctor even if you feel well.

Remember that this medicine will not cure your high blood pressure but it does help control it. Therefore, you must continue to take it as directed if you expect to lower your blood pressure and keep it down. *You may have to take high blood pressure medicine for the rest of your life.* If high blood pressure is not treated, it can cause serious problems such as heart failure, blood vessel disease, stroke, or kidney disease.

To help you remember to take your medicine, try to get into the habit of taking it at the same time each day.

Missed dose—If you miss a dose of this medicine, take it as soon as possible. Then go back to your regular dosing schedule. *If you miss two or more doses in a row, check with your doctor right away.* If your body goes without this medicine for too long, your blood pressure may go up to a dangerously high level and some unpleasant effects may occur.

Storage—To store this medicine:

- Keep out of the reach of children.
- Store away from heat and direct light.
- Do not store in the bathroom, near the kitchen sink, or in other damp places. Heat or moisture may cause the medicine to break down.
- Do not keep outdated medicine or medicine no longer needed. Be sure that any discarded medicine is out of the reach of children.

Precautions While Using This Medicine

It is important that your doctor check your progress at regular visits to make sure that this medicine is working properly.

Check with your doctor before you stop taking this medicine. Your doctor may want you to reduce gradually the amount you are taking before stopping completely.

Make sure that you have enough medicine on hand to last through weekends, holidays, or vacations. You should not miss taking any doses. You may want to ask your doctor for another written prescription to carry in your wallet or purse. You can then have it filled if you run out of medicine when you are away from home.

Before having any kind of surgery (including dental surgery) or emergency treatment, *make sure the medical doctor or dentist in charge knows that you are taking this medicine.*

Do not take other medicines unless they have been discussed with your doctor. This especially includes over-the-counter (nonprescription) medicines for appetite control, asthma, colds, cough, hay fever, or sinus problems, since they may tend to increase your blood pressure.

This medicine will add to the effects of alcohol and other CNS depressants (medicines that slow down the nervous system, possibly causing drowsiness). Some examples of CNS depressants are antihistamines or medicine for hay fever, other allergies, or colds; sedatives, tranquilizers, or sleeping medicine; prescription pain medicine or narcotics; barbiturates; medicine for seizures; muscle relaxants; or anesthetics, including some dental anesthetics. *Check with your doctor before taking any of the above while you are using this medicine.*

This medicine may cause some people to become drowsy or less alert than they are normally. This is more likely to happen when you begin to take it or when you increase the amount of medicine you are taking. *Make sure you know how you react to this medicine before you drive, use machines, or do anything else that could be dangerous if you are not alert.*

Dizziness, lightheadedness, or fainting may occur, especially when you get up from a lying or sitting position. Getting up slowly may help but if the problem continues or gets worse, check with your doctor.

The dizziness, lightheadedness, or fainting is also more likely to occur if you drink alcohol, stand for long periods of time, exercise, or if the weather is hot. Drinking alcoholic beverages may also make the drowsiness worse. While you are taking this medicine, be careful in the amount of alcohol you drink. Also, use extra care during exercise or hot weather or if you must stand for long periods of time.

This medicine may cause a loss of potassium from your body.

- To help prevent this, your doctor may want you to:
  - —eat or drink foods that have a high potassium content (for example, orange or other citrus fruit juices), or
  - —take a potassium supplement, or
  - —take another medicine to help prevent the loss of the potassium in the first place.
- It is very important to follow these directions. Also, it is important not to change your diet on your own. This is more important if you are already on a special diet (as for diabetes), or if you are taking a potassium supplement or a medicine to reduce potassium loss. Extra potassium may not be necessary and, in some cases, too much potassium could be harmful.

Check with your doctor if you become sick and have severe or continuing vomiting or diarrhea. These problems may cause you to lose additional water and potassium.

For *diabetic patients*:

- Thiazide diuretics like chlorthalidone may raise blood sugar levels. While you are using this medicine, be especially careful in testing for sugar in your urine.

A few people who take this medicine may become more sensitive to sunlight than they are normally. Exposure to sunlight, even for brief periods of time, may cause severe sunburn; skin rash, redness, itching, or discoloration; or vision changes. When you begin taking this medicine:

- Stay out of direct sunlight, especially between the hours of 10:00 a.m. and 3:00 p.m., if possible.
- Wear protective clothing, including a hat and sunglasses.
- Apply a sun block product that has a high skin protection factor (SPF) of at least 15. Some patients may require a product with a higher SPF number, especially if they have a fair complexion. If you have any questions about this, check with your doctor or pharmacist.
- Do not use a sunlamp or tanning bed or booth.

If you have a severe reaction from the sun, check with your doctor.

This medicine may cause dryness of the mouth. For temporary relief, use sugarless candy or gum, melt bits of ice in your mouth, or use a saliva substitute. However, if dry mouth continues for more than 2 weeks, check with your physician or dentist. Continuing dryness of the mouth may increase the chance of dental disease, including tooth decay, gum disease, and fungus infections.

Side Effects of This Medicine

Along with its needed effects, a medicine may cause some unwanted effects. Although not all of these side effects may occur, if they do occur they may need medical attention.

Check with your doctor immediately if any of the following side effects occur:

Signs and symptoms of overdose

Difficulty in breathing; dizziness (extreme) or faintness; pinpoint pupils of eyes; slow heartbeat; unusual tiredness or weakness (extreme)

Check with your doctor as soon as possible if any of the following side effects occur, especially since some of them may mean that your body is losing too much potassium:

Signs and symptoms of too much potassium loss

Dry mouth; increased thirst; irregular heartbeats; mood or mental changes; muscle cramps or pain; nausea or vomiting; weak pulse

Rare

Joint pain; lower back or side pain; paleness or cold feeling in fingertips and toes; skin rash or hives; sore throat and fever; stomach pain (severe) with nausea and vomiting; unusual bleeding or bruising; vivid dreams or nightmares; yellow eyes or skin

Other side effects may occur that usually do not need medical attention. These side effects may go away during treatment as your body adjusts to the medicine. However, check with your doctor if any of the following side effects continue or are bothersome:

More common

Drowsiness

Less common

Constipation; decreased sexual ability; diarrhea; dizziness or lightheadedness when getting up from a lying or sitting position; dry, itching, or burning eyes; increased sensitivity of skin to sunlight; loss of appetite; nervousness; upset stomach

After you have been using this medicine for a while, it may cause unpleasant or even harmful effects if you stop taking it too suddenly. After you stop taking this medicine, check with your doctor if any of the following occur:

Anxiety or tenseness; chest pain; fast or irregular heartbeat; headache; increased salivation; nausea; nervousness; restlessness; shaking or trembling of hands and fingers; stomach cramps; sweating; trouble in sleeping; vomiting

Other side effects not listed above may also occur in some patients. If you notice any other effects, check with your doctor.

Annual revision: July 1990

CLOTRIMAZOLE Oral†

A commonly used brand name in the U.S. is Mycelex Troches.

†Not commercially available in Canada.

Description

Clotrimazole (kloe-TRIM-a-zole) lozenges are dissolved slowly in the mouth to prevent and treat thrush. Thrush, also called candidiasis or white mouth, is a fungus infection of the mouth and throat. This medicine may also be used for other problems as determined by your doctor.

Clotrimazole is available only with your doctor's prescription, in the following dosage form:

Oral

- Lozenges (U.S.)

It is very important that you read and understand the following information. If any of it causes you special concern, check with your doctor. Also, *if you have any questions* or if you want more information about this medicine or your medical problem, *ask your doctor, nurse, or pharmacist.*

Before Using This Medicine

In deciding to use a medicine, the risks of taking the medicine must be weighed against the good it will do. This is a decision you and your doctor will make. For clotrimazole, the following should be considered:

Allergies—Tell your doctor if you have ever had any unusual or allergic reaction to clotrimazole. Also tell your doctor and pharmacist if you are allergic to any other substances, such as foods, preservatives, or dyes.

Pregnancy—Studies have not been done in humans. Studies in mice, rats, and rabbits given very high doses have not shown that clotrimazole causes birth defects. However, studies in rats and mice given high doses have shown that clotrimazole lozenges may cause other harmful effects in the fetus.

Breast-feeding—It is not known whether clotrimazole passes into breast milk. However, only small amounts of clotrimazole are absorbed into the mother's body. Clotrimazole has not been reported to cause problems in nursing babies.

Children—Although this medicine has not been shown to cause different side effects or problems in children than it does in adults, it should not be given to children under 5 years of age since they may be too young to use the lozenges safely.

Older adults—Many medicines have not been studied specifically in older people. Therefore, it may not be known whether they work exactly the same way they do in younger adults. Although there is no specific information comparing use of clotrimazole lozenges in the elderly with use in other age groups, this medicine is not expected to cause different side effects or problems in older people than it does in younger adults.

Before you begin using any new medicine (prescription or nonprescription) or if you develop any new medical problem while you are using this medicine, check with your doctor, nurse, or pharmacist.

Proper Use of This Medicine

Clotrimazole lozenges should be held in the mouth and allowed to dissolve slowly and completely, then swallowed. This may take 15 to 30 minutes. *Do not chew the lozenges or swallow them whole.*

Do not give clotrimazole lozenges to infants or children under 5 years of age. They may be too young to use the lozenges safely.

To help clear up your infection completely, *it is very important that you keep using clotrimazole for the full time of treatment,* even if your symptoms begin to clear up after a few days. Since fungus infections may be very slow to clear up, you may have to continue using this medicine every day for two weeks or more. If you stop using this medicine too soon, your symptoms may return. *Do not miss any doses.*

Dosing—The dose of clotrimazole lozenges will be different for different patients. *Follow your doctor's orders or the directions on the label.* The following information includes only the average doses of clotrimazole lozenges. *If your dose is different, do not change it* unless your doctor tells you to do so.

- For the *treatment of thrush*:
  - —Adults and children 5 years of age and older: Dissolve one 10-milligram lozenge slowly and completely in your mouth; this dose should be taken five times a day for at least fourteen days.
  - —Children up to 5 years of age: This medicine is not recommended in children under 5 years of age since they may be too young to use the lozenges safely.
- For the *prevention of thrush*:
  - —Adults and children 5 years of age and older: Dissolve one 10-milligram lozenge slowly and completely in your mouth; this dose should be taken three times a day.
  - —Children up to 5 years of age: This medicine is not recommended in children under 5 years of age since they may be too young to use the lozenges safely.

Missed dose—If you miss a dose of this medicine, take it as soon as possible. However, if it is almost time for your next dose, skip the missed dose and go back to your regular dosing schedule.

Storage—To store this medicine:

- Keep out of the reach of children.
- Store away from heat and direct light.
- Do not store in the bathroom, near the kitchen sink, or in other damp places. Heat or moisture may cause the medicine to break down.
- Do not keep outdated medicine or medicine no longer needed. Be sure that any discarded medicine is out of the reach of children.

Precautions While Using This Medicine

If your symptoms do not improve within 1 week, or if they become worse, check with your doctor.

Side Effects of This Medicine

Along with its needed effects, a medicine may cause some unwanted effects. The following side effects may go away during treatment as your body adjusts to the medicine. However, check with your doctor if any of these effects continue or are bothersome:

More common—when swallowed

Abdominal or stomach cramping or pain; diarrhea; nausea or vomiting

Other side effects not listed above may also occur in some patients. If you notice any other effects, check with your doctor.

Annual revision: 02/23/93

CLOTRIMAZOLE Topical

Some commonly used brand names are:

In the U.S.

- Lotrimin AF Cream
- Lotrimin AF Lotion
- Lotrimin AF Solution
- Lotrimin Cream
- Lotrimin Lotion
- Lotrimin Solution
- Mycelex Cream
- Mycelex Solution

In Canada

- Canesten Cream
- Canesten Solution
- Canesten Solution with Atomizer
- Clotrimaderm Cream
- Myclo Cream
- Myclo Solution
- Myclo Spray Solution
- Neo-Zol Cream

Description

Clotrimazole (kloe-TRIM-a-zole) topical preparations are used to treat fungus infections.

Some of these preparations are available only with your doctor's prescription. Others are available without a prescription; however, your doctor may have special instructions on the proper dose for your medical condition.

Clotrimazole is available in the following dosage forms:

Topical

- Cream (U.S. and Canada)
- Lotion (U.S.)
- Solution (U.S. and Canada)

It is very important that you read and understand the following information. If any of it causes you special concern, check with your doctor or pharmacist. Also, *if you have any questions* or if you want more information about this medicine or your medical problem, *ask your doctor, nurse, or pharmacist.*

Before Using This Medicine

If you are taking this medicine without a prescription, carefully read and follow any precautions on the label. For clotrimazole, the following should be considered:

Allergies—Tell your doctor if you have ever had any unusual or allergic reaction to clotrimazole. Also tell your doctor and pharmacist if you are allergic to any other substances, such as preservatives or dyes.

Pregnancy—Clotrimazole has not been studied in pregnant women during the first trimester (3 months). However, clotrimazole, used vaginally during the second and third trimesters, has not been shown to cause birth defects or other problems in humans.

Breast-feeding—It is not known whether topical clotrimazole passes into the breast milk. However, clotrimazole topical preparations have not been reported to cause problems in nursing babies.

Children—This medicine has been tested in children and, in effective doses, has not been shown to cause different side effects or problems than it does in adults.

Older adults—Many medicines have not been studied specifically in older people. Therefore, it may not be known whether they work exactly the same way they do in younger adults. Although there is no specific information comparing use of topical clotrimazole in the elderly with use in other age groups, this medicine is not expected to cause different side effects or problems in older people than it does in younger adults.

Other medicines—Although certain medicines should not be used together at all, in other cases two different medicines may be used together even if an interaction might occur. In these cases, your doctor may want to change the dose, or other precautions may be necessary. Tell your doctor and pharmacist if you are using any other topical prescription or nonprescription (over-the-counter [OTC]) medicine that is to be applied to the same area of the skin.

Before you begin using any new medicine (prescription or nonprescription) or if you develop any new medical problem while you are using this medicine, check with your doctor, nurse, or pharmacist.

Proper Use of This Medicine

Apply enough clotrimazole to cover the affected and surrounding skin areas, and rub in gently.

Keep this medicine away from the eyes.

When clotrimazole is used to treat certain types of fungus infections of the skin, an occlusive dressing (airtight covering such as, kitchen plastic wrap) should *not* be applied over the medicine. To do so may cause irritation of the skin. *Do not apply an occlusive dressing over this medicine unless you have been directed to do so by your doctor.*

To help clear up your infection completely, *it is very important that you keep using this medicine for the full time of treatment,* even if your symptoms begin to clear up after a few days. Since fungus infections may be very slow to clear up, you may have to continue using this medicine every day for several weeks or more. If you stop using this medicine too soon, your symptoms may return. *Do not miss any doses.*

Missed dose—If you do miss a dose of this medicine, apply it as soon as possible. However, if it is almost time for your next dose, skip the missed dose and go back to your regular dosing schedule.

Storage—To store this medicine:

- Keep out of the reach of children.
- Store away from heat and direct light.
- Keep the medicine from freezing.
- Do not keep outdated medicine or medicine no longer needed. Be sure that any discarded medicine is out of the reach of children.

Precautions While Using This Medicine

If your skin problem does not improve within 4 weeks, or if it becomes worse, check with your doctor.

Side Effects of This Medicine

Along with its needed effects, a medicine may cause some unwanted effects. Although not all of these side effects may occur, if they do occur they may need medical attention.

Check with your doctor as soon as possible if any of the following side effects occur:

Skin rash, hives, blistering, burning, itching, peeling, redness, stinging, swelling, or other sign of skin irritation not present before use of this medicine

Other side effects not listed above may also occur in some patients. If you notice any other effects, check with your doctor.

Annual revision: 11/21/91

CLOTRIMAZOLE AND BETAMETHASONE Topical

Some commonly used brand names are:

In the U.S.
Lotrisone

In Canada
Lotriderm

Description

Clotrimazole (kloe-TRIM-a-zole) and betamethasone (bay-ta-METH-a-sone) combination is used to treat fungus infections. Clotrimazole works by killing the fungus or preventing its growth. Betamethasone, an adrenocorticoid (cortisone-like medicine or steroid), is used to help relieve redness, swelling, itching, and other discomfort of fungus infections.

Clotrimazole and betamethasone cream is applied to the skin to treat:

- athlete's foot (ringworm of the foot; tinea pedis);
- jock itch (ringworm of the groin; tinea cruris); and
- ringworm of the body (tinea corporis).

This medicine may also be used for other fungus infections of the skin as determined by your doctor.

This medicine is available only with your doctor's prescription, in the following dosage form:

Topical

- Cream (U.S. and Canada)

It is very important that you read and understand the following information. If any of it causes you special concern, check with your doctor. Also, *if you have any questions* or if you want more information about this medicine or your medical problem, *ask your doctor, nurse, or pharmacist.*

Before Using This Medicine

In deciding to use a medicine, the risks of using the medicine must be weighed against the good it will do. This is a decision you and your doctor will make. For clotrimazole and betamethasone combination, the following should be considered:

Allergies—Tell your doctor if you have ever had any unusual or allergic reaction to this medicine or to clotrimazole (e.g., Gyne-Lotrimin, Lotrimin), betamethasone (e.g., Valisone), butoconazole (e.g., Femstat), econazole (e.g., Ecostatin, Spectazole), ketoconazole (e.g., Nizoral), miconazole (e.g., Monistat, Monistat-Derm), terconazole (e.g., Terazol 7), or to any of the other adrenocorticoids. Also tell your doctor and pharmacist if you are allergic to any other substances, such as preservatives or dyes.

Pregnancy—Clotrimazole and betamethasone combination has not been studied in pregnant women. However, for the individual medicines:

- *Clotrimazole*—Clotrimazole (e.g., Gyne-Lotrimin), used in the vagina, has not been shown to cause birth defects or other problems in studies in rats or humans. However, clotrimazole (e.g., Mycelex), given by mouth, has been shown to cause a decrease in successful pregnancies, but no birth defects, in rats and mice.
- *Betamethasone*—Studies in animals have shown that adrenocorticoids, given by mouth or by injection, may cause birth defects, even at low doses. Also, some of the stronger adrenocorticoids have been shown to cause birth defects when applied to the skin of animals.

Therefore, this medicine should not be used on large areas of the skin, in large amounts, or for a long time in pregnant patients. Before using this medicine, make sure your doctor knows if you are pregnant or if you may become pregnant.

Breast-feeding—It is not known whether topical clotrimazole and betamethasone combination passes into the breast milk, but it has not been reported to cause problems in nursing babies. However, clotrimazole and betamethasone may be absorbed into the mother's body.

- *Betamethasone*—Adrenocorticoids, given by mouth or by injection, do pass into the breast milk. They may cause unwanted effects, such as slower growth rate of nursing babies.

Children—Clotrimazole and betamethasone combination may rarely cause serious side effects. Some of these side effects may be more likely to occur in children, who may absorb greater amounts of this medicine than adults do. Long-term use in children may affect growth and development as well. Therefore, it is especially important that you discuss with the child's doctor the good that this medicine may do, as well as the risks of using it.

Older adults—Many medicines have not been studied specifically in older people. Therefore, it may not be known whether they work exactly the same way they do in younger adults or if they cause different side effects or problems in older people. There is no specific information comparing use of clotrimazole and betamethasone combination in the elderly with use in other age groups.

Other medicines—Although certain medicines should not be used together at all, in other cases two different medicines may be used together even if an interaction might occur. In these cases, your doctor may want to change the dose, or other precautions may be necessary. Tell your doctor and pharmacist if you are using any other prescription or nonprescription (over-the-counter [OTC]) medicine.

Other medical problems—The presence of other medical problems may affect the use of clotrimazole and betamethasone combination. Make sure you tell your doctor if you have any other medical problems, especially:

- Herpes or
- Vaccinia (cowpox) or
- Varicella (chickenpox) or
- Other virus infections of the skin—Betamethasone may speed up the spread of virus infections
- Tuberculosis (TB) of the skin—Betamethasone may make a TB infection worse

Before you begin using any new medicine (prescription or nonprescription) or if you develop any new medical problem while you are using this medicine, check with your doctor, nurse, or pharmacist.

Proper Use of This Medicine

Before applying this medicine, wash the affected area with soap and water, and dry thoroughly.

Do not use this medicine in the eyes.

To use:

- *Check with your doctor before using this medicine on any other skin problems.* It should not be used on bacterial or virus infections. Also, it should only be used on certain kinds of fungus infections of the skin.
- Apply a thin layer of this medicine to the affected area(s) and surrounding skin. Rub in gently and thoroughly.

The use of any kind of occlusive dressing (airtight covering, such as kitchen plastic wrap) over this medicine may increase absorption of the medicine and the chance of irritation and other side effects. Therefore, *do not bandage, wrap, or apply any occlusive dressing over this medicine* unless directed by your doctor. Also, wear loose-fitting clothing when using this medicine on the groin area. When using this medicine on the diaper area of children, *avoid tight-fitting diapers and plastic pants.*

To help clear up your skin infection completely, *keep using this medicine for the full time of treatment,* even if your symptoms have disappeared. *Do not miss any doses.* However, *do not use this medicine more often or for a longer time than your doctor ordered.* To do so may increase absorption through your skin and the chance of side effects. In addition, too much use, especially on thin skin areas (for example, face, armpits, genitals [sex organs], between the toes, groin), may result in thinning of the skin and stretch marks.

Missed dose—If you do miss a dose of this medicine, apply it as soon as possible. However, if it is almost time for your next dose, skip the missed dose and go back to your regular dosing schedule.

Storage—To store this medicine:

- Keep out of the reach of children.
- Store away from heat and direct light.
- Keep the medicine from freezing.
- Do not keep outdated medicine or medicine no longer needed. Be sure that any discarded medicine is out of the reach of children.

Precautions While Using This Medicine

If your skin infection does not improve within a few days, or if it becomes worse, check with your doctor.

To help clear up your skin infection completely and to help make sure it does not return, the following good health habits are important:

- For patients using this medicine *for athlete's foot:*

  —Carefully dry the feet, especially between the toes, after bathing.

  —Avoid wearing socks made from wool or synthetic materials (for example, rayon or nylon). Instead, wear clean, cotton socks and change them daily or more often if your feet sweat freely.

  —Wear well-ventilated shoes (for example, shoes with holes) or sandals.

  —Use a bland, absorbent powder (for example, talcum powder) or an antifungal powder freely between the toes, on the feet, and in socks and shoes once or twice a day. Be sure to use the powder after clotrimazole and betamethasone cream has been applied and has disappeared into the skin. Do not use the powder as the only treatment for your fungus infection.

  These measures will help keep the feet cool and dry.

- For patients using this medicine *for jock itch:*

  —Carefully dry the groin area after bathing.

  —Avoid wearing underwear that is tight-fitting or made from synthetic materials (for example, rayon or nylon). Instead, wear loose-fitting, cotton underwear.

  —Use a bland, absorbent powder (for example, talcum powder) or an antifungal powder freely once or twice a day. Be sure to use the powder after clotrimazole and betamethasone cream has been applied and has disappeared into the skin. Do not use the powder as the only treatment for your fungus infection.

  These measures will help reduce chafing and irritation and will also help keep the groin area cool and dry.

- For patients using this medicine *for ringworm of the body:*

  —Carefully dry yourself after bathing.

  —Avoid too much heat and humidity if possible. Try to keep moisture from building up on affected areas of the body.

  —Wear well-ventilated clothing.

  —Use a bland, absorbent powder (for example, talcum powder) or an antifungal powder freely once or twice a day. Be sure to use the powder after clotrimazole and betamethasone cream has been applied and has disappeared into the skin. Do not use the powder as the only treatment for your fungus infection.

  These measures will help keep the affected areas cool and dry.

If you have any questions about this, check with your doctor, nurse, or pharmacist.

For diabetic patients:

- *Rarely, the adrenocorticoid in this medicine may cause higher blood and urine sugar levels. This is more likely to occur if you have severe diabetes and are using large amounts of this medicine.* Check with your doctor before changing your diet or the dosage of your diabetes medicine.

Side Effects of This Medicine

Along with its needed effects, a medicine may cause some unwanted effects. Although not all of these side effects may occur, if they do occur they may need medical attention.

Check with your doctor immediately if any of the following side effects occur:

Less common

Blistering, burning, itching, peeling, dryness, redness, or other sign of skin irritation not present before use of this medicine

Additional side effects may occur if you use this medicine for a long time. Check with your doctor as soon as possible if any of the following side effects occur:

Acne or oily skin; increased hair growth, especially on the face; increased loss of hair, especially on the scalp; reddish purple lines on arms, face, legs, trunk, or groin; thinning of skin with easy bruising

Other side effects not listed above may also occur in some patients. If you notice any other effects, check with your doctor.

Annual revision: 02/10/92

CLOZAPINE Systemic

Some commonly used brand names are:

In the U.S. and Canada
Clozaril

Other
Leponex

Description

Clozapine (KLOE-za-peen) is used to treat schizophrenia in patients who have not been helped by or are unable to take other medicines.

Clozapine is only available from pharmacies that agree to participate with your doctor in a plan to monitor your blood tests. You will need to have blood tests done every week, and you will receive a 7-day supply of clozapine only if the results of your blood tests show that it is safe for you to take this medicine.

Clozapine is available in the following dosage form:

Oral
- Tablets (U.S. and Canada)

It is very important that you read and understand the following information. If any of it causes you special concern, check with your doctor. Also, *if you have any questions* or if you want more information about this medicine or your medical problem, *ask your doctor, nurse, or pharmacist.*

Before Using This Medicine

In deciding to use a medicine, the risks of taking the medicine must be weighed against the good it will do. This is a decision you and your doctor will make. For clozapine, the following should be considered:

Allergies—Tell your doctor if you have ever had any unusual or allergic reaction to clozapine. Also tell your doctor and pharmacist if you are allergic to any other substance, such as foods, preservatives, or dyes.

Pregnancy—Clozapine has not been studied in pregnant women. However, clozapine has not been shown to cause birth defects or other problems in animal studies.

Breast-feeding—Clozapine may pass into breast milk and cause sedation, decreased suckling, restlessness or irritability, seizures, or heart or blood vessel problems in nursing babies.

Children—Studies on this medicine have been done only in adult patients, and there is no specific information comparing use of clozapine in children with use in other age groups.

Older adults—Many medicines have not been tested in older people. Therefore, it may not be known whether they work exactly the same way they do in younger adults. Clozapine may be more likely to cause side effects in the elderly, including dizziness and fainting, low blood pressure, and confusion or excitement.

Other medicines—Although certain medicines should not be used together at all, in other cases 2 different medicines may be used together even if an interaction might occur. In these cases, your doctor may want to change the dose, or other precautions may be necessary. When you are taking clozapine, it is especially important that your doctor and pharmacist know if you are taking any of the following:

- Alcohol or
- Central nervous system (CNS) depressants (medicines that cause drowsiness) or
- Tricyclic antidepressants (medicine for depression)—Clozapine may cause an increase in sedation or effects on the heart, or increase the risk of seizures

- Amphotericin B by injection (e.g., Fungizone) or
- Antineoplastics (cancer medicine) or
- Antithyroid agents (medicine for overactive thyroid) or
- Azathioprine (e.g., Imuran) or
- Chlorambucil (e.g., Leukeran) or
- Chloramphenicol (e.g., Chloromycetin) or
- Colchicine or
- Cyclophosphamide (e.g., Cytoxan) or
- Flucytosine (e.g., Ancobon) or
- Interferon (e.g., Intron A, Roferon-A) or
- Mercaptopurine (e.g., Purinethol) or
- Methotrexate (e.g., Mexate) or
- Plicamycin (e.g., Mithracin) or
- Zidovudine (e.g., Retrovir)—Taking clozapine with any of these medicines may cause increased blood problems

- Lithium—Using clozapine with lithium may increase the risk of seizures, or cause confusion or body movement disorders

Other medical problems—The presence of other medical problems may affect the use of clozapine. Make sure you tell your doctor if you have any other medical problems, especially:

- Blood diseases or
- Enlarged prostate or difficult urination or
- Gastrointestinal problems or
- Heart or blood vessel problems—Clozapine may make the condition worse
- Epilepsy or other seizure disorder—Clozapine may increase the risk of seizures
- Kidney or liver disease—Higher blood levels of clozapine may occur, increasing the chance of side effects

Before you begin using any new medicine (prescription or nonprescription) or if you develop any new medical problem while you are using this medicine, check with your doctor, nurse, or pharmacist.

Proper Use of This Medicine

Take this medicine exactly as directed. Do not take more of this medicine and do not take it more often than your doctor ordered. Do not miss any doses.

This medicine has been prescribed for your current medical problem only. It must not be given to other people or used for other problems unless you are directed to do so by your doctor.

Missed dose—If you miss a dose of this medicine, take it as soon as possible. However, if it is almost time for your next dose, skip the missed dose and go back to your regular dosing schedule. Do not double doses.

Storage—To store this medicine:

- Keep out of the reach of children.
- Store away from heat and direct light.
- Do not store in the bathroom, near the kitchen sink, or in other damp places. Heat or moisture may cause the medicine to break down.
- Do not keep outdated medicine or medicine no longer needed. Be sure that any discarded medicine is out of the reach of children.

Precautions While Using This Medicine

It is important that you have your blood tests done weekly and that your doctor check your progress at regular visits. This will allow your doctor to make sure the medicine is working properly and to change the dosage if needed.

If you have been using this medicine regularly, do not stop taking it without first checking with your doctor. Your doctor may want you to reduce gradually the amount you are taking before stopping completely.

This medicine will add to the effects of alcohol and other CNS depressants (medicines that slow down the nervous system, possibly causing drowsiness). Some examples of CNS depressants are antihistamines or medicine for hay fever, other allergies, or colds; sedatives, tranquilizers, or sleeping medicine; prescription pain medicine or narcotics; barbiturates; medicine for seizures; muscle relaxants; or anesthetics, including some dental anesthetics. *Check with your doctor before taking any of the above while you are using this medicine.*

Clozapine may cause drowsiness, blurred vision or convulsions (seizures). *Do not drive, climb, swim, operate machines or do anything else that could be dangerous* while you are taking this medicine.

Dizziness, lightheadedness, or fainting may occur, especially when you get up from a lying or sitting position. Getting up slowly may help. If this problem continues or gets worse, check with your doctor.

In some patients, clozapine may cause increased watering of the mouth. Other patients, however, may get dryness of the mouth. For temporary relief of mouth dryness, use sugarless gum or candy, melt bits of ice in your mouth, or use a saliva substitute. However, if your mouth continues to feel dry for more than 2 weeks, check with your medical doctor or dentist. Continuing dryness of the mouth may increase the chance of dental disease, including tooth decay, gum disease, and fungus infections.

Side Effects of This Medicine

Along with its needed effects, a medicine may cause some unwanted effects. Although not all of these side effects may occur, if they do occur they may need medical attention.

Check with your doctor immediately if any of the following side effects occur:

More common

Fast or irregular heartbeat; fever; low blood pressure

Less common

High blood pressure

Rare

Chills; convulsions (seizures); difficult or fast breathing; increased sweating; loss of bladder control; muscle stiffness (severe); sore throat; sores, ulcers, or white spots on lips or in mouth; unusual bleeding or bruising; unusual tiredness or weakness; unusually pale skin

Check with your doctor as soon as possible if any of the following side effects occur:

More common

Dizziness or fainting

Less common

Blurred vision; confusion; restlessness or need to keep moving; trembling; unusual anxiety, nervousness, or irritability

Rare
- Absence of or decrease in movement; decreased sexual ability; difficulty in sleeping; difficulty in urinating; headache (severe or continuing); lip smacking or puckering; mental depression; puffing of cheeks; rapid or worm-like movements of tongue; uncontrolled chewing movements; uncontrolled movements of arms and legs

Symptoms of overdose
- Dizziness or fainting; drowsiness (severe); fast, slow, or irregular heartbeat; hallucinations (seeing, hearing, or feeling things that are not there); increased watering of mouth (severe); slow, irregular, or troubled breathing; unusual excitement, nervousness, or restlessness

Other side effects may occur that usually do not need medical attention. These side effects may go away during treatment as your body adjusts to the medicine. However, check with your doctor if any of the following side effects continue or are bothersome:

More common
- Constipation; dizziness or lightheadedness (mild); drowsiness; headache (mild); increased watering of mouth; nausea or vomiting; unusual weight gain

Less common
- Abdominal discomfort or heartburn; dryness of mouth

Other side effects not listed above may also occur in some patients. If you notice any other effects, check with your doctor.

Annual revision: 07/17/91
Interim revision: 03/25/92

COAL TAR Topical

Some commonly used brand names are:

In the U.S.

Alphosyl
Aquatar
Balnetar Therapeutic Tar Bath
Cutar Water Dispersible Emollient Tar
Denorex Extra Strength Medicated Shampoo
Denorex Extra Strength Medicated Shampoo with Conditioners
Denorex Medicated Shampoo
Denorex Medicated Shampoo and Conditioner
Denorex Mountain Fresh Herbal Scent Medicated Shampoo
DHS Tar Gel Shampoo
DHS Tar Shampoo
Doak Oil Forte Therapeutic Bath Treatment
Doak Oil Therapeutic Bath Treatment For All-Over Body Care
Doak Tar Lotion
Doak Tar Shampoo
Doctar Hair & Scalp Shampoo and Conditioner
Doctar Shampoo
Estar
Fototar
Ionil T Plus
Lavatar
Medotar
Pentrax Anti-Dandruff Tar Shampoo
Psorigel
PsoriNail Topical Solution
Taraphilic
Tarbonis
Tarpaste 'Doak'
T/Derm Tar Emollient
Tegrin Lotion for Psoriasis
Tegrin Medicated Cream Shampoo
Tegrin Medicated Shampoo Concentrated Gel
Tegrin Medicated Shampoo Extra Conditioning Formula
Tegrin Medicated Shampoo Herbal Formula
Tegrin Medicated Shampoo Original Formula
Tegrin Medicated Soap for Psoriasis
Tegrin Skin Cream for Psoriasis
Tersa-Tar Soapless Tar Shampoo
T/Gel Therapeutic Conditioner
T/Gel Therapeutic Shampoo
Theraplex T Shampoo
Zetar Emulsion
Zetar Medicated Antiseborrheic Shampoo

In Canada

Alphosyl
Balnetar
Denorex
Doak Oil
Doak Oil Forte
Estar
Lavatar
Liquor Carbonis Detergens
Pentrax Extra-Strength Therapeutic Tar Shampoo
Psorigel
Tar Doak
Tarpaste
Tersa-Tar Mild Therapeutic Shampoo with Protein and Conditioner
Tersa-Tar Therapeutic Shampoo
T-Gel
Zetar Emulsion
Zetar Shampoo

Description

Coal tar is used to treat eczema, psoriasis, seborrheic dermatitis, and other skin disorders.

Some of these preparations are available only with your doctor's prescription. Others are available without a prescription; however, your doctor may have special instructions on the proper use of coal tar for your medical condition.

Coal tar is available in the following dosage forms:

Topical
- Cleansing bar (U.S.)
- Cream (U.S. and Canada)
- Gel (U.S. and Canada)
- Lotion (U.S. and Canada)
- Ointment (U.S. and Canada)
- Shampoo (U.S. and Canada)
- Topical solution (U.S. and Canada)
- Topical suspension (U.S. and Canada)

It is very important that you read and understand the following information. If any of it causes you special concern, check with your doctor. Also, *if you have any questions* or if you want more information about this medicine or your medical problem, *ask your doctor, nurse, or pharmacist.*

Before Using This Medicine

If you are using this medicine without a prescription, carefully read and follow any precautions on the label. For coal tar, the following should be considered:

Allergies—Tell your doctor if you have ever had any unusual or allergic reaction to coal tar or to any other tar.

Also tell your doctor and pharmacist if you are allergic to any other substances, such as preservatives or dyes.

Pregnancy—Studies on effects in pregnancy have not been done in either humans or animals.

Breast-feeding—It is not known whether coal tar passes into the breast milk. However, this medicine has not been reported to cause problems in nursing babies.

Children—Coal tar products should not be used on infants, unless otherwise directed by your doctor. Studies on this medicine have been done only in adult patients, and there is no specific information comparing use of this medicine in children with use in other age groups.

Older adults—Many medicines have not been studied specifically in older people. Therefore, it may not be known whether they work exactly the same way they do in younger adults or if they cause different side effects or problems in older people. There is no specific information comparing use of this medicine in the elderly with use in other age groups.

Other medicines—Although certain medicines should not be used together at all, in other cases two different medicines may be used together even if an interaction might occur. In these cases, your doctor may want to change the dose, or other precautions may be necessary. Tell your doctor and pharmacist if you are using any other topical prescription or nonprescription (over-the-counter [OTC]) medicine that is to be applied to the same area of the skin.

Before you begin using any new medicine (prescription or nonprescription) or if you develop any new medical problem while you are using this medicine, check with your doctor, nurse, or pharmacist.

Proper Use of This Medicine

Use this medicine only as directed. Do not use more of it and do not use it more often than recommended on the label, unless otherwise directed by your doctor. To do so may increase the chance of side effects.

After applying coal tar, *protect the treated area from direct sunlight and do not use a sunlamp for 72 hours,* unless otherwise directed by your doctor, since a severe reaction may occur. Also, make sure you have removed all the coal tar medicine from your skin before you go back into direct sunlight or use a sunlamp.

Do not apply this medicine to infected, blistered, raw, or oozing areas of the skin.

Keep this medicine away from the eyes. If you should accidentally get some in your eyes, flush them thoroughly with water at once.

To use the *cream or ointment form* of this medicine:

- Apply enough medicine to cover the affected area, and rub in gently.

To use the *gel form* of this medicine:

- Apply enough gel to cover the affected area, and rub in gently. Allow the gel to remain on the affected area for 5 minutes, then remove excess gel by patting with a clean tissue.

To use the *shampoo form* of this medicine:

- Wet the scalp and hair with lukewarm water. Apply a generous amount of shampoo and rub into the scalp, then rinse. Apply the shampoo again, working up a rich lather, and allow to remain on the scalp for 5 minutes. Then rinse thoroughly.

To use the *nonshampoo liquid form* of this medicine:

- Some of these preparations are to be applied directly to dry or wet skin, some are to be added to lukewarm bath water, and some may be applied directly to dry or wet skin or added to lukewarm bath water. Make sure you know exactly how you should use this medicine. If you have any questions about this, check with your doctor or pharmacist.
- If this medicine is to be applied directly to the skin, apply enough to cover the affected area, and rub in gently.
- Some of these preparations contain alcohol and are flammable. Do not use near heat, near open flame, or while smoking.

Missed dose—If you miss a dose of this medicine, apply it as soon as possible. However, if it is almost time for your next dose, skip the missed dose and go back to your regular dosing schedule. Do not double doses.

Storage—To store this medicine:

- Keep out of the reach of children.
- Store away from heat and direct light.
- Keep the medicine from freezing.
- Do not keep outdated medicine or medicine no longer needed. Be sure that any discarded medicine is out of the reach of children.

Precautions While Using This Medicine

If this medicine is used on the scalp, it may temporarily discolor blond, bleached, or tinted hair.

Coal tar may stain the skin or clothing. Avoid getting it on your clothing. The stain on the skin will wear off after you stop using the medicine.

Side Effects of This Medicine

In animal studies, coal tar has been shown to increase the chance of skin cancer.

Along with its needed effects, a medicine may cause some unwanted effects. Although not all of these side effects may occur, if they do occur they may need medical attention.

Check with your doctor as soon as possible if either of the following side effects occurs:

Rare

Skin irritation not present before use of this medicine; skin rash

Other side effects may occur that usually do not need medical attention. These side effects may go away during treatment as your body adjusts to the medicine. However, check with your doctor or pharmacist if the following side effect continues or is bothersome:

More common

Stinging (mild)—especially for gel and solution dosage forms

Other side effects not listed above may also occur in some patients. If you notice any other effects, check with your doctor or pharmacist.

Annual revision: 03/04/92
Interim revision: 05/07/92

COCAINE Mucosal-Local

Description

Cocaine (KOE-kane) is a local anesthetic. It is applied to certain areas of the body (for example, the nose, mouth, or throat) to cause loss of feeling. This allows some kinds of examinations or surgery to be done without causing pain.

Cocaine can cause psychological dependence (a strong desire to continue using the medicine because of the "high" feeling it produces). This may lead to cocaine abuse (more frequent use and/or use of larger amounts of cocaine) and to an increased chance of serious side effects. Cocaine abuse has caused death from heart or breathing failure.

Use of cocaine as a local anesthetic for an examination or surgery is not likely to cause psychological dependence or other serious side effects. However, if cocaine is absorbed into the body too quickly, serious side effects can occur. Also, some people are especially sensitive to the effects of cocaine. Unwanted effects may occur in these people even with small amounts of the medicine. Before receiving cocaine as a local anesthetic, you should discuss its use with your doctor.

Cocaine is applied only by or under the immediate supervision of your doctor. It is available in the following dosage forms:

Mucosal-Local

- Crystals (U.S. and Canada)
- Solution (U.S.)

Before Receiving This Medicine

In deciding to use a medicine, the risks of taking the medicine must be weighed against the good it will do. This is a decision you and your doctor will make. For cocaine, the following should be considered:

Allergies—Tell your doctor if you have ever had any unusual or allergic reaction to cocaine. Also tell your doctor and pharmacist if you are allergic to any other substances, such as foods, preservatives, or dyes.

Pregnancy—Studies on birth defects or other problems have not been done in pregnant women receiving cocaine as a local anesthetic. However, studies in women who abused cocaine during pregnancy have shown that cocaine may cause birth defects, decreased birth weight and size, and problems affecting the baby's nervous system. These studies have also shown that too much use of cocaine may cause the baby to be born too soon, sometimes too soon to survive. Cocaine has also been shown to cause birth defects and other unwanted effects in animal studies.

Breast-feeding—Cocaine passes into the breast milk and may cause unwanted effects such as convulsions (seizures), high blood pressure, fast heartbeat, breathing problems, trembling, and unusual irritability in nursing babies. Therefore, after receiving this medicine you should stop breast-feeding your baby for about 2 days.

Children—Cocaine can cause serious side effects in any patient. Therefore, it is especially important that you discuss with the child's doctor the good that this medicine may do as well as the risks of using it.

Older adults—Side effects, including dizziness or lightheadedness or fast or irregular heartbeat, may be especially likely to occur in elderly patients, who are usually more sensitive than younger adults to the effects of cocaine.

Other medicines—Although certain medicines should not be used together at all, in other cases two different medicines may be used together even if an interaction might

occur. In these cases, your doctor may want to change the dose, or other precautions may be necessary. When you are receiving cocaine, it is especially important that your doctor and pharmacist know if you are taking any of the following:

- Amantadine (e.g., Symmetrel) or
- Amphetamines or
- Antimyasthenics (ambenonium [e.g., Mytelase], neostigmine [e.g., Prostigmin], pyridostigmine [e.g., Mestinon]) or
- Appetite suppressants (diet pills), except fenfluramine (e.g., Pondimin), or
- Beta-blockers (acebutolol [e.g., Sectral], atenolol [e.g., Tenormin], betaxolol [e.g., Kerlone], carteolol [e.g., Cartrol], labetalol [e.g., Normodyne], metoprolol [e.g., Lopressor], nadolol [e.g., Corgard], oxprenolol [e.g., Trasicor], penbutolol [e.g., Levatol], pindolol [e.g., Visken], propranolol [e.g., Inderal], sotalol [e.g., Sotacor], timolol [e.g., Blocadren]) or
- Betaxolol (ophthalmic) (e.g., Betoptic) or
- Caffeine (e.g., NoDoz) or
- Chlophedianol (e.g., Ulone) or
- Cyclophosphamide (e.g., Cytoxan) or
- Demecarium (e.g., Humorsol) or
- Echothiophate (e.g., Phospholine Iodide) or
- Guanadrel (e.g., Hylorel) or
- Guanethidine (e.g., Ismelin) or
- Isoflurophate (e.g., Floropryl) or
- Levobunolol (e.g., Betagan) or
- Levodopa (e.g., Dopar) or
- Malathion (e.g., Prioderm) or
- Medicine for asthma or other breathing problems or
- Medicine for colds, sinus problems, or hay fever or other allergies (including nose drops or sprays) or
- Methyldopa (e.g., Aldomet) or
- Methylphenidate (e.g., Ritalin) or
- Metipranolol (e.g., OptiPranolol) or
- Nabilone (e.g., Cesamet) or
- Pemoline (e.g., Cylert) or
- Thiotepa or
- Timolol (ophthalmic) (e.g., Timoptic)—The chance of serious side effects may be increased
- Monoamine oxidase (MAO) inhibitors (furazolidone [e.g., Furoxone], isocarboxazid [e.g., Marplan], phenelzine [e.g., Nardil], procarbazine [e.g., Matulane], selegiline [e.g., Eldepryl], tranylcypromine [e.g., Parnate])—Receiving cocaine while you are taking or within 2 weeks after you have taken an MAO inhibitor may increase the chance of serious side effects.

Also tell your doctor if you have recently used an insecticide (insect killer) or if you have been in an area that was recently treated with an insecticide. Some insecticides can slow the breakdown of cocaine in your body. This increases the chance of serious side effects.

Other medical problems—The presence of other medical problems may affect the use of cocaine. Make sure you tell your doctor if you have any other medical problems, especially:

- Cancer or
- Chest pain, or history of, or
- Convulsions (seizures), history of, or
- Fast or irregular heartbeat or
- Heart or blood vessel disease or
- High blood pressure or
- Liver disease or
- Myocardial infarction ("heart attack"), history of, or
- Overactive thyroid—The chance of serious side effects may be increased
- Tourette's syndrome—Cocaine can make your condition worse

Precautions After Receiving This Medicine

Cocaine and some of its metabolites (substances to which cocaine is broken down in the body) will appear in your blood and urine for several days after you have received the medicine. Tests for possible drug use will then be "positive" for cocaine. If you must have such a test within 5 days or so after receiving cocaine, be sure to tell the person in charge that you have recently received cocaine for medical reasons. It may be helpful to have written information from your doctor stating why the medicine was used, the date on which you received it, and the amount you received.

Side Effects of This Medicine

Along with its needed effects, a medicine may cause some unwanted effects. Although not all of these side effects may occur, if they do occur they may need medical attention.

After cocaine has been applied, your doctor or nurse will closely follow its effects. However, *tell your doctor or nurse immediately* if any of the following side effects occur:

Signs and symptoms of too much medicine being absorbed into the body

Abdominal or stomach pain; chills; confusion; dizziness or lightheadedness; excitement, nervousness, restlessness, or any mood or mental changes; fast or irregular heartbeat; general feeling of discomfort or illness; hallucinations (seeing, hearing, or feeling things that are not there); headache (sudden); increased sweating; nausea

Other side effects may occur that usually do not need medical attention. However, check with your doctor if the following side effects continue or are bothersome:

More common

Loss of sense of taste or smell (after application to the nose or mouth)

Other side effects not listed above may also occur in some patients. If you notice any other effects, *tell your doctor or nurse immediately*.

Annual revision: 08/08/92

COLCHICINE Systemic

Description

Colchicine (KOL-chi-seen) is used to prevent or treat attacks of gout or gouty arthritis. Some patients take it only when an attack occurs, to relieve inflammation, pain, and swelling. Other patients take small amounts of it regularly every day to prevent an attack from occurring.

Colchicine may also be used for other conditions as determined by your doctor. For some of these conditions, colchicine is taken only when an attack occurs. For other conditions, the medicine is taken regularly every day. If you are taking colchicine for one of these other conditions, the information about gout will not apply to you. However, your doctor may have other instructions for you to follow.

In addition to its helpful effects in treating your medical problem, colchicine has side effects that can be very serious. Before you take colchicine, you should discuss with your doctor the good that this medicine will do as well as the risks of using it. Make sure that you understand exactly how you are to use this medicine, and follow the instructions very carefully, to lessen the chance of unwanted effects.

This medicine is available only with your doctor's prescription, in the following dosage forms:

Oral

- Tablets (U.S. and Canada)

Parenteral

- Injection (U.S.)

It is very important that you read and understand the following information. If any of it causes you special concern, check with your doctor. Also, *if you have any questions* or if you want more information about this medicine or your medical problem, *ask your doctor, nurse, or pharmacist.*

Before Using This Medicine

In deciding to use a medicine, the risks of taking the medicine must be weighed against the good it will do. This is a decision you and your doctor will make. For colchicine, the following should be considered:

Allergies—Tell your doctor if you have ever had any unusual or allergic reaction to colchicine. Also tell your doctor and pharmacist if you are allergic to any other substances, such as foods, preservatives, or dyes.

Pregnancy—Although studies in humans have not been done, some reports have suggested that use of colchicine during pregnancy can cause harm to the fetus. Also, this medicine has been shown to cause birth defects in animal studies. Therefore, do not begin taking colchicine during pregnancy, and do not become pregnant while taking it, unless you have first discussed this problem with your doctor. Also, check with your doctor at once if you suspect that you have become pregnant while taking colchicine.

Breast-feeding—It is not known whether colchicine passes into the breast milk. However, this medicine has not been reported to cause problems in nursing babies.

Children—Studies on this medicine have been done only in adult patients and there is no specific information about the use of colchicine in children.

Older adults—Elderly people are especially sensitive to the effects of colchicine. This may increase the chance of side effects during treatment.

Other medicines—Although certain medicines should not be used together at all, in other cases two different medicines may be used together even if an interaction might occur. In these cases, your doctor may want to change the dose, or other precautions may be necessary. When you are taking colchicine, it is especially important that your doctor and pharmacist know if you are taking any of the following:

- Acyclovir (e.g., Zovirax) or
- Amphotericin B by injection (e.g., Fungizone) or
- Anticonvulsants (seizure medicine) or
- Antidiabetics, oral (diabetes medicine you take by mouth) or
- Anti-infectives by mouth or by injection (medicine for infection) or
- Antineoplastics (cancer medicine) or
- Antipsychotics (medicine for mental illness) or
- Antithyroid agents (medicine for overactive thyroid) or
- Azathioprine (e.g., Imuran) or
- Captopril (e.g., Capoten) or
- Carbamazepine (e.g., Tegretol) or
- Chloramphenicol (e.g., Chloromycetin) or
- Cyclophosphamide (e.g., Cytoxan) or
- Enalapril (e.g., Vasotec) or
- Flecainide (e.g., Tambocor) or
- Flucytosine (e.g., Ancobon) or
- Gold salts or
- Imipenem or
- Interferon (e.g., Intron A, Roferon-A) or
- Lisinopril (e.g., Prinvil, Vestril) or
- Maprotiline (e.g., Ludiomil) or
- Medicine for inflammation or pain (except narcotics) or
- Mercaptopurine (e.g., Purinethol) or
- Methotrexate (e.g., Mexate) or
- Penicillamine (e.g., Cuprimine) or
- Phenylbutazone (e.g., Butazolidin) or
- Pimozide (e.g., Orap) or
- Plicamycin (e.g., Mithracin) or
- Procainamide (e.g., Pronestyl) or
- Promethazine (e.g., Phenergan) or
- Radiation (x-ray) treatment, current or recent, or
- Sulfasalazine (e.g., Azulfidine) or

- Tocainide (e.g., Tonocard) or
- Trimeprazine (e.g., Temaril) or
- Tricyclic antidepressants (amitriptyline [e.g., Elavil], amoxapine [e.g., Asendin], clomipramine [e.g., Anafranil], desipramine [e.g., Pertofrane], doxepin [e.g., Sinequan], imipramine [e.g., Tofranil], nortriptyline [e.g., Aventyl], protriptyline [e.g., Vivactil], trimipramine [e.g., Surmontil]) or
- Zidovudine (e.g., Retrovir)—The chance of serious side effects may be increased

Other medical problems—The presence of other medical problems may affect the use of colchicine. Make sure you tell your doctor if you have any other medical problems, especially:

- Alcohol abuse or
- Blood disease or
- Heart disease or
- Intestinal disease (severe) or
- Kidney disease (severe) or
- Liver disease or
- Stomach ulcer or other stomach problems—The chance of serious side effects may be increased

Proper Use of This Medicine

For patients *taking colchicine only when an attack occurs:*

- Start taking it at the first sign of the attack for best results.
- *Stop taking this medicine as soon as the pain is relieved or at the first sign of nausea, vomiting, stomach pain, or diarrhea.* Also, stop taking colchicine when you have taken the largest amount that your doctor ordered for each attack, even if the pain is not relieved or none of these side effects occurs.
- Unless otherwise directed by your doctor, *do not take colchicine more often than every three days.*
- If you are taking colchicine for an attack of gout, and you are also taking other medicine for gout, *do not stop taking the other medicine.* Continue taking the other medicine as directed by your doctor.

For patients taking colchicine regularly to *prevent gout attacks:*

- You should increase the dose you normally take at the first sign of an attack as advised by your doctor.
- *Stop taking the larger dose of medicine as soon as the gout pain is relieved or at the first sign of nausea, vomiting, stomach pain, or diarrhea.*
- After the gout attack is over, start taking the lower dose of colchicine again as ordered by your doctor.

Take this medicine only as directed by your doctor. Do not take more of it, do not take it more often, and do not take it for a longer time than your doctor ordered. To do so may cause serious side effects. This is especially important for elderly patients, who are more sensitive than younger adults to the effects of colchicine.

Missed dose—If you are taking colchicine regularly (for example, every day) and you miss a dose of this medicine, take it as soon as possible. However, if it is almost time for your next dose, skip the missed dose and go back to your regular dosing schedule. Do not double doses.

Storage—To store this medicine:

- Keep out of the reach of children.
- Store away from heat and direct light.
- Do not store this medicine in the bathroom, near the kitchen sink, or in other damp places. Heat or moisture may cause the medicine to break down.
- Do not keep outdated medicine or medicine no longer needed. Be sure that any discarded medicine is out of the reach of children.

Precautions While Using This Medicine

If you will be taking colchicine for more than a few days at a time, your doctor should check your progress at regular visits.

Stomach problems may be more likely to occur if you drink large amounts of alcoholic beverages while taking colchicine. Also, drinking too much alcohol may increase the amount of uric acid in your blood. This may lessen the effects of colchicine when it is used to treat gout. Therefore, *do not drink alcoholic beverages while you are taking this medicine,* unless you have first checked with your doctor.

Side Effects of This Medicine

Along with its needed effects, a medicine may cause some unwanted effects. Although not all of these side effects may occur, if they do occur they may need medical attention.

Stop taking this medicine immediately if any of the following side effects occur:

More common

Diarrhea; nausea or vomiting; stomach pain

If any of these side effects continue for 3 hours or longer after you have stopped taking colchicine, check with your doctor.

Also, *check with your doctor immediately* if any of the following side effects occur:

Rare

Redness, swelling, or pain at place of injection

With long-term use

Bloody, black, or tarry stools; numbness, tingling, pain, or weakness in hands or feet; pinpoint red spots on skin; skin rash; sore throat, fever, and chills; unusual bleeding or bruising; unusual tiredness or weakness

Signs and symptoms of overdose
Bloody urine; burning feeling in stomach, throat, or skin; convulsions (seizures); diarrhea (severe or bloody); fever; mood or mental changes; muscle weakness (severe); sudden decrease in amount of urine; troubled breathing; vomiting (severe)

Other side effects may occur that usually do not need medical attention. However, check with your doctor if either of the following side effects continues or is bothersome:

Less common
Loss of appetite

With long-term use
Loss of hair

Other side effects not listed above may also occur in some patients. If you notice any other effects, check with your doctor.

Annual revision: June 1990

COLESTIPOL Oral

A commonly used brand name is:
In the U.S.
Colestid
In Canada
Colestid

Description

Colestipol (koe-LES-ti-pole) is used to lower high cholesterol levels in the blood. This may help prevent medical problems caused by cholesterol clogging the blood vessels.

Colestipol works by attaching to certain substances in the intestine. Since colestipol is not absorbed into the body, these substances also pass out of the body without being absorbed.

Colestipol may also be used for other conditions as determined by your doctor.

Colestipol is available only with your doctor's prescription, in the following dosage form:

Oral
- Powder (U.S. and Canada)

It is very important that you read and understand the following information. If any of it causes you special concern, check with your doctor. Also, *if you have any questions* or if you want more information about this medicine or your medical problem, *ask your doctor, nurse, or pharmacist.*

Before Using This Medicine

In deciding to use a medicine, the risks of taking the medicine must be weighed against the good it will do. This is a decision you and your doctor will make. For colestipol, the following should be considered:

Allergies—Tell your doctor if you have ever had any unusual or allergic reaction to colestipol. Also tell your doctor and pharmacist if you are allergic to any substances, such as foods, preservatives, or dyes.

Diet—Before prescribing medicine for your condition, your doctor will probably try to control your condition by prescribing a personal diet for you. Such a diet may be low in fats, sugars, and/or cholesterol. Many people are able to control their condition by carefully following their doctor's orders for proper diet and exercise. Medicine is prescribed only when additional help is needed and is effective only when a schedule of diet and exercise is properly followed.

Also, this medicine is less effective if you are greatly overweight. It may be very important for you to go on a reducing diet. However, check with your doctor before going on any diet.

Make certain your doctor and pharmacist know if you are on a low-sodium, low-sugar, or any other special diet.

Pregnancy—Colestipol is not absorbed into the body and is not likely to cause problems. However, it may reduce absorption of vitamins into the body. Ask your doctor whether you need to take extra vitamins.

Breast-feeding—Colestipol is not absorbed into the body and is not likely to cause problems.

Children—There is no specific information comparing use of colestipol in children with use in other age groups. However, use is not recommended in children under 2 years of age since cholesterol is needed for normal development.

Older adults—Side effects may be more likely to occur in patients over 60 years of age, who are usually more sensitive to the effects of colestipol.

Other medicines—Although certain medicines should not be used together at all, in other cases two different medicines may be used together even if an interaction might occur. In these cases, your doctor may want to change the dose, or other precautions may be necessary. When

taking colestipol it is especially important that your doctor and pharmacist know if you are taking any of the following:

- Anticoagulants (blood thinners)—The effects of the anticoagulant may be altered
- Digitalis glycosides (heart medicine) or
- Diuretics (water pills) or
- Penicillin G, taken by mouth, or
- Propranolol, taken by mouth, or
- Tetracyclines (medicine for infection), taken by mouth, or
- Thyroid hormones or
- Vancomycin, taken by mouth—Colestipol may cause these medicines to be less effective; these medicines should be taken 4 to 5 hours apart from colestipol

Other medical problems—The presence of other medical problems may affect the use of colestipol. Make sure you tell your doctor if you have any other medical problems, especially:

- Bleeding problems or
- Constipation or
- Gallstones or
- Heart or blood vessel disease or
- Hemorrhoids or
- Stomach ulcer or other stomach problems or
- Underactive thyroid—Colestipol may make these conditions worse
- Kidney disease—There is an increased risk of developing electrolyte problems
- Liver disease—Cholesterol levels may be raised

Before you begin using any new medicine (prescription or nonprescription) or if you develop any new medical problem while you are using this medicine, check with your doctor, nurse, or pharmacist.

Proper Use of This Medicine

Take this medicine exactly as directed by your doctor. Try not to miss any doses and do not take more medicine than your doctor ordered.

Follow carefully the special diet your doctor gave you. This is the most important part of controlling your condition and is necessary if the medicine is to work properly.

This medicine should never be taken in its dry form, since it could cause you to choke. Instead, always mix as follows:

- Add this medicine to 3 ounces or more of water, milk, flavored drink, or your favorite juice or carbonated drink. If you use a carbonated drink, slowly mix in the powder in a large glass to prevent too much foaming. Stir until it is completely mixed (it will *not* dissolve) before drinking. After drinking all the liquid containing the medicine, rinse the glass with a little more liquid and drink that also, to make sure you get all the medicine.
- You may also mix this medicine with milk in hot or regular breakfast cereals, or in thin soups such as tomato or chicken noodle soup. Or you may add it to some pulpy fruits such as crushed pineapple, pears, peaches, or fruit cocktail.

Missed dose—If you miss a dose of this medicine, take it as soon as possible. Then go back to your regular dosing schedule. However, if it is almost time for your next dose, skip the missed dose and go back to your regular dosing schedule. Do not double doses.

Storage—To store this medicine:

- Keep out of the reach of children.
- Store away from heat and direct light.
- Do not store in the bathroom, near the kitchen sink or in other damp places. Heat or moisture may cause the medicine to break down.
- Do not keep outdated medicine or medicine no longer needed. Be sure that any discarded medicine is out of the reach of children.

Precautions While Using This Medicine

It is very important that your doctor check your progress at regular visits. This will allow your doctor to see if the medicine is working properly to lower your cholesterol levels and to decide if you should continue to take it.

Do not stop taking this medicine without first checking with your doctor. When you stop taking this medicine, your blood cholesterol levels may increase again. Your doctor may want you to follow a special diet to help prevent this from happening.

Do not take any other medicine unless prescribed by your doctor since colestipol may interfere with other medicines.

Side Effects of This Medicine

Along with its needed effects, a medicine may cause some unwanted effects. Although not all of these side effects may occur, if they do occur they may need medical attention.

Check with your doctor immediately if either of the following side effects occurs:

Rare

Black, tarry stools; stomach pain (severe) with nausea and vomiting

Check with your doctor as soon as possible if either of the following side effects occurs:

More common

Constipation

Rare
Loss of weight (sudden)

Other side effects may occur that usually do not need medical attention. These side effects may go away during treatment as your body adjusts to the medicine. However, check with your doctor if any of the following side effects continue or are bothersome:

Less common
Belching; bloating; diarrhea; dizziness; headache; nausea or vomiting; stomach pain

Other side effects not listed above may also occur in some patients. If you notice any other effects, check with your doctor.

Additional Information

Once a medicine has been approved for marketing for a certain use, experience may show that it is also useful for other medical problems. Although these uses are not included in product labeling, colestipol is used in certain patients with the following medical conditions:

- Diarrhea caused by bile acids
- Digitalis glycoside overdose
- Excess oxalate in the urine
- Itching (pruritus) associated with partial biliary obstruction

Other than the above information, there is no additional information relating to proper use, precautions, or side effects for these uses.

Annual revision: 10/21/92

COLISTIN, NEOMYCIN, AND HYDROCORTISONE Otic

Some commonly used brand names are:

In the U.S.
Coly-Mycin S Otic

In Canada
Coly-Mycin Otic

Description

Colistin (koe-LIS-tin), neomycin (nee-oh-MYE-sin), and hydrocortisone (hye-droe-KOR-ti-sone) combination contains two antibiotics and a cortisone-like medicine. It is used in the ear to treat infections of the ear canal and to help provide relief from redness, irritation, and discomfort of certain ear problems.

Colistin, neomycin, and hydrocortisone combination is available only with your doctor's prescription, in the following dosage form:

Otic
- Suspension (U.S. and Canada)

It is very important that you read and understand the following information. If any of it causes you special concern, check with your doctor. Also, *if you have any questions* or if you want more information about this medicine or your medical problem, *ask your doctor, nurse, or pharmacist.*

Before Using This Medicine

In deciding to use a medicine, the risks of taking the medicine must be weighed against the good it will do. This is a decision you and your doctor will make. For colistin, neomycin, and hydrocortisone combination, the following should be considered:

Allergies—Tell your doctor if you have ever had any unusual or allergic reaction to this medicine or to any related antibiotics such as amikacin (e.g., Amikin), colistin by mouth or by injection (e.g., Coly-Mycin), gentamicin (e.g., Garamycin), kanamycin (e.g., Kantrex), neomycin by mouth or by injection (e.g., Mycifradin), netilmicin (e.g., Netromycin), paromomycin (e.g., Humatin), polymyxin B (e.g., Aerosporin), streptomycin, or tobramycin (e.g., Nebcin). Also tell your doctor and pharmacist if you are allergic to any other substances, such as preservatives.

Pregnancy—Colistin, neomycin, and hydrocortisone otic drops have not been shown to cause birth defects or other problems in humans.

Breast-feeding—Colistin, neomycin, and hydrocortisone otic drops have not been reported to cause problems in nursing babies.

Children—Although there is no specific information comparing use of colistin, neomycin, and hydrocortisone combination in children with use in other age groups, this medicine is not expected to cause different side effects or problems in children than it does in adults.

Older adults—Many medicines have not been studied specifically in older people. Therefore, it may not be known whether they work exactly the same way they do in younger adults. Although there is no specific information comparing use of colistin, neomycin, and hydrocortisone combination in the elderly with use in other age groups, this medicine is not expected to cause different side effects or problems in older people than it does in younger adults.

Other medicines—Although certain medicines should not be used together at all, in other cases two different medicines may be used together even if an interaction might occur. In these cases, your doctor may want to change the dose, or other precautions may be necessary. Tell your doctor and pharmacist if you are using any other prescription or nonprescription (over-the-counter [OTC]) medicine that is to be used in the ear.

Other medical problems—The presence of other medical problems may affect the use of colistin, neomycin, and hydrocortisone combination. Make sure you tell your doctor if you have any other medical problems, especially:

- Other ear infection or problem, including punctured eardrum—Use of colistin, neomycin, and hydrocortisone combination may make the condition worse or may increase the chance of side effects
- Herpes simplex—Use of hydrocortisone may make the condition worse

Before you begin using any new medicine (prescription or nonprescription) or if you develop any new medical problem while you are using this medicine, check with your doctor, nurse, or pharmacist.

Proper Use of This Medicine

Before applying this medicine, thoroughly clean the ear canal and dry it with a sterile cotton applicator.

You may warm the ear drops to body temperature (37 °C or 98.6 °F), but no higher, by holding the bottle in your hand for a few minutes before applying. If this medicine gets too warm, it may break down and not work properly.

To apply this medicine:

- Lie down or tilt the head so that the infected ear faces up. Gently pull the earlobe up and back for adults (down and back for children) to straighten the ear canal. Drop the medicine into the ear canal. Keep the ear facing up for about 5 minutes to allow the medicine to come into contact with the infection. A sterile cotton plug may be gently inserted into the ear opening to prevent the medicine from leaking out. However, your doctor may want you to keep a sterile cotton plug moistened with this medicine in your ear for the full time of treatment. If you have any questions about this, check with your doctor.

To keep the medicine as germ-free as possible, do not touch the dropper to any surface (including the ear). Also, keep the container tightly closed.

Do not use this medicine for more than 10 days unless otherwise directed by your doctor.

To help clear up your infection completely, *keep using this medicine for the full time of treatment,* even if your symptoms begin to clear up after a few days. If you stop using this medicine too soon, your symptoms may return. *Do not miss any doses.*

Missed dose—If you do miss a dose of this medicine, apply it as soon as possible. However, if it is almost time for your next dose, skip the missed dose and go back to your regular dosing schedule.

Storage—To store this medicine:

- Keep out of the reach of children.
- Store away from heat and direct light.
- Keep the medicine from freezing
- Do not keep outdated medicine or medicine no longer needed. Be sure that any discarded medicine is out of the reach of children.

Precautions While Using This Medicine

If your symptoms do not improve within 1 week, or if they become worse, check with your doctor immediately.

Side Effects of This Medicine

Along with its needed effects, a medicine may cause some unwanted effects. Although not all of these side effects may occur, if they do occur they may need medical attention.

Check with your doctor immediately if any of the following side effects occur:

More common

Itching, skin rash, redness, swelling, or other sign of irritation not present before use of this medicine

Other side effects not listed above may also occur in some patients. If you notice any other effects, check with your doctor.

Annual revision: 02/10/92
Interim revision: 04/13/92

COLONY STIMULATING FACTORS Systemic

This information applies to the following medicines:

Filgrastim (fil-GRA-stim)
Sargramostim (sar-GRAM-o-stim)

Some commonly used brand names are:

For Filgrastim

In the U.S.
Neupogen

In Canada
Neupogen

Another commonly used name is granulocyte colony stimulating factor (G-CSF).

For Sargramostim†

In the U.S.
Leukine

Another commonly used name is granulocyte-macrophage colony stimulating factor (GM-CSF).

†Not commercially available in Canada.

Description

Filgrastim and sargramostim are synthetic (man-made) versions of substances naturally produced in your body. These substances, called colony stimulating factors, help the bone marrow to make new white blood cells.

When certain cancer medicines fight your cancer cells, they also affect those white blood cells that fight infection. To help prevent infections when these cancer medicines are used, colony stimulating factors may also be given.

Colony stimulating factors are available only with your doctor's prescription, in the following dosage form:

Parenteral
- Filgrastim
  - Injection (U.S. and Canada)
- Sargramostim
  - Injection (U.S.)

It is very important that you read and understand the following information. If any of it causes you special concern, check with your doctor. Also, *if you have any questions* or if you want more information about this medicine or your medical problem, *ask your doctor, nurse, or pharmacist.*

Before Using This Medicine

In deciding to use a medicine, the risks of taking the medicine must be weighed against the good it will do. This is a decision you and your doctor will make. For colony stimulating factors, the following should be considered:

Allergies—Tell your doctor if you have ever had any unusual or allergic reaction to the colony stimulating factor. Also tell your doctor and pharmacist if you are allergic to any other substances, such as foods, preservatives, or dyes.

Pregnancy—Colony stimulating factors have not been studied in pregnant women.

- *Filgrastim*—In studies in rabbits, filgrastim did not cause birth defects but did cause internal defects, a decrease in average weight, and death of the fetus in high doses.
- *Sargramostim*—Studies on birth defects have not been done in animals.

Breast-feeding—It is not known whether colony stimulating factors pass into the breast milk. However, these medicines have not been reported to cause problems in nursing babies.

Children—Although there is no specific information comparing use of colony stimulating factors in children with use in other age groups, this medicine is not expected to cause different side effects or problems in children than it does in adults.

Older adults—Many medicines have not been studied specifically in older people. Therefore, it may not be known whether they work exactly the same way they do in younger adults. Although there is no specific information comparing use of colony stimulating factors in the elderly with use in other age groups, this medicine has been used in many elderly patients and is not expected to cause different side effects or problems in older people than it does in younger adults.

Other medicines—Although certain medicines should not be used together at all, in other cases two different medicines may be used together even if an interaction might occur. In these cases, your doctor may want to change the dose, or other precautions may be necessary. Tell your doctor and pharmacist if you are taking any other prescription or nonprescription (over-the-counter [OTC]) medicine.

Other medical problems—The presence of other medical problems may affect the use of colony stimulating factors. Make sure you tell your doctor if you have any other medical problems, especially:

- Conditions caused by inflammation or immune system problems—There is a chance these may be worsened by colony stimulating factor
- Heart disease—Risk of some unwanted effects (heart rhythm problems, retaining water) may be increased
- Kidney disease or
- Liver disease—May sometimes be worsened by colony stimulating factor
- Lung disease—Colony stimulating factor may cause shortness of breath

Before you begin using any new medicine (prescription or nonprescription) or if you develop any new medical

problem while you are using this medicine, check with your doctor, nurse, or pharmacist.

Proper Use of This Medicine

If you are injecting this medicine yourself, *use it exactly as directed by your doctor.* Do not use more or less of it, and do not use it more often than your doctor ordered. The exact amount of medicine you need has been carefully worked out. Using too much will increase the risk of side effects, while using too little may not improve your condition.

If you are injecting this medicine yourself, each package of colony stimulating factor will contain a patient instruction sheet. Read this sheet carefully and make sure you understand:

- How to prepare the injection.
- Proper use of disposable syringes.
- How to give the injection.
- How long the injection is stable.

If you have any questions about any of this, check with your doctor, nurse or pharmacist.

Missed dose—If you miss a dose of this medicine, check with your doctor.

Storage—To store this medicine:

- Keep out of the reach of children.
- Store in the refrigerator.
- Keep the medicine from freezing.
- Do not keep outdated medicine or medicine no longer needed. Ask your doctor or pharmacist how you should dispose of any medicine you do not use. Be sure that any discarded medicine is out of the reach of children.

Precautions While Using This Medicine

It is very important that your doctor check your progress at regular visits to make sure that this medicine is working properly and to check for unwanted effects.

Colony stimulating factors are used to prevent or reduce the risk of infection while you are being treated with cancer medicines. Because your body's ability to fight infection is reduced, *it is very important that you call your doctor at the first sign of any infection* (for example, if you get a fever or chills) so you can start antibiotic treatment right away.

Colony stimulating factors commonly cause mild bone pain, usually in the lower back or pelvis, about the time the white blood cells start to come back in your bone marrow. The pain is usually mild and lasts only a few days. Your doctor will probably prescribe a mild analgesic (painkiller) for you to take during that time. If you find that the analgesic is not strong enough, talk with your doctor about using something that will make you more comfortable.

Side Effects of This Medicine

Along with its needed effects, a medicine may cause some unwanted effects. Although not all of these side effects may occur, if they do occur they may need medical attention.

The side effects listed below include only those that might be caused by colony stimulating factors. To find out about other side effects that may be caused by the cancer medicines you are also receiving, look under the information about those specific medicines.

Check with your doctor as soon as possible if any of the following side effects occur:

For filgrastim

Less common

Redness or pain at the site of subcutaneous (under the skin) injection

Rare

Fever; rapid or irregular heartbeat; sores on skin; wheezing

For sargramostim

Less common

Fever; redness or pain at the site of subcutaneous (under the skin) injection; shortness of breath; swelling of feet or lower legs; weight gain (sudden)

Rare

Chest pain; rapid or irregular heartbeat; sores on skin; wheezing

Other side effects may occur that usually do not need medical attention. These side effects may go away during treatment as your body adjusts to the medicine. However, check with your doctor if any of the following side effects continue or are bothersome:

For both filgrastim and sargramostim

More common

Headache; pain in joints or muscles; pain in lower back or pelvis; skin rash or itching

Less common

Pain in arms or legs

For sargramostin only (in addition to the above)

Less common or rare

Dizziness or faintness after first dose of medicine; flushing of face after first dose of medicine; weakness

Other side effects not listed above may also occur in some patients. If you notice any other effects, check with your doctor.

Annual revision: 08/07/92
Interim revision: 04/22/93

CONDOMS

Some commonly used brand names are:

Lamb intestine condoms not containing spermicide

In the U.S.

Fourex Natural Skins
Trojan Kling-Tite Naturalamb

In Canada

Fourex Natural Skins
Trojan Kling-Tite Naturalamb

Latex condoms not containing spermicide

In the U.S.

Embrace
Excita Fiesta
Gold Circle Coin
Kimono
Lady Protex Ultra-Thin
LifeStyles Form Fitting
LifeStyles Lubricated
LifeStyles Ultra Sensitive
LifeStyles Vibra-Ribbed
Magnum Lubricated
MAXX
Mentor Lubricated
Protex Arouse
Protex Secure
Protex Touch
Ramses Non-Lubricated Reservoir End
Ramses NuFORM
Ramses Sensitol Lubricated
Saxon Ribbed Lubricated
Saxon Ultra Thin
Saxon Wet Lubricated
Sheik Fetherlite Snug-Fit
Sheik Non-Lubricated Plain End
Sheik Non-Lubricated Reservoir End
Trojan-Enz
Trojan-Enz Large Lubricated
Trojan-Enz Lubricated
Trojan Extra Strength Lubricated
Trojan Naturalube Ribbed
Trojan Plus
Trojan Ribbed
Trojans
Trojan for Women

In Canada

Conceptrol Shields
Conceptrol Supreme
Embrace
Gold Circle Coin
LifeStyles Form Fitting
LifeStyles Lubricated
LifeStyles Ultra Sensitive
LifeStyles Vibra-Ribbed
Ramses Non-lubricated
Ramses NuForm
Ramses Sensitol
Ramses Ultra
Saxon Ribbed Lubricated
Saxon Ultra Thin
Saxon Wet Lubricated
Sheik Denim
Sheik Non-Lubricated
Sheik Sensi-Creme
Trojan-Enz
Trojan-Enz Large Lubricated
Trojan-Enz Lubricated
Trojan Naturalube Ribbed
Trojan Plus
Trojan Ribbed
Trojans

Latex condoms containing nonoxynol 9 (a spermicide)

In the U.S.

Excita Extra
Kimono Plus
Koromex with Nonoxynol 9
Lady Protex with Spermicidal Lubricant
LifeStyles Extra Strength with Spermicide
LifeStyles Spermicidally Lubricated
Magnum with Spermicidal Lubricant
MAXX Plus
Mentor Plus Spermicidal Lubricant
Protex Contracept Plus with Spermicidal Lubricant
Ramses Extra with Spermicidal Lubricant
Saxon Spermicidal
Sheik Elite
Today with Spermicidal Lubricant
Trojan-Enz Large with Spermicidal Lubricant
Trojan-Enz with Spermicidal Lubricant
Trojan Plus 2
Trojan Ribbed with Spermicidal Lubricant
Trojan for Women with Spermicidal Lubricant

In Canada

LifeStyles Extra Strength with Spermicide
LifeStyles Spermicidally Lubricated
Ramses Extra
Ramses Extra-15
Ramses Ribbed
Ramses Ultra-15
Saxon Spermicidal
Sheik Elite
Sheik Excita
Trojan-Enz Large with Spermicidal Lubricant
Trojan-Enz with Spermicidal Lubricant

Description

Condoms (KON-dums) are used by a male partner during sexual intercourse as a form of birth control. Latex rubber condoms are also used during anal, vaginal, or oral sex to help protect against sexually transmitted diseases such as AIDS (HIV infection), genital herpes (herpes simplex II), gonorrhea, syphilis, chlamydia, genital warts, and hepatitis.

Condoms can be a highly effective form of birth control when they are used properly. However, pregnancy usually occurs in 12 of each 100 women during the first year of condom use. You can discuss with your doctor what your options are for birth control and the pros and cons of using each method.

Condoms work to protect against sexually transmitted diseases (STDs) and as a birth control method by acting as barrier (wall) to keep blood, semen, and other fluids from passing from one partner to the other. The germs that can cause STDs are present in these fluids. With the proper use of latex condoms, these fluids are trapped inside the condom, along with sperm and any germs that may be present.

Latex rubber condoms are preferred for the prevention of STDs. Even though lamb intestine condoms are as effective as latex condoms in preventing pregnancy, it is not known whether they are as effective as latex condoms in protecting against all of the STDs, especially AIDS. Therefore, lamb intestine condoms should be used to protect against STDs *only* if you (or your partner) are allergic or sensitive to latex rubber condoms.

The use of a spermicide along with a condom increases the condom's ability to prevent pregnancy. Also, *laboratory studies* have shown that the spermicide nonoxynol 9 kills or stops the growth of the AIDS virus (HIV) and herpes simplex I and II viruses. It was also shown to be effective against other types of germs that cause gonorrhea, chlamydia, syphilis, trichomoniasis, and other STDs. *Although this has not been proven in human studies, some scientists believe that spermicides put into the vagina or on the outside of a latex condom may kill these germs before they are able to come in contact with the vagina or rectum (lower bowel).* Spermicides also provide a back-up in case the condom breaks, slips, or leaks during sexual intercourse.

The most effective way to protect yourself against STDs (such as AIDS) is by abstinence (not having sexual intercourse) or by having only one partner and making sure that person is not already infected and is *not* going to get an STD. However, if any of these methods are not likely or possible, using latex rubber condoms with an extra spermicide product is the best way to protect yourself. This is especially important if you cannot be sure a partner does not have an STD.

The use of a condom is recommended even when you are using other methods of birth control, such as birth control pills (the Pill), the cervical cap, the contraceptive sponge, diaphragm, and the intrauterine device (IUD), since these methods do not offer any protection from STDs.

The safety of using condoms with spermicides in the rectum (lower bowel), anus, or rectal area is not known. No side effects have been reported that are different from those reported for use in the vagina. However, some studies have reported that latex condoms are more likely to break during anal intercourse.

Condoms are available without a prescription in the following product forms:

- Lamb intestine condoms (U.S. and Canada)
- Latex condoms (U.S. and Canada)
- Latex condoms and nonoxynol 9 (a spermicide) (U.S. and Canada)

If you have any questions about the following information or if you want more information about these products or the prevention of pregnancy or STDs, ask your doctor, nurse, or pharmacist.

Before Using This Product

In deciding to use condoms as a method of birth control or to prevent STDs, you need to consider the pros and cons involved with their use. This is a decision you and your sexual partner will make. The following information may help you in making your decision. Ask your doctor or pharmacist for more information if you have any questions.

Allergies—If you have ever had any unusual or allergic reaction to condoms or other rubber products, it is best to check with your doctor before using latex condoms. Also, it is a good idea to check with your doctor before using condoms with nonoxynol 9 if you have ever had an allergic or unusual reaction to spermicides.

Adolescents—These products are frequently used by teenagers and have not been shown to cause different problems than they do in adults. However, some younger or first time users may need extra counseling and information on the importance of using condoms exactly as they are supposed to be used so they will work properly.

Proper Use of This Product

Some condoms have a dry or wet lubricant applied to them. Use of a lubricant may help prevent condoms from breaking or slipping and prevent irritation to the vagina, anus, or rectum. It may be especially important to use a lubricant during anal intercourse, since some studies have shown that latex condoms break more often during anal intercourse. This is because there is greater friction (rubbing force) during anal intercourse, as compared with vaginal or oral intercourse. *If you need an extra lubricant, make sure it is a water-based product safe for use with condoms, cervical caps, or diaphragms.* Spermicides, especially gels and jellies, also provide some lubrication during sexual intercourse. *Oil-based products such as hand, face, or body cream; petroleum jelly; cooking oils or shortenings; or mineral or baby oil should not be used because they weaken the latex rubber.* (Even some products that easily rinse away with water are oil-based and should not be used.) This increases the chances of the condom breaking during sexual intercourse.

To use:

- *Before any genital contact occurs:*

  —Open the condom wrapper carefully, making sure you do not damage it before use. Always handle the unwrapped condom carefully. If the wrapper was already open, do not use the condom because the condom may be damaged or weakened.

  —Look at the unrolled condom before it is placed on the penis, to check it for any damage or defects. Occasionally, a condom may be damaged from improper storage, opening, or manufacturing. If the condom feels sticky, brittle, dried out, or gummy, do not use it. Also, check the tip for tears or holes. However, do not unroll the condom to look at it before you are ready to use it. Also, do not fill it with water to check it for leaks. Both of these actions will weaken the condom. When handling the condom, be careful also not to tear it with sharp or jagged fingernails and sharp rings or jewelry. Use a different condom if you have any doubts about any condom's quality or condition.

  —Place the unrolled condom over the tip of the erect (hard) penis. Check the condom to make sure the correct side is touching the penis. If you accidentally put on the unrolled condom with the wrong side out, it should not be used. There is a chance that germs or sperm could get on the tip of the condom. If you then reversed the condom and unrolled it correctly, your partner would be in contact with the germs or sperm.

  —Pinch the end of the condom to leave a half-inch of space for the semen to collect in. If the condom has a reservoir, pinch this reservoir to get rid of any air. Leaving this extra space will keep semen and other fluids from spilling out during intercourse.

—While still pinching the tip of the condom, completely unroll the condom down the length of the penis to its base. If the penis is uncircumcised, the foreskin should be pulled back before the condom is unrolled. To be most effective in preventing STDs, the condom must cover the entire penis.

—If you are using extra spermicide or lubricant, carefully spread some on the outside of the condom. It is a good idea to check the rest of the condom for any defects or damage at this time. A female partner should also use a spermicide inside the vagina.

- *After genital contact occurs:*

—If a condom breaks during intercourse, immediately put on a new condom. Also, apply more spermicide or lubricant.

—Immediately after ejaculation and before the penis becomes soft, firmly grasp the ring of the condom at the base of the penis. Carefully withdraw the penis to avoid tearing the condom or spilling semen. Discard the used condom properly.

—You must use a new condom each time you repeat intercourse. *Condoms should never be reused.* Spermicide or lubricant should also be re-applied outside of the new condom. A female partner should also put more spermicide in the vagina each time she has intercourse.

For females using condoms with extra spermicide:

- Condoms do not have to be used with spermicides, but the spermicide may provide a back-up in case the condom leaks or breaks.
- It is very important that the spermicide be placed properly in the vagina. It should be put deep into the vagina, directly on the cervix (opening to the uterus). The written instructions about how the product container and the applicator work, how much spermicide to use each time, and how long each application remains effective may be different for each product. Make sure you carefully read and follow the instructions that come with each product.
- *Make sure the spermicide you choose is labeled as being safe for use with latex diaphragms, cervical caps, or condoms.* Otherwise, it may cause the condom to weaken and leak or even break during intercourse.

Storage—To store:

- Store in a dark, cool, dry place. Avoid extreme temperatures and direct light. If you carry a condom with you, keep it in a wallet, loose pocket, or purse for no more than a few hours at time.
- Do not store in the bathroom or in other damp places. Heat or moisture may weaken condoms.
- Keep the product from freezing.
- Do not use outdated condoms or condoms that are clearly old or that have no date on the package. Only latex condoms with a pre-applied spermicide have an expiration date. After this time, the maker cannot guarantee the spermicide potency. Other condoms should have the date that they were made on the box. It is best if you do not buy condoms long before you use them, in case the storage has not been ideal. The best way to make sure you are using fresh condoms is to buy them only a short time before they will be used. Older condoms are more likely to break during sexual intercourse. If you have any questions about the storage and expiration dating of condoms, ask your doctor, nurse, or pharmacist.
- Be sure that any discarded condoms are out of the reach of children. Used condoms should be wrapped in tissue or paper. Discard them in the trash so that others will not accidentally handle them.

Side Effects of This Product

Condoms occasionally cause allergies or local irritation in some people. They may cause itching, burning, stinging, or a rash. These reactions could be due to the latex itself, the lubricant, or the spermicide. Changing to a different brand of condom may solve this problem. Also, using a weaker strength of vaginal spermicide (if you are using extra spermicide) may be necessary, although it will be less effective. If any of these effects continue after you have changed products, you may have an allergy to these products or an infection and should contact a doctor as soon as possible.

Very rarely, some people may have a severe allergic reaction to latex rubber. *Check with a doctor immediately* if any of the following effects occur:

Rare

For latex condoms only

Difficulty in breathing; hives; swelling of the face or inside of the throat

Also, check with a doctor as soon as possible if any of the following effects occur:

Rare

For latex condoms only

For females and males

Redness of the inside of the eyelids; skin rash, redness, swelling, irritation, local swelling, or itching that occurs each time a latex condom is used; stuffy nose after using latex condoms

For females only

Vaginal bleeding, irritation, redness, rash, dryness, or whitish discharge that occurs each time a latex condom is used (signs of vaginal allergy)

For latex condoms containing spermicide only

For females only

Bladder pain; cloudy or bloody urine; increased frequency of urination; pain on urination

Other side effects may occur that usually do not need medical attention. Using a different brand of condom may help to eliminate these effects. However, check with your doctor if any of the following side effects continue or are bothersome:

Less common

Burning, stinging, warmth, itching, or other irritation of the skin, penis, rectum, or vagina; vaginal dryness or odor

Other side effects not listed above may also occur in some people. If you notice any other effects, check with your doctor.

Annual revision: 03/04/93

COPPER SUPPLEMENTS Systemic

This information applies to the following medicines:

Copper Gluconate (KOP-er GLOO-coh-nate)
Copper Sulfate (SUL-fate)

For Copper Gluconate†

In the U.S.

Generic name product is available.

For Copper Sulfate

In the U.S.

Generic name product is available.

In Canada

Generic name product is available.

Another commonly used name for copper sulfate is cupric sulfate.

†Not commercially available in Canada.

Description

Copper supplements are used to prevent or treat copper deficiency.

The body needs copper for normal growth and health. For patients who are unable to get enough copper in their regular diet or who have a need for more copper, copper supplements may be necessary. They are generally taken by mouth but some patients may have to receive them by injection.

Lack of copper may lead to anemia and osteoporosis (weak bones).

Patients with the following conditions may be more likely to have a deficiency of copper:

- Burns
- Diarrhea
- Intestine disease
- Kidney disease
- Pancreas disease
- Stomach removal
- Stress, continuing

In addition, premature infants may need additional copper.

If any of the above apply to you, you should take copper supplements only on the advice of your physician after need has been established.

Claims that copper supplements are effective in the treatment of arthritis or skin conditions have not been proven. Use of copper supplements to cause vomiting has caused death and should be avoided.

Some preparations are available only with your doctor's prescription. Others are available without a prescription; however, your doctor may have special instructions on the proper use and dose for your condition.

Copper supplements are available in the following dosage forms:

Oral

Copper Gluconate
- Tablets (U.S.)

Parenteral

Copper Sulfate
- Injection (U.S. and Canada)

It is very important that you read and understand the following information. If any of it causes you special concern, check with your doctor or pharmacist. Also, *if you have any questions* or if you want more information about this medicine or your medical problem, *ask your doctor, nurse, pharmacist, or dietitian.*

Importance of Diet

Nutritionists recommend that, if possible, people should get all the copper they need from foods. However, some people do not get enough copper from their diets. For example, people on weight-loss diets may consume too little food to provide enough copper. Others may need more copper than normal. For such people, a copper supplement is important.

In order to get enough vitamins and minerals in your diet, it is important that you eat a balanced and varied diet. Follow carefully any diet program your doctor may recommend. For your specific vitamin and/or mineral needs, ask your doctor or dietitian for a list of appropriate foods.

Copper is found in various foods, including organ meats (especially liver), seafoods, beans, nuts, and whole-grains. Additional copper can come from drinking water from copper pipes, using copper cookware, and eating farm products sprayed with copper-containing chemicals. Copper may be decreased in foods that have high acid content and are stored in tin cans for a long time.

Experts have developed a list of recommended dietary allowances (RDA) for most vitamins and some minerals. The RDA are not an exact number but a general idea of how much you need. They do not cover amounts needed for problems caused by a serious lack of vitamins and minerals. There are no RDA for copper. The following intakes are thought to be plenty for most individuals:

- Infants and children—
  Birth to 6 months of age: 0.4 to 0.6 mg per day.
  6 months to 1 year of age: 0.6 to 0.7 mg per day.
  1 to 3 years of age: 0.7 to 1 mg per day.
  4 to 6 years of age: 1 to 1.5 mg per day.
  7 to 10 years of age: 1 to 2 mg per day.
- Adolescent males and females—1.5 to 2.5 mg per day.
- Adult males and females—1.5 to 3 mg per day.

Remember:

- The total amount of copper that you get every day includes what you get from the foods that you eat and what you may take as supplement.
- This total amount should not be greater than the above recommendations, unless ordered by your doctor.

Before Using This Dietary Supplement

If you are taking this dietary supplement without a prescription, carefully read and follow any precautions on the label. For copper supplements, the following should be considered:

Allergies—Tell your doctor and pharmacist if you are allergic to any substances, such as foods, preservatives, or dyes.

Pregnancy—It is especially important that you are receiving enough vitamins and minerals when you become pregnant and that you continue to receive the right amount of vitamins and minerals throughout your pregnancy. The healthy growth and development of the fetus depend on a steady supply of nutrients from the mother. However, taking large amounts of a dietary supplement in pregnancy may be harmful to the mother and/or fetus and should be avoided.

Breast-feeding—It is important that you receive the right amounts of vitamins and minerals so that your baby will also get the vitamins and minerals needed to grow properly. However, taking large amounts of a dietary supplement while breast-feeding may be harmful to the mother and/or baby and should be avoided.

Children—It is especially important that children receive enough copper in their diet for healthy growth and development. Although there is no specific information comparing use of copper in children with use in other age groups, this medicine is not expected to cause different side effects or problems in children than in adults.

Older adults—It is important that older people continue to receive enough copper in their daily diets.

Medicines or other dietary supplements—Although certain medicines or dietary supplements should not be used together at all, in other cases they may be used together even if an interaction might occur. In these cases, your doctor may want to change the dose, or other precautions may be necessary. When you are taking copper supplements, it is especially important that your doctor and pharmacist know if you are taking any of the following:

- Penicillamine or
- Trientine or
- Zinc supplements (taken by mouth)—Use with copper supplements may decrease the amount of copper that gets into the body; copper supplements should be taken at least 2 hours after penicillamine, trientine, or zinc supplements

Other medical problems—The presence of other medical problems may affect the use of copper supplements. Make sure you tell your doctor if you have any other medical problems, especially:

- Wilson's disease (too much copper in the body)—Copper supplements may make this condition worse

Proper Use of This Dietary Supplement

Some people believe that taking very large doses of a vitamin or mineral (called megadoses) is useful for treating certain medical problems. Studies have not proven this. Large doses should be taken only under the direction of your doctor after need has been identified.

Missed dose—If you miss taking copper supplements for one or more days there is no cause for concern, since it takes some time for your body to become seriously low in copper. However, if your doctor has recommended that you take copper try to remember to take it as directed every day.

Storage—To store this dietary supplement:

- Keep out of the reach of children.
- Store away from heat and direct light.
- Do not store in the bathroom, near the kitchen sink, or in other damp places. Heat or moisture may cause the dietary supplement to break down.
- Keep the dietary supplement from freezing. Do not refrigerate.
- Do not keep outdated dietary supplements or those no longer needed. Be sure that any discarded dietary supplement is out of the reach of children.

Precautions While Using This Dietary Supplement

Do not take copper supplements and zinc supplements at the same time. It is best to take your copper supplement 2 hours after zinc supplements, to get the full benefit of each medicine.

Side Effects of This Dietary Supplement

Along with its needed effects, a dietary supplement may cause some unwanted effects. Although copper supplements have not been reported to cause any side effects, *check with your doctor immediately* if any of the following side effects occur as a result of an overdose:

Symptoms of overdose

Black or bloody vomit; blood in urine; coma; diarrhea; dizziness or fainting; headache (severe or continuing); heartburn; loss of appetite; lower back pain; metallic taste; nausea (severe or continuing); pain or burning while urinating; vomiting; yellow eyes or skin

Other side effects not listed above may also occur in some patients. If you notice any other effects, check with your doctor.

Annual revision: 09/01/91
Interim revision: 06/25/92

CORTICOSTEROIDS Dental

This information applies to the following medicines:

Hydrocortisone (hye-droe-KOR-ti-sone)
Triamcinolone (trye-am-SIN-oh-lone)

Some commonly used brand names are:

For Hydrocortisone

In the U.S.

Orabase-HCA

Another commonly used name is cortisol.

For Triamcinolone

In the U.S.

Kenalog in Orabase
Oralone
Oracort

In Canada

Kenalog in Orabase

Description

Dental corticosteroids (kor-ti-ko-STER-oyds) are used to relieve the discomfort and redness of some mouth and gum problems. These medicines are like cortisone. They belong to the general family of medicines called steroids.

Dental corticosteroids are available only with your medical doctor's or dentist's prescription in the following dosage forms:

Dental

Hydrocortisone
- Paste (U.S.)

Triamcinolone
- Paste (U.S. and Canada)

It is very important that you read and understand the following information. If any of it causes you special concern, check with your doctor or dentist. Also, *if you have any questions* or if you want more information about this medicine or your medical problem, *ask your doctor, dentist, nurse, or pharmacist.*

Before Using This Medicine

In deciding to use a medicine, the risks of taking the medicine must be weighed against the good it will do. This is a decision you and your doctor or dentist will make. For dental corticosteroids, the following should be considered:

Allergies—Tell your doctor if you have ever had any unusual or allergic reaction to corticosteroids. Also tell your doctor and pharmacist if you are allergic to any other substances, such as foods, preservatives, or dyes.

Pregnancy—When used properly, these medicines have not been shown to cause problems in humans. Studies on birth defects with dental corticosteroids have not been done in humans. However, studies in animals have shown that topical corticosteroids, such as the hydrocortisone or triamcinolone in this medicine, when applied to the skin in large amounts or used for a long time, could cause birth defects. Studies with dental paste have not been done in animals.

Breast-feeding—When used properly, dental corticosteroids have not been reported to cause problems in nursing babies.

Children—Children and teenagers who must use this medicine should be checked often by their doctor. Dental corticosteroids may be absorbed through the lining of the mouth and, if used too often or for too long a time, may interfere with growth in children. Before using this medicine in children, you should discuss its use with your child's medical doctor or dentist.

Older adults—Although there is no specific information comparing use of dental corticosteroids in the elderly with use in other age groups, these medicines are not expected to cause different side effects or problems in older people than they do in younger adults.

Other medicines—Although certain medicines should not be used together at all, in many cases two different medicines may be used together even if an interaction might occur. In these cases, your doctor or dentist may want to change the dose, or other precautions may be necessary. Tell your doctor, dentist, and pharmacist if you are taking or using any other prescription or nonprescription (over-the-counter [OTC]) medicine.

Other medical problems—The presence of other medical problems may affect the use of dental corticosteroids. Make sure you tell your doctor or dentist if you have any other medical problems, especially:

- Diabetes mellitus (sugar diabetes)—Too much use of corticosteroids may cause a loss of control of diabetes by increasing blood and urine glucose. However, this is not likely to happen when dental corticosteroids are used for a short period of time
- Herpes sores or
- Infection or sores of the mouth or throat or
- Tuberculosis—Corticosteroids may make existing infections worse or cause new infections

Before you begin using any new medicine (prescription or nonprescription) or if you develop any new medical problem while you are using this medicine, check with your doctor, dentist, nurse, or pharmacist.

Proper Use of This Medicine

To use hydrocortisone or triamcinolone:

- Using a cotton swab, press (do not rub) a small amount of paste onto the area to be treated until the paste sticks and a smooth, slippery film forms. Do not try to spread the medicine because it will become crumbly and gritty. Apply the paste at bedtime so the medicine can work overnight. The other applications of the paste should be made following meals.

Do not use corticosteroids more often or for a longer time than your medical doctor or dentist ordered. To do so may increase the chance of absorption through the lining of the mouth and the chance of side effects.

Do not use any leftover medicine for future mouth problems without first checking with your medical doctor or dentist. This medicine should *not* be used on many kinds of bacterial, virus, or fungus infections.

Missed dose—If your medical doctor or dentist has ordered you to use this medicine according to a regular schedule and you miss a dose, use it as soon as you remember. However, if it is almost time for your next dose, skip the missed dose and go back to your regular dosing schedule.

Storage—To store this medicine:

- Keep out of the reach of children.
- Store away from heat and direct light.
- Keep the medicine from freezing.
- Do not keep outdated medicine or medicine no longer needed. Be sure that any discarded medicine is out of the reach of children.

Precautions While Using This Medicine

Check with your medical doctor or dentist:

- if your symptoms do not improve within 1 week.
- if your condition gets worse.

Side Effects of This Medicine

Along with its needed effects, a medicine may cause some unwanted effects. Although not all of these side effects may occur, if they do occur they may need medical attention.

Check with your medical doctor or dentist as soon as possible if the following side effects occur:

Signs of infection or irritation such as burning, itching, blistering, or peeling not present before use of this medicine

Other side effects not listed above may also occur in some patients. If you notice any other effects, check with your medical doctor or dentist.

Annual revision: 11/18/92

CORTICOSTEROIDS Inhalation

This information applies to the following medicines:

Beclomethasone (be-kloe-METH-a-sone)
Dexamethasone (dex-a-METH-a-sone)
Flunisolide (floo-NISS-oh-lide)
Triamcinolone (trye-am-SIN-oh-lone)

Some commonly used brand names are:

For Beclomethasone

In the U.S.

Beclovent
Vanceril

In Canada
Beclovent
Beclovent Rotacaps
Vanceril

Another commonly used name is beclometasone.

For Dexamethasone†
In the U.S.
Decadron Respihaler

For Flunisolide
In the U.S.
AeroBid
In Canada
Bronalide

For Triamcinolone
In the U.S.
Azmacort
In Canada
Azmacort

†Not commercially available in Canada.

Description

Inhalation corticosteroids (kor-ti-koe-STER-oids) are used to help prevent asthma attacks. However, they will not relieve an asthma attack that has already started. They are cortisone-like medicines. Corticosteroids also belong to the general family of medicines called steroids.

Inhalation corticosteroids are available only with your doctor's prescription, in the following dosage forms:

Oral Inhalation
Beclomethasone
- Aerosol (U.S. and Canada)
- Capsules (Canada)

Dexamethasone
- Aerosol (U.S.)

Flunisolide
- Aerosol (U.S. and Canada)

Triamcinolone
- Aerosol (U.S. and Canada)

It is very important that you read and understand the following information. If any of it causes you special concern, check with your doctor. Also, *if you have any questions* or if you want more information about this medicine or your medical problem, *ask your doctor, nurse, or pharmacist.*

Before Using This Medicine

In deciding to use a medicine, the risks of taking the medicine must be weighed against the good it will do. This is a decision you and your doctor will make. For corticosteroids, the following should be considered:

Allergies—Tell your doctor if you have ever had any unusual or allergic reaction to corticosteroids. Also tell your doctor and pharmacist if you are allergic to any other substances, such as foods, preservatives, or dyes.

Pregnancy—In one human study, use of beclomethasone inhalation did not cause birth defects or other problems. Studies on birth defects with dexamethasone, flunisolide, or triamcinolone inhalations have not been done in humans.

In animal studies, corticosteroids taken by mouth or injection during pregnancy were shown to cause birth defects. Also, too much use of corticosteroids during pregnancy may cause other unwanted effects in the infant, such as slower growth and reduced adrenal gland function.

If corticosteroids are medically necessary during pregnancy to control asthma, inhaled corticosteroids are generally considered safer than corticosteroids taken by mouth or injection. Also, use of inhaled corticosteroids may allow some patients to stop using or decrease the amount of corticosteroids taken by mouth or injection.

Breast-feeding—Dexamethasone passes into the breast milk and may cause problems in nursing babies. It may be necessary to take another medicine or to stop breast-feeding during treatment.

It is not known whether beclomethasone, flunisolide, or triamcinolone passes into the breast milk. However, these medicines have not been shown to cause problems in nursing babies.

Children—Corticosteroids taken by mouth or injection have been shown to slow or stop growth in children and cause reduced adrenal gland function. If corticosteroids are medically necessary to control asthma in a child, inhaled corticosteroids are generally considered to be safer than corticosteroids taken by mouth or injection. Most inhaled corticosteroids have not been shown to affect growth. Also, use of most inhaled corticosteroids may allow some children to stop using or decrease the amount of corticosteroids taken by mouth or injection.

Before this medicine is given to a child, you and your child's doctor should talk about the good this medicine will do as well as the risks of using it. Follow the doctor's directions very carefully to lessen the chance that these unwanted effects will occur.

Older adults—Although there is no specific information about the use of corticosteroids in the elderly, they are not expected to cause different side effects or problems in older people than they do in younger adults.

Other medicines—Although certain medicines should not be used together at all, in other cases two different medicines may be used together even if an interaction might occur. In these cases, your doctor may want to change the dose, or other precautions may be necessary. When you are using corticosteroids, it is especially important that your doctor and pharmacist know if you are taking any of the following:

- Antidiabetics, oral (diabetes medicine taken by mouth) or
- Insulin—Long-term use of dexamethasone or triamcinolone may interfere with the effects of oral antidiabetic medicines or insulin by increasing blood glucose (sugar)

levels, leading to a loss of control of diabetes mellitus (sugar diabetes)

Other medical problems—The presence of other medical problems may affect the use of corticosteroids. Make sure you tell your doctor if you have any other medical problems, especially:

For all corticosteroid aerosols
- Certain types of lung disease
- Infection of the mouth, throat, or lungs—Signs of an infection may be covered up by the use of corticosteroids, or healing of the infection may be delayed

For long-term use of dexamethasone or triamcinolone aerosols
- Bone disease or
- Colitis or
- Diabetes mellitus (sugar diabetes) or
- Diverticulitis or
- Fungus or other infection or
- Glaucoma or
- Heart disease or
- High blood pressure or
- High cholesterol levels or
- Kidney disease or kidney stones or
- Stomach ulcer or other stomach problems—These conditions may be worsened by certain side effects of dexamethasone and triamcinolone
- Heart attack (recent)—Very rarely, a serious heart condition has been reported with the use of dexamethasone or triamcinolone shortly after a heart attack
- Herpes simplex virus infection of the eye—Use of dexamethasone or triamcinolone while the eye is infected may cause a hole to form in the cornea
- Liver disease
- Myasthenia gravis—Dexamethasone or triamcinolone may cause problems in breathing
- Tuberculosis (history of)—Use of dexamethasone may cause a new tuberculosis infection
- Underactive thyroid—This condition may cause an increased effect from the dexamethasone or triamcinolone, possibly leading to toxic effects

Before you begin using any new medicine (prescription or nonprescription) or if you develop any new medical problem while you are using this medicine, check with your doctor, nurse, or pharmacist.

Proper Use of This Medicine

Inhalation corticosteroids are used with a special inhaler and usually come with patient directions. *Read the directions carefully before using.* If you do not understand the directions, or if you are not sure how to use the inhaler, check with your doctor, nurse, or pharmacist.

Do not use more of this medicine, and do not use it more often, than your doctor ordered. To do so may increase the chance of absorption into the body and the chance of unwanted effects.

In order for this medicine to help prevent asthma attacks, it must be taken every day in regularly spaced doses as ordered by your doctor. Up to four weeks may pass before you feel its full effects. However, this may take less time if you have been taking certain other medicines for your asthma.

Do not use this medicine to treat an asthma attack that has already started, because it will not work. However, continue to take this medicine at the usual time, even if you use another medicine to relieve the asthma attack.

The inhaler should be cleaned every day as directed. If you do not receive instructions with the inhaler, or if you are not certain how to clean it, check with your pharmacist.

Gargling and rinsing your mouth with water after each dose may help prevent hoarseness, throat irritation, and infection in the mouth. However, do not swallow the water after you rinse. Your doctor may also want you to use a spacer to decrease these problems. A spacer is a tube that fits on the mouthpiece of the inhaler. It makes the inhaler easier to use and allows more of the medicine to reach your lungs, rather than staying in the mouth and throat.

Missed dose—If you miss a dose of this medicine, use it as soon as possible. However, if it is almost time for your next dose, skip the missed dose and go back to your regular dosing schedule. Do not double doses.

Check with your pharmacist to see if you should save the inhaler piece that comes with this medicine. Refill units may be available at lower cost. However, remember that the inhaler is meant to be used only for the medicine that comes with it. Do not use the inhaler for any other inhalation aerosol medicine, even if the cartridge fits.

Storage—To store this medicine:
- Keep out of the reach of children.
- Store away from heat and direct light.
- Keep the medicine from getting too cold or freezing. This medicine may be less effective if the container is cold when you use it.
- Do not puncture, break, or burn the aerosol container, even after it is empty.
- Do not keep outdated medicine or medicine no longer needed. Be sure that any discarded medicine is out of the reach of children.

Precautions While Using This Medicine

Check with your doctor:
- *if you go through a period of unusual stress.*
- *if you have an asthma attack* that does not improve after you take a bronchodilator medicine.
- *if signs of mouth, throat, or lung infection occur.*

- *if your symptoms do not improve.*
- *if your condition gets worse.*

Also, *check with your doctor immediately if any of the following side effects occur* while you are using this medicine:

Abdominal or back pain
Dizziness or fainting
Fever
Muscle or joint pain
Nausea or vomiting
Prolonged loss of appetite
Shortness of breath
Unusual tiredness or weakness
Unusual weight loss

Your doctor may want you to carry a medical identification card stating that you are using this medicine and may need additional medicine during times of emergency, a severe asthma attack or other illness, or unusual stress.

Before you have any kind of surgery (including dental surgery) or emergency treatment, tell the medical doctor or dentist in charge that you are using this medicine.

For patients who are also using a bronchodilator inhalation aerosol:

- Unless otherwise directed by your doctor, use the bronchodilator aerosol first, then wait about 5 minutes before using this medicine. This allows the corticosteroid aerosol to better reach the passages of the lungs (bronchioles) because the bronchodilator opens up the bronchioles.

For patients who are also regularly taking a corticosteroid in tablet or liquid form:

- *Do not stop taking the other corticosteroid without your doctor's advice, even if your asthma seems better.* Your doctor may want you to reduce gradually the amount you are taking before stopping completely to lessen the chance of unwanted effects.
- When your doctor tells you to reduce the dose, or to stop taking the other corticosteroid, follow the directions carefully. Your body may need time to adjust to the change. The length of time this takes may depend on the amount of medicine you were taking and how long you took it. *It is especially important that your doctor check your progress at regular visits during this time.* Also, ask your doctor if there are special directions you should follow if you have a severe asthma attack, if you need any other medical or surgical treatment, or if certain side effects occur. Be certain that you understand these directions, and follow them carefully.

Side Effects of This Medicine

Along with its needed effects, a medicine may cause some unwanted effects. Although not all of these side effects may occur, if they do occur they may need medical attention.

Check with your doctor immediately if any of the following side effects occur just after you use this medicine:

Rare

Increased shortness of breath, troubled breathing, tightness in chest, or wheezing

Also, check with your doctor as soon as possible if any of the following side effects occur:

More common

Any sign of possible infection, such as chest pain, chills, fever, cough, congestion, ear pain, eye pain, red or teary eyes, runny nose, sneezing, or sore throat; creamy white, curd-like patches inside the mouth; fast or pounding heartbeat; increased susceptibility to infection; nausea or vomiting; skin rash or itching

Less common or rare

Decreased or blurred vision; difficulty in swallowing; hives; increased blood pressure; increased thirst; mental depression or other mood or mental changes; swelling of face; swelling of feet or lower legs; unusual weight gain

Additional side effects may occur after you have been using this medicine for a long time. Check with your doctor as soon as possible if any of the following side effects occur:

Acne or other skin problems; back or rib pain; bloody or black, tarry stools; fullness or rounding out of the face (moon face); frequent urination; increased thirst; irregular heartbeat; menstrual problems; muscle weakness, cramps, or pains; stomach pain or burning (severe and continuing); unusual tiredness or weakness; wounds that will not heal

Other side effects may occur that usually do not need medical attention. These side effects may go away during treatment as your body adjusts to the medicine. However, check with your doctor if any of the following side effects continue or are bothersome:

More common

Abdominal or stomach pain (mild); bloated feeling or gas; constipation; cough without other signs of infection; diarrhea; dizziness or lightheadedness; headache; heartburn or indigestion; hoarseness or other voice changes without other signs of infection; loss of appetite; loss of smell or taste sense; nervousness or restlessness; unpleasant taste

Less common or rare

Dry or irritated nose, mouth, tongue, or throat; false sense of well-being; general feeling of discomfort, illness, shakiness, or faintness; increase in appetite; increased sweating; trouble in sleeping; unexplained nosebleeds

Some of the above side effects have been reported for dexamethasone or flunisolide, but not for beclomethasone or triamcinolone. All of the inhalation corticosteroids are similar, so any of the above side effects may occur with beclomethasone or triamcinolone also, especially if large amounts are used for a long time.

Other side effects not listed above may also occur in some patients. If you notice any other effects, check with your doctor.

Annual revision: June 1990
Interim revision: 06/15/93

CORTICOSTEROIDS Nasal

This information applies to the following medicines:

Beclomethasone (be-kloe-METH-a-sone)
Dexamethasone (dex-a-METH-a-sone)†
Flunisolide (floo-NISS-oh-lide)

Some commonly used brand names are:

For Beclomethasone

In the U.S.

Beconase
Beconase AQ
Vancenase
Vancenase AQ

In Canada

Beconase
Beconase AQ
Vancenase

Another commonly used name is beclometasone.

For Dexamethasone†

In the U.S.

Decadron Turbinaire

For Flunisolide

In the U.S.

Nasalide

In Canada

Rhinalar

†Not commercially available in Canada.

Description

Nasal adrenocorticoids (a-dree-noe-KOR-ti-koids) are cortisone-like medicines. They belong to the family of medicines called steroids. These medicines are sprayed into the nose to help relieve the stuffy nose, irritation, and discomfort of hay fever, other allergies, and other nasal problems. These medicines are also used to prevent nasal polyps from growing back after they have been removed by surgery.

These medicines are available only with your doctor's prescription, in the following dosage forms:

Nasal

Beclomethasone
- Aerosol (U.S. and Canada)
- Spray (U.S. and Canada)

Dexamethasone
- Aerosol (U.S.)

Flunisolide
- Solution (U.S. and Canada)

It is very important that you read and understand the following information. If any of it causes you special concern, check with your doctor. Also, *if you have any questions* or if you want more information about this medicine or your medical problem, *ask your doctor, nurse, or pharmacist.*

Before Using This Medicine

In deciding to use a medicine, the risks of taking the medicine must be weighed against the good it will do. This is a decision you and your doctor will make. For adrenocorticoids, the following should be considered:

Allergies—Tell your doctor if you have ever had any unusual or allergic reaction to adrenocorticoids. Also tell your doctor and pharmacist if you are allergic to any other substances, such as foods, preservatives, or dyes.

Pregnancy—In one human study, use of beclomethasone oral inhalation by pregnant women did not cause birth defects or other problems. Studies on birth defects with dexamethasone or flunisolide have not been done in humans.

In animal studies, adrenocorticoids taken by mouth or injection during pregnancy were shown to cause birth defects. Also, too much use of adrenocorticoids during pregnancy may cause other unwanted effects in the infant, such as slower growth and reduced adrenal gland function.

If adrenocorticoids are medically necessary during pregnancy to control nasal problems, nasal adrenocorticoids are generally considered safer than adrenocorticoids taken by mouth or injection. Also, use of nasal adrenocorticoids may allow some patients to stop using or decrease the amount of adrenocorticoids taken by mouth or injection.

Breast-feeding—Use of dexamethasone is not recommended in nursing mothers since dexamethasone passes into the breast milk and may affect the infant's growth. It is not known whether beclomethasone or flunisolide passes into the breast milk. However, these medicines have not been reported to cause problems in nursing babies.

Children—Adrenocorticoids taken by mouth or injection have been shown to slow or stop growth in children and cause reduced adrenal gland function. If adrenocorticoids are medically necessary to control nasal problem in a child, nasal adrenocorticoids are generally considered to be safer than adrenocorticoids taken by mouth or injection. Most nasal adrenocorticoids have not been shown to affect growth. Also, use of most nasal adrenocorticoids may allow some children to stop using or decrease the amount of adrenocorticoids taken by mouth or injection. Before this medicine is given to a child, you and your child's doctor should talk about the good this medicine will do as well as the risks of using it. Follow the doctor's directions very carefully to lessen the chance that these unwanted effects will occur.

Older adults—Although there is no specific information about the use of nasal adrenocorticoids in the elderly, they are not expected to cause different side effects or problems in older people than they do in younger adults.

Other medicines—Although certain medicines should not be used together at all, in other cases two different medicines may be used together even if an interaction might occur. In these cases, your doctor may want to change the dose, or other precautions may be necessary. When you are using nasal adrenocorticoids, it is especially important that your doctor and pharmacist know if you are taking any prescription or nonprescription (over-the-counter [OTC]) medicines.

Other medical problems—The presence of other medical problems may affect the use of adrenocorticoids. Make sure you tell your doctor if you have any other medical problems, especially:

- Glaucoma—Long-term use of nasal adrenocorticoids may worsen glaucoma by increasing the pressure within the eye
- Herpes simplex (virus) infection of the eye
- Infections
- Injury to the nose (recent) or
- Nose surgery (recent) or
- Sores in the nose—Nasal adrenocorticoids may prevent proper healing of these conditions
- Liver disease
- Tuberculosis (active or history of)
- Underactive thyroid

Before you begin using any new medicine (prescription or nonprescription) or if you develop any new medical problem while you are using this medicine, check with your doctor, nurse, or pharmacist.

Proper Use of This Medicine

This medicine usually comes with patient directions. *Read them carefully before using the medicine.* Beclomethasone and dexamethasone are used with a special inhaler. If you do not understand the directions, or if you are not sure how to use the inhaler, check with your doctor, nurse, or pharmacist.

In order for this medicine to help you, it must be used regularly as ordered by your doctor. This medicine usually begins to work in about 1 week, but up to 3 weeks may pass before you feel its full effects.

Use this medicine only as directed. Do not use more of it and do not use it more often than your doctor ordered. To do so may increase the chance of absorption through the lining of the nose and the chance of unwanted effects.

Check with your doctor before using this medicine for nasal problems other than the one for which it was prescribed, since it should not be used on many bacterial, virus, or fungus nasal infections.

Save the inhaler that comes with beclomethasone or dexamethasone, since refill units may be available at lower cost.

Missed dose—If you miss a dose of this medicine and remember within an hour or so, use it right away. However, if you do not remember until later, skip the missed dose and go back to your regular dosing schedule. Do not double doses.

Storage—To store this medicine:

- Keep out of the reach of children.
- Store away from heat and direct light.
- Keep the medicine from getting too cold or freezing. This medicine may be less effective if it is too cold when you use it.
- Do not puncture, break, or burn the beclomethasone or dexamethasone aerosol container, even after it is empty.
- Do not keep outdated medicine or medicine no longer needed. Also, discard any unused flunisolide or beclomethasone solution 3 months after you open the package. Be sure that any discarded medicine is out of the reach of children.

Precautions While Using This Medicine

If you will be using this medicine for more than a few weeks, your doctor should check your progress at regular visits.

Check with your doctor:

- *if signs of a nose, sinus, or throat infection occur.*
- *if your symptoms do not improve within 7 days (for dexamethasone) or within 3 weeks (for beclomethasone or flunisolide).*
- *if your condition gets worse.*

Side Effects of This Medicine

Along with its needed effects, a medicine may cause some unwanted effects. Although not all of these side effects

may occur, if they do occur they may need medical attention.

Check with your doctor as soon as possible if any of the following side effects occur:

Less common or rare

Bloody mucus or unexplained nosebleeds; crusting, white patches, or sores inside the nose; eye pain; gradual loss of vision; headache; hives; lightheadedness or dizziness; loss of sense of taste or smell; nausea or vomiting; shortness of breath, troubled breathing, tightness in chest, or wheezing; skin rash; sore throat, cough, or hoarseness; stomach pains; stuffy nose or watery eyes (continuing); swellings on face; unusual tiredness or weakness; white patches in throat

Symptoms of overdose

Acne; fullness or rounding of the face; menstrual changes

Other side effects may occur that usually do not need medical attention. These side effects may go away during treatment as your body adjusts to the medicine. However, check with your doctor if any of the following side effects continue or are bothersome:

More common

Burning, dryness, or other irritation inside the nose (mild, lasting only a short time); increase in sneezing; irritation of throat

Not all of the side effects listed above have been reported for each of these medicines, but they have been reported for at least one of them. All of the nasal adrenocorticoids are very similar, so any of the above side effects may occur with any of these medicines.

Other side effects not listed above may also occur in some patients. If you notice any other effects, check with your doctor.

Annual revision: June 1990

CORTICOSTEROIDS Ophthalmic

This information applies to the following medicines:

Betamethasone (bay-ta-METH-a-sone)
Dexamethasone (dex-a-METH-a-sone)
Fluorometholone (flure-oh-METH-oh-lone)
Hydrocortisone (hye-droe-KOR-ti-sone)
Medrysone (ME-dri-sone)
Prednisolone (pred-NISS-oh-lone)

Some commonly used brand names are:

For Betamethasone*

In Canada

Betnesol

For Dexamethasone

In the U.S.

AK-Dex
Baldex
Decadron
Dexair
Dexotic
I-Methasone
Maxidex
Ocu-Dex

Generic name product may also be available.

In Canada

AK-Dex
Decadron
Maxidex

For Fluorometholone

In the U.S.

Fluor-Op
FML Forte
FML Liquifilm
FML S.O.P.

In Canada

Flarex
FML Forte
FML Liquifilm

For Hydrocortisone*

In Canada

Cortamed

Another commonly used name is cortisol.

For Medrysone

In the U.S.

HMS Liquifilm

In Canada

HMS Liquifilm

For Prednisolone

In the U.S.

AK-Pred
AK-Tate
Econopred
Econopred Plus
Inflamase Forte
Inflamase Mild
I-Pred
Lite Pred
Ocu-Pred
Ocu-Pred-A
Ocu-Pred Forte
Predair
Predair A
Predair Forte
Pred Forte
Pred Mild
Ultra Pred

Generic name product may also be available.

In Canada

AK-Tate
Inflamase
Inflamase Forte
Ophtho-Tate
Pred Forte
Pred Mild

*Not commercially available in the U.S.

Description

Ophthalmic adrenocorticoids (a-dree-noe-KOR-ti-koids) (cortisone-like medicines) are used to prevent permanent damage to the eye, which may occur with certain eye problems. They also provide relief from redness, irritation, and other discomfort.

Adrenocorticoids for use in the eye are available only with your doctor's prescription, in the following dosage forms:

Ophthalmic

Betamethasone

- Solution (Canada)

Dexamethasone
- Ointment (Canada)
- Solution (U.S. and Canada)
- Suspension (U.S. and Canada)

Fluorometholone
- Ointment (U.S.)
- Suspension (U.S. and Canada)

Hydrocortisone
- Ointment (Canada)

Medrysone
- Suspension (U.S. and Canada)

Prednisolone
- Solution (U.S. and Canada)
- Suspension (U.S. and Canada)

It is very important that you read and understand the following information. If any of it causes you special concern, check with your doctor. Also, *if you have any questions* or if you want more information about this medicine or your medical problem, *ask your doctor, nurse, or pharmacist.*

Before Using This Medicine

In deciding to use a medicine, the risks of taking the medicine must be weighed against the good it will do. This is a decision you and your doctor will make. For ophthalmic adrenocorticoids, the following should be considered:

Allergies—Tell your doctor if you have ever had any unusual or allergic reaction to adrenocorticoids. Also tell your doctor and pharmacist if you are allergic to any other substances, such as foods, preservatives, or dyes.

Pregnancy—Although studies on birth defects with ophthalmic adrenocorticoids have not been done in humans, these medicines have not been reported to cause birth defects or other problems. However, in animal studies, dexamethasone, fluorometholone, hydrocortisone, and prednisolone caused birth defects when applied to the eyes of pregnant animals. Also, fluorometholone and medrysone caused other unwanted effects in the animal fetus.

Breast-feeding—Ophthalmic adrenocorticoids have not been reported to cause problems in nursing babies.

Children—Children less than 2 years of age may be especially sensitive to the effects of ophthalmic adrenocorticoids. This may increase the chance of side effects. If this medicine has been ordered for a young child, you should discuss its use with your child's doctor. Be sure you follow all of the doctor's instructions very carefully.

Older adults—Although there is no specific information about the use of ophthalmic adrenocorticoids in the elderly, they are not expected to cause different side effects or problems in older people than they do in younger adults.

Other medicines—Although certain medicines should not be used together at all, in other cases two different medicines may be used together even if an interaction might occur. In these cases, your doctor may want to change the dose, or other precautions may be necessary. Tell your doctor and pharmacist if you are using any other prescription or nonprescription (over-the-counter [OTC]) ophthalmic medicine.

Other medical problems—The presence of other medical problems may affect the use of ophthalmic adrenocorticoids. Make sure you tell your doctor if you have any other medical problems, especially:

- Cataracts—Adrenocorticoids may worsen or cause cataracts
- Diabetes mellitus (sugar diabetes)—Patients with diabetes may be more likely to develop cataracts or glaucoma with the use of adrenocorticoids
- Glaucoma (or family history of)—Adrenocorticoids may worsen or cause glaucoma
- Herpes infection of the eye or
- Tuberculosis of the eye (active or history of) or
- Any other eye infection—Ophthalmic adrenocorticoids may worsen existing infections or cause new infections

Before you begin using any new medicine (prescription or nonprescription) or if you develop any new medical problem while you are using this medicine, check with your doctor, nurse, or pharmacist.

Proper Use of This Medicine

For patients who wear *contact lenses*:

- Use of ophthalmic adrenocorticoids while you are wearing contact lenses (either hard lenses or soft lenses) may increase the chance of infection. Therefore, do not apply this medicine while you are wearing contact lenses. Also, check with an ophthalmologist (eye doctor) for advice on how long to wait after applying this medicine before inserting your contact lenses. It is possible that you may be directed not to wear contact lenses at all during the entire time of treatment and for a day or two after treatment has been stopped.

For patients using an *eye drop form* of this medicine:

- If you are using a suspension form of this medicine, always shake the container very well just before applying the eye drops.
- To use:

  —First, wash your hands. With the middle finger, apply pressure to the inside corner of the eye (and continue to apply pressure for 1 or 2 minutes after the medicine has been placed in the eye). Tilt the head back and with the index finger of the same hand, pull the lower eyelid away from the eye to form a pouch. Drop the medicine into the pouch and gently close your eyes. Do not blink. Keep the eyes closed for 1 or 2 minutes to allow the medicine to come into contact with the irritation.

- If you think you did not get the drop of medicine into your eye properly, use another drop.
  —Remove any excess solution around the eye with a clean tissue, being careful not to touch the eye.
  —Immediately after using the eye drops, wash your hands to remove any medicine that may be on them.
  —To keep the medicine as germ-free as possible, do not touch the dropper or the applicator tip to any surface (including the eye). Always keep the container tightly closed.

For patients using an *ointment form* of this medicine:
- To use:
  —First, wash your hands. Then pull the lower eyelid away from the eye to form a pouch. Squeeze a thin strip of ointment into the pouch. A 1-cm (approximately ⅓ inch) strip of ointment is usually enough unless otherwise directed by your doctor. Gently close the eyes and keep them closed for 1 or 2 minutes to allow the medicine to spread over the surface of the eye and come into contact with the irritation.
  —To keep the medicine as germ-free as possible, do not touch the applicator tip to any surface (including the eye). After using the eye ointment, wipe the tip of the ointment tube with a clean tissue. Do not wash the tip with water. Always keep the tube tightly closed.

Do not use adrenocorticoids more often or for a longer time than your doctor ordered. To do so may increase the chance of side effects, especially in children 2 years of age or younger.

Do not use any leftover medicine for future eye problems without first checking with your doctor. This medicine should not be used if certain kinds of infections are present. To do so may make the infection worse and possibly lead to eye damage.

Missed dose—If you miss a dose of this medicine, apply it as soon as possible. However, if it is almost time for your next dose, skip the missed dose and go back to your regular dosing schedule.

Storage—To store this medicine:
- Keep out of the reach of children.
- Store away from heat and direct light.
- Keep the medicine from freezing.
- Do not keep outdated medicine or medicine no longer needed. Be sure that any discarded medicine is out of the reach of children.

Precautions While Using This Medicine

If you will be using this medicine for more than a few weeks, an ophthalmologist (eye doctor) should examine your eyes at regular visits to make sure it does not cause unwanted effects.

If your eye condition does not improve after 5 to 7 days, or if it becomes worse, check with your doctor.

Side Effects of This Medicine

Along with its needed effects, a medicine may cause some unwanted effects. Although not all of these side effects may occur, if they do occur they may need medical attention. Check with your doctor as soon as possible if any of the following side effects occur:

Less common or rare

Eye infection; eye pain; gradual blurring or loss of vision; increased number of floaters; nausea; seeing flashes of light; vomiting

Other side effects may occur that usually do not need medical attention. These side effects may go away during treatment as your body adjusts to the medicine. However, check with your doctor if any of the following side effects continue or are bothersome:

More frequent

Blurred vision (mild and temporary, occurs after use of ointments)

Less common or rare

Burning, stinging, redness, or watering of the eyes

Other side effects not listed may also occur in some patients. If you notice any other effects, check with your doctor.

Annual revision: 04/22/92

CORTICOSTEROIDS Otic

This information applies to the following medicines:

Betamethasone (bay-ta-METH-a-sone)
Dexamethasone (dex-a-METH-a-sone)
Hydrocortisone (hye-droe-KOR-ti-sone)

Some commonly used brand names are:

For Betamethasone*
In Canada
Betnesol

For Dexamethasone
In the U.S.
AK-Dex
Decadron
I-Methasone
In Canada
AK-Dex
Decadron

For Hydrocortisone*
In Canada
Cortamed

Another commonly used name is cortisol.

*Not commercially available in the U.S.

Description

Otic corticosteroids (kor-ti-koe-STE-roids) (cortisone-like medicines) are used in the ear to relieve the redness, itching, and swelling caused by certain ear problems.

Otic corticosteroids are available only with your doctor's prescription, in the following dosage forms:

Otic
Betamethasone
- Solution (Canada)

Dexamethasone
- Solution (U.S. and Canada)

Hydrocortisone
- Ointment (Canada)

It is very important that you read and understand the following information. If any of it causes you special concern, check with your doctor. Also, *if you have any questions* or if you want more information about this medicine or your medical problem, *ask your doctor, nurse, or pharmacist.*

Before Using This Medicine

In deciding to use a medicine, the risks of taking the medicine must be weighed against the good it will do. This is a decision you and your doctor will make. For otic corticosteroids, the following should be considered:

Allergies—Tell your doctor if you have ever had any unusual or allergic reaction to corticosteroids. Also tell your doctor and pharmacist if you are allergic to any other substances, such as certain preservatives or dyes.

Pregnancy—Otic corticosteroids have not been shown to cause birth defects or other problems in pregnant women.

Breast-feeding—Otic corticosteroids have not been reported to cause problems in nursing infants.

Children—Although there is no specific information about the use of otic corticosteroids in children, they are not expected to cause different side effects or problems in children than they do in adults.

Older adults—Although there is no specific information about the use of otic corticosteroids in the elderly, they are not expected to cause different side effects or problems in older people than they do in younger adults.

Other medical problems—The presence of other medical problems may affect the use of otic corticosteroids. Make sure you tell your doctor if you have any other medical problems, especially:

- Any other ear infection or condition (or history of)—Otic corticosteroids may worsen existing infections or cause new infections
- Punctured ear drum—Using otic corticosteroids with a punctured ear drum may damage the ear

Before you begin using any new medicine (prescription or nonprescription) or if you develop any new medical problem while you are using this medicine, check with your doctor, nurse, or pharmacist.

Proper Use of This Medicine

To use *ear drops:*

- Lie down or tilt the head so that the affected ear faces up. Gently pull the earlobe up and back for adults (down and back for children) to straighten the ear canal. Drop the medicine into the ear canal. Keep the ear facing up for several (about 5) minutes to allow the medicine to run to the bottom of the ear canal. A sterile cotton plug may be gently inserted into the ear opening to prevent the medicine from leaking out. At first, your doctor may want you to put more medicine on the cotton plug during the day to keep it moist.

To use *ear ointment:*

- Apply a small amount of ointment to the area just inside the ear canal, using a clean finger or a piece of sterile gauze. Do not use a cotton-tipped swab unless your doctor has directed you to do so and has explained exactly how to use it.

To keep the medicine as germ-free as possible, do not touch the dropper or applicator tip to any surface (including the ear). Also, keep the container tightly closed.

Do not use corticosteroids more often or for a longer time than your doctor ordered. To do so may increase the chance of side effects.

Do not use any leftover medicine for future ear problems without first checking with your doctor. This medicine should not be used if certain kinds of infections are present. To do so may make the infection worse.

Missed dose—If you miss a dose of this medicine, use it as soon as you remember. However, if it is almost time for your next dose, skip the missed dose and go back to your regular dosing schedule. Do not double doses.

Storage—To store this medicine:
- Keep out of the reach of children.
- Store away from heat and direct light.
- Keep the medicine from freezing.
- Do not keep outdated medicine or medicine no longer needed. Be sure that any discarded medicine is out of the reach of children.

Precautions While Using This Medicine

If your condition does not improve within 5 to 7 days, or if it becomes worse, check with your doctor.

Side Effects of This Medicine

Along with its needed effects, a medicine may cause some unwanted effects. The following side effects usually do not need medical attention and may go away during treatment as your body adjusts to the medicine. However, check with your doctor if either of the following side effects continues or is bothersome:

Less common
Burning or stinging of the ear

There have not been any other common or important side effects reported with this medicine. However, if you notice any unusual effects, check with your doctor.

Annual revision: 03/31/92

CORTICOSTEROIDS—Low Potency Topical

This information applies to the following medicines:
Alclometasone (al-kloe-MET-a-sone)
Clocortolone (kloe-KOR-toe-lone)
Desonide (DESS-oh-nide)
Dexamethasone (dex-a-METH-a-sone)
Flumethasone (floo-METH-a-sone)
Flurandrenolide (flure-an-DREN-oh-lide) (Drenison-¼ only)
Hydrocortisone (hye-droe-KOR-ti-sone)
Hydrocortisone acetate (hye-droe-KOR-ti-sone AS-a-tate)

Some commonly used brand names are:

For Alclometasone†
In the U.S.
Aclovate

For Clocortolone†
In the U.S.
Cloderm

For Desonide
In the U.S.
DesOwen
Tridesilon
Generic name product may also be available.
In Canada
Tridesilon

For Dexamethasone†
In the U.S.
Aeroseb-Dex
Decaderm
Decadron
Decaspray

For Flumethasone*
In Canada
Locacorten

Another commonly used name is flumetasone.

For Flurandrenolide
In Canada
Drenison-¼

For Hydrocortisone
In the U.S.
Acticort 100
Aeroseb-HC
Ala-Cort
Ala-Scalp HP
Allercort
Alphaderm
Bactine
Beta-HC
CaldeCORT Anti-Itch
Cetacort
Cortaid
Cort-Dome
Cortifair
Cortril
Delacort
Dermacort
Dermarest DriCort
DermiCort
Dermtex HC
Gly-Cort
Hi-Cor 1.0
Hi-Cor 2.5
Hydro-Tex
Hytone
LactiCare-HC
Lemoderm
Maximum Strength Cortaid
MyCort
Nutracort
Penecort
Pentacort
Rederm
S-T Cort
Synacort
Texacort
Generic name product may also be available.
In Canada
Barriere-HC
Cortate
Cortef
Emo-Cort
Emo-Cort Scalp Solution
Prevex HC
Sarna HC 1.0%
Sential
Unicort

Another commonly used name is cortisol.

For Hydrocortisone Acetate
In the U.S.
CaldeCORT Anti-Itch
CaldeCORT Light
Carmol-HC
Cortaid
Cortef Feminine Itch
Corticaine
Epifoam
FoilleCort
Gynecort
Gynecort 10
Lanacort
Lanacort 10
9-1-1
Pharma-Cort
Rhulicort
Generic name product may also be available.

In Canada

Cortacet	Cortoderm
Cortef	Hyderm
Corticreme	Novohydrocort

*Not commercially available in the U.S.
†Not commercially available in Canada.

Description

Topical corticosteroids (kor-ti-ko-STER-oyds) are used to help relieve redness, swelling, itching, and discomfort of many skin problems. These medicines are like cortisone. They belong to the general family of medicines called steroids.

Most corticosteroids are available only with your doctor's prescription. Some strengths of hydrocortisone are available without a prescription; however, your doctor may have special instructions on the proper use for your medical condition.

Topical corticosteroids are available in the following dosage forms:

Topical

Alclometasone
- Cream (U.S.)
- Ointment (U.S.)

Clocortolone
- Cream (U.S.)

Desonide
- Cream (U.S. and Canada)
- Lotion (U.S.)
- Ointment (U.S. and Canada)

Dexamethasone
- Cream (U.S.)
- Gel (U.S.)
- Topical aerosol (U.S.)

Flumethasone
- Cream (Canada)
- Ointment (Canada)

Flurandrenolide
- Cream 0.0125% (Canada)
- Ointment 0.0125% (Canada)

Hydrocortisone
- Cream (U.S. and Canada)
- Lotion (U.S. and Canada)
- Ointment (U.S. and Canada)
- Topical solution (U.S. and Canada)

Hydrocortisone acetate
- Cream (U.S. and Canada)
- Topical aerosol foam (U.S.)
- Lotion (U.S.)
- Ointment (U.S. and Canada)

It is very important that you read and understand the following information. If any of it causes you special concern, check with your doctor. Also, *if you have any questions* or if you want more information about this medicine or your medical problem, *ask your doctor, nurse, or pharmacist.*

Before Using This Medicine

In deciding to use a medicine, the risks of taking the medicine must be weighed against the good it will do. This is a decision you and your doctor will make. For topical corticosteroids, the following should be considered:

Allergies—Tell your doctor if you have ever had any unusual or allergic reaction to corticosteroids. Also tell your doctor and pharmacist if you are allergic to any other substances, such as foods, preservatives, or dyes.

Pregnancy—When used properly, these medicines have not been shown to cause problems in humans. Studies on birth defects have not been done in humans. However, studies in animals have shown that topical corticosteroids, when applied to the skin in large amounts or used for a long time, could cause birth defects.

Breast-feeding—Topical corticosteroids have not been reported to cause problems in nursing babies when used properly. However, corticosteroids should not be applied to the breasts just before nursing.

Children—Children and teenagers who must use this medicine for a long time should be checked often by their doctor. Other more potent corticosteroids are absorbed through the skin and can affect growth or cause other unwanted effects. Topical corticosteroids can also be absorbed if they are applied to large areas of skin. These effects are less likely to occur with the use of the lower potency corticosteroids. However, before using this medicine in children, you should discuss its use with your child's doctor.

Older adults—This medicine is not expected to cause different side effects or problems in older people than it does in younger adults.

Other medical problems—The presence of other medical problems may affect the use of topical corticosteroids. Make sure you tell your doctor if you have any other medical problems, especially:

- Diabetes mellitus (sugar diabetes)—Too much use of corticosteroids may cause a loss of control of diabetes by increasing blood and urine glucose. However, this is not likely to happen when topical corticosteroids are used for a short time
- Infection or sores at the place of treatment or
- Tuberculosis—Corticosteroids may make existing infections worse or cause new infections
- Skin conditions that cause thinning of skin with easy bruising—Corticosteroids may make thinning of the skin worse

Before you begin using any new medicine (prescription or nonprescription) or if you develop any new medical problem while you are using this medicine, check with your doctor, nurse, or pharmacist.

Proper Use of This Medicine

Be very careful not to get this medicine in your eyes. Wash your hands after using your finger to apply the medicine. If you accidentally get this medicine in your eyes, flush them with water.

Do not bandage or otherwise wrap the skin being treated unless directed to do so by your doctor.

If your doctor has ordered an occlusive dressing (airtight covering, such as kitchen plastic wrap or a special patch) to be applied over this medicine, make sure you know how to apply it. Since occlusive dressings increase the amount of medicine absorbed through your skin and the possibility of side effects, use them only as directed. If you have any questions about this, check with your doctor.

For patients using the *topical aerosol form* of this medicine:

- This medicine usually comes with patient directions. Read them carefully before using this medicine.
- It is important to avoid breathing in the vapors from the spray or getting them in your eyes. If you accidentally get this medicine in your eyes, flush them with water.
- Do not use near heat, near an open flame, or while smoking.

Do not use this medicine more often or for a longer time than your doctor ordered or than recommended on the package label. To do so may increase the chance of absorption through the skin and the chance of side effects.

If this medicine has been prescribed for you, it is meant to treat a specific skin problem. *Do not use it for other skin problems, and do not use nonprescription hydrocortisone for skin problems that are not listed on the package label, without first checking with your doctor.* Topical corticosteroids should not be used on many kinds of bacterial, virus, or fungus skin infections.

Missed dose—If your doctor has ordered you to use this medicine on a regular schedule and you miss a dose, apply it as soon as possible. But if it is almost time for your next dose, skip the missed dose and apply it at the next regularly scheduled time.

Storage—To store this medicine:

- Keep out of the reach of children.
- Store away from heat and direct light.
- Keep the medicine from freezing.
- Do not puncture, break, or burn aerosol containers, even after they are empty.
- Do not keep outdated medicine or medicine no longer needed. Be sure that any discarded medicine is out of the reach of children.

Precautions While Using This Medicine

Avoid using tight-fitting diapers or plastic pants on a child if this medicine is being used on the child's diaper area. Plastic pants and tight-fitting diapers may increase the chance of absorption of the medicine through the skin and the chance of side effects.

Side Effects of This Medicine

Along with its needed effects, a medicine may cause some unwanted effects. Although not all of these side effects may occur, if they do occur they may need medical attention.

Check with your doctor as soon as possible if any of the following side effects occur:

Less common or rare

Lack of healing of skin condition; skin pain, redness, itching, or pus-containing blisters; severe burning and continued itching of skin

Some side effects may occur that usually do not need medical attention. These side effects may go away during treatment as your body adjusts to the medicine. However, check with your doctor if any of the following side effects continue or are bothersome:

Less common or rare

Burning, dryness, irritation, itching, or redness of skin; increased redness or scaling of skin sores; skin rash

When the gel, solution, lotion, or aerosol form of this medicine is applied, a mild, temporary stinging may be expected.

Other side effects not listed above may also occur in some patients. If you notice any other effects, check with your doctor.

Annual revision: 11/18/92

CORTICOSTEROIDS—Medium to Very High Potency Topical

This information applies to the following medicines:

- Amcinonide (am-SIN-oh-nide)
- Beclomethasone (be-kloe-METH-a-sone)
- Betamethasone (bay-ta-METH-a-sone)
- Clobetasol (kloe-BAY-ta-sol)
- Clobetasone (kloe-BAY-ta-sone)
- Desoximetasone (des-ox-i-MET-a-sone)
- Diflorasone (dye-FLOR-a-sone)
- Diflucortolone (di-floo-KOR-toe-lone)
- Fluocinolone (floo-oh-SIN-oh-lone)
- Fluocinonide (floo-oh-SIN-oh-nide)
- Flurandrenolide (flure-an-DREN-oh-lide) (except Drenison-¼)
- Fluticasone (floo-TIK-a-sone)
- Halcinonide (hal-SIN-oh-nide)
- Halobetasol (hal-oh-BAY-ta-sol)
- Hydrocortisone butyrate (hye-droe-KOR-ti-sone bue-TEAR-ate)
- Hydrocortisone valerate (hye-droe-KOR-ti-sone val-AIR-ate)
- Mometasone (moe-MET-a-sone)
- Triamcinolone (trye-am-SIN-oh-lone)

Some commonly used brand names or other names are:

For Amcinonide

In the U.S.

Cyclocort

In Canada

Cyclocort

For Beclomethasone*

In Canada

Propaderm

Another commonly used name is beclometasone.

For Betamethasone

In the U.S.

Alphatrex
Betatrex
Beta-Val
Dermabet
Diprolene
Diprolene AF
Diprosone
Maxivate
Teladar
Uticort
Valisone
Valisone Reduced Strength
Valnac

Generic name product may also be available.

In Canada

Beben
Betacort Scalp Lotion
Betaderm
Betaderm Scalp Lotion
Betnovate
Betnovate-½
Celestoderm-V
Celestoderm-V/2
Diprolene
Diprosone
Ectosone Mild
Ectosone Regular
Ectosone Scalp Lotion
Metaderm Mild
Metaderm Regular
Novobetamet
Prevex B
Topilene
Topisone
Valisone Scalp Lotion

For Clobetasol

In the U.S.

Temovate
Temovate Scalp Application

In Canada

Dermovate
Dermovate Scalp Lotion

For Clobetasone*

In Canada

Eumovate

For Desoximetasone

In the U.S.

Topicort
Topicort LP

Generic name product may also be available.

In Canada

Topicort
Topicort Mild

For Diflorasone

In the U.S.

Florone
Florone E
Maxiflor
Psorcon

In Canada

Florone

For Diflucortolone*

In Canada

Nerisone
Nerisone Oily

For Fluocinolone

In the U.S.

Bio-Syn
Fluocet
Fluonid
Flurosyn
Synalar
Synalar-HP
Synemol

Generic name product may also be available.

In Canada

Fluoderm
Fluolar
Fluonide
Synalar
Synamol

For Fluocinonide

In the U.S.

Fluocin
Licon
Lidex
Lidex-E

Generic name product may also be available.

In Canada

Lidemol
Lidex
Lyderm
Topsyn

For Flurandrenolide

In the U.S.

Cordran
Cordran SP

Generic name product may also be available.

In Canada

Drenison

Another commonly used name is fludroxycortide.

For Fluticasone†

In the U.S.

Cutivate

For Halcinonide

In the U.S.

Halog
Halog-E

In Canada

Halog

For Halobetasol†

In the U.S.

Ultravate

For Hydrocortisone Butyrate

In the U.S.

Locoid

For Hydrocortisone Valerate

In the U.S.

Westcort

In Canada

Westcort

For Mometasone

In the U.S.

Elocon

In Canada
Elocom

For Triamcinolone
In the U.S.

Aristocort	Kenalog
Aristocort A	Kenalog-H
Delta-Tritex	Kenonel
Flutex	Triacet
Kenac	Triderm

Generic name product may also be available.

In Canada

Aristocort C	Triaderm
Aristocort D	Trianide Mild
Aristocort R	Trianide Regular
Kenalog	

*Not commercially available in the U.S.
†Not commercially available in Canada.

Description

Topical corticosteroids (kor-ti-ko-STER-oyds) are used to help relieve redness, swelling, itching, and discomfort of many skin problems. These medicines are like cortisone. They belong to the general family of medicines called steroids.

These corticosteroids are available only with your doctor's prescription. Topical corticosteroids are available in the following dosage forms:

Topical

Amcinonide
- Cream (U.S. and Canada)
- Lotion (U.S. and Canada)
- Ointment (U.S. and Canada)

Beclomethasone
- Cream (Canada)
- Lotion (Canada)
- Ointment (Canada)

Betamethasone
- Cream (U.S. and Canada)
- Gel (U.S. and Canada)
- Lotion (U.S. and Canada)
- Ointment (U.S. and Canada)
- Topical aerosol (U.S.)

Clobetasol
- Cream (U.S. and Canada)
- Ointment (U.S. and Canada)
- Solution (U.S. and Canada)

Clobetasone
- Cream (Canada)
- Ointment (Canada)

Desoximetasone
- Cream (U.S. and Canada)
- Gel (U.S. and Canada)
- Ointment (U.S.)

Diflorasone
- Cream (U.S. and Canada)
- Ointment (U.S. and Canada)

Diflucortolone
- Cream (Canada)
- Ointment (Canada)

Fluocinolone
- Cream (U.S. and Canada)
- Ointment (U.S. and Canada)
- Topical solution (U.S. and Canada)

Fluocinonide
- Cream (U.S. and Canada)
- Gel (U.S. and Canada)
- Ointment (U.S. and Canada)
- Topical solution (U.S. and Canada)

Flurandrenolide
- Cream (U.S. and Canada)
- Lotion (U.S.)
- Ointment (U.S. and Canada)
- Tape (U.S. and Canada)

Fluticasone
- Cream (U.S.)
- Ointment (U.S.)

Halcinonide
- Cream (U.S. and Canada)
- Ointment (U.S. and Canada)
- Topical solution (U.S. and Canada)

Halobetasol
- Cream (U.S.)
- Ointment (U.S.)

Hydrocortisone butyrate
- Cream (U.S.)
- Ointment (U.S.)

Hydrocortisone valerate
- Cream (U.S. and Canada)
- Ointment (U.S. and Canada)

Mometasone
- Cream (U.S. and Canada)
- Lotion (U.S. and Canada)
- Ointment (U.S. and Canada)

Triamcinolone
- Cream (U.S. and Canada)
- Lotion (U.S.)
- Ointment (U.S. and Canada)
- Topical aerosol (U.S.)

It is very important that you read and understand the following information. If any of it causes you special concern, check with your doctor. Also, *if you have any questions* or if you want more information about this medicine or your medical problem, *ask your doctor, nurse, or pharmacist.*

Before Using This Medicine

In deciding to use a medicine, the risks of taking the medicine must be weighed against the good it will do. This is a decision you and your doctor will make. For corticosteroids, the following should be considered:

Allergies—Tell your doctor if you have ever had any unusual or allergic reaction to corticosteroids. Also tell your doctor and pharmacist if you are allergic to any other substances, such as foods, preservatives, or dyes.

Pregnancy—When used properly, these medicines have not been shown to cause problems in humans. Studies on birth defects have not been done in humans. However, studies in animals have shown that topical corticosteroids, when applied to the skin in large amounts or used for a long time, could cause birth defects.

Breast-feeding—Topical corticosteroids have not been reported to cause problems in nursing babies when used properly. However, corticosteroids should not be applied to the breasts before nursing.

Children—Children and teenagers who must use this medicine should be checked often by their doctor since this medicine may be absorbed through the skin and can affect growth or cause other unwanted effects.

Older adults—Certain side effects may be more likely to occur in elderly patients since the skin of older adults may be naturally thin. These unwanted effects may include tearing of the skin or blood-containing blisters on the skin.

Other medicines—Although certain medicines should not be used together at all, in other cases two different medicines may be used together even if an interaction might occur. In these cases, your doctor may want to change the dose, or other precautions may be necessary. Tell your doctor and pharmacist if you are taking or using any other prescription or nonprescription (over-the-counter [OTC]) medicine.

Other medical problems—The presence of other medical problems may affect the use of topical corticosteroids. Make sure you tell your doctor if you have any other medical problems, especially:

- Cataracts or
- Glaucoma—Corticosteroids may make these medical problems worse, especially when stronger corticosteroids are used in the eye area
- Diabetes mellitus (sugar diabetes)—Too much use of corticosteroids may cause a loss of control of diabetes by increasing blood and urine glucose. However, this is not likely to happen when topical corticosteroids are used for a short time
- Infection or sores at the place of treatment (unless your doctor also prescribed medicine for the infection) or
- Tuberculosis—Corticosteroids may make existing infections worse or cause new infections

Before you begin using any new medicine (prescription or nonprescription) or if you develop any new medical problem while you are using this medicine, check with your doctor, nurse, or pharmacist.

Proper Use of This Medicine

Be very careful not to get this medicine in your eyes. Wash your hands after using your finger to apply the medicine. If you accidentally get this medicine in your eyes, flush them with water.

Do not bandage or otherwise wrap the skin being treated unless directed to do so by your doctor.

If your doctor has ordered an occlusive dressing (airtight covering, such as kitchen plastic wrap or a special patch) to be applied over this medicine, make sure you know how to apply it. Since occlusive dressings increase the amount of medicine absorbed through your skin and the possibility of side effects, use them only as directed. If you have any questions about this, check with your doctor.

For patients using the *topical aerosol form* of this medicine:

- This medicine usually comes with patient directions. Read them carefully before using this medicine.
- It is important to avoid breathing in the vapors from the spray or getting them in your eyes. If you accidentally get this medicine in your eyes, flush them with water.
- Do not use near heat, near an open flame, or while smoking.

For patients using *flurandrenolide tape:*

- This medicine usually comes with patient directions. Read them carefully before using this medicine.

Do not use this medicine more often or for a longer time than your doctor ordered. To do so may increase the chance of absorption through the skin and the chance of side effects. In addition, too much use, especially on areas with thinner skin (for example, face, armpits, groin), may result in thinning of the skin and stretch marks or other unwanted effects.

Do not use any leftover medicine for other skin problems without first checking with your doctor. Topical corticosteroids should not be used on many kinds of bacterial, virus, or fungus skin infections.

Missed dose—If your doctor has ordered you to use this medicine on a regular schedule and you miss a dose, apply it as soon as possible. However, if it is almost time for your next dose, skip the missed dose and apply it at the next regularly scheduled time.

Storage—To store this medicine:

- Keep out of the reach of children.
- Store away from heat and direct light.
- Keep the medicine from freezing.
- Do not puncture, break, or burn aerosol containers, even after they are empty.
- Do not keep outdated medicine or medicine no longer needed. Be sure that any discarded medicine is out of the reach of children.

Precautions While Using This Medicine

Avoid using tight-fitting diapers or plastic pants on a child if this medicine is being used on the child's diaper area. Plastic pants or tight-fitting diapers may increase the chance of absorption of the medicine through the skin and the chance of side effects.

Side Effects of This Medicine

Along with its needed effects, a medicine may cause some unwanted effects. Although not all of these side effects may occur, if they do occur they may need medical attention.

Check with your doctor as soon as possible if any of the following side effects occur:

Less frequent or rare

Blood-containing blisters on skin; increased skin sensitivity (for some brands of betamethasone lotion); lack of healing of skin condition; loss of top skin layer (for tape dosage forms); numbness in fingers; raised, dark red, wart-like spots on skin; skin pain, redness, itching or pus-containing blisters; severe burning and continued itching of skin; thinning of skin with easy bruising

Additional side effects may occur if you use this medicine improperly or for a long time. Check with your doctor if any of the following side effects occur:

Rare

Acne or oily skin; backache; blurring or loss of vision (occurs gradually if certain products have been used near the eye); burning and itching of skin with pinhead-sized red blisters; eye pain (if certain products have been used near the eye); filling or rounding out of the face; increased blood pressure; irregular heartbeat; irregular menstrual periods; irritability; irritation of skin around mouth; loss of appetite (continuing); mental depression; muscle cramps, pain, or weakness; nausea; rapid weight gain or loss; reddish purple lines (stretch marks) on arms, face, legs, trunk, or groin; skin color changes; softening of skin; stomach bloating, pain, cramping, or burning; swelling of feet or lower legs; tearing of the skin; unusual decrease in sexual desire or ability (in men); unusual increase in hair growth, especially on the face; unusual loss of hair, especially on the scalp; unusual tiredness or weakness; vomiting; weakness of the arms, legs, or trunk (severe); worsening of infections

Some side effects may occur that usually do not need medical attention. These side effects may go away during treatment as your body adjusts to the medicine. However, check with your doctor if any of the following side effects continue or are bothersome:

Less frequent or rare

Burning, dryness, irritation, itching, or redness of skin; increased redness or scaling of skin sores; skin rash

When the gel, solution, lotion, or aerosol form of this medicine is applied, a mild, temporary stinging may be expected.

Other side effects not listed above may also occur in some patients. If you notice any other effects, check with your doctor.

Annual revision: 11/18/92

CORTICOSTEROIDS AND ACETIC ACID Otic

This information applies to the following medicines:

Desonide (DESS-oh-nide) and Acetic Acid (a-SEAT-ic AS-id)
Hydrocortisone (hye-droe-KOR-ti-sone) and Acetic Acid

Some commonly used brand names are:

For Desonide and Acetic Acid
In the U.S.
Otic Tridesilon Solution

For Hydrocortisone and Acetic Acid
In the U.S.
VõSol HC
In Canada
VõSol HC

Description

Corticosteroid (kor-ti-koe-STE-roid) and acetic acid combinations are used to treat certain problems of the ear canal. They also help relieve the redness, itching, and swelling that may accompany these conditions.

These medicines may also be used for other conditions as determined by your doctor.

Corticosteroid and acetic acid combinations are available only with your doctor's prescription, in the following dosage forms:

Otic

Desonide and Acetic Acid
- Solution (U.S.)

Hydrocortisone and Acetic Acid
- Solution (U.S. and Canada)

It is very important that you read and understand the following information. If any of it causes you special concern, check with your doctor. Also, *if you have any questions* or if you want more information about this medicine or your medical problem, *ask your doctor, nurse, or pharmacist.*

Before Using This Medicine

In deciding to use a medicine, the risks of using the medicine must be weighed against the good it will do.

This is a decision you and your doctor will make. For otic corticosteroids with acetic acid, the following should be considered:

Allergies—Tell your doctor if you have ever had any unusual or allergic reaction to corticosteroids or acetic acid. Also tell your doctor and pharmacist if you are allergic to any other substances, such as certain preservatives or dyes.

Pregnancy—Corticosteroid and acetic acid combinations used in the ear have not been shown to cause birth defects or other problems in humans.

Breast-feeding—Otic corticosteroid and acetic acid combinations have not been reported to cause problems in nursing babies.

Children—Although there is no specific information comparing the use of otic corticosteroids in children with use in other age groups, this combination medicine is not expected to cause different side effects or problems in children than it does in adults.

Older adults—Although there is no specific information comparing the use of otic corticosteroids in the elderly with use in other age groups, they are not expected to cause different side effects or problems in older people than they do in younger adults.

Other medical problems—The presence of other medical problems may affect the use of otic corticosteroids. Make sure you tell your doctor if you have any other medical problems, especially:

- Any other ear infection or condition—Otic corticosteroids may worsen existing infections or cause new infections
- Punctured ear drum—Using otic corticosteroids when you have a punctured ear drum may damage the ear

Before you begin using any new medicine (prescription or nonprescription) or if you develop any new medical problem while you are using this medicine, check with your doctor, nurse, or pharmacist.

Proper Use of This Medicine

To use:

- Lie down or tilt the head so that the affected ear faces up. Gently pull the ear lobe up and back for adults (down and back for children) to straighten the ear canal. Drop the medicine into the ear canal. Keep the ear facing up for several (about 5) minutes to allow the medicine to run to the bottom of the ear canal. A sterile cotton plug may be gently inserted into the ear opening to prevent the medicine from leaking out. At first, your doctor may want you to put more medicine on the cotton plug during the day to keep it moist.

To keep the medicine as germ-free as possible, avoid touching the dropper or applicator tip to any surface as much as possible (including the ear). Also, always keep the container tightly closed.

For patients using *hydrocortisone and acetic acid ear drops:*

- *Do not wash the dropper or applicator tip,* because water may get into the medicine and make it weaker. If necessary, you may wipe the dropper or applicator tip with a clean tissue.

Do not use corticosteroids more often or for a longer time than your doctor ordered. To do so may increase the chance of side effects.

Do not use any leftover medicine for future ear problems without first checking with your doctor. This medicine should not be used if certain kinds of infections are present. To do so may make the infection worse.

Missed dose—If you miss a dose of this medicine, apply it as soon as possible. But if it is almost time for your next dose, skip the missed dose and go back to your regular dosing schedule.

Storage—To store this medicine:

- Keep out of the reach of children.
- Store away from heat and direct light.
- Keep the medicine from freezing.
- Do not keep outdated medicine or medicine no longer needed. Be sure that any discarded medicine is out of the reach of children.

Precautions While Using This Medicine

If your condition does not improve within 5 to 7 days, or if it becomes worse, check with your doctor.

Side Effects of This Medicine

Along with its needed effects, a medicine may cause some unwanted effects. The following side effects usually do not need medical attention and may go away during treatment as your body adjusts to the medicine or your condition improves. However, check with your doctor if any of the following side effects continue or are bothersome:

Less common

Stinging, itching, irritation or burning of the ear

There have not been any other side effects reported with this medicine. However, if you notice any other effects, check with your doctor.

Annual revision: 03/31/92

CORTICOSTEROIDS/CORTICOTROPIN—Glucocorticoid Effects Systemic

This information applies to the following medicines:

- Betamethasone (bay-ta-METH-a-sone)
- Corticotropin (kor-ti-koe-TROE-pin)
- Cortisone (KOR-ti-sone)
- Dexamethasone (dex-a-METH-a-sone)
- Hydrocortisone (hye-droe-KOR-ti-sone)
- Methylprednisolone (meth-ill-pred-NISS-oh-lone)
- Paramethasone (par-a-METH-a-sone)
- Prednisolone (pred-NISS-oh-lone)
- Prednisone (PRED-ni-sone)
- Triamcinolone (trye-am-SIN-oh-lone)

The following information does *not* apply to desoxycorticosterone or fludrocortisone.

Some commonly used brand names are:

For Betamethasone

In the U.S.

Celestone
Celestone Phosphate
Celestone Soluspan
Selestoject

Generic name product may also be available.

In Canada

Betnelan
Betnesol
Celestone
Celestone Soluspan

For Corticotropin

In the U.S.

Acthar
Cortrophin-Zinc
H.P. Acthar Gel

Generic name product may also be available.

In Canada

Acthar
Acthar Gel (H.P.)

Another commonly used name is ACTH.

For Cortisone

In the U.S.

Cortone Acetate

Generic name product may also be available.

In Canada

Cortone

Generic name product may also be available.

For Dexamethasone

In the U.S.

AK-Dex
Dalalone
Dalalone D.P.
Dalalone L.A.
Decadrol
Decadron
Decadron-LA
Decadron Phosphate
Decaject
Decaject-L.A.
Deronil
Dexacen-4
Dexacen LA-8
Dexamethasone Intensol
Dexasone
Dexasone-LA
Dexone
Dexone 0.5
Dexone 0.75
Dexone 1.5
Dexone 4
Dexone LA
Hexadrol
Hexadrol Phosphate
Mymethasone
Solurex
Solurex-LA

Generic name product may also be available.

In Canada

Decadron
Decadron Phosphate
Deronil
Dexasone
Hexadrol
Oradexon

Generic name product may also be available.

For Hydrocortisone

In the U.S.

A-hydroCort
Cortef
Cortenema
Cortifoam
Hydrocortone
Hydrocortone Acetate
Hydrocortone Phosphate
Solu-Cortef

In Canada

Cortef
Cortenema
Cortifoam
Solu-Cortef

Another commonly used name is cortisol.

For Methylprednisolone

In the U.S.

A-methaPred
depMedalone 40
depMedalone 80
Depoject-40
Depoject-80
Depo-Medrol
Depopred-40
Depopred-80
Depo-Predate 40
Depo-Predate 80
Duralone-40
Duralone-80
Medralone-40
Medralone-80
Medrol
Medrol Enpak
Meprolone
Rep-Pred 40
Rep-Pred 80
Solu-Medrol

Generic name product may also be available.

In Canada

Depo-Medrol
Medrol
Solu-Medrol

For Paramethasone

In the U.S.

Haldrone

For Prednisolone

In the U.S.

Articulose-50
Delta-Cortef
Hydeltrasol
Hydeltra-T.B.A.
Key-Pred 25
Key-Pred 50
Key-Pred SP
Nor-Pred T.B.A.
Pediapred
Predaject-50
Predalone 50
Predalone T.B.A.
Predate 50
Predate S
Predate TBA
Predcor-25
Predcor-50
Predcor-TBA
Predicort-50
Predicort-RP
Prelone

Generic name product may also be available.

For Prednisone

In the U.S.

Deltasone
Liquid Pred
Meticorten
Orasone 1
Orasone 5
Orasone 10
Orasone 20
Orasone 50
Prednicen-M
Prednisone Intensol
Sterapred
Sterapred DS

Generic name product may also be available.

In Canada

Apo-Prednisone
Deltasone
Winpred

Generic name product may also be available.

For Triamcinolone

In the U.S.

Amcort	Kenaject-40
Aristocort	Kenalog-10
Aristocort Forte	Kenalog-40
Artistocort Intralesional	Tac-3
Artistospan Intra-articular	Triam-A
Aristospan Intralesional	Triam-Forte
Articulose-L.A.	Triamolone 40
Cenocort A-40	Triamonide 40
Cenocort Forte	Tri-Kort
Cinalone 40	Trilog
Cinonide 40	Trilone
Kenacort	Tristoject
Kenacort Diacetate	

Generic name product may also be available.

In Canada

Aristocort	Kenacort
Artistocort Forte	Kenalog-10
Aristocort Intralesional	Kenalog-40
Aristospan Intra-articular	

Generic name product may also be available.

Description

Adrenocorticoids (a-dree-noe-KOR-ti-koids) (cortisone-like medicines) are used to provide relief for inflamed areas of the body. They lessen swelling, redness, itching, and allergic reactions. They are often used as part of the treatment for a number of different diseases, such as severe allergies or skin problems, asthma, or arthritis. Adrenocorticoids may also be used for other conditions as determined by your doctor.

Your body naturally produces certain cortisone-like hormones that are necessary to maintain good health. If your body does not produce enough, your doctor may have prescribed this medicine to help make up the difference.

Corticotropin is not an adrenocorticoid. It is a hormone that occurs naturally in the body. Corticotropin is known as an adrenocorticotropic hormone, which means it causes the adrenal glands to produce cortisone-like hormones. Corticotropin is used as a test to determine whether your adrenal glands are producing enough hormones. Also, it is sometimes used instead of adrenocorticoids to treat many of the same medical problems.

Adrenocorticoids and corticotropin are very strong medicines. In addition to their helpful effects in treating your medical problem, they have side effects that can be very serious. If your adrenal glands are not producing enough cortisone-like hormones, taking this medicine is not likely to cause problems unless you take too much of it. If you are taking this medicine to treat another medical problem, be sure that you discuss the risks and benefits of this medicine with your doctor.

These medicines are available only with your doctor's prescription, in the following dosage forms:

Oral

Betamethasone
- Syrup (U.S.)
- Tablets (U.S. and Canada)
- Effervescent tablets (Canada)
- Extended-release tablets (Canada)

Cortisone
- Tablets (U.S. and Canada)

Dexamethasone
- Elixir (U.S.)
- Oral solution (U.S.)
- Tablets (U.S. and Canada)

Hydrocortisone
- Oral suspension (U.S.)
- Tablets (U.S. and Canada)

Methylprednisolone
- Tablets (U.S. and Canada)

Paramethasone
- Tablets (U.S.)

Prednisolone
- Oral solution (U.S.)
- Syrup (U.S.)
- Tablets (U.S.)

Prednisone
- Oral solution (U.S.)
- Syrup (U.S.)
- Tablets (U.S. and Canada)

Triamcinolone
- Syrup (U.S. and Canada)
- Tablets (U.S. and Canada)

Parenteral

Betamethasone
- Injection (U.S. and Canada)

Corticotropin
- Injection (U.S. and Canada)

Cortisone
- Injection (U.S. and Canada)

Dexamethasone
- Injection (U.S. and Canada)

Hydrocortisone
- Injection (U.S. and Canada)

Methylprednisolone
- Injection (U.S. and Canada)

Prednisolone
- Injection (U.S.)

Triamcinolone
- Injection (U.S. and Canada)

Rectal

Betamethasone
- Enema (Canada)

Hydrocortisone
- Aerosol foam (U.S. and Canada)
- Enema (U.S. and Canada)

Methylprednisolone
- Enema (U.S.)

It is very important that you read and understand the following information. If any of it causes you special concern, check with your doctor. Also, *if you have any questions* or if you want more information about this medicine or your medical problem, *ask your doctor, nurse, or pharmacist.*

Before Using This Medicine

In deciding to use a medicine, the risks of taking the medicine must be weighed against the good it will do.

This is a decision you and your doctor will make. For adrenocorticoids and corticotropin, the following should be considered:

Allergies—Tell your doctor if you have ever had any unusual or allergic reaction to adrenocorticoids or corticotropin. Also tell your doctor and pharmacist if you are allergic to any other substances, such as foods, preservatives, or dyes.

Diet—If you will be using this medicine for a long time, your doctor may want you to:

- Follow a low-salt diet and/or a potassium-rich diet.
- Watch your calories to prevent weight gain.
- Add extra protein to your diet. Make certain your doctor and pharmacist know if you are already on any special diet, such as a low-sodium or low-sugar diet.

Pregnancy—Studies on birth defects with adrenocorticoids or with corticotropin have not been done in humans. However, too much use of adrenocorticoids during pregnancy may cause the baby to have problems after birth, such as slower growth. Also, studies in animals have shown that adrenocorticoids cause birth defects and that corticotropin may cause other unwanted effects in the fetus.

Breast-feeding—Adrenocorticoids pass into breast milk and may cause problems with growth or other unwanted effects in nursing babies. Depending on the amount of medicine you are taking every day, it may be necessary for you to take another medicine or to stop breast-feeding during treatment. Corticotropin has not been shown to cause problems in nursing babies.

Children—Adrenocorticoids or corticotropin may slow or stop growth in children and in growing teenagers, especially when they are used for a long time. Before this medicine is given to children or teenagers, you should discuss its use with your child's doctor and then carefully follow the doctor's instructions.

Older adults—Older patients may be more likely to develop high blood pressure or bone disease from adrenocorticoids. Women are especially at risk of developing bone disease.

Other medicines—Although certain medicines should not be used together at all, in other cases two different medicines may be used together even if an interaction might occur. In these cases, your doctor may want to change the dose, or other precautions may be necessary. When you are taking adrenocorticoids or corticotropin, it is especially important that your doctor and pharmacist know if you are taking any of the following:

- Aminoglutethimide or
- Antacids (in large amounts) or
- Barbiturates, except butalbital, or
- Carbamazepine (e.g., Tegretol) or
- Griseofulvin (e.g., Fulvicin) or
- Mitotane (e.g., Lysodren) or
- Phenylbutazone (e.g., Butazolidin) or
- Phenytoin (e.g., Dilantin) or
- Primidone (e.g., Mysoline) or
- Rifampin (e.g., Rifadin)—Use of these medicines may make corticotropin or certain adrenocorticoids less effective
- Amphotericin B by injection (e.g., Fungizone)—Adrenocorticoids and this medicine decrease the amount of potassium in the blood. Serious side effects could occur if the level of potassium gets too low
- Antidiabetics, oral (diabetes medicine taken by mouth) or
- Insulin—Adrenocorticoids may increase blood glucose (sugar) levels
- Digitalis glycosides (heart medicine)—Adrenocorticoids decrease the amount of potassium in the blood. Digitalis can cause an irregular heartbeat or other problems more commonly if the blood potassium gets too low
- Diuretics (water pills) or
- Medicine containing potassium—Using adrenocorticoids with diuretics may cause the diuretic to be less effective. Also, adrenocorticoids may increase the risk of low blood potassium, which is also a problem with certain diuretics. Potassium supplements or a different type of diuretic is used in treating high blood pressure in those people who have problems keeping their blood potassium at a normal level. Adrenocorticoids may make these medicines less able to do this
- Immunizations (vaccinations)—While you are being treated with this medicine, and even after you stop taking it, do not have any immunizations without your doctor's approval. Also, other people living in your home should not receive oral polio vaccine, since there is a chance they could pass the polio virus on to you. In addition, you should avoid close contact with other people at school or work who have recently taken oral polio vaccine
- Skin test injections—Adrenocorticoids may cause false results in skin tests
- Sodium-containing medicine—Adrenocorticoids and corticotropin cause the body to retain (keep) more salt and water. Too much sodium may cause high blood sodium, high blood pressure, and excess body water

Other medical problems—The presence of other medical problems may affect the use of adrenocorticoids and corticotropin. Make sure you tell your doctor if you have any other medical problems, especially:

- Bone disease—These medicines may worsen bone disease because they cause the body to lose more calcium
- Colitis or
- Diverticulitis or
- Stomach ulcer or other stomach or intestine problems—These medicines may cover up symptoms of a worsening stomach or intestinal condition. A patient would not know if his/her condition was getting worse and would not get medical help when needed
- Diabetes mellitus (sugar diabetes)—Adrenocorticoids may cause a loss of control of diabetes by increasing blood glucose (sugar)
- Fungus infection or any other infection or
- Herpes simplex infection of the eye or
- Infection at the place of treatment or

- Recent surgery or serious injury or
- Tuberculosis (active TB, nonactive TB, or past history of)—These medicines can cause slower healing, worsen existing infections, or cause new infections
- Glaucoma—Adrenocorticoids may cause the pressure within the eye to increase
- Heart disease or
- High blood pressure or
- Kidney disease (especially if you are receiving dialysis) or
- Kidney stones—These medicines cause the body to retain (keep) more salt and water. These conditions may be made worse by this extra body water
- High cholesterol levels—Adrenocorticoids may increase blood cholesterol levels
- Liver disease or
- Overactive thyroid or
- Underactive thyroid—With these conditions, the body may not eliminate the adrenocorticoid at the usual rate, which may change the medicine's effect
- Myasthenia gravis—When these medicines are first started, muscle weakness may occur. Your doctor may want to take special precautions because this could cause problems with breathing
- Systemic lupus erythematosus (SLE)—This condition may cause certain side effects of adrenocorticoids to occur more easily

Before you begin using any new medicine (prescription or nonprescription) or if you develop any new medical problem while you are using this medicine, check with your doctor, nurse, or pharmacist.

Proper Use of This Medicine

For patients taking this medicine by mouth:

- *Take this medicine with food* to help prevent stomach upset. If stomach upset, burning, or pain continues, check with your doctor.
- Stomach problems may be more likely to occur if you drink alcoholic beverages while being treated with this medicine. You should not drink alcoholic beverages while taking this medicine, unless you have first checked with your doctor.

For patients using this medicine rectally:

- This medicine usually comes with patient directions. Read them carefully before using this medicine.
- For patients using hydrocortisone enema:

  —Each bottle contains a single dose. Use it all, unless otherwise directed by your doctor.

  —For best results, use this medicine right after a bowel movement. Lie down on your left side when giving the enema.

  —Insert the rectal tip of the enema applicator gently to prevent damage to the rectal wall.

  —Stay on your left side for at least 30 minutes after the enema is given so the medicine can work. If you can, keep the medicine inside the rectum all night.

- For patients using hydrocortisone acetate rectal aerosol foam:

  —This medicine is used with a special applicator. Do not insert any part of the aerosol container into the rectum.

- For patients using methylprednisolone acetate for enema:

  —Each bottle contains a single dose. Use it all, unless otherwise directed by your doctor.

  —Insert the rectal tip of the enema applicator gently to prevent damage to the rectal wall.

  —If you have been directed to use this enema slowly (not all at once), shake the bottle once in a while while you are giving the enema.

  —Save your applicator. Refill units of this medicine may be available at a lower cost.

Use this medicine only as directed by your doctor. Do not use more or less of it, do not use it more often, and do not use it for a longer time than your doctor ordered. To do so may increase the chance of side effects.

Missed dose—If you miss a dose of this medicine and your dosing schedule is:

- One dose every other day—Take the missed dose as soon as possible if you remember it the same morning, then go back to your regular dosing schedule. If you do not remember the missed dose until later, wait and take it the following morning. Then skip a day and start your regular dosing schedule again.
- One dose a day—Take the missed dose as soon as possible, then go back to your regular dosing schedule. If you do not remember until the next day, skip the missed dose and do not double the next one.
- Several doses a day—Take the missed dose as soon as possible, then go back to your regular dosing schedule. If you do not remember until your next dose is due, double the next dose.

If you have any questions about this, check with your doctor, nurse, or pharmacist.

Storage—To store this medicine:

- Keep out of the reach of children.
- Store away from heat and direct light.
- Do not store tablets in the bathroom, near the kitchen sink, or in other damp places. Heat or moisture may cause the medicine to break down.
- Keep the liquid dosage forms of this medicine, including enemas, and hydrocortisone rectal aerosol foam from freezing.
- Do not puncture, break, or burn the hydrocortisone rectal aerosol foam container, even when it is empty.

- Do not keep outdated medicine or medicine no longer needed. Be sure that any discarded medicine is out of the reach of children.

Precautions While Using This Medicine

Your doctor should check your progress at regular visits. Also, your progress may have to be checked after you have stopped using this medicine, since some of the effects may continue.

Do not stop using this medicine without first checking with your doctor. Your doctor may want you to reduce gradually the amount you are using before stopping completely.

Check with your doctor if your condition reappears or worsens after the dose has been reduced or treatment with this medicine is stopped.

If you will be using adrenocorticoids or corticotropin for a long time:

- *Your doctor may want you to follow a low-salt diet and/or a potassium-rich diet.*
- Your doctor may want you to watch your calories to prevent weight gain.
- Your doctor may want you to add extra protein to your diet.
- Your doctor may want you to have your eyes examined by an ophthalmologist (eye doctor) before and also sometime later during treatment.
- Your doctor may want you to carry a medical identification card stating that you are using this medicine.

Tell the doctor in charge that you are using this medicine:

- *Before having skin tests.*
- *Before having any kind of surgery (including dental surgery) or emergency treatment.*
- *If you get a serious infection or injury.*

While you are being treated with this medicine, and after you stop taking it, *do not have any immunizations without your doctor's approval.* Also, other people living in your home should not receive oral polio vaccine, since there is a chance they could pass the polio virus on to you. In addition, you should avoid close contact with other people at school or work who have recently taken oral polio vaccine.

For *diabetic patients:*

- This medicine may affect blood sugar levels. If you notice a change in the results of your blood or urine sugar tests or if you have any questions, check with your doctor.

For patients having this medicine *injected into their joints:*

- If this medicine is injected into one of your joints, you should be careful not to put too much stress or strain on that joint for a while, even if it begins to feel better. Make sure your doctor has told you how much you are allowed to move this joint while it is healing.
- If redness or swelling occurs at the place of injection, and continues or gets worse, check with your doctor.

For patients using this medicine *rectally:*

- Check with your doctor if you notice rectal bleeding, pain, burning, itching, blistering, or any other sign of irritation not present before you started using this medicine, or if signs of infection occur.

Side Effects of This Medicine

Adrenocorticoids or corticotropin may lower your resistance to infections. Also, any infection you get may be harder to treat. Always check with your doctor as soon as possible if you notice any signs of a possible infection, such as sore throat, fever, sneezing, or coughing.

Along with its needed effects, a medicine may cause some unwanted effects. Although not all of these side effects may occur, if they do occur they may need medical attention. When this medicine is used for short periods of time, side effects usually are rare. However, check with your doctor as soon as possible if any of the following side effects occur:

Less common

Decreased or blurred vision; frequent urination; increased thirst; rectal bleeding, blistering, burning, itching, or pain not present before use of this medicine (when used rectally)

Rare

Blindness (sudden, when injected in the head or neck area); confusion; excitement; false sense of well-being; hallucinations (seeing, hearing, or feeling things that are not there); mental depression; mood swings (sudden and wide); mistaken feelings of self-importance or being mistreated; redness, swelling, pain, or other sign of allergy or infection at place of injection; restlessness

Additional side effects may occur if you take this medicine for a long time. Check with your doctor if any of the following side effects occur:

Abdominal or stomach pain or burning (continuing); acne or other skin problems; bloody or black, tarry stools; filling or rounding out of the face; irregular heartbeat; menstrual problems; muscle cramps or pain; muscle weakness; nausea; pain in back, hips, ribs, arms, shoulders, or legs; pitting, scarring, or depression of skin at place of injection; reddish purple lines on arms, face, legs, trunk, or groin; swelling of feet or lower legs; thin, shiny skin; unusual bruising; unusual tiredness or weakness; vomiting; weight gain (rapid); wounds that will not heal

Other side effects may occur that usually do not need medical attention. These side effects may go away during treatment as your body adjusts to the medicine. However,

check with your doctor if any of the following side effects continue or are bothersome:

More common

Increased appetite; indigestion; loss of appetite (for triamcinolone only); nervousness or restlessness; trouble in sleeping

Less common or rare

Darkening or lightening of skin color; dizziness; flushing of face or cheeks (after injection into the nose); headache; increased joint pain (after injection into a joint); increased sweating; lightheadedness; nosebleeds (after injection into the nose); unusual increase in hair growth on body or face

After you stop using this medicine, your body may need time to adjust. The length of time this takes depends on the amount of medicine you were using and how long you used it. If you have taken large doses of this medicine for a long time, your body may need one year to adjust. During this time, *check with your doctor immediately if any of the following side effects occur:*

Abdominal, stomach, or back pain; dizziness; fainting; fever; loss of appetite (continuing); muscle or joint pain; nausea; reappearance of disease symptoms; shortness of breath; unexplained headaches (frequent or continuing); unusual tiredness or weakness; vomiting; weight loss (rapid)

Other side effects not listed above may also occur in some patients. If you notice any other effects, check with your doctor.

Annual revision: 04/14/92

COUGH/COLD COMBINATIONS Systemic

Some commonly used brand names are:

In the U.S.—

Actagen-C Cough[41]
Actifed with Codeine Cough[41]
Adatuss D.C. Expectorant[97]
Alamine-C Liquid[28]
Alamine Expectorant[113]
Allerfrin with Codeine[41]
Ambay Cough[1]
Ambenyl Cough[1]
Ambenyl-D Decongestant Cough Formula[114]
Ambophen Expectorant[9]
Ami-Tex LA[121]
Anamine HD[23]
Anatuss[74]
Anatuss with Codeine[75]
Anti-Tuss DM Expectorant[94]
Banex[120]
Banex-LA[121]
Banex Liquid[120]
Bayaminic Expectorant[121]
Bayaminicol[27]
Baycodan[89]
Baycomine[103]
Baycomine Pediatric[103]
BayCotussend Liquid[106]
Baydec DM Drops[20]
Bayhistine DH[28]
Bayhistine Expectorant[113]
Baytussin AC[91]
Baytussin DM[94]
Benylin Expectorant Cough Formula[94]
Biphetane DC Cough[19]
Brexin[81]
Bromanate DC Cough[19]
Bromfed-AT[19b]
Bromfed-DM[19b]
Bromphen DC with Codeine Cough[19]
Broncholate[118]
Bronkotuss Expectorant[82]
Brotane DX Cough[19b]
Calcidrine[90]
Carbinoxamine Compound[20]
Carbodec DM Drops[20]
Cerose-DM[22]
Cheracol[91]
Cheracol D Cough[94]
Cheracol Plus[27]
Children's NyQuil Nighttime Cold Medicine[29]
Chlorgest-HD[23]
Citra Forte[15 44]
Co-Apap[50]
Codamine[103]
Codamine Pediatric[103]
Codan[89]
Codegest Expectorant[111]
Codehist DH[28]
Codiclear DH[97]
Codimal DH[40]
Codimal DM[39]
Codimal Expectorant[121]
Codimal PH[38]
Codistan No. 1[94]
Comtrex Multi-Symptom Cold Reliever[48]
Comtrex Daytime Caplets[108]
Comtrex Multi-Symptom Non-Drowsy Caplets[108]
Comtrex Nighttime[50]
Conar[100]
Conar-A[116]
Conar Expectorant[109]
Concentrin[114]
Conex[121]
Conex with Codeine Liquid[111]
Congess JR[122]
Congess SR[122]
Contac Jr. Children's Cold Medicine[107]
Contac Severe Cold Formula[50]
Contac Severe Cold Formula Night Strength[51]
Cophene-S[26]
Cophene-X[64]
Cophene-XP[64]
Coricidin Cough[112]
CoTylenol Cold Medication[50]
C-Tussin Expectorant[113]
DayCare[117]
Deproist Expectorant with Codeine[113]
De-Tuss[106]
Detussin Expectorant[115]
Detussin Liquid[106]
Dihistine DH[28]
Dilaudid Cough[99]
Dimacol[114]
Dimetane-DC Cough[19]
Dimetane-DX Cough[19b]
Dimetapp DM Cold and Cough[19a]
Donatussin[62]
Donatussin DC[110]
Donatussin Drops[83]
Dondril[22]
Dorcol Children's Cough[114]
Dura-Vent[121]
Efficol Cough Whip (Cough Suppressant/Decongestant)[102]
Efficol Cough Whip (Cough Suppressant/Decongestant/Antihistamine)[27]
Efficol Cough Whip (Cough Suppressant/Expectorant)[94]
Efricon Expectorant Liquid[60]
Endal-HD[23]
Entex[120]
Entex LA[121]
Entex Liquid[120]
Entex PSE[122]
Entuss-D[106 115]
Entuss Expectorant[97 98]
Entuss Pediatric Expectorant[115]
Extra Action Cough[94]
Father John's Medicine Plus[63]
Fedahist Expectorant[122]
Fedahist Expectorant Pediatric Drops[122]
Fendol[123]
2/G-DM Cough[94]
Gentab-LA[121]
Glycotuss-dM[94]
Glydeine Cough[91]
Guaifed[122]
Guaifed-PD[122]
Guaipax[121]
Guaitab[122]
Guiamid D.M. Liquid[94]
Guiatuss A.C.[91]
Guiatuss-DM[94]
Guiatussin with Codeine Liquid[91]
Halotussin-DM Expectorant[94]
Histafed C[41]
Histalet X[122]
Histatuss Pediatric[21]
Hold (Children's Formula)[102]
Hycodan[89]
Hycomine[103]
Hycomine Compound[47]
Hycomine Pediatric[103]
Hycotuss Expectorant[97]
Hydromine[103]
Hydromine Pediatric[103]
Hydropane[89]
Hydrophen[103]
Improved Sino-Tuss[46]
Iophen-C Liquid[92]
Iotuss[92]
Iotuss-DM[95]
Ipsatol Cough Formula for Children[112]
Isoclor Expectorant[113]
Kiddy Koff[112]
KIE[119]
Kolephrin/DM[49]
Kolephrin GG/DM[94]
Kolephrin NN Liquid[54]
Kophane[65]
Kophane Cough and Cold Formula[27]
Kwelcof Liquid[97]
Lanatuss Expectorant[85]
Mallergan-VC with Codeine[37]
Meda Syrup Forte[62]
Medatussin[94a]
Medatussin Plus[67a]
Medi-Flu[50]
Medi-Flu Caplets[50]
Mediquell Decongestant Formula[105]
Midahist DH[28]
Mycotussin[106]
Myhistine DH[28]
Myhistine Expectorant[113]
Myhydromine[103]
Myhydromine Pediatric[103]
Myphetane DC Cough[19]
Mytussin AC[91]
Mytussin DAC[113]
Mytussin DM[94]
Naldecon-CX Adult Liquid[111]
Naldecon-DX Adult Liquid[112]
Naldecon-DX Children's Syrup[112]
Naldecon-DX Pediatric Drops[112]
Naldecon-EX[121]
Naldecon Senior DX[94]
Nolex LA[121]
Noratuss II Liquid[114]
Normatane DC[19]
Nortussin with Codeine[91]
Novahistine DH Liquid[28]
Novahistine DMX Liquid[114]
Novahistine Expectorant[113]
Nucochem[104]
Nucochem Expectorant[113]
Nucochem Pediatric Expectorant[113]
Nucofed[104]
Nucofed Expectorant[113]
Nucofed Pediatric Expectorant[113]
NyQuil Liquicaps[50a]
NyQuil Nighttime Colds Medicine[51]
Nytime Cold Medicine Liquid[51]
Omnicol[43]
Orthoxicol Cough[27]
Par Glycerol C[92]
Par Glycerol DM[95]
PediaCare Children's Cold Relief Night Rest Cough-Cold Formula[29]
PediaCare Children's Cough-Cold Formula[29]
Pediacof Cough[61]
Pertussin AM[114]
Pertussin CS[94]
Pertussin PM[51]
Phanadex[72a]
Phanatuss[94a]
Phenameth VC with Codeine[37]
Phenergan with Codeine[5]
Phenergan with Dextromethorphan[6]
Phenergan VC with Codeine[37]

Phenhist Expectorant[113]
Phenylfenesin L.A.[121]
Pherazine VC with Codeine[37]
Polaramine Expectorant[87]
Poly-Histine-CS[19]
Poly-Histine-DM[19a]
Prometh VC with Codeine[37]
Prominic Expectorant[121]
Prominicol Cough[69]
Promist HD Liquid[30]
Pseudo-Car DM[20]
Pseudodine C Cough[41]
P-V-Tussin[13 58]
Quelidrine Cough[57]
Queltuss[94]
Remcol-C[8]
Rentamine Pediatric[21]
Rescaps-D S.R.[101]
Respaire-60 SR[122]
Respaire-120 SR[122]
Respinol-G[120]
Rhinosyn-DM[29]
Rhinosyn-DMX Expectorant[94]
Rhinosyn-X[114]
Robitussin A-C[91]
Robitussin-CF[112]
Robitussin-DAC[113]
Robitussin-DM[94]
Robitussin Night Relief[53]
Robitussin Night Relief Colds Formula Liquid[53]
Robitussin-PE[122]
Rondec-DM[20]
Rondec-DM Drops[20]
Ru-Tuss DE[122]
Ru-Tuss Expectorant[114]
Ru-Tuss with Hydrocodone Liquid[34]
Rymed[120]
Rymed Liquid[120]
Rymed-TR[122]
Ryna-C Liquid[28]
Ryna-CX Liquid[113]
Rynatuss[21]
Rynatuss Pediatric[21]
Saleto-CF[107]
Silexin Cough[94]
Sinufed Timecelles[122]
Snaplets-DM[102]
Snaplets-EX[121]
Snaplets-Multi[27]
SRC Expectorant[115]
Sudafed Cough[114]
Sudafed Severe Cold Formula Caplets[108]
Syracol Liquid[102]
TheraFlu/Flu, Cold and Cough Medicine[50]
T-Koff[24]
Tolu-Sed Cough[91]
Tolu-Sed DM Cough[94]
Triacin C Cough[41]
Triaminic-DM Cough Formula[102]
Triaminic Expectorant[121]
Triaminic Expectorant with Codeine[111]
Triaminic Nite Light[29]
Triaminicol Multi-Symptom Relief[27]
Tricodene Forte[27]
Tricodene NN[27]
Tricodene Pediatric[102]
Trifed-C Cough[41]
Trimedine Liquid[22]
Trind DM Liquid[27]
Trinex[86]
Triphenyl Expectorant[121]
Tusquelin[25]
Tuss-Ade[101]
Tussafed[20]
Tuss Allergine Modified T.D.[101]
Tussanil DH[23 76]
Tussar-2[10]
Tussar DM[29]
Tussar SF[10]
Tuss-DM[94]
Tussigon[89]
Tussionex[3a 4]
Tussi-Organidin DM Liquid[95]
Tussi-Organidin Liquid[92]
Tussirex with Codeine Liquid[78]
Tuss-LA[122]
Tusso-DM[95]
Tussogest[101]
Tuss-Ornade Liquid[101]
Tuss-Ornade Spansules[101]
Ty-Cold Cold Formula[50]
Tylenol Cold and Flu[50]
Tylenol Cold Medication[50]
Tylenol Cold Medication, Non-Drowsy[108]
Tylenol Cold Night Time[50a]
Tylenol Cough[108]
Unproco[94]
Utex-S.R.[121]
Vanex Expectorant[115]
Vanex-HD[23]
Vicks Children's Cough[94]
Vicks Formula 44 Cough Mixture[3]
Vicks Formula 44D Decongestant Cough Mixture[114]
Vicks Formula 44M Multi-symptom Cough Mixture[117]
Viro-Med[77]
Zephrex[122]
Zephrex-LA[122]

In Canada—

Actifed DM[42]
Benylin with Codeine[11]
Benylin-DM[12]
Caldomine-DH Forte[36]
Caldomine-DH Pediatric[36]
Calmylin with Codeine[11]
CoActifed[41]
CoActifed Expectorant[73]
Coricidin with Codeine[7]
Coristex-DH[33]
Coristine-DH[33]
Dimetane Expectorant[80]
Dimetane Expectorant-C[55]
Dimetane Expectorant-DC[56]
Dimetapp with Codeine[17]
Dimetapp-DM[18]
Dorcol DM[112]
Entex LA[121]
Hycomine[72]
Hycomine-S Pediatric[72]
Novahistex C[31]
Novahistex DH[33]
Novahistex DH Expectorant[68]
Novahistex DM[32]
Novahistine DH[33]
Novahistine DH Expectorant[68]
Omni-Tuss[67]
Ornade-DM 10[27]
Ornade-DM 15[27]
Ornade-DM 30[27]
Ornade Expectorant[84]
Robitussin A-C[14]
Robitussin with Codeine[14]
Sudafed DM[105]
Sudafed Expectorant[122]
Triaminic-DM Expectorant[70]
Triaminic Expectorant[88]
Triaminic Expectorant DH[71]
Triaminicin with Codeine[52]
Triaminicol DM[35]
Tylenol Cold Medication[50]
Tylenol Cold Medication, Non-Drowsy[108]
Tussaminic C Forte[34a]
Tussaminic C Pediatric[34a]
Tussaminic DH Forte[36]
Tussaminic DH Pediatric[36]
Tussionex[4]
Tuss-Ornade Spansules[26a]

Note: For quick reference the following cough/cold combinations are numbered to match the preceding corresponding brand names.

Antihistamine and antitussive combinations—

1. Bromodiphenhydramine (broe-moe-dye-fen-HYE-dra-meen) and Codeine (KOE-deen)
2. No product available
3. Chlorpheniramine (klor-fen-EER-a-meen) and Dextromethorphan (dex-troe-meth-OR-fan)

3a. Chlorpheniramine and Hydrocodone (hye-droe-KOE-done)

4. Phenyltoloxamine (fen-ill-tole-OX-a-meen) and Hydrocodone
5. Promethazine (proe-METH-a-zeen) and Codeine†
6. Promethazine and Dextromethorphan

Antihistamine, antitussive, and analgesic combinations—

7. Chlorpheniramine (klor-fen-EER-a-meen), Codeine (KOE-deen), Aspirin, and Caffeine (kaf-EEN)
8. Chlorpheniramine, Dextromethorphan (dex-troe-meth-OR-fan), and Acetaminophen (a-seat-a-MIN-oh-fen)

Antihistamine, antitussive, and expectorant combinations—

9. Bromodiphenhydramine (broe-moe-dye-fen-HYE-dra-meen), Diphenhydramine (dye-fen-HYE-dra-meen), Codeine (KOE-deen), Ammonium Chloride (a-MOE-nee-um KLOR-ide), and Potassium Guaiacolsulfonate (poe-TAS-ee-um gwye-a-kol-SUL-fon-ate)
10. Chlorpheniramine (klor-fen-EER-a-meen), Codeine, and Guaifenesin (gwye-FEN-e-sin)
11. Diphenhydramine, Codeine, and Ammonium Chloride
12. Diphenhydramine, Dextromethorphan (dex-troe-meth-OR-fan), and Ammonium Chloride
13. Phenindamine (fen-IN-da-meen), Hydrocodone (hye-droe-KOE-done), and Guaifenesin
14. Pheniramine (fen-EER-a-meen), Codeine, and Guaifenesin
15. Pheniramine, Pyrilamine (peer-ILL-a-meen), Hydrocodone, Potassium Citrate (poe-TAS-ee-um SI-trate), and Ascorbic Acid
16. No product available.

Antihistamine, decongestant, and antitussive combinations—

17. Brompheniramine (brome-fen-EER-a-meen), Phenylephrine (fen-ill-EF-rin), Phenylpropanolamine (fen-ill-proe-pa-NOLE-a-meen), and Codeine (KOE-deen)
18. Brompheniramine, Phenylephrine, Phenylpropanolamine, and Dextromethorphan (dex-troe-meth-OR-fan)
19. Brompheniramine, Phenylpropanolamine, and Codeine

19a. Brompheniramine, Phenylpropanolamine, and Dextromethorphan

19b. Brompheniramine, Pseudoephedrine (soo-doe-e-FED-rin), and Dextromethorphan

20. Carbinoxamine (kar-bi-NOX-a-meen), Pseudoephedrine, and Dextromethorphan
21. Chlorpheniramine (klor-fen-EER-a-meen), Ephedrine (e-FED-rin), Phenylephrine, and Carbetapentane (kar-bay-ta-PEN-tane)
22. Chlorpheniramine, Phenylephrine, and Dextromethorphan
23. Chlorpheniramine, Phenylephrine, and Hydrocodone (hye-droe-KOE-done)
24. Chlorpheniramine, Phenylephrine, Phenylpropanolamine, and Codeine
25. Chlorpheniramine, Phenylephrine, Phenylpropanolamine, and Dextromethorphan
26. Chlorpheniramine, Phenylephrine, Phenylpropanolamine, and Dihydrocodeine (dye-hye-droe-KOE-deen)
26a. Chlorpheniramine, Phenylpropanolamine, and Caramiphen (kar-AM-i-fen)
27. Chlorpheniramine, Phenylpropanolamine, and Dextromethorphan
28. Chlorpheniramine, Pseudoephedrine, and Codeine
29. Chlorpheniramine, Pseudoephedrine, and Dextromethorphan
30. Chlorpheniramine, Pseudoephedrine, and Hydrocodone
31. Diphenylpyraline (dye-fen-il-PEER-a-leen), Phenylephrine, and Codeine
32. Diphenylpyraline, Phenylephrine, and Dextromethorphan
33. Diphenylpyraline, Phenylephrine, and Hydrocodone
34. Pheniramine (fen-EER-a-meen), Pyrilamine (peer-ILL-a-meen), Phenylephrine, Phenylpropanolamine, and Hydrocodone
34a. Pheniramine, Pyrilamine, Phenylpropanolamine, and Codeine
35. Pheniramine, Pyrilamine, Phenylpropanolamine, and Dextromethorphan
36. Pheniramine, Pyrilamine, Phenylpropanolamine, and Hydrocodone
37. Promethazine (proe-METH-a-zeen), Phenylephrine, and Codeine
38. Pyrilamine, Phenylephrine, and Codeine
39. Pyrilamine, Phenylephrine, and Dextromethorphan
40. Pyrilamine, Phenylephrine, and Hydrocodone
41. Triprolidine (trye-PROE-li-deen), Pseudoephedrine, and Codeine
42. Triprolidine, Pseudoephedrine, and Dextromethorphan

Antihistamine, decongestant, antitussive, and analgesic combinations—

43. Chlorpheniramine (klor-fen-EER-a-meen), Phenindamine (fen-IN-da-meen), Phenylephrine (fen-ill-EF-rin), Dextromethorphan (dex-troe-meth-OR-fan), Acetaminophen (a-seat-a-MIN-oh-fen), Salicylamide (sal-i-SILL-a-mide), Caffeine (kaf-EEN), and Ascorbic (a-SKOR-bik) Acid
44. Chlorpheniramine, Pheniramine (fen-EER-a-meen), Pyrilamine (peer-ILL-a-meen), Phenylephrine, Hydrocodone (hye-droe-KOE-done), Salicylamide, Caffeine, and Ascorbic Acid
45. No product available
46. Chlorpheniramine, Phenylephrine, Dextromethorphan, Acetaminophen, and Salicylamide
47. Chlorpheniramine, Phenylephrine, Hydrocodone (hye-droe-KOE-done), Acetaminophen, and Caffeine
48. Chlorpheniramine, Phenylpropanolamine (fen-ill-proe-pa-NOLE-a-meen), Dextromethorphan, and Acetaminophen
49. Chlorpheniramine, Phenylpropanolamine, Dextromethorphan, Acetaminophen, and Caffeine
50. Chlorpheniramine, Pseudoephedrine (soo-doe-e-FED-rin), Dextromethorphan, and Acetaminophen
50a. Diphenhydramine (dye-fen-HYE-dra-meen), Pseudoephedrine, Dextromethorphan, and Acetaminophen
51. Doxylamine (dox-ILL-a-meen), Pseudoephedrine, Dextromethorphan, and Acetaminophen
52. Pheniramine, Pyrilamine, Phenylpropanolamine, Codeine, Acetaminophen, and Caffeine
53. Pyrilamine, Phenylephrine, Dextromethorphan, and Acetaminophen
54. Pyrilamine, Phenylpropanolamine, Dextromethorphan, and Sodium Salicylate (sa-LI-si-late)

Antihistamine, decongestant, antitussive, and expectorant combinations—

55. Brompheniramine (brome-fen-EER-a-meen), Phenylephrine (fen-ill-EF-rin), Phenylpropanolamine (fen-ill-proe-pa-NOLE-a-meen), Codeine (KOE-deen), and Guaifenesin (gwye-FEN-e-sin)
56. Brompheniramine, Phenylephrine, Phenylpropanolamine, Hydrocodone (hye-droe-KOE-done), and Guaifenesin
57. Chlorpheniramine, Ephedrine, Phenylephrine, Dextromethorphan (dex-troe-meth-OR-fan), Ammonium Chloride, and Ipecac (IP-e-kak)
58. Chlorpheniramine, Phenindamine (fen-IN-da-meen), Pyrilamine (peer-ILL-a-meen), Phenylephrine, Hydrocodone, and Ammonium Chloride
59. No product available
60. Chlorpheniramine, Phenylephrine, Codeine, Ammonium Chloride, Potassium Guaiacolsulfonate (poe-TAS-ee-um gwye-a-kol-SUL-fon-ate), and Sodium Citrate (SOE-dee-um SI-trate)
61. Chlorpheniramine, Phenylephrine, Codeine, and Potassium Iodide (EYE-oh-dyed)
62. Chlorpheniramine, Phenylephrine, Dextromethorphan, and Guaifenesin
63. Chlorpheniramine, Phenylephrine, Dextromethorphan, Guaifenesin, and Ammonium Chloride
64. Chlorpheniramine, Phenylephrine, Phenylpropanolamine, Carbetapentane (kar-bay-ta-PEN-tane), and Potassium Guaiacolsulfonate
65. Chlorpheniramine, Phenylpropanolamine, Dextromethorphan, and Ammonium Chloride
66. No product available
67. Chlorpheniramine, Phenyltoloxamine (fen-ill-tole-OX-a-meen), Ephedrine, Codeine, and Guaiacol Carbonate (GYWE-a-kole KAR-bone-ate)
67a. Chlorpheniramine, Phenyltoloxamine, Phenylpropanolamine, Dextromethorphan, and Guaifenesin
68. Diphenylpyraline (dye-fen-il-PEER-a-leen), Phenylephrine, Hydrocodone, and Guaifenesin
69. Pheniramine (fen-EER-a-meen), Pyrilamine, Phenylpropanolamine, Dextromethorphan, and Ammonium Chloride
70. Pheniramine, Pyrilamine, Phenylpropanolamine, Dextromethorphan, and Guaifenesin
71. Pheniramine, Pyrilamine, Phenylpropanolamine, Hydrocodone, and Guaifenesin

72. Pyrilamine, Phenylephrine, Hydrocodone, and Ammonium Chloride
72a. Pyrilamine, Phenylpropanolamine, Dextromethorphan, Guaifenesin, Potassium Citrate, and Citric Acid
73. Triprolidine (trye-PROE-li-deen), Pseudoephedrine (soo-doe-e-FED-rin), Codeine, and Guaifenesin

Antihistamine, decongestant, antitussive, expectorant, and analgesic combinations—

74. Chlorpheniramine (klor-fen-EER-a-meen), Phenylephrine (fen-ill-EF-rin), Phenylpropanolamine (fen-ill-proe-pa-NOLE-a-meen), Dextromethorphan (dex-troe-meth-OR-fan), Guaifenesin (gwye-FEN-e-sin), and Acetaminophen (a-seat-a-MIN-oh-fen)
75. Chlorpheniramine, Phenylpropanolamine, Codeine (KOE-deen), Guaifenesin, and Acetaminophen
76. Chlorpheniramine, Phenylpropanolamine, Hydrocodone (hye-droe-KOE-done), Guaifenesin, and Salicylamide (sal-i-SILL-a-mide)
77. Chlorpheniramine, Pseudoephedrine (soo-doe-e-FED-rin), Dextromethorphan, Guaifenesin, and Aspirin
78. Pheniramine (fen-EER-a-meen), Phenylephrine, Codeine, Sodium Citrate (SOE-dee-um SI-trate), Sodium Salicylate (sa-LI-sill-ate), and Caffeine (kaf-EEN)
79. No product available

Antihistamine, decongestant, and expectorant combinations—

80. Brompheniramine (brome-fen-EER-a-meen), Phenylephrine (fen-ill-EF-rin), Phenylpropanolamine (fen-ill-proe-pa-NOLE-a-meen), and Guaifenesin (gwye-FEN-e-sin)
81. Carbinoxamine (kar-bi-NOX-a-meen), Pseudoephedrine (soo-doe-e-FED-rin), and Guaifenesin
82. Chlorpheniramine (klor-fen-EER-a-meen), Ephedrine (e-FED-rin), and Guaifenesin
83. Chlorpheniramine, Phenylephrine, and Guaifenesin
84. Chlorpheniramine, Phenylpropanolamine, and Guaifenesin
85. Chlorpheniramine, Phenylpropanolamine, Guaifenesin, Sodium Citrate (SOE-dee-um SI-trate), and Citric (SI-trik) Acid
86. Chlorpheniramine, Pseudoephedrine, and Guaifenesin
87. Dexchlorpheniramine (dex-klor-fen-EER-a-meen), Pseudoephedrine, and Guaifenesin
88. Pheniramine (fen-EER-a-meen), Pyrilamine (peer-ILL-a-meen), Phenylpropanolamine, and Guaifenesin

Antitussive and anticholinergic combination—

89. Hydrocodone (hye-droe-KOE-done) and Homatropine (hoe-MA-troe-peen)†

Antitussive and expectorant combinations—

90. Codeine (KOE-deen) and Calcium Iodide (KAL-see-um EYE-oh-dyed)
91. Codeine and Guaifenesin (gwye-FEN-e-sin)
92. Codeine and Iodinated Glycerol (EYE-oh-di-nay-ted GLI-ser-ole)
93. No product available.
94. Dextromethorphan and Guaifenesin
94a. Dextromethorphan, Guaifenesin, Potassium Citrate, and Citric Acid
95. Dextromethorphan and Iodinated Glycerol
96. No product available.
97. Hydrocodone (hye-droe-KOE-done) and Guaifenesin
98. Hydrocodone and Potassium Guaiacolsulfonate
99. Hydromorphone (hye-droe-MOR-fone) and Guaifenesin

Decongestant and antitussive combinations—

100. Phenylephrine (fen-ill-EF-rin) and Dextromethorphan (dex-troe-meth-OR-fan)
101. Phenylpropanolamine (fen-ill-proe-pa-NOLE-a-meen) and Caramiphen (kar-AM-i-fen)
102. Phenylpropanolamine and Dextromethorphan
103. Phenylpropanolamine and Hydrocodone (hye-droe-KOE-done)
104. Pseudoephedrine (soo-doe-e-FED-rin) and Codeine (KOE-deen)
105. Pseudoephedrine and Dextromethorphan
106. Pseudoephedrine and Hydrocodone

Decongestant, antitussive, and analgesic combinations—

107. Phenylpropanolamine (fen-ill-proe-pa-NOLE-a-meen), Dextromethorphan (dex-troe-meth-OR-fan), and Acetaminophen (a-seat-a-MIN-oh-fen)
108. Pseudoephedrine (soo-doe-e-FED-rin), Dextromethorphan, and Acetaminophen

Decongestant, antitussive, and expectorant combinations—

109. Phenylephrine (fen-ill-EF-rin), Dextromethorphan (dex-troe-meth-OR-fan), and Guaifenesin (gwye-FEN-e-sin)
110. Phenylephrine, Hydrocodone (hye-droe-KOE-done), and Guaifenesin
111. Phenylpropanolamine (fen-ill-proe-pa-NOLE-a-meen), Codeine (KOE-deen), and Guaifenesin
112. Phenylpropanolamine, Dextromethorphan, and Guaifenesin
113. Pseudoephedrine (soo-doe-e-FED-rin), Codeine, and Guaifenesin
114. Pseudoephedrine, Dextromethorphan, and Guaifenesin
115. Pseudoephedrine, Hydrocodone, and Guaifenesin

Decongestant, antitussive, expectorant, and analgesic combinations—

116. Phenylephrine (fen-ill-EF-rin), Dextromethorphan (dex-troe-meth-OR-fan), Guaifenesin (gwye-FEN-e-sin), and Acetaminophen (a-seat-a-MIN-oh-fen)
117. Pseudoephedrine (soo-doe-e-FED-rin), Dextromethorphan, Guaifenesin, and Acetaminophen

Decongestant and expectorant combinations—

118. Ephedrine (e-FED-rin) and Guaifenesin (gwye-FEN-e-sin)
119. Ephedrine and Potassium Iodide (poe-TAS-ee-um EYE-oh-dyed)
120. Phenylephrine (fen-ill-EF-rin), Phenylpropanolamine (fen-ill-proe-pa-NOLE-a-meen), and Guaifenesin
121. Phenylpropanolamine and Guaifenesin
122. Pseudoephedrine (soo-doe-e-FED-rin) and Guaifenesin

Decongestant, expectorant, and analgesic combination—

123. Phenylephrine (fen-ill-EF-rin), Guaifenesin (gwye-FEN-e-sin), Acetaminophen (a-seat-a-MIN-oh-fen), Salicylamide and Caffeine

†Generic name product available in the U.S.

Description

Cough/cold combinations are used mainly to relieve the cough due to colds, influenza, or hay fever. They are not to be used for the chronic cough that occurs with smoking, asthma, or emphysema or when there is an unusually large amount of mucus or phlegm (pronounced flem) with the cough.

Cough/cold combination products contain more than one ingredient. For example, some products may contain an antihistamine, a decongestant, and an analgesic, in addition to a medicine for coughing. If you are treating yourself, it is important to select a product that is best for your symptoms. Also, in general, it is best to buy a product that includes only those medicines you really need. If you have questions about which product to buy, check with your pharmacist.

Since different products contain ingredients that will have different precautions and side effects, it is important that you know the ingredients of the medicine you are taking. The different kinds of ingredients that may be found in cough/cold combinations include:

Antihistamines—Antihistamines are used to relieve or prevent the symptoms of hay fever and other types of allergy. They also help relieve some symptoms of the common cold, such as sneezing and runny nose. They work by preventing the effects of a substance called histamine, which is produced by the body. Some examples of antihistamines contained in these combinations are: chlorpheniramine, diphenhydramine, pheniramine, promethazine, and triprolidine.

Decongestants—Decongestants, such as ephedrine, phenylephrine, phenylpropanolamine (also known as PPA), and pseudoephedrine, produce a narrowing of blood vessels. This leads to clearing of nasal congestion. However, this effect may also increase blood pressure in patients who have high blood pressure.

Antitussives—To help relieve coughing these combinations contain either a narcotic (codeine, dihydrocodeine, hydrocodone or hydromorphone) or a non-narcotic (carbetapentane, dextromethorphan, or noscapine) antitussive. These antitussives act directly on the cough center in the brain. Narcotics may become habit-forming, causing mental or physical dependence, if used for a long time. Physical dependence may lead to withdrawal side effects when you stop taking the medicine.

Expectorants—Guaifenesin works by loosening the mucus or phlegm in the lungs. Other ingredients added as expectorants (for example, ammonium chloride, calcium iodide, iodinated glycerol, ipecac, potassium guaiacolsulfonate, potassium iodide, and sodium citrate) have not been proven to be effective. In general, the best thing you can do to loosen mucus or phlegm is to drink plenty of water.

Analgesics—Analgesics, such as acetaminophen, aspirin, and other salicylates (such as salicylamide and sodium salicylate), are used in these combination medicines to help relieve the aches and pain that may occur with the common cold.

The use of too much acetaminophen and salicylates at the same time may cause kidney damage or cancer of the kidney or urinary bladder. This may occur if large amounts of both medicines are taken together for a long time. However, taking the recommended amounts of combination medicines that contain both acetaminophen and a salicylate for short periods of time has not been shown to cause these unwanted effects.

Anticholinergics—Anticholinergics such as homatropine may help produce a drying effect in the nose and chest.

Some of these combinations are available only with your doctor's prescription. Others are available without a prescription; however, your doctor or pharmacist may have special instructions on the proper dose of the medicine for your medical condition.

Cough/cold combinations are available in the following dosage forms:

Antihistamine and antitussive combinations—

Oral

Bromodiphenhydramine and Codeine
- Syrup (U.S.)

Chlorpheniramine and Dextromethorphan
- Oral solution (U.S.)

Chlorpheniramine and Hydrocodone
- Oral suspension (U.S.)

Phenyltoloxamine and Hydrocodone
- Capsules (Canada)
- Oral suspension (U.S. and Canada)

Promethazine and Codeine
- Syrup (U.S.)

Promethazine and Dextromethorphan
- Syrup (U.S.)

Antihistamine, antitussive, and analgesic combinations—

Oral

Chlorpheniramine, Codeine, Aspirin, and Caffeine
- Tablets (Canada)

Chlorpheniramine, Dextromethorphan, and Acetaminophen
- Capsules (U.S.)

Antihistamine, antitussive, and expectorant combinations—

Oral

Bromodiphenhydramine, Diphenhydramine, Codeine, Ammonium Chloride, and Potassium Guaiacolsulfonate
- Oral solution (U.S.)

Chlorpheniramine, Codeine, and Guaifenesin
- Syrup (U.S.)

Diphenhydramine, Codeine, and Ammonium Chloride
- Syrup (Canada)

Diphenhydramine, Dextromethorphan, and Ammonium Chloride
- Syrup (Canada)

Phenindamine, Hydrocodone, and Guaifenesin
- Tablets (U.S.)

Pheniramine, Codeine, and Guaifenesin
- Syrup (Canada)

Pheniramine, Pyrilamine, Hydrocodone, and Potassium Citrate
- Syrup (U.S.)

Antihistamine, decongestant, and antitussive combinations—
Oral

Brompheniramine, Phenylephrine, Phenylpropanolamine, and Codeine
- Tablets (Canada)

Brompheniramine, Phenylephrine, Phenylpropanolamine, and Dextromethorphan
- Elixir (Canada)
- Tablets (Canada)

Brompheniramine, Phenylpropanolamine, and Codeine
- Syrup (U.S.)

Brompheniramine, Phenylpropanolamine, and Dextromethorphan
- Syrup (U.S.)

Brompheniramine, Pseudoephedrine, and Dextromethorphan
- Syrup (U.S.)

Carbinoxamine, Pseudoephedrine, and Dextromethorphan
- Oral solution (U.S.)
- Syrup (U.S.)

Chlorpheniramine, Ephedrine, Phenylephrine, and Carbetapentane
- Oral suspension (U.S.)
- Tablets (U.S.)

Chlorpheniramine, Phenylephrine, and Dextromethorphan
- Oral solution (U.S.)
- Tablets (U.S.)

Chlorpheniramine, Phenylephrine, and Hydrocodone
- Syrup (U.S.)

Chlorpheniramine, Phenylephrine, Phenylpropanolamine, and Codeine
- Syrup (U.S.)

Chlorpheniramine, Phenylephrine, Phenylpropanolamine, and Dextromethorphan
- Syrup (U.S.)

Chlorpheniramine, Phenylephrine, Phenylpropanolamine, and Dihydrocodeine
- Syrup (U.S.)

Chlorpheniramine, Phenylpropanolamine, and Caramiphen
- Extended-release capsules (Canada)

Chlorpheniramine, Phenylpropanolamine, and Dextromethorphan
- Granules (U.S.)
- Oral gel (U.S.)
- Oral solution (U.S. and Canada)
- Syrup (U.S.)
- Tablets (U.S.)

Chlorpheniramine, Pseudoephedrine, and Codeine
- Elixir (U.S.)
- Oral solution (U.S.)
- Syrup (U.S.)

Chlorpheniramine, Pseudoephedrine, and Dextromethorphan
- Oral solution (U.S.)
- Syrup (U.S.)

Chlorpheniramine, Pseudoephedrine, and Hydrocodone
- Oral solution (U.S.)

Diphenylpyraline, Phenylephrine, and Codeine
- Oral solution (Canada)

Diphenylpyraline, Phenylephrine, and Dextromethorphan
- Syrup (Canada)

Diphenylpyraline, Phenylephrine, and Hydrocodone
- Oral solution (Canada)
- Syrup (Canada)

Pheniramine, Pyrilamine, Phenylephrine, Phenylpropanolamine, and Hydrocodone
- Oral solution (U.S.)

Pheniramine, Pyrilamine, Phenylpropanolamine, and Codeine
- Syrup (Canada)

Pheniramine, Pyrilamine, Phenylpropanolamine, and Dextromethorphan
- Syrup (Canada)

Pheniramine, Pyrilamine, Phenylpropanolamine, and Hydrocodone
- Oral solution (Canada)

Promethazine, Phenylephrine, and Codeine
- Syrup (U.S.)

Pyrilamine, Phenylephrine, and Codeine
- Syrup (U.S.)

Pyrilamine, Phenylephrine, and Dextromethorphan
- Oral solution (U.S.)

Pyrilamine, Phenylephrine, and Hydrocodone
- Syrup (U.S.)

Triprolidine, Pseudoephedrine, and Codeine
- Syrup (U.S. and Canada)
- Tablets (Canada)

Triprolidine, Pseudoephedrine, and Dextromethorphan
- Oral solution (Canada)

Antihistamine, decongestant, antitussive, and analgesic combinations—
Oral

Chlorpheniramine, Phenindamine, Phenylephrine, Dextromethorphan, Acetaminophen, Salicylamide, Caffeine, and Ascorbic Acid
- Tablets (U.S.)

Chlorpheniramine, Pheniramine, Pyrilamine, Phenylephrine, Hydrocodone, Salicylamide, Caffeine, and Ascorbic Acid
- Capsules (U.S.)

Chlorpheniramine, Phenylephrine, Dextromethorphan, Acetaminophen, and Salicylamide
- Tablets (U.S.)

Chlorpheniramine, Phenylephrine, Hydrocodone, Acetaminophen, and Caffeine
- Tablets (U.S.)

Chlorpheniramine, Phenylpropanolamine, Dextromethorphan, and Acetaminophen
- Capsules (U.S.)
- Oral solution (U.S.)
- Tablets (U.S.)

Chlorpheniramine, Phenylpropanolamine, Dextromethorphan, Acetaminophen, and Caffeine
- Capsules (U.S.)

Chlorpheniramine, Pseudoephedrine, Dextromethorphan, and Acetaminophen
- Capsules (U.S.)
- Oral solution (U.S.)
- Tablets (U.S./Canada)

Diphenhydramine, Pseudoephedrine, Dextromethorphan, and Acetaminophen
- Capsules (U.S.)
- Oral solution (U.S.)

Doxylamine, Pseudoephedrine, Dextromethorphan, and Acetaminophen
- Oral solution (U.S.)

Pheniramine, Pyrilamine, Phenylpropanolamine, Codeine, Acetaminophen, and Caffeine
- Tablets (Canada)

Pyrilamine, Phenylephrine, Dextromethorphan, and Acetaminophen
- Oral solution (U.S.)

Pyrilamine, Phenylpropanolamine, Dextromethorphan, and Sodium Salicylate
- Oral solution (U.S.)

Antihistamine, decongestant, antitussive, and expectorant combinations—
Oral

Brompheniramine, Phenylephrine, Phenylpropanolamine, Codeine, and Guaifenesin
- Syrup (Canada)

Brompheniramine, Phenylephrine, Phenylpropanolamine, Hydrocodone, and Guaifenesin
- Oral solution (Canada)

Chlorpheniramine, Ephedrine, Phenylephrine, Dextromethorphan, Ammonium Chloride, and Ipecac
- Syrup (U.S.)

Chlorpheniramine, Phenindamine, Pyrilamine, Phenylephrine, Hydrocodone, and Ammonium Chloride
- Syrup (U.S.)

Chlorpheniramine, Phenylephrine, Codeine, Ammonium Chloride, Potassium Guaiacolsulfonate, and Sodium Citrate
- Oral solution (U.S.)

Chlorpheniramine, Phenylephrine, Codeine, and Potassium Iodide
- Syrup (U.S.)

Chlorpheniramine, Phenylephrine, Dextromethorphan, and Guaifenesin
- Syrup (U.S.)

Chlorpheniramine, Phenylephrine, Dextromethorphan, Guaifenesin, and Ammonium Chloride
- Oral solution (U.S.)

Chlorpheniramine, Phenylephrine, Phenylpropanolamine, Carbetapentane, and Potassium Guaiacolsulfonate
- Capsules (U.S.)
- Syrup (U.S.)

Chlorpheniramine, Phenylpropanolamine, Dextromethorphan, and Ammonium Chloride
- Syrup (U.S.)

Chlorpheniramine, Phenyltoloxamine, Ephedrine, Codeine, and Guaiacol Carbonate
- Oral suspension (Canada)

Chlorpheniramine, Phenyltoloxamine, Phenylpropanolamine, Dextromethorphan, and Guaifenesin
- Syrup (U.S.)

Diphenylpyraline, Phenylephrine, Hydrocodone, and Guaifenesin
- Oral solution (Canada)

Pheniramine, Pyrilamine, Phenylpropanolamine, Dextromethorphan, and Ammonium Chloride
- Syrup (U.S.)

Pheniramine, Pyrilamine, Phenylpropanolamine, Dextromethorphan, and Guaifenesin
- Oral solution (Canada)

Pheniramine, Pyrilamine, Phenylpropanolamine, Hydrocodone, and Guaifenesin
- Oral solution (U.S.)

Pyrilamine, Phenylephrine, Hydrocodone, and Ammonium Chloride
- Syrup (Canada)

Pyrilamine, Phenylpropanolamine, Dextromethorphan, Guaifenesin, Potassium Citrate, and Citric Acid
- Syrup (U.S.)

Triprolidine, Pseudoephedrine, Codeine, and Guaifenesin
- Oral solution (Canada)

Antihistamine, decongestant, antitussive, expectorant, and analgesic combinations—
Oral

Chlorpheniramine, Phenylephrine, Phenylpropanolamine, Dextromethorphan, Guaifenesin, and Acetaminophen
- Syrup (U.S.)
- Tablets (U.S.)

Chlorpheniramine, Phenylpropanolamine, Codeine, Guaifenesin, and Acetaminophen
- Syrup (U.S.)
- Tablets (U.S.)

Chlorpheniramine, Phenylpropanolamine, Hydrocodone, Guaifenesin, and Salicylamide
- Tablets (U.S.)

Chlorpheniramine, Pseudoephedrine, Dextromethorphan, Guaifenesin, and Aspirin
- Tablets (U.S.)

Pheniramine, Phenylephrine, Codeine, Sodium Citrate, Sodium Salicylate, and Caffeine
- Syrup (U.S.)

Antihistamine, decongestant, and expectorant combinations—
Oral

Brompheniramine, Phenylephrine, Phenylpropanolamine, and Guaifenesin
- Syrup (Canada)

Carbinoxamine, Pseudoephedrine, and Guaifenesin
- Capsules (U.S.)
- Oral solution (U.S.)

Chlorpheniramine, Ephedrine, and Guaifenesin
- Oral solution (U.S.)

Chlorpheniramine, Phenylephrine, and Guaifenesin
- Oral solution (U.S.)

Chlorpheniramine, Phenylpropanolamine, and Guaifenesin
- Oral solution (Canada)

Chlorpheniramine, Phenylpropanolamine, Guaifenesin, Sodium Citrate, and Citric Acid
- Oral solution (U.S.)

Chlorpheniramine, Pseudoephedrine, and Guaifenesin
- Extended-release tablets (U.S.)

Dexchlorpheniramine, Pseudoephedrine, and Guaifenesin
- Oral solution (U.S.)

Pheniramine, Pyrilamine, Phenylpropanolamine, and Guaifenesin
- Oral solution (Canada)

Antitussive and anticholinergic combination—
Oral

Hydrocodone and Homatropine
- Syrup (U.S.)
- Tablets (U.S.)

Antitussive and expectorant combinations—
Oral

Codeine and Calcium Iodide
- Syrup (U.S.)

Codeine and Guaifenesin
- Oral solution (U.S.)
- Syrup (U.S.)

Codeine and Iodinated Glycerol
- Oral solution (U.S.)

Dextromethorphan and Guaifenesin
- Capsules (U.S.)
- Oral gel (U.S.)
- Lozenges (U.S.)
- Oral solution (U.S.)
- Syrup (U.S.)
- Tablets (U.S.)

Dextromethorphan, Guaifenesin, Potassium Citrate, and Citric Acid
- Syrup (U.S.)

Dextromethorphan and Iodinated Glycerol
- Oral solution (U.S.)

Hydrocodone and Guaifenesin
- Oral solution (U.S.)
- Syrup (U.S.)
- Tablets (U.S.)

Hydrocodone and Potassium Guaiacolsulfonate
- Syrup (U.S.)

Hydromorphone and Guaifenesin
- Syrup (U.S.)

Decongestant and antitussive combinations—
Oral

Phenylephrine and Dextromethorphan
- Oral suspension (U.S.)

Phenylpropanolamine and Caramiphen
- Extended-release capsules (U.S.)
- Oral solution (U.S.)

Phenylpropanolamine and Dextromethorphan
- Oral gel (U.S.)
- Granules (U.S.)
- Lozenges (U.S.)
- Oral solution (U.S.)
- Syrup (U.S.)

Phenylpropanolamine and Hydrocodone
- Oral solution (U.S.)
- Syrup (U.S.)

Pseudoephedrine and Codeine
- Capsules (U.S.)
- Syrup (U.S.)

Pseudoephedrine and Dextromethorphan
- Oral solution (Canada)
- Chewable tablets (U.S.)

Pseudoephedrine and Hydrocodone
- Oral solution (U.S.)
- Syrup (U.S.)

Decongestant, antitussive, and analgesic combinations—
Oral

Phenylpropanolamine, Dextromethorphan, and Acetaminophen
- Oral solution (U.S.)
- Tablets (U.S.)

Pseudoephedrine, Dextromethorphan, and Acetaminophen
- Oral solution (U.S.)
- Tablets (U.S./Canada)

Decongestant, antitussive, and expectorant combinations—
Oral

Phenylephrine, Dextromethorphan, and Guaifenesin
- Syrup (U.S.)

Phenylephrine, Hydrocodone, and Guaifenesin
- Syrup (U.S.)

Phenylpropanolamine, Codeine, and Guaifenesin
- Oral solution (U.S.)
- Oral suspension (U.S.)
- Syrup (U.S.)

Phenylpropanolamine, Dextromethorphan, and Guaifenesin
- Oral solution (U.S.)
- Syrup (U.S.)

Pseudoephedrine, Codeine, and Guaifenesin
- Oral solution (U.S.)
- Syrup (U.S.)

Pseudoephedrine, Dextromethorphan, and Guaifenesin
- Capsules (U.S.)
- Oral solution (U.S.)
- Syrup (U.S.)

Pseudoephedrine, Hydrocodone, and Guaifenesin
- Oral solution (U.S.)
- Tablets (U.S.)

Decongestant, antitussive, expectorant, and analgesic combinations—
Oral

Phenylephrine, Dextromethorphan, Guaifenesin, and Acetaminophen
- Tablets (U.S.)

Pseudoephedrine, Dextromethorphan, Guaifenesin, and Acetaminophen
- Oral solution (U.S.)
- Tablets (U.S.)

Decongestant and expectorant combinations—
Oral

Ephedrine and Guaifenesin
- Capsules (U.S.)
- Syrup (U.S.)

Ephedrine and Potassium Iodide
- Syrup (U.S.)

Phenylephrine, Phenylpropanolamine, and Guaifenesin
- Capsules (U.S.)
- Oral solution (U.S.)
- Tablets (U.S.)

Phenylpropanolamine and Guaifenesin
- Oral solution (U.S.)
- Syrup (U.S.)
- Extended-release tablets (U.S. and Canada)

Pseudoephedrine and Guaifenesin
- Extended-release capsules (U.S.)
- Oral solution (U.S.)
- Syrup (U.S.)
- Tablets (U.S.)
- Extended-release tablets (U.S.)

Decongestant, expectorant, and analgesic combination—
Oral

Phenylephrine, Guaifenesin, Acetaminophen, Salicylamide and Caffeine
- Tablets (U.S.)

It is very important that you read and understand the following information. If any of it causes you special concern, check with your doctor or pharmacist. Also, *if you have any questions* or if you want more information about this medicine or your medical problem, *ask your doctor, nurse, or pharmacist.*

Before Using This Medicine

If you are taking this medicine without a prescription, carefully read and follow any precautions on the label. For cough/cold combinations, the following should be considered:

Allergies—Tell your doctor if you have ever had any unusual or allergic reaction to any of the ingredients contained in this medicine. Also tell your doctor and pharmacist if you are allergic to any other substances, such as foods, preservatives, or dyes. In addition, if this medicine contains *aspirin or other salicylates*, before taking it, check with your doctor if you have ever had any unusual or allergic reaction to any of the following medicines:

Aspirin or other salicylates
Diclofenac (e.g., Voltaren)
Diflunisal (e.g., Dolobid)
Fenoprofen (e.g., Nalfon)
Floctafenine
Flurbiprofen, by mouth (e.g., Ansaid)
Ibuprofen (e.g., Motrin)
Indomethacin (e.g., Indocin)
Ketoprofen (e.g., Orudis)
Ketorolac (e.g., Toradol)
Meclofenamate (e.g., Meclomen)
Mefenamic acid (e.g., Ponstel)
Methyl salicylate (oil of wintergreen)
Naproxen (e.g., Naprosyn)
Oxyphenbutazone (e.g., Tandearil)
Phenylbutazone (e.g., Butazolidin)
Piroxicam (e.g., Feldene)
Sulindac (e.g., Clinoril)
Suprofen (e.g., Suprol)
Tiaprofenic acid (e.g., Surgam)
Tolmetin (e.g., Tolectin)
Zomepirac (e.g., Zomax)

Diet—Make certain your doctor and pharmacist know if you are on any special diet, such as a low-sodium or low-sugar diet.

Pregnancy—The occasional use of a cough/cold combination is not likely to cause problems in the fetus or in the newborn baby. However, when these medicines are used at higher doses and/or for a long time, the chance that problems might occur may increase. For the individual ingredients of these combinations, the following information should be considered before you decide to use a particular cough/cold combination:

- *Acetaminophen*—Studies on birth defects have not been done in humans. However, acetaminophen has not been shown to cause birth defects or other problems in humans.
- *Alcohol*—Some of these combination medicines contain a large amount of alcohol. Too much use of alcohol during pregnancy may cause birth defects.
- *Antihistamines*—Antihistamines have not been shown to cause problems in humans.
- *Caffeine*—Studies in humans have not shown that caffeine causes birth defects. However, studies in animals have shown that caffeine causes birth defects when given in very large doses (amounts equal to the amount of caffeine contained in 12 to 24 cups of coffee a day).
- *Codeine*—Although studies on birth defects with codeine have not been done in humans, it has not been reported to cause birth defects in humans. Codeine has not been shown to cause birth defects in animal studies, but it caused other unwanted effects. Also, regular use of narcotics during pregnancy may cause the baby to become dependent on the medicine. This may lead to withdrawal side effects after birth. In addition, narcotics may cause breathing problems in the newborn baby if taken by the mother just before delivery.
- *Hydrocodone*—Although studies on birth defects with hydrocodone have not been done in humans, it has not been reported to cause birth defects in humans. However, hydrocodone has been shown to cause birth defects in animals when given in very large doses. Also, regular use of narcotics during pregnancy may cause the baby to become dependent on the medicine. This may lead to withdrawal side effects after birth. In addition, narcotics may cause breathing problems in the newborn baby if taken by the mother just before delivery.
- *Iodides (e.g., calcium iodide and iodinated glycerol)*—Not recommended during pregnancy. Iodides have caused enlargement of the thyroid gland in the fetus and resulted in breathing problems in newborn babies whose mothers took iodides in large doses for a long period of time.
- *Phenylephrine*—Studies on birth defects with phenylephrine have not been done in either humans or animals.
- *Phenylpropanolamine*—Studies on birth defects with phenylpropanolamine have not been done in either humans or animals. However, it seems that women who take phenylpropanolamine in the weeks following delivery are more likely to suffer mental or mood changes.

- *Pseudoephedrine*—Studies on birth defects with pseudoephedrine have not been done in humans. In animal studies pseudoephedrine did not cause birth defects but did cause a decrease in average weight, length, and rate of bone formation in the animal fetus when given in high doses.
- *Salicylates (e.g., aspirin)*—Studies on birth defects in humans have been done with aspirin, but not with salicylamide or sodium salicylate. Salicylates have not been shown to cause birth defects in humans. However, salicylates have been shown to cause birth defects in animals.

  Some reports have suggested that too much use of aspirin late in pregnancy may cause a decrease in the newborn's weight and possible death of the fetus or newborn infant. However, the mothers in these reports had been taking much larger amounts of aspirin than are usually recommended. Studies of mothers taking aspirin in the doses that are usually recommended did not show these unwanted effects. However, there is a chance that regular use of salicylates late in pregnancy may cause unwanted effects on the heart or blood flow in the fetus or newborn baby.

  Use of salicylates, especially aspirin, during the last 2 weeks of pregnancy may cause bleeding problems in the fetus before or during delivery, or in the newborn baby. Also, too much use of salicylates during the last 3 months of pregnancy may increase the length of pregnancy, prolong labor, cause other problems during delivery, or cause severe bleeding in the mother before, during, or after delivery. *Do not take aspirin during the last 3 months of pregnancy unless it has been ordered by your doctor.*

Breast-feeding—If you are breast-feeding, the chance that problems might occur depends on the ingredients of the combination. For the individual ingredients of these combinations, the following apply:

- *Acetaminophen*—Acetaminophen passes into the breast milk. However, it has not been reported to cause problems in nursing babies.
- *Alcohol*—Alcohol passes into the breast milk. However, the amount of alcohol in recommended doses of this medicine does not usually cause problems in nursing babies.
- *Antihistamines*—Small amounts of antihistamines pass into the breast milk. Antihistamine-containing medicine is not recommended for use while breast-feeding since most antihistamines are especially likely to cause side effects, such as unusual excitement or irritability, in the baby. Also, since antihistamines tend to decrease the secretions of the body, the flow of breast milk may be reduced in some patients.
- *Caffeine*—Small amounts of caffeine pass into the breast milk and may build up in the nursing baby. However, the amount of caffeine in recommended doses of this medicine does not usually cause problems in nursing babies.
- *Decongestants (e.g., ephedrine, phenylephrine, phenylpropanolamine, pseudoephedrine)*—Phenylephrine and phenylpropanolamine have not been reported to cause problems in nursing babies. Ephedrine and pseudoephedrine pass into the breast milk and may cause unwanted effects in nursing babies (especially newborn and premature babies).
- *Iodides (e.g., calcium iodide and iodinated glycerol)*—These medicines pass into the breast milk and may cause unwanted effects, such as underactive thyroid, in the baby.
- *Narcotic antitussives (e.g., codeine, dihydrocodeine, hydrocodone, and hydromorphone)*—Small amounts of codeine have been shown to pass into the breast milk. However, the amount of codeine or other narcotic antitussives in recommended doses of this medicine has not been reported to cause problems in nursing babies.
- *Salicylates (e.g., aspirin)*—Salicylates pass into the breast milk. Although salicylates have not been reported to cause problems in nursing babies, it is possible that problems may occur if large amounts are taken regularly.

Children—Very young children are usually more sensitive to the effects of this medicine. *Before giving any of these combination medicines to a child, check the package label very carefully. Some of these medicines are too strong for use in children.* If you are not certain whether a specific product can be given to a child, or if you have any questions about the amount to give, check with your doctor or pharmacist, especially if it contains:

- *Antihistamines*—Nightmares, unusual excitement, nervousness, restlessness, or irritability may be more likely to occur in children taking antihistamines.
- *Decongestants (e.g., ephedrine, phenylephrine, phenylpropanolamine, pseudoephedrine)*—Increases in blood pressure may be more likely to occur in children taking decongestants. Also, mental changes may be more likely to occur in young children taking phenylpropanolamine-containing combinations.
- *Narcotic antitussives (e.g., codeine, hydrocodeine, hydrocodone, and hydromorphone)*—Breathing problems may be especially likely to occur in children younger than 2 years of age taking narcotic antitussives. Also, unusual excitement or restlessness may be more likely to occur in children receiving these medicines.
- *Salicylates (e.g., aspirin)*—*Do not give medicines containing aspirin or other salicylates to a child with a fever or other symptoms of a virus infection, especially flu or chickenpox, without first discussing its use with your child's doctor.* This is very important because salicylates may cause a serious

illness called Reye's syndrome in children with fever caused by a virus infection, especially flu or chickenpox. Also, children may be more sensitive to the aspirin or other salicylates contained in some of these medicines, especially if they have a fever or have lost large amounts of body fluid because of vomiting, diarrhea, or sweating.

Teenagers—*Do not give medicines containing aspirin or other salicylates to a teenager with a fever or other symptoms of a virus infection, especially flu or chickenpox, without first discussing its use with your child's doctor.* This is very important because salicylates may cause a serious illness called Reye's syndrome in teenagers with fever caused by a virus infection, especially flu or chickenpox.

Older adults—The elderly are usually more sensitive to the effects of this medicine, especially if it contains:

- *Antihistamines*—Confusion, difficult or painful urination, dizziness, drowsiness, feeling faint, or dryness of mouth, nose, or throat may be more likely to occur in elderly patients. Also, nightmares or unusual excitement, nervousness, restlessness, or irritability may be more likely to occur in the elderly taking antihistamines.
- *Decongestants (e.g., ephedrine, phenylephrine, phenylpropanolamine, pseudoephedrine)*—Confusion, hallucinations, drowsiness, or convulsions (seizures) may be more likely to occur in the elderly, who are usually more sensitive to the effects of this medicine. Also, increases in blood pressure may be more likely to occur in elderly persons taking decongestants.

Other medicines—Although certain medicines should not be used together at all, in other cases two different medicines may be used together even if an interaction might occur. In these cases, your doctor may want to change the dose, or other precautions may be necessary. Tell your doctor and pharmacist if you are taking *any* other prescription or nonprescription (over-the-counter [OTC]) medicine, for example, aspirin or other medicine for allergies. Some medicines may change the way this medicine affects your body. Also, the effect of other medicines may be increased or reduced by some of the ingredients in this medicine. Check with your doctor or pharmacist about which medicines you should not take with this medicine.

Other medical problems—The presence of other medical problems may affect the use of the cough/cold combination medicine. Make sure you tell your doctor if you have any other medical problems, especially:

- Alcohol abuse (or history of)—Acetaminophen-containing medicines increase the chance of liver damage; also, some of the liquid medicines contain a large amount of alcohol
- Anemia or
- Gout or
- Hemophilia or other bleeding problems or
- Stomach ulcer or other stomach problems—These conditions may become worse if you are taking a combination medicine containing aspirin or another salicylate
- Brain disease or injury or
- Colitis or
- Convulsions (seizures) (history of) or
- Diarrhea or
- Gallbladder disease or gallstones—These conditions may become worse if you are taking a combination medicine containing codeine, dihydrocodeine, hydrocodone, or hydromorphone
- Cystic fibrosis (in children)—Side effects of iodinated glycerol may be more likely in children with cystic fibrosis
- Diabetes mellitus (sugar diabetes)—Decongestants may put diabetic patients at greater risk of having heart or blood vessel disease
- Emphysema, asthma, or chronic lung disease (especially in children)—Salicylate-containing medicine may cause an allergic reaction in which breathing becomes difficult
- Enlarged prostate or
- Urinary tract blockage or difficult urination—Some of the effects of anticholinergics (e.g., homatropine) or antihistamines may make urinary problems worse
- Glaucoma—A slight increase in inner eye pressure may occur with the use of anticholinergics (e.g., homatropine) or antihistamines, which may make the condition worse
- Heart or blood vessel disease or
- High blood pressure—Decongestant-containing medicine may increase the blood pressure and speed up the heart rate; also, caffeine-containing medicine, if taken in large amounts, may speed up the heart rate
- Kidney disease—This condition may increase the chance of side effects of this medicine because the medicine may build up in the body
- Liver disease—Liver disease increases the chance of side effects because the medicine may build up in the body; also, if liver disease is severe, there is a greater chance that aspirin-containing medicine may cause bleeding
- Thyroid disease—If an overactive thyroid has caused a fast heart rate, the decongestant in this medicine may cause the heart rate to speed up further; also, if the medicine contains narcotic antitussives (e.g., codeine), iodides (e.g., iodinated glycerol), or salicylates, the thyroid problem may become worse

Proper Use of This Medicine

To help loosen mucus or phlegm in the lungs, *drink a glass of water after each dose of this medicine*, unless otherwise directed by your doctor.

Take this medicine only as directed. Do not take more of it and do not take it more often than recommended on the label, unless otherwise directed by your doctor. To do so may increase the chance of side effects.

For patients *taking the extended-release capsule or tablet form of this medicine:*

- Swallow the capsule or tablet whole.
- Do not crush, break, or chew before swallowing.

- If the capsule is too large to swallow, you may mix the contents of the capsule with applesauce, jelly, honey, or syrup and swallow without chewing.

For patients *taking a combination medicine containing an antihistamine and/or aspirin or other salicylate:*

- Take with food or a glass of water or milk to lessen stomach irritation, if necessary.

If a combination medicine containing aspirin has a strong vinegar-like odor, do not use it. This odor means the medicine is breaking down. If you have any questions about this, check with your pharmacist.

Missed dose—If you must take this medicine regularly and you miss a dose, take it as soon as possible. However, if it is almost time for your next dose, skip the missed dose and go back to your regular dosing schedule. Do not double doses.

Storage—To store this medicine:

- Keep this medicine out of the reach of children. Overdose is very dangerous in young children.
- Store away from heat and direct light.
- Do not store the capsule or tablet form of this medicine in the bathroom, near the kitchen sink, or in other damp places. Heat or moisture may cause the medicine to break down.
- Keep the liquid form of this medicine from freezing. Do not refrigerate the syrup.
- Do not keep outdated medicine or medicine no longer needed. Be sure that any discarded medicine is out of the reach of children.

Precautions While Using This Medicine

If your cough has not improved after 7 days or if you have a high fever, skin rash, continuing headache, or sore throat with the cough, check with your doctor. These signs may mean that you have other medical problems.

For patients *taking antihistamine-containing medicine:*

- Before you have any skin tests for allergies, tell the doctor in charge that you are taking this medicine. The results of the test may be affected by the antihistamine in this medicine.
- This medicine will add to the effects of alcohol and other CNS depressants (medicines that slow down the nervous system, possibly causing drowsiness). Some examples of CNS depressants are antihistamines or medicine for hay fever, other allergies, or colds; sedatives, tranquilizers, or sleeping medicine; prescription pain medicine or narcotics; barbiturates; medicine for seizures; muscle relaxants; or anesthetics, including some dental anesthetics. *Check with your doctor before taking any of the above while you are taking this medicine.*
- This medicine may cause some people to become drowsy, dizzy, or less alert than they are normally. *Make sure you know how you react to this medicine before you drive, use machines, or do anything else that could be dangerous if you are dizzy or are not alert.*
- When taking antihistamines on a regular basis, make sure your doctor knows if you are taking large amounts of aspirin at the same time (as in arthritis or rheumatism). Effects of too much aspirin, such as ringing in the ears, may be covered up by the antihistamine.
- Antihistamines may cause dryness of the mouth. For temporary relief, use sugarless candy or gum, melt bits of ice in your mouth, or use a saliva substitute. However, if your mouth continues to feel dry for more than 2 weeks, check with your medical doctor or dentist. Continuing dryness of the mouth may increase the chance of dental disease, including tooth decay, gum disease, and fungus infections.

For patients *taking decongestant-containing medicine:*

- This medicine may add to the central nervous system (CNS) stimulant and other effects of phenylpropanolamine (PPA)-containing diet aids. *Do not use medicines for diet or appetite control while taking this medicine unless you have checked with your doctor.*
- This medicine may cause some people to be nervous or restless or to have trouble in sleeping. If you have trouble in sleeping, *take the last dose of this medicine for each day a few hours before bedtime.* If you have any questions about this, check with your doctor.
- Before having any kind of surgery (including dental surgery) or emergency treatment, tell the medical doctor or dentist in charge that you are taking this medicine.

For patients *taking narcotic antitussive (codeine, dihydrocodeine, hydrocodone, or hydromorphone)–containing medicine:*

- This medicine will add to the effects of alcohol and other CNS depressants (medicines that slow down the nervous system, possibly causing drowsiness). Some examples of CNS depressants are antihistamines or medicine for hay fever, other allergies, or colds; sedatives, tranquilizers, or sleeping medicine; prescription pain medicine or narcotics; barbiturates; medicine for seizures; muscle relaxants; or anesthetics, including some dental anesthetics. *Check with your doctor before taking any of the above while you are taking this medicine.*
- This medicine may cause some people to become drowsy, dizzy, less alert than they are normally, or to feel a false sense of well-being. *Make sure you know how you react to this medicine before you drive, use machines, or do anything else that could*

be dangerous if you are dizzy or are not alert and clearheaded.

- Nausea or vomiting may occur after taking a narcotic antitussive. This effect may go away if you lie down for a while. However, if nausea or vomiting continues, check with your doctor.
- Dizziness, lightheadedness, or fainting may be especially likely to occur when you get up suddenly from a lying or sitting position. Getting up slowly may help lessen this problem.
- Before having any kind of surgery (including dental surgery) or emergency treatment, tell the medical doctor or dentist in charge that you are taking this medicine.

For patients *taking iodide (calcium iodide, iodinated glycerol, or potassium iodide)-containing medicine:*

- Make sure your doctor knows if you are planning to have any future thyroid tests. The results of the thyroid test may be affected by the iodine in this medicine.

For patients *taking analgesic-containing medicine:*

- *Check the label of all nonprescription (over-the-counter [OTC]), and prescription medicines you now take.* If any contain acetaminophen or aspirin or other salicylates, including diflunisal or bismuth subsalicylate, be especially careful. Taking them while taking a cough/cold combination medicine that already contains them may lead to overdose. If you have any questions about this, check with your doctor or pharmacist.
- Do not take aspirin-containing medicine for 5 days before any surgery, including dental surgery, unless otherwise directed by your medical doctor or dentist. Taking aspirin during this time may cause bleeding problems.

For *diabetic patients taking aspirin- or sodium salicylate–containing medicine:*

- False urine sugar test results may occur:

  —If you take 8 or more 325-mg (5-grain) doses of aspirin every day for several days in a row.

  —If you take 8 or more 325-mg (5-grain), or 4 or more 500-mg (10-grain) doses of sodium salicylate.

- Smaller doses or occasional use of aspirin or sodium salicylate usually will not affect urine sugar tests. If you have any questions about this, check with your doctor, nurse, or pharmacist, especially if your diabetes is not well controlled.

For patients *taking homatropine-containing medicine:*

- This medicine may make you sweat less, causing your body temperature to increase. *Use extra care not to become overheated during exercise or hot weather while you are taking this medicine,* since overheating may result in heat stroke. Also, hot baths or saunas may make you feel dizzy or faint while you are taking this medicine.

Side Effects of This Medicine

Along with its needed effects, a medicine may cause some unwanted effects. Although serious side effects occur rarely when this medicine is taken as recommended, they may be more likely to occur if:

- too much medicine is taken.
- it is taken in large doses.
- it is taken for a long period of time.

Get emergency help immediately if any of the following symptoms of overdose occur:

For narcotic antitussive (codeine, dihydrocodeine, hydrocodone, or hydromorphone)–containing

Cold, clammy skin; confusion (severe); convulsions (seizures); drowsiness or dizziness (severe); nervousness or restlessness (severe); pinpoint pupils of eyes; slow heartbeat; slow or troubled breathing; weakness (severe)

For acetaminophen-containing

Diarrhea; increased sweating; loss of appetite; nausea or vomiting; stomach cramps or pain; swelling or tenderness in the upper abdomen or stomach area

For salicylate-containing

Any loss of hearing; bloody urine; confusion; convulsions (seizures); diarrhea (severe or continuing); dizziness or lightheadedness; drowsiness (severe); excitement or nervousness (severe); fast or deep breathing; fever; hallucinations (seeing, hearing, or feeling things that are not there); increased sweating; nausea or vomiting (severe or continuing); shortness of breath or troubled breathing (for salicylamide only); stomach pain (severe or continuing); uncontrollable flapping movements of the hands, especially in elderly patients; unusual thirst; vision problems

For decongestant-containing

Fast, pounding, or irregular heartbeat; headache (continuing and severe); nausea or vomiting (severe); nervousness or restlessness (severe); shortness of breath or troubled breathing (severe or continuing)

Also, check with your doctor as soon as possible if any of the following side effects occur:

For all combinations

Skin rash, hives, and/or itching

For antihistamine- or anticholinergic-containing

Clumsiness or unsteadiness; convulsions (seizures); drowsiness (severe); dryness of mouth, nose, or throat (severe); flushing or redness of face; hallucinations (seeing, hearing, or feeling things that are not there); restlessness (severe); shortness of breath or troubled breathing; slow or fast heartbeat

For iodine-containing

Headache (continuing); increased watering of mouth; loss of appetite; metallic taste; skin rash, hives, or redness; sore throat; swelling of face, lips, or eyelids

For acetaminophen-containing

Unexplained sore throat and fever; unusual tiredness or weakness; yellow eyes or skin

Other side effects may occur that usually do not need medical attention. These side effects may go away during treatment as your body adjusts to the medicine. However, check with your doctor if any of the following side effects continue or are bothersome:

Constipation; decreased sweating; difficult or painful urination; dizziness or lightheadedness; drowsiness; dryness of mouth, nose, or throat; false sense of well-being; increased sensitivity of skin to sun; nausea or vomiting; nightmares; stomach pain; thickening of mucus; trouble in sleeping; unusual excitement, nervousness, restlessness, or irritability; unusual tiredness or weakness

Not all of the side effects listed above have been reported for each of these medicines, but they have been reported for at least one of them. There are some similarities among these combination medicines, so many of the above side effects may occur with any of these medicines.

Other side effects not listed above may also occur in some patients. If you notice any other effects, check with your doctor.

Annual revision: 09/03/92

CROMOLYN Inhalation

Some commonly used brand names are:

In the U.S.
Intal

In Canada
Fivent
Intal

Another commonly used name is sodium cromoglycate.

Description

Cromolyn (KROE-moe-lin) is used to prevent asthma attacks. It is also used before and during exposure to substances that cause reactions, to prevent bronchospasm (wheezing or difficulty in breathing). In addition, this medicine is used to prevent bronchospasm caused by exercise.

Cromolyn inhalation works by acting on certain cells in the body, called mast cells, to prevent them from releasing substances that cause the asthma or bronchospasm attack.

Cromolyn will not help an asthma attack that has already started. If this medicine is used during a severe attack, it may cause irritation and make the attack worse.

This medicine is available only with your doctor's prescription, in the following dosage forms:

Inhalation

- Capsules for inhalation (U.S. and Canada)
- Inhalation aerosol (U.S. and Canada)
- Inhalation solution (U.S. and Canada)

It is very important that you read and understand the following information. If any of it causes you special concern, check with your doctor. Also, *if you have any questions* or if you want more information about this medicine or your medical problem, *ask your doctor, nurse, or pharmacist.*

Before Using This Medicine

In deciding to use a medicine, the risks of taking the medicine must be weighed against the good it will do. This is a decision you and your doctor will make. For cromolyn inhalation, the following should be considered:

Allergies—Tell your doctor if you have ever had any unusual or allergic reaction to cromolyn or to inhalation aerosols. Also tell your doctor and pharmacist if you are allergic to any other substances, such as foods, preservatives, or dyes.

Diet—Make certain your doctor and pharmacist know if you are on any special diet, such as a low-sodium or low-sugar diet.

Pregnancy—Cromolyn has not been studied in pregnant women. However, studies in animals have shown that cromolyn causes a decrease in successful pregnancies and a decrease in the weight of the animal fetus when given by injection in very large amounts.

Breast-feeding—It is not known whether cromolyn passes into the breast milk. However, this medicine has not been reported to cause problems in nursing babies.

Children—Although there is no specific information about the use of cromolyn inhalation in children, it is not expected to cause different side effects or problems in children than it does in adults.

Older adults—Many medicines have not been tested in older people. Therefore, it may not be known whether

they work exactly the same way they do in younger adults. Although there is no specific information about the use of cromolyn inhalation in the elderly, it is not expected to cause different side effects or problems in older people than it does in younger adults.

Other medical problems—The presence of other medical problems may affect the use of cromolyn. Make sure you tell your doctor if you have any other medical problems, especially:

- Heart disease (or history of)—The inhalation aerosol form of cromolyn may make the condition worse
- Kidney disease or
- Liver disease—The effects of cromolyn may be increased, which may increase the chance of side effects

Before you begin using any new medicine (prescription or nonprescription) or if you develop any new medical problem while you are using this medicine, check with your doctor, nurse, or pharmacist.

Proper Use of This Medicine

Cromolyn oral inhalation is used to prevent asthma or bronchospasm (wheezing or difficulty in breathing) attacks. It will not relieve an attack that has already started. If this medicine is used during a severe attack, it may cause irritation and make the attack worse.

For patients using *cromolyn aerosol:*

- This medicine usually comes with patient directions. Read them carefully before using this medicine.
- Keep the spray away from the eyes because it may cause irritation.

For patients using *cromolyn capsules for inhalation:*

- This medicine is used with a special inhaler and usually comes with patient directions. Read the directions carefully before using.
- *Do not swallow the capsules because the medicine will not work if you swallow it.*

For patients using *cromolyn solution for inhalation:*

- Use this medicine only in a power-operated nebulizer with an adequate flow rate and equipped with a face mask or mouthpiece. Make sure you understand exactly how to use it. Hand-operated nebulizers are not suitable for use with this medicine. If you have any questions about this, check with your doctor.

Use cromolyn oral inhalation only as directed. Do not use more of it and do not use it more often than your doctor ordered. To do so may increase the chance of side effects.

For patients using *cromolyn oral inhalation* regularly (for example, every day):

- *In order for cromolyn to work properly, it must be inhaled every day in regularly spaced doses as ordered by your doctor.* Up to 4 weeks may pass before you feel the full effects of the medicine.

Missed dose—If you miss a dose of this medicine, take it as soon as possible. Then take any remaining doses for that day at regularly spaced intervals. Do not double doses.

Storage—To store this medicine:

- Keep out of the reach of children.
- Store away from heat.
- Store the capsule or solution form of this medicine away from direct light. Store the aerosol form of this medicine away from direct sunlight.
- Do not store the capsule form of this medicine in the bathroom, near the kitchen sink, or in other damp places. Heat or moisture may cause the medicine to break down.
- Keep the aerosol or solution form of this medicine from freezing.
- Do not puncture, break, or burn the aerosol container, even if it is empty.
- Do not keep outdated medicine or medicine no longer needed. Be sure that any discarded medicine is out of the reach of children.

Precautions While Using This Medicine

If your symptoms do not improve or if your condition becomes worse, check with your doctor.

If you are also taking an adrenocorticoid (cortisone-like medicine, such as cortisone or prednisone) for your asthma along with this medicine, do not stop taking the adrenocorticoid even if your asthma seems better, unless you are told to do so by your doctor.

Dryness of the mouth or throat, throat irritation, and hoarseness may occur after using this medicine. Gargling and rinsing the mouth after each dose may help prevent these effects.

Side Effects of This Medicine

Along with its needed effects, a medicine may cause some unwanted effects. Although not all of these side effects may occur, if they do occur they may need medical attention.

Check with your doctor as soon as possible if any of the following side effects occur:

Less common

Difficult or painful urination; dizziness; frequent urge to urinate; headache (severe or continuing); increased wheezing, tightness in chest, or difficulty in breathing; joint pain or swelling; muscle pain or weakness; nausea or vomiting; skin rash, hives, or itching; swelling of the face, lips, eyelids, hands, feet, or inside of mouth

Rare

Chest pain; chills; difficulty in swallowing; sweating; wheezing or difficulty in breathing (severe)

Other side effects may occur that usually do not need medical attention. These side effects may go away during treatment as your body adjusts to the medicine. However, check with your doctor if any of the following side effects continue or are bothersome:

More common

Cough; hoarseness

Less common

Dryness of the mouth or throat; sneezing; stuffy nose; throat irritation; watering of the eyes

If you are using cromolyn aerosol, you may notice an unpleasant taste. This may be expected and will go away when you stop using the medicine.

Other side effects not listed above may also occur in some patients. If you notice any other effects, check with your doctor.

Annual revision: June 1990

CROMOLYN Nasal

Some commonly used brand names are:

In the U.S.
Nasalcrom

In Canada
Rynacrom

Another commonly used name is sodium cromoglycate.

Description

Cromolyn (KROE-moe-lin) nasal solution is used in the nose to prevent or treat the symptoms (sneezing, wheezing, runny nose, itching) of seasonal (short-term) or chronic (long-term) allergic rhinitis. Cromolyn powder for nasal inhalation is used in the nose to prevent seasonal (short-term) allergic rhinitis.

This medicine works by acting on certain cells in the body, called mast cells, to prevent them from releasing substances that cause the allergic reaction.

When cromolyn is used to treat chronic (long-term) allergic rhinitis, an antihistamine and/or a nasal decongestant may be used with this medicine, especially during the first few weeks of treatment.

Nasal cromolyn is available only with your doctor's prescription, in the following dosage forms:

Nasal

- Nasal insufflation (powder for nasal inhalation) (Canada)
- Nasal solution (U.S. and Canada)

It is very important that you read and understand the following information. If any of it causes you special concern, check with your doctor. Also, *if you have any questions* or if you want more information about this medicine or your medical problem, *ask your doctor, nurse, or pharmacist.*

Before Using This Medicine

In deciding to use a medicine, the risks of using the medicine must be weighed against the good it will do. This is a decision you and your doctor will make. For nasal cromolyn, the following should be considered:

Allergies—Tell your doctor if you have ever had any unusual or allergic reaction to cromolyn. Also tell your doctor and pharmacist if you are allergic to any other substances, such as foods, preservatives, or dyes.

Pregnancy—Cromolyn has not been studied in pregnant women. However, studies in animals have shown that cromolyn causes a decrease in successful pregnancies and a decrease in the weight of the animal fetus when given by injection in very large amounts.

Breast-feeding—It is not known whether cromolyn passes into the breast milk. However, this medicine has not been reported to cause problems in nursing babies.

Children—Although there is no specific information comparing use of nasal cromolyn in children with use in other age groups, this medicine is not expected to cause different side effects or problems in children than it does in adults.

Older adults—Many medicines have not been studied specifically in older people. Therefore, it may not be known whether they work exactly the same way they do in younger adults. Although there is no specific information comparing use of nasal cromolyn in the elderly with use in other age groups, this medicine is not expected to cause different side effects or problems in older people than it does in younger adults.

Other medical problems—The presence of other medical problems may affect the use of nasal cromolyn. Make sure you tell your doctor if you have any other medical problems, especially:

- Kidney disease or
- Liver disease—The effects of cromolyn may be increased, which may increase the chance of side effects
- Polyps or growths inside the nose—Cromolyn may not work if nasal passages are blocked

Before you begin using any new medicine (prescription or nonprescription) or if you develop any new medical problem while you are using this medicine, check with your doctor, nurse, or pharmacist.

Proper Use of This Medicine

This medicine usually comes with patient directions. Read them carefully before using.

Before using this medicine, clear the nasal passages by blowing your nose.

For patients using *cromolyn nasal solution:*

- Cromolyn nasal solution is used with a special spray device. Cleaning of this device is not recommended. The spray device should be replaced every 6 months.

For patients using *cromolyn powder for nasal inhalation:*

- This medicine is used with a special inhaler. Be sure you understand exactly how to use it.

Use this medicine only as directed. Do not use more of it and do not use it more often than your doctor ordered. To do so may increase the chance of side effects.

In order for this medicine to work properly, it must be used every day in regularly spaced doses as ordered by your doctor.

For patients using cromolyn for *seasonal (short-term) allergic rhinitis:*

- Up to 1 week may pass before you begin to feel better.

For patients using cromolyn for *chronic (long-term) allergic rhinitis:*

- Up to 4 weeks may pass before you feel the full effects of this medicine.

Missed dose—If you miss a dose of this medicine, use it as soon as possible. Then use any remaining doses for that day at regularly spaced intervals. Do not double doses.

Storage—To store this medicine:

- Keep out of the reach of children.
- Store away from heat and direct light.
- Store the powder form of this medicine in a dry place. Do not store it in the bathroom, near the kitchen sink, or in other damp places. Heat or moisture may cause the medicine to break down.
- Keep the solution form of this medicine from freezing.
- Do not keep outdated medicine or medicine no longer needed. Be sure that any discarded medicine is out of the reach of children.

Precautions While Using This Medicine

If your symptoms do not improve or if your condition becomes worse, check with your doctor.

Side Effects of This Medicine

Along with its needed effects, a medicine may cause some unwanted effects. Although not all of these side effects may occur, if they do occur they may need medical attention.

Check with your doctor as soon as possible if any of the following side effects occur:

Rare

Coughing; difficulty in swallowing; nosebleed; skin rash, hives, or itching; swelling of face, lips, or eyelids; wheezing or difficulty in breathing

Other side effects may occur that usually do not need medical attention. These side effects may go away during treatment as your body adjusts to the medicine. However, check with your doctor if any of the following side effects continue or are bothersome:

More common

Burning, stinging, or irritation inside of nose; increase in sneezing

Less common

Headache; postnasal drip; unpleasant taste

Other side effects not listed above may also occur in some patients. If you notice any other effects, check with your doctor.

Annual revision: 07/16/91

CROMOLYN Ophthalmic

Some commonly used brand names are:

In the U.S.

Opticrom

In Canada

Opticrom

Vistacrom

Another commonly used name is sodium cromoglycate.

Description

Cromolyn (KROE-moe-lin) ophthalmic solution is used in the eye to treat certain disorders of the eye caused by allergies. It works by acting on certain cells, called mast cells, to prevent them from releasing substances that cause the allergic reaction.

Cromolyn is available only with your doctor's prescription, in the following dosage form:

Ophthalmic

- Ophthalmic solution (eye drops) (U.S. and Canada)

It is very important that you read and understand the following information. If any of it causes you special concern, check with your doctor. Also, *if you have any questions* or if you want more information about this medicine or your medical problem, *ask your doctor, nurse, or pharmacist*.

Before Using This Medicine

In deciding to use a medicine, the risks of using the medicine must be weighed against the good it will do. This is a decision you and your doctor will make. For ophthalmic cromolyn, the following should be considered:

Allergies—Tell your doctor if you have ever had any unusual or allergic reaction to cromolyn. Also tell your doctor and pharmacist if you are allergic to any other substances, such as foods, preservatives, or dyes.

Pregnancy—Cromolyn has not been studied in pregnant women. However, studies in animals have shown that cromolyn causes a decrease in successful pregnancies and a decrease in the weight of the animal fetus when given by injection in very large amounts. It is unlikely that cromolyn will cause problems in humans when used in the eye as directed.

Breast-feeding—It is not known whether cromolyn passes into the breast milk. However, this medicine has not been reported to cause problems in nursing babies.

Children—Although there is no specific information comparing use of ophthalmic cromolyn in children with use in other age groups, this medicine is not expected to cause different side effects or problems in children than it does in adults.

Older adults—Many medicines have not been studied specifically in older people. Therefore, it may not be known whether they work exactly the same way they do in younger adults. Although there is no specific information comparing use of ophthalmic cromolyn in the elderly with use in other age groups, this medicine is not expected to cause different side effects or problems in older people than it does in younger adults.

Before you begin using any new medicine (prescription or nonprescription) or if you develop any new medical problem while you are using this medicine, check with your doctor, nurse, or pharmacist.

Proper Use of This Medicine

To use the *eye drops:*

- First, wash your hands. Then tilt the head back and pull the lower eyelid away from the eye to form a pouch. Drop the medicine into the pouch and gently close the eyes. Do not blink. Keep the eyes closed for 1 or 2 minutes to allow the medicine to be absorbed.
- If you think you did not get the drop of medicine into your eye properly, use another drop.
- To keep the medicine as germ-free as possible, do not touch the applicator tip to any surface (including the eye). Also, keep the container tightly closed.

Use cromolyn eye drops only as directed. Do not use more of this medicine and do not use it more often than your doctor ordered. To do so may increase the chance of side effects.

In order for this medicine to work properly, it must be used every day in regularly spaced doses as ordered by your doctor. A few days may pass before you begin to feel better.

Missed dose—If you miss a dose of this medicine, apply it as soon as possible. Then go back to your regular dosing schedule.

Storage—To store this medicine:

- Keep out of the reach of children.
- Store away from heat and direct light.
- Keep the medicine from freezing.
- Do not keep outdated medicine or medicine no longer needed. Be sure that any discarded medicine is out of the reach of children.

Precautions While Using This Medicine

If your symptoms do not improve or if your condition becomes worse, check with your doctor.

Side Effects of This Medicine

Along with its needed effects, a medicine may cause some unwanted effects. Although not all of these side effects may occur, if they do occur they may need medical attention.

Check with your doctor as soon as possible if either of the following side effects occurs:

Rare

Eye irritation (including styes) not present before use of this medicine; swelling of conjunctiva (in eye) (severe)

Other side effects may occur that usually do not need medical attention. These side effects may go away during treatment as your body adjusts to the medicine. However, check with your doctor if any of the following side effects continue or are bothersome:

More common

Burning or stinging of eye (mild and temporary)

Less common or rare

Dryness or puffiness around the eye; watering or itching of eye (increased)

Other side effects not listed above may also occur in some patients. If you notice any other effects, check with your doctor.

Annual revision: 07/16/91

CROMOLYN Oral

Some commonly used brand names are:

In the U.S.

Gastrocrom

In Canada

Nalcrom

Another commonly used name is sodium cromoglycate.

Description

Cromolyn (KROE-moe-lin) is used to treat the symptoms of mastocytosis. Mastocytosis is a rare condition caused by too many mast cells in the body. These mast cells release substances that cause the symptoms of the disease, such as abdominal pain, nausea, vomiting, diarrhea, headache, flushing or itching of skin, or hives.

Cromolyn works by acting on the mast cells in the body to prevent them from releasing substances that cause the symptoms of mastocytosis.

Cromolyn is available only with your doctor's prescription, in the following dosage form:

Oral

- Capsules (U.S. and Canada)

It is very important that you read and understand the following information. If any of it causes you special concern, check with your doctor. Also, *if you have any questions* or if you want more information about this medicine or your medical problem, *ask your doctor, nurse, or pharmacist.*

Before Using This Medicine

In deciding to use a medicine, the risks of taking the medicine must be weighed against the good it will do. This is a decision you and your doctor will make. For oral cromolyn, the following should be considered:

Allergies—Tell your doctor if you have ever had any unusual or allergic reaction to cromolyn. Also tell your doctor and pharmacist if you are allergic to any other substances, such as foods, preservatives, or dyes.

Diet—Make certain your doctor and pharmacist know if you are on any special diet, such as a low-sodium diet.

Pregnancy—Cromolyn has not been studied in pregnant women. However, studies in animals have shown that cromolyn, when given by injection in very large amounts, causes a decrease in successful pregnancies and a decrease in the weight of the animal fetus.

Breast-feeding—It is not known whether cromolyn passes into the breast milk. However, this medicine has not been reported to cause problems in nursing babies.

Children—Although there is no specific information about the use of oral cromolyn in children, it is not expected to cause different side effects or problems in children than it does in adults.

Older adults—Many medicines have not been tested in older people. Therefore, it may not be known whether they work exactly the same way they do in younger adults. Although there is no specific information about the use of oral cromolyn in the elderly, it is not expected to cause different side effects or problems in older people than it does in younger adults.

Other medicines—Although certain medicines should not be used together at all, in other cases two different medicines may be used together even if an interaction might occur. In these cases, your doctor may want to change the dose, or other precautions may be necessary. When you are taking oral cromolyn, it is especially important that your doctor and pharmacist know if you are taking any other prescription or nonprescription (over-the-counter [OTC]) medicine.

Other medical problems—The presence of other medical problems may affect the use of oral cromolyn. Make sure you tell your doctor if you have any other medical problems, especially:

- Kidney disease or
- Liver disease—The effects of cromolyn may be increased, which may increase the chance of side effects

Before you begin using any new medicine (prescription or nonprescription) or if you develop any new medical

problem while you are using this medicine, check with your doctor, nurse, or pharmacist.

Proper Use of This Medicine

Unless otherwise directed by your doctor, it is best to take oral cromolyn as follows:

- Dissolve the contents of the cromolyn capsule(s) in one-half glass (4 ounces) of hot water. Stir the solution until the powder is completely dissolved and the solution is clear. Then add an equal amount (one-half glass) of cold water to the solution while stirring.
- Be sure to drink all of the solution to get the full dose of medicine.
- Do not mix this medicine with fruit juice, milk, or foods because they may keep the medicine from working as well.

Take cromolyn only as directed. Do not take more of it and do not take it more often than your doctor ordered. To do so may increase the chance of side effects.

Missed dose—If you miss a dose of this medicine, take it as soon as possible. Then take any remaining doses for that day at regularly spaced intervals. Do not double doses.

Storage—To store this medicine:

- Keep out of the reach of children.
- Store away from heat.
- Do not store the capsule form of this medicine in the bathroom, near the kitchen sink, or in other damp places. Heat or moisture may cause the medicine to break down.
- Do not keep outdated medicine or medicine no longer needed. Be sure that any discarded medicine is out of the reach of children.

Precautions While Using This Medicine

If your symptoms do not improve or if your condition becomes worse, check with your doctor.

Side Effects of This Medicine

Along with its needed effects, a medicine may cause some unwanted effects. Although not all of these side effects may occur, if they do occur they may need medical attention.

Check with your doctor immediately if any of the following side effects occur:

Rare

Coughing; difficulty in swallowing; hives or itching of skin; swelling of face, lips, or eyelids; wheezing or difficulty in breathing

Also, check with your doctor as soon as possible if the following side effect occurs:

Less common

Skin rash

Other side effects may occur that usually do not need medical attention. These side effects may go away during treatment as your body adjusts to the medicine. However, check with your doctor if any of the following side effects continue or are bothersome:

More common

Diarrhea; headache

Less common

Abdominal pain; irritability; joint pain; nausea; trouble in sleeping

Note: If the above side effects occur in patients with mastocytosis, they are usually only temporary and could be symptoms of the disease.

Other side effects not listed above may also occur in some patients. If you notice any other effects, check with your doctor.

Annual revision: August 1990

CROTAMITON Topical

Some commonly used brand names are:

In the U.S.

Eurax Cream
Eurax Lotion

In Canada

Eurax Cream

Description

Crotamiton (kroe-TAM-i-tonn) is used to treat scabies infection. It is also used to relieve the itching of certain skin conditions.

This medicine is available only with your doctor's prescription, in the following dosage forms:

Topical

- Cream (U.S. and Canada)
- Lotion (U.S.)

It is very important that you read and understand the following information. If any of it causes you special concern, check with your doctor. Also, *if you have any questions* or if you want more information about this

medicine or your medical problem, *ask your doctor, nurse, or pharmacist.*

Before Using This Medicine

In deciding to use a medicine, the risks of using the medicine must be weighed against the good it will do. This is a decision you and your doctor will make. For crotamiton, the following should be considered:

Allergies—Tell your doctor if you have ever had any unusual or allergic reaction to crotamiton. Also tell your doctor and pharmacist if you are allergic to any other substances, such as preservatives or dyes.

Pregnancy—Studies on effects in pregnancy have not been done in either humans or animals.

Breast-feeding—Topical crotamiton has not been reported to cause problems in nursing babies.

Children—Studies on this medicine have been done only in adult patients, and there is no specific information comparing use of this medicine in children with use in other age groups.

Older adults—Many medicines have not been studied specifically in older people. Therefore, it may not be known whether they work exactly the same way they do in younger adults or if they cause different side effects or problems in older people. There is no specific information comparing use of crotamiton in the elderly with use in other age groups.

Other medicines—Although certain medicines should not be used together at all, in other cases two different medicines may be used together even if an interaction might occur. In these cases, your doctor may want to change the dose, or other precautions may be necessary. Tell your doctor and pharmacist if you are using any other topical prescription or nonprescription (over-the-counter [OTC]) medicine that is to be applied to the same area of the skin.

Other medical problems—The presence of other medical problems may affect the use of crotamiton. Make sure you tell your doctor if you have any other medical problems, especially:

- Severely inflamed skin or raw oozing areas of the skin—Use of crotamiton on these areas may make the condition worse

Before you begin using any new medicine (prescription or nonprescription) or if you develop any new medical problem while you are using this medicine, check with your doctor, nurse, or pharmacist.

Proper Use of This Medicine

Keep crotamiton away from the mouth. It may be harmful if swallowed.

Use this medicine only as directed. Do not use it more often than your doctor ordered. To do so may increase the chance of side effects.

Keep crotamiton away from the eyes and other mucous membranes, such as the inside of the nose. It may cause irritation. If you should accidentally get some in your eyes, flush them thoroughly with water at once.

This medicine usually comes with patient directions. Read them carefully before using.

If you take a bath or shower before using this medicine, dry the skin well before applying crotamiton.

For patients using this medicine *for scabies:*

- Apply enough medicine to cover the entire skin surface from the chin down, and rub in well. This applies especially to folds and creases in the skin and to the hands, feet (including the soles), between fingers and toes, and moist areas (such as underarms and groin).
- Do not wash off the first coat of this medicine.
- Apply a second coat of this medicine 24 hours after the first one.
- The next day, put on freshly washed or dry-cleaned clothing and change bedding in order to prevent reinfection.
- Then, 48 hours after the second application of this medicine, take a cleansing bath to remove the medicine.
- Your sexual partner, especially, and all members of your household may need to be treated also, since the infection may spread to persons in close contact. If these persons are not being treated or if you have any questions about this, check with your doctor.

Storage—To store this medicine:

- Keep out of the reach of children.
- Store away from heat and direct light.
- Keep the medicine from freezing.
- Do not keep outdated medicine or medicine no longer needed. Be sure that any discarded medicine is out of the reach of children.

Precautions While Using This Medicine

If your condition does not improve or if it becomes worse, check with your doctor.

For patients using this medicine *for scabies:*

- To prevent reinfection or spreading of the infection to other people, good health habits are also required. These include machine washing all underwear, pajamas, sheets, pillowcases, towels, and washcloths in very hot water and drying them using the hot cycle of a dryer. Clothing or bedding that cannot be washed in this way should be dry cleaned.

Side Effects of This Medicine

Along with its needed effects, a medicine may cause some unwanted effects. Although not all of these side effects may occur, if they do occur they may need medical attention.

Check with your doctor as soon as possible if either of the following side effects occur:

Rare

Skin irritation not present before use of this medicine; skin rash

Other side effects not listed above may also occur in some patients. If you notice any other effects, check with your doctor.

Annual revision: 02/10/92

CYCLANDELATE Systemic

A commonly used brand name is Cyclospasmol.
Generic name product may also be available in the U.S.

Description

Cyclandelate (sye-KLAN-de-late) belongs to the group of medicines commonly called vasodilators. These medicines increase the size of blood vessels. Cyclandelate is used to treat problems resulting from poor blood circulation.

In the U.S., cyclandelate is available only with your doctor's prescription. It is available in the following dosage forms:

Oral

- Capsules (U.S.)
- Tablets (Canada)

It is very important that you read and understand the following information. If any of it causes you special concern, check with your doctor. Also, *if you have any questions* or if you want more information about this medicine or your medical problem, *ask your doctor, nurse, or pharmacist.*

Before Using This Medicine

In deciding to use a medicine, the risks of taking the medicine must be weighed against the good it will do. This is a decision you and your doctor will make. For cyclandelate, the following should be considered:

Allergies—Tell your doctor if you have ever had any unusual or allergic reaction to cyclandelate. Also tell your doctor and pharmacist if you are allergic to any other substances, such as foods, preservatives, or dyes.

Pregnancy—Studies on effects in pregnancy have not been done in either humans or animals.

Breast-feeding—It is not known whether cyclandelate passes into breast milk. However, cyclandelate has not been reported to cause problems in nursing babies.

Children—Studies on this medicine have been done only in adult patients, and there is no specific information comparing use of cyclandelate in children with use in other age groups.

Older adults—Many medicines have not been studied specifically in older people. Therefore, it may not be known whether they work exactly the same way they do in younger adults. Although there is no specific information comparing use of cyclandelate in the elderly with use in other age groups, this medicine is not expected to cause different side effects or problems in older people than in younger adults.

Other medicines—Although certain medicines should not be used together at all, in other cases two different medicines may be used together even if an interaction might occur. In these cases, your doctor may want to change the dose, or other precautions may be necessary. Tell your doctor and pharmacist if you are taking any other prescription or nonprescription (over-the-counter [OTC]) medicine, or if you smoke.

Other medical problems—The presence of other medical problems may affect the use of cyclandelate. Make sure you tell your doctor if you have any other medical problems, especially:

- Angina (chest pain) or
- Bleeding problems or
- Glaucoma or
- Hardening of the arteries or
- Heart attack (recent) or
- Stroke (recent)—The chance of unwanted effects may be increased

Before you begin using any new medicine (prescription or nonprescription) or if you develop any new medical problem while you are using this medicine, check with your doctor, nurse, or pharmacist.

Proper Use of This Medicine

If this medicine upsets your stomach, it may be taken with meals, milk, or antacids.

Missed dose—If you miss a dose of this medicine, take it as soon as you remember. Then go back to your regular dosing schedule. However, if it is almost time for your next dose, skip the missed dose and go back to your regular dosing schedule. Do not double doses.

Storage—To store this medicine:

- Keep out of the reach of children.
- Store away from heat and direct light.
- Do not store in the bathroom, near the kitchen sink, or in other damp places. Heat or moisture may cause the medicine to break down.
- Do not keep outdated medicine or medicine no longer needed. Be sure that any discarded medicine is out of the reach of children.

Precautions While Using This Medicine

It may take some time for this medicine to work. If you feel that the medicine is not working, do not stop taking it on your own. Instead, check with your doctor.

The helpful effects of this medicine may be decreased if you smoke.

Dizziness may occur, especially when you get up from a lying or sitting position or climb stairs. Getting up slowly may help. If this problem continues or gets worse, check with your doctor.

Side Effects of This Medicine

Along with its needed effects, a medicine may cause some unwanted effects. The following side effects may go away during treatment as your body adjusts to the medicine. However, check with your doctor if any of these effects continue or are bothersome:

Less common

Belching, heartburn, nausea, or stomach pain; dizziness; fast heartbeat; flushing of face; headache; sweating; tingling sensation in face, fingers, or toes; weakness

Other side effects not listed above may also occur in some patients. If you notice any other effects, check with your doctor.

Annual revision: 10/15/92

CYCLOBENZAPRINE Systemic

Some commonly used brand names are:

In the U.S.

Cycoflex
Flexeril

Generic name product may also be available.

In Canada

Flexeril

Description

Cyclobenzaprine (sye-kloe-BEN-za-preen) is used to help relax certain muscles in your body. It helps relieve the pain, stiffness, and discomfort caused by strains, sprains, or injuries to your muscles. However, this medicine does not take the place of rest, exercise or physical therapy, or other treatment that your doctor may recommend for your medical problem. Cyclobenzaprine acts on the central nervous system (CNS) to produce its muscle relaxant effects. Its actions on the CNS may also cause some of this medicine's side effects.

Cyclobenzaprine may also be used for other conditions as determined by your doctor.

Cyclobenzaprine is available only with your doctor's prescription, in the following dosage form:

Oral

- Tablets (U.S. and Canada)

It is very important that you read and understand the following information. If any of it causes you special concern, check with your doctor or pharmacist. Also, *if you have any questions* or if you want more information about this medicine or your medical problem, *ask your doctor, nurse, or pharmacist.*

Before Using This Medicine

In deciding to use a medicine, the risks of taking the medicine must be weighed against the good it will do. This is a decision you and your doctor will make. For cyclobenzaprine, the following should be considered:

Allergies—Tell your doctor if you have ever had any unusual or allergic reaction to cyclobenzaprine. Also tell your doctor and pharmacist if you are allergic to any other substances, such as foods, preservatives, or dyes.

Pregnancy—Studies on birth defects with cyclobenzaprine have not been done in humans. However, cyclobenzaprine has not been shown to cause birth defects or other problems in animal studies.

Breast-feeding—Although it is not known whether cyclobenzaprine passes into the breast milk, cyclobenzaprine has not been reported to cause problems in nursing babies.

Children—Studies on this medicine have been done only in adult patients, and there is no specific information comparing use of cyclobenzaprine in children with use in other age groups.

Teenagers—Studies on this medicine have been done only in adult patients, and there is no specific information comparing use of cyclobenzaprine in teenagers up to 15 years of age with use in other age groups.

Older adults—Many medicines have not been studied specifically in older people. Therefore, it may not be known whether they work exactly the same way they do in younger adults or if they cause different side effects or problems in older people. There is no specific information comparing use of cyclobenzaprine in the elderly with use in other age groups.

Other medicines—Although certain medicines should not be used together at all, in other cases two different medicines may be used together even if an interaction might occur. In these cases, your doctor may want to change the dose, or other precautions may be necessary. When you are taking cyclobenzaprine, it is especially important that your doctor and pharmacist know if you are taking any of the following:

- Central nervous system (CNS) depressants or
- Tricyclic antidepressants (amitriptyline [e.g., Elavil], amoxapine [e.g., Asendin], clomipramine [e.g., Anafranil], desipramine [e.g., Pertofrane], doxepin [e.g., Sinequan], imipramine [e.g., Tofranil], nortriptyline [e.g., Aventyl], protriptyline [e.g., Vivactil], trimipramine [e.g., Surmontil])—The chance of side effects may be increased
- Monoamine oxidase (MAO) inhibitors (furazolidone [e.g., Furoxone], isocarboxazid [e.g., Marplan], phenelzine [e.g., Nardil], procarbazine [e.g., Matulane], tranylcypromine [e.g., Parnate])—Taking cyclobenzaprine while you are taking or within 2 weeks of taking monoamine oxidase (MAO) inhibitors may increase the chance of side effects

Other medical problems—The presence of other medical problems may affect the use of cyclobenzaprine. Make sure you tell your doctor if you have any other medical problems, especially:

- Glaucoma or
- Problems with urination—Cyclobenzaprine can make your condition worse
- Heart or blood vessel disease or
- Overactive thyroid—The chance of side effects may be increased

Before you begin using any new medicine (prescription or nonprescription) or if you develop any new medical problem while you are using this medicine, check with your doctor, nurse, or pharmacist.

Proper Use of This Medicine

Take this medicine only as directed by your doctor. Do not take more of it and do not take it more often than your doctor ordered. To do so may increase the chance of serious side effects.

Missed dose—If you miss a dose of this medicine and remember within an hour or so of the missed dose, take it right away. Then go back to your regular dosing schedule. But if you do not remember until later, skip the missed dose and go back to your regular dosing schedule. Do not double doses.

Storage—To store this medicine:

- Keep out of the reach of children.
- Store away from heat and direct light.
- Do not store this medicine in the bathroom, near the kitchen sink, or in other damp places. Heat or moisture may cause the medicine to break down.
- Do not keep outdated medicine or medicine no longer needed. Be sure that any discarded medicine is out of the reach of children.

Precautions While Using This Medicine

This medicine will add to the effects of alcohol and other CNS depressants (medicines that slow down the nervous system, possibly causing drowsiness). Some examples of CNS depressants are antihistamines or medicine for hay fever, other allergies, or colds; sedatives, tranquilizers, or sleeping medicine; prescription pain medicine or narcotics; barbiturates; medicine for seizures; other muscle relaxants; or anesthetics, including some dental anesthetics. *Check with your doctor before taking any of the above while you are using this medicine.*

This medicine may cause some people to have blurred vision or to become drowsy, dizzy, or less alert than they are normally. *Make sure you know how you react to this medicine before you drive, use machines, or do anything else that could be dangerous if you are dizzy or are not alert and able to see well.*

Cyclobenzaprine may cause dryness of the mouth. For temporary relief, use sugarless candy or gum, melt bits of ice in your mouth, or use a saliva substitute. However, if your mouth continues to feel dry for more than 2 weeks, check with your medical doctor or dentist. Continuing dryness of the mouth may increase the chance of dental disease, including tooth decay, gum disease, and fungus infections.

Side Effects of This Medicine

Along with its needed effects, a medicine may cause some unwanted effects. Although not all of these side effects may occur, if they do occur they may need medical attention.

Check with your doctor immediately if any of the following side effects occur:

Rare

Fainting; swelling of face, lips, or tongue

Symptoms of overdose

Convulsions (seizures); drowsiness (severe); dry, hot, flushed skin; fast or irregular heartbeat; hallucinations (seeing, hearing, or feeling things that are not there); increase or decrease in body temperature; troubled breathing; unexplained muscle stiffness; unusual nervousness or restlessness (severe); vomiting

Also, check with your doctor as soon as possible if any of the following side effects occur:

Rare

Clumsiness or unsteadiness; confusion; mental depression or other mood or mental changes; problems in urinating; ringing or buzzing in the ears; skin rash, hives, or itching; unusual thoughts or dreams; yellow eyes or skin

Other side effects may occur that usually do not need medical attention. These side effects may go away during treatment as your body adjusts to the medicine. However, check with your doctor if any of the following side effects continue or are bothersome:

More common

Dizziness or lightheadedness; drowsiness; dryness of mouth

Less common or rare

Bloated feeling or gas, indigestion, nausea or vomiting, or stomach cramps or pain; blurred vision; constipation; decrease in blood pressure; diarrhea; excitement or nervousness; frequent urination; general feeling of discomfort or illness; headache; muscle twitching; numbness, tingling, pain, or weakness in hands or feet; pounding heartbeat; problems in speaking; trembling; trouble in sleeping; unpleasant taste or other taste changes; unusual muscle weakness; unusual tiredness

Other side effects not listed above may also occur in some patients. If you notice any other effects, check with your doctor.

Additional Information

Once a medicine has been approved for marketing for a certain use, experience may show that it is also useful for other medical problems. Although this use is not included in product labeling, cyclobenzaprine is used in certain patients with fibromyalgia syndrome (also called fibrositis or fibrositis syndrome).

There is no additional information relating to proper use, precautions, or side effects for this use of cyclobenzaprine.

Annual revision: 07/09/91

CYCLOPENTOLATE Ophthalmic

Some commonly used brand names are:

In the U.S.

Ak-Pentolate	Ocu-Pentolate
Cyclogyl	Pentolair
I-Pentolate	Spectro-Pentolate

Generic name product may also be available.

In Canada

Ak-Pentolate	Minims Cyclopentolate
Cyclogyl	

Description

Cyclopentolate (sye-kloe-PEN-toe-late) is used to dilate (enlarge) the pupil. It is used before eye examinations and to treat certain eye conditions.

This medicine is available only with your doctor's prescription, in the following dosage form:

Ophthalmic

- Ophthalmic solution (eye drops) (U.S. and Canada)

It is very important that you read and understand the following information. If any of it causes you special concern, check with your doctor. Also, *if you have any questions* or if you want more information about this medicine or your medical problem, *ask your doctor, nurse, or pharmacist*.

Before Using This Medicine

In deciding to use a medicine, the risks of using the medicine must be weighed against the good it will do. This is a decision you and your doctor will make. For cyclopentolate, the following should be considered:

Allergies—Tell your doctor if you have ever had any unusual or allergic reaction to cyclopentolate. Also tell your doctor and pharmacist if you are allergic to any other substances, such as preservatives.

Pregnancy—Cyclopentolate may be absorbed into the body. However, studies on effects in pregnancy have not been done in either humans or animals.

Breast-feeding—Cyclopentolate may be absorbed into the mother's body. It is not known whether cyclopentolate passes into the breast milk. However, cyclopentolate has not been reported to cause problems in nursing babies.

Children—Children may be especially sensitive to the effects of cyclopentolate. This may increase the chance of side effects during treatment.

Older adults—Elderly people are especially sensitive to the effects of cyclopentolate. This may increase the chance of side effects during treatment.

Other medicines—Although certain medicines should not be used together at all, in other cases two different medicines may be used together even if an interaction might occur. In these cases, your doctor may want to change the dose, or other precautions may be necessary. Tell your doctor and pharmacist if you are using any other prescription or nonprescription (over-the-counter [OTC]) medicine.

Other medical problems—The presence of other medical problems may affect the use of cyclopentolate. Make sure you tell your doctor if you have any other medical problems, especially:

- Brain damage (in children) or
- Down's syndrome (mongolism) (in children and adults) or
- Glaucoma or
- Spastic paralysis (in children)—Cyclopentolate may make the condition worse

Before you begin using any new medicine (prescription or nonprescription) or if you develop any new medical problem while you are using this medicine, check with your doctor, nurse, or pharmacist.

Proper Use of This Medicine

To use:

- First, wash your hands. With the middle finger, apply pressure to the inside corner of the eye (and continue to apply pressure for 2 or 3 minutes after the medicine has been placed in the eye). *This is especially important in infants*. Tilt the head back and with the index finger of the same hand, pull the lower eyelid away from the eye to form a pouch. Drop the medicine into the pouch and gently close the eyes. Do not blink. Keep the eyes closed for 1 or 2 minutes to allow the medicine to be absorbed.
- Immediately after using the eye drops, wash your hands to remove any medicine that may be on them. If you are using the eye drops for an infant or child, be sure to wash the infant's or child's hands also, and do not let any of the medicine get in the infant's or child's mouth.
- To keep the medicine as germ-free as possible, do not touch the applicator tip to any surface (including the eye). Also, keep the container tightly closed.

Use this medicine only as directed. Do not use more of it and do not use it more often than your doctor ordered. To do so may increase the chance of too much medicine being absorbed into the body and the chance of side effects.

Missed dose—If you miss a dose of this medicine, apply it as soon as possible. However, if it is almost time for your next dose, skip the missed dose and go back to your regular dosing schedule. Do not double doses.

Storage—To store this medicine:

- Keep out of the reach of children. Overdose of this medicine is very dangerous for infants and children.
- Store away from heat and direct light.
- Keep the medicine from freezing.
- Do not keep outdated medicine or medicine no longer needed. Be sure that any discarded medicine is out of the reach of children.

Precautions While Using This Medicine

After you apply this medicine to your eyes:

- Your pupils will become unusually large and you will have blurring of vision, especially for close objects. *Make sure your vision is clear before you drive, use machines, or do anything else that could be dangerous if you are not able to see well.*
- Your eyes will become more sensitive to light than they are normally. When you go out during the daylight hours, even on cloudy days, *wear sunglasses that block ultraviolet (UV) light to protect your eyes from sunlight and other bright lights.* Ordinary sunglasses may not protect your eyes. If you have any questions about the kind of sunglasses to wear, check with your doctor.

If these side effects continue for longer than 36 hours after you have stopped using this medicine, check with your doctor.

Side Effects of This Medicine

Along with its needed effects, a medicine may cause some unwanted effects. Although not all of these side effects may occur, if they do occur they may need medical attention.

Check with your doctor as soon as possible if any of the following side effects occur:

Symptoms of too much medicine being absorbed into the body

Clumsiness or unsteadiness; confusion; fast or irregular heartbeat; fever; flushing or redness of face; hallucinations (seeing, hearing, or feeling things that are not there); skin rash; slurred speech; swollen stomach in infants; thirst or dryness of mouth; unusual behavior, especially in children; unusual drowsiness, tiredness, or weakness

Other side effects may occur that usually do not need medical attention. These side effects may go away during treatment as your body adjusts to the medicine. However, check with your doctor if any of the following side effects continue or are bothersome:

Blurred vision; burning of eye; eye irritation not present before therapy; increased sensitivity of eyes to light

Other side effects not listed above may also occur in some patients. If you notice any other effects, check with your doctor.

Annual revision: 03/04/92

CYCLOPHOSPHAMIDE Systemic

Some commonly used brand names are:

In the U.S.

Cytoxan
Neosar

Generic name product may also be available.

In Canada

Cytoxan
Procytox

Description

Cyclophosphamide (sye-kloe-FOSS-fa-mide) belongs to the group of medicines called alkylating agents. It is used to treat some kinds of cancer.

Cyclophosphamide interferes with the growth of cancer cells, which are eventually destroyed. Since the growth of normal body cells may also be affected by cyclophosphamide, other effects will also occur. Some of these may be serious and must be reported to your doctor. Other effects, like hair loss, may not be serious but may cause concern. Some effects may not occur for months or years after the medicine is used.

Cyclophosphamide is also used for treatment of some kinds of kidney disease.

Cyclophosphamide may also be used for other conditions as determined by your doctor.

Before you begin treatment with cyclophosphamide, you and your doctor should talk about the good this medicine will do as well as the risks of using it.

Cyclophosphamide is available only with your doctor's prescription, in the following dosage forms:

Oral

- Oral solution (U.S. and Canada)
- Tablets (U.S. and Canada)

Parenteral

- Injection (U.S. and Canada)

It is very important that you read and understand the following information. If any of it causes you special concern, check with your doctor. Also, *if you have any questions* or if you want more information about this medicine or your medical problem, *ask your doctor, nurse, or pharmacist.*

Before Using This Medicine

In deciding to use a medicine, the risks of taking the medicine must be weighed against the good it will do. This is a decision you and your doctor will make. For cyclophosphamide, the following should be considered:

Allergies—Tell your doctor if you have ever had any unusual or allergic reaction to cyclophosphamide.

Pregnancy—This medicine may cause several different birth defects if either the male or female is taking it at the time of conception or if it is taken during pregnancy. In addition, many cancer medicines may cause sterility. Although sterility occurs commonly with cyclophosphamide, it is usually only temporary.

Be sure that you have discussed this with your doctor before taking this medicine. It is best to use some kind of birth control while you are taking cyclophosphamide. Tell your doctor right away if you think you have become pregnant while taking cyclophosphamide.

Breast-feeding—Cyclophosphamide passes into the breast milk. Because this medicine may cause serious side effects, breast-feeding is generally not recommended while you are taking it.

Children—This medicine has been tested in children and has not been shown to cause different side effects or problems than it does in adults.

Older adults—Many medicines have not been studied specifically in older people. Therefore, it may not be known whether they work exactly the same way they do in younger adults. Although there is no specific information comparing use of cyclophosphamide in the elderly with use in other age groups, it is not expected to cause different side effects or problems in older people than it does in younger adults.

Other medicines—Although certain medicines should not be used together at all, in other cases two different medicines may be used together even if an interaction might occur. In these cases, your doctor may want to change the dose, or other precautions may be necessary. When

taking or receiving cyclophosphamide it is especially important that your doctor and pharmacist know if you are taking any of the following:

- Amphotericin B by injection (e.g., Fungizone) or
- Antithyroid agents (medicine for overactive thyroid) or
- Chloramphenicol (e.g., Chloromycetin) or
- Colchicine or
- Flucytosine (e.g., Ancobon) or
- Ganciclovir (e.g., Cytovene) or
- Interferon (e.g., Intron A, Roferon-A) or
- Plicamycin (e.g., Mithracin) or
- Zidovudine (e.g., AZT, Retrovir) or
- If you have ever been treated with x-rays or cancer medicines—Cyclophosphamide may increase the effects of these medicines or radiation therapy on the blood
- Azathioprine (e.g., Imuran) or
- Chlorambucil (e.g., Leukeran) or
- Corticosteroids (cortisone-like medicine) or
- Cyclosporine (e.g., Sandimmune) or
- Mercaptopurine (e.g., Purinethol) or
- Muromonab-CD3 (monoclonal antibody) (e.g., Orthoclone OKT3)—There may be an increased risk of infection and development of cancer because cyclophosphamide reduces the body's ability to fight them
- Probenecid (e.g., Benemid) or
- Sulfinpyrazone (e.g., Anturane)—Cyclophosphamide may increase the amount of uric acid in the blood. Since these medicines are used to lower uric acid levels, they may not work as well in patients taking cyclophosphamide

Other medical problems—The presence of other medical problems may affect the use of cyclophosphamide. Make sure you tell your doctor if you have any other medical problems, especially:

- Chickenpox (including recent exposure) or
- Herpes zoster (shingles)—Risk of severe disease affecting other parts of the body
- Gout (history of) or
- Kidney stones—(history of)—Cyclophosphamide may increase levels of uric acid in the body, which can cause gout or kidney stones
- Infection—Cyclophosphamide can decrease your body's ability to fight infection
- Kidney disease—Effects may be increased because of slower removal of cyclophosphamide from the body
- Liver disease—The effect of cyclophosphamide may be decreased

Before you begin using any new medicine (prescription or nonprescription) or if you develop any new medical problem while you are using this medicine, check with your doctor, nurse, or pharmacist.

Proper Use of This Medicine

Take this medicine only as directed by your doctor. Do not take more or less of it, and do not take it more often than your doctor ordered. The exact amount of medicine you need has been carefully worked out. Taking too much may increase the chance of side effects, while taking too little may not improve your condition.

Cyclophosphamide is sometimes given together with certain other medicines. If you are using a combination of medicines, make sure that you take each one at the proper time and do not mix them. Ask your doctor, nurse, or pharmacist to help you plan a way to remember to take your medicines at the right times.

While you are using cyclophosphamide, it is important that you drink extra fluids so that you will pass more urine. Also, empty your bladder frequently, including at least once during the night. This will help prevent kidney and bladder problems and keep your kidneys working well. Cyclophosphamide passes from the body in the urine. If too much of it appears in the urine or if the urine stays in the bladder too long, it can cause dangerous irritation. *Follow your doctor's instructions carefully about how much fluid to drink every day.* Some patients may have to drink up to 7 to 12 cups (3 quarts) of fluid a day.

Usually it is best to take cyclophosphamide first thing in the morning, to reduce the risk of bladder problems. However, your doctor may want you to take it with food in smaller doses over the day, to lessen stomach upset or help the medicine work better. Follow your doctor's instructions carefully about when to take cyclophosphamide.

Cyclophosphamide often causes nausea, vomiting, and loss of appetite. However, it is very important that you continue to use the medicine even if you begin to feel ill. *Do not stop taking this medicine without first checking with your doctor.* Ask your doctor, nurse, or pharmacist for ways to lessen these effects.

If you vomit shortly after taking a dose of cyclophosphamide, check with your doctor. You will be told whether to take the dose again or to wait until the next scheduled dose.

Missed dose—If you miss a dose of this medicine, do not take the missed dose at all and do not double the next one. Instead, go back to your regular dosing schedule and check with your doctor.

Storage—To store this medicine:

- Keep out of the reach of children.
- Store away from heat and direct light.
- Do not store in the bathroom, near the kitchen sink, or in other damp places. Heat or moisture may cause the medicine to break down.
- Store the oral solution form of this medicine in the refrigerator. Keep it from freezing.
- Do not keep outdated medicine or medicine no longer needed. Be sure that any discarded medicine is out of the reach of children.

Precautions While Using This Medicine

It is very important that your doctor check your progress at regular visits to make sure that this medicine is working properly and to check for unwanted effects.

While you are being treated with cyclophosphamide, and after you stop treatment with it, *do not have any immunizations (vaccinations) without your doctor's approval.* Cyclophosphamide may lower your body's resistance and there is a chance you might get the infection the immunization is meant to prevent. In addition, other persons living in your house should not take oral polio vaccine since there is a chance they could pass the polio virus on to you. Also, avoid persons who have recently taken oral polio vaccine. Do not get close to them, and do not stay in the same room with them for very long. If you cannot take these precautions, you should consider wearing a protective face mask that covers the nose and mouth.

Before having any kind of surgery, including dental surgery, or emergency treatment, make sure the medical doctor or dentist in charge knows that you are taking this medicine, especially if you have taken it within the last 10 days.

Cyclophosphamide can temporarily lower the number of white blood cells in your blood, increasing the chance of getting an infection. It can also lower the number of platelets, which are necessary for proper blood clotting. If this occurs, there are certain precautions you can take, especially when your blood count is low, to reduce the risk of infection or bleeding:

- If you can, avoid people with infections. *Check with your doctor immediately* if you think you are getting an infection or if you get a fever or chills, cough or hoarseness, lower back or side pain, or painful or difficult urination.
- *Check with your doctor immediately* if you notice any unusual bleeding or bruising; black, tarry stools; blood in urine or stools; or pinpoint red spots on your skin.
- Be careful when using a regular toothbrush, dental floss, or toothpick. Your medical doctor, dentist, or nurse may recommend other ways to clean your teeth and gums. Check with your medical doctor before having any dental work done.
- Do not touch your eyes or the inside of your nose unless you have just washed your hands and have not touched anything else in the meantime.
- Be careful not to cut yourself when you are using sharp objects such as a safety razor or fingernail or toenail cutters.
- Avoid contact sports or other situations where bruising or injury could occur.

Before you have any medical tests, tell the medical doctor in charge that you are taking this medicine. The results of some tests may be affected by this medicine.

Side Effects of This Medicine

Along with their needed effects, medicines like cyclophosphamide can sometimes cause unwanted effects such as blood problems; loss of hair; problems with the lungs, heart, or bladder; and other side effects. These and others are described below. Also, because of the way these medicines act on the body, there is a chance that they might cause other unwanted effects that may not occur until months or years after the medicine is used. These may include certain types of cancer, such as leukemia or bladder cancer. Discuss these possible effects with your doctor.

Although not all of these side effects may occur, if they do occur they may need medical attention.

Stop taking this medicine and check with your doctor immediately if the following side effects occur:

With high doses and/or long-term treatment

Blood in urine; painful urination

Check with your doctor or nurse immediately if any of the following side effects occur:

Less common

Cough or hoarseness; fever or chills; lower back or side pain; painful or difficult urination

Rare

Black, tarry stools; blood in urine or stools; pinpoint red spots on skin; shortness of breath (sudden); unusual bleeding or bruising

Check with your doctor as soon as possible if any of the following side effects occur:

More common

Dizziness, confusion, or agitation; missing menstrual periods; unusual tiredness or weakness

Less common

Fast heartbeat; joint pain; shortness of breath; swelling of feet or lower legs

Rare

Frequent urination; redness, swelling, or pain at place of injection; sores in mouth and on lips; unusual thirst; yellow eyes or skin

Other side effects may occur that usually do not need medical attention. These side effects may go away during treatment as your body adjusts to the medicine. Also, your doctor or nurse may be able to tell you about ways to prevent or reduce some of these side effects. Check with your doctor or nurse if any of the following side effects continue or are bothersome or if you have any questions about them:

More common

Darkening of skin and fingernails; loss of appetite; nausea or vomiting

Less common

Diarrhea or stomach pain; flushing or redness of face; headache; increased sweating; skin rash, hives, or itching; swollen lips

Cyclophosphamide may cause a temporary loss of hair in some people. After treatment has ended, normal hair growth should return, although the new hair may be a slightly different color or texture.

After you stop using cyclophosphamide, it may still produce some side effects that need attention. During this period of time, *check with your doctor immediately* if you notice the following side effect:

Blood in urine

Other side effects not listed above may also occur in some patients. If you notice any other effects, check with your doctor.

Additional Information

Once a medicine has been approved for marketing for a certain use, experience may show that it is also useful for other medical problems. Although these uses are not included in product labeling, cyclophosphamide is used in certain patients with the following medical conditions:

- Organ transplant rejection (prevention)
- Rheumatoid arthritis
- Wegener's granulomatosis
- Systemic lupus erythematosus
- Systemic dermatomyositis or
- Multiple sclerosis

Other than the above information, there is no additional information relating to proper use, precautions, or side effects for these uses.

Annual revision: 08/17/92

CYCLOSERINE Systemic†

A commonly used brand name is Seromycin.

†Not commercially available in Canada.

Description

Cycloserine (sye-kloe-SER-een) belongs to the family of medicines called antibiotics. It is used to treat tuberculosis (TB). When cycloserine is used for TB, it is given with one or more other medicines for TB. Cycloserine may also be used for other conditions as determined by your doctor.

Cycloserine is available only with your doctor's prescription, in the following dosage form:

Oral

- Capsules (U.S.)

It is very important that you read and understand the following information. If any of it causes you special concern, check with your doctor. Also, *if you have any questions* or if you want more information about this medicine or your medical problem, *ask your doctor, nurse, or pharmacist.*

Before Using This Medicine

In deciding to use a medicine, the risks of taking the medicine must be weighed against the good it will do. This is a decision you and your doctor will make. For cycloserine, the following should be considered:

Allergies—Tell your doctor if you have ever had any unusual or allergic reaction to cycloserine. Also, tell your doctor and pharmacist if you are allergic to any other substances, such as foods, preservatives, or dyes.

Pregnancy—Cycloserine has not been shown to cause birth defects or other problems in humans. In addition, it is not known whether this medicine causes problems when taken with other TB medicines during pregnancy.

Breast-feeding—Cycloserine passes into the breast milk. However, cycloserine has not been reported to cause problems in nursing babies.

Children—Although there is no specific information comparing use of cycloserine in children with use in other age groups, this medicine is not expected to cause different side effects or problems in children than it does in adults.

Older adults—Many medicines have not been studied specifically in older people. Therefore, it may not be known whether they work exactly the same way they do in younger adults. Although there is no specific information comparing use of cycloserine in the elderly with use in other age groups, this medicine is not expected to cause different side effects or problems in older people than it does in younger adults.

Other medicines—Although certain medicines should not be used together at all, in other cases two different medicines may be used together even if an interaction might occur. In these cases, your doctor may want to change the dose, or other precautions may be necessary. When you are taking cycloserine, it is especially important that your doctor and pharmacist know if you are taking any of the following:

- Ethionamide (e.g., Trecator-SC)—Ethionamide may increase the risk of nervous system side effects, especially seizures

Other medical problems—The presence of other medical problems may affect the use of cycloserine. Make sure you tell your doctor if you have any other medical problems, especially:

- Alcohol abuse (or history of) or
- Convulsive disorders such as seizures or epilepsy—Cycloserine may increase the risk of seizures in patients who drink alcohol or have a history of seizures
- Kidney disease—Cycloserine is removed from the body through the kidneys, and patients with kidney disease may need an adjustment in dose
- Mental disorders such as mental depression, psychosis, or severe anxiety—Cycloserine may cause anxiety, mental depression, or psychosis

Before you begin using any new medicine (prescription or nonprescription) or if you develop any new medical problem while you are using this medicine, check with your doctor, nurse, or pharmacist.

Proper Use of This Medicine

Cycloserine may be taken after meals if it upsets your stomach.

To help clear up your infection completely, *it is very important that you keep taking this medicine for the full time of treatment,* even if you begin to feel better after a few weeks. If you are taking this medicine for TB, you may have to take it every day for as long as 1 to 2 years or more. If you stop taking this medicine too soon, your symptoms may return.

This medicine works best when there is a constant amount in the blood or urine. *To help keep the amount constant, do not miss any doses. Also, it is best to take the doses at evenly spaced times day and night.* For example, if you are to take 2 doses a day, the doses should be spaced about 12 hours apart. If this interferes with your sleep or other daily activities, or if you need help in planning the best times to take your medicine, check with your doctor, nurse, or pharmacist.

Missed dose—If you do miss a dose of this medicine, take it as soon as possible. This will help to keep a constant amount of medicine in the blood or urine. However, if it is almost time for your next dose, skip the missed dose and go back to your regular dosing schedule. Do not double doses.

Storage—To store this medicine:

- Keep out of the reach of children.
- Store away from heat and direct light.
- Do not store in the bathroom, near the kitchen sink, or in other damp places. Heat or moisture may cause the medicine to break down.
- Do not keep outdated medicine or medicine no longer needed. Be sure that any discarded medicine is out of the reach of children.

Precautions While Using This Medicine

It is very important that your doctor check your progress at regular visits.

If your symptoms do not improve within 2 to 3 weeks, or if they become worse, check with your doctor.

If cycloserine causes you to feel very depressed or to have thoughts of suicide, check with your doctor immediately. Your doctor will probably want to change your medicine.

This medicine may cause some people to become dizzy, drowsy, or less alert than they are normally. *Make sure you know how you react to this medicine before you drive, use machines, or do anything else that could be dangerous if you are dizzy or are not alert.* If these reactions are especially bothersome, check with your doctor.

Some of cycloserine's side effects (for example, convulsions [seizures]) may be more likely to occur if you drink alcoholic beverages regularly while you are taking this medicine. Therefore, *you should not drink alcoholic beverages while you are taking this medicine.*

Side Effects of This Medicine

Along with its needed effects, a medicine may cause some unwanted effects. Although not all of these side effects may occur, if they do occur they may need medical attention.

Check with your doctor immediately if any of the following side effects occur:

More common

Anxiety; confusion; dizziness; drowsiness; increased irritability; increased restlessness; mental depression; muscle twitching or trembling; nervousness; nightmares; other mood or mental changes; speech problems; thoughts of suicide

Less common

Convulsions (seizures); numbness, tingling, burning pain, or weakness in the hands or feet; skin rash

Other side effects may occur that usually do not need medical attention. These side effects may go away during treatment as your body adjusts to the medicine. However, check with your doctor if the following side effect continues or is bothersome:

More common

Headache

Other side effects not listed above may also occur in some patients. If you notice any other effects, check with your doctor.

Annual revision: 05/21/92

CYCLOSPORINE Systemic

A commonly used brand name in the U.S. and Canada is Sandimmune. Some other commonly used names are ciclosporin and cyclosporin A.

Description

Cyclosporine (SYE-kloe-spor-een) belongs to the group of medicines known as immunosuppressive agents. It is used to reduce the body's natural immunity in patients who receive organ (for example, kidney, liver, and heart) transplants.

When a patient receives an organ transplant, the body's white blood cells will try to get rid of (reject) the transplanted organ. Cyclosporine works by preventing the white blood cells from doing this.

Cyclosporine may also be used for other conditions, as determined by your doctor.

Cyclosporine is a very strong medicine. It may cause side effects that could be very serious, such as high blood pressure and kidney and liver problems. It may also reduce the body's ability to fight infections. You and your doctor should talk about the good this medicine will do as well as the risks of using it.

Cyclosporine is available only with your doctor's prescription, in the following dosage forms:

Oral

- Capsules (U.S. and Canada)
- Oral solution (U.S. and Canada)

Parenteral

- Injection (U.S. and Canada)

It is very important that you read and understand the following information. If any of it causes you special concern, check with your doctor. Also, *if you have any questions* or if you want more information about this medicine or your medical problem, *ask your doctor, nurse, or pharmacist.*

Before Using This Medicine

In deciding to use a medicine, the risks of taking the medicine must be weighed against the good it will do. This is a decision you and your doctor will make. For cyclosporine, the following should be considered:

Allergies—Tell your doctor if you have ever had any unusual or allergic reaction to cyclosporine.

Pregnancy—Studies have not been done in humans. However, studies in rats and rabbits have shown that cyclosporine at toxic doses (2 to 5 times the human dose) causes birth defects or death of the fetus.

Breast-feeding—Cyclosporine passes into breast milk. There is a chance that it could cause the same side effects in the baby that it does in people taking it. It may be necessary for you to stop breast-feeding during treatment. Be sure you have discussed the risks and benefits of the medicine with your doctor.

Children—This medicine has been tested in children and, in effective doses, has not been shown to cause different side effects or problems than it does in adults.

Older adults—Many medicines have not been studied specifically in older people. Therefore, it may not be known whether they work exactly the same way they do in younger adults. Although there is no specific information comparing use of cyclosporine in the elderly with use in other age groups, this medicine is not expected to cause different side effects or problems in older people than it does in younger adults.

Other medicines—Although certain medicines should not be used together at all, in other cases two different medicines may be used together even if an interaction might occur. In these cases, your doctor may want to change the dose, or other precautions may be necessary. When you are taking cyclosporine, it is especially important that your doctor and pharmacist know if you are taking any of the following:

- Amiloride or
- Spironolactone (e.g., Aldactone) or
- Triamterene (e.g., Dyrenium)—Since both cyclosporine and these medicines increase the amount of potassium in the body, potassium levels could become too high
- Androgens (male hormones) or
- Cimetidine (e.g., Tagamet) or
- Danazol (e.g., Danocrine) or
- Diltiazem (e.g., Cardizem) or

- Erythromycins (medicine for infection) or
- Estrogens (female hormones) or
- Ketoconazole (e.g., Nizoral)—May increase effects of cyclosporine by increasing the amount of this medicine in the body
- Azathioprine (e.g., Imuran) or
- Chlorambucil (e.g., Leukeran) or
- Corticosteroids (cortisone-like medicine) or
- Cyclophosphamide (e.g., Cytoxan) or
- Mercaptopurine (e.g., Purinethol) or
- Muromonab-CD3 (monoclonal antibody) (e.g., Orthoclone OKT3)—There may be an increased risk of infection and cancer because both cyclosporine and these medicines decrease the body's ability to fight them
- Lovastatin (e.g., Mevacor)—May increase the risk of kidney problems

Other medical problems—The presence of other medical problems may affect the use of cyclosporine. Make sure you tell your doctor if you have any other medical problems, especially:

- Chickenpox (including recent exposure) or
- Herpes zoster (shingles)—Risk of severe disease affecting other parts of the body
- Infection—Cyclosporine decreases the body's ability to fight infection
- Intestine problems—Effects may be decreased because cyclosporine cannot be absorbed into the body
- Kidney disease—Cyclosporine can have harmful effects on the kidney when it is taken for long periods of time
- Liver disease—Effects of cyclosporine may be increased because of slower removal from the body

Before you begin using any new medicine (prescription or nonprescription) or if you develop any new medical problem while you are using this medicine, check with your doctor, nurse, or pharmacist.

Proper Use of This Medicine

Take this medicine only as directed by your doctor. Do not take more or less of it and do not take it more often than your doctor ordered. The exact amount of medicine you need has been carefully worked out. Taking too much may increase the chance of side effects, while taking too little may not improve your condition.

To help you remember to take your medicine, try to get into the habit of taking it at the same time each day. This will also help cyclosporine work better by keeping a constant amount in the blood.

This medicine is to be taken by mouth even if it comes in a dropper bottle. The amount you should take is to be measured only with the specially marked dropper provided with your prescription. The dropper should be wiped with a clean towel after it is used, and stored in its container. If the dropper needs to be cleaned, make sure it is completely dry before using it again.

To make cyclosporine taste better, mix it in a glass container with milk, chocolate milk, or orange juice (preferably at room temperature). Do not use a wax-lined or plastic disposable container. Stir it well, then drink it immediately. After drinking all the liquid containing the medicine, rinse the glass with a little more liquid and drink that also, to make sure you get all the medicine. Dry the dropper used to measure the cyclosporine, but do not rinse it with water.

If this medicine upsets your stomach, your doctor may recommend that you take it with meals. However, check with your doctor before you decide to do this on your own.

Do not stop taking this medicine without first checking with your doctor. You may have to take medicine for the rest of your life to prevent your body from rejecting the transplant.

Missed dose—If you miss a dose of cyclosporine and remember it within 12 hours, take the missed dose as soon as you remember. However, if it is almost time for the next dose, skip the missed dose, go back to your regular dosing schedule, and check with your doctor. Do not double doses.

Storage—To store this medicine:

- Keep out of the reach of children.
- Store away from heat and direct light.
- Do not store in the bathroom, near the kitchen sink, or in other damp places. Heat or moisture may cause the medicine to break down.
- Do not store the oral solution in the refrigerator.
- Do not keep outdated medicine or medicine no longer needed. Be sure that any discarded medicine is out of the reach of children.

Precautions While Using This Medicine

It is very important that your doctor check your progress at regular visits. Your doctor will want to do laboratory tests to make sure that cyclosporine is working properly and to check for unwanted effects.

While you are being treated with cyclosporine, and after you stop treatment with it, *do not have any immunizations (vaccinations) without your doctor's approval.* Cyclosporine lowers your body's resistance and there is a chance you might get the infection the immunization is meant to prevent. In addition, other persons living in your house should not take oral polio vaccine since there is a chance they could pass the polio virus on to you. Also, avoid persons who have recently taken oral polio vaccine. Do not get close to them, and do not stay in the same room with them for very long. If you cannot take these precautions, you should consider wearing a protective face mask that covers the nose and mouth.

In some patients (usually younger patients), tenderness, swelling, or bleeding of the gums may appear soon after treatment with cyclosporine is started. Brushing and flossing your teeth carefully and regularly and massaging your gums may help prevent this. *See your dentist regularly to have your teeth cleaned. Check with your medical doctor or dentist if you have any questions about how to take care of your teeth and gums, or if you notice any tenderness, swelling, or bleeding of your gums.*

Side Effects of This Medicine

Along with its needed effects, a medicine may cause some unwanted effects. Some side effects will have signs or symptoms that you can see or feel. Your doctor will watch for others by doing certain tests.

Also, because of the way that cyclosporine acts on the body, there is a chance that it may cause effects that may not occur until years after the medicine is used. These delayed effects may include certain types of cancer, such as lymphomas or skin cancers. You and your doctor should discuss the good this medicine will do as well as the risks of using it.

Check with your doctor or nurse immediately if any of the following side effects occur:

Less common

Fever or chills; frequent urge to urinate

Rare

Blood in urine; flushing of face and neck (for injection only); wheezing or shortness of breath (for injection only)

Check with your doctor as soon as possible if any of the following side effects occur:

More common

Bleeding, tender, or enlarged gums

Less common

Convulsions (seizures)

Rare

Confusion; irregular heartbeat; numbness or tingling in hands, feet, or lips; shortness of breath or difficult breathing; stomach pain (severe) with nausea and vomiting; unexplained nervousness; unusual tiredness or weakness; weakness or heaviness of legs

This medicine may also cause the following side effects that your doctor will watch for:

More common

High blood pressure; kidney problems

Less common

Liver problems

Other side effects may occur that usually do not need medical attention. These side effects may go away during treatment as your body adjusts to the medicine. However, check with your doctor if any of the following side effects continue or are bothersome:

More common

Increase in hair growth; trembling and shaking of hands

Less common

Acne or oily skin; headache; leg cramps; nausea or vomiting

Other side effects not listed above may also occur in some patients. If you notice any other effects, check with your doctor.

Annual revision: 06/09/93

CYTARABINE Systemic

Some commonly used brand names are:

In the U.S.

Cytosar-U

Generic name product may also be available.

In Canada

Cytosar

Other commonly used names are ara-C and cytosine arabinoside.

Description

Cytarabine (sye-TARE-a-been) belongs to the group of medicines called antimetabolites. It is used to treat some kinds of cancer.

Cytarabine interferes with the growth of cancer cells, which are eventually destroyed. Since the growth of normal body cells may also be affected by cytarabine, other effects will also occur. Some of these may be serious and must be reported to your doctor. Other effects, like hair loss, may not be serious but may cause concern. Some effects may not occur for months or years after the medicine is used.

Before you begin treatment with cytarabine, you and your doctor should talk about the good this medicine will do as well as the risks of using it.

Cytarabine is to be administered only by or under the immediate supervision of your doctor. It is available in the following dosage form:

Parenteral

- Injection (U.S. and Canada)

It is very important that you read and understand the following information. If any of it causes you special concern, check with your doctor. Also, *if you have any questions* or if you want more information about this medicine or your medical problem, *ask your doctor, nurse, or pharmacist.*

Before Using This Medicine

In deciding to use a medicine, the risks of taking the medicine must be weighed against the good it will do. This is a decision you and your doctor will make. For cytarabine, the following should be considered:

Allergies—Tell your doctor if you have ever had any unusual or allergic reaction to cytarabine.

Pregnancy—This medicine may cause birth defects (such as defects of the arms, legs, or ears, which occurred in two babies) if either the male or female is taking it at the time of conception or if it is taken during pregnancy. In addition, many cancer medicines may cause sterility. Although sterility has been reported with this medicine, it is usually only temporary.

Be sure that you have discussed this with your doctor before taking this medicine. It is best to use some kind of birth control while you are receiving cytarabine. However, do not use oral contraceptives ("the Pill") since they may interfere with this medicine. Tell your doctor right away if you think you have become pregnant while receiving cytarabine.

Breast-feeding—Because cytarabine may cause serious side effects, breast-feeding is generally not recommended while you are receiving it.

Children—Although there is no specific information about the use of cytarabine in children, it is not expected to cause different side effects or problems in children than it does in adults.

Older adults—Many medicines have not been tested in older people. Therefore, it may not be known whether they work exactly the same way they do in younger adults. Although there is no specific information about the use of cytarabine in the elderly, it is not expected to cause different side effects or problems in older people than it does in younger adults.

Other medicines—Although certain medicines should not be used together at all, in other cases two different medicines may be used together even if an interaction might occur. In these cases, your doctor may want to change the dose, or other precautions may be necessary. When receiving cytarabine it is especially important that your doctor and pharmacist know if you are taking any of the following:

- Amphotericin B by injection (e.g., Fungizone) or
- Antithyroid agents (medicine for overactive thyroid) or
- Azathioprine (e.g., Imuran) or
- Chloramphenicol (e.g., Chloromycetin) or
- Colchicine or
- Flucytosine (e.g., Ancobon) or
- Interferon (e.g., Intron A, Roferon-A) or
- Plicamycin (e.g., Mithracin) or
- Zidovudine (e.g., Retrovir) or
- If you have ever been treated with x-rays or cancer medicines—Cytarabine may increase the effects of these medicines or radiation therapy on the blood
- Probenecid (e.g., Benemid) or
- Sulfinpyrazone (e.g., Anturane)—Cytarabine may raise the concentration of uric acid in the blood, which these medicines are used to lower

Other medical problems—The presence of other medical problems may affect the use of cytarabine. Make sure you tell your doctor if you have any other medical problems, especially:

- Chickenpox (including recent exposure) or
- Herpes zoster (shingles)—Risk of severe disease affecting other parts of the body
- Gout (history of) or
- Kidney stones (history of)—Cytarabine may increase levels of a chemical called uric acid in the body, which can cause gout or kidney stones
- Infection—Cytarabine can reduce immunity to infection
- Kidney disease or
- Liver disease—Effects may be increased because of slower removal of cytarabine from the body

Before you begin using any new medicine (prescription or nonprescription) or if you develop any new medical problem while you are using this medicine, check with your doctor, nurse, or pharmacist.

Proper Use of This Medicine

This medicine is sometimes given together with certain other medicines. If you are using a combination of medicines, it is important that you receive each one at the proper time. If you are taking some of these medicines by mouth, ask your doctor, nurse, or pharmacist to help you plan a way to take them at the right times.

While you are receiving this medicine, your doctor may want you to drink extra fluids so that you will pass more urine. This will help prevent kidney problems and keep your kidneys working well.

This medicine often causes nausea and vomiting. However, it is very important that you continue to receive the medicine even if you begin to feel ill. Ask your doctor, nurse, or pharmacist for ways to lessen these effects.

Precautions While Using This Medicine

It is very important that your doctor check your progress at regular visits to make sure that this medicine is working properly and to check for unwanted effects.

While you are being treated with cytarabine, and after you stop treatment with it, *do not have any immunizations (vaccinations) without your doctor's approval.* Cytarabine may lower your body's resistance and there is a chance you might get the infection the immunization is meant to prevent. In addition, other persons living in your household should not take or should not have recently taken oral polio vaccine since there is a chance they could pass the polio virus on to you. Also, avoid other persons who have taken oral polio vaccine. Do not get close to them and do not stay in the same room with them for very long. If you cannot take these precautions, you should consider wearing a protective face mask that covers the nose and mouth.

Cytarabine can lower the number of white blood cells in your blood temporarily, increasing the chance of getting an infection. It can also lower the number of platelets, which are necessary for proper blood clotting. If this occurs, there are certain precautions you can take, especially when your blood count is low, to reduce the risk of infection or bleeding:

- If you can, avoid people with infections. *Check with your doctor immediately* if you think you are getting an infection or if you get a fever or chills, cough or hoarseness, lower back or side pain, or painful or difficult urination.
- *Check with your doctor immediately* if you notice any unusual bleeding or bruising; black, tarry stools; blood in urine or stools; or pinpoint red spots on your skin.
- Be careful when using a regular toothbrush, dental floss, or toothpick. Your medical doctor, dentist, or nurse may recommend other ways to clean your teeth and gums. Check with your medical doctor before having any dental work done.
- Do not touch your eyes or the inside of your nose unless you have just washed your hands and have not touched anything else in the meantime.
- Be careful not to cut yourself when you are using sharp objects such as a safety razor or fingernail or toenail cutters.
- Avoid contact sports or other situations where bruising or injury could occur.

Side Effects of This Medicine

Along with their needed effects, medicines like cytarabine can sometimes cause unwanted effects such as blood problems and other side effects. These and others are described below. Also, because of the way these medicines act on the body, there is a chance that they might cause other unwanted effects that may not occur until months or years after the medicine is used. These delayed effects may include certain types of cancer, such as leukemia. Discuss these possible effects with your doctor.

Although not all of these side effects may occur, if they do occur they may need medical attention.

Check with your doctor or nurse immediately if any of the following side effects occur:

Less common

Black, tarry stools; blood in urine; cough or hoarseness; fever or chills; lower back or side pain; painful or difficult urination; pinpoint red spots on skin; unusual bleeding or bruising

Check with your doctor or nurse as soon as possible if any of the following side effects occur:

More common

Sores in mouth and on lips

Less common

Joint pain; numbness or tingling in fingers, toes, or face; swelling of feet or lower legs; unusual tiredness

Rare

Bone or muscle pain; chest pain; decrease in urination; difficulty in swallowing; fainting spells; general feeling of discomfort or illness or weakness; heartburn; irregular heartbeat; pain at place of injection; reddened eyes; shortness of breath; skin rash; weakness; yellow eyes or skin

Other side effects may occur that usually do not need medical attention. These side effects may go away during treatment as your body adjusts to the medicine. Also, your doctor or nurse may be able to tell you about ways to prevent or reduce some of these side effects. Check with your doctor or nurse if any of the following side effects continue or are bothersome or if you have any questions about them:

More common

Loss of appetite; nausea and vomiting

Less common or rare

Diarrhea; dizziness; headache; itching of skin; skin freckling

This medicine may cause a temporary loss of hair in some people. After treatment with cytarabine has ended, normal hair growth should return.

After you stop receiving cytarabine, it may still produce some side effects that need attention. During this period time check with your doctor if you notice any of the following:

Black, tarry stools; blood in urine or stools; cough or hoarseness; fever or chills; lower back or side pain; painful or difficult urination; pinpoint red spots on skin; unusual bleeding or bruising

Other side effects not listed above may also occur in some patients. If you notice any other effects, check with your doctor.

Annual revision: July 1990

D

DACARBAZINE Systemic

Some commonly used brand names are:

In the U.S.

DTIC-Dome

Generic name product may also be available.

In Canada

DTIC

Description

Dacarbazine (da-KAR-ba-zeen) belongs to the group of medicines called alkylating agents. It is used to treat some kinds of cancer.

Dacarbazine interferes with the growth of cancer cells, which are eventually destroyed. Since the growth of normal body cells may also be affected by dacarbazine, other effects will also occur. Some of these may be serious and must be reported to your doctor. Other effects, like hair loss, may not be serious but may cause concern. Some effects may not occur for months or years after the medicine is used.

Before you begin treatment with dacarbazine, you and your doctor should talk about the good this medicine will do as well as the risks of using it.

Dacarbazine is to be administered only by or under the immediate supervision of your doctor. It is available in the following dosage form:

Parenteral

- Injection (U.S. and Canada)

It is very important that you read and understand the following information. If any of it causes you special concern, check with your doctor. Also, *if you have any questions* or if you want more information about this medicine or your medical problem, *ask your doctor, nurse, or pharmacist.*

Before Using This Medicine

In deciding to use a medicine, the risks of taking the medicine must be weighed against the good it will do. This is a decision you and your doctor will make. For dacarbazine, the following should be considered:

Allergies—Tell your doctor if you have ever had any unusual or allergic reaction to dacarbazine.

Pregnancy—There is a chance that this medicine may cause birth defects if either the male or female is taking it at the time of conception or if it is taken during pregnancy. In addition, many cancer medicines may cause sterility, which could be permanent. Although sterility has not been reported with this medicine, the possibility should be kept in mind. Dacarbazine has caused birth defects and a decrease in successful pregnancies in animal studies involving rats and rabbits given doses several times the usual human adult dose.

Be sure that you have discussed this with your doctor before taking this medicine. It is best to use some kind of birth control while you are receiving dacarbazine. However, do not use oral contraceptives ("the Pill") since they may interfere with this medicine. Tell your doctor right away if you think you have become pregnant while receiving dacarbazine.

Breast-feeding—It is not known whether dacarbazine passes into breast milk. However, because this medicine may cause serious side effects, breast-feeding is generally not recommended while you are receiving it.

Children—Studies on this medicine have been done only in adult patients. Therefore, be sure to discuss with your child's doctor the use of this medicine in children.

Older adults—Many medicines have not been tested in older people. Therefore, it may not be known whether they work exactly the same way they do in younger adults or if they cause different side effects or problems in older people. There is no specific information about the use of dacarbazine in the elderly.

Other medicines—Although certain medicines should not be used together at all, in other cases two different medicines may be used together even if an interaction might occur. In these cases, your doctor may want to change the dose, or other precautions may be necessary. When receiving dacarbazine it is especially important that your doctor and pharmacist know if you are taking any of the following:

- Amphotericin B by injection (e.g., Fungizone) or
- Antithyroid agents (medicine for overactive thyroid) or
- Azathioprine (e.g., Imuran) or
- Chloramphenicol (e.g., Chloromycetin) or
- Colchicine or
- Flucytosine (e.g., Ancobon) or
- Interferon (e.g., Intron A, Roferon-A) or
- Plicamycin (e.g., Mithracin) or
- Zidovudine (e.g., Retrovir) or
- If you have ever been treated with x-rays or cancer medicines—Dacarbazine may increase the effects of these medicines or radiation therapy on the blood

Other medical problems—The presence of other medical problems may affect the use of dacarbazine. Make sure you tell your doctor if you have any other medical problems, especially:

- Chickenpox (including recent exposure) or
- Herpes zoster (shingles)—Risk of severe disease affecting other parts of the body
- Infection—Dacarbazine can reduce immunity to infection

- Kidney disease or
- Liver disease—Effects may be increased because of slower removal of dacarbazine from the body

Before you begin using any new medicine (prescription or nonprescription) or if you develop any new medical problem while you are using this medicine, check with your doctor, nurse, or pharmacist.

Proper Use of This Medicine

Dacarbazine is sometimes given together with certain other medicines. If you are using a combination of medicines, it is important that you receive each one at the proper time. If you are taking some of these medicines by mouth, ask your doctor, nurse, or pharmacist to help you plan a way to remember to take them at the right times.

This medicine often causes nausea, vomiting, and loss of appetite. The injection may also cause a feeling of burning or pain. However, it is very important that you continue to receive the medicine, even if you have discomfort or begin to feel ill. After 1 or 2 days, your stomach upset should lessen. Ask your doctor, nurse, or pharmacist for ways to lessen these effects.

Precautions While Using This Medicine

It is very important that your doctor check your progress at regular visits to make sure that this medicine is working properly and to check for unwanted effects.

While you are being treated with dacarbazine, and after you stop treatment with it, *do not have any immunizations (vaccinations) without your doctor's approval.* Dacarbazine may lower your body's resistance and there is a chance you might get the infection the immunization is meant to prevent. In addition, other persons living in your household should not take or should not have recently taken oral polio vaccine since there is a chance they could pass the polio virus on to you. Also, avoid other persons who have taken oral polio vaccine. Do not get close to them, and do not stay in the same room with them for very long. If you cannot take these precautions, you should consider wearing a protective face mask that covers the nose and mouth.

Dacarbazine can lower the number of white blood cells in your blood temporarily, increasing the chance of getting an infection. It can also lower the number of platelets, which are necessary for proper blood clotting. If this occurs, there are certain precautions you can take, especially when your blood count is low, to reduce the risk of infection or bleeding:

- If you can, avoid people with infections. *Check with your doctor immediately* if you think you are getting an infection or if you get a fever or chills, cough or hoarseness, lower back or side pain, or painful or difficult urination.
- *Check with your doctor immediately* if you notice any unusual bleeding or bruising; black, tarry stools; blood in urine or stools; or pinpoint red spots on your skin.
- Be careful when using a regular toothbrush, dental floss, or toothpick. Your medical doctor, dentist, or nurse may recommend other ways to clean your teeth and gums. Check with your medical doctor before having any dental work done.
- Do not touch your eyes or the inside of your nose unless you have just washed your hands and have not touched anything else in the meantime.
- Be careful not to cut yourself when you are using sharp objects such as a safety razor or fingernail or toenail cutters.
- Avoid contact sports or other situations where bruising or injury could occur.

If dacarbazine accidentally seeps out of the vein into which it is injected, it may damage some tissues and cause scarring. *Tell the doctor or nurse right away if you notice redness, pain, or swelling at the place of injection.*

Side Effects of This Medicine

Along with their needed effects, medicines like dacarbazine can sometimes cause unwanted effects such as blood problems, loss of hair, and other side effects. These and others are described below. Also, because of the way these medicines act on the body, there is a chance that they might cause other unwanted effects that may not occur until months or years after the medicine is used. These delayed effects may include certain types of cancer, such as leukemia. Discuss these possible effects with your doctor.

Although not all of these side effects may occur, if they do occur they may need medical attention.

Check with your doctor or nurse immediately if any of the following side effects occur:

More common

Redness, pain, or swelling at place of injection

Less common

Black, tarry stools; blood in urine or stools; cough or hoarseness; fever or chills; lower back or side pain; painful or difficult urination; pinpoint red spots on skin; unusual bleeding or bruising

Rare

Shortness of breath; stomach pain; swelling of face; yellow eyes or skin

Check with your doctor or nurse as soon as possible if the following side effect occurs:

Rare

Sores in mouth and on lips

Other side effects may occur that usually do not need medical attention. These side effects may go away during treatment as your body adjusts to the medicine. Also, your doctor or nurse may be able to tell you about ways to prevent or reduce some of these side effects. Check with your doctor or nurse if any of the following side effects continue or are bothersome or if you have any questions about them:

More common

Loss of appetite; nausea or vomiting (should lessen after 1 or 2 days)

Less common

Feelings of uneasiness; flushing of face; muscle pain; numbness of face

This medicine may cause a temporary loss of hair in some people. After treatment with dacarbazine has ended, normal hair growth should return.

After you stop receiving dacarbazine, it may still produce some side effects that need attention. During this period of time check with your doctor if you notice any of the following:

Black, tarry stools; blood in urine or stools; cough or hoarseness; fever or chills; lower back or side pain; painful or difficult urination; pinpoint red spots on skin; unusual bleeding or bruising

Other side effects not listed above may also occur in some patients. If you notice any other effects, check with your doctor.

Annual revision: July 1990

DACTINOMYCIN Systemic

A commonly used brand name in the U.S. and Canada is Cosmegen. Another commonly used name is actinomycin-D.

Description

Dactinomycin (dak-ti-noe-MYE-sin) belongs to the group of medicines known as antineoplastics. It is used to treat some kinds of cancer.

Dactinomycin interferes with the growth of cancer cells, which are eventually destroyed. Since the growth of normal body cells may also be affected by dactinomycin, other effects will also occur. Some of these may be serious and must be reported to your doctor. Other effects, like hair loss, may not be serious but may cause concern. Some effects may not occur for months or years after the medicine is used.

Before you begin treatment with dactinomycin, you and your doctor should talk about the good this medicine will do as well as the risks of using it.

Dactinomycin is to be administered only by or under the immediate supervision of your doctor. It is available in the following dosage form:

Parenteral

- Injection (U.S. and Canada)

It is very important that you read and understand the following information. If any of it causes you special concern, check with your doctor. Also, *if you have any questions* or if you want more information about this medicine or your medical problem, *ask your doctor, nurse, or pharmacist.*

Before Using This Medicine

In deciding to use a medicine, the risks of taking the medicine must be weighed against the good it will do. This is a decision you and your doctor will make. For dactinomycin, the following should be considered:

Allergies—Tell your doctor if you have ever had any unusual or allergic reaction to dactinomycin.

Pregnancy—There is a chance that this medicine may cause birth defects if either the male or female is receiving it at the time of conception or if it is taken during pregnancy. Studies have shown that dactinomycin causes birth defects in animals. In addition, many cancer medicines may cause sterility which could be permanent. Although sterility has not been reported with this medicine, the possibility should be kept in mind.

Be sure that you have discussed this with your doctor before receiving this medicine. It is best to use some kind of birth control while you are receiving dactinomycin. However, do not use oral contraceptives ("the Pill") since they may interfere with this medicine. Tell your doctor right away if you think you have become pregnant while receiving dactinomycin.

Breast-feeding—It is not known whether dactinomycin passes into breast milk. However, because this medicine may cause serious side effects, breast-feeding is generally not recommended while you are receiving it.

Children—Because of increased toxicity, use of dactinomycin in infants less than 6 to 12 months of age is not recommended.

Older adults—Many medicines have not been tested in older people. Therefore, it may not be known whether

they work exactly the same way they do in younger adults or if they cause different side effects or problems in older people. There is no specific information about the use of dactinomycin in the elderly.

Other medicines—Although certain medicines should not be used together at all, in other cases two different medicines may be used together even if an interaction might occur. In these cases, your doctor may want to change the dose, or other precautions may be necessary. When receiving dactinomycin it is especially important that your doctor and pharmacist know if you are taking any of the following:

- Amphotericin B by injection (e.g., Fungizone) or
- Antithyroid agents (medicine for overactive thyroid) or
- Azathioprine (e.g., Imuran) or
- Chloramphenicol (e.g., Chloromycetin) or
- Flucytosine (e.g., Ancobon) or
- Interferon (e.g., Intron A, Roferon-A) or
- Plicamycin (e.g., Mithramycin) or
- Zidovudine (e.g., Retrovir) or
- If you have ever been treated with x-rays or cancer medicine—Dactinomycin may increase the effects of these medicines or radiation therapy on the blood
- Probenecid (e.g., Benemid) or
- Sulfinpyrazone (e.g., Anturane)—Dactinomycin may increase concentrations of uric acid in the blood, which these medicines are used to lower

Other medical problems—The presence of other medical problems may affect the use of dactinomycin. Make sure you tell your doctor if you have any other medical problems, especially:

- Chickenpox (including recent exposure) or
- Herpes zoster (shingles)—Risk of severe disease affecting other parts of the body
- Gout (or history of) or
- Kidney stones—Dactinomycin may increase levels of a chemical called uric acid in the body, which can cause gout or kidney stones
- Infection—Dactinomycin can reduce immunity to infection
- Liver disease—Effects of dactinomycin may be increased

Before you begin using any new medicine (prescription or nonprescription) or if you develop any new medical problem while you are using this medicine, check with your doctor, nurse, or pharmacist.

Proper Use of This Medicine

Dactinomycin is sometimes given together with certain other medicines. If you are receiving a combination of medicines, it is important that you receive each one at the proper time. If you are taking some of these medicines by mouth, ask your doctor, nurse, or pharmacist to help you plan a way to remember to take them at the right times.

This medicine often causes nausea and vomiting. However, it is very important that you continue to receive the medicine, even if you begin to feel ill. Ask your doctor, nurse, or pharmacist for ways to lessen these effects.

Precautions While Using This Medicine

It is very important that your doctor check your progress at regular visits to make sure that this medicine is working properly and to check for unwanted effects.

While you are being treated with dactinomycin, and after you stop treatment with it, *do not have any immunizations (vaccinations) without your doctor's approval.* Dactinomycin may lower your body's resistance, and there is a chance you might get the infection the immunization is meant to prevent. In addition, other persons living in your household should not take or should not have recently taken oral polio vaccine since there is a chance they could pass the polio virus on to you. Also, avoid other persons who have taken oral polio vaccine. Do not get close to them, and do not stay in the same room with them for very long. If you cannot take these precautions, you should consider wearing a protective face mask that covers the nose and mouth.

Dactinomycin can lower the number of white blood cells in your blood temporarily, increasing the chance of getting an infection. It can also lower the number of platelets, which are necessary for proper blood clotting. If this occurs, there are certain precautions you can take, especially when your blood count is low, to reduce the risk of infection or bleeding:

- If you can, avoid people with infections. *Check with your doctor immediately* if you think you are getting an infection or if you get a fever or chills, cough or hoarseness, lower back or side pain, or painful or difficult urination.
- *Check with your doctor immediately* if you notice any unusual bleeding or bruising; black, tarry stools; blood in urine or stools; or pinpoint red spots on your skin.
- Be careful when using a regular toothbrush, dental floss, or toothpick. Your medical doctor, dentist, or nurse may recommend other ways to clean your teeth and gums. Check with your medical doctor before having any dental work done.
- Do not touch your eyes or the inside of your nose unless you have just washed your hands and have not touched anything else in the meantime.
- Be careful not to cut yourself when you are using sharp objects such as a safety razor or fingernail or toenail cutters.
- Avoid contact sports or other situations where bruising or injury could occur.

If dactinomycin accidentally seeps out of the vein into which it is injected, it may severely damage some tissues and cause scarring. *Tell the doctor or nurse right away if you notice redness, pain, or swelling at the place of injection.*

Side Effects of This Medicine

Along with their needed effects, medicines like dactinomycin can sometimes cause unwanted effects such as blood problems, loss of hair, and other side effects. These and others are described below. Also, because of the way these medicines act on the body, there is a chance that they might cause other unwanted effects that may not occur until months or years after the medicine is used. These delayed effects may include certain types of cancer, such as leukemia. Discuss these possible effects with your doctor.

Although not all of these side effects may occur, if they do occur they may need medical attention.

Check with your doctor or nurse immediately if any of the following side effects occur:

Less common

Black, tarry stools; blood in urine or stools; cough or hoarseness; fever or chills; lower back or side pain; painful or difficult urination; pinpoint red spots on skin; unusual bleeding or bruising

Rare

Pain at place of injection; wheezing

Check with your doctor or nurse as soon as possible if any of the following side effects occur:

More common

Diarrhea (continuing); difficulty in swallowing; heartburn; sores in mouth and on lips; stomach pain (continuing)

Rare

Joint pain; swelling of feet or lower legs; yellow eyes or skin

Other side effects may occur that usually do not need medical attention. These side effects may go away during treatment as your body adjusts to the medicine. Also, your doctor or nurse may be able to tell you about ways to prevent or reduce some of these side effects. Check with your doctor or nurse if any of the following side effects continue or are bothersome or if you have any questions about them:

More common

Darkening of skin; nausea and vomiting; redness of skin; skin rash or acne; unusual tiredness

This medicine often causes a temporary loss of hair, sometimes including the eyebrows. After treatment with dactinomycin has ended, normal hair growth should return.

After you stop receiving dactinomycin, it may still produce some side effects that need attention. During this period of time check with your doctor if you notice any of the following:

Black, tarry stools; blood in urine or stools; cough or hoarseness; diarrhea; fever or chills; lower back or side pain; painful or difficult urination; pinpoint red spots on skin; sores in mouth and on lips; stomach pain; unusual bleeding or bruising; yellow eyes or skin

Other side effects not listed above may also occur in some patients. If you notice any other effects, check with your doctor.

Annual revision: July 1990

DANAZOL Systemic

Some commonly used brand names are:

In the U.S.

Danocrine

Generic name product may also be available.

In Canada

Cyclomen

Description

Danazol (DA-na-zole) may be used for a number of different medical problems. These include treatment of:

- pain and/or infertility due to endometriosis;
- a tendency for females to develop cysts in the breasts (fibrocystic breast disease); or
- hereditary angioedema, which causes swelling of the face, arms, legs, throat, windpipe, bowels, or sexual organs.

Danazol may also be used for other conditions as determined by your doctor.

This medicine is available only with your doctor's prescription, in the following dosage form:

Oral

- Capsules (U.S. and Canada)

It is very important that you read and understand the following information. If any of it causes you special concern, check with your doctor. Also, *if you have any questions* or if you want more information about this medicine or your medical problem, *ask your doctor, nurse, or pharmacist.*

Before Using This Medicine

In deciding to use a medicine, the risks of taking the medicine must be weighed against the good it will do. This is a decision you and your doctor will make. For danazol, the following should be considered:

Allergies—Tell your doctor if you have ever had any unusual or allergic reaction to danazol, androgens (male hormones), or anabolic steroids. Also tell your doctor and pharmacist if you are allergic to any other substances, such as foods, preservatives, or dyes.

Pregnancy—Danazol is not recommended for use during pregnancy, since it may cause a female baby to develop certain male characteristics.

Breast-feeding—Breast-feeding is not recommended while you are taking this medicine because it may cause unwanted effects in the baby.

Children—Danazol may cause male-like changes in female children and cause premature sexual development in male children. It may also slow or stop growth in any child.

Older adults—Many medicines have not been studied specifically in older people. Therefore, it may not be known whether they work exactly the same way they do in younger adults. Although there is no specific information comparing use of danazol in the elderly with use in other age groups, danazol has effects similar to androgens (male hormones). Androgens used in older males may increase the risk of developing prostate enlargement or cancer.

Other medicines—Although certain medicines should not be used together at all, in other cases two different medicines may be used together even if an interaction might occur. In these cases, your doctor may want to change the dose, or other precautions may be necessary. When you are taking danazol, it is especially important that your doctor and pharmacist know if you are taking any of the following:

- Anticoagulants (blood thinners)—Danazol may increase the effects of these medicines and possibly increase the risk of severe bleeding

Other medical problems—The presence of other medical problems may affect the use of danazol. Make sure you tell your doctor if you have any other medical problems, especially:

- Diabetes mellitus (sugar diabetes)—Danazol may increase blood glucose levels
- Epilepsy or
- Heart disease or
- Kidney disease or
- Migraine headaches—These conditions can be made worse by the fluid retention (keeping too much body water) that can be caused by danazol
- Liver disease

Before you begin using any new medicine (prescription or nonprescription) or if you develop any new medical problem while you are using this medicine, check with your doctor, nurse, or pharmacist.

Proper Use of This Medicine

In order for danazol to help you, *it must be taken regularly for the full time of treatment* as ordered by your doctor.

Dosing—The dose of danazol will be different for different patients. *Follow your doctor's orders or the directions on the label.* The following information includes only the average doses of danazol. *If your dose is different, do not change it* unless your doctor tells you to do so.

- The number of capsules that you take depends on the strength of the medicine. Also, the number of doses you take each day, the time allowed between doses, and the length of time you take the medicine depend on the medical problems for which you are taking danazol.
- For *oral* dosage forms (capsules):
  —Adults:
  - For treatment of endometriosis: 100 to 400 milligrams two times a day.
  - For treatment of fibrocystic breast disease: 50 to 200 milligrams two times a day.
  - For prevention of attacks of hereditary angioedema: 200 milligrams two or three times a day. The dose may be lowered, depending upon your condition.

Missed dose—If you miss a dose of this medicine, take it as soon as possible. However, if it is almost time for your next dose, skip the missed dose and go back to your regular dosing schedule. Do not double doses.

Storage—To store this medicine:

- Keep out of the reach of children.
- Store away from heat and direct light.
- Do not store in the bathroom, near the kitchen sink, or in other damp places. Heat or moisture may cause the medicine to break down.
- Do not keep outdated medicine or medicine no longer needed. Be sure that any discarded medicine is out of the reach of children.

Precautions While Using This Medicine

Your doctor should check your progress at regular visits to make sure that this medicine does not cause unwanted effects.

For diabetic patients:

- This medicine may affect blood glucose levels. If you notice a change in the results of your blood or urine glucose test or if you have any questions about this, check with your doctor.

If you are taking danazol for *endometriosis* or *fibrocystic breast disease:*

- During the time you are taking danazol, your menstrual period may not be regular or you may not have a menstrual period at all. This is to be expected when you are taking this medicine. If regular menstruation does not begin within 60 to 90 days after you stop taking this medicine, check with your doctor.
- During the time you are taking danazol, you should use birth control methods that do not contain hormones. If you have any questions about this, check with your doctor, nurse, or pharmacist.
- *If you suspect that you may have become pregnant, stop taking this medicine and check with your doctor.* Continued use of danazol during pregnancy may cause male-like changes in female babies.

Danazol may cause your skin to be more sensitive to sunlight than it is normally. Exposure to sunlight, even for brief periods of time, may cause a skin rash, itching, redness, or other discoloration of the skin, or a severe sunburn. When you begin taking this medicine:

- Stay out of direct sunlight, especially between the hours of 10:00 a.m. and 3:00 p.m., if possible.
- Wear protective clothing, including a hat. Also, wear sunglasses.
- Apply a sun block product that has a skin protection factor (SPF) of a least 15. Some patients may require a product with a higher SPF number, especially if they have a fair complexion. If you have questions about this, check with your doctor or pharmacist.
- Apply a sun block lipstick that has an SPF of at least 15 to protect your lips.
- Do not use a sunlamp or tanning bed or booth.

If you have a severe reaction from the sun, check with your doctor.

Side Effects of This Medicine

Along with its needed effects, a medicine may cause some unwanted effects. Although not all of these side effects may occur, if they do occur they may need medical attention.

Check with your doctor as soon as possible if any of the following side effects occur:

For both females and males

Less common

Acne or increased oiliness of skin or hair; muscle cramps or spasms; swelling of feet or lower legs; unusual tiredness or weakness; weight gain (rapid)

Rare

Bleeding gums; bloating, pain or tenderness of abdomen or stomach; blood in urine; changes in vision; chest pain; chills; cough; dark-colored urine; diarrhea; discharge from nipple; eye pain; fast heartbeat; fever; headache; hives or other skin rashes; joint pain; light-colored stools; loss of appetite (continuing); more frequent nosebleeds; muscle aches; nausea; pain, numbness, tingling, or burning in all fingers except the smallest finger; purple- or red-colored, or other spots on body or inside the mouth or nose; sore throat; tingling, numbness, or weakness in legs, which may move upward to arms, trunk, or face; unusual bruising or bleeding; unusual tiredness, weakness, or general feeling of illness; vomiting; yellow eyes or skin

For females only

More common

Decrease in breast size; irregular menstrual periods; weight gain

Rare

Enlarged clitoris; hoarseness or deepening of voice; unnatural hair growth

For males only

Rare

Decrease in size of testicles

Other side effects may occur that usually do not need medical attention. These side effects may go away during treatment as your body adjusts to the medicine. However, check with your doctor if any of the following side effects continue or are bothersome:

For both females and males

Less common

Flushing or redness of skin; mood or mental changes; nervousness; sweating

Rare

Increased sensitivity of skin to sunlight

For females only

Less common

Burning, dryness, or itching of vagina or vaginal bleeding

Other side effects not listed above may also occur in some patients. If you notice any other effects, check with your doctor.

Additional Information

Once a medicine has been approved for marketing for a certain use, experience may show that it is also useful for other medical problems. Although these uses are not

included in product labeling, danazol is used in certain patients with the following medical conditions:

- Gynecomastia (excess breast development in males)
- Menorrhagia (excessively long menstrual periods)
- Precocious puberty in females (premature sexual development)

Other than the above information, there is no additional information relating to proper use, precautions, or side effects for these uses.

Annual revision: 02/19/93

DANTROLENE Systemic

Some commonly used brand names in the U.S. and Canada are Dantrium and Dantrium Intravenous.

Description

Dantrolene (DAN-troe-leen) is used to help relax certain muscles in your body. It relieves the spasms, cramping, and tightness of muscles caused by certain medical problems such as multiple sclerosis (MS), cerebral palsy, stroke, or injury to the spine. Dantrolene does not cure these problems, but it may allow other treatment, such as physical therapy, to be more helpful in improving your condition. Dantrolene acts directly on the muscles to produce its relaxant effects.

Dantrolene is also used to prevent or treat a medical problem called malignant hyperthermia that may occur in some people during or following surgery or anesthesia. Malignant hyperthermia consists of a group of symptoms including very high fever, fast and irregular heartbeat, and breathing problems. It is believed that the tendency to develop malignant hyperthermia is inherited.

Dantrolene has been shown to cause cancer and noncancerous tumors in some animals (but not in others) when given in large doses for a long time. It is not known whether long-term use of dantrolene causes cancer or tumors in humans. Before taking this medicine, be sure that you have discussed this with your doctor.

This medicine is available only with your doctor's prescription, in the following dosage forms:

Oral

- Capsules (U.S. and Canada)

Parenteral

- Injection (U.S. and Canada)

It is very important that you read and understand the following information. If any of it causes you special concern, check with your doctor. Also, *if you have any questions* or if you want more information about this medicine or your medical problem, *ask your doctor, nurse, or pharmacist.*

Before Using This Medicine

In deciding to use a medicine, the risks of taking the medicine must be weighed against the good it will do. This is a decision you and your doctor will make. For dantrolene, the following should be considered:

Allergies—Tell your doctor if you have ever had any unusual or allergic reaction to dantrolene. Also tell your doctor and pharmacist if you are allergic to any other substances, such as foods, preservatives, or dyes.

Pregnancy—Dantrolene has not been shown to cause birth defects or other problems in humans.

Breast-feeding—Use of dantrolene is not recommended during breast-feeding.

Children—This medicine has been tested in children 5 years of age and older and has not been shown to cause different side effects or problems than it does in adults.

Older adults—Many medicines have not been studied specifically in older people. Therefore, it may not be known whether they work exactly the same way they do in younger adults or if they cause different side effects or problems in older people. There is no specific information comparing use of dantrolene in the elderly with use in other age groups.

Other medicines—Although certain medicines should not be used together at all, in other cases two different medicines may be used together even if an interaction might occur. In these cases, your doctor may want to change the dose, or other precautions may be necessary. When you are taking dantrolene, it is especially important that your doctor and pharmacist know if you are taking any of the following:

- Acetaminophen (e.g., Tylenol) (with long-term, high-dose use) or
- Amiodarone (e.g., Cordarone) or
- Anabolic steroids (dromostanolone [e.g., Drolban], ethylestrenol [e.g., Maxibolin], nandrolone [e.g., Anabolin], oxandrolone [e.g., Anavar], oxymetholone [e.g., Anadrol], stanozolol [e.g., Winstrol]) or
- Androgens (male hormones) or
- Anti-infectives by mouth or by injection (medicine for infection) or
- Antithyroid agents (medicine for overactive thyroid) or
- Carbamazepine (e.g., Tegretol) or
- Carmustine (e.g., BiCNU) or
- Central nervous system (CNS) depressants (medicine that causes drowsiness) or
- Chloroquine (e.g., Aralen) or

- Daunorubicin (e.g., Cerubidine) or
- Disulfiram (e.g., Antabuse) or
- Divalproex (e.g., Depakote) or
- Estrogens (female hormones) or
- Etretinate (e.g., Tegison) or
- Gold salts (medicine for arthritis) or
- Hydroxychloroquine (e.g., Plaquenil) or
- Mercaptopurine (e.g., Purinethol) or
- Methotrexate (e.g., Mexate) or
- Methyldopa (e.g., Aldomet) or
- Naltrexone (e.g., Trexan) (with long-term, high-dose use) or
- Oral contraceptives (birth control pills) containing estrogen or
- Phenothiazines (acetophenazine [e.g., Tindal], chlorpromazine [e.g., Thorazine], fluphenazine [e.g., Prolixin], mesoridazine [e.g., Serentil], perphenazine [e.g., Trilafon], prochlorperazine [e.g., Compazine], promazine [e.g., Sparine], promethazine [e.g., Phenergan], thioridazine [e.g., Mellaril], trifluoperazine [e.g., Stelazine], triflupromazine [e.g., Vesprin], trimeprazine [e.g., Temaril]) or
- Phenytoin (e.g., Dilantin) or
- Plicamycin (e.g., Mithracin) or
- Tricyclic antidepressants (medicine for depression) (amitriptyline [e.g., Elavil], amoxapine [e.g., Asendin], clomipramine [e.g., Anafranil], desipramine [e.g., Pertofrane], doxepin [e.g., Sinequan], imipramine [e.g., Tofranil], nortriptyline [e.g., Aventyl], protriptyline [e.g., Vivactil], trimipramine [e.g., Surmontil]) or
- Valproic acid (e.g., Depakene)—The chance of side effects may be increased

Other medical problems—The presence of other medical problems may affect the use of dantrolene. Make sure you tell your doctor if you have any other medical problems, especially:

- Emphysema, asthma, bronchitis, or other chronic lung disease or
- Heart disease or
- Liver disease, such as hepatitis or cirrhosis (or history of)—The chance of serious side effects may be increased

Before you begin using any new medicine (prescription or nonprescription) or if you develop any new medical problem while you are using this medicine, check with your doctor, nurse, or pharmacist.

Proper Use of This Medicine

If you are unable to swallow the capsules, you may empty the number of capsules needed for one dose into a small amount of fruit juice or other liquid. Stir gently to mix the powder with the liquid before drinking. Drink the medicine right away. Rinse the glass with a little more liquid and drink that also to make sure that you have taken all of the medicine.

Dantrolene may be taken with or without food or on a full or empty stomach. However, if your doctor tells you to take the medicine a certain way, take it exactly as directed.

Take this medicine only as directed by your doctor. Do not take more of it and do not take it more often than your doctor ordered. Dantrolene may cause liver damage or other unwanted effects if too much is taken.

Dosing—The dose of dantrolene will be different for different patients. *Follow your doctor's orders or the directions on the label.* The following information includes only the average doses of dantrolene. *If your dose is different, do not change it* unless your doctor tells you to do so:

- The number of capsules that you take depends on the strength of the medicine. Also, the number of doses you take each day, the time allowed between doses, and the length of time you take the medicine depend on the medical problem for which you are taking dantrolene.
- For *oral* dosage form (capsules):
  - —For prevention or treatment of a malignant hyperthermic crisis:
    - Adults—Dose is based on body weight and must be determined by your doctor. The usual dose is 4 to 8 milligrams (mg) per kilogram (kg) (1.8 to 3.6 mg per pound) of body weight. The doctor will instruct you exactly when and how often to take your medicine.
  - —To relieve spasms:
    - Adults—To start, 25 mg once a day. The doctor may increase your dose as needed and tolerated. However, the dose is usually not more than 100 mg four times a day.
    - Children—Dose is based on body weight and must be determined by your doctor. To start, the dose is usually 0.5 mg per kg (0.23 mg per pound) of body weight twice a day. The doctor may increase the dose as needed and tolerated. However, the dose is usually not more than 3 mg per kg or 100 mg four times a day.
- For *injection* dosage form:
  - —For prevention or treatment of a malignant hyperthermia crisis:
    - Adults, teenagers, and children—Dose is based on body weight and must be determined by your doctor.

Missed dose—If you miss a dose of this medicine and remember within an hour or so of the missed dose, take it right away. Then go back to your regular dosing schedule. But if you do not remember until later, skip the missed dose and go back to your regular dosing schedule. Do not double doses.

Storage—To store this medicine:

- Keep out of the reach of children.
- Store away from heat and direct light.

- Do not store this medicine in the bathroom, near the kitchen sink, or in other damp places. Heat or moisture may cause the medicine to break down.
- Do not keep outdated medicine or medicine no longer needed. Be sure that any discarded medicine is out of the reach of children.

Precautions While Using This Medicine

If you will be taking dantrolene for a long time (for example, for several months at a time), your doctor should check your progress at regular visits. It may be necessary to have certain blood tests to check for unwanted effects while you are taking dantrolene.

This medicine will add to the effects of alcohol and other CNS depressants (medicines that slow down the nervous system, possibly causing drowsiness). Some examples of CNS depressants are antihistamines or medicine for hay fever, other allergies, or colds; sedatives, tranquilizers, or sleeping medicine; prescription pain medicine or narcotics; barbiturates; medicine for seizures; other muscle relaxants; or anesthetics, including some dental anesthetics. Therefore, *do not drink alcoholic beverages, and check with your doctor before taking any of the medicines listed above, while you are using this medicine.*

This medicine may cause drowsiness, dizziness or lightheadedness, vision problems, or muscle weakness in some people. *Make sure you know how you react to this medicine before you drive, use machines, or do anything else that could be dangerous if you are dizzy or are not alert, well-coordinated, and able to see well.*

Side Effects of This Medicine

Along with its needed effects, a medicine may cause some unwanted effects. Although not all of these side effects may occur, if they do occur they may need medical attention. Serious side effects are very rare when dantrolene is taken for a short time (for example, when it is used for a few days before, during, or after surgery or anesthesia to prevent or treat malignant hyperthermia). However, serious side effects may occur, especially when the medicine is taken for a long time.

Check with your doctor immediately if any of the following side effects occur:

Less common

Convulsions (seizures); pain, tenderness, changes in skin color, or swelling of foot or leg; shortness of breath or slow or troubled breathing

Also, check with your doctor as soon as possible if any of the following side effects occur:

Less common

Bloody or dark urine; chest pain; confusion; constipation (severe); diarrhea (severe); difficult urination; mental depression; skin rash, hives, or itching; yellow eyes or skin

Other side effects may occur that usually do not need medical attention. These side effects may go away during treatment as your body adjusts to the medicine. However, check with your doctor if any of the following side effects continue or are bothersome:

More common

Diarrhea (mild); dizziness or lightheadedness; drowsiness; general feeling of discomfort or illness; muscle weakness; nausea or vomiting; unusual tiredness

Less common

Abdominal or stomach cramps or discomfort; blurred or double vision or any change in vision; chills and fever; constipation (mild); difficulty in swallowing; frequent urge to urinate or uncontrolled urination; headache; loss of appetite; slurring of speech or other speech problems; sudden decrease in amount of urine; trouble in sleeping; unusual nervousness

Other side effects not listed above may also occur in some patients. If you notice any other effects, check with your doctor.

Annual revision: 05/10/93

DAPIPRAZOLE Ophthalmic

A commonly used brand name in the U.S. is Rev-Eyes.

Description

Dapiprazole (da-PI-pray-zole) is used in the eye to reduce the size of the pupil after certain kinds of eye examinations.

Some eye examinations are best done when your pupil (the black center of the colored part of your eye) is very large, so the doctor can see into your eye better. This medicine helps to reduce the size of your pupil back to its normal size after the eye examination.

Dapiprazole is available in the following dosage form:

Ophthalmic

- Ophthalmic solution (eye drops) (U.S.)

It is very important that you read and understand the following information. If any of it causes you special concern, check with your doctor. Also, *if you have any questions* or if you want more information about this medicine or your medical problem, *ask your doctor, nurse, or pharmacist.*

Before Using This Medicine

In deciding to use a medicine, the risks of using the medicine must be weighed against the good it will do. This is a decision you and your doctor will make. For dapiprazole, the following should be considered:

Allergies—Tell your doctor if you have ever had any unusual or allergic reaction to dapiprazole. Also tell your doctor and pharmacist if you are allergic to any other substances, such as foods, preservatives, or dyes.

Pregnancy—Dapiprazole has not been studied in pregnant women. However, dapiprazole has not been shown to cause birth defects or other problems in animal studies.

Breast-feeding—It is not known whether dapiprazole passes into the breast milk. However, this medicine has not been reported to cause problems in nursing babies.

Children—Studies on this medicine have been done only in adult patients, and there is no specific information comparing use of dapiprazole in children with use in other age groups.

Older adults—Many medicines have not been studied specifically in older people. Therefore, it may not be known whether they work exactly the same way they do in younger adults. Although there is no specific information comparing use of dapiprazole in the elderly with use in other age groups, this medicine is not expected to cause different side effects or problems in older people than it does in younger adults.

Other medicines—Although certain medicines should not be used together at all, in other cases two different medicines may be used together even if an interaction might occur. In these cases, your doctor may want to change the dose, or other precautions may be necessary. Tell your doctor and pharmacist if you are using any other ophthalmic prescription or nonprescription (over-the-counter [OTC]) medicine.

Other medical problems—The presence of other medical problems may affect the use of dapiprazole. Make sure you tell your doctor if you have any other medical problems, especially:

- Eye problems, other—Use of dapiprazole may make the condition worse

Before you begin using any new medicine (prescription or nonprescription) or if you develop any new medical problem while you are using this medicine, check with your doctor, nurse, or pharmacist.

Precautions While Using This Medicine

Even after using this medicine, you may have blurred vision or other vision problems. If any of these occur, *do not drive, use machines, or do anything else that could be dangerous if you are not able to see well.*

This medicine may cause your eyes to become more sensitive to light than they are normally. Wearing sunglasses and avoiding too much exposure to bright light may help lessen the discomfort.

Side Effects of This Medicine

Along with its needed effects, a medicine may cause some unwanted effects. Although not all of these side effects may occur, if they do occur they may need medical attention.

Check with your doctor as soon as possible if any of the following side effects occur:

Less common

Irritation (severe) or swelling of the clear part of the eye

Other side effects may occur that usually do not need medical attention. These side effects may go away during treatment as your body adjusts to the medicine. However, check with your doctor if any of the following side effects continue or are bothersome:

More common

Burning of eye when medicine is applied; redness of the white part of the eye

Less common

Blurring of vision; browache; drooping of upper eyelid; dryness of eye; headache; increased sensitivity of eye to light; itching of eye; redness of eyelid; swelling of eyelid; swelling of the membrane covering the white part of the eye; tearing of eye

Other side effects not listed above may also occur in some patients. If you notice any other effects, check with your doctor.

Annual revision: 04/13/92

DAPSONE Systemic

A commonly used brand name in Canada is Avlosulfon.
Another commonly used name is DDS.

Description

Dapsone (DAP-sone), a sulfone, belongs to the family of medicines called anti-infectives.

Dapsone is used to treat leprosy (Hansen's disease) and to help control dermatitis herpetiformis, a skin problem. When it is used to treat leprosy, dapsone may be given with one or more other medicines. Dapsone may also be used for other conditions as determined by your doctor.

Dapsone is available only with your doctor's prescription, in the following dosage form:

Oral

- Tablets (U.S. and Canada)

It is very important that you read and understand the following information. If any of it causes you special concern, check with your doctor. Also, *if you have any questions* or if you want more information about this medicine or your medical problem, *ask your doctor, nurse, or pharmacist.*

Before Using This Medicine

In deciding to use a medicine, the risks of taking the medicine must be weighed against the good it will do. This is a decision you and your doctor will make. For dapsone, the following should be considered:

Allergies—Tell your doctor if you have ever had any unusual or allergic reaction to dapsone or sulfonamides. Also tell your doctor and pharmacist if you are allergic to any other substances, such as foods, preservatives, or dyes.

Pregnancy—Studies have not been done in humans or animals. However, reports on the use of dapsone in humans have not shown that this medicine causes birth defects or other problems.

Breast-feeding—Dapsone passes into the breast milk. Dapsone may cause blood problems in nursing babies with glucose-6-phosphate dehydrogenase (G6PD) deficiency. Breast-feeding may need to be stopped because of the risks to the baby.

Children—Although there is no specific information comparing use of dapsone in children with use in other age groups, this medicine is not expected to cause different side effects or problems in children than it does in adults.

Older adults—Many medicines have not been studied specifically in older people. Therefore, it may not be known whether they work exactly the same way they do in younger adults or if they cause different side effects or problems in older people. There is no specific information comparing use of dapsone in the elderly with use in other age groups.

Other medicines—Although certain medicines should not be used together at all, in other cases two different medicines may be used together even if an interaction might occur. In these cases, your doctor may want to change the dose, or other precautions may be necessary. When you are taking dapsone, it is especially important that your doctor and pharmacist know if you are taking any of the following:

- Acetohydroxamic acid (e.g., Lithostat) or
- Antidiabetics, oral (diabetes medicine you take by mouth) or
- Furazolidone (e.g., Furoxone) or
- Methyldopa (e.g., Aldomet) or
- Nitrofurantoin (e.g., Furadantin) or
- Primaquine or
- Procainamide (e.g., Pronestyl) or
- Quinidine (e.g., Quinidex) or
- Quinine (e.g., Quinamm) or
- Sulfonamides (sulfa medicine) or
- Vitamin K (e.g., AquaMEPHYTON, Synkayvite)—Use of dapsone with these medicines may increase the chance of side effects affecting the blood
- Dideoxyinosine (e.g., ddI, Videx)—Use of dideoxyinosine with dapsone may decrease the effectiveness of dapsone

Other medical problems—The presence of other medical problems may affect the use of dapsone. Make sure you tell your doctor if you have any other medical problems, especially:

- Anemia (severe) or
- Glucose-6-phosphate dehydrogenase (G6PD) deficiency or
- Methemoglobin reductase deficiency—There is an increased risk of severe blood disorders and a decrease in red blood cell survival
- Liver disease—Dapsone may on rare occasion cause liver damage

Before you begin using any new medicine (prescription or nonprescription) or if you develop any new medical problem while you are using this medicine, check with your doctor, nurse, or pharmacist.

Proper Use of This Medicine

For patients taking dapsone for leprosy:

- To help clear up your leprosy completely or to keep it from coming back, *it is very important that you keep taking this medicine for the full time of treatment,* even if you begin to feel better after a few weeks or months. You may have to take it every day for as long as 3 years or more, or for life. If you stop taking this medicine too soon, your symptoms may return.

- This medicine works best when there is a constant amount in the blood. *To help keep the amount constant, do not miss any doses. Also, it is best to take each dose at the same time every day.* If you need help in planning the best time to take your medicine, check with your doctor, nurse, or pharmacist.
- **Missed dose**—If you do miss a dose of this medicine, take it as soon as possible. This will help keep a constant amount of medicine in the blood. However, if it is almost time for your next dose, skip the missed dose and go back to your regular dosing schedule. Do not double doses.

For patients taking dapsone for dermatitis herpetiformis:

- Your doctor may want you to follow a gluten-free diet. If you have any questions about this, check with your doctor.

Missed dose—You may skip a missed dose if it does not make your symptoms come back or get worse. If your symptoms do come back or get worse, take the missed dose as soon as possible. Then go back to your regular dosing schedule.

Storage—To store this medicine:

- Keep out of the reach of children.
- Store away from heat and direct light.
- Do not store in the bathroom, near the kitchen sink, or in other damp places. Heat or moisture may cause the medicine to break down.
- Do not keep outdated medicine or medicine no longer needed. Be sure that any discarded medicine is out of the reach of children.

Precautions While Using This Medicine

It is very important that your doctor check your progress at regular visits.

If your symptoms do not improve within 2 to 3 months (for leprosy), or within a few days (for dermatitis herpetiformis), or if they become worse, check with your doctor.

Side Effects of This Medicine

Along with its needed effects, a medicine may cause some unwanted effects. Although not all of these side effects may occur, if they do occur they may need medical attention.

Check with your doctor immediately if any of the following side effects occur:

More common

Back, leg, or stomach pains; bluish fingernails, lips, or skin; difficult breathing; fever; loss of appetite; pale skin; skin rash; unusual tiredness or weakness

Rare

Itching, dryness, redness, scaling, or peeling of the skin, or loss of hair; mood or other mental changes; numbness, tingling, pain, burning, or weakness in hands or feet; sore throat; unusual bleeding or bruising; yellow eyes or skin

Other side effects may occur that usually do not need medical attention. These side effects may go away during treatment as your body adjusts to the medicine. However, check with your doctor if any of the following side effects continue or are bothersome:

Rare

Headache; loss of appetite; nausea or vomiting; nervousness; trouble in sleeping

Other side effects not listed above may also occur in some patients. If you notice any other effects, check with your doctor.

Additional Information

Once a medicine has been approved for marketing for a certain use, experience may show that it is also useful for other medical problems. Although these uses are not specifically included in product labeling, dapsone is used in certain patients with the following medical conditions:

- Actinomycotic mycetoma
- Granuloma annulare
- Malaria (prevention of)
- Pemphigoid
- *Pneumocystis carinii* pneumonia
- Pyoderma gangrenosum
- Relapsing polychondritis
- Subcorneal pustular dermatosis
- Systemic lupus erythematosus

For patients taking this medicine for *Pneumocystis carinii* pneumonia (PCP):

- To help clear up PCP completely or to keep it from coming back, *it is very important that you keep taking this medicine for the full time of treatment.*
- If you miss a dose of this medicine, take it as soon as possible. This will help keep a constant amount of medicine in the blood. However, if it is almost time for your next dose, skip the missed dose and go back to your regular dosing schedule. Do not double doses.
- If your symptoms do not improve within 1 week, or if they become worse, check with your doctor.

Other than the above information, there is no additional information relating to proper use, precautions, or side effects for these uses.

Annual revision: 06/26/92

DAUNORUBICIN Systemic

A commonly used brand name in the U.S. and Canada is Cerubidine.

Description

Daunorubicin (daw-noe-ROO-bi-sin) belongs to the general group of medicines known as antineoplastics. It is used to treat some kinds of cancer.

Daunorubicin seems to interfere with the growth of cancer cells, which are eventually destroyed. Since the growth of normal body cells may also be affected by daunorubicin, other effects will also occur. Some of these may be serious and must be reported to your doctor. Other effects, like hair loss, may not be serious but may cause concern. Some effects may not occur for months or years after the medicine is used.

Before you begin treatment with daunorubicin, you and your doctor should talk about the good this medicine will do as well as the risks of using it.

Daunorubicin is to be administered only by or under the immediate supervision of your doctor. It is available in the following dosage form:

Parenteral
- Injection (U.S. and Canada)

It is very important that you read and understand the following information. If any of it causes you special concern, check with your doctor. Also, *if you have any questions* or if you want more information about this medicine or your medical problem, *ask your doctor, nurse, or pharmacist.*

Before Using This Medicine

In deciding to use a medicine, the risks of taking the medicine must be weighed against the good it will do. This is a decision you and your doctor will make. For daunorubicin, the following should be considered:

Allergies—Tell your doctor if you have ever had any unusual or allergic reaction to daunorubicin.

Pregnancy—This medicine may cause birth defects if either the male or female is receiving it at the time of conception or if it is taken during pregnancy. In addition, many cancer medicines may cause sterility which could be permanent. Although sterility has been reported only in male dogs with this medicine, the possibility of an effect in human males should be kept in mind.

Be sure that you have discussed this with your doctor before receiving this medicine. It is best to use some kind of birth control while you are receiving daunorubicin. However, do not use oral contraceptives ("the Pill") since they may interfere with this medicine. Tell your doctor right away if you think you have become pregnant while receiving daunorubicin.

Breast-feeding—Because daunorubicin may cause serious side effects, breast-feeding is generally not recommended while you are receiving it.

Children—Heart problems are more likely to occur in children under 2 years of age, who are usually more sensitive to the effects of daunorubicin.

Older adults—Heart problems are more likely to occur in the elderly, who are usually more sensitive to the effects of daunorubicin. The elderly may also be more likely to have blood problems.

Other medicines—Although certain medicines should not be used together at all, in other cases two different medicines may be used together even if an interaction might occur. In these cases, your doctor may want to change the dose, or other precautions may be necessary. When receiving daunorubicin it is especially important that your doctor and pharmacist know if you are taking any of the following:

- Amphotericin B by injection (e.g., Fungizone) or
- Antithyroid agents (medicine for overactive thyroid) or
- Azathioprine (e.g., Imuran) or
- Chloramphenicol (e.g., Chloromycetin) or
- Colchicine or
- Flucytosine (e.g., Ancobon) or
- Interferon (e.g., Intron A, Roferon-A) or
- Plicamycin (e.g., Mithracin) or
- Zidovudine (e.g., Retrovir) or
- If you have ever been treated with x-rays or cancer medicines—Daunorubicin may increase the effects of these medicines or radiation therapy on the blood
- Probenecid (e.g., Benemid) or
- Sulfinpyrazone (e.g., Anturane)—Daunorubicin may raise the concentration of uric acid in the blood, which these medicines are used to lower

Other medical problems—The presence of other medical problems may affect the use of daunorubicin. Make sure you tell your doctor if you have any other medical problems, especially:

- Chickenpox (including recent exposure) or
- Herpes zoster (shingles)—Risk of severe disease affecting other parts of the body
- Gout (history of) or
- Kidney stones—Daunorubicin may increase levels of a chemical called uric acid in the body, which can cause gout or kidney stones
- Heart disease—Risk of heart problems caused by daunorubicin may be increased
- Infection—Daunorubicin can reduce immunity to infection
- Kidney disease or
- Liver disease—Effects may be increased because of slower removal of daunorubicin from the body

Before you begin using any new medicine (prescription or nonprescription) or if you develop any new medical problem while you are using this medicine, check with your doctor, nurse, or pharmacist.

Proper Use of This Medicine

Daunorubicin is sometimes given together with certain other medicines. If you are using a combination of medicines, it is important that you receive each one at the proper time. If you are taking some of these medicines by mouth, ask your doctor, nurse, or pharmacist to help you plan a way to take them at the right times.

While you are receiving daunorubicin, your doctor may want you to drink extra fluids so that you will pass more urine. This will help prevent kidney problems and keep your kidneys working well.

This medicine often causes nausea and vomiting. However, it is very important that you continue to receive it, even if you begin to feel ill. Ask your doctor, nurse, or pharmacist for ways to lessen these effects.

Precautions While Using This Medicine

It is very important that your doctor check your progress at regular visits to make sure that this medicine is working properly and to check for unwanted effects.

While you are being treated with daunorubicin, and after you stop treatment with it, *do not have any immunizations (vaccinations) without your doctor's approval.* Daunorubicin may lower your body's resistance and there is a chance you might get the infection the immunization is meant to prevent. In addition, other persons living in your household should not take or should not have recently taken oral polio vaccine since there is a chance they could pass the polio virus on to you. Also, avoid other persons who have taken oral polio vaccine. Do not get close to them, and do not stay in the same room with them for very long. If you cannot take these precautions, you should consider wearing a protective face mask that covers the nose and mouth.

Daunorubicin can lower the number of white blood cells in your blood temporarily, increasing the chance of getting an infection. It can also lower the number of platelets, which are necessary for proper blood clotting. If this occurs, there are certain precautions you can take, especially when your blood count is low, to reduce the risk of infection or bleeding:

- If you can, avoid people with infections. *Check with your doctor immediately* if you think you are getting an infection or if you get a fever or chills, cough or hoarseness, lower back or side pain, or painful or difficult urination.
- *Check with your doctor immediately* if you notice any unusual bleeding or bruising; black, tarry stools; blood in urine or stools; or pinpoint red spots on your skin.
- Be careful when using a regular toothbrush, dental floss, or toothpick. Your medical doctor, dentist, or nurse may recommend other ways to clean your teeth and gums. Check with your medical doctor before having any dental work done.
- Do not touch your eyes or the inside of your nose unless you have just washed your hands and have not touched anything else in the meantime.
- Be careful not to cut yourself when you are using sharp objects such as a safety razor or fingernail or toenail cutters.
- Avoid contact sports or other situations where bruising or injury could occur.

If daunorubicin accidentally seeps out of the vein into which it is injected, it may damage some tissues and cause scarring. *Tell the doctor or nurse right away if you notice redness, pain, or swelling at the place of injection.*

Side Effects of This Medicine

Along with their needed effects, medicines like daunorubicin can sometimes cause unwanted effects such as blood problems, loss of hair, heart problems, and other side effects. These and others are described below. Also, because of the way these medicines act on the body, there is a chance that they might cause other unwanted effects that may not occur until months or years after the medicine is used. These delayed effects may include certain types of cancer, such as leukemia. Discuss these possible effects with your doctor.

Although not all of these side effects may occur, if they do occur they may need medical attention.

Check with your doctor or nurse immediately if any of the following side effects occur:

Less common

Cough or hoarseness; fever or chills; irregular heartbeat; lower back or side pain; pain at place of injection; painful or difficult urination; shortness of breath; swelling of feet and lower legs

Rare

Black, tarry stools; blood in urine or stools; pinpoint red spots on skin; unusual bleeding or bruising

Check with your doctor or nurse as soon as possible if any of the following side effects occur:

More common

Sores in mouth and on lips

Less common

Joint pain

Rare

Skin rash or itching

Other side effects may occur that usually do not need medical attention. These side effects may go away during treatment as your body adjusts to the medicine. Also, your doctor or nurse may be able to tell you about ways to prevent or reduce some of these side effects. Check with your doctor or nurse if any of the following side effects continue or are bothersome or if you have any questions about them:

More common

Nausea and vomiting

Less common or rare

Darkening or redness of skin; diarrhea

Daunorubicin causes the urine to turn reddish in color, which may stain clothes. This is not blood. It is perfectly normal and lasts for only 1 or 2 days after each dose is given.

This medicine often causes a temporary and total loss of hair. After treatment with daunorubicin has ended, normal hair growth should return.

After you stop receiving daunorubicin, it may still produce some side effects that need attention. During this period of time *check with your doctor immediately* if you notice any of the following side effects:

Irregular heartbeat; shortness of breath; swelling of feet and lower legs

Other side effects not listed above may also occur in some patients. If you notice any other effects, check with your doctor or nurse.

Annual revision: July 1990

DECONGESTANTS AND ANALGESICS Systemic

This information applies to the following medicines:

Phenylephrine (fen-ill-EF-rin) and Acetaminophen (a-seat-a-MIN-oh-fen)
Phenylpropanolamine (fen-ill-proe-pa-NOLE-a-meen) and Acetaminophen†
Phenylpropanolamine, Acetaminophen, and Aspirin (AS-pir-in)†
Phenylpropanolamine, Acetaminophen, Aspirin, and Caffeine (kaf-EEN)†
Phenylpropanolamine, Acetaminophen, Salicylamide (sal-i-SILL-a-mide), and Caffeine†
Phenylpropanolamine and Aspirin†
Pseudoephedrine (soo-doe-e-FED-rin) and Acetaminophen
Pseudoephedrine, Acetaminophen, and Caffeine†
Pseudoephedrine and Aspirin†
Pseudoephedrine, Aspirin, and Caffeine†
Pseudoephedrine and Ibuprofen (eye-byoo-PRO-fen)†

Some commonly used brand names are:

For Phenylephrine and Acetaminophen

In the U.S.

Congespirin for Children Cold Tablets

In Canada

Neo Citran Sinus Medicine

For Phenylpropanolamine and Acetaminophen†

In the U.S.

Congespirin for Children Liquid Cold Medicine
Dilotab
Genex
PhenAPAP No. 2
St. Joseph Cold Tablets for Children

For Phenylpropanolamine, Acetaminophen, and Aspirin†

In the U.S.

Rhinocaps

For Phenylpropanolamine, Acetaminophen, Aspirin, and Caffeine†

In the U.S.

Drinophen

For Phenylpropanolamine, Acetaminophen, Salicylamide, and Caffeine†

In the U.S.

Saleto D

For Phenylpropanolamine and Aspirin†

In the U.S.

BC Cold Powder Non-Drowsy Formula

For Pseudoephedrine and Acetaminophen

In the U.S.

Allerest No-Drowsiness
Coldrine
Contac Maximum Strength Sinus Caplets
Dristan Maximum Strength Caplets
Naldegesic
Ornex No Drowsiness Caplets
Sinarest No-Drowsiness
Sine-Aid
Sine-Aid Maximum Strength
Sine-Aid Maximum Strength Caplets
Sine-off Maximum Strength No Drowsiness Formula Caplets
Sinus Excedrin No Drowsiness
Sinus Excedrin No Drowsiness Caplets
Sinutab II Maximum Strength
Sinutab Maximum Strength
Sinutab Maximum Strength Without Drowsiness
Sinutab Maximum Strength Without Drowsiness Caplets
Sudafed Sinus
Maximum Strength
Sudafed Sinus Maximum Strength Caplets
Super-Anahist
Tylenol Sinus Maximum Strength
Tylenol Sinus Maximum Strength Caplets

In Canada

Sinutab No Drowsiness
Sinutab No Drowsiness Extra Strength
Tylenol Sinus Medication
Tylenol Sinus Medication Extra Strength

For Pseudoephedrine, Acetaminophen, and Caffeine†

In the U.S.

Beta-Phed

For Pseudoephedrine and Aspirin†
In the U.S.
Ursinus Inlay

For Pseudoephedrine, Aspirin, and Caffeine†
In the U.S.
Alpha-Phed

For Pseudoephedrine and Ibuprofen†
In the U.S.
CoAdvil Caplets
Dristan Sinus Caplets

†Not commercially available in Canada.

Description

Decongestant and analgesic combinations are taken by mouth to relieve sinus and nasal congestion (stuffy nose) and headache of colds, allergy, and hay fever.

Decongestants, such as phenylephrine, phenylpropanolamine (also known as PPA), and pseudoephedrine produce a narrowing of blood vessels. This leads to clearing of nasal congestion, but it may also cause an increase in blood pressure in patients who have high blood pressure.

Analgesics, such as acetaminophen, ibuprofen, and salicylates (e.g., aspirin, salicylamide), are used in these combination medicines to help relieve headache and sinus pain.

Acetaminophen and salicylates may cause kidney damage or cancer of the kidney or urinary bladder if large amounts of both medicines are taken together for a long time. However, taking the recommended amounts of combination medicines that contain both acetaminophen and a salicylate for short periods of time has not been shown to cause these unwanted effects.

These medicines are available without a prescription. However, your doctor may have special instructions on the proper dose of these medicines for your medical condition. They are available in the following dosage forms:

Oral

Phenylephrine and Acetaminophen
- For oral solution (Canada)
- Chewable tablets (U.S.)

Phenylpropanolamine and Acetaminophen
- Capsules (U.S.)
- Oral solution (U.S.)
- Tablets (U.S.)
- Chewable tablets (U.S.)

Phenylpropanolamine, Acetaminophen, and Aspirin
- Capsules (U.S.)

Phenylpropanolamine, Acetaminophen, Aspirin, and Caffeine
- Capsules (U.S.)

Phenylpropanolamine, Acetaminophen, Salicylamide, and Caffeine
- Capsules (U.S.)

Phenylpropanolamine and Aspirin
- For oral solution (U.S.)

Pseudoephedrine and Acetaminophen
- Capsules (U.S.)
- Tablets (U.S. and Canada)

Pseudoephedrine, Acetaminophen, and Caffeine
- Capsules (U.S.)

Pseudoephedrine and Aspirin
- Tablets (U.S.)

Pseudoephedrine, Aspirin, and Caffeine
- Capsules (U.S.)

Pseudoephedrine and Ibuprofen
- Tablets (U.S.)

It is very important that you read and understand the following information. If any of it causes you special concern, check with your doctor or pharmacist. Also, *if you have any questions* or if you want more information about this medicine or your medical problem, *ask your doctor, nurse, or pharmacist.*

Before Using This Medicine

If you are taking this medicine without a prescription, carefully read and follow any precautions on the label. For decongestant and analgesic combinations, the following should be considered:

Allergies—Tell your doctor if you have ever had any unusual or allergic reaction to any of the ingredients contained in this medicine.

If this medicine contains *aspirin, salicylamide,* or *ibuprofen,* before taking it, check with your doctor if you have ever had any unusual or allergic reaction to any of the following medicines:

Aspirin or other salicylates
Diclofenac (e.g., Voltaren)
Diflunisal (e.g., Dolobid)
Fenoprofen (e.g., Nalfon)
Floctafenine (e.g., Idarac)
Flurbiprofen, by mouth (e.g., Ansaid)
Ibuprofen (e.g., Motrin)
Indomethacin (e.g., Indocin)
Ketoprofen (e.g., Orudis)
Ketorolac (e.g., Toradol)
Meclofenamate (e.g., Meclomen)
Mefenamic acid (e.g., Ponstel)
Methyl salicylate (oil of wintergreen)
Naproxen (e.g., Naprosyn)
Oxyphenbutazone (e.g., Tandearil)
Phenylbutazone (e.g., Butazolidin)
Piroxicam (e.g., Feldene)
Sulindac (e.g., Clinoril)
Suprofen (e.g., Suprol)
Tiaprofenic acid (e.g., Surgam)
Tolmetin (e.g., Tolectin)
Zomepirac (e.g., Zomax)

Also tell your doctor and pharmacist if you are allergic to any other substances, such as foods, preservatives, or dyes.

Pregnancy—The occasional use of decongestant and analgesic combinations at the doses recommended on the label is not likely to cause problems in the fetus or in the newborn baby. However, when these medicines are used at higher doses and/or for a long time, the chance that problems might occur may increase. For the individual ingredients of these combinations, the following apply:

- *Alcohol*—Some of these combination medicines contain large amounts of alcohol. Too much use of alcohol during pregnancy may cause birth defects.
- *Caffeine*—Studies in humans have not shown that caffeine causes birth defects. However, studies in animals have shown that caffeine causes birth defects when given in very large doses (amounts equal to the amount of caffeine contained in 12 to 24 cups of coffee a day).
- *Ibuprofen*—Studies on birth defects have not been done in humans. However, there is a chance that ibuprofen may cause unwanted effects on the heart or blood flow of the fetus or newborn baby if it is taken regularly during the last few months of pregnancy.
- *Phenylephrine*—Studies on birth defects have not been done in either humans or animals with phenylephrine.
- *Phenylpropanolamine*—Studies on birth defects have not been done in either humans or animals with phenylpropanolamine. However, it seems that women who take phenylpropanolamine in the weeks following delivery are more likely to suffer mental or mood changes.
- *Pseudoephedrine*—Studies on birth defects with pseudoephedrine have not been done in humans. In animal studies pseudoephedrine did not cause birth defects but did cause a decrease in average weight, length, and rate of bone formation in the animal fetus when administered in high doses.
- *Salicylates (e.g., aspirin)*—Studies on birth defects in humans have been done with aspirin, but not with salicylamide. Although, salicylates have been shown to cause birth defects in animals, they have not been shown to cause birth defects in humans.

  Regular use of salicylates late in pregnancy may cause unwanted effects on the heart or blood flow in the fetus or newborn baby. Use of salicylates during the last 2 weeks of pregnancy may cause bleeding problems in the fetus before or during delivery, or in the newborn baby. Also, too much use of salicylates during the last 3 months of pregnancy may increase the length of pregnancy, prolong labor and cause other problems during delivery, or cause severe bleeding in the mother before, during, or after delivery. *Do not take aspirin during the last 3 months of pregnancy unless it has been ordered by your doctor.*

Breast-feeding—If you are breast-feeding the chance that problems might occur depends on the ingredients of the combination. For the individual ingredients of these combinations, the following apply:

- *Acetaminophen*—Acetaminophen passes into the breast milk. However, it has not been reported to cause problems in nursing babies.
- *Alcohol*—Alcohol passes into the breast milk. However, the amount of alcohol in recommended doses of this medicine does not usually cause problems in nursing babies.
- *Caffeine*—Small amounts of caffeine pass into the breast milk and may build up in the nursing baby. However, the amount of caffeine in recommended doses of this medicine does not usually cause problems in nursing babies.
- *Decongestants (e.g., phenylephrine, phenylpropanolamine, pseudoephedrine)*—Phenylephrine and phenylpropanolamine have not been shown to cause problems in nursing babies. Pseudoephedrine passes into the breast milk and may cause unwanted effects in nursing babies (especially newborn and premature babies) of mothers taking this medicine.
- *Salicylates (e.g., aspirin, salicylamide)*—Salicylates pass into the breast milk. Although salicylates have not been reported to cause problems in nursing babies, it is possible that problems may occur if large amounts are taken regularly.

Children—Very young children are usually more sensitive to the effects of this medicine. *Before giving any of these combination medicines to a child, check the package label very carefully. Some of these medicines are too strong for use in children.* If you are not certain whether a specific product can be given to a child, or if you have any questions about the amount to give, check with your doctor or pharmacist, especially if it contains:

- *Decongestants (e.g., phenylephrine, phenylpropanolamine, pseudoephedrine)*—Increases in blood pressure may be more likely to occur in children taking decongestants. Also, mental changes may be more likely to occur in young children taking phenylpropanolamine-containing combinations.
- *Salicylates (e.g., aspirin)*—*Do not give aspirin or other salicylates to a child with a fever or other symptoms of a virus infection, especially flu or chickenpox, without first discussing its use with your child's doctor.* This is very important because salicylates may cause a serious illness called Reye's syndrome in these children. Also, children may be more sensitive to the aspirin or other salicylates contained in some of these medicines, especially if they have a fever or have lost large amounts of body fluid because of vomiting, diarrhea, or sweating.

Teenagers—*Do not give aspirin or other salicylates to a teenager with a fever or other symptoms of a virus infection, especially flu or chickenpox, without first discussing its use with your child's doctor.* This is very important because salicylates may cause a serious illness called Reye's syndrome in these individuals.

Older adults—The elderly are usually more sensitive to the effects of this medicine.

Other medicines—Although certain medicines should not be used together at all, in other cases two different medicines may be used together even if an interaction might occur. In these cases, your doctor may want to change the dose, or other precautions may be necessary. Tell your doctor and pharmacist if you are taking *any* other prescription or nonprescription (over-the-counter [OTC]) medicine, for example, aspirin or other medicine for allergies. Some medicines may change the way this medicine affects your body. Also, the effect of other medicines may be increased or reduced by some of the ingredients in this medicine. Check with your doctor or pharmacist about which medicines you should not take together with this medicine.

Other medical problems—The presence of other medical problems may affect the use of decongestant and analgesic combinations. Make sure you tell your doctor if you have any other medical problems, especially:

- Alcohol abuse—Acetaminophen-containing medicine increases the chance of liver damage
- Anemia—Taking aspirin-, salicylamide-, or ibuprofen-containing medicine may make the anemia worse
- Asthma, allergies, and nasal polyps, history of—Taking salicylate- or ibuprofen-containing medicine may cause an allergic reaction in which breathing becomes difficult
- Diabetes mellitus (sugar diabetes)—The decongestant in this medicine may put the patient with diabetes at a greater risk of having heart or blood vessel disease
- Gout—Aspirin-containing medicine may make the gout worse and reduce the benefit of the medicines used for gout
- Hepatitis or other liver disease—Liver disease increases the chance of side effects because the medicine is not broken down and may build up in the body; also, if liver disease is severe there is a greater chance that aspirin-containing medicine may cause bleeding, and that ibuprofen-containing medicine may cause serious kidney damage
- Heart or blood vessel disease or
- High blood pressure—The decongestant in this medicine may cause the blood pressure to increase and may also speed up the heart rate; also, caffeine-containing medicine, if taken in large amounts may increase the heart rate; ibuprofen-containing medicine may cause the blood pressure to increase
- Hemophilia or other bleeding problems—Aspirin- or ibuprofen-containing medicine increases the chance of bleeding
- Kidney disease—The kidneys may be affected, especially if too much of this medicine is taken for a long time
- Mental illness (history of)—The decongestant in this medicine may increase the chance of mental side effects
- Overactive thyroid—If an overactive thyroid has caused a fast heart rate, the decongestant in this medicine may cause the heart rate to speed up further
- Stomach ulcer or other stomach problems—Salicylate- or ibuprofen-containing medicine may make the ulcer worse or cause bleeding of the stomach
- Systemic lupus erythematosus (SLE)—Ibuprofen-containing medicine may put the patient with SLE at a greater risk of having unwanted effects on the central nervous system and/or kidneys
- Ulcers, sores, or white spots in the mouth—This may be a sign of a serious side effect of ibuprofen-containing medicine; if you already have ulcers or sores in the mouth you and your doctor may not be able to tell when this side effect occurs

Proper Use of This Medicine

Take this medicine only as directed. Do not take more of it and do not take it more often than recommended on the label, unless otherwise directed by your doctor. To do so may increase the chance of side effects.

For *aspirin- or salicylamide-containing medicines:*

- If this medicine irritates your stomach, you may take with food or a glass of water or milk to lessen the irritation.
- *If a combination medicine containing aspirin has a strong vinegar-like odor, do not use it.* This odor means the medicine is breaking down. If you have any questions about this, check with your pharmacist.

For *ibuprofen-containing medicines:*

- To lessen stomach upset, these medicines may be taken with food or an antacid.
- Take with a full glass (8 ounces) of water. Also, do not lie down for about 15 to 30 minutes after taking the medicine. Doing so may cause irritation that may lead to trouble in swallowing.

Missed dose—If you must take this medicine regularly and you miss a dose, take it as soon as possible. However, if it is almost time for your next dose, skip the missed dose and go back to your regular dosing schedule. Do not double doses.

Storage—To store this medicine:

- Keep this medicine out of the reach of children. Overdose is very dangerous in young children.
- Store away from heat and direct light.
- Do not store the capsule or tablet form of this medicine in the bathroom, near the kitchen sink, or in other damp places. Heat or moisture may cause the medicine to break down.
- Keep the liquid form of this medicine from freezing.
- Do not keep outdated medicine or medicine no longer needed. Be sure that any discarded medicine is out of the reach of children.

Precautions While Using This Medicine

Check with your doctor if your symptoms do not improve or become worse, or if you have a high fever.

This medicine may add to the central nervous system (CNS) stimulant and other effects of phenylpropanolamine (PPA)-containing diet aids. *Do not use medicines for diet or appetite control while taking this medicine unless you have checked with your doctor.*

This medicine may cause some people to become nervous or restless or to have trouble in sleeping. If you have trouble in sleeping, *take the last dose of this medicine for each day a few hours before bedtime.* If you have any questions about this, check with your doctor.

Before having any kind of surgery (including dental surgery) or emergency treatment, tell the medical doctor or dentist in charge that you are taking this medicine.

Check the label of all over-the-counter (OTC), nonprescription, and prescription medicines you now take. If any contain acetaminophen, aspirin or other salicylates, including diflunisal or bismuth subsalicylate (e.g., Pepto-Bismol), or ibuprofen, be especially careful. This combination medicine contains acetaminophen, ibuprofen, and/or a salicylate. Therefore, taking it while taking other medicine that contains these drugs may lead to overdose. If you have any questions about this, check with your doctor or pharmacist.

Do not drink alcoholic beverages while taking this medicine. Stomach problems may be more likely to occur if you drink alcoholic beverages while you are taking aspirin or ibuprofen. Also, liver damage may be more likely to occur if you drink large amounts of alcoholic beverages while you are taking acetaminophen.

If you think that you or anyone else may have taken an overdose of this medicine, get emergency help at once. Taking an overdose of a salicylate may cause unconsciousness or death. The first sign of an aspirin overdose may be ringing or buzzing in the ears. Other signs include convulsions (seizures), hearing loss, confusion, severe drowsiness or tiredness, severe excitement or nervousness, and unusually fast or deep breathing. Signs of severe acetaminophen overdose may not appear until 2 to 4 days after the overdose is taken, but treatment to prevent liver damage or death must be started within 24 hours or less after the overdose is taken.

For patients *taking aspirin-containing medicine:*

- Do not take aspirin-containing medicine for 5 days before any surgery, including dental surgery, unless otherwise directed by your medical doctor or dentist. Taking aspirin during this time may cause bleeding problems.

For diabetic patients *taking salicylate-containing medicine:*

- False urine sugar test results may occur if you take 8 or more 325-mg (5-grain) doses of aspirin every day for several days in a row. Smaller doses or occasional use of aspirin usually will not affect urine sugar tests. If you have any questions about this, check with your doctor, nurse, or pharmacist, especially if your diabetes is not well controlled.

For patients *taking ibuprofen-containing medicine:*

- This medicine may cause some people to become confused, drowsy, dizzy, lightheaded, or less alert than they are normally. It may also cause blurred vision or other vision problems in some people. *Make sure you know how you react to this medicine before you drive, use machines, or do anything else that could be dangerous if you are dizzy or are not alert and able to see well.*

Side Effects of This Medicine

Along with its needed effects, a medicine may cause some unwanted effects. Although serious side effects occur rarely when this medicine is taken as recommended, they may be more likely to occur if:

- too much medicine is taken.
- it is taken in large doses.
- it is taken for a long period of time.

Get emergency help immediately if any of the following symptoms of overdose occur:

For all combinations

Convulsions (seizures); dizziness or lightheadedness (severe); fast, slow, or irregular heartbeat; hallucinations (seeing, hearing, or feeling things that are not there); headache (continuing and severe); increased sweating; mood or mental changes; nausea or vomiting (severe or continuing); nervousness or restlessness (severe); shortness of breath or troubled breathing; stomach cramps or pain (severe or continuing); swelling or tenderness in the upper abdomen or stomach area; trouble in sleeping

For acetaminophen-containing only

Diarrhea; loss of appetite

For aspirin- or salicylamide-containing only

Any loss of hearing; changes in behavior (in children); confusion; diarrhea (severe or continuing); drowsiness or tiredness (severe, especially in children); fast or deep breathing (especially in children); ringing or buzzing in ears (continuing); uncontrollable flapping movements of the hands, (especially in elderly patients); unexplained fever; unusual thirst; vision problems

Also, check with your doctor as soon as possible if any of the following side effects occur:

More common

Nausea, vomiting, or stomach pain (mild—for combinations containing aspirin or ibuprofen)

Less common or rare

Bloody or black, tarry stools; bloody or cloudy urine; blurred vision or any changes in vision or eyes; changes in facial skin color; changes in hearing; changes or problems with urination; difficult or painful urination;

fever; headache, severe, with fever and stiff neck; increased blood pressure; muscle cramps or pain; skin rash, hives, or itching; sores, ulcers, or white spots on lips or in mouth; swelling of face, fingers, feet, or lower legs; swollen and/or painful glands; unexplained sore throat and fever; unusual bleeding or bruising; unusual tiredness or weakness; vomiting of blood or material that looks like coffee grounds; weight gain (unusual); yellow eyes or skin

Other side effects may occur that usually do not need medical attention. These side effects may go away during treatment as your body adjusts to the medicine. However, check with your doctor if any of the following side effects continue or are bothersome:

More common

Heartburn or indigestion (for medicines containing salicylate or ibuprofen); nervousness or restlessness

Less common

Drowsiness (for medicines containing salicylamide)

Not all of the side effects listed above have been reported for each of these medicines, but they have been reported for at least one of them. There are some similarities among these combination medicines, so many of the above side effects may occur with any of these medicines.

Other side effects not listed above may also occur in some patients. If you notice any other effects, check with your doctor.

Annual revision: 11/25/91

DEFEROXAMINE Systemic

A commonly used brand name in the U.S. and Canada is Desferal. Another commonly used name is desferrioxamine.

Description

Deferoxamine (dee-fer-OX-a-meen) is used to remove excess iron from the body. This may be necessary in certain patients with anemia who must receive many blood transfusions. It is also used to treat acute iron poisoning, especially in small children.

Deferoxamine combines with iron in the bloodstream. The combination of iron and deferoxamine is then removed from the body by the kidneys. By removing the excess iron, the medicine lessens damage to various organs and tissues of the body. This medicine may be used for other conditions as determined by your doctor.

Deferoxamine is to be administered only by or under the immediate supervision of your doctor. It is available in the following dosage form:

Parenteral

- Injection (U.S. and Canada)

It is very important that you read and understand the following information. If any of it causes you special concern, check with your doctor. Also, *if you have any questions* or if you want more information about this medicine or your medical problem, *ask your doctor, nurse, or pharmacist.*

Before Receiving This Medicine

In deciding to use a medicine, the risks of taking the medicine must be weighed against the good it will do. This is a decision you and your doctor will make. For deferoxamine, the following should be considered:

Allergies—Tell your doctor if you have ever had any unusual or allergic reaction to deferoxamine. Also tell your doctor and pharmacist if you are allergic to any other substances, such as foods, preservatives, or dyes.

Pregnancy—Deferoxamine has not been shown to cause birth defects or other problems in humans. However, in animal studies this medicine caused birth defects when given in doses just above the recommended human dose. In general, deferoxamine is not recommended for women who may become pregnant or for use during early pregnancy, unless the woman's life is in danger from too much iron.

Breast-feeding—It is not known whether deferoxamine is excreted in breast milk. However, this medicine has not been reported to cause problems in nursing babies.

Children—Deferoxamine is not used for long-term treatment of children up to 3 years of age. Also, younger patients are more likely to develop hearing and vision problems with the use of deferoxamine in high doses for a long time.

Older adults—The combination of deferoxamine and vitamin C should be used with caution in older patients, since this combination may be more likely to cause heart problems in these patients than in younger adults.

Other medicines—Although certain medicines should not be used together at all, in other cases two different medicines may be used together even if an interaction might occur. In these cases, your doctor may want to change the dose, or other precautions may be necessary. When you are receiving deferoxamine, it is especially important that your doctor and pharmacist know if you are taking the following:

- Ascorbic acid (vitamin C)—Use with deferoxamine may be harmful to body tissues, especially in the elderly

Other medical problems—The presence of other medical problems may affect the use of deferoxamine. Make sure you tell your doctor if you have any other medical problems, especially:

- Kidney disease—Higher blood levels of deferoxamine may result

Before you begin using any new medicine (prescription or nonprescription) or if you develop any new medical problem while you are using this medicine, check with your doctor, nurse, or pharmacist.

Proper Use of This Medicine

Deferoxamine may sometimes be given at home to patients who do not need to be in the hospital. If you are receiving this medicine at home, *make sure you clearly understand and carefully follow your doctor's instructions.*

Storage—To store this medicine:

- Keep out of the reach of children.
- Store away from heat and direct light.
- Store the mixed medicine at room temperature for no more than one week. Do not refrigerate.
- Do not keep outdated medicine or medicine that is no longer needed. Be sure any discarded medicine is out of the reach of children.

Precautions While Receiving This Medicine

It is important that your doctor check your progress at regular visits to make sure that this medicine is working properly and to prevent unwanted effects. Certain blood and urine tests must be done regularly to allow for dosage changes.

Deferoxamine may cause some people, especially younger patients, to have hearing and vision problems within a few weeks after they start taking it. *If you notice any problems with your vision, such as blurred vision, difficulty in seeing at night, or difficulty in seeing colors, or difficulty with your hearing, check with your doctor as soon as possible.* The dose of deferoxamine may need to be adjusted.

Do not take vitamin C unless your doctor has told you to do so.

Side Effects of This Medicine

Along with its needed effects, a medicine may cause some unwanted effects. Although not all of these side effects may occur, if they do occur they may need medical attention.

Check with your doctor as soon as possible if any of the following side effects occur:

More common

Blurred vision or other problems with vision; difficulty in breathing (wheezing); convulsions (seizures); dizziness; fast heartbeat; hearing problems; pain or swelling at place of injection; redness or flushing of skin; skin rash, hives, or itching

Less common

Abdominal and muscle cramps; abdominal (stomach) discomfort; diarrhea; difficult urination; fever; leg cramps; unusual bleeding or bruising

Hearing and vision problems are more likely to occur in younger patients taking high doses and on long-term treatment.

Deferoxamine may cause the urine to turn orange-rose in color. This is to be expected while you are using this medicine.

Other side effects not listed above may also occur in some patients. If you notice any other effects, check with your doctor.

Additional Information

Once a medicine has been approved for marketing for a certain use, experience may show that it is also useful for other medical problems. Although this use is not included in product labeling, deferoxamine is used in certain patients with the following medical condition:

- Aluminum toxicity (too much aluminum in the body)

Other than the above information, there is no additional information relating to proper use, precautions, or side effects for this use.

Annual revision: 11/27/91
Interim revision: 03/04/92

DESMOPRESSIN Systemic

Some commonly used brand names are:

In the U.S.
DDAVP
Stimate

In Canada
DDAVP

Description

Desmopressin (des-moe-PRESS-in) is a hormone taken through the nose or given by injection to prevent or control the frequent urination, increased thirst, and loss of water associated with diabetes insipidus (water diabetes). It is used also to control frequent urination and increased thirst associated with certain types of brain injuries or brain surgery or bed-wetting. Desmopressin works by acting on the kidneys to reduce the flow of urine.

Desmopressin is also given by injection to treat some patients with certain bleeding problems such as hemophilia or von Willebrand's disease.

Desmopressin is available only with your doctor's prescription, in the following dosage forms:

Nasal

- Nasal solution (U.S. and Canada)

Parenteral

- Injection (U.S. and Canada)

It is very important that you read and understand the following information. If any of it causes you special concern, check with your doctor. Also, *if you have any questions* or if you want more information about this medicine or your medical problem, *ask your doctor, nurse, or pharmacist.*

Before Using This Medicine

In deciding to use a medicine, the risks of taking the medicine must be weighed against the good it will do. This is a decision you and your doctor will make. For desmopressin, the following should be considered:

Allergies—Tell your doctor if you have ever had any unusual or allergic reaction to desmopressin. Also tell your doctor and pharmacist if you are allergic to any other substances, such as foods, preservatives, or dyes.

Pregnancy—Studies have not been done in pregnant women. Desmopressin has been used before and during pregnancy to treat diabetes insipidus and has not been shown to cause birth defects.

Breast-feeding—Desmopressin passes into breast milk in very small amounts. However, it has not been reported to cause problems in nursing babies.

Children—Infants may be more sensitive to the effects of this medicine.

Older adults—Some side effects (confusion, drowsiness, continuing headache, problem with urination, weight gain) may be especially likely to occur in elderly patients, who are usually more sensitive than younger adults to the effects of desmopressin.

Other medicines—Although certain medicines should not be used together at all, in other cases two different medicines may be used together even if an interaction might occur. In these cases, your doctor may want to change the dose, or other precautions may be necessary. Tell your doctor and pharmacist if you are taking any other prescription or nonprescription (over-the-counter [OTC]) medicine.

Other medical problems—The presence of other medical problems may affect the use of desmopressin. Make sure you tell your doctor if you have any other medical problems, especially:

- Cystic fibrosis—Excess water retention and serious side effects may be more likely to occur in patients with this condition
- Heart or blood vessel disease or
- High blood pressure—Large doses of desmopressin can cause an increase in blood pressure
- Stuffy nose caused by cold or allergy—May prevent nasal desmopressin from being absorbed through the lining of the nose into the bloodstream

Before you begin using any new medicine (prescription or nonprescription) or if you develop any new medical problem while you are using this medicine, check with your doctor, nurse, or pharmacist.

Proper Use of This Medicine

For patients using the *nasal solution form* of this medicine:

- *Use this medicine only as directed.* Do not use more of it and do not use it more often than your doctor ordered. To do so may increase the chance of side effects.
- This medicine usually comes with patient directions. Read them carefully before using this medicine.

Missed dose—*For nasal solution form of this medicine:* If you miss a dose of this medicine and your dosing schedule is—

- One dose a day—Use the missed dose as soon as possible. Then go back to your regular dosing schedule. However, if you do not remember the missed dose until the next day, skip the missed dose and go back to your regular dosing schedule. Do not double doses.

- More than one dose a day—Use the missed dose as soon as possible. Then go back to your regular dosing schedule. However, if it is almost time for your next dose, skip the missed dose and go back to your regular dosing schedule. Do not double doses.

Storage—To store this medicine:
- Keep out of the reach of children.
- Store in the refrigerator. However, keep the medicine from freezing.
- Do not keep outdated medicine or medicine no longer needed. Be sure that any discarded medicine is out of the reach of children.

Side Effects of This Medicine

Along with its needed effects, a medicine may cause some unwanted effects. Although not all of these effects may occur, if they do occur they may need medical attention.

Check with your doctor immediately if any of the following side effects occur:

Confusion; convulsions (seizures); drowsiness; headache (continuing); decreased urination; weight gain (rapid)

Other side effects may occur that usually do not need medical attention. These side effects may go away during treatment as your body adjusts to the medicine. However, check with your doctor if any of the following side effects continue or are bothersome:

Less common or rare

Abdominal or stomach cramps; flushing or redness of skin; headache; nausea; pain in the vulva (genital area outside of the vagina)

With intranasal (through the nose) use

Runny or stuffy nose

With intravenous use

Pain, redness, or swelling at place of injection

Other side effects not listed above may also occur in some patients. If you notice any other effects, check with your doctor.

Annual revision: 10/26/92

DEXTROMETHORPHAN Systemic

Some commonly used brand names are:

In the U.S.

Benylin DM
Children's Hold
Delsym
Hold
Mediquell
Pertussin Cough Suppressant
Pertussin CS
Pertussin ES
Robitussin Pediatric
St. Joseph for Children
Sucrets Cough Control Formula
Trocal
Vicks Formula 44 Pediatric Formula

In Canada

Balminil D.M.
Broncho-Grippol-DM
Delsym
DM Syrup
Koffex
Neo-DM
Ornex•DM 15
Ornex•DM 30
Robidex
Sedatuss

Description

Dextromethorphan (dex-troe-meth-OR-fan) is used to relieve coughs due to colds or influenza (flu). It is not to be used for chronic cough that occurs with smoking, asthma, or emphysema or when there is an unusually large amount of mucus or phlegm with the cough.

Dextromethorphan relieves cough by acting directly on the cough center in the brain.

This medicine is available without a prescription; however, your doctor may have special instructions on the proper use of this medicine for your medical condition. It is available in the following dosage forms:

Oral
- Capsules (Canada)
- Lozenges (U.S.)
- Syrup (U.S. and Canada)
- Extended-release oral suspension (U.S. and Canada)
- Chewable tablets (U.S.)

It is very important that you read and understand the following information. If any of it causes you special concern, check with your doctor or pharmacist. Also, *if you have any questions* or if you want more information about this medicine or your medical problem, *ask your doctor, nurse, or pharmacist.*

Before Using this Medicine

If you are taking this medicine without a prescription, carefully read and follow any precautions on the label. For dextromethorphan, the following should be considered:

Allergies—Tell your doctor if you have ever had any unusual or allergic reaction to dextromethorphan. Also tell your doctor and pharmacist if you are allergic to any other substances, such as foods, sulfites or other preservatives, or dyes.

Diet—Make certain your doctor and pharmacist know if you are on a low-sodium, low-sugar, or any other special diet. Most medicines contain more than their active ingredient, and many liquid medicines contain alcohol.

Pregnancy—Dextromethorphan has not been shown to cause problems in humans.

Breast-feeding—Dextromethorphan has not been reported to cause problems in nursing babies.

Children—Although there is no specific information comparing use of dextromethorphan in children with use in other age groups, this medicine is not expected to cause different side effects or problems in children than it does in adults.

Older adults—Many medicines have not been studied specifically in older people. Therefore, it may not be known whether they work exactly the same way they do in younger adults or if they cause different side effects or problems in older people. There is no specific information comparing use of dextromethorphan in the elderly with use in other age groups.

Other medicines—Although certain medicines should not be used together at all, in other cases 2 different medicines may be used together even if an interaction might occur. In these cases, your doctor may want to change the dose, or other precautions may be necessary. When taking dextromethorphan it is especially important that your doctor and pharmacist know if you are taking any of the following:

- Central nervous system (CNS) depressants (medicines that cause drowsiness)—The depressant effects of either these medicines or dextromethorphan may be increased
- Monoamine oxidase (MAO) inhibitors (furazolidone [e.g., Furoxone], isocarboxazid [e.g., Marplan], phenelzine [e.g., Nardil], procarbazine [e.g., Matulane], tranylcypromine [e.g., Parnate])—Taking dextromethorphan if you are taking MAO inhibitors now or have taken them within the past 2 weeks may cause excited behavior, high blood pressure, and fever

Other medical problems—The presence of other medical problems may affect the use of dextromethorphan. Make sure you tell your doctor if you have any other medical problems, especially:

- Asthma—Since dextromethorphan decreases coughing, it makes it difficult to get rid of the mucous that collects in the lungs and airways during asthma
- Liver disease—Dextromethorphan may build up in the body and cause unwanted effects

Before you begin using any new medicine (prescription or nonprescription) or if you develop any new medical problem while you are using this medicine, check with your doctor, nurse, or pharmacist.

Proper Use of This Medicine

Missed dose—If you must take this medicine regularly and you miss a dose, take it as soon as possible. However, if it is almost time for your next dose, skip the missed dose and go back to your regular dosing schedule. Do not double doses.

Storage—To store this medicine:

- Store away from heat and direct light.
- Keep out of the reach of children.
- Do not store the tablet form of this medicine in the bathroom, near the kitchen sink, or in other damp places. Heat or moisture may cause the medicine to break down.
- Keep the liquid form of this medicine from freezing.
- Do not keep outdated medicine or medicine no longer needed. Be sure that any discarded medicine is out of the reach of children.

Precautions While Using This Medicine

If your cough has not improved after 7 days or if you have a high fever, skin rash, or continuing headache with the cough, check with your doctor. These signs may mean that you have other medical problems.

Side Effects of This Medicine

Along with its needed effects, a medicine may cause some unwanted effects. Although not all of these side effects may occur, if they do occur they may need medical attention.

Check with your doctor as soon as possible if any of the following side effects occur:

Symptoms of overdose

Confusion; drowsiness or dizziness; nausea or vomiting (severe); unusual excitement, nervousness, restlessness, or irritability (severe)

Other side effects may occur that usually do not need medical attention. These side effects may go away during treatment as your body adjusts to the medicine. However, check with your doctor or pharmacist if any of the following side effects continue or are bothersome:

Less common or rare

Dizziness (mild); drowsiness (mild); nausea or vomiting; stomach pain

Other side effects not listed above may also occur in some patients. If you notice any other effects, check with your doctor.

Annual revision: 05/15/91

DEXTROTHYROXINE Systemic

Some commonly used brand names are:

In the U.S.
- Choloxin

In Canada
- Choloxin

Other
- Biotirmone
- Debetrol
- Dethyrona
- Dethyrone
- Dynothel
- Eulipos
- Lisolipin
- Nadrothyron-D

Description

Dextrothyroxine (dex-troe-thye-ROX-een) is used to lower high cholesterol levels in the blood. However, it has generally been replaced by safer medicines for the treatment of high cholesterol.

Dextrothyroxine is available only with your doctor's prescription, in the following dosage form:

Oral
- Tablets (U.S. and Canada)

It is very important that you read and understand the following information. If any of it causes you special concern, check with your doctor. Also, *if you have any questions* or if you want more information about this medicine or your medical problem, *ask your doctor, nurse, or pharmacist.*

Before Using This Medicine

In deciding to use a medicine, the risks of taking the medicine must be weighed against the good it will do. This is a decision you and your doctor will make. For dextrothyroxine, the following should be considered:

Allergies—Tell your doctor if you have ever had any unusual or allergic reaction to dextrothyroxine. Also tell your doctor and pharmacist if you are allergic to any other substances, such as foods, preservatives, or dyes.

Diet—Before prescribing medicine for your condition, your doctor will probably try to control your condition by prescribing a personal diet for you. Such a diet may be low in fats, sugars, and/or cholesterol. Many people are able to control their condition by carefully following their doctor's orders for proper diet and exercise. *Medicine is prescribed only when additional help is needed* and is effective only when a schedule of diet and exercise is properly followed.

Also, this medicine is less effective if you are greatly overweight. It may be very important for you to go on a reducing diet. However, check with your doctor before going on any diet.

Make certain your doctor and pharmacist know if you are on any special diet, such as a low-sodium or low-sugar diet.

Pregnancy—Dextrothyroxine has not been studied in pregnant women. However, studies in animals have not shown that dextrothyroxine causes birth defects or other problems. Before taking this medicine, make sure your doctor knows if you are pregnant or if you may become pregnant.

Breast-feeding—It is not known whether dextrothyroxine passes into breast milk. Although most medicines pass into breast milk in small amounts, many of them may be used safely while breast-feeding. Mothers who are taking this medicine and who wish to breast-feed should discuss this with their doctor.

Children—There is no specific information comparing use of dextrothyroxine in children to use in other age groups. However, use is not recommended in children under 2 years of age since cholesterol is needed for normal development.

Older adults—Side effects are more likely to occur in the elderly, who are usually more sensitive to the effects of dextrothyroxine.

Other medicines—Although certain medicines should not be used together at all, in other cases two different medicines may be used together even if an interaction might occur. In these cases, your doctor may want to change the dose, or other precautions may be necessary. When you are taking dextrothyroxine, it is especially important that your doctor and pharmacist know if you are taking any of the following:

- Anticoagulants (blood thinners)—The effects of the anticoagulant may be altered; a change in dosage of the anticoagulant may be necessary
- Cholestyramine (e.g., Questran) or
- Colestipol (e.g., Colestid)—The effects of dextrothyroxine may decrease; these two medicines should be taken at least 4 to 5 hours before or after dextrothyroxine

Other medical problems—The presence of other medical problems may affect the use of dextrothyroxine. Make sure you tell your doctor if you have any other medical problems, especially:

- Diabetes mellitus (sugar diabetes)—Blood sugar levels may be increased
- Heart or blood vessel disease or
- High blood pressure or
- Overactive thyroid—Dextrothyroxine may make these conditions worse
- Kidney disease—Higher blood levels of dextrothyroxine may result and increase the chance of side effects
- Liver disease—May lead to an increase in cholesterol blood levels

• Underactive thyroid—There may be an increased sensitivity to the effects of dextrothyroxine

Before you begin using any new medicine (prescription or nonprescription) or if you develop any new medical problem while you are using this medicine, check with your doctor, nurse, or pharmacist.

Proper Use of This Medicine

Take this medicine exactly as directed by your doctor. Try not to miss any doses and do not take more medicine than your doctor ordered.

Remember that this medicine will not cure your cholesterol problem but it does help control it. Therefore, you must continue to take it as directed if you expect to lower your cholesterol level.

Follow carefully the special diet your doctor gave you. This is the most important part of controlling your condition, and is necessary if the medicine is to work properly.

Dosing—The dose of dextrothyroxine will be different for different patients. *Follow your doctor's orders or the directions on the label.* The following information includes only the average doses of dextrothyroxine. *If your dose is different, do not change it* unless your doctor tells you to do so:

- The number of tablets that you take depends on the strength of the medicine.
- For *oral* dosage form (tablets):
  —For treatment of high cholesterol:
    - Adults—1 to 8 milligrams (mg) a day.
    - Children up to two years of age—Use is not recommended.
    - Children two years of age and older—50 to 100 micrograms (0.05 to 0.1 mg) per kilogram of body weight a day.

Missed dose—If you miss a dose of this medicine, take it as soon as possible. However, if it is almost time for your next dose, skip the missed dose and go back to your regular dosing schedule. Do not double doses.

Storage—To store this medicine:

- Keep out of the reach of children.
- Store away from heat and direct light.
- Do not store in the bathroom, near the kitchen sink, or in other damp places. Heat or moisture may cause the medicine to break down.
- Do not keep outdated medicine or medicine no longer needed. Be sure that any discarded medicine is out of the reach of children.

Precautions While Using This Medicine

It is very important that your doctor check your progress at regular visits. This will allow your doctor to see if the medicine is working properly to lower your cholesterol levels and if you should continue to take it.

Do not stop taking this medicine without first checking with your doctor. When you stop taking this medicine, your blood cholesterol levels may increase again. Your doctor may want you to follow a special diet to help prevent this from happening.

Before having any kind of surgery (including dental surgery) or emergency treatment, *tell the medical doctor or dentist in charge that you are taking this medicine.*

Side Effects of This Medicine

Along with its needed effects, a medicine may cause some unwanted effects. Although not all of these side effects may occur, if they do occur they may need medical attention.

Check with your doctor immediately if any of the following side effects occur:

Rare

Chest pain; fast or irregular heartbeat; stomach pain (severe) with nausea and vomiting

Check with your doctor as soon as possible if the following side effects occur, since they may indicate too much medicine is being taken:

Rare

Changes in appetite; changes in menstrual periods; diarrhea; fast or irregular heartbeat; fever; hand tremors; headache; increase in urination; irritability, nervousness, or trouble in sleeping; leg cramps; shortness of breath; skin rash or itching; sweating, flushing, or increased sensitivity to heat; unusual weight loss; vomiting

Other side effects not listed above may also occur in some patients. If you notice any other effects, check with your doctor.

Annual revision: 04/22/93

DEZOCINE Systemic†

A commonly used brand name in the U.S. is Dalgan.

†Not commercially available in Canada.

Description

Dezocine (DEZ-oh-seen) belongs to the group of medicines known as narcotic analgesics (nar-KOT-ik an-al-JEE-zicks). Narcotic analgesics act in the central nervous system (CNS) to relieve pain. Some of their side effects are also caused by actions in the CNS.

Dezocine is available only with your doctor's prescription. It is available in the following dosage form:

Parenteral

- Injection (U.S.)

It is very important that you read and understand the following information. If any of it causes you special concern, check with your doctor. Also, *if you have any questions* or if you want more information about this medicine or your medical problem, *ask your doctor, nurse, or pharmacist.*

Before Using This Medicine

In deciding to use a medicine, the risks of using the medicine must be weighed against the good it will do. This is a decision you and your doctor will make. For dezocine, the following should be considered:

Allergies—Tell your doctor if you have ever had any unusual or allergic reaction to dezocine. Also tell your doctor and pharmacist if you are allergic to any other substances, such as foods, preservatives, or dyes.

Pregnancy—Studies on birth defects with dezocine have not been done in pregnant women. Dezocine did not cause birth defects in animal studies. However, the birth weights of the newborn animals were lower than normal, probably because the pregnant animals ate less than usual.

Too much use of a narcotic during pregnancy may cause the baby to become dependent on the medicine. This may lead to withdrawal side effects after birth. Also, narcotics may cause breathing problems in the newborn infant if taken just before delivery.

Breast-feeding—It is not known whether dezocine passes into the breast milk. However, it has not been reported to cause problems in nursing babies.

Children and teenagers—Studies on this medicine have been done only in adult patients, and there is no specific information about its use in patients up to 18 years of age.

Older adults—Elderly people are especially sensitive to the effects of narcotic analgesics such as dezocine. This may increase the chance of side effects, especially breathing problems, during treatment.

Other medicines—Although certain medicines should not be used together at all, in other cases two different medicines may be used together even if an interaction might occur. In these cases, your doctor may want to change the dose, or other precautions may be necessary. When you are using dezocine, it is especially important that your doctor and pharmacist know if you are taking any of the following:

- Central nervous system (CNS) depressants, including other narcotics, or
- Tricyclic antidepressants (amitriptyline [e.g., Elavil], amoxapine [e.g., Asendin], clomipramine [e.g., Anafranil], desipramine [e.g., Pertofrane], doxepin [e.g., Sinequan], imipramine [e.g., Tofranil], nortriptyline [e.g., Aventyl], protriptyline [e.g., Vivactil], trimipramine [e.g., Surmontil])—The chance of side effects may be increased
- Naltrexone (e.g., Trexan)—Dezocine may not be effective in people taking naltrexone

Other medical problems—The presence of other medical problems may affect the use of dezocine. Make sure you tell your doctor if you have any other medical problems, especially:

- Alcohol abuse, or history of, or
- Drug dependence, especially narcotic abuse, or history of, or
- Emotional problems—The chance of side effects may be increased; also, withdrawal symptoms may occur if a narcotic you are dependent on is replaced by dezocine
- Brain disease or head injury or
- Colitis or other intestinal disease or
- Diarrhea or
- Emphysema, asthma, or other chronic lung disease or
- Enlarged prostate or problems with urination—Some of the side effects of narcotic analgesics can be dangerous if these conditions are present
- Heart or blood vessel disease, severe, or
- Gallbladder disease or gallstones or
- Kidney disease or
- Liver disease or
- Underactive thyroid—The chance of side effects may be increased

Before you begin using any new medicine (prescription or nonprescription) or if you develop any new medical problem while you are using this medicine, check with your doctor, nurse, or pharmacist.

Proper Use of This Medicine

Some narcotic analgesics given by injection may be used at home by patients who do not need to be in the hospital. If you are using dezocine at home, *make sure you clearly understand and carefully follow your doctor's directions.*

Take this medicine only as directed by your doctor. Do not use more of it, do not use it more often, and do not use it for a longer time than your doctor ordered. This is especially important for elderly patients, who are more sensitive than younger adults to the effects of narcotic analgesics. If too much is taken, the medicine may become habit-forming (causing mental or physical dependence) or lead to medical problems because of an overdose.

Missed dose—If your doctor has ordered you to use dezocine according to a regular schedule and you miss a dose, use it as soon as you remember. However, if it is almost time for your next dose, skip the missed dose and go back to your regular dosing schedule. *Do not double doses.*

Storage—To store this medicine:
- Keep out of the reach of children. Overdose is very dangerous in young children.
- Store away from heat and direct light.
- Keep the medicine from freezing.
- Do not keep outdated medicine or medicine no longer needed. Be sure that any discarded medicine is out of the reach of children.

Precautions While Using This Medicine

Dezocine will add to the effects of alcohol and other CNS depressants (medicines that slow down the nervous system, possibly causing drowsiness). Some examples of CNS depressants are antihistamines or medicine for hay fever, other allergies, or colds; sedatives, tranquilizers, or sleeping medicine; other prescription pain medicines including other narcotics; barbiturates; medicine for seizures; muscle relaxants; or anesthetics, including some dental anesthetics. *Do not drink alcoholic beverages, and check with your doctor before taking any of the medicines listed above, while you are using this medicine.*

This medicine may cause some people to become drowsy, dizzy, or lightheaded. *Make sure you know how you react to this medicine before you drive, use machines, or do anything else that could be dangerous if you are dizzy or are not alert.*

Dizziness, lightheadedness, or fainting may occur, especially when you get up suddenly from a lying or sitting position. Getting up slowly may help lessen this problem. Also, lying down for a while may help relieve these effects.

Nausea or vomiting may occur, especially after the first couple of doses. This effect may go away if you lie down for a while. However, if nausea or vomiting continues, check with your doctor.

Before having any kind of surgery (including dental surgery) or emergency treatment, tell the medical doctor or dentist in charge that you are taking this medicine.

If you think you or someone else may have taken an overdose, get emergency help at once. Taking an overdose of this medicine or taking alcohol or CNS depressants with it may lead to unconsciousness or death. Signs of overdose of narcotic analgesics include convulsions (seizures), confusion, severe nervousness or restlessness, severe dizziness, severe drowsiness, slow or troubled breathing, and severe weakness.

Side Effects of This Medicine

Along with its needed effects, a medicine may cause some unwanted effects. Although not all of these side effects may occur, if they do occur they may need medical attention.

Get emergency help immediately if any of the following symptoms of overdose occur:

Cold, clammy skin; confusion, nervousness, or restlessness (severe); convulsions (seizures); dizziness (severe); drowsiness (severe); low blood pressure; pinpoint pupils of eyes; slow heartbeat; slow or troubled breathing; weakness (severe)

Also, check with your doctor as soon as possible if any of the following side effects occur:

Rare

Chest pain; coughing occurring together with breathing problems; difficult, decreased, or frequent urination; difficult, slow, or shallow breathing; increase or decrease in blood pressure; irregular heartbeat; mental depression or other mood or mental changes; skin rash or itching; swelling of face, fingers, lower legs, or feet; weight gain

Other side effects may occur that usually do not need medical attention. These side effects may go away during treatment as your body adjusts to the medicine. However, check with your doctor if any of the following side effects continue or are bothersome:

More common

Drowsiness; nausea or vomiting

Less common or rare

Abdominal or stomach pain; anxiety or crying; blurred or double vision; confusion; constipation; diarrhea; dizziness or lightheadedness; flushing or redness of skin; slurred speech

After you stop using this medicine, your body may need time to adjust. The length of time this takes depends on the amount of medicine you were using and how long you used it. During this period of time check with your doctor if you notice any of the following side effects:

Body aches; diarrhea; fast heartbeat; fever, runny nose, or sneezing; gooseflesh; increased sweating; increased yawning; loss of appetite; nausea or vomiting; nervousness, restlessness, or irritability; shivering or trembling; stomach cramps; trouble in sleeping; unusually large pupils of eyes; weakness

Other side effects not listed above may also occur in some patients. If you notice any other effects, check with your doctor.

Annual revision: 04/05/91

DIAZOXIDE Oral

A commonly used brand name in the U.S. and Canada is Proglycem.

Description

Diazoxide (dye-az-OX-ide) when taken by mouth is used in the treatment of hypoglycemia (low blood sugar). It works by preventing release of insulin from the pancreas.

Diazoxide is available only with your doctor's prescription, in the following dosage forms:

Oral

- Capsules (U.S. and Canada)
- Suspension (U.S. and Canada)

It is very important that you read and understand the following information. If any of it causes you special concern, check with your doctor. Also, *if you have any questions* or if you want more information about this medicine or your medical problem, *ask your doctor, nurse, or pharmacist.*

Before Using This Medicine

In deciding to use a medicine, the risks of taking the medicine must be weighed against the good it will do. This is a decision you and your doctor will make. For diazoxide, the following should be considered:

Allergies—Tell your doctor if you have ever had any unusual or allergic reaction to diazoxide, sulfonamides (sulfa medicine), or thiazide diuretics (certain types of water pills). Also tell your doctor and pharmacist if you are allergic to any other substances, such as foods, preservatives, or dyes.

Pregnancy—Studies have not been done in pregnant women. However, too much use of diazoxide during pregnancy may cause unwanted effects (high blood sugar, loss of hair or increased hair growth, blood problems) in the baby. Studies in animals have shown that diazoxide causes some birth defects (in the skeleton, heart, and pancreas) and other problems (delayed birth, decrease in successful pregnancies).

Breast-feeding—It is not known whether diazoxide passes into breast milk. However, this medicine has not been reported to cause problems in nursing babies.

Children—Infants are more likely to retain (keep) body water because of diazoxide. In some infants, this may lead to certain types of heart problems. Also, a few children who received diazoxide for prolonged periods (longer than 4 years) developed changes in their facial structure.

Older adults—Many medicines have not been tested in older people. Therefore, it may not be known whether they work exactly the same way they do in younger adults or if they cause different side effects or problems in older people. There is no specific information comparing use of oral diazoxide in the elderly with use in other age groups.

Other medicines—Although certain medicines should not be used together at all, in other cases two different medicines may be used together even if an interaction might occur. In these cases, your doctor may want to change the dose, or other precautions may be necessary. When you are taking diazoxide, it is especially important that your doctor and pharmacist know if you are taking any of the following:

- Amantadine (e.g., Symmetrel) or
- Antidepressants (medicine for depression) or
- Antihypertensives (high blood pressure medicine) or
- Antipsychotics (medicines for mental illness) or
- Bromocriptine (e.g., Parlodel) or
- Cyclandelate (e.g., Cyclospasmol) or
- Deferoxamine (e.g., Desferal) or
- Diuretics (water pills) or
- Hydralazine (e.g., Apresoline) or
- Isoxsuprine (e.g., Vasodilan) or
- Levobunolol (e.g., Betagan) (use in the eye) or
- Levodopa (e.g., Dopar) or
- Medicine for heart disease or
- Metipranolol (e.g., OptiPranolol) or
- Nabilone (e.g., Cesamet) (with high doses) or
- Narcotic pain medicine or
- Nicotinyl alcohol (e.g., Roniacol) or
- Nimodipine (e.g., Nimotop) or
- Nylidrin (e.g., Arlidin) or
- Papaverine (e.g., Pavabid) or
- Pentamidine (e.g., Pentam) or
- Pimozide (e.g., Orap) or
- Promethazine (e.g., Phenergan) or
- Timolol (e.g., Timoptic) (use in the eye) or
- Trimeprazine (e.g., Temaril)—Use of any of these medicines with diazoxide may cause low blood pressure

- Ethotoin (e.g., Peganone) or

- Mephenytoin (e.g., Mesantoin) or
- Phenytoin (e.g., Dilantin)—Any of these medicines and diazoxide may be less effective is they are taken at the same time

Other medical problems—The presence of other medical problems may affect the use of diazoxide. Make sure you tell your doctor if you have any other medical problems, especially:

- Angina (chest pain)
- Gout—Diazoxide may make this condition worse
- Heart attack (recent)
- Heart or blood vessel disease
- Kidney disease—The effects of diazoxide may last longer because the kidney may not be able to get the medicine out of the bloodstream as it normally would
- Liver disease
- Stroke (recent)

Before you begin using any new medicine (prescription or nonprescription) or if you develop any new medical problem while you are using this medicine, check with your doctor, nurse, or pharmacist.

Proper Use of This Medicine

Take this medicine only as directed by your doctor. Do not take more or less of it than your doctor ordered, and take it at the same time each day.

Follow carefully the special diet your doctor gave you. This is an important part of controlling your condition, and is necessary if the medicine is to work properly.

Test for sugar in your urine or blood with a diabetic urine or blood test kit as directed by your doctor. This is a convenient way to make sure your condition is being controlled, and it provides an early warning when it is not. Your doctor may also want you to test your urine for acetone.

Missed dose—If you miss a dose of this medicine, take it as soon as possible. However, if it is almost time for your next dose, skip the missed dose and go back to your regular dosing schedule. Do not double doses.

Storage—To store this medicine:

- Keep out of the reach of children.
- Store away from heat and direct light.
- Do not store in the bathroom, near the kitchen sink, or in other damp places. Heat or moisture may cause the medicine to break down.
- Keep the oral liquid form of this medicine from freezing.
- Do not keep outdated medicine or medicine no longer needed. Be sure that any discarded medicine is out of the reach of children.

Precautions While Using This Medicine

It is very important that your doctor check your progress at regular visits, especially during the first few weeks of treatment, to make sure that this medicine is working properly.

Before you have any kind of surgery, dental treatment, or emergency treatment, *tell the medical doctor or dentist in charge that you are using this medicine.*

Do not take any other medicine, unless prescribed or approved by your doctor, since some may interfere with this medicine's effects. This especially includes over-the-counter (OTC) or nonprescription medicine such as that for colds, cough, asthma, hay fever, or appetite control.

Check with your doctor right away if symptoms of high blood sugar (hyperglycemia) occur. These symptoms usually include:

Drowsiness
Flushed, dry skin
Fruit-like breath odor
Increased urination
Loss of appetite (continuing)
Unusual thirst

These symptoms may occur if the dose of the medicine is too high, or if you have a fever or infection or are experiencing unusual stress.

Check with your doctor as soon as possible also if these symptoms of low blood sugar (hypoglycemia) occur:

Anxiety
Chills
Cold sweats
Cool pale skin
Drowsiness
Excessive hunger
Fast pulse
Headache
Nausea
Nervousness
Shakiness
Unusual tiredness or weakness

Symptoms of both low blood sugar and high blood sugar must be corrected before they progress to a more serious condition. In either situation, you should check with your doctor immediately.

Side Effects of This Medicine

Along with its needed effects, a medicine may cause some unwanted effects. Although not all of these side effects may occur, if they do occur they may need medical attention.

Stop taking this medicine and get emergency help immediately if any of the following side effects occur:

Rare

Chest pain caused by exercise or activity; confusion; numbness of the hands; shortness of breath (unexplained)

Check with your doctor as soon as possible if any of the following side effects occur:

More common

Decreased urination; swelling of feet or lower legs; weight gain (rapid)

Less common

Fast heartbeat

Rare

Fever; skin rash; stiffness of arms or legs; trembling and shaking of hands and fingers; unusual bleeding or bruising

Other side effects may occur that usually do not need medical attention. These side effects may go away during treatment as your body adjusts to the medicine. However, check with your doctor if any of the following side effects continue or are bothersome:

Less common

Changes in ability to taste; constipation; increased hair growth on forehead, back, arms, and legs; loss of appetite; nausea and vomiting; stomach pain

This medicine may cause a temporary increase in hair growth in some people when it is used for a long time. After treatment with diazoxide has ended, normal hair growth should return.

Other side effects not listed above may also occur in some patients. If you notice any other effects, check with your doctor.

Annual revision: 12/15/92

DIDANOSINE Systemic

A commonly used brand name in the U.S. and Canada is Videx. Another commonly used name is ddI.

Description

Didanosine (di-DAN-oe-seen) (also known as ddI) is used in the treatment of the infection caused by the human immunodeficiency virus (HIV). HIV is the virus responsible for acquired immune deficiency syndrome (AIDS).

Didanosine (ddI) will not cure or prevent HIV infection or AIDS. It appears to slow down the destruction of the immune system caused by HIV. This may help delay the development of symptoms related to advanced HIV disease. However, it will not keep you from spreading the virus to other people. People who receive this medicine may continue to have the problems usually related to AIDS or HIV disease.

HIV infection can result in a very serious, usually fatal, disease. An estimated 1 to 1.5 million persons in the United States are currently infected with HIV. It has become one of the leading causes of death in men and women under the age of 45 and in children between 1 and 5 years of age.

HIV primarily attacks certain white blood cells and slowly, over several years, breaks down the body's immune system. When this happens, the person may develop other serious infections as well. These include fungus infections, *Pneumocystis* (noo-moe-SISS-tis) *carinii* pneumonia (PCP), and cytomegalovirus (CMV) infections, which can affect the retina of the eyes, the lungs, and the stomach and intestines. The person may also develop certain kinds of cancer, such as non-Hodgkin's lymphoma and Kaposi's sarcoma, a form of cancer usually causing purplish tumors of the skin or mouth. Didanosine may be given with other medicines to treat these problems.

Although most cases of HIV infection in the U.S. have occurred in homosexual and bisexual men, HIV infection has increased most rapidly in people exposed to the virus through heterosexual contact. Other people at risk of contracting HIV are intravenous drug users and their sexual partners, and people who received transfusions with blood or blood products contaminated with the AIDS virus and their sexual partners. Children born to mothers infected with HIV are also at risk of getting the virus.

This virus is spread from person to person by infected body fluids, such as blood, semen, vaginal fluids (including menstrual blood), and breast milk. HIV is almost always spread by the intimate exchange of these fluids that occurs during unprotected sex (vaginal, anal, and possibly oral) with someone who is infected with the virus and/or by sharing contaminated needles and syringes when injecting drugs. HIV is also spread from an infected mother to her fetus during pregnancy or childbirth, and, rarely, through breast-feeding. It is not spread by casual contact, such as touching, shaking hands, coughing, sneezing, or by routine everyday contact, such as working in the same office, going to the same school, or eating in the same restaurant.

HIV can infect people of any age, sex, race, or sexual orientation. Because symptoms may take months, or more often years, to appear, an infected person may look and feel fine. During this time a person may spread the infection to others without knowing it.

The early symptoms of HIV infection may include fever; night sweats; swollen glands in the neck, armpit, and/or groin; unexplained weight loss; profound tiredness; yeast infections in the mouth; diarrhea; continuing cough; weakness; loss of appetite; or, in women, vaginal yeast infections.

Didanosine may cause some serious side effects, including pancreatitis (inflammation of the pancreas). Symptoms of pancreatitis include stomach pain, and nausea and vomiting. Didanosine may also cause peripheral neuropathy. Symptoms of peripheral neuropathy include tingling, burning, numbness, and pain in the hands or feet. *Check with your doctor if any new health problems or symptoms occur while you are taking didanosine.*

Didanosine is available only with your doctor's prescription, in the following dosage forms:

Oral

- Oral solution (U.S.)
- Oral suspension (U.S. and Canada)
- Tablets (U.S. and Canada)

It is very important that you read and understand the following information. If any of it causes you special concern, check with your doctor. Also, *if you have any questions* or if you want more information about this medicine or your medical problem, *ask your doctor, nurse, or pharmacist.*

Before Using This Medicine

In deciding to use a medicine, the risks of taking the medicine must be weighed against the good it will do. This is a decision you and your doctor will make. For didanosine, the following should be considered:

Allergies—Tell your doctor if you have ever had any unusual or allergic reaction to didanosine. Also tell your doctor and pharmacist if you are allergic to any other substances, such as foods, preservatives, or dyes.

Diet—Make certain your doctor and pharmacist know if you are on any special diet, such as a low-sodium or low-phenylalanine diet. Didanosine chewable tablets and the oral solution packets contain a large amount of sodium.

Pregnancy—Didanosine crosses the placenta. Studies in pregnant women have not been done. However, didanosine has not been shown to cause birth defects or other problems in animal studies.

Breast-feeding—It is not known whether didanosine passes into the breast milk. However, if your baby does not already have the AIDS virus, there is a chance that you could pass it to your baby by breast-feeding. Talk to your doctor first if you are thinking about breast-feeding your baby.

Children—Didanosine can cause serious side effects in any patient. Therefore, it is especially important that you discuss with your child's doctor the good that this medicine may do as well as the risks of using it. Your child must be carefully followed, and frequently seen, by the doctor while taking didanosine.

Older adults—Didanosine has not been studied specifically in older people. Therefore, it is not known whether it causes different side effects or problems in the elderly than it does in younger adults.

Other medicines—Although certain medicines should not be used together at all, in other cases 2 different medicines may be used together even if an interaction might occur. In these cases, your doctor may want to change the dose, or other precautions may be necessary. When you are taking didanosine, it is especially important that your doctor and pharmacist know if you are taking any of the following:

- Alcohol or
- Asparaginase (e.g., Elspar) or
- Azathioprine (e.g., Imuran) or
- Estrogens (female hormones) or
- Furosemide (e.g., Lasix) or
- Methyldopa (e.g., Aldomet) or
- Pentamidine (e.g., Pentam, Pentacarinat) or
- Sulfonamides (e.g., Bactrim, Septra) or
- Sulindac (e.g., Clinoril) or
- Thiazide diuretics (e.g., Diuril, Hydrodiuril) or
- Valproic acid (e.g., Depakote)—Use of these medicines with didanosine may increase the chance of pancreatitis (inflammation of the pancreas)
- Chloramphenicol (e.g., Chloromycetin) or
- Cisplatin (e.g., Platinol) or
- Ethambutol (e.g., Myambutol) or
- Ethionamide (e.g., Trecator-SC) or
- Hydralazine (e.g., Apresoline) or
- Isoniazid (e.g., Nydrazid) or
- Lithium (e.g., Eskalith, Lithobid) or
- Metronidazole (e.g., Flagyl) or
- Nitrous oxide or
- Phenytoin (e.g., Dilantin) or
- Vincristine (e.g., Oncovin)—Use of these medicines with didanosine may increase the chance of peripheral neuropathy (tingling, burning, numbness, or pain in your hands or feet)
- Ciprofloxacin (e.g., Cipro) or
- Ketoconazole (e.g., Nizoral) or
- Norfloxacin (e.g., Noroxin) or
- Ofloxacin (e.g., Floxin) or
- Trimethoprim (e.g., Proloprim, Trimpex)—Use of these medicines with didanosine may keep these medicines from working properly; these medicines should be taken at least 2 hours before or 2 hours after taking didanosine
- Dapsone (e.g., Avlosulfon)—Use of dapsone with didanosine may increase the chance of peripheral neuropathy (tingling, burning, numbness, or pain in your hands or feet); it may also keep dapsone from working properly;

dapsone should be taken at least 2 hours before or 2 hours after taking didanosine

- Nitrofurantoin (e.g., Macrodantin)—Use of nitrofurantoin with didanosine may increase the chance of pancreatitis (inflammation of the pancreas) and peripheral neuropathy (tingling, burning, numbness, or pain in your hands or feet)
- Tetracyclines (e.g., Achromycin, Minocin)—Use of tetracyclines with didanosine may increase the chance of pancreatitis (inflammation of the pancreas); it may also keep the tetracycline from working properly; tetracyclines should be taken at least 2 hours before or 2 hours after taking didanosine

Other medical problems—The presence of other medical problems may affect the use of didanosine. Make sure you tell your doctor if you have any other medical problems, especially:

- Alcoholism, active, or
- Increased blood triglycerides or
- Pancreatitis (or a history of)—Patients with these medical problems may be at increased risk of pancreatitis (inflammation of the pancreas)

- Edema or
- Heart disease or
- High blood pressure or
- Kidney disease or
- Liver disease or
- Toxemia of pregnancy—The salt contained in the didanosine tablets and the oral solution packets may make these conditions worse
- Gout—Didanosine may cause an attack or worsen gout
- Peripheral neuropathy—Didanosine may make this condition worse
- Phenyketonuria (PKU)—Didanosine tablets contain phenylalanine, which must be restricted in patients with PKU

Before you begin using any new medicine (prescription or nonprescription) or if you develop any new medical problem while you are using this medicine, check with your doctor, nurse, or pharmacist.

Proper Use of This Medicine

Take this medicine exactly as directed by your doctor. Do not take more of it, do not take it more often, and do not take it for a longer time than your doctor ordered. Also, do not stop taking this medicine without checking with your doctor first.

Keep taking didanosine for the full time of treatment, even if you begin to feel better.

For patients taking *didanosine pediatric oral suspension:*

- Use a specially marked measuring spoon or other device to measure each dose accurately. The average household teaspoon may not hold the right amount of liquid.

For patients taking *didanosine oral solution:*

- Open the foil packet and pour its contents into approximately 1/2 glass (4 ounces) of water. Do not mix with fruit juice or other acid-containing drinks.
- Stir for approximately 2 to 3 minutes until the powder is dissolved.
- Drink at once.

For patients taking *didanosine tablets:*

- Tablets should be thoroughly chewed or crushed or mixed in 1 ounce of water before swallowing. The tablets are hard and some people may find them difficult to chew. If the tablets are mixed in water, stir well until a uniform suspension is formed and taken at once.
- Two tablets must be taken together by patients over 1 year of age. These tablets contain a special buffer to keep didanosine from being destroyed in the stomach. In order to get the correct amount of buffer, 2 tablets always need to be taken together. Infants from 6 to 12 months of age will get enough buffer from just 1 tablet.

Didanosine should be taken on an empty stomach since food may decrease the absorption in the stomach and keep it from working properly. Didanosine should be taken at least 2 hours before or 2 hours after you eat.

This medicine works best when there is a constant amount in the blood. *To help keep the amount constant, do not miss any doses.* If you need help in planning the best times to take your medicine, check with your doctor, nurse, or pharmacist.

Missed dose—If you do miss a dose of this medicine, take it as soon as possible. However, if it is almost time for your next dose, skip the missed dose and go back to your regular dosing schedule. Do not double doses.

Only take medicine that your doctor has prescribed specifically for you. Do not share your medicine with others.

Storage—To store this medicine:

- Keep out of the reach of children.
- Store away from heat and direct light.
- Do not store in the bathroom, near the kitchen sink, or in other damp places. Heat or moisture may cause the medicine to break down.
- Do not keep outdated medicine or medicine no longer needed. Be sure that any discarded medicine is out of the reach of children.

Precautions While Using This Medicine

It is very important that your doctor check your progress at regular visits.

Do not take any other medicines without checking with your doctor first. To do so may increase the chance of side effects from didanosine.

HIV may be acquired from or spread to other people through infected body fluids, including blood, vaginal fluid, or semen. *If you are infected, it is best to avoid any sexual activity involving an exchange of body fluids with other people. If you do have sex, always wear (or have your partner wear) a condom ("rubber").* Only use condoms made of latex, and *use them every time you have vaginal, anal, or oral sex.* The use of a spermicide (such as nonoxynol-9) may also help prevent transmission of HIV if it is not irritating to the vagina, rectum, or mouth. Spermicides have been shown to kill HIV in lab tests. Do not use oil-based Jelly, cold cream, baby oil, or shortening as a lubricant—these products can cause the rubber to break. Lubricants without oil, such as *K-Y jelly* or *CondomMate*, are recommended. Women may wish to carry their own condoms. Birth control pills and diaphragms will help protect against pregnancy, but they will not prevent someone from giving or getting the AIDS virus. *If you inject drugs*, get help to stop. *Do not share needles or equipment with anyone.* In some cities, more than half of the drug users are infected and sharing even 1 needle or syringe can spread the virus. If you have any questions about this, check with your doctor, nurse, or pharmacist.

Side Effects of This Medicine

Along with its needed effects, a medicine may cause some unwanted effects. Although not all of these side effects may occur, if they do occur they may need medical attention.

Check with your doctor immediately if any of the following side effects occur:

Less common

Nausea and vomiting; stomach pain; tingling, burning, numbness, and pain in the hands or feet

Rare

Convulsions (seizures); fever and chills; sore throat; skin rash and itching; unusual bleeding and bruising; unusual tiredness and weakness

Other side effects may occur that usually do not need medical attention. These side effects may go away during treatment as your body adjusts to the medicine. However, check with your doctor if any of the following side effects continue or are bothersome:

More common

Anxiety; diarrhea; difficulty in sleeping; headache; irritability; restlessness

Other side effects not listed above may also occur in some patients. If you notice any other effects, check with your doctor.

Annual revision: 06/24/92

DIETHYLCARBAMAZINE Systemic

A commonly used brand name in Canada is Hetrazan.
A generic name product may be available in the U.S.

Description

Diethylcarbamazine (dye-eth-il-kar-BAM-a-zeen) is used in the treatment of certain worm infections. It is used to treat:

- Bancroft's filariasis;
- Eosinophilic lung (tropical pulmonary eosinophilia; tropical eosinophilia);
- Loiasis; and
- River blindness (onchocerciasis).

It will not work for other kinds of worm infections (for example, pinworms or tapeworms).

Diethylcarbamazine is available only with your doctor's prescription, in the following dosage form:

Oral

- Tablets (U.S. and Canada)

It is very important that you read and understand the following information. If any of it causes you special concern, check with your doctor. Also, *if you have any questions* or if you want more information about this medicine or your medical problem, *ask your doctor, nurse, or pharmacist.*

Before Using This Medicine

In deciding to use a medicine, the risks of taking the medicine must be weighed against the good it will do. This is a decision you and your doctor will make. For diethylcarbamazine, the following should be considered:

Allergies—Tell your doctor if you have ever had any unusual or allergic reaction to diethylcarbamazine. Also tell your doctor and pharmacist if you are allergic to any other substances, such as foods, preservatives, or dyes.

Pregnancy—Treatment of pregnant patients with diethylcarbamazine should be delayed until after delivery. However, diethylcarbamazine has not been shown to cause birth defects or other problems in humans.

Breast-feeding—Diethylcarbamazine has not been reported to cause problems in nursing babies.

Children—There is no specific information comparing use of diethylcarbamazine in children with use in other age groups.

Older adults—Many medicines have not been studied specifically in older people. Therefore, it may not be known whether they work exactly the same way they do in younger adults or if they cause different side effects or problems in older people. There is no specific information comparing use of diethylcarbamazine in the elderly with use in other age groups.

Other medicines—Although certain medicines should not be used together at all, in other cases two different medicines may be used together even if an interaction might occur. In these cases, your doctor may want to change the dose, or other precautions may be necessary. Tell your doctor and pharmacist if you are taking any other prescription or nonprescription (over-the-counter [OTC]) medicine.

Other medical problems—The presence of other medical problems may affect the use of diethylcarbamazine. Make sure you tell your doctor if you have any other medical problems, especially:

- River blindness involving the eyes—Diethylcarbamazine may worsen the eye problems associated with river blindness

Before you begin using any new medicine (prescription or nonprescription) or if you develop any new medical problem while you are using this medicine, check with your doctor, nurse, or pharmacist.

Proper Use of This Medicine

Diethylcarbamazine should be taken immediately after meals.

To help clear up your infection completely, *keep taking this medicine for the full time of treatment*, even if your symptoms begin to clear up after a few days. In some patients, a second course of this medicine may be required to clear up the infection completely. If you stop taking this medicine too soon, your infection may return. *Do not miss any doses.*

Missed dose—If you do miss a dose of this medicine, take it as soon as possible. However, if it is almost time for your next dose, skip the missed dose and go back to your regular dosing schedule. Do not double doses.

Storage—To store this medicine:

- Keep out of the reach of children.
- Store away from heat and direct light.
- Do not store in the bathroom, near the kitchen sink, or in other damp places. Heat or moisture may cause the medicine to break down.
- Do not keep outdated medicine or medicine no longer needed. Be sure that any discarded medicine is out of the reach of children.

Precautions While Using This Medicine

If your symptoms do not improve within a few days, or if they become worse, check with your doctor.

For patients taking diethylcarbamazine for river blindness:

- It is important that your doctor check your progress at regular visits. This is to help make sure that the infection is cleared up completely. Also, your doctor may want you to have your eyes checked by an ophthalmologist (eye doctor).
- Diethylcarbamazine may cause loss of vision, night blindness, or tunnel vision with prolonged use. This medicine may also cause some people to become dizzy. *Make sure you know how you react to this medicine before you drive, use machines, or do anything else that could be dangerous if you are dizzy or are not alert or able to see well.* If these reactions are especially bothersome, check with your doctor.

Side Effects of This Medicine

Along with its needed effects, a medicine may cause some unwanted effects. Although not all of these side effects may occur, if they do occur they may need medical attention.

Check with your doctor immediately if any of the following side effects occur:

More common

Itching and swelling of face, especially eyes

Less common

Fever; painful and tender glands in neck, armpits, or groin; skin rash

Additional side effects may occur if you use this medicine for a long time in the treatment of river blindness. Check with your doctor as soon as possible if any of the following side effects occur:

Loss of vision; night blindness; tunnel vision

Other side effects may occur that usually do not need medical attention. These side effects may go away during treatment as your body adjusts to the medicine. However,

check with your doctor if any of the following side effects continue or are bothersome:

More common

Dizziness; headache; joint pain; unusual tiredness or weakness

Less common

Nausea or vomiting

Other side effects not listed above may also occur in some patients. If you notice any other effects, check with your doctor.

Additional Information

In addition to the above information, for patients taking diethylcarbamazine for river blindness:

- Doctors may also prescribe a corticosteroid (a cortisone-like medicine) for certain patients with river blindness, especially those with severe symptoms. This is to help reduce the inflammation caused by the death of the worms. If your doctor prescribes these two medicines together, it is important to take the corticosteroid along with diethylcarbamazine. Take them exactly as directed by your doctor. Do not miss any doses.

Annual revision: 07/22/92

DIFENOXIN AND ATROPINE Systemic†

A commonly used brand name in the U.S. is Motofen.

†Not commercially available in Canada.

Description

Difenoxin (dye-fen-OX-in) and atropine (A-troe-peen) combination medicine is used along with other measures to treat severe diarrhea. Difenoxin helps stop diarrhea by slowing down the movements of the intestines.

Since difenoxin is chemically related to some narcotics, it may be habit-forming if taken in doses that are larger than prescribed. To help prevent possible abuse, atropine (an anticholinergic) has been added. If higher-than-normal doses of the combination are taken, the atropine will cause unpleasant effects, making it unlikely that such doses will be taken again.

This medicine is available only with your doctor's prescription, in the following dosage form:

Oral

- Tablets (U.S.)

It is very important that you read and understand the following information. If any of it causes you special concern, check with your doctor. Also, *if you have any questions* or if you want more information about this medicine or your medical problem, *ask your doctor, nurse, or pharmacist.*

Before Using This Medicine

In deciding to use a medicine, the risks of taking the medicine must be weighed against the good it will do. This is a decision you and your doctor will make. For difenoxin and atropine, the following should be considered:

Allergies—Tell your doctor if you have ever had any unusual or allergic reaction to difenoxin or atropine. Also tell your doctor and pharmacist if you are allergic to any other substances, such as foods, preservatives, or dyes.

Pregnancy—Studies have not been done in humans. However, studies in rats have shown that difenoxin and atropine combination, when given in doses many times the human dose, increases the delivery time and the chance of death in the newborn.

Breast-feeding—Both difenoxin and atropine pass into the breast milk. Although it is not known how much of these drugs pass into the breast milk, large enough amounts could cause serious effects in the nursing baby. Be sure you have discussed the risks and benefits of this medicine with your doctor.

Children—This medicine should not be used in children. Children, especially very young children or children with Down's syndrome, are very sensitive to the effects of difenoxin and atropine. This may increase the chance of side effects during treatment. Also, the fluid loss caused by diarrhea may result in a severe condition. For this reason, it is very important that a sufficient amount of liquids be given to replace the fluid lost by the body. If you have any questions about this, check with your doctor, nurse, or pharmacist.

Older adults—Shortness of breath or difficulty in breathing may be more likely to occur in elderly patients, who are usually more sensitive than younger adults to the effects of difenoxin. Also, the fluid loss caused by diarrhea may result in a severe condition. For this reason, elderly persons should not take this medicine without first checking with their doctor. It is also very important that a sufficient amount of liquids be taken to replace the fluid lost by the body. If you have any questions about this, check with your doctor, nurse, or pharmacist.

Other medicines—Although certain medicines should not be used together at all, in other cases two different medicines may be used together even if an interaction might occur. In these cases, your doctor may want to change the dose, or other precautions may be necessary. When you are taking difenoxin and atropine, it is especially important that your doctor and pharmacist know if you are taking any of the following:

- Antibiotics, such as cephalosporins (e.g., Ceftin, Keflex), clindamycin (e.g., Cleocin), erythromycins (e.g., E.E.S., PCE), tetracyclines (e.g., Achromycin, Doryx)—These antibiotics may cause diarrhea. Difenoxin and atropine may make the diarrhea caused by antibiotics worse or make it last longer
- Central nervous system (CNS) depressants—Effects, such as drowsiness, of CNS depressants or of difenoxin and atropine may become greater
- Monoamine oxidase (MAO) inhibitors (furazolidone [e.g., Furoxone], isocarboxazid [e.g., Marplan], phenelzine [e.g., Nardil], procarbazine [e.g., Matulane], tranylcypromine [e.g., Parnate])—Taking difenoxin and atropine while you are taking or within 2 weeks of taking monoamine oxidase (MAO) inhibitors may cause severe side effects; these medicines should not be used together
- Naltrexone (e.g., Trexan)—Withdrawal side effects may occur in patients who have become addicted to the difenoxin in this combination medicine; also, naltrexone will make this medicine less effective against diarrhea
- Other anticholinergics (medicine to help reduce stomach acid and abdominal or stomach spasms or cramps)—Use of other anticholinergics with this combination medicine may increase the effects of the atropine in this combination; however, this is not likely to happen with the usual doses of difenoxin and atropine
- Tricyclic antidepressants (amtriptyline [e.g., Elavil], amoxapine [e.g., Asendin], clomipramine [e.g., Anafranil], desipramine [e.g., Pertofrane], doxepin [e.g., Sinequan], imipramine [e.g., Tofranil], nortriptyline [e.g., Aventyl], protriptyline [e.g., Vivactil], trimipramine [e.g., Surmontil])—Effects, such as drowsiness, of tricyclic antidepressants or difenoxin and atropine may become greater; also, taking tricyclic antidepressants with difenoxin and atropine may cause some side effects of these medicines, such as dryness of mouth, to become more severe

Other medical problems—The presence of other medical problems may affect the use of difenoxin and atropine. Make sure you tell your doctor if you have any other medical problems, especially:

- Alcohol abuse (or history of) or
- Drug abuse (history of)—There is a greater chance that this medicine may become habit-forming
- Colitis (severe)—A more serious problem of the colon may develop if you use this medicine
- Down's syndrome (mongolism) in children—Side effects may be more likely and severe in these children
- Dysentery—This condition may get worse; a different kind of treatment may be needed
- Emphysema, asthma, bronchitis, or other chronic lung disease—There is a greater chance that this medicine may cause breathing problems in patients who have any of these conditions
- Enlarged prostate or
- Urinary tract blockage or difficult urination—Problems with urination may develop with the use of this medicine
- Gallbladder disease or gallstones—Use of this medicine may cause spasms of the biliary tract and make the condition worse
- Glaucoma—Severe pain in the eye may occur with the use of this medicine; however, the chance of this happening is low
- Heart disease—This medicine may have some effects on the heart, which may make the condition worse
- Hiatal hernia—This condition may be made worse by the atropine in this medicine; however, the chance of this happening is low
- High blood pressure (hypertension)—The atropine in this medicine may cause an increase in blood pressure; however, the chance of this happening is low
- Kidney disease—The medicine may build up in the body and cause side effects
- Liver disease—The chance of central nervous system (CNS) side effects, including coma, may be greater in patients who have this condition
- Myasthenia gravis—This medicine may make the condition worse
- Overactive or underactive thyroid—Unwanted effects on breathing and heart rate may occur

Before you begin using any new medicine (prescription or nonprescription) or if you develop any new medical problem while you are using this medicine, check with your doctor, nurse, or pharmacist.

Proper Use of This Medicine

If this medicine upsets your stomach, your doctor may want you to take it with food.

Take this medicine only as directed by your doctor. Do not take more of it, do not take it more often, and do not take it for a longer time than your doctor ordered. If too much is taken, it may become habit-forming.

Importance of diet and fluids while treating diarrhea:

- *In addition to using medicine for diarrhea, it is very important that you replace the fluid lost by the body and follow a proper diet.* For the first 24 hours you should drink plenty of caffeine-free clear liquids, such as ginger ale, decaffeinated cola, decaffeinated tea, broth, and gelatin. During the next 24 hours you may eat bland foods, such as cooked cereals, bread, crackers, and applesauce. Fruits, vegetables, fried or spicy foods, bran, candy, caffeine, and alcoholic beverages may make the condition worse.

- If too much fluid has been lost by the body due to the diarrhea a serious condition may develop. Check with your doctor as soon as possible if any of the following signs of too much fluid loss occur:
  Decreased urination
  Dizziness and lightheadedness
  Dryness of mouth
  Increased thirst
  Wrinkled skin

Missed dose—If you are taking this medicine on a regular schedule and you miss a dose, take it as soon as possible. However, if it is almost time for your next dose, skip the missed dose and go back to your regular dosing schedule. Do not double doses.

Storage—To store this medicine:
- Keep out of the reach of children. Overdose is especially dangerous in children.
- Store away from heat and direct light.
- Do not store in the bathroom, near the kitchen sink, or in other damp places. Heat or moisture may cause the medicine to break down.
- Do not keep outdated medicine or medicine no longer needed. Be sure that any discarded medicine is out of the reach of children.

Precautions While Using This Medicine

Your doctor should check your progress at regular visits if you will be taking this medicine regularly for a long time.

Check with your doctor if your diarrhea does not stop after two days or if you develop a fever.

This medicine will add to the effects of alcohol and other CNS depressants (medicines that slow down the nervous system, possibly causing drowsiness). Some examples of CNS depressants are antihistamines or medicine for hay fever, other allergies, or colds; sedatives, tranquilizers, or sleeping medicine; prescription pain medicine or narcotics; barbiturates; medicine for seizures; muscle relaxants; or anesthetics, including some dental anesthetics. *Check with your doctor before taking any of the above while you are taking this medicine.*

If you think you or someone else in your home may have taken an overdose of this medicine, get emergency help at once. Taking an overdose of this medicine may lead to unconsciousness and possibly death. Signs of overdose include severe drowsiness; fast heartbeat; shortness of breath or troubled breathing; and unusual warmth, dryness, and flushing of skin.

Before having any kind of surgery (including dental surgery) or emergency treatment, tell the medical doctor or dentist in charge that you are using this medicine.

This medicine may cause some people to become dizzy, drowsy, or less alert than they are normally. Even if taken at bedtime, it may cause some people to feel drowsy or less alert on arising. *Make sure you know how you react to this medicine before you drive, use machines, or do anything else that could be dangerous if you are dizzy or are not alert.*

Side Effects of This Medicine

Along with its needed effects, a medicine may cause some unwanted effects. Although not all of these side effects may occur, if they do occur they may need medical attention.

When this medicine is used for short periods of time at low doses, side effects usually are rare. However, check with your doctor immediately if any of the following side effects are severe and occur suddenly, since they may be signs of a more severe and dangerous problem with your bowels:

Bloating; constipation; loss of appetite; stomach pain (severe) with nausea and vomiting

Check with your doctor also if any of the following effects occur, since they may be signs of an overdose of this medicine:

Blurred vision (continuing) or changes in near vision; drowsiness (severe); dryness of mouth, nose, and throat (severe); fast heartbeat; shortness of breath or troubled breathing (severe); unusual excitement, nervousness, restlessness, or irritability (especially in children); unusual warmth, dryness, and flushing of skin

Other side effects may occur that usually do not need medical attention. These side effects may go away during treatment as your body adjusts to the medicine. However, check with your doctor if any of the following side effects continue, worsen, or are bothersome:

Less common or rare

Blurred vision; confusion; difficult urination; dizziness or lightheadedness; drowsiness; dryness of skin and mouth; fever; headache; trouble in sleeping; unusual tiredness or weakness

After you stop using this medicine, your body may need time to adjust. The length of time this takes depends on the amount of medicine you were using and how long you used it. During this period of time check with your doctor if you notice any of the following side effects:

Increased sweating; muscle cramps; nausea or vomiting; shivering or trembling; stomach cramps

Other side effects not listed above may also occur in some patients. If you notice any other effects, check with your doctor.

Annual revision: 05/15/91

DIGITALIS MEDICINES Systemic

This information applies to the following medicines:

Digitoxin (di-ji-TOX-in)
Digoxin (di-JOX-in)

Some commonly used brand names are:

For Digitoxin

In the U.S.
Crystodigin

In Canada
Digitaline

Generic name product may also be available.

For Digoxin

In the U.S.
Lanoxicaps
Lanoxin

Generic name product may also be available.

In Canada
Lanoxin
Novodigoxin

Generic name product may also be available.

Description

Digitalis medicines are used to improve the strength and efficiency of the heart, or to control the rate and rhythm of the heartbeat. This leads to better blood circulation and reduced swelling of hands and ankles in patients with heart problems.

Although digitalis has been prescribed to help some patients lose weight, it should *never* be used in this way. When used improperly, digitalis can cause serious problems.

Digitalis medicines are available only with your doctor's prescription, in the following dosage forms:

Oral

Digitoxin
- Tablets (U.S. and Canada)

Digoxin
- Capsules (U.S.)
- Elixir (U.S. and Canada)
- Tablets (U.S. and Canada)

Parenteral

Digoxin
- Injection (U.S. and Canada)

It is very important that you read and understand the following information. If any of it causes you special concern, check with your doctor. Also, *if you have any questions* or if you want more information about this medicine or your medical problem, *ask your doctor, nurse, or pharmacist.*

Before Using This Medicine

In deciding to use a medicine, the risks of taking the medicine must be weighed against the good it will do. This is a decision you and your doctor will make. For digitalis medicines, the following should be considered:

Allergies—Tell your doctor if you have ever had any unusual or allergic reaction to digitalis medicines. Also tell your doctor and pharmacist if you are allergic to any other substances, such as foods, preservatives, or dyes.

Pregnancy—Digitalis medicines pass from the mother to the fetus. However, studies on effects in pregnancy have not been done in either humans or animals. Make sure your doctor knows if you are pregnant or if you may become pregnant before taking digitalis medicines.

Breast-feeding—Although small amounts of digitalis medicines pass into breast milk, they have not been reported to cause problems in nursing babies.

Children—This medicine has been tested in children and, in effective doses, has not been shown to cause different side effects or problems than it does in adults. However, the dose is very different for babies and children, and it is important to follow your doctor's instructions exactly.

Older adults—Signs and symptoms of overdose may be especially likely to occur in elderly patients, who are usually more sensitive than younger adults to the effects of digitalis medicines.

Other medicines—Although certain medicines should not be used together at all, in other cases 2 different medicines may be used together even if an interaction might occur. In these cases, your doctor may want to change the dose, or other precautions may be necessary. When you are taking or receiving digitalis medicines it is especially important that your doctor and pharmacist know if you are taking any of the following:

- Amiodarone (e.g., Cordarone)—May cause levels of digitalis medicines in the body to be higher than usual, which could lead to signs or symptoms of overdose
- Amphetamines or
- Appetite suppressants (diet pills) or
- Digitalis medicines (other) or other heart medicine or
- Medicine for asthma or other breathing problems or
- Medicine for colds, sinus problems, or hay fever or other allergies (including nose drops or sprays)—May increase the risk of heart rhythm problems
- Calcium channel blocking agents (bepridil [e.g., Bepadin, Vascor], diltiazem [e.g., Cardizem, Cardizem CD, Cardizem SR], felodipine [e.g., Plendil], flunarizine [e.g., Sibelium], isradipine [e.g., DynaCirc], nicardipine [e.g., Cardene], nifedipine [e.g., Adalat, Procardia, Procardia XL], nimodipine [e.g., Nimotop], verapamil [e.g., Calan, Calan SR, Isoptin, Isoptin SR, Verelan] or
- Propafenone—May cause levels of digitalis medicines in the body to be higher than usual, which could lead to signs or symptoms of overdose
- Cholestyramine (e.g., Questran) or
- Colestipol (e.g., Colestid) or
- Diarrhea medicine or

- Sucralfate or
- If your diet contains large amounts of fiber, such as bran—May decrease effects of digitalis medicines by keeping them from being absorbed into the body; digitalis medicines should be taken several hours apart from these
- Diuretics (water pills) or
- Other medicines that decrease the amount of potassium in the body (corticosteroids [cortisone-like medicines], alcohol, capreomycin, corticotropin, insulin, laxatives, salicylates [aspirin], vitamin B_{12}, vitamin D [high doses])—These medicines can cause hypokalemia (low levels of potassium in the body), which can increase the unwanted effects of digitalis medicines
- Potassium-containing medicines or supplements—If levels of potassium in the body become too high, there is a serious risk of heart rhythm problems being caused by digitalis medicines
- Quinidine (e.g., Quinidex)—May cause levels of digitalis medicines in the body to be higher than usual, which could lead to signs or symptoms of overdose

Other medical problems—The presence of other medical problems may affect the use of digitalis medicines. Make sure you tell your doctor if you have any other medical problems, especially:

- Heart disease or
- Lung disease (severe)—The heart may be more sensitive to the effects of digitalis medicines
- Heart rhythm problems—Digitalis glycosides may make certain heart rhythm problems worse
- Kidney disease or
- Liver disease—Effects may be increased because of slower removal of digitalis medicines from the body
- Thyroid disease—Patients with low or high thyroid gland activity may be more or less sensitive to the effects of digitalis glycosides

Before you begin using any new medicine (prescription or nonprescription) or if you develop any new medical problem while you are using this medicine, check with your doctor, nurse, or pharmacist.

Proper Use of This Medicine

To keep your heart working properly, *take this medicine exactly as directed even though you may feel well.* Do not take more of it than your doctor ordered and do not miss any doses.

For patients taking the *liquid form of digoxin:*

- This medicine is to be taken by mouth even if it comes in a dropper bottle. The amount you should take is to be measured only with the specially marked dropper.

To help you remember to take your dose of medicine, try to take it at the same time every day.

Ask your doctor about checking your pulse rate. Then, while you are taking this medicine, check your pulse regularly. If it is much slower, or faster, than your usual rate (or less than 60 beats per minute), or if it changes in rhythm or force, check with your doctor. Such changes may mean that side effects are developing.

Dosing—When you are taking digitalis medicines, it is very important that you get the exact amount of medicine that you need. The dose of digitalis medicine will be different for different patients. Your doctor will determine the proper dose of digitalis medicine for you. *Follow your doctor's orders or the directions on the label.*

After you begin taking digitalis medicines, your doctor may sometimes check your blood level of digitalis medicine to find out if your dose needs to be changed. *Do not change your dose of digitalis medicine* unless your doctor tells you to do so.

The number of capsules or tablets or teaspoonfuls of solution that you take depends on the strength of the medicine.

Missed dose—If you do miss a dose of this medicine, and you remember it within 12 hours, take it as soon as you remember. However, if you do not remember until later, do not take the missed dose at all and do not double the next one. Instead, go back to your regular dosing schedule. If you have any questions about this or if you miss doses for 2 or more days in a row, check with your doctor.

Storage—To store this medicine:

- Keep out of the reach of children.
- Store away from heat and direct light.
- Do not store in the bathroom, near the kitchen sink, or in other damp places. Heat or moisture may cause the medicine to break down.
- Keep the oral liquid form of this medicine from freezing.
- Do not keep outdated medicine or medicine no longer needed. Be sure that any discarded medicine is out of the reach of children.

Precautions While Using This Medicine

It is important that your doctor check your progress at regular visits to make sure the medicine is working properly. This will allow your doctor to make any changes in directions for taking it, if necessary.

Do not stop taking this medicine without first checking with your doctor. Stopping suddenly may cause a serious change in heart function.

Keep this medicine out of the reach of children. Digitalis medicines are a major cause of accidental poisoning in children.

Watch for signs and symptoms of overdose while you are taking digitalis medicine. Follow your doctor's directions carefully. The amount of this medicine needed to help most people is very close to the amount that could cause serious problems from overdose. Some early warning signs of overdose are loss of appetite, nausea, vomiting, diarrhea, or extremely slow heartbeat. In infants and small children, the earliest signs of overdose are changes in the rate and rhythm of the heartbeat. Children may not show the other symptoms as soon as adults.

Before having any kind of surgery (including dental surgery) or emergency treatment, tell the medical doctor or dentist in charge that you are using this medicine.

Your doctor may want you to carry a medical identification card or bracelet stating that you are taking this medicine.

Do not take any other medicine unless ordered by your doctor. Many over-the-counter (OTC) or nonprescription medicines contain ingredients that interfere with digitalis medicines or that may make your condition worse. These medicines include antacids; laxatives; asthma remedies; cold, cough, or sinus preparations; medicine for diarrhea; and reducing or diet medicines.

For patients taking the *tablet or capsule* form of this medicine:

- This medicine may look like other tablets or capsules you now take. It is very important that you do not get the medicines mixed up since this may have serious results. Ask your pharmacist for ways to avoid mix-ups with medicines that look alike.

Side Effects of This Medicine

Along with its needed effects, a medicine may cause some unwanted effects. Although not all of these side effects may occur, if they do occur they may need medical attention.

Check with your doctor as soon as possible if any of the following side effects or symptoms of overdose occur:

Rare

Skin rash or hives

Signs and symptoms of overdose (in the order in which they may occur)

Loss of appetite; nausea or vomiting; lower stomach pain; diarrhea;. unusual tiredness or weakness (extreme); slow or irregular heartbeat (may be fast heartbeat in children); blurred vision or "yellow, green, or white vision" (yellow, green, or white halo seen around objects); drowsiness; confusion or mental depression; headache; fainting

Note: Overdose symptoms in infants and small children may occur at first only as changes in the heartbeat rate or rhythm, while in adults and older children the first symptoms may be mostly stomach upset, stomach pain, loss of appetite, or unusually slow heartbeat.

Other side effects not listed above may also occur in some patients. If you notice any other effects, check with your doctor.

Annual revision: 03/10/93

DIMETHYL SULFOXIDE Mucosal

A commonly used brand name in the U.S. and Canada is Rimso-50.
Another commonly used name is DMSO.
Generic name product may also be available in the U.S.

Description

Dimethyl sulfoxide (dye-METH-il sul-FOX-ide) is a purified preparation used in the bladder to relieve the symptoms of the bladder condition called interstitial cystitis. A catheter (tube) or syringe is used to put the solution into the bladder where it is allowed to remain for about 15 minutes. Then, the solution is expelled by urinating.

Interstitial cystitis is the only human use for dimethyl sulfoxide that is approved by the U.S. Food and Drug Administration (FDA).

Claims that dimethyl sulfoxide is effective for treating various types of arthritis, ulcers in scleroderma, muscle sprains and strains, bruises, infections of the skin, burns, wounds, and mental conditions have not been proven.

Although other preparations of dimethyl sulfoxide are available for industrial and veterinary (animal) use, they must not be used by humans, because of their unknown purity. Impurities in these preparations may cause serious unwanted effects in humans. Even if dimethyl sulfoxide is applied to the skin, it is absorbed into the body through the skin and mucous membranes.

This medicine is available only with your doctor's prescription, in the following dosage form:

Topical

- Bladder irrigation (U.S. and Canada)

It is very important that you read and understand the following information. If any of it causes you special concern, check with your doctor. Also, *if you have any questions* or if you want more information about this medicine or your medical problem, *ask your doctor, nurse, or pharmacist.*

Before Using This Medicine

In deciding to use a medicine, the risks of taking the medicine must be weighed against the good it will do. This is a decision you and your doctor will make. For dimethyl sulfoxide, the following should be considered:

Allergies—Tell your doctor if you have ever had any unusual or allergic reaction to dimethyl sulfoxide. Also tell your doctor and pharmacist if you are allergic to any other substances, such as preservatives.

Pregnancy—Dimethyl sulfoxide has not been studied in pregnant women. However, some studies in animals have shown that dimethyl sulfoxide causes birth defects when used on the skin and when given in high doses by injection. Before using this medicine, make sure your doctor knows if you are pregnant or if you may become pregnant.

Breast-feeding—Dimethyl sulfoxide is absorbed into the body. It is not known whether dimethyl sulfoxide passes into the breast milk. However, this medicine has not been reported to cause problems in nursing babies.

Children—Studies on this medicine have been done only in adult patients, and there is no specific information comparing use of this medicine in children with use in other age groups.

Older adults—Many medicines have not been studied specifically in older people. Therefore, it may not be known whether they work exactly the same way they do in younger adults or if they cause different side effects or problems in older people. There is no specific information comparing use of this medicine in the elderly with use in other age groups.

Other medicines—Although certain medicines should not be used together at all, in other cases two different medicines may be used together even if an interaction might occur. In these cases, your doctor may want to change the dose, or other precautions may be necessary. Tell your doctor and pharmacist if you are using any other prescription or nonprescription (over-the-counter [OTC]) medicine.

Before you begin using any new medicine (prescription or nonprescription) or if you develop any new medical problem while you are using this medicine, check with your doctor, nurse, or pharmacist.

Side Effects of This Medicine

Along with its needed effects, a medicine may cause some unwanted effects. Although not all of these side effects may occur, if they do occur they may need medical attention.

Check with your doctor immediately if any of the following side effects occur:

Nasal congestion; shortness of breath or troubled breathing; skin rash, hives, or itching; swelling of face

Some patients may have some discomfort during the time this medicine is being put into the bladder. However, the discomfort usually becomes less each time the medicine is used.

Dimethyl sulfoxide may cause you to have a garlic-like taste within a few minutes after the medicine is put into the bladder. This effect may last for several hours. It may also cause your breath and skin to have a garlic-like odor, which may last up to 72 hours.

Other side effects not listed above may also occur in some patients. If you notice any other effects, check with your doctor.

Annual revision: 03/04/92

DINOPROST Intra-amniotic*

A commonly used brand name in Canada is Prostin F_2 Alpha.

*Not commercially available in the U.S.

Description

Dinoprost (DYE-noe-prost) is used to cause abortion during the second trimester of pregnancy. It may also be used for other purposes as determined by your doctor.

Dinoprost is to be administered only by or under the immediate care of your doctor. It is available in the following dosage form:

Parenteral

- Injection (Canada)

It is very important that you read and understand the following information. If any of it causes you special concern, check with your doctor. Also, *if you have any questions* or if you want more information about this medicine or your medical problem, *ask your doctor, nurse, or pharmacist.*

Before Receiving This Medicine

In deciding to use a medicine, the risks of taking the medicine must be weighed against the good it will do.

This is a decision you and your doctor will make. For dinoprost, the following should be considered:

Allergies—Tell your doctor if you have ever had any unusual or allergic reaction to dinoprost or other oxytocics (medicines that stimulate the uterus to contract). Also tell your doctor and pharmacist if you are allergic to any other substances, such as foods, preservatives, or dyes.

Other medicines—Although certain medicines should not be used together at all, in other cases two different medicines may be used together even if an interaction might occur. In these cases, your doctor may want to change the dose, or other precautions may be necessary. Tell your doctor if you are taking any prescription or nonprescription (over-the-counter [OTC]) medicine.

Other medical problems—The presence of other medical problems may affect the use of dinoprost. Make sure you tell your doctor if you have any other medical problems, especially:

- Anemia (history of)—In some patients, abortion with dinoprost may result in loss of blood that may require a transfusion
- Asthma (or history of) or
- Lung disease—Dinoprost may cause narrowing of the blood vessels in the lungs or narrowing of the lung passages
- Diabetes mellitus (sugar diabetes) (history of)
- Epilepsy (or history of)—Rarely, dinoprost has been reported to cause seizures in patients who have epilepsy
- Fibroid tumors of the uterus or
- Uterus surgery (history of)—There is an increased risk of rupture of the uterus
- Glaucoma—Rarely the pressure within the eye has increased and constriction of the pupils has occurred during the use of dinoprost
- Heart or blood vessel disease (or history of) or
- High blood pressure (history of) or
- Low blood pressure (history of)—Dinoprost may cause changes in heart function or blood pressure changes
- Jaundice (history of)
- Kidney disease (or history of)
- Liver disease (or history of)—The body may not get dinoprost out of the bloodstream at the usual rate, which may make the medicine work longer or cause toxic effects

Side Effects of This Medicine

Along with its needed effects, a medicine may cause some unwanted effects. Although not all of these side effects may occur, if they do occur they may need medical attention.

Tell the doctor or nurse immediately if any of the following side effects occur:

Less common or rare

Chest pain; coughing (sudden); cramping of the uterus (continuing and severe); fast heartbeat; hives; numbness in legs or other body parts; pale, cool, or blotchy skin on arms or legs; pressing or painful feeling in chest; redness and itching of skin; shortness of breath; slow or irregular heartbeat; swelling of eyelids, face, or inside of nose; tightness in chest; trouble in breathing; weak or absent pulse in arms or legs; wheezing

Also, check with the doctor or nurse as soon as possible if any of the following side effects occur:

Less common or rare

Abdominal or stomach pain (severe or continuing); blood in urine; constipation; decreased frequency of urination; difficult or painful urination; double vision or burning eyes; pain in legs, back, or shoulder; tender or mildly bloated abdomen

Other side effects may occur that usually do not need medical attention. These side effects usually go away after the medicine is stopped. However, let the doctor or nurse know if any of the following side effects continue or are bothersome:

More common

Diarrhea; nausea; stomach cramps or pain; vomiting

Less common

Anxiety; breast fullness or tenderness; burning feeling in breasts; chills or shivering; cough (continuing); dizziness; drowsiness; fever (temporary); flushing or redness of face; headache; hiccups; increased sweating; inflammation and pain at place of injection; unusual thirst

After the procedure has been completed, this procedure may still produce some side effects that need medical attention. Check with your doctor if you notice any of the following side effects:

Chills or shivering (continuing); fever (continuing); foul-smelling vaginal discharge; pain in lower abdomen; unusual increase in uterus bleeding

Other side effects not listed above may also occur in some patients. If you notice any other effects, check with your doctor or nurse.

Additional Information

Once a medicine has been approved for marketing for a certain use, experience may show that it is also useful for other medical problems. Although these uses are not specifically included in product labeling, dinoprost is used in certain patients for the following medical procedures:

- Angiography (x-ray pictures of the blood vessels)
- Inducing labor

Other than the above information, there is no additional information relating to proper use, precautions, or side effects for these uses.

Annual revision: 10/26/92

DINOPROSTONE Cervical/Vaginal

Some commonly used brand names are:

In the U.S.
Prostin E_2

In Canada
Prepidil

Description

Dinoprostone (dye-noe-PROST-one) is an oxytocic, which means it acts by causing the cervix to dilate (open) and the uterus to contract (cramp) the way it does during labor.

Dinoprostone may also be used for other purposes as determined by your doctor.

Dinoprostone is to be administered only by or under the immediate care of your doctor. It is available in the following dosage forms:

Cervical
- Gel (Canada)

Vaginal
- Gel (Canada)
- Suppositories (U.S.)

It is very important that you read and understand the following information. If any of it causes you special concern, check with your doctor. Also, *if you have any questions* or if you want more information about this medicine or your medical problem, *ask your doctor, nurse, or pharmacist.*

Before Receiving This Medicine

In deciding to use a medicine, the risks of taking the medicine must be weighed against the good it will do. This is a decision you and your doctor will make. For dinoprostone, the following should be considered:

Allergies—Tell your doctor if you have ever had any unusual or allergic reaction to dinoprostone or other oxytocics (drugs that stimulate the uterus to contract).

Other medicines—Although certain medicines should not be used together at all, in other cases two different medicines may be used together even if an interaction might occur. In these cases, your doctor may want to change the dose, or other precautions may be necessary. When you are receiving dinoprostone, it is especially important that your doctor knows if you are using any other vaginal prescription or nonprescription (over-the-counter [OTC]) medicine.

Other medical problems—The presence of other medical problems may affect the use of dinoprostone. Make sure you tell your doctor if you have any other medical problems, especially:

- Anemia (or history of)—Abortion with dinoprostone may result in loss of blood in some patients that may require a transfusion
- Asthma (or history of) or
- Lung disease—Dinoprostone may cause narrowing of the blood vessels in the lungs or narrowing of the lung passages
- Epilepsy (or history of)—Rarely, seizures have occurred with the use of dinoprostone
- Fibroid tumors of the uterus or
- Uterus surgery (history of)—There is an increased risk of rupture of the uterus
- Glaucoma—Rarely, the pressure within the eye has increased and constriction of the pupils has occurred during the use of dinoprostone
- Heart or blood vessel disease (or history of) or
- High blood pressure (or history of) or
- Low blood pressure (history of)—Dinoprostone may cause changes in heart function or blood pressure changes; 2 cases of a heart attack have occurred during the use of dinoprostone in patients with a history of heart disease
- Kidney disease (or history of) or
- Liver disease (or history of)—The body may not get dinoprostone out of the blood stream at the usual rate, which may make the dinoprostone work longer or cause an increased chance of side effects

Proper Use of This Medicine

After the suppository, cervical gel, or vaginal gel is inserted into the vagina, you will need to lie down so that the medicine can be absorbed. The length of time you must remain lying down will depend on what form of the drug you are using.

Side Effects of This Medicine

Along with its needed effects, a medicine may cause some unwanted effects. Although not all of these side effects may occur, if they do occur they may need medical attention.

Tell the doctor or nurse immediately if any of the following side effects occur:

Less common or rare

Fast or slow heartbeat; hives; increased pain of the uterus; pale, cool, blotchy skin on arms or legs; pressing or painful feeling in chest; shortness of breath; swelling of face, inside the nose, and eyelids; tightness in chest; trouble in breathing; weak or absent pulse in arms or legs; wheezing

Other side effects may occur that usually do not need medical attention. These side effects usually go away after the medicine is stopped. However, let the doctor or nurse know if any of the following side effects continue or are bothersome:

More common

Abdominal or stomach cramps; diarrhea; fever; nausea; vomiting

Less common or rare

Chills or shivering; constipation; flushing; headache; swelling of the vulva; tender or mildly bloated abdomen or stomach

This procedure may still result in some effects, which occur after the procedure is completed, that need medical attention. Check with your doctor if any of the following side effects occur:

Chills or shivering (continuing); fever (continuing); foul-smelling vaginal discharge; pain in lower abdomen; unusual increase in bleeding of the uterus

Other side effects not listed above may also occur in some patients. If you notice any other effects, check with your doctor or nurse.

Annual revision: 10/26/92

DIPHENIDOL Systemic†

A commonly used brand name in the U.S. is Vontrol.
Another commonly used name is difenidol.

†Not commercially available in Canada.

Description

Diphenidol (dye-FEN-i-dole) is used to relieve or prevent nausea, vomiting, and dizziness caused by certain medical problems.

Diphenidol is available only with your doctor's prescription in the following dosage form:

Oral

- Tablets (U.S.)

It is very important that you read and understand the following information. If any of it causes you special concern, check with your doctor. Also, *if you have any questions* or if you want more information about this medicine or your medical problem, *ask your doctor, nurse, or pharmacist.*

Before Using This Medicine

In deciding to use a medicine, the risks of taking the medicine must be weighed against the good it will do. This is a decision you and your doctor will make. For diphenidol, the following should be considered:

Allergies—Tell your doctor if you have ever had any unusual or allergic reaction to diphenidol. Also tell your doctor and pharmacist if you are allergic to any other substances, such as foods, preservatives, or dyes.

Pregnancy—Diphenidol has not been shown to cause birth defects or other problems in human or animal studies.

Breast-feeding—Diphenidol has not been reported to cause problems in nursing babies.

Children—There is no specific information comparing use of diphenidol for dizziness in children with use in other age groups. Also, there is no specific information about the use of diphenidol for nausea and vomiting in children who weigh less than 22.8 kg (50 lbs).

Older adults—Many medicines have not been studied specifically in older people. Therefore, it may not be known whether they work exactly the same way they do in younger adults or if they cause different side effects or problems in older people. There is no specific information comparing use of diphenidol in the elderly with use in other age groups.

Other medicines—Although certain medicines should not be used together at all, in other cases 2 different medicines may be used together even if an interaction might occur. In these cases, your doctor may want to change the dose, or other precautions may be necessary. When you are taking diphenidol, it is especially important that your doctor and pharmacist know if you are taking any of the following:

- Central nervous system (CNS) depressants (medicine that causes drowsiness) or
- Tricyclic antidepressants (medicine for depression)—Using these medicines with diphenidol may increase the CNS depressant effects

Other medical problems—The presence of other medical problems may affect the use of diphenidol. Make sure you tell your doctor if you have any other medical problems, especially:

- Enlarged prostate or
- Glaucoma or
- Intestinal blockage or
- Low blood pressure or
- Stomach ulcer—Diphenidol may make the condition worse
- Kidney disease or
- Urinary tract blockage—Higher blood levels of diphenidol may occur, increasing the chance of side effects

Before you begin using any new medicine (prescription or nonprescription) or if you develop any new medical problem while you are using this medicine, check with your doctor, nurse, or pharmacist.

Proper Use of This Medicine

If you are taking diphenidol to prevent nausea and vomiting, it may be taken with food or a glass of water or milk to lessen stomach irritation, unless otherwise directed by your doctor. However, if you are already suffering from nausea and vomiting, it is best to keep the stomach empty, and this medicine should be taken only with a small amount of water.

Take this medicine only as directed. Do not take more of it and do not take it more often than directed by your doctor. To do so may increase the chance of side effects.

Dosing—The dose of diphenidol will be different for different patients. *Follow your doctor's orders or the directions on the label.* The following information includes only the average doses of diphenidol. *If your dose is different, do not change it* unless your doctor tells you to do so.

- The number of tablets that you take depends on the strength of the medicine. Also, *the number of doses you take each day, the time allowed between doses, and the length of time you take the medicine depend on the medical problem for which you are taking diphenidol.*
- For *oral* dosage forms (tablets):
  —Adults: 25 to 50 milligrams (mg) every four hours as needed.
  —Children: The dose is based on body weight and must be determined by the doctor.

Missed dose—If your doctor has ordered you to take this medicine on a regular schedule and you miss a dose, take it as soon as possible. However, if it is almost time for your next dose, skip the missed dose and go back to your regular dosing schedule. Do not double doses.

Storage—To store this medicine:

- Keep out of the reach of children.
- Store away from heat and direct light.
- Do not store the tablet form of this medicine in the bathroom, near the kitchen sink, or in other damp places. Heat or moisture may cause the medicine to break down.
- Do not keep outdated medicine or medicine no longer needed. Be sure that any discarded medicine is out of the reach of children.

Precautions While Using This Medicine

This medicine will add to the effects of alcohol and other CNS depressants (medicines that slow down the nervous system, possibly causing drowsiness). Some examples of CNS depressants are antihistamines or medicine for hay fever, other allergies, or colds; sedatives, tranquilizers, or sleeping medicine; prescription pain medicine or narcotics; barbiturates; medicine for seizures; muscle relaxants; or anesthetics, including some dental anesthetics. *Check with your doctor before taking any of the above while you are using this medicine.*

This medicine may cause some people to have blurred vision or to become dizzy, drowsy or less alert than they are normally. *Make sure you know how you react to this medicine before you drive, use machines, or do anything else that could be dangerous if you are dizzy or are not alert or able to see well.*

Side Effects of This Medicine

Along with its needed effects, a medicine may cause some unwanted effects. Although not all of these side effects may occur, if they do occur they may need medical attention.

Check with your doctor as soon as possible if any of the following side effects occur:

Rare

Confusion; hallucinations (seeing, hearing, or feeling things that are not there)

Symptoms of overdose

Drowsiness (severe); shortness of breath or troubled breathing; unusual tiredness or weakness (severe)

Other side effects may occur that usually do not need medical attention. These side effects may go away during treatment as your body adjusts to the medicine. However, check with your doctor if any of the following side effects continue or are bothersome:

More common

Drowsiness

Less common or rare

Blurred vision; dizziness; dryness of mouth; headache; heartburn; nervousness, restlessness, or trouble in sleeping; skin rash; stomach upset or pain; unusual tiredness or weakness

Other side effects not listed above may also occur in some patients. If you notice any other effects, check with your doctor.

Annual revision: 04/16/93

DIPHENOXYLATE AND ATROPINE Systemic†

Some commonly used brand names are:

In the U.S.

Diphenatol	Lomotil
Lofene	Lonox
Logen	Lo-Trol
Lomanate	Nor-Mil

Generic name product may also be available.

†Not commercially available in Canada.

Description

Diphenoxylate (dye-fen-OX-i-late) and atropine (A-troe-peen) is a combination medicine used along with other measures to treat severe diarrhea. Diphenoxylate helps stop diarrhea by slowing down the movements of the intestines.

Since diphenoxylate is chemically related to some narcotics, it may be habit-forming if taken in doses that are larger than prescribed. To help prevent possible abuse, atropine (an anticholinergic) has been added. If higher than normal doses of the combination are taken, the atropine will cause unpleasant effects, making it unlikely that such doses will be taken again.

This medicine is available only with your doctor's prescription in the following dosage forms:

Oral

- Oral solution (U.S.)
- Tablets (U.S.)

It is very important that you read and understand the following information. If any of it causes you special concern, check with your doctor. Also, *if you have any questions* or if you want more information about this medicine or your medical problem, *ask your doctor, nurse, or pharmacist.*

Before Using This Medicine

In deciding to use a medicine, the risks of taking the medicine must be weighed against the good it will do. This is a decision you and your doctor will make. For diphenoxylate and atropine, the following should be considered:

Allergies—Tell your doctor if you have ever had any unusual or allergic reaction to diphenoxylate or atropine. Also tell your doctor and pharmacist if you are allergic to any other substances, such as foods, preservatives, or dyes.

Pregnancy—Studies have not been done in humans. In animal studies this medicine given in larger doses than the usual human dose has not been shown to cause birth defects. However, some studies in rats have shown that this medicine reduces the weight gain of the pregnant rat and lessens the chance of conceiving or becoming pregnant when given in doses many times the usual human dose.

Breast-feeding—Although both diphenoxylate and atropine pass into the breast milk, this medicine has not been shown to cause problems in nursing babies.

Children—This medicine should not be used in children under 2 years of age. Children, especially very young children or children with Down's syndrome, are very sensitive to the effects of diphenoxylate and atropine. This may increase the chance of side effects during treatment. Also, the fluid loss caused by diarrhea may result in a severe condition. For this reason, it is very important that a sufficient amount of liquids be given to replace the fluid lost by the body. If you have any questions about this, check with your doctor, nurse, or pharmacist.

Older adults—Shortness of breath or difficulty in breathing may be especially likely to occur in elderly patients, who are usually more sensitive than younger adults to the effects of diphenoxylate. Also, the fluid loss caused by diarrhea may result in a severe condition. For this reason, elderly persons should not take this medicine without first checking with their doctor. It is also very important that a sufficient amount of liquids be taken to replace the fluid lost by the body. If you have any questions about this, check with your doctor, nurse, or pharmacist.

Other medicines—Although certain medicines should not be used together at all, in other cases two different medicines may be used together even if an interaction might occur. In these cases, your doctor may want to change the dose, or other precautions may be necessary. When you are taking diphenoxylate and atropine, it is especially important that your doctor and pharmacist know if you are taking any of the following:

- Antibiotics, such as cephalosporins (e.g., Ceftin, Keflex), clindamycin (e.g., Cleocin), erythromycins (e.g., E.E.S., PCE), tetracyclines (e.g., Achromycin, Doryx)—These antibiotics may cause diarrhea. Diphenoxylate and atropine may make the diarrhea caused by antibiotics worse or make it last longer
- Central nervous system (CNS) depressants—Effects, such as drowsiness, of CNS depressants or of diphenoxylate and atropine may become greater
- Monoamine oxidase (MAO) inhibitors (furazolidone [e.g., Furoxone], isocarboxazid [e.g., Marplan], phenelzine [e.g., Nardil], procarbazine [e.g., Matulane], tranylcypromine [e.g., Parnate])—Taking diphenoxylate and atropine while you are taking or within 2 weeks of taking monoamine oxidase (MAO) inhibitors may cause severe side effects; these medicines should not be used together
- Naltrexone (e.g., Trexan)—Withdrawal side effects may occur in patients who have become addicted to the diphenoxylate in this combination medicine; also, naltrexone will make this medicine less effective against diarrhea

- Other anticholinergics (medicine to help reduce stomach acid and abdominal or stomach spasms or cramps)—Use of other anticholinergics with this combination medicine may increase the effects of the atropine in this combination; however, this is not likely to happen with the usual doses of diphenoxylate and atropine
- Tricyclic antidepressants (amtriptyline [e.g., Elavil], amoxapine [e.g., Asendin], clomipramine [e.g., Anafranil], desipramine [e.g., Pertofrane], doxepin [e.g., Sinequan], imipramine [e.g., Tofranil], nortriptyline [e.g., Aventyl], protriptyline [e.g., Vivactil], trimipramine [e.g., Surmontil])—Effects, such as drowsiness, of tricyclic antidepressants or diphenoxylate and atropine may become greater; also, taking tricyclic antidepressants with diphenoxylate and atropine may cause some side effects of these medicines, such as dryness of mouth, to become more severe

Other medical problems—The presence of other medical problems may affect the use of diphenoxylate and atropine. Make sure you tell your doctor if you have any other medical problems, especially:

- Alcohol abuse (or history of) or
- Drug abuse (history of)—There is a greater chance that this medicine will become habit-forming
- Colitis (severe)—A more serious problem of the colon may develop if you use this medicine
- Down's syndrome (mongolism) in children—Side effects may be more likely and severe in these children
- Dysentery—This condition may get worse; a different kind of treatment may be needed
- Emphysema, asthma, bronchitis, or other chronic lung disease—There is a greater chance that this medicine may cause serious breathing problems in patients who have any of these conditions
- Enlarged prostate or
- Urinary tract blockage or difficult urination—Severe problems with urination may develop with the use of this medicine
- Gallbladder disease or gallstones—Use of this medicine may cause spasms of the biliary tract and make the condition worse
- Glaucoma—Severe pain in the eye may occur with the use of this medicine; however, the chance of this happening is low
- Heart disease—This medicine may have some effects on the heart, which may make the condition worse
- Hiatal hernia—This condition may be made worse by the atropine in this medicine; however, the chance of this happening is low
- High blood pressure (hypertension)—The atropine in this medicine may cause an increase in blood pressure; however, the chance of this happening is low
- Kidney disease—The medicine may build up in the body and cause side effects
- Liver disease—The chance of central nervous system (CNS) side effects, including coma, may be greater in patients who have this condition
- Myasthenia gravis—This medicine may make the condition worse
- Overactive or underactive thyroid—Unwanted effects on breathing and heart rate may occur

Before you begin using any new medicine (prescription or nonprescription) or if you develop any new medical problem while you are using this medicine, check with your doctor, nurse, or pharmacist.

Proper Use of This Medicine

If this medicine upsets your stomach, your doctor may want you to take it with food.

Take this medicine only as directed by your doctor. Do not take more of it, do not take it more often, and do not take it for a longer time than your doctor ordered. If too much is taken, it may become habit-forming, or may cause overdose in a child.

For patients taking the liquid form of this medicine:

- This medicine is to be taken by mouth even if it comes in a dropper bottle. The amount to be taken is to be measured with the specially marked dropper.

Importance of diet and fluids while treating diarrhea:

- *In addition to using medicine for diarrhea, it is very important that you replace the fluid lost by the body and follow a proper diet.* For the first 24 hours you should drink plenty of caffeine-free clear liquids, such as ginger ale, decaffeinated cola, decaffeinated tea, broth, and gelatin. During the next 24 hours you may eat bland foods, such as cooked cereals, bread, crackers, and applesauce. Fruits, vegetables, fried or spicy foods, bran, candy, caffeine, and alcoholic beverages may make the condition worse.
- If too much fluid has been lost by the body due to the diarrhea a serious condition may develop. Check with your doctor as soon as possible if any of the following signs of too much fluid loss occur:

  Decreased urination
  Dizziness and lightheadedness
  Dryness of mouth
  Increased thirst
  Wrinkled skin

Missed dose—If you are taking this medicine on a regular schedule and you miss a dose, take it as soon as possible. However, if it is almost time for your next dose, skip the missed dose and go back to your regular dosing schedule. Do not double doses.

Storage—To store this medicine:

- Keep out of the reach of children since overdose is especially dangerous in children.
- Store away from heat and direct light.
- Do not store the tablet form of this medicine in the bathroom, near the kitchen sink, or in other damp places. Heat or moisture may cause the medicine to break down.

- Keep the liquid form of this medicine from freezing.
- Do not keep outdated medicine or medicine no longer needed. Be sure that any discarded medicine is out of the reach of children.

Precautions While Using This Medicine

Your doctor should check your progress at regular visits if you will be taking this medicine regularly for a long time.

Check with your doctor if your diarrhea does not stop after two days or if you develop a fever.

This medicine will add to the effects of alcohol and other CNS depressants (medicines that slow down the nervous system, possibly causing drowsiness). Some examples of CNS depressants are antihistamines or medicine for hay fever, other allergies, or colds; sedatives, tranquilizers, or sleeping medicine; prescription pain medicine or narcotics; barbiturates; medicine for seizures; muscle relaxants; or anesthetics, including some dental anesthetics. *Check with your doctor before taking any of the above while you are taking this medicine.*

If you think you or anyone else may have taken an overdose, get emergency help at once. Taking an overdose of this medicine may lead to unconsciousness and possibly death. Signs of overdose include severe drowsiness; shortness of breath or troubled breathing; fast heartbeat; and unusual warmth, dryness, and flushing of the skin.

Before having any kind of surgery (including dental surgery) or emergency treatment, tell the medical doctor or dentist in charge that you are taking this medicine.

This medicine may cause some people to become dizzy, drowsy, or less alert than they are normally. Even if taken at bedtime, it may cause some people to feel drowsy or less alert on arising. *Make sure you know how you react to this medicine before you drive, use machines, or do anything else that could be dangerous if you are dizzy or are not alert.*

Side Effects of This Medicine

Along with its needed effects, a medicine may cause some unwanted effects. Although not all of these side effects may occur, if they do occur they may need medical attention.

When this medicine is used for short periods of time at low doses, side effects usually are rare. However, check with your doctor immediately if any of the following side effects are severe and occur suddenly, since they may be signs of a more severe and dangerous problem with your bowels:

Bloating; constipation; loss of appetite; stomach pain (severe) with nausea and vomiting

Check with your doctor immediately also if the following effects occur, since they may be signs of an overdose of this medicine:

Blurred vision (continuing) or changes in near vision; drowsiness (severe); dryness of mouth, nose, and throat (severe); fast heartbeat; shortness of breath or troubled breathing (severe); unusual excitement, nervousness, restlessness, or irritability (especially in children); unusual warmth, dryness, and flushing of the skin

Other side effects may occur that usually do not need medical attention. These side effects may go away during treatment as your body adjusts to the medicine. However, check with your doctor if any of the following side effects continue, worsen, or are bothersome:

Less common or rare

Blurred vision; difficult urination; dizziness or lightheadedness; drowsiness; dryness of skin and mouth; fever; headache; mental depression; numbness of hands or feet; skin rash or itching; swelling of the gums

After you stop using this medicine, your body may need time to adjust. The length of time this takes depends on the amount of medicine you were using and how long you used it. During this time check with your doctor if you notice any of the following side effects:

Rare

Increased sweating; muscle cramps; nausea or vomiting; shivering or trembling; stomach cramps

Other side effects not listed above may also occur in some patients. If you notice any other effects, check with your doctor.

Annual revision: 05/15/91

DIPHTHERIA AND TETANUS TOXOIDS AND PERTUSSIS VACCINE ADSORBED Systemic

Some commonly used brand names in the U.S. are Acel-Imune, Tri-Immunol, and Tripedia.

Other commonly used names are acellular DTP, DTaP, DTP, DTwP, and whole-cell DTP.

Generic name product may also be available in the U.S. and Canada.

Description

Diphtheria (dif-THEER-ee-a) and Tetanus (TET-n-us) Toxoids and Pertussis (per-TUSS-iss) Vaccine (also known as DTP) is a combination immunizing agent given by injection to prevent diphtheria, tetanus, and pertussis.

Diphtheria is a serious illness that can cause breathing difficulties, heart problems, nerve damage, pneumonia, and possibly death. The risk of serious complications and death is greater in very young children and in the elderly.

Tetanus (also known as lockjaw) is a serious illness that causes convulsions (seizures) and severe muscle spasms that can be strong enough to cause bone fractures of the spine. Tetanus causes death in 30 to 40 percent of cases.

Pertussis (also known as whooping cough) is a serious disease that causes severe spells of coughing that can interfere with breathing. Pertussis can also cause pneumonia, long-lasting bronchitis, seizures, brain damage, and death.

Immunization against diphtheria, tetanus, and pertussis is recommended for all infants and children from 6 or 8 weeks of age up until their 7th birthday. Children 7 years of age and older and adults should receive immunizing agents that contain only diphtheria and tetanus toxoids and not pertussis vaccine. Persons should receive the diphtheria and tetanus injections every 10 years for the rest of their lives.

Diphtheria, tetanus, and pertussis are serious diseases that can cause life-threatening illnesses. Although some serious side effects can occur after a dose of DTP (usually from the pertussis vaccine in DTP), this rarely happens. The chance of your child catching one of these diseases and being permanently injured or dying as a result is much greater than the chance of your child getting a serious side effect from the DTP vaccine.

DTP is available in the following dosage form:

Parenteral

- Injection (U.S. and Canada)

It is very important that you read and understand the following information. If any of it causes you special concern, check with your doctor. Also, *if you have any questions* or if you want more information about this medicine or your medical problem, *ask your doctor, nurse, or pharmacist.*

Before Receiving This Vaccine

In deciding to use a medicine, the risks of taking the medicine must be weighed against the good it will do. This is a decision you and your doctor will make. For DTP, the following should be considered:

Allergies—Tell your doctor if your child has ever had any unusual or allergic reaction to diphtheria toxoid, tetanus toxoid, pertussis vaccine, or DTP. Also tell your doctor and pharmacist if your child is allergic to any other substances, such as preservatives.

Other medical problems—The presence of other medical problems may affect the use of DTP. Make sure you tell your doctor if your child has any other medical problems, especially:

- Brain disease or
- Central nervous system (CNS) disease or
- Epilepsy or
- Fever or
- Spasms or
- Seizures (convulsions)—Use of DTP may make the condition worse or may increase the chance of side effects

Precautions After Receiving This Vaccine

At the time of the DTP injection, your doctor may give your child a dose of acetaminophen (or another medicine that helps prevent fever). This is to help prevent some of the side effects of DTP. Your doctor may also want your child to take this medicine every 4 hours for 24 hours after your child receives the DTP injection. Check with your doctor if you have any questions.

Side Effects of This Vaccine

Along with its needed effects, a vaccine may cause some unwanted effects. Although not all of these side effects may occur, if they do occur they may need medical attention. *It is very important that you tell your doctor about any side effect that occurs after a dose of DTP*, even though the side effect may have gone away without treatment. Some types of side effects may mean that your child should not receive any more doses of DTP.

Get emergency help immediately if any of the following side effects occur:

Rare

Collapse; confusion; convulsions (seizures); crying for three or more hours; difficulty in breathing or swallowing; fever of 40.5 °C (105 °F) or more; headache (severe or continuing); hives; irritability (unusual); itching, especially of feet or hands; periods of unconsciousness or lack of awareness; reddening of skin, especially around ears; sleepiness (unusual and continuing); swelling of eyes, face, or inside of nose; unusual tiredness, weakness, or limpness (sudden and severe); vomiting (severe or continuing)

Other side effects may occur that usually do not need medical attention. These side effects may go away as your child's body adjusts to the vaccine. However, check with your doctor if any of the following side effects continue or are bothersome:

More common

Fever between 38 and 39 °C (100.4 and 102.2 °F) (may occur with fretfulness, drowsiness, vomiting, and loss of appetite); lump at place of injection (may be present for a few weeks after injection); redness, swelling, tenderness, or pain at place of injection

Less common

Fever between 39 and 40 °C (102.2 and 104 °F) (may occur with fretfulness, drowsiness, vomiting, and loss of appetite)

Rare

Fever between 40 and 40.5 °C (104 and 105 °F) (may occur with fretfulness, drowsiness, vomiting, and loss of appetite); skin rash; swollen glands on side of neck (following DTP injection into arm)

Other side effects not listed above may also occur in some patients. If you notice any other effects, check with your doctor.

Annual revision: 06/09/93

DIPIVEFRIN Ophthalmic

Some commonly used brand names are:

In the U.S.

Propine C Cap B.I.D.

In Canada

Propine C Cap B.I.D.
Propine C Cap Q.I.D.

Another commonly used name is dipivefrine.

Description

Dipivefrin (dye-PI-ve-frin) is used to treat certain types of glaucoma.

This medicine is available only with your doctor's prescription, in the following dosage form:

Ophthalmic

- Ophthalmic solution (eye drops) (U.S. and Canada)

It is very important that you read and understand the following information. If any of it causes you special concern, check with your doctor. Also, *if you have any questions* or if you want more information about this medicine or your medical problem, *ask your doctor, nurse, or pharmacist.*

Before Using This Medicine

In deciding to use a medicine, the risks of taking the medicine must be weighed against the good it will do. This is a decision you and your doctor will make. For dipivefrin, the following should be considered:

Allergies—Tell your doctor if you have ever had any unusual or allergic reaction to dipivefrin. Also tell your doctor and pharmacist if you are allergic to any other substances, such as preservatives.

Pregnancy—Dipivefrin has not been studied in pregnant women. However, this medication has not been shown to cause birth defects or other problems in animal studies.

Breast-feeding—Dipivefrin may be absorbed into the body, but it is not known whether dipivefrin passes into the breast milk.

Children—Although there is no specific information comparing use of this medicine in children with use in other age groups, this medicine is not expected to cause different side effects or problems in children than it does in adults.

Older adults—Many medicines have not been studied specifically in older people. Therefore, it may not be known whether they work exactly the same way they do in younger adults. Although there is no specific information comparing use of this medicine in the elderly with use in other age groups, this medicine is not expected to cause different side effects or problems in older people than it does in younger adults.

Other medicines—Although certain medicines should not be used together at all, in other cases two different medicines may be used together even if an interaction might occur. In these cases, your doctor may want to change the dose, or other precautions may be necessary. Tell your doctor and pharmacist if you are using any other prescription or nonprescription (over-the-counter [OTC]) medicine.

Other medical problems—The presence of other medical problems may affect the use of dipivefrin. Make sure you tell your doctor if you have any other medical problems, especially:

- Eye disease or problems (other)—Dipivefrin may make the condition worse

Before you begin using any new medicine (prescription or nonprescription) or if you develop any new medical problem while you are using this medicine, check with your doctor, nurse, or pharmacist.

Proper Use of This Medicine

Use this medicine only as directed. Do not use more of it and do not use it more often than your doctor ordered. To do so may increase the chance of too much medicine being absorbed into the body and the chance of side effects.

To use:

- First, wash your hands. With the middle finger, apply pressure to the inside corner of the eye (and continue to apply pressure for 1 or 2 minutes after the medicine has been placed in the eye). Tilt the head back and with the index finger of the same hand, pull the lower eyelid away from the eye to form a pouch. Drop the medicine into the pouch and gently close the eyes. Do not blink. Keep the eyes closed for 1 or 2 minutes to allow the medicine to be absorbed.
- Immediately after using the eye drops, wash your hands to remove any medicine that may be on them.
- To keep the medicine as germ-free as possible, do not touch the applicator tip to any surface (including the eye). Also, keep the container tightly closed.
- If you are using the medicine with the compliance cap (C Cap):

  —Before using the eye drops for the first time, make sure the number 1 or the correct day of the week appears in the window on the cap.

  —Remove the cap and use the eye drops as directed.

  —Replace the cap. Holding the cap between your thumb and forefinger, rotate the bottle until the cap clicks to the next station. This will tell you your next dose.

  —After every dose, rotate the bottle until the cap clicks to the position that tells you your next dose.

Missed dose—If you miss a dose of this medicine, apply the missed dose as soon as possible. However, if it is almost time for your next dose, skip the missed dose and go back to your regular dosing schedule. Do not double doses.

Storage—To store this medicine:

- Keep out of the reach of children.
- Store away from heat and direct light.
- Keep the medicine from freezing.
- Do not keep outdated medicine or medicine no longer needed. Be sure that any discarded medicine is out of the reach of children.

Precautions While Using This Medicine

Your doctor should check your eye pressure at regular visits.

Side Effects of This Medicine

Along with its needed effects, a medicine may cause some unwanted effects. Although not all of these side effects may occur, if they do occur they may need medical attention.

Check with your doctor as soon as possible if either of the following side effects occurs:

Rare—Signs and symptoms of too much medicine being absorbed into the body

Fast or irregular heartbeat; increase in blood pressure

Other side effects may occur that usually do not need medical attention. These side effects may go away during treatment as your body adjusts to the medicine. However, check with your doctor if any of the following side effects continue or are bothersome:

Less common

Burning, stinging, or other eye irritation; increased sensitivity of eyes to light

Other side effects not listed above may also occur in some patients. If you notice any other effects, check with your doctor.

Annual revision: 05/14/92

DIPYRIDAMOLE Diagnostic

Some commonly used brand names are:

In the U.S.

Dipridacot
I.V. Persantine
Persantine

Generic name product may also be available.

In Canada

Apo-Dipyridamole
Novodipiradol
Persantine

Description

Dipyridamole is used as part of a medical test that shows how well blood is flowing to your heart. The test can show your doctor whether any of the blood vessels that bring blood to the heart are blocked or in danger of becoming blocked. Your doctor can then decide on the best treatment for you. Exercise (for example, walking on a treadmill) is usually used to give your doctor this information. Dipyridamole is used instead of exercise for people who are not able to exercise at all, or cannot exercise hard enough.

For information on other uses of dipyridamole, see Dipyridamole (Therapeutic).

Dipyridamole is available only with your doctor's prescription, in the following dosage forms:

Oral
- Tablets (U.S. and Canada)

Parenteral
- Injection (U.S. and Canada)

Before Having This Test

In deciding to use a diagnostic test, any risks of the test must be weighed against the good it will do. This is a decision you and your doctor will make. Also, test results may be affected by other things. For dipyridamole, the following should be considered:

Allergies—Tell your doctor if you have ever had any unusual or allergic reaction to dipyridamole. Also tell your doctor and pharmacist if you are allergic to any other substances, such as foods, preservatives, or dyes.

Pregnancy—Although studies have not been done in pregnant women, dipyridamole has not been reported to cause birth defects or other problems. Also, dipyridamole has not been shown to cause birth defects or other problems in mice, rats, or rabbits given many times the maximum human dose.

Breast-feeding—Although dipyridamole passes into breast milk, it has not been reported to cause problems in nursing babies.

Children—This medicine has been tested only in adults, and there is no specific information comparing use of dipyridamole in children with use in other age groups.

Older adults—Dipyridamole for diagnostic use has been tested in older people. It has not been shown to cause different side effects or problems in older people than it does in younger adults.

Other medicines—Although certain medicines should not be used together at all, in other cases two different medicines may be used together even if an interaction might occur. In these cases, your doctor may want to change the dose, or other precautions may be necessary. Before you receive dipyridamole, it is especially important that your doctor knows if you are taking any of the following:
- Aminophylline (e.g., Somophyllin) or
- Caffeine (e.g., NoDoz) or
- Dyphylline (e.g., Lufyllin) or
- Oxtriphylline (e.g., Choledyl) or
- Theophylline (e.g., Somophyllin-T)—These medicines will interfere with the results of this test. Caffeine should not be taken for 8 to 12 hours before the test. It is present in many medicines (for example, stay-awake products, pain relievers, and medicines for relieving migraine headaches) and foods or beverages (for example, coffee, tea, colas or other soft drinks, cocoa, and chocolate). If you are not sure whether any medicine you are taking contains caffeine, check with your pharmacist

The other medicines listed here are used to treat asthma or other lung or breathing problems. They should not be taken for about 36 hours before the test. However, *do not stop taking the medicine on your own.* Instead, at least 3 or 4 days before the test, tell the doctor in charge of giving the test that you are taking the medicine. He or she can call the doctor who ordered the medicine for you, and together they will decide whether you should stop taking the medicine for a while
- Anticoagulants (blood thinners) or
- Aspirin or
- Carbenicillin by injection (e.g., Geopen) or
- Cefamandole (e.g., Mandol) or
- Cefoperazone (e.g., Cefobid) or
- Cefotetan (e.g., Cefotan) or
- Divalproex (e.g., Depakote) or
- Heparin or
- Inflammation or pain medicine, except narcotics, or
- Moxalactam (e.g., Moxam) or
- Pentoxifylline (e.g., Trental) or
- Plicamycin (e.g., Mithracin) or
- Sulfinpyrazone (e.g., Anturane) or
- Ticarcillin (e.g., Ticar) or
- Ticlopidine (e.g., Ticlid) or
- Valproic acid (e.g., Depakene)—The chance of bleeding may be increased

Other medical problems—The presence of other medical problems may affect the use of dipyridamole. Make sure you tell your doctor if you have any other medical problems, especially:
- Asthma or history of or
- Chest pain—The chance of side effects may be increased
- Low blood pressure—Large amounts of dipyridamole can make your condition worse

Side Effects of This Medicine

Along with its needed effects, a medicine may cause some unwanted effects. Although not all of these side effects may occur, if they do occur they may need medical attention.

While you are receiving dipyridamole, and for a while after you have received it, your doctor will closely follow its effects. If necessary, your doctor can give you a medicine that will stop any unwanted effects. *Tell your doctor right away if you notice any of the following side effects:*

More common

Chest pain

Less common or rare

Headache (severe and throbbing); shortness of breath, troubled breathing, tightness in chest, or wheezing

Other side effects may occur that usually do not need medical attention. These side effects may go away in a little while. However, check with your doctor if they continue or are bothersome:

More common

Dizziness or lightheadedness; headache

Less common

Flushing; nausea or vomiting

Other side effects not listed above may also occur in some patients. If you notice any other effects, check with your doctor.

Annual revision: 01/30/92

DIPYRIDAMOLE Therapeutic

Some commonly used brand names are:

In the U.S.

Dipridacot — Persantine

Generic name product may also be available.

In Canada

Apo-Dipyridamole — Persantine

Novodipiradol

Description

Dipyridamole (dye-peer-ID-a-mole) is used to lessen the chance of stroke or other serious medical problems that may occur when a blood vessel is blocked by blood clots. It is given only when there is a larger-than-usual chance that these problems may occur. For example, it is given to people who have had diseased heart valves replaced by mechanical valves, because dangerous blood clots are especially likely to occur in these patients. Dipyridamole works by helping to prevent dangerous blood clots from forming.

Dipyridamole may also be used for other heart and blood conditions as determined by your doctor.

Dipyridamole is also sometimes used as part of a medical test that shows how well blood is flowing to your heart. For information on this use of dipyridamole, see Dipyridamole (Diagnostic).

Dipyridamole is available only with your doctor's prescription, in the following dosage forms:

Oral

- Tablets (U.S. and Canada)

Parenteral

- Injection (Canada)

It is very important that you read and understand the following information. If any of it causes you special concern, check with your doctor. Also, *if you have any questions* or if you want more information about this medicine or your medical problem, *ask your doctor, nurse, or pharmacist.*

Before Using This Medicine

In deciding to use a medicine, the risks of taking the medicine must be weighed against the good it will do. This is a decision you and your doctor will make. For dipyridamole, the following should be considered:

Allergies—Tell your doctor if you have ever had any unusual or allergic reaction to dipyridamole. Also tell your doctor and pharmacist if you are allergic to any other substances, such as foods, preservatives, or dyes.

Pregnancy—Although studies have not been done in pregnant women, dipyridamole has not been reported to cause birth defects or other problems. Also, dipyridamole has not been shown to cause birth defects or other problems in mice, rats, or rabbits given many times the maximum human dose.

Breast-feeding—Although dipyridamole passes into breast milk, it has not been reported to cause problems in nursing babies.

Children—This medicine has been tested only in adults, and there is no specific information comparing use of dipyridamole in children with use in other age groups.

Older adults—Dipyridamole has not been studied specifically in older people taking the medicine regularly to prevent blood clots from forming. Although there is no specific information comparing this use of dipyridamole in the elderly with use in other age groups, it is not expected to cause different side effects or problems in older people than it does in younger adults.

Other medicines—Although certain medicines should not be used together at all, in other cases two different medicines may be used together even if an interaction might occur. In these cases, your doctor may want to change the dose, or other precautions may be necessary. When you are taking dipyridamole, it is especially important that your doctor and pharmacist know if you are taking any of the following:

- Anticoagulants (blood thinners) or
- Aspirin or
- Carbenicillin by injection (e.g., Geopen) or
- Cefamandole (e.g., Mandol) or
- Cefoperazone (e.g., Cefobid) or
- Cefotetan (e.g., Cefotan) or
- Divalproex (e.g., Depakote) or
- Heparin or
- Inflammation or pain medicine, except narcotics, or
- Moxalactam (e.g., Moxam) or
- Pentoxifylline (e.g., Trental) or
- Plicamycin (e.g., Mithracin) or

- Sulfinpyrazone (e.g., Anturane) or
- Ticarcillin (e.g., Ticar) or
- Ticlopidine (e.g., Ticlid) or
- Valproic acid (e.g., Depakene)—The chance of bleeding may be increased

Other medical problems—The presence of other medical problems may affect the use of dipyridamole. Make sure you tell your doctor if you have any other medical problems, especially:

- Chest pain—The chance of side effects may be increased
- Low blood pressure—Large amounts of dipyridamole can make your condition worse

Before you begin using any new medicine (prescription or nonprescription) or if you develop any new medical problem while you are using this medicine, check with your doctor, nurse, or pharmacist.

Proper Use of This Medicine

This medicine works best when there is a constant amount in the blood. To help keep the amount constant, *dipyridamole must be taken in regularly spaced doses,* as ordered by your doctor.

This medicine works best when taken with a full glass (8 ounces) of water at least 1 hour before or 2 hours after meals. However, to lessen stomach upset, your doctor may want you to take the medicine with food or milk.

Missed dose—If you miss a dose of this medicine, take it as soon as possble. However, if it is within 4 hours of your next scheduled dose, skip the missed dose and go back to your regular dosing schedule. Do not double doses.

Storage—To store this medicine:

- Keep out of the reach of children.
- Store away from heat and direct light.
- Do not store in the bathroom, near the kitchen sink, or in other damp places. Heat or moisture may cause the medicine to break down.
- Do not keep outdated medicine or medicine no longer needed. Be sure that any discarded medicine is out of the reach of children.

Precautions While Using This Medicine

Dipyridamole is sometimes used together with an anticoagulant (blood thinner) or aspirin. The combination of medicines may provide better protection against the formation of blood clots than any of the medicines used alone. However, the risk of bleeding may also be increased. To reduce the risk of bleeding:

- *Do not take aspirin, or any combination medicine containing aspirin, unless the same doctor who directed you to take dipyridamole also directs you to take aspirin.* This is especially important if you are taking an anticoagulant together with dipyridamole.
- If you have been directed to take aspirin together with dipyridamole, *take only the amount of aspirin ordered by your doctor.* If you need a medicine to relieve pain or a fever, your doctor may not want you to take extra aspirin. It is a good idea to discuss this with your doctor, so that you will know ahead of time what medicine to take.
- Your doctor should check your progress at regular visits.

Tell all medical doctors and dentists you go to that you are taking dipyridamole, and whether or not you are taking an anticoagulant (blood thinner) or aspirin together with it.

Dizziness, lightheadedness, or fainting may occur, especially when you get up from a lying or sitting position. Getting up slowly may help. If this problem continues or gets worse, check with your doctor.

Side Effects of This Medicine

Along with its needed effects, a medicine may cause some unwanted effects. Although not all of these side effects may occur, if they do occur they may need medical attention.

Check with your doctor as soon as possible if the following side effect occurs shortly after you start taking this medicine:

Less common

Skin rash or itching

Rare

Chest pain or tightness in chest

Other side effects may occur that usually do not need medical attention. These side effects may go away during treatment as your body adjusts to the medicine. However, check with your doctor if they continue or are bothersome:

More common

Dizziness

Less common

Flushing; headache; nausea or vomiting; stomach cramping; weakness

Other side effects not listed above may also occur in some patients. If you notice any other effects, check with your doctor.

Annual revision: 01/30/92

DISOPYRAMIDE Systemic

Some commonly used brand names are:

In the U.S.
- Norpace
- Norpace CR

Generic name product may also be available.

In Canada
- Norpace
- Norpace CR
- Rythmodan
- Rythmodan-LA

Description

Disopyramide (dye-soe-PEER-a-mide) is used to correct irregular heartbeats to a normal rhythm and to slow an overactive heart. This allows the heart to work more efficiently.

Disopyramide is available only with your doctor's prescription, in the following dosage forms:

Oral
- Capsules (U.S. and Canada)
- Extended-release capsules (U.S.)
- Extended-release tablets (Canada)

Parenteral
- Injection (Canada)

It is very important that you read and understand the following information. If any of it causes you special concern, check with your doctor. Also, *if you have any questions* or if you want more information about this medicine or your medical problem, *ask your doctor, nurse, or pharmacist.*

Before Using This Medicine

In deciding to use a medicine, the risks of taking the medicine must be weighed against the good it will do. This is a decision you and your doctor will make. For disopyramide, the following should be considered:

Allergies—Tell your doctor if you have ever had any unusual or allergic reaction to disopyramide. Also tell your doctor and pharmacist if you are allergic to any other substance, such as foods, preservatives, or dyes.

Pregnancy—Disopyramide has not been studied in pregnant women. However, use of disopyramide in a small number of pregnant women seems to show that this medicine may cause contractions of the uterus. Studies in animals have shown that disopyramide increases the risk of miscarriages. Before taking this medicine, make sure your doctor knows if you are pregnant or if you may become pregnant.

Breast-feeding—Disopyramide passes into breast milk.

Children—This medicine has been tested in children and has not been shown to cause different side effects or problems than it does in adults.

Older adults—Some side effects, such as difficult urination and dry mouth, may be especially likely to occur in elderly patients, who are usually more sensitive than younger adults to the effects of disopyramide.

Other medicines—Although certain medicines should not be used together at all, in other cases two different medicines may be used together even if an interaction might occur. In these cases, your doctor may want to change the dose, or other precautions may be necessary. When you are taking disopyramide, it is especially important that your doctor and pharmacist know if you are taking any of the following:

- Other heart medicine—Effects on the heart may be increased
- Pimozide (e.g., Orap)—Risk of heart rhythm problems may be increased

Other medical problems—The presence of other medical problems may affect the use of disopyramide. Make sure you tell your doctor if you have any other medical problems, especially:

- Diabetes mellitus (sugar diabetes)—Disopyramide may cause low blood sugar
- Difficult urination or
- Enlarged prostate—Disopyramide may cause difficult urination
- Glaucoma (history of) or
- Myasthenia gravis—Disopyramide may make these conditions worse
- Kidney disease or
- Liver disease—Effects may be increased because of slower removal of disopyramide from the body

Before you begin using any new medicine (prescription or nonprescription) or if you develop any new medical problem while you are using this medicine, check with your doctor, nurse, or pharmacist.

Proper Use of This Medicine

Take disopyramide exactly as directed by your doctor even though you may feel well. Do not take more medicine than ordered.

For patients taking the *extended-release capsules:*
- Swallow the capsule whole without breaking, crushing, or chewing.

For patients taking the *extended-release tablets:*
- Do not crush or chew the tablet.

This medicine works best when there is a constant amount in the blood. *To help keep the amount constant, do not miss any doses. Also, it is best to take the doses at evenly spaced times day and night.* For example, if you are to take 4 doses a day, the doses should be spaced about 6 hours apart. If this interferes with your sleep or other daily activities, or if you need help in planning the best times to take your medicine, check with your doctor, nurse, or pharmacist.

Dosing—The dose of disopyramide will be different for different patients. *Follow your doctor's orders or the directions on the label.* The following information includes only the average doses of disopyramide. *If your dose is different, do not change it* unless your doctor tells you to do so:

- The number of tablets or capsules that you take depends on the strength of the medicine.
- For *treatment* of arrhythmias:
  - —For *short-acting oral* dosage forms (capsules):
    - Adults—300 milligrams (mg) for the first dose. Then 100 to 150 mg taken every six to eight hours.
    - Children—Dose is based on body weight and age. It must be determined by your doctor. The dose is usually 6 to 30 mg per kilogram (kg) of body weight (2.73 to 13.64 mg per pound) per day. This dose is evenly divided and taken every six hours.
  - —For *long-acting oral* dosage forms (extended-release capsules or tablets):
    - Adults—200 or 300 mg every twelve hours.
    - Children—Use is not recommended.
  - —For *injection* dosage form:
    - Adults—
      - —*First few doses:* Dose is based on body weight and must be determined by your doctor. It is usually 2 mg per kg of body weight (0.91 mg per pound) injected in three divided doses, or, 2 mg per kg of body weight (0.91 mg per pound) infused over fifteen minutes.
      - —*Dose following first few doses:* Dose is based on body weight and must be determined by your doctor. It is usually 0.4 mg per kg of body weight (0.18 mg per pound) per hour given for up to twenty-four hours.
    - Children—Use is not recommended.

Missed dose—*If you do miss a dose of this medicine, take it as soon as possible unless the next scheduled dose is in less than 4 hours.* If you do not remember until later, skip the missed dose and go back to your regular dosing schedule. Do not double doses.

Storage—To store this medicine:

- Keep out of the reach of children.
- Store away from heat and direct light.
- Do not store in the bathroom, near the kitchen sink, or in other damp places. Heat or moisture may cause the medicine to break down.
- Do not keep outdated medicine or medicine no longer needed. Be sure that any discarded medicine is out of the reach of children.

Precautions While Using This Medicine

Your doctor should check your progress at regular visits to make sure the medicine is working properly.

Do not stop taking this medicine without first checking with your doctor. Stopping suddenly may cause a serious change in heart function.

Dizziness, lightheadedness, or fainting may occur, especially when you get up from a lying or sitting position. This is due to lowered blood pressure. Getting up slowly may help. This effect does not occur often at doses of disopyramide usually used; however, *make sure you know how you react to this medicine before you drive, use machines, or do anything else that could be dangerous if you are not alert.* If the problem continues or gets worse, check with your doctor.

Avoid alcoholic beverages until you have discussed their use with your doctor. Alcohol may make the low blood sugar effect worse and/or increase the possibility of dizziness or fainting.

Disopyramide may cause hypoglycemia (low blood sugar) in some people. Patients with congestive heart disease or diabetes especially should be aware of the signs of hypoglycemia. (See *Side Effects of This Medicine.*) *If these signs appear, eat or drink a food containing sugar and call your doctor right away.*

This medicine may cause blurred vision or other vision problems. If any of these occur, *do not drive, use machines, or do anything else that could be dangerous if you are not able to see well.*

Disopyramide may cause dryness of the mouth, nose, and throat. For temporary relief of mouth dryness, use sugarless candy or gum, melt bits of ice in your mouth, or use a saliva substitute. However, if dry mouth continues for more than 2 weeks, check with your medical doctor or dentist. Continuing dryness of the mouth may increase the chance of dental disease, including tooth decay, gum disease, and fungus infections.

This medicine will often make you sweat less, allowing your body temperature to increase. *Use extra care not to become overheated during exercise or hot weather while you are taking this medicine,* since overheating could possibly result in heat stroke.

Side Effects of This Medicine

Along with its needed effects, a medicine may cause some unwanted effects. Although not all of these side effects

may occur, if they do occur they may need medical attention.

Check with your doctor as soon as possible if any of the following side effects occur:

More common

Difficult urination

Less common

Chest pains; dizziness, lightheadedness, or fainting; fast or slow heartbeat; muscle weakness; shortness of breath (unexplained); swelling of feet or lower legs; weight gain (rapid)

Rare

Eye pain; mental depression; sore throat and fever; yellow eyes or skin

Signs and symptoms of hypoglycemia (low blood sugar)

Anxious feeling; chills; cold sweats; confusion; cool, pale skin; drowsiness; fast heartbeat; headache; hunger (excessive); nausea; nervousness; shakiness; unsteady walk; unusual tiredness or weakness

Other side effects may occur that usually do not need medical attention. These side effects may go away during treatment as your body adjusts to the medicine. However, check with your doctor or nurse if any of the following side effects continue or are bothersome:

More common

Dryness of mouth and throat

Less common

Bloating or stomach pain; blurred vision; constipation; decreased sexual ability; dry eyes and nose; frequent urge to urinate; loss of appetite

Other side effects not listed above may also occur in some patients. If you notice any other effects, check with your doctor.

Annual revision: 05/14/93

DISULFIRAM Systemic

A commonly used brand name in the U.S. and Canada is Antabuse. Generic name product may also be available in the U.S.

Description

Disulfiram (dye-SUL-fi-ram) is used to help overcome your drinking problem. It is not a cure for alcoholism, but rather will discourage you from drinking.

Disulfiram is available only with your doctor's prescription, in the following dosage form:

Oral

- Tablets (U.S. and Canada)

It is very important that you read and understand the following information. If any of it causes you special concern, check with your doctor. Also, *if you have any questions* or if you want more information about this medicine or your medical problem, *ask your doctor, nurse, or pharmacist.*

Before Using This Medicine

In deciding to use a medicine, the risks of taking the medicine must be weighed against the good it will do. This is a decision you and your doctor will make. For disulfiram, the following should be considered:

Allergies—Tell your doctor if you have had any unusual or allergic reactions to disulfiram, rubber, pesticides, or fungicides.

Diet—In addition to beverages, alcohol is found in many other products. Reading the list of ingredients on foods and other products before using them will help you to avoid alcohol. Do not use alcohol-containing foods such as sauces and vinegars.

Pregnancy—Disulfiram has not been studied in pregnant women. However, there have been a few reports of birth defects in infants whose mothers took disulfiram during pregnancy. Before taking this medicine, make sure your doctor knows if you are pregnant or if you may become pregnant.

Breast-feeding—Disulfiram has not been reported to cause problems in nursing babies.

Children—Studies on this medicine have been done only in adult patients, and there is no specific information comparing use of disulfiram in children with use in other age groups.

Older adults—Many medicines have not been studied specifically in older people. Therefore, it may not be known whether they work exactly the same way they do in younger adults or if they cause different side effects or problems in older people. There is no specific information comparing use of disulfiram in the elderly with use in other age groups.

Other medicines—Although certain medicines should not be used together at all, in other cases 2 different medicines may be used together even if an interaction might occur. In these cases, your doctor may want to change the dose, or other precautions may be necessary. When you are taking disulfiram, it is especially important that your doctor and pharmacist know if you are taking any of the following:

- Anticoagulants (blood thinners)—Taking disulfiram may increase the effects of anticoagulants, changing the amount you need to take
- Ethotoin (e.g., Peganone) or
- Mephenytoin (e.g., Mesantoin) or
- Phenytoin (e.g., Dilantin)—Taking these medicines with disulfiram may change the amount of anticonvulsant medicine you need to take
- Isoniazid (e.g., INH, Nydrazid)—Disulfiram may increase central nervous system (CNS) effects, such as dizziness, clumsiness, irritability, or trouble in sleeping
- Metronidazole (e.g., Flagyl) or
- Paraldehyde (e.g., Paral)—These medicines should not be taken with or within several days of disulfiram because serious side effects may occur

Ethylene dibromide or organic solvents (such as chemicals which may contain alcohol, acetaldehyde, paraldehyde, or other related chemicals used in factories and in hobbies [e.g., paint thinner])—Make sure you tell your doctor if you will come in contact with or breathe the fumes of ethylene dibromide or organic solvents while you are taking disulfiram.

Other medical problems—The presence of other medical problems may affect the use of disulfiram. Make sure you tell your doctor if you have any other medical problems, especially:

- Asthma or other lung disease, severe, or
- Diabetes mellitus (sugar diabetes) or
- Epilepsy or other seizure disorder or
- Heart or blood vessel disease or
- Kidney disease or
- Liver disease or cirrhosis of the liver or
- Underactive thyroid—A disulfiram-alcohol reaction may make the condition worse
- Depression or
- Severe mental illness—Disulfiram may make the condition worse
- Skin allergy—Disulfiram may cause an allergic reaction

Before you begin using any new medicine (prescription or nonprescription) or if you develop any new medical problem while you are using this medicine, check with your doctor, nurse, or pharmacist.

Proper Use of This Medicine

Before you take the first dose of this medicine, *make sure you have not taken any alcoholic beverage or alcohol-containing product or medicine* (for example, tonics, elixirs, and cough syrups) *during the past 12 hours.* If you are not sure about the alcohol content of medicines you may have taken, check with your doctor or pharmacist.

Take this medicine every day as directed by your doctor. The medicine is usually taken each morning. However, if it makes you drowsy, ask your doctor if you may take it at bedtime instead.

Storage—To store this medicine:

- Keep out of the reach of children.
- Store away from heat and direct light.
- Do not store in the bathroom, near the kitchen sink, or in other damp places. Heat or moisture may cause the medicine to break down.
- Do not keep outdated medicine or medicine no longer needed. Be sure that any discarded medicine is out of the reach of children.

Precautions While Using This Medicine

Do not drink any alcohol, even small amounts, while you are taking this medicine and for 14 days after you stop taking it, because the alcohol may make you very sick. In addition to beverages, alcohol is found in many other products. Reading the list of ingredients on foods and other products before using them will help you to avoid alcohol. You can also avoid alcohol if you:

- Do not use alcohol-containing foods, products, or medicines, such as elixirs, tonics, sauces, vinegars, cough syrups, mouth washes, or gargles.
- *Do not come in contact with or breathe in the fumes of chemicals that may contain alcohol, acetaldehyde, paraldehyde, or other related chemicals,* such as paint thinner, paint, varnish, or shellac.
- *Use caution when using alcohol-containing products that are applied to the skin,* such as some transdermal (stick-on patch) medicines or rubbing alcohol, back rubs, after-shave lotions, colognes, perfumes, toilet waters, or after-bath preparations. Using such products while you are taking disulfiram may cause headache, nausea, or local redness or itching because the alcohol in these products may be absorbed into your body. Before using alcohol-containing products on your skin, first test the product by applying some to a small area of your skin. Allow the product to remain on your skin for 1 or 2 hours. If no redness, itching, or other unwanted effects occur, you should be able to use the product.
- *Do not use any alcohol-containing products on raw skin or open wounds.*

Check with your doctor if you have any questions.

Some of the symptoms you may experience if you use any alcohol while taking this medicine are:

Blurred vision
Chest pain
Confusion
Dizziness or fainting
Fast or pounding heartbeat
Flushing or redness of face

Increased sweating
Nausea and vomiting
Throbbing headache
Troubled breathing
Weakness

These symptoms will last as long as there is any alcohol left in your system, from 30 minutes to several hours. On rare occasions, if you have a severe reaction or have taken a large enough amount of alcohol, a heart attack, unconsciousness, convulsions (seizures), and death may occur.

Your doctor may want you to carry an identification card stating that you are using this medicine. This card should list the symptoms most likely to occur if alcohol is taken, and the doctor, clinic, or hospital to be contacted in case of an emergency. These cards may be available from the manufacturer. Ask your doctor or pharmacist if you have any questions about this.

If you will be taking this medicine for a long period of time (for example, for several months at a time), your doctor should check your progress at regular visits.

Before buying or using any liquid prescription or nonprescription medicine, check with your pharmacist to see if it contains any alcohol.

This medicine may cause some people to become drowsy or less alert than they are normally. If this occurs, *do not drive, use machines, or do anything else that could be dangerous if you are not alert.*

Disulfiram will add to the effects of other CNS depressants (medicines that slow down the nervous system, possibly causing drowsiness). Some examples of CNS depressants are antihistamines or medicine for hay fever, other allergies, or colds; sedatives, tranquilizers, or sleeping medicine; prescription pain medicine or narcotics; barbiturates; medicine for seizures; muscle relaxants; or anesthetics, including some dental anesthetics. *Check with your doctor before taking any of the above while you are using this medicine.*

Side Effects of This Medicine

Along with its needed effects, a medicine may cause some unwanted effects. Although not all of these side effects may occur, if they do occur they may need medical attention.

Check with your doctor as soon as possible if any of the following side effects occur:

Less common

Eye pain or tenderness or any change in vision; mood or mental changes; numbness, tingling, pain, or weakness in hands or feet

Rare

Darkening of urine; light gray–colored stools; severe stomach pain; yellow eyes or skin

Other side effects may occur that usually do not need medical attention. These side effects may go away during treatment as your body adjusts to the medicine. However, check with your doctor if any of the following side effects continue or are bothersome:

More common

Drowsiness

Less common or rare

Decreased sexual ability in males; headache; metallic or garlic-like taste in mouth; skin rash; unusual tiredness

Other side effects not listed above may also occur in some patients. If you notice any other effects, check with your doctor.

Annual revision: 01/27/92

DIURETICS, LOOP Systemic

This information applies to the following medicines:

Bumetanide (byoo-MET-a-nide)
Ethacrynic Acid (eth-a-KRIN-ik AS-id)
Furosemide (fur-OH-se-mide)

Some commonly used brand names are:

For Bumetanide†
In the U.S.
Bumex

For Ethacrynic Acid
In the U.S.
Edecrin
In Canada
Edecrin

For Furosemide
In the U.S.
Lasix
Myrosemide
Generic name product may also be available.
In Canada
Apo-Furosemide
Furoside
Lasix
Lasix Special
Novosemide
Uritol
Generic name product may also be available.

†Not commercially available in Canada.

Description

Loop diuretics are given to help reduce the amount of water in the body. They work by acting on the kidneys to increase the flow of urine.

Furosemide is also used to treat high blood pressure (hypertension) in those patients who are not helped by other medicines or in those patients who have kidney problems.

High blood pressure adds to the workload of the heart and arteries. If it continues for a long time, the heart and arteries may not function properly. This can damage the blood vessels of the brain, heart, and kidneys, resulting in a stroke, heart failure, or kidney failure. High blood pressure may also increase the risk of heart attacks. These problems may be less likely to occur if blood pressure is controlled.

Loop diuretics may also be used for other conditions as determined by your doctor.

This medicine is available only with your doctor's prescription, in the following dosage forms:

Oral

Bumetanide
- Tablets (U.S.)

Ethacrynic Acid
- Oral solution (U.S. and Canada)
- Tablets (U.S. and Canada)

Furosemide
- Oral solution (U.S. and Canada)
- Tablets (U.S. and Canada)

Parenteral

Bumetanide
- Injection (U.S.)

Ethacrynic Acid
- Injection (U.S. and Canada)

Furosemide
- Injection (U.S. and Canada)

It is very important that you read and understand the following information. If any of it causes you special concern, check with your doctor. Also, *if you have any questions* or if you want more information about this medicine or your medical problem, *ask your doctor, nurse, or pharmacist.*

Before Using This Medicine

In deciding to use a medicine, the risks of taking the medicine must be weighed against the good it will do. This is a decision you and your doctor will make. For loop diuretics, the following should be considered:

Allergies—Tell your doctor if you have ever had any unusual or allergic reaction to bumetanide, ethacrynic acid, furosemide, sulfonamides (sulfa drugs), or thiazide diuretics (water pills). Also tell your doctor and pharmacist if you are allergic to any other substances, such as foods, preservatives, or dyes.

Pregnancy—Studies have not been done in pregnant women. However, studies in animals have shown this medicine to cause harmful effects.

In general, diuretics are not useful for normal swelling of feet and hands that occurs during pregnancy. Diuretics should not be taken during pregnancy unless recommended by your doctor.

Breast-feeding—This medicine has not been reported to cause problems in nursing babies. Furosemide passes into breast milk; it is not known whether bumetanide or ethacrynic acid passes into breast milk.

Children—Although there is no specific information comparing the use of loop diuretics in children with use in any other age group, they are not expected to cause different side effects in children than they do in adults.

Older adults—Dizziness, lightheadedness, or signs of too much potassium loss may be more likely to occur in the elderly, who are more sensitive to the effects of this medicine. Elderly patients may also be more likely to develop blood clots.

Other medicines—Although certain medicines should not be used together at all, in other cases two different medicines may be used together even if an interaction might occur. In these cases, your doctor may want to change the dose, or other precautions may be necessary. When you are taking loop diuretics, it is especially important that your doctor and pharmacist know if you are taking *any* other medicines.

Other medical problems—The presence of other medical problems may affect the use of loop diuretics. Make sure you tell your doctor if you have any other medical problems, especially:

- Diabetes mellitus (sugar diabetes)—Loop diuretics may increase the amount of sugar in the blood
- Diarrhea or
- Gout or
- Hearing problems or
- Pancreatitis (inflammation of the pancreas)—Loop diuretics may make these conditions worse
- Heart attack, recent—Use of loop diuretics after a recent heart attack may increase the chance of side effects
- Kidney disease (severe) or
- Liver disease—Higher blood levels of the loop diuretic may occur, which may increase the chance of side effects
- Lupus erythematosus (history of)—Ethacrynic acid and furosemide may make this condition worse

Before you begin using any new medicine (prescription or nonprescription) or if you develop any new medical problem while you are using this medicine, check with your doctor, nurse, or pharmacist.

Proper Use of This Medicine

This medicine may cause you to have an unusual feeling of tiredness when you begin to take it. You may also notice an increase in the amount of urine or in your frequency of urination. After you have taken the medicine for a while, these effects should lessen. In general, to keep the increase in urine from affecting your sleep:

- If you are to take a single dose a day, take it in the morning after breakfast.
- If you are to take more than one dose a day, take the last dose no later than 6 p.m., unless otherwise directed by your doctor.

However, it is best to plan your dose or doses according to a schedule that will least affect your personal activities and sleep. Ask your doctor, nurse, or pharmacist to help you plan the best time to take this medicine.

To help you remember to take your medicine, try to get into the habit of taking it at the same time each day.

For patients taking the *oral liquid form* of furosemide:

- This medicine is to be taken by mouth even if it comes in a dropper bottle. If this medicine does not come in a dropper bottle, use a specially marked measuring spoon or other device to measure each dose accurately, since the average household teaspoon may not hold the right amount of liquid.

For patients taking this medicine for *high blood pressure:*

- Importance of diet—When prescribing medicine for your condition, your doctor may prescribe a personal diet for you. Such a diet may be low in sodium (salt). Most people eat much more sodium than they need and too much sodium in the diet may increase blood pressure. Some foods that contain large amounts of sodium are canned soup, pickles, ketchup, green and ripe olives, relish, frankfurters, soy sauce, and carbonated beverages. Your doctor may want you to limit the amounts of these and other high-sodium foods in your diet. High blood pressure medicine is usually more effective when such a diet is properly followed.

  Also, it may be very important for you to go on a reducing diet. However, check with your doctor before changing your diet.
- Many patients who have high blood pressure will not notice any signs of the problem. In fact, many may feel normal. It is very important that you *take your medicine exactly as directed* and that you keep your appointments with your doctor even if you feel well.
- Remember that this medicine will not cure your high blood pressure but it does help control it. Therefore, you must continue to take it as directed if you expect to lower your blood pressure and keep it down. *You may have to take high blood pressure medicine for the rest of your life.* If high blood pressure is not treated, it can cause serious problems such as heart failure, blood vessel disease, stroke, or kidney disease.

If this medicine upsets your stomach, it may be taken with meals or milk. If stomach upset (nausea, vomiting, or stomach pain) continues or gets worse, or if you suddenly get severe diarrhea, check with your doctor.

Missed dose—If you miss a dose of this medicine, take it as soon as possible. However, if it is almost time for your next dose, skip the missed dose and go back to your regular dosing schedule. Do not double doses.

Storage—To store this medicine:

- Keep out of the reach of children.
- Store away from heat and direct light.
- Do not store in the bathroom, near the kitchen sink, or in other damp places. Heat or moisture may cause the medicine to break down.
- Keep the oral liquid form of this medicine from freezing.
- Do not keep outdated medicine or medicine no longer needed. Be sure that any discarded medicine is out of the reach of children.

Precautions While Using This Medicine

It is important that your doctor check your progress at regular visits to make sure that this medicine is working properly.

This medicine may cause a loss of potassium from your body:

- To help prevent this, your doctor may want you to:

  —eat or drink foods that have a high potassium content (for example, orange or other citrus fruit juices), or

  —take a potassium supplement, or

  —take another medicine to help prevent the loss of the potassium in the first place.
- It is very important to follow these directions. Also, it is important not to change your diet on your own. This is more important if you are already on a special diet (as for diabetes), or if you are taking a potassium supplement or a medicine to reduce potassium loss. Extra potassium may not be necessary and, in some cases, too much potassium could be harmful.

To prevent the loss of too much water and potassium, tell your doctor if you become sick, especially with severe or continuing nausea and vomiting or diarrhea.

Before having any kind of surgery (including dental surgery) or emergency treatment, make sure the medical doctor or dentist in charge knows that you are taking this medicine.

Dizziness, lightheadedness, or fainting may occur, especially when you get up from a lying or sitting position. This is more likely to occur in the morning. *Getting up slowly may help.* When you get up from lying down, sit on the edge of the bed with your feet dangling for 1 or

2 minutes. Then stand up slowly. If the problem continues or gets worse, check with your doctor.

The dizziness, lightheadedness, or fainting is also more likely to occur if you drink alcohol, stand for long periods of time, exercise, or if the weather is hot. *While you are taking this medicine, be careful to limit the amount of alcohol you drink. Also, use extra care during exercise or hot weather or if you must stand for long periods of time.*

For *diabetic patients:*

- This medicine may affect blood sugar levels. While you are using this medicine, be especially careful in testing for sugar in your blood or urine.

For patients taking this medicine for *high blood pressure:*

- *Do not take other medicines unless they have been discussed with your doctor.* This especially includes over-the-counter (nonprescription) medicines for appetite control, asthma, colds, cough, hay fever, or sinus problems, since they may tend to increase your blood pressure.

For patients taking *furosemide:*

- Furosemide may cause your skin to be more sensitive to sunlight than it is normally. Exposure to sunlight, even for brief periods of time, may cause a skin rash, itching, redness or other discoloration of the skin, or a severe sunburn. When you begin taking this medicine:
  —Stay out of direct sunlight, especially between the hours of 10:00 a.m. and 3:00 p.m., if possible.
  —Wear protective clothing, including a hat. Also, wear sunglasses.
  —Apply a sun block product that has a skin protection factor (SPF) of at least 15. Some patients may require a product with a higher SPF number, especially if they have a fair complexion. If you have any questions about this, check with your doctor or pharmacist.
  —Apply a sun block lipstick that has an SPF of at least 15 to protect your lips.
  —Do not use a sunlamp or tanning bed or booth.

If you have a severe reaction from the sun, check with your doctor.

Side Effects of This Medicine

Along with its needed effects, a medicine may cause some unwanted effects. Although not all of these side effects may occur, if they do occur they may need medical attention.

Check with your doctor as soon as possible if any of the following side effects occur:

Rare

Black, tarry stools; blood in urine or stools; cough or hoarseness; fever or chills; joint pain; lower back or side pain; painful or difficult urination; pinpoint red spots on skin; ringing or buzzing in ears or any loss of hearing—more common with ethacrynic acid; skin rash or hives; stomach pain (severe) with nausea and vomiting; unusual bleeding or bruising; yellow eyes or skin; yellow vision—for furosemide only

Signs and symptoms of too much potassium loss

Dryness of mouth; increased thirst; irregular heartbeat; mood or mental changes; muscle cramps or pain; nausea or vomiting; unusual tiredness or weakness; weak pulse

Other side effects may occur that usually do not need medical attention. These side effects may go away during treatment as your body adjusts to the medicine. However, check with your doctor if any of the following side effects continue or are bothersome:

More common

Dizziness or lightheadedness when getting up from a lying or sitting position

Less common or rare

Blurred vision; chest pain—with bumetanide only; confusion—with ethacrynic acid only; diarrhea—more common with ethacrynic acid; headache; increased sensitivity of skin to sunlight—with furosemide only; loss of appetite—more common with ethacrynic acid; nervousness—with ethacrynic acid only; premature ejaculation or difficulty in keeping an erection—with bumetanide only; redness or pain at place of injection; stomach cramps or pain

Other side effects not listed above may also occur in some patients. If you notice any other effects, check with your doctor.

Additional Information

Once a medicine has been approved for marketing for a certain use, experience may show that it is also useful for other medical problems. Although these uses are not included in product labeling, loop diuretics are used in certain patients with the following medical conditions:

- Hypercalcemia (too much calcium in the blood)
- Diagnostic aid for kidney disease

Other than the above information, there is no additional information relating to proper use, precautions, or side effects for these uses.

Annual revision: 08/20/91

DIURETICS, POTASSIUM-SPARING Systemic

This information applies to the following medicines:
Amiloride (a-MILL-oh-ride)
Spironolactone (speer-on-oh-LAK-tone)
Triamterene (trye-AM-ter-een)

Some commonly used brand names are:

For Amiloride
In the U.S.
Midamor
Generic name product may also be available.
In Canada
Midamor

For Spironolactone
In the U.S.
Aldactone
Generic name product may also be available.
In Canada
Aldactone
Novospiroton

For Triamterene
In the U.S.
Dyrenium
In Canada
Dyrenium

Description

Potassium-sparing diuretics are commonly used to help reduce the amount of water in the body. Unlike some other diuretics, these medicines do not cause your body to lose potassium.

Amiloride and spironolactone are also used to treat high blood pressure (hypertension). High blood pressure adds to the workload of the heart and arteries. If the condition continues for a long time, the heart and arteries may not function properly. This can damage the blood vessels of the brain, heart, and kidneys, resulting in a stroke, heart failure, or kidney failure. High blood pressure may also increase the risk of heart attacks. These problems may be less likely to occur if blood pressure is controlled.

Spironolactone is also used to help increase the amount of potassium in the body when it is getting too low.

Potassium-sparing diuretics help to reduce the amount of water in the body by acting on the kidneys to increase the flow of urine. This also helps to lower blood pressure.

These medicines can also be used for other conditions as determined by your doctor.

Potassium-sparing diuretics are available only with your doctor's prescription, in the following dosage forms:

Oral

Amiloride
- Tablets (U.S. and Canada)

Spironolactone
- Tablets (U.S. and Canada)

Triamterene
- Capsules (U.S.)
- Tablets (Canada)

It is very important that you read and understand the following information. If any of it causes you special concern, check with your doctor. Also, *if you have any questions* or if you want more information about this medicine or your medical problem, *ask your doctor, nurse, or pharmacist.*

Before Using This Medicine

In deciding to use a medicine, the risks of taking the medicine must be weighed against the good it will do. This is a decision you and your doctor will make. For potassium-sparing diuretics, the following should be considered:

Allergies—Tell your doctor if you have ever had any unusual or allergic reaction to amiloride, spironolactone, or triamterene. Also tell your doctor and pharmacist if you are allergic to any other substances, such as foods, preservatives, or dyes.

Pregnancy—Studies have not been done in pregnant women. However, this medicine has not been shown to cause birth defects or other problems in animals.

In general, diuretics are not useful for normal swelling of feet and hands that occurs during pregnancy. Diuretics should not be taken during pregnancy unless recommended by your doctor.

Breast-feeding—Although amiloride, spironolactone, and triamterene may pass into breast milk, these medicines have not been reported to cause problems in nursing babies.

Children—This medicine has been tested in children and, in effective doses, has not been shown to cause different side effects or problems in children than it does in adults.

Older adults—Signs and symptoms of too much potassium are more likely to occur in the elderly, who are more sensitive than younger adults to the effects of this medicine.

Other medicines—Although certain medicines should not be used together at all, in other cases two different medicines may be used together even if an interaction might occur. In these cases, your doctor may want to change the dose, or other precautions may be necessary. When you are taking potassium-sparing diuretics, it is especially important that your doctor and pharmacist know if you are taking any of the following:

- Angiotensin-converting enzyme (ACE) inhibitors (benazepril [e.g., Lotensin], captopril [e.g., Capoten], enalapril [e.g., Vasotec], fosinopril [e.g., Monopril], lisinopril [e.g.,

Prinivil, Zestril], quinapril [e.g., Accupril], ramipril [e.g., Altace]) or
- Cyclosporine (e.g., Sandimmune) or
- Potassium-containing medicines or supplements—Use with potassium-sparing diuretics may cause high blood levels of potassium, which may increase the chance of side effects
- Digoxin—Use with spironolactone may cause high blood levels of digoxin, which may increase the chance of side effects
- Lithium (e.g., Lithane)—Use with potassium-sparing diuretics may cause high blood levels of lithium, which may increase the chance of side effects

Other medical problems—The presence of other medical problems may affect the use of potassium-sparing diuretics. Make sure you tell your doctor if you have any other medical problems, especially:
- Diabetes mellitus (sugar diabetes) or
- Kidney disease or
- Liver disease—Higher blood levels of potassium may occur, which may increase the chance of side effects
- Gout or
- Kidney stones (history of)—Triamterene may make these conditions worse
- Menstrual problems or breast enlargement—Spironolactone may make these conditions worse

Before you begin using any new medicine (prescription or nonprescription) or if you develop any new medical problem while you are using this medicine, check with your doctor, nurse, or pharmacist.

Proper Use of This Medicine

This medicine may cause you to have an unusual feeling of tiredness when you begin to take it. You may also notice an increase in the amount of urine or in your frequency of urination. After you have taken the medicine for a while, these effects should lessen. In general, to keep the increase in urine from affecting your sleep:
- If you are to take a single dose a day, take it in the morning after breakfast.
- If you are to take more than one dose a day, take the last dose no later than 6 p.m., unless otherwise directed by your doctor.

However, it is best to plan your dose or doses according to a schedule that will least affect your personal activities and sleep. Ask your doctor, nurse, or pharmacist to help you plan the best time to take this medicine.

To help you remember to take your medicine, try to get into the habit of taking it at the same time each day.

If this medicine upsets your stomach, it may be taken with meals or milk. If stomach upset (nausea, vomiting, stomach pain or cramps) continues, check with your doctor.

For patients taking this medicine for *high blood pressure:*
- In addition to the use of the medicine your doctor has prescribed, treatment for your high blood pressure may include weight control and care in the types of foods you eat, especially foods high in sodium. Your doctor will tell you which of these are most important for you. You should check with your doctor before changing your diet.
- Many patients who have high blood pressure will not notice any signs of the problem. In fact, many may feel normal. It is very important that you *take your medicine exactly as directed* and that you keep your appointments with your doctor even if you feel well.
- Remember that this medicine will not cure your high blood pressure but it does help control it. Therefore, you must continue to take it as directed if you expect to lower your blood pressure and keep it down. *You may have to take high blood pressure medicine for the rest of your life.* If high blood pressure is not treated, it can cause serious problems such as heart failure, blood vessel disease, stroke, or kidney disease.

Missed dose—If you miss a dose of this medicine, take it as soon as possible. However, if it is almost time for your next dose, skip the missed dose and go back to your regular dosing schedule. Do not double doses.

Storage—To store this medicine:
- Keep out of the reach of children.
- Store away from heat and direct light.
- Do not store in the bathroom, near the kitchen sink, or in other damp places. Heat or moisture may cause the medicine to break down.
- Do not keep outdated medicine or medicine no longer needed. Be sure that any discarded medicine is out of the reach of children.

Precautions While Using This Medicine

It is important that your doctor check your progress at regular visits to make sure that this medicine is working properly.

This medicine does not cause a loss of potassium from your body as some other diuretics (water pills) do. Therefore, it is not necessary for you to get extra potassium in your diet, and too much potassium could even be harmful. Since salt substitutes and low-sodium milk may contain potassium, do not use them unless told to do so by your doctor.

Check with your doctor if you become sick and have severe or continuing nausea, vomiting, or diarrhea. These problems may cause you to lose additional water, which could be harmful, or to lose potassium, which could lessen the medicine's helpful effects.

Before having any kind of surgery (including dental surgery) or emergency treatment, tell the medical doctor or dentist in charge that you are taking this medicine.

Before you have any medical tests, tell the doctor in charge that you are taking this medicine. The results of some tests may be affected by this medicine.

For patients taking this medicine for *high blood pressure:*

- *Do not take other medicines unless they have been discussed with your doctor.* This especially includes over-the-counter (nonprescription) medicines for appetite control, asthma, colds, cough, hay fever, or sinus problems, since these medicines may tend to increase your blood pressure.

For patients taking *triamterene:*

- This medicine may cause your skin to be more sensitive to sunlight than it is normally. Exposure to sunlight, even for brief periods of time, may cause a skin rash, itching, redness or other discoloration of the skin, or a severe sunburn. When you begin taking this medicine:

  —Stay out of direct sunlight, especially between the hours of 10:00 a.m. and 3:00 p.m., if possible.

  —Wear protective clothing, including a hat. Also, wear sunglasses.

  —Apply a sun block product that has a skin protection factor (SPF) of at least 15. Some patients may require a product with a higher SPF number, especially if they have a fair complexion. If you have any questions about this, check with your doctor or pharmacist.

  —Apply a sun block lipstick that has an SPF of at least 15 to protect your lips.

  —Do not use a sunlamp or tanning bed or booth.

  —If you have a severe reaction from the sun, check with your doctor.

Side Effects of This Medicine

In rats, spironolactone has been found to increase the risk of tumors. It is not known if spironolactone increases the chance of tumors in humans.

Along with its needed effects, a medicine may cause some unwanted effects. Although not all of these side effects may occur, if they do occur they may need medical attention.

Check with your doctor as soon as possible if any of the following side effects occur:

Rare

For amiloride, spironolactone, and triamterene

Skin rash or itching; shortness of breath

For spironolactone and triamterene only (in addition to effects listed above)

Cough or hoarseness; fever or chills; lower back or side pain; painful or difficult urination

For triamterene only (in addition to effects listed above)

Black, tarry stools; blood in urine or stools; bright red tongue; burning, inflamed feeling in tongue; cracked corners of mouth; lower back pain (severe); pinpoint red spots on skin; unusual bleeding or bruising; weakness

Signs and symptoms of too much potassium

Confusion; irregular heartbeat; nervousness; numbness or tingling in hands, feet, or lips; shortness of breath or difficult breathing; unusual tiredness or weakness; weakness or heaviness of legs

Other side effects may occur that usually do not need medical attention. These side effects may go away during treatment as your body adjusts to the medicine. However, check with your doctor if any of the following side effects continue or are bothersome:

More common (less common with amiloride and triamterene)

Nausea and vomiting; stomach cramps and diarrhea

Less common

For amiloride, spironolactone, and triamterene

Dizziness; headache

For amiloride and spironolactone only (in addition to effects listed above)

Decreased sexual ability

For amiloride only (in addition to effects listed above)

Constipation; muscle cramps

For spironolactone only (in addition to effects listed above for spironolactone)

Breast tenderness in females; clumsiness; deepening of voice in females; enlargement of breasts in males; inability to have or keep an erection; increased hair growth in females; irregular menstrual periods; sweating

For triamterene only (in addition to effects listed above for triamterene)

Increased sensitivity of skin to sunlight

Signs and symptoms of too little sodium

Drowsiness; dryness of mouth; increased thirst; lack of energy

For *male patients:*

- Spironolactone sometimes causes enlarged breasts in males, especially when they take large doses of it for a long time. Breasts usually decrease in size gradually over several months after this medicine is stopped. If you have any questions about this, check with your doctor.

Other side effects not listed above may also occur in some patients. If you notice any other effects, check with your doctor.

Additional Information

Once a medicine has been approved for marketing for a certain use, experience may show that it is also useful for other medical problems. Although these uses are not included in product labeling, spironolactone is used in certain patients with the following medical conditions:

- Polycystic ovary syndrome
- Hirsutism, female (increased hair growth)

Other than the above information, there is no additional information relating to proper use, precautions, or side effects for this use.

Annual revision: 10/15/92

DIURETICS, POTASSIUM-SPARING, AND HYDROCHLOROTHIAZIDE Systemic

This information applies to the following medicines:

Amiloride (a-MILL-oh-ride) and Hydrochlorothiazide (hye-droe-klor-oh-THYE-a-zide)
Spironolactone (speer-on-oh-LAK-tone) and Hydrochlorothiazide
Triamterene (trye-AM-ter-een) and Hydrochlorothiazide

Some commonly used brand names are:

For Amiloride and Hydrochlorothiazide

In the U.S.
Moduretic
Generic name product may also be available.

In Canada
Moduret

For Spironolactone and Hydrochlorothiazide

In the U.S.
Aldactazide
Spirozide
Generic name product may also be available.

In Canada
Aldactazide
Novo-Spirozine

For Triamterene and Hydrochlorothiazide

In the U.S.
Dyazide
Maxzide
Generic name product may also be available.

In Canada
Apo-Triazide
Dyazide
Novo-Triamzide

Description

This medicine is a combination of two diuretics (water pills). It is commonly used to help reduce the amount of water in the body.

This combination is also used to treat high blood pressure (hypertension). High blood pressure adds to the workload of the heart and arteries. If it continues for a long time, the heart and arteries may not function properly. This can damage the blood vessels of the brain, heart, and kidneys, resulting in a stroke, heart failure, or kidney failure. High blood pressure may also increase the risk of heart attacks. These problems may be less likely to occur if blood pressure is controlled.

Diuretics help to reduce the amount of water in the body by acting on the kidneys to increase the flow of urine. This also helps to lower blood pressure.

This combination is also used to treat problems caused by too little potassium in the body.

This medicine is available only with your doctor's prescription, in the following dosage forms:

Oral

Amiloride and Hydrochlorothiazide
- Tablets (U.S. and Canada)

Spironolactone and Hydrochlorothiazide
- Tablets (U.S. and Canada)

Triamterene and Hydrochlorothiazide
- Capsules (U.S.)
- Tablets (U.S. and Canada)

It is very important that you read and understand the following information. If any of it causes you special concern, check with your doctor. Also, *if you have any questions* or if you want more information about this medicine or your medical problem, *ask your doctor, nurse, or pharmacist.*

Before Using This Medicine

In deciding to use a medicine, the risks of taking the medicine must be weighed against the good it will do. This is a decision you and your doctor will make. For potassium-sparing diuretics and hydrochlorothiazide, the following should be considered:

Allergies—Tell your doctor if you have ever had any unusual or allergic reaction to amiloride, spironolactone, triamterene, sulfonamides (sulfa drugs), bumetanide, furosemide, acetazolamide, dichlorphenamide, methazolamide, or to hydrochlorothiazide or any of the other thiazide diuretics. Also tell your doctor and pharmacist if you are allergic to any other substances, such as foods, preservatives, or dyes.

Pregnancy—When hydrochlorothiazide is used during pregnancy, it may cause side effects including jaundice, blood problems, and low potassium in the newborn infant. In addition, although this medicine has not been shown to cause birth defects, the chance always exists.

In general, diuretics are not useful for normal swelling of feet and hands that occurs during pregnancy. They should not be taken during pregnancy unless recommended by your doctor.

Breast-feeding—Although amiloride, spironolactone, triamterene, and hydrochlorothiazide may pass into breast milk, they have not been reported to cause problems in nursing babies.

Children—The medicines in this combination have been tested in children and have not been shown to cause different side effects or problems in children than they do in adults.

Older adults—Dizziness or lightheadedness and signs and symptoms of too much potassium loss may be more likely to occur in the elderly, who are more sensitive than younger adults to the effects of this medicine.

Other medicines—Although certain medicines should not be used together at all, in other cases two different medicines may be used together even if an interaction might occur. In these cases, your doctor may want to change the dose, or other precautions may be necessary. When you are taking potassium-sparing diuretics and hydrochlorothiazide, it is especially important that your doctor and pharmacist know if you are taking any of the following:

- Adrenocorticoids (cortisone-like medicine) or
- Other diuretics (water pills) or antihypertensives (high blood pressure medicine)—Use with this combination medicine may increase the chance of side effects
- Captopril (e.g., Capoten) or
- Cyclosporine (e.g., Sandimmune) or
- Enalapril (e.g., Vasotec) or
- Lisinopril (e.g., Prinivil, Zestril) or
- Potassium-containing medicines or supplements—Use with potassium-sparing diuretics may cause high blood levels of potassium, which may increase the chance of side effects
- Digitalis glycosides (heart medicine)—Use with diuretics may cause high blood levels of digoxin, which may increase the chance of side effects
- Lithium (e.g., Lithane)—Use with diuretics may cause high blood levels of lithium, which may increase the chance of side effects
- Methenamine (e.g., Mandelamine)—Use with diuretics may prevent methenamine from working properly

Other medical problems—The presence of other medical problems may affect the use of potassium-sparing diuretics and hydrochlorothiazide. Make sure you tell your doctor if you have any other medical problems, especially:

- Diabetes mellitus (sugar diabetes) or
- Kidney disease or
- Liver disease—Higher blood levels of potassium may occur, which may increase the chance of side effects
- Gout (history of) or
- Kidney stones (history of)—Triamterene may worsen these conditions
- Lupus erythematosus (history of) or
- Pancreatitis (inflammation of pancreas)—Potassium-sparing diuretics and hydrochlorothiazide may worsen these conditions
- Menstrual problems or breast enlargement—Spironolactone may worsen these conditions

Before you begin using any new medicine (prescription or nonprescription) or if you develop any new medical problem while you are using this medicine, check with your doctor, nurse, or pharmacist.

Proper Use of This Medicine

This medicine may cause you to have an unusual feeling of tiredness when you begin to take it. You may also notice an increase in the amount of urine or in your frequency of urination. After you have taken the medicine for a while, these effects should lessen. In general, to keep the increase in urine from affecting your sleep:

- If you are to take a single dose a day, take it in the morning after breakfast.
- If you are to take more than one dose a day, take the last dose no later than 6 p.m., unless otherwise directed by your doctor.

However, it is best to plan your dose or doses according to a schedule that will least affect your personal activities and sleep. Ask your doctor, nurse, or pharmacist to help you plan the best time to take this medicine.

To help you remember to take your medicine, try to get into the habit of taking it at the same time each day.

If this medicine upsets your stomach, it may be taken with meals or milk. If stomach upset (nausea, vomiting, stomach pain, or cramps) continues, check with your doctor.

For patients taking this medicine for *high blood pressure:*

- Importance of diet—When prescribing medicine for your condition, your doctor may also prescribe a personal diet for you. Such a diet may be low in sodium (salt). Most people eat much more sodium than they need and too much sodium in the diet may increase blood pressure. Some foods that contain large amounts of sodium are canned soup, pickles, ketchup, green and ripe olives, relish, frankfurters, soy sauce, and carbonated beverages. Your doctor may want you to limit the amounts of these and other high-sodium foods in your diet. High blood pressure medicine is usually more effective when such a diet is properly followed.

However, some foods low in sodium, as well as some salt substitutes, are high in potassium. If they are used together with this medicine, they may lead to too much potassium in the body. Discuss with your doctor what low-sodium foods you may use.

Also, it may be very important for you to go on a reducing diet. However, check with your doctor before changing your diet.

- Many patients who have high blood pressure will not notice any signs of the problem. In fact, many may feel normal. It is very important that you *take your medicine exactly as directed* and that you keep your appointments with your doctor even if you feel well.
- Remember that this medicine will not cure your high blood pressure but it does help control it. Therefore, you must continue to take it as directed if you expect to lower your blood pressure and keep it down. *You may have to take high blood pressure medicine for the rest of your life.* If high blood pressure is not treated, it can cause serious problems such as heart failure, blood vessel disease, stroke, or kidney disease.

Missed dose—If you miss a dose of this medicine, take it as soon as possible. However, if it is almost time for your next dose, skip the missed dose and go back to your regular dosing schedule. Do not double doses.

Storage—To store this medicine:

- Keep out of the reach of children.
- Store away from heat and direct light.
- Do not store in the bathroom, near the kitchen sink, or in other damp places. Heat or moisture may cause the medicine to break down.
- Do not keep outdated medicine or medicine no longer needed. Be sure that any discarded medicine is out of the reach of children.

Precautions While Using This Medicine

It is important that your doctor check your progress at regular visits to make sure that this medicine is working properly.

This medicine may cause a loss or increase of potassium in your body. Your doctor may have special instructions about whether or not you need to eat or drink foods or beverages that have a high potassium content (for example, orange or other citrus fruit juices), taking a potassium supplement, or using salt substitutes. Since too much potassium can be harmful, it is important not to change your diet on your own. Tell your doctor if you are already on a special diet (as for diabetes). Since salt substitutes and low-sodium milk may contain potassium, do not use them unless told to do so by your doctor. Check with your doctor, nurse, or pharmacist if you need a list of foods that are high in potassium or if you have any questions.

Check with your doctor if you become sick and have severe or continuing vomiting or diarrhea. These problems may cause you to lose additional water and potassium and lead to low blood pressure.

For *diabetic patients:*

- Hydrochlorothiazide (contained in this combination medicine) may raise blood sugar levels. While you are taking this medicine, be especially careful in testing for sugar in your blood or urine.

Potassium-sparing diuretics and hydrochlorothiazide may cause your skin to be more sensitive to sunlight than it is normally. Exposure to sunlight, even for brief periods of time, may cause a skin rash, itching, redness or other discoloration of the skin, or a severe sunburn. When you begin taking this medicine:

- Stay out of direct sunlight, especially between the hours of 10:00 a.m. and 3:00 p.m., if possible.
- Wear protective clothing, including a hat. Also, wear sunglasses.
- Apply a sun block product that has a skin protection factor (SPF) of at least 15. Some patients may require a product with a higher SPF number, especially if they have a fair complexion. If you have any questions about this, check with your doctor or pharmacist.
- Apply a sun block lipstick that has an SPF of at least 15 to protect your lips.
- Do not use a sunlamp or tanning bed or booth.

If you have a severe reaction from the sun, check with your doctor.

Before having any kind of surgery (including dental surgery) or emergency treatment, tell the medical doctor or dentist in charge that you are taking this medicine.

For patients taking *triamterene and hydrochlorothiazide combination:*

- Do not change brands of triamterene and hydrochlorothiazide without first checking with your doctor. Different products may not work the same way. If you refill your medicine and it looks different, check with your pharmacist.

For patients taking this medicine for *high blood pressure:*

- *Do not take other medicines unless they have been discussed with your doctor.* This especially includes over-the-counter (nonprescription) medicines for appetite control, asthma, colds, cough, hay fever, or sinus problems, since they may tend to increase your blood pressure.

Tell the doctor in charge that you are taking this medicine before you have any medical tests. The results of some tests may be affected by this medicine.

Side Effects of This Medicine

In rats, spironolactone has been found to increase the risk of development of tumors. However, the doses given were many times the dose of spironolactone given to humans. It is not known whether spironolactone causes tumors in humans.

Along with its needed effects, a medicine may cause some unwanted effects. Although not all of these side effects may occur, if they do occur they may need medical attention.

Check with your doctor as soon as possible if any of the following side effects occur:

Rare

Black, tarry stools; blood in urine or stools; cough or hoarseness; fever or chills; joint pain; lower back or side pain; painful or difficult urination; pinpoint red spots on skin; skin rash or hives; stomach pain (severe) with nausea and vomiting; unusual bleeding or bruising; yellow eyes or skin

Signs and symptoms of changes in potassium

Confusion; dryness of mouth; increased thirst; irregular heartbeats; mood or mental changes; muscle cramps or pain; numbness or tingling in hands, feet, or lips; shortness of breath or difficulty breathing; unusual tiredness or weakness; weak pulse; weakness or heaviness of legs

Reported for triamterene only (rare)

Bright red tongue; burning, inflamed feeling in tongue; cracked corners of mouth

Other side effects may occur that usually do not need medical attention. These side effects may go away during treatment as your body adjusts to the medicine. However, check with your doctor if any of the following side effects continue or are bothersome:

More common (less common with triamterene)

Loss of appetite; nausea and vomiting; stomach cramps and diarrhea; upset stomach

Less common

Decreased sexual ability; dizziness or lightheadedness when getting up from a lying or sitting position; headache (more common with amiloride); increased sensitivity of skin to sunlight

Reported for amiloride only (less common)

Constipation

Reported for spironolactone only (less common)

Breast tenderness in females; clumsiness; deepening of voice in females; enlargement of breasts in males; increased hair growth in females; irregular menstrual periods; sweating

Spironolactone sometimes causes enlarged breasts in males, especially when they take large doses of it for a long time. Breasts usually decrease in size gradually over several months after this medicine is stopped. If you have any questions about this, check with your doctor.

Other side effects not listed above may also occur in some patients. If you notice any other effects, check with your doctor.

Annual revision: July 1990

DIURETICS, THIAZIDE Systemic

This information applies to the following medicines:

Bendroflumethiazide (ben-droe-floo-meth-EYE-a-zide)
Benzthiazide (benz-THYE-a-zide)
Chlorothiazide (klor-oh-THYE-a-zide)
Chlorthalidone (klor-THAL-i-doan)
Cyclothiazide (sye-kloe-THYE-a-zide)
Hydrochlorothiazide (hye-droe-klor-oh-THYE-a-zide)
Hydroflumethiazide (hye-droe-floo-meth-EYE-a-zide)
Methyclothiazide (meth-ee-kloe-THYE-a-zide)
Metolazone (me-TOLE-a-zone)
Polythiazide (pol-i-THYE-a-zide)
Quinethazone (kwin-ETH-a-zone)
Trichlormethiazide (trye-klor-meth-EYE-a-zide)

Some commonly used brand names are:

For Bendroflumethiazide
In the U.S.
Naturetin
In Canada
Naturetin

For Benzthiazide†
In the U.S.
Exna
Hydrex
Generic name product may also be available.

For Chlorothiazide†
In the U.S.
Diuril
Generic name product may also be available.

For Chlorthalidone
In the U.S.
Hygroton
Thalitone
Generic name product may also be available.

In Canada
Apo-Chlorthalidone
Hygroton
Novo-Thalidone
Uridon
Generic name product may also be available.

Another commonly used name is chlortalidone.

For Cyclothiazide†
In the U.S.
Anhydron

For Hydrochlorothiazide
In the U.S.
Esidrix
Hydro-chlor
Hydro-D
HydroDIURIL
Oretic
Generic name product may also be available.
In Canada
Apo-Hydro
Diuchlor H
HydroDIURIL
Neo-Codema
Novo-Hydrazide
Urozide
Generic name product may also be available.

For Hydroflumethiazide†
In the U.S.
Diucardin
Saluron
Generic name product may also be available.

For Methyclothiazide
In the U.S.
Aquatensen
Enduron
Generic name product may also be available.
In Canada
Duretic

For Metolazone
In the U.S.
Diulo
Mykrox
Zaroxolyn
In Canada
Zaroxolyn

For Polythiazide†
In the U.S.
Renese

For Quinethazone†
In the U.S.
Hydromox

For Trichlormethiazide†
In the U.S.
Metahydrin
Naqua
Trichlorex
Generic name product may also be available.

†Not commercially available in Canada.

Description

Thiazide or thiazide-like diuretics are commonly used to treat high blood pressure (hypertension). High blood pressure adds to the workload of the heart and arteries. If it continues for a long time, the heart and arteries may not function properly. This can damage the blood vessels of the brain, heart, and kidneys, resulting in a stroke, heart failure, or kidney failure. High blood pressure may also increase the risk of heart attacks. These problems may be less likely to occur if blood pressure is controlled.

Thiazide diuretics are also used to help reduce the amount of water in the body by increasing the flow of urine. They may also be used for other conditions as determined by your doctor.

Thiazide diuretics are available only with your doctor's prescription, in the following dosage forms:

Oral

Bendroflumethiazide
- Tablets (U.S. and Canada)

Benzthiazide
- Tablets (U.S.)

Chlorothiazide
- Oral suspension (U.S.)
- Tablets (U.S.)

Chlorthalidone
- Tablets (U.S. and Canada)

Cyclothiazide
- Tablets (U.S.)

Hydrochlorothiazide
- Oral solution (U.S.)
- Tablets (U.S. and Canada)

Hydroflumethiazide
- Tablets (U.S.)

Methyclothiazide
- Tablets (U.S. and Canada)

Metolazone
- Tablets (U.S. and Canada)

Polythiazide
- Tablets (U.S.)

Quinethazone
- Tablets (U.S.)

Trichlormethiazide
- Tablets (U.S.)

Parenteral

Chlorothiazide
- Injection (U.S.)

It is very important that you read and understand the following information. If any of it causes you special concern, check with your doctor. Also, *if you have any questions* or if you want more information about this medicine or your medical problem, *ask your doctor, nurse, or pharmacist.*

Before Using This Medicine

In deciding to use a medicine, the risks of taking the medicine must be weighed against the good it will do. This is a decision you and your doctor will make. For thiazide diuretics, the following should be considered:

Allergies—Tell your doctor if you have ever had any unusual or allergic reaction to sulfonamides (sulfa drugs), bumetanide, furosemide, acetazolamide, dichlorphenamide, methazolamide, or to any of the thiazide diuretics. Also tell your doctor and pharmacist if you are allergic to any other substances, such as foods, preservatives, or dyes.

Pregnancy—When this medicine is used during pregnancy, it may cause side effects including jaundice, blood problems, and low potassium in the newborn infant. In addition, although this medicine has not been shown to cause birth defects or other problems in animals, studies have not been done in humans.

In general, diuretics are not useful for normal swelling of feet and hands that occurs during pregnancy. They should not be taken during pregnancy unless recommended by your doctor.

Breast-feeding—Thiazide diuretics pass into breast milk. These medicines also may decrease the flow of breast milk. Therefore, you should avoid use of thiazide diuretics during the first month of breast-feeding.

Children—Although there is no specific information comparing the use of thiazide diuretics in children with use in other age groups, these medicines are not expected to cause different side effects or problems in children than they do in adults. However, extra caution may be necessary in infants with jaundice, because these medicines can make the condition worse.

Older adults—Dizziness or lightheadedness and signs of too much potassium loss may be more likely to occur in the elderly, who are more sensitive than younger adults to the effects of thiazide diuretics.

Other medicines—Although certain medicines should not be used together at all, in other cases two different medicines may be used together even if an interaction might occur. In these cases, your doctor may want to change the dose, or other precautions may be necessary. When you are taking thiazide diuretics, it is especially important that your doctor and pharmacist know if you are taking any of the following:

- Cholestyramine or
- Colestipol—Use with thiazide diuretics may prevent the diuretic from working properly; take the diuretic at least 1 hour before or 4 hours after cholestyramine or colestipol
- Digitalis glycosides (heart medicine)—Use with thiazide diuretics may cause high blood levels of digoxin, which may increase the chance of side effects
- Lithium (e.g., Lithane)—Use with thiazide diuretics may cause high blood levels of lithium, which may increase the chance of side effects

Other medical problems—The presence of other medical problems may affect the use of thiazide diuretics. Make sure you tell your doctor if you have any other medical problems, especially:

- Diabetes mellitus (sugar diabetes)—Thiazide diuretics may increase the amount of sugar in the blood
- Gout (history of) or
- Lupus erythematosus (history of) or
- Pancreatitis (inflammation of the pancreas)—Thiazide diuretics may make these conditions worse
- Heart or blood vessel disease—Thiazide diuretics may cause high cholesterol levels or high triglyceride levels
- Liver disease or
- Kidney disease (severe)—Higher blood levels of the thiazide diuretic may occur, which may prevent the thiazide diuretic from working properly

Before you begin using any new medicine (prescription or nonprescription) or if you develop any new medical problem while you are using this medicine, check with your doctor, nurse, or pharmacist.

Proper Use of This Medicine

This medicine may cause you to have an unusual feeling of tiredness when you begin to take it. You may also notice an increase in the amount of urine or in your frequency of urination. After you have taken the medicine for a while, these effects should lessen. In general, to keep the increase in urine from affecting your sleep:

- If you are to take a single dose a day, take it in the morning after breakfast.
- If you are to take more than one dose a day, take the last dose no later than 6 p.m., unless otherwise directed by your doctor.

However, it is best to plan your dose or doses according to a schedule that will least affect your personal activities and sleep. Ask your doctor, nurse, or pharmacist to help you plan the best time to take this medicine.

To help you remember to take your medicine, try to get into the habit of taking it at the same time each day.

For patients taking this medicine for *high blood pressure:*

- In addition to the use of the medicine your doctor has prescribed, appropriate treatment for your high blood pressure may include weight control and care in the types of foods you eat, especially foods high in sodium. Your doctor will tell you which factors are most important for you. You should check with your doctor before changing your diet.
- Many patients who have high blood pressure will not notice any signs of the problem. In fact, many may feel normal. It is very important that you *take your medicine exactly as directed* and that you keep your appointments with your doctor even if you feel well.
- Remember that this medicine will not cure your high blood pressure but it does help control it. Therefore, you must continue to take it as directed if you expect to lower your blood pressure and keep it down. *You may have to take high blood pressure medicine for the rest of your life.* If high blood pressure is not treated, it can cause serious problems such as heart failure, blood vessel disease, stroke, or kidney disease.

For patients taking the *oral liquid form of hydrochlorothiazide,* which comes in a dropper bottle:

- This medicine is to be taken by mouth. The amount you should take is to be measured only with the specially marked dropper.

Missed dose—If you miss a dose of this medicine, take it as soon as possible. However, if it is almost time for your next dose, skip the missed dose and go back to your regular dosing schedule. Do not double doses.

Storage—To store this medicine:

- Keep out of the reach of children.
- Store away from heat and direct light.
- Do not store in the bathroom, near the kitchen sink, or in other damp places. Heat or moisture may cause the medicine to break down.
- Keep the oral liquid form of this medicine from freezing.
- Do not keep outdated medicine or medicine no longer needed. Be sure that any discarded medicine is out of the reach of children.

Precautions While Using This Medicine

It is important that your doctor check your progress at regular visits to make sure that this medicine is working properly.

This medicine may cause a loss of potassium from your body:

- To help prevent this, your doctor may want you to:
  —eat or drink foods that have a high potassium content (for example, orange or other citrus fruit juices), or
  —take a potassium supplement, or
  —take another medicine to help prevent the loss of the potassium in the first place.
- It is very important to follow these directions. Also, it is important not to change your diet on your own. This is more important if you are already on a special diet (as for diabetes), or if you are taking a potassium supplement or a medicine to reduce potassium loss. Extra potassium may not be necessary and, in some cases, too much potassium could be harmful.

Check with your doctor if you become sick and have severe or continuing vomiting or diarrhea. These problems may cause you to lose additional water and potassium.

For *diabetic patients:*

- Thiazide diuretics may raise blood sugar levels. While you are using this medicine, be especially careful in testing for sugar in your blood or urine.

Thiazide diuretics may cause your skin to be more sensitive to sunlight than it is normally. Exposure to sunlight, even for brief periods of time, may cause a skin rash, itching, redness or other discoloration of the skin, or a severe sunburn. When you begin taking this medicine:

- Stay out of direct sunlight, especially between the hours of 10:00 a.m. and 3:00 p.m., if possible.
- Wear protective clothing, including a hat. Also, wear sunglasses.
- Apply a sun block product that has a skin protection factor (SPF) of at least 15. Some patients may require a product with a higher SPF number, especially if they have a fair complexion. If you have any questions about this, check with your doctor or pharmacist.
- Apply a sun block lipstick that has an SPF of at least 15 to protect your lips.
- Do not use a sunlamp or tanning bed or booth.

If you have a severe reaction from the sun, check with your doctor.

For patients taking this medicine for *high blood pressure:*

- *Do not take other medicines unless they have been discussed with your doctor.* This especially includes over-the-counter (nonprescription) medicines for appetite control, asthma, colds, cough, hay fever, or sinus problems, since they may tend to increase your blood pressure.

Side Effects of This Medicine

Along with its needed effects, a medicine may cause some unwanted effects. Although not all of these side effects may occur, if they do occur they may need medical attention.

Check with your doctor as soon as possible if any of the following side effects occur:

Rare

Black, tarry stools; blood in urine or stools; cough or hoarseness; fever or chills; joint pain; lower back or side pain; painful or difficult urination; pinpoint red spots on skin; skin rash or hives; stomach pain (severe) with nausea and vomiting; unusual bleeding or bruising; yellow eyes or skin

Signs and symptoms of too much potassium loss

Dryness of mouth; increased thirst; irregular heartbeat; mood or mental changes; muscle cramps or pain; nausea or vomiting; unusual tiredness or weakness; weak pulse

Signs and symptoms of too much sodium loss

Confusion; convulsions; decreased mental activity; irritability; muscle cramps; unusual tiredness or weakness

Other side effects may occur that usually do not need medical attention. These side effects may go away during treatment as your body adjusts to the medicine. However, check with your doctor if any of the following side effects continue or are bothersome:

Less common

Decreased sexual ability; diarrhea; dizziness or lightheadedness when getting up from a lying or sitting position; increased sensitivity of skin to sunlight; loss of appetite; upset stomach

Other side effects not listed above may also occur in some patients. If you notice any other effects, check with your doctor.

Additional Information

Once a medicine has been approved for marketing for a certain use, experience may show that it is also useful for other medical problems. Although these uses are not specifically included in product labeling, thiazide diuretics are used in certain patients with the following medical conditions:

- Diabetes insipidus (water diabetes)
- Kidney stones (calcium-containing)

For patients taking this medicine for *diabetes insipidus (water diabetes):*

- Some thiazide diuretics are used in the treatment of diabetes insipidus (water diabetes). In patients with water diabetes, this medicine causes a decrease in the flow of urine and helps the body hold water. Thus, the information given above about increased urine flow will not apply to you.

Other than the above information, there is no additional information relating to proper use, precautions, or side effects for these uses.

Annual revision: 06/07/92

DOXAZOSIN Systemic

A commonly used brand name in the U.S. and Canada is Cardura.

Description

Doxazosin (dox-AY-zoe-sin) belongs to the general class of medicines called antihypertensives. It is used to treat high blood pressure (hypertension).

High blood pressure adds to the workload of the heart and arteries. If it continues for a long time, the heart and arteries may not function properly. This can damage the blood vessels of the brain, heart, and kidneys, resulting in a stroke, heart failure, or kidney failure. High blood pressure may also increase the risk of heart attacks. These problems may be less likely to occur if blood pressure is controlled.

Doxazosin works by relaxing blood vessels so that blood passes through them more easily. This helps to lower blood pressure.

Doxazosin is available only with your doctor's prescription, in the following dosage form:

Oral

- Tablets (U.S. and Canada)

It is very important that you read and understand the following information. If any of it causes you special concern, check with your doctor. Also, *if you have any questions* or if you want more information about this medicine or your medical problem, *ask your doctor, nurse, or pharmacist.*

Before Using This Medicine

In deciding to use a medicine, the risks of taking the medicine must be weighed against the good it will do. This is a decision you and your doctor will make. For doxazosin, the following should be considered:

Allergies—Tell your doctor if you have ever had any unusual or allergic reaction to doxazosin, prazosin, or terazosin. Also tell your doctor and pharmacist if you are allergic to any other substances, such as foods, preservatives, or dyes.

Pregnancy—Doxazosin has not been studied in pregnant women. However, studies in rats receiving oral doses of 75 times the highest recommended human dose have not shown that doxazosin causes harm to the fetus.

Breast-feeding—It is not known whether doxazosin passes into breast milk. However, this medicine has not been reported to cause problems in nursing babies.

Children—Studies on this medicine have been done only in adult patients, and there is no specific information comparing use of doxazosin in children with use in other age groups.

Older adults—Dizziness, lightheadedness, or fainting may be especially likely to occur in elderly patients, who are usually more sensitive than younger adults to the effects of doxazosin.

Other medicines—Although certain medicines should not be used together at all, in other cases two different medicines may be used together even if an interaction might occur. In these cases, your doctor may want to change the dose, or other precautions may be necessary. Tell your doctor and pharmacist if you are using any other prescription or nonprescription (over-the-counter [OTC]) medicine.

Other medical problems—The presence of other medical problems may affect the use of doxazosin. Make sure you tell your doctor if you have any other medical problems, especially:

- Liver disease—The effects of doxazosin may be increased, which may increase the chance of side effects
- Kidney disease—Possible increased sensitivity to the effects of doxazosin

Before you begin using any new medicine (prescription or nonprescription) or if you develop any new medical problem while you are using this medicine, check with your doctor, nurse, or pharmacist.

Proper Use of This Medicine

For patients *taking this medicine for high blood pressure:*

- In addition to the use of the medicine your doctor has prescribed, treatment for your high blood pressure may include weight control and care in the types of foods you eat, especially foods high in sodium. Your doctor will tell you which of these are most important for you. You should check with your doctor before changing your diet.
- Many patients who have high blood pressure will not notice any signs of the problem. In fact, many may feel normal. It is very important that you *take your medicine exactly as directed* and that you keep your appointments with your doctor even if you feel well.
- Remember that doxazosin will not cure your high blood pressure but it does help control it. Therefore, you must continue to take it as directed if you expect to lower your blood pressure and keep it down. *You may have to take high blood pressure medicine for the rest of your life.* If high blood pressure is not treated, it can cause serious problems such as heart failure, blood vessel disease, stroke, or kidney disease.

To help you remember to take your medicine, try to get into the habit of taking it at the same time each day.

Missed dose—If you miss a dose of this medicine, take it as soon as possible. However, if it is almost time for your next dose, skip the missed dose and go back to your regular dosing schedule. Do not double doses.

Storage—To store this medicine:

- Keep out of the reach of children.
- Store away from heat and direct light.
- Do not store in the bathroom, near the kitchen sink, or in other damp places. Heat or moisture may cause the medicine to break down.
- Do not keep outdated medicine or medicine no longer needed. Be sure that any discarded medicine is out of the reach of children.

Precautions While Using This Medicine

It is important that your doctor check your progress at regular visits to make sure that this medicine is working properly. This is especially important for elderly patients, who may be more sensitive to the effects of this medicine.

Do not take other medicines unless they have been discussed with your doctor. This especially includes over-the-counter (nonprescription) medicines for appetite control, asthma, colds, cough, hay fever, or sinus problems, since they may tend to increase your blood pressure.

Dizziness, lightheadedness, or sudden fainting may occur after you take this medicine, especially when you get up from a lying or sitting position. These effects are more likely to occur when you take the first dose of this medicine. Taking the first dose at bedtime may prevent problems. However, *be especially careful if you need to get up during the night.* These effects may also occur with any doses you take after the first dose. Getting up slowly may help lessen this problem. *If you feel dizzy, lie down so that you do not faint.* Then sit for a few moments before standing to prevent the dizziness from returning.

The dizziness, lightheadedness, or sudden fainting is more likely to occur if you drink alcohol, stand for a long time, exercise, or if the weather is hot. *While you are taking this medicine, be careful to limit the amount of alcohol you drink. Also, use extra care during exercise or hot weather or if you must stand for a long time.*

Doxazosin may cause some people to become drowsy or less alert than they are normally. *Make sure you know how you react to this medicine before you drive, use machines, or do anything else that could be dangerous if you are dizzy, drowsy, or are not alert.* After you have taken several doses of this medicine, these effects should lessen.

Side Effects of This Medicine

Along with its needed effects, a medicine may cause some unwanted effects. Although not all of these side effects may occur, if they do occur they may need medical attention.

Check with your doctor as soon as possible if any of the following side effects occur:

More common

Dizziness or lightheadedness

Less common

Dizziness or lightheadedness when getting up from a lying or sitting position; fainting (sudden); fast and pounding heartbeat; irregular heartbeat; shortness of breath; swelling of feet or lower legs

Other side effects may occur that usually do not need medical attention. These side effects may go away during

treatment as your body adjusts to the medicine. However, check with your doctor if any of the following side effects continue or are bothersome:

More common

Headache; unusual tiredness

Less common

Nausea; nervousness, restlessness, unusual irritability; runny nose; sleepiness or drowsiness

Other side effects not listed above may also occur in some patients. If you notice any other effects, check with your doctor.

Additional Information

Once a medicine has been approved for marketing for a certain use, experience may show that it is also useful for other medical problems. Although this use is not included in product labeling, doxazosin is used in certain patients with the following medical condition:

- Benign enlargement of the prostate

Other than the above information, there is no additional information relating to proper use, precautions, or side effects for this use.

Annual revision: 05/06/92

DOXORUBICIN Systemic

Some commonly used brand names are:

In the U.S.

Adriamycin PFS
Adriamycin RDF
Rubex
Generic name product may also be available.

In Canada

Adriamycin PFS
Adriamycin RDF

Description

Doxorubicin (dox-oh-ROO-bi-sin) belongs to the general group of medicines known as antineoplastics. It is used to treat some kinds of cancer.

Doxorubicin seems to interfere with the growth of cancer cells, which are eventually destroyed. Since the growth of normal body cells may also be affected by doxorubicin, other effects will also occur. Some of these may be serious and must be reported to your doctor. Other effects, like hair loss, may not be serious but may cause concern. Some effects may not occur for months or years after the medicine is used.

Before you begin treatment with doxorubicin, you and your doctor should talk about the good this medicine will do as well as the risks of using it.

Doxorubicin is to be administered only by or under the supervision of your doctor. It is available in the following dosage form:

Parenteral

- Injection (U.S. and Canada)

It is very important that you read and understand the following information. If any of it causes you special concern, do not decide against receiving this medicine without first checking with your doctor. Also, *if you have any questions* or if you want more information about this medicine or your medical problem, *ask your doctor, nurse or pharmacist.*

Before Using This Medicine

In deciding to use a medicine, the risks of taking the medicine must be weighed against the good it will do. This is a decision you and your doctor will make. For doxorubicin, the following should be considered:

Allergies—Tell your doctor if you have ever had any unusual or allergic reaction to doxorubicin or lincomycin.

Pregnancy—There is a chance that this medicine may cause birth defects if either the male or female is receiving it at the time of conception or if it is taken during pregnancy. Studies in rats and rabbits have shown that doxorubicin causes birth defects in the fetus and other problems (including miscarriage). In addition, many cancer medicines may cause sterility which could be permanent. Although sterility has been reported in animals and humans with this medicine, the effect is weaker in humans than in animals.

Be sure that you have discussed these possible effects with your doctor before receiving this medicine. It is best to use some kind of birth control while you are receiving doxorubicin. However, do not use oral contraceptives ("the Pill") since they may interfere with this medicine. Tell your doctor right away if you think you have become pregnant while receiving doxorubicin. Before receiving doxorubicin make sure your doctor knows if you are pregnant or if you may become pregnant.

Breast-feeding—Because doxorubicin may cause serious side effects, breast-feeding is generally not recommended while you are receiving it.

Children—Heart problems are more likely to occur in children under 2 years of age, who are usually more sensitive to the effects of doxorubicin.

Older adults—Heart problems are more likely to occur in the elderly, who are usually more sensitive to the effects of doxorubicin. The elderly may also be more likely to have blood problems.

Other medicines—Although certain medicines should not be used together at all, in other cases two different medicines may be used together even if an interaction might occur. In these cases, your doctor may want to change the dose, or other precautions may be necessary. When receiving doxorubicin it is especially important that your doctor and pharmacist know if you have ever been treated with x-rays or cancer medicines or if you are taking any of the following:

- Amphotericin B by injection (e.g., Fungizone) or
- Antithyroid agents (medicine for overactive thyroid) or
- Azathioprine (e.g., Imuran) or
- Chloramphenicol (e.g., Chloromycetin) or
- Colchicine or
- Flucytosine (e.g., Ancobon) or
- Interferon (e.g., Intron A, Roferon-A) or
- Plicamycin (e.g., Mithracin) or
- Zidovudine (e.g., Retrovir)—Doxorubicin may increase the effects of these medicines or radiation therapy on the blood
- Probenecid (e.g., Benemid) or
- Sulfinpyrazone (e.g., Anturane)—Doxorubicin may raise the concentration of uric acid in the blood, which these medicines are used to lower

Other medical problems—The presence of other medical problems may affect the use of doxorubicin. Make sure you tell your doctor if you have any other medical problems, especially:

- Chickenpox (including recent exposure) or
- Herpes zoster (shingles)—Risk of severe disease affecting other parts of the body
- Gout or
- Kidney stones—Doxorubicin may increase levels of a chemical called uric acid in the body, which can cause gout or kidney stones
- Heart disease—Risk of heart problems caused by doxorubicin may be increased
- Liver disease—Effects may be increased because of slower removal of doxorubicin from the body

Before you begin using any new medicine (prescription or nonprescription) or if you develop any new medical problem while you are using this medicine, check with your doctor, nurse, or pharmacist.

Proper Use of This Medicine

Doxorubicin is sometimes given together with certain other medicines. If you are receiving a combination of medicines, it is important that you receive each one at the proper time. If you are taking some of these medicines by mouth, ask your doctor, nurse, or pharmacist to help you plan a way to take them at the right times.

While you are using this medicine, your doctor may want you to drink extra fluids so that you will pass more urine. This will help prevent kidney problems and keep your kidneys working well.

Doxorubicin often causes nausea and vomiting. However, it is very important that you continue to receive it, even if you begin to feel ill. Ask your doctor, nurse, or pharmacist for ways to lessen these effects.

Precautions While Using This Medicine

It is very important that your doctor check your progress at regular visits to make sure that this medicine is working properly and to check for unwanted effects.

While you are being treated with doxorubicin, and after you stop treatment with it, *do not have any immunizations (vaccinations) without your doctor's approval.* Doxorubicin may lower your body's resistance, and there is a chance you might get the infection the immunization is meant to prevent. In addition, other persons living in your household should not take or should not have recently taken oral polio vaccine since there is a chance they could pass the polio virus on to you. Also, avoid other persons who have taken oral polio vaccine. Do not get close to them, and do not stay in the same room with them for very long. If you cannot take these precautions, you should consider wearing a protective face mask that covers the nose and mouth.

Doxorubicin can lower the number of white blood cells in your blood temporarily, increasing the chance of getting an infection. It can also lower the number of platelets, which are necessary for proper blood clotting. If this occurs, there are certain precautions you can take, especially when your blood count is low, to reduce the risk of infection or bleeding:

- If you can, avoid people with infections. *Check with your doctor immediately* if you think you are getting an infection or if you get a fever or chills, cough or hoarseness, lower back or side pain, or painful or difficult urination.
- *Check with your doctor immediately* if you notice any unusual bleeding or bruising; black, tarry stools; blood in urine or stools; or pinpoint red spots on your skin.
- Be careful when using a regular toothbrush, dental floss, or toothpick. Your medical doctor, dentist, or nurse may recommend other ways to clean your teeth and gums. Check with your medical doctor before having any dental work done.

- Do not touch your eyes or the inside of your nose unless you have just washed your hands and have not touched anything else in the meantime.
- Be careful not to cut yourself when you are using sharp objects such as a safety razor or fingernail or toenail cutters.
- Avoid contact sports or other situations where bruising or injury could occur.

If doxorubicin accidentally seeps out of the vein into which it is injected, it may damage some tissues and cause scarring. *Tell the doctor or nurse right away if you notice redness, pain, or swelling at the place of injection.*

Side Effects of This Medicine

Along with their needed effects, medicines like doxorubicin can sometimes cause unwanted effects such as heart problems, blood problems, loss of hair, and other side effects. These and others are described below. Also, because of the way these medicines act on the body, there is a chance that they might cause other unwanted effects that may not occur until months or years after the medicine is used. These delayed effects may include certain types of cancer, such as leukemia. Discuss these possible effects with your doctor.

Although not all of these side effects may occur, if they do occur they may need medical attention.

Check with your doctor or nurse immediately if any of the following side effects occur:

Less common

Cough or hoarseness; fast or irregular heartbeat; fever or chills; lower back or side pain; pain at place of injection; painful or difficult urination; shortness of breath; swelling of feet and lower legs

Rare

Black, tarry stools; blood in urine; pinpoint red spots on skin; unusual bleeding or bruising; wheezing

Check with your doctor or nurse as soon as possible if any of the following side effects occur:

More common

Sores in mouth and on lips

Less common

Darkening or redness of skin (after x-ray treatment); joint pain; red streaks along injected vein

Rare

Skin rash or itching

Other side effects may occur that usually do not need medical attention. These side effects may go away during treatment as your body adjusts to the medicine. Also, your doctor or nurse may be able to tell you about ways to prevent or reduce some of these side effects. Check with your doctor or nurse if any of the following side effects continue or are bothersome or if you have any questions about them:

More common

Nausea and vomiting

Less common

Darkening of soles, palms, or nails; diarrhea

Doxorubicin causes the urine to turn reddish in color, which may stain clothes. This is not blood. It is to be expected and only lasts for 1 or 2 days after each dose is given.

This medicine often causes a temporary and total loss of hair. After treatment with doxorubicin has ended, normal hair growth should return.

After you stop receiving doxorubicin, it may still produce some side effects that need attention. During this period of time, *check with your doctor or nurse immediately* if you notice any of the following side effects:

Fast or irregular heartbeat; shortness of breath; swelling of feet and lower legs

Other side effects not listed above may also occur in some patients. If you notice any other effects, check with your doctor or nurse.

Annual revision: July 1990

DRONABINOL Systemic

A commonly used brand name in the U.S. and Canada is Marinol. Another commonly used name is delta-9-tetrahydrocannabinol (THC).

Description

Dronabinol (droe-NAB-i-nol) is used to prevent the nausea and vomiting that may occur after treatment with cancer medicines. It is used only when other kinds of medicine for nausea and vomiting do not work. Dronabinol is also used to increase appetite in patients with acquired immunodeficiency syndrome (AIDS).

Dronabinol is available only with your doctor's prescription. Prescriptions cannot be refilled, and you must obtain a new prescription from your doctor each time you need this medicine. It is available in the following dosage form:

Oral

- Capsules (U.S. and Canada)

It is very important that you read and understand the following information. If any of it causes you special concern, check with your doctor. Also, *if you have any questions* or if you want more information about this medicine or your medical problem, *ask your doctor, nurse, or pharmacist.*

Before Using This Medicine

In deciding to use a medicine, the risks of taking the medicine must be weighed against the good it will do. This is a decision you and your doctor will make. For dronabinol, the following should be considered:

Allergies—Tell your doctor if you have ever had any unusual or allergic reaction to dronabinol, marijuana products, or sesame oil. Also tell your doctor and pharmacist if you are allergic to any other substances, such as foods, preservatives, or dyes.

Pregnancy—Studies have not been done in pregnant women. However, studies in animals have shown that dronabinol, given in doses many times the usual human dose, increases the risk of death of the fetus and decreases the number of live babies born.

Breast-feeding—Dronabinol passes into the breast milk. There is a possibility that the baby may become dependent on this medicine.

Children—Although there is no specific information comparing use of dronabinol in children with use in other age groups, the effects that this medicine may have on the mind may be of special concern in children. Children should be watched closely while they are taking this medicine.

Older adults—This medicine has been tested in a limited number of patients up to 82 years of age and has not been shown to cause different side effects or problems in older people than it does in younger adults. However, the effects this medicine may have on the mind may be of special concern in the elderly. Therefore, older people should be watched closely while they are taking this medicine.

Other medicines—Although certain medicines should not be used together at all, in other cases 2 different medicines may be used together even if an interaction might occur. In these cases, your doctor may want to change the dose, or other precautions may be necessary. When you are taking dronabinol, it is especially important that your doctor and pharmacist know if you are taking any of the following:

- Central nervous system (CNS) depressants (medicine that causes drowsiness) or
- Tricyclic antidepressants (medicine for depression)—Taking these medicines with dronabinol may increase the CNS depressant effects

Other medical problems—The presence of other medical problems may affect the use of dronabinol. Make sure you tell your doctor if you have any other medical problems, especially:

- Alcohol abuse (or history of) or
- Drug abuse or dependence (or history of)—Dependence on dronabinol may develop
- Heart disease or
- High blood pressure (hypertension) or
- Manic depression or
- Schizophrenia—Dronabinol may make the condition worse

Before you begin using any new medicine (prescription or nonprescription) or if you develop any new medical problem while you are using this medicine, check with your doctor, nurse, or pharmacist.

Proper Use of This Medicine

Take this medicine only as directed by your physician. Do not take more of it, do not take it more often, and do not take it for a longer time than your doctor ordered. If too much is taken, it may lead to medical problems because of an overdose.

Dosing—The dose of dronabinol will be different for different patients. *Follow your doctor's orders or the directions on the label.* The following information includes only the average doses of dronabinol. *If your dose is different, do not change it* unless your doctor tells you to do so.

The number of capsules that you take depends on the strength of the medicine. Also, *the number of doses you take each day, the time allowed between doses, and the length of time you take the medicine depend on the medical problem for which you are taking dronabinol.*

- For *oral* dosage form (capsules):
  - —For nausea and vomiting caused by cancer medicines:
    - Adults and teenagers—Dose is based on body surface area. Your doctor will tell you how much medicine to take and when to take it.
    - Children—Use and dose must be determined by your doctor.
  - —For increasing appetite in patients with AIDS:
    - Adults and teenagers—To start, 2.5 milligrams (mg) two times a day, taken before lunch and supper. Your doctor may change your dose depending on your condition. However, the dose is usually not more than 20 mg a day.

- Children—Use and dose must be determined by your doctor.

Missed dose—If you miss a dose of this medicine, take it as soon as you remember. However, if it is almost time for your next dose, skip the missed dose and go back to your regular dosing schedule. *Do not double doses.*

Storage—To store this medicine:

- Keep out of the reach of children. Overdose is very dangerous in young children.
- Store away from heat and direct light.
- Do not store this medicine in the bathroom, near the kitchen sink, or in other damp places. Heat or moisture may cause the medicine to break down.
- Keep this medicine in the refrigerator but keep it from freezing.
- Do not keep outdated medicine or medicine no longer needed. Be sure that any discarded medicine is out of the reach of children.

Precautions While Using This Medicine

Dronabinol will add to the effects of alcohol and other CNS depressants (medicines that slow down the nervous system, possibly causing drowsiness). Some examples of CNS depressants are antihistamines or medicine for hay fever, other allergies, or colds; sedatives, tranquilizers, or sleeping medicine; prescription pain medicines including other narcotics; barbiturates; medicine for seizures; muscle relaxants; or anesthetics, including some dental anesthetics. *Check with your doctor before taking any of the above while you are taking this medicine.*

This medicine may cause some people to become drowsy, dizzy, or lightheaded, or to feel a false sense of well-being. *Make sure you know how you react to this medicine before you drive, use machines, or do anything else that could be dangerous if you are dizzy or are not alert and clearheaded.*

Dizziness, lightheadedness, or fainting may occur, especially when you get up suddenly from a lying or sitting position. Getting up slowly may help lessen this problem.

If you think you or someone else may have taken an overdose of dronabinol, get emergency help at once. Taking an overdose of this medicine or taking alcohol or CNS depressants with this medicine may lead to severe mental effects. Signs of overdose include changes in mood, confusion, hallucinations, mental depression, nervousness or anxiety, and fast or pounding heartbeat.

Side Effects of This Medicine

Along with its needed effects, a medicine may cause some unwanted effects. Although not all of these side effects may occur, if they do occur they may need medical attention.

Check with your doctor or nurse immediately if any of the following side effects occur:

Less common (may also be signs of overdose)

Changes in mood; confusion; fast or pounding heartbeat; hallucinations (seeing, hearing, or feeling things that are not there); mental depression; nervousness or anxiety

Symptoms of overdose

Being forgetful; change in your sense of smell, taste, sight, sound, or touch; change in how fast you think time is passing; constipation; problems in urinating; redness of eyes; slurred speech

Other side effects may occur that usually do not need medical attention. These side effects may go away during treatment as your body adjusts to the medicine. However, check with your doctor if any of the following side effects continue or are bothersome:

More common

Clumsiness or unsteadiness; dizziness; drowsiness; trouble thinking

Less common or rare

Blurred vision or any changes in vision; dryness of mouth; feeling faint or lightheaded; restlessness; unusual tiredness or weakness

Other side effects not listed above may also occur in some patients. If you notice any other effects, check with your doctor.

Annual revision: 06/07/93

ECONAZOLE Topical

Some commonly used brand names are:

In the U.S.
Spectazole

In Canada
Ecostatin

E

Description

Econazole (e-KONE-a-zole) belongs to the family of medicines called antifungals, which are used to treat infections caused by a fungus. They work by killing the fungus or preventing its growth.

Econazole cream is applied to the skin to treat fungus infections. These include:

- ringworm of the body (tinea corporis);
- ringworm of the foot (tinea pedis; athlete's foot);
- ringworm of the groin (tinea cruris; jock itch);
- tinea versicolor (sometimes called "sun fungus"); and
- certain other fungus infections, such as Candida (Monilia) infections.

Econazole is available only with your doctor's prescription, in the following dosage form:

Topical

- Cream (U.S. and Canada)

It is very important that you read and understand the following information. If any of it causes you special concern, check with your doctor. Also, *if you have any questions* or if you want more information about this medicine or your medical problem, *ask your doctor, nurse, or pharmacist.*

Before Using This Medicine

In deciding to use a medicine, the risks of using the medicine must be weighed against the good it will do. This is a decision you and your doctor will make. For topical econazole, the following should be considered:

Allergies—Tell your doctor if you have ever had any unusual or allergic reaction to econazole. Also tell your doctor and pharmacist if you are allergic to any other substances, such as preservatives or dyes.

Pregnancy—Topical econazole has not been studied in pregnant women. Oral econazole has not been shown to cause birth defects in animal studies; however, it has been shown to cause other problems. Before using this medicine, make sure your doctor knows if you are pregnant or if you may become pregnant.

Breast-feeding—It is not known whether topical econazole passes into the breast milk. This medicine has not been reported to cause problems in nursing babies. However, econazole, when given by mouth, does pass into the milk of rats and has caused problems in the young.

Children—Although there is no specific information comparing use of this medicine in children with use in other age groups, this medicine is not expected to cause different side effects or problems in children than it does in adults.

Older adults—Many medicines have not been studied specifically in older people. Therefore, it may not be known whether they work exactly the same way they do in younger adults. Although there is no specific information comparing use of econazole in the elderly with use in other age groups, this medicine is not expected to cause different side effects or problems in older people than it does in younger adults.

Before you begin using any new medicine (prescription or nonprescription) or if you develop any new medical problem while you are using this medicine, check with your doctor, nurse, or pharmacist.

Proper Use of This Medicine

Apply enough econazole to cover the affected and surrounding skin areas, and rub in gently.

Keep this medicine away from the eyes.

When econazole is used to treat certain types of fungus infections of the skin, an occlusive dressing (airtight covering, such as kitchen plastic wrap) should *not* be applied over the medicine. To do so may cause irritation of the skin. *Do not apply an airtight covering over this medicine unless you have been directed to do so by your doctor.*

To help clear up your infection completely, *it is very important that you keep using econazole for the full time of treatment,* even if your symptoms begin to clear up after a few days. Since fungus infections may be very slow to clear up, you may have to continue using this medicine every day for several weeks or more. If you stop using this medicine too soon, your symptoms may return. *Do not miss any doses.*

Missed dose—If you do miss a dose of this medicine, apply it as soon as possible. However, if it is almost time for your next dose, skip the missed dose and go back to your regular dosing schedule.

Storage—To store this medicine:

- Keep out of the reach of children.
- Store away from heat and direct light.
- Keep the medicine from freezing.

- Do not keep outdated medicine or medicine no longer needed. Be sure that any discarded medicine is out of the reach of children.

Precautions While Using This Medicine

If your skin problem does not improve within 2 weeks or more, or if it becomes worse, check with your doctor.

To help clear up your infection completely and to help make sure it does not return, good health habits are also required.

- For patients using econazole for ringworm of the groin (tinea cruris; jock itch):
  —Avoid wearing underwear that is tight-fitting or made from synthetic materials (for example, rayon or nylon). Instead, wear loose-fitting, cotton underwear.
  —Use a bland, absorbent powder (for example, talcum powder) or an antifungal powder (for example, tolnaftate) on the skin. It is best not to use econazole cream or any other antifungal cream at the same time that you use the powder.

These measures will help reduce chafing and irritation and will also help keep the groin area cool and dry.

- For patients using econazole for ringworm of the foot (tinea pedis; athlete's foot):
  —Carefully dry the feet, especially between the toes, after bathing.
  —Avoid wearing socks made from wool or synthetic materials (for example, rayon or nylon). Instead, wear clean, cotton socks and change them daily or more often if the feet sweat freely.
  —Wear well-ventilated shoes (for example, shoes with holes) or sandals.
  —Use a bland, absorbent powder (for example, talcum powder) or an antifungal powder (for example, tolnaftate) between the toes, on the feet, and in socks and shoes freely once or twice a day. It is best not to use econazole cream or any other antifungal cream at the same time that you use the powder.

  These measures will help keep the feet cool and dry.

If you have any questions about this, check with your doctor, nurse, or pharmacist.

Side Effects of This Medicine

Along with its needed effects, a medicine may cause some unwanted effects. Although not all of these side effects may occur, if they do occur they may need medical attention.

Check with your doctor as soon as possible if any of the following side effects occur:

Less common

Burning, itching, stinging, redness, or other sign of irritation not present before use of this medicine

Other side effects not listed above may also occur in some patients. If you notice any other effects, check with your doctor.

Annual revision: 04/14/92

EFLORNITHINE Systemic†

A commonly used brand name in the U.S. is Ornidyl.

†Not commercially available in Canada.

Description

Eflornithine (ee-FLOR-ni-theen) is used to treat African sleeping sickness, a disease caused by parasites.

Eflornithine is available only with your doctor's prescription, in the following dosage form:

Parenteral

- Injection (U.S.)

It is very important that you read and understand the following information. If any of it causes you special concern, check with your doctor. Also, *if you have any questions* or if you want more information about this medicine or your medical problem, *ask your doctor, nurse, or pharmacist.*

Before Receiving This Medicine

In deciding to use a medicine, the risks of taking the medicine must be weighed against the good it will do. This is a decision you and your doctor will make. For eflornithine, the following should be considered:

Allergies—Tell your doctor if you have ever had any unusual or allergic reaction to eflornithine. Also tell your doctor and pharmacist if you are allergic to any other substances, such as foods, preservatives, or dyes.

Pregnancy—Studies have not been done in humans. However, studies in animals have shown that eflornithine causes fetal death and birth defects. Before taking this medicine, make sure your doctor knows if you are pregnant or if you may become pregnant.

Breast-feeding—It is not known whether eflornithine passes into breast milk. Be sure you have discussed the risks and benefits of the medicine if you are thinking of breast-feeding your baby.

Children—Studies on this medicine have been done only in adult patients, and there is no specific information comparing use of eflornithine in children with use in other age groups.

Older adults—Many medicines have not been studied specifically in older people. Therefore, it may not be known whether they work exactly the same way they do in younger adults or if they cause different side effects or problems in older people. There is no specific information comparing use of eflornithine in the elderly with use in other age groups.

Other medicines—Although certain medicines should not be used together at all, in other cases two different medicines may be used together even if an interaction might occur. In these cases, your doctor may want to change the dose, or other precautions may be necessary. When you are receiving eflornithine, it is especially important that your doctor and pharmacist know if you are taking any of the following:

- Amphotericin B by injection (e.g., Fungizone) or
- Antineoplastics (cancer medicine) or
- Antithyroid agents (medicine for overactive thyroid) or
- Azathioprine (e.g., Imuran) or
- Chloramphenicol (e.g., Chloromycetin) or
- Colchicine or
- Cyclophosphamide (e.g., Cytoxan) or
- Flucytosine (e.g., Ancobon) or
- Ganciclovir (e.g., Cytovene) or
- Interferon (e.g., Intron A, Roferon-A) or
- Mercaptopurine (e.g., Purinethol) or
- Methotrexate (e.g., Mexate) or
- Plicamycin (e.g., Mithracin) or
- Zidovudine (e.g., AZT, Retrovir)—Caution should be used if these medicines and eflornithine are used together; receiving eflornithine while you are using these medicines may make anemia and other blood problems worse
- Anti-infectives by mouth or by injection (medicine for infection) or
- Chloroquine (e.g., Aralen) or
- Cisplatin (e.g., Platinol) or
- Deferoxamine (e.g., Desferal) (with long-term use) or
- Hydroxychloroquine (e.g., Plaquenil) or
- Inflammation or pain medicine, except narcotics or
- Quinine (e.g., Quinamm)—Use of any of these medicines with eflornithine may increase the chance of hearing loss

Other medical problems—The presence of other medical problems may affect the use of eflornithine. Make sure you tell your doctor if you have any other medical problems, especially:

- Anemia or other blood problems—Eflornithine may cause blood problems, making the problems you already have worse
- Hearing loss—Long-term treatment with eflornithine may increase your chance of hearing loss
- Kidney disease—Patients with kidney disease may have an increased chance of side effects

Before you begin using any new medicine (prescription or nonprescription) or if you develop any new medical problem while you are using this medicine, check with your doctor, nurse, or pharmacist.

Proper Use of This Medicine

To ensure the best response, eflornithine must be given for the full time of treatment. Also, this medicine works best when there is a constant amount in the blood. To help keep the amount constant, eflornithine must be given on a regular schedule.

Precautions After Receiving This Medicine

Eflornithine can lower the number of white blood cells in your blood, increasing the chance of getting an infection. It can also lower the number of platelets, which are necessary for proper blood clotting. If this occurs, there are certain precautions you can take to reduce the risk of infection or bleeding:

- *Check with your doctor immediately* if you think you are getting an infection or if you get a fever or chills.
- *Check with your doctor immediately* if you notice any unusual bleeding or bruising; black, tarry stools; blood in urine or stools; or pinpoint red spots on your skin.
- Be careful when using a regular toothbrush, dental floss, or toothpick. Your medical doctor, dentist, or nurse may recommend other ways to clean your teeth and gums. Check with your medical doctor before having any dental work done.
- Be careful not to cut yourself when you are using sharp objects such as a safety razor or fingernail or toenail cutters.

It is very important that your doctor check your progress at regular visits. This medicine may cause blood problems.

Side Effects of This Medicine

Along with its needed effects, a medicine may cause some unwanted effects. Although not all of these side effects may occur, if they do occur they may need medical attention.

Check with your doctor immediately if any of the following side effects occur:

More common

Sore throat and fever; unusual bleeding or bruising; unusual tiredness and weakness

Rare

Convulsions (seizures); loss of hearing

Other side effects may occur that usually do not need medical attention. These side effects may go away during treatment as your body adjusts to the medicine. However, check with your doctor if any of the following side effects continue or are bothersome:

More common

Diarrhea; nausea; stomach pain; vomiting

Rare

Hair loss; headache

Other side effects not listed above may also occur in some patients. If you notice any other effects, check with your doctor.

Annual revision: 02/19/92

ENCAINIDE Systemic*†

A commonly used brand name is Enkaid.

*Not commercially available in the U.S.
†Not commercially available in Canada.

Description

Encainide (en-KAY-nide) belongs to the group of medicines known as antiarrhythmics. It is used to correct irregular heartbeats to a normal rhythm.

Encainide produces its helpful effects by slowing nerve impulses in the heart and making the heart tissue less sensitive.

There is a chance that encainide may cause new heart rhythm problems when it is used. Since it has been shown to cause severe problems in some patients, it is only used to treat serious heart rhythm problems. Discuss this possible effect with your doctor.

This medicine is available only with your doctor's prescription, in the following dosage form:

Oral

- Capsules

It is very important that you read and understand the following information. If any of it causes you special concern, check with your doctor. Also, *if you have any questions* or if you want more information about this medicine or your medical problem, *ask your doctor, nurse, or pharmacist.*

Before Using This Medicine

In deciding to use a medicine, the risks of taking the medicine must be weighed against the good it will do. This is a decision you and your doctor will make. For encainide, the following should be considered:

Allergies—Tell your doctor if you have ever had any unusual or allergic reaction to encainide. Also tell your doctor and pharmacist if you are allergic to any other substances, such as foods, preservatives, or dyes.

Pregnancy—Encainide has not been studied in pregnant women. However, this medicine has not been shown to cause birth defects or other problems in animal studies, but has been shown to reduce fertility in rats. Before taking encainide, make sure your doctor knows if you are pregnant or if you may become pregnant.

Breast-feeding—Encainide passes into the milk of some animals and may also pass into the milk of humans. However, this medicine has not been reported to cause problems in nursing babies.

Children—Studies on this medicine have been done only in adult patients. Therefore, be sure to discuss with your doctor the use of this medicine in children.

Older adults—Many medicines have not been tested in older people. Therefore, it may not be known whether they work exactly the same way they do in younger adults or if they cause different side effects or problems in older people. There is no specific information about the use of encainide in the elderly.

Other medical problems—The presence of other medical problems may affect the use of encainide. Make sure you tell your doctor if you have any other medical problems, especially:

- Diabetes mellitus—Encainide may raise blood sugar levels
- Kidney disease—Effects of encainide may be increased because of slower removal from the body
- Liver disease—Effects of encainide may be changed
- Recent heart attack—Risk of irregular heartbeats may be increased
- If you have a pacemaker—Encainide may interfere with the pacemaker and require more careful follow-up by the doctor

Before you begin using any new medicine (prescription or nonprescription) or if you develop any new medical problem while you are using this medicine, check with your doctor, nurse, or pharmacist.

Proper Use of This Medicine

Take encainide exactly as directed by your doctor, even though you may feel well. Do not take more or less of it than your doctor ordered.

This medicine works best when there is a constant amount in the blood. *To help keep the amount constant, do not miss any doses. Also, it is best to take each dose at evenly spaced times day and night.* For example, if you are to take 3 doses a day, doses should be spaced about 8 hours apart. If you need help in planning the best times to take your medicine, check with your doctor or pharmacist.

Dosing—The dose of encainide will be different for different patients. *Follow your doctor's orders or the directions on the label.* The following information includes only the average doses of encainide. *If your dose is different, do not change it* unless your doctor tells you to do so:

- For *oral* dosage form (capsules):
  - —For irregular heartbeat:
    - Adults—25 to 50 milligrams (mg) every eight hours.
    - Children—Use and dose must be determined by your doctor.

Missed dose—If you do miss a dose of encainide and remember within 4 hours, take it as soon as possible. However, if you do not remember until later, skip the missed dose and go back to your regular dosing schedule. Do not double doses.

Storage—To store this medicine:

- Keep out of the reach of children.
- Store away from heat and direct light.
- Do not store in the bathroom, near the kitchen sink, or in other damp places. Heat or moisture may cause the medicine to break down.
- Do not keep outdated medicine or medicine no longer needed. Be sure that any discarded medicine is out of the reach of children.

Precautions While Using This Medicine

It is important that your doctor check your progress at regular visits to make sure the medicine is working properly. This will allow changes to be made in the amount of medicine you are taking, if necessary.

Your doctor may want you to carry a medical identification card or bracelet stating that you are using this medicine.

Before having any kind of surgery (including dental surgery) or emergency treatment, tell the medical doctor or dentist in charge that you are taking this medicine.

Encainide may cause some people to become dizzy or light-headed. Make sure you know how you react to this medicine before you drive, use machines, or do anything else that could be dangerous if you are dizzy.

Side Effects of This Medicine

Along with its needed effects, a medicine may cause some unwanted effects. Although not all of these side effects may occur, if they do occur they may need medical attention.

Check with your doctor as soon as possible if any of the following side effects occur:

More common

Chest pain; fast or irregular heartbeat

Rare

Shortness of breath; swelling of feet or lower legs; trembling or shaking

Other side effects may occur that usually do not need medical attention. These side effects may go away during treatment as your body adjusts to the medicine. However, check with your doctor if any of the following side effects continue or are bothersome:

Less common

Blurred or double vision; dizziness; headache; nausea; pain in arms or legs; skin rash; unusual tiredness or weakness

Other side effects not listed above may also occur in some patients. If you notice any other effects, check with your doctor.

Annual revision: 06/08/93

EPINEPHRINE Ophthalmic

This information applies to the following medicines:

Epinephrine (ep-i-NEF-rin)
Epinephryl Borate (ep-i-NEF-rill BOR-ate)

Some commonly used brand names are:

Epinephrine

In the U.S.

Ayerst Epitrate
Epifrin
Glaucon
L-Epinephrine

Generic name product may also be available.

In Canada
Epifrin
Glaucon

Epinephryl Borate
In the U.S.
Epinal
Eppy/N
In Canada
Epinal
Eppy/N

Description

Ophthalmic epinephrine is used to treat certain types of glaucoma. It may also be used in eye surgery.

This medicine is available only with your doctor's prescription, in the following dosage forms:

Ophthalmic

Epinephrine
- Ophthalmic solution (eye drops) (U.S. and Canada)

Epinephryl Borate
- Ophthalmic solution (eye drops) (U.S. and Canada)

It is very important that you read and understand the following information. If any of it causes you special concern, check with your doctor. Also, *if you have any questions* or if you want more information about this medicine or your medical problem, *ask your doctor, nurse, or pharmacist.*

Before Using This Medicine

In deciding to use a medicine, the risks of taking the medicine must be weighed against the good it will do. This is a decision you and your doctor will make. For epinephrine, the following should be considered:

Allergies—Tell your doctor if you have ever had any unusual or allergic reaction to epinephrine or sulfites. Also tell your doctor and pharmacist if you are allergic to any other substances, such as preservatives.

Pregnancy—Ophthalmic epinephrine may be absorbed into the body. However, studies on effects in pregnancy have not been done in either humans or animals.

Breast-feeding—Ophthalmic epinephrine may be absorbed into the body. However, it is not known whether epinephrine passes into the breast milk.

Children—Studies on this medicine have been done only in adult patients, and there is no specific information comparing use of this medicine in children with use in other age groups.

Older adults—Many medicines have not been studied specifically in older people. Therefore, it may not be known whether they work exactly the same way they do in younger adults. Although there is no specific information comparing use of this medicine in the elderly with use in other age groups, this medicine is not expected to cause different side effects or problems in older people than it does in younger adults.

Other medicines—Although certain medicines should not be used together at all, in other cases two different medicines may be used together even if an interaction might occur. In these cases, your doctor may want to change the dose, or other precautions may be necessary. Tell your doctor and pharmacist if you are using any other prescription or nonprescription (over-the-counter [OTC]) medicine.

Other medical problems—The presence of other medical problems may affect the use of epinephrine. Make sure you tell your doctor if you have any other medical problems, especially:

- Bronchial asthma or
- Diabetes mellitus (sugar diabetes) or
- Eye disease (other) or
- Heart or blood vessel disease or
- High blood pressure or
- Overactive thyroid—Epinephrine may make the condition worse
- Dental surgery on gums—Dental surgery may include the use of epinephrine in topical or injection form. Use of ophthalmic epinephrine during this time may increase blood levels of the medicine and increase the chance of side effects

Before you begin using any new medicine (prescription or nonprescription) or if you develop any new medical problem while you are using this medicine, check with your doctor, nurse, or pharmacist.

Proper Use of This Medicine

Use this medicine only as directed. Do not use more of it and do not use it more often than your doctor ordered. To do so may increase the chance of too much medicine being absorbed into the body and the chance of side effects.

To use:

- First, wash your hands. With the middle finger, apply pressure to the inside corner of the eye (and continue to apply pressure for 1 or 2 minutes after the medicine has been placed in the eye). Tilt the head back and with the index finger of the same hand, pull the lower eyelid away from eye to form a pouch. Drop the medicine into the pouch and gently close the eyes. Do not blink. Keep the eyes closed for 1 or 2 minutes to allow the medicine to be absorbed.
- Immediately after using the eye drops, wash your hands to remove any medicine that may be on them.
- To keep the medicine as germ-free as possible, do not touch the applicator tip to any surface (including the eye). Also, keep the container tightly closed.

For patients using *epinephrine ophthalmic solution:*

- Do not use if the solution turns pinkish or brownish in color, or if it becomes cloudy.

For patients using *epinephryl borate ophthalmic solution:*

- The color of this solution may vary from colorless to amber yellow. Do not use if the solution turns dark brown or becomes cloudy.

Missed dose—If you miss a dose of this medicine, apply the missed dose as soon as possible. However, if it is almost time for your next dose, skip the missed dose and go back to your regular dosing schedule. Do not double doses.

Storage—To store this medicine:

- Keep out of the reach of children.
- Store away from heat and direct light.
- Keep the medicine from freezing.
- Do not keep outdated medicine or medicine no longer needed. Be sure that any discarded medicine is out of the reach of children.

Precautions While Using This Medicine

Your doctor should check your eye pressure at regular visits.

Side Effects of This Medicine

Along with its needed effects, a medicine may cause some unwanted effects. Although not all of these side effects may occur, if they do occur they may need medical attention.

Check with your doctor as soon as possible if any of the following side effects occur:

Less common

Blurred or decreased vision

Symptoms of too much medicine being absorbed into the body

Fast, irregular, or pounding heartbeat; feeling faint; increased sweating; paleness; trembling

Other side effects may occur that usually do not need medical attention. These side effects may go away during treatment as your body adjusts to the medicine. However, check with your doctor if any of the following side effects continue or are bothersome:

More common

Headache or browache; stinging, burning, redness, or other eye irritation; watering of eyes

Less common

Eye pain or ache

Other side effects not listed above may also occur in some patients. If you notice any other effects, check with your doctor.

Annual revision: 05/14/92

EPOETIN Systemic

Some commonly used brand names are:

In the U.S.

Epogen
Procrit

In Canada

Eprex

Other commonly used names are human erythropoietin, recombinant; EPO; and r-HuEPO.

Description

Epoetin (eh-POH-ee-tin) is a man-made version of human erythropoietin (EPO). EPO is produced naturally in the body, mostly by the kidneys. It stimulates the bone marrow to produce red blood cells. If the body does not produce enough EPO, severe anemia can occur. This often occurs in people whose kidneys are not working properly. Epoetin is used to treat severe anemia in these people.

Epoetin may also be used to prevent or treat anemia caused by other conditions, as determined by your doctor.

Epoetin is given by injection. It is available only with your doctor's prescription and is available in the following dosage form:

Parenteral

- Injection (U.S. and Canada)

It is very important that you read and understand the following information. If any of it causes you special concern, check with your doctor. Also, *if you have any questions* or if you want more information about this medicine or your medical problem, *ask your doctor, nurse, or pharmacist.*

Before Using This Medicine

In deciding to use a medicine, the risks of taking the medicine must be weighed against the good it will do.

This is a decision you and your doctor will make. For epoetin, the following should be considered:

Allergies—Tell your doctor if you have ever had any unusual or allergic reaction to epoetin or to human albumin. Also tell your doctor and pharmacist if you are allergic to any other substances, such as foods, preservatives, or dyes.

Pregnancy—Epoetin has not been reported to cause birth defects or other problems in humans. However, it did cause problems, including unwanted effects on the bones and spine, in some animal studies.

Breast-feeding—It is not known whether epoetin passes into the breast milk. However, it has not been reported to cause problems in nursing babies.

Children—There is no specific information about the use of epoetin in children up to 12 years of age.

Older adults—Epoetin has been given to elderly people. However, there is no specific information about whether epoetin works the same way it does in younger adults or whether it causes different side effects or problems in older people.

Other medicines—Although certain medicines should not be used together at all, in other cases two different medicines may be used together even if an interaction might occur. In these cases, your doctor may want to change the dose, or other precautions may be necessary. When you are taking epoetin, it is important that your doctor and pharmacist know if you are taking any other prescription or nonprescription (over-the-counter [OTC]) medicine.

Other medical problems—The presence of other medical problems may affect the use of epoetin. Make sure you tell your doctor if you have any other medical problems, especially:

- Blood clots (history of) or other problems with the blood or
- Heart or blood vessel disease or
- High blood pressure—The chance of side effects may be increased
- Bone problems or
- Sickle cell anemia—Epoetin may not work properly
- Seizures (history of)—The chance of seizures may be increased

Before you begin using any new medicine (prescription or nonprescription) or if you develop any new medical problem while you are using this medicine, check with your doctor, nurse, or pharmacist.

Proper Use of This Medicine

Epoetin is usually given by a doctor or nurse after a dialysis treatment. However, medicines given by injection are sometimes used at home. If you will be using epoetin at home, your doctor or nurse will teach you how the injections are to be given. You will also have a chance to practice giving them. *Be certain that you understand exactly how the medicine is to be injected.*

Missed dose—If you miss a dose of this medicine, use it as soon as possible. However, if it is almost time for your next dose, skip the missed dose and go back to your regular dosing schedule. Do not double doses.

Storage—To store this medicine:

- Keep out of the reach of children.
- Store in the refrigerator. However, keep the medicine from freezing.
- Do not keep outdated medicine or medicine no longer needed. Be sure that any discarded medicine is out of the reach of children.

Precautions While Using This Medicine

Epoetin sometimes causes convulsions (seizures), especially during the first 90 days of treatment. During this time, it is best to avoid driving, operating heavy machinery, or other activities that could cause a serious injury if a seizure occurs while you are performing them.

People with severe anemia usually feel very tired and sick. When epoetin begins to work, usually in about 6 weeks, most people start to feel better. Some people are able to be more active. However, epoetin only corrects anemia. It has no effect on kidney disease or any other medical problem that needs regular medical attention. Therefore, even if you are feeling much better, *it is very important that you do not miss any appointments with your doctor or any dialysis treatments.*

Many people with kidney problems need to be on a special diet. Also, people with high blood pressure (which may be caused by kidney disease or by epoetin treatment) may need to be on a special diet and/or to take medicine to keep their blood pressure under control. After their anemia has been corrected, some people feel so much better that they want to eat more than before. To keep your kidney disease or your high blood pressure from getting worse, *it is very important that you follow your special diet and take your medicines regularly,* even if you are feeling better.

In addition to epoetin, your body needs iron to make red blood cells. Your doctor may direct you to take iron supplements. He or she may also direct you to take certain vitamins that help the iron work better. *Be sure to follow your doctor's orders carefully,* because epoetin will not work properly if there is not enough iron in your body.

Side Effects of This Medicine

Along with its needed effects, a medicine may cause some unwanted effects. Although not all of these side effects

may occur, if they do occur they may need medical attention.

Check with your doctor immediately if any of the following side effects occur:

More common
Chest pain

Less common
Convulsions (seizures); shortness of breath

Also, check with your doctor as soon as possible if any of the following side effects occur:

More common
Fast heartbeat; headache; increased blood pressure; swelling of face, fingers, ankles, feet, or lower legs; vision problems; weight gain

Rare
Skin rash or hives

Other side effects may occur that usually do not need medical attention. These side effects may go away during treatment as your body adjusts to the medicine. Epoetin sometimes causes an influenza-like reaction, with symptoms such as muscle aches, bone pain, chills, shivering, and sweating, occurring about 1 or 2 hours after an injection. These symptoms usually go away within 12 hours. However, check with your doctor if this influenza-like reaction or any of the following side effects continue or are bothersome:

More common
Bone pain; diarrhea; muscle weakness (severe); nausea or vomiting; tiredness

Other side effects not listed above may also occur in some patients. If you notice any other effects, check with your doctor.

Additional Information

For patients receiving epoetin who do not have anemia caused by kidney disease:

- The information about the importance of keeping dialysis appointments and following a special diet for people with kidney problems does not apply to you. However, your doctor may have other special directions for you to follow. Be sure to follow these directions carefully, even if you feel much better after receiving epoetin for a while.

Annual revision: 07/07/92

ERGOLOID MESYLATES Systemic

Some commonly used brand names are:

In the U.S.
Gerimal
Hydergine
Hydergine LC
Generic name product may also be available.

In Canada
Hydergine

Another commonly used name is dihydrogenated ergot alkaloids.

Description

Ergoloid mesylates (ER-goe-loid MESS-i-lates) belongs to the group of medicines known as ergot alkaloids. It is used to treat some mood, behavior, or other problems that may be due to changes in the brain from Alzheimer's disease or multiple small strokes.

This medicine is different from other ergot alkaloids such as ergotamine and methysergide. It is not useful for treating migraine headache. The exact way ergoloid mesylates acts on the body is not known.

This medicine is available only with your doctor's prescription, in the following dosage forms:

Oral
- Capsules (U.S.)
- Oral solution (U.S.)
- Tablets (U.S. and Canada)

Sublingual (under-the-tongue)
- Tablets (U.S.)

It is very important that you read and understand the following information. If any of it causes you special concern, check with your doctor. Also, *if you have any questions* or if you want more information about this medicine or your medical problem, *ask your doctor, nurse, or pharmacist*.

Before Using This Medicine

In deciding to use a medicine, the risks of taking the medicine must be weighed against the good it will do. This is a decision you and your doctor will make. For ergoloid mesylates, the following should be considered:

Allergies—Tell your doctor if you have ever had any unusual or allergic reaction to ergot alkaloids. Also tell your doctor and pharmacist if you are allergic to any other substances, such as foods, preservatives, or dyes.

Other medicines—Although certain medicines should not be used together at all, in other cases 2 different medicines may be used together even if an interaction might occur. In these cases, your doctor may want to change the dose, or other precautions may be necessary. Tell your doctor and pharmacist if you are taking any other prescription or nonprescription (over-the-counter [OTC]) medicine.

Other medical problems—The presence of other medical problems may affect the use of ergoloid mesylates. Make sure you tell your doctor if you have any other medical problems, especially:

- Liver disease—Higher blood levels of ergoloid mesylates may occur, increasing the chance of side effects
- Low blood pressure or
- Other mental problems or
- Slow heartbeat—Ergoloid mesylates may make the condition worse

Before you begin using any new medicine (prescription or nonprescription) or if you develop any new medical problem while you are using this medicine, check with your doctor, nurse, or pharmacist.

Proper Use of This Medicine

Take this medicine only as directed by your doctor. Do not take more or less of it, and do not take it more often or for a longer period of time than your doctor ordered. To do so may increase the chance of unwanted effects.

For patients taking the *sublingual (under-the-tongue) tablets:*

- Dissolve the tablet under your tongue. The sublingual tablet should not be chewed or swallowed, since it works much faster when absorbed through the lining of the mouth. Do not eat, drink, or smoke while a tablet is dissolving.

Dosing—The dose of ergoloid mesylates will be different for different patients. *Follow your doctor's orders or the directions on the label.* The following information includes only the average doses of ergoloid mesylates. *If your dose is different, do not change it* unless your doctor tells you to do so.

- The number of tablets or milliliters of oral solution that you take depends on the strength of the medicine. Also, *the number of doses you take each day, the time allowed between doses, and the length of time you take the medicine depend on the medical problem for which you are taking ergoloid mesylates.*
- For *oral* dosage forms (capsules, tablets, sublingual tablets, or oral solution):
  —Adults: 1 to 2 milligrams (mg) three times a day.

Missed dose—If you miss a dose of this medicine, skip the missed dose and go back to your regular dosing schedule. Do not double doses. If you have any questions about this, or if you miss two or more doses in a row, check with your doctor.

Storage—To store this medicine:

- Keep out of the reach of children.
- Store away from heat and direct light.
- Do not store in the bathroom, near the kitchen sink, or in other damp places. Heat or moisture may cause the medicine to break down.
- Keep the oral solution from freezing.
- Do not keep outdated medicine or medicine no longer needed. Be sure that any discarded medicine is out of the reach of children.

Precautions While Using This Medicine

It is important that your doctor check your progress at regular visits to make sure this medicine is working and to check for unwanted effects.

It may take several weeks for this medicine to work. *However, do not stop taking this medicine without first checking with your doctor.*

Side Effects of This Medicine

Along with its needed effects, a medicine may cause some unwanted effects. Although not all of these side effects may occur, if they do occur they may need medical attention.

Check with your doctor as soon as possible if any of the following side effects occur:

Less common or rare

Dizziness or lightheadedness when getting up from a lying or sitting position; drowsiness; skin rash; slow pulse

Signs and symptoms of overdose

Blurred vision; dizziness; fainting; flushing; headache; loss of appetite; nausea or vomiting; stomach cramps; stuffy nose

Other side effects may occur that usually do not need medical attention. These side effects may go away during treatment as your body adjusts to the medicine. However, check with your doctor if any of the following side effects continue or are bothersome:

Less common or rare

Soreness under tongue (with sublingual use)

Other side effects not listed above may also occur in some patients. If you notice any other effects, check with your doctor.

Annual revision: 04/16/93

ERGONOVINE/METHYLERGONOVINE Systemic

This information applies to the following medicines:
Ergonovine (er-goe-NOE-veen)
Methylergonovine (meth-ill-er-goe-NOE-veen)

Some commonly used brand names are:

For Ergonovine
In the U.S.
Ergotrate
In Canada
Ergotrate Maleate
Generic name product may also be available.

Another commonly used name is ergometrine.

For Methylergonovine†
In the U.S.
Methergine

Another commonly used name is methylergometrine.

†Not commercially available in Canada.

Description

Ergonovine and methylergonovine belong to the group of medicines known as ergot alkaloids. These medicines are usually given to stop excessive bleeding that sometimes occurs after abortion or a baby is delivered. They work by causing the muscle of the uterus to contract.

Ergonovine and methylergonovine may also be used for other conditions as determined by your doctor.

These medicines are available only on prescription and are to be administered only by or under the supervision of your doctor. They are available in the following dosage forms:

Oral
Ergonovine
- Tablets (U.S. and Canada)

Methylergonovine
- Tablets (U.S.)

Parenteral
Ergonovine
- Injection (U.S. and Canada)

Methylergonovine
- Injection (U.S.)

It is very important that you read and understand the following information. If any of it causes you special concern, check with your doctor. Also, *if you have any questions* or if you want more information about this medicine or your medical problem, *ask your doctor, nurse, or pharmacist.*

Before Using This Medicine

In deciding to use a medicine, the risks of taking the medicine must be weighed against the good it will do. This is a decision you and your doctor will make. For ergonovine and methylergonovine, the following should be considered:

Allergies—Tell your doctor if you have ever had any unusual or allergic reaction to ergonovine, methylergonovine, or other ergot medicines. Also tell your doctor and pharmacist if you are allergic to any other substances, such as foods, preservatives, or dyes.

Breast-feeding—This medicine passes into the breast milk and may cause unwanted effects, such as vomiting; decreased circulation in the hands, lower legs, and feet; diarrhea; weak pulse; unstable blood pressure; or convulsions (seizures) in infants of mothers taking large doses.

Children—Although there is no specific information comparing use of ergonovine or methylergonovine in children with use in other age groups, these medicines are not expected to cause different problems in children than they do in adults.

Older adults—Many medicines have not been studied specifically in older people. Therefore, it may not be known whether they work exactly the same way they do in younger adults or if they cause different side effects or problems in older people. There is no specific information comparing use of ergonovine or methylergonovine in the elderly with use in other age groups.

Other medicines—Although certain medicines should not be used together at all, in other cases two different medicines may be used together even if an interaction might occur. In these cases, your doctor may want to change the dose, or other precautions may be necessary. When you are taking ergonovine or methylergonovine it is especially important that your doctor and pharmacist know if you are taking any of the following:

- Bromocriptine (e.g., Parlodel) or
- Other ergot alkaloids (dihydroergotamine [e.g., D.H.E. 45], ergoloid mesylates [e.g., Hydergine], ergotamine [e.g., Gynergen], methysergide [e.g., Sansert])—Use of these medicines with ergonovine or methylergonovine may increase the chance of side effects of these medicines.
- Nitrates or
- Other medicines for angina—Use of these medicines with ergonovine or methylergonovine may keep these medicines from working properly

Other medical problems—The presence of other medical problems may affect the use of ergonovine or methylergonovine. Make sure you tell your doctor if you have any other medical problems, especially:

- Angina (chest pain) or other heart problems or
- Blood vessel disease or
- High blood pressure (or history of) or
- Stroke (history of)—These medicines may cause changes in how the heart works or blood pressure changes
- Infection—Infections may cause an increased sensitivity to the effect of these medicines

- Kidney disease
- Liver disease—The body may not remove these medicines from the bloodstream at the usual rate, which may make the medicine work longer or increase the chance for side effects
- Raynaud's phenomenon—Use of these medicines may cause worsening of the blood vessel narrowing that occurs with this disease

Proper Use of This Medicine

Take this medicine only as directed by your doctor. Do not take more of it, do not take it more often, and do not take it for a longer time than your doctor ordered. If too much is taken or if it is taken for a longer time than your doctor ordered, it may cause serious effects.

Dosing—The dose of ergonovine or methylergonovine will be different for different patients. *Follow your doctor's orders or the directions on the label.* The following information includes only the average doses of ergonovine and methylergonovine. *If your dose is different, do not change it* unless your doctor tells you to do so.

For ergonovine

- For *oral* dosage forms (tablets):
  - —Adults:
    - For treatment of excessive uterine bleeding: 0.2 to 0.4 milligram, swallowed or placed under the tongue every six to twelve hours. Usually this medicine is taken for forty-eight hours or less.
- For *injection* dosage form:
  - —Adults:
    - For treatment of excessive uterine bleeding: 0.2 milligram, injected into a muscle or vein. This dose can be repeated up to five times if needed, with a two- to four-hour wait between doses.

For methylergonovine

- For *oral* dosage forms (tablets):
  - —Adults:
    - For treatment of excessive uterine bleeding: 0.2 to 0.4 milligram, taken every six to twelve hours. Usually this medicine is taken for forty-eight hours or less.
- For *injection* dosage form:
  - —Adults:
    - For treatment of excessive uterine bleeding: 0.2 milligram, injected into a muscle or vein. This dose can be repeated up to five times if needed, with a two- to four-hour wait between doses.

Missed dose—If you miss a dose of this medicine, do not take the missed dose at all and do not double the next one. Instead, go back to your regular dosing schedule. If you have any questions about this, check with your doctor.

Storage—To store this medicine:

- Keep out of the reach of children.
- Store away from heat and direct light.
- Do not store in the bathroom, near the kitchen sink, or in other damp places. Heat or moisture may cause the medicine to break down.
- Do not keep outdated medicine or medicine no longer needed. Be sure that any discarded medicine is out of the reach of children.

Precautions While Using This Medicine

If you have an infection or illness of any kind, check with your doctor before taking this medicine, since you may be more sensitive to its effects.

Side Effects of This Medicine

Along with its needed effects, a medicine may cause some unwanted effects. Although not all of these side effects may occur, if they do occur they may need medical attention.

Check with the doctor or nurse immediately if any of the following side effects occur:

Less common

Chest pain

Rare

Blurred vision; convulsions (seizures); crushing chest pain; headache (sudden and severe); irregular heartbeat; unexplained shortness of breath

Check with your doctor as soon as possible if any of the following side effects occur:

Less common

Slow heartbeat

Rare

Itching of skin; pain in arms, legs, or lower back; pale or cold hands or feet; weakness in legs

Symptoms of overdose

Bluish color of skin or inside of nose or mouth; chest pain; cool, pale, or numb arms or legs; confusion; cramping of the uterus (severe); decreased breathing rate; drowsiness; heartbeat changes; muscle pain; small pupils; tingling, itching, and cool skin; trouble in breathing; unconsciousness; unusual thirst; weak or absent pulse in arms or legs; weak pulse

With long-term use

Dry, shriveled-looking skin on hands, lower legs, or feet; false feeling of insects crawling on the skin; pain and redness in an arm or leg; paralysis of one side of the body

Other side effects may occur that usually do not need medical attention. These side effects may go away during treatment as your body adjusts to the medicine. However, check with your doctor if any of the following side effects continue or are bothersome:

More common

Cramping of the uterus; nausea; vomiting

Less common

Abdominal or stomach pain; diarrhea; dizziness; headache (mild and temporary); ringing in the ears; stuffy nose; sweating; unpleasant taste

Other side effects not listed above may also occur in some patients. If you notice any other effects, check with your doctor.

Annual revision: 06/07/93

ERGOTAMINE, BELLADONNA ALKALOIDS, AND PHENOBARBITAL Systemic

Some commonly used brand names are:

In the U.S.

Bellergal-S

In Canada

Bellergal

Bellergal Spacetabs

Description

Ergotamine (er-GOT-a-meen), belladonna alkaloids (bell-a-DON-a AL-ka-loids), and phenobarbital (feen-oh-BAR-bi-tal) combination is used to treat a variety of problems including stomach problems and some kinds of throbbing headaches. The phenobarbital in this combination medicine belongs to the group of medicines known as barbiturates.

This medicine is available only with your doctor's prescription, in the following dosage forms:

Oral

- Tablets (Canada)
- Extended-release tablets (U.S. and Canada)

It is very important that you read and understand the following information. If any of it causes you special concern, check with your doctor. Also, *if you have any questions* or if you want more information about this medicine or your medical problem, *ask your doctor, nurse, or pharmacist.*

Before Using This Medicine

In deciding to use a medicine, the risks of taking the medicine must be weighed against the good it will do. This is a decision you and your doctor will make. For ergotamine, belladonna alkaloids, and phenobarbital combination, the following should be considered:

Allergies—Tell your doctor if you have ever had any unusual or allergic reaction to ergotamine or other ergot medicines, atropine, belladonna, or barbiturates. Also tell your doctor and pharmacist if you are allergic to any other substances, such as foods, preservatives, or dyes.

Pregnancy—

- *For ergotamine*—Ergotamine is not recommended for use during pregnancy since it has been shown to increase the chance of early labor, which could result in a miscarriage.
- *For belladonna alkaloids*—Belladonna alkaloids have not been shown to cause problems in humans.
- *For phenobarbital*—Barbiturates such as phenobarbital have been shown to increase the chance of birth defects. Also, when taken during pregnancy, barbiturates may cause bleeding problems in the newborn baby. Be sure that you have discussed these problems with your doctor before taking this medicine.

Breast-feeding—

- *For ergotamine*—Ergotamine passes into the breast milk and may cause unwanted effects, such as vomiting, diarrhea, weak pulse, unstable blood pressure, or convulsions (seizures), in nursing babies whose mothers take large amounts of the medicine. Large amounts of ergotamine may also decrease the flow of breast milk.
- *For belladonna alkaloids*—Although belladonna alkaloids pass into the breast milk, the amount of belladonna alkaloids in this combination medicine has not been shown to cause problems in nursing babies. However, because the belladonna alkaloids tend to decrease the secretions of the body, it is possible that the flow of breast milk may be reduced in some patients.
- *For phenobarbital*—Phenobarbital passes into the breast milk. Taking this combination medicine two or three times a day is not likely to cause problems in nursing babies. However, larger amounts of the medicine may cause drowsiness, unusually slow heartbeat, shortness of breath, or troubled breathing in nursing babies.

Be sure that you discuss these possible problems with your doctor before taking this medicine.

Children—Children may be especially sensitive to the effects of the belladonna alkaloids and the phenobarbital in this combination medicine. This may increase the chance of side effects during treatment. Although there is no specific information about the use of ergotamine in children, it is not expected to cause different side effects or problems in children than it does in adults.

Older adults—Elderly people are especially sensitive to the effects of ergotamine, belladonna alkaloids, and barbiturates such as phenobarbital. This may increase the chance of side effects during treatment.

Other medicines—Although certain medicines should not be used together at all, in other cases two different medicines may be used together even if an interaction might occur. In these cases, your doctor may want to change the dose, or other precautions may be necessary. When you are taking this combination medicine, it is especially important that your doctor and pharmacist know if you are taking any of the following:

- Antacids or
- Diarrhea medicine containing kaolin or attapulgite—These medicines may decrease the effects of the belladonna alkaloids and the phenobarbital in this combination medicine; to prevent this, take the 2 medicines at least 1 hour apart
- Anticoagulants (blood thinners)—The phenobarbital in this combination medicine may decrease the effects of anticoagulants; a change in the dose of anticoagulant may be needed
- Antimuscarinics (medicine for abdominal or stomach spasms or cramps) or
- Central nervous system (CNS) depressants or
- Cocaine or
- Contraceptives, oral, (birth control pills) containing estrogens or progestins or
- Digitalis glycosides (heart medicine) or
- Medicines for migraine that contain ergotamine in combination with other ingredients, such as ergotamine and caffeine (e.g., Cafergot) or
- Monoamine oxidase (MAO) inhibitors (furazolidone [e.g., Furoxone], isocarboxazid [e.g., Marplan], pargyline [e.g., Eutonyl], phenelzine [e.g., Nardil], procarbazine [e.g., Matulane], tranylcypromine [e.g., Parnate] (taken currently or within the past 2 weeks) or
- Other ergot medicines (dihydroergotamine [e.g., D.H.E. 45], ergoloid mesylates [e.g., Hydergine], ergonovine [e.g., Ergotrate], methylergonovine [e.g., Methergine], methysergide [e.g., Sansert]) or
- Potassium chloride (e.g., Kay Ciel) or
- Tricyclic antidepressants (amitriptyline [e.g., Elavil], amoxapine [e.g., Asendin], clomipramine [e.g., Anafranil], desipramine [e.g., Pertofrane], doxepin [e.g., Sinequan], imipramine [e.g., Tofranil], nortriptyline [e.g., Aventyl], protriptyline [e.g., Vivactil], trimipramine [e.g., Surmontil])—The chance of serious side effects may be increased
- Ketoconazole (e.g., Nizoral)—The belladonna alkaloids in this combination medicine may reduce the effects of ketoconazole; to prevent this, take the ergotamine, belladonna alkaloids, and phenobarbital combination at least 2 hours after taking ketoconazole

Other medical problems—The presence of other medical problems may affect the use of this combination medicine. Make sure you tell your doctor if you have any other medical problems, especially:

- Asthma (or history of), emphysema, or other chronic lung disease or
- Brain damage (in children) or
- Difficult urination or
- Down's syndrome (mongolism) or
- Dry mouth (severe and continuing) or
- Enlarged prostate or
- Heart or blood vessel disease or
- High blood pressure (severe) or
- Hyperactivity (in children) or
- Infection or
- Intestinal blockage or other intestinal problems or
- Itching (severe) or
- Kidney disease or
- Liver disease or
- Overactive thyroid or
- Porphyria or
- Spastic paralysis (in children) or
- Urinary tract blockage—The chance of side effects may be increased
- Glaucoma—The belladonna alkaloids in this combination medicine may make your condition worse

Also tell your doctor if you have recently had an angioplasty (a procedure done to improve the flow of blood in a blocked blood vessel) or surgery on a blood vessel, because the chance of side effects caused by the ergotamine in this combination medicine may be increased.

Before you begin using any new medicine (prescription or nonprescription) or if you develop any new medical problem while you are using this medicine, check with your doctor, nurse, or pharmacist.

Proper Use of This Medicine

Take this medicine only as directed by your doctor. If the amount you are to take does not seem to work, do not take more than your doctor ordered. Instead, check with your doctor. Taking too much of this medicine or taking it too often may cause serious effects such as nausea and vomiting; cold, painful hands or feet; or even gangrene. Also, if too much is used, it may become habit-forming.

To take the *extended-release tablet* form of this medicine:

- Swallow the tablet whole.
- Do not crush, break, or chew the tablet before swallowing it.

Missed dose—If you miss a dose of this medicine, skip the missed dose and go back to your regular dosing schedule. Do not double doses.

Storage—To store this medicine:

- Keep out of the reach of children since overdose is especially dangerous in children.
- Store away from heat and direct light.
- Do not store in the bathroom, near the kitchen sink, or in other damp places. Heat and moisture may cause the medicine to break down.
- Do not keep outdated medicine or medicine no longer needed. Be sure that any discarded medicine is out of the reach of children.

Precautions While Using This Medicine

If you have been taking this medicine regularly, *do not stop taking it without first checking with your doctor.* Your doctor may want you to reduce gradually the amount you are using before stopping completely.

Do not take antacids or medicine for diarrhea within 1 hour of taking this medicine. Taking them too close together will make the belladonna alkaloids less effective.

This medicine will add to the effects of alcohol and other CNS depressants (medicines that slow down the nervous system, possibly causing drowsiness). Some examples of CNS depressants are antihistamines or medicine for hay fever, other allergies, or colds; sedatives, tranquilizers, or sleeping medicine; prescription pain medicine or narcotics; barbiturates; medicine for seizures; muscle relaxants; or anesthetics, including some dental anesthetics. *Check with your doctor before taking any of the above while you are taking this medicine.* Also, alcohol may make your headaches worse, so it is best to avoid alcoholic beverages while you are suffering from the headaches.

This medicine may cause some people to have blurred vision or to become drowsy, dizzy, lightheaded, or less alert than they are normally. *Make sure you know how you react to this medicine before you drive, use machines, or do anything else that could be dangerous if you are dizzy or are not alert and able to see well.*

Since smoking may increase some of the harmful effects of this medicine, it is best to avoid smoking while you are using it. If you have any questions about this, check with your doctor.

This medicine may make you more sensitive to cold temperatures, especially if you have blood circulation problems. It tends to decrease blood circulation in the skin, fingers, and toes. Dress warmly during cold weather and be careful during prolonged exposure to cold, such as in winter sports. This is especially important for elderly people, who are more likely than younger adults to already have problems with their circulation.

Belladonna alkaloids (contained in this combination medicine) will often make you sweat less, causing your body temperature to increase. *Use extra care not to become overheated during exercise or hot weather while you are taking this medicine,* as overheating may result in a heat stroke. Also, hot baths or saunas may make you feel dizzy or faint while you are taking this medicine. This is especially important in children taking this medicine.

This medicine may cause your eyes to become more sensitive to light than they are normally. Wearing sunglasses may help lessen the discomfort from bright light.

If you have a serious infection or illness of any kind, check with your doctor before taking this medicine, since you may be more sensitive to its effects.

This medicine may cause dryness of the mouth, nose and throat. For temporary relief of mouth dryness, use sugarless candy or gum, melt bits of ice in your mouth, or use a saliva substitute. However, if dry mouth continues for more than 2 weeks, check with your medical doctor or dentist. Continuing dryness of the mouth may increase the chance of dental disease, including tooth decay, gum disease, and fungus infections.

Side Effects of This Medicine

Along with its needed effects, a medicine may cause some unwanted effects. Although not all of these side effects may occur, if they do occur they may need medical attention.

Check with your doctor immediately if any of the following side effects occur since they may be symptoms of an overdose:

Blurred vision; clumsiness or unsteadiness; confusion, especially in the elderly; convulsions (seizures); dizziness (continuing); drowsiness (severe); dryness of mouth, nose, or throat (severe); excitement, nervousness, restlessness, or irritability; fast heartbeat; fever; hallucinations (seeing, hearing, or feeling things that are not there); mental depression; numbness and tingling of fingers, toes, or face; red or violet blisters on skin of hands or feet; shortness of breath or troubled breathing; slurred speech; warmth, dryness, or flushing of skin

Check with your doctor as soon as possible if any of the following side effects occur:

More common

Swelling of feet and lower legs

Less common or rare

Chest pain; eye pain; headaches, more often and/or more severe than before; pain in arms, legs, or lower back; pale or cold hands or feet; skin rash, hives, or itching; sore throat and fever; unusual bleeding or bruising; weakness in legs; yellow eyes or skin

Other side effects may occur that usually do not need medical attention. These side effects may go away during treatment as your body adjusts to the medicine. However,

check with your doctor if any of the following side effects continue or are bothersome:

More common

Constipation; decreased sweating; dizziness or lightheadedness; drowsiness; dryness of mouth, nose, throat, or skin

Less common or rare

Bloated feeling; difficult urination (especially in older men); difficulty in swallowing; increased sensitivity of eyes to sunlight; loss of memory; nausea or vomiting; reduced sweating; unusual tiredness or weakness

After you stop taking this medicine, your body may need time to adjust. The length of time this takes depends on the amount of medicine you were taking and how long you took it. During this time check with your doctor if your headaches begin again or worsen.

Other side effects not listed above may also occur in some patients. If you notice any other effects, check with your doctor.

Annual revision: June 1990

ERYTHROMYCIN Ophthalmic

A commonly used brand name in the U.S. and Canada is Ilotycin. Generic name product may also be available in the U.S.

Description

Erythromycin (eh-rith-roe-MYE-sin) belongs to the family of medicines called antibiotics. Erythromycin ophthalmic preparations are used to treat infections of the eye. They may be used with other medicines for some eye infections.

Erythromycin is available only with your doctor's prescription, in the following dosage form:

Ophthalmic

- Ophthalmic ointment (U.S. and Canada)

It is very important that you read and understand the following information. If any of it causes you special concern, check with your doctor. Also, *if you have any questions* or if you want more information about this medicine or your medical problem, *ask your doctor, nurse, or pharmacist.*

Before Using This Medicine

In deciding to use a medicine, the risks of taking the medicine must be weighed against the good it will do. This is a decision you and your doctor will make. For ophthalmic erythromycin, the following should be considered:

Allergies—Tell your doctor if you have ever had any unusual or allergic reaction to this or any of the other erythromycins. Also tell your doctor and pharmacist if you are allergic to any other substances, such as preservatives.

Pregnancy—Ophthalmic erythromycin has not been shown to cause birth defects or other problems in humans.

Breast-feeding—Ophthalmic erythromycin has not been reported to cause problems in nursing babies.

Children—Studies on this medicine have been done only in adult patients, and there is no specific information comparing use of this medicine in children with use in other age groups.

Older adults—Many medicines have not been studied specifically in older people. Therefore, it may not be known whether they work exactly the same way they do in younger adults or if they cause different side effects or problems in older people. There is no specific information comparing use of this medicine in the elderly with use in other age groups.

Before you begin using any new medicine (prescription or nonprescription) or if you develop any new medical problem while you are using this medicine, check with your doctor, nurse, or pharmacist.

Proper Use of This Medicine

To use:

- First, wash your hands. Then pull the lower eyelid away from the eye to form a pouch. Squeeze a thin strip of ointment into the pouch. A 1-cm (approximately ⅓-inch) strip of ointment is usually enough unless otherwise directed by your doctor. Gently close the eyes and keep them closed for 1 or 2 minutes to allow the medicine to come into contact with the infection.
- To keep the medicine as germ-free as possible, do not touch the applicator tip to any surface (including the eye). After using erythromycin eye ointment, wipe the tip of the ointment tube with a clean tissue and keep the tube tightly closed.

To help clear up your infection completely, *keep using this medicine for the full time of treatment,* even if your symptoms begin to clear up after a few days. If you stop using this medicine too soon, your symptoms may return. *Do not miss any doses.*

Missed dose—If you do miss a dose of this medicine, apply it as soon as possible. However, if it is almost time for your next dose, skip the missed dose and go back to your regular dosing schedule.

Storage—To store this medicine:
- Keep out of the reach of children.
- Store away from heat and direct light.
- Keep the medicine from freezing.
- Do not keep outdated medicine or medicine no longer needed. Be sure that any discarded medicine is out of the reach of children.

Precautions While Using This Medicine

If your symptoms do not improve within a few days, or if they become worse, check with your doctor.

After application, eye ointments usually cause your vision to blur for a few minutes.

Side Effects of This Medicine

Along with its needed effects, a medicine may cause some unwanted effects.

Check with your doctor as soon as possible if the following side effect occurs:

Rare

Eye irritation not present before therapy

Other side effects not listed above may also occur in some patients. If you notice any other effects, check with your doctor.

Annual revision: 06/30/92

ERYTHROMYCIN Topical

Some commonly used brand names are:

In the U.S.

Akne-Mycin	Erymax
A/T/S	Ery-Sol
Erycette	ETS
EryDerm	Staticin
Erygel	T-Stat

Generic name product may also be available.

In Canada

Sans-Acne
Staticin

Description

Erythromycin (eh-rith-roe-MYE-sin) belongs to the family of medicines called antibiotics. Erythromycin topical preparations are used on the skin to help control acne. They may be used alone or with one or more other medicines that are applied to the skin or taken by mouth for acne. They may also be used for other problems, such as skin infections, as determined by your doctor.

Erythromycin is available only with your doctor's prescription, in the following dosage forms:

Topical
- Gel (U.S.)
- Ointment (U.S.)
- Pledgets (U.S.)
- Solution (U.S. and Canada)

It is very important that you read and understand the following information. If any of it causes you special concern, check with your doctor. Also, *if you have any questions* or if you want more information about this medicine or your medical problem, *ask your doctor, nurse, or pharmacist.*

Before Using This Medicine

In deciding to use a medicine, the risks of taking the medicine must be weighed against the good it will do. This is a decision you and your doctor will make. For topical erythromycin, the following should be considered:

Allergies—Tell your doctor if you have ever had any unusual or allergic reaction to this or any of the other erythromycins. Also tell your doctor and pharmacist if you are allergic to any other substances, such as preservatives or dyes.

Pregnancy—Topical erythromycin has not been studied in pregnant women. However, this medication has not been shown to cause birth defects or other problems in animal studies.

Breast-feeding—It is not known whether topical erythromycin passes into the breast milk. Erythromycin, given by mouth or by injection, does pass into the breast milk. However, erythromycin topical preparations have not been reported to cause problems in nursing babies.

Children—Erythromycin topical solution has been tested in children 12 years of age and older and, in effective doses, has not been shown to cause different side effects or problems than it does in adults.

Older adults—Many medicines have not been studied specifically in older people. Therefore, it may not be known whether they work exactly the same way they do in younger adults. Although there is no specific information comparing use of topical erythromycin in the elderly with use in other age groups, this medicine is not expected to cause different side effects or problems in older people than it does in younger adults.

Other medicines—Although certain medicines should not be used together at all, in other cases two different medicines may be used together even if an interaction might occur. In these cases, your doctor may want to change the dose, or other precautions may be necessary. Tell your doctor and pharmacist if you are using any other topical prescription or nonprescription (over-the-counter [OTC]) medicine that is to be applied to the same area of the skin.

Before you begin using any new medicine (prescription or nonprescription) or if you develop any new medical problem while you are using this medicine, check with your doctor, nurse, or pharmacist.

Proper Use of This Medicine

Before applying this medicine, thoroughly wash the affected area with warm water and soap, rinse well, and pat dry. After washing or shaving, it is best to wait 30 minutes before applying the pledget (swab), topical gel, or topical liquid form. The alcohol in them may irritate freshly washed or shaved skin.

This medicine will not cure your acne. However, to help keep your acne under control, *keep using this medicine for the full time of treatment,* even if your symptoms begin to clear up after a few days. You may have to continue using this medicine every day for months or even longer in some cases. If you stop using this medicine too soon, your symptoms may return. *It is important that you do not miss any doses.*

Missed dose—If you do miss a dose of this medicine, apply it as soon as possible. However, if it is almost time for your next dose, skip the missed dose and go back to your regular dosing schedule.

For patients using the pledget (swab), topical gel, or topical liquid form of erythromycin:

- These forms contain alcohol and are flammable. *Do not use near heat, near open flame, or while smoking.*
- It is important that you do not use this medicine more often than your doctor ordered. It may cause your skin to become too dry or irritated.
- Also, you should avoid washing the acne-affected areas too often. This may dry your skin and make your acne worse. Washing with a mild, bland soap 2 or 3 times a day should be enough, unless you have oily skin. If you have any questions about this, check with your doctor.
- To use:

  —The topical liquid form of this medicine may come in a bottle with an applicator tip, which may be used to apply the medicine directly to the skin. Use the applicator with a dabbing motion instead of a rolling motion (not like a roll-on deodorant, for example). If the medicine does not come in an applicator bottle, you may moisten a pad with the medicine and then rub the pad over the whole affected area. Or you may also apply this medicine with your fingertips. Be sure to wash the medicine off your hands afterward.

  —Apply a thin film of medicine, using enough to cover the affected area lightly. *You should apply the medicine to the whole area usually affected by acne, not just to the pimples themselves.* This will help keep new pimples from breaking out.

  —The pledget (swab) form should be rubbed over the whole affected area. You may use extra pledgets (swabs), if needed, to cover larger areas.

  —Since these medicines contain alcohol, they may sting or burn. Therefore, *do not get these medicines in the eyes, nose, mouth, or on other mucous membranes.* Spread the medicine away from these areas when applying. If these medicines do get in the eyes, wash them out immediately, but carefully, with large amounts of cool tap water. If your eyes still burn or are painful, check with your doctor.

Storage—To store this medicine:

- Keep out of the reach of children.
- Store away from heat and direct light.
- Keep the medicine from freezing.
- Do not keep outdated medicine or medicine no longer needed. Be sure that any discarded medicine is out of the reach of children.

Precautions While Using This Medicine

If your acne does not improve within 3 to 4 weeks, or if it becomes worse, check with your doctor or pharmacist. However, treatment of acne may take up to 8 to 12 weeks before you see full improvement.

For patients using the pledget (swab), topical gel, or topical liquid form of erythromycin:

- If your doctor has ordered another medicine to be applied to the skin along with this medicine, it is best to wait at least 1 hour before you apply the second medicine. This may help keep your skin from becoming too irritated. Also, if the medicines are used too close together, they may not work properly.

- After application of this medicine to the skin, mild stinging or burning may be expected and may last up to a few minutes or more.
- This medicine may also cause the skin to become unusually dry, even with normal use. If this occurs, check with your doctor.
- You may continue to use cosmetics (make-up) while you are using this medicine for acne. However, it is best to use only "water-base" cosmetics. Also, it is best not to use cosmetics too heavily or too often. They may make your acne worse. If you have any questions about this, check with your doctor.

Side Effects of This Medicine

Along with its needed effects, a medicine may cause some unwanted effects. The following side effects may go away during treatment as your body adjusts to the medicine. However, check with your doctor if any of the following side effects continue or are bothersome:

For erythromycin ointment

Less common

Peeling; redness

For erythromycin pledget (swab), topical gel, or topical liquid form

More common

Dry or scaly skin; irritation; itching; stinging or burning feeling

Less common

Peeling; redness

Other side effects not listed above may also occur in some patients. If you notice any other effects, check with your doctor.

Annual revision: 06/23/92

ERYTHROMYCIN AND BENZOYL PEROXIDE Topical†

A commonly used brand name in the U.S. is Benzamycin.

†Not commercially available in Canada.

Description

Erythromycin (eh-rith-roe-MYE-sin) and benzoyl peroxide (BEN-zoe-ill per-OX-ide) combination is used to help control acne.

This medicine is applied to the skin. It may be used alone or with other medicines that are applied to the skin or taken by mouth for acne.

Erythromycin and benzoyl peroxide combination is available only with your doctor's prescription, in the following dosage form:

Topical

- Topical gel (U.S.)

It is very important that you read and understand the following information. If any of it causes you special concern, check with your doctor. Also, *if you have any questions* or if you want more information about this medicine or your medical problem, *ask your doctor, nurse, or pharmacist.*

Before Using This Medicine

In deciding to use a medicine, the risks of using the medicine must be weighed against the good it will do. This is a decision you and your doctor will make. For erythromycin and benzoyl peroxide combination, the following should be considered:

Allergies—Tell your doctor if you have ever had any unusual or allergic reaction to this medicine, to any of the other erythromycins, or to benzoyl peroxide (e.g., PanOxyl). Also tell your doctor and pharmacist if you are allergic to any other substances, such as preservatives or dyes.

Pregnancy—Studies on effects in pregnancy have not been done in either humans or animals. However, the benzoyl peroxide in this medicine may be absorbed into the body. Before using this medicine, make sure your doctor knows if you are pregnant or if you may become pregnant.

Breast-feeding—It is not known whether topical erythromycin or topical benzoyl peroxide passes into the breast milk. Erythromycin (e.g., E-Mycin), given by mouth or by injection, does pass into the breast milk. In addition, the benzoyl peroxide in this medicine may be absorbed into the mother's body. However, erythromycin and benzoyl peroxide combination has not been reported to cause problems in nursing babies.

Children—Studies on this medicine have been done only in adult patients, and there is no specific information comparing use of this medicine in children up to 12 years of age with use in other age groups.

Older adults—Many medicines have not been studied specifically in older people. Therefore, it may not be known whether they work exactly the same way they do in

younger adults or if they cause different side effects or problems in older people. There is no specific information comparing use of this medicine in the elderly with use in other age groups.

Other medicines—Although certain medicines should not be used together at all, in other cases two different medicines may be used together even if an interaction might occur. In these cases, your doctor may want to change the dose, or other precautions may be necessary. Tell your doctor and pharmacist if you are using any other topical prescription or nonprescription (over-the-counter [OTC]) medicine that is to be applied to the same area of the skin.

Before you begin using any new medicine (prescription or nonprescription) or if you develop any new medical problem while you are using this medicine, check with your doctor, nurse, or pharmacist.

Proper Use of This Medicine

Do not use this medicine on raw or irritated skin.

Before applying this medicine, thoroughly wash the affected area(s) with warm water and soap, rinse well, and gently pat dry. After washing or shaving, it is best to wait 30 minutes before applying the medicine. The alcohol in it may irritate freshly washed or shaved skin.

Avoid washing the acne-affected area(s) too often. This may dry your skin and make your acne worse. Washing with a mild, bland soap 2 or 3 times a day should be enough, unless you have oily skin. If you have any questions about this, check with your doctor.

To use:

- *Use this medicine only as directed.* Do not use more of it and do not use it more often than your doctor ordered. To do so may cause your skin to become too dry or irritated.
- After washing the affected area(s), you may apply this medicine with your fingertips. However, be sure to wash the medicine off your hands afterward.
- Apply and rub in a thin film of medicine, using enough to cover the affected area(s) lightly. *You should apply the medicine to the whole area usually affected by acne, not just to the pimples themselves.*
- Since this medicine contains alcohol, it may sting or burn. Therefore, *do not get this medicine in or around your eyes, nose, or mouth, or on other mucous membranes.* Spread the medicine away from these areas when applying. If this medicine does get in your eyes, wash them out immediately, but carefully, with large amounts of cool tap water. If your eyes still burn or are painful, check with your doctor.

Do not use this medicine after the expiration date on the label. The medicine may not work properly. Get a fresh supply from your pharmacist. Check with your pharmacist if you have any questions about this.

To help keep your acne under control, *keep using this medicine for the full time of treatment.* You may have to continue using this medicine every day for months or even longer in some cases.

Missed dose—If you miss a dose of this medicine, apply it as soon as possible. However, if it is almost time for your next dose, skip the missed dose and go back to your regular dosing schedule.

Storage—To store this medicine:

- Keep out of the reach of children.
- Store in the refrigerator. Heat will cause this medicine to break down. However, keep the medicine from freezing. Follow the directions on the label.
- Do not keep outdated medicine or medicine no longer needed. Be sure that any discarded medicine is out of the reach of children.

Precautions While Using This Medicine

If your acne does not improve within 3 to 4 weeks, or if it becomes worse, check with your doctor or pharmacist. However, treatment of acne may take up to 8 to 12 weeks before you see full improvement.

If your doctor has ordered another medicine to be applied to the skin along with this medicine, it is best to apply the second medicine at least 1 hour after you apply the first medicine. This may help keep your skin from becoming too irritated. Also, if the medicines are used too close together, they may not work properly.

Mild stinging or burning of the skin may be expected after this medicine is applied. These effects may last up to a few minutes or more. If irritation continues, check with your doctor. You may have to use the medicine less often. Follow your doctor's directions.

This medicine may also cause the skin to become unusually dry, even with normal use. If this occurs, check with your doctor.

This medicine may bleach hair or colored fabrics.

You may continue to use cosmetics (make-up) while you are using this medicine for acne. However, it is best to use only "oil-free" cosmetics. Also, it is best not to use cosmetics too heavily or too often. They may make your acne worse. If you have any questions about this, check with your doctor.

Side Effects of This Medicine

Along with its needed effects, a medicine may cause some unwanted effects. Although not all of these side effects

may occur, if they do occur they may need medical attention.

Check with your doctor as soon as possible if any of the following side effects occur:

Less common or rare

Burning, blistering, crusting, itching, severe redness, or swelling of the skin; painful irritation of the skin; skin rash

Symptoms of topical overdose

Burning, itching, scaling, redness, or swelling of the skin (severe)

Other side effects may occur that usually do not need medical attention. These side effects may go away during treatment as your body adjusts to the medicine. However, check with your doctor if any of the following side effects continue or are bothersome:

Less common

Dryness or peeling of the skin; feeling of warmth, mild stinging, or redness of the skin

Other side effects not listed above may also occur in some patients. If you notice any other effects, check with your doctor.

Annual revision: 06/26/92

ERYTHROMYCINS Systemic

This information applies to the following medicines:

Erythromycin Base
Erythromycin Estolate
Erythromycin Ethylsuccinate
Erythromycin Gluceptate
Erythromycin Lactobionate
Erythromycin Stearate

Some commonly used brand names are:

For Erythromycin Base

In the U.S.

E-Mycin
ERYC
Ery-Tab
PCE Dispertab
Robimycin

Generic name product may also be available.

In Canada

Apo-Erythro
Apo-Erythro-EC
E-Mycin
Erybid
ERYC-125
ERYC-250
Erythromid
Novorythro
PCE Dispertab

Generic name product may also be available.

For Erythromycin Estolate

In the U.S.

Erythrozone
Ilosone

Generic name product may also be available.

In Canada

Ilosone
Novorythro

For Erythromycin Ethylsuccinate

In the U.S.

E.E.S.
EryPed
Erythro

Generic name product may also be available.

In Canada

Apo-Erythro-ES
E.E.S.

For Erythromycin Gluceptate

In the U.S.

Ilotycin

In Canada

Ilotycin

For Erythromycin Lactobionate

In the U.S.

Erythrocin

Generic name product may also be available.

In Canada

Erythrocin

For Erythromycin Stearate

In the U.S.

Erythrocin
Erythrocot
My-E
Wintrocin
Wyamycin-S

Generic name product may also be available.

In Canada

Apo-Erythro-S
Erythrocin
Novorythro

Description

Erythromycins (eh-rith-roe-MYE-sins) are used to treat infections. Erythromycins are also used to prevent "strep" infections in patients with a history of rheumatic heart disease who may be allergic to penicillin.

These medicines may also be used to treat Legionnaires' disease and for other problems as determined by your doctor. They will not work for colds, flu, or other virus infections.

Erythromycins are available only with your doctor's prescription, in the following dosage forms:

Oral

Erythromycin Base
- Delayed-release capsules (U.S. and Canada)
- Delayed-release tablets (U.S. and Canada)
- Tablets (U.S. and Canada)

Erythromycin Estolate
- Capsules (U.S. and Canada)
- Chewable tablets (U.S.)
- Oral suspension (U.S. and Canada)
- Tablets (U.S. and Canada)

Erythromycin Ethylsuccinate
- Chewable tablets (U.S. and Canada)
- Oral suspension (U.S. and Canada)
- Tablets (U.S. and Canada)

Erythromycin Stearate
- Oral suspension (Canada)
- Tablets (U.S. and Canada)

Parenteral

Erythromycin Gluceptate
- Injection (U.S. and Canada)

Erythromycin Lactobionate
- Injection (U.S. and Canada)

It is very important that you read and understand the following information. If any of it causes you special concern, check with your doctor. Also, *if you have any questions* or if you want more information about this medicine or your medical problem, *ask your doctor, nurse, or pharmacist*.

Before Using This Medicine

In deciding to use a medicine, the risks of taking the medicine must be weighed against the good it will do. This is a decision you and your doctor will make. For erythromycins, the following should be considered:

Allergies—Tell your doctor if you have ever had any unusual or allergic reaction to erythromycins. Also tell your doctor and pharmacist if you are allergic to any other substances, such as foods, preservatives, or dyes.

Pregnancy—Erythromycin estolate has caused side effects involving the liver in some pregnant women. However, none of the erythromycins has been shown to cause birth defects or other problems in humans.

Breast-feeding—Erythromycins pass into the breast milk. However, erythromycins have not been shown to cause problems in nursing babies.

Children—This medicine has been tested in children and has not been shown to cause different side effects or problems in children than it does in adults.

Older adults—This medicine has been tested and has not been shown to cause different side effects or problems in older people than it does in younger adults.

Other medicines—Although certain medicines should not be used together at all, in other cases two different medicines may be used together even if an interaction might occur. In these cases, your doctor may want to change the dose, or other precautions may be necessary. When you are taking or receiving erythromycins, it is especially important that your doctor and pharmacist know if you are taking any of the following:

- Acetaminophen (e.g., Tylenol) (with long-term, high-dose use) or
- Amiodarone (e.g., Cordarone) or
- Anabolic steroids (nandrolone [e.g., Anabolin], oxandrolone [e.g., Anavar], oxymetholone [e.g., Anadrol], stanozolol [e.g., Winstrol]) or
- Androgens (male hormones) or
- Antithyroid agents (medicine for overactive thyroid) or
- Carmustine (e.g., BiCNU) or
- Chloroquine (e.g., Aralen) or
- Dantrolene (e.g., Dantrium) or
- Daunorubicin (e.g., Cerubidine) or
- Disulfiram (e.g., Antabuse) or
- Divalproex (e.g., Depakote) or
- Estrogens (female hormones) or
- Etretinate (e.g., Tegison) or
- Gold salts (medicine for arthritis) or
- Hydroxychloroquine (e.g., Plaquenil) or
- Mercaptopurine (e.g., Purinethol) or
- Methotrexate (e.g., Mexate) or
- Methyldopa (e.g., Aldomet) or
- Naltrexone (e.g., Trexan) (with long-term, high-dose use) or
- Oral contraceptives (birth control pills) containing estrogen or
- Other anti-infectives by mouth or by injection (medicine for infection) or
- Phenothiazines (acetophenazine [e.g., Tindal], chlorpromazine [e.g., Thorazine], fluphenazine [e.g., Prolixin], mesoridazine [e.g., Serentil], perphenazine [e.g., Trilafon], prochlorperazine [e.g., Compazine], promazine [e.g., Sparine], promethazine [e.g., Phenergan], thioridazine [e.g., Mellaril], trifluoperazine [e.g., Stelazine], triflupromazine [e.g., Vesprin], trimeprazine [e.g., Temaril]) or
- Phenytoin (e.g., Dilantin) or
- Plicamycin (e.g., Mithracin) or
- Valproic acid (e.g., Depakene)—Use of these medicines with erythromycins, especially erythromycin estolate, may increase the chance of liver problems
- Aminophylline (e.g., Somophyllin) or
- Caffeine (e.g., NoDoz) or
- Oxtriphylline (e.g., Choledyl) or
- Theophylline (e.g., Somophyllin-T, Theo-Dur)—Use of these medicines with erythromycins may increase the chance of side effects from aminophylline, caffeine, oxtriphylline, or theophylline
- Carbamazepine (e.g., Tegretol)—Use of carbamazepine with erythromycin may increase the side effects of carbamazepine or increase the chance of liver problems
- Chloramphenicol (e.g., Chloromycetin) or
- Clindamycin (e.g., Cleocin) or
- Lincomycin (e.g., Lincocin)—Use of these medicines with erythromycins may decrease their effectiveness
- Cyclosporine (e.g., Sandimmune) or
- Warfarin (e.g., Coumadin)—Use of any of these medicines with erythromycins may increase the side effects of these medicines
- Terfenadine (e.g., Seldane)—Use of terfenadine with erythromycins may cause heart problems, such as an irregular heartbeat; these medicines should not be used together

Other medical problems—The presence of other medical problems may affect the use of erythromycins. Make sure

you tell your doctor if you have any other medical problems, especially:

- Heart disease—High doses of erythromycin may increase the chance of side effects in patients with a history of an irregular heartbeat
- Liver disease—Erythromycins, especially erythromycin estolate, may increase the chance of side effects involving the liver
- Loss of hearing—High doses of erythromycins may, on rare occasion, cause hearing loss

Before you begin using any new medicine (prescription or nonprescription) or if you develop any new medical problem while you are using this medicine, check with your doctor, nurse, or pharmacist.

Proper Use of This Medicine

Erythromycins may be taken with food if they upset your stomach.

For patients taking the *oral liquid form* of this medicine:

- This medicine is to be taken by mouth even if it comes in a dropper bottle. If this medicine does not come in a dropper bottle, use a specially marked measuring spoon or other device to measure each dose accurately. The average household teaspoon may not hold the right amount of liquid.
- Do not use after the expiration date on the label. The medicine may not work properly after that date. Check with your pharmacist if you have any questions about this.

For patients taking the *chewable tablet form* of this medicine:

- Tablets must be chewed or crushed before they are swallowed.

For patients taking the *delayed-release capsule form (with enteric-coated pellets) or the delayed-release tablet form* of this medicine:

- Swallow capsules or tablets whole. Do not break or crush. If you are not sure about which type of capsule or tablet you are taking, check with your pharmacist.

To help clear up your infection completely, *keep taking this medicine for the full time of treatment,* even if you begin to feel better after a few days. *If you have a "strep" infection, you should keep taking this medicine for at least 10 days. This is especially important in "strep" infections. Serious heart problems could develop later* if your infection is not cleared up completely. Also, if you stop taking this medicine too soon, your symptoms may return.

This medicine works best when there is a constant amount in the blood. *To help keep the amount constant, do not miss any doses. Also, it is best to take the doses at evenly spaced times day and night.* For example, if you are to take 4 doses a day, the doses should be spaced about 6 hours apart. If this interferes with your sleep or other daily activities, or if you need help in planning the best times to take your medicine, check with your doctor, nurse, or pharmacist.

Missed dose—If you do miss a dose of this medicine, take it as soon as possible. This will help to keep a constant amount of medicine in the blood. However, if it is almost time for your next dose, skip the missed dose and go back to your regular dosing schedule. Do not double doses.

Storage—To store this medicine:

- Keep out of the reach of children.
- Store away from heat and direct light.
- Do not store the capsule or tablet form of erythromycins in the bathroom, near the kitchen sink, or in other damp places. Heat or moisture may cause the medicine to break down.
- Store the oral liquid form of some erythromycins in the refrigerator because heat will cause this medicine to break down. However, keep the medicine from freezing. Follow the directions on the label.
- Do not keep outdated medicine or medicine no longer needed. Be sure that any discarded medicine is out of the reach of children.

Precautions While Using This Medicine

If your symptoms do not improve within a few days, or if they become worse, check with your doctor.

Side Effects of This Medicine

Along with its needed effects, a medicine may cause some unwanted effects. Although not all of these side effects may occur, if they do occur they may need medical attention.

Check with your doctor immediately if any of the following side effects occur:

Less common–with all erythromycins
Skin rash, hives, itching

Less common–with erythromycin injection
Pain, swelling, or redness at place of injection

Less common–with erythromycin estolate (rare with other erythromycins)
Dark or amber urine; pale stools; stomach pain (severe); unusual tiredness or weakness; yellow eyes or skin

Rare (with liver or kidney disease and high doses)
Fainting (recurrent); loss of hearing (temporary)

Other side effects may occur that usually do not need medical attention. These side effects may go away during treatment as your body adjusts to the medicine. However,

check with your doctor if any of the following side effects continue or are bothersome:

More common

Abdominal or stomach cramping and discomfort; diarrhea; nausea or vomiting

Less common

Sore mouth or tongue

Other side effects not listed above may also occur in some patients. If you notice any other effects, check with your doctor.

Annual revision: 09/08/92

ERYTHROMYCIN AND SULFISOXAZOLE Systemic

Some commonly used brand names are:

In the U.S.

Eryzole
Pediazole
Sulfimycin

Generic name product may also be available.

In Canada

Pediazole

Description

Erythromycin (eh-rith-roe-MYE-sin) and sulfisoxazole (sul-fi-SOX-a-zole) is a combination antibiotic used to treat ear infections. It may also be used for other problems as determined by your doctor. It will not work for colds, flu, or other virus infections.

Erythromycin and sulfisoxazole combination is available only with your doctor's prescription, in the following dosage form:

Oral

- Suspension (U.S. and Canada)

It is very important that you read and understand the following information. If any of it causes you special concern, check with your doctor. Also, *if you have any questions* or if you want more information about this medicine or your medical problem, *ask your doctor, nurse, or pharmacist.*

Before Using This Medicine

In deciding to use a medicine, the risks of taking the medicine must be weighed against the good it will do. This is a decision you and your doctor will make. For erythromycin and sulfisoxazole, the following should be considered:

Allergies—Tell your doctor if you have ever had any unusual or allergic reaction to the erythromycins or sulfa medicines, furosemide (e.g., Lasix) or thiazide diuretics (water pills), oral antidiabetics (diabetes medicine you take by mouth), or glaucoma medicine you take by mouth (for example, acetazolamide [e.g., Diamox], dichlorphenamide [e.g., Daranide], methazolamide [e.g., Neptazane]). Also tell your doctor and pharmacist if you are allergic to any other substances, such as foods, preservatives, or dyes.

Pregnancy—Studies have not been done in humans with either erythromycins or sulfa medicines. In addition, erythromycins have not been shown to cause birth defects or other problems in humans. However, studies in mice, rats, or rabbits have shown that some sulfa medicines cause birth defects, including cleft palate and bone problems.

Breast-feeding—Erythromycins and sulfa medicines pass into the breast milk. This medicine is not recommended for use during breast-feeding. It may cause liver problems, anemia, and other unwanted effects in nursing babies, especially those with glucose-6-phosphate dehydrogenase (G6PD) deficiency.

Children—This medicine has been tested in children over the age of 2 months and has not been shown to cause different side effects or problems than it does in adults.

Older adults—This medicine is intended for use in children and is not generally used in adult patients.

Other medicines—Although certain medicines should not be used together at all, in other cases two different medicines may be used together even if an interaction might occur. In these cases, your doctor may want to change the dose, or other precautions may be necessary. When you are taking erythromycin and sulfisoxazole, it is especially important that your doctor and pharmacist know if you are taking any of the following:

- Acetaminophen (e.g., Tylenol) (with long-term, high-dose use) or
- Amiodarone (e.g., Cordarone) or
- Anabolic steroids (nandrolone [e.g., Anabolin], oxandrolone [e.g., Anavar], oxymetholone [e.g., Anadrol], stanozolol [e.g., Winstrol]) or
- Androgens (male hormones) or
- Antithyroid agents (medicine for overactive thyroid) or
- Carbamazepine (e.g., Tegretol) or
- Carmustine (e.g., BiCNU) or
- Chloroquine (e.g., Aralen) or
- Dantrolene (e.g., Dantrium) or
- Daunorubicin (e.g., Cerubidine) or
- Disulfiram (e.g., Antabuse) or
- Divalproex (e.g., Depakote) or

- Estrogens (female hormones) or
- Etretinate (e.g., Tegison) or
- Gold salts (medicine for arthritis) or
- Hydroxychloroquine (e.g., Plaquenil) or
- Mercaptopurine (e.g., Purinethol) or
- Methotrexate (e.g., Mexate) or
- Methyldopa (e.g., Aldomet) or
- Naltrexone (e.g., Trexan) (with long-term, high-dose use) or
- Oral contraceptives (birth control pills) containing estrogen or
- Other anti-infectives by mouth or by injection (medicine for infection) or
- Phenothiazines (acetophenazine [e.g., Tindal], chlorpromazine [e.g., Thorazine], fluphenazine [e.g., Prolixin], mesoridazine [e.g., Serentil], perphenazine [e.g., Trilafon], prochlorperazine [e.g., Compazine], promazine [e.g., Sparine], promethazine [e.g., Phenergan], thioridazine [e.g. Mellaril], trifluoperazine [e.g., Stelazine], triflupromazine [e.g., Vesprin], trimeprazine [e.g., Temaril]) or
- Phenytoin (e.g., Dilantin) or
- Plicamycin (e.g., Mithracin) or
- Valproic acid (e.g., Depakene)—Use of erythromycin and sulfisoxazole with any of these medicines may increase the chance of side effects affecting the liver

- Acetohydroxamic acid (e.g., Lithostat) or
- Dapsone or
- Furazolidone (e.g., Furoxone) or
- Nitrofurantion (e.g., Furadantin) or
- Primaquine or
- Procainamide (e.g., Pronestyl) or
- Quinidine (e.g., Quinidex) or
- Quinine (e.g., Quinamm) or
- Sulfoxone (e.g., Diasone)—Use of erythromycin and sulfisoxazole with these medicines may increase the chance of side effects

- Alfentanil—Long-term use of erythromycin and sulfisoxazole may increase the action of alfentanil and increase the chance of side effects

- Aminophylline (e.g., Somophyllin) or
- Caffeine (e.g., NoDoz) or
- Oxtriphylline (e.g., Choledyl) or
- Theophylline (e.g., Slo-Phyllin, Somophyllin-T, Theo-dur)—Use of erythromycin and sulfisoxazole with these medicines may increase the side effects of these medicines

- Anticoagulants (blood thinners) or
- Antidiabetics, oral (diabetes medicine you take by mouth) or
- Ethotoin (e.g., Peganone) or
- Mephenytoin (e.g., Mesantoin)—Use of erythromycin and sulfisoxazole with these medicines may increase the effects of these medicines, thereby increasing the chance of side effects

- Chloramphenicol or
- Lincomycins—Use of erythromycin and sulfisoxazole with these medicines may decrease the effectiveness of these medicines

- Methenamine (e.g., Mandelamine)—Use of erythromycin and sulfisoxazole with this medicine may, on rare occasion, increase the chance of side effects affecting the kidneys

- Oral contraceptives (birth control pills) containing estrogen—Use of erythromycin and sulfisoxazole with oral contraceptives may decrease the effectiveness of oral contraceptives, increasing the chance of breakthrough bleeding and pregnancy
- Vitamin K (e.g., AquaMEPHYTON, Synkayvite)—Patients taking erythromycin and sulfisoxazole may have an increased need for vitamin K

Other medical problems—The presence of other medical problems may affect the use of erythromycin and sulfisoxazole. Make sure you tell your doctor if you have any other medical problems, especially:

- Anemia or other blood problems or
- Glucose-6-phosphate dehydrogenase (G6PD) deficiency—Erythromycin and sulfisoxazole may increase the chance of blood problems
- Kidney disease or
- Liver disease—Patients with liver or kidney disease may have an increased chance of side effects
- Loss of hearing—High doses of erythromycin and sulfisoxazole may increase the chance for hearing loss in some patients
- Porphyria—Erythromycin and sulfisoxazole may increase the chance of a porphyria attack

Before you begin using any new medicine (prescription or nonprescription) or if you develop any new medical problem while you are using this medicine, check with your doctor, nurse, or pharmacist.

Proper Use of This Medicine

Erythromycin and sulfisoxazole combination is best taken with extra amounts of water and may be taken with food. *Additional amounts of water should be taken several times every day,* unless otherwise directed by your doctor. Drinking extra water will help to prevent some unwanted effects (e.g., kidney stones) of sulfa medicines.

Do not give this medicine to infants under 2 months of age, unless otherwise directed by your doctor. Sulfa medicines may cause liver problems in these infants.

Use a specially marked measuring spoon or other device to measure each dose accurately. The average household teaspoon may not hold the right amount of liquid.

Do not use after the expiration date on the label. The medicine may not work properly after that date. Check with your pharmacist if you have any questions about this.

To help clear up your infection completely, *keep taking this medicine for the full time of treatment,* even if you begin to feel better after a few days. If you stop taking this medicine too soon, your symptoms may return.

This medicine works best when there is a constant amount in the blood. *To help keep the amount constant, do not miss any doses. Also, it is best to take the doses at evenly spaced times day and night.* For example, if you are to take 4 doses a day, the doses should be spaced about 6 hours apart. If this interferes with your sleep or other daily activities, or if you need help in planning the best times to take your medicine, check with your doctor, nurse, or pharmacist.

Missed dose—If you do miss a dose of this medicine, take it as soon as possible. This will help to keep a constant amount of medicine in the blood. However, if it is almost time for your next dose, skip the missed dose and go back to your regular dosing schedule. Do not double the dose.

Storage—To store this medicine:

- Keep out of the reach of children.
- Store away from heat and direct light.
- Store in the refrigerator because heat will cause this medicine to break down. However, keep the medicine from freezing. Follow the directions on the label.
- Do not keep outdated medicine or medicine no longer needed. Be sure that any discarded medicine is out of the reach of children.

Precautions While Using This Medicine

It is very important that your doctor check you at regular visits for any blood problems that may be caused by this medicine, especially if you will be taking this medicine for a long time.

If your symptoms do not improve within a few days, or if they become worse, check with your doctor.

Erythromycin and sulfisoxazole may cause your skin to be more sensitive to sunlight than it is normally. Exposure to sunlight, even for brief periods of time, may cause a skin rash, itching, redness or other discoloration of the skin, or a severe sunburn. When you begin taking this medicine:

- Stay out of direct sunlight, especially between the hours of 10:00 a.m. and 3:00 p.m., if possible.
- Wear protective clothing, including a hat. Also, wear sunglasses.
- Apply a sun block product that has a skin protection factor (SPF) of at least 15. Some patients may require a product with a higher SPF number, especially if they have a fair complexion. If you have any questions about this, check with your doctor or pharmacist.
- Apply a sun block lipstick that has an SPF of at least 15 to protect your lips.
- Do not use a sunlamp or tanning bed or booth.

If you have a severe reaction from the sun, check with your doctor.

Erythromycin and sulfisoxazole combination may cause blood problems. These problems may result in a greater chance of infection, slow healing, and bleeding of the gums. Therefore, you should be careful when using regular toothbrushes, dental floss, and toothpicks. Dental work should be delayed until your blood counts have returned to normal. Check with your medical doctor or dentist if you have any questions about proper oral hygiene (mouth care) during treatment.

Side Effects of This Medicine

Along with its needed effects, a medicine may cause some unwanted effects. Although not all of these side effects may occur, if they do occur they may need medical attention.

Check with your doctor immediately if any of the following side effects occur:

More common

Itching; skin rash

Less common

Aching of joints and muscles; difficulty in swallowing; pale skin; redness, blistering, peeling, or loosening of skin; sore throat and fever; unusual bleeding or bruising; unusual tiredness or weakness; yellow eyes or skin

Rare

Blood in urine; dark or amber urine; temporary loss of hearing (with kidney disease and high doses); lower back pain; pain or burning while urinating; pale stools; severe stomach pain; swelling of front part of neck

In addition to the side effects listed above, check with your doctor as soon as possible if the following side effect occurs:

More common

Increased sensitivity to sunlight

Other side effects may occur that usually do not need medical attention. These side effects may go away during treatment as your body adjusts to the medicine. However, check with your doctor if any of the following side effects continue or are bothersome:

More common

Abdominal or stomach cramping and discomfort; diarrhea; headache; loss of appetite; nausea or vomiting

Less common

Sore mouth or tongue

Other side effects not listed above may also occur in some patients. If you notice any other effects, check with your doctor.

Additional Information

Once a medicine has been approved for marketing for a certain use, experience may show that it is also useful for other medical problems. Although this use is not specifically included in product labeling, erythromycin and sulfisoxazole combination is used in certain patients with the following medical condition:

- Sinusitis (sinus infection)

Other than the above information, there is no additional information relating to proper use, precautions, or side effects for this use.

Annual revision: 08/27/92

ESTRAMUSTINE Systemic

Some commonly used brand names are:

In the U.S.
Emcyt

In Canada
Emcyt

Other
Estracyt

Description

Estramustine (ess-tra-MUSS-teen) belongs to the general group of medicines called antineoplastics. It is used to treat some cases of prostate cancer.

Estramustine is a combination of two medicines, an estrogen and mechlorethamine. The way that estramustine works against cancer is not completely understood. However, it seems to interfere with the growth of cancer cells, which are eventually destroyed.

Estramustine is available only with your doctor's prescription, in the following dosage form:

Oral

- Capsules (U.S. and Canada)

It is very important that you read and understand the following information. If any of it causes you special concern, check with your doctor. Also, *if you have any questions* or if you want more information about this medicine or your medical problem, *ask your doctor, nurse, or pharmacist.*

Before Using This Medicine

In deciding to use a medicine, the risks of taking the medicine must be weighed against the good it will do. This is a decision you and your doctor will make. For estramustine, the following should be considered:

Allergies—Tell your doctor if you have ever had any unusual or allergic reaction to estramustine, estrogens, or mechlorethamine.

Pregnancy—There is a chance that this medicine may cause birth defects if the male is taking it at the time of conception. It may also cause permanent sterility after it has been taken for a while. Be sure that you have discussed this with your doctor before taking this medicine. Before taking estramustine, make sure your doctor knows if you intend to have children.

Older adults—Many medicines have not been studied specifically in older people. Therefore, it may not be known whether they work exactly the same way they do in younger adults or if they cause different side effects or problems in older people. There is no specific information comparing use of estramustine in the elderly with use in other age groups.

Other medicines—Although certain medicines should not be used together at all, in other cases two different medicines may be used together even if an interaction might occur. In these cases, your doctor may want to change the dose, or other precautions may be necessary. When taking estramustine it is especially important that your doctor and pharmacist know if you are taking any of the following:

- Acetaminophen (e.g., Tylenol) (with long-term, high-dose use) or
- Amiodarone (e.g., Cordarone) or
- Anabolic steroids (nandrolone [e.g., Anabolin], oxandrolone [e.g., Anavar], oxymetholone [e.g., Anadrol], stanozolol [e.g., Winstrol]) or
- Androgens (male hormones) or
- Anti-infectives by mouth or by injection (medicine for infection) or
- Antithyroid agents (medicine for overactive thyroid) or
- Carbamazepine (e.g., Tegretol) or
- Carmustine (e.g., BiCNU) or
- Chloroquine (e.g., Aralen) or
- Dantrolene (e.g., Dantrium) or
- Daunorubicin (e.g., Cerubidine) or
- Disulfiram (e.g., Antabuse) or
- Divalproex (e.g., Depakote) or
- Estrogens (female hormones) or
- Etretinate (e.g., Tegison) or
- Gold salts (medicine for arthritis) or
- Hydroxychloroquine (e.g., Plaquenil) or
- Mercaptopurine (e.g., Purinethol) or
- Methotrexate (e.g., Mexate) or
- Methyldopa (e.g., Aldomet) or
- Naltrexone (e.g., Trexan) (with long-term, high-dose use) or
- Phenothiazines (acetophenazine [e.g., Tindal], chlorpromazine [e.g., Thorazine], fluphenazine [e.g., Prolixin], mesoridazine [e.g., Serentil], perphenazine [e.g., Trilafon], prochlorperazine [e.g., Compazine], promazine [e.g., Sparine], promethazine [e.g., Phenergan], thioridazine

[e.g., Mellaril], trifluoperazine [e.g., Stelazine], triflupromazine [e.g., Vesprin], trimeprazine [e.g., Temaril]) or
- Phenytoin (e.g., Dilantin) or
- Plicamycin (e.g., Mithracin) or
- Valproic acid (e.g., Depakene)—May increase the risk of liver problems

Other medical problems—The presence of other medical problems may affect the use of estramustine. Make sure you tell your doctor if you have any other medical problems, especially:
- Asthma or
- Epilepsy or
- Mental depression (or history of) or
- Migraine headaches or
- Kidney disease—Fluid retention sometimes caused by estramustine may worsen these conditions
- Blood clots (or history of) or
- Stroke (or history of) or
- Recent heart attack or stroke—May be worsened because of blood vessel problems caused by estramustine
- Chickenpox (including recent exposure) or
- Herpes zoster (shingles)—Risk of severe disease affecting other parts of the body
- Diabetes mellitus (sugar diabetes)—Estramustine may change the amount of antidiabetic medicine needed
- Gallbladder disease (or history of)—May be worsened by estramustine
- Heart or blood vessel disease—Estramustine can cause circulation problems
- Jaundice or hepatitis (or history of) or other liver disease—Effects, including liver problems, may be increased
- Stomach ulcer—May be aggravated by estramustine

Smoking—Because smoking causes narrowing of blood vessels, it can increase the risk of serious circulation problems, which can lead to stroke or heart attack.

Before you begin using any new medicine (prescription or nonprescription) or if you develop any new medical problem while you are using this medicine, check with your doctor, nurse, or pharmacist.

Proper Use of This Medicine

Use this medicine only as directed by your doctor. Do not use more or less of it, and do not use it more often than your doctor ordered. The exact amount of medicine you need has been carefully worked out. Taking too much may increase the chance of side effects, while taking too little may not improve your condition.

Do not take estramustine within 1 hour before or 2 hours after meals or after the time you take milk, milk formulas, or other dairy products, since they may keep the medicine from working properly.

This medicine commonly causes nausea and sometimes causes vomiting. However, it may have to be taken for several weeks to months to be effective. Even if you begin to feel ill, *do not stop using this medicine without first checking with your doctor.* Ask your doctor, nurse, or pharmacist for ways to lessen these effects.

If you vomit shortly after taking a dose of estramustine, check with your doctor. You will be told whether to take the dose again or to wait until the next scheduled dose.

Missed dose—If you miss a dose of this medicine, skip the missed dose and go back to your regular dosing schedule. Do not double doses.

Storage—To store this medicine:
- Keep out of the reach of children.
- Store in the refrigerator, away from direct light.
- Do not store in the bathroom, near the kitchen sink, or in other damp places. Heat or moisture may cause the medicine to break down.
- Do not keep outdated medicine or medicine no longer needed. Be sure that any discarded medicine is out of the reach of children.

Precautions While Using This Medicine

It is very important that your doctor check your progress at regular visits to make sure that the medicine is working properly and does not cause unwanted effects.

While you are being treated with estramustine, and after you stop treatment with it, *do not have any immunizations (vaccinations) without your doctor's approval.* Estramustine may lower your body's resistance and there is a chance you might get the infection the immunization is meant to prevent. In addition, other persons living in your household should not take oral polio vaccine since there is a chance they could pass the polio virus on to you. Also, avoid persons who have recently taken oral polio vaccine. Do not get close to them and do not stay in the same room with them for very long. If you cannot take these precautions, you should consider wearing a protective face mask that covers the nose and mouth.

Side Effects of This Medicine

Along with its needed effects, a medicine may cause some unwanted effects. Although not all of these side effects may occur, if they do occur they may need medical attention.

Check with your doctor immediately if any of the following side effects occur. If your doctor is not available, go to the nearest hospital emergency room.

Rare

Black, tarry stools; blood in urine or stools; cough or hoarseness; fever or chills; headaches (severe or sudden); loss of coordination (sudden); lower back or side pain; painful or difficult urination; pains in chest, groin, or leg (especially calf of leg); pinpoint red spots on skin; shortness of breath (sudden, for no apparent reason); slurred speech (sudden); unusual bleeding or bruising; vision changes (sudden); weakness or numbness in arm or leg

Check with your doctor as soon as possible if any of the following side effects occur:

More common

Swelling of feet or lower legs

Rare

Skin rash or fever; unusual tiredness or weakness

Other side effects may occur that usually do not need medical attention. These side effects may go away during treatment as your body adjusts to the medicine. However, check with your doctor if any of the following side effects continue or are bothersome or if you have any questions about them:

More common

Breast tenderness or enlargement; decreased interest in sex; diarrhea; nausea

Less common

Trouble in sleeping; vomiting

Other side effects not listed above may also occur in some patients. If you notice any other effects, check with your doctor.

Annual revision: 08/09/92

ESTROGENS Systemic

This information applies to the following medicines:

Chlorotrianisene (klor-oh-trye-AN-i-seen)
Diethylstilbestrol (dye-eth-il-stil-BESS-trole)
Estradiol (ess-tra-DYE-ole)
Estrogens, Conjugated (ESS-troe-jenz, CON-ju-gate-ed)
Estrogens, Esterified (ess-TAIR-i-fyed)
Estrone (ESS-trone)
Estropipate (ess-troe-PI-pate)
Ethinyl Estradiol (ETH-in-il ess-tra-DYE-ole)
Quinestrol (quin-ESS-trole)

Some commonly used brand names are:

For Chlorotrianisene†

In the U.S.

TACE

For Diethylstilbestrol

In the U.S.

Stilphostrol

Generic name product may also be available.

In Canada

Honvol

Another commonly used name is DES.

For Estradiol

In the U.S.

Deladiol-40	Estra-D
Delestrogen	Estraderm
depGynogen	Estra-L 20
Depo-Estradiol	Estra-L 40
Depogen	Estro-Cyp
Dioval	Estrofem
Dioval 40	Estroject-LA
Dioval XX	Estronol-LA
Dura-Estrin	Gynogen L.A. 10
Duragen-10	Gynogen L.A. 20
Duragen-20	Gynogen L.A. 40
Duragen-40	L.A.E. 20
E-Cypionate	Valergen-10
Estrace	Valergen-20

Generic name product may also be available.

In Canada

Delestrogen	Estrace
Estraderm	Femogex

For Estrogens, Conjugated

In the U.S.

Premarin
Premarin Intravenous

In Canada

C.E.S.	Premarin Intravenous
Premarin	

Generic name product may also be available.

For Estrogens, Esterified

In the U.S.

Estratab	Menest

In Canada

Neo-Estrone

For Estrone

In the U.S.

Estroject-2	Kestrin Aqueous
Estrone '5'	Kestrone-5
Estrone-A	Theelin Aqueous
Estronol	Unigen
Gynogen	Wehgen

Generic name product may also be available.

In Canada

Femogen Forte

For Estropipate

In the U.S.

Ogen .625	Ogen 2.5
Ogen 1.25	

In Canada

Ogen

Another commonly used name is piperazine estrone sulfate.

For Ethinyl Estradiol

In the U.S.

Estinyl	Feminone

In Canada

Estinyl

For Quinestrol
In the U.S.
Estrovis

†Not commercially available in Canada.

Description

Estrogens (ESS-troe-jenz) are female hormones. They are produced by the body and are necessary for the normal sexual development of the female and for the regulation of the menstrual cycle during the childbearing years.

The ovaries begin to produce less estrogen after menopause (the change of life). This medicine is prescribed to make up for the lower amount of estrogen. This should relieve signs of menopause, such as hot flashes and unusual sweating, chills, faintness, or dizziness.

Estrogens are prescribed for several reasons:

- to provide additional hormone when the body does not produce enough of its own, as during the menopause or following certain kinds of surgery.
- in the treatment of selected cases of breast cancer in men and women.
- in the treatment of men with certain kinds of cancer of the prostate.
- to help prevent weakening of bones (osteoporosis) in women past menopause.

Estrogens may also be used for other conditions as determined by your doctor.

There is *no* medical evidence to support the belief that the use of estrogens will keep the patient feeling young, keep the skin soft, or delay the appearance of wrinkles. Nor has it been proven that the use of estrogens during the menopause will relieve emotional and nervous symptoms, unless these symptoms are caused by other menopausal symptoms, such as hot flashes or hot flushes.

Estrogens are very useful medicines. However, in addition to their helpful effects in treating your medical problem, they sometimes have side effects that could be very serious. *A paper called "Information for the Patient" should be given to you with your prescription. Read this carefully.* Also, before you use an estrogen, you and your doctor should discuss the good that it will do as well as the risks of using it.

Estrogens are available only with your doctor's prescription, in the following dosage forms:

Oral

Chlorotrianisene
- Capsules (U.S.)

Diethylstilbestrol
- Tablets (U.S. and Canada)

Estradiol
- Tablets (U.S. and Canada)

Estrogens, Conjugated
- Tablets (U.S. and Canada)

Estrogens, Esterified
- Tablets (U.S. and Canada)

Estropipate
- Tablets (U.S. and Canada)

Ethinyl Estradiol
- Tablets (U.S. and Canada)

Quinestrol
- Tablets (U.S.)

Parenteral

Diethylstilbestrol
- Injection (U.S. and Canada)

Estradiol
- Injection (U.S. and Canada)

Estrogens, Conjugated
- Injection (U.S. and Canada)

Estrone
- Injection (U.S. and Canada)

Topical

Estradiol
- Transdermal system (stick-on patch) (U.S. and Canada)

It is very important that you read and understand the following information. If any of it causes you special concern, check with your doctor. Also, *if you have any questions* or if you want more information about this medicine or your medical problem, *ask your doctor, nurse, or pharmacist.*

Before Using This Medicine

In deciding to use a medicine, the risks of taking the medicine must be weighed against the good it will do. This is a decision you and your doctor will make. For estrogens, the following should be considered:

Allergies—Tell your doctor if you have ever had any unusual or allergic reaction to estrogens. Also tell your doctor and pharmacist if you are allergic to any other substances, such as foods, preservatives, or dyes.

Pregnancy—Estrogens are not recommended for use during pregnancy, since some have been shown to cause serious birth defects in humans and animals. Some daughters of women who took diethylstilbestrol (DES) during pregnancy have developed reproductive (genital) tract problems and, rarely, cancer of the vagina or cervix (opening to the uterus) when they reached childbearing age. Some sons of women who took DES during pregnancy have developed urinary-genital tract problems.

Breast-feeding—Use of this medicine is not recommended in nursing mothers. Estrogens pass into the breast milk and their possible effect on the baby is not known.

Older adults—This medicine has been tested and has not been shown to cause different side effects or problems in older women than it does in younger women.

Other medicines—Although certain medicines should not be used together at all, in other cases two different medicines may be used together even if an interaction might occur. In these cases, your doctor may want to change the dose, or other precautions may be necessary. When you are taking estrogens, it is especially important that your doctor and pharmacist know if you are taking any of the following:

- Acetaminophen (e.g., Tylenol) (with long-term, high-dose use) or
- Amiodarone (e.g., Cordarone) or
- Anabolic steroids (nandrolone [e.g., Anabolin], oxandrolone [e.g., Anavar], oxymetholone [e.g., Anadrol], stanozolol [e.g., Winstrol]) or
- Androgens (male hormones) or
- Anti-infectives by mouth or by injection (medicine for infection) or
- Antithyroid agents (medicine for overactive thyroid) or
- Carbamazepine (e.g., Tegretol) or
- Carmustine (e.g., BiCNU) or
- Chloroquine (e.g., Aralen) or
- Dantrolene (e.g., Dantrium) or
- Daunorubicin (e.g., Cerubidine) or
- Disulfiram (e.g., Antabuse) or
- Divalproex (e.g., Depakote) or
- Etretinate (e.g., Tegison) or
- Gold salts (medicine for arthritis) or
- Hydroxychloroquine (e.g., Plaquenil) or
- Mercaptopurine (e.g., Purinethol) or
- Methotrexate (e.g., Mexate) or
- Methyldopa (e.g., Aldomet) or
- Naltrexone (e.g., Trexan) (with long-term, high-dose use) or
- Oral contraceptives (birth control pills) containing estrogen or
- Phenothiazines (acetophenazine [e.g., Tindal], chlorpromazine [e.g., Thorazine], fluphenazine [e.g., Prolixin], mesoridazine [e.g., Serentil], perphenazine [e.g., Trilafon], prochlorperazine [e.g., Compazine], promazine [e.g., Sparine], promethazine [e.g., Phenergan], thioridazine [e.g., Mellaril], trifluoperazine [e.g., Stelazine], triflupromazine [e.g., Vesprin], trimeprazine [e.g., Temaril]) or
- Phenytoin (e.g., Dilantin) or
- Plicamycin (e.g., Mithracin) or
- Valproic acid (e.g., Depakene)—Estrogens and all of these medicines can cause liver damage. Your doctor may want you to have extra blood tests that tell about your liver, if you must take any of these medicines with estrogens
- Bromocriptine (e.g., Parlodel)—Estrogens may interfere with the effects of bromocriptine
- Cyclosporine (e.g., Sandimmune)—Estrogens can increase the chance of toxic effects to the kidney or liver from cyclosporine because estrogens can interfere with the body's ability to get the cyclosporine out of the bloodstream as it normally would

Other medical problems—The presence of other medical problems may affect the use of estrogens. Make sure you tell your doctor if you have any other medical problems, especially:

For all patients

- Blood clots (or history of during previous estrogen therapy)—Estrogens may worsen blood clots or cause new clots to form
- Breast cancer (active or suspected)—Estrogens may cause growth of the tumor in some cases
- Changes in vaginal bleeding of unknown causes—Some irregular vaginal bleeding is a sign that the lining of the uterus is growing too much or is a sign of cancer of the uterus lining; estrogens may make these conditions worse
- Endometriosis—Estrogens may worsen endometriosis by causing growth of endometriosis implants
- Fibroid tumors of the uterus—Estrogens may cause fibroid tumors to increase in size
- Gallbladder disease or gallstones (or history of)—Estrogens may possibly increase the risk of gallbladder disease or gallstones
- Jaundice (or history of during pregnancy)—Estrogens may worsen or cause jaundice in these patients
- Liver disease—Toxic drug effects may occur in patients with liver disease because the body is not able to get this medicine out of the bloodstream as it normally would
- Porphyria—Estrogens can make porphyria worse

For males treated for breast or prostate cancer

- Blood clots or
- Heart or circulation disease or
- Stroke—Males with these medical problems may be more likely to have clotting problems while taking estrogens; the doses of estrogens used to treat male breast or prostate cancer have been shown to increase the chances of heart attack, phlebitis (inflamed veins) caused by a blood clot, or blood clots in the lungs

Before you begin using any new medicine (prescription or nonprescription) or if you develop any new medical problem while you are using this medicine, check with your doctor, nurse, or pharmacist.

Proper Use of This Medicine

For patients taking any of the estrogens by mouth:

- *Take this medicine only as directed by your doctor. Do not take more of it and do not take it for a longer time than your doctor ordered.* Try to take the medicine at the same time each day to reduce the possibility of side effects and to allow it to work better.
- Nausea may occur during the first few weeks after you start taking estrogens. This effect usually disappears with continued use. If the nausea is bothersome, it can usually be prevented or reduced by taking each dose with food or immediately after food.

For patients using the transdermal (stick-on patch) form of estradiol:

- This medicine comes with patient directions. Read them carefully before using this medicine.
- Wash and dry your hands thoroughly before and after handling.
- Apply the patch to a clean, dry, non-oily skin area of your abdomen (stomach) or buttocks that has little or no hair and is free of cuts or irritation.

- *Do not apply to the breasts.* Also, do not apply to the waistline or anywhere else where tight clothes may rub the patch loose.
- Press the patch firmly in place with the palm of your hand for about 10 seconds. Make sure there is good contact, especially around the edges.
- If a patch becomes loose or falls off, you may reapply it or discard it and apply a new patch.
- Each dose is best applied to a different area of skin on your abdomen so that at least 1 week goes by before the same area is used again. This will help prevent skin irritation.

Missed dose—
- For patients taking any of the estrogens by mouth: If you miss a dose of this medicine, take it as soon as possible. However, if it is almost time for your next dose, skip the missed dose and go back to your regular dosing schedule. Do not double doses.
- For patients using the transdermal (stick-on patch) form of estradiol: If you forget to apply a new patch when you are supposed to, apply it as soon as possible. However, if it is almost time for the next patch, skip the missed one and go back to your regular schedule. Do not apply more than one patch at a time.

Storage—To store this medicine:
- Keep out of the reach of children.
- Store away from heat and direct light.
- Do not store in the bathroom medicine cabinet because the heat or moisture may cause the medicine to break down.
- Keep the injectable form of this medicine from freezing.
- Do not keep outdated medicine or medicine no longer needed. Be sure that any discarded medicine is out of the reach of children.

Precautions While Using This Medicine

It is very important that your doctor check your progress at regular visits to make sure this medicine does not cause unwanted effects. These visits will usually be every year, but some doctors require them more often.

It is not yet known whether the use of estrogens increases the risk of breast cancer in women. Therefore, it is very important that you regularly check your breasts for any unusual lumps or discharge. You should also have a mammogram (x-ray pictures of the breasts) done if your doctor recommends it. Because breast cancer has occurred in men taking estrogens, regular self-breast exams and exams by your doctor for any unusual lumps or discharge should be done.

In some patients using estrogens, tenderness, swelling, or bleeding of the gums may occur. Brushing and flossing your teeth carefully and regularly and massaging your gums may help prevent this. See your dentist regularly to have your teeth cleaned. Check with your medical doctor or dentist if you have any questions about how to take care of your teeth and gums, or if you notice any tenderness, swelling, or bleeding of your gums.

If you think that you may be pregnant, stop using the medicine immediately and check with your doctor. Continued use of some estrogens during pregnancy may cause birth defects in the child. DES may also increase the risk of vaginal cancer developing in daughters when they reach childbearing age.

Do not give this medicine to anyone else. Your doctor has prescribed it only for you after studying your health record and the results of your physical examination. Estrogens may be dangerous for other people because of differences in their health and body make-up.

Side Effects of This Medicine

Discuss these possible effects with your doctor:
- The prolonged use of estrogens has been reported to increase the risk of endometrial cancer (cancer of the lining of the uterus) in women after the menopause. This risk seems to increase as the dose and the length of use increase. When estrogens are used in low doses for less than 1 year, there is less risk. The risk is also reduced if a progestin (another female hormone) is added to, or replaces part of, your estrogen dose. If the uterus has been removed by surgery (total hysterectomy), there is no risk of endometrial cancer.
- It is not yet known whether the use of estrogens increases the risk of breast cancer in women. Although some large studies show an increased risk, most studies and information gathered to date do not support this idea. Breast cancer has been reported in men taking estrogens.
- In studies with oral contraceptives (birth control pills) containing estrogens, cigarette smoking was shown to cause an increased risk of serious side effects affecting the heart or blood circulation, such as dangerous blood clots, heart attack, or stroke. The risk increased as the amount of smoking and the age of the smoker increased. Women aged 35 and over were at greatest risk when they smoked while using oral contraceptives containing estrogens. It is not known if this risk exists with the use of estrogens for symptoms of menopause. However, smoking may make estrogens less effective.

The following side effects may be caused by blood clots, which could lead to stroke, heart attack, or death. These side effects rarely occur, and, when they do occur, they occur in men treated for cancer using high doses of estrogens. *Get emergency help immediately* if any of the following side effects occur:

Rare—For males being treated for breast or prostate cancer only

Headache (sudden or severe); loss of coordination (sudden); loss of vision or change of vision (sudden); pains in chest, groin, or leg, especially in calf of leg; shortness of breath (sudden and unexplained); slurring of speech (sudden); weakness or numbness in arm or leg

Also, check with your doctor as soon as possible if any of the following side effects occur:

More common

Breast pain (in females and males); increased breast size (in females and males); swelling of feet and lower legs; weight gain (rapid)

Less common or rare

Changes in vaginal bleeding (spotting, breakthrough bleeding, prolonged or heavier bleeding, or complete stoppage of bleeding); lumps in, or discharge from, breast (in females and males); pains in stomach, side, or abdomen; uncontrolled jerky muscle movements; yellow eyes or skin

Other side effects may occur that usually do not need medical attention. These side effects may go away during treatment as your body adjusts to the medicine. However, check with your doctor if any of the following side effects continue or are bothersome:

More common

Bloating of stomach; cramps of lower stomach; loss of appetite; nausea; skin irritation or redness where skin patch was worn

Less common

Diarrhea (mild); dizziness (mild); headaches (mild); migraine headaches; problems in wearing contact lenses; unusual decrease in sexual desire (in males); unusual increase in sexual desire (in females); vomiting (usually with high doses)

Also, many women who are taking estrogens with a progestin (another female hormone) will start having monthly vaginal bleeding, similar to menstrual periods again. This effect will continue for as long as the medicine is taken. However, monthly bleeding will not occur in women who have had the uterus removed by surgery (total hysterectomy).

Other side effects not listed above may also occur in some patients. If you notice any other effects, check with your doctor.

Annual revision: 06/18/93

ESTROGENS Vaginal

This information applies to the following medicines:

Dienestrol (dye-en-ESS-trole)
Estradiol (ess-tra-DYE-ole)
Conjugated Estrogens (CON-ju-gate-ed ESS-troe-jenz)
Estrone (ESS-trone)
Estropipate (ess-troe-PI-pate)

Some commonly used brand names are:

For Dienestrol
In the U.S.
Ortho Dienestrol
Generic name product may also be available.
In Canada
Ortho Dienestrol

For Estradiol
In the U.S.
Estrace

For Conjugated Estrogens
In the U.S.
Premarin
In Canada
Premarin

For Estrone*
In Canada
Oestrilin

For Estropipate†
In the U.S.
Ogen
Generic name product may also be available.

Another commonly used name is piperazine estrone sulfate.

*Not commercially available in the U.S.
†Not commercially available in Canada.

Description

Estrogens (ESS-troe-jenz) are female hormones. They are produced by the body and are necessary for the normal sexual development of the female and for the regulation of the menstrual cycle during the childbearing years.

Uncomfortable changes may occur in vaginal tissues when the body does not produce enough estrogens, as during the menopause or following certain kinds of surgery. In order to relieve such uncomfortable conditions, estrogens are prescribed for vaginal use in the form of special creams or suppositories.

When used vaginally or on the skin, most estrogens are absorbed into the bloodstream and produce many of the same effects in the body as when they are taken by mouth or given by injection.

Estrogens are very useful medicines. However, in addition to their helpful effects in treating your medical problem, they sometimes have side effects that could be very serious. *A paper called "Information for the Patient" is given to you with your prescription. Read this carefully.* Also, you should discuss with your doctor the good that this medicine will do as well as the risks of using it.

Estrogens for vaginal use are available only with your doctor's prescription, in the following dosage forms:

Vaginal

Dienestrol
- Cream (U.S. and Canada)

Estradiol
- Cream (U.S.)

Conjugated Estrogens
- Cream (U.S. and Canada)

Estrone
- Cream (Canada)
- Suppositories (Canada)

Estropipate
- Cream (U.S.)

It is very important that you read and understand the following information. If any of it causes you special concern, check with your doctor. Also, *if you have any questions* or if you want more information about this medicine or your medical problem, *ask your doctor, nurse, or pharmacist.*

Before Using This Medicine

In deciding to use a medicine, the risks of using the medicine must be weighed against the good it will do. This is a decision you and your doctor will make. For vaginal estrogens, the following should be considered:

Allergies—Tell your doctor if you have ever had any unusual or allergic reaction to estrogens. Also tell your doctor and pharmacist if you are allergic to any other substances, such as foods, preservatives, or dyes.

Pregnancy—Estrogens are not recommended for use during pregnancy, since some have been shown to cause serious birth defects in humans and animals.

Breast-feeding—Use of this medicine is not recommended in nursing mothers. Estrogens pass into the breast milk and their possible effect on the baby is not known.

Older adults—This medicine has been tested and has not been shown to cause different side effects or problems in older people than it does in younger adults.

Other medicines—Although certain medicines should not be used together at all, in other cases two different medicines may be used together even if an interaction might occur. In these cases, your doctor may want to change the dose, or other precautions may be necessary. When you are using vaginal estrogens, it is especially important that your doctor and pharmacist know if you are taking any of the following:

- Acetaminophen (e.g., Tylenol) (with long-term, high-dose use) or
- Amiodarone (e.g., Cordarone) or
- Anabolic steroids (nandrolone [e.g., Anabolin], oxandrolone [e.g., Anavar], oxymetholone [e.g., Anadrol], stanozolol [e.g., Winstrol]) or
- Androgens (male hormones) or
- Anti-infectives by mouth or by injection (medicine for infection) or
- Antithyroid agents (medicine for overactive thyroid) or
- Carbamazepine (e.g., Tegretol) or
- Carmustine (e.g., BiCNU) or
- Chloroquine (e.g., Aralen) or
- Dantrolene (e.g., Dantrium) or
- Daunorubicin (e.g., Cerubidine) or
- Disulfiram (e.g., Antabuse) or
- Divalproex (e.g., Depakote) or
- Etretinate (e.g., Tegison) or
- Gold salts (medicine for arthritis) or
- Hydroxychloroquine (e.g., Plaquenil) or
- Mercaptopurine (e.g., Purinethol) or
- Methotrexate (e.g., Mexate) or
- Methyldopa (e.g., Aldomet) or
- Naltrexone (e.g., Trexan) (with long-term, high-dose use) or
- Oral contraceptives (birth control pills) containing estrogen or
- Phenothiazines (acetophenazine [e.g., Tindal], chlorpromazine [e.g., Thorazine], fluphenazine [e.g., Prolixin], mesoridazine [e.g., Serentil], perphenazine [e.g., Trilafon], prochlorperazine [e.g., Compazine], promazine [e.g., Sparine], promethazine [e.g., Phenergan], thioridazine [e.g., Mellaril], trifluoperazine [e.g., Stelazine], triflupromazine [e.g., Vesprin], trimeprazine [e.g., Temaril]) or
- Phenytoin (e.g., Dilantin) or
- Plicamycin (e.g., Mithracin) or
- Valproic acid (e.g., Depakene)—Estrogens and all of these medicines can cause liver damage. Your doctor may want you to have extra blood tests that tell about your liver, if you must take any of these medicines with estrogens
- Bromocriptine (e.g., Parlodel)—Estrogens may interfere with the effects of bromocriptine
- Cyclosporine (e.g., Sandimmune)—Estrogens can increase the chance of toxic effects to the kidney or liver from cyclosporine because estrogens can interfere with the body's ability to get the cyclosporine out of the bloodstream as it normally would

Other medical problems—The presence of other medical problems may affect the use of estrogens. Make sure you tell your doctor if you have any other medical problems, especially:

- Blood clots (or history of during previous estrogen therapy)—Estrogens may worsen blood clots or cause new clots to form
- Breast cancer (active or suspected)—Estrogens may cause growth of the tumor in some cases
- Changes in vaginal bleeding of unknown causes—Some irregular vaginal bleeding is a sign that the lining of the

uterus is growing too much or is a sign of cancer of the uterus lining; estrogens may make these conditions worse
- Endometriosis—Estrogens may worsen endometriosis by causing growth of endometriosis implants
- Fibroid tumors of the uterus—Estrogens may cause fibroid tumors to increase in size
- Gallbladder disease or gallstones (or history of)—Estrogens may possibly increase the risk of gallbladder disease or gallstones
- Jaundice (or history of during pregnancy)—Estrogens may worsen or cause jaundice in these patients
- Liver disease—Toxic drug effects may occur in patients with liver disease because the body is not able to get this medicine out of the bloodstream as it normally would
- Porphyria—Estrogens can worsen porphyria

Before you begin using any new medicine (prescription or nonprescription) or if you develop any new medical problem while you are using this medicine, check with your doctor, nurse, or pharmacist.

Proper Use of This Medicine

Use this medicine only as directed. Do not use more of it and do not use it for a longer time than your doctor ordered.

This medicine is often used at bedtime to increase effectiveness through better absorption. To protect your clothing while using this medicine, you may find sanitary napkins helpful.

Vaginal creams and some vaginal suppositories are inserted with a plastic dose applicator. Directions for using the applicator are included with your medicine. If you do not receive the directions or do not understand them, ask your doctor, pharmacist, or nurse for information or additional explanation.

Dosing—The dose of vaginal estrogens will be different for different women. *Follow your doctor's orders or the directions on the label.* The following information includes only the average doses of these medicines. *If your dose is different, do not change it* unless your doctor tells you to do so.

For dienestrol

- For *vaginal* dosage form (cream):
  —Adults: At first, one applicatorful of cream inserted into the vagina one to two times a day, for one to two weeks. The dosage and how often you use the medicine will likely be reduced after your condition improves. Then, usually your doctor will want you to use this medicine for three weeks of each month, with one week of no medicine between each three weeks of medicine.

For estradiol

- For *vaginal* dosage form (cream):
  —Adults: At first, 200 to 400 micrograms (0.2 to 0.4 milligrams) of estradiol inserted into the vagina once a day, for one to two weeks. The dosage and how often you use the medicine will likely be reduced after your condition improves. Then, usually your doctor will want you to use this medicine for three weeks of each month, with one week of no medicine between each three weeks of medicine.

For conjugated estrogens

- For *vaginal* dosage form (cream):
  —Adults: 1.25 to 2.5 milligrams of conjugated estrogens inserted into the vagina once a day. Usually your doctor will want you to use this medicine for three weeks of each month, with one week of no medicine between each three weeks of medicine.

For estrone

- For *vaginal* dosage form (cream):
  —Adults: 2 to 4 milligrams of estrone inserted into the vagina once a day.
- For *vaginal* dosage form (suppository):
  —Adults: 0.25 to 0.5 milligrams of estrone inserted into the vagina once a day.

For estropipate

- For *vaginal* dosage form (cream):
  —Adults: 3 to 6 milligrams of estropipate inserted into the vagina once a day. Usually your doctor will want you to use this medicine for three weeks of each month, with one week of no medicine between each three weeks of medicine.

Missed dose—If you miss a dose of this medicine and do not remember it until the next day, do not use the missed dose at all. Instead, go back to your regular dosing schedule.

Storage—To store this medicine:

- Keep out of the reach of children.
- Store away from heat and direct light.
- Keep the medicine from freezing.
- Do not keep outdated medicine or medicine no longer needed. Be sure that any discarded medicine is out of the reach of children.

Precautions While Using This Medicine

It is very important that your doctor check your progress at regular visits to make sure this medicine does not cause unwanted effects. These visits will usually be every year, but some doctors require them more often.

It is not yet known whether the use of estrogens increases the risk of breast cancer in women. Therefore, it is very important that you regularly check your breasts for any unusual lumps or discharge. You should also have a mammogram (x-ray pictures of the breasts) done if your doctor recommends it.

In some patients using estrogens, tenderness, swelling, or bleeding of the gums may occur. Brushing and flossing your teeth carefully and regularly and massaging your gums may help prevent this. See your dentist regularly to have your teeth cleaned. Check with your medical doctor or dentist if you have any questions about how to take care of your teeth and gums, or if you notice any tenderness, swelling, or bleeding of your gums.

If you think that you may be pregnant, stop using the medicine immediately and check with your doctor. Continued use of some estrogens during pregnancy may cause birth defects in the child.

Do not give this medicine to anyone else. Your doctor has prescribed it only for you after studying your health record and the results of your physical examination. Estrogens may be dangerous for other people because of differences in their health and body make-up.

Certain brands of vaginal estrogen products contain oils in the cream bases. Oils can weaken latex rubber condoms, diaphragms, or cervical caps. This increases the chances of a condom breaking during sexual intercourse. The rubber in cervical caps or diaphragms may break down faster and wear out sooner. Check with your doctor, nurse, or pharmacist to make sure the vaginal estrogen product you are using can be used with latex rubber birth control devices.

Side Effects of This Medicine

Discuss these possible effects with your doctor:

- The prolonged use of estrogens has been reported to increase the risk of endometrial cancer (cancer of the lining of the uterus) in women after the menopause. This risk seems to increase as the dose and the length of use increase. When estrogens are used in low doses for less than 1 year, there is less risk. The risk is also reduced if a progestin (another female hormone) is added to, or replaces part of, your estrogen dose. If the uterus has been removed by surgery (total hysterectomy), there is no risk of endometrial cancer.
- It is not yet known whether the use of estrogens increases the risk of breast cancer in women. Although some large studies show an increased risk, most studies and information gathered to date do not support this idea.
- In studies with oral contraceptives (birth control pills) containing estrogens, cigarette smoking was shown to cause an increased risk of serious side effects affecting the heart or blood circulation, such as dangerous blood clots, heart attack, or stroke. The risk increased as the amount of smoking and the age of the smoker increased. Women aged 35 and over were at greatest risk when they smoked while using oral contraceptives containing estrogens. It is not known if this risk exists with the use of estrogens for symptoms of menopause. However, smoking may make estrogens less effective.

Check with your doctor as soon as possible if any of the following side effects occur:

More common

Pain, tenderness, or enlargement of breasts; swelling of feet and lower legs; weight gain (rapid)

Less common or rare

Changes in vaginal bleeding (spotting, breakthrough bleeding, prolonged or heavier bleeding, or complete stoppage of bleeding); lumps in, or discharge from, breast; pains in stomach, side, or abdomen; swelling, redness, or itching around vaginal area; uncontrolled jerky muscle movements; yellow eyes or skin

Other side effects may occur that usually do not need medical attention. These side effects may go away during treatment as your body adjusts to the medicine. However, check with your doctor if any of the following side effects continue or are bothersome:

More common

Bloating of stomach; cramps of lower stomach; loss of appetite

Less common

Diarrhea (mild); dizziness (mild); headaches (mild); migraine headaches; problems in wearing contact lenses; unusual increase in sexual desire

Also, many women who are using estrogens with a progestin (another female hormone) will start having monthly vaginal bleeding, similar to menstrual periods again. This effect will continue for as long as the medicine is taken. However, monthly bleeding will not occur in women who have had the uterus removed by surgery (total hysterectomy).

Other side effects not listed above may also occur in some patients. If you notice any other effects, check with your doctor.

Annual revision: 06/16/93

ESTROGENS AND PROGESTINS Oral Contraceptives Systemic

This information applies to the following medicines:

- Ethynodiol (e-thye-noe-DYE-ole) Diacetate and Ethinyl Estradiol (ETH-in-il ess-tra-DYE-ole)
- Levonorgestrel (LEE-voe-nor-jess-trel) and Ethinyl Estradiol
- Norethindrone (nor-eth-IN-drone) Acetate and Ethinyl Estradiol
- Norethindrone and Ethinyl Estradiol
- Norethindrone and Mestranol
- Norgestrel (nor-JESS-trel) and Ethinyl Estradiol
- For information about Norethindrone (e.g., Micronor) or Norgestrel (e.g., Ovrette) when used as single-ingredient oral contraceptives, see *Progestins (Systemic)*.

Some commonly used brand names are:

For Ethynodiol Diacetate and Ethinyl Estradiol

In the U.S.

Demulen 1/35
Demulen 1/50

In Canada

Demulen 30
Demulen 50

For Levonorgestrel and Ethinyl Estradiol

In the U.S.

Levlen
Nordette
Tri-Levlen
Triphasil

In Canada

Min-Ovral
Triphasil
Triquilar

For Norethindrone Acetate and Ethinyl Estradiol

In the U.S.

Loestrin 1/20
Loestrin 1.5/30
Norlestrin 1/50
Norlestrin 2.5/50

In Canada

Loestrin 1.5/30
Minestrin 1/20
Norlestrin 1/50

For Norethindrone and Ethinyl Estradiol

In the U.S.

Brevicon
Genora 0.5/35
Genora 1/35
ModiCon
N.E.E. 1/35
N.E.E. 1/50
Nelova 0.5/35E
Nelova 1/35E
Nelova 10/11
Norcept-E 1/35
Norethin 1/35E
Norinyl 1+35
Ortho-Novum 1/35
Ortho-Novum 7/7/7
Ortho-Novum 10/11
Ovcon-35
Ovcon-50
Tri-Norinyl

In Canada

Brevicon 0.5/35
Brevicon 1/35
Ortho 0.5/35
Ortho 1/35
Ortho 7/7/7
Ortho 10/11
Synphasic

For Norethindrone and Mestranol

In the U.S.

Genora 1/50
Nelova 1/50M
Norethin 1/50M
Norinyl 1+50
Ortho-Novum 1/50

In Canada

Norinyl 1/50
Ortho-Novum 0.5
Ortho-Novum 1/50
Ortho-Novum 1/80
Ortho-Novum 2

For Norgestrel and Ethinyl Estradiol

In the U.S.

Lo/Ovral
Ovral

In Canada

Ovral

Description

Oral contraceptives are known also as the Pill, OC's, BC's, BC tablets, or birth control pills. They usually contain two types of female hormones, estrogens (ESS-troe-jenz) and progestins (proe-JESS-tins). When taken by mouth on a regular schedule, they change the hormone balance of the body, which prevents pregnancy.

Sometimes these preparations can be used in the treatment of conditions that are helped by added hormones. Oral contraceptives do not prevent or cure venereal diseases (VD), however.

Before you take an oral contraceptive, you and your doctor should discuss the benefits and risks of using these medicines. Besides surgery or not having intercourse, these medicines are the most effective method of preventing pregnancy. However, oral contraceptives sometimes have side effects that could be very serious.

To make the use of oral contraceptives as safe and reliable as possible, you should understand how and when to take them and what effects may be expected. *A paper with information for the patient will be given to you with your filled prescription, and will provide many details concerning the use of oral contraceptives. Read this paper carefully* and ask your doctor, nurse, or pharmacist if you need additional information or explanation.

Oral contraceptives are available only with your doctor's prescription, in the following dosage forms:

Oral

- Ethynodiol Diacetate and Ethinyl Estradiol
  - Tablets (U.S. and Canada)
- Levonorgestrel and Ethinyl Estradiol
  - Tablets (U.S. and Canada)
- Norethindrone Acetate and Ethinyl Estradiol
  - Tablets (U.S. and Canada)
- Norethindrone and Ethinyl Estradiol
  - Tablets (U.S. and Canada)
- Norethindrone and Mestranol
  - Tablets (U.S. and Canada)
- Norgestrel and Ethinyl Estradiol
  - Tablets (U.S. and Canada)

It is very important that you read and understand the following information. If any of it causes you special concern, check with your doctor. Also, *if you have any questions* or if you want more information about this medicine or your medical problem, *ask your doctor, nurse, or pharmacist.*

Before Using This Medicine

In deciding to use a medicine, the risks of taking the medicine must be weighed against the good it will do. This is a decision you and your doctor will make. For

estrogen and progestin birth control pills, the following should be considered:

Allergies—Tell your doctor if you have ever had any unusual or allergic reaction to estrogens or progestins. Also tell your doctor and pharmacist if you are allergic to any other substances, such as foods, preservatives, or dyes.

Pregnancy—Oral contraceptives are not recommended for use during pregnancy.

Breast-feeding—The estrogens in oral contraceptives pass into the breast milk. It is not known what effect oral contraceptives may have on the infant. Studies have shown oral contraceptives to cause tumors in humans and animals. Use of "high-dose" birth control medicines is not recommended during breast-feeding. It may be necessary for you to use another method of birth control or to stop breast-feeding while taking oral contraceptives. However, your doctor may allow you to begin using one of the "low-dose" oral contraceptives after you have been breast-feeding for a while.

Children—This medicine is frequently used for birth control in teenage females and has not been shown to cause different side effects or problems than it does in adults. However, some teenagers may need extra information on the importance of taking this medication exactly as prescribed in order for it to work.

Other medicines—Although certain medicines should not be used together at all, in other cases two different medicines may be used together even if an interaction might occur. In these cases, your doctor may want to change the dose, or other precautions may be necessary. When you are taking estrogen and progestin birth control pills, it is especially important that your doctor and pharmacist know if you are taking any of the following:

- Acetaminophen (e.g., Tylenol) (with long-term, high-dose use)
- Adrenocorticoids (cortisone-like medicine)
- Amiodarone (e.g., Cordarone)
- Anabolic steroids (nandrolone [e.g., Anabolin], oxandrolone [e.g., Anavar], oxymetholone [e.g., Anadrol], stanozolol [e.g., Winstrol])
- Androgens (male hormones)
- Anticoagulants (blood thinners)
- Anti-infectives by mouth or by injection (medicine for infection)
- Antithyroid agents (medicine for overactive thyroid)
- Barbiturates
- Bromocriptine (e.g., Parlodel)
- Carbamazepine (e.g., Tegretol)
- Carmustine (e.g., BiCNU)
- Chloroquine (e.g., Aralen)
- Dantrolene (e.g., Dantrium)
- Daunorubicin (e.g., Cerubidine)
- Disulfiram (e.g., Antabuse)
- Divalproex (e.g., Depakote)
- Estrogens (female hormones)
- Etretinate (e.g., Tegison)
- Gold salts (medicine for arthritis)
- Griseofulvin (e.g., Fulvicin)
- Hydroxychloroquine (e.g., Plaquenil)
- Mercaptopurine (e.g., Purinethol)
- Methotrexate (e.g., Mexate)
- Methyldopa (e.g., Aldomet)
- Naltrexone (e.g., Trexan) (with long-term, high-dose use)
- Phenothiazines (acetophenazine [e.g., Tindal], chlorpromazine [e.g., Thorazine], fluphenazine [e.g., Prolixin], mesoridazine [e.g., Serentil], perphenazine [e.g., Trilafon], prochlorperazine [e.g., Compazine], promazine [e.g., Sparine], promethazine [e.g., Phenergan], thioridazine [e.g., Mellaril], trifluoperazine [e.g., Stelazine], triflupromazine [e.g., Vesprin], trimeprazine [e.g., Temaril])
- Phenylbutazone (e.g., Butazolidin)
- Phenytoin (e.g., Dilantin)
- Plicamycin (e.g., Mithracin)
- Primidone (e.g., Mysoline)
- Rifampin (e.g., Rifadin)
- Tricyclic antidepressants (amitriptyline [e.g., Elavil], amoxapine [e.g., Asendin], clomipramine [e.g., Anafranil], desipramine [e.g., Pertofrane], doxepin [e.g., Sinequan], imipramine [e.g., Tofranil], nortriptyline [e.g., Aventyl], protriptyline [e.g., Vivactil], trimipramine [e.g., Surmontil])
- Valproic acid (e.g., Depakene)

Other medical problems—The presence of other medical problems may affect the use of estrogen and progestin birth control pills. Make sure you tell your doctor if you have any other medical problems, especially:

- Angina pectoris (chest pains on exertion)
- Asthma
- Blood clots (or history of)
- Bone disease
- Breast disease (not cancerous, such as fibrocystic disease [breast cysts], breast lumps, or abnormal mammograms [x-ray pictures of the breast])
- Cancer (or history of or family history of breast cancer)
- Changes in vaginal bleeding
- Diabetes mellitus (sugar diabetes)
- Endometriosis
- Epilepsy
- Fibroid tumors of the uterus
- Gallbladder disease or gallstones (or history of)
- Heart or circulation disease
- High blood cholesterol
- High blood pressure (hypertension)
- Jaundice (or history of, including jaundice during pregnancy)
- Kidney disease
- Liver disease (such as jaundice or porphyria)
- Lumps in breasts
- Mental depression (or history of)
- Migraine headaches

- Scanty or irregular menstrual periods
- Stroke (history of)
- Too much calcium in the blood
- Tuberculosis
- Varicose veins

Before you begin using any new medicine (prescription or nonprescription) or if you develop any new medical problem while you are using this medicine, check with your doctor, nurse, or pharmacist.

Proper Use of This Medicine

Take this medicine only as directed by your doctor. This medicine must be taken exactly on schedule to prevent pregnancy. Try to take the medicine at the same time each day, not more than 24 hours apart, to reduce the possibility of side effects and to provide the best protection.

Nausea may occur during the first few weeks after you start taking this medicine. This effect usually disappears with continued use. If the nausea is bothersome, it can usually be prevented or reduced by taking each dose with food or immediately after food.

Since one of the most important factors in the proper use of oral contraceptives is taking every dose exactly on schedule, you should never let your tablet supply run out. Always keep 1 extra month's supply of tablets on hand. To keep the extra month's supply from becoming too old, use it next, after the pills now being used, and replace the extra supply each month on a regular schedule. The tablets will keep well when kept dry and at room temperature (light will fade some tablet colors but will not change the medicine's effect).

Keep the tablets in the container in which you received them. Most containers aid you in keeping track of your dosage schedule.

Dosing—

- *Monophasic cycle* dosing schedule: Most available dosing schedules are of the monophasic type. If you are taking tablets of one strength (color) for 20 or 21 days, you are using a monophasic schedule. For the 28-day monophasic cycle you will also take an additional 7 inactive tablets, which are of another color.
- *Biphasic cycle* dosing schedule:

  —If you are using a biphasic 21-day schedule, you are taking tablets of one strength (color) for 10 days (the 1st phase). You then take tablets of a second strength (color) for the next 11 days (the 2nd phase). For the 28-day biphasic cycle you will also take an additional 7 inactive tablets, which are of a third color.

  —If you are using a biphasic 24-day schedule, you are taking tablets of one strength (color) for 17 days (the 1st phase). You then take tablets of a second strength (color) for the next 7 days (the 2nd phase).
- *Triphasic cycle* dosing schedule: If you are using a triphasic 21-day schedule, you are taking tablets of one strength (color) for 6 or 7 days depending on the medicine prescribed (the 1st phase). You then take tablets of a second strength (color) for the next 5 to 9 days depending on the medicine prescribed (the 2nd phase). After that, you take tablets of a third strength (color) for the next 5 to 10 days depending on the medicine prescribed (the 3rd phase). At this point, you will have taken a total of 21 tablets. For the 28-day triphasic cycle you will also take an additional 7 inactive tablets, which are of a fourth color.

It is very important that you take the tablets in the same order that they appear in the container. Tablets of different colors in the same package are also different in strength. Taking the tablets out of order may reduce the effectiveness of the medicine.

Missed dose—If you miss a dose of this medicine:

- For *monophasic* or *biphasic* cycles:

  —If you are using a 20-, 21-, or a 24-day schedule and you miss a dose of this medicine for one day, take the missed tablet as soon as you remember. If it is not remembered until the next day, take the missed tablet plus the tablet that is regularly scheduled for that day. This means that you will take 2 tablets on the same day. Then continue on your regular dosing schedule.

  —If you are using a 20-, 21-, or a 24-day schedule and you miss a dose for 2 days in a row, take 2 tablets a day for each of the next 2 days, then continue on your regular dosing schedule. In addition, you should use a second method of birth control to make sure that you are fully protected for the rest of the cycle. Report to your doctor.

  —If you are using a 20-, 21-, or a 24-day schedule and you miss a dose for 3 days or more in a row, stop taking the medicine completely and use another method of birth control until your period begins or until your doctor determines that you are not pregnant. Then restart protection with a new cycle of tablets.

  —If you are using a 28-day schedule and you miss any of the first 21 (active) tablets, follow the instructions for the 21-day schedule depending on how many doses you have missed. If you miss any of the last 7 (inactive) tablets, there is no danger of pregnancy. However, the first tablet (active) of the next month's cycle must be taken on the regularly scheduled day, in spite of any missed doses, if pregnancy is to be avoided. The active and inactive tablets are colored differently for your convenience.

- For *triphasic* cycles:

—If you are using a 21-day schedule and you miss a dose of this medicine for one day, take the missed tablet as soon as you remember. If it is not remembered until the next day, take the missed tablet plus the tablet that is regularly scheduled for that day. This means that you will take 2 tablets on the same day. Then continue on your regular dosing schedule. In addition, you should use a second method of birth control to make sure that you are fully protected for the rest of the cycle. Report to your doctor.

—If you are using a 21-day schedule and you miss a dose for 2 days in a row, take 2 tablets a day for each of the next 2 days, then continue on your regular dosing schedule. In addition, you should use a second method of birth control to make sure that you are fully protected for the rest of the cycle. Report to your doctor.

—If you are using a 21-day schedule and you miss a dose for 3 days or more in a row, stop taking the medicine completely and use another method of birth control until your period begins or until your doctor determines that you are not pregnant. Then restart protection with a new cycle of tablets.

—If you are using a 28-day schedule and you miss any of the first 21 (active) tablets, follow the instructions for the 21-day schedule depending on how many doses you have missed. If you miss any of the last 7 (inactive) tablets, there is no danger of pregnancy. However, the first tablet (active) of the next month's cycle must be taken on the regularly scheduled day, in spite of any missed doses, if pregnancy is to be avoided. The active and inactive tablets are colored differently for your convenience.

Storage—To store this medicine:

- Keep out of the reach of children.
- Store away from heat and direct light.
- Do not store in the bathroom, near the kitchen sink, or in other damp places. Heat and moisture may cause the medicine to break down.
- Do not keep outdated medicine or medicine no longer needed. Be sure that any discarded medicine is out of the reach of children.

Precautions While Using This Medicine

It is very important that your doctor check your progress at regular visits to make sure this medicine does not cause unwanted effects. These visits will usually be every 6 to 12 months, but some doctors require them more often.

When you begin to use oral contraceptives, your body will require at least 7 days to adjust before pregnancy will be prevented; therefore, you should *use a second method of birth control for the first cycle (or 3 weeks)* to ensure full protection.

Tell the medical doctor or dentist in charge that you are taking this medicine before any kind of surgery (including dental surgery) or emergency treatment, since this medicine may cause serious blood clots, heart attack, or stroke.

The following medicines may reduce the effectiveness of oral contraceptives. *You should use a second method of birth control during each cycle in which any of the following medicines are used:*

Ampicillin
Adrenocorticoids (cortisone-like medicine)
Bacampicillin
Barbiturates
Carbamazepine (e.g., Tegretol)
Chloramphenicol (e.g., Chloromycetin)
Dihydroergotamine (e.g., D.H.E. 45)
Griseofulvin (e.g., Fulvicin)
Mineral oil
Neomycin, oral
Penicillin V
Phenylbutazone (e.g., Butazolidin)
Phenytoin (e.g., Dilantin)
Primidone (e.g., Mysoline)
Rifampin (e.g., Rifadin)
Sulfonamides (sulfa medicine)
Tetracyclines (medicine for infection)
Tranquilizers
Valproic acid (e.g., Depakene)

Check with your doctor if you have any questions about this.

Vaginal bleeding of various amounts may occur between your regular menstrual periods during the first 3 months of use. This is sometimes called spotting when slight, or breakthrough bleeding when heavier. If this should occur:

- Continue on your regular dosing schedule.
- The bleeding usually stops within 1 week.
- Check with your doctor if the bleeding continues for more than 1 week.
- After you have been taking oral contraceptives on schedule and for more than 3 months, check with your doctor.

Missed menstrual periods may occur:

- if you have not taken the medicine exactly as scheduled. Pregnancy must be considered a possibility.
- if the medicine is not properly adjusted for your needs.
- if you have taken oral contraceptives for a long time, usually 2 or more years, and stop their use.

Check with your doctor if you miss any menstrual periods so that the cause may be determined.

In some patients using estrogen-containing oral contraceptives, tenderness, swelling, or bleeding of the gums may occur. Brushing and flossing your teeth carefully and regularly and massaging your gums may help prevent this. See your dentist regularly to have your teeth cleaned. Check with your medical doctor or dentist if you have any questions about how to take care of your teeth and gums, or if you notice any tenderness, swelling, or bleeding of your gums. Also, it has been shown that estrogen-containing oral contraceptives may cause a healing problem called dry socket after a tooth has been removed. If you are going to have a tooth removed, tell your dentist or oral surgeon that you are taking oral contraceptives.

Some people who take oral contraceptives may become more sensitive to sunlight than they are normally. When you begin taking this medicine, avoid too much sun and do not use a sunlamp until you see how you react to the sun, especially if you tend to burn easily. If you have a severe reaction, check with your doctor. Some people may develop brown, blotchy spots on exposed areas. These spots usually disappear gradually when the medicine is stopped.

If you wear contact lenses and notice a change in vision or are not able to wear them, check with your doctor.

If you suspect that you may have become pregnant, stop taking this medicine immediately and check with your doctor.

If you are scheduled for any laboratory tests, tell your doctor that you are taking birth control pills.

Do not give this medicine to anyone else. Your doctor has prescribed it only for you after studying your health record and the results of your physical examination. Oral contraceptives may be dangerous for other people because of differences in their health and body make-up.

Check with your doctor before taking any leftover oral contraceptives from an old prescription, especially after a pregnancy. Your old prescription may be dangerous to you now or may allow you to become pregnant if your health has changed since your last physical examination.

Side Effects of This Medicine

Discuss these possible effects with your doctor:

- Along with their needed effects, birth control tablets sometimes cause some unwanted effects such as benign (not cancerous) liver tumors, liver cancer, blood clots, heart attack, and stroke, and problems of the gallbladder, liver, and uterus. Although these effects are rare, they can be very serious and may cause death.
- *Cigarette smoking* during the use of oral contraceptives has been found to increase the risk of serious side effects affecting the heart and/or blood circulation, such as dangerous blood clots, heart attack, or stroke. The risk increases as the age of the patient and the amount of smoking increase. This risk is greater in women age 35 and over. *To reduce the risk of serious side effects, do not smoke cigarettes while using oral contraceptives.*

The following side effects may be caused by blood clots, which could lead to stroke, heart attack, or death. Although these side effects rarely occur, they require immediate medical attention. *Get emergency help immediately* if any of the following side effects occur:

Abdominal or stomach pain (sudden, severe, or continuing); coughing up blood; headache (severe or sudden); loss of coordination (sudden); loss of vision or change in vision (sudden); pains in chest, groin, or leg (especially in calf of leg); shortness of breath (sudden or unexplained); slurring of speech (sudden); weakness, numbness, or pain in arm or leg (unexplained)

Check with your doctor as soon as possible if any of the following side effects occur:

Less common or rare

Bulging eyes; changes in vaginal bleeding (spotting, breakthrough bleeding, prolonged bleeding, or complete stoppage of bleeding); double vision; fainting; frequent urge to urinate or painful urination; increased blood pressure; loss of vision (gradual, partial, or complete); lumps in, or discharge from, breast; mental depression; pains in stomach, side, or abdomen; skin rash, redness, or other skin irritation; swelling, pain, or tenderness in upper abdomen (stomach) area; unusual or dark-colored mole; vaginal discharge (thick, white, or curd-like); vaginal itching or irritation; yellow eyes or skin

Other side effects may occur that usually do not need medical attention. These side effects may go away during treatment as your body adjusts to the medicine. However, check with your doctor if any of the following side effects continue or are bothersome:

More common

Acne (usually less common after first 3 months); bloating of stomach; cramps of lower stomach; increase or decrease in appetite; nausea; swelling of ankles and feet; swelling and increased tenderness of breasts; unusual tiredness or weakness; unusual weight gain

Less common or rare

Brown, blotchy spots on exposed skin;. diarrhea (mild); dizziness; headaches or migraine headaches; increased body and facial hair; increased sensitivity to contact lenses; increased skin sensitivity to sun; irritability; some loss of scalp hair; unusual decrease or increase in sexual desire; vomiting; weight loss

Other side effects not listed above may also occur in some patients. If you notice any other effects, check with your doctor.

Annual revision: August 1990
Interim revision: 06/08/93

ETHAMBUTOL Systemic

Some commonly used brand names are:

In the U.S.
Myambutol

In Canada
Etibi
Myambutol

Description

Ethambutol (e-THAM-byoo-tole) is used to treat tuberculosis (TB). It is used with one or more other medicines for TB. This medicine may also be used for other problems as determined by your doctor.

Ethambutol is available only with your doctor's prescription, in the following dosage form:

Oral

- Tablets (U.S. and Canada)

It is very important that you read and understand the following information. If any of it causes you special concern, check with your doctor. Also, *if you have any questions* or if you want more information about this medicine or your medical problem, *ask your doctor, nurse, or pharmacist.*

Before Using This Medicine

In deciding to use a medicine, the risks of taking the medicine must be weighed against the good it will do. This is a decision you and your doctor will make. For ethambutol, the following should be considered:

Allergies—Tell your doctor if you have ever had any unusual or allergic reaction to ethambutol. Also tell your doctor and pharmacist if you are allergic to any other substances, such as foods, preservatives, or dyes.

Pregnancy—Ethambutol has not been shown to cause birth defects or other problems in humans. However, studies in animals have shown that ethambutol causes cleft palate, skull and spine defects, absence of one eye, and hare lip. In addition, it is not known whether this medicine causes problems when taken with other TB medicines.

Breast-feeding—Ethambutol passes into the breast milk. However, ethambutol has not been shown to cause problems in nursing babies.

Children—This medicine has been tested in children 13 years of age or older and has not been shown to cause different side effects or problems than it does in adults.

Older adults—Many medicines have not been studied specifically in older people. Therefore, it may not be known whether they work exactly the same way they do in younger adults. Although there is no specific information comparing use of ethambutol in the elderly with use in other age groups, this medicine is not expected to cause different side effects or problems in older people than it does in younger adults.

Other medicines—Although certain medicines should not be used together at all, in other cases two different medicines may be used together even if an interaction might occur. In these cases, your doctor may want to change the dose, or other precautions may be necessary. Tell your doctor and pharmacist if you are taking any other prescription or nonprescription (over-the-counter [OTC]) medicine.

Other medical problems—The presence of other medical problems may affect the use of ethambutol. Make sure you tell your doctor if you have any other medical problems, especially:

- Gout—Ethambutol may cause or worsen attacks of gout
- Kidney disease—Patients with kidney disease may be more likely to have side effects
- Optic neuritis (eye nerve damage)—Ethambutol may cause or worsen eye disease

Before you begin using any new medicine (prescription or nonprescription) or if you develop any new medical problem while you are using this medicine, check with your doctor, nurse, or pharmacist.

Proper Use of This Medicine

Ethambutol may be taken with food if it upsets your stomach.

To help clear up your tuberculosis (TB) completely, *it is very important that you keep taking this medicine for the full time of treatment,* even if you begin to feel better after a few weeks. You may have to take it every day for as long as 1 to 2 years or more. *It is important that you do not miss any doses.*

Missed dose—If you do miss a dose of this medicine, take it as soon as possible. However, if it is almost time for your next dose, skip the missed dose and go back to your regular dosing schedule. Do not double doses.

Storage—To store this medicine:

- Keep out of the reach of children.
- Store away from heat and direct light.
- Do not store in the bathroom, near the kitchen sink, or in other damp places. Heat or moisture may cause the medicine to break down.
- Do not keep outdated medicine or medicine no longer needed. Be sure that any discarded medicine is out of the reach of children.

Precautions While Using This Medicine

If your symptoms do not improve within 2 to 3 weeks, or if they become worse, check with your doctor.

It is very important that your doctor check your progress at regular visits.

In addition, you should *check with your doctor immediately if blurred vision, eye pain, red-green color blindness, or loss of vision occurs during treatment.* Your doctor may want you to have your eyes checked by an ophthalmologist (eye doctor). *Make sure you know how you react to this medicine before you drive, use machines, or do anything else that could be dangerous if you are not alert or able to see well.* If these reactions are especially bothersome, check with your doctor.

Side Effects of This Medicine

Along with its needed effects, a medicine may cause some unwanted effects. Although not all of these side effects may occur, if they do occur they may need medical attention.

Check with your doctor immediately if any of the following side effects occur:

Less common

Chills; pain and swelling of joints, especially big toe, ankle, or knee; tense, hot skin over affected joints

Rare

Blurred vision, eye pain, red-green color blindness, or any loss of vision (more common with high doses); fever; joint aches and pain; numbness, tingling, burning pain, or weakness in hands or feet; skin rash

Other side effects may occur that usually do not need medical attention. These side effects may go away during treatment as your body adjusts to the medicine. However, check with your doctor if any of the following side effects continue or are bothersome:

Less common

Confusion; headache; loss of appetite; nausea and vomiting; stomach pain

Other side effects not listed above may also occur in some patients. If you notice any other effects, check with your doctor.

Annual revision: 07/27/92

ETHCHLORVYNOL Systemic

A commonly used brand name in the U.S. and Canada is Placidyl. Generic name product may also be available in the U.S.

Description

Ethchlorvynol (eth-klor-VI-nole) is used to treat insomnia (trouble in sleeping). However, it has generally been replaced by other medicines for the treatment of insomnia. If ethchlorvynol is used regularly (for example, every day) to help produce sleep, it is usually not effective for more than 1 week.

This medicine is available only with your doctor's prescription, in the following dosage form:

Oral

- Capsules (U.S. and Canada)

It is very important that you read and understand the following information. If any of it causes you special concern, check with your doctor. Also, *if you have any questions* or if you want more information about this medicine or your medical problem, *ask your doctor, nurse, or pharmacist.*

Before Using This Medicine

In deciding to use a medicine, the risks of taking the medicine must be weighed against the good it will do. This is a decision you and your doctor will make. For ethchlorvynol, the following should be considered:

Allergies—Tell your doctor if you have ever had any unusual or allergic reaction to ethchlorvynol. Also tell your doctor or pharmacist if you are allergic to any other substances, such as foods, preservatives, or dyes.

Pregnancy—Ethchlorvynol has not been studied in pregnant women. However, use of ethchlorvynol during the first 6 months of pregnancy is not recommended because studies in animals have shown that high doses of ethchlorvynol increase the chance of stillbirths and decrease the chance of the newborn surviving. Taking ethchlorvynol during the last 3 months of pregnancy may cause slow heartbeat, shortness of breath, troubled breathing, or withdrawal side effects in the newborn baby.

Breast-feeding—It is not known whether ethchlorvynol passes into the breast milk.

Children—Studies on this medicine have been done only in adult patients and there is no specific information comparing use of ethchlorvynol in children with use in other age groups.

Older adults—Elderly people may be especially sensitive to the effects of ethchlorvynol. This may increase the chance of side effects during treatment.

Other medicines—Although certain medicines should not be used together at all, in other cases 2 different medicines may be used together even if an interaction might occur. In these cases, your doctor may want to change the dose, or other precautions may be necessary. When you are taking ethchlorvynol, it is especially important that your doctor and pharmacist know if you are taking any of the following:

- Anticoagulants (blood thinners)—Ethchlorvynol may change the amount of anticoagulant you need to take
- Central nervous system (CNS) depressants (medicine that causes drowsiness) or
- Tricyclic antidepressants (medicine for depression)—Using these medicines together with ethchlorvynol may increase the CNS and other depressant effects

Other medical problems—The presence of other medical problems may affect the use of ethchlorvynol. Make sure you tell your doctor if you have any other medical problems, especially:

- Alcohol abuse (or history of) or
- Drug abuse or dependence (or history of)—Dependence on ethchlorvynol may develop
- Kidney disease or
- Liver disease—Higher blood levels of ethchlorvynol may result and increase the chance of side effects
- Mental depression or
- Porphyria—Ethchlorvynol may make the condition worse

Before you begin using any new medicine (prescription or nonprescription) or if you develop any new medical problem while you are using this medicine, check with your doctor, nurse, or pharmacist.

Proper Use of This Medicine

Ethchlorvynol is best taken with food or a glass of milk to lessen the possibility of dizziness, clumsiness, or unsteadiness, which may occur shortly after you take this medicine.

Take this medicine only as directed by your doctor. Do not take more of it, do not take it more often, and do not take it for a longer time than your doctor ordered. If too much is taken, it may become habit-forming.

Dosing—The dose of ethchlorvynol will be different for different patients. *Follow your doctor's orders or the directions on the label.* The following information includes only the average doses of ethchlorvynol. *If your dose is different, do not change it* unless your doctor tells you to do so.

- For *oral* dosage forms (capsules):
  —Adults: 500 to 1000 milligrams at bedtime.
  —Children: Dose must be determined by the doctor.

Storage—To store this medicine:

- Keep out of the reach of children. Overdose of ethchlorvynol is especially dangerous in children.
- Store away from heat and direct light.
- Do not store in the bathroom, near the kitchen sink, or in other damp places. Heat or moisture may cause the medicine to break down.
- Do not keep outdated medicine or medicine no longer needed. Be sure that any discarded medicine is out of the reach of children.

Precautions While Using This Medicine

If you will be taking this medicine regularly for a long time:

- Your doctor should check your progress at regular visits.
- Do not stop taking it without first checking with your doctor. Your doctor may want you to reduce gradually the amount you are taking before stopping completely.

This medicine will add to the effects of alcohol and other CNS depressants (medicines that slow down the nervous system, possibly causing drowsiness). Some examples of CNS depressants are antihistamines or medicine for hay fever, other allergies, or colds; sedatives, tranquilizers, or sleeping medicine; prescription pain medicine or narcotics; barbiturates; medicine for seizures; muscle relaxants; or anesthetics, including some dental anesthetics. *Check with your doctor before taking any of the above while you are taking this medicine.*

If you think you or someone else may have taken an overdose of this medicine, get emergency help at once. Taking an overdose of ethchlorvynol or taking alcohol or other CNS depressants with ethchlorvynol may lead to unconsciousness and possibly death. Some signs of an overdose are continuing confusion, severe weakness, shortness of breath or slow or troubled breathing, slurred speech, staggering, and slow heartbeat.

This medicine may cause some people to become dizzy, lightheaded, drowsy, or less alert than they are normally. Even if taken at bedtime, it may cause some people to feel drowsy or less alert on arising. *Make sure you know how you react to this medicine before you drive, use machines, or do anything else that could be dangerous if you are dizzy or are not alert.*

Side Effects of This Medicine

Along with its needed effects, a medicine may cause some unwanted effects. Although not all of these side effects may occur, if they do occur they may need medical attention.

Check with your doctor as soon as possible if any of the following side effects occur:

Less common

Skin rash or hives; unusual bleeding or bruising; unusual excitement, nervousness, or restlessness

Rare

Darkening of urine; itching; pale stools; yellow eyes or skin

Symptoms of overdose

Confusion (continuing); double vision; low body temperature; numbness, tingling, pain, or weakness in hands or feet; shortness of breath or slow or troubled breathing; slow heartbeat; slurred speech; staggering; trembling; unusual movements of the eyes; weakness (severe)

Other side effects may occur that usually do not need medical attention. These side effects may go away during treatment as your body adjusts to the medicine. However, check with your doctor if any of the following side effects continue or are bothersome:

More common

Blurred vision; dizziness or lightheadedness; indigestion; nausea or vomiting; numbness of face; stomach pain; unpleasant aftertaste; unusual tiredness or weakness

Less common

Clumsiness or unsteadiness; confusion; drowsiness (daytime)

After you stop using this medicine, your body may need time to adjust. If you took this medicine in high doses or for a long time, this may take up to 2 weeks. During this period of time check with your doctor if you notice any of the following side effects:

Convulsions (seizures); hallucinations (seeing, hearing, or feeling things that are not there); muscle twitching; nausea or vomiting; restlessness, nervousness, or irritability; sweating; trembling; trouble in sleeping; weakness

Other side effects not listed above may also occur in some patients. If you notice any other effects, check with your doctor.

Annual revision: 03/09/10

ETHINAMATE Systemic†

A commonly used brand name in the U.S. is Valmid.

†Not commercially available in Canada.

Description

Ethinamate (e-THIN-a-mate) is used to treat insomnia (trouble in sleeping). However, it has generally been replaced by other medicines for the treatment of insomnia. If ethinamate is used regularly (for example, every day) to help produce sleep, it is usually not effective for more than 7 days.

This medicine is available only with your doctor's prescription, in the following dosage form:

Oral

- Capsules (U.S.)

It is very important that you read and understand the following information. If any of it causes you special concern, check with your doctor. Also, *if you have any questions* or if you want more information about this medicine or your medical problem, *ask your doctor, nurse, or pharmacist.*

Before Using This Medicine

In deciding to use a medicine, the risks of taking the medicine must be weighed against the good it will do. This is a decision you and your doctor will make. For ethinamate, the following should be considered:

Allergies—Tell your doctor if you have ever had any unusual or allergic reaction to ethinamate. Also tell your doctor or pharmacist if you are allergic to any other substances, such as foods, preservatives, or dyes.

Pregnancy—Studies on birth defects have not been done in either humans or animals.

Breast-feeding—It is not known whether ethinamate passes into the breast milk. However, this medicine has not been reported to cause problems in nursing babies.

Children—Studies on this medicine have been done only in adult patients, and there is no specific information about its use in children.

Older adults—Elderly people may be especially sensitive to the effects of ethinamate. This may increase the chance of side effects during treatment.

Other medicines—Although certain medicines should not be used together at all, in other cases 2 different medicines may be used together even if an interaction might occur. In these cases, your doctor may want to change the dose, or other precautions may be necessary. When taking ethinamate it is especially important that your doctor and pharmacist know if you are taking any of the following:

- Central nervous system (CNS) depressants, other—Using these medicines together may increase the CNS and other depressant effects

Other medical problems—The presence of other medical problems may affect the use of ethinamate. Make sure you tell your doctor if you have any other medical problems, especially:

- Alcohol abuse (or history of) or
- Drug abuse or dependence (or history of)—Dependence on ethinamate may develop
- Mental depression—Ethinamate may make the condition worse

Before you begin using any new medicine (prescription or nonprescription) or if you develop any new medical problem while you are using this medicine, check with your doctor, nurse, or pharmacist.

Proper Use of This Medicine

Take this medicine only as directed by your doctor. Do not take more of it, do not take it more often, and do not take it for a longer time than your doctor ordered. If too much is taken, it may become habit-forming.

Storage—To store this medicine:

- Keep out of the reach of children. Overdose of ethinamate is especially dangerous in children.
- Store away from heat and direct light.
- Do not store in the bathroom, near the kitchen sink, or in other damp places. Heat or moisture may cause the medicine to break down.
- Do not keep outdated medicine or medicine no longer needed. Be sure that any discarded medicine is out of the reach of children.

Precautions While Using This Medicine

If you will be taking this medicine regularly for a long time:

- Your doctor should check your progress at regular visits.
- Do not stop taking it without first checking with your doctor. Your doctor may want you to reduce gradually the amount you are taking before stopping completely.

This medicine will add to the effects of alcohol and other CNS depressants (medicines that slow down the nervous system, possibly causing drowsiness.) Some examples of CNS depressants are antihistamines or medicine for hay fever, other allergies, or colds; sedatives, tranquilizers, or sleeping medicine; prescription pain medicine or narcotics; barbiturates; medicine for seizures; muscle relaxants; or anesthetics, including some dental anesthetics. *Check with your doctor before taking any of the above while you are taking this medicine.*

If you think you or someone else may have taken an overdose of this medicine, get emergency help at once. Taking an overdose of ethinamate or taking alcohol or other CNS depressants with ethinamate may lead to unconsciousness and possibly death. Some signs of an overdose are confusion, severe weakness, shortness of breath or slow or troubled breathing, slurred speech, staggering, and slow heartbeat.

This medicine may cause some people to become drowsy or less alert than they are normally. Even if taken at bedtime, it may cause some people to feel drowsy or less alert on arising. *Make sure you know how you react to this medicine before you drive, use machines, or do anything else that could be dangerous if you are not alert.*

Side Effects of This Medicine

Along with its needed effects, a medicine may cause some unwanted effects. Although not all of these side effects may occur, if they do occur they may need medical attention.

Check with your doctor as soon as possible if any of the following side effects occur:

Less common

Skin rash; unusual excitement (especially in children)

Rare

Unusual bleeding or bruising

Symptoms of overdose

Confusion; shortness of breath or slow or troubled breathing; slow heartbeat; slurred speech; staggering; weakness (severe)

Other side effects may occur that usually do not need medical attention. These side effects may go away during treatment as your body adjusts to the medicine. However, check with your doctor if any of the following side effects continue or are bothersome:

Less common

Indigestion; nausea; stomach pain; vomiting

Rare

Drowsiness (daytime)

After you stop using this medicine, your body may need time to adjust. The length of time this takes depends on the amount of medicine you were using and how long you used it. During this period of time check with your doctor if you notice any of the following side effects:

Confusion; convulsions (seizures); hallucinations (seeing, hearing, or feeling things that are not there); restlessness, nervousness, or irritability; trembling; trouble in sleeping

Other side effects not listed above may also occur in some patients. If you notice any other effects, check with your doctor.

Annual revision: July 1990

ETHIONAMIDE Systemic†

A commonly used brand name in the U.S. is Trecator-SC.

†Not commercially available in Canada.

Description

Ethionamide (e-thye-ON-am-ide) is used with one or more other medicines to treat tuberculosis (TB). Ethionamide may also be used for other problems as determined by your doctor.

Ethionamide is available only with your doctor's prescription, in the following dosage form:

Oral

- Tablets (U.S.)

It is very important that you read and understand the following information. If any of it causes you special concern, check with your doctor. Also, *if you have any questions* or if you want more information about this medicine or your medical problem, *ask your doctor, nurse, or pharmacist.*

Before Using This Medicine

In deciding to use a medicine, the risks of taking the medicine must be weighed against the good it will do. This is a decision you and your doctor will make. For ethionamide, the following should be considered:

Allergies—Tell your doctor if you have ever had any unusual or allergic reaction to ethionamide, isoniazid (e.g., INH; Nydrazid), pyrazinamide, or niacin (e.g., Nicobid; nicotinic acid). Also tell your doctor and pharmacist if you are allergic to any other substances, such as foods, preservatives, or dyes.

Pregnancy—Use is not recommended during pregnancy. Ethionamide causes birth defects in rats and rabbits given doses greater than the usual human dose. In addition, it is not known whether this medicine causes problems when taken with other TB medicines.

Breast-feeding—It is not known whether ethionamide is excreted in breast milk. However, ethionamide has not been shown to cause problems in nursing babies.

Children—Although there is no specific information comparing use of ethionamide in children with use in other age groups, this medicine is not expected to cause different side effects or problems in children than it does in adults.

Older adults—Many medicines have not been studied specifically in older people. Therefore, it may not be known whether they work exactly the same way they do in younger adults or if they cause different side effects or problems in older people. There is no specific information comparing use of ethionamide in the elderly with use in other age groups.

Other medicines—Although certain medicines should not be used together at all, in other cases two different medicines may be used together even if an interaction might occur. In these cases, your doctor may want to change the dose, or other precautions may be necessary. When you are taking ethionamide, it is especially important that your doctor and pharmacist know if you are taking any of the following:

- Cycloserine—Use of ethionamide with cycloserine may increase the chance for nervous system side effects

Other medical problems—The presence of other medical problems may affect the use of ethionamide. Make sure you tell your doctor if you have any other medical problems, especially:

- Diabetes mellitus (sugar diabetes)—Diabetes may be harder to control in patients taking ethionamide
- Liver disease (severe)—Patients with severe liver disease may have an increased chance of side effects

Before you begin using any new medicine (prescription or nonprescription) or if you develop any new medical problem while you are using this medicine, check with your doctor, nurse, or pharmacist.

Proper Use of This Medicine

Ethionamide may be taken with or after meals if it upsets your stomach.

To help clear up your tuberculosis (TB) completely, *it is very important that you keep taking this medicine for the full time of treatment,* even if you begin to feel better after a few weeks. You may have to take it every day for 1 to 2 years or more. *It is important that you do not miss any doses.*

Your doctor may also want you to take pyridoxine (e.g., Hexa-Betalin; vitamin B_6) every day to help prevent or lessen some of the side effects of ethionamide. If so, *it is very important to take pyridoxine every day along with this medicine. Do not miss any doses.*

Missed dose—If you do miss a dose of either of these medicines, take it as soon as possible. However, if it is almost time for your next dose, skip the missed dose and go back to your regular dosing schedule. Do not double doses.

Storage—To store this medicine:

- Keep out of the reach of children.
- Store away from heat and direct light.

- Do not store in the bathroom, near the kitchen sink, or in other damp places. Heat or moisture may cause the medicine to break down.
- Do not keep outdated medicine or medicine no longer needed. Be sure that any discarded medicine is out of the reach of children.

Precautions While Using This Medicine

If your symptoms do not improve within 2 to 3 weeks, or if they become worse, check with your doctor.

It is very important that your doctor check your progress at regular visits. Also, *check with your doctor immediately if blurred vision or any loss of vision, with or without eye pain, occurs during treatment.* Your doctor may want you to have your eyes checked by an ophthalmologist (eye doctor).

This medicine may cause blurred vision or loss of vision. *Make sure you know how you react to this medicine before you drive, use machines, or do anything else that could be dangerous if you are not able to see well.* If these reactions are especially bothersome, check with your doctor.

If this medicine causes clumsiness; unsteadiness; or numbness, tingling, burning, or pain in the hands and feet, check with your doctor immediately. These may be early warning symptoms of more serious nerve problems that could develop later.

Side Effects of This Medicine

Along with its needed effects, a medicine may cause some unwanted effects. Although not all of these side effects may occur, if they do occur they may need medical attention.

Check with your doctor immediately if any of the following side effects occur:

Less common

Clumsiness or unsteadiness; confusion; mental depression; mood or other mental changes; numbness, tingling, burning, or pain in hands and feet; yellow eyes or skin

Rare

Blurred vision or loss of vision, with or without eye pain; changes in menstrual periods; coldness; decreased sexual ability (in males); difficulty in concentrating; dry, puffy skin; increased heartbeat; increased hunger; nervousness; shakiness; skin rash; swelling of front part of neck; weight gain

Other side effects may occur that usually do not need medical attention. These side effects may go away during treatment as your body adjusts to the medicine. However, check with your doctor if any of the following side effects continue or are bothersome:

More common

Dizziness (especially when getting up from a lying or sitting position); loss of appetite; metallic taste; nausea or vomiting; sore mouth

Less common or rare

Enlargement of the breasts (in males)

Other side effects not listed above may also occur in some patients. If you notice any other effects, check with your doctor.

Additional Information

Once a medicine has been approved for marketing for a certain use, experience may show that it is also useful for other medical problems. Although these uses are not included in product labeling, ethionamide is used in certain patients with the following medical conditions:

- Atypical mycobacterial infections
- Leprosy
- Tuberculosis meningitis

Other than the above information, there is no additional information relating to proper use, precautions, or side effects for these uses.

Annual revision: 08/27/92

ETIDRONATE Systemic

A commonly used brand name in the U.S. and Canada is Didronel. Another commonly used name is EHDP.

Description

Etidronate (eh-tih-DROE-nate) is used to treat Paget's disease of bone. It may also be used to treat or prevent a certain type of bone problem that may occur after hip replacement surgery or spinal injury.

Etidronate is also used to treat hypercalcemia (too much calcium in the blood) that may occur with some types of cancer.

This medicine is available only with your doctor's prescription, in the following dosage forms:

Oral

- Tablets (U.S. and Canada)

Parenteral

- Injection (U.S.)

It is very important that you read and understand the following information. If any of it causes you special concern, check with your doctor. Also, *if you have any questions* or if you want more information about this medicine or your medical problem, *ask your doctor, nurse, or pharmacist.*

Before Using This Medicine

In deciding to use a medicine, the risks of taking the medicine must be weighed against the good it will do. This is a decision you and your doctor will make. For etidronate, the following should be considered:

Allergies—Tell your doctor if you have ever had any unusual or allergic reaction to etidronate. Also tell your doctor and pharmacist if you are allergic to any other substances, such as foods, preservatives, or dyes.

Diet—Make certain your doctor and pharmacist know if your diet includes large amounts of calcium, such as milk or other dairy products, or if you are on any special diet, such as a low-sodium or low-sugar diet. Calcium in the diet may prevent the absorption of oral etidronate.

Pregnancy—Studies have not been done in humans. However, studies in rats injected with large doses of etidronate have shown that etidronate causes deformed bones in the fetus.

Breast-feeding—It is not known if etidronate passes into breast milk. However, this medicine has not been reported to cause problems in nursing babies.

Children—Some changes in bone growth may occur in children, but will usually go away when the medicine is stopped.

Older adults—When etidronate is given by injection along with a large amount of fluids, older people tend to retain (keep) the excess fluid.

Other medicines—Although certain medicines should not be used together at all, in other cases two different medicines may be used together even if an interaction might occur. In these cases, your doctor may want to change the dose, or other precautions may be necessary. When you are taking etidronate, it is especially important that your doctor and pharmacist know if you are taking any of the following:

- Antacids containing calcium, magnesium, or aluminum or
- Mineral supplements or other medicines containing calcium, iron, magnesium, or aluminum—These medicines may decrease the effects of etidronate, and should be taken at least 2 hours before or after taking etidronate

Other medical problems—The presence of other medical problems may affect the use of etidronate. Make sure you tell your doctor if you have any other medical problems, especially:

- Bone fracture, especially of arm or leg—Etidronate may increase the risk of bone fractures
- Intestinal or bowel disease—Etidronate may increase the risk of diarrhea
- Kidney disease—High blood levels of etidronate may result causing cause serious side effects

Before you begin using any new medicine (prescription or nonprescription) or if you develop any new medical problem while you are using this medicine, check with your doctor, nurse, or pharmacist.

Proper Use of This Medicine

Take etidronate with water on an empty stomach at least 2 hours before or after food (midmorning is best) or at bedtime. Food may decrease the amount of etidronate absorbed by your body.

Take etidronate only as directed. Do not take more of it, do not take it more often, and do not take it for a longer time than your doctor ordered. To do so may increase the chance of side effects.

In some patients, etidronate takes up to 3 months to work. If you feel that the medicine is not working, do not stop taking it on your own. Instead, check with your doctor.

It is important that you eat a well-balanced diet with an adequate amount of calcium and vitamin D (found in milk or other dairy products). Too much or too little of either may increase the chance of side effects while you are taking etidronate. Your doctor can help you choose the meal plan that is best for you. *However, do not take any food, especially milk, milk formulas, or other dairy products, or antacids, mineral supplements, or other medicines that are high in calcium or iron (high amounts of these minerals may also be in some vitamin preparations), magnesium, or aluminum* within 2 hours of taking etidronate. To do so may keep this medicine from working properly.

Missed dose—If you miss a dose of this medicine, take it as soon as possible. However, if it is almost time for your next dose, skip the missed dose and go back to your regular dosing schedule. Do not double doses.

Storage—To store this medicine:

- Keep out of the reach of children.
- Store away from heat and direct light.
- Do not store in the bathroom, near the kitchen sink, or in other damp places. Heat or moisture may cause the medicine to break down.
- Do not keep outdated medicine or medicine no longer needed. Be sure that any discarded medicine is out of the reach of children.

Precautions While Using This Medicine

It is important that your doctor check your progress at regular visits even if you are between treatments and are not taking this medicine. If your condition has improved and your doctor has told you to stop taking etidronate, your progress must still be checked. The results of laboratory tests or the occurrence of certain symptoms will tell your doctor if more medicine must be taken. Your doctor may want you to begin another course of treatment after you have been off the medicine for at least 3 months.

If this medicine causes you to have nausea or diarrhea and it continues, check with your doctor. The dose may need to be changed.

If bone pain occurs or worsens during treatment, check with your doctor.

Side Effects of This Medicine

Along with its needed effects, a medicine may cause some unwanted effects. Although not all of these side effects may occur, if they do occur they may need medical attention.

Check with your doctor as soon as possible if any of the following side effects occur:

More common

Bone pain or tenderness (increased, continuing, or returning—in patients with Paget's disease)

Less common

Bone fractures, especially of the thigh bone

Rare

Hives; skin rash or itching; swelling of the arms, legs, face, lips, tongue, and/or throat

Other side effects may occur that usually do not need medical attention. These side effects may go away during treatment as your body adjusts to the medicine. However, check with your doctor if any of the following side effects continue or are bothersome:

More common—at higher doses

Diarrhea; nausea

Less common—with injection

Loss of taste or metallic or altered taste

Other side effects not listed above may also occur in some patients. If you notice any other effects, check with your doctor.

Annual revision: 08/19/92

ETODOLAC Systemic†

A commonly used brand name in the U.S. is Lodine.

Another commonly used name is etodolic acid.

†Not commercially available in Canada.

Description

Etodolac (ee-TOE-doe-lac) belongs to the group of medicines called anti-inflammatory analgesics (also called nonsteroidal anti-inflammatory drugs [NSAIDs]). Etodolac is used to relieve some symptoms caused by arthritis (rheumatism), such as inflammation, swelling, stiffness, and joint pain. However, this medicine does not cure arthritis and will help you only as long as you continue to take it.

Etodolac is also used to relieve pain. It is not a narcotic and is not habit-forming. It will not cause physical or mental dependence, as narcotics can. However, etodolac is sometimes used together with a narcotic to provide better pain relief than either medicine used alone.

Etodolac may also be used to treat other conditions as determined by your doctor.

Any anti-inflammatory analgesic can cause side effects, especially when it is used for a long time or in large doses. Some of the side effects are painful or uncomfortable. Others can be more serious, resulting in the need for medical care and sometimes even death. If you will be taking this medicine for more than one or two months or in large amounts, you should discuss with your doctor the good that it can do as well as the risks of taking it. Also, it is a good idea to ask your doctor about other forms of treatment that might help to reduce the amount of etodolac that you take and/or the length of treatment.

Etodolac is available only with your medical doctor's or dentist's prescription, in the following dosage form:

Oral

- Capsules (U.S.)

It is very important that you read and understand the following information. If any of it causes you special concern, check with your doctor. Also, *if you have any questions* or if you want more information about this medicine or your medical problem, *ask your doctor, nurse, or pharmacist*.

Before Using This Medicine

In deciding to use a medicine, the risks of taking the medicine must be weighed against the good it will do. This is a decision you and your doctor will make. For etodolac, the following should be considered:

Allergies—Tell your doctor if you have ever had any unusual or allergic reaction to etodolac or to any of the following medicines:

Aspirin or other salicylates
Diclofenac (e.g., Voltaren)
Diflunisal (e.g., Dolobid)
Fenoprofen (e.g., Nalfon)
Floctafenine (e.g., Idarac)
Flurbiprofen, oral (e.g., Ansaid)
Ibuprofen (e.g., Motrin)
Indomethacin (e.g., Indocin)
Ketoprofen (e.g., Orudis)
Ketorolac (e.g., Toradol)
Meclofenamate (e.g., Meclomen)
Mefenamic acid (e.g., Ponstel)
Naproxen (e.g., Naprosyn)
Oxyphenbutazone (e.g., Tandearil)
Phenylbutazone (e.g., Butazolidin)
Piroxicam (e.g., Feldene)
Sulindac (e.g., Clinoril)
Suprofen (e.g., Suprol)
Tiaprofenic acid (e.g., Surgam)
Tolmetin (e.g., Tolectin)
Zomepirac (e.g., Zomax)

Also tell your doctor and pharmacist if you are allergic to any other substances, such as foods, preservatives, or dyes.

Pregnancy—Studies on birth defects with etodolac have not been done in pregnant women. However, etodolac has caused birth defects in animal studies.

There is a chance that regular use of any anti-inflammatory analgesic during the last few months of pregnancy may cause unwanted effects on the heart or blood flow of the fetus or newborn baby. Also, animal studies have shown that, if taken late in pregnancy, etodolac may increase the length of pregnancy, prolong labor, or cause other problems during delivery.

Breast-feeding—It is not known whether etodolac passes into the breast milk. However, it has not been reported to cause problems in nursing babies.

Children—Studies on this medicine have been done only in adult patients, and there is no specific information comparing use of etodolac in children with use in other age groups.

Older adults—This medicine has been tested and has not been shown to cause different side effects or problems in older people than it does in younger adults. However, low doses were used in these studies. Also, experience with other anti-inflammatory analgesics has shown that elderly people are more likely than younger adults to get very sick if the medicine causes stomach problems.

Other medicines—Although certain medicines should not be used together at all, in other cases two different medicines may be used together even if an interaction might occur. In these cases, your doctor may want to change the dose, or other precautions may be necessary. When you are taking etodolac, it is especially important that your doctor and pharmacist know if you are taking any of the following:

- Anticoagulants (blood thinners) or
- Cefamandole (e.g., Mandol) or
- Cefoperazone (e.g., Cefobid) or
- Cefotetan (e.g., Cefotan) or
- Heparin or
- Moxalactam (e.g., Moxam) or
- Plicamycin (e.g., Mithracin) or
- Valproic acid (e.g., Depakene)—Use of any of these medicines together with etodolac may increase the chance of bleeding
- Aspirin or other salicylates or
- Cyclosporine (e.g., Sandimmune) or
- Other inflammation or pain medicine (except narcotics), especially phenylbutazone (e.g., Butazolidin) or
- Tobacco smoking—The chance of serious side effects may be increased
- Lithium (e.g., Lithane) or
- Methotrexate (e.g., Mexate)—Higher blood levels of lithium or methotrexate and an increased chance of side effects may occur
- Probenecid (e.g., Benemid)—Higher blood levels of etodolac and an increased chance of side effects may occur

Other medical problems—The presence of other medical problems may affect the use of etodolac. Make sure you tell your doctor if you have any other medical problems, especially:

- Alcohol abuse or
- Asthma or
- Colitis, stomach ulcer, or other stomach problems, or
- Diabetes mellitus (sugar diabetes) or
- Heart disease or
- High blood pressure or
- Kidney disease or
- Liver disease or
- Systemic lupus erythematosus (SLE)—The chance of serious side effects may be increased
- Hemophilia or other bleeding problems—Etodolac may increase the chance of serious bleeding

Before you begin using any new medicine (prescription or nonprescription) or if you develop any new medical problem while you are using this medicine, check with your doctor, nurse, or pharmacist.

Proper Use of This Medicine

Etodolac may start to relieve pain a little faster if it is taken 30 minutes before meals or 2 hours after meals. However, after the first few doses, take the medicine with food or an antacid to lessen the chance of stomach upset. This is especially important if you will be taking the medicine for a long time, as for arthritis.

Take this medicine with a full glass (8 ounces) of water. Also, do not lie down for about 15 to 30 minutes after taking the medicine. This helps to prevent irritation that may lead to trouble in swallowing.

Do not take more of this medicine, do not take it more often, and do not take it for a longer time than ordered by your medical doctor or dentist. Taking too much of this medicine may increase the chance of unwanted effects, especially in elderly patients.

For patients taking this medicine for *arthritis:*

- This medicine must be taken regularly as ordered by your doctor in order for it to help you. Most anti-inflammatory analgesics usually begin to work within one week, but in severe cases up to two weeks or even longer may pass before you begin to feel better. Also, several weeks may pass before you feel the full effects of the medicine.

Missed dose—If your medical doctor or dentist has ordered you to take this medicine according to a regular schedule, and you miss a dose, take it as soon as you remember. However, if it is almost time for your next dose, skip the missed dose and go back to your regular dosing schedule. Do not double doses.

Storage—To store this medicine:

- Keep out of the reach of children.
- Store away from heat and direct light.
- Do not store this medicine in the bathroom, near the kitchen sink, or in other damp places. Heat or moisture may cause the medicine to break down.
- Do not keep outdated medicine or medicine no longer needed. Be sure that any discarded medicine is out of the reach of children.

Precautions While Using This Medicine

If you will be taking this medicine for a long time, as for arthritis (rheumatism), your doctor should check your progress at regular visits. Your doctor may want to do certain tests to find out if unwanted effects are occurring. The tests are very important because serious side effects, including ulcers or bleeding, can occur without any warning.

Stomach problems may be more likely to occur if you drink alcoholic beverages while being treated with this medicine. Therefore, *do not regularly drink alcoholic beverages while taking this medicine,* unless otherwise directed by your doctor.

Taking certain other medicines together with etodolac may increase the chance of unwanted effects. The risk will depend on how much of each medicine you take every day, and on how long you take the medicines together. Therefore, do not take acetaminophen (e.g., Tylenol) or aspirin or other salicylates together with etodolac for more than a few days, unless otherwise directed by your medical doctor or dentist. Also, *do not take any of the following medicines together with etodolac, unless your medical doctor or dentist has directed you to do so and is following your progress*:

Diclofenac (e.g., Voltaren)
Diflunisal (e.g., Dolobid)
Fenoprofen (e.g., Nalfon)
Floctafenine (e.g., Idarac)
Flurbiprofen, oral (e.g., Ansaid)
Ibuprofen (e.g., Motrin)
Indomethacin (e.g., Indocin)
Ketoprofen (e.g., Orudis)
Ketorolac (e.g., Toradol)
Meclofenamate (e.g., Meclomen)
Mefenamic acid (e.g., Ponstel)
Naproxen (e.g., Naprosyn)
Phenylbutazone (e.g., Butazolidin)
Piroxicam (e.g., Feldene)
Sulindac (e.g., Clinoril)
Tiaprofenic acid (e.g., Surgam)
Tolmetin (e.g., Tolectin)

Before having any kind of surgery (including dental surgery), tell the medical doctor or dentist in charge that you are taking this medicine.

This medicine may cause some people to become confused, drowsy, dizzy, or lightheaded. It may also cause blurred vision or other vision problems in some people. *Make sure you know how you react to this medicine before you drive, use machines, or do anything else that could be dangerous if you are dizzy or not able to see well.* If these reactions are especially bothersome, check with your doctor.

Etodolac may interfere with the results of a test that measures the amount of bilirubin (which is normally present in the body) in the urine. Before having any urine tests, be sure to tell the doctor in charge that you are taking etodolac.

For *diabetic patients:*

- Etodolac may cause some urine ketone tests to show higher-than-normal amounts of ketones in your urine. Your doctor may need to find out whether this is a false test result caused by etodolac or whether there is a problem with your diabetes. Therefore, if your test does not show a normal amount of ketones, check with your doctor. Be sure to tell the doctor that you are taking etodolac.

Etodolac may cause your eyes to become more sensitive to light than they are normally. Wearing sunglasses and avoiding too much exposure to bright light may help lessen the discomfort.

Serious side effects, including ulcers or bleeding, can occur during treatment with this medicine. Sometimes serious side effects can occur without any warning. However, possible warning signs often occur, including severe abdominal or stomach cramps, pain, or burning; black, tarry stools; severe, continuing nausea, heartburn, or indigestion; and/or vomiting of blood or material that looks like coffee grounds. *Stop taking this medicine and check with your doctor immediately if you notice any of these warning signs.*

Side Effects of This Medicine

Along with its needed effects, a medicine may cause some unwanted effects. Although not all of these side effects may occur, if they do occur they may need medical attention.

Stop taking this medicine and check with your doctor immediately if any of the following side effects occur:

Less frequent

Bloody or black, tarry stools

Rare

Abdominal or stomach pain, cramping, or burning (severe); blood in urine; fainting; hive-like swellings (large) on face, eyelids, mouth, lips, or tongue; nausea, heartburn, and/or indigestion (severe and continuing); pinpoint red spots on skin; shortness of breath, troubled breathing, wheezing, or tightness in chest; unusual bleeding or bruising; vomiting of blood or material that looks like coffee grounds

Also, check with your doctor as soon as possible if any of the following side effects occur:

Less common

Blurred vision; burning feeling in chest or stomach; fever with or without chills; frequent or painful urination; mental depression; ringing or buzzing in ears; skin rash or itching

Rare

Chest pain; decrease in amount of urine; hives; increased blood pressure; muscle cramps or pain; sores, ulcers, or white spots in mouth or on lips; sore throat (unexplained); swelling and/or tenderness in upper abdominal (stomach) area; swelling of face, fingers, feet, or lower legs; swollen and/or painful glands; unusual tiredness or weakness; weight gain; yellow eyes or skin

Other side effects may occur that usually do not need medical attention. These side effects may go away during treatment as your body adjusts to the medicine. However, check with your doctor if any of the following side effects continue or are bothersome:

More common

Abdominal or stomach cramps, pain, or discomfort (mild to moderate); bloated feeling or gas; diarrhea; dizziness; headache; indigestion or nausea; weakness

Less common or rare

Constipation; decreased appetite or loss of appetite; drowsiness; flushing; increased sensitivity of eyes to light; increased thirst; nervousness or trouble in sleeping; pounding heartbeat; vomiting

Other side effects not listed above may also occur in some patients. If you notice any other effects, check with your doctor.

Annual revision: 01/14/92

ETOPOSIDE Systemic

A commonly used brand name in the U.S. and Canada is VePesid. Another commonly used name is VP-16.

Description

Etoposide (e-TOE-poe-side) belongs to the group of medicines known as antineoplastic agents. It is used to treat cancer of the testicles and certain types of lung cancer. It is also sometimes used to treat some other kinds of cancer in both males and females.

The exact way that etoposide acts against cancer is not known. However, it seems to interfere with the growth of the cancer cells, which are eventually destroyed. Since the growth of normal body cells may also be affected by etoposide, other effects will also occur. Some of these may be serious and must be reported to your doctor. Other effects, like hair loss, may not be serious but may cause concern. Some effects may not occur for months or years after the medicine is used.

Before you begin treatment with etoposide, you and your doctor should talk about the good this medicine will do as well as the risks of using it.

This medicine is available only with your doctor's prescription, in the following dosage forms:

Oral

- Capsules (U.S. and Canada)

Parenteral

- Injection (U.S. and Canada)

It is very important that you read and understand the following information. If any of it causes you special concern, check with your doctor. Also, *if you have any questions* or if you want more information about this

medicine or your medical problem, *ask your doctor, nurse, or pharmacist.*

Before Using This Medicine

In deciding to use a medicine, the risks of taking the medicine must be weighed against the good it will do. This is a decision you and your doctor will make. For etoposide, the following should be considered:

Allergies—Tell your doctor if you have ever had any unusual or allergic reaction to etoposide.

Pregnancy—There is a good chance that this medicine will cause birth defects if it is being used at the time of conception or during pregnancy. In addition, many cancer medicines may cause sterility which could be permanent. Although sterility has not been reported with etoposide, the possibility should be kept in mind.

Be sure that you have discussed this with your doctor before receiving this medicine. It is best to use some kind of birth control while you are taking etoposide. Tell your doctor right away if you think you have become pregnant while taking etoposide. Before taking etoposide make sure your doctor knows if you are pregnant or if you may become pregnant.

Breast-feeding—Because etoposide may cause serious side effects, breast-feeding is generally not recommended while you are receiving it.

Children—Although this medicine has been used in children, there is no specific information comparing use of etoposide in children with use in other age groups.

Older adults—Many medicines have not been studied specifically in older people. Therefore, it may not be known whether they work exactly the same way they do in younger adults or if they cause different side effects or problems in older people. There is no specific information comparing use of etoposide in the elderly with use in other age groups.

Other medicines—Although certain medicines should not be used together at all, in other cases two different medicines may be used together even if an interaction might occur. In these cases, your doctor may want to change the dose, or other precautions may be necessary. When taking or receiving etoposide it is especially important that your doctor and pharmacist know if you have ever been treated with x-rays or cancer medicines or if you are taking any of the following:

- Amphotericin B by injection (e.g., Fungizone) or
- Antithyroid agents (medicine for overactive thyroid) or
- Azathioprine (e.g., Imuran) or
- Chloramphenicol (e.g., Chloromycetin) or
- Colchicine or
- Flucytosine (e.g., Ancobon) or
- Ganciclovir (e.g., Cytovene) or
- Interferon (e.g., Intron A, Roferon-A) or
- Plicamycin (e.g., Mithracin) or
- Zidovudine (e.g., AZT, Retrovir)
- If you have ever been treated with x-rays or cancer medicines—Etoposide may increase the effects of these medicines or radiation therapy on the blood

Other medical problems—The presence of other medical problems may affect the use of etoposide. Make sure you tell your doctor if you have any other medical problems, especially:

- Chickenpox (including recent exposure) or
- Herpes zoster (shingles)—Risk of severe disease affecting other parts of the body
- Infection—Etoposide can decrease your body's ability to fight infection
- Kidney disease or
- Liver disease—Effects of etoposide may be increased because of slower removal from the body

Before you begin using any new medicine (prescription or nonprescription) or if you develop any new medical problem while you are using this medicine, check with your doctor, nurse, or pharmacist.

Proper Use of This Medicine

Take etoposide only as directed by your doctor. Do not use more or less of it, and do not use it more often than your doctor ordered. The exact amount of medicine you need has been carefully worked out. Taking too much may increase the chance of side effects, while taking too little may not improve your condition.

Etoposide is sometimes given together with certain other medicines. If you are using a combination of medicines, make sure that you take each one at the proper time and do not mix them. If you are taking some of these medicines by mouth, ask your doctor, nurse, or pharmacist to help you plan a way to remember to take your medicines at the right times.

Etoposide often causes nausea, vomiting, and loss of appetite, which may be severe. However, it is very important that you continue to receive the medicine, even if you begin to feel ill. Ask your doctor, nurse, or pharmacist for ways to lessen these effects.

If you vomit shortly after taking a dose of etoposide, check with your doctor. You will be told whether to take the dose again or to wait until the next dose.

Missed dose—If you miss a dose of this medicine, do not take the missed dose at all and do not double the next one. Instead, go back to your regular dosing schedule and check with your doctor.

Storage—To store this medicine:

- Keep out of the reach of children.
- Store away from heat and direct light.

- Do not store in the bathroom, near the kitchen sink, or in other damp places. Heat or moisture may cause the medicine to break down.
- Do not keep outdated medicine or medicine no longer needed. Be sure that any discarded medicine is out of the reach of children.

Precautions While Using This Medicine

It is very important that your doctor check your progress at regular visits to make sure that etoposide is working properly and to check for unwanted effects.

While you are being treated with etoposide, and after you stop treatment with it, *do not have any immunizations (vaccinations) without your doctor's approval*. Etoposide may lower your body's resistance and there is a chance you might get the infection the immunization is meant to prevent. In addition, other persons living in your household should not take oral polio vaccine since there is a chance they could pass the polio virus on to you. Also, avoid persons who have recently taken oral polio vaccine. Do not get close to them and do not stay in the same room with them for very long. If you cannot take these precautions, you should consider wearing a protective face mask that covers the nose and mouth.

Etoposide can temporarily lower the number of white blood cells in your blood, increasing the chance of getting an infection. It can also lower the number of platelets, which are necessary for proper blood clotting. If this occurs, there are certain precautions you can take, especially when your blood count is low, to reduce the risk of infection or bleeding:

- If you can, avoid people with infections. *Check with your doctor immediately* if you think you are getting an infection or if you get a fever or chills, cough or hoarseness, lower back or side pain, or painful or difficult urination.
- *Check with your doctor immediately* if you notice any unusual bleeding or bruising; black, tarry stools; blood in urine or stools; or pinpoint red spots on your skin.
- Be careful when using a regular toothbrush, dental floss, or toothpick. Your medical doctor, dentist, or nurse may recommend other ways to clean your teeth and gums. Check with your medical doctor before having any dental work done.
- Do not touch your eyes or the inside of your nose unless you have just washed your hands and have not touched anything else in the meantime.
- Be careful not to cut yourself when you are using sharp objects such as a safety razor or fingernail or toenail cutters.
- Avoid contact sports or other situations where bruising or injury could occur.

Side Effects of This Medicine

Along with their needed effects, medicines like etoposide can sometimes cause unwanted effects such as blood problems, loss of hair, and other side effects. These and others are described below. Also, because of the way these medicines act on the body, there is a chance that they might cause other unwanted effects that may not occur until months or years after the medicine is used. These delayed effects may include certain types of cancer, such as leukemia. Discuss these possible effects with your doctor.

Although not all of these side effects may occur, if they do occur they may need medical attention.

Check with your doctor or nurse immediately if any of the following side effects occur:

Less common

Black, tarry stools; blood in urine or stools; cough or hoarseness; fever or chills; lower back or side pain; painful or difficult urination; pinpoint red spots on skin; unusual bleeding or bruising

Check with your doctor or nurse as soon as possible if any of the following side effects occur:

Less common

Sores in mouth or on lips

Rare

Difficulty in walking; fast heartbeat; numbness or tingling in fingers and toes; pain at place of injection; shortness of breath or wheezing; weakness

Other side effects may occur that usually do not need medical attention. These side effects may go away during treatment as your body adjusts to the medicine. Also, your doctor or nurse may be able to tell you about ways to prevent or reduce some of these side effects. Check with your doctor or nurse if any of the following side effects continue or are bothersome or if you have any questions about them:

More common

Loss of appetite; nausea and vomiting

Less common

Diarrhea; unusual tiredness

This medicine often causes a temporary loss of hair. After treatment with etoposide has ended, normal hair growth should return.

Other side effects not listed above may also occur in some patients. If you notice any other effects, check with your doctor or nurse.

Annual revision: 08/09/92

ETRETINATE Systemic

A commonly used brand name in the U.S. and Canada is Tegison.

Description

Etretinate (e-TRET-i-nate) is used to treat severe psoriasis. It is usually used only after other medicines have been tried and have failed to help the psoriasis.

Etretinate must not be used to treat women who are able to bear children unless other forms of treatment have been tried first and have failed. Etretinate must not be taken during pregnancy, because it causes birth defects in humans. In addition, if you take etretinate, you must plan on never having children in the future. If you are able to bear children, it is very important that you read, understand, and follow the pregnancy warnings for etretinate.

It is also recommended that etretinate not be used to treat children unless all other forms of treatment have been tried first and have failed. Etretinate may interfere with bone growth. In addition, children may be more sensitive to the side effects of the medicine.

This medicine is available only with your doctor's prescription, in the following dosage form:

Oral

- Capsules (U.S. and Canada)

It is very important that you read and understand the following information. If any of it causes you special concern, check with your doctor. Also, *if you have any questions* or if you want more information about this medicine or your medical problem, *ask your doctor, nurse, or pharmacist.*

Before Using This Medicine

In deciding to use a medicine, the risks of taking the medicine must be weighed against the good it will do. This is a decision you and your doctor will make. For etretinate, the following should be considered:

Allergies—Tell your doctor if you have ever had any unusual or allergic reaction to etretinate, isotretinoin, tretinoin, or vitamin A–like preparations. Also tell your doctor and pharmacist if you are allergic to any other substances, such as foods, preservatives, or dyes.

Pregnancy—*Etretinate must not be taken during pregnancy, because it causes birth defects in humans. In addition, since it is not known how long pregnancy should be avoided after treatment stops, you must plan on never having children if you are treated with etretinate.* If you are able to bear children, you must have a pregnancy test within 2 weeks before beginning treatment with etretinate to make sure you are not pregnant. Therapy with etretinate will then be started on the second or third day of your next normal menstrual period. *Also, etretinate must not be taken unless an effective form of contraception (birth control) is used for at least 1 month before beginning treatment. Contraception must be continued during treatment and for as long as you are able to become pregnant after etretinate is stopped. Be sure you have discussed this information with your doctor.*

Breast-feeding—It is not known whether etretinate passes into the breast milk. However, etretinate is not recommended during breast-feeding or if you plan to breast-feed in the future, because it may cause unwanted effects in nursing babies.

Children—It is recommended that etretinate not be used to treat children, unless all other forms of treatment have been tried first and have failed. Etretinate may interfere with bone growth. In addition, children may be more sensitive to the side effects of the medicine.

Older adults—Many medicines have not been tested in older people. Therefore, it may not be known whether they work exactly the same way they do in younger adults or if they cause different side effects or problems in older people. There is no specific information about the use of etretinate in the elderly.

Other medicines—Although certain medicines should not be used together at all, in other cases two different medicines may be used together even if an interaction might occur. In these cases, your doctor may want to change the dose, or other precautions may be necessary. When you are using etretinate, it is especially important that your doctor and pharmacist know if you are using any of the following:

- Abrasive or medicated soaps or cleansers or
- Cosmetics or soaps that dry the skin or
- Medicated cosmetics or "cover-ups" or
- Topical acne preparation or preparation containing a peeling agent, such as benzoyl peroxide, resorcinol, salicylic acid, sulfur, or tretinoin (vitamin A acid), or
- Topical alcohol-containing preparation, such as after-shave lotion, astringent, cologne, perfume, or shaving cream or lotion, or
- Topical medicine for the skin, other—Use of etretinate with these products will increase the chance of dryness and other irritation of the skin
- Isotretinoin (e.g., Accutane) or
- Methotrexate (e.g., Mexate) or
- Tretinoin (vitamin A acid) (e.g., Retin-A) or
- Vitamin A or any preparation containing vitamin A (e.g., Alphalin)—Use of etretinate with these products will cause an increase in side effects
- Tetracyclines (medicine for infection)—Use of etretinate may increase the chance of the side effect called pseudotumor cerebri, which is a swelling of the brain

Other medical problems—The presence of other medical problems may affect the use of etretinate. Make sure you tell your doctor if you have any other medical problems, especially:

- Alcoholism or excess use of alcohol (or history of) or
- Diabetes mellitus (sugar diabetes) (or a family history of) or
- Heart or blood vessel disease (or history of increased risk of or family history of) or
- High triglyceride (a fat-like substance) levels in the blood (history of or a family history of) or
- Severe weight problems—Use of etretinate may increase blood levels of triglyceride (a fat-like substance), which may increase the chance of heart or blood vessel problems in patients who have a family history of high triglycerides, are greatly overweight, are diabetic, or use a lot of alcohol. For persons with diabetes mellitus, use of etretinate may also change blood sugar levels
- Liver disease (or history of or family history of)—Use of etretinate may make the condition worse

Before you begin using any new medicine (prescription or nonprescription) or if you develop any new medical problem while you are using this medicine, check with your doctor, nurse, or pharmacist.

Proper Use of This Medicine

Take each dose of etretinate with milk or a fatty food. This is important because taking fats with etretinate will help your body absorb the medicine better. *However, you should follow a low-fat diet during the rest of the day* because eating a high-fat diet while you are taking this medicine may cause high triglyceride (fat-like substance) levels in the blood. This may increase the chance of heart and blood vessel disease.

It is very important that you take etretinate only as directed. Do not take more of it, do not take it more often, and do not take it for a longer period of time than your doctor ordered. To do so may increase the chance of side effects.

Missed dose—If you miss a dose of this medicine, take it as soon as possible with milk or a fatty food. However, if it is almost time for your next dose, skip the missed dose and go back to your regular dosing schedule. Do not double doses.

Storage—To store this medicine:

- Keep out of the reach of children.
- Store away from heat and direct light.
- Do not store in the bathroom, near the kitchen sink, or in other damp places. Heat or moisture may cause the medicine to break down.
- Do not keep outdated medicine or medicine no longer needed. Be sure that any discarded medicine is out of the reach of children.

Precautions While Using This Medicine

Your doctor should check your progress at regular visits to make sure this medicine does not cause unwanted effects.

Etretinate causes birth defects in humans if taken during pregnancy. In addition, it is not known how long pregnancy should be avoided after treatment stops, to prevent birth defects. Therefore, you must plan on never having children if you are treated with etretinate. For as long as you are able to become pregnant, you must use a reliable form of birth control. In addition, you must not change your birth control method unless you have checked with your doctor first. If you suspect that you may have become pregnant while taking etretinate, stop taking the medicine immediately and check with your doctor. Also, if you become pregnant at any time after you have stopped taking this medicine, check with your doctor as soon as possible. In either case, you should talk to your doctor about the risks of continuing the pregnancy.

It is not known how long etretinate stays in the blood. *Therefore, to prevent the possibility of a pregnant patient receiving your blood, you must plan on never donating blood to a blood bank if you are being treated with etretinate or if you have ever been treated with etretinate.*

Do not take vitamin A or any vitamin supplement containing vitamin A while you are taking this medicine. To do so may increase the chance of side effects.

Drinking too much alcohol while you are taking this medicine may cause high triglyceride (fat-like substance) levels in the blood. This may increase the chance of heart and blood vessel disease. Therefore, *while taking this medicine, do not drink alcoholic beverages or, at least, reduce the amount you usually drink.* If you have any questions about this, check with your doctor.

For *diabetic patients*:

- This medicine may affect blood sugar levels. If you notice a change in the results of your blood or urine sugar tests or if you have any questions, check with your doctor.

In some patients, etretinate may cause a decrease in night vision. This decrease may occur suddenly. If it does occur, *do not drive, use machines, or do anything else that could be dangerous if you are not able to see well.* Also, check with your doctor.

Etretinate may cause dryness of the eyes. Therefore, if you wear contact lenses, your eyes may be more sensitive to them while you are taking etretinate and for several weeks or longer after you stop taking it. To help relieve dryness of the eyes, check with your doctor about using an eye lubricating solution, such as artificial tears. If your eyes become inflamed, check with your doctor.

Some people who take this medicine may become more sensitive to sunlight than they are normally. When you begin taking this medicine:

- Stay out of direct sunlight, especially between the hours of 10:00 a.m. and 3:00 p.m., if possible.
- Wear protective clothing, including a hat and sunglasses.
- Apply a sun block product that has a skin protection factor (SPF) of at least 15. Some patients may require a product with a higher SPF number, especially if they have a fair complexion. If you have any questions about this, check with your doctor or pharmacist.
- Do not use a sunlamp or tanning bed or booth.

If you have a severe reaction, check with your doctor.

This medicine may cause dryness of the mouth and nose. For temporary relief of mouth dryness, use sugarless candy or gum, melt bits of ice in your mouth, or use a saliva substitute. However, if dry mouth continues for more than 2 weeks, check with your medical doctor or dentist. Continuing dryness of the mouth may increase the chance of dental disease, including tooth decay, gum disease, and fungus infections.

During the first month of treatment with etretinate, your psoriasis may seem to get worse before it gets better. There may be more redness or itching, but this usually goes away during treatment. It may take 2 or 3 months before the full effects of etretinate are seen. If irritation or other symptoms of your condition become severe, check with your doctor.

Side Effects of This Medicine

Along with its needed effects, a medicine may cause some unwanted effects. Although not all of these side effects may occur, if they do occur they may need medical attention.

Stop taking this medicine and check with your doctor immediately if any of the following side effects occur:

Less common

Blurred or double vision or other changes in vision; dark-colored urine; flu-like symptoms; yellow eyes or skin

Rare

Headache (severe or continuing); nausea and vomiting

Check with your doctor as soon as possible if any of the following side effects occur:

More common

Bone or joint pain, tenderness, or stiffness; burning, redness, itching, feeling of dryness, pain, tenderness, excessive tearing (continuing), or other sign of inflammation or irritation of eyes; cramps or pain in upper abdomen or stomach area; muscle cramps; unusual bruising

Less common

Change in hearing, earache or pain in ear, or drainage from ear

Rare

Bleeding or inflammation of gums; confusion; mental depression; mood or mental changes

Other side effects may occur that usually do not need medical attention. These side effects may go away during treatment as your body adjusts to the medicine. However, check with your doctor if any of the following side effects continue or are bothersome:

More common

Changes in appetite; chapped lips; dryness of nose or nosebleeds; dryness, redness, scaling, itching, rash, or other sign of inflammation or irritation of the skin; headache (mild); increased sensitivity to contact lenses (may occur during and after treatment); increased sensitivity of skin to sunlight; peeling of skin on fingertips, palms of hands, or soles of feet; thinning of hair; unusual thirst; unusual tiredness

Less common

Dizziness; dryness of mouth; fever; nausea (mild); redness or soreness around fingernails; loosening of the fingernails; soreness of tongue; soreness, cracking, swelling, or unusual redness of lips

Other side effects not listed above may also occur in some patients. If you notice any other effects, check with your doctor.

Annual revision: June 1990

FAT EMULSIONS Systemic

Some commonly used brand names are:

In the U.S.
- Intralipid
- Liposyn II
- Liposyn III

In Canada
- Intralipid
- Liposyn II

F-G

Description

Fat emulsions are used as dietary supplements for patients who are unable to get enough fat in their diet, usually because of certain illnesses or recent surgery. Fats are used by the body for energy and to form substances needed for normal body functions.

Fat emulsions are available by injection only with your doctor's prescription, in the following dosage form:

Parenteral
- Injection (U.S. and Canada)

It is very important that you read and understand the following information. If any of it causes you special concern, check with your doctor. Also, *if you have any questions* or if you want more information about this medicine or your medical problem, *ask your doctor, nurse, or pharmacist.*

Before Using This Medicine

In deciding to use a medicine, the risks of using the medicine must be weighed against the good it will do. This is a decision you and your doctor will make. For fat emulsions, the following should be considered:

Allergies—Tell your doctor if you have ever had any unusual or allergic reaction to eggs, soybeans, beans, peas, or fat emulsions. Also tell your doctor and pharmacist if you are allergic to any other substances, such as foods, preservatives, or dyes.

Pregnancy—Studies on effects in pregnancy have not been done in either animals or humans.

Breast-feeding—It is not known whether fat emulsions pass into the breast milk. However, this medicine has not been reported to cause problems in nursing babies.

Children—Fat emulsions may cause or worsen lung problems or jaundice if given to premature infants. Although there is no specific information comparing use of fat emulsions in older children with use in other age groups, it is not expected to cause different side effects or problems in older children than it does in adults.

Older adults—Many medicines have not been studied specifically in older people. Therefore, it may not be known whether they work exactly the same way they do in younger adults or if they cause different side effects or problems in older people. Although there is no specific information comparing use of fat emulsions in the elderly with use in other age groups, this medicine is not expected to cause different side effects or problems in older people than it does in younger adults.

Other medicines—Although certain medicines should not be used together at all, in other cases two different medicines may be used together even if an interaction might occur. In these cases, your doctor may want to change the dose, or other precautions may be necessary. Tell your doctor and pharmacist if you are using any other prescription or nonprescription (over-the-counter [OTC]) medicine.

Other medical problems—The presence of other medical problems may affect the use of fat emulsions. Make sure you tell your doctor if you have any other medical problems, especially:
- Blood problems or
- Diabetes mellitus (sugar diabetes) or
- High cholesterol levels or
- Infection or
- Jaundice or
- Kidney disease or
- Liver disease or
- Lung disease or
- Pancreas disease—Fat emulsions may make these conditions worse

Before you begin using any new medicine (prescription or nonprescription) or if you develop any new medical problem while you are using this medicine, check with your doctor, nurse, or pharmacist.

Proper Use of This Medicine

Dosing—The amount of fat emulsions to be used will be different for different patients. *Follow your doctor's orders or the directions on the label.*

Storage—To store this medicine:
- Keep out of the reach of children.
- Store away from heat and direct light.
- Do not store in the bathroom, near the kitchen sink, or in other damp places. Heat or moisture may cause the medicine to break down.
- Keep the medicine from freezing. Do not refrigerate.
- Do not keep outdated medicine or medicine no longer needed. Be sure that any discarded medicine is out of the reach of children.

Precautions While Using This Medicine

It is very important that your doctor check your progress weekly while you are receiving fat emulsions to make sure that this medicine does not cause unwanted effects.

Fat emulsions can lower your ability to fight infection. If you think you are getting an infection, check with your doctor.

Side Effects of This Medicine

Along with its needed effects, a medicine may cause some unwanted effects. Although not all of these side effects may occur, if they do occur they may need medical attention.

Check with your doctor as soon as possible if any of the following side effects occur:

More common

Chills; fever; sore throat

Rare

Bluish color of skin; chest or back pain; difficulty in breathing; headache; hives; unusual bleeding or bruising; unusual irritability; unusual tiredness or weakness; yellow eyes or skin

Other side effects may occur that usually do not need medical attention. These side effects may go away during treatment as your body adjusts to the medicine. However, check with your doctor if any of the following side effects continue or are bothersome:

More common

Redness, swelling, or pain at place of injection

Less common

Diarrhea; dizziness; flushing; nausea and vomiting

Other side effects not listed above may also occur in some patients. If you notice any other effects, check with your doctor.

Annual revision: 05/12/93

F-G

FECAL OCCULT BLOOD TEST KITS

This information applies to the following medicines:

Fecal Occult Blood Test Kits for Clinic Use
Fecal Occult Blood Test Kits for Home Use

Some commonly used brand names are:

For Clinic Use†

In the U.S.

ColoScreen
DigiWipe
Hemoccult
Hemoccult SENSA

For Home Use

In the U.S.

ColoCare
ColoScreen
ColoScreen III
ColoScreen Self-Test
EZ Detect
HemaChek
Hematest
HemaWipe
HemeSelect
Hemoccult
Hemoccult II
Hemoccult SENSA
Hemoccult II SENSA

In Canada

Colo-Rectal Test
Hematest

†Not commercially available in Canada.

Description

Fecal occult blood tests are designed to detect small, hidden amounts of blood in the bowel movement (feces). These tests are usually used to detect the small amounts of bleeding that come painlessly from cancers of the colon or rectum. These cancers may bleed without symptoms. They are frequently fatal if allowed to grow until the patient has symptoms of abdominal pain, anemia, or changes in bowel habits. Colon or rectal cancers are more likely to be cured if found in early stages.

A positive fecal occult blood test does not always mean that you have colon or rectal cancer. Rather, it means that more tests are needed to find the cause of the bleeding. Blood may come from many sources in the digestive tract, such as ulcers, diarrhea, or hemorrhoids. Other blood sources which may react include menstrual blood or blood in the urine. Some physicians will, in fact, use a fecal occult blood test to help find bleeding problems other than cancer.

Most test kits are given out when a physical examination is done. Others may be bought without a prescription in a pharmacy. Most kits also provide a toll-free number for advice on using the kits.

It is very important that you read and understand the following information. If any of it causes you special concern, check with your doctor. Also, *if you have any questions* or if you want more information about this test or your medical problem, *ask your doctor, nurse, or pharmacist*.

Before Using This Test Kit

It is important to get the best results possible from fecal occult blood test kits. Therefore, the following should be considered before you use these test kits:

Diet—Most kits recommend following a special diet. Red meats that are not completely cooked (for example, rare) may contain hemoglobin, the substance with which the test reacts. In addition, some fruits and vegetables, such as horseradish, broccoli, carrots, cauliflower, radishes, turnips, mushrooms, cucumbers, cantaloupes, and grapefruit, contain peroxidase, another chemical the test may react with. Large quantities of these foods should be avoided for 2 days before beginning testing and during the test period.

Medicines—Certain medicines may affect the results of the fecal occult blood test. Check with your doctor if you are taking any medicines, especially:

- Aspirin or other salicylates or
- Corticosteroids (cortisone-like medicine) or
- Medicine for pain and/or inflammation, except narcotics, or
- Reserpine—These medicines irritate the digestive tract and may cause bleeding that will give a positive test
- Ascorbic acid (vitamin C)—Large amounts may block a positive test reaction
- Rectal medicines—Use of rectal medicines may affect test results

Medical conditions—The presence of other medical conditions may affect the results of the fecal occult blood test. Make sure you tell your doctor if you have any other medical conditions, especially:

- Colitis or
- Constipation or
- Diarrhea or
- Diverticulitis or
- Hemorrhoids or
- Irritation of throat (severe) or
- Menstrual period or
- Nosebleeds or
- Stomach ulcer—These conditions may also cause blood to appear in the stool, resulting in a positive test

Proper Use of This Test

Check the expiration date printed on the package before purchasing. Do not use an outdated test kit. Outdated test kits will not work properly.

Read test instructions carefully. Proceed only after you understand the instructions. Most test kits include a toll-free number for consumer questions, or you may ask questions of your doctor, nurse, or pharmacist.

Stop collection/testing in the presence of diarrhea, constipation, or hemorrhoid problems, or during menstrual periods.

For bowl tests:

- Remove bowl cleanser by repeated flushing (at least 3 times) and then flush urine before bowel movement. If a continuous-cleaning product is being used, remove it from the tank system and flush several times to clear away the chemicals.
- Follow test instructions carefully for timing of reactions and watching for color changes. Use a watch or clock with a second hand. Have another person observe for color changes if you have trouble seeing.
- Complete the "control" tests as the kit directs.
- Record results with the materials provided in the kit, to be discussed with your medical doctor.

For card tests:

- Samples should be collected from 2 different areas of the feces for 3 separate bowel movements.
- Samples should be sent to the physician as soon as collected. They should not be stored for more than 5 days (14 days for *HemeSelect, Hemoccult,* and *Hemoccult SENSA*).

For wipe tests:

- Samples should be sent to the physician as soon as collected. They should not be stored for more than 5 days (14 days for *HemaWipe*).

For patients mailing test cards/slides to doctor's office or clinic:

- U.S. postal regulations prohibit mailing completed cards/slides in standard paper envelopes. Approved mailing pouches must be used.

Storage—To store this product:

- Keep out of the reach of children.
- Do not store in warm, humid conditions or in direct sunlight.

About Your Test Results

In most cases the tests are returned to the clinic or doctor's office for final development, and you will be notified if any of the tests are positive or if further testing is necessary.

A positive result means that there was some blood found in the feces. Further testing may be necessary to find the cause. It does not necessarily mean you have cancer. Only 5 to 10 percent of persons with positive fecal occult blood tests are found to have cancer.

A negative result means that no blood was found in the feces. It shows that you were not bleeding from your digestive system during the test period. However, a cancer may bleed off and on, and be missed by the test. Although it is unlikely that you have colon or rectal cancer, you should continue to watch for cancer warning signals such as changes in bowel habits or blood in the feces. You should also have a cancer check-up at regular intervals, as recommended by your health care provider.

Annual revision: 06/18/92

FENFLURAMINE Systemic

Some commonly used brand names are:

In the U.S.
- Pondimin

In Canada
- Ponderal
- Ponderal Pacaps
- Pondimin
- Pondimin Extentabs

Description

Fenfluramine (fen-FLURE-a-meen) is an appetite suppressant used in the short-term treatment of obesity. For a few weeks, fenfluramine, in combination with dieting, exercise, and changes in eating habits, can help obese patients lose weight. However, since fenfluramine's appetite-reducing effect may be temporary, it may be useful only for the first few weeks of dieting until new habits are established.

Fenfluramine may also be used for other conditions as determined by your doctor.

This medicine is available only with your doctor's prescription, in the following dosage forms:

Oral
- Extended-release capsules (Canada)
- Tablets (U.S. and Canada)
- Extended-release tablets (Canada)

It is very important that you read and understand the following information. If any of it causes you special concern, check with your doctor. Also, *if you have any questions* or if you want more information about this medicine or your medical problem, *ask your doctor, nurse, or pharmacist.*

Before Using This Medicine

In deciding to use a medicine, the risks of taking the medicine must be weighed against the good it will do. This is a decision you and your doctor will make. For fenfluramine, the following should be considered:

Allergies—Tell your doctor if you have ever had any unusual or allergic reaction to this medicine or amphetamine, dextroamphetamine, ephedrine, epinephrine, isoproterenol, metaproterenol, methamphetamine, norepinephrine, phenylephrine, phenylpropanolamine, pseudoephedrine, terbutaline, or other appetite suppressants. Also tell your doctor and pharmacist if you are allergic to any other substances, such as foods, preservatives, or dyes.

Pregnancy—Studies have not been done in pregnant women. However, animal studies have shown that fenfluramine, when given at many times the human dose, reduces fertility and may have toxic or harmful effects on the fetus.

Breast-feeding—It is not known if fenfluramine is excreted in breast milk. However, this medicine has not been reported to cause problems in nursing babies.

Children—Fenfluramine should not be used as an appetite suppressant by children under 12 years of age.

Older adults—Many medicines have not been studied specifically in older people. Therefore, it may not be known whether they work exactly the same way they do in younger adults or if they cause different side effects or problems in older people. There is no specific information comparing use of fenfluramine in the elderly to use in other age groups.

Other medicines—Although certain medicines should not be used together at all, in other cases two different medicines may be used together even if an interaction might occur. In these cases, your doctor may want to change the dose, or other precautions may be necessary. When you are taking fenfluramine, it is especially important that your doctor and pharmacist know if you are taking any of the following:

- Central nervous system (CNS) depressants or
- Tricyclic antidepressants (medicine for depression)—Using these medicines with fenfluramine may increase the CNS depressant effects
- Monoamine oxidase (MAO) inhibitors (furazolidone [e.g., Furoxone], isocarboxazid [e.g., Marplan], phenelzine [e.g., Nardil], procarbazine [e.g., Matulane], selegiline [e.g., Eldepryl], tranylcypromine [e.g., Parnate])—Taking fenfluramine while you are taking or within 2 weeks of taking monoamine oxidase (MAO) inhibitors may cause sudden extremely high blood pressure; at least 14 days should be allowed between stopping treatment with one medicine and starting treatment with the other

Other medical problems—The presence of other medical problems may affect the use of appetite suppressants. Make sure you tell your doctor if you have any other medical problems, especially:

- Alcohol abuse (or history of) or
- Drug abuse or dependence (or history of)—Dependence on fenfluramine may develop
- Diabetes mellitus (sugar diabetes)—The amount of insulin or oral antidiabetic medicine that you need to take may change
- Glaucoma or
- Heart or blood vessel disease or
- High blood pressure or
- Mental depression or
- Mental illness (severe)—Fenfluramine may make the condition worse

Proper Use of This Medicine

Take fenfluramine only as directed by your doctor. Do not take more of it, do not take it more often, and do not take it for a longer time than your doctor ordered. If too much is taken, it may become habit-forming.

If you think this medicine is not working properly after you have taken it for a few weeks, *do not increase the dose.* Instead, check with your doctor.

For patients taking the *long-acting form* of this medicine:
- These capsules or tablets are to be swallowed whole. Do not break, crush, or chew before swallowing.

Storage—To store this medicine:
- Keep out of the reach of children.
- Store away from heat and direct light.
- Do not store in the bathroom, near the kitchen sink, or in other damp places. Heat or moisture may cause the medicine to break down.
- Do not keep outdated medicine or medicine no longer needed. Be sure that any discarded medicine is out of the reach of children.

Precautions While Using This Medicine

Your doctor should check your progress at regular visits in order to make sure that this medicine does not cause unwanted effects.

Fenfluramine will add to the effects of alcohol and other CNS depressants (medicines that slow down the nervous system, possibly causing drowsiness). Some examples of CNS depressants are antihistamines or medicine for hay fever, other allergies, or colds; sedatives, tranquilizers, or sleeping medicine; prescription pain medicine or narcotics; barbiturates; medicine for seizures; muscle relaxants; or anesthetics, including some dental anesthetics. *Check with your medical doctor or dentist before taking any such depressants while you are using this medicine.*

This medicine may cause some people to have a false sense of well-being or to become dizzy, lightheaded, drowsy, or less alert than they are normally. *Make sure you know how you react to this medicine before you drive, use machines, or do anything else that could be dangerous if you are dizzy or are not alert.*

Before having any kind of surgery, dental treatment, or emergency treatment, tell the medical doctor or dentist in charge that you are using this medicine.

If you have been taking fenfluramine for a long time or in large doses and *you think you may have become mentally or physically dependent on it, check with your doctor.*
- Some signs of dependence on fenfluramine are:

  —a strong desire or need to continue taking the medicine.

  —a need to increase the dose to receive the effects of the medicine.

  —withdrawal side effects (for example, mental depression, trouble in sleeping, or nightmares when you stop taking the medicine).

For *diabetic patients:*
- This medicine may affect blood sugar levels. If you notice a change in the results of your urine or blood sugar test or if you have any questions, check with your doctor.

If you will be taking fenfluramine in large doses for a long time, *do not stop taking it without first checking with your doctor.* Your doctor may want you to reduce gradually the amount you are taking before stopping completely.

Side Effects of This Medicine

Along with its needed effects, a medicine may cause some unwanted effects. Although not all of these side effects may occur, if they do occur they may need medical attention.

Check with your doctor as soon as possible if any of the following side effects occur:

Less common

Confusion or mental depression; skin rash or hives

Rare

Difficult or troubled breathing brought on by physical effort; increased blood pressure

Symptoms of overdose

Abdominal or stomach cramps; fast breathing; fever; nausea or vomiting (severe); tremor

Other side effects may occur that usually do not need medical attention. These side effects may go away during treatment as your body adjusts to the medicine. However, check with your doctor if any of the following side effects continue or are bothersome:

More common

Diarrhea; drowsiness; dryness of mouth

Less common

Blurred vision; changes in sexual desire or decreased sexual ability; clumsiness or unsteadiness; constipation; difficult or painful urination; difficulty in talking; dizziness or lightheadedness; false sense of well-being; frequent urge to urinate or increased urination; headache; increased sweating; irritability; nausea or vomiting; nervousness or restlessness; nightmares; pounding heartbeat; stomach cramps or pain; trouble in sleeping or nightmares; unpleasant taste; unusual tiredness or weakness

After you stop using this medicine, your body may need time to adjust. The length of time this takes depends on the amount of medicine you were using and how long you used it. During this time check with your doctor if you notice any of the following side effects:

Mental depression; trouble in sleeping or nightmares

Other side effects not listed above may also occur in some patients. If you notice any other effects, check with your doctor.

Additional Information

Once a medicine has been approved for marketing for a certain use, experience may show that it is also useful for other medical problems. Although this use is not included in product labeling, fenfluramine is used in certain patients with the following medical condition:

- Infantile autism

Other than the above information, there is no additional information relating to proper use, precautions, or side effects for these uses.

Annual revision: 06/25/91

FINASTERIDE Systemic

A commonly used brand name in the in the U.S. and Canada is Proscar.

Description

Finasteride (fi-NAS-teer-ide) belongs to the group of medicines called enzyme inhibitors. It is used to treat enlargement of the prostate (benign prostatic hyperplasia or BPH), a condition that causes urinary problems in men.

Finasteride blocks an enzyme called 5-alpha-reductase, which is necessary to change testosterone to another hormone that causes the prostate to grow. As a result, the size of the prostate is decreased. The effect of finasteride on the prostate lasts only as long as the medicine is taken. If it is stopped, the prostate begins to grow again.

Oral

- Tablets (U.S. and Canada)

It is very important that you read and understand the following information. If any of it causes you special concern, check with your doctor. Also, *if you have any questions* or if you want more information about this medicine or your medical problem, *ask your doctor, nurse, or pharmacist.*

Before Using This Medicine

In deciding to use a medicine, the risks of taking the medicine must be weighed against the good it will do. This is a decision you and your doctor will make. For finasteride, the following should be considered:

Allergies—Tell your doctor if you have ever had any unusual or allergic reaction to finasteride. Also tell your doctor and pharmacist if you are allergic to any other substances, such as foods, preservatives, or dyes.

Pregnancy—Women who are or may become pregnant should not be exposed to finasteride, because it can cause changes in the genitals (sex organs) of male infants. Therefore, you should use a condom to prevent contact of your semen with your sexual partner while you are taking finasteride. Discuss with your doctor the need to stop taking finasteride if your partner wishes to become pregnant.

While you are taking finasteride, you may notice a decrease in the amount of semen when you ejaculate. This should not affect your sexual performance and is not a sign of any change in fertility.

Older adults—This medicine has been tested and has not been shown to cause different side effects or problems in older people than it does in younger adults.

Other medicines—Although certain medicines should not be used together at all, in other cases two different medicines may be used together even if an interaction might occur. In these cases, your doctor may want to change the dose, or other precautions may be necessary. When you are taking finasteride, it is especially important that your doctor and pharmacist know if you are taking any of the following:

- Amantadine (e.g., Symmetrel) or
- Amphetamines or
- Anticholinergics (medicine for abdominal or stomach spasms or cramps) or
- Antidepressants (medicine for depression) or
- Antidyskinetics (medicine for Parkinson's disease or other conditions affecting control of muscles or
- Antihistamines or
- Antipsychotics (medicine for mental illness) or
- Appetite suppressants (diet pills) or
- Buclizine (e.g., Bucladin) or
- Carbamazepine (e.g., Tegretol) or
- Cyclizine (e.g., Marezine) or
- Cyclobenzaprine (e.g., Flexerel) or
- Disopyramide (e.g., Norpace) or
- Flavoxate (e.g., Urispas) or
- Ipratropium (e.g., Atrovent) or
- Meclizine (e.g., Antivert) or
- Medicine for asthma or other breathing problems or
- Medicine for colds, sinus problems, or hay fever or other allergies (including nose drops or sprays) or
- Methylphenidate (e.g., Ritalin) or

- Orphenadrine (e.g., Norflex) or
- Oxybutynin (e.g., Ditropan)
- Procainamide (e.g., Pronestyl) or
- Promethazine (e.g., Phenergan) or
- Quinidine (e.g., Quinidex) or
- Trimeprazine (e.g., Temaril)—These medicines can cause problems with urination, which could reduce the effects of finasteride

Other medical problems—The presence of other medical problems may affect the use of finasteride. Make sure you tell your doctor if you have any other medical problems, especially:

- Liver disease—Effects of finasteride may be increased because of slower removal from the body

Before you begin using any new medicine (prescription or nonprescription) or if you develop any new medical problem while you are using this medicine, check with your doctor, nurse, or pharmacist.

Proper Use of This Medicine

To help you remember to take your medicine, try to get into the habit of taking it at the same time each day.

Remember that this medicine does not cure BPH but it does help reduce the size of the prostate. Therefore, you must continue to take it if you expect to keep the size of your prostate down. *You may have to take medicine for the rest of your life.* Do not stop taking this medicine without first discussing it with your doctor.

Finasteride tablets may be crushed to make them easier to swallow.

This medicine helps to reduce urinary problems in men with BPH. In general, it is best to avoid drinking fluids, especially coffee or alcohol, in the evening. Then your sleep will not be disturbed by your needing to urinate during the night.

Dosing—The dose of finasteride will be different for different patients. *Follow your doctor's orders or the directions on the label.* The following information includes only the average dose of finasteride. *If your dose is different, do not change it* unless your doctor tells you to do so:

- Adults: 5 mg (one tablet) once a day.

Missed dose—If you miss a dose of this medicine, take it as soon as possible. However, if it is almost time for your next dose, skip the missed dose and go back to your regular dosing schedule. Do not double doses.

Storage—To store this medicine:

- Keep out of the reach of children.
- Store away from heat and direct light.
- Do not store in the bathroom, near the kitchen sink, or in other damp places. Heat or moisture may cause the medicine to break down.
- Do not keep outdated medicine or medicine no longer needed. Be sure that any discarded medicine is out of the reach of children.

Precautions While Using This Medicine

Do not take other medicines unless they have been discussed with your doctor. This especially includes over-the-counter (nonprescription) medicines for appetite control, asthma, colds, cough, hay fever, or sinus problems. These medicines may cause problems with urination and could reduce the effects of finasteride.

Women who are or who may become pregnant should not handle crushed finasteride tablets because of the risk that it could be absorbed into the body and harm the infant.

Side Effects of This Medicine

Along with its needed effects, a medicine may cause some unwanted effects. The following side effects may go away during treatment as your body adjusts to the medicine. However, check with your doctor if any of the following side effects continue or are bothersome:

Less common or rare

Decreased libido (decreased interest in sex); decreased volume of ejaculate (amount of semen); impotence (inability to have or keep an erection)

Other side effects not listed above may also occur in some patients. If you notice any other effects, check with your doctor.

Annual revision: 03/03/93

FLAVOXATE Systemic

A commonly used brand name in the U.S. and Canada is Urispas.

Description

Flavoxate (fla-VOX-ate) belongs to the group of medicines called antispasmodics. It is taken by mouth to help decrease muscle spasms of the bladder and relieve difficult urination.

Flavoxate is available only with your doctor's prescription, in the following dosage form:

Oral

- Tablets (U.S. and Canada)

It is very important that you read and understand the following information. If any of it causes you special concern, check with your doctor. Also, *if you have any questions* or if you want more information about this medicine or your medical problem, *ask your doctor, nurse, or pharmacist.*

Before Using This Medicine

In deciding to use a medicine, the risks of taking the medicine must be weighed against the good it will do. This is a decision you and your doctor will make. For flavoxate, the following should be considered:

Allergies—Tell your doctor if you have ever had any unusual or allergic reaction to flavoxate. Also tell your doctor and pharmacist if you are allergic to any other substances, such as foods, preservatives, or dyes.

Pregnancy—Flavoxate has not been studied in pregnant women. However, flavoxate has not been shown to cause birth defects or other problems in animal studies.

Breast-feeding—Flavoxate has not been reported to cause problems in nursing babies.

Children—Although there is no specific information comparing the use of flavoxate in children with use in other age groups, this medicine is not expected to cause different side effects or problems in children than it does in adults.

Older adults—Confusion may be especially likely to occur in elderly patients, who are usually more sensitive than younger adults to the effects of flavoxate.

Other medicines—Although certain medicines should not be used together at all in other cases two different medicines may be used together even if an interaction might occur. In these cases, your doctor may want to change the dose, or other precautions may be necessary. Tell your doctor and pharmacist if you are taking any other prescription or nonprescription (over-the-counter [OTC]) medicine.

Other medical problems—The presence of other medical problems may affect the use of flavoxate. Make sure you tell your doctor if you have any other medical problems, especially:

- Bleeding (severe) or
- Glaucoma or
- Intestinal blockage or other intestinal or stomach problems or
- Urinary tract blockage—Use of flavoxate may make these conditions worse
- Enlarged prostate—Use of flavoxate may cause difficult urination

Before you begin using any new medicine (prescription or nonprescription) or if you develop any new medical problem while you are using this medicine, check with your doctor, nurse, or pharmacist.

Proper Use of This Medicine

This medicine is usually taken with water on an empty stomach. However, your doctor may want you to take it with food or milk to lessen stomach upset.

Take this medicine only as directed. Do not take more of it, do not take it more often, and do not take it for a longer time than your doctor ordered. To do so may increase the chance of side effects.

Dosing—The dose of flavoxate will be different for different patients. *Follow your doctor's orders or the directions on the label.* The following information includes only the average dose of flavoxate. *If your dose is different, do not change it* unless your doctor tells you to do so. The number of tablets that you take depends on the strength of the medicine.

- Adults and children 12 years of age and older: 100 to 200 milligrams three or four times a day.
- Children up to 12 years of age: Dose must be determined by the doctor.

Missed dose—If you miss a dose of this medicine, take it as soon as possible. However, if it is almost time for your next dose, skip the missed dose and go back to your regular dosing schedule. Do not double doses.

Storage—To store this medicine:

- Keep out of the reach of children.
- Store away from heat and direct light.
- Do not store in the bathroom, near the kitchen sink, or in other damp places. Heat or moisture may cause the medicine to break down.
- Do not keep outdated medicine or medicine no longer needed. Be sure that any discarded medicine is out of the reach of children.

Precautions While Using This Medicine

This medicine may cause your eyes to become more sensitive to light than they are normally. Wearing sunglasses may help lessen the discomfort from bright light.

This medicine may cause some people to become drowsy or have blurred vision. *Make sure you know how you react to this medicine before you drive, use machines, or do anything else that could be dangerous if you are not alert or able to see well.*

Flavoxate may make you sweat less, causing your body temperature to increase. *Use extra care not to become overheated during exercise or hot weather while you are taking this medicine,* since overheating may result in heat stroke. Also, hot baths or saunas may make you feel dizzy or faint while you are taking this medicine.

Your mouth and throat may feel very dry while you are taking this medicine. For temporary relief of mouth dryness, use sugarless candy or gum, melt bits of ice in your mouth, or use a saliva substitute. However, if your mouth continues to feel dry for more than 2 weeks, check with your medical doctor or dentist. Continuing dryness of the mouth may increase the chance of dental disease, including tooth decay, gum disease, and fungus infections.

Side Effects of This Medicine

Along with its needed effects, a medicine may cause some unwanted effects. Although not all of these side effects may occur, if they do occur they may need medical attention.

Check with your doctor as soon as possible if any of the following side effects occur:

Rare

Confusion; eye pain; skin rash or hives; sore throat and fever

Symptoms of overdose

Clumsiness or unsteadiness; dizziness (severe); drowsiness (severe); fever; flushing or redness of face; hallucinations (seeing, hearing, or feeling things that are not there); shortness of breath or troubled breathing; unusual excitement, nervousness, restlessness, or irritability

Other side effects may occur that usually do not need medical attention. These side effects may go away during treatment as your body adjusts to the medicine. However, check with your doctor if any of the following side effects continue or are bothersome:

More common

Drowsiness; dryness of mouth and throat

Less common or rare

Blurred vision; constipation; difficult urination; difficulty concentrating; dizziness; fast heartbeat; headache; increased sensitivity of eyes to light; increased sweating; nausea or vomiting; nervousness; stomach pain

Other side effects not listed above may also occur in some patients. If you notice any other effects, check with your doctor.

Annual revision: 01/18/93

FLECAINIDE Systemic

A commonly used brand name in the U.S. and Canada is Tambocor.

Description

Flecainide (FLEK-a-nide) belongs to the group of medicines known as antiarrhythmics. It is used to correct irregular heartbeats to a normal rhythm.

Flecainide produces its helpful effects by slowing nerve impulses in the heart and making the heart tissue less sensitive.

There is a chance that flecainide may cause new or make worse existing heart rhythm problems when it is used. Since it has been shown to cause severe problems in some patients, it is only used to treat serious heart rhythm problems. Discuss this possible effect with your doctor.

This medicine is available only with your doctor's prescription, in the following dosage form:

Oral

- Tablets (U.S. and Canada)

It is very important that you read and understand the following information. If any of it causes you special concern, check with your doctor. Also, *if you have any questions* or if you want more information about this medicine or your medical problem, *ask your doctor, nurse, or pharmacist.*

Before Using This Medicine

In deciding to use a medicine, the risks of taking the medicine must be weighed against the good it will do. This is a decision you and your doctor will make. For flecainide, the following should be considered:

Allergies—Tell your doctor if you have ever had any unusual or allergic reaction to flecainide, lidocaine, tocainide, or anesthetics. Also tell your doctor and pharmacist if you are allergic to any other substances, such as foods, preservatives, or dyes.

Pregnancy—Flecainide has not been studied in pregnant women. However, studies in one kind of rabbit given about 4 times the usual human dose have shown that flecainide causes birth defects. Before taking flecainide, make sure your doctor knows if you are pregnant or if you may become pregnant.

Breast-feeding—Flecainide passes into breast milk. However, this medicine has not been shown to cause problems in nursing babies.

Children—Studies on this medicine have been done only in adult patients, and there is no specific information comparing use of flecainide in children with use in other age groups.

Older adults—Elderly people are especially sensitive to the effects of flecainide. Flecainide may be more likely to cause irregular heartbeat in the elderly.

Other medicines—Although certain medicines should not be used together at all, in other cases two different medicines may be used together even if an interaction might occur. In these cases, your doctor may want to change the dose, or other precautions may be necessary. When taking flecainide it is especially important that your doctor and pharmacist know if you are taking any of the following:

- Other medicine for heart rhythm problems—Both wanted and unwanted effects on the heart may increase

Other medical problems—The presence of other medical problems may affect the use of flecainide. Make sure you tell your doctor if you have any other medical problems, especially:

- Congestive heart failure—Flecainide may make this condition worse
- Kidney disease or
- Liver disease—Effects of flecainide may be increased because of slower removal from the body
- Recent heart attack—Risk of irregular heartbeats may be increased
- If you have a pacemaker—Flecainide may interfere with the pacemaker and require more careful follow-up by the doctor

Before you begin using any new medicine (prescription or nonprescription) or if you develop any new medical problem while you are using this medicine, check with your doctor, nurse, or pharmacist.

Proper Use of This Medicine

Take flecainide exactly as directed by your doctor, even though you may feel well. Do not take more medicine than ordered.

This medicine works best when there is a constant amount in the blood. *To help keep this amount constant, do not miss any doses. Also, it is best to take the doses 12 hours apart, in the morning and at night*, unless otherwise directed by your doctor. If you need help in planning the best times to take your medicine, check with your doctor or pharmacist.

Missed dose—If you do miss a dose of flecainide and remember within 6 hours, take it as soon as possible. However, if you do not remember until later, skip the missed dose and go back to your regular dosing schedule. Do not double doses.

Storage—To store this medicine:

- Keep out of the reach of children.
- Store away from heat and direct light.
- Do not store in the bathroom, near the kitchen sink, or in other damp places. Heat or moisture may cause the medicine to break down.
- Do not keep outdated medicine or medicine no longer needed. Be sure that any discarded medicine is out of the reach of children.

Precautions While Using This Medicine

It is important that your doctor check your progress at regular visits to make sure the medicine is working properly. This will allow for changes to be made in the amount of medicine you are taking, if necessary.

Your doctor may want you to carry a medical identification card or bracelet stating that you are using this medicine.

Before having any kind of surgery (including dental surgery) or emergency treatment, tell the medical doctor or dentist in charge that you are taking this medicine.

Flecainide may cause some people to become dizzy, lightheaded, or less alert than they are normally. *Make sure you know how you react to this medicine before you drive, use machines, or do anything else that could be dangerous if you are dizzy or are not alert.*

If you have been using this medicine regularly for several weeks, do not suddenly stop using it. Check with your doctor for the best way to reduce gradually the amount you are taking before stopping completely.

Side Effects of This Medicine

Along with its needed effects, a medicine may cause some unwanted effects. Although not all of these side effects may occur, if they do occur they may need medical attention.

Check with your doctor as soon as possible if any of the following side effects occur:

Less common

Chest pain; irregular heartbeat; shortness of breath; swelling of feet or lower legs; trembling or shaking

Rare

Yellow eyes or skin

Other side effects may occur that usually do not need medical attention. These side effects may go away during

treatment as your body adjusts to the medicine. However, check with your doctor if any of the following side effects continue or are bothersome:

More common

Blurred vision or seeing spots; dizziness or lightheadedness

Less common

Anxiety or mental depression; constipation; headache; nausea or vomiting; skin rash; stomach pain or loss of appetite; unusual tiredness or weakness

Other side effects not listed above may also occur in some patients. If you notice any other effects, check with your doctor.

Annual revision: 09/24/92

FLOXURIDINE Systemic†

A commonly used brand name in the U.S. is FUDR.

Generic name product may also be available in the U.S.

†Not commercially available in Canada.

Description

Floxuridine (flox-YOOR-i-deen) belongs to the group of medicines known as antimetabolites. It is used to treat some kinds of cancer.

Floxuridine interferes with the growth of cancer cells, which are eventually destroyed. Since the growth of normal body cells may also be affected by floxuridine, other effects will also occur. Some of these may be serious and must be reported to your doctor. Other effects, like hair loss, may not be serious but may cause concern. Some effects may not occur for months or years after the medicine is used.

Before you begin treatment with floxuridine, you and your doctor should talk about the good this medicine will do as well as the risks of using it.

Floxuridine is to be administered only by or under the immediate supervision of your doctor. It is available in the following dosage form:

Parenteral

- Injection (U.S.)

It is very important that you read and understand the following information. If any of it causes you special concern, check with your doctor. Also, *if you have any questions* or if you want more information about this medicine or your medical problem, *ask your doctor, nurse, or pharmacist.*

Before Using This Medicine

In deciding to use a medicine, the risks of taking the medicine must be weighed against the good it will do. This is a decision you and your doctor will make. For floxuridine, the following should be considered:

Allergies—Tell your doctor if you have ever had any unusual or allergic reaction to floxuridine.

Pregnancy—There is a chance that this medicine may cause birth defects if either the male or female is receiving it at the time of conception or if it is taken during pregnancy. Floxuridine has been shown to cause birth defects in mice and rats. In addition, many cancer medicines may cause sterility which could be permanent. Although sterility has not been reported with this medicine, the possibility should be kept in mind.

Be sure that you have discussed this with your doctor before receiving this medicine. It is best to use some kind of birth control while you are receiving floxuridine. Tell your doctor right away if you think you have become pregnant while receiving floxuridine.

Breast-feeding—Tell your doctor if you are breast-feeding or if you intend to breast-feed during treatment with this medicine. Because floxuridine may cause serious side effects, breast-feeding is generally not recommended while you are receiving it.

Children—There is no specific information comparing use of floxuridine in children with use in other age groups.

Older adults—Many medicines have not been studied specifically in older people. Therefore, it may not be known whether they work exactly the same way they do in younger adults or if they cause different side effects or problems in older people. Although there is no specific information comparing use of floxuridine in the elderly with use in other age groups, this medicine is not expected to cause different side effects or problems in older people than it does in younger adults.

Other medicines—Although certain medicines should not be used together at all, in other cases two different medicines may be used together even if an interaction might occur. In these cases, your doctor may want to change the dose, or other precautions may be necessary. When

you are receiving floxuridine, it is especially important that your doctor and pharmacist know if you have ever been treated with x-rays or cancer medicines or if you are taking any of the following:

- Amphotericin B by injection (e.g., Fungizone) or
- Antithyroid agents (medicine for overactive thyroid) or
- Azathioprine (e.g., Imuran) or
- Chloramphenicol (e.g., Chloromycetin) or
- Colchicine or
- Flucytosine (e.g., Ancobon) or
- Ganciclovir (e.g., Cytovene) or
- Interferon (Intron A, Roferon-A) or
- Plicamycin (e.g., Mithracin) or
- Zidovudine (e.g., AZT, Retrovir)—Floxuridine may increase the effects of these medicines or radiation on the blood

Other medical problems—The presence of other medical problems may affect the use of floxuridine. Make sure you tell your doctor if you have any other medical problems, especially:

- Chickenpox (including recent exposure) or
- Herpes zoster (shingles)—Risk of severe disease affecting other parts of the body
- Hepatitis (history of)—Increased risk of hepatitis
- Kidney disease or
- Liver disease (other)—Effects of floxuridine may be increased because of slower removal from the body
- Infection—Floxuridine can decrease your body's ability to fight infection

Before you begin using any new medicine (prescription or nonprescription) or if you develop any new medical problem while you are using this medicine, check with your doctor, nurse, or pharmacist.

Proper Use of This Medicine

Floxuridine sometimes causes nausea and vomiting. *Tell your doctor if this occurs, especially if you have stomach pain.*

Precautions While Using This Medicine

It is very important that your doctor check your progress at regular visits to make sure that this medicine is working properly and to check for unwanted effects.

While you are being treated with floxuridine, and after you stop treatment with it, *do not have any immunizations (vaccinations) without your doctor's approval.* Floxuridine may lower your body's resistance and there is a chance you might get the infection the immunization is meant to prevent. In addition, other persons living in your household should not take oral polio vaccine since there is a chance they could pass the polio virus on to you. Also, avoid persons who have recently taken oral polio vaccine. Do not get close to them and do not stay in the same room with them for very long. If you cannot take these precautions, you should consider wearing a protective face mask that covers the nose and mouth.

Side Effects of This Medicine

Along with their needed effects, medicines like floxuridine can sometimes cause unwanted effects such as blood problems, inflammation of the digestive tract, liver problems, and other side effects. These and others are described below. Also, because of the way these medicines act on the body, there is a chance that they might cause other unwanted effects that may not occur until months or years after the medicine is used. These delayed effects may include certain types of cancer, such as leukemia. Discuss these possible effects with your doctor.

Although some side effects may appear only rarely, if they do occur they may need medical attention.

Check with your doctor or nurse immediately if any of the following side effects occur:

More common

Diarrhea; sores in mouth and on lips; stomach pain or cramps

Less common

Black, tarry stools; heartburn; nausea and vomiting; scaling or redness of hands or feet; swelling or soreness of the tongue

Rare

Blood in urine or stools; cough or hoarseness; fever or chills; lower back or side pain; painful or difficult urination; pinpoint red spots on skin; trouble in walking; unusual bleeding or bruising; yellow eyes or skin

Other side effects may occur that usually do not need medical attention. These side effects may go away during treatment as your body adjusts to the medicine. Also, your doctor or nurse may be able to tell you about ways to prevent or reduce some of these side effects. Check with your doctor or nurse if any of the following side effects continue or are bothersome or if you have any questions about them:

Less common or rare

Loss of appetite; skin rash or itching

This medicine sometimes causes temporary thinning of hair. After treatment with floxuridine has ended, normal hair growth should return.

Other side effects not listed above may also occur in some patients. If you notice any other effects, check with your doctor or nurse.

Annual revision: 08/09/92

FLUCONAZOLE Systemic

A commonly used brand name in the U.S. and Canada is Diflucan.

Description

Fluconazole (floo-KOE-na-zole) is used to help overcome serious fungus infections found throughout the body.

Fluconazole is available only with your doctor's prescription, in the following dosage forms:

Oral
- Tablets (U.S. and Canada)

Parenteral
- Injection (U.S. and Canada)

It is very important that you read and understand the following information. If any of it causes you special concern, check with your doctor. Also, *if you have any questions* or if you want more information about this medicine or your medical problem, *ask your doctor, nurse, or pharmacist.*

Before Using This Medicine

In deciding to use a medicine, the risks of taking the medicine must be weighed against the good it will do. This is a decision you and your doctor will make. For fluconazole, the following should be considered:

Allergies—Tell your doctor if you have ever had any unusual or allergic reaction to fluconazole or other related medicines, such as itraconazole, ketoconazole, or miconazole. Also tell your doctor and pharmacist if you are allergic to any other substances, such as foods, preservatives, or dyes.

Pregnancy—Studies have not been done in pregnant women. However, studies in some animals have shown that fluconazole taken in high doses may cause harm to the fetus. Lower doses have not been shown to cause problems.

Breast-feeding—It is not known whether fluconazole passes into breast milk.

Children—A small number of children have been safely treated with fluconazole. Be sure to discuss with your child's doctor the use of this medicine in children.

Older adults—Many medicines have not been studied specifically in older people. Therefore, it may not be known whether they work exactly the same way they do in younger adults or if they cause different side effects or problems in older people. There is no specific information comparing use of fluconazole in the elderly with use in other age groups.

Other medicines—Although certain medicines should not be used together at all, in other cases 2 different medicines may be used together even if an interaction might occur. In these cases, your doctor may want to change the dose, or other precautions may be necessary. When you are taking fluconazole, it is especially important that your doctor and pharmacist know if you are taking any of the following:

- Chlorpropamide (e.g., Diabinese) or
- Cyclosporine (e.g., Sandimmune) or
- Glipizide (e.g., Glucotrol) or
- Glyburide (e.g., DiaBeta, Micronase) or
- Phenytoin (e.g., Dilantin) or
- Tolbutamide (e.g., Orinase) or
- Warfarin (e.g., Coumadin)—Fluconazole may increase the the effects of these medicines, which may increase the chance of side effects
- Rifampin (e.g., Rifadin)—Rifampin may decrease the effects of fluconazole

Other medical problems—The presence of other medical problems may affect the use of fluconazole. Make sure you tell your doctor if you have any other medical problems, especially:

- Kidney disease—The effects of fluconazole may be increased in patients with kidney disease
- Liver disease—Patients with liver disease may have an increased chance of side effects

Before you begin using any new medicine (prescription or nonprescription) or if you develop any new medical problem while you are using this medicine, check with your doctor, nurse, or pharmacist.

Proper Use of This Medicine

To help clear up your infection completely, *keep taking this medicine for the full time of treatment,* even if you begin to feel better after a few days. Fungal infections may require many months of treatment even when all your symptoms are gone. *Do not miss any doses.*

Missed dose—If you miss a dose of this medicine, take it as soon as possible. However, if it is almost time for your next dose, skip the missed dose and go back to your regular dosing schedule. Do not double doses.

Storage—To store this medicine:
- Keep out of the reach of children.
- Store away from heat and direct light.
- Do not store in the bathroom, near the kitchen sink, or in other damp places. Heat or moisture may cause the medicine to break down.
- Do not keep outdated medicine or medicine no longer needed. Be sure that any discarded medicine is out of the reach of children.

Precautions While Using This Medicine

It is important that your doctor check your progress at regular visits. This will allow your doctor to check for any unwanted effects.

If your symptoms do not improve within a few weeks, or if they become worse, check with your doctor.

Side Effects of This Medicine

Along with its needed effects, a medicine may cause some unwanted effects. Although not all of these side effects may occur, if they do occur they may need medical attention.

Check with your doctor immediately if any of the following side effects occur:

Rare

Abdominal pain, especially on the right side under the ribs; dark or amber urine; loss of appetite; reddening, blistering, peeling, or loosening of skin and mucous membranes (insides of mouth); unusual bleeding or bruising; yellow skin or eyes

Other side effects may occur that usually do not need medical attention. These side effects may go away during treatment as your body adjusts to the medicine. However, check with your doctor if any of the following side effects continue or are bothersome:

Less common

Diarrhea; headache; nausea; stomach pain; vomiting

Other side effects not listed above may also occur in some patients. If you notice any other effects, check with your doctor.

Annual revision: 02/15/92

FLUCYTOSINE Systemic

Some commonly used brand names are:

In the U.S.

Ancobon

In Canada

Ancotil

Other commonly used names are 5-fluorocytosine and 5-FC.

Description

Flucytosine (floo-SYE-toe-seen) belongs to the group of medicines called antifungals. It is used to treat certain fungus infections.

Flucytosine is available only with your doctor's prescription, in the following dosage form:

Oral

- Capsules (U.S. and Canada)

It is very important that you read and understand the following information. If any of it causes you special concern, check with your doctor. Also, *if you have any questions* or if you want more information about this medicine or your medical problem, *ask your doctor, nurse, or pharmacist.*

Before Using This Medicine

In deciding to use a medicine, the risks of taking the medicine must be weighed against the good it will do. This is a decision you and your doctor will make. For flucytosine, the following should be considered:

Allergies—Tell your doctor if you have ever had any unusual or allergic reaction to flucytosine. Also tell your doctor and pharmacist if you are allergic to any other substances, such as foods, preservatives, or dyes.

Pregnancy—Flucytosine has not been reported to cause birth defects or other problems in humans. However, studies in rats have shown that flucytosine causes birth defects.

Breast-feeding—Flucytosine has not been reported to cause problems in nursing babies.

Children—Although there is no specific information comparing use of flucytosine in children with use in other age groups, this medicine is not expected to cause different side effects or problems in children than it does in adults.

Older adults—Many medicines have not been studied specifically in older people. Therefore, it may not be known whether they work exactly the same way they do in younger adults. Although there is no specific information comparing use of flucytosine in the elderly with use in other age groups, this medicine is not expected to cause different side effects or problems in older people than it does in younger adults.

Other medicines—Although certain medicines should not be used together at all, in other cases two different medicines may be used together even if an interaction might occur. In these cases, your doctor may want to change the dose, or other precautions may be necessary. When you are taking flucytosine, it is especially important that your doctor and pharmacist know if you are taking any of the following:

- Amphotericin B by injection (e.g., Fungizone) or
- Antineoplastics (cancer medicine) or
- Antithyroid agents (medicine for overactive thyroid) or
- Azathioprine (e.g., Imuran) or
- Chloramphenicol (e.g., Chloromycetin) or
- Colchicine or
- Cyclophosphamide (e.g., Cytoxan) or
- Ganciclovir (e.g., Cytovene) or
- Interferon (e.g., Intron A, Roferon-A) or
- Mercaptopurine (e.g., Purinethol) or
- Methotrexate (e.g., Mexate) or
- Plicamycin (e.g., Mithracin) or
- Zidovudine (e.g., AZT, Retrovir) or
- X-ray treatment—Use of flucytosine with any of these medicines may increase the chance for side effects of the blood

Other medical problems—The presence of other medical problems may affect the use of flucytosine. Make sure you tell your doctor if you have any other medical problems, especially:

- Blood disease—Flucytosine may cause blood problems
- Kidney disease—Patients with kidney disease may have an increased chance of side effects
- Liver disease—Flucytosine may cause liver side effects

Before you begin using any new medicine (prescription or nonprescription) or if you develop any new medical problem while you are using this medicine, check with your doctor, nurse, or pharmacist.

Proper Use of This Medicine

In some patients this medicine may cause nausea or vomiting. If you are taking more than 1 capsule for each dose, you may space them out over a period of 15 minutes to help lessen the nausea or vomiting. If this does not help or if you have any questions, check with your doctor.

To help clear up your infection completely, *keep taking this medicine for the full time of treatment,* even if you begin to feel better after a few days. *Do not miss any doses.*

Missed dose—If you do miss a dose of this medicine, take it as soon as possible. However, if it is almost time for your next dose, skip the missed dose and go back to your regular dosing schedule. Do not double doses.

Storage—To store this medicine:

- Keep out of the reach of children.
- Store away from heat and direct light.
- Do not store in the bathroom, near the kitchen sink, or in other damp places. Heat or moisture may cause the medicine to break down.
- Do not keep outdated medicine or medicine no longer needed. Be sure that any discarded medicine is out of the reach of children.

Precautions While Using This Medicine

Your doctor should check your progress at regular visits to make sure that this medicine does not cause unwanted effects.

Flucytosine may cause blood problems. These problems may result in a greater chance of infection, slow healing, and bleeding of the gums. Therefore, you should be careful when using regular toothbrushes, dental floss, and toothpicks. Dental work, whenever possible, should be done before you begin taking this medicine or delayed until your blood counts have returned to normal. Check with your medical doctor or dentist if you have any questions about proper oral hygiene (mouth care) during treatment.

Flucytosine may cause your skin to be more sensitive to sunlight than it is normally. Exposure to sunlight, even for brief periods of time, may cause skin rash, itching, redness, or other discoloration of the skin, or a severe sunburn. When you begin taking this medicine:

- Stay out of direct sunlight, especially between the hours of 10:00 a.m. and 3:00 p.m., if possible.
- Wear protective clothing, including a hat. Also, wear sunglasses.
- Apply a sun block product that has a skin protection factor (SPF) of at least 15. Some patients may require a product with a higher SPF number, especially if they have a fair complexion. If you have any questions about this, check with your doctor or pharmacist.
- Apply a sun block lipstick that has an SPF of at least 15 to protect your lips.
- Do not use a sunlamp or tanning bed or booth.

If you have a severe reaction from the sun, check with your doctor.

This medicine may also cause some people to become dizzy, lightheaded, drowsy, or less alert than they are normally. *Make sure you know how you react to this medicine before you drive, use machines, or do anything else that could be dangerous if you are dizzy or are not alert.* If these reactions are especially bothersome, check with your doctor.

Side Effects of This Medicine

Along with its needed effects, a medicine may cause some unwanted effects. Although not all of these side effects may occur, if they do occur they may need medical attention.

Check with your doctor immediately if any of the following side effects occur:

More common

Skin rash, redness, or itching; sore throat and fever; unusual bleeding or bruising; unusual tiredness or weakness; yellow eyes or skin

Less common

Confusion; hallucinations (seeing, hearing, or feeling things that are not there); increased sensitivity of skin to sunlight

Other side effects may occur that usually do not need medical attention. These side effects may go away during treatment as your body adjusts to the medicine. However, check with your doctor if any of the following side effects continue or are bothersome:

More common

Abdominal pain; diarrhea; loss of appetite; nausea or vomiting

Less common

Dizziness or lightheadedness; drowsiness; headache

Other side effects not listed above may also occur in some patients. If you notice any other effects, check with your doctor.

Annual revision: 07/24/92

FLUDARABINE Systemic

A commonly used brand name in the U.S. and Canada is Fludara.

Description

Fludarabine (floo-DARE-a-been) belongs to the group of medicines called antimetabolites. It is used to treat chronic lymphocytic leukemia (CLL), a type of cancer.

Fludarabine interferes with the growth of cancer cells, which are eventually destroyed. Since the growth of normal body cells may also be affected by fludarabine, other effects will also occur. Some of these may be serious and must be reported to your doctor. Other effects may not be serious but may cause concern. Some effects may not occur for months or years after the medicine is used.

Before you begin treatment with fludarabine, you and your doctor should talk about the good this medicine will do as well as the risks of using it.

Fludarabine is to be administered only by or under the immediate supervision of your doctor. It is available in the following dosage form:

Parenteral

- Injection (U.S. and Canada)

It is very important that you read and understand the following information. If any of it causes you special concern, check with your doctor. Also, *if you have any questions* or if you want more information about this medicine or your medical problem, *ask your doctor, nurse, or pharmacist.*

Before Using This Medicine

In deciding to use a medicine, the risks of taking the medicine must be weighed against the good it will do. This is a decision you and your doctor will make. For fludarabine, the following should be considered:

Allergies—Tell your doctor if you have ever had any unusual or allergic reaction to fludarabine.

Pregnancy—There is a chance that this medicine may cause birth defects if either the male or female is taking it at the time of conception or if it is taken during pregnancy. Fludarabine has been shown to cause birth defects in rats and rabbits. In addition, many cancer medicines may cause sterility which could be permanent. Although sterility has not been reported with this medicine, it does occur in animals and the possibility should be kept in mind.

Be sure that you have discussed this with your doctor before taking this medicine. It is best to use some kind of birth control while you are receiving fludarabine. Tell your doctor right away if you think you have become pregnant while receiving fludarabine.

Breast-feeding—It is not known whether fludarabine passes into breast milk. However, because this medicine may cause serious side effects, breast-feeding is generally not recommended while you are receiving it.

Children—There is no specific information about the use of fludarabine in children.

Older adults—Many medicines have not been tested in older people. Therefore, it may not be known whether they work exactly the same way they do in younger adults. Although there is no specific information about the use of fludarabine in the elderly, it is not expected to cause different side effects or problems in older people than it does in younger adults.

Other medicines—Although certain medicines should not be used together at all, in other cases two different medicines may be used together even if an interaction might occur. In these cases, your doctor may want to change the dose, or other precautions may be necessary. When receiving fludarabine it is especially important that your doctor and pharmacist know if you are taking any of the following:

- Amphotericin B by injection (e.g., Fungizone) or
- Antithyroid agents (medicine for overactive thyroid) or
- Azathioprine (e.g., Imuran) or
- Chloramphenicol (e.g., Chloromycetin) or
- Colchicine or
- Flucytosine (e.g., Ancobon) or
- Ganciclovir (e.g., Cytovene) or
- Interferon (e.g., Intron A, Roferon-A) or
- Plicamycin (e.g., Mithracin) or
- Zidovudine (e.g., AZT, Retrovir) or
- If you have ever been treated with x-rays or cancer medicines—Fludarabine may increase the effects of these medicines or radiation therapy on the blood
- Probenecid (e.g., Benemid) or
- Sulfinpyrazone (e.g., Anturane)—Fludarabine may raise the amount of uric acid in the blood. Since these medicines are used to lower uric acid levels, they may not be as effective in patients receiving fludarabine.

Other medical problems—The presence of other medical problems may affect the use of fludarabine. Make sure you tell your doctor if you have any other medical problems, especially:

- Chickenpox (including recent exposure) or
- Herpes zoster (shingles)—Risk of severe disease affecting other parts of the body
- Gout (history of) or
- Kidney stones (history of)—Fludarabine may increase levels of uric acid in the body, which can cause gout or kidney stones
- Infection—Fludarabine may decrease your body's ability to fight infection
- Kidney disease—Effects of fludarabine may be increased because of slower removal from the body

Before you begin using any new medicine (prescription or nonprescription) or if you develop any new medical problem while you are using this medicine, check with your doctor, nurse, or pharmacist.

Proper Use of This Medicine

This medicine may cause nausea and vomiting. However, it is very important that you continue to receive the medicine even if you begin to feel ill. Ask your doctor, nurse, or pharmacist for ways to lessen these effects.

Precautions While Using This Medicine

It is very important that your doctor check your progress at regular visits to make sure that this medicine is working properly and to check for unwanted effects.

While you are being treated with fludarabine, and after you stop treatment with it, *do not have any immunizations (vaccinations) without your doctor's approval.* Fludarabine may lower your body's resistance and there is a chance you might get the infection the immunization is meant to prevent. In addition, other persons living in your household should not take oral polio vaccine since there is a chance they could pass the polio virus on to you. Also, avoid persons who have recently taken oral polio vaccine. Do not get close to them and do not stay in the same room with them for very long. If you cannot take these precautions, you should consider wearing a protective face mask that covers the nose and mouth.

Fludarabine can temporarily lower the number of white blood cells in your blood, increasing the chance of getting an infection. It can also lower the number of platelets, which are necessary for proper blood clotting. If this occurs, there are certain precautions you can take, especially when your blood count is low, to reduce the risk of infection or bleeding:

- If you can, avoid people with infections. *Check with your doctor immediately* if you think you are getting an infection or if you get a fever or chills, cough or hoarseness, lower back or side pain, or painful or difficult urination.
- *Check with your doctor immediately* if you notice any unusual bleeding or bruising; black, tarry stools; blood in urine or stools; or pinpoint red spots on your skin.
- Be careful when using a regular toothbrush, dental floss, or toothpick. Your medical doctor, dentist, or nurse may recommend other ways to clean your teeth and gums. Check with your medical doctor before having any dental work done.
- Do not touch your eyes or the inside of your nose unless you have just washed your hands and have not touched anything else in the meantime.
- Be careful not to cut yourself when you are using sharp objects such as a safety razor or fingernail or toenail cutters.
- Avoid contact sports or other situations where bruising or injury could occur.

Side Effects of This Medicine

Along with their needed effects, medicines like fludarabine can sometimes cause unwanted effects such as blood problems and other side effects. These and others are described below. Also, because of the way these medicines act on the body, there is a chance that they might cause other unwanted effects that may not occur until months or years after the medicine is used. These delayed effects may include certain types of cancer. Discuss these possible effects with your doctor.

Although not all of these side effects may occur, if they do occur they may need medical attention.

Check with your doctor or nurse immediately if any of the following side effects occur:

More common

Cough or hoarseness; fever or chills; lower back or side pain; painful or difficult urination; shortness of breath

Less common

Black, tarry stools; blood in urine; pinpoint red spots on skin; unusual bleeding or bruising

Check with your doctor or nurse as soon as possible if any of the following side effects occur:

More common

Pain

Less common

Agitation or confusion; blurred vision; loss of hearing; numbness or tingling in fingers, toes, or face; sores in mouth and on lips; swelling of feet or lower legs; weakness

Other side effects may occur that usually do not need medical attention. These side effects may go away during treatment as your body adjusts to the medicine. Also, your doctor or nurse may be able to tell you about ways to prevent or reduce some of these side effects. Check with your doctor or nurse if any of the following side effects continue or are bothersome or if you have any questions about them:

More common

Diarrhea; nausea or vomiting; skin rash; unusual tiredness

Less common

Aching muscles; general feeling of discomfort or illness; headache; loss of appetite

This medicine may rarely cause a temporary loss of hair in some people. After treatment with fludarabine has ended, normal hair growth should return.

After you stop treatment with fludarabine, it may still produce some side effects that need attention. During this period of time, check with your doctor if you notice the following:

Rare

Loss of vision

Other side effects not listed above may also occur in some patients. If you notice any other effects, check with your doctor.

Annual revision: 03/23/92
Interim revision: 06/18/93

FLUDROCORTISONE Systemic

A commonly used brand name in the U.S. and Canada is Florinef.

Description

Fludrocortisone (floo-droe-KOR-tis-sone) is a corticosteroid (kor-ti-koe-STE-roid) (cortisone-like medicine). It belongs to the family of medicines called steroids. Your body naturally produces similar corticosteroids, which are necessary to maintain the balance of certain minerals and water for good health. If your body does not produce enough corticosteroids, your doctor may have prescribed this medicine to help make up the difference.

Fludrocortisone may also be used to treat other medical conditions as determined by your doctor.

Fludrocortisone is available only with your doctor's prescription, in the following dosage form:

Oral

- Tablets (U.S. and Canada)

It is very important that you read and understand the following information. If any of it causes you special concern, check with your doctor. Also, *if you have any questions* or if you want more information about this medicine or your medical problem, *ask your doctor, nurse, or pharmacist.*

Before Using This Medicine

In deciding to use a medicine, the risks of taking the medicine must be weighed against the good it will do. This is a decision you and your doctor will make. For fludrocortisone, the following should be considered:

Allergies—Tell your doctor if you have ever had any unusual or allergic reaction to fludrocortisone. Also tell your doctor and pharmacist if you are allergic to any other substances, such as foods, preservatives, or dyes.

Diet—Your doctor may want you to control the amount of sodium in your diet. When fludrocortisone is used to treat certain types of kidney diseases, too much sodium may cause high blood sodium, high blood pressure, and excess body water.

Pregnancy—Studies on birth defects in humans or animals have not been done with fludrocortisone. However, it is possible that too much use of this medicine during pregnancy may cause the baby to have an underactive adrenal gland after birth.

Breast-feeding—Fludrocortisone passes into the breast milk and may cause problems with growth or other unwanted effects in the nursing baby.

Children—Fludrocortisone may slow or stop growth in children or growing adolescents when used for a long time. The natural production of corticosteroids by the body may also be decreased by the use of this medicine. Before this medicine is given to a child or adolescent, you and your child's doctor should talk about the good this medicine will do as well as the risks of using it. Follow the doctor's directions very carefully to lessen the chance that these unwanted effects will occur.

Older adults—Many medicines have not been studied specifically in older people. Therefore, it may not be known whether they work exactly the same way they do in younger adults or if they cause different side effects or problems in older people. There is no specific information comparing the use of fludrocortisone in the elderly with its use in other age groups.

Other medicines—Although certain medicines should not be used together at all, in other cases two different medicines may be used together even if an interaction might occur. In these cases, your doctor may want to change the dose, or other precautions may be necessary. When you are taking fludrocortisone, it is especially important that your doctor and pharmacist know if you are taking any of the following:

- Acetazolamide (e.g., Diamox) or
- Amphotericin B by injection (e.g., Fungizone) or
- Azlocillin (e.g., Azlin) or
- Capreomycin (e.g., Capastat) or
- Carbenicillin by injection (e.g., Geopen) or
- Corticotropin (ACTH) or
- Dichlorphenamide (e.g., Daranide) or
- Diuretics (water pills) or
- Insulin or
- Laxatives (with overdose or chronic misuse) or
- Methazolamide (e.g., Neptazane) or
- Mezlocillin (e.g., Mezlin) or
- Piperacillin (e.g., Pipracil) or
- Salicylates or
- Sodium bicarbonate (e.g., baking soda) or
- Ticarcillin (e.g., Ticar) or
- Ticarcillin and clavulanate (e.g., Timentin) or
- Vitamin B_{12} (e.g., AlphaRedisol, Rubramin-PC) (when used in megaloblastic anemia) or
- Vitamin D—Fludrocortisone and these medicines decrease the amount of potassium in the blood, which may increase the chance of severe low blood potassium
- Alcohol—Alcohol and fludrocortisone decrease the amount of potassium in the blood, which may increase the chance of severe low blood potassium; alcohol may also make fludrocortisone less effective by causing the body to get rid of it faster
- Barbiturates or
- Carbamazepine (e.g., Tegretol) or
- Griseofulvin (e.g., Fulvicin) or
- Phenylbutazone (e.g., Butazolidin) or
- Phenytoin (e.g., Dilantin) or
- Primidone (e.g., Mysoline) or
- Rifampin (e.g., Rifadin)—Using these medicines may make fludrocortisone less effective because they cause the body to get rid of it faster
- Digitalis glycosides (heart medicine)—Fludrocortisone decreases the amount of potassium in the blood, which may increase the chance of irregular heartbeat
- Other corticosteroids (cortisone-like medicine)—Using any corticosteroid medicine with fludrocortisone will cause the body to get rid of both medicines faster. This may make either or both medicines less effective. Also, fludrocortisone and other corticosteroids decrease the amount of potassium in the blood, which may increase the chance of severe low blood potassium
- Sodium-containing medicine—When using fludrocortisone to treat certain types of kidney diseases, too much sodium may cause high blood sodium, high blood pressure, and excess body water

Other medical problems—The presence of other medical problems may affect the use of fludrocortisone. Make sure you tell your doctor if you have any other medical problems, especially:

- Bone disease—Fludrocortisone may make bone disease worse because it causes more calcium to pass into the urine
- Edema (swelling of feet or lower legs) or
- Heart disease or
- High blood pressure or
- Kidney disease—Fludrocortisone causes the body to retain (keep) more salt and water. These conditions may be made worse by this extra body water
- Liver disease or
- Thyroid disease—The body may not get fludrocortisone out of the bloodstream at the usual rate, which may increase the effect of fludrocortisone or cause more side effects

Proper Use of This Medicine

Take this medicine only as directed by your doctor. Do not take more or less of it, do not take it more often, and do not take it for a longer time than your doctor ordered. To do so may increase the chance of side effects.

Dosing—The dose of fludrocortisone will be different for different patients. *Follow your doctor's orders or the directions on the label.* The following information includes only the average doses of fludrocortisone. *If your dose is different, do not change it* unless your doctor tells you to do so.

- For *oral* dosage forms (tablets):
  —Adults
    - For adrenal gland deficiency: 50 to 200 micrograms a day.
    - For adrenogenital syndrome: 100 to 200 micrograms a day.

  —Children: For adrenal gland deficiency: 50 to 100 micrograms a day.

Missed dose—If you miss a dose of this medicine, take it as soon as you remember. However, if it is almost time for your next dose, skip the missed dose and go back to your regular dosing schedule. Do not double doses.

Storage—To store this medicine:
- Keep out of the reach of children.
- Store away from heat and direct light.
- Do not store in the bathroom, near the kitchen sink, or in other damp places. Heat or moisture may cause the medicine to break down.
- Do not keep outdated medicine or medicine no longer needed. Be sure that any discarded medicine is out of the reach of children.

Precautions While Using This Medicine

Your doctor should check your progress at regular visits to make sure this medicine does not cause unwanted effects.

If you will be using this medicine for a long time, your doctor may want you to carry a medical identification card stating that you are using this medicine.

While you are taking fludrocortisone, be careful to limit the amount of alcohol you drink.

Side Effects of This Medicine

Along with its needed effects, a medicine may cause some unwanted effects. Although not all of these side effects may occur, if they do occur they may need medical attention.

Check with your doctor immediately if any of the following side effects occur:

Less common or rare

Cough; difficulty swallowing; hives; irregular breathing or shortness of breath; irregular heartbeat; redness and itching of skin; redness of eyes; swelling of nasal passages, face, or eyelids; swollen neck veins; unusual tiredness or weakness

Check with your doctor as soon as possible if any of the following side effects occur:

Less common or rare

Dizziness; headache (severe or continuing); loss of appetite; muscle cramps or pain; nausea; swelling of feet or lower legs; weakness in arms, legs, or trunk (severe); weight gain (rapid); vomiting

Other side effects not listed above may also occur in some patients. If you notice any other effects, check with your doctor.

Additional Information

Once a medicine has been approved for marketing for a certain use, experience may show that it is also useful for other medical problems. Although these uses are not included in product labeling, fludrocortisone is used in certain patients with the following medical conditions:
- Idiopathic orthostatic hypotension (a certain type of low blood pressure)
- Too much acid in the blood, caused by kidney disease

Other than the above information, there is no additional information relating to proper use, precautions, or side effects for these uses.

Annual revision: 06/15/93

FLUOROQUINOLONES Systemic

This information applies to the following medicines:

Ciprofloxacin (sip-roe-FLOX-a-sin)
Enoxacin (en-OX-a-sin)
Lomefloxacin (loe-me-FLOX-a-sin)
Norfloxacin (nor-FLOX-a-sin)
Ofloxacin (oe-FLOX-a-sin)

Some commonly used brand names are:

For Ciprofloxacin
In the U.S.
Cipro
Cipro IV
In Canada
Cipro

For Enoxacin
In the U.S.
Penetrex
In Canada
Penetrex

For Lomefloxacin
In the U.S.
Maxaquin
In Canada
Maxaquin

For Norfloxacin
In the U.S.
Noroxin

For Ofloxacin
In the U.S.
Floxin
Floxin IV
In Canada
Floxin

Description

Fluoroquinolones (flu-roe-KWIN-a-lones) are used to treat bacterial infections in many different parts of the body. They work by killing bacteria or preventing their growth. However, these medicines will not work for colds, flu, or other virus infections. Fluoroquinolones may be used for other problems as determined by your doctor.

Fluoroquinolones are available only with your doctor's prescription, in the following dosage forms:

Oral

Ciprofloxacin
- Tablets (U.S. and Canada)

Enoxacin
- Tablets (U.S. and Canada)

Lomefloxacin
- Tablets (U.S. and Canada)

Norfloxacin
- Tablets (U.S. and Canada)

Ofloxacin
- Tablets (U.S. and Canada)

Parenteral

Ciprofloxacin
- Injection (U.S. and Canada)

Ofloxacin
- Injection (U.S.)

It is very important that you read and understand the following information. If any of it causes you special concern, check with your doctor. Also, *if you have any questions* or if you want more information about this medicine or your medical problem, *ask your doctor, nurse, or pharmacist.*

Before Using This Medicine

In deciding to use a medicine, the risks of taking the medicine must be weighed against the good it will do. This is a decision you and your doctor will make. For the fluoroquinolones, the following should be considered:

Allergies—Tell your doctor if you have ever had any unusual or allergic reaction to any of the fluoroquinolones or to any related medicines such as cinoxacin (e.g., Cinobac), or nalidixic acid (e.g., NegGram). Also tell your doctor and pharmacist if you are allergic to any other substances, such as foods, preservatives, or dyes.

Pregnancy—Studies have not been done in humans. However, use is not recommended during pregnancy since fluoroquinolones have been reported to cause bone development problems in young animals.

Breast-feeding—Some of the fluoroquinolones are known to pass into human breast milk. Since fluoroquinolones have been reported to cause bone development problems in young animals, breast-feeding is not recommended during treatment with these medicines.

Children—Use is not recommended for infants or children since fluoroquinolones have been shown to cause bone development problems in young animals. However, your doctor may choose to use one of these medicines if other medicines cannot be used.

Teenagers—Use is not recommended for teenagers up to 18 years of age since fluoroquinolones have been shown to cause bone development problems in young animals. However, your doctor may choose to use one of these medicines if other medicines cannot be used.

Older adults—These medicines have been tested and, in effective doses, have not been shown to cause different side effects or problems in older people than they do in younger adults.

Other medicines—Although certain medicines should not be used together at all, in other cases two different medicines may be used together even if an interaction might occur. In these cases, your doctor may want to change the dose, or other precautions may be necessary. When you are taking a fluoroquinolone, it is especially important that your doctor and pharmacist know if you are taking any of the following:

- Aminophylline or
- Oxtriphylline (e.g., Choledyl) or
- Theophylline (e.g., Somophyllin-T, Theodur, Elixophyllin)—Enoxacin, ciprofloxacin, and norfloxacin may increase the chance of side effects of aminophylline, oxtriphylline, or theophylline
- Antacids, aluminum-, calcium-, or magnesium-containing, or
- Iron supplements or
- Sucralfate—Antacids, iron, or sucralfate may keep any of the fluoroquinolones from working properly
- Caffeine—Enoxacin, ciprofloxacin, and norfloxacin may increase the chance of side effects of caffeine
- Didanosine (e.g., Videx, ddI)—Didanosine may keep any of the fluoroquinolones from working properly
- Warfarin (e.g., Coumadin)—Enoxacin, ciprofloxacin, and norfloxacin may increase the effect of warfarin, increasing the chance of bleeding

Other medical problems—The presence of other medical problems may affect the use of fluoroquinolones. Make sure you tell your doctor if you have any other medical problems, especially:

- Brain or spinal cord disease, including hardening of the arteries in the brain or epilepsy or other seizures—Fluoroquinolones may cause nervous system side effects
- Kidney disease or
- Kidney disease and liver disease—Patients with kidney disease (alone) or kidney disease and liver disease (together) may have an increased chance of side effects

Before you begin using any new medicine (prescription or nonprescription) or if you develop any new medical problem while you are using this medicine, check with your doctor, nurse, or pharmacist.

Proper Use of This Medicine

Do not take fluoroquinolones if you are pregnant. Do not give fluoroquinolones to infants, children, or teenagers unless otherwise directed by your doctor. These medicines have been shown to cause bone development problems in young animals.

Fluoroquinolones are best taken with a full glass (8 ounces) of water. Several additional glasses of water should be taken every day, unless you are otherwise directed by your doctor. Drinking extra water will help to prevent some unwanted effects of ciprofloxacin and norfloxacin.

Ciprofloxacin and lomefloxacin may be taken with meals or on an empty stomach.

Enoxacin, norfloxacin, and ofloxacin should be taken on an empty stomach.

To help clear up your infection completely, *keep taking your medicine for the full time of treatment,* even if you begin to feel better after a few days. If you stop taking this medicine too soon, your symptoms may return.

This medicine works best when there is a constant amount in the blood or urine. *To help keep the amount constant, do not miss any doses. Also, it is best to take the doses at evenly spaced times, day and night.* For example, if you are to take 2 doses a day, the doses should be spaced about 12 hours apart. If this interferes with your sleep or other daily activities, or if you need help in planning the best times to take your medicine, check with your doctor, nurse, or pharmacist.

Dosing—The dose of fluoroquinolones will be different for different patients. *Follow your doctor's orders or the directions on the label.* The following information includes only the average doses of fluoroquinolones. Your dose may be different if you have kidney disease. *If your dose is different, do not change it* unless your doctor tells you to do so.

The number of tablets that you take depends on the strength of the medicine. Also, *the number of doses you take each day, the time allowed between doses, and the length of time you take the medicine depend on the medical problem for which you are using a fluoroquinolone.*

For ciprofloxacin

- For *oral* dosage form (tablets):
  - —Adults: 250 to 750 milligrams (mg) every twelve hours for five to fourteen days, depending on the medical problem being treated.
  - —Children up to 18 years of age: This medicine is not recommended in infants, children, or teenagers.
- For *injection* dosage form:
  - —Adults: 200 to 400 mg every twelve hours.
  - —Children up to 18 years of age: This medicine is not recommended in infants, children, or teenagers.

For enoxacin

- For *oral* dosage form (tablets):
  - —Adults: 200 to 400 mg every twelve hours for seven to fourteen days, depending on the medical problem being treated. Gonorrhea is usually treated with a single, oral dose of 400 mg.
  - —Children up to 18 years of age: This medicine is not recommended in infants, children, or teenagers.

For lomefloxacin

- For *oral* dosage form (tablets):
  - —Adults: 400 mg once a day for ten to fourteen days, depending on the medical problem being treated.
  - —Children up to 18 years of age: This medicine is not recommended in infants, children, or teenagers.

For norfloxacin

- For *oral* dosage form (tablets):
  - —Adults: 400 mg every twelve hours for three to twenty-one days, depending on the medical problem being treated. Gonorrhea is usually treated with a single, oral dose of 800 mg.
  - —Children up to 18 years of age: This medicine is not recommended in infants, children, or teenagers.

For ofloxacin

- For *oral* dosage form (tablets):
  - —Adults: 200 to 400 mg every twelve hours for three to ten days, depending on the medical problem being treated. Gonorrhea is usually treated with a single, oral dose of 400 mg.
  - —Children up to 18 years of age: This medicine is not recommended in infants, children, or teenagers.
- For *injection* dosage form:
  - —Adults: 200 to 400 mg every twelve hours for three to ten days, depending on the medical problem being treated. Gonorrhea is usually treated with a single, oral dose of 400 mg.
  - —Children up to 18 years of age: This medicine is not recommended in infants, children, or teenagers.

Missed dose—If you miss a dose of this medicine, take it as soon as possible. This will help to keep a constant amount of medicine in the blood or urine. However, if it is almost time for your next dose, skip the missed dose and go back to your regular dosing schedule. Do not double doses.

Storage—To store this medicine:

- Keep out of the reach of children.
- Store away from heat and direct light.
- Do not store in the bathroom, near the kitchen sink, or in other damp places. Heat or moisture may cause the medicine to break down.
- Do not keep outdated medicine or medicine no longer needed. Be sure that any discarded medicine is out of the reach of children.

Precautions While Using This Medicine

If your symptoms do not improve within a few days, or if they become worse, check with your doctor.

If you are taking aluminum- or magnesium-containing antacids, or sucralfate do not take them at the same time that you take this medicine. It is best to take these medicines at least 2 hours before or 2 hours after taking norfloxacin or ofloxacin, at least 4 hours before or 2 hours after taking ciprofloxacin or lomefloxacin, and at least 8 hours before or 2 hours after taking enoxacin. These medicines may keep fluoroquinolones from working properly.

Some people who take fluoroquinolones may become more sensitive to sunlight than they are normally. Exposure to sunlight, even for brief periods of time, may cause severe sunburn; skin rash, redness, itching, or discoloration; or vision changes. When you begin taking this medicine:

- Stay out of direct sunlight, especially between the hours of 10:00 a.m. and 3:00 p.m., if possible.
- Wear protective clothing, including a hat and sunglasses.
- Apply a sun block product that has a skin protection factor (SPF) of at least 15. Some patients may require a product with a higher SPF number, especially if they have a fair complexion. If you have any questions about this, check with your doctor or pharmacist.
- Do not use a sunlamp or tanning bed or booth.

If you have a severe reaction from the sun, check with your doctor.

Fluoroquinolones may also cause some people to become dizzy, lightheaded, drowsy, or less alert than they are normally. *Make sure you know how you react to this medicine before you drive, use machines, or do anything else that could be dangerous if you are dizzy or are not alert.* If these reactions are especially bothersome, check with your doctor.

Side Effects of This Medicine

Along with its needed effects, a medicine may cause some unwanted effects. Although not all of these side effects may occur, if they do occur they may need medical attention.

Check with your doctor immediately if any of the following side effects occur:

Rare

Agitation; confusion; fever; hallucinations (seeing, hearing, or feeling things that are not there); pain at site of injection; peeling of the skin; shakiness or tremors; shortness of breath; skin rash, itching, or redness; swelling of face or neck

Other side effects may occur that usually do not need medical attention. These side effects may go away during treatment as your body adjusts to the medicine. However, check with your doctor if any of the following side effects continue or are bothersome:

More common

Abdominal or stomach pain or discomfort; diarrhea; dizziness; drowsiness; headache; lightheadedness; nausea or vomiting; nervousness; trouble in sleeping

Less frequent or rare

Increased sensitivity of skin to sunlight

Other side effects not listed above may also occur in some patients. If you notice any other effects, check with your doctor.

Annual revision: 05/20/93

FLUOROURACIL Systemic

A commonly used brand name in the U.S. and Canada is Adrucil. Generic name product may also be available in the U.S. and Canada. Another commonly used name is 5-FU.

Description

Fluorouracil (flure-oh-YOOR-a-sill) belongs to the group of medicines known as antimetabolites. It is used to treat some kinds of cancer.

Fluorouracil interferes with the growth of cancer cells, which are eventually destroyed. Since the growth of normal body cells may also be affected by fluorouracil, other effects will also occur. Some of these may be serious and must be reported to your doctor. Other effects, like hair loss, may not be serious but may cause concern. Some effects may not occur for months or years after the medicine is used.

Before you begin treatment with fluorouracil, you and your doctor should talk about the good this medicine will do as well as the risks of using it.

Fluorouracil is to be administered only by or under the immediate supervision of your doctor. It is available in the following dosage form:

Parenteral

- Injection (U.S. and Canada)

It is very important that you read and understand the following information. If any of it causes you special

concern, check with your doctor. Also, *if you have any questions* or if you want more information about this medicine or your medical problem, *ask your doctor, nurse, or pharmacist.*

Before Using This Medicine

In deciding to use a medicine, the risks of taking the medicine must be weighed against the good it will do. This is a decision you and your doctor will make. For fluorouracil, the following should be considered:

Allergies—Tell your doctor if you have ever had any unusual or allergic reaction to fluorouracil.

Pregnancy—Tell your doctor if you are pregnant or if you intend to have children. There is a chance that this medicine may cause birth defects if either the male or female is receiving it at the time of conception or if it is taken during pregnancy. Fluorouracil has been reported to cause birth defects in mice given doses slightly higher than the human dose. Also, there has been one case of a baby born with several birth defects after the mother received fluorouracil. In addition, many cancer medicines may cause sterility. Although sterility has been reported with this medicine, it is usually only temporary; the possibility should be kept in mind.

Be sure that you have discussed this with your doctor before receiving this medicine. It is best to use some kind of birth control while you are receiving fluorouracil. Tell your doctor right away if you think you have become pregnant while receiving fluorouracil.

Breast-feeding—Tell your doctor if you are breast-feeding or if you intend to breast-feed during treatment with this medicine. It is not known whether fluorouracil passes into breast milk. However, because fluorouracil may cause serious side effects, breast-feeding is generally not recommended while you are receiving it.

Children—Although there is no specific information comparing use of fluorouracil in children with use in other age groups, it is not expected to cause different side effects or problems in children than it does in adults.

Older adults—Many medicines have not been studied specifically in older people. Therefore, it may not be known whether they work exactly the same way they do in younger adults. Although there is no specific information comparing use of fluorouracil in the elderly with use in other age groups, it is not expected to cause different side effects or problems in older people than it does in younger adults.

Other medicines—Although certain medicines should not be used together at all, in other cases two different medicines may be used together even if an interaction might occur. In these cases, your doctor may want to change the dose, or other precautions may be necessary. When you are receiving fluorouracil, it is especially important that your doctor and pharmacist know if you have ever been treated with x-rays or cancer medicines or if you are taking any of the following:

- Amphotericin B by injection (e.g., Fungizone) or
- Antithyroid agents (medicine for overactive thyroid) or
- Azathioprine (e.g., Imuran) or
- Chloramphenicol (e.g., Chloromycetin) or
- Colchicine or
- Flucytosine (e.g., Ancobon) or
- Ganciclovir (e.g., Cytovene) or
- Interferon (e.g., Intron A, Roferon-A) or
- Plicamycin (e.g., Mithracin) or
- Zidovudine (e.g., AZT, Retrovir)—Fluorouracil may increase the effects of these medicines or radiation on the blood

Other medical problems—The presence of other medical problems may affect the use of fluorouracil. Make sure you tell your doctor if you have any other medical problems, especially:

- Chickenpox (including recent exposure) or
- Herpes zoster (shingles)—Risk of severe disease affecting other parts of the body
- Infection—Fluorouracil can decrease your body's ability to fight infection
- Kidney disease or
- Liver disease—Effects of fluorouracil may be increased because of slower removal from the body

Before you begin using any new medicine (prescription or nonprescription) or if you develop any new medical problem while you are using this medicine, check with your doctor, nurse, or pharmacist.

Proper Use of This Medicine

This medicine is sometimes given together with certain other medicines. If you are using a combination of medicines, it is important that you receive each one at the proper time. If you are taking some of these medicines by mouth, ask your doctor, nurse, or pharmacist to help you plan a way to remember to take them at the right times.

Fluorouracil often causes nausea and vomiting. However, it is very important that you continue to receive the medicine, even if your stomach is upset. Ask your doctor, nurse, or pharmacist for ways to lessen these effects.

Precautions While Using This Medicine

It is very important that your doctor check your progress at regular visits to make sure that this medicine is working properly and to check for unwanted effects.

While you are being treated with fluorouracil, and after you stop treatment with it, *do not have any immunizations (vaccinations) without your doctor's approval.* Fluorouracil may lower your body's resistance and there is a chance you might get the infection the immunization is meant to prevent. In addition, other persons living in your household should not take oral polio vaccine since there is a chance they could pass the polio virus on to you. Also, avoid persons who have recently taken oral polio vaccine. Do not get close to them and do not stay in the same room with them for very long. If you cannot take these precautions, you should consider wearing a protective face mask that covers the nose and mouth.

Fluorouracil can temporarily lower the number of white blood cells in your blood, increasing the chance of getting an infection. It can also lower the number of platelets, which are necessary for proper blood clotting. If this occurs, there are certain precautions you can take, especially when your blood count is low, to reduce the risk of infection or bleeding:

- If you can, avoid people with infections. *Check with your doctor immediately* if you think you are getting an infection or if you get a fever or chills, cough or hoarseness, lower back or side pain, or painful or difficult urination.
- *Check with your doctor immediately* if you notice any unusual bleeding or bruising; black, tarry stools; blood in urine or stools; or pinpoint red spots on your skin.
- Be careful when using a regular toothbrush, dental floss, or toothpick. Your medical doctor, dentist, or nurse may recommend other ways to clean your teeth and gums. Check with your medical doctor before having any dental work done.
- Do not touch your eyes or the inside of your nose unless you have just washed your hands and have not touched anything else in the meantime.
- Be careful not to cut yourself when you are using sharp objects such as a safety razor or fingernail or toenail cutters.
- Avoid contact sports or other situations where bruising or injury could occur.

Side Effects of This Medicine

Along with their needed effects, medicines like fluorouracil can sometimes cause unwanted effects such as blood problems, loss of hair, and other side effects. These and others are described below. Also, because of the way these medicines act on the body, there is a chance that they might cause other unwanted effects that may not occur until months or years after the medicine is used. These delayed effects may include certain types of cancer, such as leukemia. Discuss these possible effects with your doctor.

Although not all of these side effects may occur, if they do occur they may need medical attention.

Check with your doctor or nurse immediately if any of the following side effects occur:

More common

Diarrhea; heartburn; sores in mouth and on lips

Less common

Black, tarry stools; cough or hoarseness; fever or chills; lower back or side pain; nausea and vomiting (severe); painful or difficult urination; stomach cramps

Rare

Blood in urine or stools; pinpoint red spots on skin; unusual bleeding or bruising

Check with your doctor or nurse as soon as possible if any of the following side effects occur:

Rare

Chest pain; cough; shortness of breath; tingling of hands and feet, followed by pain, redness, and swelling; trouble with balance

Other side effects may occur that usually do not need medical attention. These side effects may go away during treatment as your body adjusts to the medicine. Also, your doctor or nurse may be able to tell you about ways to prevent or reduce some of these side effects. Check with your doctor or nurse if any of the following side effects continue or are bothersome or if you have any questions about them:

More common

Loss of appetite; nausea and vomiting; skin rash and itching; weakness

Less common

Dry or cracked skin

This medicine often causes a temporary loss of hair. After treatment with fluorouracil has ended, normal hair growth should return.

After you stop receiving fluorouracil, it may still produce some side effects that need attention. During this period of time, *check with your doctor or nurse immediately* if you notice any of the following:

Black, tarry stools; blood in urine or stools; cough or hoarseness; fever or chills; lower back or side pain; painful or difficult urination; pinpoint red spots on skin; unusual bleeding or bruising

Other side effects not listed above may also occur in some patients. If you notice any other effects, check with your doctor or nurse.

Annual revision: 08/26/92

FLUOROURACIL Topical

Some commonly used brand names are:

In the U.S.
- Efudex
- Fluoroplex

In Canada
- Efudex
- Fluoroplex

Another commonly used name is 5-FU.

Description

Fluorouracil (flure-oh-YOOR-a-sill) belongs to the group of medicines known as antimetabolites. When applied to the skin, it is used to treat certain skin problems, including cancer or conditions that could become cancerous if not treated.

Fluorouracil interferes with the growth of abnormal cells, which are eventually destroyed.

Fluorouracil is available only with your doctor's prescription, in the following dosage forms:

Topical
- Cream (U.S. and Canada)
- Topical solution (U.S. and Canada)

It is very important that you read and understand the following information. If any of it causes you special concern, check with your doctor. Also, *if you have any questions* or if you want more information about this medicine or your medical problem, *ask your doctor, nurse, or pharmacist.*

Before Using This Medicine

In deciding to use a medicine, the risks of using the medicine must be weighed against the good it will do. This is a decision you and your doctor will make. For topical fluorouracil, the following should be considered:

Allergies—Tell your doctor if you have ever had any unusual or allergic reaction to fluorouracil.

Pregnancy—Tell your doctor if you are pregnant or if you intend to become pregnant. Although fluorouracil applied to the skin has not been shown to cause problems in humans, some of it is absorbed through the skin and there is a chance that it could cause birth defects. Be sure that you have discussed this with your doctor before using this medicine.

Breast-feeding—Although fluorouracil applied to the skin has not been shown to cause problems in nursing babies, some of it is absorbed through the skin.

Children—There is no specific information comparing use of fluorouracil on the skin in children with use in other age groups.

Older adults—Many medicines have not been studied specifically in older people. Therefore, it may not be known whether they work exactly the same way they do in younger adults or if they cause different side effects or problems in older people. Although there is no specific information comparing use of fluorouracil on the skin in the elderly with use in other age groups, this medicine is not expected to cause different side effects or problems in older people than it does in younger adults.

Other medical problems—The presence of other medical problems may affect the use of fluorouracil on the skin. Make sure you tell your doctor if you have any other medical problems, especially:
- Other skin problems—May be aggravated

Before you begin using any new medicine (prescription or nonprescription) or if you develop any new medical problem while you are using this medicine, check with your doctor, nurse, or pharmacist.

Proper Use of This Medicine

Keep using this medicine for the full time of treatment. However, *do not use this medicine more often or for a longer time than your doctor ordered.* Apply enough medicine each time to cover the entire affected area with a thin layer.

After washing the area with soap and water and drying carefully, use a cotton-tipped applicator or your fingertips to apply the medicine in a thin layer to your skin.

If you apply this medicine with your fingertips, make sure you *wash your hands immediately afterwards,* to prevent any of the medicine from accidentally getting in your eyes or mouth.

Fluorouracil may cause redness, soreness, scaling, and peeling of affected skin after 1 or 2 weeks of use. This effect may last for several weeks after you stop using the medicine and is to be expected. Sometimes a pink, smooth area is left when the skin treated with this medicine heals. This area will usually fade after 1 to 2 months. Do not stop using this medicine without first checking with your doctor. If the reaction is very uncomfortable, check with your doctor.

Missed dose—If you miss a dose of this medicine, apply it as soon as you remember. However, if more than a few hours have passed, skip the missed dose and go back to your regular dosing schedule. If you miss more than one dose, check with your doctor.

Storage—To store this medicine:
- Keep out of the reach of children.
- Store away from heat and direct light.

- Do not store in the bathroom, near the kitchen sink, or in other damp places. Heat or moisture may cause the medicine to break down.
- Protect the solution from freezing.
- Do not keep outdated medicine or medicine no longer needed. Be sure that any discarded medicine is out of the reach of children.

Precautions While Using This Medicine

It is very important that your doctor check your progress at regular visits to make sure that this medicine is working properly and to check for unwanted effects.

Apply this medicine very carefully when using it on your face. Avoid getting any in your eyes, nose, or mouth.

While using this medicine, and for 1 or 2 months after you stop using it, your skin may become more sensitive to sunlight than usual and too much sunlight may increase the effect of the drug. *During this period of time:*

- Stay out of direct sunlight, especially between the hours of 10:00 a.m. and 3:00 p.m., if possible.
- Wear protective clothing, including a hat and sunglasses.
- Apply a sun block product that has a skin protection factor (SPF) of at least 15. Some patients may require a product with a higher SPF number, especially if they have a fair complexion. If you have any questions about this, check with your doctor or pharmacist.
- Do not use a sunlamp or tanning bed or booth.

If you have a severe reaction from the sun, check with your doctor.

Side Effects of This Medicine

Along with its needed effects, a medicine may cause some unwanted effects. Although not all of these side effects may occur, if they do occur they may need medical attention.

Check with your doctor immediately if the following side effects occur:

Redness and swelling of normal skin

Other side effects may occur that usually do not need medical attention. These side effects may go away during treatment as your body adjusts to the medicine. However, check with your doctor if any of the following side effects continue, worsen, or are bothersome:

More common

Burning feeling where medicine is applied; increased sensitivity of skin to sunlight; itching; oozing; skin rash; soreness or tenderness of skin

Less common or rare

Darkening of skin; scaling; watery eyes

Other side effects not listed above may also occur in some patients. If you notice any other effects, check with your doctor.

Annual revision: 06/09/93

FLUOXETINE Systemic

A commonly used brand name in the U.S. and Canada is Prozac.

Description

Fluoxetine (floo-OX-uh-teen) is used to treat mental depression.

This medicine is available only with your doctor's prescription, in the following dosage form:

Oral

- Capsules (U.S. and Canada)
- Oral Solution (U.S. and Canada)

It is very important that you read and understand the following information. If any of it causes you special concern, check with your doctor. Also, *if you have any questions* or if you want more information about this medicine or your medical problem, *ask your doctor, nurse, or pharmacist.*

Before Using This Medicine

There have been recent suggestions that the use of fluoxetine may be related to increased thoughts about suicide in a very small number of patients. More study is needed to determine if the medicine caused this effect. Be sure you discuss this, and any possible precautions you should take, with your doctor before taking fluoxetine.

In deciding to use a medicine, the risks of taking the medicine must be weighed against the good it will do. This is a decision you and your doctor will make. For fluoxetine, the following should be considered:

Allergies—Tell your doctor if you have ever had any unusual or allergic reaction to fluoxetine. Also tell your doctor and pharmacist if you are allergic to any other substances, such as foods, preservatives, or dyes.

Pregnancy—Studies have not been done in pregnant women. However, fluoxetine has not been shown to cause birth defects or other problems in animal studies.

Breast-feeding—Fluoxetine may pass into the breast milk. However, this medicine has not been reported to cause problems in nursing babies.

Children—Studies on this medicine have been done only in adult patients, and there is no specific information comparing use of fluoxetine in children with use in other age groups.

Older adults—Many medicines have not been tested in older people. Therefore, it may not be known whether they work exactly the same way they do in younger adults or if they cause different side effects or problems in older people. In studies done to date that included elderly people, fluoxetine did not cause different side effects or problems in older people than it did in younger adults.

Other medicines—Although certain medicines should not be used together at all, in other cases two different medicines may be used together even if an interaction might occur. In these cases, your doctor may want to change the dose, or other precautions may be necessary. When you are taking fluoxetine, it is especially important that your doctor and pharmacist know if you are taking any of the following:

- Anticoagulants (blood thinners) or
- Digitalis glycosides (heart medicine)—Higher or lower blood levels of these medicines or fluoxetine may occur; your doctor may need to change the dose of either medicine
- Central nervous system (CNS) depressants (medicines that cause drowsiness)—The CNS depressant effects may be increased
- Monoamine oxidase (MAO) inhibitors (furazolidone [e.g., Furoxone], isocarboxazid [e.g., Marplan], pargyline [e.g., Eutonyl], phenelzine [e.g., Nardil], procarbazine [e.g., Matulane], tranylcypromine [e.g., Parnate])—Taking fluoxetine while you are taking or within 2 weeks of taking MAO inhibitors may cause confusion, agitation, restlessness, stomach or intestinal symptoms, sudden high body temperature, extremely high blood pressure, and severe convulsions; at least 14 days should be allowed between stopping treatment with an MAO inhibitor and starting treatment with fluoxetine; if you have been taking fluoxetine, at least 5 weeks should be allowed before starting treatment with an MAO inhibitor
- Tryptophan—Taking this medicine with fluoxetine may result in increased agitation or restlessness, and stomach or intestinal problems

Other medical problems—The presence of other medical problems may affect the use of fluoxetine. Make sure you tell your doctor if you have any other medical problems, especially:

- Diabetes—The amount of insulin or oral antidiabetic medicine that you need to take may change
- Kidney disease or
- Liver disease—Higher blood levels of fluoxetine may occur, increasing the chance of side effects
- Seizure disorders (history of)—The risk of seizures may be increased

Before you begin using any new medicine (prescription or nonprescription) or if you develop any new medical problem while you are using this medicine, check with your doctor, nurse, or pharmacist.

Proper Use of This Medicine

Take this medicine only as directed by your doctor, to benefit your condition as much as possible. Do not take more of it, do not take it more often, and do not take it for a longer time than your doctor ordered.

If this medicine upsets your stomach, it may be taken with food.

Sometimes fluoxetine must be taken for up to 4 weeks or longer before you begin to feel better. Your doctor should check your progress at regular visits during this time.

Dosing—The dose of fluoxetine will be different for different patients. *Follow your doctor's orders or the directions on the label.* The following information includes only the average doses of fluoxetine. *If your dose is different, do not change it* unless your doctor tells you to do so:

- Adults: To start, usually 20 mg a day, taken as a single dose in the morning.

Missed dose—If you miss a dose of this medicine, it is not necessary to make up the missed dose. Skip the missed dose and continue with your next scheduled dose. Do not double doses.

Storage—To store this medicine:

- Keep out of the reach of children.
- Store away from heat and direct light.
- Do not store in the bathroom, near the kitchen sink, or in other damp places. Heat or moisture may cause the medicine to break down.
- Do not keep outdated medicine or medicine no longer needed. Be sure that any discarded medicine is out of the reach of children.

Precautions While Using This Medicine

It is important that your doctor check your progress at regular visits, to allow dosage adjustments and help reduce any side effects.

This medicine will add to the effects of alcohol and other CNS depressants (medicines that slow down the nervous system, possibly causing drowsiness). Some examples of

CNS depressants are antihistamines or medicine for hay fever, other allergies, or colds; sedatives, tranquilizers, or sleeping medicine; prescription pain medicine or narcotics; barbiturates; medicine for seizures; muscle relaxants; or anesthetics, including some dental anesthetics. *Check with your doctor before taking any of the above while you are using this medicine.*

If you develop a skin rash or hives, stop taking fluoxetine and check with your doctor as soon as possible.

For diabetic patients:

- This medicine may affect blood sugar levels. If you notice a change in the results of your blood or urine sugar tests or if you have any questions, check with your doctor.

This medicine may cause some people to become drowsy. *Make sure you know how you react to fluoxetine before you drive, use machines, or do anything else that could be dangerous if you are not alert.*

Dizziness, lightheadedness, or fainting may occur, especially when you get up from a lying or sitting position. Getting up slowly may help. If this problem continues or gets worse, check with your doctor.

This medicine may cause dryness of the mouth. For temporary relief, use sugarless gum or candy, melt bits of ice in your mouth, or use a saliva substitute. However, if your mouth continues to feel dry for more than 2 weeks, check with your medical doctor or dentist. Continuing dryness of the mouth may increase the chance of dental disease, including tooth decay, gum disease, and fungus infections.

Side Effects of This Medicine

Along with its needed effects, a medicine may cause some unwanted effects. Although not all of these side effects may occur, if they do occur they may need medical attention.

Check with your doctor as soon as possible if any of the following side effects occur:

Less common

Chills or fever; joint or muscle pain; skin rash, hives, or itching; trouble in breathing

Rare

Convulsions (seizures); signs of hypoglycemia (low blood sugar); including anxiety or nervousness, chills, cold sweats, confusion, cool, pale skin, difficulty in concentration, drowsiness, excessive hunger, fast heartbeat, headache, shakiness or unsteady walk, or unusual tiredness or weakness; skin rash or hives that may occur with burning or tingling in fingers, hands, or arms, chills or fever, joint or muscle pain, swelling of feet or lower legs, swollen glands, or trouble in breathing

Symptoms of overdose

Agitation and restlessness; convulsions (seizures); nausea and vomiting (severe); unusual excitement

Other side effects may occur that usually do not need medical attention. These side effects may go away during treatment as your body adjusts to the medicine. However, check with your doctor if any of the following side effects continue or are bothersome:

More common

Anxiety and nervousness; diarrhea; drowsiness; headache; increased sweating; nausea; trouble in sleeping

Less common

Abnormal dreams; change in taste; changes in vision; chest pain; constipation; cough; decreased appetite or weight loss; decreased sexual drive or ability; decrease in concentration; dizziness or lightheadedness; dryness of mouth; fast or irregular heartbeat; feeling of warmth or heat; flushing or redness of skin, especially on face and neck; frequent urination; increased appetite; menstrual pain; stomach cramps, gas, or pain; stuffy nose; tiredness or weakness; tremor; vomiting

Other side effects not listed above may also occur in some patients. If you notice any other effects, check with your doctor.

Additional Information

Once a medicine has been approved for marketing for a certain use, experience may show that it is also useful for other medical problems. Although this use is not included in product labeling, fluoxetine is used in certain patients with the following medical condition:

- Obsessive-compulsive disorder

Other than the above information, there is no additional information relating to proper use, precautions, or side effects for these uses.

Annual revision: 08/04/92

FLUTAMIDE Systemic

Some commonly used brand names are:

In the U.S.
Eulexin

In Canada
Euflex

Description

Flutamide (FLOO-ta-mide) is used to treat cancer of the prostate gland.

Flutamide belongs to the group of medicines known as antiandrogens. It blocks the effect of testosterone in the body. Giving flutamide with another medicine that decreases testosterone levels is one way of treating cancer of the prostate.

Flutamide is available only with your doctor's prescription, in the following dosage forms:

Oral

- Capsules (U.S.)
- Tablets (Canada)

It is very important that you read and understand the following information. If any of it causes you special concern, check with your doctor. Also, *if you have any questions* or if you want more information about this medicine or your medical problem, *ask your doctor, nurse, or pharmacist.*

Before Using This Medicine

In deciding to use a medicine, the risks of taking the medicine must be weighed against the good it will do. This is a decision you and your doctor will make. For flutamide, the following should be considered:

Allergies—Tell your doctor if you have ever had any unusual or allergic reaction to flutamide.

Pregnancy—This medicine causes low sperm count and the medicine it is used with causes sterility which may be permanent. If you intend to have children, be sure that you have discussed this with your doctor before taking this medicine.

Older adults—Many medicines have not been tested in older people. Therefore, it may not be known whether they work exactly the same way they do in younger adults or if they cause different side effects or problems in older people. The effects of a dose of flutamide may last a little longer in elderly patients. However, the dose that is prescribed has that taken into account. Flutamide is not expected to cause different side effects or problems in older people than in younger adults.

Proper Use of This Medicine

Take this medicine exactly as directed by your doctor. Do not use more or less of it, and do not use it more often than your doctor ordered. The exact amount of medicine you need has been carefully worked out. Taking too much may increase the chance of side effects, while taking too little may not improve your condition.

Flutamide is usually taken with another medicine. *It is very important that the two medicines be used as directed. Follow your doctor's instructions very carefully about when to use these medicines.*

Flutamide in combination therapy sometimes causes unwanted effects such as hot flashes or decreased sexual ability. It may also cause difficulty in urinating when you begin to take it. However, it is very important that you continue to take the medicine, even after you begin to feel better. *Do not stop taking this medicine without first checking with your doctor.*

If you vomit shortly after taking a dose of flutamide, check with your doctor. You will be told whether to take the dose again or to wait until the next scheduled dose.

Missed dose—If you miss a dose of this medicine, take it as soon as possible. However, if it is almost time for your next dose, skip the missed dose and go back to your regular dosing schedule. Do not double doses.

Storage—To store this medicine:

- Keep out of the reach of children.
- Store away from heat and direct light.
- Do not store in the bathroom, near the kitchen sink, or in other damp places. Heat or moisture may cause the medicine to break down.
- Do not keep outdated medicine or medicine no longer needed. Be sure that any discarded medicine is out of the reach of children.

Precautions While Using This Medicine

It is very important that your doctor check your progress at regular visits to make sure that this medicine is working properly and to check for unwanted effects.

Side Effects of This Medicine

Along with its needed effects, a medicine may cause some unwanted effects. Although not all of these side effects may occur, if they do occur they may need medical attention.

The side effects listed below are for flutamide used together with the medicine that decreases testosterone.

Check with your doctor as soon as possible if the following side effect occurs:

Rare

Yellow eyes or skin

Other side effects may occur that usually do not need medical attention. These side effects may go away during treatment as your body adjusts to the medicine. However, check with your doctor or nurse if any of the following side effects continue or are bothersome:

More common

Decrease in sexual desire or impotence; diarrhea; nausea or vomiting; sweating and feelings of warmth (sudden)

Less common

Loss of appetite; numbness or tingling of hands or feet; swelling and increased tenderness of breasts; swelling of feet or lower legs

Other side effects not listed above may also occur in some patients. If you notice any other effects, check with your doctor.

Annual revision: July 1990

FOLIC ACID Vitamin B_9 Systemic

Some commonly used brand names are:

In the U.S.

Folvite

Generic name product may also be available.

In Canada

Apo-Folic
Novo-Folacid
Folvite

Generic name product may also be available.

Another commonly used name is Vitamin B_9.

Description

Vitamins (VYE-ta-mins) are compounds that you *must* have for growth and health. They are needed in small amounts only and are usually available in the foods that you eat. Folic (FOE-lik) acid (vitamin B_9) is necessary for strong blood.

Lack of folic acid may lead to anemia (weak blood). Your doctor may treat this by prescribing folic acid for you.

Patients with the following conditions may be more likely to have a deficiency of folic acid:

- Alcoholism
- Anemia, hemolytic
- Diarrhea (continuing)
- Fever (prolonged)
- Hemodialysis
- Illness (prolonged)
- Intestinal diseases
- Liver disease
- Stress (continuing)
- Surgical removal of stomach

In addition, infants smaller than normal, breast-fed infants, or those receiving unfortified formulas (such as evaporated milk or goat's milk) may need additional folic acid.

If any of the above apply to you, you should take folic acid supplements only on the advice of your doctor after need has been established.

Some studies have found that folic acid taken by women before they become pregnant and during early pregnancy may reduce the chances of certain birth defects (neural tube defects).

Claims that folic acid and other B vitamins are effective for preventing mental problems have not been proven. Many of these treatments involve large and expensive amounts of vitamins.

Some strengths of folic acid are available only with your doctor's prescription. Others are available without a prescription. However, it may be a good idea to check with your doctor before taking folic acid on your own.

Folic acid is available in the following dosage forms:

Oral

- Tablets (U.S. and Canada)

Parenteral

- Injection (U.S. and Canada)

It is very important that you read and understand the following information. If any of it causes you special concern, check with your doctor or pharmacist. Also, *if you have any questions* or if you want more information about this dietary supplement or your medical problem, *ask your doctor, nurse, pharmacist, or dietitian.*

Importance of Diet

Vitamin supplements should be taken only if you cannot get enough vitamins in your diet; however, some diets may not contain all of the vitamins you need. This may occur with rapid weight loss, unusual diets (such as some reducing diets in which choice of foods is limited), prolonged intravenous feeding, or malnutrition. A balanced diet should provide all the vitamins you normally need.

In order to get enough vitamins and minerals in your diet, it is important that you eat a balanced and varied diet. Follow carefully any diet program your doctor may recommend. For your specific vitamin and/or mineral needs, ask your doctor for a list of appropriate foods.

Folic acid is found in various foods, including vegetables, especially green vegetables; potatoes; cereal and cereal products; fruits; and organ meats (for example, liver or kidney). It is best to eat fresh fruits and vegetables whenever possible since they contain the most vitamins. Food processing may destroy some of the vitamins. For example, heat may reduce the amount of folic acid in foods.

Vitamins alone will not take the place of a good diet and will not provide energy. Your body also needs other substances found in food such as protein, minerals, carbohydrates, and fat. Vitamins themselves often cannot work without the presence of other foods.

In some cases, it may not be possible for you to get enough food to supply you with the proper vitamins. In other cases, the amount of vitamins you need may be increased above normal. Therefore, a vitamin supplement may be needed.

Experts have developed a list of recommended dietary allowances (RDA) for most of the vitamins. The RDA are not an exact number but a general idea of how much you need. They do not cover amounts needed for problems caused by a serious lack of vitamins.

The RDA for folic acid are:

- Infants and children—
  Birth to 6 months of age: 25 micrograms (mcg) per day.
  6 months to 1 year of age: 35 mcg per day.
  1 to 3 years of age: 50 mcg per day.
  4 to 6 years of age: 75 mcg per day.
  7 to 10 years of age: 100 mcg per day.
- Adolescent and adult males—
  11 to 14 years of age: 150 mcg per day.
  15 years of age and over: 200 mcg per day.
- Adolescent and adult females—
  11 to 14 years of age: 200 mcg per day.
  15 years of age and over: 180 mcg per day.
- Pregnant females—400 mcg per day.
- Breast-feeding females—
  First 6 months: 280 mcg per day.
  Second 6 months: 260 mcg per day.

Remember:

- The total amount of each vitamin that you get every day includes what you get from the foods that you eat *and* what you may take as a supplement.
- This total amount should not be greater than the RDA, unless ordered by your doctor.

Before Using This Dietary Supplement

In deciding to use a medicine, the risks of taking the medicine must be weighed against the good it will do. This is a decision you and your doctor will make. For folic acid, the following should be considered:

Allergies—Tell your doctor if you have ever had any unusual or allergic reaction to folic acid. Also tell your doctor and pharmacist if you are allergic to any other substances, such as foods, preservatives, or dyes.

Pregnancy—It is especially important that you are receiving enough vitamins when you become pregnant and that you continue to receive the right amount of vitamins, especially folic acid, throughout your pregnancy. The healthy growth and development of the fetus depend on a steady supply of nutrients from the mother. However, taking large amounts of a dietary supplement in pregnancy may be harmful to the mother and/or fetus and should be avoided.

Your doctor may recommend that you take folic acid alone or as part of a multivitamin supplement before you become pregnant and during early pregnancy. Folic acid may reduce the chances of your baby being born with a certain type of birth defect (neural tube defects).

Breast-feeding—It is especially important that you receive the right amounts of vitamins so that your baby will also get the vitamins needed to grow properly. However, taking large amounts of a dietary supplement while breast-feeding may be harmful to the mother and/or baby and should be avoided.

Children—Normal daily requirements vary according to age. It is especially important that children receive enough vitamins in their diet for healthy growth and development. Although there is no specific information about the use of folic acid in children in doses higher than the normal daily requirements, it is not expected to cause different side effects or problems in children than in adults.

Older adults—It is important that older people continue to receive enough vitamins in their diet for good health. Although there is no specific information about the use of folic acid in older people in doses higher than the normal daily requirements, it is not expected to cause different side effects or problems in older people than in younger adults.

Medicines or other dietary supplements—Although certain dietary supplements should not be used together at all, in other cases they may be used together even if an interaction might occur. In these cases, your doctor may want to change the dose, or other precautions may be necessary. Tell your doctor and pharmacist if you are taking any other dietary supplement or any prescription or nonprescription (over-the-counter [OTC]) medicine.

Other medical problems—The presence of other medical problems may affect the use of folic acid. Make sure you tell your doctor if you have any other medical problems, especially:

- Pernicious anemia (a type of blood problem)—Taking folic acid while you have pernicious anemia may cause serious side effects. You should be sure that you do not have pernicious anemia before beginning folic acid supplementation

Proper Use of This Dietary Supplement

Some people believe that taking very large doses of vitamins (called megadoses or megavitamin therapy) is useful for treating certain medical problems. Studies have not proven this. Large doses should be taken only under the direction of your doctor after need has been identified.

Missed dose—If you miss taking a vitamin for one or more days there is no cause for concern, since it takes some time for your body to become seriously low in vitamins. However, if your doctor has recommended that you take this vitamin, try to remember to take it as directed every day.

Storage—To store this dietary supplement:

- Keep out of the reach of children.
- Store away from heat and direct light.
- Do not store in the bathroom, near the kitchen sink, or in other damp places. Heat or moisture may cause the dietary supplement to break down.
- Do not keep outdated dietary supplements or those no longer needed. Be sure that any discarded dietary supplement is out of the reach of children.

Side Effects of This Dietary Supplement

Along with its needed effects, a dietary supplement may cause some unwanted effects. Although folic acid does not usually cause any side effects, check with your doctor as soon as possible if any of the following side effects occur:

Rare

Fever; reddened skin; shortness of breath; skin rash or itching; tightness in chest; troubled breathing; wheezing

Other side effects not listed above may also occur in some patients. If you notice any other effects, check with your doctor.

Annual revision: 05/20/92

FOSCARNET Systemic

A commonly used brand name in the U.S. is Foscavir.

Other commonly used names are phosphonoformic acid and PFA.

Description

Foscarnet (foss-KAR-net) is used to treat the symptoms of cytomegalovirus (CMV) infection of the eyes in patients with acquired immune deficiency syndrome (AIDS). Foscarnet will not cure this eye infection, but it may help to control worsening of the symptoms. Foscarnet may also be used for other serious viral infections as determined by your doctor. However, it does not work in treating certain viruses, such as the common cold or the flu.

Foscarnet is administered only by or under the supervision of your doctor. It is available in the following dosage form:

Parenteral

- Injection (U.S.)

It is very important that you read and understand the following information. If any of it causes you special concern, check with your doctor. Also, *if you have any questions* or if you want more information about this medicine or your medical problem, *ask your doctor, nurse, or pharmacist.*

Before Receiving This Medicine

In deciding to use a medicine, the risks of taking the medicine must be weighed against the good it will do. This is a decision you and your doctor will make. For foscarnet, the following should be considered:

Allergies—Tell your doctor if you have ever had any unusual or allergic reaction to foscarnet. Also tell your doctor and pharmacist if you are allergic to any other substances, such as foods, preservatives, or dyes.

Pregnancy—Foscarnet has not been studied in pregnant women. However, studies in animals have shown that foscarnet causes birth defects. Before taking this medicine, make sure your doctor knows if you are pregnant or if you may become pregnant.

Breast-feeding—It is not known whether foscarnet passes into the breast milk.

Children—There is no specific information comparing use of foscarnet in children with use in other age groups. Foscarnet can cause serious side effects in any patient. Therefore, it is especially important that you discuss with the child's doctor the good that this medicine may do as well as the risks of using it.

Older adults—Many medicines have not been studied specifically in older people. Therefore, it may not be known whether they work exactly the same way they do in younger adults or if they cause different side effects or problems in older people. There is no specific information comparing use of foscarnet in the elderly with use in other age groups.

Other medicines—Although certain medicines should not be used together at all, in other cases 2 different medicines may be used together even if an interaction might occur. In these cases, your doctor may want to change the dose, or other precautions may be necessary. When you are taking foscarnet, it is especially important that your doctor and pharmacist know if you are taking any of the following:

- Carmustine (e.g., BiCNU) or
- Cisplatin (e.g., Platinol) or
- Combination pain medicine containing acetaminophen and aspirin (e.g., Excedrin) or other salicylates (with large amounts taken regularly) or
- Cyclosporine (e.g., Sandimmune) or
- Deferoxamine (e.g., Desferal) (with long-term use) or
- Gold salts (medicine for arthritis) or
- Inflammation or pain medicine, except narcotics, or
- Lithium (e.g., Lithane) or
- Methotrexate (e.g., Mexate) or
- Other anti-infectives (e.g., acyclovir by injection, amphotericin B) or
- Penicillamine (e.g., Cupramine) or
- Plicamycin (e.g., Mithracin) or
- Streptozocin (e.g., Zanosar) or
- Tiopronin (e.g., Thiola)—Use of these medicines may increase the chance of side effects affecting the kidneys
- Pentamidine (e.g., Pentam)—Use of pentamidine injection with foscarnet may lower the level of important minerals (calcium and magnesium) in the blood; it may also increase the chance of side effects affecting the kidneys

Other medical problems—The presence of other medical problems may affect the use of foscarnet. Make sure you tell your doctor if you have any other medical problems, especially:

- Anemia—Foscarnet may cause or worsen anemia
- Dehydration or
- Kidney disease—Patients who are dehydrated or have kidney disease may have an increased chance of side effects

Before you begin using any new medicine (prescription or nonprescription) or if you develop any new medical problem while you are using this medicine, check with your doctor, nurse, or pharmacist.

Proper Use of This Medicine

To ensure the best response, foscarnet must be given for the full time of treatment. Also, this medicine works best when there is a constant amount in the blood. To help keep the amount constant, foscarnet must be given on a regular schedule.

Several glasses of water should be taken every day, unless otherwise directed by your doctor. Drinking extra water will help to prevent some unwanted effects foscarnet has on the kidneys.

Precautions After Receiving This Medicine

It is very important that your doctor check your progress at regular visits. This will allow your doctor to check for possible unwanted effects.

It is also *very important that your ophthalmologist (eye doctor) check your eyes* at regular visits since it is still possible that you may have some loss of eyesight due to worsening of your retinitis. This can occur even while you are receiving foscarnet.

Side Effects of This Medicine

Along with their needed effects, medicines like foscarnet can sometimes cause serious side effects such as kidney problems; these are described below. Foscarnet may also decrease the amount of calcium in your blood, causing you to have a tingling sensation around your mouth, and pain or numbness in your hands and feet. If this occurs, especially while you are receiving the medicine, notify your doctor or nurse immediately.

Along with its needed effects, a medicine may cause some unwanted effects. Although not all of these side effects may occur, if they do occur they may need medical attention.

Check with your doctor immediately if any of the following side effects occur:

More common

Increased or decreased frequency of urination or amount of urine; increased thirst

Less common

Convulsions (seizures); fever, chills, and sore throat; muscle twitching; pain at place of injection; pain or numbness in hands or feet; tingling sensation around mouth; tremor; unusual tiredness and weakness

Rare

Sores or ulcers on the penis

Other side effects may occur that usually do not need medical attention. These side effects may go away during treatment as your body adjusts to the medicine. However,

check with your doctor if any of the following side effects continue or are bothersome:

More common

Abdominal or stomach pain; anxious feeling; confusion; dizziness; headache; loss of appetite; nausea and vomiting; unusual tiredness or weakness

Other side effects not listed above may also occur in some patients. If you notice any other effects, check with your doctor.

Additional Information

Once a medicine has been approved for marketing for a certain use, experience may show that it is also useful for other medical problems. Although these uses are not included in product labeling, foscarnet is used in certain patients with the following medical conditions:

- Cytomegalovirus infections in places other than the eyes, such as the lungs or intestines
- Herpes simplex infections of the lips and mouth that do not respond to treatment with acyclovir in patients with HIV infection
- Varicella-zoster infection (shingles) that does not respond to treatment with acyclovir in patients with HIV infection

Other than the above information, there is no additional information relating to proper use, precautions, or side effects for these uses.

Annual revision: 04/06/92

FRUCTOSE, DEXTROSE, AND PHOSPHORIC ACID Oral

A commonly used brand name in the U.S. and Canada is Emetrol.

Description

Fructose (FRUK-tose), dextrose (DEX-trose), and phosphoric (fos-FOR-ik) acid combination is used to treat nausea and vomiting. However, this combination has not been proven to be effective.

This medicine is available without a prescription; however, your doctor may have special instructions on the proper use and dose for your medical problem. Fructose, dextrose, and phosphoric acid combination is available in the following dosage form:

Oral

- Oral solution (U.S. and Canada)

It is very important that you read and understand the following information. If any of it causes you special concern, check with your doctor or pharmacist. Also, *if you have any questions* or if you want more information about this medicine or your medical problem, *ask your doctor, nurse, or pharmacist.*

Before Using This Medicine

If you are taking this medicine without a prescription, carefully read and follow any precautions on the label. For fructose, dextrose, and phosphoric acid combination, the following should be considered:

Allergies—Tell your doctor if you have ever had any unusual or allergic reaction to fructose, dextrose, or phosphoric acid.

Pregnancy—Studies on effects in pregnancy have not been done in either humans or animals.

Breast-feeding—This medicine has not been reported to cause problems in nursing babies.

Children—The fluid loss caused by vomiting may result in a severe condition, especially in children under 3 years of age. Do not give medicine for vomiting to children without first checking with their doctor.

Older adults—The fluid loss caused by vomiting may result in a severe condition. Elderly persons should not take any medicine for vomiting without first checking with their doctor.

Other medical problems—The presence of other medical problems may affect the use of fructose, dextrose, and phosphoric acid. Make sure you tell your doctor if you have any other medical problems, especially:

- Appendicitis, symptoms of, or
- Inflamed bowel, symptoms of—Make sure nausea and vomiting are not due to appendicitis or inflamed bowel before using this product. These conditions may become more severe if they are not treated by your doctor
- Diabetes mellitus—The sugars contained in this medicine may cause problems in diabetics
- Fructose intolerance, hereditary—The fructose in this medicine may cause severe side effects in patients with this condition

Before you begin using any new medicine (prescription or nonprescription) or if you develop any new medical problem while you are using this medicine, check with your doctor, nurse, or pharmacist.

Proper Use of This Medicine

For safe use of this medicine:

- Follow your doctor's instructions if this medicine was prescribed.
- Follow the manufacturer's package directions if you are treating yourself.

Do not dilute this medicine with other liquids. Also, do not drink any other liquids immediately before or after taking this medicine. To do so may keep this medicine from working properly.

Dosing—The dose of this combination product will be different for different patients. *Follow your doctor's orders or the directions on the label.* The following information includes only the average doses. *If your dose is different, do not change it* unless your doctor tells you to do so.

- For *oral* dosage form (oral solution):
  - —For *morning sickness*
    - Pregnant women: One or two tablespoonfuls upon arising and every three hours as needed.
  - —For *nausea*
    - Adults: One or two tablespoonfuls. Dose may be repeated every fifteen minutes until nausea stops. You should not take this product for more than one hour (5 doses) without checking with your doctor.
    - Children over 3 years of age: One or two teaspoonfuls. Dose may be repeated every fifteen minutes until nausea stops. This product should not be taken for more than one hour (5 doses) without checking with your doctor.
    - Children under 3 years of age: Use is not recommended.

Storage—To store this medicine:

- Keep out of the reach of children.
- Store away from heat and direct light.
- Keep the medicine from freezing.
- Do not keep outdated medicine or medicine no longer needed. Be sure that any discarded medicine is out of the reach of children.

Precautions While Using This Medicine

Check with your doctor if your nausea and vomiting continue or become worse after you have taken this medicine.

Do not take this medicine if you have any signs of appendicitis or inflamed bowel (such as stomach or lower abdominal pain, cramping, bloating, soreness, or continuing or severe nausea or vomiting). Instead, check with your doctor as soon as possible.

Side Effects of This Medicine

Along with its needed effects, a medicine may cause some unwanted effects. Although not all of these side effects may occur, if they do occur they may need medical attention.

Stop using this medicine and check with your doctor as soon as possible if any of the following side effects occur:

Signs of fructose intolerance

Fainting; swelling of face, arms, and legs; unusual bleeding; vomiting; weight loss; yellow eyes or skin

Other side effects may occur that usually do not need medical attention. These side effects may go away during treatment as your body adjusts to the medicine. However, check with your doctor if any of the following side effects continue or are bothersome:

Less common—more common with large doses

Diarrhea; stomach or abdominal pain

Other side effects not listed above may also occur in some patients. If you notice any other effects, check with your doctor.

Annual revision: 05/12/93

FURAZOLIDONE Oral†

Some commonly used brand names in the U.S. are Furoxone and Furoxone Liquid.

†Not commercially available in Canada.

Description

Furazolidone (fyoor-a-ZOE-li-done) is used to treat bacterial and protozoal (proe-toe-ZOE-al) infections. It works by killing bacteria and protozoa (tiny, one-celled animals). Some protozoa are parasites that can cause many different kinds of infections in the body.

Furazolidone is taken by mouth. It works inside the intestinal tract to treat cholera, colitis and/or diarrhea caused by bacteria, and giardiasis (jee-ar-DYE-a-siss).

This medicine is sometimes given with other medicines for bacterial infections.

Furazolidone may cause some serious side effects when taken with certain foods, beverages, or other medicines. Check with your doctor, nurse, or pharmacist for a list of products that should be avoided.

Furazolidone is available only with your doctor's prescription, in the following dosage forms:

Oral

- Oral suspension (U.S.)
- Tablets (U.S.)

It is very important that you read and understand the following information. If any of it causes you special concern, check with your doctor. Also, *if you have any questions* or if you want more information about this medicine or your medical problem, *ask your doctor, nurse, or pharmacist.*

Before Using This Medicine

In deciding to use a medicine, the risks of taking the medicine must be weighed against the good it will do. This is a decision you and your doctor will make. For furazolidone, the following should be considered:

Allergies—Tell your doctor if you have ever had any unusual or allergic reaction to furazolidone or to any related medicines such as nitrofurantoin (e.g., Furadantin) or nitrofurazone (e.g., Furacin). Also tell your doctor and pharmacist if you are allergic to any other substances, such as foods, preservatives, or dyes.

Pregnancy—Studies have not been done in humans. However, furazolidone has not been shown to cause birth defects or other problems in humans or in animals given high doses for a long time.

Breast-feeding—It is not known whether furazolidone is excreted in breast milk. However, breast-feeding is not recommended for nursing babies up to 1 month of age because furazolidone may cause anemia.

Children—Because furazolidone may cause anemia, use in infants up to 1 month of age is not recommended.

Older adults—Many medicines have not been studied specifically in older people. Therefore, it may not be known whether they work exactly the same way they do in younger adults or if they cause different side effects or problems in older people. There is no specific information comparing use of furazolidone in the elderly with use in other age groups.

Other medicines—Although certain medicines should not be used together at all, in other cases two different medicines may be used together even if an interaction might occur. In these cases, your doctor may want to change the dose, or other precautions may be necessary. When you are taking furazolidone, it is especially important that your doctor and pharmacist know if you are taking any of the following:

- Amphetamines or
- Appetite suppressants (diet pills) or
- Ephedrine (e.g., Primatene) or
- Isocarboxazid (e.g., Marplan) or
- Phenelzine (e.g., Nardil) or
- Phenylephrine (e.g., Neo-Synephrine) or
- Phenylpropanolamine (e.g., Dexatrim) or
- Procarbazine (e.g., Matulane) or
- Pseudoephedrine (e.g., Sudafed) or
- Selegiline (e.g., Eldepryl) or
- Tranylcypromine (e.g., Parnate) or
- Tricyclic antidepressants (amitriptyline [e.g., Elavil], amoxapine [e.g., Asendin], clomipramine [e.g., Anafranil], desipramine [e.g., Pertofrane], doxepin [e.g., Sinequan], imipramine [e.g., Tofranil], nortriptyline [e.g., Aventyl], protriptyline [e.g., Vivactil], trimipramine [e.g., Surmontil])—The use of furazolidone with any of these medicines may result in a severe increase in blood pressure

Other medical problems—The presence of other medical problems may affect the use of furazolidone. Make sure you tell your doctor if you have any other medical problems, especially:

- Glucose-6-phosphate dehydrogenase deficiency (lack of G6PD enzyme)—Patients with G6PD-deficiency may develop mild anemia while taking furazolidone

Before you begin using any new medicine (prescription or nonprescription) or if you develop any new medical problem while you are using this medicine, check with your doctor, nurse, or pharmacist.

Proper Use of This Medicine

Do not give furazolidone to infants up to 1 month of age, unless otherwise directed by your doctor. This medicine may cause anemia in these patients.

Furazolidone may be taken with food.

To use the *oral suspension*:

- Use a specially marked measuring spoon or other device to measure each dose accurately. The average household teaspoon may not hold the right amount of liquid.

To help clear up your infection completely, *keep taking furazolidone for the full time of treatment,* even if you begin to feel better after a few days. If you stop taking this medicine too soon, your symptoms may return. *Do not miss any doses.*

Missed dose—If you do miss a dose of this medicine, take it as soon as possible. However, if it is almost time for your next dose, skip the missed dose and go back to your regular dosing schedule. Do not double doses.

Storage—To store this medicine:
- Keep out of the reach of children.
- Store away from heat and direct light.
- Do not store the tablet form of this medicine in the bathroom, near the kitchen sink, or in other damp places. Heat or moisture may cause the medicine to break down.
- Keep the oral suspension form of this medicine from freezing.
- Do not keep outdated medicine or medicine no longer needed. Be sure that any discarded medicine is out of the reach of children.

Precautions While Using This Medicine

It is important that your doctor check your progress at regular visits. This is to check whether or not the infection is cleared up completely.

If your symptoms do not improve within a week, or if they become worse, check with your doctor.

Drinking alcoholic beverages or taking other alcohol-containing preparations (for example, elixirs, cough syrups, tonics, or injections of alcohol) while taking furazolidone may rarely cause problems. These problems include increased side effects such as redness of the face, difficult breathing, fainting, and a feeling of tightness in the chest. These side effects usually go away within 24 hours without treatment. However, these effects may occur if you drink for up to 4 days after you stop taking furazolidone. Therefore, *you should not drink alcoholic beverages or take other alcohol-containing preparations while you are taking furazolidone and for 4 days after stopping it.*

Certain foods, drinks, or other medicines may cause very dangerous reactions, such as severe high blood pressure, when taken with furazolidone. Aged or fermented foods and drinks commonly contain tyramine or other substances that increase blood pressure. To avoid such reactions, the following measures are recommended:
- *Do not eat foods that have a high tyramine content (most common in foods that are aged or fermented to increase their flavor), such as cheeses; yeast or meat extracts; fava or broad bean pods; smoked or pickled meat, poultry, or fish; fermented sausage (bologna, pepperoni, salami, summer sausage) or other fermented meat; or any overripe fruit. If a list of these foods is not given to you, ask your doctor, nurse, or pharmacist to provide one.*
- *Do not drink alcoholic beverages or alcohol-free or reduced-alcohol beer and wine.*
- Do not eat or drink large amounts of caffeine-containing food or beverages such as chocolate, coffee, tea, or cola.
- *Do not take any other medicines unless approved or prescribed by your doctor.* This includes nonprescription (over-the-counter [OTC]) appetite suppressants (diet pills) or medicine for colds, sinus problems, or hay fever or other allergies.
- *Do not take any of the above-listed foods, drinks, or medicine for at least 2 weeks after you stop taking furazolidone.* They may continue to react with this medicine during that time.
- Other foods may also contain tyramine or other substances that increase blood pressure. However, these products generally do not cause serious problems when taken with furazolidone, especially if eaten when fresh and in small amounts. These include yogurt, sour cream, cream cheese, cottage cheese, chocolate, and soy sauce. If you have any questions about this, ask your doctor, nurse, or pharmacist. Also ask for a list of foods, beverages, or medicines that may cause serious problems when taken with furazolidone.

Side Effects of This Medicine

Along with its needed effects, a medicine may cause some unwanted effects. Although not all of these side effects may occur, if they do occur they may need medical attention.

Check with your doctor immediately if any of the following side effects occur:

Rare

Fever; itching; joint pain; skin rash or redness; sore throat

Other side effects may occur that usually do not need medical attention. These side effects may go away during treatment as your body adjusts to the medicine. However, check with your doctor if any of the following side effects continue or are bothersome:

Less common

Abdominal or stomach pain; diarrhea; headache; nausea or vomiting

This medicine commonly causes dark yellow to brown discoloration of urine. This side effect does not usually need medical attention.

Other side effects not listed above may also occur in some patients. If you notice any other effects, check with your doctor.

Annual revision: 10/06/92

GADOPENTETATE Diagnostic†

A commonly used brand name in the U.S. is Magnevist.
Another commonly used name is gadopentetic acid.

†Not commercially available in Canada.

Description

Gadopentetate (gad-o-PEN-te-tate) is a paramagnetic agent. Paramagnetic agents are used to help provide a clear picture during magnetic resonance imaging (MRI). MRI is a special kind of diagnostic procedure. It uses magnets and computers to create images or "pictures" of certain areas inside the body. Unlike x-rays, it does not involve radiation.

Gadopentetate is given by injection before MRI to help diagnose problems or diseases of the brain or the spine.

Gadopentetate may also be used to diagnose other conditions as determined by your doctor.

Gadopentetate is to be used only by or under the supervision of a doctor. It is available in the following dosage form:

Parenteral
- Injection (U.S.)

It is very important that you read and understand the following information. If any of it causes you special concern, do not decide against having this test without first checking with your doctor. Also, *if you have any questions* or if you want more information about this test or your medical problem, *ask your doctor, nurse, or pharmacist.*

Before Having This Test

In deciding to use a diagnostic test, any risks of the test must be weighed against the good it will do. This is a decision you and your doctor will make. Also, test results may be affected by other things. For gadopentetate, the following should be considered:

Allergies—Tell your doctor if you have ever had any unusual or allergic reaction to contrast agents like gadopentetate. Also, tell your doctor if you are allergic to any other substances, such as foods, preservatives, or dyes.

Pregnancy—Studies have not been done in humans. However, studies in animals have shown that gadopentetate causes a delay in development of the animal fetus when given to the mother in doses many times the human dose. Also, it is not known yet what effect the magnetic field used in MRI might have on the development of the fetus. Be sure you have discussed this with your doctor.

Breast-feeding—It is not known what amount of gadopentetate passes into the breast milk. However, your doctor may want you to stop breast-feeding for some time after receiving gadopentetate. Be sure you have discussed this with your doctor.

Children—There is no specific information about the use of gadopentetate in children up to 2 years of age. However, in older children, it is not expected to cause different side effects or problems than it does in adults.

Older adults—This medicine has been tested and has not been shown to cause different side effects or problems in older people than it does in younger adults.

Other medical problems—The presence of other medical problems may affect the use of gadopentetate. Make sure you tell your doctor if you have any other medical problems, especially:

- Anemia—This condition may get worse with the use of gadopentetate
- Epilepsy—There may be an increased chance of seizures
- Kidney disease (severe)—Gadopentetate may accumulate in the body and increase the chance of side effects
- Low blood pressure—Blood pressure may become even lower

Preparation for This Test

Your doctor may have special instructions for you in preparation for your test, depending on the type of test. If you have not received such instructions or if you do not understand them, check with your doctor in advance.

Side Effects of This Medicine

Along with its needed effects, contrast agents like gadopentetate may cause some unwanted effects. Although not all of these side effects may occur, if they do occur they may need medical attention.

Less common

Convulsions (seizures); skin rash or hives; unusual tiredness or weakness; wheezing, tightness in chest, or troubled breathing

Other side effects may occur that usually do not need medical attention. These side effects may go away as your body adjusts to this agent. However, check with your doctor if any of the following side effects continue or are bothersome:

More common

Coldness at the place of injection; headache; nausea

Less common or rare

Agitation; dizziness; dryness of mouth; fever; increased watering of mouth; pain and/or burning sensation at place of injection; ringing or buzzing in ears; stomach pain; unusual warmth and flushing of skin; vomiting; weakness or tiredness

Other side effects not listed above may also occur in some patients. If you notice any other effects, check with your doctor.

Annual revision: 01/18/93
Interim revision: 03/12/93

GALLIUM NITRATE Systemic†

A commonly used brand name in the U.S. is Ganite.

†Not commercially available in Canada; however it is available by emergency drug release from the Health Protection Branch.

Description

Gallium nitrate (GAL-ee-um NYE-trate) is used to treat hypercalcemia (too much calcium in the blood) that may occur with some types of cancer.

This medicine is available only with your doctor's prescription in the following dosage form:

Parenteral

- Injection (U.S.)

It is very important that you read and understand the following information. If any of it causes you special concern, check with your doctor. Also, *if you have any questions* or if you want more information about this medicine or your medical problem, *ask your doctor, nurse, or pharmacist.*

Before Receiving This Medicine

In deciding to use a medicine, the risks of taking the medicine must be weighed against the good it will do. This is a decision you and your doctor will make. For gallium nitrate the following should be considered:

Allergies—Tell your doctor if you have ever had any unusual or allergic reaction to gallium nitrate. Also tell your doctor and pharmacist if you are allergic to any other substances, such as foods, preservatives, or dyes.

Diet—Make certain your doctor and pharmacist know if your diet includes large amounts of calcium-containing foods and/or vitamin D, such as milk or other dairy products. Calcium and vitamin D may cause the gallium nitrate to be less effective in treating high blood calcium. Also let your doctor and pharmacist know if you are on any special diet, such as a low-sodium or a low-sugar diet.

Pregnancy—Gallium nitrate has not been studied in pregnant women.

Breast-feeding—It is not known whether gallium nitrate passes into breast milk. However, this medicine is not recommended during breast-feeding, because it may cause unwanted effects in nursing babies.

Children—Studies on this medicine have been done only in adult patients, and there is no specific information comparing use of gallium nitrate in children with use in other age groups.

Older adults—Many medicines have not been studied specifically in older people. Therefore, it may not be known whether they work exactly the same way they do in younger adults or if they cause different side effects or problems in older people. There is no specific information comparing use of gallium nitrate in the elderly with use in other age groups.

Other medicines—Although certain medicines should not be used together at all, in other cases two different medicines may be used together even if an interaction might occur. In these cases, your doctor may want to change the dose, or other precautions may be necessary. When you are taking gallium nitrate, it is especially important that your doctor and pharmacist know if you are taking any of the following:

- Anti-infectives by mouth or by injection (medicine for infection) or
- Carmustine (e.g., BiCNU) or
- Cisplatin (e.g., Platinol) or
- Combination pain medicine containing acetaminophen and aspirin (e.g., Excedrin) or other salicylates (with large amounts taken regularly) or
- Cyclosporine (e.g., Sandimmune) or
- Deferoxamine (e.g., Desferal) (with long-term use) or
- Gold salts (medicine for arthritis) or
- Inflammation or pain medicine, except narcotics or
- Lithium (e.g., Lithane) or
- Methotrexate (e.g., Mexate) or
- Penicillamine (e.g., Cuprimine) or
- Plicamycin (e.g., Mithracin) or
- Streptozocin (e.g., Zanosar) or
- Tiopronin (e.g., Thiola)—Use with gallium nitrate may cause or worsen kidney problems

- Calcium-containing preparations or
- Vitamin D–containing preparations—Use with gallium nitrate may prevent gallium nitrate from working properly

Other medical problems—The presence of other medical problems may affect the use of gallium nitrate. Make

sure you tell your doctor if you have any other medical problems, especially:

- Kidney disease—Gallium nitrate may make this condition worse

Proper Use of This Medicine

Dosing—The dose of gallium nitrate will be different for different patients. *Follow your doctor's orders.*

- For *injection* dosage form:
  —For treatment of too much calcium in the blood:
    - Adults and children 12 years of age and older—The dose is based on body surface and must be determined by your doctor. Gallium nitrate is injected slowly into a vein over 24 hours, for five days. The dose may be repeated in three to four weeks.
    - Children up to 12 years of age—Use and dose have not been determined.

Storage—To store this medicine:

- Keep out of the reach of children.
- Store away from heat and direct light.
- Do not store in the bathroom, near the kitchen sink, or in other damp places. Heat or moisture may cause the medicine to break down.
- Keep the medicine from freezing. Do not refrigerate.
- Do not keep outdated medicine or medicine no longer needed. Be sure that any discarded medicine is out of the reach of children.

Precautions While Receiving This Medicine

It is important that your doctor check your progress at regular visits while you are receiving this medicine. If your condition has improved and you are no longer receiving gallium nitrate, your progress must still be checked. The results of laboratory tests or the occurrence of certain symptoms will tell your doctor if your condition is coming back.

Your doctor may want you to follow a low-calcium diet while you are receiving this medicine. If you have any questions about this, check with your doctor.

Side Effects of This Medicine

Along with its needed effects, a medicine may cause some unwanted effects. Although not all of these side effects may occur, if they do occur they may need medical attention.

More common

Blood in urine; bone pain; greatly increased or decreased frequency of urination or amount of urine; increased thirst; loss of appetite; muscle weakness; nausea or vomiting

Less common

Abdominal cramps; confusion; muscle spasms

Rare

Unusual tiredness or weakness

Other side effects may occur that usually do not need medical attention. These side effects may go away during treatment as your body adjusts to the medicine. However, check with your doctor if any of the following side effects continue or are bothersome:

More common

Diarrhea; metallic taste

Other side effects not listed above may also occur in some patients. If you notice any other effects, check with your doctor.

Annual revision: 06/15/93

GANCICLOVIR Systemic

A commonly used brand name in the U.S. and Canada is Cytovene. Another commonly used name is DHPG.

Description

Ganciclovir (gan-SYE-kloe-vir) is an antiviral. It is used to treat infections caused by viruses.

Ganciclovir is used to treat the symptoms of cytomegalovirus (CMV) infection of the eyes in people whose immune system is not working fully. This includes patients with acquired immune deficiency syndrome (AIDS). Ganciclovir will not cure this eye infection, but it may help to control worsening of the symptoms. Ganciclovir may also be used for other serious CMV infections as determined by your doctor. However, it does not work in treating certain viruses, such as the common cold or the flu.

This medicine may cause some serious side effects, including anemia and other blood problems. Before you begin treatment with ganciclovir, you and your doctor should talk about the good this medicine will do as well as the risks of using it.

Ganciclovir is to be administered by or under the supervision of your doctor. It is available in the following dosage form:

Parenteral

- Injection (U.S. and Canada)

It is very important that you read and understand the following information. If any of it causes you special concern, check with your doctor. Also, *if you have any questions* or if you want more information about this medicine or your medical problem, *ask your doctor, nurse, or pharmacist.*

Before Receiving This Medicine

In deciding to use a medicine, the risks of taking the medicine must be weighed against the good it will do. This is a decision you and your doctor will make. For ganciclovir, the following should be considered:

Allergies—Tell your doctor if you have ever had any unusual or allergic reaction to acyclovir or ganciclovir. Also tell your doctor and pharmacist if you are allergic to any other substances, such as foods, preservatives, or dyes.

Pregnancy—Use of ganciclovir during pregnancy should be avoided whenever possible since ganciclovir has caused cancer and birth defects in animal studies. The use of birth control is recommended during ganciclovir therapy. Your partner should use a condom if he is receiving ganciclovir. Animal studies have also shown that ganciclovir causes a decrease in fertility.

Breast-feeding—Breast-feeding should be stopped during treatment with this medicine because ganciclovir may cause serious unwanted effects in nursing babies.

Children—Ganciclovir can cause serious side effects in any patient. Therefore, it is especially important that you discuss with the child's doctor the good that this medicine may do as well as the risks of using it.

Older adults—Many medicines have not been studied specifically in older people. Therefore, it may not be known whether they work exactly the same way they do in younger adults or if they cause different side effects or problems in older people. There is no specific information comparing use of ganciclovir in the elderly with use in other age groups.

Other medicines—Although certain medicines should not be used together at all, in other cases 2 different medicines may be used together even if an interaction might occur. In these cases, your doctor may want to change the dose, or other precautions may be necessary. When you are taking ganciclovir, it is especially important that your doctor and pharmacist know if you are taking any of the following:

- Amphotericin B by injection (e.g., Fungizone) or
- Antineoplastics (cancer medicine) or
- Antithyroid agents (medicine for overactive thyroid) or
- Azathioprine (e.g., Imuran) or
- Chloramphenicol (e.g., Chloromycetin) or
- Colchicine or
- Cyclophosphamide (e.g., Cytoxan) or
- Flucytosine (e.g., Ancobon) or
- Interferon (e.g., Intron A, Roferon-A) or
- Mercaptopurine (e.g., Purinethol) or
- Methotrexate (e.g., Mexate) or
- Plicamycin (e.g., Mithracin) or
- Zidovudine (e.g., AZT, Retrovir)—Caution should be used if these medicines and ganciclovir are used together; receiving ganciclovir while you are using these medicines may make anemia and other blood problems worse

Other medical problems—The presence of other medical problems may affect the use of ganciclovir. Make sure you tell your doctor if you have any other medical problems, especially:

- Kidney disease—Ganciclovir may build up in the blood in patients with kidney disease, increasing the chance of side effects

Before you begin using any new medicine (prescription or nonprescription) or if you develop any new medical problem while you are using this medicine, check with your doctor, nurse, or pharmacist.

Proper Use of This Medicine

To ensure the best response, ganciclovir must be given for the full time of treatment. Also, this medicine works best when there is a constant amount in the blood. To help keep the amount constant, ganciclovir must be given on a regular schedule.

Precautions After Receiving This Medicine

Ganciclovir can lower the number of white blood cells in your blood, increasing the chance of getting an infection. It can also lower the number of platelets, which are necessary for proper blood clotting. If this occurs, there are certain precautions you can take to reduce the risk of infection or bleeding:

- *Check with your doctor immediately* if you think you are getting an infection or if you get a fever or chills.
- *Check with your doctor immediately* if you notice any unusual bleeding or bruising; black, tarry stools; blood in urine or stools; or pinpoint red spots on your skin.
- Be careful when using a regular toothbrush, dental floss, or toothpick. Your medical doctor, dentist, or nurse may recommend other ways to clean your teeth and gums. Check with your medical doctor before having any dental work done.

- Be careful not to cut yourself when you are using sharp objects such as a safety razor or fingernail or toenail cutters.

The *use of birth control is recommended for both men and women.* Women should use effective birth control methods while receiving this medicine. Men should use a condom during treatment with this medicine and for at least 90 days after treatment has been completed.

It is very important that your doctor check you at regular visits for any blood problems that may be caused by this medicine.

It is also *very important that your ophthalmologist (eye doctor) check your eyes* at regular visits since it is still possible that you may have some loss of eyesight during ganciclovir treatment.

Side Effects of This Medicine

Along with their needed effects, medicines like ganciclovir can sometimes cause serious side effects such as blood problems; these are described below. Discuss these possible effects with your doctor.

Along with its needed effects, a medicine may cause some unwanted effects. Although not all of these side effects may occur, if they do occur they may need medical attention.

Check with your doctor immediately if any of the following side effects occur:

More common

For injection into the vein only

Sore throat and fever; unusual bleeding or bruising

Less common

For injection into the vein only

Mood or other mental changes; nervousness; pain at place of injection; skin rash; tremor; unusual tiredness and weakness

For injection into the eye only

Decreased vision or any change in vision

Other side effects may occur that usually do not need medical attention. These side effects may go away during treatment as your body adjusts to the medicine. However, check with your doctor if any of the following side effects continue or are bothersome:

Less common

Abdominal or stomach pain; loss of appetite; nausea and vomiting

Other side effects not listed above may also occur in some patients. If you notice any other effects, check with your doctor.

Annual revision: 01/07/92

GEMFIBROZIL Systemic

A commonly used brand name in the U.S. and Canada is Lopid.

Description

Gemfibrozil (gem-FI-broe-zil) is used to lower cholesterol and triglyceride (fat-like substances) levels in the blood. This may help prevent medical problems caused by such substances clogging the blood vessels.

Gemfibrozil is available only with your doctor's prescription, in the following dosage forms:

Oral

- Capsules (Canada)
- Tablets (U.S. and Canada)

It is very important that you read and understand the following information. If any of it causes you special concern, check with your doctor. Also, *if you have any questions* or if you want more information about this medicine or your medical problem, *ask your doctor, nurse, or pharmacist.*

Before Using This Medicine

In addition to its helpful effects in treating your medical problem, this type of medicine may have some harmful effects.

Results of a large study using gemfibrozil seem to show that it may cause a higher rate of some cancers in humans. In addition, the action of gemfibrozil is similar to that of another medicine called clofibrate. Studies with clofibrate have suggested that it may increase the patient's risk of cancer, liver disease, pancreatitis (inflammation of the pancreas), gallstones and problems from gallbladder surgery, although it may also decrease the risk of heart attacks. Other studies have not found all of these effects.

Studies with gemfibrozil in rats found an increased risk of liver tumors when doses up to 10 times the human dose were given for a long time.

Be sure you have discussed this with your doctor before taking this medicine.

In deciding to use a medicine, the risks of taking the medicine must be weighed against the good it will do. This is a decision you and your doctor will make. For gemfibrozil, the following should be considered:

Allergies—Tell your doctor if you have ever had any unusual or allergic reaction to gemfibrozil. Also tell your doctor and pharmacist if you are allergic to any other substances, such as foods, preservatives, or dyes.

Diet—Before prescribing medicine for your condition, your doctor will probably try to control your condition by prescribing a personal diet for you. Such a diet may be low in fats, sugars, and/or cholesterol. Many people are able to control their condition by carefully following their doctor's orders for proper diet and exercise. *Medicine is prescribed only when additional help is needed* and is effective only when a schedule of diet and exercise is properly followed.

Also, this medicine is less effective if you are greatly overweight. It may be very important for you to go on a reducing diet. However, check with your doctor before going on any diet.

Make certain your doctor and pharmacist know if you are on a low-sodium, low-sugar, or any other special diet. Most medicines contain more than their active ingredient.

Pregnancy—Gemfibrozil has not been studied in pregnant women. However, studies in animals have shown that high doses of gemfibrozil may increase the number of fetal deaths, decrease birth weight, or cause some skeletal defects. Before taking this medicine, make sure your doctor knows if you are pregnant or if you may become pregnant.

Breast-feeding—It is not known whether gemfibrozil passes into breast milk. However, studies in animals have shown that high doses of gemfibrozil may increase the risk of some kinds of tumors. Therefore, you should consider this when deciding whether to breast-feed your baby while taking this medicine.

Children—There is no specific information about the use of gemfibrozil in children. However, use is not recommended in children under 2 years of age since cholesterol is needed for normal development.

Older adults—Many medicines have not been studied specifically in older people. Therefore, it may not be known whether they work exactly the same way they do in younger adults or if they cause different side effects or problems in older people. There is no specific information comparing use of gemfibrozil in the elderly with use in other age groups.

Other medicines—Although certain medicines should not be used together at all, in other cases two different medicines may be used together even if an interaction might occur. In these cases, your doctor may want to change the dose, or other precautions may be necessary. When you are taking gemfibrozil it is especially important that your doctor and pharmacist know if you are taking any of the following:

- Anticoagulants (blood thinners)—Use with gemfibrozil may increase the effect of the anticoagulant
- Lovastatin—Use with gemfibrozil may cause muscle or kidney problems or make them worse

Other medical problems—The presence of other medical problems may affect the use of gemfibrozil. Make sure you tell your doctor if you have any other medical problems, especially:

- Gallbladder disease or
- Gallstones—Gemfibrozil may make these conditions worse
- Kidney disease or
- Liver disease—Higher blood levels of gemfibrozil may result, which may increase the chance of side effects; a decrease in the dose of gemfibrozil may be needed

Before you begin using any new medicine (prescription or nonprescription) or if you develop any new medical problem while you are using this medicine, check with your doctor, nurse, or pharmacist.

Proper Use of This Medicine

Use this medicine only as directed by your doctor. Do not use more or less of it, and do not use it more often or for a longer time than your doctor ordered.

This medicine is usually taken twice a day. If you are taking 2 doses a day, it is best to take the medicine 30 minutes before your breakfast and evening meal.

Follow carefully the special diet your doctor gave you. This is the most important part of controlling your condition and is necessary if the medicine is to work properly.

Dosing—The dose of gemfibrozil will be different for different patients. *Follow your doctor's orders or the directions on the label.* The following information includes only the average doses of gemfibrozil. *If your dose is different, do not change it* unless your doctor tells you to do so:

- For *oral* dosage forms (tablets):
  —Adults: 600 milligrams two times a day to be taken thirty minutes before the morning and evening meals.

Missed dose—If you miss a dose of this medicine, take it as soon as possible. However, if it is almost time for your next dose, skip the missed dose and go back to your regular dosing schedule. Do not double doses.

Storage—To store this medicine:

- Keep out of the reach of children.
- Store away from heat and direct light.
- Do not store in the bathroom, near the kitchen sink, or in other damp places. Heat or moisture may cause the medicine to break down.

- Do not keep outdated medicine or medicine no longer needed. Be sure that any discarded medicine is out of the reach of children.

Precautions While Using This Medicine

It is very important that your doctor check your progress at regular visits. This will allow your doctor to see if the medicine is working properly to lower your cholesterol and triglyceride levels and to decide if you should continue to take it.

Do not stop taking this medication without first checking with your doctor. When you stop taking this medicine, your blood cholesterol levels may increase again. Your doctor may want you to follow a special diet to help prevent this from happening.

Side Effects of This Medicine

Along with its needed effects, a medicine may cause some unwanted effects. Although not all of these side effects may occur, if they do occur they may need medical attention.

Check with your doctor immediately if any of the following side effects occur:

Rare

Cough or hoarseness; fever or chills; lower back or side pain; painful or difficult urination; stomach pain (severe) with nausea and vomiting

Check with your doctor as soon as possible if either of the following side effects occurs:

Rare

Muscle pain; unusual tiredness or weakness

Other side effects may occur that usually do not need medical attention. These side effects may go away during treatment as your body adjusts to the medicine. However, check with your doctor if any of the following side effects continue or are bothersome:

More common

Stomach pain, gas, or heartburn

Less common

Diarrhea; nausea or vomiting; skin rash

Other side effects not listed above may also occur in some patients. If you notice any other effects, check with your doctor.

Annual revision: 05/24/93

GENTAMICIN Ophthalmic

Some commonly used brand names are:

In the U.S.

Garamycin
Genoptic Liquifilm
Genoptic S.O.P.
Gentacidin
Gentafair
Gentak
Gentrasul
Ocu-Mycin
Spectro-Genta

Generic name product may also be available.

In Canada

Alcomicin
Garamycin
Gentrasul

Another commonly used name is gentamycin.

Description

Gentamicin (jen-ta-MYE-sin) belongs to the family of medicines called antibiotics. Gentamicin ophthalmic preparations are used to treat infections of the eye.

Gentamicin is available only with your doctor's prescription, in the following dosage forms:

Ophthalmic

- Ophthalmic ointment (U.S. and Canada)
- Ophthalmic solution (eye drops) (U.S. and Canada)

It is very important that you read and understand the following information. If any of it causes you special concern, check with your doctor. Also, *if you have any questions* or if you want more information about this medicine or your medical problem, *ask your doctor, nurse, or pharmacist.*

Before Using This Medicine

In deciding to use a medicine, the risks of using the medicine must be weighed against the good it will do. This is a decision you and your doctor will make. For ophthalmic gentamicin, the following should be considered:

Allergies—Tell your doctor if you have ever had any unusual or allergic reaction to this medicine or to any related antibiotic, such as amikacin (e.g., Amikin), gentamicin by injection (e.g., Garamycin), kanamycin (e.g., Kantrex), neomycin (e.g., Mycifradin), netilmicin (e.g., Netromycin), streptomycin, or tobramycin (e.g., Nebcin). Also tell your doctor and pharmacist if you are allergic to any other substances, such as preservatives.

Pregnancy—Gentamicin ophthalmic preparations have not been shown to cause birth defects or other problems in humans.

Breast-feeding—Gentamicin ophthalmic preparations have not been reported to cause problems in nursing babies.

Children—Studies on this medicine have been done only in adult patients, and there is no specific information comparing use of this medicine in children with use in other age groups.

Older adults—Many medicines have not been studied specifically in older people. Therefore, it may not be known whether they work exactly the same way they do in younger adults or if they cause different side effects or problems in older people. There is no specific information comparing use of this medicine in the elderly with use in other age groups.

Before you begin using any new medicine (prescription or nonprescription) or if you develop any new medical problem while you are using this medicine, check with your doctor, nurse, or pharmacist.

Proper Use of This Medicine

For patients using the *eye drop form* of this medicine:

- The bottle is only partially full to provide proper drop control.
- To use:

  —First, wash your hands. Then tilt the head back and pull the lower eyelid away from the eye to form a pouch. Drop the medicine into the pouch and gently close the eyes. Do not blink. Keep the eyes closed for 1 or 2 minutes to allow the medicine to come into contact with the infection.
- If you think you did not get the drop of medicine into your eye properly, use another drop.
- To keep the medicine as germ-free as possible, do not touch the applicator tip to any surface (including the eye). Also, keep the container tightly closed.

For patients using the *eye ointment form* of this medicine:

- To apply this medicine: First, wash your hands. Then pull the lower eyelid away from the eye to form a pouch. Squeeze a thin strip of ointment into the pouch. A 1-cm (approximately ⅓-inch) strip of ointment is usually enough unless otherwise directed by your doctor. Gently close the eyes and keep them closed for 1 or 2 minutes to allow the medicine to come into contact with the infection.
- To keep the medicine as germ-free as possible, do not touch the applicator tip to any surface (including the eye). After using gentamicin eye ointment, wipe the tip of the ointment tube with a clean tissue and keep the tube tightly closed.

To help clear up your infection completely, *keep using this medicine for the full time of treatment,* even if your symptoms have disappeared. *Do not miss any doses.*

Missed dose—If you do miss a dose of this medicine, apply it as soon as possible. However, if it is almost time for your next dose, skip the missed dose and go back to your regular dosing schedule.

Storage—To store this medicine:

- Keep out of the reach of children.
- Store away from heat and direct light.
- Keep the medicine from freezing.
- Do not keep outdated medicine or medicine no longer needed. Be sure that any discarded medicine is out of the reach of children.

Precautions While Using This Medicine

If your symptoms do not improve within a few days, or if they become worse, check with your doctor.

Side Effects of This Medicine

Along with its needed effects, a medicine may cause some unwanted effects. Although not all of these side effects may occur, if they do occur they may need medical attention.

Check with your doctor immediately if any of the following side effects occur:

Less common

Itching, redness, swelling, or other sign of irritation not present before use of this medicine

Other side effects may occur that usually do not need medical attention. These side effects may go away during treatment as your body adjusts to the medicine. However, check with your doctor if either of the following side effects continues or is bothersome:

Less common

Burning or stinging

After application, eye ointments usually cause your vision to blur for a few minutes.

Other side effects not listed above may also occur in some patients. If you notice any other effects, check with your doctor.

Annual revision: 06/23/92

GENTAMICIN Otic*

A commonly used brand name in Canada is Garamycin Otic Solution*.

*Not commercially available in the U.S.

Description

Gentamicin (jen-ta-MYE-sin) belongs to the family of medicines called antibiotics. Gentamicin otic preparations are used to treat infections of the ear canal.

Gentamicin is available only with your doctor's prescription, in the following dosage form:

Otic
- Solution (Canada)

It is very important that you read and understand the following information. If any of it causes you special concern, check with your doctor. Also, *if you have any questions* or if you want more information about this medicine or your medical problem, *ask your doctor, nurse, or pharmacist.*

Before Using This Medicine

In deciding to use a medicine, the risks of using the medicine must be weighed against the good it will do. This is a decision you and your doctor will make. For gentamicin otic preparations, the following should be considered:

Allergies—Tell your doctor if you have ever had any unusual or allergic reaction to this medicine or to any related antibiotics such as amikacin (e.g., Amikin), gentamicin by injection (e.g., Garamycin), kanamycin (e.g., Kantrex), neomycin (e.g., Mycifradin), netilmicin (e.g., Netromycin), streptomycin, or tobramycin (e.g., Nebcin). Also tell your doctor and pharmacist if you are allergic to any other substances, such as preservatives.

Pregnancy—Gentamicin otic preparations have not been shown to cause birth defects or other problems in humans.

Breast-feeding—Gentamicin otic preparations have not been reported to cause problems in nursing babies.

Children—Although there is no specific information comparing use of this medicine in children with use in other age groups, this medicine is not expected to cause different side effects or problems in children than it does in adults.

Older adults—Many medicines have not been studied specifically in older people. Therefore, it may not be known whether they work exactly the same way they do in younger adults. Although there is no specific information comparing use of this medicine in the elderly with use in other age groups, this medicine is not expected to cause different side effects or problems in older people than it does in younger adults.

Other medical problems—The presence of other medical problems may affect the use of gentamicin otic preparations. Make sure you tell your doctor if you have any other medical problems, especially:
- Any other ear infection or problem (including punctured eardrum)—Use of gentamicin otic preparations in persons with this condition may lead to systemic absorption, and increase the chance of side effects

Before you begin using any new medicine (prescription or nonprescription) or if you develop any new medical problem while you are using this medicine, check with your doctor, nurse, or pharmacist.

Proper Use of This Medicine

To use:
- Lie down or tilt the head so that the infected ear faces up. Gently pull the earlobe up and back for adults (down and back for children) to straighten the ear canal. Drop the medicine into the ear canal. Keep the ear facing up for about 1 or 2 minutes to allow the medicine to come into contact with the infection. A sterile cotton plug may be gently inserted into the ear opening to prevent the medicine from leaking out.
- To keep the medicine as germ-free as possible, do not touch the applicator tip to any surface (including the ear). Also, keep the container tightly closed.

To help clear up your infection completely, *keep using this medicine for the full time of treatment,* even if your symptoms have disappeared. *Do not miss any doses.*

Missed dose—If you do miss a dose of this medicine, apply it as soon as possible. However, if it is almost time for your next dose, skip the missed dose and go back to your regular dosing schedule.

Storage—To store this medicine:
- Keep out of the reach of children.
- Store away from heat and direct light.
- Keep the medicine from freezing.
- Do not keep outdated medicine or medicine no longer needed. Be sure that any discarded medicine is out of the reach of children.

Precautions While Using This Medicine

If your symptoms do not improve within a few days, or if they become worse, check with your doctor.

Side Effects of This Medicine

Along with its needed effects, a medicine may cause some unwanted effects. Although not all of these side effects may occur, if they do occur they may need medical attention.

Check with your doctor immediately if any of the following side effects occur:

Less common

Itching, redness, swelling, or other sign of irritation not present before use of this medicine

Other side effects may occur that usually do not need medical attention. These side effects may go away during treatment as your body adjusts to the medicine. However, check with your doctor if either of the following side effects continues or is bothersome:

Less common

Burning or stinging

Other side effects not listed above may also occur in some patients. If you notice any other effects, check with your doctor.

Annual revision: 08/12/92

GENTAMICIN Topical

Some commonly used brand names are:

In the U.S.

Garamycin
G-Myticin
Gentamar

Generic name product may also be available.

In Canada

Garamycin

Description

Gentamicin (jen-ta-MYE-sin) belongs to the family of medicines called antibiotics. Gentamicin topical preparations are used to treat infections of the skin.

Gentamicin is available only with your doctor's prescription, in the following dosage forms:

Topical

- Cream (U.S. and Canada)
- Ointment (U.S. and Canada)

It is very important that you read and understand the following information. If any of it causes you special concern, check with your doctor. Also, *if you have any questions* or if you want more information about this medicine or your medical problem, *ask your doctor, nurse, or pharmacist.*

Before Using This Medicine

In deciding to use a medicine, the risks of using the medicine must be weighed against the good it will do. This is a decision you and your doctor will make. For topical gentamicin, the following should be considered:

Allergies—Tell your doctor if you have ever had any unusual or allergic reaction to this medicine or any related antibiotics, such as amikacin (e.g., Amikin), gentamicin by injection (e.g., Garamycin), kanamycin (e.g., Kantrex), neomycin (e.g., Mycifradin), netilmicin (e.g., Netromycin), streptomycin, or tobramycin (e.g., Nebcin). Also tell your doctor and pharmacist if you are allergic to any other substances, such as preservatives or dyes.

Pregnancy—Gentamicin topical preparations have not been shown to cause birth defects or other problems in humans.

Breast-feeding—Gentamicin topical preparations have not been reported to cause problems in nursing babies.

Children—This medicine has been tested in children over 1 year of age and, in effective doses, has not been shown to cause different side effects or problems than it does in adults.

Older adults—Many medicine have not been studied specifically in older people. Therefore, it may not be known whether they work exactly the same way they do in younger adults. Although there is no specific information comparing use of this medicine in the elderly with use in other age groups, this medicine is not expected to cause different side effects or problems in older people than it does in younger adults.

Other medicines—Although certain medicines should not be used together at all, in other cases two different medicines may be used together even if an interaction might occur. In these cases, your doctor may want to change the dose, or other precautions may be necessary. Tell your doctor and pharmacist if you are using any other topical prescription or nonprescription (over-the-counter [OTC]) medicine that is to be applied to the same area of the skin.

Before you begin using any new medicine (prescription or nonprescription) or if you develop any new medical problem while you are using this medicine, check with your doctor, nurse, or pharmacist.

Proper Use of This Medicine

Before applying this medicine, wash the affected area with soap and water, and dry thoroughly. Apply a small amount to the affected area and rub in gently.

After this medicine is applied, the treated area may be covered with a gauze dressing if desired.

To help clear up your infection completely, *keep using this medicine for the full time of treatment,* even though your symptoms may have disappeared. *Do not miss any doses.*

Missed dose—If you do miss a dose of this medicine, apply it as soon as possible. However, if it is almost time for your next dose, skip the missed dose and go back to your regular dosing schedule.

Storage—To store this medicine:

- Keep out of the reach of children.
- Store away from heat and direct light.
- Keep the medicine from freezing.
- Do not keep outdated medicine or medicine no longer needed. Be sure that any discarded medicine is out of the reach of children.

Precautions While Using This Medicine

If your skin problem does not improve within 1 week, or if it becomes worse, check with your doctor.

Side Effects of This Medicine

Along with its needed effects, a medicine may cause some unwanted effects. Although not all of these side effects may occur, if they do occur they may need medical attention.

Check with your doctor immediately if any of the following side effects occur:

Less common

Itching, redness, swelling, or other sign of irritation not present before use of this medicine

Other side effects not listed above may also occur in some patients. If you notice any other effects, check with your doctor.

Annual revision: 06/23/92

GENTIAN VIOLET Topical

Description

Gentian violet (JEN-shun VYE-oh-let) belongs to the group of medicines called antifungals. Topical gentian violet is used to treat some types of fungus infections inside the mouth (thrush) and of the skin.

Gentian violet is available without a prescription; however, your doctor may have special instructions on the proper use of gentian violet for your medical condition.

Gentian violet is available in the following dosage form:

Topical

- Solution (U.S.)

It is very important that you read and understand the following information. If any of it causes you special concern, check with your doctor or pharmacist. Also, *if you have any questions* or if you want more information about this medicine or your medical problem, *ask your doctor, nurse, or pharmacist.*

Before Using This Medicine

If you are using this medicine without a prescription, carefully read and follow any precautions on the label. For gentian violet, the following should be considered:

Allergies—Tell your doctor if you have ever had any unusual or allergic reaction to gentian violet. Also tell your doctor and pharmacist if you are allergic to any other substances, such as preservatives or dyes.

Pregnancy—Gentian violet topical solution has not been shown to cause birth defects or other problems in humans.

Breast-feeding—Gentian violet topical solution has not been reported to cause problems in nursing babies.

Children—Although there is no specific information comparing use of this medicine in children with use in other age groups, this medicine is not expected to cause different side effects or problems in children than it does in adults.

Older adults—Many medicine have not been studied specifically in older people. Therefore, it may not be known whether they work exactly the same way they do in younger adults. Although there is no specific information comparing use of this medicine in the elderly with use in other age groups, this medicine is not expected to cause different side effects or problems in older people than it does in younger adults.

Other medical problems—The presence of other medical problems may affect the use of gentian violet. Make sure you tell your doctor if you have any other medical problems, especially:

- Ulcerative skin condition on the face—Use of gentian violet may cause tatooing of the area

Before you begin using any new medicine (prescription or nonprescription) or if you develop any new medical problem while you are using this medicine, check with your doctor, nurse, or pharmacist.

Proper Use of This Medicine

Using a cotton swab, apply enough gentian violet to cover only the affected area.

If you are applying this medicine to affected areas in the mouth, avoid swallowing any of the medicine.

If you are using this medicine in a child's mouth, make sure you understand exactly how to apply it so that it is not swallowed. If you have any questions about this, check with your doctor, nurse, or pharmacist.

Do not apply an occlusive dressing (airtight covering such as, kitchen plastic wrap) over this medicine. It may cause irritation of the skin.

To help clear up your infection completely, *keep using this medicine for the full time of treatment,* even if your condition has improved. *Do not miss any doses.*

Missed dose—If you do miss a dose of this medicine, apply it as soon as possible. However, if it is almost time for your next dose, skip the missed dose and go back to your regular dosing schedule.

Storage—To store this medicine:

- Keep out of the reach of children.
- Store away from heat and direct light.
- Keep the medicine from freezing.
- Do not keep outdated medicine or medicine no longer needed. Be sure that any discarded medicine is out of the reach of children.

Precautions While Using This Medicine

Gentian violet will stain the skin and clothing. Avoid getting the medicine on your clothes.

Side Effects of This Medicine

Along with its needed effects, a medicine may cause some unwanted effects. Although not all of these side effects may occur, if they do occur they may need medical attention.

Check with your doctor as soon as possible if the following side effect occurs:

Skin irritation not present before use of this medicine

Other side effects not listed above may also occur in some patients. If you notice any other effects, check with your doctor.

Annual revision: 06/23/92

GENTIAN VIOLET Vaginal

A commonly used brand name in the U.S. is Genapax.

Description

Vaginal gentian violet (JEN-shun VYE-oh-let) is used to treat fungus (yeast) infections.

Vaginal gentian violet is available only with your doctor's prescription, in the following dosage form:

Vaginal

- Tampons (U.S.)

It is very important that you read and understand the following information. If any of it causes you special concern, check with your doctor. Also, *if you have any questions* or if you want more information about this medicine or your medical problem, *ask your doctor, nurse, or pharmacist.*

Before Using This Medicine

In deciding to use a medicine, the risks of using the medicine must be weighed against the good it will do. This is a decision you and your doctor will make. For gentian violet, the following should be considered:

Allergies—Tell your doctor if you have ever had any unusual or allergic reaction to gentian violet. Also tell your

doctor and pharmacist if you are allergic to any other substances, such as foods, preservatives, or dyes.

Pregnancy—Studies on effects in pregnancy have not been done in either humans or animals.

Breast-feeding—It is not known whether gentian violet, applied to the vagina, is absorbed into the body and passes into the breast milk. However, gentian violet tampons have not been reported to cause problems in nursing babies.

Children—Studies on this medicine have been done only in adult patients, and there is no specific information comparing use of vaginal gentian violet in children with use in other age groups.

Older adults—Many medicines have not been studied specifically in older people. Therefore, it may not be known whether they work exactly the same way they do in younger adults. Although there is no specific information comparing use of vaginal gentian violet in the elderly with use in other age groups, this medicine is not expected to cause different side effects or problems in older people than it does in younger adults.

Other medicines—Although certain medicines should not be used together at all, in other cases two different medicines may be used together even if an interaction might occur. In these cases, your doctor may want to change the dose, or other precautions may be necessary. Tell your doctor and pharmacist if you are using any other vaginal prescription or nonprescription (over-the-counter [OTC]) medicine.

Before you begin using any new medicine (prescription or nonprescription) or if you develop any new medical problem while you are using this medicine, check with your doctor, nurse, or pharmacist.

Proper Use of This Medicine

Gentian violet usually comes with patient directions. Read them carefully before using this medicine.

After insertion, remove the tampon from the vagina after 3 to 4 hours unless otherwise directed by your doctor.

To help clear up your infection completely, *keep using this medicine for the full time of treatment,* even though your condition may have improved. *Do not miss any doses.*

While you are using gentian violet tampons, the use of regular (non-medicated) tampons is not recommended. They will soak up the medicine that stays in the vagina after the gentian violet tampon is taken out. During your menstrual period you should wear a mini pad or sanitary napkin instead.

Missed dose—If you miss a dose of this medicine, insert it as soon as possible. However, if it is almost time for your next dose, skip the missed dose and go back to your regular dosing schedule.

Storage—To store this medicine:

- Keep out of the reach of children.
- Store away from heat and direct light.
- Do not keep outdated medicine or medicine no longer needed. Be sure that any discarded medicine is out of the reach of children.

Precautions While Using This Medicine

If your symptoms do not improve within a few days, or if they become worse, check with your doctor.

Gentian violet will stain the skin and clothing. Vaginal medicines usually will come out of the vagina during treatment. To keep the medicine from getting on your clothing, wear a minipad or sanitary napkin.

To help clear up your infection completely and to help make sure it does not return, good health habits are also needed.

- Wear cotton panties (or panties or pantyhose with cotton crotches) instead of synthetic (for example, nylon or rayon) panties.
- Wear only clean panties.

If you have any questions about this, check with your doctor, nurse, or pharmacist.

Many vaginal infections are spread by having sex. A male sexual partner may carry the germs on or in his penis. While you are using this medicine, it may be a good idea for your partner to wear a condom during sex to avoid re-infection. Also, your partner may need to be treated. *Do not stop using this medicine if you have sex during treatment.*

Some women may want to use a douche before putting each dose in the vagina. Some doctors will allow the use of a vinegar and water douche or other douche. However, others do not allow any douching. If you do use a douche, *do not overfill the vagina.* To do so may push the douche up into the uterus and possibly cause inflammation or infection. Also, *do not douche if you are pregnant since this may harm the fetus.* If you have any questions about this, check with your doctor, nurse, or pharmacist.

Side Effects of This Medicine

Along with its needed effects, a medicine may cause some unwanted effects. Although not all of these side effects may occur, if they do occur they may need medical attention.

Check with your doctor as soon as possible if any of the following side effects occur:

Vaginal burning, itching, pain, or other sign of irritation not present before use of this medicine

Other side effects not listed above may also occur in some patients. If you notice any other effects, check with your doctor.

Annual revision: 10/26/92

GLUCAGON Systemic

A commonly used brand name in the U.S. and Canada is Glucagon Emergency Kit.

Description

Glucagon (GLOO-ka-gon) belongs to the group of medicines called hormones. It is an emergency medicine used to treat severe hypoglycemia (low blood sugar) in patients with diabetes who have passed out or cannot take some form of sugar by mouth.

Glucagon is also used during x-ray tests of the stomach and bowels. Glucagon helps to improve test results by relaxing the muscles of the stomach and bowels. This also makes the testing more comfortable for the patient.

Glucagon may also be used for other conditions as determined by your doctor.

Glucagon is available only with your doctor's prescription, in the following dosage form:

Parenteral

- Injection (U.S. and Canada)

It is very important that you read and understand the following information. If any of it causes you special concern, check with your doctor. Also, *if you have any questions* or if you want more information about this medicine or your medical problem, *ask your doctor, nurse, or pharmacist.*

Before Using This Medicine

In deciding to use a medicine, the risks of taking the medicine must be weighed against the good it will do. This is a decision you and your doctor will make. For glucagon, the following should be considered:

Allergies—Tell your doctor if you have ever had any unusual or allergic reaction to glucagon or other proteins. Also, tell your doctor and pharmacist if you are allergic to any other substances, such as foods, preservatives, or dyes.

Pregnancy—Glucagon has not been studied in pregnant women. However, glucagon has not been shown to cause birth defects or other problems in animal studies.

Breast-feeding—It is not known whether glucagon passes into breast milk. However, this medicine has not been reported to cause problems in nursing babies.

Children—This medicine has been tested in children and, in effective doses, has not been shown to cause different side effects or problems than it does in adults.

Older adults—Many medicines have not been studied specifically in older people. Therefore, it may not be known whether they work exactly the same way they do in younger adults. Although there is no specific information comparing use of glucagon in the elderly with use in other age groups, it is not expected to cause different side effects or problems in older people than it does in younger adults.

Other medicines—Although certain medicines should not be used together at all, in other cases two different medicines may be used together even if an interaction might occur. In these cases, your doctor may want to change the doses or other precautions may be necessary. Tell your doctor and pharmacist if you are using any other prescription or nonprescription (over-the-counter [OTC]) medicine.

Other medical problems—The presence of other medical problems may affect the use of glucagon. Make sure you tell your doctor if you have any other medical problems, especially:

- Diabetes mellitus—When glucagon is used for test or x-ray procedures in diabetes that is well-controlled, too high blood sugar may occur; otherwise, glucagon is an important part of the management of diabetes because it is used to treat hypoglycemia (low blood sugar)
- Insulinoma (tumors of the pancreas gland that make too much insulin) (or history of)—Blood sugar concentrations may decrease
- Pheochromocytoma—Glucagon can cause high blood pressure

Before you begin using any new medicine (prescription or nonprescription) or if you develop any new medical problem while you are using this medicine, check with your doctor, nurse, or pharmacist.

Proper Use of This Medicine

Dosing—The dose of glucagon will be different for different patients. *Follow your doctor's orders or the directions on the label.* The following information includes only the average doses of glucagon. *If your dose is different, do not change it* unless your doctor tells you to do so.

- As an *emergency treatment for hypoglycemia:*
  —Adults and adolescents: 0.5 to 1 milligram. The dose may be repeated in 20 minutes if necessary.
  —Children: Dose is based on body weight (25 micrograms of glucagon per kilogram [11.4 micrograms per pound] of body weight). The dose may be repeated in 20 minutes if necessary.

Glucagon is an emergency medicine and must be used only as directed by your doctor. *Make sure that you and your family or a friend understand exactly when and how to use this medicine before it must be used.*

Some brands of glucagon come in a kit of 2 vials (one powder containing the medicine and one liquid to mix the medicine with). The contents of these 2 vials must be mixed before use. Other brands of glucagon are packaged in a kit with a vial of powder containing the medicine and a syringe filled with liquid to mix the medicine with. *Directions for mixing and injecting are in the package. Read them carefully* and ask your doctor, nurse, or pharmacist for additional explanation, if necessary.

If your glucagon kit does not already have a syringe in it, your doctor may want you to inject glucagon with the type of syringe you normally use to inject your insulin. Other patients may be told to use a different type of syringe that will allow a deeper injection. If you have any questions about the type of syringe you should be using, check with your doctor or nurse. Also, you should *regularly check to see if you have a sterile syringe and needles always available* to be used for the glucagon. It is a good idea to keep a sterile syringe taped to the glucagon carton.

Glucagon is usually mixed when an emergency occurs. However, it may be mixed ahead of time and kept in the refrigerator, ready for use. The date of mixing should then be written on the package. Mixed glucagon kept more than 48 hours (2 full days) (even if it is refrigerated) should be discarded and replaced by a fresh preparation.

Glucagon should not be mixed after the expiration date printed on the kit and on one vial. *Check the date regularly and replace the medicine before it expires.* The printed expiration date does not apply after mixing.

Storage—To store this medicine:

- Keep out of the reach of children.
- Store away from heat and direct light.
- Store the unmixed medication at room temperature.
- Do not store the unmixed or mixed medication in the bathroom, near the kitchen sink, or in other damp places. Heat or moisture may cause the medicine to break down.
- Store the mixed solution in the refrigerator for no longer than 48 hours. Do not allow it to freeze.
- Do not keep outdated medicine or medicine no longer needed. Be sure that any discarded medicine is out of the reach of children.

Precautions While Using This Medicine

Diabetic patients should be aware of the symptoms of hypoglycemia (low blood sugar). These symptoms may develop in a very short time and may result from:

- using too much insulin ("insulin reaction") or as a side effect from oral antidiabetes medicines.
- delaying or missing a scheduled snack or meal.
- sickness (especially with vomiting).
- exercising more than usual.

Unless corrected, hypoglycemia will lead to unconsciousness, convulsions (seizures), and possibly death. Early symptoms of hypoglycemia include:

Abdominal or stomach pain (mild)
Anxious feeling
Chills (continuing)
Cold sweats
Confusion
Cool pale skin
Difficulty in concentrating
Drowsiness
Excessive hunger
Fast heartbeat
Headache (continuing)
Nausea or vomiting (continuing)
Nervousness
Shakiness
Unsteady walk
Unusual tiredness or weakness
Vision changes

- Symptoms of hypoglycemia can differ from person to person. It is important that you learn your own signs of low blood sugar so that you can treat it quickly. It is a good idea also to check your blood sugar to confirm that it is low.
- *Eat or drink something containing sugar and check with your doctor right away if mild symptoms of low blood sugar (hypoglycemia) appear.* Doing this when symptoms of hypoglycemia first appear will usually prevent them from getting worse, and will probably make the use of glucagon unnecessary. Good sources of sugar include glucose tablets or gel, fruit juice, corn syrup, honey, nondiet soft drinks, or sugar cubes or table sugar (dissolved in water).
- *Tell someone to take you to your doctor or to a hospital right away if the symptoms do not improve after eating or drinking a sweet food. Do not try to drive yourself.*
- Even if you correct these symptoms by eating sugar, it is very important to call your doctor or hospital emergency service right away. Then, eat some food (such as crackers and cheese, half a sandwich, or

milk) to keep your blood sugar from going down again.
- Check your blood sugar again to make sure it is not still too low.
- *If severe symptoms such as convulsions (seizures) or unconsciousness occur, diabetics should not eat or drink anything.* There is a chance that they could choke from not swallowing correctly. Emergency medical help should be obtained immediately.

If it becomes necessary to inject glucagon in an unconscious patient, a family member or friend should know the following:
- *After injection, turn the unconscious patient on his or her side.* Glucagon may cause some patients to vomit and this position will reduce the possibility of choking.
- *Call the patient's doctor at once.*
- The patient should become conscious in less than 15 minutes after glucagon is injected into the muscle, but if not, a second dose may be given. *Get the patient to a doctor or to hospital emergency care as soon as possible,* since being unconscious too long can be harmful.
- *When the patient is conscious and can swallow, give some form of sugar.* Glucagon is not effective for much longer than 1½ hours and is *used only until the patient is able to swallow.* Fruit juice, corn syrup, honey, and sugar cubes or table sugar (dissolved in water) all work quickly. Then, if a snack or meal is not scheduled for an hour or more, the patient should also eat some crackers and cheese or half a sandwich, or drink a glass of milk. This will prevent hypoglycemia from occurring again before the next meal or snack.
- The patient or care-giver should continue to monitor the patient's blood sugar. For about 3 to 4 hours after the patient is conscious, check his or her blood sugar every hour.
- *If nausea prevents a patient from swallowing some form of sugar for an hour after glucagon is given, medical help should be obtained.*

Keep your doctor informed of any hypoglycemic episodes or use of glucagon even if the symptoms are successfully controlled and there seem to be no continuing problems. Complete information is necessary to provide the best possible treatment of any condition.

Replace your supply of glucagon as soon as possible, in case another hypoglycemic episode occurs.

You should wear a medical I.D. bracelet or chain at all times. In addition, you should carry an identification card that lists your medical conditions and medications.

Side Effects of This Medicine

Along with its needed effects, a medicine may cause some unwanted effects. Although not all of these side effects may occur, if they do occur they may need medical attention.

Get emergency help immediately if any of the following side effects occur:

Less common

Dizziness; lightheadedness; trouble in breathing

Symptoms of overdose

Irregular heartbeat; loss of appetite; muscle cramps or pain; nausea (continuing); vomiting (continuing); weakness of arms, legs, and trunk (severe)

Check with your doctor as soon as possible if any of the following side effects occur:

Less common

Skin rash or hives

Other side effects may occur that usually do not need medical attention. These side effects may go away during treatment as your body adjusts to the medicine. However, check with your doctor if any of the following side effects continue or are bothersome:

Nausea; vomiting

Other side effects not listed above may also occur in some patients. If you notice any other effects, check with your doctor.

Additional Information

Once a medicine has been approved for marketing for a certain use, experience may show that it is also useful for other medical problems. Although these uses are not included in product labeling, glucagon is used in certain patients with the following medical conditions or undergoing certain medical procedures:
- Overdose of beta-blocker medicines
- Overdose of calcium channel blockers
- Removing food or an object stuck in the esophagus
- Hysterosalpingography (x-ray examination of the uterus and fallopian tubes)

Other than the above information, there is no additional information relating to proper use, precautions, or side effects for these uses.

Annual revision: 01/13/93

GLUTETHIMIDE Systemic†

Generic name product may be available in the U.S.

†Not commercially available in Canada.

Description

Glutethimide (gloo-TETH-i-mide) is used to treat insomnia (trouble in sleeping). However, it has generally been replaced by safer and more effective medicines for the treatment of insomnia. If glutethimide is used regularly (for example, every day) to help produce sleep, it is usually not effective for more than 7 days.

This medicine is available only with your doctor's prescription, in the following dosage forms:

Oral

- Capsules (U.S.)
- Tablets (U.S.)

It is very important that you read and understand the following information. If any of it causes you special concern, check with your doctor. Also, *if you have any questions* or if you want more information about this medicine or your medical problem, *ask your doctor, nurse, or pharmacist.*

Before Using This Medicine

In deciding to use a medicine, the risks of taking the medicine must be weighed against the good it will do. This is a decision you and your doctor will make. For glutethimide the following should be considered:

Allergies—Tell your doctor if you have ever had any unusual or allergic reaction to glutethimide. Also tell your doctor or pharmacist if you are allergic to any other substances, such as foods, preservatives, or dyes.

Pregnancy—Studies of effects in pregnancy have not been done in either humans or animals. However, too much use of glutethimide during pregnancy may cause the baby to become dependent on the medicine. This may lead to withdrawal side effects after birth.

Breast-feeding—Glutethimide passes into the breast milk and may cause drowsiness in nursing babies.

Children—Studies on this medicine have been done only in adult patients and there is no specific information comparing use of glutethimide in children with use in other age groups.

Older adults—Elderly people may be especially sensitive to the effects of glutethimide. This may increase the chance of side effects during treatment.

Other medicines—Although certain medicines should not be used together at all, in other cases 2 different medicines may be used together even if an interaction might occur. In these cases, your doctor may want to change the dose, or other precautions may be necessary. When you are taking glutethimide it is especially important that your doctor and pharmacist know if you are taking any of the following:

- Anticoagulants (blood thinners)—Glutethimide may change the amount of anticoagulant you need to take
- Central nervous system (CNS) depressants, other (medicine that causes drowsiness) or
- Tricyclic antidepressants (medicine for depression)—Using these medicines together with glutethimide may increase the CNS and other depressant effects

Other medical problems—The presence of other medical problems may affect the use of glutethimide. Make sure you tell your doctor if you have any other medical problems, especially:

- Enlarged prostate or
- Intestinal blockage or
- Irregular heartbeat or
- Porphyria or
- Stomach ulcer or
- Urinary tract blockage—Glutethimide may make the condition worse
- Kidney disease—Higher blood levels of glutethimide may result and increase the chance of side effects

Before you begin using any new medicine (prescription or nonprescription) or if you develop any new medical problem while you are using this medicine, check with your doctor, nurse, or pharmacist.

Proper Use of This Medicine

Take this medicine only as directed by your doctor. Do not take more of it, do not take it more often, and do not take it for a longer time than your doctor ordered. If too much is taken, it may become habit-forming.

Dosing—The dose of glutethimide will be different for different patients. *Follow your doctor's orders or the directions on the label.* The following information includes only the average doses of glutethimide. *If your dose is different, do not change it* unless your doctor tells you to do so.

- For *oral* dosage forms (capsules or tablets):
  - —Adults: 500 milligrams (1 capsule or tablet) at bedtime.
  - —Children: Dose must be determined by the doctor.

Storage—To store this medicine:

- Keep out of the reach of children since overdose is especially dangerous in children.
- Store away from heat and direct light.

- Do not store in the bathroom, near the kitchen sink, or in other damp places. Heat or moisture may cause the medicine to break down.
- Do not keep outdated medicine or medicine no longer needed. Be sure that any discarded medicine is out of the reach of children.

Precautions While Using This Medicine

If you will be taking this medicine regularly for a long time:

- Your doctor should check your progress at regular visits.
- Do not stop taking it without first checking with your doctor. Your doctor may want you to reduce gradually the amount you are taking before stopping completely.

This medicine will add to the effects of alcohol and other CNS depressants (medicines that slow down the nervous system, possibly causing drowsiness). Some examples of CNS depressants are antihistamines or medicine for hay fever, other allergies, or colds; sedatives, tranquilizers, or sleeping medicine; prescription pain medicine or narcotics; barbiturates; medicine for seizures; muscle relaxants; or anesthetics, including some dental anesthetics. *Check with your doctor before taking any of the above while you are using this medicine.*

Before you have any medical tests, tell the doctor in charge that you are taking this medicine. The results of the metyrapone test may be affected by this medicine.

If you think you or someone else may have taken an overdose of this medicine, get emergency help at once. Taking an overdose of glutethimide or taking alcohol or other CNS depressants with glutethimide may lead to unconsciousness and possibly death. Some signs of an overdose are continuing confusion, severe weakness, shortness of breath or slow or troubled breathing, convulsions (seizures), slurred speech, staggering, and slow heartbeat.

This medicine may cause some people to become dizzy, drowsy, or less alert than they are normally. Even if taken at bedtime, it may cause some people to feel drowsy or less alert on arising. *Make sure you know how you react to this medicine before you drive, use machines, or do anything else that could be dangerous if you are dizzy or are not alert.*

Side Effects of This Medicine

Along with its needed effects, a medicine may cause some unwanted effects. Although not all of these side effects may occur, if they do occur they may need medical attention.

Check with your doctor as soon as possible if any of the following side effects occur:

Less common

Skin rash

Rare

Sore throat and fever; unusual bleeding or bruising; unusual excitement; unusual tiredness or weakness

Symptoms of overdose

Bluish coloration of skin; confusion (continuing); convulsions (seizures); fever; low body temperature; memory problems; muscle spasms or twitching; shortness of breath or slow or troubled breathing; slow heartbeat; slowness or loss of reflexes; slurred speech; staggering; trembling; trouble in concentrating; weakness (severe)

Other side effects may occur that usually do not need medical attention. These side effects may go away during treatment as your body adjusts to the medicine. However, check with your doctor if any of the following side effects continue or are bothersome:

More common

Drowsiness (daytime)

Less common

Blurred vision; clumsiness or unsteadiness; confusion; dizziness; "hangover" effect; headache; nausea; vomiting

After you stop using this medicine, your body may need time to adjust. The length of time this takes depends on the amount of medicine you were using and how long you used it. During this period of time check with your doctor if you notice any of the following side effects:

Convulsions (seizures); fast heartbeat; hallucinations (seeing, hearing, or feeling things that are not there); increased dreaming; muscle cramps or spasms; nausea or vomiting; nightmares; stomach cramps or pain; trembling; trouble in sleeping

Other side effects not listed above may also occur in some patients. If you notice any other effects, check with your doctor.

Annual revision: 05/12/93

GLYCERIN Systemic

Some commonly used brand names in the U.S. are Glyrol and Osmoglyn.

Generic name product may also be available in the U.S.

Description

Glycerin (GLI-ser-in), when taken by mouth, is used to treat certain conditions in which there is increased eye pressure, such as glaucoma. It may also be used before eye surgery to reduce pressure in the eye.

Glycerin may also be used for other conditions as determined by your doctor.

This medicine is available only with your doctor's prescription, in the following dosage form:

Oral

- Oral solution (U.S.)

It is very important that you read and understand the following information. If any of it causes you special concern, check with your doctor. Also, *if you have any questions* or if you want more information about this medicine or your medical problem, *ask your doctor, nurse, or pharmacist.*

Before Using This Medicine

In deciding to use a medicine, the risks of taking the medicine must be weighed against the good it will do. This is a decision you and your doctor will make. For glycerin, the following should be considered:

Allergies—Tell your doctor if you have ever had any unusual or allergic reaction to glycerin. Also tell your doctor and pharmacist if you are allergic to any other substances, such as foods, preservatives, or dyes.

Pregnancy—Studies have not been done in either humans or animals.

Breast-feeding—It is not known whether glycerin passes into breast milk. This medicine has not been reported to cause problems in nursing babies.

Children—Although there is no specific information comparing use of glycerin in children with use in other age groups, this medicine is not expected to cause different side effects or problems in children than it does in adults.

Older adults—Glycerin reduces water in the body, and there may be an increased risk that elderly patients taking it could become dehydrated.

Other medicines—Although certain medicines should not be used together at all, in other cases two different medicines may be used together even if an interaction might occur. In these cases, your doctor may want to change the dose, or other precautions may be necessary. Tell your doctor and pharmacist if you are taking any other prescription or nonprescription (over-the-counter [OTC]) medicine.

Other medical problems—The presence of other medical problems may affect the use of glycerin. Make sure you tell your doctor if you have any other medical problems, especially:

- Diabetes mellitus (sugar diabetes)—Use of glycerin may increase the chance of dehydration (loss of too much body water)
- Confused mental states or
- Heart disease or
- Kidney disease—Glycerin may make these conditions worse

Before you begin using any new medicine (prescription or nonprescription) or if you develop any new medical problem while you are using this medicine, check with your doctor, nurse, or pharmacist.

Proper Use of This Medicine

It is very important that you take this medicine only as directed. Do not take more of it and do not take it more often than your doctor ordered.

To improve the taste of this medicine, mix it with a small amount of unsweetened lemon, lime, or orange juice, pour over cracked ice, and sip through a straw.

Missed dose—If you miss a dose of this medicine, take it as soon as possible. However, if it is almost time for your next dose, skip the missed dose and go back to your regular dosing schedule. Do not double doses.

Storage—To store this medicine:

- Keep out of the reach of children.
- Store away from heat and direct light.
- Do not store in the bathroom, near the kitchen sink, or in other damp places. Heat or moisture may cause the medicine to break down.
- Keep the medicine from freezing.
- Do not keep outdated medicine or medicine no longer needed. Be sure that any discarded medicine is out of the reach of children.

Precautions While Using This Medicine

Your doctor should check your progress at regular visits to make sure that this medicine is working properly.

In some patients, headaches may occur when this medicine is taken. To help prevent or relieve the headache, lie down while you are taking this medicine and for a short time after taking it. If headaches become severe or continue, check with your doctor.

Side Effects of This Medicine

Along with its needed effects, a medicine may cause some unwanted effects. Although not all of these side effects may occur, if they do occur they may need medical attention.

Check with your doctor as soon as possible if either of the following side effects occurs:

Less common

Confusion

Rare

Irregular heartbeat

Other side effects may occur that usually do not need medical attention. These side effects may go away during treatment as your body adjusts to the medicine. However, check with your doctor if any of the following side effects continue or are bothersome:

More common

Headache; nausea or vomiting

Less common

Diarrhea; dizziness; dryness of mouth or increased thirst

Other side effects not listed above may also occur in some patients. If you notice any other effects, check with your doctor.

Additional Information

Once a medicine has been approved for marketing for a certain use, experience may show that it is also useful for other medical problems. Although this use is not included in product labeling, glycerin is used in certain patients with the following medical conditions:

- Cerebral edema (swelling of the brain)

Other than the above information, there is no additional information relating to proper use, precautions, or side effects for these uses.

Annual revision: 07/03/91

GOLD COMPOUNDS Systemic

This information applies to the following medicines:

Auranofin (au-RANE-oh-fin)
Aurothioglucose (aur-oh-thye-oh-GLOO-kose)
Gold Sodium Thiomalate (gold SO-dee-um thye-oh-MAH-late)

Some commonly used brand names are:

For Auranofin
In the U.S.
Ridaura
In Canada
Ridaura

For Aurothioglucose
In the U.S.
Solganal

For Gold Sodium Thiomalate
In the U.S.
Myochrysine
Generic name product may also be available.
In Canada
Myochrysine

Another commonly used name is sodium aurothiomalate.

Description

The gold compounds are used in the treatment of rheumatoid arthritis. They may also be used for other conditions as determined by your doctor.

In addition to the helpful effects of this medicine in treating your medical problem, it has side effects that can be very serious. Before you take this medicine, you should discuss with your doctor the good that this medicine will do as well as the risks of using it.

Auranofin is available only with your doctor's prescription. The other gold compounds are given by your doctor or nurse.

These medicines are available in the following dosage forms:

Oral

Auranofin
- Capsules (U.S. and Canada)

Parenteral

Aurothioglucose
- Injection (U.S.)

Gold sodium thiomalate
- Injection (U.S. and Canada)

It is very important that you read and understand the following information. If any of it causes you special concern, check with your doctor. Also, *if you have any questions* or if you want more information about this medicine or your medical problem, *ask your doctor, nurse, or pharmacist.*

Before Using This Medicine

In deciding to use a medicine, the risks of taking the medicine must be weighed against the good it will do. This is a decision you and your doctor will make. For gold compounds, the following should be considered:

Allergies—Tell your doctor if you have ever had any unusual or allergic reaction to gold or other metals, if you have received a gold compound before and developed serious side effects from it, or if any medicine you have taken has caused an allergy or a reaction that affected your blood. Also tell your doctor and pharmacist if you are allergic to any other substances, such as foods, preservatives, or dyes.

Pregnancy—Studies on birth defects with gold compounds have not been done in humans. However, studies in animals have shown that gold compounds may cause birth defects.

Breast-feeding—Aurothioglucose and gold sodium thiomalate pass into the breast milk and may cause unwanted effects in nursing babies. It is not known whether auranofin passes into the breast milk.

Children—Auranofin has been tested only in adult patients and there is no specific information about its use in children. However, aurothioglucose and gold sodium thiomalate have been tested in children and have not been shown to cause different side effects or problems than they do in adults.

Older adults—These medicines have been tested and have not been shown to cause different side effects or problems in older people than they do in younger adults.

Other medicines—Although certain medicines should not be used together at all, in other cases two different medicines may be used together even if an interaction might occur. In these cases, your doctor may want to change the dose, or other precautions may be necessary. When you are taking a gold compound, it is important that your doctor and pharmacist know if you are taking *any* other prescription or nonprescription (over-the-counter [OTC]) medicine, especially:

- Penicillamine (e.g., Cuprimine)—The chance of side effects may be increased.

Other medical problems—The presence of other medical problems may affect the use of gold compounds. Make sure you tell your doctor if you have any other medical problems, especially:

- Blood or blood vessel disease or
- Colitis or
- Kidney disease (or history of) or
- Lupus erythematosus or
- Sjögren's syndrome or
- Skin disease—The chance of unwanted effects may be increased

Before you begin using any new medicine (prescription or nonprescription) or if you develop any new medical problem while you are using this medicine, check with your doctor, nurse, or pharmacist.

Proper Use of This Medicine

In order for this medicine to work, it must be taken regularly as ordered by your doctor. Continue receiving the injections or taking auranofin even if you think the medicine is not working. You may not notice the effects of this medicine until after three to six months of regular use.

For patients taking *auranofin:*

- *Do not take more of this medicine than ordered by your doctor.* Taking too much auranofin may increase the chance of serious unwanted effects.

If you have any questions about this, check with your doctor.

Missed dose—For patients taking *auranofin:* If you miss a dose of this medicine, and your dosing schedule is—

- One dose a day—Take the missed dose as soon as possible. However, if you do not remember until the next day, skip the missed dose and go back to your regular dosing schedule. Do not double doses.
- More than one dose a day—Take the missed dose as soon as possible. However, if it is almost time for your next dose, skip the missed dose and go back to your regular dosing schedule. Do not double doses.

Storage—To store this medicine:

- Keep out of the reach of children.
- Store away from heat and direct light.
- Do not store this medicine in the bathroom, near the kitchen sink, or in other damp places. Heat or moisture may cause the medicine to break down.
- Do not keep outdated medicine or medicine no longer needed. Be sure that any discarded medicine is out of the reach of children.

Precautions While Using This Medicine

Gold compounds may cause some people to become more sensitive to sunlight than they are normally. These people may break out in a rash after being in the sun, or a skin rash that is already present may become worse. To protect yourself, it is best to:

- Stay out of direct sunlight, especially between the hours of 10:00 a.m. and 3:00 p.m., if possible.
- Wear protective clothing.
- Ask your doctor if you may apply a sun block product. Products that have a skin protection factor (SPF)

of at least 15 work best, but some patients may require a product with a higher SPF number, especially if they have a fair complexion.

- Do not use a sunlamp or tanning bed or booth.

If you have a severe reaction from the sun, check with your doctor.

For patients taking *auranofin:*

- Your doctor should check your progress at regular visits. Blood and urine tests may be needed to make certain that this medicine is not causing unwanted effects.

For patients receiving *gold injections:*

- Immediately following an injection of this medicine, side effects such as dizziness, feeling faint, flushing or redness of the face, nausea or vomiting, increased sweating, or unusual weakness may occur. These will usually go away after you lie down for a few minutes. If any of these effects continue or become worse, or if you notice any other effects within 10 minutes or so after receiving an injection, tell your doctor or nurse right away.
- Joint pain may occur for 1 or 2 days after you receive an injection of this medicine. This effect usually disappears after the first few injections. However, if this continues or is bothersome, check with your doctor.

Side Effects of This Medicine

Gold compounds have been shown to cause tumors and cancer of the kidney when given to animals in large amounts for a long time. However, these effects have not been reported in humans receiving gold compounds for arthritis. If you have any questions about this, check with your doctor.

Along with its needed effects, a medicine may cause some unwanted effects. Although not all of these side effects may occur, side effects may occur at any time during treatment with this medicine *and up to many months after treatment has ended,* and they may need medical attention.

Check with your doctor as soon as possible if any of the following side effects occur:

More common

Irritation or soreness of tongue—less common with auranofin; metallic taste—less common with auranofin; skin rash or itching; redness, soreness, swelling, or bleeding of gums—rare with auranofin; ulcers, sores, or white spots on lips or in mouth or throat

Less common

Bloody or cloudy urine; hives

Rare

Abdominal or stomach pain, cramping, or burning (severe); bloody or black, tarry stools; confusion; convulsions (seizures); coughing, hoarseness, difficulty in breathing, shortness of breath, tightness in chest, or wheezing; dark urine; decreased urination; decreased vision; difficulty in swallowing; feeling of something in the eye; fever; hair loss; hallucinations (hearing, seeing, or feeling things that are not there); irritation of nose, throat, or upper chest area, possibly with hoarseness or coughing; irritation of vagina; nausea, vomiting, or heartburn (severe and/or continuing); numbness, tingling, pain, or weakness, especially in the face, hands, arms, or feet; pale stools; painful or difficult urination; pain in lower back, side, or lower abdomen (stomach) area; pain, redness, itching, or tearing of eyes; pinpoint red spots on skin; problems with muscle coordination; red, thickened, or scaly skin; sore throat and fever with or without chills; swelling of face, fingers, ankles, lower legs, or feet; swellings (large) on face, eyelids, mouth, lips, and/or tongue; swollen and/or painful glands; unusual bleeding or bruising; unusual tiredness or weakness; vomiting of blood or material that looks like coffee grounds; yellow eyes or skin

Other side effects may occur that usually do not need medical attention. These side effects may go away during treatment as your body adjusts to the medicine. However, check with your doctor if the following side effects continue or are bothersome:

More common with auranofin; rare with injections

Abdominal or stomach cramps or pain (mild or moderate); bloated feeling, gas, or indigestion (mild or moderate); decrease or loss of appetite; diarrhea or loose stools; nausea or vomiting (mild or moderate)

Less common

Constipation—with auranofin; joint pain—with injections

Some patients receiving auranofin have noticed changes in the taste of certain foods. If you notice a metallic taste while receiving any gold compound, check with your doctor as soon as possible. If you notice any other taste changes while you are taking auranofin, it is not necessary to check with your doctor unless you find this effect especially bothersome.

Other side effects not listed above may also occur in some patients. If you notice any other effects, check with your doctor.

Annual revision: June 1990

GONADORELIN Systemic

A commonly used brand name in the U.S. and Canada is Factrel.

Other commonly used names are gonadotropin-releasing hormone, GnRH, and LHRH.

Description

Gonadorelin (goe-nad-oh-RELL-in) is a medicine that is the same as gonadotropin-releasing hormone (GnRH) that is naturally released from the hypothalamus gland. GnRH causes the pituitary gland to release other hormones (luteinizing hormone [LH] and follicle-stimulating hormone [FSH]). These other hormones control development in children and fertility in adults.

Gonadorelin is used to test how well the hypothalamus and the pituitary glands are working. It is also used to cause ovulation (release of an egg from the ovary) in women who do not have regular ovulation and menstrual periods because the hypothalamus gland does not release enough GnRH.

Gonadorelin may also be used for other conditions as determined by your doctor.

Gonadorelin is available in the following dosage form:

Parenteral

- Injection (U.S. and Canada)

It is very important that you read and understand the following information. If any of it causes you special concern, check with your doctor. Also, *if you have any questions* or if you want more information about this medicine or your medical problem, *ask your doctor, nurse, or pharmacist.*

Before Using This Medicine

In deciding to use a medicine, the risks of using the medicine must be weighed against the good it will do. This is a decision you and your doctor will make. For gonadorelin, the following should be considered:

Allergies—Tell your doctor if you have ever had any unusual or allergic reaction to gonadorelin. Also tell your doctor and pharmacist if you are allergic to any other substances, such as foods, preservatives, or dyes.

Pregnancy—Gonadorelin has not been studied in pregnant women. However, it has not been shown to cause birth defects or other problems in animal studies.

Breast-feeding—Gonadorelin has not been reported to cause problems in nursing babies.

Children—This medicine has been tested and used in children and, in effective doses, has not been shown to cause different side effects or problems in children than it does in adults.

Other medicines—Although certain medicines should not be used together at all, in other cases two different medicines may be used together even if an interaction might occur. In these cases, your doctor may want to change the dose, or other precautions may be necessary. When you are using gonadorelin, it is especially important that your doctor and pharmacist know if you are taking any other prescription or nonprescription (over-the-counter [OTC]) medicine.

Before you begin using any new medicine (prescription or nonprescription) or if you develop any new medical problem while you are using this medicine, check with your doctor, nurse, or pharmacist.

Proper Use of This Medicine

If you are having a test done with gonadorelin, one or more samples of your blood will be taken. Then gonadorelin is given by an intravenous (into a vein) or a subcutaneous (under the skin) injection. At regular times after it is given, more blood samples will be taken. Then the results of the test will be studied.

Side Effects of This Medicine

Along with its needed effects, a medicine may cause some unwanted effects. Although the following side effects usually occur rarely with the use of repeated injections, they require immediate medical attention. *Get emergency help immediately* if any of the following side effects occur:

Difficulty in breathing; flushing (continuing)

Check with your doctor as soon as possible if any of the following side effects occur:

With repeated doses

Hardening of skin around place of injection; hives; skin rash (at place of injection or over entire body)

Other side effects may occur that usually do not need medical attention. These side effects may go away during treatment as your body adjusts to the medicine. However, check with your doctor if any of the following side effects continue or are bothersome:

Less common

Abdominal or stomach discomfort; flushing (lasting only a short time); headaches; itching, pain, or swelling at place of injection; lightheadedness; nausea

Other side effects not listed above may also occur in some patients. If you notice any other effects, check with your doctor.

Additional Information

Once a medicine has been approved for marketing for a certain use, experience may show that it is also useful for other medical problems. Although not specifically included in product labeling, gonadorelin is used in certain patients with the following medical conditions:

- Delayed puberty
- Infertility in males

Other than the above information, there is no additional information relating to proper use, precautions, or side effects for these uses.

Annual revision: August 1990

GOSERELIN Systemic

A commonly used brand name in the U.S. and Canada is Zoladex.

Description

Goserelin (GOE-se-rel-in) is used to treat cancer of the prostate gland. It is usually given once a month.

Goserelin is similar to a hormone normally released from the hypothalamus gland. When given regularly, it decreases testosterone levels. Reducing the amount of testosterone in the body is one way of treating cancer of the prostate.

Goserelin is to be given only by or under the supervision of your doctor. It is injected under the skin and is available in the following dosage form:

Parenteral

- Implants (U.S. and Canada)

It is very important that you read and understand the following information. If any of it causes you special concern, check with your doctor. Also, *if you have any questions* or if you want more information about this medicine or your medical problem, *ask your doctor, nurse, or pharmacist.*

Before Using This Medicine

In deciding to use a medicine, the risks of taking the medicine must be weighed against the good it will do. This is a decision you and your doctor will make. For goserelin, the following should be considered:

Allergies—Tell your doctor if you have ever had any unusual or allergic reaction to goserelin.

Fertility—Goserelin causes sterility which may be permanent. If you intend to have children, discuss this with your doctor before receiving this medicine.

Older adults—Many medicines have not been tested in older people. Therefore, it may not be known whether they work exactly the same way they do in younger adults. Although there is no specific information comparing use of goserelin in the elderly to use in other age groups, it has been used mostly in elderly patients and is not expected to cause different side effects or problems in older people than it does in younger adults.

Before you begin using any new medicine (prescription or nonprescription) or if you develop any new medical problem while you are using this medicine, check with your doctor, nurse, or pharmacist.

Proper Use of This Medicine

Goserelin sometimes causes unwanted effects such as hot flashes or decreased sexual ability. It may also cause a temporary increase in pain, numbness or tingling of hands or feet, trouble in urinating, or weakness in your legs when you begin treatment with it. However, it is very important that you continue to receive the medicine, even after you begin to feel better. *Do not stop treatment with this medicine without first checking with your doctor.*

Missed dose—If you miss getting a dose of this medicine, get it as soon as possible.

Precautions While Using This Medicine

It is very important that your doctor check your progress at regular visits to make sure that this medicine is working properly and to check for unwanted effects.

Side Effects of This Medicine

Along with its needed effects, a medicine may cause some unwanted effects. Although not all of these side effects may occur, if they do occur they may need medical attention.

The following side effects are symptoms of a flareup of your condition that may occur during the first few days of treatment. After a few days, these symptoms should lessen. However, they may need medical attention. Check with your doctor if any of the following side effects occur or get worse:

Bone pain; numbness or tingling of hands or feet; trouble in urinating; weakness in legs

Also check with your doctor as soon as possible if any of the following side effects occur:

Less common

Chest pain; irregular heartbeat; joint pain; painful or cold hands or feet; shortness of breath; skin rash; weakness (sudden)

Other side effects may occur that usually do not need medical attention. These side effects may go away during treatment as your body adjusts to the medicine. However, check with your doctor if any of the following side effects continue or are bothersome:

More common

Decrease in sexual desire; impotence; sudden sweating and feelings of warmth ("hot flashes")

Less common

Anxiety or mental depression; constipation; diarrhea; dizziness; headache; loss of appetite; nausea or vomiting; swelling and increased tenderness of breasts; swelling of feet or lower legs; trouble in sleeping; unusual tiredness or weakness; weight gain

Other side effects not listed above may also occur in some patients. If you notice any other effects, check with your doctor.

Annual revision: July 1990

GRISEOFULVIN Systemic

Some commonly used brand names are:

In the U.S.

Fulvicin P/G	Grisactin
Fulvicin-U/F	Grisactin Ultra
Grifulvin V	Gris-PEG

In Canada

Fulvicin P/G	Grisovin-FP
Fulvicin U/F	

Description

Griseofulvin (gri-see-oh-FUL-vin) belongs to the group of medicines called antifungals. It is used to treat fungus infections of the skin, hair, fingernails, and toenails. This medicine may be taken alone or used along with medicines that are applied to the skin for fungus infections.

Griseofulvin is available only with your doctor's prescription, in the following dosage forms:

Oral

- Capsules (U.S.)
- Suspension (U.S.)
- Tablets (U.S. and Canada)

It is very important that you read and understand the following information. If any of it causes you special concern, check with your doctor. Also, *if you have any questions* or if you want more information about this medicine or your medical problem, *ask your doctor, nurse, or pharmacist.*

Before Using This Medicine

In deciding to use a medicine, the risks of taking the medicine must be weighed against the good it will do. This is a decision you and your doctor will make. For griseofulvin, the following should be considered:

Allergies—Tell your doctor if you have ever had any unusual or allergic reaction to penicillins, penicillamine (e.g., Cuprimine), or griseofulvin. Also tell your doctor and pharmacist if you are allergic to any other substances, such as foods, preservatives, or dyes.

Diet—Griseofulvin is absorbed best when it is taken with a high fat meal, such as a cheeseburger, whole milk, or ice cream. Tell your doctor if you are on a low-fat diet.

Pregnancy—Griseofulvin should not be used during pregnancy. The birth of twins that were joined together has been reported, although rarely, in women who took griseofulvin during the first 3 months of pregnancy. In addition, studies in rats and dogs have shown that griseofulvin causes birth defects and other problems.

Breast-feeding—It is not known if griseofulvin is excreted in breast milk. However, griseofulvin has not been reported to cause problems in nursing babies.

Children—This medicine has been tested in a limited number of children 2 years of age or older. In effective doses, the medicine has not been shown to cause different side effects or problems than it does in adults.

Older adults—Many medicines have not been studied specifically in older people. Therefore, it may not be known whether they work exactly the same way they do in younger adults. Although there is no specific information comparing use of griseofulvin in the elderly with use in other age groups, this medicine is not expected to cause different side effects or problems in older people than it does in younger adults.

Other medicines—Although certain medicines should not be used together at all, in other cases two different medicines may be used together even if an interaction might occur. In these cases, your doctor may want to change the dose, or other precautions may be necessary. When you are taking griseofulvin, it is especially important that your doctor and pharmacist know if you are taking any of the following:

- Anticoagulants (blood thinners)—Griseofulvin may decrease the effectiveness of anticoagulants in some patients
- Oral contraceptives (birth control pills) containing estrogen—Griseofulvin may decrease the effectiveness of birth control pills, which may result in breakthrough bleeding and unwanted pregnancies

Other medical problems—The presence of other medical problems may affect the use of griseofulvin. Make sure you tell your doctor if you have any other medical problems, especially:

- Liver disease—Griseofulvin may on rare occasion cause side effects affecting the liver
- Lupus erythematosus or lupus-like diseases—Griseofulvin may worsen lupus symptoms in patients who have lupus erythematosus or lupus-like diseases
- Porphyria—Griseofulvin may increase attacks of porphyria in patients with acute intermittent porphyria

Before you begin using any new medicine (prescription or nonprescription) or if you develop any new medical problem while you are using this medicine, check with your doctor, nurse, or pharmacist.

Proper Use of This Medicine

Griseofulvin is best taken with or after meals, especially fatty ones (for example, whole milk or ice cream). This lessens possible stomach upset and helps to clear up the infection by helping your body absorb the medicine better. *However, if you are on a low-fat diet, check with your doctor.*

For patients taking the *oral liquid form of griseofulvin:*

- Use a specially marked measuring spoon or other device to measure each dose accurately. The average household teaspoon may not hold the right amount of liquid.

To help clear up your infection completely, *keep taking this medicine for the full time of treatment,* even if you begin to feel better after a few days. *Do not miss any doses.*

Missed dose—If you do miss a dose of this medicine, take it as soon as possible. However, if it is almost time for your next dose, skip the missed dose and go back to your regular dosing schedule. Do not double doses.

Storage—To store this medicine:

- Keep out of the reach of children.
- Store away from heat and direct light.
- Do not store the capsule or tablet form of this medicine in the bathroom, near the kitchen sink, or in other damp places. Heat or moisture may cause the medicine to break down.
- Keep the oral liquid form of this medicine from freezing.
- Do not keep outdated medicine or medicine no longer needed. Be sure that any discarded medicine is out of the reach of children.

Precautions While Using This Medicine

Your doctor should check your progress at regular visits to make sure that griseofulvin does not cause unwanted effects.

Oral contraceptives (birth control pills) containing estrogen may not work properly if you take them while you are taking griseofulvin. Unplanned pregnancies may occur. You should use a different or additional means of birth control while you are taking griseofulvin and for one month after stopping griseofulvin. If you have any questions about this, check with your doctor or pharmacist.

Griseofulvin may increase the effects of alcohol. If taken with alcohol it may also cause fast heartbeat, flushing, increased sweating, or redness of the face. Therefore, if you have this reaction, do not drink alcoholic beverages while you are taking this medicine, unless you have first checked with your doctor.

This medicine may cause some people to become dizzy or less alert than they are normally. *Make sure you know how you react to this medicine before you drive, use machines, or do other things that could be dangerous if you are dizzy or are not alert.* If these reactions are especially bothersome, check with your doctor.

Griseofulvin may cause your skin to be more sensitive to sunlight than it is normally. Exposure to sunlight, even for brief periods of time, may cause a skin rash, itching, redness or other discoloration of the skin, or a severe sunburn. When you begin taking this medicine:

- Stay out of direct sunlight, especially between the hours of 10:00 a.m. and 3:00 p.m., if possible.
- Wear protective clothing, including a hat. Also, wear sunglasses.
- Apply a sun block product that has a skin protection factor (SPF) of at least 15. Some patients may require a product with a higher SPF number, especially if they have a fair complexion. If you have any questions about this, check with your doctor or pharmacist.
- Apply a sun block lipstick that has an SPF of at least 15 to protect your lips.
- Do not use a sunlamp or tanning bed or booth.

If you have a severe reaction from the sun, check with your doctor.

Side Effects of This Medicine

Griseofulvin has been shown to cause liver and thyroid tumors in some animals. *You and your doctor should discuss the good this medicine will do, as well as the risks of taking it.*

Along with its needed effects, a medicine may cause some unwanted effects. Although not all of these side effects may occur, if they do occur they may need medical attention.

Check with your doctor as soon as possible if any of the following side effects occur:

Less common

Confusion; increased sensitivity of skin to sunlight; skin rash, hives, or itching; soreness or irritation of mouth or tongue

Rare

Numbness, tingling, pain, or weakness in hands or feet; sore throat and fever; yellow eyes or skin

Other side effects may occur that usually do not need medical attention. These side effects may go away during treatment as your body adjusts to the medicine. However, check with your doctor if any of the following side effects continue or are bothersome:

More common

Headache

Less common

Diarrhea; dizziness; nausea or vomiting; stomach pain; trouble in sleeping; unusual tiredness

Other side effects not listed above may also occur in some patients. If you notice any other effects, check with your doctor.

Annual revision: 09/06/92

GROWTH HORMONE Systemic

This information applies to the following medicines:

Somatrem (SOE-ma-trem)
Somatropin (soe-ma-TROE-pin)

Some commonly used brand names are:

For Somatrem

In the U.S.
Protropin

In Canada
Protropin

For Somatropin

In the U.S.
Humatrope

In Canada
Humatrope

Other commonly used names are GH and human growth hormone (hGH).

Description

Somatrem and somatropin are man-made versions of human growth hormone. Growth hormone is naturally produced by the pituitary gland and is necessary to stimulate growth in children. If a child fails to grow normally because his or her body is not producing enough growth hormone, this medicine may be used to stimulate growth.

This medicine is available only with your doctor's prescription, in the following dosage forms:

Parenteral

Somatrem
- Injection (U.S. and Canada)

Somatropin
- Injection (U.S. and Canada)

It is very important that you read and understand the following information. If any of it causes you special concern, check with your doctor. Also, *if you have any questions* or if you want more information about this medicine or your medical problem, *ask your doctor, nurse, or pharmacist*.

Before Using This Medicine

In deciding to use a medicine, the risks of taking the medicine must be weighed against the good it will do. This is a decision you and your doctor will make. For growth hormone, the following should be considered:

Allergies—Tell your doctor if you have ever had any unusual or allergic reaction to growth hormone. Also tell your doctor and pharmacist if you are allergic to any other substances, such as foods, preservatives, or dyes.

Other medicines—Although certain medicines should not be used together at all, in other cases two different medicines may be used together even if an interaction might occur. In these cases, your doctor may want to change the dose, or other precautions may be necessary. When you are taking growth hormone, it is especially important that your doctor and pharmacist know if you are taking any of the following:

- Corticosteroids (cortisone-like medicines)—These medicines can interfere with the effects of growth hormone

Other medical problems—The presence of other medical problems may affect the use of growth hormone. Make sure you tell your doctor if you have any other medical problems, especially:

- Underactive thyroid—This condition can interfere with the effects of growth hormone

Before you begin using any new medicine (prescription or nonprescription) or if you develop any new medical problem while you are using this medicine, check with your doctor, nurse, or pharmacist.

Precautions While Using This Medicine

It is important that your doctor check your progress at regular visits.

Side Effects of This Medicine

Leukemia has been reported in a few patients after treatment with growth hormone. However, it is not definitely known whether the leukemia was caused by the growth hormone. Leukemia has also been reported in patients whose bodies do not make enough growth hormone and who have not yet been treated with man-made growth hormone. However, discuss this possible effect with your doctor.

If hGH is given to children or adults with normal growth, who do not need growth hormone, serious unwanted effects may occur because levels in the body become too high. These effects include the development of diabetes, abnormal growth of bones and internal organs such as the heart, kidneys, and liver, atherosclerosis (hardening of the arteries), and hypertension (high blood pressure).

Along with its needed effects, a medicine may cause some unwanted effects. Although not all of these side effects may occur, if they do occur they may need medical attention. When growth hormone is used to promote growth in children who have a lack of naturally produced human growth hormone, serious side effects do not usually occur. However, check with your doctor as soon as possible if any of the following side effects occur:

Rare

Limp; pain and swelling at place of injection; pain in hip or knee; skin rash or itching

Other side effects not listed above may also occur in some patients. If you notice any other effects, check with your doctor.

Annual revision: 11/18/92

GUAIFENESIN Systemic

Some commonly used brand names are:

In the U.S.

Amonidrin	Humibid L.A.
Anti-Tuss	Humibid Sprinkle
Breonesin	Hytuss
Gee-Gee	Hytuss-2X
Genatuss	Malotuss
GG-CEN	Mytussin
Glyate	Naldecon Senior EX
Glycotuss	Nortussin
Glytuss	Robafen
Guiatuss	Robitussin
Halotussin	Scot-tussin

Generic name product may also be available.

In Canada

Balminil Expectorant	Robitussin
Resyl	

Another commonly used name is glyceryl guaiacolate.

Description

Guaifenesin (gwye-FEN-e-sin) is used to relieve coughs due to colds or influenza. Guaifenesin works by loosening the mucus or phlegm (pronounced flem) in the lungs.

This medicine is not to be used for the chronic cough that occurs with smoking, asthma, or emphysema or when there is an unusually large amount of mucus or phlegm with the cough.

Guaifenesin is available without a prescription; however, your doctor may have special instructions on the proper dose of this medicine for your medical condition. It is available in the following dosage forms:

Oral

- Capsules (U.S.)
- Extended-release capsules (U.S.)
- Oral solution (U.S.)
- Syrup (U.S. and Canada)
- Tablets (U.S. and Canada)
- Extended-release tablets (U.S.)

It is very important that you read and understand the following information. If any of it causes you special concern, check with your doctor or pharmacist. Also, *if you have any questions* or if you want more information about this medicine or your medical problem, *ask your doctor, nurse, or pharmacist.*

Before Using This Medicine

If you are taking this medicine without a prescription, carefully read and follow any precautions on the label. For guaifenesin, the following should be considered:

Allergies—Tell your doctor if you have ever had any unusual or allergic reaction to guaifenesin. Also tell your doctor and pharmacist if you are allergic to any other substances, such as foods, preservatives, or dyes.

Pregnancy—Studies have not been done in either humans or animals.

Breast-feeding—Guaifenesin has not been reported to cause problems in nursing babies.

Children—Although there is no specific information comparing use of guaifenesin in children with use in other age groups, this medicine is not expected to cause different side effects or problems in children than it does in adults.

Older adults—Many medicines have not been studied specifically in older people. Therefore, it may not be known whether they work exactly the same way they do in younger adults. Although there is no specific information comparing use of guaifenesin in the elderly with use in other age groups, this medicine is not expected to cause different side effects or problems in older people than it does in younger adults.

Before you begin using any new medicine (prescription or nonprescription) or if you develop any new medical problem while you are using this medicine, check with your doctor, nurse, or pharmacist.

Proper Use of This Medicine

To help loosen mucus or phlegm in the lungs, *drink a glass of water after each dose of this medicine,* unless otherwise directed by your doctor.

For patients taking the *extended-release tablet* form of this medicine:

- Swallow the tablet whole. Do not crush, break, or chew before swallowing.

Missed dose—If you must take this medicine regularly and you miss a dose, take it as soon as possible. However, if it is almost time for your next dose, skip the missed dose and go back to your regular dosing schedule. Do not double doses.

Storage—To store this medicine:

- Keep out of the reach of children.
- Store away from heat and direct light.
- Do not store the capsule or tablet form of this medicine in the bathroom, near the kitchen sink, or in other damp places. Heat or moisture may cause the medicine to break down.
- Do not refrigerate the syrup form of this medicine.
- Do not keep outdated medicine or medicine no longer needed. Be sure that any discarded medicine is out of the reach of children.

Precautions While Using This Medicine

If your cough has not improved after 7 days or if you have a high fever, skin rash, continuing headache, or sore throat with the cough, check with your doctor. These signs may mean that you have other medical problems.

Side Effects of This Medicine

Along with its needed effects, a medicine may cause some unwanted effects. Although not all of these side effects may occur, if they do occur they may need medical attention.

Check with your doctor as soon as possible if any of the following side effects occur:

Less common or rare

Diarrhea; drowsiness; nausea or vomiting; stomach pain

Other side effects not listed above may also occur in some patients. If you notice any other effects, check with your doctor.

Annual revision: 05/15/91

GUANABENZ Systemic†

A commonly used brand name in the U.S. is Wytensin.

†Not commercially available in Canada.

Description

Guanabenz (GWAHN-a-benz) belongs to the general class of medicines called antihypertensives. It is used to treat high blood pressure (hypertension).

High blood pressure adds to the workload of the heart and arteries. If it continues for a long time, the heart and arteries may not function properly. This can damage the blood vessels of the brain, heart, and kidneys, resulting in a stroke, heart failure, or kidney failure. High blood pressure may also increase the risk of heart attacks. These problems may be less likely to occur if blood pressure is controlled.

Guanabenz works by controlling nerve impulses along certain nerve pathways. As a result, it relaxes blood vessels so that blood passes through them more easily. This helps to lower blood pressure.

Guanabenz is available only with your doctor's prescription, in the following dosage form:

Oral

- Tablets (U.S.)

It is very important that you read and understand the following information. If any of it causes you special concern, check with your doctor. Also, *if you have any questions* or if you want more information about this medicine or your medical problem, *ask your doctor, nurse, or pharmacist.*

Before Using This Medicine

In deciding to use a medicine, the risks of taking the medicine must be weighed against the good it will do. This is a decision you and your doctor will make. For guanabenz, the following should be considered:

Allergies—Tell your doctor if you have ever had any unusual or allergic reaction to guanabenz. Also tell your doctor and pharmacist if you are allergic to any other substance, such as foods, preservatives, or dyes.

Pregnancy—Guanabenz has not been studied in pregnant women. However, studies in rats have shown that guanabenz given in doses 9 to 10 times the maximum human dose caused a decrease in fertility. In addition, 3 to 6 times the maximum human dose caused birth defects (in the skeleton) in mice, and 6 to 9 times the maximum human dose caused death of the fetus in rats. Before taking this medicine, make sure your doctor knows if you are pregnant or if you may become pregnant.

Breast-feeding—It is not known whether guanabenz passes into the breast milk. However, this medicine has not been reported to cause problems in nursing babies.

Children—Studies on this medicine have been done only in adult patients, and there is no specific information comparing use of guanabenz in children with use in other age groups.

Older adults—Many medicines have not been studied specifically in older people. Therefore, it may not be known whether they work exactly the same way they do in younger adults or if they cause different side effects or problems in older people. There is no specific information comparing use of guanabenz in the elderly with use in other age groups. However, dizziness, faintness, or drowsiness may be more likely to occur in the elderly, who are usually more sensitive to the effects of guanabenz.

Other medicines—Although certain medicines should not be used together at all, in other cases two different medicines may be used together even if an interaction might occur. In these cases, your doctor may want to change the dose, or other precautions may be necessary. When you are taking guanabenz, it is especially important that your doctor and pharmacist know if you are taking any of the following:

- Beta-blockers (acebutolol [e.g., Sectral], atenolol [e.g., Tenormin], betaxolol [Kerlone], carteolol [e.g., Cartrol], labetalol [e.g., Normodyne], metoprolol [e.g., Lopressor], nadolol [e.g., Corgard], oxprenolol [e.g., Trasicor], penbutolol [e.g., Levatol], pindolol [e.g., Visken], propranolol [e.g., Inderal], sotalol [e.g., Sotacor], timolol [e.g., Blocadren])—Effects on blood pressure may be increased. Also, the risk of unwanted effects when guanabenz treatment is stopped suddenly may be increased

Other medical problems—The presence of other medical problems may affect the use of guanabenz. Make sure you tell your doctor if you have any other medical problems, especially:

- Heart or blood vessel disease—Lowering blood pressure may make some conditions worse
- Kidney disease or
- Liver disease—Effects of guanabenz may be increased because of slower removal of guanabenz from the body

Before you begin using any new medicine (prescription or nonprescription) or if you develop any new medical problem while you are using this medicine, check with your doctor, nurse, or pharmacist.

Proper Use of This Medicine

In addition to the use of the medicine your doctor has prescribed, treatment for your high blood pressure may include weight control and care in the types of foods you eat, especially foods high in sodium. Your doctor will tell you which of these are most important for you. You should check with your doctor before changing your diet.

Many patients who have high blood pressure will not notice any signs of the problem. In fact, many may feel normal. It is very important that you *take your medicine exactly as directed* and that you keep your appointments with your doctor even if you feel well.

Remember that this medicine will not cure your high blood pressure but it does help control it. Therefore, you must continue to take it as directed if you expect to lower your blood pressure and keep it down. *You may have to take high blood pressure medicine for the rest of your life.* If high blood pressure is not treated, it can cause serious problems such as heart failure, blood vessel disease, stroke, or kidney disease.

To help you remember to take your medicine, try to get into the habit of taking it at the same time each day.

Missed dose—
- If you miss a dose of this medicine, take it as soon as possible. However, if it is almost time for your next dose, skip the missed dose and go back to your regular dosing schedule. Do not double doses.
- If you miss two or more doses in a row, check with your doctor. If your body suddenly goes without this medicine, some unpleasant effects may occur. If you have any questions about this, check with your doctor.

Storage—To store this medicine:
- Keep out of the reach of children.
- Store away from heat and direct light.
- Do not store in the bathroom, near the kitchen sink, or in other damp places. Heat or moisture may cause the medicine to break down.
- Do not keep outdated medicine or medicine no longer needed. Be sure that any discarded medicine is out of the reach of children.

Precautions While Using This Medicine

It is important that your doctor check your progress at regular visits to make sure that this medicine is working properly.

Check with your doctor before you stop taking guanabenz. Your doctor may want you to reduce gradually the amount you are taking before stopping completely.

Before having any kind of surgery (including dental surgery) or emergency treatment, tell the medical doctor or dentist in charge that you are using this medicine.

Do not take other medicines unless they have been discussed with your doctor. This especially includes over-the-counter (nonprescription) medicines for appetite control, asthma, colds, cough, hay fever, or sinus problems, since they may tend to increase your blood pressure.

Guanabenz will add to the effects of alcohol and other CNS depressants (medicines that slow down the nervous system, possibly causing drowsiness). Some examples of CNS depressants are antihistamines or medicine for hay fever, other allergies, or colds; sedatives, tranquilizers, or sleeping medicine; prescription pain medicine or narcotics; barbiturates; medicine for seizures; muscle relaxants; or anesthetics, including some dental anesthetics. *Check with your doctor before taking any of the above while you are using this medicine.*

Guanabenz may cause some people to become dizzy, drowsy, or less alert than they are normally. *Make sure you know how you react to this medicine before you drive, use machines, or do anything else that could be dangerous if you are dizzy or are not alert.*

Guanabenz may cause dryness of the mouth, nose, and throat. For temporary relief of mouth dryness, use sugarless candy or gum, melt bits of ice in your mouth, or use a saliva substitute. However, if your mouth continues to feel dry for more than 2 weeks, check with your medical doctor or dentist. Continuing dryness of the mouth may increase the chance of dental disease, including tooth decay, gum disease, and fungus infections.

Side Effects of This Medicine

Along with its needed effects, a medicine may cause some unwanted effects. Although not all of these side effects may occur, if they do occur they may need medical attention.

Check with your doctor as soon as possible if any of the following side effects occur:

Signs and symptoms of overdose

Dizziness (severe); faintness; irritability; nervousness; pinpoint pupils; slow heartbeat; unusual tiredness or weakness

Other side effects may occur that usually do not need medical attention. These side effects may go away during treatment as your body adjusts to the medicine. However, check with your doctor if any of the following side effects continue or are bothersome:

More common

Dizziness; drowsiness; dryness of mouth; weakness

Less common or rare

Decreased sexual ability; headache; nausea

After you have been using this medicine for a while, unpleasant effects may occur if you stop taking it too suddenly. After you stop taking this medicine, check with your doctor if any of the following effects occur:

Anxiety or tenseness; chest pain; fast or irregular heartbeat; headache; increased salivation; increase in sweating; nausea or vomiting; nervousness or restlessness; shaking or trembling of hands or fingers; stomach cramps; trouble in sleeping

Other side effects not listed above may also occur in some patients. If you notice any other effects, check with your doctor.

Annual revision: 10/15/92

GUANADREL Systemic†

A commonly used brand name in the U.S. is Hylorel.

†Not commercially available in Canada.

Description

Guanadrel (GWAHN-a-drel) belongs to the general class of medicines called antihypertensives. It is used to treat high blood pressure (hypertension).

High blood pressure adds to the workload of the heart and arteries. If it continues for a long time, the heart and arteries may not function properly. This can damage the blood vessels of the brain, heart, and kidneys resulting in a stroke, heart failure, or kidney failure. High blood pressure may also increase the risk of heart attacks. These problems may be less likely to occur if blood pressure is controlled.

Guanadrel works by controlling nerve impulses along certain nerve pathways. As a result, it relaxes the blood vessels so that blood passes through them more easily. This helps to lower blood pressure.

Guanadrel is available only with your doctor's prescription, in the following dosage form:

Oral

- Tablets (U.S.)

It is very important that you read and understand the following information. If any of it causes you special concern, check with your doctor. Also, *if you have any questions* or if you want more information about this medicine or your medical problem, *ask your doctor, nurse, or pharmacist.*

Before Using This Medicine

In deciding to use a medicine, the risks of taking the medicine must be weighed against the good it will do. This is a decision you and your doctor will make. For guanadrel, the following should be considered:

Allergies—Tell your doctor if you have ever had any unusual or allergic reaction to guanadrel. Also tell your doctor and pharmacist if you are allergic to any other substance, such as foods, preservatives, or dyes.

Pregnancy—Guanadrel has not been studied in pregnant women. However, guanadrel has not been shown to cause birth defects or other problems in animal studies.

Breast-feeding—It is not known whether guanadrel passes into breast milk. However, it has not been reported to cause problems in nursing babies.

Children—Studies on this medicine have been done only in adult patients, and there is no specific information comparing use of guanadrel in children with use in other age groups.

Older adults—Dizziness or faintness may be more likely to occur in the elderly, who are usually more sensitive to the effects of guanadrel.

Other medicines—Although certain medicines should not be used together at all, in other cases two different medicines may be used together even if an interaction might occur. In these cases, your doctor may want to change the dose, or other precautions may be necessary. When you are taking guanadrel, it is especially important that your doctor and pharmacist know if you are taking any of the following:

- Chlorprothixene (e.g., Taractan) or
- Loxapine (e.g., Loxitane) or
- Thiothixene (e.g., Navane) or
- Tricyclic antidepressants (amitriptyline [e.g., Elavil], amoxapine [e.g., Asendin], clomipramine [e.g., Anafranil], desipramine [e.g., Pertofrane], doxepin [e.g., Sinequan], imipramine [e.g., Tofranil], nortriptyline [e.g., Aventyl], protriptyline [e.g., Vivactil], trimipramine [e.g., Surmontil]) or
- Trimeprazine (e.g., Temaril)—May decrease the effects of guanadrel on blood pressure
- Monoamine oxidase (MAO) inhibitors (furazolidone [e.g., Furoxone], isocarboxazid [e.g., Marplan], phenelzine [e.g., Nardil], procarbazine [e.g., Matulane], selegiline [e.g., Eldepryl], tranylcypromine [e.g., Parnate])—Taking guanadrel while you are taking or within 2 weeks of taking MAO inhibitors may cause a severe increase in blood pressure

Other medical problems—The presence of other medical problems may affect the use of guanadrel. Make sure you tell your doctor if you have any other medical problems, especially:

- Asthma (history of) or
- Diarrhea or
- Pheochromocytoma or
- Stomach ulcer (history of)—May be worsened by guanadrel
- Fever—Effects of guanadrel may be increased
- Heart or blood vessel disease or
- Heart attack or stroke (recent)—Lowering blood pressure may make problems resulting from these conditions worse

Before you begin using any new medicine (prescription or nonprescription) or if you develop any new medical problem while you are using this medicine, check with your doctor, nurse, or pharmacist.

Proper Use of This Medicine

In addition to the use of the medicine your doctor has prescribed, treatment for your high blood pressure may include weight control and care in the types of foods you eat, especially foods high in sodium. Your doctor will tell you which of these are most important for you. You should check with your doctor before changing your diet.

Many patients who have high blood pressure will not notice any signs of the problem. In fact, many may feel normal. It is very important that you *take your medicine exactly as directed* and that you keep your appointments with your doctor even if you feel well.

Remember that guanadrel will not cure your high blood pressure but it does help control it. Therefore, you must continue to take it as directed if you expect to lower your blood pressure and keep it down. *You may have to take high blood pressure medicine for the rest of your life.* If high blood pressure is not treated, it can cause serious problems such as heart failure, blood vessel disease, stroke, or kidney disease.

To help you remember to take your medicine, try to get into the habit of taking it at the same time each day.

Missed dose—If you miss a dose of guanadrel, take it as soon as possible. However, if it is almost time for your next dose, skip the missed dose and go back to your regular dosing schedule. Do not double doses.

Storage—To store this medicine:

- Keep out of the reach of children.
- Store away from heat and direct light.
- Do not store in the bathroom, near the kitchen sink, or in other damp places. Heat or moisture may cause the medicine to break down.
- Do not keep outdated medicine or medicine no longer needed. Be sure that any discarded medicine is out of the reach of children.

Precautions While Using This Medicine

It is important that your doctor check your progress at regular visits to make sure that this medicine is working properly.

Dizziness, lightheadedness, or fainting may occur, especially when you get up from a lying or sitting position. This may be more likely to occur in the morning. *Getting up slowly may help.* If you feel dizzy, sit or lie down. When you get up from lying down, sit on the edge of the bed with your feet dangling for 1 or 2 minutes. Then stand up slowly. If the problem continues or gets worse, check with your doctor.

The dizziness, lightheadedness, or fainting is also more likely to occur if you drink alcohol, stand for long periods of time, exercise, or if the weather is hot. *While you are taking guanadrel, be careful to limit the amount of alcohol you drink. Also, use extra care during exercise or hot weather or if you must stand for long periods of time.*

Do not take other medicines unless they have been discussed with your doctor. This especially includes over-the-counter (nonprescription) medicines for appetite control, asthma, colds, cough, hay fever, or sinus problems, since they may tend to increase your blood pressure.

Before having any kind of surgery (including dental surgery) or emergency treatment, tell the medical doctor or dentist in charge that you are taking guanadrel.

Tell your doctor if you get a fever since that may change the amount of medicine you have to take.

Side Effects of This Medicine

Along with its needed effects, a medicine may cause some unwanted effects. Although not all of these side effects may occur, if they do occur they may need medical attention.

Check with your doctor immediately if either of the following side effects occurs since they may be symptoms of an overdose:

Rare

Blurred vision; dizziness or faintness (severe)

Check with your doctor as soon as possible if any of the following side effects occur:

More common

Swelling of feet or lower legs

Less common or rare

Chest pain; shortness of breath

Other side effects may occur that usually do not need medical attention. These side effects may go away during treatment as your body adjusts to the medicine. However, check with your doctor if any of the following side effects continue or are bothersome:

More common

Difficulty in ejaculating; dizziness, lightheadedness, or fainting, especially when getting up from a lying or sitting position; drowsiness or tiredness

Less common or rare

Diarrhea or increase in bowel movements; dryness of mouth; headache; muscle pain or tremors; nighttime urination

Other side effects not listed above may also occur in some patients. If you notice any other effects, check with your doctor.

Annual revision: 10/21/92

GUANETHIDINE Systemic

Some commonly used brand names are:

In the U.S.

Ismelin

Generic name product may also be available.

In Canada

Apo-Guanethidine

Ismelin

Description

Guanethidine (gwahn-ETH-i-deen) belongs to the general class of medicines called antihypertensives. It is used to treat high blood pressure (hypertension).

High blood pressure adds to the workload of the heart and arteries. If it continues for a long time, the heart and arteries may not function properly. This can damage the blood vessels of the brain, heart, and kidneys, resulting in a stroke, heart failure, or kidney failure. High blood pressure may also increase the risk of heart attacks. These problems may be less likely to occur if blood pressure is controlled.

Guanethidine works by controlling nerve impulses along certain nerve pathways. As a result, it relaxes the blood vessels so that blood passes through them more easily. This helps to lower blood pressure.

Guanethidine is available only with your doctor's prescription, in the following dosage form:

Oral

- Tablets (U.S. and Canada)

It is very important that you read and understand the following information. If any of it causes you special concern, check with your doctor. Also, *if you have any questions* or if you want more information about this medicine or your medical problem, *ask your doctor, nurse, or pharmacist.*

Before Using This Medicine

In deciding to use a medicine, the risks of taking the medicine must be weighed against the good it will do. This is a decision you and your doctor will make. For guanethidine, the following should be considered:

Allergies—Tell your doctor if you have ever had any unusual or allergic reaction to guanethidine. Also tell your doctor and pharmacist if you are allergic to any other substance, such as foods, preservatives, or dyes.

Pregnancy—Studies on effects in pregnancy have not been done in either humans or animals.

Breast-feeding—Small amounts of guanethidine pass into breast-milk. However, this medicine has not been reported to cause problems in nursing babies.

Children—Although there is no specific information comparing use of guanethidine in children with use in other age groups, this medicine is not expected to cause different side effects or problems in children than it does in adults.

Older adults—Many medicines have not been studied specifically in older people. Therefore, it may not be known whether they work exactly the same way they do in younger adults. Although there is no specific information comparing use of guanethidine in the elderly with use in other age groups, dizziness, lightheadedness, or fainting may be more likely to occur in the elderly, who are more sensitive to the effects of guanethidine.

Other medicines—Although certain medicines should not be used together at all, in other cases two different medicines may be used together even if an interaction might occur. In these cases, your doctor may want to change the dose, or other precautions may be necessary. When you are taking guanethidine, it is especially important that your doctor and pharmacist know if you are taking any of the following:

- Antidiabetics, oral (diabetes medicine you take by mouth)—Effects may be increased by guanethidine
- Loxapine (e.g., Loxitane) or
- Thioxanthenes (chlorprothixene [e.g., Taractan], thiothixene [e.g., Navane]) or
- Tricyclic antidepressants (amitriptyline [e.g., Elavil], amoxapine [e.g., Asendin], clomipramine [e.g., Anafranil], desipramine [e.g., Pertofrane], doxepin [e.g., Sinequan], imipramine [e.g., Tofranil], nortriptyline [e.g., Aventyl], protriptyline [e.g., Vivactil], trimipramine [e.g., Surmontil]) or
- Trimeprazine (e.g., Temaril)—May decrease the effects of guanethidine on blood pressure
- Minoxidil (e.g., Loniten)—Effects on blood pressure may be greatly increased
- Monoamine oxidase (MAO) inhibitors (furazolidone [e.g., Furoxone], isocarboxazid [e.g., Marplan], phenelzine [e.g., Nardil], procarbazine [e.g., Matulane], selegiline [e.g., Eldepryl], tranylcypromine [e.g., Parnate])—Taking guanethidine while you are taking or within 2 weeks of taking MAO inhibitors may cause a severe increase in blood pressure

Other medical problems—The presence of other medical problems may affect the use of guanethidine. Make sure you tell your doctor if you have any other medical problems, especially:

- Asthma (history of) or
- Diarrhea or
- Pheochromocytoma or
- Stomach ulcer (history of)—May be worsened by guanethidine
- Diabetes mellitus (sugar diabetes)—Effects of medicine used to treat this may be increased by guanethidine
- Fever—Effects of guanethidine may be increased

- Heart or blood vessel disease or
- Heart attack or stroke (recent)—Lowering blood pressure may make problems resulting from these conditions worse
- Kidney disease—May be worsened. Also, effects of guanethidine may be increased because of slower removal of this medicine from the body
- Liver disease—Effects of guanethidine may be increased because of slower removal from the body

Before you begin using any new medicine (prescription or nonprescription) or if you develop any new medical problem while you are using this medicine, check with your doctor, nurse, or pharmacist.

Proper Use of This Medicine

In addition to the use of the medicine your doctor has prescribed, treatment for your high blood pressure may include weight control and care in the types of foods you eat, especially foods high in sodium. Your doctor will tell you which of these are most important for you. You should check with your doctor before changing your diet.

Many patients who have high blood pressure will not notice any signs of the problem. In fact, many may feel normal. It is very important that you *take your medicine exactly as directed* and that you keep your appointments with your doctor even if you feel well.

Remember that guanethidine will not cure your high blood pressure but it does help control it. Therefore, you must continue to take it as directed if you expect to lower your blood pressure and keep it down. *You may have to take high blood pressure medicine for the rest of your life.* If high blood pressure is not treated, it can cause serious problems such as heart failure, blood vessel disease, stroke, or kidney disease.

To help you remember to take your medicine, try to get into the habit of taking it at the same time each day.

Missed dose—If you miss a dose of guanethidine, take it as soon as possible. However, if it is almost time for your next dose, skip the missed dose and go back to your regular dosing schedule. Do not double doses.

Storage—To store this medicine:
- Keep out of the reach of children.
- Store away from heat and direct light.
- Do not store in the bathroom, near the kitchen sink, or in other damp places. Heat or moisture may cause the medicine to break down.
- Do not keep outdated medicine or medicine no longer needed. Be sure that any discarded medicine is out of the reach of children.

Precautions While Using This Medicine

It is important that your doctor check your progress at regular visits to make sure that this medicine is working properly.

Dizziness, lightheadedness, or fainting may occur, especially when you get up from a lying or sitting position. This is more likely to occur in the morning. *Getting up slowly may help.* When you get up from lying down, sit on the edge of the bed with your feet dangling for 1 or 2 minutes. Then stand up slowly. If the problem continues or gets worse, check with your doctor.

The dizziness, lightheadedness, or fainting is also more likely to occur if you drink alcohol, stand for long periods of time, exercise, or if the weather is hot. *While you are taking this medicine, be careful in the amount of alcohol you drink. Also, use extra care during exercise or hot weather or if you must stand for long periods of time.*

Do not take other medicines unless they have been discussed with your doctor. This especially includes over-the-counter (nonprescription) medicines for appetite control, asthma, colds, cough, hay fever, or sinus problems, since they may tend to increase your blood pressure.

Before having any kind of surgery (including dental surgery) or emergency treatment, tell the medical doctor or dentist in charge that you are taking this medicine.

Tell your doctor if you get a fever since that may change the amount of medicine you have to take.

Side Effects of This Medicine

Along with its needed effects, a medicine may cause some unwanted effects. Although not all of these side effects may occur, if they do occur they may need medical attention.

Check with your doctor as soon as possible if any of the following side effects occur:

More common

Swelling of feet or lower legs

Less common or rare

Chest pain; shortness of breath

Other side effects may occur that usually do not need medical attention. These side effects may go away during treatment as your body adjusts to the medicine. However, check with your doctor if any of the following side effects continue or are bothersome:

More common

Diarrhea or increase in bowel movements; dizziness, lightheadedness, or fainting, especially when getting up from a lying or sitting position; sexual problems in males; slow heartbeat; stuffy nose; unusual tiredness or weakness

Less common or rare

Blurred vision; drooping eyelids; dryness of mouth; headache; loss of hair on scalp; muscle pain or tremors; nausea or vomiting; nighttime urination; skin rash

Other side effects not listed above may also occur in some patients. If you notice any other effects, check with your doctor.

Annual revision: 08/05/92

GUANETHIDINE AND HYDROCHLOROTHIAZIDE Systemic

Some commonly used brand names are:

In the U.S.
Esimil

In Canada
Ismelin-Esidrix

Description

Guanethidine (gwahn-ETH-i-deen) and hydrochlorothiazide (hye-droe-klor-oh-THYE-a-zide) combination is used to treat high blood pressure (hypertension).

High blood pressure adds to the workload of the heart and arteries. If it continues for a long time, the heart and arteries may not function properly. This can damage the blood vessels of the brain, heart, and kidneys, resulting in a stroke, heart failure, or kidney failure. High blood pressure may also increase the risk of heart attacks. These problems may be less likely to occur if blood pressure is controlled.

Guanethidine works by controlling nerve impulses along certain nerve pathways. As a result, it relaxes the blood vessels so that blood passes through them more easily. The hydrochlorothiazide in this combination is a thiazide diuretic (water pill) that helps reduce the amount of water in the body by increasing the flow of urine.

Guanethidine and hydrochlorothiazide combination is available only with your doctor's prescription, in the following dosage form:

Oral

- Tablets (U.S. and Canada)

It is very important that you read and understand the following information. If any of it causes you special concern, check with your doctor. Also, *if you have any questions* or if you want more information about this medicine or your medical problem, *ask your doctor, nurse, or pharmacist.*

Before Using This Medicine

In deciding to use a medicine, the risks of taking the medicine must be weighed against the good it will do. This is a decision you and your doctor will make. For guanethidine and hydrochlorothiazide, the following should be considered:

Allergies—Tell your doctor if you have ever had any unusual or allergic reaction to guanethidine, sulfonamides (sulfa drugs), hydrochlorothiazide, bumetanide, furosemide, acetazolamide, dichlorphenamide, methazolamide, or to other thiazide diuretics (water pills). Also tell your doctor and pharmacist if you are allergic to any other substance, such as foods, preservatives, or dyes.

Pregnancy—When hydrochlorothiazide is used during pregnancy, it may cause side effects including jaundice, blood problems, and low potassium in the newborn infant. However, this medicine has not been shown to cause birth defects.

Breast-feeding—Guanethidine and hydrochlorothiazide pass into breast milk. However, this medicine has not been reported to cause problems in nursing babies.

Children—Although there is no specific information about the use of this medicine in children, it is not expected to cause different side effects or problems in children than it does in adults. However, extra caution may be necessary in infants with jaundice, because thiazide diuretics can make the condition worse.

Older adults—Dizziness, lightheadedness, fainting, or signs and symptoms of too much potassium loss may be more likely to occur in the elderly, who are more sensitive to the effects of guanethidine and hydrochlorothiazide.

Other medicines—Although certain medicines should not be used together at all, in other cases two different medicines may be used together even if an interaction might occur. In these cases, your doctor may want to change the dose, or other precautions may be necessary. When you are taking guanethidine and hydrochlorothiazide, it is especially important that your doctor and pharmacist know if you are taking any of the following:

- Antidiabetics, oral (diabetes medicine you take by mouth)—Effects may be increased by guanethidine
- Cholestyramine or
- Colestipol—Use with thiazide diuretics may prevent the diuretic from working properly; take the diuretic at least 1 hour before or 4 hours after cholestyramine or colestipol
- Digitalis glycosides (heart medicine)—Hydrochlorothiazide may cause low potassium in the blood, which can lead to symptoms of digitalis toxicity

- Lithium (e.g., Lithane)—Risk of lithium overdose, even at usual doses, may be increased
- Loxapine (e.g., Loxitane) or
- Thioxanthenes (chlorprothixene [e.g., Taractan], thiothixene [e.g., Navane]) or
- Tricyclic antidepressants (amitriptyline [e.g., Elavil], amoxapine [e.g., Asendin], clomipramine [e.g., Anafranil], desipramine [e.g., Pertofrane], doxepin [e.g., Sinequan], imipramine [e.g., Tofranil], nortriptyline [e.g., Aventyl], protriptyline [e.g., Vivactil], trimipramine [e.g., Surmontil]) or
- Trimeprazine (e.g., Temaril)—May decrease the effects of guanethidine on blood pressure
- Monoamine oxidase (MAO) inhibitors (furazolidone [e.g., Furoxone], isocarboxazid [e.g., Marplan], phenelzine [e.g., Nardil], procarbazine [e.g., Matulane], selegiline [e.g., Eldepryl], tranylcypromine [e.g., Parnate])—Taking guanethidine while you are taking or within 2 weeks of taking MAO inhibitors may cause a severe increase in blood pressure

Other medical problems—The presence of other medical problems may affect the use of guanethidine and hydrochlorothiazide. Make sure you tell your doctor if you have any other medical problems, especially:

- Asthma (history of) or
- Diarrhea or
- Pheochromocytoma or
- Stomach ulcer (history of)—May be worsened by guanethidine
- Diabetes mellitus (sugar diabetes)—Effects of medicine used to treat this may be increased by guanethidine. Hydrochlorothiazide may change the amount of diabetes medicine needed
- Fever—Effects of guanethidine may be increased
- Gout (history of)—Hydrochlorothiazide may increase the amount of uric acid in the blood, which can lead to gout
- Heart or blood vessel disease or
- Heart attack or stroke (recent)—Lowering blood pressure may make problems resulting from these conditions worse
- Kidney disease—May be worsened. Also, effects may be increased because of slower removal of guanethidine from the body
- Liver disease—Effects may be increased because of slower removal of guanethidine from the body
- Lupus erythematosus (history of)—Hydrochlorothiazide may worsen the condition
- Pancreatitis (inflammation of the pancreas)

Before you begin using any new medicine (prescription or nonprescription) or if you develop any new medical problem while you are using this medicine, check with your doctor, nurse, or pharmacist.

Proper Use of This Medicine

This medicine may cause you to have an unusual feeling of tiredness when you begin to take it. You may also notice an increase in the amount of urine or in your frequency of urination. After taking the medicine for a while, these effects should lessen. In general, in order to keep the increase in urine from affecting your sleep:

- If you are to take a single dose a day, take it in the morning after breakfast.
- If you are to take more than one dose a day, take the last dose no later than 6 p.m., unless otherwise directed by your doctor.

However, it is best to plan your dose or doses according to a schedule that will least affect your personal activities and sleep. Ask your doctor, nurse, or pharmacist to help you plan the best time to take this medicine.

In addition to the use of the medicine your doctor has prescribed, treatment for your high blood pressure may include weight control and care in the types of foods you eat, especially foods high in sodium. Your doctor will tell you which of these are most important for you. You should check with your doctor before changing your diet.

Many patients who have high blood pressure will not notice any signs of the problem. In fact, many may feel normal. It is very important that you *take your medicine exactly as directed* and that you keep your appointments with your doctor even if you feel well.

Remember that this medicine will not cure your high blood pressure but it does help control it. Therefore, you must continue to take it as directed if you expect to lower your blood pressure and keep it down. *You may have to take high blood pressure medicine for the rest of your life.* If high blood pressure is not treated, it can cause serious problems such as heart failure, blood vessel disease, stroke, or kidney disease.

To help you remember to take your medicine, try to get into the habit of taking it at the same time each day.

Missed dose—If you miss a dose of this medicine, take it as soon as possible. However, if it is almost time for your next dose, skip the missed dose and go back to your regular dosing schedule. Do not double doses.

Storage—To store this medicine:

- Keep out of the reach of children.
- Store away from heat and direct light.
- Do not store in the bathroom, near the kitchen sink, or in other damp places. Heat or moisture may cause the medicine to break down.
- Do not keep outdated medicine or medicine no longer needed. Be sure that any discarded medicine is out of the reach of children.

Precautions While Using This Medicine

It is important that your doctor check your progress at regular visits to make sure that this medicine is working properly.

Do not take other medicines unless they have been discussed with your doctor. This especially includes over-the-counter (nonprescription) medicines for appetite control, asthma, colds, cough, hay fever, or sinus problems, since they may tend to increase your blood pressure.

This medicine may cause a loss of potassium from your body.

- To help prevent this, your doctor may want you to:
  —eat or drink foods that have a high potassium content (for example, orange or other citrus fruit juices), or
  —take a potassium supplement, or
  —take another medicine to help prevent the loss of the potassium in the first place.
- It is very important to follow these directions. Also, it is important not to change your diet on your own. This is more important if you are already on a special diet (as for diabetes), or if you are taking a potassium supplement or a medicine to reduce potassium loss. Extra potassium may not be necessary and, in some cases, too much potassium could be harmful.

Check with your doctor if you become sick and have severe or continuing vomiting or diarrhea. These problems may cause you to lose additional water and potassium.

Dizziness, lightheadedness, or fainting may occur, especially when you get up from a lying or sitting position. This is more likely to occur in the morning. *Getting up slowly* may help. When you get up from lying down, sit on the edge of the bed with your feet dangling for 1 or 2 minutes. Then stand up slowly. If the problem continues or gets worse, check with your doctor.

The dizziness, lightheadedness, or fainting is also more likely to occur if you drink alcohol, stand for long periods of time or exercise, or if the weather is hot. *While you are taking this medicine, be careful in the amount of alcohol you drink. Also, use extra care during exercise or hot weather or if you must stand for long periods of time.*

For *diabetic patients*:

- This medicine may raise blood sugar levels. While you are using this medicine, be especially careful in testing for sugar in your blood or urine. If you have any questions about this, check with your doctor.

Some people who take this medicine may become more sensitive to sunlight than they are normally. Exposure to sunlight, even for brief periods of time, may cause severe sunburn; skin rash, redness, itching, or discoloration; or vision changes. When you begin taking this medicine:

- Stay out of direct sunlight, especially between the hours of 10:00 a.m. and 3:00 p.m., if possible.
- Wear protective clothing, including a hat and sunglasses.
- Apply a sun block product that has a skin protection factor (SPF) of at least 15. Some patients may require a product with a higher SPF number, especially if they have a fair complexion. If you have any questions about this, check with your doctor or pharmacist.
- Do not use a sunlamp or tanning bed or booth.

If you have a severe reaction from the sun, check with your doctor.

Tell your doctor if you get a fever since that may change the amount of medicine you have to take.

Before having any kind of surgery (including dental surgery) or emergency treatment, tell the medical doctor or dentist in charge that you are taking this medicine.

Side Effects of This Medicine

Along with its needed effects, a medicine may cause some unwanted effects. Although not all of these side effects may occur, if they do occur they may need medical attention.

Check with your doctor as soon as possible if any of the following side effects occur, especially since some of them may mean that your body is losing too much potassium:

Signs and symptoms of too much potassium loss

Dryness of mouth; increased thirst; irregular heartbeats; mood or mental changes; muscle cramps or pain; nausea or vomiting; unusual tiredness or weakness; weak pulse

Signs and symptoms of too much sodium loss

Confusion; convulsions; decreased mental activity; irritability; muscle cramps; unusual tiredness or weakness

Less common

Chest pain

Rare

Black, tarry stools; blood in urine or stools; cough or hoarseness; fever or chills; joint pain; lower back or side pain; painful or difficult urination; pinpoint red spots on skin; skin rash or hives; sore throat and fever; stomach pain (severe) with nausea and vomiting; unusual bleeding or bruising; yellow eyes or skin

Other side effects may occur that usually do not need medical attention. These side effects may go away during treatment as your body adjusts to the medicine. However, check with your doctor if any of the following side effects continue or are bothersome:

More common

Diarrhea or increase in bowel movements; dizziness, lightheadedness, or fainting, especially when getting up from a lying or sitting position; sexual problems in males; slow heartbeat; stuffy nose

Less common or rare

Blurred vision; drooping eyelids; headache; increased sensitivity of skin to sunlight; loss of appetite; loss of hair; nighttime urination

Other side effects not listed above may also occur in some patients. If you notice any other effects, check with your doctor.

Annual revision: 07/14/92

GUANFACINE Systemic†

A commonly used brand name in the U.S. is Tenex.

†Not commercially available in Canada.

Description

Guanfacine (GWAHN-fa-seen) belongs to the general class of medicines called antihypertensives. It is used to treat high blood pressure (hypertension).

High blood pressure adds to the workload of the heart and arteries. If it continues for a long time, the heart and arteries may not function properly. This can damage the blood vessels of the brain, heart, and kidneys, resulting in a stroke, heart failure, or kidney failure. High blood pressure may also increase the risk of heart attacks. These problems may be less likely to occur if blood pressure is controlled.

Guanfacine works by controlling nerve impulses along certain nerve pathways. As a result, it relaxes blood vessels so that blood passes through them more easily. This helps to lower blood pressure.

Guanfacine is available only with your doctor's prescription, in the following dosage form:

Oral

- Tablets (U.S.)

It is very important that you read and understand the following information. If any of it causes you special concern, check with your doctor. Also, *if you have any questions* or if you want more information about this medicine or your medical problem, *ask your doctor, nurse, or pharmacist.*

Before Using This Medicine

In deciding to use a medicine, the risks of taking the medicine must be weighed against the good it will do. This is a decision you and your doctor will make. For guanfacine, the following should be considered:

Allergies—Tell your doctor if you have ever had any unusual or allergic reaction to guanfacine. Also tell your doctor and pharmacist if you are allergic to any other substance, such as foods, preservatives, or dyes.

Pregnancy—Guanfacine has not been studied in pregnant women. However, guanfacine has not been shown to cause birth defects or other problems in rats or rabbits given many times the human dose. In rats and rabbits given extremely high doses (up to 200 times the human dose), there was an increase in deaths of the animal fetus.

Breast-feeding—It is not known whether guanfacine passes into breast milk. However, this medicine has not been reported to cause problems in nursing babies.

Children—Studies on this medicine have been done only in adult patients, and there is no specific information comparing use of guanfacine in children with use in other age groups.

Older adults—Dizziness, drowsiness, or faintness may be more likely to occur in the elderly, who are more sensitive to the effects of guanfacine.

Other medicines—Although certain medicines should not be used together at all, in other cases two different medicines may be used together even if an interaction might occur. In these cases, your doctor may want to change the dose, or other precautions may be necessary. Tell your doctor and pharmacist if you are taking any other prescription or nonprescription (over-the-counter [OTC]) medicine.

Other medical problems—The presence of other medical problems may affect the use of guanfacine. Make sure you tell your doctor if you have any other medical problems, especially:

- Heart disease or
- Heart attack or stroke (recent)—Lowering blood pressure may make problems resulting from these conditions worse
- Liver disease—Effects may be increased because of slower removal of guanfacine from the body
- Mental depression—Guanfacine may cause mental depression

Before you begin using any new medicine (prescription or nonprescription) or if you develop any new medical problem while you are using this medicine, check with your doctor, nurse, or pharmacist.

Proper Use of This Medicine

In addition to the use of the medicine your doctor has prescribed, treatment for your high blood pressure may include weight control and care in the types of foods you eat, especially foods high in sodium. Your doctor will tell you which of these are most important for you. You should check with your doctor before changing your diet.

Many patients who have high blood pressure will not notice any signs of the problem. In fact, many may feel normal. It is very important that you *take your medicine exactly as directed* and that you keep your appointments with your doctor even if you feel well.

Remember that this medicine will not cure your high blood pressure but it does help control it. Therefore, you must continue to use it as directed if you expect to lower your blood pressure and keep it down. *You may have to take high blood pressure medicine for the rest of your life.* If high blood pressure is not treated, it can cause serious problems such as heart failure, blood vessel disease, stroke, or kidney disease.

Take your daily dose of guanfacine at bedtime. (If you are taking more than one dose a day, take your last dose at bedtime). Taking it this way will help lessen daytime drowsiness.

Missed dose—If you miss a dose of this medicine, take it as soon as possible. However, if it is almost time for your next dose, skip the missed dose and go back to your regular dosing schedule. Do not double doses. *If you miss taking guanfacine for two or more days in a row, check with your doctor.* If your body suddenly goes without this medicine, some unwanted effects may occur. If you have any questions about this, check with your doctor.

Storage—To store this medicine:

- Keep out of the reach of children.
- Store away from heat and direct light.
- Do not store in the bathroom, near the kitchen sink, or in other damp places. Heat or moisture may cause the medicine to break down.
- Do not keep outdated medicine or medicine no longer needed. Be sure any discarded medicine is out of the reach of children.

Precautions While Using This Medicine

It is important that your doctor check your progress at regular visits to make sure this medicine is working properly.

Check with your doctor before you stop taking guanfacine. Your doctor may want you to reduce gradually the amount you are taking before stopping completely.

Make sure that you have enough guanfacine on hand to last through weekends, holidays, and vacations. You should not miss any doses. You may want to ask your doctor for another written prescription for guanfacine to carry in your wallet or purse. You can then have it filled if you run out when you are away from home.

Before having any kind of surgery (including dental surgery) or emergency treatment, tell the medical doctor or dentist in charge that you are using this medicine.

Do not take other medicines unless they have been discussed with your doctor. This especially includes over-the-counter (nonprescription) medicines for appetite control, asthma, colds, cough, hay fever, or sinus problems, since they may tend to increase your blood pressure.

Guanfacine will add to the effects of alcohol and other CNS depressants (medicines that slow down the nervous system, possibly causing drowsiness). Some examples of CNS depressants are antihistamines or medicine for hay fever, other allergies, or colds; sedatives, tranquilizers, or sleeping medicine; prescription pain medicine or narcotics; barbiturates; medicine for seizures; muscle relaxants; or anesthetics, including some dental anesthetics. *Check with your doctor before taking any of the above while you are using this medicine.*

Guanfacine may cause some people to become dizzy, drowsy, or less alert than they are normally. *Make sure you know how you react to this medicine before you drive, use machines, or do anything else that could be dangerous if you are dizzy or are not alert.*

Guanfacine may cause dryness of the mouth, nose, and throat. For temporary relief of mouth dryness, use sugarless candy or gum, melt bits of ice in your mouth, or use a saliva substitute. However, if dry mouth continues for more than 2 weeks, check with your physician or dentist. Continuing dryness of the mouth may increase the chance of dental disease, including tooth decay, gum disease, and fungus infections.

Side Effects of This Medicine

Along with its needed effects, a medicine may cause some unwanted effects. Although not all of these side effects may occur, if they do occur they may need medical attention.

Check with your doctor as soon as possible if any of the following side effects occur:

Less common

Confusion; mental depression

Signs and symptoms of overdose

Difficulty in breathing; dizziness (extreme) or faintness; slow heartbeat; unusual tiredness or weakness (severe)

Other side effects may occur that usually do not need medical attention. These side effects may go away during treatment as your body adjusts to the medicine. However, check with your doctor if any of the following side effects continue or are bothersome:

More common

Constipation; dizziness; drowsiness; dryness of mouth

Less common

Decreased sexual ability; dry, itching, or burning eyes; headache; nausea or vomiting; trouble in sleeping; unusual tiredness or weakness

After you have been using this medicine for a while, unwanted effects may occur if you stop taking it too suddenly. After you stop taking this medicine, check with your doctor if any of the following side effects occur:

Anxiety or tenseness; chest pain; fast or irregular heartbeat; headache; increased salivation; nausea or vomiting; nervousness or restlessness; shaking or trembling of hands and fingers; stomach cramps; sweating; trouble in sleeping

Other side effects not listed above may also occur in some patients. If you notice any other effects, check with your doctor.

Annual revision: 10/21/92

HAEMOPHILUS B CONJUGATE VACCINE Systemic

Some commonly used brand names are:

In the U.S.

Act-Hib	Pedvaxhib
Hibtiter	Prohibit

In Canada

Act-Hib	Pedvaxhib
Hibtiter	Prohibit

Other commonly used names are: HBOC, PRP-D, PRP-OMP, and PRP-T.

Description

Haemophilus b conjugate (hem-OFF-fil-us BEE KON-ja-gat) vaccine is an active immunizing agent used to prevent infection by *Haemophilus influenzae* type b (Hib) bacteria. The vaccine works by causing your body to produce its own protection (antibodies) against the disease.

Haemophilus b conjugate vaccine is an haemophilus b vaccine that has been prepared by adding a diphtheria-, meningococcal-, or tetanus-related substance. However, this vaccine does *not* take the place of the regular diphtheria or tetanus toxoid injections (for example, DTP, DT, or T) that children should receive, the regular tetanus toxoid or diphtheria and tetanus toxoid injections (for example T or Td) that adults should receive, or the meningococcal vaccine injection that some children and adults should receive.

Infection by *Haemophilus influenzae* type b (Hib) bacteria can cause life-threatening illnesses, such as meningitis, which affects the brain; epiglottitis, which can cause death by suffocation; pericarditis, which affects the heart; pneumonia, which affects the lungs; and septic arthritis, which affects the bones and joints. Hib meningitis causes death in 5 to 10% of children who are infected. Also, approximately 30% of children who survive Hib meningitis are left with some type of serious permanent damage, such as mental retardation, deafness, epilepsy, or partial blindness.

Immunization against Hib is recommended for all children 2 months up to 5 years of age (i.e., up to the 5th birthday).

Immunization against Hib may also be recommended for adults and children over 5 years of age with certain medical problems.

This vaccine is to be administered only by or under the supervision of your doctor or other authorized health care provider. It is available in the following dosage form:

Parenteral

- Injection (U.S. and Canada)

It is very important that you read and understand the following information. If any of it causes you special concern, check with your doctor. Also, *if you have any questions* or if you want more information about this medicine or your medical problem, *ask your doctor, nurse, or pharmacist.*

Before Receiving This Vaccine

In deciding to use a medicine, the risks of taking the medicine must be weighed against the good it will do. This is a decision you and your doctor will make. For haemophilus b conjugate vaccine, the following should be considered:

Allergies—Tell your doctor if you have ever had any unusual or allergic reaction to haemophilus b conjugate vaccine, haemophilus b polysaccharide vaccine, diphtheria or tetanus toxoid, or meningococcal vaccine. Also tell your doctor and pharmacist if you are allergic to any other substances, such as preservatives.

Pregnancy—Studies on effects in pregnancy have not been done in either humans or animals.

Breast-feeding—This vaccine has not been reported to cause problems in nursing babies.

Children—This vaccine is not recommended for children less than 2 months of age.

Older adults—Many medicines have not been studied specifically in older people. Therefore, it may not be known whether they work exactly the same way they do in younger adults. Although there is no specific information comparing use of this vaccine in the elderly with use in other age groups, this vaccine is not expected to cause different side effects or problems in older people than it does in younger adults.

Other medicines—Although certain medicines should not be used together at all, in other cases two different medicines may be used together even if an interaction might occur. In these cases, your doctor may want to change the dose, or other precautions may be necessary. Tell your doctor and pharmacist if you are using any other prescription or nonprescription (over-the-counter [OTC]) medicine.

Other medical problems—The presence of other medical problems may affect the use of haemophilus b conjugate vaccine. Make sure you tell your doctor if you have any other medical problems, especially:

- Fever or
- Serious illness—The symptoms of the condition may be confused with the possible side effects of the vaccine

After Receiving This Vaccine

This vaccine may interfere with laboratory tests that check for Hib disease. Make sure your doctor knows that you have received Hib vaccine if you are treated for a severe infection during the 2 weeks after you receive this vaccine.

Side Effects of This Vaccine

Along with its needed effects, a vaccine may cause some unwanted effects. Although not all of these side effects may occur, if they do occur they may need medical attention.

Get emergency help immediately if any of the following side effects occur:

Symptoms of allergic reactions

Difficulty in breathing or swallowing; hives; itching (especially of feet or hands); reddening of skin (especially around ears); swelling of eyes, face, or inside of nose; unusual tiredness or weakness (sudden and severe)

Check with your doctor immediately if the following side effect occurs:

Rare

Convulsions (seizures)

Other side effects may occur that usually do not need medical attention. However, check with your doctor if any of the following side effects continue or are bothersome:

More common

Fever of up to 102 °F (39 °C) (usually lasts less than 48 hours); irritability; loss of appetite; lack of interest; redness at place of injection; reduced physical activity; tenderness at place of injection; tiredness

Less common

Diarrhea; fever over 102 °F (39 °C) (usually lasts less than 48 hours); hard lump, swelling, or warm feeling at place of injection; skin rash; vomiting

Other side effects not listed above may also occur in some patients. If you notice any other effects, check with your doctor.

Annual revision: 06/21/93

HAEMOPHILUS B POLYSACCHARIDE VACCINE Systemic*†

Commonly used names are:

Haemophilus influenzae type b polysaccharide vaccine
HbPV
Hib CPS
Hib polysaccharide vaccine
PRP

*Not commercially available in the U.S.
†Not commercially available in Canada.

Description

Haemophilus b polysaccharide (hem-OFF-fil-us BEE pol-i-SAK-ka-ryd) vaccine is an active immunizing agent used to prevent infection by *Haemophilus influenzae* type b (Hib) bacteria. The vaccine works by causing your body to produce its own protection (antibodies) against the disease.

The following information applies only to the Haemophilus b polysaccharide vaccine.

Infection by *Haemophilus influenzae* type b (Hib) bacteria can cause life-threatening illnesses, such as meningitis, which affects the brain; epiglottitis, which can cause death by suffocation; pericarditis, which affects the heart; pneumonia, which affects the lungs; and septic arthritis, which affects the bones and joints. Hib meningitis causes death in 5 to 10% of children who are infected. Also, approximately 30% of children who survive Hib meningitis are left with some type of serious permanent damage, such as mental retardation, deafness, epilepsy, or partial blindness.

Immunization against Hib is recommended for all children 24 months up to 5 years of age (i.e., up to the 5th birthday). In addition, immunization is recommended for children 18 to 24 months of age, especially:

- Children attending day-care facilities.
- Children with chronic illnesses associated with increased risk of Hib disease. These illnesses include asplenia, sickle cell disease, antibody deficiency syndromes, immunosuppression, and Hodgkin's disease.
- Children 18 to 24 months of age who have already had Hib disease. These children may get the disease again if they are not immunized. Children who developed Hib disease when 24 months of age or older do not need to be immunized, since most children in this age group will develop antibodies against the disease.
- Children with human immunodeficiency virus (HIV) infection or acquired immunodeficiency syndrome (AIDS).
- Children of certain racial groups, such as American Indian and Alaskan Eskimo. Children in these groups seem to be at increased risk of Hib disease.
- Children living close together with groups of other persons. Close living conditions increase a child's risk of being exposed to persons who have Hib infection or who carry the bacteria.

It is recommended that children immunized when they were 18 to 24 months of age receive a second dose of vaccine, since these children may not produce enough antibodies to fully protect them from Hib disease. Children who were first immunized when they were 24 months of age or older do not need to be reimmunized.

This vaccine is available only from your doctor or other authorized health care provider, in the following dosage form:

Parenteral

- Injection

It is very important that you read and understand the following information. If any of it causes you special concern, check with your doctor. Also, *if you have any questions* or if you want more information about this medicine or your medical problem, *ask your doctor, nurse, or pharmacist.*

Before Receiving This Vaccine

In deciding to use a medicine, the risks of taking the medicine must be weighed against the good it will do. This is a decision you and your doctor will make. For haemophilus b polysaccharide vaccine, the following should be considered:

Allergies—Tell your doctor if you have ever had any unusual or allergic reaction to haemophilus b polysaccharide vaccine or haemophilus b conjugate vaccine. Also tell your doctor and pharmacist if you are allergic to any other substances, such as preservatives.

Children—This vaccine is not recommended for children less than 18 months of age.

Other medicines—Although certain medicines should not be used together at all, in other cases two different medicines may be used together even if an interaction might occur. In these cases, your doctor may want to change the dose, or other precautions may be necessary. Tell your doctor and pharmacist if you are using any other prescription or nonprescription (over-the-counter [OTC]) medicine.

Other medical problems—The presence of other medical problems may affect the use of haemophilus b polysaccharide vaccine. Make sure you tell your doctor if you have any other medical problems, especially:

- Fever or
- Serious illness—The symptoms of the condition may be confused with the possible side effects of the vaccine

Side Effects of This Vaccine

Along with its needed effects, a vaccine may cause some unwanted effects. Although not all of these side effects may occur, if they do occur they may need medical attention.

Get emergency help immediately if any of the following side effects occur:

Symptoms of allergic reaction

Difficulty in breathing or swallowing; hives; itching (especially of feet or hands); reddening of skin (especially around ears); swelling of eyes, face, or inside of nose; unusual tiredness or weakness (sudden and severe)

Check with your doctor immediately if the following side effect occurs:

Rare

Convulsions (seizures)

Other side effects may occur that usually do not need medical attention. However, check with your doctor if any of the following side effects continue or are bothersome:

More common

Diarrhea; fever up to 102 °F (39 °C) (usually lasts less than 48 hours); irritability; lack of appetite; lack of interest; redness at place of injection; reduced physical activity; tenderness at place of injection

Less common

Fever over 102 °F (39 °C) (usually lasts less than 48 hours); hard lump at place of injection; itching; joint aches or pains; skin rash; swelling at place of injection; trouble in sleeping; vomiting

Other side effects not listed above may also occur in some patients. If you notice any other effects, check with your doctor.

Annual revision: 06/21/93

HALOPERIDOL Systemic

Some commonly used brand names are:

In the U.S.

Haldol
Haldol Decanoate

Generic name product may also be available.

In Canada

Apo-Haloperidol
Haldol
Haldol LA
Novo-Peridol
Peridol
PMS Haloperidol

Generic name product may also be available.

Description

Haloperidol (ha-loe-PER-i-dole) is used to treat nervous, mental, and emotional conditions. It is also used to control the symptoms of Tourette's disorder. Haloperidol may also be used for other conditions as determined by your doctor.

Haloperidol is available only with your doctor's prescription, in the following dosage forms:

Oral

- Solution (U.S. and Canada)
- Tablets (U.S. and Canada)

Parenteral

- Injection (U.S. and Canada)

It is very important that you read and understand the following information. If any of it causes you special concern, check with your doctor. Also, *if you have any questions* or if you want more information about this medicine or your medical problem, *ask your doctor, nurse, or pharmacist.*

Before Using This Medicine

In deciding to use a medicine, the risks of taking the medicine must be weighed against the good it will do. This is a decision you and your doctor will make. For haloperidol, the following should be considered:

Allergies—Tell your doctor if you have ever had any unusual or allergic reaction to haloperidol. Also tell your doctor and pharmacist if you are allergic to any other substances, such as foods, preservatives, or dyes.

Pregnancy—Haloperidol has not been studied in pregnant women. However, studies in animals given 2 to 20 times the usual maximum human dose of haloperidol have shown reduced fertility, delayed delivery, cleft palate, and an increase in the number of stillbirths and newborn deaths.

Breast-feeding—Haloperidol passes into breast milk. Animal studies have shown that haloperidol in breast milk causes drowsiness and unusual muscle movements in the nursing offspring. Breast-feeding is not recommended during treatment with haloperidol.

Children—Side effects, especially muscle spasms of the neck and back, twisting movements of the body, trembling of fingers and hands, and inability to move the eyes are more likely to occur in children, who usually are more sensitive than adults to the effects of haloperidol.

Older adults—Constipation, dizziness or fainting, drowsiness, dryness of mouth, trembling of the hands and fingers, and symptoms of tardive dyskinesia (such as rapid, worm-like movements of the tongue or any other uncontrolled movements of the mouth, tongue, or jaw, and/or arms and legs) are especially likely to occur in elderly patients, who are usually more sensitive than younger adults to the effects of haloperidol.

Other medicines—Although certain medicines should not be used together at all, in other cases 2 different medicines may be used together even if an interaction might occur. In these cases, your doctor may want to change the dose, or other precautions may be necessary. When you are taking haloperidol, it is especially important that your doctor and pharmacist know if you are taking any of the following:

- Amoxapine (e.g., Asendin) or
- Metoclopramide (e.g., Reglan) or
- Metyrosine (e.g., Demser) or
- Other antipsychotics (medicine for mental illness) or
- Pemoline (e.g., Cylert) or
- Pimozide (e.g., Orap) or
- Promethazine (e.g., Phenergan) or
- Rauwolfia alkaloids (alseroxylon [e.g., Rauwiloid], deserpidine [e.g., Harmonyl], rauwolfia serpentina [e.g., Raudixin], reserpine [e.g., Serpasil]) or
- Trimeprazine (e.g., Temaril)—Taking these medicines with haloperidol may increase the frequency and severity of certain side effects
- Central nervous system (CNS) depressants (medicine that causes drowsiness) or
- Tricyclic antidepressants (medicine for depression)—Taking these medicines with haloperidol may result in increased CNS and other depressant effects, and in an increased chance of low blood pressure (hypotension)
- Epinephrine (e.g., Adrenalin)—Severe low blood pressure or irregular heartbeat may occur
- Levodopa (e.g., Dopar, Larodopa)—Haloperidol may interfere with the effects of this medicine
- Lithium (e.g., Eskalith, Lithane)—Although lithium and haloperidol are sometimes used together, their use must be closely monitored by your doctor, who may change the amount of medicine you need to take

Other medical problems—The presence of other medical problems may affect the use of haloperidol. Make sure you tell your doctor if you have any other medical problems, especially:

- Alcohol abuse—The risk of heat stroke may be increased
- Difficult urination or
- Glaucoma or
- Heart or blood vessel disease or
- Lung disease or
- Parkinson's disease—Haloperidol may make the condition worse
- Epilepsy—The risk of seizures may be increased
- Kidney disease or
- Liver disease—Higher blood levels of haloperidol may occur, increasing the chance of side effects
- Overactive thyroid—Serious unwanted effects may occur

Before you begin using any new medicine (prescription or nonprescription) or if you develop any new medical problem while you are using this medicine, check with your doctor, nurse, or pharmacist.

Proper Use of This Medicine

If this medicine upsets your stomach, it may be taken with food or milk to lessen stomach irritation.

For patients taking the *liquid form of this medicine*:

- This medicine is to be taken by mouth even if it comes in a dropper bottle. Each dose is to be measured with the specially marked dropper provided with your prescription. Do not use other droppers since they may not deliver the correct amount of medicine.
- This medicine is best taken alone. However, if necessary, it may be mixed with water. If this is done, the mixture should be taken immediately after mixing. Haloperidol should not be taken in tea or coffee, since they cause the medicine to separate out of solution.

Take this medicine only as directed by your doctor. Do not take more of it, do not take it more often, and do not take it for a longer time than your doctor ordered. This is particularly important for children or elderly patients, since they may react very strongly to this medicine.

Continue taking this medicine for the full time of treatment. *Sometimes haloperidol must be taken for several days to several weeks before its full effect is reached.*

Dosing—The dose of haloperidol will be different for different patients. *Follow your doctor's orders or the directions on the label.* The following information includes only the average doses of haloperidol. *If your dose is different, do not change it* unless your doctor tells you to do so.

- The number of tablets or teaspoonfuls of solution that you take or injections that you receive depends on the strength of the medicine. Also, *the number of doses you take each day, the time allowed between doses, and the length of time you take the medicine depend on the medical problem for which you are using haloperidol.*
- For *oral* dosage forms (solution and tablets):

  —Adults and adolescents: To start, 500 micrograms to 5 milligrams two or three times a day. Your doctor may increase your dose if needed. However, the dose is usually not more than 100 milligrams a day.

  —Children 3 to 12 years of age or weighing 15 to 40 kilograms (33 to 88 pounds): Dose is based on body weight. The usual dose is 25 to 150 micrograms per kilogram (11 to 68 micrograms per pound) a day, taken in smaller doses two or three times a day.

  —Children up to 3 years of age: Dose must be determined by the doctor.

  —Older adults: To start, 500 micrograms to 2 milligrams two or three times a day. The doctor may increase your dose if needed.
- For *short-acting injection* dosage form:

  —Adults and adolescents: To start, 2 to 5 milligrams, usually injected into a muscle. The dose may be repeated every one to eight hours, depending on your condition.

  —Children: Dose must be determined by the doctor.
- For *long-acting or depot injection* dosage form:

  —Adults and adolescents: To start, the dose is usually 10 to 15 times the daily oral dose you were taking, injected into a muscle once a month. The doctor may adjust how much of this medicine you need and how often you will need it, depending on your condition.

  —Children: Dose must be determined by the doctor.

Missed dose—If you miss a dose of this medicine, take it as soon as possible. Then take any remaining doses for that day at regularly spaced intervals. Do not double doses.

Storage—To store this medicine:

- Keep out of the reach of children.
- Store away from heat and direct light.
- Do not store the tablet form of this medicine in the bathroom, near the kitchen sink, or in other damp places. Heat or moisture may cause the medicine to break down.
- Keep the liquid form of this medicine from freezing.
- Do not keep outdated medicine or medicine no longer needed. Be sure that any discarded medicine is out of the reach of children.

Precautions While Using This Medicine

Your doctor should check your progress at regular visits, especially during the first few months of treatment with this medicine. The amount of haloperidol you take may be changed often to meet the needs of your condition. This also helps prevent side effects.

Do not stop taking this medicine without first checking with your doctor. Your doctor may want you to reduce gradually the amount you are taking before stopping completely. This will allow your body time to adjust and help avoid a worsening of your medical condition.

This medicine will add to the effects of alcohol and other CNS depressants (medicines that slow down the nervous system, possibly causing drowsiness). Some examples of CNS depressants are antihistamines or medicine for hay fever, other allergies, or colds; sedatives, tranquilizers, or sleeping medicine; prescription pain medicine or narcotics; barbiturates; medicine for seizures; muscle relaxants; or anesthetics, including some dental anesthetics. *Check with your doctor before taking any of the above while you are taking this medicine.*

This medicine may cause some people to become dizzy, drowsy, or less alert than they are normally, especially as the amount of medicine is increased. Even if you take haloperidol at bedtime, you may feel drowsy or less alert on arising. *Make sure you know how you react to this medicine before you drive, use machines, or do anything else that could be dangerous if you are dizzy or are not alert.*

Although not a problem for many patients, dizziness, lightheadedness, or fainting may occur, especially when you get up from a lying or sitting position. Getting up slowly may help. However, if the problem continues or gets worse, check with your doctor.

This medicine will often make you sweat less, causing your body temperature to increase. *Use extra care not to become overheated during exercise or hot weather while you are taking this medicine, since overheating may result in heat stroke.* Also, hot baths or saunas may make you feel dizzy or faint while you are taking this medicine.

Before using any prescription or over-the-counter (OTC) medicine for colds or allergies, check with your doctor. These medicines may increase the chance of heat stroke or other unwanted effects, such as dizziness, dry mouth, blurred vision, and constipation, while you are taking haloperidol.

Before having any kind of surgery, dental treatment, or emergency treatment, tell the medical doctor or dentist in charge that you are using this medicine. Taking haloperidol together with medicines that are used during surgery or dental or emergency treatments may increase the CNS depressant effects.

Haloperidol may cause your skin to be more sensitive to sunlight than it is normally. Exposure to sunlight, even for brief periods of time, may cause a skin rash, itching, redness or other discoloration of the skin, or a severe sunburn. When you begin taking this medicine:

- Stay out of direct sunlight, especially between the hours of 10:00 a.m. and 3:00 p.m., if possible.
- Wear protective clothing, including a hat. Also, wear sunglasses.
- Apply a sun block product that has a skin protection factor (SPF) of at least 15. Some patients may require a product with a higher SPF number, especially if they have a fair complexion. If you have any questions about this, check with your doctor or pharmacist.
- Apply a sun block lipstick that has an SPF of at least 15 to protect your lips.
- Do not use a sunlamp or tanning bed or booth.

If you have a severe reaction from the sun, check with your doctor.

Haloperidol may cause dryness of the mouth. For temporary relief, use sugarless candy or gum, melt bits of ice in your mouth, or use a saliva substitute. However, if your mouth continues to feel dry for more than 2 weeks, check with your medical doctor or dentist. Continuing dryness of the mouth may increase the chance of dental disease, including tooth decay, gum disease, and fungus infections.

If you are *receiving this medicine by injection:*

- The effects of the long-acting injection form of this medicine may last for up to 6 weeks. *The precautions and side effects information for this medicine applies during this time.*

Side Effects of This Medicine

Along with its needed effects, haloperidol can sometimes cause serious side effects. Tardive dyskinesia (a movement disorder) may occur and may not go away after you stop using the medicine. Signs of tardive dyskinesia include fine, worm-like movements of the tongue, or other uncontrolled movements of the mouth, tongue, cheeks, jaw, or arms and legs. Other serious but rare side effects may also occur. These include severe muscle stiffness, fever, unusual tiredness or weakness, fast heartbeat, difficult breathing, increased sweating, loss of bladder control, and seizures (neuroleptic malignant syndrome). *You and your doctor should discuss the good this medicine will do as well as the risks of taking it.*

Stop taking haloperidol and get emergency help immediately if any of the following side effects occur:

Rare

Convulsions (seizures); difficult or fast breathing; fast heartbeat or irregular pulse; fever (high); high or low blood pressure; increased sweating; loss of bladder control; muscle stiffness (severe); unusually pale skin; unusual tiredness or weakness

Check with your doctor as soon as possible if any of the following side effects occur:

More common

Difficulty in speaking or swallowing; inability to move eyes; loss of balance control; mask-like face; muscle spasms, especially of the neck and back; restlessness or need to keep moving (severe); shuffling walk; stiffness of arms and legs; trembling and shaking of fingers and hands; twisting movements of body; weakness of arms and legs

Less common

Decreased thirst; difficulty in urination; dizziness, lightheadedness, or fainting; hallucinations (seeing or hearing things that are not there); lip smacking or puckering; puffing of cheeks; rapid or worm-like movements of tongue; skin rash; uncontrolled chewing movements; uncontrolled movements of arms and legs

Rare

Confusion; hot, dry skin, or lack of sweating; increased blinking or spasms of eyelid; muscle weakness; sore throat and fever; uncontrolled twisting movements of neck, trunk, arms, or legs; unusual bleeding or bruising; unusual facial expressions or body positions; yellow eyes or skin

Symptoms of overdose

Difficulty in breathing (severe); dizziness (severe); drowsiness (severe); muscle trembling, jerking, stiffness, or uncontrolled movements (severe); unusual tiredness or weakness (severe)

Other side effects may occur that usually do not need medical attention. These side effects may go away during treatment as your body adjusts to the medicine. However, check with your doctor if any of the following side effects continue or are bothersome:

More common

Blurred vision; changes in menstrual period; constipation; dryness of mouth; swelling or pain in breasts (in females); unusual secretion of milk; weight gain

Less common

Decreased sexual ability; drowsiness; increased sensitivity of skin to sun (skin rash, itching, redness or other discoloration of skin, or severe sunburn); nausea or vomiting

Some side effects, such as trembling of fingers and hands, or uncontrolled movements of the mouth, tongue, and jaw, may occur after you have stopped taking this medicine. If you notice any of these effects, check with your doctor as soon as possible.

Other side effects not listed above may also occur in some patients. If you notice any other effects, check with your doctor.

Additional Information

Once a medicine has been approved for marketing for a certain use, experience may show that it is also useful for other medical problems. Although these uses are not included in product labeling, haloperidol is used in certain patients with the following medical conditions:

- Huntington's chorea (an hereditary movement disorder)
- Infantile autism
- Nausea and vomiting caused by cancer chemotherapy

Other than the above information, there is no additional information relating to proper use, precautions, or side effects for these uses.

Annual revision: 03/19/93

HALOPROGIN Topical

A commonly used brand name in the U.S. and Canada is Halotex.

Description

Haloprogin (ha-loe-PROE-jin) belongs to the group of medicines called antifungals. It is used to treat some types of fungus infections.

Haloprogin is available only with your doctor's prescription, in the following dosage forms:

Topical

- Cream (U.S. and Canada)
- Solution (U.S. and Canada)

It is very important that you read and understand the following information. If any of it causes you special concern, check with your doctor. Also, *if you have any questions* or if you want more information about this medicine or your medical problem, *ask your doctor, nurse, or pharmacist.*

Before Using This Medicine

In deciding to use a medicine, the risks of using the medicine must be weighed against the good it will do. This is a decision you and your doctor will make. For haloprogin, the following should be considered:

Allergies—Tell your doctor if you have ever had any unusual or allergic reaction to haloprogin. Also tell your doctor and pharmacist if you are allergic to any other substances, such as preservatives or dyes.

Pregnancy—Haloprogin has not been studied in pregnant women. However, this medicine has not been shown to cause birth defects or other problems in animal studies.

Breast-feeding—It is not known whether topical haloprogin is absorbed into the body and passes into the breast milk. Although most medicines pass into breast milk in small amounts, many of them may be used safely while breast-feeding. Mothers who are using this medicine and who wish to breast-feed should discuss this with their doctor.

Children—Studies on this medicine have been done only in adult patients, and there is no specific information comparing use of haloprogin in children with use in other age groups.

Older adults—Many medicines have not been studied specifically in older people. Therefore, it may not be known whether they work exactly the same way they do in

younger adults. Although there is no specific information comparing use of this medicine in the elderly with use in other age groups, this medicine is not expected to cause different side effects or problems in older people than it does in younger adults.

Before you begin using any new medicine (prescription or nonprescription) or if you develop any new medical problem while you are using this medicine, check with your doctor, nurse, or pharmacist.

Proper Use of This Medicine

Apply enough haloprogin to cover the affected area, and rub in gently.

Keep this medicine away from the eyes.

To help clear up your infection completely, *keep using this medicine for the full time of treatment,* even if your condition has improved. *Do not miss any doses.*

Dosing—The dose of topical haloprogin will be different for different patients. *Follow your doctor's orders or the directions on the label.* The following information includes only the average doses of topical haloprogin. *If your dose is different, do not change it* unless your doctor tells you to do so.

The number of doses you use each day, the time allowed between doses, and the length of time you use the medicine depend on the medical problem for which you are using topical haloprogin.

- For *cream* or *topical solution* dosage forms:
  - —For treatment of fungus infections:
    - Adults—Use 2 times a day for 2 to 4 weeks.
    - Children—Use and dose must be determined by your doctor.

Missed dose—If you miss a dose of this medicine, apply it as soon as possible. However, if it is almost time for your next dose, skip the missed dose and go back to your regular dosing schedule.

Storage—To store this medicine:

- Keep out of the reach of children.
- Store away from heat and direct light.
- Keep the medicine from freezing.
- Do not keep outdated medicine or medicine no longer needed. Be sure that any discarded medicine is out of the reach of children.

Precautions While Using This Medicine

If your skin problem does not improve within 4 weeks, or if it becomes worse, check with your doctor.

Side Effects of This Medicine

Along with its needed effects, a medicine may cause some unwanted effects. Although not all of these side effects may occur, if they do occur they may need medical attention.

Check with your doctor as soon as possible if any of the following side effects occur:

Blistering, burning, itching, or other sign of skin irritation not present before use of this medicine

When you apply the solution form of this medicine, a mild temporary stinging may be expected.

Other side effects not listed above may also occur in some patients. If you notice any other effects, check with your doctor.

Annual revision: 06/21/93

HEADACHE MEDICINES, ERGOT DERIVATIVE–CONTAINING Systemic

This information applies to the following medicines:

Dihydroergotamine (dye-hye-droe-er-GOT-a-meen)
Ergotamine (er-GOT-a-meen)
Ergotamine and Caffeine (kaf-EEN)
Ergotamine, Caffeine, and Belladonna Alkaloids (bell-a-DON-a AL-ka-loids)
Ergotamine, Caffeine, Belladonna Alkaloids, and Pentobarbital (pen-toe-BAR-bi-tal)
Ergotamine, Caffeine, and Cyclizine (SYE-kli-zeen)
Ergotamine, Caffeine, and Dimenhydrinate (dye-men-HYE-dri-nate)
Ergotamine, Caffeine, and Diphenhydramine (dye-fen-HYE-dra-mine)

Some commonly used brand names are:

For Dihydroergotamine

In the U.S.
D.H.E. 45

In Canada
Dihydroergotamine-Sandoz

For Ergotamine

In the U.S.
Ergomar
Ergostat

In Canada
Ergomar
Gynergen
Medihaler Ergotamine

For Ergotamine and Caffeine
In the U.S.
Cafergot
Cafertine
Cafetrate
Ercaf
Ergo-Caff
Gotamine
Migergot
Wigraine
Generic name product may also be available.
In Canada
Cafergot

For Ergotamine, Caffeine, and Belladonna Alkaloids*
In Canada
Wigraine

For Ergotamine, Caffeine, Belladonna Alkaloids, and Pentobarbital*
In Canada
Cafergot-PB

For Ergotamine, Caffeine, and Cyclizine*
In Canada
Megral

For Ergotamine, Caffeine, and Dimenhydrinate*
In Canada
Gravergol

For Ergotamine, Caffeine, and Diphenhydramine*
In Canada
Ergodryl

*Not commercially available in the U.S.

Description

Dihydroergotamine and ergotamine belong to the group of medicines known as ergot alkaloids. They are used to treat severe, throbbing headaches, such as migraine and cluster headaches. Dihydroergotamine and ergotamine are not ordinary pain relievers. They will not relieve any kind of pain other than throbbing headaches. Because these medicines can cause serious side effects, they are usually used for patients whose headaches are not relieved by acetaminophen, aspirin, or other pain relievers.

Dihydroergotamine and ergotamine may cause blood vessels in the body to constrict (become narrower). This effect can lead to serious side effects that are caused by a decrease in the flow of blood (blood circulation) to many parts of the body.

The caffeine present in many ergotamine-containing combinations helps ergotamine work better and faster by causing more of it to be quickly absorbed into the body. The belladonna alkaloids, cyclizine, dimenhydrinate, and diphenhydramine in some combinations help to relieve nausea and vomiting, which often occur together with the headaches. Cyclizine, dimenhydinate, diphenhydramine, and pentobarbital also help the patient relax and even sleep. This also helps relieve headaches.

Dihydroergotamine is also used for other conditions, as determined by your doctor.

These medicines are available only with your doctor's prescription, in the following dosage forms:

Oral

Ergotamine
- Inhalation aerosol (Canada)
- Sublingual tablets (U.S. and Canada)
- Tablets (Canada)

Ergotamine and Caffeine
- Tablets (U.S. and Canada)

Ergotamine, Caffeine, and Belladonna Alkaloids
- Tablets (Canada)

Ergotamine, Caffeine, Belladonna Alkaloids, and Pentobarbital
- Tablets (Canada)

Ergotamine, Caffeine, and Cyclizine
- Tablets (Canada)

Ergotamine, Caffeine, and Dimenhydrinate
- Capsules (Canada)

Ergotamine, Caffeine, and Diphenhydramine
- Capsules (Canada)

Parenteral

Dihydroergotamine
- Injection (U.S. and Canada)

Rectal

Ergotamine and Caffeine
- Suppositories (U.S. and Canada)

Ergotamine, Caffeine, and Belladonna Alkaloids
- Suppositories (Canada)

Ergotamine, Caffeine, Belladonna Alkaloids, and Pentobarbital
- Suppositories (Canada)

It is very important that you read and understand the following information. If any of it causes you special concern, check with your doctor. Also, *if you have any questions* or if you want more information about this medicine or your medical problem, *ask your doctor, nurse, or pharmacist.*

Before Using This Medicine

In deciding to use a medicine, the risks of taking the medicine must be weighed against the good it will do. This is a decision you and your doctor will make. For these headache medicines, the following should be considered:

Allergies—Tell your doctor if you have ever had any unusual or allergic reaction to atropine, belladonna, pentobarbital or other barbiturates, caffeine, cyclizine, dimenhydrinate, diphenhydramine, or an ergot medicine. Also tell your doctor and pharmacist if you are allergic to any other substances, such as foods, preservatives, or dyes.

Pregnancy—Use of dihydroergotamine or ergotamine by pregnant women may cause serious harm, including death of the fetus and miscarriage. Therefore, *these medicines should not be used during pregnancy.*

Breast-feeding—

- *For dihydroergotamine and ergotamine*: These medicines pass into the breast milk and may cause unwanted effects, such as vomiting, diarrhea, weak pulse, changes in blood pressure, or convulsions (seizures) in nursing babies. Large amounts of these medicines may also decrease the flow of breast milk.

- *For caffeine*: Caffeine passes into the breast milk. Large amounts of it may cause the baby to appear jittery or to have trouble in sleeping.
- *For belladonna alkaloids, cyclizine, dimenhydrinate, and diphenhydramine*: These medicines have drying effects. Therefore, it is possible that they may reduce the amount of breast milk in some people. Dimenhydrinate passes into the breast milk. Cylizine may also pass into the breast milk.
- *For pentobarbital*: Pentobarbital passes into the breast milk. Large amounts of it may cause unwanted effects such as drowsiness in nursing babies.

Be sure that you discuss these possible problems with your doctor before taking any of these medicines.

Children—

- *For dihydroergotamine and ergotamine*: These medicines are used to relieve severe, throbbing headaches in children 6 years of age or older. They have not been shown to cause different side effects or problems in children than they do in adults. However, these medicines can cause serious side effects in any patient. Therefore, it is especially important that you discuss with the child's doctor the good that this medicine may do as well as the risks of using it.
- *For belladonna alkaloids*: Young children, especially children with spastic paralysis or brain damage, may be especially sensitive to the effects of belladonna alkaloids. This may increase the chance of side effects during treatment.
- *For cyclizine, dimenhydrinate, diphenhydramine, and pentobarbital*: Although these medicines often cause drowsiness, some children become excited after taking them.

Older adults—

- *For dihydroergotamine and ergotamine*: The chance of serious side effects caused by decreases in blood flow is increased in elderly people receiving these medicines.
- *For belladonna alkaloids, cyclizine, dimenhydrinate, diphenhydramine, and pentobarbital*: Elderly people are more sensitive than younger adults to the effects of these medicines. This may increase the chance of side effects such as excitement, depression, dizziness, drowsiness, and confusion.

Other medicines—Although certain medicines should not be used together at all, in other cases two different medicines may be used together even if an interaction might occur. In these cases, your doctor may want to change the dose, or other precautions may be necessary. Many medicines can add to or decrease the effects of the belladonna alkaloids, caffeine, cyclizine, dimenhydrinate, diphenhydramine, or pentobarbital present in some of these headache medicines. Therefore, you should tell your doctor and pharmacist if you are taking *any* other prescription or nonprescription (over-the-counter [OTC]) medicine. This is especially important if any medicine you take causes excitement, trouble in sleeping, dryness of the mouth, dizziness, or drowsiness.

When you are taking dihydroergotamine or ergotamine, it is especially important that your doctor and pharmacist know if you are taking any of the following:

- Cocaine or
- Epinephrine by injection [e.g., Epi-Pen] or
- Other ergot medicines (ergoloid mesylates [e.g., Hydergine], ergonovine [e.g., Ergotrate], methylergonovine [e.g., Methergine], methysergide [e.g., Sansert])—The chance of serious side effects caused by dihydroergotamine or ergotamine may be increased

Other medical problems—The presence of other medical problems may affect the use of these headache medicines. Make sure you tell your doctor if you have any other medical problems, especially:

- Agoraphobia (fear of open or public places) or
- Panic attacks or
- Stomach ulcer or
- Trouble in sleeping (insomnia)—Caffeine can make your condition worse
- Diarrhea—Rectal dosage forms (suppositories) will not be effective if you have diarrhea
- Difficult urination or
- Enlarged prostate or
- Glaucoma (not well controlled) or
- Heart or blood vessel disease or
- High blood pressure (not well controlled) or
- Infection or
- Intestinal blockage or other intestinal problems or
- Itching (severe) or
- Kidney disease or
- Liver disease or
- Mental depression or
- Overactive thyroid or
- Urinary tract blockage—The chance of side effects may be increased

Also, tell your doctor if you need, or if you have recently had, an angioplasty (a procedure done to improve the flow of blood in a blocked blood vessel) or surgery on a blood vessel. The chance of serious side effects caused by dihydroergotamine or ergotamine may be increased.

Before you begin using any new medicine (prescription or nonprescription) or if you develop any new medical problem while you are using this medicine, check with your doctor, nurse, or pharmacist.

Proper Use of This Medicine

Use this medicine only as directed by your doctor. Do not use more of it, and do not use it more often, than directed. If the amount you are to use does not relieve your headache, check with your doctor. Taking too much dihydroergotamine or ergotamine, or taking it too often, may cause serious effects, especially in elderly patients. Also, if a headache medicine (especially ergotamine) is used too often for migraines, it may lose its effectiveness or even cause a type of physical dependence. If this occurs, your headaches may actually get worse.

This medicine works best if you:

- *Use it at the first sign of headache or migraine attack. If you get warning signals of a coming migraine, take it before the headache actually starts.*
- *Lie down in a quiet, dark room until you are feeling better.*

Your doctor may direct you to take another medicine to help prevent headaches. *It is important that you follow your doctor's directions, even if your headaches continue to occur.* Headache-preventing medicines may take several weeks to start working. Even after they do start working, your headaches may not go away completely. However, your headaches should occur less often, and they should be less severe and easier to relieve. This can reduce the amount of dihydroergotamine, ergotamine, or pain relievers that you need. If you do not notice any improvement after several weeks of headache-preventing treatment, check with your doctor.

For patients using *dihydroergotamine*:

- Dihydroergotamine is given only by injection. Your doctor or nurse will teach you how to inject yourself with the medicine. Be sure to follow the directions carefully. Check with your doctor or nurse if you have any problems using the medicine.

For patients using *ergotamine inhalation* [e.g., Medihaler Ergotamine]:

- This medicine comes with patient directions. Read them carefully before using the medicine, and check with your doctor or pharmacist if you have any questions.
- To use the inhaler—Remove the cap, then shake the container well. After breathing out, place the mouthpiece of the inhaler in your mouth. Aim it at the back of the throat. Breathe in; at the same time, press the vial down into the adapter. After inhaling the medicine, hold your breath as long as you can.

For patients using the *sublingual (under-the-tongue) tablets of ergotamine*:

- To use—Place the tablet under your tongue and let it remain there until it disappears. The sublingual tablet should not be chewed or swallowed, because it works faster when it is absorbed into the body through the lining of the mouth. Do not eat, drink, or smoke while the tablet is under your tongue.

For patients using *rectal suppository forms of a headache medicine*:

- If the suppository is too soft to use, chill it in the refrigerator for 30 minutes or run cold water over it before removing the foil wrapper.
- If you have been directed to use part of a suppository, you should divide the suppository into pieces that all contain the same amount of medicine. To do this, use a sharp knife and carefully cut the suppository lengthwise (from top to bottom) into pieces that are the same size. The suppository will be easier to cut if it has been kept in the refrigerator.
- To insert the suppository—First remove the foil wrapper and moisten the suppository with cold water. Lie down on your side and use your finger to push the suppository well up into the rectum.

Dosing—The dose of these headache medicines will be different for different patients. *Follow your doctor's orders or the directions on the label.* The following information includes only the average doses of these medicines. *If your dose is different, do not change it* unless your doctor tells you to do so.

For dihydroergotamine

- Adults: For relieving a migraine or cluster headache—1 mg. If your headache is not better, and no side effects are occurring, a second 1-mg dose may be used at least one hour later.
- Children 6 years of age and older: For relieving a migraine headache—It is not likely that a child will be receiving dihydrogergotamine at home. If a child needs the medicine, the dose will have to be determined by the doctor.

For ergotamine

- Some headache medicines contain only ergotamine. Some of them contain other medicines along with the ergotamine. The number of tablets, capsules, or suppositories that you need for each dose depends on the amount of ergotamine in them. The size of each dose, and the number of doses that you take, also depends on the reason you are taking the medicine and on how you react to the medicine.
- For *oral* (capsule or tablet) and *sublingual* (under-the-tongue tablet) dosage forms:
  —Adults:
    - For relieving a migraine or cluster headache—1 or 2 mg of ergotamine. If your headache is not better, and no side effects are occurring, a second dose and even a third dose may be taken; however the doses should be taken at least 30 minutes apart. People who usually need more than one dose of the medicine, and who do not get side effects from it, may be able to take a larger first dose of not more than 3 mg of ergotamine. This may provide better relief of the headache with only one dose. *The medicine should not be taken more often 2 times a week, at least five days apart.*
    - For preventing cluster headaches—The dose of ergotamine, and the number of doses you need every day, will depend on how many headaches you usually get each day. For some people, 1 or

2 mg of ergotamine once a day may be enough. Other people may need to take 1 or 2 mg of ergotamine 2 or 3 times a day.

• For all uses—*Do not take more than 6 mg of ergotamine a day in the form of capsules or tablets.*

—Children 6 years of age and older: For relieving migraine headaches—1 mg of ergotamine. If the headache is not better, and no side effects are occurring, a second dose and even a third dose may be taken; however, the doses should be taken at least 30 minutes apart. *Children should not take more than 3 mg of ergotamine a day in the form of capsules or tablets. Also, this medicine should not be taken more often than 2 times a week, at least five days apart.*

- For *rectal suppository* dosage forms:

—Adults: For relieving migraine or cluster headaches—Usually 1 mg of ergotamine, but the dose may range from half of this amount to up to 2 mg. If your headache is not better, and no side effects are occurring, a second dose and even a third dose may be used; however the doses should be taken at least 30 minutes apart. People who usually need more than one dose of the medicine, and who do not get side effects from it, may be able to use a larger first dose of not more than 3 mg. This may provide better relief of the headache with only one dose. *Adults should not use more than 4 mg of ergotamine a day in suppository form. Also, this medicine should not be used more often than 2 times a week, at least five days apart.*

—Children 6 years of age and older: For relieving migraine headaches—One-half or 1 mg of ergotamine. *Children should not receive more than 1 mg a day of ergotamine in suppository form. Also, this medicine should not be used more often than 2 times a week, at least five days apart.*

- For the *oral inhalation* dosage form:

—Adults: For relieving a migraine or cluster headache—1 spray (1 inhalation). Another inhalation may be used at least 5 minutes later, if needed. Up to a total of 6 inhalations a day may be used, at least 5 minutes apart. *This medicine should not be used more often than 2 times a week, at least five days apart.*

—Children: To be determined by the doctor.

Storage—To store this medicine:

- Keep out of the reach of children since overdose is especially dangerous in children.
- Store away from heat and direct light.
- Do not store in the bathroom, near the kitchen sink, or in other damp places. Heat or moisture may cause the medicine to break down.
- Suppositories should be stored in a cool place, but not allowed to freeze. Some manufacturers recommend keeping them in a refrigerator; others do not. Follow the directions on the package. However, cutting the suppository into smaller pieces, if you need to do so, will be easier if the suppository is kept in the refrigerator.
- Do not puncture, break, or burn the ergotamine inhalation aerosol container, even after it is empty.
- Do not keep outdated medicine or medicine no longer needed. Be sure that any discarded medicine is out of the reach of children.

Precautions While Using This Medicine

Check with your doctor:

- If your migraine headaches are worse than they were before you started using this medicine, or your headache medicine stops working as well as it did when you first started using it. This may mean that you are in danger of becoming dependent on the headache medicine. *Do not try to get better relief by increasing the dose.*
- If your migraine headaches are occurring more often than they did before you started using this medicine. This is especially important if a new headache occurs within 1 day after you took your last dose of headache medicine, or if you are having headaches every day. This may mean that you are dependent on the headache medicine. *Continuing to take this medicine will cause even more headaches later on.* Your doctor can give you advice on how to relieve the headaches.

Drinking alcoholic beverages can make headaches worse or cause new headaches to occur. People who suffer from severe headaches should probably avoid alcoholic beverages, especially during a headache.

Smoking may increase some of the harmful effects of dihydroergotamine or ergotamine. It is best to avoid smoking for several hours after taking these medicines.

Dihydroergotamine and ergotamine may make you more sensitive to cold temperatures, especially if you have blood circulation problems. They tend to decrease blood flow in the skin, fingers, and toes. Dress warmly during cold weather and be careful during prolonged exposure to cold temperatures. This is especially important for older patients, who are more likely than younger adults to already have problems with their circulation.

If you have a serious infection or illness of any kind, check with your doctor before using this medicine, since you may be more sensitive to its effects.

For patients using *ergotamine inhalation* [e.g., Medihaler Ergotamine]:

- Cough, hoarseness, or throat irritation may occur. Gargling and rinsing your mouth after each dose may help prevent the hoarseness and irritation. However, check with your doctor if these or any other side effects continue or are bothersome.

For patients taking one of the combination medicines that contains *caffeine*:

- Caffeine may interfere with the results of a test that uses dipyridamole (e.g., Persantine) to help find out how well your blood is flowing through certain blood vessels. You should not have any caffeine for at least 12 hours before the test.
- Caffeine may also interfere with some other laboratory tests. Before having any other laboratory tests, tell the person in charge if you have taken a medicine that contains caffeine.

For patients taking one of the combination medicines that contains *belladonna alkaloids, cyclizine, dimenhydrinate, diphenhydramine, or pentobarbital*:

- These medicines may cause some people to have blurred vision or to become drowsy, dizzy, lightheaded, or less alert than they are normally. These effects may be especially severe if you also take CNS depressants (medicines that slow down the nervous system, possibly causing drowsiness) together with one of these combination medicines. Some examples of CNS depressants are antihistamines or medicine for hay fever, other allergies, or colds; sedatives, tranquilizers, or sleeping medicine; prescription pain medicine or narcotics; barbiturates; medicine for seizures; muscle relaxants; and antiemetics (medicines that prevent or relieve nausea or vomiting). If you are not able to lie down for a while, *make sure you know how you react to this medicine or combination of medicines before you drive, use machines, or do anything else that could be dangerous if you are dizzy or are not alert and able to see well.*
- Belladonna alkaloids, cyclizine, dimenhydrinate, and diphenhydramine may cause dryness of the mouth, nose, and throat. For temporary relief of mouth dryness, use sugarless candy or gum, melt bits of ice in your mouth, or use a saliva substitute.
- Belladonna alkaloids may interfere with certain laboratory tests that check the amount of acid in your stomach. They should not be taken for 24 hours before the test.
- Cyclizine, dimenhydrinate, and diphenhydramine may interfere with skin tests that show whether you are allergic to certain substances. They should not be taken for 3 days before the test.

Side Effects of This Medicine

Along with its needed effects, a medicine may cause some unwanted effects. Although not all of these side effects may occur, if they do occur they may need medical attention.

Check with your doctor immediately if the following side effects occur, because they may mean that you are developing a problem with blood circulation:

Less common or rare

Anxiety or confusion (severe); change in vision; chest pain; increase in blood pressure; pain in arms, legs, or lower back, especially if pain occurs in your calves or heels while you are walking; pale, bluish-colored, or cold hands or feet (not caused by cold temperatures and occurring together with other side effects listed in this section); red or violet-colored blisters on the skin of the hands or feet

Also check with your doctor immediately if any of the following side effects occur, because they may mean that you have taken an overdose of the medicine:

Less common or rare

Convulsions (seizures); diarrhea, nausea, vomiting, or stomach pain or bloating (severe) occurring together with other signs of overdose or of problems with blood circulation; dizziness, drowsiness, or weakness (severe), occurring together with other signs of overdose or of problems with blood circulation; fast or slow heartbeat; diarrhea; headaches, more often and/or more severe than before; problems with moving bowels, occurring together with pain or discomfort in the rectum (with rectal suppositories only); shortness of breath; unusual excitement

The following side effects may go away after a little while. *Do not take any more medicine while they are present.* If any of them occur together with other signs of problems with blood circulation, *check with your doctor right away.* Even if any of the following side effects occur without other signs of problems with blood circulation, *check with your doctor if any of them continue for more than one hour*:

More common

Itching of skin; coldness, numbness, or tingling in fingers, toes, or face; weakness in legs

Also, check with your doctor as soon as possible if you notice any of the following side effects:

More common

Swelling of face, fingers, feet, or lower legs

Other side effects may occur that usually do not need medical attention. These side effects may go away after a little while. However, check with your doctor if any of the following side effects continue or are bothersome:

More common

Diarrhea, nausea, or vomiting (occurring without other signs of overdose or problems with blood circulation); dizziness or drowsiness (occurring without other signs of overdose or problems with blood circulation, especially with combinations containing cyclizine, dimenhydrinate, diphenhydramine, or pentobarbital);

nervousness or restlessness; dryness of mouth (especially with combinations containing belladonna alkaloids, cyclizine, dimenhydrinate, or diphenhydramine)

After you stop taking this medicine, your body may need time to adjust. The length of time this takes depends on the amount of medicine you were taking and how long you took it. During this time check with your doctor if your headaches begin again or worsen.

Other side effects not listed above may also occur in some patients. If you notice any other effects, check with your doctor.

Additional Information

Once a medicine has been approved for marketing for a certain use, experience may show that it is also useful for other medical problems. Although this use is not specifically included in product labeling, dihydroergotamine is sometimes used together with another medicine (heparin) to help prevent blood clots that may occur after certain kinds of surgery. It is also used to prevent or treat low blood pressure in some patients.

For patients receiving this medicine for *preventing blood clots*:

- You may need to receive this medicine two or three times a day for several days in a row. This may increase the chance of problems caused by decreased blood flow. Your doctor or nurse will be following your progress, to make sure that this medicine is not causing problems with blood circulation.

For patients using this medicine to *prevent or treat low blood pressure*:

- Take this medicine every day as directed by your doctor.
- The dose of dihydroergotamine will depend on whether the medicine is going to be injected under the skin or into a muscle, and, sometimes, on the weight of the patient. For these reasons, the dose will have to be determined by your doctor.
- Your doctor will need to check your progress at regular visits, to make sure that the medicine is working properly without causing side effects.
- This medicine is less likely to cause problems with blood circulation in patients with low blood pressure than it is in patients with normal or high blood pressure.
- In patients being treated for low blood pressure, an increase in blood pressure is the wanted effect, not a side effect that may need medical attention.

Other than the above information, there is no additional information relating to proper use, precautions, or side effects for these uses.

Annual revision: 09/08/92

HEPARIN Systemic

Some commonly used brand names are:

In the U.S.

Calciparine
Liquaemin

Generic name product may also be available.

In Canada

Calcilean
Hepalean
Calciparine
Heparin Leo

Generic name product may also be available.

Description

Heparin (HEP-a-rin) is an anticoagulant. It is used to decrease the clotting ability of the blood and help prevent harmful clots from forming in the blood vessels. This medicine is sometimes called a blood thinner, although it does not actually thin the blood. Heparin will not dissolve blood clots that have already formed, but it may prevent the clots from becoming larger and causing more serious problems.

Heparin is often used as a treatment for certain blood vessel, heart, and lung conditions. Heparin is also used to prevent blood clotting during open-heart surgery, bypass surgery, and dialysis. It is also used in low doses to prevent the formation of blood clots in certain patients, especially those who must have certain types of surgery or who must remain in bed for a long time.

Heparin is available only with your doctor's prescription, in the following dosage form:

Parenteral

- Injection (U.S. and Canada)

It is very important that you read and understand the following information. If any of it causes you special concern, check with your doctor. Also, *if you have any questions* or if you want more information about this medicine or your medical problem, *ask your doctor, nurse, or pharmacist.*

Before Using This Medicine

In deciding to use a medicine, the risks of taking the medicine must be weighed against the good it will do.

This is a decision you and your doctor will make. For heparin, the following should be considered:

Allergies—Tell your doctor if you have ever had any unusual or allergic reaction to heparin, to beef, or to pork. Also tell your doctor and pharmacist if you are allergic to any other substances, such as foods, preservatives, or dyes.

Pregnancy—Heparin has not been shown to cause birth defects or bleeding problems in the baby. However, use during the last 3 months of pregnancy or during the month following the baby's delivery may cause bleeding problems in the mother.

Breast-feeding—Heparin does not pass into the breast milk. However, heparin can rarely cause bone problems in the nursing mother. This effect has been reported to occur when heparin is used for 2 weeks or more. Be sure to discuss this with your doctor.

Children—Heparin has been tested in children and, in effective doses, has not been shown to cause different side effects or problems than it does in adults.

Older adults—Bleeding problems may be more likely to occur in elderly patients, especially women, who are usually more sensitive than younger adults to the effects of heparin.

Other medicines—Although certain medicines should not be used together at all, in other cases two different medicines may be used together even if an interaction might occur. In these cases, your doctor may want to change the dose, or other precautions may be necessary. When you are taking heparin, it is especially important that your doctor and pharmacist know if you are taking any of the following:

- Aspirin or
- Carbenicillin by injection (e.g., Geopen) or
- Dipyridamole (e.g., Persantine) or
- Divalproex (e.g., Depakote) or
- Medicine for inflammation or pain, except narcotics, or
- Medicine for overactive thyroid or
- Moxalactam (e.g., Moxam) or
- Pentoxifylline (e.g., Trental) or
- Plicamycin (e.g., Mithracin) or
- Probenecid (e.g., Benemid) or
- Sulfinpyrazone (e.g., Anturane) or
- Ticarcillin (e.g., Ticar) or
- Valproic acid (e.g., Depakene)—Using any of these medicines together with heparin may increase the risk of bleeding

Also, tell your doctor if you are now receiving any kind of medicine by intramuscular (IM) injection.

Other medical problems—The presence of other medical problems may affect the use of heparin. Make sure you tell your doctor if you have any other medical problems, especially:

- Allergies or asthma (history of)—The risk of an allergic reaction to heparin may be increased
- Blood disease or bleeding problems or
- Colitis or stomach ulcer (or history of) or
- Diabetes mellitus (sugar diabetes) (severe) or
- High blood pressure (hypertension) or
- Kidney disease or
- Liver disease or
- Tuberculosis (active)—The risk of bleeding may be increased

Also, tell your doctor if you have received heparin before and had a reaction to it called thrombocytopenia, or if new blood clots formed while you were receiving the medicine.

In addition, it is important that you tell your doctor if you have recently had any of the following conditions or medical procedures:

- Childbirth or
- Falls or blows to the body or head or
- Heavy or unusual menstrual bleeding or
- Insertion of intrauterine device (IUD) or
- Medical or dental surgery or
- Spinal anesthesia or
- X-ray (radiation) treatment—The risk of serious bleeding may be increased

Before you begin using any new medicine (prescription or nonprescription) or if you develop any new medical problem while you are using this medicine, check with your doctor, nurse, or pharmacist.

Proper Use of This Medicine

If you are using these injections at home, make sure your doctor has explained exactly how this medicine is to be given.

To obtain the best results without causing serious bleeding, *use this medicine exactly as directed by your doctor. Be certain that you are using the right amount of heparin, and that you use it according to schedule.* Be especially careful that you do not use more of it, do not use it more often, and do not use it for a longer time than your doctor ordered.

Your doctor should check your progress at regular visits. A blood test must be taken regularly to see how fast your blood is clotting so that your doctor can decide on the proper amount of heparin you should be receiving each day.

Missed dose—If you miss a dose of this medicine, use it as soon as possible. However, if it is almost time for your next dose, do not use the missed dose at all and do not double the next one. *Doubling the dose may cause bleeding.* Instead, go back to your regular dosing schedule. It is best to keep a record of each dose as you use it to avoid mistakes. Be sure to give your doctor a record of any doses you miss. If you have any questions about this, check with your doctor.

Storage—To store this medicine:

- Keep out of the reach of children.
- Store away from heat and direct light.
- Keep the medicine from freezing.
- Do not keep outdated medicine or medicine no longer needed. Be sure that any discarded medicine is out of the reach of children.

Precautions While Using This Medicine

Do not take aspirin while using this medicine. Many nonprescription (over-the-counter [OTC]) medicines and some prescription medicines contain aspirin. Check the labels of all medicines you take. Also, do not take ibuprofen unless it has been ordered by your doctor. In addition, there are many other medicines that may change the way heparin works or increase the chance of bleeding if they are used together with heparin. It is best to check with your doctor or pharmacist before taking any other medicine while you are using heparin.

Tell all medical doctors and dentists you visit that you are using this medicine.

It is recommended that you carry identification stating that you are using heparin. If you have any questions about what kind of identification to carry, check with your doctor, nurse, or pharmacist.

While you are using this medicine, it is very important that you avoid sports and other activities that may cause you to be injured. Report to your doctor any falls, blows to the body or head, or other injuries, since serious bleeding inside the body may occur without your knowing about it.

Take special care in brushing your teeth and in shaving. Use a soft toothbrush and floss gently. Also, it is best to use an electric shaver rather than a blade.

Side Effects of This Medicine

Since many things can affect the way your body reacts to this medicine, you should always watch for signs of unusual bleeding. Unusual bleeding may mean that your body is getting more heparin than it needs.

Along with its needed effects, a medicine may cause some unwanted effects. Although not all of these side effects may occur, if they do occur they may need medical attention.

Check with your doctor immediately if any of the following signs and symptoms of bleeding inside the body occur:

Abdominal or stomach pain or swelling; back pain or backaches; blood in urine; bloody or black, tarry stools; constipation; coughing up blood; dizziness; headaches (severe or continuing); joint pain, stiffness, or swelling; vomiting of blood or material that looks like coffee grounds

Also, *check with your doctor immediately* if any of the following side effects occur, since they may mean that you are having a serious allergic reaction to the medicine:

Changes in the skin color of the face; fast or irregular breathing; puffiness or swelling of the eyelids or around the eyes; shortness of breath, troubled breathing, tightness in chest, and/or wheezing; skin rash, hives, and/or itching

Also, check with your doctor as soon as possible if any of the following occur:

Bleeding from gums when brushing teeth; heavy bleeding or oozing from cuts or wounds; unexplained bruising or purplish areas on skin; unexplained nosebleeds; unusually heavy or unexpected menstrual bleeding

Other side effects that may need medical attention may occur while you are using this medicine. Check with your doctor as soon as possible if any of the following side effects occur:

Less common or rare

Back or rib pain (with long-term use only); change in skin color, especially near the place of injection or in the fingers, toes, arms, or legs; chest pain; chills and/or fever; collection of blood under skin (blood blister) at place of injection; decrease in height (with long-term use only); frequent or persistent erection; irritation, pain, redness, or ulcers at place of injection; itching and burning feeling, especially on the bottom of the feet; nausea and/or vomiting; numbness or tingling in hands or feet; pain, coldness, or blue color of skin of arms or legs; peeling of skin; runny nose; tearing of eyes; unusual hair loss (with long-term use only)

Other side effects not listed above may also occur in some patients. If you notice any other effects, check with your doctor.

Annual revision: August 1990

HEPATITIS B VACCINE RECOMBINANT Systemic

Some commonly used brand names are:

In the U.S.

Engerix-B
Recombivax HB
Recombivax HB Dialysis Formulation

In Canada

Engerix-B
Recombivax HB

Another commonly used name is HB vaccine.

Description

Hepatitis (hep-ah-ty-tiss) B vaccine recombinant is an active immunizing agent used to prevent infection by the hepatitis B virus. The vaccine works by causing your body to produce its own protection (antibodies) against the disease.

Hepatitis B vaccine recombinant is made without any human blood or blood products or any other substances of human origin and cannot give the hepatitis B virus (HBV) or the human immunodeficiency virus (HIV) to you.

HBV infection is a major cause of serious liver diseases, such as virus hepatitis and cirrhosis, and a type of liver cancer called primary hepatocellular carcinoma.

Pregnant women who have hepatitis B infection or are carriers of hepatitis B virus can give the disease to their babies when they are born. These babies often suffer serious long-term illnesses from the disease.

Immunization against hepatitis B disease is recommended for persons of all ages, including newborn babies, infants, children, and adults, who may be at increased risk of infection from hepatitis B virus. These include:

- Infants born to mothers who have hepatitis B infection or are carriers of hepatitis B.
- Sexually active homosexual and bisexual males, including those with HIV infection.
- Sexually active heterosexual persons with multiple partners.
- Persons who may be exposed to the virus by means of blood, blood products, or human bites, such as health care workers, employees in medical facilities, patients and staff of live-in facilities and day-care programs for the mentally retarded, morticians and embalmers, police and fire department personnel, and military personnel.
- Persons who have kidney disease or who undergo blood dialysis.
- Persons with blood clotting disorders who receive transfusions of clotting-factor concentrates.
- Household and sexual contacts of HBV carriers.
- Persons in areas with high risk of HBV infection, such as Alaskan Eskimos, Pacific Islanders, and refugees from Indochina, Haiti, parts of Africa, and parts of Asia; persons accepting orphans or adoptees from these areas; and travelers to these areas.
- Persons who use illegal injectable drugs and inmates of prisons.

This vaccine is available only from your doctor or other authorized health care provider, in the following dosage form:

Parenteral

- Injection (U.S. and Canada)

It is very important that you read and understand the following information. If any of it causes you special concern, check with your doctor. Also, *if you have any questions* or if you want more information about this medicine or your medical problem, *ask your doctor, nurse, or pharmacist.*

Before Receiving This Vaccine

In deciding to use a medicine, the risks of using the medicine must be weighed against the good it will do. This is a decision you and your doctor will make. For hepatitis B recombinant vaccine, the following should be considered:

Allergies—Tell your doctor if you have ever had any unusual or allergic reaction to this vaccine or to the hepatitis B vaccine made from human plasma. Also tell your doctor and pharmacist if you are allergic to any other substances, such as foods (especially baker's yeast). The vaccine is made by using baker's yeast; persons allergic to baker's yeast may also be allergic to the vaccine.

Pregnancy—Studies on effects in pregnancy have not been done in either humans or animals. However, since the vaccine does not contain contagious particles, it is not expected to cause problems during pregnancy.

Breast-feeding—It is not known whether hepatitis B vaccine passes into the breast milk. However, since the vaccine does not contain contagious particles, it is not expected to cause problems in nursing babies.

Children—Hepatitis B vaccine has been tested in newborns, infants, and children and, in effective doses, has not been shown to cause different side effects or problems than it does in adults. The vaccine strength for use in dialysis patients has been studied only in adult patients, and there is no specific information about its use in children.

Older adults—This vaccine is not expected to cause different side effects or problems in older people than it does in younger adults. However, persons over 50 years of age may not become as immune to the virus as do younger adults and may need booster doses of the vaccine.

Other medicines—Although certain medicines should not be used together at all, in other cases two different medicines may be used together even if an interaction might occur. In these cases, your doctor may want to change the dose, or other precautions may be necessary. Before you receive hepatitis B vaccine, it is especially important that your doctor and pharmacist know if you are using any other prescription or nonprescription (over-the-counter [OTC]) medicine.

Other medical problems—The presence of other medical problems may affect the use of hepatitis B vaccine. Make

sure you tell your doctor if you have any other medical problems, especially:

- Heart disease (severe) or
- Lung disease (severe)—Some of the side effects of the vaccine may make the condition worse
- Immune deficiency condition—The condition may decrease the useful effects of hepatitis B vaccine. The dose of the vaccine may need to be increased
- Severe illness with fever—The symptoms of the condition may be confused with the possible side effects of the vaccine

Before you begin using any new medicine (prescription or nonprescription) or if you develop any new medical problem while you are using this medicine, check with your doctor, nurse, or pharmacist.

Side Effects of This Medicine

Along with its needed effects, a medicine may cause some unwanted effects. Although not all of these side effects may occur, if they do occur they may need medical attention.

Get emergency help immediately if any of the following side effects occur:

Symptoms of allergic reaction—Rare

Difficulty in breathing or swallowing; hives; itching, especially of feet or hands; reddening of skin, especially around ears; swelling of eyes, face, or inside of nose; unusual tiredness or weakness (sudden and severe)

Check with your doctor as soon as possible if any of the following side effects occur:

Rare

Aches or pain in joints, fever, or skin rash or welts (may occur days to weeks following the vaccine); muscle weakness or numbness or tingling of limbs; pain or tenderness of eyes

Other side effects may occur that usually do not need medical attention. However, check with your doctor if any of the following side effects continue or are bothersome:

More common

Soreness at the place of injection

Less common

Dizziness; fever of 37.7 °C (100 °F) or over; hard lump, redness, swelling, pain, itching, purple spot, tenderness, or warmth at place of injection; headache; unusual tiredness or weakness

Rare

Aches or pain in joints or muscles; back pain or stiffness or pain in neck or shoulder; chills; diarrhea or stomach cramps or pain; feeling of bodily discomfort; increased sweating; headache (mild), sore throat, runny nose, or fever (mild); itching, welts, or skin rash; lack of appetite or decreased appetite; nausea or vomiting; sudden redness of skin; swelling of glands in armpit or neck; trouble in sleeping

Other side effects not listed above may also occur in some patients. If you notice any other effects, check with your doctor.

Annual revision: 05/10/91

HISTAMINE Diagnostic*

* Not commercially available in the U.S.

Description

Histamine (HISS-ta-meen) is used to help diagnose problems or disease of the stomach. This test determines how much acid your stomach produces.

How the stomach test is done: Before this medicine is given, the stomach contents are emptied through a tube. Then histamine is injected and, 5 minutes later, the stomach contents are emptied and tested for acidity. This procedure may be repeated several times. An antihistamine medicine may be given before the histamine is injected to prevent a possible unwanted effect.

Histamine is to be used only under the supervision of a doctor. It is available in the following dosage form:

Parenteral

- Injection (Canada)

It is very important that you read and understand the following information. If any of it causes you special concern, check with your doctor. Also, *if you have any questions* or if you want more information about this test or your medical problem, *ask your doctor, nurse, or pharmacist.*

Before Having This Test

In deciding to use a diagnostic test, any risks of the test must be weighed against the good it will do. This is a decision you and your doctor will make. Also, test results may be affected by other things. For histamine, the following should be considered:

Allergies—Tell your doctor and pharmacist if you are allergic to any substances, such as foods, preservatives, or dyes.

Pregnancy—Studies have not been done in either humans or animals.

Breast-feeding—It is not known whether histamine passes into the breast milk. However, histamine has not been reported to cause problems in nursing babies.

Children—There is no specific information comparing the use of histamine in children with use in other age groups.

Older adults—Many medicines have not been studied specifically in older people. Therefore, it may not be known whether they work exactly the same way they do in younger adults or if they cause different side effects or problems in older people. There is no specific information comparing use of histamine in the elderly with use in other age groups.

Other medicines—Although certain medicines should not be used together at all, in other cases two different medicines may be used together even if an interaction might occur. In these cases, your doctor may want to change the dose, or other precautions may be necessary. When you are receiving histamine, it is especially important that your doctor and pharmacist know if you are taking any of the following:

- Antacids or
- Anticholinergics (medicine for abdominal or stomach spasms or cramps) or
- Cimetidine (e.g., Tagamet) or
- Famotidine (e.g., Pepcid) or
- Nizatidine (e.g., Axid) or
- Omeprazole (e.g., Prilosec) or
- Ranitidine (e.g., Zantac)—These medicines decrease the effect that histamine has on the production of stomach acid, and the test may not work

Other medical problems—The presence of other medical problems may affect the use of histamine. Make sure you tell your doctor if you have any other medical problems, especially:

- Heart disease—Histamine's effect on the heart may make the condition worse
- High blood pressure (severe) or
- Low blood pressure—Histamine may increase the high blood pressure further or lower an already low blood pressure
- Kidney disease (severe)—The histamine may build up in the body and cause side effects
- Lung disease (especially asthma)—There is a chance that this test may make the condition worse; for example, an asthma attack may occur
- Pheochromocytoma—Histamine may cause serious damage to the brain and blood vessels.

Preparation For This Test

Your doctor may ask you to avoid certain medicines before the histamine test is done. *Follow your doctor's instructions carefully.* Otherwise, this test may not work and may have to be done again.

Do not eat anything for twelve hours before the test, unless otherwise directed by your doctor. Having food in the stomach may affect the interpretation of the test results.

Precautions During This Test

Do not swallow saliva during the test. The saliva may affect the results of the test.

Side Effects of This Medicine

Along with its needed effects, histamine may cause some unwanted effects. Although not all of these side effects may occur, if they do occur they may need medical attention.

Check with your doctor or nurse immediately if any of the following side effects occur:

More common

Dizziness, lightheadedness, or fainting; fast or pounding heartbeat; headache (continuing or severe); nervousness

Less common or rare

Convulsions (seizures); difficulty in breathing; flushing or redness of face

With large doses

Bluish coloration of face; blurred vision; chest discomfort or pain; decrease in blood pressure (sudden); diarrhea (severe); difficulty in breathing (severe); nausea and vomiting (severe)

Other side effects may occur that usually do not need medical attention. These side effects should go away as the effects of the medicine wear off. However, check with your doctor if any of the following side effects continue or are bothersome:

More common

Abdominal or stomach spasms or cramps; diarrhea; metallic taste; nausea or vomiting; stomach pain; swelling or redness at place of injection

Other side effects not listed above may also occur in some patients. If you notice any other effects, check with your doctor.

Annual revision: 06/02/93

HISTAMINE H_2-RECEPTOR ANTAGONISTS Systemic

This information applies to the following medicines:

Cimetidine (sye-MET-i-deen)
Famotidine (fa-MOE-ti-deen)
Nizatidine (ni-ZA-ti-deen)
Ranitidine (ra-NIT-ti-deen)

Some commonly used brand names are:

For Cimetidine

In the U.S.

Tagamet

In Canada

Apo-Cimetidine
Novocimetine
Peptol
Tagamet

For Famotidine

In the U.S.

Pepcid
Pepcid I.V.

In Canada

Pepcid
Pepcid I.V.

For Nizatidine

In the U.S.

Axid

In Canada

Axid

For Ranitidine

In the U.S.

Zantac

In Canada

Apo-Ranitidine
Zantac
Zantac-C

Description

Histamine H_2-receptor antagonists, also known as H_2-blockers, are used to treat duodenal ulcers and prevent their return. They are also used to treat gastric ulcers and in some conditions, such as Zollinger-Ellison disease, in which the stomach produces too much acid. H_2-blockers may also be used for other conditions as determined by your doctor.

H_2-blockers work by decreasing the amount of acid produced by the stomach.

They are available only with your doctor's prescription, in the following dosage forms:

Oral

Cimetidine
- Oral solution (U.S. and Canada)
- Tablets (U.S. and Canada)

Famotidine
- Oral suspension (U.S.)
- Tablets (U.S. and Canada)

Nizatidine
- Capsules (U.S. and Canada)

Ranitidine
- Capsules (Canada)
- Syrup (U.S. and Canada)
- Tablets (U.S. and Canada)

Parenteral

Cimetidine
- Injection (U.S. and Canada)

Famotidine
- Injection (U.S. and Canada)

Ranitidine
- Injection (U.S. and Canada)

It is very important that you read and understand the following information. If any of it causes you special concern, check with your doctor. Also, *if you have any questions* or if you want more information about this medicine or your medical problem, *ask your doctor, nurse, or pharmacist.*

Before Using This Medicine

In deciding to use a medicine, the risks of taking the medicine must be weighed against the good it will do. This is a decision you and your doctor will make. For H_2-blockers, the following should be considered:

Allergies—Tell your doctor if you have ever had any unusual or allergic reaction to cimetidine, famotidine, nizatidine, or ranitidine.

Pregnancy—H_2-blockers have not been studied in pregnant women. In animal studies, famotidine and ranitidine have not been shown to cause birth defects or other problems. However, one study in rats suggested that cimetidine may affect male sexual development. More studies are needed to confirm this. Also, studies in rabbits with very high doses have shown that nizatidine causes miscarriages and low birth weights. Make sure your doctor knows if you are pregnant or if you may become pregnant before taking H_2-blockers.

Breast-feeding—Cimetidine, famotidine, nizatidine, and ranitidine pass into the breast milk and may cause unwanted effects, such as decreased amount of stomach acid and increased excitement, in the nursing baby. It may be necessary for you to take another medicine or to stop breast-feeding during treatment. Be sure you have discussed the risks and benefits of the medicine with your doctor.

Children—This medicine has been tested in children and, in effective doses, has not been shown to cause different side effects or problems than it does in adults when used for short periods of time.

Older adults—Confusion and dizziness may be especially likely to occur in elderly patients, who are usually more sensitive than younger adults to the effects of H_2-blockers.

Other medicines—Although certain medicines should not be used together at all, in other cases two different medicines may be used together even if an interaction might occur. In these cases, your doctor may want to change the dose, or other precautions may be necessary. When you are taking or receiving H_2-blockers it is especially important that your doctor and pharmacist know if you are taking any of the following:

- Aminophylline (e.g., Somophyllin) or
- Anticoagulants (blood thinners) or
- Caffeine (e.g., NoDoz) or
- Metoprolol (e.g., Lopressor) or
- Oxtriphylline (e.g., Choledyl) or
- Phenytoin (e.g., Dilantin) or
- Propranolol (e.g., Inderal) or
- Theophylline (e.g., Somophyllin-T) or
- Tricyclic antidepressants (amitriptyline [e.g., Elavil], amoxapine [e.g., Asendin], clomipramine [e.g., Anafranil], desipramine [e.g., Pertofrane], doxepin [e.g., Sinequan], imipramine [e.g., Tofranil], nortriptyline [e.g., Aventyl], protriptyline [e.g., Vivactil], trimipramine [e.g., Surmontil])—Use of these medicines with cimetidine has been shown to increase the effects of cimetidine. This is less of a problem with ranitidine and has not been reported for famotidine or nizatidine. However, all of the H_2-blockers are similar, so drug interactions may occur with any of them
- Ketoconazole—H_2-blockers may decrease the effects of ketoconazole; H_2-blockers should be taken at least 2 hours after ketoconazole

Other medical problems—The presence of other medical problems may affect the use of H_2-blockers. Make sure you tell your doctor if you have any other medical problems, especially:

- Kidney disease or
- Liver disease—The H_2-blocker may build up in the bloodstream, which may increase the risk of side effects

Before you begin using any new medicine (prescription or nonprescription) or if you develop any new medical problem while you are using this medicine, check with your doctor, nurse, or pharmacist.

Proper Use of This Medicine

For patients taking:

- One dose a day—Take it at bedtime, unless otherwise directed.
- Two doses a day—Take one in the morning and one at bedtime.
- Several doses a day—Take them with meals and at bedtime for best results.

It may take several days before this medicine begins to relieve stomach pain. To help relieve this pain, antacids may be taken with the H_2-blocker, unless your doctor has told you not to use them. However, you should wait one-half to one hour between taking the antacid and the H_2-blocker.

Take this medicine for the full time of treatment, even if you begin to feel better. Also, it is important that you keep your appointments with your doctor for check-ups so that your doctor will be better able to tell you when to stop taking this medicine.

Missed dose—If you miss a dose of this medicine, take it as soon as possible. However, if it is almost time for your next dose, skip the missed dose and go back to your regular dosing schedule. Do not double doses.

Storage—To store this medicine:

- Keep out of the reach of children.
- Store away from heat and direct light.
- Do not store the tablet form of this medicine in the bathroom, near the kitchen sink, or in other damp places. Heat or moisture may cause the medicine to break down.
- Keep the liquid form of this medicine from freezing.
- Do not keep outdated medicine or medicine no longer needed. Be sure that any discarded medicine is out of the reach of children.

Precautions While Using This Medicine

Some tests may be affected by this medicine. Tell the doctor in charge that you are taking this medicine before:

- You have any skin tests for allergies.
- You have any tests to determine how much acid your stomach produces.

Remember that certain medicines, such as aspirin, and certain foods and drinks (e.g., citrus products, carbonated drinks, etc.) irritate the stomach and may make your problem worse.

Cigarette smoking tends to decrease the effect of H_2-blockers by increasing the amount of acid produced by the stomach. This is more likely to affect the stomach's nighttime production of acid. While taking H_2-blockers, stop smoking completely, or at least do not smoke after taking the last dose of the day.

Drinking alcoholic beverages while taking cimetidine or ranitidine has been reported to increase the effects of alcohol. Therefore, you should not drink alcoholic beverages while you are taking cimetidine or ranitidine.

Check with your doctor if your ulcer pain continues or gets worse.

Side Effects of This Medicine

Along with its needed effects, a medicine may cause some unwanted effects. Although not all of these side effects may occur, if they do occur they may need medical attention.

Check with your doctor as soon as possible if any of the following side effects occur:

Rare

Burning, itching, redness, skin rash; confusion; fast, pounding, or irregular heartbeat; fever; slow heartbeat; sore throat and fever; swelling; tightness in chest; unusual bleeding or bruising; unusual tiredness or weakness

Other side effects may occur that usually do not need medical attention. These side effects may go away during treatment as your body adjusts to the medicine. However, check with your doctor if any of the following side effects continue or are bothersome:

Less common or rare

Blurred vision; constipation; decreased sexual ability (especially in patients with Zollinger-Ellison disease who have received high doses of cimetidine for at least 1 year); decrease in sexual desire; diarrhea; dizziness; drowsiness; dryness of mouth or skin; headache; increased sweating; joint or muscle pain; loss of appetite; loss of hair (temporary); nausea or vomiting; ringing or buzzing in ears; skin rash; swelling of breasts or breast soreness in females and males

Not all of the side effects listed above have been reported for each of these medicines, but they have been reported for at least one of them. All of the H_2-blockers are similar, so any of the above side effects may occur with any of these medicines.

Other side effects not listed above may also occur in some patients. If you notice any other effects, check with your doctor.

Additional Information

Once a medicine has been approved for marketing for a certain use, experience may show that it is also useful for other medical problems. Although these uses are not included in product labeling, H_2-blockers are used in certain patients with the following medical conditions:

- Damage to the stomach and/or intestines due to stress or trauma
- Hives
- Pancreatic problems
- Stomach or intestinal ulcers (sores) resulting from damage caused by medication used to treat rheumatoid arthritis

Other than the above information, there is no additional information relating to proper use, precautions, or side effects for these uses.

Annual revision: 09/29/92

HMG-CoA REDUCTASE INHIBITORS Systemic

This information applies to the following medicines:

Lovastatin (LOE-va-sta-tin)
Pravastatin (PRA-va-stat-in)
Simvastatin (SIM-va-stat-in)

Some commonly used brand names are:

For Lovastatin

In the U.S.
Mevacor

In Canada
Mevacor

Another commonly used name is mevinolin.

For Pravastatin

In the U.S.
Pravachol

In Canada
Pravachol

Another commonly used name is eptastatin.

For Simvastatin

In the U.S.
Zocor

In Canada
Zocor

Other commonly used names are epistatin and synvinolin.

Description

Lovastatin, pravastatin, and simvastatin are used to lower levels of cholesterol and other fats in the blood. This may help prevent medical problems caused by cholesterol clogging the blood vessels.

These medicines belong to the group of medicines called 3-hydroxy-3-methylglutaryl coenzyme A (HMG-CoA) reductase inhibitors. They work by blocking an enzyme that is needed by the body to make cholesterol. Thus, less cholesterol is made.

HMG-CoA reductase inhibitors are available only with your doctor's prescription, in the following dosage form:

Oral

Lovastatin
- Tablets (U.S. and Canada)

Pravastatin
- Tablets (U.S. and Canada)

Simvastatin
- Tablets (U.S and Canada)

It is very important that you read and understand the following information. If any of it causes you special concern, check with your doctor. Also, *if you have any questions* or if you want more information about this

medicine or your medical problem, *ask your doctor, nurse, or pharmacist.*

Before Using This Medicine

In deciding to use a medicine, the risks of taking the medicine must be weighed against the good it will do. This is a decision you and your doctor will make. For HMG-CoA reductase inhibitors, the following should be considered:

Allergies—Tell your doctor if you have ever had any unusual or allergic reaction to HMG-CoA reductase inhibitors. Also tell your doctor and pharmacist if you are allergic to any other substances, such as foods, preservatives, or dyes.

Diet—Before prescribing medicines to lower your cholesterol, your doctor will probably try to control your condition by prescribing a personal diet for you. Such a diet may be low in fats, sugars, and/or cholesterol. Many people are able to control their condition by carefully following their doctor's orders for proper diet and exercise. *Medicine is prescribed only when additional help is needed* and is effective only when a schedule of diet and exercise is properly followed.

Also, this medicine is less effective if you are greatly overweight. It may be very important for you to go on a reducing diet. However, check with your doctor before going on any diet.

Pregnancy—Use of an HMG-CoA reductase inhibitor is not recommended during pregnancy or in a woman who plans to become pregnant in the near future. These medicines block formation of cholesterol, which is necessary for the fetus to develop properly. In addition, lovastatin has been shown to cause birth defects in animals given very high doses. Be sure you have discussed this with your doctor.

Breast-feeding—These medicines are not recommended for use during breast-feeding because they may cause unwanted effects in nursing babies.

Children—Studies on this medicine have been done only in adult patients, and there is no specific information comparing use of HMG-CoA reductase inhibitors in children with use in other age groups.

Older adults—Many medicines have not been studied specifically in older people. Therefore, it may not be known whether they work exactly the same way they do in younger adults or if they cause different side effects or problems in older people. There is no specific information comparing the use of HMG-CoA reductase inhibitors in the elderly with use in other age groups.

Other medicines—Although certain medicines should not be used together at all, in other cases two different medicines may be used together even if an interaction might occur. In these cases, your doctor may want to change the dose, or other precautions may be necessary. When you are taking HMG-CoA reductase inhibitors, it is especially important that your doctor and pharmacist know if you are taking any of the following:

- Cyclosporine (e.g., Sandimmune) or
- Gemfibrozil (e.g., Lopid) or
- Niacin—Use of these medicines with an HMG-CoA reductase inhibitor may increase the risk of developing muscle problems and kidney failure

Other medical problems—The presence of other medical problems may affect the use of HMG-CoA reductase inhibitors. Make sure you tell your doctor if you have any other medical problems, especially:

- Alcohol abuse (or history of) or
- Liver disease—Use of this medicine may make liver problems worse
- Convulsions (seizures), not well-controlled, or
- Organ transplant with immunosuppressant therapy or
- If you have recently had major surgery—Patients with these conditions may be at risk of developing problems that may lead to kidney failure

Before you begin using any new medicine (prescription or nonprescription) or if you develop any new medical problem while you are using this medicine, check with your doctor, nurse, or pharmacist.

Proper Use of This Medicine

Use this medicine only as directed by your doctor. Do not use more or less of it, and do not use it more often or for a longer time than your doctor ordered.

Remember that this medicine will not cure your condition but it does help control it. Therefore, you must continue to take it as directed if you expect to keep your cholesterol levels down.

Follow carefully the special diet your doctor gave you. This is the most important part of controlling your condition, and is necessary if the medicine is to work properly.

For patients taking *lovastatin:*

- This medicine works better when it is taken with food. If you are taking this medicine once a day, take it with the evening meal. If you are taking more than one dose a day, take each dose with a meal or snack.

Dosing—The dose of lovastatin, pravastatin, or simvastatin will be different for different patients. *Follow your doctor's orders or the directions on the label.* The following information includes only the average doses. *If your dose is different, do not change it* unless your doctor tells you to do so:

The number of tablets that you take depends on the strength of the medicine.

For lovastatin

- For *oral* dosage form (tablets):
  - —For high cholesterol:
    - Adults—20 to 80 milligrams (mg) a day taken as a single dose or in divided doses. Take with meals.
    - Children—Use is not recommended.

For pravastatin

- For *oral* dosage form (tablets):
  - —For high cholesterol:
    - Adults—10 to 40 mg once a day at bedtime.
    - Children—Use is not recommended.

For simvastatin

- For *oral* dosage form (tablets):
  - —For high cholesterol:
    - Adults—5 to 40 mg once a day in the evening.
    - Children—Use is not recommended.

Missed dose—If you miss a dose of this medicine, take it as soon as possible. However, if it is almost time for your next dose, skip the missed dose and go back to your regular dosing schedule. Do not double doses.

Storage—To store this medicine:

- Keep out of the reach of children.
- Store away from heat and direct light.
- Do not store in the bathroom, near the kitchen sink, or in other damp places. Heat or moisture may cause the medicine to break down.
- Keep the medicine from freezing. Do not refrigerate.
- Do not keep outdated medicine or medicine no longer needed. Be sure that any discarded medicine is out of the reach of children.

Precautions While Using This Medicine

It is very important that your doctor check your progress at regular visits. This will allow your doctor to see if the medicine is working properly to lower your cholesterol levels and that it does not cause unwanted effects.

Do not stop taking this medicine without first checking with your doctor. When you stop taking this medicine, your blood cholesterol levels may increase again. Your doctor may want you to follow a special diet to help prevent this from happening.

Before having any kind of surgery (including dental surgery) or emergency treatment, tell the medical doctor or dentist in charge that you are taking this medicine.

Side Effects of This Medicine

Along with its needed effects, a medicine may cause some unwanted effects. Although not all of these side effects may occur, if they do occur they may need medical attention.

Check with your doctor as soon as possible if any of the following side effects occur:

Less common

For lovastatin, pravastatin, and simvastatin

Fever; muscle aches or cramps; unusual tiredness or weakness

For lovastatin only (in addition to those listed above)

Blurred vision

Other side effects may occur that usually do not need medical attention. These side effects may go away during treatment as your body adjusts to the medicine. However, check with your doctor if any of the following side effects continue or are bothersome:

Less common

For lovastatin, pravastatin, and simvastatin

Constipation; diarrhea; dizziness; gas; heartburn; headache; nausea; skin rash; stomach pain

For lovastatin only (in addition to those listed above)

Decreased sexual ability; trouble in sleeping

Other side effects not listed above may also occur in some patients. If you notice any other effects, check with your doctor.

Annual revision: 06/18/93

HYDRALAZINE Systemic

Some commonly used brand names are:

In the U.S.

Apresoline

Generic name product may also be available.

In Canada

Apresoline

Novo-Hylazin

Description

Hydralazine (hye-DRAL-a-zeen) belongs to the general class of medicines called antihypertensives. It is used to treat high blood pressure (hypertension).

High blood pressure adds to the workload of the heart and arteries. If it continues for a long time, the heart and arteries may not function properly. This can damage the blood vessels of the brain, heart, and kidneys, resulting in a stroke, heart failure, or kidney failure. High blood pressure may also increase the risk of heart attacks. These problems may be less likely to occur if blood pressure is controlled.

Hydralazine works by relaxing blood vessels and increasing the supply of blood and oxygen to the heart while reducing its work load.

Hydralazine may also be used for other conditions as determined by your doctor.

Hydralazine is available only with your doctor's prescription, in the following dosage forms:

Oral

- Tablets (U.S. and Canada)

Parenteral

- Injection (U.S. and Canada)

It is very important that you read and understand the following information. If any of it causes you special concern, check with your doctor. Also, *if you have any questions* or if you want more information about this medicine or your medical problem, *ask your doctor, nurse, or pharmacist.*

Before Using This Medicine

In deciding to use a medicine, the risks of taking the medicine must be weighed against the good it will do. This is a decision you and your doctor will make. For hydralazine, the following should be considered:

Allergies—Tell your doctor if you have ever had any unusual or allergic reaction to hydralazine. Also tell your doctor and pharmacist if you are allergic to any other substance, such as foods, preservatives, or dyes.

Pregnancy—Hydralazine has not been studied in pregnant women. However, blood problems have been reported in infants of mothers who took hydralazine during pregnancy. In addition, studies in mice have shown that hydralazine causes birth defects (cleft palate, defects in head and face bones). These birth defects may also occur in rabbits, but do not occur in rats. Before taking this medicine, make sure your doctor knows if you are pregnant or if you may become pregnant.

Breast-feeding—It is not known whether hydralazine passes into breast milk.

Children—Although there is no specific information comparing use of hydralazine in children with use in other age groups, this medicine is not expected to cause different side effects or problems in children than it does in adults.

Older adults—Many medicines have not been studied specifically in older people. Therefore, it may not be known whether they work exactly the same way they do in younger adults. Although there is no specific information comparing use of hydralazine in the elderly with use in other age groups, this medicine is not expected to cause different side effects or problems in older people than it does in younger adults. However, dizziness or lightheadedness may be more likely to occur in the elderly, who are more sensitive to the effects of hydralazine.

Other medicines—Although certain medicines should not be used together at all, in other cases two different medicines may be used together even if an interaction might occur. In these cases, your doctor may want to change the dose, or other precautions may be necessary. When you are taking hydralazine, it is especially important that your doctor and pharmacist know if you are taking the following:

- Diazoxide (e.g., Proglycem)—Effect on blood pressure may be increased

Other medical problems—The presence of other medical problems may affect the use of hydralazine. Make sure you tell your doctor if you have any other medical problems, especially:

- Heart or blood vessel disease or
- Stroke—Lowering blood pressure may make problems resulting from these conditions worse
- Kidney disease—Effects may be increased because of slower removal of hydralazine from the body

Before you begin using any new medicine (prescription or nonprescription) or if you develop any new medical problem while you are using this medicine, check with your doctor, nurse, or pharmacist.

Proper Use of This Medicine

For patients taking this medicine *for high blood pressure:*

- In addition to the use of the medicine your doctor has prescribed, treatment for your high blood pressure may include weight control and care in the types of foods you eat, especially foods high in sodium. Your doctor will tell you which of these are most important for you. You should check with your doctor before changing your diet.
- Many patients who have high blood pressure will not notice any signs of the problem. In fact, many may feel normal. It is very important that you *take your medicine exactly as directed* and that you keep your appointments with your doctor even if you feel well.
- Remember that hydralazine will not cure your high blood pressure but it does help control it. Therefore, you must continue to take it as directed if you expect to lower your blood pressure and keep it down. *You may have to take high blood pressure medicine for the rest of your life.* If high blood pressure is not treated, it can cause serious problems such as heart failure, blood vessel disease, stroke, or kidney disease.

To help you remember to take your medicine, try to get into the habit of taking it at the same time each day.

Missed dose—If you miss a dose of this medicine, take it as soon as possible. However, if it is almost time for your next dose, skip the missed dose and go back to your regular dosing schedule. Do not double doses.

Storage—To store this medicine:

- Keep out of the reach of children.
- Store away from heat and direct light.
- Do not store in the bathroom, near the kitchen sink, or in other damp places. Heat or moisture may cause the medicine to break down.
- Do not keep outdated medicine or medicine no longer needed. Be sure that any discarded medicine is out of the reach of children.

Precautions While Using This Medicine

It is important that your doctor check your progress at regular visits to make sure that this medicine is working properly.

For patients taking this medicine *for high blood pressure:*

- *Do not take other medicines unless they have been discussed with your doctor.* This especially includes over-the-counter (nonprescription) medicines for appetite control, asthma, colds, cough, hay fever, or sinus, since they may tend to increase your blood pressure.

Hydralazine may cause some people to have headaches or to feel dizzy. *Make sure you know how you react to this medicine before you drive, use machines, or do anything else that could be dangerous if you are dizzy or are not alert.*

Side Effects of This Medicine

Along with its needed effects, a medicine may cause some unwanted effects. Although not all of these side effects may occur, if they do occur they may need medical attention.

In general, side effects with hydralazine are rare at lower doses. However, check with your doctor as soon as possible if any of the following occur:

Less common

Blisters on skin; chest pain; general feeling of discomfort or illness or weakness; joint pain; numbness, tingling, pain, or weakness in hands or feet; skin rash or itching; sore throat and fever; swelling of feet or lower legs; swelling of the lymph glands

Other side effects may occur that usually do not need medical attention. These side effects may go away during treatment as your body adjusts to the medicine. However, check with your doctor if any of the following side effects continue or are bothersome:

More common

Diarrhea; fast or irregular heartbeat; headache; loss of appetite; nausea or vomiting; pounding heartbeat

Less common

Constipation; dizziness or lightheadedness; redness or flushing of face; shortness of breath; stuffy nose; watering or irritated eyes

Other side effects not listed above may also occur in some patients. If you notice any other effects, check with your doctor.

Additional Information

Once a medicine has been approved for marketing for a certain use, experience may show that it is also useful for other medical problems. Although this use is not specifically included in product labeling, hydralazine is used in certain patients with the following medical condition:

- Congestive heart failure

Other than the above information, there is no additional information relating to proper use, precautions, or side effects for this use.

Annual revision: 06/09/92

HYDRALAZINE AND HYDROCHLOROTHIAZIDE Systemic†

Some commonly used brand names are:

In the U.S.

Apresazide	Aprozide
Apresoline-Esidrix	Hydra-zide

Generic name product may also be available.

†Not commercially available in Canada.

Description

Hydralazine (hye-DRAL-a-zeen) and hydrochlorothiazide (hye-droe-klor-oh-THYE-a-zide) combination is used to treat high blood pressure (hypertension).

High blood pressure adds to the workload of the heart and arteries. If it continues for a long time, the heart and arteries may not function properly. This can damage the blood vessels of the brain, heart, and kidneys, resulting in a stroke, heart failure, or kidney failure. High blood pressure may also increase the risk of heart attacks. These problems may be less likely to occur if blood pressure is controlled.

Hydralazine works by relaxing blood vessels and increasing the supply of blood and oxygen to the heart while reducing its work load. The hydrochlorothiazide in this combination helps reduce the amount of water in the body by acting on the kidneys to increase the flow of urine.

This medicine is available only with your doctor's prescription, in the following dosage forms:

Oral

- Capsules (U.S.)
- Tablets (U.S.)

It is very important that you read and understand the following information. If any of it causes you special concern, check with your doctor. Also, *if you have any questions* or if you want more information about this medicine or your medical problem, *ask your doctor, nurse, or pharmacist.*

Before Using This Medicine

In deciding to use a medicine, the risks of taking the medicine must be weighed against the good it will do. This is a decision you and your doctor will make. For hydralazine and hydrochlorothiazide, the following should be considered:

Allergies—Tell your doctor if you have ever had any unusual or allergic reaction to hydralazine, sulfonamides (sulfa drugs), indapamide, or any of the thiazide diuretics (water pills). Also tell your doctor and pharmacist if you are allergic to any other substance, such as foods, preservatives, or dyes.

Pregnancy—When hydrochlorothiazide is used during pregnancy, it may cause side effects including jaundice, blood problems, and low potassium in the newborn infant. Studies with hydralazine have not been done in humans. However, blood problems have been reported in infants of mothers who took hydralazine during pregnancy. In addition, studies in mice have shown that hydralazine causes birth defects (cleft palate, defects in head and face bones); these birth defects may also occur in rabbits, but do not occur in rats.

Breast-feeding—Hydrochlorothiazide passes into breast milk. However, neither hydralazine nor hydrochlorothiazide has been reported to cause problems in nursing babies.

Children—Although there is no specific information comparing use of this medicine in children with use in other age groups, this medicine is not expected to cause different side effects or problems in children than it does in adults. However, extra caution may be necessary in infants with jaundice, because thiazide diuretics can make this condition worse.

Older adults—Many medicines have not been studied specifically in older people. Therefore, it may not be known whether they work exactly the same way they do in younger adults. Although there is no specific information comparing use of hydralazine and hydrochlorothiazide combination in the elderly with use in other age groups, this medicine is not expected to cause different side effects or problems in older people than it does in younger adults. However, dizziness or lightheadedness or symptoms of too much potassium loss may be more likely to occur in the elderly, who are usually more sensitive to the effects of this medicine. Also, this medicine may reduce tolerance to cold temperatures in elderly patients.

Other medicines—Although certain medicines should not be used together at all, in other cases two different medicines may be used together even if an interaction might occur. In these cases, your doctor may want to change the dose, or other precautions may be necessary. When you are taking hydralazine and hydrochlorothiazide, it is especially important that your doctor and pharmacist know if you are taking any of the following:

- Cholestyramine or
- Colestipol—Use with thiazide diuretics may prevent the diuretic from working properly; take the diuretic at least 1 hour before or 4 hours after cholestyramine or colestipol
- Diazoxide (e.g., Proglycem)—Effect on blood pressure may be increased
- Digitalis glycosides (heart medicine)—Hydrochlorothiazide may cause low potassium in the blood, which can lead to symptoms of digitalis toxicity
- Lithium (e.g., Lithane)—Risk of lithium overdose, even at usual doses, may be increased

Other medical problems—The presence of other medical problems may affect the use of hydralazine and hydrochlorothiazide. Make sure you tell your doctor if you have any other medical problems, especially:
- Diabetes mellitus (sugar diabetes)—Hydrochlorothiazide may change the amount of diabetes medicine needed
- Gout (history of)—Hydrochlorothiazide may increase the amount of uric acid in the blood, which can lead to gout
- Heart or blood vessel disease or
- Stroke (recent)—Lowering blood pressure may make problems resulting from these conditions worse
- Kidney disease—Hydrochlorothiazide may worsen this condition. Also, the blood pressure lowering effects may be increased because of slower removal of hydralazine from the body
- Liver disease—If hydrochlorothiazide causes loss of too much water from the body, liver disease can become much worse
- Lupus erythematosus (history of)—Hydrochlorothiazide may worsen the condition
- Pancreatitis (inflammation of the pancreas)

Before you begin using any new medicine (prescription or nonprescription) or if you develop any new medical problem while you are using this medicine, check with your doctor, nurse, or pharmacist.

Proper Use of This Medicine

This medicine may cause you to have an unusual feeling of tiredness when you begin to take it. You may also notice an increase in the amount of urine or in your frequency of urination. After taking the medicine for a while, these effects should lessen. To keep the increase in urine from affecting your sleep:
- If you are to take a single dose a day, take it in the morning after breakfast.
- If you are to take more than one dose a day, take the last dose no later than 6 p.m., unless otherwise directed by your doctor.

However, it is best to plan your dose or doses according to a schedule that will least affect your personal activities and sleep. Ask your doctor, nurse, or pharmacist to help you plan the best time to take this medicine.

In addition to the use of the medicine your doctor has prescribed, treatment for your high blood pressure may include weight control and care in the types of foods you eat, especially foods high in sodium. Your doctor will tell you which of these are most important for you. You should check with your doctor before changing your diet.

Many patients who have high blood pressure will not notice any signs of the problem. In fact, many may feel normal. It is very important that you *take your medicine exactly as directed* and that you keep your appointments with your doctor even if you feel well.

Remember that this medicine will not cure your high blood pressure but it does help control it. Therefore, you must continue to take it as directed if you expect to lower your blood pressure and keep it down. *You may have to take high blood pressure medicine for the rest of your life.* If high blood pressure is not treated, it can cause serious problems such as heart failure, blood vessel disease, stroke, or kidney disease.

To help you remember to take your medicine, try to get into the habit of taking it at the same time each day.

Missed dose—If you miss a dose of this medicine, take it as soon as possible. However, if it is almost time for your next dose, skip the missed dose and go back to your regular dosing schedule. Do not double doses.

Storage—To store this medicine:
- Keep out of the reach of children.
- Store away from heat and direct light.
- Do not store in the bathroom, near the kitchen sink, or in other damp places. Heat or moisture may cause the medicine to break down.
- Do not keep outdated medicine or medicine no longer needed. Be sure that any discarded medicine is out of the reach of children.

Precautions While Using This Medicine

It is important that your doctor check your progress at regular visits to make sure that this medicine is working properly.

Do not take other medicines unless they have been discussed with your doctor. This especially includes over-the-counter (nonprescription) medicines for appetite control, asthma, colds, cough, hay fever, or sinus problems, since they may tend to increase your blood pressure.

This medicine may cause some people to have headaches or to feel dizzy. *Make sure you know how you react to this medicine before you drive, use machines, or do anything else that could be dangerous if you are dizzy or are not alert.*

Dizziness, lightheadedness, or fainting may occur, especially when you get up from a lying or sitting position. This is more likely to occur in the morning. *Getting up slowly may help.* When you get up from lying down, sit on the edge of the bed with your feet dangling for 1 or 2 minutes. Then stand up slowly. If the problem continues or gets worse, check with your doctor.

The dizziness, lightheadedness, or fainting is also more likely to occur if you drink alcohol, stand for a long time, exercise, or if the weather is hot. *While you are taking this medicine, be careful in the amount of alcohol you drink. Also, use extra care during exercise or hot weather or if you must stand for a long time.*

This medicine may cause a loss of potassium from your body.

- To help prevent this, your doctor may want you to:
  —eat or drink foods that have a high potassium content (for example, orange or other citrus fruit juices), or
  —take a potassium supplement, or
  —take another medicine to help prevent the loss of the potassium in the first place.
- It is very important to follow these directions. Also, it is important not to change your diet on your own. This is more important if you are already on a special diet (as for diabetes), or if you are taking a potassium supplement or a medicine to reduce potassium loss. Extra potassium may not be necessary and, in some cases, too much potassium could be harmful.

Check with your doctor if you become sick and have severe or continuing nausea, vomiting, or diarrhea. These problems may cause you to lose additional water and potassium.

For *diabetic patients*:

- Thiazide diuretics may raise blood sugar levels. While you are using this medicine, be especially careful in testing for sugar in your blood or urine. If you have any questions about this, check with your doctor.

Some people who take this medicine may become more sensitive to sunlight than they are normally. Exposure to sunlight, even for brief periods of time, may cause severe sunburn; skin rash, redness, itching, or discoloration; or vision changes. When you begin taking this medicine:

- Stay out of direct sunlight, especially between the hours of 10:00 a.m. and 3:00 p.m., if possible.
- Wear protective clothing, including a hat and sunglasses.
- Apply a sun block product that has a skin protection factor (SPF) of at least 15. Some patients may require a product with a higher SPF number, especially if they have a fair complexion. If you have any questions about this, check with your doctor or pharmacist.
- Do not use a sunlamp or tanning bed or booth.

If you have a severe reaction from the sun, check with your doctor.

Side Effects of This Medicine

Along with its needed effects, a medicine may cause some unwanted effects. Although not all of these side effects may occur, if they do occur they may need medical attention.

Check with your doctor as soon as possible if any of the following side effects occur:

Signs and symptoms of too much potassium loss

Dryness of mouth; increased thirst; irregular heartbeats; mood or mental changes; muscle cramps or pain; weak pulse

Signs and symptoms of too much sodium loss

Confusion; convulsions; decreased mental activity; irritability; muscle cramps; unusual tiredness or weakness

Less common

Blisters on skin; chest pain; general feeling of discomfort or illness or weakness; joint pain; numbness, tingling, pain, or weakness in hands or feet; skin rash or itching; sore throat and fever; swelling of the lymph glands

Rare

Lower back or side pain; severe stomach pain with nausea and vomiting; unusual bleeding or bruising; yellow eyes or skin

Other side effects may occur that usually do not need medical attention. These side effects may go away during treatment as your body adjusts to the medicine. However, check with your doctor if any of the following side effects continue or are bothersome:

More common

Diarrhea; fast or irregular heartbeat; headache; loss of appetite; nausea or vomiting

Less common

Constipation; decreased sexual ability; dizziness or lightheadedness, especially when getting up from a lying or sitting position; increased sensitivity of skin to sunlight; redness or flushing of face; shortness of breath with exercise or work; stuffy nose; watering or irritated eyes

Other side effects not listed above may also occur in some patients. If you notice any other effects, check with your doctor.

Annual revision: 08/24/92

HYDROCORTISONE Rectal

Some commonly used brand names are:

In the U.S.

Anucort-HC
Anusol-HC
Cort-Dome High Potency
Corticaine
Hemril-HC
Proctocort

Generic name product may also be available.

In Canada

Cortiment-10
Cortiment-40
Rectocort

Another commonly used name is cortisol.

Description

Rectal hydrocortisone (hye-droe-KOR-ti-sone) is used to help relieve swelling, itching, and discomfort of some rectal problems. Rectal hydrocortisone may also be applied to the area around the anus or rectum to relieve itching and discomfort. Hydrocortisone is a corticosteroid (kor-ti-ko-STER-oyd), which is a cortisone-like medicine. Hydrocortisone belongs to the general family of medicines called steroids.

Some hydrocortisone products for rectal use are available without a prescription; however, your doctor may have special instructions on the proper dose for your medical condition. Other hydrocortisone products for rectal use are available only with your doctor's prescription.

Rectal hydrocortisone is available in the following dosage forms:

Rectal
- Cream (U.S.)
- Ointment (Canada)
- Suppositories (U.S. and Canada)

It is very important that you read and understand the following information. If any of it causes you special concern, check with your doctor. Also, *if you have any questions* or if you want more information about this medicine or your medical problem, *ask your doctor, nurse, or pharmacist.*

Before Using This Medicine

In deciding to use rectal hydrocortisone, the risks of using it must be weighed against the good it will do. This is a decision you and possibly your doctor will make. The following information may help you in making your decision:

Allergies—If you have ever had any unusual or allergic reaction to hydrocortisone or other corticosteroids, it is best to check with your doctor before using rectal hydrocortisone.

Pregnancy—When used properly, this medicine has not been shown to cause problems in humans. Studies on birth defects with rectal hydrocortisone have not been done in humans. However, studies in animals have shown that topical corticosteroids, such as the hydrocortisone contained in this medicine, when used in large amounts or for a long time, may be absorbed through the skin and could cause birth defects.

Breast-feeding—When used properly, rectal hydrocortisone has not been reported to cause problems in nursing babies.

Children—Children and teenagers who must use this medicine should be checked often by their doctor. Hydrocortisone may be absorbed through the lining of the rectum and, rarely, may affect growth, especially if used in large amounts or for a long time. Before using this medicine in children, you should discuss its use with your child's doctor.

Older adults—Although there is no specific information comparing use of rectal hydrocortisone in the elderly with use in other age groups, this medicine is not expected to cause different side effects or problems in older people than it does in younger adults.

Other medical problems—The presence of other medical problems may affect the use of rectal hydrocortisone. Since in some cases rectal hydrocortisone should not be used, check with your doctor if you have any of the following:

- Diabetes mellitus (sugar diabetes)—Too much use of hydrocortisone may cause a loss of control of diabetes by increasing blood and urine glucose. However, this is not likely to happen when hydrocortisone is used for a short period of time
- Infection or sores at the place of treatment or
- Tuberculosis—Corticosteroids may make existing infections worse or cause new infections
- Skin conditions that cause thinning of skin with easy bruising—Corticosteroids may make thinning of the skin worse

If you develop any medical problem or begin using any new medicine (prescription or nonprescription) while you are using this medicine you may want to check with your doctor.

Proper Use of This Medicine

For patients using *hydrocortisone rectal cream or ointment:*

- If you are applying this medicine to the outer rectal area, first bathe and dry the rectal area. Then apply a small amount and rub it in gently.
- If you have been directed to insert this medicine into the rectum, first attach the plastic applicator tip onto the opened tube. Insert the applicator tip into the rectum and gently squeeze the tube to deliver the medicine. Remove the applicator tip from the tube and wash it with hot, soapy water. Replace the cap of the tube after use.

For patients using *hydrocortisone suppositories:*

- If the suppository is too soft to insert, chill it in the refrigerator for 30 minutes or run cold water over it before removing the foil wrapper.
- To insert suppository: First remove the foil wrapper and moisten the suppository with cold water. Lie down on your side and use your finger to push the suppository well up into the rectum.

Do not use rectal hydrocortisone in larger amounts, more often, or for a longer time than your doctor ordered or the package label directs. To do so may increase the chance of absorption through the lining of the rectum and the chance of side effects.

If this medicine was ordered by your doctor, do not use any leftover medicine for future rectal problems without first checking with your doctor. Also, if you are treating yourself, check with your doctor before using rectal hydrocortisone for problems other than those stated on the package, or if you suspect that an infection may be present. The medicine should not be used if many kinds of bacterial, virus, or fungus infections are present.

Missed dose—If your doctor has ordered you to use this medicine according to a regular schedule and you miss a dose, use it as soon as you remember. However, if it is almost time for your next dose, skip the missed dose and go back to your regular dosing schedule. Do not double doses.

Storage—To store this medicine:
- Keep out of the reach of children.
- Store away from heat and direct light.
- Do not store hydrocortisone suppositories in the bathroom medicine cabinet because the heat or moisture may cause the medicine to break down.
- Keep the medicine from freezing.
- Do not keep outdated medicine or medicine no longer needed. Be sure that any discarded medicine is out of the reach of children.

Precautions While Using This Medicine

Avoid using tight-fitting diapers or plastic pants on children using this medicine. Plastic pants and tight-fitting diapers may increase the chance of absorption of the medicine through the skin and the chance of side effects.

Side Effects of This Medicine

Along with its needed effects, a medicine may cause some unwanted effects. Although not all of these side effects may occur, if they do occur they may need medical attention.

Check with your doctor as soon as possible if any of the following side effects occur:

Signs of irritation or infection such as rectal bleeding, pain, burning, itching, or blistering not present before use of this medicine

Additional side effects may occur if you use this medicine for a long time. Check with your doctor as soon as possible if any of the following side effects occur:

Reddish-purple lines (stretch marks) on treated areas; thinning of skin with easy bruising

Other side effects not listed above may also occur in some patients. If you notice any other effects, check with your doctor.

Annual revision: 11/18/92

HYDROXYCHLOROQUINE Systemic

A commonly used brand name in the U.S. and Canada is Plaquenil.

Description

Hydroxychloroquine (hye-drox-ee-KLOR-oh-kwin) belongs to the family of medicines called antiprotozoals. Protozoa are tiny, one-celled animals. Some are parasites that can cause many different kinds of infections in the body.

This medicine is used to prevent and to treat malaria and to treat some conditions such as liver disease caused by protozoa. It is also used in the treatment of arthritis to help relieve inflammation, swelling, stiffness, and joint pain and to help control the symptoms of lupus erythematosus (lupus; SLE).

This medicine may be given alone or with one or more other medicines. It may also be used for other conditions as determined by your doctor.

Hydroxychloroquine is available only with your doctor's prescription, in the following dosage form:

Oral
- Tablets (U.S. and Canada)

It is very important that you read and understand the following information. If any of it causes you special concern, check with your doctor. Also, *if you have any questions* or if you want more information about this medicine or your medical problem, *ask your doctor, nurse, or pharmacist.*

Before Using This Medicine

In deciding to use a medicine, the risks of taking the medicine must be weighed against the good it will do.

This is a decision you and your doctor will make. For hydroxychloroquine, the following should be considered:

Allergies—Tell your doctor if you have ever had any unusual or allergic reaction to hydroxychloroquine or chloroquine. Also tell your doctor and pharmacist if you are allergic to any other substances, such as foods, preservatives, or dyes.

Pregnancy—Unless you are taking it for malaria or liver disease caused by protozoa, use of this medicine is not recommended during pregnancy. In animal studies, hydroxychloroquine has been shown to cause damage to the central nervous system (brain and spinal cord) of the fetus, including damage to hearing, sense of balance, bleeding inside the eyes, and other eye problems. However, when given in low doses (once a week) to prevent malaria, this medicine has not been shown to cause birth defects or other problems in pregnant women.

Breast-feeding—A very small amount of hydroxychloroquine passes into the breast milk. It has not been reported to cause problems in nursing babies to date. However, babies and children are especially sensitive to the effects of hydroxychloroquine.

Children—Children are especially sensitive to the effects of hydroxychloroquine. This may increase the chance of side effects during treatment. Overdose is especially dangerous in children. Taking as few as 3 or 4 tablets (250-mg strength) of chloroquine has resulted in death in small children. Because hydroxychloroquine is so similar to chloroquine, it is probably just as toxic.

Older adults—Many medicines have not been studied specifically in older people. Therefore, it may not be known whether they work exactly the same way they do in younger adults or if they cause different side effects or problems in older people. There is no specific information comparing use of hydroxychloroquine in the elderly with use in other age groups.

Other medicines—Although certain medicines should not be used together at all, in other cases 2 different medicines may be used together even if an interaction might occur. In these cases, your doctor may want to change the dose, or other precautions may be necessary. Tell your doctor and pharmacist if you are taking any other prescription or nonprescription (over-the-counter [OTC]) medicine.

Other medical problems—The presence of other medical problems may affect the use of hydroxychloroquine. Make sure you tell your doctor if you have any other medical problems, especially:

- Blood disease (severe)—Hydroxychloroquine may cause blood disorders
- Eye or vision problems—Hydroxychloroquine may cause serious eye side effects, especially in high doses
- Glucose-6-phosphate dehydrogenase (G6PD) deficiency—Hydroxychloroquine may cause serious blood side effects in patients with this deficiency
- Liver disease—May decrease the removal of hydroxychloroquine from the blood, increasing the chance of side effects
- Nerve or brain disease (severe), including convulsions (seizures)—Hydroxychloroquine may cause muscle weakness and, in high doses, seizures
- Porphyria—Hydroxychloroquine may worsen the symptoms of porphyria
- Psoriasis—Hydroxychloroquine may bring on severe attacks of psoriasis
- Stomach or intestinal disease (severe)—Hydroxychloroquine may cause stomach irritation

Before you begin using any new medicine (prescription or nonprescription) or if you develop any new medical problem while you are using this medicine, check with your doctor, nurse, or pharmacist.

Proper Use of This Medicine

Take this medicine with meals or milk to lessen possible stomach upset, unless otherwise directed by your doctor.

Keep this medicine out of the reach of children. Children are especially sensitive to the effects of hydroxychloroquine and overdose is especially dangerous in children. Taking as few as 3 or 4 tablets (250-mg strength) of chloroquine has resulted in death in small children. Hydroxychloroquine is probably just as dangerous.

It is very important that you *take this medicine only as directed.* Do not take more of it, do not take it more often, and do not take it for a longer time than your doctor ordered. To do so may increase the chance of serious side effects.

If you are taking this medicine to help keep you from getting malaria, *keep taking it for the full time of treatment.* If you already have malaria, you should still keep taking this medicine for the full time of treatment even if you begin to feel better after a few days. This will help to clear up your infection completely. If you stop taking this medicine too soon, your symptoms may return.

Hydroxychloroquine works best when you take it on a regular schedule. For example, if you are to take it once a week to prevent malaria, it is best to take it on the same day each week. Or if you are to take 2 doses a day, 1 dose may be taken with breakfast and the other with the evening meal. *Make sure that you do not miss any doses.* If you have any questions about this, check with your doctor, nurse, or pharmacist.

Missed dose—If you do miss a dose of this medicine, take it as soon as possible. However, if it is almost time for your next dose, skip the missed dose and go back to your regular dosing schedule. Do not double doses.

For patients taking hydroxychloroquine *to prevent malaria:*

- Your doctor may want you to start taking this medicine 1 to 2 weeks before you travel to an area where there is a chance of getting malaria. This will help you to see how you react to the medicine. Also, it will allow time for your doctor to change to another medicine if you have a reaction to this medicine.
- Also, you should keep taking this medicine while you are in the area and for 4 to 6 weeks after you leave the area. No medicine will protect you completely from malaria. However, to protect you as completely as possible, *it is important to keep taking this medicine for the full time your doctor ordered.* Also, if fever develops during your travels or within 2 months after you leave the area, *check with your doctor immediately.*

For patients taking hydroxychloroquine *for arthritis or lupus:*

- This medicine must be taken regularly as ordered by your doctor in order for it to help you. It may take up to several weeks before you begin to feel better. It may take up to 6 months before you feel the full benefit of this medicine.

For patients *unable to swallow hydroxychloroquine tablets:*

- Your pharmacist can crush the tablets and put each dose in a capsule. Contents of the capsules may then be mixed with a teaspoonful of jam, jelly, or jello. Be sure you take all the food in order to get the full dose of medicine.

Storage—To store this medicine:

- Keep out of the reach of children. Overdose of hydroxychloroquine is very dangerous in children.
- Store away from heat and direct light.
- Do not store in the bathroom, near the kitchen sink, or in other damp places. Heat or moisture may cause the medicine to break down.
- Do not keep outdated medicine or medicine no longer needed. Be sure that any discarded medicine is out of the reach of children.

Precautions While Using This Medicine

If you will be taking this medicine for a long time, *it is very important that your doctor check you at regular visits* for any blood problems or muscle weakness that may be caused by this medicine. In addition, *check with your doctor immediately if blurred vision, difficulty in reading, or any other change in vision occurs during or after treatment.* Your doctor may want you to have your eyes checked by an ophthalmologist (eye doctor).

If your symptoms do not improve within a few days (or a few weeks or months for arthritis), or if they become worse, check with your doctor.

Hydroxychloroquine may cause blurred vision, difficulty in reading, or other change in vision. It may also cause some people to become dizzy or lightheaded. *Make sure you know how you react to this medicine before you drive, use machines, or do anything else that could be dangerous if you are dizzy or are not alert or able to see well.* If these reactions are especially bothersome, check with your doctor.

Malaria is spread by mosquitoes. If you are living in, or will be traveling to, an area where there is a chance of getting malaria, the following mosquito-control measures will help to prevent infection:

- If possible, sleep under mosquito netting to avoid being bitten by malaria-carrying mosquitoes.
- Wear long-sleeved shirts or blouses and long trousers to protect your arms and legs, especially from dusk through dawn when mosquitoes are out.
- Apply mosquito repellent to uncovered areas of the skin from dusk through dawn when mosquitoes are out.

Side Effects of This Medicine

Along with its needed effects, a medicine may cause some unwanted effects. Although not all of these side effects may occur, if they do occur they may need medical attention. When this medicine is used for short periods of time, side effects usually are rare. However, when it is used for a long time and/or in high doses, side effects are more likely to occur and may be serious.

Check with your doctor immediately if any of the following side effects occur:

Less common

Blurred vision or any other change in vision—this side effect may also occur or get worse after you stop taking this medicine

Rare

Convulsions (seizures); unusual tiredness; increased muscle weakness; mood or other mental changes; ringing or buzzing in ears or any loss of hearing; sore throat and fever; unusual bleeding or bruising; weakness

Symptoms of overdose

Drowsiness; headache; increased excitability

Other side effects may occur that usually do not need medical attention. These side effects may go away during treatment as your body adjusts to the medicine. However, check with your doctor if any of the following side effects continue or are bothersome:

More common

Diarrhea; difficulty in seeing to read; headache; itching (more common in black patients); loss of appetite; nausea or vomiting; stomach cramps or pain

Less common

Bleaching of hair or increased hair loss; blue-black discoloration of skin, fingernails, or inside of mouth; dizziness or lightheadedness; nervousness or restlessness; skin rash

Other side effects not listed above may also occur in some patients. If you notice any other effects, check with your doctor.

Additional Information

Once a medicine has been approved for marketing for a certain use, experience may show that it is also useful for other medical problems. Although these uses are not included in product labeling, hydroxychloroquine is used in certain patients with the following medical conditions:

- Arthritis, juvenile
- Hypercalcemia, sarcoid-associated
- Polymorphous light eruption
- Porphyria cutanea tarda
- Urticaria, solar
- Vasculitis, chronic cutaneous

Other than the above information, there is no additional information relating to proper use, precautions, or side effects for these uses.

Annual revision: 10/06/92

HYDROXYPROPYL CELLULOSE Ophthalmic

A commonly used brand name in the U.S. and Canada is Lacrisert.

Description

Hydroxypropyl cellulose (hye-drox-ee-PROE-pil SELL-yoo-lose) belongs to the group of medicines known as artificial tears. It is inserted in the eye to relieve dryness and irritation caused by reduced tear flow that occurs in certain eye diseases.

This medicine is available only with your doctor's prescription, in the following dosage form:

Ophthalmic

- Ocular system (eye system) (U.S. and Canada)

It is very important that you read and understand the following information. If any of it causes you special concern, check with your doctor. Also, *if you have any questions* or if you want more information about this medicine or your medical problem, *ask your doctor, nurse, or pharmacist.*

Before Using This Medicine

In deciding to use a medicine, the risks of using the medicine must be weighed against the good it will do. This is a decision you and your doctor will make. For hydroxypropyl cellulose, the following should be considered:

Allergies—Tell your doctor if you have ever had any unusual or allergic reaction to hydroxypropyl cellulose. Also tell your doctor and pharmacist if you are allergic to any other substances, such as preservatives.

Pregnancy—Hydroxypropyl cellulose has not been shown to cause birth defects or other problems in humans.

Breast-feeding—Hydroxypropyl cellulose has not been reported to cause problems in nursing babies.

Children—Although there is no specific information comparing use of this medicine in children with use in other age groups, this medicine is not expected to cause different side effects or problems in children than it does in adults.

Older adults—Many medicines have not been studied specifically in older people. Therefore, it may not be known whether they work exactly the same way they do in younger adults. Although there is no specific information comparing use of this medicine in the elderly with use in other age groups, this medicine is not expected to cause different side effects or problems in older people than it does in younger adults.

Before you begin using any new medicine (prescription or nonprescription) or if you develop any new medical problem while you are using this medicine, check with your doctor, nurse, or pharmacist.

Proper Use of This Medicine

To use:

- This medicine usually comes with patient directions. Read them carefully before using this medicine. It is very important that you understand how to insert this eye system properly. If you have any questions about this, check with your doctor.
- Before opening the package containing this medicine, wash your hands thoroughly with soap and water.
- If the eye system accidentally comes out of your eye, as sometimes occurs when the eye is rubbed, do not

put it back in the eye, since it may be contaminated. Instead, insert another eye system if needed.

- You may have to use this medicine for several weeks before your eye symptoms get better.

Dosing—The dose of hydroxypropyl cellulose will be different for different patients. *Follow your doctor's orders or the directions on the label.* The following information includes only the average doses of hydroxypropyl cellulose. *If your dose is different, do not change it* unless your doctor tells you to do so.

The number of doses you use, the time allowed between doses, and the length of time you use the medicine depend on the medical problem for which you are using hydroxypropyl cellulose.

- For *eye system* dosage form:
  - —For dry eyes or eye irritation:
    - Adults and children—Place one insert in the eye each day.

Missed dose—If you forget to insert an eye system at the proper time, insert it as soon as possible. Then go back to your regular dosing schedule.

Storage—To store this medicine:

- Keep out of the reach of children.
- Store away from heat and direct light.
- Do not keep outdated medicine or medicine no longer needed. Be sure that any discarded medicine is out of the reach of children.

Precautions While Using This Medicine

This medicine may cause blurred vision for a short time after each dose is applied. *Make sure your vision is clear before you drive, use machines, or do anything else that could be dangerous if you are not able to see well.*

This medicine may also cause your eyes to become more sensitive to light than they are normally. Wearing sunglasses and avoiding too much exposure to bright light may help lessen the discomfort.

If your eye symptoms get worse or if you get new eye symptoms, remove the eye system and check with your doctor as soon as possible.

Side Effects of This Medicine

Along with its needed effects, a medicine may cause some unwanted effects. The following side effects may go away during treatment as your body adjusts to the medicine. However, check with your doctor if any of these effects continue or are bothersome:

Less common

Blurred vision; eye redness or discomfort or other irritation not present before use of this medicine; increased sensitivity of eyes to light; matting or stickiness of eyelashes; swelling of eyelids; watering of eyes

Other side effects not listed above may also occur in some patients. If you notice any other effects, check with your doctor.

Annual revision: 06/21/93

HYDROXYPROPYL METHYLCELLULOSE Ophthalmic

Some commonly used brand names are:

In the U.S.

Gonak
Goniosol
Isopto Alkaline
Isopto Plain
Isopto Tears
Just Tears
Lacril
Moisture Drops
Tearisol
Tears Naturale II
Tears Renewed
Ultra Tears

In Canada

Isopto Tears
Moisture Drops
Tears Naturale

Another commonly used name is hypromellose.

Description

Hydroxypropyl methylcellulose (hye-drox-ee-PROE-pil meth-ill-SELL-yoo-lose) belongs to the group of medicines known as artificial tears. It is used to relieve dryness and irritation caused by reduced tear flow. It helps prevent damage to the eye in certain eye diseases. Hydroxypropyl methylcellulose may also be used to moisten hard contact lenses and artificial eyes. In addition, it may be used in certain eye examinations.

Some of these preparations are available only with your doctor's prescription. Others are available without a prescription; however, your doctor may have special instructions on the proper use of this medicine for your medical problem.

Hydroxypropyl methylcellulose is available in the following dosage form:

Ophthalmic

- Ophthalmic solution (eye drops) (U.S. and Canada)

It is very important that you read and understand the following information. If any of it causes you special concern, check with your doctor or pharmacist. Also, *if you have any questions* or if you want more information about this medicine or your medical problem, *ask your doctor, nurse, or pharmacist.*

Before Using This Medicine

If you are using this medicine without a prescription, carefully read and follow any precautions on the label. For hydroxypropyl methylcellulose, the following should be considered:

Allergies—Tell your doctor if you have ever had any unusual or allergic reaction to hydroxypropyl methylcellulose. Also tell your doctor and pharmacist if you are allergic to any other substances, such as preservatives.

Pregnancy—Hydroxypropyl methylcellulose has not been shown to cause birth defects or other problems in humans.

Breast-feeding—Hydroxypropyl methylcellulose has not been reported to cause problems in nursing babies.

Children—Although there is no specific information comparing use of hydroxypropyl methylcellulose in children with use in other age groups, this medicine is not expected to cause different side effects or problems in children than it does in adults.

Older adults—Many medicine have not been studied specifically in older people. Therefore, it may not be known whether they work exactly the same way they do in younger adults. Although there is no specific information comparing use of hydroxypropyl methylcellulose in the elderly with use in other age groups, this medicine is not expected to cause different side effects or problems in older people than it does in younger adults.

Before you begin using any new medicine (prescription or nonprescription) or if you develop any new medical problem while you are using this medicine, check with your doctor, nurse, or pharmacist.

Proper Use of This Medicine

To use:

- First, wash your hands. Then tilt the head back and pull the lower eyelid away from the eye to form a pouch. Drop the medicine into the pouch and gently close the eyes. Do not blink. Keep the eyes closed for 1 or 2 minutes to allow the medicine to be absorbed.
- To keep the medicine as germ-free as possible, do not touch the applicator tip to any surface (including the eye). Also, keep the container tightly closed.

Do not use this medicine for more than 3 days, unless otherwise directed by your doctor. To do so may increase the chance of side effects.

For patients *wearing hard contact lenses*:

- Take care not to float the lens from your eye when applying this medicine. If you have any questions about this, check with your doctor, nurse, or pharmacist.

Dosing—The dose of hydroxypropyl methylcellulose will be different for different patients. *Follow your doctor's orders or the directions on the label.* The following information includes only the average doses of hydroxypropyl methylcellulose. *If your dose is different, do not change it* unless your doctor tells you to do so.

The number of doses you use each day, the time allowed between doses, and the length of time you use the medicine depend on the medical problem for which you are using hydroxypropyl methylcellulose.

- For dry eyes:
  - —For *ophthalmic solution (eye drops)* dosage form:
    - Adults and children—Use 1 drop three or four times a day.

Storage—To store this medicine:

- Keep out of the reach of children.
- Store away from heat and direct light.
- Keep the medicine from freezing.
- Do not keep outdated medicine or medicine no longer needed. Be sure that any discarded medicine is out of the reach of children.

Precautions While Using This Medicine

If you experience eye pain, changes in vision, continued redness or irritation of the eye, or if your symptoms continue or become worse, check with your doctor.

Side Effects of This Medicine

Along with its needed effects, a medicine may cause some unwanted effects. Although not all of these side effects may occur, if they do occur they may need medical attention.

Check with your doctor as soon as possible if the following side effect occurs:

Eye irritation not present before use of this medicine

Other side effects may occur that usually do not need medical attention. These side effects may go away during treatment as your body adjusts to the medicine. However,

check with your doctor or pharmacist if any of the following side effects continue or are bothersome:

Less common—more common with 1% solution

Blurred vision; matting or stickiness of eyelashes

Other side effects not listed above may also occur in some patients. If you notice any other effects, check with your doctor or pharmacist.

Annual revision: 06/21/93

HYDROXYUREA Systemic

A commonly used brand name in the U.S. and Canada is Hydrea.

Description

Hydroxyurea (hye-DROX-ee-yoo-REE-ah) belongs to the group of medicines called antimetabolites. It is used to treat some kinds of cancer.

Hydroxyurea seems to interfere with the growth of cancer cells, which are eventually destroyed. Since the growth of normal body cells may also be affected by hydroxyurea, other effects will also occur. Some of these may be serious and must be reported to your doctor. Other effects may not be serious but may cause concern. Some effects may not occur for months or years after the medicine is used.

Before you begin treatment with hydroxyurea, you and your doctor should talk about the good this medicine will do as well as the risks of using it.

Hydroxyurea is available only with your doctor's prescription, in the following dosage form:

Oral

- Capsules (U.S. and Canada)

It is very important that you read and understand the following information. If any of it causes you special concern, check with your doctor. Also, *if you have any questions* or if you want more information about this medicine or your medical problem, *ask your doctor, nurse, or pharmacist.*

Before Using This Medicine

In deciding to use a medicine, the risks of taking the medicine must be weighed against the good it will do. This is a decision you and your doctor will make. For hydroxyurea, the following should be considered:

Allergies—Tell your doctor if you have ever had any unusual or allergic reaction to hydroxyurea.

Pregnancy—Tell your doctor if you are pregnant or if you intend to have children. There is a chance that this medicine may cause birth defects if either the male or female is taking it at the time of conception or if it is taken during pregnancy. Studies have shown that hydroxyurea causes birth defects in animals. In addition, many cancer medicines may cause sterility. Although sterility seems to be only temporary with this medicine, the possibility should be kept in mind.

Be sure that you have discussed this with your doctor before taking this medicine. It is best to use some kind of birth control while you are taking hydroxyurea. Tell your doctor right away if you think you have become pregnant while taking hydroxyurea.

Breast-feeding—Tell your doctor if you are breast-feeding or if you intend to breast-feed during treatment with this medicine. Because hydroxyurea may cause serious side effects, breast-feeding is generally not recommended while you are taking it.

Children—Side effects may be likely to occur in children, who may be more sensitive to the effects of hydroxyurea.

Older adults—Side effects may be more likely to occur in the elderly, who may be more sensitive to the effects of hydroxyurea.

Other medicines—Although certain medicines should not be used together at all, in other cases two different medicines may be used together even if an interaction might occur. In these cases, your doctor may want to change the dose, or other precautions may be necessary. When you are taking hydroxyurea, it is especially important that your doctor and pharmacist know if you are taking any of the following:

- Amphotericin B by injection (e.g., Fungizone) or
- Antithyroid agents (medicine for overactive thyroid) or
- Azathioprine (e.g., Imuran) or
- Chloramphenicol (e.g., Chloromycetin) or
- Colchicine or
- Flucytosine (e.g., Ancobon) or
- Ganciclovir (e.g., Cytovene) or
- Interferon (e.g., Intron A, Roferon-A) or
- Plicamycin (e.g., Mithracin) or
- Zidovudine (e.g., AZT, Retrovir) or
- If you have ever been treated with x-rays or cancer medicines—Hydroxyurea may increase the effects of these medicines or radiation therapy on the blood

- Probenecid (e.g., Benemid) or
- Sulfinpyrazone (e.g., Anturane)—Hydroxyurea may increase the amount of uric acid in the blood. Since these

medicines are used to lower uric acid levels, they may not be as effective in patients taking hydroxyurea

Other medical problems—The presence of other medical problems may affect the use of hydroxyurea. Make sure you tell your doctor if you have any other medical problems, especially:

- Anemia—May be worsened
- Chickenpox (including recent exposure) or
- Herpes zoster (shingles)—Risk of severe disease affecting other parts of the body
- Gout or
- Kidney stones—Hydroxyurea may increase levels of uric acid in the body, which can cause gout or kidney stones
- Infection—Hydroxyurea may decrease your body's ability to fight infection
- Kidney disease—Effects may be increased because of slower removal of hydroxyurea from the body

Before you begin using any new medicine (prescription or nonprescription) or if you develop any new medical problem while you are using this medicine, check with your doctor, nurse, or pharmacist.

Proper Use of This Medicine

Take hydroxyurea only as directed by your doctor. Do not use more or less of it, and do not use it more often than your doctor ordered. The exact amount of medicine you need has been carefully worked out. Taking too much may increase the chance of side effects, while taking too little may not improve your condition.

For patients who *cannot swallow the capsules:*

- The contents of the capsule may be emptied into a glass of water and then taken immediately. Some powder may float on the surface of the water, but that is just filler from the capsule.

This medicine is sometimes given together with certain other medicines. If you are using a combination of medicines, make sure that you take each one at the right time and do not mix them. Ask your doctor, nurse, or pharmacist to help you plan a way to take your medicine at the right times.

While you are using this medicine, your doctor may want you to drink extra fluids so that you will pass more urine. This will help prevent kidney problems and keep your kidneys working well.

This medicine commonly causes nausea, vomiting, and diarrhea. However, it is very important that you continue to use the medicine, even if you begin to feel ill. Ask your doctor, nurse, or pharmacist for ways to lessen these effects.

If you vomit shortly after taking a dose of hydroxyurea, check with your doctor. You will be told whether to take the dose again or to wait until the next scheduled dose.

Missed dose—If you miss a dose of this medicine, do not take the missed dose at all and do not double the next one. Instead, go back to your regular dosing schedule and check with your doctor.

Storage—To store this medicine:

- Keep out of the reach of children.
- Store away from heat and direct light.
- Do not store in the bathroom, near the kitchen sink, or in other damp places. Heat or moisture may cause the medicine to break down.
- Do not keep outdated medicine or medicine no longer needed. Be sure that any discarded medicine is out of the reach of children.

Precautions While Using This Medicine

It is very important that your doctor check your progress at regular visits to make sure that this medicine is working properly and to check for unwanted effects.

While you are being treated with hydroxyurea, and after you stop treatment with it, *do not have any immunizations (vaccinations) without your doctor's approval.* Hydroxyurea may lower your body's resistance and there is a chance you might get the infection the immunization is meant to prevent. In addition, other persons living in your household should not take oral polio vaccine since there is a chance they could pass the polio virus on to you. Also, avoid persons who have recently taken oral polio vaccine. Do not get close to them and do not stay in the same room with them for very long. If you cannot take these precautions, you should consider wearing a protective face mask that covers the nose and mouth.

Hydroxyurea can temporarily lower the number of white blood cells in your blood, increasing the chance of getting an infection. It can also lower the number of platelets, which are necessary for proper blood clotting. If this occurs, there are certain precautions you can take, especially when your blood count is low, to reduce the risk of infection or bleeding:

- If you can, avoid people with infections. *Check with your doctor immediately* if you think you are getting an infection or if you get a fever or chills, cough or hoarseness, lower back or side pain, or painful or difficult urination.
- *Check with your doctor immediately* if you notice any unusual bleeding or bruising; black, tarry stools; blood in urine or stools; or pinpoint red spots on your skin.
- Be careful when using a regular toothbrush, dental floss, or toothpick. Your medical doctor, dentist, or nurse may recommend other ways to clean your teeth and gums. Check with your medical doctor before having any dental work done.

- Do not touch your eyes or the inside of your nose unless you have just washed your hands and have not touched anything else in the meantime.
- Be careful not to cut yourself when you are using sharp objects such as a safety razor or fingernail or toenail cutters.
- Avoid contact sports or other situations where bruising or injury could occur.

Side Effects of This Medicine

Along with their needed effects, medicines like hydroxyurea can sometimes cause unwanted effects such as blood problems and other side effects. These and others are described below. Also, because of the way these medicines act on the body, there is a chance that they might cause other unwanted effects that may not occur until months or years after the medicine is used. These delayed effects may include certain types of cancer, such as leukemia. Ask your doctor, nurse, or pharmacist for ways to lessen these effects.

Although not all of these side effects may occur, if they do occur they may need medical attention.

Check with your doctor or nurse immediately if any of the following side effects occur:

Less common

Cough or hoarseness; fever or chills; lower back or side pain; painful or difficult urination

Rare

Black, tarry stools; blood in urine or stools; pinpoint red spots on skin; unusual bleeding or bruising

Check with your doctor as soon as possible if any of the following side effects occur:

Less common

Sores in mouth and on lips

Rare

Confusion; convulsions (seizures); dizziness; hallucinations (seeing, hearing, or feeling things that are not there); headache; joint pain; swelling of feet or lower legs

Other side effects may occur that usually do not need medical attention. These side effects may go away during treatment as your body adjusts to the medicine. Also, your doctor or nurse may be able to tell you about ways to prevent or reduce some of these side effects. Check with your doctor or nurse if any of the following side effects continue or are bothersome or if you have any questions about them:

More common

Diarrhea; drowsiness; loss of appetite; nausea or vomiting

Less common

Constipation; redness of skin; skin rash and itching

After you stop taking hydroxyurea, your body may need time to adjust. The length of time this takes depends on the amount of medicine you were using and how long you used it. During this period of time check with your doctor if you notice any of the following side effects:

Black, tarry stools; blood in urine or stools; cough or hoarseness; fever or chills; lower back or side pain; painful or difficult urination; pinpoint red spots on skin; unusual bleeding or bruising

Other side effects not listed above may also occur in some patients. If you notice any other effects, check with your doctor.

Annual revision: 06/16/92

IDARUBICIN Systemic

A commonly used brand name in the U.S. and Canada is Idamycin.

Description

Idarubicin (eye-da-RUE-bi-sin) belongs to the general group of medicines known as antineoplastics. It is used to treat some kinds of cancer, including leukemia.

Idarubicin seems to interfere with the growth of cancer cells, which are eventually destroyed. Since the growth of normal body cells may also be affected by idarubicin, other effects will also occur. Some of these may be serious and must be reported to your doctor. Other effects, like hair loss, may not be serious but may cause concern. Some effects may not occur for months or years after the medicine is used.

Before you begin treatment with idarubicin, you and your doctor should talk about the good this medicine will do as well as the risks of using it.

Idarubicin is to be administered only by or under the supervision of your doctor. It is available in the following dosage form:

Parenteral

- Injection (U.S. and Canada)

It is very important that you read and understand the following information. If any of it causes you special concern, check with your doctor. Also, *if you have any questions* or if you want more information about this medicine or your medical problem, *ask your doctor, nurse or pharmacist.*

Before Using This Medicine

In deciding to use a medicine, the risks of taking the medicine must be weighed against the good it will do. This is a decision you and your doctor will make. For idarubicin, the following should be considered:

Allergies—Tell your doctor if you have ever had any unusual or allergic reaction to idarubicin.

Pregnancy—There is a chance that this medicine may cause birth defects if either the male or female is receiving it at the time of conception or if it is taken during pregnancy. Studies in rats and rabbits have shown that idarubicin causes birth defects in the fetus and other problems (including miscarriage). In addition, many cancer medicines may cause sterility which could be permanent. Although sterility has been reported only in male dogs with this medicine, the possibility of an effect in human males should be kept in mind.

Be sure that you have discussed these possible effects with your doctor before receiving this medicine. It is best to use some kind of birth control while you are receiving idarubicin. Tell your doctor right away if you think you have become pregnant while receiving idarubicin. Before receiving idarubicin make sure your doctor knows if you are pregnant or if you may become pregnant.

Breast-feeding—Because idarubicin may cause serious side effects, breast-feeding is generally not recommended while you are receiving it.

Children—There is no specific information comparing use of idarubicin in children with use in other age groups.

Older adults—Heart problems are more likely to occur in the elderly, who are usually more sensitive to the effects of idarubicin.

Other medicines—Although certain medicines should not be used together at all, in other cases two different medicines may be used together even if an interaction might occur. In these cases, your doctor may want to change the dose, or other precautions may be necessary. When you are receiving idarubicin, it is especially important that your doctor and pharmacist know if you have ever been treated with x-rays or cancer medicines or if you are taking any of the following:

- Amphotericin B by injection (e.g., Fungizone) or
- Antithyroid agents (medicine for overactive thyroid) or
- Azathioprine (e.g., Imuran) or
- Chloramphenicol (e.g., Chloromycetin) or
- Colchicine or
- Flucytosine (e.g., Ancobon) or
- Ganciclovir (e.g., Cytovene) or
- Interferon (e.g., Intron A, Roferon-A) or
- Plicamycin (e.g., Mithracin) or
- Zidovudine (e.g., AZT, Retrovir)—Idarubicin may increase the effects of these medicines or radiation therapy on the blood
- Probenecid (e.g., Benemid) or
- Sulfinpyrazone (e.g., Anturane)—Idarubicin may raise the concentration of uric acid in the blood, which these medicines are used to lower

Other medical problems—The presence of other medical problems may affect the use of idarubicin. Make sure you tell your doctor if you have any other medical problems, especially:

- Chickenpox (including recent exposure) or
- Herpes zoster (shingles)—Risk of severe disease affecting other parts of the body
- Gout or
- Kidney stones—Idarubicin may increase levels of a chemical called uric acid in the body, which can cause gout or kidney stones
- Heart disease—Risk of heart problems caused by idarubicin may be increased
- Kidney disease or
- Liver disease—Effects may be increased because of slower removal of idarubicin from the body

Before you begin using any new medicine (prescription or nonprescription) or if you develop any new medical problem while you are using this medicine, check with your doctor, nurse, or pharmacist.

Proper Use of This Medicine

Idarubicin is sometimes given together with certain other medicines. If you are receiving a combination of medicines, it is important that you receive each one at the proper time. If you are taking some of these medicines by mouth, ask your doctor, nurse, or pharmacist to help you plan a way to take them at the right times.

While you are receiving this medicine, your doctor may want you to drink extra fluids so that you will pass more urine. This will help prevent kidney problems and keep your kidneys working well.

Idarubicin often causes nausea and vomiting. However, it is very important that you continue to receive it, even if you begin to feel ill. Ask your doctor, nurse, or pharmacist for ways to lessen these effects.

Precautions While Using This Medicine

It is very important that your doctor check your progress at regular visits to make sure that this medicine is working properly and to check for unwanted effects.

While you are being treated with idarubicin, and after you stop treatment with it, *do not have any immunizations (vaccinations) without your doctor's approval.* Idarubicin may lower your body's resistance, and there is a chance you might get the infection the immunization is meant to prevent. In addition, other persons living in your household should not take or should not have recently taken oral polio vaccine since there is a chance they could pass the polio virus on to you. Also, avoid other persons who have taken oral polio vaccine. Do not get close to them, and do not stay in the same room with them for very long. If you cannot take these precautions, you should consider wearing a protective face mask that covers the nose and mouth.

Idarubicin can lower the number of white blood cells in your blood temporarily, increasing the chance of getting an infection. It can also lower the number of platelets, which are necessary for proper blood clotting. If this occurs, there are certain precautions you can take, especially when your blood count is low, to reduce the risk of infection or bleeding:

- If you can, avoid people with infections. *Check with your doctor immediately* if you think you are getting an infection or if you get a fever or chills, cough or hoarseness, lower back or side pain, or painful or difficult urination.
- *Check with your doctor immediately* if you notice any unusual bleeding or bruising; black, tarry stools; blood in urine or stools; or pinpoint red spots on your skin.
- Be careful when using a regular toothbrush, dental floss, or toothpick. Your medical doctor, dentist, or nurse may recommend other ways to clean your teeth and gums. Check with your medical doctor before having any dental work done.
- Do not touch your eyes or the inside of your nose unless you have just washed your hands and have not touched anything else in the meantime.
- Be careful not to cut yourself when you are using sharp objects such as a safety razor or fingernail or toenail cutters.
- Avoid contact sports or other situations where bruising or injury could occur.

If idarubicin accidentally seeps out of the vein into which it is injected, it may damage some tissues and cause scarring. *Tell the doctor or nurse right away if you notice redness, pain, or swelling at the place of injection.*

Side Effects of This Medicine

Along with their needed effects, medicines like idarubicin can sometimes cause unwanted effects such as heart problems, blood problems, loss of hair, and other side effects. These and others are described below. Also, because of the way these medicines act on the body, there is a chance that they might cause other unwanted effects that may not occur until months or years after the medicine is used. These delayed effects may include certain types of cancer, such as leukemia. Discuss these possible effects with your doctor.

Although not all of these side effects may occur, if they do occur they may need medical attention.

Check with your doctor or nurse immediately if any of the following side effects occur:

More common

Black, tarry stools; blood in urine or stools; cough or hoarseness; fever or chills; lower back or side pain; painful or difficult urination; pinpoint red spots on skin; unusual bleeding or bruising

Less common

Fast or irregular heartbeat; pain at place of injection; shortness of breath; swelling of feet and lower legs

Rare

Stomach pain (severe)

Check with your doctor or nurse as soon as possible if any of the following side effects occur:

More common

Sores in mouth and on lips

Less common
- Joint pain

Rare
- Skin rash or hives

Other side effects may occur that usually do not need medical attention. These side effects may go away during treatment as your body adjusts to the medicine. Also, your doctor or nurse may be able to tell you about ways to prevent or reduce some of these side effects. Check with your doctor or nurse if any of the following side effects continue or are bothersome or if you have any questions about them:

More common
- Diarrhea or stomach cramps; headache; nausea and vomiting

Less common
- Darkening or redness of skin (after x-ray treatment); numbness or tingling of fingers, toes, or face

Idarubicin causes the urine to turn reddish in color, which may stain clothes. This is not blood. It is perfectly normal and lasts for only a day or two after each dose is given.

This medicine often causes a temporary and total loss of hair. After treatment with idarubicin has ended, normal hair growth should return.

After you stop receiving idarubicin, it may still produce some side effects that need attention. During this period of time, *check with your doctor or nurse immediately* if you notice any of the following side effects:

- Fast or irregular heartbeat; shortness of breath; swelling of feet and lower legs

Other side effects not listed above may also occur in some patients. If you notice any other effects, check with your doctor or nurse.

Annual revision: 06/18/93

IDOXURIDINE Ophthalmic

Some commonly used brand names in the U.S. and Canada are Herplex Liquifilm and Stoxil.

Description

Idoxuridine (eye-dox-YOOR-i-deen) belongs to the family of medicines called antivirals. Idoxuridine is used to treat virus infections of the eye.

Idoxuridine is available only with your doctor's prescription, in the following dosage forms:

Ophthalmic
- Ophthalmic ointment (U.S. and Canada)
- Ophthalmic solution (eye drops) (U.S. and Canada)

It is very important that you read and understand the following information. If any of it causes you special concern, check with your doctor. Also, *if you have any questions* or if you want more information about this medicine or your medical problem, *ask your doctor, nurse, or pharmacist.*

Before Using This Medicine

In deciding to use a medicine, the risks of using the medicine must be weighed against the good it will do. This is a decision you and your doctor will make. For idoxuridine, the following should be considered:

Allergies—Tell your doctor if you have ever had any unusual or allergic reaction to idoxuridine or to iodine or iodine-containing preparations. Also tell your doctor and pharmacist if you are allergic to any other substances, such as preservatives.

Pregnancy—Idoxuridine ophthalmic preparations have not been shown to cause birth defects or other problems in humans. However, studies in animals have shown that idoxuridine causes protruding eyes (eyes that stick out too far) and deformed front legs in rabbits. Before using this medicine, make sure your doctor knows if you are pregnant or if you may become pregnant.

Breast-feeding—It is not known whether idoxuridine passes into the breast milk. Although most medicines pass into breast milk in small amounts, many of them may be used safely while breast-feeding. Mothers who are using this medicine and who wish to breast-feed should discuss this with their doctor.

Children—Studies on this medicine have been done only in adult patients, and there is no specific information comparing use of this medicine in children with use in other age groups.

Older adults—Many medicines have not been studied specifically in older people. Therefore, it may not be known whether they work exactly the same way they do in younger adults or if they cause different side effects or problems in older people. There is no specific information comparing use of idoxuridine in the elderly with use in other age groups.

Other medicines—Although certain medicines should not be used together at all, in other cases two different medicines may be used together even if an interaction might occur. In these cases, your doctor may want to change the dose, or other precautions may be necessary. When you are using idoxuridine, it is especially important that your doctor and pharmacist know if you are using the following:

- Eye product containing boric acid—Boric acid may interact with the idoxuridine preparation causing a gritty substance to form or may interact with the preservative in the idoxuridine preparation causing a toxic effect in the eye

Before you begin using any new medicine (prescription or nonprescription) or if you develop any new medical problem while you are using this medicine, check with your doctor, nurse, or pharmacist.

Proper Use of This Medicine

For patients using the *eye drop form* of idoxuridine:

- The bottle is only partially full to provide proper drop control.
- To use:
  —First, wash your hands. Then tilt the head back and pull the lower eyelid away from the eye to form a pouch. Drop the medicine into the pouch and gently close the eyes. Do not blink. Keep the eyes closed for 1 or 2 minutes to allow the medicine to come into contact with the infection.
  —If you think you did not get the drop of medicine into your eye properly, use another drop.
  —To keep the medicine as germ-free as possible, do not touch the applicator tip to any surface (including the eye). Also, keep the container tightly closed.

For patients using the *eye ointment form* of idoxuridine:

- To use:
  —First, wash your hands. Then pull the lower eyelid away from the eye to form a pouch. Squeeze a thin strip of ointment into the pouch. A 1-cm (approximately ⅓-inch) strip of ointment is usually enough unless otherwise directed by your doctor. Gently close the eyes and keep them closed for 1 or 2 minutes to allow the medicine to come into contact with the infection.
  —To keep the medicine as germ-free as possible, do not touch the applicator tip to any surface (including the eye). After using idoxuridine eye ointment, wipe the tip of the ointment tube with a clean tissue and keep the tube tightly closed.

Do not use this medicine more often or for a longer time than your doctor ordered. To do so may cause problems in the eyes. If you have any questions about this, check with your doctor.

To help clear up your infection completely, *keep using this medicine for the full time of treatment,* even though your symptoms may have disappeared. *Do not miss any doses.*

Dosing—The dose of idoxuridine will be different for different patients. *Follow your doctor's orders or the directions on the label.* The following information includes only the average doses of idoxuridine. *If your dose is different, do not change it* unless your doctor tells you to do so.

The number of doses you use each day, the time allowed between doses, and the length of time you use the medicine depend on the medical problem for which you are using idoxuridine.

- For virus infections of the eye:
  —For *eye ointment* dosage form:
    - Adults and children—Use every four hours during the day (five times a day).

  —For *eye solution (eye drops)* dosage form:
    - Adults and children—Use every hour during the day and every two hours during the night. After the eye condition gets better, use every two hours during the day and every four hours during the night.

Missed dose—If you miss a dose of this medicine, apply it as soon as possible. However, if it is almost time for your next dose, skip the missed dose and go back to your regular dosing schedule.

Storage—To store this medicine:

- Keep out of the reach of children.
- Store in the refrigerator or in a cool place because heat will cause this medicine to break down. However, keep the medicine from freezing. Follow the directions on the label.
- Do not keep outdated medicine or medicine no longer needed. Be sure that any discarded medicine is out of the reach of children.

Precautions While Using This Medicine

It is very important that your doctor check your progress at regular visits.

If your symptoms do not improve within a week, or if they become worse, check with your doctor.

This medicine may cause your eyes to become more sensitive to light than they are normally. Wearing sunglasses and avoiding too much exposure to bright light may help lessen the discomfort.

Side Effects of This Medicine

Along with its needed effects, a medicine may cause some unwanted effects. Although not all of these side effects

may occur, if they do occur they may need medical attention.

Check with your doctor as soon as possible if any of the following side effects occur:

Less common

Increased sensitivity of eyes to light; itching, redness, swelling, pain, or other sign of irritation not present before use of this medicine

Rare

Blurring, dimming, or haziness of vision

Other side effects may occur that usually do not need medical attention. These side effects may go away during treatment as your body adjusts to the medicine. However, check with your doctor if the following side effect continues or is bothersome:

Less common

Excess flow of tears

After application, eye ointments usually cause your vision to blur for a few minutes.

Other side effects not listed above may also occur in some patients. If you notice any other effects, check with your doctor.

Annual revision: 06/21/93

IFOSFAMIDE Systemic

A commonly used brand name in the U.S. and Canada is IFEX.

Description

Ifosfamide (eye-FOSS-fa-mide) belongs to the group of medicines called alkylating agents. It is used to treat cancer of the testicles as well as some other kinds of cancer. Another medicine, called mesna, is usually given along with ifosfamide to prevent bladder problems that can be caused by ifosfamide.

Ifosfamide interferes with the growth of cancer cells, which are eventually destroyed. Since the growth of normal body cells may also be affected by ifosfamide, other effects will also occur. Some of these may be serious and must be reported to your doctor. Other effects, like hair loss, may not be serious but may cause concern. Some effects may not occur for months or years after the medicine is used.

Before you begin treatment with ifosfamide, you and your doctor should talk about the good this medicine will do as well as the risks of using it.

Ifosfamide is to be administered only by or under the immediate supervision of your doctor. It is available in the following dosage form:

Parenteral

Injection (U.S. and Canada)

It is very important that you read and understand the following information. If any of it causes you special concern, check with your doctor. Also, *if you have any questions* or if you want more information about this medicine or your medical problem, *ask your doctor, nurse, or pharmacist.*

Before Using This Medicine

In deciding to use a medicine, the risks of taking the medicine must be weighed against the good it will do. This is a decision you and your doctor will make. For ifosfamide, the following should be considered:

Allergies—Tell your doctor if you have ever had any unusual or allergic reaction to ifosfamide.

Pregnancy—Tell your doctor if you are pregnant or if you intend to have children. There is a chance that this medicine may cause birth defects if either the male or female is taking it at the time of conception or if it is taken during pregnancy. Ifosfamide causes birth defects in animals. In addition, many cancer medicines may cause sterility which could be permanent. Although sterility has not been reported with this medicine, the possibility should be kept in mind.

Be sure that you have discussed this with your doctor before taking this medicine. It is best to use some kind of birth control while you are receiving ifosfamide. Tell your doctor right away if you think you have become pregnant while receiving ifosfamide.

Breast-feeding—Tell your doctor if you are breast-feeding or if you intend to breast-feed during treatment with this medicine. Because ifosfamide may cause serious side effects, breast-feeding is generally not recommended while you are receiving it.

Children—Although there is no specific information comparing use of ifosfamide in children with use in other age groups, this medicine is not expected to cause different side effects or problems in children than it does in adults.

Older adults—Many medicines have not been studied specifically in older people. Therefore, it may not be known whether they work exactly the same way they do in younger adults or if they cause different side effects or problems in older people. There is no specific information comparing use of ifosfamide in the elderly with use in other age groups.

Other medicines—Although certain medicines should not be used together at all, in other cases two different medicines may be used together even if an interaction might occur. In these cases, your doctor may want to change the dose, or other precautions may be necessary. When you are taking ifosfamide, it is especially important that your doctor and pharmacist know if you are taking any of the following:

- Amphotericin B by injection (e.g., Fungizone) or
- Antithyroid agents (medicine for overactive thyroid) or
- Azathioprine (e.g., Imuran) or
- Chloramphenicol (e.g., Chloromycetin) or
- Colchicine or
- Flucytosine (e.g., Ancobon) or
- Ganciclovir (e.g., Cytovene) or
- Interferon (e.g., Intron A, Roferon-A) or
- Plicamycin (e.g., Mithracin) or
- Zidovudine (e.g., AZT, Retrovir) or
- If you have ever been treated with x-rays or cancer medicines—Ifosfamide may increase the effects of these medicines or radiation therapy on the blood

Other medical problems—The presence of other medical problems may affect the use of ifosfamide. Make sure you tell your doctor if you have any other medical problems, especially:

- Chickenpox (including recent exposure) or
- Herpes zoster (shingles)—Risk of severe disease affecting other parts of the body
- Infection—Ifosfamide can decrease your body's ability to fight infection
- Kidney disease—Effects may be increased because of slower removal of ifosamide from the body
- Liver disease—Effects may be increased or decreased because the liver both makes ifosfamide work and removes it from the body

Before you begin using any new medicine (prescription or nonprescription) or if you develop any new medical problem while you are using this medicine, check with your doctor, nurse, or pharmacist.

Proper Use of This Medicine

Ifosfamide is sometimes given together with certain other medicines. If you are using a combination of medicines, make sure that you take each one at the proper time and do not mix them. Ask your doctor, nurse, or pharmacist to help you plan a way to remember to take your medicines at the right times.

While you are receiving ifosfamide, it is important that you drink extra fluids so that you will pass more urine. Also, empty your bladder frequently, including at least once during the night. This will help prevent kidney and bladder problems and keep your kidneys working well. Ifosfamide passes from the body in the urine. If too much of it appears in the urine or if the urine stays in the bladder too long, it can cause dangerous irritation. Follow your doctor's instructions carefully about how much fluid to drink every day. Some patients may have to drink up to 7 to 12 cups (3 quarts) of fluid a day.

Ifosfamide often causes nausea and vomiting. However, it is very important that you continue to receive the medicine even if you begin to feel ill. Ask your doctor, nurse, or pharmacist for ways to lessen these effects.

Precautions While Using This Medicine

It is very important that your doctor check your progress at regular visits to make sure that this medicine is working properly and to check for unwanted effects.

While you are being treated with ifosfamide, and after you stop treatment with it, *do not have any immunizations (vaccinations) without your doctor's approval.* Ifosfamide may lower your body's resistance and there is a chance you might get the infection the immunization is meant to prevent. In addition, other persons living in your house should not take oral polio vaccine since there is a chance they could pass the polio virus on to you. Also, avoid persons who have recently taken oral polio vaccine. Do not get close to them, and do not stay in the same room with them for very long. If you cannot take these precautions, you should consider wearing a protective face mask that covers the nose and mouth.

Ifosfamide can temporarily lower the number of white blood cells in your blood, increasing the chance of getting an infection. It can also lower the number of platelets, which are necessary for proper blood clotting. If this occurs, there are certain precautions you can take to reduce the risk of infection or bleeding:

- If you can, avoid people with infections. *Check with your doctor immediately* if you think you are getting an infection or if you get a fever or chills, cough or hoarseness, lower back or side pain, or painful or difficult urination.
- *Check with your doctor immediately* if you notice any unusual bleeding or bruising; black, tarry stools; blood in urine or stools; or pinpoint red spots on your skin.
- Be careful when using a regular toothbrush, dental floss, or toothpick. Your medical doctor, dentist, or nurse may recommend other ways to clean your teeth and gums. Check with your medical doctor before having any dental work done.
- Do not touch your eyes or the inside of your nose unless you have just washed your hands and have not touched anything else in the meantime.
- Be careful not to cut yourself when you are using sharp objects such as a safety razor or fingernail or toenail cutters.
- Avoid contact sports or other situations where bruising or injury could occur.

Side Effects of This Medicine

Along with their needed effects, medicines like ifosfamide can sometimes cause unwanted effects such as blood problems, loss of hair, and problems with the bladder. These and others are described below. Also, because of the way these medicines act on the body, there is a chance that they might cause other unwanted effects that may not occur until months or years after the medicine is used. These may include certain types of cancer, such as leukemia. Discuss these possible effects with your doctor.

Although not all of these side effects may occur, if they do occur they may need medical attention.

Check with your doctor immediately if any of the following side effects occur:

More common

Blood in urine; frequent urination; painful urination

Less common

Cough or hoarseness; fever or chills; lower back or side pain

Rare

Black, tarry stools; blood in stools; pinpoint red spots on skin; unusual bleeding or bruising

Check with your doctor as soon as possible if any of the following side effects occur:

More common

Agitation; confusion; hallucinations (seeing, hearing, or feeling things that are not there); unusual tiredness

Less common

Dizziness; redness, swelling, or pain at place of injection

Rare

Cough or shortness of breath; convulsions (seizures); sores in mouth and on lips

Other side effects may occur that usually do not need medical attention. These side effects may go away during treatment as your body adjusts to the medicine. Also, your doctor or nurse may be able to tell you about ways to prevent or reduce some of these side effects. Check with your doctor if any of the following side effects continue or are bothersome or if you have any questions about them:

More common

Nausea and vomiting

Ifosfamide often causes a temporary loss of hair. After treatment has ended, normal hair growth should return.

After you stop receiving ifosfamide, it may still produce some side effects that need attention. During this period of time, *check with your doctor immediately* if you notice the following side effect:

Blood in urine

Other side effects not listed above may also occur in some patients. If you notice any other effects, check with your doctor.

Annual revision: 09/09/92

IMIPENEM AND CILASTATIN Systemic

Some commonly used brand names are:

In the U.S.

Primaxin IM
Primaxin IV

In Canada

Primaxin

Description

Imipenem (i-mi-PEN-em) and cilastatin (sye-la-STAT-in) combination is used in the treatment of infections caused by bacteria. It works by killing bacteria or preventing their growth. This medicine will not work for colds, flu, or other virus infections.

Imipenem and cilastatin combination is used to treat infections in many different parts of the body. It is sometimes given with other antibiotics.

This medicine is available only with your doctor's prescription, in the following dosage form:

Parenteral

- Injection (U.S. and Canada)

It is very important that you read and understand the following information. If any of it causes you special concern, check with your doctor. Also, *if you have any questions* or if you want more information about this medicine or your medical problem, *ask your doctor, nurse, or pharmacist.*

Before Receiving This Medicine

In deciding to use a medicine, the risks of taking the medicine must be weighed against the good it will do. This is a decision you and your doctor will make. For

imipenem and cilastatin, the following should be considered:

Allergies—Tell your doctor if you have ever had any unusual or allergic reaction to imipenem and cilastatin, penicillins or cephalosporins. Also tell your doctor and pharmacist if you are allergic to any other substances, such as foods, preservatives, or dyes.

Pregnancy—Studies have not been done in humans. However, imipenem and cilastatin combination has not been reported to cause birth defects or other problems in animal studies.

Breast-feeding—It is not known whether imipenem or cilastatin passes into the breast milk. However, this medicine has not been reported to cause problems in nursing babies.

Children—This medicine has been tested in a limited number of children 12 years of age and older and, in effective doses, has not been reported to cause different side effects or problems in children than it does in adults.

Older adults—Many medicines have not been studied specifically in older people. Therefore, it may not be known whether they work exactly the same way they do in younger adults. Although there is no specific information comparing use of imipenem and cilastatin in the elderly with use in other age groups, this medicine is not expected to cause different side effects or problems in older people than it does in younger adults.

Other medicines—Although certain medicines should not be used together at all, in other cases two different medicines may be used together even if an interaction might occur. In these cases, your doctor may want to change the dose, or other precautions may be necessary. Tell your doctor and pharmacist if you are taking any other prescription or nonprescription (over-the-counter [OTC]) medicine.

Other medical problems—The presence of other medical problems may affect the use of imipenem and cilastatin. Make sure you tell your doctor if you have any other medical problems, especially:

- Central nervous system (CNS) disorders (for example, brain disease or history of seizures)—Patients with nervous system disorders, including seizures, may be more likely to have side effects
- Kidney disease—Patients with kidney disease may be more likely to have side effects

Before you begin using any new medicine (prescription or nonprescription) or if you develop any new medical problem while you are using this medicine, check with your doctor, nurse, or pharmacist.

Proper Use of This Medicine

To help clear up your infection completely, *imipenem and cilastatin combination must be given for the full time of treatment,* even if you begin to feel better after a few days. Also, this medicine works best when there is a constant amount in the blood or urine. To help keep the amount constant, it must be given on a regular schedule.

Precautions While Using This Medicine

Some patients may develop tremors or seizures while receiving this medicine. If you already have a history of seizures and you are taking anticonvulsants, you should continue to take them unless otherwise directed by your doctor.

In some patients, imipenem and cilastatin combination may cause diarrhea.

- Severe diarrhea may be a sign of a serious side effect. *Do not take any diarrhea medicine without first checking with your doctor.* Diarrhea medicines may make your diarrhea worse or make it last longer.
- For mild diarrhea, diarrhea medicine containing kaolin (e.g., Kaopectate liquid) or attapulgite (e.g., Kaopectate tablets, Diasorb) may be taken. However, other kinds of diarrhea medicine should not be taken. They may make your diarrhea worse or make it last longer.
- If you have any questions about this or if mild diarrhea continues or gets worse, check with your doctor or pharmacist.

Side Effects of This Medicine

Along with its needed effects, a medicine may cause some unwanted effects. Although not all of these side effects may occur, if they do occur they may need medical attention.

Check with your doctor or nurse immediately if any of the following side effects occur:

More common

Confusion; convulsions (seizures); dizziness; pain at place of injection; skin rash, hives, itching, fever, or wheezing; tremors

Less common

Dizziness; increased sweating; nausea or vomiting; unusual tiredness or weakness

Rare

Severe abdominal or stomach cramps and pain; watery and severe diarrhea, which may also be bloody; fever (these side effects may also occur up to several weeks after you stop receiving this medicine)

Other side effects may occur that usually do not need medical attention. These side effects may go away during treatment as your body adjusts to the medicine. However,

check with your doctor if the following side effect continues or is bothersome:

More common

Diarrhea; nausea and vomiting

Other side effects not listed above may also occur in some patients. If you notice any other effects, check with your doctor.

Annual revision: 09/08/92

IMMUNE GLOBULIN INTRAVENOUS (HUMAN) Systemic

Some commonly used brand names are:

In the U.S.

Gamimune N	Iveegam
Gammagard	Sandoglobulin
Gammar–IV	Venoglobulin–I

In Canada

Gamimune N
Iveegam

Other commonly used names are IGIV and IVIG.

Description

Immune globulin intravenous (IGIV) belongs to a group of medicines known as immunizing agents. IGIV is used to prevent or treat some illnesses that can occur when your body does not produce enough of its own immunity to prevent those diseases.

IGIV is manufactured from plasma that comes from blood that has been donated by many people. The immunity to diseases that is in the donated blood is used by your own body to increase your immunity.

IGIV is also used to treat a disorder known as idiopathic thrombocytopenic purpura (ITP). When a person has ITP, there is an increase in the breakdown of a part of the blood known as platelets. Low platelet levels in the blood increase a person's chance of bleeding or hemorrhaging. IGIV is used to increase the number of platelets in the blood to prevent this bleeding.

IGIV does not contain harmful products of hepatitis B virus, human immunodeficiency virus (HIV), acquired immunodeficiency syndrome (AIDS), or AIDS-related complex (ARC).

IGIV is available in the following dosage form:

Parenteral

- Injection (U.S. and Canada)

It is very important that you read and understand the following information. If any of it causes you special concern, check with your doctor. Also, *if you have any questions* or if you want more information about this medicine or your medical problem, *ask your doctor, nurse, or pharmacist.*

Before Using This Medicine

In deciding to use a medicine, the risks of taking the medicine must be weighed against the good it will do. This is a decision you and your doctor will make. For immune globulin intravenous (IGIV), the following should be considered:

Allergies—Tell your doctor if you have ever had any unusual or allergic reaction to intramuscular or intravenous immune globulins. Also tell your doctor and pharmacist if you are allergic to any other substances, such as foods, preservatives, or dyes.

Diet—Make certain your doctor and pharmacist know if you are on any special diet, such as a low-sodium or low-sugar diet.

Pregnancy—Studies on effects in pregnancy have not been done in either humans or animals.

Breast-feeding—It is not known whether IGIV passes into the breast milk. Although most medicines pass into breast milk in small amounts, many of them may be used safely while breast-feeding. Mothers who are using this medicine and who wish to breast-feed should discuss this with their doctor.

Children—Although there is no specific information comparing use of IGIV in children with use in other age groups, this medicine is not expected to cause different side effects or problems in children than it does in adults.

Older adults—Many medicines have not been studied specifically in older people. Therefore, it may not be known whether they work exactly the same way they do in younger adults. Although there is no specific information comparing use of IGIV in the elderly with use in other age groups, this medicine is not expected to cause different side effects or problems in older people than it does in younger adults.

Other medicines—Although certain medicines should not be used together at all, in other cases two different medicines may be used together even if an interaction might occur. In these cases, your doctor may want to change the dose, or other precautions may be necessary. Tell your doctor and pharmacist if you are using any other prescription or nonprescription (over-the-counter [OTC]) medicine.

Other medical problems—The presence of other medical problems may affect the use of IGIV. Make sure you tell your doctor if you have any other medical problems, especially:

- Agammaglobulinemia or
- Hypogammaglobulinemia—Patients with these conditions who have never received immune globulin substitution therapy or who were last treated more than 8 weeks ago may have more side effects to IGIV
- Heart problems or
- Immunoglobulin A (IgA) deficiencies—IGIV may make the conditions worse

Before you begin using any new medicine (prescription or nonprescription) or if you develop any new medical problem while you are using this medicine, check with your doctor, nurse, or pharmacist.

Proper Use of This Medicine

Dosing—The dose of IGIV will be different for different patients. Doses are based on body weight and the condition for which you are being treated. The following information includes only the average doses of IGIV. *If your dose is different, do not change it* unless your doctor tells you to do so.

- For *injection* dosage form:
  - —For immunodeficiency:
    - Adults and children—200 to 800 milligrams per kilogram (mg/kg) (90 to 360 milligrams per pound) of body weight per month, injected into a vein.
  - —For idiopathic thrombocytopenic purpura (ITP):
    - Adults and children—Either 400 milligrams per kilogram (mg/kg) (180 milligrams per pound) of body weight per day for 2 to 5 days or 1 gram per kilogram (450 milligrams per pound) of body weight per day for 1 or 2 days, injected into a vein. Doses are usually repeated every 10 to 21 days.
  - —For bacterial infection secondary to B-cell chronic lymphocytic leukemia (CLL):
    - Adults and children—400 milligrams per kilogram (mg/kg) (180 milligrams per pound) of body weight, given once every 3 or 4 weeks, injected into a vein.
  - —For any other condition: The dose will be determined by your doctor.

Side Effects of This Medicine

Along with its needed effects, a medicine may cause some unwanted effects. Although not all of these side effects may occur, if they do occur they may need medical attention.

Check with your doctor immediately if any of the following side effects occur:

Symptoms of overdose

Chest tightness; chills; dizziness; fever; nausea; redness of face; sweating; unusual tiredness or weakness; vomiting

Check with your doctor as soon as possible if any of the following side effects occur:

More common

Fast or pounding heartbeat; troubled breathing

Less common

Bluish coloring of lips or nailbeds; burning sensation in head; faintness or lightheadedness; unusual tiredness or weakness; wheezing

Other side effects may occur that usually do not need medical attention. These side effects may go away during treatment as your body adjusts to the medicine. However, check with your doctor if any of the following side effects continue or are bothersome:

More common

Backache; general feeling of discomfort or illness; headache; joint pain; muscle pain

Less common

Chest, back, or hip pain; hives; leg cramps; redness, rash, or pain at place of injection

Other side effects not listed above may also occur in some patients. If you notice any other effects, check with your doctor.

Annual revision: 06/21/93

INDAPAMIDE Systemic

Some commonly used brand names are:

In the U.S.
Lozol
In Canada
Lozide

Description

Indapamide (in-DAP-a-mide) belongs to the group of medicines known as diuretics. It is commonly used to treat high blood pressure (hypertension).

High blood pressure adds to the workload of the heart and arteries. If it continues for a long time, the heart and arteries may not function properly. This can damage the blood vessels of the brain, heart, and kidneys resulting in a stroke, heart failure, or kidney failure. High blood pressure may also increase the risk of heart attacks. These problems may be less likely to occur if blood pressure is controlled.

Indapamide is also used to help reduce the amount of water in the body by increasing the flow of urine.

Indapamide is available only with your doctor's prescription, in the following dosage form:

Oral

- Tablets (U.S. and Canada)

It is very important that you read and understand the following information. If any of it causes you special concern, check with your doctor. Also, *if you have any questions* or if you want more information about this medicine or your medical problem, *ask your doctor, nurse, or pharmacist.*

Before Using This Medicine

In deciding to use a medicine, the risks of taking the medicine must be weighed against the good it will do. This is a decision you and your doctor will make. For indapamide, the following should be considered:

Allergies—Tell your doctor if you have ever had any unusual or allergic reaction to indapamide or other sulfonamide-type medicines. Also tell your doctor and pharmacist if you are allergic to any other substances, such as foods, preservatives, or dyes.

Pregnancy—Indapamide has not been studied in pregnant women. However, indapamide has not been shown to cause birth defects or other problems in animal studies.

In general, diuretics are not useful for normal swelling of feet and hands that occurs during pregnancy. Diuretics should not be taken during pregnancy unless recommended by your doctor.

Breast-feeding—It is not known whether indapamide passes into breast milk. However, this medicine has not been reported to cause problems in nursing babies.

Children—Studies on this medicine have been done only in adult patients, and there is no specific information comparing use of indapamide in children with use in other age groups.

Older adults—Dizziness or lightheadedness and signs and symptoms of too much potassium loss are more likely to occur in the elderly, who are usually more sensitive than younger adults to the effects of indapamide.

Other medicines—Although certain medicines should not be used together at all, in other cases two different medicines may be used together even if an interaction might occur. In these cases, your doctor may want to change the dose, or other precautions may be necessary. When you are taking indapamide, it is especially important that your doctor and pharmacist know if you are taking any of the following:

- Digitalis glycosides (heart medicine)—Use with indapamide may increase the chance of side effects of digitalis glycosides
- Lithium (e.g., Lithane)—Use with indapamide may cause high blood levels of lithium, which may increase the chance of side effects

Other medical problems—The presence of other medical problems may affect the use of indapamide. Make sure you tell your doctor if you have any other medical problems, especially:

- Diabetes mellitus (sugar diabetes) or
- Gout (history of)—Indapamide may make these conditions worse
- Kidney disease—May prevent indapamide from working properly
- Liver disease—Higher blood levels of indapamide may occur, which may increase the chance of side effects

Before you begin using any new medicine (prescription or nonprescription) or if you develop any new medical problem while you are using this medicine, check with your doctor, nurse, or pharmacist.

Proper Use of This Medicine

Indapamide may cause you to have an unusual feeling of tiredness when you begin to take it. You may also notice an increase in the amount of urine or in your frequency of urination. After taking the medicine for a while, these effects should lessen. In general, to keep the increase in urine from affecting your sleep:

- If you are to take a single dose a day, take it in the morning after breakfast.
- If you are to take more than one dose a day, take the last dose no later than 6 p.m., unless otherwise directed by your doctor.

However, it is best to plan your dose or doses according to a schedule that will least affect your personal activities and sleep. Ask your doctor, nurse, or pharmacist to help you plan the best time to take this medicine.

To help you remember to take indapamide, try to get into the habit of taking it at the same time each day.

For patients taking indapamide for *high blood pressure:*

- In addition to the use of the medicine your doctor has prescribed, treatment for your high blood pressure may include weight control and care in the types of foods you eat, especially foods high in sodium. Your doctor will tell you which of these are most important for you. You should check with your doctor before changing your diet.

- Many patients who have high blood pressure will not notice any signs of the problem. In fact, many may feel normal. It is very important that you *take your medicine exactly as directed* and that you keep your appointments with your doctor even if you feel well.
- Remember that this medicine will not cure your high blood pressure but it does help control it. Therefore, you must continue to take it as directed if you expect to lower your blood pressure and keep it down. *You may have to take high blood pressure medicine for the rest of your life.* If high blood pressure is not treated, it can cause serious problems such as heart failure, blood vessel disease, stroke, or kidney disease.

Dosing—The dose of indapamide will be different for different patients. *Follow your doctor's orders or the directions on the label.* The following information includes only the average doses of indapamide. *If your dose is different, do not change it* unless your doctor tells you to do so:

- For *oral* dosage forms (tablets):
  —Adults: 2.5 to 5 milligrams once a day.

Missed dose—If you miss a dose of this medicine, take it as soon as possible. However, if it is almost time for your next dose, skip the missed dose and go back to your regular dosing schedule. Do not double doses.

Storage—To store this medicine:

- Keep out of the reach of children.
- Store away from heat and direct light.
- Do not store in the bathroom, near the kitchen sink, or in other damp places. Heat or moisture may cause the medicine to break down.
- Do not keep outdated medicine or medicine no longer needed. Be sure that any discarded medicine is out of the reach of children.

Precautions While Using This Medicine

It is important that your doctor check your progress at regular visits to make sure that indapamide is working properly.

This medicine may cause a loss of potassium from your body:

- To help prevent this, your doctor may want you to:
  —eat or drink foods that have a high potassium content (for example, orange or other citrus fruit juices), or
  —take a potassium supplement, or
  —take another medication to help prevent the loss of the potassium in the first place.
- It is very important to follow these directions. Also, it is important not to change your diet on your own. This is more important if you are already on a special diet (as for diabetes), or if you are taking a potassium supplement or a medicine to reduce potassium loss. Extra potassium may not be necessary and, in some cases, too much potassium could be harmful.

Check with your doctor if you become sick and have severe or continuing vomiting or diarrhea. These problems may cause you to lose additional water and potassium.

For patients taking this medicine for *high blood pressure:*

- *Do not take other medicines unless they have been discussed with your doctor.* This especially includes over-the-counter (nonprescription) medicines for appetite control, asthma, colds, hay fever, or sinus problems, since they may tend to increase your blood pressure.

Side Effects of This Medicine

Along with its needed effects, a medicine may cause some unwanted effects. Although not all of these side effects may occur, if they do occur they may need medical attention.

Check with your doctor as soon as possible if any of the following side effects occur:

Dryness of mouth; increased thirst; irregular heartbeat; mood or mental changes; muscle cramps or pain; nausea or vomiting; unusual tiredness or weakness; weak pulse

Rare

Skin rash, itching, or hives

Other side effects may occur that usually do not need medical attention. These side effects may go away during treatment as your body adjusts to the medicine. However, check with your doctor if any of the following side effects continue or are bothersome:

Less common or rare

Diarrhea; dizziness or lightheadedness, especially when getting up from a lying or sitting position; headache; loss of appetite; trouble in sleeping; stomach upset

Other side effects not listed above may also occur in some patients. If you notice any other effects, check with your doctor.

Annual revision: 01/20/93

INFLUENZA VIRUS VACCINE Systemic

Some commonly used brand names are:

In the U.S.
- Flu-Imune
- Fluzone
- Fluogen

Generic name product may also be available.

In Canada
- Fluviral
- Fluzone

Another commonly used name is flu vaccine.

Description

Influenza (in-floo-EN-za) Virus Vaccine is an active immunizing agent given by injection each year. It is also known as a "Flu shot." The vaccine helps to prevent infection by influenza viruses.

There are many kinds of influenza viruses, but not all will cause problems in any given year. Therefore, before the influenza vaccine for each year is produced, the World Health Organization (WHO) and the U.S. and Canadian Public Health Services decide which influenza viruses will be most likely to cause influenza infection that year. Then they include the antigens to these viruses in the influenza vaccine made available. Usually, both the U.S. and Canada use the same influenza vaccine; however, they are not required to do so.

It is necessary to receive an influenza vaccine injection each year, since influenza infections are usually caused by viruses with different antigens each year and because the immunity gained by the vaccine lasts less than a year.

Influenza is a virus infection of the throat, bronchial tubes, and lungs. Influenza infection causes fever, chills, cough, headache, and muscle aches and pains in your back, arms, and legs. In addition, adults and children weakened by other diseases or medical conditions and persons 65 years of age and over, even if they are healthy, may get a much more serious illness and may have to be treated in a hospital. Each year thousands of persons die as a result of an influenza infection.

The best way to help prevent influenza infection is to get an influenza vaccination each year, usually in early November. Immunization against influenza is recommended for everyone, including infants 6 months of age and over, all children, and all adults.

This vaccine is available only from your doctor or other authorized health care provider, in the following dosage form:

Parenteral
- Injection (U.S. and Canada)

It is very important that you read and understand the following information. If any of it causes you special concern, check with your doctor. Also, *if you have any questions* or if you want more information about this medicine or your medical problem, *ask your doctor, nurse, or pharmacist.*

Before Receiving This Vaccine

In deciding to use a medicine, the risks of taking the medicine must be weighed against the good it will do. This is a decision you and your doctor will make. For influenza vaccine, the following should be considered:

Allergies—Tell your doctor if you have ever had any unusual or allergic reaction to influenza vaccine or to antibiotics, such as gentamicin sulfate, streptomycin sulfate, or other aminoglycosides. Influenza vaccine available in the U.S. or Canada may contain these antibiotics. Also tell your doctor and pharmacist if you are allergic to any other substances, such as foods (especially eggs) or preservatives (especially sodium bisulfite or thimerosal). Influenza vaccine is grown in the fluids of chick embryos.

Pregnancy—Influenza vaccine has not been shown to cause birth defects or other problems in humans.

Breast-feeding—Influenza vaccine has not been reported to cause problems in nursing babies.

Children—Use is not recommended for infants up to 6 months of age. In addition, only the split-virus vaccine should be given to children 6 months up to 13 years of age. Also, some side effects of the vaccine, such as fever, unusual tiredness or weakness, or aches or pains in muscles, are more likely to occur in infants and children, who are usually more sensitive than adults to the effects of influenza vaccine

Older adults—This vaccine is not expected to cause different side effects or problems in older persons than it does in younger adults. However, elderly persons may not become as immune to head and upper chest influenza infections as younger adults, although the vaccine may still be effective in preventing lower chest influenza infections and other complications of influenza.

Other medicines—Although certain medicines should not be used together at all, in other cases two different medicines may be used together even if an interaction might occur. In these cases, your doctor may want to change the dose, or other precautions may be necessary. Tell your doctor and pharmacist if you are using any other prescription or nonprescription (over-the-counter [OTC]) medicine.

Other medical problems—The presence of other medical problems may affect the use of influenza vaccine. Make

sure you tell your doctor if you have any other medical problems, especially:

- Bronchitis, pneumonia, or other illness involving lungs or bronchial tubes—Use of influenza vaccine may make the condition worse
- Convulsions (seizures) caused by fever (history of)—Fever, a possible side effect of the vaccine, may cause the condition to occur again
- Guillain-Barré syndrome (GBS) (history of)—Use of influenza vaccine may reactivate the condition
- Severe illness with fever—The symptoms of the condition may be confused with the possible side effects of the vaccine

Before you begin using any new medicine (prescription or nonprescription) or if you develop any new medical problem while you are using this medicine, check with your doctor, nurse, or pharmacist.

Proper Use of This Vaccine

Dosing—The dose of influenza vaccine will be different for different patients. *Follow your doctor's orders*. The following information includes only the average doses of influenza vaccine.

- For *injection* dosage form:
  - —To help prevent influenza infection:
    - Adults and children 6 months of age and older—One injection each year.

Side Effects of This Vaccine

In 1976, a number of persons who received the "swine flu" influenza vaccine developed Guillain-Barré syndrome (GBS). Most of these persons were over 25 years of age. Although only 10 out of one million persons receiving the vaccine actually developed GBS, this number was 6 times more than would normally have been expected. Most of the persons who got GBS recovered completely from the paralysis it caused.

It is assumed that the "swine flu" virus included in the 1976 vaccine caused the problem, but this has not been proven. Since that time, the "swine flu" virus has not been used in influenza vaccines, and there has been no recurrence of GBS associated with influenza vaccinations.

Along with its needed effects, a vaccine may cause some unwanted effects. Although not all of these side effects may occur, if they do occur they may need medical attention.

Get emergency help immediately if any of the following side effects occur:

Symptoms of allergic reaction

Difficulty in breathing or swallowing; hives; itching, especially of feet or hands; reddening of skin, especially around ears; swelling of eyes, face, or inside of nose; unusual tiredness or weakness (sudden and severe)

Other side effects may occur that usually do not need medical attention. However, check with your doctor if any of the following side effects continue or are bothersome:

More common

Tenderness, redness, or hard lump at place of injection

Less common

Fever, general feeling of discomfort or illness, or aches or pains in muscles

Other side effects not listed above may also occur in some patients. If you notice any other effects, check with your doctor.

Annual revision: 06/21/93

INSULIN Systemic

This information applies to the following medicines:

Insulin (IN-su-lin)
Insulin Human
Buffered Insulin Human
Isophane (EYE-so-fayn) Insulin
Isophane Insulin, Human
Isophane Insulin and Insulin
Isophane Insulin, Human and Insulin Human
Insulin Zinc
Insulin Zinc, Human
Extended Insulin Zinc
Extended Insulin Zinc, Human
Prompt Insulin Zinc
Protamine (PRO-tah-meen) Zinc Insulin

Some commonly used brand names are:

For Insulin

In the U.S.

Regular (Concentrated) Iletin II, U-500
Regular Iletin I
Regular Iletin II
Regular Insulin
Velosulin

Another commonly used name is regular insulin.

For Insulin Human

In the U.S.

Humulin R
Novolin R
Velosulin Human

For Buffered Insulin Human
In the U.S.
Humulin BR

For Isophane Insulin
In the U.S.
Insulatard NPH
NPH Iletin I
NPH Iletin II
NPH Insulin

Another commonly used name is NPH insulin.

For Isophane Insulin, Human
In the U.S.
Humulin N
Insulatard NPH Human
Novolin N

For Isophane Insulin and Insulin
In the U.S.
Mixtard

For Isophane Insulin, Human and Insulin Human
In the U.S.
Humulin 70/30
Mixtard Human 70/30
Novolin 70/30

For Insulin Zinc
In the U.S.
Lente Iletin I
Lente Iletin II
Lente Insulin

Another commonly used name is lente insulin.

For Insulin Zinc, Human
In the U.S.
Humulin L
Novolin L

For Extended Insulin Zinc
In the U.S.
Ultralente Iletin I
Ultralente Insulin

Another commonly used name is ultralente insulin.

For Extended Insulin Zinc, Human
In the U.S.
Humulin U
Ultralente

For Prompt Insulin Zinc
In the U.S.
Semilente Iletin I
Semilente Insulin

Another commonly used name is semilente insulin.

For Protamine Zinc Insulin
In the U.S.
Protamine Zinc & Iletin I
Protamine Zinc & Iletin II

Another commonly used name is PZI insulin.

Description

Insulin (IN-su-lin) is a hormone that helps the body turn the food we eat into energy. This occurs whether we make our own insulin in the pancreas gland or take it by injection.

Diabetes mellitus (sugar diabetes) is a condition where the body does not make enough insulin to meet its needs or does not properly use the insulin it makes.

Insulin can be obtained from beef or pork pancreas glands or from new processes that produce human insulin. All types of insulin must be injected because, if taken by mouth, insulin is destroyed by chemical reactions in the stomach.

One or more injections of insulin a day may be needed to control your diabetes. Insulin is usually injected before meals or at bedtime. Your doctor will discuss the number of injections you will need, the kind of insulin to use, the correct dose, and the right time to take it.

A prescription is not necessary to purchase most insulin. However, your doctor must first determine your insulin needs and provide you with special instructions for control of your diabetes. Insulin is available in the following dosage forms:

Parenteral

Insulin
- Injection (U.S.)

Insulin Human
- Injection (U.S.)

Buffered Insulin Human
- Injection (U.S.)

Isophane Insulin
- Injection (U.S.)

Isophane Insulin, Human
- Injection (U.S.)

Isophane Insulin, Human, and Insulin Human
- Injection (U.S.)

Insulin Zinc
- Injection (U.S.)

Insulin Zinc, Human
- Injection (U.S.)

Extended Insulin Zinc
- Injection (U.S.)

Extended Insulin Zinc, Human
- Injection (U.S.)

Prompt Insulin Zinc
- Injection (U.S.)

Protamine Zinc Insulin
- Injection (U.S.)

It is very important that you read and understand the following information. If any of it causes you special concern, check with your doctor. Also, *if you have any questions* or if you want more information about this medicine or your medical problem, *ask your doctor, nurse, or pharmacist.*

Before Using This Medicine

In deciding to use a medicine, the risks of taking the medicine must be weighed against the good it will do. This is a decision you and your doctor will make. For insulin, the following should be considered:

Allergies—Tell your doctor if you have ever had any unusual or allergic reaction to insulin. Also tell your doctor and pharmacist if you are allergic to any other substances, such as foods, preservatives, or dyes.

Diet—If you have insulin-dependent diabetes (type I), your doctor will prescribe both insulin and a personalized meal plan for you. Such a diet is low in fat and simple sugars such as table sugar, and sweet foods and beverages. This meal plan is also high in complex carbohydrates (starchy foods) such as cereals, grains, bread, pasta or noodles, starchy vegetables, and dried beans, peas, or lentils. The daily number of calories in this meal plan should be adjusted by your doctor or a registered dietitian to help you reach and maintain a healthy body weight. In addition, meals and snacks are arranged to meet the energy needs of your body at different times of the day. *It is very important that you carefully follow your meal plan.*

Pregnancy—Your requirements for insulin change during pregnancy. Because it is especially important for the health of both you and the baby that your blood sugar be closely controlled, be sure to tell your doctor if you suspect you are pregnant or if you are planning to become pregnant.

Breast-feeding—Insulin does not pass into breast milk and will not affect the nursing infant.

Other medicines—Although certain medicines should not be used together at all, in other cases two different medicines may be used together even if an interaction might occur. In these cases, your doctor may want to change the dose, or other precautions may be necessary. When using insulin, it is especially important that your doctor and pharmacist know if you are taking any of the following:

- Adrenocorticoids (e.g., prednisone or other cortisone-like medicines)—Your dose of either medicine may need to be adjusted because the adrenocorticoids may interfere with insulin and thus increase your blood sugar
- Beta-blockers—Beta-blockers may increase the risk of developing either high or low blood sugar levels. Also, they can mask symptoms of low blood sugar (such as rapid pulse). Because of this, a person with diabetes might not recognize low blood sugar and might not take immediate steps to treat it. Beta-blockers can also cause a low blood sugar level to last longer than it would have normally

Other medical problems—The presence of other medical problems may affect the dose of insulin you need. Be sure to tell your doctor if you have any other medical problems, especially:

- Infections or
- Kidney disease or
- Liver disease or
- Thyroid disease—These conditions may change your daily insulin dose

Before you begin using any new medicine (prescription or nonprescription) or if you develop any new medical problem while you are using this medicine, check with your doctor, nurse, or pharmacist.

Proper Use of This Medicine

Make sure you have the type and strength of insulin that your doctor ordered for you. You may find that keeping an insulin label with you is helpful when buying insulin supplies. The concentration (strength) of insulin is measured by units, and is sometimes expressed in terms such as U-100 insulin.

Insulin doses are measured and given with specially marked insulin syringes. These syringes come in 3 sizes: 30 units, 50 units, and 100 units. Your insulin syringe will allow you to measure the units of insulin that have been prescribed for you, and allow you to easily read the measuring scale.

There are several important steps that will help you successfully prepare your insulin injection. To draw the insulin up into the syringe correctly, you need to follow these steps:

- Wash your hands.
- If your insulin is the intermediate- or long-acting kind (cloudy), be sure that it is completely mixed. Mix the insulin by slowly rolling the bottle between your hands or gently tipping the bottle over a few times.
- Never shake the bottle vigorously (hard).
- Do not use the insulin if it looks lumpy or grainy, seems unusually thick, sticks to the bottle, or seems to be even a little discolored. Do not use the insulin if it contains crystals or if the bottle looks frosted. Regular insulin (short-acting) should be used only if it is clear and colorless.
- Remove the colored protective cap on the bottle. Do *not* remove the rubber stopper.
- Wipe the top of the bottle with an alcohol swab.
- Remove the needle cover of the insulin syringe.
- Draw air into the syringe by pulling back on the plunger. The amount of air should be equal to your insulin dose.
- Gently push the needle through the top of the rubber stopper.
- Push plunger in all the way, to inject air into the bottle.
- Turn the bottle with syringe upside down in one hand. Be sure the tip of the needle is covered by the insulin. With your other hand, draw the plunger back slowly to draw the correct dose of insulin into the syringe.
- Check the insulin in the syringe for air bubbles. To remove air bubbles, push the insulin slowly back into the bottle and draw up your dose again.
- Check your dose again.
- Remove the needle from the bottle and re-cover the needle.

If you are mixing more than 1 type of insulin in the same syringe, you also need to know about the following:

- When mixing regular insulin with another type of insulin, *always* draw the regular insulin into the syringe first. When mixing 2 types of insulins other than regular insulin, it does not matter in what order you draw them.

- After you decide on a certain order for drawing up your insulin, you should use the same order each time.
- Some mixtures of insulins have to be injected immediately. Others may be stable for longer periods of time, which means that you can wait before you inject the mixture. Check with your doctor, nurse, or pharmacist to find out which type you have.
- If your mixture is stable and you mixed it ahead of time, gently turn the filled syringe back and forth to remix the insulins before you inject them. Do not shake the syringe.

After you have your syringe prepared, you are ready to inject the insulin into your body. To do this:

- Clean the site where the injection is to be made with an alcohol swab, and let the area dry.
- Inject the insulin into fatty tissue. Injection sites include your thighs, abdomen (stomach area), upper arms, or buttocks. Generally, insulin is absorbed into the bloodstream most evenly from the abdomen. If you are either thin or greatly overweight, you may be given special instructions for giving yourself insulin injections.
- Pinch up a large area of skin and hold it firmly. With your other hand, hold the syringe like a pencil. Push the needle straight into the pinched-up skin at a 90-degree angle. Be sure the needle is all the way in. Drawing back on the syringe each time to check for blood (also called routine aspiration) is not necessary.
- Push the plunger all the way down, using less than 5 seconds to inject the dose. Hold an alcohol swab near the needle and pull the needle straight out of the skin.
- Press the swab against the injection site for several seconds. Do not rub.

For patients using *disposable syringes:*

- Manufacturers of disposable syringes recommend that they be used only once, because the sterility of a reused syringe cannot be guaranteed. However, some patients prefer to reuse a syringe until its needle becomes dull. Most insulins have chemicals added that keep them from growing the bacteria that are usually found on the skin. Because of this, some patients may decide to reuse a disposable syringe. However, the syringe should be thrown away when the needle becomes dull, has been bent, or has come into contact with any surface other than the cleaned and swabbed area of skin. Also, if you plan to reuse a syringe, the needle must be recapped after each use. Check with your doctor, nurse, or pharmacist to find out the best way to reuse syringes.
- Laws in some states require that used insulin syringes and needles be destroyed. Be careful when you recap, bend, or break a needle, because these actions increase the chances of a needle-stick injury. It is best to put used syringes and needles in a disposable container that is puncture-resistant or to use a needle-clipping device. The chances of a syringe being reused by someone else is lower if the plunger is taken out of the barrel and broken in half when you dispose of a syringe.

For patients using *a glass syringe and metal needle:*

- This type of syringe and needle may be used repeatedly if it is sterilized each time. You should get an instruction sheet that tells you how to do this. If you need more information on this, ask your doctor, nurse, or pharmacist.

For patients using *an insulin-infusion pump:*

- Regular insulin is the only insulin product that should be used with insulin infusion pumps.
- Do not use the insulin injection if it looks lumpy, cloudy, unusually thick, or even slightly discolored, or if it contains crystals. Use the insulin only if it is clear and colorless.
- Do not mix the buffered regular insulin injection with any other insulin. If you do, crystals may form that will block the pump catheter. Also, the potency of the insulin may change.
- It is important to follow the pump manufacturer's directions on how to load the syringe and/or pump reservoir. Your correct insulin dose may not be given if loading is not done correctly.
- Check the infusion tubing and infusion-site dressing often for improper insulin infusion, as your physician or nurse recommends.

Storage—Storage and expiration date:

- When buying insulin, always check the package expiration date to make sure the insulin will be used before it expires.
- This expiration date applies *only* when the insulin has been stored in the refrigerator. Expiration is much shorter if the insulin is left unrefrigerated. Do not use insulin after the expiration date stated on the label even if the bottle has never been opened. Check with your pharmacist about a possible exchange of bottles.
- An unopened bottle of insulin should be refrigerated until needed. It should never be frozen. Remove the insulin from the refrigerator and allow it to reach room temperature before injecting.
- An insulin bottle in use may be kept at room temperature for up to 1 month. Insulin that has been kept at room temperature for longer than a month should be thrown away.
- Do not expose insulin to extremely hot temperatures or to sunlight. Do not leave insulin in the hot summer sun or in a hot closed car. Extreme heat will cause insulin to become less effective much more quickly.

Precautions While Using This Medicine

It is very important that your doctor check your progress at regular visits, especially during the first few weeks of insulin treatment.

It is very important to follow carefully any instructions from your health care team about:

- Alcohol—Drinking alcohol may cause severe low blood sugar. Discuss this with your health care team.
- Tobacco—If you have been smoking for a long time and suddenly stop, your dosage of insulin may need to be reduced. If you decide to quit, tell your doctor first.
- Meal plan—To be successful in your treatment, you must closely follow the diet your doctor or dietitian prescribed for you. Do not miss or delay your meals.
- Exercise—Ask your doctor what kind of exercise to do, the best time to do it, and how much you should do daily.
- Blood tests—This is the best way to tell whether your diabetes is being controlled properly. Blood sugar testing is a useful guide to help you and your health care team adjust your insulin dose, meal plan, and exercise schedule.
- Urine ketone tests—You will also be asked at certain times to test for acetone, which is an acid that may be released from your bloodstream into your urine when your blood glucose is too high.
- Injection sites—If you carefully select and rotate the sites where you give your insulin injections, you may be able to prevent skin problems. Also, the insulin may be better absorbed into the bloodstream.
- Other medicines—Do not take other medicines unless they have been discussed with your doctor. This especially includes nonprescription medicines such as aspirin, and those for appetite control, asthma, colds, cough, hay fever, or sinus problems.

Insulin can cause low blood sugar (also called insulin reaction or hypoglycemia). Symptoms of low blood sugar are:

Anxious feeling
Cold sweats
Confusion
Cool pale skin
Difficulty in concentration
Drowsiness
Excessive hunger
Headache
Nausea
Nervousness
Rapid pulse
Shakiness
Unusual tiredness or weakness
Vision changes

- Different people may feel different symptoms of low blood sugar (hypoglycemia). It is important that you learn the symptoms of low blood sugar that you usually have so that you can treat it quickly.
- The symptoms of hypoglycemia (low blood sugar) may develop quickly and may result from:
  —delaying or missing a scheduled meal or snack.
  —exercising more than usual.
  —drinking a significant amount of alcohol.
  —taking certain medicines.
  —using too much insulin.
  —sickness (especially with vomiting or diarrhea).
- Eating some form of quick-acting sugar when symptoms of hypoglycemia first appear will usually prevent them from getting worse. Good sources of sugar include:

  Glucose tablets or gel that you can buy
  A restaurant sugar packet
  Fruit juice (4 to 6 ounces or one-half cup)
  Corn syrup (1 tablespoon)
  Honey (1 tablespoon)
  Regular (non-diet) soft drinks (4 to 6 ounces or one-half cup)
  Sugar cubes (6 one-half-inch sized) or table sugar (dissolved in water)
- Do not use chocolate because its fat slows down the sugar entering into the bloodstream.
- If a snack is not scheduled for an hour or more you should also eat some crackers and cheese, or a half a sandwich, or ice cream, or a peanut butter cookie, or drink an 8 ounce glass of milk.
- Symptoms of low blood sugar must be treated before they lead to unconsciousness (passing out). Glucagon is also used in emergency situations such as unconsciousness. Have a glucagon kit available, along with a syringe and needle, and know how to prepare and use it. Members of your household should know how and when to use it, also. Check the expiration date of the glucagon and remind yourself when to buy a new kit. If your kit has expired, ask your pharmacist to exchange it for a new one.

Hyperglycemia (high blood sugar) is another problem related to uncontrolled diabetes. If you have any symptoms of high blood sugar, you need to contact your health care team right away. If it is not treated, severe hyperglycemia can lead to ketoacidosis (diabetic coma) and death. The symptoms of hyperglycemia appear more slowly than those of low blood sugar and usually include:

Increased urination
Unusual thirst
Dry mouth
Drowsiness
Flushed, dry skin
Fruit-like breath odor
Loss of appetite
Stomach ache, nausea, or vomiting
Tiredness
Troubled breathing (rapid and deep)
Increased blood sugar level

- Symptoms of ketoacidosis (diabetic coma) that need immediate hospitalization include:

  Flushed, dry skin
  Fruit-like breath odor
  Stomach ache, nausea, or vomiting
  Troubled breathing (rapid and deep)

- Hyperglycemia (high blood sugar) symptoms may occur if you:

  —have a fever, diarrhea, or infection.
  —do not take enough insulin.
  —skip a dose of insulin.
  —do not exercise as much as usual.
  —overeat or do not follow your meal plan.

- Your doctor may recommend changes in your insulin dose or meal plan to avoid hyperglycemia. Symptoms of high blood sugar must be corrected before they progress to more serious conditions. Check with your doctor often to make sure you are controlling your blood sugar.

In case of emergency—There may be a time when you need emergency help for a problem caused by your diabetes. You need to be prepared for these emergencies. It is a good idea to:

- Wear a medical identification (I.D.) bracelet or neck chain at all times. Also, carry an I.D. card in your wallet or purse that says that you have diabetes and lists all of your medicines.
- Keep an extra supply of insulin and syringes with needles on hand.
- Have a glucagon kit and a syringe and needle available and know how to prepare and use it if severe hypoglycemia (low blood sugar) occurs.
- Keep some kind of quick-acting sugar handy to treat hypoglycemia (low blood sugar) symptoms.

In case of illness:

- When you become ill with a cold, fever, or the flu, you need to take your usual insulin dose, even if you feel too sick to eat. This is especially true if you have nausea, vomiting, or diarrhea. Infection usually increases your need for insulin. Call your doctor for specific instructions.
- Continue taking your insulin and try to stay on your regular meal plan. However, if you have trouble eating solid food, drink fruit juices, non-diet soft drinks, or clear soups, or eat small amounts of bland foods. A dietitian or your doctor can give you a list of foods and the amounts to use for sick days.
- Test your blood sugar level at least every 4 hours while you are awake and check your urine for acetone. If acetone is present, call your doctor at once. If you have severe or prolonged vomiting, check with your doctor. Even when you start feeling better, let your doctor know how you are doing.

Travel—If you take a few special precautions when you travel, you are less likely to have problems related to your diabetes during trips away from home. It is a good idea to:

- Carry a recent prescription from your doctor for your diabetes medicine and also for the type of syringe and needles you use.
- Do not make major changes in your meal plan or medicine schedule without advice from your health care team.
- Carry your diabetic supplies on your person or in a purse or briefcase to reduce the possibility of loss.
- Carry snack foods with you in case of delays between meals.
- Make allowances for changing time zones and keep your meal times as close to usual as possible.
- In hot climates, use an insulated container for your insulin.
- When traveling to foreign countries, it is advisable to pack enough diabetic supplies to last until you return home and to have extra or reserve supplies kept separate from your main supplies.
- Carry a letter from your doctor with all the details of your diabetes and medicines you need, including your need for syringes.
- When carrying a large quantity of diabetic supplies, divide them throughout your hand-carried luggage to avoid problems if something is lost, and to avoid possible freezing in airplane storage areas.

Annual revision: September 1990
Interim revision: 06/28/93

INTERFERON, GAMMA Systemic†

A commonly used brand name in the U.S. is Actimmune.

†Not commercially available in Canada.

Description

Gamma interferon (in-ter-FEER-on) is a synthetic (man-made) version of a substance naturally produced by cells in the body to help fight infections and tumors. Gamma interferon is used to treat chronic granulomatous disease.

Gamma interferon is available only with your doctor's prescription, in the following dosage form:

Parenteral

- Injection (U.S.)

It is very important that you read and understand the following information. If any of it causes you special concern, check with your doctor. Also, *if you have any questions* or if you want more information about this medicine or your medical problem, *ask your doctor, nurse, or pharmacist.*

Before Using This Medicine

In deciding to use a medicine, the risks of taking the medicine must be weighed against the good it will do. This is a decision you and your doctor will make. For gamma interferon, the following should be considered:

Allergies—Tell your doctor if you have ever had any unusual or allergic reaction to gamma interferon.

Pregnancy—Gamma interferon has not been studied in pregnant women. However, in monkeys given 100 times the human dose of gamma interferon and in mice, there was an increase in deaths of the fetus. Also, in mice, toxic doses of gamma interferon caused bleeding of the uterus.

Breast-feeding—It is not known whether gamma interferon passes into the breast milk. However, because this medicine may cause serious side effects, breast-feeding may not be recommended while you are receiving it. Discuss with your doctor whether or not you should breast-feed while you are are receiving gamma interferon.

Children—Studies on this medicine have been done mostly in children and is not expected to cause different side effects or problems than it does in adults.

Older adults—Many medicines have not been studied specifically in older people. Therefore, it may not be known whether they work exactly the same way they do in younger adults or if they cause different side effects or problems in older people. There is no specific information comparing use of gamma interferon in the elderly with use in other age groups.

Other medicines—Although certain medicines should not be used together at all, in other cases two different medicines may be used together even if an interaction might occur. In these cases, your doctor may want to change the dose, or other precautions may be necessary. Tell your doctor and pharmacist if you are taking any other prescription or nonprescription (over-the-counter [OTC]) medicine.

Other medical problems—The presence of other medical problems may affect the use of gamma interferon. Make sure you tell your doctor if you have any other medical problems, especially:

- Convulsions (seizures) or
- Mental problems (or history of)—Risk of problems affecting the central nervous system may be increased
- Heart disease or
- Multiple sclerosis or
- Systemic lupus erythematosus—May be worsened by gamma interferon

Before you begin using any new medicine (prescription or nonprescription) or if you develop any new medical problem while you are using this medicine, check with your doctor, nurse, or pharmacist.

Proper Use of This Medicine

If you are injecting this medicine yourself, *use it exactly as directed by your doctor.* Do not use more or less of it, and do not use it more often than your doctor ordered. The exact amount of medicine you need has been carefully worked out. Using too much will increase the risk of side effects, while using too little may not improve your condition.

Each package of gamma interferon contains a patient instruction sheet. Read this sheet carefully and make sure you understand:

- How to prepare the injection.
- Proper use of disposable syringes.
- How to give the injection.
- How long the injection is stable.

If you have any questions about any of this, check with your doctor, nurse, or pharmacist.

While you are using gamma interferon, your doctor may want you to drink extra fluids. This will help prevent low blood pressure due to loss of too much water.

Gamma interferon often causes flu-like symptoms, which can be severe. This effect is less likely to cause problems if you inject your gamma interferon at bedtime.

Missed dose—If you miss a dose of this medicine, do not give the missed dose at all and do not double the next one. Check with your doctor for further instructions.

Storage—To store this medicine:

- Keep out of the reach of children.
- Store in the refrigerator.
- Keep the medicine from freezing.
- Do not keep outdated medicine or medicine no longer needed. Ask your doctor or pharmacist how you should dispose of any medicine you do not use. Be sure that any discarded medicine is out of the reach of children.

Precautions While Using This Medicine

It is very important that your doctor check your progress at regular visits to make sure that this medicine is working properly and to check for unwanted effects.

This medicine commonly causes a flu-like reaction, with aching muscles, fever and chills, and headache. To prevent problems from your temperature going too high, your doctor may ask you to take acetaminophen before each dose of gamma interferon. You may also need to take it after a dose to bring your temperature down. *Follow your doctor's instructions carefully about taking your temperature, and how much and when to take the acetaminophen.*

Side Effects of This Medicine

Along with its needed effects, a medicine may cause some unwanted effects. Although not all of these side effects may occur, if they do occur they may need medical attention.

Check with your doctor as soon as possible if any of the following side effects occur:

Rare

Black, tarry stools; blood in urine or stools; confusion; cough or hoarseness; loss of balance control; lower back or side pain; mask-like face; painful or difficult urination; pinpoint red spots on skin; shuffling walk; stiffness of arms or legs; trembling and shaking of hands and fingers; trouble in speaking or swallowing; trouble in thinking or concentrating; trouble in walking; unusual bleeding or bruising

Other side effects may occur that usually do not need medical attention. These side effects may go away during treatment as your body adjusts to the medicine. However, check with your doctor if any of the following side effects continue or are bothersome:

More common

Aching muscles; diarrhea; fever and chills; general feeling of discomfort or illness; headache; nausea or vomiting; skin rash; unusual tiredness

Less common

Back pain; dizziness; joint pain; loss of appetite; weight loss

Other side effects not listed above may also occur in some patients. If you notice any other effects, check with your doctor.

Annual revision: 06/04/92

INTERFERONS, ALPHA Systemic

This information applies to the following medicines:

Interferon Alfa-2a, Recombinant
Interferon Alfa-2b, Recombinant
Interferon Alfa-n1 (lns)
Interferon Alfa-n3

Some commonly used brand names are:

For Interferon Alfa-2a, Recombinant
In the U.S.
Roferon-A
In Canada
Roferon-A

For Interferon Alfa-2b, Recombinant
In the U.S.
Intron A
In Canada
Intron A

For Interferon Alfa-n1 (lns)*
In Canada
Wellferon

For Interferon Alfa-n3†
In the U.S.
Alferon N

*Not commercially available in the U.S.
†Not commercially available in Canada.

Description

Interferons (in-ter-FEER-ons) are substances naturally produced by cells in the body to help fight infections and tumors. They may also be synthetic (man-made) versions of these substances. Alpha interferons are used to treat hairy cell leukemia and AIDS-related Kaposi's sarcoma. They are also used to treat laryngeal papillomatosis (growths in the respiratory tract) in children, genital warts, and some kinds of hepatitis.

Alpha interferons may also be used for other conditions as determined by your doctor.

Alpha interferons are available only with your doctor's prescription, in the following dosage form:

Parenteral

Interferon Alfa-2a, Recombinant
- Injection (U.S. and Canada)

Interferon Alfa-2b, Recombinant
- Injection (U.S. and Canada)

Interferon Alfa-n1 (lns)
- Injection (Canada)

Interferon Alfa-n3
- Injection (U.S.)

It is very important that you read and understand the following information. If any of it causes you special concern, check with your doctor. Also, *if you have any questions* or if you want more information about this medicine or your medical problem, *ask your doctor, nurse, or pharmacist.*

Before Using This Medicine

In deciding to use a medicine, the risks of taking the medicine must be weighed against the good it will do. This is a decision you and your doctor will make. For interferons, the following should be considered:

Allergies—Tell your doctor if you have ever had any unusual or allergic reaction to alpha interferon.

Pregnancy—Alpha interferons have not been shown to cause birth defects or other problems in humans. However, in monkeys given 20 to 500 times the human dose of recombinant interferon alfa-2a or 90 to 180 times the usual dose of recombinant interferon alfa-2b there was an increase in deaths of the fetus.

Breast-feeding—It is not known whether alpha interferons pass into the breast milk. However, because this medicine may cause serious side effects, breast-feeding may not be recommended while you are receiving it. Discuss with your doctor whether or not you should breast-feed while you are are receiving alpha interferon.

Children—There is no specific information comparing use of alpha interferon for cancer or genital warts in children with use in other age groups.

Teenagers—Alpha interferons may cause changes in the menstrual cycle. Discuss this possible effect with your doctor.

Older adults—Some side effects of alpha interferons (chest pain, irregular heartbeat, unusual tiredness, confusion, mental depression, trouble in thinking or concentrating) may be more likely to occur in the elderly, who are usually more sensitive to the effects of alpha interferons.

Other medicines—Although certain medicines should not be used together at all, in other cases two different medicines may be used together even if an interaction might occur. In these cases, your doctor may want to change the dose, or other precautions may be necessary. Tell your doctor and pharmacist if you are taking any other prescription or nonprescription (over-the-counter [OTC]) medicine.

Other medical problems—The presence of other medical problems may affect the use of alpha interferons. Make sure you tell your doctor if you have any other medical problems, especially:

- Bleeding problems—May be worsened by recombinant interferon alfa-2b
- Chickenpox (including recent exposure) or
- Herpes zoster (shingles)—Risk of severe disease affecting other parts of the body
- Convulsions (seizures) or
- Mental problems (or history of)—Risk of problems affecting the central nervous system may be increased
- Diabetes mellitus (sugar diabetes) or
- Heart attack (recent) or
- Heart disease or
- Kidney disease or
- Liver disease or
- Lung disease—May be worsened by alpha interferons
- Problems with overactive immune system—Alpha interferons make the immune system even more active
- Thyroid disease—Recombinant interferon alfa-2b can cause thyroid problems when it is used to treat hepatitis

Before you begin using any new medicine (prescription or nonprescription) or if you develop any new medical problem while you are using this medicine, check with your doctor, nurse, or pharmacist.

Proper Use of This Medicine

If you are injecting this medicine yourself, *use it exactly as directed by your doctor.* Do not use more or less of it, and do not use it more often than your doctor ordered. The exact amount of medicine you need has been carefully worked out. Using too much will increase the risk of side effects, while using too little may not improve your condition.

Each package of alpha interferon contains a patient instruction sheet. Read this sheet carefully and make sure you understand:

- How to prepare the injection.
- Proper use of disposable syringes.
- How to give the injection.
- How long the injection is stable.

If you have any questions about any of this, check with your doctor, nurse, or pharmacist.

While you are using alpha interferon, your doctor may want you to drink extra fluids. This will help prevent low blood pressure due to loss of too much water.

Alpha interferons often cause unusual tiredness, which can be severe. This effect is less likely to cause problems if you inject your interferon at bedtime.

Missed dose—If you miss a dose of this medicine, do not give the missed dose at all and do not double the next one. Check with your doctor for further instructions.

Storage—To store this medicine:

- Keep out of the reach of children.
- Store in the refrigerator.
- Keep the medicine from freezing.
- Do not keep outdated medicine or medicine no longer needed. Ask your doctor or pharmacist how you should dispose of any medicine you do not use. Be sure that any discarded medicine is out of the reach of children.

Precautions While Using This Medicine

It is very important that your doctor check your progress at regular visits to make sure that this medicine is working properly and to check for unwanted effects.

Do not change to another brand of alpha interferon without checking with your physician. Different kinds of alpha interferon have different doses. If you refill your medicine and it looks different, check with your pharmacist.

This medicine will add to the effects of alcohol and other CNS depressants (medicines that slow down the nervous system, possibly causing drowsiness). Some examples of CNS depressants are antihistamines or medicine for hay fever, other allergies, or colds; sedatives, tranquilizers, or sleeping medicine; prescription pain medicine or narcotics; barbiturates; medicine for seizures; muscle relaxants; or anesthetics, including some dental anesthetics. *Check with your doctor before taking any of the above while you are using this medicine.*

Alpha interferon may cause some people to become unusually tired or dizzy, or less alert than they are normally. *Make sure you know how you react to this medicine before you drive, use machines, or do anything else that could be dangerous if you are dizzy or if you are not alert.*

This medicine commonly causes a flu-like reaction, with aching muscles, fever and chills, and headache. To prevent problems from your temperature going too high, your doctor may ask you to take acetaminophen before each dose of interferon. You may also need to take it after a dose to bring your temperature down. *Follow your doctor's instructions carefully about taking your temperature, and how much and when to take the acetaminophen.*

Alpha interferon can lower the number of white blood cells in your blood temporarily, increasing the chance of getting an infection. It can also lower the number of platelets, which are necessary for proper blood clotting. If this occurs, there are certain precautions you can take, especially when your blood count is low, to reduce the risk of infection or bleeding:

- If you can, avoid people with infections. *Check with your doctor immediately* if you think you are getting an infection or if you get a fever or chills, cough or hoarseness, lower back or side pain, or painful or difficult urination.
- *Check with your doctor immediately* if you notice any unusual bleeding or bruising; black, tarry stools; blood in urine or stools; or pinpoint red spots on your skin.
- Be careful when using a regular toothbrush, dental floss, or toothpick. Your medical doctor, dentist, or nurse may recommend other ways to clean your teeth and gums. Check with your medical doctor before having any dental work done.
- Do not touch your eyes or the inside of your nose unless you have just washed your hands and have not touched anything else in the meantime.
- Be careful not to cut yourself when you are using sharp objects such as a safety razor or fingernail or toenail cutters.
- Avoid contact sports or other situations where bruising or injury could occur.

Side Effects of This Medicine

Along with its needed effects, a medicine may cause some unwanted effects. Although not all of these side effects may occur, if they do occur they may need medical attention.

Because this medicine is used for many different conditions and in many different doses, the actual frequency of side effects may vary. In general, side effects are less common with low doses than with high doses. Also, when alpha interferon is used for genital warts, very little of it gets into the rest of the body, so side effects are generally less common than in other conditions.

Check with your doctor as soon as possible if any of the following side effects occur:

Less common

Confusion; mental depression; nervousness; numbness or tingling of fingers, toes, and face; trouble in sleeping; trouble in thinking or concentrating

Rare

Black, tarry stools; blood in urine or stools; chest pain; cough or hoarseness; fever or chills (beginning after 3 weeks of treatment); irregular heartbeat; lower back or side pain; painful or difficult urination; pinpoint red spots on skin; unusual bleeding or bruising

Other side effects may occur that usually do not need medical attention. These side effects may go away during

treatment as your body adjusts to the medicine. However, check with your doctor if any of the following side effects continue or are bothersome:

More common

Aching muscles; change in taste or metallic taste; fever and chills (should lessen after the first 1 or 2 weeks of treatment); general feeling of discomfort or illness; headache; loss of appetite; nausea and vomiting; skin rash; unusual tiredness

Less common or rare

Back pain; blurred vision; diarrhea; dizziness; dryness of mouth; dry skin or itching; increased sweating; joint pain; leg cramps; sores in mouth and on lips; weight loss

Alpha interferon may cause a temporary loss of some hair. After treatment has ended, normal hair growth should return.

Other side effects not listed above may also occur in some patients. If you notice any other effects, check with your doctor.

Additional Information

Once a medicine has been approved for marketing for a certain use, experience may show that it is also useful for other medical problems. Although these uses are not included in product labeling, alpha interferons are used in certain patients with the following medical conditions:

- Bladder cancer
- Cervical cancer
- Chronic myelocytic leukemia
- Kidney cancer
- Laryngeal papillomatosis (growths on larynx)
- Lymphomas, non-Hodgkin's
- Malignant melanoma
- Multiple myeloma
- Mycosis fungoides

Other than the above information, there is no additional information relating to proper use, precautions, or side effects for these uses.

Annual revision: 01/16/92
Interim revision: 04/17/93

INULIN Diagnostic

Generic name product available in the U.S.

Description

Inulin (IN-yoo-lin) is used as a test to help diagnose problems or disease of the kidneys. This test determines how well your kidneys are working.

Inulin passes out of the body entirely in the urine. Measuring the amount of inulin in the blood after it has been given can help the doctor determine if the kidneys are working properly.

How test is done: Inulin is given through an intravenous infusion (run into a vein). Several times during the test, blood and sometimes urine samples are taken. A tube called a catheter may be placed in your bladder to help take the urine samples. The amount of inulin in your blood or urine is measured. Then the results of the test are studied.

Inulin is to be used only under the supervision of a doctor. It is available in the following dosage form:

Parenteral

- Injection (U.S.)

It is very important that you read and understand the following information. If any of it causes you special concern, check with your doctor. Also, *if you have any questions* or if you want more information about this test or your medical problem, *ask your doctor, nurse, or pharmacist*.

Before Having This Test

In deciding to use a diagnostic test, the risks of the test must be weighed against the good it will do. This is a decision you and your doctor will make. Also, test results may be affected by other things. For inulin, the following should be considered:

Allergies—Tell your doctor if you have ever had any unusual or allergic reaction to inulin. Also tell your doctor if you are allergic to any other substances, such as foods, preservatives, or dyes.

Pregnancy—Inulin has not been shown to cause birth defects or other problems in humans.

Breast-feeding—Inulin has not been reported to cause problems in nursing babies.

Children—This medicine has been used in children. In effective doses, inulin has not been shown to cause different side effects or problems than it does in adults.

Older adults—Many medicines have not been studied specifically in older people. Therefore, it may not be known whether they work exactly the same way they do in younger adults. Although there is no specific information comparing the use of inulin in the elderly with use in other age groups, this medicine is not expected to cause different side effects or problems in older people than it does in younger adults.

Other medical problems—The presence of other medical problems may affect the use of inulin. Make sure you tell your doctor if you have any other medical problems, especially:

- Heart disease or
- Liver disease or
- Underactive adrenal gland or
- Underactive thyroid—These conditions may affect the inulin test results by reducing the amount of inulin that is cleared from the blood

Side Effects of This Medicine

Along with its needed effects, a medicine may cause some unwanted effects. Although inulin does not usually cause any side effects, check with your doctor if you notice any unusual effects.

Annual revision: 09/27/91

IOBENGUANE, RADIOIODINATED Therapeutic*†

A commonly used name for iobenguane is meta-iodobenzylguanidine or mIBG.

*Not commercially available in the U.S.
†Not commercially available in Canada.

Description

Radioiodinated iobenguane is a radiopharmaceutical (ray-dee-oh-far-ma-SOO-ti-kal). Radiopharmaceuticals are radioactive agents, which may be used to find and treat certain diseases or to study the function of the body's organs.

Radioiodinated iobenguane is used to treat certain kinds of cancer of the adrenal glands.

When very small doses of radioiodinated iobenguane are given, the radioactivity taken up by the adrenal gland helps find tumors of the adrenal glands. An image of the gland on film or on a computer screen can be provided to help with the diagnosis.

The information that follows applies only to the use of radioiodinated iobenguane in treating cancer of the adrenal gland.

Radioiodinated iobenguane is to be given only by or under the direct supervision of a doctor with specialized training in nuclear medicine. Radioiodinated iobenguane is available in the following dosage form:

Parenteral

- Injection

It is very important that you read and understand the following information. If any of it causes you special concern, check with your doctor. Also, *if you have any questions* or if you want more information about this medicine or your medical problem, *ask your doctor, nurse, or pharmacist.*

Before Using This Medicine

In deciding to use a medicine, the risks of taking the medicine must be weighed against the good it will do. This is a decision you and your doctor will make. For radioiodinated iobenguane, the following should be considered:

Pregnancy—This radiopharmaceutical is not recommended for use during pregnancy. This is to avoid exposing the fetus to harmful levels of radiation.

Breast-feeding—Some radiopharmaceuticals pass into the breast milk and may expose the baby to radiation. If you must receive radioiodinated iobenguane, it may be necessary for you to stop breast-feeding after receiving it. Be sure you have discussed this with your doctor.

Children and adolescents—Children and adolescents are especially sensitive to the effects of radiation. This may increase the chance of side effects during and after treatment. Be sure you have discussed this with your doctor.

Older adults—Radioiodinated iobenguane has been used in older people and has not been shown to cause different side effects or problems in older people than it does in younger adults.

Other medicines—Although certain medicines should not be used together at all, in other cases two different medicines may be used together even if an interaction might occur. In these cases, your doctor may want to change the dose, or other precautions may be necessary. When you are receiving radioiodinated iobenguane, it is especially important that your doctor knows if you are taking any of the following:

- Amphetamines or
- Appetite suppressants (diet pills) or
- Calcium channel blocking agents (diltiazem [e.g., Cardizem], nicardipine [e.g., Cardene], nifedipine [e.g., Procardia], verapamil [e.g., Calan]) or

- Cocaine or
- Guanethidine (e.g., Ismelin) or
- Haloperidol (e.g., Haldol) or
- Labetalol (e.g., Normodyne) or
- Loxapine (e.g., Loxitane) or
- Medicines for colds, sinus problems, or hay fever or other allergies (including nose drops or sprays) or
- Phenothiazines (acetophenazine [e.g., Tindal], chlorpromazine [e.g., Thorazine], fluphenazine [e.g., Prolixin], mesoridazine [e.g., Serentil], perphenazine [e.g., Trilafon], prochlorperazine [e.g., Compazine], promazine [e.g., Sparine], promethazine [e.g., Phenergan], thioridazine [e.g., Mellaril], trifluoperazine [e.g., Stelazine], triflupromazine [e.g., Vesprin], trimeprazine [e.g., Temaril]) or
- Reserpine (e.g., Serpasil) or
- Thiothixene (e.g., Navane) or
- Tricyclic antidepressants (amitriptyline [e.g., Elavil], amoxapine [e.g., Asendin], clomipramine [e.g., Anafranil], desipramine [e.g., Pertofrane], doxepin [e.g., Sinequan], imipramine [e.g., Tofranil], nortriptyline [e.g., Aventyl], protriptyline [e.g., Vivactil], trimipramine [e.g., Surmontil])—These medicines may keep the affected organ or tissue from getting the amount of radioiodinated iobenguane it needs to fight the disease

Other medical problems—The presence of other medical problems may affect the use of radioiodinated iobenguane. Make sure you tell your doctor if you have any other medical problems.

Preparation for This Treatment

Your doctor may have special instructions for you in preparation for your treatment. If you have not received such instructions or you do not understand them, check with your doctor in advance.

This radiopharmaceutical contains radioactive iodine, which may be taken up in your thyroid. To protect your thyroid, your doctor will prescribe a medicine (e.g., potassium iodide or SSKI) that contains non-radioactive iodine. You must take this medicine before starting treatment with radioiodinated iobenguane and continue taking it after treatment for as long as your doctor tells you.

Side Effects of This Medicine

Along with its needed effects, a medicine may cause some unwanted effects. Although not all of these side effects may occur, if they do occur they may need medical attention.

Check with your doctor as soon as possible if any of the following side effects occur after treatment for tumors of the adrenal gland:

Rare

Pale skin; sore throat and fever; unusual bleeding or bruising; unusual tiredness or weakness

Other side effects may occur that usually do not need medical attention. These side effects may go away during treatment as your body adjusts to the medicine. However, check with your doctor if the following side effects continue or are bothersome:

Less common or rare

Flushing of skin; nausea; slight and temporary increase in blood pressure

Other side effects not listed above may also occur in some patients. If you notice any other effects, check with your doctor.

Annual revision: 05/05/93

IODINATED GLYCEROL Systemic

Some commonly used brand names are:

In the U.S.

Iophen
Organic-1
Organidin

Generic name product may also be available.

In Canada

Organidin

Description

Iodinated glycerol (EYE-oh-di-nay-ted GLI-ser-ole) is used to thin and loosen mucus secretions. It is used in the treatment of respiratory tract conditions such as asthma, bronchitis, emphysema, sinusitis, and cystic fibrosis.

Iodinated glycerol is available only with your doctor's prescription, in the following dosage forms:

Oral

- Elixir (U.S. and Canada)
- Oral solution (U.S. and Canada)
- Tablets (U.S. and Canada)

It is very important that you read and understand the following information. If any of it causes you special concern, check with your doctor. Also, *if you have any questions* or if you want more information about this medicine or your medical problem, *ask your doctor, nurse, or pharmacist.*

Before Using This Medicine

In deciding to use a medicine, the risks of taking the medicine must be weighed against the good it will do. This is a decision you and your doctor will make. For iodinated glycerol, the following should be considered:

Allergies—Tell your doctor if you have ever had any unusual or allergic reaction to iodinated glycerol, iodine, or iodine-containing preparations. Also tell your doctor and pharmacist if you are allergic to any other substances, such as foods, preservatives, or dyes.

Pregnancy—Iodinated glycerol is not recommended for use during pregnancy because it may cause enlargement of the thyroid gland in the fetus and result in breathing problems.

Breast-feeding—Iodinated glycerol is not recommended for use in nursing mothers because it may cause skin rash and thyroid problems in the baby.

Children—Swelling of the neck (goiter or enlarged thyroid gland) may be especially likely to occur in children with cystic fibrosis. These patients are usually more sensitive than adults to this effect of iodinated glycerol.

Older adults—Many medicines have not been studied specifically in older people. Therefore, it may not be known whether they work exactly the same way they do in younger adults or if they cause different side effects or problems in older people. There is no specific information comparing use of iodinated glycerol in the elderly with use in other age groups.

Other medicines—Although certain medicines should not be used together at all, in other cases two different medicines may be used together even if an interaction might occur. In these cases, your doctor may want to change the dose, or other precautions may be necessary. When you are taking iodinated glycerol, it is especially important that your doctor and pharmacist know if you are taking any of the following:

- Antithyroid agents (medicine for overactive thyroid) or
- Lithium (e.g., Lithane)—Taking these medicines with iodinated glycerol may increase the chance of goiter or an underactive thyroid

Other medical problems—The presence of other medical problems may affect the use of iodinated glycerol. Make sure you tell your doctor if you have any other medical problems, especially:

- Acne (teenage)—Iodinated glycerol may make the condition worse
- Cystic fibrosis (in children)—Iodinated glycerol may increase the chance of goiter in these patients
- Thyroid disease (or history of)—Iodinated glycerol may increase the chance of goiter in patients with an overactive thyroid; also, prolonged use of iodinated glycerol may result in an underactive thyroid

Before you begin using any new medicine (prescription or nonprescription) or if you develop any new medical problem while you are using this medicine, check with your doctor, nurse, or pharmacist.

Proper Use of This Medicine

For patients taking the *oral solution form of iodinated glycerol*:

- This medicine is to be taken by mouth even if it comes in a dropper bottle.
- Take this medicine mixed in water or another liquid. Be sure to drink all of the liquid to get the full dose of medicine.

To help thin and loosen mucus in the lungs, *drink a glass of water after each dose of this medicine* unless otherwise directed by your doctor.

Take iodinated glycerol only as directed. Do not take more of it, do not take it more often, and do not take it for a longer time than your doctor ordered. To do so may increase the chance of side effects.

Missed dose—If you miss a dose of this medicine, take it as soon as possible. However, if it is almost time for your next dose, skip the missed dose and go back to your regular dosing schedule. Do not double doses.

Storage—To store this medicine:

- Keep out of the reach of children.
- Store away from heat and direct light.
- Do not store the tablet form of this medicine in the bathroom, near the kitchen sink, or in other damp places. Heat or moisture may cause the medicine to break down.
- Keep the liquid form of this medicine from freezing.
- Do not keep outdated medicine or medicine no longer needed. Be sure that any discarded medicine is out of the reach of children.

Precautions While Using This Medicine

Your doctor should check your progress at regular visits to make sure this medicine is working properly and does not cause unwanted effects.

Side Effects of This Medicine

Along with its needed effects, a medicine may cause some unwanted effects. Although not all of these side effects may occur, if they do occur they may need medical attention.

Check with your doctor as soon as possible if any of the following side effects occur:

Rare

Chills or fever; headache (continuing); joint pain; loss of appetite; pain on chewing or swallowing; skin rash, hives, or redness; sore throat; swelling of face, lips, or eyelids; tenderness or swelling below or in front of ear

With long-term use

Burning of mouth and throat; dry skin; headache (severe); increased watering of the mouth; irritation of eyes or swelling of eyelids; metallic taste; runny nose, sneezing, and other symptoms of head cold; soreness of teeth and gums; swelling around the eyes; swelling of neck; unusual sensitivity to cold; unusual tiredness or weakness; unusual weight gain

Other side effects may occur that usually do not need medical attention. These side effects may go away during treatment as your body adjusts to the medicine. However, check with your doctor if any of the following side effects continue or are bothersome:

More common

Diarrhea; nausea or vomiting; stomach pain

Other side effects not listed above may also occur in some patients. If you notice any other effects, check with your doctor.

Annual revision: 08/07/91

IODINE, STRONG Systemic

Another commonly used name in the U.S. and Canada is Lugol's solution.

Description

Strong iodine (EYE-oh-dine) is used to treat overactive thyroid, iodine deficiency, and to protect the thyroid gland from the effects of radiation from radioactive forms of iodine. It may be used before and after administration of a radioactive medicine containing radioactive iodine or after accidental exposure to radiation (for example, from nuclear power plant accidents). It may also be used for other conditions as determined by your doctor.

Strong iodine is available only with your doctor's prescription, in the following dosage form:

Oral

- Oral solution (U.S. and Canada)

It is very important that you read and understand the following information. If any of it causes you special concern, check with your doctor. Also, *if you have any questions* or if you want more information about this medicine or your medical problem, *ask your doctor, nurse, or pharmacist.*

Before Using This Medicine

In deciding to use a medicine, the risks of taking the medicine must be weighed against the good it will do. This is a decision you and your doctor will make. For strong iodine, the following should be considered:

Allergies—Tell your doctor if you have ever had any unusual or allergic reaction to iodine or potassium iodide. Also tell your doctor and pharmacist if you are allergic to any substances, such as foods, preservatives, or dyes.

Pregnancy—Taking strong iodine during pregnancy may cause thyroid problems or goiter in the newborn infant.

Breast-feeding—Strong iodine may cause skin rash and thyroid problems in nursing babies.

Children—Strong iodine may cause skin rash and thyroid problems in infants.

Older adults—Many medicines have not been studied specifically in older people. Therefore, it may not be known whether they work exactly the same way they do in younger adults. Although there is no specific information comparing use of strong iodine in the elderly with use in other age groups, this medicine is not expected to cause different side effects or problems in older people than it does in younger adults.

Other medicines—Although certain medicines should not be used together at all, in other cases two different medicines may be used together even if an interaction might occur. In these cases, your doctor may want to change the dose, or other precautions may be necessary. When you are taking strong iodine, it is especially important that your doctor and pharmacist know if you are taking any of the following:

- Amiloride (e.g., Midamor) or
- Spironolactone (e.g., Aldactone) or
- Triamterene (e.g., Dyrenium)—Use of these medicines with strong iodine may increase the amount of potassium in the blood and increase the chance of side effects
- Antithyroid agents (medicine for overactive thyroid) or
- Lithium (e.g., Lithane)—Use of these medicines with strong iodine may increase the chance of side effects

Other medical problems—The presence of other medical problems may affect the use of strong iodine. Make sure

you tell your doctor if you have any other medical problems, especially:

- Bronchitis or
- Other lung conditions—Use of strong iodine may make this condition worse
- Hyperkalemia (too much potassium in the blood) or
- Kidney disease—Use of strong iodine may increase the amount of potassium in the blood and increase the chance of side effects

Before you begin using any new medicine (prescription or nonprescription) or if you develop any new medical problem while you are using this medicine, check with your doctor, nurse, or pharmacist.

Proper Use of This Medicine

For patients taking this medicine for *radiation exposure:*

- Take this medicine only when directed to do so by state or local public health authorities.
- Take this medicine once a day for 10 days, unless otherwise directed by public health authorities. *Do not take more of it and do not take it more often than directed.* Taking more of the medicine will not protect you better and may result in a greater chance of side effects.

If strong iodine upsets your stomach, *take it after meals or with food or milk* unless otherwise directed by your doctor. If stomach upset (nausea, vomiting, stomach pain, or diarrhea) continues, check with your doctor.

This medicine is to be taken by mouth even if it comes in a dropper bottle.

Do not use this solution if it turns brownish yellow.

Take strong iodine in a full glass (8 ounces) of water or in fruit juice, milk, or broth to improve the taste and lessen stomach upset. Be sure to drink all of the liquid to get the full dose of medicine.

If crystals form in strong iodine solution, they may be dissolved by warming the closed container of solution in warm water and then gently shaking the container.

Missed dose—If you miss a dose of this medicine, take it as soon as possible. However, if it is almost time for your next dose, skip the missed dose and go back to your regular dosing schedule. Do not double doses.

Storage—To store this medicine:

- Keep out of the reach of children.
- Store away from heat and direct light.
- Do not store in the bathroom, near the kitchen sink, or in other damp places.
- Keep the medicine from freezing. Do not refrigerate.
- Do not keep outdated medicine or medicine no longer needed. Be sure that any discarded medicine is out of the reach of children.

Precautions While Using This Medicine

Your doctor should check your progress at regular visits to make sure that this medicine does not cause unwanted effects.

For patients on a low-potassium diet:

- *This medicine contains potassium.* Check with your doctor or pharmacist before you take this medicine.

Side Effects of This Medicine

Along with its needed effects, a medicine may cause some unwanted effects. Although not all of these side effects may occur, if they do occur they may need medical attention. When this medicine is used for a short time at low doses, side effects usually are rare.

Check with your doctor as soon as possible if any of the following side effects occur:

Less common

Hives; joint pain; swelling of the arms, face, legs, lips, tongue, and/or throat; swelling of the lymph glands

With long-term use

Burning of mouth or throat; confusion; headache (severe); increased watering of mouth; irregular heartbeat; metallic taste; numbness, tingling, pain, or weakness in hands or feet; soreness of teeth and gums; stomach upset; symptoms of head cold; unusual tiredness; weakness or heaviness of legs

Other side effects may occur that usually do not need medical attention. These side effects may go away during treatment as your body adjusts to the medicine. However, check with your doctor if any of the following side effects continue or are bothersome:

Less common

Diarrhea; nausea or vomiting; stomach pain

Other side effects not listed above may also occur in some patients. If you notice any other effects, check with your doctor.

Annual revision: 04/15/92

IODOQUINOL Oral

Some commonly used brand names are:

In the U.S.

Diquinol
Yodoquinol
Yodoxin

Generic name product may also be available.

In Canada

Diodoquin
Yodoxin

Another commonly used name is diiodohydroxyquin.

Description

Iodoquinol (eye-oh-doe-KWIN-ole) belongs to the group of medicines called antiprotozoals. Although sometimes used to treat other types of infection, it is used most often in the treatment of intestinal infections.

Iodoquinol is available only with your doctor's prescription, in the following dosage form:

Oral

- Tablets (U.S. and Canada)

It is very important that you read and understand the following information. If any of it causes you special concern, check with your doctor. Also, *if you have any questions* or if you want more information about this medicine or your medical problem, *ask your doctor, nurse, or pharmacist.*

Before Using This Medicine

In deciding to use a medicine, the risks of taking the medicine must be weighed against the good it will do. This is a decision you and your doctor will make. For iodoquinol, the following should be considered:

Allergies—Tell your doctor if you have ever had any unusual or allergic reaction to iodoquinol, chloroxine (e.g., Capitrol), clioquinol (e.g., Vioform), iodine, pamaquine, pentaquine, or primaquine. Also tell your doctor and pharmacist if you are allergic to any other substances, such as foods, preservatives, or dyes.

Pregnancy—Iodoquinol has not been reported to cause birth defects or other problems in humans.

Breast-feeding—Iodoquinol has not been reported to cause problems in nursing babies.

Children—Children may be more likely to develop side effects, especially if given high doses for a long time.

Older adults—Many medicines have not been studied specifically in older people. Therefore, it may not be known whether they work exactly the same way they do in younger adults or if they cause different side effects or problems in older people. There is no specific information comparing use of iodoquinol in the elderly with use in other age groups.

Other medicines—Although certain medicines should not be used together at all, in other cases two different medicines may be used together even if an interaction might occur. In these cases, your doctor may want to change the dose, or other precautions may be necessary. Tell your doctor and pharmacist if you are taking any other prescription or nonprescription (over-the-counter [OTC]) medicine.

Other medical problems—The presence of other medical problems may affect the use of iodoquinol. Make sure you tell your doctor if you have any other medical problems, especially:

- Eye disease—Iodoquinol may cause side effects affecting the eye or make eye disease worse
- Kidney disease or
- Liver disease or
- Thyroid disease—Patients with kidney disease, liver disease, or thyroid disease may have an increased chance of side effects

Before you begin using any new medicine (prescription or nonprescription) or if you develop any new medical problem while you are using this medicine, check with your doctor, nurse, or pharmacist.

Proper Use of This Medicine

Take this medicine after meals to lessen possible stomach upset, unless otherwise directed by your doctor.

If these tablets are too large to swallow whole, they may be crushed and mixed with a small amount of applesauce or chocolate syrup.

To help clear up your infection completely, *keep taking this medicine for the full time of treatment,* even if you begin to feel better after a few days. *Do not miss any doses.*

Missed dose—If you do miss a dose of this medicine, take it as soon as possible. However, if it is almost time for your next dose, skip the missed dose and go back to your regular dosing schedule. Do not double doses.

Storage—To store this medicine:

- Keep out of the reach of children.
- Store away from heat and direct light.
- Do not store in the bathroom, near the kitchen sink, or in other damp places. Heat or moisture may cause the medicine to break down.
- Do not keep outdated medicine or medicine no longer needed. Be sure that any discarded medicine is out of the reach of children.

Precautions While Using This Medicine

This medicine may cause blurred vision or loss of vision. *Make sure you know how you react to this medicine before you drive, use machines, or do anything else that could be dangerous if you are not able to see well.* If these reactions are especially bothersome, check with your doctor.

If you must have thyroid function tests, make sure the doctor knows that you are taking this medicine or have taken it within the past 6 months.

Side Effects of This Medicine

Along with its needed effects, a medicine may cause some unwanted effects. Although not all of these side effects may occur, if they do occur they may need medical attention.

Check with your doctor immediately if any of the following side effects occur:

Less common

Fever or chills; skin rash, hives, or itching; swelling of neck

With long-term use of high doses—especially in children

Blurred vision or any change in vision; clumsiness or unsteadiness; decreased vision or eye pain; increased weakness; muscle pain; numbness, tingling, pain, or weakness in hands or feet

Other side effects may occur that usually do not need medical attention. These side effects may go away during treatment as your body adjusts to the medicine. However, check with your doctor if any of the following side effects continue or are bothersome:

More common

Diarrhea; nausea or vomiting; stomach pain

Less common

Headache; itching of the rectal area

Blurred vision or any change in vision; decreased vision; eye pain; or numbness, tingling, pain, or weakness in hands or feet may be more likely to occur in children, especially with long-term use of high doses.

Other side effects not listed above may also occur in some patients. If you notice any other effects, check with your doctor.

Annual revision: 10/06/92

IPECAC Oral

Available in the U.S. and Canada as generic name product.

Description

Ipecac (IP-e-kak) is used in the emergency treatment of certain kinds of poisoning. It is used to cause vomiting of the poison.

Only the syrup form of ipecac should be used. A bottle of ipecac labeled as being Ipecac Fluidextract or Ipecac Tincture should not be used. These dosage forms are too strong and may cause serious side effects or death. Only ipecac syrup contains the proper strength of ipecac for treating poisonings.

Ordinarily, this medicine should not be used if strychnine, corrosives such as alkalies (lye) and strong acids, or petroleum distillates such as kerosene, gasoline, coal oil, fuel oil, paint thinner, or cleaning fluid have been swallowed, since it may cause seizures, additional injury to the throat, or pneumonia.

Ipecac should not be used to cause vomiting as a means of losing weight. If used regularly for this purpose, serious heart problems or even death may occur.

This medicine in amounts of more than 1 ounce is available only with your doctor's prescription. It is available in ½- and 1-ounce bottles without a prescription. However, before using ipecac syrup, call your doctor, a poison control center, or an emergency room for advice.

Oral

- Syrup (U.S. and Canada)

It is very important that you read and understand the following information. If any of it causes you special concern, check with your doctor or pharmacist. Also, *if you have any questions* or if you want more information about this medicine or your medical problem, *ask your doctor, nurse, or pharmacist.*

Before Using This Medicine

Before using this medicine to cause vomiting in poisoning, call a poison control center, your doctor, or an emergency room for advice. It is a good idea to have these telephone numbers readily available. In addition, before you use ipecac, the following should be considered:

Pregnancy—Studies with ipecac have not been done in either humans or animals.

Children—Infants and very young children are at a greater risk of choking with their own vomit (or getting vomit in their lungs). Therefore, it is especially important to call a poison control center, a doctor, or an emergency room for instructions before giving ipecac to an infant or young child.

Older adults—This medicine has been tested and has not been shown to cause different side effects or problems in older people than it does in younger adults.

Other medical problems—If you have heart disease. There is an increased risk of heart problems such as unusually fast heartbeat if the ipecac is not vomited.

Proper Use of This Medicine

It is very important that you take this medicine only as directed. Do not take more of it and do not take it more often than recommended on the label, unless otherwise directed. When too much ipecac is used, it can cause damage to the heart and other muscles, and may even cause death.

Do not give this medicine to unconscious or very drowsy persons, since the vomited material may enter the lungs and cause pneumonia.

To help this medicine cause vomiting of the poison, adults should drink 1 full glass (8 ounces) of water and children should drink ½ to 1 full glass (4 to 8 ounces) of water immediately after taking this medicine. Water may be given first in the case of a small or scared child.

Do not take this medicine with milk, milk products, or with carbonated beverages. Milk or milk products may prevent this medicine from working properly, and carbonated beverages may cause swelling of the stomach.

If vomiting does not occur within 20 minutes after you have taken the first dose of this medicine, take a second dose. If vomiting does not occur after you have taken the second dose, you must immediately see your doctor or go to an emergency room.

If you have been told to take both this medicine and activated charcoal to treat the poisoning, *do not take the activated charcoal until after you have taken this medicine to cause vomiting and vomiting has stopped. This takes usually about 30 minutes.*

Storage—To store this medicine:

- Keep out of the reach of children since overdose is very dangerous in children.
- Store away from heat and direct light.
- Keep the syrup from freezing.
- Do not keep outdated medicine or medicine no longer needed. Be sure that any discarded medicine is out of the reach of children.
- Do not keep a bottle of ipecac that has been opened. Ipecac may evaporate over a period of time. It is best to replace it with a new one.

Side Effects of This Medicine

Along with its needed effects, a medicine may cause some unwanted effects. Although side effects usually do not occur with recommended doses of ipecac, if they do occur they may need medical attention.

Check with your doctor as soon as possible if any of the following side effects occur:

Symptoms of overdose (may also occur if ipecac is taken regularly)

Diarrhea; fast or irregular heartbeat; nausea or vomiting (continuing more than 30 minutes); stomach cramps or pain; troubled breathing; unusual tiredness or weakness; weakness, aching, and stiffness of muscles, especially those of the neck, arms, and legs

Other side effects not listed above may also occur in some patients. If you notice any other effects, check with your doctor.

Annual revision: 07/03/91

IPRATROPIUM Inhalation

A commonly used brand name in the U.S. and Canada is Atrovent.

Description

Ipratropium (i-pra-TROE-pee-um) belongs to the group of medicines called bronchodilators (medicines that open up the bronchial tubes [air passages] of the lungs). It is used to control the symptoms of lung diseases, such as chronic bronchitis and emphysema.

Ipratropium may also be used for other conditions as determined by your doctor.

Ipratropium is available only with your doctor's prescription, in the following dosage forms:

Inhalation

- Inhalation aerosol (U.S. and Canada)
- Inhalation solution (Canada)

It is very important that you read and understand the following information. If any of it causes you special concern, check with your doctor. Also, *if you have any questions* or if you want more information about this medicine or your medical problem, *ask your doctor, nurse, or pharmacist.*

Before Using This Medicine

In deciding to use a medicine, the risks of taking the medicine must be weighed against the good it will do. This is a decision you and your doctor will make. For ipratropium, the following should be considered:

Allergies—Tell your doctor if you have ever had any unusual or allergic reaction to ipratropium, atropine, belladonna, hyoscyamine, or scopolamine or to other inhalation aerosol medicines. Also tell your doctor and pharmacist if you are allergic to any other substances, such as foods, preservatives, or dyes.

Pregnancy—Studies have not been done in pregnant women. Although ipratropium has not been shown to cause birth defects in animals, it has been shown to cause fetal death and a slight decrease in successful pregnancies when the medicine was given to rats in very high doses.

Breast-feeding—It is not known whether ipratropium passes into the breast milk. However, this medicine has not been reported to cause problems in nursing babies.

Children—Although there is no specific information about the use of ipratropium in children, it is not expected to cause different side effects or problems in children than it does in adults.

Older adults—Many medicines have not been tested in older people. Therefore, it may not be known whether they work exactly the same way they do in younger adults or if they cause different side effects or problems in older people. There is no specific information about the use of ipratropium in the elderly.

Other medicines—Although certain medicines should not be used together at all, in other cases two different medicines may be used together even if an interaction might occur. In these cases, your doctor may want to change the dose, or other precautions may be necessary. When you are taking ipratropium, it is especially important that your doctor and pharmacist know if you are taking any other prescription or nonprescription (over-the-counter [OTC]) medicine.

Other medical problems—The presence of other medical problems may affect the use of ipratropium. Make sure you tell your doctor if you have any other medical problems, especially:

- Difficult urination or
- Enlarged prostate—Ipratropium may make the condition worse

Before you begin using any new medicine (prescription or nonprescription) or if you develop any new medical problem while you are using this medicine, check with your doctor, nurse, or pharmacist.

Proper Use of This Medicine

Ipratropium usually comes with patient directions. Read them carefully before using this medicine.

For patients using *ipratropium inhalation aerosol*:

- If you are directed to use more than 1 inhalation of this medicine for each dose, allow 1 minute between the inhalations in order to receive the full effect of the medicine.

For patients using *ipratropium inhalation solution*:

- If you are using ipratropium inhalation solution in a nebulizer, make sure you understand exactly how to use it. If you have any questions about this, check with your doctor or pharmacist.

It is very important that you use ipratropium only as directed. Do not use more of it and do not use it more often than your doctor ordered. To do so may increase the chance of serious side effects.

Keep the spray or solution away from the eyes because it may cause irritation. Also, if the medicine gets in the eyes, it may cause blurred vision for a short time.

Missed dose—If you miss a dose of this medicine, use it as soon as possible. However, if it is almost time for your next dose, skip the missed dose and go back to your regular dosing schedule. Do not double doses.

Storage—To store this medicine:

- Keep out of the reach of children.
- Store away from heat and direct sunlight.
- Keep the medicine from freezing.
- Do not puncture, break, or burn the container, even if it is empty.
- Do not keep outdated medicine or medicine no longer needed. Be sure that any discarded medicine is out of the reach of children.

Precautions While Using This Medicine

Check with your doctor at once if your symptoms do not improve within 30 minutes after using a dose of this medicine or if your condition gets worse.

For patients using *ipratropium inhalation aerosol*:

- If you are also using another bronchodilator inhalation aerosol, use the other bronchodilator inhalation aerosol first, then wait about 5 minutes before using this medicine, unless otherwise directed by your doctor. This allows the ipratropium to better reach the passages of the lungs (bronchioles) because the other bronchodilator inhalation aerosol opens up the bronchioles.

- If you are also using an adrenocorticoid inhalation aerosol or cromolyn inhalation aerosol, use the ipratropium inhalation aerosol first, then wait about 5 minutes before using the adrenocorticoid aerosol or cromolyn aerosol, unless otherwise directed by your doctor. This allows the adrenocorticoid or cromolyn to better reach the passages of the lungs (bronchioles) because the ipratropium inhalation aerosol opens up the bronchioles.

For patients using *ipratropium inhalation solution*:

- *If you are also using cromolyn inhalation solution, do not mix this solution with the ipratropium inhalation solution for use in a nebulizer.* To do so will cause the solution to become cloudy and prevent the cromolyn from working properly.

Ipratropium may cause dryness of the mouth or throat. For temporary relief of mouth dryness, use sugarless candy or gum, melt bits of ice in your mouth, or use a saliva substitute. However, if dry mouth continues for more than 2 weeks, check with your medical doctor or dentist. Continuing dryness of the mouth may increase the chance of dental disease, including tooth decay, gum disease, and fungus infections.

Side Effects of This Medicine

Along with its needed effects, a medicine may cause some unwanted effects. Although not all of these side effects may occur, if they do occur they may require medical attention.

Check with your doctor as soon as possible if any of the following side effects occur:

Rare

Skin rash or hives; ulcers or sores in mouth and on lips

Other side effects may occur that usually do not need medical attention. These side effects may go away during treatment as your body adjusts to the medicine. However, check with your doctor if any of the following side effects continue or are bothersome:

More common

Cough or dryness of mouth or throat; headache or dizziness; nervousness; stomach upset or nausea

Less common or rare

Blurred vision or other changes in vision; difficult urination; metallic or unpleasant taste; pounding heartbeat; stuffy nose; trembling; trouble in sleeping; unusual tiredness or weakness

Other side effects not listed above may also occur in some patients. If you notice any other effects, check with your doctor.

Annual revision: August 1990

IRON SUPPLEMENTS Systemic

This information applies to the following medicines:

Ferrous Fumarate (FER-us FYOO-ma-rate)
Ferrous Gluconate (FER-us GLOO-koe-nate)
Ferrous Sulfate (FER-us SUL-fate)
Iron Dextran (DEX-tran)
Iron-Polysaccharide (pol-i-SAK-a-ride)
Iron Sorbitol (SOR-bi-tole)

Some commonly used brand names are:

For Ferrous Fumarate

In the U.S.

Femiron
Feostat
Feostat Drops
Fumasorb
Fumerin
Hemocyte
Ircon
Palmiron
Span-FF

Generic name product may also be available.

In Canada

Neo-Fer
Novofumar
Palafer
Palafer Pediatric Drops

For Ferrous Gluconate

In the U.S.

Fergon
Ferralet
Simron

Generic name product may also be available.

In Canada

Apo-Ferrous Gluconate
Fertinic
Novoferrogluc

Generic name product may also be available.

For Ferrous Sulfate

In the U.S.

Feosol
Fer-In-Sol
Fer-In-Sol Drops
Fer-In-Sol Syrup
Fer-Iron Drops
Fero-Gradumet
Ferospace
Ferralyn Lanacaps
Ferra-TD
Mol-Iron
Slow Fe

Generic name product may also be available.

In Canada

Apo-Ferrous Sulfate
Fer-In-Sol Drops
Fer-In-Sol Syrup
Fero-Grad
Novoferrosulfa
PMS Ferrous Sulfate
Slow Fe

Generic name product may also be available.

For Iron Dextran

In the U.S.

InFeD

In Canada
Imferon

For Iron-Polysaccharide†
In the U.S.
Hytinic
Niferex
Niferex-150
Nu-Iron
Nu-Iron 150

For Iron Sorbitol*
In Canada
Jectofer

*Not commercially available in the U.S.
†Not commercially available in Canada.

Description

Iron is a mineral that the body needs to produce red blood cells. When the body does not get enough iron, it cannot produce the number of normal red blood cells needed to keep you in good health. This condition is called iron deficiency (iron shortage) or iron deficiency anemia.

Although many people in the U.S. get enough iron from their diet, some must take additional amounts to meet their needs. For example, iron is sometimes lost with slow or small amounts of bleeding in the body that you would not be aware of and which can only be detected by your doctor. Your doctor can determine if you have an iron deficiency, what is causing the deficiency, and if an iron supplement is necessary.

Lack of iron may lead to unusual tiredness, shortness of breath, a decrease in physical performance, learning problems in children, and may increase your chance of getting an infection.

Patients with the following conditions may be more likely to have a deficiency of iron:

- Bleeding problems
- Burns
- Hemodialysis
- Intestinal diseases
- Stomach removal

In addition, premature infants and those receiving unfortified formulas may need additional iron.

If any of the above apply to you, you should take iron supplements only on the advice of your doctor after need has been established.

Some iron preparations are available only with your doctor's prescription. Others are available without a prescription; however, your doctor may have special instructions on the proper use and dose for your condition.

Iron supplements are available in the following dosage forms:

Oral

Ferrous Fumarate
- Capsules (Canada)
- Extended-release capsules (U.S.)
- Solution (U.S. and Canada)
- Suspension (U.S. and Canada)
- Tablets (U.S. and Canada)
- Chewable tablets (U.S.)

Ferrous Gluconate
- Capsules (U.S.)
- Elixir (U.S.)
- Syrup (Canada)
- Tablets (U.S. and Canada)

Ferrous Sulfate
- Capsules (U.S.)
- Extended-release capsules (U.S. and Canada)
- Elixir (U.S.)
- Solution (U.S. and Canada)
- Tablets (U.S. and Canada)
- Enteric-coated tablets (U.S. and Canada)
- Extended-release tablets (U.S. and Canada)

Iron-Polysaccharide
- Capsules (U.S.)
- Elixir (U.S.)
- Tablets (U.S.)

Parenteral

Iron Dextran
- Injection (U.S. and Canada)

Iron Sorbitol
- Injection (Canada)

It is very important that you read and understand the following information. If any of it causes you special concern, check with your doctor or pharmacist. Also, *if you have any questions* or if you want more information about this dietary supplement or your medical problem, *ask your doctor, nurse, pharmacist, or dietitian.*

Importance of Diet

Many nutritionists recommend that, if possible, people should get all the iron they need from foods. However, many people do not get enough iron from food. For example, people on weight-loss diets may consume too little food to provide enough iron. Others may need more iron than normal. For such people, an iron supplement is important.

In order to get enough vitamins and minerals in your diet, it is important that you eat a balanced and varied diet. Follow carefully any diet program your doctor may recommend. For your specific vitamin and/or mineral needs, ask your doctor or dietitian for a list of appropriate foods.

Experts have developed a list of Recommended Dietary Allowances (RDA) of iron. The RDA are not an exact number but a general idea of how much you need every day. The RDA do not cover amounts needed for problems caused by a serious lack of iron.

The daily RDA for iron are as follows (Note that the RDA are expressed as an actual amount of iron. The drug form [e.g., ferrous fumarate, ferrous gluconate, ferrous sulfate] has a different strength):

- Infants and children—
  Birth to 6 months of age: 6 milligrams (mg) per day.
  6 months to 10 years of age: 10 mg per day.
- Adolescent and adult males—
  11 to 18 years of age: 12 mg per day.
  19 years of age and over: 10 mg per day.
- Adolescent and adult females—
  11 to 50 years of age: 15 mg per day.
  51 years of age and over: 10 mg per day.
- Pregnant females—30 mg per day.
- Breast-feeding females—15 mg per day.

Iron is found in the diet in two forms—heme iron, which is well absorbed and nonheme iron, which is poorly absorbed. The best dietary source of absorbable iron (heme iron) is lean red meat. Chicken, turkey, and fish are also sources of iron, but they contain less than red meat. Foods rich in vitamin C (e.g., citrus fruits and fresh vegetables) eaten with small amounts of heme iron-containing foods, such as meat, may increase the amount of iron absorbed from cereals, beans, and other vegetables, which contain poorly absorbed iron (nonheme iron). Some foods (e.g., milk, eggs, spinach, fiber, coffee, tea) may decrease the amount of nonheme iron absorbed from foods. Additional iron may be added to food from cooking in iron pots.

Before Using This Dietary Supplement

If you are taking this dietary supplement without a prescription, carefully read and follow any precautions on the label. For iron supplements, the following should be considered:

Allergies—Tell your doctor if you have ever had any unusual or allergic reaction to iron medicine. Also tell your doctor and pharmacist if you are allergic to any other substances, such as foods, preservatives, or dyes.

Pregnancy—During the first 3 months of pregnancy, a proper diet usually provides enough iron. However, during the last 6 months, in order to meet the increased needs of the developing baby, an iron supplement may be recommended by your doctor. However, taking large amounts of a dietary supplement in pregnancy may be harmful to the mother and/or fetus and should be avoided.

Breast-feeding—Iron normally is present in breast milk in small amounts. When prescribed by a doctor, iron preparations are not known to cause problems during breast-feeding. However, nursing mothers are advised to check with their doctor before taking iron supplements or any other medication. Taking large amounts of a dietary supplement while breast-feeding may be harmful to the mother and/or infant and should be avoided.

Children—Iron supplements, when prescribed by your doctor, are not expected to cause different side effects in children than they do in adults. However, it is important to follow the directions carefully, since iron overdose in children is especially dangerous.

Older adults—Elderly people sometimes do not absorb iron as easily as younger adults and may need a larger dose. If you think you need to take an iron supplement, check with your doctor first. Only your doctor can decide if you need an iron supplement and how much you should take.

Medicines or other dietary supplements—Although certain medicines or dietary supplements should not be used together at all, in other cases they may be used together even if an interaction might occur. In these cases, your doctor may want to change the dose, or other precautions may be necessary. When you are taking iron supplements, it is especially important that your doctor and pharmacist know if you are taking any of the following:

- Acetohydroxamic acid (e.g., Lithostat)—Use with iron supplements may cause either medicine to be less effective
- Dimercaprol—Iron supplements and dimercaprol may combine in the body to form a harmful chemical
- Etidronate or
- Tetracyclines (taken by mouth) (medicine for infection)—Use with iron supplements may make these medicines less effective; iron supplements should be taken 2 hours after etidronate or tetracycline

Other medical problems—The presence of other medical problems may affect the use of iron supplements. Make sure you tell your doctor if you have any other medical problems, especially:

- Arthritis (rheumatoid) or
- Asthma or allergies—The injected form of iron may make these conditions worse
- Blood disease (other than iron-deficiency anemia) or
- Colitis or other intestinal problems or
- Stomach ulcer—Iron supplements may make these conditions worse
- Kidney infection or
- Liver disease—Higher blood levels of the iron supplement may occur, which may increase the chance of side effects

Proper Use of This Dietary Supplement

After you start using this dietary supplement, continue to return to your doctor to see if you are benefiting from the iron. Some blood tests may be necessary for this.

Iron is best taken on an empty stomach, with water or fruit juice (adults: full glass or 8 ounces; children: ½ glass or 4 ounces), about 1 hour before or 2 hours after meals. However, to lessen the possibility of stomach upset, iron may be taken with food or immediately after meals.

For safe and effective use of iron supplements:

- Follow your doctor's instructions if this dietary supplement was prescribed.

- Follow the manufacturer's package directions if you are treating yourself. If you think you still need iron after taking it for 1 or 2 months, check with your doctor.

Liquid forms of iron supplement tend to stain the teeth. To prevent, reduce, or remove these stains:

- Mix each dose in water, fruit juice, or tomato juice. You may use a drinking tube or straw to help keep the iron supplement from getting on the teeth.
- When doses of liquid iron supplement are to be given by dropper, the dose may be placed well back on the tongue and followed with water or juice.
- Iron stains on teeth can usually be removed by brushing with baking soda (sodium bicarbonate) or medicinal peroxide (hydrogen peroxide 3%).

Missed dose—If you miss a dose of this dietary supplement, skip the missed dose and go back to your regular dosing schedule. Do not double doses.

Storage—To store this dietary supplement:

- Keep out of the reach of children because iron overdose is especially dangerous in children. As few as 3 or 4 adult iron tablets can cause serious poisoning in small children. Vitamin-iron products for use during pregnancy and flavored vitamins with iron often cause iron overdose in small children.
- Store away from heat and direct light.
- Do not store in the bathroom, near the kitchen sink, or in other damp places. Heat or moisture may cause the dietary supplement to break down.
- Keep the liquid form of this dietary supplement from freezing.
- Do not keep outdated dietary supplements or those no longer needed. Be sure that any discarded dietary supplement is out of the reach of children.

Precautions While Using This Dietary Supplement

When iron is combined with certain foods it may lose much of its value. If you are taking iron, the following foods should be avoided or only taken in very small amounts for at least 1 hour before or 2 hours after you take iron:

Cheese and yogurt
Eggs
Milk
Spinach
Tea or coffee
Whole-grain breads and cereals and bran

Do not take iron supplements and antacids or calcium supplements at the same time. It is best to space doses of these 2 products 1 to 2 hours apart, to get the full benefit from each medicine or dietary supplement.

If you are taking iron supplement *without a doctor's prescription:*

- Do not take iron supplements by mouth if you are receiving iron injections. To do so may result in iron poisoning.
- Do not regularly take large amounts of iron for longer than 6 months without checking with your doctor. People differ in their need for iron, and those with certain medical conditions can gradually become poisoned by taking too much iron over a period of time. Also, unabsorbed iron can mask the presence of blood in the stool, which may delay discovery of a serious condition.
- Your total daily intake of iron must be considered, not just the amount contained in iron supplements. Iron-fortified bread, cereals, and other foods must be added for the total amount.

If you have been taking a long-acting or coated iron tablet and your stools have *not* become black, check with your doctor. The tablets may not be breaking down properly in your stomach, and you may not be receiving enough iron.

It is important to keep iron preparations out of the reach of children. Keep a 1-ounce bottle of *syrup* of ipecac available at home to be taken in case of an iron overdose emergency when a doctor, poison control center, or emergency room orders its use.

If you think you or anyone else has taken an overdose of iron medicine:

- *Immediate medical attention is very important.*
- *Call your doctor, a poison control center, or the nearest hospital emergency room at once.* Always keep these phone numbers readily available.
- *Follow any instructions given to you.* If syrup of ipecac has been ordered and given, do not delay going to the emergency room while waiting for the ipecac syrup to empty the stomach, since it may require 20 to 30 minutes to show results.
- *Go to the emergency room without delay.*
- *Take the container of iron medicine with you.*

Early signs of iron overdose may not appear for up to 60 minutes or more. Do not delay going to the emergency room while waiting for signs to appear.

Side Effects of This Dietary Supplement

Along with its needed effects, a dietary supplement may cause some unwanted effects. Although not all of these effects may occur, if they do occur they may need medical attention.

Check with your doctor if any of the following side effects occur:

More common—with the injection only

Backache or muscle pain; chills; dizziness; fever with increased sweating; headache; metallic taste; nausea or vomiting; numbness, pain, or tingling of hands or feet; pain or redness at injection site; skin rash or hives; troubled breathing

More common—when taken by mouth only

Abdominal or stomach pain, cramping, or soreness (continuing)

Less common or rare—when taken by mouth only

Chest or throat pain, especially when swallowing; stools with signs of blood (red or black color)

Early symptoms of iron overdose

Diarrhea (may contain blood); nausea; stomach pain or cramping (sharp); vomiting, severe (may contain blood)

Note: Symptoms of iron overdose may not occur for up to 60 minutes or more after the overdose was taken. By this time you should have had emergency room treatment. Do not delay going to emergency room while waiting for signs to appear.

Late symptoms of iron overdose

Bluish-colored lips, fingernails, and palms of hands; convulsions (seizures); drowsiness; pale, clammy skin; unusual tiredness or weakness; weak and fast heartbeat

Other side effects may occur that usually do not need medical attention. These side effects may go away during treatment as your body adjusts to the dietary supplement. However, check with your doctor if any of the following side effects continue or are bothersome:

More common

Constipation; diarrhea; nausea; vomiting

Less common

Darkened urine; heartburn

Stools commonly become dark green or black when iron preparations are taken by mouth. This is caused by unabsorbed iron and is harmless. However, in rare cases, black stools of a sticky consistency may occur along with other side effects such as red streaks in the stool, cramping, soreness, or sharp pains in the stomach or abdominal area. Check with your doctor immediately if these side effects appear.

If you have been receiving injections of iron, you may notice a brown discoloration of your skin. This color usually fades within several weeks or months.

Other side effects not listed above may also occur in some patients. If you notice any other effects, check with your doctor.

Annual revision: 04/16/92
Interim revision: 06/29/92

ISOMETHEPTENE, DICHLORALPHENAZONE, AND ACETAMINOPHEN Systemic

Some commonly used brand names are:

In the U.S.

Amidrine	Migquin
I.D.A.	Migratine
Iso-Acetazone	Migrazone
Isocom	Migrend
Midchlor	Migrex
Midrin	Mitride
Migrapap	

Description

Isometheptene (eye-soe-meth-EP-teen), dichloralphenazone (dye-klor-al-FEN-a-zone), and acetaminophen (a-seat-a-MIN-oh-fen) combination is used to treat certain kinds of headaches, such as "tension" headaches and migraine headaches. This combination is not used regularly (for example, every day) to prevent headaches. It should be taken only after headache pain begins, or after a warning sign that a migraine is coming appears. Isometheptene helps to relieve throbbing headaches, but it is not an ordinary pain reliever. Dichloralphenazone helps you to relax, and acetaminophen relieves pain.

This medicine is available only with your doctor's prescription, in the following dosage form:

Oral

- Capsules (U.S.)

It is very important that you read and understand the following information. If any of it causes you special concern, check with your doctor. Also, *if you have any questions* or if you want more information about this medicine or your medical problem, *ask your doctor, nurse, or pharmacist.*

Before Using This Medicine

In deciding to use a medicine, the risks of taking the medicine must be weighed against the good it will do. This is a decision you and your doctor will make. For this combination medicine, the following should be considered:

Allergies—Tell your doctor if you have ever had any unusual or allergic reaction to acetaminophen or to this combination medicine. Also tell your doctor and pharmacist if you are allergic to any other substances, such as foods, preservatives, or dyes.

Pregnancy—Studies with this combination medicine have not been done in either humans or animals.

Breast-feeding—Acetaminophen passes into the breast milk in small amounts. However, this medicine has not been shown to cause problems in nursing babies.

Children—Studies with this medicine have been done only in adult patients, and there is no specific information about its use in children.

Older adults—Many medicines have not been tested in older people. Therefore, it may not be known whether they work exactly the same way they do in younger adults or if they cause different side effects or problems in older people. There is no specific information comparing use of this combination medicine in the elderly with use in other age groups.

Other medicines—Although certain medicines should not be used together at all, in other cases two different medicines may be used together even if an interaction might occur. In these cases, your doctor may want to change the dose, or other precautions may be necessary. When you are taking this combination medicine, it is especially important that your doctor and pharmacist know if you are taking any of the following:

- Monoamine oxidase (MAO) inhibitors (furazolidone [e.g., Furoxone], isocarboxazid [e.g., Marplan], phenelzine [e.g., Nardil], procarbazine [e.g., Matulane], selegiline [e.g., Eldepryl], tranylcypromine [e.g., Parnate])—Taking this combination medicine while you are taking or within 2 weeks of taking a monoamine oxidase (MAO) inhibitor may increase the chance of side effects

Other medical problems—The presence of other medical problems may affect the use of this medicine. Make sure you tell your doctor if you have any other medical problems, especially:

- Alcohol abuse or
- Heart attack (recent) or
- Heart or blood vessel disease or
- Kidney disease or
- Liver disease or
- Stroke (recent) or
- Virus infection of the liver (viral hepatitis)—The chance of side effects may be increased
- Glaucoma, not well controlled, or
- High blood pressure (hypertension), not well controlled—The isometheptene in this combination medicine may make these conditions worse

Before you begin using any new medicine (prescription or nonprescription) or if you develop any new medical problem while you are using this medicine, check with your doctor, nurse, or pharmacist.

Proper Use of This Medicine

Take this medicine only as directed by your doctor. Do not take more of it, do not take it more often than directed, and do not take it every day for several days in a row. If the amount you are to take does not relieve your headache, check with your doctor. If a headache medicine is used too often, it may lose its effectiveness or even cause a type of physical dependence. If this occurs, your headaches may actually get worse. Also, taking too much acetaminophen can cause liver damage.

This medicine works best if you:

- *Take it as soon as the headache begins.* If you get warning signals of a migraine, take this medicine as soon as you are sure that the migraine is coming. This may even stop the headache pain from occurring.
- *Lie down in a quiet, dark room until you are feeling better.*

People who get a lot of headaches may need to take a different medicine to help prevent headaches. *It is important that you follow your doctor's directions, even if your headaches continue to occur.* Headache-preventing medicines may take several weeks to start working. Even after they do start working, your headaches may not go away completely. However, your headaches should occur less often, and they should be less severe and easier to relieve, than before. This will reduce the amount of headache relievers that you need. If you do not notice any improvement after several weeks of headache-preventing treatment, check with your doctor.

Dosing—The dose of this combination medicine will be different for different patients. *Follow your doctor's orders or the directions on the label.* The following information includes only the average doses of this medicine. *If your dose is different, do not change it unless your doctor tells you to do so.*

- *For "tension" headaches:*

  —Adults: 1 or 2 capsules every 4 hours, as needed. Not more than 8 capsules a day.

  —Children: Dose must be determined by the doctor.
- *For migraine headaches:*

  —Adults: 2 capsules for the first dose, then 1 capsule every hour, as needed. Not more than 5 capsules in 12 hours.

  —Children: Dose must be determined by the doctor.

Storage—To store this medicine:

- Keep out of the reach of children.
- Store away from heat and direct light.
- Do not store in the bathroom, near the kitchen sink, or in other damp places. Heat and moisture may cause the medicine to break down.
- Do not keep outdated medicine or medicine no longer needed. Be sure that any discarded medicine is out of the reach of children.

Precautions While Using This Medicine

Check with your doctor:

- *If the medicine stops working as well as it did when you first started using it.* This may mean that you are in danger of becoming dependent on the medicine. *Do not try to get better relief by increasing the dose.*
- *If you are having headaches more often than you did before you started using this medicine.* This is especially important if a new headache occurs within 1 day after you took your last dose of headache medicine, headaches begin to occur every day, or a headache continues for several days in a row. This may mean that you are dependent on the medicine. *Continuing to take this medicine will cause even more headaches later on.* Your doctor can give you advice on how to relieve the headaches.

Check the labels of all nonprescription (over-the-counter [OTC]) and prescription medicines you now take. Taking other medicines that contain acetaminophen together with this medicine may lead to an overdose. If you have any questions about this, check with your doctor or pharmacist.

This medicine may cause some people to become drowsy, dizzy, or less alert than they are normally. These effects may be especially severe if you also take CNS depressants (medicines that slow down the nervous system, possibly causing drowsiness) together with this medicine. Some examples of CNS depressants are antihistamines or medicine for hay fever, other allergies, or colds; sedatives, tranquilizers, or sleeping medicine; prescription pain medicine or narcotics; barbiturates; medicine for seizures; muscle relaxants; antiemetics (medicines that prevent or relieve nausea or vomiting), and anesthetics. If you are not able to lie down for a while, *make sure you know how you react to this medicine or combination of medicines before you drive, use machines, or do anything else that could be dangerous if you are drowsy or dizzy or are not alert.*

Do not drink alcoholic beverages while taking this medicine. To do so may increase the chance of liver damage caused by acetaminophen, especially if you drink large amounts of alcoholic beverages regularly. Also, because drinking alcoholic beverages may make your headaches worse or cause new headaches to occur, people who often get headaches should probably avoid alcohol.

Side Effects of This Medicine

Along with its needed effects, a medicine may cause some unwanted effects. Although not all of these side effects may occur, if they do occur they may need medical attention.

Check with your doctor as soon as possible if any of the following side effects occur:

Less common

Unusual tiredness or weakness

Rare

Black, tarry stools; blood in urine or stools; pinpoint red spots on skin; skin rash, hives, or itching; sore throat and fever; unusual bleeding or bruising; yellow eyes or skin

Symptoms of dependence on this medicine

Headaches, more severe and/or more frequent than before

Symptoms of acetaminophen overdose

Diarrhea; increased sweating; loss of appetite; nausea or vomiting; pain, tenderness, and/or swelling in the upper abdominal (stomach) area; stomach cramps or pain

Other side effects may occur that usually do not need medical attention. These side effects may go away during treatment as your body adjusts to the medicine. However, check with your doctor if any of the following side effects continue or are bothersome:

More common

Drowsiness

Rare

Dizziness; fast or irregular heartbeat

Other side effects not listed above may also occur in some patients. If you notice any other effects, check with your doctor.

Annual revision: 08/18/92

ISONIAZID Systemic

Some commonly used brand names are:

In the U.S.

Laniazid
Nydrazid
Tubizid

Generic name product may also be available.

In Canada

Isotamine
PMS Isoniazid

Another commonly used name is INH.

Description

Isoniazid (eye-soe-NYE-a-zid) is used to prevent or treat tuberculosis (TB). It may be given alone to prevent, or, in combination with other medicines, to treat TB. This medicine may also be used for other problems as determined by your doctor.

This medicine may cause some serious side effects, including damage to the liver. Liver damage is more likely to occur in patients over 50 years of age. *You and your doctor should talk about the good this medicine will do, as well as the risks of taking it.*

Isoniazid is available only with your doctor's prescription, in the following dosage forms:

Oral

- Syrup (U.S. and Canada)
- Tablets (U.S. and Canada)

Parenteral

- Injection (U.S.)

It is very important that you read and understand the following information. If any of it causes you special concern, check with your doctor. Also, *if you have any questions* or if you want more information about this medicine or your medical problem, *ask your doctor, nurse, or pharmacist.*

Before Using This Medicine

In deciding to use a medicine, the risks of taking the medicine must be weighed against the good it will do. This is a decision you and your doctor will make. For isoniazid, the following should be considered:

Allergies—Tell your doctor if you have ever had any unusual or allergic reaction to isoniazid, ethionamide (e.g., Trecator-SC), pyrazinamide, or niacin (e.g., Nicobid, nicotinic acid). Also tell your doctor and pharmacist if you are allergic to any other substances, such as foods, preservatives, or dyes.

Diet—Make certain your doctor and pharmacist know if you are on a low-sodium, low-sugar, or any other special diet. Most medicines contain more than their active ingredient, and many liquid medicines contain alcohol.

Pregnancy—Isoniazid has not been shown to cause birth defects or other problems in humans or animals. However, studies in rats and rabbits have shown that isoniazid may increase the risk of fetal death. In addition, it is not known whether this medicine causes problems when taken with other TB medicines.

Breast-feeding—Isoniazid passes into the breast milk. However, isoniazid has not been reported to cause problems in nursing babies.

Children—Isoniazid can cause serious side effects in any patient. Therefore, it is especially important that you discuss with the child's doctor the good that this medicine may do as well as the risks of using it.

Older adults—Hepatitis may be especially likely to occur in older patients, who are usually more sensitive than younger adults to the effects of isoniazid.

Other medicines—Although certain medicines should not be used together at all, in other cases two different medicines may be used together even if an interaction might occur. In these cases, your doctor may want to change the dose, or other precautions may be necessary. When you are taking or receiving isoniazid it is especially important that your doctor and pharmacist know if you are taking any of the following:

- Acetaminophen (e.g., Tylenol) (with long-term, high-dose use) or
- Amiodarone (e.g., Cordarone) or
- Anabolic steroids (nandrolone [e.g., Anabolin], oxandrolone [e.g., Anavar], oxymetholone [e.g., Anadrol], stanozolol [e.g., Winstrol]) or
- Androgens (male hormones) or
- Antithyroid agents (medicine for overactive thyroid) or
- Carmustine (e.g., BiCNU) or
- Chloroquine (e.g., Aralen) or
- Dantrolene (e.g., Dantrium) or
- Daunorubicin (e.g., Cerubidine) or
- Disulfiram (e.g., Antabuse) or
- Divalproex (e.g., Depakote) or
- Estrogens (female hormones) or
- Etretinate (e.g., Tegison) or
- Gold salts (medicine for arthritis) or
- Hydroxychloroquine (e.g., Plaquenil) or
- Mercaptopurine (e.g., Purinethol) or
- Methotrexate (e.g., Mexate) or
- Methyldopa (e.g., Aldomet) or
- Naltrexone (e.g., Trexan) (with long-term, high-dose use) or
- Oral contraceptives (birth control pills) containing estrogen or
- Other anti-infectives by mouth or by injection (medicine for infection) or
- Phenothiazines (acetophenazine [e.g., Tindal], chlorpromazine [e.g., Thorazine], fluphenazine [e.g., Prolixin], mesoridazine [e.g., Serentil], perphenazine [e.g., Trilafon], prochlorperazine [e.g., Compazine], promazine [e.g., Sparine], promethazine [e.g., Phenergan], thioridazine

[e.g., Mellaril], trifluoperazine [e.g., Stelazine], triflupromazine [e.g., Vesprin], trimeprazine [e.g., Temaril]) or
- Plicamycin (e.g., Mithracin) or
- Valproic acid (e.g., Depakene)—These medicines may increase the chance of liver damage if taken with isoniazid
- Carbamazepine (e.g., Tegretol) or
- Phenytoin (e.g., Dilantin)—These medicines may increase the chance of liver damage if taken with isoniazid. There may also be an increased chance of side effects of carbamazepine and phenytoin
- Disulfiram (e.g., Antabuse)—This medicine may increase the chance of liver damage and side effects, such as dizziness, lack of coordination, irritability, and trouble in sleeping
- Ketoconazole (e.g., Nizoral) or
- Rifampin (e.g., Rifadin)—Use of these medicines with isoniazid can lower the blood levels of ketoconazole or rifampin, decreasing their effects

Other medical problems—The presence of other medical problems may affect the use of isoniazid. Make sure you tell your doctor if you have any other medical problems, especially:
- Alcohol abuse (or history of) or
- Liver disease—There may be an increased chance of hepatitis with daily drinking of alcohol or in patients with liver disease
- Kidney disease (severe)—There may be an increased chance of side effects in patients with severe kidney disease
- Seizure disorders such as epilepsy—There may be an increased incidence of seizures (convulsions) in some patients

Before you begin using any new medicine (prescription or nonprescription) or if you develop any new medical problem while you are using this medicine, check with your doctor, nurse, or pharmacist.

Proper Use of This Medicine

If you are taking isoniazid by mouth and it upsets your stomach, take it with food. Antacids may also help. However, do not take aluminum-containing antacids within 1 hour of taking isoniazid. They may keep this medicine from working properly.

For patients taking the *oral liquid form* of isoniazid:
- Use a specially marked measuring spoon or other device to measure each dose accurately. The average household teaspoon may not hold the right amount of liquid.

To help clear up your tuberculosis (TB) completely, *it is very important that you keep taking this medicine for the full time of treatment*, even if you begin to feel better after a few weeks. You may have to take it every day for as long as 6 months to 2 years. *It is important that you do not miss any doses.*

Your doctor may also want you to take pyridoxine (e.g., Hexa-Betalin, vitamin B_6) every day to help prevent or lessen some of the side effects of isoniazid. This is not usually needed in children, who receive enough pyridoxine in their diet. If it is needed, *it is very important to take pyridoxine every day along with this medicine. Do not miss any doses.*

Missed dose—If you do miss a dose of this medicine, take it as soon as possible. However, if it is almost time for your next dose, skip the missed dose and go back to your regular dosing schedule. Do not double doses.

Storage—To store this medicine:
- Keep out of the reach of children.
- Store away from heat and direct light.
- Do not store the tablet form of this medicine in the bathroom, near the kitchen sink, or in other damp places. Heat or moisture may cause the medicine to break down.
- Keep the oral liquid form of this medicine from freezing.
- Do not keep outdated medicine or medicine no longer needed. Be sure that any discarded medicine is out of the reach of children.

Precautions While Using This Medicine

It is very important that your doctor check your progress at regular visits. Also, *check with your doctor immediately if blurred vision or loss of vision, with or without eye pain, occurs during treatment*. Your doctor may want you to have your eyes checked by an ophthalmologist (eye doctor).

If your symptoms do not improve within 2 to 3 weeks, or if they become worse, check with your doctor.

Certain foods such as cheese (Swiss or Cheshire) or fish (tuna, skipjack, or Sardinella) may rarely cause reactions in some patients taking isoniazid. Check with your doctor if redness or itching of the skin, hot feeling, fast or pounding heartbeat, sweating, chills or clammy feeling, headache, or lightheadedness occurs while you are taking this medicine.

Liver problems may be more likely to occur if you drink alcoholic beverages regularly while you are taking this medicine. Also, the regular use of alcohol may keep this medicine from working properly. Therefore, *you should strictly limit the amount of alcoholic beverages you drink while you are taking this medicine.*

If this medicine causes you to feel very tired or very weak; or causes clumsiness; unsteadiness; a loss of appetite; nausea; numbness, tingling, burning, or pain in the hands and feet; or vomiting, check with your doctor immediately. These may be early warning signs of more serious liver or nerve problems that could develop later.

For diabetic patients:

- *This medicine may cause false test results with some urine sugar tests.* Check with your doctor before changing your diet or the dosage of your diabetes medicine.

Side Effects of This Medicine

Along with its needed effects, a medicine may cause some unwanted effects. Although not all of these side effects may occur, if they do occur they may need medical attention.

Check with your doctor immediately if any of the following side effects occur:

More common

Clumsiness or unsteadiness; dark urine; loss of appetite; nausea or vomiting; numbness, tingling, burning, or pain in hands and feet; unusual tiredness or weakness; yellow eyes or skin

Rare

Blurred vision or loss of vision, with or without eye pain; convulsions (seizures); fever and sore throat; joint pain; mental depression; mood or other mental changes; skin rash; unusual bleeding or bruising

Other side effects may occur that usually do not need medical attention. These side effects may go away during treatment as your body adjusts to the medicine. However, check with your doctor if any of the following side effects continue or are bothersome:

More common

Diarrhea; stomach pain

For injection form

Irritation at the place of injection

Dark urine and yellowing of the eyes or skin (signs of liver problems) are more likely to occur in patients over 50 years of age.

Other side effects not listed above may also occur in some patients. If you notice any other effects, check with your doctor.

Additional Information

Once a medicine has been approved for marketing for a certain use, experience may show that it is also useful for other medical problems. Although these uses are not included in product labeling, isoniazid is used in certain patients with the following medical conditions:

- Tuberculous meningitis
- Nontuberculous mycobacterial infections

Other than the above information, there is no additional information relating to proper use, precautions, or side effects for these uses.

Annual revision: 10/06/92

ISOPROTERENOL AND PHENYLEPHRINE Systemic

Some commonly used brand names are:

In the U.S.

Duo-Medihaler

In Canada

Duo-Medihaler

Isuprel-Neo Mistometer

Description

Isoproterenol (eye-soe-proe-TER-e-nole) and phenylephrine (fen-ill-EF-rin) combination medicine is used to treat bronchial asthma, bronchitis, emphysema, and other lung diseases. It relieves wheezing, shortness of breath, and troubled breathing.

This medicine is available only with your doctor's prescription, in the following dosage form:

Inhalation

- Inhalation aerosol (U.S. and Canada)

It is very important that you read and understand the following information. If any of it causes you special concern, check with your doctor. Also, *if you have any questions* or if you want more information about this medicine or your medical problem, *ask your doctor, nurse, or pharmacist.*

Before Using This Medicine

In deciding to use a medicine, the risks of taking the medicine must be weighed against the good it will do. This is a decision you and your doctor will make. For isoproterenol and phenylephrine combination, the following should be considered:

Allergies—Tell your doctor if you have ever had any unusual or allergic reaction to isoproterenol and phenylephrine or to medicines like them, such as amphetamines, ephedrine, epinephrine, metaproterenol, norepinephrine, phenylpropanolamine, pseudoephedrine, or terbutaline, or to other inhalation aerosol medicines. Also tell your

doctor and pharmacist if you are allergic to any other substances, such as foods, preservatives, or dyes.

Pregnancy—Studies on effects in pregnancy with isoproterenol and phenylephrine have not been done in either humans or animals. However, use of phenylephrine during late pregnancy or during labor may cause a lack of oxygen and slow heartbeat in the fetus.

Breast-feeding—It is not known whether isoproterenol and phenylephrine pass into the breast milk. However, this combination medicine has not been reported to cause problems in nursing babies.

Children—Studies on isoproterenol and phenylephrine combination have been done only in adult patients, and there is no specific information about its use in children.

Older adults—Many medicines have not been tested in older people. Therefore, it may not be known whether they work exactly the same way they do in younger adults or if they cause different side effects or problems in older people. There is no specific information about the use of isoproterenol and phenylephrine combination in the elderly.

Other medicines—Although certain medicines should not be used together at all, in other cases two different medicines may be used together even if an interaction might occur. In these cases, your doctor may want to change the dose, or other precautions may be necessary. When you are taking isoproterenol and phenylephrine combination, it is especially important that your doctor and pharmacist know if you are taking any of the following:

- Beta-blockers (acebutolol [e.g., Sectral], atenolol [e.g., Tenormin], betaxolol [e.g., Kerlone], carteolol [e.g., Cartrol], labetalol [e.g., Normodyne], metoprolol [e.g., Lopressor], nadolol [e.g., Corgard], oxprenolol [e.g., Trasicor], penbutolol [e.g., Levatol], pindolol [e.g., Visken], propranolol [e.g., Inderal], sotalol [e.g., Sotacor], timolol [e.g., Blocadren])—Taking these medicines with isoproterenol and phenylephrine combination may prevent either medicine from working properly
- Cocaine—The effects of phenylephrine (contained in this combination medicine) may be increased
- Digitalis glycosides (heart medicine)—Taking these medicines with isoproterenol and phenylephrine combination may increase the chance of irregular heartbeat
- Ergoloid mesylates (e.g., Hydergine) or
- Ergotamine (e.g., Cafergot, Gynergen)—The effects of either these medicines or phenylephrine (contained in this combination medicine) may be increased
- Maprotiline (e.g., Ludiomil) or
- Tricyclic antidepressants (amitriptyline [e.g., Elavil], amoxapine [e.g., Asendin], clomipramine (e.g., Anafranil), desipramine [e.g., Pertofrane], doxepin [e.g., Sinequan], imipramine [e.g., Tofranil], nortriptyline [e.g., Aventyl], protriptyline [e.g., Vivactil], trimipramine [e.g., Surmontil])—Taking isoproterenol and phenylephrine combination with these medicines may increase the effects on the heart, possibly resulting in fast or irregular heartbeat, severe high blood pressure, or fever
- Methyldopa (e.g., Aldomet)—The effects of methyldopa may be decreased; also, the effects of phenylephrine (contained in this combination medicine) may be increased
- Monoamine oxidase (MAO) inhibitors (furazolidone [e.g., Furoxone], isocarboxazid [e.g., Marplan], pargyline [e.g., Eutonyl], phenelzine [e.g., Nardil], procarbazine [e.g., Matulane], tranylcypromine [e.g., Parnate])—Taking phenylephrine (contained in this combination medicine) while you are taking or within 2 weeks of taking monoamine oxidase (MAO) inhibitors may increase the effects of phenylephrine, possibly resulting in serious side effects

Other medical problems—The presence of other medical problems may affect the use of isoproterenol and phenylephrine combination. Make sure you tell your doctor if you have any other medical problems, especially:

- Diabetes mellitus (sugar diabetes)
- Heart or blood vessel disease or
- High blood pressure—The condition may become worse
- Overactive thyroid—The chance of side effects may be increased

Before you begin using any new medicine (prescription or nonprescription) or if you develop any new medical problem while you are using this medicine, check with your doctor, nurse, or pharmacist.

Proper Use of This Medicine

This medicine usually comes with patient directions. Read them carefully before using this medicine.

Keep spray away from the eyes.

Do not take more than 2 inhalations of this medicine at any one time, unless otherwise directed by your doctor. Allow 1 to 5 minutes after the first inhalation to make certain that a second inhalation is necessary.

Save your applicator. Refill units of this medicine may be available.

Use this medicine only as directed. Do not use more of it and do not use it more often than your doctor ordered. To do so may increase the chance of serious side effects. Isoproterenol inhalation preparations have been reported to cause death when too much of the medicine was used.

Storage—To store this medicine:

- Keep out of the reach of children.
- Store away from heat and direct sunlight.
- Keep the medicine from freezing.
- Do not puncture, break, or burn container, even if it is empty.
- Do not keep outdated medicine or medicine no longer needed. Be sure that any discarded medicine is out of the reach of children.

Precautions While Using This Medicine

If you still have trouble breathing after using this medicine, or if your condition becomes worse, check with your doctor at once.

If you are also using the inhalation aerosol form of an adrenocorticoid (cortisone-like medicine, such as beclomethasone, dexamethasone, flunisolide, or triamcinolone) or ipratropium, *use the isoproterenol and phenylephrine inhalation aerosol first and then wait about 5 minutes before using the adrenocorticoid or ipratropium inhalation aerosol*, unless otherwise directed by your doctor. This will allow the adrenocorticoid or ipratropium inhalation aerosol to better reach the passages of the lungs (bronchioles) after isoproterenol and phenylephrine inhalation aerosol opens them.

Side Effects of This Medicine

Along with its needed effects, a medicine may cause some unwanted effects. Although not all of these side effects may occur, if they do occur they may need medical attention.

Check with your doctor as soon as possible if any of the following side effects occur:

Rare

Chest pain; irregular heartbeat

Symptoms of overdose

Chest pain (continuing or severe); dizziness or lightheadedness (continuing or severe); fast, slow, or pounding heartbeat (continuing); headache (continuing or severe); increase in blood pressure; irregular heartbeat (continuing or severe); nausea or vomiting (continuing or severe); sensation of fullness in head; tingling in hands or feet; trembling (severe); unusual anxiety, nervousness, or restlessness; weakness (severe)

Other side effects may occur that usually do not need medical attention. These side effects may go away during treatment as your body adjusts to the medicine. However, check with your doctor if any of the following side effects continue or are bothersome:

More common

Nervousness; restlessness; trouble in sleeping

Less common

Dizziness or lightheadedness; fast or pounding heartbeat; flushing or redness of face or skin; headache; increased sweating; nausea or vomiting; trembling; weakness

This medicine may cause the saliva to turn pinkish to red in color. This is to be expected while you are using this medicine.

Other side effects not listed above may also occur in some patients. If you notice any other effects, check with your doctor.

Annual revision: August 1990

ISOTRETINOIN Systemic

Some commonly used brand names are:

In the U.S.

Accutane

In Canada

Accutane Roche

Description

Isotretinoin (eye-soe-TRET-i-noyn) is used to treat severe, disfiguring cystic acne. It should be used only after other acne medicines have been tried and have failed to help the acne. Isotretinoin may also be used to treat other skin diseases as determined by your doctor.

Isotretinoin must not be used to treat women who are able to bear children unless other forms of treatment have been tried first and have failed. Isotretinoin must not be taken during pregnancy, because it causes birth defects in humans. If you are able to bear children, it is very important that you read, understand, and follow the pregnancy warnings for isotretinoin.

This medicine is available only with your doctor's prescription and should be prescribed only by a doctor who has special knowledge in the diagnosis and treatment of severe, uncontrollable cystic acne.

Isotretinoin is available in the following dosage form:

Oral

- Capsules (U.S. and Canada)

It is very important that you read and understand the following information. If any of it causes you special concern, check with your doctor. Also, *if you have any questions* or if you want more information about this medicine or your medical problem, *ask your doctor, nurse, or pharmacist.*

Before Using This Medicine

Isotretinoin comes with patient information. It is very important that you read and understand this information. Be sure to ask your doctor about anything you do not understand.

In deciding to use a medicine, the risks of taking the medicine must be weighed against the good it will do. This is a decision you and your doctor will make. For isotretinoin, the following should be considered:

Allergies—Tell your doctor if you have ever had any unusual or allergic reaction to isotretinoin, etretinate, tretinoin, or vitamin A preparations. Also tell your doctor and pharmacist if you are allergic to any other substances, such as foods, preservatives, or dyes.

Pregnancy—*Isotretinoin must not be taken during pregnancy, because it causes birth defects in humans. In addition, isotretinoin must not be taken if there is a chance that you may become pregnant during treatment or within one month following treatment.* Women who are able to have children must have a pregnancy blood test within 2 weeks before beginning treatment with isotretinoin to make sure they are not pregnant. Treatment with isotretinoin will then be started on the second or third day of the woman's next normal menstrual period. In addition, you must have a pregnancy blood test each month while you are taking this medicine and one month after treatment is completed. Also, *isotretinoin must not be taken unless an effective form of contraception (birth control) has been used for at least 1 month before the beginning of treatment. Contraception must be continued during the period of treatment, which is up to 20 weeks, and for 1 month after isotretinoin is stopped. Be sure you have discussed this information with your doctor. In addition, you will be asked to sign an informed consent form stating that you understand the above information.*

Breast-feeding—It is not known whether isotretinoin passes into the breast milk. However, isotretinoin is not recommended during breast-feeding, because it may cause unwanted effects in nursing babies.

Children—Children may be especially sensitive to the effects of isotretinoin. This may increase the chance of side effects during treatment.

Older adults—Many medicines have not been tested in older people. Therefore, it may not be known whether they work exactly the same way they do in younger adults or if they cause different side effects or problems in older people. There is no specific information about the use of isotretinoin in the elderly.

Other medicines—Although certain medicines should not be used together at all, in other cases two different medicines may be used together even if an interaction might occur. In these cases, your doctor may want to change the dose, or other precautions may be necessary. When you are using isotretinoin, it is especially important that your doctor and pharmacist know if you are using any of the following:

- Etretinate (e.g., Tegison) or
- Tretinoin (vitamin A acid) (e.g., Retin-A) or
- Vitamin A or any preparation containing vitamin A—Use of isotretinoin with these medicines will result in an increase in side effects
- Tetracyclines (medicine for infection)—Use of isotretinoin with these medicines may increase the chance of a side effect called pseudotumor cerebri, which is a swelling of the brain

Other medical problems—The presence of other medical problems may affect the use of isotretinoin. Make sure you tell your doctor if you have any other medical problems, especially:

- Alcoholism or excess use of alcohol (or history of) or
- Diabetes mellitus (sugar diabetes) (or a family history of) or
- Family history of high triglyceride (a fat-like substance) levels in the blood or
- Severe weight problems—Use of isotretinoin may increase blood levels of triglyceride (a fat-like substance), which may increase the chance of heart or blood vessel problems in patients who have a family history of high triglycerides, are greatly overweight, are diabetic, or use a lot of alcohol. For persons with diabetes mellitus, use of isotretinoin may also change blood sugar levels

Before you begin using any new medicine (prescription or nonprescription) or if you develop any new medical problem while you are using this medicine, check with your doctor, nurse, or pharmacist.

Proper Use of This Medicine

It is very important that you take isotretinoin only as directed. Do not take more of it, do not take it more often, and do not take it for a longer time than your doctor ordered. To do so may increase the chance of side effects.

Missed dose—If you miss a dose of this medicine, take it as soon as possible. However, if it is almost time for your next dose, skip the missed dose and go back to your regular dosing schedule. Do not double doses.

Storage—To store this medicine:

- Keep out of the reach of children.
- Store away from heat and direct light.
- Do not store in the bathroom, near the kitchen sink, or in other damp places. Heat or moisture may cause the medicine to break down.
- Do not keep outdated medicine or medicine no longer needed. Be sure that any discarded medicine is out of the reach of children.

Precautions While Using This Medicine

Your doctor should check your progress at regular visits to make sure this medicine does not cause unwanted effects.

Isotretinoin causes birth defects in humans if taken during pregnancy. Therefore, if you suspect that you may have become pregnant, stop taking this medicine immediately and check with your doctor.

Do not donate blood to a blood bank while you are taking isotretinoin or for 30 days after you stop taking it. This is to prevent the possibility of a pregnant patient receiving the blood.

Do not take vitamin A or any vitamin supplement containing vitamin A while taking this medicine, unless otherwise directed by your doctor. To do so may increase the chance of side effects.

Drinking too much alcohol while taking this medicine may cause high triglyceride (fat-like substance) levels in the blood and possibly increase the chance of unwanted effects on the heart and blood vessels. Therefore, *while taking this medicine, it is best that you do not drink alcoholic beverages or that you at least reduce the amount you usually drink.* If you have any questions about this, check with your doctor.

For diabetic patients:

- This medicine may affect blood sugar levels. If you notice a change in the results of your blood or urine sugar tests or if you have any questions, check with your doctor.

In some patients, isotretinoin may cause a decrease in night vision. This decrease may occur suddenly. If it does occur, *do not drive, use machines, or do anything else that could be dangerous if you are not able to see well.* Also, check with your doctor.

Isotretinoin may cause dryness of the eyes. Therefore, if you wear contact lenses, your eyes may be more sensitive to them during the time you are taking isotretinoin and for up to about 2 weeks after you stop taking it. To help relieve dryness of the eyes, check with your doctor about using an eye lubricating solution, such as artificial tears. If eye inflammation occurs, check with your doctor.

Some people who take this medicine may become more sensitive to sunlight than they are normally. When you first begin taking this medicine, avoid too much sun and do not use a sunlamp until you see how you react to the sun, especially if you tend to burn easily. If you have a severe reaction, check with your doctor.

Isotretinoin may cause dryness of the mouth and nose. For temporary relief of mouth dryness, use sugarless candy or gum, melt bits of ice in your mouth, or use a saliva substitute. However, if dry mouth continues for more than 2 weeks, check with your medical doctor or dentist. Continuing dryness of the mouth may increase the chance of dental disease, including tooth decay, gum disease, and fungus infections.

For patients taking isotretinoin for acne:

- When you begin taking isotretinoin, your acne may seem to get worse before it gets better. If irritation or other symptoms of your condition become severe, check with your doctor.

Side Effects of This Medicine

Along with its needed effects, a medicine may cause some unwanted effects. Although not all of these side effects may occur, if they do occur they may need medical attention.

Check with your doctor as soon as possible if any of the following side effects occur:

More common

Burning, redness, itching, or other sign of eye inflammation; nosebleeds; scaling, redness, burning, pain, or other sign of inflammation of lips

Less common

Mental depression; skin infection or rash

Rare

Abdominal or stomach pain (severe); bleeding or inflammation of gums; blurred vision or other changes in vision; diarrhea (severe); headache (severe or continuing); mood changes; nausea and vomiting; pain or tenderness of eyes; rectal bleeding; yellow eyes or skin

Other side effects may occur that usually do not need medical attention. These side effects may go away during treatment as your body adjusts to the medicine. However, check with your doctor if any of the following side effects continue or are bothersome:

More common

Dryness of mouth or nose; dryness or itching of skin

Less common

Dryness of eyes; headache (mild); increased sensitivity of skin to sunlight; pain, tenderness, or stiffness in muscles, bones, or joints; peeling of skin on palms of hands or soles of feet; stomach upset; thinning of hair; unusual tiredness

Other side effects not listed above may also occur in some patients. If you notice any other effects, check with your doctor.

Annual revision: June 1990

ISOXSUPRINE Systemic

A commonly used brand name in the U.S. and Canada is Vasodilan. Generic name product may also be available in the U.S.

Description

Isoxsuprine (eye-SOX-syoo-preen) belongs to the group of medicines called vasodilators. Vasodilators increase the size of blood vessels. Isoxsuprine is used to treat problems resulting from poor blood circulation.

It may also be used for other conditions as determined by your doctor.

Isoxsuprine is available only with your doctor's prescription, in the following dosage forms:

Oral

- Tablets (U.S. and Canada)

Parenteral

- Injection (Canada)

It is very important that you read and understand the following information. If any of it causes you special concern, check with your doctor or pharmacist. Also, *if you have any questions* or if you want more information about this medicine or your medical problem, *ask your doctor, nurse, or pharmacist.*

Before Using This Medicine

In deciding to use a medicine, the risks of taking the medicine must be weighed against the good it will do. This is a decision you and your doctor will make. For isoxsuprine, the following should be considered:

Allergies—Tell your doctor if you have ever had any unusual or allergic reaction to isoxsuprine. Also tell your doctor and pharmacist if you are allergic to any other substances, such as foods, preservatives, or dyes.

Pregnancy—Isoxsuprine has not been shown to cause birth defects in humans. However, isoxsuprine given shortly before delivery may cause fast heartbeat and other problems (low blood sugar, bowel problems, low blood pressure) in the newborn.

Breast-feeding—Isoxsuprine has not been reported to cause problems in nursing babies.

Older adults—Many medicines have not been studied specifically in older people. Therefore, it may not be known whether they work exactly the same way they do in younger adults or if they cause different side effects or problems in older people. There is no specific informaiton comparing use of isoxsuprine in the elderly with use in other age groups. However, isoxsuprine may reduce tolerance to cold temperatures in elderly patients.

Other medicines—Although certain medicines should not be used together at all, in other cases two different medicines may be used together even if an interaction might occur. In these cases, your doctor may want to change the dose, or other precautions may be necessary. Tell your doctor and pharmacist if you are taking any other prescription or nonprescription (over-the-counter [OTC]) medicine, or if you smoke.

Other medical problems—The presence of other medical problems may affect the use of isoxsuprine. Make sure you tell your doctor if you have any other medical problems, especially:

- Angina (chest pain) or
- Bleeding problems or
- Glaucoma or
- Hardening of the arteries or
- Heart attack (recent) or
- Stroke (recent)—The chance of side effects may be increased

Before you begin using any new medicine (prescription or nonprescription) or if you develop any new medical problem while you are using this medicine, check with your doctor, nurse, or pharmacist.

Proper Use of This Medicine

If this medicine upsets your stomach, it may be taken with meals, milk, or antacids.

Missed dose—If you miss a dose of this medicine, take it as soon as possible. However, if it is almost time for your next dose, skip the missed dose and go back to your regular dosing schedule. Do not double doses.

Storage—To store this medicine:

- Keep out of the reach of children.
- Store away from heat and direct light.
- Do not store in the bathroom, near the kitchen sink, or in other damp places. Heat or moisture may cause the medicine to break down.
- Do not keep outdated medicine or medicine no longer needed. Be sure that any discarded medicine is out of the reach of children.

Precautions While Using This Medicine

It may take some time for this medicine to work. If you feel that the medicine is not working, do not stop taking it on your own. Instead, check with your doctor.

The helpful effects of this medicine may be decreased if you smoke. If you have any questions about this, check with your doctor.

Dizziness may occur, especially when you get up from a lying or sitting position or climb stairs. Getting up slowly may help. If this problem continues or gets worse, check with your doctor.

Side Effects of This Medicine

Along with its needed effects, a medicine may cause some unwanted effects. Although not all of these side effects may occur, if they do occur they may need medical attention.

Check with your doctor as soon as possible if any of the following side effects occur:

Rare

Chest pain; dizziness or faintness (more common for injection); fast heartbeat (more common for injection); shortness of breath; skin rash

Other side effects may occur that usually do not need medical attention. These side effects may go away during treatment as your body adjusts to the medicine. However, check with your doctor if the following side effects continue or are bothersome:

Less common

Nausea or vomiting (more common for injection)

Other side effects not listed above may also occur in some patients. If you notice any other effects, check with your doctor.

Additional Information

Although this use is not included in U.S. product labeling, isoxsuprine is used in certain women to stop premature labor.

In addition to the above information, the following information applies when this medicine is used to stop premature labor:

- Before you begin treatment with this medicine, tell your doctor if you have any of the following medical problems:
  Asthma
  Diabetes mellitus (sugar diabetes)
  Heart disease
  High blood pressure
  Overactive thyroid
- *Check with your doctor immediately:*
  —if your contractions begin again or your water breaks.
  —if you notice chest pain or shortness of breath while taking isoxsuprine.

Annual revision: 07/06/92

IVERMECTIN Systemic*†

A commonly used brand name is Mectizan.

*Not commercially available in the U.S.
†Not commercially available in Canada.

Description

Ivermectin (eye-ver-MEK-tin) is used in the treatment of certain worm infections. It is used to treat river blindness (onchocerciasis), filariasis, and strongyloidiasis. It may be used for some other kinds of worm infections.

Ivermectin appears to work by paralyzing and then killing the offspring of adult worms. It may also slow down the rate at which adult worms reproduce. This results in fewer worms in the skin, blood, and eyes.

Ivermectin is available only with your doctor's prescription, in the following dosage form:

Oral

- Tablets (International)

It is very important that you read and understand the following information. If any of it causes you special concern, check with your doctor. Also, *if you have any questions* or if you want more information about this medicine or your medical problem, ***ask your doctor, nurse, or pharmacist.***

Before Using This Medicine

In deciding to use a medicine, the risks of taking the medicine must be weighed against the good it will do. This is a decision you and your doctor will make. For ivermectin, the following should be considered:

Allergies—Tell your doctor if you have ever had any unusual or allergic reaction to ivermectin. Also tell your doctor and pharmacist if you are allergic to any other substances, such as foods, preservatives, or dyes.

Pregnancy—Although studies have not been done in humans, use is not recommended during pregnancy. Studies in rats and rabbits, given 7 or 8 times the usual human dose for several days, have not shown that ivermectin causes birth defects or other problems. However, studies in mice, given 5 times the usual human dose, have shown that ivermectin causes birth defects. Studies in other animals have also shown that this medicine may harm the fetus.

Breast-feeding—Ivermectin is excreted in breast milk. However, it has not been reported to cause problems in nursing babies.

Children—This medicine has been tested in a limited number of children 5 years of age or older and, in effective doses, has not been reported to cause different side effects or problems in children than it does in adults.

Older adults—Many medicines have not been studied specifically in older people. Therefore, it may not be known whether they work exactly the same way they do in younger adults or if they cause different side effects or problems in older people. There is no specific information comparing use of ivermectin in the elderly with use in other age groups.

Other medicines—Although certain medicines should not be used together at all, in other cases two different medicines may be used together even if an interaction might occur. In these cases, your doctor may want to change the dose, or other precautions may be necessary. Tell your doctor and pharmacist if you are taking any other prescription or nonprescription (over-the-counter [OTC]) medicine.

Before you begin using any new medicine (prescription or nonprescription) or if you develop any new medical problem while you are using this medicine, check with your doctor, nurse, or pharmacist.

Proper Use of This Medicine

Ivermectin is best taken as a single dose with a full glass (8 ounces) of water on an empty stomach (1 hour before breakfast), unless otherwise directed by your doctor.

To help clear up your infection, *take this medicine exactly as directed.* Your doctor may want you to take another dose every 6 to 12 months.

Your doctor may also prescribe a corticosteroid (a cortisone-like medicine) for certain patients with river blindness, especially those with severe symptoms. This is to help reduce the inflammation caused by the death of the worms. If your doctor prescribes these two medicines together, it is important to take the corticosteroid along with ivermectin. Take them exactly as directed by your doctor. Do not miss any doses.

Storage—To store this medicine:

- Keep out of the reach of children.
- Store away from heat and direct light.
- Do not store in the bathroom, near the kitchen sink, or in other damp places. Heat or moisture may cause the medicine to break down.
- Do not keep outdated medicine or medicine no longer needed. Be sure that any discarded medicine is out of the reach of children.

Precautions While Using This Medicine

It is important that your doctor check your progress at regular visits. This is to help make sure that the infection is cleared up completely. In addition, if you have river blindness (onchocerciasis), your doctor may want you to have your eyes checked by an ophthalmologist (eye doctor).

If your symptoms become worse, check with your doctor.

This medicine may cause some people to become lightheaded. *Make sure you know how you react to this medicine before you drive, use machines, or do anything else that could be dangerous if you are lightheaded.* If these reactions occur, check with your doctor.

Side Effects of This Medicine

Along with its needed effects, a medicine may cause some unwanted effects. The following side effects may go away during treatment as your body adjusts to the medicine. However, check with your doctor if any of the following side effects continue or are bothersome:

Less common

Dizziness; fever; headache; joint or muscle pain; painful and tender glands in neck, armpits, or groin; skin rash or itching; unusual tiredness or weakness

Rare

Lightheadedness while standing up

Other side effects not listed above may also occur in some patients. If you notice any other effects, check with your doctor.

Annual revision: 10/06/92

KANAMYCIN Oral†

A commonly used brand name in the U.S. is Kantrex.

†Not commercially available in Canada.

Description

Oral kanamycin (kan-a-MYE-sin) belongs to the family of medicines called antibiotics. It is used before surgery affecting the bowel to help prevent infection during surgery.

Kanamycin is available only with your doctor's prescription, in the following dosage form:

Oral
- Capsules (U.S.)

It is very important that you read and understand the following information. If any of it causes you special concern, check with your doctor. Also, *if you have any questions* or if you want more information about this medicine or your medical problem, *ask your doctor, nurse, or pharmacist.*

Before Using This Medicine

In deciding to use a medicine, the risks of taking the medicine must be weighed against the good it will do. This is a decision you and your doctor will make. For oral kanamycin, the following should be considered:

Allergies—Tell your doctor if you have ever had any unusual or allergic reaction to oral kanamycin or to any related antibiotics such as amikacin (e.g., Amikin), gentamicin (e.g., Garamycin), kanamycin by injection (e.g., Kantrex), neomycin (e.g., Mycifradin), netilmicin (e.g., Netromycin), streptomycin, or tobramycin (e.g., Nebcin). Also tell your doctor and pharmacist if you are allergic to any other substances, such as foods, preservatives, or dyes.

Pregnancy—Oral kanamycin has not been reported to cause birth defects or other problems in humans.

Breast-feeding—Oral kanamycin has not been reported to cause problems in nursing babies.

Children—Although there is no specific information comparing use of oral kanamycin in children with use in other age groups, this medicine is not expected to cause different side effects or problems in children than it does in adults.

Older adults—Many medicines have not been studied specifically in older people. Therefore, it may not be known whether they work exactly the same way they do in younger adults or if they cause different side effects or problems in older people. There is no specific information comparing use of oral kanamycin in the elderly with use in other age groups.

Other medicines—Although certain medicines should not be used together at all, in other cases two different medicines may be used together even if an interaction might occur. In these cases, your doctor may want to change the dose, or other precautions may be necessary. Tell your doctor or pharmacist if you are taking any other prescription or nonprescription (over-the-counter [OTC]) medicine.

Other medical problems—The presence of other medical problems may affect the use of oral kanamycin. Make sure you tell your doctor if you have any other medical problems, especially:

- Blockage of the bowel—Oral kanamycin should never be used in patients who have a blockage of the bowel
- Eighth-cranial-nerve disease (loss of hearing and/or balance)—Use of oral kanamycin may increase problems related to hearing and/or balance
- Kidney disease or
- Ulcers of the bowel—Use of kanamycin in patients with either condition may cause an increase in side effects

Before you begin using any new medicine (prescription or nonprescription) or if you develop any new medical problem while you are using this medicine, check with your doctor, nurse, or pharmacist.

Proper Use of This Medicine

This medicine may be taken on a full or empty stomach.

Keep taking this medicine for the full time of treatment. Do not miss any doses.

Missed dose—For patients taking *oral kanamycin before any surgery affecting the bowel:*

- If you do miss a dose of this medicine, take it as soon as possible. However, if it is almost time for your next dose, skip the missed dose and go back to your regular dosing schedule. Do not double doses.

Storage—To store this medicine:

- Keep out of the reach of children.
- Store away from heat and direct light.
- Do not store in the bathroom, near the kitchen sink, or in other damp places. Heat and moisture may cause the medicine to break down.
- Do not keep outdated medicine or medicine no longer needed. Be sure that any discarded medicine is out of the reach of children.

Side Effects of This Medicine

Along with its needed effects, a medicine may cause some unwanted effects. Although not all of these side effects may occur, if they do occur they may need medical attention.

Check with your doctor immediately if any of the following side effects occur:

Rare—with long-term use and high doses

Any loss of hearing; clumsiness; dizziness; greatly decreased frequency of urination or amount of urine; increased thirst; ringing or buzzing or a feeling of fullness in the ears; unsteadiness

Other side effects may occur that usually do not need medical attention. These side effects may go away during treatment as your body adjusts to the medicine. However, check with your doctor if any of the following side effects continue or are bothersome:

More common

Diarrhea; nausea or vomiting

Rare—with prolonged treatment

Increased amount of gas; light-colored, frothy, fatty-appearing stools

Other side effects not listed above may also occur in some patients. If you notice any other effects, check with your doctor.

Annual revision: 09/08/92

KAOLIN AND PECTIN Oral

Some commonly used brand names are:

In the U.S.

Kao-tin K-P
Kapectolin K-Pek
K-C

Generic product may also be available.

In Canada

Donnagel-MB Kao-Con

Description

Kaolin (KAY-oh-lin) and pectin (PEK-tin) combination medicine is used to treat diarrhea.

Kaolin is a clay-like powder believed to work by adsorbing the bacteria or germ that may be causing the diarrhea.

This medicine is available without a prescription; however, the product's directions and warnings should be carefully followed. In addition, your doctor may have special instructions on the proper dose or use of kaolin and pectin combination medicine for your medical condition. Kaolin and pectin combination is available in the following dosage form:

Oral

- Oral suspension (U.S. and Canada)

It is very important that you read and understand the following information. If any of it causes you special concern, check with your doctor or pharmacist. Also, *if you have any questions* or if you want more information about this medicine or your medical problem, *ask your doctor, nurse, or pharmacist.*

Before Using This Medicine

If you are taking this medicine without a prescription, carefully read and follow any precautions on the label. For kaolin and pectin combination, the following should be considered:

Pregnancy—This medicine is not absorbed into the body and is not likely to cause problems.

Breast-feeding—This medicine is not absorbed into the body and is not likely to cause problems.

Children—The fluid loss caused by diarrhea may result in a severe condition. For this reason, antidiarrheals must not be given to young children (under 3 years of age) without first checking with their doctor. In older children with diarrhea, antidiarrheals may be used, but it is also very important that a sufficient amount of liquids be given to replace the fluid lost by the body. If you have any questions about this, check with your doctor, nurse, or pharmacist.

Older adults—The fluid loss caused by diarrhea may result in a severe condition. For this reason, elderly persons with diarrhea, in addition to using an antidiarrheal, must receive a sufficient amount of liquids to replace the fluid lost by the body. If you have any questions about this, check with your doctor, nurse, or pharmacist.

Other medicines—Although certain medicines should not be used together at all, in other cases two different medicines may be used together even if an interaction might occur. In these cases, your doctor may want to change the dose, or other precautions may be necessary. Tell your doctor and pharmacist if you are taking any other prescription or nonprescription (over-the-counter [OTC]) medicine.

Other medical problems—The presence of other medical problems may affect the use of kaolin and pectin. Make

sure you tell your doctor if you have any other medical problems, especially:

- Dysentery—This condition may get worse; a different kind of treatment may be needed

Before you begin using any new medicine (prescription or nonprescription) or if you develop any new medical problem while you are using this medicine, check with your doctor, nurse, or pharmacist.

Proper Use of This Medicine

Take this medicine, following the directions in the product package, after each loose bowel movement until the diarrhea is controlled, unless otherwise directed by your doctor.

Importance of diet and fluid intake while treating diarrhea:

- *In addition to using medicine for diarrhea, it is very important that you replace the fluid lost by the body and follow a proper diet.* For the first 24 hours you should drink plenty of clear liquids, such as ginger ale, decaffeinated cola, decaffeinated tea, broth, and gelatin. During the next 24 hours you may eat bland foods, such as cooked cereals, bread, crackers, and applesauce. Fruits, vegetables, fried or spicy foods, bran, candy, and caffeine and alcoholic beverages may make the condition worse.
- If too much fluid has been lost by the body due to the diarrhea, a serious condition may develop. Check with your doctor as soon as possible if any of the following signs of too much fluid loss occur:
  - Decreased urination
  - Dizziness and lightheadedness
  - Dryness of mouth
  - Increased thirst
  - Wrinkled skin

Storage—To store this medicine:

- Keep out of the reach of children.
- Store away from heat and direct light.
- Keep this medicine from freezing.
- Do not keep outdated medicine or medicine no longer needed. Be sure that any discarded medicine is out of the reach of children.

Precautions While Using This Medicine

Check with your doctor if your diarrhea does not stop after 1 or 2 days or if you develop a fever.

If you are taking any other medicine, do not take it within 2 to 3 hours of kaolin and pectin. Taking the medicines together may prevent the other medicine from being absorbed by your body. If you have any questions about this, check with your doctor, nurse, or pharmacist.

Side Effects of This Medicine

Along with its needed effects, a medicine may cause some unwanted effects. No serious side effects have been reported for this medicine. However, this medicine may cause constipation in some patients, especially if they take a lot of it. Check with your doctor as soon as possible if constipation continues or is bothersome.

Other side effects not listed above may also occur in some patients. If you notice any other effects, check with your doctor.

Annual revision: 07/29/91

KAOLIN, PECTIN, BELLADONNA ALKALOIDS, AND OPIUM Systemic†

Some commonly used brand names are:

In the U.S.

Amogel PG
Donnagel-PG
Donnapectolin-PG
Kapectolin PG
Quiagel PG

†Not commercially available in Canada.

Description

Kaolin (KAY-oh-lin), pectin (PEK-tin), belladonna alkaloids (bell-a-DON-a AL-ka-loyds), and opium (OH-pee-um) combination medicine is used to treat diarrhea.

In some states, this medicine is available without a prescription. However, the product's directions and warnings should be carefully followed. In addition, your doctor may have special instructions on the proper dose or use of this medicine for your medical condition. This medicine is available in the following dosage form:

Oral

- Oral suspension (U.S.)

It is very important that you read and understand the following information. If any of it causes you special concern, check with your doctor or pharmacist. Also, *if you have any questions* or if you want more information about this medicine or your medical problem, *ask your doctor, nurse, or pharmacist.*

Before Using This Medicine

If you are taking this medicine without a prescription, carefully read and follow any precautions on the label. For kaolin, pectin, belladonna alkaloids, and opium, the following should be considered:

Allergies—Tell your doctor if you have ever had any unusual or allergic reaction to any of the belladonna alkaloids (atropine, hyoscyamine, scopolamine) or medicines like morphine, codeine, or papaverine. Also, tell your doctor or pharmacist if you are allergic to any other substances, such as foods, preservatives, or dyes.

Pregnancy—This medicine has not been shown to cause problems in humans. However, too much use of opium (contained in this combination medicine) during pregnancy may cause the baby to become dependent on the medicine. This may lead to withdrawal side effects after birth.

Breast-feeding—This medicine has not been reported to cause problems in nursing babies.

Children—Children are especially sensitive to the effects of belladonna alkaloids and opium (contained in this combination medicine). This may increase the chance of side effects during treatment. Also, the fluid loss caused by the diarrhea may result in a severe condition. For these reasons, do not give this medicine for diarrhea to young children (under 6 years of age) without first checking with their doctor. In older children with diarrhea, medicine for diarrhea may be used, but it is also very important that a sufficient amount of liquids be given to replace the fluid lost by the body. If you have any questions about this, check with your doctor, nurse, or pharmacist.

Older adults—Elderly people are especially sensitive to the effects of belladonna alkaloids and opium (contained in this combination medicine). This may increase the chance of side effects during treatment. Also, the fluid loss caused by the diarrhea may result in a severe condition. For this reason, elderly persons should not take this medicine without first checking with their doctor. It is also very important that a sufficient amount of liquids be taken to replace the fluid lost by the body. If you have any questions about this, check with your doctor, nurse, or pharmacist.

Other medicines—Although certain medicines should not be used together at all, in other cases two different medicines may be used together even if an interaction might occur. In these cases, your doctor may want to change the dose, or other precautions may be necessary. When you are taking belladonna alkaloids and opium (contained in this combination medicine), it is especially important that your doctor and pharmacist know if you are taking any of the following:

- Central nervous system (CNS) depressants—Effects, such as drowsiness, of CNS depressants or of belladonna alkaloids and opium may become greater
- Ketoconazole [e.g., Nizoral]—Use of this medicine with ketoconazole may decrease the effectiveness of ketoconazole
- Monoamine oxidase (MAO) inhibitors (furazolidone [e.g., Furoxone], isocarboxazid [e.g., Marplan], phenelzine [e.g., Nardil], procarbazine [e.g., Matulane], tranylcypromine [e.g., Parnate])—Taking belladonna alkaloids while you are taking or within 2 weeks of taking MAO inhibitors may cause an increase in the effects of belladonna alkaloids
- Naltrexone (e.g., Trexan)—Withdrawal side effects may occur in patients who have become addicted to the opium in this combination medicine; also, naltrexone will make this medicine less effective against diarrhea
- Potassium chloride (e.g., Kay Ciel)—Use with belladonna alkaloids may worsen stomach and intestinal problems caused by potassium

Other medical problems—The presence of other medical problems may affect the use of this medicine. Make sure you tell your doctor if you have any other medical problems, especially:

- Alcohol or drug abuse or dependence (history of)—There is a greater chance that this medicine may become habit-forming
- Brain damage (children) or
- Down's syndrome (mongolism) or
- Spastic paralysis (children)—The effects of belladonna alkaloids may be increased
- Colitis or other intestinal disease—A more serious condition may develop with the use of this medicine
- Difficult urination or
- Dryness of the mouth (severe and continuing) or
- Emphysema, asthma, bronchitis, or other chronic lung disease or
- Enlarged prostate or
- Gallbladder disease or gallstones or
- Glaucoma or
- Heart disease or
- Hiatal hernia or
- Irregular heartbeat—The belladonna alkaloids contained in this medicine may make these conditions worse
- Dysentery—This condition may get worse; a different kind of treatment may be needed
- Kidney disease or
- Liver disease—Higher blood levels of the belladonna alkaloids and opium may result, increasing the chance of side effects
- Underactive thyroid—This medicine may cause central nervous system (CNS) depression and breathing problems in patients with this condition

Before you begin using any new medicine (prescription or nonprescription) or if you develop any new medical problem while you are using this medicine, check with your doctor, nurse, or pharmacist.

Proper Use of This Medicine

If this medicine upsets your stomach, you may take it with food.

Take this medicine only as directed on the label or as ordered by your doctor. Do not take more of it, do not take it more often, and do not take it for a long time. If too much is taken, it may become habit-forming.

Importance of diet and fluids while treating diarrhea:

- *In addition to using medicine for diarrhea, it is very important that you replace the fluid lost by the body and follow a proper diet.* For the first 24 hours you should drink plenty of caffeine-free clear liquids, such as ginger ale, decaffeinated cola, decaffeinated tea, broth, and gelatin. During the next 24 hours you may eat bland foods, such as cooked cereals, bread, crackers, and applesauce. Fruits, vegetables, fried or spicy foods, bran, candy, caffeine, and alcoholic beverages may make the condition worse.
- If too much fluid has been lost by the body due to the diarrhea, a serious condition may develop. Check with your doctor as soon as possible if any of the following signs of too much fluid loss occur:

  Decreased urination
  Dizziness and lightheadedness
  Dryness of mouth
  Increased thirst
  Wrinkled skin

Storage—To store this medicine:

- Keep out of the reach of children since overdose is especially dangerous in children.
- Store away from heat and direct light.
- Keep this medicine from freezing.
- Do not keep outdated medicine or medicine no longer needed. Be sure that any discarded medicine is out of the reach of children.

Precautions While Using This Medicine

Check with your doctor if your diarrhea does not stop after 1 or 2 days or if you develop a fever.

This medicine will add to the effects of alcohol and other CNS depressants (medicines that slow down the nervous system, possibly causing drowsiness). Some examples of CNS depressants are antihistamines or medicine for hay fever, other allergies, or colds; sedatives, tranquilizers, or sleeping medicine; prescription pain medicine or narcotics; barbiturates; medicine for seizures; muscle relaxants; or anesthetics, including some dental anesthetics. *Check with your doctor before taking any of the above while you are taking this medicine.*

This medicine may cause some people to become dizzy, drowsy, or less alert than they are normally. Even if taken at bedtime, it may cause some people to feel drowsy or less alert on arising. *Make sure you know how you react to this medicine before you drive, use machines, or do anything else that could be dangerous if you are dizzy or are not alert.*

This medicine may cause your eyes to become more sensitive to light than they are normally. Wearing sunglasses and avoiding too much exposure to bright light may help lessen the discomfort.

This medicine may make you sweat less, causing your body temperature to increase. *Use extra care not to become overheated during exercise or hot weather while you are taking this medicine,* since overheating may result in heat stroke. Also, hot baths or saunas may make you feel dizzy or faint while you are taking this medicine.

This medicine may cause dryness of the mouth, nose, and throat. For temporary relief, use sugarless candy or gum, melt bits of ice in your mouth, or use a saliva substitute. However, if your mouth continues to feel dry for more than 2 weeks, check with your medical doctor or dentist. Continuing dryness of the mouth may increase the chance of dental disease, including tooth decay, gum disease, and fungus infections.

Side Effects of This Medicine

Along with its needed effects, a medicine may cause some unwanted effects. Although not all of these side effects appear very often, when they do occur they may need medical attention.

Check with your doctor immediately if any of the following side effects are severe and occur suddenly since they may be signs of a more severe and dangerous problem with your bowels:

Rare

Bloating; constipation; loss of appetite; stomach pain (severe) with nausea and vomiting

Also, check with your doctor as soon as possible if the following effects occur:

Rare

Eye pain; hallucinations (seeing, hearing, or feeling things that are not there); shortness of breath; skin rash or itching; slow heartbeat; troubled breathing

Other side effects may occur that usually do not need medical attention. These side effects may go away during treatment as your body adjusts to the medicine. However, check with your doctor if any of the following side effects continue or are bothersome:

More common with large doses

Confusion; constipation; decreased sweating; difficult urination; dizziness; drowsiness; dryness of mouth, nose, throat, or skin; faintness; fast heartbeat; headache; increased sweating; lightheadedness; redness or flushing of face; unusual tiredness or weakness

Less common

Blurred vision; decreased sexual ability; increased sensitivity of eyes to sunlight; loss of memory (especially in the elderly); nervousness; reduced sense of taste

Other side effects not listed above may also occur in some patients. If you notice any other effects, check with your doctor.

Annual revision: 05/15/91

KAOLIN, PECTIN, AND PAREGORIC Systemic

Some commonly used brand names are:

In the U.S.
- Kapectolin with Paregoric
- Parepectolin

In Canada
- Donnagel-PG

Description

Kaolin (KAY-oh-lin), pectin (PEK-tin), and paregoric (par-e-GOR-ik) combination medicine is used to treat diarrhea.

In some states, this medicine is available without a prescription; however, the product's directions and warnings should be carefully followed. In addition, your doctor may have special instructions on the proper dose or use of this medicine for your medical condition. It is available in the following dosage form:

Oral
- Oral suspension (U.S. and Canada)

It is very important that you read and understand the following information. If any of it causes you special concern, check with your doctor or pharmacist. Also, *if you have any questions* or if you want more information about this medicine or your medical problem, *ask your doctor, nurse, or pharmacist.*

Before Using This Medicine

If you are taking this medicine without a prescription, carefully read and follow any precautions on the label. For kaolin, pectin, and paregoric, the following should be considered:

Allergies—If you have ever had an unusual or allergic reaction to morphine, codeine, or papaverine. Also, tell your doctor or pharmacist if you are allergic to any other substances, such as foods, preservatives, or dyes.

Pregnancy—This medicine has not been shown to cause problems in humans. However, too much use of opium preparations such as paregoric (contained in this combination medicine) during pregnancy may cause the baby to become dependent on the medicine. This may lead to withdrawal side effects after birth.

Breast-feeding—Although the paregoric in this medicine passes into breast milk, it has not been reported to cause problems in nursing babies.

Children—Children are especially sensitive to the effects of paregoric (contained in this combination medicine). This may increase the chance of side effects during treatment. Also, the fluid loss caused by the diarrhea may result in a severe condition. For this reason, antidiarrheals must not be given to young children (under 3 years of age) without first checking with their doctor. In older children with diarrhea, antidiarrheals may be used, but it is also very important that a sufficient amount of liquids be given to replace the fluid lost by the body. If you have any questions about this, check with your doctor, nurse, or pharmacist.

Older adults—Elderly people are especially sensitive to the effects of paregoric (contained in this combination medicine). This may increase the chance of side effects during treatment. Also, the fluid loss caused by the diarrhea may result in a severe condition. For this reason, elderly persons should not take this medicine without first checking with their doctor. It is also very important that a sufficient amount of liquids be taken to replace the fluid lost by the body. If you have any questions about this, check with your doctor, nurse, or pharmacist.

Other medicines—Although certain medicines should not be used together at all, in other cases two different medicines may be used together even if an interaction might occur. In these cases, your doctor may want to change the dose, or other precautions may be necessary. When you are taking this medicine, it is especially important that your doctor and pharmacist know if you are taking any of the following:

- Central nervous system (CNS) depressants—Effects, such as drowsiness, of CNS depressants or of paregoric may become greater

Other medical problems—The presence of other medical problems may affect the use of this medicine. Make sure you tell your doctor if you have any other medical problems, especially:

- Alcohol or drug abuse or dependence (history of)—There is a greater chance that this medicine may become habit-forming
- Colitis or other intestinal disease—A more serious condition may develop with the use of this medicine

- Diarrhea caused by antibiotics—This medicine may make the diarrhea caused by antibiotics worse or make it last longer
- Difficult urination or
- Emphysema, asthma, bronchitis, or other chronic lung disease, or
- Enlarged prostate or
- Gallbladder disease or gallstones or
- Heart disease or
- Irregular heartbeat—The paregoric contained in this medicine may make these conditions worse
- Dysentery—This condition may get worse; a different kind of treatment may be needed
- Kidney disease or
- Liver disease—In patients with kidney or liver disease, paregoric may accumulate in the body; smaller doses of this medicine may be needed
- Underactive thyroid—This medicine may cause central nervous system (CNS) depression and breathing problems in patients with this condition

Before you begin using any new medicine (prescription or nonprescription) or if you develop any new medical problem while you are using this medicine, check with your doctor, nurse, or pharmacist.

Proper Use of This Medicine

If this medicine upsets your stomach, you may take it with food.

Take this medicine only as directed on the label or as ordered by your doctor. Do not take more of it, do not take it more often, and do not take it for a long time. If too much is taken, it may become habit-forming.

Importance of diet and fluid intake while treating diarrhea:

- *In addition to using medicine for diarrhea, it is very important that you replace the fluid lost by the body and follow a proper diet.* For the first 24 hours you should drink plenty of clear liquids, such as ginger ale, decaffeinated cola, decaffeinated tea, broth, and gelatin. During the next 24 hours you may eat bland foods, such as cooked cereals, bread, crackers, and applesauce. Fruits, vegetables, fried or spicy foods, bran, candy, and caffeine and alcoholic beverages may make the condition worse.
- If too much fluid has been lost by the body due to the diarrhea a serious condition may develop. Check with your doctor as soon as possible if any of the following signs of too much fluid loss occur:

  Decreased urination
  Dizziness and lightheadedness
  Dryness of mouth
  Increased thirst
  Wrinkled skin

Storage—To store this medicine:

- Keep out of the reach of children since overdose is especially dangerous in children.
- Store away from heat and direct light.
- Do not store this medicine in the refrigerator. If it does get cold and you notice any solid particles in it, throw it away.
- Keep this medicine from freezing.
- Keep the container for this medicine tightly closed to prevent the alcohol from evaporating and the medicine from becoming stronger.
- Do not keep outdated medicine or medicine no longer needed. Be sure that any discarded medicine is out of the reach of children.

Precautions While Using This Medicine

Check with your doctor if your diarrhea does not stop after 1 or 2 days or if you develop a fever.

This medicine will add to the effects of alcohol and other CNS depressants (medicines that slow down the nervous system, possibly causing drowsiness). Some examples of CNS depressants are antihistamines or medicine for hay fever, other allergies, or colds; sedatives, tranquilizers, or sleeping medicine; prescription pain medicine or narcotics; barbiturates; medicine for seizures; muscle relaxants; or anesthetics, including some dental anesthetics. *Check with your doctor before taking any of the above while you are taking this medicine.*

This medicine may cause some people to become dizzy, drowsy, or less alert than they are normally. Even if taken at bedtime, it may cause some people to feel drowsy or less alert on arising. *Make sure you know how you react to this medicine before you drive, use machines, or do anything else that could be dangerous if you are dizzy or are not alert.*

Side Effects of This Medicine

Along with its needed effects, a medicine may cause some unwanted effects. Although not all of these side effects appear very often, when they do occur they may require medical attention. *Check with your doctor immediately* if any of the following side effects are severe and occur suddenly since they may indicate a more severe and dangerous problem with your bowels:

Rare

Bloating; constipation (severe); loss of appetite; stomach pain (severe) with nausea and vomiting

Also, check with your doctor as soon as possible if the following effects occur:

Rare

Decreased blood pressure; fast heartbeat; increased sweating; mental depression; redness or flushing of face; shortness of breath, wheezing, or troubled breathing; skin rash, hives, or itching

Other side effects may occur that usually do not need medical attention. These side effects may go away during treatment as your body adjusts to the medicine. However, check with your doctor if any of the following side effects continue or are bothersome:

More common with large doses

Constipation; difficult or painful urination or frequent urge to urinate; dizziness, feeling faint, lightheadedness, unusual tiredness or weakness; drowsiness; nervousness or restlessness

Other side effects not listed above may also occur in some patients. If you notice any other effects, check with your doctor.

Annual revision: 06/12/91

KETOCONAZOLE Systemic

A commonly used brand name in the U.S. and Canada is Nizoral.

Description

Ketoconazole (kee-toe-KON-a-zole) is used to treat fungus infections. It may be given alone or with other medicines that are used on the skin for fungus infections. This medicine may also be used for other problems as determined by your doctor.

Ketoconazole is available only with your doctor's prescription, in the following dosage forms:

Oral

- Suspension (Canada)
- Tablets (U.S. and Canada)

It is very important that you read and understand the following information. If any of it causes you special concern, check with your doctor. Also, *if you have any questions* or if you want more information about this medicine or your medical problem, *ask your doctor, nurse, or pharmacist.*

Before Using This Medicine

In deciding to use a medicine, the risks of taking the medicine must be weighed against the good it will do. This is a decision you and your doctor will make. For ketoconazole, the following should be considered:

Allergies—Tell your doctor if you have ever had any unusual or allergic reaction to ketoconazole, or other related medicines, such as fluconazole, miconazole, or itraconazole. Also tell your doctor and pharmacist if you are allergic to any other substances, such as foods, preservatives, or dyes.

Pregnancy—Studies have not been done in humans. However, studies in rats given doses 10 times the highest recommended human dose have shown that ketoconazole causes webbed toes or fewer toes than normal. When given in higher doses, ketoconazole may also cause other problems in the fetus. Ketoconazole has also been shown to cause difficult labor in rats given doses slightly higher than the highest recommended human dose.

Breast-feeding—Ketoconazole passes into the breast milk and may increase the chance of brain problems in nursing babies. Therefore, you should stop breast-feeding when you begin taking ketoconazole, during treatment, and for 24 to 48 hours after you have finished taking the medicine. During this time the breast milk should be squeezed out or sucked out with a breast pump and thrown away. After the 24 to 48 hours, you may go back to breast-feeding, as directed by your doctor.

Children—This medicine has been tested in a limited number of children 2 years of age and older. In effective doses, the medicine has not been shown to cause different side effects or problems in children than it does in adults.

Older adults—Many medicines have not been studied specifically in older people. Therefore, it may not be known whether they work exactly the same way they do in younger adults or if they cause different side effects or problems in older people. There is no specific information comparing use of ketoconazole in the elderly with use in other age groups.

Other medicines—Although certain medicines should not be used together at all, in other cases two different medicines may be used together even if an interaction might occur. In these cases, your doctor may want to change the dose, or other precautions may be necessary. When you are taking ketoconazole, it is especially important that your doctor and pharmacist know if you are taking any of the following:

- Acetaminophen (e.g., Tylenol) (with long-term, high-dose use) or
- Amiodarone (e.g., Cordarone) or
- Anabolic steroids (nandrolone [e.g., Anabolin], oxandrolone [e.g., Anavar], oxymetholone [e.g., Anadrol], stanozolol [e.g., Winstrol]) or
- Androgens (male hormones) or
- Antithyroid agents (medicine for overactive thyroid) or
- Carmustine (e.g., BiCNU) or
- Chloroquine (e.g., Aralen) or
- Dantrolene (e.g., Dantrium) or

- Daunorubicin (e.g., Cerubidine) or
- Disulfiram (e.g., Antabuse) or
- Divalproex (e.g., Depakote) or
- Estrogens (female hormones) or
- Etretinate (e.g., Tegison) or
- Gold salts (medicine for arthritis) or
- Hydroxychloroquine (e.g., Plaquenil) or
- Mercaptopurine (e.g., Purinethol) or
- Methotrexate (e.g., Mexate) or
- Methyldopa (e.g., Aldomet) or
- Naltrexone (e.g., Trexan) (with long-term, high-dose use) or
- Oral contraceptives (birth control pills) containing estrogen or
- Other anti-infectives by mouth or by injection (medicine for infection) or
- Phenothiazines (acetophenazine [e.g., Tindal], chlorpromazine [e.g., Thorazine], fluphenazine [e.g., Prolixin], mesoridazine [e.g., Serentil], perphenazine [e.g., Trilafon], prochlorperazine [e.g., Compazine], promazine [e.g., Sparine], promethazine [e.g., Phenergan], thioridazine [e.g., Mellaril], trifluoperazine [e.g., Stelazine], triflupromazine [e.g., Vesprin], trimeprazine [e.g., Temaril]) or
- Phenytoin (e.g., Dilantin) or
- Plicamycin (e.g., Mithracin) or
- Valproic acid (e.g., Depakene)—Use of these medicines with ketoconazole may increase the chance of side effects affecting the liver
- Amantadine (e.g., Symmetrel) or
- Antacids or
- Anticholinergics (medicine for abdominal or stomach spasms or cramps) or
- Antidepressants (medicine for depression) or
- Antidyskinetics (medicine for Parkinson's disease or other conditions affecting control of muscles) or
- Antihistamines or
- Antipsychotics (medicine for mental illness) or
- Buclizine (e.g., Bucladin) or
- Cimetidine (e.g., Tagamet) or
- Cyclizine (e.g., Marezine) or
- Cyclobenzaprine (e.g., Flexeril) or
- Disopyramide (e.g., Norpace) or
- Famotidine (e.g., Pepcid) or
- Flavoxate (e.g., Urispas) or
- Ipratropium (e.g., Atrovent) or
- Meclizine (e.g., Antivert) or
- Methylphenidate (e.g., Ritalin) or
- Nizatidine (e.g., Axid) or
- Omeprazole (e.g., Prilosac) or
- Orphenadrine (e.g., Norflex) or
- Oxybutynin (e.g., Ditropan) or
- Procainamide (e.g., Pronestyl) or
- Promethazine (e.g., Phenergan) or
- Quinidine (e.g., Quinidex) or
- Ranitidine (e.g., Zantac) or
- Trimeprazine (e.g., Temaril)—Use of any of these medicines with ketoconazole may decrease the effects of ketoconazole
- Carbamazepine (e.g., Tegretol)—Use of carbamazepine with ketoconazole may decrease the effects of ketoconazole or increase side effects affecting the liver
- Cyclosporine (e.g., Sandimmune)—Use with ketoconazole may increase the chance of side effects of cyclosporine
- Dideoxyinosine (e.g., ddI, Videx)—Use of dideoxyinosine with ketoconazole may decrease the effects of ketoconazole
- Isoniazid or
- Rifampin—Use of isoniazid or rifampin with ketoconazole may decrease the effects of ketoconazole
- Terfenadine (e.g., Seldane)—Use of terfenadine with ketoconazole may increase the chance for heart problems, such as an irregular heartbeat

Other medical problems—The presence of other medical problems may affect the use of ketoconazole. Make sure you tell your doctor if you have any other medical problems, especially:

- Achlorhydria (absence of stomach acid) or
- Hypochlorhydria (decreased amount of stomach acid)—Ketoconazole may not be absorbed from the stomach as well in patients who have low or no stomach acid
- Alcohol abuse (or history of) or
- Liver disease—Alcohol abuse or liver disease may increase the chance of side effects caused by ketoconazole

Before you begin using any new medicine (prescription or nonprescription) or if you develop any new medical problem while you are using this medicine, check with your doctor, nurse, or pharmacist.

Proper Use of This Medicine

This medicine may be taken with a meal or snack.

For patients taking the *oral liquid form of ketoconazole:*

- Use a specially marked measuring spoon or other device to measure each dose accurately. The average household teaspoon may not hold the right amount of liquid.

If you have achlorhydria (absence of stomach acid) or hypochlorhydria (decreased amount of stomach acid), your doctor may want you to dissolve each tablet in a teaspoonful of weak hydrochloric acid solution to help you absorb the medicine better. Your doctor or pharmacist can prepare the solution for you. After you dissolve the tablet in the acid solution, add this mixture to a small amount (1 or 2 teaspoonfuls) of water in a glass. Drink the mixture through a plastic or glass drinking straw. Place the straw behind your teeth, as far back in your mouth as you can. This will keep the acid from harming your teeth. Be sure to drink all the liquid to get the full dose of medicine. Then drink about ½ glass of water, swish it around in your mouth, and swallow it.

To help clear up your infection completely, *it is very important that you keep taking this medicine for the full time of treatment,* even if your symptoms begin to clear up or you begin to feel better after a few days. Since fungus infections may be very slow to clear up, you may have to continue taking this medicine every day for as long as 6 months to a year or more. Some fungus infections never clear up completely and require continuous treatment. If you stop taking this medicine too soon, your symptoms may return.

This medicine works best when there is a constant amount in the blood or urine. *To help keep the amount constant, do not miss any doses. Also, it is best to take each dose at the same time every day.* If you need help in planning the best time to take your medicine, check with your doctor, nurse, or pharmacist.

Missed dose—If you do miss a dose of this medicine, take it as soon as possible. This will help to keep a constant amount of medicine in the blood or urine. However, if it is almost time for your next dose, skip the missed dose and go back to your regular dosing schedule. Do not double doses.

Storage—To store this medicine:

- Keep out of the reach of children.
- Store away from heat and direct light.
- Do not store the tablet form of this medicine in the bathroom, near the kitchen sink, or in other damp places. Heat or moisture may cause the medicine to break down.
- Keep the oral liquid form of this medicine from freezing.
- Do not keep outdated medicine or medicine no longer needed. Be sure that any discarded medicine is out of the reach of children.

Precautions While Using This Medicine

It is important that your doctor check your progress at regular visits. This will allow your doctor to check for any unwanted effects.

If your symptoms do not improve within a few weeks, or if they become worse, check with your doctor.

If you are taking antacids, cimetidine (e.g., Tagamet), famotidine (e.g., Pepcid), nizatidine (e.g., Axid), ranitidine (e.g., Zantac), or omeprazole (e.g., Prilosec), while you are taking ketoconazole, take them at least 2 hours after you take ketoconazole. If you take these medicines at the same time that you take ketoconazole, they will keep ketoconazole from working properly.

Liver problems may be more likely to occur if you drink alcoholic beverages while you are taking this medicine. Alcoholic beverages may also cause stomach pain, nausea, vomiting, headache, or flushing or redness of the face. Other alcohol-containing preparations (for example, elixirs, cough syrups, tonics) may also cause problems. These problems may occur for at least a day after you stop taking ketoconazole. Therefore, *you should not drink alcoholic beverages while you are taking this medicine and for at least a day after you stop taking it.*

This medicine may cause your eyes to become more sensitive to light than they are normally. Wearing sunglasses and avoiding too much exposure to bright light may help lessen the discomfort.

This medicine may also cause some people to become dizzy, drowsy, or less alert than they are normally. *Make sure you know how you react to this medicine before you drive, use machines, or do anything else that could be dangerous if you are dizzy or are not alert.* If these reactions are especially bothersome, check with your doctor.

Side Effects of This Medicine

Along with its needed effects, a medicine may cause some unwanted effects. Although not all of these effects may occur, if they do occur they may need medical attention.

Check with your doctor immediately if any of the following side effects occur:

Rare

Dark or amber urine; loss of appetite; pale stools; skin rash or itching; stomach pain; unusual tiredness or weakness; yellow eyes or skin

Other side effects may occur that usually do not need medical attention. These side effects may go away during treatment as your body adjusts to the medicine. However, check with your doctor if any of the following side effects continue or are bothersome:

Less common

Diarrhea; nausea or vomiting

Rare

Decreased sexual ability in males; dizziness; drowsiness; enlargement of the breasts in males; headache; increased sensitivity of the eyes to light; irregular menstrual periods

Other side effects not listed above may also occur in some patients. If you notice any other effects, check with your doctor.

Annual revision: 09/21/92

KETOCONAZOLE Topical

Some commonly used brand names in the U.S. and Canada are Nizoral Cream and Nizoral Shampoo.

Description

Ketoconazole (kee-toe-KOE-na-zole) is used to treat infections caused by a fungus or yeast. It works by killing the fungus or yeast or preventing its growth.

Ketoconazole cream is used to treat:

- Athlete's foot (tinea pedis; ringworm of the foot);
- Ringworm of the body (tinea corporis);
- Ringworm of the groin (tinea cruris; jock itch);
- Seborrheic dermatitis;
- "Sun fungus" (tinea versicolor; pityriasis versicolor); and
- Yeast infection of the skin (cutaneous candidiasis).

Ketoconazole shampoo is used to treat dandruff.

This medicine may also be used for other fungus infections of the skin as determined by your doctor.

Ketoconazole is available only with your doctor's prescription, in the following dosage forms:

Topical
- Cream (U.S. and Canada)
- Shampoo (U.S. and Canada)

It is very important that you read and understand the following information. If any of it causes you special concern, check with your doctor. Also, *if you have any questions* or if you want more information about this medicine or your medical problem, *ask your doctor, nurse, or pharmacist.*

Before Using This Medicine

In deciding to use a medicine, the risks of using the medicine must be weighed against the good it will do. This is a decision you and your doctor will make. For topical ketoconazole, the following should be considered:

Allergies—Tell your doctor if you have ever had any unusual or allergic reaction to ketoconazole, miconazole or other imidazoles, or sulfites. The cream form of ketoconazole contains sulfites. Also tell your doctor and pharmacist if you are allergic to any other substances, such as preservatives or dyes.

Pregnancy—Ketoconazole has not been studied in pregnant women. However, studies in animals have shown that ketoconazole causes birth defects or other problems. Before using this medicine, make sure your doctor knows if you are pregnant or if you may become pregnant.

Breast-feeding—It is not known whether topical ketoconazole, used on a regular basis, is absorbed into the mother's body enough to pass into the breast milk. However, this medicine was not absorbed through the skin after a single dose. Therefore, it is unlikely to cause problems in nursing babies.

Children—Studies on this medicine have been done only in adult patients, and there is no specific information comparing use of this medicine in children with use in other age groups.

Older adults—Many medicines have not been studied specifically in older people. Therefore, it may not be known whether they work exactly the same way they do in younger adults or if they cause different side effects or problems in older people. There is no specific information comparing use of topical ketoconazole in the elderly with use in other age groups.

Other medicines—Although certain medicines should not be used together at all, in other cases two different medicines may be used together even if an interaction might occur. In these cases, your doctor may want to change the dose, or other precautions may be necessary. Tell your doctor and pharmacist if you are using any other prescription or nonprescription (over-the-counter [OTC]) medicine.

Before you begin using any new medicine (prescription or nonprescription) or if you develop any new medical problem while you are using this medicine, check with your doctor, nurse, or pharmacist.

Proper Use of This Medicine

Keep this medicine away from the eyes.

For patients using the *cream form* of this medicine:

- Apply enough ketoconazole cream to cover the affected and surrounding skin areas, and rub in gently.
- To help clear up your infection completely, *it is very important that you keep using ketoconazole cream for the full time of treatment,* even if your symptoms begin to clear up after a few days. Since fungus or yeast infections may be very slow to clear up, you may have to continue using this medicine every day for up to several weeks. If you stop using this medicine too soon, your symptoms may return. *Do not miss any doses.*

For patients using the *shampoo form* of this medicine:

- Wet your hair and scalp well with water.
- Apply enough shampoo to work up a good lather and gently massage it over your entire scalp for about 1 minute.

- Rinse your hair and scalp with warm water.
- Repeat application, then leave the shampoo on your scalp for 3 minutes more.
- Rinse your hair and scalp well with warm water, and dry your hair.

Dosing—The dose of topical ketoconazole will be different for different patients. *Follow your doctor's orders or the directions on the label.* The following information includes only the average doses of topical ketoconazole. *If your dose is different, do not change it* unless your doctor tells you to do so.

The number of doses you use each day, the time allowed between doses, and the length of time you use the medicine depend on the medical problem for which you are using topical ketoconazole.

- For *cream* dosage form:
  —For cutaneous candidiasis, tinea corporis, tinea cruris, tinea pedis, or pityriasis versicolor:
    - Adults—Apply once a day to the affected skin and surrounding area.
    - Children—Use and dose must be determined by your doctor.

  —For seborrheic dermatitis:
    - Adults—Apply two times a day to the affected skin and surrounding area.
    - Children—Use and dose must be determined by your doctor.
- For *shampoo* dosage form:
  —For dandruff:
    - Adults—Use every 4 days for 4 weeks. Then use once every 1 or 2 weeks to keep dandruff under control.
    - Children—Use and dose must be determined by your doctor.

Missed dose—If you miss a dose of this medicine, apply it as soon as possible. However, if it is almost time for your next dose, skip the missed dose and go back to your regular dosing schedule.

Storage—To store this medicine:

- Keep out of the reach of children.
- Store away from heat and direct light.
- Keep the medicine from freezing.
- Do not keep outdated medicine or medicine no longer needed. Be sure that any discarded medicine is out of the reach of children.

Precautions While Using This Medicine

For patients using the *cream form* of this medicine:

- If your skin problem does not improve within 2 to 4 weeks, or if it becomes worse, check with your doctor.
- *To help clear up your infection completely and to help make sure it does not return, good health habits are also required.*
- For patients using ketoconazole cream for *athlete's foot* (tinea pedis; ringworm of the foot), the following instructions will help keep the feet cool and dry.

  —Avoid wearing socks made from wool or synthetic materials (for example, rayon or nylon). Instead, wear clean, cotton socks and change them daily or more often if your feet sweat a lot.

  —Wear sandals or well-ventilated shoes (for examples, shoes with holes).

  —Use a bland, absorbent powder (for example, talcum powder) or an antifungal powder between the toes, on the feet, and in socks and shoes one or two times a day. It is best to use the powder between the times you use ketoconazole cream.

  If you have any questions about these instructions, check with your doctor, nurse, or pharmacist.
- For patients using ketoconazole cream for *ringworm of the groin* (tinea cruris; jock itch), the following instructions will help reduce chafing and irritation and will also help keep the groin area cool and dry.

  —Avoid wearing underwear that is tight-fitting or made from synthetic materials (for example, rayon or nylon). Instead, wear loose-fitting, cotton underwear.

  —Use a bland, absorbent powder (for example, talcum powder) or an antifungal powder on the skin. It is best to use the powder between the times you use ketoconazole cream.

  If you have any questions about these instructions, check with your doctor, nurse or pharmacist.

Side Effects of This Medicine

Along with its needed effects, a medicine may cause some unwanted effects. Although not all of these side effects may occur, if they do occur they may need medical attention.

Check with your doctor as soon as possible if any of the following side effects occur:

More common

Itching, stinging, or irritation not present before use of this medicine

Other side effects not listed above may also occur in some patients. If you notice any other effects, check with your doctor.

Annual revision: 06/21/93

KETOROLAC Systemic

Some commonly used brand names are:

In the U.S.
Toradol*IM* Toradol*ORAL*

In Canada
Toradol Toradol*IM*

Description

Ketorolac (kee-TOE-role-ak) is used to relieve pain. It belongs to the group of medicines called anti-inflammatory analgesics. Ketorolac is not a narcotic and is not habit-forming. It will not cause physical or mental dependence, as narcotics can. However, ketorolac is sometimes used together with a narcotic to provide better pain relief than either medicine used alone.

Ketorolac is available only with your doctor's prescription, in the following dosage forms:

Oral
- Tablets (U.S. and Canada)

Parenteral
- Injection (U.S. and Canada)

It is very important that you read and understand the following information. If any of it causes you special concern, check with your doctor. Also, *if you have any questions* or if you want more information about this medicine or your medical problem, *ask your doctor, nurse, or pharmacist.*

Before Using This Medicine

In deciding to use a medicine, the risks of taking the medicine must be weighed against the good it will do. This is a decision you and your doctor will make. For ketorolac, the following should be considered:

Allergies—Tell your doctor if you have ever had any unusual or allergic reaction to ketorolac or to any of the following medicines:

Aspirin or other salicylates
Diclofenac (e.g., Voltaren)
Diflunisal (e.g., Dolobid)
Etodolac (e.g., Lodine)
Fenoprofen (e.g., Nalfon)
Floctafenine (e.g., Idarac)
Flurbiprofen, oral (e.g., Ansaid)
Ibuprofen (e.g., Motrin)
Indomethacin (e.g., Indocin)
Ketoprofen (e.g., Orudis)
Meclofenamate (e.g., Meclomen)
Mefenamic acid (e.g., Ponstel)
Nabumetone (e.g., Relafen)
Naproxen (e.g., Naprosyn)
Oxaprozin (e.g., Daypro)
Oxyphenbutazone (e.g., Tandearil)
Phenylbutazone (e.g., Butazolidin)
Piroxicam (e.g., Feldene)
Sulindac (e.g., Clinoril)
Suprofen (e.g., Suprol)
Tenoxicam (e.g., Mobiflex)
Tiaprofenic acid (e.g., Surgam)
Tolmetin (e.g., Tolectin)
Zomepirac (e.g., Zomax)

Also tell your doctor and pharmacist if you are allergic to any other substances, such as foods, preservatives, or dyes.

Pregnancy—Studies on birth defects with ketorolac have not been done in pregnant women. However, it crosses the placenta. There is a chance that regular use of ketorolac during the last few months of pregnancy may cause unwanted effects on the heart or blood flow of the fetus or newborn baby. Ketorolac has not been shown to cause birth defects in animal studies. However, animal studies have shown that, if taken late in pregnancy, ketorolac may increase the length of pregnancy, prolong labor, or cause other problems during delivery.

Breast-feeding—Small amounts of ketorolac pass into the breast milk. Mothers who are taking this medicine and who wish to breast-feed should discuss this with their doctor.

Children—Studies on this medicine have been done only in adult patients, and there is no specific information comparing use of ketorolac in children with use in other age groups.

Older adults—Stomach or intestinal problems, swelling of the face, feet, or lower legs, or sudden decrease in the amount of urine, may be especially likely to occur in elderly patients, who are usually more sensitive than younger adults to the effects of anti-inflammatory analgesics such as ketorolac. Also, elderly people are more likely than younger adults to get very sick if the medicine causes stomach problems. Studies in older adults have shown that ketorolac stays in the body longer than it does in younger people. Your doctor will consider this when deciding on how much ketorolac should be given for each dose and how often it should be given.

Other medicines—Although certain medicines should not be used together at all, in other cases two different medicines may be used together even if an interaction might occur. In these cases, your doctor may want to change the dose, or other precautions may be necessary. When you are using ketorolac, it is especially important that your doctor and pharmacist know if you are taking any of the following:

- Anticoagulants (blood thinners) or
- Cefamandole (e.g., Mandol) or
- Cefoperazone (e.g., Cefobid) or
- Cefotetan (e.g., Cefotan) or
- Heparin or
- Moxalactam (e.g., Moxam) or

- Plicamycin (e.g., Mithracin) or
- Valproic acid (e.g., Depakene)—Use of any of these medicines together with ketorolac may increase the chance of bleeding
- Aspirin or other salicylates or
- Other medicine for inflammation or pain, except narcotics—The chance of serious side effects may be increased
- Lithium (e.g., Lithane) or
- Methotrexate (e.g., Mexate)—Higher blood levels of lithium or methotrexate and an increased chance of side effects may occur
- Probenecid (e.g., Benemid)—Higher blood levels of ketorolac and an increased chance of side effects may occur

Other medical problems—The presence of other medical problems may affect the use of ketorolac. Make sure you tell your doctor if you smoke tobacco or if you have any other medical problems, especially:

- Alcohol abuse or
- Diabetes mellitus (sugar diabetes) or
- Edema (swelling of face, fingers, feet or lower legs caused by too much fluid in the body) or
- Kidney disease or
- Liver disease (severe) or
- Systemic lupus erythematosus (SLE)—The chance of serious side effects may be increased
- Asthma or
- Colitis, stomach ulcer, or other stomach problems or
- Heart disease or
- High blood pressure—Ketorolac may make your condition worse
- Hemophilia or other bleeding problems—Ketorolac may increase the chance of serious bleeding

Before you begin using any new medicine (prescription or nonprescription) or if you develop any new medical problem while you are using this medicine, check with your doctor, nurse, or pharmacist.

Proper Use of This Medicine

For patients taking *ketorolac tablets:*

- To lessen stomach upset, ketorolac tablets should be taken with food (a meal or a snack) or with an antacid. However, your doctor may want you to take the first few doses 30 minutes before meals or 2 hours after meals. This helps the medicine work a little faster when you first begin to take it.
- Take this medicine with a full glass of water. Also, do not lie down for about 15 to 30 minutes after taking it. This helps to prevent irritation that may lead to trouble in swallowing.

For patients using *ketorolac injection*:

- Medicines given by injection are sometimes used at home. If you will be using ketorolac at home, your doctor or nurse will teach you how the injections are to be given. You will also have a chance to practice giving injections. *Be certain that you understand exactly how the medicine is to be injected.*

For safe and effective use of this medicine, do not use more of it, do not use it more often, and do not use it for a longer time than ordered by your doctor. Using too much of this medicine increases the chance of unwanted effects, especially in elderly patients.

Dosing—The dose of ketorolac will be different for different patients. *Follow your doctor's orders or the directions on the label.* The following information includes only the average doses of ketorolac. *If your dose is different, do not change it* unless your doctor tells you to do so.

- For *oral* dosage form (tablets):
  - —For pain:
    - Adults—One 10-milligram (mg) tablet four times a day, four to six hours apart. Your doctor may want you to take two tablets for the first dose only. This helps the medicine start working a little faster.
    - Children—Use and dose must be determined by your doctor.
- For *injection* dosage form:
  - —For pain:
    - Adults—15 or 30 mg four times a day, at least 4 to 6 hours apart. This amount of medicine may be contained in 1 mL or in one-half (0.5) mL of the injection, depending on the strength. Sometimes, larger amounts are used for the first dose only. This helps the medicine start working a little faster.
    - Children—Use and dose must be determined by your doctor.

Missed dose—If you have been directed to use this medicine according to a regular schedule, and you miss a dose, use it as soon as possible. However, if it is almost time for your next dose, skip the missed dose and go back to your regular dosing schedule. Do not double doses.

Storage—To store this medicine:

- Keep out of the reach of children.
- Store away from heat and direct light.
- Do not store ketorolac tablets in the bathroom, near the kitchen sink, or in other damp places. Heat or moisture may cause the medicine to break down.
- Keep the injection form of ketorolac from freezing. Do not store it in the refrigerator.
- Do not keep outdated medicine or medicine no longer needed. Be sure that any discarded medicine is out of the reach of children.

Precautions While Using This Medicine

Taking certain other medicines together with ketorolac may increase the chance of unwanted effects. The risk will depend on how much of each medicine you take every day, and on how long you take the medicines together. Therefore, do not take acetaminophen (e.g., Tylenol) or aspirin or other salicylates together with ketorolac for more than a few days, unless otherwise directed by your medical doctor or dentist. Also, *do not take any of the following medicines together with ketorolac, unless your medical doctor or dentist has directed you to do so and is following your progress*:

- Diclofenac (e.g., Voltaren)
- Diflunisal (e.g., Dolobid)
- Etodolac (e.g., Lodine)
- Fenoprofen (e.g., Nalfon)
- Floctafenine (e.g., Idarac)
- Flurbiprofen, oral (e.g., Ansaid)
- Ibuprofen (e.g., Motrin)
- Indomethacin (e.g., Indocin)
- Ketoprofen (e.g., Orudis)
- Meclofenamate (e.g., Meclomen)
- Mefenamic acid (e.g., Ponstel)
- Nabumetone (e.g., Relafen)
- Naproxen (e.g., Naprosyn)
- Oxaprozin (e.g., Daypro)
- Phenylbutazone (e.g., Butazolidin)
- Piroxicam (e.g., Feldene)
- Sulindac (e.g., Clinoril)
- Tenoxicam (e.g., Mobiflex)
- Tiaprofenic acid (e.g., Surgam)
- Tolmetin (e.g., Tolectin)

Ketorolac may cause some people to become dizzy or drowsy. If either of these side effects occurs, *do not drive, use machines, or do anything else that could be dangerous if you are not alert.*

Side Effects of This Medicine

Along with its needed effects, a medicine may cause some unwanted effects. Although not all of these side effects may occur, if they do occur they may need medical attention.

Stop using this medicine and check with your doctor immediately if any of the following side effects occur:

Rare

Bleeding or crusting sores on lips; blue lips and fingernails; chest pain; convulsions; fainting; shortness of breath, fast, irregular, noisy or troubled breathing, tightness in chest, and/or wheezing; vomiting of blood or material that looks like coffee grounds

Also, check with your doctor as soon as possible if any of the following side effects occur:

Less common

Swelling of face, fingers, lower legs, ankles, and/or feet; weight gain (unusual)

Rare

Abdominal or stomach pain, cramping, or burning (severe); bleeding from rectum or bloody or black, tarry stools; bloody or cloudy urine; bruising (not at place of injection) or small red spots on skin; burning, red, tender, thick, scaly, or peeling skin; decrease in amount of urine (sudden); fever with or without chills or sore throat; hallucinations (seeing, hearing, or feeling things that are not there); hives or itching of skin; increased blood pressure; increased sweating; muscle cramps or pain; nausea, heartburn, and/or indigestion (severe and continuing); nosebleeds; pain in lower back and/or side; puffiness or swelling of the eyelids or around the eyes; skin rash; sores, ulcers, or white spots on lips or in mouth; swollen and/or painful glands; swollen tongue; thirst (continuing); unusual tiredness or weakness

Other side effects may occur that usually do not need medical attention. These side effects may go away during treatment as your body adjusts to the medicine. However, check with your doctor if any of the following side effects continue or are bothersome:

More common

Abdominal or stomach pain (mild or moderate); bruising at place of injection; drowsiness; indigestion; nausea

Less common or rare

Bloating or gas; burning or pain at place of injection; constipation; diarrhea; dizziness; feeling of fullness in abdominal or stomach area; headache; increased sweating; vomiting

Other side effects not listed above may also occur in some patients. If you notice any other effects, check with your doctor.

Annual revision: 05/14/93

LAXATIVES Oral

Some commonly used brand names and other names are:

In the U.S.—

Afko-Lube[43]
Afko-Lube Lax[37]
Agoral[24]
Agoral Marshmallow[24]
Agoral Plain[22]
Agoral Raspberry[24]
Alaxin[44]
Alophen[33]
Alphamul[31]
Bilagog[17]
Bilax[39]
Bisac-Evac[26]
Black-Draught[27]
Black-Draught Lax-Senna[34]
Caroid Laxative[30]
Carter's Little Pills[26]
Cholac[13]
Cholan-HMB[32]
Chronulac[13]
Cillium[5]
Citrate of magnesia[14]
Citroma[14]
Citro-Nesia[14]
Citrucel Orange Flavor[3]
Citrucel Sugar-Free Orange Flavor[3]
Colace[43]
Colax[41]
Cologel[3]
Constilac[13]
Constulose[13]
Correctol[41]
Correctol Extra Gentle[43]
Dacodyl[26]
Decholin[32]
Deficol[26]
Dialose[43]
Dialose Plus[41]
Diocto[43]
Diocto-C[37]
Diocto-K[43]
Diocto-K Plus[37]
Dioctyl sodium sulfosuccinate[43]
Dioeze[43]
Diosuccin[43]
Dio-Sul[43]
Diothron[37]
Disanthrol[37]
Disolan[41]
Disolan Forte[11]
Disonate[43]
Disoplex[12]
Di-Sosul[43]
Di-Sosul Forte[37]
Docucal-P[41]
Docu-K Plus[37]
Doss[43]
Doxidan[41]
Doxinate[43]
DSMC Plus[37]
D-S-S[43]
D-S-S plus[37]
Dulcolax[26]
Duosol[43]
Duphalac[13]
Effer-syllium[6]
Emulsoil[31]
Enulose[13]
Epsom salts[17]
Equalactin[4]
Espotabs[33]
Evac-U-Gen[33]
Evac-U-Lax[33]
Ex-Lax[33]
Ex-Lax Maximum Relief Formula[33]
Ex-Lax Pills[33]
Extra Gentle Ex-Lax[41]
Feen-a-Mint[41]
Feen-a-Mint Gum[33]
Feen-a-Mint Pills[41]
Fiberall[6]
Fibercon[4]
FiberNorm[4]
Fleet Flavored Castor Oil[31]
Fleet Laxative[26]
Fleet Phospho-Soda[18]
Fletcher's Castoria[34]
Generlac[13]
Gentlax S[42]
Gentle Nature[35]
Haley's M-O[19]
Hepahydrin[32]
Hydrocil Instant[6]
Kasof[43]
Kellogg's Castor Oil[31]
Kondremul Plain[22]
Kondremul with Cascara[23]
Kondremul with Phenolphthalein[24]
Konsyl[5]
Konsyl-D[6]
Konsyl-Orange[6]
Laxinate 100[43]
Liqui-Doss[22]
Liquid petrolatum[22]
Mag-Ox 400[16]
Maltsupex[1]
Maox[16]
Medilax[33]
Metamucil[6]
Metamucil Apple Crisp Fiber Wafers[6]
Metamucil Cinnamon Spice Fiber Wafers[6]
Metamucil Orange Flavor[6]
Metamucil Sugar-Free, Lemon-Lime Flavor[6]
Metamucil Sugar-Free, Orange Flavor[6]
Metamucil Sunrise Smooth, Citrus Flavor[6]
Metamucil Sunrise Smooth, Orange Flavor[6]
Metamucil Sunrise Smooth Sugar-Free, Citrus Flavor[6]
Metamucil Sunrise Smooth Sugar-Free, Orange Flavor[6]
Metamucil Sunrise Smooth Sugar-Free, Regular Flavor[6]
Milkinol[22]
Mitrolan[4]
Modane[33]
Modane Bulk[6]
Modane Soft[43]
Molatoc[43]
Molatoc-CST[37]
Naturacil[5]
Nature's Remedy[29]
Neo-Cultol[22]
Neolax[39]
Neoloid[31]
Nujol[22]
Nytilax[35]
Perdiem[8]
Perdiem Plain[5]
Peri-Colace[37]
Petrogalar Plain[22]
Phenolax[33]
Phenolphthalein Petrogalar[24]
Phillips' Gelcaps[41]
Phillips' LaxCaps[41]
Phillips' Milk of Magnesia[15]
Poloxalkol[44]
Portalac[13]
Pro-Cal-Sof[43]
Pro-Lax[6]
Prompt[10]
Pro-Sof[43]
Pro-Sof Liquid Concentrate[43]
Pro-Sof Plus[37]
Purge[31]
Regulace[37]
Regulax SS[43]
Reguloid Natural[6]
Reguloid Orange[6]
Regutol[43]
Sal hepatica[18]
Senexon[34]
Senokot[34]
Senokot-S[42]
Senolax[34]
Serutan[6]
Serutan Toasted Granules[7]
Siblin[5]
Stulex[43]
Surfak[43]
Syllact[5]
Syllamalt[2]
Trilax[40]
Versabran[6]
V-Lax[6]
X-Prep Liquid[34]
Zymenol[22]

In Canada—

Agarol[21]
Bisacolax[26]
Chronulac[13]
Citro-Mag[14]
Colace[43]
Doss[38]
Doxidan[41]
Dulcodos[36]
Dulcolax[26]
Ex-Lax[33]
Ex-Lax Pills[33]
Extra Gentle Ex-Lax[41]
Fibrepur[6]
Glysennid[35]
Karacil[6]
Kondremul[22]
Lactulax[13]
Lansoÿl[22]
Laxit[26]
Magnolax[20]
Metamucil[6]
Metamucil Instant Mix, Orange Flavor[6]
Metamucil Orange Flavor[6]
Metamucil Sugar Free[6]
Metamucil Sugar-Free, Orange Flavor[6]
Mitrolan[4]
Peri-Colace[37]
Phillips' Magnesia Tablets[15]
Phillips' Milk of Magnesia[15]
Prodiem[9]
Prodiem Plain[6]
Regulex[43]
Regulex-D[38]
Senokot[34]
Senokot-S[42]
Siblin[5]

Note: For quick reference the following laxatives are numbered to match the corresponding brand names.

Bulk-forming laxatives—

1. Malt Soup Extract
2. Malt Soup Extract and Psyllium (SILL-i-yum)
3. Methylcellulose (meth-ill-SELL-yoo-lose)‡
4. Polycarbophil (pol-i-KAR-boe-fil)
5. Psyllium
6. Psyllium Hydrophilic Mucilloid (hye-droe-FILL-ik MYOO-sill-oid)
7. Psyllium Hydrophilic Mucilloid and Carboxymethylcellulose (kar-box-ee-meth-ill-SELL-yoo-lose)

Bulk-forming and stimulant combinations—

8. Psyllium and Senna
9. Psyllium Hydrophilic Mucilloid and Senna
10. Psyllium Hydrophilic Mucilloid and Sennosides

Bulk-forming, stimulant, and stool softener (emollient) combinations—

11. Carboxymethylcellulose, Casanthranol (ka-SAN-thra-nole), and Docusate (DOK-yoo-sate)

Bulk-forming and stool softener (emollient) combinations—

12. Carboxymethylcellulose and Docusate

Hyperosmotic laxatives—Lactulose:

13. Lactulose

Hyperosmotic laxatives—Saline:

14. Magnesium Citrate (mag-NEE-zhum SI-trate)‡
15. Magnesium Hydroxide‡
16. Magnesium Oxide
17. Magnesium Sulfate (SUL-fate)‡
18. Sodium Phosphate (SOE-dee-um FOS-fate)‡

Hyperosmotic and lubricant combinations—

19. Milk of Magnesia and Mineral Oil
20. Milk of Magnesia, Mineral Oil, and Glycerin

Hyperosmotic, lubricant, and stimulant combinations—

21. Mineral Oil, Glycerin, and Phenolphthalein (fee-nole-THAY-leen)

Lubricant laxatives—

22. Mineral Oil‡

Lubricant and stimulant combinations—

23. Mineral Oil and Cascara (kas-KAR-a) Sagrada
24. Mineral Oil and Phenolphthalein
25. Product not available

Stimulant laxatives—

26. Bisacodyl (bis-a-KOE-dill)‡
27. Casanthranol

28. Cascara Sagrada‡
29. Cascara Sagrada and Aloe
30. Cascara Sagrada and Phenolphthalein
31. Castor (KAS-tor) Oil‡
32. Dehydrocholic (dee-hye-droe-KOE-lik) Acid‡
33. Phenolphthalein
34. Senna
35. Sennosides

Stimulant and stool softener (emollient) combinations—

36. Bisacodyl and Docusate
37. Casanthranol and Docusate‡
38. Danthron and Docusate
39. Dehydrocholic Acid and Docusate
40. Dehydrocholic Acid, Docusate, and Phenolphthalein
41. Docusate and Phenolphthalein
42. Senna and Docusate

Stool softener (emollient) laxatives—

43. Docusate‡
44. Poloxamer 188 (pol-OX-a-mer)

‡Generic name product may also be available.

Description

Oral laxatives are medicines taken by mouth to encourage bowel movements to relieve constipation.

There are several different types of oral laxatives and they work in different ways. Since directions for use are different for each type, it is important to know which one you are taking. The different types of oral laxatives include:

Bulk-formers—Bulk-forming laxatives are not digested but absorb liquid in the intestines and swell to form a soft, bulky stool. The bowel is then stimulated normally by the presence of the bulky mass. Some bulk-forming laxatives, like psyllium and polycarbophil, may be prescribed by your doctor to treat diarrhea.

Hyperosmotics—Hyperosmotic laxatives encourage bowel movements by drawing water into the bowel from surrounding body tissues. This provides a soft stool mass and increased bowel action.

There are two types of hyperosmotic laxatives taken by mouth—the saline and the lactulose types. The *saline type* is often called "salts." They are used for rapid emptying of the lower intestine and bowel. They are not used for long-term or repeated correction of constipation. With smaller doses than those used for the laxative effect, some saline laxatives are used as antacids. The information that follows applies only to their use as laxatives. Sodium phosphate may also be prescribed for other conditions as determined by your doctor.

The *lactulose type* is a special sugar-like laxative that works the same way as the saline type. However, it produces results much more slowly and is often used for long-term treatment of chronic constipation. Lactulose may sometimes be used in the treatment of certain medical conditions to reduce the amount of ammonia in the blood. It is available only with your doctor's prescription.

Lubricants—Lubricant laxatives, such as mineral oil, taken by mouth encourage bowel movements by coating the bowel and the stool mass with a waterproof film. This keeps moisture in the stool. The stool remains soft and its passage is made easier.

Stimulants—Stimulant laxatives, also known as contact laxatives, encourage bowel movements by acting on the intestinal wall. They increase the muscle contractions that move along the stool mass. Stimulant laxatives are a popular type of laxative for self-treatment. However, they also are more likely to cause side effects. One of the stimulant laxatives, dehydrocholic acid, may also be used for treating certain conditions of the biliary tract.

Stool softeners (emollients)—Stool softeners encourage bowel movements by helping liquids mix into the stool and prevent dry, hard stool masses. This type of laxative has been said not to *cause* a bowel movement but instead *allows* the patient to have a bowel movement without straining.

Combinations—There are many products that you can buy for constipation that contain more than one type of laxative. For example, a product may contain both a stool softener and a stimulant laxative. In general, combination products may be more likely to cause side effects because of the multiple ingredients. In addition, they may not offer any advantage over products containing only one type of laxative. *If you are taking a combination laxative, make certain you know the proper use and precautions for each of the different ingredients.*

Most laxatives (except saline laxatives) may be used to provide relief:

- during pregnancy.
- for a few days after giving birth.
- during preparation for examination or surgery.
- for constipation of bedfast patients.
- for constipation caused by other medicines.
- following surgery when straining should be avoided.
- following a period of poor eating habits or a lack of physical exercise in order to develop normal bowel function (bulk-forming laxatives only).
- for some medical conditions that may be made worse by straining, for example:
  - Heart disease
  - Hemorrhoids
  - Hernia (rupture)
  - High blood pressure (hypertension)
  - History of stroke

Saline laxatives have more limited uses and may be used to provide rapid results:

- during preparation for examination or surgery.
- for elimination of food or drugs from the body in cases of poisoning or overdose.
- for simple constipation that happens on occasion (although another type of laxative may be preferred).
- in supplying a fresh stool sample for diagnosis.

Most laxatives are available without a prescription; however, your doctor may have special instructions for the proper use and dose for your medical condition. They are available in the following dosage forms:

Oral

Bulk-forming laxatives—

Malt Soup Extract
- Powder (U.S.)
- Oral solution (U.S.)
- Tablets (U.S.)

Malt Soup Extract and Psyllium
- Powder (U.S.)

Methylcellulose
- Capsules (U.S.)
- Granules (U.S.)
- Powder (U.S.)
- Oral solution (U.S.)
- Tablets (U.S.)

Polycarbophil
- Tablets (U.S.)
- Chewable tablets (U.S. and Canada)

Psyllium
- Caramels (U.S.)
- Granules (U.S. and Canada)
- Powder (U.S.)

Psyllium Hydrophilic Mucilloid
- Granules (Canada)
- Powder (U.S. and Canada)
- Effervescent powder (U.S. and Canada)
- Wafers (U.S.)

Psyllium Hydrophilic Mucilloid and Carboxymethylcellulose
- Granules (U.S.)

Bulk-forming and stimulant combinations—

Psyllium and Senna
- Granules (U.S.)

Psyllium Hydrophilic Mucilloid and Senna
- Granules (Canada)

Psyllium Hydrophilic Mucilloid and Sennosides
- Powder (U.S.)

Bulk-forming, stimulant, and stool softener (emollient) combination—

Carboxymethylcellulose, Casanthranol, and Docusate
- Capsules (U.S.)

Bulk-forming and stool softener (emollient) combination—

Carboxymethylcellulose and Docusate
- Capsules (U.S.)

Hyperosmotic laxative—Lactulose:

Lactulose
- Solution (U.S. and Canada)

Hyperosmotic laxatives—Saline:

Magnesium Citrate
- Oral solution (U.S. and Canada)

Magnesium Hydroxide
- Milk of magnesia (U.S. and Canada)
- Tablets (U.S. and Canada)

Magnesium Oxide
- Tablets (U.S.)

Magnesium Sulfate
- Crystals (U.S.)
- Tablets (U.S.)

Sodium Phosphate
- Effervescent powder (U.S.)
- Oral solution (U.S.)

Hyperosmotic and lubricant combinations—

Milk of Magnesia and Mineral Oil
- Emulsion (U.S.)

Milk of Magnesia, Mineral Oil, and Glycerin
- Emulsion (Canada)

Hyperosmotic, lubricant, and stimulant combination—

Mineral Oil, Glycerin, and Phenolphthalein
- Emulsion (Canada)

Lubricant laxatives—

Mineral Oil
- Oil (U.S. and Canada)
- Emulsion (U.S. and Canada)
- Gel (U.S. and Canada)
- Oral suspension (U.S.)

Lubricant and stimulant combinations—

Mineral Oil and Cascara Sagrada
- Emulsion (U.S.)

Mineral Oil and Phenolphthalein
- Emulsion (U.S.)
- Oral suspension (U.S.)

Stimulant laxatives—

Bisacodyl
- Tablets (U.S. and Canada)

Casanthranol
- Syrup (U.S.)

Cascara Sagrada
- Fluidextract (U.S.)
- Tablets (U.S.)

Cascara Sagrada and Aloe
- Tablets (U.S.)

Cascara Sagrada and Phenolphthalein
- Tablets (U.S.)

Castor Oil
- Oil (U.S. and Canada)
- Emulsion (U.S.)

Dehydrocholic Acid
- Tablets (U.S.)

Phenolphthalein
- Chewing gum (U.S.)
- Tablets (U.S. and Canada)
- Chewable tablets (U.S. and Canada)
- Wafers (U.S.)

Senna
- Granules (U.S. and Canada)
- Oral solution (U.S.)
- Syrup (U.S. and Canada)
- Tablets (U.S. and Canada)

Sennosides
- Tablets (U.S. and Canada)

Stimulant and stool softener (emollient) combinations—

Bisacodyl and Docusate
- Tablets (Canada)

Casanthranol and Docusate
- Capsules (U.S. and Canada)
- Syrup (U.S.)
- Tablets (U.S.)

Danthron and Docusate
- Capsules (Canada)
- Tablets (Canada)

Dehydrocholic Acid and Docusate
- Capsules (U.S.)
- Tablets (U.S.)

Dehydrocholic Acid, Docusate, and Phenolphthalein
- Capsules (U.S.)

Docusate and Phenolphthalein
- Capsules (U.S. and Canada)
- Tablets (U.S. and Canada)
- Chewable tablets (U.S.)

Senna and Docusate
- Tablets (U.S. and Canada)

Stool softener (emollient) laxatives—

Docusate
- Capsules (U.S. and Canada)
- Oral solution (U.S. and Canada)
- Syrup (U.S. and Canada)
- Tablets (U.S.)

Poloxamer 188 (pol-OX-a-mer)
- Capsules (U.S.)

It is very important that you read and understand the following information. If any of it causes you special concern, check with your doctor or pharmacist. Also, *if you have any questions* or if you want more information about this medicine or your medical problem, *ask your doctor, nurse, or pharmacist.*

Before Using This Medicine

Importance of diet, fluids, and exercise to prevent constipation—Laxatives are to be used to provide short-term relief only, unless otherwise directed by a doctor. A proper diet containing roughage (whole grain breads and cereals, bran, fruit, and green, leafy vegetables), with 6 to 8 full glasses (8 ounces each) of liquids each day, and daily exercise are most important in maintaining healthy bowel function. Also, for individuals who have problems with constipation, foods such as pastries, puddings, sugar, candy, cake, and cheese may make the constipation worse.

If you are taking this medicine without a prescription, carefully read and follow any precautions on the label. For oral laxatives, the following should be considered:

Allergies—Tell your doctor if you have ever had any unusual or allergic reaction to laxatives. Also tell your doctor and pharmacist if you are allergic to any other substances, such as foods, preservatives, or dyes.

Diet—Make certain your doctor and pharmacist know if you are on any special diet, such as a low-sodium or low-sugar diet. Some laxatives have large amonts of sodium or sugars in them.

Pregnancy—Although laxatives are often used during pregnancy, some types are better than others. Stool softeners (emollient) laxatives and bulk-forming laxatives are probably used most often. If you are using a laxative during pregnancy, remember that:

- Some laxatives (in particular, the bulk-formers) contain a large amount of sodium or sugars, which may have possible unwanted effects such as increasing blood pressure or causing water to be held in the body.
- Saline laxatives containing magnesium, potassium, or phosphates may have to be avoided if your kidney function is not normal.
- Mineral oil is usually not used during pregnancy because of possible unwanted effects on the mother or infant. Mineral oil may interfere with the absorption of nutrients and vitamins in the mother. Also, if taken for a long time during pregnancy, mineral oil may cause severe bleeding in the newborn infant.
- Stimulant laxatives may cause unwanted effects in the expectant mother if improperly used. Castor oil in particular should not be used as it may cause contractions of the womb.

Breast-feeding—Laxatives containing cascara, danthron, and phenolphthalein may pass into the breast milk. Although the amount of laxative in the milk is generally thought to be too small to cause problems in the baby, your doctor should be told if you plan to use such laxatives. Some reports claim that diarrhea has been caused in the infant.

Children—*Laxatives should not be given to young children (up to 6 years of age) unless prescribed by their doctor.* Since children usually cannot describe their symptoms very well, they should be checked by a doctor before being given a laxative. The child may have a condition that needs other treatment. If so, laxatives will not help, and may even cause unwanted effects or make the condition worse.

Mineral oil should not be given to young children (up to 6 years of age) because a form of pneumonia may be caused by the inhalation of oil droplets into the lungs.

Also, bisacodyl tablets should not be given to children up to 6 years of age because if chewed they may cause stomach irritation.

Older adults—Mineral oil should not be taken by bedridden elderly persons because a form of pneumonia may be caused by the inhalation of oil droplets into the lungs. Also, stimulant laxatives (e.g., bisacodyl, casanthranol, or phenolphthalein), if taken too often, may worsen weakness, lack of coordination, or dizziness and lightheadedness.

Other medicines—Although certain medicines should not be used together at all, in other cases two different medicines may be used together even if an interaction might occur. In these cases, your doctor may want to change the dose, or other precautions may be necessary. When you are taking oral laxatives, it is especially important that your doctor and pharmacist know if you are taking any of the following:

- Anticoagulants, oral (blood thinners you take by mouth) or
- Digitalis glycosides (heart medicine)—The use of magnesium-containing laxatives may reduce the effects of these medicines
- Ciprofloxacin (e.g., Cipro) or
- Etidronate (e.g., Didronel) or
- Sodium polysterene sulfonate—Use of magnesium-containing laxatives will keep these medicines from working
- Tetracyclines taken by mouth (medicine for infection)—Use of bulk-forming or magnesium-containing laxatives will keep the tetracycline medicine from working

Other medical problems—The presence of other medical problems may affect the use of oral laxatives. Make sure you tell your doctor if you have any other medical problems, especially:

- Appendicitis (or signs of) or
- Rectal bleeding of unknown cause—These conditions need immediate attention by a doctor
- Colostomy or
- Intestinal blockage or
- Ileostomy—The use of laxatives may create other problems if these conditions are present
- Diabetes mellitus (sugar diabetes)—Diabetic patients should be careful since some laxatives contain large amounts of sugars, such as dextrose, galactose, and/or sucrose
- Heart disease or
- High blood pressure—Some laxatives contain large amounts of sodium, which may make these conditions worse
- Kidney disease—Magnesium and potassium (contained in some laxatives) may build up in the body if kidney disease is present; a serious condition may develop
- Swallowing difficulty—Mineral oil should not be used since it may get into the lungs by accident and cause pneumonia; also, bulk-forming laxatives may get lodged in the esophagus of patients who have difficulty in swallowing

Before you begin using any new medicine (prescription or nonprescription) or if you develop any new medical problem while you are using this medicine, check with your doctor, nurse, or pharmacist.

Proper Use of This Medicine

For safe and effective use of your laxative:

- Follow your doctor's instructions if this laxative was prescribed.
- Follow the manufacturer's package directions if you are treating yourself.

With all kinds of laxatives, at least 6 to 8 glasses (8 ounces each) of liquids should be taken each day. This will help make the stool softer.

For *patients taking laxatives containing a bulk-forming ingredient:*

- Do not try to swallow in the dry form. Take with liquid.
- To allow bulk-forming laxatives to work properly and to prevent intestinal blockage, it is necessary to drink plenty of fluids during their use. Each dose should be taken in or with a full glass (8 ounces) or more of cold water or fruit juice. This will provide enough liquid for the laxative to work properly. A second glass of water or juice by itself is often recommended with each dose for best effect and to avoid side effects.
- When taking a product that contains only a bulk-forming ingredient, results often may be obtained in 12 hours. However, this may not occur for some individuals until after 2 or 3 days.

For *patients taking laxatives containing a stool softener (emollient):*

- Liquid forms may be taken in milk or fruit juice to improve flavor.
- When taking a product that contains only a stool softener, results usually occur 1 to 2 days after the first dose. However, this may not occur for some individuals until after 3 to 5 days.

For *patients taking laxatives containing a hyperosmotic ingredient:*

- Each dose should be taken in or with a full glass (8 ounces) or more of cold water or fruit juice. This will provide enough liquid for the laxative to work properly. A second glass of water or juice by itself is often recommended with each dose for best effect and, in the case of saline laxatives, to prevent you from becoming dehydrated.
- The unpleasant taste produced by some hyperosmotic laxatives may be improved by following each dose with citrus fruit juice or citrus-flavored carbonated beverage.
- Lactulose may not produce laxative results for 24 to 48 hours.
- Saline laxatives usually produce results within ½ to 3 hours following a dose. When a larger dose is taken on an empty stomach, the results are quicker. When a smaller dose is taken with food, the results are delayed. Therefore, large doses of saline laxatives are usually not taken late in the day on an empty stomach.

For *patients taking laxatives containing mineral oil:*

- Mineral oil should not be taken within 2 hours of meals because of possible interference with food digestion and absorption of nutrients and vitamins.

- Mineral oil is usually taken at bedtime (but not while lying down) for convenience and because it requires about 6 to 8 hours to produce results.

For *patients taking laxatives containing a stimulant ingredient:*

- Stimulant laxatives are usually taken on an empty stomach for rapid effect. Results are slowed if taken with food.
- Many stimulant laxatives (but not castor oil) are often taken at bedtime to produce results the next morning (although some may require 24 hours or more).
- *Castor oil* is not usually taken late in the day because its results occur within 2 to 6 hours.
- The unpleasant taste of *castor oil* may be improved by chilling in the refrigerator for at least an hour and then stirring the dose into a full glass of cold orange juice just before it is taken. Also, flavored preparations of castor oil are available.
- *Bisacodyl tablets* are specially coated to allow them to work properly without causing irritation and/or nausea. To protect this coating, do not chew, crush, or take the tablets within an hour of milk or antacids.
- Because of the way *phenolphthalein* works in the body, a single dose may cause a laxative effect in some people for up to 3 days.

Storage—To store this medicine:

- Keep out of the reach of children.
- Store away from heat and direct light.
- Do not store the capsule, tablet, granules, or powder form of this medicine in the bathroom, near the kitchen sink, or in other damp places. Heat or moisture may cause the medicine to break down.
- Keep the liquid form of this medicine from freezing.
- Do not keep outdated medicine or medicine no longer needed. Be sure that any discarded medicine is out of the reach of children.

Precautions While Using This Medicine

Do not take any type of laxative:

- *if you have signs of appendicitis or inflamed bowel* (such as stomach or lower abdominal pain, cramping, bloating, soreness, nausea, or vomiting). Instead, check with your doctor as soon as possible.
- *for more than 1 week* unless your doctor has prescribed or ordered a special schedule for you. This is true even when you have had no results from the laxative.
- *within 2 hours of taking other medicine* because the desired effect of the other medicine may be reduced.
- *if you do not need it,* as for the common cold, "to clean out your system," or as a "tonic to make you feel better."
- *if you miss a bowel movement for a day or two.*
- *if you develop a skin rash* while taking a laxative or if you had a rash the last time you took it. Instead, check with your doctor.

If you notice a sudden change in bowel habits or function that lasts longer than 2 weeks, or that keeps returning off and on, check with your doctor before using a laxative. This will allow the cause of your problem to be determined before it may become more serious.

The "laxative habit"—Laxative products are overused by many people. Such a practice often leads to dependence on the laxative action to produce a bowel movement. In severe cases, overuse of some laxatives has caused damage to the nerves, muscles, and tissues of the intestines and bowel. If you have any questions about the use of laxatives, check with your doctor or pharmacist.

Many laxatives often contain large amounts of sugars, carbohydrates, and sodium. If you are on a low-sugar, low-caloric, or low-sodium diet, check with your doctor or pharmacist before using a laxative.

For *patients taking laxatives containing mineral oil:*

- Mineral oil should not be taken often or for long periods of time because:
  —gradual build-up in body tissues may create additional problems.
  —the use of mineral oil may interfere with the body's ability to absorb certain food nutrients and vitamins A, D, E, and K.
- Large doses of mineral oil may cause some leakage from the rectum. The use of absorbent pads or a decrease in dose may be necessary to prevent the soiling of clothing.
- Do not take mineral oil within 2 hours of a stool softener (emollient laxative). The stool softener may increase the amount of mineral oil absorbed.

For *patients taking laxatives containing a stimulant ingredient:*

- Stimulant laxatives are most often associated with:
  —overuse and the laxative habit.
  —skin rashes.
  —intestinal cramping after dosing (especially if taken on an empty stomach).
  —potassium loss.

Side Effects of This Medicine

Along with its needed effects, a medicine may cause some unwanted effects. Although not all of these side effects may occur, if they do occur they may need medical attention.

Check with your doctor as soon as possible if any of the following side effects occur:

For bulk-forming–containing

Difficulty in breathing; intestinal blockage; skin rash or itching; swallowing difficulty (feeling of lump in throat)

For hyperosmotic-containing

Confusion; dizziness or lightheadedness; irregular heartbeat; muscle cramps; unusual tiredness or weakness

For stimulant-containing

Confusion; irregular heartbeat; muscle cramps; pink to red coloration of alkaline urine and stools (for phenolphthalein only); pink to red, red to violet, or red to brown coloration of alkaline urine (for cascara, danthron, and/or senna only); skin rash; unusual tiredness or weakness; yellow to brown coloration of acid urine (for cascara, phenolphthalein, and/or senna only)

For stool softener (emollient)–containing

Skin rash

Other side effects may occur that usually do not need medical attention. These side effects are less common and may go away during treatment as your body adjusts to the medicine. However, check with your doctor if any of the following side effects continue or are bothersome:

For hyperosmotic-containing

Cramping; diarrhea; gas; increased thirst

For lubricant-containing

Skin irritation surrounding rectal area

For stimulant-containing

Belching; cramping; diarrhea; nausea

For stool softener (emollient)–containing

Stomach and/or intestinal cramping; throat irritation (liquid forms only)

Other side effects not listed above may also occur in some patients. If you notice any other effects, check with your doctor.

Additional Information

Once a medicine has been approved for marketing for a certain use, experience may show that it is also useful for other medical problems. Although this use is not included in product labeling, psyllium hydrophilic mucilloid is used in certain patients with high cholesterol (hypercholesterolemia).

For patients taking psyllium hydrophilic mucilloid for *high cholesterol*:

- Importance of diet—Before prescribing medicine for your condition, your doctor will probably try to control your condition by prescribing a personal diet for you. Such a diet may be low in fats, sugars, and/or cholesterol. Many people are able to control their condition by carefully following their doctor's orders for proper diet and exercise. Medicine is prescribed only when additional help is needed. *Follow carefully the special diet your doctor gave you,* since the medicine is effective only when a schedule of diet and exercise is properly followed.
- Do not try to swallow the powder form of this medicine in the dry form. Mix with liquid following the directions in the package.
- Remember that this medicine will not cure your cholesterol problem but it will help control it. Therefore, you must continue to take it as directed by your doctor if you expect to lower your cholesterol level.

Other than the above information, there is no additional information relating to proper use, precautions, or side effects for this use.

Annual revision: 06/25/93

LAXATIVES Rectal

This information applies to the following medicines:

Carbon dioxide–releasing laxatives—
- Potassium Bitartrate and Sodium Bicarbonate (SOE-dee-um bye-KAR-boe-nate)

Hyperosmotic laxatives—
- Glycerin (GLI-ser-in)
- Sodium Phosphates (soe-dee-um FOS-fates)

Lubricant laxatives—
- Mineral Oil

Stimulant laxatives—
- Bisacodyl (bis-a-KOE-dill)
- Senna

Stool softeners (emollient laxatives)—
- Docusate (DOK-yoo-sate)

Some commonly used brand names are:

For Bisacodyl

In the U.S.

Bisco-Lax
Clysodrast
Dacodyl
Deficol
Dulcolax
Fleet Bisacodyl
Fleet Bisacodyl Prep
Fleet Laxative
Theralax

Generic name product may also be available.

In Canada

Bisacolax
Dulcolax
Laxit

Generic name product may also be available.

For Docusate

In the U.S.

Therevac Plus
Therevac-SB

For Glycerin
In the U.S.
Fleet Babylax — Sani-Supp
Generic name product may also be available.
In Canada
Generic name product may also be available.

For Mineral Oil
In the U.S.
Fleet Enema Mineral Oil
In Canada
Fleet Enema Mineral Oil

For Potassium Bitartrate and Sodium Bicarbonate
In the U.S.
Ceo-Two

For Senna
In the U.S.
Senokot
In Canada
Senokot

For Sodium Phosphates
In the U.S.
Fleet Enema
In Canada
Fleet Enema

Description

Rectal laxatives are used as enemas or suppositories to produce bowel movements in a short time.

There are several different types of rectal laxatives and they work in different ways. Since directions for use are different for each type, it is important to know which one you are taking. The different types of rectal laxatives include:

Carbon dioxide–releasing—Carbon dioxide–releasing laxatives are suppositories that encourage bowel movements by forming carbon dioxide, a gas. This gas pushes against the intestinal wall, causing contractions that move along the stool mass.

Hyperosmotic—Hyperosmotic laxatives draw water into the bowel from surrounding body tissues. This provides a soft stool mass and increased bowel action.

Lubricant—Mineral oil coats the bowel and the stool mass with a waterproof film. This keeps moisture in the stool. The stool remains soft and its passage is made easier.

Stimulants—Stimulant laxatives, also known as contact laxatives, act on the intestinal wall. They increase the muscle contractions that move along the stool mass.

Stool softeners (emollients)—Stool softeners (emollient laxatives) encourage bowel movements by helping liquids mix into the stool and prevent dry, hard stool masses. This type of laxative has been said not to *cause* a bowel movement but instead *allows* the patient to have a bowel movement without straining.

Rectal laxatives may provide relief in a number of situations such as:

- before giving birth.
- for a few days after giving birth.
- preparation for examination or surgery.
- to aid in developing normal bowel function following a period of poor eating habits or a lack of physical exercise (glycerin suppositories only).
- following surgery when straining should be avoided.
- constipation caused by other medicines.

Some of these laxatives are available only with your doctor's prescription. Others are available without a prescription; however, your doctor may have special instructions for the proper use and dose for your medical condition. They are available in the following dosage forms:

Rectal

Bisacodyl
- Enema (U.S. and Canada)
- Suppositories (U.S. and Canada)
- Powder for enema (U.S.)

Docusate
- Enema (U.S.)

Glycerin
- Enema (U.S.)
- Suppositories (U.S. and Canada)

Mineral Oil
- Enema (U.S. and Canada)

Potassium Bitartrate and Sodium Bicarbonate
- Suppositories (U.S.)

Senna
- Suppositories (U.S. and Canada)

Sodium Phosphates
- Enema (U.S. and Canada)

It is very important that you read and understand the following information. If any of it causes you special concern, check with your doctor or pharmacist. Also, *if you have any questions* or if you want more information about this medicine or your medical problem, *ask your doctor, nurse, or pharmacist.*

Before Using This Medicine

Importance of diet, fluids, and exercise to prevent constipation—Laxatives are to be used to provide short-term relief only, unless otherwise directed by your doctor. A proper diet containing roughage (whole grain breads and cereals, bran, fruit, and green, leafy vegetables), with 6 to 8 full glasses (8 ounces each) of liquids each day, and daily exercise are most important in maintaining healthy bowel function. Also, for individuals who have problems with constipation, foods such as pastries, puddings, sugar, candy, cake, and cheese may make the constipation worse.

If you are using this medicine without a prescription, carefully read and follow any precautions on the label. For rectal laxatives, the following should be considered:

Allergies—Tell your doctor if you have ever had any unusual or allergic reaction to rectal laxatives. Also tell your doctor and pharmacist if you are allergic to any other substances, such as preservatives or dyes.

Children—*Laxatives should not be given to young children (up to 6 years of age) unless prescribed by their doctor.* Since children cannot usually describe their symptoms very well, they should be checked by a doctor before being given a laxative. The child may have a condition that needs other treatment. If so, laxatives will not help and may even cause unwanted effects or make the condition worse.

Also, weakness, increased sweating, and convulsions (seizures) may be especially likely to occur in children receiving enemas or rectal solutions, since they may be more sensitive than adults to their effects.

Older adults—Weakness, increased sweating, and convulsions (seizures) may be especially likely to occur in elderly patients, since they may be more sensitive than younger adults to the effects of rectal laxatives.

Other medical problems—The presence of other medical problems may affect the use of rectal laxatives. Make sure you tell your doctor if you have any other medical problems, especially:

- Appendicitis (or signs of) or
- Rectal bleeding of unknown cause—These conditions need immediate attention by a doctor
- Intestinal blockage—The use of laxatives may create other problems if this condition is present

Before you begin using any new medicine (prescription or nonprescription) or if you develop any new medical problem while you are using this medicine, check with your doctor, nurse, or pharmacist.

Proper Use of This Medicine

For safe and effective use of laxatives:

- Follow your doctor's orders if this laxative was prescribed.
- Follow the manufacturer's package directions if you are treating yourself.

For patients using *the enema form* of this medicine:

- This medicine usually comes with patient directions. Read them carefully before using this medicine.
- Lubricate anus with petroleum jelly before inserting the enema applicator.
- Gently insert the rectal tip of the enema applicator to prevent damage to the rectal wall.
- Results often may be obtained with:
  - —bisacodyl enema in 15 minutes to 1 hour.
  - —docusate enema in 2 to 15 minutes.
  - —glycerin enema in 15 minutes to 1 hour.
  - —mineral oil enema in 2 to 15 minutes.
  - —senna enema in 30 minutes, but may not occur for some individuals for up to 2 hours.
  - —sodium phosphates enema in 2 to 5 minutes.

For patients using *the suppository form* of this medicine:

- If the suppository is too soft to insert, chill the suppository in the refrigerator for 30 minutes or run cold water over it, before removing the foil wrapper.
- To insert suppository: First remove the foil wrapper and moisten the suppository with cold water. Lie down on your side and use your finger to push the suppository well up into the rectum.
- Results often may be obtained with:
  - —bisacodyl suppositories in 15 minutes to 1 hour.
  - —carbon dioxide–releasing suppositories in 5 to 30 minutes.
  - —glycerin suppositories in 15 minutes to 1 hour.
  - —senna suppositories in 30 minutes, but may not occur for some individuals for up to 2 hours.

Storage—To store this medicine:

- Keep out of the reach of children.
- Store away from heat and direct light.
- Do not store in the bathroom, near the kitchen sink, or in other damp places. Heat or moisture may cause the medicine to break down.
- Do not keep outdated medicine or medicine no longer needed. Be sure that any discarded medicine is out of the reach of children.

Precautions While Using This Medicine

Do not use any type of laxative:

- *if you have signs of appendicitis or inflamed bowel* (such as stomach or lower abdominal pain, cramping, bloating, soreness, nausea, or vomiting). Instead, check with your doctor as soon as possible.
- *more often than your doctor prescribed. This is true even when you have had no results from the laxative.*
- *if you do not need it,* as for the common cold, "to clean out your system," or as a "tonic to make you feel better."
- *if you miss a bowel movement for a day or two.*

If you notice a sudden change in bowel habits or function that lasts longer than 2 weeks, or keeps returning off and on, check with your doctor before using a laxative. This will allow the cause of your problem to be determined before it becomes more serious.

The "laxative habit"—Laxative products are overused by many people. Such a practice often leads to dependence on the laxative action to produce a bowel movement. In severe cases, overuse of some laxatives has caused damage to the nerves, muscles, and tissues of the intestines and bowel. If you have any questions about the use of laxatives, check with your doctor or pharmacist.

For patients using *the enema form* of this medicine:

- *Check with your doctor if you notice rectal bleeding, blistering, pain, burning, itching, or other sign of irritation not present before you started using this medicine.*

For patients using *the suppository form* of this medicine:

- Do not lubricate the suppository with mineral oil or petroleum jelly before inserting into the rectum. To do so may affect the way the suppository works. Moisten only with water.

Side Effects of This Medicine

Along with its needed effects, a medicine may cause some unwanted effects. Although not all of these side effects may occur, if they do occur they may need medical attention.

Check with your doctor as soon as possible if any of the following side effects occur:

Less common

Rectal bleeding, blistering, burning, itching, or pain (with enemas only)

Other side effects may occur that usually do not need medical attention. These side effects may go away during treatment as your body adjusts to the medicine. However, check with your doctor if the following side effect continues or is bothersome:

Less common

Skin irritation surrounding rectal area

Other side effects not listed above may also occur in some patients. If you notice any other effects, check with your doctor.

Annual revision: 06/25/93

LEUCOVORIN Systemic

A commonly used brand name in the U.S. is Wellcovorin.
Generic name product may also be available in the U.S. and Canada.
Other commonly used names are citrovorum factor and folinic acid.

Description

Leucovorin (loo-koe-VOR-in) is used as an antidote to the harmful effects of methotrexate (a cancer medicine) that is given in high doses. It is used also to prevent or treat certain kinds of anemia. Leucovorin acts the same way in the body as folic acid, which may be low in these patients.

Leucovorin is also used along with fluorouracil (a cancer medicine) to treat cancer of the colon (bowel).

Leucovorin is available only with a prescription and is to be given only by or under the supervision of your doctor. It is available in the following dosage forms:

Oral

- Tablets (U.S. and Canada)

Parenteral

- Injection (U.S. and Canada)

It is very important that you read and understand the following information. If any of it causes you special concern, check with your doctor. Also, *if you have any questions* or if you want more information about this medicine or your medical problem, *ask your doctor, nurse, or pharmacist.*

Before Using This Medicine

In deciding to use a medicine, the risks of taking the medicine must be weighed against the good it will do. This is a decision you and your doctor will make. For leucovorin, the following should be considered:

Allergies—Tell your doctor if you have ever had any unusual or allergic reaction to leucovorin. Also tell your doctor and pharmacist if you are allergic to any other substance, such as foods, sulfites or other preservatives, or dyes.

Pregnancy—Studies on effects in pregnancy have not been done in either humans or animals.

Breast-feeding—It is not known whether leucovorin passes into the breast milk. However, it has not been reported to cause problems in nursing babies.

Children—In children with seizures, leucovorin may increase the number of seizures that occur.

Older adults—Many medicines have not been studied specifically in older people. Therefore, it may not be known whether they work exactly the same way they do in

younger adults or if they cause different side effects or problems in older people. There is no specific information comparing use of leucovorin in the elderly with use in other age groups.

Other medicines—Although certain medicines should not be used together at all, in other cases two different medicines may be used together even if an interaction might occur. In these cases, your doctor may want to change the dose, or other precautions may be necessary. Tell your doctor and pharmacist if you are taking any other prescription or nonprescription (over-the-counter [OTC]) medicine.

Other medical problems—The presence of other medical problems may affect the use of leucovorin. If you are taking leucovorin as an antidote to methotrexate, make sure you tell your doctor if you have any other medical problems, especially:

- Kidney disease—Levels of methotrexate may be increased because of its slower removal from the body, so the dose of leucovorin may not be enough to block the unwanted effects of methotrexate
- Nausea and vomiting—Not enough leucovorin may be absorbed into the body to block the unwanted effects of methotrexate

Before you begin using any new medicine (prescription or nonprescription) or if you develop any new medical problem while you are using this medicine, check with your doctor, nurse, or pharmacist.

Proper Use of This Medicine

It is very important that you *take leucovorin exactly as directed,* especially when it is being taken to counteract the harmful effects of cancer medicine. *Do not miss any doses. Also, it is best to take the doses at evenly spaced times day and night.* For example, if you are to take 4 doses a day, the doses should be spaced about 6 hours apart. If this interferes with your sleep or other daily activities, or if you need help in planning the best times to take your medicine, check with your doctor, nurse, or pharmacist.

Do not stop taking leucovorin without checking with your doctor. It is very important that you get exactly the right amount.

Missed dose—If you miss a dose of leucovorin or if you vomit shortly after taking a dose, *check with your doctor right away.* Your doctor may want you to take extra leucovorin to make up for what you missed. Do not take more medicine on your own, however, since it is very important that you receive just the right dose at the right time.

Storage—To store this medicine:

- Keep out of the reach of children.
- Store away from heat and direct light.
- Do not store in the bathroom, near the kitchen sink, or in other damp places. Heat or moisture may cause the medicine to break down.
- Do not keep outdated medicine or medicine no longer needed. Be sure that any discarded medicine is out of the reach of children.

Side Effects of This Medicine

Along with its needed effects, a medicine may cause some unwanted effects. Leucovorin usually does not cause any side effects. However, *check with your doctor immediately* if any of the following side effects occur shortly after you receive this medicine:

Skin rash, hives, or itching; wheezing

Other side effects not listed above may also occur in some patients. If you notice any other effects, check with your doctor.

Annual revision: 07/23/92

LEUPROLIDE Systemic

Some commonly used brand names in the U.S. and Canada are Lupron and Lupron Depot.

Another commonly used name is leuprorelin.

Description

Leuprolide (loo-PROE-lide) may be used for a number of different medical problems. These include treatment of:

- cancer of the prostate gland in men;
- pain and/or infertility due to endometriosis in women.

Leuprolide is similar to a hormone normally released from the hypothalamus gland.

When given regularly to men, leuprolide decreases testosterone levels. Reducing the amount of testosterone in the body is one way of treating cancer of the prostate.

When given regularly to women, leuprolide decreases estrogen levels. Reducing the amount of estrogen in the body is one way of treating endometriosis.

Leuprolide is available only with your doctor's prescription, in the following dosage form:

Parenteral

- Injection (U.S. and Canada)

It is very important that you read and understand the following information. If any of it causes you special concern, check with your doctor. Also, *if you have any questions* or if you want more information about this medicine or your medical problem, *ask your doctor, nurse, or pharmacist.*

Before Using This Medicine

In deciding to use a medicine, the risks of taking the medicine must be weighed against the good it will do. This is a decision you and your doctor will make. For leuprolide, the following should be considered:

Allergies—Tell your doctor if you have ever had any unusual or allergic reaction to leuprolide, buserelin, gonadorelin, histrelin, or nafarelin.

Pregnancy—Tell your doctor if you intend to have children.

- For men: Leuprolide may cause sterility which probably is only temporary. Be sure that you have discussed this with your doctor before receiving this medicine.
- For women: There is a chance that leuprolide may cause birth defects if it is taken after you become pregnant. It could also cause a miscarriage if taken during pregnancy. *Stop using this medicine and tell your doctor immediately if you think you have become pregnant* while receiving this medicine.

Older adults—Many medicines have not been studied specifically in older people. Therefore, it may not be known whether they work exactly the same way they do in younger adults. Although there is no specific information comparing use of leuprolide in the elderly to use in other age groups, it is not expected to cause different side effects or problems in older people than it does in younger adults.

Other medical problems—The presence of other medical problems may affect the use of leuprolide. Make sure you tell your doctor if you have any other medical problems, especially:

- Bleeding from the vagina with unknown cause (for use in endometriosis)
- Problems in passing urine (for use for cancer of the prostate)—May get worse for a short time after leuprolide treatment is started

Proper Use of This Medicine

Leuprolide comes with patient directions. Read these instructions carefully.

Use the syringes provided in the kit. Other syringes may not provide the correct dose. These disposable syringes and needles are already sterilized and designed to be used one time only and then discarded. If you have any questions about the use of disposable syringes, check with your doctor, nurse, or pharmacist.

Use this medicine only as directed by your doctor. Do not use more or less of it, and do not use it more often than your doctor ordered. The exact amount of medicine you need has been carefully worked out. Using too much may increase the chance of side effects, while using too little may not improve your condition.

For patients receiving leuprolide for *endometriosis*:

- Leuprolide sometimes causes unwanted effects such as hot flashes or decreased interest in sex. It may also cause a temporary increase in pain when you first begin to use it. However, it is very important that you continue to use the medicine, even after you begin to feel better. *Do not stop using this medicine without first checking with your doctor.*

For patients receiving leuprolide for *cancer of the prostate:*

- Leuprolide sometimes causes unwanted effects such as hot flashes or decreased sexual ability. It may also cause a temporary increase in pain or difficulty in urinating, as well as temporary numbness or tingling of hands or feet or weakness when you first begin to use it. However, it is very important that you continue to use the medicine, even after you begin to feel better. *Do not stop using this medicine without first checking with your doctor.*

Dosing—The dose of leuprolide will be different for different patients. *Follow your doctor's orders or the directions on the label.* The following information includes only the average doses of leuprolide. *If your dose is different, do not change it* unless your doctor tells you to do so:

- For injection dosage form:
  - —For *endometriosis:*
    - Adults—3.75 milligrams (mg) injected into the muscle once a month.
  - —For *cancer of the prostate:*
    - Adults—
      1 mg injected under the skin once a day or
      7.5 mg injected into the muscle once a month.

Missed dose—If you are using this medicine every day and you miss a dose, give it as soon as possible. However, if you do not remember until the next day, skip the missed dose and go back to your regular dosing schedule. Do not double doses.

Storage—To store this medicine:

- Keep out of the reach of children.
- Store away from heat and direct light.

- Keep the medicine from freezing.
- Do not keep outdated medicine or medicine no longer needed. Dispose of used syringes properly in the container provided. Be sure that any discarded medicine is out of the reach of children.

Precautions While Using This Medicine

It is very important that your doctor check your progress at regular visits to make sure that this medicine is working properly and to check for unwanted effects.

For patients receiving leuprolide for *endometriosis:*

- During the time you are receiving leuprolide, your menstrual period may not be regular or you may not have a menstrual period at all. This is to be expected when being treated with this medicine. If regular menstruation does not begin within 60 to 90 days after you stop receiving this medicine, check with your doctor.
- During the time you are receiving leuprolide, you should use birth control methods which do not contain hormones. If you have any questions about this, check with your doctor, nurse, or pharmacist.
- *If you suspect you may have become pregnant, stop using this medicine and check with your doctor.* There is a chance that continued use of leuprolide during pregnancy could cause birth defects or a miscarriage.

Side Effects of This Medicine

Along with its needed effects, a medicine may cause some unwanted effects. Some side effects will have signs or symptoms that you can see or feel. Your doctor may watch for others by doing certain tests.

The following side effects may be caused by blood clots but occur only rarely. However, they require immediate medical attention. *Get emergency help immediately* if any of the following side effects occur:

For males only

Rare

Pains in groin or legs (especially in calves of legs); shortness of breath (sudden)

Check with your doctor as soon as possible if any of the following side effects occur:

For both females and males

Less common

Fast or irregular heartbeat

For females only

Less common

Deepening of voice; increased hair growth

For males only

Less common

Chest pain

Other side effects may occur that usually do not need medical attention. These side effects may go away during treatment as your body adjusts to the medicine. However, check with your doctor if any of the following side effects continue or are bothersome:

For both females and males

More common

Sudden sweating and feelings of warmth ("hot flashes")

Less common

Blurred vision; burning, itching, redness, or swelling at place of injection; dizziness; headache; nausea or vomiting; numbness or tingling of hands or feet; swelling of feet or lower legs; trouble in sleeping; weight gain

For females only

More common

Light, irregular vaginal bleeding; stopping of menstrual periods

Less common

Burning, dryness, or itching of vagina; decreased interest in sex; increased tenderness of breasts; mood changes; pelvic pain

For males only

Less common

Bone pain; constipation; decreased size of testicles; impotence or decreased interest in sex; loss of appetite; swelling and increased tenderness of breasts

Other side effects not listed above may also occur in some patients. If you notice any other effects, check with your doctor.

Annual revision: 06/25/93

LEVAMISOLE Systemic

A commonly used brand name in the U.S. and Canada is Ergamisol.

Description

Levamisole (lee-VAM-i-sole) is used with another cancer medicine (fluorouracil) to help make it work better against cancer of the colon.

Levamisole is available only with your doctor's prescription in the following dosage form:

Oral

- Tablets (U.S. and Canada)

It is very important that you read and understand the following information. If any of it causes you special concern, check with your doctor. Also, *if you have any questions* or if you want more information about this medicine or your medical problem, *ask your doctor, nurse, or pharmacist.*

Before Using This Medicine

In deciding to use a medicine, the risks of taking the medicine must be weighed against the good it will do. This is a decision you and your doctor will make. For levamisole, the following should be considered:

Allergies—Tell your doctor if you have ever had any unusual or allergic reaction to levamisole or to any other medicines.

Pregnancy—Levamisole has not been studied in pregnant women. However, studies in rats and rabbits have not shown that levamisole causes birth defects or other problems.

Breast-feeding—It is not known whether levamisole passes into the breast milk in humans, although it passes into cows' milk. However, this medicine has not been reported to cause problems in nursing babies.

Children—Studies on this medicine have been done only in adult patients, and there is no specific information comparing use of levamisole in children with use in other age groups.

Older adults—Many medicines have not been studied specifically in older people. Therefore, it may not be known whether they work exactly the same way they do in younger adults or if they cause different side effects or problems in older people. Although there is no specific information comparing use of levamisole in the elderly with use in other age groups, this medicine has been used in elderly patients and is not expected to cause different side effects or problems in older people than it does in younger adults.

Other medicines—Although certain medicines should not be used together at all, in other cases two different medicines may be used together even if an interaction might occur. In these cases, your doctor may want to change the dose, or other precautions may be necessary. Tell your doctor and pharmacist if you are taking any other prescription or nonprescription (over-the-counter [OTC]) medicine.

Other medical problems—The presence of other medical problems may affect the use of levamisole. Make sure you tell your doctor if you have any other medical problems, especially:

- Infection—Levamisole may decrease your body's ability to fight infection

Before you begin using any new medicine (prescription or nonprescription) or if you develop any new medical problem while you are using this medicine, check with your doctor, nurse, or pharmacist.

Proper Use of This Medicine

Take this medicine only as directed by your doctor. Do not take more or less of it, and do not take it more often than your doctor ordered. The exact amount of medicine you need has been carefully worked out. Taking too much may increase the chance of side effects, while taking too little may not improve your condition.

If you vomit shortly after taking a dose of levamisole, check with your doctor. You will be told whether to take the dose again or to wait until the next scheduled dose.

Missed dose—If you miss a dose of this medicine, do not take the missed dose at all and do not double the next one. Instead, go back to your regular dosing schedule and check with your doctor.

Storage—To store this medicine:

- Keep out of the reach of children.
- Store away from heat and direct light.
- Do not store in the bathroom, near the kitchen sink, or in other damp places. Heat or moisture may cause the medicine to break down.
- Do not keep outdated medicine or medicine no longer needed. Be sure that any discarded medicine is out of the reach of children.

Precautions While Using This Medicine

It is very important that your doctor check your progress at regular visits to make sure that this medicine is working properly and to check for unwanted effects.

Side Effects of This Medicine

Along with its needed effects, a medicine may cause some unwanted effects. Although not all of these side effects may occur, if they do occur they may need medical attention.

Check with your doctor immediately if any of the following side effects occur:

Less common

Fever or chills; unusual feeling of discomfort or weakness

Rare

Black, tarry stools; blood in urine or stools; cough or hoarseness; lower back or side pain; painful or difficult urination; pinpoint red spots on skin; unusual bleeding or bruising

Check with your doctor as soon as possible if the following side effects occur:

Less common

Sores in mouth and on lips

Rare

Blurred vision; confusion; convulsions (seizures); lip smacking or puffing; numbness, tingling, or pain in face, hands, or feet; paranoia (feelings of persecution); puffing of cheeks; rapid or worm-like movements of tongue; trembling or shaking; trouble in walking; uncontrolled movements of arms and legs

Other side effects may occur that usually do not need medical attention. These side effects may go away during treatment as your body adjusts to the medicine. Also, your doctor or nurse may be able to tell you about ways to prevent or reduce some of these side effects. However, check with your doctor if any of the following side effects continue or are bothersome:

More common

Diarrhea; metallic taste; nausea

Less common

Anxiety or nervousness; dizziness; headache; mental depression; nightmares; pain in joints or muscles; skin rash or itching; trouble in sleeping; unusual tiredness or sleepiness; vomiting

Levamisole may cause a temporary loss of hair in some people. After treatment has ended, normal hair growth should return.

Other side effects not listed above may also occur in some patients. If you notice any other effects, check with your doctor.

Annual revision: 08/12/92

LEVOCARNITINE Systemic†

Some commonly used brand names in the U.S. are Carnitor and VitaCarn. Another commonly used name is L-Carnitine.

†Not commercially available in Canada.

Description

Levocarnitine (lee-voe-KAR-ni-teen) is a substance that helps the cells use fat to produce energy needed by the body. It is needed in small amounts only and is usually available in the foods that you eat. Lack of carnitine can lead to liver, heart, and muscle problems. Your doctor may treat lack of carnitine by prescribing levocarnitine for you.

Carnitine comes in two forms. Levocarnitine (L-Carnitine) should not be confused with the D,L-carnitine form (labeled as "vitamin B_T"). Only the L-form of carnitine is used by the body. The D,L-form does not help the body use fat and can actually interfere with and cause a lack of levocarnitine.

Certain levocarnitine products have been specifically approved by the U.S. Food and Drug Administration for drug use and are available only with your doctor's prescription. Other levocarnitine products are sold without a prescription as food supplements.

Levocarnitine is available in the following dosage forms:

Oral

- Capsules (U.S.)
- Solution (U.S.)
- Tablets (U.S.)

It is very important that you read and understand the following information. If any of it causes you special concern, check with your doctor or pharmacist. Also, *if you have any questions* or if you want more information about this dietary supplement or your medical problem, *ask your doctor, nurse, pharmacist, or dietitian.*

Before Using This Dietary Supplement

If you are taking this dietary supplement without a prescription, carefully read and follow any precautions on the label. For levocarnitine, the following should be considered:

Allergies—Tell your doctor or pharmacist if you are allergic to any substances, such as foods, preservatives, or dyes.

Pregnancy—Studies have not been done in humans. However, levocarnitine has not been shown to cause birth defects or other problems in animal studies. Normal healthy fetal growth and development may depend on a steady supply of nutrients such as levocarnitine from mother to fetus.

Breast-feeding—Levocarnitine has not been shown to cause problems in nursing babies. It normally is present in breast milk, even in women not taking supplements of it, because it is obtained from the diet.

Children—Although there is no specific information comparing use of levocarnitine in children with use in other age groups, this dietary supplement is not expected to cause different side effects or problems in children than it does in adults.

Older adults—Many dietary supplements have not been studied specifically in older people. Therefore, it may not be known whether they work exactly the same way they do in younger adults. Although there is no specific information comparing use of levocarnitine in the elderly with use in other age groups, this medicine is not expected to cause different side effects or problems in older people than it does in younger adults.

Medicines or other dietary supplements—Although certain medicines or dietary supplements should not be used together at all, in other cases they may be used together even if an interaction might occur. In these cases, your doctor may want to change the dose, or other precautions may be necessary. Tell your doctor and pharmacist if you are taking any other dietary supplement or any prescription or nonprescription (over-the-counter [OTC]) medicine.

Proper Use of This Dietary Supplement

Take levocarnitine with or just after meals. Also, if you are taking it in liquid form, drink it slowly. It will be less likely to upset your stomach if you take it this way.

This dietary supplement is also less likely to cause unwanted effects when there is a constant amount in the blood. If you are taking more than one dose a day, take the doses at evenly spaced times throughout the day. Doses should be spaced at least 3 to 4 hours apart. If you need help in planning the best times to take your dietary supplement, check with your doctor or pharmacist.

Missed dose—If you miss a dose of this dietary supplement, skip the missed dose and go back to your regular dosing schedule. Do not double doses. Taking doses too close together may increase stomach upset.

Storage—To store this dietary supplement:

- Keep out of the reach of children.
- Store away from heat and direct light.
- Do not store in the bathroom, near the kitchen sink, or in other damp places. Heat or moisture may cause the dietary supplement to break down.
- Keep the oral solution form of this dietary supplement from freezing. Do not refrigerate.
- Do not keep outdated dietary supplements or those no longer needed. Be sure that any discarded dietary supplement is out of the reach of children.

Precautions While Using This Dietary Supplement

Do not change brands or dosage forms of levocarnitine without first checking with your doctor. Different products may not work in the same way. If you refill your dietary supplement and it looks different, check with your pharmacist.

Side Effects of This Dietary Supplement

Along with its needed effects, a dietary supplement may cause some unwanted effects. The following side effects may go away during treatment as your body adjusts to the medicine. However, check with your doctor if any of these effects continue or are bothersome:

More common

Body odor; diarrhea or stomach cramps; nausea or vomiting

Other side effects not listed above may also occur in some patients. If you notice any other effects, check with your doctor.

Additional Information

Once a medicine or dietary supplement has been approved for marketing for a certain use, experience may show that it is also useful for other medical problems. Although this use is not included in product labeling, levocarnitine is used in certain patients with the following medical condition:

- Carnitine deficiency that results from treatment with valproic acid

Other than the above information, there is no additional information relating to proper use, precautions, or side effects for this use.

Annual revision: 03/04/92
Interim revision: 08/10/92

LEVODOPA Systemic

This information applies to the following medicines:

Carbidopa and Levodopa (KAR-bi-doe-pa and LEE-voe-doe-pa)
Levodopa

Some commonly used brand names are:

For Carbidopa and Levodopa

In the U.S.
Sinemet
Sinemet CR

In Canada
Sinemet
Sinemet CR

For Levodopa

In the U.S.
Dopar
Larodopa

In Canada
Larodopa

Description

Levodopa is used alone or in combination with carbidopa to treat Parkinson's disease, sometimes referred to as shaking palsy or paralysis agitans. Some patients require the combination of medicine, while others benefit from levodopa alone. By improving muscle control, this medicine allows more normal movements of the body.

Levodopa alone or in combination is available only with your doctor's prescription. It is available in the following dosage forms:

Oral

Carbidopa and Levodopa
- Tablets (U.S. and Canada)
- Extended-release tablets (U.S. and Canada)

Levodopa
- Capsules (U.S.)
- Tablets (U.S. and Canada)

It is very important that you read and understand the following information. If any of it causes you special concern, check with your doctor or pharmacist. Also, *if you have any questions* or if you want more information about this medicine or your medical problem, *ask your doctor, nurse, or pharmacist.*

Before Using This Medicine

In deciding to use a medicine, the risks of taking the medicine must be weighed against the good it will do. This is a decision you and your doctor will make. For levodopa and for carbidopa and levodopa combination, the following should be considered:

Allergies—Tell your doctor if you have ever had any unusual or allergic reaction to levodopa alone or in combination with carbidopa. Also tell your doctor and pharmacist if you are allergic to any other substances, such as foods, preservatives, or dyes.

Diet—Since protein may interfere with the body's response to levodopa, high protein diets should be avoided. Intake of normal amounts of protein should be spaced equally throughout the day.

For patients taking levodopa by itself:
- Pyridoxine (vitamin B_6) has been found to reduce the effects of levodopa when levodopa is taken by itself. This does not happen with the combination of carbidopa and levodopa. *If you are taking levodopa by itself, do not take vitamin products containing vitamin B_6 during treatment, unless prescribed by your doctor.*
- Large amounts of pyridoxine are also contained in some foods such as avocado, bacon, beans, beef liver, dry skim milk, oatmeal, peas, pork, sweet potato, tuna, and certain health foods. Check with your doctor about how much of these foods you may have in your diet while you are taking levodopa. Also, ask your doctor or pharmacist for help when selecting vitamin products.

Pregnancy—Studies have not been done in pregnant women. However, studies in animals have shown that levodopa affects the baby's growth both before and after birth if given during pregnancy in doses many times the human dose. Also, studies in rabbits have shown that levodopa, alone or in combination with carbidopa, causes birth defects.

Breast-feeding—Levodopa and carbidopa pass into the breast milk and may cause unwanted side effects in the nursing baby. Also, levodopa may reduce the flow of breast milk.

Children—Studies on this medicine have been done only in adult patients, and there is no specific information comparing use of levodopa or carbidopa in children with use in other age groups.

Older adults—Elderly people are especially sensitive to the effects of levodopa. This may increase the chance of side effects during treatment.

Other medicines—Although certain medicines should not be used together at all, in other cases 2 different medicines may be used together even if an interaction might occur. In these cases, your doctor may want to change the dose, or other precautions may be necessary. When you are taking levodopa or carbidopa and levodopa combination, it is especially important that your doctor and pharmacist know if you are taking any of the following:
- Cocaine—Cocaine use by individuals taking levodopa, alone or in combination with carbidopa, may cause an irregular heartbeat
- Ethotoin (e.g., Peganone) or
- Haloperidol (e.g., Haldol) or
- Mephenytoin (e.g., Mesantoin) or
- Phenothiazines (acetophenazine [e.g., Tindal], chlorpromazine [e.g., Thorazine], fluphenazine [e.g., Prolixin],

mesoridazine [e.g., Serentil], perphenazine [e.g., Trilafon], prochlorperazine [e.g., Compazine], promazine [e.g., Sparine], promethazine [e.g., Phenergan], thioridazine [e.g., Mellaril], trifluoperazine [e.g., Stelazine], triflupromazine [e.g., Vesprin], trimeprazine [e.g., Temaril]) or

- Phenytoin (e.g., Dilantin)—Taking these medicines with levodopa may lessen the effects of levodopa
- Monoamine oxidase (MAO) inhibitors (furazolidone [e.g., Furoxone], isocarboxazid [e.g., Marplan], phenelzine [e.g., Nardil], procarbazine [e.g., Matulane], tranylcypromine [e.g., Parnate])—Taking levodopa while you are taking or within 2 weeks of taking monoamine oxidase (MAO) inhibitors may cause sudden extremely high blood pressure; at least 14 days should be allowed between stopping treatment with one medicine and starting treatment with the other medicine
- Pyridoxine (vitamin B_6, e.g., Hexa-Betalin), present in some foods and vitamin formulas (for levodopa used alone)—Pyridoxine reverses the effects of levodopa
- Selegiline—Dosage of levodopa or carbidopa and levodopa combination may need to be decreased

Other medical problems—The presence of other medical problems may affect the use of levodopa. Make sure you tell your doctor if you have any other medical problems, especially:

- Diabetes mellitus (sugar diabetes)—The amount of insulin or antidiabetic medicine that you need to take may change
- Emphysema, asthma, bronchitis, or other chronic lung disease or
- Glaucoma or
- Heart or blood vessel disease or
- Hormone problems or
- Melanoma (a type of skin cancer) (or history of) or
- Mental illness—Levodopa may make the condition worse
- Kidney disease or
- Liver disease—Higher blood levels of levodopa may occur, increasing the chance of side effects
- Seizure disorders, such as epilepsy (history of)—The risk of seizures may be increased
- Stomach ulcer (history of)—The ulcer may occur again

Before you begin using any new medicine (prescription or nonprescription) or if you develop any new medical problem while you are using this medicine, check with your doctor, nurse, or pharmacist.

Proper Use of This Medicine

It is best not to take this medicine with or after food, especially high-protein food, since food may decrease levodopa's effect. However, *to lessen possible stomach upset, your doctor may want you to take food shortly after taking this medicine (about 15 minutes after)*. If stomach upset is severe or continues, check with your doctor.

Take this medicine only as directed. Do not take more or less of it, and do not take it more often than your doctor ordered.

For patients taking *carbidopa and levodopa extended-release tablets*:

- Swallow the tablet whole without crushing or chewing, unless your doctor tells you not to. If your doctor tells you to, you may break the tablet in half.

Some people must take this medicine for several weeks or months before full benefit is received. *Do not stop taking it even if you do not think it is working.* Instead, check with your doctor.

Missed dose—If you miss a dose of this medicine, take it as soon as possible. However, if your next scheduled dose is within 2 hours, skip the missed dose and go back to your regular dosing schedule. Do not double doses.

Storage—To store this medicine:

- Keep out of the reach of children.
- Store away from heat and direct light.
- Do not store in the bathroom, near the kitchen sink, or in other damp places. Heat or moisture may cause the medicine to break down.
- Do not keep outdated medicine or medicine no longer needed. Be sure that any discarded medicine is out of the reach of children.

Precautions While Using This Medicine

Before having any kind of surgery (including dental surgery) or emergency treatment, tell the medical doctor or dentist in charge that you are taking this medicine.

For *diabetic patients*:

- This medicine may cause test results for urine sugar or ketones to be wrong. Check with your doctor before depending on home tests using the paper-strip or tablet method.

This medicine may cause some people to become drowsy or less alert than they are normally. *Make sure you know how you react to this medicine before you drive, use machines, or do anything else that could be dangerous if you are not alert.*

Dizziness, lightheadedness, or fainting may occur, especially when you get up from a lying or sitting position. Getting up slowly may help. If the problem continues or gets worse, check with your doctor.

For patients taking levodopa by itself:

- Pyridoxine (vitamin B_6) has been found to reduce the effects of levodopa when levodopa is taken by itself. This does not happen with the combination of carbidopa and levodopa. *If you are taking levodopa by itself, do not take vitamin products containing vitamin B_6 during treatment, unless prescribed by your doctor.*
- Large amounts of pyridoxine are also contained in some foods such as avocado, bacon, beans, beef liver,

dry skim milk, oatmeal, peas, pork, sweet potato, tuna, and certain health foods. Check with your doctor about how much of these foods you may have in your diet while you are taking levodopa. Also, ask your doctor or pharmacist for help when selecting vitamin products.

As your condition improves and your body movements become easier, *be careful not to overdo physical activities. Injuries resulting from falls may occur.* Physical activities must be increased gradually to allow your body to adjust to changing balance, circulation, and coordination. *This is especially important in the elderly.*

After taking this medicine for long periods of time, such as a year or more, some patients suddenly lose the ability to move. Their muscles do not seem to work. This loss of movement may last from a few minutes to several hours. The patient then is able to move as before. This condition may unexpectedly occur again and again. If you should have this problem, sometimes called the "on-off" effect, check with your doctor.

Side Effects of This Medicine

Along with its needed effects, a medicine may cause some unwanted effects. Although not all of these side effects may occur, if they do occur they may need medical attention.

Check with your doctor as soon as possible if any of the following side effects occur:

More common

Mental depression; mood or mental changes (such as aggressive behavior); unusual and uncontrolled movements of the body

Less common—more common when levodopa is used alone

Difficult urination; dizziness or lightheadedness when getting up from a lying or sitting position; irregular heartbeat; nausea or vomiting (severe or continuing); spasm or closing of eyelids (not more common when levodopa is used alone)

Rare

High blood pressure; stomach pain; unusual tiredness or weakness

Other side effects may occur that usually do not need medical attention. These side effects may go away during treatment as your body adjusts to the medicine. However, check with your doctor if any of the following side effects continue or are bothersome:

More common

Anxiety, confusion, or nervousness (especially in elderly patients receiving other medicine for Parkinson's disease)

Less common

Constipation (more common when levodopa is used alone); diarrhea; dryness of mouth; flushing of skin; headache; loss of appetite; muscle twitching; nightmares (more common when levodopa is used alone); trouble in sleeping

This medicine may sometimes cause the urine and sweat to be darker in color than usual. The urine may at first be reddish, then turn to nearly black after being exposed to air. Some bathroom cleaning products will produce a similar effect when in contact with urine containing this medicine. This is to be expected during treatment with this medicine.

Other side effects not listed above may also occur in some patients. If you notice any other effects, check with your doctor.

Annual revision: 08/18/92

LIDOCAINE—For Self-Injection Systemic†

A commonly used brand name in the U.S. is LidoPen.

This information does *not* apply to any other dosage forms or brand names of lidocaine.

†Not commercially available in Canada.

Description

Lidocaine (LYE-doe-kane) belongs to the group of medicines called antiarrhythmics. It is used to change an abnormal rhythm in the heart back to normal. Lidocaine produces its helpful effects by slowing abnormal nerve impulses in the heart and reducing irritability of heart tissues.

Lidocaine is usually given by a doctor or nurse when a rapid effect is needed. However, this dosage form has been prescribed by your doctor as part of the early management of a heart attack when certain abnormal heart rhythms occur. It is designed to be used by the patient under instructions from a doctor.

This form of lidocaine is available only with your doctor's prescription and *is to be administered only under direct orders from your doctor.* It is available in the following dosage form:

Parenteral

- Injection (U.S.)

It is very important that you read and understand the following information. If any of it causes you special concern, check with your doctor. Also, *if you have any questions* or if you want more information about this medicine or your medical problem, *ask your doctor, nurse, or pharmacist.*

Before Using This Medicine

In deciding to use a medicine, the risks of taking the medicine must be weighed against the good it will do. This is a decision you and your doctor will make. For lidocaine, the following should be considered:

Allergies—Tell your doctor if you have ever had any unusual or allergic reaction to lidocaine, flecainide, tocainide, or anesthetics.

Pregnancy—Lidocaine has not been studied in pregnant women. However, this medicine may reduce the blood supply to the unborn baby.

Breast-feeding—It is not known whether lidocaine passes into breast milk. However, this medicine has not been reported to cause problems in nursing babies.

Children—Although there is no specific information comparing use of lidocaine in children with use in other age groups, this medicine is not expected to cause different side effects or problems in children than it does in adults.

Older adults—Elderly people are especially sensitive to the effects of lidocaine. This may increase the chance of side effects during treatment.

Other medicines—Although certain medicines should not be used together at all, in other cases two different medicines may be used together even if an interaction might occur. In these cases, your doctor may want to change the dose, or other precautions may be necessary. When receiving lidocaine it is especially important that your doctor and pharmacist know if you are taking any of the following:

- Ethotoin (e.g., Peganone) or
- Mephenytoin (e.g., Mesantoin) or
- Phenytoin (e.g., Dilantin)—Risk of slow heartbeat may be increased. Other effects of lidocaine may be decreased because these medicines may cause it to be removed from the body more quickly

Other medical problems—The presence of other medical problems may affect the use of lidocaine. Make sure you tell your doctor if you have any other medical problems, especially:

- Congestive heart failure or
- Kidney disease or
- Liver disease—Effects may be increased because of slower removal of lidocaine from the body

Before you begin using any new medicine (prescription or nonprescription) or if you develop any new medical problem while you are using this medicine, check with your doctor, nurse, or pharmacist.

Proper Use of This Medicine

This medicine should be kept within easy reach, along with your doctor's telephone number. Check the expiration date on the lidocaine regularly. Replace the medicine before it expires.

Be familiar with possible symptoms of a heart attack and how to recognize them. If they occur, *telephone your doctor immediately.* The special device your doctor gave you will transmit your electrocardiogram (ECG or EKG) over the telephone. Your doctor will look at your ECG and tell you whether you need to use this medicine.

Lidocaine comes with patient directions. Read them carefully before you actually need to use this medicine. Then, when an emergency arises, you will know how to inject the lidocaine.

To use the lidocaine self-injector:

- Remove the gray safety cap.
- Place the black end of the self-injector on the thickest part of your thigh and press hard until the injector functions. You should feel a needle prick.
- Hold the device firmly in place for 10 seconds, then remove it. Massage the injection area for 10 seconds.

Storage—To store this medicine:

- Keep out of the reach of children.
- Store away from heat and direct light.
- Keep the medicine from freezing.

Precautions While Using This Medicine

Do not administer this injection unless instructed to do so by your doctor. Your doctor is trained to read the electrocardiogram and decide whether an arrhythmia is occurring.

Unless it is absolutely necessary, *do not attempt to drive after using this medicine.* Follow your doctor's instructions about what to do next, including going to the doctor's office or hospital emergency room, if necessary.

Side Effects of This Medicine

Along with its needed effects, a medicine may cause some unwanted effects. Although not all of these side effects

may occur, if they do occur they may need medical attention.

Check with your doctor immediately if any of the following side effects occur:

Rare

Convulsions (seizures); difficulty in breathing; itching; skin rash; swelling of skin

Check with your doctor as soon as possible if any of the following side effects occur:

Signs and symptoms of overdose

Blurred or double vision; dizziness (severe) or fainting; nausea or vomiting; ringing in ears; slow heartbeat; tremors or twitching

Other side effects may occur that usually do not need medical attention. However, check with your doctor if the following side effects continue or are bothersome:

Less common or rare

Anxiety or nervousness; dizziness; drowsiness; feelings of coldness, heat, or numbness; pain at place of injection

Other side effects not listed above may also occur in some patients. If you notice any other effects, check with your doctor.

Annual revision: 10/21/92

LINCOMYCIN Systemic

A commonly used brand name is:

In the U.S.
Lincocin
Lincorex

In Canada
Lincocin

Description

Lincomycin belongs to the family of medicines called antibiotics. These medicines are used to treat infections. They will not work for colds, flu, or other virus infections.

Lincomycin is available only with your doctor's prescription, in the following dosage forms:

Oral

- Capsules (U.S. and Canada)

Parenteral

- Injection (U.S. and Canada)

It is very important that you read and understand the following information. If any of it causes you special concern, check with your doctor. Also, *if you have any questions* or if you want more information about this medicine or your medical problem, *ask your doctor, nurse, or pharmacist.*

Before Using This Medicine

In deciding to use a medicine, the risks of taking the medicine must be weighed against the good it will do. This is a decision you and your doctor will make. For lincomycin, the following should be considered:

Allergies—Tell your doctor if you have ever had any unusual or allergic reaction to lincomycin, clindamycin, or doxorubicin. Also tell your doctor and pharmacist if you are allergic to any other substances, such as foods, preservatives, or dyes.

Pregnancy—Lincomycin has not been reported to cause birth defects or other problems in humans.

Breast-feeding—Lincomycin passes into the breast milk. However, lincomycin has not been reported to cause problems in nursing babies.

Children—Lincomycin has been used in children 1 month of age or older and has not been reported to cause different side effects or problems than it does in adults.

Older adults—Many medicines have not been studied specifically in older people. Therefore, it may not be known whether they work exactly the same way they do in younger adults or if they cause different side effects or problems in older people. There is no specific information comparing use of lincomycin in the elderly with use in other age groups.

Other medicines—Although certain medicines should not be used together at all, in other cases two different medicines may be used together even if an interaction might occur. In these cases, your doctor may want to change the dose, or other precautions may be necessary. When you are taking lincomycin, it is especially important that your doctor and pharmacist know if you are taking any of the following:

- Chloramphenicol (e.g., Chloromycetin) or
- Diarrhea medicine containing kaolin or attapulgite or
- Erythromycins (medicine for infection)—Taking these medicines along with lincomycin may decrease the effects of lincomycin
- Diarrhea medicine, such as loperamide (Imodium A-D)—Patients who take diarrhea medicine, such as loperamide (Imodium A-D) or diphenyoxylate and atropine (Lomotil), may worsen diarrhea that is a side effect of lincomycin

Other medical problems—The presence of other medical problems may affect the use of lincomycin. Make sure

you tell your doctor if you have any other medical problems, especially:

- Kidney disease (severe) or
- Liver disease (severe)—Severe kidney or liver disease may increase blood levels of this medicine, increasing the chance of side effects
- Stomach or intestinal disease, history of (especially colitis, including colitis caused by antibiotics, or enteritis)—Patients with a history of stomach or intestinal disease may have an increased chance of side effects

Before you begin using any new medicine (prescription or nonprescription) or if you develop any new medical problem while you are using this medicine, check with your doctor, nurse, or pharmacist.

Proper Use of This Medicine

Lincomycin is best taken with a full glass (8 ounces) of water on an empty stomach (either 1 hour before or 2 hours after meals), unless otherwise directed by your doctor.

To help clear up your infection completely, *keep taking this medicine for the full time of treatment,* even if you begin to feel better after a few days. *If you have a "strep" infection, you should keep taking this medicine for at least 10 days. This is especially important in "strep" infections. Serious heart problems could develop later* if your infection is not cleared up completely. Also, if you stop taking this medicine too soon, your symptoms may return.

This medicine works best when there is a constant amount in the blood. *To help keep the amount constant, do not miss any doses. Also, it is best to take each dose at evenly spaced times day and night.* For example, if you are to take 4 doses a day, doses should be spaced about 6 hours apart. If this interferes with your sleep or other daily activities, or if you need help in planning the best times to take your medicine, check with your doctor, nurse, or pharmacist.

Missed dose—If you do miss a dose of this medicine, take it as soon as possible. This will help to keep a constant amount of medicine in the blood. However, if it is almost time for your next dose, skip the missed dose and go back to your regular dosing schedule. Do not double doses.

Storage—To store this medicine:

- Keep out of the reach of children.
- Store away from heat and direct light.
- Do not store the capsule form of this medicine in the bathroom, near the kitchen sink, or in other damp places. Heat or moisture may cause the medicine to break down.
- Do not keep outdated medicine or medicine no longer needed. Be sure that any discarded medicine is out of the reach of children.

Precautions While Using This Medicine

It is important that your doctor check your progress at regular visits.

If your symptoms do not improve within a few days, or if they become worse, check with your doctor.

In some patients, lincomycin may cause diarrhea.

- Severe diarrhea may be a sign of a serious side effect. *Do not take any diarrhea medicine without first checking with your doctor.* Diarrhea medicines may make your diarrhea worse or make it last longer.
- For mild diarrhea, diarrhea medicine containing attapulgite (e.g., Kaopectate tablets, Diasorb) may be taken. However, kaolin or attapulgite may keep lincomycin from being absorbed into the body. Therefore, these diarrhea medicines should be taken at least 2 hours before or 3 to 4 hours after you take lincomycin by mouth. Other kinds of diarrhea medicine should not be taken. They may make your diarrhea worse or make it last longer.
- If you have any questions about this or if mild diarrhea continues or gets worse, check with your doctor or pharmacist.

Before having surgery (including dental surgery) with a general anesthetic, tell the medical doctor or dentist in charge that you are taking lincomycin.

Side Effects of This Medicine

Along with its needed effects, a medicine may cause some unwanted effects. Although not all of these side effects may occur, if they do occur they may need medical attention.

Check with your doctor immediately if any of the following side effects occur:

More common

Abdominal or stomach cramps and pain (severe); abdominal tenderness; diarrhea (watery and severe), which may also be bloody; fever

Note: The above side effects may also occur up to several weeks after you stop taking this medicine.

Less common

Skin rash, redness, and itching; sore throat and fever; unusual bleeding and bruising

Other side effects may occur that usually do not need medical attention. These side effects may go away during treatment as your body adjusts to the medicine. However, check with your doctor if any of the following side effects continue or are bothersome:

More common

Diarrhea (mild); nausea and vomiting; stomach pain

Less common

Itching of rectal or genital (sex organ) areas

Other side effects not listed above may also occur in some patients. If you notice any other effects, check with your doctor.

Annual revision: 10/06/92

LINDANE Topical

Some commonly used brand names are:

In the U.S.

Bio-Well	Kwell
GBH	Kwildane
G-well	Scabene
Kildane	Thionex

Generic name product may also be available.

In Canada

GBH	PMS Lindane
Kwellada	

Another commonly used name for lindane is gamma benzene hexachloride.

Description

Lindane (LIN-dane), formerly known as gamma benzene hexachloride, is an insecticide and is used to treat scabies and lice infestations.

Lindane cream and lotion are usually used to treat only scabies infestation. Lindane shampoo is used to treat only lice infestations.

Lindane is available only with your doctor's prescription, in the following dosage forms:

Topical

- Cream (U.S. and Canada)
- Lotion (U.S. and Canada)
- Shampoo (U.S. and Canada)

It is very important that you read and understand the following information. If any of it causes you special concern, check with your doctor. Also, *if you have any questions* or if you want more information about this medicine or your medical problem, *ask your doctor, nurse, or pharmacist.*

Before Using This Medicine

In deciding to use a medicine, the risks of using the medicine must be weighed against the good it will do. This is a decision you and your doctor will make. For lindane, the following should be considered:

Allergies—Tell your doctor if you have ever had any unusual or allergic reaction to lindane. Also tell your doctor and pharmacist if you are allergic to any other substances, such as preservatives or dyes.

Pregnancy—Lindane is absorbed through the skin and could possibly cause toxic effects on the central nervous system (CNS) of the unborn baby. *Use lindane only as directed by your doctor. Do not use more of it, do not use it more often, and do not use it for a longer time than your doctor ordered. In addition, you should not be treated with lindane more than twice during your pregnancy.*

Breast-feeding—Lindane is absorbed through the mother's skin and is present in breast milk. Even though lindane has not been reported to cause problems in nursing babies, you should use another method of feeding your baby for 2 days after you use lindane. Be sure you have discussed this with your doctor.

Children—Infants and children are especially sensitive to the effects of lindane. This may increase the chance of side effects during treatment. In addition, use of lindane is not recommended in premature infants.

Older adults—Absorption of lindane may be increased in the elderly. This may increase the chance of problems during treatment with this medicine.

Other medicines—Although certain medicines should not be used together at all, in other cases two different medicines may be used together even if an interaction might occur. In these cases, your doctor may want to change the dose, or other precautions may be necessary. When you are using lindane, it is especially important that your doctor and pharmacist know if you are using any other prescription or nonprescription (over-the-counter [OTC]) medicine.

Other medical problems—The presence of other medical problems may affect the use of lindane. Make sure you tell your doctor if you have any other medical problems, especially:

- Seizure disorder—Use of lindane may make the condition worse
- Skin rash or raw or broken skin—Condition may increase the absorption of lindane and the chance of side effects

Before you begin using any new medicine (prescription or nonprescription) or if you develop any new medical problem while you are using this medicine, check with your doctor, nurse, or pharmacist.

Proper Use of This Medicine

Lindane is poisonous. Keep it away from the mouth because it is harmful and may be fatal if swallowed.

Use lindane only as directed by your doctor. Do not use more of it, do not use it more often, and do not use it for a longer time than your doctor ordered. To do so may increase the chance of absorption through the skin and the chance of lindane poisoning.

Keep lindane away from the eyes. If you should accidentally get some in your eyes, flush them thoroughly with water at once and contact your doctor.

Do not use lindane on open wounds, such as cuts or sores on the skin or scalp. To do so may increase the chance of lindane poisoning.

When applying lindane to another person, you should wear plastic disposable or rubber gloves, especially if you are pregnant or are breast-feeding. This will prevent lindane from being absorbed through your skin. If you have any questions about this, check with your doctor.

Lindane usually comes with patient directions. Read them carefully before using lindane.

Your sexual partner or partners, especially, and all members of your household may need to be treated also, since the infestation may spread to persons in close contact. If these persons have not been checked for an infestation or if you have any questions about this, check with your doctor.

To use the *cream or lotion form of lindane for scabies:*

- If your skin has any cream, lotion, ointment, or oil on it, wash, rinse, and dry your skin well before applying lindane.
- If you take a warm bath or shower before using lindane, dry the skin well before applying it.
- Apply enough lindane to your dry skin to cover the entire skin surface from the neck down, including the soles of your feet, and rub in well.
- Leave lindane on for no more than 8 hours, then remove by washing thoroughly.

To use the *shampoo form of lindane for lice:*

- If your hair has any cream, lotion, ointment, or oil-based product on it, shampoo, rinse, and dry your hair and scalp well before applying lindane.
- If you apply this shampoo in the shower or in the bathtub, make sure the shampoo is not allowed to run down on other parts of your body. Also, do not apply this shampoo in a bathtub where the shampoo may run into the bath water in which you are sitting. To do so may increase the chance of absorption through the skin. When you rinse out the shampoo, be sure to thoroughly rinse your entire body also to remove any shampoo that may have gotten on it.
- Apply enough shampoo to your dry hair (1 ounce or less for short hair, 1½ ounces for medium length hair, and 2 ounces or less for long hair) to thoroughly wet the hair and skin or scalp of the affected and surrounding hairy areas.
- Thoroughly rub the shampoo into the hair and skin or scalp and allow to remain in place for 4 minutes. Then, use just enough water to work up a good lather.
- Rinse thoroughly and dry with a clean towel.
- When the hair is dry, comb with a fine-toothed comb to remove any remaining nits (eggs) or nit shells.
- *Do not use as a regular shampoo.*

Storage—To store this medicine:

- Keep out of the reach of children.
- Store away from heat and direct light.
- Keep lindane from freezing.
- Do not keep outdated lindane or lindane no longer needed. Be sure that any discarded lindane is out of the reach of children.

Precautions While Using This Medicine

To help prevent reinfestation or spreading of the infestation to other persons:

- For scabies—All recently worn underwear and pajamas and used sheets, pillow cases, and towels should be washed in very hot water or dry-cleaned.
- For lice—All recently worn clothing and used bed linens and towels should be washed in very hot water or dry-cleaned.

Side Effects of This Medicine

In infants and children, the risk of lindane being absorbed through the skin and causing unwanted side effects is greater than in adults. In premature newborn infants, use of lindane is not recommended, because lindane may be more likely to be absorbed through their skin than through the skin of older infants. You should discuss these possible effects with your doctor.

Along with its needed effects, a medicine may cause some unwanted effects. Although not all of these side effects may occur, if they do occur they may need medical attention.

Check with your doctor as soon as possible if any of the following side effects occur:

Rare

Skin irritation not present before use of lindane; skin rash

Symptoms of lindane poisoning

Convulsions (seizures); dizziness, clumsiness, or unsteadiness; fast heartbeat; muscle cramps; nervousness, restlessness, or irritability; vomiting

After you stop using lindane, itching may occur and continue for 1 to several weeks. If this continues longer or is bothersome, check with your doctor.

Other side effects not listed above may also occur in some patients. If you notice any other effects, check with your doctor.

Annual revision: August 1990

LITHIUM Systemic

Some commonly used brand names are:

In the U.S.

- Cibalith-S
- Eskalith
- Eskalith CR
- Lithane
- Lithobid
- Lithonate
- Lithotabs

Generic name product may also be available.

In Canada

- Carbolith
- Duralith
- Lithane
- Lithizine

Description

Lithium (LITH-ee-um) is used to treat the manic stage of bipolar disorder (manic-depressive illness). Manic-depressive patients experience severe mood changes, ranging from an excited or manic state (for example, unusual anger or irritability or a false sense of well-being) to depression or sadness. Lithium is used to reduce the frequency and severity of manic states. Lithium may also reduce the frequency and severity of depression in bipolar disorder.

It is not known how lithium works to stabilize a person's mood. However, it does act on the central nervous system. It helps you to have more control over your emotions and helps you cope better with the problems of living.

It is important that you and your family understand all the effects of lithium. These effects depend on your individual condition and response and the amount of lithium you use. You also must know when to contact your doctor if there are problems with the medicine's use. Lithium may also be used for other conditions as determined by your doctor.

This medicine is available only with your doctor's prescription, in the following dosage forms:

Oral

- Capsules (U.S. and Canada)
- Slow-release capsules (Canada)
- Syrup (U.S.)
- Tablets (U.S. and Canada)
- Extended-release tablets (U.S. and Canada)

It is very important that you read and understand the following information. If any of it causes you special concern, check with your doctor. Also, *if you have any questions* or if you want more information about this medicine or your medical problem, *ask your doctor, nurse, or pharmacist.*

Before Using This Medicine

In deciding to use a medicine, the risks of taking the medicine must be weighed against the good it will do. This is a decision you and your doctor will make. For lithium, the following should be considered:

Allergies—Tell your doctor if you have ever had any unusual or allergic reaction to lithium. Also tell your doctor and pharmacist if you are allergic to any other substances, such as foods, preservatives, or dyes.

Diet—Make certain your doctor, nurse, and pharmacist know if you are on a low-sodium or low-salt diet. Too little salt in your diet could lead to serious side effects.

Pregnancy—Lithium is not recommended for use during pregnancy, especially during the first 3 months. Studies have shown that lithium may rarely cause thyroid problems and heart or blood vessel defects in the baby. It has also been shown to cause muscle weakness and severe drowsiness in newborn babies of mothers taking lithium near time of delivery.

Breast-feeding—Lithium passes into the breast milk. It has been reported to cause unwanted effects such as muscle weakness, lowered body temperature, and heart problems in nursing babies. Before taking this medicine, be sure you have discussed with your doctor the risks and benefits of breast-feeding.

Children—Lithium may cause weakened bones in children during treatment.

Older adults—Unusual thirst, an increase in amount of urine, diarrhea, drowsiness, loss of appetite, muscle weakness, trembling, slurred speech, nausea or vomiting, goiter, or symptoms of underactive thyroid are especially likely to occur in elderly patients, who are often more sensitive than younger adults to the effects of lithium.

Other medicines—Although certain medicines should not be used together at all, in other cases 2 different medicines may be used together even if an interaction might occur. In these cases, your doctor may want to change the dose, or other precautions may be necessary. When you are taking lithium, it is especially important that your doctor and pharmacist know if you are taking any of the following:

- Antipsychotics (medicine for mental illness)—Blood levels of both medicines may change, increasing the chance of serious side effects
- Diuretics (water pills) or
- Inflammation or pain medicine, except narcotics—Higher blood levels of lithium may occur, increasing the chance of serious side effects
- Medicine for asthma, bronchitis, emphysema, sinusitis, or cystic fibrosis that contains the following:
  Calcium iodide or
  Iodinated glycerol or
  Potassium iodide—Unwanted effects on the thyroid gland may occur

Other medical problems—The presence of other medical problems may affect the use of lithium. Make sure you tell your doctor if you have any other medical problems, especially:

- Brain disease or
- Schizophrenia—You may be especially sensitive to lithium, and mental effects (such as increased confusion) may occur
- Diabetes mellitus (sugar diabetes)—Lithium may increase the blood levels of insulin; the dose of insulin you need to take may change
- Difficult urination or
- Infection (severe, occurring with fever, prolonged sweating, diarrhea, or vomiting) or
- Kidney disease—Higher blood levels of lithium may occur, increasing the chance of serious side effects
- Epilepsy or
- Goiter or other thyroid disease, or
- Heart disease or
- Parkinson's disease or
- Psoriasis—Lithium may make the condition worse
- Leukemia (history of)—Lithium may cause the leukemia to occur again

Before you begin using any new medicine (prescription or nonprescription) or if you develop any new medical problem while you are using this medicine, check with your doctor, nurse, or pharmacist.

Proper Use of This Medicine

Take this medicine after a meal or snack. Doing so will reduce stomach upset, tremors, or weakness and may also prevent a laxative effect.

For patients taking the *long-acting or slow-release form* of lithium:

- Swallow the tablet or capsule whole.
- Do not break, crush, or chew before swallowing.

For patients taking the *syrup form* of lithium:

- Dilute the syrup in fruit juice or another flavored beverage before taking.

During treatment with lithium, drink 2 or 3 quarts of water or other fluids each day, and use a normal amount of salt in your food, unless otherwise directed by your doctor.

Take this medicine exactly as directed. Do not take more or less of it, do not take it more or less often, and do not take it for a longer time than your doctor ordered. To do so may increase the chance of unwanted effects.

Sometimes lithium must be taken for 1 to several weeks before you begin to feel better.

In order for lithium to work properly, it must be taken every day in regularly spaced doses as ordered by your doctor. This is necessary to keep a constant amount of lithium in your blood. To help keep the amount constant, do not miss any doses and *do not stop taking the medicine even if you feel better.*

Dosing—The dose of lithium will be different for different patients. *Follow your doctor's orders or the directions on the label.* The following information includes only the average doses of lithium. *If your dose is different, do not change it* unless your doctor tells you to do so.

- The number of capsules or tablets or teaspoonfuls of syrup that you take depends on the strength of the medicine. Also, *the number of doses you take each day, the time allowed between doses, and the length of time you take the medicine depend on the medical problem for which you are using lithium.*
- For *short-acting oral* dosage forms (capsules, tablets, syrup):
  —Adults and adolescents: To start, 300 to 600 milligrams three times a day.
  —Children up to 12 years of age: The dose is based on body weight. To start, the usual dose is 15 to 20 milligrams per kilogram of body weight (6.8 to 9 milligrams per pound) a day, given in smaller doses two or three times during the day.
- For *long-acting oral* dosage forms (slow-release capsules, extended-release tablets):
  —Adults and adolescents: 300 to 600 milligrams three times a day, or 450 to 900 milligrams two times a day.
  —Children up to 12 years of age: Dose must be determined by the doctor.

Missed dose—If you miss a dose of this medicine, take it as soon as possible. However, if it is within 4 hours (about 6 hours for extended-release tablets or slow-release capsules) of your next dose, skip the missed dose and go back to your regular dosing schedule. Do not double doses.

Storage—To store this medicine:

- Keep out of the reach of children.
- Store away from heat and direct light.
- Do not store in the bathroom, near the kitchen sink, or in other damp places. Heat or moisture may cause the medicine to break down.
- Keep the syrup form of this medicine from freezing.
- Do not keep outdated medicine or medicine no longer needed. Be sure that any discarded medicine is out of the reach of children.

Precautions While Using This Medicine

Your doctor should check your progress at regular visits to make sure that the medicine is working properly and that possible side effects are avoided. Laboratory tests may be necessary.

Lithium may not work properly if you drink large amounts of caffeine-containing coffee, tea, or colas.

This medicine may cause some people to become dizzy, drowsy, or less alert than they are normally. *Make sure you know how you react to this medicine before you drive, use machines, or do anything else that could be dangerous if you are dizzy or are not alert.*

Use extra care in hot weather and during activities that cause you to sweat heavily, such as hot baths, saunas, or exercising. The loss of too much water and salt from your body could lead to serious side effects from this medicine.

If you have an infection or illness that causes heavy sweating, vomiting, or diarrhea, check with your doctor. The loss of too much water and salt from your body could lead to serious side effects from lithium.

Do not go on a diet to lose weight and do not make a major change in your diet without first checking with your doctor. Improper dieting could cause the loss of too much water and salt from your body and could lead to serious side effects from this medicine.

For patients taking the *slow-release capsules or the extended-release tablets*:

- Do not use this medicine interchangeably with other lithium products.

It is important that you and your family know the early symptoms of lithium overdose or toxicity and when to call the doctor.

Side Effects of This Medicine

Along with its needed effects, a medicine may cause some unwanted effects. Although not all of these side effects may occur, if they do occur they may need medical attention.

Check with your doctor immediately if any of the following side effects occur:

Early symptoms of overdose or toxicity

Diarrhea; drowsiness; loss of appetite; muscle weakness; nausea or vomiting; slurred speech; trembling

Late symptoms of overdose or toxicity

Blurred vision; clumsiness or unsteadiness; confusion; convulsions (seizures); dizziness; increase in amount of urine; trembling (severe)

Check with your doctor as soon as possible if any of the following side effects occur:

Less common

Fainting; fast or slow heartbeat; irregular pulse; troubled breathing (especially during hard work or exercise); unusual tiredness or weakness; weight gain

Rare

Blue color and pain in fingers and toes; coldness of arms and legs; dizziness; eye pain; headache; noises in the ears; vision problems

Signs of low thyroid function

Dry, rough skin; hair loss; hoarseness; mental depression; sensitivity to cold; swelling of feet or lower legs; swelling of neck; unusual excitement

Other side effects may occur that usually do not need medical attention. These side effects may go away during treatment as your body adjusts to the medicine. However, check with your doctor if any of the following side effects continue or are bothersome:

More common

Increased frequency of urination or loss of bladder control—more common in women than in men, usually beginning 2 to 7 years after start of treatment; increased thirst; nausea (mild); trembling of hands (slight)

Less common

Acne or skin rash; bloated feeling or pressure in the stomach; muscle twitching (slight)

Other side effects not listed above may also occur in some patients. If you notice any other effects, check with your doctor.

Additional Information

Once a medicine has been approved for marketing for a certain use, experience may show that it is also useful for other medical problems. Although these uses are not

included in product labeling, lithium is used in certain patients with the following medical conditions:

- Cluster headaches
- Mental depression
- Neutropenia (a blood condition in which there is a decreased number of a certain type of white blood cells)

Other than the above information, there is no additional information relating to proper use, precautions, or side effects for these uses.

Annual revision: 03/09/93

LOMUSTINE Systemic

A commonly used brand name in the U.S. and Canada is CeeNU. Another commonly used name is CCNU.

Description

Lomustine (loe-MUS-teen) belongs to the group of medicines known as alkylating agents. It is used to treat some kinds of cancer.

Lomustine interferes with the growth of cancer cells, which are eventually destroyed. Since the growth of normal body cells may also be affected by lomustine, other effects will also occur. Some of these may be serious and must be reported to your doctor. Other effects, like hair loss, may not be serious but may cause concern. Some effects may not occur for months or years after the medicine is used.

Before you begin treatment with lomustine, you and your doctor should talk about the good this medicine will do as well as the risks of using it.

Lomustine is available only with your doctor's prescription, in the following dosage form:

Oral

- Capsules (U.S. and Canada)

It is very important that you read and understand the following information. If any of it causes you special concern, check with your doctor. Also, *if you have any questions* or if you want more information about this medicine or your medical problem, *ask your doctor, nurse, or pharmacist.*

Before Using This Medicine

In deciding to use a medicine, the risks of taking the medicine must be weighed against the good it will do. This is a decision you and your doctor will make. For lomustine, the following should be considered:

Allergies—Tell your doctor if you have ever had any unusual or allergic reaction to lomustine.

Pregnancy—Tell your doctor if you are pregnant or if you intend to have children. There is a chance that this medicine may cause birth defects if either the male or female is taking it at the time of conception or if it is taken during pregnancy. Lomustine causes birth defects in rats and causes toxic or harmful effects in the fetus of rats and rabbits at doses about the same as the human dose. In addition, many cancer medicines may cause sterility which could be permanent. Sterility has been reported in animals and humans with this medicine.

Be sure that you have discussed this with your doctor before taking this medicine. It is best to use some kind of birth control while you are taking lomustine. Tell your doctor right away if you think you have become pregnant while taking lomustine.

Breast-feeding—Tell your doctor if you are breast-feeding or if you intend to breast-feed during treatment with this medicine. Because lomustine may cause serious side effects, breast-feeding is generally not recommended while you are receiving it.

Children—Although there is no specific information comparing use of lomustine in children with use in other age groups, this medicine is not expected to cause different side effects or problems in children than it does in adults.

Older adults—Many medicines have not been studied specifically in older people. Therefore, it may not be known whether they work exactly the same way they do in younger adults or if they cause different side effects or problems in older people. There is no specific information comparing use of lomustine in the elderly with use in other age groups.

Other medicines—Although certain medicines should not be used together at all, in other cases two different medicines may be used together even if an interaction might occur. In these cases, your doctor may want to change the dose, or other precautions may be necessary. When you are taking lomustine, it is especially important that your doctor and pharmacist know if you have ever been treated with x-rays or cancer medicines or if you are taking any of the following:

- Amphotericin B by injection (e.g., Fungizone) or
- Antithyroid agents (medicine for overactive thyroid) or
- Azathioprine (e.g., Imuran) or
- Chloramphenicol (e.g., Chloromycetin) or
- Colchicine or
- Flucytosine (e.g., Ancobon) or

- Ganciclovir (e.g., Cytovene) or
- Interferon (e.g., Intron A, Roferon-A) or
- Plicamycin (e.g., Mithracin) or
- Zidovudine (e.g., AZT, Retrovir)—Lomustine may increase the effects of these medicines or radiation therapy on the blood

Other medical problems—The presence of other medical problems may affect the use of lomustine. Make sure you tell your doctor if you have any other medical problems, especially:

- Chickenpox (including recent exposure) or
- Herpes zoster (shingles)—Risk of severe disease affecting other parts of the body
- Infection—Lomustine can decrease your body's ability to fight infection
- Kidney disease—Effects of lomustine may be increased because of slower removal from the body
- Lung disease—Risk of lung problems caused by lomustine may be increased

Before you begin using any new medicine (prescription or nonprescription) or if you develop any new medical problem while you are using this medicine, check with your doctor, nurse, or pharmacist.

Proper Use of This Medicine

Take this medicine only as directed by your doctor. Do not take more or less of it than your doctor ordered. The exact amount of medicine you need has been carefully worked out. Taking too much may increase the chance of side effects, while taking too little may not improve your condition.

In order that you receive the proper dose of lomustine, there may be two or more different types of capsules in the container. This is not an error. It is important that you take all of the capsules in the container as one dose so that you receive the right dose of the medicine.

This medicine is sometimes given together with certain other medicines. If you are using a combination of medicines, make sure that you take each one at the right time and do not mix them. Ask your doctor, nurse, or pharmacist to help you plan a way to remember to take your medicines at the right times.

Nausea and vomiting occur often after lomustine is taken, but usually last less than 24 hours. Loss of appetite may last for several days. This medicine is best taken on an empty stomach at bedtime so that it will cause less stomach upset. Ask your doctor, nurse, or pharmacist for other ways to lessen these effects.

If you vomit shortly after taking a dose of lomustine, check with your doctor. You may be told to take the dose again.

Precautions While Using This Medicine

It is important that your doctor check your progress at regular visits to make sure that this medicine is working properly and to check for unwanted effects.

While you are being treated with lomustine, and after you stop treatment with it, *do not have any immunizations (vaccinations) without your doctor's approval.* Lomustine may lower your body's resistance and there is a chance you might get the infection the immunization is meant to prevent. In addition, other persons living in your household should not take oral polio vaccine since there is a chance they could pass the polio virus on to you. Also, avoid persons who have recently taken oral polio vaccine. Do not get close to them, and do not stay in the same room with them for very long. If you cannot take these precautions, you should consider wearing a protective face mask that covers the nose and mouth.

Lomustine can temporarily lower the number of white blood cells in your blood, increasing the chance of getting an infection. It can also lower the number of platelets, which are necessary for proper blood clotting. If this occurs, there are certain precautions you can take, especially when your blood count is low, to reduce the risk of infection or bleeding:

- If you can, avoid people with infections. *Check with your doctor immediately* if you think you are getting an infection or if you get a fever or chills, cough or hoarseness, lower back or side pain, or painful or difficult urination.
- *Check with your doctor immediately* if you notice any unusual bleeding or bruising; black, tarry stools; blood in urine or stools; or pinpoint red spots on your skin.
- Be careful when using a regular toothbrush, dental floss, or toothpick. Your medical doctor, dentist, or nurse may recommend other ways to clean your teeth and gums. Check with your medical doctor before having any dental work done.
- Do not touch your eyes or the inside of your nose unless you have just washed your hands and have not touched anything else in the meantime.
- Be careful not to cut yourself when you are using sharp objects such as a safety razor or fingernail or toenail cutters.
- Avoid contact sports or other situations where bruising or injury could occur.

Side Effects of This Medicine

Along with their needed effects, medicines like lomustine can sometimes cause unwanted effects such as blood problems, loss of hair, and other side effects; these are described below. Also, because of the way these medicines act on the body, there is a chance that they might cause other unwanted effects that may not occur until months or years after the medicine is used. These delayed effects may include certain types of cancer, such as leukemia. Discuss these possible effects with your doctor.

Although not all of these side effects may occur, if they do occur they may need medical attention.

Check with your doctor or nurse immediately if any of the following side effects occur:

Less common

Black, tarry stools; blood in urine or stools; cough or hoarseness; fever or chills; lower back or side pain; painful or difficult urination; pinpoint red spots on skin; unusual bleeding or bruising

Check with your doctor as soon as possible if any of the following side effects occur:

Less common

Awkwardness; confusion; decrease in urination; slurred speech; sores in mouth and on lips; swelling of feet or lower legs; unusual tiredness or weakness

Rare

Cough; shortness of breath

Other side effects may occur that usually do not need medical attention. These side effects may go away during treatment as your body adjusts to the medicine. Also, your doctor or nurse may be able to tell you about ways to prevent or reduce some of these side effects. Check with your doctor or nurse if any of the following side effects continue or are bothersome or if you have any questions about them:

More common

Loss of appetite
Nausea and vomiting (usually last less than 24 hours)

Less common

Darkening of skin; diarrhea; skin rash and itching

This medicine may cause a temporary loss of hair in some people. After treatment with lomustine has ended, normal hair growth should return.

After you stop using this medicine, it may still produce some side effects that need attention. During this period of time, check with your doctor if you notice any of the following side effects:

Black, tarry stools; blood in urine or stools; cough or hoarseness; fever or chills; lower back or side pain; painful or difficult urination; pinpoint red spots on skin; unusual bleeding or bruising

Other side effects not listed above may also occur in some patients. If you notice any other effects, check with your doctor.

Annual revision: 08/09/92

LOPERAMIDE Oral

Some commonly used brand names are:

In the U.S.

Imodium
Imodium A-D
Imodium A-D Caplets

In Canada

Imodium

Description

Loperamide (loe-PER-a-mide) is a medicine used along with other measures to treat diarrhea. Loperamide helps stop diarrhea by slowing down the movements of the intestines.

In the U.S., loperamide capsules are available only with your doctor's prescription, while the liquid form and the tablet form are available without a prescription. In Canada, all the dosage forms are available without a prescription.

Loperamide is available in the following dosage forms:

Oral

- Capsules (U.S. and Canada)
- Oral solution (U.S. and Canada)
- Tablets (U.S. and Canada)

It is very important that you read and understand the following information. If any of it causes you special concern, check with your doctor or pharmacist. Also, *if you have any questions* or if you want more information about this medicine or your medical problem, *ask your doctor, nurse, or pharmacist.*

Before Using This Medicine

If you are taking this medicine without a prescription, carefully read and follow any precautions on the label. For loperamide, the following should be considered:

Allergies—Tell your doctor if you have ever had any unusual or allergic reaction to loperamide. Also tell your doctor and pharmacist if you are allergic to any other substances, such as foods, preservatives, or dyes.

Pregnancy—Studies have not been done in humans. However, studies in animals have not shown that loperamide causes cancer or birth defects or lessens the chances of becoming pregnant when given in doses many times the human dose.

Breast-feeding—It is not known whether loperamide passes into the breast milk. However, this medicine has not been reported to cause problems in nursing babies.

Children—This medicine should not be used in children under 2 years of age. Children, especially very young children, are very sensitive to the effects of loperamide. This may increase the chance of side effects during treatment. Also, the fluid loss caused by diarrhea may result in a severe condition. For these reasons, do not give medicine for diarrhea to young children without first checking with their doctor. In older children with diarrhea, medicine for diarrhea may be used, but it is also very important that a sufficient amount of liquids be given to replace the fluid lost by the body. If you have any questions about this, check with your doctor, nurse, or pharmacist.

Older adults—The fluid loss caused by diarrhea may result in a severe condition. For this reason, elderly persons with diarrhea, in addition to using medicine for diarrhea, must receive a sufficient amount of liquids to replace the fluid lost by the body. If you have any questions about this, check with your doctor, nurse, or pharmacist.

Other medicines—Although certain medicines should not be used together at all, in other cases two different medicines may be used together even if an interaction might occur. In these cases, your doctor may want to change the dose, or other precautions may be necessary. When you are taking loperamide, it is especially important that your doctor and pharmacist know if you are taking any of the following:

- Antibiotics such as cephalosporins (e.g., Ceftin, Keflex), clindamycin (e.g., Cleocin), erythromycins (e.g., E.E.S., PCE), tetracyclines (e.g., Achromycin, Doryx)—These antibiotics may cause diarrhea; loperamide may make the diarrhea caused by antibiotics worse or make it last longer
- Narcotic pain medicine—There is a greater chance that severe constipation may occur if loperamide is used together with narcotic pain medicine

Other medical problems—The presence of other medical problems may affect the use of loperamide. Make sure you tell your doctor if you have any other medical problems, especially:

- Colitis (severe)—A more serious problem of the colon may develop if you use this medicine
- Dysentery—This condition may get worse; a different kind of treatment may be needed
- Liver disease—The chance of severe central nervous system (CNS) side effects may be greater in patients with liver disease

Before you begin using any new medicine (prescription or nonprescription) or if you develop any new medical problem while you are using this medicine, check with your doctor, nurse, or pharmacist.

Proper Use of This Medicine

For safe and effective use of this medicine:

- *Follow your doctor's instructions if this medicine was prescribed.*
- Follow the manufacturer's package directions if you are treating yourself.

Importance of diet and fluid intake while treating diarrhea:

- *In addition to using medicine for diarrhea, it is very important that you replace the fluid lost by the body and follow a proper diet.* For the first 24 hours, you should drink plenty of caffeine-free clear liquids, such as ginger ale, decaffeinated cola, decaffeinated tea, broth, and gelatin. During the next 24 hours you may eat bland foods, such as cooked cereals, bread, crackers, and applesauce. Fruits, vegetables, fried or spicy foods, bran, candy, caffeine, and alcoholic beverages may make the condition worse.
- If too much fluid has been lost by the body due to the diarrhea, a serious condition may develop. Check with your doctor as soon as possible if any of the following signs of too much fluid loss occur:

  Decreased urination
  Dizziness and lightheadedness
  Dryness of mouth
  Increased thirst
  Wrinkled skin

Missed dose—If you must take this medicine regularly and you miss a dose, skip the missed dose and go back to your regular dosing schedule. Do not double doses.

Storage—To store this medicine:

- Keep out of the reach of children
- Store away from heat and direct light.
- Do not store the capsule or tablet form of this medicine in the bathroom, near the kitchen sink, or in other damp places. Heat or moisture may cause the medicine to break down.
- Keep the liquid form of this medicine from freezing.
- Do not keep outdated medicine or medicine no longer needed. Be sure that any discarded medicine is out of the reach of children.

Precautions While Using This Medicine

Loperamide should not be used for more than 2 days, unless directed by your doctor. If you will be taking this medicine regularly for a long time, your doctor should check your progress at regular visits.

Check with your doctor if your diarrhea does not stop after two days or if you develop a fever.

Side Effects of This Medicine

Along with its needed effects, a medicine may cause some unwanted effects. *When this medicine is used for short periods of time at low doses, side effects usually are rare.*

However, check with your doctor immediately if any of the following side effects are severe and occur suddenly since they may be signs of a more severe and dangerous problem with your bowels:

Rare

Bloating; constipation; loss of appetite; stomach pain (severe) with nausea and vomiting

Also, check with your doctor as soon as possible if the following side effect occurs:

Rare

Skin rash

Other side effects may occur that usually do not need medical attention. These side effects may go away during treatment as your body adjusts to the medicine. However, check with your doctor if any of the following side effects continue or are bothersome:

Rare

Drowsiness or dizziness; dryness of mouth

Other side effects not listed above may also occur in some patients. If you notice any other effects, check with your doctor.

Annual revision: 05/15/91

LOXAPINE Systemic

Some commonly used brand names are:

In the U.S.

Loxitane
Loxitane C
Loxitane IM

Generic name product may also be available.

In Canada

Loxapac

Description

Loxapine (LOX-a-peen) is used to treat nervous, mental, and emotional conditions.

Loxapine is available only with your doctor's prescription, in the following dosage forms:

Oral

- Solution (U.S. and Canada)
- Capsules (U.S.)
- Tablets (Canada)

Parenteral

- Injection (U.S. and Canada)

It is very important that you read and understand the following information. If any of it causes you special concern, check with your doctor. Also, *if you have any questions* or if you want more information about this medicine or your medical problem, *ask your doctor, nurse, or pharmacist.*

Before Using This Medicine

In deciding to use a medicine, the risks of taking the medicine must be weighed against the good it will do. This is a decision you and your doctor will make. For loxapine, the following should be considered:

Allergies—Tell your doctor if you have ever had any unusual or allergic reaction to loxapine or amoxapine. Also tell your doctor and pharmacist if you are allergic to any other substances, such as foods, preservatives, or dyes.

Pregnancy—Loxapine has not been shown to cause birth defects or other problems in humans. However, animal studies have shown unwanted effects in the fetus.

Breast-feeding—It is not known if loxapine passes into breast milk.

Children—Studies on this medicine have been done only in adult patients, and there is no specific information comparing use of loxapine in children with use in other age groups.

Older adults—Elderly patients are usually more sensitive than younger adults to the effects of loxapine. Constipation, dizziness or fainting, drowsiness, dry mouth, trembling of the hands and fingers, and symptoms of tardive dyskinesia (such as rapid, worm-like movements of the tongue or any other uncontrolled movements of the mouth, tongue, or jaw, and/or arms and legs) are especially likely to occur in elderly patients.

Other medicines—Although certain medicines should not be used together at all, in other cases 2 different medicines may be used together even if an interaction might occur. In these cases, your doctor may want to change the dose, or other precautions may be necessary. When you are taking loxapine, it is especially important that

your doctor and pharmacist know if you are taking any of the following:

- Amoxapine (e.g., Asendin) or
- Methyldopa (e.g., Aldomet) or
- Metoclopramide (e.g., Reglan) or
- Metyrosine (e.g., Demser) or
- Other antipsychotics (medicine for mental illness) or
- Pemoline (e.g., Cylert) or
- Pimozide (e.g., Orap) or
- Promethazine (e.g., Phenergan) or
- Rauwolfia alkaloids (alseroxylon [e.g., Rauwiloid], deserpidine [e.g., Harmonyl], rauwolfia serpentina [e.g., Raudixin], reserpine [e.g., Serpasil]) or
- Trimeprazine (e.g., Temaril)—Taking these medicines with loxapine may increase the chance and seriousness of some side effects
- Central nervous system (CNS) depressants (medicine that causes drowsiness) or
- Tricyclic antidepressants (medicine for depression)—Taking these medicines with loxapine may increase the CNS depressant effects
- Guanadrel (e.g., Hylorel) or
- Guanethidine (e.g., Ismelin)—Loxapine may decrease the effects of these medicines

Other medical problems—The presence of other medical problems may affect the use of loxapine. Make sure you tell your doctor if you have any other medical problems, especially:

- Alcohol abuse—CNS depressant effects may be increased
- Difficult urination or
- Enlarged prostate or
- Glaucoma (or predisposition to) or
- Parkinson's disease—Loxapine may make the condition worse
- Heart or blood vessel disease—An increased risk of low blood pressure (hypotension) or changes in the rhythm of your heart may occur
- Liver disease—Higher blood levels of loxapine may occur, increasing the chance of side effects
- Seizure disorders—Loxapine may increase the risk of seizures

Before you begin using any new medicine (prescription or nonprescription) or if you develop any new medical problem while you are using this medicine, check with your doctor, nurse, or pharmacist.

Proper Use of This Medicine

This medicine may be taken with food or a full glass (8 ounces) of water or milk to reduce stomach irritation.

For patients taking the *oral solution*:

- Measure the solution only with the dropper provided by the manufacturer. This will give a more accurate dose.

The liquid medicine must be mixed with orange juice or grapefruit juice just before you take it to make it easier to take.

Do not take more of this medicine, do not take it more often, and do not take it for a longer time than your doctor ordered. To do so may increase the chance of unwanted effects.

Dosing—The dose of loxapine will be different for different patients. *Follow your doctor's orders or the directions on the label.* The following information includes only the average doses of loxapine. *If your dose is different, do not change it* unless your doctor tells you to do so:

- The number of capsules or tablets or amount of solution that you take depends on the strength of the medicine. Also, *the number of doses you take each day, the time allowed between doses, and the length of time you take the medicine depend on the medical problem for which you are taking loxapine.*
- For *oral* dosage forms (capsules, oral solution, or tablets):
  —Adults: To start, 10 milligrams taken two times a day. Your doctor may increase your dose if needed.
  —Children up to 16 years of age: The dose must be determined by the doctor.
- For *injection* dosage form:
  —Adults: 12.5 to 50 milligrams every four to six hours, injected into a muscle.
  —Children up to 16 years of age: The dose must be determined by the doctor.

Missed dose—If you miss a dose of this medicine, take it as soon as possible. However, if it is within one hour of your next dose, skip the missed dose and go back to your regular dosing schedule. Do not double doses.

Storage—To store this medicine:

- Keep out of the reach of children.
- Store away from heat and direct light.
- Do not store the capsule or tablet form of this medicine in the bathroom, near the kitchen sink, or in other damp places. Heat or moisture may cause the medicine to break down.
- Keep the liquid form of this medicine from freezing.
- Do not keep outdated medicine or medicine no longer needed. Be sure that any discarded medicine is out of the reach of children.

Precautions While Using This Medicine

Your doctor should check your progress at regular visits, especially during the first few months of treatment with this medicine. The amount of loxapine you take may be changed often to meet the needs of your condition and to help avoid side effects.

Do not stop taking this medicine without first checking with your doctor. Your doctor may want you to reduce gradually the amount you are taking before stopping completely. This will allow your body time to adjust and to keep your condition from becoming worse.

This medicine will add to the effects of alcohol and other CNS depressants (medicines that slow down the nervous system, possibly causing drowsiness). Some examples of CNS depressants are antihistamines or medicine for hay fever, other allergies, or colds; sedatives, tranquilizers, or sleeping medicine; prescription pain medicine or narcotics; barbiturates; medicine for seizures; or anesthetics, including some dental anesthetics. *Check with your doctor before taking any of the above while you are taking this medicine.*

Do not take this medicine within two hours of taking antacids or medicine for diarrhea. Taking loxapine and antacids or medicine for diarrhea too close together may make this medicine less effective.

This medicine may cause some people to become drowsy or less alert than they are normally, especially as the amount of medicine is increased. Even if you take this medicine at bedtime, you may feel drowsy or less alert on arising. *Make sure you know how you react to this medicine before you drive, use machines, or do anything else that could be dangerous if you are not alert.*

Although it is not a problem for most patients, dizziness, lightheadedness, or fainting may occur, especially when you get up from a lying or sitting position. Getting up slowly may help. However, if the problem continues or gets worse, check with your doctor.

Loxapine may cause your skin to be more sensitive to sunlight than it is normally. Exposure to sunlight, even for brief periods of time, may cause a skin rash, itching, redness or other discoloration of the skin, or a severe sunburn. When you begin taking this medicine:

- Stay out of direct sunlight, especially between the hours of 10:00 a.m. and 3:00 p.m., if possible.
- Wear protective clothing, including a hat. Also, wear sunglasses.
- Apply a sun block product that has a skin protection factor (SPF) of at least 15. Some patients may require a product with a higher SPF number, especially if they have a fair complexion. If you have any questions about this, check with your doctor or pharmacist.
- Apply a sun block lipstick that has an SPF of at least 15 to protect your lips.
- Do not use a sunlamp or tanning bed or booth.

If you have a severe reaction from the sun, check with your doctor.

Loxapine may cause dryness of the mouth. For temporary relief, use sugarless candy or gum, melt bits of ice in your mouth, or use a saliva substitute. However, if your mouth continues to feel dry for more than 2 weeks, check with your medical doctor or dentist. Continuing dryness of the mouth may increase the chance of dental disease, including tooth decay, gum disease, and fungus infections.

Before having any kind of surgery, dental treatment, or emergency treatment, tell the medical doctor or dentist in charge that you are taking this medicine. Taking loxapine together with medicines that are used during surgery or dental or emergency treatments may increase the CNS depressant effects.

Side Effects of This Medicine

Along with its needed effects, loxapine can sometimes cause serious side effects. Tardive dyskinesia (a movement disorder) may occur and may not go away after you stop using the medicine. Signs of tardive dyskinesia include fine, worm-like movements of the tongue, or other uncontrolled movements of the mouth, tongue, cheeks, jaw, or arms and legs. Other serious but rare side effects may also occur. These include severe muscle stiffness, fever, unusual tiredness or weakness, fast heartbeat, difficult breathing, increased sweating, loss of bladder control, and seizures (neuroleptic malignant syndrome). *You and your doctor should discuss the good this medicine will do as well as the risks of taking it.*

Stop taking loxapine and get emergency help immediately if any of the following side effects occur:

Rare

Convulsions (seizures); difficult or fast breathing; fast heartbeat or irregular pulse; fever (high); high or low blood pressure; increased sweating; loss of bladder control; muscle stiffness (severe); unusually pale skin; unusual tiredness or weakness

Check with your doctor immediately if any of the following side effects occur:

More common

Lip smacking or puckering; puffing of cheeks; rapid or fine, worm-like movements of tongue; uncontrolled chewing movements; uncontrolled movements of arms or legs

Also, check with your doctor as soon as possible if any of the following side effects occur:

More common (occurring with increase of dosage)

Difficulty in speaking or swallowing; loss of balance control; mask-like face; restlessness or desire to keep moving; shuffling walk; slowed movements; stiffness of arms and legs; trembling and shaking of fingers and hands

Less common

Constipation (severe); difficult urination; inability to move eyes; muscle spasms, especially of the neck and back; skin rash; twisting movements of the body

Rare

Sore throat and fever; increased blinking or spasms of eyelid; uncontrolled twisting movements of neck, trunk, arms, or legs; unusual bleeding or bruising; unusual facial expressions or body positions; yellow eyes or skin

Symptoms of overdose

Dizziness (severe); drowsiness (severe); muscle trembling, jerking, stiffness, or uncontrolled movements (severe); troubled breathing (severe); unusual tiredness or weakness (severe)

Other side effects may occur that usually do not need medical attention. These side effects may go away during treatment as your body adjusts to the medicine. However, check with your doctor if any of the following side effects continue or are bothersome:

More common

Blurred vision; confusion; dizziness, lightheadedness, or fainting; drowsiness; dryness of mouth

Less common

Constipation (mild); decreased sexual ability; enlargement of breasts (males and females); headache; increased sensitivity of skin to sun; missing menstrual periods; nausea or vomiting; trouble in sleeping; unusual secretion of milk; weight gain

Certain side effects of this medicine may occur after you have stopped taking it. Check with your doctor as soon as possible if you notice any of the following effects after you have stopped taking loxapine:

Dizziness; nausea and vomiting; rapid or worm-like movements of the tongue; stomach upset or pain; trembling of fingers and hands; uncontrolled chewing movements

Other side effects not listed above may also occur in some patients. If you notice any other effects, check with your doctor.

Additional Information

Once a medicine has been approved for marketing for a certain use, experience may show that it is also useful for other medical problems. Although this use is not included in product labeling, loxapine is used in certain patients with the following medical condition:

- Anxiety associated with mental depression

Other than the above information, there is no additional information relating to proper use, precautions, or side effects for this use.

Annual revision: 01/29/93

LYPRESSIN Systemic

A commonly used brand name in the U.S. is Diapid.

Description

Lypressin (lye-PRESS-in) is a hormone used to prevent or control the frequent urination, increased thirst, and loss of water associated with diabetes insipidus (water diabetes).

Lypressin is available only with your doctor's prescription, in the following dosage form:

Nasal

- Nasal spray (U.S.)

It is very important that you read and understand the following information. If any of it causes you special concern, check with your doctor. Also, *if you have any questions* or if you want more information about this medicine or your medical problem, *ask your doctor, nurse, or pharmacist.*

Before Using This Medicine

In deciding to use a medicine, the risks of taking the medicine must be weighed against the good it will do. This is a decision you and your doctor will make. For lypressin, the following should be considered:

Allergies—Tell your doctor if you have ever had any unusual or allergic reaction to lypressin or vasopressin. Also tell your doctor and pharmacist if you are allergic to any other substances, such as foods, preservatives, or dyes.

Pregnancy—Studies on the effects in pregnancy have not been done in either humans or animals.

Breast-feeding—It is not known whether lypressin passes into breast milk. However, this medicine has not been reported to cause problems in nursing babies.

Children—Although there is no specific information comparing use of lypressin in children with use in other age groups, this medicine is not expected to cause different side effects or problems in children than it does in adults.

Older adults—Many medicines have not been studied specifically in older people. Therefore, it may not be known whether they work exactly the same way they do in younger adults or if they cause different side effects or problems in older people. There is no specific information comparing use of lypressin in the elderly with use in other age groups.

Other medicines—Although certain medicines should not be used together at all, in other cases two different medicines may be used together even if an interaction might occur. In these cases, your doctor may want to change the dose, or other precautions may be necessary. Tell your doctor and pharmacist if you are taking any other prescription or nonprescription (over-the-counter [OTC]) medicine.

Other medical problems—The presence of other medical problems may affect the use of lypressin. Make sure you tell your doctor if you have any other medical problems, especially:

- Hay fever or other allergies or
- Infection of ears, lungs, nose, or throat or
- Stuffy nose—May prevent nasal lypressin from being absorbed into the bloodstream, through the lining of the nose
- High blood pressure—Lypressin may increase blood pressure

M

Before you begin using any new medicine (prescription or nonprescription) or if you develop any new medical problem while you are using this medicine, check with your doctor, nurse, or pharmacist.

Proper Use of This Medicine

Use this medicine only as directed. Do not use more of it and do not use it more often than your doctor ordered. To do so may increase the chance of unwanted effects.

To use:

- Blow nose gently. Hold the bottle in an upright position. With head upright, spray the medicine into each nostril by squeezing the bottle quickly and firmly. Do not lie down when spraying this medicine.

Rinse the tip of the bottle with hot water, taking care not to suck water into the bottle, and dry with a clean tissue. Replace the cap right after use.

Dosing—The dose of lypressin will be different for different patients. *Follow your doctor's orders or the directions on the label.* The following information includes only the average doses of lypressin. *If your dose is different, do not change it* unless your doctor tells you to do so.

- For *nasal* dosage forms:
  - —Adults: One or two sprays in each nostril four times a day.
  - —Children six weeks of age and older: One or two sprays in each nostril four times a day.
  - —Children less than six weeks of age: Use is generally not recommended.

Missed dose—If you miss a dose of this medicine, use it as soon as possible. However, if it is almost time for your next dose, skip the missed dose and go back to your regular dosing schedule. Do not double doses.

Storage—To store this medicine:

- Keep out of the reach of children.
- Store away from heat and direct light.
- Do not store in the bathroom, near the kitchen sink, or in other damp places. Heat or moisture may cause the medicine to break down.
- Keep the medicine from freezing.
- Do not keep outdated medicine or medicine no longer needed. Be sure that any discarded medicine is out of the reach of children.

Side Effects of This Medicine

Along with its needed effects, a medicine may cause some unwanted effects. Although not all of these effects may occur, if they do occur they may need medical attention.

Check with your doctor immediately if any of the following side effects occur since they may be signs or symptoms of too much fluid in the body or overdose:

Coma; confusion; convulsions (seizures); drowsiness; headache (continuing); problems with urination; weight gain

Check with your doctor as soon as possible if any of the following side effects occur:

Rare

Cough (continuing); feeling of tightness in chest; shortness of breath or troubled breathing

Other side effects may occur that usually do not need medical attention. These side effects may go away during treatment as your body adjusts to the medicine. However, check with your doctor if any of the following side effects continue or are bothersome:

Less common or rare

Abdominal or stomach cramps; headache; heartburn; increased bowel movements; irritation or pain in the eye; itching, irritation, or sores inside nose; runny or stuffy nose

Other side effects not listed above may also occur in some patients. If you notice any other effects, check with your doctor.

Annual revision: 07/01/93

MAFENIDE Topical

A commonly used brand name in the U.S. and Canada is Sulfamylon.

Description

Mafenide (MA-fe-nide), a sulfa medicine, is used to prevent and treat bacterial or fungus infections. It works by preventing growth of the fungus or bacteria.

Mafenide cream is applied to the skin and/or burned area(s) to prevent and treat bacterial or fungus infections that may occur in burns.

Other medicines are used along with this medicine for burns. Patients with severe burns or burns over a large area of the body must be treated in a hospital.

This medicine is available only with your doctor's prescription, in the following dosage form:

Topical

- Cream (U.S. and Canada)

It is very important that you read and understand the following information. If any of it causes you special concern, check with your doctor. Also, *if you have any questions* or if you want more information about this medicine or your medical problem, *ask your doctor, nurse, or pharmacist.*

Before Using This Medicine

In deciding to use a medicine, the risks of taking the medicine must be weighed against the good it will do. This is a decision you and your doctor will make. For mafenide, the following should be considered:

Allergies—Tell your doctor if you have ever had any unusual or allergic reaction to mafenide, acetazolamide (e.g., Diamox), oral antidiabetics (diabetes medicine you take by mouth), dichlorphenamide (e.g., Daranide), furosemide (e.g., Lasix), methazolamide (e.g., Neptazane), other sulfa medicines, or thiazide diuretics (water pills). Also tell your doctor and pharmacist if you are allergic to any other substances, such as preservatives or dyes.

Pregnancy—Studies on effects in pregnancy have not been done in either humans or animals. However, use is not recommended in women during their child-bearing years unless the burn area covers more than 20% of the total body surface. In addition, sulfa medicines may increase the chance of liver problems in newborn infants and should not be used near the due date of the pregnancy.

Breast-feeding—Mafenide, when used on skin and/or burns, is absorbed into the mother's body. It is not known whether it passes into the breast milk. Sulfa medicines given by mouth do pass into the breast milk, and may cause liver problems, anemia (iron-poor blood), and other unwanted effects in nursing babies, especially those with glucose-6-phosphate dehydrogenase deficiency (lack of G6PD enzyme). Therefore, caution is recommended when using mafenide.

Children—Use is not recommended in premature or newborn infants up to 2 months of age. Sulfa medicines may cause liver problems in these infants.

Older adults—Many medicines have not been tested in older people. Therefore, it may not be known whether they work exactly the same way they do in younger adults or if they cause different side effects or problems in older people. There is no specific information about the use of mafenide in the elderly.

Other medical problems—The presence of other medical problems may affect the use of mafenide. Make sure you tell your doctor if you have any other medical problems, especially:

- Blood problems—Use of mafenide may make the condition worse
- Glucose-6-phosphate dehydrogenase deficiency (lack of G6PD enzyme)—Use of mafenide in persons with this condition may result in hemolytic anemia
- Kidney problems or
- Lung problems or
- Metabolic acidosis—Use of mafenide in persons with any of these conditions may increase the risk of a side effect called metabolic acidosis

Before you begin using any new medicine (prescription or nonprescription) or if you develop any new medical problem while you are using this medicine, check with your doctor, nurse, or pharmacist.

Proper Use of This Medicine

To use:

- Before applying this medicine, cleanse the affected area(s). Remove dead or burned skin and other debris.
- Wear a sterile glove to apply this medicine. Apply a thin layer (about 1/16 inch) of mafenide to the affected area(s). Keep the affected area(s) covered with the medicine at all times.
- If this medicine is rubbed off the affected area(s) by moving around or if it is washed off during bathing, showering, or the use of a whirlpool bath, reapply the medicine.
- After this medicine has been applied, the treated area(s) may be covered with a dressing or left uncovered as desired.

To help clear up your skin and/or burn infection completely, *keep using mafenide for the full time of treatment*. You should keep using this medicine until the burn area has healed or is ready for skin grafting. *Do not miss any doses.*

Missed dose—If you do miss a dose of this medicine, apply it as soon as possible. However, if it is almost time for your next dose, skip the missed dose and go back to your regular dosing schedule.

Storage—To store this medicine:
- Keep out of the reach of children.
- Store away from heat and direct light.
- Keep the medicine from freezing.
- Do not keep outdated medicine or medicine no longer needed. Be sure that any discarded medicine is out of the reach of children.

Precautions While Using This Medicine

It is important that your doctor check your progress at regular visits.

If your skin infection or burn does not improve within a few days or weeks (for more serious burns or burns over larger areas), or if it becomes worse, check with your doctor.

Side Effects of This Medicine

Along with its needed effects, a medicine may cause some unwanted effects. Although not all of these side effects may occur, if they do occur they may need medical attention.

Check with your doctor immediately if any of the following side effects occur:

Less common

Itching; skin rash or redness; swelling of face or skin; wheezing or troubled breathing

Rare

Bleeding or oozing of skin; drowsiness; nausea; rapid, deep breathing

Other side effects may occur that usually do not need medical attention. These side effects may go away during treatment as your body adjusts to the medicine. However, check with your doctor if any of the following side effects continue or are bothersome:

More common

Pain or burning feeling on treated area(s)

Other side effects not listed above may also occur in some patients. If you notice any other effects, check with your doctor.

Annual revision: July 1990

MAGNESIUM SUPPLEMENTS Systemic

This information applies to the following medicines:

Magnesium Chloride (mag-NEE-zhum KLOR-ide)
Magnesium Citrate (SIH-trayt)
Magnesium Gluceptate (gloo-SEP-tate)
Magnesium Gluconate (GLOO-ko-nate)
Magnesium Hydroxide (hye-DROX-ide)
Magnesium Lactate (LAK-tate)
Magnesium Oxide (OX-ide)
Magnesium Pidolate (PID-o-late)
Magnesium Sulfate (SUL-fate)

Some commonly used brand names are:

For Magnesium Chloride†

In the U.S.

Slow-Mag

Generic name product may also be available.

For Magnesium Citrate

In the U.S.

Citroma
Citro-Nesia

Generic name product may also be available.

In Canada

Citro-Mag

For Magnesium Gluceptate*

In Canada

Magnesium-Rougier

Another commonly used name is magnesium glucoheptonate.

For Magnesium Gluconate†

In the U.S.

Generic name product is available.

In Canada

Maglucate

For Magnesium Hydroxide

In the U.S.

Concentrated Phillips' Milk of Magnesia
Phillips' Milk of Magnesia

Generic name product is available.

In Canada

Phillips' Milk of Magnesia

Generic name product may also be available.

For Magnesium Lactate†

In the U.S.

Mag-Tab SR

Generic name product may also be available.

For Magnesium Oxide

In the U.S.

Mag-Ox
Maox
Uro-Mag

Generic name product may also be available.

In Canada

Generic name product is available.

For Magnesium Pidolate*
In Canada
Mag 2
Another commonly used name is magnesium pyroglutamate.

Magnesium Sulfate
In the U.S.
Generic name product is available.
In Canada
Generic name product is available.

*Not commercially available in the U.S.
†Not commercially available in Canada.

Description

Magnesium is used as a dietary supplement for patients who are deficient in magnesium. Although a balanced diet usually supplies all the magnesium a person needs, magnesium supplements may be needed by patients who have lost magnesium because of illness or treatment with certain medicines.

Lack of magnesium may lead to irritability, muscle weakness, and irregular heartbeat.

Some magnesium preparations are available only with your doctor's prescription. Others are available without a prescription; however, your doctor may have special instructions on the proper dose for your medical condition. You should take magnesium supplements only under the supervision of your doctor.

Magnesium supplements are available in the following dosage forms:

Oral

Magnesium Chloride
- Tablets (U.S.)

Magnesium Citrate
- Oral solution (U.S. and Canada)

Magnesium Gluceptate
- Oral solution (Canada)

Magnesium Gluconate
- Tablets (U.S. and Canada)

Magnesium Hydroxide
- Chewable tablets (U.S. and Canada)
- Oral solution (U.S. and Canada)

Magnesium Lactate
- Extended-release tablets (U.S.)

Magnesium Oxide
- Capsules (U.S.)
- Tablets (U.S. and Canada)

Magnesium Pidolate
- Powder for oral solution (Canada)

Magnesium Sulfate
- Crystals (U.S.)

Parenteral

Magnesium Chloride
- Injection (U.S.)

Magnesium Sulfate
- Injection (U.S. and Canada)

It is very important that you read and understand the following information. If any of it causes you special concern, check with your doctor. Also, *if you have any questions* or if you want more information about this medicine or your medical problem, *ask your doctor, nurse, or pharmacist.*

Importance of Diet

Many nutritionists recommend that, if possible, people should get all the magnesium they need from foods. However, some people may not get enough magnesium from food. For example, people on weight-loss diets may consume too little food to provide enough magnesium. Others may lose magnesium from the body because of illness or treatment with certain medicines. For such people, a magnesium supplement, taken under a doctor's care, is important.

In order to get enough vitamins and minerals in your diet, it is important that you eat a balanced and varied diet. Follow carefully any diet program your doctor may recommend. For your specific vitamin and/or mineral needs, ask your doctor or dietitian for a list of appropriate foods.

The best dietary sources of magnesium include green leafy vegetables, nuts, peas, beans, and cereal grains in which the germ or outer layers have not been removed. Hard water has been found to contain more magnesium than soft water. A diet high in fat may cause less magnesium to be absorbed. Cooking may decrease the magnesium content of food.

Experts have developed Recommended Dietary Allowances (RDA) for vitamins and other nutrients, based on the amount you need for good health. RDA cover the needs of most healthy people. They do not cover the needs of those who require extra vitamins or nutrients because of disease or serious lack of good nutrition. RDA should not be thought of as the amount of vitamins or other nutrients you need every day. Instead, they are the amounts you should eat on an average over time.

The RDA for magnesium are:
- Infants and children—
  Birth to 6 months of age: 40 milligrams (mg) per day.
  6 months to 1 year of age: 60 mg per day.
  1 to 3 years of age: 80 mg per day.
  4 to 6 years of age: 120 mg per day.
  7 to 10 years of age: 170 mg per day.
- Adolescent and adult males—
  11 to 14 years of age: 270 mg per day.
  15 to 18 years of age: 400 mg per day.
  19 years of age and over: 350 mg per day.
- Adolescent and adult females—
  11 to 14 years of age: 280 mg per day.
  15 to 18 years of age: 300 mg per day.
  19 years of age and over: 280 mg per day.
- Pregnant females—320 mg per day.

- Breast-feeding females—
  First 6 months: 355 mg per day.
  Second 6 months: 340 mg per day.

Remember:

- The total amount of magnesium that you get every day includes what you get from food *and* what you may take as a supplement.
- The total intake of magnesium averaged over several days need not be greater than twice the RDA, unless ordered by your doctor. In some cases, excessive amounts of magnesium may be harmful.

Before Using This Dietary Supplement

If you are taking this dietary supplement without a prescription, carefully read and follow any precautions on the label. For magnesium supplements, the following should be considered:

Allergies—Tell your doctor if you have ever had any unusual or allergic reaction to magnesium. Also tell your doctor and pharmacist if you are allergic to any other substances, such as foods, preservatives, or dyes.

Pregnancy—It is especially important that you are receiving enough vitamins and minerals when you become pregnant and that you continue to receive the right amount of vitamins and minerals throughout your pregnancy. The healthy growth and development of the fetus depend on a steady supply of nutrients from the mother. However, taking large amounts of dietary supplements during pregnancy may be harmful to the mother and/or fetus and should be avoided.

Breast-feeding—It is especially important that you receive the right amount of vitamins and minerals so that your baby will also get the vitamins and minerals needed to grow properly. However, taking large amounts of a dietary supplement while breast-feeding may be harmful to the mother and/or baby and should be avoided.

Children—Although there is no specific information comparing use of oral magnesium in children with use in other age groups, dietary supplements are not expected to cause different side effects in children than they do in adults.

Older adults—Many dietary supplements have not been studied specifically in older people. Therefore, it may not be known whether they work exactly the same way they do in younger adults or if they cause different side effects, or problems in older people. There is no specific information comparing use of magnesium in the elderly with use in other age groups.

Studies have shown that older adults may have lower blood levels of magnesium than younger adults. Your doctor may recommend that you take a magnesium supplement.

Medicines or other dietary supplements—Although certain medicines or other dietary supplements should not be used together at all, in other cases they may be used together even if an interaction might occur. In these cases, your doctor may want to change the dose, or other precautions may be necessary. When you are taking magnesium, it is especially important that your doctor and pharmacist know if you are taking any of the following:

- Cellulose sodium phosphate—Use with magnesium supplements may prevent cellulose sodium phosphate from working properly; magnesium supplements should be taken at least 1 hour before or after cellulose sodium phosphate
- Magnesium-containing medications, other, including magnesium enemas—Use with magnesium supplements may cause high blood levels of magnesium, which may increase the chance of side effects
- Sodium polystyrene sulfonate—Use with magnesium supplements may cause the magnesium supplement to be less effective
- Tetracyclines, oral—Use with magnesium supplements may prevent the tetracycline from working properly; magnesium supplements should be taken at least 1 to 3 hours before or after oral tetracycline

Other medical problems—The presence of other medical problems may affect the use of magnesium. Make sure you tell your doctor if you have any other medical problems, especially:

- Heart disease—Magnesium supplements may make this condition worse
- Kidney problems—Magnesium supplements may increase the risk of hypermagnesemia (too much magnesium in the blood), which could cause serious side effects; your doctor may need to change your dose.

Proper Use of This Dietary Supplement

Magnesium supplements should be taken with meals. Taking magnesium supplements on an empty stomach may cause diarrhea.

For patients taking the *extended-release form* of this dietary supplement:

- Swallow the tablets whole. Do not chew or suck on the tablet.
- Some tablets may be broken or crushed and sprinkled on applesauce or other soft food. However, check with your doctor or pharmacist first, since this should not be done for most tablets.

For patients taking the *powder form* of this dietary supplement:

- Pour powder into a glass.
- Add water and stir.

Missed dose—If you miss taking your magnesium supplement for one or more days there is no cause for concern, since it takes some time for your body to become seriously low in magnesium. However, if your doctor has recommended that you take magnesium, try to remember to take it as directed every day.

Storage—To store this dietary supplement:
- Keep out of the reach of children.
- Store away from heat and direct light.
- Do not store in the bathroom, near the kitchen sink, or in other damp places. Heat or moisture may cause the dietary supplement to break down.
- Keep the dietary supplement from freezing. Do not refrigerate.
- Do not keep dietary supplements that are outdated or are no longer needed. Be sure that any discarded dietary supplement is out of the reach of children.

Side Effects of This Dietary Supplement

Along with its needed effects, a dietary supplement may cause some unwanted effects. Although not all of these side effects may occur, if they do occur they may need medical attention.

Check with your doctor immediately if any of the following side effects occur:

Rare (with injectable magnesium only)

Dizziness or fainting; flushing; irritation and pain at injection site—for intramuscular administration only; muscle paralysis; troubled breathing

Symptoms of overdose (rare in patients with normal kidney function)

Blurred or double vision; coma; dizziness or fainting; drowsiness (severe); increased or decreased urination; slow heartbeat; troubled breathing

Other side effects may occur that usually do not need medical attention. These side effects may go away during treatment as your body adjusts to the medicine. However, check with your doctor if the following side effect continues or is bothersome:

Less common (with oral magnesium)

Diarrhea

Other side effects not listed above may also occur in some patients. If you notice any other effects, check with your doctor.

Annual revision: 12/03/92
Interim revision: 03/28/93

MALATHION Topical

Some commonly used brand names are:

In the U.S.
Ovide

In Canada
Prioderm

Other
Derbac-M
Suleo-M

Description

Malathion (mal-a-THYE-on) belongs to the group of medicines known as pediculicides (medicines that kill lice).

Malathion is applied to the hair and scalp to treat head lice infections. It acts by killing both the lice and their eggs.

This medicine is available only with your doctor's prescription, in the following dosage form:

Topical
- Lotion (U.S. and Canada)

It is very important that you read and understand the following information. If any of it causes you special concern, check with your doctor. Also, *if you have any questions* or if you want more information about this medicine or your medical problem, *ask your doctor, nurse, or pharmacist.*

Before Using This Medicine

In deciding to use a medicine, the risks of taking the medicine must be weighed against the good it will do. This is a decision you and your doctor will make. For malathion, the following should be considered:

Allergies—Tell your doctor if you have ever had any unusual or allergic reaction to malathion. Also tell your doctor and pharmacist if you are allergic to any other substances, such as preservatives or dyes.

Pregnancy—Malathion may be absorbed through the skin. Although it has not been studied in pregnant women, malathion has not been shown to cause birth defects or other problems in animal studies.

Breast-feeding—Malathion may be absorbed through the mother's skin. Although it is not known whether malathion passes into the breast milk, this medicine has not been reported to cause problems in nursing babies.

Children—This medicine has been tested in children 2 years of age and older and, in effective doses, has not been shown to cause different side effects or problems than it does in adults. There is no specific information about its use in children less than 2 years of age.

Older adults—Many medicines have not been tested in older people. Therefore, it may not be known whether they work exactly the same way they do in younger adults or if they cause different side effects or problems in older people. There is no specific information about the use of malathion in the elderly.

Other medicines—Although certain medicines should not be used together at all, in other cases two different medicines may be used together even if an interaction might occur. In these cases, your doctor may want to change the dose, or other precautions may be necessary. When you are using malathion, it is especially important that your doctor and pharmacist know if you are using any of the following:

- Antimyasthenics (ambenonium, neostigmine, pyridostigmine) or
- Demecarium, echothiophate, or isoflurophate eye medicine—Use of malathion with these medicines may increase the chance of side effects

Other medical problems—The presence of other medical problems may affect the use of malathion. Make sure you tell your doctor if you have any other medical problems, especially:

- Anemia (severe) or
- Brain surgery, recent, or
- Liver disease or
- Malnutrition—These conditions may increase the chance of some side effects of malathion
- Asthma or
- Epilepsy or other seizure disorders or
- Heart disease or
- Myasthenia gravis or other nerve/muscle disease or
- Parkinson's disease or
- Stomach ulcer or other stomach or intestinal problems—Use of malathion may make the condition worse

Before you begin using any new medicine (prescription or nonprescription) or if you develop any new medical problem while you are using this medicine, check with your doctor, nurse, or pharmacist.

Proper Use of This Medicine

Malathion is a poisonous medicine. Keep it away from the mouth because it is harmful if swallowed.

Use this medicine only as directed by your doctor. Do not use more of it, do not use it more often, and do not use it for a longer time than your doctor ordered. To do so may increase the chance of absorption through the skin and the chance of malathion poisoning.

To use:

- Apply malathion by sprinkling on dry hair and rubbing in until the hair and scalp are thoroughly moistened.
- Immediately after using this medicine, wash your hands to remove any medicine that may be on them.
- Allow the hair to dry naturally. Use no heat (as from a hair dryer) and leave the hair uncovered.
- After the medicine has been allowed to remain on the hair and scalp for 8 to 12 hours, *wash the hair with a nonmedicated shampoo and then rinse thoroughly.*
- After rinsing, use a fine-toothed comb to remove the dead lice and eggs from the hair.

Keep this medicine away from the eyes. If you should accidentally get some in your eyes, flush them thoroughly with water at once.

This medicine is flammable. Do not use near heat, near open flame, or while smoking.

Head lice can be easily transferred from one person to another by direct contact with clothing, hats, scarves, bedding, towels, washcloths, hairbrushes and combs, or hairs from infected persons. Therefore, *all household members of your family should be examined for head lice and receive treatment if they are found to be infected.* If you have any questions about this, check with your doctor.

Storage—To store this medicine:

- Keep out of the reach of children.
- Store away from heat and direct light.
- Keep the medicine from freezing.
- Do not keep outdated medicine or medicine no longer needed. Be sure that any discarded medicine is out of the reach of children.

Precautions While Using This Medicine

To prevent reinfection or the spreading of the infection to other people, good health habits are also required. These include the following:

- Wash all clothing, bedding, towels, and washcloths in very hot water or dry clean them.
- Wash all hairbrushes and combs in very hot soapy water and do not share them with other people.
- Clean the house or room by thorough vacuuming.

If you have any questions about this, check with your doctor.

Breathing in even small amounts of carbamate- or organophosphate-type insecticides or pesticides (for example, carbaryl [Sevin], demeton [Systox], diazinon, malathion, parathion, ronnel [Trolene]) may add to the effects of this medicine. Farmers, gardeners, residents of communities undergoing insecticide or pesticide spraying or dusting, workers in plants manufacturing such products, or other persons exposed to such poisons should protect themselves by wearing a mask over the nose and mouth, changing clothes frequently, and washing hands often while using this medicine.

Side Effects of This Medicine

Along with its needed effects, a medicine may cause some unwanted effects. Although not all of these side effects may occur, if they do occur they may need medical attention.

Check with your doctor as soon as possible if any of the following side effects occur:

Rare

Skin rash

When malathion is applied to the skin in recommended doses, symptoms of poisoning have not been reported. However, the chance may exist, especially if the skin is broken. *Symptoms of malathion poisoning* include:

Abdominal or stomach cramps; anxiety or restlessness; clumsiness or unsteadiness; confusion or mental depression; convulsions (seizures); diarrhea; difficult or labored breathing; dizziness; drowsiness; increased sweating; increased watering of mouth or eyes; loss of bowel or bladder control; muscle twitching of eyelids, face, and neck; pinpoint pupils; slow heartbeat; trembling; unusual weakness

Other side effects may occur that usually do not need medical attention. These side effects may go away during treatment as your body adjusts to the medicine. However, check with your doctor if either of the following side effects continues or is bothersome:

Less common or rare

Stinging or irritation of scalp

Other side effects not listed above may also occur in some patients. If you notice any other effects, check with your doctor.

Annual revision: July 1990

MANGANESE SUPPLEMENTS Systemic

This information applies to the following medicines:

Manganese Gluconate (MAN-ga-nees GLOO-coh-nate)
Manganese Sulfate (SUL-fate)

Some commonly used brand names are:

For Manganese Gluconate

In the U.S.

Generic name product is available.

In Canada

Generic name product is available.

For Manganese Sulfate

In the U.S.

Generic name product is available.

In Canada

Generic name product is available.

Description

Manganese supplements are used to prevent or treat manganese deficiency.

The body needs manganese for normal growth and health. For patients who are unable to get enough manganese in their regular diet or who have a need for more manganese, manganese supplements may be necessary.

Manganese deficiency has not been reported in humans. Lack of manganese in animals has been found to cause improper formation of bone and cartilage, may decrease the body's ability to use sugar properly, and may cause growth problems.

Some manganese preparations are available only with your doctor's prescription. Others are available without a prescription; however, your doctor may have special instructions on the proper use and dose for your condition.

Manganese supplements are available in the following dosage forms:

Oral

Manganese Gluconate

- Tablets (U.S. and Canada)

Parenteral

Manganese Sulfate

- Injection (U.S. and Canada)

It is very important that you read and understand the following information. If any of it causes you special concern, check with your doctor or pharmacist. Also, *if you have any questions* or if you want more information about this dietary supplement or your medical problem, *ask your doctor, nurse, pharmacist, or dietitian.*

Importance of Diet

Many nutritionists recommend that, if possible, people should get all the manganese they need from foods. However, some people may not get enough manganese from their diet. For such people, a manganese supplement is important.

In order to get enough vitamins and minerals in your regular diet, it is important that you eat a balanced and varied diet. Follow carefully any diet program your doctor may recommend. For your specific vitamin and/or mineral needs, ask your doctor or dietitian for a list of appropriate foods.

Manganese is found in whole grains, cereal products, lettuce, dry beans, and peas.

Experts have developed a list of recommended dietary allowances (RDA) for most vitamins and some minerals. The RDA are not an exact number but a general idea of how much you need. They do not cover amounts needed for problems caused by serious lack of vitamins and minerals.

Because a lack of manganese is rare, there are no RDA for it. The following intakes are thought to be plenty for most individuals:

- Infants and children—
  Birth to 6 months of age: 0.3 to 0.6 milligrams (mg) per day.
  6 months to 1 year of age: 0.6 to 1 mg per day.
  1 to 3 years of age: 1 to 1.5 mg per day.
  4 to 6 years of age: 1.5 to 2 mg per day.
  7 to 10 years of age: 2 to 3 mg per day.
- Adolescents and adults—2 to 5 mg per day.

Before Using This Dietary Supplement

If you are taking this dietary supplement without a prescription, carefully read and follow any precautions on the label. For manganese, the following should be considered:

Allergies—Tell your doctor if you have ever had any unusual or allergic reaction to manganese. Also tell your doctor and pharmacist if you are allergic to any other substances, such as foods, preservatives, or dyes.

Pregnancy—It is especially important that you are receiving enough vitamins and minerals when you become pregnant and that you continue to receive the right amount of vitamins and minerals throughout your pregnancy. The healthy growth and development of the fetus depend on a steady supply of nutrients from the mother. However, taking large amounts of a dietary supplement in pregnancy may be harmful to the mother and/or fetus and should be avoided.

Breast-feeding—It is important that you receive the right amounts of vitamins and minerals so that your baby will also get the vitamins and minerals needed to grow properly. However, taking large amounts of a dietary supplement while breast-feeding may be harmful to the mother and/or baby and should be avoided.

Children—It is especially important that children receive enough manganese in their diet for healthy growth and development. Although there is no specific information about the use of manganese in children in doses higher than normal daily requirements, it is not expected to cause different side effects or problems in children than it does in adults.

Older adults—It is important that older people continue to receive enough vitamins and minerals in their diet for good health. Manganese has been tested and has not been shown to cause different side effects or problems in older people than it does in younger adults.

Medicines or other dietary supplements—Although certain medicines or dietary supplements should not be used together at all, in other cases they may be used together even if an interaction might occur. In these cases, your doctor may want to change the dose, or other precautions may be necessary. Tell your doctor and pharmacist if you are taking any other dietary supplement or any prescription or nonprescription (over-the-counter [OTC]) medicines.

Other medical problems—The presence of other medical problems may affect the use of manganese. Make sure you tell your doctor if you have any other medical problems, especially:

- Biliary disease or
- Liver disease—Taking manganese supplements may cause high blood levels of manganese, and dosage of manganese may have to be changed

Proper Use of This Dietary Supplement

Some people believe that taking very large doses of a vitamin or mineral (called megadoses) is useful for treating certain medical problems. Studies have not proven this. Large doses should be taken only under the direction of your doctor after need has been identified.

Missed dose—If you miss taking manganese supplements for one or more days there is no cause for concern, since it takes some time for your body to become seriously low in manganese. However, if your doctor has recommended that you take manganese, try to remember to take it as directed every day.

Storage—To store this dietary supplement:

- Keep out of the reach of children.
- Store away from heat and direct light.
- Do not store in the bathroom, near the kitchen sink, or in other damp places. Heat or moisture may cause the dietary supplement to break down.

- Keep the dietary supplement from freezing. Do not refrigerate.
- Do not keep outdated dietary supplements or those no longer needed. Be sure that any discarded dietary supplement is out of the reach of children.

Side Effects of This Dietary Supplement

No side effects have been reported for manganese. However, check with your doctor if you notice any unusual effects while you are taking it.

Annual revision: 02/01/92
Interim revision: 08/07/92

MAPROTILINE Systemic

A commonly used brand name in the U.S. and Canada is Ludiomil.

Generic name product may also be available in the U.S.

Description

Maprotiline (ma-PROE-ti-leen) belongs to the group of medicines known as tetracyclic antidepressants or "mood elevators." It is used to relieve mental depression, including anxiety that sometimes occurs with depression.

Maprotiline is available only with your doctor's prescription, in the following dosage form:

Oral

- Tablets (U.S. and Canada)

It is very important that you read and understand the following information. If any of it causes you special concern, check with your doctor. Also, *if you have any questions* or if you want more information about this medicine or your medical problem, *ask your doctor, nurse, or pharmacist.*

Before Using This Medicine

In deciding to use a medicine, the risks of taking the medicine must be weighed against the good it will do. This is a decision you and your doctor will make. For maprotiline, the following should be considered:

Allergies—Tell your doctor if you have ever had any unusual or allergic reaction to maprotiline or tricyclic antidepressants. Also tell your doctor and pharmacist if you are allergic to any other substances, such as foods, preservatives, or dyes.

Pregnancy—Maprotiline has not been studied in pregnant women. However, this medicine has not been shown to cause birth defects or other problems in animal studies.

Breast-feeding—Maprotiline passes into the breast milk. However, this medicine has not been reported to cause problems in nursing babies.

Children—Studies on this medicine have been done only in adult patients, and there is no specific information comparing use of maprotiline in children with use in other age groups.

Older adults—Drowsiness, dizziness or lightheadedness; confusion; vision problems; dryness of mouth; constipation; and difficulty in urinating may be especially likely to occur in elderly patients, who are usually more sensitive than younger adults to the effects of maprotiline.

Other medicines—Although certain medicines should not be used together at all, in other cases 2 different medicines may be used together even if an interaction might occur. In these cases, your doctor may want to change the dose, or other precautions may be necessary. When you are taking maprotiline, it is especially important that your doctor and pharmacist know if you are taking any of the following:

- Amphetamines or
- Appetite suppressants (diet pills) or
- Medicine for asthma or other breathing problems or
- Medicine for colds, sinus problems, or hay fever or other allergies (including nose drops or sprays)—Using these medicines with maprotiline may cause serious unwanted effects on your heart and blood pressure
- Central nervous system (CNS) depressants—Taking these medicines with maprotiline may increase the CNS depressant effects
- Monoamine oxidase (MAO) inhibitors (furazolidone [e.g., Furoxone], isocarboxazid [e.g., Marplan], phenelzine [e.g., Nardil], procarbazine [e.g., Matulane], selegiline [e.g., Eldepryl], tranylcypromine [e.g., Parnate])—Taking maprotiline while you are taking or within 2 weeks of taking monoamine oxidase (MAO) inhibitors may cause very serious side effects, such as sudden high body temperature, extremely high blood pressure, and severe convulsions; at least 14 days should be allowed between stopping treatment with one medicine and starting treatment with the other

Other medical problems—The presence of other medical problems may affect the use of maprotiline. Make sure you tell your doctor if you have any other medical problems, especially:

- Alcohol abuse or
- Seizure disorders (including epilepsy)—The risk of seizures may be increased
- Asthma or
- Difficult urination or
- Enlarged prostate or
- Glaucoma or
- Mental illness (severe) or
- Stomach or intestinal problems—Maprotiline may make the condition worse
- Heart or blood vessel disease or
- Overactive thyroid—Serious effects on your heart may occur
- Liver disease—Higher blood levels of maprotiline may occur, increasing the chance of side effects

Before you begin using any new medicine (prescription or nonprescription) or if you develop any new medical problem while you are using this medicine, check with your doctor, nurse, or pharmacist.

Proper Use of This Medicine

Take this medicine only as directed by your doctor to benefit your condition as much as possible. Do not take more of it, do not take it more often, and do not take it for a longer time than your doctor ordered.

Sometimes this medicine must be taken for up to two or three weeks before you begin to feel better. Your doctor should check your progress at regular visits.

Missed dose—If you miss a dose of this medicine and your dosing schedule is:

- One dose a day at bedtime—Do not take the missed dose in the morning since it may cause disturbing side effects during waking hours. Instead, check with your doctor.
- More than one dose a day—Take the missed dose as soon as possible. Then go back to your regular dosing schedule. However, if it is almost time for your next dose, skip the missed dose and go back to your regular dosing schedule. Do not double doses. If you have any questions about this, check with your doctor.

Storage—To store this medicine:

- Keep out of the reach of children.
- Store away from heat and direct light.
- Do not store in the bathroom, near the kitchen sink, or in other damp places. Heat or moisture may cause the medicine to break down.
- Do not keep outdated medicine or medicine no longer needed. Be sure that any discarded medicine is out of the reach of children.

Precautions While Using This Medicine

It is very important that your doctor check your progress at regular visits. This will allow your dosage to be changed if necessary and will help to reduce side effects.

This medicine will add to the effects of alcohol and other CNS depressants (medicines that slow down the nervous system, possibly causing drowsiness). Some examples of CNS depressants are antihistamines or medicine for hay fever, other allergies, or colds; sedatives, tranquilizers, or sleeping medicine; prescription pain medicine or narcotics; barbiturates; medicine for seizures; or anesthetics, including some dental anesthetics. *Check with your doctor before taking any of the above while you are using this medicine.*

This medicine may cause blurred vision, especially during the first few weeks of treatment. It may also cause some people to become drowsy or less alert than they are normally. *If these effects occur, do not drive, use machines, or do anything else that could be dangerous if you are not alert or able to see well.*

Dizziness, lightheadedness, or fainting may occur, especially when you get up from a lying or sitting position. Getting up slowly may help. If this problem continues or gets worse, check with your doctor.

Maprotiline may cause dryness of the mouth. For temporary relief, use sugarless gum or candy, melt bits of ice in your mouth, or use a saliva substitute. However, if your mouth continues to feel dry for more than 2 weeks, check with your medical doctor or dentist. Continuing dryness of the mouth may increase the chance of dental disease, including tooth decay, gum disease, and fungus infections.

Before having any kind of surgery, dental treatment, or emergency treatment, tell the medical doctor or dentist in charge that you are using this medicine.

Do not stop taking this medicine without first checking with your doctor. Your doctor may want you to reduce gradually the amount you are taking before stopping completely. This will allow your body to adjust properly and will reduce the possibility of unwanted effects.

Side Effects of This Medicine

Along with its needed effects, a medicine may cause some unwanted effects. Although not all of these side effects may occur, if they do occur they may need medical attention.

Check with your doctor as soon as possible if any of the following side effects occur:

More common

Skin rash, redness, swelling, or itching

Less common

Constipation (severe); convulsions (seizures); nausea or vomiting; shakiness or trembling; unusual excitement

Rare

Breast enlargement—in males and females; confusion (especially in the elderly); difficulty in urinating; fainting; hallucinations (seeing, hearing, or feeling things that are not there); inappropriate secretion of milk—in females; irregular heartbeat (pounding, racing, skipping); sore throat and fever; swelling of testicles; yellow eyes or skin

Symptoms of overdose

Convulsions (seizures); dizziness (severe); drowsiness (severe); fast or irregular heartbeat; fever; muscle stiffness or weakness (severe); restlessness or agitation; trouble in breathing; vomiting

Other side effects may occur that usually do not need medical attention. These side effects may go away during treatment as your body adjusts to the medicine. However, check with your doctor if any of the following side effects continue or are bothersome:

More common

Blurred vision; decreased sexual ability; dizziness or lightheadedness (especially in the elderly); drowsiness; dryness of mouth; headache; increased or decreased sexual drive; tiredness or weakness

Less common

Constipation (mild); diarrhea; heartburn; increased appetite and weight gain; increased sensitivity of skin to sunlight; increased sweating; trouble in sleeping; weight loss

After you stop taking this medicine, your body will need time to adjust. This usually takes about 3 to 10 days. Continue to follow the precautions listed above during this period of time.

Other side effects not listed above may also occur in some patients. If you notice any other effects, check with your doctor.

Additional Information

Once a medicine has been approved for marketing for a certain use, experience may show that it is also useful for other medical problems. Although this use in not included in product labeling, maprotiline is used in certain patients with the following medical condition:

- Chronic neurogenic pain (a certain type of pain that is continuing)

Other than the above information, there is no additional information relating to proper use, precautions, or side effects for these uses.

Annual revision: 07/29/91

MEASLES VIRUS VACCINE LIVE Systemic

A commonly used brand name in the U.S. and Canada is Attenuvax. Generic name product may also be available in Canada.

Description

Measles (MEE-zills) Virus Vaccine Live is an immunizing agent used to prevent infection by the measles virus. It works by causing your body to produce its own protection (antibodies) against the virus. This vaccine does not protect you against German measles (Rubella). A separate immunization is needed for that type of measles.

The following information applies only to the vaccine made from the more attenuated line of Enders' attenuated Edmonston strain of measles virus. Different types of measles vaccine may be available in countries other than the U.S. and Canada.

Measles (also known as coughing measles, hard measles, morbilli, red measles, rubeola, and ten-day measles) is an infection that is easily spread from one person to another. Infection with measles can cause serious problems, such as pneumonia, ear infections, sinus problems, convulsions (seizures), brain damage, and possibly death. The risk of serious complications and death is greater for adults and infants than for children and adolescents.

Immunization against measles is recommended for everyone 15 months of age (in Canada, 12 months of age) up to persons born in 1957. In addition, there may be special reasons why children from 6 months of age up to 15 months of age (up to 12 months of age in Canada) may also require measles vaccine.

Immunization against measles is not usually recommended for infants younger than 12 months of age, unless the risk of their getting a measles infection is high. This is because antibodies they received from their mothers before birth may interfere with the effectiveness of the vaccine. Children who were immunized against measles before 12 months of age should be immunized twice again.

You can be considered to be immune to measles only if you received 2 doses of measles vaccine starting on or after your first birthday and have the medical record to prove it, if you have a doctor's diagnosis of a previous measles infection, or if you have had a blood test showing immunity to measles.

This vaccine is available only from your doctor or other authorized health care provider, in the following dosage form:

Parenteral

- Injection (U.S. and Canada)

It is very important that you read and understand the following information. If any of it causes you special concern, check with your doctor. Also, *if you have any questions* or if you want more information about this medicine or your medical problem, *ask your doctor, nurse, or pharmacist.*

Before Receiving This Vaccine

In deciding to use a medicine, the risks of taking the medicine must be weighed against the good it will do. This is a decision you and your doctor will make. For measles vaccine, the following should be considered:

Allergies—Tell your doctor if you have ever had any unusual or allergic reaction to measles vaccine or to any form of the antibiotic neomycin or streptomycin. Also tell your doctor and pharmacist if you are allergic to any other substances, such as foods (especially eggs) or preservatives. The measles vaccine available in the U.S. and Canada is grown in a chick embryo cell culture.

Pregnancy—Although studies on effects in pregnancy have not been done in humans and problems have not been shown to occur, use of measles vaccine during pregnancy, or becoming pregnant within 3 months after receiving measles vaccine, is not recommended. Since the natural measles infection has been shown to increase the chance of birth defects and other problems, it is thought that the live virus vaccine might cause similar problems.

Breast-feeding—It is not known whether measles vaccine passes into the breast milk. However, this vaccine has not been reported to cause problems in nursing babies.

Children—In the U.S., measles vaccine is usually not recommended for infants up to 15 months of age. In Canada, use is not recommended for infants up to 12 months of age. In special cases, such as children traveling outside the U.S. or children living in high risk areas, measles vaccine may be given to children as young as 6 months of age.

Other medicines—Although certain medicines should not be used together at all, in other cases two different medicines may be used together even if an interaction might occur. In these cases, your doctor may want to change the dose, or other precautions may be necessary. Before you receive measles vaccine, it is especially important that your doctor and pharmacist know if you have received any of the following:

- Any other live virus vaccines in the last month or if you intend to within the next month—Live virus vaccines should be given at the same time or at least 1 month apart, so they do not interfere with the useful effects of one another
- Blood transfusions or other blood products or gamma globulin or other globulins in the last 3 months or if you intend to within the next 2 weeks—These products may reduce the useful effect of the vaccine
- Treatment with x-rays or cancer medicines—Treatment may increase the action of the vaccine, causing an increase in vaccine side effects, or treatment may interfere with the useful effect of the vaccine

Other medical problems—The presence of other medical problems may affect the use of measles vaccine. Make sure you tell your doctor if you have any other medical problems, especially:

- Brain or head injury or
- Convulsions (seizures) due to fever (history of)—Fever, a side effect of measles vaccine, may make the condition worse
- Immune deficiency condition (or family history of)—Condition may increase the chance and severity of side effects of the vaccine and/or may decrease the useful effects of the vaccine
- Severe illness with fever—The symptoms of the condition may be confused with the possible side effects of the vaccine
- Tuberculosis—Use of measles vaccine may make the condition worse or may interfere with the tuberculin skin test

Before you begin using any new medicine (prescription or nonprescription) or if you develop any new medical problem while you are using this medicine, check with your doctor, nurse, or pharmacist.

Precautions After Receiving This Vaccine

Do not become pregnant for 3 months after receiving measles vaccine without first checking with your doctor. There is a chance that this vaccine may cause birth defects.

Tell your doctor that you have received this vaccine:

- If you are to receive a tuberculin skin test within 6 weeks after receiving this medicine. The results of the test may be affected by this vaccine.
- If you are to receive any other live virus vaccines within 1 month after receiving this vaccine.
- If you are to receive blood transfusions or other blood products within 2 weeks after receiving this vaccine.
- If you are to receive gamma globulin or other globulins within 2 weeks after receiving this vaccine.

Side Effects of This Vaccine

Along with its needed effects, a vaccine may cause some unwanted effects. Although not all of these side effects may occur, if they do occur they may need medical attention.

Get emergency help immediately if any of the following side effects occur:

Symptoms of allergic reaction

Difficulty in breathing or swallowing; hives; itching, especially of feet or hands; reddening of skin, especially around ears; swelling of eyes, face, or inside of nose; unusual tiredness or weakness (sudden and severe)

Check with your doctor as soon as possible if any of the following side effects occur:

More common

Fever over 103 °F (39.4 °C)

Rare

Bruising or purple spots on skin; confusion; convulsions (seizures); double vision; headache (severe or continuing); irritability; stiff neck; swelling of glands in neck; vomiting

Other side effects may occur that usually do not need medical attention. However, check with your doctor if any of the following side effects continue or are bothersome:

More common

Burning or stinging at place of injection; fever of 100 °F (37.7 °C) or less

Less common

Fever between 100 and 103 °F (37.7 and 39.4 °C); itching, swelling, redness, tenderness, or hard lump at place of injection; skin rash

Fever or skin rash may occur from 5 to 12 days after vaccination and usually lasts several days.

Some side effects, such as fever over 103 °F (39.4 °C), swelling of glands in neck, or swelling, blistering, or pain at place of injection, may be more frequent, be more severe, or last longer in persons who received inactivated (killed) measles vaccine (available in the U.S. from 1963 to 1967 and in Canada until 1970). If any of these side effects occur, check with your doctor as soon as possible.

Other side effects not listed above may also occur in some patients. If you notice any other effects, check with your doctor.

Annual revision: August 1990

MEBENDAZOLE Systemic

Some commonly used brand names are:

In the U.S.
Vermox

In Canada
Vermox

Other
Mebendacin
Mebutar
Nemasole

Description

Mebendazole (me-BEN-da-zole) belongs to the family of medicines called anthelmintics (ant-hel-MIN-tiks). Anthelmintics are medicines used in the treatment of worm infections.

Mebendazole is used to treat:

- Common roundworms (ascariasis);
- Hookworm infections (uncinariasis);
- Pinworms (enterobiasis; oxyuriasis);
- Whipworms (trichuriasis); and
- More than one worm infection at a time.

This medicine may also be used for other worm infections as determined by your doctor.

Mebendazole works by keeping the worm from absorbing sugar (glucose). This gradually causes loss of energy and death of the worm.

Mebendazole is available only with your doctor's prescription, in the following dosage form:

Oral

- Chewable tablets (U.S. and Canada)

It is very important that you read and understand the following information. If any of it causes you special concern, check with your doctor. Also, *if you have any questions* or if you want more information about this medicine or your medical problem, *ask your doctor, nurse, or pharmacist.*

Before Using This Medicine

In deciding to use a medicine, the risks of taking the medicine must be weighed against the good it will do. This is a decision you and your doctor will make. For mebendazole, the following should be considered:

Allergies—Tell your doctor if you have ever had any unusual or allergic reaction to mebendazole. Also tell your doctor and pharmacist if you are allergic to any other substances, such as foods, preservatives, or dyes.

Pregnancy—Mebendazole is not recommended for use during pregnancy. It has been shown to cause birth defects and other problems in rats given a single dose, which was several times the usual human dose. However, mebendazole did not cause birth defects or other problems in women who took this medicine during the first 3 months of pregnancy. Be sure you have discussed this with your doctor.

Breast-feeding—It is not known whether mebendazole passes into the breast milk. However, this medicine has not been reported to cause problems in nursing babies.

Children—This medicine has been tested in a limited number of children 2 years of age or older and, in effective doses, has not been shown to cause different side effects or problems in children than it does in adults.

Older adults—Many medicines have not been studied specifically in older people. Therefore, it may not be known whether they work exactly the same way they do in younger adults or if they cause different side effects or problems in older people. There is no specific information comparing use of mebendazole in the elderly with use in other age groups.

Other medicines—Although certain medicines should not be used together at all, in other cases two different medicines may be used together even if an interaction might occur. In these cases, your doctor may want to change the dose, or other precautions may be necessary. Tell your doctor and pharmacist if you are taking any prescription or nonprescription (over-the-counter [OTC]) medicine.

Other medical problems—The presence of other medical problems may affect the use of mebendazole. Make sure you tell your doctor if you have any other medical problems, especially:

- Crohn's disease or
- Liver disease or
- Ulcerative colitis—Patients with these diseases may have an increased chance of side effects from mebendazole

Before you begin using any new medicine (prescription or nonprescription) or if you develop any new medical problem while you are using this medicine, check with your doctor, nurse, or pharmacist.

Proper Use of This Medicine

Mebendazole usually comes with patient directions. Read them carefully before using this medicine.

No special preparations (for example, special diets, fasting, other medicines, laxatives, or enemas) are necessary before, during, or immediately after taking mebendazole.

Mebendazole tablets may be chewed, swallowed whole, or crushed and mixed with food.

For patients taking *mebendazole for hookworms, roundworms, or whipworms:*

- To help clear up your infection completely, *take this medicine exactly as directed by your doctor for the full time of treatment.* In some patients a second course of this medicine may be required to clear up the infection completely. *Do not miss any doses.*

For patients taking *mebendazole for pinworms:*

- To help clear up your infection completely, *take this medicine exactly as directed by your doctor.* A second course of this medicine is usually required to clear up the infection completely.
- Pinworms may be easily passed from one person to another, especially in a household. Therefore, all household members may have to be treated at the same time. This helps to prevent infection or reinfection of other household members. Also, all household members may have to be treated again in 2 to 3 weeks to clear up the infection completely.

For patients taking mebendazole for infections in which *high doses* are needed:

- *Mebendazole is best taken with meals, especially fatty ones (for example, meals that include whole milk or ice cream).* This helps to clear up the infection by helping your body absorb the medicine better. *However, if you are on a low-fat diet, check with your doctor.*

Missed dose—If you do miss a dose of this medicine, take it as soon as possible. However, if it is almost time for your next dose, skip the missed dose and go back to your regular dosing schedule. Do not double doses.

Storage—To store this medicine:

- Keep out of the reach of children.
- Store away from heat and direct light.
- Do not store in the bathroom, near the kitchen sink, or in other damp places. Heat or moisture may cause the medicine to break down.
- Do not keep outdated medicine or medicine no longer needed. Be sure that any discarded medicine is out of the reach of children.

Precautions While Using This Medicine

It is important that your doctor check your progress at regular visits, especially in infections in which high doses are needed. This is to make sure that the infection is cleared up completely and to allow your doctor to check for any unwanted effects.

If your symptoms do not improve within a few days, or if they become worse, check with your doctor.

For patients taking *mebendazole for pinworms:*

- In some patients, pinworms may return after treatment with mebendazole. Washing (not shaking) all bedding and nightclothes (pajamas) after treatment may help to prevent this.
- Some doctors may also recommend other measures to help keep your infection from returning. If you

have any questions about this, check with your doctor.

For patients taking *mebendazole for hookworms or whipworms:*

- In hookworm and whipworm infections anemia may occur. Therefore, your doctor may want you to take iron supplements to help clear up the anemia. If so, it is important to take iron every day while you are being treated for hookworms or whipworms; do not miss any doses. Your doctor may also want you to keep taking iron supplements for up to 6 months after you stop taking mebendazole. If you have any questions about this, check with your doctor.

Side Effects of This Medicine

Along with its needed effects, a medicine may cause some unwanted effects. Although not all of these side effects may occur, if they do occur they may need medical attention.

Check with your doctor as soon as possible if any of the following side effects occur:

Rare

Fever; skin rash or itching; sore throat and fever; unusual tiredness and weakness

Other side effects may occur that usually do not need medical attention. These side effects may go away during treatment as your body adjusts to the medicine. However, check with your doctor if any of the following side effects continue or are bothersome:

Less common

Abdominal or stomach pain or upset; diarrhea; nausea or vomiting

Rare

Dizziness; hair loss; headache

Other side effects not listed above may also occur in some patients. If you notice any other effects, check with your doctor.

Annual revision: 10/06/92

MECAMYLAMINE Systemic†

A commonly used brand name in the U.S. is Inversine.

†Not commercially available in Canada.

Description

Mecamylamine (mek-a-MILL-a-meen) belongs to the general class of medicines called antihypertensives. It is used to treat high blood pressure (hypertension).

High blood pressure adds to the workload of the heart and arteries. If it continues for a long time, the heart and arteries may not function properly. This can damage the blood vessels of the brain, heart, and kidneys, resulting in a stroke, heart failure, or kidney failure. High blood pressure may also increase the risk of heart attacks. These problems may be less likely to occur if blood pressure is controlled.

Mecamylamine works by controlling impulses along certain nerve pathways. As a result, it relaxes blood vessels so that blood passes through them more easily. This helps to lower blood pressure.

Mecamylamine is available only with your doctor's prescription, in the following dosage form:

Oral

- Tablets (U.S.)

It is very important that you read and understand the following information. If any of it causes you special concern, check with your doctor. Also, *if you have any questions* or if you want more information about this medicine or your medical problem, *ask your doctor, nurse, or pharmacist.*

Before Using This Medicine

In deciding to use a medicine, the risks of taking the medicine must be weighed against the good it will do. This is a decision you and your doctor will make. For mecamylamine, the following should be considered:

Allergies—Tell your doctor if you have ever had any unusual or allergic reaction to mecamylamine. Also tell your doctor and pharmacist if you are allergic to any other substances, such as foods, preservatives, or dyes.

Pregnancy—Studies on effects in pregnancy have not been done in either humans or animals. However, in general, use of this medicine during pregnancy is not recommended because pregnant women may be more sensitive to its effects. In addition, mecamylamine may cause bowel problems in the unborn baby.

Breast-feeding—It is not known whether mecamylamine passes into breast milk. However, this medicine has not been reported to cause problems in nursing babies.

Children—Studies on this medicine have been done only in adult patients, and there is no specific information comparing use of mecamylamine in children with use in other age groups.

Older adults—Dizziness or lightheadedness may be more likely to occur in the elderly, who are more sensitive to the effects of mecamylamine.

Other medicines—Although certain medicines should not be used together at all, in many cases two different medicines may be used together even if an interaction might occur. In these cases, changes in dose or other precautions may be necessary. When taking mecamylamine it is especially important that your doctor and pharmacist know if you are taking any of the following:

- Antibiotics or
- Sulfonamides (sulfa medicine)—Patients with chronic pyelonephritis being treated with these medications should not be treated with mecamylamine
- Antimyasthenics (ambenonium [e.g., Mytelase], neostigmine [e.g., Prostigmin], pyridostigmine [e.g., Mestinon])—Effects of these medicines may be decreased by mecamylamine
- Urinary alkalizers (medicine that makes the urine less acid, such as acetazolamide [e.g., Diamox], calcium- and/or magnesium-containing antacids, dichlorphenamide [e.g., Daranide], methazolamide [e.g., Neptazane], potassium or sodium citrate and/or citric acid, sodium bicarbonate [baking soda])—Effects of mecamylamine may be increased because these medicines cause it to be removed more slowly from the body

Other medical problems—The presence of other medical problems may affect the use of mecamylamine. Make sure you tell your doctor if you have any other medical problems, especially:

- Bladder or prostate problems—Mecamylamine may interfere with urination
- Bowel problems—Patients with bowel problems who take mecamylamine may be at inceased risk for serious bowel side effects of mecamylamine
- Diarrhea or
- Fever or infection or
- Nausea or vomiting—Effects of mecamylamine on blood pressure may be increased
- Glaucoma—Mecamylamine may make this condition worse
- Heart or blood vessel disease or
- Heart attack or stroke (recent)—Lowering of blood pressure by mecamylamine may make problems resulting from these conditions worse
- Kidney disease—Effects of mecamylamine may be increased because of slower removal of mecamylamine from the body

Before you begin using any new medicine (prescription or nonprescription) or if you develop any new medical problem while you are using this medicine, check with your doctor, nurse, or pharmacist.

Proper Use of This Medicine

In addition to the use of the medicine your doctor has prescribed, treatment for your high blood pressure may include weight control and care in the types of foods you eat, especially foods high in sodium. Your doctor will tell you which of these are most important for you. You should check with your doctor before changing your diet.

Many patients who have high blood pressure will not notice any signs of the problem. In fact, many may feel normal. *It is very important that you take your medicine exactly as directed and that you keep your appointments with your doctor* even if you feel well.

Remember that this medicine will not cure your high blood pressure but it does help control it. Therefore, you must continue to take it as directed if you expect to lower your blood pressure and keep it down. *You may have to take high blood pressure medicine for the rest of your life.* If high blood pressure is not treated, it can cause serious problems such as heart failure, blood vessel disease, stroke, or kidney disease.

To help you remember to take your medicine, try to get into the habit of taking it at the same time each day.

Dosing—The dose of mecamylamine will be different for different patients. *Follow your doctor's orders or the directions on the label.* The following information includes only the average doses of mecamylamine. *If your dose is different, do not change it* unless your doctor tells you to do so:

- For *oral* dosage forms (tablets):
  - —Adults: 2.5 milligrams two times a day to 25 milligrams three times a day.

Missed dose—If you miss a dose of this medicine, take it as soon as possible. Then go back to your regular dosing schedule. *If you miss two or more doses in a row, check with your doctor right away.* If your body goes without this medicine for too long, your blood pressure may go up to a dangerously high level.

Storage—To store this medicine:

- Keep out of the reach of children.
- Store away from heat and direct light.
- Do not store in the bathroom, near the kitchen sink, or in other damp places. Heat or moisture may cause the medicine to break down.
- Do not keep outdated medicine or medicine no longer needed. Be sure that any discarded medicine is out of the reach of children.

Precautions While Using This Medicine

It is important that your doctor check your progress at regular visits to make sure that this medicine is working properly.

Check with your doctor before you stop taking this medicine. Your doctor may want you to reduce gradually the amount you are taking before stopping completely.

Make sure that you have enough medicine on hand to last through weekends, holidays, or vacations. You should not miss taking any doses. You may want to ask your doctor for another written prescription for mecamylamine to carry in your wallet or purse. You can then have it filled if you run out of medicine when you are away from home.

Do not take other medicines unless they have been discussed with your doctor. This especially includes over-the-counter (nonprescription) medicines for appetite control, asthma, colds, cough, hay fever, or sinus problems, since they may tend to increase your blood pressure.

Dizziness, lightheadedness, or fainting may occur, especially when you get up from a lying or sitting position. This is more likely to occur in the morning. *Getting up slowly may help.* When you get up from lying down, sit on the edge of the bed with your feet dangling for one or two minutes. Then stand up slowly. If you feel dizzy, sit or lie down. If the problem continues or gets worse, check with your doctor.

The dizziness, lightheadedness, or fainting is also more likely to occur if you drink alcohol, stand for a long time, exercise, or if the weather is hot. *While you are taking this medicine, be careful to limit the amount of alcohol you drink. Also, use extra care during exercise or hot weather or if you must stand for a long time.*

Sodium bicarbonate (commonly known as baking soda) may cause you to get a greater than normal effect from this medicine. To prevent problems, check with your doctor or pharmacist before using an antacid or medicine for heartburn since some of these contain sodium bicarbonate.

Tell your doctor if you get a fever or infection since that may change the amount of medicine you have to take.

Mecamylamine may cause dryness of the mouth, nose, and throat. For temporary relief of mouth dryness, use sugarless candy or gum, melt bits of ice in your mouth, or use a saliva substitute. However, if your mouth continues to feel dry for more than 2 weeks, check with your medical doctor or dentist. Continuing dryness of the mouth may increase the chance of dental disease, including tooth decay, gum disease, and fungus infections.

Before having any kind of surgery (including dental surgery) or emergency treatment, tell the medical doctor or dentist in charge that you are taking this medicine.

Side Effects of This Medicine

Along with its needed effects, a medicine may cause some unwanted effects. Although not all of these side effects may occur, if they do occur they may need medical attention.

Check with your doctor as soon as possible if any of the following side effects occur:

More common

Dizziness or lightheadedness, especially when getting up from a lying or sitting position

Less common

Difficult urination

Rare

Bloating and frequent loose stools; confusion or excitement; constipation (severe); convulsions (seizures); mental depression; shortness of breath; trembling; uncontrolled movements of face, hands, arms, or legs

Other side effects may occur that usually do not need medical attention. These side effects may go away during treatment as your body adjusts to the medicine. However, check with your doctor if any of the following side effects continue or are bothersome:

More common

Constipation; drowsiness; unusual tiredness

Less common or rare

Blurred vision; decreased sexual ability or interest in sex; dryness of mouth; enlarged pupils; loss of appetite; nausea and vomiting; weakness

Other side effects not listed above may also occur in some patients. If you notice any other effects, check with your doctor.

Annual revision: 01/20/93

MECHLORETHAMINE Systemic

A commonly used brand name in the U.S. and Canada is Mustargen. Another commonly used name is nitrogen mustard.

Description

Mechlorethamine (me-klor-ETH-a-meen) belongs to the group of medicines called alkylating agents. It is used to treat some kinds of cancer as well as some noncancerous conditions.

Mechlorethamine interferes with the growth of cancer cells, which are eventually destroyed. Since the growth of normal body cells may also be affected by mechlorethamine, other effects will also occur. Some of these may be serious and must be reported to your doctor. Other effects, like hair loss, may not be serious but may cause concern. Some effects may not occur for months or years after the medicine is used.

Before you begin treatment with mechlorethamine, you and your doctor should talk about the good this medicine will do as well as the risks of using it.

Mechlorethamine is to be administered only by or under the immediate supervision of your doctor. It is available in the following dosage form:

Parenteral

- Injection (U.S. and Canada)

It is very important that you read and understand the following information. If any of it causes you special concern, check with your doctor. Also, *if you have any questions* or if you want more information about this medicine or your medical problem, *ask your doctor, nurse, or pharmacist.*

Before Using This Medicine

In deciding to use a medicine, the risks of taking the medicine must be weighed against the good it will do. This is a decision you and your doctor will make. For mechlorethamine, the following should be considered:

Allergies—Tell your doctor if you have ever had any unusual or allergic reaction to mechlorethamine, including a reaction if it was applied to the skin.

Pregnancy—Tell your doctor if you are pregnant or if you intend to have children. This medicine may cause birth defects if either the male or female is receiving it at the time of conception or if it is used during pregnancy. In addition, many cancer medicines may cause sterility which could be permanent. Sterility has been reported with mechlorethamine and the possibility should be kept in mind.

Be sure that you have discussed this with your doctor before receiving this medicine. It is best to use some kind of birth control while you are receiving mechlorethamine. Tell your doctor right away if you think you have become pregnant while receiving mechlorethamine.

Breast-feeding—Tell your doctor if you are breast-feeding or if you intend to breast-feed during treatment with this medicine. Because mechlorethamine may cause serious side effects, breast-feeding is generally not recommended while you are receiving it.

Children—Although there is no specific information about the use of mechlorethamine in children, it is not expected to cause different side effects or problems in children than it does in adults.

Older adults—Many medicines have not been tested in older people. Therefore, it may not be known whether they work exactly the same way they do in younger adults or if they cause different side effects or problems in older people. There is no specific information about the use of mechlorethamine in the elderly.

Other medicines—Although certain medicines should not be used together at all, in other cases two different medicines may be used together even if an interaction might occur. In these cases, your doctor may want to change the dose, or other precautions may be necessary. When you are receiving mechlorethamine, it is especially important that your doctor and pharmacist know if you are taking any of the following:

- Amphotericin B by injection (e.g., Fungizone) or
- Antithyroid agents (medicine for overactive thyroid) or
- Azathioprine (e.g., Imuran) or
- Chloramphenicol (e.g., Chloromycetin) or
- Colchicine or
- Flucytosine (e.g., Ancobon) or
- Interferon (e.g., Intron A, Roferon-A) or
- Plicamycin (e.g., Mithracin) or
- Zidovudine (e.g., Retrovir) or
- If you have ever been treated with x-rays or cancer medicines—Mechlorethamine may increase the effects of these medicines or radiation therapy on the blood
- Probenecid (e.g., Benemid) or
- Sulfinpyrazone (e.g., Anturane)—Mechlorethamine may raise the concentration of uric acid in the blood, which these medicines are used to lower

Other medical problems—The presence of other medical problems may affect the use of mechlorethamine. Make sure you tell your doctor if you have any other medical problems, especially:

- Chickenpox (including recent exposure) or
- Herpes zoster (shingles)—Risk of severe disease affecting other parts of the body
- Gout or
- Kidney stones—Mechlorethamine may increase levels of a chemical called uric acid in the body, which can cause gout and kidney stones
- Infection—Mechlorethamine can reduce immunity to infection

Before you begin using any new medicine (prescription or nonprescription) or if you develop any new medical problem while you are using this medicine, check with your doctor, nurse, or pharmacist.

Proper Use of This Medicine

Mechlorethamine is sometimes given together with certain other medicines. If you are using a combination of medicines, it is important that you receive each one at the proper time. If you are taking some of these medicines by mouth, ask your doctor, nurse, or pharmacist to help you plan a way to take them at the right times.

While you are using this medicine, your doctor may want you to drink extra fluids so that you will pass more urine. This will help prevent kidney problems and keep your kidneys working well.

Mechlorethamine often causes nausea and vomiting, which usually last only 8 to 24 hours. It is very important that you continue to receive the medicine, even if you begin to feel ill. Ask your doctor, nurse, or pharmacist for ways to lessen these effects.

Precautions While Using This Medicine

It is very important that your doctor check your progress at regular visits to make sure that this medicine is working properly and to check for unwanted effects.

While you are being treated with mechlorethamine, and after you stop treatment with it, *do not have any immunizations (vaccinations) without your doctor's approval.* Mechlorethamine may lower your body's resistance and there is a chance you might get the infection the immunization is meant to prevent. In addition, other persons living in your household should not take or should not have recently taken oral polio vaccine since there is a chance they could pass the polio virus on to you. Also, avoid other persons who have taken oral polio vaccine. Do not get close to them, and do not stay in the same room with them for very long. If you cannot take these precautions, you should consider wearing a protective face mask that covers the nose and mouth.

Mechlorethamine can lower the number of white blood cells in your blood temporarily, increasing the chance of getting an infection. It can also lower the number of platelets, which are necessary for proper blood clotting. If this occurs, there are certain precautions you can take, especially when your blood count is low, to reduce the risk of infection or bleeding:

- If you can, avoid people with infections. *Check with your doctor immediately* if you think you are getting an infection or if you get a fever or chills, cough or hoarseness, lower back or side pain, or painful or difficult urination.
- *Check with your doctor immediately* if you notice any unusual bleeding or bruising; black, tarry stools; blood in urine or stools; or pinpoint red spots on your skin.
- Be careful when using a regular toothbrush, dental floss, or toothpick. Your medical doctor, dentist, or nurse may recommend other ways to clean your teeth and gums. Check with your medical doctor before having any dental work done.
- Do not touch your eyes or the inside of your nose unless you have just washed your hands and have not touched anything else in the meantime.
- Be careful not to cut yourself when you are using sharp objects such as a safety razor or fingernail or toenail cutters.
- Avoid contact sports or other situations where bruising or injury could occur.

If mechlorethamine accidentally seeps out of the vein into which it is injected, it may damage some tissues and cause scarring. *Tell the doctor or nurse right away if you notice redness, pain, or swelling at the place of injection.*

Side Effects of This Medicine

Along with their needed effects, medicines like mechlorethamine can sometimes cause blood problems, loss of hair, and other side effects. These and others are described below. Also, because of the way these medicines act on the body, there is a chance that they might cause other effects that may not occur until months or years after these medicine is used. These delayed effects may include certain types of cancer, such as leukemia. Discuss these possible effects with your doctor.

Although not all of these side effects may occur, if they do occur they may need medical attention.

Check with your doctor or nurse immediately if any of the following side effects occur:

Less common

Black, tarry stools; blood in urine or stools; cough or hoarseness; fever or chills; lower back or side pain; pain or redness at place of injection; painful or difficult urination; pinpoint red spots on skin; unusual bleeding or bruising

Rare

Shortness of breath, itching, or wheezing

Check with your doctor or nurse as soon as possible if any of the following side effects occur:

More common

Missing menstrual periods; painful rash

Less common

Dizziness; joint pain; loss of hearing; ringing in ears; swelling of feet or lower legs

Rare

Numbness, tingling, or burning of fingers, toes, or face; sores in mouth and on lips; yellow eyes or skin

Other side effects may occur that usually do not need medical attention. These side effects may go away during treatment as your body adjusts to the medicine. Also, your doctor or nurse may be able to tell you about ways to prevent or reduce some of these side effects. Check with your doctor or nurse if any of the following side effects continue or are bothersome or if you have any questions about them:

More common

Nausea and vomiting (usually lasts only 8 to 24 hours)

Less common

Confusion; diarrhea; drowsiness; headache; loss of appetite; metallic taste; weakness

This medicine may cause a temporary loss of hair in some people. After treatment with mechlorethamine has ended, normal hair growth should return.

After you stop receiving mechlorethamine, it may still produce some side effects that need attention. During this period of time, check with your doctor if you notice any of the following side effects:

Black, tarry stools; blood in urine or stools; cough or hoarseness; fever or chills; lower back or side pain; painful or difficult urination; pinpoint red spots on skin; unusual bleeding or bruising

Other side effects not listed above may also occur in some patients. If you notice any other effects, check with your doctor.

Annual revision: August 1990
Interim revision: 07/29/93

MECHLORETHAMINE Topical*†

Another commonly used name is nitrogen mustard.

*Not commercially available in the U.S.
†Not commercially available in Canada.

Description

Mechlorethamine (me-klor-ETH-a-meen) belongs to the group of medicines called alkylating agents. It is used to treat certain skin conditions that could turn to cancer if left untreated.

Mechlorethamine interferes with the growth of problem cells, which are eventually destroyed. However, there is also a chance that mechlorethamine can cause some kinds of skin cancer, especially after it has been used for several years.

Before you begin treatment with mechlorethamine, you and your doctor should talk about the good this medicine will do as well as the risks of using it.

Mechlorethamine is available only with your doctor's prescription, in the following dosage forms:

Topical

- Ointment (U.S. and Canada)
- Topical solution (U.S. and Canada)

It is very important that you read and understand the following information. If any of it causes you special concern, check with your doctor. Also, *if you have any questions* or if you want more information about this medicine or your medical problem, *ask your doctor, nurse, or pharmacist.*

Before Using This Medicine

In deciding to use a medicine, the risks of taking the medicine must be weighed against the good it will do. This is a decision you and your doctor will make. For mechlorethamine applied to the skin, the following should be considered:

Allergies—Tell your doctor if you have ever had any unusual or allergic reaction to mechlorethamine.

Pregnancy—Although mechlorethamine applied to the skin has not been shown to cause problems in humans, some of it may be absorbed through the skin.

Breast-feeding—Although mechlorethamine applied to the skin has not been shown to cause problems in nursing babies, some of it may be absorbed through the skin. Because this medicine can cause serious side effects, breast-feeding is generally not recommended while you are using it.

Children—There is no specific information about use of mechlorethamine on the skin in children.

Older adults—Many medicines have not been tested in older people. Therefore, it may not be known whether they work exactly the same way they do in younger adults or if they cause different side effects or problems in older people. There is no specific information about the use of mechlorethamine on the skin in the elderly.

Before you begin using any new medicine (prescription or nonprescription) or if you develop any new medical problem while you are using this medicine, check with your doctor, nurse, or pharmacist.

Proper Use of This Medicine

Mechlorethamine may be used either as a solution or as an ointment. If you are using the solution, it must be mixed just before you use it since it breaks down quickly. *Mix the solution carefully according to your doctor's or pharmacists's directions.*

When preparing the solution, remember:

- Do not use the mechlorethamine if the solution is discolored or if droplets of water appear in the vial.
- Avoid inhaling the powder or any vapors. If some of the powder or solution accidentally gets on your skin, *immediately* wash that area of skin. Use a large amount of water and continue to wash for at least 15 minutes. If eye contact occurs, use an eyewash recommended by your doctor. Keep this eyewash on hand. *Follow carefully any other instructions your doctor may have given you.*
- All equipment used must be specially cleaned, even if it is to be thrown away. *Follow carefully your doctor's instructions* for doing this, using the special solution recommended.

Take a shower and rinse carefully just before you apply mechlorethamine solution or ointment, unless otherwise directed by your doctor. Make sure your skin is completely dry before applying the ointment. Do not shower again until the next treatment.

Apply the solution or ointment all over the body, until the entire amount for a dose is used up. Wear rubber or plastic gloves if you are using your hands. To apply the solution, a 2-inch-wide soft brush or gauze may be used instead. Let the solution dry.

Mechlorethamine should be applied more lightly to the groin, armpits, inside the bends of the elbows, and behind the knees. These areas are more likely to get irritated.

Avoid contact with the eyes, nose, or mouth, unless otherwise directed by your doctor.

Mechlorethamine is usually applied once a day. However, follow your doctor's instructions. Continue to use the medicine as long as you are told to. This may be months or years. However, do not use this medicine more often or for a longer time than ordered. To do so may increase the chance of unwanted effects.

Missed dose—If you miss a dose of this medicine, go back to your regular dosing schedule and check with your doctor. Do not change the amount you are using unless directed to do so by your doctor.

Storage—To store this medicine:

- Keep out of the reach of children.
- Store away from heat and direct light. This applies to either the ointment or the vials of mechlorethamine used to make the solution. The solution should not be stored but instead should be freshly made just before it is used.
- Do not store in the bathroom, near the kitchen sink, or in other damp places. Heat or moisture may cause the medicine to break down.
- Do not keep outdated medicine or medicine no longer needed. Be sure that any discarded medicine is out of the reach of children.

Precautions While Using This Medicine

It is very important that your doctor check your progress at regular visits to make sure that mechlorethamine is working properly and to check for unwanted effects.

Side Effects of This Medicine

Along with its needed effects, a medicine may cause some unwanted effects. When mechlorethamine is applied to the skin, it does not usually cause the same effects as when it is given by injection. *However, stop using this medicine and check with your doctor immediately* if the following side effects occur:

Hives; shortness of breath (sudden); skin rash or itching; sore, reddened skin

Check with your doctor also if you develop dry skin. There may be a lotion or ointment that you can use to help this. However, do not use anything else on your skin unless directed by your doctor.

Your skin color may darken after you have used this medicine for a while. The effect will go away after you have stopped using the medicine.

Other side effects not listed above may also occur in some patients. If you notice any other effects, check with your doctor.

Annual revision: August 1990

MECLIZINE/BUCLIZINE/CYCLIZINE Systemic

Some commonly used brand names are:

For Buclizine†
In the U.S.
Bucladin-S Softabs

For Cyclizine
In the U.S.
Marezine
In Canada
Marzine

For Meclizine

In the U.S.

Antivert	D-Vert 15
Antivert/25	D-Vert 30
Antivert/50	Meni-D
Bonine	Ru-Vert M

Generic name product may also be available.

In Canada

Bonamine

†Not commercially available in Canada.

Description

Buclizine (BYOO-kli-zeen), cyclizine (SYE-kli-zeen), and meclizine (MEK-li-zeen) are used to prevent and treat nausea, vomiting, and dizziness associated with motion sickness, and dizziness caused by other medical problems.

Some of these preparations are available only with your doctor's prescription. Others are available without a prescription; however, your doctor may have special instructions on the proper dose of the medicine for your medical condition. They are available in the following dosage forms:

Oral

Buclizine
- Chewable tablets (U.S.)

Cyclizine
- Tablets (U.S.)

Meclizine
- Capsules (U.S.)
- Tablets (U.S. and Canada)
- Chewable tablets (U.S.)

Parenteral

Cyclizine
- Injection (U.S. and Canada)

It is very important that you read and understand the following information. If any of it causes you special concern, check with your doctor or pharmacist. Also, *if you have any questions* or if you want more information about this medicine or your medical problem, *ask your doctor, nurse, or pharmacist.*

Before Using This Medicine

If you are taking this medicine without a prescription, carefully read and follow any precautions on the label. For buclizine, cyclizine, and meclizine, the following should be considered:

Allergies—Tell your doctor if you have ever had any unusual or allergic reaction to buclizine, cyclizine, or meclizine. Also tell your doctor and pharmacist if you are allergic to any other substances, such as foods, preservatives, or dyes.

Pregnancy—These medicines have not been shown to cause birth defects or other problems in humans. However, studies in animals have shown that buclizine, cyclizine, and meclizine given in doses many times the usual human dose cause birth defects, such as cleft palate.

Breast-feeding—Although these medicines may pass into the breast milk, they have not been reported to cause problems in nursing babies. However, since these medicines tend to decrease the secretions of the body, it is possible that the flow of breast milk may be reduced in some patients.

Children—There is no specific information comparing use of buclizine, cyclizine, and meclizine in children with use in other age groups. However, children may be especially sensitive to the anticholinergic effects (e.g., dryness of mouth, nose, and throat) of these medicines.

Older adults—There is no specific information comparing use of buclizine, cyclizine, and meclizine in the elderly with use in other age groups. However, older people may be especially sensitive to the anticholinergic effects (e.g., dryness of mouth, nose, and throat) of these medicines.

Other medicines—Although certain medicines should not be used together at all, in other cases two different medicines may be used together even if an interaction might occur. In these cases, your doctor may want to change the dose, or other precautions may be necessary. When you are taking buclizine, cyclizine, or meclizine, it is especially important that your doctor and pharmacist know if you are taking the following:

- Alcohol or
- Central nervous system (CNS) depressants, other (medicines that cause drowsiness)—Use with buclizine, cyclizine, or meclizine may increase the side effects of either medicine

Other medical problems—The presence of other medical problems may affect the use of buclizine, cyclizine, or meclizine. Make sure you tell your doctor if you have any other medical problems, especially:

- Enlarged prostate or
- Glaucoma or
- Intestinal blockage or
- Urinary tract blockage—Buclizine, cyclizine, or meclizine may make these conditions worse
- Heart failure—Cyclizine may make the condition worse

Before you begin using any new medicine (prescription or nonprescription) or if you develop any new medical problem while you are using this medicine, check with your doctor, nurse, or pharmacist.

Proper Use of This Medicine

Take this medicine with food or a glass of water or milk to lessen stomach irritation, if necessary.

This medicine is used to relieve or prevent the symptoms of motion sickness or dizziness caused by other medical problems. Take it only as directed. Do not take more of it or take it more often than stated on the label or ordered by your doctor. To do so may increase the chance of side effects.

For patients taking this medicine for *motion sickness:*

- Take buclizine or cyclizine at least 30 minutes before you begin to travel.
- Take meclizine at least 1 hour before you begin to travel.

Missed dose—If you must take this medicine regularly and you miss a dose, take the missed dose as soon as possible. However, if it is almost time for your next dose, skip the missed dose and go back to your regular dosing schedule. Do not double doses.

Storage—To store this medicine:

- Keep out of the reach of children.
- Store away from heat and direct light.
- Do not store the tablets in the bathroom, near the kitchen sink, or in other damp places. Heat or moisture may cause the medicine to break down.
- Do not keep outdated medicine or medicine no longer needed. Be sure that any discarded medicine is out of the reach of children.

Precautions While Using This Medicine

Tell the doctor in charge that you are taking this medicine before you have any skin tests for allergies. The results of the test may be affected by this medicine.

Buclizine, cyclizine, or meclizine will add to the effects of alcohol and other CNS depressants (medicines that slow down the nervous system, possibly causing drowsiness). Some examples of CNS depressants are antihistamines or medicine for hay fever, other allergies, or colds; sedatives, tranquilizers, or sleeping medicine; prescription pain medicine or narcotics; barbiturates; medicine for seizures; muscle relaxants; or anesthetics, including some dental anesthetics. *Check with your doctor before taking any of the above while you are using this medicine.*

This medicine may cause some people to become drowsy or less alert than they are normally. *Make sure you know how you react to this medicine before you drive, use machines, or do anything else that could be dangerous if you are not alert.*

Buclizine, cyclizine, and meclizine may cause dryness of the mouth. For temporary relief use sugarless candy or gum, melt bits of ice in your mouth, or use a saliva substitute. However, if your mouth continues to feel dry for more than 2 weeks, check with your medical doctor or dentist. Continuing dryness of the mouth may increase the chance of dental disease, including tooth decay, gum disease, and fungus infections.

Side Effects of This Medicine

Along with its needed effects, a medicine may cause some unwanted effects. The following side effects may go away during treatment as your body adjusts to the medicine; however, check with your doctor if they continue or are bothersome:

More common

Drowsiness

Less common or rare

Blurred vision; constipation; difficult or painful urination; dizziness; dryness of mouth, nose, and throat; fast heartbeat; headache; loss of appetite; nervousness, restlessness, or trouble in sleeping; skin rash; upset stomach

Not all of the side effects listed above have been reported for each of these medicines, but they have been reported for at least one of them. Buclizine, cyclizine, and meclizine are similar, so any of the above side effects may occur with any of these medicines.

Other side effects not listed above may also occur in some patients. If you notice any other effects, check with your doctor.

Annual revision: 12/02/92

MEFLOQUINE Systemic†

A commonly used brand name in the U.S. is Lariam.

†Not commercially available in Canada.

Description

Mefloquine (ME-floe-kwin) is used to prevent or treat malaria. It works by killing malaria parasites (tiny, one-celled animals) or preventing their growth.

Mefloquine will not actually prevent you from becoming infected with malaria. However, it will prevent the development of symptoms of malaria in people who are living in, or will be traveling to, an area where there is a chance of getting malaria. This medicine may also be used to treat malaria in patients who have already developed symptoms of malaria. Mefloquine may be taken alone or with other medicines for malaria.

This medicine may cause some serious side effects. Therefore, it is usually used only to prevent the symptoms of malaria or to treat serious malaria infections in areas where it is known that other medicines may not work.

Mefloquine is available only with your doctor's prescription, in the following dosage form:

Oral

- Tablets (U.S.)

It is very important that you read and understand the following information. If any of it causes you special concern, check with your doctor. Also, *if you have any questions* or if you want more information about this medicine or your medical problem, *ask your doctor, nurse, or pharmacist.*

Before Using This Medicine

In deciding to use a medicine, the risks of taking the medicine must be weighed against the good it will do. This is a decision you and your doctor will make. For mefloquine, the following should be considered:

Allergies—Tell your doctor if you have ever had any unusual or allergic reaction to mefloquine, quinidine (e.g., Quinidex), quinine (e.g., Quinamm), or any related medicines. Also tell your doctor and pharmacist if you are allergic to any other substances, such as foods, preservatives, or dyes.

Pregnancy—Mefloquine has not been studied in pregnant women, and its use is not recommended during pregnancy. Studies in animals have shown that mefloquine may cause birth defects and other problems.

However, mefloquine has been used in some women in the second and third trimesters of pregnancy. It is important to prevent malaria since if a pregnant woman gets malaria, there is an increased chance of premature births, stillbirths, and abortion.

It is best if pregnant women can avoid traveling to areas where there is a chance of getting malaria. However, if travel is necessary and mefloquine is used, women who may become pregnant should use effective birth control measures while taking this medicine and for 2 months after taking the last dose.

Breast-feeding—Mefloquine passes into the breast milk in small amounts.

Children—Studies on mefloquine use in children have shown that this medicine causes side effects in children like those seen in adults, e.g., nausea, vomiting, and dizziness. Its use is not recommended in infants and children up to 2 years of age or those weighing up to 15 kg (33 pounds).

Older adults—Many medicines have not been studied specifically in older people. Therefore, it may not be known whether they work exactly the same way they do in younger adults or if they cause different side effects or problems in older people. There is no specific information comparing use of mefloquine in the elderly with use in other age groups.

Other medicines—Although certain medicines should not be used together at all, in other cases two different medicines may be used together even if an interaction might occur. In these cases, your doctor may want to change the dose, or other precautions may be necessary. When you are taking mefloquine, it is especially important that your doctor and pharmacist know if you are taking any of the following:

- Bepridil (e.g., Vascor) or
- Beta-adrenergic blocking agents (acebutolol [e.g., Sectral], atenolol [e.g., Tenormin], betaxolol [e.g., Kerlone], carteolol [e.g., Cartrol], labetalol [e.g., Normodyne], metoprolol [e.g., Lopressor], nadolol [e.g., Corgard], oxprenolol [e.g., Trasicor], penbutolol [e.g., Levatol], pindolol [e.g., Visken], propranolol [e.g., Inderal], sotalol [e.g., Sotacor], timolol [e.g., Blocadren]) or
- Diltiazem (e.g., Cardizem) or
- Flunarizine (e.g., Sibelium) or
- Isradipine (e.g., DynaCirc) or
- Nicardipine (e.g., Cardene) or
- Nifedipine (e.g., Procardia) or
- Nimodipine (e.g., Nimotop) or
- Quinidine (e.g., Quinidex) or
- Quinine (e.g., Quinamm) or
- Verapamil (e.g., Calan)—Use of these medicines together with mefloquine may result in slow heartbeat and other heart problems; also, an increased chance of convulsions (seizures) may occur when quinine is taken together with mefloquine
- Chloroquine (e.g., Aralen)—Use of chloroquine with mefloquine may increase the chance of convulsions (seizures)
- Divalproex (e.g., Depakote) or
- Valproic acid (e.g., Depakene)—Use of these medicines together with mefloquine may result in low blood levels of valproic acid and an increased chance of convulsions (seizures)
- Typhoid vaccine, oral (e.g., Vivotif Vaccine)—Use of the oral typhoid vaccine with mefloquine may keep the vaccine from working properly

Other medical problems—The presence of other medical problems may affect the use of mefloquine. Make sure you tell your doctor if you have any other medical problems, especially:

- Convulsions (seizures) or
- Epilepsy or
- Heart block or
- Psychiatric (mental) disorders, history of—Mefloquine may make these conditions worse

Before you begin using any new medicine (prescription or nonprescription) or if you develop any new medical problem while you are using this medicine, check with your doctor, nurse, or pharmacist.

Proper Use of This Medicine

Do not give this medicine to infants and children up to 2 years of age or to those weighing less than 15 kg (33 pounds).

Mefloquine is best taken with a full glass (8 ounces) of water and with food, unless otherwise directed by your doctor.

For patients taking *mefloquine* to *prevent the symptoms of malaria:*

- Your doctor will want you to start taking this medicine 1 week before you travel to an area where there is a chance of getting malaria. This will help you to see how you react to the medicine. Also, it will allow time for your doctor to prescribe another medicine for you if you have a reaction to this medicine.
- Also, you should keep taking this medicine while you are in the area and for 4 weeks after you leave the area. No medicine will protect you completely from malaria. However, to protect you as completely as possible, *it is important that you keep taking this medicine for the full time your doctor ordered.* Also, if fever or "flu-like" symptoms develop during your travels or within 2 to 3 months after you leave the area, *check with your doctor immediately.*
- This medicine works best when you take it on a regular schedule. For example, if you are to take it once a week, it is best to take it on the same day each week. *Do not miss any doses.* If you have any questions about this, check with your doctor, nurse, or pharmacist.

For patients taking *mefloquine* to *treat malaria:*

- To help clear up your infection completely, *take this medicine exactly as directed by your doctor.*

Missed dose—If you do miss a dose of this medicine, take it as soon as possible. This will help to keep you taking your medicine on a regular schedule. However, if it is almost time for your next dose, skip the missed dose and go back to your regular dosing schedule. Do not double doses.

Storage—To store this medicine:

- Keep out of the reach of children.
- Store away from heat and direct light.
- Do not store in the bathroom, near the kitchen sink, or in other damp places. Heat or moisture may cause the medicine to break down.
- Do not keep outdated medicine or medicine no longer needed. Be sure that any discarded medicine is out of the reach of children.

Precautions While Using This Medicine

Mefloquine may cause vision problems. It may also cause some people to become dizzy or lightheaded or to have hallucinations (seeing, hearing, or feeling things that are not there). *Make sure you know how you react to this medicine before you drive, use machines, or do anything else that could be dangerous if you are dizzy or are not alert or able to see well.* This is especially important for people whose jobs require fine coordination. If these reactions are especially bothersome, check with your doctor.

Malaria is spread by the bite of certain kinds of infected female mosquitoes. If you are living in, or will be traveling to, an area where there is a chance of getting malaria, the following mosquito-control measures will help to prevent infection:

- If possible, sleep under mosquito netting to avoid being bitten by malaria-carrying mosquitoes.
- Wear long-sleeved shirts or blouses and long trousers to protect your arms and legs, especially from dusk through dawn when mosquitoes are out.
- Apply mosquito repellant, preferably one containing DEET, to uncovered areas of the skin from dusk through dawn when mosquitoes are out.
- Using a pyrethrum-containing flying insect spray to kill mosquitoes in living and sleeping quarters during evening and nighttime hours.

If you are taking quinidine (e.g., Quinidex) or quinine (e.g., Quinamm) talk to your doctor before you take mefloquine. While you are taking mefloquine, take mefloquine at least 12 hours after the last dose of quinidine or quinine. Taking mefloquine and either of these medicines at the same time may result in a greater chance of serious side effects.

For patients taking *mefloquine* to *treat malaria:*

- If your symptoms do not improve within a few days, or if they become worse, check with your doctor.

Side Effects of This Medicine

Along with its needed effects, a medicine may cause some unwanted effects. Although not all of these side effects may occur, if they do occur they may need medical attention.

Check with your doctor immediately if any of the following side effects occur:

Rare
- Anxiety; confusion; convulsions (seizures); hallucinations (seeing, hearing, or feeling things that are not there); mental depression; mood or mental changes; restlessness; slow heartbeat

Other side effects may occur that usually do not need medical attention. These side effects may go away during treatment as your body adjusts to the medicine. However, check with your doctor if any of the following side effects continue or are bothersome:

More common
- Abdominal or stomach pain; diarrhea; difficulty concentrating; dizziness; headache; lightheadedness; loss of appetite; nausea or vomiting; trouble in sleeping; visual changes

Other side effects not listed above may also occur in some patients. If you notice any other effects, check with your doctor.

Annual revision: 10/06/92

MELPHALAN Systemic

A commonly used brand name in the U.S. and Canada is Alkeran. Other commonly used names are L-PAM and phenylalanine mustard.

Description

Melphalan (MEL-fa-lan) belongs to the group of medicines called alkylating agents. It is used to treat some kinds of cancer.

Melphalan interferes with the growth of cancer cells, which are eventually destroyed. Since the growth of normal body cells may also be affected by melphalan, other effects will also occur. Some of these may be serious and must be reported to your doctor. Other effects may not be serious but may cause concern. Some effects may not occur for months or years after the medicine is used.

Before you begin treatment with melphalan, you and your doctor should talk about the good this medicine will do as well as the risks of using it.

Melphalan is available only with your doctor's prescription, in the following dosage form:

Oral
- Tablets (U.S. and Canada)

It is very important that you read and understand the following information. If any of it causes you special concern, check with your doctor. Also, *if you have any questions* or if you want more information about this medicine or your medical problem, *ask your doctor, nurse, or pharmacist.*

Before Using This Medicine

In deciding to use a medicine, the risks of taking the medicine must be weighed against the good it will do. This is a decision you and your doctor will make. For melphalan, the following should be considered:

Allergies—Tell your doctor if you have ever had any unusual or allergic reaction to melphalan or chlorambucil.

Pregnancy—Tell your doctor if you are pregnant or if you intend to have children. There is a chance that this medicine may cause birth defects if either the male or female is taking it at the time of conception or if it is taken during pregnancy. In addition, many cancer medicines may cause sterility which could be permanent. Sterility has been reported with melphalan and the possibility should be kept in mind.

Be sure that you have discussed this with your doctor before taking this medicine. It is best to use some kind of birth control while you are taking melphalan. Tell your doctor right away if you think you have become pregnant while taking melphalan.

Breast-feeding—Tell your doctor if you are breast-feeding or if you intend to breast-feed during treatment with this medicine. Because melphalan may cause serious side effects, breast-feeding is generally not recommended while you are taking it.

Children—There is no specific information about the use of melphalan in children.

Older adults—Many medicines have not been tested in older people. Therefore, it may not be known whether they work exactly the same way they do in younger adults or if they cause different side effects or problems in older people. There is no specific information about the use of melphalan in the elderly.

Other medicines—Although certain medicines should not be used together at all, in other cases two different medicines may be used together even if an interaction might occur. In these cases, your doctor may want to change the dose, or other precautions may be necessary. When you are taking melphalan, it is especially important that your doctor and pharmacist know if you are taking any of the following:

- Amphotericin B by injection (e.g., Fungizone) or
- Antithyroid agents (medicine for overactive thyroid) or
- Azathioprine (e.g., Imuran) or
- Chloramphenicol (e.g., Chloromycetin) or
- Colchicine or

- Flucytosine (e.g., Ancobon) or
- Interferon (e.g., Intron A, Roferon-A) or
- Plicamycin (e.g., Mithracin) or
- Zidovudine (e.g., Retrovir) or
- If you have ever been treated with x-rays or cancer medicines—Melphalan may increase the effects of these medicines or radiation therapy on the blood
- Probenecid (e.g., Benemid) or
- Sulfinpyrazone (e.g., Anturane)—Melphalan may raise the concentration of uric acid in the blood, which these medicines are used to lower

Other medical problems—The presence of other medical problems may affect the use of melphalan. Make sure you tell your doctor if you have any other medical problems, especially:

- Chickenpox (including recent exposure) or
- Herpes zoster (shingles)—Risk of severe disease affecting other parts of the body
- Gout (history of) or
- Kidney stones (history of)—Melphalan may increase levels of a chemical called uric acid in the body, which can cause gout or kidney stones
- Infection—Melphalan can reduce immunity to infection
- Kidney disease

Before you begin using any new medicine (prescription or nonprescription) or if you develop any new medical problem while you are using this medicine, check with your doctor, nurse, or pharmacist.

Proper Use of This Medicine

Take melphalan only as directed by your doctor. Do not take more or less of it, do not take it more often, and do not take it for a longer time than your doctor ordered. The exact amount of medicine you need has been carefully worked out. Taking too much may increase the chance of side effects, while taking too little may not improve your condition.

This medicine is sometimes given together with certain other medicines. If you are using a combination of medicines, make sure that you take each one at the proper time and do not mix them. Ask your doctor, nurse, or pharmacist to help you plan a way to remember to take your medicine at the right times.

While you are using melphalan, your doctor may want you to drink extra fluids so that you will pass more urine. This will help prevent kidney problems and keep your kidneys working well.

This medicine often causes nausea, vomiting, and loss of appetite. However, it may have to be taken for several months to be effective. Even if you begin to feel ill, *do not stop using this medicine without first checking with your doctor.* Ask your doctor, nurse, or pharmacist for ways to lessen these effects.

If you vomit shortly after taking a dose of melphalan, check with your doctor. You will be told whether to take the dose again or to wait until the next scheduled dose.

Missed dose—If you miss a dose of this medicine, do not take the missed dose at all and do not double the next one. Instead, go back to your regular dosing schedule and check with your doctor.

Storage—To store this medicine:

- Keep out of the reach of children.
- Store in the original glass container away from heat and direct light.
- Do not store in the bathroom, near the kitchen sink, or in other damp places. Heat or moisture may cause the medicine to break down.
- Do not keep outdated medicine or medicine no longer needed. Be sure that any discarded medicine is out of the reach of children.

Precautions While Using This Medicine

It is very important that your doctor check your progress at regular visits to make sure that this medicine is working properly and to check for unwanted effects.

While you are being treated with melphalan, and after you stop treatment with it, *do not have any immunizations (vaccinations) without your doctor's approval.* Melphalan may lower your body's resistance and there is a chance you might get the infection the immunization is meant to prevent. In addition, other persons living in your household should not take or should not have recently taken oral polio vaccine since there is a chance they could pass the polio virus on to you. Also, avoid other persons who have taken oral polio vaccine. Do not get close to them and do not stay in the same room with them for very long. If you cannot take these precautions, you should consider wearing a protective face mask that covers the nose and mouth.

Melphalan can lower the number of white blood cells in your blood temporarily, increasing the chance of getting an infection. It can also lower the number of platelets, which are necessary for proper blood clotting. If this occurs, there are certain precautions you can take, especially when your blood count is low, to reduce the risk of infection or bleeding:

- If you can, avoid people with infections. *Check with your doctor immediately* if you think you are getting an infection or if you get a fever or chills, cough or hoarseness, lower back or side pain, or painful or difficult urination.
- *Check with your doctor immediately* if you notice any unusual bleeding or bruising; black, tarry stools; blood in urine or stools; or pinpoint red spots on your skin.

- Be careful when using a regular toothbrush, dental floss, or toothpick. Your medical doctor, dentist, or nurse may recommend other ways to clean your teeth and gums. Check with your medical doctor before having any dental work done.
- Do not touch your eyes or the inside of your nose unless you have just washed your hands and have not touched anything else in the meantime.
- Be careful not to cut yourself when you are using sharp objects such as a safety razor or fingernail or toenail cutters.
- Avoid contact sports or other situations where bruising or injury could occur.

Side Effects of This Medicine

Along with their needed effects, medicines like melphalan can sometimes cause unwanted effects such as blood problems and other side effects. These and others are described below. Also, because of the way these medicines act on the body, there is a chance that they might cause other unwanted effects that may not occur until months or years after the medicine is used. These delayed effects may include certain types of cancer, such as leukemia. Discuss these possible effects with your doctor.

Although not all of these side effects may occur, if they do occur they may need medical attention.

Check with your doctor immediately if any of the following side effects occur:

Less common

Black, tarry stools; blood in urine or stools; cough or hoarseness; fever or chills; lower back or side pain; painful or difficult urination; pinpoint red spots on skin; skin rash or itching (sudden); unusual bleeding or bruising

Check with your doctor as soon as possible if any of the following side effects occur:

Less common or rare

Joint pain; sores in mouth and on lips; swelling of feet or lower legs

Other side effects may occur that usually do not need medical attention. These side effects may go away during treatment as your body adjusts to the medicine. Also, your doctor or nurse may be able to tell you about ways to prevent or reduce some of these side effects. Check with your doctor or nurse if the following side effects continue or are bothersome or if you have any questions about them:

Less common

Nausea and vomiting

After you stop taking melphalan, it may still produce some side effects that need attention. During this period of time, check with your doctor if you notice any of the following side effects:

Black, tarry stools; blood in urine or stools; cough or hoarseness; fever or chills; lower back or side pain; painful or difficult urination; pinpoint red spots on skin; unusual bleeding or bruising

Other side effects not listed above may also occur in some patients. If you notice any other effects, check with your doctor.

Annual revision: August 1990
Interim revision: 07/29/93

MENINGOCOCCAL POLYSACCHARIDE VACCINE Systemic

A commonly used brand name in the U.S. and Canada is Menomune-A/C/Y/W-135

Description

Meningococcal polysaccharide (ma-nin-ja-KOK-kal poli-SAK-ka-ryd) vaccine is an active immunizing agent used to prevent infection by certain groups of meningococcal bacteria. The vaccine works by causing your body to produce its own protection (antibodies) against the disease.

The following information applies only to the meningococcal vaccine used for meningococcal bacteria groups A, C, Y, and W-135. These groups cause approximately 50% of meningococcal meningitis cases in the U.S. The vaccine will not protect against infection caused by other meningococcal bacteria groups, such as Group B.

Meningococcal infection can cause life-threatening illnesses, such as meningococcal meningitis, which affects the brain, and meningococcemia, which affects the blood. Approximately 10% of persons with meningococcal meningitis and 20% of persons with meningococcemia die. These diseases are more likely to occur in young children and in persons with certain diseases or conditions that make them more susceptible to a meningococcal infection or more likely to develop serious problems from a meningococcal infection.

Immunization against meningococcal disease is recommended for persons 2 years of age or older who are at risk of getting the disease because:

- they have certain diseases or conditions that make them more susceptible to a meningococcal infection or more likely to develop serious problems from a meningococcal infection.

- they are living in, working in, or visiting an area where there is a high possibility of getting meningococcal disease.

Usually a person needs to receive meningococcal vaccine only once. However, additional injections may be needed for young children who remain at high risk of meningococcal disease.

Meningococcal polysaccharide vaccine is available only from your doctor or other authorized health care providers, in the following dosage form:

Parenteral

- Injection (U.S. and Canada)

It is very important that you read and understand the following information. If any of it causes you special concern, check with your doctor. Also, *if you have any questions* or if you want more information about this medicine or your medical problem, *ask your doctor, nurse, or pharmacist.*

Before Receiving This Vaccine

In deciding to use a medicine, the risks of taking the medicine must be weighed against the good it will do. This is a decision you and your doctor will make. For meningococcal vaccine, the following should be considered:

Allergies—Tell your doctor if you have ever had any unusual or allergic reaction to meningococcal vaccine. Also tell your doctor and pharmacist if you are allergic to any other substances, such as food (especially lactose) or preservatives. This vaccine contains lactose.

Pregnancy—Meningococcal vaccine has not been shown to cause birth defects or other problems in humans.

Breast-feeding—It is not known whether meningococcal vaccine passes into the breast milk. However, the vaccine has not been reported to cause problems in nursing babies.

Children—This vaccine has been tested in children and, in effective doses, has not been shown to cause different side effects or problems than it does in adults.

Older adults—Many medicines have not been tested in older people. Therefore, it may not be known whether they work exactly the same way they do in younger adults. Although there is no specific information about the use of this vaccine in the elderly, it is not expected to cause different side effects or problems in older people than it does in younger adults.

Other medicines—Although certain medicines should not be used together at all, in other cases two different medicines may be used together even if an interaction might occur. In these cases, your doctor may want to change the dose, or other precautions may be necessary. Before you receive meningococcal vaccine, it is especially important that your doctor and pharmacist know if you have received any of the following:

- Treatment with x-rays, cancer medicines, or immunosuppressive agents (agents that reduce the body's natural immunity)—Condition may lessen the useful effect of the vaccine

Other medical problems—The presence of other medical problems may affect the use of meningococcal vaccine. Make sure you tell your doctor if you have any other medical problems, especially:

- Severe illness with fever—The symptoms of the condition may be confused with the possible side effects of the vaccine

Side Effects of This Vaccine

Along with its needed effects, a vaccine may cause some unwanted effects. Although not all of these side effects may occur, if they do occur they may need medical attention.

Get emergency help immediately if any of the following side effects occur:

Symptoms of allergic reactions

Difficulty in breathing or swallowing; hives; itching, especially of feet or hands; reddening of skin, especially around ears; swelling of eyes, face, or inside of nose; unusual tiredness or weakness (sudden and severe)

Other side effects may occur that usually do not need medical attention. However, check with your doctor if any of the following side effects continue or are bothersome:

More common

Redness at place of injection—may last 1 or 2 days; tenderness, soreness, or pain at place of injection

Less common

Chills; feeling of body discomfort; fever over 100 °F (37.8 °C); hard lump at place of injection; headache; tiredness or weakness

Other side effects not listed above may also occur in some patients. If you notice any other effects, check with your doctor.

Annual revision: August 1990

MENOTROPINS Systemic

A commonly used brand name in the U.S. and Canada is Pergonal. Another commonly used name is human menopausal gonadotropins (HMG).

Description

Menotropins (men-oh-TROE-pins) are a mixture of follicle-stimulating hormone (FSH) and luteinizing hormone (LH) that are naturally produced by the pituitary gland.

Use in females:

FSH is primarily responsible for stimulating growth of the ovarian follicle, which includes the developing egg, the cells surrounding the egg that produce the hormones needed to support a pregnancy, and the fluid around the egg. As the follicle grows, an increasing amount of the hormone estrogen is produced by the cells in the follicle and released into the bloodstream. Estrogen causes the endometrium (lining of the uterus) to thicken before ovulation occurs. The higher blood levels of estrogen will also tell the hypothalamus and pituitary gland to slow the production and release of FSH.

LH also helps to increase the amount of estrogen produced by the follicle cells. However, its main function is to cause ovulation. The sharp rise in the blood level of LH that triggers ovulation is called the LH surge. After ovulation, the group of hormone-producing follicle cells become the corpus luteum, which will produce estrogen and large amounts of another hormone, progesterone. Progesterone causes the endometrium to mature so that it can support implantation of the fertilized egg or embryo. If implantation of a fertilized egg does not occur, the levels of estrogen and progesterone decrease, the endometrium sloughs off, and menstruation occurs.

Menotropins are usually given in combination with human chorionic gonadotropin (hCG). The actions of hCG are almost the same as those of LH. It is given to simulate the natural LH surge. This results in ovulation at an expected time.

Many women choosing treatment with menotropins have already tried clomiphene (e.g., Serophene) and have not been able to conceive yet. Menotropins may also be used to cause the ovary to produce several follicles, which can then be harvested for use in gamete intrafallopian transfer (GIFT) or *in vitro* fertilization (IVF).

Use in males:

Menotropins are used to stimulate the production of sperm in some forms of male infertility.

Menotropins are to be given only by or under the supervision of your doctor. It is available in the following dosage form:

Parenteral

- Injection (U.S. and Canada)

It is very important that you read and understand the following information. If any of it causes you special concern, check with your doctor. Also, *if you have any questions* or if you want more information about this medicine or your medical problem, *ask your doctor, nurse, or pharmacist.*

Before Using This Medicine

In deciding to use a medicine, the risks of taking the medicine must be weighed against the good it will do. This is a decision you and your doctor will make. For menotropins, the following should be considered:

Allergies—Tell your doctor if you have ever had any unusual or allergic reaction to menotropins. Also tell your doctor and pharmacist if you are allergic to any other substances, such as foods, preservatives, or dyes.

Pregnancy—If you become pregnant as a result of using this medicine, there is an increased chance of a multiple pregnancy.

Other medicines—Although certain medicines should not be used together at all, in other cases two different medicines may be used together even if an interaction might occur. In these cases, your doctor may want to change the dose, or other precautions may be necessary. Tell your doctor and pharmacist if you are taking any other prescription or nonprescription (over-the-counter [OTC]) medicine.

Other medical problems—The presence of other medical problems may affect the use of menotropins. Make sure you tell your doctor if you have any other medical problems, especially:

- Cyst on ovary—Menotropins can cause further growth of cysts on the ovary
- Unusual vaginal bleeding—Some irregular vaginal bleeding is a sign that the endometrium is growing too rapidly, possibly of endometrial cancer, or some hormone imbalances; the increases in estrogen production caused by menotropins can make these problems worse. If a hormonal imbalance is present, it should be treated before the beginning of menotropins therapy

Before you begin using any new medicine (prescription or nonprescription) or if you develop any new medical problem while you are using this medicine, check with your doctor, nurse, or pharmacist.

Precautions While Using This Medicine

It is very important that your doctor check your progress at regular visits to make sure that the medicine is working properly and to check for unwanted effects. Your doctor will likely want to watch the development of the ovarian follicle(s) by measuring the amount of estrogen in your bloodstream and by checking the size of the follicle(s) with ultrasound examinations.

For females only:

- If your doctor has asked you to record your basal body temperatures (BBTs) daily, make sure that you do this every day. It is important that intercourse take place around the time of ovulation to give you the best chance of becoming pregnant. *Follow your doctor's instructions carefully.*

Side Effects of This Medicine

Along with its needed effects, a medicine may cause some unwanted effects. Although not all of these side effects may occur, if they do occur they may need medical attention.

Check with your doctor as soon as possible if any of the following side effects occur:

For females only

More common

Bloating (mild); pain, swelling, or irritation at place of injection; rash at place of injection or on body; stomach or pelvic pain

Less common or rare

Abdominal or stomach pain (severe); bloating (moderate to severe); decreased amount of urine; feeling of indigestion; nausea, vomiting, or diarrhea (continuing or severe); pelvic pain (severe); shortness of breath; swelling of the lower legs; weight gain (rapid)

For males only

More common

Dizziness; fainting; headache; irregular heartbeat; loss of appetite; more frequent nosebleeds; shortness of breath

Other side effects may occur that usually do not need medical attention. These side effects may go away during treatment as your body adjusts to the medicine. However, check with your doctor if the following side effect continues or is bothersome:

For males only

Less common

Enlargement of breasts

After you stop using this medicine, your body may need time to adjust. The length of time this takes depends on the amount of medicine you were using and how long you used it. During this period of time check with your doctor if you notice any of the following side effects:

For females only

Abdominal or stomach pain (severe); bloating (moderate to severe); decreased amount of urine; feeling of indigestion; nausea, vomiting, or diarrhea (continuing or severe); pelvic pain (severe); shortness of breath; weight gain (rapid)

Other side effects not listed above may also occur in some patients. If you notice any other effects, check with your doctor.

Annual revision: 07/07/92

MEPROBAMATE Systemic

Some commonly used brand names are:

In the U.S.

Equanil	'Miltown'-400
Meprospan 200	'Miltown'-600
Meprospan 400	Probate
'Miltown'-200	Trancot

Generic name product may also be available.

In Canada

Apo-Meprobamate	Meprospan-400
Equanil	Miltown

Description

Meprobamate (me-proe-BA-mate) is used to relieve nervousness or tension. This medicine should not be used for nervousness or tension caused by the stress of everyday life.

Meprobamate is available only with your doctor's prescription, in the following dosage forms:

Oral

- Extended-release capsules (U.S. and Canada)
- Tablets (U.S. and Canada)

It is very important that you read and understand the following information. If any of it causes you special concern, check with your doctor. Also, *if you have any questions* or if you want more information about this medicine or your medical problem, *ask your doctor, nurse, or pharmacist.*

Before Using This Medicine

In deciding to use a medicine, the risks of taking the medicine must be weighed against the good it will do. This is a decision you and your doctor will make. For meprobamate, the following should be considered:

Allergies—Tell your doctor if you have ever had any unusual or allergic reaction to meprobamate or to medicines like meprobamate such as carbromal, carisoprodol, mebutamate, or tybamate. Also tell your doctor and pharmacist if you are allergic to any other substances, such as foods, preservatives, or dyes.

Pregnancy—Meprobamate has been reported to increase the chance of birth defects if taken during the first 3 months of pregnancy.

Breast-feeding—Meprobamate passes into the breast milk and may cause drowsiness in babies of mothers taking this medicine.

Children—Studies on this medicine have been done only in adult patients, and there is no specific information comparing use of meprobamate in children with use in other age groups.

Older adults—Elderly people may be especially sensitive to the effects of meprobamate. This may increase the chance of side effects during treatment.

Other medicines—Although certain medicines should not be used together at all, in other cases two different medicines may be used together even if an interaction might occur. In these cases, your doctor may want to change the dose, or other precautions may be necessary. When you are taking meprobamate, it is especially important that your doctor and pharmacist know if you are taking any of the following:

- Central nervous system (CNS) depressants (medicines that cause drowsiness) or
- Tricyclic antidepressants (medicine for depression)—Taking these medicines with meprobamate may increase the CNS depressant effects

Other medical problems—The presence of other medical problems may affect the use of meprobamate. Make sure you tell your doctor if you have any other medical problems, especially:

- Alcohol abuse (or history of) or
- Drug abuse or dependence (or history of)—Dependence on meprobamate may develop
- Epilepsy—The risk of seizures may be increased
- Kidney disease or
- Liver disease—Higher blood levels of meprobamate may occur, increasing the chance of side effects
- Porphyria—Meprobamate may make the condition worse

Before you begin using any new medicine (prescription or nonprescription) or if you develop any new medical problem while you are using this medicine, check with your doctor, nurse, or pharmacist.

Proper Use of This Medicine

Take this medicine only as directed by your doctor. Do not take more of it, do not take it more often, and do not take it for a longer time than your doctor ordered. If too much is taken, it may become habit-forming.

Dosing—The dose of meprobamate will be different for different patients. *Follow your doctor's orders or the directions on the label.* The following information includes only the average doses of meprobamate. *If your dose is different, do not change it* unless your doctor tells you to do so:

- For *regular (short-acting)* tablets:
  —Adults and children 12 years of age and older: 400 milligrams three or four times a day, or 600 milligrams two times a day.
  —Children 6 to 12 years of age: 100 to 200 milligrams two or three times a day.
  —Children up to 6 years of age: Dose must be determined by the doctor.
- For *long-acting* dosage forms (extended-release tablets):
  —Adults and children 12 years of age or older: 400 to 800 milligrams two times a day, in the morning and at bedtime.
  —Children 6 to 12 years of age: 200 milligrams two times a day, in the morning and at bedtime.
  —Children up to 6 years of age: Dose must be determined by the doctor.

Missed dose—If you miss a dose of this medicine and remember within an hour or so of the missed dose, take it right away. However, if you do not remember until later, skip the missed dose and go back to your regular dosing schedule. Do not double doses.

Storage—To store this medicine:

- Keep out of the reach of children. Overdose of meprobamate is very dangerous in children.
- Store away from heat and direct light.
- Do not store in the bathroom, near the kitchen sink, or in other damp places. Heat or moisture may cause the medicine to break down.
- Do not keep outdated medicine or medicine no longer needed. Be sure that any discarded medicine is out of the reach of children.

Precautions While Using This Medicine

If you will be taking this medicine regularly for a long time:

- Your doctor should check your progress at regular visits.
- Check with your doctor at least every 4 months to make sure you need to continue taking this medicine.

If you will be taking this medicine in large doses or for a long time, do not stop taking it without first checking with your doctor. Your doctor may want you to reduce gradually the amount you are taking before stopping completely.

This medicine will add to the effects of alcohol and other CNS depressants (medicines that slow down the nervous system, possibly causing drowsiness). Some examples of CNS depressants are antihistamines or medicine for hay fever, other allergies, or colds; sedatives, tranquilizers, or sleeping medicine; prescription pain medicine or narcotics; barbiturates; medicine for seizures; muscle relaxants; or anesthetics, including some dental anesthetics. *Check with your doctor before taking any of the above while you are taking this medicine.*

Before you have any medical tests, tell the medical doctor in charge that you are taking this medicine. The results of some tests, such as the metyrapone test and the phentolamine test, may be affected by this medicine.

If you think you or someone else may have taken an overdose of this medicine, get emergency help at once. Taking an overdose of meprobamate or taking alcohol or other CNS depressants with meprobamate may lead to unconsciousness and possibly death. Some signs of an overdose are severe confusion, drowsiness, or weakness; shortness of breath or slow or troubled breathing; slurred speech; staggering; and slow heartbeat.

This medicine may cause some people to become dizzy, lightheaded, drowsy, or less alert than they are normally. Even if taken at bedtime, it may cause some people to feel drowsy or less alert on arising. *Make sure you know how you react to this medicine before you drive, use machines, or do anything else that could be dangerous if you are dizzy or are not alert.*

Meprobamate may cause dryness of the mouth. For temporary relief, use sugarless candy or gum, melt bits of ice in your mouth, or use a saliva substitute. However, if your mouth continues to feel dry for more than 2 weeks, check with your medical doctor or dentist. Continuing dryness of the mouth may increase the chance of dental disease, including tooth decay, gum disease, and fungus infections.

Side Effects of This Medicine

Along with its needed effects, a medicine may cause some unwanted effects. Although not all of these side effects may occur, if they do occur they may need medical attention.

Check with your doctor as soon as possible if any of the following side effects occur:

Less common

Skin rash, hives, or itching

Rare

Confusion; fast, pounding, or irregular heartbeat; sore throat and fever; unusual bleeding or bruising; unusual excitement; wheezing, shortness of breath, or troubled breathing

Symptoms of overdose

Confusion (severe); dizziness or lightheadedness (continuing); drowsiness (severe); shortness of breath or slow or troubled breathing; slow heartbeat; slurred speech; staggering; weakness (severe)

Other side effects may occur that usually do not need medical attention. These side effects may go away during treatment as your body adjusts to the medicine. However, check with your doctor if any of the following side effects continue or are bothersome:

More common

Clumsiness or unsteadiness; drowsiness

Less common

Blurred vision or change in near or distant vision; diarrhea; dizziness or lightheadedness; false sense of well-being; headache; nausea or vomiting; unusual tiredness or weakness

After you stop using this medicine, your body may need time to adjust. If you took this medicine in high doses or for a long time, this may take about 2 days. During this period of time check with your doctor if you notice any of the following side effects:

Clumsiness or unsteadiness; confusion; convulsions (seizures); hallucinations (seeing, hearing, or feeling things that are not there); increased dreaming; muscle twitching; nausea or vomiting; nervousness or restlessness; nightmares; trembling; trouble in sleeping

Other side effects not listed above may also occur in some patients. If you notice any other effects, check with your doctor.

Annual revision: 01/13/93

MEPROBAMATE AND ASPIRIN Systemic

Some commonly used brand names are:

In the U.S.

- Epromate-M
- Equagesic
- Heptogesic
- Meprogesic
- Meprogesic Q
- Micrainin

Generic name product may also be available.

In Canada

- Equagesic‡

‡In Canada, Equagesic also contains ethoheptazine citrate.

Description

Meprobamate (me-proe-BA-mate) and aspirin (AS-pir-in) combination is used to relieve pain, anxiety, and tension in certain disorders or diseases.

This medicine is available only with your doctor's prescription, in the following dosage form:

Oral

- Tablets (U.S. and Canada)

It is very important that you read and understand the following information. If any of it causes you special concern, check with your doctor. Also, *if you have any questions* or if you want more information about this medicine or your medical problem, *ask your doctor, nurse, or pharmacist.*

Before Using This Medicine

In deciding to use a medicine, the risks of taking the medicine must be weighed against the good it will do. This is a decision you and your doctor will make. For meprobamate and aspirin combination, the following should be considered:

Allergies—Tell your doctor if you have ever had any unusual or allergic reaction to meprobamate or to medicines like meprobamate such as carbromal, carisoprodol, mebutamate, or tybamate, or to aspirin or other salicylates, including methyl salicylate (oil of wintergreen), or to any of the following medicines:

- Diclofenac (e.g., Voltaren)
- Diflunisal (e.g., Dolobid)
- Etodolac (e.g., Lodine)
- Fenoprofen (e.g., Nalfon)
- Floctafenine (e.g., Idarac)
- Flurbiprofen, oral (e.g., Ansaid)
- Ibuprofen (e.g., Motrin)
- Indomethacin (e.g., Indocin)
- Ketoprofen (e.g., Orudis)
- Ketorolac (e.g., Toradol)
- Meclofenamate (e.g., Meclomen)
- Mefenamic acid (e.g., Ponstel)
- Naproxen (e.g., Naprosyn)
- Oxyphenbutazone (e.g., Tandearil)
- Phenylbutazone (e.g., Butazolidin)
- Piroxicam (e.g., Feldene)
- Sulindac (e.g., Clinoril)
- Suprofen (e.g., Suprol)
- Tiaprofenic acid (e.g., Surgam)
- Tolmetin (e.g., Tolectin)
- Zomepirac (e.g., Zomax)

Also tell your doctor and pharmacist if you are allergic to any other substances, such as foods, preservatives, or dyes.

Pregnancy—Meprobamate (contained in this combination medicine) has been reported to increase the chance of birth defects if taken during the first 3 months of pregnancy.

Studies in humans have not shown that aspirin (contained in this combination medicine) causes birth defects. However, studies in animals have shown that aspirin causes birth defects. Some reports have suggested that too much use of aspirin late in pregnancy may cause a decrease in the newborn's weight and possible death of the fetus or newborn infant. However, the mothers in these reports had been taking much larger amounts of aspirin than are usually recommended. Studies of mothers taking aspirin in the doses that are usually recommended did not show these unwanted effects. However, regular use of aspirin late in pregnancy may cause unwanted effects on the heart or blood flow in the fetus or in the newborn infant. Also, use of aspirin during the last 2 weeks of pregnancy may cause bleeding problems in the fetus before or during delivery or in the newborn infant. In addition, too much use of aspirin during the last 3 months of pregnancy may increase the length of pregnancy, prolong labor, cause other problems during delivery, or cause severe bleeding in the mother before, during, or after delivery.

Breast-feeding—Meprobamate (contained in this combination medicine) passes into the breast milk and may cause drowsiness in babies of mothers taking this medicine. Although aspirin (contained in this combination medicine) passes into the breast milk, it has not been shown to cause problems in nursing babies.

Children—*Do not give a medicine containing aspirin to a child with a fever or other symptoms of a virus infection, especially flu or chickenpox, without first discussing this with your child's doctor.* This is very important because aspirin may cause a serious illness called Reye's syndrome in children with fever caused by a virus infection, especially flu or chickenpox. Children who do not have a virus infection may also be more sensitive to the effects of aspirin (contained in this combination medicine), especially if they have a fever or have lost large amounts of body fluid because of vomiting, diarrhea, or sweating. This may increase the chance of side effects during treatment.

Teenagers—*Teenagers with fever or other symptoms of a virus infection, especially flu or chickenpox, should check with a doctor before taking this medicine.* The aspirin in this combination medicine may cause a serious illness called Reye's syndrome in teenagers with fever caused by a virus infection, especially flu or chickenpox.

Older adults—Elderly people may be especially sensitive to the effects of meprobamate and aspirin. This may increase the chance of side effects during treatment.

Other medicines—Although certain medicines should not be used together at all, in other cases two different medicines may be used together even if an interaction might occur. In these cases, your doctor may want to change the dose, or other precautions may be necessary. When you are taking meprobamate and aspirin combination, it is especially important that your doctor and pharmacist know if you are taking any of the following:

- Anticoagulants (blood thinners) or
- Carbenicillin by injection (e.g., Geopen) or
- Cefamandole (e.g., Mandol) or
- Cefoperazone (e.g., Cefobid) or
- Cefotetan (e.g., Cefotan) or
- Dipyridamole (e.g., Persantine) or
- Divalproex (e.g., Depakote) or
- Heparin or
- Inflammation or pain medicine, except narcotics, or
- Moxalactam (e.g., Moxam) or
- Pentoxifylline (e.g., Trental) or
- Plicamycin (e.g., Mithracin) or
- Ticarcillin (e.g., Ticar) or
- Valproic acid (e.g., Depakene)—Taking these medicines together with aspirin may increase the chance of bleeding
- Antidiabetics, oral (diabetes medicine you take by mouth)—Aspirin may increase the effects of the antidiabetic medicine; a change in dose may be needed if meprobamate and aspirin combination is taken regularly
- Central nervous system (CNS) depressants (medicine that causes drowsiness) or
- Tricyclic antidepressants (medicine for depression)—Taking these medicines with meprobamate and aspirin combination may increase the CNS depressant effects
- Methotrexate (e.g., Mexate)—The chance of serious side effects may be increased
- Probenecid (e.g., Benemid)—Aspirin may keep probenecid from working properly in the treatment of gout
- Sulfinpyrazone (e.g., Anturane)—Aspirin may keep sulfinpyrazone from working properly in the treatment of gout; also, there may be an increased chance of bleeding
- Urinary alkalizers (medicine that makes the urine less acid, such as acetazolamide [e.g., Diamox], calcium- and/or magnesium-containing antacids, dichlorphenamide [e.g., Daranide], methazolamide [e.g., Neptazane], potassium or sodium citrate and/or citric acid, sodium bicarbonate [baking soda])—These medicines may make aspirin less effective by causing it to be removed from the body more quickly
- Vancomycin (e.g., Vancocin)—Hearing loss may occur and may lead to deafness

Other medical problems—The presence of other medical problems may affect the use of meprobamate and aspirin combination. Make sure you tell your doctor if you have any other medical problems, especially:

- Alcohol abuse (or history of) or
- Drug abuse or dependence (or history of)—Dependence on meprobamate may develop
- Anemia or
- Stomach ulcer or other stomach problems—Aspirin may make your condition worse
- Asthma, allergies, and nasal polyps (history of) or
- Kidney disease or
- Liver disease—The chance of side effects may be increased.
- Epilepsy—The risk of seizures may be increased
- Gout—Aspirin may make this condition worse and may also lessen the effects of some medicines used to treat gout
- Hemophilia or other bleeding problems—The chance of bleeding may be increased by aspirin
- Porphyria—Meprobamate may make the condition worse

Before you begin using any new medicine (prescription or nonprescription) or if you develop any new medical problem while you are using this medicine, check with your doctor, nurse, or pharmacist.

Proper Use of This Medicine

Take this medicine with food or a full glass (8 ounces) of water to lessen stomach irritation.

If this combination medicine containing aspirin has a strong vinegar-like odor, do not use it. This odor means the medicine is breaking down. If you have any questions about this, check with your pharmacist.

Take this medicine only as directed by your doctor. Do not take more of it, do not take it more often, and do not take it for a longer time than your doctor ordered. If too much meprobamate is taken, it may become habit-forming. Also, taking too much aspirin may cause stomach problems or lead to medical problems because of an overdose.

Dosing—The dose of meprobamate and aspirin combination will be different for different patients. *Follow your doctor's orders or the directions on the label.* The following information includes only the average doses of meprobamate and aspirin combination. *If your dose is different, do not change it* unless your doctor tells you to do so:

- Adults—Oral, 1 or 2 tablets three or four times a day, as needed.
- Children up to 12 years of age: Use is not recommended.

Storage—To store this medicine:
- Keep this medicine out of the reach of children. Overdose of meprobamate is very dangerous in children.
- Store away from heat and direct light.
- Do not store in the bathroom, near the kitchen sink, or in other damp places. Heat or moisture may cause the medicine to break down.
- Do not keep outdated medicine or medicine no longer needed. Be sure that any discarded medicine is out of the reach of children.

Precautions While Using This Medicine

If you will be taking this medicine regularly for a long time:
- Your doctor should check your progress at regular visits.
- Check with your doctor at least every 4 months to make sure you need to continue taking this medicine.

If you will be taking this medicine in large doses or for a long time, do not stop taking it without first checking with your doctor. Your doctor may want you to reduce gradually the amount you are taking before stopping completely.

Check the labels of all nonprescription (over-the-counter [OTC]) and prescription medicines you now take. If any contain aspirin or other salicylates (including bismuth subsalicylate [e.g., Pepto-Bismol]), be especially careful. Taking or using any of these medicines while taking this combination medicine containing aspirin may lead to overdose. If you have any questions about this, check with your doctor or pharmacist.

This medicine will add to the effects of alcohol and other CNS depressants (medicines that slow down the nervous system, possibly causing drowsiness). Some examples of CNS depressants are antihistamines or medicine for hay fever, other allergies, or colds; sedatives, tranquilizers, or sleeping medicine; prescription pain medicine or narcotics; barbiturates; medicine for seizures; muscle relaxants; or anesthetics, including some dental anesthetics. *Check with your doctor before taking any of the above while you are taking this medicine.*

Stomach problems may be more likely to occur if you drink alcoholic beverages while being treated with this medicine, especially if you are taking the medicine in high doses or for a long time. Check with your doctor if you have any questions about this.

Too much use of this medicine together with certain other medicines may increase the chance of stomach problems. Therefore, do not regularly take this medicine together with any of the following medicines, unless directed to do so by your medical doctor or dentist:

Acetaminophen (e.g., Tylenol)
Diclofenac (e.g., Voltaren)
Diflunisal (e.g., Dolobid)
Etodolac (e.g., Lodine)
Fenoprofen (e.g., Nalfon)
Floctafenine (e.g., Idarac)
Flurbiprofen (oral) (e.g., Ansaid)
Ibuprofen (e.g., Motrin)
Indomethacin (e.g., Indocin)
Ketoprofen (e.g., Orudis)
Ketorolac (e.g., Toradol)
Meclofenamate (e.g., Meclomen)
Mefenamic acid (e.g., Ponstel)
Naproxen (e.g., Naprosyn)
Phenylbutazone (e.g., Butazolidin)
Piroxicam (e.g., Feldene)
Sulindac (e.g., Clinoril)
Tiaprofenic acid (e.g., Surgam)
Tolmetin (e.g., Tolectin)

If you are taking a laxative containing cellulose, do not take it within 2 hours of taking this medicine. Taking these medicines close together may make this medicine less effective by preventing the aspirin (contained in this combination medicine) from being absorbed by your body.

For diabetic patients:
- False urine sugar test results may occur if you take 8 or more 325-mg (5-grain) doses of aspirin (contained in this combination medicine) every day for several days in a row. Smaller doses or occasional use of aspirin usually will not affect urine sugar tests. If you have any questions about this, check with your doctor, especially if your diabetes is not well controlled.

Before you have any medical tests, tell the medical doctor in charge that you are taking this medicine. The results of some tests, such as the metyrapone test and the phentolamine test, may be affected by this medicine.

If you plan to have surgery, including dental surgery, do not take aspirin (contained in this combination medicine) for 5 days before the surgery, unless otherwise directed by your medical doctor or dentist. Taking aspirin during this time may cause bleeding problems.

If you think you or someone else may have taken an overdose of this medicine, get emergency help at once. Taking an overdose of this medicine or taking alcohol or other CNS depressants with it may lead to unconsciousness and possibly death. Some signs of an overdose are continuing ringing or buzzing in ears; any hearing loss; severe confusion, drowsiness, or weakness; shortness of breath or slow or troubled breathing; staggering; and slow heartbeat.

This medicine may cause some people to become dizzy, lightheaded, drowsy, or less alert than they are normally. *Make sure you know how you react to this medicine before you drive, use machines, or do anything else that could be dangerous if you are dizzy or are not alert.*

Meprobamate (contained in this combination medicine) may cause dryness of the mouth. For temporary relief, use sugarless candy or gum, melt bits of ice in your mouth, or use a saliva substitute. However, if your mouth continues to feel dry for more than 2 weeks, check with your medical doctor or dentist. Continuing dryness of the mouth may increase the chance of dental disease, including tooth decay, gum disease, and fungus infections.

Side Effects of This Medicine

Along with its needed effects, a medicine may cause some unwanted effects. Although not all of these side effects may occur, if they do occur they may need medical attention.

Check with your doctor immediately if any of the following side effects occur:

Rare

Wheezing, shortness of breath, troubled breathing, or tightness in chest

Symptoms of overdose

Any loss of hearing; bloody urine; confusion (severe); convulsions (seizures); diarrhea (severe or continuing); dizziness or lightheadedness (continuing); drowsiness (severe); fast or deep breathing; hallucinations (seeing, hearing, or feeling things that are not there); headache (severe or continuing); increased sweating; nausea or vomiting (continuing); nervousness or excitement (severe); ringing or buzzing in ears (continuing); slow heartbeat; slurred speech; staggering; stomach pain (severe or continuing); unexplained fever; unusual or uncontrolled flapping movements of the hands, especially in elderly patients; unusual thirst; vision problems; weakness (severe)

Symptoms of overdose in children

Changes in behavior; drowsiness or tiredness (severe); fast or deep breathing

Also, check with your doctor as soon as possible if any of the following side effects occur:

Rare

Bloody or black, tarry stools; confusion; skin rash, hives, or itching; sore throat and fever; unusual bleeding or bruising; unusual excitement; unusual tiredness or weakness; vomiting of blood or material that looks like coffee grounds

Other side effects may occur that usually do not need medical attention. These side effects may go away during treatment as your body adjusts to the medicine. However, check with your doctor if any of the following side effects continue or are bothersome:

More common

Drowsiness; heartburn or indigestion; nausea with or without vomiting; stomach pain (mild)

Less common

Blurred vision or change in near or distant vision; dizziness or lightheadedness; headache

After you stop using this medicine, your body may need time to adjust. The length of time this takes depends on the amount of medicine you were using and how long you used it. During this period of time check with your doctor if you notice any of the following side effects:

Clumsiness or unsteadiness; confusion; convulsions (seizures); hallucinations (seeing, hearing, or feeling things that are not there); increased dreaming; muscle twitching; nausea or vomiting; nervousness or restlessness; nightmares; trembling; trouble in sleeping

Other side effects not listed above may also occur in some patients. If you notice any other effects, check with your doctor.

Annual revision: 01/13/93

MERCAPTOPURINE Systemic

A commonly used brand name in the U.S. and Canada is Purinethol. Another commonly used name is 6-MP.

Description

Mercaptopurine (mer-kap-toe-PYOOR-een) belongs to the group of medicines known as antimetabolites. It is used to treat some kinds of cancer.

Mercaptopurine interferes with the growth of cancer cells, which are eventually destroyed. Since the growth of normal body cells may also be affected by mercaptopurine, other effects will also occur. Some of these may be serious and must be reported to your doctor. Other effects may not be serious but may cause concern. Some effects may not occur for months or years after the medicine is used.

Before you begin treatment with mercaptopurine, you and your doctor should talk about the good this medicine will do as well as the risks of using it.

Mercaptopurine may also be used for other conditions as determined by your doctor.

Mercaptopurine is available only with your doctor's prescription, in the following dosage form:

Oral

- Tablets (U.S. and Canada)

It is very important that you read and understand the following information. If any of it causes you special concern, check with your doctor. Also, *if you have any questions* or if you want more information about this medicine or your medical problem, *ask your doctor, nurse, or pharmacist.*

Before Using This Medicine

In deciding to use a medicine, the risks of taking the medicine must be weighed against the good it will do. This is a decision you and your doctor will make. For mercaptopurine, the following should be considered:

Allergies—Tell your doctor if you have ever had any unusual or allergic reaction to mercaptopurine.

Pregnancy—Tell your doctor if you are pregnant or if you intend to have children. There is a chance that this medicine may cause birth defects if either the male or female is taking it at the time of conception or if it is taken during pregnancy. However, studies have not been done in humans. Mercaptopurine has been shown to cause damage to the fetus in rats and increases the risk of miscarriage or premature births in humans. In addition, many cancer medicines may cause sterility which could be permanent. Although this has not been reported with this medicine, the possibility should be kept in mind.

Be sure that you have discussed this with your doctor before taking this medicine. It is best to use some kind of birth control while you are taking mercaptopurine. Tell your doctor right away if you think you have become pregnant while taking mercaptopurine.

Breast-feeding—Tell your doctor if you are breast-feeding or if you intend to breast-feed during treatment with this medicine. Because mercaptopurine may cause serious side effects, breast-feeding is generally not recommended while you are taking it.

Children—Although there is no specific information about the use of mercaptopurine in children, it is not expected to cause different side effects or problems in children than it does in adults.

Older adults—Many medicines have not been tested in older people. Therefore, it may not be known whether they work exactly the same way they do in younger adults or if they cause different side effects or problems in older people. There is no specific information about the use of mercaptopurine in the elderly.

Other medicines—Although certain medicines should not be used together at all, in other cases two different medicines may be used together even if an interaction might occur. In these cases, your doctor may want to change the dose, or other precautions may be necessary. When you are taking mercaptopurine, it is especially important that your doctor and pharmacist know if you are taking any of the following:

- Acetaminophen (e.g., Tylenol) (with long-term, high-dose use) or
- Amiodarone (e.g., Cordarone) or
- Anabolic steroids (dromostanolone [e.g., Drolban], ethylestrenol [e.g., Maxibolin], nandrolone [e.g., Anabolin], oxandrolone [e.g., Anavar], oxymetholone [e.g., Anadrol], stanozolol [e.g., Winstrol]) or
- Androgens (male hormones) or
- Anti-infectives by mouth or by injection (medicine for infection) or
- Carbamazepine (e.g., Tegretol) or
- Chloroquine (e.g., Aralen) or
- Dantrolene (e.g., Dantrium) or
- Disulfiram (e.g., Antabuse) or
- Divalproex (e.g., Depakote) or
- Estrogens (female hormones) or
- Etretinate (e.g., Tegison) or
- Gold salts or
- Hydroxychloroquine (e.g., Plaquenil) or
- Methyldopa (e.g., Aldomet) or
- Naltrexone (e.g., Trexan) (with long-term, high-dose use) or
- Oral contraceptives (birth control pills) containing estrogen or
- Phenothiazines (acetophenazine [e.g., Tindal], chlorpromazine [e.g., Thorazine], fluphenazine [e.g., Prolixin], mesoridazine [e.g., Serentil], perphenazine [e.g., Trilafon], prochlorperazine [e.g., Compazine], promazine [e.g., Sparine], promethazine [e.g., Phenergan], thioridazine [e.g., Mellaril], trifluoperazine [e.g., Stelazine], triflupromazine [e.g., Vesprin], trimeprazine [e.g., Temaril]) or
- Phenytoin (e.g., Dilantin) or
- Valproic acid (e.g., Depakene)—Risk of unwanted effects on the liver may be increased
- Adrenocorticoids (cortisone-like medicine) or
- Cyclosporine (e.g., Sandimmune) or
- Muromonab-CD3 (monoclonal antibody) (e.g., Orthoclone OKT3)—There may be an increased risk of infection and development of cancer because mercaptopurine reduces the body's immunity
- Allopurinol (e.g., Zyloprim)—Effects of mercaptopurine may be increased because allopurinol blocks its removal from the body
- Amphotericin B by injection (e.g., Fungizone) or
- Antithyroid agents (medicine for overactive thyroid) or
- Azathioprine (e.g., Imuran) or
- Chloramphenicol (e.g., Chloromycetin) or
- Colchicine or
- Flucytosine (e.g., Ancobon) or
- Interferon (e.g., Intron A, Roferon-A) or
- Plicamycin (e.g., Mithracin) or
- Zidovudine (e.g., Retrovir) or
- If you have ever been treated with x-rays or cancer medicines—Mercaptopurine may increase the effects of these medicines or radiation therapy on the blood
- Probenecid (e.g., Benemid) or

- Sulfinpyrazone (e.g., Anturane)—Mercaptopurine may raise the concentration of uric acid in the blood, which these medicines are used to lower

Other medical problems—The presence of other medical problems may affect the use of mercaptopurine. Make sure you tell your doctor if you have any other medical problems, especially:

- Chickenpox (including recent exposure) or
- Herpes zoster (shingles)—Risk of severe disease affecting other parts of the body
- Gout (history of) or
- Kidney stones (history of)—Mercaptopurine may increase levels of a chemical called uric acid in the body, which can cause gout or kidney stones
- Infection—Mercaptopurine can reduce immunity to infection
- Kidney disease or
- Liver disease—Effects may be increased because of slower removal of mercaptopurine from the body

Before you begin using any new medicine (prescription or nonprescription) or if you develop any new medical problem while you are using this medicine, check with your doctor, nurse, or pharmacist.

Proper Use of This Medicine

Use this medicine only as directed by your doctor. Do not use more or less of it, and do not use it more often than your doctor ordered. The exact amount of medicine you need has been carefully worked out. Taking too much may increase the chance of side effects, while taking too little may not improve your condition.

Mercaptopurine is often given together with certain other medicines. If you are using a combination of medicines, make sure that you take each one at the right time and do not mix them. Ask your doctor, nurse, or pharmacist to help you plan a way to remember to take your medicines at the right times.

While you are using mercaptopurine, your doctor may want you to drink extra fluids so that you will pass more urine. This will help prevent kidney problems and keep your kidneys working well.

If you vomit shortly after taking a dose of mercaptopurine, check with your doctor. You will be told whether to take the dose again or to wait until the next scheduled dose.

Missed dose—If you miss a dose of this medicine, do not take the missed dose at all and do not double the next one. Instead, go back to your regular dosing schedule and check with your doctor.

Storage—To store this medicine:

- Keep out of the reach of children.
- Store away from heat and direct light.
- Do not store in the bathroom, near the kitchen sink, or in other damp places. Heat or moisture may cause the medicine to break down.
- Do not keep outdated medicine or medicine no longer needed. Be sure that any discarded medicine is out of the reach of children.

Precautions While Using This Medicine

It is very important that your doctor check your progress at regular visits to make sure that this medicine is working properly and to check for unwanted effects.

Avoid alcoholic beverages until you have discussed their use with your doctor. Alcohol may increase the harmful effects of this medicine.

While you are being treated with mercaptopurine, and after you stop treatment with it, *do not have any immunizations (vaccinations) without your doctor's approval.* Mercaptopurine may lower your body's resistance and there is a chance you might get the infection the immunization is meant to prevent. In addition, other persons living in your household should not take or should not have recently taken oral polio vaccine since there is a chance they could pass the polio virus on to you. Also, avoid other persons who have taken oral polio vaccine. Do not get close to them and do not stay in the same room with them for very long. If you cannot take these precautions, you should consider wearing a protective face mask that covers the nose and mouth.

Mercaptopurine can lower the number of white blood cells in your blood temporarily, increasing the chance of getting an infection. It can also lower the number of platelets, which are necessary for proper blood clotting. If this occurs, there are certain precautions you can take, especially when your blood count is low, to reduce the risk of infection or bleeding:

- If you can, avoid people with infections. *Check with your doctor immediately* if you think you are getting an infection or if you get a fever or chills, cough or hoarseness, lower back or side pain, or painful or difficult urination.
- *Check with your doctor immediately* if you notice any unusual bleeding or bruising; black, tarry stools; blood in urine or stools; or pinpoint red spots on your skin.
- Be careful when using a regular toothbrush, dental floss, or toothpick. Your medical doctor, dentist, or nurse may recommend other ways to clean your teeth and gums. Check with your medical doctor before having any dental work done.
- Do not touch your eyes or the inside of your nose unless you have just washed your hands and have not touched anything else in the meantime.

- Be careful not to cut yourself when you are using sharp objects such as a safety razor or fingernail or toenail cutters.
- Avoid contact sports or other situations where bruising or injury could occur.

Tell the doctor in charge that you are taking this medicine before you have any medical tests. The results of tests for the amount of sugar or uric acid in the blood measured by a machine called a sequential multiple analyzer (SMA) may be affected by this medicine.

Side Effects of This Medicine

Along with their needed effects, medicines like mercaptopurine can sometimes cause unwanted effects such as blood problems, liver problems, and other side effects. These and others are described below. Also, because of the way these medicines act on the body, there is a chance that they might cause other unwanted effects that may not occur until months or years after the medicine is used. These delayed effects may include certain types of cancer, such as leukemia. Discuss these possible effects with your doctor.

Although not all of these side effects may occur, if they do occur they may need medical attention.

Check with your doctor immediately if any of the following side effects occur:

Less common

Black, tarry stools; blood in urine or stools; cough or hoarseness; fever or chills; lower back or side pain; painful or difficult urination; pinpoint red spots on skin; unusual bleeding or bruising

Check with your doctor as soon as possible if any of the following side effects occur:

More common

Unusual tiredness or weakness; yellow eyes or skin

Less common

Joint pain; loss of appetite; nausea and vomiting; swelling of feet or lower legs

Rare

Sores in mouth and on lips

Other side effects may occur that usually do not need medical attention. These side effects may go away during treatment as your body adjusts to the medicine. Also, your doctor or nurse may be able to tell you about ways to prevent or reduce some of these side effects. Check with your doctor or nurse if any of the following side effects continue or are bothersome or if you have any questions about them:

Less common

Darkening of skin; diarrhea; headache; skin rash and itching; weakness

After you stop taking mercaptopurine, it may still produce some side effects that need attention. During this period of time, check with your doctor if you notice any of the following side effects:

Black, tarry stools; blood in urine or stools; cough or hoarseness; fever or chills; lower back or side pain; painful or difficult urination; pinpoint red spots on skin; unusual bleeding or bruising; yellow eyes or skin

Other side effects not listed above may also occur in some patients. If you notice any other effects, check with your doctor.

Annual revision: August 1990
Interim revision: 07/29/93

MESALAMINE Rectal

Some commonly used brand names are:

In the U.S.
Rowasa

In Canada
Salofalk

Other commonly used names are 5-aminosalicylic acid, 5-ASA, and mesalazine.

Description

Mesalamine (me-SAL-a-meen) is used to treat inflammatory bowel disease, such as ulcerative colitis. This medicine works inside the bowel by helping to reduce the inflammation and other symptoms.

Mesalamine is available only with your doctor's prescription. It is available in the following dosage forms:

Rectal
- Enema (U.S. and Canada)
- Suppositories (U.S. and Canada)

It is very important that you read and understand the following information. If any of it causes you special concern, check with your doctor. Also, *if you have any questions* or if you want more information about this medicine or your medical problem, *ask your doctor, nurse, or pharmacist.*

Before Using This Medicine

In deciding to use a medicine, the risks of using the medicine must be weighed against the good it will do. This is a decision you and your doctor will make. For mesalamine, the following should be considered:

Allergies—Tell your doctor if you have ever had any unusual or allergic reaction to mesalamine, olsalazine, sulfasalazine, or salicylates (e.g., aspirin). Also tell your doctor and pharmacist if you are allergic to any other substances, such as foods, preservatives, or dyes.

Pregnancy—Studies have not been done in humans. However, mesalamine has not been shown to cause birth defects or other problems in animal studies.

Breast-feeding—It is not known whether mesalamine passes into the breast milk.

Children—Studies on this medicine have been done only in adult patients, and there is no specific information comparing use of mesalamine in children with use in other age groups.

Older adults—Many medicines have not been studied specifically in older people. Therefore, it may not be known whether they work exactly the same way they do in younger adults or if they cause different side effects or problems in older people. There is no specific information comparing use of mesalamine in the elderly with use in other age groups.

Other medicines—Although certain medicines should not be used together at all, in other cases two different medicines may be used together even if an interaction might occur. In these cases, your doctor may want to change the dose, or other precautions may be necessary. Tell your doctor and pharmacist if you are taking any other medicines.

Other medical problems—The presence of other medical problems may affect the use of mesalamine. Make sure you tell your doctor if you have any other medical problems, especially:

- Kidney disease—The use of mesalamine may cause further damage to the kidneys

Before you begin using any new medicine (prescription or nonprescription) or if you develop any new medical problem while you are using this medicine, check with your doctor, nurse, or pharmacist.

Proper Use of This Medicine

This medicine usually comes with patient directions. Read them carefully before using this medicine.

For best results, empty your bowel just before using this rectal enema.

Keep using this medicine for the full time of treatment even if you begin to feel better after a few days. *Do not miss any doses.*

Missed dose—If you do miss a dose of this medicine, use it as soon as possible if you remember it that same night. However, if you do not remember it until the next morning, skip the missed dose and go back to your regular dosing schedule.

Storage—To store this medicine:

- Keep out of the reach of children.
- Store away from heat and direct light.
- Keep the enema from freezing.
- Keep the suppositories at room temperature.
- Do not keep outdated medicine or medicine no longer needed. Be sure that any discarded medicine is out of the reach of children.

Precautions While Using This Medicine

It is important that your doctor check your progress at regular visits.

Check with your doctor if you notice rectal bleeding, blistering, pain, burning, itching, or other sign of irritation not present before you started using this medicine.

Side Effects of This Medicine

Along with its needed effects, a medicine may cause some unwanted effects. Although not all of these side effects may occur, if they do occur they may need medical attention.

Stop using this medicine and check with your doctor immediately if any of the following side effects occur:

Rare

Abdominal or stomach cramps or pain (severe); bloody diarrhea; fever; headache (severe); skin rash

Also, check with your doctor as soon as possible if the following side effect occurs:

Rare

Rectal irritation

Other side effects may occur that usually do not need medical attention. These side effects may go away during treatment as your body adjusts to the medicine. However, check with your doctor if the following side effects continue or are bothersome:

More common

Abdominal or stomach cramps or pain (mild); gas or flatulence; headache (mild); nausea

Less common or rare

Loss of hair

Other side effects not listed above may also occur in some patients. If you notice any other effects, check with your doctor.

Annual revision: 06/28/91

MESNA Systemic

Some commonly used brand names are:

In the U.S.
MESNEX

In Canada
Uromitexan

Description

Mesna is used to reduce the harmful effects of some cancer medicines on the bladder.

Mesna is to be given only by or under the immediate supervision of your doctor. It is available in the following dosage form:

Parenteral

- Injection (U.S. and Canada)

It is very important that you read and understand the following information. If any of it causes you special concern, check with your doctor. Also, *if you have any questions* or if you want more information about this medicine or your medical problem, *ask your doctor, nurse, or pharmacist.*

Before Using This Medicine

In deciding to use a medicine, the risks of taking the medicine must be weighed against the good it will do. This is a decision you and your doctor will make. For mesna, the following should be considered:

Allergies—Tell your doctor if you have ever had any unusual or allergic reaction to mesna.

Pregnancy—Mesna has not been shown to cause birth defects or other problems in humans.

Breast-feeding—It is not known whether mesna passes into the breast milk. However, this medicine has not been reported to cause problems in nursing babies.

Children—Although there is no specific information comparing use of mesna in children with use in other age groups, this medicine is not expected to cause different side effects or problems in children than it does in adults.

Older adults—Many medicines have not been studies specifically in older people. Therefore, it may not be known whether they work exactly the same way they do in younger adults or if they cause different side effects or problems in older people. There is no specific information comparing use of mesna in the elderly with use in other age groups.

Before you begin using any new medicine (prescription or nonprescription) or if you develop any new medical problem while you are using this medicine, check with your doctor, nurse, or pharmacist.

Side Effects of This Medicine

Along with its needed effects, a medicine may cause some unwanted effects. Although not all of these side effects may occur, if they do occur they may need medical attention.

Check with your doctor as soon as possible if either of the following side effects occur:

Rare

Skin rash or itching

Other side effects may occur that usually do not need medical attention. These side effects may go away during treatment as your body adjusts to the medicine. However, check with your doctor if any of the following side effects continue or are bothersome:

Less common

Diarrhea; nausea or vomiting; unpleasant taste

Other side effects not listed above may also occur in some patients. If you notice any other effects, check with your doctor.

Annual revision: 08/09/92

METHACHOLINE Inhalation†

A commonly used brand name in the U.S. is Provocholine.

†Not commercially available in Canada.

Description

Methacholine (METH-a-koe-leen) is used to help find out whether a patient has asthma.

Before the test with methacholine inhalation is given, another test will be done to find out how well your lungs are working.

How test is done: Although there are 5 different strengths of methacholine solution that may be used in this test, not all of them may be necessary. It depends on how you react to each increasing strength of solution during the test. The weakest strength solution is used first. It is placed in a nebulizer and 5 inhalations are taken by mouth. After 3 to 5 minutes, a test will be done to determine what effect the medicine had on your lungs. Each time the test dose is repeated, a stronger solution will be used. During this test, wheezing and difficulty in breathing may occur. If these effects do occur, your doctor may give you a bronchodilator (medicine that opens up the bronchial tubes [air passages] of the lungs) by inhalation to relieve the discomfort.

Methacholine is to be used only by or under the immediate supervision of a doctor. It is available in the following dosage form:

Inhalation

- Inhalation solution (U.S.)

It is very important that you read and understand the following information. If any of it causes you special concern, check with your doctor. Also, *if you have any questions* or if you want more information about this test or your medical problem, *ask your doctor, nurse, or pharmacist.*

Before Having This Test

In deciding to use a diagnostic test, any risks of the test must be weighed against the good it will do. This is a decision you and your doctor will make. Also, test results may be affected by other things. For methacholine, the following should be considered:

Allergies—Tell your doctor if you have ever had any unusual or allergic reaction to methacholine or to similar medicines, such as ambenonium, bethanechol, neostigmine, and pyridostigmine. Also tell your doctor and pharmacist if you are allergic to any other substances, such as foods, preservatives, or dyes.

Pregnancy—Studies on birth defects have not been done in either humans or animals. However, if the test is necessary, women who are able to bear children should be given the test within 10 days after the beginning of the last menstrual period or within 2 weeks after a pregnancy test has shown they are not pregnant.

Breast-feeding—It is not known whether methacholine passes into the breast milk.

Children—Although there is no specific information about the use of methacholine in children, it is not expected to cause different side effects or problems in children than it does in adults.

Older adults—Many medicines have not been tested in older people. Therefore, it may not be known whether they work exactly the same way they do in younger adults or if they cause different side effects or problems in older people. There is no specific information about the use of methacholine in the elderly.

Other medicines—Although certain medicines should not be used together at all, in other cases two different medicines may be used together even if an interaction might occur. In these cases, your doctor may want to change the dose, or other precautions may be necessary. When you are using methacholine, it is especially important that your doctor and pharmacist know if you are taking or using any of the following:

- Adrenocorticoids (cortisone-like medicine) or
- Anticholinergics (medicine for abdominal or stomach spasms or cramps) or
- Cromolyn (e.g., Intal) or
- Medicine for breathing problems, colds, sinus problems, or hay fever or other allergies (including nose drops or sprays) or
- Smoking tobacco—These medicines or smoking tobacco may affect the results of this test
- Beta-blockers (acebutolol [e.g., Sectral], atenolol [e.g., Tenormin], betaxolol [e.g., Kerlone], carteolol [e.g., Cartrol], labetalol [e.g., Normodyne], metoprolol [e.g., Lopressor], nadolol [e.g., Corgard], oxprenolol [e.g., Trasicor], penbutolol [e.g., Levatol], pindolol [e.g., Visken], propranolol [e.g., Inderal], sotalol [e.g., Sotacor], timolol [e.g., Blocadren])—These medicines may increase the reaction to the methacholine test

Other medical problems—The presence of other medical problems may affect the use of methacholine . Make sure you tell your doctor if you have any other medical problems, especially:

- Asthma (or if any member of your family has asthma), hay fever, allergic rhinitis, wheezing, chronic lung disease, or respiratory virus illness—Methacholine may cause severe difficulty in breathing
- Epilepsy or
- Heart or blood vessel disease or
- Stomach ulcer or

- Thyroid disease or
- Urinary tract blockage—Use of methacholine may make the condition worse

Preparation for This Test

Unless otherwise directed by your doctor:

- *For 24 hours before the test, do not take any extended-release capsule or tablet form of aminophylline, oxtriphylline, or theophylline. For 12 hours before the test, do not use any other medicine,* especially anticholinergics (medicine for abdominal or stomach spasms or cramps) or medicine for breathing problems, sinus problems, or hay fever or other allergies (including nose drops or sprays). To do so may affect the results of this test.

Side Effects of This Medicine

Along with its needed effects, a medicine may cause some unwanted effects. Although not all of these side effects may occur, if they do occur they may need medical attention.

Check with your doctor or nurse immediately if any of the following side effects occur:

Wheezing, tightness in chest, or difficulty in breathing (continuing or severe)

Other side effects may occur that usually do not need medical attention. These side effects should go away as the effects of the medicine wear off. However, check with your doctor if any of the following side effects continue or are bothersome:

Less common or rare

Headache or lightheadedness; irritation of throat; itching

Other side effects not listed above may also occur in some patients. If you notice any other effects, check with your doctor.

Annual revision: August 1990

METHENAMINE Systemic

Some commonly used brand names are:

In the U.S.

Hiprex
Urex
Mandelamine

Generic name product may also be available.

In Canada

Hip-Rex
Mandelamine

Description

Methenamine (meth-EN-a-meen) belongs to the family of medicines called anti-infectives. It is used to help prevent and treat infections of the urinary tract. Methenamine is available only with your doctor's prescription, in the following dosage forms:

Oral

- Enteric-coated tablets (U.S.)
- Granules for oral solution (U.S.)
- Oral suspension (U.S.)
- Tablets (U.S. and Canada)

It is very important that you read and understand the following information. If any of it causes you special concern, check with your doctor. Also, *if you have any questions* or if you want more information about this medicine or your medical problem, *ask your doctor, nurse, or pharmacist.*

Before Using This Medicine

In deciding to use a medicine, the risks of taking the medicine must be weighed against the good it will do. This is a decision you and your doctor will make. For methenamine, the following should be considered:

Allergies—Tell your doctor if you have ever had any unusual or allergic reaction to methenamine. Also tell your doctor and pharmacist if you are allergic to any other substances, such as foods, preservatives, or dyes.

Pregnancy—Methenamine has not been studied in either humans or animals. However, individual case reports on the use of methenamine during pregnancy have not shown that this medicine causes birth defects or other problems in humans.

Breast-feeding—Methenamine passes into the breast milk. However, methenamine has not been reported to cause problems in nursing babies.

Children—Although there is no special information comparing use of methenamine in children with use in other age groups, this medicine is not expected to cause different side effects or problems in children than it does in adults.

Older adults—Many medicines have not been studied specifically in older people. Therefore, it may not be known whether they work exactly the same way they do in younger adults or if they cause different side effects or problems in older people. There is no specific information

comparing use of methenamine in the elderly with use in other age groups.

Other medicines—Although certain medicines should not be used together at all, in other cases two different medicines may be used together even if an interaction might occur. In these cases, your doctor may want to change the dose, or other precautions may be necessary. When you are taking methenamine, it is especially important that your doctor and pharmacist know if you are taking any of the following:

- Thiazide diuretics (water pills) or
- Urinary alkalizers (medicine that makes the urine less acid, such as acetazolamide [e.g., Diamox], calcium- and/or magnesium-containing antacids, dichlorphenamide [e.g., Daranide], methazolamide [e.g., Neptazane], potassium or sodium citrate and/or citric acid, sodium bicarbonate [baking soda])—Use of methenamine with any of these medicines may decrease the effectiveness of methenamine

Other medical problems—The presence of other medical problems may affect the use of methenamine. Make sure you tell your doctor if you have any other medical problems, especially:

- Dehydration (severe) or
- Kidney disease (severe)—Patients with severe kidney disease who take methenamine may have an increase in side effects that affect the kidneys
- Liver disease (severe)—Patients with severe liver disease who take methenamine may have an increase in symptoms of their liver disease

Before you begin using any new medicine (prescription or nonprescription) or if you develop any new medical problem while you are using this medicine, check with your doctor, nurse, or pharmacist.

Proper Use of This Medicine

Before you start taking this medicine, check your urine with phenaphthazine paper or another test to see if it is acid. *Your urine must be acidic (pH 5.5 or below) for this medicine to work properly.* If you have any questions about this, check with your doctor, nurse, or pharmacist.

The following changes in your diet may help make your urine more acid; however, check with your doctor first if you are on a special diet (for example, for diabetes). Avoid most fruits (especially citrus fruits and juices), milk and other dairy products, and other foods that make the urine less acid. Also, avoid antacids unless otherwise directed by your doctor. Eating more protein and foods such as cranberries (especially cranberry juice with vitamin C added), plums, or prunes may also help. If your urine is still not acid enough, check with your doctor.

If this medicine causes nausea or upset stomach, it may be taken after meals and at bedtime.

For patients taking the *dry granule form of this medicine:*

- Dissolve the contents of each packet in 2 to 4 ounces of cold water immediately before taking. Stir well. Be sure to drink all the liquid to get the full dose of medicine.

For patients taking the *oral liquid form of this medicine:*

- Use a specially marked measuring spoon or other device to measure each dose accurately. The average household teaspoon may not hold the right amount of liquid.

For patients taking the *enteric-coated tablet form of this medicine:*

- Swallow tablets whole. Do not break, crush, or take if chipped.

To help clear up your infection completely, *keep taking this medicine for the full time of treatment,* even if you begin to feel better after a few days. *Do not miss any doses.*

Missed dose—If you do miss a dose of this medicine, take it as soon as possible. However, if it is almost time for your next dose, skip the missed dose and go back to your regular dosing schedule. Do not double doses.

Storage—To store this medicine:

- Keep out of the reach of children.
- Store away from heat and direct light.
- Do not store the dry granule or tablet form of this medicine in the bathroom, near the kitchen sink, or in other damp places. Heat or moisture may cause the medicine to break down.
- Keep the oral liquid form of this medicine from freezing.
- Do not keep outdated medicine or medicine no longer needed. Be sure that any discarded medicine is out of the reach of children.

Precautions While Using This Medicine

If your symptoms do not improve within a few days, or if they become worse, check with your doctor.

Side Effects of This Medicine

Along with its needed effects, a medicine may cause some unwanted effects. Although not all of these side effects may occur, if they do occur they may need medical attention.

Check with your doctor immediately if any of the following side effects occur:

Less common

Skin rash

Rare
Blood in urine; lower back pain; pain or burning while urinating

Other side effects may occur that usually do not need medical attention. These side effects may go away during treatment as your body adjusts to the medicine. However, check with your doctor if any of the following side effects continue or are bothersome:

Less common
Nausea and vomiting

Other side effects not listed above may also occur in some patients. If you notice any other effects, check with your doctor.

Annual revision: 10/20/92

METHOTREXATE—For Cancer Systemic

Some commonly used brand names in the U.S. are:

Folex	Mexate
Folex PFS	Mexate-AQ

Generic name product may also be available in the U.S. and Canada.
Another commonly used name is amethopterin.

Description

Methotrexate (meth-o-TREX-ate) belongs to the group of medicines known as antimetabolites. It is used to treat some kinds of cancer.

Methotrexate blocks an enzyme needed by the cell to live. This interferes with the growth of cancer cells, which are eventually destroyed. Since the growth of normal body cells may also be affected by methotrexate, other effects will also occur. Some of these may be serious and must be reported to your doctor. Other effects, like hair loss, may not be serious but may cause concern. Some effects may not occur for months or years after the medicine is used.

Before you begin treatment with methotrexate, you and your doctor should talk about the good this medicine will do as well as the risks of using it.

Methotrexate is available only with your doctor's prescription, in the following dosage forms:

Oral
- Tablets (U.S. and Canada)

Parenteral
- Injection (U.S. and Canada)

It is very important that you read and understand the following information. If any of it causes you special concern, check with your doctor. Also, *if you have any questions* or if you want more information about this medicine or your medical problem, *ask your doctor, nurse, or pharmacist.*

Before Using This Medicine

In deciding to use a medicine, the risks of taking the medicine must be weighed against the good it will do. This is a decision you and your doctor will make. For methotrexate, the following should be considered:

Allergies—Tell your doctor if you have ever had any unusual or allergic reaction to methotrexate.

Pregnancy—Tell your doctor if you are pregnant or if you intend to have children. There is a good chance that this medicine may cause birth defects if either the male or female is taking it at the time of conception or if it is taken during pregnancy. Methotrexate may cause harm or even death of the fetus. In addition, many cancer medicines may cause sterility which could be permanent. Although sterility is probably rare with this medicine, the possibility should be kept in mind.

Be sure that you have discussed this with your doctor before taking this medicine. It is best to use some kind of birth control while you are taking methotrexate. However, do not use oral contraceptives ("the Pill") since they may interfere with this medicine. Tell your doctor right away if you think you have become pregnant while taking methotrexate.

Breast-feeding—Tell your doctor if you are breast-feeding or if you intend to breast-feed during treatment with this medicine. Because methotrexate may cause serious side effects, breast-feeding is generally not recommended while you are taking it.

Children—Newborns and other infants may be more sensitive to the effects of methotrexate. However, in other children it is not expected to cause different side effects or problems than it does in adults.

Older adults—Side effects may be more likely to occur in the elderly, who are usually more sensitive to the effects of methotrexate.

Other medicines—Although certain medicines should not be used together at all, in other cases two different medicines may be used together even if an interaction might occur. In these cases, your doctor may want to change the dose, or other precautions may be necessary. When you are taking methotrexate, it is especially important that your doctor and pharmacist know if you are taking any other prescription or nonprescription (over-the-counter [OTC]) medicine. They should also be told if you have ever been treated with x-rays or cancer medicines or if you drink alcohol.

Other medical problems—The presence of other medical problems may affect the use of methotrexate. Make sure you tell your doctor if you have any other medical problems, especially:

- Alcohol abuse (or history of)—Increased risk of unwanted effects on the liver
- Chickenpox (including recent exposure) or
- Herpes zoster (shingles)—Risk of severe disease affecting other parts of the body
- Colitis
- Disease of the immune system
- Gout (history of) or
- Kidney stones (or history of)—Methotrexate may increase levels of a chemical called uric acid in the body, which can cause gout or kidney stones
- Infection—Methotrexate can reduce immunity to infection
- Intestine blockage or
- Kidney disease or
- Liver disease—Effects may be increased because of slower removal of methotrexate from the body
- Mouth sores or inflammation or
- Stomach ulcer—May be worsened

Before you begin using any new medicine (prescription or nonprescription) or if you develop any new medical problem while you are using this medicine, check with your doctor, nurse, or pharmacist.

Proper Use of This Medicine

Take this medicine only as directed by your doctor. Do not take more or less of it, and do not take it more often than your doctor ordered. The exact amount of medicine you need has been carefully worked out. Taking too much may increase the chance of side effects, while taking too little may not improve your condition.

Methotrexate is often given together with certain other medicines. If you are using a combination of medicines, make sure that you take each one at the proper time and do not mix them. Ask your doctor, nurse, or pharmacist to help you plan a way to remember to take your medicines at the right times.

While you are using methotrexate, your doctor may want you to drink extra fluids so that you will pass more urine. This will help the drug to pass from the body, and will prevent kidney problems and keep your kidneys working well.

Methotrexate commonly causes nausea and vomiting. Even if you begin to feel ill, *do not stop using this medicine without first checking with your doctor.* Ask your doctor, nurse, or pharmacist for ways to lessen these effects.

If you vomit shortly after taking a dose of methotrexate, check with your doctor. You will be told whether to take the dose again or to wait until the next scheduled dose.

Missed dose—If you miss a dose of this medicine, do not take the missed dose at all and do not double the next one. Instead, go back to your regular dosing schedule and check with your doctor.

Storage—To store this medicine:

- Keep out of the reach of children.
- Store away from heat and direct light.
- Do not store in the bathroom, near the kitchen sink, or in other damp places. Heat or moisture may cause the medicine to break down.
- Do not keep outdated medicine or medicine no longer needed. Be sure that any discarded medicine is out of the reach of children.

Precautions While Using This Medicine

It is very important that your doctor check your progress at regular visits to make sure that this medicine is working properly and to check for unwanted effects.

Do not drink alcohol while using this medicine. Alcohol can increase the chance of liver problems.

Some patients who take methotrexate may become more sensitive to sunlight than they are normally. When you first begin taking methotrexate, avoid too much sun and do not use a sunlamp until you see how you react to the sun, especially if you tend to burn easily. In case of a severe burn, check with your doctor.

Do not take medicine for inflammation or pain (aspirin or other salicylates, diclofenac, diflunisal, fenoprofen, ibuprofen, indomethacin, ketoprofen, meclofenamate, mefenamic acid, naproxen, phenylbutazone, piroxicam, sulindac, suprofen, tolmetin) without first checking with your doctor. These medicines may increase the effects of methotrexate, which could be harmful.

While you are being treated with methotrexate, and after you stop treatment with it, *do not have any immunizations (vaccinations) without your doctor's approval.* Methotrexate may lower your body's resistance and there is a chance you might get the infection the immunization is meant to prevent. In addition, other persons living in your household should not take or should not have recently taken oral polio vaccine since there is a chance they could pass the polio virus on to you. Also, avoid other persons who have taken oral polio vaccine. Do not get close to them, and do not stay in the same room with them for very long. If you cannot take these precautions, you should consider wearing a protective face mask that covers the nose and mouth.

Methotrexate can lower the number of white blood cells in your blood temporarily, increasing the chance of getting an infection. It can also lower the number of platelets, which are necessary for proper blood clotting. If this occurs, there are certain precautions you can take, especially when your blood count is low, to reduce the risk of infection or bleeding:

- If you can, avoid people with infections. *Check with your doctor immediately* if you think you are getting an infection or if you get a fever or chills, cough or hoarseness, lower back or side pain, or painful or difficult urination.
- *Check with your doctor immediately* if you notice any unusual bleeding or bruising; black, tarry stools; blood in urine or stools; or pinpoint red spots on your skin.
- Be careful when using a regular toothbrush, dental floss, or toothpick. Your medical doctor, dentist, or nurse may recommend other ways to clean your teeth and gums. Check with your medical doctor before having any dental work done.
- Do not touch your eyes or the inside of your nose unless you have just washed your hands and have not touched anything else in the meantime.
- Be careful not to cut yourself when you are using sharp objects such as a safety razor or fingernail or toenail cutters.
- Avoid contact sports or other situations where bruising or injury could occur.

Side Effects of This Medicine

Along with their needed effects, medicines like methotrexate can sometimes cause unwanted effects such as blood problems, kidney problems, stomach or liver problems, loss of hair, and other side effects. These and others are described below. Also, because of the way these medicines act on the body, there is a chance that they might cause other unwanted effects that may not occur until months or years after the medicine is used. These delayed effects may include certain types of cancer, such as leukemia. Discuss these possible effects with your doctor.

Although not all of these side effects may occur, if they do occur they may need medical attention.

Check with your doctor immediately if any of the following side effects occur:

More common

Black, tarry stools; bloody vomit; diarrhea; reddening of skin; sores in mouth and on lips; stomach pain

Less common

Blood in urine or stools; blurred vision; confusion; convulsions (seizures); cough or hoarseness; fever or chills; lower back or side pain; painful or difficult urination; pinpoint red spots on skin; shortness of breath; swelling of feet or lower legs; unusual bleeding or bruising

Check with your doctor as soon as possible if any of the following side effects occur:

Less common

Back pain; dark urine; dizziness; drowsiness; headache; joint pain; unusual tiredness or weakness; yellow eyes or skin

Other side effects may occur that usually do not need medical attention. These side effects may go away during treatment as your body adjusts to the medicine. Also, your doctor or nurse may be able to tell you about ways to prevent or reduce some of these side effects. Check with your doctor or nurse if any of the following side effects continue or are bothersome or if you have any questions about them:

More common

Loss of appetite; nausea or vomiting

Less common

Acne; boils; pale skin; skin rash or itching

This medicine may cause a temporary loss of hair in some people. After treatment with methotrexate has ended, normal hair growth should return.

After you stop using methotrexate, it may still produce some side effects that need attention. During this period of time, check with your doctor as soon as possible if you notice any of the following side effects:

Back pain; blurred vision; confusion; convulsions (seizures); dizziness; drowsiness; fever; headache; unusual tiredness or weakness

Other side effects not listed above may also occur in some patients. If you notice any other effects, check with your doctor.

Annual revision: August 1990

METHOTREXATE—For Noncancerous Conditions Systemic

Some commonly used brand names in the U.S. are:

In the U.S.

- Folex
- Folex PFS
- Mexate
- Mexate-AQ
- Rheumatrex

In Canada

- Rheumatrex

Generic name product may also be available in the U.S. and Canada.

Another commonly used name is amethopterin.

Description

Methotrexate (meth-o-TREX-ate) belongs to the group of medicines known as antimetabolites. It is used to treat psoriasis and rheumatoid arthritis. It may also be used for other conditions as determined by your doctor.

Methotrexate blocks an enzyme needed by the cell to live. This interferes with the growth of certain cells, such as skin cells in psoriasis that are growing rapidly. Since the growth of normal body cells may also be affected by methotrexate, other effects will also occur. Some of these may be serious and must be reported to your doctor. Other effects, like hair loss, may not be serious but may cause concern. Some effects may not occur for months or years after the medicine is used.

Before you begin treatment with methotrexate, you and your doctor should talk about the good this medicine will do as well as the risks of using it.

Methotrexate is available only with your doctor's prescription, in the following dosage forms:

Oral

- Tablets (U.S. and Canada)

Parenteral

- Injection (U.S. and Canada)

It is very important that you read and understand the following information. If any of it causes you special concern, check with your doctor. Also, *if you have any questions* or if you want more information about this medicine or your medical problem, *ask your doctor, nurse, or pharmacist.*

Before Using This Medicine

In deciding to use a medicine, the risks of taking the medicine must be weighed against the good it will do. This is a decision you and your doctor will make. For methotrexate, the following should be considered:

Allergies—Tell your doctor if you have ever had any unusual or allergic reaction to methotrexate.

Pregnancy—There is a good chance that this medicine may cause birth defects if either the male or female is taking it at the time of conception or if it is taken during pregnancy. Methotrexate may cause harm or even death of the fetus. In addition, this medicine may rarely cause temporary sterility.

Methotrexate is not recommended during pregnancy. Be sure that you have discussed this with your doctor before taking this medicine. It is best to use some kind of birth control while you are taking methotrexate. Tell your doctor right away if you think you have become pregnant while taking methotrexate.

Breast-feeding—Tell your doctor if you are breast-feeding or if you intend to breast-feed during treatment with this medicine. Because methotrexate may cause serious side effects, breast-feeding is generally not recommended while you are taking it.

Children—Newborns and other infants may be more sensitive to the effects of methotrexate. However, in other children it is not expected to cause different side effects or problems than it does in adults.

Older adults—Side effects may be more likely to occur in the elderly, who are usually more sensitive to the effects of methotrexate.

Other medicines—Although certain medicines should not be used together at all, in other cases two different medicines may be used together even if an interaction might occur. In these cases, your doctor may want to change the dose, or other precautions may be necessary. When you are taking methotrexate, it is especially important that your doctor and pharmacist know if you are taking any other prescription or nonprescription (over-the-counter [OTC]) medicine. They should also be told if you have ever been treated with x-rays or cancer medicines or if you drink alcohol.

Other medical problems—The presence of other medical problems may affect the use of methotrexate. Make sure you tell your doctor if you have any other medical problems, especially:

- Alcohol abuse (or history of)—Increased risk of unwanted effects on the liver
- Chickenpox (including recent exposure) or
- Herpes zoster (shingles)—Risk of severe disease affecting other parts of the body
- Colitis
- Disease of the immune system
- Infection—Methotrexate can reduce immunity to infection
- Intestine blockage or
- Kidney disease or
- Liver disease—Effects may be increased because of slower removal of methotrexate from the body
- Mouth sores or inflammation or
- Stomach ulcer—May be worsened

Before you begin using any new medicine (prescription or nonprescription) or if you develop any new medical

problem while you are using this medicine, check with your doctor, nurse, or pharmacist.

Proper Use of This Medicine

Take this medicine only as directed by your doctor. Do not take more or less of it, and do not take it more often than your doctor ordered. The exact amount of medicine you need has been carefully worked out. Taking too much may increase the chance of side effects, while taking too little may not improve your condition.

Methotrexate may cause nausea. Even if you begin to feel ill, *do not stop using this medicine without first checking with your doctor.* Ask your doctor, nurse, or pharmacist for ways to lessen these effects. If you begin vomiting, check with your doctor.

If you vomit shortly after taking a dose of methotrexate, check with your doctor. You will be told whether to take the dose again or to wait until the next scheduled dose.

Missed dose—If you miss a dose of this medicine, do not take the missed dose at all and do not double the next one. Instead, go back to your regular dosing schedule and check with your doctor.

Storage—To store this medicine:
- Keep out of the reach of children.
- Store away from heat and direct light.
- Do not store in the bathroom, near the kitchen sink, or in other damp places. Heat or moisture may cause the medicine to break down.
- Do not keep outdated medicine or medicine no longer needed. Be sure that any discarded medicine is out of the reach of children.

Precautions While Using This Medicine

It is very important that your doctor check your progress at regular visits to make sure that this medicine is working properly and to check for unwanted effects.

Do not drink alcohol while using this medicine. Alcohol can increase the chance of liver problems.

Some patients who take methotrexate may become more sensitive to sunlight than they are normally. When you first begin taking methotrexate, avoid too much sun and do not use a sunlamp until you see how you react to the sun, especially if you tend to burn easily. In case of a severe burn, check with your doctor. This is especially important if you are taking this medicine for psoriasis because sunlight can make the psoriasis worse.

Do not take medicine for inflammation or pain (aspirin or other salicylates, diclofenac, diflunisal, fenoprofen, ibuprofen, indomethacin, ketoprofen, meclofenamate, mefenamic acid, naproxen, phenylbutazone, piroxicam, sulindac, suprofen, tolmetin) without first checking with your doctor. These medicines may increase the effects of methotrexate, which could be harmful.

While you are being treated with methotrexate, and after you stop treatment with it, *do not have any immunizations (vaccinations) without your doctor's approval.* Methotrexate may lower your body's resistance and there is a chance you might get the infection the immunization is meant to prevent. In addition, other persons living in your household should not take or should not have recently taken oral polio vaccine since there is a chance they could pass the polio virus on to you. Also, avoid other persons who have taken oral polio vaccine. Do not get close to them, and do not stay in the same room with them for very long. If you cannot take these precautions, you should consider wearing a protective face mask that covers the nose and mouth.

Methotrexate can lower the number of white blood cells in your blood temporarily, increasing the chance of getting an infection. It can also lower the number of platelets, which are necessary for proper blood clotting. If this occurs, there are certain precautions you can take, especially when your blood count is low, to reduce the risk of infection or bleeding:
- If you can, avoid people with infections. *Check with your doctor immediately* if you think you are getting an infection or if you get a fever or chills, cough or hoarseness, lower back or side pain, or painful or difficult urination.
- *Check with your doctor immediately* if you notice any unusual bleeding or bruising; black, tarry stools; blood in urine or stools; or pinpoint red spots on your skin.
- Be careful when using a regular toothbrush, dental floss, or toothpick. Your medical doctor, dentist, or nurse may recommend other ways to clean your teeth and gums. Check with your medical doctor before having any dental work done.
- Do not touch your eyes or the inside of your nose unless you have just washed your hands and have not touched anything else in the meantime.
- Be careful not to cut yourself when you are using sharp objects such as a safety razor or fingernail or toenail cutters.
- Avoid contact sports or other situations where bruising or injury could occur.

Side Effects of This Medicine

Along with their needed effects, medicines like methotrexate can sometimes cause unwanted effects such as blood problems, kidney problems, stomach or liver problems, loss of hair, and other side effects. These and others are described below. Also, because of the way these medicines act on the body, there is a chance that they might cause other unwanted effects that may not occur until months or years after the medicine is used. These delayed effects may include certain types of cancer, such as leukemia. Discuss these possible effects with your doctor.

Although not all of these side effects may occur, if they do occur they may need medical attention.

Check with your doctor immediately if any of the following side effects occur:

Less common

Diarrhea; reddening of skin; sores in mouth and on lips; stomach pain

Rare

Black, tarry stools; blood in urine or stools; blurred vision; convulsions (seizures); cough or hoarseness; fever or chills; lower back or side pain; painful or difficult urination; pinpoint red spots on skin; shortness of breath; unusual bleeding or bruising

Check with your doctor as soon as possible if any of the following side effects occur:

Rare

Back pain; dark urine; dizziness; drowsiness; headache; unusual tiredness or weakness; yellow eyes or skin

Other side effects may occur that usually do not need medical attention. These side effects may go away during treatment as your body adjusts to the medicine. Also, your doctor or nurse may be able to tell you about ways to prevent or reduce some of these side effects. Check with your doctor or nurse if any of the following side effects continue or are bothersome or if you have any questions about them:

Less common or rare

Acne; boils; loss of appetite; nausea or vomiting; pale skin; skin rash or itching

This medicine may cause a temporary loss of hair in some people. After treatment with methotrexate has ended, normal hair growth should return.

Other side effects not listed above may also occur in some patients. If you notice any other effects, check with your doctor.

Additional Information

Once a medicine has been approved for marketing for a certain use, experience may show that it is also useful for other medical problems. Although these uses are not included in product labeling, methotrexate is used in certain patients with the following medical conditions:

- Psoriatic arthritis
- Systemic dermatomyositis

Other than the above information, there is no additional information relating to proper use, precautions, or side effects for these uses.

Annual revision: August 1990
Interim revision: 07/08/93

METHOXSALEN Systemic

Some commonly used brand names are:

In the U.S.
8-MOP
Oxsoralen-Ultra

In Canada
Oxsoralen
Ultra MOP

Description

Methoxsalen (meth-OX-a-len) belongs to the group of medicines called psoralens. It is used along with ultraviolet light (found in sunlight and some special lamps) in a treatment called PUVA to treat vitiligo, a disease in which skin color is lost, and psoriasis, a skin condition associated with red and scaly patches.

Methoxsalen is also used with ultraviolet light in the treatment of white blood cells. This treatment is called photopheresis and is used to treat the skin problems associated with mycosis fungoides, which is a type of lymphoma.

Methoxsalen may also be used for other conditions as determined by your doctor.

This medicine is available only with your doctor's prescription, in the following dosage forms:

Oral

- Hard gelatin capsules (U.S. and Canada)
- Soft gelatin capsules (U.S. and Canada)

It is very important that you read and understand the following information. If any of it causes you special concern, check with your doctor. Also, *if you have any questions* or if you want more information about this medicine or your medical problem, *ask your doctor, nurse, or pharmacist.*

Before Using This Medicine

Methoxsalen is a very strong medicine that increases the skin's sensitivity to sunlight. In addition to causing serious sunburns if not properly used, it has been reported to increase the chance of skin cancer and cataracts. Also, like too much sunlight, PUVA can cause premature aging of the skin. Therefore, methoxsalen should be used only as directed and it should *not* be used simply for suntanning. Before using this medicine, be sure that you have discussed its use with your doctor.

In deciding to use a medicine, the risks of using the medicine must be weighed against the good it will do. This is a decision you and your doctor will make. For methoxsalen, the following should be considered:

Allergies—Tell your doctor if you have ever had any unusual or allergic reaction to methoxsalen. Also tell your doctor and pharmacist if you are allergic to any other substances, such as foods, preservatives, or dyes.

Diet—Eating certain foods while you are taking methoxsalen may increase your skin's sensitivity to sunlight. To help prevent this, avoid eating limes, figs, parsley, parsnips, mustard, carrots, and celery while you are being treated with this medicine.

Pregnancy—Studies on effects in pregnancy have not been done in either humans or animals.

Breast-feeding—It is not known whether methoxsalen passes into breast milk. However, this medicine has not been reported to cause problems in nursing babies.

Children—Some of the side effects are more likely to occur in children up to 12 years of age, since these children may be more sensitive to the effects of methoxsalen.

Older adults—Many medicines have not been tested in older people. Therefore, it may not be known whether they work exactly the same way they do in younger adults or if they cause different side effects or problems in older people. There is no specific information about the use of methoxsalen in the elderly.

Other medicines—Although certain medicines should not be used together at all, in other cases two different medicines may be used together even if an interaction might occur. In these cases, your doctor may want to change the dose, or other precautions may be necessary. When you are using methoxsalen, it is especially important that your doctor and pharmacist know if you are using the following:

- Recent treatment with x-rays or cancer medicines or plans to have x-rays in the near future—Increases the chance of side effects from treatment with PUVA

Other medical problems—The presence of other medical problems may affect the use of methoxsalen. Make sure you tell your doctor if you have any other medical problems, especially:

- Allergy to sunlight (or family history of) or
- Infection or
- Lupus erythematosus or
- Porphyria or
- Skin cancer (history of) or
- Skin conditions (other) or
- Stomach problems—Use of PUVA may make the condition worse
- Eye problems, such as cataracts or loss of the lens of the eye—The light treatment may make the condition worse or may cause damage to the eye
- Heart or blood vessel disease (severe)—The heat or prolonged standing associated with each light treatment may make the condition worse
- Liver disease—Condition may cause increased blood levels of the medicine and cause an increase in side effects

Before you begin using any new medicine (prescription or nonprescription) or if you develop any new medical problem while you are using this medicine, check with your doctor, nurse, or pharmacist.

Proper Use of This Medicine

Methoxsalen usually comes with patient directions. Read them carefully before using this medicine.

This medicine may take 6 to 8 weeks to really help your condition. *Do not increase the amount of methoxsalen you are taking or spend extra time in the sunlight or under an ultraviolet lamp.* This will not make the medicine act any more quickly and may result in a serious burn.

If this medicine upsets your stomach:

- Patients taking the hard gelatin capsules may take them with food or milk.
- Patients taking the soft gelatin capsules may take them with low fat food or low fat milk.

Missed dose—If you are late in taking, or miss taking, a dose of this medicine, notify your doctor so your light treatment can be rescheduled. Remember that exposure to sunlight or ultraviolet light must take place a certain number of hours *after* you take the medicine or it will not work. For patients taking the hard gelatin capsules, this is 2 to 4 hours. For patients taking the soft gelatin capsules, this is 1½ to 2 hours. If you have any questions about this, check with your doctor.

Storage—To store this medicine:

- Keep out of the reach of children.
- Store away from heat and direct light.
- Do not store in the bathroom, near the kitchen sink, or in other damp places. Heat or moisture may cause the medicine to break down.
- Do not keep outdated medicine or medicine no longer needed. Be sure that any discarded medicine is out of the reach of children.

Precautions While Using This Medicine

Your doctor should check your progress at regular visits to make sure this medicine is working and that it does not cause unwanted effects. Eye examinations should be included.

This medicine increases the sensitivity of your skin and lips to sunlight. Therefore, *exposure to the sun, even through window glass or on a cloudy day, could cause a serious burn.* If you must go out during the daylight hours:

- *Before each treatment, cover your skin for at least 24 hours* by wearing protective clothing, such as long-sleeved shirts, full-length slacks, wide-brimmed hat, and gloves. In addition, *protect your lips with a special sun block lipstick that has a protection factor of at least 15.* Check with your doctor before using sun block products on other parts of your body before a treatment, since sun block products should not be used on the areas of your skin that are to be treated.
- *After each treatment, cover your skin for at least 8 hours* by wearing protective clothing. In addition, use a sun block product that has a protection factor of at least 15 on your lips and on those areas of your body that cannot be covered.

If you have any questions about this, check with your doctor or pharmacist.

Your skin may continue to be sensitive to sunlight for some time after treatment with this medicine. Use extra caution for at least 48 hours following each treatment if you plan to spend any time in the sun. In addition, do not sunbathe anytime during your course of treatment with methoxsalen.

For 24 hours after you take each dose of methoxsalen, your eyes should be protected during daylight hours with special wraparound sunglasses that totally block or absorb ultraviolet light (ordinary sunglasses are not adequate). This is to prevent cataracts. Your doctor will tell you what kind of sunglasses to use. These glasses should be worn even in indirect light, such as light coming through window glass or on a cloudy day.

This medicine may cause your skin to become dry or itchy. *However, check with your doctor before applying anything to your skin to treat this problem.*

Side Effects of This Medicine

Along with its needed effects, a medicine may cause some unwanted effects. Although not all of these side effects may occur, if they do occur they may need medical attention.

Check with your doctor immediately if you think you have taken an overdose or if any of the following side effects occur, since they may indicate a serious burn:

Blistering and peeling of skin; reddened, sore skin; swelling (especially of feet or lower legs)

Other side effects may occur that usually do not need medical attention. These side effects may go away during treatment as your body adjusts to the medicine. However, check with your doctor if any of the following side effects continue for more than 48 hours or are bothersome:

More common

Itching of skin; nausea

Less common

Dizziness; headache; leg cramps; mental depression; nervousness; skin rash; trouble in sleeping

Treatment with this medicine usually causes a slight reddening of your skin 24 to 48 hours after the treatment. This is an expected effect and is no cause for concern. However, check with your doctor right away if your skin becomes sore and red or blistered.

There is an increased risk of developing skin cancer after use of methoxsalen. You should check your body regularly and show your doctor any skin sores that do not heal, new skin growths, and skin growths that have changed in the way they look or feel.

Premature aging of the skin may occur as a result of prolonged methoxsalen therapy. This effect is permanent and is similar to what happens when a person sunbathes for long periods of time.

Other side effects not listed above may also occur in some patients. If you notice any other effects, check with your doctor.

Annual revision: August 1990

METHOXSALEN Topical

Some commonly used brand names are:

In the U.S.
Oxsoralen Lotion

In Canada
Oxsoralen Lotion
UltraMOP Lotion

Description

Methoxsalen (meth-OX-a-len) belongs to the group of medicines called psoralens. It is used along with ultraviolet light (found in sunlight and some special lamps) in a treatment called PUVA to treat vitiligo, a disease in which skin color is lost. Methoxsalen may also be used for other conditions as determined by your doctor.

Methoxsalen is available only with a prescription and is to be administered by or under the direct supervision of your doctor, in the following dosage form:

Topical

- Topical solution (U.S. and Canada)

It is very important that you read and understand the following information. If any of it causes you special concern, check with your doctor. Also, *if you have any questions* or if you want more information about this medicine or your medical problem, *ask your doctor, nurse, or pharmacist.*

Before Using This Medicine

Methoxsalen is a very strong medicine that increases the skin's sensitivity to sunlight. In addition to causing serious sunburns if not properly used, it has been reported to increase the chance of skin cancer. Also, like too much sunlight, PUVA can cause premature aging of the skin. Therefore, methoxsalen should be used only as directed and should *not* be used simply for suntanning. Before using this medicine, be sure that you have discussed its use with your doctor.

In deciding to use a medicine, the risks of using the medicine must be weighed against the good it will do. This is a decision you and your doctor will make. For topical methoxsalen, the following should be considered:

Allergies—Tell your doctor if you have ever had any unusual or allergic reaction to methoxsalen. Also tell your doctor and pharmacist if you are allergic to any other substances, such as foods, preservatives, or dyes.

Diet—Eating certain foods while you are using methoxsalen may increase your skin's sensitivity to sunlight. To help prevent this, avoid eating limes, figs, parsley, parsnips, mustard, carrots, and celery while you are being treated with this medicine.

Pregnancy—Studies on effects in pregnancy have not been done in either humans or animals.

Breast-feeding—It is not known whether methoxsalen passes into breast milk. However, methoxsalen has not been reported to cause problems in nursing babies.

Children—Studies on this medicine have been done only in adult patients, and there is no specific information about its use in children.

Older adults—Many medicines have not been tested in older people. Therefore, it may not be known whether they work exactly the same way they do in younger adults or if they cause different side effects or problems in older people. There is no specific information about the use of topical methoxsalen in the elderly.

Other medicines—Although certain medicines should not be used together at all, in other cases two different medicines may be used together even if an interaction might occur. In these cases, your doctor may want to change the dose, or other precautions may be necessary. When you are using topical methoxsalen, it is especially important that your doctor and pharmacist know if you are using the following:

- Recent treatment with x-rays or cancer medicines or plans to have x-rays in the near future—Increases the chance of side effects from treatment with PUVA

Other medical problems—The presence of other medical problems may affect the use of topical methoxsalen. Make sure you tell your doctor if you have any other medical problems, especially:

- Allergy to sunlight (or family history of) or
- Infection or
- Lupus erythematosus or
- Porphyria or
- Skin cancer (history of) or
- Skin conditions (other)—Use of PUVA may make the condition worse
- Heart or blood vessel disease (severe)—The heat or prolonged standing associated with each light treatment may make the condition worse

Before you begin using any new medicine (prescription or nonprescription) or if you develop any new medical problem while you are using this medicine, check with your doctor, nurse, or pharmacist.

Precautions While Using This Medicine

It is important that you visit your doctor as directed for treatments and to have your progress checked.

This medicine increases the sensitivity of the treated areas of your skin to sunlight. Therefore, *exposure to the sun, even through window glass or on a cloudy day, could cause a serious burn.* After each light treatment, thoroughly wash the treated areas of your skin. Also, if you must go out during daylight hours, cover the treated areas of your skin for at least 12 to 48 hours following treatment by wearing protective clothing or a sun block product that has a skin protection factor (SPF) of at least 15. Some patients may require a product with a higher SPF number, especially if they have a fair complexion. If you have any questions about this, check with your doctor or pharmacist.

The treated areas of your skin may continue to be sensitive to sunlight for some time after treatment with this medicine. Use extra caution for at least 72 hours following each treatment if you plan to spend any time in the sun. In addition, do not sunbathe anytime during your course of treatment with methoxsalen.

This medicine may cause your skin to become dry or itchy. *However, check with your doctor before applying anything to your skin to treat this problem.*

Side Effects of This Medicine

Along with its needed effects, a medicine may cause some unwanted effects. Although not all of these side effects may occur, if they do occur they may need medical attention.

Check with your doctor immediately if any of the following side effects occur, since they may indicate a serious burn:

Blistering and peeling of skin; reddened, sore skin; swelling, especially of the feet or lower legs

There is an increased risk of developing skin cancer after use of methoxsalen. You should check the treated areas of your body regularly and show your doctor any skin sores that do not heal, new skin growths, and skin growths that have changed in the way they look or feel.

Premature aging of the skin may occur as a result of prolonged methoxsalen therapy. This effect is permanent and is similar to what happens when a person sunbathes for long periods of time.

Other side effects not listed above may also occur in some patients. If you notice any other effects, check with your doctor.

Annual revision: August 1990

METHYLDOPA Systemic

Some commonly used brand names are:

In the U.S.

Aldomet

Generic name product may also be available.

In Canada

Aldomet
Apo-Methyldopa
Dopamet
Novomedopa

Generic name product may also be available.

Description

Methyldopa (meth-ill-DOE-pa) belongs to the general class of medicines called antihypertensives. It is used to treat high blood pressure (hypertension).

High blood pressure adds to the workload of the heart and arteries. If it continues for a long time, the heart and arteries may not function properly. This can damage the blood vessels of the brain, heart, and kidneys, resulting in a stroke, heart failure, or kidney failure. High blood pressure may also increase the risk of heart attacks. These problems may be less likely to occur if blood pressure is controlled.

Methyldopa works by controlling impulses along certain nerve pathways. As a result, it relaxes blood vessels so that blood passes through them more easily. This helps to lower blood pressure.

Methyldopa is available only with your doctor's prescription, in the following dosage forms:

Oral

- Oral suspension (U.S.)
- Tablets (U.S. and Canada)

Parenteral

- Injection (U.S. and Canada)

It is very important that you read and understand the following information. If any of it causes you special concern, check with your doctor. Also, *if you have any questions* or if you want more information about this medicine or your medical problem, *ask your doctor, nurse, or pharmacist.*

Before Using This Medicine

In deciding to use a medicine, the risks of taking the medicine must be weighed against the good it will do. This is a decision you and your doctor will make. For methyldopa, the following should be considered:

Allergies—Tell your doctor if you have ever had any unusual or allergic reaction to methyldopa. Also tell your doctor and pharmacist if you are allergic to any other substances, such as foods, sulfites or other preservatives, or dyes. Some methyldopa products may contain sulfites. Your doctor, nurse, or pharmacist can help you avoid products that may cause a problem.

Pregnancy—Methyldopa has not been studied in pregnant women in the first and second trimesters (the first 6 months of pregnancy). However, studies in pregnant women during the third trimester (the last 3 months of pregnancy) have not shown that methyldopa causes birth defects or other problems.

Breast-feeding—Although methyldopa passes into breast milk, it has not been reported to cause problems in nursing babies.

Children—Although there is no specific information comparing use of methyldopa in children with use in other age groups, this medicine is not expected to cause different side effects or problems in children than it does in adults.

Older adults—Dizziness or lightheadedness and drowsiness may be more likely to occur in the elderly, who are more sensitive to the effects of methyldopa.

Other medicines—Although certain medicines should not be used together at all, in other cases two different medicines may be used together even if an interaction might occur. In these cases, your doctor may want to change the dose, or other precautions may be necessary. When taking methyldopa, it is especially important that your doctor and pharmacist know if you are taking any of the following:

- Monoamine oxidase (MAO) inhibitors (furazolidone [e.g., Furoxone], isocarboxazid [e.g., Marplan], phenelzine [e.g., Nardil], procarbazine [e.g., Matulane], selegiline [e.g., Eldepryl], tranylcypromine [e.g., Parnate])—Taking methyldopa while you are taking or within 2 weeks of taking MAO inhibitors may cause nervousness in patients receiving MAO inhibitors; headache, severe high blood pressure, and hallucinations have been reported

Other medical problems—The presence of other medical problems may affect the use of methyldopa. Make sure you tell your doctor if you have any other medical problems, especially:

- Angina (chest pain)—Methyldopa may worsen the condition
- Kidney disease or
- Liver disease—Effects of methyldopa may be increased because of slower removal from the body
- Mental depression (history of)—Methyldopa can cause mental depression
- Parkinson's disease—Methyldopa may worsen condition
- Pheochromocytoma—Methyldopa may interfere with tests for the condition; in addition, there have been reports of increased blood pressure
- If you have taken methyldopa in the past and developed liver problems

Before you begin using any new medicine (prescription or nonprescription) or if you develop any new medical problem while you are using this medicine, check with your doctor, nurse, or pharmacist.

Proper Use of This Medicine

In addition to the use of the medicine your doctor has prescribed, treatment for your high blood pressure may include weight control and care in the types of foods you eat, especially foods high in sodium. Your doctor will tell you which of these are most important for you. You should check with your doctor before changing your diet.

Many patients who have high blood pressure will not notice any signs of the problem. In fact, many may feel normal. It is very important that you *take your medicine exactly as directed* and that you keep your appointments with your doctor even if you feel well.

Remember that methyldopa will not cure your high blood pressure but it does help control it. Therefore, you must continue to take it as directed if you expect to lower your blood pressure and keep it down. *You may have to take high blood pressure medicine for the rest of your life.* If high blood pressure is not treated, it can cause serious problems such as heart failure, blood vessel disease, stroke, or kidney disease.

To help you remember to take your medicine, try to get into the habit of taking it at the same time each day.

Missed dose—If you miss a dose of this medicine, take it as soon as possible. However, if it is almost time for your next dose, skip the missed dose and go back to your regular dosing schedule. Do not double doses.

Storage—To store this medicine:

- Keep out of the reach of children.
- Store away from heat and direct light.
- Do not store in the bathroom, near the kitchen sink, or in other damp places. Heat or moisture may cause the medicine to break down.
- Keep the oral liquid form of this medicine from freezing.
- Do not keep outdated medicine or medicine no longer needed. Be sure that any discarded medicine is out of the reach of children.

Precautions While Using This Medicine

It is important that your doctor check your progress at regular visits to make sure that this medicine is working properly.

Do not take other medicines unless they have been discussed with your doctor. This especially includes over-the-counter (nonprescription) medicines for appetite control, asthma, colds, cough, hay fever, or sinus problems, since they may tend to increase your blood pressure.

If you have a fever and there seems to be no reason for it, check with your doctor. This is especially important during the first few weeks you take methyldopa, since fever may be a sign of a serious reaction to this medicine.

Before having any kind of surgery (including dental surgery) or emergency treatment, make sure the medical doctor or dentist in charge knows that you are taking this medicine.

Methyldopa may cause some people to become drowsy or less alert than they are normally. This is more likely to happen when you begin to take it or when you increase the amount of medicine you are taking. *Make sure you know how you react to this medicine before you drive, use machines, or do anything else that could be dangerous if you are not alert.*

Dizziness, lightheadedness, or fainting may occur, especially when you get up from a lying or sitting position. Getting up slowly may help, but if the problem continues or gets worse, check with your doctor.

Methyldopa may cause dryness of the mouth. For temporary relief, use sugarless candy or gum, melt bits of ice in your mouth, or use a saliva substitute. However, if your mouth continues to feel dry for more than 2 weeks, check with your medical doctor or dentist. Continuing dryness of the mouth may increase the chance of dental disease, including tooth decay, gum disease, and fungus infections.

Tell the doctor in charge that you are taking this medicine before you have any medical tests. The results of some tests may be affected by this medicine.

Side Effects of This Medicine

Along with its needed effects, a medicine may cause some unwanted effects. Although not all of these side effects may occur, if they do occur they may need medical attention.

Check with your doctor immediately if the following side effect occurs:

Less common

Fever, shortly after starting to take this medicine

Check with your doctor as soon as possible if any of the following side effects occur:

More common

Swelling of feet or lower legs

Less common

Mental depression or anxiety; nightmares or unusually vivid dreams

Rare

Dark or amber urine; diarrhea or stomach cramps (severe or continuing); fever, chills, troubled breathing, and fast heartbeat; general feeling of discomfort or illness or weakness; joint pain; pale stools; skin rash or itching; stomach pain (severe) with nausea and vomiting; tiredness or weakness after having taken this medicine for several weeks (continuing); yellow eyes or skin

Other side effects may occur that usually do not need medical attention. These side effects may go away during treatment as your body adjusts to the medicine. However, check with your doctor if any of the following side effects continue or are bothersome:

More common

Drowsiness; dryness of mouth; headache

Less common

Decreased sexual ability or interest in sex; diarrhea; dizziness or lightheadedness when getting up from a lying or sitting position; nausea or vomiting; numbness, tingling, pain, or weakness in hands or feet; slow heartbeat; stuffy nose; swelling of breasts or unusual milk production

Other side effects not listed above may also occur in some patients. If you notice any other effects, check with your doctor.

Annual revision: 08/05/92

METHYLDOPA AND THIAZIDE DIURETICS Systemic

This information applies to the following medicines:

Methyldopa (meth-ill-DOE-pa) and Chlorothiazide (klor-oh-THYE-a-zide)

Methyldopa and Hydrochlorothiazide (hye-droe-klor-oh-THYE-a-zide)

Some commonly used brand names are:

For Methyldopa and Chlorothiazide

In the U.S.

Aldoclor

Generic name product may also be available.

In Canada

Supres

For Methyldopa and Hydrochlorothiazide

In the U.S.

Aldoril

Generic name product may also be available.

In Canada

Aldoril

Novodoparil

PMS Dopazide

Description

Combinations of methyldopa and a thiazide diuretic (chlorothiazide or hydrochlorothiazide) are used to treat high blood pressure (hypertension).

High blood pressure adds to the workload of the heart and arteries. If it continues for a long time, the heart and arteries may not function properly. This can damage the blood vessels of the brain, heart, and kidneys, resulting in a stroke, heart failure, or kidney failure. High blood pressure may also increase the risk of heart attacks. These problems may be less likely to occur if blood pressure is controlled.

Methyldopa works by controlling nerve impulses along certain nerve pathways. As a result, it relaxes blood vessels so that blood passes through them more easily. Thiazide diuretics help reduce the amount of water in the body by increasing the flow of urine. These actions help to lower blood pressure.

This medicine is available only with your doctor's prescription, in the following dosage forms:

Oral

Methyldopa and Chlorothiazide
- Tablets (U.S. and Canada)

Methyldopa and Hydrochlorothiazide
- Tablets (U.S. and Canada)

It is very important that you read and understand the following information. If any of it causes you special concern, check with your doctor. Also, *if you have any questions* or if you want more information about this medicine or your medical problem, *ask your doctor, nurse, or pharmacist.*

Before Using This Medicine

In deciding to use a medicine, the risks of taking the medicine must be weighed against the good it will do. This is a decision you and your doctor will make. For methyldopa and thiazide diuretics, the following should be considered:

Allergies—Tell your doctor if you have ever had any unusual or allergic reaction to methyldopa, sulfonamides (sulfa drugs), bumetanide, furosemide, indapamide, acetazolamide, dichlorphenamide, methazolamide, or thiazide diuretics (water pills). Also tell your doctor and pharmacist if you are allergic to any other substances, such as foods, sulfites or other preservatives, or dyes.

Pregnancy—Studies in humans have not shown that methyldopa causes birth defects or other problems. However, when thiazide diuretics are used during pregnancy, they may cause side effects including jaundice, blood problems, and low potassium in the newborn infant. Thiazide diuretics have not been shown to cause birth defects.

Breast-feeding—This medicine passes into breast milk. Thiazide diuretics may decrease the flow of breast milk. Therefore, you should avoid use of thiazide diuretics during the first month of breast-feeding.

Children—Although there is no specific information comparing use of this medicine in children with use in other age groups, it is not expected to cause different side effects or problems in children than it does in adults.

Older adults—Dizziness or lightheadedness, drowsiness, or signs of too much potassium loss may be more likely to occur in the elderly, who are more sensitive to the effects of methyldopa and thiazide diuretics.

Other medicines—Although certain medicines should not be used together at all, in other cases two different medicines may be used together even if an interaction might occur. In these cases, your doctor may want to change the dose, or other precautions may be necessary. When you are taking methyldopa and thiazide diuretics, it is especially important that your doctor and pharmacist know if you are taking any of the following:

- Digitalis glycosides (heart medicine)—Thiazide diuretics may cause low potassium in the blood, which can lead to symptoms of digitalis toxicity
- Lithium (e.g., Lithane)—Risk of lithium overdose, even at usual doses, may be increased
- Monoamine oxidase (MAO) inhibitors (furazolidone [e.g., Furoxone], isocarboxazid [e.g., Marplan], phenelzine [e.g., Nardil], procarbazine [e.g., Matulane], selegiline [e.g., Eldepryl], tranylcypromine [e.g., Parnate])—Taking methyldopa while you are taking or within 2 weeks of taking MAO inhibitors may cause nervousness; headache, severe high blood pressure, and hallucinations have been reported

Other medical problems—The presence of other medical problems may affect the use of methyldopa and thiazide diuretics. Make sure you tell your doctor if you have any other medical problems, especially:

- Angina (chest pain)—Methyldopa may worsen the condition
- Diabetes mellitus (sugar diabetes)—Thiazide diuretics may change the amount of diabetes medicine needed
- Gout (history of)—Thiazide diuretics may increase the amount of uric acid in the blood, which can lead to gout
- High cholesterol—Thiazide diuretics may raise cholesterol levels
- Kidney disease—Effects of methyldopa and thiazide diuretics may be increased because of slower removal from the body. If severe, thiazide diuretics may not work
- Liver disease—Effects of methyldopa may be increased because of slower removal from the body. If thiazide diuretics cause loss of too much water from the body, liver disease can become much worse
- Lupus erythematosus (history of)—Thiazide diuretics may worsen the condition
- Mental depression (history of)—Methyldopa can cause mental depression
- Pancreatitis (inflammation of the pancreas)
- Parkinson's disease—Methyldopa may worsen the condition
- Pheochromocytoma—Methyldopa may interfere with tests for the condition; in addition, there have been reports of increased blood pressure
- If you have taken methyldopa in the past and developed liver problems

Before you begin using any new medicine (prescription or nonprescription) or if you develop any new medical problem while you are using this medicine, check with your doctor, nurse, or pharmacist.

Proper Use of This Medicine

In addition to the use of the medicine your doctor has prescribed, appropriate treatment for your high blood pressure may include weight control and care in the types of foods you eat, especially foods high in sodium. Your doctor will tell you which factors are most important for you. You should check with your doctor before changing your diet.

Many patients who have high blood pressure will not notice any signs of the problem. In fact, many may feel normal. It is very important *that you take your medicine exactly as directed* and that you keep your appointments with your doctor even if you feel well.

Remember that this medicine will not cure your high blood pressure but it does help control it. Therefore, you must continue to take it as directed if you expect to lower your blood pressure and keep it down. *You may have to take high blood pressure medicine for the rest of your life.* If high blood pressure is not treated, it can cause serious problems such as heart failure, blood vessel disease, stroke, or kidney disease.

This medicine may cause you to have an unusual feeling of tiredness when you begin to take it. You may also notice an increase in the amount of urine or in your frequency of urination. After taking the medicine for a while, these effects should lessen. In general, to keep the increase in urine from affecting your sleep:

- If you are to take a single dose a day, take it in the morning after breakfast.
- If you are to take more than one dose a day, take the last dose no later than 6 p.m., unless otherwise directed by your doctor.

However, it is best to plan your dose or doses according to a schedule that will least affect your personal activities and sleep. Ask your doctor, nurse, or pharmacist to help you plan the best time to take this medicine.

To help you remember to take your medicine, try to get into the habit of taking it at the same time each day.

Dosing—The dose of methyldopa and thiazide diuretic combinations will be different for different patients. *Follow your doctor's orders or the directions on the label.* The following information includes only the average doses of methyldopa and thiazide diuretic combinations. *If your dose is different, do not change it* unless your doctor tells you to do so:

- For methyldopa and chlorothiazide *oral* dosage form (tablets):
  - —Adults: Two to four tablets a day, taken as a single dose or in divided doses.
  - —Children: Dose must be determined by your doctor.
- For methyldopa and hydrochlorothiazide *oral* dosage form (tablets):
  - —Adults: Two to four tablets a day, taken as a single dose or in divided doses.
  - —Children: Dose must be determined by your doctor.

Missed dose—If you miss a dose of this medicine, take it as soon as possible. However, if it is almost time for your next dose, skip the missed dose and go back to your regular dosing schedule. Do not double doses.

Storage—To store this medicine:

- Keep out of the reach of children.
- Store away from heat and direct light.
- Do not store in the bathroom, near the kitchen sink, or in other damp places. Heat or moisture may cause the medicine to break down.
- Do not keep outdated medicine or medicine no longer needed. Be sure that any discarded medicine is out of the reach of children.

Precautions While Using This Medicine

It is important that your doctor check your progress at regular visits to make sure that this medicine is working properly.

Do not take other medicines unless they have been discussed with your doctor. This especially includes over-the-counter (nonprescription) medicines for appetite control, asthma, colds, cough, hay fever, or sinus problems, since they may tend to increase your blood pressure.

This medicine may cause a loss of potassium from your body:

- To help prevent this, your doctor may want you to:
  - —eat or drink foods that have a high potassium content (for example, orange or other citrus fruit juices), or
  - —take a potassium supplement, or
  - —take another medicine to help prevent the loss of the potassium in the first place.
- It is very important to follow these directions. Also, it is important not to change your diet on your own. This is more important if you are already on a special diet (as for diabetes), or if you are taking a potassium supplement or a medicine to reduce potassium loss. Extra potassium may not be necessary and, in some cases, too much potassium could be harmful.

Check with your doctor if you become sick and have severe or continuing vomiting or diarrhea. These problems may cause you to lose additional water and potassium.

Before having any kind of surgery (including dental surgery) or emergency treatment, tell the medical doctor or dentist in charge that you are taking this medicine.

If you have a fever and there seems to be no reason for it, check with your doctor. This is especially important during the first few weeks you take this medicine since fever may be a sign of a serious reaction to methyldopa.

This medicine may cause some people to become drowsy or less alert than they are normally. This is more likely to happen when you begin to take it or when you increase the amount of medicine you are taking. *Make sure you know how you react to this medicine before you drive, use machines, or do anything else that could be dangerous if you are not alert.*

Dizziness, lightheadedness, or fainting may occur, especially when you get up from a lying or sitting position. Getting up slowly may help, but if the problem continues or gets worse, check with your doctor.

The dizziness, lightheadedness, or fainting is also more likely to occur if you drink alcohol, stand for long periods of time, exercise, or if the weather is hot. Drinking alcoholic beverages may also make the drowsiness worse. *While you are taking this medicine, be careful in the amount of alcohol you drink.* Also, use extra care during exercise or hot weather or if you must stand for long periods of time.

For *diabetic patients*:

- This medicine may raise blood sugar levels. While you are using this medicine, be especially careful in testing for sugar in your urine. If you have any questions about this, check with your doctor.

This medicine may cause dryness of the mouth. For temporary relief, use sugarless candy or gum, melt bits of ice in your mouth, or use a saliva substitute. However, if your mouth continues to feel dry for more than 2 weeks, check with your medical doctor or dentist. Continuing dryness of the mouth may increase the chance of dental disease, including tooth decay, gum disease, and fungus infections.

Thiazide diuretics may cause your skin to be more sensitive to sunlight than it is normally. Exposure to sunlight, even for brief periods of time, may cause a skin rash, itching, redness or other discoloration of the skin, or a severe sunburn. When you begin taking this medicine:

- Stay out of direct sunlight, especially between the hours of 10:00 a.m. and 3:00 p.m., if possible.
- Wear protective clothing, including a hat. Also, wear sunglasses.
- Apply a sun block product that has a skin protection factor (SPF) of at least 15. Some patients may require a product with a higher SPF number, especially if they have a fair complexion. If you have any questions about this, check with your doctor or pharmacist.
- Apply a sun block lipstick that has an SPF of at least 15 to protect your lips.
- Do not use a sunlamp or tanning bed or booth.

If you have a severe reaction from the sun, check with your doctor.

Before you have any medical tests, tell the doctor in charge that you are taking this medicine. The results of some tests may be affected by this medicine.

Side Effects of This Medicine

Along with its needed effects, a medicine may cause some unwanted effects. Although not all of these side effects may occur, if they do occur they may need medical attention.

Check with your doctor immediately if the following side effect occurs:

Rare

Unexplained fever shortly after starting to take this medicine

Check with your doctor as soon as possible if any of the following side effects occur, especially since some of them may mean that your body is losing too much potassium:

Signs and symptoms of too much potassium loss

Dry mouth; increased thirst; irregular heartbeats; muscle cramps or pain; nausea or vomiting; unusual tiredness or weakness; weak pulse

Less common

Mental depression or anxiety; nightmares or unusually vivid dreams

Rare

Cough or hoarseness; dark or amber urine; diarrhea or stomach cramps (severe or continuing); fever, chills, troubled breathing, and fast heartbeat; general feeling of discomfort or illness or weakness; joint pain; lower back or side pain; painful or difficult urination; pale stools; skin rash, hives, or itching; stomach pain (severe) with nausea and vomiting; tiredness or weakness after having taken this medicine for several weeks (continuing); yellow eyes or skin

Other side effects may occur that usually do not need medical attention. These side effects may go away during treatment as your body adjusts to the medicine. However, check with your doctor if any of the following side effects continue or are bothersome:

More common

Dizziness or lightheadedness when getting up from a lying or sitting position; drowsiness; dryness of mouth; headache

Less common

Decreased sexual ability or interest in sex; diarrhea; increased sensitivity of skin to sunlight (skin rash, itching, redness or other discoloration of skin or severe sunburn after exposure to sunlight); loss of appetite; numbness, tingling, pain, or weakness in hands or feet; slow heartbeat; stuffy nose; swelling of breasts or unusual milk production

Other side effects not listed above may also occur in some patients. If you notice any other effects, check with your doctor.

Annual revision: 04/13/93

METHYLPHENIDATE Systemic

Some commonly used brand names are:

In the U.S.

Ritalin
Ritalin-SR

Generic name product may also be available.

In Canada

PMS-Methylphenidate
Ritalin
Ritalin SR

Description

Methylphenidate (meth-ill-FEN-i-date) belongs to the group of medicines called central stimulants. It is used to treat children with attention-deficit hyperactivity disorder (ADHD).

Methylphenidate works by increasing attention and decreasing restlessness in children who are overactive, cannot concentrate for very long or are easily distracted, and are emotionally unstable. This medicine is used as part of a total treatment program that also includes social, educational, and psychological treatment.

Methylphenidate is also used in the treatment of narcolepsy (uncontrollable desire for sleep or sudden attacks of deep sleep).

This medicine is available only with a doctor's prescription. Prescriptions cannot be refilled. A new written prescription must be obtained from your doctor each time you or your child needs this medicine.

Methylphenidate is available in the following dosage forms:

Oral

- Tablets (U.S. and Canada)
- Extended-release tablets (U.S. and Canada)

It is very important that you read and understand the following information. If any of it causes you special concern, check with your doctor. Also, *if you have any questions* or if you want more information about this medicine or your medical problem, *ask your doctor, nurse, or pharmacist.*

Before Using This Medicine

In deciding to use a medicine, the risks of taking the medicine must be weighed against the good it will do. This is a decision you and your doctor will make. For methylphenidate, the following should be considered:

Allergies—Tell your doctor if you have ever had any unusual or allergic reaction to methylphenidate. Also tell your doctor and pharmacist if you are allergic to any other substances, such as foods, preservatives, or dyes.

Pregnancy—Studies on effects in pregnancy have not been done in either humans or animals.

Breast-feeding—It is not known whether methylphenidate passes into breast milk.

Children—Loss of appetite, trouble in sleeping, stomach pain, and weight loss, may be especially likely to occur in children, who are usually more sensitive than adults to the effects of methylphenidate. Also, there have been reports of children's growth rate being slowed when methylphenidate was used for a long time. Some doctors recommend drug-free periods during treatment with methylphenidate.

Older adults—Many medicines have not been studied specifically in older people. Therefore, it may not be known whether they work exactly the same way they do in younger adults or if they cause different side effects or problems in older people. There is no specific information comparing use of methylphenidate in the elderly with use in other age groups.

Other medicines—Although certain medicines should not be used together at all, in other cases 2 different medicines may be used together even if an interaction might occur. In these cases, your doctor may want to change the dose, or other precautions may be necessary. When you are taking methylphenidate, it is especially important that your doctor and pharmacist know if you are taking any of the following:

- Amantadine (e.g., Symmetrel) or
- Amphetamines or
- Appetite suppressants (diet pills), except fenfluramine (e.g., Pondimin) or
- Caffeine (e.g., NoDoz) or
- Chlophedianol (e.g., Ulone) or
- Cocaine or
- Medicine for asthma or other breathing problems or

- Medicine for colds, sinus problems, hay fever or other allergies (including nose drops or sprays) or
- Nabilone (e.g., Cesamet) or
- Pemoline (e.g., Cylert)—Using these medicines with methylphenidate may cause severe nervousness, irritability, trouble in sleeping, or possibly irregular heartbeat or seizures
- Monoamine oxidase (MAO) inhibitors (furazolidone [e.g., Furoxone], isocarboxazid [e.g., Marplan], phenelzine [e.g., Nardil], procarbazine [e.g., Matulane], selegiline at doses more than 10 milligrams a day [e.g., Eldepryl], tranylcypromine [e.g., Parnate])—Taking methylphenidate while you are taking or within 2 weeks of taking MAO inhibitors may cause sudden extremely high blood pressure and severe convulsions; at least 14 days should be allowed between stopping treatment with one medicine and starting treatment with the other
- Pimozide (e.g., Orap)—The cause of tics may be masked

Other medical problems—The presence of other medical problems may affect the use of methylphenidate. Make sure you tell your doctor if you have any other medical problems, especially:

- Alcohol abuse (or history of) or
- Drug abuse or dependence (or history of)—Dependence on methylphenidate may develop
- Epilepsy or other seizure disorders—The risk of convulsions (seizures) may be increased
- Gilles de la Tourette's disorder (or history of) or
- Glaucoma or
- High blood pressure or
- Psychosis or
- Severe anxiety, agitation, tension, or depression or
- Tics (other than Tourette's disorder)—Methylphenidate may make the condition worse

Before you begin using any new medicine (prescription or nonprescription) or if you develop any new medical problem while you are using this medicine, check with your doctor, nurse, or pharmacist.

Proper Use of This Medicine

Take this medicine only as directed by your doctor. Do not take more of it, do not take it more often, and do not take it for a longer time than your doctor ordered. If too much is taken, it may become habit-forming.

Take this medicine about 30 to 45 minutes before meals. To do so will help it to work better.

If you are taking the long-acting form of this medicine:

- These tablets are to be swallowed whole. Do not break, crush, or chew before swallowing.

To help prevent trouble in sleeping, take the last dose of this medicine for each day before 6 p.m., unless otherwise directed by your doctor.

If you think this medicine is not working properly after you have taken it for several weeks, *do not increase the dose.* Instead, check with your doctor.

Dosing—The dose of methylphenidate will be different for different patients. *Follow your doctor's orders or the directions on the label.* The following information includes only the average doses of methylphenidate. *If your dose is different, do not change it* unless your doctor tells you to do so.

- The number of tablets that you take depends on the strength of the medicine. Also, *the number of doses you take each day, the time allowed between doses, and the length of time you take the medicine depend on the medical problem for which you are using methylphenidate.*
- For *short-acting oral* dosage forms (tablets):
  —Adults and adolescents: 5 to 20 milligrams two or three times a day, taken thirty to forty-five minutes before meals.
  —Children 6 years of age and over: To start, 5 milligrams two times a day, before breakfast and lunch. Your doctor may increase your dose if needed by 5 to 10 milligrams a week until symptoms improve or a maximum dose is reached.
  —Children up to 6 years of age: The dose must be determined by the doctor.
- For *long-acting oral* dosage forms (extended-release tablets):
  —Adults and adolescents: 20 milligrams one to three times a day, spaced eight hours apart, and taken on an empty stomach.
  —Children 6 years of age and over: 20 milligrams one to three times a day, spaced eight hours apart, and taken on an empty stomach.
  —Children up to 6 years of age: The dose must be determined by the doctor.

Missed dose—If you miss a dose of this medicine, take it as soon as possible. Then take any remaining doses for that day at regularly spaced intervals. Do not double doses.

Storage—To store this medicine:

- Keep out of the reach of children.
- Store away from heat and direct light.
- Do not store in the bathroom, near the kitchen sink, or in other damp places. Heat or moisture may cause the medicine to break down.
- Do not keep outdated medicine or medicine no longer needed. Be sure that any discarded medicine is out of the reach of children.

Precautions While Using This Medicine

Your doctor should check your progress at regular visits to make sure that this medicine does not cause unwanted effects.

If you will be taking this medicine in large doses for a long time, *do not stop taking it without first checking with your doctor*. Your doctor may want you to reduce gradually the amount you are taking before stopping completely.

If you have been using this medicine for a long time and you think you may have become mentally or physically dependent on it, check with your doctor. Some signs of dependence on methylphenidate are:

- A strong desire or need to continue taking the medicine.
- A need to increase the dose to receive the effects of the medicine.
- Withdrawal side effects (for example, mental depression, unusual behavior, or unusual tiredness or weakness) occurring after the medicine is stopped.

Side Effects of This Medicine

Along with its needed effects, a medicine may cause some unwanted effects. Although not all of these side effects may occur, if they do occur they may need medical attention.

Check with your doctor as soon as possible if any of the following side effects occur:

More common

Fast heartbeat

Less common

Bruising; chest pain; fever; joint pain; skin rash or hives; uncontrolled movements of the body

Rare

Blurred vision or any change in vision; convulsions (seizures); sore throat and fever; unusual tiredness or weakness

With long-term use

Mood or mental changes; weight loss

Symptoms of overdose

Agitation; confusion; convulsions (seizures); delirium or hallucinations; dryness of mouth; false sense of well-being; fast, pounding, or irregular heartbeat; fever and sweating; headache (severe); increased blood pressure; muscle twitching; trembling or tremors; vomiting

Other side effects may occur that usually do not need medical attention. These side effects may go away during treatment as your body adjusts to the medicine. However, check with your doctor if any of the following side effects continue or are bothersome:

More common

Loss of appetite; nervousness; trouble in sleeping

Less common

Dizziness; drowsiness; headache; nausea; stomach pain

After you stop using this medicine, your body may need time to adjust. The length of time this takes depends on the amount of medicine you were using and how long you used it. During this period of time check with your doctor if you notice any of the following side effects:

Mental depression (severe); unusual behavior; unusual tiredness or weakness

Other side effects not listed above may also occur in some patients. If you notice any other effects, check with your doctor.

Annual revision: 03/09/93

METHYPRYLON Systemic

A commonly used brand name in the U.S. and Canada is Noludar.

Description

Methyprylon (meth-i-PRYE-lon) is used to treat insomnia (trouble in sleeping). However, it has generally been replaced by other medicines for the treatment of insomnia. If methyprylon is used regularly (for example, every day) to help produce sleep, it may not be effective for more than 1 week.

This medicine is available only with your doctor's prescription, in the following dosage forms:

Oral

- Capsules (U.S. and Canada)
- Tablets (U.S.)

It is very important that you read and understand the following information. If any of it causes you special concern, check with your doctor. Also, *if you have any questions* or if you want more information about this medicine or your medical problem, *ask your doctor, nurse, or pharmacist*.

Before Using This Medicine

In deciding to use a medicine, the risks of taking the medicine must be weighed against the good it will do.

This is a decision you and your doctor will make. For methyprylon, the following should be considered:

Allergies—Tell your doctor if you have ever had any unusual or allergic reaction to methyprylon. Also tell your doctor and pharmacist if you are allergic to any other substances, such as foods, preservatives, or dyes.

Pregnancy—Methyprylon has not been studied in pregnant women. However, it has not been shown to cause birth defects or other problems in animal studies.

Breast-feeding—It is not known whether methyprylon passes into the breast milk. However, this medicine has not been reported to cause problems in nursing babies.

Children—Studies on this medicine have been done only in adult patients and there is no specific information about its use in children.

Older adults—Elderly people may be especially sensitive to the effects of methyprylon. This may increase the chance of side effects during treatment.

Other medicines—Although certain medicines should not be used together at all, in other cases two different medicines may be used together even if an interaction might occur. In these cases, your doctor may want to change the dose, or other precautions may be necessary. When you are taking methyprylon, it is especially important that your doctor and pharmacist know if you are taking any of the following:

- Central nervous system (CNS) depressants, other—Using these medicines with methyprylon may increase the CNS and other depressant effects

Other medical problems—The presence of other medical problems may affect the use of methyprylon. Make sure you tell your doctor if you have any other medical problems, especially:

- Kidney disease or
- Liver disease—Higher blood levels of methyprylon may occur, increasing the chance of side effects
- Porphyria—Methyprylon may make the condition worse

Before you begin using any new medicine (prescription or nonprescription) or if you develop any new medical problem while you are using this medicine, check with your doctor, nurse, or pharmacist.

Proper Use of This Medicine

Take this medicine only as directed by your doctor. Do not take more of it, do not take it more often, and do not take it for a longer time than your doctor ordered. If too much is taken, it may become habit-forming.

Storage—To store this medicine:

- Keep out of the reach of children. Overdose of methyprylon is especially dangerous in children.
- Store away from heat and direct light.
- Do not store in the bathroom, near the kitchen sink, or in other damp places. Heat or moisture may cause the medicine to break down.
- Do not keep outdated medicine or medicine no longer needed. Be sure that any discarded medicine is out of the reach of children.

Precautions While Using This Medicine

If you will be taking this medicine regularly for a long time:

- Your doctor should check your progress at regular visits.
- Do not stop taking it without first checking with your doctor. Your doctor may want you to reduce gradually the amount you are taking before stopping completely.

This medicine will add to the effects of alcohol and other CNS depressants (medicines that slow down the nervous system, possibly causing drowsiness). Some examples of CNS depressants are antihistamines or medicine for hay fever, other allergies, or colds; sedatives, tranquilizers, or sleeping medicine; prescription pain medicine or narcotics; barbiturates; medicine for seizures; muscle relaxants; or anesthetics, including some dental anesthetics. *Check with your doctor before taking any of the above while you are taking this medicine.*

If you think you or someone else may have taken an overdose of this medicine, get emergency help at once. Taking an overdose of methyprylon or taking alcohol or other CNS depressants with methyprylon may lead to unconsciousness and possibly death. Some signs of an overdose are confusion, fast heartbeat, severe weakness, shortness of breath or slow or troubled breathing, and staggering.

This medicine may cause some people to become dizzy, drowsy, or less alert than they are normally. Even if taken at bedtime, it may cause some people to feel drowsy or less alert on arising. *Make sure you know how you react to this medicine before you drive, use machines, or do anything else that could be dangerous if you are dizzy or are not alert.*

Side Effects of This Medicine

Along with its needed effects, a medicine may cause some unwanted effects. Although not all of these side effects may occur, if they do occur they may need medical attention.

Check with your doctor as soon as possible if any of the following side effects occur:

Less common
Skin rash; unusual excitement

Rare

Fever (unexplained); mental depression; ulcers or sores in mouth or throat (continuing); unusual bleeding or bruising

Symptoms of overdose

Confusion; drowsiness (severe); fast heartbeat; shortness of breath or slow or troubled breathing; staggering; swelling of feet or lower legs; weakness (severe)

Other side effects may occur that usually do not need medical attention. These side effects may go away during treatment as your body adjusts to the medicine. However, check with your doctor if any of the following side effects continue or are bothersome:

More common

Dizziness; drowsiness (daytime) (mild); headache

Less common or rare

Blurred or double vision; clumsiness or unsteadiness; constipation; diarrhea; nausea; unusual weakness; vomiting

After you stop using this medicine, your body may need time to adjust. The length of time this takes depends on the amount of medicine you were using and how long you used it. During this period of time check with your doctor if you notice any of the following side effects:

Confusion; convulsions (seizures); hallucinations (seeing, hearing, or feeling things that are not there); increased dreaming; increased sweating; nausea or vomiting; nightmares; restlessness or nervousness; stomach cramps; trembling; trouble in sleeping; unusual weakness

Other side effects not listed above may also occur in some patients. If you notice any other effects, check with your doctor.

Annual revision: August 1990

METHYSERGIDE Systemic

A commonly used brand name in the U.S. and Canada is Sansert.

Description

Methysergide (meth-i-SER-jide) belongs to the group of medicines known as ergot alkaloids. It is used to prevent migraine headaches and some kinds of throbbing headaches. It is not used to treat an attack once it has started. The exact way methysergide acts on the body is not known.

This medicine is available only with your doctor's prescription, in the following dosage form:

Oral

- Tablets (U.S. and Canada)

It is very important that you read and understand the following information. If any of it causes you special concern, check with your doctor. Also, *if you have any questions* or if you want more information about this medicine or your medical problem, *ask your doctor, nurse, or pharmacist.*

Before Using This Medicine

In deciding to use a medicine, the risks of taking the medicine must be weighed against the good it will do. This is a decision you and your doctor will make. For methysergide, the following should be considered:

Allergies—Tell your doctor if you have ever had any unusual or allergic reaction to methysergide or to other ergot medicines. Also tell your doctor and pharmacist if you are allergic to any other substances, such as foods, preservatives, or dyes.

Pregnancy—Studies with methysergide have not been done in either humans or animals.

Breast-feeding—This medicine passes into the breast milk and may cause unwanted effects such as vomiting, diarrhea, weak pulse, unstable blood pressure, and convulsions (seizures) in nursing babies.

Children—Methysergide can cause serious side effects in any patient. Therefore, it is especially important that you discuss with the child's doctor the good that this medicine may do as well as the risks of using it.

Older adults—Elderly people are especially sensitive to the effects of methysergide. This may increase the chance of side effects during treatment.

Other medicines—Although certain medicines should not be used together at all, in other cases two different medicines may be used together even if an interaction might occur. In these cases, your doctor may want to change the dose, or other precautions may be necessary. When you are taking methysergide, it is important that your doctor and pharmacist know if you are using any other prescription or nonprescription (over-the-counter [OTC]) medicine, or if you smoke.

Other medical problems—The presence of other medical problems may affect the use of methysergide. Make sure you tell your doctor if you have any other medical problems, especially:

- Arthritis or
- Heart or blood vessel disease or
- Infection or
- Itching (severe) or
- Kidney disease or
- Liver disease or
- Lung disease—The chance of serious side effects may be increased
- High blood pressure or
- Stomach ulcer—Methysergide can make your condition worse

Before you begin using any new medicine (prescription or nonprescription) or if you develop any new medical problem while you are using this medicine, check with your doctor, nurse, or pharmacist.

Proper Use of This Medicine

Take this medicine only as directed by your doctor. If the amount you are to take does not prevent your headaches from occurring as often as before, do not take more than your doctor ordered. Instead, check with your doctor. Taking too much of this medicine or taking it too frequently may cause serious effects such as nausea and vomiting; cold, painful hands or feet; or even gangrene.

If this medicine upsets your stomach, it may be taken with meals or milk. If stomach upset continues or is severe, check with your doctor.

Missed dose—If you miss a dose of this medicine, skip the missed dose and go back to your regular dosing schedule. Do not double doses.

Storage—To store this medicine:
- Keep out of the reach of children.
- Store away from heat and direct light.
- Do not store in the bathroom, near the kitchen sink, or in other damp places. Heat or moisture may cause the medicine to break down.
- Do not keep outdated medicine or medicine no longer needed. Be sure that any discarded medicine is out of the reach of children.

Precautions While Using This Medicine

If you have been taking this medicine regularly, *do not stop taking it without first checking with your doctor.* Your doctor may want you to reduce gradually the amount you are using before stopping completely. If you stop taking it suddenly, your headaches may return or worsen.

Your doctor will tell you how long you should take this medicine. Usually it is not taken for longer than 6 months at a time. *If the doctor tells you to stop taking the medicine for a while, do not continue to take it.* If your body does not get a rest from the medicine, it can have harmful effects.

This medicine may cause some people to become dizzy, lightheaded, drowsy, or less alert than they are normally. Even if taken at bedtime, it may cause some people to feel drowsy or less alert on arising. *Make sure you know how you react to this medicine before you drive, use machines, or do anything else that could be dangerous if you are dizzy or are not alert.*

If dizziness occurs, get up slowly after lying or sitting down. If the problem continues or gets worse, check with your doctor.

Since drinking alcoholic beverages may make headaches worse, it is best to avoid alcohol while you are suffering from them. If you have any questions about this, check with your doctor.

Since smoking may increase some of the harmful effects of this medicine, it is best to avoid smoking while you are using it. If you have any questions about this, check with your doctor.

This medicine may make you more sensitive to cold temperatures, especially if you have blood circulation problems. It tends to decrease blood circulation in the skin, fingers, and toes. Dress warmly during cold weather and be careful during prolonged exposure to cold, such as in winter sports. This is especially important for elderly people, who are more likely than younger adults to already have problems with their circulation.

Check with your doctor if a serious infection or illness of any kind occurs while you are taking methysergide, since an infection may make you more sensitive to the medicine's effects.

Side Effects of This Medicine

Along with its needed effects, a medicine may cause some unwanted effects. Although not all of these side effects may occur, if they do occur they may need medical attention.

Check with your doctor immediately if any of the following side effects occur:

Chest pain or tightness in chest; difficult or painful urination; dizziness (severe); fever or chills; increase or decrease (large) in the amount of urine; leg cramps; pain in arms, legs, groin, lower back, or side; pale or cold hands or feet; shortness of breath or difficult breathing; swelling of hands, ankles, feet, or lower legs

Check with your doctor as soon as possible if the following side effects occur:

More common

Abdominal or stomach pain; itching; numbness and tingling of fingers, toes, or face; weakness in the legs

Less common or rare

Changes in vision; clumsiness or unsteadiness; cough or hoarseness; excitement or difficulty in thinking; fast or slow heartbeat; feeling of being outside the body;

hallucinations (seeing, hearing, or feeling things that are not there); loss of appetite or weight loss; mental depression; nightmares; raised red spots on skin; redness or flushing of face; skin rash

Other side effects may occur that usually do not need medical attention. These side effects may go away during treatment as your body adjusts to the medicine. However, check with your doctor if any of the following side effects continue or are bothersome:

More common

Diarrhea; dizziness or lightheadedness, especially when you get up from a lying or sitting position; drowsiness; nausea or vomiting

Less common or rare

Constipation; heartburn; trouble in sleeping

After you stop using this medicine, your body may need time to adjust. The length of time this takes depends on the amount of medicine you were using and how long you used it. During this time check with your doctor if your headaches begin again or worsen.

Other side effects not listed above may also occur in some patients. If you notice any other effects, check with your doctor.

Annual revision: July 1990

METOCLOPRAMIDE Systemic

Some commonly used brand names are:

In the U.S.

Clopra
Octamide
Octamide PFS
Reclomide
Reglan

Generic name product may also be available.

In Canada

Apo-Metoclop
Emex
Maxeran
Reglan

Description

Metoclopramide (met-oh-KLOE-pra-mide) is a medicine that increases the movements or contractions of the stomach and intestines. When given by injection it is used to help diagnose certain problems of the stomach and/or intestines. It is also used by injection to prevent the nausea and vomiting that may occur after treatment with anticancer medicines. Another medicine may be used with metoclopramide to prevent side effects that may occur when metoclopramide is used with anticancer medicines.

When taken by mouth, metoclopramide is used to treat the symptoms of a certain type of stomach problem called diabetic gastroparesis. It relieves symptoms such as nausea, vomiting, continued feeling of fullness after meals, and loss of appetite. Metoclopramide is also used, for a short time, to treat symptoms such as heartburn in patients who suffer esophageal injury from a backward flow of gastric acid into the esophagus.

Metoclopramide may also be used for other conditions as determined by your doctor.

Metoclopramide is available only with your doctor's prescription. It is available in the following dosage forms:

Oral

- Tablets (U.S. and Canada)
- Syrup (U.S. and Canada)

Parenteral

- Injection (U.S. and Canada)

It is very important that you read and understand the following information. If any of it causes you special concern, check with your doctor. Also, *if you have any questions* or if you want more information about this medicine or your medical problem, *ask your doctor, nurse, or pharmacist.*

Before Using This Medicine

In deciding to use a medicine, the risks of taking the medicine must be weighed against the good it will do. This is a decision you and your doctor will make. For metoclopramide, the following should be considered:

Allergies—Tell your doctor if you have ever had any unusual or allergic reaction to metoclopramide, procaine, or procainamide. Also tell your doctor and pharmacist if you are allergic to any other substances, such as foods, preservatives, or dyes.

Pregnancy—Not enough studies have been done in humans to determine metoclopramide's safety during pregnancy. However, metoclopramide has not been shown to cause birth defects or other problems in animal studies.

Breast-feeding—Although metoclopramide passes into the breast milk, it has not been shown to cause problems in nursing babies.

Children—Muscle spasms, especially of jaw, neck, and back, and tic-like (jerky) movements of head and face may be especially likely to occur in children, who are usually more sensitive than adults to the effects of metoclopramide. Premature and full-term infants may develop blood problems if given high doses of metoclopramide.

Older adults—Shuffling walk and trembling and shaking of hands may be especially likely to occur in elderly patients after they have taken metoclopramide over a long time.

Other medicines—Although certain medicines should not be used together at all, in other cases 2 different medicines may be used together even if an interaction might occur. In these cases, your doctor may want to change the dose, or other precautions may be necessary. When you are taking metoclopramide, it is especially important that your doctor and pharmacist know if you are taking the following:

- Central nervous system (CNS) depressants (medicine that causes drowsiness)—Use with metoclopramide may cause severe drowsiness

Other medical problems—The presence of other medical problems may affect the use of metoclopramide. Make sure you tell your doctor if you have any other medical problems, especially:

- Abdominal or stomach bleeding or
- Asthma or
- High blood pressure or
- Intestinal blockage or
- Parkinson's disease—Metoclopramide may make these conditions worse
- Epilepsy—Metoclopramide may increase the risk of having a seizure
- Kidney disease (severe) or
- Liver disease (severe)—Higher blood levels of metoclopramide may result, possibly increasing the chance of side effects

Before you begin using any new medicine (prescription or nonprescription) or if you develop any new medical problem while you are using this medicine, check with your doctor, nurse, or pharmacist.

Proper Use of This Medicine

Take this medicine 30 minutes before meals and at bedtime, unless otherwise directed by your doctor.

Take metoclopramide only as directed. Do not take more of it, do not take it more often, and do not take it for a longer time than your doctor ordered. To do so may increase the chance of side effects.

Missed dose—If you miss a dose of this medicine, take it as soon as possible. However, if it is almost time for your next dose, skip the missed dose and go back to your regular dosing schedule. Do not double doses.

Storage—To store this medicine:

- Keep out of the reach of children.
- Store away from heat and direct light.
- Do not store the tablet form of this medicine in the bathroom, near the kitchen sink, or in other damp places. Heat or moisture may cause the medicine to break down.
- Keep the syrup form of this medicine from freezing.
- Do not keep outdated medicine or medicine no longer needed. Be sure that any discarded medicine is out of the reach of children.

Precautions While Using This Medicine

This medicine will add to the effects of alcohol and other CNS depressants (medicines that slow down the nervous system, possibly causing drowsiness). Some examples of CNS depressants are antihistamines or medicine for hay fever, other allergies, or colds; sedatives, tranquilizers, or sleeping medicine; prescription pain medicine or narcotics; barbiturates; medicine for seizures; muscle relaxants; or anesthetics, including some dental anesthetics. *Check with your doctor before taking any of the above while you are using this medicine.*

This medicine may cause some people to become dizzy, lightheaded, drowsy, or less alert than they are normally. *Make sure you know how you react to this medicine before you drive, use machines, or do anything else that could be dangerous if you are dizzy or are not alert.*

Side Effects of This Medicine

Along with its needed effects, a medicine may cause some unwanted effects. Although not all of these side effects may occur, if they do occur they may need medical attention.

Check with your doctor as soon as possible if any of the following side effects occur:

Rare

Chills; difficulty in speaking or swallowing; dizziness or fainting; fast or irregular heartbeat; fever; general feeling of tiredness or weakness; headache (severe or continuing); increase in blood pressure; lip smacking or puckering; loss of balance control; mask-like face; rapid or worm-like movements of tongue; shuffling walk; sore throat; stiffness of arms or legs; trembling and shaking of hands and fingers; uncontrolled chewing movements; uncontrolled movements of arms and legs

With high doses—may occur within minutes of receiving a dose of metoclopramide and last for 2 to 24 hours

Aching or discomfort in lower legs; panic-like sensation; sensation of crawling in legs; unusual nervousness, restlessness, or irritability

Symptoms of overdose—may also occur rarely with usual doses, especially in children and young adults, and with high doses used to treat the nausea and vomiting caused by anticancer medicines

Confusion; drowsiness (severe)

Other side effects may occur that usually do not need medical attention. These side effects may go away during treatment as your body adjusts to the medicine. However, check with your doctor if any of the following side effects continue or are bothersome:

More common

Diarrhea—with high doses; drowsiness; restlessness

Less common or rare

Breast tenderness and swelling; changes in menstruation; constipation; depression; increased flow of breast milk; nausea; skin rash; trouble in sleeping; unusual dryness of mouth; unusual irritability

Other side effects not listed above may also occur in some patients. If you notice any other effects, check with your doctor.

Additional Information

Once a medicine has been approved for marketing for a certain use, experience may show that it is also useful for other medical problems. Although these uses are not included in product labeling, metoclopramide is used in certain patients with the following medical conditions:

- Failure of the stomach to empty its contents
- Nausea and vomiting caused by other medicines
- Persistent hiccups
- Prevention of aspirating fluid into the lungs during surgery
- Vascular headaches

Other than the above information, there is no additional information relating to proper use, precautions, or side effects for these uses.

Annual revision: 05/20/92

METRONIDAZOLE Systemic

Some commonly used brand names are:

In the U.S.

- Flagyl
- Flagyl I.V.
- Flagyl I.V. RTU
- Metric 21
- Metro I.V.
- Protostat

Generic name product may also be available.

In Canada

- Apo-Metronidazole
- Flagyl
- Novonidazol
- Trikacide

Generic name product may also be available.

Description

Metronidazole (me-troe-NI-da-zole) is used to treat infections. It may also be used for other problems as determined by your doctor. It will not work for colds, flu, or other virus infections.

Metronidazole is available only with your doctor's prescription, in the following dosage forms:

Oral

- Capsules (Canada)
- Tablets (U.S. and Canada)

Parenteral

- Injection (U.S. and Canada)

It is very important that you read and understand the following information. If any of it causes you special concern, check with your doctor. Also, *if you have any questions* or if you want more information about this medicine or your medical problem, *ask your doctor, nurse, or pharmacist.*

Before Using This Medicine

In deciding to use a medicine, the risks of taking the medicine must be weighed against the good it will do. This is a decision you and your doctor will make. For metronidazole, the following should be considered:

Allergies—Tell your doctor if you have ever had any unusual or allergic reaction to metronidazole. Also tell your doctor and pharmacist if you are allergic to any other substances, such as foods, preservatives, or dyes.

Pregnancy—Studies have not been done in humans. Metronidazole has not been shown to cause birth defects in animal studies; however, use is not recommended during the first trimester of pregnancy.

Breast-feeding—Use is not recommended in nursing mothers since metronidazole passes into the breast milk and may cause unwanted effects in the baby. However, in some infections your doctor may want you to stop breast-feeding and take this medicine for a short time. During this time the breast milk should be squeezed out or sucked out with a breast pump and thrown away. One or two days after you finish taking this medicine, you may go back to breast-feeding.

Children—Metronidazole has been used in children and, in effective doses, has not been shown to cause different side effects or problems in children than it does in adults.

Older adults—Many medicines have not been studied specifically in older people. Therefore, it may not be known whether they work exactly the same way they do in

younger adults or if they cause different side effects or problems in older people. There is no specific information comparing use of metronidazole in the elderly with use in other age groups.

Other medicines—Although certain medicines should not be used together at all, in other cases two different medicines may be used together even if an interaction might occur. In these cases, your doctor may want to change the dose, or other precautions may be necessary. When you are taking metronidazole, it is especially important that your doctor and pharmacist know if you are taking any of the following:

- Anticoagulants (blood thinners)—Patients taking anticoagulants with metronidazole may have an increased chance of bleeding
- Disulfiram (e.g., Antabuse)—Patients taking disulfiram with metronidazole may have an increase in side effects affecting the central nervous system

Other medical problems—The presence of other medical problems may affect the use of metronidazole. Make sure you tell your doctor if you have any other medical problems, especially:

- Blood disease or a history of blood disease—Metronidazole may make the condition worse
- Central nervous system (CNS) disease, including epilepsy—Metronidazole may increase the chance of seizures (convulsions) or other CNS side effects
- Heart disease—Metronidazole by injection may make heart disease worse
- Liver disease, severe—Patients with severe liver disease may have an increase in side effects

Before you begin using any new medicine (prescription or nonprescription) or if you develop any new medical problem while you are using this medicine, check with your doctor, nurse, or pharmacist.

Proper Use of This Medicine

If this medicine upsets your stomach, it may be taken with meals or a snack. If stomach upset (nausea, vomiting, stomach pain, or diarrhea) continues, check with your doctor.

To help clear up your infection completely, *keep taking this medicine for the full time of treatment,* even if you begin to feel better after a few days. If you stop taking this medicine too soon, your symptoms may return.

In some kinds of infections, this medicine works best when there is a constant amount in the blood. *To help keep the amount constant, do not miss any doses. Also, it is best to take the doses at evenly spaced times, day and night.* For example, if you are to take 4 doses a day, the doses should be spaced about 6 hours apart. If this interferes with your sleep or other daily activities, or if you need help in planning the best times to take your medicine, check with your doctor, nurse, or pharmacist.

Missed dose—If you do miss a dose of this medicine, take it as soon as possible. This will help to keep a constant amount of medicine in the blood. However, if it is almost time for your next dose, skip the missed dose and go back to your regular dosing schedule. Do not double doses.

Storage—To store this medicine:

- Keep out of the reach of children.
- Store away from heat and direct light.
- Do not store the capsule or tablet form of this medicine in the bathroom, near the kitchen sink, or in other damp places. Heat or moisture may cause the medicine to break down.
- Do not keep outdated medicine or medicine no longer needed. Be sure that any discarded medicine is out of the reach of children.

Precautions While Using This Medicine

If your symptoms do not improve within a few days, or if they become worse, check with your doctor.

Drinking alcoholic beverages while taking this medicine may cause stomach pain, nausea, vomiting, headache, or flushing or redness of the face. Other alcohol-containing preparations (for example, elixirs, cough syrups, tonics) may also cause problems. These problems may last for at least a day after you stop taking metronidazole. Also, this medicine may cause alcoholic beverages to taste different. Therefore, *you should not drink alcoholic beverages or take other alcohol-containing preparations while you are taking this medicine and for at least a day after stopping it.*

Metronidazole may cause dryness of the mouth, an unpleasant or sharp metallic taste, and a change in taste sensation. For temporary relief of dry mouth, use sugarless candy or gum, melt bits of ice in your mouth, or use a saliva substitute. However, if your mouth continues to feel dry for more than 2 weeks, check with your medical doctor or dentist. Continuing dryness of the mouth may increase the chance of dental disease, including tooth decay, gum disease, and fungus infections.

This medicine may also cause some people to become dizzy or lightheaded. *Make sure you know how you react to this medicine before you drive, use machines, or do anything else that could be dangerous if you are dizzy or are not alert.* If these reactions are especially bothersome, check with your doctor.

If you are taking this medicine for trichomoniasis (an infection of the sex organs in males and females), your doctor may want to treat your sexual partner at the same time you are being treated, even if he or she has no symptoms. Also, it may be desirable to use a condom (prophylactic) during intercourse. These measures will help keep you from getting the infection back again from your partner. If you have any questions about this, check with your doctor.

Side Effects of This Medicine

Along with its needed effects, a medicine may cause some unwanted effects. Although not all of these side effects may occur, if they do occur they may need medical attention.

Check with your doctor immediately if any of the following side effects occur:

Less common

Numbness, tingling, pain, or weakness in hands or feet

Rare

Convulsions (seizures)

Also, check with your doctor as soon as possible if any of the following side effects occur:

Less common

Any vaginal irritation, discharge, or dryness not present before use of this medicine; clumsiness or unsteadiness; mood or other mental changes; skin rash, hives, redness, or itching; sore throat and fever; stomach and back pain (severe)

For injection form

Pain, tenderness, redness, or swelling over vein in which the medicine is given

Other side effects may occur that usually do not need medical attention. These side effects may go away during treatment as your body adjusts to the medicine. However, check with your doctor if any of the following side effects continue or are bothersome:

More common

Diarrhea; dizziness or lightheadedness; headache; loss of appetite; nausea or vomiting; stomach pain or cramps

Less common or rare

Change in taste sensation; dryness of mouth; unpleasant or sharp metallic taste

In some patients metronidazole may cause dark urine. This is only temporary and will go away when you stop taking this medicine.

Other side effects not listed above may also occur in some patients. If you notice any other effects, check with your doctor.

Additional Information

Once a medicine has been approved for marketing for a certain use, experience may show that it is also useful for other medical problems. Although these uses are not included in product labeling, metronidazole is used in certain patients with the following medical conditions:

- Antibiotic-associated colitis
- Bacterial vaginosis
- Balantidiasis
- Dental infections
- Gastritis or ulcer due to *Helicobacter pylori*
- Giardiasis
- Inflammatory bowel disease

For patients taking this medicine for *giardiasis*:

- After treatment, it is important that your doctor check whether or not the infection in your intestinal tract has been cleared up completely.

Other than the above information, there is no additional information relating to proper use, precautions, or side effects for this use.

Annual revision: 10/20/92

METRONIDAZOLE Topical†

A commonly used brand name in the U.S. is MetroGel.

†Not commercially available in Canada.

Description

Topical metronidazole (me-troe-NI-da-zole) is applied to the skin in adults to help control rosacea (roe-ZAY-she-ah), also known as acne rosacea and "adult acne." This medicine helps to reduce the redness of the skin and the number of pimples, usually found on the face, in patients with rosacea.

Topical metronidazole is available only with your doctor's prescription, in the following dosage form:

Topical

- Topical gel (U.S.)

It is very important that you read and understand the following information. If any of it causes you special concern, check with your doctor. Also, *if you have any questions* or if you want more information about this medicine or your medical problem, *ask your doctor, nurse, or pharmacist.*

Before Using This Medicine

In deciding to use a medicine, the risks of taking the medicine must be weighed against the good it will do. This is a decision you and your doctor will make. For topical metronidazole, the following should be considered:

Allergies—Tell your doctor if you have ever had any unusual or allergic reaction to metronidazole. Also tell your doctor and pharmacist if you are allergic to any other substances, such as preservatives or dyes.

Pregnancy—Topical metronidazole has not been studied in pregnant women. However, metronidazole given by mouth (e.g., Flagyl) has not been shown to cause birth defects or other problems in animal studies.

Breast-feeding—Topical metronidazole is absorbed into the mother's body only in small amounts. The small amounts of this medicine that are absorbed are unlikely to cause serious problems in nursing babies.

Children—Rosacea is usually considered an adult disease. Therefore, topical metronidazole is not generally used in children.

Older adults—Many medicines have not been tested in older people. Therefore, it may not be known whether they work exactly the same way they do in younger adults or if they cause different side effects or problems in older people. There is no specific information about the use of topical metronidazole in the elderly.

Before you begin using any new medicine (prescription or nonprescription) or if you develop any new medical problem while you are using this medicine, check with your doctor, nurse, or pharmacist.

Proper Use of This Medicine

Do not use this medicine in or near the eyes. Watering of the eyes may occur when the medicine is used too close to the eyes.

If this medicine does get into your eyes, wash them out immediately, but carefully, with large amounts of cool tap water. If your eyes still burn or are painful, check with your doctor.

Before applying this medicine, thoroughly wash the affected area(s) with a mild, nonirritating cleanser, rinse well, and gently pat dry.

To use:

- After washing the affected area(s), apply this medicine with your fingertips. However, be sure to wash the medicine off your hands afterward.
- Apply and rub in a thin film of medicine, using enough to cover the affected area(s) lightly. *You should apply the medicine to the whole area usually affected by rosacea, not just to the pimples themselves.*

To help keep your rosacea under control, *keep using this medicine for the full time of treatment.* You may have to continue using this medicine every day for 9 weeks or longer. *Do not miss any doses.*

Missed dose—If you do miss a dose of this medicine, apply it as soon as possible. However, if it is almost time for your next dose, skip the missed dose and go back to your regular dosing schedule.

Storage—To store this medicine:

- Keep out of the reach of children.
- Store away from heat and direct light.
- Keep the medicine from freezing.
- Do not keep outdated medicine or medicine no longer needed. Be sure that any discarded medicine is out of the reach of children.

Precautions While Using This Medicine

If your rosacea does not improve within 3 weeks, or if it becomes worse, check with your doctor. However, treatment of rosacea may take up to 9 weeks or longer before you see full improvement.

Stinging or burning of the skin may be expected after this medicine is applied. These effects may last up to a few minutes or more. If irritation continues, check with your doctor. You may have to use the medicine less often or stop using it altogether. Follow your doctor's directions.

You may continue to use cosmetics (make-up) while you are using this medicine for rosacea. However, it is best to use only "oil-free" cosmetics. Also, it is best not to use cosmetics too heavily or too often. They may make your rosacea worse. If you have any questions about this, check with your doctor.

Side Effects of This Medicine

Along with its needed effects, a medicine may cause some unwanted effects. The following side effects may go away during treatment as your body adjusts to the medicine. However, check with your doctor if any of these effects continue or are bothersome:

Less common

Dry skin; redness or other sign of skin irritation not present before use of this medicine; stinging or burning of the skin; watering of eyes

Other side effects not listed above may also occur in some patients. If you notice any other effects, check with your doctor.

Annual revision: June 1990

METYRAPONE Systemic

A commonly used brand name is:

In the U.S.
Metopirone

In Canada
Metopirone

Description

Metyrapone (me-TEER-a-pone) is used in the diagnosis of certain problems of the adrenal glands. These glands are located near the kidneys. The adrenal glands produce a steroid chemical called cortisol (hydrocortisone) that helps the body respond to stress or illness. From the results of a metyrapone test, your doctor will be able to tell if your adrenal glands produce the correct amount of cortisol under stress or during illnesses.

How test is done: Metyrapone is taken by mouth in one or more doses the day before the testing is done. The next day, blood and/or urine samples are taken. A tube called a catheter may be placed in your bladder to help take the urine sample. The amount of hormones in your blood or urine is measured. Then the results of the test are studied.

Metyrapone may also be used for other conditions as determined by your doctor.

Metyrapone is available only with your doctor's prescription, in the following dosage form:

Oral

- Tablets (U.S. and Canada)

It is very important that you read and understand the following information. If any of it causes you special concern, check with your doctor. Also, *if you have any questions* or if you want more information about this medicine or your medical problem, *ask your doctor, nurse, or pharmacist.*

Before Using This Medicine

In deciding to use a medicine, the risks of taking the medicine must be weighed against the good it will do. This is a decision you and your doctor will make. For metyrapone, the following should be considered:

Allergies—Tell your doctor if you have ever had any unusual or allergic reaction to metyrapone. Also, tell your doctor and pharmacist if you are allergic to any other substances, such as foods, preservatives, or dyes.

Pregnancy—Metyrapone has not been fully studied in pregnant women. However, some small studies have shown that metyrapone can affect the production of chemicals by the pituitary and adrenal glands of the fetus. Also, the large amounts of estrogen produced by your body during pregnancy may cause false results in metyrapone testing. Before you take metyrapone, make sure your doctor knows if you are pregnant or if you may become pregnant.

Breast-feeding—It is not known whether metyrapone passes into the breast milk. However, use of metyrapone is not recommended during breast-feeding because it may cause unwanted effects in nursing babies.

Children—This medicine has been tested in children and has not been shown to cause different side effects or problems in children than it does in adults.

Older adults—Although there is no specific information about the use of metyrapone in the elderly, it is not expected to cause different side effects or problems in older people than it does in younger adults.

Other medicines—Although certain medicines should not be used together at all, in other cases 2 different medicines may be used together even if an interaction might occur. In these cases, your doctor may want to change the dose, or other precautions may be necessary. When you are taking metyrapone, it is especially important that your doctor and pharmacist know if you are also taking any other medicines, since many medicines can cause false results in metyrapone testing. This may result in a wrong diagnosis. It is especially important that your doctor know if you are taking any of the following:

- Alcohol (with chronic use)
- Barbiturates
- Carbamazepine (e.g., Tegretol)
- Corticosteroids (cortisone-like medicine)
- Estrogens (female hormones)
- Griseofulvin (e.g., Fulvicin)

- Oral contraceptives (birth control pills) containing estrogen
- Phenylbutazone (e.g., Butazolidin)
- Phenytoin (e.g., Dilantin)
- Primidone (e.g., Mysoline)
- Rifampin (e.g., Rifadin)

Other medical problems—The presence of other medical problems may affect the use of metyrapone. Make sure you tell your doctor if you have any other medical problems, especially:

- Breast cancer or
- Diabetes mellitus (sugar diabetes) or
- Heart disease or
- Liver disease or
- Low blood sugar or
- Thyroid disease—These conditions may cause false results in metyrapone testing and result in a wrong diagnosis
- Excessive body hair in females—Long-term use may increase growth of body hair
- Porphyria—Metyrapone may worsen active cases of porphyria
- Underactive adrenal or pituitary gland—Metyrapone may severely reduce the amount of certain hormones produced by the adrenal glands; these hormones are needed to respond to stress or illness

Before you begin using any new medicine (prescription or nonprescription) or if you develop any new medical problem while you are using this medicine, check with your doctor, nurse, or pharmacist.

Proper Use of This Medicine

Metyrapone may cause nausea and vomiting, especially if taken in larger doses. Taking each dose with food or milk or immediately after eating may lessen this effect.

Before you have any medical tests, tell the doctor in charge that you are taking this medicine. The results of some tests may be affected by this medicine.

Missed dose—If you are taking metyrapone every day to treat Cushing's syndrome and you miss a dose, take it as soon as possible. However, if it is almost time for your next dose, skip the missed dose and go back to your regular dosing schedule. Do not double doses. If you are taking metyrapone for a test procedure and you miss a dose, contact your physician. Missing doses or taking them on the wrong schedule may cause false test results.

Storage—To store this medicine:

- Keep out of the reach of children.
- Store away from heat and direct light.
- Do not store in the bathroom, near the kitchen sink, or in other damp places. Heat or moisture may cause the medicine to break down.
- Do not keep outdated medicine or medicine no longer needed. Be sure that any discarded medicine is out of the reach of children.

Precautions While Using This Medicine

This medicine may cause some people to become dizzy, lightheaded, drowsy, or less alert than they are normally. Even if taken at bedtime, it may cause some people to feel drowsy or less alert on arising. *Make sure you know how you react to this medicine before you drive, use machines, or do anything else that could be dangerous if you are dizzy or are not alert.*

Side Effects of This Medicine

Along with its needed effects, a medicine may cause some unwanted effects. Although not all of these side effects may occur, if they do occur they may need medical attention.

Check with your doctor immediately if any of the following side effects occur:

Rare (with long-term use)

Irregular heartbeat

Check with your doctor as soon as possible if any of the following side effects occur:

Less common

Skin rash

Rare (usually with long-term use)

Enlargement of clitoris; muscle cramps or pain; sore throat or fever; swelling of feet or lower legs; unusual bleeding or bruising; unusual tiredness or weakness; weight gain (rapid)

Symptoms of overdose

Abdominal or stomach pain (severe); confusion; decrease in consciousness; diarrhea (severe); nausea (severe); nervousness; unusual thirst; vomiting (severe); weakness (sudden)

Other side effects may occur that usually do not need medical attention. These side effects may go away during treatment as your body adjusts to the medicine. However, check with your doctor if any of the following side effects continue or are bothersome:

More common

Dizziness; drowsiness; headache; lightheadedness; nausea

Rare

Confusion or mental slowing; excessive hair growth; greater-than-normal loss of scalp hair; increased sweating; loss of appetite; upper abdominal or stomach pain; vomiting; worsening of acne

Other side effects not listed above may also occur in some patients. If you notice any other effects, check with your doctor.

Additional Information

Once a medicine has been approved for marketing for a certain use, experience may show that it is also useful

for other medical problems. Although this use is not included in product labeling, metyrapone is used in certain patients with the following medical condition:

- Cushing's syndrome (diagnosis and treatment)

Since treatment for Cushing's syndrome may require longer therapy, side effects are more likely to occur.

Annual revision: 07/08/92

METYROSINE Systemic†

A commonly used brand name in the U.S. is Demser.

†Not commercially available in Canada.

Description

Metyrosine (me-TYE-roe-seen) belongs to the general class of medicines called antihypertensives. It is used to treat high blood pressure (hypertension) caused by a disease called pheochromocytoma (a noncancerous tumor of the adrenal gland).

Metyrosine reduces the amount of certain chemicals in the body. When these chemicals are present in large amounts, they cause high blood pressure.

Metyrosine is available only with your doctor's prescription, in the following dosage form:

Oral

- Capsules (U.S.)

It is very important that you read and understand the following information. If any of it causes you special concern, check with your doctor. Also, *if you have any questions* or if you want more information about this medicine or your medical problem, *ask your doctor, nurse, or pharmacist.*

Before Using This Medicine

In deciding to use a medicine, the risks of taking the medicine must be weighed against the good it will do. This is a decision you and your doctor will make. For metyrosine, the following should be considered:

Allergies—Tell your doctor if you have ever had any unusual or allergic reaction to metyrosine. Also tell your doctor and pharmacist if you are allergic to any other substances, such as foods, sulfites or other preservatives, or dyes.

Pregnancy—Studies on effects in pregnancy have not been done in either humans or animals.

Breast-feeding—It is not known whether metyrosine passes into breast milk. However, this medicine has not been reported to cause problems in nursing babies.

Children—Studies on this medicine have been done only in adult patients, and there is no specific information comparing use of metyrosine in children with use in other age groups.

Older adults—Many medicines have not been studied specifically in older people. Therefore, it may not be known whether they work exactly the same way they do in younger adults or if they cause different side effects or problems in older people. There is no specific information comparing use of metyrosine in the elderly with use in other age groups.

Other medicines—Although certain medicines should not be used together at all, in other cases two different medicines may be used together even if an interaction might occur. In these cases, your doctor may want to change the dose, or other precautions may be necessary. Tell your doctor or pharmacist if you are taking any other prescription or nonprescription (over-the-counter [OTC]) medicine.

Other medical problems—The presence of other medical problems may affect the use of metyrosine. Make sure you tell your doctor if you have any other medical problems, especially:

- Kidney disease or
- Liver disease—Effects of metyrosine may be increased because of slower removal from the body
- Mental depression (or history of) or
- Parkinson's disease—Metyrosine may make these conditions worse

Before you begin using any new medicine (prescription or nonprescription) or if you develop any new medical problem while you are using this medicine, check with your doctor, nurse, or pharmacist.

Proper Use of This Medicine

Take this medicine only as directed by your doctor. Do not take more or less of it than your doctor ordered.

To help you remember to take your medicine, try to get into the habit of taking it at the same times each day.

Dosing—The dose of metyrosine will be different for different patients. *Follow your doctor's orders or the directions on the label.* The following information includes only the average doses of metyrosine. *If your dose is*

different, do not change it unless your doctor tells you to do so:
- For *oral* dosage forms (capsules):
  —Adults and children 12 years of age and older: 1000 milligrams to 3000 milligrams (1 to 3 grams) a day, divided into four doses.

Missed dose—If you miss a dose of this medicine, take it as soon as possible. However, if it is almost time for your next dose, skip the missed dose and go back to your regular dosing schedule. Do not double doses.

Storage—To store this medicine:
- Keep out of the reach of children.
- Store away from heat and direct light.
- Do not store in the bathroom, near the kitchen sink, or in other damp places. Heat or moisture may cause the medicine to break down.
- Do not keep outdated medicine or medicine no longer needed. Be sure that any discarded medicine is out of the reach of children.

Precautions While Using This Medicine

It is important that your doctor check your progress at regular visits to make sure that this medicine is working properly and to check for unwanted effects.

While taking this medicine, it is important that you drink plenty of fluids and urinate often. This will help prevent kidney problems and keep your kidneys working well. If you have any questions about how much you should drink, check with your doctor.

This medicine will add to the effects of alcohol and other CNS depressants (medicines that slow down the nervous system, possibly causing drowsiness). Some examples of CNS depressants are antihistamines or medicine for hay fever, other allergies, or colds; sedatives, tranquilizers, or sleeping medicine; prescription pain medicine or narcotics; barbiturates; medicine for seizures; tricyclic antidepressants (medicine for depression); muscle relaxants; or anesthetics, including some dental anesthetics. *Check with your doctor before taking any of the above while you are taking this medicine.*

Before having any kind of surgery (including dental surgery), tell the medical doctor or dentist in charge that you are taking this medicine.

This medicine may cause most people to become drowsy or less alert than they are normally. *Make sure you know how you react to this medicine before you drive, use machines, or do anything else that could be dangerous if you are not alert.*

Side Effects of This Medicine

Along with its needed effects, a medicine may cause some unwanted effects. Although not all of these side effects may occur, if they do occur they may need medical attention.

Check with your doctor as soon as possible if any of the following side effects occur:

More common

Diarrhea; drooling; trembling and shaking of hands and fingers; trouble in speaking

Less common

Anxiety; confusion; hallucinations (seeing, hearing, or feeling things that are not there); mental depression

Rare

Black, tarry stools; blood in urine or stools; unusual bleeding or bruising; muscle spasms, especially of neck and back; painful urination; pinpoint red spots on skin; restlessness; shortness of breath; shuffling walk; skin rash and itching; swelling of feet or lower legs; tic-like (jerky) movements of head, face, mouth, and neck; unusual tiredness or weakness

Other side effects may occur that usually do not need medical attention. These side effects may go away during treatment as your body adjusts to the medicine. However, check with your doctor if any of the following side effects continue or are bothersome:

More common

Drowsiness

Less common

Decreased sexual ability in men; dryness of mouth; nausea, vomiting, or stomach pain; stuffy nose; swelling of breasts or unusual milk production

After you stop taking this medicine, it may still produce some side effects that need attention. During this period of time check with your doctor if you notice the following side effect:

Diarrhea

Also, after you stop taking this medicine, you may have feelings of increased energy or you may have trouble sleeping. However, these effects should last only for two or three days.

Other side effects not listed above may also occur in some patients. If you notice any other effects, check with your doctor.

Annual revision: 01/20/93

MEXILETINE Systemic

A commonly used brand name in the U.S. and Canada is Mexitil.

Description

Mexiletine (MEX-i-le-teen) belongs to the group of medicines known as antiarrhythmics. It is used to correct irregular heartbeats to a normal rhythm.

Mexiletine produces its helpful effects by slowing nerve impulses in the heart and making the heart tissue less sensitive.

Mexiletine is available only with your doctor's prescription, in the following dosage form:

Oral

- Capsules (U.S. and Canada)

It is very important that you read and understand the following information. If any of it causes you special concern, check with your doctor. Also, *if you have any questions* or if you want more information about this medicine or your medical problem, *ask your doctor, nurse, or pharmacist.*

Before Using This Medicine

In deciding to use a medicine, the risks of taking the medicine must be weighed against the good it will do. This is a decision you and your doctor will make. For mexiletine, the following should be considered:

Allergies—Tell your doctor if you have ever had any unusual or allergic reaction to mexiletine, lidocaine, or tocainide. Also tell your doctor and pharmacist if you are allergic to any other substance, such as foods, preservatives, or dyes.

Pregnancy—Mexiletine has not been studied in pregnant women. However, studies in animals have shown that mexiletine causes a decrease in successful pregnancies but no birth defects. Before taking this medicine, make sure your doctor knows if you are pregnant or if you may become pregnant.

Breast-feeding—Mexiletine passes into breast milk. Because this medicine may cause serious side effects, breast-feeding is generally not recommended while you are receiving it. Be sure you have discussed this with your doctor before taking mexiletine.

Children—Studies on this medicine have been done only in adult patients, and there is no specific information comparing use of mexiletine in children with use in other age groups.

Older adults—Many medicines have not been studied specifically in older people. Therefore, it may not be known whether they work exactly the same way they do in younger adults or if they cause different side effects or problems in older people. There is no specific information comparing use of mexiletine in the elderly with use in other age groups.

Other medicines—Although certain medicines should not be used together at all, in other cases two different medicines may be used together even if an interaction might occur. In these cases, your doctor may want to change the dose, or other precautions may be necessary. Tell your doctor and pharmacist if you are taking any other prescription or nonprescription (over-the-counter [OTC]) medicine.

Smoking—Smoking may decrease the effects of mexiletine.

Other medical problems—The presence of other medical problems may affect the use of mexiletine. Make sure you tell your doctor if you have any other medical problems, especially:

- Congestive heart failure or
- Low blood pressure—Mexiletine may make these conditions worse
- Heart attack (severe) or
- Liver disease—Effects may last longer because of slower removal of mexiletine from the body
- Seizures (history of)—Mexiletine can cause seizures

Before you begin using any new medicine (prescription or nonprescription) or if you develop any new medical problem while you are using this medicine, check with your doctor, nurse, or pharmacist.

Proper Use of This Medicine

Take mexiletine exactly as directed by your doctor, even though you may feel well. Do not take more medicine than ordered.

To lessen the possibility of stomach upset, mexiletine should be taken with food or immediately after meals or with milk or an antacid.

This medicine works best when there is a constant amount in the blood. *To help keep this amount constant, do not miss any doses. Also it is best to take the doses at evenly spaced times day and night.* For example, if you are to take 3 doses a day, the doses should be spaced about 8 hours apart. If this interferes with your sleep or other daily activities, or if you need help in planning the best times to take your medicine, check with your doctor, nurse, or pharmacist.

Missed dose—If you miss a dose of this medicine and remember within 4 hours, take it as soon as possible. Then go back to your regular dosing schedule. However, if you do not remember until later, skip the missed dose and go back to your regular dosing schedule. Do not double doses.

Storage—To store this medicine:

- Keep out of the reach of children.
- Store away from heat and direct light.
- Do not store in the bathroom, near the kitchen sink, or in other damp places. Heat or moisture may cause the medicine to break down.
- Do not keep outdated medicine or medicine no longer needed. Be sure that any discarded medicine is out of the reach of children.

Precautions While Using This Medicine

It is important that your doctor check your progress at regular visits to make sure the medicine is working properly. This will allow for changes to be made in the amount of medicine you are taking, if necessary.

Your doctor may want you to carry a medical identification card or bracelet stating that you are using this medicine.

Before having any kind of surgery (including dental surgery) or emergency treatment, tell the medical doctor or dentist in charge that you are taking this medicine.

Mexiletine may cause some people to become dizzy, lightheaded, or less alert than they are normally. *Make sure you know how you react to this medicine before you drive, use machines, or do anything else that could be dangerous if you are dizzy or are not alert.*

Side Effects of This Medicine

Along with its needed effects, a medicine may cause some unwanted effects. Although not all of these side effects may occur, if they do occur they may need medical attention.

Check with your doctor as soon as possible if any of the following side effects occur:

Less common

Chest pain; fast or irregular heartbeat; shortness of breath

Rare

Convulsions (seizures); fever or chills; unusual bleeding or bruising

Other side effects may occur that usually do not need medical attention. These side effects may go away during treatment as your body adjusts to the medicine. However, check with your doctor if any of the following side effects continue or are bothersome:

More common

Dizziness or lightheadedness; heartburn; nausea and vomiting; nervousness; trembling or shaking of the hands; unsteadiness or difficulty in walking

Less common

Blurred vision; confusion; constipation or diarrhea; headache; numbness or tingling of fingers and toes; ringing in the ears; skin rash; slurred speech; trouble in sleeping; unusual tiredness or weakness

Other side effects not listed above may also occur in some patients. If you notice any other effects, check with your doctor.

Annual revision: 10/06/92

MICONAZOLE Systemic†

A commonly used brand name in the U.S. is Monistat I.V.

†Not commercially available in Canada.

Description

Miconazole (mi-KON-a-zole) belongs to the group of medicines called antifungals. It is used to treat certain fungus infections.

Miconazole is available only with your doctor's prescription, in the following dosage form:

Parenteral

- Injection (U.S.)

It is very important that you read and understand the following information. If any of it causes you special concern, check with your doctor. Also, *if you have any questions* or if you want more information about this medicine or your medical problem, *ask your doctor, nurse, or pharmacist.*

Before Receiving This Medicine

In deciding to use a medicine, the risks of taking the medicine must be weighed against the good it will do. This is a decision you and your doctor will make. For miconazole, the following should be considered:

Allergies—Tell your doctor if you have ever had any unusual or allergic reaction to miconazole, or other related medicines, such as fluconazole, ketoconazole, or itraconazole. Also tell your doctor and pharmacist if you are allergic to any other substances, such as foods, preservatives, or dyes.

Pregnancy—Studies have not been done in humans. However, miconazole has not been shown to cause birth defects or other problems in studies in rats and rabbits.

Breast-feeding—Miconazole has not been reported to cause problems in nursing babies.

Children—This medicine has been tested in a limited number of children 1 year of age or older and, in effective doses, has not been reported to cause different side effects or problems in children than it does in adults.

Older adults—Many medicines have not been studied specifically in older people. Therefore, it may not be known whether they work exactly the same way they do in younger adults or if they cause different side effects or problems in older people. There is no specific information comparing use of intravenous miconazole in the elderly with use in other age groups.

Other medicines—Although certain medicines should not be used together at all, in other cases two different medicines may be used together even if an interaction might occur. In these cases, your doctor may want to change the dose, or other precautions may be necessary. When you are receiving miconazole, it is especially important that your doctor and pharmacist know if you are taking any of the following:

- Isoniazid (e.g., INH, Nydrazid) or
- Rifampin (e.g., Rifadin)—Use of these medicines with miconazole may decrease the effects of miconazole

Before you begin using any new medicine (prescription or nonprescription) or if you develop any new medical problem while you are using this medicine, check with your doctor, nurse, or pharmacist.

Side Effects of This Medicine

Along with its needed effects, a medicine may cause some unwanted effects. Although not all of these side effects may occur, if they do occur they may need medical attention.

Check with your doctor as soon as possible if any of the following side effects occur:

More common

Fever and chills; redness, swelling, or pain at place of injection; skin rash or itching

Less common or rare

Unusual bleeding or bruising; unusual tiredness or weakness

Other side effects may occur that usually do not need medical attention. These side effects may go away during treatment as your body adjusts to the medicine. However, check with your doctor if any of the following side effects continue or are bothersome:

More common

Diarrhea; loss of appetite; nausea or vomiting

Less common

Drowsiness; flushing or redness of face or skin

Other side effects not listed above may also occur in some patients. If you notice any other effects, check with your doctor.

Annual revision: 10/20/92

MICONAZOLE Topical

Some commonly used brand names in the U.S. and Canada are Micatin and Monistat-Derm.

Description

Miconazole (mi-KON-a-zole) belongs to the group of medicines called antifungals. Topical miconazole is used to treat some types of fungus infections.

Some of these preparations may be available without a prescription; however, your doctor may have special instructions on the proper use of these medicines for your medical problem. Others are available only with your doctor's prescription.

Topical miconazole is available in the following dosage forms:

Topical

- Aerosol powder (U.S.)
- Aerosol solution (U.S.)
- Cream (U.S. and Canada)
- Lotion (U.S. and Canada)
- Powder (U.S.)

It is very important that you read and understand the following information. If any of it causes you special concern, check with your doctor or pharmacist. Also, *if you have any questions* or if you want more information about this medicine or your medical problem, *ask your doctor, nurse, or pharmacist.*

Before Using This Medicine

If you are taking this medicine without a prescription, carefully read and follow any precautions on the label. For miconazole, the following should be considered:

Allergies—Tell your doctor if you have ever had any unusual or allergic reaction to miconazole. Also tell your doctor and pharmacist if you are allergic to any other substances, such as preservatives or dyes.

Pregnancy—Miconazole topical preparations have not been shown to cause birth defects or other problems in humans.

Breast-feeding—Miconazole topical preparations have not been reported to cause problems in nursing babies.

Children—Although there is no specific information about the use of topical miconazole in children, it is not expected to cause different side effects or problems in children than it does in adults.

Older adults—Many medicines have not been tested in older people. Therefore, it may not be known whether they work exactly the same way they do in younger adults. Although there is no specific information about the use of topical miconazole in the elderly, it is not expected to cause different side effects or problems in older people than it does in younger adults.

Other medicines—Although certain medicines should not be used together at all, in other cases two different medicines may be used together even if an interaction might occur. In these cases, your doctor may want to change the dose, or other precautions may be necessary. When you are using miconazole, it is important that your doctor and pharmacist know if you are using any other topical prescription or nonprescription (over-the-counter [OTC]) medicine that is to be applied to the same area of the skin.

Before you begin using any new medicine (prescription or nonprescription) or if you develop any new medical problem while you are using this medicine, check with your doctor, nurse, or pharmacist.

Proper Use of This Medicine

Keep this medicine away from the eyes.

Apply enough miconazole to cover the affected area, and rub in gently.

To use the *aerosol powder form* of miconazole:

- Shake well before using.
- From a distance of 6 to 10 inches, spray the powder on the affected areas. If it is used on the feet, spray it between the toes, on the feet, and in the socks and shoes.
- Do not inhale the powder.
- Do not use near heat, near open flame, or while smoking.

To use the *powder form* of miconazole:

- If the powder is used on the feet, sprinkle it between the toes, on the feet, and in the socks and shoes.

To use the *aerosol solution form* of miconazole:

- Shake well before using.
- From a distance of 4 to 6 inches, spray the solution on the affected areas. If it is used on the feet, spray it between the toes and on the feet.
- Do not inhale the vapors from the spray.
- Do not use near heat, near open flame, or while smoking.

When miconazole is used to treat certain types of fungus infections of the skin, an occlusive dressing (airtight covering such as, kitchen plastic wrap) should *not* be applied over this medicine. To do so may cause irritation of the skin. *Do not apply an occlusive dressing over this medicine unless you have been directed to do so by your doctor.*

To help clear up your infection completely, *keep using this medicine for the full time of treatment,* even if your condition has improved. *Do not miss any doses.*

Missed dose—If you do miss a dose of this medicine, apply it as soon as possible. However, if it is almost time for your next dose, skip the missed dose and go back to your regular dosing schedule.

Storage—To store this medicine:

- Keep out of the reach of children.
- Store away from heat and direct light.
- Do not store the powder form of this medicine in the bathroom, near the kitchen sink, or in other damp places. Heat or moisture may cause the medicine to break down.
- Keep the cream, lotion, and aerosol solution forms of this medicine from freezing.
- Do not puncture, break, or burn the aerosol powder or aerosol solution container.
- Do not keep outdated medicine or medicine no longer needed. Be sure that any discarded medicine is out of the reach of children.

Precautions While Using This Medicine

If your skin problem does not improve within 4 weeks, or if it becomes worse, check with your doctor or pharmacist.

Side Effects of This Medicine

Along with its needed effects, a medicine may cause some unwanted effects. Although not all of these side effects may occur, if they do occur they may need medical attention.

Check with your doctor as soon as possible if any of the following side effects occur:

Skin rash, blistering, burning, redness, or other sign of skin irritation not present before use of this medicine

Other side effects not listed above may also occur in some patients. If you notice any other effects, check with your doctor.

Annual revision: May 1990

MIDAZOLAM Systemic

A commonly used brand name in the U.S. and Canada is Versed.

Description

Midazolam (mid-AY-zoe-lam) is used to produce sleepiness or drowsiness and to relieve anxiety before surgery or certain procedures. It is also used to produce loss of consciousness before and during surgery.

Midazolam is given only by or under the immediate supervision of a doctor trained to use this medicine. If you will be receiving midazolam during surgery, your doctor or anesthesiologist will give you the medicine and closely follow your progress.

Midazolam is available in the following dosage form:

Parenteral

- Injection (U.S. and Canada)

It is very important that you read and understand the following information. If any of it causes you special concern, check with your doctor. Also, *if you have any questions* or if you want more information about this medicine or your medical problem, *ask your doctor, nurse, or pharmacist.*

Before Receiving This Medicine

In deciding to use a medicine, the risks of taking the medicine must be weighed against the good it will do. This is a decision you and your doctor will make. For midazolam, the following should be considered:

Allergies—Tell your doctor if you have ever had any unusual or allergic reaction to midazolam or other benzodiazepines (such as alprazolam [e.g., Xanax], bromazepam [e.g., Lectopam], chlordiazepoxide [e.g., Librium], clonazepam [e.g., Klonopin], diazepam [e.g., Valium], estazolam [e.g., ProSom], flurazepam [e.g., Dalmane], halazepam [e.g., Paxipam], ketazolam [e.g., Loftran], lorazepam [e.g., Ativan], nitrazepam [e.g., Mogadon], oxazepam [e.g., Serax], prazepam [e.g., Centrax], quazepam [e.g., Doral], temazepam [e.g., Restoril], triazolam [e.g., Halcion]). Also, tell your doctor and pharmacist if you are allergic to any other substances, such as foods, preservatives, or dyes.

Pregnancy—Midazolam is not recommended for use during pregnancy because it may cause birth defects. Other benzodiazepines, such as chlordiazepoxide (e.g., Librium) and diazepam (e.g., Valium) that are related chemically and in action to midazolam, have been reported to increase the chance of birth defects when used during the first 3 months of pregnancy. Also, use of midazolam during pregnancy, especially during the last few days, may cause drowsiness, slow heartbeat, shortness of breath, or troubled breathing in the newborn infant. In addition, receiving midazolam just before or during labor may cause weakness in the newborn infant.

Breast-feeding—It is not known whether midazolam passes into the breast milk. However, this medicine has not been reported to cause problems in nursing babies.

Children—Although there is no specific information comparing use of midazolam in children with use in other age groups, this medicine is not expected to cause different side effects or problems in children than it does in adults.

Older Adults—Elderly people are especially sensitive to the effects of midazolam. This may increase the chance of side effects during the use of this medicine. Also, time to complete recovery after midazolam is given may be slower in the elderly than in younger adults.

Other medicines—Although certain medicines should not be used together at all, in other cases 2 different medicines may be used together even if an interaction might occur. In these cases, your doctor may want to change the dose, or other precautions may be necessary. When you are receiving midazolam, it is especially important that your doctor and pharmacist know if you are taking any of the following:

- Central nervous system (CNS) depressants (medicine that causes drowsiness)—The CNS depressant and other effects of either these medicines or midazolam may be increased; also, the effects of midazolam may be prolonged

Other medical problems—The presence of other medical problems may affect the use of midazolam. Make sure you tell your doctor if you have any other medical problems, especially:

- Heart disease or
- Kidney disease or
- Liver disease or
- Obesity (overweight)—The effects of midazolam may be prolonged
- Lung disease or
- Myasthenia gravis or other muscle and nerve disease—Midazolam may make the condition worse

Before you begin using any new medicine (prescription or nonprescription) or if you develop any new medical problem while you are using this medicine, check with your doctor, nurse, or pharmacist.

Precautions After Receiving This Medicine

For patients going home within 24 hours after receiving midazolam:

- Midazolam may cause some people to feel drowsy, tired, or weak for one or two days after it has been given. It may also cause problems with coordination and one's ability to think. Therefore, *do not drive, use machines, or do anything else that could be dangerous if you are not alert* until the effects of the medicine have disappeared or until the day after you receive midazolam, whichever period of time is longer.
- *Do not drink alcoholic beverages or take other CNS depressants (medicines that slow down the nervous system, possibly causing drowsiness) for about 24 hours after you have received midazolam, unless otherwise directed by your doctor.* To do so may add to the effects of the medicine. Some examples of CNS depressants are antihistamines or medicine for hay fever, other allergies, or colds; other sedatives, tranquilizers, or sleeping medicine; prescription pain medicine or narcotics; medicine for seizures; and muscle relaxants.

Side Effects of This Medicine

Some side effects may occur that usually do not need medical attention. The following side effects may go away as the effects of midazolam wear off. However, check with your doctor if any of the following side effects continue or are bothersome:

Less common or rare

Blurred vision or other changes in vision; coughing; dizziness, lightheadedness, or feeling faint; drowsiness (prolonged); headache; hiccups; nausea or vomiting; numbness, tingling, pain, or weakness in hands or feet; redness, pain, lump or hardness, or muscle stiffness at place of injection

Other side effects not listed above may also occur in some patients. If you notice any other effects, check with your doctor.

Annual revision: 11/11/91

MINOXIDIL Systemic

A commonly used brand name in the U.S. and Canada is Loniten. Generic name product may also be available in the U.S.

Description

Minoxidil (mi-NOX-i-dill) belongs to the general class of medicines called antihypertensives. It is used to treat high blood pressure (hypertension).

High blood pressure adds to the workload of the heart and arteries. If it continues for a long time, the heart and arteries may not function properly. This can damage the blood vessels of the brain, heart, and kidneys, resulting in a stroke, heart failure, or kidney failure. High blood pressure may also increase the risk of heart attacks. These problems may be less likely to occur if blood pressure is controlled.

Minoxidil works by relaxing blood vessels so that blood passes through them more easily. This helps to lower blood pressure.

Minoxidil has other effects that could be bothersome for some patients. These include increased hair growth, weight gain, fast heartbeat, and chest pain. Before you take this medicine, be sure that you have discussed the use of it with your doctor.

Minoxidil is being applied to the scalp in liquid form by some balding men to stimulate hair growth. However, improper use of liquids made from minoxidil tablets can result in minoxidil being absorbed into the body, where it may cause unwanted effects on the heart and blood vessels.

Minoxidil is available only with your doctor's prescription, in the following dosage form:

Oral

- Tablets (U.S. and Canada)

It is very important that you read and understand the following information. If any of it causes you special concern, check with your doctor. Also, *if you have any questions* or if you want more information about this medicine or your medical problem, *ask your doctor, nurse, or pharmacist.*

Before Using This Medicine

In deciding to use a medicine, the risks of taking the medicine must be weighed against the good it will do. This is a decision you and your doctor will make. For minoxidil, the following should be considered:

Allergies—Tell your doctor if you have ever had any unusual or allergic reaction to minoxidil. Also tell your doctor and pharmacist if you are allergic to any other substances, such as foods, preservatives, or dyes.

Pregnancy—Minoxidil has not been studied in pregnant women. However, there have been reports of babies born with extra thick or dark hair on their bodies after the mothers took minoxidil during pregnancy. Discuss this possible effect with your doctor.

Studies in rats found a decreased rate of conception, and studies in rabbits at 5 times the human dose have shown a decrease in successful pregnancies. Minoxidil did not cause birth defects in rats or rabbits.

Breast-feeding—Although minoxidil passes into breast milk, it has not been reported to cause problems in nursing babies.

Children—Although there is no specific information comparing use of minoxidil in children with use in other age groups, this medicine is not expected to cause different side effects or problems in children than it does in adults.

Older adults—Elderly patients may be more sensitive to the effects of minoxidil. In addition, minoxidil may reduce tolerance to cold temperatures in elderly patients.

Other medicines—Although certain medicines should not be used together at all, in other cases two different medicines may be used together even if an interaction might occur. In these cases, your doctor may want to change the dose, or other precautions may be necessary. When taking minoxidil it is especially important that your doctor and pharmacist know if you are taking any of the following:

- Guanethidine (e.g., Ismelin) or
- Nitrates (medicine for angina)—Severe lowered blood pressure may occur

Other medical problems—The presence of other medical problems may affect the use of minoxidil. Make sure you tell your doctor if you have any other medical problems, especially:

- Angina (chest pain)—Minoxidil may make this condition worse
- Heart attack or stroke (recent)—Lowering blood pressure may make problems resulting from heart attack or stroke worse
- Heart or blood vessel disease—Minoxidil can cause fluid buildup, which can cause problems
- Kidney disease—Effects may be increased because of slower removal of minoxidil from the body
- Pheochromocytoma—Minoxidil may cause the tumor to be more active

Before you begin using any new medicine (prescription or nonprescription) or if you develop any new medical problem while you are using this medicine, check with your doctor, nurse, or pharmacist.

Proper Use of This Medicine

In addition to the use of the medicine your doctor has prescribed, treatment for your high blood pressure may include weight control and care in the types of foods you eat, especially foods high in sodium. Your doctor will tell you which of these are most important for you. You should check with your doctor before changing your diet.

Many patients who have high blood pressure will not notice any signs of the problem. In fact, many may feel normal. It is very important that you *take your medicine exactly as directed* and that you keep your appointments with your doctor even if you feel well.

Remember that minoxidil will not cure your high blood pressure but it does help control it. Therefore, you must continue to take it as directed if you expect to lower your blood pressure and keep it down. *You may have to take high blood pressure medicine for the rest of your life.* If high blood pressure is not treated, it can cause serious problems such as heart failure, blood vessel disease, stroke, or kidney disease.

To help you remember to take your medicine, try to get into the habit of taking it at the same time each day.

This medicine is usually given together with certain other medicines. If you are using a combination of drugs, make sure that you take each medicine at the proper time and do not mix them. Ask your doctor, nurse, or pharmacist to help you plan a way to remember to take your medicines at the right time.

Dosing—The dose of minoxidil will be different for different patients. *Follow your doctor's orders or the directions on the label.* The following information includes only the average doses of minoxidil. *If your dose is different, do not change it* unless your doctor tells you to do so:

- For *oral* dosage forms (tablets):
  —Adults and children over 12 years of age: 5 to 40 milligrams taken as a single dose or in divided doses.
  —Children up to 12 years of age: 200 micrograms to 1 milligram per kilogram of body weight a day to be taken as a single dose or in divided doses.

Missed dose—If you miss a dose of this medicine and remember it within a few hours, take it when you remember. However, if you do not remember until the next day, skip the missed dose and go back to your regular dosing schedule. Do not double doses.

Storage—To store this medicine:

- Keep out of the reach of children.
- Store away from heat and direct light.
- Do not store in the bathroom, near the kitchen sink, or in other damp places. Heat or moisture may cause the medicine to break down.
- Do not keep outdated medicine or medicine no longer needed. Be sure that any discarded medicine is out of the reach of children.

Precautions While Using This Medicine

It is important that your doctor check your progress at regular visits to make sure that this medicine is working properly.

Ask your doctor about checking your pulse rate before and after taking minoxidil. Then, while you are taking this medicine, *check your pulse regularly while you are resting.* If it increases by 20 beats or more a minute, check with your doctor right away.

While you are taking minoxidil, *weigh yourself every day.* A weight gain of 2 to 3 pounds (about 1 kg) in an adult is normal and should be lost with continued treatment. However, if you suddenly gain 5 pounds (2 kg) or more (for a child, 2 pounds [1 kg] or more) or if you notice swelling of your feet or lower legs, check with your doctor right away.

Do not take other medicines unless they have been discussed with your doctor. This especially includes over-the-counter (nonprescription) medicines for appetite control, asthma, colds, cough, hay fever, or sinus problems, since they may tend to increase your blood pressure.

Side Effects of This Medicine

Along with its needed effects, a medicine may cause some unwanted effects. Although not all of these side effects may occur, if they do occur they may need medical attention.

Check with your doctor immediately if any of the following side effects occur:

More common

Fast or irregular heartbeat; weight gain (rapid) of more than 5 pounds (2 pounds in children)

Less common

Chest pain; shortness of breath

Check with your doctor as soon as possible if any of the following side effects occur:

More common

Bloating; flushing or redness of skin; swelling of feet or lower legs

Less common

Numbness or tingling of hands, feet, or face

Rare

Skin rash and itching

Other side effects may occur that usually do not need medical attention. These side effects may go away during treatment as your body adjusts to the medicine. However, check with your doctor if any of the following side effects continue or are bothersome:

More common

Increase in hair growth, usually on face, arms, and back

Less common or rare

Breast tenderness in males and females; headache

This medicine causes a temporary increase in hair growth in most people. Hair may grow longer and darker in both men and women. This may first be noticed on the face several weeks after you start taking minoxidil. Later, new hair growth may be noticed on the back, arms, legs, and scalp. Talk to your doctor about shaving or using a hair remover during this time. After treatment with minoxidil has ended, the hair will stop growing, although it may take several months for the new hair growth to go away.

Other side effects not listed above may also occur in some patients. If you notice any other effects, check with your doctor.

Annual revision: 05/26/93

MINOXIDIL Topical

A commonly used brand name in the U.S. and Canada is Rogaine. Generic name product may also be available in Canada.

Description

Minoxidil (mi-NOX-i-dill) applied to the scalp is used to stimulate hair growth in men and women with a certain type of baldness. The exact way that it works is not known.

If hair growth is going to occur with the use of minoxidil, it usually occurs after the medicine has been used for about 4 months and lasts only as long as the medicine continues to be used. The new hair will be lost within a few months after minoxidil treatment is stopped.

This medicine is available only with your doctor's prescription, in the following dosage form:

Topical
- Topical solution (U.S. and Canada)

It is very important that you read and understand the following information. If any of it causes you special concern, check with your doctor. Also, *if you have any questions* or if you want more information about this medicine or your medical problem, *ask your doctor, nurse, or pharmacist.*

Before Using This Medicine

In deciding to use a medicine, the risks of using the medicine must be weighed against the good it will do. This is a decision you and your doctor will make. For topical minoxidil, the following should be considered:

Allergies—Tell your doctor if you have ever had any unusual or allergic reaction to minoxidil. Also tell your doctor and pharmacist if you are allergic to any other substances, such as preservatives or dyes.

Pregnancy—Topical minoxidil has not been studied in pregnant women. However, some studies in animals have shown that minoxidil, when given by mouth, causes problems during pregnancy, although the studies have not shown that the medicine causes birth defects. Before using this medicine, make sure your doctor knows if you are pregnant or if you may become pregnant.

Breast-feeding—It is not known whether topical minoxidil passes into breast milk. However, minoxidil, taken by mouth, does pass into breast milk. Minoxidil is not recommended during breast-feeding, because it may cause problems in nursing babies.

Older adults—Many medicines have not been studied specifically in older people. Therefore, it may not be known whether they work exactly the same way they do in younger adults or if they cause different side effects or problems in older people. There is no specific information comparing use of minoxidil on the scalp in the elderly with use in other age groups.

Other medicines—Although certain medicines should not be used together at all, in other cases two different medicines may be used together even if an interaction might occur. In these cases, your doctor may want to change the dose, or other precautions may be necessary. When you are using topical minoxidil, it is especially important that your doctor and pharmacist know if you are taking any other prescription or nonprescription (over-the-counter [OTC]) medicine or if you are using any of the following on your scalp:

- Adrenocorticoids (cortisone-like medicine) or
- Petrolatum (e.g., Vaseline) or
- Tretinoin (e.g., Retin A)—Use of these products on your scalp may cause too much topical minoxidil to be absorbed into the body and may increase the chance of side effects

- Minoxidil, systemic (e.g., Loniten)—Use of topical minoxidil with minoxidil taken by mouth for high blood pressure may increase the chance of side effects

Other medical problems—The presence of other medical problems may affect the use of topical minoxidil. Make sure you tell your doctor if you have any other medical problems, especially:

- Any other skin problems or an irritation or a sunburn on the scalp—The condition may cause too much topical minoxidil to be absorbed into the body and may increase the chance of side effects

- Heart disease or
- Hypertension (high blood pressure)—The condition may get worse if too much medicine is absorbed into the body

Before you begin using any new medicine (prescription or nonprescription) or if you develop any new medical problem while you are using this medicine, check with your doctor, nurse, or pharmacist.

Proper Use of This Medicine

This medicine usually comes with patient instructions. It is important that you read the instructions carefully.

It is very important that you use this medicine only as directed. Do not use more of it and do not use it more often than your doctor ordered. To do so may increase the chance of it being absorbed through the skin. For the same reason, do not apply minoxidil to other parts of your body. Absorption into the body may affect the heart and blood vessels and cause unwanted effects.

Do not use any other skin products on the same skin area on which you use minoxidil.

To apply minoxidil solution:

- Shampoo your hair each morning before applying minoxidil. Make sure your hair and scalp are completely dry before applying this medicine.
- Apply the amount prescribed to the area of the scalp being treated, beginning in the center of the area. Follow your doctor's instructions on how to apply the solution, using the applicator provided.
- Immediately after using this medicine, wash your hands to remove any medicine that may be on them.
- Do not use a hairdryer to dry the scalp after you apply minoxidil solution. Blowing with a hairdryer on the scalp may make the treatment less effective.
- If you are using this medicine at bedtime, do not go to bed until at least 30 minutes after you use it. That way, less of the medicine will rub off on the pillowcase.

If your scalp becomes abraded, irritated, or sunburned, check with your doctor before applying minoxidil.

Keep this medicine away from the eyes, nose, and mouth. If you should accidentally get some in your eyes, nose, or mouth, flush the area thoroughly with cool tap water. If you are using the pump spray, be careful not to breathe the spray in.

Missed dose—If you miss a dose of this medicine, go back to your regular dosing schedule. Do not double doses.

Storage—To store this medicine:

- Keep out of the reach of children.
- Store away from heat and direct light.
- Keep the medicine from freezing.
- Do not keep outdated medicine or medicine no longer needed. Be sure that any discarded medicine is out of the reach of children.

Precautions While Using This Medicine

It is important that your doctor check your progress at regular visits to make sure that this medicine is working properly and to check for unwanted effects.

Tell your doctor if you notice itching, redness, or burning of your scalp after you apply minoxidil. If the itching, redness, or burning is severe, wash the medicine off and check with your doctor before using it again.

Side Effects of This Medicine

Along with its needed effects, a medicine may cause some unwanted effects. Although not all of these side effects may occur, if they do occur they may need medical attention.

Check with your doctor as soon as possible if any of the following side effects occur:

Less common

Itching or skin rash

Rare

Blurred vision or other change in vision; burning of scalp; decrease of sexual ability or desire; dizziness; increased hair loss; lightheadedness; soreness at root of hair; swelling of face

Signs and symptoms of too much medicine being absorbed into the body—Rare

Chest pain; fast or irregular heartbeat; flushing; headache; numbness or tingling of hands, feet, or face; swelling of face, hands, feet, or lower legs; weight gain (rapid)

Other side effects may occur that usually do not need medical attention. These side effects may go away during treatment as your body adjusts to the medicine. However, check with your doctor if either of the following side effects continues or is bothersome:

Less common

Dry or flaking skin; reddened skin

Other side effects not listed above may also occur in some patients. If you notice any other effects, check with your doctor.

Annual revision: 04/14/92

MISOPROSTOL Systemic

A commonly used brand name in the U.S. and Canada is Cytotec.

Description

Misoprostol (mye-soe-PROST-ole) is taken to prevent stomach ulcers in patients taking anti-inflammatory drugs, including aspirin. Misoprostol may also be used for other conditions as determined by your doctor.

Misoprostol helps the stomach protect itself against acid damage. It also decreases the amount of acid produced by the stomach.

This medicine is available only with your doctor's prescription, in the following dosage form:

Oral

- Tablets (U.S. and Canada)

It is very important that you read and understand the following information. If any of it causes you special

concern, check with your doctor. Also, *if you have any questions* or if you want more information about this medicine or your medical problem, *ask your doctor, nurse, or pharmacist.*

Before Using This Medicine

In deciding to use a medicine, the risks of taking the medicine must be weighed against the good it will do. This is a decision you and your doctor will make. For misoprostol, the following should be considered:

Allergies—Tell your doctor if you have ever had any unusual or allergic reaction to misoprostol. Also tell your doctor and pharmacist if you are allergic to any other substances, such as foods, preservatives, or dyes.

Pregnancy—*Misoprostol must not be used during pregnancy.* It has been shown to cause contractions and bleeding of the uterus. Misoprostol may also cause miscarriage.

Before starting to take this medicine you must have had a negative pregnancy test within the previous 2 weeks. Also, you must start taking misoprostol only on the second or third day of your next normal menstrual period. In addition, it will be necessary that you use an effective form of birth control while taking this medicine. Be sure that you have discussed this with your doctor before taking this medicine.

Breast-feeding—It is not known whether misoprostol passes into breast milk. However, misoprostol is not recommended for use during breast-feeding because it may cause diarrhea in nursing babies.

Children—Studies on this medicine have been done only in adult patients, and there is no specific information comparing use of misoprostol in children with use in other age groups.

Older adults—This medicine has been tested and has not been shown to cause different side effects or problems in older people than it does in younger adults.

Other medicines—Although certain medicines should not be used together at all, in other cases two different medicines may be used together even if an interaction might occur. In these cases, your doctor may want to change the dose, or other precautions may be necessary. Tell your doctor and pharmacist if you are taking any other prescription or nonprescription (over-the-counter [OTC]) medicine.

Other medical problems—The presence of other medical problems may affect the use of misoprostol. Make sure you tell your doctor if you have any other medical problems, especially:

- Blood vessel disease—Medicines similar to misoprostol have been shown to make this condition worse
- Epilepsy (uncontrolled)—Medicines similar to misoprostol have been shown to cause convulsions (seizures)

Before you begin using any new medicine (prescription or nonprescription) or if you develop any new medical problem while you are using this medicine, check with your doctor, nurse, or pharmacist.

Proper Use of This Medicine

Misoprostol is best taken with or after meals and at bedtime, unless otherwise directed by your doctor.

Missed dose—If you miss a dose of this medicine, take it as soon as possible. However, if it is almost time for your next dose, skip the missed dose and go back to your regular dosing schedule. Do not double doses.

Storage—To store this medicine:

- Keep out of the reach of children.
- Store away from heat and direct light.
- Do not store in the bathroom, near the kitchen sink, or in other damp places. Heat or moisture may cause the medicine to break down.
- Do not keep outdated medicine or medicine no longer needed. Be sure that any discarded medicine is out of the reach of children.

Precautions While Using This Medicine

Misoprostol may cause miscarriage if taken during pregnancy. Therefore, if you suspect that you may have become pregnant, stop taking this medicine immediately and check with your doctor.

This medicine may cause diarrhea in some people. The diarrhea will usually disappear within a few days as your body adjusts to the medicine. However, check with your doctor if the diarrhea is severe and/or does not stop after a week. Your doctor may have to lower the dose of misoprostol you are taking.

Side Effects of This Medicine

Along with its needed effects, a medicine may cause some unwanted effects. Some side effects may occur that usually do not need medical attention. These side effects may go away during treatment as your body adjusts to the medicine. However, check with your doctor if any of the following side effects continue or are bothersome:

More common

Abdominal or stomach pain (mild); diarrhea

Less common or rare

Bleeding from vagina; constipation; cramps in lower abdomen or stomach area; gas; headache; nausea and/or vomiting

Other side effects not listed above may also occur in some patients. If you notice any other effects, check with your doctor.

Additional Information

Once a medicine has been approved for marketing for a certain use, experience may show that it is also useful for other medical problems. Although this use is not included in product labeling, misoprostol is used in certain patients with the following medical condition:

- Duodenal ulcers

For patients taking this medicine for *duodenal ulcers*:

- Antacids may be taken with misoprostol, if needed, to help relieve stomach pain, unless you are otherwise directed by your doctor. However, do not take magnesium-containing antacids, since they may cause diarrhea or worsen the diarrhea that is sometimes caused by misoprostol.
- Take this medicine for the full time of treatment, even if you begin to feel better. Also, it is important that you keep your appointments with your doctor so that your doctor will be better able to tell you when to stop taking this medicine.
- *Misoprostol is not normally taken for more than 4 weeks when used to treat duodenal ulcers.* However, your doctor may order treatment for a second 4-week period if needed.

Other than the above information, there is no additional information relating to proper use, precautions, or side effects for these uses.

Annual revision: 04/14/92

MITOMYCIN Systemic

A commonly used brand name in the U.S. and Canada is Mutamycin.

Description

Mitomycin (mye-toe-MYE-sin) belongs to the group of medicines known as antineoplastics. It is used to treat some kinds of cancer.

Mitomycin interferes with the growth of cancer cells, which are eventually destroyed. Since the growth of normal body cells may also be affected by mitomycin, other effects will also occur. Some of these may be serious and must be reported to your doctor. Other effects, like hair loss, may not be serious but may cause concern. Some effects may not occur for months or years after the medicine is used.

Before you begin treatment with mitomycin, you and your doctor should talk about the good this medicine will do as well as the risks of using it.

Mitomycin is to be administered only by or under the immediate supervision of your doctor. It is available in the following dosage form:

Parenteral

- Injection (U.S. and Canada)

It is very important that you read and understand the following information. If any of it causes you special concern, check with your doctor. Also, *if you have any questions* or if you want more information about this medicine or your medical problem, *ask your doctor, nurse, or pharmacist.*

Before Using This Medicine

In deciding to use a medicine, the risks of taking the medicine must be weighed against the good it will do. This is a decision you and your doctor will make. For mitomycin, the following should be considered:

Allergies—Tell your doctor if you have ever had any unusual or allergic reaction to mitomycin.

Pregnancy—Tell your doctor if you are pregnant or if you intend to have children. There is a chance that this medicine may cause birth defects if either the male or female is taking it at the time of conception or if it is taken during pregnancy. Studies have shown that mitomycin causes birth defects in animals. In addition, many cancer medicines may cause sterility which could be permanent. Although sterility has not been reported with this medicine, the possibility should be kept in mind.

Be sure that you have discussed this with your doctor before taking this medicine. It is best to use some kind of birth control while you are receiving mitomycin. Tell your doctor right away if you think you have become pregnant while receiving mitomycin.

Breast-feeding—Tell your doctor if you are breast-feeding or if you intend to breast-feed during treatment with this medicine. Because mitomycin may cause serious side effects, breast-feeding is generally not recommended while you are receiving it.

Children—Although there is no specific information about the use of mitomycin in children, it is not expected to cause different side effects or problems in children than it does in adults.

Older adults—Many medicines have not been tested in older people. Therefore, it may not be known whether they work exactly the same way they do in younger adults or if they cause different side effects or problems in older people. There is no specific information about the use of mitomycin in the elderly.

Other medicines—Although certain medicines should not be used together at all, in other cases two different medicines may be used together even if an interaction might occur. In these cases, your doctor may want to change the dose, or other precautions may be necessary. When you are receiving mitomycin, it is especially important that your doctor and pharmacist know if you have ever been treated with x-rays or cancer medicines or if you are taking any of the following:

- Amphotericin B by injection (e.g., Fungizone) or
- Antithyroid agents (medicine for overactive thyroid) or
- Azathioprine (e.g., Imuran) or
- Chloramphenicol (e.g., Chloromycetin) or
- Colchicine or
- Flucytosine (e.g., Ancobon) or
- Interferon (e.g., Intron A, Roferon-A) or
- Plicamycin (e.g., Mithracin) or
- Zidovudine (e.g., Retrovir)—Mitomycin may increase the effects of these medicines or radiation therapy on the blood

Other medical problems—The presence of other medical problems may affect the use of mitomycin. Make sure you tell your doctor if you have any other medical problems, especially:

- Bleeding problems
- Chickenpox (including recent exposure) or
- Herpes zoster (shingles)—Risk of severe disease affecting other parts of the body
- Infection—Mitomycin can reduce immunity to infection
- Kidney disease—May be worsened

Before you begin using any new medicine (prescription or nonprescription) or if you develop any new medical problem while you are using this medicine, check with your doctor, nurse, or pharmacist.

Proper Use of This Medicine

Mitomycin is usually given together with certain other medicines. If you are using a combination of medicines, it is important that you receive each one at the proper time. If you are taking some of these medicines by mouth, ask your doctor, nurse, or pharmacist to help you plan a way to remember to take them at the right times.

This medicine often causes nausea, vomiting, and loss of appetite. However, it is very important that you continue to receive the medicine, even if you begin to feel ill. Ask your doctor, nurse, or pharmacist for ways to lessen these effects.

Precautions While Using This Medicine

It is very important that your doctor check your progress at regular visits to make sure that this medicine is working properly and to check for unwanted effects.

While you are being treated with mitomycin, and after you stop treatment with it, *do not have any immunizations (vaccinations) without your doctor's approval.* Mitomycin may lower your body's resistance and there is a chance you might get the infection the immunization is meant to prevent. In addition, other persons living in your household should not take or should not have recently taken oral polio vaccine since there is a chance they could pass the polio virus on to you. Also, avoid other persons who have taken oral polio vaccine. Do not get close to them, and do not stay in the same room with them for very long. If you cannot take these precautions, you should consider wearing a protective face mask that covers the nose and mouth.

Mitomycin can lower the number of white blood cells in your blood temporarily, increasing the chance of getting an infection. It can also lower the number of platelets, which are necessary for proper blood clotting. If this occurs, there are certain precautions you can take, especially when your blood count is low, to reduce the risk of infection or bleeding:

- If you can, avoid people with infections. *Check with your doctor immediately* if you think you are getting an infection or if you get a fever or chills, cough or hoarseness, lower back or side pain, or painful or difficult urination.
- *Check with your doctor immediately* if you notice any unusual bleeding or bruising; black, tarry stools; blood in urine or stools; or pinpoint red spots on your skin.
- Be careful when using a regular toothbrush, dental floss, or toothpick. Your medical doctor, dentist, or nurse may recommend other ways to clean your teeth and gums. Check with your medical doctor before having any dental work done.
- Do not touch your eyes or the inside of your nose unless you have just washed your hands and have not touched anything else in the meantime.
- Be careful not to cut yourself when you are using sharp objects such as a safety razor or fingernail or toenail cutters.
- Avoid contact sports or other situations where bruising or injury could occur.

If mitomycin accidentally seeps out of the vein into which it is injected, it may damage the skin and cause scarring. In some patients, this may occur weeks or even months after this medicine is given. *Tell the doctor or nurse right away if you notice redness, pain, or swelling at the place of injection or anywhere else on your skin.*

Side Effects of This Medicine

Along with their needed effects medicines like mitomycin can sometimes cause unwanted effects such as blood problems, loss of hair, and other side effects. These and others are described below. Also, because of the way these medicines act on the body, there is a chance that they might cause other unwanted effects that may not occur until months or years after the medicine is used. These delayed effects may include certain types of cancer, such as leukemia. Discuss these possible effects with your doctor.

Although not all of these side effects may occur, if they do occur they may need medical attention.

Check with your doctor or nurse immediately if any of the following side effects occur:

Less common

Black, tarry stools; blood in urine or stools; cough or hoarseness; fever or chills; lower back or side pain; painful or difficult urination; pinpoint red spots on skin; unusual bleeding or bruising

Rare

Redness or pain, especially at place of injection

Check with your doctor as soon as possible if any of the following side effects occur:

Less common

Cough; decreased urination; shortness of breath; sores in mouth and on lips; swelling of feet or lower legs

Rare

Bloody vomit

Other side effects may occur that usually do not need medical attention. These side effects may go away during treatment as your body adjusts to the medicine. Also, your doctor or nurse may be able to tell you about ways to prevent or reduce some of these side effects. Check with your doctor if any of the following side effects continue or are bothersome or if you have any questions about them:

More common

Loss of appetite; nausea and vomiting

Less common

Numbness or tingling in fingers and toes; purple-colored bands on nails; skin rash; unusual tiredness or weakness

Mitomycin sometimes causes a temporary loss of hair. After treatment has ended, normal hair growth should return.

After you stop receiving mitomycin, it may still produce some side effects that need attention. During this period of time, *check with your doctor immediately* if you notice the following:

Blood in urine

Also, check with your doctor if you notice any of the following:

Black, tarry stools; blood in stools; cough or hoarseness; decreased urination; fever or chills; lower back or side pain; painful or difficult urination; pinpoint red spots on skin; red or painful skin; shortness of breath; swelling of feet or lower legs; unusual bleeding or bruising

Other side effects not listed above may also occur in some patients. If you notice any other effects, check with your doctor.

Annual revision: June 1990
Interim revision: 07/30/93

MITOTANE Systemic

A commonly used brand name in the U.S. and Canada is Lysodren.

Description

Mitotane (MYE-toe-tane) is a medicine that acts on a part of the body called the adrenal cortex. It is used to treat some kinds of cancer that affect the adrenal cortex. Also, it is sometimes used when the adrenal cortex is overactive without being cancerous.

Mitotane reduces the amounts of adrenocorticoids (cortisone-like hormones) produced by the adrenal cortex. These steroids are important for various functions of the body, including growth. However, too much of these steroids can cause problems.

Mitotane is available only with your doctor's prescription, in the following dosage form:

Oral

- Tablets (U.S. and Canada)

It is very important that you read and understand the following information. If any of it causes you special concern, check with your doctor. Also, *if you have any questions* or if you want more information about this medicine or your medical problem, *ask your doctor, nurse, or pharmacist.*

Before Using This Medicine

In deciding to use a medicine, the risks of taking the medicine must be weighed against the good it will do.

This is a decision you and your doctor will make. For mitotane, the following should be considered:

Allergies—Tell your doctor if you have ever had any unusual or allergic reaction to mitotane. Also tell your doctor and pharmacist if you are allergic to any other substance, such as foods, preservatives, or dyes.

Pregnancy—Mitotane has not been shown to cause problems in humans.

Breast-feeding—Although it is not known whether mitotane passes into the breast milk, it has not been reported to cause problems in nursing babies.

Children—Although there is no specific information about the use of mitotane in children, it is not expected to cause different side effects or problems in children than it does in adults.

Older adults—Many medicines have not been tested in older people. Therefore, it may not be known whether they work exactly the same way they do in younger adults or if they cause different side effects or problems in older people. There is no specific information about the use of mitotane in the elderly.

Other medicines—Although certain medicines should not be used together at all, in other cases two different medicines may be used together even if an interaction might occur. In these cases, your doctor may want to change the dose, or other precautions may be necessary. When you are taking mitotane, it is especially important that your doctor and pharmacist know if you are taking any of the following:

- Central nervous system (CNS) depressants—CNS depressant effects may be increased

Other medical problems—The presence of other medical problems may affect the use of mitotane. Make sure you tell your doctor if you have any other medical problems, especially:

- Infection
- Liver disease—Effects may be increased because of slower removal of mitotane from the body

Before you begin using any new medicine (prescription or nonprescription) or if you develop any new medical problem while you are using this medicine, check with your doctor, nurse, or pharmacist.

Proper Use of This Medicine

Take mitotane only as directed by your doctor. Do not take more or less of it, and do not take it more often than your doctor ordered.

Do not stop taking this medicine without first checking with your doctor. To do so may increase the chance of unwanted effects.

Missed dose—If you miss a dose of this medicine, take the missed dose as soon as you remember it. However, if it is almost time for the next dose, skip the missed dose and do not double the next one. Instead, go back to your regular dosing schedule and check with your doctor.

Storage—To store this medicine:

- Keep out of the reach of children.
- Store away from heat and direct light.
- Do not store in the bathroom, near the kitchen sink, or in other damp places. Heat or moisture may cause the medicine to break down.
- Do not keep outdated medicine or medicine no longer needed. Be sure that any discarded medicine is out of the reach of children.

Precautions While Using This Medicine

It is very important that your doctor check your progress at regular visits to make sure this medicine is working properly and to check for unwanted effects.

Your doctor may want you to carry an identification card stating that you are taking this medicine.

This medicine will add to the effects of alcohol and other CNS depressants (medicines that slow down the nervous system, possibly causing drowsiness). Some examples of CNS depressants are antihistamines or medicine for hay fever, other allergies, or colds; sedatives, tranquilizers, or sleeping medicine; prescription pain medicine or narcotics; barbiturates; medicine for seizures; tricyclic antidepressants (medicine for depression); muscle relaxants; or anesthetics, including some dental anesthetics. *Check with your doctor before taking any of the above while you are using this medicine.*

This medicine may cause some people to become dizzy, drowsy, or less alert than they are normally. *Make sure you know how you react to this medicine before you drive, use machines, or do anything else that could be dangerous if you are dizzy or are not alert.*

Check with your doctor right away if you get an injury, infection, or illness of any kind. This medicine may weaken your body's defenses against infection or inflammation.

Side Effects of This Medicine

Along with its needed effects, a medicine may cause some unwanted effects. Although not all of these side effects may occur, if they do occur they may need medical attention.

Check with your doctor as soon as possible if any of the following side effects occur:

More common

Darkening of skin; diarrhea; dizziness; drowsiness; loss of appetite; mental depression; nausea and vomiting; skin rash; unusual tiredness

Less common

Blood in urine; blurred vision; double vision

Rare

Shortness of breath; wheezing

Other side effects may occur that usually do not need medical attention. These side effects may go away during treatment as your body adjusts to the medicine. However, check with your doctor or nurse if any of the following side effects continue or are bothersome:

Less common

Aching muscles; dizziness or lightheadedness when getting up from a lying or sitting position; fever; flushing or redness of skin; muscle twitching

Other side effects not listed above may also occur in some patients. If you notice any other effects, check with your doctor.

Annual revision: August 1990

MITOXANTRONE Systemic

A commonly used brand name in the U.S. and Canada is Novantrone.

Description

Mitoxantrone (mye-toe-ZAN-trone) belongs to the general group of medicines known as antineoplastics. It is used to treat some kinds of cancer.

Mitoxantrone seems to interfere with the growth of cancer cells, which are eventually destroyed. Since the growth of normal body cells may also be affected by mitoxantrone, other effects will also occur. Some of these may be serious and must be reported to your doctor. Other effects, like hair loss, may not be serious but may cause concern. Some effects may not occur for months or years after the medicine is used.

Before you begin treatment with mitoxantrone, you and your doctor should talk about the good this medicine will do as well as the risks of using it.

Mitoxantrone is to be administered only by or under the immediate supervision of your doctor. It is available in the following dosage form:

Parenteral

- Injection (U.S. and Canada)

It is very important that you read and understand the following information. If any of it causes you special concern, check with your doctor. Also, *if you have any questions* or if you want more information about this medicine or your medical problem, *ask your doctor, nurse, or pharmacist.*

Before Using This Medicine

In deciding to use a medicine, the risks of taking the medicine must be weighed against the good it will do. This is a decision you and your doctor will make. For mitoxantrone, the following should be considered:

Allergies—Tell your doctor if you have ever had any unusual or allergic reaction to mitoxantrone.

Pregnancy—Tell your doctor if you are pregnant or if you intend to have children. There is a chance that this medicine may cause birth defects if either the male or female is receiving it at the time of conception or if it is taken during pregnancy. Mitoxantrone has been reported to cause low birth weight and slow growth of the kidney in rats and premature birth in rabbits. In addition, many cancer medicines may cause sterility which could be permanent. Although sterility has not been reported with this medicine, the possibility should be kept in mind.

Be sure that you have discussed this with your doctor before receiving this medicine. It is best to use some kind of birth control while you are receiving mitoxantrone. Tell your doctor right away if you think you have become pregnant while receiving mitoxantrone.

Breast-feeding—if you are breast-feeding or if you intend to breast-feed during treatment with this medicine. Because mitoxantrone may cause serious side effects, breast-feeding is generally not recommended while you are receiving it.

Children—There is no specific information about the use of mitoxantrone in children.

Older adults—Many medicines have not been tested in older people. Therefore, it may not be known whether they work exactly the same way they do in younger adults or if they cause different side effects or problems in older people. There is no specific information about the use of mitoxantrone in the elderly.

Other medicines—Although certain medicines should not be used together at all, in other cases two different medicines may be used together even if an interaction might occur. In these cases, your doctor may want to change the dose, or other precautions may be necessary. When you are receiving mitoxantrone, it is especially important that your doctor and pharmacist know if you are taking any of the following:

- Amphotericin B by injection (e.g., Fungizone) or
- Antithyroid agents (medicine for overactive thyroid) or
- Chloramphenicol (e.g., Chloromycetin) or
- Colchicine or
- Flucytosine (e.g., Ancobon) or
- Interferon (e.g., Intron A, Roferon-A) or
- Plicamycin (e.g., Mithracin) or
- Zidovudine (e.g., Retrovir) or
- If you have been treated with x-rays or cancer medicines—Mitoxantrone may increase the effects of these medicines or radiation therapy on the blood
- Probenecid (e.g., Benemid) or
- Sulfinpyrazone (e.g., Anturane)—Mitoxantrone may increase the concentration of uric acid in the blood, which these medicines are used to lower

Other medical problems—The presence of other medical problems may affect the use of mitoxantrone. Make sure you tell your doctor if you have any other medical problems, especially:

- Chickenpox (including recent exposure) or
- Herpes zoster (shingles)—Risk of severe disease affecting other parts of the body
- Gout (history of) or
- Kidney stones—Mitoxantrone may increase levels of a chemical called uric acid in the body, which can cause gout or kidney stones
- Heart disease—Risk of heart problems caused by mitoxantrone may be increased
- Infection—Mitoxantrone can reduce immunity to infection
- Liver disease—Effects may be increased because of slower removal of mitoxantrone from the body

Before you begin using any new medicine (prescription or nonprescription) or if you develop any new medical problem while you are using this medicine, check with your doctor, nurse, or pharmacist.

Proper Use of This Medicine

Mitoxantrone is sometimes given together with certain other medicines. If you are using a combination of medicines, it is important that you receive each one at the proper time. If you are taking some of these medicines by mouth, ask your doctor, nurse, or pharmacist to help you plan a way to take them at the right times.

While you are receiving mitoxantrone, your doctor may want you to drink extra fluids so that you will pass more urine. This will help prevent kidney problems and keep your kidneys working well.

Mitoxantrone often causes nausea and vomiting. However, it is very important that you continue to receive the medicine, even if your stomach is upset. Ask your doctor, nurse, or pharmacist for ways to lessen these effects.

Precautions While Using This Medicine

It is very important that your doctor check your progress at regular visits to make sure that this medicine is working properly and to check for unwanted effects.

While you are being treated with mitoxantrone, and after you stop treatment with it, *do not have any immunizations (vaccinations) without your doctor's approval.* Mitoxantrone may lower your body's resistance and there is a chance you might get the infection the immunization is meant to prevent. In addition, other persons living in your household should not take or should not have recently taken oral polio vaccine since there is a chance they could pass the polio virus on to you. Also, avoid other persons who have taken oral polio vaccine. Do not get close to them and do not stay in the same room with them for very long. If you cannot take these precautions, you should consider wearing a protective face mask that covers the nose and mouth.

Tell your doctor right away if you think you have become pregnant while receiving mitoxantrone. There is a chance that it may cause birth defects or other problems if it is used during pregnancy.

Mitoxantrone can lower the number of white blood cells in your blood temporarily, increasing the chance of getting an infection. It can also lower the number of platelets, which are necessary for proper blood clotting. If this occurs, there are certain precautions you can take, especially when your blood count is low, to reduce the risk of infection or bleeding:

- If you can, avoid people with infections. *Check with your doctor immediately* if you think you are getting an infection or if you get a fever or chills, cough or hoarseness, lower back or side pain, or painful or difficult urination.
- *Check with your doctor immediately* if you notice any unusual bleeding or bruising; black, tarry stools; blood in urine or stools; or pinpoint red spots on your skin.
- Be careful when using a regular toothbrush, dental floss, or toothpick. Your medical doctor, dentist, or nurse may recommend other ways to clean your teeth and gums. Check with your medical doctor before having any dental work done.
- Do not touch your eyes or the inside of your nose unless you have just washed your hands and have not touched anything else in the meantime.
- Be careful not to cut yourself when you are using sharp objects such as a safety razor or fingernail or toenail cutters.

• Avoid contact sports or other situations where bruising or injury could occur.

Side Effects of This Medicine

Along with their needed effects, medicines like mitoxantrone can sometimes cause unwanted effects such as blood problems, loss of hair, and other side effects. These and others are described below. Also, because of the way these medicines act on the body, there is a chance that they might cause other unwanted effects that may not occur until months or years after the medicine is used. These delayed effects may include certain types of cancer, such as leukemia. Discuss these possible effects with your doctor.

Although not all of these side effects may occur, if they do occur they may need medical attention.

Check with your doctor or nurse immediately if any of the following side effects occur:

More common

Black, tarry stools; cough or shortness of breath

Less common

Blood in urine or stools; fast or irregular heartbeat; fever or chills; lower back or side pain; painful or difficult urination; pinpoint red spots on skin; swelling of feet and lower legs; unusual bleeding or bruising

Check with your doctor or nurse as soon as possible if any of the following side effects occur:

More common

Sores in mouth and on lips; stomach pain

Less common

Decrease in urination; seizures; sore, red eyes; yellow eyes or skin

Rare

Blue skin at place of injection; pain or redness at place of injection; skin rash

Other side effects may occur that usually do not need medical attention. These side effects may go away during treatment as your body adjusts to the medicine. Also, your doctor or nurse may be able to tell you about ways to prevent or reduce some of these side effects. Check with your doctor or nurse if any of the following side effects continue or are bothersome:

More common

Diarrhea; headache; nausea and vomiting

Mitoxantrone may cause the urine to turn a blue-green color. It may also cause the whites of the eyes to turn a blue color. These effects are normal and last for only 1 or 2 days after each dose is given.

This medicine often causes a temporary loss of hair. After treatment with mitoxantrone has ended, normal hair growth should return.

Other side effects not listed above may also occur in some patients. If you notice any other effects, check with your doctor or nurse.

Annual revision: 06/02/92
Interim revision: 07/30/93

MOLINDONE Systemic†

Some commonly used brand names in the U.S. are Moban and Moban Concentrate.

†Not commercially available in Canada.

Description

Molindone (moe-LIN-done) is used to treat nervous, mental, and emotional conditions.

Molindone is available only with your doctor's prescription, in the following dosage forms:

Oral

- Solution (U.S.)
- Tablets (U.S.)

It is very important that you read and understand the following information. If any of it causes you special concern, check with your doctor. Also, *if you have any questions* or if you want more information about this medicine or your medical problem, *ask your doctor, nurse, or pharmacist.*

Before Using This Medicine

In deciding to use a medicine, the risks of taking the medicine must be weighed against the good it will do. This is a decision you and your doctor will make. For molindone, the following should be considered:

Allergies—Tell your doctor if you have ever had any unusual or allergic reaction to molindone, phenothiazines, thioxanthenes, haloperidol, or loxapine. Also tell your doctor and pharmacist if you are allergic to any other substances, such as foods, preservatives, or dyes.

Pregnancy—Molindone has not been shown to cause birth defects or other problems in humans. However, studies in mice have shown a slight decrease in successful pregnancies.

Breast-feeding—It is not known if molindone passes into breast milk.

Children—Studies on this medicine have been done only in adult patients, and there is no specific information comparing use of molindone in children with use in other age groups.

Older adults—Elderly patients are usually more sensitive than younger adults to the effects of molindone. Constipation, dizziness or lightheadedness, drowsiness, dryness of mouth, trembling of the hands and fingers, and symptoms of tardive dyskinesia (such as rapid, worm-like movements of the tongue or any other uncontrolled movements of the mouth, tongue, or jaw, and/or arms and legs) are especially likely to occur in elderly patients.

Other medicines—Although certain medicines should not be used together at all, in other cases 2 different medicines may be used together even if an interaction might occur. In these cases, your doctor may want to change the dose, or other precautions may be necessary. When you are taking molindone, it is especially important that your doctor and pharmacist know if you are taking any of the following:

- Amoxapine (e.g., Asendin) or
- Methyldopa (e.g., Aldomet) or
- Metoclopramide (e.g., Reglan) or
- Metyrosine (e.g., Demser) or
- Other antipsychotics (medicine for mental illness) or
- Pemoline (e.g., Cylert) or
- Pimozide (e.g., Orap) or
- Promethazine (e.g., Phenergan) or
- Rauwolfia alkaloids (alseroxylon [e.g., Rauwiloid], deserpidine [e.g., Harmonyl], rauwolfia serpentina [e.g., Raudixin], reserpine [e.g., Serpasil]) or
- Trimeprazine (e.g., Temaril)—Taking these medicines with molindone may increase the chance and seriousness of some side effects
- Central nervous system (CNS) depressants (medicine that causes drowsiness) or
- Tricyclic antidepressants (medicine for depression)—Taking these medicines with molindone may increase the CNS depressant effects
- Lithium (e.g., Eskalith, Lithane)—The chance of serious side effects may be increased

Other medical problems—The presence of other medical problems may affect the use of molindone. Make sure you tell your doctor if you have any other medical problems, especially:

- Brain tumor or
- Intestinal blockage—Molindone may interfere with the diagnosis of these conditions
- Difficult urination or
- Enlarged prostate or
- Glaucoma or
- Liver disease or
- Parkinson's disease—Molindone may make the condition worse

Before you begin using any new medicine (prescription or nonprescription) or if you develop any new medical problem while you are using this medicine, check with your doctor, nurse, or pharmacist.

Proper Use of This Medicine

Molindone should be taken with food or a full glass (8 ounces) of water or milk to reduce stomach irritation.

The liquid form of molindone may be taken undiluted or mixed with milk, water, fruit juice, or carbonated beverages.

Take this medicine only as directed by your doctor. Do not take more of it, do not take it more often, and do not take it for a longer time than your doctor ordered. To do so may increase the chance of side effects.

Sometimes this medicine must be taken for several weeks before its full effect is reached in the treatment of certain mental and emotional conditions.

Dosing—The dose of molindone will be different for different patients. *Follow your doctor's orders or the directions on the label.* The following information includes only the average doses of molindone. *If your dose is different, do not change it* unless your doctor tells you to do so.

- The number of tablets or amount of solution that you take depends on the strength of the medicine. Also, *the number of doses you take each day, the time allowed between doses, and the length of time you take the medicine depend on the medical problem for which you are using molindone.*
- For *oral* dosage forms (solution or tablets):

  —Adults: To start, 50 to 75 milligrams a day, taken in smaller doses three or four times during the day. For maintenance, the dose you take will depend on your condition and may be from 15 to 225 milligrams a day, taken in smaller doses three or four times during the day.

  —Children up to 12 years of age: The dose must be determined by the doctor.

Missed dose—If you miss a dose of this medicine, take it as soon as possible. However, if it is within 2 hours of your next dose, skip the missed dose and go back to your regular dosing schedule. Do not double doses.

Storage—To store this medicine:

- Keep out of the reach of children.
- Store away from heat and direct light.
- Do not store the tablets in the bathroom, near the kitchen sink, or in other damp places. Heat or moisture may cause the medicine to break down.
- Keep the liquid form of this medicine from freezing

- Do not keep outdated medicine or medicine no longer needed. Be sure that any discarded medicine is out of the reach of children.

Precautions While Using This Medicine

Your doctor should check your progress at regular visits. This will allow the dosage of the medicine to be adjusted when necessary and also will reduce the possibility of side effects.

Do not stop taking this medicine without first checking with your doctor. Your doctor may want you to reduce gradually the amount you are taking before stopping completely.

Do not take molindone within 1 or 2 hours of taking antacids or medicine for diarrhea. Taking them too close together may make molindone less effective.

This medicine will add to the effects of alcohol and other CNS depressants (medicines that slow down the nervous system, possibly causing drowsiness). Some examples of CNS depressants are antihistamines or medicine for hay fever, other allergies, or colds; sedatives, tranquilizers, or sleeping medicine; prescription pain medicine or narcotics; barbiturates; medicine for seizures; muscle relaxants; or anesthetics, including some dental anesthetics. *Check with your doctor before taking any of the above while you are using this medicine.*

Molindone may cause some people to become drowsy or less alert than they are normally, especially during the first few weeks the medicine is being taken. Even if you take this medicine only at bedtime, you may feel drowsy or less alert on arising. *Make sure you know how you react to this medicine before you drive, use machines, or do anything else that could be dangerous if you are not alert.*

Dizziness or lightheadedness may occur, especially when you get up from a lying or sitting position. Getting up slowly may help. If the problem continues or gets worse, check with your doctor.

These medicines may make you sweat less, causing your body temperature to increase. *Use extra care not to become overheated during exercise or hot weather while you are taking this medicine, since overheating may result in heat stroke.* Also, hot baths or saunas may make you feel dizzy or faint while you are taking this medicine.

Molindone may cause dryness of the mouth. For temporary relief, use sugarless candy or gum, melt bits of ice in your mouth, or use a saliva substitute. However, if your mouth continues to feel dry for more than 2 weeks, check with your medical doctor or dentist. Continuing dryness of the mouth may increase the chance of dental disease, including tooth decay, gum disease, and fungus infection.

Side Effects of This Medicine

Along with its needed effects, molindone can sometimes cause serious side effects. Tardive dyskinesia (a movement disorder) may occur and may not go away after you stop using the medicine. Symptoms of tardive dyskinesia include fine, worm-like movements of the tongue, or other uncontrolled movements of the mouth, tongue, cheeks, jaw, or arms and legs. Other serious but rare side effects may also occur. These include severe muscle stiffness, fever, unusual tiredness or weakness, fast heartbeat, difficult breathing, increased sweating, loss of bladder control, and seizures (neuroleptic malignant syndrome). *You and your doctor should discuss the good this medicine will do as well as the risks of taking it.*

Stop taking molindone and get emergency help immediately if any of the following side effects occur:

Rare

Convulsions (seizures); difficult or fast breathing; fast heartbeat or irregular pulse; fever (high); high or low (irregular) blood pressure; increased sweating; loss of bladder control; muscle stiffness (severe); unusually pale skin; unusual tiredness or weakness

Also, check with your doctor as soon as possible if any of the following side effects occur:

More common

Difficulty in talking or swallowing; inability to move eyes; lip smacking or puckering; loss of balance control; mask-like face; muscle spasms, especially of the neck and back; puffing of cheeks; rapid or worm-like movements of tongue; restlessness or need to keep moving (severe); shuffling walk; stiffness of arms and legs; trembling and shaking of hands; twisting movements of body; uncontrolled movements of arms and legs; unusual chewing movements

Less common

Mental depression

Rare

Confusion; hot, dry skin, or lack of sweating; muscle weakness; skin rash; yellow eyes or skin

Other side effects may occur that usually do not need medical attention. These side effects may go away during treatment as your body adjusts to the medicine. However, check with your doctor if any of the following side effects continue or are bothersome:

More common

Blurred vision; constipation; decreased sweating; difficult urination; dizziness or lightheadedness, especially when getting up suddenly from a lying or sitting position; drowsiness; dryness of mouth; headache; nausea; stuffy nose

Less common

Changes in menstrual periods; decreased sexual ability; false sense of well-being; swelling of breasts; unusual secretion of milk

Some side effects may occur after you have stopped taking this medicine. Check with your doctor as soon as possible if you notice any of the following effects:

Lip smacking or puckering; puffing of cheeks; rapid or worm-like movements of tongue; uncontrolled chewing movements; uncontrolled movements of arms and legs

Other side effects not listed above may also occur in some patients. If you notice any other effects, check with your doctor.

Annual revision: 03/19/93

MOLYBDENUM SUPPLEMENTS Systemic†

A commonly used brand name in the U.S. is Molypen.

Generic name product may also be available.

†Not commercially available in Canada.

Description

The body needs molybdenum for normal growth and health. For patients who are unable to get enough molybdenum in their regular diet or who have a need for more molybdenum, molybdenum supplements may be necessary. They are generally taken by mouth in multivitamin/mineral products but some patients may have to receive them by injection.

A deficiency of molybdenum is rare. However, if the body does not get enough molybdenum, certain enzymes needed by the body are affected. This may lead to a build up of unwanted substances in some people.

Injectable molybdenum is administered only by or under the supervision of your doctor. This medicine is available in the following dosage forms:

Oral

Molybdenum is available orally as part of a multivitamin/mineral combination.

Parenteral

- Injection (U.S.)

It is very important that you read and understand the following information. If any of it causes you special concern, check with your doctor or pharmacist. Also, *if you have any questions* or if you want more information about this dietary supplement or your medical problem, *ask your doctor, nurse, pharmacist, or dietitian.*

Importance of Diet

Many nutritionists recommend that, if possible, people should get all the molybdenum they need from foods. However, some people do not get enough molybdenum from their diet. For example, people on weight-loss diets may consume too little food to provide enough molybdenum. Others may need more molybdenum than normal. For such people, a molybdenum supplement is important.

In order to get enough vitamins and minerals in your regular diet, it is important that you eat a balanced and varied diet. Follow carefully any diet program your doctor may recommend. For your specific vitamin and/or mineral needs, ask your doctor or dietitian for a list of appropriate foods.

The amount of molybdenum in foods depends on the soil in which the food is grown. Some soils have more molybdenum than others. Peas, beans, cereal products, leafy vegetables, and low-fat milk are good sources of molybdenum.

Experts have developed a list of recommended dietary allowances (RDA) for most vitamins and some minerals. The RDA are not an exact number but a general idea of how much you need. They do not cover amounts needed for problems caused by serious lack of vitamins and minerals.

Because a lack of molybdenum is rare, there are no RDA for it. The following intakes are thought to be plenty for most individuals:

Infants and children—
- Birth to 6 months of age: 15–30 micrograms (mcg) per day.
- 6 months to 1 year of age: 20–40 mcg per day.
- 1 to 3 years of age: 25–50 mcg per day.
- 4 to 6 years of age: 30–75 mcg per day.
- 7 to 10 years of age: 50–150 mcg per day.

Adolescents and adults—75–250 mcg per day.

Before Using This Dietary Supplement

In deciding to use a dietary supplement, the risks of taking the dietary supplement must be weighed against the good it will do. This is a decision you and your doctor will make. For molybdenum, the following should be considered:

Allergies—Tell your doctor if you have ever had any unusual or allergic reaction to molybdenum. Also tell your doctor and pharmacist if you are allergic to any other substances, such as foods, preservatives, or dyes.

Pregnancy—It is especially important that you are receiving enough vitamins and minerals when you become pregnant and that you continue to receive the right amount of vitamins and minerals throughout your pregnancy. The healthy growth and development of the fetus depend on a steady supply of nutrients from the mother. However, taking large amounts of a dietary supplement in pregnancy may be harmful to the mother and/or fetus and should be avoided.

Breast-feeding—It is important that you receive the right amounts of vitamins and minerals so that your baby will also get the vitamins and minerals needed to grow properly. However, taking large amounts of a dietary supplement while breast-feeding may be harmful to the mother and/or baby and should be avoided.

Children—It is especially important that children receive enough molybdenum in their diet for healthy growth and development.

Older adults—It is important that older people continue to receive enough vitamins in their diet for good health.

Medicines or other dietary supplements—Although certain medicines or dietary supplements should not be used together at all, in other cases they may be used together even if an interaction might occur. In these cases, your doctor may want to change the dose, or other precautions may be necessary. Tell your doctor and pharmacist if you are taking any other dietary supplement or any prescription or nonprescription (over-the-counter [OTC]) medicine.

Other medical problems—The presence of other medical problems may affect the use of molybdenum. Make sure you tell your doctor if you have any other medical problems, especially:

- Copper deficiency—Molybdenum may make this condition worse
- Kidney diease or
- Liver disease—These conditions may cause higher blood levels of molybdenum, which may increase the chance of unwanted effects

Proper Use of This Dietary Supplement

Molybdenum is available orally only as part of a multivitamin/mineral product.

Some people believe that taking very large doses of a vitamin or mineral (called megadoses) is useful for treating certain medical problems. Studies have not proven this. Large doses should be taken only under the direction of your doctor after need has been identified.

Missed dose—If you miss taking your multivitamin containing molybdenum for one or more days there is no cause for concern, since it takes some time for your body to become seriously low in molybdenum. However, if your doctor has recommended that you take molybdenum, try to remember to take it as directed every day.

Storage—To store this dietary supplement:

- Keep out of the reach of children.
- Store away from heat and direct light.
- Do not store in the bathroom, near the kitchen sink, or in other damp places. Heat or moisture may cause the dietary supplement to break down.
- Keep the dietary supplement from freezing. Do not refrigerate.
- Do not keep outdated dietary supplements or those no longer needed. Be sure that any discarded dietary supplement is out of the reach of children.

Precautions While Using This Dietary Supplement

Large amounts of molybdenum may cause your body to lose copper. Your doctor may recommend that you take a copper supplement while on molybdenum therapy.

Side Effects of This Dietary Supplement

Along with its needed effects, a dietary supplement may cause some unwanted effects. Although molybdenum has not been reported to cause any side effects, *check with your doctor immediately* if any of the following side effects occur as a result of a molybdenum overdose:

Symptoms of overdose

Joint pain; side, lower back, or stomach pain; swelling of feet or lower legs

Other side effects not listed above may also occur in some patients. If you notice any other effects, check with your doctor.

Annual revision: 03/02/92
Interim revision: 07/31/92

MONOOCTANOIN Local†

A commonly used brand name in the U.S. is Moctanin.

†Not commercially available in Canada.

Description

Monooctanoin (mono-OCK-ta-noyn) is used to dissolve cholesterol gallstones. Gallstones, which are found in the gallbladder or bile duct, sometimes remain in the bile duct even after the gallbladder has been removed by surgery. These stones may be too large to pass out of the body on their own. A catheter or tube is used to put the solution of monooctanoin into the bile duct where it will come in contact with the gallstone or galistones and dissolve them. This is done for a period of 1 to 3 weeks.

Monooctanoin is available only with your doctor's prescription. It is available in the following dosage form:

Local

- Irrigation (U.S.)

It is very important that you read and understand the following information. If any of it causes you special concern, check with your doctor. Also, *if you have any questions* or if you want more information about this medicine or your medical problem, *ask your doctor, nurse, or pharmacist.*

Before Using This Medicine

In deciding to use a medicine, the risks of taking the medicine must be weighed against the good it will do. This is a decision you and your doctor will make. For monooctanoin, the following should be considered:

Allergies—Tell your doctor if you have ever had any unusual or allergic reaction to monooctanoin or any vegetable oils. Also, tell your doctor if you are allergic to any other substances, such as foods, preservatives, or dyes.

Pregnancy—Studies with this medicine have not been done in either humans or animals.

Breast-feeding—It is not known whether monooctanoin passes into the breast milk. However, this medicine has not been reported to cause problems in nursing babies.

Children—Studies on this medicine have been done only in adult patients, and there is no specific information comparing use of monooctanoin in children with use in other age groups.

Older adults—Many medicines have not been studied specifically in older people. Therefore, it may not be known whether they work exactly the same way they do in younger adults or if they cause different side effects or problems in older people. There is no specific information comparing use of monooctanoin in the elderly with use in other age groups.

Other medical problems—The presence of other medical problems may affect the use of monooctanoin. Make sure you tell your doctor if you have any other medical problems, especially:

- Biliary tract problems (other) or
- Jaundice or
- Pancreatitis (inflammation of the pancreas)—Monooctanoin may make these conditions worse
- Duodenal ulcer (recent) or
- Intestinal problems—Monooctanoin may make these conditions worse and may increase the chance of bleeding
- Liver disease (severe)—Unwanted effects may occur if the liver is not working properly

Before you begin using any new medicine (prescription or nonprescription) or if you develop any new medical problem while you are using this medicine, check with your doctor, nurse, or pharmacist.

Side Effects of This Medicine

Along with its needed effects, a medicine may cause some unwanted effects. Although not all of these side effects appear very often, when they do occur they may require medical attention.

Check with your doctor as soon as possible if any of the following side effects occur:

Less common or rare

Abdominal or stomach pain (severe); back pain (severe); drowsiness (severe); fever, chills, or sore throat; nausea (continuing); shortness of breath (severe)

Other side effects may occur that usually do not need medical attention. These side effects may go away during treatment as your body adjusts to the medicine. However, check with your doctor if any of the following side effects continue or are bothersome:

More common

Abdominal or stomach pain (mild) or burning sensation

Less common or rare

Back pain (mild); diarrhea; flushing or redness of face; loss of appetite; metallic taste; nausea or vomiting

Other side effects not listed above may also occur in some patients. If you notice any other effects, check with your doctor.

Annual revision: 08/16/91

MORICIZINE Systemic†

A commonly used brand name in the U.S. is Ethmozine.

†Not commercially available in Canada.

Description

Moricizine (mor-IH-siz-een) belongs to the group of medicines known as antiarrhythmics. It is used to correct irregular or rapid heartbeats to a normal rhythm by making the heart tissue less sensitive.

There is a chance that moricizine may cause new or make worse existing heart rhythm problems when it is used. Since other antiarrhythmic medicines have been shown to cause severe problems in some patients, moricizine is only used to treat serious heart rhythm problems. Discuss this possible effect with your doctor.

This medicine is available only with your doctor's prescription, in the following dosage form:

Oral

- Tablets (U.S.)

It is very important that you read and understand the following information. If any of it causes you special concern, check with your doctor. Also, *if you have any questions* or if you want more information about this medicine or your medical problem, *ask your doctor, nurse, or pharmacist.*

Before Using This Medicine

In deciding to use a medicine, the risks of taking the medicine must be weighed against the good it will do. This is a decision you and your doctor will make. For moricizine, the following should be considered:

Allergies—Tell your doctor if you have ever had any unusual or allergic reaction to moricizine. Also tell your doctor and pharmacist if you are allergic to any other substances, such as foods, preservatives, or dyes.

Pregnancy—Moricizine has not been studied in pregnant women. However, this medicine has not been shown to cause birth defects or other problems in animal studies, although it affected weight gain in some animals. Before taking moricizine, make sure your doctor knows if you are pregnant or if you may become pregnant.

Breast-feeding—Moricizine passes into the milk of some animals and may also pass into the milk of humans. However, this medicine has not been reported to cause problems in nursing babies.

Children—Studies on this medicine have been done only in adult patients, and there is no specific information comparing use of moricizine in children with use in other age groups.

Older adults—Many medicines have not been studied specifically in older people. Therefore, it may not be known whether they work exactly the same way they do in younger adults or if they cause different side effects or problems in older people. There is no specific information comparing use of moricizine in the elderly with use in other age groups, although the risk of some unwanted effects may be increased.

Other medicines—Although certain medicine should not be used together at all, in other cases two different medicines may be used together even if an interaction might occur. In these cases, your doctor may want to change the dose, or other precautions may be necessary. Tell your doctor and pharmacist if you are taking any other prescription or nonprescription (over-the-counter [OTC]) medicine.

Other medical problems—The presence of other medical problems may affect the use of moricizine. Make sure you tell your doctor if you have any other medical problems, especially:

- Kidney disease or
- Liver disease—Effects may be increased because of slower removal of moricizine from the body
- Heart disease or
- Recent heart attack or
- If you have a pacemaker—Risk of irregular heartbeats may be increased

Before you begin using any new medicine (prescription or nonprescription) or if you develop any new medical problem while you are using this medicine, check with your doctor, nurse, or pharmacist.

Proper Use of This Medicine

Take moricizine exactly as directed by your doctor, even though you may feel well. Do not take more or less of it than your doctor ordered.

This medicine works best when there is a constant amount in the blood. *To help keep the amount constant, do not miss any doses. Also, it is best to take each dose at evenly spaced times day and night.* For example, if you are to take 3 doses a day, doses should be spaced about 8 hours apart. If you need help in planning the best times to take your medicine, check with your doctor or pharmacist.

Missed dose—If you do miss a dose of moricizine and remember within 4 hours, take it as soon as possible. However, if you do not remember until later, skip the missed dose and go back to your regular dosing schedule. Do not double doses.

Storage—To store this medicine:

- Keep out of the reach of children.
- Store away from heat and direct light.
- Do not store in the bathroom, near the kitchen sink, or in other damp places. Heat or moisture may cause the medicine to break down.
- Do not keep outdated medicine or medicine no longer needed. Be sure that any discarded medicine is out of the reach of children.

Precautions While Using This Medicine

It is important that your doctor check your progress at regular visits to make sure the medicine is working properly. This will allow changes to be made in the amount of medicine you are taking, if necessary.

Your doctor may want you to carry a medical identification card or bracelet stating that you are using this medicine.

Before having any kind of surgery (including dental surgery) or emergency treatment, tell the medical doctor or dentist in charge that you are taking this medicine.

Moricizine may cause some people to become dizzy or lightheaded. Make sure you know how you react to this medicine before you drive, use machines, or do anything else that could be dangerous if you are dizzy.

Side Effects of This Medicine

Along with its needed effects, a medicine may cause some unwanted effects. Although not all of these side effects may occur, if they do occur they may need medical attention.

Check with your doctor as soon as possible if any of the following side effects occur:

Less common

Chest pain; fast or irregular heartbeat; shortness of breath; swelling of feet or lower legs

Rare

Fever (sudden, high)

Other side effects may occur that usually do not need medical attention. These side effects may go away during treatment as your body adjusts to the medicine. However, check with your doctor if any of the following side effects continue or are bothersome:

More common

Dizziness

Less common

Blurred vision; diarrhea; dryness of mouth; headache; nausea or vomiting; nervousness; numbness or tingling in arms or legs or around mouth; pain in arms or legs; stomach pain; trouble in sleeping; unusual tiredness or weakness

Other side effects not listed above may also occur in some patients. If you notice any other effects, check with your doctor.

Annual revision: 09/27/92

MUMPS VIRUS VACCINE LIVE Systemic

A commonly used brand name in the U.S. and Canada is Mumpsvax.

Description

Mumps Virus Vaccine Live is an active immunizing agent used to prevent infection by the mumps virus. It works by causing your body to produce its own protection (antibodies) against the virus.

The following information applies only to the Jeryl Lynn strain of mumps vaccine. Different types of mumps vaccines may be available in countries other than the U.S. and Canada.

Mumps is an infection that can cause serious problems, such as encephalitis and meningitis, which affect the brain. In addition, adolescent boys and men are very susceptible to a condition called orchitis, which causes pain and swelling in the testicles and scrotum and, in rare cases, sterility. Also, mumps infection can cause spontaneous abortion in women during the first three months of pregnancy.

Although immunization against mumps is recommended for everyone (children, adolescents, and adults) born in or after 1957, it is especially important for:

- persons born between 1967 and 1977.
- children 12 months of age and older, including school-age children, children in day-care centers, and children of pregnant women who have not yet received their own mumps vaccination.
- boys nearing the age of puberty, adolescent boys, and men.
- women of child-bearing age who are not pregnant.
- persons vaccinated during the years 1950 through 1978 (especially during the years 1950 through 1967)

- with either the inactivated (killed) mumps vaccine or with an unknown type of mumps vaccine.
- persons traveling outside the U.S.

Immunization against mumps is not recommended for infants younger than 12 months of age, because antibodies they received from their mothers before birth may interfere with the effectiveness of the vaccine. Children who were immunized against mumps before 12 months of age should be immunized again.

If the mumps vaccine is going to be given in a combination immunization that includes measles vaccine, the person to be immunized should be at least 15 months old to make sure the measles vaccine is effective.

You can be considered to be immune to mumps only if you:

- received mumps vaccine on or after your first birthday and have the medical record to prove it, or
- have a doctor's diagnosis of a previous mumps infection, or
- have had a laboratory test that shows that you are immune to mumps.

This vaccine is available only from your doctor or other authorized health care provider, in the following dosage form:

Parenteral

- Injection (U.S. and Canada)

It is very important that you read and understand the following information. If any of it causes you special concern, check with your doctor. Also, *if you have any questions* or if you want more information about this medicine or your medical problem, *ask your doctor, nurse, or pharmacist.*

Before Receiving This Vaccine

In deciding to use a medicine, the risks of taking the medicine must be weighed against the good it will do. This is a decision you and your doctor will make. For mumps vaccine, the following should be considered:

Allergies—Tell your doctor if you have ever had any unusual or allergic reaction to mumps vaccine or to any form of the antibiotic neomycin. Also tell your doctor and pharmacist if you are allergic to any other substances, such as foods (especially eggs) or preservatives. The mumps vaccine available in the U.S. and Canada is grown in a chick embryo cell culture.

Pregnancy—Tell your doctor if you are now pregnant or if you may become pregnant within 3 months after receiving this medicine. Studies on effects in pregnancy have not been done in either humans or animals. However, use during pregnancy is not recommended, because mumps vaccine may infect the placenta, although the vaccine has not been shown to infect the fetus or to cause birth defects.

Breast-feeding—Mumps vaccine has not been reported to cause problems in nursing babies.

Children—Use is not recommended for infants up to 12 months of age.

Other medicines—Although certain medicines should not be used together at all, in other cases two different medicines may be used together even if an interaction might occur. In these cases, your doctor may want to change the dose, or other precautions may be necessary. Before receiving mumps vaccine, it is especially important that your doctor and pharmacist know if you have received any of the following:

- Any other live virus vaccine in the last month or intention to within the next month—One live virus vaccine may decrease the useful effect of the other live virus vaccine
- Blood transfusions or other blood products or gamma globulin or other globulins in the last 3 months or intention to within the next 2 weeks—The useful effects of either these products or the mumps vaccine may be decreased
- Treatment with x-rays or cancer medicines—May decrease the useful effect of mumps vaccine

Other medical problems—The presence of other medical problems may affect the use of mumps vaccine. Make sure you tell your doctor if you have any other medical problems, especially:

- Immune deficiency condition (or family history of)—The condition may decrease the useful effect of the vaccine or may increase the risk and severity of side effects
- Serious illness with fever—The symptoms of the illness may be confused with the possible side effects of the vaccine
- Tuberculosis—Mumps vaccine will interfere with the results of the skin test for tuberculosis for 4 or more weeks

Before you begin using any new medicine (prescription or nonprescription) or if you develop any new medical problem while you are using this medicine, check with your doctor, nurse, or pharmacist.

Precautions After Receiving This Vaccine

Do not become pregnant for 3 months after receiving mumps vaccine without first checking with your doctor. There is a chance that this vaccine may cause problems during pregnancy.

Tell your doctor that you have received this vaccine:

- if you are to receive a tuberculin skin test within 6 weeks after receiving this vaccine. The results of the test may be affected by this vaccine.
- if you are to receive any other live virus vaccines within 1 month after receiving this vaccine.
- if you are to receive blood transfusions or other blood products within 2 weeks after receiving this vaccine.

- if you are to receive gamma globulin or other globulins within 2 weeks after receiving this vaccine.

Side Effects of This Vaccine

Along with its needed effects, a medicine may cause some unwanted effects. Although not all of these side effects may occur, if they do occur they may need medical attention.

Get emergency help immediately if any of the following side effects occur:

Symptoms of allergic reaction

Difficulty in breathing or swallowing; hives; itching, especially of feet or hands; reddening of skin, especially around ears; swelling of eyes, face, or inside of nose; unusual tiredness or weakness (sudden and severe)

Check with your doctor as soon as possible if any of the following side effects occur:

Rare

Bruising or purple spots on skin; confusion; convulsions (seizures); fever over 103 °F (39.4 °C); headache (severe or continuing); irritability; pain, tenderness, or swelling in testicles and scrotum (in adolescent boys and men); stiff neck; vomiting

Other side effects may occur that usually do not need medical attention. However, check with your doctor if any of the following side effects continue or are bothersome:

More common

Burning or stinging at place of injection

Less common or rare

Fever of 100 °F (37.7 °C) or less; itching, swelling, redness, tenderness, or hard lump at place of injection; skin rash; swollen glands on side of face or neck

Other side effects not listed above may also occur in some patients. If you notice any other effects, check with your doctor.

Annual revision: September 1990

MUPIROCIN Topical

A commonly used brand name in the U.S. and Canada is Bactroban. Another commonly used name is pseudomonic acid.

Description

Mupirocin (myoo-PEER-oh-sin) is used to treat bacterial infections. It works by killing bacteria or preventing their growth.

Mupirocin ointment is applied to the skin to treat impetigo. It may also be used for other bacterial skin infections as determined by your doctor.

Mupirocin is available in the U.S. only with your doctor's prescription. It is available in Canada without a prescription; however, your doctor may have special instructions on the proper use of this medicine for your medical problem. Mupirocin is available in the following dosage form:

Topical

- Ointment (U.S. and Canada)

It is very important that you read and understand the following information. If any of it causes you special concern, check with your doctor. Also, *if you have any questions* or if you want more information about this medicine or your medical problem, *ask your doctor, nurse, or pharmacist.*

Before Using This Medicine

In deciding to use a medicine, the risks of taking the medicine must be weighed against the good it will do. This is a decision you and your doctor will make. For topical mupirocin, the following should be considered:

Allergies—Tell your doctor if you have ever had any unusual or allergic reaction to mupirocin. Also tell your doctor and pharmacist if you are allergic to any other substances, such as preservatives or dyes.

Pregnancy—Topical mupirocin has not been studied in pregnant women. However, this medication has not been shown to cause birth defects or other problems in animal studies.

Breast-feeding—It is not known whether topical mupirocin passes into the breast milk. However, this medicine is unlikely to pass into the breast milk in large amounts, since very little mupirocin is absorbed into the mother's body when applied to the skin.

Children—Studies on this medicine have been done only in adult patients, and there is no specific information about its use in children.

Older adults—Many medicines have not been tested in older people. Therefore, it may not be known whether they work exactly the same way they do in younger adults or if they cause different side effects or problems in older people. There is no specific information about the use of mupirocin in the elderly.

Before you begin using any new medicine (prescription or nonprescription) or if you develop any new medical problem while you are using this medicine, check with your doctor, nurse, or pharmacist.

Proper Use of This Medicine

Do not use this medicine in the eyes.

To use:

- Before applying this medicine, wash the affected area(s) with soap and water, and dry thoroughly. Then apply a small amount to the affected area(s) and rub in gently.
- After applying this medicine, the treated area(s) may be covered with a gauze dressing if desired.

To help clear up your skin infection completely, keep using mupirocin for the full time of treatment, even if your symptoms have disappeared. *Do not miss any doses.*

Missed dose—If you do miss a dose of this medicine, apply it as soon as possible. However, if it is almost time for your next dose, skip the missed dose and go back to your regular dosing schedule.

Storage—To store this medicine:

- Keep out of the reach of children.
- Store away from heat and direct light.
- Keep the medicine from freezing.
- Do not keep outdated medicine or medicine no longer needed. Be sure that any discarded medicine is out of the reach of children.

Precautions While Using This Medicine

If your skin infection does not improve within 3 to 5 days, or if it becomes worse, check with your doctor or pharmacist.

Side Effects of This Medicine

Along with its needed effects, a medicine may cause some unwanted effects. The following side effects may go away during treatment as your body adjusts to the medicine. However, check with your doctor if any of these effects continue or are bothersome:

Less common

Dry skin; skin rash, redness, swelling, burning, itching, stinging, or pain

Other side effects not listed above may also occur in some patients. If you notice any other effects, check with your doctor.

Annual revision: June 1990

MUROMONAB-CD3 Systemic

A commonly used brand name in the U.S. and Canada is Orthoclone OKT3.

Description

Muromonab (myoor-oh-MON-ab)-CD3 is a monoclonal antibody. It is used to reduce the body's natural immunity in patients who receive organ (for example, kidney) transplants.

When a patient receives an organ transplant, the body's white blood cells will try to get rid of (reject) the transplanted organ. Muromonab-CD3 works by preventing the white blood cells from doing this.

The effect of muromonab-CD3 on the white blood cells may also reduce the body's ability to fight infections. Before you begin treatment, you and your doctor should talk about the good this medicine will do as well as the risks of using it.

Muromonab-CD3 is to be administered only by or under the immediate supervision of your doctor. It is available in the following dosage form:

Parenteral

- Injection (U.S. and Canada)

It is very important that you read and understand the following information. If any of it causes you special concern, check with your doctor. Also, *if you have any questions* or if you want more information about this medicine or your medical problem, *ask your doctor, nurse, or pharmacist.*

Before Using This Medicine

In deciding to use a medicine, the risks of taking the medicine must be weighed against the good it will do. This is a decision you and your doctor will make. For muromonab-CD3, the following should be considered:

Allergies—Tell your doctor if you have ever had any unusual or allergic reaction to muromonab-CD3 or to rodents (such as mice or rats). Muromonab-CD3 is grown in a mouse cell culture. Also tell your doctor and pharmacist if you are allergic to any other substance, such as preservatives.

Pregnancy—Studies have not been done in either humans or animals.

Breast-feeding—Muromonab-CD3 has not been reported to cause problems in nursing babies. However, it may be necessary for you to stop breast-feeding during treatment. Be sure you have discussed the risks and benefits of the medicine with your doctor.

Children—Although there is no specific information comparing use of muromonab-CD3 in children with use in other age groups, this medicine is not expected to cause different side effects or problems in children than it does in adults.

Older adults—Many medicines have not been studied specifically in older people. Therefore, it may not be known whether they work exactly the same way they do in younger adults or if they cause different side effects or problems in older people. There is no specific information comparing use of muromonab-CD3 in the elderly with use in other age groups.

Other medicines—Although certain medicines should not be used together at all, in other cases two different medicines may be used together even if an interaction might occur. In these cases, your doctor may want to change the dose, or other precautions may be necessary. When you are receiving muromonab-CD3, it is especially important that your doctor and pharmacist know if you are taking any of the following:

- Azathioprine (e.g., Imuran) or
- Chlorambucil (e.g., Leukeran) or
- Corticosteroids (cortisone-like medicine) or
- Cyclophosphamide (e.g., Cytoxan) or
- Cyclosporine (e.g., Sandimmune) or
- Mercaptopurine (e.g., Purinethol)—There may be an increased risk of infection and development of cancer because muromonab-CD3 reduces the body's ability to fight them

Other medical problems—The presence of other medical problems may affect the use of muromonab-CD3. Make sure you tell your doctor if you have any other medical problems, especially:

- Chickenpox (including recent exposure) or
- Herpes zoster (shingles)—Risk of severe disease affecting other parts of the body
- Infection—Muromonab-CD3 decreases your body's ability to fight infection

Before you begin using any new medicine (prescription or nonprescription) or if you develop any new medical problem while you are using this medicine, check with your doctor, nurse, or pharmacist.

Precautions While Using This Medicine

It is very important that your doctor check your progress at regular visits to make sure that this medicine is working properly and to check for unwanted effects.

While you are being treated with muromonab-CD3 and after you stop treatment with it, *do not have any immunizations (vaccinations) without your doctor's approval.* Muromonab-CD3 may lower your body's resistance and there is a chance you might get the infection the immunization is meant to prevent. In addition, other persons living in your house should not take oral polio vaccine since there is a chance they could pass the polio virus on to you. Also, avoid persons who have recently taken oral polio vaccine. Do not get close to them and do not stay in the same room with them for very long. If you cannot take these precautions, you should consider wearing a protective face mask that covers the nose and mouth.

Treatment with muromonab-CD3 may also increase the chance of getting other infections. If you can, avoid people with colds or other infections. If you think you are getting a cold or other infection, check with your doctor.

This medicine commonly causes chest pain, dizziness, fever and chills, shortness of breath, stomach upset, and trembling within a few hours after the first dose. These effects should be much less after the second dose and should not occur after that. However, *check with your doctor or nurse immediately* if you have severe shortness of breath after the first dose or if the effects continue.

Side Effects of This Medicine

Along with its needed effects, a medicine may cause some unwanted effects. Because of the way that muromonab-CD3 acts on the body, there is a chance that it may cause effects that may not occur until years after the medicine is used. These delayed effects may include certain types of cancer, such as lymphomas. Discuss these possible effects with your doctor.

Although not all of these side effects may occur, if they do occur, they may need medical attention.

Check with your doctor or nurse immediately if the following side effect occurs with the first dose of this medicine:

Less common

Shortness of breath (severe)

Check with your doctor as soon as possible if any of the following side effects occur within the first 2 or 3 days after a dose:

More common

Chest pain; diarrhea; dizziness or faintness; fever and chills; headache; nausea and vomiting; rapid or irregular heartbeat; shortness of breath or wheezing; trembling and shaking of hands

Less common

Stiff neck; unusual sensitivity of eyes to light

Rare

Confusion; convulsions (seizures); hallucinations (seeing, hearing, or feeling things that are not there); unusual tiredness

After you stop using this medicine, it may still produce some side effects that need medical attention. During this period of time check with your doctor if you notice the following side effects:

Fever and chills

Other side effects not listed above may also occur in some patients. If you notice any other effects, check with your doctor.

Annual revision: 08/09/92

N

NABILONE Systemic*

A commonly used brand name in Canada is Cesamet.

*Not commercially available in the U.S.

Description

Nabilone (NAB-i-lone) is chemically related to marijuana. It is used to prevent the nausea and vomiting that may occur after treatment with cancer medicines. It is used only when other kinds of medicine for nausea and vomiting do not work.

Nabilone is available only with your doctor's prescription. Prescriptions cannot be refilled and you must obtain a new prescription from your doctor each time you need this medicine. Nabilone is available in the following dosage form:

Oral

- Capsules (Canada)

It is very important that you read and understand the following information. If any of it causes you special concern, check with your doctor. Also, *if you have any questions* or if you want more information about this medicine or your medical problem, *ask your doctor, nurse, or pharmacist.*

Before Using This Medicine

In deciding to use a medicine, the risks of taking the medicine must be weighed against the good it will do. This is a decision you and your doctor will make. For nabilone, the following should be considered:

Allergies—Tell your doctor if you have ever had any unusual or allergic reaction to nabilone or marijuana products. Also tell your doctor and pharmacist if you are allergic to any other substances, such as foods, preservatives, or dyes.

Pregnancy—Studies have not been done in pregnant women. However, studies in animals have shown a decrease in successful pregnancies and a decrease in the number of live babies born, when nabilone was given in doses many times the usual human dose.

Breast-feeding—It is not known whether nabilone passes into the breast milk. However, nabilone is not recommended during breast-feeding because other medicines similar to nabilone that pass into the breast milk have been shown to cause unwanted effects in the nursing baby.

Children—Studies on this medicine have been done only in adult patients, and there is no specific information comparing use of nabilone in children with use in other age groups.

Older adults—Fast or pounding heartbeat, feeling faint or lightheaded, and unusual tiredness or weakness may be especially likely to occur in elderly patients, who are usually more sensitive than younger adults to the effects of nabilone. Also, the effects this medicine may have on the mind may be of special concern in the elderly. Therefore, older people should be watched closely while taking this medicine.

Other medicines—Although certain medicines should not be used together at all, in other cases 2 different medicines may be used together even if an interaction might occur. In these cases, your doctor may want to change the dose, or other precautions may be necessary. When you are taking nabilone, it is especially important that your doctor and pharmacist know if you are taking any of the following:

- Central nervous system (CNS) depressants (medicine that causes drowsiness) or
- Tricyclic antidepressants (medicine for depression)—Taking these medicines with nabilone may increase the CNS depressant effects

N

Other medical problems—The presence of other medical problems may affect the use of nabilone. Make sure you tell your doctor if you have any other medical problems, especially:

- Alcohol abuse (or history of) or
- Drug abuse or dependence (or history of)—Dependence on nabilone may develop
- Heart disease or
- High blood pressure or
- Low blood pressure or
- Manic depression or
- Schizophrenia—Nabilone may make the condition worse
- Liver disease (severe)—Higher blood levels of nabilone may occur, increasing the chance of side effects

Before you begin using any new medicine (prescription or nonprescription) or if you develop any new medical problem while you are using this medicine, check with your doctor, nurse, or pharmacist.

Proper Use of This Medicine

Take this medicine only as directed by your doctor. Do not take more of it, do not take it more often, and do not take it for a longer time than your doctor ordered. If too much is taken, it may lead to other medical problems because of an overdose.

Dosing—The dose of nabilone will be different for different patients. *Follow your doctor's orders or the directions on the label.* The following information includes only the average doses of nabilone. *If your dose is different, do not change it* unless your doctor tells you to do so.

- For *oral* dosage forms (capsules):
  —For nausea and vomiting caused by cancer medicines:
    - Adults and teenagers—Usually 1 or 2 milligrams (mg) twice a day. Your doctor will tell you how and when to take this medicine while you are taking your cancer medicine.
    - Children—Use and dose must be determined by your doctor.

Missed dose—If you miss a dose of this medicine, take it as soon as you remember. However, if it is almost time for your next dose, skip the missed dose and go back to your regular dosing schedule. *Do not double doses.*

Storage—To store this medicine:
- Keep out of the reach of children.
- Store away from heat and direct light.
- Do not store this medicine in the bathroom, near the kitchen sink, or in other damp places. Heat or moisture may cause the medicine to break down.
- Do not keep outdated medicine or medicine no longer needed. Be sure that any discarded medicine is out of the reach of children.

Precautions While Using This Medicine

Nabilone will add to the effects of alcohol and other central nervous system (CNS) depressants (medicines that slow down the nervous system, possibly causing drowsiness). Some examples of CNS depressants are antihistamines or medicine for hay fever, other allergies, or colds; sedatives, tranquilizers, or sleeping medicine; prescription pain medicines including other narcotics; barbiturates; medicine for seizures; muscle relaxants; or anesthetics, including some dental anesthetics. *Check with your doctor before taking any of the above while you are taking this medicine.*

If you think you or someone else may have taken an overdose, get emergency help at once. Taking an overdose of this medicine or taking alcohol or CNS depressants with this medicine may cause severe mental effects. Symptoms of overdose include changes in mood; confusion; difficulty in breathing; dizziness (severe) or fainting; hallucinations (seeing, hearing, or feeling things that are not there); increase in blood pressure; mental depression; nervousness or anxiety; fast, slow, irregular, or pounding heartbeat; and unusual tiredness or weakness (severe).

This medicine may cause some people to become drowsy, dizzy, or lightheaded, or to feel a false sense of well-being. *Make sure you know how you react to this medicine before you drive, use machines, or do anything else that could be dangerous if you are dizzy or are not alert and clearheaded.*

Dizziness, lightheadedness, or fainting may occur, especially when you get up suddenly from a lying or sitting position. Getting up slowly may help lessen this problem.

Nabilone may cause dryness of the mouth. For temporary relief, use sugarless candy or gum, melt bits of ice in your mouth, or use a saliva substitute. However, if your mouth continues to feel dry for more than 2 weeks, check with your medical doctor or dentist. Continuing dryness of the mouth may increase the chance of dental disease, including tooth decay, gum disease, and fungus infections.

Side Effects of This Medicine

Along with its needed effects, a medicine may cause some unwanted effects. Although not all of these side effects may occur, if they do occur they may need medical attention.

Check with your doctor or nurse immediately if any of the following side effects occur:

Symptoms of overdose

Changes in mood; confusion; difficulty in breathing; dizziness (severe) or fainting; fast, slow, irregular, or pounding heartbeat; hallucinations (seeing, hearing, or feeling things that are not there); increase in blood pressure; mental depression; nervousness or anxiety; unusual tiredness or weakness (severe)

Other side effects may occur that usually do not need medical attention. These side effects may go away during treatment as your body adjusts to the medicine. However, check with your doctor if any of the following side effects continue or are bothersome:

More common

Clumsiness or unsteadiness; difficulty concentrating; dizziness; drowsiness; dryness of mouth; false sense of well-being; headache

Less common or rare

Blurred vision or any changes in vision; dizziness or lightheadedness, especially when getting up from a lying or sitting position—more common with high doses; loss of appetite; muscle pain or weakness

Other side effects not listed above may also occur in some patients. If you notice any other effects, check with your doctor.

Annual revision: 06/17/93

NABUMETONE Systemic†

A commonly used brand name in the U.S. is Relafen.

†Not commercially available in Canada.

Description

Nabumetone (na-BYOO-me-tone) belongs to the group of medicines called anti-inflammatory analgesics (also called nonsteroidal anti-inflammatory drugs [NSAIDs]). Nabumetone is used to relieve symptoms caused by arthritis (rheumatism), such as inflammation, swelling, stiffness, and joint pain. However, this medicine does not cure arthritis and will help you only as long as you continue to take it.

Any anti-inflammatory analgesic can cause side effects, especially when it is used for a long time or in large doses. Some of the side effects are painful or uncomfortable. Others can be more serious, resulting in the need for medical care, and sometimes even death. Nabumetone may be less likely than other anti-inflammatory analgesics to cause serious stomach or intestinal problems, such as ulcers. However, if you will be taking this medicine for more than one or two months or in large amounts, you should discuss with your doctor the good that it can do as well as the risks of taking it. Also, it is a good idea to ask your doctor about other forms of treatment that might help to reduce the amount of nabumetone that you take and/or the length of treatment.

Nabumetone is available only with your doctor's prescription, in the following dosage form:

Oral

- Tablets (U.S.)

It is very important that you read and understand the following information. If any of it causes you special concern, check with your doctor. Also, *if you have any questions* or if you want more information about this medicine or your medical problem, *ask your doctor, nurse, or pharmacist.*

Before Using This Medicine

In deciding to use a medicine, the risks of taking the medicine must be weighed against the good it will do. This is a decision you and your doctor will make. For nabumetone, the following should be considered:

Allergies—Tell your doctor if you have ever had any unusual or allergic reaction to nabumetone or to any of the following medicines:

Aspirin or other salicylates
Diclofenac (e.g., Voltaren)
Diflunisal (e.g., Dolobid)
Etodolac (e.g., Lodine)
Fenoprofen (e.g., Nalfon)
Floctafenine (e.g., Idarac)
Flurbiprofen, oral (e.g., Ansaid)
Ibuprofen (e.g., Motrin)
Indomethacin (e.g., Indocin)
Ketoprofen (e.g., Orudis)
Ketorolac (e.g., Toradol)
Meclofenamate (e.g., Meclomen)
Mefenamic acid (e.g., Ponstel)
Naproxen (e.g., Naprosyn)
Oxyphenbutazone (e.g., Tandearil)
Phenylbutazone (e.g., Butazolidin)
Piroxicam (e.g., Feldene)
Sulindac (e.g., Clinoril)
Suprofen (e.g., Suprol)
Tenoxicam (e.g., Mobiflex)
Tiaprofenic acid (e.g., Surgam)
Tolmetin (e.g., Tolectin)
Zomepirac (e.g., Zomax)

Also tell your doctor and pharmacist if you are allergic to any other substances, such as foods, preservatives, or dyes.

Pregnancy—Studies on birth defects with nabumetone have not been done in pregnant women. Nabumetone did not cause birth defects in animal studies, but it did cause other unwanted effects.

There is a chance that regular use of an anti-inflammatory analgesic during the last few months of pregnancy may cause unwanted effects on the heart or blood flow of the fetus or newborn baby. Also, taking an anti-inflammatory analgesic late in pregnancy may increase the length of pregnancy, prolong labor, or cause other problems during delivery.

Breast-feeding—It is not known whether nabumetone passes into the breast milk. However, it has not been reported to cause problems in nursing babies.

Children—Studies on this medicine have been done only in adult patients, and there is no specific information comparing use of nabumetone in children with use in other age groups.

Older adults—This medicine has been tested and has not been shown to cause different side effects or problems in older people than it does in younger adults. However, experience with other anti-inflammatory analgesics has shown that elderly people are more likely than younger adults to get very sick if the medicine causes stomach problems.

Other medicines—Although certain medicines should not be used together at all, in other cases two different medicines may be used together even if an interaction might occur. In these cases, your doctor may want to change the dose, or other precautions may be necessary. When you are taking nabumetone, it is especially important that

your doctor and pharmacist know if you are taking any of the following:

- Cyclosporine (e.g., Sandimmune) or
- Lithium (e.g., Lithane) or
- Methotrexate (e.g., Mexate)—Higher blood levels of these medicines and an increased chance of side effects may occur
- Probenecid (e.g., Benemid)—Higher blood levels of nabumetone and an increased chance of side effects may occur

Other medical problems—The presence of other medical problems may affect the use of nabumetone. Make sure you tell your doctor if you have any other medical problems, especially:

- Alcohol abuse or
- Colitis, stomach ulcer, or other stomach problems or
- Tobacco smoking—The chance of serious stomach problems may be increased
- Asthma or
- Diabetes mellitus (sugar diabetes) or
- Heart disease or
- High blood pressure or
- Kidney disease or
- Liver disease or
- Systemic lupus erythematosus (SLE)—The chance of serious side effects may be increased
- Hemophilia or other bleeding problems—Nabumetone may increase the chance of serious bleeding

Before you begin using any new medicine (prescription or nonprescription) or if you develop any new medical problem while you are using this medicine, check with your doctor, nurse, or pharmacist.

Proper Use of This Medicine

Nabumetone should be taken with food or an antacid to help prevent stomach upset. Also, taking nabumetone together with food or milk helps the medicine to be absorbed into your body.

Nabumetone must be taken regularly as ordered by your doctor in order for it to help you. Most anti-inflammatory analgesics usually begin to work within one week, but in severe cases up to two weeks or even longer may pass before you begin to feel better. Also, several weeks may pass before you feel the full effects of the medicine.

Do not take more of this medicine, do not take it more often, and do not take it for a longer time than ordered by your doctor. Taking too much of this medicine may increase the chance of unwanted effects.

Dosing—The dose of nabumetone will be different for different patients. *Follow your doctor's orders or the directions on the label.* The following information includes only the average doses of nabumetone. *If your dose is different, do not change it* unless your doctor tells you to do so.

- Adults: Nabumetone is usually taken one or two times a day. At first, most people take 1000 mg a day (two 500-mg tablets once a day or one 500-mg tablet two times a day). Some people may need 1500 mg a day (one 750-mg tablet two times a day) or even 2000 mg a day (two 500-mg tablets two times a day). In general, people need more medicine during a "flare-up" than they do between "flare-ups" of arthritis symptoms. Therefore, your dose may need to be changed as your condition changes.
- Children: If nabumetone is needed by a child, the dose will have to be determined by the doctor.

Missed dose—If you miss a dose of this medicine, take it as soon as you remember. However, if it is almost time for your next dose, skip the missed dose and go back to your regular dosing schedule. Do not double doses.

Storage—To store this medicine:

- Keep out of the reach of children.
- Store away from heat and direct light.
- Do not store this medicine in the bathroom, near the kitchen sink, or in other damp places. Heat or moisture may cause the medicine to break down.
- Do not keep outdated medicine or medicine no longer needed. Be sure that any discarded medicine is out of the reach of children.

Precautions While Using This Medicine

If you will be taking this medicine for a long time, as for arthritis (rheumatism), your doctor should check your progress at regular visits.

Stomach problems may be more likely to occur if you drink alcoholic beverages while being treated with this medicine. Therefore, *do not regularly drink alcoholic beverages while taking this medicine,* unless otherwise directed by your doctor.

Taking certain other medicines together with nabumetone may increase the chance of unwanted effects. The risk will depend on how much of each medicine you take every day, and on how long you take the medicines together. Therefore, do not take acetaminophen (e.g., Tylenol) or aspirin or other salicylates together with nabumetone for more than a few days, unless otherwise directed by your doctor. Also, *do not take any of the following medicines together with nabumetone, unless your doctor has directed you to do so and is following your progress*:

Diclofenac (e.g., Voltaren)
Diflunisal (e.g., Dolobid)
Etodolac (e.g., Lodine)
Fenoprofen (e.g., Nalfon)
Floctafenine (e.g., Idarac)
Flurbiprofen, oral (e.g., Ansaid)
Ibuprofen (e.g., Motrin)
Indomethacin (e.g., Indocin)

Ketoprofen (e.g., Orudis)
Ketorolac (e.g., Toradol)
Meclofenamate (e.g., Meclomen)
Mefenamic acid (e.g., Ponstel)
Naproxen (e.g., Naprosyn)
Phenylbutazone (e.g., Butazolidin)
Piroxicam (e.g., Feldene)
Sulindac (e.g., Clinoril)
Tenoxicam (e.g., Mobiflex)
Tiaprofenic acid (e.g., Surgam)
Tolmetin (e.g., Tolectin)

This medicine may cause some people to become drowsy, dizzy, or lightheaded. It may also cause vision problems in some people. *Make sure you know how you react to this medicine before you drive, use machines, or do anything else that could be dangerous if you are dizzy or not able to see well.* If these reactions are especially bothersome, check with your doctor.

Nabumetone may cause your skin to be more sensitive to sunlight than it is normally. Exposure to sunlight, even for brief periods of time, may cause a skin rash, itching, blisters, redness or other discoloration of the skin, or a severe sunburn. When you begin taking this medicine:

- Stay out of direct sunlight, especially between the hours of 10:00 a.m. and 3:00 p.m., if possible.
- Wear protective clothing, including a hat. Also, wear sunglasses.
- Apply a sun block product that has a skin protection factor (SPF) of at least 15. Some patients may require a product with a higher SPF number, especially if they have a fair complexion. If you have any questions about this, check with your doctor or pharmacist.
- Apply a sun block lipstick that has an SPF of at least 15 to protect your lips.
- Do not use a sunlamp or tanning bed or booth.

If you have a severe reaction from the sun, check with your doctor.

Serious side effects, including ulcers or bleeding, can occur during treatment with this medicine. Sometimes serious side effects occur without any warning. However, possible warning signs often occur, including severe abdominal or stomach cramps, pain, or burning; black, tarry stools; severe, continuing nausea, heartburn, or indigestion; and/or vomiting of blood or material that looks like coffee grounds. *Stop taking this medicine and check with your doctor immediately if you notice any of these warning signs.*

Side Effects of This Medicine

Along with its needed effects, a medicine may cause some unwanted effects. Although not all of these side effects may occur, if they do occur they may need medical attention.

Stop taking this medicine and check with your doctor immediately if any of the following side effects occur:

Rare

Abdominal or stomach pain, cramping, or burning (severe); bloody or black, tarry stools; large, hive-like swellings on face, eyelids, mouth, lips, or tongue; nausea, heartburn, and/or indigestion (severe and continuing); shortness of breath, troubled breathing, tightness in chest, and/or wheezing; spitting blood; vomiting of blood or material that looks like coffee grounds

Also, check with your doctor as soon as possible if any of the following side effects occur:

More common

Ringing or buzzing in ears; skin rash or itching; swelling of face, fingers, hands, feet, or lower legs

Less common

Burning feeling in throat, chest, or stomach; sores, ulcers, or white spots on lips or in mouth

Rare

Abdominal or stomach pain, diarrhea, or nausea (mild); blisters on skin; bloody or cloudy urine; change in vision; difficulty in swallowing, hives; mental depression; muscle pain, cramps, and/or weakness; sudden decrease in amount of urine; unusual tiredness or weakness; yellow eyes or skin; weight gain

Other side effects may occur that usually do not need medical attention. These side effects may go away during treatment as your body adjusts to the medicine. However, check with your doctor if any of the following side effects continue or are bothersome:

More common

Abdominal or stomach pain (mild to moderate); bloated feeling or gas; constipation; diarrhea; dizziness; headache; indigestion or nausea

Less common or rare

Drowsiness; dryness of mouth; increased sweating; nervousness; tiredness; trouble in sleeping; vomiting

Other side effects not listed above may also occur in some patients. If you notice any other effects, check with your doctor.

Annual revision: 11/16/92

NAFARELIN Systemic

A commonly used brand name in the U.S. and Canada is Synarel.

Description

Nafarelin (NAF-a-re-lin) is used to treat endometriosis. Endometriosis is a condition in which tissue similar to the lining of the uterus implants in other places in a woman's pelvis area. These growths increase in response to estrogen. Nafarelin works by stopping the production of estrogen by the ovaries.

Nafarelin is usually only used in those women who cannot or do not want to take danazol (e.g., Danocrine), oral contraceptives (birth control pills), or a progestin (another type of female hormone) or choose not to undergo surgery. Danazol and nafarelin work equally well for pain caused by endometriosis, but each has different types of side effects. Danazol is similar to testosterone. Because of this, it causes side effects such as acne, oily skin or hair, rapid weight gain, decreased breast size, enlarged clitoris, hoarseness or deepening of the voice, and unnatural hair growth. Most of the side effects of nafarelin are related to the lower amount of estrogen in the bloodstream. This includes a temporary thinning of the bones that occurs with a continued shortage of estrogen. Because it is not yet known if repeating therapy with nafarelin can increase a woman's risk of osteoporosis (brittle bones) and an increased risk of broken bones in later life, nafarelin therapy is usually only used for short periods of time (a few months) and is generally not repeated.

Nasal

- Spray solution (U.S. and Canada)

It is very important that you read and understand the following information. If any of it causes you special concern, check with your doctor. Also, *if you have any questions* or if you want more information about this medicine or your medical problem, *ask your doctor, nurse, or pharmacist.*

Before Using This Medicine

In deciding to use a medicine, the risks of taking the medicine must be weighed against the good it will do. This is a decision you and your doctor will make. For nafarelin, the following should be considered:

Allergies—Tell your doctor if you have ever had any unusual or allergic reaction to nafarelin. Also tell your doctor and pharmacist if you are allergic to any other substances, such as foods, preservatives, or dyes.

Pregnancy—Nafarelin is not recommended during pregnancy. Nafarelin has not been studied in pregnant women. Some animal studies showed an increase in stillbirths and decreases in fetal weight, which would be expected from the changes in hormones caused by nafarelin. Because of this, you and your partner should use a birth control method that does not contain hormones, such as condoms, a diaphragm, or a cervical cap, with a spermicide. If you suspect that you may have become pregnant, stop taking this medicine and check with your doctor.

Breast-feeding—It is not known whether nafarelin passes into the breast milk.

Other medicines—Although certain medicines should not be used together at all, in other cases two different medicines may be used together even if an interaction might occur. In these cases, your doctor may want to change the dose, or other precautions may be necessary. When you are taking nafarelin, it is especially important that your doctor and pharmacist know if you are taking the following:

- Nasal decongestant sprays—It is not known whether nasal decongestant sprays can decrease the amount of nafarelin that enters the bloodstream through the lining of the nose. For this reason, you should allow at least 30 minutes to pass before you use a nasal decongestant spray after using nafarelin

Other medical problems—The presence of other medical problems may affect the use of nafarelin. Make sure you tell your doctor if you have any other medical problems, especially:

- Other conditions that increase the chances for osteoporosis (brittle bones)—Since nafarelin causes a temporary thinning of the bones, it is important that your doctor know if you already have an increased risk of osteoporosis. Some things that can increase your risk for having osteoporosis include cigarette smoking, alcohol abuse, taking or drinking a lot of caffeine, and a family history of osteoporosis or easily broken bones. Some medicines, such as adrenocorticoids (cortisone-like medicines) or anticonvulsants (seizure medicine), can also cause thinning of the bones

Before you begin using any new medicine (prescription or nonprescription) or if you develop any new medical problem while you are using this medicine, check with your doctor, nurse, or pharmacist.

Proper Use of This Medicine

You will be given a fact sheet with your prescription for nafarelin that explains how to use the pump spray bottle. If you have any questions about using the pump spray, ask your doctor, nurse, or pharmacist.

To use *nafarelin spray:*

- Before you use each new bottle of nafarelin, the spray pump needs to be started. To do this, point the bottle away from you and pump the bottle firmly about 7 times. A spray should come out by the seventh time you pump the spray bottle. *This only needs to be done once for each new bottle of nafarelin.* Be careful not to breathe in this spray. You could inhale extra doses of nafarelin, since the medicine is dissolved in the spray.

- Before you take your daily doses of nafarelin, blow your nose gently. Hold your head forward a little. Put the spray tip into one nostril. Aim the tip toward the back and outside of your nostril. You do not need to put the tip too far into your nose.
- Close your other nostril off by pressing on the outside of your nose with a finger. Then, sniff in the spray as you pump the bottle once.
- Take the spray bottle out of your nose. Tilt your head back for a few seconds, to let the spray get onto the back of your nose.
- Repeat these steps for each dose of medicine.
- Each time you use the spray bottle, wipe off the tip with a clean tissue or cloth. Keep the blue safety clip and plastic cap on the bottle when you are not using it.
- Every 3 or 4 days you should clean the tip of the spray bottle. To do this, hold the bottle sideways. Rinse the tip with warm water, while wiping the tip with your finger or soft cloth for about 15 seconds. Dry the tip with a soft cloth or tissue. Replace the cap right after use. Be careful not to get water into the bottle, since this could dilute the medicine.

Missed dose—If you miss a dose of this medicine, take it as soon as possible. However, if it is almost time for your next dose, skip the missed dose and go back to your regular dosing schedule. Do not double doses.

Storage—To store this medicine:

- Keep out of the reach of children.
- The bottle should be stored standing upright, with the tip up.
- Store away from heat and direct light.
- Keep the medicine from freezing. Do not refrigerate.
- Do not keep outdated medicine or medicine no longer needed. Be sure that any discarded medicine is out of the reach of children.

Precautions While Using This Medicine

Your doctor should check your progress at regular visits to make sure that this medicine is working properly and to check for unwanted effects.

Using nafarelin can cause dryness of the vagina. If this is uncomfortable, especially during sex, there are several water-based vaginal lubricant products that you can use. Using a lubricant may also help to prevent soreness or damage to the vagina from sex. If you decide to use a lubricant during sex and you are using condoms, a cervical cap, or a diaphragm, make sure the lubricant you choose will not damage the birth control device. Some products contain oils, which can break down latex rubber and cause any of these types of birth control devices to rip or tear.

Side Effects of This Medicine

In some animal studies, nafarelin was shown to increase the chance of certain types of tumors. The doses given were higher and were used longer than those used in humans. These effects have not been found in humans using recommended doses.

Along with its needed effects, a medicine may cause some unwanted effects. Although not all of these side effects may occur, if they do occur they may need medical attention.

Check with your doctor as soon as possible if any of the following side effects occur:

More common

Light vaginal bleeding between regular menstrual periods, which does not need the use of a pad or tampon ("spotting"); longer or heavier menstrual periods; vaginal bleeding between regular menstrual periods, which may need the use of a pad or tampon ("breakthrough bleeding")

Rare

Allergic reaction (shortness of breath, chest pain, hives); joint pain; pelvic or lower abdomen bloating or tenderness (mild); unexpected or excess flow of milk

Other side effects may occur that usually do not need medical attention. Some of these side effects may go away during treatment as your body adjusts to the medicine. However, check with your doctor if any of the following side effects continue or are bothersome:

More common

Lower estrogen in the bloodstream (acne, decreased sex drive, dryness of the vagina, hot flashes, pain during sex, decreased breast size, palpitations, oily skin); stopping of menstrual periods

Less common or rare

Breast pain; headache (mild and transient); irritated or runny nose; mental depression (mild and transient); mood swings; skin rash; weight changes

Other side effects not listed above may also occur in some patients. If you notice any other effects, check with your doctor.

Annual revision: 10/26/92

NAFTIFINE Topical†

A commonly used brand name in the U.S. is Naftin.

†Not commercially available in Canada.

Description

Naftifine (NAF-ti-feen) is used to treat fungus infections. It works by killing the fungus or preventing its growth.

Naftifine cream is applied to the skin to treat:

- athlete's foot (ringworm of the feet; tinea pedis);
- jock itch (ringworm of the groin; tinea cruris); and
- ringworm of the body (tinea corporis).

This medicine may also be used for other fungus infections of the skin as determined by your doctor.

Naftifine is available only with your doctor's prescription, in the following dosage form:

Topical

- Cream (U.S.)

It is very important that you read and understand the following information. If any of it causes you special concern, check with your doctor. Also, *if you have any questions* or if you want more information about this medicine or your medical problem, *ask your doctor, nurse, or pharmacist.*

Before Using This Medicine

In deciding to use a medicine, the risks of taking the medicine must be weighed against the good it will do. This is a decision you and your doctor will make. For topical naftifine, the following should be considered:

Allergies—Tell your doctor if you have ever had any unusual or allergic reaction to naftifine. Also tell your doctor and pharmacist if you are allergic to any other substances, such as preservatives or dyes.

Pregnancy—Topical naftifine has not been studied in pregnant women. However, naftifine, when given by mouth, has not been shown to cause birth defects or other problems in animal studies.

Breast-feeding—Topical naftifine is absorbed into the body in small amounts. However, it is not known whether naftifine passes into the breast milk. In addition, this medicine has not been reported to cause problems in nursing babies.

Children—Studies on this medicine have been done only in adult patients, and there is no specific information about its use in children.

Older adults—Many medicines have not been tested in older people. Therefore, it may not be known whether they work exactly the same way they do in younger adults or if they cause different side effects or problems in older people. There is no specific information about the use of naftifine in the elderly.

Before you begin using any new medicine (prescription or nonprescription) or if you develop any new medical problem while you are using this medicine, check with your doctor, nurse, or pharmacist.

Proper Use of This Medicine

Keep this medicine away from the eyes, nose, mouth, or other mucous membranes.

To use:

- Apply enough naftifine to cover the affected skin and surrounding areas, and rub in gently.
- After applying naftifine, wash your hands to remove any medicine that may be on them.

To help clear up your skin infection completely, *keep using naftifine for the full time of treatment.* You should keep using this medicine for 1 to 2 weeks after your symptoms have disappeared. If you stop using this medicine too soon, your symptoms may return. *Do not miss any doses.*

Missed dose—If you do miss a dose of this medicine, apply it as soon as possible. However, if it is almost time for your next dose, skip the missed dose and go back to your regular dosing schedule.

Storage—To store this medicine:

- Keep out of the reach of children.
- Store away from heat and direct light.
- Keep the medicine from freezing.
- Do not keep outdated medicine or medicine no longer needed. Be sure that any discarded medicine is out of the reach of children.

Precautions While Using This Medicine

If your skin infection does not improve within 4 weeks, or if it becomes worse, check with your doctor.

To help clear up your skin infection completely and to help make sure it does not return, the following good health habits are important:

- *For patients using naftifine for athlete's foot*, these measures will help keep the feet cool and dry:
  —Carefully dry the feet, especially between the toes, after bathing.
  —Avoid wearing socks made from wool or synthetic materials (for example, rayon or nylon). Instead,

wear clean, cotton socks and change them daily or more often if your feet sweat freely.

—Wear well-ventilated shoes (for example, shoes with holes) or sandals.

—Use a bland, absorbent powder (for example, talcum powder) or an antifungal powder freely between the toes, on the feet, and in socks and shoes once or twice a day. Be sure to use the powder after naftifine cream has been applied and has disappeared into the skin. Do not use the powder as the only treatment for your fungus infection.

- *For patients using naftifine for jock itch*, these measures will help reduce chafing and irritation and will also help keep the groin area cool and dry:

  —Carefully dry the groin area after bathing.

  —Avoid wearing underwear that is tight-fitting or made from synthetic materials (for example, rayon or nylon). Instead, wear loose-fitting, cotton underwear.

  —Use a bland, absorbent powder (for example, talcum powder) or an antifungal powder freely once or twice a day. Be sure to use the powder after naftifine cream has been applied and has disappeared into the skin. Do not use the powder as the only treatment for your fungus infection.

- *For patients using naftifine for ringworm of the body*, these measures will help keep the affected areas cool and dry:

  —Carefully dry yourself after bathing.

  —Avoid too much heat and humidity if possible. Try to keep moisture from building up on affected areas of the body.

  —Wear well-ventilated clothing.

  —Use a bland, absorbent powder (for example, talcum powder) or an antifungal powder freely once or twice a day. Be sure to use the powder after naftifine cream has been applied and has disappeared into the skin. Do not use the powder as the only treatment for your fungus infection.

If you have any questions about this, check with your doctor, nurse, or pharmacist.

Side Effects of This Medicine

Along with its needed effects, a medicine may cause some unwanted effects. The following side effects may go away during treatment as your body adjusts to the medicine. However, check with your doctor if any of these effects continue or are bothersome:

More common

Burning or stinging feeling on treated area(s)

Less common

Dry skin; itching, redness, or other sign of skin irritation not present before use of this medicine

Other side effects not listed above may also occur in some patients. If you notice any other effects, check with your doctor.

Annual revision: June 1990

NALIDIXIC ACID Systemic

A commonly used brand name in the U.S. and Canada is NegGram.

Description

Nalidixic (nal-i-DIX-ik) acid is used to treat infections of the urinary tract. It may be used for other problems as determined by your doctor.

Nalidixic acid is available only with your doctor's prescription, in the following dosage forms:

Oral

- Suspension (U.S.)
- Tablets (U.S. and Canada)

It is very important that you read and understand the following information. If any of it causes you special concern, check with your doctor. Also, *if you have any questions* or if you want more information about this medicine or your medical problem, *ask your doctor, nurse, or pharmacist.*

Before Using This Medicine

In deciding to use a medicine, the risks of taking the medicine must be weighed against the good it will do. This is a decision you and your doctor will make. For nalidixic acid, the following should be considered:

Allergies—Tell your doctor if you have ever had any unusual or allergic reaction to nalidixic acid, or to any related medicines such as cinoxacin (e.g., Cinobac), ciprofloxacin (e.g., Cipro), enoxacin (e.g. Penetrex), lomefloxacin (e.g., Maxaquin), norfloxacin (e.g., Noroxin), or ofloxacin (e.g., Floxin). Also tell your doctor and pharmacist if you are allergic to any other substances, such as foods, preservatives, or dyes.

Pregnancy—Studies have not been done in humans. However, use is not recommended during pregnancy since nalidixic acid has been shown to cause bone development problems in young animals.

Breast-feeding—Nalidixic acid passes into the breast milk. This medicine may cause blood problems in nursing babies with glucose-6-phosphate dehydrogenase (G6PD) deficiency. However, problems in other nursing babies have not been reported.

Children—This medicine is not recommended for use in infants up to 3 months of age since nalidixic acid has been shown to cause bone problems in young animals.

Older adults—This medicine has been studied in a limited number of elderly patients and has not been shown to cause different side effects or problems in older people than it does in younger adults.

Other medicines—Although certain medicines should not be used together at all, in other cases two different medicines may be used together even if an interaction might occur. In these cases, your doctor may want to change the dose, or other precautions may be necessary. When you are taking nalidixic acid, it is especially important that your doctor and pharmacist know if you are taking any of the following:

- Anticoagulants (blood thinners)—Patients taking nalidixic acid with anticoagulants may have an increased chance of bleeding

Other medical problems—The presence of other medical problems may affect the use of nalidixic acid. Make sure you tell your doctor if you have any other medical problems, especially:

- Convulsive disorders, history of (seizures, epilepsy) or
- Hardening of the arteries in the brain (severe)—Patients with these medical problems may have an increased chance of side effects affecting the nervous system
- Glucose-6-phosphate dehydrogenase (G6PD) deficiency—Patients with G6PD deficiency may have an increased chance of side effects affecting the blood
- Kidney disease (severe) or
- Liver disease—Patients with liver disease or severe kidney disease may have an increase in side effects

Before you begin using any new medicine (prescription or nonprescription) or if you develop any new medical problem while you are using this medicine, check with your doctor, nurse, or pharmacist.

Proper Use of This Medicine

Do not give this medicine to infants or children unless otherwise directed by your doctor. It has been shown to cause bone problems in young animals and may cause these problems in children.

Nalidixic acid is best taken with a full glass (8 ounces) of water on an empty stomach (either 1 hour before or 2 hours after meals). However, if this medicine causes nausea or upset stomach, it may be taken with food or milk.

For patients taking the *oral liquid form* of this medicine:

- Use a specially marked measuring spoon or other device to measure each dose accurately. The average household teaspoon may not hold the right amount of liquid.

To help clear up your infection completely, *keep taking this medicine for the full time of treatment,* even if you begin to feel better after a few days. *Do not miss any doses.*

Dosing—The dose of nalidixic acid will be different for different patients. *Follow your doctor's orders or the directions on the label.* The following information includes only the average doses of nalidixic acid. *If your dose is different, do not change it* unless your doctor tells you to do so.

- The number of tablets or teaspoonfuls of suspension that you take depends on the strength of the medicine. Also, *the number of doses you take each day, the time allowed between doses, and the length of time you take the medicine depend on the medical problem for which you are taking nalidixic acid.*
- For *oral* dosage forms (oral suspension or tablets):
  —Adults and children 12 years of age and older: 1 gram (g) every six hours for one to two weeks to start; then, 500 milligrams (mg) every six hours.
  —Children 3 months to 12 years of age: The dose is based on body weight and must be determined by the doctor.
  —Infants up to 3 months of age: This medicine is not recommended in infants up to 3 months of age since nalidixic acid has been shown to cause bone problems in young animals.

Missed dose—If you do miss a dose of this medicine, take it as soon as possible. However, if it is almost time for your next dose, skip the missed dose and go back to your regular dosing schedule. Do not double doses.

Storage—To store this medicine:

- Keep out of the reach of children.
- Store away from heat and direct light.
- Do not store the tablet form of this medicine in the bathroom, near the kitchen sink, or in other damp places. Heat or moisture may cause the medicine to break down.
- Keep the oral liquid form of this medicine from freezing.
- Do not keep outdated medicine or medicine no longer needed. Be sure that any discarded medicine is out of the reach of children.

Precautions While Using This Medicine

If you will be taking this medicine for more than 2 weeks, your doctor should check your progress at regular visits.

If your symptoms do not improve within 2 days, or if they become worse, check with your doctor.

This medicine may cause blurred vision or other vision problems. It may also cause some people to become dizzy, drowsy, or less alert than they are normally. *Make sure you know how you react to this medicine before you drive, use machines, or do anything else that could be dangerous if you are dizzy or are not alert or able to see well.* If these reactions are especially bothersome, check with your doctor.

Nalidixic acid may cause your skin to be more sensitive to sunlight than it is normally. Exposure to sunlight, even for brief periods of time, may cause a skin rash, itching, redness or other discoloration of the skin, or a severe sunburn. When you begin taking this medicine:

- Stay out of direct sunlight, especially between the hours of 10:00 a.m. and 3:00 p.m., if possible.
- Wear protective clothing, including a hat. Also, wear sunglasses.
- Apply a sun block product that has a skin protection factor (SPF) of at least 15. Some patients may require a product with a higher SPF number, especially if they have a fair complexion. If you have any questions about this, check with your doctor or pharmacist.
- Apply a sun block lipstick that has an SPF of at least 15 to protect your lips.
- Do not use a sunlamp or tanning bed or booth.

If you have a severe reaction from the sun, check with your doctor.

For diabetic patients:

- *This medicine may cause false test results with some urine glucose (sugar) tests.* Check with your doctor before changing your diet or the dosage of your diabetes medicine.

Side Effects of This Medicine

Along with its needed effects, a medicine may cause some unwanted effects. Although not all of these side effects may occur, if they do occur they may need medical attention.

Check with your doctor immediately if any of the following side effects occur:

More common

Blurred or decreased vision; change in color vision; double vision; halos around lights; overbright appearance of lights

Rare

Bulging of fontanel (soft spot) on top of head of an infant; convulsions (seizures); dark or amber urine; hallucinations (seeing, hearing, or feeling things that are not there); headache (severe); mood or other mental changes; pale skin; pale stools; skin rash and itching; sore throat and fever; stomach pain (severe); unusual bleeding or bruising; unusual tiredness or weakness; yellow eyes or skin

Other side effects may occur that usually do not need medical attention. These side effects may go away during treatment as your body adjusts to the medicine. However, check with your doctor if any of the following side effects continue or are bothersome:

More common

Diarrhea; dizziness; drowsiness; headache; nausea or vomiting; stomach pain

Less common

Increased sensitivity of skin to sunlight

Other side effects not listed above may also occur in some patients. If you notice any other effects, check with your doctor.

Annual revision: 05/14/93

NALTREXONE Systemic

A commonly used brand name in the U.S. is Trexan.

Description

Naltrexone (nal-TREX-zone) is used to help narcotic addicts who have stopped taking narcotics to stay drug-free. The medicine is not a cure for addiction. It is used as part of an overall program that may include counseling, attending support group meetings, and other treatment recommended by your doctor.

Naltrexone is not a narcotic. It works by blocking the effects of narcotics, especially the "high" feeling that makes you want to use them. It will not produce any narcotic-like effects or cause mental or physical dependence.

Naltrexone will cause withdrawal symptoms in people who are physically dependent on narcotics. Therefore, naltrexone treatment is started after you are no longer dependent on narcotics. The length of time this takes may depend on which narcotic you took, the amount you took, and how long you took it. Before you start taking this medicine, be sure to tell your doctor if you think you are still having withdrawal symptoms.

Naltrexone is available only with your doctor's prescription, in the following dosage form:

Oral

- Tablets (U.S.)

It is very important that you read and understand the following information. If any of it causes you special concern, check with your doctor. Also, *if you have any questions* or if you want more information about this medicine or your medical problem, *ask your doctor, nurse, or pharmacist.*

Before Using This Medicine

In deciding to use a medicine, the risks of taking the medicine must be weighed against the good it will do. This is a decision you and your doctor will make. For naltrexone, the following should be considered:

Allergies—Tell your doctor if you have ever had any unusual or allergic reaction to naltrexone. Also tell your doctor and pharmacist if you are allergic to any other substances, such as foods, preservatives, or dyes.

Pregnancy—Studies on birth defects with naltrexone have not been done in humans. Studies in animals have shown that naltrexone causes unwanted effects when given in very large doses.

Breast-feeding—It is not known whether naltrexone passes into the breast milk. However, this medicine has not been reported to cause problems in nursing babies.

Children—Naltrexone has been tested only in adult patients and there is no specific information about its use in patients up to 18 years of age.

Older adults—Many medicines have not been tested in older people. Therefore, it may not be known whether they work exactly the same way they do in younger adults or if they cause different side effects or problems in older people. There is no specific information about the use of naltrexone in the elderly.

Other medical problems—The presence of other medical problems may affect the use of naltrexone. Make sure you tell your doctor if you have any other medical problems, especially:

- Hepatitis or other liver disease—The chance of side effects may be increased

Before you begin using any new medicine (prescription or nonprescription) or if you develop any new medical problem while you are using this medicine, check with your doctor, nurse, or pharmacist.

Proper Use of This Medicine

Take naltrexone regularly as ordered by your doctor. It may be helpful to have someone else, such as a family member, doctor, or nurse, give you each dose as scheduled.

Missed dose—If you miss a dose of this medicine, and your regular dosing schedule is:

- One tablet every day:

  —Take the missed dose as soon as possible. However, if you do not remember until the next day, skip the missed dose and go back to your regular dosing schedule. Do not double the next day's dose.

- One tablet every weekday and two tablets on Saturday:

  —If you miss a weekday dose, follow the directions for one tablet every day.

  —If you miss the Saturday dose, take it as soon as possible. However, if you do not remember until Sunday, take one tablet on Sunday. Then go back to your regular dosing schedule on Monday.

- Two tablets every other day:

  —Take two tablets as soon as you remember, then skip a day, then go back to taking the medicine every other day; or

  —Take two tablets as soon as possible if you remember the same day. However, if you do not remember until the next day, take one tablet the next day. Then go back to your regular dosing schedule.

- Two tablets on Monday and Wednesday and three tablets on Friday:

  —If you miss one of the Monday or Wednesday doses, take it as soon as possible. However, if you do not remember until the next day, take one tablet the next day. Then go back to your regular dosing schedule.

  —If you miss the Friday dose, take it as soon as possible if you remember the same day. However, if you do not remember until Saturday, take two tablets on Saturday. If you do not remember until Sunday, take one tablet on Sunday. Then go back to your regular dosing schedule on Monday.

- Three tablets every three days:

  —Take three tablets as soon you remember, then skip two days, then go back to taking the medicine every three days; or

  —Take three tablets as soon as possible if you remember the same day. However, if you do not remember until the next day, take two tablets, then skip a day and go back to your regular dosing schedule. If you do not remember until the second day, take one tablet. Then go back to your regular dosing schedule.

Storage—To store this medicine:
- Keep out of the reach of children.
- Store away from heat and direct light.
- Do not store this medicine in the bathroom, near the kitchen sink, or in other damp places. Heat or moisture may cause the medicine to break down.
- Do not keep outdated medicine.

Precautions While Using This Medicine

It is very important that your doctor check your progress at regular visits. Your doctor may want to do certain blood tests to see if the medicine is causing unwanted effects.

Remember that use of naltrexone is only part of your treatment. *Be sure that you follow all of your doctor's orders, including seeing your therapist and/or attending support group meetings on a regular basis.*

Do not try to overcome the effects of naltrexone by taking very large amounts of narcotics. To do so may cause coma or death.

Naltrexone also blocks the useful effects of narcotics. *Always use a non-narcotic medicine to treat pain, diarrhea, or cough.* If you have any questions about the proper medicine to use, check with your doctor, nurse, or pharmacist.

Never share this medicine with anyone else. This is especially important if the other person is using narcotics because naltrexone will cause withdrawal symptoms.

Tell all medical doctors, dentists, and pharmacists you go to that you are taking naltrexone.

It is recommended that you carry identification stating that you are taking naltrexone. Identification cards may be available from your doctor.

Side Effects of This Medicine

Along with its needed effects, a medicine may cause some unwanted effects. Although not all of these side effects may occur, if they do occur they may need medical attention.

Check with your doctor as soon as possible if any of the following side effects occur:

More common

Skin rash

Rare

Abdominal or stomach pain (severe); blurred vision or aching, burning, or swollen eyes; confusion; discomfort while urinating and/or frequent urination; earache; fever; hallucinations (seeing, hearing, or feeling things that are not there); increased blood pressure; itching; mental depression or other mood or mental changes; nosebleeds (unexplained); pain, tenderness, or color changes in legs or feet; ringing or buzzing in ears; shortness of breath; swelling of face, feet, or lower legs; swollen glands; weight gain

Other side effects may occur that usually do not need medical attention. These side effects may go away during treatment as your body adjusts to the medicine. However, check with your doctor if any of the following side effects continue or are bothersome:

More common

Abdominal or stomach cramping or pain (mild or moderate); anxiety, nervousness, restlessness, and/or trouble in sleeping; headache; joint or muscle pain; nausea or vomiting; unusual tiredness

Less common or rare

Chills; constipation; cough, hoarseness, runny or stuffy nose, sinus problems, sneezing, and/or sore throat; diarrhea; dizziness; fast or pounding heartbeat; increased thirst; irritability; loss of appetite; sexual problems in males

Other side effects not listed above, possibly including withdrawal symptoms, may also occur in some patients. If you notice any other effects, check with your doctor.

Annual revision: June 1990

NAPHAZOLINE Ophthalmic

Some commonly used brand names are:

In the U.S.

Ak-Con	Muro's Opcon
Albalon	Nafazair
Allerest	Naphcon
Clear Eyes Lubricating Eye Redness Reliever	Naphcon Forte
Comfort Eye Drops	Ocu-Zoline Sterile Ophthalmic Solution
Degest 2	VasoClear
Estivin II	VasoClear A
I-Naphline	Vasocon Regular

Generic name product may also be available.

In Canada

Ak-Con	Naphcon Forte
Albalon Liquifilm	Vasocon

Description

Naphazoline (naf-AZ-oh-leen) is used to relieve redness due to minor eye irritations, such as those caused by colds, dust, wind, smog, pollen, swimming, or wearing contact lenses.

Some of these preparations are available only with your doctor's prescription. Others are available without a prescription; however, your doctor may have special instructions on the proper use of this medicine for your medical problem.

Naphazoline is available in the following dosage form:

Ophthalmic

- Ophthalmic solution (eye drops) (U.S. and Canada)

It is very important that you read and understand the following information. If any of it causes you special concern, check with your doctor. Also, *if you have any questions* or if you want more information about this medicine or your medical problem, *ask your doctor, nurse, or pharmacist.*

Before Using This Medicine

If you are using this medicine without a prescription, carefully read and follow any precautions on the label. For ophthalmic naphazoline, the following should be considered:

Allergies—Tell your doctor if you have ever had any unusual or allergic reaction to naphazoline. Also tell your doctor and pharmacist if you are allergic to any other substances, such as preservatives.

Pregnancy—This medicine may be absorbed into the body. However, studies on effects in pregnancy have not been done in either humans or animals.

Breast-feeding—Naphazoline may be absorbed into the mother's body. However, this medicine has not been reported to cause problems in nursing babies.

Children—Use by infants and children is not recommended, since they are especially sensitive to the effects of naphazoline.

Older adults—Many medicines have not been studied specifically in older people. Therefore, it may not be known whether they work exactly the same way they do in younger adults or if they cause different side effects or problems in older people. There is no specific information comparing use of naphazoline in the elderly with use in other age groups.

Other medicines—Although certain medicines should not be used together at all, in other cases two different medicines may be used together even if an interaction might occur. In these cases, your doctor may want to change the dose, or other precautions may be necessary. Tell your doctor and pharmacist if you are using any other prescription or nonprescription (over-the-counter [OTC]) medicine.

Other medical problems—The presence of other medical problems may affect the use of ophthalmic naphazoline. Make sure you tell your doctor if you have any other medical problems, especially:

- Diabetes mellitus (sugar diabetes) or
- Heart disease or
- High blood pressure or
- Overactive thyroid—Use of ophthalmic naphazoline may make the condition worse
- Eye disease, infection, or injury—The symptoms of the condition may be confused with possible side effects of ophthalmic naphazoline

Before you begin using any new medicine (prescription or nonprescription) or if you develop any new medical problem while you are using this medicine, check with your doctor, nurse, or pharmacist.

Proper Use of This Medicine

Do not use naphazoline ophthalmic solution if it becomes cloudy or changes color.

Naphazoline should not be used in infants and children. It may cause severe slowing down of the central nervous system (CNS), which may lead to unconsciousness. It may also cause a severe decrease in body temperature.

Use this medicine only as directed. Do not use more of it, do not use it more often, and do not use it for more than 72 hours, unless otherwise directed by your doctor. To do so may make your eye redness and irritation worse and may also increase the chance of side effects.

To use:

- First, wash your hands. With the middle finger, apply pressure to the inside corner of the eye (and continue to apply pressure for 1 or 2 minutes after the medicine has been placed in the eye). Tilt the head back and with the index finger of the same hand, pull the lower eyelid away from the eye to form a pouch. Drop the medicine into the pouch and gently close the eyes. Do not blink. Keep the eyes closed for 1 or 2 minutes to allow the medicine to be absorbed.
- To keep the medicine as germ-free as possible, do not touch the applicator tip to any surface (including the eye). Also, keep the container tightly closed.

Storage—To store this medicine:

- Keep out of the reach of children.
- Store away from heat and direct light.
- Keep the medicine from freezing.
- Do not keep outdated medicine or medicine no longer needed. Be sure that any discarded medicine is out of the reach of children.

Precautions While Using This Medicine

If eye pain or change in vision occurs or if redness or irritation of the eye continues, gets worse, or lasts for more than 72 hours, stop using the medicine and check with your doctor.

Side Effects of This Medicine

Along with its needed effects, a medicine may cause some unwanted effects. Although not all of these side effects may occur, if they do occur they may need medical attention.

When this medicine is used for short periods of time at recommended doses, side effects usually are rare. However, check with your doctor as soon as possible if any of the following occur:

With overuse or long-term use

Increase in eye irritation

Symptoms of too much medicine being absorbed into the body

Dizziness; headache; increased sweating; nausea; nervousness; weakness

Symptoms of overdose

Decrease in body temperature; drowsiness; slow heartbeat; weakness (severe)

Other side effects may occur that usually do not need medical attention. These side effects may go away during treatment as your body adjusts to the medicine. However, check with your doctor or pharmacist if either of the following side effects continues or is bothersome:

Less common or rare

Blurred vision; large pupils

Other side effects not listed above may also occur in some patients. If you notice any other effects, check with your doctor or pharmacist.

Annual revision: 05/14/92

NARCOTIC ANALGESICS—For Pain Relief Systemic

This information applies to the following medicines:

Buprenorphine (byoo-pre-NOR-feen)
Butorphanol (byoo-TOR-fa-nole)
Codeine (KOE-deen)
Hydrocodone (hye-droe-KOE-done)
Hydromorphone (hye-droe-MOR-fone)
Levorphanol (lee-VOR-fa-nole)
Meperidine (me-PER-i-deen)
Methadone (METH-a-done)
Morphine (MOR-feen)
Nalbuphine (NAL-byoo-feen)
Opium Injection (OH-pee-um)
Oxycodone (ox-i-KOE-done)
Oxymorphone (ox-i-MOR-fone)
Pentazocine (pen-TAZ-oh-seen)
Propoxyphene (proe-POX-i-feen)

This information does *not* apply to Opium Tincture or Paregoric.

Some commonly used brand names are:

For Buprenorphine
In the U.S.
Buprenex

For Butorphanol
In the U.S.
Stadol
In Canada
Stadol

For Codeine
In the U.S.
Available by generic name.
In Canada
Paveral
Generic name product may also be available.

For Hydrocodone*
In Canada
Hycodan‡
Robidone

For Hydromorphone
In the U.S.
Dilaudid
Dilaudid-HP
Generic name product may also be available.
In Canada
Dilaudid
Dilaudid-HP

Another commonly used name is dihydromorphinone.

For Levorphanol
In the U.S.
Levo-Dromoran
Generic name product may also be available.
In Canada
Levo-Dromoran

Another commonly used name is levorphan.

For Meperidine
In the U.S.
Demerol
Generic name product may also be available.
In Canada
Demerol
Generic name product may also be available.

Another commonly used name is pethidine.

For Methadone§
In the U.S.
Dolophine
Methadose
Generic name product may also be available.

For Morphine
In the U.S.
Astramorph
Astramorph PF
Duramorph
M S Contin
MSIR
RMS Uniserts
Roxanol
Roxanol 100
Roxanol SR
Generic name product may also be available.
In Canada
Epimorph
Morphine H.P.
Morphitec
M.O.S.
M.O.S.-S.R.
M S Contin
Roxanol
Statex
Generic name product may also be available.

For Nalbuphine
In the U.S.
Nubain
Generic name product may also be available.
In Canada
Nubain

For Opium
In the U.S.
Pantopon
In Canada
Pantopon
Another commonly used name is papaveretum.

For Oxycodone
In the U.S.
Roxicodone
In Canada
Supeudol

For Oxymorphone
In the U.S.
Numorphan
In Canada
Numorphan

For Pentazocine
In the U.S.
Talwin
Talwin-Nx
In Canada
Talwin

For Propoxyphene
In the U.S.
Darvon
Darvon-N
Dolene
Doraphen
Doxaphene
Profene
Pro Pox
Propoxycon
Generic name product may also be available.
In Canada
Darvon-N
Novopropoxyn
642
Another commonly used name is dextropropoxyphene.

---

*Not commercially available in the U.S.

‡For Canadian product only. In the U.S., *Hycodan* also contains homatropine; in Canada, *Hycodan* contains only hydrocodone.

§In Canada, methadone is available only through doctors who have received special approval to prescribe it.

Description

Narcotic (nar-KOT-ik) analgesics (an-al-JEE-zicks) are used to relieve pain. Some of these medicines are also used just before or during an operation to help the anesthetic work better. Codeine and hydrocodone are also used to relieve coughing. Methadone is also used to help some people control their dependence on heroin or other narcotics. Narcotic analgesics may also be used for other conditions as determined by your doctor.

Narcotic analgesics act in the central nervous system (CNS) to relieve pain. Some of their side effects are also caused by actions in the CNS.

If a narcotic is used for a long time, it may become habit-forming (causing mental or physical dependence). Physical dependence may lead to withdrawal side effects when you stop taking the medicine.

These medicines are available only with your medical doctor's or dentist's prescription. For some of them, prescriptions cannot be refilled and you must obtain a new prescription from your medical doctor or dentist each time you need the medicine. In addition, other rules and regulations may apply when methadone is used to treat narcotic dependence.

These medicines are available in the following dosage forms:

Oral

Codeine
- Oral solution (U.S. and Canada)
- Tablets (U.S. and Canada)

Hydrocodone
- Syrup (Canada)
- Tablets (Canada)

Hydromorphone
- Tablets (U.S. and Canada)

Levorphanol
- Tablets (U.S. and Canada)

Meperidine
- Syrup (U.S.)
- Tablets (U.S. and Canada)

Methadone
- Oral concentrate (U.S.)
- Oral solution (U.S.)
- Tablets (U.S.)
- Dispersible tablets (U.S.)

Morphine
- Oral solution (U.S. and Canada)
- Syrup (Canada)
- Tablets (U.S. and Canada)
- Extended-release tablets (U.S. and Canada)

Oxycodone
- Oral solution (U.S.)
- Tablets (U.S. and Canada)

Pentazocine
- Tablets (Canada)

Pentazocine and Naloxone
- Tablets (U.S.)

Propoxyphene
- Capsules (U.S. and Canada)
- Oral suspension (U.S.)
- Tablets (U.S. and Canada)

Parenteral

Buprenorphine
- Injection (U.S.)

Butorphanol
- Injection (U.S. and Canada)

Codeine
- Injection (U.S. and Canada)

Hydromorphone
- Injection (U.S. and Canada)

Levorphanol
- Injection (U.S. and Canada)

Meperidine
- Injection (U.S. and Canada)

Methadone
- Injection (U.S.)

Morphine
- Injection (U.S. and Canada)

Nalbuphine
- Injection (U.S. and Canada)

Opium
- Injection (U.S. and Canada)

Oxymorphone
- Injection (U.S. and Canada)

Pentazocine
- Injection (U.S. and Canada)

Rectal

Hydromorphone
- Suppositories (U.S. and Canada)

Morphine
- Suppositories (U.S. and Canada)

Oxycodone
- Suppositories (Canada)

Oxymorphone
- Suppositories (U.S. and Canada)

It is very important that you read and understand the following information. If any of it causes you special concern, check with your doctor. Also, *if you have any questions* or if you want more information about this medicine or your medical problem, *ask your doctor, nurse, or pharmacist.*

Before Using This Medicine

In deciding to use a medicine, the risks of taking the medicine must be weighed against the good it will do. This is a decision you and your doctor will make. For narcotic analgesics, the following should be considered:

Allergies—Tell your doctor if you have ever had any unusual or allergic reaction to any of the narcotic analgesics. Also tell your doctor and pharmacist if you are allergic to any other substances, such as foods, preservatives, or dyes.

Pregnancy—Although studies on birth defects with narcotic analgesics have not been done in pregnant women, these medicines have not been reported to cause birth defects. However, hydrocodone, hydromorphone, and morphine caused birth defects in animals when given in very large doses. Buprenorphine and codeine did not cause birth defects in animal studies, but they caused other unwanted effects. Butorphanol, nalbuphine, pentazocine, and propoxyphene did not cause birth defects in animals. There is no information about whether other narcotic analgesics cause birth defects in animals.

Too much use of a narcotic during pregnancy may cause the baby to become dependent on the medicine. This may lead to withdrawal side effects after birth. Also, some of these medicines may cause breathing problems in the newborn infant if taken just before delivery.

Breast-feeding—Most narcotic analgesics have not been reported to cause problems in nursing babies. However, when the mother is taking large amounts of methadone (in a methadone maintenance program), the nursing baby may become dependent on the medicine. Also, butorphanol, codeine, meperidine, morphine, opium, and propoxyphene pass into the breast milk.

Children—Breathing problems may be especially likely to occur in children younger than 2 years of age. These children are usually more sensitive than adults to the effects of narcotic analgesics. Also, unusual excitement or restlessness may be more likely to occur in children receiving these medicines.

Older adults—Elderly people are especially sensitive to the effects of narcotic analgesics. This may increase the chance of side effects, especially breathing problems, during treatment.

Other medicines—Although certain medicines should not be used together at all, in other cases two different medicines may be used together even if an interaction might occur. In these cases, your doctor may want to change the dose, or other precautions may be necessary. When you are taking a narcotic analgesic, it is especially important that your doctor and pharmacist know if you are taking any of the following:

- Carbamazepine (e.g., Tegretol)—Propoxyphene may increase the blood levels of carbamazepine, which increases the chance of serious side effects
- Central nervous system (CNS) depressants or
- Monoamine oxidase (MAO) inhibitors (furazolidone [e.g., Furoxone], isocarboxazid [e.g., Marplan], pargyline [e.g., Eutonyl], phenelzine [e.g., Nardil], procarbazine [e.g., Matulane], tranylcypromine [e.g., Parnate] (taken currently or within the past 2 weeks) or
- Tricyclic antidepressants (amitriptyline [e.g., Elavil], amoxapine [e.g., Asendin], clomipramine [e.g., Anafranil], desipramine [e.g., Pertofrane], doxepin [e.g., Sinequan], imipramine [e.g., Tofranil], nortriptyline [e.g., Aventyl], protriptyline [e.g., Vivactil], trimipramine [e.g., Surmontil])—The chance of side effects may be increased; the combination of meperidine (e.g., Demerol) and MAO inhibitors is especially dangerous
- Naltrexone (e.g., Trexan)—Narcotics will not be effective in people taking naltrexone
- Rifampin (e.g., Rifadin)—Rifampin decreases the effects of methadone and may cause withdrawal symptoms in people who are dependent on methadone

- Zidovudine (e.g., AZT, Retrovir)—Morphine may increase the blood levels of zidovudine and increase the chance of serious side effects

Other medical problems—The presence of other medical problems may affect the use of narcotic analgesics. Make sure you tell your doctor if you have any other medical problems, especially:

- Alcohol abuse, or history of, or
- Drug dependence, especially narcotic abuse, or history of, or
- Emotional problems—The chance of side effects may be increased; also, withdrawal symptoms may occur if a narcotic you are dependent on is replaced by buprenorphine, butorphanol, nalbuphine, or pentazocine
- Brain disease or head injury or
- Emphysema, asthma, or other chronic lung disease or
- Enlarged prostate or problems with urination or
- Gallbladder disease or gallstones—Some of the side effects of narcotic analgesics can be dangerous if these conditions are present
- Colitis or
- Heart disease or
- Kidney disease or
- Liver disease or
- Underactive thyroid—The chance of side effects may be increased
- Convulsions (seizures), history of—Some of the narcotic analgesics can cause convulsions

Before you begin using any new medicine (prescription or nonprescription) or if you develop any new medical problem while you are using this medicine, check with your doctor, nurse, or pharmacist.

Proper Use of This Medicine

Some narcotic analgesics given by injection may be given at home to patients who do not need to be in the hospital. If you are using an injection form of this medicine at home, *make sure you clearly understand and carefully follow your doctor's instructions.*

To take the *syrup form of meperidine:*

- Unless otherwise directed by your medical doctor or dentist, *take this medicine mixed with a half glass (4 ounces) of water* to lessen the numbing effect of the medicine on your mouth and throat.

To take the *oral liquid forms of methadone:*

- *This medicine may have to be mixed with water or another liquid before you take it.* Read the label carefully for directions. If you have any questions about this, check with your doctor, nurse, or pharmacist.

To take the *dispersible tablet form of methadone:*

- *These tablets must be stirred into water or fruit juice just before each dose is taken. Read the label carefully for directions.* If you have any questions about this, check with your doctor, nurse, or pharmacist.

To take *oral liquid forms of morphine:*

- This medicine may be mixed with a glass of fruit juice just before you take it, if desired, to improve the taste.

To take *long-acting morphine tablets:*

- *These tablets must be swallowed whole.* Do not break, crush, or chew them before swallowing.

To use *suppositories:*

- If the suppository is too soft to insert, chill it in the refrigerator for 30 minutes or run cold water over it before removing the foil wrapper.
- To insert the suppository: First remove the foil wrapper and moisten the suppository with cold water. Lie down on your side and use your finger to push the suppository well up into the rectum.

Take this medicine only as directed by your medical doctor or dentist. Do not take more of it, do not take it more often, and do not take it for a longer time than your medical doctor or dentist ordered. This is especially important for young children and elderly patients, who are especially sensitive to the effects of narcotic analgesics. If too much is taken, the medicine may become habit-forming (causing mental or physical dependence) or lead to medical problems because of an overdose.

If you think this medicine is not working properly after you have been taking it for a few weeks, *do not increase the dose.* Instead, check with your doctor.

Missed dose—If your medical doctor or dentist has ordered you to take this medicine according to a regular schedule and you miss a dose, take it as soon as you remember. However, if it is almost time for your next dose, skip the missed dose and go back to your regular dosing schedule. *Do not double doses.*

Storage—To store this medicine:

- Keep out of the reach of children. Overdose is very dangerous in young children.
- Store away from heat and direct light.
- Do not store tablets or capsules in the bathroom, near the kitchen sink, or in other damp places. Heat or moisture may cause the medicine to break down.
- Store hydromorphone, oxycodone, or oxymorphone suppositories in the refrigerator.
- Keep liquid (including injections) and suppository forms of the medicine from freezing.
- Do not keep outdated medicine or medicine no longer needed. Be sure that any discarded medicine is out of the reach of children.

Precautions While Using This Medicine

If you will be taking this medicine for a long time (for example, for several months at a time), your doctor should check your progress at regular visits.

Narcotic analgesics will add to the effects of alcohol and other CNS depressants (medicines that slow down the nervous system, possibly causing drowsiness). Some examples of CNS depressants are antihistamines or medicine for hay fever, other allergies, or colds; sedatives, tranquilizers, or sleeping medicine; other prescription pain medicines including other narcotics; barbiturates; medicine for seizures; muscle relaxants; or anesthetics, including some dental anesthetics. *Do not drink alcoholic beverages, and check with your medical doctor or dentist before taking any of the medicines listed above, while you are using this medicine.*

This medicine may cause some people to become drowsy, dizzy, or lightheaded, or to feel a false sense of well-being. *Make sure you know how you react to this medicine before you drive, use machines, or do anything else that could be dangerous if you are dizzy or are not alert and clearheaded.*

Dizziness, lightheadedness, or fainting may occur, especially when you get up suddenly from a lying or sitting position. Getting up slowly may help lessen this problem.

Nausea or vomiting may occur, especially after the first couple of doses. This effect may go away if you lie down for a while. However, if nausea or vomiting continues, check with your medical doctor or dentist. Lying down for a while may also help relieve some other side effects, such as dizziness or lightheadedness, that may occur.

Before having any kind of surgery (including dental surgery) or emergency treatment, tell the medical doctor or dentist in charge that you are taking this medicine.

Narcotic analgesics may cause dryness of the mouth. For temporary relief, use sugarless candy or gum, melt bits of ice in your mouth, or use a saliva substitute. However, if dry mouth continues for more than 2 weeks, check with your dentist. Continuing dryness of the mouth may increase the chance of dental disease, including tooth decay, gum disease, and fungus infections.

If you have been taking this medicine regularly for several weeks or more, *do not suddenly stop using it without first checking with your doctor.* Your doctor may want you to reduce gradually the amount you are taking before stopping completely, in order to lessen the chance of withdrawal side effects.

If you think you or someone else may have taken an overdose, get emergency help at once. Taking an overdose of this medicine or taking alcohol or CNS depressants with this medicine may lead to unconsciousness or death. Signs of overdose include convulsions (seizures), confusion, severe nervousness or restlessness, severe dizziness, severe drowsiness, slow or troubled breathing, and severe weakness.

Side Effects of This Medicine

Along with its needed effects, a medicine may cause some unwanted effects. Although not all of these side effects may occur, if they do occur they may need medical attention.

Get emergency help immediately if any of the following symptoms of overdose occur:

Cold, clammy skin; confusion; convulsions (seizures); dizziness (severe); drowsiness (severe); low blood pressure; nervousness or restlessness (severe); pinpoint pupils of eyes; slow heartbeat; slow or troubled breathing; weakness (severe)

Also, check with your doctor as soon as possible if any of the following side effects occur:

Less common or rare

Dark urine (for propoxyphene only); fast, slow, or pounding heartbeat; feelings of unreality; hallucinations (seeing, hearing, or feeling things that are not there); hives, itching, or skin rash; increased sweating (more common with hydrocodone, meperidine, and methadone); irregular breathing; mental depression or other mood or mental changes; pale stools (for propoxyphene only); redness or flushing of face (more common with hydrocodone, meperidine, and methadone); ringing or buzzing in the ears; shortness of breath, wheezing, or troubled breathing; swelling of face; trembling or uncontrolled muscle movements; unusual excitement or restlessness (especially in children); yellow eyes or skin (for propoxyphene only)

Other side effects may occur that usually do not need medical attention. These side effects may go away during treatment as your body adjusts to the medicine. However, check with your doctor if any of the following side effects continue or are bothersome:

More common

Dizziness, lightheadedness, or feeling faint; drowsiness; nausea or vomiting

Less common or rare

Blurred or double vision or other changes in vision; constipation (more common with long-term use and with codeine); decrease in amount of urine; difficult or painful urination; dry mouth; false sense of well-being; frequent urge to urinate; general feeling of discomfort or illness; headache; loss of appetite; nervousness or restlessness; nightmares or unusual dreams; redness, swelling, pain, or burning at place of injection; stomach cramps or pain; trouble in sleeping; unusual tiredness or weakness

After you stop using this medicine, your body may need time to adjust. The length of time this takes depends on the amount of medicine you were using and how long you used it. During this period of time check with your doctor if you notice any of the following side effects:

Body aches; diarrhea; fast heartbeat; fever, runny nose, or sneezing; gooseflesh; increased sweating; increased yawning; loss of appetite; nausea or vomiting; nervousness, restlessness, or irritability; shivering or trembling; stomach cramps; trouble in sleeping; unusually large pupils of eyes; weakness

Other side effects not listed above may also occur in some patients. If you notice any other effects, check with your doctor.

Annual revision: July 1990

NARCOTIC ANALGESICS—For Surgery and Obstetrics Systemic

This information applies to the following medicines:

- Alfentanil (al-FEN-ta-nil)
- Buprenorphine (byoo-pre-NOR-feen)
- Butorphanol (byoo-TOR-fa-nole)
- Fentanyl (FEN-ta-nil)
- Meperidine (me-PER-i-deen)
- Morphine (MOR-feen)
- Nalbuphine (NAL-byoo-feen)
- Sufentanil (soo-FEN-ta-nil)

Some commonly used brand names are:

For Alfentanil

In the U.S.
Alfenta

In Canada
Alfenta

For Buprenorphine

In the U.S.
Buprenex

For Butorphanol

In the U.S.
Stadol

In Canada
Stadol

For Fentanyl

In the U.S.
Sublimaze
Generic name product may also be available.

In Canada
Sublimaze

For Meperidine

In the U.S.
Demerol
Generic name product may also be available.

In Canada
Demerol
Generic name product may also be available.

Another commonly used name is pethidine.

For Morphine

In the U.S.
Astramorph
Astramorph PF
Duramorph
Generic name product may also be available.

In Canada
Epimorph
Generic name product may also be available.

For Nalbuphine

In the U.S.
Nubain
Generic name product may also be available.

In Canada
Nubain

For Sufentanil

In the U.S.
Sufenta

In Canada
Sufenta

Description

Narcotic analgesics (nar-KOT-ik an-al-JEE-zicks) are given to relieve pain before and during surgery (including dental surgery) or during labor and delivery. These medicines may also be given before or together with an anesthetic (either a general anesthetic or a local anesthetic), even when the patient is not in pain, to help the anesthetic work better.

When a narcotic analgesic is used for surgery or obstetrics (labor and delivery), it will be given by or under the immediate supervision of a medical doctor or dentist, or by a specially trained nurse, in the doctor's office or in a hospital.

The following information applies only to these special uses of narcotic analgesics. If you are taking or receiving a narcotic analgesic to relieve pain after surgery, or for any other reason, ask your doctor, nurse, or pharmacist for additional information about the medicine and its use.

These medicines are available in the following dosage forms:

Parenteral

Alfentanil
- Injection (U.S. and Canada)

Buprenorphine
- Injection (U.S.)

Butorphanol
- Injection (U.S. and Canada)

Fentanyl
- Injection (U.S. and Canada)

Meperidine
- Injection (U.S. and Canada)

Morphine
- Injection (U.S. and Canada)

Nalbuphine
- Injection (U.S. and Canada)

Sufentanil
- Injection (U.S. and Canada)

Before Receiving This Medicine

In deciding to use a medicine, the risks of using the medicine must be weighed against the good it will do. This is a decision you and your doctor will make. For narcotic analgesics, the following should be considered:

Allergies—Tell your doctor if you have ever had any unusual or allergic reaction to a narcotic analgesic. Also tell your doctor and pharmacist if you are allergic to any other substances, such as foods, preservatives, or dyes.

Pregnancy—Although studies on birth defects have not been done in pregnant women, these medicines have not been reported to cause birth defects. However, in animal studies, many narcotics have caused birth defects or other unwanted effects when they were given for a long time in amounts that were large enough to cause harmful effects in the mother.

Use of a narcotic during labor and delivery sometimes causes drowsiness or breathing problems in the newborn baby. If this happens, your doctor or nurse can give the baby another medicine that will overcome these effects. Narcotics are usually not used during the delivery of a premature baby.

Breast-feeding—Some narcotics have been shown to pass into the breast milk. However, these medicines have not been reported to cause problems in nursing babies.

Children—Children younger than 2 years of age may be especially sensitive to the effects of narcotic analgesics. This may increase the chance of side effects.

Older adults—Elderly people are especially sensitive to the effects of narcotic analgesics. This may increase the chance of side effects.

Other medicines—Although certain medicines should not be used together at all, in other cases two different medicines may be used together even if an interaction might occur. In these cases, it may be necessary to change the dose, or other precautions may be necessary. It is very important that you tell the person in charge if you are taking:

- Any other medicine, prescription or nonprescription (over-the-counter [OTC]), or
- "Street" drugs, such as amphetamines ("uppers"), barbiturates ("downers"), cocaine (including "crack"), marijuana, phencyclidine (PCP, "angel dust"), and heroin or other narcotics—Serious side effects may occur if anyone gives you an anesthetic without knowing that you have taken another medicine

Other medical problems—The presence of other medical problems may affect the use of narcotic analgesics. Make sure you tell your doctor if you have *any* other medical problems.

Precautions After Receiving This Medicine

For patients going home within a few hours after surgery:

- Narcotic analgesics and other medicines that may be given with them during surgery may cause some people to feel drowsy, tired, or weak for up to a few days after they have been given. Therefore, for at least 24 hours (or longer if necessary) after receiving this medicine, *do not drive, use machines, or do anything else that could be dangerous if you are dizzy or are not alert.*
- Unless otherwise directed by your medical doctor or dentist, *do not drink alcoholic beverages or take other CNS depressants (medicines that slow down the nervous system, possibly causing drowsiness) for about 24 hours after you have received this medicine.* To do so may add to the effects of the narcotic analgesic. Some examples of CNS depressants are antihistamines or medicine for hay fever, other allergies, or colds; sedatives, tranquilizers, or sleeping medicine; prescription pain medicine or narcotics; barbiturates; medicine for seizures; and muscle relaxants.

Side Effects of This Medicine

Along with its needed effects, a medicine may cause some unwanted effects. Before you leave the hospital or doctor's office, your doctor or nurse will closely follow the effects of this medicine. However, some effects may continue, or may not be noticed until later.

The following side effects usually do not need medical attention. They will gradually go away as the effects of the medicine wear off. However, check with your medical doctor or dentist if any of the following side effects continue or are bothersome:

More common

Dizziness, lightheadedness, or feeling faint; drowsiness; nausea or vomiting; unusual tiredness or weakness

Less common or rare

Blurred or double vision or other vision problems; confusion; constipation; difficult or painful urination; dryness of mouth; general feeling of discomfort or illness; headache; mental depression or other mood or mental changes; nightmares or unusual dreams

Other side effects not listed above may also occur in some patients. If you notice any other effects, check with your doctor.

Annual revision: July 1990

NARCOTIC ANALGESICS AND ACETAMINOPHEN Systemic

This information applies to the following medicines:

Acetaminophen (a-seat-a-MIN-oh-fen) and Codeine (KOE-deen)
Acetaminophen, Codeine, and Caffeine (kaf-EEN)
Dihydrocodeine (dye-hye-droe-KOE-deen), Acetaminophen, and Caffeine
Hydrocodone (hye-droe-KOE-done) and Acetaminophen
Meperidine (me-PER-i-deen) and Acetaminophen
Oxycodone (ox-i-KOE-done) and Acetaminophen
Pentazocine (pen-TAZ-oh-seen) and Acetaminophen
Propoxyphene (proe-POX-i-feen) and Acetaminophen

Some commonly used brand names are:

For Acetaminophen and Codeine

In the U.S.

Acetaco
Aceta with Codeine
Capital with Codeine
M-Gesic
Myapap with Codeine
Phenaphen with Codeine No.2‡
Phenaphen with Codeine No.3‡
Phenaphen with Codeine No.4‡
Phenaphen-650 with Codeine
Proval
Pyregesic-C
Tylaprin with Codeine
Tylenol with Codeine
Tylenol with Codeine No.1
Tylenol with Codeine No.2
Tylenol with Codeine No.3
Tylenol with Codeine No.4
Ty-Pap with Codeine
Ty-Tab with Codeine No.2
Ty-Tab with Codeine No.3
Ty-Tab with Codeine No.4

Generic name product may also be available.

In Canada

Empracet-30
Empracet-60
Emtec-30
Lenoltec with Codeine No.4
Rounox and Codeine 15
Rounox and Codeine 30
Rounox and Codeine 60
Tylenol with Codeine No.4

Another commonly used name is APAP with codeine.

For Acetaminophen, Codeine, and Caffeine

In the U.S.

Codalan No.1
Codalan No.2
Codalan No.3

In Canada

Atasol-8
Atasol-15
Atasol-30
Codamin #2
Codamin #3
Codaminophen
Exdol-8
Exdol-15
Exdol-30
Lenoltec with Codeine No.1
Lenoltec with Codeine No.2
Lenoltec with Codeine No.3
Novogesic C8
Novogesic C15
Novogesic C30
Tylenol No.1
Tylenol No.1 Forte
Tylenol with Codeine
Tylenol with Codeine No.2
Tylenol with Codeine No.3
Veganin

Generic name product may also be available.

For Dihydrocodeine, Acetaminophen, and Caffeine†

In the U.S.

Compal

Another commonly used name is drocode, acetaminophen, and caffeine.

For Hydrocodone and Acetaminophen†

In the U.S.

Allay
Amacodone
Anexsia
Anexsia 7.5
Anodynos DHC
Anolor DH 5
Bancap-HC
Co-Gesic
Dolacet
Duocet
Duradyne DHC
HY-5
Hycomed
Hycopap
Hyco-Pap
Hydrocet
Hydrogesic
HY-PHEN
Lorcet-HD
Lorcet Plus
Lortab
Lortab 5
Lortab 7
Megagesic
Norcet
Norcet 7.5
Polygesic
Propain-HC
Rogesic No.3
Senefen III
Ultragesic
Vapocet
Vicodin
Vicodin ES
Zydone

Generic name product may also be available.

Another commonly used name is hydrocodone with APAP.

For Meperidine and Acetaminophen†

In the U.S.

Demerol-APAP

For Oxycodone and Acetaminophen

In the U.S.

Percocet
Roxicet
Roxicet 5/500
Tylox

Generic name product may also be available.

In Canada

Endocet
Oxycocet
Percocet
Percocet-Demi

Another commonly used name is oxycodone with APAP.

For Pentazocine and Acetaminophen†

In the U.S.

Talacen

For Propoxyphene and Acetaminophen†

In the U.S.

Darvocet-N 50
Darvocet-N 100
Dolene-AP-65
Doxapap-N
D-Rex 65
E-Lor
Genagesic
Propacet 100
Pro Pox with APAP
Wygesic

Generic name product may also be available.

Another commonly used name is propoxyphene with APAP.

†Not commercially available in Canada.
‡In Canada, *Phenaphen with Codeine* is different from the product with that name in the U.S. The Canadian product contains phenobarbital, ASA, and codeine.

Description

Combination medicines containing narcotic (nar-KOT-ik) analgesics (an-al-JEE-zicks) and acetaminophen are used to relieve pain. A narcotic analgesic and acetaminophen used together may provide better pain relief than either medicine used alone. In some cases, relief of pain may come at lower doses of each medicine.

Narcotic analgesics act in the central nervous system (CNS) to relieve pain. Many of their side effects are also caused by actions in the CNS. When narcotics are used for a long time, your body may get used to them so that larger amounts are needed to relieve pain. This is called tolerance to the medicine. Also, when narcotics are used for a long time or in large doses, they may become habit-forming (causing mental or physical dependence). Physical dependence may lead to withdrawal symptoms when you stop taking the medicine.

Acetaminophen does not become habit-forming when taken for a long time or in large doses, but it may cause other unwanted effects, including liver damage, if too much is taken.

In the U.S., these medicines are available only with your medical doctor's or dentist's prescription. In Canada, some acetaminophen, codeine, and caffeine combinations are available without a prescription.

These medicines are available in the following dosage forms:

Oral

Acetaminophen and Codeine
- Capsules (U.S.)
- Elixir (U.S. and Canada)
- Oral suspension (U.S.)
- Tablets (U.S. and Canada)

Acetaminophen, Codeine, and Caffeine
- Capsules (Canada)
- Tablets (U.S. and Canada)

Dihydrocodeine, Acetaminophen, and Caffeine
- Capsules (U.S.)

Hydrocodone and Acetaminophen
- Capsules (U.S.)
- Oral solution (U.S.)
- Tablets (U.S.)

Meperidine and Acetaminophen
- Tablets (U.S.)

Oxycodone and Acetaminophen
- Capsules (U.S.)
- Oral solution (U.S.)
- Tablets (U.S. and Canada)

Pentazocine and Acetaminophen
- Tablets (U.S.)

Propoxyphene and Acetaminophen
- Capsules (U.S.)
- Tablets (U.S.)

It is very important that you read and understand the following information. If any of it causes you special concern, check with your doctor. Also, *if you have any questions* or if you want more information about this medicine or your medical problem, *ask your doctor, nurse, or pharmacist.*

Before Using This Medicine

In deciding to use a medicine, the risks of taking the medicine must be weighed against the good it will do. This is a decision you and your doctor will make. For narcotic analgesic and acetaminophen combinations, the following should be considered:

Allergies—Tell your doctor if you have ever had any unusual or allergic reaction to acetaminophen or to a narcotic analgesic. Also tell your doctor and pharmacist if you are allergic to any other substances, such as foods, preservatives, or dyes.

Pregnancy—
- *For acetaminophen*: Although studies on birth defects with acetaminophen have not been done in pregnant women, it has not been reported to cause birth defects or other problems.
- *For narcotic analgesics*: Although studies on birth defects with narcotic analgesics have not been done in pregnant women, they have not been reported to cause birth defects. However, hydrocodone caused birth defects in animal studies when very large doses were used. Codeine did not cause birth defects in animals, but it caused slower development of bones and other toxic or harmful effects in the fetus. Pentazocine and propoxyphene did not cause birth defects in animals. There is no information about whether dihydrocodeine, meperidine, or oxycodone cause birth defects in animals.

  Too much use of a narcotic during pregnancy may cause the fetus to become dependent on the medicine. This may lead to withdrawal side effects in the newborn baby. Also, some of these medicines may cause breathing problems in the newborn baby if taken just before or during delivery.
- *For caffeine:* Studies in humans have not shown that caffeine (contained in some of these combination medicines) causes birth defects. However, studies in animals have shown that caffeine causes birth defects when given in very large doses (amounts equal to those present in 12 to 24 cups of coffee a day).

Breast-feeding—Acetaminophen, codeine, meperidine, and propoxyphene pass into the breast milk. It is not known whether other narcotic analgesics pass into the breast milk. However, these medicines have not been reported to cause problems in nursing babies.

Children—Breathing problems may be especially likely to occur when narcotic analgesics are given to children younger than 2 years of age. These children are usually more sensitive than adults to the effects of narcotic analgesics. Also, unusual excitement or restlessness may be more likely to occur in children receiving these medicines.

Acetaminophen has been tested in children and has not been shown to cause different side effects or problems in children than it does in adults.

Older adults—Elderly people are especially sensitive to the effects of narcotic analgesics. This may increase the chance of side effects, especially breathing problems, during treatment.

Acetaminophen has been tested and has not been shown to cause different side effects or problems in older people than it does in younger adults.

Other medicines—Although certain medicines should not be used together at all, in other cases two different medicines may be used together even if an interaction might occur. In these cases, your doctor may want to change the dose, or other precautions may be necessary. When you are taking a narcotic analgesic and acetaminophen combination, it is especially important that your doctor and pharmacist know if you are taking any of the following:

- Carbamazepine (e.g., Tegretol)—Propoxyphene may increase the blood levels of carbamazepine, which increases the chance of serious side effects
- Central nervous system (CNS) depressants or
- Monoamine oxidase (MAO) inhibitors (furazolidone [e.g., Furoxone], isocarboxazid [e.g., Marplan], pargyline [e.g., Eutonyl], phenelzine [e.g., Nardil], procarbazine [e.g., Matulane], tranylcypromine [e.g., Parnate]) (taken currently or within the past 2 weeks) or
- Tricyclic antidepressants (amitriptyline [e.g., Elavil], amoxapine [e.g., Asendin], clomipramine [e.g., Anafranil], desipramine [e.g., Pertofrane], doxepin [e.g., Sinequan], imipramine [e.g., Tofranil], nortriptyline [e.g., Aventyl], protriptyline [e.g., Vivactil], trimipramine [e.g., Surmontil])—Taking these medicines together with a narcotic analgesic may increase the chance of serious side effects
- Naltrexone (e.g., Trexan)—Naltrexone keeps narcotic analgesics from working to relieve pain; people taking naltrexone should take pain relievers that do not contain a narcotic
- Zidovudine (e.g., AZT, Retrovir)—Acetaminophen may increase the blood levels of zidovudine, which increases the chance of serious side effects

Other medical problems—The presence of other medical problems may affect the use of narcotic analgesic and acetaminophen combinations. Make sure you tell your doctor if you have any other medical problems, especially:

- Alcohol and/or other drug abuse, or history of, or
- Brain disease or head injury or
- Colitis or
- Convulsions (seizures), history of, or
- Emotional problems or mental illness or
- Emphysema, asthma, or other chronic lung disease or
- Hepatitis or other liver disease or
- Kidney disease or
- Underactive thyroid—The chance of serious side effects may be increased
- Enlarged prostate or problems with urination or
- Gallbladder disease or gallstones—Some of the effects of narcotic analgesics may be especially serious in people with these medical problems
- Heart disease—Caffeine (present in some of these combination medicines) can make some kinds of heart disease worse

Before you begin using any new medicine (prescription or nonprescription) or if you develop any new medical problem while you are using this medicine, check with your doctor, nurse, or pharmacist.

Proper Use of This Medicine

Take this medicine only as directed by your medical doctor or dentist. Do not take more of it, do not take it more often, and do not take it for a longer time than your medical doctor or dentist ordered. This is especially important for young children and elderly patients, who may be more sensitive than other people to the effects of narcotic analgesics. If too much of a narcotic analgesic is taken, it may become habit-forming (causing mental or physical dependence) or lead to medical problems because of an overdose. Taking too much acetaminophen may cause liver damage.

If you think that this medicine is not working properly after you have been taking it for a few weeks, *do not increase the dose.* Instead, check with your medical doctor or dentist.

Missed dose—If your medical doctor or dentist has ordered you to take this medicine according to a regular schedule and you miss a dose, take it as soon as you remember. However, if it is almost time for your next dose, skip the missed dose and go back to your regular dosing schedule. *Do not double doses.*

Storage—To store this medicine:

- Keep out of the reach of children. Overdose is very dangerous in young children.
- Store away from heat and direct light.
- Do not store tablets or capsules in the bathroom, near the kitchen sink, or in other damp places. Heat or moisture may cause the medicine to break down.
- Keep the liquid forms of this medicine from freezing.
- Do not keep outdated medicine or medicine no longer needed. Be sure that any discarded medicine is out of the reach of children.

Precautions While Using This Medicine

If you will be taking this medicine for a long time (for example, for several months at a time), or in high doses, your doctor should check your progress at regular visits.

Check the labels of all nonprescription (over-the-counter [OTC]) and prescription medicines you now take. If any contain acetaminophen or a narcotic be especially careful, since taking them while taking this medicine may lead to overdose. If you have any questions about this, check with your medical doctor, dentist, or pharmacist.

The narcotic analgesic in this medicine will add to the effects of alcohol and other CNS depressants (medicines that slow down the nervous system, possibly causing drowsiness). Some examples of CNS depressants are antihistamines or medicine for hay fever, other allergies, or colds; sedatives, tranquilizers, or sleeping medicine; other prescription pain medicine or narcotics; barbiturates; medicine for seizures; muscle relaxants; or anesthetics, including some dental anesthetics. Also, there may be a greater risk of liver damage if large amounts of alcoholic beverages are used while you are taking acetaminophen. *Do not drink alcoholic beverages, and check with your medical doctor or dentist before taking any of the medicines listed above, while you are using this medicine.*

Too much use of the acetaminophen in this combination medicine together with certain other medicines may increase the chance of unwanted effects. The risk will depend on how much of each medicine you take every day, and on how long you take the medicines together. If your doctor directs you to take these medicines together on a regular basis, follow his or her directions carefully. However, do not take this medicine together with any of the following medicines for more than a few days, unless your doctor has directed you to do so and is following your progress:

- Aspirin or other salicylates
- Diclofenac (e.g., Voltaren)
- Diflunisal (e.g., Dolobid)
- Fenoprofen (e.g., Nalfon)
- Floctafenine (e.g., Idarac)
- Flurbiprofen, oral (e.g., Ansaid)
- Ibuprofen (e.g., Motrin)
- Indomethacin (e.g., Indocin)
- Ketoprofen (e.g., Orudis)
- Ketorolac (e.g., Toradol)
- Meclofenamate (e.g., Meclomen)
- Mefenamic acid (e.g., Ponstel)
- Naproxen (e.g., Naprosyn)
- Phenylbutazone (e.g., Butazolidin)
- Piroxicam (e.g., Feldene)
- Sulindac (e.g., Clinoril)
- Tiaprofenic acid (e.g., Surgam)
- Tolmetin (e.g., Tolectin)

This medicine may cause some people to become drowsy, dizzy, or lightheaded, or to feel a false sense of well-being. *Make sure you know how you react to this medicine before you drive, use machines, or do anything else that could be dangerous if you are dizzy or are not alert and clearheaded.*

Dizziness, lightheadedness, or fainting may occur, especially when you get up suddenly from a lying or sitting position. Getting up slowly may help lessen this problem.

Nausea or vomiting may occur, especially after the first couple of doses. This effect may go away if you lie down for a while. However, if nausea or vomiting continues, check with your medical doctor or dentist. Lying down for a while may also help relieve some other side effects, such as dizziness or lightheadedness, that may occur.

Before having any kind of surgery (including dental surgery) or emergency treatment, tell the medical doctor or dentist in charge that you are taking this medicine.

Narcotic analgesics may cause dryness of the mouth. For temporary relief, use sugarless candy or gum, melt bits of ice in your mouth, or use a saliva substitute. However, if dry mouth continues for more than 2 weeks, check with your dentist. Continuing dryness of the mouth may increase the chance of dental disease, including tooth decay, gum disease, and fungus infections.

If you have been taking this medicine regularly for several weeks or more, *do not suddenly stop taking it without first checking with your doctor.* Your doctor may want you to reduce gradually the amount you are taking before stopping completely, to lessen the chance of withdrawal side effects. This will depend on which of these medicines you have been taking, and the amount you have been taking every day.

If you think you or someone else may have taken an overdose of this medicine, get emergency help at once. Taking an overdose of this medicine or taking alcohol or CNS depressants with this medicine may lead to unconsciousness or death. Signs of overdose of narcotics include convulsions (seizures), confusion, severe nervousness or restlessness, severe dizziness, severe drowsiness, shortness of breath or troubled breathing, and severe weakness. Signs of severe acetaminophen overdose may not occur until several days after the overdose is taken.

Side Effects of This Medicine

Along with its needed effects, a medicine may cause some unwanted effects. Although not all of these side effects may occur, if they do occur they may need medical attention.

Get emergency help immediately if any of the following symptoms of overdose occur:

Cold, clammy skin; confusion (severe); convulsions (seizures); diarrhea; dizziness (severe); drowsiness (severe); increased sweating; low blood pressure; nausea or vomiting (continuing); nervousness or restlessness (severe); pinpoint pupils of eyes; shortness of breath or unusually slow or troubled breathing; slow heartbeat; stomach cramps or pain; weakness (severe)

Also, check with your doctor as soon as possible if any of the following side effects occur:

Less common or rare

Black, tarry stools; bloody or cloudy urine; confusion; dark urine; difficult or painful urination; fast, slow, or pounding heartbeat; frequent urge to urinate; hallucinations (seeing, hearing, or feeling things that are not there); increased sweating; irregular breathing or wheezing; mental depression; pain in lower back and/or side (severe and/or sharp); pale stools; pinpoint red spots on skin; redness or flushing of face; ringing or buzzing in ears; skin rash, hives, or itching; sore throat and fever; sudden decrease in amount of urine; swelling of face; trembling or uncontrolled muscle movements; unusual bleeding or bruising; unusual excitement (especially in children); yellow eyes or skin

Other side effects may occur that usually do not need medical attention. These side effects may go away during treatment as your body adjusts to the medicine. However, check with your medical doctor or dentist if any of the following side effects continue or are bothersome:

More common

Dizziness, lightheadedness, or feeling faint; drowsiness; nausea or vomiting; unusual tiredness or weakness

Less common or rare

Blurred or double vision or other changes in vision; constipation (more common with long-term use and with codeine or meperidine); dry mouth; false sense of well-being; general feeling of discomfort or illness; headache; loss of appetite; nervousness or restlessness; nightmares or unusual dreams; trouble in sleeping

Although not all of the side effects listed above have been reported for all of these combination medicines, they have been reported for at least one of them. However, since all of the narcotic analgesics are very similar, any of the above side effects may occur with any of these medicines.

After you stop using this medicine, your body may need time to adjust. The length of time this takes depends on which of these medicines you were taking, the amount of medicine you were using, and how long you used it. During this time check with your doctor if you notice any of the following side effects:

Body aches; diarrhea; fast heartbeat; fever, runny nose, or sneezing; gooseflesh; increased sweating; increased yawning; loss of appetite; nausea or vomiting; nervousness, restlessness, or irritability; shivering or trembling; stomach cramps; trouble in sleeping; weakness

Other side effects not listed above may also occur in some patients. If you notice any other effects, check with your doctor.

Annual revision: July 1990

NARCOTIC ANALGESICS AND ASPIRIN Systemic

This information applies to the following medicines:

Aspirin, Caffeine, and Dihydrocodeine (dye-hye-droe-KOE-deen)
Aspirin (AS-pir-in) and Codeine (KOE-deen)
Aspirin, Codeine, and Caffeine (kaf-EEN)
Aspirin, Codeine, and Caffeine, Buffered
Hydrocodone (hye-droe-KOE-done) and Aspirin
Hydrocodone, Aspirin, and Caffeine
Oxycodone (ox-i-KOE-done) and Aspirin
Pentazocine (pen-TAZ-oh-seen) and Aspirin
Propoxyphene (proe-POX-i-feen) and Aspirin
Propoxyphene, Aspirin, and Caffeine

Some commonly used brand names are:

For Aspirin, Caffeine, and Dihydrocodeine†

In the U.S.

Synalgos-DC

Generic name product may also be available.

Other commonly used names are dihydrocodeine compound and drocode and aspirin.

For Aspirin and Codeine

In the U.S.

Emcodeine No.2 | Empirin with Codeine No.2
Emcodeine No.3 | Empirin with Codeine No.3
Emcodeine No.4 | Empirin with Codeine No.4

Generic name product may also be available.

In Canada‡

Coryphen with Codeine

For Aspirin, Codeine, and Caffeine*

In Canada‡

A.C.&C. | 222 Forte
Anacin with Codeine | 222
Ancasal 8 | 282
Ancasal 15 | 292
Ancasal 30 | 293
C2 with Codeine

For Aspirin, Codeine, and Caffeine, Buffered*

In Canada‡

C2 Buffered with Codeine

For Hydrocodone and Aspirin†

In the U.S.

Azdone | Lortab ASA

For Hydrocodone, Aspirin, and Caffeine†

In the U.S.

Damason-P

For Oxycodone and Aspirin

In the U.S.

Percodan | Roxiprin
Percodan-Demi

Generic name product may also be available.

In Canada‡

Endodan | Percodan
Oxycodan | Percodan-Demi

For Pentazocine and Aspirin†

In the U.S.

Talwin Compound

For Propoxyphene and Aspirin
In the U.S.
Darvon with A.S.A.
Darvon-N with A.S.A.
In Canada‡
Darvon-N with A.S.A.

For Propoxyphene, Aspirin, and Caffeine
In the U.S.
Bexophene
Cotanal-65
Darvon Compound
Darvon Compound-65
Doraphen Compound-65
Doxaphene Compound
Margesic A-C
Pro Pox Plus
Generic name product may also be available.
In Canada‡
Darvon-N Compound
Novopropoxyn Compound
692

Another commonly used name is propoxyphene hydrochloride compound.

*Not commercially available in the U.S.
†Not commercially available in Canada.
‡In Canada, *Aspirin* is a brand name. Acetylsalicylic acid is the generic name in Canada. ASA, a synonym for acetylsalicylic acid, is the term that commonly appears on Canadian product labels.

Description

Combination medicines containing narcotic (nar-KOT-ik) analgesics (an-al-JEE-zicks) and aspirin are used to relieve pain. A narcotic analgesic and aspirin used together may provide better pain relief than either medicine used alone. In some cases, relief of pain may come at lower doses of each medicine.

Narcotic analgesics act in the central nervous system (CNS) to relieve pain. Many of their side effects are also caused by actions in the CNS. When narcotics are used for a long time, your body may get used to them so that larger amounts are needed to relieve pain. This is called tolerance to the medicine. Also, when narcotics are used for a long time or in large doses, they may become habit-forming (causing mental or physical dependence). Physical dependence may lead to withdrawal symptoms when you stop taking the medicine.

Aspirin does not become habit-forming when taken for a long time or in large doses, but it may cause other unwanted effects if too much is taken.

In the U.S., these medicines are available only with your medical doctor's or dentist's prescription. In Canada, some strengths of aspirin, codeine, and caffeine combination are available without a prescription.

These medicines are available in the following dosage forms:

Oral
Aspirin, Caffeine, and Dihydrocodeine
- Capsules (U.S.)

Aspirin and Codeine
- Tablets (U.S. and Canada)

Aspirin, Codeine, and Caffeine
- Tablets (Canada)

Aspirin, Codeine, and Caffeine, Buffered
- Tablets (Canada)

Hydrocodone and Aspirin
- Tablets (U.S.)

Hydrocodone, Aspirin, and Caffeine
- Tablets (U.S.)

Oxycodone and Aspirin
- Tablets (U.S. and Canada)

Pentazocine and Aspirin
- Tablets (U.S.)

Propoxyphene and Aspirin
- Capsules (U.S. and Canada)
- Tablets (U.S.)

Propoxyphene, Aspirin, and Caffeine
- Capsules (U.S. and Canada)
- Tablets (Canada)

It is very important that you read and understand the following information. If any of it causes you special concern, check with your doctor. Also, *if you have any questions* or if you want more information about this medicine or your medical problem, *ask your doctor, nurse, or pharmacist.*

Before Using This Medicine

In deciding to use a medicine, the risks of taking the medicine must be weighed against the good it will do. This is a decision you and your doctor will make. For narcotic analgesic and aspirin combinations, the following should be considered:

Allergies—Tell your doctor if you have ever had any unusual or allergic reaction to a narcotic analgesic, aspirin or other salicylates, including methyl salicylate (oil of wintergreen), or any of the following medicines:

Diclofenac (e.g., Voltaren)
Diflunisal (e.g., Dolobid)
Fenoprofen (e.g., Nalfon)
Floctafenine (e.g., Idarac)
Flurbiprofen, oral (e.g., Ansaid)
Ibuprofen (e.g., Motrin)
Indomethacin (e.g., Indocin)
Ketoprofen (e.g., Orudis)
Ketorolac (e.g., Toradol)
Meclofenamate (e.g., Meclomen)
Mefenamic acid (e.g., Ponstel)
Naproxen (e.g., Naprosyn)
Oxyphenbutazone (e.g., Tandearil)
Phenylbutazone (e.g., Butazolidin)
Piroxicam (e.g., Feldene)
Sulindac (e.g., Clinoril)
Suprofen (e.g., Suprol)
Tiaprofenic acid (e.g., Surgam)
Tolmetin (e.g., Tolectin)
Zomepirac (e.g., Zomax)

Also tell your doctor and pharmacist if you are allergic to any other substances, such as foods, preservatives, or dyes.

Pregnancy—

- *For aspirin*: Studies in humans have not shown that aspirin causes birth defects. However, studies in animals have shown that aspirin causes birth defects.

Some reports have suggested that too much use of aspirin late in pregnancy may cause a decrease in the newborn's weight and possible death of the fetus or newborn baby. However, the mothers in these reports had been taking much larger amounts of aspirin than are usually recommended. Studies of mothers taking aspirin in the doses that are usually recommended did not show these effects. However, regular use of aspirin late in pregnancy may cause unwanted effects on the heart or blood flow in the fetus or in the newborn baby. Also, use of aspirin during the last 2 weeks of pregnancy may cause bleeding problems in the fetus before or during delivery or in the newborn baby.

Too much use of aspirin during the last 3 months of pregnancy may increase the length of pregnancy, prolong labor, cause other problems during delivery, or cause severe bleeding in the mother before, during, or after delivery. *Do not take aspirin during the last 3 months of pregnancy unless it has been ordered by your doctor.*

- *For narcotic analgesics*: Although studies on birth defects with narcotic analgesics have not been done in pregnant women, they have not been reported to cause birth defects. However, hydrocodone caused birth defects in animal studies when given in very large doses. Codeine did not cause birth defects in animals, but it caused slower development of bones and other toxic or harmful effects on the fetus. Pentazocine and propoxyphene did not cause birth defects in animals. There is no information about whether dihydrocodeine or oxycodone causes birth defects in animals.

  Too much use of a narcotic during pregnancy may cause the fetus to become dependent on the medicine. This may lead to withdrawal side effects in the newborn baby. Also, some of these medicines may cause breathing problems in the newborn baby if taken just before or during delivery.
- *For caffeine*: Studies in humans have not shown that caffeine (contained in some of these combination medicines) causes birth defects. However, studies in animals have shown that caffeine causes birth defects when given in very large doses (amounts equal to those present in 12 to 24 cups of coffee a day).

Breast-feeding—These combination medicines have not been reported to cause problems in nursing babies. However, aspirin, caffeine, codeine, and propoxyphene pass into the breast milk. It is not known whether dihydrocodeine, hydrocodone, oxycodone, or pentazocine passes into the breast milk.

Children—*Do not give a medicine containing aspirin to a child or a teenager with a fever or other symptoms of a virus infection, especially flu or chickenpox, without first discussing its use with your child's doctor.* This is very important because aspirin may cause a serious illness called Reye's syndrome in children with fever caused by a virus infection, especially flu or chickenpox. Children who do not have a virus infection may also be more sensitive to the effects of aspirin, especially if they have a fever or have lost large amounts of body fluid because of vomiting, diarrhea, or sweating. This may increase the chance of side effects during treatment.

The narcotic analgesic in this combination medicine can cause breathing problems, especially in children younger than 2 years of age. These children are usually more sensitive than adults to the effects of narcotic analgesics. Also, unusual excitement or restlessness may be more likely to occur in children receiving these medicines.

Older adults—Elderly people are especially sensitive to the effects of aspirin and of narcotic analgesics. This may increase the chance of side effects, especially breathing problems caused by narcotic analgesics, during treatment.

Other medicines—Although certain medicines should not be used together at all, in other cases two different medicines may be used together even if an interaction might occur. In these cases, your doctor may want to change the dose, or other precautions may be necessary. When you are taking a narcotic analgesic and aspirin combination, it is especially important that your doctor and pharmacist know if you are taking any of the following:

- Anticoagulants (blood thinners) or
- Carbenicillin by injection (e.g., Geopen) or
- Cefamandole (e.g., Mandol) or
- Cefoperazone (e.g., Cefobid) or
- Cefotetan (e.g., Cefotan) or
- Dipyridamole (e.g., Persantine) or
- Divalproex (e.g., Depakote) or
- Heparin or
- Medicine for inflammation or pain, except narcotics, or
- Moxalactam (e.g., Moxam) or
- Pentoxifylline (e.g., Trental) or
- Plicamycin (e.g., Mithracin) or
- Ticarcillin (e.g., Ticar) or
- Valproic acid (e.g., Depakene)—Taking these medicines together with aspirin may increase the chance of bleeding
- Antidiabetics, oral (diabetes medicine you take by mouth)—Aspirin may increase the effects of the antidiabetic medicine; a change in the dose of the antidiabetic medicine may be needed if aspirin is taken regularly
- Carbamazepine (e.g., Tegretol)—Propoxyphene can increase the blood levels of carbamazepine, which increases the chance of serious side effects
- Central nervous system (CNS) depressants or
- Diarrhea medicine or
- Methotrexate (e.g., Mexate) or
- Tricyclic antidepressants (amitriptyline [e.g., Elavil], amoxapine [e.g., Asendin], clomipramine [e.g., Anafranil], desipramine [e.g., Pertofrane], doxepin [e.g., Sinequan], imipramine [e.g., Tofranil], nortriptyline [e.g., Aventyl], protriptyline [e.g., Vivactil], trimipramine [e.g., Surmontil]) or
- Vancomycin (e.g., Vancocin)—The chance of side effects may be increased

- Naltrexone (e.g., Trexan)—Naltrexone keeps narcotic analgesics from working to relieve pain; people taking naltrexone should use pain relievers that do not contain a narcotic
- Probenecid (e.g., Benemid) or
- Sulfinpyrazone (e.g., Anturane)—Aspirin can keep these medicines from working as well for treating gout; also, use of sulfinpyrazone and aspirin together may increase the chance of bleeding
- Urinary alkalizers (medicine that makes the urine less acid, such as acetazolamide [e.g., Diamox], calcium- and/or magnesium-containing antacids, dichlorphenamide [e.g., Daranide], methazolamide [e.g., Neptazane], potassium or sodium citrate and/or citric acid, sodium bicarbonate [baking soda])—These medicines may make aspirin less effective by causing it to be removed from the body more quickly
- Zidovudine (e.g., AZT, Retrovir)—Higher blood levels of zidovudine and an increased chance of serious side effects may occur

Other medical problems—The presence of other medical problems may affect the use of narcotic analgesic and aspirin combinations. Make sure you tell your doctor if you have any other medical problems, especially:

- Alcohol and/or other drug abuse, or history of, or
- Asthma, allergies, and nasal polyps (history of) or
- Brain disease or head injury or
- Colitis or
- Convulsions (seizures), history of, or
- Emotional problems or mental illness or
- Emphysema or other chronic lung disease or
- Kidney disease or
- Liver disease or
- Underactive thyroid—The chance of serious side effects may be increased
- Anemia or
- Overactive thyroid or
- Stomach ulcer or other stomach problems—Aspirin may make these conditions worse
- Enlarged prostate or problems with urination or
- Gallbladder disease or gallstones—Narcotic analgesics have side effects that may be dangerous if these medical problems are present
- Gout—Aspirin can make this condition worse and can also lessen the effects of some medicines used to treat gout
- Heart disease—Large amounts of aspirin and caffeine (present in some of these combination medicines) can make some kinds of heart disease worse
- Hemophilia or other bleeding problems or
- Vitamin K deficiency—Aspirin increases the chance of serious bleeding

Before you begin using any new medicine (prescription or nonprescription) or if you develop any new medical problem while you are using this medicine, check with your doctor, nurse, or pharmacist.

Proper Use of This Medicine

Take this medicine with food or a full glass (8 ounces) of water to lessen stomach irritation.

Do not take this medicine if it has a strong vinegar-like odor. This odor means the aspirin in it is breaking down. If you have any questions about this, check with your doctor or pharmacist.

Take this medicine only as directed by your medical doctor or dentist. Do not take more of it, do not take it more often, and do not take it for a longer time than your medical doctor or dentist ordered. This is especially important for children and elderly patients, who are usually more sensitive to the effects of these medicines. If too much of a narcotic analgesic is taken, it may become habit-forming (causing mental or physical dependence) or lead to medical problems because of an overdose. Also, taking too much aspirin may cause stomach problems or lead to medical problems because of an overdose.

If you think that this medicine is not working as well after you have been taking it for a few weeks, *do not increase the dose.* Instead, check with your medical doctor or dentist.

Missed dose—If your medical doctor or dentist has ordered you to take this medicine according to a regular schedule and you miss a dose, take it as soon as you remember. However, if it is almost time for your next dose, skip the missed dose and go back to your regular dosing schedule. *Do not double doses.*

Storage—To store this medicine:

- Keep out of the reach of children. Overdose is very dangerous in young children.
- Store away from heat and direct light.
- Do not store this medicine in the bathroom, near the kitchen sink, or in other damp places. Heat or moisture may cause the medicine to break down.
- Do not keep outdated medicine or medicine no longer needed. Be sure that any discarded medicine is out of the reach of children.

Precautions While Using This Medicine

If you will be taking this medicine for a long time (for example, for several months at a time), your doctor should check your progress at regular visits.

Check the labels of all nonprescription (over-the-counter [OTC]) and prescription medicines you now take. If any contain a narcotic, aspirin, or other salicylates, be especially careful, since taking them while taking this medicine may lead to overdose. If you have any questions about this, check with your physician, dentist, or pharmacist.

This medicine will add to the effects of alcohol and other CNS depressants (medicines that slow down the nervous system, possibly causing drowsiness). Some examples of CNS depressants are antihistamines or medicine for hay fever, other allergies, or colds; sedatives, tranquilizers, or sleeping medicine; other prescription pain medicine or narcotics; barbiturates; medicine for seizures; muscle relaxants; or anesthetics, including some dental anesthetics. Also, stomach problems may be more likely to occur if you drink alcoholic beverages while you are taking aspirin. *Do not drink alcoholic beverages, and check with your medical doctor or dentist before taking any of the medicines listed above, while you are using this medicine.*

Taking acetaminophen or certain other medicines together with the aspirin in this combination medicine may increase the chance of unwanted effects. The risk will depend on how much of each medicine you take every day, and on how long you take the medicines together. If your doctor directs you to take these medicines together on a regular basis, follow his or her directions carefully. However, do not take acetaminophen or any of the following medicines together with this combination medicine for more than a few days, unless your doctor has directed you to do so and is following your progress:

Diclofenac (e.g., Voltaren)
Diflunisal (e.g., Dolobid)
Fenoprofen (e.g., Nalfon)
Floctafenine (e.g., Idarac)
Flurbiprofen, oral (e.g., Ansaid)
Ibuprofen (e.g., Motrin)
Indomethacin (e.g., Indocin)
Ketoprofen (e.g., Orudis)
Ketorolac (e.g., Toradol)
Meclofenamate (e.g., Meclomen)
Mefenamic acid (e.g., Ponstel)
Naproxen (e.g., Naprosyn)
Phenylbutazone (e.g., Butazolidin)
Piroxicam (e.g., Feldene)
Sulindac (e.g., Clinoril)
Tiaprofenic acid (e.g., Surgam)
Tolmetin (e.g., Tolectin)

This medicine may cause some people to become drowsy, dizzy, or lightheaded, or to feel a false sense of well-being. *Make sure you know how you react to this medicine before you drive, use machines, or do anything else that could be dangerous if you are dizzy or are not alert and clearheaded.*

Dizziness, lightheadedness, or fainting may occur, especially when you get up suddenly from a lying or sitting position. Getting up slowly may help lessen this problem.

Nausea or vomiting may occur, especially after the first couple of doses. This effect may go away if you lie down for a while. However, if nausea or vomiting continues, check with your doctor. Lying down for a while may also help some other side effects, such as dizziness or lightheadedness.

Before having any kind of surgery (including dental surgery) or emergency treatment, tell the medical doctor or dentist in charge that you are taking this medicine.

Do not take this medicine for 5 days before any surgery, including dental surgery, unless otherwise directed by your medical doctor or dentist. Taking aspirin during this time may cause bleeding problems.

If you are taking one of the combination medicines containing buffered aspirin, and you are also taking a tetracycline antibiotic, do not take the two medicines within 3 to 4 hours of each other. Taking them too close together may prevent the tetracycline from being absorbed by your body. If you have any questions about this, check with your doctor or pharmacist.

For *diabetic patients:*

- False urine sugar test results may occur if you are regularly taking 8 or more 325-mg (5-grain) or 5 or more 500-mg doses of aspirin a day. Smaller amounts or occasional use of aspirin usually will not affect urine sugar tests. If you have any questions about this, check with your doctor, nurse, or pharmacist, especially if your diabetes is not well controlled.

Narcotic analgesics may cause dryness of the mouth. For temporary relief, use sugarless candy or gum, melt bits of ice in your mouth, or use a saliva substitute. However, if dry mouth continues for more than 2 weeks, check with your dentist. Continuing dryness of the mouth may increase the chance of dental disease, including tooth decay, gum disease, and fungus infections.

If you have been taking this medicine regularly for several weeks or more, *do not suddenly stop using it without first checking with your doctor.* Depending on which of these medicines you have been taking, and the amount you have been taking every day, your doctor may want you to reduce gradually the amount you are taking before stopping completely, to lessen the chance of withdrawal side effects.

If you think you or someone else may have taken an overdose of this medicine, get emergency help at once. Taking an overdose of this medicine or taking alcohol or CNS depressants with this medicine may lead to unconsciousness or death. Signs of overdose of this medicine include convulsions (seizures); hearing loss; confusion; ringing or buzzing in the ears; severe excitement, nervousness, or restlessness; severe dizziness, severe drowsiness, shortness of breath or troubled breathing, and severe weakness.

Side Effects of This Medicine

Along with its needed effects, a medicine may cause some unwanted effects. Although not all of these side effects may occur, if they do occur they may need medical attention.

Get emergency help immediately if any of the following symptoms of overdose occur:

Any loss of hearing; bloody urine; cold, clammy skin; confusion (severe); convulsions (seizures); diarrhea (severe or continuing); dizziness or lightheadedness (severe); drowsiness (severe); excitement, nervousness, or restlessness (severe); fever; hallucinations (seeing, hearing, or feeling things that are not there); headache (severe or continuing); increased sweating; increased thirst; low blood pressure; nausea or vomiting (severe or continuing); pinpoint pupils of eyes; ringing or buzzing in the ears; shortness of breath or unusually slow or troubled breathing; slow heartbeat; stomach pain (severe or continuing); uncontrollable flapping movements of the hands (especially in elderly patients); vision problems; weakness (severe)

Also, check with your doctor as soon as possible if any of the following side effects occur:

Less common or rare

Bloody or black, tarry stools; confusion; dark urine; fast, slow, or pounding heartbeat; increased sweating (more common with hydrocodone); irregular breathing; mental depression; pale stools; redness or flushing of face (more common with hydrocodone); skin rash, hives, or itching; stomach pain (severe); swelling of face; tightness in chest or wheezing; trembling or uncontrolled muscle movements; unusual excitement (especially in children); unusual tiredness or weakness; vomiting of blood or material that looks like coffee grounds; yellow eyes or skin

Other side effects may occur that usually do not need medical attention. These side effects may go away during treatment as your body adjusts to the medicine. However, check with your doctor if any of the following side effects continue or are bothersome:

More common

Dizziness, lightheadedness, or feeling faint; drowsiness; heartburn or indigestion; nausea or vomiting; stomach pain (mild)

Less common or rare

Blurred or double vision or other changes in vision; constipation (more common with long-term use and with codeine); difficult, painful, or decreased urination; dryness of mouth; false sense of well-being; frequent urge to urinate; general feeling of discomfort or illness; headache; loss of appetite; nervousness or restlessness; nightmares or unusual dreams; trouble in sleeping; unusual tiredness; unusual weakness

Although not all of the side effects listed above have been reported for all of these medicines, they have been reported for at least one of them. However, since all of the narcotic analgesics are very similar, any of the above side effects may occur with any of these medicines.

After you stop using this medicine, your body may need time to adjust. The length of time this takes depends on which of these medicines you were taking, the amount of medicine you were using, and how long you used it. During this period of time check with your doctor if you notice any of the following side effects:

Body aches; diarrhea; fever, runny nose, or sneezing; gooseflesh; increased sweating; increased yawning; loss of appetite; nausea or vomiting; nervousness, restlessness, or irritability; shivering or trembling; stomach cramps; trouble in sleeping; weakness

Other side effects not listed above may also occur in some patients. If you notice any other effects, check with your medical doctor or dentist.

Annual revision: July 1990

NATAMYCIN Ophthalmic

A commonly used brand name in the U.S. is Natacyn.
Another commonly used name is pimaricin.

Description

Natamycin (na-ta-MYE-sin) belongs to the group of medicines called antifungals. It is used to treat some types of fungus infections of the eye.

Natamycin is available only with your doctor's prescription, in the following dosage form:

Ophthalmic

- Ophthalmic suspension (eye drops) (U.S.)

It is very important that you read and understand the following information. If any of it causes you special concern, check with your doctor. Also, *if you have any questions* or if you want more information about this medicine or your medical problem, *ask your doctor, nurse, or pharmacist.*

Before Using This Medicine

In deciding to use a medicine, the risks of taking the medicine must be weighed against the good it will do. This is a decision you and your doctor will make. For ophthalmic natamycin, the following should be considered:

Allergies—Tell your doctor if you have ever had any unusual or allergic reaction to natamycin. Also tell your doctor and pharmacist if you are allergic to any other substances, such as preservatives.

Pregnancy—Natamycin has not been shown to cause birth defects or other problems in humans.

Breast-feeding—Natamycin has not been reported to cause problems in nursing babies.

Children—Studies on this medicine have been done only in adult patients, and there is no specific information about its use in children.

Older adults—Many medicines have not been tested in older people. Therefore, it may not be known whether they work exactly the same way they do in younger adults or if they cause different side effects or problems in older people. There is no specific information about the use of natamycin in the elderly.

Before you begin using any new medicine (prescription or nonprescription) or if you develop any new medical problem while you are using this medicine, check with your doctor, nurse, or pharmacist.

Proper Use of This Medicine

The bottle is only partially full to provide proper drop control.

To use:

- First, wash your hands. Then tilt the head back and pull the lower eyelid away from the eye to form a pouch. Drop the medicine into the pouch and gently close the eyes. Do not blink. Keep the eyes closed for 1 or 2 minutes to allow the medicine to come into contact with the infection.
- If you think you did not get the drop of medicine into your eye properly, use another drop.
- To keep the medicine as germ-free as possible, do not touch the applicator tip to any surface (including the eye). Also, keep the container tightly closed.

To help clear up your eye infection completely, *keep using this medicine for the full time of treatment,* even if your condition has improved. *Do not miss any doses.*

Missed dose—If you do miss a dose of this medicine, apply it as soon as possible. Then go back to your regular dosing schedule.

Storage—To store this medicine:

- Keep out of the reach of children.
- Store away from heat and direct light.
- Keep the medicine from freezing.
- Do not keep outdated medicine or medicine no longer needed. Be sure that any discarded medicine is out of the reach of children.

Precautions While Using This Medicine

Your doctor should check your progress at regular visits.

If your symptoms do not improve within 7 to 10 days, or if they become worse, check with your doctor.

Side Effects of This Medicine

Along with its needed effects, a medicine may cause some unwanted effects. Although not all of these side effects may occur, if they do occur they may need medical attention.

Check with your doctor as soon as possible if the following side effect occurs:

Eye irritation not present before use of this medicine

Other side effects not listed above may also occur in some patients. If you notice any other effects, check with your doctor.

Annual revision: June 1990

NEOMYCIN Ophthalmic*

*Not commercially available in the U.S.

Description

Neomycin (nee-oh-MYE-sin) belongs to the family of medicines called antibiotics. Neomycin ophthalmic preparations are used to treat infections of the eye.

Neomycin is available only with your doctor's prescription, in the following dosage form:

Ophthalmic

- Ophthalmic ointment

It is very important that you read and understand the following information. If any of it causes you special concern, check with your doctor. Also, *if you have any questions* or if you want more information about this medicine or your medical problem, *ask your doctor, nurse, or pharmacist.*

Before Using This Medicine

In deciding to use a medicine, the risks of taking the medicine must be weighed against the good it will do. This is a decision you and your doctor will make. For

neomycin ophthalmic preparations, the following should be considered:

Allergies—Tell your doctor if you have ever had any unusual or allergic reaction to this medicine or to any related antibiotic, such as amikacin (e.g., Amikin), gentamicin (e.g., Garamycin), kanamycin (e.g., Kantrex), netilmicin (e.g., Netromycin), streptomycin, or tobramycin (e.g., Nebcin). Also tell your doctor and pharmacist if you are allergic to any other substances, such as preservatives.

Pregnancy—Neomycin ophthalmic preparations have not been shown to cause birth defects or other problems in humans.

Breast-feeding—Neomycin ophthalmic preparations have not been reported to cause problems in nursing babies.

Children—Studies on this medicine have been done only in adult patients, and there is no specific information about its use in children.

Older adults—Many medicines have not been tested in older people. Therefore, it may not be known whether they work exactly the same way they do in younger adults or if they cause different side effects or problems in older people. There is no specific information about the use of neomycin in the elderly.

Before you begin using any new medicine (prescription or nonprescription) or if you develop any new medical problem while you are using this medicine, check with your doctor, nurse, or pharmacist.

Proper Use of This Medicine

To use:

- First, wash your hands. Then pull the lower eyelid away from the eye to form a pouch. Squeeze a thin strip of ointment into the pouch. A 1-cm (approximately ⅓-inch) strip of ointment is usually enough unless otherwise directed by your doctor. Gently close the eyes and keep them closed for 1 or 2 minutes to allow the medicine to come into contact with the infection.
- To keep the medicine as germ-free as possible, do not touch the applicator tip to any surface (including the eye). After using neomycin eye ointment, wipe the tip of the ointment tube with a clean tissue and keep the tube tightly closed.

To help clear up your infection completely, *keep using this medicine for the full time of treatment,* even if your symptoms have disappeared. *Do not miss any doses.*

Missed dose—If you do miss a dose of this medicine, apply it as soon as possible. However, if it is almost time for your next dose, skip the missed dose and go back to your regular dosing schedule.

Storage—To store this medicine:

- Keep out of the reach of children.
- Store away from heat and direct light.
- Keep the medicine from freezing.
- Do not keep outdated medicine or medicine no longer needed. Be sure that any discarded medicine is out of the reach of children.

Precautions While Using This Medicine

If your symptoms do not improve within a few days, or if they become worse, check with your doctor.

Side Effects of This Medicine

Along with its needed effects, a medicine may cause some unwanted effects. Although not all of these side effects may occur, if they do occur they may need medical attention.

Check with your doctor immediately if any of the following side effects occur:

More common

Itching, rash, redness, swelling, or other sign of irritation not present before use of this medicine

Other side effects may occur that usually do not need medical attention. These side effects may go away during treatment as your body adjusts to the medicine. However, check with your doctor if either of the following side effects continues or is bothersome:

Less common

Burning or stinging

After application, eye ointments may be expected to cause your vision to blur for a few minutes.

Other side effects not listed above may also occur in some patients. If you notice any other effects, check with your doctor.

Annual revision: June 1990

NEOMYCIN Oral

A commonly used brand name in the U.S. and Canada is Mycifradin. Generic name product may also be available in the U.S.

Description

Oral neomycin (nee-oh-MYE-sin) is used to help lessen the symptoms of hepatic coma, a complication of liver disease. In addition, it may be used with another medicine before any surgery affecting the bowels to help prevent infection during surgery.

Neomycin is available only with your doctor's prescription, in the following dosage forms:

Oral
- Solution (U.S. and Canada)
- Tablets (U.S. and Canada)

It is very important that you read and understand the following information. If any of it causes you special concern, check with your doctor. Also, *if you have any questions* or if you want more information about this medicine or your medical problem, *ask your doctor, nurse, or pharmacist.*

Before Using This Medicine

In deciding to use a medicine, the risks of taking the medicine must be weighed against the good it will do. This is a decision you and your doctor will make. For oral neomycin, the following should be considered:

Allergies—Tell your doctor if you have ever had any unusual or allergic reaction to oral neomycin, or to any related antibiotics such as amikacin (e.g., Amikin), gentamicin (e.g., Garamycin), kanamycin (e.g., Kantrex), neomycin by injection (e.g., Mycifradin), netilmicin (e.g., Netromycin), streptomycin, or tobramycin (e.g., Nebcin). Also tell your doctor and pharmacist if you are allergic to any other substances, such as foods, preservatives, or dyes.

Pregnancy—Studies have shown that neomycin may damage the infant's kidneys. In addition, some reports have shown that related medicines, especially streptomycin and tobramycin (e.g., Nebcin), may damage the infant's hearing and sense of balance. Be sure you have discussed this with your doctor.

Breast-feeding—It is not known whether neomycin passes into the breast milk. However, neomycin has not been reported to cause problems in nursing babies.

Children—Damage to hearing, sense of balance, and kidneys is more likely to occur in premature infants and neonates, who are more sensitive than adults to the effects of neomycin.

Older adults—Serious side effects, such as damage to hearing, sense of balance, and kidneys may occur in elderly patients, who are usually more sensitive than younger adults to the effects of neomycin.

Other medicines—Although certain medicines should not be used together at all, in other cases two different medicines may be used together even if an interaction might occur. In these cases, your doctor may want to change the dose, or other precautions may be necessary. Tell your doctor and pharmacist if you are taking any other prescription or nonprescription (over-the-counter [OTC]) medicine.

Other medical problems—The presence of other medical problems may affect the use of oral neomycin. Make sure you tell your doctor if you have any other medical problems, especially:

- Blockage of the bowel
- Eighth-cranial-nerve disease (loss of hearing and/or balance)—Oral neomycin may increase the chance of hearing loss and/or balance problems
- Kidney disease—Patients with kidney disease may have an increased chance of side effects
- Myasthenia gravis or
- Parkinson's disease—Patients with myasthenia gravis or Parkinson's disease may have an increased chance of developing muscular weakness
- Ulcers of the bowel—Patients with ulcers of the bowel may have an increased chance of side effects since more neomycin may be absorbed by the body

Before you begin using any new medicine (prescription or nonprescription) or if you develop any new medical problem while you are using this medicine, check with your doctor, nurse, or pharmacist.

Proper Use of This Medicine

This medicine may be taken on a full or empty stomach.

For patients taking the *oral liquid form* of neomycin:
- Use a specially marked measuring spoon or other device to measure each dose accurately. The average household teaspoon may not hold the right amount of liquid.

Keep taking this medicine for the full time of treatment. Do not miss any doses.

Missed dose—If you do miss a dose of this medicine, take it as soon as possible. However, if it is almost time for your next dose, skip the missed dose and go back to your regular dosing schedule. Do not double doses.

Storage—To store this medicine:

- Keep out of the reach of children.
- Store away from heat and direct light.
- Do not store the tablet form of this medicine in the bathroom, near the kitchen sink, or in other damp places. Heat or moisture may cause the medicine to break down.
- Keep the oral liquid form of this medicine from freezing.
- Do not keep outdated medicine or medicine no longer needed. Be sure that any discarded medicine is out of the reach of children.

Side Effects of This Medicine

Along with its needed effects, a medicine may cause some unwanted effects. Although not all of these side effects may occur, if they do occur they may need medical attention.

Check with your doctor immediately if any of the following side effects occur:

Rare

Any loss of hearing; clumsiness; diarrhea; difficulty in breathing; dizziness; drowsiness; greatly decreased frequency of urination or amount of urine; increased amount of gas; increased thirst; light-colored, frothy, fatty-appearing stools; ringing or buzzing or a feeling of fullness in the ears; skin rash; unsteadiness; weakness

Other side effects may occur that usually do not need medical attention. These side effects may go away during treatment as your body adjusts to the medicine. However, check with your doctor if any of the following side effects continue or are bothersome:

More common

Irritation or soreness of the mouth or rectal area; nausea or vomiting

Other side effects not listed above may also occur in some patients. If you notice any other effects, check with your doctor.

Annual revision: 10/20/92

NEOMYCIN Topical

A commonly used brand name in the U.S. and Canada is Myciguent. Generic name product may also be available in the U.S.

Description

Neomycin (nee-oh-MYE-sin) belongs to the family of medicines called antibiotics. Neomycin topical preparations are used to help prevent infections of the skin. This medicine may be used for other problems as determined by your doctor.

Neomycin topical preparations are available without a prescription; however, your doctor may have special instructions on the proper use of topical neomycin for your medical problem.

Topical neomycin is available in the following dosage forms:

Topical

- Cream (U.S.)
- Ointment (U.S. and Canada)

It is very important that you read and understand the following information. If any of it causes you special concern, check with your doctor. Also, *if you have any questions* or if you want more information about this medicine or your medical problem, *ask your doctor, nurse, or pharmacist.*

Before Using This Medicine

In deciding to use a medicine, the risks of using the medicine must be weighed against the good it will do. This is a decision you and your doctor will make. For topical neomycin, the following should be considered:

Allergies—Tell your doctor if you have ever had any unusual or allergic reaction to this medicine or to any related antibiotic, such as amikacin (e.g., Amikin), gentamicin (e.g., Garamycin), kanamycin (e.g., Kantrex), neomycin by mouth or by injection (e.g., Mycifradin), netilmicin (e.g., Netromycin), streptomycin, or tobramycin (e.g., Nebcin). Also tell your doctor and pharmacist if you are allergic to any other substances, such as preservatives or dyes.

Pregnancy—Neomycin topical preparations have not been shown to cause birth defects or other problems in humans.

Breast-feeding—Neomycin topical preparations have not been reported to cause problems in nursing babies.

Children—Studies on this medicine have been done only in adult patients, and there is no specific information about its use in children.

Older adults—Many medicines have not been tested in older people. Therefore, it may not be known whether they work exactly the same way they do in younger adults or if they cause different side effects or problems in older people. There is no specific information about the use of topical neomycin in the elderly.

Other medicines—Although certain medicines should not be used together at all, in other cases two different medicines may be used together even if an interaction might occur. In these cases, your doctor may want to change the dose, or other precautions may be necessary. Tell your doctor and pharmacist if you are using any other topical prescription or nonprescription (over-the-counter [OTC]) medicine that is to be applied to the same area of the skin.

Before you begin using any new medicine (prescription or nonprescription) or if you develop any new medical problem while you are using this medicine, check with your doctor, nurse, or pharmacist.

Proper Use of This Medicine

If you are using this medicine without a prescription, do not use it to treat deep wounds, puncture wounds, serious burns, or raw areas without first checking with your doctor or pharmacist.

Do not use this medicine in the eyes.

Before applying this medicine, wash the affected area with soap and water, and dry thoroughly.

For patients using the *cream form* of this medicine:
- Apply a generous amount of cream to the affected area, and rub in gently until the cream disappears.

For patients using the *ointment form* of this medicine:
- Apply a generous amount of ointment to the affected area, and rub in gently.

After applying this medicine, the treated area may be covered with a gauze dressing if desired.

To help clear up your infection completely, *keep using this medicine for the full time of treatment,* even if your symptoms have disappeared. *Do not miss any doses.*

Missed dose—If you do miss a dose of this medicine, apply it as soon as possible. However, if it is almost time for your next dose, skip the missed dose and go back to your regular dosing schedule.

Storage—To store this medicine:
- Keep out of the reach of children.
- Store away from heat and direct light.
- Keep the medicine from freezing.
- Do not keep outdated medicine or medicine no longer needed. Be sure that any discarded medicine is out of the reach of children.

Precautions While Using This Medicine

If your skin problem does not improve within 1 week, or if it becomes worse, check with your doctor or pharmacist.

Side Effects of This Medicine

Along with its needed effects, a medicine may cause some unwanted effects. Although not all of these side effects may occur, if they do occur they may need medical attention.

Check with your doctor immediately if any of the following side effects occur:

More common

Itching, rash, redness, swelling, or other sign of irritation not present before use of this medicine

Rare

Any loss of hearing

Other side effects not listed above may also occur in some patients. If you notice any other effects, check with your doctor.

Annual revision: June 1990

NEOMYCIN AND POLYMYXIN B Topical†

A commonly used brand name in the U.S. is Neosporin Cream‡.

†Not commercially available in Canada.
‡In Canada, Neosporin cream also contains gramicidin.

Description

Neomycin (nee-oh-MYE-sin) and polymyxin (pol-i-MIX-in) B combination is used to prevent bacterial infections. It works by killing bacteria.

Neomycin and polymyxin B cream is applied to the skin to prevent minor bacterial skin infections. It may also be used for other problems as determined by your doctor.

This medicine is available without a prescription; however, your doctor may have special instructions on the proper use of this medicine for your medical problem.

Neomycin and polymyxin B combination is available in the following dosage form:

Topical
- Cream (U.S.)

It is very important that you read and understand the following information. If any of it causes you special concern, check with your doctor. Also, *if you have any questions* or if you want more information about this medicine or your medical problem, *ask your doctor, nurse, or pharmacist.*

Before Using This Medicine

If you are using this medicine without a prescription, carefully read and follow any precautions on the label. For neomycin and polymyxin B topical preparations, the following should be considered:

Allergies—Tell your doctor if you have ever had any unusual or allergic reaction to neomycin and polymyxin B combination or to any related antibiotic: Amikacin (e.g., Amikin), colistimethate (e.g., Coly-Mycin M), colistin (e.g., Coly-Mycin S), gentamicin (e.g., Garamycin), kanamycin (e.g., Kantrex), neomycin by mouth or by injection (e.g., Mycifradin), netilmicin (e.g., Netromycin), paromomycin (e.g., Humatin), polymyxin B by injection (e.g., Aerosporin), streptomycin, or tobramycin (e.g., Nebcin). Also, tell your doctor and pharmacist if you are allergic to any other substances, such as preservatives or dyes.

Pregnancy—Neomycin and polymyxin B topical preparations have not been shown to cause birth defects or other problems in humans.

Breast-feeding—Neomycin and polymyxin B topical preparations have not been reported to cause problems in nursing babies.

Children—Studies on this medicine have been done only in adult patients, and there is no specific information about its use in children.

Older adults—Many medicines have not been tested in older people. Therefore, it may not be known whether they work exactly the same way they do in younger adults or if they cause different side effects or problems in older people. There is no specific information about the use of neomycin and polymyxin B combination in the elderly.

Other medicines—Although certain medicines should not be used together at all, in other cases two different medicines may be used together even if an interaction might occur. In these cases, your doctor may want to change the dose, or other precautions may be necessary. When you are using neomycin and polymyxin B topical preparations, it is important that your doctor and pharmacist know if you are using any other topical prescription or nonprescription (over-the-counter [OTC]) medicine that is to be applied to the same area of the skin.

Before you begin using any new medicine (prescription or nonprescription) or if you develop any new medical problem while you are using this medicine, check with your doctor, nurse, or pharmacist.

Proper Use of This Medicine

If you are using this medicine without a prescription, *do not use it to treat deep wounds, puncture wounds, animal bites, serious burns, or raw areas* without first checking with your doctor or pharmacist.

Do not use this medicine in the eyes.

To use:
- Before applying this medicine, wash the affected area(s) with soap and water, and dry thoroughly.
- Apply a small amount of this medicine to the affected area(s) and rub in gently.
- After applying this medicine, the treated area(s) may be covered with a gauze dressing if desired.

Do not use this medicine for longer than 1 week or on large areas of the skin, unless otherwise directed by your doctor. To do so may increase the chance of side effects.

To help clear up your skin infection completely, *keep using this medicine for the full time of treatment,* even if your symptoms have disappeared. *Do not miss any doses.*

Missed dose—If you do miss a dose of this medicine, apply it as soon as possible. However, if it is almost time for your next dose, skip the missed dose and go back to your regular dosing schedule.

Storage—To store this medicine:
- Keep out of the reach of children.
- Store away from heat and direct light.
- Keep the medicine from freezing.
- Do not keep outdated medicine or medicine no longer needed. Be sure that any discarded medicine is out of the reach of children.

Precautions While Using This Medicine

If your skin infection does not improve within 1 week, or if it becomes worse, check with your doctor or pharmacist.

Side Effects of This Medicine

Along with its needed effects, a medicine may cause some unwanted effects. Although not all of these side effects

may occur, if they do occur they may need medical attention.

Check with your doctor immediately if any of the following side effects occur:

More common

Itching, skin rash, redness, swelling, pain, or other sign of skin irritation not present before use of this medicine

Rare

Loss of hearing

Other side effects not listed above may also occur in some patients. If you notice any other effects, check with your doctor.

Annual revision: June 1990

NEOMYCIN, POLYMYXIN B, AND BACITRACIN Ophthalmic

Some commonly used brand names are:

In the U.S.

Ak-Spore
Mycitracin
Neocidin
Neosporin Ophthalmic Ointment
Neotal
Neotricin Ophthalmic Ointment
Ocu-Spor-B
Ocusporin
Ocutricin
Ophthalmic
Regasporin
Spectro-Sporin
Tri-Thalmic

Generic name product may also be available.

Description

Neomycin (nee-oh-MYE-sin), polymyxin (pol-i-MIX-in) B, and bacitracin (bass-i-TRAY-sin) combination antibiotic medicine is used to treat infections of the eye.

Neomycin, polymyxin B, and bacitracin combination is available only with your doctor's prescription, in the following dosage form:

Ophthalmic

- Ophthalmic ointment (U.S.)

It is very important that you read and understand the following information. If any of it causes you special concern, check with your doctor. Also, *if you have any questions* or if you want more information about this medicine or your medical problem, *ask your doctor, nurse, or pharmacist.*

Before Using This Medicine

In deciding to use a medicine, the risks of taking the medicine must be weighed against the good it will do. This is a decision you and your doctor will make. For neomycin, polymyxin B, and bacitracin ophthalmic preparations, the following should be considered:

Allergies—Tell your doctor if you have ever had any unusual or allergic reaction to this medicine or to any related antibiotic, such as amikacin (e.g., Amikin), colistimethate (e.g., Coly-Mycin M), colistin (e.g., Coly-Mycin S), gentamicin (e.g., Garamycin), kanamycin (e.g., Kantrex), netilmicin (e.g., Netromycin), paromomycin (e.g., Humatin), streptomycin, or tobramycin (e.g., Nebcin). Also tell your doctor and pharmacist if you are allergic to any other substances, such as preservatives or dyes.

Pregnancy—Neomycin, polymyxin B, and bacitracin ophthalmic preparations have not been shown to cause birth defects or other problems in humans.

Breast-feeding—Neomycin, polymyxin B, and bacitracin ophthalmic preparations have not been reported to cause problems in nursing babies.

Children—Studies on this medicine have been done only in adult patients, and there is no specific information about its use in children.

Older adults—Many medicines have not been tested in older people. Therefore, it may not be known whether they work exactly the same way they do in younger adults or if they cause different side effects or problems in older people. There is no specific information about the use of neomycin, polymyxin B, and bacitracin combination in the elderly.

Before you begin using any new medicine (prescription or nonprescription) or if you develop any new medical problem while you are using this medicine, check with your doctor, nurse, or pharmacist.

Proper Use of This Medicine

To use:

- First, wash your hands. Then pull the lower eyelid away from the eye to form a pouch. Squeeze a thin strip of ointment into the pouch. A 1-cm (approximately ⅓-inch) strip of ointment is usually enough unless otherwise directed by your doctor. Gently close the eyes and keep them closed for 1 or 2 minutes to allow the medicine to come into contact with the infection.
- To keep the medicine as germ-free as possible, do not touch the applicator tip to any surface (including

the eye). After using neomycin, polymyxin B, and bacitracin eye ointment, wipe the tip of the ointment tube with a clean tissue and keep the tube tightly closed.

To help clear up your infection completely, *keep using this medicine for the full time of treatment,* even if your symptoms have disappeared. *Do not miss any doses.*

Missed dose—If you do miss a dose of this medicine, apply it as soon as possible. However, if it is almost time for your next dose, skip the missed dose and go back to your regular dosing schedule.

Storage—To store this medicine:
- Keep out of the reach of children.
- Store away from heat and direct light.
- Keep the medicine from freezing.
- Do not keep outdated medicine or medicine no longer needed. Be sure that any discarded medicine is out of the reach of children.

Precautions While Using This Medicine

If your symptoms do not improve within a few days, or if they become worse, check with your doctor.

Side Effects of This Medicine

Along with its needed effects, a medicine may cause some unwanted effects. Although not all of these side effects may occur, if they do occur they may need medical attention.

Check with your doctor immediately if any of the following side effects occur:

More common

Itching, rash, redness, swelling, or other sign of irritation not present before use of this medicine

After application, eye ointments usually cause your vision to blur for a few minutes.

Other side effects not listed above may also occur in some patients. If you notice any other effects, check with your doctor.

Annual revision: June 1990

NEOMYCIN, POLYMYXIN B, AND BACITRACIN Topical

Some commonly used brand names in the U.S. are:

Bactine First Aid Antibiotic
Foille
Mycitracin
Neosporin Ointment
Neosporin Maximum Strength Ointment
Topisporin

Generic name product may also be available in the U.S.

Description

Neomycin (nee-oh-MYE-sin), polymyxin (pol-i-MIX-in) B, and bacitracin (bass-i-TRAY-sin) is a combination antibiotic medicine used to help prevent infections of the skin.

Neomycin, polymyxin B, and bacitracin combination is available without a prescription; however, your doctor may have special instructions on the proper use of this medicine for your medical problem.

Topical neomycin, polymyxin B, and bacitracin combination is available in the following dosage form:

Topical
- Ointment (U.S.)

It is very important that you read and understand the following information. If any of it causes you special concern, check with your doctor. Also, *if you have any questions* or if you want more information about this medicine or your medical problem, *ask your doctor, nurse, or pharmacist.*

Before Using This Medicine

If you are using this medicine without a prescription, carefully read and follow any precautions on the label. For topical neomycin, polymyxin B, and bacitracin combination, the following should be considered:

Allergies—Tell your doctor if you have ever had any unusual or allergic reaction to this medicine or to any related antibiotic, such as amikacin (e.g., Amikin), colistimethate (e.g., Coly-Mycin M), colistin (e.g., Coly-Mycin S), gentamicin (e.g., Garamycin), kanamycin (e.g., Kantrex), neomycin by mouth or by injection (e.g., Mycifradin), netilmicin (e.g., Netromycin), paromomycin (e.g., Humatin), polymyxin B by injection (e.g., Aerosporin), streptomycin, or tobramycin (e.g., Nebcin). Also tell your doctor and pharmacist if you are allergic to any other substances, such as preservatives or dyes.

Pregnancy—Neomycin, polymyxin B, and bacitracin topical preparations have not been shown to cause birth defects or other problems in humans.

Breast-feeding—Neomycin, polymyxin B, and bacitracin topical preparations have not been reported to cause problems in nursing babies.

Children—Studies on this medicine have been done only in adult patients, and there is no specific information about its use in children.

Older adults—Many medicines have not been tested in older people. Therefore, it may not be known whether they work exactly the same way they do in younger adults or if they cause different side effects or problems in older people. There is no specific information about the use of topical neomycin, polymyxin B, and bacitracin combination in the elderly.

Other medicines—Although certain medicines should not be used together at all, in other cases two different medicines may be used together even if an interaction might occur. In these cases, your doctor may want to change the dose, or other precautions may be necessary. When you are using topical neomycin, polymyxin B, and bacitracin combination, it is especially important that your doctor and pharmacist know if you are using any other prescription or nonprescription (over-the-counter [OTC]) medicine.

Before you begin using any new medicine (prescription or nonprescription) or if you develop any new medical problem while you are using this medicine, check with your doctor, nurse, or pharmacist.

Proper Use of This Medicine

If you are using this medicine without a prescription, do not use it to treat deep wounds, puncture wounds, serious burns, or raw areas without first checking with your doctor or pharmacist.

Do not use this medicine in the eyes.

Before applying this medicine, wash the affected area with soap and water, and dry thoroughly.

After applying this medicine, the treated area may be covered with a gauze dressing if desired.

To help clear up your infection completely, *keep using this medicine for the full time of treatment,* even if your symptoms have disappeared. *Do not miss any doses.*

Missed dose—If you do miss a dose of this medicine, apply it as soon as possible. However, if it is almost time for your next dose, skip the missed dose and go back to your regular dosing schedule.

Storage—To store this medicine:
- Keep out of the reach of children.
- Store away from heat and direct light.
- Keep the medicine from freezing.
- Do not keep outdated medicine or medicine no longer needed. Be sure that any discarded medicine is out of the reach of children.

Precautions While Using This Medicine

If your skin problem does not improve within 1 week, or if it becomes worse, check with your doctor or pharmacist.

Side Effects of This Medicine

Along with its needed effects, a medicine may cause some unwanted effects. Although not all of these side effects may occur, if they do occur they may need medical attention.

Check with your doctor immediately if any of the following side effects occur:

More common

Itching, skin rash, redness, swelling, or other sign of irritation not present before use of this medicine

Rare

Any loss of hearing

Other side effects not listed above may also occur in some patients. If you notice any other effects, check with your doctor.

Annual revision: June 1990

NEOMYCIN, POLYMYXIN B, AND GRAMICIDIN Ophthalmic

Some commonly used brand names are:

In the U.S.

- Ak-Spore
- Bio-Triple
- Neocidin
- Neosporin Ophthalmic Solution
- Neotricin Ophthalmic Solution
- Ocu-Spor-G
- Ocutricin
- P.N. Ophthalmic
- Tribiotic
- Tri-Ophthalmic

Generic name product may also be available.

Description

Neomycin (nee-oh-MYE-sin), polymyxin (pol-i-MIX-in) B, and gramicidin (gram-i-SYE-din) is a combination antibiotic medicine used to treat infections of the eye.

Neomycin, polymyxin B, and gramicidin combination is available only with your doctor's prescription, in the following dosage form:

Ophthalmic

- Ophthalmic solution (eye drops) (U.S.)

It is very important that you read and understand the following information. If any of it causes you special concern, check with your doctor. Also, *if you have any questions* or if you want more information about this medicine or your medical problem, *ask your doctor, nurse, or pharmacist.*

Before Using This Medicine

In deciding to use a medicine, the risks of taking the medicine must be weighed against the good it will do. This is a decision you and your doctor will make. For neomycin, polymyxin B, and gramicidin ophthalmic drops, the following should be considered:

Allergies—Tell your doctor if you have ever had any unusual or allergic reaction to this medicine or to any related antibiotic, such as amikacin (e.g., Amikin), colistimethate (e.g., Coly-Mycin M), colistin (e.g., Coly-Mycin S), gentamicin (e.g., Garamycin), kanamycin (e.g., Kantrex), netilmicin (e.g., Netromycin), paromomycin (e.g., Humatin), streptomycin, or tobramycin (e.g., Nebcin). Also tell your doctor and pharmacist if you are allergic to any other substances, such as preservatives.

Pregnancy—Neomycin, polymyxin B, and gramicidin combination has not been shown to cause birth defects or other problems in humans.

Breast-feeding—Neomycin, polymyxin B, and gramicidin combination has not been reported to cause problems in nursing babies.

Children—Studies on this medicine have been done only in adult patients, and there is no specific information about its use in children.

Older adults—Many medicines have not been tested in older people. Therefore, it may not be known whether they work exactly the same way they do in younger adults or if they cause different side effects or problems in older people. There is no specific information about the use of neomycin, polymyxin B, and gramicidin combination in the elderly.

Before you begin using any new medicine (prescription or nonprescription) or if you develop any new medical problem while you are using this medicine, check with your doctor, nurse, or pharmacist.

Proper Use of This Medicine

The bottle is only partially full to provide proper drop control.

To use:

- First, wash your hands. Then tilt the head back and pull the lower eyelid away from the eye to form a pouch. Drop the medicine into the pouch and gently close the eyes. Do not blink. Keep the eyes closed for 1 or 2 minutes to allow the medicine to come into contact with the infection.
- If you think you did not get the drop of medicine into your eye properly, use another drop.
- To keep the medicine as germ-free as possible, do not touch the applicator tip or dropper to any surface (including the eye). Also, keep the container tightly closed.

To help clear up your infection completely, *keep using this medicine for the full time of treatment,* even if your symptoms have disappeared. *Do not miss any doses.*

Missed dose—If you do miss a dose of this medicine, apply it as soon as possible. However, if it is almost time for your next dose, skip the missed dose and go back to your regular dosing schedule.

Storage—To store this medicine:

- Keep out of the reach of children.
- Store away from heat and direct light.
- Keep the medicine from freezing.
- Do not keep outdated medicine or medicine no longer needed. Be sure that any discarded medicine is out of the reach of children.

Precautions While Using This Medicine

If your symptoms do not improve within a few days, or if they become worse, check with your doctor.

Side Effects of This Medicine

Along with its needed effects, a medicine may cause some unwanted effects. Although not all of these side effects may occur, if they do occur they may need medical attention.

Check with your doctor immediately if any of the following side effects occur:

More common

Itching, rash, redness, swelling, or other sign of irritation not present before use of this medicine

Other side effects may occur that usually do not need medical attention. These side effects may go away during treatment as your body adjusts to the medicine. However, check with your doctor if either of the following side effects continues or is bothersome:

Less common

Burning or stinging

Other side effects not listed above may also occur in some patients. If you notice any other effects, check with your doctor.

Annual revision: June 1990

NEOMYCIN, POLYMYXIN B, AND HYDROCORTISONE Ophthalmic

Some commonly used brand names are:

In the U.S.

Ak-Spore H.C.
Bacticort
Cobiron
Cortisporin Ophthalmic Suspension
Cortomycin
Hydromycin
I-Neocort
Ocutricin HC
Triple-Gen

Generic name product may also be available.

In Canada

Cortisporin Ophthalmic Suspension

Description

Neomycin (nee-oh-MYE-sin), polymyxin (pol-i-MIX-in) B, and hydrocortisone (hye-droe-KOR-ti-sone) is a combination antibiotic and cortisone-like medicine. It is used to treat infections of the eye and to help provide relief from redness, irritation, and discomfort of certain eye problems.

Neomycin, polymyxin B, and hydrocortisone combination is available only with your doctor's prescription, in the following dosage form:

Ophthalmic

- Ophthalmic suspension (eye drops) (U.S. and Canada)

It is very important that you read and understand the following information. If any of it causes you special concern, check with your doctor. Also, *if you have any questions* or if you want more information about this medicine or your medical problem, *ask your doctor, nurse, or pharmacist.*

Before Using This Medicine

In deciding to use a medicine, the risks of using the medicine must be weighed against the good it will do. This is a decision you and your doctor will make. For neomycin, polymyxin B, and hydrocortisone ophthalmic drops, the following should be considered:

Allergies—Tell your doctor if you have ever had any unusual or allergic reaction to this medicine or to any related antibiotic, such as amikacin (e.g., Amikin), colistimethate (e.g., Coly-Mycin M), colistin (e.g., Coly-Mycin S), gentamicin (e.g., Garamycin), kanamycin (e.g., Kantrex), netilmicin (e.g., Netromycin), paromomycin (e.g., Humatin), streptomycin, or tobramycin (e.g., Nebcin). Also tell your doctor and pharmacist if you are allergic to any other substances, such as preservatives.

Pregnancy—Neomycin, polymyxin B, and hydrocortisone ophthalmic preparations have not been studied in pregnant women. However, studies in animals have shown that topical corticosteroids cause birth defects. Before using this medicine, make sure your doctor knows if you are pregnant or if you may become pregnant.

Breast-feeding—Neomycin, polymyxin B, and hydrocortisone ophthalmic drops have not been reported to cause problems in nursing babies.

Children—Studies on this medicine have been done only in adult patients, and there is no specific information comparing use in children with use in other age groups.

Older adults—Many medicines have not been studied specifically in older people. Therefore, it may not be known whether they work exactly the same way they do in younger adults or if they cause different side effects or problems in older people. There is no specific information comparing use of ophthalmic neomycin, polymyxin B, and hydrocortisone combination in the elderly with use in other age groups.

Other medical problems—The presence of other medical problems may affect the use of neomycin, polymyxin B, and hydrocortisone ophthalmic drops. Make sure you tell your doctor if you have any other medical problems, especially:

- Any other eye infection or condition—Use of neomycin, polymyxin B, and hydrocortisone ophthalmic drops may make the condition worse

Before you begin using any new medicine (prescription or nonprescription) or if you develop any new medical problem while you are using this medicine, check with your doctor, nurse, or pharmacist.

Proper Use of This Medicine

The bottle is only partially full to provide proper drop control.

To use:

- First, wash your hands. Then tilt the head back and pull the lower eyelid away from the eye to form a pouch. Drop the medicine into the pouch and gently close the eyes. Do not blink. Keep the eyes closed for 1 or 2 minutes to allow the medicine to come into contact with the infection.
- If you think you did not get the drop of medicine into your eye properly, use another drop.
- To keep the medicine as germ-free as possible, do not touch the applicator tip to any surface (including the eye). Also, keep the container tightly closed.

To help clear up your infection completely, *keep using this medicine for the full time of treatment,* even if your symptoms have disappeared. *Do not miss any doses.*

Dosing—The dose of ophthalmic neomycin, polymyxin B, and hyrdocortisone combination will be different for different patients. *Follow your doctor's orders or the directions on the label.* The following information includes only the average doses of ophthalmic neomycin, polymyxin B, and hydrocortisone combination. *If your dose is different, do not change it* unless your doctor tells you to do so.

The number of doses you use each day, the time allowed between doses, and the length of time you use the medicine depend on the medical problem for which you are using ophthalmic neomycin, polymyxin B, and hydrocortisone combination.

- For eye infection:
  - —For *ophthalmic suspension* dosage forms:
    - Adults and children—One drop every three to four hours.

Missed dose—If you miss a dose of this medicine, apply it as soon as possible. However, if it is almost time for your next dose, skip the missed dose and go back to your regular dosing schedule.

Do not use any leftover medicine for future eye problems without checking with your doctor first. This medicine should not be used on many different kinds of infection.

Storage—To store this medicine:

- Keep out of the reach of children.
- Store away from heat and direct light.
- Keep the medicine from freezing.
- Do not keep outdated medicine or medicine no longer needed. Be sure that any discarded medicine is out of the reach of children.

Precautions While Using This Medicine

If you will be using this medicine for a long time (for example, longer than 6 weeks), your doctor should check your eyes at regular visits.

If your symptoms do not improve within a few days, or if they become worse, check with your doctor.

Side Effects of This Medicine

Along with its needed effects, a medicine may cause some unwanted effects. Although not all of these side effects may occur, if they do occur they may need medical attention.

Check with your doctor immediately if any of the following side effects occur:

More common

Itching, rash, redness, swelling, or other sign of irritation not present before use of this medicine

Other side effects may occur that usually do not need medical attention. These side effects may go away during treatment as your body adjusts to the medicine. However, check with your doctor if either of the following side effects continues or is bothersome:

Less common

Burning or stinging

Other side effects not listed above may also occur in some patients. If you notice any other effects, check with your doctor.

Annual revision: 07/01/93

NEOMYCIN, POLYMYXIN B, AND HYDROCORTISONE Otic

Some commonly used brand names are:

In the U.S.

Cortisporin
LazerSporin-C
Octicair
Ortega Otic-M
Otocort
Otoreid-HC
Pediotic

Generic name product may also be available.

In Canada

Cortisporin

Description

Neomycin (nee-oh-MYE-sin), polymyxin (pol-i-MIX-in) B, and hydrocortisone (hye-droe-KOR-ti-sone) is a combination antibiotic and cortisone-like medicine. It is used to treat infections of the ear canal and to help provide relief from redness, irritation, and discomfort of certain ear problems.

Neomycin, polymyxin B, and hydrocortisone combination is available only with your doctor's prescription, in the following dosage forms:

Otic

- Solution (U.S.)
- Suspension (U.S. and Canada)

It is very important that you read and understand the following information. If any of it causes you special concern, check with your doctor. Also, *if you have any questions* or if you want more information about this medicine or your medical problem, *ask your doctor, nurse, or pharmacist.*

Before Using This Medicine

In deciding to use a medicine, the risks of using the medicine must be weighed against the good it will do. This is a decision you and your doctor will make. For neomycin, polymyxin B, and hydrocortisone otic preparations, the following should be considered:

Allergies—Tell your doctor if you have ever had any unusual or allergic reaction to this medicine or to any related antibiotic, such as amikacin (e.g., Amikin), colistimethate (e.g., Coly-Mycin M), colistin (e.g., Coly-Mycin S), gentamicin (e.g., Garamycin), kanamycin (e.g., Kantrex), neomycin by mouth or by injection (e.g., Mycifradin), netilmicin (e.g., Netromycin), paromomycin (e.g., Humatin), polymyxin B by injection (e.g., Aerosporin), streptomycin, or tobramycin (e.g., Nebcin). Also tell your doctor and pharmacist if you are allergic to any other substances, such as preservatives or dyes.

Pregnancy—Neomycin, polymyxin B, and hydrocortisone otic preparations have not been studied in pregnant women. However, studies in animals have shown that topical adrenocorticoids cause birth defects. Before using this medicine, make sure your doctor knows if you are pregnant or if you may become pregnant.

Breast-feeding—Neomycin, polymyxin B, and hydrocortisone otic preparations have not been reported to cause problems in nursing babies.

Children—Although there is no specific information about the use of otic neomycin, polymyxin B, and hydrocortisone combination in children, it is not expected to cause different side effects or problems in children than it does in adults.

Older adults—Many medicines have not been tested in older people. Therefore, it may not be known whether they work exactly the same way they do in younger adults or if they cause different side effects or problems in older people. There is no specific information about the use of otic neomycin, polymyxin B, and hydrocortisone combination in the elderly.

Other medical problems—The presence of other medical problems may affect the use of neomycin, polymyxin B, and hydrocortisone otic preparations. Make sure you tell your doctor if you have any other medical problems, especially:

- Any other ear infection or condition (including punctured eardrum)—Use of neomycin, polymyxin B, and hydrocortisone otic preparations may make the condition worse

Before you begin using any new medicine (prescription or nonprescription) or if you develop any new medical problem while you are using this medicine, check with your doctor, nurse, or pharmacist.

Proper Use of This Medicine

You may warm the ear drops to body temperature (37 °C or 98.6 °F), but no higher, by holding the bottle in your hand for a few minutes before applying. If the medicine gets too warm, it may break down and not work at all.

To use:

- Lie down or tilt the head so that the infected ear faces up. Gently pull the earlobe up and back for adults (down and back for children) to straighten the ear canal. Drop the medicine into the ear canal. Keep the ear facing up for about 5 minutes to allow the medicine to come into contact with the infection. A sterile cotton plug may be gently inserted into the ear opening to prevent the medicine from leaking out. However, your doctor may want you to keep a sterile cotton plug moistened with this medicine in your ear for the full time of treatment. If you have any questions about this, check with your doctor.
- To keep the medicine as germ-free as possible, do not touch the dropper to any surface (including the ear). Also, keep the container tightly closed.

To help clear up your infection completely, *keep using this medicine for the full time of treatment,* even if your symptoms have disappeared. *Do not miss any doses.*

Missed dose—If you do miss a dose of this medicine, apply it as soon as possible. However, if it is almost time for your next dose, skip the missed dose and go back to your regular dosing schedule.

Do not use this medicine for more than 10 days unless otherwise directed by your doctor.

Storage—To store this medicine:

- Keep out of the reach of children.
- Store away from heat and direct light.
- Keep the medicine from freezing.
- Do not keep outdated medicine or medicine no longer needed. Be sure that any discarded medicine is out of the reach of children.

Precautions While Using This Medicine

If your symptoms do not improve within 1 week, or if they become worse, check with your doctor.

Side Effects of This Medicine

Along with its needed effects, a medicine may cause some unwanted effects. Although not all of these side effects may occur, if they do occur they may need medical attention.

Check with your doctor immediately if any of the following side effects occur:

More common

Itching, skin rash, redness, swelling, or other sign of irritation not present before use of this medicine

Other side effects not listed above may also occur in some patients. If you notice any other effects, check with your doctor.

Annual revision: June 1990

NIACIN—For High Cholesterol Systemic

Some commonly used brand names are:

In the U.S.

- Endur-Acin
- Nia-Bid
- Niac
- Niacels
- Niacor
- Nico-400
- Nicobid
- Nicolar
- Nicotinex Elixir
- Slo-Niacin
- Tega-Span

Generic name product may also be available.

In Canada

- Tri-B3

Generic name product may also be available.

Other commonly used names are nicotinic acid or vitamin B_3.

Description

Niacin (NYE-a-sin) is used to help lower high cholesterol and fat levels in the blood. This may help prevent medical problems caused by cholesterol and fat clogging the blood vessels.

Some strengths of niacin are available only with your doctor's prescription. Others are available without a prescription, since niacin is also a vitamin. However, it is best to take it only under your doctor's direction so that you can be sure you are taking the correct dose.

Niacin for use in the treatment of high cholesterol is available in the following dosage forms:

Oral

- Extended-release capsules (U.S. and Canada)
- Solution (U.S.)
- Tablets (U.S. and Canada)
- Extended-release tablets (U.S.)

It is very important that you read and understand the following information. If any of it causes you special concern, check with your doctor or pharmacist. Also, *if you have any questions* or if you want more information about this medicine or your medical problem, *ask your doctor, nurse, or pharmacist.*

Before Using This Medicine

If you are taking this medicine without a prescription, carefully read and follow any precautions on the label. For niacin, the following should be considered:

Allergies—Tell your doctor if you have ever had any unusual or allergic reaction to niacin. Also tell your doctor and pharmacist if you are allergic to any other substances, such as foods, preservatives, or dyes.

Diet—Before prescribing medicine for your condition, your doctor will probably try to control your condition by prescribing a personal diet for you. Such a diet may be low in fats, sugars, and/or cholesterol. Many people are able to control their condition by carefully following their doctor's orders for proper diet and exercise. *Medicine is prescribed only when additional help is needed* and is effective only when a schedule of diet and exercise is properly followed.

Also, this medicine is less effective if you are greatly overweight. It may be very important for you to go on a reducing diet. However, check with your doctor before going on any diet.

Make certain your doctor and pharmacist know if you are on any special diet, such as a low-sodium or low-sugar diet.

Pregnancy—Studies have not been done in either humans or animals.

Breast-feeding—Niacin has not been reported to cause problems in nursing babies.

Children—There is no specific information comparing the use of niacin for high cholesterol in children with use in other age groups. However, use is not recommended in children under 2 years of age since cholesterol is needed for normal development.

Older adults—Many medicines have not been studied specifically in older people. Therefore, it may not be known whether they work exactly the same way they do in younger adults or if they cause different side effects or problems in older people. Although there is no specific information comparing the use of niacin for high cholesterol in the elderly with use in other age groups, it is not expected to cause different side effects or problems in older people than in younger adults.

Other medicines—Although certain medicines should not be used together at all, in other cases two different medicines may be used together even if an interaction might occur. In these cases, your doctor may want to change the dose, or other precautions may be necessary. Tell your doctor and pharmacist if you are using any other prescription or nonprescription (over-the-counter [OTC]) medicine.

Other medical problems—The presence of other medical problems may affect the use of niacin. Make sure you tell your doctor if you have any other medical problems, especially:

- Bleeding problems or
- Diabetes mellitus (sugar diabetes) or
- Glaucoma or
- Gout or
- Liver disease or
- Low blood pressure or
- Stomach ulcer—Niacin may make these conditions worse

Before you begin using any new medicine (prescription or nonprescription) or if you develop any new medical problem while you are using this medicine, check with your doctor, nurse, or pharmacist.

Proper Use of This Medicine

Use this medicine only as directed by your doctor. Do not use more or less of it, do not use it more often, and do not use it for a longer time than your doctor ordered. To do so may increase the chance of unwanted effects.

Remember that niacin will not cure your condition but it does help control it. Therefore, you must continue to take it as directed if you expect to keep your cholesterol levels down.

Follow carefully the special diet your doctor gave you. This is the most important part of controlling your condition, and is necessary if the medicine is to work properly.

If this medicine upsets your stomach, it may be taken with meals or milk. If stomach upset (nausea or diarrhea) continues, check with your doctor.

For patients taking the *extended-release capsule form* of this medicine:

- Swallow the capsule whole. Do not crush, break, or chew before swallowing. However, if the capsule is too large to swallow, you may mix the contents of the capsule with jam or jelly and swallow without chewing.

For patients taking the *extended-release tablet form* of this medicine:

- Swallow the tablet whole. If the tablet is scored, it may be broken, but not crushed or chewed, before being swallowed.

Missed dose—If you miss a dose of this medicine, take it as soon as possible. However, if it is almost time for your next dose, skip the missed dose and go back to your regular dosing schedule. Do not double doses.

Storage—To store this medicine:

- Keep out of the reach of children.
- Store away from heat and direct light.
- Do not store in the bathroom, near the kitchen sink, or in other damp places. Heat or moisture may cause the medicine to break down.
- Keep the liquid form of this medicine from freezing.
- Do not keep outdated medicine or medicine no longer needed. Be sure that any discarded medicine is out of the reach of children.

Precautions While Using This Medicine

It is very important that your doctor check your progress at regular visits. This will allow your doctor to see if the medicine is working properly to lower your cholesterol and triglyceride (fat) levels and if you should continue to take it.

Do not stop taking niacin without first checking with your doctor. When you stop taking this medicine, your blood cholesterol levels may increase again. Your doctor may want you to follow a special diet to help prevent this from happening.

This medicine may cause you to feel dizzy or faint, especially when you get up from a lying or sitting position. Getting up slowly may help. This effect should lessen after a week or two as your body gets used to the medicine. However, if the problem continues or gets worse, check with your doctor.

Side Effects of This Medicine

Along with its needed effects, a medicine may cause some unwanted effects. Although not all of these side effects may occur, if they do occur they may need medical attention. *Check with your doctor immediately* if any of the following side effects occur:

Less common

With prolonged use of extended-release niacin

Darkening of urine; light gray-colored stools; loss of appetite; severe stomach pain; yellow eyes or skin

Other side effects may occur that usually do not need medical attention. These side effects may go away during treatment as your body adjusts to the medicine. However, check with your doctor if any of the following side effects continue or are bothersome:

Less common

Feeling of warmth; flushing or redness of skin, especially on face and neck; headache

With high doses

Diarrhea; dizziness or faintness; dryness of skin; fever; frequent urination; itching of skin; joint pain; muscle aching or cramping; nausea or vomiting; side, lower back, or stomach pain; swelling of feet or lower legs; unusual thirst; unusual tiredness or weakness; unusually fast, slow, or irregular heartbeat

Other side effects not listed above may also occur in some patients. If you notice any other effects, check with your doctor or pharmacist.

Annual revision: 11/09/91

NIACIN (Vitamin B_3) Systemic

Some commonly used brand names are:

In the U.S.

- Endur-Acin
- Nia-Bid
- Niac
- Niacels
- Niacor
- Nico-400
- Nicobid
- Nicolar
- Nicotinex Elixir
- Slo-Niacin
- Tega-Span

Generic name product may also be available.

In Canada

- Tri-B3

Generic name product may also be available.

Other commonly used names are niacinamide (nye-a-SIN-a-mide), nicotinic acid, nicotinamide, or vitamin B_3.

Description

Vitamins (VYE-ta-mins) are compounds that you *must* have for growth and health. They are needed in small amounts only and are usually available in the foods that you eat. Niacin (NYE-a-sin) is necessary for many normal functions of the body, including normal tissue metabolism. It may have other effects as well.

Lack of niacin may lead to a condition called pellagra, with diarrhea, stomach problems, skin problems, sores in the mouth, anemia (weak blood), and mental problems. Your doctor may treat this by prescribing niacin for you.

Patients with the following conditions may be more likely to have a lack of niacin:

- Cancer
- Diabetes mellitus (sugar diabetes)
- Diarrhea (prolonged)
- Fever (prolonged)
- Hartnup disease
- Infection (prolonged)
- Intestinal problems
- Liver disease
- Mouth or throat sores
- Overactive thyroid
- Pancreas disease
- Stomach ulcer
- Stress (prolonged)
- Surgical removal of stomach

If any of the above apply to you, you should take niacin supplements only on the advice of your physician after need has been established.

Claims that niacin is effective for treatment of acne, alcoholism, unwanted effects of drug abuse, leprosy, motion sickness, muscle problems, poor circulation, and mental problems, and for prevention of heart attacks, have not been proven. Many of these treatments involve large and expensive amounts of vitamins.

Some strengths of niacin are available only with your doctor's prescription. Others are available without a prescription. However, it may be a good idea to check with your doctor or pharmacist before taking niacin on your own.

This medicine is available in the following dosage forms:

Oral

Niacin
- Extended-release capsules (U.S. and Canada)
- Solution (U.S.)
- Tablets (U.S. and Canada)
- Extended-release tablets (U.S.)

Niacinamide
- Capsules (U.S.)
- Tablets (U.S. and Canada)

Parenteral

Niacin
- Injection (U.S.)

Niacinamide
- Injection (U.S.)

It is very important that you read and understand the following information. If any of it causes you special concern, check with your doctor or pharmacist. Also, *if you have any questions* or if you want more information about this dietary supplement or your medical problem, *ask your doctor, nurse, pharmacist, or dietitian.*

Importance of Diet

Vitamin supplements should be taken only if you cannot get enough vitamins in your diet; however, some diets may not contain all of the vitamins you need. This may occur with rapid weight loss, unusual diets (such as some reducing diets in which choice of foods is very limited), prolonged intravenous feeding, or malnutrition. A balanced diet should provide all the vitamins you normally need.

In order to get enough vitamins and minerals in your diet, it is important that you eat a balanced and varied diet. Follow carefully any diet program your doctor may recommend. For your specific vitamin and/or mineral needs, ask your doctor for a list of appropriate foods.

Niacin is found in meats, eggs, and milk and dairy products. Little niacin is lost from foods during ordinary cooking.

Vitamins alone will not take the place of a good diet and will not provide energy. Your body also needs other substances found in food such as protein, minerals, carbohydrates, and fat. Vitamins themselves often cannot work without the presence of other foods.

In some cases, it may not be possible for you to get enough food to supply you with the proper vitamins. In other cases, the amount of vitamins you need may be increased above normal. Therefore, a vitamin supplement may be needed.

Experts have developed a list of recommended dietary allowances (RDA) for most of the vitamins. The RDA are not an exact number but a general idea of how much you need. They do not cover amounts needed for problems caused by a serious lack of vitamins.

The RDA for niacin are:

- Infants and children—
  Birth to 6 months of age: 5 mg per day.
  6 months to 1 year of age: 6 mg per day.
  1 to 3 years of age: 9 mg per day.
  4 to 6 years of age: 12 mg per day.
  7 to 10 years of age: 13 mg per day.
- Adolescent and adult males—
  11 to 14 years of age: 17 mg per day.
  15 to 18 years of age: 20 mg per day.
  19 to 50 years of age: 19 mg per day.
  50 years of age and over: 15 mg per day.
- Adolescent and adult females—
  11 to 50 years of age: 15 mg per day.
  50 years of age and over: 13 mg per day.
- Pregnant females—17 mg per day.
- Lactating females—20 mg per day.

Remember:

- The total amount of each vitamin that you get every day includes what you get from the foods that you eat *and* what you may take as a supplement.
- Your total amount should not be greater than the RDA, unless ordered by your doctor. Taking too much niacin over a period of time may cause unwanted effects such as high blood sugar, peptic ulcer, gout, heart problems, or liver problems.

Before Using This Dietary Supplement

If you are taking this dietary supplement without a prescription, carefully read and follow any precautions on the label. For niacin or niacinamide, the following should be considered:

Allergies—Tell your doctor if you have ever had any unusual or allergic reaction to niacin or niacinamide. Also tell your doctor and pharmacist if you are allergic to any other substances, such as foods, preservatives, or dyes.

Pregnancy—It is especially important that you are receiving enough vitamins when you become pregnant and that you continue to receive the right amount of vitamins throughout your pregnancy. The healthy growth and development of the fetus depend on a steady supply of nutrients from the mother. However, taking large amounts of a dietary supplement in pregnancy may be harmful to the mother and/or fetus and should be avoided.

Breast-feeding—It is especially important that you receive the right amounts of vitamins so that your baby will also get the vitamins needed to grow properly. However, taking large amounts of a dietary supplement while breast-feeding may be harmful to the mother and/or baby and should be avoided.

Children—Normal daily requirements vary according to age. It is especially important that children receive enough vitamins in their diet for healthy growth and development. Although there is no specific information about the use of niacin in children in doses higher than the normal daily requirements, it is not expected to cause different side effects or problems in children than in adults.

Older adults—It is important that older people continue to receive enough vitamins in their diet for good health.

Medicines or other dietary supplements—Although certain medicines or dietary supplements should not be used together at all, in other cases they may be used together even if an interaction might occur. In these cases, your doctor may want to change the dose, or other precautions may be necessary. Tell your doctor and pharmacist if you are using any other dietary supplement or any prescription or nonprescription (over-the-counter [OTC]) medicine.

Other medical problems—The presence of other medical problems may affect the use of niacin or niacinamide. Make sure you tell your doctor if you have any other medical problems, especially:

- Bleeding problems or
- Diabetes mellitus (sugar diabetes) or
- Glaucoma or
- Gout or
- Liver disease or
- Low blood pressure or
- Stomach ulcer—Niacin or niacinamide may make these conditions worse

Proper Use of This Dietary Supplement

Some people believe that taking very large doses of vitamins (called megadoses or megavitamin therapy) is useful for treating certain medical problems. Studies have not proven this. Large doses should be taken only under the direction of your doctor after need has been identified.

If this dietary supplement upsets your stomach, it may be taken with meals or milk. If stomach upset (nausea or diarrhea) continues, check with your doctor.

For patients taking the *extended-release capsule form* of this dietary supplement:

- Swallow the capsule whole. Do not crush, break, or chew before swallowing. However, if the capsule is too large to swallow, you may mix the contents of the capsule with jam or jelly and swallow without chewing.

For patients taking the *extended-release tablet form* of this dietary supplement:

- Swallow the tablet whole. If the tablet is scored, it may be broken, but not crushed or chewed, before being swallowed.

Missed dose—If you miss taking a vitamin for one or more days there is no cause for concern, since it takes some time for your body to become seriously low in vitamins. However, if your doctor has recommended that you take this vitamin, try to remember to take it as directed every day.

Storage—To store this dietary supplement:

- Keep out of the reach of children.
- Store away from heat and direct light.
- Do not store in the bathroom, near the kitchen sink, or in other damp places. Heat or moisture may cause the dietary supplement to break down.
- Keep the liquid form of this dietary supplement from freezing.
- Do not keep outdated dietary supplements or those no longer needed. Be sure that any discarded dietary supplement is out of the reach of children.

Precautions While Using This Dietary Supplement

This dietary supplement may cause you to feel dizzy or faint, especially when you get up from a lying or sitting position. Getting up slowly may help. This effect should lessen after a week or two as your body gets used to the dietary supplement. However, if the problem continues or gets worse, check with your doctor.

Side Effects of This Dietary Supplement

Along with its needed effects, a dietary supplement may cause some unwanted effects. Although not all of these side effects may occur, if they do occur they may need medical attention.

Check with your doctor immediately if any of the following side effects occur:

With injection only

Skin rash or itching; wheezing

With prolonged use of extended-release niacin

Darkening of urine; light gray-colored stools; loss of appetite; severe stomach pain; yellow eyes or skin

Other side effects may occur that usually do not need medical attention. These side effects may go away during treatment as your body adjusts to the dietary supplement. However, check with your doctor or pharmacist if any of the following side effects continue or are bothersome:

Less common—with niacin only

Feeling of warmth; flushing or redness of skin, especially on face and neck; headache

With high doses

Diarrhea; dizziness or faintness; dryness of skin; fever; frequent urination; itching of skin; joint pain; muscle aching or cramping; nausea or vomiting; side, lower back, or stomach pain; swelling of feet or lower legs; unusual thirst; unusual tiredness or weakness; unusually fast, slow, or irregular heartbeat

Other side effects not listed above may also occur in some patients. If you notice any other effects, check with your doctor or pharmacist.

Annual revision: 11/09/91
Interim revision: 08/07/92

NICLOSAMIDE Oral†

A commonly used brand name in the U.S. is Niclocide.

†Not commercially available in Canada.

Description

Niclosamide (ni-KLOE-sa-mide) belongs to the family of medicines called anthelmintics (ant-hel-MIN-tiks). Anthelmintics are medicines used in the treatment of worm infections.

Niclosamide is used to treat broad or fish tapeworm, dwarf tapeworm, and beef tapeworm infections. Niclosamide may also be used for other tapeworm infections as determined by your doctor. It will not work for other types of worm infections (for example, pinworms or roundworms).

Niclosamide works by killing tapeworms on contact. The killed worms are then passed in the stool. However, you may not notice them since they are sometimes destroyed in the intestine.

Niclosamide is available only with your doctor's prescription, in the following dosage form:

Oral

- Chewable tablets (U.S.)

It is very important that you read and understand the following information. If any of it causes you special concern, check with your doctor. Also, *if you have any questions* or if you want more information about this medicine or your medical problem, *ask your doctor, nurse, or pharmacist.*

Before Using This Medicine

In deciding to use a medicine, the risks of taking the medicine must be weighed against the good it will do. This is a decision you and your doctor will make. For niclosamide, the following should be considered:

Allergies—Tell your doctor if you have ever had any unusual or allergic reaction to niclosamide. Also tell your doctor and pharmacist if you are allergic to any other substances, such as foods, preservatives, or dyes.

Pregnancy—Studies have not been done in pregnant women. However, niclosamide has not been shown to cause birth defects or other problems in rats and rabbits given 25 times the usual human dose or in mice given 12 times the usual human dose.

Breast-feeding—It is not known whether niclosamide passes into the breast milk. However, this medicine has not been reported to cause problems in nursing babies.

Children—This medicine has been tested in a limited number of children 2 years of age or older and, in effective doses, has not been reported to cause different side effects or problems in children than it does in adults.

Older adults—Many medicines have not been studied specifically in older people. Therefore, it may not be known whether they work exactly the same way they do in younger adults or if they cause different side effects or problems in older people. There is no specific information comparing use of niclosamide in the elderly with use in other age groups.

Other medicines—Although certain medicines should not be used together at all, in other cases two different medicines may be used together even if an interaction might occur. In these cases, your doctor may want to change the dose, or other precautions may be necessary. Tell your doctor and pharmacist if you are taking any other prescription or nonprescription (over-the-counter [OTC]) medicine.

Before you begin using any new medicine (prescription or nonprescription) or if you develop any new medical problem while you are using this medicine, check with your doctor, nurse, or pharmacist.

Proper Use of This Medicine

No special preparations (for example, special diets, fasting, other medicines, laxatives, or enemas) are necessary before, during, or immediately after taking niclosamide.

Niclosamide may be taken on an empty stomach (either 1 hour before or 2 hours after a meal). However, to prevent stomach upset, it is best taken after a light meal (for example, breakfast).

Niclosamide tablets should be thoroughly chewed or crushed and then swallowed with a small amount of water. If this medicine is being given to a young child, the tablets should be crushed to a fine powder and mixed with a small amount of water to form a paste.

For patients taking this medicine for *beef tapeworms or broad or fish tapeworms:*

- To help clear up your infection completely, *take this medicine exactly as directed by your doctor.* Usually one dose is enough. However, in some patients a second dose of this medicine may be required to clear up the infection completely.

For patients taking this medicine for *dwarf tapeworms:*

- To help clear up your infection completely, *keep taking this medicine for the full time of treatment (usually 7 days),* even if your symptoms begin to clear up after a few days. In some patients, a second course of this medicine may be required to clear up the infection completely. If you stop taking this medicine too soon, your infection may return. *Do not miss any doses.* Some patients with tapeworm infections may not notice any symptoms or may have only mild symptoms.

Missed dose—If you do miss a dose of this medicine, take it as soon as possible. However, if it is almost time for your next dose, skip the missed dose and go back to your regular dosing schedule. Do not double doses.

Storage—To store this medicine:

- Keep out of the reach of children.
- Store away from heat and direct light.
- Do not store in the bathroom, near the kitchen sink, or in other damp places. Heat or moisture may cause the medicine to break down.
- Do not keep outdated medicine or medicine no longer needed. Be sure that any discarded medicine is out of the reach of children.

Precautions While Using This Medicine

It is important that your doctor check your progress at regular visits. This is to make sure that the infection is cleared up completely.

If your symptoms do not improve within a few days, or if they become worse, check with your doctor.

Side Effects of This Medicine

Along with its needed effects, a medicine may cause some unwanted effects. The following side effects may go away during treatment as your body adjusts to the medicine. However, check with your doctor if any of the following side effects continue or are bothersome:

Less common

Abdominal or stomach cramps or pain; diarrhea; loss of appetite; nausea or vomiting

Rare

Unpleasant taste; dizziness or lightheadedness; drowsiness; itching of the rectal area; skin rash

Other side effects not listed above may also occur in some patients. If you notice any other effects, check with your doctor.

Annual revision: 10/20/92

NICOTINE Systemic

Some commonly used brand names are:

In the U.S.

Habitrol
Nicoderm
Nicorette
Nicotrol
ProStep

In Canada

Habitrol
Nicoderm
Nicorette

Description

Nicotine (NIK-o-teen), in a flavored chewing gum or a skin patch, is used to help you stop smoking. It is used for up to 12 to 20 weeks as part of a supervised stop-smoking program. These programs may include education, counseling, and psychological support. Using nicotine replacement products without taking part in a supervised stop-smoking program has not been shown to be effective.

- As you chew nicotine gum, nicotine passes through the lining of your mouth and into your body.
- When you wear a nicotine patch, nicotine passes through your skin into your bloodstream.

This nicotine takes the place of nicotine that you would otherwise get from smoking. In this way, the withdrawal effects of not smoking are less severe. Then, as your body adjusts to not smoking, the use of the nicotine gum is decreased gradually, or the strength of the patches is decreased over a few weeks. Finally, use is stopped altogether.

Children, pregnant women, and nonsmokers should not use nicotine gum or patches because of unwanted effects.

Nicotine gum and patches are available only with your doctor's prescription, in the following dosage forms:

Oral

- Chewing gum tablets (U.S. and Canada)

Topical

- Transdermal (stick-on) skin patch (U.S. and Canada)

It is very important that you read and understand the following information. If any of it causes you special concern, check with your doctor or pharmacist. Also, *if you have any questions* or if you want more information about this medicine or your medical problem, *ask your doctor, nurse, or pharmacist.*

Before Using This Medicine

In deciding to use a medicine, the risks of taking the medicine must be weighed against the good it will do.

This is a decision you and your doctor will make. For nicotine gum, the following should be considered:

Allergies—Tell your doctor if you have ever had any unusual or allergic reaction to nicotine. Also tell your doctor and pharmacist if you are allergic to any other substances, such as foods, preservatives, or dyes. If you plan to use the nicotine patches, tell your doctor if you have ever had a rash or irritation from adhesive tape or bandages.

Pregnancy—Nicotine, whether from smoking or from the gum or patches, is not recommended during pregnancy. Studies in humans show that miscarriages have occurred in pregnant women using nicotine replacement products. In addition, studies in animals have shown that nicotine can cause harmful effects in the fetus.

Breast-feeding—Nicotine passes into breast milk and may cause unwanted effects in the baby. It may be necessary for you to stop breast-feeding during treatment.

Children—Small amounts of nicotine can cause serious harm in children. Even used nicotine patches contain enough nicotine to cause problems in children.

Older adults—Nicotine gum and patches have been used in a limited number of patients 60 years of age or older, and have not been shown to cause different side effects or problems in older people than in younger adults.

Other medicines—Although certain medicines should not be used together at all, in other cases 2 different medicines may be used together even if an interaction might occur. In these cases, your doctor may want to change the dose, or other precautions may be necessary. When you are using nicotine gum or patches, it is especially important that your doctor and pharmacist know if you are taking any of the following:

- Aminophylline (e.g., Somophyllin) or
- Insulin or
- Oxtriphylline (e.g., Choledyl) or
- Propoxyphene (e.g., Darvon) or
- Propranolol (e.g., Inderal) or
- Theophylline (e.g., Somophyllin-T)—Stopping smoking may increase the effects of these medicines; the amount of medicine you need to take may change

Other medical problems—The presence of other medical problems may affect the use of nicotine gum or patches. Make sure you tell your doctor if you have any other medical problems, especially:

- Dental problems (with gum only) or
- Diabetes mellitus (sugar diabetes) or
- Heart or blood vessel disease or
- High blood pressure or
- Inflammation of mouth or throat (with gum only) or
- Irritated skin (with patches only) or
- Overactive thyroid or
- Pheochromocytoma (PCC) or
- Stomach ulcer or
- Temporomandibular (jaw) joint disorder (TMJ) (with gum only)—Nicotine gum or patches may make the condition worse

Before you begin using any new medicine (prescription or nonprescription) or if you develop any new medical problem while you are using this medicine, check with your doctor, nurse, or pharmacist.

Proper Use of This Medicine

For patients using the *chewing gum tablets:*

- Nicotine gum usually comes with patient directions. *Read the directions carefully before using this medicine.*
- *When you feel the urge to smoke, chew one piece of gum very slowly* until you taste it or feel a slight tingling in your mouth. Stop chewing, and place ("park") the chewing gum tablet between your cheek and gum until the taste or tingling is almost gone. Then chew slowly until you taste it again. Continue chewing and stopping ("parking") in this way for about 30 minutes in order to get the full dose of nicotine.
- *Do not chew too fast*, do not chew more than one piece at a time, and do not chew a piece of gum too soon after another. To do so may cause unwanted side effects or an overdose. Also, slower chewing will reduce the possibility of belching.
- *Use nicotine gum exactly as directed by your doctor.* Remember that it is also important to participate in a stop-smoking program during treatment. This may make it easier for you to stop smoking.
- As your urge to smoke becomes less frequent, *gradually reduce the number of pieces of gum you chew each day* until you are chewing one or two pieces a day. This may be possible within 2 to 3 months.
- *Remember to carry nicotine gum with you at all times* in case you feel the sudden urge to smoke. One cigarette may be enough to start you on the smoking habit again.
- Using hard sugarless candy between doses of gum may help to relieve the discomfort in your mouth.

For patients using the *transdermal system (skin patch):*

- *Use this medicine exactly as directed by your doctor.* It will work only if applied correctly. *This medicine usually comes with patient instructions. Read them carefully before using this product.* Remember that it is also important to participate in a stop-smoking program during treatment. This may make it easier for you to stop smoking.
- Do not remove the patch from its sealed pouch until you are ready to put it on your skin. The patch may not work as well if it is unwrapped too soon.
- Do not try to trim or cut the adhesive patch to adjust the dosage. Check with your doctor if you think the medicine is not working as it should.
- Apply the patch to a clean, dry area of skin on your upper arm, chest, or back. Choose an area that is

not very oily, has little or no hair, and is free of scars, cuts, burns, or any other skin irritations.

- Press the patch firmly in place with the palm of your hand for about 10 seconds. Make sure there is good contact with your skin, especially around the edges of the patch.
- The patch should stay in place even when you are showering, bathing, or swimming. Apply a new patch if one falls off.
- Rinse your hands with plain water after you have finished applying the patch to your skin. Nicotine on your hands could get into your eyes and nose and cause stinging, redness, or more serious problems. Using soap to wash your hands will increase the amount of nicotine that passes through your skin.
- After 16 or 24 hours, depending on which product you are using, remove the patch. Choose a different place on your skin to apply the next patch. Do not put a new patch in the same place for at least one week. Do not leave the patch on for more than 24 hours. It will not work as well after that time and it may irritate your skin.
- After removing a used patch, fold the patch in half with the sticky sides together. Place the folded, used patch in its protective pouch or in aluminum foil. Make sure to dispose of it out of the reach of children and pets.
- Try to change the patch at the same time each day. If you want to change the time when you put on your patch, just remove the patch you are wearing and put on a new patch. After that, apply a fresh patch at the new time each day.

Storage—To store this medicine:

- Keep out of the reach of children because even small doses of nicotine can cause serious harm in children.
- Store away from heat and direct light.
- Do not store in the bathroom, near the kitchen sink, or in other damp places. Heat or moisture may cause the medicine to break down.
- Do not keep outdated medicine or medicine no longer needed. Be sure that any discarded medicine is out of the reach of children and pets.

Precautions While Using This Medicine

Your doctor should check your progress at regular visits to make sure that the nicotine gum or patches are working properly and that possible side effects are avoided.

Do not smoke during treatment with nicotine gum or patches because of the risk of nicotine overdose.

Nicotine should not be used in pregnancy. If there is a possibility you might become pregnant, you may want to use some type of birth control. If you think you may have become pregnant, stop taking this medicine immediately and check with your doctor.

Nicotine products must be kept out of the reach of children and pets. Even used nicotine patches contain enough nicotine to cause problems in children. If a child chews or swallows one or more pieces of nicotine gum, contact your doctor or poison control center at once. If a child puts on a nicotine patch or plays with a patch that is out of the sealed pouch, take it away from the child and contact your doctor or poison control center at once.

For patients using the *chewing gum tablets:*

- *Do not chew more than 30 pieces of gum a day.* Chewing too many pieces may be harmful because of the risk of overdose.
- *Do not use nicotine gum for longer than 6 months.* To do so may result in physical dependence on the nicotine.
- *If the gum sticks to your dental work, stop using it and check with your medical doctor or dentist.* Dentures or other dental work may be damaged because nicotine gum is stickier and harder to chew than ordinary gum.

For patients using the *transdermal system (skin patch)*:

- Mild itching, burning, or tingling may occur when the patch is first applied, and should go away within an hour. After a patch is removed, the skin underneath it may be somewhat red. It should not remain red for more than a day. *If you get a skin rash from the patch, or if the skin becomes swollen or very red, call your doctor.* Do not put on a new patch. If you become allergic to the nicotine in the patch, you could get sick from using cigarettes or other products that contain nicotine.
- *Do not use nicotine patches for longer than 12 to 20 weeks* (depending on the product) if you have stopped smoking, because continuing use of nicotine in any form can be harmful and addictive.

Side Effects of This Medicine

Along with its needed effects, a medicine may cause some unwanted effects. Although not all of these side effects may occur, if they do occur they may need medical attention.

Check with your doctor as soon as possible if any of the following side effects occur:

More common

Injury to mouth, teeth, or dental work—with chewing gum only

Rare

Irregular heartbeat; rash or hives; redness, swelling, and itching at the site of application of the patch that lasts longer than 1 day

Symptoms of overdose (may occur in the following order)

Nausea and/or vomiting; increased watering of mouth (severe); abdominal or stomach pain (severe); diarrhea (severe); cold sweat; headache (severe); dizziness (severe); drooling; disturbed hearing and vision; confusion; weakness (severe); fainting; low blood pressure; difficulty in breathing (severe); fast, weak, or irregular heartbeat; convulsions (seizures)

Other side effects may occur that usually do not need medical attention. These side effects may go away during treatment as your body adjusts to the medicine. However, check with your doctor if any of the following side effects continue or are bothersome:

More common

Belching—with chewing gum only; fast heartbeat; headache (mild); increased appetite; increased watering of mouth (mild)—with chewing gum only; jaw muscle ache—with chewing gum only; redness, itching, and/or burning at site of application of patch—usually stops within an hour; sore mouth or throat—with chewing gum only

Less common or rare

Constipation; coughing (increased); diarrhea; dizziness or lightheadedness (mild); drowsiness; dryness of mouth; hiccups—with chewing gum only; hoarseness—with chewing gum only; irritability or nervousness; loss of appetite; menstrual pain; muscle or joint pain; stomach upset or indigestion (mild); sweating (increased); trouble in sleeping or unusual dreams

Other side effects not listed above may also occur in some patients. If you notice any other effects, check with your doctor.

Annual revision: 09/08/92

NICOTINYL ALCOHOL Systemic*

A commonly used brand name in Canada is Roniacol.

*Not commercially available in the U.S.

Description

Nicotinyl (nik-oh-TIN-ill) alcohol belongs to the group of medicines called vasodilators. Vasodilators increase the size of blood vessels and are used to treat problems resulting from poor blood circulation.

Nicotinyl alcohol is available without a prescription, in the following dosage form:

Oral

- Extended-release tablets (Canada)

It is very important that you read and understand the following information. If any of it causes you special concern, check with your doctor or pharmacist. Also, *if you have any questions* or if you want more information about this medicine or your medical problem, *ask your doctor, nurse, or pharmacist.*

Before Using This Medicine

If you are taking this medicine without a prescription, carefully read and follow any precautions on the label. For nicotinyl alcohol, the following should be considered:

Allergies—Tell your doctor if you have ever had any unusual or allergic reaction to nicotinyl alcohol. Also tell your doctor and pharmacist if you are allergic to any other substances, such as foods, preservatives, or dyes.

Pregnancy—Studies on effects in pregnancy have not been done in either humans or animals.

Breast-feeding—It is not known whether nicotinyl alcohol passes into breast milk. However, this medicine has not been reported to cause problems in nursing babies.

Older adults—Many medicines have not been studied specifically in older people. Therefore, it may not be known whether they work exactly the same way they do in younger adults or if they cause different side effects or problems in older people. There is no specific information comparing use of nicotinyl alcohol in the elderly with use in other age groups. However, nicotinyl alcohol may reduce tolerance to cold temperatures in elderly patients.

Other medicines—Although certain medicines should not be used together at all, in other cases two different medicines may be used together even if an interaction might occur. In these cases, your doctor may want to change the dose, or other precautions may be necessary. Tell your doctor and pharmacist if you are taking any other prescription or nonprescription (over-the-counter [OTC]) medicine, or if you smoke.

Other medical problems—The presence of other medical problems may affect the use of nicotinyl alcohol. Make sure you tell your doctor if you have any other medical problems, especially:

- Angina (chest pain) or
- Diabetes mellitus (sugar diabetes) or
- Heart attack (recent) or
- Stomach ulcer
- Stroke (recent)—Nicotinyl alcohol can make your condition worse

- Glaucoma or
- High cholesterol levels—The chance of side effects may be increased

Before you begin using any new medicine (prescription or nonprescription) or if you develop any new medical problem while you are using this medicine, check with your doctor, nurse, or pharmacist.

Proper Use of This Medicine

Nicotinyl alcohol tablets should be swallowed whole. Do not break, crush, or chew the tablets before swallowing them.

Dosing—The dose of nicotinyl alcohol will be different for different patients. *Follow your doctor's orders or the directions on the label.* The following information includes only the average doses of nicotinyl alcohol. *If your dose is different, do not change it* unless your doctor tells you to do so:

- For *oral* dosage forms (tablets):
  - —Adults: 150 to 300 milligrams two times a day, taken in the morning and evening.

Missed dose—If you miss a dose of this medicine, take it as soon as you remember. However, if it is almost time for your next dose, skip the missed dose and go back to your regular dosing schedule. Do not double doses.

Storage—To store this medicine:

- Keep out of the reach of children.
- Store away from heat and direct light.
- Do not store in the bathroom, near the kitchen sink, or in other damp places. Heat or moisture may cause the medicine to break down.
- Do not keep outdated medicine or medicine no longer needed. Be sure that any discarded medicine is out of the reach of children.

Precautions While Using This Medicine

It may take some time for this medicine to work. If you feel that the medicine is not working, do not stop taking it on your own. Instead, check with your doctor.

The helpful effects of this medicine may be decreased if you smoke.

Side Effects of This Medicine

Along with its needed effects, a medicine may cause some unwanted effects. Although not all of these side effects may occur, if they do occur they may need medical attention.

Check with your doctor as soon as possible if any of the following side effects occur:

Rare

Swelling of feet or lower legs; yellow eyes or skin

Other side effects may occur that usually do not need medical attention. These side effects may go away during treatment as your body adjusts to the medicine. However, check with your doctor if any of the following side effects continue or are bothersome:

More common

Flushing; warmth or tingling

Less common or rare

Diarrhea; dizziness or faintness; increased hair loss; nausea and vomiting; skin rash

Other side effects not listed above may also occur in some patients. If you notice any other effects, check with your doctor.

Annual revision: 04/06/93

NITRATES—Lingual Aerosol Systemic

This information applies to nitroglycerin oral spray.

A commonly used brand name in the U.S. and Canada is Nitrolingual. Another commonly used name is glyceryl trinitrate.

Description

Nitrates (NYE-trates) are used to treat the symptoms of angina (chest pain). Depending on the type of dosage form and how it is taken, nitrates are used to treat angina in three ways:

- to relieve an attack that is occurring by using the medicine when the attack begins;
- to prevent attacks from occurring by using the medicine just before an attack is expected to occur; or
- to reduce the number of attacks that occur by using the medicine regularly on a long-term basis.

When used as a lingual (in the mouth) spray, nitroglycerin is used either to relieve the pain of angina attacks or to prevent an expected angina attack.

Nitroglycerin works by relaxing blood vessels and increasing the supply of blood and oxygen to the heart while reducing its work load.

Nitroglycerin as discussed here is available only with your doctor's prescription, in the following dosage form:

Oral

- Lingual aerosol (U.S. and Canada)

It is very important that you read and understand the following information. If any of it causes you special concern, check with your doctor. Also, *if you have any questions* or if you want more information about this medicine or your medical problem, *ask your doctor, nurse, or pharmacist.*

Before Using This Medicine

In deciding to use a medicine, the risks of taking the medicine must be weighed against the good it will do. This is a decision you and your doctor will make. For nitroglycerin lingual aerosol, the following should be considered:

Allergies—Tell your doctor if you have ever had any unusual or allergic reaction to nitrates or nitrites. Also tell your doctor and pharmacist if you are allergic to any other substance, such as certain foods, preservatives, or dyes.

Pregnancy—Studies have not been done in humans. However, nitroglycerin has not been shown to cause problems.

Breast-feeding—It is not known whether this medicine passes into breast milk. However, nitroglycerin has not been reported to cause problems in nursing babies.

Children—There is no specific information about the use of nitrates in children.

Older adults—Dizziness or lightheadedness may be more likely to occur in the elderly, who may be more sensitive to the effects of nitrates.

Other medicines—Although certain medicines should not be used together at all, in other cases two different medicines may be used together even if an interaction might occur. In these cases, your doctor may want to change the dose, or other precautions may be necessary. When you are taking nitroglycerin, it is especially important that your doctor and pharmacist know if you are taking any of the following:

- Antihypertensives (high blood pressure medicine) or
- Other heart medicine—May increase the effects of nitroglycerin on blood pressure

Other medical problems—The presence of other medical problems may affect the use of nitroglycerin. Make sure you tell your doctor if you have any other medical problems, especially:

- Anemia (severe)
- Glaucoma—May be worsened by nitroglycerin
- Head injury (recent) or
- Stroke (recent)—Nitroglycerin may increase pressure in the brain, which can make problems worse
- Heart attack (recent)—Nitroglycerin may lower blood pressure, which can aggravate problems associated with heart attack
- Kidney disease or
- Liver disease—Effects may be increased because of slower removal of nitroglycerin from the body
- Overactive thyroid

Before you begin using any new medicine (prescription or nonprescription) or if you develop any new medical problem while you are using this medicine, check with your doctor, nurse, or pharmacist.

Proper Use of This Medicine

Use nitroglycerin spray exactly as directed by your doctor. It will work only if used correctly.

This medicine usually comes with patient instructions. Read them carefully before you actually need to use it. Then, if you need the medicine quickly, you will know how to use it.

To use nitroglycerin lingual spray:

- Remove the plastic cover. *Do not shake the container.*
- Hold the container upright. With the container held close to your mouth, press the button to spray onto or under your tongue. *Do not inhale the spray.*
- Release the button and close your mouth. Avoid swallowing immediately after using the spray.

For patients using nitroglycerin oral spray *to relieve the pain of an angina attack:*

- *When you begin to feel an attack of angina starting (chest pains or a tightness or squeezing in the chest), sit down. Then use 1 or 2 sprays as directed by your doctor.* This medicine works best when you are standing or sitting. However, since you may become dizzy, lightheaded, or faint soon after using a spray, it is safer to sit rather than stand while the medicine is working. If you become dizzy or faint while sitting, take several deep breaths and bend forward with your head between your knees.
- Remain calm and you should feel better in a few minutes.
- *This medicine usually gives relief in less than 5 minutes.* However, if the pain is not relieved, use a second spray. If the pain continues for another 5 minutes, a third spray may be used. *If you still have the chest pains after a total of 3 sprays in a 15-minute period, contact your doctor or go to a hospital emergency room immediately.*

For patients using nitroglycerin oral spray *to prevent an expected angina attack:*

- You may prevent anginal chest pains for up to 1 hour by using a spray 5 to 10 minutes before expected emotional stress or physical exertion that in the past seemed to bring on an attack.

Storage—To store this medicine:
- Keep out of the reach of children.
- Store away from heat and direct light.
- Keep the medicine from freezing.
- Do not puncture, break, or burn the aerosol container, even after it is empty.
- Do not keep outdated medicine or medicine no longer needed. Be sure that any discarded medicine is out of the reach of children.

Precautions While Using This Medicine

If you have been using this medicine regularly for several weeks, do not suddenly stop using it. Stopping suddenly may bring on attacks of angina. Check with your doctor for the best way to reduce gradually the amount you are using before stopping completely.

Dizziness, lightheadedness, or faintness may occur, especially when you get up quickly from a lying or sitting position. Getting up slowly may help. If you feel dizzy, sit or lie down.

The dizziness, lightheadedness, or fainting is also more likely to occur if you drink alcohol, stand for long periods of time, exercise, or if the weather is hot. *While you are taking this medicine, be careful in the amount of alcohol you drink. Also, use extra care during exercise or hot weather or if you must stand for long periods of time.*

After using a dose of this medicine you may get a headache that lasts for a short time. This is a common side effect, which should become less noticeable after you have used the medicine for a while. If this effect continues or if the headaches are severe, check with your doctor.

Side Effects of This Medicine

Along with its needed effects, a medicine may cause some unwanted effects. Although not all of these side effects may occur, if they do occur they may need medical attention.

Check with your doctor as soon as possible if any of the following side effects occur:

Rare

Blurred vision; dry mouth; headache (severe or prolonged); skin rash

Signs and symptoms of overdose (in the order in which they may occur)

Bluish-colored lips, fingernails, or palms of hands; dizziness (extreme) or fainting; feeling of extreme pressure in head; shortness of breath; unusual tiredness or weakness; weak and fast heartbeat; fever; convulsions (seizures)

Other side effects may occur that usually do not need medical attention. These side effects may go away during treatment as your body adjusts to the medicine. However, check with your doctor if any of the following side effects continue or are bothersome:

More common

Dizziness or lightheadedness, especially when getting up from a lying or sitting position; fast pulse; flushing of face and neck; headache; nausea or vomiting; restlessness

Other side effects not listed above may also occur in some patients. If you notice any other effects, check with your doctor.

Annual revision: August 1990

NITRATES—Oral Systemic

This information applies to the following medicines:

Erythrityl Tetranitrate (e-RI-thri-till tet-ra-NYE-trate)
Isosorbide Dinitrate (eye-soe-SOR-bide dye-NYE-trate)
Nitroglycerin (nye-troe-GLI-ser-in)
Pentaerythritol Tetranitrate (pen-ta-er-ITH-ri-tole tet-ra-NYE-trate)

Note: This information does *not* apply to amyl nitrite or mannitol hexanitrate.

Some commonly used brand names are:

For Erythrityl Tetranitrate

In the U.S. and Canada

Cardilate

Some other commonly used names are eritrityl tetranitrate and erythritol tetranitrate.

For Isosorbide Dinitrate

In the U.S.

Dilatrate-SR
Iso-Bid
Isonate
Isorbid
Isordil
Isotrate
Sorbitrate
Sorbitrate SA

Generic name product may also be available.

In Canada

Apo-ISDN
Cedocard-SR
Coronex
Isordil
Novosorbide

For Nitroglycerin

In the U.S.

Klavikordal
Niong
Nitro-Bid
Nitrocap
Nitrocap T.D.
Nitrocine
Nitroglyn
Nitrolin
Nitronet
Nitrong
Nitrospan

Generic name product may also be available.

In Canada
Nitrong SR

Another commonly used name is glyceryl trinitrate.

For Pentaerythritol Tetranitrate

In the U.S.

Duotrate	Pentylan
Naptrate	Peritrate
Pentritol	Peritrate SA

Generic name product may also be available.

In Canada

Peritrate	Peritrate SA
Peritrate Forte	

Some other commonly used names are pentaerythrityl tetranitrate and P.E.T.N.

Description

Nitrates (NYE-trates) are used to treat the symptoms of angina (chest pain). Depending on the type of dosage form and how it is taken, nitrates are used to treat angina in three ways:

- to relieve an attack that is occurring by using the medicine when the attack begins;
- to prevent attacks from occurring by using the medicine just before an attack is expected to occur; or
- to reduce the number of attacks that occur by using the medicine regularly on a long-term basis.

When taken orally and swallowed, nitrates are used to reduce the number of angina attacks that occur. They do not act fast enough to relieve the pain of an angina attack.

Nitrates work by relaxing blood vessels and increasing the supply of blood and oxygen to the heart while reducing its work load.

Nitrates may also be used for other conditions as determined by your doctor.

The nitrates discussed here are available only with your doctor's prescription, in the following dosage forms:

Oral

Erythrityl tetranitrate
- Tablets (U.S. and Canada)

Isosorbide dinitrate
- Capsules (U.S.)
- Extended-release capsules (U.S.)
- Tablets (U.S. and Canada)
- Chewable tablets (U.S.)
- Extended-release tablets (U.S. and Canada)

Nitroglycerin
- Extended-release capsules (U.S.)
- Extended-release tablets (U.S. and Canada)

Pentaerythritol tetranitrate
- Extended-release capsules (U.S.)
- Tablets (U.S. and Canada)
- Extended-release tablets (U.S. and Canada)

It is very important that you read and understand the following information. If any of it causes you special concern, check with your doctor. Also, *if you have any questions* or if you want more information about this medicine or your medical problem, *ask your doctor, nurse, or pharmacist.*

Before Using This Medicine

In deciding to use a medicine, the risks of taking the medicine must be weighed against the good it will do. This is a decision you and your doctor will make. For nitrates, the following should be considered:

Allergies—Tell your doctor if you have ever had any unusual or allergic reaction to nitrates or nitrites. Also tell your doctor and pharmacist if you are allergic to any other substance, such as certain foods, preservatives, or dyes.

Pregnancy—Although nitrates have not been shown to cause problems in humans, studies in rabbits given large doses of isosorbide dinitrate have shown adverse effects on the fetus. Studies have not been done with erythrityl tetranitrate, nitroglycerin, or pentaerythrityl tetranitrate.

Breast-feeding—It is not known whether this medicine passes into breast milk. However, nitrates have not been reported to cause problems in nursing babies.

Children—There is no specific information about the use of nitrates in children.

Older adults—Dizziness or lightheadedness may be more likely to occur in the elderly, who may be more sensitive to the effects of nitrates.

Other medicines—Although certain medicines should not be used together at all, in other cases two different medicines may be used together even if an interaction might occur. In these cases, your doctor may want to change the dose, or other precautions may be necessary. When you are taking nitrates, it is especially important that your doctor and pharmacist know if you are taking any of the following:

- Antihypertensives (high blood pressure medicine) or
- Other heart medicine—May increase the effects of nitrates on blood pressure

Other medical problems—The presence of other medical problems may affect the use of nitroglycerin. Make sure you tell your doctor if you have any other medical problems, especially:

- Anemia (severe)
- Glaucoma—May be worsened by nitrates
- Head injury (recent) or
- Stroke (recent)—Nitrates may increase pressure in the brain, which can make problems worse
- Heart attack (recent)—Nitrates may lower blood pressure, which can aggravate problems associated with heart attack
- Kidney disease or
- Liver disease—Effects may be increased because of slower removal of nitroglycerin from the body
- Overactive thyroid

Before you begin using any new medicine (prescription or nonprescription) or if you develop any new medical problem while you are using this medicine, check with your doctor, nurse, or pharmacist.

Proper Use of This Medicine

Take this medicine exactly as directed by your doctor. It will work only if taken correctly.

This form of nitrate is used to reduce the number of angina attacks. In most cases, it will not relieve an attack that has already started, because it works too slowly (the extended-release form releases medicine gradually over a 6-hour period to provide its effect for 8 to 10 hours). Check with your doctor if you need a fast-acting medicine to relieve the pain of an angina attack.

Take this medicine with a full glass (8 ounces) of water on an empty stomach. If taken either 1 hour before or 2 hours after meals, it will start working sooner.

Extended-release capsules and tablets are not to be broken, crushed, or chewed before they are swallowed. If broken up, they will not release the medicine properly.

Missed dose—If you are taking this medicine regularly and you miss a dose, take it as soon as possible. However, if the next scheduled dose is within 2 hours (or within 6 hours for extended-release capsules or tablets), skip the missed dose and go back to your regular dosing schedule. Do not double doses.

Storage—To store this medicine:

- Keep out of the reach of children.
- Store away from heat and direct light.
- Do not store in the bathroom, near the kitchen sink, or in other damp places. Heat or moisture may cause the medicine to break down.
- Do not keep outdated medicine or medicine no longer needed. Be sure that any discarded medicine is out of the reach of children.

Precautions While Using This Medicine

If you have been taking this medicine regularly for several weeks or more, do not suddenly stop using it. Stopping suddenly may bring on attacks of angina. Check with your doctor for the best way to reduce gradually the amount you are taking before stopping completely.

Dizziness, lightheadedness, or faintness may occur, especially when you get up quickly from a lying or sitting position. Getting up slowly may help. If you feel dizzy, sit or lie down.

The dizziness, lightheadedness, or fainting is also more likely to occur if you drink alcohol, stand for long periods of time, exercise, or if the weather is hot. *While you are taking this medicine, be careful in the amount of alcohol you drink. Also, use extra care during exercise or hot weather or if you must stand for long periods of time.*

After taking a dose of this medicine you may get a headache that lasts for a short time. This is a common side effect, which should become less noticeable after you have taken the medicine for a while. If this effect continues, or if the headaches are severe, check with your doctor.

For patients taking the *extended-release dosage forms of isosorbide dinitrate or pentaerythritol tetranitrate:*

- Partially dissolved tablets have been found in the stools of a few patients taking the extended-release tablets. Be alert to this possibility, especially if you have frequent bowel movements, diarrhea, or digestive problems. Notify your doctor if any such tablets are discovered. The tablets must be properly digested to provide the correct dose of medicine.

Side Effects of This Medicine

Along with its needed effects, a medicine may cause some unwanted effects. Although not all of these side effects may occur, if they do occur they may need medical attention.

Check with your doctor as soon as possible if any of the following side effects occur:

Rare

Blurred vision; dry mouth; headache (severe or prolonged); skin rash

Signs and symptoms of overdose (in the order in which they may occur)

Bluish-colored lips, fingernails, or palms of hands; dizziness (extreme) or fainting; feeling of extreme pressure in head; shortness of breath; unusual tiredness or weakness; weak and fast heartbeat; fever; convulsions (seizures)

Other side effects may occur that usually do not need medical attention. These side effects may go away during treatment as your body adjusts to the medicine. However, check with your doctor if any of the following side effects continue or are bothersome:

More common

Dizziness or lightheadedness, especially when getting up from a lying or sitting position; fast pulse; flushing of face and neck; headache; nausea or vomiting; restlessness

Other side effects not listed above may also occur in some patients. If you notice any other effects, check with your doctor.

Annual revision: August 1990

NITRATES—Sublingual, Chewable, or Buccal Systemic

This information applies to the following medicines:

Erythrityl Tetranitrate (e-RI-thri-till tet-ra-NYE-trate)
Isosorbide Dinitrate (eye-soe-SOR-bide dye-NYE-trate)
Nitroglycerin (nye-troe-GLI-ser-in)

Note: This information does *not* apply to amyl nitrite or pentaerythritol tetranitrate.

Some commonly used brand names are:

For Erythrityl Tetranitrate
In the U.S. and Canada
Cardilate

Some other commonly used names are eritrityl tetranitrate and erythritol tetranitrate.

For Isosorbide Dinitrate
In the U.S.
Isonate
Isorbid
Isordil
Sorbitrate
Generic name product may also be available.

In Canada
Apo-ISDN
Coronex
Isordil

For Nitroglycerin
In the U.S.
Nitrogard
Nitrostat
Generic name product may also be available.

In Canada
Nitrogard SR
Nitrostat
Generic name product may also be available.

Another commonly used name is glyceryl trinitrate.

Description

Nitrates (NYE-trates) are used to treat the symptoms of angina (chest pain). Depending on the type of dosage form and how it is taken, nitrates are used to treat angina in three ways:

- to relieve an attack that is occurring by using the medicine when the attack begins;
- to prevent attacks from occurring by using the medicine just before an attack is expected to occur; or
- to reduce the number of attacks that occur by using the medicine regularly on a long-term basis.

Nitrates are available in different forms. Sublingual nitrates are generally placed under the tongue where they dissolve and are absorbed through the lining of the mouth. Some can also be used buccally, being placed under the lip or in the cheek. The chewable dosage forms, after being chewed and held in the mouth before swallowing, are absorbed in the same way. *It is important to remember that each dosage form is different and that the specific directions for each type must be followed if the medicine is to work properly.*

Nitrates that are used *to relieve the pain* of an angina attack include:

- sublingual nitroglycerin;
- buccal nitroglycerin;
- sublingual isosorbide dinitrate; and
- chewable isosorbide dinitrate.

Those that can be used *to prevent expected attacks* of angina include:

- sublingual nitroglycerin;
- buccal nitroglycerin;
- sublingual erythrityl tetranitrate;
- sublingual isosorbide dinitrate; and
- chewable isosorbide dinitrate.

Products that are used regularly on a long-term basis *to reduce the number of attacks* that occur include:

- buccal nitroglycerin;
- oral/sublingual erythrityl tetranitrate; and
- chewable isosorbide dinitrate; and
- sublingual isosorbide dinitrate.

Nitrates work by relaxing blood vessels and increasing the supply of blood and oxygen to the heart while reducing its work load.

Nitrates may also be used for other conditions as determined by your doctor.

The nitrates discussed here are available only with your doctor's prescription, in the following dosage forms:

Buccal
Nitroglycerin
- Tablets (U.S. and Canada)

Chewable
Isosorbide dinitrate
- Tablets (U.S.)

Sublingual
Erythrityl tetranitrate
- Tablets (U.S. and Canada)

Isosorbide dinitrate
- Tablets (U.S. and Canada)

Nitroglycerin
- Tablets (U.S. and Canada)

It is very important that you read and understand the following information. If any of it causes you special concern, check with your doctor. Also, *if you have any questions* or if you want more information about this medicine or your medical problem, *ask your doctor, nurse, or pharmacist.*

Before Using This Medicine

In deciding to use a medicine, the risks of taking the medicine must be weighed against the good it will do.

This is a decision you and your doctor will make. For nitrates, the following should be considered:

Allergies—Tell your doctor if you have ever had any unusual or allergic reaction to nitrates or nitrites. Also tell your doctor and pharmacist if you are allergic to any other substance, such as certain foods, preservatives, or dyes.

Pregnancy—Although nitrates have not been shown to cause problems in humans, studies in rabbits given large doses of isosorbide dinitrate have shown adverse effects on the fetus. Studies have not been done with erythrityl tetranitrate, nitroglycerin, or pentaerythrityl tetranitrate.

Breast-feeding—It is not known whether this medicine passes into breast milk. However, nitrates have not been reported to cause problems in nursing babies.

Children—There is no specific information about the use of nitrates in children.

Older adults—Dizziness or lightheadedness may be more likely to occur in the elderly, who may be more sensitive to the effects of nitrates.

Other medicines—Although certain medicines should not be used together at all, in other cases two different medicines may be used together even if an interaction might occur. In these cases, your doctor may want to change the dose, or other precautions may be necessary. When you are taking nitrates, it is especially important that your doctor and pharmacist know if you are taking any of the following:

- Antihypertensives (high blood pressure medicine) or
- Other heart medicine—May increase the effects of nitrates on blood pressure

Other medical problems—The presence of other medical problems may affect the use of nitroglycerin. Make sure you tell your doctor if you have any other medical problems, especially:

- Anemia (severe)
- Glaucoma—May be worsened by nitrates
- Head injury (recent) or
- Stroke (recent)—Nitrates may increase pressure in the brain, which can make problems worse
- Heart attack (recent)—Nitrates may lower blood pressure, which can aggravate problems associated with heart attack
- Kidney disease or
- Liver disease—Effects may be increased because of slower removal of nitroglycerin from the body
- Overactive thyroid

Before you begin using any new medicine (prescription or nonprescription) or if you develop any new medical problem while you are using this medicine, check with your doctor, nurse, or pharmacist.

Proper Use of This Medicine

Take this medicine exactly as directed by your doctor. It will work only if taken correctly.

Sublingual tablets should not be chewed, crushed, or swallowed. They work much faster when absorbed through the lining of the mouth. Place the tablet under the tongue, between the lip and gum, or between the cheek and gum and let it dissolve there. Do not eat, drink, smoke, or use chewing tobacco while a tablet is dissolving.

Buccal extended-release tablets should not be chewed, crushed, or swallowed. They are designed to release a dose of nitroglycerin over a period of hours, not all at once.

- Allow the tablet to dissolve slowly in place between the upper lip and gum (above the front teeth), or between the cheek and upper gum. If food or drink is to be taken during the 3 to 5 hours when the tablet is dissolving, place the tablet between the *upper* lip and gum, above the front teeth. If you have dentures, you may place the tablet anywhere between the cheek and gum.
- Touching the tablet with your tongue or drinking hot liquids may cause the tablet to dissolve faster.
- Do not go to sleep while a tablet is dissolving because it could slip down your throat and cause choking.
- If you accidentally swallow the tablet, replace it with another one.
- Do not use chewing tobacco while a tablet is in place.

Chewable tablets must be chewed well and held in the mouth for about 2 minutes before you swallow them. This will allow the medicine to be absorbed through the lining of the mouth.

For patients using *nitroglycerin or isosorbide dinitrate to relieve the pain of an angina attack*:

- *When you begin to feel an attack of angina starting (chest pains or a tightness or squeezing in the chest), sit down. Then place a tablet in your mouth, either sublingually or buccally, or chew a chewable tablet.* This medicine works best when you are standing or sitting. However, since you may become dizzy, lightheaded, or faint soon after using a tablet, it is safer to sit rather than stand while the medicine is working. If you become dizzy or faint while sitting, take several deep breaths and bend forward with your head between your knees.
- Remain calm and you should feel better in a few minutes.
- *This medicine usually gives relief in 1 to 5 minutes.* However, if the pain is not relieved, and you are using:

  —Sublingual tablets, either sublingually or buccally: Use a second tablet. If the pain continues for another 5 minutes, a third tablet may be used. *If you still have the chest pains after a total of 3 tablets in a 15-minute period, contact your doctor or go to a hospital emergency room immediately.*

—Buccal extended-release tablets: *Use a sublingual (under the tongue) nitroglycerin tablet and check with your doctor.* Do not use another buccal tablet since the effects of a buccal tablet last for several hours.

For patients using *nitroglycerin, erythrityl tetranitrate, or isosorbide dinitrate to prevent an expected angina attack:*

- You may prevent anginal chest pains for up to 1 hour (6 hours for the extended-release nitroglycerin tablet) by using a buccal or sublingual tablet or chewing a chewable tablet 5 to 10 minutes before expected emotional stress or physical exertion that in the past seemed to bring on an attack.

For patients using *isosorbide dinitrate or extended-release buccal nitroglycerin regularly on a long-term basis to reduce the number of angina attacks that occur:*

- Chewable or sublingual isosorbide dinitrate and buccal extended-release nitroglycerin tablets can be used either to prevent angina attacks or to help relieve an attack that has already started.

Missed dose—For patients using isosorbide dinitrate or extended-release buccal nitroglycerin regularly on a long-term basis to reduce the number of angina attacks that occur:

- If you miss a dose of this medicine, use it as soon as possible. However, if the next scheduled dose is within 2 hours, skip the missed dose and go back to your regular dosing schedule. Do not double doses.

Stability and storage—

For sublingual nitroglycerin

- When properly stored, sublingual nitroglycerin tablets retain their strength until the expiration date printed on the original label. However, because of patient usage, changing temperature and moisture, shaking, and repeated bottle opening, the tablets may be good for only 3 to 6 months. The "stabilized" sublingual tablets may stay good for a longer period of time but require the same care in storage and use.
- Some people think they should test the strength of their sublingual nitroglycerin tablets by looking for a tingling or burning sensation, a feeling of warmth or flushing, or a headache, after a tablet has been dissolved under the tongue. This kind of testing is not completely reliable since some patients may be unable to detect these effects. In addition, newer, stabilized sublingual nitroglycerin tablets are less likely to produce these detectable effects.
- To help keep the nitroglycerin tablets at full strength:

  —keep the medicine in the original glass, screw-cap bottle. For patients who wish to carry a small number of tablets with them for emergency use, a specially designed container is available. However, only containers specifically labeled as suitable for use with nitroglycerin sublingual tablets should be used.

  —remove the cotton plug that comes in the bottle and *do not* put it back.

  —*put the cap on the bottle quickly and tightly after each use.*

  —to select a tablet for use, pour several into the bottle cap, take one, and pour the others back into the bottle. Try not to hold them in the palm of your hand because they may pick up moisture and crumble.

  —do not keep other medicines in the same bottle with the nitroglycerin since they will weaken the nitroglycerin effect.

  —keep the medicine handy at all times but try not to carry the bottle close to the body. Medicine may lose strength because of body warmth. Instead, carry the tightly closed bottle in your purse or the pocket of a jacket or other loose-fitting clothing whenever possible.

  —store the bottle of nitroglycerin tablets in a cool, dry place. Storage at average room temperature away from direct heat or direct sunlight is best. Do not store in the refrigerator or in a bathroom medicine cabinet because the moisture usually present in these areas may cause the tablets to crumble if the container is not tightly closed. Do not keep the tablets in your automobile glove compartment.
- Keep out of the reach of children.
- Do not keep outdated medicine or medicine no longer needed. Be sure that any discarded medicine is out of the reach of children.

For erythrityl tetranitrate, isosorbide dinitrate, and buccal extended-release nitroglycerin

- These forms of nitrates are more stable than sublingual nitroglycerin.
- Keep out of the reach of children.
- Store away from heat and direct light.
- Do not store in the bathroom, near the kitchen sink, or in other damp places. Heat or moisture may cause the medicine to break down.
- Do not keep outdated medicine or medicine no longer needed. Be sure that any discarded medicine is out of the reach of children.

Precautions While Using This Medicine

If you have been taking this medicine regularly for several weeks, do not suddenly stop using it. Stopping suddenly may bring on attacks of angina. Check with your doctor for the best way to reduce gradually the amount you are taking before stopping completely.

Dizziness, lightheadedness, or faintness may occur, especially when you get up quickly from a lying or sitting position. Getting up slowly may help. If you feel dizzy, sit or lie down.

The dizziness, lightheadedness, or fainting is also more likely to occur if you drink alcohol, stand for long periods of time, exercise, or if the weather is hot. *While you are taking this medicine, be careful in the amount of alcohol you drink. Also, use extra care during exercise or hot weather or if you must stand for long periods of time.*

After taking a dose of this medicine you may get a headache that lasts for a short time. This is a common side effect, which should become less noticeable after you have taken the medicine for a while. If this effect continues or if the headaches are severe, check with your doctor.

Side Effects of This Medicine

Along with its needed effects, a medicine may cause some unwanted effects. Although not all of these side effects may occur, if they do occur they may need medical attention.

Check with your doctor as soon as possible if any of the following side effects occur:

Rare

Blurred vision; dry mouth; headache (severe or prolonged); skin rash

Signs and symptoms of overdose (in the order in which they may occur)

Bluish-colored lips, fingernails, or palms of hands; dizziness (extreme) or fainting; feeling of extreme pressure in head; shortness of breath; unusual tiredness or weakness; weak and fast heartbeat; fever; convulsions (seizures)

Other side effects may occur that usually do not need medical attention. These side effects may go away during treatment as your body adjusts to the medicine. However, check with your doctor if any of the following side effects continue or are bothersome:

More common

Dizziness or lightheadedness, especially when getting up from a lying or sitting position; fast pulse; flushing of face and neck; headache; nausea or vomiting; restlessness

Other side effects not listed above may also occur in some patients. If you notice any other effects, check with your doctor.

Annual revision: August 1990

NITRATES—Topical Systemic

This information applies to nitroglycerin ointment and transdermal patches.

Some commonly used brand names are:

For nitroglycerin ointment

In the U.S.

Nitro-Bid
Nitrol
Nitrong
Nitrostat

Generic name product may also be available.

In Canada

Nitro-Bid
Nitrol
Nitrong

Another commonly used name is glyceryl trinitrate.

For nitroglycerin transdermal patches

In the U.S.

Deponit
Nitrocine
Nitrodisc
Nitro-Dur
Nitro-Dur II
NTS
Transderm-Nitro

Generic name product may also be available.

In Canada

Transderm-Nitro

Another commonly used name is glyceryl trinitrate.

Description

Nitrates (NYE-trates) are used to treat the symptoms of angina (chest pain). Depending on the type of dosage form and how it is taken, nitrates are used to treat angina in three ways:

- to relieve an attack that is occurring by using the medicine when the attack begins;
- to prevent attacks from occurring by using the medicine just before an attack is expected to occur; or
- to reduce the number of attacks that occur by using the medicine regularly on a long-term basis.

When applied to the skin, nitrates are used to reduce the number of angina attacks that occur. The only nitrate available for this purpose is topical nitroglycerin (nye-troe-GLI-ser-in).

Topical nitroglycerin is absorbed through the skin. It works by relaxing blood vessels and increasing the supply of blood and oxygen to the heart while reducing its work load. This helps prevent future angina attacks from occurring.

Topical nitroglycerin may also be used for other conditions as determined by your doctor.

Nitroglycerin as discussed here is available only with your doctor's prescription, in the following dosage forms:

Topical
- Ointment (U.S. and Canada)
- Transdermal (stick-on) patch (U.S. and Canada)

It is very important that you read and understand the following information. If any of it causes you special concern, check with your doctor. Also, *if you have any questions* or if you want more information about this medicine or your medical problem, *ask your doctor, nurse, or pharmacist.*

Before Using This Medicine

In deciding to use a medicine, the risks of taking the medicine must be weighed against the good it will do. This is a decision you and your doctor will make. For nitroglycerin applied to the skin, the following should be considered:

Allergies—Tell your doctor if you have ever had any unusual or allergic reaction to nitrates or nitrites. Also tell your doctor and pharmacist if you are allergic to any other substance, such as certain foods, preservatives, or dyes.

Pregnancy—Studies have not been done in humans. However, nitroglycerin has not been shown to cause problems.

Breast-feeding—It is not known whether this medicine passes into breast milk. However, nitroglycerin has not been reported to cause problems in nursing babies.

Children—There is no specific information about the use of nitrates in children.

Older adults—Dizziness or lightheadedness may be more likely to occur in the elderly, who may be more sensitive to the effects of nitrates.

Other medicines—Although certain medicines should not be used together at all, in other cases two different medicines may be used together even if an interaction might occur. In these cases, your doctor may want to change the dose, or other precautions may be necessary. When you are using nitroglycerin, it is especially important that your doctor and pharmacist know if you are taking any of the following:

- Antihypertensives (high blood pressure medicine) or
- Other heart medicine—May increase the effects of nitroglycerin on blood pressure

Other medical problems—The presence of other medical problems may affect the use of nitroglycerin. Make sure you tell your doctor if you have any other medical problems, especially:

- Anemia (severe)
- Glaucoma—May be worsened by nitroglycerin
- Head injury (recent) or
- Stroke (recent)—Nitroglycerin may increase pressure in the brain, which can make problems worse
- Heart attack (recent)—Nitroglycerin may lower blood pressure, which can aggravate problems associated with heart attack
- Kidney disease or
- Liver disease—Effects may be increased because of slower removal of nitroglycerin from the body
- Overactive thyroid

Before you begin using any new medicine (prescription or nonprescription) or if you develop any new medical problem while you are using this medicine, check with your doctor, nurse, or pharmacist.

Proper Use of This Medicine

Use nitroglycerin exactly as directed by your doctor. It will work only if applied correctly.

The ointment and transdermal forms of nitroglycerin are used to reduce the number of angina attacks. They will not relieve an attack that has already started because they work too slowly. Check with your doctor if you need a fast-acting medicine to relieve the pain of an angina attack.

This medicine usually comes with patient instructions. Read them carefully before using.

For patients using the *ointment* form of this medicine:

- Before applying a new dose of ointment, remove any ointment remaining on the skin from a previous dose. This will allow the fresh ointment to release the nitroglycerin properly.
- This medicine comes with dose-measuring papers. Use them to measure the length of ointment squeezed from the tube and to apply the ointment to the skin. *Do not rub or massage the ointment into the skin; just spread in a thin, even layer, covering an area of the same size each time it is applied.*
- Apply the ointment to skin that has little or no hair.
- Apply each dose of ointment to a different area of skin to prevent irritation or other skin problems.
- If your doctor has ordered an occlusive dressing (airtight covering, such as kitchen plastic wrap) to be applied over this medicine, make sure you know how to apply it. Since occlusive dressings increase the amount of medicine absorbed through the skin and the possibility of side effects, use them only as directed. If you have any questions about this, check with your doctor, nurse, or pharmacist.

For patients using the *transdermal (stick-on patch) system:*

- Do not try to trim or cut the adhesive patch to adjust the dosage. Check with your doctor if you think the medicine is not working as it should.
- Apply the patch to a clean, dry skin area with little or no hair and free of scars, cuts, or irritation. Remove the previous patch before applying a new one.
- Apply a new patch if the first one becomes loose or falls off.
- Apply each dose to a different area of skin to prevent skin irritation or other problems.

Missed dose—

- For patients using the *ointment* form of this medicine: If you miss a dose of this medicine, apply it as soon as possible unless the next scheduled dose is within 2 hours. Then go back to your regular dosing schedule. Do not increase the amount used.
- For patients using the *transdermal (stick-on patch) system*: If you miss a dose of this medicine, apply it as soon as possible. Then go back to your regular dosing schedule.

Storage—

- To store the *ointment* form of this medicine:
  —Keep out of the reach of children.
  —Store the tube of nitroglycerin ointment in a cool place and keep it tightly closed.
  —Do not keep outdated medicine or medicine no longer needed. Be sure that any discarded medicine is out of the reach of children.
- To store the *transdermal (stick-on patch) system*:
  —Keep out of the reach of children.
  —Store away from heat and direct light.
  —Do not store in the bathroom, near the kitchen sink, or in other damp places. Heat or moisture may cause the medicine to break down.
  —Do not keep outdated medicine or medicine no longer needed. Be sure that any discarded medicine is out of the reach of children.

Precautions While Using This Medicine

If you have been using nitroglycerin regularly for several weeks or more, do not suddenly stop using it. Stopping suddenly may bring on attacks of angina. Check with your doctor for the best way to reduce gradually the amount you are using before stopping completely.

Dizziness, lightheadedness, or faintness may occur, especially when you get up quickly from a lying or sitting position. Getting up slowly may help. If you feel dizzy, sit or lie down.

The dizziness, lightheadedness, or fainting is also more likely to occur if you drink alcohol, stand for long periods of time, exercise, or if the weather is hot. *While you are taking this medicine, be careful in the amount of alcohol you drink. Also, use extra care during exercise or hot weather or if you must stand for long periods of time.*

After using a dose of this medicine you may get a headache that lasts for a short time. This is a common side effect, which should become less noticeable after you have used the medicine for a while. If this effect continues, or if the headaches are severe, check with your doctor.

Side Effects of This Medicine

Along with its needed effects, a medicine may cause some unwanted effects. Although not all of these side effects may occur, if they do occur they may need medical attention.

Check with your doctor as soon as possible if any of the following side effects occur:

Rare

Blurred vision; dry mouth; headache (severe or prolonged)

Signs and symptoms of overdose (in the order in which they may occur)

Bluish-colored lips, fingernails, or palms of hands; dizziness (extreme) or fainting; feeling of extreme pressure in head; shortness of breath; unusual tiredness or weakness; weak and fast heartbeat; fever; convulsions (seizures)

Other side effects may occur that usually do not need medical attention. These side effects may go away during treatment as your body adjusts to the medicine. However, check with your doctor if any of the following side effects continue or are bothersome:

More common

Dizziness or lightheadedness, especially when getting up from a lying or sitting position; fast pulse; flushing of face and neck; headache; nausea or vomiting; restlessness

Less common

Sore, reddened skin

Other side effects not listed above may also occur in some patients. If you notice any other effects, check with your doctor.

Annual revision: August 1990

NITROFURANTOIN Systemic

Some commonly used brand names are:

In the U.S.

Furadantin	Macrobid
Furalan	Macrodantin
Furatoin	Nitrofuracot

Generic name product may also be available.

In Canada

Apo-Nitrofurantoin	Macrodantin

Description

Nitrofurantoin (nye-troe-fyoor-AN-toyn) belongs to the family of medicines called anti-infectives. It is used to treat infections of the urinary tract. It may also be used for other conditions as determined by your doctor.

Nitrofurantoin is available only with your doctor's prescription, in the following dosage forms:

Oral

- Capsules (U.S. and Canada)
- Extended-release Capsules (U.S.)
- Oral Suspension (U.S.)
- Tablets (U.S. and Canada)

It is very important that you read and understand the following information. If any of it causes you special concern, check with your doctor. Also, *if you have any questions* or if you want more information about this medicine or your medical problem, *ask your doctor, nurse, or pharmacist.*

Before Using This Medicine

In deciding to use a medicine, the risks of taking the medicine must be weighed against the good it will do. This is a decision you and your doctor will make. For nitrofurantoin, the following should be considered:

Allergies—Tell your doctor if you have ever had any unusual or allergic reaction to nitrofurantoin or to any related medicines such as furazolidone (e.g., Furoxone) or nitrofurazone (e.g., Furacin). Also tell your doctor and pharmacist if you are allergic to any other substances, such as foods, preservatives, or dyes.

Pregnancy—Nitrofurantoin should not be used if you are within a week or 2 of your delivery date or during labor and delivery. It may cause problems in the infant.

Breast-feeding—Nitrofurantoin passes into the breast milk in small amounts and may cause problems in nursing babies, especially those with glucose-6-phosphate dehydrogenase (G6PD) deficiency.

Children—Infants up to 1 month of age should not be given this medicine because they are especially sensitive to the effects of nitrofurantoin.

Older adults—Elderly people may be more sensitive to the effects of nitrofurantoin. This may increase the chance of side effects during treatment.

Other medicines—Although certain medicines should not be used together at all, in other cases two different medicines may be used together even if an interaction might occur. In these cases, your doctor may want to change the dose, or other precautions may be necessary. When you are taking nitrofurantoin, it is especially important that your doctor and pharmacist know if you are taking any of the following:

- Acetohydroxamic acid (e.g., Lithostat) or
- Antidiabetics, oral (diabetes medicine you take by mouth) or
- Dapsone or
- Furazolidone (e.g., Furoxone) or
- Methyldopa (e.g., Aldomet) or
- Primaquine or
- Procainamide (e.g., Pronestyl) or
- Quinidine (e.g., Quinidex) or
- Sulfonamides (sulfa medicine) or
- Sulfoxone (e.g., Diasone) or
- Vitamin K (e.g., AquaMEPHYTON, Synkayvite)—Patients who take nitrofurantoin with any of these medicines may have an increase in side effects affecting the blood
- Carbamazepine (e.g., Tegretol) or
- Chloroquine (e.g., Aralen) or
- Cisplatin (e.g., Platinol) or
- Cytarabine (e.g., Cytosar-U) or
- Diphtheria, tetanus, and pertussis (DTP) vaccine or
- Disulfiram (e.g., Antabuse) or
- Ethotoin (e.g., Peganone) or
- Hydroxychloroquine (e.g., Plaquenil) or
- Lindane, topical (e.g., Kwell) or
- Lithium (e.g., Lithane) or
- Mephenytoin (e.g., Mesantoin) or
- Mexiletine (e.g., Mexitil) or
- Other anti-infectives by mouth or by injection (medicine for infection) or
- Pemoline (e.g., Cylert) or
- Phenytoin (e.g., Dilantin) or
- Pyridoxine (e.g., Hexa-Betalin) (with long-term, high-dose use) or
- Vincristine (e.g., Oncovin)—Patients who take nitrofurantoin with any of these medicines, or who have received a DTP vaccine within the last 30 days or are going to receive a DTP may have an increase in side effects affecting the nervous system
- Probenecid (e.g., Benemid) or
- Sulfinpyrazone (e.g., Anturane)—Patients who take nitrofurantoin with any of these medicines may have an increase in side effects
- Quinine (e.g., Quinamm)—Patients who take nitrofurantoin with quinine may have an increase in side effects affecting the blood and the nervous system

Other medical problems—The presence of other medical problems may affect the use of nitrofurantoin. Make sure

you tell your doctor if you have any other medical problems, especially:

- Glucose-6-phosphate dehydrogenase (G6PD) deficiency—Nitrofurantoin may cause anemia in patients with G6PD deficiency
- Kidney disease (other than infection)—The chance of side effects of this medicine may be increased and the medicine may be less effective in patients with kidney disease
- Lung disease or
- Nerve damage—Patients with lung disease or nerve damage may have an increase in side effects when they take nitrofurantoin

Before you begin using any new medicine (prescription or nonprescription) or if you develop any new medical problem while you are using this medicine, check with your doctor, nurse, or pharmacist.

Proper Use of This Medicine

Do not give this medicine to infants up to 1 month of age.

Nitrofurantoin is best taken with food or milk. This may lessen stomach upset and help your body absorb the medicine better.

For patients taking the *oral liquid form of this medicine:*

- Shake the oral liquid forcefully before each dose to help make it pour more smoothly and to be sure the medicine is evenly mixed.
- Use a specially marked measuring spoon or other device to measure each dose accurately. The average household teaspoon may not hold the right amount of liquid.
- Nitrofurantoin may be mixed with water, milk, fruit juices, or infants' formulas. If it is mixed with other liquids, take the medicine immediately after mixing. Be sure to drink all the liquid in order to get the full dose of medicine.

For patients taking the *extended-release capsule* form of this medicine:

- Swallow the capsules whole.
- Do not open, crush, or chew the capsules before swallowing them.

To help clear up your infection completely, *keep taking this medicine for the full time of treatment,* even if you begin to feel better after a few days. *Do not miss any doses.*

Dosing—The dose of nitrofurantoin will be different for different patients. *Follow your doctor's orders or the directions on the label.* The following information includes only the average doses of nitrofurantoin. *If your dose is different, do not change it* unless your doctor tells you to do so.

- For the *capsule, oral suspension, and tablet* dosage forms:

  —Adults and adolescents: 50 to 100 mg every six hours.

  —Children 1 month of age and older: Dose is based on body weight and will be determined by your doctor.

  —Children up to 1 month of age: Use is not recommended.

- For the *extended-release capsule* dosage form:

  —Adults and children 12 years of age and older: 100 mg every twelve hours for seven days.

  —Children up to 12 years of age: Dose must be determined by the doctor.

Missed dose—If you do miss a dose of this medicine, take it as soon as possible. However, if it is almost time for your next dose, skip the next dose and go back to your regular dosing schedule. Do not double doses.

Storage—To store this medicine:

- Keep out of the reach of children.
- Store away from heat and direct light.
- Do not store the capsule or tablet form of this medicine in the bathroom, near the kitchen sink, or in other damp places. Heat or moisture may cause the medicine to break down.
- Keep the oral liquid form of this medicine from freezing.
- Do not keep outdated medicine or medicine no longer needed. Be sure that any discarded medicine is out of the reach of children.

Precautions While Using This Medicine

It is important that your doctor check your progress at regular visits if you will be taking this medicine for a long time.

If your symptoms do not improve within a few days, or if they become worse, check with your doctor.

For *diabetic patients:*

- *This medicine may cause false test results with some urine sugar tests.* Check with your doctor before changing your diet or the dosage of your diabetes medicine.

Side Effects of This Medicine

Along with its needed effects, a medicine may cause some unwanted effects. Although not all of these side effects may occur, if they do occur they may need medical attention.

Check with your doctor immediately if any of the following side effects occur:

More common

Chest pain; chills; cough; fever; troubled breathing

Less common

Dizziness; drowsiness; headache; numbness, tingling, or burning of face or mouth; sore throat and fever; unusual muscle weakness; unusual tiredness or weakness

Rare

Itching; joint pain; pale skin; skin rash; yellow eyes or skin

Other side effects may occur that usually do not need medical attention. These side effects may go away during treatment as your body adjusts to the medicine. However, check with your doctor if any of the following side effects continue or are bothersome:

More common

Abdominal or stomach pain or upset; diarrhea; loss of appetite; nausea or vomiting

This medicine may cause the urine to become rust-yellow to brown. This side effect does not require medical attention.

Other side effects not listed above may also occur in some patients. If you notice any other effects, check with your doctor.

Annual revision: 01/19/93

NORFLOXACIN Ophthalmic

Some commonly used brand names are:

In the U.S.
Chibroxin

In Canada
Noroxin

Description

Norfloxacin (nor-FLOX-a-sin) is an antibiotic. The ophthalmic preparation is used to treat infections of the eye.

Norfloxacin is available only with your doctor's prescription, in the following dosage form:

Ophthalmic

- Ophthalmic solution (eye drops) (U.S. and Canada)

It is very important that you read and understand the following information. If any of it causes you special concern, check with your doctor. Also, *if you have any questions* or if you want more information about this medicine or your medical problem, *ask your doctor, nurse, or pharmacist.*

Before Using This Medicine

In deciding to use a medicine, the risks of taking the medicine must be weighed against the good it will do. This is a decision you and your doctor will make. For ophthalmic norfloxacin, the following should be considered:

Allergies—Tell your doctor if you have ever had any unusual or allergic reaction to norfloxacin or to any related medicines, such as cinoxacin (e.g., Cinobac), ciprofloxacin (e.g., Cipro), ofloxacin (e.g., Floxin), or nalidixic acid (e.g., NegGram). Also tell your doctor and pharmacist if you are allergic to any other substances, such as foods, preservatives, or dyes.

Pregnancy—Studies have not been done in humans. However, norfloxacin taken by mouth can cause bone problems in young animals. Since it is not known whether ophthalmic norfloxacin can cause bone problems in infants, use is not recommended during pregnancy.

Breast-feeding—It is not known whether ophthalmic norfloxacin passes into the breast milk. Low doses of norfloxacin taken by mouth do not pass into breast milk, but other related medicines do. Also, norfloxacin taken by mouth can cause bone problems in young animals. Since it is not known whether ophthalmic norfloxacin can cause bone problems in infants, use is not recommended in nursing mothers.

Children—Use is not recommended in infants and children up to 1 year of age. Norfloxacin taken by mouth has been shown to cause bone problems in young animals. It is not known whether ophthalmic norfloxacin can cause bone problems in infants. In children 1 year of age and older, this medicine is not expected to cause different side effects or problems than it does in adults.

Older adults—Many medicines have not been studied specifically in older people. Therefore, it may not be known whether they work exactly the same way they do in younger adults. Although there is no specific information comparing use of ophthalmic norfloxacin in the elderly with use in other age groups, this medicine is not expected to cause different side effects or problems in older people than it does in younger adults.

Other medicines—Although certain medicines should not be used together at all, in other cases two different medicines may be used together even if an interaction might occur. In these cases, your doctor may want to change the dose, or other precautions may be necessary. Tell your doctor and pharmacist if you are taking or using any prescription or nonprescription (over-the-counter [OTC]) medicine.

Before you begin using any new medicine (prescription or nonprescription) or if you develop any new medical problem while you are using this medicine, check with your doctor, nurse, or pharmacist.

Proper Use of This Medicine

To use:

- First, wash your hands. Then tilt the head back and pull the lower eyelid away from the eye to form a pouch. Drop the medicine into the pouch and gently close the eyes. Do not blink. Keep the eyes closed for 1 or 2 minutes to allow the medicine to come into contact with the infection.
- If you think you did not get the drop of medicine into your eye properly, use another drop.
- To keep the medicine as germ-free as possible, do not touch the applicator tip to any surface (including the eye). Also, keep the container tightly closed.

Dosing—The dose of ophthalmic norfloxacin will be different for different patients. *Follow your doctor's orders or the directions on the label.* The following information includes only the average doses of ophthalmic norfloxacin. *If your dose is different, do not change it* unless your doctor tells you to do so:

- For infants and children up to 1 year of age: Use is not recommended.
- For adults and children 1 year of age and over: Place 1 drop in each eye four times a day for 7 days.

To help clear up your infection completely, *keep using this medicine for the full time of treatment,* even if your symptoms begin to clear up after a few days. If you stop using this medicine too soon, your symptoms may return. *Do not miss any doses.*

Missed dose—If you do miss a dose of this medicine, apply it as soon as possible. However, if it is almost time for your next dose, skip the missed dose and go back to your regular dosing schedule.

Storage—To store this medicine:

- Keep out of the reach of children.
- Store away from heat and direct light.
- Keep the medicine from freezing.
- Do not keep outdated medicine or medicine no longer needed. Be sure that any discarded medicine is out of the reach of children.

Precautions While Using This Medicine

If your symptoms do not improve within a few days, or if they become worse, check with your doctor.

This medicine may cause your eyes to become more sensitive to light than they are normally. Wearing sunglasses and avoiding too much exposure to bright light may help lessen the discomfort.

Side Effects of This Medicine

Along with its needed effects, a medicine may cause some unwanted effects. Although not all of these side effects may occur, if they do occur they may need medical attention.

Check with your doctor immediately if any of the following side effects occur:

Rare

Skin rash or other sign of allergic reaction

Other side effects may occur that usually do not need medical attention. These side effects may go away during treatment as your body adjusts to the medicine. However, check with your doctor if any of the following side effects continue or are bothersome:

More common

Burning or other eye discomfort

Less common

Bitter taste following use in the eye; swelling of the membrane covering the white part of the eye; redness of the lining of the eyelids; increased sensitivity of eye to light

Other side effects not listed above may also occur in some patients. If you notice any other effects, check with your doctor.

Annual revision: 09/02/92

NYLIDRIN Systemic*

Some commonly used brand names are:

In Canada

Arlidin
Arlidin Forte
PMS Nylidrin

*Not commercially available in the U.S.

Description

Nylidrin (NYE-li-drin) belongs to the group of medicines called vasodilators. Vasodilators increase the size of blood vessels. Nylidrin is used to treat problems due to poor blood circulation.

Nylidrin is available only with your doctor's prescription, in the following dosage form:

Oral

- Tablets (Canada)

It is very important that you read and understand the following information. If any of it causes you special concern, check with your doctor. Also, *if you have any questions* or if you want more information about this medicine or your medical problem, *ask your doctor, nurse, or pharmacist.*

Before Using This Medicine

In deciding to use a medicine, the risks of taking the medicine must be weighed against the good it will do. This is a decision you and your doctor will make. For nylidrin, the following should be considered:

Allergies—Tell your doctor if you have ever had any unusual or allergic reaction to nylidrin. Also tell your doctor and pharmacist if you are allergic to any other substances, such as foods, preservatives, or dyes.

Pregnancy—Studies on effects in pregnancy have have not been done in either humans or animals.

Breast-feeding—It is not known whether nylidrin passes into breast milk. Although most medicines pass into breast milk in small amounts, many of them may be used safely while breast-feeding. Mothers who are taking this medicine and who wish to breast-feed should discuss this with their doctor.

Older adults—Many medicines have not been studied specifically in older people. Therefore, it may not be known whether they work exactly the same way they do in younger adults or if they cause different side effects or problems in older people. There is no specific information comparing use of nylidrin in the elderly with use in other age groups. However, nylidrin may reduce tolerance to cold temperatures in elderly patients.

Other medicines—Although certain medicines should not be used together at all, in other cases two different medicines may be used together even if an interaction might occur. In these cases, your doctor may want to change the dose, or other precautions may be necessary. Tell your doctor and pharmacist if you are taking any other prescription or nonprescription (over-the-counter [OTC]) medicine, or if you smoke.

Other medical problems—The presence of other medical problems may affect the use of nylidrin. Make sure you tell your doctor if you have any other medical problems, especially:

- Angina (chest pain) or
- Fast heartbeat or
- Heart attack (recent) or other heart disease or
- Overactive thyroid gland or
- Stomach ulcer—Nylidrin may make these conditions worse

Before you begin using any new medicine (prescription or nonprescription) or if you develop any new medical problem while you are using this medicine, check with your doctor, nurse, or pharmacist.

Proper Use of This Medicine

Nylidrin may cause you to have a fast or pounding heartbeat. To keep this from affecting your sleep, do not take the last dose of the day at bedtime. Instead, it is best to plan your dose or doses according to a schedule that will least affect your sleep. Ask your doctor, nurse, or pharmacist to help you plan the best time to take this medicine.

Dosing—The dose of nylidrin will be different for different patients. *Follow your doctor's orders or the directions on the label.* The following information includes only the average doses of nylidrin. *If your dose is different, do not change it* unless your doctor tells you to do so:

- For *oral* dosage form (tablets):
  —Adults: 3 to 12 milligrams (mg) three or four times a day.

Missed dose—If you miss a dose of this medicine, take the missed dose as soon as you remember. However, if it is almost time for the next dose, skip the missed dose and go back to your regular dosing schedule. Do not double doses.

Storage—To store this medicine:

- Keep out of the reach of children.
- Store away from heat and direct light.
- Do not store in the bathroom, near the kitchen sink, or in other damp places. Heat or moisture may cause the medicine to break down.

- Do not keep outdated medicine or medicine no longer needed. Be sure that any discarded medicine is out of the reach of children.

Precautions While Using This Medicine

It may take some time for this medicine to work. If you feel that the medicine is not working, do not stop taking it on your own. Instead, check with your doctor.

The helpful effects of this medicine may be decreased if you smoke. If you have any questions about this, check with your doctor.

Side Effects of This Medicine

Along with its needed effects, a medicine may cause some unwanted effects. Although not all of these side effects may occur, if they do occur they may need medical attention.

Check with your doctor as soon as possible if any of the following side effects occur:

Less common

Dizziness; fast or irregular heartbeat; weakness or tiredness (continuing)

Signs and symptoms of overdose

Blurred vision; chest pain; decrease in urination or inability to urinate; fever; metallic taste

Other side effects may occur that usually do not need medical attention. These side effects may go away during treatment as your body adjusts to the medicine. However, check with your doctor if any of the following side effects continue or are bothersome:

Less common

Chilliness; flushing or redness of face; headache; nausea and vomiting; nervousness; trembling

Other side effects not listed above may also occur in some patients. If you notice any other effects, check with your doctor.

Annual revision: 05/14/93

NYSTATIN Oral

Some commonly used brand names are:

In the U.S.

Mycostatin
Nystex
Nilstat

Generic name product may also be available.

In Canada

Mycostatin
Nilstat
Nadostine
PMS Nystatin

Description

Nystatin (nye-STAT-in) belongs to the group of medicines called antifungals. The dry powder, lozenge (pastille), and liquid forms of this medicine are used to treat fungus infections in the mouth.

Nystatin is available only with your doctor's prescription, in the following dosage forms:

Oral

- Lozenges (Pastilles) (U.S.)
- Oral suspension (U.S. and Canada)
- Powder for oral suspension (U.S. and Canada)
- Tablets (U.S. and Canada)

It is very important that you read and understand the following information. If any of it causes you special concern, check with your doctor. Also, *if you have any questions* or if you want more information about this medicine or your medical problem, *ask your doctor, nurse, or pharmacist*.

Before Using This Medicine

In deciding to use a medicine, the risks of taking the medicine must be weighed against the good it will do. This is a decision you and your doctor will make. For nystatin, the following should be considered:

Allergies—Tell your doctor if you have ever had any unusual or allergic reaction to nystatin. Also tell your doctor and pharmacist if you are allergic to any other substances, such as foods, preservatives, or dyes.

Pregnancy—Studies in humans have not shown that oral nystatin causes birth defects or other problems.

Breast-feeding—Oral nystatin has not been reported to cause problems in nursing babies.

Children—This medicine has been tested in children and has not been reported to cause different side effects or problems in children than it does in adults. However, since children up to 5 years of age may be too young to use the lozenges (pastilles) or tablets safely, the oral suspension dosage form is best for this age group.

Older adults—Many medicines have not been studied specifically in older people. Therefore, it may not be known whether they work exactly the same way they do in younger adults or if they cause different side effects or problems in older people. There is no specific information

comparing use of oral nystatin in the elderly with use in other age groups.

Before you begin using any new medicine (prescription or nonprescription) or if you develop any new medical problem while you are using this medicine, check with your doctor, nurse, or pharmacist.

Proper Use of This Medicine

For patients taking the *dry powder form of nystatin*:

- Add about 1/8 teaspoonful of dry powder to about 4 ounces of water immediately before taking. Stir well.
- After it is mixed, take this medicine by dividing the whole amount (4 ounces) into several portions. Hold each portion of the medicine in your mouth or swish it around in your mouth for as long as possible, gargle, and swallow. Be sure to use all the liquid to get the full dose of medicine.

For patients taking the *lozenge (pastille) form of nystatin*:

- Nystatin lozenges (pastilles) should be held in the mouth and allowed to dissolve slowly and completely. This may take 15 to 30 minutes. Also, the saliva should be swallowed during this time. *Do not chew or swallow the lozenges whole.*
- *Do not give nystatin lozenges (pastilles) to infants or children up to 5 years of age.* They may be too young to use the lozenges safely.

For patients taking the *oral liquid form of nystatin*:

- This medicine is to be taken by mouth even if it comes in a dropper bottle. If it does come in a dropper bottle, use the specially marked dropper to measure each dose accurately.
- Take this medicine by placing one-half of the dose in each side of your mouth. Hold the medicine in your mouth or swish it around in your mouth for as long as possible, then gargle and swallow.

Patients with full or partial dentures may need to soak their dentures nightly in nystatin for oral suspension to eliminate the fungus from the dentures. In rare cases when this does not eliminate the fungus, it may be necessary to have new dentures made.

To help clear up your infection completely, *keep taking this medicine for the full time of treatment,* even if your condition has improved. *Do not miss any doses.*

Dosing—The dose of nystatin will be different for different patients. *Follow your doctor's orders or the directions on the label.* The following information includes only the average doses of nystatin. *If your dose is different, do not change it* unless your doctor tells you to do so.

- The number of lozenges, tablets, or milliliters (mL) of suspension that you take depends on the strength of the medicine. Also, *the number of doses you take each day, the time allowed between doses, and the length of time you take the medicine depend on the medical problem for which you are taking nystatin.*
- For the *lozenge (pastille) and tablet* dosage forms:
  —Adults and children 5 years of age and older: 1 or 2 lozenges or tablets three to five times a day for up to fourteen days.

  —Children up to 5 years of age: Children this young may not be able to use the lozenges or tablets safely. The oral suspension is better for this age group.
- For the *suspension* dosage form:
  —Adults and children 5 years of age and older: 4 to 6 milliliters (mL) (about 1 teaspoonful) four times a day.

  —For older infants: 2 mL four times a day.

  —For premature and low-birth-weight infants: 1 mL four times a day.

Missed dose—If you do miss a dose of this medicine, take it as soon as possible. However, if it is almost time for your next dose, skip the missed dose and go back to your regular dosing schedule. Do not double doses.

Storage—To store this medicine:

- Keep out of the reach of children.
- Store away from heat and direct light.
- Do not store the tablet or dry powder form of this medicine in the bathroom, near the kitchen sink, or in other damp places. Heat or moisture may cause the medicine to break down.
- Store the lozenge (pastille) form in the refrigerator. Heat will cause this medicine to break down.
- Keep the oral liquid form of this medicine from freezing.
- Do not keep outdated medicine or medicine no longer needed. Be sure that any discarded medicine is out of the reach of children.

Side Effects of This Medicine

Along with its needed effects, a medicine may cause some unwanted effects. The following side effects may go away during treatment as your body adjusts to the medicine. However, check with your doctor if any of the following side effects continue or are bothersome:

Less common

Diarrhea; nausea or vomiting; stomach pain

Other side effects not listed above may also occur in some patients. If you notice any other effects, check with your doctor.

Additional Information

Once a medicine has been approved for marketing for a certain use, experience may show that it is also useful

for other medical problems. Although this use is not included in product labeling, nystatin is used in certain patients with the following medical condition:

- Candidiasis, oral (fungus infection of the mouth) (prevention)

Other than the above information, there is no additional information relating to proper use, precautions, or side effects for this use.

Annual revision: 01/19/93

NYSTATIN Topical

Some commonly used brand names are:

In the U.S.

Mycostatin	Nystex
Nilstat	

Generic name product may also be available.

In Canada

Mycostatin	Nilstat
Nadostine	Nyaderm

Description

Nystatin (nye-STAT-in) belongs to the group of medicines called antifungals. Topical nystatin is used to treat some types of fungus infections.

Nystatin is available only with your doctor's prescription, in the following dosage forms:

Topical

- Cream (U.S. and Canada)
- Ointment (U.S. and Canada)
- Topical powder (U.S. and Canada)

It is very important that you read and understand the following information. If any of it causes you special concern, check with your doctor. Also, *if you have any questions* or if you want more information about this medicine or your medical problem, *ask your doctor, nurse, or pharmacist.*

Before Using This Medicine

In deciding to use a medicine, the risks of taking the medicine must be weighed against the good it will do. This is a decision you and your doctor will make. For nystatin, the following should be considered:

Allergies—Tell your doctor if you have ever had any unusual or allergic reaction to nystatin. Also tell your doctor and pharmacist if you are allergic to any other substances, such as preservatives or dyes.

Pregnancy—Nystatin topical preparations have not been shown to cause birth defects or other problems in humans.

Breast-feeding—It is not known whether nystatin passes into the breast milk. However, this medicine has not been reported to cause problems in nursing babies.

Children—This medicine has been tested in children and, in effective doses, has not been shown to cause different side effects or problems than it does in adults.

Older adults—Many medicines have not been tested in older people. Therefore, it may not be known whether they work exactly the same way they do in younger adults or if they cause different side effects or problems in older people. There is no specific information about the use of topical nystatin in the elderly.

Other medicines—Although certain medicines should not be used together at all, in other cases two different medicines may be used together even if an interaction might occur. In these cases, your doctor may want to change the dose, or other precautions may be necessary. When you are using nystatin, it is important that your doctor and pharmacist know if you are using any other topical prescription or nonprescription (over-the-counter [OTC]) medicine that is to be applied to the same area of the skin.

Before you begin using any new medicine (prescription or nonprescription) or if you develop any new medical problem while you are using this medicine, check with your doctor, nurse, or pharmacist.

Proper Use of This Medicine

Apply enough nystatin to cover the affected area.

For patients using the *powder form* of this medicine on the feet:

- Sprinkle the powder between the toes, on the feet, and in socks and shoes.

The use of any kind of occlusive dressing (airtight covering, such as kitchen plastic wrap) over this medicine may increase the chance of irritation. Therefore, *do not bandage, wrap, or apply any occlusive dressing over this medicine* unless directed to do so by your doctor. When using this medicine on the diaper area of children, *avoid tight-fitting diapers and plastic pants.*

To help clear up your infection completely, *keep using this medicine for the full time of treatment,* even if your condition has improved. *Do not miss any doses.*

Missed dose—If you do miss a dose of this medicine, apply it as soon as possible. Then go back to your regular dosing schedule.

Storage—To store this medicine:
- Keep out of the reach of children.
- Store away from heat and direct light.
- Do not store the powder form of this medicine in the bathroom, near the kitchen sink, or in other damp places. Heat or moisture may cause the medicine to break down.
- Keep the cream and ointment forms of this medicine from freezing.
- Do not keep outdated medicine or medicine no longer needed. Be sure that any discarded medicine is out of the reach of children.

Side Effects of This Medicine

Along with its needed effects, a medicine may cause some unwanted effects. Although not all of these side effects may occur, if they do occur they may need medical attention.

Check with your doctor as soon as possible if the following side effect occurs:

Skin irritation not present before use of this medicine

Other side effects not listed above may also occur in some patients. If you notice any other effects, check with your doctor.

Annual revision: May 1990

NYSTATIN Vaginal

Some commonly used brand names are:

In the U.S.

Mycostatin	Nilstat

Generic name product may also be available.

In Canada

Mycostatin	Nilstat
Nadostine	Nyaderm

Description

Nystatin (nye-STAT-in) belongs to the group of medicines called antifungals. Vaginal nystatin is used to treat fungus infections of the vagina. Nystatin vaginal cream or tablets may also be used for other problems as determined by your doctor.

Nystatin is available only with your doctor's prescription, in the following dosage forms:

Vaginal
- Cream (Canada)
- Tablets (U.S. and Canada)

It is very important that you read and understand the following information. If any of it causes you special concern, check with your doctor. Also, *if you have any questions* or if you want more information about this medicine or your medical problem, *ask your doctor, nurse, or pharmacist.*

Before Using This Medicine

In deciding to use a medicine, the risks of taking the medicine must be weighed against the good it will do. This is a decision you and your doctor will make. For nystatin, the following should be considered:

Allergies—Tell your doctor if you have ever had any unusual or allergic reaction to nystatin. Also tell your doctor and pharmacist if you are allergic to any other substances, such as foods, preservatives, or dyes.

Pregnancy—Studies have not been done in animals. However, nystatin vaginal tablets have not been shown to cause birth defects or other problems in humans.

Breast-feeding—It is not known whether nystatin passes into breast milk. However, this medicine has not been reported to cause problems in nursing babies.

Children—Studies on this medicine have been done only in adults, and there is no specific information comparing use of vaginal nystatin in children with use in other age groups.

Older adults—Many medicines have not been studied specifically in older people. Therefore, it may not be known whether they work exactly the same way they do in younger adults or if they cause different side effects or problems in older people. There is no specific information comparing the use of vaginal nystatin in the elderly with use in other age groups.

Other medicines—Although certain medicines should not be used together at all, in other cases two different medicines may be used together even if an interaction might occur. In these cases, your doctor may want to change the dose, or other precautions may be necessary. Tell your doctor and pharmacist if you are using any other vaginal prescription or nonprescription (over-the-counter [OTC]) medicine.

Before you begin using any new medicine (prescription or nonprescription) or if you develop any new medical problem while you are using this medicine, check with your doctor, nurse, or pharmacist.

Proper Use of This Medicine

Nystatin usually comes with patient directions. Read them carefully before using this medicine.

This medicine is usually inserted into the vagina with an applicator. However, if you are pregnant, check with your doctor before using the applicator to insert the vaginal tablet.

To help clear up your infection completely, *keep using this medicine for the full time of treatment,* even if your condition has improved. Also, keep using this medicine even if you begin to menstruate during the time of treatment. *Do not miss any doses.*

Missed dose—If you do miss a dose of this medicine, insert it as soon as possible. However, if it is almost time for your next dose, skip the missed dose and go back to your regular dosing schedule.

Storage—To store this medicine:

- Keep out of the reach of children.
- Store away from heat and direct light.
- Do not store in the bathroom, near the kitchen sink, or in other damp places. Heat or moisture may cause the medicine to break down.
- Do not keep outdated medicine or medicine no longer needed. Be sure that any discarded medicine is out of the reach of children.

Precautions While Using This Medicine

To help cure the infection and to help prevent reinfection, good health habits are required.

- Wear cotton panties (or panties or pantyhose with cotton crotches) instead of synthetic (for example, nylon, rayon) underclothes.
- Wear freshly laundered underclothes.

If you have any questions about this, check with your doctor, nurse, or pharmacist.

If you have any questions about douching or intercourse during the time of treatment with nystatin, check with your doctor.

Since there may be some vaginal drainage while you are using this medicine, a sanitary napkin may be worn to protect your clothing.

Side Effects of This Medicine

Along with its needed effects, a medicine may cause some unwanted effects. Although not all of these side effects may occur, if they do occur they may need medical attention.

Check with your doctor as soon as possible if the following side effect occurs:

Rare

Vaginal irritation not present before use of this medicine

Other side effects not listed above may also occur in some patients. If you notice any other effects, check with your doctor.

Annual revision: 09/08/92

NYSTATIN AND TRIAMCINOLONE Topical

Some commonly used brand names in the U.S. are:

Dermacomb	Myco-Triacet II
Myco II	Mykacet
Mycobiotic II	Mykacet II
Mycogen II	Mytrex
Mycolog II	Tristatin II

Generic name product may also be available.

Description

Nystatin (nye-STAT-in) and triamcinolone (trye-am-SIN-oh-lone) combination contains an antifungal and an adrenocorticoid (a-dree-noe-KOR-ti-koid) (cortisone-like medicine).

Antifungals are used to treat infections caused by a fungus. They work by killing the fungus or preventing its growth. This medicine will not work for other kinds of infections. Adrenocorticoids belong to the family of medicines called steroids. They are used to help relieve redness, swelling, itching, and other discomfort of many skin problems.

This medicine is used to treat certain fungus infections, such as Candida (Monilia), and to help relieve the discomfort of the infection.

Topical adrenocorticoids may rarely cause some serious side effects. Some of the side effects may be more likely to occur in children. *Before using this medicine in children, be sure to talk to your doctor about these problems, as well as the good this medicine may do.*

Nystatin and triamcinolone combination is available only with your doctor's prescription, in the following dosage forms:

Topical

- Cream (U.S.)
- Ointment (U.S.)

It is very important that you read and understand the following information. If any of it causes you special concern, check with your doctor. Also, *if you have any questions* or if you want more information about this medicine or your medical problem, *ask your doctor, nurse, or pharmacist.*

Before Using This Medicine

In deciding to use a medicine, the risks of taking the medicine must be weighed against the good it will do. This is a decision you and your doctor will make. For nystatin and triamcinolone combination, the following should be considered:

Allergies—Tell your doctor if you have ever had any unusual or allergic reaction to nystatin or triamcinolone. Also tell your doctor and pharmacist if you are allergic to any other substances, such as preservatives or dyes.

Pregnancy—Nystatin and triamcinolone combination has not been studied in pregnant women. However, studies in animals have shown that adrenocorticoids given by mouth or by injection may cause birth defects, even at low doses. Also, some of the stronger adrenocorticoids have been shown to cause birth defects when applied to the skin of animals. Therefore, this medicine should not be used on large areas of skin, in large amounts, or for a long time in pregnant patients. Before taking this medicine, make sure your doctor knows if you are pregnant or if you may become pregnant.

Breast-feeding—It is not known whether nystatin or triamcinolone passes into the breast milk. Although this combination medicine has not been reported to cause problems in humans, topical adrenocorticoids may be absorbed into the body. Also, adrenocorticoids given by mouth or by injection do pass into the breast milk and may cause unwanted effects, such as interfering with nursing babies' growth.

Children—Children may be especially sensitive to the effects of topical nystatin and triamcinolone combination. This may increase the chance of side effects during treatment. Therefore, it is especially important that you discuss with your child's doctor the good that this medicine may do as well as the risks of using it.

Older adults—Many medicines have not been tested in older people. Therefore, it may not be known whether they work exactly the same way they do in younger adults. Although there is no specific information about the use of topical nystatin and triamcinolone combination in the elderly, it is not expected to cause different side effects or problems in older people than it does in younger adults.

Other medicines—Although certain medicines should not be used together at all, in other cases two different medicines may be used together even if an interaction might occur. In these cases, your doctor may want to change the dose, or other precautions may be necessary. When you are using nystatin and triamcinolone combination, it is especially important that your doctor and pharmacist know if you are using any other prescription or nonprescription (over-the-counter [OTC]) medicine.

Other medical problems—The presence of other medical problems may affect the use of nystatin and triamcinolone combination. Make sure you tell your doctor if you have any other medical problems, especially:

- Herpes
- Vaccinia (cowpox)
- Varicella (chickenpox)
- Other virus infections of the skin—Triamcinolone may speed up the spread of virus infections
- Tuberculosis (TB) of the skin—Triamcinolone may make a TB infection worse

Before you begin using any new medicine (prescription or nonprescription) or if you develop any new medical problem while you are using this medicine, check with your doctor, nurse, or pharmacist.

Proper Use of This Medicine

Do not use this medicine in or around the eyes.

Check with your doctor before using this medicine on any other skin problems. It should not be used on bacterial or virus infections. Also, it should only be used on certain fungus infections of the skin.

Apply a thin layer of this medicine to the affected area and rub in gently and thoroughly.

The use of any kind of airtight covering over this medicine may increase absorption of the medicine and the chance of irritation and other side effects. Therefore, *do not bandage, wrap, or apply any airtight covering or other occlusive dressing (for example, kitchen plastic wrap) over this medicine* unless directed to do so by your doctor. Also, wear loose-fitting clothing when using this medicine on the groin area. When using this medicine on the diaper area of children, *avoid tight-fitting diapers and plastic pants.*

To help clear up your infection completely, *keep using this medicine for the full time of treatment,* even if your symptoms have disappeared. *Do not miss any doses.*

However, *do not use this medicine more often or for a longer time than your doctor ordered.* To do so may increase absorption through your skin and the chance of side effects. In addition, too much use, especially on thin skin areas (for example, face, armpits, groin), may result in thinning of the skin and stretch marks.

Missed dose—If you do miss a dose of this medicine, apply it as soon as possible. However, if it is almost time for your next dose, skip the missed dose and go back to your regular dosing schedule.

Storage—To store this medicine:

- Keep out of the reach of children.
- Store away from heat and direct light.
- Keep the medicine from freezing.
- Do not keep outdated medicine or medicine no longer needed. Be sure that any discarded medicine is out of the reach of children.

Precautions While Using This Medicine

To help clear up your infection completely and to help make sure it does not return, good health habits are also required. Keep the affected area as cool and dry as possible.

If your skin problem does not improve within 2 or 3 weeks, or if it becomes worse, check with your doctor.

The adrenocorticoid in this medicine may be absorbed through the skin and may be more likely to cause side effects in children. Long-term use may affect growth and development as well. *Children who must use this medicine should be followed closely by their doctor.*

For diabetic patients:

- *Although rare, the adrenocorticoid in this medicine may cause higher blood and urine sugar levels, especially if you have severe diabetes and are using large amounts of this medicine.* Check with your doctor before changing your diet or the dosage of your diabetes medicine.

Side Effects of This Medicine

Along with its needed effects, a medicine may cause some unwanted effects. Although not all of these side effects may occur, if they do occur they may need medical attention.

Check with your doctor immediately if any of the following side effects occur:

Rare

Blistering, burning, itching, peeling, dryness, or other sign of irritation not present before use of this medicine

Additional side effects may occur if you use this medicine for a long time. Check with your doctor as soon as possible if any of the following side effects occur:

Acne or oily skin; increased hair growth, especially on the face; increased loss of hair, especially on the scalp; reddish purple lines on arms, face, legs, trunk, or groin; thinning of skin with easy bruising

Many of the above side effects are more likely to occur in children, who may absorb greater amounts of this medicine.

Other side effects not listed above may also occur in some patients. If you notice any other effects, check with your doctor.

Annual revision: May 1990

OCTREOTIDE Systemic

A commonly used brand name in the U.S. and Canada is Sandostatin.

Description

Octreotide (oak-TREE-oh-tide) is used to treat the severe diarrhea and other symptoms that occur with certain intestinal tumors. It does not cure the tumor but it helps the patient live a more normal life. Octreotide may also be used for other medical conditions as determined by your doctor.

Octreotide is available only with your doctor's prescription, in the following dosage form:

Parenteral
- Injection (U.S. and Canada)

It is very important that you read and understand the following information. If any of it causes you special concern, check with your doctor. Also, *if you have any questions* or if you want more information about this medicine or your medical problem, *ask your doctor, nurse, or pharmacist.*

O

Before Using This Medicine

In deciding to use a medicine, the risks of using the medicine must be weighed against the good it will do. This is a decision you and your doctor will make. For octreotide, the following should be considered:

Allergies—Tell your doctor if you have ever had any unusual or allergic reaction to octreotide. Also tell your doctor and pharmacist if you are allergic to any other substances, such as foods, preservatives, or dyes.

Pregnancy—Studies have not been done in humans. However, studies in rats and rabbits have not shown that octreotide causes birth defects or other problems, even when given in doses many times the human dose.

Breast-feeding—It is not known whether octreotide passes into the breast milk. However, octreotide has not been reported to cause problems in nursing babies.

Children—This medicine has been tested in a limited number of children as young as 1 month of age and has not been shown to cause different side effects or problems than it does in adults.

Older adults—This medicine has been used in persons up to 83 years of age and has not been shown to cause different side effects or problems in older people than it does in younger adults.

Other medicines—Although certain medicines should not be used together at all, in other cases two different medicines may be used together even if an interaction might occur. In these cases, your doctor may want to change the dose, or other precautions may be necessary. When you are taking octreotide, it is especially important that your doctor and pharmacist know if you are taking any of the following:

- Antidiabetics, oral (diabetes medicine you take by mouth) or
- Glucagon or
- Insulin—Octreotide may cause high or low blood sugar; your doctor may need to change the dose of your diabetes medicine
- Growth hormone—Octreotide may cause high or low blood sugar; your doctor may need to change the dose of this medicine

Other medical problems—The presence of other medical problems may affect the use of octreotide. Make sure you tell your doctor if you have any other medical problems, especially:

- Diabetes mellitus (sugar diabetes)—Octreotide may cause high or low blood sugar; your doctor may need to change the dose of your diabetes medicine
- Gallbladder disease or gallstones (or history of)—This medicine may increase the chance of having gallstones
- Kidney disease (severe)—If you have this condition, octreotide may remain longer in the body; your doctor may need to change the dose of your medicine

Proper Use Of This Medicine

To control the symptoms of your medical problem, this medicine must be taken daily in evenly spaced doses as ordered by your doctor. He or she will tell you how much octreotide you need to take each day and how to divide the doses through the day. *Make sure that you understand exactly how to use this medicine.*

Octreotide is packaged in a kit containing an ampul opener, alcohol swabs, and ampuls of the medicine. *Directions on how to use the medicine are in the package. Read them carefully* and ask your doctor, nurse, or pharmacist for additional explanation, if necessary.

Missed dose—If you miss a dose of this medicine, use it as soon as you remember it. However, if it is almost time for the next dose, skip the missed dose and go back to your regular dosing schedule. Do not double doses. Although you will not be harmed by forgetting a dose, the symptoms that you are trying to control (for example, diarrhea) may reappear. To be able to control your symptoms, your doses should be evenly spaced over a period of 24 hours. If you have any questions about this, check with your doctor, nurse, or pharmacist.

Storage—To store this medicine:
- Keep out of the reach of children.
- Store the ampuls of octreotide in the refrigerator until they are to be used. Remove the ampul that is

going to be used from the refrigerator and allow it to reach room temperature before using it. Using octreotide at room temperature will help lessen the burning sensation that some people feel when injecting octreotide. Ampuls may be kept at room temperature for the day they will be used; however, they should not be kept at room temperature for longer than 24 hours.

- Do not keep outdated medicine or medicine no longer needed. Be sure that any discarded medicine and syringes are out of the reach of children.

Precautions While Using This Medicine

It is very important that your doctor check your progress at regular visits to make sure that this medicine is working properly and to check for unwanted effects.

It is very important to follow any instructions from your doctor about the careful selection and rotation of injection sites on your body. This will help prevent skin problems, such as irritation.

Side Effects of This Medicine

Along with its needed effects, a medicine may cause some unwanted effects. Although these problems are rare, patients using octreotide may develop symptoms of high blood sugar (hyperglycemia) or low blood sugar (hypoglycemia). *If any of the following symptoms of hyperglycemia or hypoglycemia occur, stop using octreotide and check with your doctor right away:*

Symptoms of hyperglycemia usually include:

Drowsiness; dry mouth; flushed, dry skin; fruit-like breath odor; increased urination; loss of appetite; stomachache, nausea, or vomiting; troubled breathing (rapid and deep); unusual thirst; unusual tiredness; weight loss (rapid)

Early symptoms of hypoglycemia include:

Anxious feeling; chills; cool pale skin; difficulty in concentrating; headache; hunger; nausea; nervousness; shakiness; sweating; unusual tiredness; weakness

Other side effects may occur that usually do not need medical attention. These side effects may go away during treatment as your body adjusts to the medicine. However, check with your doctor if any of the following side effects continue or are bothersome:

More common

Abdominal or stomach pain or discomfort; diarrhea; nausea and vomiting; pain, stinging, tingling, or burning sensation at place of injection, with redness and swelling

Less common or rare

Dizziness or lightheadedness; unusual tiredness or weakness; headache; redness or flushing of face; swelling of feet and lower legs

Other side effects not listed above may also occur in some patients. If you notice any other effects, check with your doctor.

Additional Information

Once a medicine has been approved for marketing for a certain use, experience may show that it is also useful for other medical problems. Although this use is not included in product labeling, octreotide is used in certain patients with the following medical conditions:

- Acromegaly (enlargement of the face, hands, and feet because of too much growth hormone)
- Acquired immune deficiency syndrome (AIDS)–related diarrhea
- Insulin-producing tumors of the pancreas

Other than the above information, there is no additional information relating to proper use, precautions, or side effects for these uses.

Annual revision: 12/15/92

OLSALAZINE Oral

A commonly used brand name in the U.S. and Canada is Dipentum. Other commonly used names are sodium azodisalicylate and azodisal sodium.

Description

Olsalazine (ole-SAL-a-zeen) is used in patients who have had ulcerative colitis to prevent the condition from occurring again. It works inside the bowel by helping to reduce the inflammation and other symptoms of the disease.

Olsalazine is available only with your doctor's prescription, in the following dosage form:

Oral

- Capsules (U.S. and Canada)

It is very important that you read and understand the following information. If any of it causes you special

concern, check with your doctor. Also, *if you have any questions* or if you want more information about this medicine or your medical problem, *ask your doctor, nurse, or pharmacist.*

Before Using This Medicine

In deciding to use a medicine, the risks of taking the medicine must be weighed against the good it will do. This is a decision you and your doctor will make. For olsalazine, the following should be considered:

Allergies—Tell your doctor if you have ever had any unusual or allergic reaction to olsalazine, mesalamine, or any salicylates (for example, aspirin). Also tell your doctor and pharmacist if you are allergic to any other substances, such as foods, preservatives, or dyes.

Pregnancy—Studies have not been done in humans. However, studies in rats have shown that olsalazine causes birth defects and other problems at doses 5 to 20 times the human dose. Before taking this medicine, make sure your doctor knows if you are pregnant or if you may become pregnant.

Breast-feeding—It is not known whether olsalazine passes into the breast milk.

Children—Studies on this medicine have been done only in adult patients, and there is no specific information comparing use of olsalazine in children with use in other age groups.

Older adults—Many medicines have not been studied specifically in older people. Therefore, it may not be known whether they work exactly the same way they do in younger adults. Although there is no specific information comparing use of olsalazine in the elderly with use in other age groups, this medicine is not expected to cause different side effects or problems in older people than it does in younger adults.

Other medicines—Although certain medicines should not be used together at all, in other cases two different medicines may be used together even if an interaction might occur. In these cases, your doctor may want to change the dose, or other precautions may be necessary. When you are using olsalazine, it is especially important that your doctor and pharmacist know if you are taking any other medicines.

Other medical problems—The presence of other medical problems may affect the use of olsalazine. Make sure you tell your doctor if you have any other medical problems, especially:

- Kidney disease—The use of olsalazine may cause further damage to the kidneys

Before you begin using any new medicine (prescription or nonprescription) or if you develop any new medical problem while you are using this medicine, check with your doctor, nurse, or pharmacist.

Proper Use of This Medicine

Olsalazine is best taken with food, to lessen stomach upset and diarrhea. If stomach or intestinal problems continue or are bothersome, check with your doctor.

Keep taking this medicine for the full time of treatment, even if you begin to feel better after a few days. *Do not miss any doses.*

Missed dose—If you do miss a dose of this medicine, take it as soon as possible. However, if it is almost time for your next dose, skip the missed dose and go back to your regular dosing schedule. Do not double doses.

Storage—To store this medicine:

- Keep out of the reach of children.
- Store away from heat and direct light.
- Do not store this medicine in the bathroom, near the kitchen sink, or in other damp places. Heat or moisture may cause the medicine to break down.
- Do not keep outdated medicine or medicine no longer needed. Be sure that any discarded medicine is out of the reach of children.

Precautions While Using This Medicine

It is very important that your doctor check your progress at regular visits, especially if you will be taking it for a long time. Olsalazine may cause blood problems.

Side Effects of This Medicine

Along with its needed effects, a medicine may cause some unwanted effects. Although not all of these side effects may occur, if they do occur they may need medical attention.

Check with your doctor as soon as possible if any of the following side effects occur:

Rare

Bloody diarrhea; fever; pale skin; skin rash; sore throat; unusual bleeding or bruising; unusual tiredness or weakness; yellow eyes or skin

Other side effects may occur that usually do not need medical attention. These side effects may go away during treatment as your body adjusts to the medicine. However, check with your doctor if any of the following side effects continue or are bothersome:

More common

Abdominal or stomach pain or upset; diarrhea; loss of appetite; nausea or vomiting

Less common

Aching joints and muscles; acne; anxiety or depression, drowsiness or dizziness; headache; insomnia

Other side effects not listed above may also occur in some patients. If you notice any other effects, check with your doctor.

Annual revision: 05/13/91

OMEPRAZOLE Systemic

Some commonly used brand names are:

In the U.S.

Prilosec

In Canada

Losec

Description

Omeprazole (o-MEP-ra-zole) is used to treat certain conditions in which there is too much acid in the stomach. It is used to treat duodenal ulcers and gastroesophageal reflux disease, a condition in which the acid in the stomach washes back up into the esophagus. Omeprazole is also used to treat Zollinger-Ellison disease, a condition in which the stomach produces too much acid. It may also be used for other conditions as determined by your doctor.

Omeprazole works by decreasing the amount of acid produced by the stomach.

This medicine is available only with your doctor's prescription.

Oral

- Delayed-release capsules (U.S. and Canada)

It is very important that you read and understand the following information. If any of it causes you special concern, check with your doctor. Also, *if you have any questions* or if you want more information about this medicine or your medical problem, *ask your doctor, nurse, or pharmacist.*

Before Using This Medicine

In deciding to use a medicine, the risks of taking the medicine must be weighed against the good it will do. This is a decision you and your doctor will make. For omeprazole, the following should be considered:

Allergies—Tell your doctor if you have ever had any unusual or allergic reaction to omeprazole. Also tell your doctor and pharmacist if you are allergic to any other substances, such as foods, preservatives, or dyes.

Pregnancy—Studies have not been done in humans. However, studies in animals have shown that omeprazole may cause harm to the fetus.

Breast-feeding—Omeprazole may pass into the breast milk. Since this medicine has been shown to cause unwanted effects, such as tumors and cancer in animals, it may be necessary for you to take another medicine or to stop breast-feeding during treatment. Be sure you have discussed the risks and benefits of the medicine with your doctor.

Children—There is no specific information comparing the use of omeprazole in children with use in other age groups.

Older adults—Many medicines have not been studied specifically in older people. Therefore, it may not be known whether they work exactly the same way they do in younger adults or if they cause different side effects or problems in older people. There is no specific information comparing use of omeprazole in the elderly with use in other age groups.

Other medicines—Although certain medicines should not be used together at all, in other cases two different medicines may be used together even if an interaction might occur. In these cases, your doctor may want to change the dose, or other precautions may be necessary. When you are taking omeprazole, it is especially important that your doctor and pharmacist know if you are taking any of the following:

- Anticoagulants (blood thinners) or
- Diazepam (e.g., Valium) or
- Phenytoin (e.g., Dilantin)—Use with omeprazole may cause high blood levels of these medicines, which may increase the chance of side effects

Other medical problems—The presence of other medical problems may affect the use of omeprazole. Make sure you tell your doctor if you have any other medical problems, especially:

- Liver disease or a history of liver disease—This condition may cause omeprazole to build up in the body

Before you begin using any new medicine (prescription or nonprescription) or if you develop any new medical problem while you are using this medicine, check with your doctor, nurse, or pharmacist.

Proper Use of This Medicine

Take omeprazole immediately before a meal, preferably in the morning.

It may take several days before this medicine begins to relieve stomach pain. To help relieve this pain, antacids may be taken with omeprazole, unless your doctor has told you not to use them.

Swallow the capsule whole. Do not crush, break, chew, or open the capsule.

Take this medicine for the full time of treatment, even if you begin to feel better. Also, keep your appointments with your doctor for check-ups so that your doctor will be better able to tell you when to stop taking this medicine.

Missed dose—If you miss a dose of this medicine, take it as soon as possible. However, if it is almost time for your next dose, skip the missed dose and go back to your regular dosing schedule. Do not double doses.

Storage—To store this medicine:

- Keep out of the reach of children.
- Store away from heat and direct light.
- Do not store in the bathroom, near the kitchen sink, or in other damp places. Heat or moisture may cause the medicine to break down.
- Do not keep outdated medicine or medicine no longer needed. Be sure that any discarded medicine is out of the reach of children.

Precautions While Using This Medicine

If your condition does not improve, or if it becomes worse, check with your doctor.

Side Effects of This Medicine

Along with its needed effects, a medicine may cause some unwanted effects. Although not all of these side effects may occur, if they do occur they may need medical attention.

Check with your doctor as soon as possible if any of the following side effects occur:

Rare

Bloody or cloudy urine; continuing ulcers or sores in mouth; difficult, burning, or painful urination; frequent urge to urinate; sore throat and fever; unusual bleeding or bruising; unusual tiredness or weakness

Other side effects may occur that usually do not need medical attention. These side effects may go away during treatment as your body adjusts to the medicine. However, check with your doctor if any of the following side effects continue or are bothersome:

More common

Abdominal or stomach pain

Less common

Chest pain; constipation; diarrhea or loose stools; dizziness; gas; headache; heartburn; muscle pain; nausea and vomiting; skin rash or itching; unusual drowsiness; unusual tiredness

Other side effects not listed above may also occur in some patients. If you notice any other effects, check with your doctor.

Additional Information

Once a medicine has been approved for marketing for a certain use, experience may show that it is also useful for other medical problems. Although this use is not included in product labeling, omeprazole is used in certain patients with the following medical condition:

- Gastric ulcer

Other than the above information, there is no additional information relating to proper use, precautions, or side effects for these uses.

Annual revision: 02/25/92

ONDANSETRON Systemic†

A commonly used brand name in the U.S. is Zofran.

†Not commercially available in Canada.

Description

Ondansetron (on-DAN-se-tron) is used to prevent the nausea and vomiting that may occur after treatment with anti-cancer medicines.

Ondansetron is to be given only by or under the immediate supervision of your doctor. It is available in the following dosage form:

Parenteral

- Injection (U.S.)

It is very important that you read and understand the following information. If any of it causes you special

concern, check with your doctor. Also, *if you have any questions* or if you want more information about this medicine or your medical problem, *ask your doctor, nurse, or pharmacist.*

Before Using This Medicine

In deciding to use a medicine, the risks of taking the medicine must be weighed against the good it will do. This is a decision you and your doctor will make. For ondansetron, the following should be considered:

Allergies—Tell your doctor if you have ever had any unusual or allergic reaction to ondansetron. Also tell your doctor and pharmacist if you are allergic to any other substances, such as foods, preservatives, or dyes.

Pregnancy—Ondansetron has not been studied in pregnant women. However, this medicine has not been shown to cause birth defects or other problems in animal studies.

Breast-feeding—It is not known whether ondansetron passes into the breast milk.

Children—This medicine has been tested in a limited number of children 4 years of age or older. In effective doses, the medicine has not been shown to cause different side effects or problems than it does in adults.

Older adults—This medicine has been tested in a limited number of patients 65 years of age or older and has not been shown to cause different side effects or problems in older people than it does in younger adults.

Other medicines—Although certain medicines should not be used together at all, in other cases two different medicines may be used together even if an interaction might occur. In these cases, your doctor may want to change the dose, or other precautions may be necessary. Tell your doctor and pharmacist if you are taking any other prescription or nonprescription (over-the-counter [OTC]) medicine.

Side Effects of This Medicine

Along with its needed effects, a medicine may cause some unwanted effects. Although not all of these side effects may occur, if they do occur they may need medical attention.

Check with your doctor or nurse immediately if any of the following side effects occur:

Rare

Shortness of breath; tightness in chest; troubled breathing; wheezing

Other side effects may occur that usually do not need medical attention. These side effects may go away during treatment as your body adjusts to the medicine. However, check with your doctor if any of the following side effects continue or are bothersome:

More common

Constipation; diarrhea; fever and/or chills; headache

Less common

Abdominal pain or stomach cramps; dizziness or lightheadedness; drowsiness; dryness of mouth; skin rash; unusual tiredness or weakness

Other side effects not listed above may also occur in some patients. If you notice any other effects, check with your doctor.

Annual revision: 07/16/91

OPIUM PREPARATIONS Systemic

This information applies to the following medicines:

Opium Tincture (OH-pee-um)
Paregoric (par-e-GOR-ik)

Some commonly used names are:

For Opium Tincture
In the U.S.
Laudanum
In Canada
Laudanum

For Paregoric
In the U.S.
Camphorated Opium Tincture
In Canada
Camphorated Opium Tincture

Description

Opium preparations are used along with other measures to treat severe diarrhea. These medicines belong to the group of medicines called narcotics. If too much of a narcotic is taken, it may become habit-forming, causing mental or physical dependence. Physical dependence may lead to withdrawal side effects when you stop taking the medicine.

Opium preparations are available only with your doctor's prescription, in the following dosage forms:

Oral

Opium Tincture
- Oral liquid (U.S. and Canada)

Paregoric
- Oral liquid (U.S. and Canada)

It is very important that you read and understand the following information. If any of it causes you special concern, check with your doctor. Also, *if you have any questions* or if you want more information about this medicine or your medical problem, *ask your doctor, nurse, or pharmacist.*

Before Using This Medicine

In deciding to use a medicine, the risks of taking the medicine must be weighed against the good it will do. This is a decision you and your doctor will make. For opium preparations, the following should be considered:

Allergies—Tell your doctor if you have ever had any unusual or allergic reaction to morphine, codeine, or papaverine. Also tell your doctor and pharmacist if you are allergic to any other substances, such as foods, preservatives, or dyes.

Pregnancy—Opium preparations have not been studied in pregnant women. However, morphine (contained in these medicines) has caused birth defects in animals when given in very large doses.

Regular use of opium preparations during pregnancy may cause the fetus to become dependent on the medicine. This may lead to withdrawal side effects in the newborn baby. Also, these medicines may cause breathing problems in the newborn baby, especially if they are taken just before delivery.

Breast-feeding—Opium preparations have not been reported to cause problems in nursing babies.

Children—Breathing problems may be especially likely to occur in children up to 2 years of age, who are usually more sensitive than adults to the effects of opium preparations.

Older adults—Breathing problems may be especially likely to occur in elderly patients, who are usually more sensitive than younger adults to the effects of opium preparations.

Other medicines—Although certain medicines should not be used together at all, in other cases two different medicines may be used together even if an interaction might occur. In these cases, your doctor may want to change the dose, or other precautions may be necessary. When you are taking an opium preparation, it is especially important that your doctor and pharmacist know if you are taking any of the following:

- Anticholinergics (medicine for abdominal or stomach spasms or cramps) or
- Central nervous system (CNS) depressants, especially other narcotics, or
- Other diarrhea medicine or
- Tricyclic antidepressants (amitriptyline [e.g., Elavil], amoxapine [e.g., Asendin], clomipramine [e.g., Anafranil], desipramine [e.g., Pertofrane], doxepin [e.g., Sinequan], imipramine [e.g., Tofranil], nortriptyline [e.g., Aventyl], protriptyline [e.g., Vivactil], trimipramine [e.g., Surmontil])—The chance of side effects is increased
- Naltrexone (e.g., Trexan)—Naltrexone blocks the effects of opium preparations and makes them less effective in treating diarrhea

Other medical problems—The presence of other medical problems may affect the use of opium preparations. Make sure you tell your doctor if you have any other medical problems, especially:

- Alcohol or other drug abuse (or history of) or
- Colitis or
- Heart disease or
- Kidney disease or
- Liver disease or
- Underactive thyroid—The chance of side effects may be increased
- Brain disease or head injury or
- Emphysema, asthma, bronchitis, or other chronic lung disease or
- Enlarged prostate or problems with urination or
- Gallbladder disease or gallstones—Some of the side effects of opium preparations can be dangerous if these conditions are present
- Convulsions (seizures), history of—Opium can rarely cause convulsions

Before you begin using any new medicine (prescription or nonprescription) or if you develop any new medical problem while you are using this medicine, check with your doctor, nurse, or pharmacist.

Proper Use of This Medicine

This medicine is to be taken by mouth even if it comes in a dropper bottle. The amount you should take is to be measured with the special dropper provided with your prescription and diluted with water just before you take each dose. This will cause the medicine to turn milky in color, but it will still work.

If your prescription does not come in a dropper bottle and the directions on the bottle say to take it by the teaspoonful, it is not necessary to dilute it before using.

If this medicine upsets your stomach, your doctor may want you to take it with food.

Take this medicine only as directed by your doctor. Do not take more of it, do not take it more often, and do not take it for a longer time than your doctor ordered. This is especially important for young children and for elderly patients, who are especially sensitive to the effects of opium preparations. If too much is taken, this medicine may become habit-forming (causing mental or physical dependence) or lead to problems because of an overdose.

Missed dose—If you miss a dose of this medicine, take it as soon as you remember. However, if it is almost time for your next dose, skip the missed dose and go back to your regular dosing schedule. *Do not double doses.*

Storage—To store this medicine:
- Keep out of the reach of children. Overdose is very dangerous in young children.
- Store away from heat and direct light.
- Keep the container for this medicine tightly closed to prevent the alcohol from evaporating and the medicine from becoming stronger.
- Do not store this medicine in the refrigerator or allow the medicine to freeze. If it does get cold and you notice any solid particles in it, throw it away.
- Do not keep outdated medicine or medicine no longer needed. Be sure that any discarded medicine is out of the reach of children.

Precautions While Using This Medicine

Check with your doctor if your diarrhea does not stop after 1 or 2 days or if you develop a fever.

This medicine will add to the effects of alcohol and other CNS depressants (medicines that slow down the nervous system, possibly causing drowsiness). Some examples of CNS depressants are antihistamines or medicine for hay fever, other allergies, or colds; sedatives, tranquilizers, or sleeping medicine; prescription pain medicine or other narcotics; barbiturates; medicine for seizures; muscle relaxants; or anesthetics, including some dental anesthetics. *Do not drink alcoholic beverages, and check with your doctor before taking any of the medicines listed above, while you are taking this medicine.*

This medicine may cause some people to become drowsy, dizzy, lightheaded, or less alert than they are normally. Even if taken at bedtime, it may cause some people to feel drowsy or less alert on arising. *Make sure you know how you react to this medicine before you drive, use machines, or do anything else that could be dangerous if you are dizzy or are not alert.*

Dizziness, lightheadedness, or fainting may be especially likely to occur when you get up suddenly from a lying or sitting position. Getting up slowly may help lessen this problem. If you feel very dizzy, lightheaded, or faint after taking this medicine, lying down for a while may help.

If you have been taking this medicine regularly for several weeks or more, *do not stop using it without first checking with your doctor.* Your doctor may want you to reduce gradually the amount you are using before stopping completely, to lessen the chance of withdrawal side effects.

If you think you or someone else may have taken an overdose, get emergency help at once. Taking an overdose of this medicine or taking alcohol or other CNS depressants with this medicine may lead to unconsciousness and possibly death. Signs of overdose include convulsions (seizures), confusion, severe nervousness or restlessness, severe dizziness, severe drowsiness, slow or irregular breathing, and severe weakness.

Side Effects of This Medicine

Along with its needed effects, a medicine may cause some unwanted effects. Although not all of these side effects may occur, if they do occur they may need medical attention.

Get emergency help immediately if any of the following symptoms of overdose occur:

Cold, clammy skin; confusion; convulsions (seizures); dizziness (severe); drowsiness (severe); low blood pressure; nervousness or restlessness (severe); pinpoint pupils of eyes; slow heartbeat; slow or irregular breathing; weakness (severe)

Also, *check with your doctor immediately* if any of the following side effects are severe and occur suddenly since they may indicate a more severe and dangerous problem with your bowels:

Rare

Bloating; constipation; loss of appetite; nausea or vomiting; stomach cramps or pain

In addition, check with your doctor as soon as possible if any of the following side effects occur:

Rare

Fast heartbeat; increased sweating; mental depression; redness or flushing of face; shortness of breath, wheezing, or troubled breathing; skin rash, hives, or itching; slow heartbeat

Other side effects may occur that usually do not need medical attention. These side effects may go away during treatment as your body adjusts to the medicine. However, check with your doctor if any of the following side effects continue or are bothersome:

More common with large doses

Difficult or painful urination; dizziness, lightheadedness, or feeling faint; drowsiness; frequent urge to urinate; nervousness or restlessness; unusual decrease in amount of urine; unusual tiredness or weakness

After you stop using this medicine, your body may need time to adjust. The length of time this takes depends on the amount of medicine you were using and how long you used it. During this period of time check with your doctor if you notice any of the following side effects:

Body aches; diarrhea; fever, runny nose, or sneezing; gooseflesh; increased sweating; increased yawning; loss of appetite; nausea or vomiting; nervousness, restlessness, or irritability; shivering or trembling; stomach cramps; trouble in sleeping; unusually large pupils of eyes; weakness (severe)

Other side effects not listed above may also occur in some patients. If you notice any other effects, check with your doctor.

Annual revision: 10/05/92

ORPHENADRINE Systemic

Some commonly used brand names are:

In the U.S.

Banflex	Myotrol
Blanex	Neocyten
Disipal	Noradex
Flexagin	Norflex
Flexain	O-Flex
Flexoject	Orflagen
Flexon	Orfro
K-Flex	Orphenate
Marflex	Tega-Flex
Myolin	

Generic name product may also be available.

In Canada

Disipal	Norflex

Description

Orphenadrine (or-FEN-a-dreen) is used to help relax certain muscles in your body and relieve the pain and discomfort caused by strains, sprains, or other injury to your muscles. One form of orphenadrine is also used to relieve trembling caused by Parkinson's disease. However, this medicine does not take the place of rest, exercise or physical therapy, or other treatment that your doctor may recommend for your medical problem.

Orphenadrine acts in the central nervous system (CNS) to produce its muscle relaxant effects. Orphenadrine also has other actions (anticholinergic) that produce its helpful effects in Parkinson's disease. Orphenadrine's CNS and anticholinergic actions may also be responsible for some of its side effects.

In the U.S., this medicine is available only with your doctor's prescription. In Canada, it may be available without a prescription. It is available in the following dosage forms:

Oral

- Tablets (U.S. and Canada)
- Extended-release tablets (U.S. and Canada)

Parenteral

- Injection (U.S. and Canada)

It is very important that you read and understand the following information. If any of it causes you special concern, check with your doctor. Also, *if you have any questions* or if you want more information about this medicine or your medical problem, *ask your doctor, nurse, or pharmacist.*

Before Using This Medicine

In deciding to use a medicine, the risks of taking the medicine must be weighed against the good it will do. This is a decision you and your doctor will make. For orphenadrine, the following should be considered:

Allergies—Tell your doctor if you have ever had any unusual or allergic reaction to orphenadrine. Also tell your doctor and pharmacist if you are allergic to any other substances, such as foods, preservatives, or dyes.

Pregnancy—Orphenadrine has not been reported to cause birth defects or other problems in humans.

Breast-feeding—It is not known whether orphenadrine passes into the breast milk. However, orphenadrine has not been reported to cause problems in nursing babies.

Children—Studies on this medicine have been done only in adult patients, and there is no specific information about its use in children.

Older adults—Many medicines have not been tested in older people. Therefore, it may not be known whether they work exactly the same way they do in younger adults or if they cause different side effects or problems in older people. There is no specific information about the use of orphenadrine in the elderly.

Other medicines—Although certain medicines should not be used together at all, in other cases two different medicines may be used together even if an interaction might occur. In these cases, your doctor may want to change the dose, or other precautions may be necessary. When you are taking orphenadrine, it is especially important that your doctor and pharmacist know if you are taking any of the following:

- Central nervous system (CNS) depressants
- Tricyclic antidepressants (amitriptyline [e.g., Elavil], amoxapine [e.g., Asendin], clomipramine [e.g., Anafranil], desipramine [e.g., Pertofrane], doxepin [e.g., Sinequan], imipramine [e.g., Tofranil], nortriptyline [e.g., Aventyl], protriptyline [e.g., Vivactil], trimipramine [e.g.,

Surmontil])—The chance of side effects may be increased

Other medical problems—The presence of other medical problems may affect the use of orphenadrine. Make sure you tell your doctor if you have any other medical problems, especially:

- Disease of the digestive tract, especially esophagus disease, stomach ulcer, or intestinal blockage, or
- Enlarged prostate or
- Fast or irregular heartbeat or
- Glaucoma or
- Myasthenia gravis or
- Urinary tract blockage—Orphenadrine has side effects that may be harmful to people with these conditions
- Heart disease or
- Kidney disease or
- Liver disease—The chance of side effects may be increased

Before you begin using any new medicine (prescription or nonprescription) or if you develop any new medical problem while you are using this medicine, check with your doctor, nurse, or pharmacist.

Proper Use of This Medicine

Missed dose—If you miss a dose of this medicine and remember within an hour or so of the missed dose, take it right away. But if you do not remember until later, skip the missed dose and go back to your regular dosing schedule. Do not double doses.

Storage—To store this medicine:

- Keep out of the reach of children.
- Store away from heat and direct light.
- Do not store this medicine in the bathroom, near the kitchen sink, or in other damp places. Heat or moisture may cause the medicine to break down.
- Do not keep outdated medicine or medicine no longer needed. Be sure that any discarded medicine is out of the reach of children.

Precautions While Using This Medicine

If you will be taking this medicine for a long time (for example, more than a few weeks), your doctor should check your progress at regular visits.

This medicine may add to the effects of alcohol and other CNS depressants (medicines that slow down the nervous system, possibly causing drowsiness). Some examples of CNS depressants are antihistamines or medicine for hay fever, other allergies, or colds; sedatives, tranquilizers, or sleeping medicine; prescription pain medicine or narcotics; barbiturates; medicine for seizures; other muscle relaxants; or anesthetics, including some dental anesthetics. *Do not drink alcoholic beverages, and check with your doctor before taking any of the medicines listed above, while you are using this medicine.*

This medicine may cause some people to have blurred vision or to become drowsy, dizzy, lightheaded, faint, or less alert than they are normally. It may also cause muscle weakness in some people. *Make sure you know how you react to this medicine before you drive, use machines, or do anything else that could be dangerous if you are dizzy or are not alert and able to see well.*

Orphenadrine may cause dryness of the mouth. For temporary relief, use sugarless candy or gum, melt bits of ice in your mouth, or use a saliva substitute. However, if dry mouth continues for more than 2 weeks, check with your dentist. Continuing dryness of the mouth may increase the chance of dental disease, including tooth decay, gum disease, and fungus infections.

Side Effects of This Medicine

Along with its needed effects, a medicine may cause some unwanted effects. Although not all of these side effects may occur, if they do occur they may need medical attention.

Check with your doctor as soon as possible if any of the following side effects occur:

Less common

Decreased urination; eye pain; fainting; fast or pounding heartbeat

Rare

Hallucinations (seeing, hearing, or feeling things that are not there); shortness of breath, troubled breathing, tightness in chest, and/or wheezing; skin rash, hives, itching, or redness; sores, ulcers, or white spots on lips or in mouth; swollen and/or painful glands; unusual bruising or bleeding; unusual tiredness or weakness

Other side effects may occur that usually do not need medical attention. These side effects may go away during treatment as your body adjusts to the medicine. However, check with your doctor if any of the following side effects continue or are bothersome:

More common

Dryness of mouth

Less common or rare

Abdominal or stomach cramps or pain; blurred or double vision or other vision problems; confusion; constipation; difficult urination; dizziness or lightheadedness; drowsiness; excitement, irritability, nervousness, or restlessness; headache; muscle weakness; nausea or vomiting; trembling; unusually large pupils of eyes

Other side effects not listed above may also occur in some patients. If you notice any other effects, check with your doctor.

Annual revision: August 1990

ORPHENADRINE AND ASPIRIN Systemic

Some commonly used brand names are:

In the U.S.

Norgesic	N3 Gesic
Norgesic Forte	N3 Gesic Forte
Norphadrine	Orphenagesic
Norphadrine Forte	Orphenagesic Forte

In Canada‡

Norgesic	Norgesic Forte

‡In Canada, *Aspirin* is a brand name. Acetylsalicylic acid is the generic name in Canada. ASA, a synonym for acetylsalicylic acid, is the term that commonly appears on Canadian product labels.

Description

Orphenadrine (or-FEN-a-dreen) and aspirin (AS-pir-in) combination is used to help relax certain muscles in your body and relieve the pain and discomfort caused by strains, sprains, or other injury to your muscles. However, this medicine does not take the place of rest, exercise, or other treatment that your doctor may recommend for your medical problem.

Orphenadrine acts in the central nervous system (CNS) to produce its muscle relaxant effects. Actions in the CNS may also be responsible for some of its side effects. Orphenadrine also has other actions (antimuscarinic) that may be responsible for some of its side effects.

This combination medicine also contains caffeine (kaf-EEN).

In the U.S., this combination medicine is available only with your doctor's prescription. In Canada, it is available without a prescription.

These medicines are available in the following dosage forms:

Oral

- Tablets (U.S. and Canada)

It is very important that you read and understand the following information. If any of it causes you special concern, check with your doctor. Also, *if you have any questions* or if you want more information about this medicine or your medical problem, *ask your doctor, nurse, or pharmacist.*

Before Using This Medicine

In deciding to use a medicine, the risks of taking the medicine must be weighed against the good it will do. This is a decision you and your doctor will make. For orphenadrine and aspirin combination, the following should be considered:

Allergies—Tell your doctor if you have ever had any unusual or allergic reaction to orphenadrine, caffeine, aspirin or other salicylates including methyl salicylate (oil of wintergreen), or to any of the following medicines:

Diclofenac (e.g., Voltaren)
Diflunisal (e.g., Dolobid)
Fenoprofen (e.g., Nalfon)
Floctafenine (e.g., Idarac)
Flurbiprofen, oral (e.g., Ansaid)
Ibuprofen (e.g., Motrin)
Indomethacin (e.g., Indocin)
Ketoprofen (e.g., Orudis)
Ketorolac (e.g., Toradol)
Meclofenamate (e.g., Meclomen)
Mefenamic acid (e.g., Ponstel)
Naproxen (e.g., Naprosyn)
Oxyphenbutazone (e.g., Tandearil)
Phenylbutazone (e.g., Butazolidin)
Piroxicam (e.g., Feldene)
Sulindac (e.g., Clinoril)
Suprofen (e.g., Suprol)
Tiaprofenic acid (e.g., Surgam)
Tolmetin (e.g., Tolectin)
Zomepirac (e.g., Zomax)

Also tell your doctor and pharmacist if you are allergic to any other substances, such as foods, preservatives, or dyes.

Pregnancy—

- *For aspirin:* Studies in humans have not shown that aspirin causes birth defects. However, aspirin has caused birth defects in animal studies.

  Some reports have suggested that too much use of aspirin late in pregnancy may cause a decrease in the newborn's weight and possible death of the fetus or newborn baby. However, the mothers in these reports had been taking much larger amounts of aspirin than are usually recommended. Studies of mothers taking aspirin in the doses that are usually recommended did not show these unwanted effects.

  Regular use of aspirin late in pregnancy may cause unwanted effects on the heart or blood flow in the fetus or in the newborn baby. Also, use of aspirin during the last 2 weeks of pregnancy may cause bleeding problems in the fetus before or during delivery or in the newborn baby. In addition, too much use of aspirin during the last 3 months of pregnancy may increase the length of pregnancy, prolong labor, cause other problems during delivery, or cause severe bleeding in the mother before, during, or after delivery. *Do not take aspirin during the last 3 months of pregnancy unless it has been ordered by your doctor.*
- *For orphenadrine:* Orphenadrine has not been reported to cause birth defects or other problems in humans.

Breast-feeding—This medicine has not been shown to cause problems in nursing babies. However, aspirin passes into the breast milk. Also, caffeine passes into the breast milk in small amounts. It is not known whether orphenadrine passes into the breast milk.

Children—*Do not give a medicine containing aspirin to a child or a teenager with a fever or other symptoms of a virus infection, especially flu or chickenpox, without first discussing its use with your child's doctor.* This is very important because aspirin may cause a serious illness called Reye's syndrome in children with fever caused by a virus infection, especially flu or chickenpox. Children who do not have a virus infection may also be more sensitive to the effects of aspirin, especially if they have a fever or have lost large amounts of body fluid because of vomiting, diarrhea, or sweating. This may increase the chance of side effects during treatment.

There is no specific information about the use of orphenadrine in children.

Older adults—Elderly people are especially sensitive to the effects of aspirin. This may increase the chance of side effects during treatment.

There is no specific information about the use of orphenadrine in the elderly.

Other medicines—Although certain medicines should not be used together at all, in other cases two different medicines may be used together even if an interaction might occur. In these cases, your doctor may want to change the dose, or other precautions may be necessary. When you are taking orphenadrine and aspirin combination, it is especially important that your doctor and pharmacist know if you are taking any of the following:

- Anticoagulants (blood thinners) or
- Carbenicillin by injection (e.g., Geopen) or
- Cefamandole (e.g., Mandol) or
- Cefoperazone (e.g., Cefobid) or
- Cefotetan (e.g., Cefotan) or
- Dipyridamole (e.g., Persantine) or
- Divalproex (e.g., Depakote) or
- Heparin or
- Medicine for inflammation or pain, except narcotics, or
- Moxalactam (e.g., Moxam) or
- Pentoxifylline (e.g., Trental) or
- Plicamycin (e.g., Mithracin) or
- Ticarcillin (e.g., Ticar) or
- Valproic acid (e.g., Depakene)—Taking these medicines together with aspirin may increase the chance of bleeding
- Anticholinergics (medicine for abdominal or stomach spasms or cramps) or
- Central nervous system (CNS) depressants or
- Methotrexate (e.g., Mexate) or
- Tricyclic antidepressants (amitriptyline [e.g., Elavil], amoxapine [e.g., Asendin], clomipramine [e.g., Anafranil], desipramine [e.g., Pertofrane], doxepin [e.g., Sinequan], imipramine [e.g., Tofranil], nortriptyline [e.g., Aventyl], protriptyline [e.g., Vivactil], trimipramine [e.g., Surmontil]) or
- Vancomycin (e.g., Vancocin)—The chance of side effects may be increased
- Antidiabetics, oral (diabetes medicine you take by mouth)—Aspirin may increase the effects of the antidiabetic medicine; a change in dose may be needed if aspirin is taken regularly
- Probenecid (e.g., Benemid) or
- Sulfinpyrazone (e.g., Anturane)—Aspirin can keep these medicines from working properly for treating gout; also, taking aspirin together with sulfinpyrazone may increase the chance of bleeding
- Urinary alkalizers (medicine that makes the urine less acid, such as acetazolamide [e.g., Diamox], dichlorphenamide [e.g., Daranide], methazolamide [e.g., Neptazane], potassium or sodium citrate and/or citric acid)—These medicines may make aspirin less effective by causing it to be removed from the body more quickly
- Zidovudine (e.g., AZT; Retrovir)—Aspirin may increase the blood levels of zidovudine, which increases the chance of serious side effects

Other medical problems—The presence of other medical problems may affect the use of orphenadrine and aspirin combination. Make sure you tell your doctor if you have any other medical problems, especially:

- Anemia or
- Overactive thyroid or
- Stomach ulcer or other stomach problems—Aspirin may make your condition worse
- Asthma, allergies, and nasal polyps, history of or
- Glucose-6-phosphate dehydrogenase (G6PD) deficiency or
- Kidney disease or
- Liver disease—The chance of side effects may be increased
- Disease of the digestive tract, especially esophagus disease or intestinal blockage, or
- Enlarged prostate or
- Fast or irregular heartbeat or
- Glaucoma or
- Myasthenia gravis or
- Urinary tract blockage—Orphenadrine has side effects that may be harmful to people with these conditions
- Gout—Aspirin can make this condition worse and can also lessen the effects of some medicines used to treat gout
- Heart disease—The chance of some side effects may be increased. Also, the caffeine present in this combination medicine can make your condition worse
- Hemophilia or other bleeding problems or
- Vitamin K deficiency—Aspirin may increase the chance of bleeding

Before you begin using any new medicine (prescription or nonprescription) or if you develop any new medical problem while you are using this medicine, check with your doctor, nurse, or pharmacist.

Proper Use of This Medicine

Take this medicine with food or a full glass (8 ounces) of water to lessen stomach irritation.

Do not take this medicine if it has a strong vinegar-like odor. This odor means the aspirin in it is breaking down.

If you have any questions about this, check with your doctor or pharmacist.

Do not take more of this medicine than your doctor ordered to lessen the chance of side effects or overdose.

Missed dose—If you miss a dose of this medicine and remember within an hour or so of the missed dose, take it right away. But if you do not remember until later, skip the missed dose and go back to your regular dosing schedule. Do not double doses.

Storage—To store this medicine:

- Keep out of the reach of children. Overdose of aspirin is especially dangerous in young children.
- Store away from heat and direct light.
- Do not store this medicine in the bathroom, near the kitchen sink, or in other damp places. Heat or moisture may cause the medicine to break down.
- Do not keep outdated medicine or medicine no longer needed. Be sure that any discarded medicine is out of the reach of children.

Precautions While Using This Medicine

If you will be taking this medicine for a long time (for example, more than a few weeks), your doctor should check your progress at regular visits.

Check the labels of all nonprescription (over-the-counter [OTC]) and prescription medicines you now take. If any contain orphenadrine or aspirin or other salicylates be especially careful, since taking them while taking this medicine may lead to overdose. If you have any questions about this, check with your doctor or pharmacist.

Too much use of acetaminophen or certain other medicines together with the aspirin in this combination medicine may increase the chance of unwanted effects. The risk depends on how much of each medicine you take every day, and on how long you take the medicines together. If your doctor directs you to take these medicines together on a regular basis, follow his or her directions carefully. However, do not take acetaminophen or any of the following medicines together with this combination medicine for more than a few days, unless your doctor has directed you to do so and is following your progress:

Diclofenac (e.g., Voltaren)
Diflunisal (e.g., Dolobid)
Fenoprofen (e.g., Nalfon)
Floctafenine (e.g., Idarac)
Flurbiprofen, oral (e.g., Ansaid)
Ibuprofen (e.g., Motrin)
Indomethacin (e.g., Indocin)
Ketoprofen (e.g., Orudis)
Ketorolac (e.g., Toradol)
Meclofenamate (e.g., Meclomen)
Mefenamic acid (e.g., Ponstel)
Naproxen (e.g., Naprosyn)
Phenylbutazone (e.g., Butazolidin)
Piroxicam (e.g., Feldene)
Sulindac (e.g., Clinoril)
Tiaprofenic acid (e.g., Surgam)
Tolmetin (e.g., Tolectin)

For *diabetic patients:*

- The aspirin in this combination medicine may cause false urine sugar test results if you are regularly taking 6 or more of the regular-strength tablets or 3 or more of the double-strength tablets of this medicine a day. Smaller doses or occasional use of aspirin usually will not affect urine sugar tests. If you have any questions about this, check with your doctor, nurse, or pharmacist, especially if your diabetes is not well controlled.

Do not take this medicine for 5 days before any surgery, including dental surgery, unless otherwise directed by your medical doctor or dentist. Taking aspirin during this time may cause bleeding problems.

The orphenadrine in this combination medicine may add to the effects of alcohol and other CNS depressants (medicines that slow down the nervous system, possibly causing drowsiness). Some examples of CNS depressants are antihistamines or medicine for hay fever, other allergies, or colds; sedatives, tranquilizers, or sleeping medicine; prescription pain medicine or narcotics; barbiturates; medicine for seizures; other muscle relaxants; or anesthetics, including some dental anesthetics. Also, stomach problems may be more likely to occur if you drink alcoholic beverages while you are taking aspirin. *Do not drink alcoholic beverages, and check with your doctor before taking any of the medicines listed above, while you are using this medicine.*

This medicine may cause some people to have blurred vision or to become drowsy, dizzy, lightheaded, faint, or less alert than they are normally. *Make sure you know how you react to this medicine before you drive, use machines, or do anything else that could be dangerous if you are dizzy or are not alert.*

Dryness of the mouth may occur while you are taking this medicine. For temporary relief, use sugarless candy or gum, melt bits of ice in your mouth, or use a saliva substitute. However, if dry mouth continues for more than 2 weeks, check with your dentist. Continuing dryness of the mouth may increase the chance of dental disease, including tooth decay, gum disease, and fungus infections.

If you think that you or someone else may have taken an overdose of this medicine, get emergency help at once. Taking an overdose of this medicine may cause unconsciousness or death. Signs of overdose include convulsions (seizures), hearing loss, confusion, ringing or buzzing in the ears, severe drowsiness or tiredness, severe excitement or nervousness, and fast or deep breathing.

Side Effects of This Medicine

Along with its needed effects, a medicine may cause some unwanted effects. Although not all of these side effects may occur, if they do occur they may need medical attention.

Get emergency help immediately if any of the following symptoms of overdose occur:

Any loss of hearing; bloody urine; confusion; convulsions (seizures); diarrhea; dizziness or lightheadedness (severe); drowsiness (severe); excitement or nervousness (severe); fast or deep breathing; hallucinations (seeing, hearing, or feeling things that are not there); headache (severe or continuing); increased sweating; nausea or vomiting (severe or continuing); ringing or buzzing in the ears (continuing); uncontrollable flapping movements of the hands, especially in elderly patients; unexplained fever; unusual thirst; vision problems

Symptoms of overdose in children

Changes in behavior; drowsiness or tiredness (severe); fast or deep breathing

Also, check with your doctor as soon as possible if any of the following side effects occur:

Less common or rare

Abdominal or stomach pain, cramping, or burning (severe); bloody or black, tarry stools; decreased urination; eye pain; fainting; fast or pounding heartbeat; shortness of breath, troubled breathing, tightness in chest, or wheezing; skin rash, hives, itching, or redness; sores, ulcers, or white spots on lips or in mouth; swollen and/or painful glands; unusual bleeding or bruising; unusual tiredness or weakness; vomiting of blood or material that looks like coffee grounds

Other side effects may occur that usually do not need medical attention. These side effects may go away during treatment as your body adjusts to the medicine. However, check with your doctor if any of the following side effects continue or are bothersome:

More common

Abdominal or stomach cramps, pain, or discomfort (mild to moderate); dryness of mouth; heartburn or indigestion; nausea or vomiting (mild)

Less common

Blurred or double vision or other vision problems; confusion; constipation; difficult urination; dizziness or lightheadedness; drowsiness; excitement, nervousness, or restlessness; headache; muscle weakness; trembling; unusually large pupils of eyes

Other side effects not listed above may also occur in some patients. If you notice any other effects, check with your doctor.

Annual revision: July 1990

OVULATION PREDICTION TEST KITS FOR HOME USE

Some commonly used brand names are:

In the U.S.

Clearplan
First Response
Fortel
OvuKit
OvuQuick

Description

Ovulation prediction kits are used to help a woman know when she is most likely to ovulate. This is helpful in timing sexual intercourse for becoming pregnant. It may be useful for couples who are having problems conceiving or are concerned about the timing of a pregnancy. A medical doctor may also recommend the use of this type of kit for timing artificial insemination or for fertility problems. *These tests are not intended for contraceptive (birth control) use.*

Ovulation is the release of an egg from the ovary. It normally occurs once a month in about the middle of the menstrual cycle. The egg can be fertilized only for about 48 hours (24 hours is best), so this is the only time during the menstrual cycle that a woman can become pregnant. Ovulation is controlled by luteinizing hormone (LH). The amount of LH present in the blood and urine is very small during most of the menstrual cycle but rises suddenly for a short time near the middle of the menstrual cycle. This sharp rise, the LH surge, usually causes ovulation within about 30 hours. A woman is most likely to become pregnant if she has sexual intercourse within the first 24 hours after detecting the LH surge.

Ovulation prediction test kits test for this large amount of LH in the urine. A change in color of the test pad or liquid will occur if enough LH is in the urine. Correctly using an ovulation prediction test kit is more accurate for predicting ovulation than measuring daily basal body temperature.

Before Using This Test Kit

It is important to get the best results possible from ovulation prediction test kits while you are using them. Therefore, the following should be considered by you and possibly by your doctor before you decide to use these test kits:

Diet—Drinking large amounts of fluids such as water or alcohol can dilute your urine. This may interfere with test results and lead to improper timing of intercourse.

Medicines—Certain medicines may affect the results of your testing. Check with your doctor if you are taking any medicines, especially:

- Anticonvulsants (seizure medicine) or
- Birth control pills or
- Estrogens (female hormones) or
- Medicine for mental problems or
- Menotropins or
- Progestins (another type of female hormone)—The use of these medicines may interfere with testing for the rise in LH that comes before ovulation and could result in improper timing of intercourse
- Clomiphene—Clomiphene changes the pattern of LH release; your doctor may recommend a different way to use the test kits

Medical conditions—The presence of other medical conditions may affect the results of your testing. Check with your doctor if you have any medical conditions, especially:

- Cysts of the ovaries or
- Decreased function of the ovaries
- Endometriosis or
- Menopause (change of life) or
- Pregnancy or
- Thyroid disease or
- Urinary tract infection—These conditions may interfere with testing for the rise in LH that comes before ovulation and could result in improper timing of intercourse

Also, if you have vision problems (such as color-blindness or poor vision), you will need someone to help you in reading your test results.

Before you begin using any new medicine (prescription or nonprescription) or if you develop any new medical condition while you are using these test kits, it is a good idea to check with your doctor, nurse, or pharmacist.

Proper Use of This Test Kit

Ovulation prediction test kits test for a large amount of LH in the urine. A change in color of the test pad or liquid will occur if enough LH is in the urine.

These kits contain enough chemicals to perform 6 to 9 tests. The woman tests her urine daily, usually starting 2 to 3 days before ovulation is expected, according to her usual menstrual cycle length. If your menstrual cycles are unpredictable or irregular, ask your doctor about the best time to perform the tests.

To use:

- Your doctor may give you instructions on using the kit. If not, follow the test kit instructions carefully. The printed instructions on the proper use of ovulation prediction kits may be different for each brand.
- Collect a urine sample according to the written package instructions or your doctor's instructions. If you do not have time to test your urine right away, it may be stored according to the test kit instructions. Refrigeration of the urine may interfere with the test results.
- Choose a well-lighted area with normal room temperature and humidity. Perform the test on a clean, dry working surface with a cold water faucet nearby. You will also need a watch, timer, or clock that can measure in seconds.
- Be careful not to touch the testing areas. Skin oils or perspiration may affect the test results. It is also important that you use clean, dry test kit materials. Traces of old test chemicals or soaps may affect test reactions if materials are reused.
- At the end of the timing period compare the color of the test to the color chart on the package.
- Record your test results to discuss with your doctor, nurse, or pharmacist.

Storage—To store this product:

- Keep out of the reach of children. Test chemicals can be poisonous if swallowed.
- Store the kit in a cool, dry place, away from heat, moisture, and direct sunlight. Heat-exposed or chilled test kits will not work properly.
- Keep the product from freezing.
- Before purchasing, check the date printed on the package that tells you when the kit is too old to use (expiration date). Do not use an outdated test kit. Outdated test kits will not work properly.
- Discard used tests in the trash. Liquids may be poured down the drain or flushed in the toilet.

About Your Test Results

Your best chance of becoming pregnant is by having intercourse or being artificially inseminated within 24 hours of detecting the LH surge. Each cycle may have a slightly different time of ovulation, or ovulation may not even occur in some cycles. Couples who have problems conceiving should always consult a doctor for advice and medical evaluation, especially if it takes longer than 6 to 12 months for the woman to become pregnant.

If you have any other questions about your results or the use of ovulation prediction test kits, ask your doctor, nurse, or pharmacist. Also, most kits also provide a toll-free number for advice on using the kits.

Annual revision: 10/08/91

OXAMNIQUINE Systemic†

A commonly used brand name in the U.S. is Vansil.

†Not commercially available in Canada.

Description

Oxamniquine (ox-AM-ni-kwin) is used to treat a certain kind of worm infection (blood fluke), also known as snail fever, Manson's schistosomiasis (shis-toe-soe-MYE-a-siss), or bilharziasis (bil-har-ZYE-a-siss). It will not work for other kinds of worm infections (for example, pinworms or roundworms).

Oxamniquine is available only with your doctor's prescription, in the following dosage form:

Oral

- Capsules (U.S.)

It is very important that you read and understand the following information. If any of it causes you special concern, check with your doctor. Also, *if you have any questions* or if you want more information about this medicine or your medical problem, *ask your doctor, nurse, or pharmacist.*

Before Using This Medicine

In deciding to use a medicine, the risks of taking the medicine must be weighed against the good it will do. This is a decision you and your doctor will make. For oxamniquine, the following should be considered:

Allergies—Tell your doctor if you have ever had any unusual or allergic reaction to oxamniquine. Also tell your doctor and pharmacist if you are allergic to any other substances, such as foods, preservatives, or dyes.

Pregnancy—Studies have not been done in humans. Studies in animals have shown that oxamniquine may harm the unborn animal when it is given in high doses. However, there have been no reports of problems with the pregnancies or babies of pregnant women who took oxamniquine.

Breast-feeding—It is not known whether oxamniquine passes into the breast milk. However, this medicine has not been reported to cause problems in nursing babies.

Children—This medicine has been used in children, and, in effective doses, has not been shown to cause different side effects or problems in children than it does in adults.

Older adults—Many medicines have not been studied specifically in older people. Therefore, it may not be known whether they work exactly the same way they do in younger adults or if they cause different side effects or problems in older people. There is no specific information comparing use of oxamniquine in the elderly with use in other age groups.

Other medicines—Although certain medicines should not be used together at all, in other cases two different medicines may be used together even if an interaction might occur. In these cases, your doctor may want to change the dose, or other precautions may be necessary. Tell your doctor and pharmacist if you are taking any other prescription or nonprescription (over-the-counter [OTC]) medicine.

Other medical problems—The presence of other medical problems may affect the use of oxamniquine. Make sure you tell your doctor if you have any other medical problems, especially:

- History of epilepsy or other medical problems that cause convulsions—Patients with a history of epilepsy may be more likely to have side effects

Before you begin using any new medicine (prescription or nonprescription) or if you develop any new medical problem while you are using this medicine, check with your doctor, nurse, or pharmacist.

Proper Use of This Medicine

No special preparations (for example, special diets, fasting, other medicines, laxatives, or enemas) are necessary before, during, or immediately after taking oxamniquine.

Take this medicine after meals to lessen the chance of side effects such as stomach upset, drowsiness, or dizziness, unless otherwise directed by your doctor.

To help clear up your infection completely, *take this medicine exactly as directed by your doctor for the full time of treatment. Do not miss any doses.*

Dosing—The dose of oxamniquine will be different for different patients. *Follow your doctor's orders or the directions on the label.* The following information includes only the average doses of oxamniquine. *If your dose is different, do not change it* unless your doctor tells you to do so.

- For the treatment of schistosomiasis:
  —Adults and children over 30 kg (66 pounds): Dose is based on body weight and will be determined by your doctor. This dose is taken one or two times a day for one to three days.
  —Children up to 30 kg (66 pounds): Dose is based on body weight and will be determined by your doctor. This dose is taken two times a day for one day.

Missed dose—If you do miss a dose of this medicine, take it as soon as possible. However, if it is almost time for your next dose, skip the missed dose and go back to your regular dosing schedule. Do not double doses.

Storage—To store this medicine:
- Keep out of the reach of children.
- Store away from heat and direct light.
- Do not store in the bathroom, near the kitchen sink, or in other damp places. Heat or moisture may cause the medicine to break down.
- Do not keep outdated medicine or medicine no longer needed. Be sure that any discarded medicine is out of the reach of children.

Precautions While Using This Medicine

It is important that your doctor check your progress at regular visits.

If your symptoms do not improve after you take this medicine for the full time of treatment, or if they become worse, check with your doctor.

This medicine may cause some people to become dizzy, drowsy, or less alert than they are normally. *Make sure you know how you react to this medicine before you drive, use machines, or do anything else that could be dangerous if you are dizzy or are not alert.* If these reactions are especially bothersome, check with your doctor.

Side Effects of This Medicine

Along with its needed effects, a medicine may cause some unwanted effects. Although not all of these side effects may occur, if they do occur they may need medical attention.

Check with your doctor immediately if any of the following side effects occur:

Rare

Convulsions (seizures); fever; hallucinations (seeing, hearing, or feeling things that are not there); skin rash or hives

Other side effects may occur that usually do not need medical attention. These side effects may go away during treatment as your body adjusts to the medicine. However, check with your doctor if any of the following side effects continue or are bothersome:

More common

Dizziness; drowsiness; headache

Less common

Abdominal or stomach pain; diarrhea; loss of appetite; nausea or vomiting

This medicine may cause the urine to turn reddish orange. This side effect does not require medical attention.

Other side effects not listed above may also occur in some patients. If you notice any other effects, check with your doctor.

Annual revision: 01/19/93

OXAPROZIN Systemic†

A commonly used brand name in the U.S. is Daypro.

†Not commercially available in Canada.

Description

Oxaprozin (ox-a-PROE-zin) belongs to the group of medicines called anti-inflammatory analgesics (also called nonsteroidal anti-inflammatory drugs [NSAIDs]). Oxaprozin is used to relieve some symptoms caused by arthritis (rheumatism), such as inflammation, swelling, stiffness, and joint pain. However, this medicine does not cure arthritis and will help you only as long as you continue to take it.

Any anti-inflammatory analgesic can cause side effects, especially when it is used for a long time or in large doses. Some of the side effects are painful or uncomfortable. Others can be more serious, resulting in the need for medical care and sometimes even in death. If you will be taking this medicine for more than 1 or 2 months or in large amounts, you should discuss with your doctor the good that it can do as well as the risks of taking it.

Also, it is a good idea to ask your doctor about other forms of treatment that might help to reduce the amount of oxaprozin that you take and/or the length of treatment.

Oxaprozin is available only with your doctor's prescription, in the following dosage form:

Oral

- Tablets (U.S.)

It is very important that you read and understand the following information. If any of it causes you special concern, check with your doctor. Also, *if you have any questions* or if you want more information about this medicine or your medical problem, *ask your doctor, nurse, or pharmacist.*

Before Using This Medicine

In deciding to use a medicine, the risks of taking the medicine must be weighed against the good it will do. This is a decision you and your doctor will make. For oxaprozin, the following should be considered:

Allergies—Tell your doctor if you have ever had any unusual or allergic reaction to oxaprozin or to any of the following medicines:

Aspirin or other salicylates
Diclofenac (e.g., Voltaren)
Diflunisal (e.g., Dolobid)
Etodolac (e.g., Lodine)
Fenoprofen (e.g., Nalfon)
Floctafenine (e.g., Idarac)
Flurbiprofen, oral (e.g., Ansaid)
Ibuprofen (e.g., Motrin)
Indomethacin (e.g., Indocin)
Ketoprofen (e.g., Orudis)
Ketorolac (e.g., Toradol)
Meclofenamate (e.g., Meclomen)
Mefenamic acid (e.g., Ponstel)
Nabumetone (e.g., Relafen)
Naproxen (e.g., Naprosyn)
Oxyphenbutazone (e.g., Tandearil)
Phenylbutazone (e.g., Butazolidin)
Piroxicam (e.g., Feldene)
Sulindac (e.g., Clinoril)
Suprofen (e.g., Suprol)
Tenoxicam (e.g., Mobiflex)
Tiaprofenic acid (e.g., Surgam)
Tolmetin (e.g., Tolectin)
Zomepirac (e.g., Zomax)

Also tell your doctor and pharmacist if you are allergic to any other substances, such as foods, preservatives, or dyes.

Pregnancy—Studies on birth defects with oxaprozin have not been done in pregnant women. However, oxaprozin has caused birth defects in animal studies.

There is a chance that regular use of any anti-inflammatory analgesic during the last few months of pregnancy may cause unwanted effects on the heart or blood flow of the fetus or newborn baby. Also, animal studies have shown that, if taken late in pregnancy, oxaprozin may increase the length of pregnancy, prolong labor, or cause other problems during delivery.

Breast-feeding—It is not known whether oxaprozin passes into the breast milk. Although most medicines pass into breast milk in small amounts, many of them may be used safely while breast-feeding. Mothers who are taking this medicine and who wish to breast-feed should discuss this with their doctor.

Children—Oxaprozin has been used in children with arthritis. However, there is no specific information comparing use of this medicine in children with use in other age groups.

Older adults—Studies in elderly patients have shown that some side effects may be more likely to occur in elderly patients, who are usually more sensitive than younger adults to the effects of anti-inflammatory analgesics. Also, elderly people are more likely than younger adults to get very sick if the medicine causes stomach problems.

Other medicines—Although certain medicines should not be used together at all, in other cases two different medicines may be used together even if an interaction might occur. In these cases, your doctor may want to change the dose, or other precautions may be necessary. When you are taking oxaprozin, it is especially important that your doctor and pharmacist know if you are taking any of the following:

- Anticoagulants (blood thinners) or
- Cefamandole (e.g., Mandol) or
- Cefoperazone (e.g., Cefobid) or
- Cefotetan (e.g., Cefotan) or
- Heparin or
- Moxalactam (e.g., Moxam) or
- Plicamycin (e.g., Mithracin) or
- Valproic acid (e.g., Depakene)—Use of any of these medicines together with oxaprozin may increase the chance of bleeding
- Aspirin or other salicylates or
- Cyclosporine (e.g., Sandimmune) or
- Other inflammation or pain medicine (except narcotics)—The chance of serious side effects may be increased
- Lithium (e.g., Lithane) or
- Methotrexate (e.g., Mexate)—Higher blood levels of lithium or methotrexate and an increased chance of side effects may occur
- Probenecid (e.g., Benemid)—Higher blood levels of oxaprozin and an increased chance of side effects may occur

Other medical problems—The presence of other medical problems may affect the use of oxaprozin. Make sure you tell your doctor if you smoke tobacco or if you have any other medical problems, especially:

- Alcohol abuse or
- Asthma or
- Colitis, stomach ulcer, or other stomach problems, or
- Diabetes mellitus (sugar diabetes) or
- Heart disease or

- High blood pressure or
- Kidney disease or
- Liver disease or
- Systemic lupus erythematosus (SLE)—The chance of serious side effects may be increased
- Hemophilia or other bleeding problems—Oxaprozin may increase the chance of serious bleeding

Before you begin using any new medicine (prescription or nonprescription) or if you develop any new medical problem while you are using this medicine, check with your doctor, nurse, or pharmacist.

Proper Use of This Medicine

Oxaprozin should be taken with food or an antacid to lessen the chance of stomach upset. This is especially important if you will be taking the medicine for a long time.

Take this medicine with a full glass (8 ounces) of water. Also, do not lie down for about 15 to 30 minutes after taking the medicine. This helps to prevent irritation that may lead to trouble in swallowing.

This medicine must be taken regularly as ordered by your doctor in order for it to help you. Most anti-inflammatory analgesics usually begin to work within a week, but in severe cases up to 2 weeks or even longer may pass before you begin to feel better. Several weeks more may pass before you feel the full effects of the medicine.

Do not take more of this medicine, do not take it more often, and do not take it for a longer time than ordered by your medical doctor or dentist. Taking too much of this medicine may increase the chance of unwanted effects, especially in elderly patients.

Dosing—The dose of oxaprozin will be different for different patients. *Follow your doctor's orders or the directions on the label.* The following information includes only the average doses of oxaprozin. *If your dose is different, do not change it* unless your doctor tells you to do so.

- For the *oral* dosage form (tablets):
  - —For arthritis:
    - Adults—At first, most people will take one or two 600-milligram (mg) tablets of oxaprozin once a day. A larger amount is sometimes given for the first dose only. If you get side effects after taking the whole amount at one time, your doctor may want you to take smaller amounts two or even three times a day. Some people may need a higher dose of up to 1800 mg a day. This larger dose should be divided into smaller amounts that are taken two or three times a day. In general, people need more medicine during a "flare-up" than they do between "flare-ups" of arthritis symptoms. Therefore, your dose may need to be changed as your condition changes.
    - Children—Use and dose must be determined by your doctor. The dose depends on the child's weight as well as on the child's condition.

Missed dose—If you miss a dose of this medicine, and you remember it within an hour or two after the dose should have been taken, take it right away. If you do not remember until later, skip the missed dose and go back to your regular dosing schedule. Do not double doses.

Storage—To store this medicine:

- Keep out of the reach of children.
- Store away from heat and direct light.
- Do not store this medicine in the bathroom, near the kitchen sink, or in other damp places. Heat or moisture may cause the medicine to break down.
- Do not keep outdated medicine or medicine no longer needed. Be sure that any discarded medicine is out of the reach of children.

Precautions While Using This Medicine

If you will be taking this medicine for a long time, your doctor should check your progress at regular visits. Your doctor may want to do certain tests to find out if unwanted effects are occurring. The tests are very important because serious side effects, including ulcers or bleeding, can occur without any warning.

Stomach problems may be more likely to occur if you drink alcoholic beverages while being treated with this medicine. Therefore, *do not regularly drink alcoholic beverages while taking this medicine,* unless otherwise directed by your doctor.

Taking certain other medicines together with oxaprozin may increase the chance of unwanted effects. The risk will depend on how much of each medicine you take every day, and on how long you take the medicines together. Therefore, do not take acetaminophen (e.g., Tylenol) or aspirin or other salicylates together with oxaprozin for more than a few days, unless otherwise directed by your medical doctor or dentist. Also, *do not take any of the following medicines together with oxaprozin, unless your medical doctor or dentist has directed you to do so and is following your progress*:

Diclofenac (e.g., Voltaren)
Diflunisal (e.g., Dolobid)
Etodolac (e.g., Lodine)
Fenoprofen (e.g., Nalfon)
Floctafenine (e.g., Idarac)
Flurbiprofen, oral (e.g., Ansaid)
Ibuprofen (e.g., Motrin)
Indomethacin (e.g., Indocin)
Ketoprofen (e.g., Orudis)
Ketorolac (e.g., Toradol)
Meclofenamate (e.g., Meclomen)
Mefenamic acid (e.g., Ponstel)
Nabumetone (e.g., Relafen)
Naproxen (e.g., Naprosyn)

Phenylbutazone (e.g., Butazolidin)
Piroxicam (e.g., Feldene)
Sulindac (e.g., Clinoril)
Tenoxicam (e.g., Mobiflex)
Tiaprofenic acid (e.g., Surgam)
Tolmetin (e.g., Tolectin)

Oxaprozin may increase bleeding during and after surgery. Before having any kind of surgery (including dental surgery) or emergency treatment, tell the medical doctor or dentist in charge that you are taking this medicine. It is best to discuss the use of oxaprozin with your doctor or dentist when your surgery is first being planned. It may be necessary for you to stop taking the medicine for a while.

This medicine may cause some people to become drowsy. It may also cause blurred vision in some people. *Make sure you know how you react to this medicine before you drive, use machines, or do anything else that could be dangerous if you are drowsy or are not able to see well.* If these reactions are especially bothersome, check with your doctor.

Some people who take oxaprozin may become more sensitive to sunlight than they are normally. Exposure to sunlight, even for brief periods of time, may cause a skin rash. When you begin taking this medicine:

- Stay out of direct sunlight, especially between the hours of 10:00 a.m. and 3:00 p.m., if possible.
- Wear protective clothing, including a hat.
- Apply a sun block product that has a skin protection factor (SPF) of at least 15. Some patients may require a product with a higher SPF number, especially if they have a fair complexion. If you have any questions about this, check with your doctor or pharmacist.
- Do not use a sunlamp or tanning bed or booth.

If you have a severe reaction from the sun, check with your doctor.

Serious side effects, including ulcers or bleeding, can occur during treatment with this medicine. Sometimes serious side effects can occur without any warning. However, possible warning signs often occur, including severe abdominal or stomach cramps, pain, or burning; black, tarry stools; severe, continuing nausea, heartburn, or indigestion; and/or vomiting of blood or material that looks like coffee grounds. *Stop taking this medicine and check with your doctor immediately if you notice any of these warning signs.*

Side Effects of This Medicine

Along with its needed effects, a medicine may cause some unwanted effects. Although not all of these side effects may occur, if they do occur they may need medical attention.

Stop taking this medicine and check with your doctor immediately if any of the following side effects occur:

Rare

Abdominal or stomach pain, cramping, or burning (severe); bloody urine, bloody or black, tarry stools, or any other bleeding; nausea, heartburn, and/or indigestion (severe and continuing); shortness of breath, troubled breathing, wheezing, or tightness in chest; vomiting of blood or material that looks like coffee grounds

Also, check with your doctor as soon as possible if any of the following side effects occur:

More common

Skin rash

Less common

Difficult, frequent or painful urination; mental depression; ringing or buzzing in ears

Rare

Blurred vision; bruising; cloudy urine; cough or hoarseness; fever with or without chills; hives or itching of skin; increased blood pressure; pain in lower back or side; pain, redness, irritation, and/or swelling in or around the eyes; pinpoint red spots on skin; sores, ulcers, or white spots on lips or in mouth; sudden decrease in amount of urine; swelling and/or tenderness in upper abdominal or stomach area; swelling of face, fingers, feet, and/or lower legs; swollen and/or painful glands; unusual bleeding or bruising; thirst (continuing); unusual tiredness or weakness; weight gain; yellow eyes or skin

Oxaprozin stays in the body for a long time. Therefore, side effects may continue to occur for a while after treatment has been stopped. Check with your doctor if any of the above side effects occur within a few weeks after you have stopped taking the medicine.

Other side effects may occur that usually do not need medical attention. These side effects may go away during treatment as your body adjusts to the medicine. However, check with your doctor if any of the following side effects continue or are bothersome:

More common

Constipation; diarrhea; indigestion; nausea

Less common

Abdominal or stomach cramps, pain, or discomfort (mild to moderate); bloated feeling or gas; confusion; drowsiness; loss of appetite; trouble in sleeping; vomiting

Other side effects not listed above may also occur in some patients. If you notice any other effects, check with your doctor.

Annual revision: 07/13/93

OXICONAZOLE Topical†

A commonly used brand name in the U.S. is Oxistat.

†Not commercially available in Canada.

Description

Oxiconazole (ox-i-KON-a-zole) is used to treat infections caused by a fungus. It works by killing the fungus or preventing its growth.

Oxiconazole is applied to the skin to treat:

- ringworm of the body (tinea corporis);
- ringworm of the foot (tinea pedis; athlete's foot); and
- ringworm of the groin (tinea cruris; jock itch).

Oxiconazole is available only with your doctor's prescription, in the following dosage forms:

Topical

- Cream (U.S.)
- Lotion (U.S.)

It is very important that you read and understand the following information. If any of it causes you special concern, check with your doctor. Also, *if you have any questions* or if you want more information about this medicine or your medical problem, *ask your doctor, nurse, or pharmacist.*

Before Using This Medicine

In deciding to use a medicine, the risks of using the medicine must be weighed against the good it will do. This is a decision you and your doctor will make. For oxiconazole, the following should be considered:

Allergies—Tell your doctor if you have ever had any unusual or allergic reaction to oxiconazole. Also tell your doctor and pharmacist if you are allergic to any other substances, such as foods, preservatives, or dyes.

Pregnancy—Oxiconazole has not been studied in pregnant women. However, this medication has not been shown to cause birth defects or other problems in animal studies.

Breast-feeding—Topical oxiconazole passes into breast milk. Mothers who are using this medicine and who wish to breast-feed should discuss this with their doctor.

Children—Although there is no specific information comparing use of topical oxiconazole in children with use in other age groups, this medicine is not expected to cause different side effects or problems in children than it does in adults.

Older adults—Many medicines have not been studied specifically in older people. Therefore, it may not be known whether they work excactly the same way they do in younger adults. Although there is no specific information comparing use of topical oxiconazole in the elderly with use in other age groups, this medicine is not expected to cause different side effects or problems in older people than it does in younger adults.

Other medicines—Although certain medicines should not be used together at all, in other cases two different medicines may be used together even if an interaction might occur. In these cases, your doctor may want to change the dose, or other precautions may be necessary. Tell your doctor and pharmacist if you are using any other topical prescription or nonprescription (over-the-counter [OTC]) medicine that is to be applied to the same area of the skin.

Before you begin using any new medicine (prescription or nonprescription) or if you develop any new medical problem while you are using this medicine, check with your doctor, nurse, or pharmacist.

Proper Use of This Medicine

Apply enough oxiconazole to cover the affected and surrounding skin areas and rub in gently.

Keep this medicine away from the eyes. Also, do not use it in the vagina.

To help clear up your infection completely, *it is very important that you keep using oxiconazole for the full time of treatment,* even if your symptoms begin to clear up after a few days. Since fungus infections may be very slow to clear up, you may have to continue using this medicine every day for several weeks or more. If you stop using this medicine too soon, your symptoms may return. *Do not miss any doses.*

Dosing—The dose of topical oxiconazole will be different for different patients. *Follow your doctor's orders or the directions on the label.* The following information includes only the average doses of topical oxiconazole. *If your dose is different, do not change it* unless your doctor tells you to do so.

The number of doses you use each day, the time allowed between doses, and the length of time you use the medicine depend on the medical problem for which you are using topical oxiconazole.

- For *cream* or *lotion* dosage form:
  - —For ringworm of the body or groin:
    - Adults and children—Use 1 or 2 times a day for at least 2 weeks.
  - —For athlete's foot:
    - Adults and children—Use 1 or 2 times a day for at least 4 weeks.

Missed dose—If you miss a dose of this medicine, use it as soon as possible. However, if it is almost time for your next dose, skip the missed dose and go back to your regular dosing schedule.

Storage—To store this medicine:
- Keep out of the reach of children.
- Store away from heat and direct light.
- Keep the medicine from freezing. Do not refrigerate.
- Do not keep outdated medicine or medicine no longer needed. Be sure that any discarded medicine is out of the reach of children.

Precautions While Using This Medicine

If your skin problem does not improve within 2 to 4 weeks, or if it becomes worse, check with your doctor.

To help clear up your infection completely and to help make sure it does not return, good health habits are also required. The following measures will help reduce chaffing and irritation and will also help keep the area cool and dry.

- *For patient using oxiconazole for ringworm of the groin:*
  —Avoid wearing underwear that is tight-fitting or made from synthetic materials (for example, rayon or nylon). Instead, wear loose-fitting, cotton underwear.
  —Use a bland, absorbent powder (for example, talcum powder) or an antifungal powder on the skin. It is best to use the powder between the times you use oxiconazole.
- *For patients using oxiconazole for ringworm of the foot:*
  —Carefully dry the feet, especially between the toes, after bathing.
  —Avoid wearing socks made from wool or synthetic materials (for example, rayon or nylon). Instead, wear clean, cotton socks and change them daily or more often if the feet sweat a lot.
  —Wear sandals or other well-ventilated shoes.
  —Use a bland, absorbent powder (for example, talcum powder) or an antifungal powder between the toes, on the feet, and in socks and shoes 1 or 2 times a day. It is best to use the powder between the times you use oxiconazole.

If you have any questions about these measures, check with your doctor, nurse, or pharmacist.

Side Effects of This Medicine

Along with its needed effects, a medicine may cause some unwanted effects. Although not all of these side effects may occur, if they do occur they may need medical attention.

Check with your doctor as soon as possible if the following side effect occurs:

Rare
Rash

Other side effects may occur that usually do not need medical attention. These side effects may go away during treatment as your body adjusts to the medicine. However, check with your doctor if any of the following side effects continue or are bothersome:

Less common
Burning, stinging, itching, redness, or other sign of irritation not present before use of this medicine

Other side effects not listed above may also occur in some patients. If you notice any other effects, check with your doctor.

Annual revision: 07/06/93

OXTRIPHYLLINE AND GUAIFENESIN Systemic

Some commonly used brand names are:

In the U.S.
Brondecon
Brondelate

In Canada
Choledyl Expectorant

Description

Oxtriphylline (ox-TRYE-fi-lin) and guaifenesin (gwye-FEN-e-sin) combination is used to treat the symptoms of bronchial asthma, chronic bronchitis, emphysema, and other lung diseases. This medicine relieves cough, wheezing, shortness of breath, and troubled breathing. It works by opening up the bronchial tubes (air passages) of the lungs and increasing the flow of air through them.

This medicine is available only with your doctor's prescription, in the following dosage forms:

Oral
- Elixir (U.S. and Canada)
- Tablets (U.S. and Canada)

It is very important that you read and understand the following information. If any of it causes you special concern, check with your doctor. Also, *if you have any questions* or if you want more information about this medicine or your medical problem, *ask your doctor, nurse, or pharmacist.*

Before Using This Medicine

In deciding to use a medicine, the risks of taking the medicine must be weighed against the good it will do. This is a decision you and your doctor will make. For oxtriphylline and guaifenesin combination, the following should be considered:

Allergies—Tell your doctor if you have ever had any unusual or allergic reaction to aminophylline, caffeine, dyphylline, oxtriphylline, theobromine, or theophylline. Also tell your doctor and pharmacist if you are allergic to any other substances, such as foods, preservatives, or dyes.

Diet—Make certain your doctor and pharmacist know if you are on any special diet, such as a low-sodium or low-sugar diet or a high-protein, low-carbohydrate or low-protein, high-carbohydrate diet. A high-protein, low-carbohydrate diet may decrease the effects of oxtriphylline; a low-protein, high-carbohydrate diet may increase the effects of oxtriphylline.

Avoid eating or drinking large amounts of caffeine-containing foods or beverages, such as chocolate, cocoa, tea, coffee, and cola drinks, because they may increase the central nervous system (CNS) stimulant effects of oxtriphylline.

Also, eating charcoal broiled foods every day while taking oxtriphylline may keep this medicine from working properly.

Pregnancy—Studies on birth defects have not been done in humans. However, some studies in animals have shown that oxtriphylline causes birth defects when given in doses many times the human dose. Also, use of oxtriphylline during pregnancy may cause unwanted effects such as fast heartbeat, jitteriness, irritability, gagging, vomiting, and breathing problems in the newborn infant. Guaifenesin has not been shown to cause birth defects or other problems in humans.

Breast-feeding—Theophylline passes into the breast milk and may cause irritability, fretfulness, or trouble in sleeping in babies of mothers taking oxtriphylline. Guaifenesin has not been reported to cause problems in nursing babies.

Children—The side effects of oxtriphylline are more likely to occur in newborn infants, who are usually more sensitive to the effects of this medicine.

Although there is no specific information about the use of guaifenesin in children, it is not expected to cause different side effects or problems in children than it does in adults.

Older adults—The side effects of oxtriphylline are more likely to occur in elderly patients, who are usually more sensitive than younger adults to the effects of this medicine.

Although there is no specific information about the use of guaifenesin in the elderly, it is not expected to cause different side effects or problems in older people than it does in younger adults.

Other medicines—Although certain medicines should not be used together at all, in other cases two different medicines may be used together even if an interaction might occur. In these cases, your doctor may want to change the dose, or other precautions may be necessary. When you are taking oxtriphylline and guaifenesin combination, it is especially important that your doctor and pharmacist know if you are taking any of the following:

- Beta-blockers (acebutolol [e.g., Sectral], atenolol [e.g., Tenormin], betaxolol [e.g., Betoptic, Kerlone], carteolol [e.g., Cartrol], labetalol [e.g., Normodyne], levobunolol [e.g., Betagan], metoprolol [e.g., Lopressor], nadolol [e.g., Corgard], oxprenolol [e.g., Trasicor], penbutolol [e.g., Levatol], pindolol [e.g., Visken], propranolol [e.g., Inderal], sotalol [e.g., Sotacor], timolol [e.g., Blocadren, Timoptic])—Use of these medicines with oxtriphylline may prevent either the beta-blocker or oxtriphylline from working properly
- Cimetidine (e.g., Tagamet) or
- Ciprofloxacin (e.g., Cipro) or
- Erythromycin (e.g., E-Mycin) or
- Nicotine chewing gum (e.g., Nicorette) or
- Norfloxacin (e.g., Noroxin) or
- Ranitidine (e.g., Zantac) or
- Troleandomycin (e.g., TAO)—These medicines may increase the effects of oxtriphylline
- Phenytoin (e.g., Dilantin)—The effects of phenytoin may be decreased by oxtriphylline
- Smoking tobacco or marijuana—If you smoke or have smoked (tobacco or marijuana) regularly within the last 2 years, the amount of medicine you need may vary, depending on how much and how recently you have smoked

Other medical problems—The presence of other medical problems may affect the use of oxtriphylline and guaifenesin combination. Make sure you tell your doctor if you have any other medical problems, especially:

- Alcohol abuse (or history of) or
- Fever or
- Liver disease or
- Respiratory infections, such as influenza (flu)—The effects of oxtriphylline may be increased
- Diarrhea—The absorption of oxtriphylline may be decreased; therefore, the effects of this medicine may be decreased
- Enlarged prostate or
- Heart disease or

- High blood pressure or
- Stomach ulcer (or history of) or other stomach problems—Oxtriphylline may make the condition worse
- Fibrocystic breast disease—Symptoms of this disease may be increased by oxtriphylline
- Overactive thyroid—The effects of oxtriphylline may be decreased

Before you begin using any new medicine (prescription or nonprescription) or if you develop any new medical problem while you are using this medicine, check with your doctor, nurse, or pharmacist.

Proper Use of This Medicine

This medicine works best when taken with a glass of water on an empty stomach (either 30 minutes to 1 hour before meals or 2 hours after meals) since that way it will get into the blood sooner. However, in some cases your doctor may want you to take this medicine with meals or right after meals to lessen stomach upset. If you have any questions about how you should be taking this medicine, check with your doctor.

Take this medicine only as directed by your doctor. Do not take more of it, do not take it more often, and do not take it for a longer time than your doctor ordered. To do so may increase the chance of serious side effects.

In order for this medicine to help your medical problem, it must be taken every day in regularly spaced doses as ordered by your doctor. This is necessary to keep a constant amount of the medicine in the blood. To help keep the amount constant, do not miss any doses.

Missed dose—If you do miss a dose of this medicine, take it as soon as possible. However, if it is almost time for your next dose, skip the missed dose and go back to your regular dosing schedule. Do not double doses.

Storage—To store this medicine:

- Keep out of the reach of children.
- Store away from heat and direct light.
- Do not store the tablet form of this medicine in the bathroom, near the kitchen sink, or in other damp places. Heat or moisture may cause the medicine to break down.
- Keep the liquid form of this medicine from freezing.
- Do not keep outdated medicine or medicine no longer needed. Be sure that any discarded medicine is out of the reach of children.

Precautions While Using This Medicine

Your doctor should check your progress at regular visits, especially for the first few weeks after you begin using this medicine. A blood test may be taken to help your doctor decide whether the dose of this medicine should be changed.

The oxtriphylline in this medicine may add to the central nervous system stimulant effects of caffeine-containing foods or beverages such as chocolate, cocoa, tea, coffee, and cola drinks. *Avoid eating or drinking large amounts of these foods or beverages while taking this medicine.* If you have any questions about this, check with your doctor.

Do not eat charcoal-broiled foods every day while taking this medicine since these foods may keep the medicine from working properly.

Check with your doctor at once if you develop symptoms of influenza (flu) or a fever since either of these may increase the chance of side effects with this medicine.

Also, *check with your doctor if diarrhea occurs* because the dose of this medicine may need to be changed.

Side Effects of This Medicine

Along with its needed effects, a medicine may cause some unwanted effects. Although not all of these side effects may occur, if they do occur they may need medical attention.

Check with your doctor as soon as possible if any of the following side effects occur:

Less common

Heartburn and/or vomiting

Symptoms of overdose

Bloody or black, tarry stools; confusion or change in behavior; convulsions (seizures); diarrhea; dizziness or lightheadedness; fast breathing; fast, pounding, or irregular heartbeat; flushing or redness of face; headache; increased urination; irritability; loss of appetite; muscle twitching; nausea (continuing or severe) or vomiting; stomach cramps or pain; trembling; trouble in sleeping; unusual tiredness or weakness; vomiting blood or material that looks like coffee grounds

Other side effects may occur that usually do not need medical attention. These side effects may go away during treatment as your body adjusts to the medicine. However, check with your doctor if any of the following side effects continue or are bothersome:

More common

Nausea; nervousness or restlessness

Other side effects not listed above may also occur in some patients. If you notice any other effects, check with your doctor.

Annual revision: September 1990

OXYBUTYNIN Systemic

A commonly used brand name in the U.S. and Canada is Ditropan. Generic name product may also be available in the U.S.

Description

Oxybutynin (ox-i-BYOO-ti-nin) belongs to the group of medicines called antispasmodics. It helps decrease muscle spasms of the bladder and the frequent urge to urinate caused by these spasms.

Oxybutynin is available only with your doctor's prescription, in the following dosage forms:

Oral

- Syrup (U.S. and Canada)
- Tablets (U.S. and Canada)

It is very important that you read and understand the following information. If any of it causes you special concern, check with your doctor. Also, *if you have any questions* or if you want more information about this medicine or your medical problem, *ask your doctor, nurse, or pharmacist.*

Before Using This Medicine

In deciding to use a medicine, the risks of taking the medicine must be weighed against the good it will do. This is a decision you and your doctor will make. For oxybutynin, the following should be considered:

Allergies—Tell your doctor if you have ever had any unusual or allergic reaction to oxybutynin. Also tell your doctor and pharmacist if you are allergic to any other substances, such as foods, preservatives, or dyes.

Pregnancy—Oxybutynin has not been studied in pregnant women. However, it has not been shown to cause birth defects or other problems in animal studies.

Breast-feeding—Oxybutynin has not been reported to cause problems in nursing babies. However, since this medicine tends to decrease the secretions of the body, it is possible that the flow of breast milk may be reduced in some patients.

Children—There is no specific information about the use of oxybutynin in children under 5 years of age. In older children, oxybutynin is not expected to cause different side effects or problems than it does in adults.

Older adults—Elderly people are especially sensitive to the effects of oxybutynin. This may increase the chance of side effects during treatment.

Other medicines—Although certain medicines should not be used together at all, in other cases two different medicines may be used together even if an interaction might occur. In these cases, your doctor may want to change the dose, or other precautions may be necessary. When you are taking oxybutynin, it is especially important that your doctor and pharmacist know if you are taking any of the following:

- Amantadine (e.g., Symmetrel) or
- Anticholinergics (medicine for abdominal or stomach spasms or cramps) or
- Antidepressants (medicine for depression) or
- Antidyskinetics (medicine for Parkinson's disease or other conditions affecting control of muscles) or
- Antihistamines or
- Antipsychotics (medicine for mental illness) or
- Buclizine (e.g., Bucladin) or
- Carbamazepine (e.g., Tegretol) or
- Cyclizine (e.g., Marezine) or
- Cyclobenzaprine (e.g., Flexeril) or
- Disopyramide (e.g., Norpace) or
- Flavoxate (e.g., Urispas) or
- Ipratropium (e.g., Atrovent) or
- Meclizine (e.g., Antivert) or
- Methylphenidate (e.g., Ritalin) or
- Orphenadrine (e.g., Norflex) or
- Procainamide (e.g., Pronestyl) or
- Promethazine (e.g., Phenergan) or
- Quinidine (e.g., Quinidex) or
- Trimeprazine (e.g., Temaril)—Taking oxybutynin with these medicines may increase the effects of either medicine

Other medical problems—The presence of other medical problems may affect the use of oxybutynin. Make sure you tell your doctor if you have any other medical problems, especially:

- Bleeding (severe)—Oxybutynin may increase heart rate, which may make this condition worse
- Colitis (severe) or
- Dryness of mouth (severe and continuing) or
- Enlarged prostate or
- Glaucoma or
- Heart disease or
- Hiatal hernia or
- High blood pressure (hypertension) or
- Intestinal blockage or other intestinal or stomach problems or
- Myasthenia gravis or
- Toxemia of pregnancy or
- Urinary tract blockage or problems with urination—Oxybutynin may make these conditions worse
- Kidney disease or
- Liver disease—Higher blood levels of oxybutynin may occur, which increases the chance of side effects
- Overactive thyroid—Oxybutynin may further increase heart rate

Before you begin using any new medicine (prescription or nonprescription) or if you develop any new medical problem while you are using this medicine, check with your doctor, nurse, or pharmacist.

Proper Use of This Medicine

This medicine is usually taken with water on an empty stomach. However, your doctor may want you to take it with food or milk to lessen stomach upset.

Take this medicine only as directed. Do not take more of it, do not take it more often, and do not take it for a longer time than your doctor ordered. To do so may increase the chance of side effects.

Dosing—The dose of oxybutynin will be different for different patients. *Follow your doctor's orders or the directions on the label.* The following information includes only the average doses of oxybutynin. *If your dose is different, do not change it* unless your doctor tells you to do so.

- For *oral* dosage forms (syrup or tablets):
  - —For treatment of bladder problems:
    - Adults and children 12 years of age and over—5 milligrams (mg) two or three times a day.
    - Children up to 5 years of age—Use and dose have not been determined.
    - Children 5 to 12 years of age—5 mg two or three times a day. The dose is usually not more than 15 mg a day.

Missed dose—If you miss a dose of this medicine, take it as soon as possible. However, if it is almost time for your next dose, skip the missed dose and go back to your regular dosing schedule. Do not double doses.

Storage—To store this medicine:
- Keep out of the reach of children.
- Store away from heat and direct light.
- Do not store the tablet form of this medicine in the bathroom, near the kitchen sink, or in other damp places. Heat or moisture may cause the medicine to break down.
- Keep the syrup form of this medicine from freezing.
- Do not keep outdated medicine or medicine no longer needed. Be sure that any discarded medicine is out of the reach of children.

Precautions While Using This Medicine

This medicine will add to the effects of alcohol and other CNS depressants (medicines that slow down the nervous system, possibly causing drowsiness). Some examples of CNS depressants are antihistamines or medicine for hay fever, other allergies, or colds; sedatives, tranquilizers, or sleeping medicine; prescription pain medicine or narcotics; barbiturates; medicine for seizures; muscle relaxants; or anesthetics, including some dental anesthetics. *Check with your doctor before taking any of the above while you are using this medicine.*

This medicine may cause your eyes to become more sensitive to light than they are normally. Wearing sunglasses and avoiding too much exposure to bright light may help lessen the discomfort.

This medicine may cause some people to become drowsy or have blurred vision. *Make sure you know how you react to this medicine before you drive, use machines, or do anything else that could be dangerous if you are not alert or able to see well.*

Oxybutynin may make you sweat less, causing your body temperature to increase. *Use extra care not to become overheated during exercise or hot weather while you are taking this medicine,* since overheating may result in heat stroke. Also, hot baths or saunas may make you feel dizzy or faint while you are taking this medicine.

Your mouth, nose, and throat may feel very dry while you are taking this medicine. For temporary relief of mouth dryness, use sugarless candy or gum, melt bits of ice in your mouth, or use a saliva substitute. However, if your mouth continues to feel dry for more than 2 weeks, check with your medical doctor or dentist. Continuing dryness of the mouth may increase the chance of dental disease, including tooth decay, gum disease, and fungus infections.

Side Effects of This Medicine

Along with its needed effects, a medicine may cause some unwanted effects. Although not all of these side effects may occur, if they do occur they may need medical attention.

Check with your doctor as soon as possible if any of the following side effects occur:

Rare

Eye pain; skin rash or hives

Symptoms of overdose

Clumsiness or unsteadiness; confusion; dizziness; drowsiness (severe); fast heartbeat; fever; flushing or redness of face; hallucinations (seeing, hearing, or feeling things that are not there); shortness of breath or troubled breathing; unusual excitement, nervousness, restlessness, or irritability

Other side effects may occur that usually do not need medical attention. These side effects may go away during treatment as your body adjusts to the medicine. However, check with your doctor if any of the following side effects continue or are bothersome:

More common

Constipation; decreased sweating; drowsiness; dryness of mouth, nose, and throat

Less common or rare

Blurred vision; decreased flow of breast milk; decreased sexual ability; difficult urination; difficulty in swallowing; headache; increased sensitivity of eyes to light; nausea or vomiting; trouble in sleeping; unusual tiredness or weakness

Other side effects not listed above may also occur in some patients. If you notice any other effects, check with your doctor.

Annual revision: 06/16/93

OXYMETAZOLINE Nasal

Some commonly used brand names are:

In the U.S.

- Afrin Children's Strength 12 Hour Nose Drops
- Afrin Children's Strength Nose Drops
- Afrin 12 Hour Nasal Spray
- Afrin 12 Hour Nose Drops
- Afrin Menthol Nasal Spray
- Afrin Nasal Spray
- Afrin Nasal Spray Pump
- Afrin Nose Drops
- Allerest 12 Hour Nasal Spray
- Coricidin Nasal Mist
- Dristan Long Lasting Menthol Nasal Spray
- Dristan Long Lasting Nasal Pump Spray
- Dristan Long Lasting Nasal Spray
- Dristan Long Lasting Nasal Spray 12 Hour Metered Dose Pump
- Duramist Plus Up To 12 Hours Decongestant Nasal Spray
- Duration 12 Hour Nasal Spray Pump
- Neo-Synephrine 12 Hour Nasal Spray
- Neo-Synephrine 12 Hour Nasal Spray Pump
- Neo-Synephrine 12 Hour Nose Drops
- Neo-Synephrine 12 Hour Vapor Nasal Spray
- Nostrilla 12 Hour Nasal Decongestant
- Nostril Nasal Decongestant Mild
- Nostril Nasal Decongestant Regular
- NTZ Long Acting Decongestant Nasal Spray
- NTZ Long Acting Decongestant Nose Drops
- Sinarest 12 Hour Nasal Spray
- Vicks Sinex 12-Hour Formula Decongestant Nasal Spray
- Vicks Sinex 12-Hour Formula Decongestant Ultra Fine Mist
- Vicks Sinex Long-Acting 12 Hour Nasal Spray
- 4-Way Long Acting Nasal Spray

In Canada

- Nafrine Decongestant Nasal Drops
- Nafrine Decongestant Nasal Spray
- Nafrine Decongestant Pediatric Nasal Spray/Drops

Description

Oxymetazoline (ox-i-met-AZ-oh-leen) is used for the temporary relief of nasal congestion or stuffiness caused by hay fever or other allergies, colds, or sinus trouble.

This medicine may also be used for other conditions as determined by your doctor.

This medicine is available without a prescription; however, your doctor may have special instructions on the proper use or dose for your medical condition.

Oxymetazoline is available in the following dosage forms:

Nasal

- Nasal drops (U.S. and Canada)
- Nasal spray (U.S. and Canada)

It is very important that you read and understand the following information. If any of it causes you special concern, check with your doctor. Also, *if you have any questions* or if you want more information about this medicine or your medical problem, *ask your doctor, nurse, or pharmacist.*

Before Using This Medicine

If you are using this medicine without a prescription, carefully read and follow any precautions on the label. For oxymetazoline, the following should be considered:

Allergies—Tell your doctor if you have ever had any unusual or allergic reaction to oxymetazoline or any other nasal decongestant. Also tell your doctor and pharmacist if you are allergic to any other substances, such as foods, preservatives, or dyes.

Pregnancy—The medication may be absorbed into the body. However, oxymetazoline has not been shown to cause birth defects or other problems in humans.

Breast-feeding—Oxymetazoline may be absorbed into the body. However, oxymetazoline has not been reported to cause problems in nursing babies.

Children—Children may be especially sensitive to the effects of oxymetazoline. This may increase the chance of side effects during treatment.

Older adults—Many medicines have not been tested in older people. Therefore, it may not be known whether they work exactly the same way they do in younger adults or if they cause different side effects or problems in older people. There is no specific information about the use of oxymetazoline in the elderly.

Other medicines—Although certain medicines should not be used together at all, in other cases two different medicines may be used together even if an interaction might occur. In these cases, your doctor may want to change the dose, or other precautions may be necessary. When you are using oxymetazoline, it is especially important that your doctor and pharmacist know if you are taking any other prescription or nonprescription (over-the-counter [OTC]) medicine.

Other medical problems—The presence of other medical problems may affect the use of oxymetazoline. Make sure you tell your doctor if you have any other medical problems, especially:

- Diabetes mellitus (sugar diabetes)
- Heart or blood vessel disease or
- High blood pressure—Oxymetazoline may make the condition worse
- Overactive thyroid

Before you begin using any new medicine (prescription or nonprescription) or if you develop any new medical problem while you are using this medicine, check with your doctor, nurse, or pharmacist.

Proper Use of This Medicine

To use the *nose drops*:

- Blow your nose gently. Tilt the head back while standing or sitting up, or lie down on a bed and hang the head over the side. Place the drops into each nostril and keep the head tilted back for a few minutes to allow the medicine to spread throughout the nose.
- Rinse the dropper with hot water and dry with a clean tissue. Replace the cap right after use.
- To avoid spreading the infection, do not use the container for more than one person.

To use the *nose spray*:

- Blow your nose gently. With the head upright, spray the medicine into each nostril. Sniff briskly while squeezing the bottle quickly and firmly. For best results, spray once into each nostril, wait 3 to 5 minutes to allow the medicine to work, then blow the nose gently and thoroughly. Repeat until the complete dose is used.
- Rinse the tip of the spray bottle with hot water, taking care not to suck water into the bottle, and dry with a clean tissue. Replace the cap right after use.
- To avoid spreading the infection, do not use the container for more than one person.

Use this medicine only as directed. Do not use more of it, do not use it more often, and do not use it for longer than 3 days without first checking with your doctor. To do so may make your runny or stuffy nose worse and may also increase the chance of side effects.

Missed dose—If you are using this medicine on a regular schedule and you miss a dose, use it right away if you remember within an hour or so of the missed dose. However, if you do not remember until later, skip the missed dose and go back to your regular dosing schedule. Do not double doses.

Storage—To store this medicine:

- Keep out of the reach of children.
- Store away from heat and direct light.
- Keep the medicine from freezing.
- Do not keep outdated medicine or medicine no longer needed. Be sure that any discarded medicine is out of the reach of children.

Side Effects of This Medicine

Along with its needed effects, a medicine may cause some unwanted effects. Although not all of these side effects may occur, if they do occur they may need medical attention.

When this medicine is used for short periods of time at low doses, side effects usually are rare. However, check with your doctor as soon as possible if any of the following occur:

Increase in runny or stuffy nose

Symptoms of too much medicine being absorbed into the body

Fast, irregular, or pounding heartbeat; headache or lightheadedness; nervousness; trembling; trouble in sleeping

The above side effects are more likely to occur in children because there is a greater chance in children that too much of this medicine may be absorbed into the body.

Other side effects may occur that usually do not need medical attention. These side effects may go away during treatment as your body adjusts to the medicine. However, check with your doctor or pharmacist if any of the following side effects continue or are bothersome:

Burning, dryness, or stinging on inside of nose; sneezing

Other side effects not listed above may also occur in some patients. If you notice any other effects, check with your doctor or pharmacist.

Annual revision: August 1990

OXYMETAZOLINE Ophthalmic

Some commonly used brand names are:

In the U.S.
- OcuClear
- Visine L.R.

In Canada
- OcuClear

Description

Oxymetazoline (ox-i-met-AZ-oh-leen) is used to relieve redness due to minor eye irritations, such as those caused by colds, dust, wind, smog, pollen, swimming, or wearing contact lenses.

Oxymetazoline is available without a prescription; however, your doctor may have special instructions on the proper use of this medicine for your medical condition.

Oxymetazoline is available in the following dosage form:

Ophthalmic

- Ophthalmic solution (eye drops) (U.S. and Canada)

It is very important that you read and understand the following information. If any of it causes you special concern, check with your doctor or pharmacist. Also, *if you have any questions* or if you want more information about this medicine or your medical problem, *ask your doctor, nurse, or pharmacist.*

Before Using This Medicine

If you are taking this medicine without a prescription, carefully read and follow any precautions on the label. For ophthalmic oxymetazoline, the following should be considered:

Allergies—Tell your doctor if you have ever had any unusual or allergic reaction to oxymetazoline or to any other decongestant used in the eye. Also tell your doctor and pharmacist if you are allergic to any other substances, such as preservatives.

Pregnancy—Studies in humans have not shown that oxymetazoline causes birth defects or other problems in humans.

Breast-feeding—Oxymetazoline may be absorbed into the body. However, oxymetazoline has not been shown to cause problems in nursing babies.

Children—Check with your doctor before using oxymetazoline eye drops in children up to 6 years of age. Eye redness in children can occur with illnesses, such as allergies, fevers, colds, and measles, that may require medical attention.

Older adults—Many medicines have not been studied specifically in older people. Therefore, it may not be known whether they work exactly the same way they do in younger adults or if they cause different side effects or problems in older people. There is no specific information comparing use of oxymetazoline in the elderly with use in other age groups.

Other medicines—Although certain medicines should not be used together at all, in other cases two different medicines may be used together even if an interaction might occur. In these cases, your doctor may want to change the dose, or other precautions may be necessary. Tell your doctor and pharmacist if you are using any other prescription or nonprescription (over-the-counter [OTC]) medicine.

Other medical problems—The presence of other medical problems may affect the use of ophthalmic oxymetazoline. Make sure you tell your doctor if you have any other medical problems, especially:

- Eye disease, infection, or injury—This medicine may mask the symptoms of these conditions
- Heart or blood vessel disease or
- High blood pressure or
- Overactive thyroid—If absorbed into the body, this medicine may cause side effects that may make the medical problem worse
- Use of soft contact lenses—Because of the preservative in this medicine, some eye conditions may get worse if this medicine is used on top of soft contact lenses

Before you begin using any new medicine (prescription or nonprescription) or if you develop any new medical problem while you are using this medicine, check with your doctor, nurse, or pharmacist.

Proper Use of This Medicine

Do not use oxymetazoline ophthalmic solution if it becomes cloudy or changes color.

To use:

- First, wash your hands. With the middle finger, apply pressure to the inside corner of the eye (and continue to apply pressure for 1 or 2 minutes after the medicine has been placed in the eye). Tilt the head back and with the index finger of the same hand, pull the lower eyelid away from the eye to form a pouch. Drop the medicine into the pouch and gently close the eyes. Do not blink. Keep the eyes closed for 1 or 2 minutes to allow the medicine to be absorbed.
- To keep the medicine as germ-free as possible, do not touch the applicator tip to any surface (including the eye). Also, keep the container tightly closed.

Use this medicine only as directed. Do not use more of it, do not use it more often, and do not use it for more than 72 hours, unless otherwise directed by your doctor.

To do so may make your eye irritation worse and may also increase the chance of side effects.

Storage—To store this medicine:

- Keep out of the reach of children.
- Store away from heat and direct light.
- Keep the medicine from freezing.
- Do not keep outdated medicine or medicine no longer needed. Be sure that any discarded medicine is out of the reach of children.

Precautions While Using This Medicine

If eye pain or change in vision occurs or if redness or irritation of the eye continues, gets worse, or lasts for more than 72 hours, stop using the medicine and check with your doctor.

Side Effects of This Medicine

Along with its needed effects, a medicine may cause some unwanted effects. Although not all of these side effects may occur, if they do occur they may need medical attention.

When this medicine is used for short periods of time at low doses, side effects usually are rare.

Check with your doctor as soon as possible if any of the following side effects occur:

With overuse or long-term use

Increase in irritation or redness of eyes

Symptoms of too much medicine being absorbed into the body

Fast, irregular, or pounding heartbeat; headache or lightheadedness; nervousness; trembling; trouble in sleeping

Other side effects not listed above may also occur in some patients. If you notice any other effects, check with your doctor.

Annual revision: 04/29/92

OXYTOCIN Systemic

Some commonly used brand names are:

In the U.S.

Pitocin
Syntocinon

Generic name product may also be available.

In Canada

Syntocinon

Description

Oxytocin (ox-i-TOE-sin) is a hormone used to help start or continue labor and to control bleeding after delivery. It is also sometimes used to help milk secretion in breast-feeding.

Oxytocin may also be used for other conditions as determined by your doctor.

In general, oxytocin should not be used to start labor unless there are specific medical reasons. Be sure you have discussed this with your doctor before receiving this medicine.

Oxytocin is available only with your doctor's prescription, in the following dosage forms:

Nasal

- Solution (U.S. and Canada)

Parenteral

- Injection (U.S. and Canada)

It is very important that you read and understand the following information. If any of it causes you special concern, check with your doctor. Also, *if you have any questions* or if you want more information about this medicine or your medical problem, *ask your doctor, nurse, or pharmacist.*

Before Using This Medicine

In deciding to use a medicine, the risks of taking the medicine must be weighed against the good it will do. This is a decision you and your doctor will make. For oxytocin, the following should be considered:

Allergies—Tell your doctor if you have ever had any unusual or allergic reaction to oxytocin. Also tell your doctor and pharmacist if you are allergic to any other substances, such as foods, preservatives, or dyes.

Breast-feeding—Although very small amounts of this medicine pass into breast milk, it has not been reported to cause problems in nursing babies.

Other medicines—Although certain medicines should not be used together at all, in other cases two different medicines may be used together even if an interaction might occur. In these cases, your doctor may want to change the dose, or other precautions may be necessary. Tell your doctor and pharmacist if you are taking any other prescription or nonprescription (over-the-counter [OTC]) medicine.

Other medical problems—The presence of other medical problems may affect the use of oxytocin. Make sure you tell your doctor if you have any other medical problems, especially:

- Heart disease
- Hypertension
- Kidney disease

Before you begin using any new medicine (prescription or nonprescription) or if you develop any new medical problem while you are using this medicine, check with your doctor, nurse, or pharmacist.

Proper Use of This Medicine

For patients using the *nasal spray* form of this medicine:

- This medicine usually comes with directions for use. Read them carefully before using.

Storage—To store this medicine:

- Keep out of the reach of children.
- Store away from heat and direct light.
- Protect the medicine from freezing.
- Do not keep outdated medicine or medicine no longer needed. Be sure that any discarded medicine is out of the reach of children.

P

Precautions While Using This Medicine

Oxytocin nasal spray may not help milk secretion in some breast-feeding women. Call your doctor if this medicine is not working.

Side Effects of This Medicine

Oxytocin can be very useful for helping labor. However, there are certain risks with using it. Oxytocin causes contractions of the uterus. In women who are unusually sensitive to its effects, these contractions may become too strong. In rare cases, this may lead to tearing of the uterus. Also, if contractions are too strong, the supply of blood and oxygen to the fetus may be decreased.

Oxytocin has been reported to cause irregular heartbeat and increase bleeding after delivery in some women. It has also been reported to cause jaundice in some newborn infants.

Along with its needed effects, a medicine may cause some unwanted effects. Although not all of these side effects may occur, if they do occur they may need medical attention:

Rare (with use of injection)

Confusion; convulsions (seizures); difficulty in breathing; dizziness; fast or irregular heartbeat; headache (continuing or severe); hives; pelvic or abdominal pain (severe); skin rash or itching; vaginal bleeding (increased or continuing); weakness; weight gain (rapid)

Rare (with use of nasal spray)

Convulsions (seizures); mental disturbances; unexpected bleeding or contractions of the uterus

Other side effects may occur that usually do not need medical attention. However, check with your doctor if any of the following side effects continue or are bothersome:

Rare (with use of injection)

Nausea; vomiting

Rare (with use of nasal spray)

Nasal irritation; runny nose; tearing of the eyes

Other side effects not listed above may also occur in some patients. If you notice any other effects, check with your doctor.

Additional information

Once a medicine has been approved for marketing for a certain use, experience may show that it is also useful for other medical problems. Although this use is not included in product labeling, oxytocin is used in certain patients for the following:

- Testing the ability of the placenta to support a pregnancy

Other than the above information, there is no additional information relating to proper use, precautions, or side effects for this use.

Annual revision: 07/14/93

PAMIDRONATE Systemic

A commonly used brand name in the U.S. and Canada is Aredia. Another commonly used name is APD.

Description

Pamidronate (pa-mi-DROE-nate) is used to treat hypercalcemia (too much calcium in the blood) that may occur with some types of cancer. This medicine may be used for other conditions as determined by your doctor.

This medicine is to be administered only by or under the supervision of your doctor. It is available in the following dosage form:

Parenteral

- Injection (U.S. and Canada)

It is very important that you read and understand the following information. If any of it causes you special concern, check with your doctor. Also, *if you have any questions* or if you want more information about this medicine or your medical problem, *ask your doctor, nurse, or pharmacist.*

Before Receiving This Medicine

In deciding to use a medicine, the risks of receiving the medicine must be weighed against the good it will do. This is a decision you and your doctor will make. For pamidronate, the following should be considered:

Allergies—Tell your doctor if you have ever had any unusual or allergic reaction to pamidronate or etidronate. Also tell your doctor and pharmacist if you are allergic to any other substances, such as foods, preservatives, or dyes.

Pregnancy—Studies have not been done in humans. However, studies in rats given higher doses of oral pamidronate have shown that the medicine may decrease fertility, increase the length of pregnancy, and cause death of the baby rat.

Breast-feeding—It is not known if pamidronate passes into breast milk.

Children—Studies on this medicine have been done only in adult patients, and there is no specific information comparing use of pamidronate in children with use in other age groups.

Older adults—When pamidronate is given along with a large amount of fluids, older people tend to retain (keep) the excess fluid.

Other medicines—Although certain medicines should not be used together at all, in other cases two different medicines may be used together even if an interaction might occur. In these cases, your doctor may want to change the dose, or other precautions may be necessary. When you are receiving pamidronate, it is especially important that your doctor and pharmacist know if you are taking any of the following:

- Calcium-containing preparations or
- Vitamin D–containing preparations—Use with pamidronate may keep pamidronate from working properly

Other medical problems—The presence of other medical problems may affect the use of pamidronate. Make sure you tell your doctor if you have any other medical problems, especially:

- Heart problems—The increased amount of fluid may make this condition worse
- Kidney problems—Pamidronate may build up in the bloodstream, which may increase the chance of unwanted effects

Before you begin using any new medicine (prescription or nonprescription) or if you develop any new medical problem while you are using this medicine, check with your doctor, nurse, or pharmacist.

Proper Use of This Medicine

Dosing—The dose of pamidronate will be different for different patients. *Follow your doctor's orders.* The following information includes only the average doses of pamidronate.

- For *injectable* dosage form:
  —For treating hypercalcemia (too much calcium in the blood):
  - Adults: 30 to 90 mg in a solution to be given over 4 to 24 hours into a vein.
  - Children: Use is not recommended.

Precautions While Receiving This Medicine

It is important that your doctor check your progress at regular visits after you have received pamidronate. If your condition has improved, your progress must still be checked. The results of laboratory tests or the occurrence of certain symptoms will tell your doctor if your condition is coming back and a second treatment is needed.

For patients using this medicine for *hypercalcemia (too much calcium in the blood):*

- Your doctor may want you to follow a low-calcium diet. If you have any questions about this, check with your doctor.

Side Effects of This Medicine

Along with its needed effects, a medicine may cause some unwanted effects. Although not all of these side effects

P

may occur, if they do occur they may need medical attention.

Check with your doctor as soon as possible if any of the following side effects occur:

More common

Abdominal cramps; chills; confusion; fever; muscle spasms; sore throat

Note: Abdominal cramps, confusion, and muscle spasms are less common when pamidronate is given in doses of 60 mg or less.

Other side effects may occur that usually do not need medical attention. These side effects may go away during treatment as your body adjusts to the medicine. However, check with your doctor if any of the following side effects continue or are bothersome:

More common—at higher doses

Nausea; pain and swelling at place of injection

Less common

Muscle stiffness

Other side effects not listed above may also occur in some patients. If you notice any other effects, check with your doctor.

Additional Information

Once a medicine has been approved for marketing for a certain use, experience may show that it is also useful for other medical problems. Although these uses are not included in product labeling, pamidronate is used in certain patients with the following medical conditions:

- Bone metastases
- Paget's disease of bone

Other than the above information, there is no additional information relating to proper use, precautions, or side effects for these uses.

Annual revision: 06/02/93

PANCREATIN, PEPSIN, BILE SALTS, HYOSCYAMINE, ATROPINE, SCOPOLAMINE, AND PHENOBARBITAL Systemic

A commonly used brand name in the U.S. and Canada is Donnazyme.

Description

Pancreatin (PAN-kree-a-tin), pepsin (PEP-sin), bile salts, hyoscyamine (hye-oh-SYE-a-meen), atropine (A-troe-peen), scopolamine (skoe-POL-a-meen), and phenobarbital (fee-noe-BAR-bi-tal) combination is used to relieve indigestion in certain conditions in which the body does not produce enough of the enzymes needed for the complete digestion of food.

This medicine is available only with your doctor's prescription, in the following dosage form:

Oral

- Tablets (U.S. and Canada)

It is very important that you read and understand the following information. If any of it causes you special concern, check with your doctor. Also, *if you have any questions* or if you want more information about this medicine or your medical problem, *ask your doctor, nurse, or pharmacist.*

Before Using This Medicine

In deciding to use a medicine, the risks of taking the medicine must be weighed against the good it will do. This is a decision you and your doctor will make. For this combination medicine, the following should be considered:

Allergies—Tell your doctor if you have ever had any unusual or allergic reaction to any of the belladonna alkaloids such as atropine, hyoscyamine, or scopolamine; to pancrelipase, pancreatin, or beef or pork products; or to barbiturates. Also tell your doctor and pharmacist if you are allergic to any other substances, such as foods, preservatives, or dyes.

Pregnancy—Studies have not been done in either humans or animals.

Breast-feeding—This medicine has not been reported to cause problems in nursing babies. However, the chance always exists since traces of the belladonna alkaloids and phenobarbital (contained in this combination medicine) pass into the breast milk. Also, because the belladonna alkaloids tend to decrease the secretions of the body, it is possible that the flow of breast milk may be reduced in some patients.

Children—Children are especially sensitive to the effects of belladonna alkaloids and barbiturates (contained in this combination medicine). This may increase the chance of side effects during treatment.

Older adults—Confusion or memory loss, drowsiness, unusual excitement or agitation may be more likely to occur in the elderly, who are usually more sensitive than younger adults to the effects of belladonna alkaloids and barbiturates (contained in this combination medicine).

Other medicines—Although certain medicines should not be used together at all, in other cases two different medicines may be used together even if an interaction might occur. In these cases, your doctor may want to change the dose, or other precautions may be necessary. When you are taking this combination medicine, it is especially important that your doctor and pharmacist know if you are taking any of the following:

- Alcohol or
- Central nervous system (CNS) depressants—Taking this combination medicine with CNS depressants may increase the effects of either medicine
- Antacids or
- Diarrhea medicine containing kaolin or attapulgite—Use of these medicines with this combination medicine may prevent this combination medicine from working properly; these medicines and this combination medicine should be taken 2 hours apart
- Anticoagulants, coumarin- or indandione-type (blood thinners) or
- Digitalis glycosides (heart medicine) or
- Ketoconazole (e.g., Nizoral)—Use of digitalis glycosides, anticoagulants, or ketoconazole with this combination medicine may prevent the digitalis glycoside, anticoagulant, or ketoconazole from working properly
- Potassium chloride (e.g., Kay Ciel)—Use of potassium chloride with this combination medicine may make stomach and intestine problems caused by potassium worse

Other medical problems—The presence of other medical problems may affect the use of this combination medicine. Make sure you tell your doctor if you have any other medical problems, especially:

- Bleeding (severe)—The belladonna alkaloids in this combination medicine may increase heart rate, which may make this condition worse
- Colitis or
- Difficult urination or problems with urination or
- Dryness of mouth (severe and continuing) or
- Enlarged prostate or
- Fast heartbeat or
- Glaucoma or
- Heart disease or
- Hernia or
- High blood pressure (hypertension) or
- Intestinal blockage or other intestinal or stomach problems or
- Myasthenia gravis or
- Porphyria (or history of) or
- Urinary tract blockage—This combination medicine may make these conditions worse
- Drug abuse or history of—The phenobarbital in this combination may be habit-forming
- Kidney disease or
- Liver disease—Higher blood levels of this combination medicine may occur, which increases the chance of side effects
- Overactive thyroid—The belladonna alkaloids in this combination medicine may further increase heart rate

Before you begin using any new medicine (prescription or nonprescription) or if you develop any new medical problem while you are using this medicine, check with your doctor, nurse, or pharmacist.

Proper Use of This Medicine

Take this medicine with or after meals unless otherwise directed by your doctor.

Take this medicine only as directed by your doctor. Do not take more or less of it, do not take it more often, and do not take it for a longer period of time than your doctor ordered. If too much is used, it may increase the chance of side effects and it may also become habit-forming.

Importance of diet—When prescribing this medicine for your condition, your doctor may also prescribe a personal diet for you. Follow carefully the special diet your doctor gave you. This is most important and necessary for the medicine to work properly and to avoid indigestion.

Swallow the tablets without chewing, to avoid mouth irritation.

Missed dose—If you miss a dose of this medicine, take it as soon as possible. However, if it is almost time for your next dose, skip the missed dose and go back to your regular dosing schedule. Do not double doses.

Storage—To store this medicine:

- Keep out of the reach of children. Overdose is especially dangerous in young children.
- Store away from heat and direct light.
- Do not store the tablet form of this medicine in the bathroom, near the kitchen sink, or in other damp places. The heat or moisture may cause the medicine to break down.
- Do not keep outdated medicine or medicine no longer needed. Be sure that any discarded medicine is out of the reach of children.

Precautions While Using This Medicine

This medicine will add to the effects of alcohol and other CNS depressants (medicines that slow down the nervous system, possibly causing drowsiness). Some examples of CNS depressants are antihistamines or medicine for hay fever, other allergies, or colds; sedatives, tranquilizers, or sleeping medicine; prescription pain medicine or narcotics; barbiturates; medicine for seizures; muscle relaxants; or anesthetics, including some dental anesthetics. *Check with your doctor before taking any of the above while you are using this medicine.*

This medicine may cause your eyes to become more sensitive to light than they are normally. Wearing sunglasses and avoiding too much exposure to bright light may help lessen the discomfort from bright light.

This medicine may cause some people to have blurred vision or to become drowsy, dizzy, or less alert than they are normally. *Make sure you know how you react to this medicine before you drive, use machines, or do anything else that could be dangerous if you are dizzy or are not alert and able to see well.*

Belladonna alkaloids will often make you sweat less, causing your body temperature to increase. *Use extra care not to become overheated during exercise or hot weather while you are taking this medicine,* since overheating may result in heat stroke. Also, hot baths or saunas may make you feel dizzy or faint while you are taking this medicine.

The belladonna alkaloids in this medicine may cause dryness of the mouth, nose, and throat. For temporary relief of mouth dryness, use sugarless candy or gum, melt bits of ice in your mouth, or use a saliva substitute. However, if your mouth continues to feel dry for more than 2 weeks, check with your medical doctor or dentist. Continuing dryness of the mouth may increase the chance of dental disease, including tooth decay, gum disease, and fungus infections.

Side Effects of This Medicine

Along with its needed effects, a medicine may cause some unwanted effects. Although not all of these side effects appear very often, when they do occur they may require medical attention.

Check with your doctor as soon as possible if any of the following side effects occur:

Rare

Blood in urine; diarrhea; eye pain; joint pain; nausea or vomiting; skin rash or hives; sore throat and fever; stomach cramps or pain; swelling of feet or lower legs; unusual bleeding or bruising; yellow eyes or skin

Symptoms of overdose

Clumsiness, unsteadiness, or staggering; confusion (especially in the elderly); dizziness; fever; flushing or redness of face; hallucinations (seeing, hearing, or feeling things that are not there); shortness of breath or troubled breathing; slow or fast heartbeat; unusual excitement, nervousness, restlessness, or irritability

Other side effects may occur that usually do not need medical attention. These side effects may go away during treatment as your body adjusts to the medicine. However, check with your doctor if any of the following side effects continue or are bothersome:

More common

Constipation; decreased sweating; drowsiness; dryness of mouth, nose, and throat

Less common or rare

Blurred vision; decreased flow of breast milk; decreased sexual ability; difficult urination (especially in older men); difficulty in swallowing; headache; increased sensitivity of eyes to light; trouble in sleeping; unusual tiredness or weakness

Other side effects not listed above may also occur in some patients. If you notice any other effects, check with your doctor.

Annual revision: 04/15/92

PANCRELIPASE Systemic

Some commonly used brand names are:

In the U.S.

- Cotazym
- Cotazym-S
- Enzymase-16
- Ilozyme
- Ku-Zyme HP
- Pancoate
- Pancrease
- Pancrease MT 4
- Pancrease MT 10
- Pancrease MT 16
- Protilase
- Ultrase MT 12
- Ultrase MT 20
- Ultrase MT 24
- Viokase
- Zymase

In Canada

- Cotazym
- Cotazym-65 B
- Cotazym E.C.S. 8
- Cotazym E.C.S. 20
- Pancrease
- Pancrease MT 4
- Pancrease MT 10
- Pancrease MT 16

Another commonly used name is lipancreatin.

Description

Pancrelipase (pan-kre-LI-pase) is used to help digestion in certain conditions in which the pancreas is not working properly. It may also be used for other conditions as determined by your doctor.

Pancrelipase contains the enzymes needed for the digestion of proteins, starches, and fats.

Pancrelipase is available only with your doctor's prescription, in the following dosage forms:

Oral

- Capsules (U.S. and Canada)
- Delayed-release capsules (U.S. and Canada)
- Powder (U.S.)
- Tablets (U.S.)

It is very important that you read and understand the following information. If any of it causes you special concern, check with your doctor. Also, *if you have any questions* or if you want more information about this medicine or your medical problem, *ask your doctor, nurse, or pharmacist.*

Before Using This Medicine

In deciding to use a medicine, the risks of taking the medicine must be weighed against the good it will do. This is a decision you and your doctor will make. For pancrelipase, the following should be considered:

Allergies—Tell your doctor if you have ever had any unusual or allergic reaction to pancrelipase, pancreatin, or pork products. Also tell your doctor and pharmacist if you are allergic to any other substances, such as foods, preservatives, or dyes.

Pregnancy—Studies have not been done in either humans or animals.

Breast-feeding—Pancrelipase has not been reported to cause problems in nursing babies.

Children—This medicine has been tested in children 6 months of age or older and has not been shown to cause different side effects or problems than it does in adults.

Older adults—Many medicines have not been studied specifically in older people. Therefore, it may not be known whether they work exactly the same way they do in younger adults. Although there is no specific information comparing use of pancrelipase in the elderly with use in other age groups, this medicine is not expected to cause different side effects or problems in older people than it does in younger adults.

Other medicines—Although certain medicines should not be used together at all, in other cases two different medicines may be used together even if an interaction might occur. In these cases, your doctor may want to change the dose, or other precautions may be necessary. Tell your doctor and pharmacist if you are taking any other prescription or nonprescription (over-the-counter [OTC]) medicine.

Other medical problems—The presence of other medical problems may affect the use of pancrelipase. Make sure you tell your doctor if you have any other medical problems, especially:

- Pancreatitis (sudden, severe inflammation of the pancreas)—Pancrelipase may make this condition worse

Before you begin using any new medicine (prescription or nonprescription) or if you develop any new medical problem while you are using this medicine, check with your doctor, nurse, or pharmacist.

Proper Use of This Medicine

Take this medicine before or with meals and snacks, unless otherwise directed by your doctor.

When prescribing this medicine for your condition, your doctor may also prescribe a personal diet for you. Follow carefully the special diet your doctor gave you. This is most important and necessary for the medicine to work properly and to avoid indigestion.

For patients taking the *tablet form* of this medicine:

- *Swallow the tablets quickly with some liquid, without chewing,* to avoid mouth irritation.

For patients taking the *capsules containing the enteric-coated spheres:*

- Swallow the capsule whole.
- Do not crush, break, or chew before swallowing.
- When given to children, the capsule may be opened and sprinkled on a small amount of liquid or soft food that can be swallowed without chewing, such as applesauce or gelatin. However, it should not be mixed with alkaline foods, such as milk and ice cream, which may reduce its effect.

Missed dose—If you miss a dose of this medicine, take it as soon as possible. However, if it is almost time for your next dose, skip the missed dose and go back to your regular dosing schedule. Do not double doses.

Storage—To store this medicine:

- Keep out of the reach of children.
- Store away from heat and direct light.
- Do not store the capsule, powder, or tablet form of this medicine in the bathroom, near the kitchen sink, or in other damp places. Heat or moisture may cause the medicine to break down.
- Do not keep outdated medicine or medicine no longer needed. Be sure that any discarded medicine is out of the reach of children.

Precautions While Using This Medicine

Your doctor may recommend that you take pancrelipase with another medicine, such as certain antacids or anti-ulcer medicines. However, antacids that contain calcium carbonate and/or magnesium hydroxate may not let the pancrelipase work properly and should be avoided.

Do not change brands or dosage forms of pancrelipase without first checking with your doctor. Different products may not work in the same way. If you refill your medicine and it looks different, check with your pharmacist.

For patients taking the *capsules containing the powder:*

- If the capsules are opened to mix with food, be careful not to breathe in the powder. To do so may cause harmful effects such as stuffy nose, shortness of breath, troubled breathing, wheezing, or tightness in chest.

For patients taking the *powder form* of this medicine:

- Avoid breathing in the powder. To do so may cause harmful effects such as stuffy nose, shortness of breath, troubled breathing, wheezing, or tightness in chest.

Side Effects of This Medicine

Along with its needed effects, a medicine may cause some unwanted effects. Although not all of these side effects may occur, if they do occur they may need medical attention.

Check with your doctor as soon as possible if any of the following side effects occur:

Rare

Skin rash or hives

With high doses

Diarrhea; intestinal blockage; nausea; stomach cramps or pain

With very high doses

Blood in urine; joint pain; swelling of feet or lower legs

With powder dosage form or powder from opened capsules—if breathed in

Shortness of breath; stuffy nose; tightness in chest; troubled breathing; wheezing

With tablets—if held in mouth

Irritation of the mouth

Other side effects not listed above may also occur in some patients. If you notice any other effects, check with your doctor.

Annual revision: 02/13/92

PANTOTHENIC ACID (Vitamin B_5) Systemic

Other commonly used names are vitamin B_5 and calcium pantothenate. Generic name product may also be available in the U.S. and Canada.

Description

Vitamins (VYE-ta-mins) are compounds that you *must* have for growth and health. They are needed in only small amounts and are usually available in the foods that you eat. Pantothenic acid (vitamin B_5) is necessary for normal metabolism.

No problems have been found that are due to a lack of pantothenic acid alone. However, a lack of one B vitamin usually goes along with a lack of others, so pantothenic acid is often included in B complex products.

Claims that pantothenic acid is effective for treatment of nerve damage, breathing problems, itching and other skin problems, and poisoning with some other drugs; for getting rid of or preventing gray hair; for preventing arthritis, allergies, and birth defects; or for improving mental ability have not been proven.

Pantothenic acid is available without a prescription. However, it may be a good idea to check with your doctor before taking any on your own. If you take more than you need, it will simply be lost from your body.

This vitamin is available in the following dosage forms:

Oral

Calcium pantothenate

- Tablets (U.S. and Canada)

Pantothenic acid

- Tablets (U.S.)

It is very important that you read and understand the following information. If any of it causes you special concern, check with your doctor or pharmacist. Also, *if you have any questions* or if you want more information about this dietary supplement or your medical problem, *ask your doctor, nurse, pharmacist, or dietitian.*

Importance of Diet

Vitamin supplements should be taken only if you cannot get enough vitamins in your diet; however, some diets may not contain all of the vitamins you need. You may not be getting enough vitamins because of rapid weight loss, unusual diets (such as some reducing diets in which choice of foods is very limited), prolonged intravenous feeding, or malnutrition. A balanced diet should provide all the vitamins you normally need.

In order to get enough vitamins and minerals in your diet, it is important that you eat a balanced and varied diet.

Follow carefully any diet program your doctor may recommend. For your specific vitamin and/or mineral needs, ask your doctor or dietitian for a list of appropriate foods.

Pantothenic acid is found in various foods including peas and beans (except green beans), lean meat, poultry, fish, and whole-grain cereals. Little pantothenic acid is lost from foods with ordinary cooking.

Vitamins alone will not take the place of a good diet and will not provide energy. Your body also needs other substances found in food—protein, minerals, carbohydrates, and fat.

In some cases, it may not be possible for you to get enough food to supply you with the proper vitamins. In other cases, the amount of vitamins you need may be increased above normal. Therefore, a vitamin supplement may be needed.

Experts have developed a list of recommended dietary allowances (RDA) for most of the vitamins. The RDA are not an exact number but a general idea of how much you need. They do not cover amounts needed for problems caused by a serious lack of vitamins. Because lack of pantothenic acid is so rare, there are no RDA for this vitamin. However, it is thought that 4 to 7 mg for adults and adolescents and 3 to 4 mg of pantothenic acid for children is enough.

Before Using This Dietary Supplement

If you are taking this dietary supplement without a prescription, carefully read and follow any precautions on the label. For pantothenic acid, the following should be considered:

Allergies—Tell your doctor and pharmacist if you are allergic to any substances, such as foods, preservatives, or dyes.

Pregnancy—It is especially important that you are receiving enough vitamins when you become pregnant and that you continue to receive the right amount of vitamins throughout your pregnancy. The healthy growth and development of the fetus depend on a steady supply of nutrients from the mother. However, taking large amounts of a nutritional supplement during pregnancy may be harmful to the mother and/or fetus and should be avoided.

Breast-feeding—It is especially important that you receive the right amounts of vitamins so that your baby will also get the vitamins needed to grow properly. However, taking large amounts of a nutritional supplement while breast-feeding may be harmful to the mother and/or baby and should be avoided.

Children—Normal daily requirements vary according to age. It is especially important that children receive enough vitamins in their diet for healthy growth and development. There is no specific information about the use of pantothenic acid in children in doses higher than the normal daily requirements.

Older adults—It is important that older people continue to receive enough vitamins in their diet for good health. There is no specific information about the use of pantothenic acid in older people in doses higher than the normal daily requirements.

Other medicines or dietary supplements—Although certain medicines or dietary supplements should not be used together at all, in other cases two different medicines or dietary supplements may be used together even if an interaction might occur. In these cases, your doctor may want to change the dose, or other precautions may be necessary. Tell your doctor and pharmacist if you are taking any other prescription, nonprescription (over-the-counter [OTC]) medicine, or dietary supplements.

Proper Use of This Dietary Supplement

Some people believe that taking very large doses of vitamins (called megadoses or megavitamin therapy) is useful for treating certain medical problems. Studies have not proven this. Large doses should be taken only under the direction of your doctor after need has been identified.

Missed dose—If you miss taking a vitamin for one or more days there is no cause for concern, since it takes some time for your body to become seriously low in vitamins. However, if your doctor has recommended that you take this vitamin, try to remember to take it as directed every day.

Storage—To store this dietary supplement:

- Keep out of the reach of children.
- Store away from heat and direct light.
- Do not store in the bathroom, near the kitchen sink, or in other damp places. Heat or moisture may cause the dietary supplement to break down.
- Do not keep outdated dietary supplements or those no longer needed. Be sure that any discarded dietary supplement is out of the reach of children.

Side Effects of This Dietary Supplement

Along with its needed effects, a dietary supplement may cause some unwanted effects. Although pantothenic acid does not usually cause any side effects, check with your doctor if you notice any unusual effects while you are taking it.

Annual revision: 07/16/92

PAPAVERINE Intracavernosal

Generic name product available in the U.S. and Canada.

Description

Papaverine (pa-PAV-er-een) belongs to the group of medicines called vasodilators. Vasodilators cause blood vessels to expand, thereby increasing blood flow. Papaverine is used to produce erections in some impotent men. When papaverine is injected into the penis (intracavernosal), it increases blood flow to the penis, which results in an erection.

Papaverine injection should not be used as a sexual aid by men who are not impotent. If the medicine is not used properly, permanent damage to the penis and loss of the ability to have erections could result.

Papaverine is available only with your doctor's prescription, in the following dosage form:

Parenteral

- Injection (U.S. and Canada)

It is very important that you read and understand the following information. If any of it causes you special concern, check with your doctor. Also, *if you have any questions* or if you want more information about this medicine or your medical problem, *ask your doctor, nurse, or pharmacist.*

Before Using This Medicine

In deciding to use a medicine, the risks of taking the medicine must be weighed against the good it will do. This is a decision you and your doctor will make. For papaverine, the following should be considered:

Allergies—Tell your doctor if you have ever had any unusual or allergic reaction to papaverine. Also tell your doctor and pharmacist if you are allergic to any other substances, such as foods, preservatives, or dyes.

Older adults—Many medicines have not been studied specifically in older people. Therefore, it may not be known whether they work exactly the same way they do in younger adults or if they cause different side effects or problems in older people. Although there is no specific information comparing the use of papaverine for impotence in the elderly with use in other age groups, this medicine is not expected to cause different side effects or problems in older people than it does in younger adults.

Other medicines—Although certain medicines should not be used together at all, in other cases two different medicines may be used together even if an interaction might occur. In these cases, your doctor may want to change the dose, or other precautions may be necessary. Tell your doctor and pharmacist if you are taking any other prescription or nonprescription (over-the-counter [OTC]) medicine.

Other medical problems—The presence of other medical problems may affect the use of papaverine. Make sure you tell your doctor if you have any other medical problems, especially:

- Bleeding problems—These conditions increase the risk of bleeding at the place of injection
- Liver disease—Papaverine can cause liver damage when it is given in ways that allow it to get into the bloodstream (by mouth or by injection into a muscle, a vein, or an artery); when papaverine is given by intracavernosal injection, liver damage is much less likely because the medicine enters the bloodstream very slowly
- Priapism (history of) or
- Sickle cell disease—Patients with these conditions have an increased risk of priapism (erection lasting longer than 4 hours) while using papaverine

Before you begin using any new medicine (prescription or nonprescription) or if you develop any new medical problem while you are using this medicine, check with your doctor, nurse, or pharmacist.

Proper Use of This Medicine

To give papaverine injection:

- Cleanse the injection site with alcohol. Using a sterile needle, *inject the medicine slowly and directly into the base of the penis as instructed by your doctor. Papaverine should not be injected just under the skin.* The injection is usually not painful, although you may feel some tingling in the tip of your penis. If the injection is very painful or you notice bruising or swelling at the place of injection, that means you have been injecting the medicine under the skin. Stop, withdraw the needle, and reposition it properly before continuing with the injection.
- After you have completed the injection, put pressure on the place of injection to prevent bruising. Then massage your penis as instructed by your doctor. This helps the medicine spread to all parts of the penis, so that it will work better.

This medicine usually begins to work in about 10 minutes. You should attempt intercourse within 2 hours after injecting the medicine.

Storage—To store this medicine:

- Keep out of the reach of children.
- Store away from heat and direct light.
- Keep the medicine from freezing.

Precautions While Using This Medicine

Use papaverine injection exactly as directed by your doctor. Do not use more of it and do not use it more often than ordered. If too much is used, the erection may become so strong that it lasts too long and does not reverse when it should. This condition is called priapism, and it can be very dangerous. If the effect is not reversed, the blood supply to the penis may be cut off and permanent damage may occur.

Contact your doctor immediately if the erection lasts for longer than 4 hours or if it becomes painful. This may be a sign of priapism and must be treated right away to prevent permanent damage.

If you notice bleeding at the site when you inject papaverine, put pressure on the spot until the bleeding stops. If it doesn't stop, check with your doctor.

It is important for you to examine your penis regularly. Check with your doctor if you find a lump where the medicine has been injected or if you notice that your penis is becoming curved. These may be signs that unwanted tissue is growing (called fibrosis), which should be seen by your doctor.

Side Effects of This Medicine

Along with its needed effects, a medicine may cause some unwanted effects. Although not all of these side effects may occur, if they do occur they may need medical attention.

Check with your doctor immediately if the following side effect occurs:

Rare

Erection continuing for more than 4 hours, or painful erection

Check with your doctor as soon as possible if the following side effects occur:

Rare

Dizziness; lumps in the penis

Other side effects may occur that usually do not need medical attention. These side effects may go away during treatment as your body adjusts to the medicine. However, check with your doctor if any of the following side effects continue or are bothersome:

Less common or rare

Bruising or bleeding at place of injection; burning (mild) along penis; difficulty in ejaculating; swelling at place of injection

Papaverine injected into the penis may cause tingling at the tip of the penis. This is no cause for concern.

Other side effects not listed above may also occur in some patients. If you notice any other effects, check with your doctor.

Annual revision: 08/06/92

PAPAVERINE Systemic

Some commonly used brand names are:

In the U.S.

Cerespan	Pavagen
Genabid	Pavarine
Pavabid	Pavased
Pavabid HP	Pavatine
Pavacels	Pavatym
Pavacot	Paverolan

Generic name product may also be available in the U.S. and Canada.

Description

Papaverine (pa-PAV-er-een) belongs to the group of medicines called vasodilators. Vasodilators cause blood vessels to expand, thereby increasing blood flow. This medicine is used to treat problems resulting from poor blood circulation.

Papaverine is available only with your doctor's prescription, in the following dosage forms:

Oral

- Extended-release capsules (U.S.)
- Tablets (U.S. and Canada)

Parenteral

- Injection (U.S. and Canada)

It is very important that you read and understand the following information. If any of it causes you special concern, check with your doctor. Also, *if you have any questions* or if you want more information about this medicine or your medical problem, *ask your doctor, nurse, or pharmacist.*

Before Using This Medicine

In deciding to use a medicine, the risks of taking the medicine must be weighed against the good it will do. This is a decision you and your doctor will make. For papaverine, the following should be considered:

Allergies—Tell your doctor if you have ever had any unusual or allergic reaction to papaverine. Also tell your

doctor and pharmacist if you are allergic to any other substances, such as foods, preservatives, or dyes.

Pregnancy—Studies on effects in pregnancy have not been done in either humans or animals.

Breast-feeding—It is not known whether papaverine passes into the breast milk. However, this medicine has not been reported to cause problems in nursing babies.

Children—Although there is no specific information comparing use of papaverine in children with use in other age groups, this medicine is not expected to cause different side effects or problems in children than it does in adults.

Older adults—Papaverine may reduce tolerance to cold temperatures in elderly patients.

Other medicines—Although certain medicines should not be used together at all, in other cases two different medicines may be used together even if an interaction might occur. In these cases, your doctor may want to change the dose, or other precautions may be necessary. Tell your doctor and pharmacist if you are taking any other prescription or nonprescription (over-the-counter [OTC]) medicine, or if you smoke.

Other medical problems—The presence of other medical problems may affect the use of papaverine. Make sure you tell your doctor if you have any other medical problems, especially:

- Angina (chest pain) or
- Glaucoma or
- Heart disease or
- Myocardial infarction ("heart attack"), recent, or
- Stroke, recent—The chance of unwanted effects may be increased

Before you begin using any new medicine (prescription or nonprescription) or if you develop any new medical problem while you are using this medicine, check with your doctor, nurse, or pharmacist.

Proper Use of This Medicine

If this medicine upsets your stomach, it may be taken with meals, milk, or antacids.

For patients taking the *extended-release capsule* form of this medicine:

- Swallow the capsules whole. Do not crush, break, or chew before swallowing. However, if the capsule is too large to swallow, you may mix the contents with jam or jelly and swallow without chewing.

Dosing—The dose of papaverine will be different for different patients. *Follow your doctor's orders or the directions on the label.* The following information includes only the average doses of papaverine. *If your dose is different, do not change it* unless your doctor tells you to do so:

- For *oral* dosage form (extended-release capsules):
  - —Adults: 150 milligrams (mg) every twelve hours. The dose may be increased to 150 mg every eight hours or 300 mg every twelve hours.
- For *oral* dosage form (tablets):
  - —Adults: 100 to 300 mg three to five times a day.
- For *injection* dosage form:
  - —Adults: 30 to 120 mg every three hours injected slowly into the muscle or vein.
  - —Children: 1.5 mg per kilogram (0.68 mg per pound) of body weight four times a day injected into the muscle or vein.

Missed dose—If you miss a dose of this medicine, take it as soon as you remember. However, if it is almost time for the next dose, skip the missed dose and go back to your regular dosing schedule. Do not double doses.

Storage—To store this medicine:

- Keep out of the reach of children.
- Store away from heat and direct light.
- Do not store in the bathroom, near the kitchen sink, or in other damp places. Heat or moisture may cause the medicine to break down.
- Do not keep outdated medicine or medicine no longer needed. Be sure that any discarded medicine is out of the reach of children.

Precautions While Using This Medicine

It may take some time for this medicine to work. If you feel that the medicine is not working, do not stop taking it on your own. Instead, check with your doctor.

The helpful effects of this medicine may be decreased if you smoke. If you have any questions about this, check with your doctor.

Dizziness may occur, especially when you get up from a lying or sitting position or climb stairs. Getting up slowly may help. If this problem continues or gets worse, check with your doctor.

Side Effects of This Medicine

Along with its needed effects, a medicine may cause some unwanted effects. Although not all of these side effects may occur, if they do occur they may need medical attention.

Check with your doctor as soon as possible if any of the following side effects occur:

Symptoms of overdose

Blurred or double vision; drowsiness; weakness

Rare

Yellow eyes or skin

Other side effects may occur after papaverine is given by injection. Check with your doctor if you notice any redness, swelling, or pain at the place of injection.

Other side effects that usually do not need medical attention may occur soon after an injection of this medicine. They usually go away after a little while. However, check with your doctor if any of the following side effects continue or are bothersome:

Deep breathing; dizziness; fast heartbeat; flushing of face

Other side effects not listed above may also occur in some patients. If you notice any other effects, check with your doctor.

Annual revision: 04/13/93

PARALDEHYDE Systemic

A commonly used brand name in the U.S. is Paral.

Generic name product may also be available in the U.S. and Canada.

Description

Paraldehyde (par-AL-de-hyde) is used to treat certain convulsive disorders. It also has been used in the treatment of alcoholism and in the treatment of nervous and mental conditions to calm or relax patients who are nervous or tense and to produce sleep. However, this medicine has generally been replaced by safer and more effective medicines for the treatment of alcoholism and in the treatment of nervous and mental conditions.

This medicine is available only with your doctor's prescription, in the following dosage forms:

Oral

- Oral liquid (U.S. and Canada)

Parenteral

- Injection (Canada)

Rectal

- Rectal liquid (U.S. and Canada)

It is very important that you read and understand the following information. If any of it causes you special concern, check with your doctor. Also, *if you have any questions* or if you want more information about this medicine or your medical problem, *ask your doctor, nurse, or pharmacist.*

Before Using This Medicine

In deciding to use a medicine, the risks of taking the medicine must be weighed against the good it will do. This is a decision you and your doctor will make. For paraldehyde, the following should be considered:

Allergies—Tell your doctor if you have ever had any unusual or allergic reaction to paraldehyde. Also tell your doctor and pharmacist if you are allergic to any other substances, such as foods, preservatives, or dyes.

Pregnancy—Paraldehyde crosses the placenta. Studies on birth defects have not been done in either humans or animals. Use of paraldehyde during labor may cause breathing problems in the newborn infant.

Breast-feeding—Paraldehyde has not been reported to cause problems in nursing babies.

Children—Although there is no specific information comparing use of paraldehyde in children with use in other age groups, this medicine is not expected to cause different side effects or problems in children than it does in adults.

Older adults—Many medicines have not been studied specifically in older people. Therefore, it may not be known whether they work exactly the same way they do in younger adults or if they cause different side effects or problems in older people. There is no specific information comparing use of paraldehyde in the elderly with use in other age groups.

Other medicines—Although certain medicines should not be used together at all, in other cases 2 different medicines may be used together even if an interaction might occur. In these cases, your doctor may want to change the dose, or other precautions may be necessary. When you are taking paraldehyde, it is especially important that your doctor and pharmacist know if you are taking any of the following:

- Central nervous system (CNS) depressants (medicine that causes drowsiness) or
- Tricyclic antidepressants (medicine for depression)—CNS depressant effects may be increased
- Disulfiram (e.g., Antabuse)—Higher blood levels of paraldehyde may occur, increasing the chance of side effects

Other medical problems—The presence of other medical problems may affect the use of paraldehyde. Make sure you tell your doctor if you have any other medical problems, especially:

- Alcohol abuse (or history of) or
- Drug abuse or dependence (or history of)—Dependence on paraldehyde may develop

- Colitis—Paraldehyde used rectally may make the condition worse.
- Emphysema, asthma, bronchitis, or other chronic lung disease, or
- Liver disease—Higher blood levels of paraldehyde may occur, increasing the chance of side effects
- Gastroenteritis (stomach flu) or
- Stomach ulcer—Paraldehyde taken by mouth may make the condition worse.

Before you begin using any new medicine (prescription or nonprescription) or if you develop any new medical problem while you are using this medicine, check with your doctor, nurse, or pharmacist.

Proper Use of This Medicine

Use this medicine only as directed by your doctor. Do not use more of it, do not use it more often, and do not use it for a longer time than your doctor ordered. If too much is used, the medicine may become habit-forming.

Do not use if liquid turns brownish in color or if it has a strong vinegar-like odor, since this means the paraldehyde is breaking down. If you have any questions about this, check with your doctor or pharmacist.

For patients taking this medicine by mouth:

- *Do not use a plastic spoon, plastic glass, or any other plastic container to take this medicine,* since paraldehyde may react with the plastic. Use a metal spoon or glass container.
- *Take this medicine mixed in a glass of milk or iced fruit juice* to improve the taste and odor and to lessen stomach upset.

For patients using this medicine rectally:

- *Do not use paraldehyde in any plastic container* since it may react with the plastic.
- Before using paraldehyde rectally, make sure you understand exactly how to use it. Paraldehyde may need to be diluted. If you have any questions about this, check with your doctor or pharmacist.

Keep this medicine away from the eyes and avoid getting it on the skin and clothing.

Keep this medicine away from heat, open flame, and sparks.

Dosing—The dose of paraldehyde will be different for different patients. *Follow your doctor's orders or the directions on the label.* The following information includes only the average doses of paraldehyde. *If your dose is different, do not change it* unless your doctor tells you to do so.

- The amount of paraldehyde that you take depends on the strength of the medicine. Also, *the number of doses you take each day, the time allowed between doses, and the length of time you take the medicine depend on the medical problem for which you are taking paraldehyde.*
- For *oral and rectal* dosage forms (liquid):
  - —Adults: Dose must be determined by your doctor.
  - —Children: Dose is based on body weight, and must be determined by the doctor.
- For *injection* dosage form:
  - —Adults: Dose must be determined by your doctor. It will be injected into a muscle or a vein.
  - —Children: Dose is based on body weight, and must be determined by the doctor.

Missed dose—If you are taking this medicine regularly (for example, every day) and you miss a dose, take it right away if you remember within an hour or so of the missed dose. However, if you do not remember until later, skip the missed dose and go back to your regular dosing schedule. Do not double doses.

Storage—To store this medicine:

- Keep out of the reach of children.
- Store away from heat and direct light.
- Keep the medicine from freezing.
- Do not keep outdated medicine or medicine no longer needed. Be sure that any discarded medicine is out of the reach of children.

Precautions While Using This Medicine

If you will be using this medicine regularly for a long time:

- Your doctor should check your progress at regular visits.
- Do not stop using it without first checking with your doctor. Your doctor may want you to reduce gradually the amount you are using before stopping completely.

This medicine will add to the effects of alcohol and other CNS depressants (medicines that slow down the nervous system, possibly causing drowsiness). Some examples of CNS depressants are antihistamines or medicine for hay fever, other allergies, or colds; sedatives, tranquilizers, or sleeping medicine; prescription pain medicine or narcotics; barbiturates; medicine for seizures; muscle relaxants; or anesthetics, including some dental anesthetics. *Check with your doctor before taking any of the above while you are using this medicine.*

Before you have any medical tests, tell the medical doctor in charge that you are taking this medicine. The results of some tests, such as the metyrapone test and the phentolamine test, may be affected by this medicine.

If you think you or someone else may have taken an overdose of this medicine, get emergency help at once. Taking an overdose of paraldehyde or taking alcohol or other CNS depressants with paraldehyde may lead to unconsciousness and possibly death. Some signs of an overdose are confusion, muscle tremors, nausea or vomiting (continuing or severe), severe stomach cramps, severe weakness, shortness of breath or slow or troubled breathing, and slow heartbeat.

This medicine may cause some people to become drowsy or less alert than they are normally. Even if taken at bedtime, it may cause some people to feel drowsy or less alert on arising. *Make sure you know how you react to this medicine before you drive, use machines, or do anything else that could be dangerous if you are not alert.*

Side Effects of This Medicine

Along with its needed effects, a medicine may cause some unwanted effects. Although not all of these side effects may occur, if they do occur they may need medical attention.

Check with your doctor as soon as possible if any of the following side effects occur:

More common

Coughing (with injection only); skin rash

Less common

Redness, swelling, or pain at injection site

With long-term use

Yellow eyes or skin

Symptoms of overdose

Cloudy urine; confusion; decreased urination; fast and deep breathing; muscle tremors; nausea or vomiting (continuing or severe); nervousness, restlessness, or irritability; shortness of breath or slow or troubled breathing; slow heartbeat; stomach cramps (severe); weakness (severe)

Other side effects may occur that usually do not need medical attention. These side effects may go away during treatment as your body adjusts to the medicine. However, check with your doctor if any of the following side effects continue or are bothersome:

More common

Drowsiness; nausea or vomiting (when taken by mouth); stomach pain (when taken by mouth); unpleasant breath odor

Less common

Clumsiness or unsteadiness; dizziness; "hangover" effect

After you stop using this medicine, your body may need time to adjust. The length of time this takes depends on the amount of medicine you were using and how long you used it. During this period of time check with your doctor if you notice any of the following side effects:

Convulsions (seizures); hallucinations (seeing, hearing, or feeling things that are not there); increased sweating; muscle cramps; nausea and vomiting; stomach cramps; trembling

Paraldehyde will cause your breath to have a strong unpleasant odor. This effect will last until about one day after you have stopped using this medicine.

Other side effects not listed above may also occur in some patients. If you notice any other effects, check with your doctor.

Annual revision: 03/19/93

PEGADEMASE Systemic†

A commonly used brand name in the U.S. is Adagen.

Other commonly used names are PEG-ADA and PEG-adenosine deaminase.

†Not commercially available in Canada.

Description

Pegademase contains an enzyme called adenosine deaminase (ADA). It is used to treat children who do not have a properly developed immune system because of a lack of ADA in the body.

Pegademase is to be given only by or under the supervision of your doctor. It is available in the following dosage form:

Parenteral

- Injection (U.S.)

It is very important that you read and understand the following information. If any of it causes you special concern, check with your doctor. Also, *if you have any questions* or if you want more information about this medicine or your medical problem, *ask your doctor, nurse, or pharmacist.*

Before Using This Medicine

In deciding to use a medicine, the risks of taking the medicine must be weighed against the good it will do. This is a decision you and your doctor will make. For pegademase, the following should be considered:

Allergies—Tell your doctor if you have ever had any unusual or allergic reaction to pegademase. Also tell your doctor and pharmacist if you are allergic to any other substances, such as foods, preservatives, or dyes.

Other medicines—Although certain medicines should not be used together at all, in other cases two different medicines may be used together even if an interaction might occur. In these cases, your doctor may want to change the dose, or other precautions may be necessary. When you are receiving pegademase, it is especially important that your doctor and pharmacist know if you are taking any other medicine.

Other medical problems—The presence of other medical problems may affect the use of pegademase. Make sure you tell your doctor if you have any other medical problems, especially:

- Blood clotting problems—Injection may cause bleeding

Before you begin using any new medicine (prescription or nonprescription) or if you develop any new medical problem while you are using this medicine, check with your doctor, nurse, or pharmacist.

Proper Use of This Medicine

If you miss getting a dose of this medicine, get it as soon as possible.

Precautions While Using This Medicine

It is very important that you continue to receive treatment with pegademase. Treatment must be continued for life. Do not stop treatment with pegademase without checking with your doctor. If regular treatment is not continued, the immune system will break down and serious infections may occur.

Side Effects of This Medicine

Along with its needed effects, a medicine may cause some unwanted effects. Pegademase does not usually cause any side effects. However, check with your doctor if pain at the place of injection occurs and continues or is bothersome.

Other side effects not listed above may also occur in some patients. If you notice any other effects, check with your doctor.

Annual revision: September 1990

PEMOLINE Systemic

Some commonly used brand names are:

In the U.S.
- Cylert
- Cylert Chewable

In Canada
- Cylert

Description

Pemoline (PEM-oh-leen) belongs to the group of medicines called central nervous system (CNS) stimulants. It is used to treat children with attention-deficit hyperactivity disorder (ADHD).

Pemoline increases attention and decreases restlessness in children who are overactive, cannot concentrate for very long or are easily distracted, and are emotionally unstable. This medicine is used as part of a total treatment program that also includes social, educational, and psychological treatment.

Pemoline is available only with your doctor's prescription, in the following dosage forms:

Oral
- Tablets (U.S. and Canada)
- Chewable tablets (U.S.)

It is very important that you read and understand the following information. If any of it causes you special concern, check with your doctor. Also, *if you have any questions* or if you want more information about this medicine or your medical problem, *ask your doctor, nurse, or pharmacist.*

Before Using This Medicine

In deciding to use a medicine, the risks of taking the medicine must be weighed against the good it will do. This is a decision you and your doctor will make. For pemoline, the following should be considered:

Allergies—Tell your doctor if you have ever had any unusual or allergic reaction to pemoline. Also tell your doctor and pharmacist if you are allergic to any other substances, such as foods, preservatives, or dyes.

Pregnancy—Pemoline has not been shown to cause birth defects or other problems in humans. However, studies in animals given large doses of pemoline have shown that pemoline causes an increase in stillbirths and decreased survival of the offspring after birth.

Breast-feeding—It is not known if pemoline is excreted in breast milk.

Children—Slowed growth rate in children who received pemoline for a long period of time have been reported. Some doctors recommend drug-free periods during treatment with pemoline.

Other medicines—Although certain medicines should not be used together at all, in other cases 2 different medicines may be used together even if an interaction might occur. In these cases, your doctor may want to change the dose, or other precautions may be necessary. Tell your doctor and pharmacist if you are taking any other prescription or nonprescription (over-the-counter [OTC]) medicine.

Other medical problems—The presence of other medical problems may affect the use of pemoline. Make sure you tell your doctor if you have any other medical problems, especially:

- Gilles de la Tourette's disorder or other tics or
- Mental illness (severe) or
- Liver disease—Pemoline may make the condition worse
- Kidney disease—Higher blood levels of pemoline may occur, increasing the chance of side effects

Before you begin using any new medicine (prescription or nonprescription) or if you develop any new medical problem while you are using this medicine, check with your doctor, nurse, or pharmacist.

Proper Use of This Medicine

For patients taking the *chewable tablet form* of this medicine:

- These tablets must be chewed before swallowing. Do not swallow whole.

Sometimes this medicine must be taken for 3 to 4 weeks before improvement is noticed.

Take pemoline only as directed by your doctor. Do not take more of it, do not take it more often, and do not take it for a longer time than your doctor ordered. If too much is taken, it may become habit-forming.

Dosing—The dose of pemoline will be different for different patients. *Follow your doctor's orders or the directions on the label.* The following information includes only the average doses of pemoline. *If your dose is different, do not change it* unless your doctor tells you to do so.

- The number of tablets that you take depends on the strength of the medicine. Also, *the number of doses you take each day, the time allowed between doses, and the length of time you take the medicine depend on the medical problem for which you are taking pemoline.*
- For *oral* or *chewable* dosage forms (tablets):
  —Children 6 years of age and over: To start, 37.5 milligrams (mg) every morning. Your doctor may increase your dose if needed. However, the dose is usually not more than 112.5 mg a day.
  —Children up to 6 years of age: Dose must be determined by the doctor.

Missed dose—If you miss a dose of this medicine, take it as soon as possible. Then go back to your regular dosing schedule. But if you do not remember the missed dose until the next day, skip it and go back to your regular dosing schedule. Do not double doses.

Storage—To store this medicine:

- Keep out of the reach of children.
- Store away from heat and direct light.
- Do not store in the bathroom, near the kitchen sink, or in other damp places. Heat or moisture may cause the medicine to break down.
- Do not keep outdated medicine or medicine no longer needed. Be sure that any discarded medicine is out of the reach of children.

Precautions While Using This Medicine

Your doctor should check your progress at regular visits to make sure that this medicine does not cause unwanted effects.

If you will be taking this medicine in large doses for a long time, do not stop taking it without first checking with your doctor. Your doctor may want you to reduce gradually the amount you are taking before stopping completely.

This medicine may cause some people to become dizzy or less alert than they are normally. *Make sure you know how you react to this medicine before you ride a bicycle or do anything else that could be dangerous if you are dizzy or are not alert.*

If you have been using this medicine for a long time and you think you may have become mentally or physically dependent on it, check with your doctor. Some signs of dependence on pemoline are:

- a strong desire or need to continue taking the medicine.
- a need to increase the dose to receive the effects of the medicine.
- withdrawal side effects (for example, mental depression, unusual behavior, or unusual tiredness or weakness) occurring after the medicine is stopped.

Side Effects of This Medicine

Along with their needed effects, medicines like pemoline, when used for a long time, have been reported to slow the growth rate of children. Some doctors recommend drug-free periods during treatment with pemoline. Pemoline may also cause unwanted effects on behavior in children with severe emotional problems.

Although not all of these side effects may occur, if they do occur they may need medical attention.

Check with your doctor as soon as possible if any of the following side effects occur:

Rare

Yellow eyes or skin

Symptoms of overdose

Agitation; confusion; convulsions (seizures); false sense of well-being; fast heartbeat; hallucinations (seeing, hearing, or feeling things that are not there); headache (severe); high blood pressure; high fever with sweating; large pupils; muscle trembling or twitching; nervousness or restlessness; uncontrolled movements of the eyes or other parts of the body; vomiting

Other side effects may occur that usually do not need medical attention. These side effects may go away during treatment as your body adjusts to the medicine. However, check with your doctor if any of the following side effects continue or are bothersome:

More common

Loss of appetite; trouble in sleeping; weight loss

Less common

Dizziness; drowsiness; increased irritability; mental depression; nausea; skin rash; stomach ache

After you stop using this medicine, your body may need time to adjust. The length of time this takes depends on the amount of medicine you were using and how long you used it. During this period of time check with your doctor if you notice any of the following side effects:

Mental depression (severe); unusual behavior; unusual tiredness or weakness

Other side effects not listed above may also occur in some patients. If you notice any other effects, check with your doctor.

Annual revision: 04/16/93

PENICILLAMINE Systemic

Some commonly used brand names in the U.S. and Canada are Cuprimine and Depen.

Description

Penicillamine (pen-i-SILL-a-meen) is used in the treatment of medical problems such as Wilson's disease (too much copper in the body) and rheumatoid arthritis. Also, it is used to prevent kidney stones. Penicillamine may also be used for other conditions as determined by your doctor.

In addition to the helpful effects of this medicine, it has side effects that can be very serious. Before you take penicillamine, be sure that you have discussed the use of it with your doctor.

This medicine is available only with your doctor's prescription, in the following dosage forms:

Oral

- Capsules (U.S. and Canada)
- Tablets (U.S. and Canada)

It is very important that you read and understand the following information. If any of it causes you special concern, check with your doctor. Also, *if you have any questions* or if you want more information about this medicine or your medical problem, *ask your doctor, nurse, or pharmacist.*

Before Using This Medicine

In deciding to use a medicine, the risks of taking the medicine must be weighed against the good it will do. This is a decision you and your doctor will make. For penicillamine, the following should be considered:

Allergies—Tell your doctor if you have ever had any unusual or allergic reaction to penicillin or to penicillamine. Also tell your doctor and pharmacist if you are allergic to any other substances, such as foods, preservatives, or dyes.

Pregnancy—Penicillamine may cause birth defects if taken during pregnancy.

Breast-feeding—Penicillamine has not been reported to cause problems in nursing babies.

Children—Although there is no specific information about the use of penicillamine in children, it is not expected to cause different side effects or problems in children than it does in adults.

Older adults—Sore throat and fever, with or without chills; sores, ulcers, or white spots on the lips or in the mouth; shortness of breath, troubled breathing, tightness in the chest, and/or wheezing; swollen and/or painful glands; black, tarry stools; blood in urine or stools; pinpoint red spots on skin; cough or hoarseness; lower back or side pain; painful or difficult urination; unusual bleeding or bruising; and unusual tiredness or weakness may be especially likely to occur in elderly patients, who are usually more sensitive than younger adults to some of the effects of penicillamine.

Other medicines—Although certain medicines should not be used together at all, in other cases two different medicines may be used together even if an interaction might occur. In these cases, your doctor may want to change the dose, or other precautions may be necessary. When you are taking penicillamine, it is important that your doctor and pharmacist know if you are taking *any* other prescription or nonprescription (over-the-counter [OTC]) medicine, especially gold compounds.

Other medical problems—The presence of other medical problems may affect the use of penicillamine. Make sure you tell your doctor if you have any other medical problems, especially:

- Blood disease caused by penicillamine treatment, history of, or
- Kidney disease or history of (only for patients with rheumatoid arthritis)—The chance of side effects may be increased

Before you begin using any new medicine (prescription or nonprescription) or if you develop any new medical problem while you are using this medicine, check with your doctor, nurse, or pharmacist.

Proper Use of This Medicine

Since penicillamine is taken in different ways for different medical problems, it is very important that you understand exactly why you are taking this medicine and how to take it. See below for information on specific medical problems. If you have any questions about this, check with your doctor.

For patients taking this medicine to *prevent kidney stones:*

- You should drink 2 full glasses (8 ounces each) of water at bedtime and another 2 full glasses (8 ounces each) during the night.
- It is very important that you follow any special instructions from your doctor, such as following a low-methionine diet. If you have any questions about this, check with your doctor.

For patients taking this medicine for *rheumatoid arthritis:*

- Take this medicine on an empty stomach (at least 1 hour before meals or 2 hours after meals) and at least 1 hour before or after any other food, milk, or medicine.
- After you begin taking this medicine, 2 to 3 months may pass before you feel its effects. It is very important that you keep taking the medicine, even if you do not feel better, in order to give it time to work.

For patients taking this medicine for *Wilson's disease:*

- Take this medicine on an empty stomach (at least ½ to 1 hour before meals or 2 hours after meals).
- It is very important that you follow any special instructions from your doctor, such as following a low-copper diet. If you have any questions about this, check with your doctor.
- After you begin taking this medicine, 1 to 3 months may pass before you notice any improvement in your condition.

For patients taking this medicine for *lead poisoning:*

- Take this medicine on an empty stomach (2 hours before meals or at least 3 hours after meals).

For *all patients:*

- *Take this medicine regularly as directed. Do not stop taking it without first checking with your doctor,* since stopping the medicine and then restarting it may increase the possibility of side effects.

Missed dose—If you miss a dose of this medicine and your dosing schedule is:

- One dose a day—Take the missed dose as soon as possible. But if you do not remember the missed dose until the next day, skip the missed dose and go back to your regular dosing schedule. Do not double the next day's dose.
- Two doses a day—Take the missed dose as soon as possible. However, if it is almost time for your next dose, skip the missed dose and go back to your regular dosing schedule. Do not double doses.
- More than two doses a day—If you remember within an hour or so of the missed dose, take it right away. But if you do not remember until later, skip the missed dose and go back to your regular dosing schedule. Do not double doses.

If you have any questions about this, check with your doctor.

Storage—To store this medicine:

- Keep out of the reach of children.
- Store away from heat and direct light.
- Do not store this medicine in the bathroom, near the kitchen sink, or in other damp places. Heat or moisture may cause the medicine to break down.
- Do not keep outdated medicine or medicine no longer needed. Be sure that any discarded medicine is out of the reach of children.

Precautions While Using This Medicine

Your doctor should check your progress at regular visits to make sure that this medicine does not cause unwanted effects.

Before having any kind of surgery (including dental surgery), tell the medical doctor or dentist in charge that you are taking this medicine.

If you are taking iron preparations, or vitamin preparations containing iron, do not take them within 2 hours of the time you take this medicine. Taking the 2 medicines too close together may keep the penicillamine from working properly.

Side Effects of This Medicine

Along with its needed effects, a medicine may cause some unwanted effects. Although not all of these side effects may occur, if they do occur they may need medical attention.

Check with your doctor as soon as possible if any of the following side effects occur:

More common

Fever; joint pain; skin rash, hives, or itching; swollen and/or painful glands; ulcers, sores, or white spots on lips or in mouth

Less common

Bloody or cloudy urine; shortness of breath, troubled breathing, tightness in chest, or wheezing; sore throat and fever with or without chills; swelling of face, feet, or lower legs; unusual bleeding or bruising; unusual tiredness or weakness; weight gain

Rare

Abdominal or stomach pain (severe); blisters on skin; bloody or black, tarry stools; chest pain; coughing or hoarseness; dark urine; difficulty in breathing, chewing, talking, or swallowing; eye pain, blurred or double vision, or any change in vision; general feeling of discomfort or illness or weakness; lower back or side pain; muscle weakness; painful or difficult urination; pale stools; pinpoint red spots on skin; redness, tenderness, itching, burning, or peeling of skin; red or irritated eyes; red, thick, or scaly skin; ringing or buzzing in the ears; spitting blood; yellow eyes or skin

Other side effects may occur that usually do not need medical attention. These side effects may go away during treatment as your body adjusts to the medicine. However, check with your doctor if any of the following side effects continue or are bothersome:

More common

Diarrhea; lessening or loss of taste sense; loss of appetite; nausea or vomiting; stomach pain (mild)

Other side effects not listed above may also occur in some patients. If you notice any other effects, check with your doctor.

Annual revision: July 1990

PENICILLINS Systemic

This information applies to the following medicines:

- Amoxicillin (a-mox-i-SILL-in)
- Amoxicillin and Clavulanate (klav-yoo-LAN-ate)
- Ampicillin (am-pi-SILL-in)
- Ampicillin and Sulbactam (sul-BAK-tam)
- Azlocillin (az-loe-SILL-in)
- Bacampicillin (ba-kam-pi-SILL-in)
- Carbenicillin (kar-ben-i-SILL-in)
- Cloxacillin (klox-a-SILL-in)
- Cyclacillin (sye-kla-SILL-in)
- Dicloxacillin (dye-klox-a-SILL-in)
- Methicillin (meth-i-SILL-in)
- Mezlocillin (mez-loe-SILL-in)
- Nafcillin (naf-SILL-in)
- Oxacillin (ox-a-SILL-in)
- Penicillin G (pen-i-SILL-in)
- Penicillin V
- Piperacillin (pi-PER-a-sill-in)
- Ticarcillin (tye-kar-SILL-in)
- Ticarcillin and Clavulanate

Some commonly used brand names and other names are:

For Amoxicillin

In the U.S.

Amoxil, Larotid, Polymox, Trimox, Wymox

Generic name product may also be available.

In Canada

Amoxil, Apo-Amoxi, Novamoxin, Nu-Amoxi

Another commonly used name for amoxicillin is amoxicilline.

For Amoxicillin and Clavulanate

In the U.S.

Augmentin

In Canada

Clavulin

For Ampicillin

In the U.S.

Omnipen, Omnipen-N, Polycillin, Polycillin-N, Principen

Generic name product may also be available.

In Canada

Ampicin, Apo-Ampi, Novo Ampicillin, Nu-Ampi, Penbritin

For Ampicillin and Sulbactam†

In the U.S.

Unasyn

For Azlocillin†

In the U.S.

Azlin

For Bacampicillin
In the U.S.
Spectrobid
In Canada
Penglobe

For Carbenicillin
In the U.S.
Geocillin
Geopen
In Canada
Geopen Oral
Pyopen

Another commonly used name for carbenicillin indanyl sodium is carindacillin.

For Cloxacillin
In the U.S.
Cloxapen
Tegopen
Generic name product may also be available.
In Canada
Apo-Cloxi
Novocloxin
Nu-Cloxi
Orbenin
Tegopen

For Cyclacillin†
In the U.S.
Generic name product may also be available.

Another commonly used name for cyclacillin is ciclacillin.

For Dicloxacillin†
In the U.S.
Dycill
Dynapen
Pathocil
Generic name product may also be available.

For Methicillin†
In the U.S.
Staphcillin

Another commonly used name for methicillin is meticillin.

For Mezlocillin†
In the U.S.
Mezlin

For Nafcillin
In the U.S.
Nafcil
Nallpen
Unipen
Generic name product may also be available.
In Canada
Unipen

For Oxacillin†
In the U.S.
Bactocill
Prostaphlin
Generic name product may also be available.

For Penicillin G
In the U.S.
Bicillin L-A
Crysticillin 300 AS
Pentids
Pfizerpen
Pfizerpen-AS
Wycillin
Generic name product may also be available.
In Canada
Ayercillin
Bicillin L-A
Crystapen
Megacillin
Wycillin
Generic name product may also be available.

Another commonly used name for penicillin G benzathine is benzathine benzylpenicillin.

For Penicillin V
In the U.S.
Beepen-VK
Betapen-VK
Ledercillin VK
Pen Vee K
Robicillin VK
V-Cillin K
Veetids
Generic name product may also be available.
In Canada
Apo-Pen-VK
Ledercillin
Nadopen-V 200
Nadopen-V 400
Nadopen-VK
Novopen-VK
Nu-Pen-VK
Pen Vee
PVF
PVF K
V-Cillin K
VC-K

Another commonly used name for penicillin V is phenoxymethylpenicillin.

For Piperacillin
In the U.S.
Pipracil
In Canada
Pipracil

For Ticarcillin
In the U.S.
Ticar
In Canada
Ticar

For Ticarcillin and Clavulanate
In the U.S.
Timentin
In Canada
Timentin

†Not commercially available in Canada.

Description

Penicillins are used in the treatment of bacterial infections. They work by killing bacteria or preventing their growth.

There are several different kinds of penicillins. Each is used to treat different kinds of bacterial infections. One kind of penicillin usually may not be used in place of another.

Penicillins are used to treat bacterial infections in many different parts of the body. They are sometimes given with other antibacterial medicines. Carbenicillin taken by mouth is used only to treat bacterial infections of the urinary tract and prostate gland. Penicillin G and penicillin V are also used to prevent "strep" infections in patients with a history of rheumatic heart disease. Piperacillin is given by injection to prevent bacterial infections before, during, and after surgery also. Some of the penicillins may also be used for other problems as determined by your doctor. However, none of the penicillins will work for colds, flu, or other virus infections.

Penicillins are available only with your doctor's prescription, in the following dosage forms:

Oral

Amoxicillin
- Capsules (U.S. and Canada)
- Oral suspension (U.S. and Canada)
- Chewable tablets (U.S. and Canada)

Amoxicillin and Clavulanate
- Oral suspension (U.S. and Canada)
- Tablets (U.S. and Canada)
- Chewable tablets (U.S.)

Ampicillin
- Capsules (U.S. and Canada)
- Oral suspension (U.S. and Canada)

Bacampicillin
- Oral suspension (U.S.)
- Tablets (U.S. and Canada)

Carbenicillin
- Tablets (U.S. and Canada)

Cloxacillin
- Capsules (U.S. and Canada)
- Oral solution (U.S. and Canada)

Cyclacillin
- Tablets (U.S.)

Dicloxacillin
- Capsules (U.S.)
- Oral suspension (U.S.)

Nafcillin
- Capsules (U.S.)
- Oral solution (U.S.)
- Tablets (U.S.)

Oxacillin
- Capsules (U.S.)
- Oral solution (U.S.)

Penicillin G Benzathine
- Oral suspension (Canada)

Penicillin G Potassium
- Oral solution (U.S.)
- Tablets (U.S. and Canada)

Penicillin V Benzathine
- Oral suspension (Canada)

Penicillin V Potassium
- Oral solution (U.S. and Canada)
- Tablets (U.S. and Canada)

Parenteral

Ampicillin
- Injection (U.S. and Canada)

Ampicillin and Sulbactam
- Injection (U.S.)

Azlocillin
- Injection (U.S.)

Carbenicillin
- Injection (U.S. and Canada)

Cloxacillin
- Injection (Canada)

Methicillin
- Injection (U.S.)

Mezlocillin
- Injection (U.S.)

Nafcillin
- Injection (U.S. and Canada)

Oxacillin
- Injection (U.S.)

Penicillin G Benzathine
- Injection (U.S. and Canada)

Penicillin G Potassium
- Injection (U.S. and Canada)

Penicillin G Procaine
- Injection (U.S. and Canada)

Penicillin G Sodium
- Injection (U.S. and Canada)

Piperacillin
- Injection (U.S. and Canada)

Ticarcillin
- Injection (U.S. and Canada)

Ticarcillin and Clavulanate
- Injection (U.S. and Canada)

It is very important that you read and understand the following information. If any of it causes you special concern, check with your doctor. Also, *if you have any questions* or if you want more information about this medicine or your medical problem, *ask your doctor, nurse, or pharmacist.*

Before Using This Medicine

In deciding to use a medicine, the risks of taking the medicine must be weighed against the good it will do. This is a decision you and your doctor will make. For penicillins, the following should be considered:

Allergies—Tell your doctor if you have ever had any unusual or allergic reaction to any of the penicillins, cephalosporins, griseofulvin (e.g., Fulvicin), or penicillamine (e.g., Cuprimine). Also tell your doctor and pharmacist if you are allergic to any other substances, such as foods, preservatives, or dyes, or procaine (e.g., Novocain) or other ester-type anesthetics (medicines that cause numbing) if you are receiving penicillin G procaine.

Pregnancy—Studies have not been done in pregnant women. However, penicillins have not been shown to cause birth defects or other problems in animals given more than 25 times the usual human dose.

Breast-feeding—Most penicillins pass into the breast milk. Even though only small amounts may pass into breast milk, allergic reactions, diarrhea, fungus infections, and skin rash may occur in nursing babies.

Children—Many penicillins have been used in children and, in effective doses, are not expected to cause different side effects or problems in children than they do in adults.

Older adults—Penicillins have been used in the elderly and have not been shown to cause different side effects or problems in older people than they do in younger adults.

Other medicines—Although certain medicines should not be used together at all, in other cases two different medicines may be used together even if an interaction might occur. In these cases, your doctor may want to change the dose, or other precautions may be necessary. When you are taking a penicillin, it is especially important that your doctor and pharmacist know if you are taking any of the following:

- Amiloride (e.g., Midamor) or
- Captopril (e.g., Capoten) or
- Enalapril (e.g., Vasotec) or
- Lisinopril (e.g., Prinivil, Zestril) or
- Potassium-containing medicine or

- Spironolactone (e.g., Aldactone) or
- Triamterene (e.g., Dyrenium)—Use of these medicines with penicillin G by injection may cause an increase in side effects
- Anticoagulants (blood thinners) or
- Dipyridamole (e.g., Persantine) or
- Divalproex (e.g., Depakote) or
- Heparin (e.g., Panheprin) or
- Inflammation or pain medicine (except narcotics) or
- Moxalactam (e.g., Moxam) or
- Pentoxifylline (e.g., Trental) or
- Plicamycin (e.g., Mithracin) or
- Sulfinpyrazone (e.g., Anturane) or
- Valproic acid (e.g., Depakene)—Use of these medicines with carbenicillin or ticarcillin may increase the chance of bleeding
- Cholestyramine (e.g., Questran) or
- Colestipol (e.g., Colestid)—Use of these medicines with oral penicillin G may prevent penicillin G from working properly
- Oral contraceptives (birth control pills) containing estrogen—Use of ampicillin, bacampicillin, or penicillin V with estrogen-containing oral contraceptives may prevent oral contraceptives from working properly, increasing the chance of pregnancy
- Probenecid (e.g., Benemid)—Probenecid increases the blood level of many penicillins. Although your doctor may give you probenecid with a penicillin to treat some infections, in other cases, this effect may be unwanted and may increase the chance of side effects

Other medical problems—The presence of other medical problems may affect the use of penicillins. Make sure you tell your doctor if you have any other medical problems, especially:

- Allergy, general (such as asthma, eczema, hay fever, hives), history of—Patients with a history of general allergies may be more likely to have a severe reaction to penicillins if an allergy develops
- Bleeding problems, history of—Patients with a history of bleeding problems may have an increased chance of bleeding when receiving carbenicillin or ticarcillin
- Kidney disease—Patients with kidney disease may have an increased chance of side effects
- Mononucleosis, infectious ("mono")—Patients with infectious mononucleosis may have an increased chance of skin rash
- Stomach or intestinal disease, history of (especially colitis, including colitis caused by antibiotics, or enteritis)—Patients with a history of stomach or intestinal disease may be more likely to develop colitis while taking penicillins

Before you begin using any new medicine (prescription or nonprescription) or if you develop any new medical problem while you are using this medicine, check with your doctor, nurse, or pharmacist.

Proper Use of This Medicine

Penicillins (except bacampicillin tablets, amoxicillin, amoxicillin and clavulanate combination, and penicillin V) are best taken with a full glass (8 ounces) of water on an empty stomach (either 1 hour before or 2 hours after meals) unless otherwise directed by your doctor.

For patients taking *amoxicillin, amoxicillin and clavulanate combination, and penicillin V:*

- Amoxicillin, amoxicillin and clavulanate combination, and penicillin V may be taken on a full or empty stomach.
- The *liquid form of amoxicillin* may also be taken straight or mixed with formulas, milk, fruit juice, water, ginger ale, or other cold drinks. If mixed with other liquids, take immediately after mixing. Be sure to drink all the liquid to get the full dose of medicine.

For patients taking *bacampicillin:*

- The liquid form of this medicine is best taken with a full glass (8 ounces) of water on an empty stomach (either 1 hour before or 2 hours after meals) unless otherwise directed by your doctor.
- The tablet form of this medicine may be taken on a full or empty stomach.

For patients taking *penicillin G by mouth:*

- Do not drink acidic fruit juices (for example, orange or grapefruit juice) or other acidic beverages within 1 hour of taking penicillin G since this may keep the medicine from working properly.

For patients taking the *oral liquid form of penicillins:*

- This medicine is to be taken by mouth even if it comes in a dropper bottle. If this medicine does not come in a dropper bottle, use a specially marked measuring spoon or other device to measure each dose accurately. The average household teaspoon may not hold the right amount of liquid.
- Do not use after the expiration date on the label. The medicine may not work properly after that date. If you have any questions about this, check with your pharmacist.

For patients taking the *chewable tablet form of penicillins:*

- Tablets should be chewed or crushed before they are swallowed.

To help clear up your infection completely, *keep taking this medicine for the full time of treatment*, even if you begin to feel better after a few days. *If you have a "strep" infection, you should keep taking this medicine for at least 10 days. This is especially important in "strep" infections. Serious heart problems could develop later* if your infection is not cleared up completely. Also, if you stop taking this medicine too soon, your symptoms may return.

This medicine works best when there is a constant amount in the blood or urine. *To help keep the amount constant, do not miss any doses. Also, it is best to take the doses at evenly spaced times, day and night.* For example, if you are to take 4 doses a day, the doses should be spaced about 6 hours apart. If this interferes with your sleep or other daily activities, or if you need help in planning the best times to take your medicine, check with your doctor, nurse, or pharmacist.

Missed dose—If you do miss a dose of this medicine, take it as soon as possible. This will help to keep a constant amount of medicine in the blood or urine. However, if it is almost time for your next dose, skip the missed dose and go back to your regular dosing schedule. Do not double doses.

Storage—To store this medicine:

- Keep out of the reach of children.
- Store away from heat and direct light.
- Do not store the capsule or tablet form of penicillins in the bathroom, near the kitchen sink, or in other damp places. Heat or moisture may cause the medicine to break down.
- Store the oral liquid form of penicillins in the refrigerator because heat will cause this medicine to break down. However, keep the medicine from freezing. Follow the directions on the label.
- Do not keep outdated medicine or medicine no longer needed. Be sure that any discarded medicine is out of the reach of children.

Precautions While Using This Medicine

If your symptoms do not improve within a few days, or if they become worse, check with your doctor.

If you have ever had an allergic reaction to any of the penicillins, your doctor may want you to carry a medical identification (ID) card or wear a medical ID bracelet stating this.

In some patients, penicillins may cause diarrhea.

- Severe diarrhea may be a sign of a serious side effect. *Do not take any diarrhea medicine without first checking with your doctor.* Diarrhea medicines may make your diarrhea worse or make it last longer.
- For mild diarrhea, diarrhea medicine containing kaolin or attapulgite (e.g., Kaopectate tablets, Diasorb) may be taken. However, other kinds of diarrhea medicine should not be taken. They may make your diarrhea worse or make it last longer.
- If you have any questions about this or if mild diarrhea continues or gets worse, check with your doctor or pharmacist.

Oral contraceptives (birth control pills) containing estrogen may not work properly if you take them while you are taking ampicillin, bacampicillin, or penicillin V. Unplanned pregnancies may occur. You should use a different or additional means of birth control while you are taking any of these penicillins. If you have any questions about this, check with your doctor or pharmacist.

For *diabetic patients:*

- *Amoxicillin, amoxicillin and clavulanate combination, ampicillin, ampicillin and sulbactam combination, bacampicillin, and penicillin G may cause false test results with some urine sugar tests.* Check with your doctor before changing your diet or the dosage of your diabetes medicine.

Tell the doctor in charge that you are taking this medicine before you have any medical tests. The results of some tests may be affected by this medicine.

Side Effects of This Medicine

Along with its needed effects, a medicine may cause some unwanted effects. Although not all of these side effects may occur, if they do occur they may need medical attention.

Stop taking this medicine and get emergency help immediately if any of the following side effects occur:

Rare (may be less common with some penicillins)

Difficulty in breathing; lightheadedness; skin rash, hives, itching, or wheezing

In addition to the side effects mentioned above, *check with your doctor immediately* if any of the following side effects occur:

Rare (may be more common with some penicillins)

Abdominal or stomach cramps and pain (severe); abdominal bloating; blood in urine; convulsions (seizures); decreased amount of urine; diarrhea (watery and severe), which may also be bloody; fever; joint pain; sore throat and fever; unusual bleeding or bruising (some of the above side effects may also occur up to several weeks after you stop taking any of these medicines)

Other side effects may occur that usually do not need medical attention. These side effects may go away during treatment as your body adjusts to the medicine. However, check with your doctor if any of the following side effects continue or are bothersome:

More common (may be less common with some penicillins)

Diarrhea (mild); nausea or vomiting; sore mouth or tongue

Overdose is very unlikely to occur with penicillins. However, if you think that you or someone else, especially a child, has taken too much, check with your doctor. Severe diarrhea, nausea, or vomiting may need to be treated.

Other side effects not listed above may also occur in some patients. If you notice any other effects, check with your doctor.

Annual revision: 09/30/91

PENTAGASTRIN Diagnostic

A commonly used brand name in the U.S. and Canada is Peptavlon.

Description

Pentagastrin (pen-ta-GAS-trin) is a testing agent used to help diagnose problems or disease of the stomach. This test determines how much acid your stomach produces.

How the test is done: The pentagastrin is injected beneath the skin. Ten or 15 minutes later, the contents of the stomach are emptied and tested for the amount of the contents and the amount of acid in the contents. The procedure may be repeated several times.

Pentagastrin is used only under the supervision of a doctor. It is available in the following dosage form:

Parenteral
- Injection (U.S. and Canada)

It is very important that you read and understand the following information. If any of it causes you special concern, check with your doctor. Also, *if you have any questions* or if you want more information about this test or your medical problem, *ask your doctor, nurse, or pharmacist.*

Before Having This Test

In deciding to use a diagnostic test, any risks of the test must be weighed against the good it will do. This is a decision you and your doctor will make. Also, test results may be affected by other things. For pentagastrin, the following should be considered:

Allergies—Tell your doctor if you have ever had any unusual or allergic reaction to pentagastrin. Also tell your doctor and pharmacist if you are allergic to any other substances, such as foods, preservatives, or dyes.

Pregnancy—Studies on effects in pregnancy have not been done in either humans or animals.

Breast-feeding—It is not known whether pentagastrin passes into the breast milk. Although most medicines pass into breast milk in small amounts, many of them may be used safely while breast-feeding. Mothers who are receiving this diagnostic test and wish to breast-feed should discuss this with their doctor.

Children—Studies on this medicine have been done only in adult patients, and there is no specific information comparing use of pentagastrin in children with use in other age groups.

Older adults—Many medicines have not been studied specifically in older people. Therefore, it may not be known whether they work exactly the same way they do in younger adults or if they cause different side effects or problems in older people. There is no specific information comparing use of pentagastrin in the elderly with use in other age groups.

Other medicines—Although certain medicines should not be used together at all, in other cases two different medicines may be used together even if an interaction might occur. In these cases, your doctor may want to change the dose, or other precautions may be necessary. When you will be given pentagastrin, it is especially important that your doctor and pharmacist know if you are taking any of the following:

- Antacids or
- Anticholinergics (medicine for abdominal or stomach spasms or cramps) or
- Cimetidine (e.g., Tagamet) or
- Famotidine (e.g., Pepcid) or
- Nizatidine (e.g., Axid) or
- Omeprazole (e.g., Prilosec) or
- Ranitidine (e.g., Zantac)—These medicines decrease the effect that pentagastrin has on the production of stomach acid, and the test may not work

Other medical problems—The presence of other medical problems may affect the use of pentagastrin. Make sure you tell your doctor if you have any other medical problems, especially:

- Gallbladder problems or
- Liver disease or
- Pancreatitis (inflammation of the pancreas) (severe) or
- Stomach ulcer (severe or bleeding)—Pentagastrin may make these conditions worse

Preparation For This Test

Unless otherwise directed by your doctor:

- Do not eat anything beginning the night before and do not drink anything for at least four hours before

the test. Having food or liquid in the stomach may affect the interpretation of the test results.
- Do not take antacids on the morning of the test. To do so may decrease the effect of pentagastrin and affect the test results.
- For 24 hours before the test, do not take any anticholinergics (medicine for abdominal or stomach spasms or cramps), cimetidine, famotidine, nizatidine, ranitidine, or any other medicine that decreases stomach acid. Do not take omeprazole for 96 hours (4 days) before the test.

Side Effects of This Medicine

Along with its needed effects, pentagastrin may cause some unwanted effects. Although the side effects usually are rare, when they do occur they may require medical attention.

Check with your doctor or nurse immediately if either of the following side effects occurs:

Rare

Skin rash or hives

Other side effects may occur that usually do not need medical attention. These side effects should go away as the effects of the medicine wear off. However, check with your doctor if any of the following side effects continue or are bothersome:

More common (usually disappear within 15 minutes after injection)

Gas; nausea or vomiting; stomach pain; urge to have bowel movement

Less common or rare

Blurred vision; chills; dizziness, faintness, or lightheadedness; drowsiness; fast heartbeat; feeling of heaviness of arms and legs; headache; increased sweating; numbness, tingling, pain, or weakness in hands or feet; shortness of breath; unusual tiredness; unusual warmth or flushing of skin

Other side effects not listed above may also occur in some patients. If you notice any other effects, check with your doctor.

Annual revision: 07/14/93

PENTAMIDINE Inhalation

Some commonly used brand names are:

In the U.S.

NebuPent

In Canada

Pentacarinat

Pneumopent

Description

Pentamidine (pen-TAM-i-deen) is used to try to prevent pneumocystis (noo-moe-SISS-tis) pneumonia (PCP), a very serious type of pneumonia. This type of pneumonia occurs commonly in patients whose immune systems are not working normally, such as patients with acquired immune deficiency syndrome (AIDS). Inhaled pentamidine does not prevent illness in parts of the body outside the lungs. This medicine may also be used for other conditions as determined by your doctor.

Pentamidine is available only with your doctor's prescription, in the following dosage form:

Inhalation

- Inhalation solution (U.S. and Canada)

It is very important that you read and understand the following information. If any of it causes you special concern, check with your doctor. Also, *if you have any questions* or if you want more information about this medicine or your medical problem, *ask your doctor, nurse, or pharmacist.*

Before Using This Medicine

In deciding to use a medicine, the risks of taking the medicine must be weighed against the good it will do. This is a decision you and your doctor will make. For pentamidine inhalation, the following should be considered:

Allergies—Tell your doctor if you have ever had any unusual or allergic reaction to pentamidine inhalation. Also tell your doctor and pharmacist if you are allergic to any other substances, such as foods, preservatives, or dyes.

Pregnancy—Studies on birth defects have not been done in humans. However, studies in rabbits, given doses by injection much larger than humans would absorb into their bloodstream through the lungs, have shown an increase in miscarriages and bone defects in the fetus.

Breast-feeding—It is not known whether pentamidine passes into breast milk. However, pentamidine has not been reported to cause problems in nursing babies.

Children—Studies on this medicine have been done only in adult patients, and there is no specific information comparing use of pentamidine inhalation in children with use in other age groups. However, pentamidine inhalation is recommended in children 5 years of age and older who cannot tolerate other medicines.

Older adults—Many medicines have not been studied specifically in older people. Therefore, it may not be known whether they work exactly the same way they do in younger adults or if they cause different side effects or problems in older people. There is no specific information comparing use of pentamidine inhalation in the elderly with use in other age groups.

Other medicines—Although certain medicines should not be used together at all, in other cases two different medicines may be used together even if an interaction might occur. In these cases, your doctor may want to change the dose, or other precautions may be necessary. Tell your doctor and pharmacist if you are taking any other prescription or nonprescription (over-the-counter [OTC]) medicine.

Other medical problems—The presence of other medical problems may affect the use of pentamidine inhalation. Make sure you tell your doctor if you have any other medical problems, especially:

- Asthma—Patients with asthma may have an increase in coughing or difficulty in breathing while receiving pentamidine inhalation

Before you begin using any new medicine (prescription or nonprescription) or if you develop any new medical problem while you are using this medicine, check with your doctor, nurse, or pharmacist.

Proper Use of This Medicine

To help prevent the development or return of pneumocystis pneumonia, you must receive pentamidine inhalation on a regular basis, even if you are feeling well.

Missed dose—If you miss a dose of this medicine, receive your treatment as soon as possible.

Precautions While Using This Medicine

If you are also using the inhalation form of a bronchodilator (medicine used to help relieve breathing problems), use the pentamidine inhalation at least 5 to 10 minutes after the bronchodilator, unless otherwise directed by your doctor. This will help to reduce the possibility of side effects. Do not use the bronchodilator or any medicine other than pentamidine in the nebulizer.

A bitter or metallic taste may occur during use of this medicine. Sucking on a hard candy after each treatment can help reduce this problem.

Cigarette smoking can increase the chance of coughing and difficulty in breathing during pentamidine inhalation therapy.

Side Effects of This Medicine

On rare occasions, pneumocystis infections have occurred in parts of the body outside the lungs in patients receiving pentamidine inhalation therapy. You should discuss this possible problem with your doctor.

Along with its needed effects, a medicine may cause some unwanted effects. Although not all of these side effects may occur, if they do occur they may need medical attention.

Check with your doctor or nurse immediately if any of the following side effects occur:

More common

Burning pain, dryness, or sensation of lump in throat; chest pain or congestion; coughing; difficulty in breathing; difficulty in swallowing; skin rash; wheezing

Rare

Nausea and vomiting; pain in upper abdomen, possibly radiating to the back; pain in side of chest (severe); shortness of breath (sudden and severe)

Rare—with daily treatment doses only

Anxiety; chills; cold sweats; cool, pale skin; decreased urination; headache; increased hunger; loss of appetite; nausea and vomiting; nervousness; shakiness; stomach pain; unusual tiredness

Other side effects not listed above may also occur in some patients. If you notice any other effects, check with your doctor.

Annual revision: 03/03/92

PENTAMIDINE Systemic

Some commonly used brand names are:

In the U.S.
Pentam 300

In Canada
Pentacarinat

Description

Pentamidine (pen-TAM-i-deen) is used to treat protozoal infections. It works by killing protozoa (tiny, one-celled animals) or preventing their growth. Some protozoa are parasites that can cause many different kinds of infections in the body.

Pentamidine is also used to treat pneumocystis (noo-moe-SISS-tis) pneumonia (PCP), a very serious kind of pneumonia. This particular kind of pneumonia occurs commonly in patients whose immune system is not working normally, such as cancer patients, transplant patients, and patients with acquired immune deficiency syndrome (AIDS). This medicine may also be used for other conditions as determined by your doctor.

Pentamidine may cause some serious side effects. Before you begin treatment with pentamidine, you and your doctor should talk about the good this medicine will do as well as the risks of using it.

Pentamidine is to be administered only by or under the immediate supervision of your doctor, and is available in the following dosage form:

Parenteral

- Injection (U.S. and Canada)

It is very important that you read and understand the following information. If any of it causes you special concern, check with your doctor. Also, *if you have any questions* or if you want more information about this medicine or your medical problem, *ask your doctor, nurse, or pharmacist.*

Before Receiving This Medicine

In deciding to use a medicine, the risks of taking the medicine must be weighed against the good it will do. This is a decision you and your doctor will make. For pentamidine, the following should be considered:

Allergies—Tell your doctor if you have ever had any unusual or allergic reaction to pentamidine. Also tell your doctor and pharmacist if you are allergic to any other substances, such as foods, preservatives, or dyes.

Diet—Make certain your doctor and pharmacist know if you are on a low-sodium, low-sugar, or any other special diet. Since most medicines contain more than their active ingredient, some products may have to be avoided.

Pregnancy—Pentamidine has not been studied in pregnant women. However, studies in rabbits have shown an increase in miscarriages and bone defects in the fetus.

Breast-feeding—It is not known whether pentamidine passes into breast milk. However, because of the risk of side effects in the newborn, breast-feeding is not recommended during treatment with this medicine.

Children—Although pentamidine has not been widely used in children, this medicine is not expected to cause different side effects or problems in children than it does in adults.

Older adults—Many medicines have not been studied specifically in older people. Therefore, it may not be known whether they work exactly the same way they do in younger adults or if they cause different side effects or problems in older people. There is no specific information comparing use of pentamidine in the elderly with use in other age groups.

Other medicines—Although certain medicines should not be used together at all, in other cases two different medicines may be used together even if an interaction might occur. In these cases, your doctor may want to change the dose, or other precautions may be necessary. When you are receiving pentamidine, it is especially important that your doctor and pharmacist know if you are taking any of the following:

- Amphotericin B by injection (e.g., Fungizone) or
- Antithyroid agents (medicine for overactive thyroid) or
- Azathioprine (e.g., Imuran) or
- Chloramphenicol (e.g., Chloromycetin) or
- Colchicine or
- Cyclophosphamide (e.g., Cytoxan) or
- Flucytosine (e.g., Ancobon) or
- Ganciclovir (e.g., Cytovene) or
- Interferon (e.g., Intron A, Roferon-A) or
- Mercaptopurine (e.g., Purinethol) or
- X-ray treatment or
- Zidovudine (e.g., AZT, Retrovir) or
- If you have ever been treated with x-rays or cancer medicine—When taken with pentamidine, these medicines may increase the chance of damage to your blood cells
- Carmustine (e.g., BiCNU) or
- Cisplatin (e.g., Platinol) or
- Combination pain medicine containing acetaminophen and aspirin (e.g., Excedrin) or other salicylates (with large amounts taken regularly) or
- Cyclosporine (e.g., Sandimmune) or
- Deferoxamine (e.g., Desferal) (with long-term use) or
- Gold salts (medicine for arthritis) or
- Inflammation or pain medicine (except narcotics) or
- Lithium (e.g., Lithane) or
- Other anti-infectives by mouth or by injection (medicine for infection) or
- Penicillamine (e.g., Cuprimine) or
- Streptozocin (e.g., Zanosar) or
- Tiopronin (e.g., Thiola)—When taken with pentamidine, these medicines may increase the chance of kidney damage
- Didanosine (e.g., ddI, Videx)—When taken with pentamidine, didanosine may increase the chance of pancreatitis
- Foscarnet (e.g., Foscavir)—When given with pentamidine, foscarnet may increase the chance of kidney damage
- Methotrexate (e.g., Mexate) or
- Plicamycin (e.g., Mithracin)—When taken with pentamidine, these medicines may increase the chance of damage to your blood cells and to your kidney

Other medical problems—The presence of other medical problems may affect the use of pentamidine. Make sure you tell your doctor if you have any other medical problems, especially:

- Anemia or
- Heart disease or
- History of bleeding disorders or
- Hypotension (low blood pressure) or

- Kidney disease or
- Liver disease—Pentamidine may make these conditions worse
- Diabetes mellitus (sugar diabetes) or
- Hypoglycemia (low blood sugar)—Pentamidine may increase or decrease blood sugar levels and may disturb control of sugar diabetes

Before you begin using any new medicine (prescription or nonprescription) or if you develop any new medical problem while you are using this medicine, check with your doctor, nurse, or pharmacist.

Proper Use of This Medicine

To help clear up your infection completely, *pentamidine must be given for the full time of treatment,* even if you begin to feel better after a few days. Also, this medicine works best when there is a constant amount in the blood. To help keep the amount constant, pentamidine must be given on a regular schedule.

Dosing—The dose of pentamidine will be different for different patients. *Follow your doctor's orders or the directions on the label.* The following information includes only the average doses of pentamidine. *If your dose is different, do not change it* unless your doctor tells you to do so.

- For *injection* dosage form:
  - —For *Pneumocystis carinii* pneumonia (PCP):
    - Adults and children—Dose is based on body weight and must be determined by your doctor. The usual dose is 4 milligrams (mg) per kilogram (8.8 mg per pound) of body weight given once a day for fourteen to twenty-one days. It is injected slowly into a vein over a one- to two-hour period of time.

Precautions While Using This Medicine

Some patients may develop sudden, severe low blood pressure after a dose of pentamidine. Therefore, you should be lying down while you are receiving this medicine. Also, your doctor may want to check your blood pressure while you are receiving pentamidine and several times afterward until your blood pressure is stable.

Pentamidine can lower the number of white blood cells in your blood, increasing the chance of getting certain infections. It can also lower the number of platelets, which are necessary for proper blood clotting. If these problems occur, there are certain precautions you can take to reduce the risk of infection or bleeding:

- *Check with your doctor immediately* if you think you are getting a cold or other infection.
- *Check with your doctor immediately* if you notice any unusual bleeding or bruising.
- Be careful when using regular toothbrushes, dental floss, or toothpicks. Your medical doctor, dentist, or nurse may recommend other ways to clean your teeth and gums. Check with your medical doctor before having any dental work done.
- Avoid using a safety razor. Use an electric shaver instead. Also, be careful when using fingernail or toenail cutters.

Side Effects of This Medicine

Pentamidine may cause some serious side effects, including heart problems, low blood pressure, low or high blood sugar, and other blood problems. *You and your doctor should discuss the good this medicine will do as well as the risks of receiving it.*

Along with its needed effects, a medicine may cause some unwanted effects. Although not all of these side effects may occur, if they do occur they may need medical attention.

Check with your doctor or nurse immediately if any of the following side effects occur:

More common

Decrease in urination; sore throat and fever; unusual bleeding or bruising

Signs of diabetes mellitus or high blood sugar

Drowsiness; flushed, dry skin; fruit-like breath odor; increased thirst; increased urination; loss of appetite

Signs of low blood sugar

Anxiety; chills; cold sweats; cool, pale skin; headache; increased hunger; nausea; nervousness; shakiness

Signs of low blood pressure

Blurred vision; confusion; dizziness; fainting or lightheadedness; unusual tiredness or weakness

Note: *Signs of diabetes mellitus or high blood sugar, or signs of low blood sugar* may also occur up to several months after you stop receiving this medicine.

Less common

Fever; pain in upper abdomen; pain, redness, and/or hardness at place of injection; rapid or irregular pulse; skin rash, redness, or itching

Other side effects may occur that usually do not need medical attention. These side effects may go away during treatment as your body adjusts to the medicine. However, check with your doctor if any of the following side effects continue or are bothersome:

More common

Diarrhea; loss of appetite; nausea and vomiting

Gastrointestinal disturbances, such as nausea and vomiting, or loss of appetite, are common minor side effects seen in pentamidine treatment. However, if you have these problems, and at the same time have sharp pain in the upper abdomen, or an unusual decrease in urine output, check with your doctor immediately.

Pentamidine may also cause an unpleasant metallic taste. This side effect is to be expected and does not require medical attention.

Other side effects not listed above may also occur in some patients. If you notice any other effects, check with your doctor.

Additional Information

Once a medicine has been approved for marketing for a certain use, experience may show that it is also useful for other medical problems. Although these uses are not included in product labeling, pentamidine is used in certain patients with the following medical conditions:

- Leishmaniasis, cutaneous
- Leishmaniasis, visceral (kala-azar)
- Trypanosomiasis, African (African sleeping sickness)

If you are living in or will be traveling to an area where there is a chance of getting kala-azar or African sleeping sickness, the following measures will help to prevent either disease:

- If possible, sleep under fine-mesh netting to avoid being bitten by sandflies (which carry kala-azar) or tsetse flies (which carry African sleeping sickness).
- Wear long-sleeved shirts or blouses and long trousers to protect your arms and legs, especially at dusk or during evening hours when sandflies are out. Since tsetse flies can bite through thin clothing, it is best to wear clothing made from fairly heavy material to protect arms and legs.
- Apply insect repellant to uncovered areas of the skin when sandflies or tsetse flies are out.

Other than the above information, there is no additional information relating to proper use, precautions, or side effects for these uses.

Annual revision: 07/14/93

PENTOSTATIN Systemic

A commonly used brand name in the U.S. and Canada is Nipent.
Other commonly used names are 2′-deoxycoformycin and 2′DCF.

Description

Pentostatin (PEN-toe-stat-in) belongs to the group of medicines called antimetabolites. It is used to treat hairy cell leukemia.

Pentostatin interferes with the growth of cancer cells, which are eventually destroyed. Since the growth of normal body cells may also be affected by pentostatin, other effects will also occur. Some of these may be serious and must be reported to your doctor. Other effects may not be serious but may cause concern. Some effects may not occur for months or years after the medicine is used.

Before you begin treatment with pentostatin, you and your doctor should talk about the good this medicine will do as well as the risks of using it.

Pentostatin is to be administered only by or under the immediate supervision of your doctor. It is available in the following dosage form:

Parenteral

- Injection (U.S. and Canada)

It is very important that you read and understand the following information. If any of it causes you special concern, check with your doctor. Also, *if you have any questions* or if you want more information about this medicine or your medical problem, *ask your doctor, nurse, or pharmacist.*

Before Using This Medicine

In deciding to use a medicine, the risks of taking the medicine must be weighed against the good it will do. This is a decision you and your doctor will make. For pentostatin, the following should be considered:

Allergies—Tell your doctor if you have ever had any unusual or allergic reaction to pentostatin.

Pregnancy—There is a chance that this medicine may cause birth defects if either the male or female is taking it at the time of conception or if it is taken during pregnancy. Pentostatin has been shown to cause birth defects in rats and mice. In addition, many cancer medicines may cause sterility which could be permanent. Although sterility has not been reported with this medicine, it does occur in animals and the possibility should be kept in mind.

Be sure that you have discussed this with your doctor before taking this medicine. It is best to use some kind of birth control while you are receiving pentostatin. Tell your doctor right away if you think you have become pregnant while receiving pentostatin.

Breast-feeding—It is not known whether pentostatin passes into breast milk. However, because this medicine may cause serious side effects, breast-feeding is generally not recommended while you are receiving it.

Children—There is no specific information comparing use of pentostatin in children with use in other age groups.

Older adults—Many medicines have not been studied specifically in older people. Therefore, it may not be known whether they work exactly the same way they do in younger adults. Although there is no specific information comparing use of pentostatin in the elderly with use in other adults, this medicine is not expected to cause different side effects or problems in older people than it does in younger adults.

Other medicines—Although certain medicines should not be used together at all, in other cases two different medicines may be used together even if an interaction might occur. In these cases, your doctor may want to change the dose, or other precautions may be necessary. When you are receiving pentostatin, it is especially important that your doctor and pharmacist know if you are taking any of the following:

- Amphotericin B by injection (e.g., Fungizone) or
- Antithyroid agents (medicine for overactive thyroid) or
- Azathioprine (e.g., Imuran) or
- Chloramphenicol (e.g., Chloromycetin) or
- Colchicine or
- Flucytosine (e.g., Ancobon) or
- Ganciclovir (e.g., Cytovene) or
- Interferon (e.g., Intron A, Roferon-A) or
- Plicamycin (e.g., Mithracin) or
- Zidovudine (e.g., AZT, Retrovir) or
- If you have ever been treated with x-rays or cancer medicines—Pentostatin may increase the effects of these medicines or radiation therapy on the blood
- Probenecid (e.g., Benemid) or
- Sulfinpyrazone (e.g., Anturane)—Pentostatin may raise the amount of uric acid in the blood. Since these medicines are used to lower uric acid levels, they may not be as effective in patients receiving pentostatin

Other medical problems—The presence of other medical problems may affect the use of pentostatin. Make sure you tell your doctor if you have any other medical problems, especially:

- Chickenpox (including recent exposure) or
- Herpes zoster (shingles)—Risk of severe disease affecting other parts of the body
- Gout (history of) or
- Kidney stones (history of)—Pentostatin may increase levels of uric acid in the body, which can cause gout or kidney stones
- Infection—Pentostatin may decrease your body's ability to fight infection
- Kidney disease—Effects of pentostatin may be increased because of slower removal from the body

Before you begin using any new medicine (prescription or nonprescription) or if you develop any new medical problem while you are using this medicine, check with your doctor, nurse, or pharmacist.

Proper Use of This Medicine

This medicine often causes nausea and vomiting. However, it is very important that you continue to receive the medicine even if you begin to feel ill. Ask your doctor, nurse, or pharmacist for ways to lessen these effects.

Precautions While Using This Medicine

It is very important that your doctor check your progress at regular visits to make sure that this medicine is working properly and to check for unwanted effects.

While you are being treated with pentostatin, and after you stop treatment with it, *do not have any immunizations (vaccinations) without your doctor's approval.* Pentostatin may lower your body's resistance and there is a chance you might get the infection the immunization is meant to prevent. In addition, other persons living in your household should not take oral polio vaccine since there is a chance they could pass the polio virus on to you. Also, avoid persons who have taken oral polio vaccine. Do not get close to them and do not stay in the same room with them for very long. If you cannot take these precautions, you should consider wearing a protective face mask that covers the nose and mouth.

Pentostatin can lower the number of white blood cells in your blood temporarily, increasing the chance of getting an infection. It can also lower the number of platelets, which are necessary for proper blood clotting. If this occurs, there are certain precautions you can take, especially when your blood count is low, to reduce the risk of infection or bleeding:

- If you can, avoid people with infections. *Check with your doctor immediately* if you think you are getting an infection or if you get a fever or chills, cough or hoarseness, lower back or side pain, or painful or difficult urination.
- *Check with your doctor immediately* if you notice any unusual bleeding or bruising; black, tarry stools; blood in urine or stools; or pinpoint red spots on your skin.
- Be careful when using a regular toothbrush, dental floss, or toothpick. Your medical doctor, dentist, or nurse may recommend other ways to clean your teeth and gums. Check with your medical doctor before having any dental work done.
- Do not touch your eyes or the inside of your nose unless you have just washed your hands and have not touched anything else in the meantime.
- Be careful not to cut yourself when you are using sharp objects such as a safety razor or fingernail or toenail cutters.
- Avoid contact sports or other situations where bruising or injury could occur.

Side Effects of This Medicine

Along with its needed effects, a medicine may cause some unwanted effects. Some side effects will have signs or symptoms that you can see or feel. Your doctor may watch for others by doing certain tests.

Also, because of the way these medicines act on the body, there is a chance that they might cause other unwanted effects that may not occur until months or years after the medicine is used. These delayed effects may include certain types of cancer. Discuss these possible effects with your doctor.

Check with your doctor or nurse immediately if any of the following side effects occur:

More common
- Cough or hoarseness; fever or chills; lower back or side pain; painful or difficult urination

Less common
- Black, tarry stools; blood in urine or stools; chest pain; pinpoint red spots on skin; unusual bleeding or bruising

Check with your doctor or nurse as soon as possible if any of the following side effects occur:

More common
- Pain; skin rash or itching (sudden); unusual tiredness

Less common
- Anxiety or nervousness; changes in vision; confusion; cramps in lower legs; mental depression; nosebleed; numbness or tingling of hands or feet; shortness of breath; sleepiness; sore, red eyes; sores in mouth or on lips; stomach pain; swelling of feet or lower legs; trouble in sleeping

This medicine may also cause the following side effects that your doctor will watch for:

More common
- Anemia; liver problems; low platelet counts

Less common
- Kidney problems

Other side effects may occur that usually do not need medical attention. These side effects may go away during treatment as your body adjusts to the medicine. Also, your doctor or nurse may be able to tell you about ways to prevent or reduce some of these side effects. Check with your doctor or nurse if any of the following side effects continue or are bothersome or if you have any questions about them:

More common
- Diarrhea; headache; loss of appetite; muscle pain; nausea and vomiting; skin rash

Less common
- Back pain; bloating or gas; constipation; dry skin; general feeling of discomfort or illness; itching; joint pain; weakness; weight loss

Other side effects not listed above may also occur in some patients. If you notice any other effects, check with your doctor.

Annual revision: 05/06/93

PENTOXIFYLLINE Systemic

A commonly used brand name in the U.S. and Canada is Trental. Another commonly used name is oxypentifylline.

Description

Pentoxifylline (pen-tox-IF-i-lin) improves the flow of blood through blood vessels. It is used to reduce leg pain caused by poor blood circulation. Pentoxifylline makes it possible to walk farther before having to rest because of leg cramps.

Pentoxifylline is available only with your doctor's prescription, in the following dosage form:

Oral
- Extended-release tablets (U.S. and Canada)

It is very important that you read and understand the following information. If any of it causes you special concern, check with your doctor. Also, *if you have any questions* or if you want more information about this medicine or your medical problem, *ask your doctor, nurse, or pharmacist.*

Before Using This Medicine

In deciding to use a medicine, the risks of taking the medicine must be weighed against the good it will do. This is a decision you and your doctor will make. For pentoxifylline, the following should be considered:

Allergies—Tell your doctor if you have ever had any unusual or allergic reaction to pentoxifylline or to other xanthines such as aminophylline, caffeine, dyphylline, ethylenediamine (contained in aminophylline), oxtriphylline, theobromine, or theophylline. Also tell your doctor and pharmacist if you are allergic to any other substances, such as foods, preservatives, or dyes.

Pregnancy—Pentoxifylline has not been studied in pregnant women. Studies in animals have not shown that it causes birth defects. However, at very high doses it has caused other harmful effects. Before taking this medicine, make sure your doctor knows if you are pregnant or if you may become pregnant.

Breast-feeding—Pentoxifylline passes into breast milk. The medicine has not been reported to cause problems in nursing babies. However, pentoxifylline has caused noncancerous tumors in animals when given for a long time in doses much larger than those used in humans. Therefore, your doctor may not want you to breast-feed while taking it. Be sure that you discuss the risks and benefits of this medicine with your doctor.

Children—Studies on this medicine have been done only in adult patients, and there is no specific information comparing use of pentoxifylline in children with use in other age groups.

Older adults—Side effects may be more likely to occur in the elderly, who are usually more sensitive than younger adults to the effects of pentoxifylline.

Other medicines—Although certain medicines should not be used together at all, in other cases two different medicines may be used together even if an interaction might occur. In these cases, your doctor may want to change the dose, or other precautions may be necessary. When you are taking pentoxifylline, it is important that your doctor and pharmacist know if you are taking any other prescription or nonprescription (over-the-counter [OTC]) medicine, or if you smoke tobacco.

Other medical problems—The presence of other medical problems may affect the use of pentoxifylline. Make sure you tell your doctor if you have any other medical problems, especially:

- Any condition in which there is a risk of bleeding (e.g., recent stroke)—Pentoxifylline may make the condition worse
- Kidney disease or
- Liver disease—The chance of side effects may be increased

Before you begin using any new medicine (prescription or nonprescription) or if you develop any new medical problem while you are using this medicine, check with your doctor, nurse, or pharmacist.

Proper Use of This Medicine

Swallow the tablet whole. Do not crush, break, or chew it before swallowing.

Pentoxifylline should be taken with meals to lessen the chance of stomach upset. Taking an antacid with the medicine may also help.

Dosing—The dose of pentoxifylline will be different for different patients. *Follow your doctor's orders or the directions on the label.* The following information includes only the average doses of pentoxifylline. *If your dose is different, do not change it* unless your doctor tells you to do so.

- For *oral* dosage form (extended-release tablets):
  - —For peripheral vascular disease (circulation problems):
    - Adults—400 milligrams (mg) two to three times a day, taken with meals.
    - Children—Use must be determined by your doctor.

Missed dose—If you miss a dose of this medicine, take it as soon as possible. However, if it is almost time for your next dose, skip the missed dose and go back to your regular dosing schedule. Do not double doses.

Storage—To store this medicine:

- Keep out of the reach of children.
- Store away from heat and direct light.
- Do not store in the bathroom, near the kitchen sink, or in other damp places. Heat or moisture may cause the medicine to break down.
- Do not keep outdated medicine or medicine no longer needed. Be sure that any discarded medicine is out of the reach of children.

Precautions While Using This Medicine

It may take several weeks for this medicine to work. If you feel that pentoxifylline is not working, do not stop taking it on your own. Instead, check with your doctor.

Smoking tobacco may worsen your condition since nicotine may further narrow your blood vessels. Therefore, it is best to avoid smoking.

Side Effects of This Medicine

Along with its needed effects, a medicine may cause some unwanted effects. Although not all of these side effects may occur, if they do occur they may need medical attention.

Check with your doctor as soon as possible if any of the following side effects occur:

Rare

Chest pain; irregular heartbeat

Signs and symptoms of overdose (in the order in which they may occur)

Drowsiness; flushing; faintness; unusual excitement; convulsions (seizures)

Other side effects may occur that usually do not need medical attention. These side effects may go away during treatment as your body adjusts to the medicine. However, check with your doctor if any of the following side effects continue or are bothersome:

Less common

Dizziness; headache; nausea or vomiting; stomach discomfort

Other side effects not listed above may also occur in some patients. If you notice any other effects, check with your doctor.

Annual revision: 07/13/93

PERGOLIDE Systemic

A commonly used brand name in the U.S. and Canada is Permax.

Description

Pergolide (PER-go-lide) belongs to the group of medicines known as ergot alkaloids. It is used with levodopa or with carbidopa and levodopa combination to treat people who have Parkinson's disease. It works by stimulating certain parts of the central nervous system (CNS) that are involved in this disease.

Pergolide is available only with your doctor's prescription, in the following dosage form:

Oral

- Tablets (U.S. and Canada)

It is very important that you read and understand the following information. If any of it causes you special concern, check with your doctor. Also, *if you have any questions* or if you want more information about this medicine or your medical problem, *ask your doctor, nurse, or pharmacist.*

Before Using This Medicine

In deciding to use a medicine, the risks of taking the medicine must be weighed against the good it will do. This is a decision you and your doctor will make. For pergolide, the following should be considered:

Allergies—Tell your doctor if you have ever had any unusual or allergic reaction to pergolide or other ergot medicines such as ergotamine. Also tell your doctor and pharmacist if you are allergic to any other substances, such as foods, preservatives, or dyes.

Pregnancy—Studies have not been done in pregnant women. However, pergolide has not been shown to cause birth defects or other problems in animal studies.

Breast-feeding—This medicine may stop milk from being produced.

Children—Studies on this medicine have been done only in adult patients, and there is no specific information about its use in children.

Older adults—This medicine has been tested and has not been shown to cause different side effects or problems in older people than it does in younger adults.

Other medicines—Although certain medicines should not be used together at all, in other cases 2 different medicines may be used together even if an interaction might occur. In these cases, your doctor may want to change the dose, or other precautions may be necessary. When you are taking pergolide, it is especially important that your doctor and pharmacist know if you are taking any other prescription or nonprescription (over-the-counter [OTC]) medicine.

Other medical problems—The presence of other medical problems may affect the use of pergolide. Make sure you tell your doctor if you have any other medical problems, especially:

- Heart disease or
- Mental problems (history of)—Pergolide may make the condition worse

Before you begin using any new medicine (prescription or nonprescription) or if you develop any new medical problem while you are using this medicine, check with your doctor, nurse, or pharmacist.

Proper Use of This Medicine

If pergolide upsets your stomach, it may be taken with meals. If stomach upset continues, check with your doctor.

Dosing—The dose of pergolide will be different for different patients. *Follow your doctor's orders or the directions on the label.* The following information includes only the average doses of pergolide. *If your dose is different, do not change it* unless your doctor tells you to do so.

- The number of tablets that you take depends on the strength of the medicine. Also, *the number of doses you take each day, the time allowed between doses, and the length of time you take the medicine depend on the medical problem for which you are taking pergolide.*

- For *oral* dosage forms (tablets):
  —Adults: 50 micrograms a day for the first two days. The dose may be increased every three days as needed. However, the usual dose is not more than 5000 micrograms.

Missed dose—If you miss a dose of this medicine, take it as soon as you remember it. However, if it is almost time for your next dose, skip the missed dose and go back to your regular dosing schedule. Do not double doses.

Storage—To store this medicine:
- Keep out of the reach of children.
- Store away from heat and direct light.
- Do not store in the bathroom, near the kitchen sink, or in other damp places. Heat or moisture may cause the medicine to break down.
- Do not keep outdated medicine or medicine no longer needed. Be sure that any discarded medicine is out of the reach of children.

Precautions While Using This Medicine

It is important that your doctor check your progress at regular visits, to make sure that this medicine is working and to check for unwanted effects.

This medicine may cause some people to become drowsy, dizzy, or less alert than they are normally. *Make sure you know how you react to this medicine before you drive, use machines, or do anything else that could be dangerous if you are dizzy or are not alert.*

Dizziness, lightheadedness, or fainting may occur after the first doses of pergolide, especially when you get up from a lying or sitting position. Getting up slowly may help. Taking the first dose at bedtime or when you are able to lie down may also lessen problems. If the problem continues or gets worse, check with your doctor.

Pergolide may cause dryness of the mouth. For temporary relief, use sugarless candy or gum, melt bits of ice in your mouth, or use a saliva substitute. However, if your mouth continues to feel dry for more than 2 weeks, check with your medical doctor or dentist. Continuing dryness of the mouth may increase the chance of dental disease, including tooth decay, gum disease, and fungus infections.

It may take several weeks for pergolide to work. Do not stop taking this medicine or reduce the amount you are taking without first checking with your doctor.

Side Effects of This Medicine

Along with its needed effects, a medicine may cause some unwanted effects. Although not all of these side effects may occur, if they do occur they may need medical attention.

Check with your doctor immediately if any of the following side effects occur:

Rare

Chest pain (severe); convulsions (seizures); fainting; fast heartbeat; headache (severe or continuing); increased sweating; nausea and vomiting (continuing or severe); nervousness; unexplained shortness of breath; vision changes, such as blurred vision or temporary blindness; weakness (sudden)

Also, check with your doctor as soon as possible if any of the following side effects occur:

More common

Confusion; hallucinations (seeing, hearing, or feeling things that are not there); pain or burning while urinating; uncontrolled movements of the body, such as the face, tongue, arms, hands, head, and upper body

Less common

High blood pressure

Other side effects may occur that usually do not need medical attention. These side effects may go away during treatment as your body adjusts to the medicine. However, check with your doctor if any of the following side effects continue or are bothersome:

More common

Abdominal or stomach pain; constipation; dizziness or lightheadedness, especially when getting up from a lying or sitting position; drowsiness; lower back pain; nausea; runny nose; weakness

Less common

Chills; diarrhea; dryness of mouth; loss of appetite; swelling of the face; vomiting

Other side effects not listed above may also occur in some patients. If you notice any other effects, check with your doctor.

Annual revision: 03/19/93

PERMETHRIN Topical

A commonly used brand name in the U.S. is Nix Cream Rinse.

Description

Permethrin (per-METH-rin) is used to treat head lice infections. It acts by destroying both the lice and their eggs.

This medicine is available only with your doctor's prescription, in the following dosage form:

Topical
- Lotion (U.S.)

It is very important that you read and understand the following information. If any of it causes you special concern, check with your doctor. Also, *if you have any questions* or if you want more information about this medicine or your medical problem, *ask your doctor, nurse, or pharmacist.*

Before Using This Medicine

In deciding to use a medicine, the risks of using the medicine must be weighed against the good it will do. This is a decision you and your doctor will make. For topical permethrin, the following should be considered:

Allergies—Tell your doctor if you have ever had any unusual or allergic reaction to permethrin; to other synthetic pyrethroids, such as those found in household insecticides; to pyrethrins or chrysanthemums; or to veterinary insecticides containing permethrin. Also tell your doctor and pharmacist if you are allergic to any other substances, such as preservatives or dyes.

Pregnancy—Permethrin has not been studied in pregnant women. However, this medication has not been shown to cause birth defects or other problems in animal studies.

Breast-feeding—It is not known whether permethrin passes into the breast milk. However, animal studies have shown that permethrin can cause tumors. Be sure you have discussed the risks and benefits of the medicine with your doctor.

Children—Studies on this medicine have been done only in adult patients, and there is no specific information about its use in children.

Older adults—Many medicines have not been tested in older people. Therefore, it may not be known whether they work exactly the same way they do in younger adults or if they cause different side effects or problems in older people. There is no specific information about the use of topical permethrin in the elderly.

Other medical problems—The presence of other medical problems may affect the use of topical permethrin. Make sure you tell your doctor if you have other medical problems, especially:

- Severe inflammation of the scalp—Use of permethrin may make the condition worse

Before you begin using any new medicine (prescription or nonprescription) or if you develop any new medical problem while you are using this medicine, check with your doctor, nurse, or pharmacist.

Proper Use of This Medicine

Keep this medicine away from the eyes. If you should accidentally get some in your eyes, flush them thoroughly with water at once.

Permethrin lotion comes in a container that holds only one treatment. Use as much of the medicine as you need and discard any remaining lotion properly.

To use:
- Shampoo the hair and scalp using regular shampoo.
- Thoroughly rinse and towel dry the hair and scalp.
- Allow hair to air dry for a few minutes.
- Shake the permethrin lotion well before applying.
- Thoroughly wet the hair and scalp with the permethrin lotion. Be sure to cover the areas behind the ears and on the back of the neck also. Allow the lotion to remain in place for 10 minutes.
- Then, rinse the hair and scalp thoroughly and dry with a clean towel.
- When the hair is dry, you may want to comb the hair with a fine-toothed comb to remove any remaining nits (eggs) or nit shells.

Head lice can be easily transferred from one person to another by direct contact with clothing, hats, scarves, bedding, towels, washcloths, hairbrushes and combs, or hairs from infected persons. Therefore, *all members of your household should be examined for head lice and should receive treatment if they are found to be infected.* If you have any questions about this, check with your doctor.

Storage—To store this medicine:
- Keep out of the reach of children.
- Store away from heat and direct light.
- Keep this medicine from freezing. Do not refrigerate.
- Do not keep outdated medicine or medicine no longer needed. Be sure that any discarded medicine is out of the reach of children.

Precautions While Using This Medicine

To prevent reinfection or spreading of the infection to other people, good health habits are required. These include the following:

- Machine wash all clothing (including hats, scarves, and coats), bedding, towels, and washcloths in very hot water and dry them by using the hot cycle of a dryer for at least 20 minutes. Clothing or bedding that cannot be washed should be dry cleaned or sealed in an airtight plastic bag for 2 weeks.
- Shampoo all wigs and hairpieces.
- Wash all hairbrushes and combs in very hot soapy water (above 130 °F) for 5 to 10 minutes and do not share them with other people.
- Clean the house or room by thoroughly vacuuming upholstered furniture, rugs, and floors.
- Wash all toys in very hot soapy water (above 130 °F) for 5 to 10 minutes or seal in an airtight plastic bag for 2 weeks. This is especially important for stuffed toys used on the bed.

Side Effects of This Medicine

Along with its needed effects, a medicine may cause some unwanted effects. Although not all of these side effects may occur, if they do occur they may need medical attention.

Check with your doctor if any of the following side effects continue or are bothersome:

Less common or rare

Itching, redness, swelling, burning, numbness, rash, stinging, or tingling of the scalp

Other side effects not listed above may also occur in some patients. If you notice any other effects, check with your doctor.

Annual revision: June 1990

PERPHENAZINE AND AMITRIPTYLINE Systemic

Some commonly used brand names are:

In the U.S.

Etrafon
Etrafon-A
Etrafon-Forte
Triavil

Generic name product may also be available.

In Canada

Elavil Plus
Etrafon
Etrafon-A
Etrafon-D
Etrafon-F
PMS Levazine
Triavil

Description

Perphenazine (per-FEN-a-zeen) and amitriptyline (a-mee-TRIP-ti-leen) combination is used to treat certain mental and emotional conditions.

This combination is available only with your doctor's prescription, in the following dosage form:

Oral

- Tablets (U.S. and Canada).

It is very important that you read and understand the following information. If any of it causes you special concern, check with your doctor. Also, *if you have any questions* or if you want more information about this medicine or your medical problem, *ask your doctor, nurse, or pharmacist.*

Before Using This Medicine

In deciding to use a medicine, the risks of taking the medicine must be weighed against the good it will do. This is a decision you and your doctor will make. For perphenazine and amitriptyline combination, the following should be considered:

Allergies—Tell your doctor if you have ever had any unusual or allergic reaction to perphenazine (e.g., Trilafon) or other phenothiazines (such as acetophenazine [e.g., Tindal], chlorpromazine [e.g., Thorazine], fluphenazine [e.g., Prolixin], mesoridazine [e.g., Serentil], prochlorperazine [e.g., Compazine], promazine [e.g., Sparine], promethazine [e.g., Phenergan], thioridazine [e.g., Mellaril], trifluoperazine [e.g., Stelazine], triflupromazine [e.g., Vesprin], trimeprazine [e.g., Temaril]) or to amitriptyline (e.g., Elavil) or other tricyclic antidepressants (such as amoxapine [e.g., Asendin], clomipramine [e.g., Anafranil], desipramine [e.g., Pertofrane], doxepin [e.g., Sinequan], imipramine [e.g., Tofranil], nortriptyline [e.g., Aventyl], protriptyline [e.g., Vivactil], trimipramine [e.g., Surmontil]). Also tell your doctor and pharmacist if you are allergic to any other substances, such as foods, preservatives, or dyes.

Pregnancy—Studies have not been done in pregnant women. However, perphenazine and amitriptyline combination has not been shown to cause birth defects in animal studies. Side effects such as jaundice and muscle tremors have occurred in some newborn babies when their mothers received other phenothiazines during pregnancy.

Breast-feeding—Perphenazine and amitriptyline combination passes into the breast milk. However, it has not been reported to cause problems in nursing babies.

Children—Certain side effects, such as muscle spasms of the face, neck, and back, tic-like or twitching movements, inability to move the eyes, twisting of the body, or weakness of the arms and legs, are more likely to occur in children, who are usually more sensitive than adults to some of the side effects of perphenazine and amitriptyline combination.

Older adults—Confusion, vision problems, dizziness or fainting, drowsiness, dryness of mouth, constipation, problems in urinating, trembling of the hands and fingers, and symptoms of tardive dyskinesia (such as uncontrolled movements of the mouth, tongue, jaw, arms, and/or legs) are especially likely to occur in elderly patients. Older patients are usually more sensitive than younger adults to the effects of perphenazine and amitriptyline combination.

Other medicines—Although certain medicines should not be used together at all, in other cases 2 different medicines may be used together even if an interaction might occur. In these cases, your doctor may want to change the dose, or other precautions may be necessary. When you are taking perphenazine and amitriptyline combination, it is especially important that your doctor and pharmacist know if you are taking any of the following:

- Amphetamines or
- Appetite suppressants (diet pills) or
- Medicine for asthma or other breathing problems or
- Medicine for colds, sinus problems, or hay fever or other allergies (including nose drops and sprays)—Using these medicines with perphenazine and amitriptyline combination may increase the risk of serious effects on the heart
- Antithyroid agents (medicine for overactive thyroid) or
- Cimetidine (e.g., Tagamet) or
- Methyldopa (e.g., Aldomet) or
- Metoclopramide (e.g., Reglan) or
- Metyrosine (e.g., Demser) or
- Pemoline (e.g., Cylert) or
- Pimozide (e.g., Orap) or
- Promethazine (e.g., Phenergan) or
- Rauwolfia alkaloids (alseroxylon [e.g., Rauwiloid], deserpidine [e.g., Harmonyl], rauwolfia serpentina [e.g., Raudixin], reserpine [e.g., Serpasil]) or
- Trimeprazine (e.g., Temaril)—Taking these medicines with perphenazine and amitriptyline combination may increase the risk of serious side effects
- Central nervous system (CNS) depressants (medicines that cause drowsiness)—Taking these medicines with perphenazine and amitriptyline combination may increase the CNS depressant effects
- Epinephrine (e.g., Adrenalin)—Severe low blood pressure (hypotension) and fast heartbeat may occur if epinephrine is used with perphenazine and amitriptyline combination
- Levodopa (e.g., Dopar)—Perphenazine may prevent levodopa from working properly in the treatment of Parkinson's disease
- Lithium (e.g., Lithane)—The amount of medicine you need to take may change
- Metrizamide—When this dye is used for myelograms during the use of perphenazine and amitriptyline combination, there is an increased risk of seizures
- Monoamine oxidase (MAO) inhibitors (furazolidone [e.g., Furoxone], isocarboxazid [e.g., Marplan], phenelzine [e.g., Nardil], procarbazine [e.g., Matulane], selegiline [e.g., Eldepryl], tranylcypromine [e.g., Parnate])—Taking amitriptyline while you are taking or within 2 weeks of taking monoamine oxidase (MAO) inhibitors may cause sudden high body temperature, extremely high blood pressure, and severe convulsions; however, sometimes certain of these medicines may be used together under close supervision by your doctor

Other medical problems—The presence of other medical problems may affect the use of perphenazine and amitriptyline combination. Make sure you tell your doctor if you have any other medical problems, especially:

- Alcohol abuse—Certain side effects such as heat stroke may be more likely to occur
- Asthma (history of) or other lung disease or
- Bipolar disorder (manic-depressive illness) or
- Blood disease or
- Breast cancer or
- Difficult urination or
- Enlarged prostate or
- Epilepsy or other seizure disorders or
- Glaucoma or
- Heart or blood vessel disease or
- Mental illness (severe) or
- Parkinson's disease or
- Stomach or intestinal problems—Perphenazine and amitriptyline combination may make the condition worse
- Kidney disease or
- Liver disease—Higher blood levels of perphenazine and amitriptyline may occur, increasing the chance of side effects
- Overactive thyroid—Perphenazine and amitriptyline combination may cause an increased chance of serious effects on the heart
- Reye's syndrome—There may be an increased chance of unwanted effects on the liver

Before you begin using any new medicine (prescription or nonprescription) or if you develop any new medical problem while you are using this medicine, check with your doctor, nurse, or pharmacist.

Proper Use of This Medicine

To lessen stomach upset, take this medicine immediately after meals or with food, unless your doctor has told you to take it on an empty stomach.

Do not take more of this medicine and do not take it more often than your doctor ordered. This is particularly important for elderly patients, since they are more sensitive to the effects of this medicine.

Sometimes perphenazine and amitriptyline combination must be taken for several weeks before its full effect is reached.

Missed dose—If you miss a dose of this medicine, take it as soon as possible. However, if it is within 2 hours of your next dose, skip the missed dose and go back to your regular dosing schedule. Do not double doses.

Storage—To store this medicine:

- Keep out of the reach of children. Overdose of perphenazine and amitriptyline combination is especially dangerous in young children.
- Store away from heat and direct light.
- Do not store in the bathroom, near the kitchen sink, or in other damp places. Heat or moisture may cause the medicine to break down.
- Do not keep outdated medicine or medicine no longer needed. Be sure that any discarded medicine is out of the reach of children.

Precautions While Using This Medicine

Your doctor should check your progress at regular visits to allow dose adjustments and help reduce side effects.

Do not stop taking this medicine without first checking with your doctor. Your doctor may want you to reduce gradually the amount you are taking before stopping completely. This is to prevent side effects and to prevent your condition from becoming worse.

Do not take this medicine within two hours of taking antacids or medicine for diarrhea. Taking these products too close together may make this medicine less effective.

This medicine will add to the effects of alcohol and other CNS depressants (medicines that slow down the nervous system, possibly causing drowsiness). Some examples of CNS depressants are antihistamines or medicine for hay fever, other allergies, or colds; sedatives, tranquilizers, or sleeping medicine; prescription pain medicine or narcotics barbiturates; medicine for seizures; or anesthetics, including some dental anesthetics. *Check with your doctor before taking any of the above while you are using this medicine.*

Before having any kind of surgery, dental treatment, or emergency treatment, tell the medical doctor or dentist in charge that you are taking this medicine.

This medicine may cause some people to become drowsy or less alert than they are normally, especially during the first few weeks of treatment. Even if this medicine is taken only at bedtime, it may cause some people to feel drowsy or less alert on arising. *Make sure you know how you react to this medicine before you drive, use machines, or do anything else that could be dangerous if you are not alert.*

Dizziness, lightheadedness, or fainting may occur, especially when you get up from a lying or sitting position. Getting up slowly may help. If the problem continues or gets worse, check with your doctor.

This medicine may make you sweat less, causing your body temperature to increase. *Use extra care not to become overheated during exercise or hot weather while you are taking this medicine,* since overheating may result in heat stroke. Also, hot baths or saunas may make you feel dizzy or faint.

Perphenazine and amitriptyline combination may cause dryness of the mouth. For temporary relief, use sugarless gum or candy, melt bits of ice in your mouth, or use a saliva substitute. However, if your mouth continues to feel dry for more than 2 weeks, check with your medical doctor or dentist. Continuing dryness of the mouth may increase the chance of dental disease, including tooth decay, gum disease, and fungus infections.

Perphenazine may cause your skin to be more sensitive to sunlight than it is normally. Exposure to sunlight, even for brief periods of time, may cause a skin rash, itching, redness or other discoloration of the skin, or a severe sunburn. When you begin taking this medicine:

- Stay out of direct sunlight, especially between the hours of 10:00 a.m. and 3:00 p.m., if possible.
- Wear protective clothing, including a hat. Also, wear sunglasses.
- Apply a sun block product that has a skin protection factor (SPF) of at least 15. Some patients may require a product with a higher SPF number, especially if they have a fair complexion. If you have any questions about this, check with your doctor or pharmacist.
- Apply a sun block lipstick that has an SPF of at least 15 to protect your lips.
- Do not use a sunlamp or tanning bed or booth.

If you have a severe reaction from the sun, check with your doctor.

Side Effects of This Medicine

Along with its needed effects, perphenazine (included in this combination medicine) can sometimes cause serious side effects. Tardive dyskinesia (a movement disorder) may occur and may not go away after you stop using the medicine. Signs of tardive dyskinesia include fine, worm-like movements of the tongue, or other uncontrolled movements of the mouth, tongue, cheeks, jaw, or arms and legs. Other serious but rare side effects may also occur. These include severe muscle stiffness, fever, unusual tiredness or weakness, fast heartbeat, difficult breathing, increased sweating, loss of bladder control, and seizures (neuroleptic malignant syndrome). *You and your doctor should discuss the good this medicine will do as well as the risks of taking it.*

Stop taking this medicine and get emergency help immediately if any of the following side effects occur:

Rare

Convulsions (seizures); difficulty in breathing; fast heartbeat; fever; high or low blood pressure; increased sweating; loss of bladder control; muscle stiffness (severe); unusual tiredness or weakness; unusually pale skin

Also, check with your doctor as soon as possible if any of the following side effects occur:

More common

Blurred vision or any change in vision; difficulty in speaking or swallowing; fainting; inability to move eyes; lip smacking or puckering; loss of balance control; mask-like face; muscle spasms, especially of face, neck, and back; nervousness, restlessness, or need to keep moving; puffing of cheeks; rapid or fine, worm-like movements of tongue; shuffling walk; stiffness of arms and legs; trembling and shaking of fingers and hands; tic-like or twitching movements; twisting movements of body; uncontrolled chewing movements; uncontrolled movements of arms or legs; weakness of arms and legs

Less common

Confusion; constipation; difficult urination; eye pain; hallucinations (seeing, hearing, or feeling things that are not there); increased skin sensitivity to sun; shakiness; slow pulse or irregular heartbeat

Rare

Abdominal or stomach pain; aching muscles or joints; back or leg pain; fever and chills; hair loss; hot, dry skin or lack of sweating; irritability; loss of appetite; muscle weakness or twitching; nausea, vomiting, or diarrhea; nosebleeds; prolonged, painful, inappropriate penile erection; ringing, buzzing, or other unexplained noises in ears; skin discoloration; skin rash and itching; sore throat and fever; swelling of face and tongue; swelling of testicles; unusual bleeding or bruising; yellow eyes or skin

Symptoms of overdose

Agitation; confusion; convulsions (seizures); drowsiness (severe); enlarged pupils; fast, slow, or irregular heartbeat; fever; hallucinations (seeing, hearing, or feeling things that are not there); shortness of breath or troubled breathing; unusual tiredness or weakness (severe); vomiting (severe)

Other side effects may occur that usually do not need medical attention. These side effects may go away during treatment as your body adjusts to the medicine. However, check with your doctor if any of the following side effects continue or are bothersome:

More common

Decreased sweating; dizziness; drowsiness; dryness of mouth; headache; increased appetite for sweets; nasal congestion; tiredness or weakness (mild); unpleasant taste; weight gain (unusual)

Less common

Changes in menstrual period; decreased sexual ability; heartburn; increased sweating; swelling or pain in breasts or unusual secretion of milk

After you stop using this medicine, your body may need time to adjust. The length of time this takes depends on the amount of medicine you are using and how long you used it. During this time, check with your doctor if you notice any of the following symptoms:

Dizziness; nausea or vomiting; stomach pain; trembling of fingers and hands; symptoms of tardive dyskinesia, including lip smacking or puckering, puffing of cheeks, rapid or fine, worm-like movements of tongue, uncontrolled chewing movements, or uncontrolled movements of arms or legs

Other side effects may occur if the medicine is stopped suddenly or stopped after long-term treatment. Check with your doctor if you notice any of the following symptoms:

Diarrhea; headache; irritability; restlessness; trouble in sleeping, with vivid dreams; unusual excitement

Other side effects not listed above may also occur in some patients. If you notice any other effects, check with your doctor.

Annual revision: 01/27/92

PHENACEMIDE Systemic†

Some commonly used brand names are:

In the U.S.

Phenurone

Other

Epiclase
Phetylureum

Another commonly used name is phenacetylcarbamide.

---

†Not commercially available in Canada.

Description

Phenacemide (fe-NASS-e-mide) is used to control certain seizures in the treatment of epilepsy. This medicine acts on the central nervous system (CNS) to reduce the number and severity of seizures.

Phenacemide is available only with your doctor's prescription in the following dosage form:

Oral

- Tablets (U.S.)

It is very important that you read and understand the following information. If any of it causes you special concern, check with your doctor. Also, *if you have any questions* or if you want more information about this medicine or your medical problem, *ask your doctor, nurse, or pharmacist.*

Before Using This Medicine

In deciding to use a medicine, the risks of taking the medicine must be weighed against the good it will do. This is a decision you and your doctor will make. For phenacemide, the following should be considered:

Allergies—Tell your doctor if you have ever had any unusual or allergic reaction to phenacemide or any other anticonvulsant medicines in the past. Also tell your doctor and pharmacist if you are allergic to any other substances, such as foods, preservatives, or dyes.

Pregnancy—Phenacemide has been reported to cause birth defects when taken by the mother during pregnancy. However, this medicine may be necessary to control seizures in some pregnant patients. Be sure you have discussed this with your doctor. In addition, when taken during pregnancy, phenacemide may cause a bleeding problem in the mother during delivery and in the newborn. This may be prevented by giving vitamin K to the mother 1 month before and during delivery, and to the baby immediately after birth.

Breast-feeding—It is not known whether this medicine passes into breast milk.

Children—Although there is no specific information comparing use of phenacemide in children with use in other age groups, this medicine is not expected to cause different side effects or problems than it does in adults.

Older adults—Many medicines have not been studied specifically in older people. Therefore, it may not be known whether they work exactly the same way they do in younger adults. Although there is no specific information comparing use of phenacemide in the elderly with use in other age groups, this medicine is not expected to cause different side effects or problems in older people than it does in younger adults.

Other medicines—Although certain medicines should not be used together at all, in other cases 2 different medicines may be used together even if an interaction might occur. In these cases, your doctor may want to change the dose, or other precautions may be necessary. When you are taking phenacemide, it is especially important that your doctor and pharmacist know if you are taking the following:

- Other anticonvulsants—Use of phenacemide may increase the chance of serious side effects

Other medical problems—The presence of other medical problems may affect the use of phenacemide. Make sure you tell your doctor if you have any other medical problems, especially:

- Blood disease or
- Kidney disease or
- Liver disease or
- Personality disorder (mental illness)—Phenacemide may make the condition worse

Before you begin using any new medicine (prescription or nonprescription) or if you develop any new medical problem while you are using this medicine, check with your doctor, nurse, or pharmacist.

Proper Use of This Medicine

To control your medical problem, *take this medicine every day* exactly as ordered by your doctor. Do not take more or less of it than your doctor ordered. To help you remember to take the medicine at the correct times, try to get into the habit of taking it at the same times each day.

Dosing—The dose of phenacemide will be different for different patients. *Follow your doctor's orders or the directions on the label.* The following information includes only the average doses of phenacemide. *If your dose is different, do not change it* unless your doctor tells you to do so:

- Adults—Oral, to start, 500 milligrams three times a day. After one week, your doctor may add an additional 500 milligram dose to be taken upon arising if needed. In the third week, your doctor may add another 500 milligram dose to be taken at bedtime if needed. Your doctor may increase your dose further. However, the dose is usually not more than 5000 milligrams a day.
- Children 5 years of age and older—Oral, to start, 250 milligrams three times a day. The doctor may increase the dose further. However, the dose is usually not more than 1500 milligrams a day.
- Children up to 5 years of age—Dose must be determined by the doctor.

Missed dose—If you miss a dose of this medicine, take it as soon as possible. However, if it is almost time for your next dose, skip the missed dose and go back to your regular dosing schedule. Do not double doses.

Storage—To store this medicine:

- Keep out of the reach of children.
- Store away from heat and direct light.

- Do not store in the bathroom, near the kitchen sink, or in other damp places. Heat or moisture may cause the medicine to break down.
- Do not keep outdated medicine or medicine no longer needed. Be sure that any discarded medicine is out of the reach of children.

Precautions While Using This Medicine

Your doctor should check your progress at regular visits, especially during the first few months of treatment with this medicine. During this time, the amount of medicine you are taking may have to be changed often to meet your individual needs.

If you have been taking phenacemide regularly, do not stop taking it without first checking with your doctor. Your doctor may want you to decrease gradually the amount you are taking before stopping completely. This will help reduce the possibility of seizures.

Be sure to tell your doctor as soon as possible if you have a sore throat, fever, or general feeling of tiredness, or if you notice any unusual bleeding or bruising, such as reddish or purplish spots on skin, or recurring nosebleeds or bleeding gums.

Also, be sure to tell your doctor as soon as possible if you or your family notice any changes in your behavior or mood, such as aggressiveness, depression, or a decreased interest in your surroundings.

This medicine will add to the effects of alcohol and other CNS depressants (medicines that slow down the nervous system, possibly causing drowsiness). Some examples of CNS depressants are antihistamines or medicine for hay fever, other allergies, or colds; sedatives, tranquilizers, or sleeping medicine; prescription pain medicine or narcotics; barbiturates; other medicine for seizures; muscle relaxants; or anesthetics, including some dental anesthetics. *Check with your doctor before taking any of the above while you are using this medicine.*

This medicine may cause some people to become dizzy or drowsy. *Make sure your know how you react to this medicine before you drive, use machines, or do anything else that could be dangerous if you are dizzy or are not alert.*

Side Effects of This Medicine

Phenacemide may cause some serious side effects, including behavior or mental changes, blood problems, liver problems, or kidney problems. You and your doctor should discuss the good this medicine will do as well as the risks of receiving it.

Check with your doctor as soon as possible if any of the following side effects occur:

More common

Behavior or mood changes

Rare

Blood in urine; dark-colored urine; difficulty in breathing, shortness of breath, wheezing, or tightness in chest; drowsiness; flu-like symptoms (fever with or without chills, headache, body ache); nausea or vomiting; skin rash; sore throat and fever; swelling of face, feet, or lower legs; swollen or painful glands; unusual bleeding or bruising; unusual tiredness or weakness; weight gain; white spots, sores, or ulcers on lips, or in mouth or throat; yellow eyes or skin

Symptoms of overdose (in the order in which they may occur)

Unusual excitement, nervousness, or irritability; clumsiness or unsteadiness; drowsiness (severe)

Other side effects may occur that usually do not need medical attention. These side effects may go away during treatment as your body adjusts to the medicine. However, check with your doctor if any of the following side effects continue or are bothersome:

More common

Drowsiness; headache; loss of appetite

Less common or rare

Dizziness; fever; muscle pain; pounding heartbeat; tingling, burning, or prickly sensations; trouble in sleeping; unusual tiredness or weakness; weight loss

Other side effects not listed above may also occur in some patients. If you notice any other effects, check with your doctor.

Annual revision: 03/09/93

PHENAZOPYRIDINE Systemic

Some commonly used brand names are:

In the U.S.

Azo-Standard
Baridium
Eridium
Geridium
Phenazodine
Pyridiate
Pyridium
Urodine
Urogesic
Viridium

Generic name product may also be available.

In Canada

Phenazo
Pyridium

Description

Phenazopyridine (fen-az-oh-PEER-i-deen) is used to relieve the pain, burning, and discomfort caused by infection or irritation of the urinary tract. It is not an antibiotic and will not cure the infection itself.

In the U.S., phenazopyridine is available only with your doctor's prescription. In Canada, it is available without a prescription. It is available in the following dosage form:

Oral

- Tablets (U.S. and Canada)

It is very important that you read and understand the following information. If any of it causes you special concern, check with your doctor or pharmacist. Also, *if you have any questions* or if you want more information about this medicine or your medical problem, *ask your doctor, nurse, or pharmacist.*

Before Using This Medicine

In deciding to use a medicine, the risks of taking the medicine must be weighed against the good it will do. This is a decision you and your doctor will make. For phenazopyridine, the following should be considered:

Allergies—Tell your doctor if you have ever had any unusual or allergic reaction to phenazopyridine. Also tell your doctor and pharmacist if you are allergic to any other substances, such as foods, preservatives, or dyes.

Pregnancy—Phenazopyridine has not been studied in pregnant women. However, phenazopyridine has not been shown to cause birth defects in animal studies.

Breast-feeding—It is not known whether phenazopyridine passes into the breast milk. However, phenazopyridine has not been reported to cause problems in nursing babies.

Children—Although there is no specific information comparing use of phenazopyridine in children with use in other age groups, it is not expected to cause different side effects or problems in children than it does in adults.

Older adults—Many medicines have not been studied specifically in older people. Therefore, it may not be known whether they work exactly the same way they do in younger adults. Although there is no specific information comparing use of phenazopyridine in the elderly with use in other age groups, this medicine is not expected to cause different side effects or problems in older people than it does in younger adults.

Other medicines—Although certain medicines should not be used together at all, in other cases two different medicines may be used together even if an interaction might occur. In these cases, your doctor may want to change the dose, or other precautions may be necessary. Tell your doctor and pharmacist if you are taking any other prescription or nonprescription (over-the-counter [OTC]) medicine).

Other medical problems—The presence of other medical problems may affect the use of phenazopyridine. Make sure you tell your doctor if you have any other medical problems, especially:

- Glucose-6-phosphate dehydrogenase (G6PD) deficiency or
- Hepatitis or
- Kidney disease—The chance of side effects may be increased.

Before you begin using any new medicine (prescription or nonprescription) or if you develop any new medical problem while you are using this medicine, check with your doctor, nurse, or pharmacist.

Proper Use of This Medicine

This medicine is best taken with food or after eating a meal or a snack to lessen stomach upset.

Do not use any leftover medicine for future urinary tract problems without first checking with your doctor. An infection may require additional medicine.

Missed dose—If you miss a dose of this medicine, take it as soon as you remember. However, if it is almost time for your next dose, skip the missed dose and go back to your regular dosing schedule. Do not double doses.

Storage—To store this medicine:

- Keep out of the reach of children.
- Store away from heat and direct light.
- Do not store this medicine in the bathroom, near the kitchen sink, or in other damp places. Heat or moisture may cause the medicine to break down.
- Do not keep outdated medicine or medicine no longer needed. Be sure that any discarded medicine is out of the reach of children.

Precautions While Using This Medicine

Check with your doctor if symptoms such as bloody urine, difficult or painful urination, frequent urge to urinate, or sudden decrease in the amount of urine appear or become worse while you are taking this medicine.

Phenazopyridine causes the urine to turn reddish orange. This is to be expected while you are using it. This effect is harmless and will go away after you stop taking the medicine. Also, the medicine may stain clothing.

For *patients who wear soft contact lenses:*

- It is best not to wear soft contact lenses while being treated with this medicine. Phenazopyridine may cause discoloration or staining of contact lenses. It may not be possible to remove the stain.

For *diabetic patients:*

- This medicine may cause false test results with urine sugar tests and urine ketone tests. If you have any questions about this, check with your doctor, nurse, or pharmacist, especially if your diabetes is not well controlled.

Before you have any medical tests, tell the person in charge that you are taking this medicine. The results of some tests may be affected by this medicine.

Side Effects of This Medicine

Along with its needed effects, a medicine may cause some unwanted effects. Although not all of these side effects may occur, if they do occur they may need medical attention.

Check with your doctor as soon as possible if any of the following side effects occur:

Rare

Blue or blue-purple color of skin; fever and confusion; shortness of breath, tightness in chest, wheezing, or troubled breathing; skin rash; sudden decrease in the amount of urine; swelling of face, fingers, feet, and/or lower legs; unusual tiredness or weakness; weight gain; yellow eyes or skin

Other side effects may occur that usually do not need medical attention. These side effects may go away during treatment as your body adjusts to the medicine. However, check with your doctor if any of the following side effects continue or are bothersome:

Less common or rare

Dizziness; headache; indigestion; stomach cramps or pain

Other side effects not listed above may also occur in some patients. If you notice any other effects, check with your doctor.

Annual revision: 06/08/92

PHENOLSULFONPHTHALEIN Diagnostic

Some commonly used names are phenol red and PSP.

Description

Phenolsulfonphthalein (fee-nole-sul-fon-THAY-leen) is used as a test to help diagnose problems or disease of the kidneys. This test determines how well your kidneys are working.

Phenolsulfonphthalein passes out of the body almost entirely in the urine. Measuring the amount of phenolsulfonphthalein in the urine can help the doctor determine if the kidneys are working properly.

How test is done: After you have emptied your bladder, phenolsulfonphthalein will be given by injection. Then you will be asked to empty your bladder into a container one or more times after the medicine is given. The amount of this medicine in your urine will be measured. Then the results of the test will be studied.

It is very important that you *empty the bladder completely* and collect all the urine when you are asked to do so. If any urine is left behind or lost, it will change the results of the test.

Phenolsulfonphthalein is to be used only under the supervision of a doctor. It is available in the following dosage form:

Parenteral

- Injection (U.S.)

It is very important that you read and understand the following information. If any of it causes you special concern, check with your doctor. Also, *if you have any questions* or if you want more information about this test or your medical problem, *ask your doctor, nurse, or pharmacist.*

Before Having This Test

In deciding to use a diagnostic test, any risks of the test must be weighed against the good it will do. This is a decision you and your doctor will make. Also, test results may be affected by other things. For phenolsulfonphthalein, the following should be considered:

Allergies—Tell your doctor if you have ever had any unusual or allergic reaction to phenolsulfonphthalein. Also tell your doctor if you are allergic to any other substances, such as foods, preservatives, or dyes.

Pregnancy—Studies have not been done in either humans or animals.

Breast-feeding—It is not known whether phenolsulfonphthalein passes into the breast milk. This medicine has not been reported to cause problems in nursing babies.

Children—Although there is no specific information comparing use of phenolsulfonphthalein in children with use in other age groups, phenolsulfonphthalein is not expected to cause different side effects or problems in children than it does in adults.

Older adults—Many medicines have not been studied specifically in older people. Therefore, it may not be known whether they work exactly the same way they do in younger adults. Although there is no specific information comparing use of phenolsulfonphthalein in the elderly with use in other age groups, this medicine is not expected to cause different side effects or problems in older people than it does in younger adults.

Other medicines—Although certain medicines should not be used together at all, in other cases two different medicines may be used together even if an interaction might occur. In these cases, your doctor may want to change the dose, or other precautions may be necessary. When you are taking phenolsulfonphthalein, it is especially important that your doctor and pharmacist know if you are taking any of the following:

- Aspirin or other salicylates or
- Atropine or
- Diuretics (water pills) or
- Penicillins or
- Probenecid (e.g., Benemid) or
- Sulfinpyrazone (e.g., Anturane) or
- Sulfonamides (sulfa medicine)—Use of any of these medicines at the same time as phenolsulfonphthalein may affect the test results

Other medical problems—The presence of other medical problems may affect the use of phenolsulfonphthalein. Make sure you tell your doctor if you have any other medical problems, especially:

- Gout or
- Liver disease or
- Multiple myeloma (a kind of cancer)—These conditions may affect how fast the body gets rid of the phenolsulfonphthalein
- Heart or blood vessel disease or
- Kidney disease (severe)—Patients with these conditions are at greater risk of becoming ill because of the large amount of liquids that must be taken for this test

Preparation for This Test

Your doctor will ask you to drink a certain amount of water a little while before this test is done. *Follow your doctor's instructions carefully*. Otherwise, this test may not work and may have to be done again.

Side Effects of This Medicine

Along with its needed effects, a medicine may cause some unwanted effects. Although this medicine usually does not cause any side effects, *tell your doctor or nurse immediately if you notice wheezing or skin rash or itching shortly after it is given.*

Other side effects not listed above may also occur in some patients. If you notice any other effects, check with your doctor.

Annual revision: 10/07/91

PHENOTHIAZINES Systemic

This information applies to the following medicines:

Acetophenazine (a-set-oh-FEN-a-zeen)
Chlorpromazine (klor-PROE-ma-zeen)
Fluphenazine (floo-FEN-a-zeen)
Mesoridazine (mez-oh-RID-a-zeen)
Methotrimeprazine (meth-oh-trim-EP-ra-zeen)
Pericyazine (pair-ee-SYE-a-zeen)
Perphenazine (per-FEN-a-zeen)
Pipotiazine (pip-oh-TYE-a-zeen)
Prochlorperazine (proe-klor-PAIR-a-zeen)
Promazine (PROE-ma-zeen)
Thiopropazate (thye-oh-PROE-pa-zayt)
Thioproperazine (thye-oh-proe-PAIR-a-zeen)
Thioridazine (thye-oh-RID-a-zeen)
Trifluoperazine (trye-floo-oh-PAIR-a-zeen)
Triflupromazine (trye-floo-PROE-ma-zeen)

Note: This information does *not* apply to Ethopropazine, Promethazine, Propiomazine, and Trimeprazine.

Some commonly used brand names are:

For Acetophenazine†
In the U.S.
Tindal

For Chlorpromazine
In the U.S.
Ormazine
Thorazine
Thorazine Concentrate
Thorazine Spansule
Thor-Prom

Generic name product may also be available.

In Canada
Chlorpromanyl-5
Chlorpromanyl-20
Chlorpromanyl-40
Largactil
Largactil Liquid
Largactil Oral Drops
Novo-Chlorpromazine

Generic name product may also be available.

For Fluphenazine
In the U.S.
Permitil
Permitil Concentrate
Prolixin
Prolixin Concentrate
Prolixin Decanoate
Prolixin Enanthate

Generic name product may also be available.

In Canada
Apo-Fluphenazine
Modecate
Modecate Concentrate
Moditen Enanthate
Moditen HCl
Moditen HCl-H.P.
Permitil

For Mesoridazine
In the U.S.
Serentil
Serentil Concentrate
In Canada
Serentil

For Methotrimeprazine
In the U.S.
Levoprome
In Canada
Nozinan
Nozinan Liquid
Nozinan Oral Drops

For Pericyazine*
In Canada
Neuleptil

For Perphenazine
In the U.S.
Trilafon
Trilafon Concentrate
Generic name product may also be available.
In Canada
Apo-Perphenazine
PMS Perphenazine
Trilafon
Trilafon Concentrate
Generic name product may also be available.

For Pipotiazine*
In Canada
Piportil L_4

For Prochlorperazine
In the U.S.
Compa-Z
Compazine
Compazine Spansule
Cotranzine
Ultrazine-10
Generic name product may also be available.
In Canada
PMS Prochlorperazine
Prorazin
Stemetil
Stemetil Liquid
Generic name product may also be available.

For Promazine
In the U.S.
Primazine
Prozine-50
Sparine
Generic name product may also be available.
In Canada
Generic name product may be available.

For Thiopropazate*
In Canada
Dartal

For Thioproperazine*
In Canada
Majeptil

For Thioridazine
In the U.S.
Mellaril
Mellaril Concentrate
Mellaril-S
Generic name product may also be available.
In Canada
Apo-Thioridazine
Mellaril
Novo-Ridazine
PMS Thioridazine

For Trifluoperazine
In the U.S.
Stelazine
Stelazine Concentrate
Generic name product may also be available.
In Canada
Apo-Trifluoperazine
Novo-Flurazine
PMS Trifluoperazine
Solazine
Stelazine
Stelazine Concentrate
Terfluzine
Terfluzine Concentrate

For Triflupromazine†
In the U.S.
Vesprin

*Not commercially available in the U.S.
†Not commercially available in Canada.

Description

Phenothiazines (FEE-noe-THYE-a-zeens) are used to treat nervous, mental, and emotional disorders. Some are used also to control anxiety or agitation in certain patients, severe nausea and vomiting, severe hiccups, and moderate to severe pain in some hospitalized patients. Chlorpromazine is also used in the treatment of certain types of porphyria, and with other medicines in the treatment of tetanus. Phenothiazines may also be used for other conditions as determined by your doctor.

Phenothiazines are available only with your doctor's prescription in the following dosage forms:

Oral

Acetophenazine
- Tablets (U.S.)

Chlorpromazine
- Extended-release capsules (U.S.)
- Oral concentrate (U.S. and Canada)
- Syrup (U.S. and Canada)
- Tablets (U.S. and Canada)

Fluphenazine
- Elixir (U.S. and Canada)
- Oral solution (U.S.)
- Tablets (U.S. and Canada)

Mesoridazine
- Oral solution (U.S.)
- Tablets (U.S. and Canada)

Methotrimeprazine
- Oral solution (Canada)
- Syrup (Canada)
- Tablets (Canada)

Pericyazine
- Capsules (Canada)
- Oral solution (Canada)

Perphenazine
- Oral solution (U.S. and Canada)
- Syrup (Canada)
- Tablets (U.S. and Canada)

Prochlorperazine
- Extended-release capsules (U.S.)
- Syrup (U.S. and Canada)
- Tablets (U.S. and Canada)

Promazine
- Tablets (U.S.)

Thiopropazate
- Tablets (Canada)

Thioproperazine
- Tablets (Canada)

Thioridazine
- Oral solution (U.S. and Canada)
- Oral suspension (U.S. and Canada)
- Tablets (U.S. and Canada)

Trifluoperazine
- Oral solution (U.S. and Canada)
- Syrup (Canada)
- Tablets (U.S. and Canada)

Parenteral

Chlorpromazine
- Injection (U.S. and Canada)

Fluphenazine
- Injection (U.S. and Canada)

Mesoridazine
- Injection (U.S.)

Methotrimeprazine
- Injection (U.S. and Canada)

Perphenazine
- Injection (U.S. and Canada)

Pipotiazine
- Injection (Canada)

Prochlorperazine
- Injection (U.S. and Canada)

Promazine
- Injection (U.S. and Canada)

Trifluoperazine
- Injection (U.S. and Canada)

Triflupromazine
- Injection (U.S.)

Rectal

Chlorpromazine
- Suppositories (U.S. and Canada)

Prochlorperazine
- Suppositories (U.S. and Canada)

It is very important that you read and understand the following information. If any of it causes you special concern, check with your doctor. Also, *if you have any questions* or if you want more information about this medicine or your medical problem, *ask your doctor, nurse, or pharmacist.*

Before Using This Medicine

In deciding to use a medicine, the risks of taking the medicine must be weighed against the good it will do. This is a decision you and your doctor will make. For phenothiazines, the following should be considered:

Allergies—Tell your doctor if you have ever had any unusual or allergic reaction to phenothiazines. Also tell your doctor and pharmacist if you are allergic to any other substances, such as foods, preservatives, or dyes.

Pregnancy—Although studies have not been done in pregnant women, some side effects, such as jaundice and muscle tremors and other movement disorders, have occurred in a few newborns whose mothers received phenothiazines close to the time of delivery. Studies in animals have shown that chlorpromazine and trifluoperazine, given in doses many times the usual human dose, may cause birth defects.

Breast-feeding—Phenothiazines pass into the breast milk and may cause drowsiness and a greater chance of unusual muscle movement in the nursing baby.

Children—Certain side effects, such as muscle spasms of the face, neck, and back, tic-like or twitching movements, inability to move the eyes, twisting of the body, or weakness of the arms and legs, are more likely to occur in children, especially those with severe illness or dehydration. Children are usually more sensitive than adults to some of the side effects of phenothiazines.

Older adults—Constipation, dizziness or fainting, drowsiness, dryness of mouth, trembling of the hands and fingers, and symptoms of tardive dyskinesia (such as rapid, worm-like movements of the tongue or any other uncontrolled movements of the mouth, tongue, or jaw, and/or arms and legs) are especially likely to occur in elderly patients, who are usually more sensitive than younger adults to the effects of phenothiazines.

Other medicines—Although certain medicines should not be used together at all, in other cases 2 different medicines may be used together even if an interaction might occur. In these cases, your doctor may want to change the dose, or other precautions may be necessary. When you are taking phenothiazines, it is especially important that your doctor and pharmacist know if you are taking any of the following:

- Amantadine (e.g., Symmetrel) or
- Antihypertensives (high blood pressure medicine) or
- Bromocriptine (e.g., Parlodel) or
- Deferoxamine (e.g., Desferal) or
- Diuretics (water pills) or
- Levobunolol (e.g., Betagan) or
- Medicine for heart disease or
- Metipranolol (e.g., OptiPranolol)
- Nabilone (e.g., Cesamet) (with high doses) or
- Narcotic pain medicine or
- Nimodipine (e.g., Nimotop) or
- Other antipsychotics (medicine for mental illness) or
- Pentamidine (e.g., Pentam) or
- Pimozide (e.g., Orap)
- Promethazine (e.g., Phenergan) or
- Trimeprazine (e.g., Temaril)—Severe low blood pressure may occur
- Antidepressants (medicine for depression)—The risk of serious side effects may be increased
- Antithyroid agents (medicine for overactive thyroid) or
- Central nervous system (CNS) depressants (medicines that cause drowsiness)—There may be an increased chance of blood problems
- Epinephrine (e.g., Adrenalin)—Severe low blood pressure and fast heartbeat may occur

- Levodopa (e.g., Dopar)—Phenothiazines may prevent levodopa from working properly in the treatment of Parkinson's disease
- Lithium (e.g., Lithane, Lithizine)—The amount of medicine you need to take may change
- Methyldopa (e.g., Aldomet) or
- Metoclopramide (e.g., Reglan) or
- Metyrosine (e.g. Demser) or
- Pemoline (e.g., Cylert) or
- Rauwolfia alkaloids (alseroxylon [e.g., Rauwiloid], deserpidine [e.g., Harmonyl], rauwolfia serpentina [e.g., Raudixin], reserpine [e.g., Serpasil])—Taking these medicines with phenothiazines may increase the chance and severity of certain side effects
- Metrizamide—When this dye is used for myelograms, the risk of seizures may be increased

Other medical problems—The presence of other medical problems may affect the use of phenothiazines. Make sure you tell your doctor if you have any other medical problems, especially:

- Alcohol abuse—Certain side effects such as heat stroke may be more likely to occur
- Blood disease or
- Breast cancer or
- Difficult urination or
- Enlarged prostate or
- Glaucoma or
- Heart or blood vessel disease or
- Lung disease or
- Parkinson's disease or
- Seizure disorders or
- Stomach ulcers—Phenothiazines may make the condition worse
- Liver disease—Higher blood levels of phenothiazines may occur, increasing the chance of side effects
- Reye's syndrome—There may be an increased chance of unwanted effects on the liver

Before you begin using any new medicine (prescription or nonprescription) or if you develop any new medical problem while you are using this medicine, check with your doctor, nurse, or pharmacist.

Proper Use of This Medicine

For patients taking this medicine *by mouth:*

- This medicine may be taken with food or a full glass (8 ounces) of water or milk to reduce stomach irritation.
- *If your medicine comes in a dropper bottle,* measure each dose with the special dropper provided with your prescription and dilute it in ½ a glass (4 ounces) of orange or grapefruit juice or water.
- If you are taking the *extended-release capsule form* of this medicine, each dose should be swallowed whole. Do not break, crush, or chew before swallowing.

For patients using the *suppository form* of this medicine:

- If the suppository is too soft to insert, chill it in the refrigerator for 30 minutes or run cold water over it before removing the foil wrapper.
- To insert the suppository: First remove the foil wrapper and moisten the suppository with cold water. Lie down on your side and use your finger to push the suppository well up into the rectum.

Do not take more of this medicine and do not take it more often than your doctor ordered. This is particularly important for children or elderly patients, since they may react very strongly to this medicine.

Sometimes this medicine must be taken for several weeks before its full effect is reached when it is used to treat mental and emotional conditions.

Missed dose—If you miss a dose of this medicine and your dosing schedule is:

- One dose a day: Take the missed dose as soon as possible. Then go back to your regular dosing schedule. However, if you do not remember the missed dose until the next day, skip it and go back to your regular dosing schedule. Do not double doses.
- More than one dose a day: If you remember within an hour or so of the missed dose, take it right away. However, if you do not remember until later, skip the missed dose and go back to your regular dosing schedule. Do not double doses.

If you have any questions about this, check with your doctor.

Storage—To store this medicine:

- Keep out of the reach of children.
- Store away from heat and direct light.
- Do not store the capsule or tablet form of this medicine in the bathroom, near the kitchen sink, or in other damp places. Heat or moisture may cause the medicine to break down.
- Keep the liquid form of this medicine from freezing.
- Do not keep outdated medicine or medicine no longer needed. Be sure that any discarded medicine is out of the reach of children.

Precautions While Using This Medicine

Your doctor should check your progress at regular visits, especially during the first few months of treatment with this medicine. This will allow your dosage to be changed if necessary to meet your needs.

Do not stop taking this medicine without first checking with your doctor. Your doctor may want you to reduce gradually the amount you are taking before stopping completely. This is to prevent side effects and to keep your condition from becoming worse.

Do not take this medicine within two hours of taking antacids or medicine for diarrhea. Taking these products too close together may make this medicine less effective.

This medicine will add to the effects of alcohol and other CNS depressants (medicines that slow down the nervous system, possibly causing drowsiness). Some examples of CNS depressants are antihistamines or medicine for hay fever, other allergies, or colds; sedatives, tranquilizers, or sleeping medicine; prescription pain medicine or narcotics; barbiturates; medicine for seizures; muscle relaxants; or anesthetics, including some dental anesthetics. *Check with your doctor before taking any of the above while you are using this medicine.*

Before using any prescription or over-the-counter (OTC) medicine for colds or allergies, check with your doctor. These medicines may increase the chance of heat stroke or other unwanted effects, such as dizziness, dry mouth, blurred vision, and constipation, while you are taking a phenothiazine.

Before you have any medical tests, tell the medical doctor in charge that you are taking this medicine. The results of some tests (such as electrocardiogram [ECG] readings, certain pregnancy tests, the metyrapone test, and urine bilirubin tests) may be affected by this medicine.

Before having any kind of surgery, dental treatment, or emergency treatment, tell the medical doctor or dentist in charge that you are using this medicine.

This medicine may cause some people to become drowsy or less alert than they are normally. Even if this medicine is taken only at bedtime, it may cause some people to feel drowsy or less alert on arising. *Make sure you know how you react to this medicine before you drive, use machines, or do anything else that could be dangerous if you are not alert.*

Phenothiazines may cause blurred vision, difficulty in reading, or other changes in vision, especially during the first few weeks of treatment. Do not drive, use machines, or do anything else that could be dangerous if you are not able to see well. *If the problem continues or gets worse, check with your doctor.*

Dizziness, lightheadedness, or fainting may occur, especially when you get up from a lying or sitting position. Getting up slowly may help. If the problem continues or gets worse, check with your doctor.

This medicine may make you sweat less, causing your body temperature to increase. *Use extra care not to become overheated during exercise or hot weather while you are taking this medicine,* since overheating may result in heat stroke. Also, hot baths or saunas may make you feel dizzy or faint while you are taking this medicine.

This medicine may also make you more sensitive to cold temperatures. Dress warmly during cold weather. Be careful during prolonged exposure to cold, such as in winter sports or swimming in cold water.

Phenothiazines may cause dryness of the mouth. For temporary relief, use sugarless candy or gum, melt bits of ice in your mouth, or use a saliva substitute. However, if your mouth continues to feel dry for more than 2 weeks, check with your medical doctor or dentist. Continuing dryness of the mouth may increase the chance of dental disease, including tooth decay, gum disease, and fungus infections.

Phenothiazines may cause your skin to be more sensitive to sunlight than it is normally. Exposure to sunlight, even for brief periods of time, may cause a skin rash, itching, redness or other discoloration of the skin, or a severe sunburn. When you begin taking this medicine:

- Stay out of direct sunlight, especially between the hours of 10:00 a.m. and 3:00 p.m., if possible.
- Wear protective clothing, including a hat. Also, wear sunglasses.
- Apply a sun block product that has a skin protection factor (SPF) of at least 15. Some patients may require a product with a higher SPF number, especially if they have a fair complexion. If you have any questions about this, check with your doctor or pharmacist.
- Apply a sun block lipstick that has an SPF of at least 15 to protect your lips.
- Do not use a sunlamp or tanning bed or booth.

If you have a severe reaction from the sun, check with your doctor.

Phenothiazines may cause your eyes to be more sensitive to sunlight than they are normally. Exposure to sunlight over a period of time (several months to years) may cause blurred vision, change in color vision, or difficulty in seeing at night. When you go out during the daylight hours, even on cloudy days, wear sunglasses that block ultraviolet (UV) light. Ordinary sunglasses may not protect your eyes. If you have any questions about the kind of sunglasses to wear, check with your medical doctor or eye doctor.

If you are taking a liquid form of this medicine, avoid getting it on your skin or clothing because it may cause a skin rash or other irritation.

If you are receiving this medicine by injection:

- The effects of the long-acting injection form of this medicine may last for up to 12 weeks. *The precautions and side effects information for this medicine applies during this time.*

Side Effects of This Medicine

Along with their needed effects, phenothiazines can sometimes cause serious side effects. Tardive dyskinesia (a movement disorder) may occur and may not go away after you stop using the medicine. Signs of tardive dyskinesia include fine, worm-like movements of the tongue, or other uncontrolled movements of the mouth, tongue, cheeks, jaw, or arms and legs. Other serious but rare side effects may also occur. These include severe muscle stiffness, fever, unusual tiredness or weakness, fast heartbeat, difficult breathing, increased sweating, loss of bladder control, and seizures (neuroleptic malignant syndrome). *You and your doctor should discuss the good this medicine will do as well as the risks of taking it.*

Stop taking this medicine and check with your doctor immediately if any of the following side effects occur:

Rare

Convulsions (seizures); difficult or fast breathing; fast heartbeat or irregular pulse; fever; high or low blood pressure; increased sweating; loss of bladder control; muscle stiffness (severe); unusually pale skin; unusual tiredness or weakness

Check with your doctor immediately if any of the following side effects occur:

More common

Lip smacking or puckering; puffing of cheeks; rapid or fine, worm-like movements of tongue; uncontrolled chewing movements; uncontrolled movements of arms or legs

Also, check with your doctor as soon as possible if any of the following side effects occur:

More common

Blurred vision, change in color vision, or difficulty in seeing at night; difficulty in speaking or swallowing; fainting; inability to move eyes; loss of balance control; mask-like face; muscle spasms (especially of face, neck, and back); restlessness or need to keep moving; shuffling walk; stiffness of arms or legs; tic-like or twitching movements; trembling and shaking of hands and fingers; twisting movements of body; weakness of arms and legs

Less common

Difficulty in urinating; skin rash; sunburn (severe)

Rare

Abdominal or stomach pains; aching muscles and joints; confusion; fever and chills; hot, dry skin or lack of sweating; muscle weakness; nausea, vomiting, or diarrhea; painful, inappropriate penile erection (continuing); skin discoloration (tan or blue-gray); skin itching (severe); sore throat and fever; unusual bleeding or bruising; yellow eyes or skin

Other side effects may occur that usually do not need medical attention. These side effects may go away during treatment as your body adjusts to the medicine. However, check with your doctor if any of the following side effects continue or are bothersome:

More common

Constipation; decreased sweating; dizziness; drowsiness; dryness of mouth; nasal congestion

Less common

Changes in menstrual period; decreased sexual ability; increased sensitivity of skin to sunlight (skin rash, itching, redness or other discoloration of skin, or severe sunburn); swelling or pain in breasts; unusual secretion of milk; weight gain (unusual)

After you stop using this medicine, your body may need time to adjust. The length of time this takes depends on the amount of medicine you are using and how long you used it. During this time, check with your doctor if you notice dizziness, nausea and vomiting, stomach pain, trembling of the fingers and hands, or any of the following symptoms of tardive dyskinesia:

Lip smacking or puckering; puffing of cheeks; rapid or fine, worm-like movements of tongue; uncontrolled chewing movements; uncontrolled movements of arms or legs

Although not all of the side effects listed above have been reported for all of these medicines, they have been reported for at least one of them. However, since all of the phenothiazines are very similar, any of the above side effects may occur with any of these medicines.

Other side effects not listed above may also occur in some patients. If you notice any other effects, check with your doctor.

Additional Information

Once a medicine has been approved for marketing for a certain use, experience may show that it is also useful for other medical problems. Although these uses are not included in product labeling, phenothiazines are used in certain patients with the following medical conditions:

- Chronic neurogenic pain (certain continuing pain conditions)
- Huntington's chorea (hereditary movement disorder)

Other than the above information, there is no additional information relating to proper use, precautions, or side effects for these uses.

Annual revision: 03/16/92

PHENOXYBENZAMINE Systemic

A commonly used brand name in the U.S. is Dibenzyline.

Description

Phenoxybenzamine (fen-ox-ee-BEN-za-meen) belongs to the general class of medicines called antihypertensives. It is used to treat high blood pressure (hypertension) due to a disease called pheochromocytoma.

Phenoxybenzamine blocks the effects of certain chemicals in the body. When these chemicals are present in large amounts, they cause high blood pressure.

Phenoxybenzamine may also be used for other conditions as determined by your doctor.

Phenoxybenzamine is available only with your doctor's prescription, in the following dosage form:

Oral

- Capsules (U.S.)

It is very important that you read and understand the following information. If any of it causes you special concern, check with your doctor. Also, *if you have any questions* or if you want more information about this medicine or your medical problem, *ask your doctor, nurse, or pharmacist.*

Before Using This Medicine

In deciding to use a medicine, the risks of taking the medicine must be weighed against the good it will do. This is a decision you and your doctor will make. For phenoxybenzamine, the following should be considered:

Allergies—Tell your doctor if you have ever had any unusual or allergic reaction to phenoxybenzamine. Also, tell your doctor and pharmacist if you are allergic to any other substances, such as foods, preservatives, or dyes.

Pregnancy—Phenoxybenzamine has not been studied in pregnant women or animals. Make sure your doctor knows if you are pregnant or if you may become pregnant before taking phenoxybenzamine.

Breast-feeding—It is not known whether phenoxybenzamine passes into breast milk. However, this medicine has not been reported to cause problems in nursing babies.

Children—Although there is no specific information about the use of phenoxybenzamine in children, it is not expected to cause different side effects or problems in children than it does in adults.

Older adults—Dizziness or lightheadedness may be more likely to occur in the elderly, who are more sensitive to the effects of phenoxybenzamine. In addition, phenoxybenzamine may reduce tolerance to cold temperatures in elderly patients.

Other medicines—Although certain medicines should not be used together at all, in other cases two different medicines may be used together even if an interaction might occur. In these cases, your doctor may want to change the dose, or other precautions may be necessary. Tell your doctor and pharmacist if you are taking any other prescription or nonprescription (over-the-counter [OTC]) medicine.

Other medical problems—The presence of other medical problems may affect the use of phenoxybenzamine. Make sure you tell your doctor if you have any other medical problems, especially:

- Angina (chest pain) or
- Heart or blood vessel disease—Some kinds may be worsened by phenoxybenzamine
- Kidney disease—Effects may be increased
- Lung infection—Symptoms such as stuffy nose may be worsened
- Recent heart attack or stroke—Lowering blood pressure may make problems resulting from stroke or heart attack worse

Before you begin using any new medicine (prescription or nonprescription) or if you develop any new medical problem while you are using this medicine, check with your doctor, nurse, or pharmacist.

Proper Use of This Medicine

To help you remember to take your medicine, try to get into the habit of taking it at the same time each day.

Missed dose—If you miss a dose of this medicine, take it as soon as you remember. However, if it is almost time for your next dose, skip the missed dose and go back to your regular dosing schedule. Do not double doses.

Storage—To store this medicine:

- Keep out of the reach of children.
- Store away from heat and direct light.
- Do not store in the bathroom, near the kitchen sink, or in other damp places. Heat or moisture may cause the medicine to break down.
- Do not keep outdated medicine or medicine no longer needed. Be sure that any discarded medicine is out of the reach of children.

Precautions While Using This Medicine

It is important that your doctor check your progress at regular visits to make sure that this medicine is working properly and to check for unwanted effects.

Do not take other medicines unless they have been discussed with your doctor. This especially includes over-the-counter (nonprescription) medicines for appetite control, asthma, colds, cough, hay fever, or sinus problems, since they may interfere with the effects of this medicine.

Phenoxybenzamine may cause some people to become dizzy, drowsy, or less alert than they are normally. This is more likely to happen when you begin to take it or when you increase the amount of medicine you are taking. *Make sure you know how you react to this medicine before you drive, use machines, or do anything else that could be dangerous if you are dizzy or not alert.*

Dizziness, lightheadedness, or fainting may occur, especially when you get up from a lying or sitting position. Getting up slowly may help, but if the problem continues or gets worse, check with your doctor.

The dizziness, lightheadedness, or fainting is also more likely to occur if you drink alcohol, stand for a long time, exercise, or if the weather is hot. *While you are taking this medicine, be careful in the amount of alcohol you drink. Also, use extra care during exercise or hot weather or if you must stand for a long time.*

Before having any kind of surgery (including dental surgery) or emergency treatment, *tell the medical doctor or dentist in charge that you are using this medicine.*

Phenoxybenzamine may cause dryness of the mouth, nose, and throat. For temporary relief of mouth dryness, use sugarless candy or gum, melt bits of ice in your mouth, or use a saliva substitute. However, if dry mouth continues for more than 2 weeks, check with your medical doctor or dentist. Continuing dryness of the mouth may increase the chance of dental disease, including tooth decay, gum disease, and fungus infections.

Side Effects of This Medicine

In rats and mice, phenoxybenzamine has been found to increase the risk of development of malignant tumors. It is not known if phenoxybenzamine increases the chance of tumors in humans.

Along with its needed effects, a medicine may cause some unwanted effects. The following side effects may go away as your body adjusts to the medicine. However, check with your doctor if any of these effects continue or are bothersome:

More common

Dizziness or lightheadedness, especially when getting up from a lying or sitting position; fast heartbeat; pinpoint pupils; stuffy nose

Less common

Confusion; drowsiness; dryness of mouth; headache; lack of energy; sexual problems in males; unusual tiredness or weakness

Other side effects not listed above may also occur in some patients. If you notice any other effects, check with your doctor.

Additional Information

Once a medicine has been approved for marketing for a certain use, experience may show that it is also useful for other medical problems. Although this use is not included in product labeling, phenoxybenzamine is used in certain patients with the following medical condition:

- Benign prostatic hypertrophy

Other than the above information, there is no additional information relating to proper use, precautions, or side effects for this use.

Annual revision: 09/20/92

PHENTOLAMINE AND PAPAVERINE Intracavernosal

Some commonly used brand names for phentolamine are:

In the U.S.

Regitine

Generic name product may also be available.

In Canada

Rogitine

Generic name product may also be available.

Description

Phentolamine (fen-TOLE-a-meen) given by injection causes blood vessels to expand, thereby increasing blood flow. When it is used in combination with papaverine (pa-PAV-er-een), another medicine that has this effect, and is injected into the penis (intracavernosal), it increases blood flow to the penis, which results in an erection. This combination is used to treat some men who are impotent.

This medicine should not be used as a sexual aid by men who are not impotent. If the medicine is not used properly, permanent damage to the penis and loss of the ability to have erections could result.

Phentolamine and papaverine are available only with your doctor's prescription, in the following dosage form:

Parenteral

- Injection (U.S. and Canada)

It is very important that you read and understand the following information. If any of it causes you special concern, check with your doctor. Also, *if you have any questions* or if you want more information about this medicine or your medical problem, *ask your doctor, nurse, or pharmacist.*

Before Using This Medicine

In deciding to use a medicine, the risks of taking the medicine must be weighed against the good it will do. This is a decision you and your doctor will make. For papaverine and phentolamine, the following should be considered:

Allergies—Tell your doctor if you have ever had any unusual or allergic reaction to papaverine or phentolamine. Also tell your doctor and pharmacist if you are allergic to any other substances, such as foods, preservatives, or dyes.

Older adults—Many medicines have not been studied specifically in older people. Therefore, it may not be known whether they work exactly the same way they do in younger adults or if they cause different side effects or problems in older people. Although there is no specific information comparing the use of phentolamine and papaverine for impotence in the elderly, it is not expected to cause different side effects or problems in older people than it does in younger adults.

Other medicines—Although certain medicines should not be used together at all, in other cases two different medicines may be used together even if an interaction might occur. In these cases, your doctor may want to change the dose, or other precautions may be necessary. Tell your doctor and pharmacist if you are taking any other prescription or nonprescription (over-the-counter [OTC]) medicine.

Other medical problems—The presence of other medical problems may affect the use of papaverine and phentolamine. Make sure you tell your doctor if you have any other medical problems, especially:

- Bleeding problems—These conditions increase the risk of bleeding at the place of injection
- Liver disease—Papaverine can cause liver damage when it is given in ways that allow it to get into the bloodstream (by mouth or by injection into a muscle, a vein, or an artery); when papaverine is given by intracavernosal injection, liver damage is much less likely because the medicine enters the bloodstream very slowly
- Priapism (history of) or
- Sickle cell disease—Patients with these conditions have an increased risk of priapism (erection lasting longer than 4 hours) while using papaverine and phentolamine

Before you begin using any new medicine (prescription or nonprescription) or if you develop any new medical problem while you are using this medicine, check with your doctor, nurse, or pharmacist.

Proper Use of This Medicine

To give the injection:

- Cleanse the injection site with alcohol. Using a sterile needle, *inject the medicine slowly and directly into the base of the penis as instructed by your doctor. It should not be injected just under the skin.* The injection is usually not painful, although you may feel some tingling in the tip of your penis. If the injection is very painful or you notice bruising or swelling at the place of injection, that means you are injecting the medicine under the skin. Stop, withdraw the needle, and reposition it properly before continuing with the injection.
- After you have completed the injection, put pressure on the place of injection to prevent bruising. Then massage your penis as instructed by your doctor. This helps the medicine spread to all parts of the penis, so that it will work better.

This medicine usually begins to work in about 10 minutes. You should attempt intercourse within 2 hours after injecting the medicine.

Storage—To store this medicine:

- Keep out of the reach of children.
- Store away from heat and direct light.
- Keep the medicine from freezing.

Precautions While Using This Medicine

Use the injection exactly as directed by your doctor. Do not use more of it and do not use it more often than ordered. If too much is used, the erection may become so strong that it lasts too long and does not reverse when it should. This condition is called priapism, and it can be very dangerous. If the effect is not reversed, the blood supply to the penis may be cut off and permanent damage may occur.

Contact your doctor immediately if the erection lasts for longer than 4 hours or if it becomes painful. This may be a sign of priapism and must be treated right away to prevent permanent damage.

If you notice bleeding at the site when you inject the medicine, put pressure on the spot until the bleeding stops. If it doesn't stop, check with your doctor.

It is important for you to examine your penis regularly. Check with your doctor if you find a lump where the medicine has been injected or if you notice that your penis is becoming curved. These may be signs that unwanted tissue is growing (called fibrosis), which should be seen by your doctor.

Side Effects of This Medicine

Along with its needed effects, a medicine may cause some unwanted effects. Although not all of these side effects may occur, if they do occur they may need medical attention.

Check with your doctor immediately if the following side effects occur:

Rare

Erection continuing for more than 4 hours, or painful erection

Check with your doctor as soon as possible if the following side effects occur:

Rare

Dizziness; lumps in the penis

Other side effects may occur that usually do not need medical attention. These side effects may go away during treatment as your body adjusts to the medicine. However, check with your doctor if any of the following side effects continue or are bothersome:

Less common or rare

Bruising or bleeding at place of injection; burning (mild) along penis; difficulty in ejaculating; swelling at place of injection

Phentolamine and papaverine injected into the penis may cause tingling at the tip of the penis. This is no cause for concern.

Other side effects not listed above may also occur in some patients. If you notice any other effects, check with your doctor.

Annual revision: 09/20/92

PHENYLEPHRINE Nasal

Some commonly used brand names are:

In the U.S.

Alconefrin 12	Nostril
Alconefrin 25	Rhinall
Alconefrin 50	Rhinall-10 Children's Flavored Nose Drops
Doktors	St. Joseph
Duration	Vicks Sinex
Neo-Synephrine	

Generic name product may also be available.

In Canada

Neo-Synephrine

Description

Phenylephrine (fen-ill-EF-rin) is used for the temporary relief of congestion or stuffiness in the nose caused by hay fever or other allergies, colds, or sinus trouble. It may also be used in ear infections to relieve congestion.

This medicine may also be used for other conditions as determined by your doctor.

This medicine is available without a prescription; however, your doctor may have special instructions on the proper use or dose for your medical condition.

Phenylephrine is available in the following dosage forms:

Nasal

- Nasal jelly (U.S.)
- Nasal drops (U.S. and Canada)
- Nasal spray (U.S. and Canada)

It is very important that you read and understand the following information. If any of it causes you special concern, check with your doctor or pharmacist. Also, *if you have any questions* or if you want more information about this medicine or your medical problem, *ask your doctor, nurse, or pharmacist.*

Before Using This Medicine

If you are using this medicine without a prescription, carefully read and follow any precautions on the label. For nasal phenylephrine, the following should be considered:

Allergies—Tell your doctor if you have ever had any unusual or allergic reaction to phenylephrine or to any other nasal decongestant. Also tell your doctor and pharmacist if you are allergic to any other substances, such as foods, preservatives, or dyes.

Pregnancy—Nasal phenylephrine may be absorbed into the body. However, nasal phenylephrine has not been shown to cause birth defects or other problems in humans.

Breast-feeding—Nasal phenylephrine may be absorbed into the body. However, it is not known whether phenylephrine passes into the breast milk. This medicine has not been reported to cause problems in nursing babies.

Children—Children may be especially sensitive to the effects of nasal phenylephrine. This may increase the chance of side effects during treatment.

Older adults—Many medicines have not been tested in older people. Therefore, it may not be known whether they work exactly the same way they do in younger adults or if they cause different side effects or problems in older people. There is no specific information about the use of nasal phenylephrine in the elderly.

Other medicines—Although certain medicines should not be used together at all, in other cases two different medicines may be used together even if an interaction might occur. In these cases, your doctor may want to change the dose, or other precautions may be necessary. When you are using nasal phenylephrine, it is especially important that your doctor and pharmacist know if you are using any other prescription or nonprescription (over-the-counter [OTC]) medicine.

Other medical problems—The presence of other medical problems may affect the use of nasal phenylephrine. Make sure you tell your doctor if you have any other medical problems, especially:

- Diabetes mellitus (sugar diabetes)
- Heart or blood vessel disease or
- High blood pressure—Nasal phenylephrine may make the condition worse
- Overactive thyroid

Before you begin using any new medicine (prescription or nonprescription) or if you develop any new medical problem while you are using this medicine, check with your doctor, nurse, or pharmacist.

Proper Use of This Medicine

To use the *nose drops:*

- Blow your nose gently. Tilt the head back while standing or sitting up, or lie down on a bed and hang head over the side. Place the drops into each nostril and keep the head tilted back for a few minutes to allow the medicine to spread throughout the nose.
- Rinse the dropper with hot water and dry with a clean tissue. Replace the cap right after use.
- To avoid spreading the infection, do not use the container for more than one person.

To use the *nose spray:*

- Blow your nose gently. With the head upright, spray the medicine into each nostril. Sniff briskly while squeezing the bottle quickly and firmly. For best results, spray once or twice into each nostril and wait 3 to 5 minutes to allow the medicine to work. Then, blow your nose gently and thoroughly. Repeat until the complete dose is used.
- Rinse the tip of the spray bottle with hot water, taking care not to suck water into the bottle, and dry with a clean tissue. Replace the cap right after use.
- To avoid spreading the infection, do not use the container for more than one person.

To use the *nose jelly:*

- Blow your nose gently. Wash your hands before applying the medicine. With your finger, place a small amount of jelly (about the size of a pea) up each nostril. Sniff it well back into the nose.
- Wipe the tip of the tube with a clean, damp tissue and replace the cap right after use.

Use this medicine only as directed. Do not use more of it, do not use it more often, and do not use it for longer than 3 days without first checking with your doctor. To do so may make your runny or stuffy nose worse and may also increase the chance of side effects.

Missed dose—If you are using this medicine on a regular schedule and you miss a dose, use it right away if you remember within an hour or so of the missed dose. However, if you do not remember until later, skip the missed dose and go back to your regular dosing schedule. Do not double doses.

Storage—To store this medicine:

- Keep out of the reach of children.
- Store away from heat and direct light.
- Keep the medicine from freezing.
- Do not keep outdated medicine or medicine no longer needed. Be sure that any discarded medicine is out of the reach of children.

Side Effects of This Medicine

Along with its needed effects, a medicine may cause some unwanted effects. Although not all of these side effects may occur, if they do occur they may need medical attention.

When this medicine is used for short periods of time at low doses, side effects usually are rare. However, check with your doctor as soon as possible if any of the following occur:

Increase in runny or stuffy nose

Symptoms of too much medicine being absorbed into the body

Fast, irregular, or pounding heartbeat; headache or dizziness; increased sweating; nervousness; paleness; trembling; trouble in sleeping

Note: The above side effects are more likely to occur in children because there is a greater chance that too much of this medicine may be absorbed into the body.

Other side effects may occur that usually do not need medical attention. These side effects may go away during treatment as your body adjusts to the medicine. However, check with your doctor or pharmacist if any of the following side effects continue or are bothersome:

Burning, dryness, or stinging of inside of nose

Other side effects not listed above may also occur in some patients. If you notice any other effects, check with your doctor or pharmacist.

Annual revision: September 1990

PHENYLEPHRINE Ophthalmic

Some commonly used brand names are:

In the U.S.

- Ak-Dilate
- Ak-Nefrin
- Dilatair
- I-Phrine
- Isopto Frin
- Mydfrin
- Neo-Synephrine
- Ocugestrin
- Ocu-Phrin Sterile Eye Drops
- Ocu-Phrin Sterile Ophthalmic Solution
- Prefrin Liquifilm
- Relief Eye Drops for Red Eyes

Generic name product may also be available.

In Canada

- Ak-Dilate
- Minims Phenylephrine
- Mydfrin
- Prefrin Liquifilm
- Spersaphrine

Description

Ophthalmic phenylephrine (fen-ill-EF-rin) in strengths of 2.5 and 10% is used to dilate (enlarge) the pupil. It is used before eye examinations, before and after eye surgery, and to treat certain eye conditions. These preparations are available only with your doctor's prescription.

Ophthalmic phenylephrine in the strength of 0.12% is used to relieve redness due to minor irritations of the eye, such as those caused by allergy, dust, smoke, wind, and other irritants. This preparation is available without a prescription; however, your doctor may have special instructions on the proper use of phenylephrine for your eye problem.

Phenylephrine is available in the following dosage form:

Ophthalmic

- Ophthalmic solution (eye drops) (U.S. and Canada)

It is very important that you read and understand the following information. If any of it causes you special concern, check with your doctor or pharmacist. Also, *if you have any questions* or if you want more information about this medicine or your medical problem, *ask your doctor, nurse, or pharmacist.*

Before Using This Medicine

In deciding to use a medicine, the risks of taking the medicine must be weighed against the good it will do. This is a decision you and your doctor will make. For phenylephrine, the following should be considered:

Allergies—Tell your doctor if you have ever had any unusual or allergic reaction to phenylephrine or to sulfites. Also tell your doctor and pharmacist if you are allergic to any other substances, such as preservatives.

Pregnancy—Ophthalmic phenylephrine may be absorbed into the body. However, studies on effects in pregnancy have not been done in either humans or animals.

Breast-feeding—Ophthalmic phenylephrine may be absorbed into the mother's body. However, it is not known whether phenylephrine passes into the breast milk. This medicine has not been reported to cause problems in nursing babies.

Children—Children may be especially sensitive to the effects of phenylephrine. This may increase the chance of side effects during treatment. In addition, the 10% strength is not recommended for use in infants. Also, the 2.5 and 10% strengths are not recommended for use in low birth weight infants.

Older adults—Repeated use of 2.5 or 10% phenylephrine may increase the chance of problems during treatment with this medicine. In addition, heart and blood vessel problems have occurred more often in elderly patients than in younger adults.

Other medicines—Although certain medicines should not be used together at all, in other cases two different medicines may be used together even if an interaction might occur. In these cases, your doctor may want to change the dose, or other precautions may be necessary. Tell your doctor and pharmacist if you are using any other prescription or nonprescription (over-the-counter [OTC]) medicine.

Other medical problems—The presence of other medical problems may affect the use of phenylephrine. Make sure you tell your doctor if you have any other medical problems, especially:

- Diabetes mellitus (sugar diabetes) or
- Heart or blood vessel disease or
- High blood pressure—The 2.5 and 10% strengths of phenylephrine may make the condition worse

- Idiopathic orthostatic hypotension (low blood pressure of a certain kind)—Use of this medicine may cause a large increase in blood pressure to occur

Before you begin using any new medicine (prescription or nonprescription) or if you develop any new medical problem while you are using this medicine, check with your doctor, nurse, or pharmacist.

Proper Use of This Medicine

Do not use if the solution turns brown or becomes cloudy.

To use:

- First, wash your hands. With the middle finger, apply pressure to the inside corner of the eye (and continue to apply pressure for 2 or 3 minutes after the medicine has been placed in the eye). Tilt the head back and with the index finger of the same hand, pull the lower eyelid away from eye to form a pouch. Drop the medicine into the pouch and gently close the eyes. Do not blink. Keep the eyes closed for 1 or 2 minutes to allow the medicine to be absorbed.
- Immediately after using the eye drops, wash your hands to remove any medicine that may be on them.
- To keep the medicine as germ-free as possible, do not touch the applicator tip to any surface (including the eye). Also, keep the container tightly closed.

For patients using the *2.5 or 10% eye drops:*

- *It is very important that you use this medicine only as directed.* Do not use more of it and do not use it more often than your doctor ordered. To do so may increase the chance of too much medicine being absorbed into the body and the chance of side effects. *This is especially important when this medicine is used in children or in patients with heart disease or high blood pressure,* since high doses of this medicine may cause an irregular heartbeat and an increase in blood pressure.

Missed dose—If you are using the 2.5 or 10% eye drops and you miss a dose of this medicine, apply it as soon as possible. However, if it is almost time for your next dose, skip the missed dose and go back to your regular dosing schedule. Do not double doses.

Storage—To store this medicine:

- Keep out of the reach of children.
- Store away from heat and direct light.
- Keep the medicine from freezing.
- Do not keep outdated medicine or medicine no longer needed. Be sure that any discarded medicine is out of the reach of children.

Precautions While Using This Medicine

If eye pain or change in vision occurs or if redness or irritation of the eye continues, gets worse, or lasts for more than 72 hours, stop using the medicine and check with your doctor.

For patients using the *2.5 or 10% eye drops:*

- After you apply this medicine to your eyes, your pupils will become unusually large. This will cause your eyes to become more sensitive to light than they are normally. *When you go out during the daylight hours, even on cloudy days, wear sunglasses that block ultraviolet (UV) light to protect your eyes from sunlight and other bright lights.* Ordinary sunglasses may not protect your eyes. If you have any questions about the kind of sunglasses to wear, check with your doctor. Also, if this effect continues for longer than 12 hours after you have stopped using this medicine, check with your doctor.

Side Effects of This Medicine

Along with its needed effects, a medicine may cause some unwanted effects. Although not all of these side effects may occur, if they do occur they may need medical attention.

Check with your doctor as soon as possible if any of the following side effects occur:

Symptoms of too much medicine being absorbed into the body—Less common with 10% solution; rare with 2.5% or weaker solution

Dizziness; fast, irregular, or pounding heartbeat; increased sweating; increase in blood pressure; paleness; trembling

Other side effects may occur that usually do not need medical attention. These side effects may go away during treatment as your body adjusts to the medicine. However, check with your doctor if any of the following side effects continue or are bothersome:

More common with 2.5 or 10% solution

Burning or stinging of eyes; headache or browache; sensitivity of eyes to light; watering of eyes

Less common

Eye irritation not present before use of this medicine

Other side effects not listed above may also occur in some patients. If you notice any other effects, check with your doctor.

Annual revision: 05/14/92

PHENYLPROPANOLAMINE Systemic†

Some commonly used brand names are:

In the U.S.—

Acutrim 16 Hour	Dexatrim Maximum Strength Caplets
Acutrim Late Day	Dexatrim Maximum Strength Pre-Meal Caplets
Acutrim II Maximum Strength	Diet-Aid Maximum Strength
Control	Efed II Yellow
Dex-A-Diet Maximum Strength	Phenyldrine
Dex-A-Diet Maximum Strength Caplets	Prolamine
Dexatrim	Propagest
Dexatrim Maximum Strength	Rhindecon
	Stay Trim Diet Gum
	Unitrol

Generic name product may also be available.

Another commonly used name is PPA.

†Not commercially available in Canada.

Description

Phenylpropanolamine (fen-ill-proe-pa-NOLE-a-meen), commonly known as PPA, is used as a nasal decongestant or as an appetite suppressant. It acts on many different parts of the body. PPA produces effects that may be helpful or harmful. This depends on a patient's individual condition and response and the amount of medicine taken.

Phenylpropanolamine clears nasal congestion (stuffy nose) by narrowing or constricting the blood vessels. However, this same action may cause an increase in blood pressure in patients who have hypertension (high blood pressure).

Phenylpropanolamine also decreases appetite. However, the way PPA and similar medicines do this is unclear. Stimulation of the central nervous system (CNS) may be a major reason. For a few weeks, phenylpropanolamine in combination with dieting, exercise, and changes in eating habits can help obese patients lose weight. However, this appetite-reducing effect is only temporary, and is useful only for the first few weeks of dieting until new eating habits are established.

Phenylpropanolamine has caused serious side effects (even death) when too much was taken.

There are a number of products on the market that contain only phenylpropanolamine. Other products contain PPA along with added ingredients. The information that follows is for PPA alone. There may be additional information for the combination products. Read the label of the product you are using. If you have questions or if you want more information about the other ingredients, check with your doctor or pharmacist.

Some preparations containing PPA are available only with your doctor's prescription. Others are available without a prescription; however, your doctor may have special instructions on the proper use of this medicine.

Phenylpropanolamine is available in the following dosage forms:

Oral

- Capsules (U.S.)
- Extended-release capsules (U.S.)
- Tablets (U.S.)
- Chewing gum tablets (U.S.)
- Extended-release tablets (U.S.)

It is very important that you read and understand the following information. If any of it causes you special concern, check with your doctor or pharmacist. Also, *if you have any questions* or if you want more information about this medicine or your medical problem, *ask your doctor, nurse, or pharmacist.*

Before Using This Medicine

If you are taking this medicine without a prescription, carefully read and follow any precautions on the label. For phenylpropanolamine, the following should be considered:

Allergies—Tell your doctor if you have ever had any unusual or allergic reaction to phenylpropanolamine or to amphetamine, dextroamphetamine, ephedrine, epinephrine, isoproterenol, metaproterenol, methamphetamine, norepinephrine, phenylephrine, pseudoephedrine, or terbutaline. Also tell your doctor and pharmacist if you are allergic to any other substances, such as foods, preservatives, or dyes.

Pregnancy—Phenylpropanolamine has not been shown to cause birth defects in humans. However, it seems that women who take phenylpropanolamine in the weeks following delivery are more likely to suffer mental or mood changes.

Breast-feeding—Phenylpropanolamine has not been reported to cause problems in nursing babies.

Children—Mental changes may be more likely to occur in young children taking phenylpropanolamine than in adults. Phenylpropanolamine should not be used for weight control in children under the age of 12 years. Children 12 to 18 years old should not take phenylpropanolamine for weight control unless its use is ordered and supervised by a doctor.

Older adults—Many medicines have not been studied specifically in older people. Therefore, it may not be known whether they work exactly the same way they do in younger adults or if they cause different side effects or problems in older people. There is no specific information comparing use of phenylpropanolamine in the elderly with use in other age groups.

Other medicines—Although certain medicines should not be used together at all, in other cases 2 different medicines may be used together even if an interaction might occur. In these cases, your doctor may want to change the dose, or other precautions may be necessary. When you are taking phenylpropanolamine, it is especially important that your doctor and pharmacist know if you are taking any of the following:

- Amantadine (e.g., Symmetrel) or
- Amphetamines or
- Caffeine (e.g., NoDoz) or
- Chlophedianol (e.g., Ulone) or
- Cocaine or
- Medicine for asthma or other breathing problems or
- Methylphenidate (e.g., Ritalin) or
- Nabilone (e.g., Cesamet) or
- Other appetite suppressants (diet pills) or
- Other medicine for colds, sinus problems, or hay fever or other allergies (including nose drops or sprays) or
- Pemoline (e.g., Cylert)—Using these medicines while taking phenylpropanolamine may cause severe nervousness, irritability, trouble in sleeping, or possibly irregular heartbeat or seizures
- Beta-blockers (acebutolol [e.g., Sectral], atenolol [e.g., Tenormin], betaxolol [e.g., Kerlone], carteolol [e.g., Cartrol], labetalol [e.g., Normodyne], metoprolol [e.g., Lopressor], nadolol [e.g., Corgard], oxprenolol [e.g., Trasicor], penbutolol [e.g., Levatol], pindolol [e.g., Visken], propranolol [e.g., Inderal], sotalol [e.g., Sotacor], timolol [e.g., Blocadren])—Taking these medicines with phenylpropanolamine may cause serious high blood pressure (hypertension) and other effects on the heart
- Digitalis glycosides (heart medicine)—Changes in the rhythm of your heart may occur
- Monoamine oxidase (MAO) inhibitors (furazolidone [e.g., Furoxone], isocarboxazid [e.g., Marplan], phenelzine [e.g., Nardil], procarbazine [e.g., Matulane], tranylcypromine [e.g., Parnate])—Taking phenylpropanolamine while you are taking or within 2 weeks of taking MAO inhibitors may cause sudden high body temperature, extremely high blood pressure, and severe convulsions; at least 14 days should be allowed between stopping treatment with one medicine and starting treatment with the other
- Rauwolfia alkaloids (alseroxylon [e.g., Rauwiloid], deserpidine [e.g., Harmonyl], rauwolfia serpentina [e.g., Raudixin], reserpine [e.g., Serpasil])—Phenylpropanolamine may not work properly when taken with rauwolfia alkaloids

Other medical problems—The presence of other medical problems may affect the use of phenylpropanolamine. Make sure you tell your doctor if you have any other medical problems, especially:

- Diabetes mellitus (sugar diabetes)—Phenylpropanolamine may cause an increase in blood glucose levels
- Enlarged prostate or
- Glaucoma or
- High blood pressure—Phenylpropanolamine may make the condition worse
- Heart or blood vessel disease (including a history of heart attack or stroke) or
- Overactive thyroid—Serious effects on the heart may occur

Before you begin using any new medicine (prescription or nonprescription) or if you develop any new medical problem while you are using this medicine, check with your doctor, nurse, or pharmacist.

Proper Use of This Medicine

For patients taking an *extended-release form* of this medicine:

- Swallow the capsule or tablet whole.
- Do not break, crush, or chew the capsule or tablet before swallowing it.
- Take only once a day after breakfast.

Take phenylpropanolamine (PPA) only as directed. Do not take more of it, do not take it more often, and do not take it for a longer time than directed. To do so may increase the chance of side effects.

If PPA causes trouble in sleeping, take the last dose for each day a few hours before bedtime. If you are taking an extended-release form of this medicine, take your daily dose at least 12 hours before bedtime.

Missed dose—For patients taking phenylpropanolamine *for nasal congestion:* If you miss a dose, take it as soon as possible. However, if it is within 2 hours (or 12 hours for extended-release forms) of your next dose, skip the missed dose and go back to your regular dosing schedule. Do not double doses.

Storage—To store this medicine:

- Keep out of the reach of children.
- Store away from heat and direct light.
- Do not store in the bathroom, near the kitchen sink, or in other damp places. Heat or moisture may cause the medicine to break down.
- Do not keep outdated medicine or medicine no longer needed. Be sure that any discarded medicine is out of the reach of children.

Precautions While Using This Medicine

Do not drink large amounts of caffeine-containing coffee, tea, or colas while you are taking this medicine. To do so may cause unwanted effects.

For patients taking this medicine *for nasal congestion:*

- *If cold symptoms do not improve within 7 days or if you also have a high fever, check with your doctor.* These signs may mean that you have other medical problems.

Side Effects of This Medicine

Along with its needed effects, a medicine may cause some unwanted effects. Although not all of these side effects may occur, if they do occur they may need medical attention.

Check with your doctor as soon as possible if any of the following side effects occur:

Rare

Headache (severe)—may suggest serious side effects could occur; increased blood pressure; painful or difficult urination; tightness in chest

Early symptoms of overdose

Abdominal or stomach pain; fast, pounding, or irregular heartbeat; headache (severe); increased sweating not associated with exercise; nausea and vomiting (severe); nervousness (severe); restlessness (severe)

Late symptoms of overdose

Confusion; convulsions (seizures); fast breathing; fast and irregular pulse; hallucinations (seeing, hearing, or feeling things that are not there); hostile behavior; muscle trembling

Other side effects may occur that usually do not need medical attention. These side effects may go away during treatment as your body adjusts to the medicine. However, check with your doctor if any of the following side effects continue or are bothersome:

Less common—more common with high doses

Dizziness; dryness of nose or mouth; false sense of well-being; headache (mild); nausea (mild); nervousness (mild); restlessness (mild); trouble in sleeping

Other side effects not listed above may also occur in some patients. If you notice any other effects, check with your doctor.

Additional Information

Once a medicine has been approved for marketing for a certain use, experience may show that it is also useful for other medical problems. Although this use is not included in product labeling, phenylpropanolamine is used in certain patients with the following medical conditions:

- Urinary stress incontinence (loss of bladder control when you cough, sneeze, or laugh)

Other than the above information, there is no additional information relating to proper use, precautions, or side effects for these uses.

Annual revision: 06/05/91
Interim revision: 06/24/91

PHOSPHATES Systemic

This information applies to the following medicines:

Potassium Phosphates (poe-TASS-ee-um FOS-fates)
Potassium Phosphate, Monobasic
Potassium and Sodium (SOE-dee-um) Phosphates
Sodium Phosphates

Some commonly used brand names are:

For Potassium Phosphates

In the U.S.

K-Phos Original
Neutra-Phos-K

Generic name product may also be available.

In Canada

Generic name product may be available.

For Potassium and Sodium Phosphates

In the U.S.

K-Phos M. F.
K-Phos Neutral
K-Phos No. 2
Neutra-Phos
Uro-KP-Neutral

In Canada

Uro-KP-Neutral

For Sodium Phosphates†

In the U.S.

Generic name product may be available.

†Not commercially available in Canada.

Description

Phosphates are used as dietary supplements for patients who are unable to get enough phosphorus in their regular diet, usually because of certain illnesses or diseases. Phosphate is the drug form (salt) of phosphorus. Some phosphates are used to make the urine more acid, which helps treat certain urinary tract infections. Some phosphates are used to prevent the formation of calcium stones in the urinary tract.

Some of these preparations are available only with your doctor's prescription. Others are available without a prescription; however, your doctor may have special instructions on the proper dose of this medicine for your medical condition. You should take phosphates only under the supervision of your doctor.

Phosphates are available in the following dosage forms:

Oral

Potassium Phosphates

- Capsules for solution (U.S.)
- Powder for solution (U.S.)
- Tablets for solution (U.S.)

Potassium and Sodium Phosphates
- Capsules for solution (U.S.)
- Powder for solution (U.S.)
- Tablets for solution (U.S. and Canada)

Parenteral

Potassium Phosphates
- Injection (U.S. and Canada)

Sodium Phosphates
- Injection (U.S.)

It is very important that you read and understand the following information. If any of it causes you special concern, check with your doctor. Also, *if you have any questions* or if you want more information about this medicine or your medical problem, *ask your doctor, nurse, or pharmacist.*

Importance of Diet

Many nutritionists recommend that, if possible, people should get all the phosphorus they need from foods. However, many people do not get enough phosphorus from food. For example, people on weight-loss diets may consume too little food to provide enough phosphorus. Others may lose phosphorus from the body because of illness or treatment with certain medicines. For such people, a phosphate supplement, given under your physician's care, is important.

In order to get enough vitamins and minerals in your diet, it is important that you eat a balanced and varied diet. Follow carefully any diet program your doctor may recommend. For your specific vitamin and/or mineral needs, ask your doctor for a list of appropriate foods.

The best dietary sources of phosphorus include dairy products, meat, poultry, fish, and cereal products.

Experts have developed a list of recommended dietary allowances (RDA) for most of the vitamins and some minerals. The RDA are not an exact number but a general idea of how much you need. They do not cover amounts needed for problems caused by a serious lack of vitamins or minerals.

The RDA for phosphorus are:
- Infants and children—
  Birth to 6 months of age: 400 mg per day.
  6 months to 1 year of age: 500 mg per day.
  1 to 10 years of age: 800 mg per day.
- Adolescent and adult males—
  11 to 24 years of age: 1200 mg per day.
  25 years of age and over: 800 mg per day.
- Adolescent and adult females—
  11 to 24 years of age: 1200 mg per day.
  25 years of age and over: 800 mg per day.
- Pregnant females—1200 mg per day.
- Breast-feeding females—1200 mg per day.

Remember:
- The total amount of phosphorus that you get every day includes what you get from food *and* what you may take as a supplement. Read the labels of processed foods, products such as certain soft drinks may contain phosphorus.
- Your total intake of phosphorus need not be greater than the recommended amounts, unless ordered by your doctor. In some cases, excessive amounts of phosphorus may be harmful.

Before Using This Medicine

In deciding to use a medicine, the risks of taking the medicine must be weighed against the good it will do. This is a decision you and your doctor will make. For phosphates the following should be considered:

Allergies—Tell your doctor if you have ever had any unusual or allergic reaction to potassium, sodium, or phosphates. Also, tell your doctor and pharmacist if you are allergic to any other substances, such as foods, preservatives, or dyes.

Pregnancy—It is especially important that you are receiving enough vitamins and minerals when you become pregnant and that you continue to receive the right amount of vitamins and minerals throughout your pregnancy. The healthy growth and development of the fetus depend on a steady supply of nutrients from the mother. However, taking large amounts of a nutritional supplement in pregnancy may be harmful to the mother and/or fetus and should be avoided.

Breast-feeding—It is especially important that you receive the right amount of vitamins and minerals so that your baby will also get the vitamins and minerals needed to grow properly. However, taking large amounts of a nutritional supplement while breast-feeding may be harmful to the mother and/or baby and should be avoided.

Children—Although there is no specific information comparing use of oral phosphates in children with use in other age groups, these medicines are not expected to cause different side effects in children than they do in adults. However, use of enemas that contain phosphates in children has resulted in high blood levels of phosphorus.

Older adults—Many medicines have not been studied specifically in older people. Therefore, it may not be known whether they work exactly the same way they do in younger adults or if they cause different side effects or problems in older people. There is no specific information comparing use of phosphates in the elderly with use in other age groups.

Other medicines—Although certain medicines should not be used together at all, in other cases two different medicines may be used together even if an interaction might occur. In these cases, your doctor may want to change the dose, or other precautions may be necessary. When you are taking phosphates, it is especially important that your doctor and pharmacist know if you are taking any of the following:

- Adrenocorticoids (cortisone-like medicine)—Use with sodium-containing phosphates may increase the risk of edema
- Amiloride (e.g., Midamor) or
- Captopril or
- Cyclosporine
- Digitalis glycosides (heart medicine) or
- Enalapril (e.g., Vasotec) or
- Heparin (e.g., Panheprin), with long-term use, or
- Lisinopril (e.g., Prinivil; Zestril) or
- Medicine for inflammation or pain (except narcotics) or
- Other potassium-containing medicine or
- Salt substitutes, low-salt foods, or milk or
- Spironolactone (e.g., Aldactone) or
- Triamterene (e.g., Dyrenium)—Use with potassium-containing phosphates may increase the risk of hyperkalemia (too much potassium in the blood), possibly leading to serious side effects
- Antacids—Use with phosphates may prevent the phosphate from working properly
- Calcium-containing medicine, including antacids and calcium supplements—Use with phosphates may prevent the phosphate from working properly; calcium deposits may form in tissues
- Phosphate-containing medications, other, including phosphate enemas—Use with sodium or potassium phophates may cause high blood levels of phosphorus which may increase the chance of side effects
- Sodium-containing medicines (other)—Use with sodium phosphates may cause your body to retain (keep) water

Other medical problems—The presence of other medical problems may affect the use of phosphates. Make sure you tell your doctor if you have any other medical problems, especially:

- Dehydration or
- Underactive adrenal glands—Potassium-containing phosphates may increase the risk of hyperkalemia (too much potassium in the blood)
- Edema (swelling in feet or lower legs or fluid in lungs) or
- High blood pressure or
- Liver disease or
- Toxemia of pregnancy—Sodium-containing phosphates may make these conditions worse
- Burns, severe or
- Heart disease or
- Pancreatitis (inflammation of the pancreas) or
- Rickets or
- Softening of bones or
- Underactive parathyroid glands—Sodium- or potassium-containing phosphates may make these conditions worse
- High blood levels of phosphate (hyperphosphatemia)—Use of phosphates may make this condition worse
- Infected kidney stones—Phosphates may make this condition worse
- Kidney disease—Sodium-containing phosphates may make this condition worse; potassium-containing phosphates may increase the risk of hyperkalemia (too much potassium in the blood)
- Myotonia congenita—Potassium-containing phosphates may increase the risk of hyperkalemia (too much potassium in the blood), and make this condition worse

Before you begin using any new medicine (prescription or nonprescription) or if you develop any new medical problem while you are using this medicine, check with your doctor, nurse, or pharmacist.

Proper Use of This Medicine

For patients taking the *tablet form* of this medicine:

- *Do not swallow the tablet.* Before taking, dissolve the tablet in ¾ to 1 glass (6 to 8 ounces) of water. Let the tablet soak in water for 2 to 5 minutes and then stir until completely dissolved.

For patients using the *capsule form* of this medicine:

- *Do not swallow the capsule.* Before taking, mix the contents of 1 capsule in one-third glass (about 2½ ounces) of water or juice or the contents of 2 capsules in two-thirds glass (about 5 ounces) of water and stir well until dissolved.

For patients using the *powder form* of this medicine:

- Add the entire contents of 1 bottle (2¼ ounces) to enough warm water to make 1 gallon of solution *or* the contents of one packet to enough warm water to make 1/3 of a glass (about 2.5 ounces) of solution. Shake the container for 2 or 3 minutes or until all the powder is dissolved.
- Do not dilute solution further.
- This solution may be chilled to improve the flavor; do not allow it to freeze.
- Discard unused solution after 60 days.

Take this medicine immediately after meals or with food to lessen possible stomach upset or laxative action.

To help prevent kidney stones, *drink at least a full glass (8 ounces) of water every hour during waking hours,* unless otherwise directed by your doctor.

Take this medicine only as directed. Do not take more of it and do not take it more often than recommended on the label, unless otherwise directed by your doctor.

Missed dose—If you miss a dose of this medicine, take it as soon as possible. However, if it is within 1 or 2 hours of your next dose, skip the missed dose and go back to your regular dosing schedule. Do not double doses.

Storage—To store this medicine:

- Keep out of the reach of children.
- Store away from heat and direct light.
- Do not store the capsule, tablet, or powder form of this medicine in the bathroom, near the kitchen sink,

or in other damp places. Heat or moisture may cause the medicine to break down.

- Keep the liquid form of this medicine from freezing.
- Do not keep outdated medicine or medicine no longer needed. Be sure that any discarded medicine is out of the reach of children.

Precautions While Using This Medicine

Your doctor should check your progress at regular visits to make sure that this medicine does not cause unwanted effects.

Do not take iron supplements within 1 to 2 hours of taking this medicine. To do so may keep the iron from working properly.

For patients taking potassium phosphate-containing medicines:

- Check with your doctor before starting any strenuous physical exercise, especially if you are out of condition and are taking other medication. Exercise and certain medicines may increase the amount of potassium in the blood.

For patients on a *potassium-restricted diet:*

- This medicine may contain a large amount of potassium. If you have any questions about this, check with your doctor or pharmacist.
- Do not use salt substitutes and low-salt milk unless told to do so by your doctor. They may contain potassium.

For patients on a sodium-restricted diet:

- This medicine may contain a large amount of sodium. If you have any questions about this, check with your doctor or pharmacist.

Side Effects of This Medicine

Along with its needed effects, a medicine may cause some unwanted effects. Although not all of these side effects may occur, if they do occur they may need medical attention.

Check with your doctor as soon as possible if any of the following side effects occur:

Less common or rare

Confusion; convulsions (seizures); decrease in amount of urine or in frequency of urination; fast, slow, or irregular heartbeat; headache or dizziness; increased thirst; muscle cramps; numbness, tingling, pain, or weakness in hands or feet; numbness or tingling around lips; shortness of breath or troubled breathing; swelling of feet or lower legs; tremor; unexplained anxiety; unusual tiredness or weakness; weakness or heaviness of legs; weight gain

Other side effects may occur that usually do not need medical attention. These side effects may go away during treatment as your body adjusts to the medicine. However, check with your doctor if any of the following side effects continue or are bothersome:

Diarrhea; nausea or vomiting; stomach pain

Other side effects not listed above may also occur in some patients. If you notice any other effects, check with your doctor.

Annual revision: 04/16/92

PHYSOSTIGMINE Ophthalmic†

Some commonly used brand names in the U.S. are Eserine Salicylate, Eserine Sulfate, and Isopto Eserine.

Generic name product may also be available in the U.S.

†Not commercially available in Canada.

Description

Physostigmine (fi-zoe-STIG-meen) is used to treat certain types of glaucoma.

This medicine is available only with your doctor's prescription, in the following dosage forms:

Ophthalmic

- Ophthalmic ointment (U.S.)
- Ophthalmic solution (eye drops) (U.S.)

It is very important that you read and understand the following information. If any of it causes you special concern, check with your doctor. Also, *if you have any questions* or if you want more information about this medicine or your medical problem, *ask your doctor, nurse, or pharmacist.*

Before Using This Medicine

In deciding to use a medicine, the risks of taking the medicine must be weighed against the good it will do.

This is a decision you and your doctor will make. For physostigmine, the following should be considered:

Allergies—Tell your doctor if you have ever had any unusual or allergic reaction to physostigmine. Also tell your doctor and pharmacist if you are allergic to any other substances, such as preservatives.

Pregnancy—Ophthalmic physostigmine may be absorbed into the body. However, studies on effects in pregnancy have not been done in either humans or animals.

Breast-feeding—Ophthalmic physostigmine may be absorbed into the mother's body. However, physostigmine has not been reported to cause problems in nursing babies.

Children—Although there is no specific information comparing use of this medicine in children with use in other age groups, it is not expected to cause different side effects or problems in children than it does in adults.

Older adults—Many medicines have not been studied specifically in older people. Therefore, it may not be known whether they work exactly the same way they do in younger adults or if they cause different side effects or problems in older people. Although there is no specific information comparing use of physostigmine in the elderly with use in other age groups, it is not expected to cause different side effects or problems in older people than it does in younger adults.

Other medicines—Although certain medicines should not be used together at all, in other cases two different medicines may be used together even if an interaction might occur. In these cases, your doctor may want to change the dose, or other precautions may be necessary. Tell your doctor and pharmacist if you are using any other prescription or nonprescription (over-the-counter [OTC]) medicine.

Other medical problems—The presence of other medical problems may affect the use of physostigmine. Make sure you tell your doctor if you have any other medical problems, especially:

- Eye disease or problems (other)—Physostigmine may make the condition worse

Before you begin using any new medicine (prescription or nonprescription) or if you develop any new medical problem while you are using this medicine, check with your doctor, nurse, or pharmacist.

Proper Use of This Medicine

To use the *ophthalmic solution (eye drops) form* of this medicine:

- Do not use if the solution becomes discolored.
- First, wash your hands. With the middle finger, apply pressure to the inside corner of the eye (and continue to apply pressure for 1 or 2 minutes after the medicine has been placed in the eye). Tilt the head back and with the index finger of the same hand, pull the lower eyelid away from the eye to form a pouch. Drop the medicine into the pouch and gently close the eyes. Do not blink. Keep the eyes closed for 1 or 2 minutes to allow the medicine to be absorbed.
- Immediately after using the eye drops, wash your hands to remove any medicine that may be on them.
- To keep the medicine as germ-free as possible, do not touch the applicator tip to any surface (including the eye). Also, keep the container tightly closed.

To use the *ointment form* of this medicine:

- First, wash your hands. Pull the lower eyelid away from the eye to form a pouch. Squeeze a thin strip of ointment into the pouch. A 1-cm (approximately 1/3-inch) strip of ointment is usually enough unless otherwise directed by your doctor. Gently close the eyes and keep them closed for 1 or 2 minutes to allow the medicine to be absorbed.
- Immediately after using the eye ointment, wash your hands to remove any medicine that may be on them.
- To keep the medicine as germ-free as possible, do not touch the applicator tip to any surface (including the eye). After using the eye ointment, wipe the tip of the ointment tube with a clean tissue and keep the tube tightly closed.

Use this medicine only as directed. Do not use more of it and do not use it more often than your doctor ordered. To do so may increase the chance of too much medicine being absorbed into the body and the chance of side effects.

Dosing—The dose of ophthalmic physostigmine will be different for different patients. *Follow your doctor's orders or the directions on the label.* The following information includes only the average doses of ophthalmic physostigmine. *If your dose is different, do not change it* unless your doctor tells you to do so.

The number of doses you use each day, the time allowed between doses, and the length of time you use the medicine depend on the medical problem for which you are using ophthalmic physostigmine.

- For glaucoma:
  - —For *ophthalmic ointment* dosage form:
    - Adults and children—Use in each eye one to three times a day.
  - —For *ophthalmic solution (eye drops)* dosage form:
    - Adults and children—One drop in each eye up to four times a day.

Missed dose—If you miss a dose of this medicine and your dosing schedule is:

- One dose a day—Apply the missed dose as soon as possible. However, if you do not remember the missed dose until the next day, skip the missed dose and go back to your regular dosing schedule. Do not double doses.

- More than one dose a day—Apply the missed dose as soon as possible. However, if it is almost time for your next dose, skip the missed dose and go back to your regular dosing schedule. Do not double doses.

Storage—To store this medicine:

- Keep out of the reach of children.
- Store away from heat and direct light.
- Keep the medicine from freezing.
- Do not keep outdated medicine or medicine no longer needed. Be sure that any discarded medicine is out of the reach of children.

Precautions While Using This Medicine

Your doctor should check your eye pressure at regular visits.

For a short time after you apply this medicine, your vision may be blurred or there may be a change in your near or distant vision, especially at night. *Make sure your vision is clear before you drive, use machines, or do anything else that could be dangerous if you are not able to see well.*

Side Effects of This Medicine

Along with its needed effects, a medicine may cause some unwanted effects. Although not all of these side effects may occur, if they do occur they may need medical attention.

Check with your doctor as soon as possible if any of the following side effects occur:

Symptoms of too much medicine being absorbed into the body

Increased sweating; loss of bladder control; muscle weakness; nausea, vomiting, diarrhea, or stomach cramps or pain; shortness of breath, tightness in chest, or wheezing; slow or irregular heartbeat; unusual tiredness or weakness; watering of mouth

Other side effects may occur that usually do not need medical attention. These side effects may go away during treatment as your body adjusts to the medicine. However, check with your doctor if any of the following side effects continue or are bothersome:

More common

Blurred vision or change in near or distant vision; eye pain

Less common

Burning, redness, stinging, or other eye irritation; headache or browache; twitching of eyelids; watering of eyes

Other side effects not listed above may also occur in some patients. If you notice any other effects, check with your doctor.

Annual revision: 07/01/93

PILOCARPINE Ophthalmic

Some commonly used brand names are:

In the U.S.

Adsorbocarpine	Pilocar
Akarpine	Pilokair
I-Pilocarpine	Pilopine HS
Isopto Carpine	Piloptic-1
Ocu-Carpine	Piloptic-2
Ocusert Pilo-20	Piloptic-4
Ocusert Pilo-40	Pilostat
Pilagan	Spectro-Pilo

Generic name product may also be available.

In Canada

Isopto Carpine	Pilopine HS
Minims Pilocarpine	Pilostat
Miocarpine	P.V. Carpine Liquifilm
Ocusert Pilo-20	Spersacarpine
Ocusert Pilo-40	

Description

Pilocarpine (pye-loe-KAR-peen) is used to treat glaucoma and other eye conditions.

This medicine is available only with your doctor's prescription, in the following dosage forms:

Ophthalmic

- Ocular system (eye insert) (U.S. and Canada)
- Ophthalmic gel (eye gel) (U.S. and Canada)
- Ophthalmic solution (eye drops) (U.S. and Canada)

It is very important that you read and understand the following information. If any of it causes you special concern, check with your doctor. Also, *if you have any questions* or if you want more information about this medicine or your medical problem, *ask your doctor, nurse, or pharmacist.*

Before Using This Medicine

In deciding to use a medicine, the risks of taking the medicine must be weighed against the good it will do.

This is a decision you and your doctor will make. For pilocarpine, the following should be considered:

Allergies—Tell your doctor if you have ever had any unusual or allergic reaction to pilocarpine. Also tell your doctor and pharmacist if you are allergic to any other substances, such as preservatives

Pregnancy—Ophthalmic pilocarpine may be absorbed into the body. However, studies on effects in pregnancy have not been done in either humans or animals.

Breast-feeding—Ophthalmic pilocarpine may be absorbed into the body. However, it is not known whether pilocarpine passes into the breast milk. Although most medicines pass into breast milk in small amounts, many of them may be used safely while breast-feeding. Mothers who are using this medicine and who wish to breast-feed should discuss this with their doctor.

Children—Although there is no specific information comparing use of this medicine in children with use in other age groups, pilocarpine is not expected to cause different side effects or problems in children than it does in adults.

Older adults—Many medicines have not been studied specifically in older people. Therefore, it may not be known whether they work exactly the same way they do in younger adults or if they cause different side effects or problems in older people. Although there is no specific information comparing use of pilocarpine in the elderly with use in other age groups, this medicine is not expected to cause different side effects or problems in older people than it does in younger adults.

Other medicines—Although certain medicines should not be used together at all, in other cases two different medicines may be used together even if an interaction might occur. In these cases, your doctor may want to change the dose, or other precautions may be necessary. Tell your doctor and pharmacist if you are using any other prescription or nonprescription (over-the-counter [OTC]) medicine.

Other medical problems—The presence of other medical problems may affect the use of pilocarpine. Make sure you tell your doctor if you have any other medical problems, especially:

- Asthma or
- Eye disease or problems (other)—Pilocarpine may make the condition worse

Before you begin using any new medicine (prescription or nonprescription) or if you develop any new medical problem while you are using this medicine, check with your doctor, nurse, or pharmacist.

Proper Use of This Medicine

To use the *eye drop form* of pilocarpine:

- First, wash your hands. With the middle finger, apply pressure to the inside corner of the eye (and continue to apply pressure for 1 or 2 minutes after the medicine has been placed in the eye). Tilt the head back and with the index finger of the same hand, pull the lower eyelid away from the eye to form a pouch. Drop the medicine into the pouch and gently close the eyes. Do not blink. Keep the eyes closed for 1 or 2 minutes to allow the medicine to be absorbed.
- Immediately after using the eye drops, wash your hands to remove any medicine that may be on them.
- To keep the medicine as germ-free as possible, do not touch the applicator tip to any surface (including the eye). Also, keep the container tightly closed.

To use the *eye gel form* of pilocarpine:

- First, wash your hands. Pull the lower eyelid away from the eye to form a pouch. Squeeze a thin strip of gel into the pouch. A 1½-cm (approximately ½-inch) strip of gel is usually enough unless otherwise directed by your doctor. Gently close the eyes and keep them closed for 1 or 2 minutes to allow the medicine to be absorbed.
- Immediately after using the eye gel, wash your hands to remove any medicine that may be on them.
- To keep the medicine as germ-free as possible, do not touch the applicator tip to any surface (including the eye). After using the eye gel, wipe the tip of the gel tube with a clean tissue and keep the tube tightly closed.

To use the *eye insert form* of pilocarpine:

- This medicine usually comes with patient directions. Read them carefully before using this medicine.
- If you think this medicine unit may be damaged, do not use it. If you have any questions about this, check with your doctor or pharmacist.
- If the unit seems to be releasing too much medicine into your eye, remove it and replace with a new unit. If you have any questions about this, check with your doctor.

Use this medicine only as directed. Do not use more of it and do not use it more often than your doctor ordered. To do so may increase the chance of too much medicine being absorbed into the body and the chance of side effects.

Dosing—The dose of ophthalmic pilocarpine will be different for different patients. *Follow the doctor's orders or the directions on the label.* The following information includes only the average doses of ophthalmic pilocarpine. *If your dose is different, do not change it unless your doctor tells you to do so.*

The number of doses you use each day, the time allowed between doses, and the length of time you use the medicine depend on the medical problem for which you are using ophthalmic pilocarpine.

- For *eye insert* dosage form:
  - —For glaucoma:
    - Adults and children—Insert one ocular system every seven days.
    - Infants—Use is generally not recommended.
- For *eye gel* dosage form:
  - —For glaucoma:
    - Adults and adolescents—Use once a day at bedtime.
    - Children—Use is generally not recommended.
- For *eye drop* dosage form:
  - —For chronic glaucoma:
    - Adults and children—One drop one to four times a day.
  - —For acute angle-closure glaucoma:
    - Adults and children—One drop every five to ten minutes for three to six doses. Then one drop every one to three hours until eye pressure is reduced.

Missed dose—
- For patients using the *eye drop form* of pilocarpine: If you miss a dose of this medicine, apply it as soon as possible. However, if it is almost time for your next dose, skip the missed dose and go back to your regular dosing schedule. Do not double doses.
- For patients using the *eye gel form* of pilocarpine: If you miss a dose of this medicine, apply it as soon as possible. However, if you do not remember the missed dose until the next day, skip the missed dose and go back to your regular dosing schedule. Do not double doses.
- For patients using the *eye insert form* of pilocarpine: If you forget to replace the eye insert at the proper time, replace it as soon as possible. Then go back to your regular dosing schedule.

Storage—To store this medicine:
- Keep out of the reach of children.
- Store away from heat and direct light.
- Store the eye system form of this medicine in the refrigerator. However, keep the medicine from freezing.
- Store the 5-gram size of the gel form of this medicine in the refrigerator. Store the 3.5-gram size at room temperature.
- Keep the gel or solution form of this medicine from freezing.
- Do not keep outdated medicine or medicine no longer needed. Be sure that any discarded medicine is out of the reach of children.

Precautions While Using This Medicine

Your doctor should check your eye pressure at regular visits.

For patients using the *eye drop or gel form* of this medicine:
- For a short time after you apply this medicine, your vision may be blurred or there may be a change in your near or far vision, especially at night. *Make sure your vision is clear before you drive, use machines, or do anything else that could be dangerous if you are not able to see well.*

For patients using the *eye insert form* of this medicine:
- For the first several hours after you insert this unit in the eye, your vision may be blurred or there may be a change in your near or far vision, especially at night. Therefore, insert this unit in the eye at bedtime, unless otherwise directed by your doctor. If this unit is inserted in the eye at any other time of the day, *make sure your vision is clear before you drive, use machines, or do anything else that could be dangerous if you are not able to see well.*

Side Effects of This Medicine

Along with its needed effects, a medicine may cause some unwanted effects. Although not all of these side effects may occur, if they do occur they may need medical attention.

Check with your doctor as soon as possible if any of the following side effects occur:

Symptoms of too much medicine being absorbed into the body

Increased sweating; muscle tremors; nausea, vomiting, or diarrhea; troubled breathing or wheezing; watering of mouth

Less common or rare

Eye pain

Other side effects may occur that usually do not need medical attention. These side effects may go away during treatment as your body adjusts to the medicine. However, check with your doctor if any of the following side effects continue or are bothersome:

More common

Blurred vision or change in near or far vision; decrease in night vision

Less common

Eye irritation; headache or browache

Other side effects not listed above may also occur in some patients. If you notice any other effects, check with your doctor.

Annual revision: 07/01/93

PIMOZIDE Systemic

A commonly used brand name in the U.S. and Canada is Orap.

Description

Pimozide (PIM-oh-zide) is used to treat the symptoms of Tourette's syndrome. It is meant only for patients with severe symptoms who cannot take or have not been helped by other medicine.

Pimozide works in the central nervous system to help control the vocal outbursts and uncontrolled, repeated movements of the body (tics) that interfere with normal life. It will not completely cure the tics, but will help to reduce their number and severity.

Pimozide may also be used for other conditions as determined by your doctor.

This medicine is available only with your doctor's prescription, in the following dosage form:

Oral

- Tablets (U.S. and Canada)

It is very important that you read and understand the following information. If any of it causes you special concern, check with your doctor. Also, *if you have any questions* or if you want more information about this medicine or your medical problem, *ask your doctor, nurse, or pharmacist.*

Before Using This Medicine

In deciding to use a medicine, the risks of taking the medicine must be weighed against the good it will do. This is a decision you and your doctor will make. For pimozide, the following should be considered:

Allergies—Tell your doctor if you have ever had any unusual or allergic reaction to pimozide, haloperidol, loxapine, molindone, phenothiazines, or thioxanthenes. Also tell your doctor and pharmacist if you are allergic to any other substances, such as foods, preservatives, or dyes.

Pregnancy—Studies in rats and rabbits given more than the usual human dose of pimozide have shown fewer pregnancies, slowed development of the fetus, and toxic effects in the mother and fetus.

Breast-feeding—It is not known whether pimozide passes into breast milk.

Children—Children are especially sensitive to the effects of pimozide. This may increase the chance of side effects during treatment. Pimozide should not be used in children for any medical problem other than Tourette's syndrome.

Older adults—Constipation, dizziness or fainting, drowsiness, dryness of mouth, and trembling of the hands and fingers, and symptoms of tardive dyskinesia (such as rapid, worm-like movements of the tongue or any other uncontrolled movements of the mouth, tongue, or jaw, and/or arms and legs) may be especially likely to occur in the elderly, who are usually more sensitive than younger adults to the effects of pimozide.

Other medicines—Although certain medicines should not be used together at all, in other cases 2 different medicines may be used together even if an interaction might occur. In these cases, your doctor may want to change the dose, or other precautions may be necessary. When you are taking pimozide, it is especially important that your doctor and pharmacist know if you are taking any of the following:

- Amoxapine (e.g., Asendin) or
- Methyldopa (e.g., Aldomet) or
- Metoclopramide (e.g., Reglan) or
- Metyrosine (e.g., Demser) or
- Promethazine (e.g., Phenergan) or
- Rauwolfia alkaloids (alseroxylon [e.g., Rauwiloid], deserpidine [e.g., Harmonyl], rauwolfia serpentina [e.g., Raudixin], reserpine [e.g., Serpasil]) or
- Trimeprazine (e.g., Temaril)—Taking these medicines with pimozide may increase the chance of serious side effects
- Amphetamines or
- Methylphenidate (e.g., Ritalin) or
- Pemoline (e.g., Cylert)—Taking these medicines with pimozide may cover up the cause of tics
- Anticholinergics (medicine for abdominal or stomach spasms or cramps)—Taking these medicines with pimozide may cause an increased chance of certain side effects, such as dryness of mouth, constipation, and unusual excitement
- Antipsychotics (medicine for mental illness) or
- Disopyramide (e.g., Norpace) or
- Maprotiline (e.g., Ludiomil) or
- Procainamide (e.g., Pronestyl) or
- Quinidine (e.g., Quinidex) or
- Tricyclic antidepressants (medicine for depression)—Taking these medicines with pimozide may increase the chance of serious effects on the rhythm of your heart
- Central nervous system (CNS) depressants—Using these medicines with pimozide may increase the CNS depressant effects

Other medical problems—The presence of other medical problems may affect the use of pimozide. Make sure you tell your doctor if you have any other medical problems, especially:

- Breast cancer (history of) or
- Heart disease—Pimozide may make the condition worse
- Kidney disease or
- Liver disease—Higher blood levels of pimozide may occur, increasing the chance of side effects
- Tics other than those caused by Tourette's syndrome—Pimozide should not be used because of the risk of serious side effects

Before you begin using any new medicine (prescription or nonprescription) or if you develop any new medical problem while you are using this medicine, check with your doctor, nurse, or pharmacist.

Proper Use of This Medicine

Use pimozide only as directed by your doctor. Do not use more of it, do not use it more often, and do not use it for a longer time than your doctor ordered. To do so may increase the chance of side effects.

Dosing—The dose of pimozide will be different for different patients. *Follow your doctor's orders or the directions on the label.* The following information includes only the average doses of pimozide. *If your dose is different, do not change it* unless your doctor tells you to do so.

- The number of tablets that you take depends on the strength of the medicine. Also, *the number of doses you take each day, the time allowed between doses, and the length of time you take the medicine depend on the medical problem for which you are using pimozide.*
- For *oral* dosage forms (tablets):
  —Adults and adolescents: To start, 1 to 2 milligrams (mg) a day. Your doctor may increase your dose if needed. However, the dose is usually not more than 10 mg a day.
  —Children up to 12 years of age: Dose must be determined by the doctor.

Missed dose—If you miss a dose of this medicine, take it as soon as possible. Then take any remaining doses for that day at regularly spaced times. Do not double doses.

Storage—To store this medicine:

- Keep out of the reach of children.
- Store away from heat and direct light.
- Do not store in the bathroom, near the kitchen sink, or in other damp places. Heat or moisture may cause the medicine to break down.
- Do not keep outdated medicine or medicine no longer needed. Be sure that any discarded medicine is out of the reach of children.

Precautions While Using This Medicine

Your doctor should check your progress at regular visits, especially during the first few months of treatment with this medicine. The amount of pimozide you take may be changed often to meet the needs of your condition and to help avoid unwanted effects.

Do not suddenly stop taking this medicine without first checking with your doctor. Your doctor may want you to reduce gradually the amount you are taking before stopping completely. This will allow your body time to adjust and help to avoid worsening of your medical condition.

This medicine will add to the effects of alcohol and other CNS depressants (medicines that slow down the nervous system, possibly causing drowsiness). Some examples of CNS depressants are antihistamines or medicine for hay fever, other allergies, or colds; sedatives, tranquilizers, or sleeping medicine; prescription pain medicine or narcotics; barbiturates; medicine for seizures; muscle relaxants; or anesthetics, including some dental anesthetics. *Check with your doctor before taking any of the above while you are using this medicine.*

This medicine may cause some people to become drowsy or less alert or to have blurred vision or muscle stiffness, especially as the amount of medicine is increased. Even if you take pimozide at bedtime, you may feel drowsy or less alert on arising. *Make sure you know how you react to this medicine before you drive, use machines, or do anything else that could be dangerous if you are not alert or able to see well or if you do not have good muscle control.*

Although not a problem for many patients, dizziness, lightheadedness, or fainting may occur, especially when you get up from a sitting or lying position. Getting up slowly may help. If the problem continues or gets worse, check with your doctor.

Before having any kind of surgery, dental treatment, or emergency treatment, tell the medical doctor or dentist in charge that you are using this medicine. Taking pimozide together with medicines that are used during surgery or dental or emergency treatment may increase the CNS depressant effects.

Pimozide may cause dryness of the mouth. For temporary relief, use sugarless gum or candy, melt bits of ice in your mouth, or use a saliva substitute. However, if your mouth continues to feel dry for more than 2 weeks, check with your medical doctor or dentist. Continuing dryness of the mouth may increase the chance of dental disease, including tooth decay, gum disease, and fungus infections.

Side Effects of This Medicine

Along with its needed effects, pimozide can sometimes cause serious side effects. Tardive dyskinesia (a movement disorder) may occur and may not go away after you stop using the medicine. Signs of tardive dyskinesia include fine, worm-like movements of the tongue, or other uncontrolled movements of the mouth, tongue, cheeks, jaw, or arms and legs. Other serious but rare side effects may also occur. These include severe muscle stiffness, fever, unusual tiredness or weakness, fast heartbeat, difficult breathing, increased sweating, loss of bladder control, and seizures (neuroleptic malignant syndrome). *You and your doctor should discuss the good this medicine will do as well as the risks of taking it.*

Stop taking pimozide and get emergency help immediately if any of the following side effects occur:

Rare

Convulsions (seizures); difficult or fast breathing; fast heartbeat or irregular pulse; fever (high); high or low (irregular) blood pressure; increased sweating; loss of bladder control; muscle stiffness (severe); tiredness or weakness; unusually pale skin

Symptoms of overdose

Drowsiness or dizziness (severe); muscle trembling, jerking, or stiffness (severe); troubled breathing (severe); uncontrolled movements (severe); unusual tiredness or weakness (severe)

Check with your doctor as soon as possible if any of the following side effects occur:

More common

Difficulty in speaking or swallowing; loss of balance control; mask-like face; mood or behavior changes; restlessness or need to keep moving; shuffling walk; slowed movements; stiffness of arms and legs; trembling and shaking of fingers and hands

Less common or rare

Inability to move eyes; increased blinking or spasms of eyelid; lip smacking or puckering; muscle spasms, especially of the face, neck, or back; puffing of cheeks; rapid or worm-like movements of tongue; sore throat and fever; uncontrolled chewing movements; uncontrolled twisting movements of neck, trunk, arms, or legs; unusual bleeding or bruising; unusual facial expressions or body positions; yellow eyes or skin

Other side effects may occur that usually do not need medical attention. These side effects may go away during treatment as your body adjusts to the medicine. However, check with your doctor if any of the following side effects continue or are bothersome:

More common

Blurred vision or other vision problems; constipation; dizziness, lightheadedness, or fainting (especially when getting up from a lying or sitting position); drowsiness; dryness of mouth; skin rash, itching, or discoloration; swelling or soreness of breasts; unusual secretion of milk

Less common

Decreased sexual ability; diarrhea; headache; loss of appetite and weight; mental depression; nausea or vomiting; swelling of the face

After you stop using pimozide, it may still produce some side effects that need attention. During this period of time, check with your doctor as soon as possible if you notice any of the following side effects:

Lip smacking or puckering; puffing of cheeks; rapid or worm-like movements of the tongue; uncontrolled chewing movements; uncontrolled movements of the arms and legs

Other side effects not listed above may also occur in some patients. If you notice any other effects, check with your doctor.

Annual revision: 04/16/93

PLICAMYCIN Systemic†

A commonly used brand name in the U.S. is Mithracin.

Another commonly used name is mithramycin.

†Not commercially available in Canada.

Description

Plicamycin (plye-ka-MYE-sin) belongs to the group of medicines known as antineoplastics. It may be used to treat certain types of cancer. It is also used to treat hypercalcemia or hypercalciuria (too much calcium in the blood or urine) that may occur with some types of cancer.

Plicamycin is to be administered by or under the immediate care of your doctor. It is available only with a prescription, in the following dosage form:

Parenteral

- Injection (U.S.)

Plicamycin may also be used for other conditions as determined by your doctor.

It is very important that you read and understand the following information. If any of it causes you special concern, check with your doctor. Also, *if you have any questions* or if you want more information about this medicine or your medical problem, *ask your doctor, nurse, or pharmacist.*

Before Receiving This Medicine

Plicamycin is a very strong medicine. In addition to its helpful effects in treating your medical problem, it has side effects that could be very serious. Before you receive this medicine, be sure that you have discussed its use with your doctor.

In deciding to use a medicine, the risks of taking the medicine must be weighed against the good it will do. This is a decision you and your doctor will make. For plicamycin, the following should be considered:

Allergies—Tell your doctor if you have ever had any unusual or allergic reaction to plicamycin. Also tell your doctor and pharmacist if you are allergic to any other substances, such as foods, preservatives, or dyes.

Pregnancy—Plicamycin is not recommended for use during pregnancy. There is a possibility that it may be harmful to the fetus.

Breast-feeding—It is not known whether plicamycin passes into the breast milk.

Children—Studies on this medicine have not been done in children; however, plicamycin can cause serious side effects in any patient. Therefore, it is especially important that you discuss with the child's doctor the good that this medicine may do as well as the risks of using it.

Older adults—Many medicines have not been studied specifically in older people. Therefore, it may not be known whether they work exactly the same way they do in younger adults or if they cause different side effects or problems in older people. There is no specific information comparing use of plicamycin in the elderly with use in other age groups.

Other medicines—Although certain medicines should not be used together at all, in other cases two different medicines may be used together even if an interaction might occur. In these cases, your doctor may want to change the dose, or other precautions may be necessary. Tell your doctor and pharmacist if you are taking *any* other medicines or are having x-ray treatments.

Other medical problems—The presence of other medical problems may affect the use of plicamycin. Make sure you tell your doctor if you have any other medical problems, especially:

- Bleeding problems—Use of plicamycin may increase the risk of bleeding
- Blood disease or
- Kidney disease or
- Liver disease—Use of plicamycin may make these conditions worse
- Chickenpox (including recent exposure) or
- Herpes zoster (shingles)—Use of plicamycin may make your reaction to either of these conditions worse

Before you begin using any new medicine (prescription or nonprescription) or if you develop any new medical problem while you are receiving this medicine, check with your doctor, nurse, or pharmacist.

Proper Use of This Medicine

Plicamycin sometimes causes nausea, vomiting, and loss of appetite. However, it is very important that you continue to receive the medicine, even if you begin to feel ill. If you have any questions about this, check with your doctor.

Precautions After Receiving This Medicine

It is very important that your doctor check your progress daily while you are receiving plicamycin to make sure that this medicine does not cause unwanted effects.

Your doctor may want you to follow a low-calcium, low-vitamin D diet. If you have any questions about this, check with your doctor.

Do not take aspirin or large amounts of any other preparations containing aspirin, other salicylates, or acetaminophen without first checking with your doctor. These medicines may increase the effects of plicamycin.

While you are being treated with plicamycin, and after you stop treatment with it, *do not have any immunizations (vaccinations) without your doctor's approval.* Plicamycin may lower your body's resistance and there is a chance you might get the infection the immunization is meant to prevent. In addition, other persons living in your household should not take or have recently taken oral polio vaccine since there is a chance they could pass the polio virus on to you. Also, avoid other persons who have taken oral polio vaccine. Do not get close to them, and do not stay in the same room with them for very long. If you cannot take these precautions, you should consider wearing a protective face mask that covers the nose and mouth.

Plicamycin can lower the number of white blood cells in your blood temporarily, increasing the chance of getting an infection. It can also lower the number of platelets, which are necessary for proper blood clotting. If this occurs, there are certain precautions your doctor may ask you to take, especially when your blood count is low, to reduce the risk of infection of bleeding:

- If you can, avoid people with infections. *Check with your doctor immediately* if you think you are getting an infection or if you get a fever or chills.
- *Check with your doctor immediately* if you notice any unusual bleeding or bruising.
- Be careful when using a regular toothbrush, dental floss, or toothpick. Your medical doctor, dentist, or nurse may recommend other ways to clean your teeth and gums. Check with your medical doctor before having any dental work done.
- Do not touch your eyes or the inside of your nose unless you have just washed your hands and have not touched anything else in the meantime.
- Be careful not to cut yourself when you are using sharp objects such as a safety razor or fingernail or toenail cutters.
- Avoid contact sports or other situations where bruising or injury could occur.

Side Effects of This Medicine

Along with its needed effects, a medicine may cause some unwanted effects. Although not all of these side effects may occur, if they do occur they may need medical attention.

Check with your doctor or nurse immediately if any of the following side effects occur:

Less common

Muscle and abdominal cramps

Symptoms of overdose

Bloody or black, tarry stools; flushing or redness or swelling of face; nosebleed; skin rash or small red spots on skin; sore throat and fever; unusual bleeding or bruising; vomiting of blood; yellow eyes or skin

Other side effects may occur that usually do not need medical attention. These side effects may go away during treatment as your body adjusts to the medicine. However, check with your doctor if any of the following side effects continue or are bothersome:

More common

Diarrhea; irritation or soreness of mouth; loss of appetite; nausea or vomiting—may occur 1 to 2 hours after the injection is started and continue for 12 to 24 hours

Less common

Drowsiness; fever; headache; mental depression; pain, redness, soreness, or swelling at place of injection; unusual tiredness or weakness

After you stop using plicamycin, it may still produce some side effects that need attention. During this period of time check with your doctor if you notice any of the following side effects:

Bloody or black, tarry stools; nosebleed; sore throat and fever; unusual bleeding or bruising; vomiting of blood

Other side effects not listed above may also occur in some patients. If you notice any other effects, check with your doctor.

Additional Information

Once a medicine has been approved for marketing for a certain use, experience may show that it is also useful for other medical problems. Although this use is not included in product labeling, plicamycin is used in certain patients with the following medical condition:

- Paget's disease of the bone

Other than the above information, there is no additional information relating to proper use, precautions, or side effects for these uses.

Annual revision: 09/14/92

PNEUMOCOCCAL VACCINE POLYVALENT Systemic

Some commonly used brand names are:

In the U.S.

Pneumovax 23
Pnu-Imune 23

In Canada

Pneumovax 23

Description

Pneumococcal (NEU-mo-KOK-al) vaccine polyvalent is an active immunizing agent used to prevent infection by pneumococcal bacteria. It works by causing your body to produce its own protection (antibodies) against the disease.

The following information applies only to the polyvalent 23 pneumococcal vaccine. Other polyvalent pneumococcal vaccines may be available in countries other than the U.S.

Pneumococcal infection can cause serious problems, such as pneumonia, which affects the lungs; meningitis, which affects the brain; bacteremia, which is a severe infection in the blood; and possibly death. These problems are more likely to occur in older adults and persons with certain diseases or conditions that make them more susceptible to a pneumococcal infection or more apt to develop serious problems from a pneumococcal infection.

Immunization against pneumococcal disease is recommended for:

- older adults, especially those 50 years of age and older.
- adults and children 2 years of age or older with chronic illnesses.
- persons with human immunodeficiency virus (HIV) infection, either with or without symptoms.
- persons with spleen problems or without spleens and persons who are to have their spleens removed.
- persons with sickle cell disease.
- persons who are waiting for organ transplants.
- persons who will be treated with x-rays or cancer medicines.

- persons in nursing homes and orphanages.
- persons who will be traveling outside the U.S. and who have certain diseases or conditions that make them more susceptible to pneumococcal infection or more likely to develop serious problems from pneumococcal infection.
- persons who are bedridden.

Immunization against pneumococcal infection is not recommended for infants and children younger than 2 years of age, because these persons cannot produce enough antibodies to the vaccine to protect them against a pneumococcal infection.

Pneumococcal vaccine is usually given only once to each person. Additional injections are not given, except in special cases, because of the possibility of more frequent and more severe side effects.

This vaccine is available only from your doctor or other authorized health care providers, in the following dosage form:

Parenteral
- Injection (U.S. and Canada)

It is very important that you read and understand the following information. If any of it causes you special concern, check with your doctor. Also, *if you have any questions* or if you want more information about this medicine or your medical problem, *ask your doctor, nurse, or pharmacist.*

Before Receiving This Vaccine

In deciding to use a medicine, the risks of taking the medicine must be weighed against the good it will do. This is a decision you and your doctor will make. For pneumococcal vaccine, the following should be considered:

Allergies—Tell your doctor if you have ever had any unusual or allergic reaction to pneumococcal vaccine. Also tell your doctor and pharmacist if you are allergic to any other substances, such as preservatives.

Pregnancy—Studies on effects in pregnancy have not been done in either humans or animals. However, if the vaccine is needed, it should be given after the first three months of pregnancy and only to women who have certain diseases or conditions that make them more susceptible to a pneumococcal infection or more likely to develop serious problems from a pneumococcal infection.

Breast-feeding—It is not known whether pneumococcal vaccine passes into the breast milk. However, this vaccine has not been reported to cause problems in nursing babies.

Children—Use of pneumococcal vaccine is not recommended in infants and children younger than 2 years of age. In children 2 years of age and older, this vaccine is not expected to cause different side effects or problems than it does in adults.

Older adults—This vaccine is not expected to cause different side effects or problems in older people than it does in younger adults.

Other medicines—Although certain medicines should not be used together at all, in other cases two different medicines may be used together even if an interaction might occur. In these cases, your doctor may want to change the dose, or other precautions may be necessary. Before you receive pneumococcal vaccine, it is especially important that your doctor and pharmacist know if you have received any of the following:

- Pneumococcal vaccine injection of any kind in the past—May increase the chance and severity of side effects

Other medical problems—The presence of other medical problems may affect the use of pneumococcal vaccine. Make sure you tell your doctor if you have any other medical problems, especially:

- Severe illness with fever—The symptoms of the illness may be confused with possible side effects of the vaccine
- Thrombocytopenic purpura (blood disorder)—Use of pneumococcal vaccine may make the condition worse

Before you begin using any new medicine (prescription or nonprescription) or if you develop any new medical problem while you are using this medicine, check with your doctor, nurse, or pharmacist.

Precautions After Receiving This Vaccine

If you have more than one doctor, be sure they all know that you have received pneumococcal vaccine polyvalent 23 so that they can put the information in your medical records. *This vaccine is usually given only once* to each person, except in special cases.

Side Effects of This Medicine

Along with its needed effects, a medicine may cause some unwanted effects. Although not all of these side effects may occur, if they do occur they may need medical attention.

Get emergency help immediately if any of the following side effects occur:

Symptoms of allergic reaction

Difficulty in breathing or swallowing; hives; itching, especially of feet or hands; reddening of skin, especially around ears; swelling of eyes, face, or inside of nose; unusual tiredness or weakness (sudden and severe)

Check with your doctor as soon as possible if the following side effect occurs:

Rare

Fever over 102 °F (39 °C)

Other side effects may occur that usually do not need medical attention. However, check with your doctor if any of the following side effects continue or are bothersome:

More common

Redness, soreness, hard lump, swelling, or pain at place of injection

Less common or rare

Aches or pain in joints or muscles; fever of 101 °F (38.3 °C) or less; skin rash; swollen glands; unusual tiredness or weakness; vague feeling of bodily discomfort

Side effects may be more common and more severe if this is not the first time you have received pneumococcal vaccine. Check with your doctor as soon as possible if you do have a severe reaction.

Other side effects not listed above may also occur in some patients. If you notice any other effects, check with your doctor.

Annual revision: September 1990

PODOPHYLLUM Topical

A commonly used brand name in the U.S. is Podofin.

Description

Podophyllum (pode-oh-FILL-um) is used to remove benign (not cancer) growths, such as certain kinds of warts. It works by destroying the tissue of the growth.

A few hours after podophyllum is applied to a wart, the wart becomes blanched (loses all color). In 24 to 48 hours, the medicine causes death of the tissue. After about 72 hours, the wart begins to slough or come off and gradually disappears.

Podophyllum is usually applied only in a doctor's office because it is a poison and can cause serious side effects if not used properly. However, your doctor may ask you to apply this medicine at home. If you do apply it at home, be sure you understand exactly how to use it.

Podophyllum is available only with your doctor's prescription, in the following dosage form:

Topical

- Topical solution (U.S.)

It is very important that you read and understand the following information. If any of it causes you special concern, check with your doctor. Also, *if you have any questions* or if you want more information about this medicine or your medical problem, *ask your doctor, nurse, or pharmacist.*

Before Using This Medicine

In deciding to use a medicine, the risks of taking the medicine must be weighed against the good it will do. This is a decision you and your doctor will make. For podophyllum, the following should be considered:

Allergies—Tell your doctor if you have ever had any unusual or allergic reaction to podophyllum or benzoin. Also tell your doctor and pharmacist if you are allergic to any other substances, such as preservatives or dyes.

Pregnancy—Topical podophyllum is absorbed through the skin. It should not be used during pregnancy, since it may cause birth defects or other harmful effects in the fetus.

Breast-feeding—Topical podophyllum is absorbed through the skin. However, it has not been reported to cause problems in nursing babies.

Children—There is no specific information about the use of podophyllum in children.

Older adults—Many medicines have not been tested in older people. Therefore, it may not be known whether they work exactly the same way they do in younger adults or if they cause different side effects or problems in older people. There is no specific information about the use of podophyllum in the elderly.

Other medicines—Although certain medicines should not be used together at all, in other cases two different medicines may be used together even if an interaction might occur. In these cases, your doctor may want to change the dose, or other precautions may be necessary. When you are using podophyllum, it is especially important that your doctor and pharmacist know if you are using any other prescription or nonprescription (over-the-counter [OTC]) medicine.

Other medical problems—The presence of other medical problems may affect the use of podophyllum. Make sure

you tell your doctor if you have any other medical problems, especially:

- Crumbling or bleeding warts or warts that have recently had surgery on them—Using podophyllum on these warts may increase the chance of absorption of the medicine through the skin

Before you begin using any new medicine (prescription or nonprescription) or if you develop any new medical problem while you are using this medicine, check with your doctor, nurse, or pharmacist.

Proper Use of This Medicine

Podophyllum is a poison. Keep it away from the mouth because it is harmful if swallowed.

Also, *keep podophyllum away from the eyes and other mucous membranes,* such as the inside of the nose. This medicine may cause severe irritation. If you get some in your eyes, immediately flush the eyes with water for 15 minutes. If you get some on your normal skin, thoroughly wash the skin with soap and water to remove the medicine. However, if this medicine contains tincture of benzoin, it may be removed more easily from the skin by swabbing with rubbing alcohol.

This medicine may contain alcohol and therefore may be flammable. *Do not use near heat, near open flame, or while smoking.*

Use podophyllum only as directed. Do not use more of it, do not use it more often, and do not use it for a longer period of time than your doctor ordered. To do so may increase the chance of too much medicine being absorbed into the body and the chance of side effects.

Do not use podophyllum on moles or birthmarks. To do so may cause severe irritation.

Also, *do not apply this medicine to crumbling or bleeding warts or to warts that have recently had surgery on them.* To do so may increase the chance of absorption through the skin.

To use:

- Podophyllum can cause severe irritation of normal skin. Therefore, apply petrolatum around the affected area before you apply podophyllum, and/or apply talcum powder to the treated area immediately after you apply podophyllum. This is to prevent the medicine from spreading to the normal skin.
- Use a toothpick or a cotton-tipped or glass applicator to apply this medicine. Apply one drop at a time, allowing time for drying between drops, until the affected area is covered.
- After podophyllum is applied, allow it to remain on the affected area for 1 to 6 hours as directed by your doctor. Then, remove the medicine by thoroughly washing the affected area with soap and water. If this medicine contains tincture of benzoin, it may be removed more easily by swabbing the affected area with rubbing alcohol. However, this may be more irritating than washing with soap and water.
- Immediately after applying this medicine, wash your hands to remove any medicine that may be on them.

Missed dose—If you miss a dose of this medicine, apply it as soon as possible. Then go back to your regular dosing schedule.

Storage—To store this medicine:

- Keep out of the reach of children.
- Store away from heat and direct light.
- Do not store in the bathroom, near the kitchen sink, or in other damp places. Heat or moisture may cause the medicine to break down.
- Do not keep outdated medicine or medicine no longer needed. Be sure that any discarded medicine is out of the reach of children.

Side Effects of This Medicine

Along with its needed effects, a medicine may cause some unwanted effects. Although not all of these side effects may occur, if they do occur they may need medical attention.

Check with your doctor immediately if any of the following side effects occur:

Early symptoms of too much medicine being absorbed into the body

Abdominal or stomach pain; clumsiness or unsteadiness; confusion; decreased or loss of reflexes; diarrhea (may be severe and continuing); excitement, irritability, or nervousness; hallucinations (seeing, hearing, or feeling things that are not there); muscle weakness; nausea or vomiting; sore throat and fever; unusual bleeding or bruising

Delayed symptoms of too much medicine being absorbed into the body

Constipation; convulsions (seizures); difficult or painful urination; difficulty in breathing; dizziness or lightheadedness, especially when getting up from a lying or sitting position; drowsiness; fast heartbeat; numbness, tingling, pain, or weakness in hands or feet (may not occur for about 2 weeks after medicine is used); pain in upper abdomen or stomach (mild, dull, and continuing)

Also, check with your doctor as soon as possible if any of the following side effects occur:

Redness, burning, or other irritation of affected area; skin rash or itching

Other side effects not listed above may also occur in some patients. If you notice any other effects, check with your doctor.

Annual revision: September 1990

POLIOVIRUS VACCINE Systemic

This information applies to the following medicines:
Poliovirus Vaccine Inactivated
Poliovirus Vaccine Inactivated Enhanced Potency
Poliovirus Vaccine Live Oral

Some commonly used brand names are:

For Poliovirus Vaccine Inactivated
In the U.S.
Generic name product may be available.
In Canada
Generic name product may be available.

Other commonly used names are IPV and Salk vaccine.

For Poliovirus Vaccine Inactivated Enhanced Potency
In the U.S.
Poliovax
Generic name product may also be available.
In Canada
Generic name product may be available.

Other commonly used names are enhanced-potency IPV and N-IPV.

For Poliovirus Vaccine Live Oral
In the U.S.
Orimune
In Canada
Generic name product may be available.

Other commonly used names are OPV, Sabin vaccine, and TOPV.

Description

Poliovirus (POE-lee-oh VYE-russ) vaccine is an active immunizing agent used to prevent poliomyelitis (polio). It works by causing your body to produce its own protection (antibodies) against the virus that causes polio.

There are two types of polio vaccine that are given by injection, poliovirus vaccine inactivated (IPV) and poliovirus vaccine inactivated enhanced potency (enhanced-potency IPV). The type of vaccine that is given by mouth is called poliovirus vaccine live oral (OPV).

Polio is a very serious infection that causes paralysis of the muscles, including the muscles that enable you to walk and breathe. A polio infection may leave a person unable to breathe without the help of an iron lung, unable to walk without leg braces, or confined to a wheelchair. There is no cure for polio.

Immunization against polio is recommended for all infants from age 6 to 12 weeks, all children, all adolescents up to 18 years of age, and certain adults, including:

- Persons traveling outside the U.S. to countries where polio is uncontrolled, whether or not they have been vaccinated against polio in the past.
- All adults who may be exposed to polio, whether or not they have been vaccinated against polio in the past.
- Adults who have not been vaccinated or who have not had the complete series of vaccinations against polio and who live in households in which children are to be given the oral polio vaccine (OPV).
- Employees in day-care centers and group homes for children, such as orphanages.
- Employees in medical facilities, such as hospitals and doctors' offices.
- Laboratory workers handling samples that may contain polioviruses.

Immunization against polio is not recommended for infants younger than 6 weeks of age, because antibodies they received from their mothers before birth may interfere with the effectiveness of the vaccine. Infants who were immunized against polio before 6 weeks of age should receive the complete series of polio immunization.

This vaccine is available only from your doctor or other authorized health care provider, in the following dosage forms:

Oral
- Oral solution (U.S. and Canada)

Parenteral
- Injection (U.S. and Canada)

It is very important that you read and understand the following information. If any of it causes you special concern, check with your doctor. Also, *if you have any questions* or if you want more information about this medicine or your medical problem, *ask your doctor, nurse, or pharmacist.*

Before Receiving This Vaccine

For a while after you are immunized, there is a very small risk (1 in 5 million) that any persons living in your household who have not yet been immunized against polio or who have or had an immune deficiency condition may develop poliomyelitis (polio) from being around you. Talk to your doctor if you have any questions about this.

In deciding to use a medicine, the risks of taking the medicine must be weighed against the good it will do. This is a decision you and your doctor will make. For polio vaccine, the following should be considered:

Allergies—Tell your doctor if you have ever had any unusual or allergic reaction to polio vaccine or to neomycin, penicillin, polymyxin B, or streptomycin. The polio vaccines available in the U.S. may contain neomycin and streptomycin. The polio vaccines available in Canada may contain neomycin, penicillin, polymyxin B, and/or streptomycin. Also tell your doctor and pharmacist if you are allergic to any other substances, such as foods, preservatives, or dyes.

Diet—Make certain your doctor and pharmacist know if you are on any special diet, such as a low-sugar diet, because the oral solution form of polio vaccine may be given to you on a sugar cube.

Pregnancy—Studies on effects in pregnancy have not been done in either humans or animals. However, this vaccine has not been shown to cause birth defects or other problems in humans. Although it is not recommended for all pregnant women, polio vaccine is given to pregnant women at great risk of catching polio.

Breast-feeding—It is not known whether polio vaccine passes into the breast milk. However, this vaccine has not been reported to cause problems in nursing babies.

Children—Use is not recommended for infants up to 6 weeks of age. For infants and children 6 weeks of age and older, poliovirus vaccine is not expected to cause different side effects or problems than it does in adults.

Older adults—This vaccine is not expected to cause different side effects or problems in older persons than it does in younger adults.

Other medicines—Although certain medicines should not be used together at all, in other cases two different medicines may be used together even if an interaction might occur. In these cases, your doctor may want to change the dose, or other precautions may be necessary. Before you receive polio vaccine, it is especially important that your doctor and pharmacist know if you are receiving or have received any of the following:

- Treatment with x-rays, cancer medicines, or high doses of steroids—May reduce the useful effect of the vaccine

Other medical problems—The presence of other medical problems may affect the use of polio vaccine. Make sure you tell your doctor if you have any other medical problems, especially:

- Diarrhea or
- Virus infection or
- Vomiting—The condition may reduce the useful effect of the vaccine
- Fever or
- Illness (severe) or
- Weakness (severe)—The symptoms of the condition may be confused with possible side effects of the vaccine
- Immune deficiency condition (or family history of)—The condition may increase the chance of side effects of the vaccine

Before you begin using any new medicine (prescription or nonprescription) or if you develop any new medical problem while you are using this medicine, check with your doctor, nurse, or pharmacist.

Precautions After Receiving This Vaccine

Tell your doctor that you have received this vaccine if you are to receive any other live virus vaccines within 1 month after receiving this vaccine.

Side Effects of This Vaccine

In very rare instances (approximately 1 case in 3.2 million doses), healthy persons who have taken the oral vaccine (OPV) and healthy persons who are close contacts of adults or children who have taken OPV have been infected by the polio virus and have become paralyzed. No paralysis caused by polio infection has occurred with the injected vaccine (IPV) since 1955.

Along with its needed effects, a vaccine may cause some unwanted effects. Although not all of these side effects may occur, if they do occur they may need medical attention.

Get emergency help immediately if any of the following side effects occur:

Symptoms of allergic reaction

Difficulty in breathing or swallowing; hives; itching, especially of feet or hands; reddening of skin, especially around ears; swelling of eyes, face, or inside of nose; unusual tiredness or weakness (sudden and severe)

Other side effects may occur that usually do not need medical attention. However, check with your doctor if any of the following side effects continue or are bothersome:

Less common

Fever over 101.3 °F (38.5 °C) (with injection); itching or skin rash (with injection); redness, soreness, hard lump, tenderness, or pain at the place of injection (with injection)

Other side effects not listed above may also occur in some patients. If you notice any other effects, check with your doctor.

Annual revision: September 1990

POLYETHYLENE GLYCOL AND ELECTROLYTES Local

Some commonly used brand names are:

In the U.S.

Colovage	GoLYTELY
Colyte	Nulytely
Colyte-flavored	OCL

In Canada

Colyte	Peglyte
GoLYTELY	

Description

The polyethylene glycol (pol-ee-ETH-i-leen GLYE-col) (PEG) and electrolytes solution is used to clean the colon (large bowel or lower intestine) before certain tests or surgery of the colon. The PEG-electrolyte solution is usually taken by mouth. However, sometimes it is given in the hospital through a nasogastric tube (a tube inserted through the nose).

The PEG-electrolyte solution acts like a laxative. It causes liquid stools or mild diarrhea. In this way, it flushes all solid material from the colon, so the doctor can have a clear view of the colon.

The PEG-electrolyte solution is available only with your doctor's prescription. It is available in the following dosage forms:

Oral

- Oral solution (U.S. and Canada)
- Powder for oral solution (U.S. and Canada)

It is very important that you read and understand the following information. If any of it causes you special concern, check with your doctor. Also, *if you have any questions* or if you want more information about this medicine or your medical problem, *ask your doctor, nurse, or pharmacist.*

Before Using This Medicine

In deciding to use a medicine, the risks of taking the medicine must be weighed against the good it will do. This is a decision you and your doctor will make. For the PEG-electrolyte solution, the following should be considered:

Allergies—Tell your doctor if you have ever had any unusual or allergic reaction to PEG. Also tell your doctor and pharmacist if you are allergic to any other substances, such as foods, preservatives, or dyes.

Pregnancy—Studies on effects in pregnancy have not been done in either humans or animals. Before taking the PEG-electrolyte solution or having a colon examination, make sure your doctor knows if you are pregnant.

Breast-feeding—The PEG-electrolyte solution has not been reported to cause problems in nursing babies.

Children—Although there is no specific information comparing use of PEG-electrolyte solution in children with use in other age groups, this medicine is not expected to cause different side effects or problems in children than it does in adults.

Older adults—This medicine has been tested and has not been shown to cause different side effects or problems in older people than it does in younger adults.

Other medicines—Although certain medicines should not be used together at all, in other cases two different medicines may be used together even if an interaction might occur. In these cases, your doctor may want to change the dose, or other precautions may be necessary. Tell your doctor and pharmacist if you are taking any of the following:

- Any other oral medicines—Any medicines taken within 1 hour of the PEG-electrolyte solution may be flushed from the body and not have an effect

Other medical problems—The presence of other medical problems may affect the use of PEG-electrolyte solution. Make sure you tell your doctor if you have any other medical problems, especially:

- Blockage or obstruction of the intestine or
- Paralytic ileus or
- Perforated bowel or
- Toxic colitis or
- Toxic megacolon—PEG-electrolyte solution may make these conditions worse; in some cases the colon may rip open or tear

Before you begin using any new medicine (prescription or nonprescription) or if you develop any new medical problem while you are using this medicine, check with your doctor, nurse, or pharmacist.

Proper Use of This Medicine

Your doctor may have special instructions for you, depending on the type of test you are going to have. If you have not received such instructions or if you do not understand them, check with your doctor in advance.

Take the PEG-electrolyte solution exactly as directed. Otherwise, the test you are going to have may not work and may have to be done again.

Do not eat anything for at least 3 hours before taking the PEG-electrolyte solution. If you do so, the colon may not get completely clean. If you are drinking the PEG-electrolyte solution the evening before the test, you may drink clear liquids (e.g., water, ginger ale, decaffeinated cola, decaffeinated tea, broth, gelatin) up until the time of the test. However, check first with your doctor.

For patients *using the powder form of this medicine:*

- *The powder must be mixed with water before it is used.* Add lukewarm water to the fill mark on the bottle.
- *Shake well* until all the ingredients are dissolved.
- Do not add any other ingredients, such as flavoring, to the solution.
- After you mix the solution, you must use it within 48 hours.

Dosing—*Follow your doctor's orders or the directions on the label.* The following information includes only the usual amount taken of PEG-electrolyte solution. *If your dose is different, do not change it* unless your doctor tells you to do so:

- Drink one full glass (8 ounces) of the PEG-electrolyte solution *rapidly* every 10 minutes. If you sip small amounts of the solution, it will not work as well.
- It will take close to 3 hours to drink all of the PEG-electrolyte solution. The first bowel movement may start an hour or so after you start drinking the solution. *Continue drinking all the solution to get the best results,* unless otherwise directed by your doctor.

Storage—To store this medicine:

- Keep out of the reach of children.
- Store away from heat and direct light.
- Store the solution in the refrigerator to improve the taste. However, keep the medicine from freezing.
- Do not keep any leftover solution. Be sure that any discarded medicine is out of the reach of children.

Side Effects of This Medicine

Along with its needed effects, a medicine may cause some unwanted effects. Although not all of these side effects may occur, if they do occur they may need medical attention.

Check with your doctor as soon as possible if the following side effect occurs:

Rare

Skin rash

Other side effects may occur that usually do not need medical attention. These side effects may go away as your body adjusts to the medicine. However, check with your doctor or pharmacist if any of the following side effects continue or are bothersome:

More common

Bloating; nausea

Less common

Abdominal or stomach cramps; irritation of the anus; vomiting

Other side effects not listed above may also occur in some patients. If you notice any other effects, check with your doctor or pharmacist.

Annual revision: 10/05/92

POTASSIUM IODIDE Systemic

Some commonly used brand names are:

In the U.S.

Pima

Generic name product may also be available.

In Canada

Thyro-Block*

Other commonly used names are KI and SSKI.

*Not commercially available in the U.S.; however, potassium iodide tablets are available to government and public health organizations for use in radiation emergencies.

Description

Potassium iodide (poe-TAS-ee-um EYE-oh-dide) is used to treat overactive thyroid and to protect the thyroid gland from the effects of radiation from inhaled or swallowed radioactive iodine. It may be used before and after administration of medicine containing radioactive iodine or after accidental exposure to radioactive iodine (for example, from nuclear power plant accidents that involved release of radioactivity to the environment). It may also be used for other problems as determined by your doctor.

Potassium iodide is taken by mouth. It may be taken as an oral solution, syrup, uncoated tablet, or enteric-coated tablet. However, the enteric-coated tablet form may cause serious side effects and its use is generally not recommended.

Some brands of the oral solution are available without a prescription. Use them only as directed by state or local public health authorities in case of a radiation emergency. Other forms and strengths of potassium iodide are available only with your doctor's prescription.

Potassium iodide is available in the following dosage forms:

Oral

- Enteric-coated tablets (U.S.)
- Oral solution (U.S.)
- Syrup (U.S.)
- Tablets (Canada)

It is very important that you read and understand the following information. If any of it causes you special concern, check with your doctor. Also, *if you have any questions* or if you want more information about this medicine or your medical problem, *ask your doctor, nurse, or pharmacist.*

Before Using This Medicine

In deciding to use a medicine, the risks of taking the medicine must be weighed against the good it will do. This is a decision you and your doctor will make. For potassium iodide, the following should be considered:

Allergies—Tell your doctor if you have ever had any unusual or allergic reaction to potassium iodide, iodine, or iodine-containing foods. Also tell your doctor and pharmacist if you are allergic to any substances, such as foods, preservatives, or dyes.

Pregnancy—Taking potassium during pregnancy may cause thyroid problems or goiter in the newborn infant.

Breast-feeding—Potassium iodide passes into the breast milk and may cause skin rash and thyroid problems in nursing babies.

Children—Potassium iodide may cause skin rash and thyroid problems in infants.

Older adults—Many medicines have not been studied specifically in older people. Therefore, it may not be known whether they work exactly the same way they do in younger adults. Although there is no specific information comparing use of potassium iodide in the elderly with use in other age groups, this medicine is not expected to cause different side effects or problems in older people than in younger adults.

Other medicines—Although certain medicines should not be used together at all, in other cases two different medicines may be used together even if an interaction might occur. In these cases, your doctor may want to change the dose, or other precautions may be necessary. When you are taking potassium iodide, it is especially important that your doctor and pharmacist know if you are taking any of the following:

- Amiloride (e.g., Midamor) or
- Spironolactone (e.g., Aldactone) or
- Triamterene (e.g., Dyrenium)—Use of these medicines with potassium iodide may increase the amount of potassium in the blood and increase the chance of side effects
- Antithyroid agents (medicine for overactive thyroid) or
- Lithium (e.g., Lithane)—Use of these medicines with potassium iodide may increase the chance of side effects

Other medical problems—The presence of other medical problems may affect the use of potassium iodide. Make sure you tell your doctor if you have any other medical problems, especially:

- High blood levels of potassium (hyperkalemia) or
- Myotonia congenita or
- Tuberculosis—Potassium iodine may make these conditions worse
- Kidney disease—May cause an increase of potassium in the blood
- Overactive thyroid (unless you are taking this medicine for this medical problem)—Prolonged use of potassium iodine may be harmful to the thyroid gland

Before you begin using any new medicine (prescription or nonprescription) or if you develop any new medical problem while you are using this medicine, check with your doctor, nurse, or pharmacist.

Proper Use of This Medicine

For patients taking this medicine for *radiation exposure:*

- Take this medicine only when directed to do so by state or local public health authorities.
- Take this medicine once a day for 10 days, unless otherwise directed by public health authorities. *Do not take more of it and do not take it more often than directed.* Taking more of the medicine will not protect you better and may result in a greater chance of side effects.

If potassium iodide upsets your stomach, *take it after meals or with food or milk* unless otherwise directed by your doctor. If stomach upset (nausea, vomiting, stomach pain, or diarrhea) continues, check with your doctor.

For patients taking the *oral solution form* of this medicine:

- This medicine is to be taken by mouth even if it comes in a dropper bottle.
- Do not use if solution turns brownish yellow.
- Take potassium iodide in a full glass (8 ounces) of water or in fruit juice, milk, or broth to improve the taste and lessen stomach upset. Be sure to drink all of the liquid to get the full dose of medicine.
- If crystals form in potassium iodide solution, they may be dissolved by warming the closed container of solution in warm water and then gently shaking the container.

For patients taking the *uncoated tablet form* of this medicine:

- Before taking, dissolve each tablet in ½ glass (4 ounces) of water or milk. Be sure to drink all of the liquid to get the full dose of medicine.

Missed dose—If you miss a dose of this medicine, take it as soon as possible. However, if it is almost time for your next dose, skip the missed dose and go back to your regular dosing schedule. Do not double doses.

Storage—To store this medicine:

- Keep out of the reach of children.
- Store away from heat and direct light.
- Do not store the tablet form of this medicine in the bathroom, near the kitchen sink, or in other damp places. Heat or moisture may cause the medicine to break down.
- Keep the oral liquid forms of this medicine from freezing. Do not refrigerate.
- Do not keep outdated medicine or medicine no longer needed. Be sure that any discarded medicine is out of the reach of children.

Precautions While Using This Medicine

Your doctor should check your progress at regular visits to make sure that this medicine does not cause unwanted effects.

For patients on a low-potassium diet:

- *This medicine contains potassium.* Check with your doctor or pharmacist before you take this medicine.

Side Effects of This Medicine

Along with its needed effects, a medicine may cause some unwanted effects. Although not all of these side effects may occur, if they do occur they may need medical attention. When this medicine is used for a short time at low doses, side effects usually are rare.

Check with your doctor as soon as possible if any of the following side effects occur:

Less common

Hives; joint pain; swelling of arms, face, legs, lips, tongue, and/or throat; swelling of lymph glands

With long-term use

Burning of mouth or throat; confusion; headache (severe); increased watering of mouth; irregular heartbeat; metallic taste; numbness, tingling, pain or weakness in hands or feet; soreness of teeth and gums; sores on skin; symptoms of head cold; unusual tiredness; weakness or heaviness of legs

Other side effects may occur that usually do not need medical attention. These side effects may go away during treatment as your body adjusts to the medicine. However, check with your doctor if any of the following side effects continue or are bothersome:

Less common

Diarrhea; nausea or vomiting; stomach pain

Other side effects not listed above may also occur in some patients. If you notice any other effects, check with your doctor.

Additional Information

Once a medicine has been approved for marketing for a certain use, experience may show that it is also useful for other medical problems. Although these uses are not included in product labeling, potassium iodide is used in certain patients with the following medical conditions:

- To prepare the thyroid gland before a thyroid operation
- Iodine deficiency
- Certain skin conditions caused by fungus

In addition to the above information, for patients taking this medicine for a fungus infection:

- *Keep taking it for the full course of treatment,* even if you begin to feel better after a few days. This will help clear up your infection completely. *Do not miss any doses.*

Other than the above information, there is no additional information relating to proper use, precautions, or side effects for these uses.

Annual revision: 04/14/92

POTASSIUM SUPPLEMENTS Systemic

This information applies to the following medicines:

Potassium Acetate (poe-TAS-ee-um AS-a-tate)
Potassium Bicarbonate (bi-KAR-bo-nate)
Potassium Bicarbonate and Potassium Chloride (KLOR-ide)
Potassium Bicarbonate and Potassium Citrate (SIH-trayt)
Potassium Chloride
Potassium Chloride, Potassium Bicarbonate, and Potassium Citrate
Potassium Gluconate (GLOO-ko-nate)
Potassium Gluconate and Potassium Chloride
Potassium Gluconate and Potassium Citrate
Trikates (TRI-kates)

Some commonly used brand names are:

For Potassium Acetate

In the U.S.

Generic name product is available.

In Canada

Generic name product is available.

For Potassium Bicarbonate
In the U.S.
K+ Care ET
K-Ide
Klor-Con/EF
K-Lyte
In Canada
K-Lyte

For Potassium Bicarbonate and Potassium Chloride
In the U.S.
Klorvess
Klorvess Effervescent Granules
K-Lyte/Cl
K-Lyte/Cl 50
In Canada
Neo-K
Potassium-Sandoz

For Potassium Bicarbonate and Potassium Citrate†
In the U.S.
Effer-K
K-Lyte DS

For Potassium Chloride
In the U.S.
Cena-K
Gen-K
K+ 10
Kaochlor 10%
Kaochlor S-F 10%
Kaon-Cl
Kaon-Cl-10
Kaon-Cl 20% Liquid
Kato
Kay Ciel
K+ Care
K-Dur
K-Ide
K-Lease
K-Lor
Klor-Con 8
Klor-Con 10
Klor-Con Powder
Klor-Con/25 Powder
Klorvess 10% Liquid
Klotrix
K-Lyte/Cl Powder
K-Norm
K-Tab
Micro-K
Micro-K 10
Micro-K LS
Potage
Potasalan
Rum-K
Slow-K
Ten-K

Generic name product may also be available.

In Canada
Apo-K
K-10
Kalium Durules
Kaochlor-10
Kaochlor-20
KCL 5%
K-Dur
K-Long
K-Lor
K-Lyte/Cl
Micro-K
Micro-K 10
Novolente-K
Roychlor-10%
Slow-K

Generic name product may also be available.

For Potassium Chloride, Potassium Bicarbonate, and Potassium Citrate†
In the U.S.
Kaochlor-Eff

For Potassium Gluconate
In the U.S.
Kaon
Kaylixir
K-G Elixir

Generic name product may also be available.

In Canada
Kaon
Potassium-Rougier

For Potassium Gluconate and Potassium Chloride†
In the U.S.
Kolyum

For Potassium Gluconate and Potassium Citrate†
In the U.S.
Twin-K

For Trikates†
In the U.S.
Tri-K

Generic name product may also be available.

Another commonly used name for trikates is potassium triplex.

†Not commercially available in Canada.

Description

Potassium is needed to maintain good health. Although a balanced diet usually supplies all the potassium a person needs, potassium supplements may be needed by patients who do not have enough potassium in their regular diet or have lost too much potassium because of illness or treatment with certain medicines.

There is no evidence that potassium supplements are useful in the treatment of high blood pressure.

Lack of potassium may cause muscle weakness, irregular heartbeat, mood changes, or nausea and vomiting.

Some forms of potassium may be available in stores without a prescription. Since too much potassium may cause health problems, you should take potassium supplements only if directed by your doctor. Potassium supplements are available with your doctor's prescription in the following dosage forms:

Oral

Potassium Bicarbonate
- Tablets for solution (U.S. and Canada)

Potassium Bicarbonate and Potassium Chloride
- Powder for solution (U.S. and Canada)
- Tablets for solution (U.S. and Canada)

Potassium Bicarbonate and Potassium Citrate
- Tablets for solution (U.S.)

Potassium Chloride
- Extended-release capsules (U.S. and Canada)
- Solution (U.S. and Canada)
- Powder for solution (U.S. and Canada)
- Powder for suspension (U.S.)
- Extended-release tablets (U.S. and Canada)

Potassium Chloride, Potassium Bicarbonate, and Potassium Citrate
- Tablets for solution (U.S.)

Potassium Gluconate
- Elixir (U.S. and Canada)
- Tablets (U.S.)

Potassium Gluconate and Potassium Chloride
- Solution (U.S.)
- Powder for solution (U.S.)

Potassium Gluconate and Potassium Citrate
- Solution (U.S.)

Trikates
- Solution (U.S.)

Parenteral

Potassium Acetate
- Injection (U.S. and Canada)

Potassium Chloride
- Concentrate for injection (U.S. and Canada)

It is very important that you read and understand the following information. If any of it causes you special concern, check with your doctor. Also, *if you have any questions* or if you want more information about this medicine or your medical problem, *ask your doctor, nurse, or pharmacist.*

Importance of Diet

Many nutritionists recommend that, if possible, people get the potassium they need from the foods they eat. However, many people do not get enough potassium from their diets. For example, people on weight-loss diets may consume too little food to get enough potassium. Others may lose potassium from the body because of illness or treatment with certain medicines. For such people, a potassium supplement, given under a doctor's supervision, is important.

In order to get enough vitamins and minerals in your diet, it is important that you eat a balanced and varied diet. Follow carefully any diet program your doctor may recommend. For your specific vitamin and/or mineral needs, ask your doctor for a list of appropriate foods.

The following table includes some potassium-rich foods.

Food (amount)	Milligrams of potassium	Milli-equivalents of potassium
Acorn squash, cooked (1 cup)	896	23
Potato with skin, baked (1 long)	844	22
Spinach, cooked (1 cup)	838	21
Lentils, cooked (1 cup)	731	19
Kidney beans, cooked (1 cup)	713	18
Split peas, cooked (1 cup)	710	18
White navy beans, cooked (1 cup)	669	17
Butternut squash, cooked (1 cup)	583	15
Watermelon (1/16)	560	14
Raisins (½ cup)	553	14
Yogurt, low-fat, plain (1 cup)	531	14
Orange juice, frozen (1 cup)	503	13
Brussel sprouts, cooked (1 cup)	494	13
Zucchini, cooked, sliced (1 cup)	456	12
Banana (medium)	451	12
Collards, frozen, cooked (1 cup)	427	11
Cantaloupe (¼)	412	11
Milk, low-fat 1% (1 cup)	348	9
Broccoli, frozen, cooked (1 cup)	332	9

Experts have developed a list of recommended dietary allowances (RDA) for most of the vitamins and some minerals. The RDA are not an exact number but a general idea of how much you need. They do not cover amounts needed for problems caused by a serious lack of vitamins or minerals. Because lack of potassium is rare, there are no RDA for this mineral. However, it is thought that 1600 to 2000 mg (40 to 50 mEq) per day for adults is adequate.

Remember:
- The total amount of potassium that you get every day includes what you get from food *and* what you may take as a supplement. Read the labels of processed foods. Many foods now have added potassium.
- Your total intake of potassium should not be greater than the recommended amounts, unless ordered by your doctor. In some cases, too much potassium may cause muscle weakness, confusion, irregular heartbeat, or difficult breathing.

Before Using This Medicine

In deciding to use a medicine, the risks of taking the medicine must be weighed against the good it will do. This is a decision you and your doctor will make. For potassium supplements, the following should be considered:

Allergies—Tell your doctor if you have ever had any unusual or allergic reaction to potassium preparations. Also tell your doctor and pharmacist if you are allergic to any other substances, such as foods, preservatives, or dyes.

Pregnancy—Potassium supplements have not been shown to cause problems in humans.

Breast-feeding—Potassium supplements pass into breast milk. However, this medicine has not been reported to cause problems in nursing babies.

Children—Although there is no specific information comparing use of potassium supplements in children with use in other age groups, they are not expected to cause different side effects or problems in children than they do in adults.

Older adults—Many medicines have not been studied specifically in older people. Therefore, it may not be known whether they work exactly the same way they do in younger adults. Although there is no specific information comparing use of potassium supplements in the elderly with use in other age groups, they are not expected to cause different side effects or problems in older people than they do in younger adults.

Older adults may be at a greater risk of developing high blood levels of potassium (hyperkalemia).

Other medicines—Although certain medicines should not be used together at all, in other cases two different medicines may be used together even if an interaction might occur. In these cases, your doctor may want to change the dose, or other precautions may be necessary. When you are taking potassium supplements, it is especially important that your doctor and pharmacist know if you are taking any of the following:
- Amantadine (e.g., Symmetrel) or
- Anticholinergics (medicine for abdominal or stomach spasms or cramps) or

- Antidepressants (medicine for depression) or
- Antidyskinetics (medicine for Parkinson's disease or other conditions affecting control of muscles) or
- Antihistamines or
- Antipsychotic medicine (medicine for mental illness) or
- Buclizine (e.g., Bucladin) or
- Carbamazepine (e.g., Tegretol) or
- Cyclizine (e.g., Marezine) or
- Cyclobenzaprine (e.g., Flexeril) or
- Disopyramide (e.g., Norpace) or
- Flavoxate (e.g., Urispas) or
- Ipratropium (e.g., Atrovent) or
- Meclizine (e.g., Antivert) or
- Methylphenidate (e.g., Ritalin) or
- Orphenadrine (e.g., Norflex) or
- Oxybutynin (e.g., Ditropan) or
- Procainamide (e.g., Pronestyl) or
- Promethazine (e.g., Phenergan) or
- Quinidine (e.g., Quinidex) or
- Trimeprazine (e.g., Temaril)—Use with potassium supplements may cause or worsen certain stomach or intestine problems
- Angiotensin-converting enzyme (ACE) inhibitors (benazepril [e.g., Lotensin], captopril [e.g., Capoten], enalapril [e.g., Vasotec], fosinopril [e.g., Monotril], lisinopril [e.g., Prinivil, Zestril], quinapril [e.g., Accupril], ramipril [e.g., Altace]) or
- Amiloride (e.g., Midamor) or
- Beta-adrenergic blocking agents (acebutolol [e.g., Sectral], atenolol [e.g., Tenormin], betaxolol [e.g., Kerlone], carteolol [e.g., Cartrol], labetalol [e.g., Normodyne], metoprolol [e.g., Lopressor], nadolol [e.g., Corgard], oxprenolol [e.g., Trasicor], penbutolol [e.g., Levatol], pindolol [e.g., Visken], propranolol [e.g., Inderal], sotalol [e.g., Sotacor], timolol [e.g., Blocadren]) or
- Heparin (e.g., Panheprin) or
- Inflammation or pain medicine (except narcotics) or
- Potassium-containing medicines (other) or
- Salt substitutes, low-salt foods, or milk or
- Spironolactone (e.g., Aldactone) or
- Triamterene (e.g., Dyrenium)—Use with potassium supplements may further increase potassium blood levels, which may cause or worsen heart problems
- Digitalis glycosides (heart medicine)—Use with potassium supplements may make heart problems worse
- Thiazide diuretics (water pills)—If you have been taking a potassium supplement and a thiazide diuretic together, stopping the thiazide diuretic may cause hyperkalemia (high blood levels of potassium)

Other medical problems—The presence of other medical problems may affect the use of potassium supplements. Make sure you tell your doctor if you have any other medical problems, especially:

- Addison's disease (underactive adrenal glands) or
- Dehydration (excessive loss of body water, continuing or severe)
- Diabetes mellitus or
- Kidney disease—Potassium supplements may increase the risk of hyperkalemia (high blood levels of potassium), which may worsen or cause heart problems in patients with these conditions
- Diarrhea (continuing or severe)—The loss of fluid in combination with potassium supplements may cause kidney problems, which may increase the risk of hyperkalemia (high blood levels of potassium)
- Heart disease—Potassium supplements may make this condition worse
- Intestinal or esophageal blockage—Potassium supplements may damage the intestines
- Stomach ulcer—Potassium supplements may make this condition worse

Before you begin using any new medicine (prescription or nonprescription) or if you develop any new medical problem while you are using this medicine, check with your doctor, nurse, or pharmacist.

Proper Use of This Medicine

For patients taking the *liquid form* of this medicine:

- This medicine *must be diluted* in at least one-half glass (4 ounces) of cold water or juice to reduce its possible stomach-irritating or laxative effect.
- If you are on a salt (sodium)-restricted diet, check with your doctor before using tomato juice to dilute your medicine. Tomato juice has a high salt content.

For patients taking the *soluble granule, soluble powder, or soluble tablet form* of this medicine:

- This medicine must be completely dissolved in at least one-half glass (4 ounces) of cold water or juice to reduce its possible stomach-irritating or laxative effect.
- Allow any "fizzing" to stop before taking the dissolved medicine.
- If you are on a salt (sodium)-restricted diet, check with your doctor before using tomato juice to dilute your medicine. Tomato juice has a high salt content.

For patients taking the *extended-release tablet form* of this medicine:

- Swallow the tablets whole with a full (8-ounce) glass of water. Do not chew or suck on the tablet.
- Some tablets may be broken or crushed and sprinkled on applesauce or other soft food. However, check with your doctor or pharmacist first, since this should not be done for most tablets.
- If you have trouble swallowing tablets or if they seem to stick in your throat, check with your doctor. When this medicine is not properly released, it can cause irritation that may lead to ulcers.

For patients taking the *extended-release capsule form* of this medicine:

- Do not crush or chew the capsule. Swallow the capsule whole with a full (8-ounce) glass of water.
- Some capsules may be opened and the contents sprinkled on applesauce or other soft food. However,

check with your doctor or pharmacist first, since this should not be done for most capsules.

Take this medicine immediately after meals or with food to lessen possible stomach upset or laxative action.

Take this medicine only as directed by your doctor. Do not take more of it, do not take it more often, and do not take it for a longer time than your doctor ordered. *This is especially important if you are also taking both diuretics (water pills) and digitalis medicines for your heart.*

Missed dose—If you miss a dose of this medicine and remember within 2 hours, take the missed dose right away with food or liquids. Then go back to your regular dosing schedule. However, if you do not remember until later, skip the missed dose and go back to your regular dosing schedule. Do not double doses.

Storage—To store this medicine:

- Keep out of the reach of children.
- Store away from heat and direct light.
- Do not store in the bathroom, near the kitchen sink, or in other damp places. Heat or moisture may cause the medicine to break down.
- Keep the liquid form of this medicine from freezing.
- Do not keep outdated medicine or medicine no longer needed. Be sure that any discarded medicine is out of the reach of children.

Precautions While Using This Medicine

Your doctor should check your progress at regular visits to make sure the medicine is working properly and that possible side effects are avoided. Laboratory tests may be necessary.

Do not use salt substitutes, eat low-sodium foods, especially some breads and canned foods, or drink low-sodium milk unless you are told to do so by your doctor, since these products may contain potassium. It is important to read the labels carefully on all low-sodium food products.

Check with your doctor before starting any physical exercise program, especially if you are out of condition and are taking any other medicine. Exercise and certain medicines may increase the amount of potassium in the blood.

Check with your doctor at once if you notice blackish stools or other signs of stomach or intestinal bleeding. This medicine may cause such a condition to become worse, especially when taken in tablet form.

Side Effects of This Medicine

Along with its needed effects, a medicine may cause some unwanted effects. Although not all of these side effects may occur, if they do occur they may need medical attention.

Stop taking this medicine and check with your doctor immediately if any of the following side effects occur:

Less common

Confusion; irregular or slow heartbeat; numbness or tingling in hands, feet, or lips; shortness of breath or difficult breathing; unexplained anxiety; unusual tiredness or weakness; weakness or heaviness of legs

Also, check with your doctor if any of the following side effects occur:

Rare

Abdominal or stomach pain, cramping, or soreness (continuing); chest or throat pain, especially when swallowing; stools with signs of blood (red or black color)

Other side effects may occur that usually do not need medical attention. These side effects may go away during treatment as your body adjusts to the medicine. However, check with your doctor if any of the following side effects continue or are bothersome:

More common

Diarrhea; nausea; stomach pain, discomfort, or gas (mild); vomiting

Sometimes you may see what appears to be a whole tablet in the stool after taking certain extended-release potassium chloride tablets. This is to be expected. Your body has absorbed the potassium from the tablet and the shell is then expelled.

Other side effects not listed above may also occur in some patients. If you notice any other effects, check with your doctor.

Annual revision: 07/16/92

PRAZIQUANTEL Systemic†

A commonly used brand name in the U.S. is Biltricide. Another brand name is Cysticide.

†Not commercially available in Canada.

Description

Praziquantel (pray-zi-KWON-tel) belongs to the family of medicines called anthelmintics (ant-hel-MIN-tiks).

Anthelmintics are used in the treatment of worm infections.

Praziquantel is used to treat blood fluke infections. These are also known as snail fever, schistosomiasis (shis-toe-soe-MYE-a-siss), or bilharziasis (bil-har-ZYE-a-siss). Praziquantel may also be used for other worm infections as determined by your doctor. However, it will not work for pinworms or other roundworms.

Praziquantel works by causing severe spasms and paralysis of the worms' muscles. Some kinds of worms are then passed in the stool. However, you may not notice them since they are sometimes completely destroyed in the intestine.

Praziquantel is available only with your doctor's prescription, in the following dosage form:

Oral

- Tablets (U.S.)

It is very important that you read and understand the following information. If any of it causes you special concern, check with your doctor. Also, *if you have any questions* or if you want more information about this medicine or your medical problem, *ask your doctor, nurse, or pharmacist.*

Before Using This Medicine

In deciding to use a medicine, the risks of taking the medicine must be weighed against the good it will do. This is a decision you and your doctor will make. For praziquantel, the following should be considered:

Allergies—Tell your doctor if you have ever had any unusual or allergic reaction to praziquantel. Also tell your doctor and pharmacist if you are allergic to any other substances, such as foods, preservatives, or dyes.

Pregnancy—Studies have not been done in humans. Studies in rats and rabbits given up to 40 times the usual human dose have not shown that praziquantel causes birth defects. However, praziquantel has been shown to cause a greater chance of miscarriage in rats given 3 times the human dose.

Breast-feeding—Praziquantel passes into the breast milk. You should stop breast-feeding on the day you begin taking praziquantel. Do not restart breast-feeding until 72 hours after treatment is completed. During this time the breast milk should be squeezed out or sucked out with a breast pump and thrown away.

Children—This medicine has been tested in a limited number of children 4 years of age or older and, in effective doses, has not been reported to cause different side effects or problems in children over 4 years of age than it does in adults.

Older adults—Many medicines have not been studied specifically in older people. Therefore, it may not be known whether they work exactly the same way they do in younger adults or if they cause different side effects or problems in older people. There is no specific information comparing use of praziquantel in the elderly with use in other age groups.

Other medicines—Although certain medicines should not be used together at all, in other cases two different medicines may be used together even if an interaction might occur. In these cases, your doctor may want to change the dose, or other precautions may be necessary. Tell your doctor and pharmacist if you are taking any other prescription or nonprescription (over-the-counter [OTC]) medicine.

Other medical problems—The presence of other medical problems may affect the use of praziquantel. Make sure you tell your doctor if you have any other medical problems, especially:

- Liver disease—Patients with moderate to severe liver disease may have an increased chance of side effects
- Worm cysts in the eye—The death of worm cysts in the eye caused by praziquantel may cause damage to the eyes

Before you begin using any new medicine (prescription or nonprescription) or if you develop any new medical problem while you are using this medicine, check with your doctor, nurse, or pharmacist.

Proper Use of This Medicine

No special preparations (for example, special diets, fasting, other medicines, laxatives, or enemas) are necessary before, during, or immediately after taking praziquantel.

Praziquantel has a bitter taste that may cause gagging or vomiting. The bitter taste may be more noticeable if the tablets are held in the mouth or chewed. Therefore, *do not chew praziquantel tablets.* Swallow them whole with a small amount of liquid during meals.

To help clear up your infection completely, *take this medicine exactly as directed by your doctor for the full time of treatment. Do not miss any doses.*

Dosing—The dose of praziquantel will be different for different patients. *Follow your doctor's orders or the directions on the label.* The following information includes only the average doses of praziquantel. *If your dose is different, do not change it* unless your doctor tells you to do so.

- *The number of doses you take each day, the time allowed between doses, and the length of time you take the medicine depend on the medical problem for which you are taking praziquantel.*

- For the treatment of clonorchiasis (Chinese or Oriental liver fluke) and opisthorchiasis (liver flukes):
  - —Adults and children 4 years of age and older: Dose is based on body weight and will be determined by your doctor. This dose is taken three times a day for one day.
  - —Children up to 4 years of age: Dose must be determined by the doctor.
- For the treatment of schistosomiasis:
  - —Adults and children 4 years of age and older: Dose is based on body weight and will be determined by your doctor. This dose is taken two or three times a day for one day.
  - —Children up to 4 years of age: Dose must be determined by the doctor.

Missed dose—If you do miss a dose of this medicine, take it as soon as possible. However, if it is almost time for your next dose, skip the missed dose and go back to your regular dosing schedule. Do not double doses.

Storage—To store this medicine:
- Keep out of the reach of children.
- Store away from heat and direct light.
- Do not store in the bathroom, near the kitchen sink, or in other damp places. Heat or moisture may cause the medicine to break down.
- Do not keep outdated medicine or medicine no longer needed. Be sure that any discarded medicine is out of the reach of children.

Precautions While Using This Medicine

It is important that your doctor check your progress after treatment. This is to make sure that the infection is cleared up completely.

If your symptoms do not improve after you have taken this medicine for the full time of treatment, or if they become worse, check with your doctor.

This medicine may cause some people to become dizzy, drowsy, or less alert than they are normally. If any of these side effects occur, *do not drive, use machines, or do anything else that could be dangerous if you are dizzy or are not alert* while you are taking praziquantel and for 24 hours after you stop taking it.

Side Effects of This Medicine

Along with its needed effects, a medicine may cause some unwanted effects. The following side effects may go away during treatment as your body adjusts to the medicine. However, check with your doctor if any of the following side effects continue or are bothersome:

More common

Abdominal or stomach cramps or pain; bloody diarrhea; dizziness; drowsiness; fever; headache; increased sweating; loss of appetite; general feeling of discomfort or illness; nausea or vomiting

Less common

Skin rash, hives, or itching

Other side effects not listed above may also occur in some patients. If you notice any other effects, check with your doctor.

Additional Information

Once a medicine has been approved for marketing for a certain use, experience may show that it is also useful for other medical problems. Although these uses are not included in product labeling, praziquantel is used in certain patients with the following medical conditions:
- Some kinds of fluke infections
- Some kinds of tapeworm infections

Other than the above information, there is no additional information relating to proper use, precautions, or side effects for these uses.

Annual revision: 03/23/93

PRAZOSIN Systemic

A commonly used brand name in the U.S. and Canada is Minipress. Generic name product may also be available in the U.S.

Description

Prazosin (PRA-zoe-sin) belongs to the general class of medicines called antihypertensives. It is used to treat high blood pressure (hypertension).

High blood pressure adds to the workload of the heart and arteries. If it continues for a long time, the heart and arteries may not function properly. This can damage the blood vessels of the brain, heart, and kidneys, resulting in a stroke, heart failure, or kidney failure. High blood pressure may also increase the risk of heart attacks. These problems may be less likely to occur if blood pressure is controlled.

Prazosin works by relaxing blood vessels so that blood passes through them more easily. This helps to lower blood pressure.

Prazosin may also be used for other conditions as determined by your doctor.

Prazosin is available only with your doctor's prescription, in the following dosage forms:

Oral
- Capsules (U.S.)
- Tablets (Canada)

It is very important that you read and understand the following information. If any of it causes you special concern, check with your doctor. Also, *if you have any questions* or if you want more information about this medicine or your medical problem, *ask your doctor, nurse, or pharmacist.*

Before Using This Medicine

In deciding to use a medicine, the risks of taking the medicine must be weighed against the good it will do. This is a decision you and your doctor will make. For prazosin, the following should be considered:

Allergies—Tell your doctor if you have ever had any unusual or allergic reaction to prazosin, doxazosin, or terazosin. Also tell your doctor and pharmacist if you are allergic to any other substance, such as foods, preservatives, or dyes.

Pregnancy—Limited use of prazosin to control high blood pressure in pregnant women has not shown that prazosin causes birth defects or other problems. Studies in animals given many times the highest recommended human dose of prazosin also have not shown that prazosin causes birth defects. However, in rats given many times the highest recommended human dose, lower birth weights were seen.

Breast-feeding—Prazosin passes into breast milk in small amounts. However, it has not been reported to cause problems in nursing babies.

Children—Studies on this medicine have been done only in adult patients, and there is no specific information comparing use of prazosin in children with use in other age groups.

Older adults—Dizziness, lightheadedness, or fainting (especially when getting up from a lying or sitting position) may be more likely to occur in the elderly, who are more sensitive to the effects of prazosin. In addition, prazosin may reduce tolerance to cold temperatures in elderly patients.

Other medicines—Although certain medicines should not be used together at all, in other cases two different medicines may be used together even if an interaction might occur. In these cases, your doctor may want to change the dose, or other precautions may be necessary. Tell your doctor and pharmacist if you are taking any other prescription or nonprescription (over-the-counter [OTC]) medicine.

Other medical problems—The presence of other medical problems may affect the use of prazosin. Make sure you tell your doctor if you have any other medical problems, especially:
- Angina (chest pain)—Prazosin may make this condition worse
- Heart disease (severe)—Prazosin may make this condition worse
- Kidney disease—Possible increased sensitivity to the effects of prazosin

Before you begin using any new medicine (prescription or nonprescription) or if you develop any new medical problem while you are using this medicine, check with your doctor, nurse, or pharmacist.

Proper Use of This Medicine

For patients *taking this medicine for high blood pressure:*
- In addition to the use of the medicine your doctor has prescribed, treatment for your high blood pressure may include weight control and care in the types of foods you eat, especially foods high in sodium. Your doctor will tell you which of these are most important for you. You should check with your doctor before changing your diet.
- Many patients who have high blood pressure will not notice any signs of the problem. In fact, many may feel normal. It is very important that you *take your medicine exactly as directed* and that you keep your appointments with your doctor even if you feel well.
- Remember that prazosin will not cure your high blood pressure but it does help control it. Therefore, you must continue to take it as directed if you expect to lower your blood pressure and keep it down. *You may have to take high blood pressure medicine for the rest of your life.* If high blood pressure is not treated, it can cause serious problems such as heart failure, blood vessel disease, stroke, or kidney disease.

To help you remember to take your medicine, try to get into the habit of taking it at the same time each day.

Missed dose—If you miss a dose of this medicine, take it as soon as possible. However, if it is almost time for your next dose, skip the missed dose and go back to your regular dosing schedule. Do not double doses.

Storage—To store this medicine:
- Keep out of the reach of children.
- Store away from heat and direct light.

- Do not store in the bathroom, near the kitchen sink, or in other damp places. Heat or moisture may cause the medicine to break down.
- Do not keep outdated medicine or medicine no longer needed. Be sure that any discarded medicine is out of the reach of children.

Precautions While Using This Medicine

It is important that your doctor check your progress at regular visits to make sure that this medicine is working properly.

For patients *taking this medicine for high blood pressure:*

- *Do not take other medicines unless they have been discussed with your doctor.* This especially includes over-the-counter (nonprescription) medicines for appetite control, asthma, colds, cough, hay fever, or sinus problems, since they may tend to make prazosin less effective.

Dizziness, lightheadedness, or sudden fainting may occur after you take this medicine, especially when you get up from a lying or sitting position. These effects are more likely to occur when you take the first dose of this medicine. Taking the first dose at bedtime may prevent problems. However, *be especially careful if you need to get up during the night.* These effects may also occur with any doses you take after the first dose. Getting up slowly may help lessen this problem. *If you feel dizzy, lie down so that you do not faint.* Then sit for a few moments before standing to prevent the dizziness from returning.

The dizziness, lightheadedness, or fainting is more likely to occur if you drink alcohol, stand for a long time, exercise, or if the weather is hot. *While you are taking this medicine, be careful to limit the amount of alcohol you drink. Also, use extra care during exercise or hot weather or if you must stand for a long time.*

Prazosin may cause some people to become drowsy or less alert than they are normally. *Make sure you know how you react to this medicine before you drive, use machines, or do anything else that could be dangerous if you are dizzy, drowsy, or are not alert.* After you have taken several doses of this medicine, these effects should lessen.

Side Effects of This Medicine

Along with its needed effects, a medicine may cause some unwanted effects. Although not all of these side effects may occur, if they do occur they may need medical attention.

Check with your doctor as soon as possible if any of the following side effects occur:

More common

Dizziness or lightheadedness, especially when getting up from a lying or sitting position; fainting (sudden)

Less common

Loss of bladder control; pounding heartbeat; swelling of feet or lower legs

Rare

Chest pain; painful inappropriate erection of penis (continuing); shortness of breath

Other side effects may occur that usually do not need medical attention. These side effects may go away during treatment as your body adjusts to the medicine. However, check with your doctor if any of the following side effects continue or are bothersome:

More common

Drowsiness; headache; lack of energy

Less common

Dryness of mouth; nervousness; unusual tiredness or weakness

Rare

Nausea; frequent urge to urinate

Other side effects not listed above may also occur in some patients. If you notice any other effects, check with your doctor.

Additional Information

Once a medicine has been approved for marketing for a certain use, experience may show that it is also useful for other medical problems. Although these uses are not included in product labeling, prazosin is used in certain patients with the following medical conditions:

- Congestive heart failure
- Ergot alkaloid poisoning
- Pheochromocytoma
- Raynaud's disease
- Benign enlargement of the prostate

Other than the above information, there is no additional information relating to proper use, precautions, or side effects for these uses.

Annual revision: 06/09/92

PRAZOSIN AND POLYTHIAZIDE Systemic†

A commonly used brand name in the U.S. is Minizide.

†Not commercially available in Canada.

Description

Prazosin (PRA-zoe-sin) and polythiazide (pol-i-THYE-a-zide) combination is used in the treatment of high blood pressure (hypertension).

High blood pressure adds to the workload of the heart and arteries. If it continues for a long time, the heart and arteries may not function properly. This can damage the blood vessels of the brain, heart, and kidneys resulting in a stroke, heart failure, or kidney failure. High blood pressure may also increase the risk of heart attacks. These problems may be less likely to occur if blood pressure is controlled.

Prazosin works by relaxing blood vessels so that blood passes through them more easily. The polythiazide in this combination is a thiazide diuretic (water pill) that helps to reduce the amount of water in the body by increasing the flow of urine. Both of these actions help to lower blood pressure.

This medicine is available only with your doctor's prescription, in the following dosage form:

Oral

- Capsules (U.S.)

It is very important that you read and understand the following information. If any of it causes you special concern, check with your doctor. Also, *if you have any questions* or if you want more information about this medicine or your medical problem, *ask your doctor, nurse, or pharmacist.*

Before Using This Medicine

In deciding to use a medicine, the risks of taking the medicine must be weighed against the good it will do. This is a decision you and your doctor will make. For prazosin and polythiazide, the following should be considered:

Allergies—Tell your doctor if you have ever had any unusual or allergic reaction to prazosin, sulfonamides (sulfa drugs), bumetanide, furosemide, acetazolamide, dichlorphenamide, methazolamide, or any of the thiazide diuretics. Also tell your doctor and pharmacist if you are allergic to any other substance, such as foods, preservatives, or dyes.

Pregnancy—When polythiazide (contained in this combination medicine) is used during pregnancy, it may cause side effects including jaundice, blood problems, and low potassium in the newborn infant. The combination of prazosin and polythiazide has not been shown to cause birth defects.

Breast-feeding—Polythiazide passes into breast milk. Prazosin passes into breast milk in small amounts. However, prazosin and polythiazide combination has not been reported to cause problems in nursing babies.

Children—Although there is no specific information about the use of this medicine in children, it is not expected to cause different side effects or problems in children than it does in adults. However, extra caution may be necessary in infants with jaundice, because these medicines can make the condition worse.

Older adults—Dizziness, lightheadedness, or fainting or symptoms of too much potassium loss may be more likely to occur in the elderly, who are more sensitive to the effects of prazosin and polythiazide. In addition, this medicine may reduce tolerance to cold temperatures in elderly patients.

Other medicines—Although certain medicines should not be used together at all, in other cases two different medicines may be used together even if an interaction might occur. In these cases, your doctor may want to change the dose, or other precautions may be necessary. When you are taking prazosin and polythiazide, it is especially important that your doctor and pharmacist know if you are taking any of the following:

- Cholestyramine or
- Colestipol—Use with thiazide diuretics may prevent the diuretic from working properly; take the diuretic at least 1 hour before or 4 hours after cholestyramine or colestipol
- Digitalis glycosides (heart medicine)—Polythiazide may cause low potassium in the blood, which can lead to symptoms of digitalis toxicity
- Lithium (e.g., Lithane)—Risk of lithium overdose, even at usual doses, may be increased

Other medical problems—The presence of other medical problems may affect the use of prazosin and polythiazide. Make sure you tell your doctor if you have any other medical problems, especially:

- Angina (chest pain) or
- Heart disease (severe)—Prazosin may make these conditions worse
- Diabetes mellitus (sugar diabetes)—Polythiazide may increase the amount of sugar in the blood
- Gout (history of) or
- Lupus erythematosus (history of) or
- Pancreatitis (inflammation of the pancreas)—Thiazide diuretics may make these conditions worse
- Kidney disease—Effects of this combination medicine may be increased because of increased sensitivity to the effects of prazosin and slower removal of polythiazide from the body. If kidney disease is severe, polythiazide may not work

- Liver disease—If polythiazide causes loss of too much water from the body, liver disease can become much worse

Before you begin using any new medicine (prescription or nonprescription) or if you develop any new medical problem while you are using this medicine, check with your doctor, nurse, or pharmacist.

Proper Use of This Medicine

In addition to the use of the medicine your doctor has prescribed, treatment for your high blood pressure may include weight control and care in the types of foods you eat, especially foods high in sodium. Your doctor will tell you which of these are most important for you. You should check with your doctor before changing your diet.

Many patients who have high blood pressure will not notice any signs of the problem. In fact, many may feel normal. It is very important that you *take your medicine exactly as directed* and that you keep your appointments with your doctor even if you feel well.

Remember that this medicine will not cure your high blood pressure but it does help control it. Therefore, you must continue to take it as directed if you expect to lower your blood pressure and keep it down. *You may have to take high blood pressure medicine for the rest of your life.* If high blood pressure is not treated, it can cause serious problems such as heart failure, blood vessel disease, stroke, or kidney disease.

This medicine may cause you to have an unusual feeling of tiredness when you begin to take it. You may also notice an increase in the amount of urine or in your frequency of urination. After taking the medicine for a while, these effects should lessen.

It is best to plan your dose or doses according to a schedule that will least affect your personal activities and sleep. Ask your doctor, nurse, or pharmacist to help you plan the best time to take this medicine.

To help you remember to take your medicine, try to get into the habit of taking it at the same time each day.

Missed dose—If you miss a dose of this medicine, take it as soon as possible. However, if it is almost time for your next dose, skip the missed dose and go back to your regular dosing schedule. Do not double doses.

Storage—To store this medicine:

- Keep out of the reach of children.
- Store away from heat and direct light.
- Do not store in the bathroom, near the kitchen sink, or in other damp places. Heat or moisture may cause the medicine to break down.
- Do not keep outdated medicine or medicine no longer needed. Be sure that any discarded medicine is out of the reach of children.

Precautions While Using This Medicine

It is important that your doctor check your progress at regular visits to make sure this medicine is working properly.

Do not take other medicines unless they have been discussed with your doctor. This especially includes over-the-counter (nonprescription) medicine for appetite control, asthma, colds, cough, hay fever, or sinus problems, since they may tend to increase your blood pressure.

This medicine may cause a loss of potassium from your body.

- To help prevent this, your doctor may want you to:
  —eat or drink foods that have a high potassium content (for example, orange or other citrus fruit juices), or
  —take a potassium supplement, or
  —take another medicine to help prevent the loss of the potassium in the first place.
- It is very important to follow these directions. Also, it is important not to change your diet on your own. This is more important if you are already on a special diet (as for diabetes), or if you are taking a potassium supplement or a medicine to reduce potassium loss. Extra potassium may not be necessary and, in some cases, too much potassium could be harmful.

Check with your doctor if you become sick and have severe or continuing vomiting or diarrhea. These problems may cause you to lose additional water and potassium.

Dizziness, lightheadedness, or sudden fainting may occur after you take this medicine, especially when you get up from a lying or sitting position. These effects are more likely to occur when you take the first dose of this medicine. Taking the first dose at bedtime may prevent problems. However, *be especially careful if you need to get up during the night.* These effects may also occur with any doses you take after the first dose. Getting up slowly may help lessen this problem. *If you feel dizzy, lie down so that you do not faint.* Then sit for a few moments before standing to prevent the dizziness from returning.

Make sure you know how you react to this medicine before you drive, use machines, or do anything else that could be dangerous if you are dizzy or are not alert. After you have taken several doses of this medicine, these effects should lessen.

The dizziness, lightheadedness, or fainting is also more likely to occur if you drink alcohol, stand for a long time, exercise, or if the weather is hot. *While you are taking this medicine, be careful to limit the amount of alcohol you drink. Also, use extra care during exercise or hot weather or if you must stand for a long time.*

For *diabetic patients*:

- Polythiazide (contained in this combination medicine) may raise blood sugar levels. While you are using this medicine, be especially careful in testing for sugar in your blood or urine. If you have any questions about this, check with your doctor.

Some people who take this medicine may become more sensitive to sunlight than they are normally. Exposure to sunlight, even for brief periods of time, may cause a skin rash, itching, redness or other discoloration of the skin, or a severe sunburn. When you begin taking this medicine:

- Stay out of direct sunlight, especially between the hours of 10:00 a.m. and 3:00 p.m., if possible.
- Wear protective clothing, including a hat and sunglasses.
- Apply a sun block product that has a skin protection factor (SPF) of at least 15. Some patients may require a product with a higher SPF number, especially if they have a fair complexion. If you have any questions about this, check with your doctor or pharmacist.
- Do not use a sunlamp or tanning bed or booth.
- Apply a sun block lipstick that has an SPF of at least 15 to protect your lips.

If you have a severe reaction from the sun, check with your doctor.

Side Effects of This Medicine

Along with its needed effects, a medicine may cause some unwanted effects. Although not all of these side effects may occur, if they do occur they may need medical attention.

Check with your doctor as soon as possible if any of the following side effects occur, especially since some of them may mean that your body is losing too much potassium:

Signs and symptoms of too much potassium loss

Dryness of mouth (severe); increased thirst; irregular heartbeat (continuing); mood or mental changes; muscle cramps or pain; nausea or vomiting; unusual tiredness or weakness; weak pulse

Signs and symptoms of too much sodium loss

Confusion; convulsions; decreased mental activity; irritability; muscle cramps; unusual tiredness or weakness

More common

Dizziness or lightheadedness, especially when getting up from a lying or sitting position; sudden fainting

Less common

Inability to control urination; irregular heartbeat; pounding heartbeat; swelling of feet or lower legs; weight gain

Rare

Black, tarry stools; blood in urine or stools; chest pain; cough or hoarseness; fever or chills; joint pain; lower back or side pain; painful or difficult urination; painful, inappropriate erection of penis, continuing; pinpoint red spots on skin; shortness of breath; skin rash or hives; stomach pain (severe) with nausea and vomiting; unusual bleeding or bruising; yellow eyes or skin

Other side effects may occur that usually do not need medical attention. These side effects may go away during treatment as your body adjusts to the medicine. However, check with your doctor if any of the following side effects continue or are bothersome:

Less common

Decreased sexual ability; diarrhea; drowsiness; headache; increased sensitivity of skin to sunlight; lack of energy; loss of appetite; nervousness; stomach upset or pain

Rare

Frequent urge to urinate; nausea

Other side effects not listed above may also occur in some patients. If you notice any other effects, check with your doctor.

Annual revision: 07/21/92

PREGNANCY TEST KITS FOR HOME USE

Some commonly used brand names are:

In the U.S.

Advance
Answer
Answer II
Answer Plus
Answer Plus II
Answer Quick & Simple
ClearBlue Pregnancy Test
Daisy 2
e.p.t. Stick-test
Fact Plus
First Response 5 Minute Pregnancy Test
PTK Plus
Q-test

Description

Pregnancy test kits may be purchased without a prescription for use in the home. The materials in the kit are designed to detect a hormone, human chorionic gonadotropin (HCG), in the urine.

HCG is produced by the fertilized egg (ovum) when it implants in the woman's uterus, and can be found in the urine 1 to 2 weeks after the fertilized ovum is implanted in the uterus. HCG helps make the hormones necessary for pregnancy and disappears from the woman's urine and blood when pregnancy is over. Therefore, it is seen as a way to tell when pregnancy has occurred.

Test kits can usually detect a pregnancy as early as 1 day after the first missed period should have started. Many kits contain enough materials for 2 tests, and advise that a second test be performed 7 days later if the first test is negative.

It is important to have the pregnancy confirmed by a health care professional as soon as a woman thinks she is pregnant. The pregnancy due date should be determined. Early prenatal care benefits both the mother and baby by checking for possible problems in the pregnancy. Also, women should avoid drugs, tobacco, alcohol, x-rays, and other treatments that can be harmful to the fetus.

Before Using This Test Kit

It is important to get the correct result from a home pregnancy test kit. Therefore, the following should be considered by you and possibly your doctor before you decide to use one of these test kits:

Medicines—Certain medicines may affect your pregnancy test and cause a false result. Check with your doctor if you are taking any medicines, especially:

- Anticonvulsants (seizure medicine)
- Medicine for mental problems

Medical conditions—The presence of certain medical conditions may affect your pregnancy test and cause a false test result. Check with your doctor if you have any medical conditions, especially:

- Abortion (incomplete or recent)
- Cancer
- Certain problems of the ovaries
- Delivery of a baby (recent)
- Endometriosis
- Menopause (change of life)
- Pregnancy (abnormal or tubal)
- Thyroid disease
- Urinary tract infection

Also, if you have vision problems (such as color-blindness or poor vision), you will need someone to help you in reading your test results

Proper Use of This Test Kit

Check the expiration date printed on the package before purchasing. Do not use an outdated test kit. Outdated test kits will not work properly.

To use:

- Read and follow the test kit instructions carefully. Be careful not to skip or rush any steps.
- Collect a urine sample in a clean, dry container according to the written package instructions. Pregnancy tests are best done on the first morning urine.
- Choose a well-lighted area with normal room temperature and humidity. Perform the test on a clean, dry working surface with a cold water faucet nearby. You will also need a watch, timer, or clock that can measure in seconds.
- Be careful not to touch the areas of the kit where you will put urine. Skin oils or perspiration may affect the test results. It is also important that you use clean, dry test materials. If no container comes with the test kit, use one that is clean and dry. Traces of old test chemicals or soaps may affect test reactions if materials are reused.
- At the end of the timing period, compare the color of the test with the color chart on the package. The test colors will begin to fade after this period has passed or as the test paper begins to dry.
- Record your test results and the date you did the test, to discuss your results with your doctor.

Storage—To store this product:

- Keep out of the reach of children. Test kit chemicals can be poisonous if swallowed.
- Store these test kits in their original containers. Keep the container tightly closed.
- Keep in a cool, dry place, away from heat, humidity (such as the bathroom or shower area), and direct sunlight. Heat-exposed test kits will not work properly.
- Do not refrigerate this product. Keep the kit from freezing.
- Discard used tests in the trash. Liquids may be poured down the drain or flushed in the toilet. Be sure that any discarded test kit is out of the reach of children.

About Your Test Results

Notify your doctor if the pregnancy test is positive, so that you can begin regular prenatal care.

If the test is negative, retest your urine after 7 days. If the test results are still negative after the second test and you still have not started your menstrual period, you should still see your doctor.

If you have any other questions about your results or about the use of pregnancy test kits, ask your doctor or pharmacist. Also, most kits have a toll-free number for advice on using them.

Annual revision: 07/20/93

PRIMAQUINE Systemic

Generic name product may be available in the U.S. and Canada.

Description

Primaquine (PRIM-a-kween) belongs to the group of medicines called antiprotozoals. It is used in the treatment of malaria.

Primaquine is available only with your doctor's prescription, in the following dosage form:

Oral

- Tablets (U.S. and Canada)

It is very important that you read and understand the following information. If any of it causes you special concern, check with your doctor. Also, *if you have any questions* or if you want more information about this medicine or your medical problem, *ask your doctor, nurse, or pharmacist.*

Before Using This Medicine

In deciding to use a medicine, the risks of taking the medicine must be weighed against the good it will do. This is a decision you and your doctor will make. For primaquine, the following should be considered:

Allergies—Tell your doctor if you have ever had any unusual or allergic reaction to primaquine or iodoquinol (e.g., Yodoxin). Also tell your doctor and pharmacist if you are allergic to any other substances, such as foods, preservatives, or dyes.

Pregnancy—Primaquine is not recommended for use during pregnancy.

Breast-feeding—It is not known if primaquine is excreted in breast milk. However, primaquine has not been reported to cause problems in nursing babies.

Children—Although there is no specific information comparing use of primaquine in children with use in other age groups, this medicine is not expected to cause different side effects or problems in children than it does in adults.

Older adults—Many medicines have not been studied specifically in older people. Therefore, it may not be known whether they work exactly the same way they do in younger adults or if they cause different side effects or problems in older people. There is no specific information comparing use of primaquine in the elderly with use in other age groups.

Other medicines—Although certain medicines should not be used together at all, in other cases two different medicines may be used together even if an interaction might occur. In these cases, your doctor may want to change the dose, or other precautions may be necessary. When you are taking primaquine it is especially important that your doctor and pharmacist know if you are taking any of the following:

- Acetohydroxamic acid (e.g., Lithostat) or
- Antidiabetics, oral (diabetes medicine you take by mouth) or
- Dapsone or
- Furazolidone (e.g., Furoxone) or
- Methyldopa (e.g., Aldomet) or
- Nitrofurantoin (e.g., Furadantin) or
- Procainamide (e.g., Pronestyl) or
- Quinacrine (e.g., Atabrine) or
- Quinidine (e.g., Quinidex) or
- Quinine (e.g., Quinamm) or
- Sulfonamides (sulfa medicine) or
- Sulfoxone (e.g., Diasone) or
- Vitamin K (e.g., AquaMEPHYTON, Synkayvite)—Taking these medicines with primaquine may increase the chance of side effects affecting the blood

Other medical problems—The presence of other medical problems may affect the use of primaquine. Make sure you tell your doctor if you have any other medical problems, especially:

- Family or personal history of favism or hemolytic anemia or
- Glucose-6-phosphate dehydrogenase (G6PD) deficiency or
- Nicotinamide adenine dinucleotide (NADH) methemoglobin reductase deficiency—Patients with any of these medical problems who take primaquine may have an increased chance of side effects affecting the blood

Before you begin using any new medicine (prescription or nonprescription) or if you develop any new medical problem while you are using this medicine, check with your doctor, nurse, or pharmacist.

Proper Use of This Medicine

If this medicine upsets your stomach, it may be taken with meals or antacids. If stomach upset (nausea, vomiting, or stomach pain) continues, check with your doctor.

If you are taking primaquine for malaria, *keep taking it for the full time of treatment* to help prevent or completely clear up the infection. *Do not miss any doses.*

Dosing—The dose of primaquine will be different for different patients. *Follow your doctor's orders or the directions on the label.* The following information includes only the average doses of primaquine. *If your dose is different, do not change it* unless your doctor tells you to do so.

- The number of tablets that you take depends on the strength of the medicine. Also, *the number of doses you take each day, the time allowed between doses, and the length of time you take the medicine depend on the medical problem for which you are taking primaquine.*

- For the *treatment of malaria*:

  —Adults and older children: 26.3 mg of primaquine phosphate (which equals 15 mg of primaquine base) once a day for fourteen days.

  —Younger children: Dose is based on body weight and must be determined by the doctor.

Missed dose—If you do miss a dose of this medicine, take it as soon as possible. However, if it is almost time for your next dose, skip the missed dose and go back to your regular dosing schedule. Do not double doses.

Storage—To store this medicine:
- Keep out of the reach of children.
- Store away from heat and direct light.
- Do not store in the bathroom, near the kitchen sink, or in other damp places. Heat or moisture may cause the medicine to break down.
- Do not keep outdated medicine or medicine no longer needed. Be sure that any discarded medicine is out of the reach of children.

Precautions While Using This Medicine

Your doctor should check your progress at regular visits to make sure that primaquine is not causing blood problems.

Side Effects of This Medicine

Along with its needed effects, a medicine may cause some unwanted effects. Although not all of these side effects may occur, if they do occur they may need medical attention.

Check with your doctor immediately if any of the following side effects occur:

More common

Back, leg, or stomach pains; dark urine; fever; loss of appetite; pale skin; unusual tiredness or weakness

Less common

Bluish fingernails, lips, or skin; dizziness or lightheadedness; difficulty breathing

Rare

Sore throat and fever

Other side effects may occur that usually do not need medical attention. These side effects may go away during treatment as your body adjusts to the medicine. However, check with your doctor if any of the following side effects continue or are bothersome:

More common

Nausea or vomiting; stomach pain or cramps

Other side effects not listed above may also occur in some patients. If you notice any other effects, check with your doctor.

Additional Information

Once a medicine has been approved for marketing for a certain use, experience may show that it is also useful for other medical problems. Although this use is not included in product labeling, primaquine is used in certain patients with the following medical condition:
- *Pneumocystis carinii* pneumonia (PCP)

Other than the above information, there is no additional information relating to proper use, precautions, or side effects for this use.

Annual revision: 01/19/93

PRIMIDONE Systemic

Some commonly used brand names are:

In the U.S.

Myidone
Mysoline
Generic name product may also be available.

In Canada

Apo-Primidone
Mysoline
PMS Primidone
Sertan
Generic name product may also be available.

Description

Primidone (PRYE-mih-done) belongs to the group of medicines called anticonvulsants. It is used in the treatment of epilepsy to manage certain types of seizures. Primidone may be used alone or in combination with other anticonvulsants. It acts by controlling nerve impulses in the brain.

Primidone is available only with your doctor's prescription, in the following dosage forms:

Oral

- Suspension (U.S.)
- Tablets (U.S. and Canada)
- Chewable tablets (Canada)

It is very important that you read and understand the following information. If any of it causes you special concern, check with your doctor. Also, *if you have any questions* or if you want more information about this medicine or your medical problem, *ask your doctor, nurse, or pharmacist.*

Before Using This Medicine

In deciding to use a medicine, the risks of taking the medicine must be weighed against the good it will do. This is a decision you and your doctor will make. For primidone, the following should be considered:

Allergies—Tell your doctor if you have ever had any unusual or allergic reaction to primidone or to any barbiturate medicine (for example, amobarbital, butabarbital, pentobarbital, phenobarbital, secobarbital). Also tell your doctor and pharmacist if you are allergic to any other substances, such as foods, preservatives, or dyes.

Pregnancy—Although most mothers who take medicine for seizure control deliver normal babies, there are reports of increased birth defects when these medicines are used during pregnancy. Newborns whose mothers were taking primidone during pregnancy have been reported to have bleeding problems. It is not definitely known if any of these medicines are the cause of such problems.

Breast-feeding—Primidone passes into the breast milk and may cause unusual drowsiness in nursing babies. It may be necessary for you to take another medicine or to stop breast-feeding during treatment. Be sure you have discussed the risks and benefits of the medicine with your doctor.

Children—Unusual excitement or restlessness may occur in children, who are usually more sensitive than adults to these effects of primidone.

Older adults—Unusual excitement or restlessness may occur in elderly patients, who are usually more sensitive than younger adults to these effects of primidone.

Other medicines—Although certain medicines should not be used together at all, in other cases 2 different medicines may be used together even if an interaction might occur. In these cases, your doctor may want to change the dose, or other precautions may be necessary. When you are taking primidone it is especially important that your doctor and pharmacist know if you are taking any of the following:

- Adrenocorticoids (cortisone-like medicines) or
- Anticoagulants (blood thinners)—Use with primidone may decrease the effects of these medications, and the amount of medicine you need to take may change
- Central nervous system (CNS) depressants (medicine that causes drowsiness)—Using these medicines with primidone may increase the CNS and other depressant effects
- Oral contraceptives (birth control pills) containing estrogen—Primidone may decrease the effectiveness of these oral contraceptives, and you may need to change to a different type of birth control
- Other anticonvulsants (seizure medicine)—A change in the pattern of seizures may occur; close monitoring of blood levels of both medications is recommended. Use of valproic acid with primidone may cause increased CNS depression and other serious side effects
- Monoamine oxidase (MAO) inhibitors (furazolidone [e.g., Furoxone], isocarboxazid [e.g., Marplan], phenelzine [e.g., Nardil], procarbazine [e.g., Matulane], selegiline [e.g., Eldepryl], tranylcypromine [e.g., Parnate])—Taking primidone while you are taking or within 2 weeks of taking monoamine oxidase (MAO) inhibitors may prolong the effects of primidone and may change the pattern of seizures

Other medical problems—The presence of other medical problems may affect the use of primidone. Make sure you tell your doctor if you have any other medical problems, especially:

- Asthma, emphysema, or chronic lung disease—Primidone may cause serious problems in breathing
- Hyperactivity (in children) or
- Kidney disease or
- Liver disease—Primidone may make the condition worse
- Porphyria—Primidone should not be used when this medical problem exists because it may make the condition worse

Before you begin using any new medicine (prescription or nonprescription) or if you develop any new medical problem while you are using this medicine, check with your doctor, nurse, or pharmacist.

Proper Use of This Medicine

Take primidone every day in regularly spaced doses as ordered by your doctor. This will provide the proper amount of medicine needed to prevent seizures.

Missed dose—If you miss a dose of this medicine, take it as soon as possible. However, if it is within an hour of your next dose, skip the missed dose and go back to your regular dosing schedule. Do not double doses.

Storage—To store this medicine:

- Keep out of the reach of children.
- Store away from heat and direct light.
- Do not store the tablet form of this medicine in the bathroom, near the kitchen sink, or in other damp places. Heat or moisture may cause the medicine to break down.
- Keep the liquid form of this medicine from freezing.

- Do not keep outdated medicine or medicine no longer needed. Be sure that any discarded medicine is out of the reach of children.

Precautions While Using This Medicine

It is very important that your doctor check your progress at regular visits, especially during the first few months of treatment with primidone. This will allow your doctor to adjust the amount of medicine you are taking to meet your needs.

If you have been taking primidone regularly for several weeks, you should not suddenly stop taking it. Your doctor may want you to reduce gradually the amount you are taking before stopping completely.

Before you have any medical tests, tell the medical doctor in charge that you are taking this medicine. The results of some tests (such as the metyrapone and phentolamine tests) may be affected by this medicine.

Before having any kind of surgery, dental treatment, or emergency treatment, tell the medical doctor or dentist in charge that you are using this medicine.

This medicine will add to the effects of alcohol and other CNS depressants (medicines that slow down the nervous system, possibly causing drowsiness). Some examples of CNS depressants are antihistamines or medicine for hay fever, other allergies, or colds; sedatives, tranquilizers, or sleeping medicine; prescription pain medicine or narcotics; barbiturates; medicine for seizures; muscle relaxants; or anesthetics, including some dental anesthetics. *Check with your doctor before taking any of the above while you are using this medicine.*

Primidone may cause some people to become dizzy, lightheaded, drowsy, or less alert than they are normally. Even if taken at bedtime, it may cause some people to feel drowsy or less alert on arising. *Make sure you know how you react to this medicine before you drive, use machines, or do anything else that could be dangerous if you are dizzy or are not alert.*

Oral contraceptives (birth control pills) containing estrogen may not work properly if you take them while you are taking primidone. Unplanned pregnancies may occur. You should use a different or additional means of birth control while you are taking primidone. If you have any questions about this, check with your doctor or pharmacist.

Side Effects of This Medicine

Along with its needed effects, a medicine may cause some unwanted effects. Although not all of these side effects may occur, if they do occur they may need medical attention.

Check with your doctor if any of the following side effects occur:

Less common

Unusual excitement or restlessness (especially in children and in the elderly)

Rare

Skin rash; unusual tiredness or weakness

Symptoms of overdose

Confusion; continuous, uncontrolled back-and-forth and/or rolling eye movements; double vision; shortness of breath or troubled breathing

Other side effects may occur that usually do not need medical attention. These side effects may go away during treatment as your body adjusts to the medicine. However, check with your doctor if any of the following side effects continue or are bothersome:

More common

Clumsiness or unsteadiness; dizziness

Less common

Decreased sexual ability; drowsiness; loss of appetite; mood or mental changes; nausea or vomiting

Other side effects not listed above may also occur in some patients. If you notice any other effects, check with your doctor.

Additional Information

Once a medicine has been approved for marketing for a certain use, experience may show that it is also useful for other medical problems. Although this use is not included in product labeling, primidone is used in certain patients with the following medical conditions:

- Essential tremor

Other than the above information, there is no additional information relating to proper use, precautions, or side effects for these uses.

Annual revision: 01/27/92

PROBENECID Systemic

Some commonly used brand names are:

In the U.S.

Benemid Probalan

Generic name product may also be available.

In Canada

Benemid Benuryl

Description

Probenecid (proe-BEN-e-sid) is used in the treatment of chronic gout or gouty arthritis. These conditions are caused by too much uric acid in the blood. The medicine works by removing the extra uric acid from the body. Probenecid does not cure gout, but after you have been taking it for a few months it will help prevent gout attacks. This medicine will help prevent gout attacks only as long as you continue to take it.

Probenecid is also used to prevent or treat other medical problems that may occur if too much uric acid is present in the body.

Probenecid is sometimes used with certain kinds of antibiotics to make them more effective in the treatment of infections.

Probenecid is available only with your doctor's prescription, in the following dosage form:

Oral

- Tablets (U.S. and Canada)

It is very important that you read and understand the following information. If any of it causes you special concern, check with your doctor. Also, *if you have any questions* or if you want more information about this medicine or your medical problem, *ask your doctor, nurse, or pharmacist.*

Before Using This Medicine

In deciding to use a medicine, the risks of taking the medicine must be weighed against the good it will do. This is a decision you and your doctor will make. For probenecid, the following should be considered:

Allergies—Tell your doctor if you have ever had any unusual or allergic reaction to probenecid. Also tell your doctor and pharmacist if you are allergic to any other substances, such as foods, preservatives, or dyes.

Pregnancy—Probenecid has not been shown to cause birth defects or other problems in humans.

Breast-feeding—Probenecid has not been reported to cause problems in nursing babies.

Children—Probenecid has been tested in children 2 to 14 years of age for use together with antibiotics. It has not been shown to cause different side effects or problems than it does in adults. Studies on the effects of probenecid in patients with gout have been done only in adults. Gout is very rare in children.

Older adults—Many medicines have not been studied specifically in older people. Therefore, it may not be known whether they work exactly the same way they do in younger adults. There is no specific information comparing use of probenecid in the elderly with use in other age groups.

Other medicines—Although certain medicines should not be used together at all, in other cases two different medicines may be used together even if an interaction might occur. In these cases, your doctor may want to change the dose, or other precautions may be necessary. When you are taking probenecid, it is especially important that your doctor and pharmacist know if you are taking any of the following:

- Antineoplastics (cancer medicine)—The chance of serious side effects may be increased
- Aspirin or other salicylates—These medicines may keep probenecid from working properly for treating gout, depending on the amount of aspirin or other salicylate that you take and how often you take it
- Heparin—Probenecid may increase the effects of heparin, which increases the chance of side effects
- Indomethacin (e.g., Indocin) or
- Ketoprofen (e.g., Orudis) or
- Methotrexate (e.g., Mexate)—Probenecid may increase the blood levels of these medicines, which increases the chance of side effects
- Medicine for infection, including tuberculosis or virus infection—Probenecid may increase the blood levels of many of these medicines. In some cases, this is a desired effect and probenecid may be used to help the other medicine work better. However, the chance of side effects is sometimes also increased
- Nitrofurantoin (e.g., Furadantin)—Probenecid may keep nitrofurantoin from working properly
- Zidovudine (e.g., AZT, Retrovir)—Probenecid increases the blood level of zidovudine and may allow lower doses of zidovudine to be used. However, the chance of side effects is also increased

Other medical problems—The presence of other medical problems may affect the use of probenecid. Make sure you tell your doctor if you have any other medical problems, especially:

- Blood disease or
- Cancer being treated by antineoplastics (cancer medicine) or radiation (x-rays) or
- Kidney disease or stones (or history of) or
- Stomach ulcer (history of)—The chance of side effects may be increased

Before you begin using any new medicine (prescription or nonprescription) or if you develop any new medical

problem while you are using this medicine, check with your doctor, nurse, or pharmacist.

Proper Use of This Medicine

If probenecid upsets your stomach, it may be taken with food. If this does not work, an antacid may be taken. If stomach upset (nausea, vomiting, or loss of appetite) continues, check with your doctor.

For patients taking probenecid *for gout:*

- After you begin to take probenecid, gout attacks may continue to occur for a while. However, if you take this medicine regularly as directed by your doctor, the attacks will gradually become less frequent and less painful than before. After you have been taking probenecid for several months, they may stop completely.
- This medicine will help prevent gout attacks but it will not relieve an attack that has already started. *Even if you take another medicine for gout attacks, continue to take this medicine also.* If you have any questions about this, check with your doctor.

For patients taking probenecid *for gout or to help remove uric acid from the body:*

- When you first begin taking probenecid, the amount of uric acid in the kidneys is greatly increased. This may cause kidney stones or other kidney problems in some people. To help prevent this, your doctor may want you to drink at least 10 to 12 full glasses (8 ounces each) of fluids each day, or to take another medicine to make your urine less acid. It is important that you follow your doctor's instructions very carefully.

Dosing—The dose of probenecid will be different for different patients. *Follow your doctor's orders or the directions on the label.* The following information includes only the average doses of probenecid. *If your dose is different, do not change it* unless your doctor tells you to do so.

- *For treating gout or removing uric acid from the body:*
  —Adults: 250 mg (one-half of a 500-mg tablet) two times a day for about one week, then 500 mg (one tablet) two times a day for a few weeks. After this, the dose will depend on the amount of uric acid in your blood or urine. Most people need 2, 3, or 4 tablets a day, but some people may need higher doses.
  —Children: It is not likely that probenecid will be needed to treat gout or to remove uric acid from the body in children. If a child needs this medicine, however, the dose would have to be determined by the doctor.
- *For helping antibiotics work better:*
  —Adults: The amount of probenecid will depend on the condition being treated. Sometimes, only one dose of 2 tablets is needed. Other times, the dose will be 1 tablet four times a day.
  —Children: The dose will have to be determined by the doctor. It depends on the child's weight, as well as on the condition being treated. Older children and teenagers may need the same amount as adults.

Missed dose—If you are taking probenecid regularly and you miss a dose, take the missed dose as soon as possible. However, if you do not remember until it is almost time for the next dose, skip the missed dose and go back to your regular dosing schedule. Do not double doses.

Storage—To store this medicine:

- Keep out of the reach of children.
- Store away from heat and direct light.
- Do not store this medicine in the bathroom, near the kitchen sink, or in other damp places. Heat or moisture may cause the medicine to break down.
- Do not keep outdated medicine or medicine no longer needed. Be sure that any discarded medicine is out of the reach of children.

Precautions While Using This Medicine

If you will be taking probenecid for more than a few weeks, your doctor should check your progress at regular visits.

Before you have any medical tests, tell the person in charge that you are taking this medicine. The results of some tests may be affected by probenecid.

For *diabetic patients:*

- Probenecid may cause false test results with copper sulfate urine sugar tests (Clinitest®), but not with glucose enzymatic urine sugar tests (Clinistix®). If you have any questions about this, check with your doctor or pharmacist.

For patients taking probenecid *for gout or to help remove uric acid from the body:*

- Taking aspirin or other salicylates may lessen the effects of probenecid. This will depend on the dose of aspirin or other salicylate that you take, and on how often you take it. Also, drinking too much alcohol may increase the amount of uric acid in the blood and lessen the effects of this medicine. Therefore, *do not take aspirin or other salicylates or drink alcoholic beverages while taking this medicine,* unless you have first checked with your doctor.

Side Effects of This Medicine

Along with its needed effects, a medicine may cause some unwanted effects. Although not all of these side effects may occur, if they do occur they may need medical attention.

The following side effects may mean that you are having an allergic reaction to this medicine. *Check with your doctor immediately* if any of the following side effects occur:

Rare

Fast or irregular breathing; puffiness or swellings of the eyelids or around the eyes; shortness of breath, troubled breathing, tightness in chest, or wheezing; changes in the skin color of the face occurring together with any of the other side effects listed here; or skin rash, hives, or itching occurring together with any of the other side effects listed here

Also, check with your doctor as soon as possible if any of the following side effects occur:

Less common

Bloody urine; difficult or painful urination; lower back or side pain (especially if severe or sharp); skin rash, hives, or itching (occurring without other signs of an allergic reaction)

Rare

Cloudy urine; cough or hoarseness; fast or irregular breathing; fever; pain in back and/or ribs; sores, ulcers, or white spots on lips or in mouth; sore throat and fever with or without chills; sudden decrease in the amount of urine; swelling of face, fingers, feet, and/or lower legs; swollen and/or painful glands; unusual bleeding or bruising; unusual tiredness or weakness; yellow eyes or skin; weight gain

Other side effects may occur that usually do not need medical attention. These side effects may go away during treatment as your body adjusts to the medicine. However, check with your doctor if any of the following side effects continue or are bothersome:

More common

Headache; joint pain, redness, or swelling; loss of appetite; nausea or vomiting (mild)

Less common

Dizziness; flushing or redness of face (occurring without any signs of an allergic reaction); frequent urge to urinate; sore gums

Other side effects not listed above may also occur in some patients. If you notice any other effects, check with your doctor.

Annual revision: 09/01/92

PROBENECID AND COLCHICINE Systemic

Some commonly used brand names are:

In the U.S.

ColBenemid
Col-Probenecid
Proben-C

Generic name product may also be available.

Description

Probenecid (proe-BEN-e-sid) and colchicine (KOL-chi-seen) combination is used to treat gout or gouty arthritis.

The probenecid in this medicine helps to prevent gout attacks by removing extra uric acid from the body. The colchicine in this medicine also helps to prevent gout attacks. Although colchicine may also be used to relieve an attack of gout, this requires more colchicine than this combination medicine contains. Probenecid and colchicine combination does not cure gout. This medicine will help prevent gout attacks only as long as you continue to take it.

Probenecid and colchicine combination is available only with your doctor's prescription, in the following dosage form:

Oral

- Tablets (U.S.)

It is very important that you read and understand the following information. If any of it causes you special concern, check with your doctor. Also, *if you have any questions* or if you want more information about this medicine or your medical problem, *ask your doctor, nurse, or pharmacist.*

Before Using This Medicine

In deciding to use a medicine, the risks of taking the medicine must be weighed against the good it will do. This is a decision you and your doctor will make. For probenecid and colchicine combination, the following should be considered:

Allergies—Tell your doctor if you have ever had any unusual or allergic reaction to probenecid or to colchicine. Also tell your doctor and pharmacist if you are allergic to any other substances, such as foods, preservatives, or dyes.

Pregnancy—Probenecid has not been shown to cause birth defects or other problems in humans. Although studies with colchicine have not been done in pregnant women, some reports have suggested that use of colchicine during pregnancy can cause harm to the fetus. Also, studies in animals have shown that colchicine causes birth defects. Therefore, do not begin taking this medicine during pregnancy, and do not become pregnant while taking it, unless you have first discussed this problem with your doctor. Also, check with your doctor immediately if you suspect that you have become pregnant while taking this medicine.

Breast-feeding—This medicine has not been reported to cause problems in nursing babies.

Children—Studies on this combination medicine have been done only in adult patients, and there is no specific information about its use in children.

Older adults—Elderly people are especially sensitive to the effects of colchicine. This may increase the chance of side effects during treatment.

There is no specific information comparing use of probenecid in the elderly with use in other age groups.

Other medicines—Although certain medicines should not be used together at all, in other cases two different medicines may be used together even if an interaction might occur. In these cases, your doctor may want to change the dose, or other precautions may be necessary. When you are taking probenecid and colchicine combination, it is especially important that your doctor and pharmacist know if you are taking any of the following:

- Acyclovir (e.g., Zovirax) or
- Amphotericin B by injection (e.g., Fungizone) or
- Anticonvulsants (seizure medicine) or
- Antidiabetics, oral (diabetes medicine you take by mouth) or
- Antineoplastics (cancer medicine) or
- Antipsychotics (medicine for mental illness) or
- Antithyroid agents (medicine for overactive thyroid) or
- Azathioprine (e.g., Imuran) or
- Captopril (e.g., Capoten) or
- Carbamazepine (e.g., Tegretol) or
- Cyclophosphamide (e.g., Cytoxan) or
- Enalapril (e.g., Vasotec) or
- Flecainide (e.g., Tambocor) or
- Flucytosine (e.g., Ancobon) or
- Ganciclovir (e.g., Cytovene) or
- Gold salts (medicine for arthritis) or
- Imipenem or
- Inflammation or pain medicine (except narcotics) or
- Interferon (e.g., Intron A, Roferon-A) or
- Lisinopril (e.g., Prinvil, Zestril) or
- Maprotiline (e.g., Ludiomil) or
- Mercaptopurine (e.g., Purinethol) or
- Methotrexate (e.g., Mexate) or
- Penicillamine (e.g., Cuprimine) or
- Pimozide (e.g., Orap) or
- Plicamycin (e.g., Mithracin) or
- Procainamide (e.g., Pronestyl) or
- Promethazine (e.g., Phenergan) or
- Ramipril (e.g., Altace) or
- Sulfasalazine (e.g., Azulfidine) or
- Tiopronin (e.g., Thiola) or
- Tocainide (e.g., Tonocard) or
- Tricyclic antidepressants (amitriptyline [e.g., Elavil], amoxapine [e.g., Asendin], clomipramine [e.g., Anafranil], desipramine [e.g., Pertofrane], doxepin [e.g., Sinequan], imipramine [e.g., Tofranil], nortriptyline [e.g., Aventyl], protriptyline [e.g., Vivactil], trimipramine [e.g., Surmontil]) or
- Trimeprazine (e.g., Temaril) or
- Zidovudine (e.g., AZT, Retrovir)—Taking any of these medicines together with colchicine may increase the chance of serious side effects. Also, the chance of serious side effects may be increased when antineoplastics (cancer medicine), methotrexate, or zidovudine are taken together with probenecid
- Aspirin or other salicylates, including bismuth subsalicylate (e.g., Pepto-Bismol)—These medicines may keep probenecid from working properly for treating gout, depending on the amount of aspirin or other salicylate that you take and how often you take it
- Heparin—Probenecid may increase the effects of heparin, which increases the chance of side effects
- Indomethacin (e.g., Indocin) or
- Ketoprofen (e.g., Orudis)—Probenecid may increase the blood levels of these medicines, which increases the chance of side effects
- Medicine for infection, including tuberculosis or virus infection—Probenecid may increase the blood levels of many of these medicines, which may increase the chance of side effects. Also, the chance of serious side effects may be increased when some of these medicines are taken together with colchicine
- Nitrofurantoin (e.g., Furadantin)—Probenecid may keep nitrofurantoin from working properly

Other medical problems—The presence of other medical problems may affect the use of probenecid and colchicine combination. Make sure you tell your doctor if you have any other medical problems, especially:

- Alcohol abuse or
- Blood disease or
- Cancer being treated by antineoplastics (cancer medicine) or radiation (x-rays) or
- Heart disease (severe) or
- Intestinal disease (severe) or
- Kidney disease or stones (or history of) or
- Liver disease or
- Stomach ulcer or other stomach problems (or history of)—The chance of serious side effects may be increased

Before you begin using any new medicine (prescription or nonprescription) or if you develop any new medical problem while you are using this medicine, check with your doctor, nurse, or pharmacist.

Proper Use of This Medicine

If this medicine upsets your stomach, it may be taken with food. If this does not work, an antacid may be taken.

If stomach upset (nausea, vomiting, loss of appetite, or stomach pain) continues, check with your doctor.

Take this medicine only as directed by your doctor. Do not take more of it and do not take it more often than your doctor ordered. The colchicine in this combination medicine may cause serious side effects if too much is taken.

After you begin to take this medicine, gout attacks may continue to occur for a while. However, if you take this medicine regularly as directed by your doctor, the attacks will gradually become less frequent and less painful than before. After you have been taking this medicine for several months, they may stop completely.

This medicine will help prevent gout attacks but it will not relieve an attack that has already started. *Even if you take another medicine for gout attacks, continue to take this medicine also.*

When you first begin taking this medicine, the amount of uric acid in the kidneys is greatly increased. This may cause kidney stones or other kidney problems in some people. To help prevent this, your doctor may want you to drink at least 10 to 12 full glasses (8 ounces each) of fluids each day, or to take another medicine to make your urine less acid. It is important that you follow your doctor's instructions very carefully.

Missed dose—If you miss a dose of this medicine, take it as soon as possible. However, if it is almost time for your next dose, skip the missed dose and go back to your regular dosing schedule. Do not double doses.

Storage—To store this medicine:

- Keep out of the reach of children.
- Store away from heat and direct light.
- Do not store this medicine in the bathroom, near the kitchen sink, or in other damp places. Heat or moisture may cause the medicine to break down.
- Do not keep outdated medicine or medicine no longer needed. Be sure that any discarded medicine is out of the reach of children.

Precautions While Using This Medicine

Your doctor should check your progress at regular visits while you are taking this medicine.

Before you have any medical tests, tell the person in charge that you are taking this medicine. The results of some tests may be affected by probenecid or by colchicine.

For *diabetic patients:*

- The probenecid in this combination medicine may cause false test results with copper sulfate urine sugar tests (e.g., Clinitest®), but not with glucose enzymatic urine sugar tests (e.g., Clinistix®). If you have any questions about this, check with your doctor or pharmacist.

Taking aspirin or other salicylates may lessen the effects of the probenecid in this combination medicine. This will depend on the dose of aspirin or other salicylate that you take, and on how often you take it. Also, drinking large amounts of alcoholic beverages may increase the chance of stomach problems and may increase the amount of uric acid in your blood. *Therefore, do not take aspirin or other salicylates or drink alcoholic beverages while you are taking this medicine,* unless you have first checked with your doctor.

For patients taking 4 tablets or more of this medicine a day:

- *Stop taking this medicine immediately and check with your doctor as soon as possible if severe diarrhea, nausea or vomiting, or stomach pain occurs while you are taking this medicine.*

Side Effects of This Medicine

Along with its needed effects, a medicine may cause some unwanted effects. Although not all of these side effects may occur, if they do occur they may need medical attention.

The following side effects may mean that you are having an allergic reaction to this medicine. *Check with your doctor immediately* if any of the following side effects occur:

Rare

Fast or irregular breathing; puffiness or swelling of the eyelids or around the eyes; shortness of breath, troubled breathing, tightness in chest, or wheezing; changes in the skin color of the face occurring together with any of the other side effects listed here; or skin rash, hives, or itching occurring together with any of the other side effects listed here

Also check with your doctor immediately if any of the following side effects occur:

Symptoms of overdose

Bloody urine; burning feeling in stomach, throat, or skin; convulsions (seizures); diarrhea (severe or bloody); fever; mood or mental changes; muscle weakness (severe); nausea or vomiting (severe and continuing); sudden decrease in amount of urine; troubled or difficult breathing

Also, check with your doctor as soon as possible if any of the following side effects occur:

Less common

Difficult or painful urination; lower back or side pain (especially if severe or sharp); skin rash, hives, or itching (occurring without other signs of an allergic reaction)

Rare

Black or tarry stools; cloudy urine; cough or hoarseness; fast or irregular breathing; numbness, tingling, pain, or weakness in hands or feet; pinpoint red spots on skin; sores, ulcers, or white spots on lips or in mouth; sore throat, fever, and chills; sudden decrease in the amount of urine; swelling of face, fingers, feet, and/or lower legs; swollen and/or painful glands; unusual bleeding or bruising; unusual tiredness or weakness; yellow eyes or skin; weight gain

Other side effects may occur that usually do not need medical attention. These side effects may go away during treatment as your body adjusts to the medicine. However, check with your doctor if any of the following side effects continue or are bothersome:

More common

Diarrhea (mild); headache; loss of appetite; nausea or vomiting (mild); stomach pain

Less common

Dizziness; flushing or redness of face (occurring without any signs of an allergic reaction); frequent urge to urinate; sore gums; unusual loss of hair

Other side effects not listed above may also occur in some patients. If you notice any other effects, check with your doctor.

Annual revision: 09/09/92

PROBUCOL Systemic

Some commonly used brand names are:

In the U.S.
Lorelco

In Canada
Lorelco

Other
Bifenabid
Lesterol
Lurselle
Panesclerina
Superlipid

Description

Probucol (PROE-byoo-kole) is used to lower levels of cholesterol (a fat-like substance) in the blood. This may help prevent medical problems caused by cholesterol clogging the blood vessels.

Probucol is available only with your doctor's prescription, in the following dosage form:

Oral
- Tablets (U.S. and Canada)

It is very important that you read and understand the following information. If any of it causes you special concern, check with your doctor. Also, *if you have any questions* or if you want more information about this medicine or your medical problem, *ask your doctor, nurse, or pharmacist.*

Before Using This Medicine

In deciding to use a medicine, the risks of taking the medicine must be weighed against the good it will do. This is a decision you and your doctor will make. For probucol, the following should be considered:

Allergies—Tell your doctor if you have ever had any unusual or allergic reaction to probucol. Also tell your doctor and pharmacist if you are allergic to any other substances, such as foods, preservatives, or dyes.

Diet—Before prescribing medicine for your condition, your doctor will probably try to control your condition by prescribing a personal diet for you. Such a diet may be low in fats, sugars, and/or cholesterol. Many people are able to control their condition by carefully following their doctor's orders for proper diet and exercise. Medicine is prescribed only when additional help is needed and is effective only when a schedule of diet and exercise is properly followed.

Also, this medicine is less effective if you are greatly overweight. It may be very important for you to go on a reducing diet. However, check with your doctor before going on any diet.

Make certain your doctor and pharmacist know if you are on a low-sodium, low-sugar, or any other special diet.

Pregnancy—Probucol has not been studied in pregnant women. However, it has not been shown to cause birth defects or other problems in rats or rabbits.

Breast-feeding—It is not known whether probucol passes into the breast milk. However, this medicine is not recommended for use during breast-feeding because it may cause unwanted effects in nursing babies.

Children—There is no specific information about the use of probucol in children. However, use is not recommended in children under 2 years of age since cholesterol is needed for normal development.

Older adults—Many medicines have not been studied specifically in older people. Therefore, it may not be known whether they work exactly the same way they do in younger adults or if they cause different side effects or problems in older people. There is no specific information comparing use of probucol in the elderly with use in other age groups.

Other medicines—Although certain medicines should not be used together at all, in other cases two different medicines may be used together even if an interaction might occur. In these cases, your doctor may want to change the dose, or other precautions may be necessary. Tell your doctor and pharmacist if you are taking any other prescription or nonprescription (over-the-counter [OTC]) medicine.

Other medical problems—The presence of other medical problems may affect the use of probucol. Make sure you tell your doctor if you have any other medical problems, especially:

- Gallbladder disease or gallstones or
- Heart disease—Probucol may make these conditions worse
- Liver disease—Higher blood levels of probucol may result, which may increase the chance of side effects

Before you begin using any new medicine (prescription or nonprescription) or if you develop any new medical problem while you are using this medicine, check with your doctor, nurse, or pharmacist.

Proper Use of This Medicine

Many patients who have high cholesterol levels will not notice any signs of the problem. In fact, many may feel normal. *Take this medicine exactly as directed by your doctor, even though you may feel well.* Try not to miss any doses and do not take more medicine than your doctor ordered.

Remember that this medicine will not cure your condition but it does help control it. Therefore, you must continue to take it as directed if you expect to keep your cholesterol levels down.

Follow carefully the special diet your doctor gave you. This is the most important part of controlling your condition, and is necessary if the medicine is to work properly.

This medicine works better when taken with meals.

Dosing—The dose of probucol will be different for different patients. *Follow your doctor's orders or the directions on the label.* The following information includes only the average doses of probucol. *If your dose is different, do not change it* unless your doctor tells you to do so:

- The number of tablets that you take depends on the strength of the medicine.
- For *oral* dosage form (tablets):
  —Adults: 500 milligrams two times a day taken with the morning and evening meals.
  —Children:
    - Up to 2 years of age—Use is not recommended.
    - 2 years of age and over—Dose must be determined by your doctor.

Missed dose—If you miss a dose of this medicine, take it as soon as possible. However, if it is almost time for your next dose, skip the missed dose and go back to your regular dosing schedule. Do not double doses.

Storage—To store this medicine:

- Keep out of the reach of children.
- Store away from heat and direct light.
- Do not store in the bathroom, near the kitchen sink, or in other damp places. Heat or moisture may cause the medicine to break down.
- Do not keep outdated medicine or medicine no longer needed. Be sure that any discarded medicine is out of the reach of children.

Precautions While Using This Medicine

It is very important that your doctor check your progress at regular visits. This will allow your doctor to see if the medicine is working properly to lower your cholesterol levels and to decide if you should continue to take it.

Do not stop taking this medicine without first checking with your doctor. When you stop taking this medicine, your blood fat levels may increase again. Your doctor may want you to follow a special diet to help prevent this.

Side Effects of This Medicine

Along with its needed effects, a medicine may cause some unwanted effects. Although not all of these side effects may occur, if they do occur they may need medical attention.

Check with your doctor as soon as possible if any of the following side effects occur:

More common

Dizziness or fainting; fast or irregular heartbeat

Rare

Swellings on face, hands, or feet, or in mouth; unusual bleeding or bruising; unusual tiredness or weakness

Other side effects may occur that usually do not need medical attention. These side effects may go away during treatment as your body adjusts to the medicine. However, check with your doctor if any of the following side effects continue or are bothersome:

More common

Bloating; diarrhea; nausea and vomiting; stomach pain

Less common

Headache; numbness or tingling of fingers, toes, or face

Other side effects not listed above may also occur in some patients. If you notice any other effects, check with your doctor.

Annual revision: 04/13/93

PROCAINAMIDE Systemic

Some commonly used brand names are:

In the U.S.

Procan SR	Pronestyl
Promine	Pronestyl-SR

Generic name product may also be available.

In Canada

Procan SR	Pronestyl-SR
Pronestyl	

Generic name product may also be available.

Description

Procainamide (proe-KANE-a-mide) is used to correct irregular heartbeats to a normal rhythm and to slow an overactive heart. This allows the heart to work more efficiently. Procainamide produces its beneficial effects by slowing nerve impulses in the heart and reducing sensitivity of heart tissues.

Procainamide is available only with your doctor's prescription, in the following dosage forms:

Oral

- Capsules (U.S. and Canada)
- Tablets (U.S.)
- Extended-release tablets (U.S. and Canada)

Parenteral

- Injection (U.S. and Canada)

It is very important that you read and understand the following information. If any of it causes you special concern, check with your doctor. Also, *if you have any questions* or if you want more information about this medicine or your medical problem, *ask your doctor, nurse, or pharmacist.*

Before Using This Medicine

In deciding to use a medicine, the risks of taking the medicine must be weighed against the good it will do. This is a decision you and your doctor will make. For procainamide, the following should be considered:

Allergies—Tell your doctor if you have ever had any unusual or allergic reaction to procainamide, procaine, or any other "caine-type" medicine. Also tell your doctor and pharmacist if you are allergic to any other substance, such as foods, preservatives, or dyes.

Pregnancy—Procainamide has not been studied in pregnant women. However, it has been used in some pregnant women and has not been shown to cause problems. Before taking this medicine, make sure your doctor knows if you are pregnant or if you may become pregnant.

Breast-feeding—Procainamide passes into breast milk.

Children—Procainamide has been used in a limited number of children. In effective doses, the medicine has not been shown to cause different side effects or problems than it does in adults.

Older adults—Dizziness or lightheadedness is more likely to occur in the elderly, who are usually more sensitive to the effects of this medicine.

Other medicines—Although certain medicines should not be used together at all, in other cases two different medicines may be used together even if an interaction might occur. In these cases, your doctor may want to change the dose, or other precautions may be necessary. When you are taking procainamide, it is especially important that your doctor and pharmacist know if you are taking any of the following:

- Antiarrhythmics (medicines for heart rhythm problems), other—Effects on the heart may be increased
- Antihypertensives (high blood pressure medicine)—Effects on blood pressure may be increased
- Antimyasthenics (ambenonium [e.g., Mytelase], neostigmine [e.g., Prostigmin], pyridostigmine [e.g., Mestinon])—Effects may be blocked by procainamide
- Pimozide (e.g., Orap)—May increase the risk of heart rhythm problems

Other medical problems—The presence of other medical problems may affect the use of procainamide. Make sure you tell your doctor if you have any other medical problems, especially:

- Asthma—Possible allergic reaction
- Kidney disease or
- Liver disease—Effects may be increased because of slower removal of procainamide from the body
- Lupus erythematosus (history of)—Procainamide may cause the condition to become active
- Myasthenia gravis—Procainamide may increase muscle weakness

Before you begin using any new medicine (prescription or nonprescription) or if you develop any new medical problem while you are using this medicine, check with your doctor, nurse, or pharmacist.

Proper Use of This Medicine

Take procainamide exactly as directed by your doctor, even though you may feel well. Do not take more medicine than ordered.

Procainamide should be taken with a glass of water on an empty stomach 1 hour before or 2 hours after meals so that it will be absorbed more quickly. However, to lessen stomach upset, your doctor may want you to take the medicine with food or milk.

For patients taking the *extended-release tablets:*

- Swallow the tablet whole without breaking, crushing, or chewing it.

This medicine works best when there is a constant amount in the blood. *To help keep the amount constant, do not miss any doses. Also, it is best to take the doses at evenly spaced times day and night.* For example, if you are to take 6 doses a day, the doses should be spaced about 4 hours apart. If this interferes with your sleep or other daily activities, or if you need help in planning the best times to take your medicine, check with your doctor, nurse, or pharmacist.

Dosing—The dose of procainamide will be different for different patients. *Follow your doctor's orders or the directions on the label.* The following information includes only the average doses of procainamide. *If your dose is different, do not change it* unless your doctor tells you to do so.

The number of capsules or tablets that you take depends on the strength of the medicine.

- For *regular (short-acting) oral* dosage forms (capsules or tablets):
  - —For atrial arrhythmias (fast or irregular heartbeat):
    - Adults—500 milligrams (mg) to 1000 mg (1 gram) every four to six hours.
    - Children—12.5 mg per kilogram (5.68 mg per pound) of body weight four times a day.
  - —For ventricular arrhythmias (fast or irregular heartbeat):
    - Adults—50 mg per kilogram (22.73 mg per pound) of body weight per day divided into eight doses taken every three hours.
    - Children—12.5 mg per kilogram (5.68 mg per pound) of body weight four times a day.
- For *long-acting oral* dosage form (extended-release tablets):
  - —For atrial arrhythmias (fast or irregular heartbeat):
    - Adults—1000 mg (1 gram) every six hours.
    - Children—Use is not recommended.
  - —For ventricular arrhythmias (fast or irregular heartbeat):
    - Adults—50 mg per kilogram (22.73 mg per pound) of body weight per day divided into four doses taken every six hours.
- For *injection* dosage form:
  - —For arrhythmias (fast or irregular heartbeat):
    - Adults—
      - —*First few doses:* May be given intramuscularly (into the muscle) at 50 mg per kilogram (22.73 mg per pound) of body weight per day in divided doses every three hours; or may be given intravenously (into the vein) by slowly injecting 100 mg (mixed in fluid) every five minutes or infusing 500 to 600 mg (mixed in fluid) over a twenty-five to thirty minute period.
      - —*Doses after the first few doses:* 2 to 6 mg (mixed in fluid) per minute infused into the vein.
    - Children—Dose must be determined by your doctor.

Missed dose—If you miss a dose of this medicine and remember within 2 hours (4 hours if you are taking the long-acting tablets), take it as soon as possible. However, if you do not remember until later, skip the missed dose and go back to your regular dosing schedule. Do not double doses.

Storage—To store this medicine:

- Keep out of the reach of children.
- Store away from heat and direct light.
- Do not store in the bathroom, refrigerator, near the kitchen sink, or in other damp places. Moisture usually present in these areas may cause the medicine to break down. Keep the container tightly closed and store in a dry place.
- Do not keep outdated medicine or medicine no longer needed. Be sure that any discarded medicine is out of the reach of children.

Precautions While Using This Medicine

It is important that your doctor check your progress at regular visits to make sure the medicine is working properly. This will allow necessary changes in the amount of medicine you are taking, which also may help reduce side effects.

Do not stop taking this medicine without first checking with your doctor. Stopping it suddenly may cause a serious change in the activity of your heart. Your doctor may want you to reduce gradually the amount you are taking before stopping completely.

Before having any kind of surgery (including dental surgery) or emergency treatment, tell the medical doctor or dentist in charge that you are taking this medicine.

Your doctor may want you to carry a medical identification card or bracelet stating that you are taking this medicine.

Dizziness or lightheadedness may occur, especially in elderly patients and when large doses are used. *Elderly patients should use extra care to avoid falling. Make sure you know how you react to this medicine before you drive, use machines, or do anything else that could be dangerous if you are dizzy or are not alert.*

Tell the doctor in charge that you are taking this medicine before you have any medical tests. The results of some tests may be affected by this medicine.

Side Effects of This Medicine

Along with its needed effects, a medicine may cause some unwanted effects. Although not all of these side effects may occur, if they do occur they may need medical attention.

Check with your doctor as soon as possible if any of the following side effects occur:

Less common

Fever and chills; joint pain or swelling; pains with breathing; skin rash or itching

Rare

Confusion; fever or sore mouth, gums, or throat; hallucinations (seeing, hearing, or feeling things that are not there); mental depression; unusual bleeding or bruising; unusual tiredness or weakness

Signs and symptoms of overdose

Confusion; decrease in urination; dizziness (severe) or fainting; drowsiness; fast or irregular heartbeat; nausea and vomiting

Other side effects may occur that usually do not need medical attention. These side effects may go away during treatment as your body adjusts to the medicine. However, check with your doctor if any of the following side effects continue or are bothersome:

More common

Diarrhea; loss of appetite

Less common

Dizziness or lightheadedness

The medicine in the extended-release tablets is contained in a special wax form (matrix). The medicine is slowly released, after which the wax matrix passes out of the body. Sometimes it may be seen in the stool. This is normal and is no cause for concern.

Other side effects not listed above may also occur in some patients. If you notice any other effects, check with your doctor.

Annual revision: 08/04/93

PROCARBAZINE Systemic

Some commonly used brand names are:

In the U.S.

Matulane

In Canada

Natulan

Description

Procarbazine (pro-KAR-ba-zeen) belongs to the group of medicines known as alkylating agents. It is used to treat some kinds of cancer.

Procarbazine is thought to interfere with the growth of cancer cells which are eventually destroyed. It also blocks the action of a chemical substance in the central nervous system called monoamine oxidase (MAO), but this is probably not related to its effect against cancer. Since the growth of normal body cells may also be affected by procarbazine, other effects will also occur. Some of these may be serious and must be reported to your doctor. Other effects, like hair loss, may not be serious but may cause concern. Some effects may not occur for months or years after the medicine is used.

Before you begin treatment with procarbazine, you and your doctor should talk about the good this medicine will do as well as the risks of using it.

Procarbazine is available only with your doctor's prescription, in the following dosage form:

Oral

- Capsules (U.S. and Canada)

It is very important that you read and understand the following information. If any of it causes you special concern, check with your doctor. Also, *if you have any questions* or if you want more information about this medicine or your medical problem, ***ask your doctor, nurse, or pharmacist.***

Before Using This Medicine

In deciding to use a medicine, the risks of taking the medicine must be weighed against the good it will do. This is a decision you and your doctor will make. For procarbazine, the following should be considered:

Allergies—Tell your doctor if you have ever had any unusual or allergic reaction to procarbazine.

Pregnancy—Tell your doctor if you are pregnant or if you intend to have children. This medicine may cause birth defects or premature birth if either the male or female is taking it at the time of conception or if it is taken during pregnancy. Procarbazine causes birth defects frequently in animals. In addition, many cancer medicines may cause sterility which could be permanent. Although sterility has not been reported with this medicine, procarbazine does affect production of sperm and the possibility should be kept in mind.

Be sure that you have discussed this with your doctor before taking this medicine. It is best to use some kind of birth control while you are taking procarbazine. Tell your doctor right away if you think you have become pregnant while taking procarbazine.

Breast-feeding—Tell your doctor if you are breast-feeding or if you intend to breast-feed during treatment with this medicine. Because procarbazine may cause serious side effects, breast-feeding is generally not recommended while you are taking it.

Children—Although there is no specific information about the use of procarbazine in children, it is not expected to cause different side effects or problems in children than it does in adults.

Older adults—Side effects may be more likely to occur in elderly patients, who are usually more sensitive to the effects of procarbazine.

Other medicines—Although certain medicines should not be used together at all, in other cases two different medicines may be used together even if an interaction might occur. In these cases, your doctor may want to change the dose, or other precautions may be necessary. When you are taking procarbazine, it is especially important that your doctor and pharmacist know if you are taking any of the following:

- Amantadine (e.g., Symmetrel) or
- Anticholinergics (medicine to help reduce stomach acid and for abdominal or stomach spasms or cramps) or
- Antidiabetics, oral (diabetes medicine you take by mouth) or
- Antidyskinetics (medicine for Parkinson's disease or other conditions affecting control of muscles) or
- Antihistamines or
- Antipsychotics (medicine for mental illness) or
- Buclizine (e.g., Bucladin) or
- Central nervous system (CNS) depressants or
- Cyclizine (e.g., Marezine) or
- Disopyramide (e.g., Norpace) or
- Flavoxate (e.g., Urispas) or
- Insulin or
- Ipratropium (e.g., Atrovent) or
- Meclizine (e.g., Antivert) or
- Orphenadrine (e.g., Norflex) or
- Oxybutynin (e.g., Ditropen) or
- Procainamide (e.g., Pronestyl) or
- Promethazine (e.g., Phenergan) or
- Quinidine (e.g., Quinidex) or
- Trimeprazine (e.g., Temaril)—Effects of these medicines may be increased by procarbazine
- Amphetamines or
- Appetite suppressants (diet pills) or
- Dextromethorphan (e.g., Delsym) or
- Levodopa (e.g., Dopar) or
- Medicine for asthma or other breathing problems or
- Medicine for colds, sinus problems, or hay fever or other allergies (including nose drops or sprays) or
- Methyldopa (e.g., Aldomet) or
- Methylphenidate (e.g., Ritalin) or
- Narcotic pain medicine—Taking any of these medicines while you are taking or within 2 weeks of taking procarbazine may cause a severe high blood pressure reaction
- Amphotericin B by injection (e.g., Fungizone) or
- Antithyroid agents (medicine for overactive thyroid) or
- Azathioprine (e.g., Imuran) or
- Chloramphenicol (e.g., Chloromycetin) or
- Colchicine or
- Flucytosine (e.g., Ancobon) or
- Interferon (e.g., Intron A, Roferon-A) or
- Plicamycin (e.g., Mithracin) or
- Zidovudine (e.g., Retrovir) or
- If you have ever been treated with x-rays or cancer medicines—Procarbazine may increase the effects of these medicines or radiation therapy on the blood
- Buspirone (e.g., BuSpar)—Risk of increased blood pressure
- Carbamazepine (e.g., Tegretol) or
- Cyclobenzaprine (e.g., Flexeril) or
- Maprotiline (e.g., Ludiomil) or
- Monoamine oxidase (MAO) inhibitors (furazolidone [e.g., Furoxone], isocarboxazid [e.g., Marplan], pargyline [e.g., Eutonyl], phenelzine [e.g., Nardil], procarbazine [e.g., Matulane], tranylcypromine [e.g., Parnate]) or
- Tricyclic antidepressants (amitriptyline [e.g., Elavil], amoxapine [e.g., Asendin], clomipramine [e.g., Anafranil], desipramine [e.g., Pertofrane], doxepin [e.g., Sinequan], imipramine [e.g., Tofranil], nortriptyline [e.g., Aventyl], protriptyline [e.g., Vivactil], trimipramine [e.g., Surmontil])—Taking procarbazine while you are taking or within 2 weeks of taking any of these medicines may cause a severe high blood pressure reaction
- Cocaine—Use of cocaine while you are taking or within 2 weeks of taking procarbazine may cause a severe high blood pressure reaction
- Fluoxetine (e.g., Prozac)—Taking this medicine while you are taking or within 2 weeks of taking procarbazine may cause a severe high blood pressure reaction or may lead to confusion, agitation, restlessness, and stomach problems
- Guanadrel (e.g., Hylorel) or
- Guanethidine (e.g., Ismelin) or
- Rauwolfia alkaloids (alseroxylon [e.g., Rauwiloid], deserpidine [e.g., Harmonyl], rauwolfia serpentina [e.g., Raudixin], reserpine [e.g., Serpasil])—Taking these medicines while you are taking or within 1 week of taking procarbazine may cause a severe high blood pressure reaction

Other medical problems—The presence of other medical problems may affect the use of procarbazine. Make sure you tell your doctor if you have any other medical problems, especially:

- Alcoholism
- Angina (chest pain) or

- Heart or blood vessel disease or
- Heart attack or stroke (recent)—Lowered blood pressure caused by procarbazine may make problems associated with some of these conditions worse
- Chickenpox (including recent exposure) or
- Herpes zoster (shingles)—Risk of severe disease affecting other parts of the body
- Diabetes mellitus (sugar diabetes)—Procarbazine may change the amount of diabetes medicine needed
- Epilepsy—Procarbazine may change the seizures
- Headaches (severe or frequent)—You may not realize when a severe headache is caused by a dangerous reaction to procarbazine
- Infection—Procarbazine can reduce immunity to infection
- Kidney disease—Effects may be increased because of slower removal of procarbazine from the body
- Liver disease—Procarbazine can cause severe liver disease to become much worse
- Mental illness (or history of)—Some cases of mental illness may be worsened
- Overactive thyroid—Increased risk of dangerous reaction to procarbazine
- Parkinson's disease—May be worsened
- Pheochromocytoma—Blood pressure may be affected

Before you begin using any new medicine (prescription or nonprescription) or if you develop any new medical problem while you are using this medicine, check with your doctor, nurse, or pharmacist.

Proper Use of This Medicine

Use this medicine only as directed by your doctor. Do not use more or less of it and do not use it more often than your doctor ordered. The exact amount of medicine you need has been carefully worked out. Taking too much may increase the chance of side effects while taking too little may not improve your condition.

Procarbazine is sometimes given together with certain other medicines. If you are using a combination of medicines, make sure that you take each one at the right time and do not mix them. Ask your doctor, nurse, or pharmacist to help you plan a way to take your medicines at the right times.

Procarbazine commonly causes nausea and vomiting. Even if you begin to feel ill, *do not stop using this medicine without first checking with your doctor.* Ask your doctor, nurse, or pharmacist for ways to lessen these effects.

If you vomit shortly after taking a dose of procarbazine, check with your doctor. You will be told whether to take the dose again or to wait until the next scheduled dose.

Missed dose—If you miss a dose of this medicine and you remember it within a few hours, take it as soon as you remember it. However, if several hours have passed or if it is almost time for the next dose, skip the missed dose and go back to your regular dosing schedule and check with your doctor. Do not double doses.

Storage—To store this medicine:

- Keep out of the reach of children.
- Store away from heat and direct light.
- Do not store in the bathroom, near the kitchen sink, or in other damp places. Heat or moisture may cause the medicine to break down.
- Do not keep outdated medicine or medicine no longer needed. Be sure that any discarded medicine is out of the reach of children.

Precautions While Using This Medicine

It is very important that your doctor check your progress at regular visits to make sure that this medicine is working properly and to check for unwanted effects.

Check with your doctor or hospital emergency room immediately if severe headache, stiff neck, chest pains, fast heartbeat, or nausea and vomiting occur while you are taking this medicine. These may be symptoms of a serious high blood pressure reaction that should have a doctor's attention.

When taken with certain foods, drinks, or other medicines, procarbazine can cause very dangerous reactions such as sudden high blood pressure. To avoid such reactions, *obey the following rules of caution:*

- Do not eat foods that have a high tyramine content (most common in foods that are aged or fermented to increase their flavor), such as cheeses, yeast or meat extracts, fava or broad bean pods, smoked or pickled meat, poultry, or fish, fermented sausage (bologna, pepperoni, salami, and summer sausage) or other unfresh meat, or any overripe fruit. If a list of these foods and beverages is not given to you, ask your doctor, nurse, or pharmacist to provide one.
- Do not drink alcoholic beverages or alcohol-free or reduced-alcohol beer or wine.
- Do not eat or drink large amounts of caffeine-containing food or beverages, such as chocolate, coffee, tea, or cola.
- Do not take any other medicine unless approved or prescribed by your doctor. This especially includes over-the-counter (OTC) or nonprescription medicine such as that for colds (including nose drops or sprays), cough, asthma, hay fever, appetite control; "keep awake" products; or products that make you sleepy.

After you stop using this medicine you must continue to obey the rules of caution concerning food, drink, and other medication for at least 2 weeks since procarbazine may continue to react with certain foods or other medicines for up to 14 days after you stop taking it.

This medicine will add to the effects of alcohol and other CNS depressants (medicines that slow down the nervous system, possibly causing drowsiness). Some examples of CNS depressants are antihistamines or medicine for hay fever, other allergies, or colds; sedatives, tranquilizers, or sleeping medicine; prescription pain medicine or narcotics; barbiturates; medicine for seizures; muscle relaxants; or anesthetics, including some dental anesthetics. *Check with your doctor before taking any of the above while you are using this medicine.*

This medicine may cause some people to become drowsy or less alert than they are normally. Make sure you know how you react to this medicine before you drive, use machines, or do anything else that could be dangerous if you are not alert.

While you are being treated with procarbazine, and after you stop treatment with it, *do not have any immunizations (vaccinations) without your doctor's approval.* Procarbazine may lower your body's resistance and there is a chance you might get the infection the immunization is meant to prevent. In addition, other persons living in your household should not take or should not have recently taken oral polio vaccine since there is a chance they could pass the polio virus on to you. Also, avoid persons who have taken oral polio vaccine. Do not get close to them and do not stay in the same room with them for very long. If you cannot take these precautions, you should consider wearing a protective face mask that covers the nose and mouth.

Procarbazine can lower the number of white blood cells in your blood temporarily, increasing the chance of getting an infection. It can also lower the number of platelets, which are necessary for proper blood clotting. If this occurs, there are certain precautions you can take, especially when your blood count is low, to reduce the risk of infection or bleeding:

- If you can, avoid people with infections. *Check with your doctor immediately* if you think you are getting an infection or if you get a fever or chills, cough or hoarseness, lower back or side pain, or painful or difficult urination.
- *Check with your doctor immediately* if you notice any unusual bleeding or bruising; black, tarry stools; blood in urine or stools; or pinpoint red spots on your skin.
- Be careful when using a regular toothbrush, dental floss, or toothpick. Your medical doctor, dentist, or nurse may recommend other ways to clean your teeth and gums. Check with your medical doctor before having any dental work done.
- Do not touch your eyes or the inside of your nose unless you have just washed your hands and have not touched anything else in the meantime.
- Be careful not to cut yourself when you are using sharp objects such as a safety razor or fingernail or toenail cutters.
- Avoid contact sports or other situations where bruising or injury could occur.

For *diabetic patients:*

- Procarbazine may affect blood sugar levels. While you are using this medicine, be especially careful in testing for sugar in your blood or urine.

If you are going to have surgery (including dental surgery) or emergency treatment tell the medical doctor or dentist in charge that you are using this medicine or have used it within the past 2 weeks.

Your doctor may want you to carry an identification card stating that you are using this medicine.

Side Effects of This Medicine

Along with their needed effects, medicines like procarbazine can sometimes cause unwanted effects such as blood problems, loss of hair, high blood pressure reactions, and other side effects. These and others are described below. Also, because of the way these medicines act on the body, there is a chance that they might cause other unwanted effects that may not occur until months or years after the medicine is used. These delayed effects may include certain types of cancer, such as leukemia. Discuss these possible effects with your doctor.

Although not all of these side effects may occur, if they do occur they may need medical attention.

Stop taking this medicine and check with your doctor immediately if the following side effects occur. If your doctor is not available, go to the nearest hospital emergency room.

Rare

Chest pain (severe); enlarged pupils of eyes; fast or slow heartbeat; headache (severe); increased sensitivity of eyes to light; increased sweating (possibly with fever or cold, clammy skin); stiff or sore neck

Check with your doctor immediately if any of the following side effects occur:

Less common

Black, tarry stools; blood in urine or stools; bloody vomit; cough or hoarseness; fever or chills; lower back or side pain; painful or difficult urination; pinpoint red spots on skin; unusual bleeding or bruising

Check with your doctor as soon as possible if any of the following side effects occur:

More common

Confusion; convulsions (seizures); cough; hallucinations (seeing, hearing, or feeling things that are not there); missing menstrual periods; shortness of breath; thickening of bronchial secretions; tiredness or weakness (continuing)

Less common

Diarrhea; sores in mouth and on lips; tingling or numbness of fingers or toes; unsteadiness or awkwardness; yellow eyes or skin

Rare

Fainting; skin rash, hives, or itching; wheezing

Other side effects may occur that usually do not need medical attention. These side effects may go away during treatment as your body adjusts to the medicine. Also, your doctor or nurse may be able to tell you about ways to prevent or reduce some of these side effects. Check with your doctor or nurse if any of the following side effects continue or are bothersome or if you have any questions about them:

More common

Drowsiness; muscle or joint pain; muscle twitching; nausea and vomiting; nervousness; nightmares; trouble in sleeping; unusual tiredness or weakness

Less common

Constipation; darkening of skin; difficulty in swallowing; dizziness or lightheadedness when getting up from a lying or sitting position; dry mouth; feeling of warmth and redness in face; headache; loss of appetite; mental depression

This medicine may cause a temporary loss of hair in some people. After treatment with procarbazine has ended, normal hair growth should return.

Other side effects not listed above may also occur in some patients. If you notice any other effects, check with your doctor.

Annual revision: August 1990
Interim revision: 08/05/93

PROGESTINS Systemic

This information applies to the following medicines:

Hydroxyprogesterone (hye-drox-ee-proe-JESS-te-rone)
Medroxyprogesterone (me-DROX-ee-proe-JESS-te-rone)
Megestrol (me-JESS-trole)
Norethindrone (nor-eth-IN-drone)
Norgestrel (nor-JESS-trel)
Progesterone (proe-JESS-ter-one)

Some commonly used brand names are:

For Hydroxyprogesterone†

In the U.S.

Delta-Lutin
Duralutin
Gesterol LA 250
Hy/Gestrone
Hylutin
Hyprogest 250
Pro-Depo
Prodrox
Pro-Span

Generic name product may also be available.

For Medroxyprogesterone

In the U.S.

Amen
Curretab
Cycrin
Depo-Provera
Provera

Generic name product may also be available.

In Canada

Depo-Provera
Provera

For Megestrol

In the U.S.

Megace

Generic name product may also be available.

In Canada

Megace

For Norethindrone

In the U.S.

Aygestin
Micronor
Norlutate
Norlutin
Nor-QD

In Canada

Micronor
Norlutate

Another commonly used name is norethisterone.

For Norgestrel†

In the U.S.

Ovrette

For Progesterone

In the U.S.

Gesterol 50
Progestaject

Generic name product may also be available.

In Canada

PMS-Progesterone

†Not commercially available in Canada.

Description

Progestins (proe-JESS-tins) are sometimes called female hormones. They are produced by the body and are necessary during the childbearing years for the development of the milk-producing glands, and for the proper regulation of the menstrual cycle.

Progestins are prescribed for several reasons:

- for the proper regulation of the menstrual cycle.
- to treat a certain type of disorder of the uterus known as endometriosis.
- to prevent pregnancy, when used in birth-control pills.
- to help treat selected cases of cancer of the breast, kidney, or uterus.
- for testing the body's production of certain hormones.

Progestins may also be used for other conditions as determined by your doctor.

Progestins should not be used in pregnancy tests or in most cases of threatened miscarriage, since there have been some reports that these medications may cause harmful effects on the fetus. However, progesterone is sometimes used in a few patients to treat a certain type of infertility. These patients are given progesterone because their bodies do not produce enough natural progesterone to support a pregnancy. Progesterone is used if this problem has not responded well to other types of treatment.

To make the use of a progestin as safe and reliable as possible, you should understand how and when to take it and what effects may be expected. A paper with information for the patient may be given to you with your filled prescription, and will provide many details concerning most uses of this medicine. Read this paper carefully and ask your doctor, nurse, or pharmacist if you need additional information or explanation.

Progestins are available only with your doctor's prescription, in the following dosage forms:

Oral

Medroxyprogesterone
- Tablets (U.S. and Canada)

Megestrol
- Tablets (U.S. and Canada)

Norethindrone
- Tablets (U.S. and Canada)

Norgestrel
- Tablets (U.S.)

Parenteral

Hydroxyprogesterone
- Injection (U.S.)

Medroxyprogesterone
- Injection (U.S. and Canada)

Progesterone
- Injection (U.S. and Canada)

Rectal

Progesterone
- Suppositories

Vaginal

Progesterone
- Suppositories

It is very important that you read and understand the following information. If any of it causes you special concern, check with your doctor. Also, *if you have any questions* or if you want more information about this medicine or your medical problem, *ask your doctor, nurse, or pharmacist.*

Before Using This Medicine

In deciding to use a medicine, the risks of taking the medicine must be weighed against the good it will do. This is a decision you and your doctor will make. For progestins, the following should be considered:

Allergies—Tell your doctor if you have ever had any unusual or allergic reaction to progestins. Also tell your doctor and pharmacist if you are allergic to any other substances, such as foods, preservatives, or dyes.

Pregnancy—Progestins are not recommended for use during pregnancy since there have been some reports that these medications may cause harmful effects on the fetus. However, progesterone is sometimes used in a few patients to treat a certain type of infertility. These patients are given progesterone because their bodies do not produce enough natural progesterone to support a pregnancy. Progesterone is used if this problem has not responded well to other types of treatment.

Breast-feeding—Progestins pass into the breast milk and may cause unwanted effects in the nursing baby. It may be necessary for you to take another medicine or to stop breast-feeding during treatment.

Children—Studies on this medicine have been done only in adults, and there is no specific information about its use in children.

Older adults—This medicine has been tested and has not been shown to cause different side effects or problems in older people than it does in younger adults.

Other medicines—Although certain medicines should not be used together at all, in other cases two different medicines may be used together even if an interaction might occur. In these cases, your doctor may want to change the dose, or other precautions may be necessary. When you are taking a progestin, it is especially important that your doctor and pharmacist know if you are taking any of the following:

- Bromocriptine (e.g., Parlodel)

Other medical problems—The presence of other medical problems may affect the use of progestins. Make sure you tell your doctor if you have any other medical problems, especially:

- Asthma
- Blood clots (or history of)
- Cancer (or history of)
- Changes in vaginal bleeding
- Diabetes mellitus (sugar diabetes)
- Epilepsy
- Heart or circulation disease
- High blood cholesterol
- Kidney disease
- Liver or gallbladder disease
- Mental depression (or history of)
- Migraine headaches
- Stroke (or history of)

Before you begin using any new medicine (prescription or nonprescription) or if you develop any new medical

problem while you are using this medicine, check with your doctor, nurse, or pharmacist.

Proper Use of This Medicine

Take this medicine only as directed by your doctor. Do not take more of it and do not take it for a longer time than your doctor ordered. To do so may increase the chance of side effects. Try to take the medicine at the same time each day to reduce the possibility of side effects and to allow it to work better. When used for birth control, this medicine should be taken every day of the year, with doses taken 24 hours apart without interruption.

For patients using the rectal suppository form of this medicine:
- If the suppository is too soft to insert, chill it in the refrigerator for 30 minutes.
- To insert the suppository: Moisten the suppository with cold water. Lie down on your side and use your finger to push the suppository well up into the rectum.

For patients using the vaginal suppository form of this medicine:
- Use as directed by your doctor.

Missed dose—If you miss a dose of this medicine:
- If you are *not* taking this medicine for birth control, take the missed dose as soon as possible. However, if it is almost time for your next dose, skip the missed dose and go back to your regular dosing schedule. Do not double doses.
- *If you are taking this medicine for birth control,* the safest thing to do when you miss 1 day's dose is to stop taking the medicine immediately and use another method of birth control until your period begins or until your doctor determines that you are not pregnant. This procedure is different from the one used after missed doses of birth control tablets that contain more than one hormone.

Storage—To store this medicine:
- Keep out of the reach of children.
- Store away from heat and direct light.
- Do not store in the bathroom medicine cabinet because the heat or moisture may cause the medicine to break down.
- Keep the injectable form of this medicine from freezing.
- Do not keep outdated medicine or medicine no longer needed. Be sure that any discarded medicine is out of the reach of children.

Precautions While Using This Medicine

It is very important that your doctor check your progress at regular visits. This will allow your dosage to be adjusted to your changing needs, and will allow any unwanted effects to be detected. These visits will usually be every 6 to 12 months, but some doctors require them more often.

Check with your doctor right away:
- if vaginal bleeding continues for an unusually long time.
- if your menstrual period has not started within 45 days of your last period.
- *if you suspect that you may have become pregnant. You should stop taking this medicine immediately,* since there have been some reports that these medications may cause harmful effects on the fetus when used during pregnancy. However, progesterone is sometimes used during early pregnancy to treat a certain type of infertility.

If you are scheduled for any laboratory tests, tell your doctor that you are taking a progestin.

In some patients, tenderness, swelling, or bleeding of the gums may occur. Brushing and flossing your teeth carefully and regularly and massaging your gums may help prevent this. See your dentist regularly to have your teeth cleaned. Check with your medical doctor or dentist if you have any questions about how to take care of your teeth and gums, or if you notice any tenderness, swelling, or bleeding of your gums.

If you are taking this medicine for birth control:
- *When you begin to use birth control tablets,* your body will require time to adjust before pregnancy will be prevented; therefore, you should *use a second method of birth control for at least the first 3 weeks to ensure full protection.*
- Since one of the most important factors in the proper use of birth control tablets is taking every dose exactly on schedule, you should make sure you never run out of tablets. Therefore, always keep 1 extra month's supply of tablets on hand. To keep the extra month's supply from becoming too old, use it next, after the pills now being used, and replace the extra supply each month on a regular schedule. The tablets will keep well when kept dry and at room temperature (light will fade some tablet colors but will not change the tablets' effect).
- Keep the tablets in the container in which you received them. Most containers aid you in keeping track of dosage schedule.
- Your doctor has prescribed this medicine only for you after studying your health record and the results of your physical examination. Use of the tablets by other persons may be dangerous because of differences in health and body make-up. Therefore, do not

give your birth control tablets to anyone else, and do not take tablets prescribed for someone else. Also, check with your doctor before taking any leftover birth control tablets from an old prescription, especially after a pregnancy. This medicine may be dangerous if your health has changed since your last physical examination.

Side Effects of This Medicine

Along with their needed effects, progestins sometimes cause some unwanted effects such as blood clots, heart attacks, and strokes, and problems of the liver and eyes. Although these effects are rare, they can be very serious and may cause death.

The following side effects may be caused by blood clots. Although not all of these side effects may occur, if they do occur they need immediate medical attention. *Get emergency help immediately* if any of the following side effects occur:

Headache (severe or sudden); loss of coordination (sudden); loss of vision or change in vision (sudden); pains in chest, groin, or leg (especially in calf of leg); shortness of breath (sudden); slurred speech (sudden); weakness, numbness, or pain in arm or leg

Also, check with your doctor as soon as possible if any of the following side effects occur:

More common

Changes in vaginal bleeding (spotting, breakthrough bleeding, prolonged or complete stoppage of bleeding)

Less common or rare

Bulging eyes; discharge from breasts; double vision; loss of vision (gradual, partial, or complete); mental depression; pains in stomach, side, or abdomen; skin rash or itching; yellow eyes or skin

Other side effects may occur that usually do not need medical attention. These side effects may go away during treatment as your body adjusts to the medicine. However, check with your doctor if any of the following side effects continue or are bothersome:

More common

Changes in appetite; changes in weight; pain or irritation at injection site (with progesterone); swelling of ankles and feet; unusual tiredness or weakness

Less common or rare

Acne; brown, blotchy spots on exposed skin; fever; increased body and facial hair; increased breast tenderness; nausea; some loss of scalp hair; trouble in sleeping

Other side effects not listed above may also occur in some patients. If you notice any other effects, check with your doctor.

Annual revision: September 1990
Interim revision: 08/16/93

PROPAFENONE Systemic

A commonly used brand name in the U.S. and Canada is Rythmol.

Description

Propafenone (proe-pa-FEEN-none) belongs to the group of medicines known as antiarrhythmics. It is used to correct irregular heartbeats to a normal rhythm.

Propafenone produces its helpful effects by slowing nerve impulses in the heart and making the heart tissue less sensitive.

There is a chance that propafenone may cause new or make worse existing heart rhythm problems when it is used. Since similar medicines have been shown to cause severe problems in some patients, propafenone is only used to treat serious heart rhythm problems. Discuss this possible effect with your doctor.

This medicine is available only with your doctor's prescription, in the following dosage form:

Oral

- Tablets (U.S. and Canada)

It is very important that you read and understand the following information. If any of it causes you special concern, check with your doctor. Also, *if you have any questions* or if you want more information about this medicine or your medical problem, *ask your doctor, nurse, or pharmacist.*

Before Using This Medicine

In deciding to use a medicine, the risks of taking the medicine must be weighed against the good it will do. This is a decision you and your doctor will make. For propafenone, the following should be considered:

Allergies—Tell your doctor if you have ever had any unusual or allergic reaction to propafenone. Also tell your doctor and pharmacist if you are allergic to any other substances, such as foods, preservatives, or dyes.

Pregnancy—Propafenone has not been studied in pregnant women. Although this medicine has not been shown to cause birth defects in animal studies, it has been shown to reduce fertility in monkeys, dogs, and rabbits. In addition, in rats it caused decreased growth in the infant and deaths of mothers and infants. Before taking propafenone, make sure your doctor knows if you are pregnant or if you may become pregnant.

Breast-feeding—Propafenone passes into breast milk. However, this medicine has not been reported to cause problems in nursing babies.

Children—Propafenone can cause serious side effects in any patient. Therefore, it is especially important that you discuss with the child's doctor the good that this medicine may do as well as the risks of using it.

Older adults—Many medicines have not been studied specifically in older people. Therefore, it may not be known whether they work exactly the same way they do in younger adults or if they cause different side effects or problems in older people. There is no specific information comparing use of propafenone in the elderly with use in other age groups.

Other medicines—Although certain medicines should not be used together at all, in other cases two different medicines may be used together even if an interaction might occur. In these cases, your doctor may want to change the dose, or other precautions may be necessary. When you are taking propafenone it is especially important that your doctor and pharmacist know if you are taking either of the following:

- Digoxin (e.g., Lanoxin) or
- Warfarin (e.g., Coumadin)—Effects of these medicines may be increased when used with propafenone

Other medical problems—The presence of other medical problems may affect the use of propafenone. Make sure you tell your doctor if you have any other medical problems, especially:

- Asthma or
- Bronchitis or
- Emphysema—Propafenone can increase trouble in breathing
- Bradycardia (unusually slow heartbeat)—There is a risk of further decreased heart function
- Congestive heart failure—Propafenone may make this condition worse
- Kidney disease or
- Liver disease—Effects of propafenone may be increased because of slower removal from the body
- Recent heart attack—Risk of irregular heartbeat may be increased
- If you have a pacemaker—Propafenone may interfere with the pacemaker and require more careful follow-up by the doctor

Before you begin using any new medicine (prescription or nonprescription) or if you develop any new medical problem while you are using this medicine, check with your doctor, nurse, or pharmacist.

Proper Use of This Medicine

Take propafenone exactly as directed by your doctor, even though you may feel well. Do not take more or less of it than your doctor ordered.

This medicine works best when there is a constant amount in the blood. *To help keep the amount constant, do not miss any doses. Also, it is best to take each dose at evenly spaced times day and night.* For example, if you are to take 3 doses a day, doses should be spaced about 8 hours apart. If you need help in planning the best times to take your medicine, check with your doctor or pharmacist.

Dosing—The dose of propafenone will be different for different patients. *Follow your doctor's orders or the directions on the label.* The following information includes only the average doses of propafenone. *If your dose is different, do not change it* unless your doctor tells you to do so:

- The number of tablets that you take depends on the strength of the medicine.
- For *oral* dosage forms (tablets):

  —Adults: 150 milligrams every eight hours; may be increased to 225 milligrams every eight hours or 300 mg every twelve hours; up to 300 mg every eight hours.

Missed dose—If you do miss a dose of propafenone and remember within 4 hours, take it as soon as possible. However, if you do not remember until later, skip the missed dose and go back to your regular dosing schedule. Do not double doses.

Storage—To store this medicine:

- Keep out of the reach of children.
- Store away from heat and direct light.
- Do not store in the bathroom, near the kitchen sink, or in other damp places. Heat or moisture may cause the medicine to break down.
- Do not keep outdated medicine or medicine no longer needed. Be sure that any discarded medicine is out of the reach of children.

Precautions While Using This Medicine

It is important that your doctor check your progress at regular visits to make sure the medicine is working properly. This will allow changes to be made in the amount of medicine you are taking, if necessary.

Your doctor may want you to carry a medical identification card or bracelet stating that you are using this medicine.

Before having any kind of surgery (including dental surgery) or emergency treatment, tell the medical doctor or dentist in charge that you are taking this medicine.

Propafenone may cause some people to become dizzy or lightheaded. Make sure you know how you react to this medicine before you drive, use machines, or do anything else that could be dangerous if you are dizzy.

Side Effects of This Medicine

Along with its needed effects, a medicine may cause some unwanted effects. Although not all of these side effects may occur, if they do occur they may need medical attention.

Check with your doctor as soon as possible if any of the following side effects occur:

More common

Fast or irregular heartbeat

Less common

Chest pain; shortness of breath; swelling of feet or lower legs

Rare

Fever or chills; joint pain; low blood pressure; slow heartbeat; trembling or shaking

Other side effects may occur that usually do not need medical attention. These side effects may go away during treatment as your body adjusts to the medicine. However, check with your doctor if any of the following side effects continue or are bothersome:

More common

Change in taste or bitter or metallic taste; dizziness

Less common

Blurred vision; constipation or diarrhea; dryness of mouth; headache; nausea and/or vomiting; skin rash; unusual tiredness or weakness

Other side effects not listed above may also occur in some patients. If you notice any other effects, check with your doctor.

Annual revision: 10/07/92

PROPIOMAZINE Systemic†

A commonly used brand name in the U.S. is Largon.

†Not commercially available in Canada.

Description

Propiomazine (proe-pee-OH-ma-zeen) is used to produce sleepiness or drowsiness and to relieve anxiety before or during surgery or certain procedures. It is also used with analgesics (pain medicine) during labor to produce drowsiness and relieve anxiety.

Propiomazine is given only by or under the immediate supervision of a medical doctor or dentist trained to use this medicine. If you will be receiving propiomazine during surgery, your doctor or anesthesiologist will give you the medicine and closely follow your progress.

Propiomazine is available in the following dosage form:

Parenteral

- Injection (U.S.)

It is very important that you read and understand the following information. If any of it causes you special concern, check with your doctor. Also, *if you have any questions* or if you want more information about this medicine or your medical problem, *ask your doctor, nurse, or pharmacist.*

Before Receiving This Medicine

In deciding to use a medicine, the risks of taking the medicine must be weighed against the good it will do. This is a decision you and your doctor will make. For propiomazine, the following should be considered:

Allergies—Tell your doctor if you have ever had any unusual or allergic reaction to propiomazine or to other phenothiazines (such as acetophenazine, chlorpromazine, fluphenazine, mesoridazine, perphenazine, prochlorperazine, promazine, promethazine, thioridazine, trifluoperazine, triflupromazine, trimeprazine). Also tell your doctor and pharmacist if you are allergic to any other substances, such as foods, preservatives, or dyes.

Pregnancy—Propiomazine has not been shown to cause problems in pregnant women.

Breast-feeding—Propiomazine has not been reported to cause problems in nursing babies.

Children—Although there is no specific information comparing use of propiomazine in children with use in other age groups, this medicine is not expected to cause different side effects or problems in children than it does in adults.

Older adults—Many medicines have not been studied specifically in older people. Therefore, it may not be known whether they work exactly the same way they do in younger adults or if they cause different side effects or problems in older people. There is no specific information

comparing use of propiomazine in the elderly with use in other age groups.

Other medicines—Although certain medicines should not be used together at all, in other cases 2 different medicines may be used together even if an interaction might occur. In these cases, your doctor may want to change the dose, or other precautions may be necessary. When you are taking propiomazine, it is especially important that your doctor and pharmacist know if you are taking any of the following:

- Central nervous system (CNS) depressants (medicine that causes drowsiness) or
- Tricyclic antidepressants (medicine for depression)—Taking these medicines with propiomazine will cause an increase in CNS depressant effects

Before you begin using any new medicine (prescription or nonprescription) or if you develop any new medical problem while you are using this medicine, check with your doctor, nurse, or pharmacist.

Precautions After Receiving This Medicine

For patients going home within 24 hours after receiving propiomazine:

- Propiomazine may cause some people to feel drowsy, tired, or weak for up to one or two days after it has been given. It may also cause problems with coordination and one's ability to think. Therefore, *do not drive, use machines, or do other things that could be dangerous if you are not alert* until the effects of the medicine have disappeared or until the day after receiving propiomazine, whichever period of time is longer.
- *Do not drink alcoholic beverages or take other CNS depressants (medicines that slow down the nervous system, possibly causing drowsiness) for about 24 hours after you have received propiomazine, unless otherwise directed by your doctor.* To do so may add to the effects of the medicine. Some examples of CNS depressants are antihistamines or medicine for hay fever, other allergies, or colds; other sedatives, tranquilizers, or sleeping medicine; prescription pain medicine or narcotics; medicine for seizures; and muscle relaxants.

Side Effects of This Medicine

Along with its needed effects, a medicine may cause some unwanted effects. Although not all of these side effects may occur, if they do occur they may need medical attention.

Check with your doctor immediately if any of the following side effects occur:

Rare

Convulsions (seizures); difficult or unusually fast breathing; fast or irregular heartbeat or pulse; fever (high); high or low blood pressure; loss of bladder control; muscle stiffness (severe); unusual increase in sweating; unusually pale skin; unusual tiredness or weakness

Also, check with your doctor as soon as possible if the following side effect occurs:

Redness, swelling, or pain at place of injection

Other side effects may occur that usually do not need medical attention. The following side effects may go away as the effects of propiomazine wear off. However, check with your doctor if any of the following side effects continue or are bothersome:

More common

Dizziness; drowsiness (prolonged); dryness of mouth

Less common

Confusion; diarrhea; nausea or vomiting; restlessness; skin rash; stomach pain

Other side effects not listed above may also occur in some patients. If you notice any other effects, check with your doctor.

Annual revision: 04/16/93

PROTIRELIN Diagnostic

Some commonly used brand names are:

In the U.S.
Relefact TRH
Thypinone

In Canada
Relefact TRH

Description

Protirelin (proe-TYE-re-lin) is used to test the response of the anterior pituitary gland in people who may have certain medical conditions involving the thyroid gland. Testing with this medicine may help to identify the problem or may ensure that the dose of medicine being used is correct.

Protirelin stimulates release of a hormone called thyroid-stimulating hormone or TSH from the anterior pituitary gland. TSH then stimulates the thyroid gland. By measuring the amount of TSH in the blood after protirelin is given, the doctor can determine how well the anterior pituitary is working.

How test is done: First, a sample of your blood is taken. Then protirelin is given by injection. A little while after it is given, one or more blood samples are taken. Then the results of the test are studied. You will be asked to lie down before, during, and for 15 minutes after the test. This is to prevent dizziness and possible fainting.

Protirelin is to be used only under the supervision of a doctor. It is available in the following dosage form:

Parenteral

- Injection (U.S. and Canada)

It is very important that you read and understand the following information. If any of it causes you special concern, check with your doctor. Also, *if you have any questions* or if you want more information about this test or your medical problem, *ask your doctor, nurse, or pharmacist.*

Before Having This Test

In deciding to use a diagnostic test, any risks of the test must be weighed against the good it will do. This is a decision you and your doctor will make. Also, test results may be affected by other things. For protirelin, the following should be considered:

Allergies—Tell your doctor if you have ever had any unusual or allergic reaction to protirelin. Also tell your doctor and pharmacist if you are allergic to any other substances, such as foods, preservatives, or dyes.

Pregnancy—Studies have not been done in humans. However, studies in rabbits have shown that protirelin increases the chance of death of the fetus when given in doses 1½ and 6 times the human dose.

Breast-feeding—Protirelin has not been reported to cause problems in nursing babies. However, it may cause extra swelling of the breasts and leaking of milk for up to 2 or 3 days after it is given.

Children—This medicine has been tested in children and, in effective doses, has not been shown to cause different side effects or problems in children than it does in adults.

Older adults—This medicine has been tested and has not been shown to cause different side effects or problems in older people than it does in younger adults.

Other medicines—Although certain medicines should not be used together at all, in other cases two different medicines may be used together even if an interaction might occur. In these cases, your doctor may want to change the dose, or other precautions may be necessary. Tell your doctor and pharmacist if you are taking any other prescription or nonprescription (over-the-counter [OTC]) medicine.

Other medical problems—The presence of other medical problems may affect the use of protirelin. Make sure you tell your doctor if you have any other medical problems, especially:

- Heart or blood vessel disease or
- High blood pressure or
- Stroke (history of)—Sudden changes in blood pressure caused by protirelin may put patients with these conditions at greater risk
- Kidney disease—Test results may be affected if patient has kidney disease

Preparation for This Test

Your doctor may ask you not to eat for several hours before the test or to eat a low-fat meal before the test. This will not be necessary for all patients. If it is necessary for you, *follow your doctor's instructions carefully*. Otherwise, this test may not work and may have to be done again.

Side Effects of This Medicine

Along with its needed effects, a medicine may cause some unwanted effects. Check with your doctor or nurse as soon as possible if either of the following side effects occurs:

Rare

Fainting

For patients with pituitary tumors—Rare

Loss of vision (temporary)

Protirelin commonly causes some side effects just after it is given. Usually they last for only a few minutes. However, check with your doctor if any of the following side effects continue or are bothersome:

More common

Flushing or redness of skin; frequent urge to urinate; headache (sometimes severe); lightheadedness; nausea; stomach pain; unpleasant taste in mouth or dryness of mouth

Less common

Anxiety; drowsiness; pressure in the chest or tightness in throat; sweating; tingling

Other side effects not listed above may also occur in some patients. If you notice any other effects, check with your doctor.

Annual revision: 09/19/91

PSEUDOEPHEDRINE Systemic

Some commonly used brand names are:

In the U.S.

Afrinol Repetabs	Halofed Adult Strength
AlleRid	Myfedrine
Cenafed	NeoFed
Children's Sudafed Liquid	Novafed
Chlor-Trimeton Non-Drowsy Formula	PediaCare Infants' Oral Decongestant Drops
Decofed	Pseudo
DeFed-60	Pseudogest
Dorcol Children's Decongestant Liquid	SinuStat
	Sudafed
Drixoral Non-Drowsy Formula	Sudafed 60
	Sudafed 12 Hour
Genaphed	Sudrin
Halofed	Sufedrin

Generic name product may also be available.

In Canada

Congestac N.D. Caplets	Otrivin
Eltor 120	Pseudofrin
Maxenal	Robidrine
Ornex Cold	Sudafed

Description

Pseudoephedrine (soo-doe-e-FED-rin) is used to relieve nasal or sinus congestion caused by the common cold, sinusitis, and hay fever and other respiratory allergies. It is also used to relieve ear congestion caused by ear inflammation or infection.

Some of these preparations are available only with your doctor's prescription. Others are available without a prescription; however, your doctor may have special instructions on the proper dose of pseudoephedrine for your medical condition.

Pseudoephedrine is available in the following dosage forms:

Oral

- Capsules (U.S. and Canada)
- Extended-release capsules (U.S. and Canada)
- Oral solution (U.S. and Canada)
- Syrup (U.S. and Canada)
- Tablets (U.S. and Canada)
- Extended-release tablets (U.S.)

It is very important that you read and understand the following information. If any of it causes you special concern, check with your doctor or pharmacist. Also, *if you have any questions* or if you want more information about this medicine or your medical problem, *ask your doctor, nurse, or pharmacist.*

Before Using This Medicine

If you are taking this medicine without a prescription, carefully read and follow any precautions on the label. For pseudoephedrine, the following should be considered:

Allergies—Tell your doctor if you have ever had any unusual or allergic reaction to pseudoephedrine or similar medicines, such as albuterol, amphetamines, ephedrine, epinephrine, isoproterenol, metaproterenol, norepinephrine, phenylephrine, phenylpropanolamine, or terbutaline. Also tell your doctor and pharmacist if you are allergic to any other substances, such as foods, preservatives, or dyes.

Pregnancy—Studies on birth defects have not been done in humans. However, pseudoephedrine has not been shown to cause birth defects in animal studies. Studies in animals have shown that pseudoephedrine causes a reduction in average weight, length, and rate of bone formation in the animal fetus.

Breast-feeding—Pseudoephedrine passes into the breast milk and may cause unwanted effects in nursing babies (especially newborn and premature babies).

Children—Pseudoephedrine may be more likely to cause side effects in infants, especially newborn and premature infants, than in older children and adults.

Older adults—Many medicines have not been tested in older people. Therefore, it may not be known whether they work exactly the same way they do in younger adults or if they cause different side effects or problems in older people. There is no specific information about the use of pseudoephedrine in the elderly.

Other medicines—Although certain medicines should not be used together at all, in other cases two different medicines may be used together even if an interaction might occur. In these cases, your doctor may want to change the dose, or other precautions may be necessary. When you are taking pseudoephedrine, it is especially important that your doctor and pharmacist know if you are taking any of the following:

- Beta-blockers (acebutolol [e.g., Sectral], atenolol [e.g., Tenormin], betaxolol [e.g., Kerlone], carteolol [e.g., Cartrol], labetalol [e.g., Normodyne], metoprolol [e.g., Lopressor], nadolol [e.g., Corgard], oxprenolol [e.g., Trasicor], penbutolol [e.g., Levatol], pindolol [e.g., Visken], propranolol [e.g., Inderal], sotalol [e.g., Sotacor], timolol [e.g., Blocadren])—Pseudoephedrine may decrease the effect of these medicines; also, taking pseudoephedrine with beta-blockers may increase the chance of side effects
- Cocaine—Using cocaine with pseudoephedrine may increase the effects of either one of these medicines on the heart and increase the chance of side effects
- Monoamine oxidase (MAO) inhibitors (furazolidone [e.g., Furoxone], isocarboxazid [e.g., Marplan], pargyline [e.g., Eutonyl], phenelzine [e.g., Nardil], procarbazine [e.g., Matulane], tranylcypromine [e.g., Parnate])—Taking pseudoephedrine while you are taking or within 2 weeks of taking monoamine oxidase (MAO) inhibitors may increase the chance of serious side effects

Other medical problems—The presence of other medical problems may affect the use of pseudoephedrine. Make

sure you tell your doctor if you have any other medical problems, especially:

- Diabetes mellitus (sugar diabetes)
- Enlarged prostate or
- Heart or blood vessel disease or
- High blood pressure—Pseudoephedrine may make the condition worse
- Overactive thyroid

Before you begin using any new medicine (prescription or nonprescription) or if you develop any new medical problem while you are using this medicine, check with your doctor, nurse, or pharmacist.

Proper Use of This Medicine

For patients taking *pseudoephedrine extended-release capsules:*

- Swallow the capsule whole. However, if the capsule is too large to swallow, you may mix the contents of the capsule with jam or jelly and swallow without chewing.
- Do not crush, break, or chew before swallowing.

For patients taking *pseudoephedrine extended-release tablets:*

- Swallow the tablet whole.
- Do not break, crush, or chew before swallowing.

To help prevent trouble in sleeping, *take the last dose of pseudoephedrine for each day a few hours before bedtime.* If you have any questions about this, check with your doctor.

Take this medicine only as directed. Do not take more of it and do not take it more often than recommended on the label, unless otherwise directed by your doctor. To do so may increase the chance of side effects.

Missed dose—If you miss a dose of this medicine and you remember within an hour or so of the missed dose, take it right away. However, if you do not remember until later, skip the missed dose and go back to your regular dosing schedule. Do not double doses.

Storage—To store this medicine:

- Keep out of the reach of children.
- Store away from heat and direct light.
- Do not store the capsule or tablet form of this medicine in the bathroom, near the kitchen sink, or in other damp places. Heat or moisture may cause the medicine to break down.
- Keep the liquid form of this medicine from freezing.
- Do not keep outdated medicine or medicine no longer needed. Be sure that any discarded medicine is out of the reach of children.

Precautions While Using This Medicine

If symptoms do not improve within 5 days or if you also have a high fever, check with your doctor since these signs may mean that you have other medical problems.

Side Effects of This Medicine

Along with its needed effects, a medicine may cause some unwanted effects. Although not all of these side effects may occur, if they do occur they may need medical attention.

Check with your doctor as soon as possible if any of the following side effects occur:

Rare—more common with high doses

Convulsions (seizures); hallucinations (seeing, hearing, or feeling things that are not there); irregular or slow heartbeat; shortness of breath or troubled breathing

Symptoms of overdose

Convulsions (seizures); fast breathing; hallucinations (seeing, hearing, or feeling things that are not there); increase in blood pressure; irregular heartbeat (continuing); shortness of breath or troubled breathing (severe or continuing); slow or fast heartbeat (severe or continuing); unusual nervousness, restlessness, or excitement

Other side effects may occur that usually do not need medical attention. These side effects may go away during treatment as your body adjusts to the medicine. However, check with your doctor or pharmacist if any of the following side effects continue or are bothersome:

More common

Nervousness; restlessness; trouble in sleeping

Less common

Difficult or painful urination; dizziness or lightheadedness; fast or pounding heartbeat; headache; increased sweating; nausea or vomiting; trembling; troubled breathing; unusual paleness; weakness

Other side effects not listed above may also occur in some patients. If you notice any other effects, check with your doctor or pharmacist.

Annual revision: September 1990
Interim revision(s): 05/19/92

PYRANTEL Oral

Some commonly used brand names are:

In the U.S.

- Antiminth
- Reese's Pinworm Medicine

Generic name product may also be available.

In Canada

- Combantrin

Other

- Aut
- Cobantril
- Helmex
- Lombriareu
- Trilombrin

Description

Pyrantel (pi-RAN-tel) belongs to the family of medicines called anthelmintics (ant-hel-MIN-tiks). Anthelmintics are used in the treatment of worm infections.

Pyrantel is used to treat:

- common roundworms (ascariasis);
- pinworms (enterobiasis; oxyuriasis); and
- more than one worm infection at a time.

This medicine may also be used for other worm infections as determined by your doctor.

Pyrantel works by paralyzing the worms. They are then passed in the stool.

Pyrantel is available in the following dosage forms:

Oral

- Oral suspension (U.S. and Canada)
- Tablets (Canada)

It is very important that you read and understand the following information. If any of it causes you special concern, check with your doctor. Also, *if you have any questions* or if you want more information about this medicine or your medical problem, *ask your doctor, nurse, or pharmacist.*

Before Using This Medicine

In deciding to use a medicine, the risks of taking the medicine must be weighed against the good it will do. This is a decision you and your doctor will make. For pyrantel, the following should be considered:

Allergies—Tell your doctor if you have ever had any unusual or allergic reaction to pyrantel. Also tell your doctor and pharmacist if you are allergic to any other substances, such as foods, preservatives, or dyes.

Pregnancy—Studies have not been done in pregnant women. However, pyrantel has not been reported to cause birth defects or other problems in animal studies.

Breast-feeding—Only small amounts of pyrantel are absorbed into the body. Pyrantel has not been reported to cause problems in nursing babies.

Children—This medicine has been tested in a limited number of children 2 years of age or older and, in effective doses, has not been reported to cause different side effects or problems in children than it does in adults.

Older adults—Many medicines have not been studied specifically in older people. Therefore, it may not be known whether they work exactly the same way they do in younger adults or if they cause different side effects or problems in older people. There is no specific information comparing use of pyrantel in the elderly with use in other age groups.

Other medicines—Although certain medicines should not be used together at all, in other cases two different medicines may be used together even if an interaction might occur. In these cases, your doctor may want to change the dose, or other precautions may be necessary. When you are taking pyrantel, it is especially important that your doctor and pharmacist know if you are taking any of the following:

- Piperazine (e.g., Entacyl)—Using pyrantel and piperazine together may decrease the effectiveness of pyrantel

Before you begin using any new medicine (prescription or nonprescription) or if you develop any new medical problem while you are using this medicine, check with your doctor, nurse, or pharmacist.

Proper Use of This Medicine

No special preparations (for example, special diets, fasting, other medicines, laxatives, or enemas) are necessary before, during, or immediately after you take pyrantel.

For patients taking pyrantel *oral suspension:*

- Use a specially marked measuring spoon or other device to measure each dose accurately. The average household teaspoon may not hold the right amount of liquid.

To help clear up your infection completely, *take this medicine exactly as directed by your doctor.* In some infections a second dose of this medicine may be required to clear up the infection completely.

For patients taking pyrantel for *pinworms:*

- Pinworms may be easily passed from one person to another, especially among persons in the same household. Therefore, all household members may have to be treated at the same time to prevent their infection or reinfection. Also, all household members may have to be treated again in 2 to 3 weeks to clear up the infection completely.

Dosing—The dose of pyrantel will be different for different patients. *Follow your doctor's orders or the directions on the label.* The following information includes only the average doses of pyrantel. *If your dose is different, do not change it* unless your doctor tells you to do so.

- The number of tablets or teaspoonfuls of suspension that you take depends on the strength of the medicine. Also, *the number of doses you take each day, the time allowed between doses, and the length of time you take the medicine depend on the medical problem for which you are taking pyrantel.*
- For *oral* dosage forms (oral suspension or tablets):
  —Adults and children 2 years of age and older: Dose is based on body weight and will be determined by your doctor. It is taken as a single dose and may need to be repeated in two to three weeks.

Storage—To store this medicine:

- Keep out of the reach of children.
- Store away from heat and direct light.
- Keep the liquid form of this medicine from freezing.
- Do not keep outdated medicine or medicine no longer needed. Be sure that any discarded medicine is out of the reach of children.

Precautions While Using This Medicine

If your symptoms do not improve within a few days, or if they become worse, check with your doctor.

This medicine may cause some people to become dizzy, drowsy, or less alert than they are normally. *Make sure you know how you react to this medicine before you drive, use machines, or do anything else that could be dangerous if you are dizzy or are not alert.* If these reactions are especially bothersome, check with your doctor.

For patients taking pyrantel for *pinworms:*

- In some patients, pinworms may return after treatment with pyrantel. Washing (not shaking) all bedding and nightclothes (pajamas) after treatment may help to prevent this.
- Some doctors may also recommend other measures to help keep your infection from returning. If you have any questions about this, check with your doctor.

Side Effects of This Medicine

Along with its needed effects, a medicine may cause some unwanted effects. Although not all of these side effects may occur, if they do occur they may need medical attention.

Check with your doctor as soon as possible if any of the following side effects occur:

Rare

Skin rash

Other side effects may occur that usually do not need medical attention. These side effects may go away during treatment as your body adjusts to the medicine. However, check with your doctor if any of the following side effects continue or are bothersome:

Less common

Abdominal or stomach cramps or pain; diarrhea; dizziness; drowsiness; headache; loss of appetite; nausea or vomiting; trouble in sleeping

Other side effects not listed above may also occur in some patients. If you notice any other effects, check with your doctor.

Additional Information

Once a medicine has been approved for marketing for a certain use, experience may show that it is also useful for other medical problems. Although this use is not included in product labeling, pyrantel is used in certain patients with the following medical condition:

- Hookworm infection

For patients taking this medicine for *hookworm infection:*

- Anemia (iron-poor blood) may occur in patients with hookworm infections. Therefore, your doctor may want you to take iron supplements to help clear up the anemia. If so, it is important to take iron every day while you are being treated for hookworms. Do not miss any doses. Your doctor may also want you to keep taking iron supplements for up to 6 months after you stop taking pyrantel. If you have any questions about this, check with your doctor.

Other than the above information, there is no additional information relating to proper use, precautions, or side effects for this use.

Annual revision: 01/19/93

PYRAZINAMIDE Systemic

Some commonly used brand names in Canada are PMS Pyrazinamide and Tebrazid.

Available in the U.S. as generic name product.

Description

Pyrazinamide (peer-a-ZIN-a-mide) belongs to the family of medicines called anti-infectives. It is used, along with one or more other medicines, to treat tuberculosis (TB).

Pyrazinamide is available only with your doctor's prescription, in the following dosage form:

Oral

- Tablets (U.S. and Canada)

It is very important that you read and understand the following information. If any of it causes you special concern, check with your doctor. Also, *if you have any questions* or if you want more information about this medicine or your medical problem, *ask your doctor, nurse, or pharmacist.*

Before Using This Medicine

In deciding to use a medicine, the risks of taking the medicine must be weighed against the good it will do. This is a decision you and your doctor will make. For pyrazinamide, the following should be considered:

Allergies—Tell your doctor if you have ever had any unusual or allergic reaction to pyrazinamide or to ethionamide (e.g., Trecator-SC), isoniazid (e.g., INH, Nydrazid), or niacin (e.g., Nicobid, nicotinic acid). Also tell your doctor and pharmacist if you are allergic to any other substances, such as foods, preservatives, or dyes.

Pregnancy—Studies on effects in pregnancy have not been done in either humans or animals. In addition, it is not known whether this medicine causes problems when taken with other TB medicines.

Breast-feeding—Pyrazinamide passes into the breast milk in small amounts.

Children—Pyrazinamide has been used in children and, in effective doses, has not been reported to cause different side effects or problems in children than it does in adults.

Older adults—Many medicines have not been studied specifically in older people. Therefore, it may not be known whether they work exactly the same way they do in younger adults. Although there is no specific information comparing pyrazinamide in the elderly with use in other age groups, this medicine is not expected to cause different side effects or problems in older people than it does in younger adults.

Other medicines—Although certain medicines should not be used together at all, in other cases two different medicines may be used together even if an interaction might occur. In these cases, your doctor may want to change the dose, or other precautions may be necessary. Tell your doctor and pharmacist if you are taking any other prescription or nonprescription (over-the-counter [OTC]) medicine.

Other medical problems—The presence of other medical problems may affect the use of pyrazinamide. Make sure you tell your doctor if you have any other medical problems, especially:

- Gout (history of)—Pyrazinamide may worsen or cause a gout attack in patients with a history of gout
- Liver disease (severe)—Patients with severe liver disease who take pyrazinamide may have an increase in side effects

Before you begin using any new medicine (prescription or nonprescription) or if you develop any new medical problem while you are using this medicine, check with your doctor, nurse, or pharmacist.

Proper Use of This Medicine

To help clear up your TB completely, *it is important that you keep taking this medicine for the full time of treatment,* even if you begin to feel better after a few weeks. *It is important that you do not miss any doses.*

Dosing—The dose of pyrazinamide will be different for different patients. *Follow your doctor's orders or the directions on the label.* The following information includes only the average doses of pyrazinamide. *If your dose is different, do not change it* unless your doctor tells you to do so.

- For *tuberculosis (TB)*:
  —Adults and children: Dose is based on body weight. The usual dose is 15 to 30 milligrams of pyrazinamide per kilogram (6.8 to 13.6 milligrams per pound) of body weight. This medicine is taken once a day and must be taken along with other medicines used to treat TB.

Missed dose—If you miss a dose of this medicine, take it as soon as possible. However, if it is almost time for your next dose, skip the missed dose and go back to your regular dosing schedule. Do not double doses.

Storage—To store this medicine:

- Keep out of the reach of children.
- Store away from heat and direct light.
- Do not store in the bathroom, near the kitchen sink, or in other damp places. Heat or moisture may cause the medicine to break down.

- Do not keep outdated medicine or medicine no longer needed. Be sure that any discarded medicine is out of the reach of children.

Precautions While Using This Medicine

It is very important that your doctor check your progress at regular visits.

If your symptoms do not improve within 2 to 3 weeks, or if they become worse, check with your doctor.

For diabetic patients:

- *This medicine may cause false test results with urine ketone tests.* Check with your doctor before changing your diet or the dosage of your diabetes medicine.

Side Effects of This Medicine

Along with its needed effects, a medicine may cause some unwanted effects. Although not all of these side effects may occur, if they do occur they may need medical attention.

Check with your doctor immediately if any of the following side effects occur:

More common

Pain in large and small joints

Rare

Loss of appetite; pain and swelling of joints, especially big toe, ankle, and knee; tense, hot skin over affected joints; unusual tiredness or weakness; yellow eyes or skin

Other side effects may occur that usually do not need medical attention. These side effects may go away during treatment as your body adjusts to the medicine. However, check with your doctor if any of the following side effects continue or are bothersome:

Rare

Itching; skin rash

Other side effects not listed above may also occur in some patients. If you notice any other effects, check with your doctor.

Annual revision: 02/23/93

PYRETHRINS AND PIPERONYL BUTOXIDE Topical

Some commonly used brand names are:

In the U.S.

A-200 Gel Concentrate
A-200 Shampoo Concentrate
Barc
Blue
Licetrol
Pronto Lice Killing Shampoo Kit
Pyrinyl
R & C
Rid
Tisit
Tisit Blue
Tisit Shampoo
Triple X

In Canada

R & C

Description

Medicine containing pyrethrins (pye-REE-thrins) is used to treat head, body, and pubic lice infections. This medicine is absorbed by the lice and destroys them by acting on their nervous systems. It does not affect humans in this way. The piperonyl butoxide (pye-PEER-i-nil byoo-TOX-ide) is included to make the pyrethrins more effective in killing the lice. This combination medicine is known as a pediculicide (pe-DIK-yoo-li-side).

This medicine is available without a prescription; however, your doctor may have special instructions on the proper use of this medicine for your medical condition.

Pyrethrins and piperonyl butoxide combination medicine is available in the following dosage forms:

Topical

- Gel (U.S.)
- Solution shampoo (U.S. and Canada)
- Topical solution (U.S.)

It is very important that you read and understand the following information. If any of it causes you special concern, check with your doctor or pharmacist. Also, *if you have any questions* or if you want more information about this medicine or your medical problem, *ask your doctor, nurse, or pharmacist.*

Before Using This Medicine

If you are using this medicine without a prescription, carefully read and follow any precautions on the label. For pyrethrins and piperonyl butoxide combination, the following should be considered:

Allergies—Tell your doctor if you have ever had any unusual or allergic reaction to pyrethrins, piperonyl butoxide, ragweed, chrysanthemum plants, or kerosene or other petroleum products. Also tell your doctor and pharmacist if you are allergic to any other substances, such as preservatives or dyes.

Pregnancy—Pyrethrins and piperonyl butoxide may be absorbed through the skin. However, this medicine has not been shown to cause birth defects or other problems in humans when used on the skin.

Breast-feeding—Pyrethrins and piperonyl butoxide combination may be absorbed through the mother's skin. It is not known whether pyrethrins and piperonyl butoxide combination passes into the breast milk. Although most medicines pass into breast milk in small amounts, many of them may be used safely while breast-feeding. Mothers who are using this medicine and who wish to breast-feed should discuss this with their doctor.

Children—Although there is no specific information comparing use of pyrethrins and piperonyl butoxide combination in children with use in other age groups, this medicine is not expected to cause different side effects or problems in children than it does in adults.

Older adults—Many medicines have not been studied specifically in older people. Therefore, it may not be known whether they work exactly the same way they do in younger adults. Although there is no specific information comparing use of pyrethrins and piperonyl butoxide combination medicine in the elderly with use in other age groups, this medicine is not expected to cause different side effects or problems in older people than it does in younger adults.

Other medical problems—The presence of other medical problems may affect the use of pyrethrins and piperonyl butoxide combination. Make sure you tell your doctor if you have any other medical problems, especially:

- Inflammation of the skin (severe)—Use of pyrethrins and piperonyl butoxide combination may make the condition worse

Before you begin using any new medicine (prescription or nonprescription) or if you develop any new medical problem while you are using this medicine, check with your doctor, nurse, or pharmacist.

Proper Use of This Medicine

Pyrethrins and piperonyl butoxide combination medicine usually comes with patient directions. Read them carefully before using this medicine.

Use this medicine only as directed. Do not use more of it and do not use it more often than recommended on the label. To do so may increase the chance of absorption through the skin and the chance of side effects.

Keep pyrethrins and piperonyl butoxide combination medicine away from the mouth and do not inhale it. This medicine is harmful if swallowed or inhaled.

To lessen the chance of inhaling this medicine, apply it in a well-ventilated room (for example, one with free flowing air or with a fan turned on).

Keep this medicine away from the eyes and other mucous membranes, such as the inside of the nose, because it may cause irritation. If you accidentally get some in your eyes, flush them thoroughly with water at once.

Do not apply this medicine to the eyelashes or eyebrows. If they become infected with lice, check with your doctor.

To use the *gel or solution form* of this medicine:

- Apply enough medicine to thoroughly wet the dry hair and scalp or skin. Allow the medicine to remain on the affected areas for exactly 10 minutes.
- Then, thoroughly wash the affected areas with warm water and soap or regular shampoo. Rinse thoroughly and dry with a clean towel.

To use the *shampoo form* of this medicine:

- Apply enough medicine to thoroughly wet the dry hair and scalp or skin. Allow the medicine to remain on the affected areas for exactly 10 minutes.
- Then use a small amount of water and work shampoo into the hair and scalp or skin until a lather forms. Rinse thoroughly and dry with a clean towel.

After rinsing and drying, use a nit removal comb (special fine-toothed comb, usually included with this medicine) to remove the dead lice and eggs (nits) from hair.

Immediately after using this medicine, wash your hands to remove any medicine that may be on them.

This medicine should be used again in 7 to 10 days after the first treatment in order to kill any newly hatched lice.

Lice can easily move from one person to another by close body contact. This can happen also by direct contact with such things as clothing, hats, scarves, bedding, towels, washcloths, hairbrushes and combs, or the hair of infected persons. Therefore, *all members of your household should be examined for lice and receive treatment if they are found to be infected.*

To use this medicine for *pubic (crab) lice:*

- Your sexual partner may also need to be treated, since the infection may spread to persons in close contact. If your partner is not being treated or if you have any questions about this, check with your doctor.

Dosing—The dose of pyrethrins and piperonyl butoxide combination will be different for different patients. *Follow your doctor's orders or the directions on the label.* The following information includes only the average doses of pyrethrins and piperonyl butoxide combination. *If your dose is different, do not change it* unless your doctor tells you to do so.

- For *topical* dosage forms (gel, solution shampoo, and topical solution):
  - —For head, body, or pubic lice:
    - Adults and children—Use one time, then repeat one time in seven to ten days.

Storage—To store this medicine:

- Keep out of the reach of children.
- Store away from heat and direct light.
- Keep the medicine from freezing.
- Do not keep outdated medicine or medicine no longer needed. Be sure that any discarded medicine is out of the reach of children.

Precautions While Using This Medicine

To prevent reinfection or spreading of the infection to other people, good health habits are also required. These include the following:

- For *head lice*

  —Machine wash all clothing (including hats, scarves, and coats), bedding, towels, and washcloths in very hot water and dry them by using the hot cycle of a dryer for at least 20 minutes. Clothing or bedding that cannot be washed should be dry-cleaned or sealed in a plastic bag for 2 weeks.

  —Shampoo all wigs and hairpieces.

  —Wash all hairbrushes and combs in very hot soapy water (above 130 °F) for 5 to 10 minutes and do not share them with other people.

  —Clean the house or room by thoroughly vacuuming upholstered furniture, rugs, and floors.
- For *body lice*

  —Machine wash all clothing, bedding, towels, and washcloths in very hot water and dry them by using the hot cycle of a dryer for at least 20 minutes. Clothing or bedding that cannot be washed should be dry-cleaned or sealed in a plastic bag for 2 weeks.

  —Clean the house or room by thoroughly vacuuming upholstered furniture, rugs, and floors.
- For *pubic lice*

  —Machine wash all clothing (especially underwear), bedding, towels, and washcloths in very hot water and dry them by using the hot cycle of a dryer for at least 20 minutes. Clothing or bedding that cannot be washed should be dry-cleaned or sealed in a plastic bag for 2 weeks.

  —Scrub toilet seats frequently.

Side Effects of This Medicine

Along with its needed effects, a medicine may cause some unwanted effects. Although not all of these side effects may occur, if they do occur they may need medical attention.

Check with your doctor as soon as possible if any of the following side effects occur:

Less common or rare

Skin irritation not present before use of this medicine; skin rash or infection; sneezing (sudden attacks of); stuffy or runny nose; wheezing or difficulty in breathing

Other side effects not listed above may also occur in some patients. If you notice any other effects, check with your doctor or pharmacist.

Annual revision: 07/26/93

PYRIDOXINE (Vitamin B_6) Systemic

Some commonly used brand names are:

In the U.S.

Beesix
Rodex
Vitabee 6

Generic name product may also be available.

In Canada

Hexa-Betalin

Generic name product is available.

Description

Vitamins (VYE-ta-mins) are compounds that you *must* have for growth and health. They are needed in small amounts only and are usually available in the foods that you eat. Pyridoxine (peer-i-DOX-een) (vitamin B_6) is necessary for normal metabolism.

Patients with the following conditions may be more likely to have a deficiency of pyridoxine:

- Alcoholism
- Burns
- Diarrhea
- Dialysis
- Heart disease
- Intestinal problems
- Liver disease
- Overactive thyroid
- Stress, long-term illness, or serious injury
- Surgical removal of stomach

In addition, infants receiving unfortified formulas such as evaporated milk may need additional pyridoxine.

If any of the above apply to you, you should take pyridoxine only on the advice of your doctor after need has been established.

Lack of pyridoxine may lead to anemia (weak blood), nerve damage, seizures, skin problems, and sores in the mouth. Your doctor may treat these problems by prescribing pyridoxine for you.

Claims that pyridoxine is effective for treatment of acne and other skin problems, alcohol intoxication, asthma, hemorrhoids, kidney stones, mental problems, migraine headaches, morning sickness, and menstrual problems, or to stimulate appetite or milk production have not been proven.

Oral forms of pyridoxine are available without a prescription. However, it may be a good idea to check with your doctor before taking any on your own.

Pyridoxine is available in the following dosage forms:

Oral

- Extended-release capsules (U.S.)
- Tablets (U.S. and Canada)

Parenteral

- Injection (U.S. and Canada)

It is very important that you read and understand the following information. If any of it causes you special concern, check with your doctor or pharmacist. Also, *if you have any questions* or if you want more information about this dietary supplement or your medical problem, *ask your doctor, nurse, pharmacist, or dietitian.*

Importance of Diet

Vitamin supplements should be taken only if you cannot get enough vitamins in your diet; however, some diets may not contain all of the vitamins you need. You may not be getting enough vitamins because of rapid weight loss, unusual diets (such as some reducing diets in which choice of foods is very limited), prolonged intravenous feeding, or malnutrition. A balanced diet should provide all the vitamins you normally need.

In order to get enough vitamins and minerals in your diet, it is important that you eat a balanced and varied diet. Follow carefully any diet program your doctor may recommend. For your specific vitamin and/or mineral needs, ask your doctor or dietitian for a list of appropriate foods.

Pyridoxine is found in various foods, including meats, bananas, lima beans, egg yolks, peanuts, and whole-grain cereals. Pyridoxine is not lost from food during ordinary cooking, although some other forms of vitamin B$_6$ are.

Vitamins alone will not take the place of a good diet and will not provide energy. Your body also needs other substances found in food such as protein, minerals, carbohydrates, and fat. Vitamins themselves often cannot work without the presence of other foods.

In some cases, it may not be possible for you to get enough food to supply you with the proper vitamins. In other cases, the amount of vitamins you need may be increased above normal. Therefore, a vitamin supplement may be needed.

Experts have developed a list of recommended dietary allowances (RDA) for most of the vitamins. The RDA are not an exact number but a general idea of how much you need. They do not cover amounts needed for problems caused by a serious lack of vitamins.

The RDA for pyridoxine are:

- Infants and children—
  - Birth to 6 months of age: 0.3 milligrams (mg) per day.
  - 6 months to 1 year of age: 0.6 mg per day.
  - 1 to 3 years of age: 1 mg per day.
  - 4 to 6 years of age: 1.1 mg per day.
  - 7 to 10 years of age: 1.4 mg per day.
- Adolescent and adult males—
  - 11 to 14 years of age: 1.7 mg per day.
  - 15 years of age and over: 2 mg per day.
- Adolescent and adult females—
  - 11 to 14 years of age: 1.4 mg per day.
  - 15 to 18 years of age: 1.5 mg per day.
  - 19 years of age and over: 1.6 mg per day.
- Pregnant females—2.2 mg per day.
- Breast-feeding females—2.1 mg per day.

Remember:

- The total amount of each vitamin that you get every day includes what you get from the foods that you eat *and* what you may take as a supplement.
- This total amount should not be greater than the RDA, unless ordered by your doctor.

Before Using This Dietary Supplement

If you are taking this dietary supplement without a prescription, carefully read and follow any precautions on the label. For pyridoxine, the following should be considered:

Allergies—Tell your doctor if you have ever had any unusual or allergic reaction to pyridoxine. Also tell your doctor and pharmacist if you are allergic to any other substances, such as foods, preservatives, or dyes.

Pregnancy—It is especially important that you are receiving enough vitamins when you become pregnant and that you continue to receive the right amount of vitamins throughout your pregnancy. The healthy growth and development of the fetus depend on a steady supply of nutrients from the mother. However, excessive doses of pyridoxine taken during pregnancy may cause the infant to become dependent on pyridoxine.

Breast-feeding—It is especially important that you receive the right amounts of vitamins so that your baby will also get the vitamins needed to grow properly. You should also check with your doctor if you are giving your baby an unfortified formula. In that case, the baby must get the vitamins needed some other way. However, taking large amounts of a dietary supplement while breast-feeding may be harmful to the mother and/or baby and should be avoided.

Children—Normal daily requirements vary according to age. It is especially important that children receive enough vitamins in their diet for healthy growth and development. Although there is no specific information about the use of pyridoxine in children in doses higher than the normal daily requirements, it is not expected to cause different side effects or problems in children than in adults.

Older adults—It is important that older people continue to receive enough vitamins in their diet for good health. Although there is no specific information about the use of pyridoxine in older people in doses higher than the normal daily requirements, it is not expected to cause different side effects or problems in older people than in younger adults.

Medicines or other dietary supplements—Although certain medicines or dietary supplements should not be used together at all, in other cases they may be used together even if an interaction might occur. In these cases, your doctor may want to change the dose, or other precautions may be necessary. When you are taking pyridoxine, it is especially important that your doctor and pharmacist know if you are taking the following:

- Levodopa (e.g., Larodopa)—Use with pyridoxine may prevent the levodopa from working properly

Proper Use of This Dietary Supplement

Do not take more than the recommended daily amount. Taking too much pyridoxine may cause harmful effects, such as nerve damage, which may appear as clumsiness, or numbness of hands or feet. Some people believe that taking very large doses of vitamins (called megadoses or megavitamin therapy) is useful for treating certain medical problems. Studies have not proven this. Large doses should be taken only under the direction of your doctor after need has been identified.

To use the *extended-release capsule form* of this dietary supplement:

- Swallow the capsule whole.
- Do not crush, break, or chew before swallowing.
- If the capsule is too large to swallow, you may mix the contents of the capsule with jam or jelly and swallow without chewing.

Missed dose—If you miss taking a vitamin for 1 or more days there is no cause for concern, since it takes some time for your body to become seriously low in vitamins. However, if your doctor has recommended that you take this vitamin, try to remember to take it as directed every day.

Storage—To store this dietary supplement:

- Keep out of the reach of children.
- Store away from heat and direct light.
- Do not store the capsule or tablet form of this medicine in the bathroom, near the kitchen sink, or in other damp places. Heat or moisture may cause the dietary supplement to break down.
- Do not keep outdated dietary supplements or those no longer needed. Be sure that any discarded medicine is out of the reach of children.

Side Effects of This Dietary Supplement

Along with its needed effects, a dietary supplement may cause some unwanted effects. Although pyridoxine does not usually cause any side effects at usual doses, check with your doctor as soon as possible if you notice either of the following side effects:

With large doses

Clumsiness; numbness of hands or feet

Also check with your doctor if you notice any other unusual effects while you are taking pyridoxine.

Annual revision: 09/21/92

PYRIMETHAMINE Systemic

A commonly used brand name in the U.S. and Canada is Daraprim.

Description

Pyrimethamine (peer-i-METH-a-meen) is an antiprotozoal (an-tee-proe-toe-ZOE-al) medicine. Antiprotozoals work by killing protozoa (tiny, one-celled animals) or preventing their growth. Some protozoa are parasites that can cause many different kinds of infections in the body.

This medicine is used with one or more other medicines to treat malaria and toxoplasmosis (tok-soe-plaz-MOE-siss). This medicine may also be used for other problems as determined by your doctor.

Pyrimethamine is available only with your doctor's prescription, in the following dosage form:

Oral

- Tablets (U.S. and Canada)

It is very important that you read and understand the following information. If any of it causes you special concern, check with your doctor. Also, *if you have any questions* or if you want more information about this medicine or your medical problem, *ask your doctor, nurse, or pharmacist.*

Before Using This Medicine

In deciding to use a medicine, the risks of taking the medicine must be weighed against the good it will do. This is a decision you and your doctor will make. For pyrimethamine, the following should be considered:

Allergies—Tell your doctor if you have ever had any unusual or allergic reaction to pyrimethamine. Also tell your doctor and pharmacist if you are allergic to any other substances, such as foods, preservatives, or dyes.

Pregnancy—Studies in humans have not shown that pyrimethamine causes birth defects. Also, use in pregnant women has not shown pyrimethamine to cause birth defects. However, use is not generally recommended during the first 3 to 4 months of pregnancy. Studies in animals have shown that pyrimethamine may cause birth defects, anemia, or other problems, especially when given in large doses.

Breast-feeding—Pyrimethamine passes into the breast milk. However, problems in nursing babies have not been reported.

Children—Pyrimethamine has been used in children and, in effective doses, has not been shown to cause different side effects or problems in children than it does in adults.

Older adults—Many medicines have not been studied specifically in older people. Therefore, it may not be known whether they work exactly the same way they do in younger adults or if they cause different side effects or problems in older people. There is no specific information comparing use of pyrimethamine in the elderly with use in other age groups.

Other medicines—Although certain medicines should not be used together at all, in other cases two different medicines may be used together even if an interaction might occur. In these cases, your doctor may want to change the dose, or other precautions may be necessary. When you are taking pyrimethamine, it is especially important that your doctor and pharmacist know if you are taking any of the following:

- Amphotericin B by injection (e.g., Fungizone) or
- Antineoplastics (cancer medicine) or
- Antithyroid agents (medicine for overactive thyroid) or
- Azathioprine (e.g., Imuran) or
- Chloramphenicol (e.g., Chloromycetin) or
- Colchicine or
- Cyclophosphamide (e.g., Cytoxan) or
- Flucytosine (e.g., Ancobon) or
- Ganciclovir (e.g., Cytovene) or
- Interferon (e.g., Intron A, Roferon-A) or
- Mercaptopurine (e.g., Purinethol) or
- Methotrexate (e.g., Mexate) or
- Plicamycin (e.g., Mithracin) or
- Zidovudine (e.g., AZT, Retrovir)—Use of these medicines together with pyrimethamine may increase the chance of side effects affecting the blood

Other medical problems—The presence of other medical problems may affect the use of pyrimethamine. Make sure you tell your doctor if you have any other medical problems, especially:

- Anemia or other blood problems—High doses of pyrimethamine may make these conditions worse
- Liver disease—Patients with liver disease may have an increased chance of side effects
- Seizure disorders, such as epilepsy—High doses of pyrimethamine may increase the chance of convulsions (seizures)

Before you begin using any new medicine (prescription or nonprescription) or if you develop any new medical problem while you are using this medicine, check with your doctor, nurse, or pharmacist.

Proper Use of This Medicine

Keep this medicine out of the reach of children. Overdose is especially dangerous.

If this medicine upsets your stomach or causes vomiting, it may be taken with meals or a snack.

If you are taking this medicine to *treat malaria*, take the number of tablets your doctor told you to take (up to 3) once, as a single dose, along with other medicine your doctor gave you. If you develop a fever and are not near a medical facility, and are taking this medicine to treat what you think may possibly be malaria, take the number of tablets your doctor told you to take (up to 3) once, as a single dose.

This medicine works best when you take it on a regular schedule. If you are to take 2 doses a day, one dose may be taken with breakfast and the other one with the evening meal. *Make sure that you do not miss any doses.* If you have any questions about this, check with your doctor, nurse, or pharmacist.

Dosing—The dose of pyrimethamine will be different for different patients. *Follow your doctor's orders or the directions on the label.* The following information includes only the average doses of pyrimethamine. *If your dose is different, do not change it* unless your doctor tells you to do so.

- *The number of doses you take each day, the time allowed between doses, and the length of time you take the medicine depend on the medical problem for which you are taking pyrimethamine.*
- For the treatment of *malaria*:
  —Adults and adolescents: 75 milligrams of pyrimethamine together with 1.5 grams of sulfadoxine as a single dose. These 2 medicines may also be taken with other medicine. This will be determined by your doctor.
  —Children: Dose is based on body weight and will be determined by the doctor. Pyrimethamine taken together with other medicines.
- For the treatment of *toxoplasmosis*:
  —Adults and adolescents: 25 to 200 milligrams of pyrimethamine taken together with other medicines for several weeks. The proper dose for you must be determined by the doctor.
  —Children: Dose is based on body weight and must be determined by the doctor.

Missed dose—If you do miss a dose of this medicine, take it as soon as possible. This will help to keep you taking your medicine on a regular schedule. However, if it is almost time for your next dose, skip the missed dose and go back to your regular dosing schedule. Do not double doses.

Storage—To store this medicine:

- Keep out of the reach of children. Overdose is very dangerous.
- Store away from heat and direct light.
- Do not store in the bathroom, near the kitchen sink, or in other damp places. Heat or moisture may cause the medicine to break down.
- Do not keep outdated medicine or medicine no longer needed. Be sure that any discarded medicine is out of the reach of children.

Precautions While Using This Medicine

It is very important that your doctor check you at regular visits for any blood problems that may be caused by this medicine, especially if you will be taking this medicine in high doses for toxoplasmosis.

If your symptoms do not improve within a few days or if they become worse, check with your doctor.

If this medicine causes anemia, your doctor may want you to take leucovorin (e.g., folinic acid, Wellcovorin) to help clear up the anemia. If so, it is important to take the leucovorin every day while you are taking this medicine. Do not miss any doses.

Pyrimethamine, especially in high doses, may cause blood problems. These problems may result in a greater chance of certain infections, slow healing, and bleeding of the gums. Therefore, you should be careful when using regular toothbrushes, dental floss, and toothpicks. Dental work should be delayed until your blood counts have returned to normal. Check with your medical doctor or dentist if you have any questions about proper oral hygiene (mouth care) during treatment.

Side Effects of This Medicine

Along with its needed effects, a medicine may cause some unwanted effects. Although not all of these side effects may occur, if they do occur they may need medical attention.

Check with your doctor immediately if any of the following side effects occur:

More common with high doses

Change in or loss of taste; fever and sore throat; soreness, swelling, or burning of tongue; unusual bleeding or bruising; unusual tiredness or weakness

Rare

Skin rash

Symptoms of overdose

Abdominal or stomach pain; convulsions (seizures); increased excitability; vomiting (severe and continuing)

Other side effects may occur that usually do not need medical attention. These side effects may go away during treatment as your body adjusts to the medicine. However, check with your doctor if either of the following side effects continues or is bothersome:

More common with high doses

Diarrhea; loss of appetite; nausea; vomiting

Other side effects not listed above may also occur in some patients. If you notice any other effects, check with your doctor.

Additional Information

Once a medicine has been approved for marketing for a certain use, experience may show that it is also useful for other medical problems. Although these uses are not included in product labeling, pyrimethamine is used in certain patients with the following medical conditions:

- Isosporiasis (treatment and prevention)
- *Pneumocystis carinii* pneumonia (treatment)

For patients taking this medicine for *Pneumocystis carinii* pneumonia:

- Pyrimethamine is used in combination with other medicines for mild to moderate pneumonia in patients who cannot take standard treatment.

Other than the above information, there is no additional information relating to proper use, precautions, or side effects for these uses.

Annual revision: 01/19/93

PYRITHIONE Topical

Some commonly used brand names are:

In the U.S.

- Danex
- DHS Zinc Dandruff Shampoo
- Head & Shoulders Antidandruff Cream Shampoo Normal to Dry Formula
- Head & Shoulders Antidandruff Cream Shampoo Normal to Oily Formula
- Head & Shoulders Antidandruff Lotion Shampoo Normal to Dry Formula
- Head & Shoulders Antidandruff Lotion Shampoo Normal to Oily Formula
- Head & Shoulders Antidandruff Lotion Shampoo 2 in 1 (Complete Dandruff Shampoo plus Conditioner in One) Formula
- Head & Shoulders Dry Scalp Conditioning Formula Lotion Shampoo
- Head & Shoulders Dry Scalp Regular Formula Lotion Shampoo
- Head & Shoulders Dry Scalp 2 in 1 (Dry Scalp Shampoo Plus Conditioner in One) Formula Lotion Shampoo
- Sebex
- Sebulon
- Zincon Dandruff Lotion Shampoo
- ZNP Bar Shampoo
- ZNP Shampoo

In Canada

- Dan-Gard
- Sebulon

Description

Pyrithione (peer-i-THYE-one) is used to help control the symptoms of dandruff and seborrheic dermatitis of the scalp.

This medicine is available without a prescription; however, your doctor may have special instructions on the proper use of this medicine for your medical condition.

Pyrithione is available in the following dosage forms:

Topical

- Bar shampoo (U.S.)
- Cream shampoo (U.S.)
- Lotion shampoo (U.S. and Canada)

It is very important that you read and understand the following information. If any of it causes you special concern, check with your doctor or pharmacist. Also, *if you have any questions* or if you want more information about this medicine or your medical problem, *ask your doctor, nurse, or pharmacist.*

Before Using This Medicine

If you are using this medicine without a prescription, carefully read and follow any precautions on the label. For pyrithione, the following should be considered:

Allergies—Tell your doctor if you have ever had any unusual or allergic reaction to pyrithione. Also tell your doctor and pharmacist if you are allergic to any other substances, such as preservatives or dyes.

Pregnancy—Pyrithione has not been shown to cause birth defects or other problems in humans.

Breast-feeding—Pyrithione has not been reported to cause problems in nursing babies.

Children—Although there is no specific information comparing use of pyrithione in children with use in other age groups, this medicine is not expected to cause different side effects or problems in children than it does in adults.

Older adults—Many medicines have not been studied specifically in older people. Therefore, it may not be known whether they work exactly the same way they do in younger adults. Although there is no specific information comparing use of pyrithione in the elderly with use in other age groups, this medicine is not expected to cause different side effects or problems in older people than it does in younger adults.

Other medicines—Although certain medicines should not be used together at all, in other cases two different medicines may be used together even if an interaction might

occur. In these cases, your doctor may want to change the dose, or other precautions may be necessary. Tell your doctor and pharmacist if you are using any other topical prescription or nonprescription (over-the-counter [OTC]) medicine that is to be applied to the same area of the skin.

Before you begin using any new medicine (prescription or nonprescription) or if you develop any new medical problem while you are using this medicine, check with your doctor, nurse, or pharmacist.

Proper Use of This Medicine

For best results, use this medicine at least 2 times a week or as directed by your doctor.

To use:

- Before applying this shampoo, wet the hair and scalp with lukewarm water.
- Apply enough shampoo to the scalp to work up a lather and rub in well, then rinse.
- Apply the shampoo again and rinse thoroughly.

Keep this medicine away from the eyes. If you should accidentally get some in your eyes, flush them thoroughly with water.

Dosing—The dose of pyrithione will be different for different patients. *Follow your doctor's orders or the directions on the label.* The following information includes only the average dose of pyrithione. *If your dose is different, do not change it* unless your doctor tells you to do so:

- For *topical* dosage forms (bar shampoo, cream shampoo, and lotion shampoo):
  - —For dandruff and seborrheic dermatitis of the scalp:
    - Adults and children—Use as a shampoo on the scalp 2 times a week.

Missed dose—If you miss a dose of this medicine, use it as soon as possible. However, if it is almost time for your next dose, skip the missed dose and go back to your regular dosing schedule.

Storage—To store this medicine:

- Keep out of the reach of children.
- Store away from heat and direct light.
- Keep the medicine from freezing.
- Do not keep outdated medicine or medicine no longer needed. Be sure that any discarded medicine is out of the reach of children.

Precautions While Using This Medicine

If your condition does not get better after regular use of this medicine, or if it gets worse, check with your doctor.

Side Effects of This Medicine

Along with its needed effects, a medicine may cause some unwanted effects. Although not all of these side effects may occur, if they do occur they may need medical attention.

Check with your doctor as soon as possible if the following side effect occurs:

Less common or rare

Irritation of skin

Other side effects not listed above may also occur in some patients. If you notice any other effects, check with your doctor or pharmacist.

Annual revision: 07/26/93

PYRVINIUM Oral*

A commonly used brand name in Canada is Vanquin.

Another commonly used name is viprynium.

*Not commercially available in the U.S.

Description

Pyrvinium (peer-VIN-ee-um) is used to treat pinworms (enterobiasis). It will not work for other types of worm infections (for example, roundworms or tapeworms).

Pyrvinium is available only with your doctor's prescription, in the following dosage forms:

Oral

- Oral suspension (Canada)

It is very important that you read and understand the following information. If any of it causes you special concern, check with your doctor. Also, *if you have any questions* or if you want more information about this medicine or your medical problem, *ask your doctor, nurse, or pharmacist.*

Before Using This Medicine

In deciding to use a medicine, the risks of taking the medicine must be weighed against the good it will do. This is a decision you and your doctor will make. For pyrvinium, the following should be considered:

Allergies—Tell your doctor if you have ever had any unusual or allergic reaction to pyrvinium. Also tell your doctor and pharmacist if you are allergic to any other substances, such as foods, preservatives, or dyes.

Pregnancy—Pyrvinium has not been studied in pregnant women or animals. However, pyrvinium has not been reported to cause birth defects or other problems in humans.

Breast-feeding—Pyrvinium has not been reported to cause problems in nursing babies.

Children—Pyrvinium has been studied in children and, in effective doses, has not been reported to cause different side effects or problems in children than it does in adults. However, because of limited experience, caution is recommended in children weighing less than 10 kilograms (22 pounds). Older children are more likely to have stomach upset after receiving large doses.

Older adults—Many medicines have not been studied specifically in older people. Therefore, it may not be known whether they work exactly the same way they do in younger adults. Although there is no specific information comparing use of pyrvinium in the elderly with use in other age groups, this medicine is not expected to cause different side effects or problems in older people than it does in younger adults.

Other medicines—Although certain medicines should not be used together at all, in other cases two different medicines may be used together even if an interaction might occur. In these cases, your doctor may want to change the dose, or other precautions may be necessary. Tell your doctor and pharmacist if you are taking any other prescription or nonprescription (over-the-counter [OTC]) medicine.

Other medical problems—The presence of other medical problems may affect the use of pyrvinium. Make sure you tell your doctor if you have any other medical problems, especially:

- Inflammatory bowel disease—Patients with inflammatory bowel disease may have an increased chance of side effects

Before you begin using any new medicine (prescription or nonprescription) or if you develop any new medical problem while you are using this medicine, check with your doctor, nurse, or pharmacist.

Proper Use of This Medicine

No special preparations (for example, special diets, fasting, other medicines, laxatives, or enemas) are necessary before, during, or immediately after you take pyrvinium.

Use a specially marked measuring spoon or other device to measure each dose accurately. The average household teaspoon may not hold the right amount of liquid.

Pinworms may be easily passed from one person to another, especially among persons in the same household. Therefore, all household members may have to be treated at the same time to prevent their infection or reinfection. Also, all household members may have to be treated again in 2 to 3 weeks to clear up the infection completely. Make sure each family member takes the correct amount, since the dose may be different for each person.

To help clear up your infection completely, *take this medicine exactly as directed by your doctor.* Read the instructions on the label and follow them carefully. The amount of medicine you need is based on your weight. You must take the exact amount if the medicine is going to work. A second course of pyrvinium is usually required to clear up the infection completely.

Dosing—The dose of pyrvinium will be different for different patients. *Follow your doctor's orders or the directions on the label.* The following information includes only the average doses of pyrvinium. *If your dose is different, do not change it* unless your doctor tells you to do so.

- For the *oral suspension* dosage form:
  - —Adults and children: Dose is based on body weight and will be determined by your doctor. It is taken as a single dose and is repeated in 2 to 3 weeks.

Storage—To store this medicine:

- Keep out of the reach of children.
- Store away from heat and direct light.
- Do not store in the bathroom, near the kitchen sink, or in other damp places. Heat or moisture may cause the medicine to break down.
- Do not freeze oral suspension.
- Do not keep outdated medicine or medicine no longer needed. Be sure that any discarded medicine is out of the reach of children.

Precautions While Using This Medicine

If your symptoms do not improve within a few days, or if they become worse, check with your doctor.

Pyrvinium may cause your skin to be more sensitive to sunlight than it is normally. Exposure to sunlight, even for brief periods of time, may cause a skin rash, itching, redness or other discoloration of the skin, or a severe sunburn. For a day or two after taking this medicine:

- Stay out of direct sunlight, especially between the hours of 10:00 a.m. and 3:00 p.m., if possible.
- Wear protective clothing, including a hat. Also, wear sunglasses.
- Apply a sun block product that has a skin protection factor (SPF) of at least 15. Some patients may require a product with a higher SPF number, especially if they have a fair complexion. If you have any questions about this, check with your doctor or pharmacist.
- Apply a sunblock lipstick that has an SPF of at least 15 to protect your lips.
- Do not use a sunlamp or tanning bed or booth.

If you have a severe reaction from the sun, check with your doctor.

In some patients, pinworms may return after treatment with pyrvinium. Washing (not shaking) all bedding and nightclothes (pajamas) after treatment may help to prevent this. Some doctors may also recommend other measures to help keep your infection from returning. If you have any questions about this, check with your doctor.

Side Effects of This Medicine

Along with its needed effects, a medicine may cause some unwanted effects. Although not all of these side effects may occur, if they do occur they may need medical attention.

Check with your doctor as soon as possible if the following side effect occurs:

Rare

Skin rash

Other side effects may occur that usually do not need medical attention. These side effects may go away during treatment as your body adjusts to the medicine. However, check with your doctor if any of the following side effects continue or are bothersome:

Rare

Diarrhea; increased sensitivity of skin to sunlight; nausea and vomiting; stomach cramps

This medicine is a dye and will *color your stools red.* This color is not harmful and will disappear in a few days. Pyrvinium may also stain clothing red. If vomiting occurs, the vomit will be red in color.

Other side effects not listed above may also occur in some patients. If you notice any other effects, check with your doctor.

Annual revision: 01/19/93

QUINACRINE Systemic

A commonly used brand name in the U.S. and Canada is Atabrine. Another commonly used name is mepacrine.

Description

Quinacrine (KWIN-a-kreen) is used to treat giardiasis (jee-ar-DYE-a-siss), a protozoal infection of the intestinal tract. This medicine may also be used for other conditions as determined by your doctor.

Quinacrine is available only with your doctor's prescription, in the following dosage form:

Oral

- Tablets (U.S. and Canada)

It is very important that you read and understand the following information. If any of it causes you special concern, check with your doctor. Also, *if you have any questions* or if you want more information about this medicine or your medical problem, *ask your doctor, nurse, or pharmacist.*

Before Using This Medicine

In deciding to use a medicine, the risks of taking the medicine must be weighed against the good it will do. This is a decision you and your doctor will make. For quinacrine, the following should be considered:

Allergies—Tell your doctor if you have ever had any unusual or allergic reaction to quinacrine. Also tell your doctor and pharmacist if you are allergic to any other substances, such as foods, preservatives, or dyes.

Pregnancy—Use of quinacrine to treat giardiasis in a pregnant woman should be delayed until after delivery as long as the woman is not experiencing symptoms of the disease.

Breast-feeding—Quinacrine is excreted in breast milk. However, quinacrine has not been reported to cause problems in nursing babies.

Children—Quinacrine can cause serious side effects in any patient. Therefore, it is especially important that you discuss with the child's doctor the good that this medicine may do as well as the risks of using it.

Older adults—Many medicines have not been studied specifically in older people. Therefore, it may not be known whether they work exactly the same way they do in younger adults. Although there is no specific information comparing use of quinacrine in the elderly with use in other age groups, this medicine is not expected to cause different side effects or problems in older people than it does in younger adults.

Other medicines—Although certain medicines should not be used together at all, in other cases two different medicines may be used together even if an interaction might occur. In these cases, your doctor may want to change the dose, or other precautions may be necessary. When you are taking quinacrine, it is especially important that your doctor and pharmacist know if you are taking any of the following:

- Primaquine—Use with quinacrine may increase the chance of side effects from primaquine

Other medical problems—The presence of other medical problems may affect the use of quinacrine. Make sure you tell your doctor if you have any other medical problems, especially:

- Mental illness (severe) (history of)—Quinacrine may cause mood or other mental changes in some patients
- Porphyria—Quinacrine may make porphyria worse
- Psoriasis—Quinacrine may cause an attack of psoriasis or make psoriasis worse

Before you begin using any new medicine (prescription or nonprescription) or if you develop any new medical problem while you are using this medicine, check with your doctor, nurse, or pharmacist.

Proper Use of This Medicine

Quinacrine is best taken after meals with a full glass (8 ounces) of water, tea, or fruit juice, unless otherwise directed by your doctor.

For patients *unable to swallow tablets or unable to tolerate bitter taste:*

- The tablets may be crushed and mixed with jam, honey, or chocolate syrup or placed in empty gelatin capsules to cover up the bitter taste. Be sure to take all the food so that you get the full dose of medicine.

To help clear up your infection completely, *keep taking quinacrine for the full time of treatment,* even if you begin to feel better after a few days. If you stop taking this medicine too soon, your symptoms may return. *Do not miss any doses.*

Dosing—The dose of quinacrine will be different for different patients. *Follow your doctor's orders or the directions on the label.* The following information includes only the average doses of quinacrine. *If your dose is different, do not change it* unless your doctor tells you to do so.

- For the *tablet* dosage form:
  —Adults and older children: 100 milligrams three times a day for five to seven days.

Q-R

—Younger children: Dose is based on body weight and will be determined by the doctor. The dose is taken three times a day for five to seven days.

Missed dose—If you do miss a dose of this medicine, take it as soon as possible. However, if it is almost time for your next dose, skip the missed dose and go back to your regular dosing schedule. Do not double doses.

Storage—To store this medicine:
- Keep out of the reach of children.
- Store away from heat and direct light.
- Do not store in the bathroom, near the kitchen sink, or in other damp places. Heat or moisture may cause the medicine to break down.
- Do not keep outdated medicine or medicine no longer needed. Be sure that any discarded medicine is out of the reach of children.

Precautions While Using This Medicine

It is important that your doctor check your progress at different times. This is to check whether or not the infection is cleared up completely.

If your symptoms do not improve within a few days, or if they become worse, check with your doctor.

Quinacrine may cause some people to become dizzy. *Make sure you know how you react to this medicine before you drive, use machines, or do anything else that could be dangerous if you are dizzy or are not alert.* If this reaction is especially bothersome, check with your doctor.

Side Effects of This Medicine

Along with its needed effects, a medicine may cause some unwanted effects. Although not all of these side effects may occur, if they do occur they may need medical attention. When this medicine is used for a short time, side effects are not generally serious. However, if this medicine is used for a long time and/or in high doses, other more serious side effects may occur.

Check with your doctor immediately if any of the following side effects occur:

Less common

Hallucinations (seeing, hearing, or feeling things that are not there); irritability; mood or other mental changes; nervousness; nightmares; skin rash, redness, itching, or peeling

Symptoms of overdose

Convulsions (seizures); fainting; irregular heartbeat

Other side effects may occur that usually do not need medical attention. These side effects may go away during treatment as your body adjusts to the medicine. However, check with your doctor if any of the following side effects continue or are bothersome:

More common

Abdominal or stomach cramps; diarrhea; dizziness; headache; loss of appetite; nausea or vomiting

Quinacrine is a dye-like medicine and commonly causes *yellow discoloration of the skin or urine.* This side effect is only *temporary* and will go away when you stop taking this medicine.

Other side effects not listed above may also occur in some patients. If you notice any other effects, check with your doctor.

Additional Information

Once a medicine has been approved for marketing for a certain use, experience may show that it is also useful for other medical problems. Although this use is not included in product labeling, quinacrine is used in certain patients with the following medical condition:
- Discoid lupus erythematosus

Other than the above information, there is no additional information relating to proper use, precautions, or side effects for this use.

Annual revision: 02/01/93

QUINIDINE Systemic

Some commonly used brand names are:

In the U.S.

Cardioquin
Cin-Quin
Duraquin
Quinaglute Dura-tabs
Quinalan
Quinidex Extentabs
Quinora

Generic name product may also be available.

In Canada

Apo-Quinidine
Cardioquin
Novoquinidin
Quinaglute Dura-tabs
Quinate
Quinidex Extentabs

Generic name product may also be available.

Description

Quinidine (KWIN-i-deen) is most often used to correct certain irregular heartbeats to a normal rhythm and to slow an overactive heart. It is also sometimes used for other conditions as determined by your doctor.

Quinidine acts directly on the heart tissues to make them less responsive. It also slows impulses along special nerve networks to the heart. This allows the heart to work more efficiently.

Do not confuse this medicine with *quinine*, which, although related, has different medical uses.

Quinidine is available only with your doctor's prescription, in the following dosage forms:

Oral
- Capsules (U.S.)
- Tablets (U.S. and Canada)
- Extended-release tablets (U.S. and Canada)

Parenteral
- Injection (U.S. and Canada)

It is very important that you read and understand the following information. If any of it causes you special concern, check with your doctor. Also, *if you have any questions* or if you want more information about this medicine or your medical problem, *ask your doctor, nurse, or pharmacist.*

Before Using This Medicine

In deciding to use a medicine, the risks of taking the medicine must be weighed against the good it will do. This is a decision you and your doctor will make. For quinidine, the following should be considered:

Allergies—Tell your doctor if you have ever had any unusual or allergic reaction to quinidine or quinine. Also tell your doctor and pharmacist if you are allergic to any other substance, such as foods, preservatives, or dyes.

Pregnancy—Although studies have not been done in either humans or animals, a closely related medicine, quinine, has been shown to cause birth defects of the nervous system, fingers, and toes and decreased hearing in the infant. Quinine also may cause contractions of the uterus.

Breast-feeding—Although quinidine passes into the breast milk, it has not been reported to cause problems in nursing babies.

Children—There is no specific information about the use of quinidine in children. Use of the extended-release tablets in children is not recommended.

Older adults—Many medicines have not been tested in older people. Therefore, it may not be known whether they work exactly the same way they do in younger adults. Although there is no specific information about the use of quinidine in the elderly, it is not expected to cause different side effects or problems in older people than it does in younger adults.

Other medicines—Although certain medicines should not be used together at all, in other cases two different medicines may be used together even if an interaction might occur. In these cases, your doctor may want to change the dose, or other precautions may be necessary. When you are taking quinidine, it is especially important that your doctor and pharmacist know if you are taking any of the following:

- Anticoagulants (blood thinners)—Risk of bleeding may be increased
- Other heart medicine (especially digoxin)—Effects on the heart may be increased
- Pimozide (e.g., Orap)—Risk of heart rhythm problems may be increased
- Urinary alkalizers (medicine that makes the urine less acid, such as acetazolamide [e.g., Diamox], calcium- and/or magnesium-containing antacids, dichlorphenamide [e.g., Daranide], methazolamide [e.g., Neptazane], potassium or sodium citrate and/or citric acid, sodium bicarbonate [baking soda])—Effects may be increased because levels of quinidine in the body may be increased

Other medical problems—The presence of other medical problems may affect the use of quinidine. Make sure you tell your doctor if you have any other medical problems, especially:

- Asthma or emphysema—Possible allergic reaction
- Blood disease
- Infection
- Kidney disease or
- Liver disease—Effects may be increased because of slower removal of quinidine from the body
- Myasthenia gravis—Muscle weakness may be increased
- Overactive thyroid
- Psoriasis

Before you begin using any new medicine (prescription or nonprescription) or if you develop any new medical problem while you are using this medicine, check with your doctor, nurse, or pharmacist.

Proper Use of This Medicine

Take quinidine with a full glass (8 ounces) of water on an empty stomach 1 hour before or 2 hours after meals so that it will be absorbed more quickly. However, to lessen stomach upset, your doctor may want you to take the medicine with food or milk.

For patients taking the *extended-release tablet* form of this medicine:
- These tablets are to be swallowed whole.
- Do not break, crush, or chew before swallowing.

Take quinidine exactly as directed by your doctor even though you may feel well. Do not take more medicine than ordered and do not miss any doses.

Missed dose—If you do miss a dose of this medicine and remember within 2 hours of the missed dose, take it as soon as possible. However, if you do not remember until later, skip the missed dose and go back to your regular dosing schedule. Do not double doses.

Storage—To store this medicine:
- Keep out of the reach of children.
- Store away from heat and direct light.
- Do not store in the bathroom, near the kitchen sink, or in other damp places. Heat or moisture may cause the medicine to break down.
- Do not keep outdated medicine or medicine no longer needed. Be sure that any discarded medicine is out of the reach of children.

Precautions While Using This Medicine

It is very important that your doctor check your progress at regular visits to make sure that the quinidine is working properly and does not cause unwanted effects.

Do not stop taking this medicine without first checking with your doctor, to avoid possible worsening of your condition.

Before having any kind of surgery (including dental surgery) or emergency treatment, tell the medical doctor or dentist in charge that you are taking this medicine.

Your doctor may want you to carry a medical identification card or bracelet stating that you are using this medicine.

Some people who are unusually sensitive to this medicine may have side effects after the first dose or first few doses. Check with your doctor right away if the following side effects occur: breathing difficulty, changes in vision, dizziness, fever, headache, ringing in ears, or skin rash.

Side Effects of This Medicine

Along with its needed effects, a medicine may cause some unwanted effects. Although not all of these side effects may occur, if they do occur they may need medical attention.

Check with your doctor immediately if any of the following side effects occur:

Less common

Blurred vision or any change in vision; dizziness, lightheadedness, or fainting; fever; headache (severe); ringing or buzzing in the ears or any loss of hearing; skin rash, hives, or itching; wheezing, shortness of breath, or troubled breathing

Rare

Fast heartbeat; unusual bleeding or bruising; unusual tiredness or weakness

Other side effects may occur that usually do not need medical attention. These side effects may go away during treatment as your body adjusts to the medicine. However, check with your doctor if any of the following side effects continue or are bothersome:

More common

Bitter taste; diarrhea; flushing of skin with itching; loss of appetite; nausea or vomiting; stomach pain or cramping

Less common

Confusion

Other side effects not listed above may also occur in some patients. If you notice any other effects, check with your doctor.

Additional Information

Once a medicine has been approved for marketing for a certain use, experience may show that it is also useful for other medical problems. Although this use is not included in product labeling, quinidine is used in certain patients with the following medical condition:
- Malaria

Other than the above information, there is no additional information relating to proper use, precautions, or side effects for these uses.

Annual revision: August 1990

QUININE Systemic

Some commonly used brand names are:

In the U.S.

Legatrin
Quin-260
Quin-amino
Quinamm
Quindan
Quiphile
Q-vel

Generic name product may also be available.

In Canada

Novoquinine

Generic name product may also be available.

Description

Quinine (KWYE-nine) is used to treat malaria. This medicine is usually given with one or more other medicines for malaria.

Quinine is also used to prevent and treat nighttime leg cramps. It may also be used for other problems as determined by your doctor. Do not confuse quinine with *quinidine*, a different medicine that is used for heart problems.

Some quinine products for use in nighttime leg cramps are available only with your doctor's prescription; others are available without a prescription.

Quinine is available in the following dosage forms:

Oral

- Capsules (U.S. and Canada)
- Tablets (U.S.)

It is very important that you read and understand the following information. If any of it causes you special concern, check with your doctor. Also, *if you have any questions* or if you want more information about this medicine or your medical problem, *ask your doctor, nurse, or pharmacist.*

Before Using This Medicine

In deciding to use a medicine, the risks of taking the medicine must be weighed against the good it will do. This is a decision you and your doctor will make. For quinine, the following should be considered:

Allergies—Tell your doctor if you have ever had any unusual or allergic reaction to quinine, quinidine (e.g., Quinidex), or to dietary items that contain quinine, such as tonic water or bitter lemon. Also tell your doctor and pharmacist if you are allergic to any other substances, such as foods, preservatives, or dyes.

Pregnancy—Quinine has been used for the treatment of malaria in pregnant women. Treatment is important because if a pregnant woman gets malaria, there is an increased chance of premature births, stillbirths, and abortion. However, quinine has been shown to cause birth defects in rabbits and guinea pigs and has also been shown to cause rare birth defects, stillbirths, and other problems in humans. In addition, quinine has been shown to cause miscarriage when taken in large amounts.

Breast-feeding—Quinine passes into the breast milk in small amounts. However, this medicine has not been reported to cause problems in nursing babies.

Children—This medicine has been used to treat malaria in children and, in effective doses, has not been shown to cause different side effects or problems in children than it does in adults.

Older adults—Many medicines have not been studied specifically in older people. Therefore, it may not be known whether they work exactly the same way they do in younger adults or if they cause different side effects or problems in older people. There is no specific information comparing use of quinine in the elderly with use in other age groups.

Other medicines—Although certain medicines should not be used together at all, in other cases two different medicines may be used together even if an interaction might occur. In these cases, your doctor may want to change the dose, or other precautions may be necessary. When you are taking quinine, it is especially important that your doctor and pharmacist know if you are taking the following:

- Mefloquine (e.g., Larium)—Use of mefloquine with quinine may increase the chance of side effects

Other medical problems—The presence of other medical problems may affect the use of quinine. Make sure you tell your doctor if you have any other medical problems, especially:

- Blackwater fever, history of, or
- Glucose-6-phosphate dehydrogenase (G6PD) deficiency or
- Purpura, or history of (purplish or brownish red discoloration of skin)—Patients with a history of blackwater fever, G6PD deficiency, or purpura may have an increased risk of side effects affecting the blood
- Heart disease—Quinine can cause side effects of the heart, usually at higher doses
- Hypoglycemia—Quinine may cause low blood sugar
- Myasthenia gravis—Quinine may increase muscle weakness in patients with myasthenia gravis

Before you begin using any new medicine (prescription or nonprescription) or if you develop any new medical problem while you are using this medicine, check with your doctor, nurse, or pharmacist.

Proper Use of This Medicine

Take this medicine only as directed. Do not take more of it, do not take it more often, and do not take it for a longer time than recommended on the label, unless otherwise directed by your doctor. To do so may increase the chance of side effects.

Take this medicine with or after meals to lessen possible stomach upset, unless otherwise directed by your doctor. If you are to take this medicine at bedtime, take it with a snack or with a glass of water, milk, or other beverage.

For patients *taking quinine for malaria:*

- To help clear up your infection completely, *keep taking this medicine for the full time of treatment,* even if you begin to feel better after a few days. If you stop taking this medicine too soon, your symptoms may return. *Do not miss any doses.*

Dosing—The dose of quinine will be different for different patients. *Follow your doctor's orders or the directions on the label.* The following information includes only the average doses of quinine. *If your dose is different, do not change it* unless your doctor tells you to do so.

- The number of capsules or tablets that you take depends on the strength of the medicine. Also, *the number of doses you take each day, the time allowed between doses, and the length of time you take the medicine depend on the medical problem for which you are taking quinine.*
- For treatment of *malaria:*
  —Adults and older children: 600 to 650 mg every eight hours for at least three days. This medicine must be taken with other medicine to treat malaria.
  —Younger children: Dose must be determined by the doctor.
- For prevention and treatment of *leg cramps:*
  —Adults: 200 to 300 mg taken at bedtime.
  —Children: Dose has not been determined.

Missed dose—If you do miss a dose of this medicine, take it as soon as possible. However, if it is almost time for your next dose, skip the missed dose and go back to your regular dosing schedule. Do not double doses.

Storage—To store this medicine:

- Keep out of the reach of children.
- Store away from heat and direct light.
- Do not store in the bathroom, near the kitchen sink, or in other damp places. Heat or moisture may cause the medicine to break down.
- Do not keep outdated medicine or medicine no longer needed. Be sure that any discarded medicine is out of the reach of children.

Precautions While Using This Medicine

Quinine may cause blurred vision or a change in color vision. *Make sure you know how you react to this medicine before you drive, use machines, or do anything else that could be dangerous if you are not able to see well.* If these reactions are especially bothersome, check with your doctor.

Side Effects of This Medicine

Along with its needed effects, a medicine may cause some unwanted effects. Although not all of these side effects may occur, if they do occur they may need medical attention.

Check with your doctor immediately if any of the following side effects occur:

Rare

Anxiety; back, leg, or stomach pains; cold sweats; cool, pale skin; fever and chills; headache; increased hunger; loss of appetite; muscle aches; nausea and vomiting; nervousness; pale skin; pale stools; shakiness; skin rash, redness, hives, or itching; sore throat and fever; stomach pain; sweating; unusual bleeding or bruising; unusual tiredness or weakness; wheezing, shortness of breath, or difficult breathing; yellow skin and eyes

Signs and symptoms of overdose

Blindness; confusion; convulsions (seizures); decreased vision; irregular heartbeat; lightheadedness

Other side effects may occur that usually do not need medical attention. These side effects may go away during treatment as your body adjusts to the medicine. However, check with your doctor if any of the following side effects continue or are bothersome:

More common

Abdominal or stomach cramps or pain; blurred vision or change in color vision; diarrhea; headache (severe); nausea and vomiting; ringing or buzzing in ears or loss of hearing (usually temporary)

Other side effects not listed above may also occur in some patients. If you notice any other effects, check with your doctor.

Annual revision: 02/23/93

RADIOPAQUE AGENTS Diagnostic

This information applies to the following medicines:

- Diatrizoates (dye-a-tri-ZOE-ates)
- Iodipamide (eye-oh-DI-pa-mide)
- Iohexol (eye-oh-HEX-ole)
- Iopamidol (eye-oh-PA-mi-dole)
- Iothalamate (eye-oh-thal-A-mate)
- Ioversol (eye-oh-VER-sole)
- Ioxaglate (eye-OX-a-glate)
- Metrizamide (me-TRI-za-mide)

Used in diagnosis of:	Generic names:
Biliary tract problems	Diatrizoates Iodipamide Iohexol Iothalamate
Blood vessel diseases	Diatrizoates Iohexol Iopamidol Iothalamate Ioversol Ioxaglate Metrizamide
Blood vessel diseases of the brain	Diatrizoates Iohexol Iopamidol Iothalamate Ioversol Ioxaglate
Blood vessel diseases of the heart	Diatrizoates Iohexol Iopamidol Iothalamate Ioversol Ioxaglate Metrizamide
Brain diseases and tumors	Diatrizoates Iohexol Iopamidol Iothalamate Ioversol Ioxaglate Metrizamide
Breast lesions	Diatrizoates
Heart disease	Diatrizoates Iohexol Iopamidol Iothalamate Ioversol Ioxaglate Metrizamide
Impaired flow of cerebrospinal fluid in brain	Iohexol Iopamidol Metrizamide
Kidney diseases	Diatrizoates Iothalamate Ioversol Ioxaglate
Joint diseases	Diatrizoates Iohexol Iothalamate Ioxaglate Metrizamide
Liver diseases	Diatrizoates Iohexol Iothalamate Ioversol Ioxaglate
Pancreas disease	Diatrizoates Iohexol Iothalamate Ioversol Ioxaglate
Spinal disk diseases	Diatrizoates
Spleen diseases	Diatrizoates Iothalamate
Stomach and intestinal problems	Diatrizoates Iohexol
Urinary tract problems	Diatrizoates Iohexol Iopamidol Iothalamate Ioversol Ioxaglate Metrizamide

Description

Radiopaque agents are drugs used to help diagnose certain medical problems. They contain iodine, which absorbs x-rays. Depending on how they are given, radiopaque agents build up in a particular area of the body. The resulting high level of iodine allows the x-rays to make a "picture" of the area.

Radiopaque agents are taken by mouth or given by enema or injection. X-rays are then used to check if there are any problems with the stomach, intestines, kidneys, or other parts of the body.

Some radiopaque agents, such as iohexol, iopamidol, and metrizamide are given by injection into the spinal canal. X-rays are then used to help diagnose problems or diseases in the head, spinal canal, and nervous system.

Radiopaque agents are to be used only by or under the direct supervision of a doctor.

It is very important that you read and understand the following information. If any of it causes you special concern, check with your doctor. Also, *if you have any questions* or if you want more information about this test or your medical problem, *ask your doctor, nurse, or pharmacist.*

Before Having This Test

In deciding to use a diagnostic test, any risks of the test must be weighed against the good it will do. This is a decision you and your doctor will make. Also, test results may be affected by other things. For radiopaque agents, the following should be considered:

Allergies—Tell your doctor if you have ever had any unusual or allergic reaction to iodine, to products containing iodine (for example, iodine-containing foods such as seafood, cabbage, kale, rape [turnip-like vegetable], turnips, or iodized salt), or to any radiopaque agent. Also tell your doctor if you are allergic to any other substance, such as sulfites or other preservatives.

Pregnancy—Studies have not been done in humans with most of the radiopaque agents. However, iohexol, iopamidol, iothalamate, ioversol, ioxaglate, and metrizamide have not been shown to cause birth defects or other problems in animal studies. Some of the radiopaque agents, such as diatrizoates have, on rare occasions, caused hypothyroidism (underactive thyroid) in the baby when they were taken late in the pregnancy. Also, x-rays of the abdomen are usually not recommended during pregnancy. This is to avoid exposing the fetus to radiation. Be sure you have discussed this with your doctor.

Breast-feeding—Although some of these radiopaque agents pass into the breast milk, they have not been shown to cause problems in nursing babies. However, it may be necessary for you to stop breast-feeding temporarily after receiving a radiopaque agent. Be sure you have discussed this with your doctor.

Children—Children, especially those with other medical problems, may be especially sensitive to the effects of radiopaque agents. This may increase the chance of side effects.

Older adults—Elderly people are especially sensitive to the effects of radiopaque agents. This may increase the chance of side effects.

Other medical problems—The presence of other medical problems may affect the use of radiopaque agents. Make sure you tell your doctor if you have any other medical problems, especially:

- Asthma, hay fever, or other allergies (history of)—If you have a history of these conditions, the risk of having a reaction, such as an allergic reaction to the radiopaque agent, is greater
- Diabetes mellitus (sugar diabetes)—There is a greater risk of having kidney problems
- High blood pressure (severe) or
- Pheochromocytoma (PCC)—Injection of the radiopaque agent may cause a dangerous rise in blood pressure
- Kidney disease (severe)—More serious kidney problems may develop; also, the radiopaque agent may build up in the body and cause side effects
- Liver disease—The radiopaque agent may build up in the body and cause side effects
- Multiple myeloma (bone cancer)—Serious kidney problems may develop in patients with this condition
- Overactive thyroid—A sudden increase in symptoms, such as fast heartbeat or palpitations, unusual tiredness or weakness, nervousness, excessive sweating, or muscle weakness may occur
- Sickle cell disease—The radiopaque agent may promote the formation of abnormal blood cells

Preparation For This Test

Your doctor may have special instructions for you in preparation for your test. He or she might prescribe a special diet or use of a laxative, depending on the type of test. If you have not received such instructions or if you do not understand them, check with your doctor in advance.

For some tests your doctor may tell you not to eat for several hours before having the test. This is to prevent any food from coming back up and entering your lungs during the test. You may be allowed to drink small amounts of clear liquids; however, check first with your doctor.

Precautions After Having This Test

Make sure your doctor knows if you are planning to have any thyroid tests in the near future. Even after several weeks or months the results of the thyroid test may be affected by the iodine in this agent.

Side Effects of This Medicine

Along with their needed effects, radiopaque agents can sometimes cause serious effects such as severe allergic reactions or heart problems. These effects may occur almost immediately or a few minutes after the radiopaque agent is given. Although these serious side effects appear only rarely, your doctor or nurse will be prepared to give you immediate medical attention if needed. If you have any questions about this, check with your doctor.

Check with your doctor as soon as possible if the following side effects occur:

With injection into the spinal canal

Rare

Hallucinations (seeing hearing, or feeling things that are not there); paralysis of one side of body or of legs and arms

Other side effects may occur that usually do not need medical attention. These side effects may go away as your body adjusts to this agent. However, check with your doctor if any of the following side effects continue or are bothersome:

With oral or rectal use

Less common

Diarrhea or laxative effect

With injection into a vein or an artery

More common

Unusual warmth and flushing of skin

Less common

Chills; dizziness or lightheadedness; headache; nausea or vomiting; pain or burning at the place of injection; sweating; unusual or metallic taste; unusual thirst

With injection into the spinal canal

More common

Backache; dizziness; headache (mild to moderate); nausea and vomiting (mild to moderate); stiffness of neck

Less common or rare

Difficult urination; drowsiness; headache (severe); increased sensitivity of eyes to light; increased sweating; loss of appetite; ringing or buzzing in ears; unusual tiredness or weakenss

Not all of the side effects listed above have been reported for each of these agents, but they have been reported for at least one of them. There are some similarities among these agents, so many of the above side effects may occur with any of them.

Other side effects not listed above may also occur in some patients. If you notice any other effects, check with your doctor.

Annual revision: August 1990

RADIOPAQUE AGENTS Diagnostic, Mucosal

This information applies to the following medicines:

Diatrizoate and Iodipamide (dye-a-tri-ZOE-ate and eye-oh-DI-pa-mide)
Diatrizoates
Iohexol (eye-oh-HEX-ole)
Iothalamate (eye-oh-thal-A-mate)
Ioxaglate (eye-OX-a-glate)

Used in diagnosis of:	Generic names:
Urinary tract diseases	Diatrizoates Iohexol Iothalamate
Uterus and fallopian tube diseases	Diatrizoate and Iodipamide Diatrizoates Iohexol Ioxaglate

Description

Radiopaque agents are drugs used to help diagnose certain medical problems. They contain iodine, which absorbs x-rays. Depending on how the radiopaque agent is given, it builds up in certain areas of the body. The resulting high level of iodine allows the x-rays to make a "picture" of the area.

A catheter or syringe is used to put the solution of the radiopaque agent into the bladder or ureters to help diagnose problems or diseases of the kidneys or other areas of the urinary tract. It may also be placed into the uterus and fallopian tubes to help diagnose problems or disease of those organs. After the test is done, the patient expels most of the solution by urinating (after bladder or ureter studies) or from the vagina (after uterine or fallopian tube studies).

Radiopaque agents are to be used only by or under the supervision of a doctor.

It is very important that you read and understand the following information. If any of it causes you special concern, check with your doctor. Also, *if you have any questions* or if you want more information about this test or your medical problem, *ask your doctor, nurse, or pharmacist.*

Before Having This Test

In deciding to use a diagnostic test, any risks of the test must be weighed against the good it will do. This is a decision you and your doctor will make. Also, test results may be affected by other things. For radiopaque agents the following should be considered:

Allergies—Tell your doctor if you have ever had any unusual or allergic reaction to iodine, to products containing iodine (for example, iodine-containing foods, such as seafoods, cabbage, kale, rape [turnip-like vegetable], turnips, or iodized salt), or to other radiopaque agents. Also tell your doctor if you are allergic to any other substance, such as sulfites or other preservatives.

Pregnancy—Studies on effects in pregnancy when radiopaque agents are instilled into the bladder or ureters have not been done in women. Studies in animals have been done only with iothalamate, which has not been shown to cause birth defects or other problems.

Diagnostic tests of the uterus and fallopian tubes using radiopaque agents are not recommended during pregnancy or for at least 6 months after a pregnancy has ended. The test may cause other problems, such as infection in the uterus.

Also, radiopaque agents containing iodine have, on rare occasions, caused hypothyroidism (underactive thyroid) in the baby when they were injected late in the pregnancy. In addition, x-rays of the abdomen during pregnancy may have harmful effects on the fetus. Make sure your doctor knows if you are pregnant or if you suspect that you may be pregnant when you are to receive this radiopaque agent.

Breast-feeding—Although small amounts of radiopaque agents are absorbed into the body and may pass into the breast milk, these agents have not been shown to cause problems in nursing babies.

Children—Although there is no specific information about the use of radiopaque agents in children they are not expected to cause different side effects or problems in children than they do in adults when used in the bladder or ureters. There is no specific information about the use of radiopaque agents in children for studies of the uterus or fallopian tubes.

Older adults—Many medicines have not been tested in older people. Therefore, it may not be known whether they work exactly the same way they do in younger adults. Although there is no specific information about the use of radiopaque agents for instillation into the bladder or ureters or into the uterus and fallopian tubes in the elderly, they are not expected to cause different side effects or problems in older people than they do in younger adults.

Other medical problems—The presence of other medical problems may affect the use of radiopaque agents. Make sure you tell your doctor if you have any other medical problems, especially:

- Asthma, hay fever, or other allergies (history of)—If you have a history of these conditions, there is a greater chance of having a reaction, such as an allergic reaction, to the radiopaque agent
- Enlarged prostate or
- Kidney disease (severe)—There may be blockage that makes it difficult or impossible to put the solution of the radiopaque agent into the bladder or ureters
- Genital tract infection or
- Urinary tract infection—The risk of complications is greater in patients with these conditions
- Pelvic inflammatory disease (severe)—The condition may be aggravated by this test

Preparation for This Test

Your doctor may have special instructions for you in preparation for your test, such as the need for a special diet or for a laxative, enema, or vaginal douche depending on the kind of test you are having done. If you have not received such instructions or if you do not understand them, check with your doctor in advance.

For your comfort and for best test results, you may be instructed to urinate just before the procedure.

Precautions After Having This Test

Make sure your doctor knows if you are planning to have any thyroid tests in the near future. Even after several weeks the results of the thyroid test may be affected by the iodine in this agent.

Side Effects of This Medicine

Along with its needed effects, radiopaque agents can cause serious side effects such as allergic reactions. These effects may occur almost immediately or a few minutes after the radiopaque agent is given. Although these serious side effects appear only rarely, your doctor or nurse will be prepared to give you immediate medical attention if needed. If you have any questions about this, check with your doctor.

Check with your doctor or nurse immediately if any of the following side effects occur:

Less common

Abdominal or stomach pain and discomfort (severe); backache

Other side effects may occur that usually do not need medical attention. These side effects should go away as the effects of the radiopaque agent wear off. However, check with your doctor if any of the following side effects continue or are bothersome:

More common

Abdominal or stomach pain and discomfort

Less common

Chills; fever; nausea and vomiting

Other side effects not listed above may also occur in some patients. If you notice any other effects, check with your doctor.

Annual revision: August 1990

RADIOPHARMACEUTICALS Diagnostic

This information applies to the following medicines when used for diagnosis:

- Ammonia N 13 (a-MOE-nya)
- Cyanocobalamin Co 57 (sye-an-oh-koe-BAL-a-min)
- Ferrous Citrate Fe 59 (FER-us SI-trate)
- Fludeoxyglucose F 18 (flu-dee-ox-ee-GLOO-kose)
- Gallium Citrate Ga 67 (GAL-ee-um)
- Indium In 111 Oxyquinoline (IN-dee-um ox-i-KWIN-oh-leen)
- Indium In 111 Pentetate (PEN-te-tate)
- Indium In 111 Satumomab Pendetide
- Iobenguane, Radioiodinated
- Iodohippurate Sodium I 123 (eye-oh-doe-HIP-yoor-ate SOE-dee-um)
- Iodohippurate Sodium I 131
- Iofetamine I 123 (eye-oh-FET-a-meen)
- Iothalamate Sodium I 125 (eye-oh-thal-A-mate)
- Krypton Kr 81m (KRIP-tonn)
- Radioiodinated Albumin (ray-dee-oh-EYE-oh-din-nay-ted al-BYOO-min)
- Rubidium Rb 82 (roo-BID-ee-um)
- Sodium Chromate Cr 51 (KROE-mate)
- Sodium Iodide I 123 (EYE-oh-dyed)
- Sodium Iodide I 131
- Sodium Pertechnetate Tc 99m (per-TEK-ne-tate)
- Technetium Tc 99m Albumin (tek-NEE-see-um al-BYOO-min)
- Technetium Tc 99m Albumin Aggregated
- Technetium Tc 99m Disofenin (DYE-so-fen-in)
- Technetium Tc 99m Exametazime (ex-a-MET-a-zeem)
- Technetium Tc 99m Gluceptate (gloo-SEP-tate)
- Technetium Tc 99m Lidofenin (lye-doe-FEN-in)
- Technetium Tc 99m Mebrofenin (ME-bro-fen-in)
- Technetium Tc 99m Medronate (ME-droe-nate)
- Technetium Tc 99m Mertiatide (meer-TYE-a-tide)
- Technetium Tc 99m Oxidronate (OX-i-dron-ate)
- Technetium Tc 99m Pentetate (PEN-te-tate)
- Technetium Tc 99m Pyrophosphate (peer-oh-FOS-fate)
- Technetium Tc 99m (Pyro- and trimeta-) Phosphates
- Technetium Tc 99m Sestamibi (SES-ta-mi-bi)
- Technetium Tc 99m Succimer (SUX-sim-mer)
- Technetium Tc 99m Sulfur Colloid
- Technetium Tc 99m Teboroxime (te-boe-ROX-eem)
- Thallous Chloride Tl 201 (THA-luss KLOR-ide)
- Xenon Xe 127 (ZEE-non)
- Xenon Xe 133

Used in diagnosis of:	Generic names:
Abscess and infection	Gallium Citrate Ga 67 Indium In 111 Oxyquinoline
Biliary tract blockage	Technetium Tc 99m Disofenin Technetium Tc 99m Lidofenin Technetium Tc 99m Mebrofenin
Blood volume studies	Radioiodinated Albumin Sodium Chromate Cr 51
Blood vessel diseases	Sodium Pertechnetate Tc 99m
Blood vessel diseases of the brain	Ammonia N 13 Iofetamine I 123 Technetium Tc 99m Exametazime Xenon Xe 133
Bone diseases	Technetium Tc 99m Medronate Technetium Tc 99m Oxidronate Technetium Tc 99m Pyrophosphate Technetium Tc 99m (Pyro- and trimeta-) Phosphates
Bone marrow diseases	Sodium Chromate Cr 51 Technetium Tc 99m Sulfur Colloid
Brain diseases and tumors	Fludeoxyglucose F 18 Iofetamine I 123 Sodium Pertechnetate Tc 99m Technetium Tc 99m Exametazime Technetium Tc 99m Gluceptate Technetium Tc 99m Pentetate
Cancer; tumors	Fludeoxyglucose F 18 Gallium Citrate Ga 67 Indium In 111 Satumomab Pendetide Iobenguane, Radioiodinated
Disorders of iron metabolism and absorption	Ferrous Citrate Fe 59
Heart disease	Ammonia N 13 Fludeoxyglucose F 18 Rubidium Rb 82 Sodium Pertechnetate Tc 99m Technetium Tc 99m Albumin Technetium Tc 99m Sestamibi Technetium Tc 99m Teboroxime Thallous Chloride Tl 201
Heart muscle damage (infarct)	Ammonia N 13 Fludeoxyglucose F 18 Rubidium Rb 82 Technetium Tc 99m Pyrophosphate Technetium Tc 99m (Pyro- and trimeta-) Phosphates Technetium Tc 99m Sestamibi Technetium Tc 99m Teboroxime Thallous Chloride Tl 201
Impaired flow of cerebrospinal fluid in brain	Indium In 111 Pentetate
Kidney diseases	Iodohippurate Sodium I 123 Iodohippurate Sodium I 131 Iothalamate Sodium I 125 Technetium Tc 99m Gluceptate Technetium Tc 99m Mertiatide Technetium Tc 99m Pentetate Technetium Tc 99m Succimer
Liver diseases	Ammonia N 13 Fludeoxyglucose F 18 Technetium Tc 99m Disofenin Technetium Tc 99m Lidofenin Technetium Tc 99m Mebrofenin Technetium Tc 99m Sulfur Colloid

Used in diagnosis of:	Generic names:
Lung diseases	Krypton Kr 81m Technetium Tc 99m Albumin Aggregated Technetium Tc 99m Pentetate Xenon Xe 127 Xenon Xe 133
Parathyroid diseases; parathyroid cancer	Technetium Tc 99m Sestamibi Thallous Chloride Tl 201
Pernicious anemia; improper absorption of vitamin B_{12} from intestines	Cyanocobalamin Co 57
Red blood cell diseases	Sodium Chromate Cr 51
Salivary gland diseases	Sodium Pertechnetate Tc 99m
Spleen diseases	Sodium Chromate Cr 51 Technetium Tc 99m Sulfur Colloid
Stomach and intestinal bleeding	Sodium Chromate Cr 51 Sodium Pertechnetate Tc 99m Technetium Tc 99m (Pyro- and trimeta-) Phosphates Technetium Tc 99m Sulfur Colloid
Stomach problems	Technetium Tc 99m Sulfur Colloid
Tear duct blockage	Sodium Pertechnetate Tc 99m
Thyroid diseases; thyroid cancer	Fludeoxyglucose F 18 Iobenguane, Radioiodinated Sodium Iodide I 123 Sodium Iodide I 131 Sodium Pertechnetate Tc 99m Technetium Tc 99m Sestamibi
Urinary bladder diseases	Sodium Pertechnetate Tc 99m

Description

Radiopharmaceuticals (ray-dee-oh-far-ma-SOO-ti-kals) are agents used to diagnose certain medical problems or treat certain diseases. They may be given to the patient in several different ways. For example, they may be given by mouth, given by injection, or placed into the eye or into the bladder.

Radiopharmaceuticals are radioactive agents. However, when small amounts are used, the radiation your body receives is very low and is considered safe. When larger amounts of these agents are given to treat disease, there may be different effects on the body.

When radiopharmaceuticals are used to help diagnose medical problems, only small amounts are given to the patient. The radiopharmaceutical is then taken up by an organ of the body (which organ depends on what radiopharmaceutical is used and how it has been given). Then the radioactivity is detected, and pictures produced, by special imaging equipment. These pictures allow the nuclear medicine doctor to study how the organ is functioning.

Some radiopharmaceuticals are used in larger amounts to treat certain kinds of cancer and other diseases. In those cases, the radioactive agent is taken up in the cancerous area and destroys the affected tissue. *The information that follows applies only to radiopharmaceuticals when used in small amounts to diagnose medical problems.*

Radiopharmaceuticals are to be given only by or under the direct supervision of a doctor with specialized training in nuclear medicine.

It is very important that you read and understand the following information. If any of it causes you special concern, do not decide against having this test without first checking with your doctor. Also, *if you have any questions* or if you want more information about this test or your medical problem, *ask your doctor, nuclear medicine physician and/or technologist, nuclear pharmacist, or nurse.*

Before Having This Test

In deciding to use a diagnostic test, any risks of the test must be weighed against the good it will do. This is a decision you and your doctor will make. Also, test results may be affected by other things. For radiopharmaceuticals, the following should be considered:

Allergies—If you will be receiving albumin in the form of radioiodinated albumin, technetium Tc 99m albumin aggregated, or technetium Tc 99m albumin for your test, tell your doctor if you have ever had any unusual or allergic reaction to products containing human serum albumin.

Also tell your doctor if you are allergic to any other substance, such as foods, preservatives, or dyes.

Pregnancy—Radiopharmaceuticals usually are not recommended for use during pregnancy. This is to avoid exposing the fetus to radiation. However, some radiopharmaceuticals may be used for diagnostic tests, but it is necessary to inform your doctor if you are pregnant so the doctor may reduce the radiation dose to the baby. This is especially important with radiopharmaceuticals that contain radioactive iodine, which can go to the baby's thyroid gland and, in high enough concentration, may cause thyroid damage. Be sure you have discussed this with your doctor.

Breast-feeding—Some radiopharmaceuticals pass into the breast milk and may expose the baby to radiation. If you must receive a radiopharmaceutical, it may be necessary for you to stop breast-feeding for some time after receiving it. Be sure you have discussed this with your doctor.

Children—For most radiopharmaceuticals, the amount of radiation used for a diagnostic test is very low and considered safe. However, be sure you have discussed with your doctor the benefit versus the risk of exposing your child to radiation.

Older adults—Many medicines have not been tested in older people. Therefore, it may not be known whether they work exactly the same way they do in younger adults or if they cause different side effects or problems in older people. Although there is no specific information comparing use of most radiopharmaceuticals in the elderly with use in other age groups, problems would not be expected to occur. However, it is a good idea to check with your doctor if you notice any unusual effects after receiving a radiopharmaceutical.

Other medicines—Although certain medicines should not be used together at all, in other cases two different medicines may be used together even if an interaction might occur. In these cases, your doctor may want to change the dose, or other precautions may be necessary. When you are going to receive a radiopharmaceutical, it is especially important that your doctor know if you are taking any other prescription or nonprescription (over-the-counter [OTC]) medicine.

In addition, if you will be receiving radioactive iodine (sodium iodide I 123, sodium iodide I 131) or sodium pertechnetate Tc 99m for a thyroid test, it is especially important that your doctor know if you have been taking iodine through other medicine or foods. For example, the results of your test may be affected if:

- you are taking iodine-containing medicines, including certain multivitamins and cough syrups.
- you eat large amounts of iodine-containing foods, such as iodized salt, seafood, cabbage, kale, rape (turnip-like vegetable), or turnips.
- you have had an x-ray test recently for which you were given a special dye that contained iodine.

Other medical problems—The presence of other medical problems may affect the use of radiopharmaceuticals. Make sure you tell your doctor if you have any other medical problems.

Preparation for This Test

The nuclear medicine doctor may have special instructions for you in preparation for your test. For example, before some tests you must fast for several hours, or the results of the test may be affected. For other tests you should drink plenty of liquids and urinate often to lessen the amount of radiation to your bladder. If you do not understand the instructions you receive or if you have not received any instructions, check with the nuclear medicine doctor in advance.

Dosing—The dosages of radiopharmaceuticals will be different for different patients and depend on the type of test. The amount of radioactivity of a radiopharmaceutical is expressed in units called becquerels or curies. Radiopharmaceutical dosages given may be as small as 0.185 megabecquerels (5 microcuries) or as high as 1295 megabecquerels (35 millicuries). The radiation received from these dosages may be about the same as, or even less than, the radiation received from an x-ray study of the same organ.

Precautions After Having This Test

There are usually no special precautions to observe for radiopharmaceuticals when they are used in small amounts for diagnosis.

Some radiopharmaceuticals may accumulate in your bladder. Therefore, to increase the flow of urine and lessen the amount of radiation to your bladder, your doctor may instruct you to drink plenty of liquids and urinate often after certain tests.

For patients receiving *radioactive iodine (iodohippurate sodium I 123, iodohippurate sodium I 131, iofetamine I 123, iothalamate I 125, radioiodinated albumin, or radiodiodinated iobenguane)*:

- Make sure your doctor knows if you are planning to have any future thyroid tests. Even after several weeks, the results of the thyroid test may be affected by the iodine solution that may be given before the radiopharmaceutical.

Side Effects of This Medicine

Along with its needed effects, a medicine may cause some unwanted effects. When radiopharmaceuticals are used in very small doses to study an organ of the body, side effects are rare and usually involve an allergic reaction. These effects may occur almost immediately or a few minutes after the radiopharmaceutical is given. It may be helpful to note the time when you first notice any side effect. Your doctor, nuclear medicine physician and/or technologist, or nurse will be prepared to give you immediate medical attention if needed.

Check with your doctor or nurse immediately if any of the following side effects occur:

Rare

Chills; difficulty breathing; drowsiness (severe); fainting; fast heartbeat; fever; flushing or redness of skin; headache (severe); nausea or vomiting; skin rash, hives, or itching; stomach pain; swelling of throat, hands, or feet

Other side effects not listed above may also occur in some patients. If you notice any other effects, note the time when they start and check with your doctor.

Annual revision: 08/16/93

RAUWOLFIA ALKALOIDS Systemic

This information applies to the following medicines:

Deserpidine (de-SER-pi-deen)
Rauwolfia Serpentina (rah-WOOL-fee-a ser-pen-TEE-na)
Reserpine (re-SER-peen)

Some commonly used brand names are:

For Deserpidine†
In the U.S.
Harmonyl

For Rauwolfia Serpentina†
In the U.S.
Raudixin
Rauval
Rauverid
Wolfina
Generic name product may also be available.

For Reserpine
In the U.S.
Serpalan
Generic name product may also be available.
In Canada
Novoreserpine
Reserfia
Serpasil
Generic name product may also be available.

†Not commercially available in Canada.

Description

Rauwolfia alkaloids belong to the general class of medicines called antihypertensives. They are used to treat high blood pressure (hypertension).

High blood pressure adds to the workload of the heart and arteries. If it continues for a long time, the heart and arteries may not function properly. This can damage the blood vessels of the brain, heart, and kidneys, resulting in a stroke, heart failure, or kidney failure. High blood pressure may also increase the risk of heart attacks. These problems may be less likely to occur if blood pressure is controlled.

Rauwolfia alkaloids work by controlling nerve impulses along certain nerve pathways. As a result, they act on the heart and blood vessels to lower blood pressure.

Rauwolfia alkaloids may also be used to treat other conditions as determined by your doctor.

These medicines are available only with your doctor's prescription, in the following dosage forms:

Oral

Deserpidine
- Tablets (U.S.)

Rauwolfia Serpentina
- Tablets (U.S.)

Reserpine
- Tablets (U.S. and Canada)

It is very important that you read and understand the following information. If any of it causes you special concern, check with your doctor. Also, *if you have any questions* or if you want more information about this medicine or your medical problem, *ask your doctor, nurse, or pharmacist.*

Before Using This Medicine

In deciding to use a medicine, the risks of taking the medicine must be weighed against the good it will do. This is a decision you and your doctor will make. For rauwolfia alkaloids, the following should be considered:

Allergies—Tell your doctor if you have ever had any unusual or allergic reaction to rauwolfia alkaloids. Also tell your doctor and pharmacist if you are allergic to any other substance, such as foods, preservatives, or dyes.

Pregnancy—Rauwolfia alkaloids have not been studied in pregnant women. However, too much use of rauwolfia alkaloids during pregnancy may cause unwanted effects (difficult breathing, low temperature, loss of appetite) in the baby. In rats, use of rauwolfia alkaloids during pregnancy causes birth defects and in guinea pigs decreases newborn survival rates. Before taking this medicine, make sure your doctor knows if you are pregnant or if you may become pregnant.

Breast-feeding—Rauwolfia alkaloids pass into breast milk and may cause unwanted effects (difficult breathing, low temperature, loss of appetite) in infants of mothers taking large doses of this medicine. Be sure you have discussed this with your doctor before taking this medicine.

Children—Although there is no specific information comparing use of rauwolfia alkaloids in children with use in other age groups, rauwolfia alkaloids are not expected to cause different side effects or problems in children than they do in adults.

Older adults—Many medicines have not been studied specifically in older people. Therefore, it may not be known whether they work exactly the same way they do in younger adults. Although there is no specific information comparing use of rauwolfia alkaloids in the elderly with use in other age groups, dizziness or drowsiness may be more likely to occur in the elderly, who are more sensitive to the effects of rauwolfia alkaloids.

Other medicines—Although certain medicines should not be used together at all, in other cases two different medicines may be used together even if an interaction might occur. In these cases, your doctor may want to change the dose, or other precautions may be necessary. When you are taking rauwolfia alkaloids, it is especially important that your doctor and pharmacist know if you are taking any of the following:

- Monoamine oxidase (MAO) inhibitors (furazolidone [e.g., Furoxone], isocarboxazid [e.g., Marplan], phenelzine [e.g., Nardil], procarbazine [e.g., Matulane], selegiline [e.g.,

Eldepryl], tranylcypromine [e.g., Parnate])—Taking a rauwolfia alkaloid while you are taking or within 2 weeks of taking MAO inhibitors may increase the risk of central nervous system depression or may cause a severe high blood pressure reaction

Other medical problems—The presence of other medical problems may affect the use of rauwolfia alkaloids. Make sure you tell your doctor if you have any other medical problems, especially:

- Allergies or other breathing problems such as asthma—Rauwolfia alkaloids can cause breathing problems
- Epilepsy
- Gallstones or
- Stomach ulcer or
- Ulcerative colitis—Rauwolfia alkaloids increase activity of the stomach, which may make the condition worse
- Heart disease—Rauwolfia alkaloids can cause heart rhythm problems or slow heartbeat
- Kidney disease—Some patients may not do well when blood pressure is lowered by rauwolfia alkaloids
- Mental depression (or history of)—Rauwolfia alkaloids cause mental depression
- Parkinson's disease—Rauwolfia alkaloids can cause parkinsonism-like effects
- Pheochromocytoma

Before you begin using any new medicine (prescription or nonprescription) or if you develop any new medical problem while you are using this medicine, check with your doctor, nurse, or pharmacist.

Proper Use of This Medicine

For patients taking this medicine *for high blood pressure*:

- In addition to the use of the medicine your doctor has prescribed, treatment for your high blood pressure may include weight control and care in the types of foods you eat, especially foods high in sodium. Your doctor will tell you which of these are most important for you. You should check with your doctor before changing your diet.
- Many patients who have high blood pressure will not notice any signs of the problem. In fact, many may feel normal. It is very important that you *take your medicine exactly as directed* and that you keep your appointments with your doctor even if you feel well.
- Remember that this medicine will not cure your high blood pressure but it does help control it. Therefore, you must continue to take it as directed if you expect to lower your blood pressure and keep it down. *You may have to take high blood pressure medicine for the rest of your life.* If high blood pressure is not treated, it can cause serious problems such as heart failure, blood vessel disease, stroke, or kidney disease.

To help you remember to take your medicine, try to get into the habit of taking it at the same time each day.

This medicine is sometimes given together with certain other medicines. If you are using a combination of drugs, make sure that you take each medicine at the proper time and do not mix them. Ask your doctor, nurse, or pharmacist to help you plan a way to remember to take your medicines at the right times.

If this medicine upsets your stomach, it may be taken with meals or milk. If stomach upset (nausea, vomiting, stomach cramps or pain) continues or gets worse, check with your doctor.

Missed dose—If you miss a dose of this medicine, do not take the missed dose at all and do not double the next one. Instead, go back to your regular dosing schedule.

Storage—To store this medicine:

- Keep out of the reach of children.
- Store away from heat and direct light.
- Do not store in the bathroom, near the kitchen sink, or in other damp places. Heat or moisture may cause the medicine to break down.
- Do not keep outdated medicine or medicine no longer needed. Be sure that any discarded medicine is out of the reach of children.

Precautions While Using This Medicine

It is important that your doctor check your progress at regular visits to make sure that this medicine is working properly.

For patients taking this medicine *for high blood pressure*:

- *Do not take other medicines unless they have been discussed with your doctor.* This especially includes over-the-counter (nonprescription) medicines for appetite control, asthma, colds, cough, hay fever, or sinus problems, since they may tend to increase your blood pressure.

Before having any kind of surgery (including dental surgery) or emergency treatment, *tell the medical doctor or dentist in charge that you are taking this medicine.*

In some patients, this medicine may cause mental depression. *Tell your doctor right away:*

- if you or anyone else notices unusual changes in your mood.
- if you start having early-morning sleeplessness or unusually vivid dreams or nightmares.

This medicine will add to the effects of alcohol and other CNS depressants (medicines that slow down the nervous system, possibly causing drowsiness). Some examples of CNS depressants are antihistamines or medicine for hay fever, other allergies, or colds; sedatives, tranquilizers, or sleeping medicine; prescription pain medicine or narcotics; barbiturates; medicine for seizures; muscle relaxants; or anesthetics, including some dental anesthetics. *Check with your doctor before taking any of the above while you are using this medicine.*

This medicine may cause some people to become drowsy or less alert than they are normally. This is more likely to happen when you begin to take it or when you increase the amount of medicine you are taking. *Make sure you know how you react to this medicine before you drive, use machines, or do anything else that could be dangerous if you are not alert.*

This medicine may cause dryness of the mouth. For temporary relief, use sugarless candy or gum, melt bits of ice in your mouth, or use a saliva substitute. However, if dry mouth continues for more than 2 weeks, check with your medical doctor or dentist. Continuing dryness of the mouth may increase the chance of dental disease, including tooth decay, gum disease, and fungus infections.

This medicine often causes stuffiness in the nose. However, do not use nasal decongestant medicines without first checking with your doctor or pharmacist.

Side Effects of This Medicine

Suggestions that rauwolfia alkaloids may increase the risk of breast cancer occurring later have not been proven. However, rats and mice given 100 to 300 times the human dose had an increased number of tumors.

Along with its needed effects, a medicine may cause some unwanted effects. Although not all of these side effects may occur, if they do occur they may need medical attention.

Check with your doctor immediately if any of the following side effects occur:

Less common

Drowsiness or faintness; impotence or decreased sexual interest; lack of energy or weakness; mental depression or inability to concentrate; nervousness or anxiety; vivid dreams or nightmares or early-morning sleeplessness

Check with your doctor as soon as possible if any of the following side effects occur:

More common

Dizziness

Less common

Black, tarry stools; bloody vomit; chest pain; headache; irregular heartbeat; shortness of breath; slow heartbeat; stomach cramps or pain

Rare

Painful or difficult urination; skin rash or itching; stiffness; trembling and shaking of hands and fingers; unusual bleeding or bruising

Signs and symptoms of overdose

Dizziness or drowsiness (severe); flushing of skin; pinpoint pupils of eyes; slow pulse

Other side effects may occur that usually do not need medical attention. These side effects may go away during treatment as your body adjusts to the medicine. However, check with your doctor if any of the following side effects continue or are bothersome:

More common

Diarrhea; dryness of mouth; loss of appetite; nausea and vomiting; stuffy nose

Less common

Swelling of feet and lower legs

After you stop using this medicine, it may still produce some side effects that need attention. During this period of time *check with your doctor immediately* if you notice any of the following side effects:

Drowsiness or faintness; impotence or decreased sexual interest; irregular or slow heartbeat; lack of energy or weakness; mental depression or inability to concentrate; nervousness or anxiety; vivid dreams or nightmares or early-morning sleeplessness

Other side effects not listed above may also occur in some patients. If you notice any other effects, check with your doctor.

Additional Information

Once a medicine has been approved for marketing for a certain use, experience may show that it is also useful for other medical problems. Although this use is not included in product labeling, reserpine is used in certain patients with the following medical condition:

- Raynaud's disease

Other than the above information, there is no additional information relating to proper use, precautions, or side effects for these uses.

Annual revision: 07/28/92

RAUWOLFIA ALKALOIDS AND THIAZIDE DIURETICS Systemic

This information applies to the following medicines:

Deserpidine (de-SER-pi-deen) and Hydrochlorothiazide (hye-droe-klor-oh-THYE-a-zide)
Deserpidine and Methyclothiazide (meth-i-kloe-THYE-a-zide)
Rauwolfia Serpentina (rah-WOOL-fee-a ser-pen-TEE-na) and Bendroflumethiazide (ben-droe-floo-meth-EYE-a-zide)
Reserpine (re-SER-peen) and Chlorothiazide (klor-oh-THYE-a-zide)
Reserpine and Chlorthalidone (klor-THAL-i-done)
Reserpine and Hydrochlorothiazide
Reserpine and Hydroflumethiazide (hye-droe-floo-meth-EYE-a-zide)
Reserpine and Methyclothiazide
Reserpine and Polythiazide (pol-i-THYE-a-zide)
Reserpine and Trichlormethiazide (trye-klor-meth-EYE-a-zide)

Some commonly used brand names are:

For Deserpidine and Hydrochlorothiazide†
In the U.S.
Oreticyl
Oreticyl Forte

For Deserpidine and Methyclothiazide
In the U.S.
Enduronyl
Enduronyl Forte
Generic name product may also be available.
In Canada
Dureticyl

For Rauwolfia Serpentina and Bendroflumethiazide†
In the U.S.
Rauzide

For Reserpine and Chlorothiazide†
In the U.S.
Diupres
Diurigen with Reserpine
Generic name product may also be available.

For Reserpine and Chlorthalidone†
In the U.S.
Demi-Regroton
Regroton

For Reserpine and Hydrochlorothiazide
In the U.S.
Hydropres
Hydrosine
Hydrotensin
Mallopres
Generic name product may also be available.
In Canada
Hydropres

For Reserpine and Hydroflumethiazide
In the U.S.
Hydropine
Hydropine H.P.
Salazide
Salutensin
Salutensin-Demi
Generic name product may also be available.
In Canada
Salutensin

For Reserpine and Methyclothiazide†
In the U.S.
Diutensen-R

For Reserpine and Polythiazide†
In the U.S.
Renese-R

For Reserpine and Trichlormethiazide†
In the U.S.
Diurese-R
Metatensin
Naquival
Generic name product may also be available.

†Not commercially available in Canada.

Description

Rauwolfia alkaloid and thiazide diuretic combinations are used in the treatment of high blood pressure (hypertension).

High blood pressure adds to the workload of the heart and arteries. If it continues for a long time, the heart and arteries may not function properly. This can damage the blood vessels of the brain, heart, and kidneys, resulting in a stroke, heart failure, or kidney failure. High blood pressure may also increase the risk of heart attacks. These problems may be less likely to occur if blood pressure is controlled.

Rauwolfia alkaloids work by controlling nerve impulses along certain nerve pathways. As a result, they act on the heart and blood vessels to lower blood pressure. Thiazide diuretics help to reduce the amount of water in the body by increasing the flow of urine. This also helps to lower blood pressure.

These medicines are available only with your doctor's prescription, in the following dosage forms:

Oral

Deserpidine and Hydrochlorothiazide
- Tablets (U.S.)

Deserpidine and Methyclothiazide
- Tablets (U.S. and Canada)

Rauwolfia Serpentina and Bendroflumethiazide
- Tablets (U.S.)

Reserpine and Chlorothiazide
- Tablets (U.S.)

Reserpine and Chlorthalidone
- Tablets (U.S.)

Reserpine and Hydrochlorothiazide
- Tablets (U.S. and Canada)

Reserpine and Hydroflumethiazide
- Tablets (U.S. and Canada)

Reserpine and Methyclothiazide
- Tablets (U.S.)

Reserpine and Polythiazide
- Tablets (U.S.)

Reserpine and Trichlormethiazide
- Tablets (U.S.)

It is very important that you read and understand the following information. If any of it causes you special concern, check with your doctor. Also, *if you have any questions* or if you want more information about this medicine or your medical problem, *ask your doctor, nurse, or pharmacist.*

Before Using This Medicine

In deciding to use a medicine, the risks of taking the medicine must be weighed against the good it will do. This is a decision you and your doctor will make. For rauwolfia alkaloids and thiazide diuretics, the following should be considered:

Allergies—Tell your doctor if you have ever had any unusual or allergic reaction to sulfonamides (sulfa drugs), thiazide diuretics (water pills), or rauwolfia alkaloids. Also tell your doctor and pharmacist if you are allergic to any other substance, such as foods, preservatives, or dyes.

Pregnancy—Too much use of thiazide diuretics (contained in this combination medicine) during pregnancy may cause unwanted effects including jaundice, blood problems, and low potassium in the baby. Too much use of rauwolfia alkaloids may cause difficult breathing, low temperature, and loss of appetite in the baby. This medicine has not been shown to cause birth defects in humans. In rats, use of rauwolfia alkaloids during pregnancy decreases newborn survival rates. Be sure that you have discussed this with your doctor before taking this medicine.

Breast-feeding—Rauwolfia alkaloids pass into breast milk and may cause unwanted effects (difficult breathing, low temperature, loss of appetite) in infants of mothers taking it in large doses. Thiazide diuretics also pass into breast milk. Be sure you have discussed this with your doctor before taking this medicine.

Children—Although there is no specific information comparing use of these medicines in children with use in other age groups, these medicines are not expected to cause different side effects or problems in children than they do in adults.

Older adults—Many medicines have not been studied specifically in older people. Therefore, it may not be known whether they work exactly the same way they do in younger adults. Although there is no specific information comparing use of rauwolfia alkaloid and thiazide diuretic combinations in the elderly with use in other age groups, this medicine is not expected to cause different side effects or problems in older people than it does in younger adults. However, drowsiness, dizziness, or faintness or symptoms of too much potassium loss may be more likely to occur in the elderly, who are more sensitive to the effects of rauwolfia alkaloids and thiazide diuretics.

Other medicines—Although certain medicines should not be used together at all, in other cases two different medicines may be used together even if an interaction might occur. In these cases, your doctor may want to change the dose, or other precautions may be necessary. When you are taking rauwolfia alkaloids and thiazide diuretics, it is especially important that your doctor and pharmacist know if you are taking any of the following:

- Cholestyramine or
- Colestipol—Use with thiazide diuretics may prevent the diuretic from working properly; take the diuretic at least 1 hour before or 4 hours after cholestyramine or colestipol
- Digitalis glycosides (heart medicine)—Thiazide diuretics may cause low potassium in the blood, which can lead to symptoms of digitalis toxicity
- Lithium (e.g., Lithane)—Risk of lithium overdose, even at usual doses, may be increased
- Monoamine oxidase (MAO) inhibitors (furazolidone [e.g., Furoxone], isocarboxazid [e.g., Marplan], phenelzine [e.g., Nardil], procarbazine [e.g., Matulane], selegiline [e.g., Eldepryl], tranylcypromine [e.g., Parnate])—Taking a rauwolfia alkaloid while you are taking or within 2 weeks of taking MAO inhibitors may increase the risk of central nervous system depression or may cause a severe high blood pressure reaction

Other medical problems—The presence of other medical problems may affect the use of rauwolfia alkaloids and thiazide diuretics. Make sure you tell your doctor if you have any other medical problems, especially:

- Allergies or other breathing problems such as asthma—Rauwolfia alkaloids can cause breathing problems
- Diabetes mellitus (sugar diabetes)—Thiazide diuretics may change the amount of diabetes medicine needed
- Epilepsy
- Gallstones or
- Stomach ulcer or
- Ulcerative colitis—Rauwolfia alkaloids increase activity of the stomach, which may make the condition worse
- Gout (history of)—Thiazide diuretics may increase the amount of uric acid in the blood, which can lead to gout
- Heart disease—Rauwolfia alkaloids can cause heart rhythm problems or slow heartbeat
- Kidney disease—Some patients may not do well when blood pressure is lowered by this medicine. If kidney disease is severe, thiazide diuretics may not work
- Liver disease—If thiazide diuretics cause loss of too much water from the body, liver disease can become much worse
- Lupus erythematosus (history of)—Thiazide diuretics may worsen the condition
- Mental depression (or history of)—Rauwolfia alkaloids cause mental depression
- Pancreatitis (inflammation of pancreas)
- Parkinson's disease—Rauwolfia alkaloids can cause parkinsonism-like effects
- Pheochromocytoma

Before you begin using any new medicine (prescription or nonprescription) or if you develop any new medical problem while you are using this medicine, check with your doctor, nurse, or pharmacist.

Proper Use of This Medicine

In addition to the use of the medicine your doctor has prescribed, treatment for your high blood pressure may include weight control and care in the types of foods you eat, especially foods high in sodium. Your doctor will tell you which of these are most important for you. You should check with your doctor before changing your diet.

Many patients who have high blood pressure will not notice any signs of the problem. In fact, many may feel normal. It is very important that you *take your medicine exactly as directed* and that you keep your appointments with your doctor even if you feel well.

Remember that this medicine will not cure your high blood pressure but it does help control it. Therefore, you must continue to take it as directed if you expect to lower your blood pressure and keep it down. *You may have to take high blood pressure medicine for the rest of your life.* If high blood pressure is not treated, it can cause serious problems such as heart failure, blood vessel disease, stroke, or kidney disease.

This medicine may cause you to have an unusual feeling of tiredness when you begin to take it. You may also notice an increase in the amount of urine or in your frequency of urination. After you have taken the medicine for a while, these effects should lessen. In general, to keep the increase in urine from affecting your sleep:

- If you are to take a single dose a day, take it in the morning after breakfast.
- If you are to take more than one dose a day, take the last dose no later than 6 p.m., unless otherwise directed by your doctor.

However, it is best to plan your dose or doses according to a schedule that will least affect your personal activities and sleep. Ask your doctor, nurse, or pharmacist to help you plan the best time to take this medicine.

To help you remember to take your medicine, try to get into the habit of taking it at the same time each day.

If this medicine upsets your stomach, it may be taken with meals or milk. If stomach upset (nausea, vomiting, stomach pain or cramps) continues, check with your doctor.

Missed dose—If you miss a dose of this medicine, take it as soon as possible. However, if it is almost time for your next dose, skip the missed dose and go back to your regular dosing schedule. Do not double doses.

Storage—To store this medicine:

- Keep out of the reach of children.
- Store away from heat and direct light.
- Do not store in the bathroom, near the kitchen sink, or in other damp places. Heat or moisture may cause the medicine to break down.
- Do not keep outdated medicine or medicine no longer needed. Be sure that any discarded medicine is out of the reach of children.

Precautions While Using This Medicine

It is important that your doctor check your progress at regular visits to make sure that this medicine is working properly.

Do not take other medicines unless they have been discussed with your doctor. This especially includes over-the-counter (nonprescription) medicines for appetite control, asthma, colds, cough, hay fever, or sinus problems, since they may tend to increase your blood pressure.

Before having any kind of surgery (including dental surgery), or emergency treatment, *tell the medical doctor or dentist in charge that you are taking this medicine.*

This medicine may cause a loss of potassium from your body.

- To help prevent this, your doctor may want you to:
  —eat or drink foods that have a high potassium content (for example, orange or other citrus fruit juices), or
  —take a potassium supplement, or
  —take another medicine to help prevent the loss of the potassium in the first place.
- It is very important to follow these directions. Also, it is important not to change your diet on your own. This is more important if you are already on a special diet (as for diabetes), or if you are taking a potassium supplement or a medicine to reduce potassium loss. Extra potassium may not be necessary and, in some cases, too much potassium could be harmful.

Check with your doctor if you become sick and have severe or continuing vomiting or diarrhea. These problems may cause you to lose additional water and potassium.

This medicine may cause some people to become drowsy or less alert than they are normally. This is more likely to happen when you begin to take it or when you increase the amount of medicine you are taking. *Make sure you know how you react to this medicine before you drive, use machines, or do anything else that could be dangerous if you are not alert.*

Dizziness, lightheadedness, or fainting may occur, especially when you get up from a lying or sitting position. This is more likely to occur in the morning. Getting up slowly may help. When you get up from lying down, sit on the edge of the bed with your feet dangling for 1 or 2 minutes. Then stand up slowly. If the problem continues or gets worse, check with your doctor.

The dizziness, lightheadedness, or fainting is also more likely to occur if you drink alcohol, stand for a long time, exercise, or if the weather is hot. *While you are taking this medicine, be careful to limit the amount of alcohol you drink. Also, use extra care during exercise or hot weather or if you must stand for a long time.*

In some patients, this medicine may cause mental depression. *Tell your doctor right away:*

- if you or anyone else notices unusual changes in your moods.
- if you start having early-morning sleeplessness or unusually vivid dreams or nightmares.

This medicine will add to the effects of alcohol and other CNS depressants (medicines that slow down the nervous system, possibly causing drowsiness). Some examples of CNS depressants are antihistamines or medicine for hay fever, other allergies, or colds; sedatives, tranquilizers, or sleeping medicine; prescription pain medicine or narcotics; barbiturates; medicine for seizures; muscle relaxants; or anesthetics, including dental anesthetics. *Check with your doctor before taking any of the above while you are taking this medicine.*

For *diabetic patients*:

- This medicine may raise blood sugar levels. While you are using this medicine, be especially careful in testing for sugar in your urine. If you have any questions about this, check with your doctor.

Some people who take this medicine may become more sensitive to sunlight than they are normally. Exposure to sunlight, even for brief periods of time, may cause severe sunburn; skin rash, redness, itching, or discoloration; or vision changes. When you begin taking this medicine:

- Stay out of direct sunlight, especially between the hours of 10:00 a.m. and 3:00 p.m., if possible.
- Wear protective clothing, including a hat and sunglasses.
- Apply a sun block product that has a skin protection factor (SPF) of at least 15. Some patients may require a product with a higher SPF number, especially if they have a fair complexion. If you have any questions about this, check with your doctor or pharmacist.
- Do not use a sunlamp or tanning bed or booth.

If you have a severe reaction from the sun, check with your doctor.

This medicine often causes stuffiness in the nose. However, do not use nasal decongestant medicines without first checking with your doctor or pharmacist.

This medicine may cause dryness of the mouth. For temporary relief, use sugarless candy or gum, melt bits of ice in your mouth, or use a saliva substitute. However, if dry mouth continues for more than 2 weeks, check with your medical doctor or dentist. Continuing dryness of the mouth may increase the chance of dental disease, including tooth decay, gum disease, and fungus infections.

Side Effects of This Medicine

Suggestions that rauwolfia alkaloids may increase the risk of breast cancer occurring later have not been proven. However, rats and mice given 100 to 300 times the human dose had an increased risk of tumors.

Along with its needed effects, a medicine may cause some unwanted effects. Although not all of these side effects may occur, if they do occur they may need medical attention.

Check with your doctor immediately if any of the following side effects occur:

Less common

Drowsiness or faintness; impotence or decreased sexual interest; lack of energy or weakness; mental depression or inability to concentrate; nervousness or anxiety; vivid dreams or nightmares or early-morning sleeplessness

Check with your doctor as soon as possible if any of the following side effects occur:

Less common

Black, tarry stools; bloody vomit; chest pain; headache; irregular or slow heartbeat; joint pain; shortness of breath

Rare

Painful or difficult urination; skin rash or itching; sore throat and fever; stiffness; stomach pain (severe) with nausea and vomiting; trembling and shaking of hands and fingers; unusual bleeding or bruising; yellow eyes or skin

Symptoms of too much potassium loss or overdose

Dry mouth; increased thirst; muscle cramps or pain; nausea or vomiting

Other signs and symptoms of overdose

Dizziness or drowsiness, severe; flushing of skin; pinpoint pupils of eyes; slow pulse

Other side effects may occur that usually do not need medical attention. These side effects may go away during treatment as your body adjusts to the medicine. However, check with your doctor if any of the following side effects continue or are bothersome:

More common

Diarrhea; dizziness, especially when getting up from a lying or sitting position; loss of appetite; stuffy nose

After you stop using this medicine, it may still produce some side effects that need attention. During this period of time *check with your doctor immediately* if you notice any of the following side effects:

Drowsiness or faintness; impotence or decreased sexual interest; irregular or slow heartbeat; lack of energy or weakness; mental depression or inability to concentrate; nervousness or anxiety; vivid dreams or nightmares or early-morning sleeplessness

Other side effects not listed above may also occur in some patients. If you notice any other effects, check with your doctor.

Annual revision: 09/22/92

RESERPINE, HYDRALAZINE, AND HYDROCHLOROTHIAZIDE Systemic

Some commonly used brand names are:

In the U.S.

Cam-Ap-Es	Ser-Ap-Es
Cherapas	Serpazide
Ser-A-Gen	Tri-Hydroserpine
Seralazide	Unipres

Generic name product may also be available.

In Canada

Ser-Ap-Es

Description

Reserpine (re-SER-peen), hydralazine (hye-DRAL-a-zeen), and hydrochlorothiazide (hye-droe-KLOR-oh-THYE-a-zide) combinations are used to treat high blood pressure (hypertension).

High blood pressure adds to the workload of the heart and arteries. If it continues for a long time, the heart and arteries may not function properly. This can damage the blood vessels of the brain, heart, and kidneys, resulting in a stroke, heart failure, or kidney failure. High blood pressure may also increase the risk of heart attacks. These problems may be less likely to occur if blood pressure is controlled.

Reserpine works by controlling nerve impulses along certain nerve pathways. As a result, it acts on the heart and blood vessels to lower blood pressure. Hydralazine works by relaxing blood vessels and increasing the supply of blood to the heart while reducing its work load. Hydrochlorothiazide is a thiazide diuretic (water pill) that helps to reduce the amount of water in the body by increasing the flow of urine. This also helps to lower blood pressure.

This medicine is available only with your doctor's prescription, in the following dosage form:

Oral

- Tablets (U.S. and Canada)

It is very important that you read and understand the following information. If any of it causes you special concern, check with your doctor. Also, *if you have any questions* or if you want more information about this medicine or your medical problem, *ask your doctor, nurse, or pharmacist.*

Before Using This Medicine

In deciding to use a medicine, the risks of taking the medicine must be weighed against the good it will do. This is a decision you and your doctor will make. For reserpine, hydralazine, and hydrochlorothiazide, the following should be considered:

Allergies—Tell your doctor if you have ever had any unusual or allergic reaction to hydralazine, sulfonamides (sulfa drugs), thiazide diuretics (water pills), or rauwolfia alkaloids. Also tell your doctor and pharmacist if you are allergic to any other substance, such as foods, preservatives, or dyes.

Pregnancy—Too much use of reserpine and hydrochlorothiazide during pregnancy may cause unwanted effects (jaundice, blood problems, low potassium, difficult breathing, low temperatures, and loss of appetite) in the baby. In rats, rauwolfia alkaloids (like reserpine) decrease newborn survival rates.

Studies with hydralazine have not been done in humans. However, studies in mice have shown that hydralazine causes birth defects (cleft palate, defects in head and face bones); these birth defects may also occur in rabbits, but do not occur in rats. Be sure that you have discussed this with your doctor before taking this medicine.

Breast-feeding—Reserpine passes into breast milk and may cause unwanted effects (difficult breathing, low temperature, loss of appetite) in infants of mothers taking large doses of it. Hydrochlorothiazide also passes into breast milk. Be sure you have discussed this with your doctor before taking this medicine.

Children—Although there is no specific information comparing use of this medicine in children with use in other age groups, this medicine is not expected to cause different side effects or problems in children than it does in adults.

Older adults—Many medicines have not been studied specifically in older people. Therefore, it may not be known whether they work exactly the same way they do in younger adults. Although there is no specific information comparing use of reserpine, hydralazine, and hydrochlorothiazide combination in the elderly with use in other age groups, this medicine is not expected to cause different side effects or problems in older people than it does in younger adults. However, drowsiness, dizziness, or faintness, or symptoms of too much potassium loss may be more likely to occur in the elderly, who are usually more sensitive to the effects of this medicine. Also, this medicine may reduce tolerance to cold temperatures in elderly patients.

Other medicines—Although certain medicines should not be used together at all, in other cases two different medicines may be used together even if an interaction might occur. In these cases, your doctor may want to change the dose, or other precautions may be necessary. When you are taking this medicine, it is especially important that your doctor and pharmacist know if you are taking any of the following:

- Cholestyramine or
- Colestipol—Use with thiazide diuretics may prevent the diuretic from working properly; take the diuretic at least 1 hour before or 4 hours after cholestyramine or colestipol
- Diazoxide (e.g., Proglycem)—Effect on blood pressure may be increased
- Digitalis glycosides (heart medicine)—Hydrochlorothiazide may cause low potassium in the blood, which can lead to symptoms of digitalis toxicity
- Lithium (e.g., Lithane)—Risk of lithium overdose, even at usual doses, may be increased
- Monoamine oxidase (MAO) inhibitors (furazolidone [e.g., Furoxone], isocarboxazid [e.g., Marplan], phenelzine [e.g., Nardil], procarbazine [e.g., Matulane], selegiline [e.g., Eldepryl], tranylcypromine [e.g., Parnate])—Taking a rauwolfia alkaloid while you are taking or within 2 weeks of taking MAO inhibitors may increase the risk of central nervous system depression or may cause a severe high blood pressure reaction

Other medical problems—The presence of other medical problems may affect the use of this medicine. Make sure you tell your doctor if you have any other medical problems, especially:

- Allergies or other breathing problems such as asthma—Reserpine can cause breathing problems
- Diabetes mellitus (sugar diabetes)—Hydrochlorothiazide may change the amount of diabetes medicine needed
- Epilepsy
- Gallstones or
- Stomach ulcer or
- Ulcerative colitis—Reserpine increases activity of the stomach, which may make the condition worse
- Gout (history of)—Hydrochlorothiazide may increase the amount of uric acid in the blood, which can lead to gout
- Heart disease—Reserpine can cause heart rhythm problems or slow heartbeat. Lowering blood pressure may worsen some conditions
- Kidney disease—Some patients may not do well when blood pressure is lowered by this medicine. Effects of hydralazine may be increased because of slower removal from the body. If kidney disease is severe, hydrochlorothiazide may not work
- Liver disease—If hydrochlorothiazide causes loss of too much water from the body, liver disease can become much worse
- Lupus erythematosus (history of)—Hydrochlorothiazide may worsen the condition
- Mental depression (or history of)—Reserpine causes mental depression
- Pancreatitis (inflammation of pancreas)
- Parkinson's disease—Reserpine can cause parkinsonism-like effects
- Pheochromocytoma
- Stroke (recent)—Lowering blood pressure may make problems resulting from this condition worse

Before you begin using any new medicine (prescription or nonprescription) or if you develop any new medical problem while you are using this medicine, check with your doctor, nurse, or pharmacist.

Proper Use of This Medicine

In addition to the use of the medicine your doctor has prescribed, treatment for your high blood pressure may include weight control and care in the types of foods you eat, especially foods high in sodium. Your doctor will tell you which of these are most important for you. You should check with your doctor before changing your diet.

Many patients who have high blood pressure will not notice any signs of the problem. In fact, many may feel normal. It is very important that you *take your medicine exactly as directed* and that you keep your appointments with your doctor even if you feel well.

Remember that this medicine will not cure your high blood pressure but it does help control it. Therefore, you must continue to take it as directed if you expect to lower your blood pressure and keep it down. *You may have to take high blood pressure medicine for the rest of your life.* If high blood pressure is not treated, it can cause serious problems such as heart failure, blood vessel disease, stroke, or kidney disease.

This medicine may cause you to have an unusual feeling of tiredness when you begin to take it. You may also notice an increase in the amount of urine or in your frequency of urination. After you have taken the medicine for a while, these effects should lessen. In general, to keep the increase in urine from affecting your sleep:

- If you are to take a single dose a day, take it in the morning after breakfast.
- If you are to take more than one dose a day, take the last dose no later than 6 p.m., unless otherwise directed by your doctor.

However, it is best to plan your dose or doses according to a schedule that will least affect your personal activities and sleep. Ask your doctor, nurse, or pharmacist to help you plan the best time to take this medicine.

To help you remember to take your medicine, try to get into the habit of taking it at the same time each day.

If this medicine upsets your stomach, it may be taken with meals or milk. If stomach upset (nausea, vomiting, stomach pain or cramps) continues, check with your doctor.

Missed dose—If you miss a dose of this medicine, take it as soon as possible. However, if it is almost time for your next dose, skip the missed dose and go back to your regular dosing schedule. Do not double doses.

Storage—To store this medicine:
- Keep out of the reach of children.
- Store away from heat and direct light.
- Do not store in the bathroom, near the kitchen sink, or in other damp places. Heat or moisture may cause the medicine to break down.
- Do not keep outdated medicine or medicine no longer needed. Be sure that any discarded medicine is out of the reach of children.

Precautions While Using This Medicine

It is important that your doctor check your progress at regular visits to make sure that this medicine is working properly.

Do not take other medicines unless they have been discussed with your doctor. This especially includes over-the-counter (nonprescription) medicines for appetite control, asthma, colds, cough, hay fever, or sinus problems, since they may tend to increase your blood pressure.

Before having any kind of surgery (including dental surgery), or emergency treatment, *make sure the medical doctor or dentist in charge knows that you are taking this medicine.*

This medicine may cause some people to have headaches or to feel dizzy or drowsy. *Make sure you know how you react to this medicine before you drive, use machines, or do anything else that could be dangerous if you are dizzy or are not alert.*

Dizziness, lightheadedness, or fainting may occur, especially when you get up from a lying or sitting position. This is more likely to occur in the morning. *Getting up slowly may help.* When you get up from lying down, sit on the edge of the bed with your feet dangling for 1 or 2 minutes. Then stand up slowly. If the problem continues or gets worse, check with your doctor.

The dizziness, lightheadedness, or fainting is also more likely to occur if you drink alcohol, stand for a long time, exercise, or if the weather is hot. *While you are taking this medicine, be careful to limit the amount of alcohol you drink. Also, use extra care during exercise or hot weather or if you must stand for a long time.*

In some patients, this medicine may cause mental depression. *Tell your doctor right away:*
- if you or anyone else notices unusual changes in your mood.
- if you start having early-morning sleeplessness or unusually vivid dreams or nightmares.

This medicine will add to the effects of alcohol and other CNS depressants (medicines that slow down the nervous system, possibly causing drowsiness). Some examples of CNS depressants are antihistamines or medicine for hay fever, other allergies, or colds; sedatives, tranquilizers, or sleeping medicine; prescription pain medicine or narcotics; barbiturates; medicine for seizures; muscle relaxants; or anesthetics, including dental anesthetics. *Check with your doctor before taking any of the above while you are taking this medicine.*

This medicine may cause a loss of potassium from your body.
- To help prevent this, your doctor may want you to:
  —eat or drink foods that have a high potassium content (for example, orange or other citrus fruit juices), or
  —take a potassium supplement, or
  —take another medicine to help prevent the loss of the potassium in the first place.
- It is very important to follow these directions. Also, it is important not to change your diet on your own. This is more important if you are already on a special diet (as for diabetes), or if you are taking a potassium supplement or a medicine to reduce potassium loss. Extra potassium may not be necessary and, in some cases, too much potassium could be harmful.

Check with your doctor if you become sick and have severe or continuing nausea, vomiting, or diarrhea. These problems may cause you to lose additional water and potassium.

For *diabetic patients:*
- This medicine may raise blood sugar levels. While you are using this medicine, be especially careful in testing for sugar in your urine. If you have any questions about this, check with your doctor.

Some people who take this medicine may become more sensitive to sunlight than they are normally. Exposure to sunlight, even for brief periods of time, may cause severe sunburn; skin rash, redness, itching, or discoloration; or vision changes. When you begin taking this medicine:
- Stay out of direct sunlight, especially between the hours of 10:00 a.m. and 3:00 p.m., if possible.
- Wear protective clothing, including a hat and sunglasses.
- Apply a sun block product that has a skin protection factor (SPF) of at least 15. Some patients may require a product with a higher SPF number, especially if they have a fair complexion. If you have

any questions about this, check with your doctor or pharmacist.

- Do not use a sunlamp or tanning bed or booth.

If you have a severe reaction from the sun, check with your doctor.

This medicine often causes stuffiness in the nose. However, do not use nasal decongestant medicines without first checking with your doctor or pharmacist.

This medicine may cause dryness of the mouth. For temporary relief, use sugarless candy or gum, melt bits of ice in your mouth, or use a saliva substitute. However, if dry mouth continues for more than 2 weeks, check with your medical doctor or dentist. Continuing dryness of the mouth may increase the chance of dental disease, including tooth decay, gum disease, and fungus infections.

Side Effects of This Medicine

Suggestions that rauwolfia alkaloids may increase the risk of breast cancer occurring later have not been proven. However, rats and mice given 100 to 300 times the human dose had an increased number of tumors.

Along with its needed effects, a medicine may cause some unwanted effects. Although not all of these side effects may occur, if they do occur they may need medical attention.

Check with your doctor immediately if any of the following side effects occur:

More common

General feeling of discomfort or illness or weakness

Less common

Drowsiness or faintness; impotence or decreased sexual interest; lack of energy or weakness; mental depression or inability to concentrate; nervousness or anxiety; vivid dreams or nightmares or early-morning sleeplessness

Check with your doctor as soon as possible if any of the following side effects occur:

Signs and symptoms of too much potassium loss

Dryness of mouth; increased thirst; irregular heartbeat; mood or mental changes; muscle cramps or pain; weak pulse

Signs and symptoms of too much sodium loss

Confusion; convulsions; decreased mental activity; irritability; muscle cramps; unusual tiredness or weakness

Less common

Black, tarry stools; blisters on skin; bloody vomit; chest pain; fever and sore throat; headache; irregular heartbeat; joint pain; numbness, tingling, pain, or weakness in hands or feet; shortness of breath; skin rash or itching; slow heartbeat; stomach cramps or pain; swelling of lymph glands

Rare

Lower back or side pain; painful or difficult urination; stiffness; stomach pain (severe) with nausea and vomiting; trembling and shaking of hands and fingers; unusual bleeding or bruising; yellow eyes or skin

Signs and symptoms of overdose

Dizziness or drowsiness (severe); dryness of mouth; flushing of skin; increased thirst; muscle cramps or pain; nausea or vomiting (severe); pinpoint pupils of eyes; slow pulse

Other side effects may occur that usually do not need medical attention. These side effects may go away during treatment as your body adjusts to the medicine. However, check with your doctor if any of the following side effects continue or are bothersome:

More common

Diarrhea; dizziness, especially when getting up from a lying or sitting position; loss of appetite; nausea or vomiting; stuffy nose

Less common

Constipation; flushing or redness of skin; increased sensitivity of skin to sunlight; swelling of feet and lower legs; watering or irritated eyes

After you stop using this medicine, it may still produce some side effects that need attention. During this period of time *check with your doctor immediately* if you notice any of the following side effects:

Drowsiness or faintness; general feeling of discomfort or illness or weakness; impotence or decreased sexual interest; irregular heartbeat; mental depression or inability to concentrate; nervousness or anxiety; vivid dreams or nightmares or early-morning sleeplessness

Other side effects not listed above may also occur in some patients. If you notice any other effects, check with your doctor.

Annual revision: 09/22/92

RESORCINOL Topical

A commonly used brand name in the U.S. is RA.

Description

Resorcinol (re-SOR-si-nole) is used to treat acne, seborrheic dermatitis, eczema, psoriasis, and other skin disorders. It is also used to treat corns, calluses, and warts.

Resorcinol works by helping to remove hard, scaly, or roughened skin.

Some of these preparations are available only with your doctor's prescription. Others are available without a prescription; however, your doctor may have special instructions on the proper use of resorcinol for your medical condition.

Resorcinol is available in the following dosage forms:

Topical
- Lotion (U.S.)
- Ointment (U.S. and Canada)

It is very important that you read and understand the following information. If any of it causes you special concern, check with your doctor or pharmacist. Also, *if you have any questions* or if you want more information about this medicine or your medical problem, *ask your doctor, nurse, or pharmacist.*

Before Using This Medicine

If you are using this medicine without a prescription, carefully read and follow any precautions on the label. For resorcinol, the following should be considered:

Allergies—Tell your doctor if you have ever had any unusual or allergic reaction to resorcinol. Also tell your doctor and pharmacist if you are allergic to any other substances, such as preservatives or dyes.

Pregnancy—Resorcinol may be absorbed through the mother's skin. However, topical resorcinol has not been shown to cause birth defects or other problems in humans.

Breast-feeding—This medicine may be absorbed through the mother's skin. However, topical resorcinol has not been reported to cause problems in nursing babies.

Children—Resorcinol may be absorbed through the skin and should not be used on large areas of the bodies of infants and children. In addition, resorcinol should not be used on wounds, since doing so may cause a blood disease called methemoglobinemia.

Older adults—Many medicines have not been studied specifically in older people. Therefore, it may not be known whether they work exactly the same way they do in younger adults. Although there is no specific information comparing use of resorcinol in the elderly with use in other age groups, this medicine is not expected to cause different side effects or problems in older people than it does in younger adults.

Other medicines—Although certain medicines should not be used together at all, in other cases two different medicines may be used together even if an interaction might occur. In these cases, your doctor may want to change the dose, or other precautions may be necessary. Tell your doctor and pharmacist if you are using any other prescription or nonprescription (over-the-counter [OTC]) medicine.

Before you begin using any new medicine (prescription or nonprescription) or if you develop any new medical problem while you are using this medicine, check with your doctor, nurse, or pharmacist.

Proper Use of This Medicine

It is very important that you use this medicine only as directed. Do not use more of it, do not use it more often, and do not use it for a longer time than your doctor ordered. To do so may increase the chance of absorption through the skin and the chance of resorcinol poisoning.

Apply enough resorcinol to cover the affected areas, and rub in gently.

Immediately after using this medicine, wash your hands to remove any medicine that may be on them.

Keep this medicine away from the eyes. If you should accidentally get some in your eyes, flush them thoroughly with water.

Dosing—The dose of resorcinol will be different for different patients. *Follow your doctor's orders or the directions on the label.* The following information includes only the average doses of resorcinol. *If your dose is different, do not change it* unless your doctor tells you to do so.

- For *lotion* dosage form:
  - —For acne, seborrheic dermatitis, eczema, or psoriasis:
    - Adults and children—Use as needed.
- For *ointment* dosage form:
  - —For acne, seborrheic dermatitis, eczema, psoriasis, corns, calluses, or warts:
    - Adults and children—Use and dose must be determined by the doctor.

Missed dose—If you miss a dose of this medicine, apply it as soon as possible. However, if it is almost time for your next dose, skip the missed dose and go back to your regular dosing schedule. Do not double doses.

Storage—To store this medicine:

- Keep out of the reach of children.
- Store away from heat and direct light.
- Keep the medicine from freezing.
- Do not keep outdated medicine or medicine no longer needed. Be sure that any discarded medicine is out of the reach of children.

Precautions While Using This Medicine

When using resorcinol, do not use any of the following preparations on the same affected area as this medicine, unless otherwise directed by your doctor:

Abrasive soaps or cleansers
Alcohol-containing preparations
Any other topical acne preparation or preparation containing a peeling agent (for example, benzoyl peroxide, salicylic acid, sulfur, or tretinoin [vitamin A acid])
Cosmetics or soaps that dry the skin
Medicated cosmetics
Other topical medicine for the skin

To use any of the above preparations on the same affected area as resorcinol may cause severe irritation of the skin.

This medicine may darken light-colored hair.

Side Effects of This Medicine

Along with its needed effects, a medicine may cause some unwanted effects. Although not all of these side effects may occur, if they do occur they may need medical attention.

Check with your doctor as soon as possible if any of the following side effects occur:

Less common or rare

Skin irritation not present before use of this medicine

Symptoms of resorcinol poisoning

Diarrhea, nausea, stomach pain, or vomiting; dizziness; drowsiness; headache (severe or continuing); nervousness or restlessness; slow heartbeat, shortness of breath, or troubled breathing; sweating; unusual tiredness or weakness

Other side effects may occur that usually do not need medical attention. These side effects may go away during treatment as your body adjusts to the medicine. However, check with your doctor if the following side effect continues or is bothersome:

More common

Redness and peeling of skin (may occur after a few days)

Other side effects not listed above may also occur in some patients. If you notice any other effects, check with your doctor.

Annual revision: 07/26/93

RESORCINOL AND SULFUR Topical

Some commonly used brand names are:

In the U.S.

Acnomel Acne Cream
Bensulfoid Cream
Clearasil Adult Care Medicated Blemish Cream
Clearasil Adult Care Medicated Blemish Stick
Night Cast Special Formula Mask-lotion
Rezamid Acne Treatment
Sulforcin

In Canada

Acne-Aid Gel
Acnomel Cake
Acnomel Cream
Acnomel Vanishing Cream
Rezamid Lotion

Description

Resorcinol and sulfur (re-SOR-si-nole and SUL-fur) combination is used to treat acne and similar skin conditions.

This medicine is available without a prescription; however, your doctor may have special instructions on the proper use of this medicine for your medical condition.

Resorcinol and sulfur combination is available in the following dosage forms:

Topical

- Cake (Canada)
- Cream (U.S. and Canada)
- Gel (Canada)
- Lotion (U.S. and Canada)
- Stick (U.S.)

It is very important that you read and understand the following information. If any of it causes you special concern, check with your doctor or pharmacist. Also, *if you have any questions* or if you want more information about this medicine or your medical problem, *ask your doctor, nurse, or pharmacist.*

Before Using This Medicine

If you are using this medicine without a prescription, carefully read and follow any precautions on the label.

For resorcinol and sulfur combination, the following should be considered:

Allergies—Tell your doctor if you have ever had any unusual or allergic reaction to resorcinol or sulfur. Also tell your doctor and pharmacist if you are allergic to any other substances, such as preservatives or dyes.

Pregnancy—Resorcinol may be absorbed through the mother's skin. However, topical resorcinol and sulfur combination has not been shown to cause birth defects or other problems in humans.

Breast-feeding—Resorcinol may be absorbed through the mother's skin. However, topical resorcinol and sulfur combination has not been reported to cause problems in nursing babies.

Children—Resorcinol may be absorbed through the skin and should not be used on large areas of the bodies of infants and children. In addition, resorcinol should not be used on wounds, since doing so may cause a blood disease called methemoglobinemia.

Older adults—Many medicines have not been studied specifically in older people. Therefore, it may not be known whether they work exactly the same way they do in younger adults or if they cause different side effects or problems in older people. There is no specific information comparing use of resorcinol and sulfur in the elderly with use in other age groups.

Other medicines—Although certain medicines should not be used together at all, in other cases two different medicines may be used together even if an interaction might occur. In these cases, your doctor may want to change the dose, or other precautions may be necessary. Tell your doctor and pharmacist if you are using any other prescription or nonprescription (over-the-counter [OTC]) medicine.

Before you begin using any new medicine (prescription or nonprescription) or if you develop any new medical problem while you are using this medicine, check with your doctor, nurse, or pharmacist.

Proper Use of This Medicine

Use this medicine only as directed. Do not use more of it and do not use it more often than recommended on the label, unless otherwise directed by your doctor. To do so may increase the chance of absorption through the skin and the chance of resorcinol poisoning.

Before using this medicine, wash the affected areas thoroughly and gently pat dry. Then apply a small amount to the affected areas and spread on gently, but do not rub in.

Immediately after using this medicine, wash your hands to remove any medicine that may be on them.

Keep this medicine away from the eyes. If you should accidentally get some in your eyes, flush them thoroughly with water.

Dosing—The dose of resorcinol and sulfur combination will be different for different patients. *Follow your doctor's orders or the directions on the label.* The following information includes only the average doses of resorcinol and sulfur combination. *If your dose is different, do not change it* unless your doctor tells you to do so.

- For acne and similar skin conditions:
  - —For *cake* dosage form:
    - Adults and children—Use two or three times a day.
  - —For *cream* dosage form:
    - Adults and children—Use one to three times a day.
  - —For *gel and stick* dosage forms:
    - Adults and children—Use as needed.
  - —For *lotion* dosage form:
    - Adults and children—Use two times a day.

Missed dose—If you miss a dose of this medicine, apply it as soon as possible. However, if it is almost time for your next dose, skip the missed dose and go back to your regular dosing schedule. Do not double doses.

Storage—To store this medicine:

- Keep out of the reach of children.
- Store away from heat and direct light.
- Keep the medicine from freezing.
- Do not keep outdated medicine or medicine no longer needed. Be sure that any discarded medicine is out of the reach of children.

Precautions While Using This Medicine

When using resorcinol and sulfur combination, do not use any of the following preparations on the same affected area as this medicine, unless otherwise directed by your doctor:

Abrasive soaps or cleansers
Alcohol-containing preparations
Any other topical acne preparation or preparation containing a peeling agent (for example, benzoyl peroxide, salicylic acid, or tretinoin [vitamin A acid])
Cosmetics or soaps that dry the skin
Medicated cosmetics
Other topical medicine for the skin

To use any of the above preparations on the same affected area as this medicine may cause severe irritation of the skin.

Do not use any topical mercury-containing preparation, such as ammoniated mercury ointment, on the same affected area as this medicine. To do so may cause a foul odor, may be irritating to the skin, and may stain the skin black. If you have any questions about this, check with your doctor or pharmacist.

This medicine (depending on the product you are using) may darken light-colored hair. If you have any questions about this, check with your doctor or pharmacist.

Side Effects of This Medicine

Along with its needed effects, a medicine may cause some unwanted effects. Although not all of these side effects may occur, if they do occur they may need medical attention.

Check with your doctor as soon as possible if the following side effect occurs:

Less common or rare

Skin irritation not present before use of this medicine

Symptoms of resorcinol poisoning

Diarrhea, nausea, stomach pain, or vomiting; dizziness; drowsiness; headache (severe or continuing); nervousness or restlessness; slow heartbeat, shortness of breath, or troubled breathing; sweating; unusual tiredness or weakness

Other side effects may occur that usually do not need medical attention. However, check with your doctor or pharmacist if the following side effects continue or are bothersome:

More common

Redness and peeling of skin (may occur after a few days)

Less common

Unusual dryness of skin

Other side effects not listed above may also occur in some patients. If you notice any other effects, check with your doctor or pharmacist.

Annual revision: 07/26/93

RIBAVIRIN Systemic

Some commonly used brand names are:

In the U.S.
Virazole

In Canada
Virazole

Other
Virazid

Another commonly used name is tribavirin.

Description

Ribavirin (rye-ba-VYE-rin) is used to treat severe virus pneumonia in infants and young children. It is given by oral inhalation (breathing in the medicine as a fine mist through the mouth), using a special nebulizer (sprayer) attached to an oxygen hood or tent or face mask.

This medicine may also be used for other virus infections as determined by your doctor. However, it will not work for certain viruses, such as the common cold.

Ribavirin is to be administered only by or under the immediate supervision of your doctor, in the following dosage form:

Inhalation

- Aerosol (U.S. and Canada)

It is very important that you read and understand the following information. If any of it causes you special concern, check with your doctor. Also, *if you have any questions* or if you want more information about this medicine or your medical problem, *ask your doctor, nurse, or pharmacist.*

Before Receiving This Medicine

In deciding to use a medicine, the risks of taking the medicine must be weighed against the good it will do. This is a decision you and your doctor will make. For ribavirin, the following should be considered:

Allergies—Tell your doctor if you or your child has ever had any unusual or allergic reaction to ribavirin aerosol. Also tell your doctor and pharmacist if you or your child is allergic to any other substances, such as foods, preservatives, or dyes.

Pregnancy—Ribavirin aerosol is not usually prescribed for teenagers or adults. However, women who are pregnant or may become pregnant may be exposed to ribavirin that is given off in the air if they spend time at the patient's bedside while ribavirin is being given. Although studies have not been done in humans, ribavirin has been shown to cause birth defects and other problems in certain animal studies. Be sure you have discussed this with your doctor.

Breast-feeding—Ribavirin aerosol is not usually prescribed for teenagers or adults. However, ribavirin passes into the breast milk of animals and has been shown to cause problems in nursing animals and their young.

Children—This medicine has been tested in children, and, when used as it should be and in effective doses, has not been shown to cause serious side effects or problems.

Older adults—Ribavirin aerosol is not usually prescribed for use in elderly patients.

Before you begin using any new medicine (prescription or nonprescription) or if you develop any new medical problem while you are using this medicine, check with your doctor, nurse, or pharmacist.

Proper Use of This Medicine

To help clear up your infection completely, *ribavirin must be given for the full time of treatment,* even if you or your child begins to feel better after a few days. Also, this medicine works best when there is a constant amount in the lungs. To help keep the amount constant, ribavirin must be given on a regular or continuous schedule.

Dosing—The dose of ribavirin will be different for different patients. *Follow your doctor's orders or the directions.* The following information includes only the average doses of ribavirin. *If your dose is different, do not change it* unless your doctor tells you to do so.

- For the *inhalation* dosage form:
  - —Adults and adolescents: Dose has not been determined since this medicine is not usually prescribed for teenagers or adults.
  - —Infants and children: Dose must be determined by the doctor.

Side Effects of This Medicine

Along with its needed effects, a medicine may cause some unwanted effects. The following side effects may go away during treatment as your body adjusts to the medicine. However, check with your doctor if any of the following side effects continue or are bothersome:

Rare

Headache; itching, redness, or swelling of eye; skin rash or irritation

Other side effects not listed above may also occur in some patients. If you notice any other effects, check with your doctor.

Additional Information

Once a medicine has been approved for marketing for a certain use, experience may show that it is also useful for other medical problems. Although these uses are not included in product labeling, ribavirin is used in certain patients with the following medical conditions:

- Influenza A and B (given by aerosol inhalation)
- Lassa fever (either given orally or by injection)

For patients taking this medicine by mouth or injection for *Lassa fever*:

- *Check with your doctor immediately* if any of the following side effects occur:

  More common

  Unusual tiredness and weakness
- Other side effects may occur that usually do not need medical attention. The following side effects may go away during treatment as your body adjusts to the medicine. However, check with your doctor if any of the following side effects continue or are bothersome:

  Less common

  Fatigue; headache; loss of appetite; nausea; trouble in sleeping

Other than the above information, there is no additional information relating to proper use, precautions, or side effects for these uses.

Annual revision: 02/23/93

RIBOFLAVIN (Vitamin B_2) Systemic

Generic name product is available in the U.S. and Canada.

Description

Vitamins (VYE-ta-mins) are compounds that you *must* have for growth and health. They are needed in small amounts only and are usually available in the foods that you eat. Riboflavin (RYE-boe-flay-vin) (vitamin B_2) is necessary for normal metabolism.

Lack of riboflavin may lead to itching and burning eyes, sensitivity of eyes to light, sore tongue, itching and peeling skin on the nose and scrotum, and sores in the mouth. Your doctor may treat this condition by prescribing riboflavin for you.

Patients with the following conditions may be more likely to have a deficiency of riboflavin:

- Alcoholism
- Burns

- Cancer
- Diarrhea (continuing)
- Fever (continuing)
- Illness (continuing)
- Infection
- Intestinal diseases
- Liver disease
- Overactive thyroid
- Serious injury
- Stress (continuing)
- Surgical removal of stomach

In addition, riboflavin may be given to infants with high blood levels of bilirubin (hyperbilirubinemia).

If any of the above apply to you, you should take riboflavin supplements only on the advice of your doctor after need has been established.

Claims that riboflavin is effective for treatment of acne, some kinds of anemia (weak blood), migraine headaches, and muscle cramps have not been proven.

Oral forms of riboflavin are available without a prescription. However, it may be a good idea to check with your doctor before taking riboflavin on your own. If you take more than you need, it will simply be lost from your body.

Riboflavin is available in the following dosage form:

Oral

- Tablets (U.S. and Canada)

It is very important that you read and understand the following information. If any of it causes you special concern, check with your doctor or pharmacist. Also, *if you have any questions* or if you want more information about this medicine or your medical problem, *ask your doctor, nurse, or pharmacist.*

Importance of Diet

Vitamin supplements should be taken only if you cannot get enough vitamins in your diet; however, some diets may not contain all of the vitamins you need. You may not be getting enough vitamins because of rapid weight loss, unusual diets (such as some reducing diets in which choice of foods is very limited), prolonged intravenous feeding, or malnutrition. A balanced diet should provide all the vitamins you normally need.

In order to get enough vitamins and minerals in your diet, it is important that you eat a balanced and varied diet. Follow carefully any diet program your doctor may recommend. For your specific vitamin and/or mineral needs, ask your doctor for a list of appropriate foods.

Riboflavin is found in various foods, including milk and dairy products, fish, meats, green leafy vegetables, and whole grain and enriched cereals and bread. It is best to eat fresh fruits and vegetables whenever possible since they contain the most vitamins. Food processing may destroy some of the vitamins, although little riboflavin is lost from foods during ordinary cooking.

Vitamins alone will not take the place of a good diet and will not provide energy. Your body also needs other substances found in food such as protein, minerals, carbohydrates, and fat. Vitamins themselves often cannot work without the presence of other foods.

In some cases it may not be possible for you to get enough food to supply you with the proper vitamins. In other cases, the amount of vitamins you need may be increased above normal. Therefore, a vitamin supplement may be needed.

Experts have developed a list of recommended dietary allowances (RDA) for most of the vitamins. The RDA are not an exact number but a general idea of how much you need. They do not cover amounts needed for problems caused by a serious lack of vitamins.

The RDA for riboflavin are:

- Infants and children—
  - Birth to 6 months of age: 0.4 milligrams (mg) per day.
  - 6 months to 1 year of age: 0.5 mg per day.
  - 1 to 3 years of age: 0.8 mg per day.
  - 4 to 6 years of age: 1.1 mg per day.
  - 7 to 10 years of age: 1.2 mg per day.
- Adolescent and adult males—
  - 11 to 14 years of age: 1.5 mg per day.
  - 15 to 18 years of age: 1.8 mg per day.
  - 19 to 50 years of age: 1.7 mg per day.
  - 51 years of age and over: 1.4 mg per day.
- Adolescent and adult females—
  - 11 to 50 years of age: 1.3 mg per day.
  - 51 years of age and over: 1.2 mg per day.
- Pregnant females: 1.6 mg per day.
- Breast-feeding females:
  - First 6 months: 1.6 mg per day.
  - Second 6 months: 1.7 mg per day.

Remember:

- The total amount of each vitamin that you get every day includes what you get from the foods that you eat *and* what you may take as a supplement.
- Your total amount should not be greater than the RDA, unless ordered by your doctor.

Before Using This Dietary Supplement

If you are taking this dietary supplement without a prescription, carefully read and follow any precautions on the label. For riboflavin, the following should be considered:

Allergies—Tell your doctor and pharmacist if you are allergic to any substances, such as foods, preservatives, or dyes.

Pregnancy—It is especially important that you are receiving enough vitamins when you become pregnant and that you continue to receive the right amounts of vitamins throughout your pregnancy. The healthy growth and development of the fetus depend on a steady supply of nutrients from the mother. However, taking large amounts of a dietary supplement in pregnancy may be harmful to the mother and/or fetus and should be avoided.

Breast-feeding—It is especially important that you receive the right amounts of vitamins so that your baby will also get the vitamins needed to grow properly. However, taking large amounts of a dietary supplement while breast-feeding may be harmful to the mother and/or baby and should be avoided.

Children—Normal daily requirements vary according to age. It is especially important that children receive enough vitamins in their diet for healthy growth and development. Although there is no specific information about the use of riboflavin in children in doses higher than the normal daily requirements, it is not expected to cause different side effects or problems in children than in adults.

Older adults—It is important that older people continue to receive enough vitamins in their diet for good health. Although there is no specific information about the use of riboflavin in older people in doses higher than the normal daily requirements, it is not expected to cause different side effects or problems in older people than in younger adults.

Other medicines or dietary supplements—Although certain medicines or dietary supplements should not be used together at all, in other cases two different medicines or dietary supplements may be used together even if an interaction might occur. In these cases, your doctor may want to change the dose, or other precautions may be necessary. Tell your doctor and pharmacist if you are taking any other dietary supplements or prescription or nonprescription (over-the-counter [OTC]) medicine.

Proper Use of This Dietary Supplement

Some people believe that taking very large doses of vitamins (called megadoses or megavitamin therapy) is useful for treating certain medical problems. Studies have not proven this. Large doses should be taken only under the direction of your doctor after need has been identified.

Missed dose—If you miss taking a vitamin for 1 or more days there is no cause for concern, since it takes some time for your body to become seriously low in vitamins. However, if your doctor has recommended that you take this vitamin, try to remember to take it as directed every day.

Storage—To store this dietary supplement:

- Keep out of the reach of children.
- Store away from heat and direct light.
- Do not store in the bathroom, near the kitchen sink, or in other damp places. Heat or moisture may cause the dietary supplement to break down.
- Do not keep outdated dietary supplements or those no longer needed. Be sure that any discarded dietary supplement is out of the reach of children.

Side Effects of This Dietary Supplement

Along with its needed effects, a dietary supplement may cause some unwanted effects. Riboflavin may cause urine to have a more yellow color than normal, especially if large doses are taken. This is to be expected and is no cause for alarm. Usually, however, riboflavin does not cause any side effects. Check with your doctor if you notice any other unusual effects while you are using it.

Annual revision: 08/22/92

RIFAMPIN Systemic

Some commonly used brand names are:

In the U.S.
- Rifadin
- Rifadin IV
- Rimactane

In Canada
- Rifadin
- Rimactane
- Rofact

Another commonly used name is rifampicin.

Description

Rifampin (rif-AM-pin) is used to treat selected bacterial infections.

Rifampin is used with one or more other medicines to treat tuberculosis (TB). Rifampin is also taken alone by patients who may carry meningitis bacteria in their nose and throat (without feeling sick) and may spread these bacteria to others. This medicine may also be used for other problems as determined by your doctor. However, rifampin will not work for colds, flu, or other virus infections.

Rifampin is available only with your doctor's prescription, in the following dosage forms:

Oral
- Capsules (U.S. and Canada)

Parenteral
- Injection (U.S.)

It is very important that you read and understand the following information. If any of it causes you special concern, check with your doctor. Also, *if you have any questions* or if you want more information about this medicine or your medical problem, *ask your doctor, nurse, or pharmacist.*

Before Using This Medicine

In deciding to use a medicine, the risks of taking the medicine must be weighed against the good it will do. This is a decision you and your doctor will make. For rifampin, the following should be considered:

Allergies—Tell your doctor if you have ever had any unusual or allergic reaction to rifampin. Also tell your doctor and pharmacist if you are allergic to any other substances, such as foods, preservatives, or dyes.

Pregnancy—Rifampin has caused bleeding in newborn babies and mothers when it was taken during the last weeks of pregnancy. Studies in rodents have shown that rifampin given in high doses causes birth defects, usually backbone problems (spina bifida) and cleft palate. In addition, it is not known whether this medicine causes problems when taken with other TB medicines.

Breast-feeding—Rifampin passes into the breast milk. However, rifampin has not been reported to cause problems in nursing babies.

Children—This medicine has been tested in children and, in effective doses, has not been shown to cause different side effects or problems in children than it does in adults.

Older adults—Many medicines have not been studied specifically in older people. Therefore, it may not be known whether they work exactly the same way they do in younger adults. Although there is no specific information comparing use of rifampin in the elderly with use in other age groups, this medicine is not expected to cause different side effects or problems in older people than it does in younger adults.

Other medicines—Although certain medicines should not be used together at all, in other cases two different medicines may be used together even if an interaction might occur. In these cases, your doctor may want to change the dose, or other precautions may be necessary. When you are taking rifampin, it is especially important that your doctor and pharmacist know if you are taking any of the following:

- Acetaminophen (e.g., Tylenol) (with long-term, high-dose use) or
- Amiodarone (e.g., Cordarone) or
- Anabolic steroids (nandrolone [e.g., Anabolin], oxandrolone [e.g., Anavar], oxymetholone [e.g., Anadrol], stanozolol [e.g., Winstrol]) or
- Androgens (male hormones) or
- Antithyroid agents (medicine for overactive thyroid) or
- Carbamazepine (e.g., Tegretol) or
- Carmustine (e.g., BiCNU) or
- Chloroquine (e.g., Aralen) or
- Dantrolene (e.g., Dantrium) or
- Daunorubicin (e.g., Cerubidine) or
- Disulfiram (e.g., Antabuse) or
- Divalproex (e.g., Depakote) or
- Etretinate (e.g., Tegison) or
- Gold salts (medicine for arthritis) or
- Hydroxychloroquine (e.g., Plaquenil) or
- Isoniazid (e.g., INH, Nydrazid) or
- Mercaptopurine (e.g., Purinethol) or
- Methotrexate (e.g., Mexate) or
- Methyldopa (e.g., Aldomet) or
- Naltrexone (e.g., Trexan) (with long-term, high-dose use) or
- Other anti-infectives by mouth or by injection (medicine for infection) or
- Phenothiazines (acetophenazine [e.g., Tindal], chlorpromazine [e.g., Thorazine], fluphenazine [e.g., Prolixin], mesoridazine [e.g., Serentil], perphenazine [e.g., Trilafon], prochlorperazine [e.g., Compazine], promazine [e.g., Sparine], promethazine [e.g., Phenergan], thioridazine [e.g., Mellaril], trifluoperazine [e.g., Stelazine], triflupromazine [e.g., Vesprin], trimeprazine [e.g., Temaril]) or
- Plicamycin (e.g., Mithracin) or
- Valproic acid (e.g., Depakene)—These medicines may increase the chance of liver damage if taken with rifampin
- Anticoagulants (blood thinners) or
- Aminophylline (e.g., Somophyllin) or
- Antidiabetics, oral (diabetes medicine you take by mouth), or
- Chloramphenicol or
- Corticosteroids (cortisone-like medicine) or
- Digitalis glycosides (heart medicine) or
- Disopyramide (e.g., Norpace) or
- Fluconazole (e.g., Diflucan) or
- Ketoconazole (e.g., Nizoral) or
- Methadone (e.g., Dolophine) or
- Mexiletine (e.g., Mexitil) or
- Oxtriphylline (e.g., Choledyl) or
- Quinidine (e.g., Quinidex) or
- Theophylline (e.g., Theo-dur, Somophyllin-T) or
- Tocainide (e.g., Tonocard) or
- Verapamil (e.g., Calan)—Rifampin may decrease the effects of these medicines
- Estramustine (e.g., EMCYT) or
- Estrogens (female hormones) or

- Oral contraceptives (birth control pills) containing estrogen or
- Phenytoin (e.g., Dilantin)—Rifampin may decrease the effects of these medicines. If you are taking oral contraceptives, this may increase the chance of pregnancy. These medicines may also increase the chance of liver damage if taken with rifampin

Other medical problems—The presence of other medical problems may affect the use of rifampin. Make sure you tell your doctor if you have any other medical problems, especially:

- Alcohol abuse (or history of) or
- Liver disease—There may be an increased chance of side effects affecting the liver in patients with a history of alcohol abuse or liver disease

Before you begin using any new medicine (prescription or nonprescription) or if you develop any new medical problem while you are using this medicine, check with your doctor, nurse, or pharmacist.

Proper Use of This Medicine

Rifampin is best taken with a full glass (8 ounces) of water on an empty stomach (either 1 hour before or 2 hours after a meal). However, if this medicine upsets your stomach, your doctor may want you to take it with food.

For *patients unable to swallow capsules:*

- Contents of the capsules may be mixed with applesauce or jelly. Be sure to take all the food to get the full dose of medicine.
- Your pharmacist can prepare an oral liquid form of this medicine if needed. The liquid form may be kept at room temperature or in the refrigerator. Follow the directions on the label. Shake the bottle well before using. Do not use after the expiration date on the label. The medicine may not work properly after that date. In addition, use a specially marked measuring spoon or other device to measure each dose accurately. The average household teaspoon may not hold the right amount of liquid.

To help clear up your tuberculosis (TB) completely, *it is very important that you keep taking this medicine for the full time of treatment,* even if you begin to feel better after a few weeks. You may have to take it every day for as long as 1 to 2 years or more. *It is important that you do not miss any doses.*

Dosing—The dose of rifampin will be different for different patients. *Follow your doctor's orders or the directions on the label.* The following information includes only the average doses of rifampin. *If your dose is different, do not change it* unless your doctor tells you to do so.

- The number of capsules that you take depends on the strength of the medicine. Also, *the number of doses you take each day, the time allowed between doses, and the length of time you take the medicine depend on the medical problem for which you are taking rifampin.*
- For the treatment of *tuberculosis (TB)*:
  - —Adults and older children: 600 milligrams once a day, taken with other medicines to treat tuberculosis.
  - —Infants and children: Dose is based on body weight and will be determined by your doctor. Rifampin is taken once a day with other medicines to treat tuberculosis.
- For the treatment of patients who *carry meningitis bacteria*:
  - —Adults and older children: 600 milligrams two times a day for two days.
  - —Children 1 month of age and older: Dose is based on body weight and will be determined by your doctor. It is taken twice a day for two days.
  - —Infants up to 1 month of age: Dose is based on body weight and will be determined by your doctor. It is taken twice a day for two days.

Missed dose—If you do miss a dose of this medicine, take it as soon as possible. However, if it is almost time for your next dose, skip the missed dose and go back to your regular dosing schedule. Do not double doses. *If this medicine is taken on an irregular schedule, side effects may occur more often and may be more serious than usual.* If you have any questions about this, check with your doctor or pharmacist.

Storage—To store this medicine:

- Keep out of the reach of children.
- Store away from heat and direct light.
- Do not store in the bathroom, near the kitchen sink, or in other damp places. Heat or moisture may cause the medicine to break down.
- Do not keep outdated medicine or medicine no longer needed. Be sure that any discarded medicine is out of the reach of children.

Precautions While Using This Medicine

It is very important that your doctor check your progress at regular visits.

If your symptoms do not improve within 2 to 3 weeks, or if they become worse, check with your doctor.

Oral contraceptives (birth control pills) containing estrogen may not work properly if you take them while you are taking rifampin. Unplanned pregnancies may occur. You should use a different means of birth control while you are taking rifampin. If you have any questions about this, check with your doctor or pharmacist.

Liver problems may be more likely to occur if you drink alcoholic beverages regularly while you are taking this medicine. Also, the regular use of alcohol may keep this medicine from working properly. Therefore, *you should not drink alcoholic beverages while you are taking this medicine.*

If this medicine causes you to feel very tired or very weak or causes a loss of appetite, nausea, or vomiting, stop taking it and check with your doctor immediately. These may be early warning signs of more serious problems that could develop later.

Rifampin will cause the urine, stool, saliva, sputum, sweat, and tears to turn reddish orange to reddish brown. This is to be expected while you are taking this medicine. This effect may cause soft contact lenses to become permanently discolored. Standard cleaning solutions may not take out all the discoloration. Therefore, *it is best not to wear soft contact lenses while taking this medicine.* Hard contact lenses are not discolored by rifampin. If you have any questions about this, check with your doctor.

Rifampin can lower the number of white blood cells in your blood temporarily, increasing the chance of getting an infection. It can also lower the number of platelets, which are necessary for proper blood clotting. These problems may result in a greater chance of getting certain infections, slow healing, and bleeding of the gums. Be careful when using a regular toothbrush, dental floss, or a toothpick. Dental work should be delayed until your blood counts have returned to normal. Check with your medical doctor or dentist if you have any questions about proper oral hygiene (mouth care) during treatment.

Before you have any medical tests, tell the doctor in charge that you are taking this medicine. The results of some tests may be affected by this medicine.

Side Effects of This Medicine

Along with its needed effects, a medicine may cause some unwanted effects. Although not all of these side effects may occur, if they do occur they may need medical attention.

Check with your doctor immediately if any of the following side effects occur:

Less common

Chills; difficult breathing; dizziness; fever; headache; itching; muscle and bone pain; shivering; skin rash and redness

Rare

Bloody or cloudy urine; greatly decreased frequency of urination or amount of urine; loss of appetite; nausea or vomiting; sore throat; unusual bleeding or bruising; unusual tiredness or weakness; yellow eyes or skin

Signs and symptoms of overdose

Itching over the whole body; reddish orange color of skin, mouth, and eyeballs; swelling around the eyes or the whole face

Other side effects may occur that usually do not need medical attention. These side effects may go away during treatment as your body adjusts to the medicine. However, check with your doctor if any of the following side effects continue or are bothersome:

More common

Diarrhea; stomach cramps

Less common

Sore mouth or tongue

This medicine commonly causes reddish orange to reddish brown discoloration of urine, stools, saliva, sputum, sweat, and tears. This side effect does not usually need medical attention. However, tears that have been discolored by this medicine may also discolor soft contact lenses.

Other side effects not listed above may also occur in some patients. If you notice any other effects, check with your doctor.

Additional Information

Once a medicine has been approved for marketing for a certain use, experience may show that it is also useful for other medical problems. Although these uses are not included in product labeling, rifampin is used in certain patients with the following medical conditions:

- Leprosy (Hansen's disease)
- Prevention of the spread of the influenza virus to young children

Other than the above information, there is no additional information relating to proper use, precautions, or side effects for these uses.

Annual revision: 01/19/93

RIFAMPIN AND ISONIAZID Systemic†

A commonly used brand name in the U.S. is Rifamate.
Another commonly used name is rifampicin and isoniazid.

†Not commercially available in Canada.

Description

Rifampin (rif-AM-pin) and isoniazid (eye-soe-NYE-a-zid) is a combination antibiotic and anti-infective medicine. It is used to treat tuberculosis (TB). It may be taken alone or with one or more other medicines for TB.

Rifampin and isoniazid combination is available only with your doctor's prescription, in the following dosage form:

Oral

- Capsules (U.S.)

It is very important that you read and understand the following information. If any of it causes you special concern, check with your doctor. Also, *if you have any questions* or if you want more information about this medicine or your medical problem, *ask your doctor, nurse, or pharmacist.*

Before Using This Medicine

In deciding to use a medicine, the risks of taking the medicine must be weighed against the good it will do. This is a decision you and your doctor will make. For rifampin and isoniazid combination, the following should be considered:

Allergies—Tell your doctor if you have ever had any unusual or allergic reaction to ethionamide (e.g., Trecator-SC), pyrazinamide, niacin (e.g., Nicobid, nicotinic acid), rifampin (e.g., Rifadin), or isoniazid (e.g., INH, Nydrazid). Also tell your doctor and pharmacist if you are allergic to any other substances, such as foods, preservatives, or dyes.

Pregnancy—Rifampin has caused bleeding in newborn babies and mothers when it was taken during the last weeks of pregnancy. Rifampin and isoniazid combination has not been shown to cause birth defects or other problems in humans. However, studies in rodents have shown that rifampin given in high doses causes birth defects, usually backbone problems (spina bifida) and cleft palate. Studies in rats and rabbits have shown that isoniazid may kill the fetus. In addition, it is not known whether this medicine causes problems when taken with other TB medicines.

Breast-feeding—Rifampin and isoniazid both pass into the breast milk. However, rifampin and isoniazid have not been reported to cause problems in nursing babies.

Children—Rifampin and isoniazid combination is not recommended for use in children.

Older adults—Dark urine and yellowing of the eyes or skin are more likely to occur in patients over 50 years of age who are taking isoniazid-containing medicines.

Other medicines—Although certain medicines should not be used together at all, in other cases two different medicines may be used together even if an interaction might occur. In these cases, your doctor may want to change the dose, or other precautions may be necessary. When you are taking rifampin and isoniazid combination, it is especially important that your doctor and pharmacist know if you are taking any of the following:

- Acetaminophen (e.g., Tylenol) (with long-term, high-dose use) or
- Amiodarone (e.g., Cordarone) or
- Anabolic steroids (nandrolone [e.g., Anabolin], oxandrolone [e.g., Anavar], oxymetholone [e.g., Anadrol], stanozolol [e.g., Winstrol]) or
- Androgens (male hormones) or
- Antithyroid agents (medicine for overactive thyroid) or
- Carbamazepine (e.g., Tegretol) or
- Carmustine (e.g., BiCNU) or
- Chloroquine (e.g., Aralen) or
- Dantrolene (e.g., Dantrium) or
- Daunorubicin (e.g., Cerubidine) or
- Disulfiram (e.g., Antabuse) or
- Divalproex (e.g., Depakote) or
- Etretinate (e.g., Tegison) or
- Gold salts (medicine for arthritis) or
- Hydroxychloroquine (e.g., Plaquenil) or
- Isoniazid (e.g., INH, Nydrazid) or
- Mercaptopurine (e.g., Purinethol) or
- Methyldopa (e.g., Aldomet) or
- Naltrexone (e.g., Trexan) (with long-term, high-dose use) or
- Other anti-infectives by mouth or by injection (medicine for infection) or
- Phenothiazines (acetophenazine [e.g., Tindal], chlorpromazine [e.g., Thorazine], fluphenazine [e.g., Prolixin], mesoridazine [e.g., Serentil], perphenazine [e.g., Trilafon], prochlorperazine [e.g., Compazine], promazine [e.g., Sparine], promethazine [e.g., Phenergan], thioridazine [e.g., Mellaril], trifluoperazine [e.g., Stelazine], triflupromazine [e.g., Vesprin], trimeprazine [e.g., Temaril]) or
- Plicamycin (e.g., Mithracin) or
- Valproic acid (e.g., Depakene)—These medicines may increase the chance of liver damage if taken with rifampin and isoniazid combination
- Aminophylline (e.g., Somophyllin) or
- Anticoagulants (blood thinners) or
- Antidiabetics, oral (diabetes medicine you take by mouth) or
- Chloramphenicol or
- Corticosteroids (cortisone-like medicine) or
- Digitalis glycosides (heart medicine) or
- Disopyramide (e.g., Norpace) or
- Estramustine (e.g., EMCYT) or
- Fluconazole (e.g., Diflucan) or
- Ketoconazole (e.g., Nizoral) or

- Methadone (e.g., Dolophine) or
- Methotrexate (e.g., Mexate) or
- Mexiletine (e.g., Mexitil) or
- Oxtriphylline (e.g., Choledyl) or
- Quinidine (e.g., Quinidex) or
- Theophylline (e.g., Theo-dur, Somophyllin-T) or
- Tocainide (e.g., Tonocard) or
- Verapamil (e.g., Calan)—Rifampin and isoniazid combination may decrease the effects of these medicines
- Disulfiram (e.g., Antabuse)—This medicine may increase the chance of liver damage and side effects, such as dizziness, lack of coordination, irritability, and inability to sleep
- Estrogens (female hormones) or
- Oral contraceptives (birth control pills) containing estrogen or
- Phenytoin (e.g., Dilantin)—Rifampin and isoniazid combination may decrease the effects of these medicines. If you are taking oral contraceptives, this may increase the chance of pregnancy. These medicines may also increase the chance of liver damage if taken with rifampin and isoniazid combination

Other medical problems—The presence of other medical problems may affect the use of rifampin and isoniazid combination. Make sure you tell your doctor if you have any other medical problems, especially:

- Alcohol abuse (or history of) or
- Liver disease—There may be an increased chance of getting hepatitis if you take this medicine and drink alcohol daily
- Convulsive disorders such as seizures or epilepsy—Rifampin and isoniazid combination may increase the frequency of seizures (convulsions) in some patients
- Kidney disease (severe)—There may be an increased chance of side effects in patients with severe kidney disease

Before you begin using any new medicine (prescription or nonprescription) or if you develop any new medical problem while you are using this medicine, check with your doctor, nurse, or pharmacist.

Proper Use of This Medicine

If this medicine upsets your stomach, take it with food. Antacids may also help. However, do not take aluminum-containing antacids within 1 hour of the time you take rifampin and isoniazid combination. They may keep this medicine from working properly.

To help clear up your tuberculosis (TB) completely, *it is very important that you keep taking this medicine for the full time of treatment,* even if you begin to feel better after a few weeks. You may have to take it every day for as long as 1 to 2 years or more. *It is important that you do not miss any doses.*

Your doctor may also want you to take pyridoxine (e.g., Hexa-Betalin, vitamin B_6) every day to help prevent or lessen some of the side effects of isoniazid. If it is needed, *it is very important to take pyridoxine every day along with this medicine. Do not miss any doses.*

Dosing—The dose of rifampin and isoniazid combination will be different for different patients. *Follow your doctor's orders or the directions on the label.* The following information includes only the average doses of rifampin and isoniazid combination. *If your dose is different, do not change it* unless your doctor tells you to do so.

- For the *tablet* dosage form:
  —Adults and older children: 600 milligrams of rifampin and 300 milligrams of isoniazid once a day.
  —Children—This medicine is not recommended for use in children.

Missed dose—If you do miss a dose of this medicine, take it as soon as possible. However, if it is almost time for your next dose, skip the missed dose and go back to your regular dosing schedule. Do not double doses. *If rifampin and isoniazid combination is taken on an irregular schedule, side effects may occur more often and may be more serious than usual.* If you have any questions about this, check with your doctor or pharmacist.

Storage—To store this medicine:

- Keep out of the reach of children.
- Store away from heat and direct light.
- Do not store in the bathroom, near the kitchen sink, or in other damp places. Heat or moisture may cause the medicine to break down.
- Do not keep outdated medicine or medicine no longer needed. Be sure that any discarded medicine is out of the reach of children.

Precautions While Using This Medicine

It is very important that your doctor check your progress at regular visits. In addition, you should *check with your doctor immediately if blurred vision or loss of vision, with or without eye pain, occurs during treatment.* He or she may want you to have your eyes checked by an ophthalmologist (eye doctor).

If your symptoms do not improve within 2 to 3 weeks, or if they become worse, check with your doctor.

Oral contraceptives (birth control pills) containing estrogen may not work properly if you take them while you are taking rifampin and isoniazid combination. Unplanned pregnancies may occur. You should use a different means of birth control while you are taking this medicine. If you have any questions about this, check with your doctor or pharmacist.

Liver problems may be more likely to occur if you drink alcoholic beverages regularly while you are taking this medicine. Also, the regular use of alcohol may keep this medicine from working properly. Therefore, *you should strictly limit the amount of alcoholic beverages you drink while you are taking this medicine.*

Certain foods such as cheese (Swiss or Cheshire) or fish (tuna, skipjack, or Sardinella) may rarely cause reactions in some patients taking isoniazid-containing medicines. Check with your doctor if redness or itching of the skin, hot feeling, fast or pounding heartbeat, sweating, chills or clammy feeling, headache, or lightheadedness occurs while you are taking this medicine.

This medicine will cause the urine, stool, saliva, sputum, sweat, and tears to turn reddish orange to reddish brown. This is to be expected while you are taking this medicine. This effect may cause soft contact lenses to become permanently discolored. Standard cleaning solutions may not take out all the discoloration. Therefore, *it is best not to wear soft contact lenses while taking this medicine.* Hard contact lenses are not discolored by this medicine. If you have any questions about this, check with your doctor.

If this medicine causes you to feel very tired or very weak; or causes clumsiness; unsteadiness; a loss of appetite; nausea; numbness, tingling, burning, or pain in the hands and feet; or vomiting, stop taking it and check with your doctor immediately. These may be early warning symptoms of more serious liver or nerve problems that could develop later.

Rifampin and isoniazid combination may cause blood problems. These problems may result in a greater chance of certain infections, slow healing, and bleeding of the gums. Therefore, you should be careful when using regular toothbrushes, dental floss, and toothpicks. Dental work should be delayed until your blood counts have returned to normal. Check with your medical doctor or dentist if you have any questions about proper oral hygiene (mouth care) during treatment.

Side Effects of This Medicine

Along with its needed effects, a medicine may cause some unwanted effects. Although not all of these side effects may occur, if they do occur they may need medical attention.

Check with your doctor immediately if any of the following side effects occur:

More common

Clumsiness or unsteadiness; dark urine; loss of appetite; nausea or vomiting; numbness, tingling, burning, or pain in hands and feet; unusual tiredness or weakness; yellow eyes or skin

Less common

Chills; difficult breathing; dizziness; fever; headache; itching; muscle and bone pain; shivering; skin rash and redness

Rare

Bloody or cloudy urine; blurred vision or loss of vision, with or without eye pain; convulsions (seizures); depression; greatly decreased frequency of urination or amount of urine; joint pain; mood or mental changes; sore throat; unusual bruising or bleeding

Other side effects may occur that usually do not need medical attention. These side effects may go away during treatment as your body adjusts to the medicine. However, check with your doctor if any of the following side effects continue or are bothersome:

More common

Diarrhea; stomach cramps or upset

Less common

Sore mouth or tongue

This medicine commonly causes reddish orange to reddish brown discoloration of urine, stools, saliva, sputum, sweat, and tears. This side effect does not usually require medical attention. However, tears that have been discolored by this medicine may also discolor soft contact lenses (see *Precautions While Using This Medicine*).

Dark urine and yellowing of the eyes or skin (signs of liver problems) are more likely to occur in patients over 50 years of age.

Other side effects not listed above may also occur in some patients. If you notice any other effects, check with your doctor.

Annual revision: 01/19/93

RITODRINE Systemic

A commonly used brand name in the U.S. and Canada is Yutopar.
Generic name product may be available in the U.S.

Description

Ritodrine (RI-toe-dreen) is used to stop premature labor. It is available only with your doctor's prescription and is to be administered only by or under the supervision of your doctor.

Ritodrine is available in the following dosage forms:

Oral

- Tablets (U.S. and Canada)

Parenteral
- Injection (U.S. and Canada)

It is very important that you read and understand the following information. If any of it causes you special concern, check with your doctor. Also, *if you have any questions* or if you want more information about this medicine or your medical problem, *ask your doctor, nurse, or pharmacist.*

Before Using This Medicine

In deciding to use a medicine, the risks of taking the medicine must be weighed against the good it will do. This is a decision you and your doctor will make. For ritodrine, the following should be considered:

Allergies—Tell your doctor if you have ever had any unusual or allergic reaction to ritodrine. Also tell your doctor and pharmacist if you are allergic to any other substances, such as foods, preservatives, or dyes.

Other medicines—Although certain medicines should not be used together at all, in other cases two different medicines may be used together even if an interaction might occur. In these cases, your doctor may want to change the dose, or other precautions may be necessary. When you are taking ritodrine, it is especially important that your doctor and pharmacist know if you are taking any of the following:

- Corticosteroids (cortisone-like medicines)—There is an increased chance of fluid in the lungs when these medicines and ritodrine are used together
- Beta-adrenergic blocking agents (acebutolol [e.g., Sectral], atenolol [e.g., Tenormin], betaxolol [e.g., Kerlone], carteolol [e.g., Cartrol], labetalol [e.g., Normodyne], metoprolol [e.g., Lopressor], nadolol [e.g., Corgard], oxprenolol [e.g., Trasicor], penbutolol [e.g., Levatol], pindolol [e.g., Visken], propranolol [e.g., Inderal], sotalol [e.g., Sotacor], timolol [e.g., Blocadren])—Ritodrine may be less effective if it is used with any of these medicines

Other medical problems—The presence of other medical problems may affect the use of ritodrine. Make sure you tell your doctor if you have any other medical problems, especially:

- Asthma
- Diabetes mellitus (sugar diabetes)—Ritodrine may make this condition worse
- Heart disease or
- Overactive thyroid—Use of ritodrine may cause serious effects on the heart, including irregular heartbeat
- High blood pressure (hypertension)
- Migraine headaches (or history of)—Rarely, use of ritodrine may cause problems with blood circulation in the brain

Before you begin using any new medicine (prescription or nonprescription) or if you develop any new medical problem while you are using this medicine, check with your doctor, nurse, or pharmacist.

Proper Use of This Medicine

Dosing—The dose of ritodrine will be different for different women. *Follow your doctor's orders or the directions on the label.* The following information includes only the average doses of ritodrine. *If your dose is different, do not change it* unless your doctor tells you to do so.

- For *injection* dosage forms:
  —Adults: 50 to 350 micrograms per minute, injected into a vein.
- For *oral* dosage forms (tablets):
  —Adults: In the first twenty-four hours after the doctor stops your intravenous ritodrine, your dose may be as high as 10 milligrams (mg) every two hours. After that, the dose is usually 10 to 20 mg every four to six hours. Your doctor may want you to take oral ritodrine up until it is time for you to deliver your baby.

Missed dose—If you miss a dose of this medicine and remember within an hour or so of the missed dose, take it right away. However, if you do not remember until later, skip the missed dose and go back to your regular dosing schedule. Do not double doses.

Storage—To store this medicine:
- Keep out of the reach of children.
- Store away from heat and direct light.
- Do not store in the bathroom, near the kitchen sink, or in other damp places. Heat or moisture may cause the medicine to break down.
- Do not keep outdated medicine or medicine no longer needed. Be sure that any discarded medicine is out of the reach of children.

Precautions While Using This Medicine

Check with your doctor right away if your contractions begin again or your water breaks.

Do not take other medicines unless they have been discussed with your doctor. This especially includes over-the-counter (nonprescription) medicines for appetite control, asthma, colds, cough, hay fever, or sinus problems since they may increase the unwanted effects of this medicine.

Side Effects of This Medicine

Along with its needed effects, a medicine may cause some unwanted effects. Although not all of these side effects

may occur, if they do occur they may need medical attention.

Tell your doctor or nurse immediately if either of the following side effects occurs while you are receiving this medicine by injection:

Rare

Chest pain or tightness; shortness of breath

Check with your doctor or nurse as soon as possible if the following side effects occur:

More common

Fast or irregular heartbeat

Rare

Yellow eyes or skin

Symptoms of overdose

Fast or irregular heartbeat (severe); nausea or vomiting (severe); nervousness or trembling (severe); shortness of breath (severe)

Other side effects may occur that usually do not need medical attention. These side effects may go away during treatment as your body adjusts to the medicine. However, check with your doctor if any of the following side effects continue or are bothersome:

More common

Trembling

Less common

Anxiety; emotional upset; headache—more common with injection; jitteriness, nervousness, or restlessness; nausea and vomiting; reddened skin—injection only; skin rash

Other side effects not listed above may also occur in some patients. If you notice any other effects, check with your doctor.

Annual revision: 07/28/93

RUBELLA VIRUS VACCINE LIVE Systemic

Some commonly used brand names are:

In the U.S.

Meruvax II

In Canada

Meruvax II

Generic name product may also be available.

Description

Rubella (rue-BELL-a) Virus Vaccine Live is an active immunizing agent used to prevent infection by the rubella virus. It works by causing your body to produce its own protection (antibodies) against the virus.

The following information applies only to the Wistar RA 27/3 strain of rubella vaccine. Different types of rubella vaccines may be available in countries other than the U.S. and Canada.

Rubella (also known as German measles) is a serious infection that causes miscarriages, stillbirths, or birth defects in unborn babies when pregnant women get the disease. While immunization against rubella is recommended for everyone, it is especially important for women of child-bearing age.

Immunization against rubella is also important for employees in medical facilities, persons in colleges and in the military, persons traveling outside the U.S., children of pregnant women who have not yet received their own rubella immunization, and all children 12 months of age and older, including school-age children.

Immunization against rubella is not recommended for infants younger than 12 months of age, because antibodies they received from their mothers before birth may interfere with the effectiveness of the vaccine. Children who were immunized against rubella before 12 months of age should be immunized again.

If the rubella vaccine is going to be given in a combination immunization that includes measles vaccine, the child to be immunized should be at least 15 months old to make sure the measles vaccine is effective.

You can be considered to be immune to rubella only if you received rubella vaccine on or after your first birthday and have the medical record to prove it or if you have had a blood test showing immunity to rubella. A past history of having a rubella infection is not used to prove immunity, because the signs of rubella infection are not reliable enough to be certain that you have had the disease.

Since vaccination with rubella vaccine may not provide protection for everyone, you may want to ask your doctor to check your immunity to the rubella virus 6 to 8 weeks following your vaccination. This may be especially important if you are a woman of child-bearing age who intends to become pregnant in the future.

This vaccine is available only from your doctor or other authorized health care providers, in the following dosage form:

Parenteral

- Injection (U.S. and Canada)

It is very important that you read and understand the following information. If any of it causes you special concern, check with your doctor. Also, *if you have any questions* or if you want more information about this

medicine or your medical problem, *ask your doctor, nurse, or pharmacist.*

Before Receiving This Vaccine

In deciding to use a medicine, the risks of taking the medicine must be weighed against the good it will do. This is a decision you and your doctor will make. For rubella vaccine, the following should be considered:

Allergies—Tell your doctor if you have ever had any unusual or allergic reaction to rubella vaccine or to the antibiotic neomycin or polymyxin B. Also tell your doctor and pharmacist if you are allergic to any other substances, such as preservatives.

Pregnancy—Tell your doctor if you are pregnant or if you may become pregnant within 3 months after receiving this vaccine. Although studies have not been done in either humans or animals, use during pregnancy is not recommended, because rubella vaccine crosses the placenta. However, the Centers for Disease Control observed over 200 women who received the vaccine within 3 months before or after becoming pregnant and those women gave birth to normal babies.

Breast-feeding—Rubella vaccine may pass into the breast milk and may cause mild rubella infection in nursing babies. However, studies have not shown that this infection causes any problems.

Children—Use is not recommended for infants younger than 12 months of age. This medicine has been tested in older infants and children and, in effective doses, has not been shown to cause different side effects or problems than it does in adults.

Other medicines—Although certain medicines should not be used together at all, in other cases two different medicines may be used together even if an interaction might occur. In these cases, your doctor may want to change the dose, or other precautions may be necessary. Before you receive rubella vaccine, it is especially important that your doctor and pharmacist know if you have received any of the following:

- Treatment with x-rays or cancer medicines—Treatment may interfere with the useful effect of the vaccine

Other medical problems—The presence of other medical problems may affect the use of rubella vaccine. Make sure you tell your doctor if you have any other medical problems, especially:

- Immune deficiency condition (or family history of)—Condition may increase the chance and severity of side effects of the vaccine and/or may decrease the useful effects of the vaccine
- Severe illness with fever—The symptoms of the condition may be confused with the possible side effects of the vaccine
- Tuberculosis—Use of rubella vaccine may interfere with the tuberculin skin test

Precautions After Receiving This Vaccine

Do not become pregnant for 3 months after receiving rubella vaccine without first checking with your doctor. There is a chance that this vaccine may cause birth defects.

Tell your doctor that you have received this vaccine:

- if you are to receive a tuberculin skin test within 8 weeks after receiving this vaccine. The results of the test may be affected by this vaccine.
- if you are to receive any other live virus vaccines within 1 month after receiving this vaccine.
- if you are to receive blood transfusions or other blood products within 2 weeks after receiving this vaccine.
- if you are to receive gamma globulin or other globulins within 2 weeks after receiving this vaccine.

Side Effects of This Vaccine

Along with its needed effects, a vaccine may cause some unwanted effects. Although not all of these side effects may occur, if they do occur they may need medical attention.

Get emergency help immediately if any of the following side effects occur:

Symptoms of allergic reaction

Difficulty in breathing or swallowing; hives; itching, especially of feet or hands; reddening of skin, especially around ears; swelling of eyes, face, or inside of nose; unusual tiredness or weakness (sudden and severe)

Check with your doctor as soon as possible if any of the following side effects occur:

Less common

Pain or tenderness of eyes

Rare

Bruising or purple spots on skin; confusion; convulsions (seizures); headache (severe or continuing); pain, numbness, or tingling of hands, arms, legs, or feet; stiff neck; unusual irritability; vomiting

Other side effects may occur that usually do not need medical attention. However, check with your doctor if any of the following side effects continue or are bothersome:

More common

Burning or stinging at place of injection; skin rash; swelling of glands in neck

Less common

Aches or pain in joints; headache (mild), sore throat, runny nose, or fever; itching, swelling, redness, tenderness, or hard lump at place of injection; nausea; vague feeling of bodily discomfort

The above side effects (especially aches or pain in joints) are more likely to occur in adults, particularly women.

Some of the above side effects may not occur until 1 to 4 weeks after immunization and usually last less than 1 week.

Check with your doctor as soon as possible if any of the following side effects occur:

Pain, numbness, or tingling of hands, arms, legs, or feet; pain or tenderness of eyes

In addition, check with your doctor if any of the following side effects continue or are bothersome:

Headache (mild), sore throat, runny nose, or fever; swelling of glands in neck; vague feeling of bodily discomfort

Also, aches or pain in joints may not occur until 1 to 10 weeks after immunization and usually last less than 1 week. Check with your doctor if either of these side effects continues or is bothersome.

Other side effects not listed above may also occur in some patients. If you notice any other effects, check with your doctor.

Annual revision: September 1990

SALICYLATES Systemic

This information applies to the following medicines:

Aspirin (AS-pir-in)
Aspirin and Caffeine (kaf-EEN)
Buffered Aspirin
Choline Salicylate (KOE-leen sa-LI-si-late)
Choline and Magnesium (mag-NEE-zhum) Salicylates
Magnesium Salicylate
Salsalate (SAL-sa-late)
Sodium Salicylate

Some commonly used brand names are:

For Aspirin

In the U.S.

Aspergum
Bayer Aspirin
Easprin
Ecotrin
Empirin
8-Hour Bayer Timed-Release
Halfprin
Measurin
Norwich Aspirin
St. Joseph Adult Chewable Aspirin
Therapy Bayer
ZORprin

Generic name product may also be available.

In Canada

Apo-Asa
Apo-Asen
Arthrinol
Arthrisin
Artria S.R.
Aspergum
Aspirin
Astrin
Bayer Timed-Release Arthritic Pain Formula
Coryphen
Ecotrin
Entrophen
Headstart
Novasen
Riphen
Sal-Adult
Sal-Infant
Supasa
Triaphen

Generic name product may also be available.

Other commonly used names for aspirin are acetylsalicylic acid and ASA. Because Aspirin is a brand name in Canada, ASA is the term that commonly appears on Canadian product labels.

For Aspirin and Caffeine

In the U.S.

Anacin
APAC Improved
P-A-C Revised Formula

Generic name product may also be available.

In Canada

Anacin
C2
Instantine
Nervine
217
217 Strong

Other commonly used names for aspirin are acetylsalicylic acid and ASA. Because Aspirin is a brand name in Canada, ASA is the term that commonly appears on Canadian product labels.

For Buffered Aspirin

In the U.S.

Arthritis Pain Formula
Ascriptin
Ascriptin A/D
Buffaprin
Bufferin
Buffinol
Cama Arthritis Pain Reliever
Magnaprin
Magnaprin Arthritis Strength
Maprin
Maprin I-B

Generic name product may also be available.

In Canada

APF Arthritic Pain Formula
Bufferin

Other commonly used names for aspirin are acetylsalicylic acid and ASA. Because Aspirin is a brand name in Canada, ASA is the term that commonly appears on Canadian product labels.

Note: Some of the buffered aspirin products listed above may be identified on the label as Aspirin (or ASA), Alumina, and Magnesia.

For Buffered Aspirin and Caffeine*

In Canada

C2 Buffered

Other commonly used names for aspirin are acetylsalicylic acid and ASA. Because Aspirin is a brand name in Canada, ASA is the term that commonly appears on Canadian product labels.

For Choline Salicylate

In the U.S.

Arthropan

For Choline and Magnesium Salicylates

In the U.S.

Tricosal
Trilisate

In Canada

Trilisate

Another commonly used name is choline magnesium trisalicylate.

For Magnesium Salicylate

In the U.S.

Doan's
Magan
Mobidin

In Canada

Back-Ese
Doan's

For Salsalate

In the U.S.

Amigesic
Diagen
Disalcid
Mono-Gesic
Salcylic Acid
Salflex
Salgesic
Salsitab

Generic name product may also be available.

Another commonly used name is salicylsalicylic acid.

For Sodium Salicylate

In the U.S.

Uracel

Generic name product may also be available.

In Canada

Dodd's Pills

*Not commercially available in the U.S.

Description

Salicylates are used to relieve pain and reduce fever. Most salicylates are also used to relieve some symptoms caused by arthritis (rheumatism), such as swelling, stiffness, and joint pain. However, they do not cure arthritis and will help you only as long as you continue to take them.

Aspirin may also be used to lessen the chance of heart attack, stroke, or other problems that may occur when a blood vessel is blocked by blood clots. Aspirin helps prevent dangerous blood clots from forming. However, this effect of aspirin may increase the chance of serious bleeding in some people. Therefore, aspirin should be used for this purpose only when your doctor decides, after studying your medical condition and history, that the danger of blood clots is greater than the risk of bleeding. *Do not take aspirin to prevent blood clots or a heart attack unless it has been ordered by your doctor.*

Salicylates may also be used for other conditions as determined by your doctor.

The caffeine present in some of these products may provide additional relief of headache pain or faster pain relief.

Some salicylates are available only with your medical doctor's or dentist's prescription. Others are available without a prescription; however, your medical doctor or dentist may have special instructions on the proper dose of these medicines for your medical condition.

These medicines are available in the following dosage forms:

Oral

Aspirin
- Capsules (U.S.)
- Delayed-release (enteric-coated) capsules (Canada)
- Tablets (U.S. and Canada)
- Chewable tablets (U.S. and Canada)
- Chewing gum tablets (U.S. and Canada)
- Delayed-release (enteric-coated) tablets (U.S. and Canada)
- Dispersible tablets (Canada)
- Extended-release tablets (U.S. and Canada)

Aspirin and Caffeine
- Capsules (Canada)
- Tablets (U.S. and Canada)

Buffered Aspirin
- Tablets (U.S. and Canada)

Buffered Aspirin and Caffeine
- Tablets (Canada)

Choline Salicylate
- Oral solution (U.S.)

Choline and Magnesium Salicylates
- Oral solution (U.S.)
- Tablets (U.S. and Canada)

Magnesium Salicylate
- Tablets (U.S. and Canada)

Salsalate
- Capsules (U.S.)
- Tablets (U.S.)

Sodium Salicylate
- Tablets (U.S. and Canada)
- Delayed-release (enteric-coated) tablets (U.S.)

Rectal

Aspirin
- Suppositories (U.S. and Canada)

It is very important that you read and understand the following information. If any of it causes you special concern, check with your doctor. Also, *if you have any questions* or if you want more information about this medicine or your medical problem, *ask your doctor, nurse, or pharmacist.*

Before Using This Medicine

If you are taking this medicine without a prescription, carefully read and follow any precautions on the label. For salicylates, the following should be considered:

Allergies—Tell your doctor if you have ever had any unusual or allergic reaction to aspirin or other salicylates, including methyl salicylate (oil of wintergreen), or to any of the following medicines:

Diclofenac (e.g., Voltaren)
Diflunisal (e.g., Dolobid)
Fenoprofen (e.g., Nalfon)
Floctafenine (e.g., Idarac)
Flurbiprofen, oral (e.g., Ansaid)
Ibuprofen (e.g., Motrin)
Indomethacin (e.g., Indocin)
Ketoprofen (e.g., Orudis)
Ketorolac (e.g., Toradol)
Meclofenamate (e.g., Meclomen)
Mefenamic acid (e.g., Ponstel)
Naproxen (e.g., Naprosyn)
Oxyphenbutazone (e.g., Tandearil)
Phenylbutazone (e.g., Butazolidin)
Piroxicam (e.g., Feldene)
Sulindac (e.g., Clinoril)
Suprofen (e.g., Suprol)
Tiaprofenic acid (e.g., Surgam)
Tolmetin (e.g., Tolectin)
Zomepirac (e.g., Zomax)

Also tell your doctor and pharmacist if you are allergic to any other substances, such as foods, preservatives, or dyes.

Diet—Make certain your doctor and pharmacist know if you are on a low-sodium diet. Regular use of large amounts of sodium salicylate (as for arthritis) can add a large amount of sodium to your diet. Sodium salicylate contains 46 mg of sodium in each 325-mg tablet and 92 mg of sodium in each 650-mg tablet.

Pregnancy—Salicylates have not been shown to cause birth defects in humans. Studies on birth defects in humans have been done with aspirin but not with other salicylates. However, salicylates caused birth defects in animal studies.

Some reports have suggested that too much use of aspirin late in pregnancy may cause a decrease in the newborn's weight and possible death of the fetus or newborn infant. However, the mothers in these reports had been taking much larger amounts of aspirin than are usually recommended. Studies of mothers taking aspirin in the doses that are usually recommended did not show these unwanted effects. However, there is a chance that regular use of salicylates late in pregnancy may cause unwanted effects on the heart or blood flow in the fetus or in the newborn infant.

S

Use of salicylates, especially aspirin, during the last 2 weeks of pregnancy may cause bleeding problems in the fetus before or during delivery or in the newborn infant. Also, too much use of salicylates during the last 3 months of pregnancy may increase the length of pregnancy, prolong labor, cause other problems during delivery, or cause severe bleeding in the mother before, during, or after delivery. *Do not take aspirin during the last 3 months of pregnancy unless it has been ordered by your doctor.*

Studies in humans have not shown that caffeine (present in some aspirin products) causes birth defects. However, studies in animals have shown that caffeine causes birth defects when given in very large doses (amounts equal to those present in 12 to 24 cups of coffee a day).

Breast-feeding—Salicylates pass into the breast milk. Although salicylates have not been reported to cause problems in nursing babies, it is possible that problems may occur if large amounts are taken regularly, as for arthritis (rheumatism).

Caffeine passes into the breast milk in small amounts.

Children—*Do not give aspirin or other salicylates to a child or a teenager with a fever or other symptoms of a virus infection, especially flu or chickenpox, without first discussing its use with your child's doctor.* This is very important because salicylates may cause a serious illness called Reye's syndrome in children and teenagers with fever caused by a virus infection, especially flu or chickenpox.

Some children may need to take aspirin or another salicylate regularly (as for arthritis). However, your child's doctor may want to stop the medicine for a while if a fever or other symptoms of a virus infection occur. Discuss this with your child's doctor, so that you will know ahead of time what to do if your child gets sick.

Children who do not have a virus infection may also be more sensitive to the effects of salicylates, especially if they have a fever or have lost large amounts of body fluid because of vomiting, diarrhea, or sweating. This may increase the chance of side effects during treatment.

Older adults—Elderly people are especially sensitive to the effects of salicylates. This may increase the chance of side effects during treatment.

Other medicines—Although certain medicines should not be used together at all, in other cases two different medicines may be used together even if an interaction might occur. In these cases, your doctor may want to change the dose, or other precautions may be necessary. When you are taking a salicylate, it is especially important that your doctor and pharmacist know if you are taking any of the following:

- Anticoagulants (blood thinners) or
- Carbenicillin by injection (e.g., Geopen) or
- Cefamandole (e.g., Mandol) or
- Cefoperazone (e.g., Cefobid) or
- Cefotetan (e.g., Cefotan) or
- Dipyridamole (e.g., Persantine) or
- Divalproex (e.g., Depakote) or
- Heparin or
- Medicine for inflammation or pain, except narcotics, or
- Moxalactam (e.g., Moxam) or
- Pentoxifylline (e.g., Trental) or
- Plicamycin (e.g., Mithracin) or
- Ticarcillin (e.g., Ticar) or
- Valproic acid (e.g., Depakene)—Taking these medicines together with a salicylate, especially aspirin, may increase the chance of bleeding
- Antidiabetics, oral (diabetes medicine you take by mouth)—Salicylates may increase the effects of the antidiabetic medicine; a change in dose may be needed if a salicylate is taken regularly
- Ketoconazole (e.g., Nizoral) or
- Tetracyclines (medicine for infection), taken by mouth—The antacids present in buffered aspirin products can keep the ketoconazole or tetracycline from working properly if taken too close to them. Also, the magnesium present in choline and magnesium salicylates (e.g., Trilisate) or magnesium salicylate (e.g., Doan's) can keep the tetracycline from working properly if taken too close to it
- Methotrexate (e.g., Mexate) or
- Vancomycin (e.g., Vancocin)—The chance of serious side effects may be increased
- Probenecid (e.g., Benemid)—Salicylates can keep probenecid from working properly for treating gout
- Sulfinpyrazone (e.g., Anturane)—Salicylates can keep sulfinpyrazone from working properly for treating gout; also, taking a salicylate, especially aspirin, with sulfinpyrazone may increase the chance of bleeding
- Urinary alkalizers (medicine that makes the urine less acid, such as acetazolamide [e.g., Diamox], calcium- and/or magnesium-containing antacids, dichlorphenamide [e.g., Daranide], methazolamide [e.g., Neptazane], potassium or sodium citrate and/or citric acid, sodium bicarbonate [baking soda])—These medicines may make the salicylate less effective by causing it to be removed from the body more quickly
- Zidovudine (e.g., AZT, Retrovir)—Aspirin may increase the blood levels of zidovudine, which increases the chance of serious side effects

Other medical problems—The presence of other medical problems may affect the use of salicylates. Make sure you tell your doctor if you have any other medical problems, especially:

- Anemia or
- Overactive thyroid or
- Stomach ulcer or other stomach problems—Salicylates may make your condition worse
- Asthma, allergies, and nasal polyps (history of) or
- Glucose-6-phosphate dehydrogenase (G6PD) deficiency or
- High blood pressure (hypertension) or
- Kidney disease or
- Liver disease—The chance of side effects may be increased.

- Gout—Salicylates can make this condition worse and can also lessen the effects of some medicines used to treat gout
- Heart disease—The chance of some side effects may be increased. Also, the caffeine present in some aspirin products can make some kinds of heart disease worse
- Hemophilia or other bleeding problems—The chance of bleeding may be increased, especially with aspirin

Before you begin using any new medicine (prescription or nonprescription) or if you develop any new medical problem while you are using this medicine, check with your doctor, nurse, or pharmacist.

Proper Use of This Medicine

Take this medicine after meals or with food (except for enteric-coated capsules or tablets and aspirin suppositories) to lessen stomach irritation.

Take tablet or capsule forms of this medicine with a full glass (8 ounces) of water. Also, do not lie down for about 15 to 30 minutes after swallowing the medicine. This helps to prevent irritation that may lead to trouble in swallowing.

For patients taking *aspirin (including buffered aspirin and/or products containing caffeine):*

- *Do not use any product that contains aspirin if it has a strong, vinegar-like odor.* This odor means the medicine is breaking down. If you have any questions about this, check with your doctor or pharmacist.
- If you are to take any medicine that contains aspirin within 7 days after having your tonsils removed, a tooth pulled, or other dental or mouth surgery, be sure to swallow the aspirin whole. Do not chew aspirin during this time.
- Do not place any medicine that contains aspirin directly on a tooth or gum surface. This may cause a burn.
- There are several different forms of aspirin or buffered aspirin tablets. If you are using:

  —*chewable aspirin tablets,* they may be chewed, dissolved in liquid, crushed, or swallowed whole.

  —*dispersible aspirin tablets,* they are to be dissolved in the mouth before swallowing. If your mouth is too dry, sip a little water to help dissolve the medicine.

  —*delayed-release (enteric-coated) aspirin tablets,* they must be swallowed whole. Do not crush them or break them up before taking.

  —*extended-release (long-acting) aspirin tablets,* check with your pharmacist as to how they should be taken. Some may be broken up (but must not be crushed) before swallowing if you cannot swallow them whole. Others should not be broken up and must be swallowed whole.

To use *aspirin suppositories:*

- If the suppository is too soft to insert, chill it in the refrigerator for 30 minutes or run cold water over it before removing the foil wrapper.
- To insert the suppository: First remove the foil wrapper and moisten the suppository with cold water. Lie down on your side and use your finger to push the suppository well up into the rectum.

To take *choline and magnesium salicylates (e.g., Trilisate) oral solution:*

- The liquid may be mixed with fruit juice just before taking.
- Drink a full glass (8 ounces) of water after taking the medicine.

To take *enteric-coated sodium salicylate tablets:*

- The tablets must be swallowed whole. Do not crush them or break them up before taking.

Unless otherwise directed by your medical doctor or dentist:

- Do not take more of this medicine than recommended on the label, to lessen the chance of side effects.
- Children up to 12 years of age should not take this medicine more than 5 times a day.

When used for arthritis (rheumatism), this medicine must be taken regularly as ordered by your doctor in order for it to help you. Up to 2 to 3 weeks or longer may pass before you feel the full effects of this medicine.

Missed dose—If your medical doctor or dentist has ordered you to take this medicine according to a regular schedule and you miss a dose, take it as soon as you remember. However, if it is almost time for your next dose, skip the missed dose and go back to your regular dosing schedule. Do not double doses.

Storage—To store this medicine:

- Keep out of the reach of children. Overdose is very dangerous in young children.
- Store away from heat and direct light.
- Do not store tablets or capsules in the bathroom, near the kitchen sink, or in other damp places. Heat or moisture may cause the medicine to break down.
- Keep liquid forms of this medicine from freezing.
- Store aspirin suppositories in a cool place. It is usually best to keep them in the refrigerator, but keep them from freezing.
- Do not keep outdated medicine or medicine no longer needed. Be sure that any discarded medicine is out of the reach of children.

Precautions While Using This Medicine

Check the labels of all nonprescription (over-the-counter [OTC]) and prescription medicines you now take. If any contain aspirin or other salicylates, including bismuth subsalicylate (e.g., Pepto-Bismol), be especially careful. Also, be especially careful if you regularly use a shampoo or other medicine for your skin that contains salicylic acid or any other salicylate. Using other salicylate-containing products while taking this medicine may lead to overdose. If you have any questions about this, check with your doctor or pharmacist.

If you will be taking salicylates for a long time (more than 5 days in a row for children or 10 days in a row for adults) or in large amounts, *your doctor should check your progress at regular visits.*

Check with your medical doctor or dentist:

- If you are taking this medicine to relieve pain and the pain lasts for more than 10 days (5 days for children) or if the pain gets worse, if new symptoms occur, or if redness or swelling is present. These could be signs of a serious condition that needs medical or dental treatment.
- If you are taking this medicine to bring down a fever, and the fever lasts for more than 3 days or returns, if the fever gets worse, if new symptoms occur, or if redness or swelling is present. These could be signs of a serious condition that needs treatment.
- If you are taking this medicine for a sore throat, and the sore throat is very painful, lasts for more than 2 days, or occurs together with or is followed by fever, headache, skin rash, nausea, or vomiting.
- If you are taking this medicine regularly, as for arthritis (rheumatism), and you notice a ringing or buzzing in your ears or severe or continuing headaches. These are often the first signs that too much salicylate is being taken. Your doctor may want to change the amount of medicine you are taking every day.

For patients taking *aspirin to lessen the chance of heart attack, stroke, or other problems caused by blood clots:*

- *Take only the amount of aspirin ordered by your doctor.* If you need a medicine to relieve pain, a fever, or arthritis, your doctor may not want you to take extra aspirin. It is a good idea to discuss this with your doctor, so that you will know ahead of time what medicine to take.
- *Do not stop taking this medicine for any reason without first checking with the doctor who directed you to take it.*

Taking certain other medicines together with a salicylate may increase the chance of unwanted effects. The risk will depend on how much of each medicine you take every day, and on how long you take the medicines together. If your doctor directs you to take these medicines together on a regular basis, follow his or her directions carefully. However, *do not take any of the following medicines together with a salicylate for more than a few days, unless your doctor has directed you to do so and is following your progress*:

Acetaminophen (e.g., Tylenol)
Diclofenac (e.g., Voltaren)
Diflunisal (e.g., Dolobid)
Fenoprofen (e.g., Nalfon)
Floctafenine (e.g., Idarac)
Flurbiprofen, oral (e.g., Ansaid)
Ibuprofen (e.g., Motrin)
Indomethacin (e.g., Indocin)
Ketoprofen (e.g., Orudis)
Ketorolac (e.g., Toradol)
Meclofenamate (e.g., Meclomen)
Mefenamic acid (e.g., Ponstel)
Naproxen (e.g., Naprosyn)
Phenylbutazone (e.g., Butazolidin)
Piroxicam (e.g., Feldene)
Sulindac (e.g., Clinoril)
Tiaprofenic acid (e.g., Surgam)
Tolmetin (e.g., Tolectin)

For *diabetic patients:*

- False urine sugar test results may occur if you are regularly taking large amounts of salicylates, such as:

  —*Aspirin:* 8 or more 325-mg (5-grain), or 4 or more 500-mg or 650-mg (10-grain), or 3 or more 800-mg (or higher strength), doses a day.

  —*Buffered aspirin or*
  —*Sodium salicylate:* 8 or more 325-mg (5-grain), or 4 or more 500-mg or 650-mg (10-grain), doses a day.

  —*Choline salicylate:* 4 or more teaspoonfuls (each teaspoonful containing 870 mg) a day.

  —*Choline and magnesium salicylates:* 5 or more 500-mg tablets or teaspoonfuls, 4 or more 750-mg tablets, or 2 or more 1000-mg tablets, a day.

  —*Magnesium salicylate:* 7 or more 325-mg, or 4 or more 500-mg (or higher strength), tablets a day.

  —*Salsalate:* 4 or more 500-mg doses, or 3 or more 750-mg doses, a day.
- Smaller doses or occasional use of salicylates usually will not affect urine sugar tests. However, check with your doctor, nurse, or pharmacist (especially if your diabetes is not well-controlled) if:

  —you are not sure how much salicylate you are taking every day.

  —you notice any change in your urine sugar test results.

  —you have any other questions about this possible problem.

Do not take aspirin for 5 days before any surgery, including dental surgery, unless otherwise directed by your medical doctor or dentist. Taking aspirin during this time may cause bleeding problems.

For patients taking *buffered aspirin, choline and magnesium salicylates (e.g., Trilisate), or magnesium salicylate (e.g., Doan's):*

- If you are also taking a tetracycline antibiotic, do not take the 2 medicines within 3 to 4 hours of each other. Taking them too close together may prevent the tetracycline from being absorbed by your body.
- If you are also taking ketoconazole, do not take buffered aspirin within 3 hours of the ketoconazole. Taking them too close together may prevent the ketoconazole from being absorbed by your body.
- If you have any questions about this, check with your doctor or pharmacist.

If you are taking a laxative containing cellulose, take the salicylate at least 2 hours before or after you take the laxative. Taking these medicines too close together may lessen the effects of the salicylate.

For patients taking this medicine by mouth:

- Stomach problems may be more likely to occur if you drink alcoholic beverages while being treated with this medicine, especially if you are taking it in high doses or for a long time. Check with your doctor if you have any questions about this.

For patients using *aspirin suppositories:*

- Aspirin suppositories may cause irritation of the rectum. Check with your doctor if this occurs.

Salicylates may interfere with the results of some medical tests. Before you have any medical tests, tell the doctor in charge if you have taken any of these medicines within the past week. If possible, it is best to check with the doctor first, to find out whether the medicine may be taken during the week before the test.

For patients taking one of the products that contains *caffeine:*

- Caffeine may interfere with the result of a test that uses dipyridamole (e.g., Persantine) to help find out how well your blood is flowing through certain blood vessels. Therefore, you should not have any caffeine for at least 4 hours before the test.

If you think that you or anyone else may have taken an overdose, get emergency help at once. Taking an overdose of these medicines may cause unconsciousness or death. Signs of overdose include convulsions (seizures), hearing loss, confusion, ringing or buzzing in the ears, severe drowsiness or tiredness, severe excitement or nervousness, and fast or deep breathing.

Side Effects of This Medicine

Along with its needed effects, a medicine may cause some unwanted effects. When this medicine is used for short periods of time at low doses, side effects usually are rare. Although not all of the following side effects may occur, if they do occur they may need medical attention.

Get emergency help immediately if any of the following side effects occur:

Any loss of hearing; bloody urine; confusion; convulsions (seizures); diarrhea (severe or continuing); difficulty in swallowing; dizziness, lightheadedness, or feeling faint (severe); drowsiness (severe); excitement or nervousness (severe); fast or deep breathing; flushing, redness, or other change in skin color; hallucinations (seeing, hearing, or feeling things that are not there); increased sweating; increased thirst; nausea or vomiting (severe or continuing); shortness of breath, troubled breathing, tightness in chest, or wheezing; stomach pain (severe or continuing); swelling of eyelids, face, or lips; unexplained fever; uncontrollable flapping movements of the hands (especially in elderly patients); vision problems

Symptoms of overdose in children

Changes in behavior; drowsiness or tiredness (severe); fast or deep breathing

Also, check with your doctor as soon as possible if any of the following side effects occur:

Less common or rare

Abdominal or stomach pain, cramping, or burning (severe); bloody or black, tarry stools; headache (severe or continuing); ringing or buzzing in ears (continuing); skin rash, hives, or itching; unusual tiredness or weakness; vomiting of blood or material that looks like coffee grounds

Other side effects may occur that usually do not need medical attention. These side effects may go away during treatment as your body adjusts to the medicine. However, check with your doctor or pharmacist if any of the following side effects continue or are bothersome:

More common

Abdominal or stomach cramps, pain, or discomfort (mild to moderate); heartburn or indigestion; nausea or vomiting

Less common

Trouble in sleeping, nervousness, or jitters (only for products containing caffeine)

Other side effects not listed above may also occur in some patients. If you notice any other effects, check with your doctor.

Annual revision: August 1990

SALICYLIC ACID Topical

Some commonly used brand names are:

In the U.S.

Antinea
Buf-Puf Acne Cleansing Bar with Vitamin E
Calicylic Creme
Clearasil Clearstick Maximum Strength Topical Solution
Clearasil Clearstick Regular Strength Topical Solution
Clearasil Double Textured Pads Maximum Strength
Clearasil Double Textured Pads Regular Strength
Clearasil Medicated Deep Cleanser Topical Solution
Clear Away
Clear by Design Medicated Cleansing Pads
Compound W Gel
Compound W Liquid
Duofilm
Duoplant Topical Solution
Freezone
Gordofilm
Hydrisalic
Ionax Astringent Skin Cleanser Topical Solution
Ionil Plus Shampoo
Ionil Shampoo
Keralyt
Keratex Gel
Lactisol
Listerex Golden Scrub Lotion
Listerex Herbal Scrub Lotion
Mediplast
Noxzema Anti-Acne Gel
Noxzema Anti-Acne Pads Maximum Strength
Noxzema Anti-Acne Pads Regular Strength
Occlusal-HP Topical Solution
Occlusal Topical Solution
Off-Ezy Topical Solution Corn & Callus Remover Kit
Off-Ezy Topical Solution Wart Removal Kit
Oxy Clean Medicated Cleanser
Oxy Clean Medicated Pads Maximum Strength
Oxy Clean Medicated Pads Regular Strength
Oxy Clean Medicated Pads Sensitive Skin
Oxy Night Watch Maximum Strength Lotion
Oxy Night Watch Sensitive Skin Lotion
Paplex
Paplex Ultra
Propa pH Medicated Acne Cream Maximum Strength
Propa pH Medicated Cleansing Pads Maximum Strength
Propa pH Medicated Cleansing Pads Sensitive Skin
Propa pH Perfectly Clear Skin Cleanser Topical Solution Normal/Combination Skin
Propa pH Perfectly Clear Skin Cleanser Topical Solution Oily Skin
Propa pH Perfectly Clear Skin Cleanser Topical Solution Sensitive Skin Formula
P&S
Salac
Salacid
Sal-Acid Plaster
Salactic Film Topical Solution
Sal-Clens Plus Shampoo
Sal-Clens Shampoo
Saligel
Salonil
Sal-Plant Gel Topical Solution
Sebucare
Stri-Dex Dual Textured Pads Maximum Strength
Stri-Dex Dual Textured Pads Regular Strength
Stri-Dex Dual Textured Pads Sensitive Skin
Stri-Dex Maximum Strength Pads
Stri-Dex Regular Strength Pads
Stri-Dex Super Scrub Pads
Trans-Plantar
Trans-Ver-Sal
Verukan-HP Topical Solution
Verukan Topical Solution
Viranol
Viranol Ultra
Wart-Off Topical Solution
X-Seb

Generic name product may also be available.

In Canada

Compound W Gel
Compound W Liquid
Cuplex Gel
Occlusal-HP Topical Solution
Occlusal Topical Solution
Oxy Clean Extra Strength Medicated Pads
Oxy Clean Extra Strength Cleanser Topical Solution
Oxy Clean Medicated Soap
Oxy Clean Regular Strength Medicated Cleanser Topical Solution
Oxy Clean Regular Strength Medicated Pads
Oxy Clean Sensitive Skin Cleanser Topical Solution
Oxy Clean Sensitive Skin Pads
Oxy Night Watch Night Time Acne Medication Extra Strength Lotion
Oxy Night Watch Night Time Acne Medication Regular Strength Lotion
Oxy Sensitive Skin Vanishing Formula Lotion
Salac
Tersac Cleansing Gel
Trans-Ver-Sal

Description

Salicylic acid (sal-i-SILL-ik AS-id) is used to treat many skin disorders, such as acne, dandruff, psoriasis, seborrheic dermatitis of the skin and scalp, calluses, corns, common warts, and plantar warts, depending on the dosage form and strength of the preparation.

Some of these preparations are available only with your doctor's prescription. Others are available without a prescription; however, your doctor may have special instructions on the proper use of salicylic acid for your medical condition.

Salicylic acid is available in the following dosage forms:

Topical

- Cream (U.S.)
- Gel (U.S. and Canada)
- Lotion (U.S. and Canada)
- Ointment (U.S.)
- Pads (U.S. and Canada)
- Plaster (U.S. and Canada)
- Shampoo (U.S.)
- Soap (U.S. and Canada)
- Topical solution (U.S. and Canada)

It is very important that you read and understand the following information. If any of it causes you special concern, check with your doctor or pharmacist. Also, *if you have any questions* or if you want more information about this medicine or your medical problem, *ask your doctor, nurse, or pharmacist.*

Before Using This Medicine

If you are using this medicine without a prescription, carefully read and follow any precautions on the label. For salicylic acid, the following should be considered:

Allergies—Tell your doctor if you have ever had any unusual or allergic reaction to salicylic acid. Also tell your doctor and pharmacist if you are allergic to any other substances, such as preservatives or dyes.

Pregnancy—This medicine may be absorbed through the mother's skin. Salicylic acid has not been studied in pregnant women. However, studies in animals have shown that salicylic acid causes birth defects when given orally in doses about 6 times the highest dose recommended for topical use in humans. Before using this medicine, make sure your doctor knows if you are pregnant or if you may become pregnant, especially if you will be using salicylic acid on large areas of your body.

Breast-feeding—Salicylic acid may be absorbed through the mother's skin. However, topical salicylic acid has not been reported to cause problems in nursing babies.

Children—Young children may be at increased risk of unwanted effects because of increased absorption of salicylic acid through the skin. Also, young children may be more likely to get skin irritation from salicylic acid. Salicylic acid should not be applied to large areas of the body, used for long periods of time, or used under occlusive dressing (air-tight covering, such as kitchen plastic wrap) in infants and children.

Older adults—Elderly people are more likely to have age-related blood vessel disease. This may increase the chance of problems during treatment with this medicine.

Other medicines—Although certain medicines should not be used together at all, in other cases two different medicines may be used together even if an interaction might occur. In these cases, your doctor may want to change the dose, or other precautions may be necessary. Tell your doctor and pharmacist if you are using any other prescription or nonprescription (over-the-counter [OTC]) medicine.

Other medical problems—The presence of other medical problems may affect the use of salicylic acid, especially if you are using a 5% or stronger salicylic acid preparation. Make sure you tell your doctor if you have any other medical problems, especially:

- Blood vessel disease
- Diabetes mellitus (sugar diabetes)—Use of this medicine may cause severe redness or ulceration, especially on the hands or feet
- Inflammation, irritation, or infection of the skin—Use of this medicine may cause severe irritation if applied to inflamed, irritated, or infected area of the skin

Before you begin using any new medicine (prescription or nonprescription) or if you develop any new medical problem while you are using this medicine, check with your doctor, nurse, or pharmacist.

Proper Use of This Medicine

It is very important that you use this medicine only as directed. Do not use more of it, do not use it more often, and do not use it for a longer time than recommended on the label, unless otherwise directed by your doctor. To do so may increase the chance of absorption through the skin and the chance of salicylic acid poisoning.

If your doctor has ordered an occlusive dressing (airtight covering, such as kitchen plastic wrap) to be applied over this medicine, make sure you know how to apply it. Since an occlusive dressing will increase the amount of medicine absorbed through your skin and the possibility of salicylic acid poisoning, use it only as directed. If you have any questions about this, check with your doctor.

Keep this medicine away from the eyes and other mucous membranes, such as the mouth and inside of the nose. If you should accidentally get some in your eyes or on other mucous membranes, immediately flush them with water for 15 minutes.

To use the *cream, lotion, or ointment form* of salicylic acid:

- Apply enough medicine to cover the affected area, and rub in gently.

To use the *gel form* of salicylic acid:

- Before using salicylic acid gel, apply wet packs to the affected areas for at least 5 minutes. If you have any questions about this, check with your doctor or pharmacist.
- Apply enough gel to cover the affected areas, and rub in gently.

To use the *pad form* of salicylic acid:

- Wipe the pad over the affected areas.
- Do not rinse off medicine after treatment.

To use the *plaster form* of salicylic acid for warts, corns, or calluses:

- This medicine comes with patient instructions. Read them carefully before using.
- *Do not use this medicine on irritated skin or on any area that is infected or reddened. Also, do not use this medicine if you are a diabetic or if you have poor blood circulation.*
- *Do not use this medicine on warts with hair growing from them or on warts on the face, in or on the genital (sex) organs, or inside the nose or mouth. Also do not use on moles or birthmarks.* To do so may cause severe irritation.
- Wash the area to be treated and dry thoroughly. Warts may be soaked in warm water for 5 minutes before drying.
- Cut the plaster to fit the wart, corn, or callus and apply.
- For corns and calluses:
  —Repeat every 48 hours as needed for up to 14 days, or as directed by your doctor, until the corn or callus is removed.
  —Corns or calluses may be soaked in warm water for 5 minutes to help in their removal.
- For warts:
  —Depending on the product, either:
  - Apply plaster and repeat every 48 hours as needed, or

• Apply plaster at bedtime, leave in place for at least 8 hours, remove plaster in the morning, and repeat every 24 hours as needed.
  —Repeat for up to 12 weeks as needed, or as directed by your doctor, until wart is removed.
• If discomfort gets worse during treatment or continues after treatment, or if the wart spreads, check with your doctor.

To use the *shampoo form* of salicylic acid:
• Before applying this medicine, wet the hair and scalp with lukewarm water. Apply enough medicine to work up a lather and rub well into the scalp for 2 or 3 minutes, then rinse. Apply the medicine again and rinse thoroughly.

To use the *soap form* of salicylic acid:
• Work up a lather with the soap, using hot water, and scrub the entire affected area with a washcloth or facial sponge or mitt.
• If you are to use this soap in a foot bath, work up rich suds in hot water and soak the feet for 10 to 15 minutes. Then pat dry without rinsing.

To use the *topical solution form* of salicylic acid for acne:
• Wet a cotton ball or pad with the topical solution and wipe the affected areas.
• Do not rinse off medicine after treatment.

To use the *topical solution form* of salicylic acid for warts, corns, or calluses:
• This medicine comes with patient instructions. Read them carefully before using.
• *This medicine is flammable. Do not use it near heat or open flame or while smoking.*
• *Do not use this medicine on irritated skin or on any area that is infected or reddened. Also, do not use this medicine if you are a diabetic or if you have poor blood circulation.*
• *Do not use this medicine on warts with hair growing from them or on warts on the face, in or on the genital (sex) organs, or inside the nose or mouth. Also do not use on moles or birthmarks.* To do so may cause severe irritation.
• Avoid breathing in the vapors from the medicine.
• Wash the area to be treated and dry thoroughly. Warts may be soaked in warm water for 5 minutes before drying.
• Apply the medicine one drop at a time to completely cover each wart, corn, or callus. Let dry.
• For warts—Repeat one or two times a day as needed for up to 12 weeks, or as directed by your doctor, until wart is removed.
• For corns and calluses—Repeat one or two times a day as needed for up to 14 days, or as directed by your doctor, until the corn or callus is removed.
• Corns and calluses may be soaked in warm water for 5 minutes to help in their removal.
• If discomfort gets worse during treatment or continues after treatment, or if the wart spreads, check with your doctor.

Unless your hands are being treated, wash them immediately after applying this medicine to remove any medicine that may be on them.

Dosing—The dose of salicylic acid will be different for different patients. *Follow your doctor's orders or the directions on the label.* The following information includes only the average doses of salicylic acid. *If your dose is different, do not change it* unless your doctor tells you to do so.

• For *cream* dosage form:
  —For corns and calluses:
    • Adults and children—Use the 2 to 10% cream as needed. Use the 25 to 60% cream one time every three to five days.
• For *gel* dosage form:
  —For acne:
    • Adults and children—Use the 0.5 to 5% gel one time a day.
  —For psoriasis:
    • Adults and children—Use the 5% gel one time a day.
  —For common warts:
    • Adults and children—Use the 5 to 26% gel one time a day.
• For *lotion* dosage form:
  —For acne:
    • Adults and children—Use the 1 to 2% lotion one to three times a day.
  —For dandruff and antiseborrhic dermatitis of the scalp:
    • Adults and children—Use the 1.8 to 2% lotion on the scalp one or two times a day.
• For *ointment* dosage form:
  —For acne:
    • Adults and children—Use the 3 to 6% ointment as needed.
  —For psoriasis and seborrheic dermatitis:
    • Adults and children—Use the 3 to 10% ointment as needed.
  —For common warts:
    • Adults and children—Use the 3 to 10% ointment as needed. Use the 25 to 60% ointment one time every three to five days.
• For *pads* dosage form:
  —For acne:
    • Adults and children—Use one to three times a day.

- For *plaster* dosage form:
  - —For corns, calluses, common warts, or plantar warts:
    - Adults and children—Use one time a day or one time every other day.
- For *shampoo* dosage form:
  - —For dandruff or seborrheic dermatitis of the scalp:
    - Adults and children—Use on the scalp one or two times a week.
- For *soap* dosage form:
  - —For acne:
    - Adults and children—Use as needed.
- For *topical solution* dosage form:
  - —For acne:
    - Adults and children—Use the 0.5 to 2% topical solution one to three times a day.
  - —For common warts and plantar warts:
    - Adults and children—Use the 5 to 27% topical solution one or two times a day.
  - —For corns and calluses:
    - Adults and children—Use the 12 to 27% topical solution one or two times a day.

Missed dose—If you miss a dose of this medicine, apply it as soon as possible. However, if it is almost time for your next dose, skip the missed dose and go back to your regular dosing schedule.

Storage—To store this medicine:
- Keep out of the reach of children.
- Store away from heat and direct light.
- Keep the medicine from freezing.
- Do not keep outdated medicine or medicine no longer needed. Be sure that any discarded medicine is out of the reach of children.

Precautions While Using This Medicine

When using salicylic acid, do not use any of the following preparations on the same affected area as this medicine, unless otherwise directed by your doctor:

Abrasive soaps or cleansers
Alcohol-containing preparations
Any other topical acne preparation or preparation containing a peeling agent (for example, benzoyl peroxide, resorcinol, sulfur, or tretinoin [vitamin A acid])
Cosmetics or soaps that dry the skin
Medicated cosmetics
Other topical medicine for the skin

To use any of the above preparations on the same affected area as salicylic acid may cause severe irritation of the skin.

Side Effects of This Medicine

Along with its needed effects, a medicine may cause some unwanted effects. Although not all of these side effects may occur, if they do occur they may need medical attention.

Check with your doctor as soon as possible if any of the following side effects occur:

Less common or rare

Skin irritation not present before use of this medicine (moderate or severe)

Symptoms of salicylic acid poisoning

Confusion; dizziness; headache (severe or continuing); rapid breathing; ringing or buzzing in ears (continuing)

Other side effects may occur that usually do not need medical attention. However, check with your doctor if any of the following side effects continue or are bothersome:

More common

Skin irritation not present before use of this medicine (mild); stinging

Other side effects not listed above may also occur in some patients. If you notice any other effects, check with your doctor or pharmacist.

Annual revision: 07/26/93

SALICYLIC ACID AND SULFUR Topical

Some commonly used brand names are:

In the U.S.

Acno	Sastid (AL) Scrub
Acnotex	Sastid Plain Shampoo and Acne Wash
Aveeno Cleansing Bar	Sastid Soap
Creamy SS Shampoo	Sebasorb Liquid
Fostex Regular Strength Medicated Cleansing Bar	Sebex
Fostex Regular Strength Medicated Cleansing Cream (for face and scalp)	Sebulex Antiseborrheic Treatment and Conditioning Shampoo
Meted Maximum Strength Anti-Dandruff Shampoo with Conditioners	Sebulex Antiseborrheic Treatment Shampoo
Night Cast Regular Formula Mask-lotion	Sebulex Cream Medicated Shampoo
Pernox Lemon Medicated Scrub Cleanser	Sebulex Medicated Dandruff Shampoo with Conditioners
Pernox Lotion Lathering Abradant Scrub Cleanser	Sebulex Regular Medicated Dandruff Shampoo
Pernox Lotion Lathering Scrub Cleanser	Therac Lotion
Pernox Regular Medicated Scrub Cleanser	Vanseb Cream Dandruff Shampoo
	Vanseb Lotion Dandruff Shampoo

Generic name product may also be available.

In Canada

Aveeno Acne Bar	Pernox Lemon Medicated Scrub Cleanser
Fostex Medicated Cleansing Bar	Pernox Regular Medicated Scrub Cleanser
Fostex Medicated Cleansing Cream (for face and scalp)	Sastid Soap
Fostex Medicated Cleansing Liquid	Sebulex Conditioning Suspension Shampoo
Meted Maximum Strength Anti-Dandruff Shampoo with Conditioners	Sebulex Lotion Shampoo
Night Cast R	Sebulex Medicated Shampoo
	Sulsal Soap

Description

Salicylic acid (sal-i-SILL-ik AS-id) and sulfur (SUL-fur) combination is used to treat acne and other skin disorders and dandruff and other scalp disorders, such as seborrheic dermatitis.

This medicine is available without a prescription; however, your doctor may have special instructions on the proper use of this medicine for your medical condition.

Salicylic acid and sulfur combination is available in the following dosage forms:

Topical

- Cleansing cream (U.S. and Canada)
- Lotion (U.S. and Canada)
- Cleansing lotion (U.S. and Canada)
- Cream shampoo (U.S. and Canada)
- Lotion shampoo (U.S. and Canada)
- Suspension shampoo (U.S. and Canada)
- Bar soap (U.S. and Canada)
- Cleansing suspension (U.S. and Canada)
- Topical suspension (U.S.)

It is very important that you read and understand the following information. If any of it causes you special concern, check with your doctor or pharmacist. Also, *if you have any questions* or if you want more information about this medicine or your medical problem, *ask your doctor, nurse, or pharmacist.*

Before Using This Medicine

If you are using this medicine without a prescription, carefully read and follow any precautions on the label. For salicylic acid and sulfur combination, the following should be considered:

Allergies—Tell your doctor if you have ever had any unusual or allergic reaction to salicylic acid or sulfur. Also tell your doctor and pharmacist if you are allergic to any other substances, such as preservatives or dyes.

Pregnancy—Salicylic acid and sulfur combination has not been studied in pregnant women. However, for the individual medicines:

- *Salicylic acid*—Salicylic acid may be absorbed through the mother's skin. Studies with topical salicylic acid have not been done in humans. However, studies in animals have shown that salicylic acid causes birth defects when given orally in doses about 6 times the highest dose recommended for topical use in humans.
- *Sulfur*—Topical sulfur has not been shown to cause birth defects or other problems in humans.

Before using this medicine, make sure your doctor knows if you are pregnant or if you may become pregnant.

Breast-feeding—Salicylic acid may be absorbed through the mother's skin. However, topical salicylic acid and sulfur combination has not been reported to cause problems in nursing babies.

Children—Young children may be at increased risk of unwanted effects because of increased absorption of salicylic acid through the skin. Products containing salicylic acid should not be applied to large areas of the body or used for long periods of time in infants and children.

Older adults—Many medicines have not been studied specifically in older people. Therefore, it may not be known whether they work exactly the same way they do in younger adults or if they cause different side effects or problems in older people. There is no specific information comparing use of salicylic acid and sulfur combination in the elderly with use in other age groups.

Other medicines—Although certain medicines should not be used together at all, in other cases two different medicines may be used together even if an interaction might

occur. In these cases, your doctor may want to change the dose, or other precautions may be necessary. Tell your doctor and pharmacist if you are using any other topical prescription or nonprescription (over-the-counter [OTC]) medicine that is to be applied to the same area of the skin.

Before you begin using any new medicine (prescription or nonprescription) or if you develop any new medical problem while you are using this medicine, check with your doctor, nurse, or pharmacist.

Proper Use of This Medicine

Use this medicine only as directed. Do not use more of it and do not use it more often than recommended on the label, unless otherwise directed by your doctor.

Immediately after using this medicine, wash your hands to remove any medicine that may be on them.

Keep this medicine away from the eyes. If you should accidentally get some in your eyes, flush them thoroughly with water.

To use the *skin cleanser form* of this medicine:

- After wetting the skin, apply this medicine with your fingertips or a wet sponge and rub in gently to work up a lather. Then rinse thoroughly and pat dry.

To use the *lotion or topical suspension form* of this medicine:

- Apply a small amount of this medicine to the affected areas, and rub in gently.

To use the *shampoo form* of this medicine:

- Wet the hair and scalp with lukewarm water. Then apply enough medicine to work up a lather and rub into the scalp. Continue rubbing the lather into the scalp for several minutes or allow it to remain on the scalp for about 5 minutes, depending on the product being used, then rinse. Apply the medicine again and rinse thoroughly.

To use the *bar soap form* of this medicine:

- After wetting the skin, use this medicine to wash the face and other affected areas. Then rinse thoroughly and pat dry.

Dosing—The dose of salicylic acid and sulfur combination will be different for different patients. *Follow your doctor's orders or the directions on the label.* The following information includes only the average doses of salicylic acid and sulfur combination. *If your dose is different, do not change it* unless your doctor tells you to do so.

- For acne or oily skin:
  - —For *bar soap and cleansing cream* dosage forms:
    - Adults and children—Use on the skin two or three times a day.
  - —For *cleansing suspension, lotion, and topical suspension* dosage forms:
    - Adults and children—Use on the skin one or two times a day.
  - —For *cleansing lotion* dosage form:
    - Adults and children—Use on the skin one to three times a day.
- For dandruff and seborrheic dermatitis of the scalp:
  - —For *cream shampoo, lotion shampoo, and suspension shampoo* dosage forms:
    - Adults and children—Use on the scalp one or two times a week.

Missed dose—If you miss a dose of this medicine, apply or use it as soon as possible. However, if it is almost time for your next dose, skip the missed dose and go back to your regular dosing schedule.

Storage—To store this medicine:

- Keep out of the reach of children.
- Store away from heat and direct light.
- Keep the medicine from freezing.
- Do not keep outdated medicine or medicine no longer needed. Be sure that any discarded medicine is out of the reach of children.

Precautions While Using This Medicine

When using salicylic acid and sulfur combination medicine, do not use any of the following preparations on the same affected area as this medicine, unless otherwise directed by your doctor:

Abrasive soaps or cleansers
Alcohol-containing preparations
Any other topical acne preparation or preparation containing a peeling agent (for example, benzoyl peroxide, resorcinol, or tretinoin [vitamin A acid])
Cosmetics or soaps that dry the skin
Medicated cosmetics
Other topical medicine for the skin

To use any of the above preparations on the same affected area as salicylic acid and sulfur combination medicine may cause severe irritation of the skin.

Do not use any topical mercury-containing preparation, such as ammoniated mercury ointment, on the same affected area as this medicine. To do so may cause a foul odor, may be irritating to the skin, and may stain the skin black. If you have any questions about this, check with your doctor or pharmacist.

Taking large doses of aspirin or other salicylates (including diflunisal) while using topical salicylic acid (contained in this medicine) may lead to overdose. If you have any questions about this, check with your doctor or pharmacist.

Side Effects of This Medicine

Along with its needed effects, a medicine may cause some unwanted effects. Although not all of these side effects may occur, if they do occur they may need medical attention.

Check with your doctor as soon as possible if the following side effect occurs:

Skin irritation not present before use of this medicine

Other side effects may occur that usually do not need medical attention. However, check with your doctor or pharmacist if the following side effects continue or are bothersome:

Redness and peeling of skin (may occur after a few days); unusual dryness of skin

Other side effects not listed above may also occur in some patients. If you notice any other effects, check with your doctor or pharmacist.

Annual revision: 07/26/93

SALICYLIC ACID, SULFUR, AND COAL TAR Topical

Some commonly used brand names are:

In the U.S.

Sebex-T Tar Shampoo
Vanseb-T
Sebutone

In Canada

Sebutone

Description

Salicylic acid (sal-i-SILL-ik AS-id), sulfur (SUL-fur), and coal tar combination is used to treat dandruff, seborrheic dermatitis, and psoriasis of the scalp.

This medicine is available without a prescription; however, your doctor may have special instructions on the proper use of this medicine for your medical condition.

Salicylic acid, sulfur, and coal tar combination is available in the following dosage forms:

Topical

- Cream shampoo (U.S.)
- Lotion shampoo (U.S. and Canada)

It is very important that you read and understand the following information. If any of it causes you special concern, check with your doctor or pharmacist. Also, *if you have any questions* or if you want more information about this medicine or your medical problem, *ask your doctor, nurse, or pharmacist.*

Before Using This Medicine

If you are using this medicine without a prescription, carefully read and follow any precautions on the label. For salicylic acid, sulfur, and coal tar combination, the following should be considered:

Allergies—Tell your doctor if you have ever had any unusual or allergic reaction to salicylic acid, sulfur, or coal tar. Also tell your doctor and pharmacist if you are allergic to any other substances, such as preservatives or dyes.

Pregnancy—Salicylic acid, sulfur, and coal tar combination has not been studied in pregnant women. However, for the individual medicines:

- *Salicylic acid*—Salicylic acid may be absorbed through the mother's skin. Studies with topical salicylic acid have not been done in humans. However, studies in animals have shown that salicylic acid causes birth defects when given orally in doses about 6 times the highest dose recommended for topical use in humans.
- *Sulfur*—Sulfur has not been shown to cause birth defects or other problems in humans.
- *Coal tar*—Studies with coal tar on effects in pregnancy have not been done in either humans or animals.

Breast-feeding—Salicylic acid may be absorbed through the mother's skin. However, topical salicylic acid, sulfur, and coal tar combination has not been reported to cause problems in nursing babies.

Children—Young children may be at increased risk of unwanted effects because of increased absorption of salicylic acid through the skin. Medicines containing salicylic acid should not be applied to large areas of the body or used for long periods of time in infants and children.

Older adults—Many medicines have not been studied specifically in older people. Therefore, it may not be known whether they work exactly the same way they do in younger adults or if they cause different side effects or problems in older people. There is no specific information comparing use of salicylic acid, sulfur, and coal tar combination medicine in the elderly with use in other age groups.

Other medicines—Although certain medicines should not be used together at all, in other cases two different medicines may be used together even if an interaction might occur. In these cases, your doctor may want to change the dose, or other precautions may be necessary. Tell your doctor and pharmacist if you are using any other topical prescription or nonprescription (over-the-counter [OTC]) medicine that is to be applied to the same area of the skin.

Before you begin using any new medicine (prescription or nonprescription) or if you develop any new medical problem while you are using this medicine, check with your doctor, nurse, or pharmacist.

Proper Use of This Medicine

Use this medicine only as directed. Do not use it more often than recommended on the label, unless otherwise directed by your doctor.

Keep this medicine away from the eyes. If you should accidentally get some in your eyes, flush them thoroughly with water.

Before using this medicine, wet the hair and scalp with lukewarm water. Then apply a generous amount to the scalp and work up a rich lather. Rub the lather into the scalp for 5 minutes, then rinse. Apply the medicine again and rinse thoroughly.

Immediately after using this medicine, wash your hands to remove any medicine that may be on them.

Dosing—The dose of salicylic acid, sulfur, and coal tar combination will be different for different patients. *Follow your doctor's orders or the directions on the label.* The following information includes only the average doses of salicylic acid, sulfur, and coal tar combination. *If your dose is different, do not change it* unless your doctor tells you to do so.

- For dandruff, seborrheic dermatitis, and psoriasis of the scalp:
  —For *cream shampoo and lotion shampoo* dosage forms:
    - Adults and children—Use on the scalp one or two times a week.

Missed dose—If you miss a dose of this medicine, apply it as soon as possible. However, if it is almost time for your next dose, skip the missed dose and go back to your regular dosing schedule.

Storage—To store this medicine:
- Keep out of the reach of children.
- Store away from heat and direct light.
- Keep the medicine from freezing.
- Do not keep outdated medicine or medicine no longer needed. Be sure that any discarded medicine is out of the reach of children.

Precautions While Using This Medicine

Do not use any topical mercury-containing preparation, such as ammoniated mercury ointment, on the same affected area as this medicine. To do so may cause a foul odor, may be irritating to the skin, and may stain the skin black. If you have any questions about this, check with your doctor or pharmacist.

This medicine may temporarily discolor blond, bleached, or tinted hair.

Side Effects of This Medicine

In animal studies, coal tar (contained in this combination medicine) has been shown to increase the chance of skin cancer.

Along with its needed effects, a medicine may cause some unwanted effects. Although not all of these side effects may occur, if they do occur they may need medical attention.

Check with your doctor as soon as possible if the following side effect occurs:

Skin irritation not present before use of this medicine

Other side effects not listed above may also occur in some patients. If you notice any other effects, check with your doctor or pharmacist.

Annual revision: 07/26/93

SELEGILINE Systemic

Some commonly used brand names are:

In the U.S.
Eldepryl

In Canada
Eldepryl
SD Deprenyl

Other
Jumex
Jumexal
Juprenil
Movergan
Procythol

Other commonly used names are deprenil and deprenyl.

Description

Selegiline (seh-LEDGE-ah-leen) is used in combination with levodopa or levodopa and carbidopa combination to treat Parkinson's disease, sometimes called shaking palsy or paralysis agitans. This medicine works to increase and extend the effects of levodopa, and may help to slow the progress of Parkinson's disease.

Selegiline is available only with your doctor's prescription, in the following dosage form:

Oral

- Tablets (U.S. and Canada)

It is very important that you read and understand the following information. If any of it causes you special concern, check with your doctor. Also, *if you have any questions* or if you want more information about this medicine or your medical problem, *ask your doctor, nurse, or pharmacist.*

Before Using This Medicine

In deciding to use a medicine, the risks of taking the medicine must be weighed against the good it will do. This is a decision you and your doctor will make. For selegiline, the following should be considered:

Allergies—Tell your doctor if you have ever had any unusual or allergic reaction to selegiline. Also tell your doctor and pharmacist if you are allergic to any other substances, such as foods, preservatives, or dyes.

Pregnancy—Selegiline has not been studied in pregnant women. However, this medicine has not been shown to cause birth defects or other problems in animal studies.

Breast-feeding—It is not known whether selegiline passes into the breast milk.

Children—Studies on this medicine have been done only in adult patients and there is no specific information about its use in children. Therefore, be sure to discuss with your doctor the use of this medicine in children.

Older adults—In studies done to date that included elderly people, selegiline did not cause different side effects or problems in older people than it did in younger adults.

Other medicines—Although certain medicines should not be used together at all, in other cases 2 different medicines may be used together even if an interaction might occur. In these cases, your doctor may want to change the dose, or other precautions may be necessary. When you are taking selegiline, it is especially important that your doctor and pharmacist know if you are taking any of the following:

- Fluoxetine (e.g., Prozac) or
- Meperidine (e.g., Demerol)—Using these medicines together may increase the chance of serious side effects

Other medical problems—The presence of other medical problems may affect the use of selegiline. Make sure you tell your doctor if you have any other medical problems, especially:

- Stomach ulcer (history of)—Selegiline may make the condition worse

Before you begin using any new medicine (prescription or nonprescription) or if you develop any new medical problem while you are using this medicine, check with your doctor, nurse, or pharmacist.

Proper Use of This Medicine

Take this medicine only as directed by your doctor. Do not take more of it, do not take it more often, and do not take it for a longer time than your doctor ordered.

Dosing—The dose of selegiline will be different for different patients. Your doctor will determine the proper dose of selegiline for you. *Follow your doctor's orders or the directions on the label.*

For the treatment of Parkinson's disease, the usual dose of selegiline is 5 mg two times a day, taken with breakfast and lunch. Some patients may need less than this.

Missed dose—If you miss a dose of this medicine, take it as soon as possible. However, if you do not remember the missed dose until late afternoon or evening, skip the missed dose and go back to your regular dosing schedule. Do not double doses.

Storage—To store this medicine:

- Keep out of the reach of children.
- Store away from heat and direct light.
- Do not store in the bathroom, near the kitchen sink, or in other damp places. Heat or moisture may cause the medicine to break down.
- Do not keep outdated medicine or medicine no longer needed. Be sure that any discarded medicine is out of the reach of children.

Precautions While Using This Medicine

When selegiline is taken at doses of 10 mg or less per day for the treatment of Parkinson's disease, there are no restrictions on food or beverages you eat or drink. However, the chance exists that dangerous reactions, such as sudden high blood pressure, may occur if doses higher than those used for Parkinson's disease are taken with certain foods, beverages, or other medicines. These foods, beverages, and medicines include:

- Foods that have a high tyramine content (most common in foods that are aged or fermented to increase their flavor), such as cheeses; fava or broad bean pods; yeast or meat extracts; smoked or pickled meat, poultry, or fish; fermented sausage (bologna, pepperoni, salami, summer sausage) or other fermented meat; sauerkraut; or any overripe fruit. If a list of these foods and beverages is not given to you, ask your doctor, nurse, or pharmacist to provide one.
- Alcoholic beverages or alcohol-free or reduced-alcohol beer and wine.
- Large amounts of caffeine-containing food or beverages such as coffee, tea, cola, or chocolate.
- Any other medicine unless approved or prescribed by your doctor. This especially includes nonprescription (over-the-counter [OTC]) medicine, such as that for colds (including nose drops or sprays), cough, asthma, hay fever, and appetite control; "keep awake" products; or products that make you sleepy.

Also, for at least 2 weeks after you stop taking this medicine, these foods, beverages, and other medicines may continue to react with selegiline if it was taken in doses higher than those usually used for Parkinson's disease.

Check with your doctor or hospital emergency room immediately if severe headache, stiff neck, chest pains, fast heartbeat, or nausea and vomiting occur while you are taking this medicine. These may be symptoms of a serious side effect that should have a doctor's attention.

Dizziness, lightheadedness, or fainting may occur, especially when you get up from a lying or sitting position. Getting up slowly may help. If the problem continues or gets worse, check with your doctor.

Selegiline may cause dryness of the mouth. For temporary relief, use sugarless candy or gum, melt bits of ice in your mouth, or use a saliva substitute. However, if your mouth continues to feel dry for more than 2 weeks, check with your medical doctor or dentist. Continuing dryness of the mouth may increase the chance of dental disease, including tooth decay, gum disease, and fungus infections.

Side Effects of This Medicine

When you start taking selegiline in addition to levodopa or carbidopa and levodopa combination, you may experience an increase in side effects. If this occurs, your doctor may gradually reduce the amount of levodopa or carbidopa and levodopa combination you take.

Along with its needed effects, a medicine may cause some unwanted effects. Although not all of these side effects may occur, if they do occur they may need medical attention.

Stop taking this medicine and get emergency help immediately if any of the following side effects occur:

Symptoms of unusually high blood pressure (caused by reaction of higher than usual doses of selegiline with restricted foods or medicines)

Chest pain (severe); enlarged pupils; fast or slow heartbeat; headache (severe); increased sensitivity of eyes to light; increased sweating (possibly with fever or cold, clammy skin); nausea and vomiting (severe); stiff or sore neck

Check with your doctor as soon as possible if any of the following side effects occur:

More common

Increase in unusual movements of body; mood or other mental changes

Less common or rare

Bloody or black, tarry stools; severe stomach pain; or vomiting of blood or material that looks like coffee grounds; difficulty in speaking; loss of balance control; uncontrolled movements, especially of face, neck, and back; restlessness or desire to keep moving; or twisting movements of body; difficult or frequent urination; dizziness or lightheadedness, especially when getting up from a lying or sitting position; hallucinations (seeing, hearing, or feeling things that are not there); irregular heartbeat; lip smacking or puckering, puffing of cheeks, rapid or worm-like movements of tongue, uncontrolled chewing movements, uncontrolled movements of arms and legs; swelling of feet or lower legs; wheezing, difficulty in breathing, or tightness in chest

Symptoms of overdose

Agitation or irritability; chest pain; convulsions (seizures); difficulty opening mouth or lockjaw; dizziness (severe) or fainting; fast or irregular pulse (continuing); high fever; high or low blood pressure; increased sweating (possibly with fever or cold, clammy skin); severe spasm where the head and heels are bent backward and the body arched forward; troubled breathing

Other side effects may occur that usually do not need medical attention. These side effects may go away during treatment as your body adjusts to the medicine. However, check with your doctor if any of the following side effects continue or are bothersome:

More common

Abdominal or stomach pain; dizziness or feeling faint; dryness of mouth; nausea or vomiting; trouble in sleeping

Less common or rare

Anxiety, nervousness, or restlessness; blurred or double vision; body ache or back or leg pain; burning of lips, mouth, or throat; chills; constipation or diarrhea;

drowsiness; headache; heartburn; high or low blood pressure; inability to move; slow or difficult urination; frequent urge to urinate; increased sensitivity of skin to light; increased sweating; irritability (temporary); loss of appetite or weight loss; memory problems; muscle cramps or numbness of fingers or toes; pounding or fast heartbeat; red, raised, or itchy skin; ringing or buzzing in ears; slowed movements; uncontrolled closing of eyelids; taste changes; unusual feeling of well-being; unusual tiredness or weakness

With doses higher than 10 mg a day

Clenching, gnashing, or grinding teeth; sudden jerky movements of body

Other side effects not listed above may also occur in some patients. If you notice any other effects, check with your doctor.

Annual revision: 09/30/92

SELENIUM SULFIDE Topical

Some commonly used brand names are:

In the U.S.

- Exsel Lotion Shampoo
- Glo-Sel
- Head & Shoulders Intensive Treatment Conditioning Formula Dandruff Lotion Shampoo
- Head & Shoulders Intensive Treatment Regular Formula Dandruff Lotion Shampoo
- Head & Shoulders Intensive Treatment 2 in 1 (Persistent Dandruff Shampoo plus Conditioner in One) Formula Dandruff Lotion Shampoo
- Selsun
- Selsun Blue Dry Formula
- Selsun Blue Extra Conditioning Formula
- Selsun Blue Extra Medicated Formula
- Selsun Blue Oily Formula
- Selsun Blue Regular Formula

Generic name product may also be available.

In Canada

- Selsun
- Selsun Blue
- Selsun Blue Extra Conditioning Formula
- Versel Lotion

Description

Selenium sulfide (se-LEE-nee-um SUL-fide) 1% and 2.5% strengths are used on the scalp to help control the symptoms of dandruff and seborrheic dermatitis.

Selenium sulfide 2.5% strength is used also on the body to treat tinea versicolor (a type of fungus infection of the skin).

In the United States, the 2.5% strength is available only with your doctor's prescription. The 1% strength is available without a prescription; however, your doctor may have special instructions on the proper use of this medicine for your medical problem.

Selenium sulfide is available in the following dosage form:

Topical

- Lotion (U.S. and Canada)

It is very important that you read and understand the following information. If any of it causes you special concern, check with your doctor or pharmacist. Also, *if you have any questions* or if you want more information about this medicine or your medical problem, *ask your doctor, nurse, or pharmacist.*

Before Using This Medicine

If you are using this medicine without a prescription, carefully read and follow any precautions on the label. For selenium sulfide, the following should be considered:

Allergies—Tell your doctor if you have ever had any unusual or allergic reaction to selenium sulfide. Also tell your doctor and pharmacist if you are allergic to any other substances, such as preservatives or dyes.

Pregnancy—

- *For use on the scalp:* Selenium sulfide has not been shown to cause birth defects or other problems in humans.
- *For use on the body:* Selenium sulfide should not be used if you are pregnant or if you may become pregnant. The medicine may be absorbed into your body and may affect your baby.

Breast-feeding—Selenium sulfide has not been reported to cause problems in nursing babies.

Children—There is no specific information comparing use of selenium sulfide in infants and children with use in other age groups; however, this medicine is not expected to cause different side effects or problems in children than it does in adults.

Older adults—Many medicines have not been studied specifically in older people. Therefore, it may not be known whether they work exactly the same way they do in younger adults. Although there is no specific information comparing use of selenium sulfide in the elderly with use in other age groups, this medicine is not expected to cause different side effects or problems in older people than it does in younger adults.

Other medicines—Although certain medicines should not be used together at all, in other cases two different medicines may be used together even if an interaction might occur. In these cases, your doctor may want to change the dose, or other precautions may be necessary. Tell your doctor and pharmacist if you are using any other topical prescription or nonprescription (over-the-counter [OTC]) medicine that is to be applied to the same area of the skin.

Other medical problems—The presence of other medical problems may affect the use of selenium sulfide. Make sure you tell your doctor if you have any other medical problems, especially:

- Blistered, raw, or oozing areas on your scalp or body—Use of this medicine on these areas may increase the chance of absorption through the skin

Before you begin using any new medicine (prescription or nonprescription) or if you develop any new medical problem while you are using this medicine, check with your doctor, nurse, or pharmacist.

Proper Use of This Medicine

If you are using the 2.5% strength of selenium sulfide: Use this medicine only as directed. Do not use it more often than recommended on the label, unless otherwise directed by your doctor.

If you are using the 1% strength of selenium sulfide: For best results, use this medicine at least 2 times a week or as directed by your doctor.

To use selenium sulfide for *dandruff or seborrheic dermatitis of the scalp:*

- Before using this medicine, wet the hair and scalp with lukewarm water.
- Apply enough medicine (1 or 2 teaspoonfuls) to the scalp to work up a lather. Allow the lather to remain on the scalp for 2 to 3 minutes, then rinse.
- Apply the medicine again and rinse well.
- If this medicine is used on light or blond, gray, or chemically treated (bleached, tinted, permanent-waved) hair, rinse your hair well for at least 5 minutes after using the medicine to lessen the chance of hair discoloration.
- After treatment, wash your hands well.

To use selenium sulfide for *tinea versicolor of the body:*

- Apply the medicine to the affected areas of your body, except for your face and genitals (sex organs).
- Work up a lather using a small amount of water.
- Allow the medicine to remain on your skin for 10 minutes.
- Rinse your body well to remove all the medicine.

Do not use this medicine if blistered, raw, or oozing areas are present on your scalp or the area of your body that is to be treated, unless otherwise directed by your doctor.

Keep this medicine away from the eyes. If you should accidentally get some in your eyes, flush them thoroughly with water.

Dosing—The dose of selenium sulfide will be different for different patients. *Follow your doctor's orders or the directions on the label.* The following information includes only the average doses of selenium sulfide. *If your dose is different, do not change it* unless your doctor tells you to do so.

- For *lotion* dosage form:
  - —For dandruff or seborrheic dermatitis:
    - Adults and children—If you are using the 1% lotion, use on the scalp two times a week. If you are using the 2.5% lotion, use on the scalp two times a week for two weeks, then use one time a week or less often.
    - Infants—Use and dose must be determined by your doctor.
  - —For tinea versicolor:
    - Adults and children—Use the 2.5% lotion on the body one time a day for seven days.
    - Infants—Use and dose must be determined by your doctor.

Missed dose—If you miss a dose of this medicine, use it as soon as possible. However, if it is almost time for your next dose, skip the missed dose and go back to your regular dosing schedule.

Storage—To store this medicine:

- Keep out of the reach of children.
- Store away from heat and direct light.
- Keep the medicine from freezing.
- Do not keep outdated medicine or medicine no longer needed. Be sure that any discarded medicine is out of the reach of children.

Precautions While Using This Medicine

If your condition does not get better after regular use of this medicine, or if it gets worse, check with your doctor.

Side Effects of This Medicine

Along with its needed effects, a medicine may cause some unwanted effects. Although not all of these side effects may occur, if they do occur they may need medical attention.

Check with your doctor as soon as possible if the following side effect occurs:

Less common or rare

Skin irritation

Other side effects may occur that usually do not need medical attention. Check with your doctor or pharmacist if any of the following side effects continue or are bothersome:

More common

Unusual dryness or oiliness of hair or scalp

Less common

Increase in normal hair loss

Other side effects not listed above may also occur in some patients. If you notice any other effects, check with your doctor or pharmacist.

Annual revision: 07/26/93

SELENIUM SUPPLEMENTS Systemic

This information applies to the following medicines:

Selenious Acid (se-LEE-nee-us as-id)
Selenium (se-LEE-nee-um)

Some commonly used brand names are:

For Selenious Acid†

In the U.S.

Sele-Pak
Selepen
Generic name product may also be available.

For Selenium

In the U.S.

Available as generic name product.

In Canada

Available as generic name product.

†Not commercially available in Canada.

Description

Selenium supplements are used to prevent or treat selenium deficiency.

The body needs selenium for normal growth and health. For patients who are unable to get enough selenium in their regular diet or who have need for more selenium, selenium supplements may be necessary.

Lack of selenium may lead to changes in fingernails, muscle weakness, and heart problems.

Selenium deficiency in the United States is rare. Patients receiving total parenteral nutrition (TPN) for long periods of time may need selenium. Selenium deficiency is a problem in areas of the world where the soil contains little selenium.

Although selenium is being used to prevent certain types of cancer, there is not enough information to show that this is effective.

Some selenium preparations are available only with your doctor's prescription. Others are available without a prescription; however, your doctor may have special instructions on the proper use and dose for your condition.

Selenium supplements are available as part of a multivitamin/mineral complex or alone in the following dosage forms:

Oral

Selenium
- Tablets (U.S. and Canada)

Parenteral

Selenious Acid
- Injection (U.S.)

It is very important that you read and ufnderstand the following information. If any of it causes you special concern, check with your doctor. Also, *if you have any questions* or if you want more information about this dietary supplement or your medical problem, *ask your doctor, nurse, pharmacist, or dietitian.*

Importance of Diet

Many nutritionists recommend that, if possible, people should get all the selenium they need from foods. However, some people do not get enough selenium from their diets. For such people, a selenium supplement is important.

In order to get enough vitamins and minerals in your regular diet, it is important that you eat a balanced and varied diet. Follow carefully any diet program your doctor may recommend. For your specific vitamin and/or mineral needs, ask your doctor or dietitian for a list of appropriate foods.

Selenium is found in seafood, liver, lean red meat, and grains grown in soil that is rich in selenium.

Experts have developed a list of recommended dietary allowances (RDA) of selenium. The RDA are not an exact number but a general idea of how much you need every day. They do not cover amounts needed for problems caused by a serious lack of selenium.

The RDA for selenium are as follows:

- Infants and children—
  - Birth to 6 months of age: 10 micrograms (mcg) a day.
  - 6 months to 1 year of age: 15 mcg a day.
  - 1 to 6 years of age: 20 mcg a day.
  - 7 to 10 years of age: 30 mcg a day.
- Adolescent and adult males—
  - 11 to 14 years of age: 40 mcg a day.
  - 15 to 18 years of age: 50 mcg a day.
  - 19 years of age and over: 70 mcg a day.
- Adolescent and adult females—
  - 11 to 14 years of age: 45 mcg a day.
  - 15 to 18 years of age: 50 mcg a day.
  - 19 years of age and over: 55 mcg a day.
- Pregnant females—65 mcg a day.
- Breast-feeding females—75 mcg a day.

Remember:

- The total amount of selenium that you get every day includes what you get from the food that you eat *and* what you may take as a supplement.
- This total amount should not be greater than the RDA, unless ordered by your doctor.

Before Using This Dietary Supplement

If you are taking this dietary supplement without a prescription, carefully read and follow any precautions on the label. For selenium supplements, the following should be considered:

Allergies—Tell your doctor if you have ever had any unusual or allergic reaction to selenious acid or selenium. Also tell your doctor and pharmacist if you are allergic to any other substances, such as foods, preservatives, or dyes.

Pregnancy—It is especially important that you are receiving enough vitamins and minerals when you become pregnant and that you continue to receive the right amount of vitamins and minerals throughout your pregnancy. The healthy growth and development of the fetus depend on a steady supply of nutrients from the mother. However, taking large amounts of a dietary supplement in pregnancy may be harmful to the mother and/or fetus and should be avoided.

Breast-feeding—It is important that you receive the right amounts of vitamins and minerals so that your baby will also get the vitamins and minerals needed to grow properly. However, taking large amounts of a dietary supplement while breast-feeding may be harmful to the mother and/or baby and should be avoided.

Children—It is especially important that children receive enough selenium in their diet for healthy growth and development. Although there is no specific information comparing use of selenium in children with use in other age groups, this medicine is not expected to cause different side effects or problems in children than it does in adults.

Older adults—It is important that older people continue to receive enough selenium in their daily diets.

Medicines or dietary supplements—Although certain medicines should not be used together at all, in other cases or dietary supplements may be used together even if an interaction might occur. In these cases, your doctor may want to change the dose, or other precautions may be necessary. Tell your doctor and pharmacist if you are taking any other dietary supplement or any nonprescription (over-the-counter [OTC]) or prescription medicine.

Proper Use of This Dietary Supplement

Some people believe that taking very large doses of a vitamin or mineral (called megadoses) is useful for treating certain medical problems. Studies have not proven this. Large doses should be taken only under the direction of your doctor after need has been identified.

Missed dose—If you miss taking selenium supplements for one or more days there is no cause for concern, since it takes some time for your body to become seriously low in selenium. However, if your doctor has recommended that you take selenium, try to remember to take it as directed every day.

Storage—To store this dietary supplement:

- Keep out of the reach of children.
- Store away from heat and direct light.
- Do not store in the bathroom, near the kitchen sink, or in other damp places. Heat or moisture may cause the dietary supplement to break down.
- Keep the dietary supplement from freezing. Do not refrigerate.
- Do not keep outdated dietary supplement or those no longer needed. Be sure that any discarded dietary supplement is out of the reach of children.

Side Effects of This Dietary Supplement

Along with its needed effects, a dietary supplement may cause some unwanted effects. Although selenium supplements have not been reported to cause any side effects, check with your doctor immediately if any of the following side effects occur as a result of an overdose:

Symptoms of overdose
Diarrhea; fingernail weakening; garlic odor of breath and sweat; hair loss; irritability; itching of skin; metallic taste; nausea and vomiting; unusual tiredness and weakness

Other side effects not listed above may also occur in some patients. If you notice any other effects, check with your doctor.

Annual revision: 04/16/92
Interim revision: 06/06/92

SERTRALINE Systemic

A commonly used brand name in the U.S. and Canada is Zoloft.

Description

Sertraline (SER-tral-leen) is used to treat mental depression.

This medicine is available only with your doctor's prescription, in the following dosage form:

Oral
- Capsules (Canada)
- Tablets (U.S.)

It is very important that you read and understand the following information. If any of it causes you special concern, check with your doctor. Also, *if you have any questions* or if you want more information about this medicine or your medical problem, *ask your doctor, nurse, or pharmacist.*

Before Using This Medicine

In deciding to use a medicine, the risks of taking the medicine must be weighed against the good it will do. This is a decision you and your doctor will make. For sertraline, the following should be considered:

Allergies—Tell your doctor if you have ever had any unusual or allergic reaction to sertraline. Also tell your doctor and pharmacist if you are allergic to any other substances, such as foods, preservatives, or dyes.

Pregnancy—Studies have not been done in pregnant women. However, studies in animals have shown that sertraline may cause delayed development and decreased survival rates of offspring when given in doses many times the usual human dose. Before taking this medicine, make sure your doctor knows if you are pregnant or if you may become pregnant.

Breast-feeding—It is not known whether sertraline is excreted in breast milk.

Children—Studies on this medicine have been done only in adult patients, and there is no specific information comparing use of sertraline in children with use in other age groups.

Older adults—In studies done to date that have included elderly people, sertraline did not cause different side effects or problems in older people than it did in younger adults.

Other medicines—Although certain medicines should not be used together at all, in other cases two different medicines may be used together even if an interaction might occur. In these cases, your doctor may want to change the dose, or other precautions may be necessary. When you are taking sertraline, it is especially important that your doctor and pharmacist know if you are taking any of the following:

- Digitoxin (e.g., Crystodigin) or
- Warfarin (e.g., Coumadin)—Higher or lower blood levels of these medicines or sertraline may occur, which may increase the chance of unwanted effects; your doctor may need to change the dose of either these medicines or sertraline
- Monoamine oxidase (MAO) inhibitors (furazolidone [e.g., Furoxone], isocarboxazid [e.g., Marplan], phenelzine [e.g., Nardil], procarbazine [e.g., Matulane], selegiline [e.g., Eldepryl], tranylcypromine [e.g., Parnate])—Taking sertraline while you are taking or within 2 weeks of taking MAO inhibitors may cause confusion, agitation, restlessness, stomach or intestinal symptoms, sudden high body temperature, extremely high blood pressure, and severe convulsions; at least 14 days should be allowed between stopping treatment with one medicine and starting treatment with the other

Other medical problems—The presence of other medical problems may affect the use of sertraline. Make sure you tell your doctor if you have any other medical problems, especially:

- Drug abuse or dependence (or history of)—Because sertraline is a new drug, it is not known if it could become habit-forming, causing mental or physical dependence
- Kidney disease, severe, or
- Liver disease—Higher blood levels of sertraline may occur, increasing the chance of side effects

Before you begin using any new medicine (prescription or nonprescription) or if you develop any new medical problem while you are using this medicine, check with your doctor, nurse, or pharmacist.

Proper Use of This Medicine

Take this medicine only as directed by your doctor, to benefit your condition as much as possible. Do not take more of it, do not take it more often, and do not take it for a longer time than your doctor ordered.

You may have to take sertraline for up to 4 weeks or longer before you begin to feel better. Your doctor should check your progress at regular visits during this time.

This medicine should always be taken at the same time in relation to meals and snacks to make sure that it is absorbed in the same way.

Dosing—The dose of sertraline will be different for different patients. *Follow your doctor's orders or the directions on the label.* The following information includes only the average doses of sertraline. *If your dose is different, do not change it* unless your doctor tells you to do so.

- The number of capsules or tablets that you take depends on the strength of the medicine and the medical problem for which you are taking sertraline.
- For *oral* dosage forms (capsules or tablets):
  —Adults: To start, usually 50 milligrams once a day, taken either in the morning or evening. Your doctor may gradually increase your dose if needed.
  —Children: Dose must be determined by the doctor.
  —Older adults: To start, usually 12.5 to 25 milligrams once a day, taken either in the morning or evening. Your doctor may gradually increase your dose if needed.

Missed dose—Because sertraline may be given to different patients at different times of the day, you and your doctor should discuss what to do about any missed doses.

Storage—To store this medicine:

- Keep out of the reach of children.
- Store away from heat and direct light.
- Do not store in the bathroom, near the kitchen sink, or in other damp places. Heat or moisture may cause the medicine to break down.
- Do not keep outdated medicine or medicine no longer needed. Be sure that any discarded medicine is out of the reach of children.

Precautions While Using This Medicine

It is important that your doctor check your progress at regular visits, to allow for changes in your dose and to help reduce any side effects.

This medicine could possibly add to the effects of alcohol and other CNS depressants (medicines that slow down the nervous system, possibly causing drowsiness). Some examples of CNS depressants are antihistamines or medicine for hay fever, other allergies, or colds; sedatives, tranquilizers, or sleeping medicine; prescription pain medicine or narcotics; barbiturates; medicine for seizures; muscle relaxants; or anesthetics, including some dental anesthetics. *Check with your doctor before taking any of the above while you are using this medicine.*

This medicine may cause some people to become drowsy. *Make sure you know how you react to sertraline before you drive, use machines, or do anything else that could be dangerous if you are not alert.*

This medicine may cause dryness of the mouth. For temporary relief, use sugarless gum or candy, melt bits of ice in your mouth, or use a saliva substitute. However, if your mouth continues to feel dry for more than 2 weeks, check with your medical doctor or dentist. Continuing dryness of the mouth may increase the chance of dental disease, including tooth decay, gum disease, and fungus infections.

Side Effects of This Medicine

Along with its needed effects, a medicine may cause some unwanted effects. Although not all of these side effects may occur, if they do occur they may need medical attention.

Check with your doctor as soon as possible if any of the following side effects occur:

Less common or rare

Fast talking and excited feelings or actions that are out of control; fever; skin rash, hives, or itching

Other side effects may occur that usually do not need medical attention. These side effects may go away during treatment as your body adjusts to the medicine. However, check with your doctor if any of the following side effects continue or are bothersome:

More common

Decreased appetite or weight loss; decreased sexual drive or ability; diarrhea; drowsiness; dryness of mouth; headache; nausea; stomach or abdominal cramps, gas, or pain; tiredness or weakness; tremor; trouble in sleeping

Less common

Anxiety, agitation, nervousness or restlessness; changes in vision, including blurred vision; constipation; fast or irregular heartbeat; flushing or redness of skin, with feeling of warmth or heat; increased appetite; vomiting

Other side effects not listed above may also occur in some patients. If you notice any other effects, check with your doctor.

Annual revision: 03/19/93

SILVER SULFADIAZINE Topical

Some commonly used brand names are:

In the U.S.
- Flint SSD
- Sildimac
- Silvadene
- SSD
- SSD AF
- Thermazene

In Canada
- Flamazine

Description

Silver sulfadiazine (SILL-ver sul-fa-DYE-a-zeen), a sulfa medicine, is used to prevent and treat bacterial or fungus infections. It works by killing the fungus or bacteria.

Silver sulfadiazine cream is applied to the skin and/or burned area(s) to prevent and treat bacterial or fungus infections that may occur in burns. This medicine may also be used for other problems as determined by your doctor.

Other medicines are used along with this medicine for burns. Patients with severe burns or burns over a large area of the body must be treated in a hospital.

Silver sulfadiazine is available only with your doctor's prescription, in the following dosage form:

Topical
- Cream (U.S. and Canada)

It is very important that you read and understand the following information. If any of it causes you special concern, check with your doctor. Also, *if you have any questions* or if you want more information about this medicine or your medical problem, *ask your doctor, nurse, or pharmacist.*

Before Using This Medicine

In deciding to use a medicine, the risks of using the medicine must be weighed against the good it will do. This is a decision you and your doctor will make. For silver sulfadiazine, the following should be considered:

Allergies—Tell your doctor if you have ever had any unusual or allergic reaction to silver sulfadiazine or to any of the following medicines:
- Acetazolamide (e.g., Diamox)
- Antidiabetics, oral (diabetes medicine you take by mouth)
- Dichlorphenamide (e.g., Daranide)
- Furosemide (e.g., Lasix)
- Methazolamide (e.g., Neptazane)
- Sulfonamides, other (sulfa medicine)
- Thiazide diuretics (water pills)

Also tell your doctor and pharmacist if you are allergic to any other substances, such as preservatives or dyes.

Pregnancy—Studies have not been done in humans. However, sulfa medicines may increase the chance of liver problems in newborn infants. Silver sulfadiazine has not been shown to cause birth defects or other problems in studies in rabbits treated with 3 to 10 times the usual amount of silver sulfadiazine.

Breast-feeding—It is not known whether silver sulfadiazine applied to the skin and/or burns passes into the breast milk. However, silver sulfadiazine may be absorbed into the body when used on skin and/or burns. Sulfa medicines given by mouth do pass into the breast milk. They may cause liver problems, anemia (iron-poor blood), and other unwanted effects in nursing babies, especially those with glucose-6-phosphate dehydrogenase deficiency (lack of G6PD enzyme). Therefore, caution is recommended when using this medicine in nursing women.

Children—Use is not recommended in premature or newborn infants up to 1 month of age. Sulfa medicines may cause liver problems in these infants. Although there is no specific information comparing use of silver sulfadiazine in older infants and children with use in other age groups, this medicine is not expected to cause different side effects or problems in older infants and children than it does in adults.

Older adults—Many medicines have not been studied specifically in older people. Therefore, it may not be known whether they work exactly the same way they do in younger adults or if they cause different side effects or problems in older people. There is no specific information comparing use of silver sulfadiazine in the elderly with use in other age groups.

Other medicines—Although certain medicines should not be used together at all, in other cases two different medicines may be used together even if an interaction might occur. In these cases, your doctor may want to change the dose, or other precautions may be necessary. When you are taking silver sulfadiazine, it is especially important that your doctor and pharmacist know if you are taking any of the following:
- Collagenase (e.g., Santyl) or
- Papain (e.g., Panafil) or
- Sutilains (e.g., Travase)—Silver sulfadiazine may prevent these enzymes from working properly

Other medical problems—The presence of other medical problems may affect the use of silver sulfadiazine. Make sure you tell your doctor if you have any other medical problems, especially:
- Blood problems or
- Glucose-6-phosphate dehydrogenase deficiency (lack of G6PD enzyme)—Use of this medicine may cause blood problems or make them worse
- Kidney disease or
- Liver disease—In persons with these conditions, use may result in higher blood levels of this medicine; a smaller dose may be needed

- Porphyria—Use of this medicine may result in a severe attack of porphyria

Before you begin using any new medicine (prescription or nonprescription) or if you develop any new medical problem while you are using this medicine, check with your doctor, nurse, or pharmacist.

Proper Use of This Medicine

This medicine should not be used on premature or newborn infants up to 1 month of age, unless otherwise directed by your doctor. It may cause liver problems in these infants.

To use:

- Before applying this medicine, cleanse the affected area(s). Remove dead or burned skin and other debris.
- Wear a sterile glove to apply this medicine. Apply a thin layer (about 1/16 inch) of silver sulfadiazine to the affected area(s). Keep the affected area(s) covered with the medicine at all times.
- If this medicine is rubbed off the affected area(s) by moving around or if it is washed off during bathing, showering, or the use of a whirlpool bath, reapply the medicine.
- After this medicine has been applied, the treated area(s) may be covered with a dressing or left uncovered as desired.

To help clear up your skin and/or burn infection completely, *keep using silver sulfadiazine for the full time of treatment.* You should keep using this medicine until the burned area has healed or is ready for skin grafting. *Do not miss any doses.*

Dosing—The dose of silver sulfadiazine will be different for different patients. *Follow your doctor's orders or the directions on the label.* The following information includes only the average doses of silver sulfadiazine. *If your dose is different, do not change it* unless your doctor tells you to do so.

- For *topical* dosage form (cream):
  —For burn wound infections:
  - Adults and children 1 month of age and older—Use one or two times a day.
  - Premature and newborn infants up to 1 month of age—Use and dose must be determined by the doctor.

Missed dose—If you miss a dose of this medicine, apply it as soon as possible. However, if it is almost time for your next dose, skip the missed dose and go back to your regular dosing schedule.

Storage—To store this medicine:

- Keep out of the reach of children.
- Store away from heat and direct light.
- Keep the medicine from freezing.
- Do not keep outdated medicine or medicine no longer needed. Be sure that any discarded medicine is out of the reach of children.

Precautions While Using This Medicine

It is important that your doctor check your progress at regular visits.

If your skin infection or burn does not improve within a few days or weeks (for more serious burns or burns over larger areas), or if it becomes worse, check with your doctor.

This medicine may rarely stain skin brownish gray.

Side Effects of This Medicine

Along with its needed effects, a medicine may cause some unwanted effects. Although not all of these side effects may occur, if they do occur they may need medical attention.

Check with your doctor as soon as possible if the following side effect occurs:

Rare

Increased sensitivity of skin to sunlight, especially in patients with burns on large areas

Other side effects may occur that usually do not need medical attention. These side effects may go away during treatment as your body adjusts to the medicine. However, check with your doctor if any of the following side effects continue or are bothersome:

More common

Burning feeling on treated area(s)

Less common or rare

Brownish-gray skin discoloration; itching or skin rash

Other side effects not listed above may also occur in some patients. If you notice any other effects, check with your doctor.

Annual revision: 07/26/93

SIMETHICONE Oral

Some commonly used brand names are:

In the U.S.

- Extra Strength Gas-X
- Gas Relief
- Gas-X
- Maximum Strength Gas Relief
- Maximum Strength Phazyme
- Mylanta Gas
- Mylanta Gas Maximum Strength
- Mylanta Gas Regular Strength
- Mylicon Drops
- Phazyme

Generic name product may also be available.

In Canada

- Ovol
- Ovol-40
- Ovol-80
- Phazyme 55
- Phazyme 95

Description

Simethicone (si-METH-i-kone) is used to relieve the painful symptoms of too much gas in the stomach and intestines.

Simethicone may also be used for other conditions as determined by your doctor.

Simethicone is available without a prescription; however, your doctor may have special instructions on the proper use and dose for your medical problem. It is available in the following dosage forms:

Oral

- Capsules (U.S.)
- Oral suspension (U.S. and Canada)
- Tablets (U.S. and Canada)
- Chewable tablets (U.S. and Canada)

It is very important that you read and understand the following information. If any of it causes you special concern, check with your doctor or pharmacist. Also, *if you have any questions* or if you want more information about this medicine or your medical problem, *ask your doctor, nurse, or pharmacist.*

Before Using This Medicine

In deciding to use a medicine, the risks of taking the medicine must be weighed against the good it will do. This is a decision you and your doctor will make. For simethicone, the following should be considered:

Allergies—Tell your doctor if you have ever had any unusual or allergic reaction to simethicone. Also tell your doctor and pharmacist if you are allergic to any other substances, such as foods, preservatives, or dyes.

Diet—Avoid foods that seem to increase gas. Chew food thoroughly and slowly. Reduce air swallowing by avoiding fizzy, carbonated drinks. Do not smoke before meals. Develop regular bowel habits and exercise regularly. Make certain your doctor and pharmacist know if you are on a low-sodium, low-sugar, or any other special diet. Most medicines contain more than their active ingredient.

Pregnancy—Simethicone is not absorbed into the body and is not likely to cause problems.

Breast-feeding—Simethicone has not been reported to cause problems in nursing babies.

Children—This medicine has been tested in children and, in effective doses, has not been shown to cause different side effects or problems than it does in adults.

Older adults—Many medicines have not been studied specifically in older people. Therefore, it may not be known whether they work exactly the same way they do in younger adults. There is no specific information comparing use of simethicone in the elderly with use in other age groups.

Before you begin using any new medicine (prescription or nonprescription) or if you develop any new medical problem while you are using this medicine, check with your doctor, nurse, or pharmacist.

Proper Use of This Medicine

For effective use of simethicone:

- Follow your doctor's instructions if this medicine was prescribed.
- Follow the manufacturer's package directions if you are treating yourself.

Take this medicine after meals and at bedtime for best results.

For patients taking the *chewable tablet* form of this medicine:

- It is important that you chew the tablets thoroughly before you swallow them. This is to allow the medicine to work faster and more completely.

For patients taking the *oral liquid* form of this medicine:

- This medicine is to be taken by mouth even if it comes in a dropper bottle. The amount you should take is to be measured with the specially marked dropper.

Dosing—The dose of simethicone will be different for different patients. *Follow your doctor's orders or the directions on the label.* The following information includes only the average doses of simethicone. *If your dose is different, do not change it* unless your doctor tells you to do so.

- For symptoms of too much gas:
  - —For *oral* dosage forms (capsules or tablets):
    - Adults and children 12 years of age and older—40 to 125 milligrams (mg) four times a day, after meals and at bedtime. The dose should not be more than 500 mg in 24 hours.
    - Children up to 12 years of age—Dose must be determined by the doctor.
  - —For *oral* dosage form (suspension):
    - Adults and children 12 years of age and older—40 mg four times a day, before meals and at bedtime. The dose should not be more than 500 mg in 24 hours.
    - Children up to 12 years of age—Dose must be determined by the doctor.

Missed dose—If you must take this medicine regularly and you miss a dose, take it as soon as possible. However, if it is almost time for your next dose, skip the missed dose and go back to your regular dosing schedule. Do not double doses.

Storage—To store this medicine:

- Keep out of the reach of children.
- Store away from heat and direct light.
- Do not store the tablet form of this medicine in the bathroom, near the kitchen sink, or in other damp places. Heat or moisture may cause the medicine to break down.
- Keep the liquid form of this medicine from freezing.
- Do not keep outdated medicine or medicine no longer needed. Be sure that any discarded medicine is out of the reach of children.

Side Effects of This Medicine

There have not been any common or important side effects reported with this medicine. However, if you notice any side effects, check with your doctor.

Additional Information

Once a medicine has been approved for marketing for a certain use, experience may show that it is also useful for other medical problems. Although these uses are not included in product labeling, simethicone is used in certain patients before the following tests:

- Before a gastroscopy
- Before a radiography of the bowel

Other than the above information, there is no additional information relating to proper use, precautions, or side effects for these uses.

Annual revision: 06/16/93

SKELETAL MUSCLE RELAXANTS Systemic

This information applies to the following medicines:

Carisoprodol (kar-eye-soe-PROE-dole)
Chlorphenesin (klor-FEN-e-sin)
Chlorzoxazone (klor-ZOX-a-zone)
Metaxalone (me-TAX-a-lone)
Methocarbamol (meth-oh-KAR-ba-mole)

This information does *not* apply to the following medicines: Baclofen, cyclobenzaprine, dantrolene, diazepam, and orphenadrine.

Some commonly used brand names are:

For Carisoprodol

In the U.S.

Rela
Sodol
Soma
Soprodol
Soridol

Generic name product may also be available.

In Canada

Soma

For Chlorphenesin

In the U.S.

Maolate

For Chlorzoxazone

In the U.S.

Paraflex
Parafon Forte DSC

Generic name product may also be available.

For Metaxalone

In the U.S.

Skelaxin

For Methocarbamol

In the U.S.

Carbacot
Delaxin
Marbaxin
Robamol
Robaxin
Robomol
Skelex

Generic name product may also be available.

In Canada

Robaxin

Description

Skeletal muscle relaxants are used to relax certain muscles in your body and relieve the pain and discomfort caused by strains, sprains, or other injury to your muscles. However, these medicines do not take the place of rest, exercise or physical therapy, or other treatment that your doctor may recommend for your medical problem. Methocarbamol also has been used to relieve some of the muscle problems caused by tetanus.

Skeletal muscle relaxants act in the central nervous system (CNS) to produce their muscle relaxant effects. Their actions in the CNS may also produce some of their side effects.

In the U.S., these medicines are available only with your doctor's prescription. In Canada, some of these medicines are available without a prescription.

These medicines are available in the following dosage forms:

Oral

- Carisoprodol
  - Tablets (U.S. and Canada)
- Chlorphenesin
  - Tablets (U.S.)
- Chlorzoxazone
  - Tablets (U.S.)
- Metaxalone
  - Tablets (U.S.)
- Methocarbamol
  - Tablets (U.S. and Canada)

Parenteral

- Methocarbamol
  - Injection (U.S. and Canada)

It is very important that you read and understand the following information. If any of it causes you special concern, check with your doctor. Also, *if you have any questions* or if you want more information about this medicine or your medical problem, *ask your doctor, nurse, or pharmacist.*

Before Using This Medicine

In deciding to use a medicine, the risks of taking the medicine must be weighed against the good it will do. This is a decision you and your doctor will make. For the skeletal muscle relaxants, the following should be considered:

Allergies—Tell your doctor if you have ever had any unusual or allergic reaction to any of the skeletal muscle relaxants or to carbromal, mebutamate, meprobamate (e.g., Equanil), or tybamate. Also tell your doctor and pharmacist if you are allergic to any other substances, such as foods, preservatives, or dyes.

Pregnancy—Although skeletal muscle relaxants have not been shown to cause birth defects or other problems, studies on birth defects have not been done in pregnant women. Studies in animals with metaxalone have not shown that it causes birth defects.

Breast-feeding—Carisoprodol passes into the breast milk and may cause drowsiness or stomach upset in nursing babies. Chlorphenesin, chlorzoxazone, metaxalone, and methocarbamol have not been shown to cause problems in nursing babies. However, methocarbamol passes into the breast milk in small amounts. It is not known whether chlorphenesin, chlorzoxazone, or metaxalone passes into the breast milk.

Children—Chlorzoxazone has been tested in children and has not been shown to cause different side effects or problems than it does in adults.

Although there is no specific information about the use of carisoprodol in children, it is not expected to cause different side effects or problems in children than it does in adults.

There is no specific information about the use of other skeletal muscle relaxants in children.

Older adults—Many medicines have not been tested in older people. Therefore, it may not be known whether they work exactly the same way they do in younger adults or if they cause different side effects or problems in older people. There is no specific information about the use of skeletal muscle relaxants in the elderly.

Other medicines—Although certain medicines should not be used together at all, in other cases two different medicines may be used together even if an interaction might occur. In these cases, your doctor may want to change the dose, or other precautions may be necessary. When you are taking a skeletal muscle relaxant, it is especially important that your doctor and pharmacist know if you are taking any of the following:

- Central nervous system (CNS) depressants or
- Tricyclic antidepressants (amitriptyline [e.g., Elavil], amoxapine [e.g., Asendin], clomipramine [e.g., Anafranil], desipramine [e.g., Pertofrane], doxepin [e.g., Sinequan], imipramine [e.g., Tofranil], nortriptyline [e.g., Aventyl], protriptyline [e.g., Vivactil], trimipramine [e.g., Surmontil])—The chance of side effects may be increased

Other medical problems—The presence of other medical problems may affect the use of a skeletal muscle relaxant. Make sure you tell your doctor if you have any other medical problems, especially:

- Allergies, history of, or
- Blood disease caused by an allergy or reaction to any other medicine, history of, or
- Drug abuse or dependence, or history of, or
- Kidney disease or
- Liver disease or
- Porphyria—Depending on which of the skeletal muscle relaxants you take, the chance of side effects may be increased; your doctor can choose a muscle relaxant that is less likely to cause problems
- Epilepsy—Convulsions may be more likely to occur if methocarbamol is given by injection

Before you begin using any new medicine (prescription or nonprescription) or if you develop any new medical problem while you are using this medicine, check with your doctor, nurse, or pharmacist.

Proper Use of This Medicine

Chlorzoxazone, metaxalone, or methocarbamol tablets may be crushed and mixed with a little food or liquid if needed to make the tablets easier to swallow.

Missed dose—If you miss a dose of this medicine and remember within an hour or so of the missed dose, take it right away. But if you do not remember until later, skip the missed dose and go back to your regular dosing schedule. Do not double doses.

Storage—To store this medicine:

- Keep out of the reach of children.
- Store away from heat and direct light.
- Do not store this medicine in the bathroom, near the kitchen sink, or in other damp places. Heat or moisture may cause the medicine to break down.
- Do not keep outdated medicine or medicine no longer needed. Be sure that any discarded medicine is out of the reach of children.

Precautions While Using This Medicine

If you will be taking this medicine for a long time (for example, more than a few weeks), your doctor should check your progress at regular visits.

This medicine will add to the effects of alcohol and other CNS depressants (medicines that slow down the nervous system, possibly causing drowsiness). Some examples of CNS depressants are antihistamines or medicine for hay fever, other allergies, or colds; sedatives, tranquilizers, or sleeping medicine; prescription pain medicine or narcotics; barbiturates; medicine for seizures; other muscle relaxants; or anesthetics, including some dental anesthetics. *Do not drink alcoholic beverages, and check with your doctor before taking any of the medicines listed above, while you are using this medicine.*

Skeletal muscle relaxants may cause blurred vision or clumsiness or unsteadiness in some people. They may also cause some people to feel drowsy, dizzy, lightheaded, faint, or less alert than they are normally. *Make sure you know how you react to this medicine before you drive, use machines, or do anything else that could be dangerous if you are dizzy or are not alert, well-coordinated, and able to see well.*

For *diabetic patients:*

- Metaxalone (e.g., Skelaxin) may cause false test results with one type of test for sugar in your urine. If your urine sugar test shows an unusually large amount of sugar, or if you have any questions about this, check with your doctor, nurse, or pharmacist. This is especially important if your diabetes is not well controlled.

Side Effects of This Medicine

Along with its needed effects, a medicine may cause some unwanted effects. Although not all of these side effects may occur, if they do occur they may need medical attention.

Check with your doctor as soon as possible if any of the following side effects occur:

Less common

Fainting; fast heartbeat; fever; hive-like swellings (large) on face, eyelids, mouth, lips, and/or tongue; mental depression; shortness of breath, troubled breathing, tightness in chest, and/or wheezing; skin rash, hives, itching, or redness; slow heartbeat (methocarbamol injection only); stinging or burning of eyes; stuffy nose and red or bloodshot eyes

Rare

Blood in urine; bloody or black, tarry stools; convulsions (seizures) (methocarbamol injection only); cough or hoarseness; fast or irregular breathing; lower back or side pain; muscle cramps or pain (not present before treatment or more painful than before treatment); painful or difficult urination; pain, tenderness, heat, redness, or swelling over a blood vessel (vein) in arm or leg (methocarbamol injection only); pinpoint red spots on skin; puffiness or swelling of the eyelids or around the eyes; sores, ulcers, or white spots on lips or in mouth; sore throat and fever with or without chills; swollen and/or painful glands; unusual bruising or bleeding; unusual tiredness or weakness; vomiting of blood or material that looks like coffee grounds; yellow eyes or skin

Other side effects may occur that usually do not need medical attention. These side effects may go away during treatment as your body adjusts to the medicine. However, check with your doctor if any of the following side effects continue or are bothersome:

More common

Blurred or double vision or any change in vision; dizziness or lightheadedness; drowsiness

Less common or rare

Abdominal or stomach cramps or pain; clumsiness or unsteadiness; confusion; constipation; diarrhea; excitement, nervousness, restlessness, or irritability; flushing or redness of face; headache; heartburn; hiccups; muscle weakness; nausea or vomiting; pain or peeling of skin at place of injection (methocarbamol only); trembling; trouble in sleeping; uncontrolled movements of eyes (methocarbamol injection only)

Although not all of the side effects listed above have been reported for all of these medicines, they have been reported for at least one of them. However, since all of these skeletal muscle relaxants have similar effects, it is possible that any of the above side effects may occur with any of these medicines.

In addition to the other side effects listed above, chlorzoxazone may cause your urine to turn orange or reddish purple. Methocarbamol may cause your urine to turn black, brown, or green. This effect is harmless and will go away when you stop taking the medicine. However, if you have any questions about this, check with your doctor.

Other side effects not listed above may also occur in some patients. If you notice any other effects, check with your doctor.

Annual revision: August 1990
Interim revision: 08/17/93

SODIUM BENZOATE AND SODIUM PHENYLACETATE Systemic†

A commonly used brand name in the U.S. is Ucephan.

†Not commercially available in Canada.

Description

Sodium benzoate (SOE-dee-um BEN-zo-ate) and sodium phenylacetate (fen-ill-AH-seh-tate) combination is used to treat a condition caused by too much ammonia in the blood (hyperammonemia). This medicine works by causing less ammonia to be produced by the body.

Ammonia is formed from the breakdown of protein in the body. If the ammonia cannot be removed by the body, then a buildup may cause serious unwanted effects.

Sodium benzoate and sodium phenylacetate combination is available only with your doctor's prescription in the following dosage form:

Oral

- Oral solution (U.S.)

It is very important that you read and understand the following information. If any of it causes you special concern, check with your doctor. Also, *if you have any questions* or if you want more information about this medicine or your medical problem, *ask your doctor, nurse, or pharmacist.*

Before Using This Medicine

In deciding to use a medicine, the risks of taking the medicine must be weighed against the good it will do. This is a decision you and your doctor will make. For sodium benzoate and sodium phenylacetate combination, the following should be considered:

Allergies—Tell your doctor if you have ever had any unusual or allergic reaction to sodium benzoate or sodium phenylacetate. Also tell your doctor and pharmacist if you are allergic to any other substances, such as foods, preservatives, or dyes.

Pregnancy—Sodium benzoate and sodium phenylacetate combination has not been studied in pregnant women or animals.

Breast-feeding—It is not known whether sodium benzoate and sodium phenylacetate combination passes into the breast milk. Although most medicines pass into breast milk in small amounts, many of them may be used safely while breast-feeding. Mothers who are taking this medicine and who wish to breast-feed should discuss this with their doctor.

Children—Sodium benzoate and sodium phenylacetate may cause serious unwanted effects if given to infants of low birthweight.

Older adults—Many medicines have not been studied specifically in older people. Therefore, it may not be known whether they work exactly the same way they do in younger adults or if they cause different side effects or problems in older people. There is no specific information comparing the use of sodium benzoate and sodium phenylacetate in the elderly with use in other age groups.

Other medicines—Although certain medicines should not be used together at all, in other cases two different medicines may be used together even if an interaction might occur. In these cases, your doctor may want to change the dose, or other precautions may be necessary. When you are taking sodium benzoate and sodium phenylacetate combination, it is especially important that your doctor and pharmacist know if you are taking the following:

- Penicillins—Use with penicillins may keep the sodium benzoate and sodium phenylacetate combination from working properly

Other medical problems—The presence of other medical problems may affect the use of sodium benzoate and sodium phenylacetate combination. Make sure you tell your doctor if you have any other medical problems, especially:

- Edema (swelling) or
- Heart disease or
- Kidney disease or
- Toxemia of pregnancy—Increased retention of water may make these conditions worse

Before you begin using any new medicine (prescription or nonprescription) or if you develop any new medical problem while you are using this medicine, check with your doctor, nurse, or pharmacist.

Proper Use of This Medicine

This medicine should be added to infant formula or milk and given immediately after mixing. Sodium benzoate and sodium phenylacetate should not be mixed with other beverages (especially acidic beverages such as tea or coffee), since they may cause the medicine to separate out.

Take this medicine with meals.

It is important that you follow any special instructions from your doctor, such as following a low protein diet. If you have any questions about this, check with your doctor.

Dosing—The dose of this combination medicine will be different for different patients. *Follow your doctor's orders or the directions on the label.* The following information includes only the average dose of this combination medicine. *If your dose is different, do not change it* unless your doctor tells you to do so.

- For *oral* dosage form (solution):
  —Treatment of too much ammonia in the blood:
    - Adults and children—The dose is based on body weight and must be determined by the doctor. It is usually 2.5 milliliters (mL) per kilogram (1.1 mL per pound) a day, given in three to six divided doses. The dose is usually no more than 100 mL a day.

Missed dose—If you miss a dose of this medicine, take it as soon as possible. However, if it is almost time for your next dose, skip the missed dose and go back to your regular dosing schedule. Do not double doses.

Storage—To store this medicine:

- Keep out of the reach of children.
- Store away from heat and direct light.
- Do not store in the bathroom, near the kitchen sink, or in other damp places. Heat or moisture may cause the medicine to break down.
- Keep the medicine from freezing. Do not refrigerate.
- Do not keep outdated medicine or medicine no longer needed. Be sure that any discarded medicine is out of the reach of children.

Precautions While Using This Medicine

Your doctor should check your progress at regular visits to make sure that this medicine is working properly.

Side Effects of This Medicine

Along with its needed effects, a medicine may cause some unwanted effects. Although not all of these side effects may occur, if they do occur they may need medical attention.

Stop taking this medicine and get emergency help immediately if any of the following side effects occur:

Symptoms of overdose

Continual vomiting; feeling of faintness; rapid fall in blood pressure; shortness of breath or troubled breathing; unusual drowsiness; unusual irritability

Other side effects may occur that usually do not need medical attention. These side effects may go away during treatment as your body adjusts to the medicine. However, check with your doctor if either of the following side effects continue or are bothersome:

More common

Nausea or vomiting

Other side effects not listed above may also occur in some patients. If you notice any other effects, check with your doctor.

Annual revision: 07/15/93

SODIUM BICARBONATE Systemic

Some commonly used brand names are:

In the U.S.

Arm and Hammer Pure Baking Soda
Bell/ans
Citrocarbonate
Soda Mint

Generic name product may also be available.

In Canada

Citrocarbonate

Generic name product may also be available.

Description

Sodium bicarbonate (SOE-dee-um bye-KAR-boe-nate), also known as baking soda, is used to relieve heartburn, sour stomach, or acid indigestion by neutralizing excess stomach acid. When used for this purpose, it is said to belong to the group of medicines called antacids. It may be used to treat the symptoms of stomach or duodenal ulcers. Sodium bicarbonate is also used to make the blood and urine more alkaline in certain conditions.

Antacids should not be given to young children (up to 6 years of age) unless prescribed by their doctor. Since children cannot usually describe their symptoms very well, a doctor should check the child before giving this medicine. The child may have a condition that needs other treatment. If so, antacids will not help and may even cause unwanted effects or make the condition worse.

Sodium bicarbonate for oral use is available without a prescription; however, your doctor may have special instructions on the proper use and dose for your medical problem. Sodium bicarbonate is available in the following dosage forms:

Oral
- Effervescent powder (U.S. and Canada)
- Oral powder (U.S. and Canada)
- Tablets (U.S. and Canada)

Parenteral
- Injection (U.S. and Canada)

It is very important that you read and understand the following information. If any of it causes you special concern, check with your doctor or pharmacist. Also, *if you have any questions* or if you want more information about this medicine or your medical problem, *ask your doctor, nurse, or pharmacist.*

Before Using This Medicine

If you are taking this medicine without a prescription, carefully read and follow any precautions on the label. For sodium bicarbonate, the following should be considered:

Allergies—Tell your doctor if you have ever had any unusual or allergic reaction to sodium bicarbonate. Also tell your doctor and pharmacist if you are allergic to any other substances, such as foods, preservatives, or dyes.

Pregnancy—Sodium bicarbonate is absorbed by the body and although it has not been shown to cause problems, the chance always exists. In addition, medicines containing sodium should usually be avoided if you tend to retain (keep) body water.

Breast-feeding—It is not known whether sodium bicarbonate passes into the breast milk. However, this medicine has not been reported to cause problems in nursing babies.

Children—Antacids should not be given to young children (up to 6 years of age) unless prescribed by a physician. This medicine may not help and may even worsen some conditions, so make sure that your child's problem should be treated with this medicine before you use it.

Older adults—Many medicines have not been studied specifically in older people. Therefore, it may not be known whether they work exactly the same way they do in younger adults or if they cause different side effects or problems in older people. There is no specific information comparing use of sodium bicarbonate in the elderly with use in other age groups.

Other medicines—Although certain medicines should not be used together at all, in other cases two different medicines may be used together even if an interaction might occur. In these cases, your doctor may want to change the dose, or other precautions may be necessary. When you are taking sodium bicarbonate, it is especially important that your doctor and pharmacist know if you are taking any of the following:

- Ketoconazole (e.g., Nizoral) or
- Tetracyclines (medicine for infection) taken by mouth—Use with sodium bicarbonate may result in lower blood levels of these medicines, possibly decreasing their effectiveness
- Mecamylamine (e.g., Inversine)—Use with sodium bicarbonate may increase the effects of mecamylamine
- Methenamine (e.g., Mandelamine)—Use with sodium bicarbonate may reduce the effects of methenamine

Other medical problems—The presence of other medical problems may affect the use of sodium bicarbonate. Make sure you tell your doctor if you have any other medical problems, especially:

- Appendicitis or
- Intestinal or rectal bleeding—Oral forms of sodium bicarbonate may make these conditions worse
- Edema (swelling of feet or lower legs) or
- Heart disease or
- High blood pressure (hypertension)
- Kidney disease or
- Liver disease or
- Problems with urination or
- Toxemia of pregnancy—Sodium bicarbonate may cause the body to retain (keep) water, which may make these conditions worse

Proper Use of This Medicine

For safe and effective use of sodium bicarbonate:

- Follow your doctor's instructions if this medicine was prescribed.
- Follow the manufacturer's package directions if you are treating yourself.

For patients *taking this medicine for a stomach ulcer:*

- *Take it exactly as directed and for the full time of treatment as ordered by your doctor,* to obtain maximum relief of your symptoms.
- Take it 1 and 3 hours after meals and at bedtime for best results, unless otherwise directed by your doctor.

If you must take this medicine regularly and you miss a dose, take it as soon as possible. However, if it is almost time for your next dose, skip the missed dose and go back to your regular dosing schedule. Do not double doses.

Storage—To store this medicine:

- Keep out of the reach of children.
- Store away from heat and direct light.
- Do not store the powder or tablet form of this medicine in the bathroom, near the kitchen sink, or in other damp places. Heat or moisture may cause the medicine to break down.
- Do not keep outdated medicine or medicine no longer needed. Be sure that any discarded medicine is out of the reach of children.

Precautions While Using This Medicine

If this medicine has been ordered by your doctor and if you will be taking it regularly for a long time, your doctor should check your progress at regular visits. This is to make sure the medicine does not cause unwanted effects.

Do not take sodium bicarbonate:

- *Within 1 to 2 hours of taking other medicine by mouth.* To do so may keep the other medicine from working properly.
- *For a long period of time.* To do so may increase the chance of side effects.

For patients on a *sodium-restricted diet*:

- This medicine contains a large amount of sodium. If you have any questions about this, check with your doctor or pharmacist.

For patients *taking this medicine as an antacid*:

- *Do not take this medicine if you have any signs of appendicitis* (such as stomach or lower abdominal pain, cramping, bloating, soreness, nausea, or vomiting). Instead, check with your doctor as soon as possible.
- *Do not take this medicine with large amounts of milk or milk products.* To do so may increase the chance of side effects.
- *Do not take sodium bicarbonate for more than 2 weeks* or if the problem comes back often. Instead, check with your doctor. Antacids should be used only for occasional relief, unless otherwise directed by your doctor.

Side Effects of This Medicine

Along with its needed effects, a medicine may cause some unwanted effects. Although the following side effects occur very rarely when this medicine is taken as recommended, they may be more likely to occur if it is taken:

- In large doses.
- For a long time.
- By patients with kidney disease.

Check with your doctor as soon as possible if any of the following side effects occur:

Frequent urge to urinate; headache (continuing); loss of appetite (continuing); mood or mental changes; muscle pain or twitching; nausea or vomiting; nervousness or restlessness; slow breathing; swelling of feet or lower legs; unpleasant taste; unusual tiredness or weakness

Other side effects may occur that usually do not need medical attention. These side effects may go away during treatment as your body adjusts to the medicine. However, check with your doctor if any of the following side effects continue or are bothersome:

Less common

Increased thirst; stomach cramps

Other side effects not listed above may also occur in some patients. If you notice any other effects, check with your doctor.

Annual revision: 02/03/92

SODIUM CHLORIDE Intra-amniotic

Description

Sodium chloride (SOE-dee-um KLOR-ide) as a 20% solution is given by injection into the uterus to cause abortion. It is to be administered only by or under the immediate care of your doctor. It is available in the following dosage form:

Parenteral

- Injection (U.S. and Canada)

It is very important that you read and understand the following information. If any of it causes you special concern, check with your doctor. Also, *if you have any questions* or if you want more information about this medicine or your medical problem, *ask your doctor, nurse, or pharmacist.*

Before Receiving This Medicine

In deciding to use a medicine, the risks of taking the medicine must be weighed against the good it will do.

This is a decision you and your doctor will make. For sodium chloride, the following should be considered:

Allergies—Tell your doctor if you have ever had any unusual or allergic reaction to sodium chloride. Also, tell your doctor and pharmacist if you are allergic to any other substances, such as foods, preservatives, or dyes.

Teenagers—Although there is no specific information comparing use of sodium chloride in adolescent females with use in other age groups, this medicine is not expected to cause different side effects or problems in adolescent females than it does in adults.

Other medicines—Although certain medicines should not be used together at all, in other cases two different medicines may be used together even if an interaction might occur. In these cases, your doctor may want to change the dose, or other precautions may be necessary. Tell your doctor and pharmacist if you are taking any other prescription or nonprescription (over-the-counter [OTC]) medicine.

Other medical problems—The presence of other medical problems may affect the use of sodium chloride. Make sure you tell your doctor if you have any other medical problems, especially:

- Bleeding problems
- Epilepsy
- Fibroid tumors of the uterus
- Heart or blood vessel disease
- High blood pressure (hypertension)
- Kidney disease

Proper Use of This Medicine

Unless otherwise directed by your doctor, drink at least 2 liters (about 2 quarts) of fluids the day that this procedure is to be done.

Side Effects of This Medicine

Along with its needed effects, a medicine may cause some unwanted effects. Although not all of these effects may occur, if they do occur they may need medical attention.

Check with your doctor or nurse immediately if any of the following side effects occur during the time that the injection is being given:

Less common

Burning pain in lower abdomen; confusion; feeling of heat; feeling of warmth in lips and tongue; headache (severe); nervousness; numbness of the fingertips; pain in lower back, pelvis, or stomach; ringing in the ears; thirst (sudden) or salty taste

Other side effects may occur that usually do not need medical attention. These side effects usually go away after the medicine is stopped. However, let the doctor or nurse know if either of the following side effects continues or is bothersome:

More common

Fever; flushing or redness of face

After the procedure is completed, this procedure may still produce some side effects that need medical attention. Check with your doctor if you notice any of the following side effects:

Chills or shivering; fever; foul-smelling vaginal discharge; increase in bleeding from the uterus; pain in lower abdomen

Other side effects not listed above may also occur in some patients. If you notice any other effects, check with your doctor or nurse.

Annual revision: 07/28/93

SODIUM FLUORIDE Systemic

Some commonly used brand names are:

In the U.S.

Fluoritab	Karidium
Fluorodex	Luride
Flura	Luride-SF
Flura-Drops	Pediaflor

Generic name product may also be available.

In Canada

Fluor-A-Day	Pedi-Dent
Fluotic	Solu-Flur
Karidium	

Description

Fluoride has been found to be helpful in reducing the number of cavities in the teeth. It is usually present naturally in drinking water. However, some areas of the country do not have a high enough level in the water to prevent cavities. To make up for this, extra fluorides may be added to the diet. Some children may require both dietary fluorides and topical fluoride treatments by the dentist. Use of a fluoride toothpaste or rinse may be helpful as well.

Taking fluorides does not replace good dental habits. These include eating a good diet, brushing and flossing teeth often, and having regular dental checkups.

Fluoride may also be used for other conditions as determined by your medical doctor or dentist.

This medicine is available only with your medical doctor's or dentist's prescription, in the following dosage forms:

Oral

- Oral solution (U.S. and Canada)
- Tablets (U.S. and Canada)
- Chewable tablets (U.S. and Canada)

It is very important that you read and understand the following information. If any of it causes you special concern, check with your medical doctor or dentist. Also, *if you have any questions* or if you want more information about this medicine or your problem, *ask your medical doctor, dentist, nurse, or pharmacist.*

Importance of Diet

Nutritionists recommend that, if possible, people should get all the fluoride they need from foods and or drinking water that has fluoride added to it. However, some people do not get enough fluoride from their diets. For these people, a fluoride supplement may be necessary.

In order to get enough vitamins and minerals in your regular diet, it is important that you eat a balanced and varied diet. Follow carefully any diet program your doctor may recommend. For your specific vitamin and/or minerals needs, ask your doctor for a list of appropriate foods.

Experts have developed a list of recommended dietary allowances (RDA) for most vitamins and some minerals. The RDA are not an exact number but a general idea of how much you need. They do not cover amounts needed for problems caused by a serious lack of vitamins and minerals. There are no RDA for fluoride. The following intakes are thought to be plenty for most individuals:

- Infants and children—
  Birth to 6 months of age: 0.1 to 0.5 mg a day.
  1 to 3 years of age: 0.5 to 1.5 mg a day.
  4 to 6 years of age: 1 to 2.5 mg a day.
  7 to 10 years of age: 1.5 to 2.5 mg a day.
- Adolescent and adult men and women: 1.5 to 4 mg a day.

People get needed fluoride from fish that are eaten with their bones, tea, and drinking water that has fluoride added to it. Food that is cooked in water containing fluoride or in Teflon-coated pans also provides fluoride. However, foods cooking in aluminium pans provide less fluoride.

Remember:

- The total amount of fluoride you get every day includes what you get from the foods and beverages that you eat and what you may take as a supplement.
- This total amount *should not* be greater than the above recommendations, unless ordered by your doctor. Taking too much fluoride can cause serious problems to the teeth and bones.

Before Using This Medicine

In deciding to use a medicine, the risks of taking the medicine must be weighed against the good it will do. This is a decision you and your medical doctor or dentist will make. For sodium fluoride, the following should be considered:

Allergies—Tell your medical doctor, dentist, and pharmacist if you are allergic to any other substances, such as foods, preservatives, or dyes.

Pregnancy—Sodium fluoride occurs naturally in water and has not been shown to cause problems in infants of mothers who drank fluoridated water or took appropriate doses of supplements.

Breast-feeding—Small amounts of sodium fluoride pass into breast milk.

Children—Doses of sodium fluoride that are too large or are taken for a long time may cause bone problems and teeth discoloration in children.

Older adults—Older people are more likely to have joint pain, kidney problems, or stomach ulcers which may be made worse by taking large doses of sodium fluoride. You should check with your doctor.

Other medicines—Although certain medicines should not be used together at all, in other cases two different medicines may be used together even if an interaction might occur. In these cases, your medical doctor or dentist may want to change the dose, or other precautions may be necessary. Tell your medical doctor, dentist, and pharmacist if you are taking/using any other prescription or nonprescription (over-the-counter [OTC]) medicine.

Other medical problems—The presence of other medical problems may affect the use of sodium fluoride. Make sure you tell your medical doctor or dentist if you have any other medical problems, especially:

- Brown, white, or black discoloration of teeth or
- Joint pain or
- Kidney problems (severe) or
- Stomach ulcer—Sodium fluoride may make these conditions worse

Before you begin using any new medicine (prescription or nonprescription) or if you develop any new medical problem while you are using this medicine, check with your medical doctor, dentist, nurse, or pharmacist.

Proper Use of This Medicine

Take this medicine only as directed by your medical doctor or dentist. Do not take more of it and do not take it more often than ordered. Taking too much fluoride over a period of time may cause unwanted effects.

For patients taking the *chewable tablet form* of this medicine:

- Tablets should be chewed or crushed before they are swallowed.
- This medicine works best if it is taken at bedtime, after the teeth have been thoroughly brushed. Do not eat or drink for at least 15 minutes after taking sodium fluoride.

For patients taking the *oral liquid form* of this medicine:

- This medicine is to be taken by mouth even though it comes in a dropper bottle. The amount to be taken is to be measured with the specially marked dropper.
- *Always store this medicine in the original plastic container.* Fluoride will affect glass and should not be stored in glass containers.
- This medicine may be dropped directly into the mouth or mixed with cereal, fruit juice, or other food. However, if this medicine is mixed with foods or beverages that contain calcium, the amount of sodium fluoride that is absorbed may be reduced.

Missed dose—If you miss a dose of this medicine, take it as soon as you remember. However, if it is almost time for the next dose, skip the missed dose and go back to your regular dosing schedule. Do not double doses. If you have any questions about this, check with your medical doctor or dentist.

Storage—To store this medicine:

- Keep out of the reach of children, since overdose is especially dangerous in children.
- Store away from heat and direct light.
- Do not store in the bathroom, near the kitchen sink, or in other damp places. Heat or moisture may cause the medicine to break down.
- Protect the oral liquid from freezing.
- Do not keep outdated medicine or medicine no longer needed. Be sure that any discarded medicine is out of the reach of children.

Precautions While Using This Medicine

The level of fluoride present in the water is different in different parts of the U.S. If you move to another area, check with a medical doctor or dentist in the new area as soon as possible to see if this medicine is still needed or if the dose needs to be changed. Also, check with your medical doctor or dentist if you change infant feeding habits (e.g., breast-feeding to infant formula), drinking water (e.g., city water to nonfluoridated bottled water), or filtration (e.g., tap water to filtered tap water).

Do not take calcium supplements or aluminum hydroxide–containing products and sodium fluoride at the same time. It is best to space doses of these two products 2 hours apart, to get the full benefit from each medicine.

Inform your medical doctor or dentist as soon as possible if you notice white, brown, or black spots on the teeth. These are signs of too much fluoride in children when it is given during periods of tooth development.

Side Effects of This Medicine

Along with its needed effects, a medicine may cause some unwanted effects. Although not all of these side effects may occur, if they do occur they may need medical attention.

Check with your doctor as soon as possible if any of the following side effects occur(s):

Sores in mouth and on lips (rare)

Sodium fluoride in drinking water or taken as a supplement does not usually cause any side effects. However, *taking an overdose of fluoride may cause serious problems.*

Stop taking this medicine and check with your medical doctor or dentist immediately if any of the following side effects occur, as they may be symptoms of severe overdose:

Black, tarry stools; bloody vomit; diarrhea; drowsiness; faintness; increased watering of mouth; nausea or vomiting; shallow breathing; stomach cramps or pain; tremors; unusual excitement; watery eyes; weakness

Check with your medical doctor or dentist as soon as possible if the following side effects occur, as some may be early symptoms of possible chronic overdose:

Pain and aching of bones; stiffness; white, brown, or black discoloration of teeth—occur only during periods of tooth development in children

Other side effects not listed above may also occur in some patients. If you notice any other effects, check with your medical doctor or dentist.

Annual revision: 07/17/92

SODIUM IODIDE Systemic†

A commonly used brand name in the U.S. is Iodopen.

†Not commercially available in Canada.

Description

Sodium iodide is used to prevent or treat iodine deficiency.

The body needs iodine for normal growth and health. For patients who are unable to get enough iodine in their regular diet or who have a need for more iodine, sodium iodide may be necessary.

Iodine deficiency in the United States is rare because iodine is added to table salt. Most people get enough salt from the foods they eat, without adding salt to their meals. Iodine deficiency is a problem in other areas of the world.

Lack of iodine may lead to thyroid problems, mental problems, hearing loss, and goiter.

Sodium iodide is available by itself only as an injection, which is given by your doctor or under your doctor's supervision. Some multivitamin/mineral preparations that contain sodium iodide are available without your doctors prescription.

Sodium iodide is available in the following dosage form:

Parenteral

Sodium Iodide
- Injection (U.S.)

It is very important that you read and understand the following information. If any of it causes you special concern, check with your doctor. Also, *if you have any questions* or if you want more information about this medicine or your medical problem, *ask your doctor, nurse, or pharmacist.*

Importance of Diet

Nutritionists recommend that, if possible, people should get all the iodine they need from foods. However, some people may not get enough iodine from their diets. Others may need more iodine than normal. For such people, an iodine supplement is important.

In order to get enough vitamins and minerals in your diet, it is important that you eat a balanced and varied diet. Follow carefully any diet program your doctor may recommend. For your specific vitamin and/or mineral needs, ask your doctor for a list of appropriate foods.

Iodine is found in various foods, including seafood, small amounts of iodized salt, and vegetables grown in iodine-rich soils. Iodine-containing mist from the ocean is another important source of iodine, since iodine is absorbed by the skin. Iodized salt provides 76 mcg of iodine per gram of salt.

Experts have developed a list of recommended dietary allowances (RDA) for most vitamins and some minerals. The RDA are not an exact number but a general idea of how much you need. They do not cover amounts needed for problems caused by a serious lack of vitmains and minerals.

The RDA for iodine are:

Infants and children—
- Birth to 6 months of age: 40 micrograms (mcg) a day.
- 6 months to 1 year of age: 50 mcg a day.
- 1 to 3 years of age: 70 mcg a day.
- 4 to 6 years of age: 90 mcg a day.
- 7 to 10 years of age: 120 mcg a day.

Adolescent and adult males—150 mcg a day.
Adolescent and adult females—150 mcg a day.
Pregnant females—175 mcg a day.
Breast-feeding females—200 mcg a day.

Remember:
- The total amount of iodine that you get every day includes what you get from the foods that you eat *and* what you may take as a supplement.
- This total amount should not be greater than the RDA, unless ordered by your doctor.

Before Using This Medicine

In deciding to use a medicine, the risks of taking the medicine must be weighed against the good it will do. This is a decision you and your doctor will make. For sodium iodide, the following should be considered:

Allergies—Tell your doctor if you have ever had any unusual or allergic reaction to iodine, iodine-containing foods, or sodium iodide. Also tell your doctor and pharmacist if you are allergic to any other substances, such as foods, preservatives, or dyes.

Pregnancy—It is especially important that you are receiving enough vitamins and minerals when you become pregnant and that you continue to receive the right amount of vitamins and minerals throughout your pregnancy. The healthy growth and development of the fetus depend on a steady supply of nutrients from the mother. A deficiency of iodine in the mother may cause nerve or growth problems for the fetus. Taking high doses of sodium iodide may cause thyroid problems or goiter in the newborn infant.

Breast-feeding—It is important that you receive the right amounts of vitamins and minerals so that your baby will also get the vitamins and minerals needed to grow properly. Taking high doses of sodium iodide may cause skin rash and thyroid problems in nursing babies.

Children—It is especially important that children receive enough iodine in their diet for healthy growth and development. However, high doses of sodium iodide may cause skin rash and thyroid problems in infants.

Older adults—It is important that older people continue to receive enough iodine in their daily diets.

Other medicines—Although certain medicines should not be used together at all, in other cases two different medicines may be used together even if an interaction might occur. In these cases, your doctor may want to change the dose, or other precautions may be necessary. When you are taking sodium iodide, it is especially important that your doctor and pharmacist know if you are taking any of the following:

- Antithyroid agents (medicine for overactive thyroid)—These medicines may prevent sodium iodide from working properly
- Iodine-containing medicines, other—Use of these medicines with sodium iodide may increase blood levels of iodine, which may increase the chance of side effects
- Lithium (e.g., Lithane)—Use of this medicine with sodium iodide may increase the chance of side effects

Other medical problems—The presence of other medical problems may affect the use of sodium iodide. Make sure you tell your doctor if you have any other medical problems, especially:

- Kidney disease—Use of sodium iodide may increase the amount of iodine in the blood and increase the chance of side effects
- Thyroid disease—This condition may increase the chance of side effects of sodium iodide
- Tuberculosis—Use of sodium iodide may make this condition worse

Before you begin using any new medicine (prescription or nonprescription) or if you develop any new medical problem while you are using this medicine, check with your doctor, nurse, or pharmacist.

Proper Use of This Medicine

Some people believe that taking very large doses of a vitamin or mineral (called megadoses) is useful for treating certain medical problems. Studies have not proven this. Large doses should be taken only under the direction of your doctor after need has been identified.

Missed dose—If you miss taking sodium iodide for one or more days there is no cause for concern, since it takes some time for your body to become seriously low in iodine. However, if your doctor has recommended that you take iodine try to remember to use it as directed every day.

Storage—To store this medicine:

- Keep out of the reach of children.
- Store away from heat and direct light.
- Do not store in the bathroom, near the kitchen sink, or in other damp places. Heat or moisture may cause the medicine to break down.
- Keep the medicine from freezing. Do not refrigerate.
- Do not keep outdated medicine or medicine no longer needed. Be sure that any discarded medicine is out of the reach of children.

Precautions While Using This Medicine

Many other products contain iodine. For example, iodine is absorbed through the skin from some skin cleansers (e.g., povidone-iodine). It may be especially important that infants and small children not receive large amounts of iodine. Check with your doctor before using any other products that contain iodine while you are using this medicine.

Side Effects of This Medicine

Along with its needed effects, a medicine may cause some unwanted effects. Although not all of these side effects may occur, if they do occur they may need medical attention. When this medicine is used at low doses, side effects are rare.

Check with your doctor as soon as possible if any of the following side effects occur:

Less common

Hives; joint pain; swelling of arms, face, legs, lips, tongue, and/or throat; swelling of lymph glands

With long-term use

Burning of mouth or throat; headache (severe); increased watering of mouth; metallic taste; skin sores; soreness of teeth and gums; stomach irritation

Other side effects not listed above may also occur in some patients. If you notice any other effects, check with your doctor.

Additional Information

Once a medicine has been approved for marketing for a certain use, experience may show that it is also useful for other medical problems. Although this use is not included in product labeling, injections of sodium iodide are used in certain patients with the following medical condition:

- Thyrotoxicosis crisis (severe overactive thyroid)

Other than the above information, there is no additional information relating to proper use, precautions, or side effects for this use.

Annual revision: 02/26/92

SODIUM IODIDE I 131 Therapeutic

Description

Sodium iodide (EYE-oh-dyed) I 131 (radioactive iodine) is a radiopharmaceutical (ray-dee-oh-far-ma-SOO-ti-kal). Radiopharmaceuticals are radioactive agents, which may be used to treat certain diseases or to study the function of the body's organs.

Sodium iodide I 131 is used to treat an overactive thyroid gland and certain kinds of thyroid cancer. It builds up mainly in the thyroid gland. Large doses of sodium iodide I 131 are usually used after thyroid cancer surgery to destroy any remaining diseased thyroid tissue.

When very small doses are given, a measure of the radioactivity taken up by the gland helps determine the function of the thyroid gland. Also, an image of the organ on paper or a computer print out can be provided.

The information that follows applies only to the use of sodium iodide I 131 in treating an overactive or cancerous thyroid gland.

Sodium iodide I 131 is to be given only by or under the direct supervision of a doctor with specialized training in nuclear medicine. It is available in the following dosage forms:

Oral

- Capsules (U.S. and Canada)
- Solution (U.S. and Canada)

It is very important that you read and understand the following information. If any of it causes you special concern, check with your doctor. Also, *if you have any questions* or if you want more information about this medicine or your medical problem, *ask your doctor, nurse, or pharmacist.*

Before Using This Medicine

In deciding to use a medicine, the risks of taking the medicine must be weighed against the good it will do. This is a decision you and your doctor will make. For sodium iodide I 131, the following should be considered:

Diet—If you eat large amounts of iodine-containing foods, such as iodized salt and seafoods, or cabbage, kale, rape (turnip-like vegetable), or turnips, the iodine contained in these foods will reduce the amount of this radiopharmaceutical that your thyroid gland will accept. Avoid these foods for at least 2 weeks before the treatment with radioactive iodine.

Pregnancy—Sodium iodide I 131 is not recommended for use during pregnancy. This is to avoid exposing the fetus to radiation. Also, it may cause the newborn baby to have an underactive thyroid gland. Be sure you have discussed this with your doctor.

Breast-feeding—Sodium iodide I 131 passes into the breast milk and may cause unwanted effects, such as underactive thyroid, in the nursing baby. If you must receive this radiopharmaceutical, it may be necessary for you to stop breast-feeding. Be sure you have discussed this with your doctor.

Children—Children and adolescents are especially sensitive to the effects of radiation. This may increase the chance of side effects during and after treatment. Also, the younger the patient is at the time of treatment, the greater the chance of later developing an underactive thyroid gland. Be sure you have discussed this with your doctor.

Older adults—Sodium iodide I 131 has been used in older people and has not been shown to cause different side effects or problems in older people than it does in younger adults.

Other medicines/tests—If you have had an x-ray test recently for which you were given a radiopaque agent that contained iodine. The iodine contained in the radiopaque agent will reduce the amount of sodium iodide I 131 that your thyroid gland will accept.

Other medical problems—The presence of other medical problems may affect the use of sodium iodide I 131. Make sure you tell your doctor if you have any other medical problems, especially:

- Diarrhea or
- Vomiting—May indicate a more serious condition and treatment may aggravate symptoms
- Iodine deficiency—The thyroid gland will take more of the sodium iodide I 131 than it would normally take
- Kidney disease—Elimination of radioactive iodine from the body may decrease

- If you have heart disease and are receiving sodium iodide I 131 to treat an overactive thyroid—The radiation may worsen the thyroid condition if antithyroid medicine and/or beta-blockers, such as propranolol, are not given before and after treatment

Before you begin using any new medicine (prescription or nonprescription) or if you develop any new medical problem while you are using this medicine, check with your doctor, nuclear medicine physician and/or technologist, nuclear pharmacist, or nurse.

Proper Use of This Medicine

Your doctor may have special instructions for you in preparation for your test or treatment. If you have not received such instructions or you do not understand them, check with your doctor in advance.

Precautions After Using This Medicine

There are no special precautions when this drug is used in very small doses to help study the activity of the thyroid. However, if you are receiving sodium iodide I 131 for an overactive thyroid or cancer of the thyroid, *follow these guidelines for 48 to 72 hours* after receiving the medicine, to help reduce the chance of contaminating other persons:

- *Do not kiss anyone, or handle or use another person's eating or drinking utensils, toothbrush, or bathroom glass.*
- *Do not engage in any sexual activities.*
- *Do not sit close to others and do not hold children in your lap for long periods of time.*
- Sleep alone.
- *Wash the tub and sink after each use (including after brushing teeth).*
- *Wash your hands after using the toilet.*
- Use a separate towel and washcloth.
- Wash your clothes, bed linens, and eating utensils separately.
- Sodium iodide I 131 is passed in the urine. To prevent contamination of your home environment, *flush the toilet twice after urination.*

To increase the flow of urine and lessen the amount of radioactive iodine in your body, drink plenty of liquids.

Side Effects of This Medicine

Studies have not shown that sodium iodide I 131 increases the chance of cancer or other long-term problems. When used to treat an overactive thyroid gland or cancer of the thyroid, sodium iodide I 131 may cause the patient to have an underactive thyroid gland after treatment. Before receiving this medicine, be sure you have discussed its use with your doctor.

Along with its needed effects, a medicine may cause some unwanted effects. Although not all of these side effects may occur, if they do occur they may need medical attention.

When this drug is used in very small doses to help study the function of the gland, side effects are rare. However, check with your doctor as soon as possible if any of the following side effects occur after treatment for overactive thyroid or cancer of the thyroid:

In treatment of overactive thyroid or cancer of the thyroid

Symptoms of an underactive thyroid

Changes in menstrual periods; clumsiness; coldness; drowsiness; dry, puffy skin; headache; listlessness; muscle aches; thinning of hair (temporary)—may occur 2 to 3 months after treatment; unusual tiredness or weakness; weight gain

Rare

In treatment of overactive thyroid

Unusual irritability; unusual tiredness

In treatment of cancer of the thyroid

Fever, chills, and sore throat; unusual bleeding or bruising

Other side effects may occur that usually do not need medical attention. These side effects may go away during treatment as your body adjusts to the medicine. However, check with your doctor if any of the following side effects continue or are bothersome:

Less common

In treatment of overactive thyroid or cancer of the thyroid

Neck tenderness or swelling; sore throat

In treatment of cancer of the thyroid

Loss of taste (temporary); nausea and vomiting (temporary); tenderness of salivary glands

Other side effects not listed above may also occur in some patients. If you notice any other effects, check with your doctor.

Annual revision: August 1990

SODIUM PHOSPHATE P 32 Therapeutic

Description

Sodium phosphate (SOE-dee-um FOS-fate) P 32 is a radiopharmaceutical (ray-dee-oh-far-ma-SOO-ti-kal). Radiopharmaceuticals are radioactive agents that may be used to treat certain diseases or to study the activity of the body's organs.

Sodium phosphate P 32 is used to treat certain kinds of cancer. In this case, the radioactive agent builds up in the cancerous area and destroys the affected tissue. This radiopharmaceutical may also be used for other conditions as determined by your doctor.

Sodium phosphate P 32 is to be given only by or under the direct supervision of a doctor with specialized training in nuclear medicine. It is available in the following dosage form:

Parenteral

- Solution (U.S. and Canada)

It is very important that you read and understand the following information. If any of it causes you special concern, check with your doctor. Also, *if you have any questions* or if you want more information about this medicine or your medical problem, *ask your doctor, nurse, or pharmacist.*

Before Using This Medicine

In deciding to use a medicine, the risks of taking the medicine must be weighed against the good it will do. This is a decision you and your doctor will make. For sodium phosphate P 32, the following should be considered:

Allergies—Tell your doctor if you have ever had any unusual or allergic reaction to sodium phosphate P 32. Also tell your doctor if you are allergic to any other substances, such as foods, preservatives, or dyes.

Pregnancy—Studies have not been done in either humans or animals. However, to avoid exposing the fetus to radiation, sodium phosphate P 32 is not recommended for use during pregnancy. Be sure you have discussed this with your doctor.

Breast-feeding—Sodium phosphate may pass into the breast milk. If you must receive this radiopharmaceutical, it will be necessary for you to stop breast-feeding during treatment. Be sure you have discussed this with your doctor.

Children—Studies on this medicine have been done only in adult patients, and there is no specific information about its use in children. However, children are especially sensitive to the effects of radiation. This may increase the chance of side effects during and after treatment.

Older adults—Older adults are especially sensitive to the effects of radiation. This may increase the chance of side effects during and after treatment.

Other medicines—Although certain medicines should not be used together at all, in other cases two different medicines may be used together even if an interaction might occur. In these cases, your doctor may want to change the dose, or other precautions may be necessary. When you are receiving sodium phosphate P 32, it is especially important that your doctor know if you are taking any other prescription or nonprescription (over-the-counter [OTC]) medicine.

Other medical problems—The presence of other medical problems may affect the use of sodium phosphate P 32. Make sure you tell your doctor if you have any other medical problems.

Proper Use of This Medicine

Your doctor may have special instructions for you in preparation for your treatment. If you do not understand them or if you have not received such instructions, check with your doctor in advance.

Dosing—The doses of radiopharmaceuticals will be different for different patients and for the different types of treatments. The amount of radioactivity of a radiopharmaceutical is expressed in units called becquerels or curies. Usual adult doses of sodium phosphate P 32 range from 37 megabecquerels (1 millicurie) to 185 megabecquerels (5 millicuries). The dose you receive depends on your size, age, and blood test measurements (blood counts). The amount of radiation received by the body to treat a disease is many times higher than from any diagnostic test, such as x-rays and nuclear medicine scans. Repeated doses may be necessary, depending on the kind of disease you have and how your body is responding to treatment.

Side Effects of This Medicine

Along with its needed effects, a medicine may cause some unwanted effects. When sodium phosphate P 32 is used at recommended doses, side effects usually are rare. However, blood problems, such as anemia or a decrease in the number of white blood cells, may occur in some patients.

Also, the following side effects may occur in patients with bone cancer receiving sodium phosphate P 32 for the relief of bone pain:

More common

Diarrhea, fever, nausea, vomiting

Other side effects not listed above may also occur in some patients. If you notice any other effects, check with your doctor.

Annual revision: 07/16/93

SPECTINOMYCIN Systemic

A commonly used brand name in the U.S. and Canada is Trobicin.

Description

Spectinomycin (spek-ti-noe-MYE-sin) is used to treat most types of gonorrhea. It is given by injection into a muscle. It is sometimes given with other medicines for gonorrhea and related infections.

Spectinomycin may be used in patients who are allergic to penicillins, cephalosporins, or probenecid (e.g., Benemid). This medicine is also used to treat recent sexual partners of patients who have gonorrhea. However, spectinomycin will not work for gonorrhea of the throat, syphilis, colds, flu, or other virus infections.

Spectinomycin is available only with your doctor's prescription, in the following dosage form:

Parenteral

- Injection (U.S. and Canada)

It is very important that you read and understand the following information. If any of it causes you special concern, check with your doctor. Also, *if you have any questions* or if you want more information about this medicine or your medical problem, *ask your doctor, nurse, or pharmacist.*

Before Receiving This Medicine

In deciding to use a medicine, the risks of taking the medicine must be weighed against the good it will do. This is a decision you and your doctor will make. For spectinomycin, the following should be considered:

Allergies—Tell your doctor if you have ever had any unusual or allergic reaction to spectinomycin. Also tell your doctor and pharmacist if you are allergic to any other substances, such as foods, preservatives, or dyes.

Pregnancy—Studies have not been done in humans. However, spectinomycin has been recommended for the treatment of gonorrhea and related infections in pregnant patients who are allergic to penicillins, cephalosporins, or probenecid (e.g., Benemid). In addition, studies in animals have not shown that spectinomycin causes birth defects or other problems.

Breast-feeding—It is not known if spectinomycin passes into breast milk. However, spectinomycin has not been reported to cause problems in nursing babies.

Children—This medicine has been used in a limited number of children. In effective doses, the medicine has not been shown to cause different side effects or problems than it does in adults. However, use in infants is not recommended.

Older adults—Many medicines have not been studied specifically in older people. Therefore, it may not be known whether they work exactly the same way they do in younger adults. Although there is no specific information comparing use of spectinomycin in the elderly with use in other age groups, this medicine is not expected to cause different side effects or problems in older people than it does in younger adults.

Other medicines—Although certain medicines should not be used together at all, in other cases two different medicines may be used together even if an interaction might occur. In these cases, your doctor may want to change the dose, or other precautions may be necessary. Tell your doctor and pharmacist if you are taking any other prescription or nonprescription (over-the-counter [OTC]) medicine.

Before you begin using any new medicine (prescription or nonprescription) or if you develop any new medical problem while you are using this medicine, check with your doctor, nurse, or pharmacist.

Proper Use of This Medicine

Spectinomycin is given by injection into a muscle. To help clear up your gonorrhea completely, usually only one dose is needed. However, in some infections a second dose of this medicine may be required.

Gonorrhea and related infections are spread by having sex with an infected partner. Therefore, it may be desirable that the male sexual partner wear a condom (prophylactic) during intercourse to prevent infection. Also, it may be necessary for your partner to be treated at the same time you are being treated. This will help to avoid passing the infection back and forth.

Dosing—The dose of spectinomycin will be different for different patients. The following information includes only the average doses of spectinomycin.

- For *cervical, rectal, or urethral gonorrhea*:
  —Adults and children 45 kilograms of body weight (99 pounds) and over: 2 grams injected into a muscle as a single dose.
  —Children up to 45 kilograms of body weight (99 pounds): 40 milligrams per kilogram of body weight injected into a muscle as a single dose.
  —Infants: Use is not recommended.

Precautions After Receiving This Medicine

If your symptoms do not improve within a few days, or if they become worse, check with your doctor.

This medicine may cause some people to become dizzy. *Make sure you know how you react to this medicine before you drive, use machines, or do anything else that could be dangerous if you are dizzy.* If this reaction is especially bothersome, check with your doctor.

Side Effects of This Medicine

Along with its needed effects, a medicine may cause some unwanted effects. Although not all of these side effects may occur, if they do occur they may need medical attention.

Check with your doctor as soon as possible if any of the following side effects occur:

Rare

Chills or fever; itching or redness of the skin

Other side effects may occur that usually do not need medical attention. These side effects may go away during treatment as your body adjusts to the medicine. However, check with your doctor if any of these effects continue or are bothersome:

Less common

Dizziness; nausea and vomiting; pain at the place of injection; stomach cramps

Other side effects not listed above may also occur in some patients. If you notice any other effects, check with your doctor.

Annual revision: 02/23/93

SPERMICIDES Vaginal

This information applies to the following medicines:

Benzalkonium (benz-al-KOE-nee-um) Chloride
Nonoxynol (no-NOX-i-nole) 9
Octoxynol (awk-TOX-i-nole) 9

Some commonly used brand names are:

For Benzalkonium Chloride*

In Canada

Pharmatex

For Nonoxynol 9

In the U.S.

Because
Conceptrol Contraceptive Inserts
Conceptrol Gel
Delfen
Emko
Encare
Gynol II Extra Strength Contraceptive Jelly
Gynol II Original Formula Contraceptive Jelly
Koromex Crystal Clear Gel
Koromex Foam
Koromex Jelly
Ortho-Creme
Pre-Fil
Ramses Crystal Clear Gel
Semicid
Shur-Seal
Today
VCF

In Canada

Delfen
Emko
Ramses Contraceptive Foam
Ramses Contraceptive Vaginal Jelly
Today

Another commonly used name is nonoxinol 9.

For Octoxynol 9

In the U.S.

Koromex Cream
Ortho-Gynol

In Canada

Ortho-Gynol

Another commonly used name is octoxinol.

*Not commercially available in the U.S.

Description

Vaginal spermicides are a type of contraceptive (birth control). These products are inserted into the vagina *before* any genital contact occurs or sexual intercourse begins. They work by damaging and killing sperm in the vagina. Therefore, sperm are not able to travel from the vagina into the uterus and fallopian tubes, where fertilization usually takes place.

Vaginal spermicides when used alone are much less effective in preventing pregnancy than birth control pills or the IUD or spermicides used with another form of birth control such as the condom, cervical cap, diaphragm, or sponge. *Studies have shown that when spermicides are used alone, pregnancy usually occurs in 21 of each 100 women during the first year of spermicide use*. The number of pregnancies is reduced when spermicides are used with another method, especially the condom. Discuss with a doctor what your options are for birth control and the risks and benefits of each method.

Laboratory studies have shown that nonoxynol 9 kills or stops the growth of the AIDS virus (HIV) and herpes simplex I and II viruses. It was also shown to be effective against other types of organisms that cause gonorrhea, chlamydia, syphilis, trichomoniasis, and other sexually transmitted diseases (venereal disease, VD, STDs). Benzalkonium chloride also killed the AIDS virus in laboratory studies. Although this has *not* been proven in *human* studies, some scientists *believe* that if spermicides are put into the vagina or on the inside and outside of a latex (rubber) condom, they *may* kill these germs before they are able to come in contact with the vagina or rectum (lower bowel).

The most effective way to protect yourself against STDs (such as AIDS) is by abstinence (not having sexual intercourse) or by having one partner you can be sure is not already infected or is not going to get an STD. However, if either of these methods is not likely or possible, using latex (rubber) condoms with a spermicide is the best way of protecting yourself.

The use of a spermicide is recommended even when you are using nonbarrier methods of birth control such as birth control pills (the Pill) or intrauterine devices (IUDs), since these do not offer any protection from STDs.

The safety of using spermicides in the rectum (lower bowel), anus, or rectal area is not known. However, no side effects or problems have been reported that are different from those reported for use in the vagina.

Vaginal spermicides are available without a prescription, in the following dosage forms:

Vaginal

Benzalkonium chloride
- Suppositories (Canada)

Nonoxynol 9
- Cream (U.S. and Canada)
- Film (U.S.)
- Foam (U.S. and Canada)
- Gel (U.S.)
- Jelly (U.S. and Canada)
- Sponge (U.S. and Canada)
- Suppositories (U.S.)

Octoxynol 9
- Cream (U.S.)
- Jelly (U.S. and Canada)

It is very important that you read and understand the following information. If any of it causes you special concern, check with your doctor or pharmacist. Also, *if you have any questions* or if you want more information about this medicine or your medical problem, *ask your doctor, nurse, or pharmacist.*

Before Using This Medicine

In deciding to use vaginal spermicides, the risks of using them must be weighed against the good they will do. This is a decision you and possibly your doctor will make. The following information may help you in making your decision:

Allergies—If you have ever had any unusual or allergic reaction to benzalkonium chloride, nonoxynol 9, or octoxynol 9, it is best to check with your doctor before using vaginal spermicides.

Pregnancy—Many studies have shown that the use of vaginal spermicides does not increase the risk of birth defects or miscarriage.

Breast-feeding—It is not known if vaginal spermicides pass into breast milk in humans. However, their use has not been reported to cause problems in nursing babies.

Adolescents—These products have been used by teenagers and have not been shown to cause different side effects or problems than they do in adults. However, some younger users may need extra counseling and information on the importance of using spermicides exactly as they are supposed to be used so they will work properly.

Other medicines—Although certain medicines should not be used together at all, in other cases 2 different medicines may be used together even if an interaction might occur. In these cases, your doctor may want you to use the spermicide differently or other precautions may be necessary. When using vaginal spermicides, it is especially important that your doctor or pharmacist know if you are using any of the following:

- Salicylates used on the skin (e.g., some types of ointments for muscle aches) or
- Sulfonamides (sulfa medicine) for use in the vagina or
- Chemicals or substances such as aluminum, citrate, cotton, hydrogen peroxide, lanolin, iodides, nitrates, permanganates, some forms of silver, soaps, detergents, or tartrates—Benzalkonium chloride may not work if it comes in direct contact with these as well as many other chemicals
- Vaginal medicines, douches, or rinsing—For spermicides to work properly to prevent pregnancy, they must stay in contact with the sperm in the vagina for at least 6 or 8 hours (depending upon which brand of spermicide you use) after sexual intercourse. *Vaginal douching is not necessary after use of these medicines.* Douching too soon (even with just water) may stop the spermicide from working. Washing or rinsing the vaginal or rectal area may also make the spermicide ineffective in helping to prevent sexually transmitted diseases

Medical problems—The presence of certain medical problems may affect the use of vaginal spermicides. Since in some cases spermicides should not be used, check with your doctor if you have any of the following:

- Allergies, irritations, or infections of the genitals—Using vaginal spermicides may cause moderate to severe irritation in these conditions. Also, benzalkonium suppositories may be less effective in women with vaginal infections
- Conditions or medical problems where it is important that pregnancy does not occur—Vaginal spermicides when used alone are much less effective than birth control pills or the IUD or spermicides used with another form of birth control such as the condom, cervical cap, diaphragm, or sponge. Discuss with your doctor what your options are for birth control and the risks and benefits of each method.
- During the menstrual period or
- Recent childbirth or abortion or
- Toxic-shock syndrome (history of)—The cervical cap, contraceptive sponge, or diaphragm should not be used in these cases because there is an increased risk of toxic-shock syndrome; your doctor may recommend that you use condoms with a spermicide instead during your menstrual period
- Sores on the genitals (sex organs) or
- Irritation of the vagina—It is not known whether spermicides can cause breaks in the skin that could increase the chances of getting a sexually transmitted disease, especially AIDS. Discuss this with a doctor if you have any questions

If you develop any medical problem or begin using any new medicine (prescription or nonprescription) while you are using this medicine, you may want to check with your doctor.

Proper Use of This Medicine

It is very important that the spermicide be placed properly in the vagina. It should be put deep into the vagina, directly on the cervix (opening to the uterus). The written instructions about how the product container and the applicator work, how much spermicide to use each time, and how long each application remains effective may be different for each product. Make sure you carefully read and follow the instructions that come with each product.

Make sure the spermicide you choose is labeled as being safe for use with latex diaphragms, cervical caps, or condoms. Otherwise, it may cause the diaphragm, cervical cap, or condom to weaken and leak or even break during intercourse. If there is a leak or break during intercourse, it may be a good idea for a female partner to immediately place more spermicide in the vagina.

Spermicides, especially gels and jellies, provide some lubrication during sexual intercourse. *If you need an extra lubricant, make sure it is a water-based product safe for use with condoms, cervical caps, or diaphragms.* Oil-based products such as hand, face, or body cream; petroleum jelly; cooking oils or shortenings; or baby oil should *not* be used because they weaken the latex rubber. (Even some products that easily rinse away with water are oil-based and should not be used.) Use of oil-based products increases the chances of the condom breaking during sexual intercourse. These products can also cause the rubber in cervical caps or diaphragms to break down faster and wear out sooner.

For patients using spermicides with a cervical cap:

- *To be most effective at preventing pregnancy, the cervical cap must always be used with a spermicide.* Both must be used every time you have sexual intercourse.
- Before inserting the cervical cap, inspect it for holes, tears, or cracks. If there are holes or defects, the cervical cap will not work effectively, even with a spermicide. It must be replaced.
- Before you put the cap over the cervix (opening to the uterus), a spermicide cream, foam, gel, or jelly should be put into the cup of the cap. Follow the manufacturer's directions on how long before sexual intercourse you may apply the spermicide. Fill the cap one-third full with spermicide.
- To insert the cervical cap, squeeze the rim between your thumb and forefinger so that it is narrow enough to fit into the vagina. While in a comfortable position, push the cervical cap as deeply into the vagina as it will go. Release the rim and press it into place around the cervix with your finger. The rim should be round again and be directly on the cervix. The cap is held onto the cervix by suction.
- Some doctors may recommend that you put more spermicide into the vagina each time you repeat sexual intercourse using a cervical cap. You should also check to make sure the cap is in the proper position on the cervix before and after each time you have intercourse. You may wear the cervical cap for up to 48 hours (2 days).
- *Do not remove the cap if it has been less than 8 hours since the last time you had sexual intercourse.* For the cervical cap to be most effective at preventing pregnancy, it must remain in the vagina for at least 8 hours after sexual intercourse.
- To remove the cervical cap, use 1 or 2 fingers to push the rim away from the cervix. This will break the suction seal with the cervix. Then gently pull the cap out of the vagina.

For patients using spermicides with condoms:

- Condoms do not have to be used with spermicides, but the spermicide may provide a back-up in case the condom breaks or leaks.
- Spread some spermicide on the outside of the condom, after it is unrolled over the penis. It is even more important that a female partner also use a spermicide inside the vagina.
- Each time you repeat intercourse, a new condom must be used. *Condoms should never be reused.* Spermicide should also be applied outside of the new

condom. A female partner must also put more spermicide in the vagina for each time she has intercourse.

For patients using spermicides with a diaphragm:

- *To be most effective at preventing pregnancy, diaphragms must always be used with a spermicide.* Some women may choose to insert a diaphragm every night, to avoid the chance of unprotected sexual intercourse and unplanned pregnancy happening.
- Inspect the diaphragm for holes by holding it up to a light. If there are holes or defects, the diaphragm will not work effectively, even with a spermicide. It must be replaced.
- Before you put the diaphragm over the cervix (opening to the uterus), a spermicide cream, foam, gel, or jelly should be put into the cup of the diaphragm. Follow the manufacturer's directions on how much spermicide to use and how long before sexual intercourse you may apply the spermicide. Also, spread some spermicide all around the rim of the diaphragm that will be touching the cervix. Some doctors also advise spreading more spermicide on the outside of the cup of the diaphragm.
- To insert the diaphragm, squeeze the rim between your thumb and forefinger so that it is narrow enough to fit into the vagina. While in a comfortable position, push the diaphragm as deeply into the vagina as it will go. (Some women use a special applicator that makes it easier to insert the diaphragm.) Release the rim. The diaphragm rim should be round again and be directly on the cervix.
- Each time you repeat sexual intercourse, you should put more spermicide into the vagina. *Do not remove the diaphragm if it has been less than 6 or 8 hours (depending upon which brand of spermicide you use) since the last sexual intercourse.* For the diaphragm to be most effective at preventing pregnancy, it must remain in the vagina for at least 6 or 8 hours (depending upon which brand of spermicide you use) after sexual intercourse. Be careful not to move the diaphragm out of place while you are applying more spermicide.
- Do not wear the diaphragm for more than 24 hours, since doing so increases the risk of getting toxic-shock syndrome or a urinary tract (bladder) infection.
- To remove the diaphragm, hook one finger over the rim nearest the front. Pull the diaphragm downward and out of the vagina.

For patients using the contraceptive sponge:

- Before the sponge is inserted, activate the spermicide by wetting the sponge with clean water and squeezing it. When you insert the sponge, it should be very wet and foamy when it is squeezed.
- Fold the sponge in half so that the dimple side is facing up and the removal loop is facing down. Carefully insert the sponge into the vagina. Push it deeply into the vagina so that the dimple side fits directly onto the cervix (the opening to the uterus) and the removal loop is on the side of the sponge that faces out of the vagina.
- It is not necessary to use more spermicide during the 24 hours the sponge is in the correct position in the vagina, regardless of how many times you have sexual intercourse. You may also bathe or swim while the sponge is in the vagina.
- *For the sponge to be most effective at preventing pregnancy, it must remain in the vagina for at least 6 hours after the last intercourse. Do not wear the sponge for longer than 30 hours, since doing so increases the risk of getting toxic-shock syndrome.*
- Sometimes the sponge can move from its proper place during urination or a bowel movement. If the sponge moves away from its proper place on the cervix but does not come out of the vagina, use one finger to move it back into place. If the sponge comes completely out of the vagina, discard it. Then immediately wet a new sponge and insert it. Using a new sponge is necessary only if it has been less than 6 hours since the last sexual intercourse.
- To remove the contraceptive sponge, hook one finger through the removal loop and gently pull the sponge out of the vagina. *Contact a doctor immediately if you have problems removing the sponge.* Examples are tearing of the sponge or loop, breaking off pieces of the sponge in the vagina, or scratching or injuring the vagina. The chances of your getting toxic-shock syndrome may be increased if any of these things happen.

Storage—To store this medicine:

- Keep out of the reach of children.
- Store away from heat and direct light.
- Do not store in the bathroom, near the kitchen sink, or in other damp places. Heat or moisture may cause the medicine to break down.
- Do not refrigerate.
- Do not keep outdated products or products no longer needed. Be sure that any discarded products are out of the reach of children.

Precautions While Using This Medicine

During use of spermicides, either partner may notice burning, stinging, warmth, itching, or other irritation of the skin, sex organs, anus, or rectum. Using a weaker strength of vaginal spermicide or one with different ingredients may be necessary. If you are using benzalkonium chloride suppositories, it may help to wet them before they are inserted into the vagina. If any of these effects continue after you have changed products, you may have an allergy to these products or an infection and should contact a doctor as soon as possible.

Side Effects of This Medicine

Along with its needed effects, a medicine may cause some unwanted effects. Although not all of these side effects may occur, if they do occur they may need medical attention.

Check with a doctor *immediately* if any of the following side effects occur:

Rare

For the cervical cap, contraceptive sponge, or diaphragm only

Signs of toxic-shock syndrome such as:

Chills; confusion; dizziness; fever; lightheadedness; muscle aches; sunburn-like rash that is followed by peeling of the skin; unusual redness of the inside of the nose, mouth, throat, vagina, or insides of the eyelids

Also, check with a doctor as soon as possible if any of the following side effects occur:

Rare

For females and males

Skin rash, redness, irritation, or itching that does not subside or go away within a short period of time

For females only

Signs of urinary tract infection or vaginal allergy or infection such as:

Cloudy or bloody urine; increased frequency of urination; pain in the bladder or lower abdomen; pain on urination; thick, white, or curd-like vaginal discharge—with use of the cervical cap, contraceptive sponge, or diaphragm only; vaginal irritation, redness, rash, dryness, or whitish discharge

Other side effects may occur that usually do not need medical attention. However, check with a doctor if any of the following side effects continue or are bothersome:

Less common

Vaginal discharge (temporary)—for creams, foams, and suppositories; vaginal dryness or odor

Also, either partner may notice burning, stinging, warmth, itching, or other irritation of the skin, sex organs, anus, or rectum. Using a weaker strength of vaginal spermicide or one with different ingredients may be necessary. If you are using benzalkonium chloride suppositories, it may help to wet them before they are inserted into the vagina. If any of these effects continue after you have changed products, it is possible that you may have an infection and you should contact a doctor as soon as possible.

Other side effects not listed above may also occur in some people. If you notice any other effects, check with your doctor.

Annual revision: 07/28/93

STREPTOZOCIN Systemic

A commonly used brand name in the U.S. and Canada is Zanosar.

Description

Streptozocin (strep-toe-ZOE-sin) belongs to the group of medicines known as alkylating agents. It is used to treat cancer of the pancreas.

Streptozocin seems to interfere with the growth of cancer cells, which are eventually destroyed. It also directly affects the way the pancreas works. Since the growth of normal body cells may also be affected by streptozocin, other effects will also occur. Some of these may be serious and must be reported to your doctor. Other effects may not be serious but may cause concern. Some effects may not occur for months or years after the medicine is used.

Before you begin treatment with streptozocin, you and your doctor should talk about the good this medicine will do as well as the risks of using it.

Streptozocin is to be given only by or under the immediate supervision of your doctor. It is available in the following dosage form:

Parenteral

- Injection (U.S. and Canada)

It is very important that you read and understand the following information. If any of it causes you special concern, check with your doctor. Also, *if you have any questions* or if you want more information about this medicine or your medical problem, *ask your doctor, nurse, or pharmacist.*

Before Using This Medicine

In deciding to use a medicine, the risks of taking the medicine must be weighed against the good it will do.

This is a decision you and your doctor will make. For streptozocin, the following should be considered:

Allergies—Tell your doctor if you have ever had any unusual or allergic reaction to streptozocin.

Pregnancy—Tell your doctor if you are pregnant or if you intend to have children. There is a chance that this medicine may cause birth defects if either the male or the female is receiving it at the time of conception or if it is taken during pregnancy. Studies in rats and rabbits have shown that streptozocin causes birth defects or miscarriage. In addition, many cancer medicines may cause sterility which could be permanent. Although this has not been reported with this medicine, the possibility should be kept in mind.

Be sure that you have discussed this with your doctor before receiving this medicine. It is best to use some kind of birth control while you are receiving streptozocin. Tell your doctor right away if you think you have become pregnant while receiving streptozocin.

Breast-feeding—Tell your doctor if you are breast-feeding or if you intend to breast-feed during treatment with this medicine. Because streptozocin may cause serious side effects, breast-feeding is generally not recommended while you are receiving it.

Children—There is no specific information comparing use of streptozocin in children with use in other age groups.

Older adults—Many medicines have not been studies specifically in older people. Therefore, it may not be known whether they work exactly the same way they do in younger adults or if they cause different side effects or problems in older people. There is no specific information comparing use of streptozocin in the elderly with use in other age groups.

Other medicines—Although certain medicines should not be used together at all, in other cases two different medicines may be used together even if an interaction might occur. In these cases, your doctor may want to change the dose, or other precautions may be necessary. When you are receiving streptozocin, it is especially important that your doctor and pharmacist know if you are taking any of the following:

- Anti-infectives by mouth or by injection (medicine for infection) or
- Carmustine (e.g., BiCNU) or
- Cisplatin (e.g., Platinol) or
- Combination pain medicine containing acetaminophen and aspirin (e.g., Excedrin) or other salicylates (with large amounts taken regularly) or
- Cyclosporine (e.g., Sandimmune) or
- Deferoxamine (e.g., Desferal) (with long-term use) or
- Gold salts (medicine for arthritis) or
- Inflammation or pain medicine except narcotics or
- Lithium (e.g., Lithane) or
- Methotrexate (e.g., Mexate) or
- Penicillamine (e.g., Cuprimine) or
- Plicamycin (e.g., Mithracin) or
- Tiopronin (e.g., Thiola)—Increased risk of harmful effects on the kidney
- Phenytoin (e.g., Dilantin)—May interfere with the effects of streptozocin

Other medical problems—The presence of other medical problems may affect the use of streptozocin. Make sure you tell your doctor if you have any other medical problems, especially:

- Chickenpox (including recent exposure) or
- Herpes zoster (shingles)—Risk of severe disease affecting other parts of the body
- Diabetes mellitus (sugar diabetes)—May be worsened
- Infection—Streptozocin can decrease your body's ability to fight infection
- Kidney disease or
- Liver disease—Effects of streptozocin may be increased because of slower removal from the body

Before you begin using any new medicine (prescription or nonprescription) or if you develop any new medical problem while you are using this medicine, check with your doctor, nurse, or pharmacist.

Proper Use of This Medicine

While you are receiving streptozocin, your doctor may want you to drink extra fluids so that you will pass more urine. This will help prevent kidney problems and keep your kidneys working well.

This medicine usually causes nausea and vomiting, which may be severe. However, it is very important that you continue to receive the medicine, even if you begin to feel ill. Ask your doctor, nurse, or pharmacist for ways to lessen these effects.

Precautions While Using This Medicine

It is very important that your doctor check your progress at regular visits to make sure that this medicine is working properly and to check for any unwanted effects.

While you are being treated with streptozocin, and after you stop treatment with it, *do not have any immunizations (vaccinations) without your doctor's approval.* Streptozocin may lower your body's resistance and there is a chance you might get the infection the immunization is meant to prevent. In addition, other people living in your household should not take oral polio vaccine since there is a chance they could pass the polio virus on to you. Also, avoid persons who have recently taken oral polio vaccine. Do not get close to them and do not stay in the same room with them for very long. If you cannot take these precautions, you should consider wearing a protective face mask that covers the nose and mouth.

If streptozocin accidentally seeps out of the vein into which it is injected, it may damage some tissues and cause scarring. *Tell the doctor or nurse right away if you notice redness, pain, or swelling at the place of injection.*

Side Effects of This Medicine

Along with their needed effects, medicines like streptozocin can sometimes cause unwanted effects such as kidney problems and other side effects. These and others are described below. Also, because of the way these medicines act on the body, there is a chance that they might cause other unwanted effects that may not occur until months or years after the medicine is used. These delayed effects may include certain types of cancer, such as leukemia. Streptozocin has been shown to cause tumors (some cancerous) in animals. Discuss these possible effects with your doctor.

Although not all of these side effects may occur, if they do occur they may need medical attention.

Check with your doctor or nurse immediately if any of the following side effects occur shortly after the medicine is given:

Less common

Anxiety, nervousness, or shakiness; chills, cold sweats, or cool, pale skin; drowsiness or unusual tiredness or weakness; fast pulse; headache; pain or redness at place of injection; unusual hunger

Check with your doctor immediately if the following side effects occur any time while you are being treated with this medicine:

Rare

Black, tarry stools; blood in urine or stools; cough or hoarseness; fever or chills; lower back or side pain; painful or difficult urination; pinpoint red spots on skin; unusual bleeding or bruising

Check with your doctor or nurse as soon as possible if any of the following side effects occur:

More common

Swelling of feet or lower legs; unusual decrease in urination

Other side effects may occur that usually do not need medical attention. These side effects may go away during treatment as your body adjusts to the medicine. Also, your doctor or nurse may be able to tell you about ways to prevent or reduce some of these side effects. Check with your doctor or nurse if any of the following side effects continue or are bothersome or if you have any questions about them:

More common

Nausea and vomiting (usually occurs within 2 to 4 hours after receiving dose and may be severe)

Less common

Diarrhea

After you stop receiving streptozocin, your body may need time to adjust. The length of time this takes depends on the amount of medicine you were using and how long you used it. During this period of time, check with your doctor if you notice either of the following side effects:

More common

Decrease in urination; swelling of feet or lower legs

Other side effects not listed above may also occur in some patients. If you notice any other effects, check with your doctor.

Annual revision: 08/26/92

SUCCIMER Systemic†

A commonly used brand name in the U.S. is Chemet.

Other commonly used names are dimercaptosuccinic acid and DMSA.

†Not commercially available in Canada.

Description

Succimer (SUX-i-mer) is used to remove excess lead from the body. It is used to treat acute lead poisoning, especially in small children.

Succimer combines with lead in the bloodstream. The combination of lead and succimer is then removed from the body by the kidneys. By removing the excess lead, the medicine lessens damage to various organs and tissues of the body.

Oral

Capsules (U.S.)

It is very important that you read and understand the following information. If any of it causes you special concern, check with your doctor. Also, *if you have any questions* or if you want more information about this medicine or your medical problem, *ask your doctor, nurse, or pharmacist.*

Before Using This Medicine

In deciding to use a medicine, the risks of taking the medicine must be weighed against the good it will do.

This is a decision you and your doctor will make. For succimer, the following should be considered:

Allergies—Tell your doctor if you have ever had any unusual or allergic reaction to succimer. Also, tell your doctor and pharmacist if you are allergic to any other substances, such as foods, preservatives, or dyes.

Pregnancy—Studies have not been done in humans. However, some studies in animals have shown that succimer causes birth defects.

Breast-feeding—It is not known whether succimer is excreted in breast milk.

Children—This medicine has been tested in children over the age of 1 year and, in effective doses, has not been shown to cause different side effects or problems than it does in adults.

Older adults—Many medicines have not been studied specifically in older people. Therefore, it may not be known whether they work exactly the same way they do in younger adults or if they cause different side effects or problems in older people. There is no specific information comparing use of succimer in the elderly with use in other age groups.

Other medical problems—The presence of other medical problems may affect the use of succimer. Make sure you tell your doctor if you have any other medical problems, especially:

- Dehydration or
- Kidney disease—Higher blood levels of succimer may result and your doctor may need to change your dose

Before you begin using any new medicine (prescription or nonprescription) or if you develop any new medical problem while you are using this medicine, check with your doctor, nurse, or pharmacist.

Proper Use of This Medicine

Children who have too much lead in their bodies should be removed from the lead-containing environment (for example, home, school, or other areas where the child has been exposed to lead) until the lead has been removed from the environment.

Your doctor may want to put your child in the hospital while he or she is receiving succimer. This will allow the doctor to check your child's condition while the lead can be removed from the child's environment.

When opening your bottle of succimer, you may notice an unpleasant odor. However, this is a normal odor for these capsules and does not affect the medicine's working properly.

If the capsules cannot be swallowed, the contents of the capsule may be sprinkled on food and eaten immediately. The contents may also be given on a spoon and followed by a fruit drink.

Dosing—The dose of succimer will be different for different patients. *Follow your doctor's orders or the directions on the label.*

- For the *oral* dosage form (capsules):
  —For treatment of lead poisoning:
    - For adults and children 12 years of age and older—Dose is based on body weight. The usual dose is 10 milligrams (mg) of succimer per kilogram (4.5 mg per pound) of body weight every eight hours for five days.
    - For children up to 12 years of age—Dose is based on body weight. The usual dose is 10 mg of succimer per kilogram (4.5 mg per pound) of body weight every eight hours for five days. The same dose is then given every twelve hours for the next fourteen days, for a total of nineteen days of therapy.

Missed dose—If you miss a dose of this medicine, take it as soon as possible. However, if it is almost time for your next dose, skip the missed dose and go back to your regular dosing schedule. Do not double doses.

Storage—To store this medicine:

- Keep out of the reach of children.
- Store away from heat and direct light.
- Do not store in the bathroom, near the kitchen sink, or in other damp places. Heat or moisture may cause the medicine to break down.
- Keep the medicine from freezing. Do not refrigerate.
- Do not keep outdated medicine or medicine no longer needed. Be sure that any discarded medicine is out of the reach of children.

Precautions While Using This Medicine

It is important that your doctor check your progress at regular visits to make sure that this medicine is working properly and to prevent unwanted effects. Certain blood and urine tests must be done regularly to make sure you are taking the correct dose of succimer.

Side Effects of This Medicine

Along with its needed effects, a medicine may cause some unwanted effects. Although not all of these side effects may occur, if they do occur they may need medical attention.

Check with your doctor as soon as possible if the following side effect occurs:

Less common

Fever and chills

Other side effects may occur that usually do not need medical attention. These side effects may go away during

treatment as your body adjusts to the medicine. However, check with your doctor if any of the following side effects continue or are bothersome:

More common

Diarrhea; loose stools; loss of appetite; nausea and vomiting; skin rash

Succimer may cause your urine, sweat, and feces to have an unpleasant odor.

Other side effects not listed above may also occur in some patients. If you notice any other effects, check with your doctor.

Annual revision: 06/22/93

SUCRALFATE Oral

Some commonly used brand names are:

In the U.S.

Carafate

In Canada

Sulcrate

Description

Sucralfate (soo-KRAL-fate) is used to treat and prevent duodenal ulcers. This medicine may also be used for other conditions as determined by your doctor.

Sucralfate works by forming a "barrier" or "coating" over the ulcer. This protects the ulcer from the acid of the stomach, allowing it to heal. Sucralfate contains an aluminum salt.

This medicine is available only with your doctor's prescription, in the following dosage form:

Oral

- Oral suspension (Canada)
- Tablets (U.S. and Canada)

It is very important that you read and understand the following information. If any of it causes you special concern, check with your doctor. Also, *if you have any questions* or if you want more information about this medicine or your medical problem, *ask your doctor, nurse, or pharmacist.*

Before Using This Medicine

In deciding to use a medicine, the risks of taking the medicine must be weighed against the good it will do. This is a decision you and your doctor will make. For sucralfate, the following should be considered:

Allergies—Tell your doctor if you have ever had any unusual or allergic reaction to sucralfate. Also, tell your doctor and pharmacist if you are allergic to any other substances, such as foods, preservatives, or dyes.

Pregnancy—Studies have not been done in humans. However, sucralfate has not been shown to cause birth defects or other problems in animal studies.

Breast-feeding—Sucralfate has not been shown to cause problems in nursing babies.

Children—This medicine has been tested in a limited number of children. In effective doses, the medicine has not been shown to cause different side effects or problems than it does in adults.

Older adults—Many medicines have not been studied specifically in older people. Therefore, it may not be known whether they work exactly the same way they do in younger adults. Although there is no specific information comparing the use of sucralfate in the elderly with use in other age groups, this medicine is not expected to cause different side effects or problems in older people than it does in younger adults.

Other medicines—Although certain medicines should not be used together at all, in other cases two different medicines may be used together even if an interaction might occur. In these cases, your doctor may want to change the dose, or other precautions may be necessary. When you are taking sucralfate, it is especially important that your doctor and pharmacist know if you are taking the following:

- Ciprofloxacin or
- Digoxin or
- Norfloxacin or
- Ofloxacin or
- Phenytoin or
- Theophylline—Sucralfate may prevent these medicines from working properly

Other medical problems—The presence of other medical problems may affect the use of sucralfate. Make sure you tell your doctor if you have any other medical problems, especially:

- Gastrointestinal tract obstruction disease—Sucralfate may bind with other foods and drugs and cause obstruction of the gastrointestinal tract
- Kidney failure—Use may lead to a toxic increase of aluminum blood levels

Before you begin using any new medicine (prescription or nonprescription) or if you develop any new medical

problem while you are using this medicine, check with your doctor, nurse, or pharmacist.

Proper Use of This Medicine

Sucralfate is best taken with water on an empty stomach 1 hour before meals and at bedtime, unless otherwise directed by your doctor.

Take this medicine for the full time of treatment, even if you begin to feel better. Also, it is important that you keep your doctor's appointments for check-ups so that your doctor will be better able to tell you when to stop taking this medicine.

Missed dose—If you miss a dose of this medicine, take it as soon as possible. However, if it is almost time for your next dose, skip the missed dose and go back to your regular dosing schedule. Do not double doses.

Storage—To store this medicine:
- Keep out of the reach of children.
- Store away from heat and direct light.
- Do not store in the bathroom, near the kitchen sink, or in other damp places. Heat or moisture may cause the medicine to break down.
- Keep the liquid form of this medicine from freezing. Do not refrigerate.
- Do not keep outdated medicine or medicine no longer needed. Be sure that any discarded medicine is out of the reach of children.

Precautions While Using This Medicine

Antacids may be taken with sucralfate to help relieve any stomach pain, unless your doctor has told you not to use them. *However, antacids should not be taken within 30 minutes before or after sucralfate.* Taking these medicines too close together may keep sucralfate from working properly.

Side Effects of This Medicine

Along with its needed effects, a medicine may cause some unwanted effects. Some side effects may occur that usually do not need medical attention. These side effects may go away during treatment as your body adjusts to the medicine. *Check with your doctor immediately* if any of the following side effects occur:

Signs of aluminum toxicity

Drowsiness; convulsions (seizures)

Check with your doctor as soon as possible if any of the following side effects continue or are bothersome:

More common

Constipation

Less common or rare

Backache; diarrhea; dizziness or lightheadedness; dryness of mouth; indigestion; nausea; skin rash, hives, or itching; stomach cramps or pain

Other side effects not listed above may also occur in some patients. If you notice any other effects, check with your doctor.

Additional Information

Once a medicine has been approved for marketing for a certain use, experience may show that it is also useful for other medical problems. Although these uses are not included in product labeling, sucralfate is used in certain patients with the following medical conditions:
- Gastric ulcers
- Gastroesophageal reflux disease (a condition in which stomach acid washes back into the esophagus)
- Stomach or intestinal ulcers resulting from stress or trauma damage or from damage caused by medication used to treat rheumatoid arthritis

Other than the above information, there is no additional information relating to proper use, precautions, or side effects for these uses.

Annual revision: 03/24/92

SULFADOXINE AND PYRIMETHAMINE Systemic

A commonly used brand name in the U.S. and Canada is Fansidar.

Description

Sulfadoxine (sul-fa-DOX-een), a sulfa medicine, and pyrimethamine (peer-i-METH-a-meen) combination is used to treat malaria. This medicine may also be used to prevent malaria in people who are living in, or will be traveling to, an area where there is a chance of getting malaria. Sulfadoxine and pyrimethamine combination may also be taken with other medicines for malaria, or may be used for other problems as determined by your doctor.

Since sulfadoxine and pyrimethamine combination may cause some serious side effects, it is usually used only to prevent or treat serious malaria infections in areas where it is known that other medicines may not work.

This medicine is available only with your doctor's prescription, in the following dosage form:

Oral

- Tablets (U.S. and Canada)

It is very important that you read and understand the following information. If any of it causes you special concern, check with your doctor. Also, *if you have any questions* or if you want more information about this medicine or your medical problem, *ask your doctor, nurse, or pharmacist.*

Before Using This Medicine

In deciding to use a medicine, the risks of taking the medicine must be weighed against the good it will do. This is a decision you and your doctor will make. For sulfadoxine and pyrimethamine combination, the following should be considered:

Allergies—Tell your doctor if you have ever had any unusual or allergic reaction to sulfa medicines, furosemide (e.g., Lasix) or thiazide diuretics (water pills), oral antidiabetics (diabetes medicine you take by mouth), glaucoma medicine you take by mouth (acetazolamide [e.g., Diamox], dichlorphenamide [e.g., Daranide], methazolamide [e.g., Neptazane]), or pyrimethamine (e.g., Daraprim). Also tell your doctor and pharmacist if you are allergic to any other substances, such as foods, preservatives, or dyes.

Pregnancy—Studies have not been done in pregnant women. However, use is not recommended during pregnancy. Studies in rats have shown that sulfadoxine and pyrimethamine combination may cause birth defects and anemia. Also, women who travel to an area where there is a chance of getting malaria, and who may be taking sulfadoxine and pyrimethamine combination, should not become pregnant.

Breast-feeding—Sulfadoxine and pyrimethamine pass into the breast milk. This medicine is not recommended for use during breast-feeding. It may cause liver problems, anemia, and other unwanted effects in nursing babies.

Children—Sulfadoxine and pyrimethamine combination should not be used in infants up to 2 months of age.

Older adults—Many medicines have not been studied specifically in older people. Therefore, it may not be known whether they work exactly the same way they do in younger adults or if they cause different side effects or problems in older people. There is no specific information comparing use of sulfadoxine and pyrimethamine combination in the elderly with use in other age groups.

Other medicines—Although certain medicines should not be used together at all, in other cases two different medicines may be used together even if an interaction might occur. In these cases, your doctor may want to change the dose, or other precautions may be necessary. When you are taking sulfadoxine and pyrimethamine combination, it is especially important that your doctor and pharmacist know if you are taking any of the following:

- Acetaminophen (e.g., Tylenol) (with long-term, high-dose use) or
- Amiodarone (e.g., Cordarone) or
- Anabolic steroids (dromostanolone [e.g., Drolban], ethylestrenol [e.g., Maxibolin], nandrolone [e.g., Anabolin], oxandrolone [e.g., Anavar], oxymetholone [e.g., Anadrol], stanozolol [e.g., Winstrol]) or
- Androgens (male hormones) or
- Carbamazepine (e.g., Tegretol) or
- Carmustine (e.g., BiCNU) or
- Chloroquine (e.g., Aralen) or
- Dantrolene (e.g., Dantrium) or
- Daunorubicin (e.g., Cerubidine) or
- Disulfiram (e.g., Antabuse) or
- Divalproex (e.g., Depakote) or
- Estrogens (female hormones) or
- Etretinate (e.g., Tegison) or
- Gold salts (medicine for arthritis) or
- Hydroxychloroquine (e.g., Plaquenil) or
- Naltrexone (e.g., Trexan) (with long-term, high-dose use) or
- Oral contraceptives (birth control pills) containing estrogen or
- Other anti-infectives by mouth or by injection (medicine for infection) or
- Phenothiazines (acetophenazine [e.g., Tindal], chlorpromazine [e.g., Thorazine], fluphenazine [e.g., Prolixin], mesoridazine [e.g., Serentil], perphenazine [e.g., Trilafon], prochlorperazine [e.g., Compazine], promazine [e.g., Sparine], promethazine [e.g., Phenergan], thioridazine [e.g., Mellaril], trifluoperazine [e.g., Stelazine], triflupromazine [e.g., Vesprin], trimeprazine [e.g., Temaril]) or
- Phenytoin (e.g., Dilantin) or
- Valproic acid (e.g., Depakene)—Use of sulfadoxine and pyrimethamine combination with these medicines may increase the chance of side effects affecting the liver
- Acetohydroxamic acid (e.g., Lithostat) or
- Amphotericin B by injection (e.g., Fungizone) or
- Antidiabetics, oral (diabetes medicine you take by mouth) or
- Antineoplastics (cancer medicine) or
- Azathioprine (e.g., Imuran) or
- Chloramphenicol (e.g., Chloromycetin) or
- Colchicine or
- Cyclophosphamide (e.g., Cytoxan) or
- Dapsone or
- Flucytosine (e.g., Ancobon) or
- Furazolidone (e.g., Furoxone) or
- Ganciclovir (e.g., Cytovene) or
- Interferon (e.g., Intron A, Roferon-A) or
- Nitrofurantoin (e.g., Furadantin) or
- Primaquine or
- Procainamide (e.g., Pronestyl) or
- Quinidine (e.g., Quinidex) or

- Quinine (e.g., Quinamm) or
- Sulfoxone (e.g., Diasone) or
- Vitamin K (e.g., AquaMEPHYTON, Synkayvite) or
- Zidovudine (e.g., AZT, Retrovir)—Use of sulfadoxine and pyrimethamine combination with these medicines may increase the chance of side effects affecting the blood
- Antithyroid agents (medicine for overactive thyroid) or
- Mercaptopurine (e.g., Purinethol) or
- Methotrexate (e.g., Mexate) or
- Methyldopa (e.g., Aldomet) or
- Plicamycin (e.g., Mithracin)—Use of sulfadoxine and pyrimethamine combination with these medicines may increase the chance of side effects affecting the liver and the blood

Other medical problems—The presence of other medical problems may affect the use of sulfadoxine and pyrimethamine combination. Make sure you tell your doctor if you have any other medical problems, especially:

- Anemia or other blood problems—Patients with these problems may have an increase in side effects involving the blood
- Kidney disease or
- Liver disease—Patients with kidney and/or liver disease may have an increased chance of side effects
- Porphyria—This medicine may cause an attack of porphyria
- Seizure disorders, such as epilepsy—High doses of this medicine may increase the chance of convulsions (seizures)

Before you begin using any new medicine (prescription or nonprescription) or if you develop any new medical problem while you are using this medicine, check with your doctor, nurse, or pharmacist.

Proper Use of This Medicine

Do not give this medicine to infants under 2 months of age unless otherwise directed by your doctor. Also, *keep this medicine out of the reach of children.* Overdose is especially dangerous in children.

Sulfa-containing medicines are best taken with a full glass (8 ounces) of water. Several additional glasses of water should be taken every day, unless otherwise directed by your doctor. Drinking extra water will help to prevent some unwanted effects (e.g., kidney stones) of this medicine. If this medicine upsets your stomach or causes vomiting, it may be taken with meals or a snack.

For patients taking this medicine *to prevent malaria:*

- Your doctor may want you to start taking this medicine 1 to 2 weeks before you travel to an area where there is a chance of getting malaria. This will help you to see how you react to the medicine. Also, it will allow time for your doctor to change your medicine if you have a reaction to this medicine.
- Also, you should keep taking this medicine while you are in the area and for 4 weeks after you leave the area. No medicine will protect you completely from malaria. However, to protect you as completely as possible, *it is important that you keep taking this medicine for the full time your doctor ordered.* Also, if fever develops during your travels or within 2 months after you leave the area, *check with your doctor immediately.*
- This medicine works best when you take it on a regular schedule. For example, if you are to take it once a week, it is best to take it on the same day each week. *Do not miss any doses.* If you have any questions about this, check with your doctor, nurse, or pharmacist.

For patients taking this medicine *to treat malaria:*

- To help clear up your infection completely, *take this medicine exactly as directed by your doctor.*

For patients taking this medicine *to self-treat presumptive malaria:*

- After you take this medicine to self-treat presumptive malaria, you should continue to take your other medicine for malaria once a week.

Dosing—The dose of sulfadoxine and pyrimethamine combination will be different for different patients. *Follow your doctor's orders or the directions on the label.* The following information includes only the average doses of sulfadoxine and pyrimethamine combination. *If your dose is different, do not change it* unless your doctor tells you to do so.

- For *treatment* of malaria:
  - —Adults and teenagers: 3 tablets as a single dose on the third day of quinine therapy.
  - —Children: Dose is based on body weight and must be determined by your doctor.
- For *self-treatment of presumed malaria*:
  - —Adults and teenagers: 3 tablets as a single dose when you get a fever and medical care is not available.
  - —Children: Dose is based on body weight and must be determined by your doctor. The dose may range from ¼ tablet to 3 tablets taken as a single dose.
- For *prevention* of malaria:
  - —Adults and teenagers: 1 tablet once every seven days, or 2 tablets once every fourteen days.
  - —Children: Dose is based on body weight and must be determined by your doctor. The dose may range from ½ tablet to ¾ tablet taken once every seven days, or ¼ tablet to 1½ tablets taken once every fourteen days.

Missed dose—For patients taking this medicine *to prevent malaria:* If you do miss a dose of this medicine, take it as soon as possible. This will help to keep you taking your medicine on a regular schedule. However, if it is almost time for your next dose, skip the missed dose and go back to your regular dosing schedule. Do not double doses.

Storage—To store this medicine:

- Keep out of the reach of children. Overdose of sulfadoxine and pyrimethamine combination is very dangerous in children.
- Store away from heat and direct light.
- Do not store in the bathroom, near the kitchen sink, or in other damp places. Heat or moisture may cause the medicine to break down.
- Do not keep outdated medicine or medicine no longer needed. Be sure that any discarded medicine is out of the reach of children.

Precautions While Using This Medicine

If this medicine causes skin rash, itching, redness, sores in the mouth or on the genitals (sex organs), or sore throat, check with your doctor immediately. These may be early warning signs of more serious skin or related problems that could develop later.

Malaria is spread by mosquitoes. If you are living in, or will be traveling to, an area where there is a chance of getting malaria, the following mosquito-control measures will help to prevent infection:

- If possible, sleep under mosquito netting to avoid being bitten by malaria-carrying mosquitoes.
- Wear long-sleeved shirts or blouses and long trousers to protect your arms and legs, especially from dusk through dawn when mosquitoes are out.
- Apply mosquito repellant to uncovered areas of the skin from dusk through dawn when mosquitoes are out.

For patients taking this medicine *to prevent malaria:*

- *It is very important that your doctor check your progress at regular visits.* This medicine may cause blood problems, especially if it is taken for a long time.
- If this medicine causes anemia, your doctor may want you to take leucovorin (e.g., folinic acid, Wellcovorin) to help clear up the anemia. If so, it is important to take the leucovorin every day while you are taking this medicine. Do not miss any doses.
- Sulfadoxine and pyrimethamine combination may cause blood problems. These problems may result in a greater chance of certain infections, slow healing, and bleeding of the gums. Therefore, you should be careful when using regular toothbrushes, dental floss, and toothpicks. Dental work should be delayed until your blood counts have returned to normal. Check with your medical doctor or dentist if you have any questions about proper oral hygiene (mouth care) during treatment.
- Sulfadoxine and pyrimethamine combination may cause your skin to be more sensitive to sunlight than it is normally. Exposure to sunlight, even for brief periods of time, may cause a skin rash, itching, redness or other discoloration of the skin, or a severe sunburn. When you begin taking this medicine:

  —Stay out of direct sunlight, especially between the hours of 10:00 a.m. and 3:00 p.m., if possible.

  —Wear protective clothing, including a hat. Also, wear sunglasses.

  —Apply a sun block product that has a skin protection factor (SPF) of at least 15. Some patients may require a product with a higher SPF number, especially if they have a fair complexion. If you have any questions about this, check with your doctor or pharmacist.

  —Apply a sun block lipstick that has an SPF of at least 15 to protect your lips.

  —Do not use a sunlamp or tanning bed or booth.

  If you have a severe reaction from the sun, check with your doctor.

For patients taking this medicine *to self-treat presumed malaria:*

- Seek medical help as soon as possible, especially if your symptoms do not improve within 48 hours.

Side Effects of This Medicine

Along with its needed effects, a medicine may cause some unwanted effects. Although not all of these side effects may occur, if they do occur they may need medical attention.

Check with your doctor immediately if any of the following side effects occur:

More common

Change in or loss of taste; fever and sore throat; skin rash; soreness, redness, swelling, burning, or stinging of tongue; unusual bleeding or bruising; unusual tiredness or weakness

Less common

Aching of joints and muscles; redness, blistering, peeling, or loosening of skin; yellow eyes or skin

Rare

Blood in urine; lower back pain; pain or burning while urinating; swelling of front part of neck

Symptoms of overdose

Bleeding or bruising (severe); clumsiness or unsteadiness; convulsions (seizures); loss of appetite (severe); sore throat and fever (severe); tiredness or weakness (severe); trembling; vomiting (severe)

Also, check with your doctor as soon as possible if the following side effect occurs:

More common

Increased sensitivity of skin to sunlight

Other side effects may occur that usually do not need medical attention. These side effects may go away during treatment as your body adjusts to the medicine. However, check with your doctor if any of the following side effects continue or are bothersome:

More common

Diarrhea; headache; nausea or vomiting; nervousness; stomach pain

Other side effects not listed above may also occur in some patients. If you notice any other effects, check with your doctor.

Additional Information

Once a medicine has been approved for marketing for a certain use, experience may show that it is also useful for other medical problems. Although this use is not included in product labeling, sulfadoxine and pyrimethamine combination is used in certain patients with the following medical condition:

- Isosporiasis (prevention)

Other than the above information, there is no additional information relating to proper use, precautions, or side effects for this use.

Annual revision: 02/23/93

SULFAMETHOXAZOLE AND TRIMETHOPRIM Systemic

Some commonly used brand names are:

In the U.S.

Bactrim	Sulfatrim
Bactrim DS	Sulfatrim DS
Cotrim	Sulfoxaprim
Cotrim DS	Sulfoxaprim DS
Septra	Triazole
Septra DS	Triazole DS
Sulfamethoprim	Trimeth-Sulfa
Sulfamethoprim DS	Trisulfam
Sulfaprim	Uroplus DS
Sulfaprim DS	Uroplus SS

Generic name product may also be available.

In Canada

Apo-Sulfatrim	Nu-Cotrimox
Apo-Sulfatrim DS	Nu-Cotrimox DS
Bactrim	Roubac
Bactrim DS	Septra
Novotrimel	Septra DS
Novotrimel DS	

Some other commonly used names are cotrimoxazole and SMZ-TMP.

Description

Sulfamethoxazole and trimethoprim (sul-fa-meth-OX-a-zole and trye-METH-oh-prim) combination is used to treat infections, such as bronchitis, middle ear infection, urinary tract infection, traveler's diarrhea, and *Pneumocystis carinii* pneumonia (PCP). It will not work for colds, flu, or other virus infections. It may also be used for other conditions as determined by your doctor.

Sulfamethoxazole and trimethoprim combination is available only with your doctor's prescription, in the following dosage forms:

Oral

- Oral suspension (U.S. and Canada)
- Tablets (U.S. and Canada)

Parenteral

- Injection (U.S. and Canada)

It is very important that you read and understand the following information. If any of it causes you special concern, check with your doctor. Also, *if you have any questions* or if you want more information about this medicine or your medical problem, *ask your doctor, nurse, or pharmacist.*

Before Using This Medicine

In deciding to use a medicine, the risks of taking the medicine must be weighed against the good it will do. This is a decision you and your doctor will make. For sulfamethoxazole and trimethoprim combination, the following should be considered:

Allergies—Tell your doctor if you have ever had any unusual or allergic reaction to sulfa medicines, furosemide (e.g., Lasix) or thiazide diuretics (water pills), oral antidiabetics (diabetes medicine you take by mouth), glaucoma medicine you take by mouth (for example, acetazolamide [e.g., Diamox], dichlorphenamide [e.g., Daranide], methazolamide [e.g., Neptazane]), or trimethoprim (e.g., Trimpex). Also tell your doctor and pharmacist if you are allergic to any other substances, such as foods, preservatives, or dyes.

Pregnancy—Sulfamethoxazole and trimethoprim combination has not been reported to cause birth defects or other problems in humans. However, studies in mice, rats, and rabbits have shown that some sulfonamides cause birth defects, including cleft palate and bone problems. Studies in rabbits have also shown that trimethoprim causes birth defects, as well as a decrease in the number of successful pregnancies.

Breast-feeding—Sulfamethoxazole and trimethoprim pass into the breast milk. This medicine is not recommended for use during breast-feeding. It may cause liver problems, anemia, and other unwanted effects in nursing babies, especially those with glucose-6-phosphate dehydrogenase (G6PD) deficiency.

Children—This medicine should not be given to infants under 2 months of age unless directed by the child's doctor, because it may cause brain problems.

Older adults—Elderly people are especially sensitive to the effects of sulfamethoxazole and trimethoprim combination. Severe skin problems and blood problems may be more likely to occur in the elderly. These problems may also be more likely to occur in patients who are taking diuretics (water pills) along with this medicine.

Other medicines—Although certain medicines should not be used together at all, in other cases two different medicines may be used together even if an interaction might occur. In these cases, your doctor may want to change the dose, or other precautions may be necessary. When you are taking sulfamethoxazole and trimethoprim combination, it is especially important that your doctor and pharmacist know if you are taking any of the following:

- Acetaminophen (e.g., Tylenol) (with long-term, high-dose use) or
- Amiodarone (e.g., Cordarone) or
- Anabolic steroids (nandrolone [e.g., Anabolin], oxandrolone [e.g., Anavar], oxymetholone [e.g., Anadrol], stanozolol [e.g., Winstrol]) or
- Androgens (male hormones) or
- Antithyroid agents (medicine for overactive thyroid) or
- Carbamazepine (e.g., Tegretol) or
- Carmustine (e.g., BiCNU) or
- Chloroquine (e.g., Aralen) or
- Dantrolene (e.g., Dantrium) or
- Daunorubicin (e.g., Cerubidine) or
- Disulfiram (e.g., Antabuse) or
- Divalproex (e.g., Depakote) or
- Estrogens (female hormones) or
- Etretinate (e.g., Tegison) or
- Gold salts (medicine for arthritis) or
- Hydroxychloroquine (e.g., Plaquenil) or
- Mercaptopurine (e.g., Purinethol) or
- Naltrexone (e.g., Trexan) (with long-term, high-dose use) or
- Oral contraceptives (birth control pills) containing estrogens or
- Other anti-infectives by mouth or by injection (medicine for infection) or
- Phenothiazines (acetophenazine [e.g., Tindal], chlorpromazine [e.g., Thorazine], fluphenazine [e.g., Prolixin], mesoridazine [e.g., Serentil], perphenazine [e.g., Trilafon], prochlorperazine [e.g., Compazine], promazine [e.g., Sparine], promethazine [e.g., Phenergan], thioridazine [e.g., Mellaril], trifluoperazine [e.g., Stelazine], triflupromazine [e.g., Vesprin], trimeprazine [e.g., Temaril]) or
- Plicamycin (e.g., Mithracin) or
- Valproic acid (e.g., Depakene)—Use of sulfamethoxazole and trimethoprim combination with these medicines may increase the chance of side effects affecting the liver
- Acetohydroxamic acid (e.g., Lithostat) or
- Dapsone or
- Furazolidone (e.g., Furoxone) or
- Nitrofurantoin (e.g., Furadantin) or
- Primaquine or
- Procainamide (e.g., Pronestyl) or
- Quinidine (e.g., Quinidex) or
- Quinine (e.g., Quinamm)—Use of sulfamethoxazole and trimethoprim combination with these medicines may increase the chance of side effects affecting the blood
- Anticoagulants (blood thinners) or
- Ethotoin (e.g., Peganone) or
- Mephenytoin (e.g., Mesantoin)—Use of sulfamethoxazole and trimethoprim combination with these medicines may increase the chance of side effects of these medicines
- Antidiabetics, oral (diabetes medicine you take by mouth)—Use of oral antidiabetics with sulfamethoxazole and trimethoprim combination may increase the chance of side effects affecting the blood and/or the side effects of the oral antidiabetics
- Methenamine (e.g., Mandelamine)—Use of methenamine with sulfamethoxazole and trimethoprim combination may increase the chance of side effects of the sulfamethoxazole
- Methyldopa (e.g., Aldomet)—Use of methyldopa with sulfamethoxazole and trimethoprim combination may increase the chance of side effects affecting the liver and/or the blood
- Methotrexate (e.g., Mexate) or
- Phenytoin (e.g., Dilantin)—Use of these medicines with sulfamethoxazole and trimethoprim combination may increase the chance of side effects affecting the liver and/or the side effects of these medicines

Other medical problems—The presence of other medical problems may affect the use of sulfamethoxazole and trimethoprim combination. Make sure you tell your doctor if you have any other medical problems, especially:

- Anemia or other blood problems or
- Glucose-6-phosphate dehydrogenase (G6PD) deficiency—Patients with these problems may have an increase in side effects affecting the blood
- Kidney disease or
- Liver disease—Patients with kidney and/or liver disease may have an increased chance of side effects
- Porphyria—This medicine may bring on an attack of porphyria

Before you begin using any new medicine (prescription or nonprescription) or if you develop any new medical problem while you are using this medicine, check with your doctor, nurse, or pharmacist.

Proper Use of This Medicine

Sulfamethoxazole and trimethoprim combination is best taken with a full glass (8 ounces) of water. Several additional glasses of water should be taken every day, unless otherwise directed by your doctor. Drinking extra water will help to prevent some unwanted effects (e.g., kidney stones) of sulfonamides.

For patients taking the *oral liquid form* of this medicine:

- Use a specially marked measuring spoon or other device to measure each dose accurately. The average household teaspoon may not hold the right amount of liquid.

To help clear up your infection completely, *keep taking this medicine for the full time of treatment,* even if you begin to feel better after a few days. If you stop taking this medicine too soon, your symptoms may return.

This medicine works best when there is a constant amount in the blood or urine. *To help keep the amount constant, do not miss any doses. Also, it is best to take the doses at evenly spaced times day and night.* For example, if you are to take 4 doses a day, the doses should be spaced about 6 hours apart. If this interferes with your sleep or other daily activities, or if you need help in planning the best times to take your medicine, check with your doctor, nurse, or pharmacist.

Missed dose—If you do miss a dose of this medicine, take it as soon as possible. This will help to keep a constant amount of medicine in the blood or urine. However, if it is almost time for your next dose, skip the missed dose and go back to your regular dosing schedule. Do not double doses.

Storage—To store this medicine:

- Keep out of the reach of children.
- Store away from heat and direct light.
- Do not store the tablet form of this medicine in the bathroom, near the kitchen sink, or in other damp places. Heat or moisture may cause the medicine to break down.
- Keep the oral liquid form of this medicine from freezing.
- Do not keep outdated medicine or medicine no longer needed. Be sure that any discarded medicine is out of the reach of children.

Precautions While Using This Medicine

It is very important that your doctor check your progress at regular visits. This medicine may cause blood problems, especially if it is taken for a long time.

If your symptoms do not improve within a few days, or if they become worse, check with your doctor.

Sulfamethoxazole and trimethoprim combination may cause blood problems. These problems may result in a greater chance of certain infections, slow healing, and bleeding of the gums. Therefore, you should be careful when using regular toothbrushes, dental floss, and toothpicks. Dental work should be delayed until your blood counts have returned to normal. Check with your medical doctor or dentist if you have any questions about proper oral hygiene (mouth care) during treatment.

Sulfamethoxazole and trimethoprim combination may cause your skin to be more sensitive to sunlight than it is normally. Exposure to sunlight, even for brief periods of time, may cause a skin rash, itching, redness or other discoloration of the skin, or a severe sunburn. When you begin taking this medicine:

- Stay out of direct sunlight, especially between the hours of 10:00 a.m. and 3:00 p.m., if possible.
- Wear protective clothing, including a hat. Also, wear sunglasses.
- Apply a sun block product that has a skin protection factor (SPF) of at least 15. Some patients may require a product with a higher SPF number, especially if they have a fair complexion. If you have any questions about this, check with your doctor or pharmacist.
- Apply a sun block lipstick that has an SPF of at least 15 to protect your lips.
- Do not use a sunlamp or tanning bed or booth.

If you have a severe reaction from the sun, check with your doctor.

This medicine may also cause some people to become dizzy. *Make sure you know how you react to this medicine before you drive, use machines, or do anything else that could be dangerous if you are dizzy or are not alert.* If this reaction is especially bothersome, check with your doctor.

Side Effects of This Medicine

Along with its needed effects, a medicine may cause some unwanted effects. Although not all of these side effects may occur, if they do occur they may need medical attention.

Check with your doctor immediately if any of the following side effects occur:

More common

Itching; skin rash

Less common

Aching of joints and muscles; difficulty in swallowing; pale skin; redness, blistering, peeling, or loosening of skin; sore throat and fever; unusual bleeding or bruising; unusual tiredness or weakness; yellow eyes or skin

Rare

Blood in urine; bluish fingernails, lips, or skin; difficult breathing; greatly increased or decreased frequency of urination or amount of urine; increased thirst; lower back pain; pain or burning while urinating; swelling of front part of neck

Also, check with your doctor as soon as possible if the following side effect occurs:

More common

Increased sensitivity of skin to sunlight

Other side effects may occur that usually do not need medical attention. These side effects may go away during treatment as your body adjusts to the medicine. However, check with your doctor if any of the following side effects continue or are bothersome:

More common

Diarrhea; dizziness; headache; loss of appetite; nausea or vomiting

Other side effects not listed above may also occur in some patients. If you notice any other effects, check with your doctor.

Additional Information

Once a medicine has been approved for marketing for a certain use, experience may show that it is also useful for other medical problems. Although these uses are not included in product labeling, sulfamethoxazole and trimethoprim combination is used in certain patients with the following medical conditions:

- Bile infections
- Bone and joint infections
- *Pneumocystis carinii* pneumonia (PCP) (for prevention)
- Sexually transmitted diseases, such as gonorrhea
- Sinus infections
- Urinary tract infections (for prevention)

Other than the above information, there is no additional information relating to proper use, precautions, or side effects for these uses.

Annual revision: 09/30/92

SULFAPYRIDINE Systemic

A commonly used brand name in Canada is Dagenan.
Generic name product may also be available in the U.S. and Canada.

Description

Sulfapyridine (sul-fa-PEER-i-deen) is a sulfa medicine. It is used to help control dermatitis herpetiformis (Duhring's disease), a skin problem. It may also be used for other problems as determined by your doctor. However, this medicine will not work for any kind of infection as other sulfa medicines do.

This medicine may cause some serious side effects. *Before using this medicine, be sure to talk to your doctor about these problems, as well as the good this medicine will do.*

Sulfapyridine is available only with your doctor's prescription, in the following dosage form:

Oral

- Tablets (U.S. and Canada)

It is very important that you read and understand the following information. If any of it causes you special concern, check with your doctor. Also, *if you have any questions* or if you want more information about this medicine or your medical problem, *ask your doctor, nurse, or pharmacist.*

Before Using This Medicine

In deciding to use a medicine, the risks of taking the medicine must be weighed against the good it will do. This is a decision you and your doctor will make. For sulfapyridine, the following should be considered:

Allergies—Tell your doctor if you have ever had any unusual or allergic reaction to sulfa medicines, furosemide (e.g., Lasix) or thiazide diuretics (water pills), oral antidiabetics (diabetes medicine you take by mouth), glaucoma medicine you take by mouth (acetazolamide [e.g., Diamox], dichlorphenamide [e.g., Daranide], methazolamide [e.g., Neptazane]), or pyrimethamine (e.g., Daraprim). Also tell your doctor and pharmacist if you are allergic to any other substances, such as foods, preservatives, or dyes.

Pregnancy—Studies have not been done in humans. Studies in rats and mice have shown that some sulfa medicines, given by mouth in high doses, cause birth defects, including cleft palate and bone problems. In addition, sulfa medicines may cause liver problems in newborn infants. Therefore, use is not recommended during pregnancy.

Breast-feeding—Sulfapyridine passes into the breast milk. This medicine may cause liver problems in nursing babies. In addition, it may cause blood problems in nursing babies with glucose-6-phosphate dehydrogenase (G6PD) deficiency (lack of G6PD enzyme). Therefore, use is not recommended in nursing women.

Children—Use of this medicine is not recommended since dermatitis herpetiformis usually does not occur in children.

Older adults—Many medicines have not been studied specifically in older people. Therefore, it may not be known whether they work exactly the same way they do in younger adults or if they cause different side effects or problems in older people. There is no specific information comparing the use of sulfapyridine in the elderly with use in other age groups.

Other medicines—Although certain medicines should not be used together at all, in other cases two different medicines may be used together even if an interaction might occur. In these cases, your doctor may want to change the dose, or other precautions may be necessary. When you are taking sulfapyridine, it is especially important that your doctor and pharmacist know if you are taking any of the following:

- Acetaminophen (e.g., Tylenol) (with long-term, high-dose use) or
- Amiodarone (e.g., Cordarone) or
- Anabolic steroids (nandrolone [e.g., Anabolin], oxandrolone [e.g., Anavar], oxymetholone [e.g., Anadrol], stanozolol [e.g., Winstrol]) or
- Androgens (male hormones) or
- Antithyroid agents (medicine for overactive thyroid) or
- Carbamazepine (e.g., Tegretol) or
- Carmustine (e.g., BiCNU) or
- Chloroquine (e.g., Aralen) or
- Dantrolene (e.g., Dantrium) or
- Daunorubicin (e.g., Cerubidine) or
- Disulfiram (e.g., Antabuse) or
- Divalproex (e.g., Depakote) or
- Estrogens (female hormones) or
- Etretinate (e.g., Tegison) or
- Gold salts (medicine for arthritis) or
- Hydroxychloroquine (e.g., Plaquenil) or
- Mercaptopurine (e.g., Purinethol) or
- Naltrexone (e.g., Trexan) (with long-term, high-dose use) or
- Oral contraceptives (birth control pills) containing estrogen or
- Other anti-infectives by mouth or by injection (medicine for infection) or
- Phenothiazines (acetophenazine [e.g., Tindal], chlorpromazine [e.g., Thorazine], fluphenazine [e.g., Prolixin], mesoridazine [e.g., Serentil], perphenazine [e.g., Trilafon], prochlorperazine [e.g., Compazine], promazine [e.g., Sparine], promethazine [e.g., Phenergan], thioridazine [e.g., Mellaril], trifluoperazine [e.g., Stelazine], triflupromazine [e.g., Vesprin], trimeprazine [e.g., Temaril]) or
- Plicamycin (e.g., Mithracin) or
- Valproic acid (e.g., Depakene)—Use of sulfapyridine with these medicines may increase the chance of side effects affecting the liver
- Acetohydroxamic acid (e.g., Lithostat) or
- Dapsone or
- Furazolidone (e.g., Furoxone) or
- Nitrofurantoin (e.g., Furadantin) or
- Primaquine or
- Procainamide (e.g., Pronestyl) or
- Quinidine (e.g., Quinidex) or
- Quinine (e.g., Quinamm) or
- Sulfoxone (e.g., Diasone) or
- Vitamin K (e.g., AquaMEPHYTON, Synkayvite)—Use of sulfapyridine with these medicines may increase the chance of side effects affecting the blood
- Anticoagulants (blood thinners) or
- Ethotoin (e.g., Peganone) or
- Mephenytoin (e.g., Mesantoin)—Use of sulfapyridine with these medicines may increase the chance of side effects of these medicines
- Antidiabetics, oral (diabetes medicine you take by mouth)—Use of oral antidiabetics with sulfapyridine may increase the chance of side effects affecting the blood and/or the side effects or oral antidiabetics
- Methotrexate (e.g., Mexate)—Use of methotrexate with sulfapyridine may increase the chance of side effects affecting the liver and/or the side effects of methotrexate
- Methyldopa (e.g., Aldomet)—Use of methyldopa with sulfapyridine may increase the chance of side effects affecting the liver and/or the blood
- Phenytoin (e.g., Dilantin)—Use of phenytoin with sulfapyridine may increase the chance of side effects affecting the liver and/or the side effects of phenytoin

Other medical problems—The presence of other medical problems may affect the use of sulfapyridine. Make sure you tell your doctor if you have any other medical problems, especially:

- Blood problems or
- Glucose-6-phosphate dehydrogenase deficiency (lack of G6PD enzyme)—Patients with these problems may have an increase in side effects affecting the blood
- Kidney disease or
- Liver disease—Patients with kidney disease or liver disease may have an increased chance of side effects
- Porphyria—Use of sulfapyridine may cause an attack of porphyria

Before you begin using any new medicine (prescription or nonprescription) or if you develop any new medical problem while you are using this medicine, check with your doctor, nurse, or pharmacist.

Proper Use of This Medicine

Each dose of sulfapyridine should be taken with a full glass (8 ounces) of water. Several additional glasses of water should be taken every day, unless otherwise directed by your doctor. Drinking extra water will help to prevent some unwanted effects (e.g., kidney stones) of the sulfa medicine.

For patients taking sulfapyridine *for dermatitis herpetiformis:*

- Your doctor may want you to follow a strict, gluten-free diet.
- You may have to use this medicine regularly for 6 months to a year before you can reduce the dose of sulfapyridine or stop it altogether. If you have any questions about this, check with your doctor.

Dosing—The dose of sulfapyridine will be different for different patients. *Follow your doctor's orders or the directions on the label.* The following information includes only the average doses of sulfapyridine. Your dose may be different if you have kidney disease. *If your dose is different, do not change it* unless your doctor tells you to do so.

- For *dermatitis herpetiformis*:
  —Adults and adolescents: 250 milligrams to 1 gram four times a day until improvement occurs. After improvement has occurred, the dose should then be reduced by 250 to 500 milligrams every three days until there are no symptoms; that dose should be taken once daily.
  —Children: Use is not recommended, because children usually do not get this condition.

Missed dose—For patients taking sulfapyridine *for dermatitis herpetiformis:* You may skip a missed dose if this does not make your symptoms return or get worse. If your symptoms do return or get worse, take the missed dose as soon as possible. Then go back to your regular dosing schedule.

Storage—To store this medicine:

- Keep out of the reach of children.
- Store away from heat and direct light.
- Do not store in the bathroom, near the kitchen sink, or in other damp places. Heat or moisture may cause the medicine to break down.
- Do not keep outdated medicine or medicine no longer needed. Be sure that any discarded medicine is out of the reach of children.

Precautions While Using This Medicine

It is very important that your doctor check your progress at regular visits. This medicine may cause blood problems, especially if it is taken for a long time.

If your symptoms do not improve within a few days, or if they become worse, check with your doctor.

Sulfapyridine may cause blood problems. These problems may result in a greater chance of certain infections, slow healing, and bleeding of the gums. Therefore, you should be careful when using regular toothbrushes, dental floss, and toothpicks. Dental work should be delayed until your blood counts have returned to normal. Check with your medical doctor or dentist if you have any questions about proper oral hygiene (mouth care) during treatment.

Sulfapyridine may cause your skin to be more sensitive to sunlight than it is normally. Exposure to sunlight, even for brief periods of time, may cause a skin rash, itching, redness or other discoloration of the skin, or a severe sunburn. When you begin taking this medicine:

- Stay out of direct sunlight, especially between the hours of 10:00 A.M. and 3:00 P.M., if possible.
- Wear protective clothing, including a hat. Also, wear sunglasses.
- Apply a sun block product that has a skin protection factor (SPF) of at least 15. Some patients may require a product with a higher SPF number, especially if they have a fair complexion. If you have any questions about this, check with your doctor or pharmacist.
- Apply a sun block lipstick that has an SPF of at least 15 to protect your lips.
- Do not use a sunlamp or tanning bed or booth.

You may still be more sensitive to sunlight or sunlamps for many months after stopping this medicine. *If you have a severe reaction from the sun, check with your doctor.*

Tell the doctor in charge that you are taking this medicine before you have any medical tests. The results of the bentiromide (e.g., Chymex) test for pancreas function are affected by this medicine.

Side Effects of This Medicine

Along with its needed effects, a medicine may cause some unwanted effects. Although not all of these side effects may occur, if they do occur they may need medical attention.

Check with your doctor immediately if any of the following side effects occur:

More common

Fever; headache (continuing); itching; skin rash

Less common

Aching of joints and muscles; difficulty in swallowing; pale skin; redness, blistering, peeling, or loosening of skin; sore throat; unusual bleeding or bruising; unusual tiredness or weakness; yellow eyes or skin

Rare

Blood in urine; lower back pain; pain or burning while urinating; swelling of front part of neck

Also, check with your doctor as soon as possible if the following side effect occurs:

More common

Increased sensitivity of skin to sunlight

Other side effects may occur that usually do not need medical attention. These side effects may go away during treatment as your body adjusts to the medicine. However, check with your doctor if any of the following side effects continue or are bothersome:

More common

Diarrhea; loss of appetite; nausea or vomiting

Other side effects not listed above may also occur in some patients. If you notice any other effects, check with your doctor.

Additional Information

Once a medicine has been approved for marketing for a certain use, experience may show that it is also useful for other medical problems. Although these uses are not included in product labeling, sulfapyridine is used in certain patients with the following medical conditions:

- Pemphigoid
- Pyoderma gangrenosum
- Subcorneal pustular dermatitis

Other than the above information, there is no additional information relating to proper use, precautions, or side effects for these uses.

Annual revision: 02/01/93

SULFASALAZINE Systemic

Some commonly used brand names are:

In the U.S.

Azulfidine	Azulfidine EN-Tabs

Generic name product may also be available.

In Canada

PMS Sulfasalazine	Salazopyrin EN-Tabs
PMS Sulfasalazine E.C.	S.A.S.-500
Salazopyrin	S.A.S. Enteric-500

Other commonly used names are salazosulfapyridine and salicylazosulfapyridine.

Description

Sulfasalazine (sul-fa-SAL-a-zeen), a sulfa medicine, is used to prevent and treat inflammatory bowel disease, such as ulcerative colitis. It works inside the bowel by helping to reduce the inflammation and other symptoms of the disease. Sulfasalazine is sometimes given with other medicines to treat inflammatory bowel disease. However, this medicine will not work for all kinds of infection the way other sulfa medicines do.

Sulfasalazine is available only with your doctor's prescription, in the following dosage forms:

Oral

- Enteric-coated tablets (U.S. and Canada)
- Oral suspension (U.S.)
- Tablets (U.S. and Canada)

It is very important that you read and understand the following information. If any of it causes you special concern, check with your doctor. Also, *if you have any questions* or if you want more information about this medicine or your medical problem, *ask your doctor, nurse, or pharmacist.*

Before Using This Medicine

In deciding to use a medicine, the risks of taking the medicine must be weighed against the good it will do. This is a decision you and your doctor will make. For sulfasalazine, the following should be considered:

Allergies—Tell your doctor if you have ever had any unusual or allergic reaction to any of the sulfa medicines, furosemide (e.g., Lasix) or thiazide diuretics (water pills), oral antidiabetics (diabetes medicine you take by mouth), glaucoma medicine you take by mouth (for example, acetazolamide [e.g., Diamox], dichlorphenamide [e.g., Daranide], methazolamide [e.g., Neptazane]), or salicylates (for example, aspirin). Also tell your doctor and pharmacist if you are allergic to any other substances, such as foods, preservatives, or dyes.

Pregnancy—Studies have not been done in humans. However, reports on women who took sulfasalazine during pregnancy have not shown that it causes birth defects or other problems. In addition, sulfasalazine has not been shown to cause birth defects in studies in rats and rabbits given doses of up to 6 times the human dose.

Breast-feeding—Sulfa medicines pass into the breast milk in small amounts. They may cause unwanted effects in nursing babies with glucose-6-phosphate dehydrogenase (G6PD) deficiency.

Children—Sulfasalazine should not be used in children up to 2 years of age because it may cause brain problems. However, sulfasalazine has not been shown to cause different side effects or problems in children over the age of 2 than it does in adults.

Older adults—Many medicines have not been studied specifically in older people. Therefore, it may not be known whether they work exactly the same way they do in younger adults or if they cause different side effects or problems in older people. There is no specific information comparing use of sulfasalazine in the elderly with use in other age groups.

Other medicines—Although certain medicines should not be used together at all, in other cases two different medicines may be used together even if an interaction might

occur. In these cases, your doctor may want to change the dose, or other precautions may be necessary. When you are taking sulfasalazine, it is especially important that your doctor and pharmacist know if you are taking any of the following:

- Acetaminophen (e.g., Tylenol) (with long-term, high-dose use) or
- Amiodarone (e.g., Cordarone) or
- Anabolic steroids (nandrolone [e.g., Anabolin], oxandrolone [e.g., Anavar], oxymetholone [e.g., Anadrol], stanozolol [e.g., Winstrol]) or
- Androgens (male hormones) or
- Antithyroid agents (medicine for overactive thyroid) or
- Carbamazepine (e.g., Tegretol) or
- Carmustine (e.g., BiCNU) or
- Chloroquine (e.g., Aralen) or
- Dantrolene (e.g., Dantrium) or
- Daunorubicin (e.g., Cerubidine) or
- Disulfiram (e.g., Antabuse) or
- Divalproex (e.g., Depakote) or
- Estrogens (female hormones) or
- Etretinate (e.g., Tegison) or
- Gold salts (medicine for arthritis) or
- Hydroxychloroquine (e.g., Plaquenil) or
- Mercaptopurine (e.g., Purinethol) or
- Naltrexone (e.g., Trexan) (with long-term, high-dose use) or
- Oral contraceptives (birth control pills) containing estrogen or
- Other anti-infectives by mouth or by injection (medicine for infection) or
- Phenothiazines (acetophenazine [e.g., Tindal], chlorpromazine [e.g., Thorazine], fluphenazine [e.g., Prolixin], mesoridazine [e.g., Serentil], perphenazine [e.g., Trilafon], prochlorperazine [e.g., Compazine], promazine [e.g., Sparine], promethazine [e.g., Phenergan], thioridazine [e.g., Mellaril], trifluoperazine [e.g., Stelazine], triflupromazine [e.g., Vesprin], trimeprazine [e.g., Temaril]) or
- Plicamycin (e.g., Mithracin) or
- Valproic acid (e.g., Depakene)—Use of sulfasalazine with these medicines may increase the chance of side effects affecting the liver

- Acetohydroxamic acid (e.g., Lithostat) or
- Dapsone or
- Furazolidone (e.g., Furoxone) or
- Nitrofurantoin (e.g., Furadantin) or
- Primaquine or
- Procainamide (e.g., Pronestyl) or
- Quinidine (e.g., Quinidex) or
- Quinine (e.g., Quinamm) or
- Sulfoxone (e.g., Diasone) or
- Vitamin K (e.g., AquaMEPHYTON, Synkayvite)—Use of sulfasalazine with these medicines may increase the chance of side effects affecting the blood

- Anticoagulants (blood thinners) or
- Ethotoin (e.g., Peganone) or
- Mephenytoin (e.g., Mesantoin)—Use of sulfasalazine with these medicines may increase the chance of side effects of these medicines

- Antidiabetics, oral (diabetes medicine you take by mouth)—Use of oral antidiabetics with sulfasalazine may increase the chance of side effects affecting the blood and/or the side effects or oral antidiabetics
- Methotrexate (e.g., Mexate)—Use of methotrexate with sulfasalazine may increase the chance of side effects affecting the liver and/or the side effects of methotrexate
- Methyldopa (e.g., Aldomet)—Use of methyldopa with sulfasalazine may increase the chance of side effects affecting the liver and/or the blood
- Phenytoin (e.g., Dilantin)—Use of phenytoin with sulfasalazine may increase the chance of side effects affecting the liver and/or the side effects of phenytoin

Other medical problems—The presence of other medical problems may affect the use of sulfasalazine. Make sure you tell your doctor if you have any other medical problems, especially:

- Blood problems or
- Glucose-6-phosphate dehydrogenase deficiency (lack of G6PD enzyme)—Patients with these problems may have an increase in side effects affecting the blood

- Kidney disease or
- Liver disease—Patients with kidney disease or liver disease may have an increased chance of side effects

- Porphyria—Use of sulfasalazine may cause an attack of porphyria

Before you begin using any new medicine (prescription or nonprescription) or if you develop any new medical problem while you are using this medicine, check with your doctor, nurse, or pharmacist.

Proper Use of This Medicine

Do not give sulfasalazine to infants up to 2 years of age, unless otherwise directed by your doctor. It may cause brain problems.

Sulfasalazine is best taken after meals or with food to lessen stomach upset. If stomach upset continues or is bothersome, check with your doctor.

Each dose of sulfasalazine should also be taken with a full glass (8 ounces) of water. Several additional glasses of water should be taken every day, unless otherwise directed by your doctor. Drinking extra water will help to prevent some unwanted effects (e.g., kidney stones) of the sulfa medicine.

For patients taking the *enteric-coated tablet form* of this medicine:

- Swallow tablets whole. Do not break or crush.

Keep taking this medicine for the full time of treatment, even if you begin to feel better after a few days. *Do not miss any doses.*

Missed dose—If you do miss a dose of this medicine, take it as soon as possible. However, if it is almost time for your next dose, skip the missed dose and go back to your regular dosing schedule. Do not double doses.

Storage—To store this medicine:
- Keep out of the reach of children.
- Store away from heat and direct light.
- Do not store the tablet form of this medicine in the bathroom, near the kitchen sink, or in other damp places. Heat or moisture may cause the medicine to break down.
- Keep the oral liquid form of this medicine from freezing.
- Do not keep outdated medicine or medicine no longer needed. Be sure that any discarded medicine is out of the reach of children.

Precautions While Using This Medicine

It is very important that your doctor check your progress at regular visits. This medicine may cause blood problems, especially if it is taken for a long time.

If your symptoms (including diarrhea) do not improve within a month or 2, or if they become worse, check with your doctor.

Sulfasalazine may cause blood problems. These problems may result in a greater chance of certain infections, slow healing, and bleeding of the gums. Therefore, you should be careful when using regular toothbrushes, dental floss, and toothpicks. Dental work should be delayed until your blood counts have returned to normal. Check with your medical doctor or dentist if you have any questions about proper oral hygiene (mouth care) during treatment.

Sulfasalazine may cause your skin to be more sensitive to sunlight than it is normally. Exposure to sunlight, even for brief periods of time, may cause a skin rash, itching, redness or other discoloration of the skin, or a severe sunburn. When you begin taking this medicine:
- Stay out of direct sunlight, especially between the hours of 10:00 a.m. and 3:00 p.m., if possible.
- Wear protective clothing, including a hat. Also, wear sunglasses.
- Apply a sun block product that has a skin protection factor (SPF) of at least 15. Some patients may require a product with a higher SPF number, especially if they have a fair complexion. If you have any questions about this, check with your doctor or pharmacist.
- Apply a sun block lipstick that has an SPF of at least 15 to protect your lips.
- Do not use a sunlamp or tanning bed or booth.

If you have a severe reaction from the sun, check with your doctor.

This medicine may also cause some people to become dizzy. *Make sure you know how you react to this medicine before you drive, use machines, or do anything else that could be dangerous if you are dizzy.* If this reaction is especially bothersome, check with your doctor.

Before you have any medical tests, tell the doctor in charge that you are taking this medicine. The results of the bentiromide (e.g., Chymex) test for pancreas function are affected by this medicine.

Side Effects of This Medicine

Along with its needed effects, a medicine may cause some unwanted effects. Although not all of these side effects may occur, if they do occur they may need medical attention.

Check with your doctor immediately if any of the following side effects occur:

More common

Aching of joints and muscles; headache (continuing); itching; skin rash

Less common

Back, leg, or stomach pains; difficulty in swallowing; fever and sore throat; pale skin; redness, blistering, peeling, or loosening of skin; unusual bleeding or bruising; unusual tiredness or weakness; yellow eyes or skin

Rare

Bloody diarrhea, fever, and rash; cough; difficult breathing

Also, check with your doctor as soon as possible if the following side effect occurs:

More common

Increased sensitivity of skin to sunlight

Other side effects may occur that usually do not need medical attention. These side effects may go away during treatment as your body adjusts to the medicine. However, check with your doctor if any of the following side effects continue or are bothersome:

More common

Abdominal or stomach pain or upset; diarrhea; dizziness; loss of appetite; nausea or vomiting

In some patients this medicine may also cause the urine or skin to become orange-yellow. This side effect does not need medical attention.

Other side effects not listed above may also occur in some patients. If you notice any other effects, check with your doctor.

Additional Information

Once a medicine has been approved for marketing for a certain use, experience may show that it is also useful for other medical problems. Although these uses are not

included in product labeling, sulfasalazine is used in certain patients with the following medical conditions:
- Ankylosing spondylitis
- Rheumatoid arthritis

Other than the above information, there is no additional information relating to proper use, precautions, or side effects for these uses.

Annual revision: 08/22/91

SULFINPYRAZONE Systemic

Some commonly used brand names are:

In the U.S.
Anturane
Generic name product may also be available.

In Canada
Anturan
Apo-Sulfinpyrazone
Novopyrazone

Description

Sulfinpyrazone (sul-fin-PEER-a-zone) is used in the treatment of chronic gout (gouty arthritis), which is caused by too much uric acid in the blood. The medicine works by removing the extra uric acid from the body. Sulfinpyrazone does not cure gout, but after you have been taking it for a few months it may help prevent gout attacks. This medicine will help prevent gout attacks only as long as you continue to take it.

Sulfinpyrazone is sometimes used to prevent or treat other medical problems that may occur if too much uric acid is present in the body.

Sulfinpyrazone may also be used for other conditions as determined by your doctor.

Sulfinpyrazone is available only with your doctor's prescription, in the following dosage forms:

Oral
- Capsules (U.S.)
- Tablets (U.S. and Canada)

It is very important that you read and understand the following information. If any of it causes you special concern, check with your doctor. Also, *if you have any questions* or if you want more information about this medicine or your medical problem, *ask your doctor, nurse, or pharmacist.*

Before Using This Medicine

In deciding to use a medicine, the risks of taking the medicine must be weighed against the good it will do. This is a decision you and your doctor will make. For sulfinpyrazone, the following should be considered:

Allergies—Tell your doctor if you have ever had any unusual or allergic reaction to sulfinpyrazone or to aspirin, oxyphenbutazone (e.g., Tandearil), or phenylbutazone (e.g., Butazolidin), or other anti-inflammatory analgesics (medicines used for pain and/or inflammation). Also tell your doctor and pharmacist if you are allergic to any other substances, such as foods, preservatives, or dyes.

Pregnancy—Sulfinpyrazone has not been reported to cause problems in humans.

Breast-feeding—It is not known whether sulfinpyrazone passes into the breast milk.

Children—Studies on this medicine have been done only in adult patients, and there is no specific information comparing use of sulfinpyrazone in children with use in other age groups.

Older adults—Many medicines have not been studied specifically in older people. Therefore, it may not be known whether they work exactly the same way they do in younger adults or if they cause different side effects or problems in older people. There is no specific information comparing use of sulfinpyrazone in the elderly with use in other age groups.

Other medicines—Although certain medicines should not be used together at all, in other cases two different medicines may be used together even if an interaction might occur. In these cases, your doctor may want to change the dose, or other precautions may be necessary. When you are taking sulfinpyrazone, it is especially important that your doctor and pharmacist know if you are taking any of the following:
- Anticoagulants (blood thinners) or
- Carbenicillin by injection (e.g., Geopen) or
- Cefamandole (e.g., Mandol) or
- Cefoperazone (e.g., Cefobid) or
- Cefotetan (e.g., Cefotan) or
- Dipyridamole (e.g., Persantine) or
- Divalproex (e.g., Depakote) or
- Heparin (e.g., Panheprin) or
- Inflammation or pain medicine, except narcotics, or
- Moxalactam (e.g., Moxam) or
- Pentoxifylline (e.g., Trental) or
- Plicamycin (e.g., Mithracin) or
- Ticarcillin (e.g., Ticar) or
- Valproic acid (e.g., Depakene)—Use of these medicines together with sulfinpyrazone may increase the chance of bleeding
- Antineoplastics (cancer medicine)—The chance of serious side effects may be increased

- Aspirin or other salicylates, including bismuth subsalicylate (e.g., Pepto Bismol)—These medicines may keep sulfinpyrazone from working properly in treating gout, depending on the amount of aspirin or other salicylate that you take and how often you take it. Taking sulfinpyrazone and aspirin together may also increase the chance of bleeding
- Nitrofurantoin (e.g., Furadantin)—Sulfinpyrazone may keep nitrofurantoin from working properly

Other medical problems—The presence of other medical problems may affect the use of sulfinpyrazone. Make sure you tell your doctor if you have any other medical problems, especially:

- Blood disease (or history of) or
- Cancer being treated by antineoplastics (cancer medicine) or radiation (x-rays) or
- Kidney stones (or history of) or other kidney disease or
- Stomach ulcer or other stomach or intestinal problems (or history of)—The chance of serious side effects may be increased; also, sulfinpyrazone may not work properly for treating gout if some kinds of kidney disease are present

Before you begin using any new medicine (prescription or nonprescription) or if you develop any new medical problem while you are using this medicine, check with your doctor, nurse, or pharmacist.

Proper Use of This Medicine

If sulfinpyrazone upsets your stomach, it may be taken with food. If this does not work, an antacid may be taken. If stomach upset (nausea, vomiting, or stomach pain) continues, check with your doctor.

In order for sulfinpyrazone to help you, it must be taken regularly as ordered by your doctor.

When you first begin taking sulfinpyrazone, the amount of uric acid in the kidneys is greatly increased. This may cause kidney stones in some people. To help prevent this, your doctor may want you to drink at least 10 to 12 full glasses (8 ounces each) of fluids each day, or to take another medicine to make your urine less acid. *It is important that you follow your doctor's instructions very carefully.*

For patients taking sulfinpyrazone for *gout:*

- After you begin to take sulfinpyrazone, gout attacks may continue to occur for a while. However, if you take this medicine regularly as directed by your doctor, the attacks will gradually become less frequent and less painful. After you have been taking sulfinpyrazone for several months, they may stop completely.
- Sulfinpyrazone helps to prevent gout attacks. It will not relieve an attack that has already started. *Even if you take another medicine for gout attacks, continue to take this medicine also.*

Dosing—The dose of sulfinpyrazone will be different for different patients. *Follow your doctor's orders or the directions on the label.* The following information includes only the average doses of sulfinpyrazone. *If your dose is different, do not change it* unless your doctor tells you to do so.

- *For treating gout or removing uric acid from the body:*
  —Adults: The starting dose of sulfinpyrazone is usually 100 mg or 200 mg a day (one-half of a 100-mg tablet two times a day, one 100-mg tablet one or two times a day, or one 200-mg capsule or tablet once a day). Then, the dose is usually increased by 100 mg or 200 mg every few days, up to 800 mg a day. Starting with a low dose and increasing the dose gradually helps prevent kidney stones and other side effects. After a while, the dose may be changed again, depending on the amount of uric acid in your blood or urine.

  —Children: It is not likely that sulfinpyrazone will be needed to treat gout or remove uric acid from the body in children. However, if a child needs this medicine, the dose would have to be determined by the doctor.

Missed dose—If you miss a dose of this medicine, take it as soon as possible. However, if is almost time for your next dose, skip the missed dose and go back to your regular dosing schedule. Do not double doses.

Storage—To store this medicine:

- Keep out of the reach of children.
- Store away from heat and direct light.
- Do not store this medicine in the bathroom, near the kitchen sink, or in other damp places. Heat or moisture may cause the medicine to break down.
- Do not keep outdated medicine or medicine no longer needed. Be sure that any discarded medicine is out of the reach of children.

Precautions While Using This Medicine

Your doctor should check your progress at regular visits to make sure that this medicine does not cause unwanted effects.

Before you have any medical tests, tell the person in charge that you are taking this medicine. The results of some tests may be affected by sulfinpyrazone.

For patients taking sulfinpyrazone for *gout or to help remove uric acid from the body:*

- Taking aspirin or other salicylates may lessen the effects of sulfinpyrazone. This will depend on the dose of aspirin or other salicylate that you take, and on how often you take it. Also, drinking too much alcohol may increase the amount of uric acid in the blood and lessen the effects of sulfinpyrazone. Therefore, *do not take aspirin or other salicylates or drink alcoholic beverages while taking this medicine,* unless you have first checked with your doctor.

Side Effects of This Medicine

Along with its needed effects, a medicine may cause some unwanted effects. Although not all of these side effects may occur, if they do occur they may need medical attention.

Check with your doctor immediately if any of the following side effects occur:

Rare

Shortness of breath, troubled breathing, tightness in chest, and/or wheezing; sores, ulcers, or white spots on lips or in mouth; sore throat and fever with or without chills; swollen and/or painful glands; unusual bleeding or bruising

Symptoms of overdose

Clumsiness or unsteadiness; convulsions (seizures); diarrhea; nausea or vomiting (severe or continuing); stomach pain (severe or continuing); difficulty in breathing

Also, check with your doctor as soon as possible if any of the following side effects occur:

More common

Lower back and/or side pain; painful urination (possibly with blood)

Less common

Skin rash

Rare

Bloody or black, tarry stools; fever; increased blood pressure; pinpoint red spots on skin; sudden decrease in amount of urine; swelling of face, fingers, feet, and/or lower legs; unusual tiredness or weakness; vomiting of blood or material that looks like coffee grounds; weight gain

Other side effects may occur that usually do not need medical attention. These side effects may go away during treatment as your body adjusts to the medicine. However, check with your doctor if any of the following side effects continue or are bothersome:

More common

Joint pain, redness, and/or swelling; nausea or vomiting; stomach pain

Other side effects not listed above may also occur in some patients. If you notice any other effects, check with your doctor.

Annual revision: 01/19/93

SULFONAMIDES Ophthalmic

This information applies to the following medicines:

Sulfacetamide (sul-fa-SEE-ta-mide)
Sulfisoxazole (sul-fi-SOX-a-zole)

Some commonly used brand names are:

For Sulfacetamide

In the U.S.

Ak-Sulf
Bleph-10
Cetamide
Isopto-Cetamide
I-Sulfacet
Ocu-Sul-10
Ocu-Sul-15
Ocu-Sul-30
Ocusulf-10
Ophthacet
Sodium Sulamyd
Spectro-Sulf
Steri-Units Sulfacetamide
Sulf-10
Sulfair
Sulfair 10
Sulfair 15
Sulfair Forte
Sulfamide
Sulten-10

Generic name product may also be available.

In Canada

Ak-Sulf
Bleph-10
Cetamide
Isopto-Cetamide
Sodium Sulamyd
Sulfex

For Sulfisoxazole

In the U.S.

Gantrisin

Another commonly used name is sulfafurazole.

Description

Sulfonamides (sul-FON-a-mides) or sulfa medicines belong to the family of medicines called anti-infectives. Sulfonamide ophthalmic preparations are used to treat infections of the eye.

Sulfonamides are available only with your doctor's prescription, in the following dosage forms:

Ophthalmic

Sulfacetamide
- Ophthalmic ointment (U.S. and Canada)
- Ophthalmic solution (eye drops) (U.S. and Canada)

Sulfisoxazole
- Ophthalmic ointment (U.S.)
- Ophthalmic solution (eye drops) (U.S.)

It is very important that you read and understand the following information. If any of it causes you special concern, check with your doctor. Also, *if you have any questions* or if you want more information about this medicine or your medical problem, *ask your doctor, nurse, or pharmacist.*

Before Using This Medicine

In deciding to use a medicine, the risks of using the medicine must be weighed against the good it will do. This is a decision you and your doctor will make. For sulfonamide ophthalmic preparations, the following should be considered:

Allergies—Tell your doctor if you have ever had any unusual or allergic reaction to any of the sulfa medicines; furosemide (e.g., Lasix) or thiazide diuretics (water pills); oral antidiabetics (diabetes medicine you take by mouth); or glaucoma medicine you take by mouth (for example, acetazolamide [e.g., Diamox], dichlorphenamide [e.g., Daranide], or methazolamide [e.g., Neptazane]). Also tell your doctor and pharmacist if you are allergic to any other substances, such as preservatives.

Pregnancy—Sulfonamide ophthalmic preparations have not been shown to cause birth defects or other problems in humans.

Breast-feeding—Sulfonamide ophthalmic preparations have not been reported to cause problems in nursing babies.

Children—Studies on sulfonamide ophthalmic preparations have been done only in adult patients, and there is no specific information comparing use in children with use in other age groups.

Older adults—Many medicines have not been studied specifically in older people. Therefore, it may not be known whether they work exactly the same way they do in younger adults or if they cause different side effects or problems in older people. There is no specific information comparing use of sulfonamides in the elderly with use in other age groups.

Other medicines—Although certain medicines should not be used together at all, in other cases two different medicines may be used together even if an interaction might occur. In these cases, your doctor may want to change the dose, or other precautions may be necessary. When you are taking sulfonamide ophthalmic preparations, it is especially important that your doctor and pharmacist know if you are using any of the following:

- Silver preparations, such as silver nitrate or mild silver protein for the eye—Sulfonamide ophthalmic preparations should not be used with silver ophthalmic preparations, since a chemical reaction may occur.

Before you begin using any new medicine (prescription or nonprescription) or if you develop any new medical problem while you are using this medicine, check with your doctor, nurse, or pharmacist.

Proper Use of This Medicine

For patients using the *eye drop form* of sulfonamides:

- The bottle is only partially full to provide proper drop control.
- To use:

  —First, wash your hands. Then tilt the head back and pull the lower eyelid away from the eye to form a pouch. Drop the medicine into the pouch and gently close the eyes. Do not blink. Keep the eyes closed for 1 or 2 minutes to allow the medicine to come into contact with the infection.

  —If you think you did not get the drop of medicine into your eye properly, use another drop.

  —To keep the medicine as germ-free as possible, do not touch the applicator tip to any surface (including the eye). Also, keep the container tightly closed.

For patients using the *eye ointment form* of sulfonamides:

- To use:

  —First, wash your hands. Then pull the lower eyelid away from the eye to form a pouch. Squeeze a thin strip of ointment into the pouch. A 1.25- to 2.5-cm (approximately ½- to 1-inch) strip of ointment is usually enough unless otherwise directed by your doctor. Gently close the eyes and keep them closed for 1 or 2 minutes to allow the medicine to come into contact with the infection.

  —To keep the medicine as germ-free as possible, do not touch the applicator tip to any surface (including the eye). After using sulfonamides eye ointment, wipe the tip of the ointment tube with a clean tissue and keep the tube tightly closed.

To help clear up your infection completely, *keep using this medicine for the full time of treatment,* even if your symptoms have disappeared. *Do not miss any doses.*

Dosing—The dose of ophthalmic sulfonamides will be different for different patients. *Follow your doctor's orders or the directions on the label.* The following information includes only the average doses of ophthalmic sulfonamides. *If your dose is different, do not change it* unless your doctor tells you to do so.

The number of doses you use each day, the time allowed between doses, and the length of time you use the medicine depend on the medical problem for which you are using ophthalmic sulfonamides.

For sulfacetamide

- For eye infections:
  - —For *ophthalmic* dosage forms (ointment):
    - Adults and adolescents—Use four times a day and at bedtime.
    - Children—Use and dose must be determined by your doctor.
  - —For *ophthalmic* dosage forms (solution):
    - Adults and adolescents—One drop every one to three hours during the day and less often during the night.
    - Children—Use and dose must be determined by your doctor.

For sulfisoxazole

- For eye infections:
  - —For *ophthalmic* dosage forms (ointment):
    - Adults and children—Use one to three times a day and at bedtime.
  - —For *ophthalmic* dosage forms (solution):
    - Adults and adolescents—One drop three or more times a day.
    - Children—
      - —Infants up to 2 months of age: Use and dose must be determined by your doctor.
      - —Infants and children 2 months of age and older: One drop three or more times a day.

Missed dose—If you miss a dose of this medicine, apply it as soon as possible. However, if it is almost time for your next dose, skip the missed dose and go back to your regular dosing schedule.

Storage—To store this medicine:

- Keep out of the reach of children.
- Store away from heat and direct light.
- Keep sulfacetamide eye drops in a cool place. Keep all dosage forms of these medicines from freezing.
- Do not keep outdated medicine or medicine no longer needed. Be sure that any discarded medicine is out of the reach of children.

Precautions While Using This Medicine

After application, eye ointments usually cause your vision to blur for a few minutes.

After application of this medicine to the eye, occasional stinging or burning may be expected.

If your symptoms do not improve within a few days, or if they become worse, check with your doctor.

Side Effects of This Medicine

Along with its needed effects, a medicine may cause some unwanted effects. Although not all of these side effects may occur, if they do occur they may need medical attention.

Check with your doctor as soon as possible if any of the following side effects occur:

More common

Itching, redness, swelling, or other sign of irritation not present before use of this medicine

Other side effects not listed above may also occur in some patients. If you notice any other effects, check with your doctor.

Annual revision: 07/01/93

SULFONAMIDES Systemic

This information applies to the following medicines:

Sulfacytine (sul-fa-SYE-teen)
Sulfadiazine (sul-fa-DYE-a-zeen)
Sulfamethizole (sul-fa-METH-a-zole)
Sulfamethoxazole (sul-fa-meth-OX-a-zole)
Sulfisoxazole (sul-fi-SOX-a-zole)

Some commonly used brand names are:

For Sulfacytine†
In the U.S.
Renoquid

For Sulfadiazine†
In the U.S.
Generic name product may be available.

For Sulfamethizole†
In the U.S.
Thiosulfil Forte

For Sulfamethoxazole
In the U.S.
Gantanol
Generic name product may also be available.
In Canada
Apo-Sulfamethoxazole Gantanol

For Sulfisoxazole
In the U.S.
Gantrisin
Generic name product may be available.
In Canada
Novosoxazole

Another commonly used name is sulfafurazole.

†Not commercially available in Canada.

Description

Sulfonamides (sul-FON-a-mides) or sulfa medicines are used to treat infections. They will not work for colds, flu, or other virus infections.

Sulfonamides are available only with your doctor's prescription, in the following dosage forms:

Oral

Sulfacytine
- Tablets (U.S.)

Sulfadiazine
- Tablets (U.S.)

Sulfamethizole
- Tablets (U.S.)

Sulfamethoxazole
- Oral suspension (U.S.)
- Tablets (U.S. and Canada)

Sulfisoxazole
- Oral suspension (U.S.)
- Syrup (U.S.)
- Tablets (U.S. and Canada)

It is very important that you read and understand the following information. If any of it causes you special concern, check with your doctor. Also, *if you have any questions* or if you want more information about this medicine or your medical problem, *ask your doctor, nurse, or pharmacist.*

Before Using This Medicine

In deciding to use a medicine, the risks of taking the medicine must be weighed against the good it will do. This is a decision you and your doctor will make. For sulfonamides, the following should be considered:

Allergies—Tell your doctor if you have ever had any unusual or allergic reaction to sulfa medicines, furosemide (e.g., Lasix) or thiazide diuretics (water pills), oral antidiabetics (diabetes medicine you take by mouth), glaucoma medicine you take by mouth (for example, acetazolamide [e.g., Diamox], dichlorphenamide [e.g., Daranide], or methazolamide [e.g., Neptazane]). Also tell your doctor and pharmacist if you are allergic to any other substances, such as foods, preservatives, or dyes.

Pregnancy—Studies have not been done in pregnant women. However, studies in mice, rats, and rabbits have shown that some sulfonamides cause birth defects, including cleft palate and bone problems.

Breast-feeding—Sulfonamides pass into the breast milk. This medicine is not recommended for use during breast-feeding. It may cause liver problems, anemia, and other unwanted effects in nursing babies, especially those with glucose-6-phosphate dehydrogenase (G6PD) deficiency.

Children—Sulfonamides should not be given to infants under 2 months of age unless directed by the child's doctor, because they may cause brain problems. Sulfacytine should not be given to children up to the age of 14.

Older adults—Elderly people are especially sensitive to the effects of sulfonamides. Severe skin problems and blood problems may be more likely to occur in the elderly. These problems may also be more likely to occur in patients who are taking diuretics (water pills) along with this medicine.

Other medicines—Although certain medicines should not be used together at all, in other cases two different medicines may be used together even if an interaction might occur. In these cases, your doctor may want to change the dose, or other precautions may be necessary. When you are taking sulfonamides, it is especially important that your doctor and pharmacist know if you are taking any of the following:

- Acetaminophen (e.g., Tylenol) (with long-term, high-dose use) or
- Amiodarone (e.g., Cordarone) or
- Anabolic steroids (nandrolone [e.g., Anabolin], oxandrolone [e.g., Anavar], oxymetholone [e.g., Anadrol], stanozolol [e.g., Winstrol]) or
- Androgens (male hormones) or
- Antithyroid agents (medicine for overactive thyroid) or
- Carbamazepine (e.g., Tegretol) or
- Carmustine (e.g., BiCNU) or
- Chloroquine (e.g., Aralen) or
- Dantrolene (e.g., Dantrium) or
- Daunorubicin (e.g., Cerubidine) or
- Disulfiram (e.g., Antabuse) or
- Divalproex (e.g., Depakote) or
- Estrogens (female hormones) or
- Etretinate (e.g., Tegison) or
- Gold salts (medicine for arthritis) or
- Hydroxychloroquine (e.g., Plaquenil) or
- Mercaptopurine (e.g., Purinethol) or
- Naltrexone (e.g., Trexan) (with long-term, high-dose use) or
- Oral contraceptives (birth control pills) containing estrogens or
- Other anti-infectives by mouth or by injection (medicine for infection) or
- Phenothiazines (acetophenazine [e.g., Tindal], chlorpromazine [e.g., Thorazine], fluphenazine [e.g., Prolixin], mesoridazine [e.g., Serentil], perphenazine [e.g., Trilafon], prochlorperazine [e.g., Compazine], promazine [e.g., Sparine], promethazine [e.g., Phenergan], thioridazine [e.g., Mellaril], trifluoperazine [e.g., Stelazine], triflupromazine [e.g., Vesprin], trimeprazine [e.g., Temaril]) or
- Plicamycin (e.g., Mithracin) or
- Valproic acid (e.g., Depakene)—Use of sulfonamides with these medicines may increase the chance of side effects affecting the liver

- Acetohydroxamic acid (e.g., Lithostat) or
- Dapsone or
- Furazolidone (e.g., Furoxone) or
- Nitrofurantoin (e.g., Furadantin) or
- Primaquine or
- Procainamide (e.g., Pronestyl) or
- Quinidine (e.g., Quinidex) or
- Quinine (e.g., Quinamm) or
- Sulfoxone (e.g., Diasone)—Use of sulfonamides with these medicines may increase the chance of side effects affecting the blood

- Anticoagulants (blood thinners) or
- Ethotoin (e.g., Peganone) or
- Mephenytoin (e.g., Mesantoin)—Use of sulfonamides with these medicines may increase the chance of side effects of these medicines

- Antidiabetics, oral (diabetes medicine you take by mouth)—Use of oral antidiabetics with sulfonamides may increase the chance of side effects affecting the blood and/or the side effects of oral antidiabetics

- Methenamine (e.g., Mandelamine)—Use of this medicine with sulfonamides may increase the chance of side effects of sulfonamides
- Methyldopa (e.g., Aldomet)—Use of methyldopa with sulfonamides may increase the chance of side effects affecting the liver and/or the blood
- Methotrexate (e.g., Mexate) or
- Phenytoin (e.g., Dilantin)—Use of these medicines with sulfonamides may increase the chance of side effects affecting the liver and/or the side effects of these medicines

Other medical problems—The presence of other medical problems may affect the use of sulfonamides. Make sure you tell your doctor if you have any other medical problems, especially:

- Anemia or other blood problems or
- Glucose-6-phosphate dehydrogenase (G6PD) deficiency—Patients with these problems may have an increase in side effects affecting the blood
- Kidney disease or
- Liver disease—Patients with kidney and/or liver disease may have an increased chance of side effects
- Porphyria—This medicine may bring on an attack of porphyria

Before you begin using any new medicine (prescription or nonprescription) or if you develop any new medical problem while you are using this medicine, check with your doctor, nurse, or pharmacist.

Proper Use of This Medicine

Sulfonamides are best taken with a full glass (8 ounces) of water. Several additional glasses of water should be taken every day, unless otherwise directed by your doctor. Drinking extra water will help to prevent some unwanted effects (e.g., kidney stones) of sulfonamides.

For patients taking the *oral liquid form* of this medicine:

- Use a specially marked measuring spoon or other device to measure each dose accurately. The average household teaspoon may not hold the right amount of liquid.

To help clear up your infection completely, *keep taking this medicine for the full time of treatment,* even if you begin to feel better after a few days. If you stop taking this medicine too soon, your symptoms may return.

This medicine works best when there is a constant amount in the blood or urine. *To help keep the amount constant, do not miss any doses. Also, it is best to take the doses at evenly spaced times day and night.* For example, if you are to take 4 doses a day, the doses should be spaced about 6 hours apart. If this interferes with your sleep or other daily activities, or if you need help in planning the best times to take your medicine, check with your doctor, nurse, or pharmacist.

Missed dose—If you do miss a dose of this medicine, take it as soon as possible. This will help to keep a constant amount of medicine in the blood or urine. However, if it is almost time for your next dose, skip the missed dose and go back to your regular dosing schedule. Do not double doses.

Storage—To store this medicine:

- Keep out of the reach of children.
- Store away from heat and direct light.
- Do not store the tablet form of this medicine in the bathroom, near the kitchen sink, or in other damp places. Heat or moisture may cause the medicine to break down.
- Keep the oral liquid forms of this medicine from freezing.
- Do not keep outdated medicine or medicine no longer needed. Be sure that any discarded medicine is out of the reach of children.

Precautions While Using This Medicine

It is very important that your doctor check your progress at regular visits. This medicine may cause blood problems, especially if it is taken for a long time.

If your symptoms do not improve within a few days, or if they become worse, check with your doctor.

Sulfonamides may cause blood problems. These problems may result in a greater chance of certain infections, slow healing, and bleeding of the gums. Therefore, you should be careful when using regular toothbrushes, dental floss, and toothpicks. Dental work should be delayed until your blood counts have returned to normal. Check with your medical doctor or dentist if you have any questions about proper oral hygiene (mouth care) during treatment.

Sulfonamides may cause your skin to be more sensitive to sunlight than it is normally. Exposure to sunlight, even for brief periods of time, may cause a skin rash, itching, redness or other discoloration of the skin, or a severe sunburn. When you begin taking this medicine:

- Stay out of direct sunlight, especially between the hours of 10:00 a.m. and 3:00 p.m., if possible.
- Wear protective clothing, including a hat. Also, wear sunglasses.
- Apply a sun block product that has a skin protection factor (SPF) of at least 15. Some patients may require a product with a higher SPF number, especially if they have a fair complexion. If you have any questions about this, check with your doctor or pharmacist.
- Apply a sun block lipstick that has an SPF of at least 15 to protect your lips.
- Do not use a sunlamp or tanning bed or booth.

If you have a severe reaction from the sun, check with your doctor.

This medicine may also cause some people to become dizzy. *Make sure you know how you react to this medicine before you drive, use machines, or do anything else that could be dangerous if you are dizzy or are not alert.* If this reaction is especially bothersome, check with your doctor.

Side Effects of This Medicine

Along with its needed effects, a medicine may cause some unwanted effects. Although not all of these side effects may occur, if they do occur they may need medical attention.

Check with your doctor immediately if any of the following side effects occur:

More common

Itching; skin rash

Less common

Aching of joints and muscles; difficulty in swallowing; pale skin; redness, blistering, peeling, or loosening of skin; sore throat and fever; unusual bleeding or bruising; unusual tiredness or weakness; yellow eyes or skin

Rare

Blood in urine; greatly increased or decreased frequency of urination or amount of urine; increased thirst; lower back pain; pain or burning while urinating; swelling of front part of neck

Also, check with your doctor as soon as possible if the following side effect occurs:

More common

Increased sensitivity of skin to sunlight

Other side effects may occur that usually do not need medical attention. These side effects may go away during treatment as your body adjusts to the medicine. However, check with your doctor if any of the following side effects continue or are bothersome:

More common

Diarrhea; dizziness; headache; loss of appetite; nausea or vomiting; tiredness

Other side effects not listed above may also occur in some patients. If you notice any other effects, check with your doctor.

Annual revision: 10/10/92

SULFONAMIDES Vaginal

This information applies to the following medicines:

Sulfanilamide (sul-fa-NILL-a-mide)
Sulfanilamide, Aminacrine (am-in-AK-rin), and Allantoin (al-AN-toyn)
Triple Sulfa (TRI-pel SUL-fa)

Some commonly used brand names are:

For Sulfanilamide

In the U.S.

AVC
Vagitrol

For Sulfanilamide, Aminacrine, and Allantoin*

In Canada

AVC

For Triple Sulfa

In the U.S.

Sulfa-Gyn
Sulnac
Sultrin
Trysul
V.V.S.

Generic name product may also be available.

In Canada

Sultrin

Another commonly used name for triple sulfa is sulfathiazole, sulfacetamide, and sulfabenzamide.

*Not commercially available in the U.S.

Description

Sulfonamides (sul-FON-a-mides), or sulfa medicines, are used to treat bacterial infections. They work by killing bacteria or preventing their growth.

Vaginal sulfonamides are used to treat bacterial infections. These medicines may also be used for other problems as determined by your doctor.

Vaginal sulfonamides are available only with your doctor's prescription, in the following dosage forms:

Vaginal

Sulfanilamide
- Cream (U.S.)
- Suppositories (U.S.)

Sulfanilamide, Aminacrine, and Allantoin
- Cream (Canada)
- Suppositories (Canada)

Triple Sulfa
- Cream (U.S. and Canada)
- Tablets (U.S.)

It is very important that you read and understand the following information. If any of it causes you special concern, check with your doctor. Also, *if you have any questions* or if you want more information about this medicine or your medical problem, *ask your doctor, nurse, or pharmacist.*

Before Using This Medicine

In deciding to use a medicine, the risks of using the medicine must be weighed against the good it will do.

This is a decision you and your doctor will make. For vaginal sulfonamides, the following should be considered:

Allergies—Tell your doctor if you have ever had any unusual or allergic reaction to any of the sulfa medicines, furosemide (e.g., Lasix) or thiazide diuretics (water pills), oral antidiabetics (diabetes medicine you take by mouth), or glaucoma medicine you take by mouth (for example, acetazolamide [e.g., Diamox], dichlorphenamide [e.g., Daranide], or methazolamide [e.g., Neptazane]). Also tell your doctor and pharmacist if you are allergic to any other substances, such as foods, preservatives, or dyes.

Pregnancy—Studies have not been done in humans. However, vaginal sulfonamides are absorbed through the vagina into the bloodstream and appear in the bloodstream of the fetus. Studies in rats and mice given high doses by mouth have shown that certain sulfonamides cause birth defects.

Breast-feeding—Vaginal sulfonamides are absorbed through the vagina into the bloodstream and pass into the breast milk. Use is not recommended in nursing mothers. Vaginal sulfonamides may cause liver problems in nursing babies. These medicines may also cause anemia in nursing babies with glucose-6-phosphate dehydrogenase (G6PD) deficiency.

Children—Studies on this medicine have been done only in adult patients and there is no specific information comparing the use of vaginal sulfonamides in children with use in other age groups.

Older adults—Many medicines have not been studied specifically in older people. Therefore, it may not be known whether they work exactly the same way they do in younger adults or if they cause different side effects or problems in older people. There is no specific information comparing the use of vaginal sulfonamides in the elderly with use in other age groups.

Other medicines—Although certain medicines should not be used together at all, in other cases two different medicines may be used together even if an interaction might occur. In these cases, your doctor may want to change the dose, or other precautions may be necessary. Tell your doctor and pharmacist if you are taking or using any other prescription or nonprescription (over-the-counter [OTC]) medicine.

Other medical problems—The presence of other medical problems may affect the use of vaginal sulfonamides. Make sure you tell your doctor if you have any other medical problems, especially:

- Glucose-6-phosphate dehydrogenase (G6PD) deficiency—Anemia (a blood problem) can occur if sulfonamides are used
- Kidney disease
- Porphyria—Sulfonamides can cause porphyria attacks

Before you begin using any new medicine (prescription or nonprescription) or if you develop any new medical problem while you are using this medicine, check with your doctor, nurse, or pharmacist.

Proper Use of This Medicine

Vaginal sulfonamides usually come with patient directions. Read them carefully before using this medicine.

This medicine is usually inserted into the vagina with an applicator. However, if you are pregnant, check with your doctor before using the applicator.

To help clear up your infection completely, *it is very important that you keep using this medicine for the full time of treatment*, even if your symptoms begin to clear up after a few days. If you stop using this medicine too soon, your symptoms may return. *Do not miss any doses.* Also, *do not stop using this medicine if your menstrual period starts during the time of treatment.*

Missed dose—If you do miss a dose of this medicine, insert it as soon as possible. However, if it is almost time for your next dose, skip the missed dose and go back to your regular dosing schedule.

Storage—To store this medicine:

- Keep out of the reach of children.
- Store away from heat and direct light.
- Do not store the vaginal tablet or vaginal suppository form of this medicine in the bathroom, near the kitchen sink, or in other damp places. Heat or moisture may cause the medicine to break down.
- Keep the vaginal cream and vaginal suppository forms of this medicine from freezing.
- Do not keep outdated medicine or medicine no longer needed. Be sure that any discarded medicine is out of the reach of children.

Precautions While Using This Medicine

If your symptoms do not improve within a few days, or if they become worse, check with your doctor.

Vaginal medicines usually will slowly work their way out of the vagina during treatment. Also, aminacrine-containing vaginal sulfonamides may stain underclothing. To keep the medicine from soiling or staining your clothing, a sanitary napkin may be worn. Minipads, clean paper tissues, or paper diapers may also be used. However, the use of tampons is not recommended since they may soak up too much of the medicine. In addition, tampons may be more likely to slip out of the vagina if you use them during treatment with this medicine.

To help clear up your infection completely and to help make sure it does not return, good health habits are also required.

- Wear cotton panties (or panties or pantyhose with cotton crotches) instead of synthetic (for example, nylon or rayon) underclothes.
- Wear only freshly washed underclothes.

If you have any questions about this, check with your doctor, nurse, or pharmacist.

Many vaginal infections are spread by sexual intercourse. The male sexual partner may carry the fungus or other organism in his reproductive tract. Therefore, it may be desirable that your partner wear a condom (prophylactic) during intercourse to keep the infection from returning. Also, it may be necessary for your partner to be treated at the same time you are being treated to avoid passing the infection back and forth. In addition, *do not stop using this medicine if you have intercourse during treatment.*

Some patients who use vaginal medicines may prefer to use a douche for cleansing purposes before inserting the next dose of medicine. Some doctors recommend a vinegar and water or other douche. However, others do not recommend douching at all. If you do use a douche, *do not overfill the vagina with douche solution.* To do so may force the solution up into the uterus (womb) and may cause inflammation or infection. Also, *do not douche if you are pregnant since this may harm the fetus.* If you have any questions about this or which douche products are best for you, check with your doctor, nurse, or pharmacist.

Side Effects of This Medicine

Studies in rats have shown that long-term use of sulfonamides may cause cancer of the thyroid gland. In addition, studies in rats have shown that sulfonamides may increase the chance of goiters (noncancerous tumors of the thyroid gland).

Along with its needed effects, a medicine may cause some unwanted effects. Although not all of these side effects may occur, if they do occur they may need medical attention.

Check with your doctor immediately if any of the following side effects occur:

Less common

Itching, burning, skin rash, redness, swelling, or other sign of irritation not present before use of this medicine

Other side effects may occur that usually do not need medical attention. These side effects may go away during treatment as your body adjusts to the medicine. However, check with your doctor if either of the following side effects continues or is bothersome:

Less common or rare

Rash or irritation of penis of sexual partner

Other side effects not listed above may also occur in some patients. If you notice any other effects, check with your doctor.

Annual revision: 07/22/92

SULFONAMIDES AND PHENAZOPYRIDINE Systemic

This information applies to the following medicines:

Sulfamethoxazole (sul-fa-meth-OX-a-zole) and Phenazopyridine (fen-az-oh-PEER-i-deen)

Sulfisoxazole (sul-fi-SOX-a-zole) and Phenazopyridine

Some commonly used brand names are:

For Sulfamethoxazole and Phenazopyridine†

In the U.S.

Azo Gantanol
Azo-Sulfamethoxazole

Generic name product may also be available.

For Sulfisoxazole and Phenazopyridine

In the U.S.

Azo Gantrisin
Azo-Sulfisoxazole
Azo-Truxazole
Sul-Azo

Generic name product may also be available.

In Canada

Azo Gantrisin

†Not commercially available in Canada.

Description

Sulfonamides and phenazopyridine, combination products containing a sulfa medicine and a urinary pain reliever, are used to treat infections of the urinary tract and to help relieve the pain, burning, and irritation of these infections.

Sulfonamides and phenazopyridine combinations are available only with your doctor's prescription, in the following dosage forms:

Oral

Sulfamethoxazole and Phenazopyridine
- Tablets (U.S.)

Sulfisoxazole and Phenazopyridine
- Tablets (U.S. and Canada)

It is very important that you read and understand the following information. If any of it causes you special concern, check with your doctor. Also, *if you have any*

questions or if you want more information about this medicine or your medical problem, *ask your doctor, nurse, or pharmacist.*

Before Using This Medicine

In deciding to use a medicine, the risks of taking the medicine must be weighed against the good it will do. This is a decision you and your doctor will make. For sulfonamides and phenazopyridine, the following should be considered:

Allergies—Tell your doctor if you have ever had any unusual or allergic reaction to any of the sulfa medicines, furosemide (e.g., Lasix) or thiazide diuretics (water pills), oral antidiabetics (diabetes medicine you take by mouth), glaucoma medicine you take by mouth (for example, acetazolamide [e.g., Diamox], dichlorphenamide [e.g., Daranide], or methazolamide [e.g., Neptazane]), or phenazopyridine (e.g., Pyridium). Also tell your doctor and pharmacist if you are allergic to any other substances, such as foods, preservatives, or dyes.

Pregnancy—Studies have not been done in humans. Studies in mice, rats, and rabbits have shown that some sulfonamides cause birth defects, including cleft palate and bone problems. In addition, sulfa medicines may cause liver problems in newborn infants. Therefore, use is not recommended during pregnancy. Phenazopyridine has not been shown to cause birth defects in animal studies.

Breast-feeding—Sulfonamides pass into the breast milk. This medicine is not recommended for use during breast-feeding. It may cause liver problems, anemia, and other unwanted effects in nursing babies, especially those with glucose-6-phosphate dehydrogenase (G6PD) deficiency.

Children—This medicine has been tested in a limited number of children 12 years of age or older. In effective doses, the medicine has not been shown to cause different side effects or problems in children than it does in adults.

Older adults—Elderly people are especially sensitive to the effects of sulfonamides. Severe skin problems and blood problems may be more likely to occur in the elderly. These problems may also be more likely to occur in patients who are taking diuretics (water pills) along with this medicine.

Other medicines—Although certain medicines should not be used together at all, in other cases two different medicines may be used together even if an interaction might occur. In these cases, your doctor may want to change the dose, or other precautions may be necessary. When you are taking sulfonamides and phenazopyridine, it is especially important that your doctor and pharmacist know if you are taking any of the following:

- Acetaminophen (e.g., Tylenol) (with long-term, high-dose use) or
- Amiodarone (e.g., Cordarone) or
- Anabolic steroids (nandrolone [e.g., Anabolin], oxandrolone [e.g., Anavar], oxymetholone [e.g., Anadrol], stanozolol [e.g., Winstrol]) or
- Androgens (male hormones) or
- Antithyroid agents (medicine for overactive thyroid) or
- Carbamazepine (e.g., Tegretol) or
- Carmustine (e.g., BiCNU) or
- Chloroquine (e.g., Aralen) or
- Dantrolene (e.g., Dantrium) or
- Daunorubicin (e.g., Cerubidine) or
- Disulfiram (e.g., Antabuse) or
- Divalproex (e.g., Depakote) or
- Estrogens (female hormones) or
- Etretinate (e.g., Tegison) or
- Gold salts (medicine for arthritis) or
- Hydroxychloroquine (e.g., Plaquenil) or
- Mercaptopurine (e.g., Purinethol) or
- Naltrexone (e.g., Trexan) (with long-term, high-dose use) or
- Oral contraceptives (birth control pills) containing estrogen or
- Other anti-infectives by mouth or by injection (medicine for infection) or
- Phenothiazines (acetophenazine [e.g., Tindal], chlorpromazine [e.g., Thorazine], fluphenazine [e.g., Prolixin], mesoridazine [e.g., Serentil], perphenazine [e.g., Trilafon], prochlorperazine [e.g., Compazine], promazine [e.g., Sparine], promethazine [e.g., Phenergan], thioridazine [e.g., Mellaril], trifluoperazine [e.g., Stelazine], triflupromazine [e.g., Vesprin], trimeprazine [e.g., Temaril]) or
- Plicamycin (e.g., Mithracin) or
- Valproic acid (e.g., Depakene)—Use of sulfonamides and phenazopyridine combination with these medicines may increase the chance of side effects affecting the liver

- Acetohydroxamic acid (e.g., Lithostat) or
- Dapsone or
- Furazolidone (e.g., Furoxone) or
- Nitrofurantoin (e.g., Furadantin) or
- Primaquine or
- Procainamide (e.g., Pronestyl) or
- Quinidine (e.g., Quinidex) or
- Quinine (e.g., Quinamm) or
- Sulfoxone (e.g., Diasone) or
- Vitamin K (e.g., AquaMEPHYTON, Synkayvite)—Use of sulfonamides and phenazopyridine combination with these medicines may increase the chance of side effects affecting the blood

- Anticoagulants (blood thinners) or
- Ethotoin (e.g., Peganone) or
- Heparin or
- Mephenytoin (e.g., Mesantoin)—Use of sulfonamides and phenazopyridine combination with these medicines may increase the chance of side effects of these medicines

- Antidiabetics, oral (diabetes medicine you take by mouth)—Use of oral antidiabetics with sulfonamides and phenazopyridine combination may increase the chance of side effects affecting the blood and/or the side effects of oral antidiabetics

- Methenamine (e.g., Mandelamine) or
- Methenamine-containing medicines (e.g., Urised)—Use of these medicines with sulfonamides and phenazopyridine combination may increase the chance of side effects of the sulfonamides

- Methotrexate (e.g., Mexate)—Use of methotrexate with sulfonamides and phenazopyridine combination may increase the chance of side effects affecting the liver and/or the side effects of methotrexate
- Methyldopa (e.g., Aldomet)—Use of methyldopa with sulfonamides and phenazopyridine combination may increase the chance of side effects affecting the liver and/or the blood
- Phenytoin (e.g., Dilantin)—Use of phenytoin with sulfonamides and phenazopyridine combination may increase the chance of side effects affecting the liver and/or the side effects of phenytoin

Other medical problems—The presence of other medical problems may affect the use of sulfonamides and phenazopyridine. Make sure you tell your doctor if you have any other medical problems, especially:

- Anemia or other blood problems or
- Glucose-6-phosphate dehydrogenase deficiency (lack of G6PD enzyme)—Patients with these problems may have an increase in side effects affecting the blood
- Hepatitis or other liver disease or
- Kidney disease—Patients with kidney disease or liver disease may have an increased chance of side effects
- Porphyria—Use of sulfonamides may bring on an attack of porphyria

Before you begin using any new medicine (prescription or nonprescription) or if you develop any new medical problem while you are using this medicine, check with your doctor, nurse, or pharmacist.

Proper Use of This Medicine

Sulfonamides and phenazopyridine combinations are best taken with a full glass (8 ounces) of water. Several additional glasses of water should be taken every day, unless otherwise directed by your doctor. Drinking extra water will help to prevent some unwanted effects (e.g., kidney stones) of the sulfonamide. This medicine may be taken with meals or following meals if it upsets your stomach.

To help clear up your infection completely, *keep taking this medicine for the full time of treatment,* even if you begin to feel better after a few days. If you stop taking this medicine too soon, your symptoms may return.

This medicine works best when there is a constant amount in the urine. *To help keep the amount constant, do not miss any doses. Also, it is best to take the doses at evenly spaced times, day and night.* For example, if you are to take 4 doses a day, the doses should be spaced about 6 hours apart. If this interferes with your sleep or other daily activities, or if you need help in planning the best times to take your medicine, check with your doctor, nurse, or pharmacist.

Dosing—The dose of sulfonamides and phenazopyridine combination may be different for different patients. *Follow your doctor's orders or the directions on the label.* The following information includes only the average doses of sulfonamides and phenazopyridine combination. Your dose may be different if you have kidney disease. *If your dose is different, do not change it* unless your doctor tells you to do so.

- For *sulfamethoxazole and phenazopyridine combination*:
  —Adults and children 12 years of age and older: 2 grams of sulfamethoxazole and 400 mg of phenazopyridine for the first dose, then 1 gram of sulfamethoxazole and 200 mg of phenazopyridine every twelve hours for up to two days.
  —Children up to 12 years of age: This medication is not recommended.
- For *sulfisoxazole and phenazopyridine combination*:
  —Adults and children 12 years of age and older: 2 to 3 grams of sulfisoxazole and 200 to 300 mg of phenazopyridine for the first dose, then 1 gram of sulfisoxazole and 100 mg of phenazopyridine every twelve hours for up to two days.
  —Children up to 12 years of age: This medication is not recommended.

Missed dose—If you miss a dose of this medicine, take it as soon as possible. This will help to keep a constant amount of medicine in the urine. However, if it is almost time for your next dose, skip the missed dose and go back to your regular dosing schedule. Do not double doses.

Storage—To store this medicine:

- Keep out of the reach of children.
- Store away from heat and direct light.
- Do not store in the bathroom, near the kitchen sink, or in other damp places. Heat or moisture may cause the medicine to break down.
- Do not keep outdated medicine or medicine no longer needed. Be sure that any discarded medicine is out of the reach of children.

Precautions While Using This Medicine

If your symptoms do not improve within a few days, or if they become worse, check with your doctor.

Sulfonamides may cause blood problems. These problems may result in a greater chance of certain infections, slow healing, and bleeding of the gums. Therefore, you should be careful when using regular toothbrushes, dental floss, and toothpicks. Dental work should be delayed until your blood counts have returned to normal. Check with your medical doctor or dentist if you have any questions about proper oral hygiene (mouth care) during treatment.

Sulfonamides may cause your skin to be more sensitive to sunlight than it is normally. Exposure to sunlight, even for brief periods of time, may cause a skin rash, itching, redness or other discoloration of the skin, or a severe sunburn. When you begin taking this medicine:

- Stay out of direct sunlight, especially between the hours of 10:00 a.m. and 3:00 p.m., if possible.
- Wear protective clothing, including a hat. Also, wear sunglasses.
- Apply a sun block product that has a skin protection factor (SPF) of at least 15. Some patients may require a product with a higher SPF number, especially if they have a fair complexion. If you have any questions about this, check with your doctor or pharmacist.
- Apply a sun block lipstick that has an SPF of at least 15 to protect your lips.
- Do not use a sunlamp or tanning bed or booth.

If you have a severe reaction, check with your doctor.

This medicine may also cause some people to become dizzy. *Make sure you know how you react to this medicine before you drive, use machines, or do anything else that could be dangerous if you are dizzy or are not alert.* If this reaction is especially bothersome, check with your doctor.

This medicine causes the urine to turn reddish orange. This is to be expected while you are using this medicine and is not harmful. Also, the medicine may stain clothing. If you have any questions about removing the stain, check with your doctor or pharmacist.

For diabetic patients:

- *This medicine may cause false test results with some urine sugar tests and urine ketone tests.* Check with your doctor before changing your diet or the dosage of your diabetes medicine.

Side Effects of This Medicine

Along with its needed effects, a medicine may cause some unwanted effects. Although not all of these side effects may occur, if they do occur they may need medical attention.

Check with your doctor immediately if any of the following side effects occur:

More common

Itching; skin rash

Less common

Aching of joints and muscles; blue or blue-purple discoloration of skin; difficulty in swallowing; pale skin; redness, blistering, peeling, or loosening of skin; shortness of breath; sore throat and fever; unusual bleeding or bruising; unusual tiredness or weakness; yellow eyes or skin

Rare

Blood in urine; greatly increased or decreased frequency of urination or amount of urine; increased thirst; lower back pain; pain or burning while urinating; swelling of front part of neck

In addition to the side effects listed above, check with your doctor as soon as possible if the following side effect occurs:

More common

Increased sensitivity of skin to sunlight

Other side effects may occur that usually do not need medical attention. These side effects may go away during treatment as your body adjusts to the medicine. However, check with your doctor if any of the following side effects continue or are bothersome:

More common

Diarrhea; dizziness; headache; loss of appetite; nausea or vomiting; tiredness

Less common

Indigestion; stomach cramps or pain

This medicine causes the urine to become reddish orange. This side effect does not require medical attention.

Other side effects not listed above may also occur in some patients. If you notice any other effects, check with your doctor.

Annual revision: 02/01/93

SULFUR Topical

Some commonly used brand names are:

In the U.S.

Cuticura Ointment
Finac
Fostex Regular Strength Medicated Cover-Up
Fostril Lotion
Lotio Alsulfa
Sulpho-Lac

Generic name product may also be available.

In Canada

Fostex CM
Fostril Cream

Generic name product may also be available.

Description

Sulfur (SUL-fur) is used to treat many kinds of skin disorders. Sulfur cream, lotion, ointment, and bar soap are used to treat acne. Sulfur ointment is used to treat seborrheic dermatitis and scabies. Sulfur may also be used for other conditions as determined by your doctor.

Some of these preparations are available only with your doctor's prescription. Others are available without a prescription; however, your doctor may have special instructions on the proper use of sulfur for your medical condition.

Sulfur is available in the following dosage forms:

Topical

- Cream (U.S. and Canada)
- Lotion (U.S.)
- Ointment (U.S.)
- Bar soap (U.S. and Canada)

It is very important that you read and understand the following information. If any of it causes you special concern, check with your doctor or pharmacist. Also, *if you have any questions* or if you want more information about this medicine or your medical problem, *ask your doctor, nurse, or pharmacist.*

Before Using This Medicine

If you are using this medicine without a prescription, carefully read and follow any precautions on the label. For topical sulfur preparations, the following should be considered:

Allergies—Tell your doctor if you have ever had any unusual or allergic reaction to sulfur. Also tell your doctor and pharmacist if you are allergic to any other substances, such as preservatives or dyes.

Pregnancy—Topical sulfur has not been shown to cause birth defects or other problems in humans.

Breast-feeding—Topical sulfur has not been reported to cause problems in nursing babies.

Children—Although there is no specific information comparing use of this medicine in children with use in other age groups, this medicine is not expected to cause different side effects or problems in children than it does in adults.

Older adults—Many medicines have not been studied specifically in older people. Therefore, it may not be known whether they work exactly the same way they do in younger adults or if they cause different side effects or problems in older people. There is no specific information comparing use of sulfur in the elderly with use in other age groups.

Other medicines—Although certain medicines should not be used together at all, in other cases two different medicines may be used together even if an interaction might occur. In these cases, your doctor may want to change the dose, or other precautions may be necessary. Tell your doctor and pharmacist if you are using any other topical prescription or nonprescription (over-the-counter [OTC]) medicine that is to be applied to the same area of the skin.

Before you begin using any new medicine (prescription or nonprescription) or if you develop any new medical problem while you are using this medicine, check with your doctor, nurse, or pharmacist.

Proper Use of This Medicine

Use this medicine only as directed. Do not use it more often and do not use it for a longer period of time than recommended on the label, unless otherwise directed by your doctor.

Keep this medicine away from the eyes. If you should accidentally get some in your eyes, flush them thoroughly with water.

To use the *cream or lotion form* of this medicine:

- Before applying the medicine, wash the affected areas with soap and water and dry thoroughly. Then apply enough medicine to cover the affected areas and rub in gently.

To use the *ointment form* of this medicine for *seborrheic dermatitis:*

- Before applying the medicine, wash the affected areas with soap and water and dry thoroughly. Then apply enough medicine to cover the affected areas and rub in gently.

To use the *ointment form* of this medicine for *scabies:*

- Before applying the medicine, wash your entire body with soap and water and dry thoroughly.
- At bedtime, apply enough medicine to cover your entire body from the neck down and rub in gently. Leave the medicine on your body for 24 hours.
- Before applying the medicine again, you may wash your entire body.
- 24 hours after the last treatment with this medicine, it is important that you thoroughly wash your entire body again.

To use the *soap form* of this medicine:

- Work up a rich lather with the soap, using warm water. Wash the affected areas and rinse thoroughly. Apply again, and rub in gently for a few minutes. Remove excess lather with a towel or tissue without rinsing.

Missed dose—If you miss a dose of this medicine, apply or use it as soon as possible. However, if it is almost time for your next dose, skip the missed dose and go back to your regular dosing schedule.

Storage—To store this medicine:

- Keep out of the reach of children.
- Store away from heat and direct light.
- Keep the cream, lotion, and ointment forms of this medicine from freezing.
- Do not keep outdated medicine or medicine no longer needed. Be sure that any discarded medicine is out of the reach of children.

Precautions While Using This Medicine

When using sulfur, do not use any of the following preparations on the same affected area as this medicine, unless otherwise directed by your doctor:

Abrasive soaps or cleansers
Alcohol-containing preparations
Any other topical acne preparation or preparation containing a peeling agent (for example, benzoyl peroxide, resorcinol, salicylic acid, or tretinoin [vitamin A acid])
Cosmetics or soaps that dry the skin
Medicated cosmetics
Other topical medicine for the skin

To use any of the above preparations on the same affected area as sulfur may cause severe irritation of the skin.

Do not use any topical mercury-containing preparation, such as ammoniated mercury ointment, on the same area as this medicine. To do so may cause a foul odor, may be irritating to the skin, and may stain the skin black. If you have any questions about this, check with your doctor or pharmacist.

Side Effects of This Medicine

Along with its needed effects, a medicine may cause some unwanted effects. Although not all of these side effects may occur, if they do occur they may need medical attention.

Check with your doctor as soon as possible if the following side effect occurs:

Skin irritation not present before use of this medicine

Other side effects may occur that usually do not need medical attention. However, check with your doctor or pharmacist if the following side effect continues or is bothersome:

Redness and peeling of skin (may occur after a few days)

Other side effects not listed above may also occur in some patients. If you notice any other effects, check with your doctor or pharmacist.

Annual revision: 01/15/92

SULFURATED LIME Topical

Some commonly used brand names are:

In the U.S.
Vlemasque
Generic name product may also be available.

In Canada
Vlemasque

Another commonly used name is Vleminckx's solution.

Description

Sulfurated (SUL-fur-ay-ted) lime is used to treat acne, scabies, and other skin disorders.

This medicine is available without a prescription; however, your doctor may have special instructions on the proper use of this medicine for your medical problem.

Sulfurated lime is available in the following dosage forms:

Topical

- Mask (U.S. and Canada)
- Topical solution (U.S.)

It is very important that you read and understand the following information. If any of it causes you special concern, check with your doctor or pharmacist. Also, *if you have any questions* or if you want more information about this medicine or your medical problem, *ask your doctor, nurse, or pharmacist.*

Before Using This Medicine

If you are using this medicine without a prescription, carefully read and follow any precautions on the label. For sulfurated lime, the following should be considered:

Allergies—Tell your doctor if you have ever had any unusual or allergic reaction to sulfurated lime. Also tell your doctor and pharmacist if you are allergic to any other substances, such as preservatives or dyes.

Pregnancy—Sulfurated lime has not been shown to cause birth defects or other problems in humans.

Breast-feeding—Sulfurated lime has not been reported to cause problems in nursing babies.

Children—Although there is no specific information comparing use of sulfurated lime in children with use in other age groups, this medicine is not expected to cause different side effects or problems in children than it does in adults.

Older adults—Many medicines have not been studied specifically in older people. Therefore, it may not be known whether they work exactly the same way they do in younger adults or if they cause different side effects or problems in older people. There is no specific information comparing use of sulfurated lime in the elderly with use in other age groups.

Other medicines—Although certain medicines should not be used together at all, in other cases two different medicines may be used together even if an interaction might occur. In these cases, your doctor may want to change the dose, or other precautions may be necessary. Tell your doctor and pharmacist if you are using any other topical prescription or nonprescription (over-the-counter [OTC]) medicine that is to be applied to the same area of the skin.

Before you begin using any new medicine (prescription or nonprescription) or if you develop any new medical problem while you are using this medicine, check with your doctor, nurse, or pharmacist.

Proper Use of This Medicine

Use this medicine only as directed. Do not use more of it, do not use it more often, and do not use it for a longer period of time than recommended on the label, unless otherwise directed by your doctor.

Keep this medicine away from the eyes. If you should accidentally get some in your eyes, flush them thoroughly with water.

To use the *topical solution form* of sulfurated lime for wet dressings, as a soak, or in a bath:

- Sulfurated lime solution must be diluted before you use it on your skin for wet dressings, as a soak, or in a bath. Make sure you understand exactly how you should use this solution. If you have any questions about this, check with your doctor or pharmacist.
- Before diluting and/or applying this solution, remove all jewelry and metallic ornaments, since the solution may discolor metals. Also, avoid getting this solution on metal spoons or bath fixtures.

To use the *mask form* of sulfurated lime:

- Apply a generous amount of this medicine over the entire face and neck, unless otherwise directed by your doctor.
- Allow the medicine to remain on the affected areas for 20 to 25 minutes.
- Remove the medicine with lukewarm water, using a gentle circular motion. Then, pat the skin dry.

Missed dose—If you miss a dose of this medicine, apply it as soon as possible. However, if it is almost time for your next dose, skip the missed dose and go back to your regular dosing schedule.

Storage—To store this medicine:

- Keep out of the reach of children.
- Store away from heat and direct light.
- Keep the medicine from freezing.
- Do not keep outdated medicine or medicine no longer needed. Be sure that any discarded medicine is out of the reach of children.

Precautions While Using This Medicine

When using sulfurated lime, do not use any of the following preparations on the same affected area as this medicine, unless otherwise directed by your doctor:

Abrasive soaps or cleansers
Alcohol-containing preparations
Any other topical acne preparation or preparation containing a peeling agent (for example, benzoyl peroxide, resorcinol, salicylic acid, sulfur, or tretinoin [vitamin A acid])
Cosmetics or soaps that dry the skin
Medicated cosmetics
Other topical medicine for the skin

To use any of the above preparations on the same affected area as sulfurated lime may cause severe irritation of the skin.

Do not use any topical mercury-containing preparation, such as ammoniated mercury ointment on the same affected area as this medicine. To do so may cause a foul odor, may be irritating to the skin, and may stain the skin black. If you have any questions about this, check with your doctor.

Side Effects of This Medicine

Along with its needed effects, a medicine may cause some unwanted effects. Although not all of these side effects may occur, if they do occur they may need medical attention.

Check with your doctor as soon as possible if the following side effect occurs:

Skin irritation not present before use of this medicine

Other side effects may occur that usually do not need medical attention. However, check with your doctor or pharmacist if the following side effects continue or are bothersome:

Redness and peeling of skin (may occur after a few days); unusual dryness of skin

Other side effects not listed above may also occur in some patients. If you notice any other effects, check with your doctor or pharmacist.

Annual revision: 11/05/91

SUMATRIPTAN Systemic

A commonly used brand name in the U.S. and Canada is Imitrex.

Description

Sumatriptan (soo-ma-TRIP-tan) is used to treat severe migraine headaches. Many people find that their headaches go away completely after they take sumatriptan. Other people find that their headaches are much less painful, and that they are able to go back to their normal activities even though their headaches are not completely gone. Sumatriptan often relieves other symptoms that occur together with a migraine headache, such as nausea, vomiting, sensitivity to light, and sensitivity to sound.

Sumatriptan is not an ordinary pain reliever. It will not relieve any kind of pain other than migraine headaches. This medicine is usually used for people whose headaches are not relieved by acetaminophen, aspirin, or other pain relievers.

Sumatriptan is available only with your doctor's prescription, in the following dosage forms:

Oral

- Tablets (Canada)

Parenteral

- Injection (U.S. and Canada)

It is very important that you read and understand the following information. If any of it causes you special concern, check with your doctor. Also, *if you have any questions* or if you want more information about this medicine or your medical problem, *ask your doctor, nurse, or pharmacist.*

Before Using This Medicine

In deciding to use a medicine, the risks of using the medicine must be weighed against the good it will do. This is a decision you and your doctor will make. For sumatriptan, the following should be considered:

Allergies—Tell your doctor if you have ever had any unusual or allergic reaction to sumatriptan. Also tell your doctor and pharmacist if you are allergic to any other substances, such as foods, preservatives, or dyes.

Pregnancy—Sumatriptan has not been studied in pregnant women. However, in some animal studies, sumatriptan caused harmful effects on the fetus. These unwanted effects usually occurred when sumatriptan was given in amounts that were large enough to cause harmful effects in the mother.

Breast-feeding—It is not known whether sumatriptan passes into human breast milk. However, it has been found in the breast milk of animals. Breast-feeding mothers should discuss the risks and benefits of this medicine with their doctors.

Children—Studies on this medicine have been done only in adult patients, and there is no specific information comparing use of sumatriptan in children with use in other age groups.

Teenagers—Studies on this medicine have been done only in patients 18 years of age or older, and there is no specific information comparing use of sumatriptan in younger teenagers with use in other age groups.

Older adults—This medicine has been tested in a limited number of patients between 60 and 65 years of age. It did not cause different side effects or problems in these patients than it did in younger adults. However, there is no specific information comparing use of sumatriptan in patients older than 65 years of age with use in younger adults.

Other medicines—Although certain medicines should not be used together at all, in other cases two different medicines may be used together even if an interaction might occur. In these cases, your doctor may want to change the dose, or other precautions may be necessary. Tell your doctor and pharmacist if you are taking any other prescription or nonprescription (over-the-counter [OTC]) medicine, especially other prescription medicine for migraine headaches, or if you smoke tobacco.

Other medical problems—The presence of other medical problems may affect the use of sumatriptan. Make sure you tell your doctor if you have any other medical problems, especially:

- Angina (chest pain) or
- Fast or irregular heartbeat or
- Heart or blood vessel disease or
- High blood pressure or
- Kidney disease or

- Liver disease or
- Stroke (history of)—The chance of side effects may be increased

Before you begin using any new medicine (prescription or nonprescription) or if you develop any new medical problem while you are using this medicine, check with your doctor, nurse, or pharmacist.

Proper Use of This Medicine

To relieve your migraine as soon as possible, use sumatriptan at the first sign that the headache is coming. If you get warning signals of a coming migraine (an aura), you may use the medicine before the headache pain actually starts. However, even if you do not use sumatriptan until your migraine has been present for several hours, the medicine will still work.

Lying down in a quiet, dark room for a while after you use this medicine may help relieve your migraine.

If you are not much better in 1 or 2 hours after an injection of sumatriptan, or in 2 to 4 hours after a tablet is taken, *do not use any more of this medicine for the same migraine.* A migraine that is not relieved by the first dose of sumatriptan probably will not be relieved by a second dose, either. Ask your doctor ahead of time about other medicine to be taken if sumatriptan does not work. However, even if sumatriptan does not relieve one migraine, it may still relieve the next one.

If you feel much better after a dose of sumatriptan, but your headache comes back or gets worse after a while, you may use more sumatriptan. However, *use this medicine only as directed by your doctor. Do not use more of it, and do not use it more often, than directed.* Using too much sumatriptan may increase the chance of side effects.

Your doctor may direct you to take another medicine to help prevent headaches. *It is important that you follow your doctor's directions, even if your headaches continue to occur.* Headache-preventing medicines may take several weeks to start working. Even after they do start working, your headaches may not go away completely. However, your headaches should occur less often, and they should be less severe and easier to relieve. This can reduce the amount of sumatriptan or pain relievers that you need. If you do not notice any improvement after several weeks of headache-preventing treatment, check with your doctor.

For patients taking *sumatriptan tablets*:

- Sumatriptan tablets are to be swallowed whole. *Do not break, crush, or chew the tablets before swallowing them.*

For patients using *sumatriptan injection*:

- This medicine comes with patient directions. *Read them carefully before using the medicine,* and check with your doctor or pharmacist if you have any questions.
- Your doctor or nurse will teach you how to inject yourself with the medicine. *Be sure to follow the directions carefully. Check with your doctor or nurse if you have any problems using the medicine.*
- After you have finished injecting the medicine, be sure to follow the precautions in the patient directions about safely discarding the empty cartridge and the needle. Always return the empty cartridge and needle to their container before discarding them. Do not throw away the autoinjector unit, because refills are available.

Dosing—The dose of sumatriptan will be different for different patients. *Follow your doctor's orders or the directions on the label.* The following information includes only the average doses of sumatriptan. *If your dose is different, do not change it* unless your doctor tells you to do so.

- For *oral* dosage form (tablets):
  —For migraine headaches:
  - Adults—One 100-milligram (mg) tablet. Another 100-mg tablet may be taken one or two times more, if necessary, if the migraine comes back after being relieved. *Do not take more than three 100-mg tablets in any twenty-four-hour period.*
  - Children—Use and dose must be determined by your doctor.
- For *parenteral* dosage form (injection):
  —For migraine headaches:
  - Adults—6 mg. One more 6-mg dose may be injected, if necessary, if the migraine comes back after being relieved. However, the second injection should not be given any sooner than one hour after the first one. *Do not use more than two 6-mg injections in forty-eight hours (two days).*
  - Children—Use and dose must be determined by your doctor.

Storage—To store this medicine:

- Keep out of the reach of children since overdose is especially dangerous in children.
- Store away from heat and direct light.
- Do not store tablets in the bathroom, near the kitchen sink, or in other damp places. Heat or moisture may cause the medicine to break down.
- Keep the injection form of sumatriptan from freezing.
- Do not keep outdated medicine or medicine no longer needed. Be sure that any discarded medicine is out of the reach of children.

Precautions While Using This Medicine

Check with your doctor if you have used sumatriptan for 3 headaches, and have not had good relief. Also, check with your doctor if your migraine headaches are worse, or if they are occurring more often, than before you started using sumatriptan.

Drinking alcoholic beverages can make headaches worse or cause new headaches to occur. People who suffer from severe headaches should probably avoid alcoholic beverages, especially during a headache.

Some people feel drowsy or dizzy during or after a migraine, or after taking sumatriptan to relieve a migraine. As long as you are feeling drowsy or dizzy, *do not drive, use machines, or do anything else that could be dangerous if you are dizzy or are not alert.*

Side Effects of This Medicine

Along with its needed effects, a medicine may cause some unwanted effects. Most side effects of sumatriptan are milder and occur less often with the tablets than with the injection. Although not all of these side effects may occur, if they do occur they may need medical attention.

Stop using this medicine and check with your doctor immediately if any of the following side effects occur:

Rare

Chest pain (severe); swelling of eyelids, face, or lips; wheezing

Check with your doctor right away if any of the following side effects continue for more than 1 hour. Even if they go away in less than 1 hour, *check with your doctor before using any more sumatriptan if any of the following side effects occur*:

Less common

Chest pain (mild); heaviness, tightness, or pressure in chest and/or neck

Also check with your doctor as soon as possible if any of the following side effects occur:

Less common

Difficulty in swallowing; pounding heartbeat; skin rash or bumps on skin

Other side effects may occur that usually do not need medical attention. Some of the following effects, such as nausea, vomiting, drowsiness, dizziness, and general feeling of illness or tiredness often occur during or after a migraine, even when sumatriptan has not been used. Most of the side effects caused by sumatriptan go away within a short time (less than 1 hour after an injection or 2 hours after a tablet). However, check with your doctor if any of the following side effects continue or are bothersome:

More common

Burning, pain, or redness at place of injection; feeling of burning, warmth, heat, numbness, tightness, or tingling; discomfort in jaw, mouth, tongue, throat, nose, or sinuses; dizziness; drowsiness; feeling cold, "strange," or weak; flushing; lightheadedness; muscle aches, cramps, or stiffness; nausea or vomiting

Less common or rare

Anxiety; general feeling of illness or tiredness; vision changes

Other side effects not listed above may also occur in some patients. If you notice any other effects, check with your doctor.

Annual revision: 07/01/93

TAMOXIFEN Systemic

Some commonly used brand names are:

In the U.S.

Nolvadex

In Canada

Alpha-Tamoxifen	Tamofen
Nolvadex	Tamone
Nolvadex-D	Tamoplex
Novo-Tamoxifen	

Description

Tamoxifen (ta-MOX-i-fen) is a medicine that blocks the effects of the hormone estrogen in the body. It is used to treat some cases of breast cancer.

The exact way that tamoxifen works against cancer is not known but it may be related to the way it blocks the effects of estrogen on the body.

Before you begin treatment with tamoxifen, you and your doctor should talk about the good this medicine will do as well as the risks of using it.

Tamoxifen is available only with your doctor's prescription, in the following dosage forms:

Oral

- Tablets (U.S. and Canada)
- Enteric-coated tablets (Canada)

It is very important that you read and understand the following information. If any of it causes you special concern, check with your doctor. Also, *if you have any questions* or if you want more information about this medicine or your medical problem, *ask your doctor, nurse, or pharmacist.*

T

Before Using This Medicine

In deciding to use a medicine, the risks of taking the medicine must be weighed against the good it will do. This is a decision you and your doctor will make. For tamoxifen, the following should be considered:

Allergies—Tell your doctor if you have ever had any unusual or allergic reaction to tamoxifen.

Pregnancy—Tell your doctor if you are pregnant or if you intend to become pregnant. Tamoxifen has been shown to cause miscarriages, birth defects, death of the fetus, and vaginal bleeding. Studies in rats and rabbits have also shown that tamoxifen causes miscarriages, death of the fetus, and slowed learning.

Be sure that you have discussed this with your doctor before taking this medicine. It is best to use some kind of birth control while you are taking tamoxifen. However, do not use oral contraceptives ("the Pill") since they may interfere with this medicine. Tell your doctor right away if you think you have become pregnant while taking tamoxifen.

Breast-feeding—Because this medicine may cause serious side effects, breast-feeding is generally not recommended while you are taking it.

Older adults—Many medicines have not been studied specifically in older people. Therefore, it may not be known whether they work exactly the same way they do in younger adults. Although there is no specific information comparing use of tamoxifen in the elderly with use in other age groups, this medicine is not expected to cause different side effects or problems in older people than it does in younger adults.

Other medicines—Although certain medicines should not be used together at all, in other cases two different medicines may be used together even if an interaction might occur. In these cases, your doctor may want to change the dose, or other precautions may be necessary. Tell your doctor and pharmacist if you are taking any other prescription or nonprescription (over-the-counter [OTC]) medicine.

Other medical problems—The presence of other medical problems may affect the use of tamoxifen. Make sure you tell your doctor if you have any other medical problems, especially:

- Cataracts or other eye problems—Tamoxifen may also cause these problems

Before you begin using any new medicine (prescription or nonprescription) or if you develop any new medical problem while you are using this medicine, check with your doctor, nurse, or pharmacist.

Proper Use of This Medicine

Use this medicine only as directed by your doctor. Do not use more or less of it, and do not use it more often than your doctor ordered. The exact amount of medicine you need has been carefully worked out. Taking too much may increase the chance of side effects, while taking too little may not improve your condition.

For patients taking *enteric-coated tamoxifen tablets:*

- The tablets must be swallowed whole. Do not crush them or break them up before taking.

Tamoxifen commonly causes nausea and vomiting. However, it may have to be taken for several weeks or months to be effective. Even if you begin to feel ill, *do not stop using this medicine without first checking with your doctor.* Ask your doctor, nurse, or pharmacist for ways to lessen these effects.

If you vomit shortly after taking a dose of tamoxifen, check with your doctor. You will be told whether to take the dose again or to wait until the next scheduled dose.

Missed dose—If you miss a dose of this medicine, do not take the missed dose at all and do not double the next one. Instead, go back to your regular dosing schedule and check with your doctor.

Storage—To store this medicine:

- Keep out of the reach of children.
- Store away from heat and direct light.
- Do not store in the bathroom, near the kitchen sink, or in other damp places. Heat or moisture may cause the medicine to break down.
- Do not keep outdated medicine or medicine no longer needed. Be sure that any discarded medicine is out of the reach of children.

Precautions While Using This Medicine

It is very important that your doctor check your progress at regular visits to make sure that this medicine is working properly and to check for unwanted effects.

Tamoxifen may make you more fertile. It is best to use some type of birth control while you are taking it. However, do not use oral contraceptives (the "Pill") since they may change the effects of tamoxifen. Tell your doctor right away if you think you have become pregnant while taking this medicine.

For patients taking *enteric-coated tamoxifen tablets:*

- If you are also taking an antacid, take this medicine at least 1 or 2 hours before or after taking the antacid. Taking the two medicines too close together may cause the enteric coating to dissolve too early. This may increase the risk of unwanted effects from tamoxifen.

Side Effects of This Medicine

Along with its needed effects, a medicine may cause some unwanted effects. Some side effects will have signs or symptoms that you can see or feel. Your doctor will watch for others by doing certain tests.

Also, because of the way this medicine acts on the body, there is a chance that it might cause other unwanted effects that may not occur until months or years after the medicine is used. Tamoxifen has been reported to increase the chance of cancer of the uterus (womb) in some women taking it. Discuss this possible effect with your doctor.

Check with your doctor as soon as possible if any of the following side effects occur:

Rare

Blurred vision; confusion; pain or swelling in legs; shortness of breath; vaginal bleeding; weakness or sleepiness; yellow eyes or skin

This medicine may also cause the following side effect that your doctor will watch for:

Less common or rare

Liver problems

Other side effects may occur that usually do not need medical attention. These side effects may go away during treatment as your body adjusts to the medicine. Also, your doctor or nurse may be able to tell you about ways to prevent or reduce some of these side effects. Check with your doctor or nurse if any of the following side effects continue or are bothersome or if you have any questions about them:

More common

Hot flashes; nausea and/or vomiting; weight gain

Less common

Bone pain; changes in menstrual period; headache; itching in genital area; skin rash or dryness; vaginal discharge

Other side effects not listed above may also occur in some patients. If you notice any other effects, check with your doctor.

Annual revision: 08/19/92
Interim revision(s): 06/26/93; 08/05/93

T

TERAZOSIN Systemic

A commonly used brand name in the U.S. and Canada is Hytrin.

Description

Terazosin (ter-AY-zoe-sin) belongs to the general class of medicines called antihypertensives. It is used to treat high blood pressure (hypertension).

High blood pressure adds to the workload of the heart and arteries. If it continues for a long time, the heart and arteries may not function properly. This can damage the blood vessels of the brain, heart, and kidneys, resulting in a stroke, heart failure, or kidney failure. High blood pressure may also increase the risk of heart attacks. These problems may be less likely to occur if blood pressure is controlled.

Terazosin works by relaxing blood vessels so that blood passes through them more easily. This helps to lower blood pressure.

Terazosin is available only with your doctor's prescription, in the following dosage form:

Oral

- Tablets (U.S. and Canada)

It is very important that you read and understand the following information. If any of it causes you special concern, check with your doctor. Also, *if you have any questions* or if you want more information about this medicine or your medical problem, *ask your doctor, nurse, or pharmacist.*

Before Using This Medicine

In deciding to use a medicine, the risks of taking the medicine must be weighed against the good it will do. This is a decision you and your doctor will make. For terazosin, the following should be considered:

Allergies—Tell your doctor if you have ever had any unusual or allergic reaction to terazosin, prazosin, or doxazosin. Also tell your doctor and pharmacist if you are allergic to any other substances, such as foods, preservatives, or dyes.

Pregnancy—Studies have not been done in humans. Studies in animals given many times the highest recommended human dose have not shown that terazosin causes birth defects. However, these studies have shown a decrease in successful pregnancies.

Breast-feeding—It is not known whether terazosin passes into breast milk. However, this medicine has not been reported to cause problems in nursing babies.

Children—Studies on this medicine have been done only in adult patients, and there is no specific information comparing use of terazosin in children with use in other age groups.

Older adults—Dizziness, lightheadedness, or fainting (especially when getting up from a lying or sitting position) may be more likely to occur in the elderly, who are more sensitive to the effects of terazosin.

Other medicines—Although certain medicines should not be used together at all, in other cases two different medicines may be used together even if an interaction might occur. In these cases, your doctor may want to change the dose, or other precautions may be necessary. Tell your doctor and pharmacist if you are taking any other prescription or nonprescription (over-the-counter [OTC]) medicine.

Other medical problems—The presence of other medical problems may affect the use of terazosin. Make sure you tell your doctor if you have any other medical problems, especially:

- Angina (chest pain)—Terazosin may make this condition worse
- Heart disease (severe)—Terazosin may make this condition worse
- Kidney disease—Possible increased sensitivity to the effects of terazosin

Before you begin using any new medicine (prescription or nonprescription) or if you develop any new medical problem while you are using this medicine, check with your doctor, nurse, or pharmacist.

Proper Use of This Medicine

For patients *taking this medicine for high blood pressure:*

- In addition to the use of the medicine your doctor has prescribed, treatment for your high blood pressure may include weight control and care in the types of foods you eat, especially foods high in sodium. Your doctor will tell you which of these are most important for you. You should check with your doctor before changing your diet.
- Many patients who have high blood pressure will not notice any signs of the problem. In fact, many may feel normal. It is very important that you *take your medicine exactly as directed* and that you keep your appointments with your doctor even if you feel well.
- Remember that terazosin will not cure your high blood pressure but it does help control it. Therefore, you must continue to take it as directed if you expect to lower your blood pressure and keep it down. *You may have to take high blood pressure medicine for the rest of your life.* If high blood pressure is not treated, it can cause serious problems such as heart failure, blood vessel disease, stroke, or kidney disease.

To help you remember to take your medicine, try to get into the habit of taking it at the same time each day.

Missed dose—If you miss a dose of this medicine, take it as soon as possible the same day. However, if you do not remember the missed dose until the next day, skip the missed dose and go back to your regular dosing schedule. Do not double doses.

Storage—To store this medicine:

- Keep out of the reach of children.
- Store away from heat and direct light.
- Do not store in the bathroom, near the kitchen sink, or in other damp places. Heat or moisture may cause the medicine to break down.

- Do not keep outdated medicine or medicine no longer needed. Be sure that any discarded medicine is out of the reach of children.

Precautions While Using This Medicine

It is important that your doctor check your progress at regular visits to make sure that this medicine is working properly.

For patients *taking this medicine for high blood pressure:*

- *Do not take other medicines unless they have been discussed with your doctor.* This especially includes over-the-counter (nonprescription) medicines for appetite control, asthma, colds, cough, hay fever, or sinus problems, since they may tend to increase your blood pressure.

Dizziness, lightheadedness, or sudden fainting may occur after you take this medicine, especially when you get up from a lying or sitting position. These effects are more likely to occur when you take the first dose of this medicine. Taking the first dose at bedtime may prevent problems. However, *be especially careful if you need to get up during the night.* These effects may also occur with any doses you take after the first dose. Getting up slowly may help lessen this problem. *If you feel dizzy, lie down so that you do not faint.* Then sit for a few moments before standing to prevent the dizziness from returning.

The dizziness, lightheadedness, or fainting is more likely to occur if you drink alcohol, stand for long periods of time, exercise, or if the weather is hot. *While you are taking this medicine, be careful to limit the amount of alcohol you drink. Also, use extra care during exercise or hot weather or if you must stand for long periods of time.*

Terazosin may cause some people to become drowsy or less alert than they are normally. *Make sure you know how you react to this medicine before you drive, use machines, or do anything else that could be dangerous if you are dizzy, drowsy, or are not alert.* After you have taken several doses of this medicine, these effects should lessen.

Side Effects of This Medicine

Along with its needed effects, a medicine may cause some unwanted effects. Although not all of these side effects may occur, if they do occur they may need medical attention.

Check with your doctor as soon as possible if any of the following side effects occur:

More common

Dizziness

Less common

Chest pain; dizziness or lightheadedness, when getting up from a lying or sitting position; fainting (sudden); fast or irregular heartbeat; pounding heartbeat; shortness of breath; swelling of feet or lower legs

Rare

Weight gain

Other side effects may occur that usually do not need medical attention. These side effects may go away during treatment as your body adjusts to the medicine. However, check with your doctor if any of the following side effects continue or are bothersome:

More common

Headache; unusual tiredness or weakness

Less common

Back or joint pain; blurred vision; drowsiness; nausea and vomiting; stuffy nose

Other side effects not listed above may also occur in some patients. If you notice any other effects, check with your doctor.

Additional Information

Once a medicine has been approved for marketing for a certain use, experience may show that it is also useful for other medical problems. Although this use is not included in product labeling, terazosin is used in certain patients with the following medical condition:

- Benign enlargement of the prostate

Other than the above information, there is no additional information relating to proper use, precautions, or side effects for this use.

Annual revision: 06/26/92

TERBINAFINE Topical†

A commonly used brand name in the U.S. is Lamisil.

†Not commercially available in Canada.

Description

Terbinafine (TER-bin-a-feen) is used to treat infections caused by a fungus. It works by killing the fungus or preventing its growth.

Terbinafine is applied to the skin to treat:
- ringworm of the body (tinea corporis);
- ringworm of the foot (tinea pedis; athlete's foot); and
- ringworm of the groin (tinea cruris; jock itch).

Terbinafine is available only with your doctor's prescription, in the following dosage form:

Topical
- Cream (U.S.)

It is very important that you read and understand the following information. If any of it causes you special concern, check with your doctor. Also, *if you have any questions* or if you want more information about this medicine or your medical problem, *ask your doctor, nurse, or pharmacist.*

Before Using This Medicine

In deciding to use a medicine, the risks of using the medicine must be weighed against the good it will do. This is a decision you and your doctor will make. For terbinafine, the following should be considered:

Allergies—Tell your doctor if you have ever had any unusual or allergic reaction to terbinafine. Also tell your doctor and pharmacist if you are allergic to any other substances, such as foods, preservatives, or dyes.

Pregnancy—Terbinafine has not been studied in pregnant women. However, terbinafine has not been shown to cause birth defects or other problems in animal studies.

Breast-feeding—Oral terbinafine passes into the breast milk. It is not known whether topical terbinafine passes into breast milk. Although most medicines pass into breast milk in small amounts, many of them may be used safely while breast-feeding. Mothers who are using this medicine and who wish to breast-feed should discuss this with their doctor.

Children—Studies on this medicine have been done only in adult patients, and there is no specific information comparing use of terbinafine in children under the age of 12 with use in other age groups.

Older adults—Many medicines have not been studied specifically in older people. Therefore, it may not be known whether they work exactly the same way they do in younger adults. Although there is no specific information comparing use of terbinafine in the elderly with use in other age groups, this medicine is not expected to cause different side effects or problems in older people than it does in younger adults.

Other medicines—Although certain medicines should not be used together at all, in other cases two different medicines may be used together even if an interaction might occur. In these cases, your doctor may want to change the dose, or other precautions may be necessary. Tell your doctor and pharmacist if you are using any other topical prescription or nonprescription (over-the-counter [OTC]) medicine that is to be applied to the same area of the skin.

Before you begin using any new medicine (prescription or nonprescription) or if you develop any new medical problem while you are using this medicine, check with your doctor, nurse, or pharmacist.

Proper Use of This Medicine

Apply enough terbinafine to cover the affected and surrounding skin areas and rub in gently.

Keep this medicine away from the eyes.

Do not apply an occlusive dressing (airtight covering, such as a tight bandage or plastic kitchen wrap) over this medicine unless you have been directed to do so by your doctor.

Dosing—The dose of terbinafine will be different for different patients. *Follow your doctor's orders or the directions on the label.* The following information includes only the average doses of terbinafine. *If your dose is different, do not change it* unless your doctor tells you to do so:

The number of doses you use each day, the time allowed between doses, and the length of time you use the medicine depend on the medical problem for which you are using terbinafine.

- For *topical* dosage form (cream):
  - —For tinea corporis or tinea cruris:
    - Adults and children 12 years of age and over—Use one or two times a day.
    - Infants and children up to 12 years of age—Use and dose must be determined by your doctor.
  - —For tinea pedis:
    - Adults and children 12 years of age and over—Use two times a day.

- Infants and children up to 12 years of age—Use and dose must be determined by your doctor.

To help clear up your infection completely, it *is very important that you keep using terbinafine for the full time of treatment,* even if your symptoms begin to clear up after a few days. Since fungus infections may be very slow to clear up, you may have to continue using this medicine every day for several weeks or more. If you stop using this medicine too soon, your symptoms may return. *Do not miss any doses.*

Missed dose—If you do miss a dose of this medicine, apply it as soon as possible. However, if it is almost time for your next dose, skip the missed dose and go back to your regular dosing schedule.

Storage—To store this medicine:

- Keep out of the reach of children.
- Store away from heat and direct light.
- Keep the medicine from freezing.
- Do not keep outdated medicine or medicine no longer needed. Be sure that any discarded medicine is out of the reach of children.

Precautions While Using This Medicine

If your skin problem does not improve within 4 weeks, or if it becomes worse, check with your doctor.

To help clear up your infection completely and to help make sure it does not return, good health habits are also needed. The following measures will help reduce chafing and irritation and will also help keep the area cool and dry.

- *For patients using terbinafine for ringworm of the body:*
  —Carefully dry yourself after bathing.
  —Avoid too much heat and humidity if possible. Try to keep moisture from building up on affected areas of the body.
  —Wear well-ventilated, loose-fitting clothing.
  —Use a bland, absorbent powder (for example, talcum powder) once or twice a day. Be sure to use the powder after terbinafine cream has been applied and has disappeared into the skin.
- *For patients using terbinafine for ringworm of the groin:*
  —Avoid wearing underwear that is tight-fitting or made from synthetic (man-made) materials (for example, rayon or nylon). Instead, wear loose-fitting, cotton underwear.
  —Use a bland, absorbent powder (for example, talcum powder) on the skin. It is best to use the powder between the times you use terbinafine.
- *For patients using terbinafine for ringworm of the foot:*
  —Carefully dry the feet, especially between the toes, after bathing.
  —Avoid wearing socks made from wool or synthetic materials (for example, rayon or nylon). Instead, wear clean, cotton socks and change them daily or more often if the feet sweat a lot.
  —Wear sandals or well-ventilated shoes (for example, shoes with holes).
  —Use a bland, absorbent powder (for example, talcum powder) between the toes, on the feet, and in socks and shoes once or twice a day. It is best to use the powder between the times you use terbinafine.

If you have any questions about these measures, check with your doctor, nurse, or pharmacist.

Side Effects of This Medicine

Along with its needed effects, a medicine may cause some unwanted effects. Although not all of these side effects may occur, if they do occur they may need medical attention.

Check with your doctor or pharmacist as soon as possible if any of the following side effects occur:

Rare

Redness, itching, burning, blistering, swelling, oozing, or other signs of skin irritation not present before use of this medicine

Other side effects not listed above may also occur in some patients. If you notice any other effects, check with your doctor.

Annual revision: 07/29/93

TERIPARATIDE Systemic†

A commonly used brand name in the U.S. is Parathar.

†Not commercially available in Canada.

Description

Teriparatide (terr-ih-PAR-a-tyd) is synthetic human parathyroid hormone used by injection as a test to help diagnose problems of the parathyroid gland. This test determines whether you have hypoparathyroidism or a type of pseudohypoparathyroidism.

How this test is done: Before the medicine is given, at least three blood and urine samples will be collected and tested. Teriparatide is then injected into an arm vein over a 10-minute period, and blood and urine samples are collected and tested again. Teriparatide causes changes in the amounts of certain chemicals in the urine. These changes will help determine which hypoparathyroid problem you have.

Teriparatide is to be used only by or under the supervision of a doctor, in the following dosage form:

Parenteral
- Injection (U.S.)

It is very important that you read and understand the following information. If any of it causes you special concern, check with your doctor. Also, *if you have any questions* or if you want more information about this medicine or your medical problem, *ask your doctor, nurse, or pharmacist.*

Before Having This Test

In deciding to use a diagnostic test, any risks of the test must be weighed against the good it will do. This is a decision you and your doctor will make. For teriparatide, the following should be considered:

Allergies—Tell your doctor if you have ever had any unusual or allergic reaction to peptides, gelatin, or teriparatide. Also tell your doctor and pharmacist if you are allergic to any other substances, such as foods, preservatives, or dyes.

Pregnancy—Teriparatide has not been shown to cause birth defects or other problems in humans.

Breast-feeding—It is not known whether teriparatide passes into the breast milk. However, teriparatide is not recommended during breast-feeding, because it may cause unwanted effects in nursing babies.

Children—This medicine has not been shown to cause different side effects or problems in children over 3 years of age than it does in adults.

Older adults—Many medicines have not been studied specifically in older people. Therefore, it may not be known whether they work exactly the same way they do in younger adults. Although there is no specific information comparing use of teriparatide in the elderly with use in other age groups, this medicine is not expected to cause different side effects or problems in older people than it does in younger adults.

Other medicines—Although certain medicines should not be used together at all, in other cases two different medicines may be used together even if an interaction might occur. In these cases, your doctor may want to change the dose, or other precautions may be necessary. Tell your doctor and pharmacist if you are taking any other prescription or nonprescription (over-the-counter [OTC]) medicine.

Before you begin using any new medicine (prescription or nonprescription) or if you develop any new medical problem while you are using this medicine, check with your doctor, nurse, or pharmacist.

Preparation for This Test

Follow your doctor's instructions carefully. Otherwise, this test may not work well and may have to be done again.

Unless otherwise directed by your doctor:

- Do not eat or drink anything but water after 8:00 p.m. the night before the test. Food may affect the test results.
- Starting about 2½ hours before the test, drink about 6 or 7 ounces of water every 30 minutes until the test is finished. This is to be sure there is enough urine for testing.

Side Effects of This Medicine

Along with its needed effects, a medicine may cause some unwanted effects. Check with your doctor as soon as possible if any of the following side effects occur:

Symptoms of overdose

Constipation; headache; loss of appetite; muscle weakness

Other side effects may occur that usually do not need medical attention. These side effects may go away after the test as your body adjusts to the medicine. However, check with your doctor if any of the following side effects continue or are bothersome:

Rare

Abdominal or stomach cramps; diarrhea; metallic taste; nausea; pain at the place of injection during or following injection; tingling feeling in hands and feet; urge for bowel movement

Other side effects not listed above may also occur in some patients. If you notice any other effects, check with your doctor.

Annual revision: 06/22/92

TESTOLACTONE Systemic†

A commonly used brand name in the U.S. is Teslac.

†Not commercially available in Canada.

Description

Testolactone (tess-toe-LAK-tone) belongs to the general group of medicines called antineoplastics. It is used to treat some cases of breast cancer in females.

Testolactone is available only with your doctor's prescription, in the following dosage form:

Oral

- Tablets (U.S.)

It is very important that you read and understand the following information. If any of it causes you special concern, check with your doctor. Also, *if you have any questions* or if you want more information about this medicine or your medical problem, *ask your doctor, nurse, or pharmacist.*

Before Using This Medicine

In deciding to use a medicine, the risks of taking the medicine must be weighed against the good it will do. This is a decision you and your doctor will make. For testolactone, the following should be considered:

Allergies—Tell your doctor if you have ever had any unusual or allergic reaction to testolactone.

Pregnancy—Studies have not been done in humans. However, studies in rats at doses 2.5 to 7.5 times the human dose have shown that testolactone causes an increase in the number of fetus and infant deaths and abnormal growth.

Breast-feeding—It is not known whether testolactone passes into breast milk. However, this medicine has not been reported to cause problems in nursing babies.

Older adults—Many medicines have not been studied specifically in older people. Therefore, it may not be known whether they work exactly the same way they do in younger adults or if they cause different side effects or problems in older people. There is no specific information comparing use of testolactone in the elderly with use in other age groups.

Other medicines—Although certain medicines should not be used together at all, in other cases two different medicines may be used together even if an interaction might occur. In these cases, your doctor may want to change the dose, or other precautions may be necessary. Tell your doctor and pharmacist if you are taking any other prescription or nonprescription (over-the-counter [OTC]) medicine.

Other medical problems—The presence of other medical problems may affect the use of testolactone. Make sure you tell your doctor if you have any other medical problems, especially:

- Heart or kidney disease

Before you begin using any new medicine (prescription or nonprescription) or if you develop any new medical problem while you are using this medicine, check with your doctor, nurse, or pharmacist.

Proper Use of This Medicine

Use this medicine only as directed by your doctor. Do not use more or less of it, and do not use it more often than your doctor ordered. The exact amount of medicine you need has been carefully worked out. Taking too much may increase the chance of side effects, while taking too little may not improve your condition.

Testolactone sometimes causes nausea and vomiting. However, it may have to be taken for several weeks or months to be effective. Even if you begin to feel ill, *do not stop using this medicine without first checking with your doctor.* Ask your doctor, nurse, or pharmacist for ways to lessen these effects.

If you vomit shortly after taking a dose of testolactone, check with your doctor. You will be told whether to take the dose again or to wait until the next scheduled dose.

Missed dose—If you miss a dose of this medicine, take it as soon as you remember. However, if it is almost time for the next dose, skip the missed dose and go back to your regular dosing schedule. Do not double doses. If you miss two or more doses in a row, check with your doctor.

Storage—To store this medicine:

- Keep out of the reach of children.
- Store away from heat and direct light.
- Do not store in the bathroom, near the kitchen sink, or in other damp places. Heat or moisture may cause the medicine to break down.
- Do not keep outdated medicine or medicine no longer needed. Be sure that any discarded medicine is out of the reach of children.

Precautions While Using This Medicine

It is very important that your doctor check your progress at regular visits to make sure that this medicine is working properly and to check for unwanted effects.

Side Effects of This Medicine

Along with its needed effects, a medicine may cause some unwanted effects. Although not all of these side effects may occur, if they do occur they may need medical attention.

Check with your doctor as soon as possible if the following side effect occurs:

Less common

Numbness or tingling of fingers, toes, or face

Other side effects may occur that usually do not need medical attention. These side effects may go away during treatment as your body adjusts to the medicine. Also, your doctor or nurse may be able to tell you about ways to prevent or reduce some of these side effects. Check with your doctor or nurse if any of the following side effects continue or are bothersome or if you have any questions about them:

Less common

Diarrhea; loss of appetite; nausea or vomiting; pain or swelling in feet or lower legs; swelling or redness of tongue

Other side effects not listed above may also occur in some patients. If you notice any other effects, check with your doctor.

Annual revision: 08/04/92

TETANUS TOXOID Systemic

Description

Tetanus (TET-n-us) Toxoid is used to prevent tetanus (also known as lockjaw). Tetanus is a serious illness that causes convulsions (seizures) and severe muscle spasms that can be strong enough to cause bone fractures of the spine. Tetanus causes death in 30 to 40 percent of cases.

Immunization against tetanus is recommended for all infants from 6 or 8 weeks of age and older, all children, and all adults. Immunization against tetanus consists first of a series of either 3 or 4 injections, depending on which type of tetanus toxoid you receive. In addition, it is very important that you get a booster injection every 10 years for the rest of your life. Also, if you get a wound that is unclean or hard to clean, you may need an emergency booster injection if it has been more than 5 years since your last booster. In recent years, two-thirds of all tetanus cases have been in persons 50 years of age and older. A tetanus infection in the past does not make you immune to tetanus in the future.

This vaccine is available only from your doctor or other authorized health care provider, in the following dosage form:

Parenteral

- Injection (U.S. and Canada)

It is very important that you read and understand the following information. If any of it causes you special concern, check with your doctor. Also, *if you have any questions* or if you want more information about this medicine or your medical problem, *ask your doctor, nurse, or pharmacist.*

Before Receiving This Vaccine

In deciding to receive this medicine, the risks of receiving the medicine must be weighed against the good it will do. This is a decision you and your doctor will make. For tetanus toxoid, the following should be considered:

Allergies—Tell your doctor if you have ever had any unusual or allergic reaction to tetanus toxoid. Also tell your doctor and pharmacist if you are allergic to any other substances, such as preservatives.

Pregnancy—This vaccine has not been shown to cause birth defects or other problems in humans. Vaccination of a pregnant woman can prevent her newborn baby from getting tetanus at birth.

Breast-feeding—It is not known whether tetanus toxoid passes into the breast milk. However, this vaccine has not been reported to cause problems in nursing babies.

Children—Use is not recommended for infants up to 6 weeks of age.

Older adults—This vaccine is not expected to cause different side effects or problems in older people than it does in younger adults. However, the vaccine may be slightly less effective in older persons than in younger adults.

Other medicines—Although certain medicines should not be used together at all, in other cases two different medicines may be used together even if an interaction might occur. In these cases, your doctor may want to change the dose, or other precautions may be necessary. Before you receive tetanus toxoid, it is especially important that your doctor and pharmacist know if you are using any prescription or nonprescription (over-the-counter [OTC]) medicine.

Other medical problems—The presence of other medical problems may affect the use of tetanus toxoid. Make sure you tell your doctor if you have any other medical problems, especially:

- A severe reaction or a fever greater than 103 °F (39.4 °C) following a previous dose of tetanus toxoid—May increase the chance of side effects with future doses of tetanus toxoid; be sure your doctor knows about this before you receive the next dose of tetanus toxoid
- Bronchitis, pneumonia, or other illness involving lungs or bronchial tubes, or
- Severe illness with fever—Possible side effects from tetanus toxoid may be confused with the symptoms of the condition

Side Effects of This Vaccine

Along with its needed effects, a vaccine may cause some unwanted effects. Although not all of these side effects may occur, if they do occur they may need medical attention.

Get emergency help immediately if any of the following side effects occur:

Symptoms of allergic reaction

Difficulty in breathing or swallowing; hives; itching, especially of feet or hands; reddening of skin, especially around ears; swelling of eyes, face, or inside of nose; unusual tiredness or weakness (sudden and severe)

Check with your doctor as soon as possible if any of the following side effects occur:

Rare

Confusion; convulsions (seizures); fever over 103 °F (39.4 °C); headache (severe or continuing); sleepiness (excessive); swelling, blistering, or pain at place of injection (severe or continuing); swelling of glands in armpit; unusual irritability; vomiting (severe or continuing)

Other side effects may occur that usually do not need medical attention. However, check with your doctor if any of the following side effects continue or are bothersome:

More common

Redness or hard lump at place of injection

Less common

Chills, fever, irritability, or unusual tiredness; pain, tenderness, itching, or swelling at place of injection; skin rash

Other side effects not listed above may also occur in some patients. If you notice any other effects, check with your doctor.

Annual revision: September 1990

TETRACYCLINES Ophthalmic

This information applies to the following medicines:

Chlortetracycline (klor-te-tra-SYE-kleen)
Tetracycline (te-tra-SYE-kleen)

Some commonly used brand names are:

Chlortetracycline

In the U.S.
Aureomycin

In Canada
Aureomycin

Tetracycline

In the U.S.
Achromycin

In Canada
Achromycin

Description

Tetracyclines belong to the family of medicines called antibiotics. Tetracycline ophthalmic preparations are used to treat infections of the eye. They may also be used along with other medicines that are taken by mouth for infections of the eye.

Tetracyclines are available only with your doctor's prescription, in the following dosage forms:

Ophthalmic

Chlortetracycline

- Ophthalmic ointment (U.S. and Canada)

Tetracycline
- Ophthalmic ointment (U.S. and Canada)
- Ophthalmic suspension (eye drops) (U.S.)

It is very important that you read and understand the following information. If any of it causes you special concern, check with your doctor. Also, *if you have any questions* or if you want more information about this medicine or your medical problem, *ask your doctor, nurse, or pharmacist.*

Before Using This Medicine

In deciding to use a medicine, the risks of using the medicine must be weighed against the good it will do. This is a decision you and your doctor will make. For tetracycline ophthalmic preparations, the following should be considered:

Allergies—Tell your doctor if you have ever had any unusual or allergic reaction to tetracycline or chlortetracycline or to any related antibiotics, such as demeclocycline (e.g., Declomycin), doxycycline (e.g., Vibramycin), methacycline (e.g., Rondomycin), minocycline (e.g., Minocin), or oxytetracycline (e.g., Terramycin). Also tell your doctor and pharmacist if you are allergic to any other substances, such as preservatives.

Pregnancy—Tetracycline ophthalmic preparations have not been shown to cause birth defects or other problems in humans.

Breast-feeding—Tetracycline ophthalmic preparations have not been reported to cause problems in nursing babies.

Children—Although there is no specific information comparing use of ophthalmic tetracyclines in children with use in other age groups, they are not expected to cause different side effects or problems in children than they do in adults.

Older adults—Many medicines have not been studied specifically in older people. Therefore, it may not be known whether they work exactly the same way they do in younger adults or if they cause different side effects or problems in older people. There is no specific information comparing use of tetracyclines in the elderly with use in other age groups.

Other medicines—Although certain medicines should not be used together at all, in other cases two different medicines may be used together even if an interaction might occur. In these cases, your doctor may want to change the dose, or other precautions may be necessary. Tell your doctor and pharmacist if you are using any other prescription or nonprescription (over-the-counter [OTC]) medicine that is to be used in the eye.

Before you begin using any new medicine (prescription or nonprescription) or if you develop any new medical problem while you are using this medicine, check with your doctor, nurse, or pharmacist.

Proper Use of This Medicine

For patients using the *eye drop form* of tetracyclines:
- The bottle is only partially full to provide proper drop control.
- To use:

  —First, wash your hands. Then tilt the head back and pull the lower eyelid away from the eye to form a pouch. Drop the medicine into the pouch and gently close the eyes. Do not blink. Keep the eyes closed for 1 or 2 minutes to allow the medicine to come into contact with the infection.

  —If you think you did not get the drop of medicine into your eye properly, use another drop.

  —To keep the medicine as germ-free as possible, do not touch the applicator tip to any surface (including the eye). Also, keep the container tightly closed.

For patients using the *eye ointment form* of tetracyclines:
- To use:

  —First, wash your hands. Then pull the lower eyelid away from the eye to form a pouch. Squeeze a thin strip of ointment into the pouch. A 1-cm (approximately ⅓-inch) strip of ointment is usually enough unless otherwise directed by your doctor. Gently close the eyes and keep them closed for 1 or 2 minutes to allow the medicine to come into contact with the infection.

  —To keep the medicine as germ-free as possible, do not touch the applicator tip to any surface (including the eye). After using tetracyclines eye ointment, wipe the tip of the ointment tube with a clean tissue and keep the tube tightly closed.

To help clear up your infection completely, *keep using this medicine for the full time of treatment,* even if your symptoms have disappeared. *Do not miss any doses.*

Dosing—The dose of ophthalmic tetracyclines will be different for different patients. *Follow your doctor's orders or the directions on the label.* The following information includes only the average doses of ophthalmic tetracyclines. *If your dose is different, do not change it unless your doctor tells you to do so.*

The number of doses you use each day, the time allowed between doses, and the length of time you use the medicine depend on the medical problem for which you are using ophthalmic tetracyclines.

- *For eye infections:*

  —*For ophthalmic ointment* dosage forms:
  - Adults and children—Use every two to four hours.

—For *ophthalmic suspension* dosage form:
- Adults and children—One drop every six to twelve hours.

Missed dose—If you miss a dose of this medicine, apply it as soon as possible. However, if it is almost time for your next application, skip the missed dose and go back to your regular dosing schedule.

Storage—To store this medicine:
- Keep out of the reach of children.
- Store away from heat and direct light.
- Keep the medicine from freezing.
- Do not keep outdated medicine or medicine no longer needed. Be sure that any discarded medicine is out of the reach of children.

Precautions While Using This Medicine

After application, this medicine usually causes your vision to blur for a few minutes.

If your symptoms do not improve within a few days, or if they become worse, check with your doctor.

Side Effects of This Medicine

There have not been any common or important side effects reported with this medicine. However, if you notice any unusual effects, check with your doctor.

Annual revision: 07/01/93

TETRACYCLINES Systemic

This information applies to the following medicines:

Demeclocycline (dem-e-kloe-SYE-kleen)
Doxycycline (dox-i-SYE-kleen)
Minocycline (mi-noe-SYE-kleen)
Oxytetracycline (ox-i-te-tra-SYE-kleen)
Tetracycline (te-tra-SYE-kleen)

Some commonly used brand names are:

For Demeclocycline

In the U.S.
Declomycin

In Canada
Declomycin

For Doxycycline

In the U.S.
Doryx
Doxy
Doxy-Caps
Monodox
Vibramycin
Vibra-Tabs

Generic name product may also be available.

In Canada
Apo-Doxy
Doryx
Doxycin
Novodoxylin
Vibramycin
Vibra-Tabs

For Minocycline

In the U.S.
Minocin

Generic name product may also be available.

In Canada
Minocin

For Oxytetracycline

In the U.S.
Terramycin
Tija

Generic name product may also be available.

For Tetracycline

In the U.S.
Achromycin
Achromycin V
Panmycin
Robitet
Sumycin
Tetracyn

Generic name product may also be available.

In Canada
Achromycin
Achromycin V
Apo-Tetra
Novotetra
Nu-Tetra
Tetracyn

Description

Tetracyclines are used to treat infections and to help control acne. Demeclocycline and doxycycline may also be used for other problems as determined by your doctor. Tetracyclines will not work for colds, flu, or other virus infections.

Tetracyclines are available only with your doctor's prescription, in the following dosage forms:

Oral

Demeclocycline
- Capsules (U.S.)
- Tablets (U.S. and Canada)

Doxycycline
- Capsules (U.S. and Canada)
- Delayed-release capsules (U.S. and Canada)
- Oral suspension (U.S.)
- Tablets (U.S. and Canada)

Minocycline
- Capsules (U.S. and Canada)
- Oral suspension (U.S.)
- Tablets (U.S.)

Oxytetracycline
- Capsules (U.S.)

Tetracycline
- Capsules (U.S. and Canada)
- Oral suspension (U.S. and Canada)
- Tablets (U.S. and Canada)

Parenteral

Doxycycline
- Injection (U.S. and Canada)

Minocycline
- Injection (U.S.)

Oxytetracycline
- Injection (U.S.)

Tetracycline
- Injection (U.S. and Canada)

It is very important that you read and understand the following information. If any of it causes you special concern, check with your doctor. Also, *if you have any questions* or if you want more information about this medicine or your medical problem, *ask your doctor, nurse, or pharmacist.*

Before Using This Medicine

In deciding to use a medicine, the risks of taking the medicine must be weighed against the good it will do. This is a decision you and your doctor will make. For tetracyclines, the following should be considered:

Allergies—Tell your doctor if you have ever had any unusual or allergic reaction to any of the tetracyclines or combination medicines containing a tetracycline. Also tell your doctor and pharmacist if you are allergic to any other substances, such as foods, preservatives, or dyes. In addition, if you are going to be given oxytetracycline or tetracycline by injection, tell your doctor if you have ever had an unusual or allergic reaction to "caine-type" anesthetics.

Pregnancy—Use is not recommended during the last half of pregnancy. Tetracyclines may cause the unborn infant's teeth to become discolored and may slow down the growth of the infant's teeth and bones if they are taken during that time. In addition, liver problems may occur in pregnant women, especially those receiving high doses by injection into a vein.

Breast-feeding—Use is not recommended since tetracyclines pass into the breast milk. They may cause the nursing baby's teeth to become discolored and may slow down the growth of the baby's teeth and bones. They may also cause increased sensitivity of nursing babies' skin to sunlight and fungus infections of the mouth and vagina. In addition, minocycline may cause dizziness, lightheadedness, or unsteadiness in nursing babies.

Children—Tetracyclines may cause permanent discoloration of teeth and slow down the growth of bones. These medicines should not be given to children up to 8 years of age unless directed by the child's doctor.

Older adults—Many medicines have not been studied specifically in older people. Therefore, it may not be known whether they work exactly the same way they do in younger adults or if they cause different side effects or problems in older people. There is no specific information comparing use of tetracyclines in the elderly with use in other age groups.

Other medicines—Although certain medicines should not be used together at all, in other cases two different medicines may be used together even if an interaction might occur. In these cases, your doctor may want to change the dose, or other precautions may be necessary. When you are taking tetracyclines, it is especially important that your doctor and pharmacist know if you are taking any of the following:

- Antacids or
- Calcium supplements such as calcium carbonate or
- Cholestyramine (e.g., Questran) or
- Choline and magnesium salicylates (e.g., Trilisate) or
- Colestipol (e.g., Colestid) or
- Iron-containing medicine or
- Laxatives (magnesium-containing) or
- Magnesium salicylate (e.g., Magan)—Use of these medicines with tetracyclines may decrease the effect of tetracyclines
- Oral contraceptives (birth control pills) containing estrogen—Use of birth control pills with tetracyclines may decrease the effect of the birth control pills and increase the chance of unwanted pregnancy

Other medical problems—The presence of other medical problems may affect the use of tetracyclines. Make sure you tell your doctor if you have any other medical problems, especially:

- Diabetes insipidus (water diabetes)—Demeclocycline may make the condition worse
- Kidney disease (does not apply to doxycycline or minocycline)—Patients with kidney disease may have an increased chance of side effects
- Liver disease—Patients with liver disease may have an increased chance of side effects if they use doxycycline or minocycline

Before you begin using any new medicine (prescription or nonprescription) or if you develop any new medical problem while you are using this medicine, check with your doctor, nurse, or pharmacist.

Proper Use of This Medicine

Do not give tetracyclines to infants or children up to 8 years of age unless directed by your doctor. Tetracyclines may cause permanently discolored teeth and other problems in this age group.

Do not take milk, milk formulas, or other dairy products within 1 to 2 hours of the time you take tetracyclines (except doxycycline and minocycline) by mouth. They may keep this medicine from working properly.

If this medicine has changed color or tastes or looks different, has become outdated (old), has been stored incorrectly (too warm or too damp area or place), do not use it. To do so may cause *serious side effects.* Discard the medicine. If you have any questions about this, check with your doctor or pharmacist.

Tetracyclines should be taken with a full glass (8 ounces) of water to prevent irritation of the esophagus (tube between the throat and stomach) or stomach. In addition, most tetracyclines (except doxycycline and minocycline) are best taken on an empty stomach (either 1 hour before or 2 hours after meals). However, if this medicine upsets your stomach, your doctor may want you to take it with food.

For patients taking the *oral liquid form* of this medicine:

- Use a specially marked measuring spoon or other device to measure each dose accurately. The average household teaspoon may not hold the right amount of liquid.
- Do not use after the expiration date on the label since the medicine may not work properly after that date. Check with your pharmacist if you have any questions about this.

For patients taking *doxycycline or minocycline:*

- These medicines may be taken with food or milk if they upset your stomach.
- Swallow the capsule (with enteric-coated pellets) form of doxycycline whole. Do not break or crush.

To help clear up your infection completely, *keep taking this medicine for the full time of treatment*, even if you begin to feel better after a few days. If you stop taking this medicine too soon, your symptoms may return.

This medicine works best when there is a constant amount in the blood or urine. *To help keep the amount constant, do not miss any doses. Also, it is best to take the doses at evenly spaced times day and night.* For example, if you are to take 4 doses a day, the doses should be spaced about 6 hours apart. If this interferes with your sleep or other daily activities, or if you need help in planning the best times to take your medicine, check with your doctor, nurse, or pharmacist.

Missed dose—If you do miss a dose of this medicine, take it as soon as possible. This will help to keep a constant amount of medicine in the blood or urine. However, if it is almost time for your next dose, skip the missed dose and go back to your regular dosing schedule. Do not double doses.

Storage—To store this medicine:

- Keep out of the reach of children.
- Store away from heat and direct light.
- Do not store the capsule or tablet form of this medicine in the bathroom, near the kitchen sink, or in other damp places. Heat or moisture may cause the medicine to break down.
- Keep the oral liquid forms of this medicine from freezing.
- Do not keep outdated medicine or medicine no longer needed. Be sure that any discarded medicine is out of the reach of children.

Precautions While Using This Medicine

If your symptoms do not improve within a few days (or a few weeks or months for acne patients), or if they become worse, check with your doctor.

Do not take antacids; calcium supplements such as calcium carbonate; *choline and magnesium salicylates combination (e.g., Trilisate); magnesium salicylate (e.g., Magan); magnesium-containing laxatives* such as Epsom salt; *or sodium bicarbonate* (baking soda) within 1 to 2 hours of the time you take any of the tetracyclines by mouth. In addition, *do not take iron preparations* (including vitamin preparations that contain iron) within 2 to 3 hours of the time you take tetracyclines by mouth. To do so may keep this medicine from working properly.

Oral contraceptives (birth control pills) containing estrogen may not work properly if you take them while you are taking tetracyclines. Unplanned pregnancies may occur. You should use a different or additional means of birth control while you are taking tetracyclines. If you have any questions about this, check with your doctor or pharmacist.

Before having surgery (including dental surgery) with a general anesthetic, tell the medical doctor or dentist in charge that you are taking a tetracycline. This does not apply to doxycycline, however.

Tetracyclines may cause your skin to be more sensitive to sunlight than it is normally. Exposure to sunlight, even for brief periods of time, may cause a skin rash, itching, redness or other discoloration of the skin, or a severe sunburn. When you begin taking this medicine:

- Stay out of direct sunlight, especially between the hours of 10:00 a.m. and 3:00 p.m., if possible.
- Wear protective clothing, including a hat. Also, wear sunglasses.
- Apply a sun block product that has a skin protection factor (SPF) of at least 15. Some patients may require a product with a higher SPF number, especially if they have a fair complexion. If you have any questions about this, check with your doctor or pharmacist.
- Apply a sun block lipstick that has an SPF of at least 15 to protect your lips.
- Do not use a sunlamp or tanning bed or booth.

You may still be more sensitive to sunlight or sunlamps for 2 weeks to several months or more after stopping this medicine. *If you have a severe reaction, check with your doctor.*

For patients taking *minocycline:*

- Minocycline may also cause some people to become dizzy, lightheaded, or unsteady. *Make sure you know how you react to this medicine before you drive, use machines, or do anything else that could be dangerous if you are dizzy or are not alert.* If these reactions are especially bothersome, check with your doctor.

Side Effects of This Medicine

Along with its needed effects, a medicine may cause some unwanted effects. In some infants and children, tetracyclines may cause the teeth to become discolored. Even though this may not happen right away, check with your doctor as soon as possible if you notice this effect or if you have any questions about it.

For all tetracyclines

More common

Increased sensitivity of skin to sunlight (rare with minocycline)

Rare

Abdominal pain; bulging fontanel (soft spot on head) of infants; headache; loss of appetite; nausea and vomiting; yellowing skin; visual changes

For demeclocycline only

Less common

Greatly increased frequency of urination or amount of urine; increased thirst; unusual tiredness or weakness

For minocycline only

Less common

Pigmentation (darker color or discoloration) of skin and mucous membranes

Other side effects may occur that usually do not need medical attention. These side effects may go away during treatment as your body adjusts to the medicine. However, check with your doctor if any of the following side effects continue or are bothersome:

For all tetracyclines

More common

Cramps or burning of the stomach; diarrhea; nausea or vomiting

Less common

Itching of the rectal or genital (sex organ) areas; sore mouth or tongue

For minocycline only

More common

Dizziness, lightheadedness, or unsteadiness

In some patients tetracyclines may cause the tongue to become darkened or discolored. This effect is only temporary and will go away when you stop taking this medicine.

Other side effects not listed above may also occur in some patients. If you notice any other effects, check with your doctor.

Additional Information

Once a medicine has been approved for marketing for a certain use, experience may show that it is also useful for other medical problems. Although these uses are not included in product labeling, tetracyclines are used in certain patients with the following medical conditions:

- Syndrome of inappropriate antidiuretic hormone (SIADH) (for demeclocycline)
- Traveler's diarrhea (for doxycyline)

For patients taking this medicine for *SIADH:*

- Some doctors may prescribe demeclocycline for certain patients who retain (keep) more body water than usual. Although demeclocycline works like a diuretic (water pill) in these patients, it will not work that way in other patients who may need a diuretic.

For patients taking this medicine for *Traveler's diarrhea:*

- Some doctors may prescribe doxycycline by mouth to help prevent or treat traveler's diarrhea. It is usually given daily for three weeks to prevent traveler's diarrhea. If you have any questions about this, check with your doctor.

Other than the above information, there is no additional information relating to proper use, precautions, or side effects for these uses.

Annual revision: 08/30/92

TETRACYCLINES Topical

This information applies to the following medicines:

Chlortetracycline (klor-te-tra-SYE-kleen)
Meclocycline (me-kloe-SYE-kleen)
Tetracycline (te-tra-SYE-kleen)

Some commonly used brand names are:

For Chlortetracycline

In the U.S.

Aureomycin

In Canada

Aureomycin

For Meclocycline

In the U.S.

Meclan

For Tetracycline

In the U.S.

Achromycin
Topicycline

In Canada

Achromycin

Description

Tetracyclines belong to the family of medicines called antibiotics. The topical ointment forms are used to treat infections of the skin. Meclocycline cream and the topical liquid form of tetracycline are used to help control acne. They may be used alone or with one or more other medicines which are applied to the skin or taken by mouth for acne.

Topical ointment forms of the tetracyclines are available without a prescription; however, your doctor may have special instructions on the proper use of these medicines for your medical problem. Meclocycline cream and the topical liquid form of tetracycline are available only with your doctor's prescription.

Topical tetracycline is available in the following dosage forms:

Topical

Chlortetracycline
- Ointment (U.S. and Canada)

Meclocycline
- Cream (U.S.)

Tetracycline
- Ointment (U.S. and Canada)
- Topical solution (U.S.)

It is very important that you read and understand the following information. If any of it causes you special concern, check with your doctor or pharmacist. Also, *if you have any questions* or if you want more information about this medicine or your medical problem, *ask your doctor, nurse, or pharmacist.*

Before Using This Medicine

In deciding to use a medicine, the risks of using the medicine must be weighed against the good it will do. This is a decision you and your doctor will make. For topical tetracyclines, the following should be considered:

Allergies—Tell your doctor if you have ever had any unusual or allergic reaction to topical tetracyclines or to any related antibiotics, such as chlortetracycline for the eye (e.g., Aureomycin); demeclocycline (e.g., Declomycin); doxycycline (e.g., Vibramycin); methacycline (e.g., Rondomycin); minocycline (e.g., Minocin); oxytetracycline (e.g., Terramycin); or tetracycline by mouth or by injection (e.g., Achromycin). In addition, if you are to use the cream form of meclocycline, tell your doctor if you have ever had any unusual or allergic reaction to formaldehyde. Also tell your doctor and pharmacist if you are allergic to any other substances, such as preservatives or dyes.

Pregnancy—Studies have not been done in humans. In studies in rats and rabbits, chlortetracycline and tetracycline topical preparations have not been shown to cause birth defects or other problems. However, studies in rabbits have shown meclocycline to cause a slight delay in bone formation.

Breast-feeding—It is not known whether tetracycline topical preparations, applied to the mother's skin, are absorbed into the body and pass into the breast milk. However, this medicine has not been reported to cause problems in nursing babies.

Children—Tetracycline topical solution has been tested on a limited number of children 11 years of age or older and has not been shown to cause different side effects or problems in children than it does in adults. Although there is no specific information about the use of topical chlortetracycline or topical meclocycline in children, they are not expected to cause different side effects or problems in children than they do in adults.

Older adults—Many medicines have not been tested in older people. Therefore, it may not be known whether they work exactly the same way they do in younger adults or if they cause different side effects or problems in older people. There is no specific information about the use of topical tetracyclines in the elderly.

Other medicines—Although certain medicines should not be used together at all, in other cases two different medicines may be used together even if an interaction might occur. In these cases, your doctor may want to change the dose, or other precautions may be necessary. When you are using topical tetracyclines, it is important that your doctor and pharmacist know if you are using any other topical prescription or nonprescription (over-the-counter [OTC]) medicine that is to be applied to the same area of the skin.

Before you begin using any new medicine (prescription or nonprescription) or if you develop any new medical problem while you are using this medicine, check with your doctor, nurse, or pharmacist.

Proper Use of This Medicine

For patients using the *cream form or topical liquid form* of this medicine for acne:

- The cream or topical liquid form of this medicine will not cure your acne. However, to help keep your acne under control, *keep using this medicine for the full time of treatment,* even if your symptoms begin to clear up after a few days. You may have to continue using this medicine every day for months or even longer in some cases. If you stop using this medicine too soon, your symptoms may return. *It is important that you do not miss any doses.*

For patients using the *cream form* of this medicine for acne:

- Do not get this medicine on your clothing since it may stain.

- Before applying this medicine, thoroughly wash the affected area with warm water and soap, rinse well, and pat dry.
- To use:
  —Apply a thin film of medicine, using enough to cover the affected area lightly. *You should apply the medicine to the whole area usually affected by acne, not just to the pimples themselves.* This will help keep new pimples from breaking out.
  —Do not get this medicine in the eyes, nose, mouth, or on other mucous membranes. Spread the medicine away from these areas when applying.

For patients using the *topical liquid form* of this medicine for acne:

- Do not get this medicine on your clothing since it may stain.
- This medicine usually comes with patient instructions. Read these instructions carefully before using this medicine.
- The liquid form contains alcohol and is flammable. *Do not use near heat, near open flame, or while smoking.*
- Do not use after the expiration date on the label. The medicine may not work properly. Check with your pharmacist if you have any questions about this.
- The presence of the floating plastic plug in the liquid means that the medicine has been mixed properly. *Do not remove the plastic plug.*
- It is important that you do not use this medicine more often than your doctor ordered. It may cause your skin to become too dry or irritated.
- Before applying this medicine, thoroughly wash the affected area with warm water and soap, rinse well, and pat dry. After washing or shaving, it is best to wait 30 minutes before applying this medicine. The alcohol in it may irritate freshly washed or shaved skin.
- However, you should avoid washing the acne-affected areas too often. This may dry your skin and make your acne worse. Washing with a mild, bland soap 2 or 3 times a day should be enough, unless you have oily skin. If you have any questions about this, check with your doctor.
- To use:
  —This medicine comes in a bottle with an applicator tip which may be used to apply the medicine directly to the skin. Use the applicator with a dabbing motion instead of a rolling motion (not like a roll-on deodorant, for example). Tilt the bottle and press the tip firmly against your skin. If needed, you can make the medicine flow faster from the applicator tip by slightly increasing the pressure against the skin. If the medicine flows too fast, use less pressure.
  —Apply a generous amount of medicine, using enough so that the skin feels wet all over. After applying the medicine with the applicator, use your fingertips to spread the medicine around evenly and rub it into your skin. A second coat may be needed to completely cover the affected areas. Be sure to wash the medicine off your hands afterward.
  —*You should apply the medicine to the whole area usually affected by acne, not just to the pimples themselves.* This will help keep new pimples from breaking out.
  —Since this medicine contains alcohol, it will sting or burn. Therefore, *do not get this medicine in the eyes, nose, mouth, or on other mucous membranes.* Spread the medicine away from these areas when applying. If this medicine does get in the eyes, wash them out immediately, but carefully, with large amounts of cool tap water. If your eyes still burn or are painful, check with your doctor.
- The bottle contains about an 8-week supply of medicine if used only on the face and neck or about a 4-week supply if used on the face and neck plus other affected areas.

For patients using the *topical ointment form* of this medicine:

- To help clear up your infection completely, *keep using this medicine for the full time of treatment,* even if your symptoms begin to clear up after a few days. If you stop using this medicine too soon, your symptoms may return. *Do not miss any doses.*
- If you do miss a dose of this medicine, apply it as soon as possible. However, if it is almost time for your next dose, skip the missed dose and go back to your regular dosing schedule.
- Do not get this medicine on your clothing since it may stain.
- If you are using this medicine without a prescription, do not use it to treat deep wounds, puncture wounds, or serious burns without first checking with your doctor or pharmacist.
- Do not get this medicine in the eyes.
- Before applying this medicine, thoroughly wash the affected area with warm water and soap, rinse well, and dry completely.
- After applying this medicine, you may cover the treated area with a gauze dressing if you wish.

Missed dose—For patients using the *cream form or topical liquid form* of this medicine: If you miss a dose of this medicine, apply it as soon as possible. However, if it is almost time for your next dose, skip the missed dose and go back to your regular dosing schedule.

Storage—To store this medicine:

- Keep out of the reach of children.
- Store away from heat and direct light.

- Keep the medicine from freezing.
- Do not keep outdated medicine or medicine no longer needed. Be sure that any discarded medicine is out of the reach of children.

Precautions While Using This Medicine

For patients using either the *cream form or the topical liquid form* of this medicine for acne:

- Some people may notice improvement in their acne within 4 to 6 weeks. However, if there is no improvement in your acne after you have used this medicine for 6 to 8 weeks or if it becomes worse, check with your doctor or pharmacist. The treatment of acne may take up to 8 to 12 weeks before full improvement is seen.
- If your doctor has ordered another medicine to be applied to the skin along with this medicine, it is best to wait at least 1 hour before you apply the second medicine. This may help keep your skin from becoming too irritated. Also, if the medicines are used too close together, they may not work properly.
- The liquid form of this medicine may also cause the skin to become unusually dry, even with normal use. If this occurs, check with your doctor.
- This medicine may cause faint yellowing of the skin, especially around hair roots. This may be more easily seen in people with light complexions. The color may be removed by washing. However, the medicine should be left on the skin as long as possible. Do not wash immediately after applying the medicine. This will keep the medicine from working properly. If the yellow color is bothersome during the daytime, the medicine may be applied after school or work and again at bedtime, unless otherwise directed by your doctor.
- Treated areas of the skin may glow bright yellow under "black" (ultraviolet or UV) light such as that used in some discos. To help reduce or avoid this, apply the medicine later in the evening or wash it off before exposure to "black" light.
- You may continue to use cosmetics (make-up) while you are using this medicine for acne. However, it is best to use only "water-base" cosmetics. Also, it is best not to use cosmetics too heavily or too often. They may make your acne worse. If you have any questions about this, check with your doctor.

For patients using the *topical ointment form* of this medicine:

- If your skin infection does not improve within 2 weeks, or if it becomes worse, check with your doctor or pharmacist.

Side Effects of This Medicine

Along with its needed effects, a medicine may cause some unwanted effects. Although not all of these side effects may occur, if they do occur they may need medical attention.

Check with your doctor as soon as possible if any of the following side effects occur:

Less common

Pain, redness, swelling, or other sign of irritation not present before use of this medicine

Other side effects may occur that usually do not need medical attention. These side effects may go away during treatment as your body adjusts to the medicine. However, check with your doctor if any of the following side effects continue or are bothersome:

More common—For topical liquid form only

Dry or scaly skin; stinging or burning feeling

More common—For cream and topical liquid forms only

Faint yellowing of the skin, especially around hair roots

Other side effects not listed above may also occur in some patients. If you notice any other effects, check with your doctor.

Annual revision: September 1990

THEOPHYLLINE, EPHEDRINE, GUAIFENESIN, AND BARBITURATES Systemic

This information applies to the following medicines:

Theophylline (thee-OFF-i-lin), Ephedrine (e-FED-rin), Guaifenesin (gwye-FEN-e-sin), and Butabarbital (byoo-ta-BAR-bi-tal)

Theophylline, Ephedrine, Guaifenesin, and Phenobarbital (fee-noe-BAR-bi-tal)

Some commonly used brand names are:

In the U.S.

Bronkolixir
Bronkotabs
Guaiphed
Mudrane GG
Quibron Plus

Description

Theophylline, ephedrine, guaifenesin, and barbiturates (bar-BI-tyoo-rates) combination is used to treat the symptoms of bronchial asthma, chronic bronchitis, emphysema, and other lung diseases. This medicine relieves cough, wheezing, shortness of breath, and troubled breathing. It works by opening up the bronchial tubes (air passages) of the lungs and increasing the flow of air through them.

Some of these preparations are available only with your doctor's prescription. Others are available without a prescription; however, your doctor may have special instructions on the proper use of this medicine for your medical condition.

Theophylline, ephedrine, guaifenesin, and barbiturates combination is available in the following dosage forms:

Oral

- Capsules (U.S.)
- Elixir (U.S.)
- Tablets (U.S.)

It is very important that you read and understand the following information. If any of it causes you special concern, check with your doctor. Also, *if you have any questions* or if you want more information about this medicine or your medical problem, *ask your doctor, nurse, or pharmacist.*

Before Using This Medicine

If you are taking this medicine without a prescription, carefully read and follow any precautions on the label. For theophylline, ephedrine, guaifenesin, and barbiturates combination medicine, the following should be considered:

Allergies—Tell your doctor if you have ever had any unusual or allergic reaction to aminophylline, caffeine, dyphylline, oxtriphylline, theobromine, or theophylline; ephedrine or medicines like ephedrine such as albuterol, amphetamines, epinephrine, isoproterenol, metaproterenol, norepinephrine, phenylephrine, phenylpropanolamine, pseudoephedrine, or terbutaline; or barbiturates. Also tell your doctor and pharmacist if you are allergic to any other substances, such as foods, preservatives, or dyes.

Diet—Make certain your doctor and pharmacist know if you are on any special diet, such as a low-sodium or low-sugar diet or a high-protein, low-carbohydrate or low-protein, high-carbohydrate diet. A high-protein, low-carbohydrate diet may decrease the effects of theophylline; a low-protein, high-carbohydrate diet may increase the effects of theophylline.

Avoid eating or drinking large amounts of caffeine-containing foods or beverages, such as chocolate, cocoa, tea, coffee, and cola drinks, because they may increase the central nervous system (CNS) stimulant effects of theophylline.

Also, eating charcoal broiled foods every day while taking theophylline may keep this medicine from working properly.

Pregnancy—Studies with theophylline on birth defects have not been done in humans. However, some studies in animals have shown that theophylline causes birth defects when given in doses many times the human dose. Also, use of theophylline during pregnancy may cause unwanted effects such as fast heartbeat, jitteriness, irritability, gagging, vomiting, and breathing problems in the newborn infant.

Studies with ephedrine on birth defects have not been done in either humans or animals.

Barbiturates taken during pregnancy have been shown to increase the chance of birth defects in humans. Also, taking barbiturates regularly during the last 3 months of pregnancy may cause the baby to become dependent on the medicine. This may lead to withdrawal side effects in the baby after birth. In addition, one study in humans has suggested that barbiturates taken during pregnancy may increase the chance of brain tumors in the baby.

Guaifenesin has not been shown to cause birth defects or other problems in humans.

Breast-feeding—The theophylline, ephedrine, and barbiturate in this combination medicine pass into the breast milk and may cause unwanted effects such as drowsiness, irritability, fretfulness, or trouble in sleeping in babies of mothers taking this medicine. Guaifenesin has not been reported to cause problems in nursing babies.

Children—Newborn infants may be especially sensitive to the effects of theophylline, ephedrine, guaifenesin, and barbiturates combination medicine. This may increase the chance of side effects during treatment.

Older adults—Elderly people 55 years of age or older may be especially sensitive to the effects of theophylline, ephedrine, guaifenesin, and barbiturates combination medicine. This may increase the chance of side effects during treatment.

Other medicines—Although certain medicines should not be used together at all, in other cases two different medicines may be used together even if an interaction might occur. In these cases, your doctor may want to change the dose, or other precautions may be necessary. When you are taking theophylline, ephedrine, guaifenesin, and barbiturates combination medicine, it is especially important that your doctor and pharmacist know if you are taking any of the following:

- Adrenocorticoids (cortisone-like medicine) or
- Anticoagulants (blood thinners) or
- Corticotropin—The effects of these medicines may be decreased by the barbiturate in this combination medicine
- Beta-blockers (acebutolol [e.g., Sectral], atenolol [e.g., Tenormin], betaxolol [e.g., Betoptic, Kerlone], carteolol [e.g., Cartrol], labetalol [e.g., Normodyne], levobunolol [e.g., Betagan], metoprolol [e.g., Lopressor], nadolol [e.g., Corgard], oxprenolol [e.g., Trasicor], penbutolol [e.g., Levatol], pindolol [e.g., Visken], propranolol [e.g., Inderal], sotalol [e.g., Sotacor], timolol [e.g., Blocadren,

Timoptic])—Use of these medicines with this combination medicine may prevent either the beta-blocker or this combination medicine from working properly
- Central nervous system (CNS) depressants—The effects of these medicines or the barbiturate in this combination medicine may be increased
- Cimetidine (e.g., Tagamet) or
- Ciprofloxacin (e.g., Cipro) or
- Erythromycin (e.g., E-Mycin) or
- Nicotine chewing gum (e.g., Nicorette) or
- Norfloxacin (e.g., Noroxin) or
- Ranitidine (e.g., Zantac) or
- Troleandomycin (e.g., TAO)—These medicines may increase the effects of theophylline
- Cocaine or
- Ergoloid mesylates (e.g., Hydergine) or
- Ergotamine (e.g., Gynergen)—The effects of these medicines on the heart and blood vessels may be increased by ephedrine
- Digitalis glycosides (heart medicine)—Use of digitalis glycosides with this combination medicine may increase the chance of irregular heartbeat
- Monoamine oxidase (MAO) inhibitors (furazolidone [e.g., Furoxone], isocarboxazid [e.g., Marplan], pargyline [e.g., Eutonyl], phenelzine [e.g., Nardil], procarbazine [e.g., Matulane], tranylcypromine [e.g., Parnate])—Taking ephedrine while you are taking or within 2 weeks of taking monoamine oxidase (MAO) inhibitors may increase the chance of serious side effects
- Oral contraceptives (birth control pills) containing estrogen—Barbiturates may decrease the birth control effects of these medicines; use of another method of birth control may be necessary while you are taking this combination medicine
- Phenytoin—The effects of phenytoin may be decreased by theophylline
- Smoking tobacco or marijuana—If you smoke or have smoked (tobacco or marijuana) regularly within the last 2 years, the amount of medicine you need may vary, depending on how much and how recently you have smoked

Other medical problems—The presence of other medical problems may affect the use of theophylline, ephedrine, guaifenesin, and barbiturates combination medicine. Make sure you tell your doctor if you have any other medical problems, especially:

- Alcohol abuse or
- Fever or
- Liver disease or
- Respiratory infections, such as influenza (flu)—The effects of theophylline may be increased
- Diabetes mellitus (sugar diabetes)—Ephedrine may make the condition worse; your doctor may need to change the dose of your diabetes medicine
- Diarrhea—The absorption of theophylline may be decreased; therefore, the effects of this medicine may be decreased
- Enlarged prostate or
- Heart or blood vessel disease or
- High blood pressure or
- Hyperactivity (in children) or
- Stomach ulcer (or history of) or other stomach problems or
- Underactive adrenal gland—This combination medicine may make the condition worse
- Fibrocystic breast disease—Symptoms of this disease may be increased by theophylline
- Kidney disease—The effects of phenobarbital may be increased
- Overactive thyroid—The effects of theophylline may be decreased
- Pain—The barbiturate in this combination medicine may cause unusual excitement in the presence of pain
- Porphyria (or history of)—The barbiturate in this combination medicine may make the symptoms of this disease worse

Before you begin using any new medicine (prescription or nonprescription) or if you develop any new medical problem while you are using this medicine, check with your doctor, nurse, or pharmacist.

Proper Use of This Medicine

This medicine works best when taken with a glass of water on an empty stomach (either 30 minutes to 1 hour before meals or 2 hours after meals) since that way it will get into the blood sooner. However, in some cases your doctor may want you to take this medicine with meals or right after meals to lessen stomach upset. If you have any questions about how you should be taking this medicine, check with your doctor.

Take this medicine only as directed. Do not take more of it and do not take it more often than recommended on the label, unless otherwise directed by your doctor. To do so may increase the chance of serious side effects. Also, if too much is taken, the barbiturate in this medicine may become habit-forming.

In order for this medicine to help your medical problem, it must be taken every day in regularly spaced doses as recommended. This is necessary to keep a constant amount of this medicine in the blood. To help keep the amount constant, do not miss any doses.

Missed dose—If you do miss a dose of this medicine, take it as soon as possible. However, if it is almost time for your next dose, skip the missed dose and go back to your regular dosing schedule. Do not double doses.

Storage—To store this medicine:

- Keep out of the reach of children.
- Store away from heat and direct light.
- Do not store the capsule or tablet form of this medicine in the bathroom, near the kitchen sink, or in other damp places. Heat or moisture may cause the medicine to break down.
- Keep the liquid form of this medicine from freezing.

- Do not keep outdated medicine or medicine no longer needed. Be sure that any discarded medicine is out of the reach of children.

Precautions While Using This Medicine

The theophylline in this medicine may add to the central nervous system (CNS) stimulant effects of caffeine-containing foods or beverages such as chocolate, cocoa, tea, coffee, and cola drinks. *Avoid eating or drinking large amounts of these foods or beverages while taking this medicine.* If you have any questions about this, check with your doctor.

The barbiturate in this medicine will add to the effects of alcohol and other CNS depressants (medicines that slow down the nervous system, possibly causing drowsiness). Some examples of CNS depressants are antihistamines or medicine for hay fever, other allergies, or colds; sedatives, tranquilizers, or sleeping medicine; prescription pain medicine or narcotics; barbiturates; medicine for seizures; muscle relaxants; or anesthetics, including some dental anesthetics. *Check with your doctor before taking any of the above while you are using this medicine.*

Do not eat charcoal-broiled foods every day while taking this medicine since these foods may keep the medicine from working properly.

Check with your doctor at once if you develop symptoms of influenza (flu) or a fever, since either of these may increase the chance of side effects with this medicine.

Also, *check with your doctor if diarrhea occurs* because the dose of this medicine may need to be changed.

This medicine may cause some people to become dizzy, lightheaded, drowsy, or less alert than they are normally. *Make sure you know how you react to this medicine before you drive, use machines, or do anything else that could be dangerous if you are dizzy or are not alert.*

Side Effects of This Medicine

Along with its needed effects, a medicine may cause some unwanted effects. Although not all of these side effects may occur, if they do occur they may need medical attention.

Check with your doctor as soon as possible if any of the following side effects occur:

Less common

Heartburn and/or vomiting

Symptoms of overdose

Bloody or black, tarry stools; chest pain; convulsions (seizures); diarrhea; dizziness or lightheadedness; fast, pounding, or irregular heartbeat; hallucinations (seeing, hearing, or feeling things that are not there); increase or decrease in blood pressure; irritability; loss of appetite; mood or mental changes; muscle twitching; nausea (continuing or severe) or vomiting; stomach cramps or pain; trembling; trouble in sleeping; unusual tiredness or weakness; vomiting blood or material that looks like coffee grounds

Other side effects may occur that usually do not need medical attention. These side effects may go away during treatment as your body adjusts to the medicine. However, check with your doctor or pharmacist if any of the following side effects continue or are bothersome:

More common

Drowsiness; headache; nausea; nervousness or restlessness

Less common

Difficult or painful urination; feeling of warmth; flushing or redness of face

Other side effects not listed above may also occur in some patients. If you notice any other effects, check with your doctor.

Annual revision: October 1990

THEOPHYLLINE, EPHEDRINE, AND HYDROXYZINE Systemic

Some commonly used brand names are:

In the U.S.

Hydrophed
Hydrophed D.F.
Marax
Marax-DF
T.E.H.
Theozine

Generic name product may also be available.

Description

Theophylline (thee-OFF-i-lin), ephedrine (e-FED-rin), and hydroxyzine (hye-DROX-i-zeen) combination medicine is used to treat the symptoms of bronchial asthma, chronic bronchitis, emphysema, and other lung diseases. This medicine relieves cough, wheezing, shortness of breath, and troubled breathing. It works by opening up the bronchial tubes (air passages) of the lungs and increasing the flow of air through them.

This medicine is available only with your doctor's prescription, in the following dosage forms:

Oral

- Syrup (U.S.)
- Tablets (U.S.)

It is very important that you read and understand the following information. If any of it causes you special concern, check with your doctor. Also, *if you have any questions* or if you want more information about this medicine or your medical problem, *ask your doctor, nurse, or pharmacist.*

Before Using This Medicine

In deciding to use a medicine, the risks of taking the medicine must be weighed against the good it will do. This is a decision you and your doctor will make. For theophylline, ephedrine, and hydroxyzine combination medicine, the following should be considered:

Allergies—Tell your doctor if you have ever had any unusual or allergic reaction to aminophylline, caffeine, dyphylline, oxtriphylline, theobromine, or theophylline; ephedrine or medicines like ephedrine such as albuterol, amphetamines, epinephrine, isoproterenol, metaproterenol, norepinephrine, phenylephrine, phenylpropanolamine, pseudoephedrine, or terbutaline; or hydroxyzine. Also tell your doctor and pharmacist if you are allergic to any other substances, such as foods, preservatives, or dyes.

Diet—Make certain your doctor and pharmacist know if you are on any special diet, such as a low-sodium or low-sugar diet or a high-protein, low-carbohydrate or low-protein, high-carbohydrate diet. A high-protein, low-carbohydrate diet may decrease the effects of theophylline; a low-protein, high-carbohydrate diet may increase the effects of theophylline.

Avoid eating or drinking large amounts of caffeine-containing foods or beverages, such as chocolate, cocoa, tea, coffee, and cola drinks, because they may increase the central nervous system (CNS) stimulant effects of theophylline.

Also, eating charcoal broiled foods every day while taking theophylline may keep this medicine from working properly.

Pregnancy—Studies with theophylline on birth defects have not been done in humans. However, some studies in animals have shown that theophylline causes birth defects when given in doses many times the human dose. Also, use of theophylline during pregnancy may cause unwanted effects such as fast heartbeat, jitteriness, irritability, gagging, vomiting, and breathing problems in the newborn infant.

Studies with ephedrine on birth defects have not been done in either humans or animals.

Hydroxyzine is not recommended during the first months of pregnancy because it has been shown to cause birth defects in rats when given in doses up to many times the usual human dose.

Breast-feeding—Theophylline and ephedrine pass into the breast milk and may cause unwanted effects such as irritability, fretfulness, or trouble in sleeping in babies of mothers taking this medicine. Hydroxyzine has not been reported to cause problems in nursing babies.

Children—Theophylline, ephedrine, and hydroxyzine combination medicine is not recommended for use in children up to 2 years of age. Although there is no specific information about the use of theophylline, ephedrine, and hydroxyzine combination medicine in children 2 years of age and older, it is not expected to cause different side effects or problems in these children than it does in adults.

Older adults—Elderly people 55 years of age or older may be especially sensitive to the effects of theophylline, ephedrine, and hydroxyzine combination medicine. This may increase the chance of side effects during treatment.

Other medicines—Although certain medicines should not be used together at all, in other cases two different medicines may be used together even if an interaction might occur. In these cases, your doctor may want to change the dose, or other precautions may be necessary. When you are taking theophylline, ephedrine, and hydroxyzine combination medicine, it is especially important that your doctor and pharmacist know if you are taking any of the following:

- Beta-blockers (acebutolol [e.g., Sectral], atenolol [e.g., Tenormin], betaxolol [e.g., Betoptic, Kerlone], carteolol [e.g., Cartrol], labetalol [e.g., Normodyne], levobunolol [e.g., Betagan], metoprolol [e.g., Lopressor], nadolol [e.g., Corgard], oxprenolol [e.g., Trasicor], penbutolol [e.g., Levatol], pindolol [e.g., Visken], propranolol [e.g., Inderal], sotalol [e.g., Sotacor], timolol [e.g., Blocadren, Timoptic])—Use of these medicines with this combination medicine may prevent either the beta-blocker or this medicine from working properly
- Central nervous system (CNS) depressants—The effects of these medicines or hydroxyzine may be increased
- Cimetidine (e.g., Tagamet) or
- Ciprofloxacin (e.g., Cipro) or
- Erythromycin (e.g., E-Mycin) or
- Nicotine chewing gum (e.g., Nicorette) or
- Norfloxacin (e.g., Noroxin) or
- Ranitidine (e.g., Zantac) or
- Troleandomycin (e.g., TAO)—These medicines may increase the effects of theophylline
- Cocaine or
- Ergoloid mesylates (e.g., Hydergine) or
- Ergotamine (e.g., Gynergen)—The effects of these medicines on the heart and blood vessels may be increased by ephedrine

- Digitalis glycosides (heart medicine)—Use of these medicines with ephedrine may increase the chance of irregular heartbeat
- Monoamine oxidase (MAO) inhibitors (furazolidone [e.g., Furoxone], isocarboxazid [e.g., Marplan], pargyline [e.g., Eutonyl], phenelzine [e.g., Nardil], procarbazine [e.g., Matulane], tranylcypromine [e.g., Parnate])—Taking ephedrine while you are taking or within 2 weeks of taking monoamine oxidase (MAO) inhibitors may increase the chance of serious side effects
- Phenytoin—The effects of phenytoin may be decreased by theophylline
- Smoking tobacco or marijuana—If you smoke or have smoked (tobacco or marijuana) regularly within the last 2 years, the amount of medicine you need may vary, depending on how much and how recently you have smoked

Other medical problems—The presence of other medical problems may affect the use of theophylline, ephedrine, and hydroxyzine combination medicine. Make sure you tell your doctor if you have any other medical problems, especially:

- Alcohol abuse or
- Fever or
- Liver disease or
- Respiratory infections, such as influenza (flu)—The effects of theophylline may be increased
- Diabetes mellitus (sugar diabetes)—Ephedrine may make the condition worse; your doctor may need to change the dose of your diabetes medicine
- Diarrhea—The absorption of theophylline may be decreased; therefore, the effects of this medicine may be decreased
- Enlarged prostate or
- Heart or blood vessel disease or
- High blood pressure or
- Stomach ulcer (or history of) or other stomach problems—This combination medicine may make the condition worse
- Fibrocystic breast disease—Symptoms of this disease may be increased by theophylline
- Overactive thyroid—The effects of theophylline may be decreased

Before you begin using any new medicine (prescription or nonprescription) or if you develop any new medical problem while you are using this medicine, check with your doctor, nurse, or pharmacist.

Proper Use of This Medicine

This medicine works best when taken with a glass of water on an empty stomach (either 30 minutes to 1 hour before meals or 2 hours after meals) since that way it will get into the blood sooner. However, in some cases your doctor may want you to take this medicine with meals or right after meals to lessen stomach upset. If you have any questions about how you should be taking this medicine, check with your doctor.

Take this medicine only as directed. Do not take more of it and do not take it more often than your doctor ordered. To do so may increase the chance of serious side effects.

In order for this medicine to help your medical problem, it must be taken every day in regularly spaced doses as ordered by your doctor. This is necessary to keep a constant amount of this medicine in the blood. To help keep the amount constant, do not miss any doses.

Missed dose—If you do miss a dose of this medicine, take it as soon as possible. However, if it is almost time for your next dose, skip the missed dose and go back to your regular dosing schedule. Do not double doses.

Storage—To store this medicine:

- Keep out of the reach of children.
- Store away from heat and direct light.
- Do not store the tablet form of this medicine in the bathroom, near the kitchen sink, or in other damp places. Heat or moisture may cause the medicine to break down.
- Keep the syrup form of this medicine from freezing.
- Do not keep outdated medicine or medicine no longer needed. Be sure that any discarded medicine is out of the reach of children.

Precautions While Using This Medicine

The theophylline in this medicine may add to the central nervous system stimulant effects of caffeine-containing foods or beverages such as chocolate, cocoa, tea, coffee, and cola drinks. *Avoid eating or drinking large amounts of these foods or beverages while taking this medicine.* If you have any questions about this, check with your doctor.

The hydroxyzine in this medicine will add to the effects of alcohol and CNS depressants (medicines that slow down the nervous system, possibly causing drowsiness). Some examples of CNS depressants are antihistamines or medicine for hay fever, other allergies, or colds; sedatives, tranquilizers, or sleeping medicine; prescription pain medicine or narcotics; barbiturates; medicine for seizures; muscle relaxants; or anesthetics, including dental anesthetics. *Check with your doctor before taking any of the above while you are taking this medicine.*

Do not eat charcoal-broiled foods every day while taking this medicine since these foods may keep the medicine from working properly.

Check with your doctor at once if you develop symptoms of influenza (flu) or a fever, since either of these may increase the chance of side effects with this medicine.

Also, *check with your doctor if diarrhea occurs* because the dose of this medicine may need to be changed.

This medicine may cause some people to become dizzy, lightheaded, drowsy, or less alert than they are normally. *Make sure you know how you react to this medicine before you drive, use machines, or do anything else that could be dangerous if you are dizzy or are not alert.*

Side Effects of This Medicine

Along with its needed effects, a medicine may cause some unwanted effects. Although not all of these side effects may occur, if they do occur they may need medical attention.

Check with your doctor as soon as possible if any of the following side effects occur:

Less common

Heartburn and/or vomiting

Symptoms of overdose

Bloody or black, tarry stools; chest pain; convulsions (seizures); diarrhea; dizziness or lightheadedness; fast, pounding, or irregular heartbeat; hallucinations (seeing, hearing, or feeling things that are not there); increase or decrease in blood pressure; irritability; loss of appetite; mood or mental changes; muscle twitching; nausea (continuing or severe) or vomiting; stomach cramps or pain; trembling; trouble in sleeping; unusual tiredness or weakness; vomiting blood or material that looks like coffee grounds

Other side effects may occur that usually do not need medical attention. These side effects may go away during treatment as your body adjusts to the medicine. However, check with your doctor if any of the following side effects continue or are bothersome:

More common

Drowsiness; headache; nausea; nervousness or restlessness

Less common

Difficult or painful urination; feeling of warmth; flushing or redness of face

Other side effects not listed above may also occur in some patients. If you notice any other effects, check with your doctor.

Annual revision: October 1990

THEOPHYLLINE, EPHEDRINE, AND PHENOBARBITAL Systemic

Some commonly used brand names are:

In the U.S.

Azma Aid	Tedrigen
Phedral C.T.	Theodrine
Primatene "P" Formula	Theodrine Pediatric
Tedral	Theofed
Tedral SA	Theofedral

Generic name product may also be available.

In Canada

Tedral

Description

Theophylline (thee-OFF-i-lin), ephedrine (e-FED-rin), and phenobarbital (fee-noe-BAR-bi-tal) combination is used to treat the symptoms of bronchial asthma, asthmatic bronchitis, and other lung diseases. This medicine relieves cough, wheezing, shortness of breath, and troubled breathing. It works by opening up the bronchial tubes (air passages) of the lungs and increasing the flow of air through them.

Some preparations of this medicine are available only with your doctor's prescription. Others are available without a prescription; however, your doctor may have special instructions on the proper dose of this medicine for your medical condition.

Theophylline, ephedrine, and phenobarbital combination is available in the following dosage forms:

Oral

- Elixir (U.S. and Canada)
- Suspension (U.S.)
- Tablets (U.S. and Canada)
- Extended-release tablets (U.S.)

It is very important that you read and understand the following information. If any of it causes you special concern, check with your doctor. Also, *if you have any questions* or if you want more information about this medicine or your medical problem, *ask your doctor, nurse, or pharmacist.*

Before Using This Medicine

If you are taking this medicine without a prescription, carefully read and follow any precautions on the label. For theophylline, ephedrine, and phenobarbital combination medicine, the following should be considered:

Allergies—Tell your doctor if you have ever had any unusual or allergic reaction to aminophylline, caffeine, dyphylline, oxtriphylline, theobromine, or theophylline; to ephedrine or medicines like ephedrine such as albuterol, amphetamines, epinephrine, isoproterenol, metaproterenol, norepinephrine, phenylephrine, phenylpropanolamine, pseudoephedrine, or terbutaline; or to barbiturates. Also tell your doctor and pharmacist if you are allergic to any other substances, such as foods, preservatives, or dyes.

Diet—Make certain your doctor and pharmacist know if you are on any special diet, such as a low-sodium or low-sugar diet or a high-protein, low-carbohydrate or low-protein, high-carbohydrate diet. A high-protein, low-carbohydrate diet may decrease the effects of theophylline; a low-protein, high-carbohydrate diet may increase the effects of theophylline.

Avoid eating or drinking large amounts of caffeine-containing foods or beverages, such as chocolate, cocoa, tea, coffee, and cola drinks, because they may increase the central nervous system (CNS) stimulant effects of theophylline.

Also, eating charcoal broiled foods every day while taking theophylline may keep this medicine from working properly.

Pregnancy—Studies with theophylline on birth defects have not been done in humans. However, some studies in animals have shown that theophylline causes birth defects when given in doses many times the human dose. Also, use of theophylline during pregnancy may cause unwanted effects such as fast heartbeat, jitteriness, irritability, gagging, vomiting, and breathing problems in the newborn infant.

Studies with ephedrine on birth defects have not been done in either humans or animals.

Phenobarbital taken during pregnancy has been shown to increase the chance of birth defects in humans. Also, taking phenobarbital regularly during the last 3 months of pregnancy may cause the baby to become dependent on the medicine. This may lead to withdrawal side effects in the baby after birth. In addition, one study in humans has suggested that phenobarbital taken during pregnancy may increase the chance of brain tumors in the baby.

Breast-feeding—Theophylline, ephedrine, and phenobarbital pass into the breast milk and may cause unwanted effects such as drowsiness, irritability, fretfulness, or trouble in sleeping in nursing babies of mothers taking this medicine.

Children—Newborn infants may be especially sensitive to the effects of theophylline, ephedrine, and phenobarbital combination medicine. This may increase the chance of side effects during treatment.

Older adults—Elderly people 55 years of age or older may be especially sensitive to the effects of theophylline, ephedrine, and phenobarbital combination medicine. This may increase the chance of side effects during treatment.

Other medicines—Although certain medicines should not be used together at all, in other cases two different medicines may be used together even if an interaction might occur. In these cases, your doctor may want to change the dose, or other precautions may be necessary. When you are taking theophylline, ephedrine, and phenobarbital combination medicine, it is especially important that your doctor and pharmacist know if you are taking any of the following:

- Adrenocorticoids (cortisone-like medicine) or
- Anticoagulants (blood thinners) or
- Corticotropin—The effects of these medicines may be decreased by phenobarbital

- Beta-blockers (acebutolol [e.g., Sectral], atenolol [e.g., Tenormin], betaxolol [e.g., Betoptic, Kerlone], carteolol [e.g., Cartrol], labetalol [e.g., Normodyne], levobunolol [e.g., Betagan], metoprolol [e.g., Lopressor], nadolol [e.g., Corgard], oxprenolol [e.g., Trasicor], penbutolol [e.g., Levatol], pindolol [e.g., Visken], propranolol [e.g., Inderal], sotalol [e.g., Sotacor], timolol [e.g., Blocadren, Timoptic])—Use of these medicines with this combination medicine may prevent either the beta-blocker or this combination medicine from working properly

- Central nervous system (CNS) depressants—The effects of these medicines or phenobarbital may be increased
- Cimetidine (e.g., Tagamet) or
- Ciprofloxacin (e.g., Cipro) or
- Erythromycin (e.g., E-Mycin) or
- Nicotine chewing gum (e.g., Nicorette) or
- Norfloxacin (e.g., Noroxin) or
- Ranitidine (e.g., Zantac) or
- Troleandomycin (e.g., TAO)—These medicines may increase the effects of theophylline

- Cocaine or
- Ergoloid mesylates (e.g., Hydergine) or
- Ergotamine (e.g., Gynergen)—The effects of these medicines on the heart and blood vessels may be increased by ephedrine

- Digitalis glycosides (heart medicine)—Use of digitalis glycosides with this combination medicine may increase the chance of irregular heartbeat

- Monoamine oxidase (MAO) inhibitors (furazolidone [e.g., Furoxone], isocarboxazid [e.g., Marplan], pargyline [e.g., Eutonyl], phenelzine [e.g., Nardil], procarbazine [e.g., Matulane], tranylcypromine [e.g., Parnate])—Taking ephedrine while you are taking or within 2 weeks of taking monoamine oxidase (MAO) inhibitors may increase the chance of serious side effects

- Oral contraceptives (birth control pills) containing estrogen—Phenobarbital may decrease the birth control effects of these medicines; use of another method of birth control may be necessary while you are taking this combination medicine

- Phenytoin—The effects of phenytoin may be decreased by theophylline

- Smoking tobacco or marijuana—If you smoke or have smoked (tobacco or marijuana) regularly within the last 2 years, the amount of medicine you need may vary, depending on how much and how recently you have smoked

Other medical problems—The presence of other medical problems may affect the use of theophylline, ephedrine, and phenobarbital combination medicine. Make sure you tell your doctor if you have any other medical problems, especially:

- Alcohol abuse or
- Fever or
- Liver disease or
- Respiratory infections, such as influenza (flu)—The effects of theophylline may be increased
- Diabetes mellitus (sugar diabetes)—Ephedrine may make the condition worse; your doctor may need to change the dose of your diabetes medicine
- Diarrhea—The absorption of theophylline may be decreased; therefore, the effects of this medicine may be decreased
- Enlarged prostate or
- Heart or blood vessel disease or
- High blood pressure or
- Hyperactivity (in children) or
- Stomach ulcer (or history of) or other stomach problems or
- Underactive adrenal gland—This combination medicine may make the condition worse
- Fibrocystic breast disease—Symptoms of this disease may be increased by theophylline
- Kidney disease—The effects of phenobarbital may be increased
- Overactive thyroid—The effects of theophylline may be decreased
- Pain—Phenobarbital may cause unusual excitement in the presence of pain
- Porphyria (or history of)—Phenobarbital may make the symptoms of this disease worse

Before you begin using any new medicine (prescription or nonprescription) or if you develop any new medical problem while you are using this medicine, check with your doctor, nurse, or pharmacist.

Proper Use of This Medicine

For patients taking the *extended-release tablet* form of this medicine:

- Swallow the tablet whole. Do not crush, break, or chew before swallowing.

This medicine works best when taken with a glass of water on an empty stomach (either 30 minutes to 1 hour before meals or 2 hours after meals) since that way it will get into the blood sooner. However, in some cases your doctor may want you to take this medicine with meals or right after meals to lessen stomach upset. If you have any questions about how you should be taking this medicine, check with your doctor.

Take this medicine only as directed. Do not take more of it and do not take it more often than recommended on the label, unless otherwise directed by your doctor. To do so may increase the chance of serious side effects. Also, if too much is taken, the phenobarbital in this medicine may become habit-forming.

In order for this medicine to help your medical problem, it must be taken every day in regularly spaced doses as recommended. This is necessary to keep a constant amount of this medicine in the blood. To help keep the amount constant, do not miss any doses.

Missed dose—If you do miss a dose of this medicine, take it as soon as possible. However, if it is almost time for your next dose, skip the missed dose and go back to your regular dosing schedule. Do not double doses.

Storage—To store this medicine:

- Keep out of the reach of children.
- Store away from heat and direct light.
- Do not store the tablet form of this medicine in the bathroom, near the kitchen sink, or in other damp places. Heat or moisture may cause the medicine to break down.
- Keep the liquid form of this medicine from freezing.
- Do not keep outdated medicine or medicine no longer needed. Be sure that any discarded medicine is out of the reach of children.

Precautions While Using This Medicine

The theophylline in this medicine may add to the central nervous system stimulant effects of caffeine-containing foods or beverages such as chocolate, cocoa, tea, coffee, and cola drinks. *Avoid eating or drinking large amounts of these foods or beverages while taking this medicine.* If you have any questions about this, check with your doctor.

The phenobarbital in this combination medicine will add to the effects of alcohol and other CNS depressants (medicines that slow down the nervous system, possibly causing drowsiness). Some examples of CNS depressants are antihistamines or medicine for hay fever, other allergies, or colds; sedatives, tranquilizers, or sleeping medicine; prescription pain medicine or narcotics; barbiturates; medicine for seizures; muscle relaxants; or anesthetics, including some dental anesthetics. *Check with your doctor before taking any of the above while you are using this medicine.*

Do not eat charcoal-broiled foods every day while taking this medicine since these foods may keep the medicine from working properly.

Check with your doctor at once if you develop symptoms of influenza (flu) or a fever since either of these may increase the chance of side effects with this medicine.

Also, *check with your doctor if diarrhea occurs* because the dose of this medicine may need to be changed.

This medicine may cause some people to become dizzy, lightheaded, drowsy, or less alert than they are normally. *Make sure you know how you react to this medicine before you drive, use machines, or do anything else that could be dangerous if you are dizzy or are not alert.*

Side Effects of This Medicine

Along with its needed effects, a medicine may cause some unwanted effects. Although not all of these side effects may occur, if they do occur they may need medical attention.

Check with your doctor as soon as possible if any of the following side effects occur:

Less common

Heartburn and/or vomiting

Symptoms of overdose

Bloody or black, tarry stools; chest pain; convulsions (seizures); diarrhea; dizziness or lightheadedness; fast, pounding, or irregular heartbeat; hallucinations (seeing, hearing, or feeling things that are not there); increase or decrease in blood pressure; irritability; loss of appetite; mood or mental changes; muscle twitching; nausea (continuing or severe) or vomiting; stomach cramps or pain; trembling; trouble in sleeping; unusual tiredness or weakness; vomiting blood or material that looks like coffee grounds

Other side effects may occur that usually do not need medical attention. These side effects may go away during treatment as your body adjusts to the medicine. However, check with your doctor or pharmacist if any of the following side effects continue or are bothersome:

More common

Drowsiness; headache; nausea; nervousness or restlessness

Less common

Difficult or painful urination; feeling of warmth; flushing or redness of face

Other side effects not listed above may also occur in some patients. If you notice any other effects, check with your doctor.

Annual revision: October 1990

THEOPHYLLINE AND GUAIFENESIN Systemic

Some commonly used brand names are:

In the U.S.

- Asbron G
- Asbron G Inlay-Tabs
- Bronchial
- Elixophyllin-GG
- Glyceryl-T
- Lanophyllin-GG
- Mudrane GG-2
- Q-B
- Quiagen
- Quibron
- Quibron-300
- Slo-Phyllin GG
- Synophylate-GG
- Theocolate
- Theolate

Generic name product may also be available.

Another commonly used name is theophylline and glyceryl guaiacolate.

Description

Theophylline (thee-OFF-i-lin) and guaifenesin (gwye-FEN-e-sin) combination is used to treat the symptoms of bronchial asthma, chronic bronchitis, emphysema, and other lung diseases. This medicine relieves cough, wheezing, shortness of breath, and troubled breathing. It works by opening up the bronchial tubes (air passages) of the lungs and increasing the flow of air through them.

This medicine is available only with your doctor's prescription, in the following dosage forms:

Oral

- Capsules (U.S.)
- Elixir (U.S.)
- Oral solution (U.S.)
- Syrup (U.S.)
- Tablets (U.S.)

It is very important that you read and understand the following information. If any of it causes you special concern, check with your doctor. Also, *if you have any questions* or if you want more information about this medicine or your medical problem, ***ask your doctor, nurse, or pharmacist.***

Before Using This Medicine

In deciding to use a medicine, the risks of taking the medicine must be weighed against the good it will do. This is a decision you and your doctor will make. For theophylline and guaifenesin combination medicine, the following should be considered:

Allergies—Tell your doctor if you have ever had any unusual or allergic reaction to aminophylline, caffeine, dyphylline, oxtriphylline, theobromine, or theophylline. Also tell your doctor and pharmacist if you are allergic to any other substances, such as foods, preservatives, or dyes.

Diet—Make certain your doctor and pharmacist know if you are on any special diet, such as a low-sodium or low-sugar diet or a high-protein, low-carbohydrate or low-protein, high-carbohydrate diet. A high-protein, low-carbohydrate diet may decrease the effects of theophylline;

a low-protein, high-carbohydrate diet may increase the effects of theophylline.

Avoid eating or drinking large amounts of caffeine-containing foods or beverages, such as chocolate, cocoa, tea, coffee, and cola drinks, because they may increase the central nervous system (CNS) stimulant effects of theophylline.

Also, eating charcoal broiled foods every day while taking theophylline may keep this medicine from working properly.

Pregnancy—Studies on birth defects have not been done in humans. However, some studies in animals have shown that theophylline causes birth defects when given in doses many times the human dose. Also, use of theophylline during pregnancy may cause unwanted effects such as fast heartbeat, jitteriness, irritability, gagging, vomiting, and breathing problems in the newborn infant. Guaifenesin has not been shown to cause birth defects or other problems in humans.

Breast-feeding—Theophylline passes into the breast milk and may cause irritability, fretfulness, or trouble in sleeping in babies of mothers taking this medicine. Guaifenesin has not been reported to cause problems in nursing babies.

Children—The side effects of theophylline are more likely to occur in newborn infants, who are usually more sensitive to the effects of this medicine.

Although there is no specific information about the use of guaifenesin in children, it is not expected to cause different side effects or problems in children than it does in adults.

Older adults—The side effects of theophylline are more likely to occur in elderly patients 55 years of age and older, who are usually more sensitive than younger adults to the effects of this medicine.

Although there is no specific information about the use of guaifenesin in the elderly, it is not expected to cause different side effects or problems in older people than it does in younger adults.

Other medicines—Although certain medicines should not be used together at all, in other cases two different medicines may be used together even if an interaction might occur. In these cases, your doctor may want to change the dose, or other precautions may be necessary. When you are taking theophylline and guaifenesin combination medicine, it is especially important that your doctor and pharmacist know if you are taking any of the following:

- Beta-blockers (acebutolol [e.g., Sectral], atenolol [e.g., Tenormin], betaxolol [e.g., Betoptic, Kerlone], carteolol [e.g., Cartrol], labetalol [e.g., Normodyne], levobunolol [e.g., Betagan], metoprolol [e.g., Lopressor], nadolol [e.g., Corgard], oxprenolol [e.g., Trasicor], penbutolol [e.g., Levatol], pindolol [e.g., Visken], propranolol [e.g., Inderal], sotalol [e.g., Sotacor], timolol [e.g., Blocadren, Timoptic])—Use of these medicines with theophylline may prevent either the beta-blocker or theophylline from working properly
- Cimetidine (e.g., Tagamet) or
- Ciprofloxacin (e.g., Cipro) or
- Erythromycin (e.g., E-Mycin) or
- Nicotine chewing gum (e.g., Nicorette) or
- Norfloxacin (e.g., Noroxin) or
- Ranitidine (e.g., Zantac) or
- Troleandomycin (e.g., TAO)—These medicines may increase the effects of theophylline
- Phenytoin (e.g., Dilantin)—The effects of phenytoin may be decreased by theophylline
- Smoking tobacco or marijuana—If you smoke or have smoked (tobacco or marijuana) regularly within the last 2 years, the amount of medicine you need may vary, depending on how much and how recently you have smoked

Other medical problems—The presence of other medical problems may affect the use of theophylline and guaifenesin combination medicine. Make sure you tell your doctor if you have any other medical problems, especially:

- Alcohol abuse or
- Fever or
- Liver disease or
- Respiratory infections, such as influenza (flu)—The effects of theophylline may be increased
- Diarrhea—The absorption of theophylline may be decreased; therefore, the effects of this medicine may be decreased
- Enlarged prostate or
- Heart disease or
- High blood pressure or
- Stomach ulcer (or history of) or other stomach problems—Theophylline may make the condition worse
- Fibrocystic breast disease—Symptoms of this disease may be increased by theophylline
- Overactive thyroid—The effects of theophylline may be decreased

Before you begin using any new medicine (prescription or nonprescription) or if you develop any new medical problem while you are using this medicine, check with your doctor, nurse, or pharmacist.

Proper Use of This Medicine

This medicine works best when taken with a glass of water on an empty stomach (either 30 minutes to 1 hour before meals or 2 hours after meals) since that way it will get into the blood sooner. However, in some cases your doctor may want you to take this medicine with meals or right after meals to lessen stomach upset. If you have any questions about how you should be taking this medicine, check with your doctor.

Take this medicine only as directed. Do not take more of it, do not take it more often, and do not take it for a longer time than your doctor ordered. To do so may increase the chance of serious side effects.

In order for this medicine to help your medical problem, it must be taken every day in regularly spaced doses as ordered by your doctor. This is necessary to keep a constant amount of this medicine in the blood. To help keep the amount constant, do not miss any doses.

Missed dose—If you do miss a dose of this medicine, take it as soon as possible. However, if it is almost time for your next dose, skip the missed dose and go back to your regular dosing schedule. Do not double doses.

Storage—To store this medicine:

- Keep out of the reach of children.
- Store away from heat and direct light.
- Do not store the capsule or tablet form of this medicine in the bathroom, near the kitchen sink, or in other damp places. Heat or moisture may cause the medicine to break down.
- Keep the liquid form of this medicine from freezing.
- Do not keep outdated medicine or medicine no longer needed. Be sure that any discarded medicine is out of the reach of children.

Precautions While Using This Medicine

Your doctor should check your progress at regular visits, especially for the first few weeks after you begin taking this medicine. A blood test may be taken to help your doctor decide whether the dose of this medicine should be changed.

The theophylline in this medicine may add to the central nervous system stimulant effects of caffeine-containing foods or beverages such as chocolate, cocoa, tea, coffee, and cola drinks. *Avoid eating or drinking large amounts of these foods or beverages while taking this medicine.* If you have any questions about this, check with your doctor.

Do not eat charcoal-broiled foods every day while taking this medicine since these foods may keep the medicine from working properly.

Check with your doctor at once if you develop symptoms of influenza (flu) or a fever since either of these may increase the chance of side effects with this medicine.

Also, *check with your doctor if diarrhea occurs* because the dose of this medicine may need to be changed.

Side Effects of This Medicine

Along with its needed effects, a medicine may cause some unwanted effects. Although not all of these side effects may occur, if they do occur they may need medical attention.

Check with your doctor as soon as possible if any of the following side effects occur:

Less common

Heartburn and/or vomiting

Symptoms of overdose of theophylline

Bloody or black, tarry stools; confusion or change in behavior; convulsions (seizures); diarrhea; dizziness or lightheadedness; fast breathing; fast, pounding, or irregular heartbeat; flushing or redness of face; headache; increased urination; irritability; loss of appetite; muscle twitching; nausea (continuing or severe) or vomiting; stomach cramps or pain; trembling; trouble in sleeping; unusual tiredness or weakness; vomiting blood or material that looks like coffee grounds

Other side effects may occur that usually do not need medical attention. These side effects may go away during treatment as your body adjusts to the medicine. However, check with your doctor if any of the following side effects continue or are bothersome:

More common

Nausea; nervousness or restlessness

Other side effects not listed above may also occur in some patients. If you notice any other effects, check with your doctor.

Annual revision: October 1990

THIABENDAZOLE Systemic†

Some commonly used brand names are:

In the U.S.

Mintezol

Other

Foldan
Minzolum
Triasox

†Not commercially available in Canada.

Description

Thiabendazole (thye-a-BEN-da-zole) belongs to the family of medicines called anthelmintics (ant-hel-MIN-tiks). Anthelmintics are medicines used in the treatment of worm infections.

Thiabendazole is used to treat:

- creeping eruption (cutaneous larva migrans);
- pork worms (trichinosis);
- threadworms (strongyloidiasis); and
- visceral larva migrans (toxocariasis).

This medicine may also be used for other worm infections as determined by your doctor.

Thiabendazole is available only with your doctor's prescription, in the following dosage forms:

Oral

- Chewable tablets (U.S.)
- Oral suspension (U.S.)

It is very important that you read and understand the following information. If any of it causes you special concern, check with your doctor. Also, *if you have any questions* or if you want more information about this medicine or your medical problem, *ask your doctor, nurse, or pharmacist.*

Before Using This Medicine

In deciding to use a medicine, the risks of taking the medicine must be weighed against the good it will do. This is a decision you and your doctor will make. For thiabendazole, the following should be considered:

Allergies—Tell your doctor if you have ever had any unusual or allergic reaction to thiabendazole. Also tell your doctor and pharmacist if you are allergic to any other substances, such as foods, preservatives, or dyes.

Pregnancy—Studies have not been done in humans. In addition, thiabendazole has not been shown to cause birth defects or other problems in studies in rabbits, rats, and mice given 2½ to 15 times the usual human dose. However, another study in mice given 10 times the usual human dose has shown that thiabendazole causes cleft palate (a split in the roof of the mouth) and bone defects.

Breast-feeding—It is not known whether thiabendazole passes into human breast milk. However, this medicine has not been reported to cause problems in nursing babies.

Children—This medicine has been tested in children over 13.6 kg of body weight (30 pounds). In effective doses, it has not been reported to cause different side effects or problems in children than it does in adults.

Older adults—Many medicines have not been studied specifically in older people. Therefore, it may not be known whether they work exactly the same way they do in younger adults or if they cause different side effects or problems in older people. There is no specific information comparing use of thiabendazole in the elderly with use in other age groups.

Other medicines—Although certain medicines should not be used together at all, in other cases two different medicines may be used together even if an interaction might occur. In these cases, your doctor may want to change the dose, or other precautions may be necessary. When you are taking thiabendazole, it is especially important that your doctor and pharmacist know if you are taking any of the following:

- Theophylline—Patients taking thiabendazole and theophylline together may have an increased chance of theophylline side effects

Other medical problems—The presence of other medical problems may affect the use of thiabendazole. Make sure you tell your doctor if you have any other medical problems, especially:

- Kidney disease or
- Liver disease—Patients with kidney and/or liver disease may have an increased chance of side effects

Before you begin using any new medicine (prescription or nonprescription) or if you develop any new medical problem while you are using this medicine, check with your doctor, nurse, or pharmacist.

Proper Use of This Medicine

No special preparations (for example, special diets, fasting, other medicines, laxatives, or enemas) are necessary before, during, or immediately after treatment with thiabendazole.

Thiabendazole is best taken after meals (breakfast and evening meal). This helps to prevent some common side effects such as nausea, vomiting, dizziness, or loss of appetite.

Doctors may also prescribe a corticosteroid (a cortisone-like medicine) for certain patients with *pork worms (trichinosis)*, especially for those with severe symptoms. This is to help reduce the inflammation caused by the pork worm larvae. If your doctor prescribes these 2 medicines together, it is important to take the corticosteroid along with thiabendazole. Take them exactly as directed by your doctor. Do not miss any doses.

For patients taking the *oral liquid form* of thiabendazole:

- Use a specially marked measuring spoon or other device to measure each dose accurately. The average household teaspoon may not hold the right amount of liquid.

For patients taking the *chewable tablet form* of thiabendazole:

- Tablets should be chewed or crushed before they are swallowed.

To help clear up your infection completely, *take this medicine exactly as directed by your doctor for the full time of treatment.* In some patients a second course of this medicine may be required to clear up the infection completely. *Do not miss any doses.*

Dosing—The dose of thiabendazole will be different for different patients. *Follow your doctor's orders or the directions on the label.* The following information includes only the average doses of thiabendazole. *If your dose is different, do not change it* unless your doctor tells you to do so.

- The number of tablets or teaspoonfuls of suspension that you take depends on the strength of the medicine. Also, *the number of doses you take each day, the time allowed between doses, and the length of time you take the medicine depend on the medical problem for which you are taking thiabendazole.*
- For *oral* dosage forms (oral suspension or tablets):
  —Adults and children over 13.6 kilograms (30 pounds) of body weight:
  - For *cutaneous larva migrans* and *strongyloidiasis*: Dose is based on body weight and will be determined by your doctor. The dose is taken two times a day for two days.
  - For *trichinosis*: Dose is based on body weight and will be determined by your doctor. The dose is taken two times a day for two to four days.
  - For *visceral larva migrans*: Dose is based on body weight and will be determined by your doctor. The dose is taken two times a day for five to seven days.

  —Children up to 13.6 kilograms (30 pounds) of body weight: Dose must be determined by the doctor.

Missed dose—If you do miss a dose of this medicine, take it as soon as possible. However, if it is almost time for your next dose, skip the missed dose and go back to your regular dosing schedule. Do not double doses.

Storage—To store this medicine:

- Keep out of the reach of children.
- Store away from heat and direct light.
- Do not store the chewable tablet form of this medicine in the bathroom, near the kitchen sink, or in other damp places. Heat or moisture may cause the medicine to break down.
- Keep the oral liquid form of this medicine from freezing.
- Do not keep outdated medicine or medicine no longer needed. Be sure that any discarded medicine is out of the reach of children.

Precautions While Using This Medicine

It is important that your doctor check your progress at regular visits. This is to make sure that the infection is cleared up completely.

Thiabendazole may cause blurred vision or yellow vision. It may also cause some people to become dizzy, drowsy, or less alert than they are normally. *Make sure you know how you react to this medicine before you drive, use machines, or do anything else that could be dangerous if you are dizzy or are not alert or able to see well.* If these reactions are especially bothersome, check with your doctor.

Good health habits are required to help prevent reinfection. These include the following:

- For creeping eruption (cutaneous larva migrans) or visceral larva migrans (toxocariasis):
  —Keep dogs and cats off beaches and bathing areas.

  —Treat household pets for worms (deworm) regularly.

  —Cover children's sandboxes when not being used. These measures help to prevent contamination of the sand or soil by worm larvae from the animals' wastes. This helps to keep children from picking up the larvae when they put their hands in their mouths after touching contaminated sand or soil.
- For pork worms (trichinosis):
  —Cook all pork, pork-containing products, and game at not less than 140 °F (60 °C) until well done (not pink in the center) before eating. This will kill any trichinosis larvae that may be in the meat.

Side Effects of This Medicine

Along with its needed effects, a medicine may cause some unwanted effects. Although not all of these side effects may occur, if they do occur they may need medical attention.

Check with your doctor immediately if any of the following side effects occur:

More common

Confusion; diarrhea (severe); hallucinations (seeing, hearing, and feeling things that are not there); irritability; loss of appetite; nausea and vomiting (severe); numbness or tingling in the hands or feet

Less common

Skin rash or itching

In addition to the side effects mentioned above, check with your doctor as soon as possible if any of the following side effects occur:

Rare

Aching of joints and muscles; blurred or yellow vision; chills; convulsions (seizures); dark urine; fever; lower back pain; pain or burning while urinating; pale stools; redness, blistering, peeling, or loosening of skin; unusual feeling in the eyes; unusual tiredness or weakness; yellow eyes and skin

Other side effects may occur that usually do not need medical attention. These side effects may go away during treatment as your body adjusts to the medicine. However,

check with your doctor if any of the following side effects continue or are bothersome:

More common

Dizziness; drowsiness; dryness of eyes and mouth; headache; ringing or buzzing in the ears

This medicine may cause the urine to have an asparagus-like or other unusual odor while you are taking it and for about 24 hours after you stop taking it. This side effect does not need medical attention.

Other side effects not listed above may also occur in some patients. If you notice any other effects, check with your doctor.

Additional Information

Once a medicine has been approved for marketing for a certain use, experience may show that it is also useful for other medical problems. Although these uses are not included in product labeling, thiabendazole is used in certain patients with the following medical conditions:

- Capillariasis
- Dracunculiasis
- Trichostrongyliasis

Other than the above information, there is no additional information relating to proper use, precautions, or side effects for these uses.

Annual revision: 02/01/93

THIABENDAZOLE Topical*

*Not commercially available in the U.S.

Description

Thiabendazole (thye-a-BEN-da-zole) belongs to the family of medicines called anthelmintics (ant-hel-MIN-tiks). Anthelmintics are medicines used in the treatment of worm infections.

Thiabendazole topical preparations are used to treat cutaneous larva migrans (creeping eruption). Cutaneous larva migrans is caused by dog and cat hookworm larvae. These larvae cause slowly moving burrows or tunnels in the skin. This may result in itching, redness, or inflammation around the end of the burrows or tunnels.

Thiabendazole is available only with your doctor's prescription, in the following dosage form:

Topical

- Topical suspension

It is very important that you read and understand the following information. If any of it causes you special concern, check with your doctor. Also, *if you have any questions* or if you want more information about this medicine or your medical problem, *ask your doctor, nurse, or pharmacist.*

Before Using This Medicine

In deciding to use a medicine, the risks of using the medicine must be weighed against the good it will do. This is a decision you and your doctor will make. For topical thiabendazole, the following should be considered:

Allergies—Tell your doctor if you have ever had any unusual or allergic reaction to thiabendazole. Also tell your doctor and pharmacist if you are allergic to any other substances, such as preservatives or dyes.

Pregnancy—Thiabendazole may be absorbed through the skin. However, thiabendazole topical preparations have not been shown to cause birth defects or other problems in humans.

Breast-feeding—Thiabendazole may be absorbed through the mother's skin. However, thiabendazole topical preparations have not been shown to cause problems in nursing babies.

Children—Although there is no specific information about the use of thiabendazole in children, it is not expected to cause different side effects or problems in children than it does in adults.

Older adults—Many medicines have not been tested in older people, Therefore, it may not be known whether they work exactly the same way they do in younger adults. Although there is no specific information about the use of thiabendazole in the elderly, it is not expected to cause different side effects or problems in older people than it does in younger adults.

Other medicines—Although certain medicines should not be used together at all, in other cases two different medicines may be used together even if an interaction might occur. In these cases, your doctor may want to change the dose, or other precautions may be necessary. When you are using thiabendazole, it is important that your doctor and pharmacist know if you are using any other topical prescription or nonprescription (over-the-counter [OTC]) medicine that is to be applied to the same area of the skin.

Before you begin using any new medicine (prescription or nonprescription) or if you develop any new medical problem while you are using this medicine, check with your doctor, nurse, or pharmacist.

Proper Use of This Medicine

Apply thiabendazole directly to, and about 5 to 7.5 cm (2 to 3 inches) around, the slowly moving end of each burrow or tunnel being made by the larva of the worm in the skin.

To help clear up your infection completely, *use this medicine exactly as directed by your doctor for the full time of treatment. Do not miss any doses.*

Missed dose—If you do miss a dose of this medicine, apply it as soon as possible. However, if it is almost time for your next dose, skip the missed dose and go back to your regular dosing schedule.

Storage—To store this medicine:

- Keep out of the reach of children.
- Store away from heat and direct light.
- Keep the medicine from freezing.
- Do not keep outdated medicine or medicine no longer needed. Be sure that any discarded medicine is out of the reach of children.

Precautions While Using This Medicine

If your skin problem does not improve within a few days, or if the burrow or tunnel continues to get longer, check with your doctor.

Side Effects of This Medicine

There have not been any common or important side effects reported with this medicine when used on the skin. However, if you notice any side effects, check with your doctor.

Annual revision: September 1990

THIAMINE (Vitamin B_1) Systemic

Some commonly used brand names are:

In the U.S.

Betalin S
Biamine

Generic name product may also be available.

In Canada

Betaxin
Bewon

Generic name product may also be available.

Description

Vitamins (VYE-ta-mins) are compounds that you *must* have for growth and health. They are needed in small amounts only and are usually available in the foods that you eat. Thiamine (THYE-a-min) (vitamin B_1) is necessary for normal metabolism.

Patients with the following conditions may be more likely to have a deficiency of thiamine:

- Alcoholism
- Burns
- Diarrhea (continuing)
- Fever (continuing)
- Illness (continuing)
- Intestinal disease
- Liver disease
- Overactive thyroid
- Stress (continuing)
- Surgical removal of stomach

Also, the following groups of people may have a deficiency of thiamine:

- Patients using an artificial kidney (on hemodialysis)
- Individuals who do heavy manual labor on a daily basis

If any of the above apply to you, you should take thiamine supplements only on the advice of your doctor after need has been established.

Lack of thiamine may lead to a condition called beriberi. Signs of beriberi include loss of appetite, constipation, muscle weakness, pain or tingling in arms or legs, and possible swelling of feet or lower legs. In addition, if severe, lack of thiamine may cause mental depression, memory problems, weakness, shortness of breath, and fast heartbeat. Your doctor may treat this by prescribing thiamine for you.

Thiamine may also be used for other conditions as determined by your doctor.

Claims that thiamine is effective for treatment of skin problems, chronic diarrhea, tiredness, mental problems, multiple sclerosis, nerve problems, and ulcerative colitis (a disease of the intestines), or as an insect repellant or to stimulate appetite have not been proven.

Oral forms of thiamine are available without a prescription. However, it may be a good idea to check with your doctor before taking thiamine on your own.

Thiamine is available in the following dosage forms:

Oral

- Elixir (Canada)
- Tablets (U.S. and Canada)

Parenteral

- Injection (U.S. and Canada)

It is very important that you read and understand the following information. If any of it causes you special concern, check with your doctor or pharmacist. Also, *if you have any questions* or if you want more information about this dietary supplement or your medical problem, *ask your doctor, nurse, pharmacist, or dietitian.*

Importance of Diet

Vitamin supplements should be taken only if you cannot get enough vitamins in your diet; however, some diets may not contain all of the vitamins you need. You may not be getting enough vitamins because of rapid weight loss, unusual diets (such as some reducing diets in which choice of foods is limited), prolonged intravenous feeding, or malnutrition. A balanced diet should provide all the vitamins you normally need.

In order to get enough vitamins and minerals in your diet, it is important that you eat a balanced and varied diet. Follow carefully any diet program your doctor may recommend. For your specific vitamin and/or mineral needs, ask your doctor or dietitian for a list of appropriate foods.

Thiamine is found in various foods, including cereals (whole-grain and enriched), peas, beans, nuts, and meats (especially pork and beef). Some thiamine in foods is lost with cooking.

Vitamins alone will not take the place of a good diet and will not provide energy. Your body also needs other substances found in food such as protein, minerals, carbohydrates, and fat. Vitamins themselves often cannot work without the presence of other foods.

In some cases, it may not be possible for you to get enough food to supply you with the proper vitamins. In other cases, the amount of vitamins you need may be increased above normal. Therefore, a vitamin supplement may be needed.

Experts have developed a list of recommended dietary allowances (RDA) for most of the vitamins. The RDA are not an exact number but a general idea of how much you need. They do not cover amounts needed for problems caused by a serious lack of vitamins.

The RDA for thiamine are:

- Infants and children—
  - Birth to 6 months of age: 0.3 milligrams (mg) per day.
  - 6 months to 1 year of age: 0.4 mg per day.
  - 1 to 3 years of age: 0.7 mg per day.
  - 4 to 6 years of age: 0.9 mg per day.
  - 7 to 10 years of age: 1 mg per day.
- Adolescent and adult males—
  - 11 to 14 years of age: 1.1 mg per day.
  - 15 to 50 years of age: 1.5 mg per day.
  - 51 years of age and over: 1.2 mg per day.
- Adolescent and adult females—
  - 11 to 50 years of age: 1.1 mg per day.
  - 51 years of age and over: 1 mg per day.
- Pregnant females—1.5 mg per day.
- Breast-feeding females—1.6 mg per day.

Remember:

- The total amount of each vitamin that you get every day includes what you get from the foods that you eat *and* what you may take as a supplement.
- Your total amount should not be greater than the RDA, unless ordered by your doctor.

Before Using This Dietary Supplement

If you are taking this dietary supplement without a prescription, carefully read and follow any precautions on the label. For thiamine, the following should be considered:

Allergies—Tell your doctor if you have ever had any unusual or allergic reaction to thiamine. Also tell your doctor and pharmacist if you are allergic to any other substances, such as foods, preservatives, or dyes.

Pregnancy—It is especially important that you are receiving enough vitamins when you become pregnant and that you continue to receive the right amount of vitamins throughout your pregnancy. The healthy growth and development of the fetus depend on a steady supply of nutrients from the mother. However, taking large amounts of a dietary supplement in pregnancy may be harmful to the mother and/or fetus and should be avoided.

Breast-feeding—It is especially important that you receive the right amounts of vitamins so that your baby will also get the vitamins needed to grow properly. However, taking large amounts of a dietary supplement while breast-feeding may be harmful to the mother and/or baby and should be avoided.

Children—Normal daily requirements vary according to age. It is especially important that children receive enough vitamins in their diet for healthy growth and development. Although there is no specific information about the use of thiamine in children in doses higher than the normal daily requirements, it is not expected to cause different side effects or problems in children than in adults.

Older adults—It is important that older people continue to receive enough vitamins in their diet for good health. Studies have shown that older adults may have lower blood levels of thiamine than younger adults. Your doctor may recommend that you take a vitamin supplement that contains thiamine.

Medicines or other dietary supplements—Although certain medicines or dietary supplements should not be used together at all, in other cases they may be used together even if an interaction might occur. In these cases, your doctor may want to change the dose, or other precautions may be necessary. Tell your doctor and pharmacist if you are taking any other dietary supplement or prescription or nonprescription (over-the-counter [OTC]) medicine.

Proper Use of This Dietary Supplement

Some people believe that taking very large doses of vitamins (called megadoses or megavitamin therapy) is useful for treating certain medical problems. Studies have not proven this. Large doses should be taken only under the direction of your doctor after need has been identified.

Missed dose—If you miss taking a vitamin for 1 or more days there is no cause for concern, since it takes some time for your body to become seriously low in vitamins. However, if your doctor has recommended that you take this vitamin, try to remember to take it as directed every day.

Storage—To store this dietary supplement:

- Keep out of the reach of children.
- Store away from heat and direct light.
- Do not store in the bathroom, near the kitchen sink, or in other damp places. Heat or moisture may cause the dietary supplement to break down.
- Keep the oral liquid form of this dietary supplement from freezing.
- Do not keep outdated dietary supplements or those no longer needed. Be sure that any discarded dietary supplement is out of the reach of children.

Side Effects of This Dietary Supplement

Along with its needed effects, a dietary supplement may cause some unwanted effects. Although not all of these side effects may occur, if they do occur they may need medical attention.

Check with your doctor immediately if any of the following side effects occur:

Rare—Soon after receiving injection only

Coughing; difficulty in swallowing; hives; itching of skin; swelling of face, lips, or eyelids; wheezing or difficulty in breathing

Other side effects not listed above may also occur in some patients. If you notice any other effects, check with your doctor.

Additional Information

Once a medicine or dietary supplement has been approved for marketing for a certain use, experience may show that it is also useful for other medical problems. Although this use is not included in product labeling, thiamine is used in certain patients with the following medical conditions:

- Enzyme deficiency diseases such as encephalomyelopathy, maple syrup urine disease, pyruvate carboxylase, and hyperalaninemia

Other than the above information, there is no additional information relating to proper use, precautions, or side effects for these uses.

Annual revision: 06/24/92

THIETHYLPERAZINE Systemic

Some commonly used brand names are:

In the U.S.

Norzine
Torecan

In Canada

Torecan

Description

Thiethylperazine (thye-eth-il-PER-a-zeen) is a phenothiazine medicine. It is used to treat nausea and vomiting.

This medicine is available only with your doctor's prescription in the following dosage forms:

Oral

- Tablets (U.S. and Canada)

Parenteral
- Injection (U.S. and Canada)

Rectal
- Suppositories (U.S.)

It is very important that you read and understand the following information. If any of it causes you special concern, check with your doctor. Also, *if you have any questions* or if you want more information about this medicine or your medical problem, *ask your doctor, nurse, or pharmacist.*

Before Using This Medicine

In deciding to use a medicine, the risks of taking the medicine must be weighed against the good it will do. This is a decision you and your doctor will make. For thiethylperazine, the following should be considered:

Allergies—Tell your doctor if you have ever had any unusual or allergic reaction to thiethylperazine or other phenothiazine medicines. Also tell your doctor and pharmacist if you are allergic to any other substances, such as foods, preservatives, or dyes.

Pregnancy—Thiethylperazine is not recommended during pregnancy. Other phenothiazine medicines have been reported to cause unwanted effects, such as jaundice and muscle tremors and other movement disorders, in newborn babies whose mothers took these medicines during pregnancy.

Breast-feeding—It is not known if thiethylperazine passes into the breast milk. However, thiethylperazine is not recommended for use during breast-feeding because there is the chance that it may cause unwanted effects in nursing babies.

Children—Children are usually more sensitive than adults to the effects of phenothiazine medicines such as thiethylperazine. Certain side effects, such as muscle spasms of the face, neck, and back, tic-like or twitching movements, inability to move the eyes, twisting of the body, or weakness of the arms and legs, are more likely to occur in children, especially those with severe illness or dehydration.

Older adults—Elderly patients are usually more sensitive to the effects of phenothiazine medicines such as thiethylperazine. Confusion; difficult or painful urination; dizziness; drowsiness; feeling faint; or dryness of mouth, nose, or throat may be more likely to occur in elderly patients. Also, nightmares or unusual excitement, nervousness, restlessness, or irritability may be more likely to occur in elderly patients. In addition, uncontrolled movements may be more likely to occur in elderly patients taking thiethylperazine.

Other medicines—Although certain medicines should not be used together at all, in other cases two different medicines may be used together even if an interaction might occur. In these cases, your doctor may want to change the dose, or other precautions may be necessary. When you are taking thiethylperazine, it is especially important that your doctor and pharmacist know if you are taking any of the following:

- Amoxapine (e.g., Asendin) or
- Antipsychotics (medicine for mental illness) or
- Methyldopa (e.g., Aldomet) or
- Metoclopramide (e.g., Reglan) or
- Metyrosine (e.g., Demser) or
- Pemoline (e.g., Cylert) or
- Pimozide (e.g., Orap) or
- Promethazine (e.g., Phenergan) or
- Rauwolfia alkaloids (alseroxylon [e.g., Rauwiloid], deserpidine [e.g., Harmonyl], rauwolfia serpentina [e.g., Raudixin], reserpine [e.g., Serpasil]) or
- Trimeprazine (e.g., Temaril)—Side effects of these medicines, such as uncontrolled body movements, may become more severe and frequent if they are used together with thiethylperazine
- Central nervous system (CNS) depressants (medicine that causes drowsiness) or
- Tricyclic antidepressants (medicine for depression)—CNS depressant effects of these medicines or thiethylperazine, such as drowsiness, may be increased in severity; also, taking maprotiline or tricyclic antidepressants may cause some side effects of these medicines, such as dryness of mouth, to become more severe
- Contrast agents, injected into spinal canal—If you are having an x-ray test of the head, spinal canal, or nervous system for which you are going to receive an injection into the spinal canal, thiethylperazine may increase your chance of having seizures
- Epinephrine—Side effects, such as low blood pressure and fast or racing heartbeat, may occur more often or may be more severe
- Levodopa—When used together with thiethylperazine, the levodopa may not work as it should
- Quinidine—Unwanted effects on the heart may occur or become more severe

Other medical problems—The presence of other medical problems may affect the use of thiethylperazine. Make sure you tell your doctor if you have any other medical problems, especially:

- Alcohol abuse—This medicine, if taken together with alcohol, may lower the blood pressure and cause CNS depressant effects, such as severe drowsiness
- Asthma attack or
- Other lung diseases—Thiethylperazine may cause secretions to become thick so that it might be difficult to cough them up, for example, during an asthma attack
- Blood disease or
- Heart or blood vessel disease—These medicines may cause more serious conditions to develop
- Difficult urination or
- Enlarged prostate—This medicine may cause urinary problems to get worse

- Glaucoma—This medicine may cause an increase in inner eye pressure
- Liver disease—Thiethylperazine may accumulate in the body, increasing the chance of side effects, such as muscle spasms
- Parkinson's disease or
- Seizure disorders—The chance of thiethylperazine causing seizures or uncontrolled movements is greater when these conditions are present

Before you begin using any new medicine (prescription or nonprescription) or if you develop any new medical problem while you are using this medicine, check with your doctor, nurse, or pharmacist.

Proper Use of This Medicine

Thiethylperazine is used only to relieve or prevent nausea and vomiting. *Use it only as directed. Do not use more of it and do not use it more often than your doctor ordered.* To do so may increase the chance of side effects.

For patients *taking this medicine by mouth:*

- This medicine may be taken with food or a full glass (8 ounces) of water or milk to reduce stomach irritation.

For patients using the *suppository form of this medicine:*

- To insert suppository: First, remove foil wrapper and moisten the suppository with cold water. Lie down on your side and use your finger to push the suppository well up into the rectum. If the suppository is too soft to insert, chill it in the refrigerator for 30 minutes or run cold water over it before removing the foil wrapper.

Dosing—The dose of thiethylperazine will be different for different patients. *Follow your doctor's orders or the directions on the label.* The following information includes only the average doses of thiethylperazine. *If your dose is different, do not change it* unless your doctor tells you to do so.

The number of doses you take each day, the time allowed between doses, and the length of time you take the medicine depend on the medical problem for which you are taking thiethylperazine.

- For nausea and vomiting:
  - —For *oral* dosage form (tablets):
    - Adults—10 milligrams (mg) one to three times a day.
    - Children—Use and dose must be determined by your doctor.
  - —For *injection* dosage form:
    - Adults—10 mg one to three times a day, injected into a muscle.
    - Children—Use and dose must be determined by your doctor.
  - —For *rectal* dosage form (suppositories):
    - Adults—10 mg one to three times a day.
    - Children—Use and dose must be determined by your doctor.

Missed dose—If you are taking this medicine regularly and you miss a dose, take it as soon as possible. However, if it is almost time for your next dose, skip the missed dose and go back to your regular dosing schedule. Do not double doses.

Storage—To store this medicine:

- Keep out of the reach of children, since overdose may be very dangerous in children.
- Store away from heat and direct light.
- Do not store the tablet form of this medicine in the bathroom medicine cabinet, near the kitchen sink, or in other damp places. Heat or moisture may cause the medicine to break down.
- Do not keep outdated medicine or medicine no longer needed. Be sure that any discarded medicine is out of the reach of children.

Precautions While Using This Medicine

If you are going to be taking this medicine for a long time, your doctor should check your progress at regular visits, especially during the first few months of treatment with this medicine. This will allow your dosage to be changed if necessary to meet your needs.

Thiethylperazine will add to the effects of alcohol and other CNS depressants (medicines that slow down the nervous system, possibly causing drowsiness). Some examples of CNS depressants are antihistamines or medicine for hay fever, other allergies, or colds; sedatives, tranquilizers, or sleeping medicine; prescription pain medicine or narcotics; barbiturates; medicine for seizures; muscle relaxants; or anesthetics, including some dental anesthetics. *Check with your doctor before taking any of the above while you are using this medicine.*

This medicine may cause some people to have blurred vision or to become dizzy, lightheaded, drowsy, or less alert than they are normally. *Make sure you know how you react to this medicine before you drive, use machines, or do anything else that could be dangerous if you are dizzy or are not alert or able to see well.*

Dizziness, lightheadedness, or fainting may occur, especially when you get up from a lying or sitting position. Getting up slowly may help. If the problem continues or gets worse, check with your doctor.

When using thiethylperazine on a regular basis, make sure your doctor knows if you are taking large amounts of aspirin or other salicylates at the same time (as for arthritis or rheumatism). Effects of too much aspirin, such as ringing in the ears, may be covered up by this medicine.

Thiethylperazine may cause dryness of the mouth, nose, and throat. For temporary relief of mouth dryness, use sugarless candy or gum, melt bits of ice in your mouth, or use a saliva substitute. However, if your mouth continues to feel dry for more than 2 weeks, check with your medical doctor or dentist. Continuing dryness of the mouth may increase the chance of dental disease, including tooth decay, gum disease, and fungus infections.

Side Effects of This Medicine

Along with its needed effects, a medicine may cause some unwanted effects. Although not all of these side effects may occur, if they do occur they may need medical attention.

Check with your doctor immediately if any of the following side effects occur:

Less common or rare

Lip smacking or puckering; puffing of cheeks; rapid or fine, worm-like movements of tongue; uncontrolled chewing movements; uncontrolled movements of arms or legs

Also, check with your doctor as soon as possible if any of the following side effects occur:

Less common or rare

Abdominal or stomach pains; aching muscles and joints; blurred vision, change in color vision, or difficulty in seeing at night; confusion (especially in the elderly); convulsions (seizures); difficulty in speaking or swallowing; fast heartbeat; fever and chills; inability to move eyes; loss of balance control; mask-like face; muscle spasms (especially of face, neck, and back); nausea, vomiting, or diarrhea; shuffling walk; skin itching (severe); sore throat and fever; stiffness of arms or legs; swelling of arms, hands, and face; tic-like or twitching movements; trembling and shaking of hands and fingers; twisting movements of body; unusual bleeding or bruising; unusual tiredness or weakness; weakness of arms and legs; yellow eyes or skin

Other side effects may occur that usually do not need medical attention. These side effects may go away during treatment as your body adjusts to the medicine. However, check with your doctor if any of the following side effects continue or are bothersome:

More common

Drowsiness or dizziness

Less common or rare

Constipation; decreased sweating; dryness of mouth, nose and throat; feeling faint; fever; headache; lightheadedness; nightmares (continuing); ringing or buzzing in ears; skin rash; unusual excitement, nervousness, restlessness, or irritability

Other side effects not listed above may also occur in some patients. If you notice any other effects, check with your doctor.

Annual revision: 06/17/93

THIOGUANINE Systemic

A commonly used brand name in Canada is Lanvis.
Generic name product available in the U.S.

Description

Thioguanine (thye-oh-GWON-een) belongs to the group of medicines known as antimetabolites. It is used to treat some kinds of cancer.

Thioguanine interferes with the growth of cancer cells, which are eventually destroyed. Since the growth of normal body cells may also be affected by thioguanine, other effects will also occur. Some of these may be serious and must be reported to your doctor. Other effects may not be serious but may cause concern. Some effects may not occur for months or years after the medicine is used.

Before you begin treatment with thioguanine, you and your doctor should talk about the good this medicine will do as well as the risks of using it.

Thioguanine is available only with your doctor's prescription, in the following dosage form:

Oral

- Tablets (U.S. and Canada)

It is very important that you read and understand the following information. If any of it causes you special concern, check with your doctor. Also, *if you have any questions* or if you want more information about this medicine or your medical problem, *ask your doctor, nurse, or pharmacist.*

Before Using This Medicine

In deciding to use a medicine, the risks of taking the medicine must be weighed against the good it will do.

This is a decision you and your doctor will make. For thioguanine, the following should be considered:

Allergies—Tell your doctor if you have ever had any unusual or allergic reaction to thioguanine.

Pregnancy—Tell your doctor if you are pregnant or if you intend to have children. There is a chance that this medicine may cause birth defects if either the male or female is taking it at the time of conception or if it is taken during pregnancy. In addition, many cancer medicines may cause sterility which could be permanent. Although this has not been reported with this medicine, the possibility should be kept in mind.

Be sure that you have discussed this with your doctor before taking this medicine. It is best to use some kind of birth control while you are taking thioguanine. Tell your doctor right away if you think you have become pregnant while taking thioguanine.

Breast-feeding—Tell your doctor if you are breast-feeding or if you intend to breast-feed during treatment with this medicine. Because thioguanine may cause serious side effects, breast-feeding is generally not recommended while you are receiving it.

Children—Although there is no specific information about the use of thioguanine in children, it is not expected to cause different side effects or problems in children than it does in adults.

Older adults—Many medicines have not been tested in older people. Therefore, it may not be known whether they work exactly the same way they do in younger adults or if they cause different side effects or problems in older people. There is no specific information about the use of thioguanine in the elderly.

Other medicines—Although certain medicines should not be used together at all, in other cases two different medicines may be used together even if an interaction might occur. In these cases, your doctor may want to change the dose, or other precautions may be necessary. When you are taking thioguanine, it is especially important that your doctor and pharmacist know if you are taking any of the following:

- Antithyroid agents (medicine for overactive thyroid) or
- Azathioprine (e.g., Imuran) or
- Chloramphenicol (e.g., Chloromycetin) or
- Colchicine or
- Flucytosine (e.g., Ancobon) or
- Interferon (e.g., Intron A, Roferon-A) or
- Plicamycin (e.g., Mithracin) or
- Zidovudine (e.g., Retrovir) or
- If you have ever been treated with x-rays or cancer medicines—Thioguanine may increase the effects of these medicines or radiation therapy on the blood
- Probenecid (e.g., Benemid) or
- Sulfinpyrazone (e.g., Anturane)—Thioguanine may increase the concentration of uric acid in the blood, which these medicines are used to lower

Other medical problems—The presence of other medical problems may affect the use of thioguanine. Make sure you tell your doctor if you have any other medical problems, especially:

- Chickenpox (including recent exposure) or
- Herpes zoster (shingles)—Risk of severe disease affecting other parts of the body
- Gout (history of) or
- Kidney stones (history of)—Thioguanine may increase levels of uric acid in the body, which can cause gout or kidney stones
- Infection—Thioguanine can reduce immunity to infection
- Kidney disease or
- Liver disease—Effects may be increased because of slower removal of thioguanine from the body

Before you begin using any new medicine (prescription or nonprescription) or if you develop any new medical problem while you are using this medicine, check with your doctor, nurse, or pharmacist.

Proper Use of This Medicine

Take this medicine only as directed by your doctor. Do not take more or less of it, and do not take it more often than your doctor ordered. The exact amount of medicine you need has been carefully worked out. Taking too much may increase the chance of side effects, while taking too little may not improve your condition.

Thioguanine is sometimes given together with certain other medicines. If you are using a combination of medicines, make sure that you take each one at the right time and do not mix them. Ask your doctor, nurse, or pharmacist to help you plan a way to take your medicine at the right times.

While you are using thioguanine, your doctor may want you to drink extra fluids so that you will pass more urine. This will help prevent kidney problems and keep your kidneys working well.

Thioguanine sometimes causes nausea and vomiting. However, it is very important that you continue to take this medicine, even if you begin to feel ill. *Do not stop taking this medicine without first checking with your doctor.* Ask your doctor, nurse, or pharmacist for ways to lessen these effects.

If you vomit shortly after taking a dose of thioguanine, check with your doctor. You will be told whether to take the dose again or to wait until the next scheduled dose.

Missed dose—If you miss a dose of this medicine, do not take the missed dose at all and do not double the next one. Instead, go back to your regular dosing schedule and check with your doctor.

Storage—To store this medicine:

- Keep out of the reach of children.
- Store away from heat and direct light.
- Do not store in the bathroom, near the kitchen sink, or in other damp places. Heat or moisture may cause the medicine to break down.
- Do not keep outdated medicine or medicine no longer needed. Be sure that any discarded medicine is out of the reach of children.

Precautions While Using This Medicine

It is very important that your doctor check your progress at regular visits to make sure that this medicine is working properly and to check for unwanted effects.

While you are being treated with thioguanine, and after you stop treatment with it, *do not have any immunizations (vaccinations) without your doctor's approval*. Thioguanine may lower your body's resistance and there is a chance you might get the infection the immunization is meant to prevent. Other people living in your household should not take or should not have recently taken oral polio vaccine since there is a chance they could pass the polio virus on to you. Also, avoid other persons who have taken oral polio vaccine. Do not get close to them and do not stay in the same room with them for very long. If you cannot take these precautions, you should consider wearing a protective face mask that covers the nose and mouth.

Thioguanine can lower the number of white blood cells in your blood temporarily, increasing the chance of getting an infection. It can also lower the number of platelets, which are necessary for proper blood clotting. If this occurs, there are certain precautions you can take, especially when your blood count is low, to reduce the risk of infection or bleeding:

- If you can, avoid people with infections. *Check with your doctor immediately* if you think you are getting an infection or if you get a fever or chills, cough or hoarseness, lower back or side pain, or painful or difficult urination.
- *Check with your doctor immediately* if you notice any unusual bleeding or bruising; black, tarry stools; blood in urine or stools; or pinpoint red spots on your skin.
- Be careful when using a regular toothbrush, dental floss, or toothpick. Your medical doctor, dentist, or nurse may recommend other ways to clean your teeth and gums. Check with your medical doctor before having any dental work done.
- Do not touch your eyes or the inside of your nose unless you have just washed your hands and have not touched anything else in the meantime.
- Be careful not to cut yourself when you are using sharp objects such as a safety razor or fingernail or toenail cutters.
- Avoid contact sports or other situations where bruising or injury could occur.

Side Effects of This Medicine

Along with their needed effects, medicines like thioguanine can sometimes cause unwanted effects such as blood problems and other side effects. These and others are described below. Also, because of the way these medicines act on the body, there is a chance that they might cause other unwanted effects that may not occur until months or years after the medicine is used. These delayed effects may include certain types of cancer, such as leukemia. Discuss these possible effects with your doctor.

Although not all of these side effects may occur, if they do occur they may need medical attention.

Check with your doctor immediately if any of the following side effects occur:

Less common

Black, tarry stools; blood in urine or stools; cough or hoarseness; fever or chills; lower back or side pain; painful or difficult urination; pinpoint red spots on skin; unusual bleeding or bruising

Check with your doctor as soon as possible if any of the following side effects occur:

Less common

Joint pain; swelling of feet or lower legs; unsteadiness when walking

Rare

Sores in mouth and on lips; yellow eyes or skin

Other side effects may occur that usually do not need medical attention. These side effects may go away during treatment as your body adjusts to the medicine. Also, your doctor or nurse may be able to tell you about ways to prevent or reduce some of these side effects. Check with your doctor or nurse if any of the following side effects continue or are bothersome or if you have any questions about them:

Less common

Diarrhea; loss of appetite; nausea and vomiting; skin rash or itching

After you stop taking thioguanine, it may still produce some side effects that need attention. During this period of time, check with your doctor if you notice any of the following side effects:

Black, tarry stools; blood in urine or stools; cough or hoarseness; fever or chills; lower back or side pain; painful or difficult urination; pinpoint red spots on skin; unusual bleeding or bruising

Other side effects not listed above may also occur in some patients. If you notice any other effects, check with your doctor.

Annual revision: September 1990
Interim revision: 08/11/93

THIOTEPA Systemic

Generic name product available in the U.S. and Canada.

Description

Thiotepa (thye-oh-TEP-a) belongs to the group of medicines called alkylating agents. It is used to treat some kinds of cancer.

Thiotepa interferes with the growth of cancer cells, which are eventually destroyed. Since the growth of normal body cells may also be affected by thiotepa, other effects will also occur. Some of these may be serious and must be reported to your doctor. Other effects, like hair loss, may not be serious but may cause concern. Some effects do not occur for months or years after the medicine is used.

Before you begin treatment with thiotepa, you and your doctor should talk about the good this medicine will do as well as the risks of using it.

Thiotepa is to be administered only by or under the immediate supervision of your doctor. It is available in the following dosage form:

Parenteral

- Injection (U.S. and Canada)

It is very important that you read and understand the following information. If any of it causes you special concern, check with your doctor. Also, *if you have any questions* or if you want more information about this medicine or your medical problem, *ask your doctor, nurse, or pharmacist.*

Before Using This Medicine

In deciding to use a medicine, the risks of taking the medicine must be weighed against the good it will do. This is a decision you and your doctor will make. For thiotepa, the following should be considered:

Allergies—Tell your doctor if you have ever had any unusual or allergic reaction to thiotepa.

Pregnancy—Tell your doctor if you are pregnant or if you intend to have children. There is a chance that this medicine may cause birth defects if either the male or female is using it at the time of conception or if it is used during pregnancy. Studies have shown that thiotepa causes birth defects in humans. In addition, many cancer medicines may cause sterility which could be permanent. Although this is uncommon with this medicine, the possibility should be kept in mind.

Be sure that you have discussed this with your doctor before using this medicine. It is best to use some kind of birth control while you are receiving thiotepa. Tell your doctor right away if you think you have become pregnant while receiving thiotepa.

Breast-feeding—Tell your doctor if you intend to breast-feed. Because this medicine may cause serious side effects, breast-feeding is generally not recommended while you are receiving it. It is not known whether thiotepa passes into the breast milk.

Children—There is no specific information about the use of thiotepa in children.

Older adults—Many medicines have not been tested in older people. Therefore, it may not be known whether they work exactly the same way they do in younger adults or if they cause different side effects or problems in older people. There is no specific information about the use of thiotepa in the elderly.

Other medicines—Although certain medicines should not be used together at all, in other cases two different medicines may be used together even if an interaction might occur. In these cases, your doctor may want to change the dose, or other precautions may be necessary. When you are receiving thiotepa, it is especially important that your doctor and pharmacist know if you are taking any of the following:

- Antithyroid agents (medicine for overactive thyroid) or
- Azathioprine (e.g., Imuran) or
- Chloramphenicol (e.g., Chloromycetin) or
- Colchicine or
- Flucytosine (e.g., Ancobon) or
- Interferon (e.g., Intron A, Roferon-A) or
- Plicamycin (e.g., Mithracin) or
- Zidovudine (e.g., Retrovir) or
- If you have ever been treated with x-rays or cancer medicines—Thiotepa may increase the effects of these medicines or radiation therapy on the blood
- Probenecid (e.g., Benemid) or
- Sulfinpyrazone (e.g., Anturane)—Thiotepa may increase the concentration of uric acid in the blood, which these medicines are used to lower

Other medical problems—The presence of other medical problems may affect the use of thiotepa. Make sure you tell your doctor if you have any other medical problems, especially:

- Chickenpox (including recent exposure) or
- Herpes zoster (shingles)—Risk of severe disease affecting other parts of the body
- Gout (history of) or
- Kidney stones (history of)—Thiotepa may increase levels of uric acid in the body, which can cause gout or kidney stones
- Infection—Thiotepa can reduce immunity to infection
- Kidney disease or
- Liver disease—Effects may be increased because of slower removal of thiotepa from the body

Before you begin using any new medicine (prescription or nonprescription) or if you develop any new medical problem while you are using this medicine, check with your doctor, nurse, or pharmacist.

Proper Use of This Medicine

While you are using thiotepa, your doctor may want you to drink extra fluids so that you will pass more urine. This will help prevent kidney problems and keep your kidneys working well.

Thiotepa sometimes causes nausea, vomiting, and loss of appetite. However, it is very important that you continue to receive the medicine, even if you begin to feel ill. Ask your doctor, nurse, or pharmacist for ways to lessen these effects.

Precautions While Using This Medicine

It is very important that your doctor check your progress at regular visits to make sure that this medicine is working properly and to check for unwanted effects.

Before having any kind of surgery, including dental surgery, make sure the medical doctor or dentist in charge knows that you are taking this medicine.

While you are being treated with thiotepa, and after you stop treatment with it, *do not have any immunizations (vaccinations) without your doctor's approval.* Thiotepa may lower your body's resistance and there is a chance you might get the infection the immunization is meant to prevent. Other people living in your household should not take or should not have recently taken oral polio vaccine since there is a chance they could pass the polio virus on to you. Also, avoid other persons who have taken oral polio vaccine. Do not get close to them and do not stay in the same room with them for very long. If you cannot take these precautions, you should consider wearing a protective face mask that covers the nose and mouth.

Thiotepa can lower the number of white blood cells in your blood temporarily, increasing the chance of getting an infection. It can also lower the number of platelets, which are necessary for proper blood clotting. If this occurs, there are certain precautions you can take, especially when your blood count is low, to reduce the risk of infection or bleeding:

- If you can, avoid people with infections. *Check with your doctor immediately* if you think you are getting an infection or if you get a fever or chills, cough or hoarseness, lower back or side pain, or painful or difficult urination.
- *Check with your doctor immediately* if you notice any unusual bleeding or bruising; black, tarry stools; blood in urine or stools; or pinpoint red spots on your skin.
- Be careful when using a regular toothbrush, dental floss, or toothpick. Your medical doctor, dentist, or nurse may recommend other ways to clean your teeth and gums. Check with your medical doctor before having any dental work done.
- Do not touch your eyes or the inside of your nose unless you have just washed your hands and have not touched anything else in the meantime.
- Be careful not to cut yourself when you are using sharp objects such as a safety razor or fingernail or toenail cutters.
- Avoid contact sports or other situations where bruising or injury could occur.

Side Effects of This Medicine

Along with their needed effects, medicines like thiotepa can sometimes cause unwanted effects such as blood problems, loss of hair, and other side effects. These and others are described below. Also, because of the way these medicines act on the body, there is a chance that they might cause other unwanted effects that may not occur until months or years after the medicine is used. These delayed effects may include certain types of cancer, such as leukemia. Discuss these possible effects with your doctor.

Although not all of these side effects may occur, if they do occur they may need medical attention.

Check with your doctor or nurse immediately if any of the following side effects occur:

Less common

Black, tarry stools; blood in urine or stools; cough or hoarseness; fever or chills; lower back or side pain; painful or difficult urination; pinpoint red spots on skin; unusual bleeding or bruising

Rare

Skin rash; tightness of throat; wheezing

Check with your doctor or nurse as soon as possible if any of the following side effects occur:

Less common

Joint pain; pain at place of injection or instillation; swelling of feet or lower legs

Rare

Sores in mouth and on lips

Other side effects may occur that usually do not need medical attention. These side effects may go away during treatment as your body adjusts to the medicine. Also, your doctor or nurse may be able to tell you about ways to prevent or reduce some of these side effects. Check with your doctor or nurse if any of the following side effects continue or are bothersome or if you have any questions about them:

Less common

Dizziness; hives; loss of appetite; missing menstrual periods; nausea and vomiting

This medicine may cause a temporary loss of hair in some people. After treatment with thiotepa has ended, normal hair growth should return.

After you stop receiving thiotepa, it may still produce some side effects that need attention. During this period of time, check with your doctor if you notice any of the following:

Black, tarry stools; blood in urine or stools; cough or hoarseness; fever or chills; lower back or side pain; painful or difficult urination; pinpoint red spots on skin; unusual bleeding or bruising

Other side effects not listed above may also occur in some patients. If you notice any other effects, check with your doctor.

Annual revision: September 1990
Interim revision: 08/11/93

THIOXANTHENES Systemic

This information applies to the following medicines:

Chlorprothixene (klor-proe-THIX-een)
Flupenthixol (floo-pen-THIX-ole)
Thiothixene (thye-oh-THIX-een)

Some commonly used brand names are:

For Chlorprothixene†
In the U.S.
Taractan

For Flupenthixol*
In Canada
Fluanxol
Fluanxol Depot

For Thiothixene
In the U.S.
Navane
Thiothixene HCl Intensol
Generic name product may also be available.
In Canada
Navane

*Not commercially available in the U.S.
†Not commercially available in Canada.

Description

This medicine belongs to the family of medicines known as thioxanthenes (thye-oh-ZAN-theens). It is used in the treatment of nervous, mental, and emotional conditions. Improvement in such conditions is thought to result from the effect of the medicine on nerve pathways in specific areas of the brain.

Thioxanthene medicines are available only with your doctor's prescription, in the following dosage forms:

Oral

Chlorprothixene
- Suspension (U.S.)
- Tablets (U.S.)

Flupenthixol
- Tablets (Canada)

Thiothixene
- Capsules (U.S. and Canada)
- Solution (U.S.)

Parenteral

Chlorprothixene
- Injection (U.S.)

Flupenthixol
- Injection (Canada)

Thiothixene
- Injection (U.S.)

It is very important that you read and understand the following information. If any of it causes you special concern, check with your doctor. Also, ***if you have any questions*** or if you want more information about this medicine or your medical problem, ***ask your doctor, nurse, or pharmacist.***

Before Using This Medicine

In deciding to use a medicine, the risks of taking the medicine must be weighed against the good it will do. This is a decision you and your doctor will make. For thioxanthenes, the following should be considered:

Allergies—Tell your doctor if you have ever had any unusual or allergic reaction to thioxanthene or to phenothiazine medicines. Also tell your doctor and pharmacist if you are allergic to any other substances, such as foods, preservatives, or dyes.

Pregnancy—Studies have not been done in pregnant women. Although animal studies have not shown that thioxanthenes cause birth defects, the studies have shown that these medicines cause a decrease in fertility and fewer successful pregnancies.

Breast-feeding—It is not known if thioxanthenes pass into the breast milk. However, similar medicines for nervous, mental, or emotional conditions do pass into breast milk and may cause drowsiness and increase the risk of other problems in the nursing baby. Be sure you have discussed the risks and benefits of this medicine with your doctor.

Children—Certain side effects, such as muscle spasms of the face, neck, and back, tic-like or twitching movements, inability to move the eyes, twisting of the body, or weakness of the arms and legs, are more likely to occur in children, who are usually more sensitive than adults to the side effects of thioxanthenes.

Older adults—Constipation, dizziness or fainting, drowsiness, dryness of mouth, trembling of the hands and fingers, and symptoms of tardive dyskinesia (such as rapid, worm-like movements of the tongue or any other uncontrolled movements of the mouth, tongue, or jaw, and/or arms and legs) are especially likely to occur in elderly patients, who are usually more sensitive than younger adults to the effects of thioxanthenes.

Other medicines—Although certain medicines should not be used together at all, in other cases 2 different medicines may be used together even if an interaction might occur. In these cases, your doctor may want to change the dose, or other precautions may be necessary. When you are taking thioxanthenes, it is especially important that your doctor and pharmacist know if you are taking any of the following:

- Amoxapine (e.g., Asendin) or
- Methyldopa (e.g., Aldomet) or
- Metoclopramide (e.g., Reglan) or
- Metyrosine (e.g., Demser) or
- Other antipsychotics (medicine for mental illness) or
- Pemoline (e.g., Cylert) or
- Pimozide (e.g., Orap) or
- Promethazine (e.g., Phenergan) or
- Rauwolfia alkaloids (alseroxylon [e.g., Rauwiloid], deserpidine [e.g., Harmonyl], rauwolfia serpentina [e.g., Raudixin], reserpine [e.g., Serpasil]) or
- Trimeprazine (e.g., Temaril)—Taking these medicines with thioxanthenes may increase the chance and severity of certain side effects
- Central nervous system (CNS) depressants (medicine that causes drowsiness) or
- Tricyclic antidepressants (medicine for depression)—Taking these medicines with thioxanthenes may add to the CNS depressant effects
- Epinephrine (e.g., Adrenalin)—Severe low blood pressure (hypotension) and fast heartbeat may occur if epinephrine is used with thioxanthenes
- Levodopa (e.g., Sinemet)—Thioxanthenes may keep levodopa from working properly in the treatment of Parkinson's disease
- Quinidine (e.g., Quinidex)—Unwanted effects on your heart may occur

Other medical problems—The presence of other medical problems may affect the use of thioxanthenes. Make sure you tell your doctor if you have any other medical problems, especially:

- Alcohol abuse—Drinking alcohol will add to the central nervous system (CNS) depressant effects of thioxanthenes
- Blood disease or
- Enlarged prostate or
- Glaucoma or
- Heart or blood vessel disease or
- Lung disease or
- Parkinson's disease or
- Stomach ulcers or
- Urination problems—Thioxanthenes may make the condition worse
- Liver disease—Higher blood levels of thioxanthenes may occur, increasing the chance of side effects
- Reye's syndrome—The risk of liver problems may be increased
- Seizure disorders—The risk of seizures may be increased

Before you begin using any new medicine (prescription or nonprescription) or if you develop any new medical problem while you are using this medicine, check with your doctor, nurse, or pharmacist.

Proper Use of This Medicine

This medicine may be taken with food or a full glass (8 ounces) of water or milk to reduce stomach irritation.

For patients taking *thiothixene oral solution:*

- This medicine must be diluted before you take it. Just before taking, measure the dose with the specially marked dropper. Mix the medicine with a full glass of water, milk, tomato or fruit juice, soup, or carbonated beverage.

Do not take more of this medicine or take it more often than your doctor ordered. This is particularly important when this medicine is given to children, since they may react very strongly to its effects.

Sometimes this medicine must be taken for several weeks before its full effect is reached.

Dosing—The dose of these medicines will be different for different patients. *Follow your doctor's orders or the directions on the label.* The following information includes only the average doses of these medicines. *If your dose is different, do not change it* unless your doctor tells you to do so.

The number of capsules or tablets or the amount of liquid that you take depends on the strength of the medicine. Also, the number of doses you take each day, the time allowed between doses, and the length of time you take the medicine depend on the medical problem for which you are taking thioxanthenes.

For chlorprothixene

- For treatment of psychosis:
  - —*Oral* dosage forms (suspension or tablets):
    - Adults and teenagers—25 to 50 milligrams (mg) three or four times a day.
    - Children 6 to 12 years of age—10 to 25 mg three or four times a day.
    - Children up to 6 years of age—Use and dose must be determined by your doctor.
  - —*Injection* dosage form:
    - Adults and teenagers—25 to 50 mg, injected into a muscle, three or four times a day.
    - Children up to 12 years of age—Use and dose must be determined by your doctor.

For flupenthixol

- For treatment of psychosis:
  - —*Oral* dosage form (tablets):
    - Adults—To start, 1 milligram (mg) three times a day. Your doctor may increase your dose if needed, depending on your condition.
    - Children— Use and dose must be determined by your doctor.
  - —*Long-acting injection* dosage form:
    - Adults—To start, 20 to 40 milligrams (mg) injected into a muscle. Your doctor will determine whether your dose needs to be changed, depending on your condition.
    - Children—Use and dose must be determined by your doctor.

For thiothixene

- For treatment of psychosis:
  - —*Oral* dosage forms (capsules and solution):
    - Adults and teenagers—To start, 2 milligrams (mg) three times a day, or 5 mg two times a day. Your doctor may increase your dose if needed. However, the dose is usually not more than 60 mg a day.
    - Children up to 12 years of age—Use and dose must be determined by your doctor.
  - —*Injection* dosage form:
    - Adults and teenagers—4 milligrams (mg), injected into a muscle, two to four times a day. Your doctor may increase your dose if needed. However, the dose is usually not more than 30 mg a day.
    - Children up to 12 years of age—Use and dose must be determined by your doctor.

Missed dose—If you miss a dose of this medicine, take it as soon as possible. However, if it is within 2 hours of your next dose, skip the missed dose and go back to your regular dosing schedule. Do not double doses.

Storage—To store this medicine:

- Keep out of the reach of children.
- Store away from heat and direct light.
- Do not store the capsule or tablet form of this medicine in the bathroom, near the kitchen sink, or in other damp places. Heat or moisture may cause the medicine to break down.
- Keep the liquid form of this medicine from freezing.
- Do not keep outdated medicine or medicine no longer needed. Be sure that any discarded medicine is out of the reach of children.

Precautions While Using This Medicine

Your doctor should check your progress at regular visits. This will allow the dosage of the medicine to be adjusted when necessary and also will reduce the possibility of side effects.

Do not stop taking this medicine without first checking with your doctor. Your doctor may want you to gradually reduce the amount you are taking before stopping completely. This is to prevent side effects and to prevent your condition from becoming worse.

This medicine will add to the effects of alcohol and other CNS depressants (medicines that slow down the nervous system, possibly causing drowsiness). Some examples of CNS depressants are antihistamines or medicine for hay fever, other allergies, or colds; sedatives, tranquilizers, or sleeping medicine; prescription pain medicine or narcotics; barbiturates; medicine for seizures; muscle relaxants; or anesthetics, including some dental anesthetics. *Check with your doctor before taking any such depressants while you are using this medicine.*

Do not take this medicine within an hour of taking antacids or medicine for diarrhea. Taking them too close together may make this medicine less effective.

Before having any kind of surgery, dental treatment, or emergency treatment, tell the medical doctor or dentist in charge that you are using this medicine. Taking thioxanthenes together with medicines that are used during surgery or dental or emergency treatments may increase the CNS depressant effects.

This medicine may cause some people to become drowsy or less alert than they are normally, especially during the first few weeks the medicine is being taken. Even if you take this medicine only at bedtime, you may feel drowsy or less alert on arising. *Make sure you know how you react to this medicine before you drive, use machines, or do anything else that could be dangerous if you are not alert.*

Dizziness, lightheadedness, or fainting may occur while you are taking this medicine, especially when you get up from a lying or sitting position. Getting up slowly may help. If the problem continues or gets worse, check with your doctor.

This medicine may make you sweat less, causing your body temperature to increase. *Use extra care not to become overheated during exercise or hot weather while you are taking this medicine,* since overheating may result in heat stroke. Also, hot baths or saunas may make you feel dizzy or faint while you are taking this medicine.

Thioxanthenes may cause your skin to be more sensitive to sunlight than it is normally. Exposure to sunlight, even for brief periods of time, may cause a skin rash, itching, redness or other discoloration of the skin, or a severe sunburn. When you begin taking this medicine:

- Stay out of direct sunlight, especially between the hours of 10:00 a.m. and 3:00 p.m., if possible.
- Wear protective clothing, including a hat. Also, wear sunglasses.
- Apply a sun block product that has a skin protection factor (SPF) of at least 15. Some patients may require a product with a higher SPF number, especially if they have a fair complexion. If you have any questions about this, check with your doctor or pharmacist.
- Apply a sun block lipstick that has an SPF of at least 15 to protect your lips.
- Do not use a sunlamp or tanning bed or booth.

If you have a severe reaction from the sun, check with your doctor.

This medicine may cause dryness of the mouth. For temporary relief, use sugarless gum or candy, melt bits of ice in your mouth, or use a saliva substitute. However, if your mouth continues to feel dry for more than 2 weeks, check with your medical doctor or dentist. Continuing dryness of the mouth may increase the chance of dental disease, including tooth decay, gum disease, and fungus infections.

If you are taking a liquid form of this medicine, *try to avoid spilling it on your skin or clothing.* Skin rash and irritation have been caused by similar medicines.

If you are receiving this medicine by injection:

- The effects of the long-acting injection form of this medicine may last for up to 3 weeks. *The precautions and side effects information for this medicine applies during this period of time.*

Side Effects of This Medicine

Along with their needed effects, thioxanthenes can sometimes cause serious side effects. Tardive dyskinesia (a movement disorder) may occur and may not go away after you stop using the medicine. Signs of tardive dyskinesia include fine, worm-like movements of the tongue, or other uncontrolled movements of the mouth, tongue, cheeks, jaw, or arms and legs. Other serious but rare side effects may also occur. Some of these side effects, including severe muscle stiffness, fever, unusual tiredness or weakness, fast heartbeat, difficult breathing, increased sweating, loss of bladder control, and seizures, may be the sign of a condition called neuroleptic malignant syndrome. *You and your doctor should discuss the good this medicine will do as well as the risks of taking it.*

Although not all of these side effects may occur, if they do occur they may need medical attention.

Stop taking this medicine and get emergency help immediately if any of the following side effects occur:

Rare

Convulsions (seizures); difficulty in breathing; fast heartbeat; high fever; high or low (irregular) blood pressure; increased sweating; loss of bladder control; muscle stiffness (severe); unusually pale skin; unusual tiredness

Also, check with your doctor as soon as possible if any of the following side effects occur:

More common

Difficulty in talking or swallowing; inability to move eyes; lip smacking or puckering; loss of balance control; mask-like face; muscle spasms, especially of the neck and back; puffing of cheeks; rapid or worm-like movements of tongue; restlessness or need to keep moving (severe); shuffling walk; stiffness of arms and legs; trembling and shaking of fingers and hands; twisting movements of body; uncontrolled chewing movements; uncontrolled movements of the arms and legs

Less common

Blurred vision or other eye problems; difficult urination; fainting; skin discoloration; skin rash

Rare

Hot, dry skin or lack of sweating; increased blinking or spasms of eyelid; muscle weakness; sore throat and fever; uncontrolled twisting movements of neck, trunk, arms, or legs; unusual bleeding or bruising; unusual facial expressions or body positions; yellow eyes or skin

Symptoms of overdose

Difficulty in breathing (severe); dizziness (severe); drowsiness (severe); muscle trembling, jerking, stiffness, or uncontrolled movements (severe); small pupils; unusual excitement; unusual tiredness or weakness (severe)

Other side effects may occur that usually do not need medical attention. These side effects may go away during treatment as your body adjusts to the medicine. However, check with your doctor if any of the following side effects continue or are bothersome:

More common

Constipation; decreased sweating; dizziness, lightheadedness, or fainting; drowsiness (mild); dryness of mouth;

increased appetite and weight; increased sensitivity of skin to sunlight (skin rash, itching, redness or other discoloration of skin, or severe sunburn); stuffy nose

Less common

Changes in menstrual period; decreased sexual ability; swelling of breasts (in males and females); unusual secretion of milk

After you stop taking this medicine your body may need time to adjust, especially if you took this medicine in high doses or for a long time. If you stop taking it too quickly, the following withdrawal effects may occur and should be reported to your doctor:

Dizziness; nausea and vomiting; stomach pain; trembling of fingers and hands; uncontrolled, continuing movements of mouth, tongue, or jaw

Although not all of the side effects listed above have been reported for all thioxanthenes, they have been reported for at least one of them. However, since these medicines are very similar, any of the above side effects may occur with any of them.

Other side effects not listed above may also occur in some patients. If you notice any other effects, check with your doctor.

Annual revision: 06/17/93

THROMBOLYTIC AGENTS Systemic

This information applies to the following medicines:

Alteplase, Recombinant (AL-ti-plase)
Streptokinase (strep-toe-KYE-nase)
Urokinase (yoor-oh-KYE-nase)

Anistreplase (e.g., Eminase), another thrombolytic agent, is not included in the following information. See Anistreplase (Systemic) for information about that medicine.

Some commonly used brand names are:

For Alteplase, Recombinant

In the U.S.
Activase

In Canada
Activase rt-PA

Other commonly used names are tissue-type plasminogen activator (recombinant), t-PA, and rt-PA.

For Streptokinase

In the U.S.
Kabikinase
Streptase

In Canada
Streptase

For Urokinase

In the U.S.
Abbokinase
Abbokinase Open-Cath

Description

Thrombolytic agents are used to break up (lyse) or dissolve blood clots that have formed in certain blood vessels. These medicines are most likely to be used when a blood clot seriously lessens the flow of blood to certain parts of the body.

Thrombolytic agents are also used to dissolve blood clots that form in tubes that are placed into the body. The tubes allow treatments (such as dialysis or injections into a vein) to be given over a long period of time. When used to clear these tubes, the medicine is placed directly into the tube. It is not injected into the body. However, some may get into the body and cause unwanted effects.

These medicines are used only in a hospital. They are given by or under the direct supervision of a doctor.

These medicines are available in the following dosage forms:

Parenteral

Alteplase, Recombinant
- Injection (U.S. and Canada)

Streptokinase
- Injection (U.S. and Canada)

Urokinase
- Injection (U.S.)

It is very important that you read and understand the following information. If any of it causes you special concern, check with your doctor. Also, *if you have any questions* or if you want more information about this medicine or your medical problem, *ask your doctor, nurse, or pharmacist.*

Before Receiving This Medicine

In deciding to use a medicine, the risks of using the medicine must be weighed against the good it will do. This is a decision you and your doctor will make. For thrombolytic agents, the following should be considered:

Allergies—Tell your doctor if you have ever had any unusual or allergic reaction to alteplase, anistreplase, streptokinase, or urokinase. Also tell your doctor and pharmacist if you are allergic to any other substances, such as foods, preservatives, or dyes.

Pregnancy—Tell your doctor if you are pregnant or if you have recently delivered a baby. Studies in pregnant women have not shown that streptokinase causes miscarriage or birth defects or other problems in the fetus or newborn baby. However, there is a slight chance that use of a thrombolytic agent during the first 5 months of pregnancy may cause a miscarriage.

Studies on birth defects with alteplase have not been done in either pregnant women or animals. Studies on birth defects with urokinase have not been done in pregnant women. However, studies in animals have not shown that urokinase causes birth defects or other problems.

Use of a thrombolytic agent soon after the birth of a baby may cause serious bleeding in the mother.

Breast-feeding—It is not known whether thrombolytic agents pass into the breast milk. However, these medicines have not been reported to cause problems in nursing babies.

Children—Although there is no specific information about the use of thrombolytic agents in children, these medicines are not expected to cause different side effects or other problems in children than they do in adults.

Older adults—The need for treatment with a thrombolytic agent (instead of other kinds of treatment) may be increased in elderly patients with blood clots. However, the chance of bleeding may also be increased. It is especially important that you discuss the use of this medicine with your doctor.

Other medicines—Although certain medicines should not be used together at all, in other cases two different medicines may be used together even if an interaction might occur. In these cases, your doctor may want to change the dose, or other precautions may be necessary. Before you receive a thrombolytic agent, it is especially important that your doctor know if you are taking any of the following:

- Anticoagulants (blood thinners) or
- Aspirin or
- Carbenicillin by injection (e.g., Geopen) or
- Cefamandole (e.g., Mandol) or
- Cefoperazone (e.g., Cefobid) or
- Cefotetan (e.g., Cefotan) or
- Dipyridamole (e.g., Persantine) or
- Divalproex (e.g., Depakote) or
- Heparin or
- Medicine for inflammation or pain (except narcotics) or
- Moxalactam (e.g., Moxam) or
- Pentoxifylline (e.g., Trental) or
- Plicamycin (e.g., Mithracin) or
- Sulfinpyrazone (e.g., Anturane) or
- Ticarcillin (e.g., Ticar) or
- Valproic acid (e.g., Depakene)—The chance of bleeding may be increased

Also, tell your doctor if you have had an injection of anistreplase (e.g., Eminase) or streptokinase within the past year, because, if you have, streptokinase may not work properly. Your doctor may decide to use alteplase or urokinase instead.

Other medical problems—The presence of other medical problems may affect the use of thrombolytic agents. Make sure you tell your doctor if you have any other medical problems, especially:

- Blood disease, bleeding problems, or a history of bleeding in any part of the body or
- Brain disease or tumor or
- Colitis or stomach ulcer (or history of) or
- Heart or blood vessel disease or
- High blood pressure or
- Stroke (or history of) or
- Tuberculosis (TB) (active)—The chance of serious bleeding may be increased
- Streptococcal ("strep") infection (recent)—Streptokinase may not work properly after a streptococcal infection; your doctor may decide to use a different thrombolytic agent

Also, tell your doctor if you have recently had any of the following conditions:

- Falls or blows to the body or head or any other injury or
- Injections into a blood vessel or
- Placement of any tube into the body or
- Surgery, including dental surgery—The chance of serious bleeding may be increased

Precautions While Receiving This Medicine

Thrombolytic agents can cause bleeding that usually is not serious. However, serious bleeding may occur in some people. *To help prevent serious bleeding, follow any instructions given by your doctor or nurse very carefully. Also, move around as little as possible, and do not get out of bed on your own, while receiving this medicine.*

Side Effects of This Medicine

Along with its needed effects, a medicine may cause some unwanted effects. Although not all of these side effects may occur, if they do occur they may need medical attention.

Tell your doctor or nurse immediately if any of the following side effects occur:

More common

Bleeding or oozing from cuts or around the place of injection; fast, slow, or irregular heartbeat; fever

Less common or rare

Flushing or redness of skin; headache (mild); muscle pain (mild); nausea; shortness of breath, troubled breathing, tightness in chest, or wheezing; skin rash, itching, or hives; swelling of eyes, face, lips, or tongue

Symptoms of bleeding inside the body

Abdominal or stomach pain or swelling; back pain or backaches; blood in urine; bloody or black, tarry stools; constipation; coughing up blood; dizziness; headaches (sudden, severe, or continuing); joint pain, stiffness, or swelling; muscle pain or stiffness (severe or continuing); nosebleeds; unexpected or unusually heavy bleeding from vagina; vomiting of blood or material that looks like coffee grounds

Other side effects not listed above may also occur in some patients. If you notice any other effects, check with your doctor.

Annual revision: August 1990

THYROID HORMONES Systemic

This information applies to the following medicines:

- Levothyroxine (lee-voe-thye-ROX-een)
- Liothyronine (lye-oh-THYE-roe-neen)
- Liotrix (LYE-oh-trix)
- Thyroglobulin (thye-roe-GLOB-yoo-lin)
- Thyroid (THYE-roid)

Note: This information does *not* apply to Thyrotropin.

Some commonly used brand names are:

For Levothyroxine

In the U.S.

Levoid
Levothroid
Levoxine
Synthroid

Generic name product may also be available.

In Canada

Eltroxin
Synthroid

For Liothyronine

In the U.S.

Cytomel

Generic name product may also be available.

In Canada

Cytomel

For Liotrix

In the U.S.

Euthroid
Thyrolar

In Canada

Thyrolar

For Thyroglobulin*

In Canada

Proloid

For Thyroid

In the U.S. and Canada

Generic name product available.

*Not commercially available in the U.S.

Description

Thyroid medicines belong to the general group of medicines called hormones. They are used when the thyroid gland does not produce enough hormone. They are also used to help decrease the size of enlarged thyroid glands (known as goiter) and to treat thyroid cancer.

These medicines are available only with your doctor's prescription, in the following dosage forms:

Oral

Levothyroxine
- Tablets (U.S. and Canada)

Liothyronine
- Tablets (U.S. and Canada)

Liotrix
- Tablets (U.S. and Canada)

Thyroglobulin
- Tablets (Canada)

Thyroid
- Tablets (U.S. and Canada)
- Enteric-coated tablets (U.S.)

Parenteral

Levothyroxine
- Injection (U.S. and Canada)

It is very important that you read and understand the following information. If any of it causes you special concern, check with your doctor. Also, *if you have any questions* or if you want more information about this medicine or your medical problem, *ask your doctor, nurse, or pharmacist.*

Before Using This Medicine

In deciding to use a medicine, the risks of taking the medicine must be weighed against the good it will do. This is a decision you and your doctor will make. For thyroid hormones, the following should be considered:

Allergies—Tell your doctor if you have ever had any unusual or allergic reaction to thyroid hormones. Also tell your doctor and pharmacist if you are allergic to any other substances, such as foods, preservatives, or dyes.

Pregnancy—It is essential that your baby receive the right amount of thyroid for normal development. You may need to take different amounts while you are pregnant. In addition, you may respond differently than usual to some tests. Your doctor should check your progress at regular visits while you are pregnant.

Breast-feeding—Use of proper amounts of thyroid hormones by mothers has not been shown to cause problems in nursing babies.

Children—Thyroid hormones have been tested in children and have not been shown to cause different side effects or problems in children than they do in adults.

Older adults—This medicine has been tested and has not been shown to cause different side effects or problems in older people than it does in younger adults. However, a different dose may be needed in the elderly. Therefore, it is important to take the medicine only as directed by the doctor.

Other medicines—Although certain medicines should not be used together at all, in other cases two different medicines may be used together even if an interaction might occur. In these cases, your doctor may want to change the dose, or other precautions may be necessary. When you are taking thyroid hormones, it is especially important that your doctor and pharmacist know if you are taking any of the following:

- Amphetamines
- Anticoagulants (blood thinners)
- Appetite suppressants (diet pills)
- Cholestyramine (e.g., Questran)
- Colestipol (e.g., Colestid)
- Medicine for asthma or other breathing problems
- Medicine for colds, sinus problems, or hay fever or other allergies (including nose drops or sprays)

Other medical problems—The presence of other medical problems may affect the use of thyroid hormones. Make sure you tell your doctor if you have any other medical problems especially:

- Diabetes mellitus (sugar diabetes)
- Hardening of the arteries
- Heart disease
- High blood pressure
- Overactive thyroid (history of)
- Underactive adrenal gland
- Underactive pituitary gland

Before you begin using any new medicine (prescription or nonprescription) or if you develop any new medical problem while you are using this medicine, check with your doctor, nurse, or pharmacist.

Proper Use of This Medicine

Use this medicine only as directed by your doctor. Do not use more or less of it, and do not use it more often than your doctor ordered. Your doctor has prescribed the exact amount your body needs and if you take different amounts, you may experience symptoms of an overactive or underactive thyroid. Take it at the same time each day to make sure it always has the same effect.

If your condition is due to a lack of thyroid hormone, you may have to take this medicine for the rest of your life. It is very important that you *do not stop taking this medicine without first checking with your doctor.*

Missed dose—If you miss a dose of this medicine, take it as soon as possible. However, if it is almost time for your next dose, skip the missed dose and go back to your regular dosing schedule. Do not double doses. If you miss 2 or more doses in a row or if you have any questions about this, check with your doctor.

Storage—To store this medicine:

- Keep out of the reach of children.
- Store away from heat and direct light.
- Do not store in the bathroom, near the kitchen sink, or in other damp places. Heat or moisture may cause the medicine to break down.
- Do not keep outdated medicine or medicine no longer needed. Be sure that any discarded medicine is out of the reach of children.

Precautions While Using This Medicine

It is very important that your doctor check your progress at regular visits, to make sure that this medicine is working properly.

If you have certain kinds of heart disease, this medicine may cause chest pain or shortness of breath when you exert yourself. If these occur, do not overdo exercise or physical work. If you have any questions about this, check with your doctor.

Before having any kind of surgery (including dental surgery) or emergency treatment, *tell the medical doctor or dentist in charge that you are taking this medicine.*

Do not take any other medicine unless prescribed by your doctor. Some medicines may increase or decrease the effects of thyroid on your body and cause problems in controlling your condition. Also, thyroid hormones may change the effects of other medicines.

Side Effects of This Medicine

Along with its needed effects, a medicine may cause some unwanted effects. Although not all of these side effects may occur, if they do occur they may need medical attention.

Check with your doctor as soon as possible if any of the following side effects occur since they may indicate an overdose or an allergic reaction:

Rare

Headache (severe) in children; skin rash or hives

Signs and symptoms of overdose

Chest pain; fast or irregular heartbeat; shortness of breath

For patients taking this medicine for underactive thyroid:

- This medicine usually takes several weeks to have a noticeable effect on your condition. Until it begins to work, you may experience no change in your symptoms. Check with your doctor if the following symptoms continue:

  Clumsiness; coldness; constipation; dry, puffy skin; listlessness; muscle aches; sleepiness; tiredness; weakness; weight gain

Other effects may occur if the dose of the medicine is not exactly right. These side effects will go away when the dose is corrected. Check with your doctor if any of the following symptoms occur:

Changes in appetite; changes in menstrual periods; diarrhea; fever; hand tremors; headache; increased sensitivity to heat; irritability; leg cramps; nervousness; sweating; trouble in sleeping; vomiting; weight loss

Other side effects not listed above may also occur in some patients. If you notice any other effects, check with your doctor.

Annual revision: 05/22/92

THYROTROPIN Systemic

A commonly used brand name in the U.S. and Canada is Thytropar.

Description

Thyrotropin (thye-roe-TROE-pin) is used in a test to determine how well your thyroid is working. It may also be used for other conditions as determined by your doctor.

Thyrotropin is to be administered only by or under the immediate supervision of your doctor. It is available in the following dosage form:

Parenteral

- Injection (U.S. and Canada)

It is very important that you read and understand the following information. If any of it causes you special concern, check with your doctor. Also, *if you have any questions* or if you want more information about this medicine or your medical problem, *ask your doctor, nurse, or pharmacist.*

Before Using This Medicine

In deciding to use a medicine, the risks of taking the medicine must be weighed against the good it will do. This is a decision you and your doctor will make. For thyrotropin, the following should be considered:

Allergies—Tell your doctor if you have ever received thyrotropin or ever had any unusual or allergic reaction to thyrotropin. Also tell your doctor and pharmacist if you are allergic to any other substances, such as foods, preservatives, or dyes.

Pregnancy—Studies on effects in pregnancy have not been done in either humans or animals.

Breast-feeding—It is not known whether thyrotropin passes into breast milk. However, this medicine has not been reported to cause problems in nursing babies.

Children—This medicine has been tested in children and has not been shown to cause different side effects or problems than it does in adults.

Older adults—Many medicines have not been studied specifically in the elderly. Therefore, it may not be known whether they work exactly the same way they do in younger adults. Although, there is no specific information comparing the use of thyrotropin in the elderly with use in other age groups, this medicine is not expected to cause different side effects or problems in older people than it does in younger adults.

Other medicines—Although certain medicines should not be used together at all, in other cases two different medicines may be used together even if an interaction might occur. In these cases, your doctor may want to change the dose, or other precautions may be necessary. When you are receiving thyrotropin, it is especially important that your doctor and pharmacist know if you are taking any of the following:

- Thyroid hormones—You may not respond as strongly to thyrotropin if you have been taking thyroid hormones regularly

Other medical problems—The presence of other medical problems may affect the use of thyrotropin. Make sure you tell your doctor if you have any other medical problems, especially:

- Hardening of the arteries or
- Heart disease or
- High blood pressure—Thyrotropin increases body metabolism and causes the heart to work harder, which may make these conditions worse

- Untreated underactive adrenal gland or
- Untreated underactive pituitary gland—Use of thyrotropin may severely worsen these conditions

Before you begin using any new medicine (prescription or nonprescription) or if you develop any new medical problem while you are using this medicine, check with your doctor, nurse, or pharmacist.

Proper Use of This Medicine

For your doctor to properly treat your medical condition, *you must receive every dose of this medicine.* After the last dose, the doctor may want to perform certain tests that are very important.

Side Effects of This Medicine

Along with its needed effects, a medicine may cause some unwanted effects. Although not all of these side effects may occur, if they do occur they may need medical attention.

Check with your doctor immediately if any of the following side effects occur:

Rare—more common in patients who have received thyrotropin previously

Faintness; itching; redness or swelling at place of injection; skin rash; tightness of throat; wheezing

Other effects may occur if the dose of the medicine is not exactly right. Check with your doctor as soon as possible if any of the following symptoms occur:

Chest pain; fast or irregular heartbeat; irritability; nervousness; shortness of breath; sweating

Other side effects may occur that usually do not need medical attention. These side effects may go away during treatment as your body adjusts to the medicine. However, check with your doctor if any of the following side effects continue or are bothersome:

More common

Flushing of face; frequent urge to urinate; headache; nausea and vomiting; stomach discomfort

Other side effects not listed above may also occur in some patients. If you notice any other effects, check with your doctor.

Annual revision: 01/31/92

TICLOPIDINE Systemic

A commonly used brand name in the U.S. and Canada is Ticlid.

Description

Ticlopidine (tye-KLOE-pi-deen) is used to lower the chance of having a stroke. It is given to people who have already had a stroke and to people with certain medical problems that may lead to a stroke. Because ticlopidine can cause serious side effects, especially during the first 3 months of treatment, it is used mostly for people who cannot take aspirin to prevent strokes.

A stroke may occur when a blood vessel in the brain is blocked by a blood clot. Ticlopidine lessens the chance that a harmful blood clot will form, by preventing certain cells in the blood from clumping together. This effect of ticlopidine may also increase the chance of serious bleeding in some people.

This medicine is available in the following dosage forms:

Oral

- Tablets (U.S. and Canada)

It is very important that you read and understand the following information. If any of it causes you special concern, check with your doctor. Also, *if you have any questions* or if you want more information about this medicine or your medical problem, *ask your doctor, nurse, or pharmacist.*

Before Using This Medicine

In deciding to use a medicine, the risks of taking the medicine must be weighed against the good it will do. This is a decision you and your doctor will make. For ticlopidine, the following should be considered:

Allergies—Tell your doctor if you have ever had any unusual or allergic reaction to ticlopidine. Also tell your doctor and pharmacist if you are allergic to any other substances, such as foods, preservatives, or dyes.

Pregnancy—Studies with ticlopidine have not been done in pregnant women. This medicine did not cause birth defects in animal studies. However, it caused other unwanted effects in animal studies when it was given in amounts that were large enough to cause harmful effects in the mother.

Breast-feeding—It is not known whether ticlopidine passes into the breast milk.

Children—There is no specific information comparing use of ticlopidine in children with use in other age groups.

Older adults—This medicine has been tested and has not been shown to cause different side effects or problems in older people than it does in younger adults.

Other medicines—Although certain medicines should not be used together at all, in other cases two different medicines may be used together even if an interaction might occur. In these cases, your doctor may want to change the dose, or other precautions may be necessary. When you are taking ticlopidine, it is especially important that your doctor and pharmacist know if you are taking any of the following:

- Anticoagulants (blood thinners) or
- Aspirin or
- Heparin (e.g., Hepalean, Liquaemin)—The chance of serious bleeding may be increased

Other medical problems—The presence of other medical problems may affect the use of ticlopidine. Make sure you tell your doctor if you have any other medical problems, especially:

- Blood disease—The chance of serious side effects may be increased
- Blood clotting problems, such as hemophilia, or
- Liver disease (severe) or
- Stomach ulcers—The chance of serious bleeding may be increased
- Kidney disease (severe)—Ticlopidine is removed from the body more slowly when the kidneys are not working properly. This may increase the chance of side effects.

Before you begin using any new medicine (prescription or nonprescription) or if you develop any new medical problem while you are using this medicine, check with your doctor, nurse, or pharmacist.

Proper Use of This Medicine

Ticlopidine should be taken with food. This increases the amount of medicine that is absorbed into the body. It may also lessen the chance of stomach upset.

Take this medicine only as directed by your doctor. Ticlopidine will not work properly if you take less of it than directed. Taking more ticlopidine than directed may increase the chance of serious side effects without increasing the helpful effects.

Dosing—*Follow your doctor's orders or the directions on the label.* The following dose was used, and found effective, in studies. However, some people may need a different dose. *If your dose is different, do not change it* unless your doctor tells you to do so:

- For adults—1 tablet (250 mg) two times a day, with food.
- For children—It is not likely that ticlopidine would be used to help prevent strokes in children. If a child needs this medicine, however, the dose would have to be determined by the doctor.

Missed dose—If you miss a dose of this medicine, take it as soon as possible. However, if it is almost time for your next dose, skip the missed dose and go back to your regular dosing schedule. Do not double doses.

Storage—To store this medicine:

- Keep out of the reach of children.
- Store away from heat and direct light.
- Do not store in the bathroom, near the kitchen sink, or in other damp places. Heat or moisture may cause the medicine to break down.
- Do not keep outdated medicine or medicine no longer needed. Be sure that any discarded medicine is out of the reach of children.

Precautions While Using This Medicine

It is very important that blood tests be done every 2 weeks for the first 3 months of treatment with ticlopidine. The tests are needed to find out whether certain side effects are occurring. Finding these side effects early helps to prevent them from becoming serious. Your doctor will arrange for the blood tests to be done. *Be sure that you do not miss any appointments for these tests.* You will probably not need to have your blood tested so often after the first 3 months of treatment, because the side effects are less likely to occur after that time.

Tell all medical doctors, dentists, nurses, and pharmacists you go to that you are taking this medicine. Ticlopidine may increase the risk of serious bleeding during an operation or some kinds of dental work. Therefore, treatment may have to be stopped about 10 days to 2 weeks before the operation or dental work is done.

Ticlopidine may cause serious bleeding, especially after an injury. Sometimes, bleeding inside the body can occur without your knowing about it. Ask your doctor whether there are certain activities you should avoid while taking this medicine (for example, sports that can cause injuries). *Also, check with your doctor immediately if you are injured while being treated with this medicine.*

Check with your doctor immediately if you notice any of the following side effects:

- Bruising or bleeding, especially bleeding that is hard to stop.
- Any sign of infection, such as fever, chills, or sore throat.
- Sores, ulcers, or white spots in the mouth.

After you stop taking ticlopidine, the chance of bleeding may continue for 1 or 2 weeks. During this period of time, continue to follow the same precautions that you followed while you were taking the medicine.

Side Effects of This Medicine

Along with its needed effects, a medicine may cause some unwanted effects. Although not all of these side effects may occur, if they do occur they may need medical attention.

Check with your doctor immediately if any of the following side effects occur:

Less common or rare

Abdominal or stomach pain (severe) or swelling; back pain; blood in eyes; blood in urine; bloody or black, tarry stools; bruising or purple areas on skin; coughing up blood; decreased alertness; dizziness; fever, chills, or sore throat; headache (severe or continuing); joint pain or swelling; nosebleeds; pinpoint red spots on skin; sores, ulcers, or white spots in mouth; paralysis or problems with coordination; stammering or other difficulty in speaking; unusually heavy bleeding or oozing from cuts or wounds; unusually heavy or unexpected menstrual bleeding; vomiting of blood or material that looks like coffee grounds

Also, check with your doctor as soon as possible if any of the following side effects occur:

More common

Skin rash

Less common or rare

Hives or itching of skin; ringing or buzzing in ears; yellow eyes or skin

Other side effects may occur that usually do not need medical attention. These side effects may go away during treatment as your body adjusts to the medicine. However, check with your doctor if any of the following side effects continue or are bothersome:

More common

Abdominal or stomach pain (mild); bloating or gas; diarrhea; nausea

Less common

Indigestion; vomiting

Other side effects not listed above may also occur in some patients. If you notice any other effects, check with your doctor.

Annual revision: 07/22/92

TIOPRONIN Systemic†

Some commonly used brand names are:

In the U.S.

Thiola

Other

Capen
Captimer
Epatiol
Mucolysin
Sutilan
Thiosol
Tioglis
Vincol

†Not commercially available in Canada.

Description

Tiopronin (tye-oh-PRO-nin) is used to prevent kidney stones, which may develop due to too much cystine in the urine (cystinuria). This medicine works by removing the extra cystine from the body.

In addition to the helpful effects of this medicine, it has side effects that can be very serious. Before you take tiopronin, be sure that you have discussed its use with your doctor.

Tiopronin is available only with your doctor's prescription, in the following dosage form:

Oral

- Tablets (U.S.)

It is very important that you read and understand the following information. If any of it causes you special concern, check with your doctor. Also, *if you have any questions* or if you want more information about this medicine or your medical problem, *ask your doctor, nurse, or pharmacist.*

Before Using This Medicine

In deciding to use a medicine, the risks of taking the medicine must be weighed against the good it will do. This is a decision you and your doctor will make. For tiopronin, the following should be considered:

Allergies—Tell your doctor if you have ever had any unusual or allergic reaction to penicillamine or tiopronin. Also tell your doctor and pharmacist if you are allergic to any other substances, such as foods, preservatives, or dyes.

Diet—It is important that you follow any special instructions from your doctor, such as following a low-methionine diet. Methionine is found in animal proteins such as milk, eggs, cheese, and fish. Also, make certain your doctor and pharmacist know if you are on any special diet, such as a low-sodium or low-sugar diet.

Pregnancy—Studies have not been done in humans. However, studies in animals have shown that tiopronin may cause problems during pregnancy and harmful effects on the fetus.

Breast-feeding—Tiopronin may pass into the breast milk. This medicine is not recommended during breast-feeding because it may cause unwanted effects in nursing babies.

Children—Although there is no specific information comparing use of tiopronin in children with use in other age groups, this medicine is not expected to cause different side effects or problems in children than it does in adults.

Older adults—Many medicines have not been studied specifically in older people. Therefore, it may not be known whether they work exactly the same way they do in younger adults or if they cause different side effects or problems in older people. Although there is no specific information comparing the use of tiopronin in the elderly with use in other age groups, this medicine is not expected to cause different side effects or problems in older people than it does in younger adults.

Other medicines—Although certain medicines should not be used together at all, in other cases two different medicines may be used together even if an interaction might occur. In these cases, your doctor may want to change the dose, or other precautions may be necessary. Tell your doctor and pharmacist if you are taking any other prescription or nonprescription (over-the-counter [OTC]) medicine.

Other medical problems—The presence of other medical problems may affect the use of tiopronin. Make sure you tell your doctor if you have any other medical problems, especially:

- Blood problems (or a history of) or
- Kidney disease (or a history of) or
- Liver disease—Tiopronin may make these conditions worse

Before you begin using any new medicine (prescription or nonprescription) or if you develop any new medical problem while you are using this medicine, check with your doctor, nurse, or pharmacist.

Proper Use of This Medicine

Take this medicine on an empty stomach (at least 30 minutes before meals or 2 hours after meals).

You should drink 2 full glasses (8 ounces each) of water with each meal and at bedtime. You should also drink another 2 full glasses during the night.

It is important that you follow any special instructions from your doctor, such as following a low-methionine diet. Methionine is found in animal proteins such as milk, eggs, cheese, and fish. If you have any questions about this, check with your doctor.

Take this medicine regularly as directed. Do not stop taking it without first checking with your doctor, since stopping the medicine and then restarting it may increase the chance of side effects.

Missed dose—If you of this medicine, take it as soon as possible. However, if it is almost time for your next dose, skip the missed dose and go back to your regular dosing schedule. Do not double doses.

Storage—To store this medicine:

- Keep out of the reach of children.
- Store away from heat and direct light.
- Do not store in the bathroom, near the kitchen sink, or in other damp places. Heat or moisture may cause the medicine to break down.
- Do not keep outdated medicine or medicine no longer needed. Be sure that any discarded medicine is out of the reach of children.

Precautions While Using This Medicine

Your doctor should check your progress at regular visits to make sure that this medicine is working properly and does not cause unwanted effects.

Side Effects of This Medicine

Along with its needed effects, a medicine may cause some unwanted effects. Although not all of these side effects may occur, if they do occur they may need medical attention.

Check with your doctor immediately if any of the following side effects occur:

More common

Yellow skin or eyes

Less common

Muscle pain; sore throat and fever; unusual bleeding or bruising

Check with your doctor as soon as possible if any of the following side effects occur:

More common

Pain, swelling, or tenderness of the skin; skin rash, hives or itching; ulcers or sores in mouth

Less common

Bloody or cloudy urine; chills; difficulty in breathing; high blood pressure; hoarseness; joint pain; swelling of feet or lower legs; tenderness of glands; unusual bleeding

Rare

Chest pain; cough; difficulty in chewing, talking, or swallowing; double vision; general feeling of discomfort, illness, or weakness; muscle weakness; spitting up blood; swelling of lymph glands

Other side effects may occur that usually do not need medical attention. These side effects may go away during treatment as your body adjusts to the medicine. However,

check with your doctor if any of the following side effects continue or are bothersome:

More common

Abdominal or stomach pain; bloating or gas; diarrhea or soft stools; loss of appetite; nausea and vomiting; warts; wrinkling or peeling or unusually dry skin

Less common

Changes in taste or smell

Other side effects not listed above may also occur in some patients. If you notice any other effects, check with your doctor.

Annual revision: 05/19/92

TOBRAMYCIN Ophthalmic

A commonly used brand name in the U.S. and Canada is Tobrex.

Description

Ophthalmic tobramycin (toe-bra-MYE-sin) is used in the eye to treat bacterial infections of the eye. Tobramycin works by killing bacteria.

Ophthalmic tobramycin may be used alone or with other medicines for eye infections. Either the drops or ointment form of this medicine may be used alone during the day. In addition, both forms may be used together, with the drops being used during the day and the ointment at night.

Tobramycin ophthalmic preparations are available only with your doctor's prescription, in the following dosage forms:

Ophthalmic

- Ophthalmic ointment (U.S. and Canada)
- Ophthalmic solution (eye drops) (U.S. and Canada)

It is very important that you read and understand the following information. If any of it causes you special concern, check with your doctor. Also, *if you have any questions* or if you want more information about this medicine or your medical problem, *ask your doctor, nurse, or pharmacist*.

Before Using This Medicine

In deciding to use a medicine, the risks of using the medicine must be weighed against the good it will do. This is a decision you and your doctor will make. For ophthalmic tobramycin, the following should be considered:

Allergies—Tell your doctor if you have ever had any unusual or allergic reaction to ophthalmic tobramycin or to any related medicines, such as amikacin (e.g., Amikin), gentamicin (e.g., Garamycin), kanamycin (e.g., Kantrex), neomycin (e.g., Mycifradin), netilmicin (e.g., Netromycin), streptomycin, or tobramycin by injection (e.g., Nebcin). Also tell your doctor and pharmacist if you are allergic to any other substances, such as preservatives.

Pregnancy—Studies have not been done in humans. However, tobramycin ophthalmic preparations have not been shown to cause birth defects or other problems in animals given high doses.

Breast-feeding—Tobramycin ophthalmic preparations may be absorbed into the eye. However, tobramycin is unlikely to pass into the breast milk in large amounts and little would be absorbed by the infant. Therefore, this medicine is unlikely to cause serious problems in nursing babies.

Children—This medicine has been tested in children and, in effective doses, has not been shown to cause different side effects or problems than it does in adults.

Older adults—Many medicines have not been studied specifically in older people. Therefore, it may not be known whether they work exactly the same way they do in younger adults or if they cause different side effects or problems in older people. There is no specific information comparing use of ophthalmic tobramycin in the elderly with use in other age groups.

Other medicines—Although certain medicines should not be used together at all, in other cases two different medicines may be used together even if an interaction might occur. In these cases, your doctor may want to change the dose, or other precautions may be necessary. Tell your doctor and pharmacist if you are using any other prescription or nonprescription (over-the-counter [OTC]) medicine that is to be used in the eye.

Before you begin using any new medicine (prescription or nonprescription) or if you develop any new medical problem while you are using this medicine, check with your doctor, nurse, or pharmacist.

Proper Use of This Medicine

For patients using tobramycin *ophthalmic solution (eye drops):*

- The bottle is only partially full to provide proper drop control.
- To use:
  —First, wash your hands. Then tilt the head back and pull the lower eyelid away from the eye to form a pouch. Drop the medicine into the pouch and gently close the eyes. Do not blink. Keep the eyes closed for 1 or 2 minutes to allow the medicine to come into contact with the infection.
  —If you think you did not get the drop of medicine into your eye properly, use another drop.
  —To keep the medicine as germ-free as possible, do not touch the applicator tip to any surface (including the eye). Also, keep the container tightly closed.
- If your doctor ordered two different ophthalmic solutions to be used together, wait at least 5 minutes between the times you apply the medicines. This will help to keep the second medicine from "washing out" the first one.

For patients using tobramycin *ophthalmic ointment (eye ointment):*

- To use:
  —First, wash your hands. Then pull the lower eyelid away from the eye to form a pouch. Squeeze a thin strip of ointment into the pouch. A 1.25-cm (approximately ½-inch) strip of ointment is usually enough unless otherwise directed by your doctor. Gently close the eyes and keep them closed for 1 or 2 minutes to allow the medicine to come into contact with the infection.
  —To keep the medicine as germ-free as possible, do not touch the applicator tip to any surface (including the eye). After using tobramycin eye ointment, wipe the tip of the ointment tube with a clean tissue and keep the tube tightly closed.

To help clear up your eye infection completely, *keep using tobramycin for the full time of treatment,* even if your symptoms have disappeared. *Do not miss any doses.*

Dosing—The dose of ophthalmic tobramycin will be different for different patients. *Follow your doctor's orders or the directions on the label.* The following information includes only the average dose of ophthalmic tobramycin. *If your dose is different, do not change it* unless your doctor tells you to do so.

The number of doses you use each day, the time allowed between doses, and the length of time you use the medicine depend on the medical problem for which you are using ophthalmic tobramycin.

- For *ophthalmic ointment* dosage forms:
  —For mild to moderate infections:
    - Adults and children—Use every eight to twelve hours.

  —For severe infections:
    - Adults and children—Use every three to four hours until improvement occurs.
- For *ophthalmic solution (eye drops)* dosage forms:
  —For mild to moderate infections:
    - Adults and children—One drop every four hours.

  —For severe infections:
    - Adults and children—One drop every hour until improvement occurs.

Missed dose—If you miss a dose of this medicine, apply it as soon as possible. However, if it is almost time for your next dose, skip the missed dose and go back to your regular dosing schedule.

Storage—To store this medicine:

- Keep out of the reach of children.
- Store away from heat and direct light.
- Keep the medicine from freezing.
- Do not keep outdated medicine or medicine no longer needed. Be sure that any discarded medicine is out of the reach of children.

Precautions While Using This Medicine

If your eye infection does not improve within a few days, or if it becomes worse, check with your doctor.

Side Effects of This Medicine

Along with its needed effects, a medicine may cause some unwanted effects. Although not all of these side effects may occur, if they do occur they may need medical attention.

Check with your doctor immediately if any of the following side effects occur:

Less common

Itching, redness, swelling, or other sign of eye or eyelid irritation not present before use of this medicine

Symptoms of overdose

Increased watering of the eyes; itching, redness, or swelling of the eyes or eyelids

Other side effects may occur that usually do not need medical attention. These side effects may go away during treatment as your body adjusts to the medicine. However,

check with your doctor if either of the following side effects continues or is bothersome:

Less common

Burning or stinging of the eyes

Eye ointments usually cause your vision to blur for a few minutes after application.

Other side effects not listed above may also occur in some patients. If you notice any other effects, check with your doctor.

Annual revision: 07/01/93

TOCAINIDE Systemic

A commonly used brand name in the U.S. and Canada is Tonocard.

Description

Tocainide (toe-KAY-nide) belongs to the group of medicines known as antiarrhythmics. It is used to correct irregular heartbeats to a normal rhythm.

Tocainide produces its helpful effects by slowing nerve impulses in the heart and making the heart tissue less sensitive.

Tocainide is available only with your doctor's prescription, in the following dosage form:

Oral

- Tablets (U.S. and Canada)

It is very important that you read and understand the following information. If any of it causes you special concern, check with your doctor. Also, *if you have any questions* or if you want more information about this medicine or your medical problem, *ask your doctor, nurse, or pharmacist*.

Before Using This Medicine

In deciding to use a medicine, the risks of taking the medicine must be weighed against the good it will do. This is a decision you and your doctor will make. For tocainide, the following should be considered:

Allergies—Tell your doctor if you have ever had any unusual or allergic reaction to tocainide or anesthetics. Also tell your doctor and pharmacist if you are allergic to any other substance, such as foods, preservatives, or dyes.

Pregnancy—Tocainide has not been shown to cause birth defects or other problems in humans. Studies in animals have shown that high doses of tocainide may increase the possibility of death in the animal fetus, although it has not been shown to cause birth defects.

Breast-feeding—It is not known whether tocainide passes into breast milk. However, this medicine has not been reported to cause problems in nursing babies.

Children—Studies on this medicine have been done only in adult patients and there is no specific information comparing use of tocainide in children with use in other age groups.

Older adults—Dizziness or lightheadedness may be more likely to occur in the elderly, who are usually more sensitive to the effects of tocainide.

Other medicines—Although certain medicines should not be used together at all, in other cases two different medicines may be used together even if an interaction might occur. In these cases, your doctor may want to change the dose, or other precautions may be necessary. Tell your doctor and pharmacist know if you are taking any other prescription or nonprescription (over-the-counter [OTC]) medicine.

Other medical problems—The presence of other medical problems may affect the use of tocainide. Make sure you tell your doctor if you have any other medical problems, especially:

- Congestive heart failure—Tocainide may make this condition worse
- Kidney disease or
- Liver disease—Effects may be increased because of slower removal of tocainide from the body

Before you begin using any new medicine (prescription or nonprescription) or if you develop any new medical problem while you are using this medicine, check with your doctor, nurse, or pharmacist.

Proper Use of This Medicine

Take tocainide exactly as directed by your doctor, even though you may feel well. Do not take more medicine than ordered.

If tocainide upsets your stomach, your doctor may advise you to take it with food or milk.

This medicine works best when there is a constant amount in the blood. *To help keep the amount constant, do not miss any doses. Also, it is best to take the doses at evenly spaced times day and night.* For example, if you are to take 3 doses a day, the doses should be spaced about

8 hours apart. If this interferes with your sleep or other daily activities, or if you need help in planning the best times to take your medicine, check with your doctor, nurse, or pharmacist.

Missed dose—If you miss a dose of tocainide and remember within 4 hours, take it as soon as possible. Then go back to your regular dosing schedule. However, if you do not remember until later, skip the missed dose and go back to your regular dosing schedule. Do not double doses.

Storage—To store this medicine:

- Keep out of the reach of children.
- Store away from heat and direct light.
- Do not store in the bathroom, near the kitchen sink, or in other damp places. Heat or moisture may cause the medicine to break down.
- Do not keep outdated medicine or medicine no longer needed. Be sure that any discarded medicine is out of the reach of children.

Precautions While Using This Medicine

It is important that your doctor check your progress at regular visits to make sure the medicine is working properly. This will allow changes to be made in the amount of medicine you are taking, if necessary.

Your doctor may want you to carry a medical identification card or bracelet stating that you are using this medicine.

Tocainide may cause some people to become dizzy, lightheaded, or less alert than they are normally. *Make sure you know how you react to this medicine before you drive, use machines, or do anything else that could be dangerous if you are dizzy or are not alert.*

Before having any kind of surgery (including dental surgery) or emergency treatment, tell the medical doctor or dentist in charge that you are taking this medicine.

Side Effects of This Medicine

Along with its needed effects, a medicine may cause some unwanted effects. Although not all of these side effects may occur, if they do occur they may need medical attention.

Check with your doctor as soon as possible if any of the following side effects occur:

Less common

Trembling or shaking

Rare

Blisters on skin; cough or shortness of breath; fever or chills; irregular heartbeats; peeling or scaling of skin; skin rash (severe); sores in mouth; unusual bleeding or bruising

Other side effects may occur that usually do not need medical attention. These side effects may go away during treatment as your body adjusts to the medicine. However, check with your doctor if any of the following side effects continue or are bothersome:

More common

Dizziness or lightheadedness; loss of appetite; nausea

Less common

Blurred vision; confusion; headache; nervousness; numbness or tingling of fingers and toes; skin rash; sweating; vomiting

Other side effects not listed above may also occur in some patients. If you notice any other effects, check with your doctor.

Annual revision: 08/06/92

TOLNAFTATE Topical

Some commonly used brand names are:

In the U.S.

Aftate for Athlete's Foot Aerosol Spray Liquid
Aftate for Athlete's Foot Aerosol Spray Powder
Aftate for Athlete's Foot Gel
Aftate for Athlete's Foot Sprinkle Powder
Aftate for Jock Itch Aerosol Spray Powder
Aftate for Jock Itch Gel
Aftate for Jock Itch Sprinkle Powder
Genaspore Cream
NP-27 Cream
NP-27 Powder
NP-27 Solution
NP-27 Spray Powder
Tinactin Aerosol Liquid
Tinactin Aerosol Powder
Tinactin Antifungal Deodorant Powder Aerosol
Tinactin Cream
Tinactin Jock Itch Cream
Tinactin Jock Itch Spray Powder
Tinactin Powder
Tinactin Solution
Ting Antifungal Cream
Ting Antifungal Powder
Ting Antifungal Spray Liquid
Ting Antifungal Spray Powder
Zeasorb-AF Powder

Generic name product may also be available.

In Canada

Pitrex Cream
Tinactin Aerosol Liquid
Tinactin Aerosol Powder
Tinactin Cream
Tinactin Jock Itch Aerosol Powder
Tinactin Jock Itch Cream
Tinactin Plus Aerosol Powder
Tinactin Plus Powder
Tinactin Powder
Tinactin Solution

Description

Tolnaftate (tole-NAF-tate) belongs to the group of medicines called antifungals. It is used to treat some types of fungus infections. It may also be used together with medicines taken by mouth for fungus infections.

Tolnaftate is available without a prescription; however, your doctor may have special instructions on the proper use of tolnaftate for your medical problem.

Tolnaftate is available in the following dosage forms:

Topical

- Aerosol powder (U.S. and Canada)
- Aerosol solution (U.S. and Canada)
- Cream (U.S. and Canada)
- Gel (U.S.)
- Powder (U.S. and Canada)
- Topical solution (U.S. and Canada)

It is very important that you read and understand the following information. If any of it causes you special concern, check with your doctor or pharmacist. Also, *if you have any questions* or if you want more information about this medicine or your medical problem, *ask your doctor, nurse, or pharmacist.*

Before Using This Medicine

If you are taking this medicine without a prescription, carefully read and follow any precautions on the label. For tolnaftate, the following should be considered:

Allergies—Tell your doctor if you have ever had any unusual or allergic reaction to tolnaftate. Also tell your doctor and pharmacist if you are allergic to any other substances, such as preservatives or dyes.

Pregnancy—Tolnaftate topical preparations have not been shown to cause birth defects or other problems in humans.

Breast-feeding—Tolnaftate topical preparations have not been reported to cause problems in nursing babies.

Children—Tolnaftate should not be used on children up to 2 years of age, unless otherwise directed by your doctor. Although there is no specific information comparing use of tolnaftate in children 2 years of age and older with use in other age groups, this medicine is not expected to cause different side effects or problems in children 2 years of age and older than it does in adults.

Older adults—Many medicines have not been studied specifically in older people. Therefore, it may not be known whether they work exactly the same way they do in younger adults or if they cause different side effects or problems in older people. There is no specific information comparing use of tolnaftate in the elderly with use in other age groups.

Other medicines—Although certain medicines should not be used together at all, in other cases two different medicines may be used together even if an interaction might occur. In these cases, your doctor may want to change the dose, or other precautions may be necessary. Tell your doctor and pharmacist if you are using any other topical prescription or nonprescription (over-the-counter [OTC]) medicine that is to be applied to the same area of the skin.

Before you begin using any new medicine (prescription or nonprescription) or if you develop any new medical problem while you are using this medicine, check with your doctor, nurse, or pharmacist.

Proper Use of This Medicine

Before applying tolnaftate, wash the affected area and dry thoroughly. Then apply enough medicine to cover the affected area.

Keep this medicine away from the eyes.

For patients using the *powder form* of this medicine:

- If the powder is used on the feet, sprinkle it between toes, on feet, and in socks and shoes.

For patients using the *aerosol powder form* of this medicine:

- Shake well before using.
- From a distance of 6 to 10 inches, spray the powder on the affected areas. If it is used on the feet, spray it between toes, on feet, and in socks and shoes.
- Do not inhale the powder.
- Do not use near heat, near open flame, or while smoking.

For patients using the *solution form* of this medicine:

- If tolnaftate solution becomes a solid, it may be dissolved by warming the closed container of medicine in warm water.

For patients using the *aerosol solution form* of this medicine:

- Shake well before using.
- From a distance of 6 inches, spray the solution on the affected areas. If it is used on the feet, spray between toes and on feet.
- Do not inhale the vapors from the spray.
- Do not use near heat, near open flame, or while smoking.

To help clear up your infection completely, *keep using this medicine for 2 weeks after burning, itching, or other symptoms have disappeared,* unless otherwise directed by your doctor. *Do not miss any doses.*

Missed dose—If you do miss a dose of this medicine, apply it as soon as possible. Then go back to your regular dosing schedule.

Storage—To store this medicine:

- Keep out of the reach of children.
- Store away from heat and direct light.
- Do not store the powder form of this medicine in the bathroom, near the kitchen sink, or in other damp

places. Heat or moisture may cause the medicine to break down.

- Keep the medicine from freezing.
- Do not puncture, break, or burn the aerosol powder or aerosol solution container.
- Do not keep outdated medicine or medicine no longer needed. Be sure that any discarded medicine is out of the reach of children.

Precautions While Using This Medicine

If your skin problem does not improve within 4 weeks, or if it becomes worse, check with your doctor or pharmacist.

To help prevent reinfection after the period of treatment with this medicine, the powder or spray powder form of this medicine may be used each day after bathing and carefully drying the affected area.

Side Effects of This Medicine

Along with its needed effects, a medicine may cause some unwanted effects. Although not all of these side effects may occur, if they do occur they may need medical attention.

Check with your doctor or pharmacist as soon as possible if the following side effect occurs:

Skin irritation not present before use of this medicine

When you apply the aerosol solution form of this medicine, a mild temporary stinging may be expected.

Other side effects not listed above may also occur in some patients. If you notice any other effects, check with your doctor or pharmacist.

Annual revision: 11/05/91
Interim revision: 02/03/92

TRAZODONE Systemic

Some commonly used brand names are:

In the U.S.
Desyrel
Trazon
Trialodine

Generic name product may also be available.

In Canada
Desyrel

Description

Trazodone (TRAZ-oh-done) belongs to the group of medicines known as antidepressants or "mood elevators." It is used to relieve mental depression and depression that sometimes occurs with anxiety.

Trazodone is available only with your doctor's prescription, in the following dosage form:

Oral

- Tablets (U.S. and Canada)

It is very important that you read and understand the following information. If any of it causes you special concern, check with your doctor. Also, *if you have any questions* or if you want more information about this medicine or your medical problem, *ask your doctor, nurse, or pharmacist.*

Before Using This Medicine

In deciding to use a medicine, the risks of taking the medicine must be weighed against the good it will do. This is a decision you and your doctor will make. For trazodone, the following should be considered:

Allergies—Tell your doctor if you have ever had any unusual or allergic reaction to trazodone. Also tell your doctor and pharmacist if you are allergic to any other substances, such as foods, preservatives, or dyes.

Pregnancy—Studies have not been done in pregnant women. However, studies in animals have shown that trazodone causes birth defects and a decrease in the number of successful pregnancies when given in doses many times larger than human doses.

Breast-feeding—Trazodone passes into breast milk.

Children—Studies on this medicine have been done only in adult patients, and there is no specific information comparing use of trazodone in children with use in other age groups.

Older adults—Drowsiness, dizziness, confusion, vision problems, dryness of mouth, and constipation may be more likely to occur in the elderly, who are usually more sensitive to the effects of trazodone.

Other medicines—Although certain medicines should not be used together at all, in other cases two different medicines may be used together even if an interaction might occur. In these cases, your doctor may want to change the dose, or other precautions may be necessary. When you are taking trazodone, it is especially important that

your doctor and pharmacist know if you are taking any of the following:

- Antihypertensives (high blood pressure medicine)—Taking these medicines with trazodone may result in low blood pressure (hypotension); the amount of medicine you need to take may change
- Central nervous system (CNS) depressants (medicine that causes drowsiness) or
- Tricyclic antidepressants (medicine for depression)—Taking these medicines with trazodone may add to the CNS depressant effects

Other medical problems—The presence of other medical problems may affect the use of trazodone. Make sure you tell your doctor if you have any other medical problems, especially:

- Alcohol abuse (or history of)—Drinking alcohol with trazodone will increase the central nervous system (CNS) depressant effects
- Heart disease—Trazodone may make the condition worse
- Kidney disease or
- Liver disease—Higher blood levels of trazodone may occur, increasing the chance of side effects

Before you begin using any new medicine (prescription or nonprescription) or if you develop any new medical problem while you are using this medicine, check with your doctor, nurse, or pharmacist.

Proper Use of This Medicine

To lessen stomach upset and to reduce dizziness and lightheadedness, take this medicine with or shortly after a meal or light snack, even for a daily bedtime dose, unless your doctor has told you to take it on an empty stomach.

Take trazodone only as directed by your doctor, to benefit your condition as much as possible.

Sometimes trazodone must be taken for up to 4 weeks before you begin to feel better, although most people notice improvement within 2 weeks.

Dosing—The dose of trazodone will be different for different patients. *Follow your doctor's orders or the directions on the label.* The following information includes only the average doses of trazodone. *If your dose is different, do not change it* unless your doctor tells you to do so:

- Adults—Oral, to start, 50 milligrams per dose taken three times a day, or 75 milligrams per dose taken two times a day. Your doctor may increase your dose if needed.
- Children 6 to 18 years of age—Oral. Your doctor will tell you what dose to take based on your body weight.
- Children up to 6 years of age—Dose must be determined by the doctor.
- Elderly patients—Oral, to start, 25 milligrams per dose taken three times a day. Your doctor may increase your dose if needed.

Missed dose—If you miss a dose of this medicine, take it as soon as possible. However, if it is within 4 hours of your next dose, skip the missed dose and go back to your regular dosing schedule. Do not double doses.

Storage—To store this medicine:

- Keep out of the reach of children.
- Store away from heat and direct light.
- Do not store in the bathroom, near the kitchen sink, or in other damp places. Heat or moisture may cause the medicine to break down.
- Do not keep outdated medicine or medicine no longer needed. Be sure that any discarded medicine is out of the reach of children.

Precautions While Using This Medicine

It is very important that your doctor check your progress at regular visits. This will allow your doctor to check the medicine's effects and to change the dose if needed.

Do not stop taking this medicine without first checking with your doctor. To prevent a possible return of your medical problem, your doctor may want you to reduce gradually the amount of medicine you are using before you stop completely.

Before having any kind of surgery, dental treatment, or emergency treatment, tell the medical doctor or dentist in charge that you are using this medicine. Taking trazodone together with medicines that are used during surgery or dental or emergency treatments may increase the CNS depressant effects.

This medicine will add to the effects of alcohol and other CNS depressants (medicines that slow down the nervous system, possibly causing drowsiness). Some examples of CNS depressants are antihistamines or medicine for hay fever, other allergies, or colds; sedatives, tranquilizers, or sleeping medicine; prescription pain medicine or narcotics; barbiturates; medicine for seizures; muscle relaxants; or anesthetics, including some dental anesthetics. *Check with your doctor before taking any of the above while you are using this medicine.*

This medicine may cause some people to become drowsy or less alert than they are normally. *Make sure you know how you react to this medicine before you drive, use machines, or do anything else that could be dangerous if you are not alert.*

Dizziness, lightheadedness, or fainting may occur, especially when you get up from a lying or sitting position. Getting up slowly may help. If this problem continues or gets worse, check with your doctor.

Trazodone may cause dryness of the mouth. For temporary relief, use sugarless gum or candy, melt bits of ice in your mouth, or use a saliva substitute. However, if your mouth continues to feel dry for more than 2 weeks, check with your medical doctor or dentist. Continuing dryness of the mouth may increase the chance of dental disease, including tooth decay, gum disease, and fungus infections.

Side Effects of This Medicine

Along with its needed effects, a medicine may cause some unwanted effects. Although not all of these side effects may occur, if they do occur they may need medical attention.

Stop taking this medicine and check with your doctor immediately if the following side effect occurs:

Rare

Painful, inappropriate erection of the penis, continuing

Also, check with your doctor as soon as possible if any of the following side effects occur:

Less common

Confusion; muscle tremors

Rare

Fainting; fast or slow heartbeat; skin rash; unusual excitement

Symptoms of overdose

Drowsiness; loss of muscle coordination; nausea and vomiting

Other side effects may occur that usually do not need medical attention. These side effects may go away during treatment as your body adjusts to the medicine. However, check with your doctor if any of the following side effects continue or are bothersome:

More common

Dizziness or lightheadedness; drowsiness; dryness of mouth (usually mild); headache; nausea and vomiting; unpleasant taste

Less common

Blurred vision; constipation; diarrhea; muscle aches or pains; unusual tiredness or weakness

Other side effects not listed above may also occur in some patients. If you notice any other effects, check with your doctor.

Annual revision: 01/13/93

TRETINOIN Topical

Some commonly used brand names are:

In the U.S.
- Retin-A
- Retin-A Regimen Kit

In Canada
- Retin-A
- Stieva-A
- Stieva-A Forte
- Vitamin A Acid

Another commonly used name is retinoic acid.

Description

Tretinoin (TRET-i-noyn) is used to treat certain types of acne. It may also be used to treat other skin diseases as determined by your doctor.

Although tretinoin is being used to treat skin that has been damaged by long time exposure to sunlight, there is not enough information to show that this treatment is safe and effective.

Tretinoin is available only with your doctor's prescription, in the following dosage forms:

Topical

- Cream (U.S. and Canada)
- Gel (U.S. and Canada)
- Topical solution (U.S. and Canada)

It is very important that you read and understand the following information. If any of it causes you special concern, check with your doctor. Also, *if you have any questions* or if you want more information about this medicine or your medical problem, *ask your doctor, nurse, or pharmacist.*

Before Using This Medicine

In deciding to use a medicine, the risks of taking the medicine must be weighed against the good it will do. This is a decision you and your doctor will make. For tretinoin, the following should be considered:

Allergies—Tell your doctor if you have ever had any unusual or allergic reaction to etretinate, isotretinoin, tretinoin, or vitamin A preparations. Also tell your doctor and pharmacist if you are allergic to any other substances, such as preservatives or dyes.

Pregnancy—Tretinoin has not been studied in pregnant women. Topical tretinoin has been shown to cause some delayed bone development in some animal fetuses. Before using this medicine, make sure your doctor knows if you are pregnant or if you may become pregnant.

Breast-feeding—It is not known whether tretinoin passes into the breast milk. However, this medicine has not been reported to cause problems in nursing babies.

Children—Studies on this medicine have been done only in adult patients, and there is no specific information comparing use of this medicine in children with use in other age groups.

Older adults—Many medicines have not been studied specifically in older people. Therefore, it may not be known whether they work exactly the same way they do in younger adults or if they cause different side effects or problems in older people. There is no specific information comparing use of tretinoin in the elderly with use in other age groups.

Other medicines—Although certain medicines should not be used together at all, in other cases two different medicines may be used together even if an interaction might occur. In these cases, your doctor may want to change the dose, or other precautions may be necessary. Tell your doctor and pharmacist if you are using any other topical prescription or nonprescription (over-the-counter [OTC]) medicine that is to be applied to the same area of the skin.

Other medical problems—The presence of other medical problems may affect the use of tretinoin. Make sure you tell your doctor if you have any other medical problems, especially:

- Eczema or
- Sunburn—Use of this medicine may cause or increase the irritation associated with these problems

Before you begin using any new medicine (prescription or nonprescription) or if you develop any new medical problem while you are using this medicine, check with your doctor, nurse, or pharmacist.

Proper Use of This Medicine

It is very important that you use this medicine only as directed. Do not use more of it, do not use it more often, and do not use it for a longer time than your doctor ordered. To do so may cause irritation of the skin.

Do not apply this medicine to windburned or sunburned skin or on open wounds.

Do not use this medicine in or around the eyes or mouth, or inside of the nose. Spread the medicine away from these areas when applying.

This medicine usually comes with patient directions. Read them carefully before using the medicine.

Before applying tretinoin, wash the skin with a mild or nonallergic type of soap and warm water; then gently pat dry. Wait 20 to 30 minutes before applying this medicine to make sure the skin is completely dry.

To use the *cream or gel form* of this medicine:

- Apply enough medicine to cover the affected areas, and rub in gently.

To use the *solution form* of this medicine:

- Using your fingertips, a gauze pad, or a cotton swab, apply enough tretinoin solution to cover the affected areas. If you use a gauze pad or a cotton swab for applying the medicine, avoid getting it too wet, to prevent the medicine from running into areas not intended for treatment.

Missed dose—If you miss a dose of this medicine, skip the missed dose and go back to your regular dosing schedule. Do not double doses.

Storage—To store this medicine:

- Keep out of the reach of children.
- Store away from heat and direct light.
- Keep the medicine from freezing.
- Do not keep outdated medicine or medicine no longer needed. Be sure that any discarded medicine is out of the reach of children.

Precautions While Using This Medicine

During the first 2 or 3 weeks you are using tretinoin, your acne may seem to get worse before it gets better. However, you should not stop using tretinoin unless irritation or other symptoms become severe. If you have any questions about this, check with your doctor.

You should avoid washing your face too often. Washing it with a mild bland soap 2 or 3 times a day should be enough, unless you are otherwise directed by your doctor.

When using tretinoin, do not use any of the following preparations on the same affected area as this medicine, unless otherwise directed by your doctor:

Abrasive soaps or cleansers
Alcohol-containing preparations
Any other topical acne preparation or preparation containing a peeling agent (for example, benzoyl peroxide, resorcinol, salicylic acid, or sulfur)
Cosmetics or soaps that dry the skin
Medicated cosmetics
Other topical medicine for the skin

To use any of the above preparations on the same affected area as tretinoin may cause severe irritation of the skin.

You may use cosmetics (nonmedicated) while being treated with tretinoin, unless otherwise directed by your doctor. However, the areas to be treated must be washed thoroughly before the medicine is applied.

During treatment with this medicine, *avoid exposing the treated areas to too much sunlight or overuse of a sunlamp*, since the skin may be more prone to sunburn.

If exposure to too much sunlight cannot be avoided while you are using this medicine, use sunscreen preparations or wear protective clothing over the treated areas.

Some people who use this medicine may become more sensitive to wind and cold temperatures than they are normally. *When you first begin using this medicine, use protection against wind or cold until you see how you react.* If you notice severe skin irritation, check with your doctor.

Side Effects of This Medicine

In some animal studies, tretinoin has been shown to cause skin tumors to develop faster when the treated area is exposed to ultraviolet light (sunlight or artificial sunlight of a sunlamp). It is not known if tretinoin causes skin tumors to develop faster in humans.

Along with its needed effects, a medicine may cause some unwanted effects. Although not all of these side effects may occur, if they do occur they may need medical attention.

Check with your doctor as soon as possible if any of the following side effects occur:

Blistering, crusting, severe burning or redness, or swelling of skin; darkening or lightening of the treated skin

Other side effects may occur that usually do not need medical attention. These side effects may go away during treatment as your body adjusts to the medicine. However, check with your doctor if any of the following side effects continue or are bothersome:

Feeling of warmth on skin; peeling of skin (may occur after a few days); stinging (mild) or redness of skin

The side effects of tretinoin will go away after you stop using the medicine. However, the side effect of darkening or lightening of the skin may take several months before it goes away.

Other side effects not listed above may also occur in some patients. If you notice any other effects, check with your doctor.

Annual revision: 01/15/92

TRIENTINE Systemic†

A commonly used brand name in the U.S. is Syprine.

Another commonly used name is trien.

†Not commercially available in Canada.

Description

Trientine (TRYE-en-teen) is used to treat Wilson's disease, a disease in which there is too much copper in the body.

This medicine combines with excess copper in the body and may prevent your body from absorbing the copper in the foods you eat. Removing copper from the body prevents damage to the liver, brain, and other organs. The combination of copper and trientine is then easily removed by the kidneys and it passes from the body in urine.

Trientine is available only with your doctor's prescription, in the following dosage form:

Oral

- Capsules (U.S.)

It is very important that you read and understand the following information. If any of it causes you special concern, check with your doctor. Also, *if you have any questions* or if you want more information about this medicine or your medical problem, *ask your doctor, nurse, or pharmacist.*

Before Using This Medicine

In deciding to use a medicine, the risks of taking the medicine must be weighed against the good it will do. This is a decision you and your doctor will make. For trientine, the following should be considered:

Pregnancy—Trientine has not been shown to cause birth defects or other problems in humans. However, it has been shown to cause birth defects in rats.

Breast-feeding—It is not known whether trientine passes into the breast milk. This medicine has not been reported to cause problems in nursing babies.

Children—Anemia is especially likely to occur in children during treatment with trientine.

Older adults—Many medicines have not been studied specifically in older people. Therefore, it may not be known whether they work exactly the same way they do in younger adults or if they cause different side effects or problems in older people. There is no specific information comparing use of trientine in the elderly with use in other age groups.

Other medicines—Although certain medicines should not be used together at all, in other cases two different medicines may be used together even if an interaction might occur. In these cases, your doctor may want to change the dose, or other precautions may be necessary. When

you are taking trientine, it is especially important that your doctor and pharmacist know if you are taking:

- Copper supplements or
- Iron supplements or other medicine containing minerals (contained in some vitamin combination products)—Use of these medicines with trientine may decrease the effects of trientine; iron supplements or other medicines containing minerals should be given 2 hours before or after trientine

Other medical problems—The presence of other medical problems may affect the use of trientine. Make sure you tell your doctor if you have any other medical problems, especially:

- Iron-deficiency—Trientine may make this condition worse

Before you begin using any new medicine (prescription or nonprescription) or if you develop any new medical problem while you are using this medicine, check with your doctor, nurse, or pharmacist.

Proper Use of This Medicine

Take trientine with water. The capsule should be swallowed whole. It must not be opened, crushed, or chewed.

Take this medicine on an empty stomach (at least 1 hour before or 2 hours after meals) and at least 1 hour before or after any other medicine, food, or milk. This will allow trientine to be better absorbed by your body.

Trientine will not cure Wilson's disease, but it will help remove the excess copper from your body. Therefore, *you must continue to take this medicine regularly, as directed. You may have to take trientine for the rest of your life.* If Wilson's disease is not treated continually, it can cause severe liver damage and can cause death. *Do not stop taking this medicine without first checking with your doctor.*

It is very important for you to follow any special instructions from your doctor, such as following a low-copper diet. You may need to avoid foods known to be high in copper, such as chocolate, mushrooms, liver, molasses, broccoli, cereals enriched with copper, shellfish, organ meats, and nuts. If you have any questions about this, check with your doctor.

Take this medicine only as directed by your doctor. Do not take more or less of it and do not take it more often than your doctor ordered. If too much is used, it may increase the chance of side effects.

Missed dose—If you miss a dose of this medicine, double the next dose. Do not make up more than one missed dose at a time.

Storage—To store this medicine:

- Keep out of the reach of children.
- Store sealed, unopened bottles of trientine in the refrigerator, but not in the freezer. Before opening a sealed bottle, let it stand at room temperature for about 6 hours. Keep it at room temperature after opening it.
- Do not store in the bathroom, near the kitchen sink, or in other damp places. Heat or moisture may cause the medicine to break down.
- Do not keep outdated medicine or medicine no longer needed. Be sure that any discarded medicine is out of the reach of children.

Precautions While Using This Medicine

Your doctor should check your progress at regular visits to make sure trientine is working properly and to check for unwanted effects. Laboratory tests may be needed. This will allow your doctor to change your dose, if necessary.

During the first month of treatment, you may need to take your temperature each night. *Tell your doctor if you develop a fever or skin rash.*

Do not take copper or iron preparations or any other mineral supplements within 2 hours of taking trientine. This includes any vitamin preparation that contains minerals.

If a capsule breaks open and the contents touch your skin, wash the area right away with water. Trientine may cause a rash.

Side Effects of This Medicine

Along with its needed effects, a medicine may cause some unwanted effects. Although not all of these side effects may occur, if they do occur they may need medical attention.

Check with your doctor as soon as possible if any of the following side effects occur:

More common—Symptoms of anemia

Unusually pale skin; unusual tiredness

Note: The above signs of anemia are more likely to occur in children, menstruating women, and pregnant women, who usually need more iron than other patients. If these signs appear during trientine treatment, your doctor will need to do some tests.

Rare

Fever; general feeling of discomfort, illness, or weakness; joint pain; skin rash, blisters, hives, or itching; swollen glands

Other side effects not listed above may also occur in some patients. If you notice any other effects, check with your doctor.

Annual revision: 09/17/92

TRIFLURIDINE Ophthalmic

A commonly used brand name in the U.S. and Canada is Viroptic. Another commonly used name is trifluorothymidine.

Description

Trifluridine (trye-FLURE-i-deen) ophthalmic preparations are used to treat virus infections of the eye.

Trifluridine is available only with your doctor's prescription, in the following dosage form:

Ophthalmic

- Ophthalmic solution (eye drops) (U.S. and Canada)

It is very important that you read and understand the following information. If any of it causes you special concern, check with your doctor. Also, *if you have any questions* or if you want more information about this medicine or your medical problem, *ask your doctor, nurse, or pharmacist.*

Before Using This Medicine

In deciding to use a medicine, the risks of using the medicine must be weighed against the good it will do. This is a decision you and your doctor will make. For trifluridine, the following should be considered:

Allergies—Tell your doctor if you have ever had any unusual or allergic reaction to trifluridine. Also tell your doctor and pharmacist if you are allergic to any other substances, such as preservatives.

Pregnancy—Studies have not been done in humans. When injected into developing chick embryos, trifluridine has been shown to cause birth defects. However, studies in rats and rabbits have not shown that trifluridine causes birth defects, although it did cause delayed bone formation in rats and rabbits and death in unborn rabbits.

Breast-feeding—It is unlikely that trifluridine, used in the eyes, is absorbed into the mother's body and passes into the breast milk. In addition, trifluridine has not been reported to cause problems in nursing babies.

Children—Although there is no specific information comparing the use of trifluridine in children with use in other age groups, it is not expected to cause different side effects or problems in children than it does in adults.

Older adults—Many medicines have not been studied specifically in older people. Therefore, it may not be known whether they work exactly the same way they do in younger adults or if they cause different side effects or problems in older people. There is no specific information comparing the use of trifluridine in the elderly with use in other age groups.

Other medicines—Although certain medicines should not be used together at all, in other cases two different medicines may be used together even if an interaction might occur. In these cases, your doctor may want to change the dose, or other precautions may be necessary. Tell your doctor and pharmacist if you are using any other prescription or nonprescription (over-the-counter [OTC]) medicine that is to be used in the eye.

Before you begin using any new medicine (prescription or nonprescription) or if you develop any new medical problem while you are using this medicine, check with your doctor, nurse, or pharmacist.

Proper Use of This Medicine

The bottle is only partially full to provide proper drop control.

To use:

- First, wash your hands. Then tilt the head back and pull the lower eyelid away from the eye to form a pouch. Drop the medicine into the pouch and gently close the eyes. Do not blink. Keep the eyes closed for 1 or 2 minutes to allow the medicine to come into contact with the infection.
- If you think you did not get the drop of medicine into your eye properly, use another drop.
- To keep the medicine as germ-free as possible, do not touch the applicator tip to any surface (including the eye). Also, keep the container tightly closed.

Do not use this medicine more often or for a longer time than your doctor ordered. To do so may cause problems in the eyes. If you have any questions about this, check with your doctor.

To help clear up your infection completely, *keep using this medicine for the full time of treatment,* even if your symptoms have disappeared. *Do not miss any doses.*

Dosing—The dose of ophthalmic trifluridine will be different for different patients. *Follow your doctor's orders or the directions on the label.* The following information includes only the average doses of ophthalmic trifluridine. *If your dose is different, do not change it unless your doctor tells you to do so.*

The number of doses you use each day, the time allowed between doses, and the length of time you use the medicine depend on the medical problem for which you are using ophthalmic trifluridine.

- For *ophthalmic solution* dosage forms:
  - —For virus eye infection:
    - Adults and children—One drop every two hours while you are awake. After healing has occurred, the dose may be reduced for seven more days to one drop every four hours (at least 5 doses a day) while you are awake.

Missed dose—If you miss a dose of this medicine, apply it as soon as possible. However, if it is almost time for your next dose, skip the missed dose and go back to your regular dosing schedule.

Storage—To store this medicine:

- Keep out of the reach of children.
- Store in the refrigerator because heat will cause this medicine to break down. However, keep the medicine from freezing. Follow the directions on the label.
- Do not keep outdated medicine or medicine no longer needed. Be sure that any discarded medicine is out of the reach of children.

Precautions While Using This Medicine

It is very important that you keep your appointment with your doctor. If your symptoms become worse, check with your doctor sooner.

Side Effects of This Medicine

Along with its needed effects, a medicine may cause some unwanted effects. Although not all of these side effects may occur, if they do occur they may need medical attention.

Check with your doctor as soon as possible if any of the following side effects occur:

Rare

Blurred vision or other change in vision; dryness of eye; irritation of eye; itching, redness, swelling, or other sign of irritation not present before use of this medicine

Other side effects may occur that usually do not need medical attention. These side effects may go away during treatment as your body adjusts to the medicine. However, check with your doctor if either of the following side effects continues or is bothersome:

More common

Burning or stinging

Other side effects not listed above may also occur in some patients. If you notice any other effects, check with your doctor.

Annual revision: 07/01/93

TRILOSTANE Systemic†

A commonly used brand name in the U.S. is Modrastane.

†Not commercially available in Canada.

Description

Trilostane (TRYE-loe-stane) is used in the treatment of Cushing's syndrome. It is normally used in short-term treatment until permanent therapy is possible.

In Cushing's syndrome, the adrenal gland overproduces steroids. Although steroids are important for various functions of the body, too much can cause problems. Trilostane reduces the amount of steroids produced by the adrenal gland.

Trilostane is available only with your doctor's prescription, in the following dosage form:

Oral

- Capsules (U.S.)

It is very important that you read and understand the following information. If any of it causes you special concern, check with your doctor. Also, *if you have any questions* or if you want more information about this medicine or your medical problem, *ask your doctor, nurse, or pharmacist.*

Before Using This Medicine

In deciding to use a medicine, the risks of taking the medicine must be weighed against the good it will do.

This is a decision you and your doctor will make. For trilostane, the following should be considered:

Allergies—Tell your doctor if you have ever had any unusual or allergic reaction to trilostane. Also tell your doctor and pharmacist if you are allergic to any other substance, such as foods, preservatives, or dyes.

Pregnancy—Use of trilostane is not recommended during pregnancy. It has been shown to cause serious problems, including miscarriage, in humans. Trilostane has also been shown to cause birth defects in animals.

Breast-feeding—It is not known whether trilostane passes into breast milk. However, this medicine has not been reported to cause problems in nursing babies.

Children—There is no specific information about the use of trilostane in children.

Older adults—Many medicines have not been tested in older people. Therefore, it may not be known whether they work exactly the same way they do in younger adults or if they cause different side effects or problems in older people. There is no specific information about the use of trilostane in the elderly.

Other medicines—Although certain medicines should not be used together at all, in other cases two different medicines may be used together even if an interaction might occur. In these cases, your doctor may want to change the dose, or other precautions may be necessary. When you are taking trilostane, it is especially important that your doctor and pharmacist know if you are taking any other prescription or nonprescription (over-the-counter [OTC]) medicine.

Other medical problems—The presence of other medical problems may affect the use of trilostane. Make sure you tell your doctor if you have any other medical problems, especially:

- Infection or
- Injury (recent serious)—Trilostane may weaken the body's normal defenses
- Kidney disease
- Liver disease

Before you begin using any new medicine (prescription or nonprescription) or if you develop any new medical problem while you are using this medicine, check with your doctor, nurse, or pharmacist.

Proper Use of This Medicine

Take trilostane only as directed by your doctor. Do not take more or less of it, and do not take it more often than your doctor ordered.

Missed dose—If you miss a dose of this medicine, take it as soon as possible. However, if it is almost time for your next dose, skip the missed dose and go back to your regular dosing schedule. Do not double doses.

Storage—To store this medicine:

- Keep out of the reach of children.
- Store away from heat and direct light.
- Do not store in the bathroom, near the kitchen sink, or in other damp places. Heat or moisture may cause the medicine to break down.
- Do not keep outdated medicine or medicine no longer needed. Be sure that any discarded medicine is out of the reach of children.

Precautions While Using This Medicine

It is very important that your doctor check your progress at regular visits to make sure that trilostane is working properly and does not cause unwanted effects.

Check with your doctor right away if you get an injury, infection, or illness of any kind. This medicine may weaken your body's normal defenses.

Before having any kind of surgery (including dental surgery) or emergency treatment, tell the medical doctor or dentist in charge that you are taking trilostane.

Your doctor may want you to carry a medical identification card or wear a bracelet stating that you are taking this medicine.

Side Effects of This Medicine

Along with its needed effects, a medicine may cause some unwanted effects. Although not all of these side effects may occur, if they do occur they may need medical attention.

Check with your doctor as soon as possible if any of the following side effects occur:

Rare

Darkening of skin; drowsiness or tiredness; loss of appetite; mental depression; skin rash; vomiting

Other side effects may occur that usually do not need medical attention. These side effects may go away during treatment as your body adjusts to the medicine. However, check with your doctor or nurse if any of the following side effects continue or are bothersome:

More common

Diarrhea; stomach pain or cramps

Less common

Aching muscles; belching or bloating; burning mouth or nose; dizziness or lightheadedness; fever; flushing; headache; increase in salivation; nausea; watery eyes

Other side effects not listed above may also occur in some patients. If you notice any other effects, check with your doctor.

Annual revision: September 1990

TRIMETHOBENZAMIDE Systemic†

Some commonly used brand names are:

In the U.S.

Arrestin	T-Gen
Benzacot	Ticon
Bio-Gan	Tigan
Stemetic	Tiject-20
Tebamide	Triban
Tegamide	Tribenzagan

Generic name product may also be available.

†Not commercially available in Canada.

Description

Trimethobenzamide (trye-meth-oh-BEN-za-mide) is used to treat nausea and vomiting.

This medicine is available only with your doctor's prescription in the following dosage forms:

Oral

- Capsules (U.S.)

Parenteral

- Injection (U.S.)

Rectal

- Suppositories (U.S.)

It is very important that you read and understand the following information. If any of it causes you special concern, check with your doctor. Also, *if you have any questions* or if you want more information about this medicine or your medical problem, *ask your doctor, nurse, or pharmacist.*

Before Using This Medicine

In deciding to use a medicine, the risks of taking the medicine must be weighed against the good it will do. This is a decision you and your doctor will make. For trimethobenzamide, the following should be considered:

Allergies—Tell your doctor if you have ever had any unusual or allergic reaction to trimethobenzamide, or if you are allergic or sensitive to benzocaine or other local anesthetics (the suppository form of this medicine contains benzocaine). Also tell your doctor and pharmacist if you are allergic to any other substances, such as foods, preservatives, or dyes.

Pregnancy—Studies have not been done in pregnant women. However, although studies in animals have not shown that trimethobenzamide causes birth defects, it has been shown to increase the chance of a miscarriage.

Breast-feeding—It is not known whether trimethobenzamide passes into breast milk. Although most medicines pass into breast milk in small amounts, many of them may be used safely while breast-feeding. Mothers who are taking this medicine and who wish to breast-feed should discuss this with their doctor.

Children—This medicine should not be used to treat nausea and vomiting in children unless otherwise directed by your doctor. Some side effects may be more serious in children.

Older adults—Many medicines have not been studied specifically in older people. Therefore, it may not be known whether they work exactly the same way they do in younger adults or if they cause different side effects or problems in older people. There is no specific information comparing use of trimethobenzamide in the elderly with use in other age groups.

Other medicines—Although certain medicines should not be used together at all, in other cases 2 different medicines may be used together even if an interaction might occur. In these cases, your doctor may want to change the dose, or other precautions may be necessary. When you are using trimethobenzamide, it is especially important that your doctor and pharmacist know if you are taking any of the following:

- Central nervous system (CNS) depressants (medicine that causes drowsiness) or
- Tricyclic antidepressants (medicine for depression)—Taking these medicines with trimethobenzamide may cause increased CNS depressant or other serious effects

Other medical problems—The presence of other medical problems may affect the use of trimethobenzamide. Make sure you tell your doctor if you have any other medical problems, especially:

- High fever or
- Intestinal infection—Using trimethobenzamide may result in serious side effects

Before you begin using any new medicine (prescription or nonprescription) or if you develop any new medical

problem while you are using this medicine, check with your doctor, nurse, or pharmacist.

Proper Use of This Medicine

Do not use this medicine to treat nausea and vomiting in children unless otherwise directed by your doctor. If you are giving this medicine to a child, be especially careful not to give more than is prescribed since side effects may be more serious in children.

Trimethobenzamide is used only to relieve or prevent nausea and vomiting. Use it only as directed. Do not use more of it and do not use it more often than your doctor ordered. To do so may increase the chance of side effects.

To insert the *rectal suppository form* of this medicine:

- First, remove foil wrapper and moisten the suppository with cold water. Lie down on your side and use your finger to push the suppository well up into the rectum. If the suppository is too soft to insert, chill it in the refrigerator for 30 minutes or run cold water over it before removing the foil wrapper.
- Wash your hands with soap and water.

Dosing—The dose of trimethobenzamide will be different for different patients. *Follow your doctor's orders or the directions on the label.* The following information includes only the average doses of trimethobenzamide. *If your dose is different, do not change it* unless your doctor tells you to do so.

- The number of capsules that you take, or suppositories that you use, depends on the strength of the medicine. Also, *the number of doses you take each day, the time allowed between doses, and the length of time you take the medicine depend on the medical problem for which you are taking trimethobenzamide.*
- For *oral* dosage form (capsules):
  —For nausea and vomiting:
  - Adults and children 12 years of age and older—250 milligrams (mg) three or four times a day as needed.
  - Children—Dose is based on body weight and must be determined by your doctor. The usual dose is 15 mg per kilogram (6.8 mg per pound). The dose is usually not more than 200 mg three or four times a day as needed.
- For *rectal* dosage form (suppositories):
  —For nausea and vomiting:
  - Adults and children 12 years of age and older—200 mg three or four times a day as needed.
  - Children—Dose is based on body weight and must be determined by your doctor. The usual dose is 15 mg per kilogram (6.8 mg per pound). The dose is usually not more than 200 mg three or four times a day as needed.
- For *injection* dosage form:
  —For nausea and vomiting:
  - Adults and children 12 years of age and older—200 mg three or four times a day as needed, injected into a muscle.
  - Children—Dose must be determined by your doctor.

Missed dose—If you must use this medicine regularly and you miss a dose, use it as soon as possible. However, if it is almost time for your next dose, skip the missed dose and go back to your regular dosing schedule. Do not double doses.

Storage—To store this medicine:

- Keep out of the reach of children.
- Store away from heat and direct light.
- Do not store the capsule form of this medicine in the bathroom, near the kitchen sink, or in other damp places. Heat or moisture may cause the medicine to break down.
- Do not keep outdated medicine or medicine no longer needed. Be sure that any discarded medicine is out of the reach of children.

Precautions While Using This Medicine

Trimethobenzamide will add to the effects of alcohol and other CNS depressants (medicines that slow down the nervous system, possibly causing drowsiness). Some examples of CNS depressants are antihistamines or medicine for hay fever, other allergies, or colds; sedatives, tranquilizers, or sleeping medicine; prescription pain medicine or narcotics; barbiturates; medicine for seizures; muscle relaxants; or anesthetics, including some dental anesthetics. *Check with your doctor before taking any of the above while you are using this medicine.*

This medicine may cause some people to become dizzy, lightheaded, drowsy, or less alert than they are normally. *Make sure you know how you react to this medicine before you drive, use machines, or do anything else that could be dangerous if you are dizzy or are not alert.*

When using trimethobenzamide on a regular basis, make sure your doctor knows if you are taking large amounts of aspirin or other salicylates at the same time (as for arthritis or rheumatism). Effects of too much aspirin, such as ringing in the ears, may be covered up by this medicine.

Side Effects of This Medicine

Along with its needed effects, a medicine may cause some unwanted effects. Although not all of these side effects

may occur, if they do occur they may need medical attention.

Check with your doctor as soon as possible if any of the following side effects occur:

Rare

Body spasm, with head and heels bent backward and body bowed forward; convulsions (seizures); mental depression; shakiness or tremors; skin rash; sore throat and fever; unusual tiredness; vomiting (severe or continuing); yellow eyes or skin

Other side effects may occur that usually do not need medical attention. These side effects may go away during treatment as your body adjusts to the medicine. However, check with your doctor if any of the following side effects continue or are bothersome:

More common

Drowsiness

Less common

Blurred vision; diarrhea; dizziness; headache; muscle cramps

Other side effects not listed above may also occur in some patients. If you notice any other effects, check with your doctor.

Annual revision: 05/12/93

TRIMETHOPRIM Systemic

Some commonly used brand names are:

In the U.S.

Proloprim Trimpex

Generic name product may also be available.

In Canada

Proloprim

Description

Trimethoprim (trye-METH-oh-prim) is used to treat infections of the urinary tract. It may also be used for other problems as determined by your doctor. It will not work for colds, flu, or other virus infections.

Trimethoprim is available only with your doctor's prescription, in the following dosage form:

Oral

- Tablets (U.S. and Canada)

It is very important that you read and understand the following information. If any of it causes you special concern, check with your doctor. Also, *if you have any questions* or if you want more information about this medicine or your medical problem, *ask your doctor, nurse, or pharmacist.*

Before Using This Medicine

In deciding to use a medicine, the risks of taking the medicine must be weighed against the good it will do. This is a decision you and your doctor will make. For trimethoprim, the following should be considered:

Allergies—Tell your doctor if you have ever had any unusual or allergic reaction to trimethoprim. Also tell your doctor and pharmacist if you are allergic to any other substances, such as foods, preservatives, or dyes.

Pregnancy—Studies have not been done in humans. Studies in rats have shown that trimethoprim causes birth defects. Studies in rabbits have shown that trimethoprim causes a decrease in the number of successful pregnancies. However, in the few reports where trimethoprim was taken by pregnant women, trimethoprim has not been reported to cause birth defects or other problems in humans.

Breast-feeding—Trimethoprim passes into the breast milk. However, this medicine has not been reported to cause serious problems in nursing babies.

Children—This medicine has been used in a limited number of children 2 months of age or older, and tested in children 12 years of age or older. In effective doses, the medicine has not been shown to cause different side effects or problems in children than it does in adults.

Older adults—Elderly people may be more sensitive to the effects of trimethoprim. Blood problems may be more likely to occur in elderly patients who are taking diuretics (water pills) along with this medicine.

Other medicines—Although certain medicines should not be used together at all, in other cases two different medicines may be used together even if an interaction might occur. In these cases, your doctor may want to change the dose, or other precautions may be necessary. When you are taking trimethoprim, it is especially important that your doctor and pharmacist know if you are taking any of the following:

- Anticonvulsants (seizure medicine) or
- Methotrexate (e.g., Mexate) or
- Pyrimethamine (e.g., Daraprim) or
- Triamterene (e.g., Dyrenium)—Use of these medicines with trimethoprim may increase the chance of side effects effecting the blood

Other medical problems—The presence of other medical problems may affect the use of trimethoprim. Make sure you tell your doctor if you have any other medical problems, especially:

- Anemia—Patients with anemia may have an increased chance of side effects affecting the blood
- Kidney disease—Patients with kidney disease may have an increased chance of side effects

Before you begin using any new medicine (prescription or nonprescription) or if you develop any new medical problem while you are using this medicine, check with your doctor, nurse, or pharmacist.

Proper Use of This Medicine

Do not give this medicine to infants or children under 12 years of age unless otherwise directed by your doctor.

Trimethoprim may be taken on an empty stomach or, if it upsets your stomach, it may be taken with food.

To help clear up your infection completely, *keep taking this medicine for the full time of treatment* even if you begin to feel better after a few days. If you stop taking this medicine too soon, your symptoms may return.

This medicine works best when there is a constant amount in the body. *To help keep the amount constant, do not miss any doses. Also, it is best to take the doses at evenly spaced times day and night.* For example, if you are to take 2 doses a day, the doses should be spaced about 12 hours apart. If this interferes with your sleep or other daily activities, or if you need help in planning the best times to take your medicine, check with your doctor, nurse, or pharmacist.

Dosing—The dose of trimethoprim will be different for different patients. *Follow your doctor's orders or the directions on the label.* The following information includes only the average doses of trimethoprim. Your dose may be different if you have kidney disease. *If your dose is different, do not change it* unless your doctor tells you to do so.

- The number of tablets that you take depends on the strength of the medicine. Also, *the number of doses you take each day, the time allowed between doses, and the length of time you take the medicine depend on the medical problem for which you are taking trimethoprim.*
- For the *treatment of urinary tract infections:*
  - —Adults and children 12 years of age and older: 100 milligrams every twelve hours for ten days, or 200 milligrams once a day for ten days.
  - —Children up to 12 years of age: Dose must be determined by the doctor.

Missed dose—If you do miss a dose of this medicine, take it as soon as possible. This will help to keep a constant amount of medicine in the body. However, if it is almost time for your next dose, skip the missed dose and go back to your regular dosing schedule. Do not double doses.

Storage—To store this medicine:

- Keep out of the reach of children.
- Store away from heat and direct light.
- Do not store in the bathroom, near the kitchen sink, or in other damp places. Heat or moisture may cause the medicine to break down.
- Do not keep outdated medicine or medicine no longer needed. Be sure that any discarded medicine is out of the reach of children.

Precautions While Using This Medicine

It is important that your doctor check your progress at regular visits if you will be taking this medicine for a long time. This will allow your doctor to check for any unwanted effects that may be caused by this medicine.

If your symptoms do not improve within a few days, or if they become worse, check with your doctor.

If this medicine causes anemia, your doctor may want you to take folic acid (a vitamin) every day to help clear up the anemia. If so, it is important to take folic acid every day along with this medicine; do not miss any doses.

Trimethoprim may cause blood problems. These problems may result in a greater chance of certain infections, slow healing, and bleeding of the gums. Therefore, you should be careful when using regular toothbrushes, dental floss, and toothpicks. Dental work should be delayed until your blood counts have returned to normal. Check with your medical doctor or dentist if you have any questions about proper oral hygiene (mouth care) during treatment.

Side Effects of This Medicine

Along with its needed effects, a medicine may cause some unwanted effects. Although not all of these side effects may occur, if they do occur they may need medical attention.

Check with your doctor immediately if any of the following side effects occur:

Rare

Bluish fingernails, lips, or skin; difficult breathing; headache; general feeling of discomfort or illness; nausea; neck stiffness; pale skin; skin rash or itching; sore throat and fever; unusual bleeding or bruising; unusual tiredness or weakness; signs of Stevens-Johnson syndrome, such as aching joints and muscles; redness, blistering, peeling, or loosening of skin; unusual tiredness or weakness

Other side effects may occur that usually do not need medical attention. These side effects may go away during

treatment as your body adjusts to the medicine. However, check with your doctor if any of the following side effects continue or are bothersome:

Less common

Diarrhea; headache; loss of appetite; nausea or vomiting; stomach cramps or pain

Other side effects not listed above may also occur in some patients. If you notice any other effects, check with your doctor.

Additional Information

Once a medicine has been approved for marketing for a certain use, experience may show that it is also useful for other medical problems. Although these uses are not included in product labeling, trimethoprim is used in certain patients for the following medical conditions:

- Prevention of urinary tract infections
- Treatment of *Pneumocystis carinii* pneumonia (PCP)

For patients taking this medicine for *prevention of urinary tract infections*:

- Your doctor may have prescribed this medicine to *prevent* infections of the urinary tract. It is usually given once a day and may be given for a long time for this purpose. If you have any questions about this, check with your doctor.

Other than the above information, there is no additional information relating to proper use, precautions, or side effects for these uses.

Annual revision: 02/23/93

TRIOXSALEN Systemic

A commonly used brand name in the U.S. and Canada is Trisoralen. Another commonly used name is trioxysalen.

Description

Trioxsalen (trye-OX-sa-len) belongs to the group of medicines called psoralens. It is used along with ultraviolet light (found in sunlight and some special lamps) in a treatment called PUVA to treat vitiligo, a disease in which skin color is lost. Trioxsalen may also be used for other conditions as determined by your doctor.

Trioxsalen is available only with your doctor's prescription, in the following dosage form:

Oral

- Tablets (U.S. and Canada)

It is very important that you read and understand the following information. If any of it causes you special concern, check with your doctor. Also, *if you have any questions* or if you want more information about this medicine or your medical problem, *ask your doctor, nurse, or pharmacist*.

Before Using This Medicine

Trioxsalen is a very strong medicine that increases the skin's sensitivity to sunlight. In addition to causing serious sunburns if not properly used, it has been reported to increase the chance of skin cancer and cataracts. Also, like too much sunlight, PUVA can cause premature aging of the skin. Therefore, trioxsalen should be used only as directed and it should *not* be used simply for suntanning.

Before using this medicine, be sure that you have discussed its use with your doctor.

In deciding to use a medicine, the risks of taking the medicine must be weighed against the good it will do. This is a decision you and your doctor will make. For trioxsalen, the following should be considered:

Allergies—Tell your doctor if you have ever had any unusual or allergic reaction to trioxsalen. Also tell your doctor and pharmacist if you are allergic to any other substances, such as preservatives or dyes.

Pregnancy—Studies have not been done in either humans or animals.

Breast-feeding—Trioxsalen has not been reported to cause problems in nursing babies.

Children—Although there is no specific information about the use of trioxsalen in children, it is not expected to cause different side effects or problems in children than it does in adults.

Older adults—Many medicines have not been tested in older people. Therefore, it may not be known whether they work exactly the same way they do in younger adults or if they cause different side effects or problems in older people. There is no specific information about the use of trioxsalen in the elderly.

Other medicines—Although certain medicines should not be used together at all, in other cases two different medicines may be used together even if an interaction might occur. In these cases, your doctor may want to change the dose, or other precautions may be necessary. When you are using trioxsalen, it is especially important that your doctor and pharmacist know if you are using any other prescription or nonprescription (over-the-counter [OTC]) medicine.

Other medical problems—The presence of other medical problems may affect the use of trioxsalen. Make sure you tell your doctor if you have any other medical problems, especially:

- Allergy to sunlight (family history of) or
- Lupus erythematosus or
- Porphyria or
- Other conditions that make you more sensitive to light—These conditions make you more sensitive to light, and this medicine will make the condition worse
- Eye problems, such as cataracts or loss of the lens of the eyes—Use of this medicine may make your cataracts or other eye problems worse; having no lens in your eye may increase the side effects of this medicine
- Heart or blood vessel disease (severe)—The heat from the light treatment may make the condition worse
- Infection or
- Stomach problems—Use of this medicine may make the condition worse
- Melanoma or other skin cancer (history of) or
- Recent treatment with x-rays or cancer medicines or plans to have x-rays in the near future—May increase your chance of skin cancer

Before you begin using any new medicine (prescription or nonprescription) or if you develop any new medical problem while you are using this medicine, check with your doctor, nurse, or pharmacist.

Proper Use of This Medicine

This medicine may take several weeks or months to help your condition. *Do not increase the amount of trioxsalen you are taking or spend extra time in the sunlight or under an ultraviolet lamp.* This will not make the medicine act any more quickly and may result in a serious burn.

If this medicine upsets your stomach, it may be taken with meals or milk.

Missed dose—If you are late in taking, or miss taking, a dose of this medicine, notify your doctor so your light treatment can be rescheduled. Remember that exposure to sunlight or ultraviolet light must take place 2 to 4 hours *after* you take the medicine or it will not work. If you have any questions about this, check with your doctor.

Storage—To store this medicine:

- Keep out of the reach of children.
- Store away from heat and direct light.
- Do not store in the bathroom, near the kitchen sink, or in other damp places. Heat or moisture may cause the medicine to break down.
- Do not keep outdated medicine or medicine no longer needed. Be sure that any discarded medicine is out of the reach of children.

Precautions While Using This Medicine

Your doctor should check your progress at regular visits to make sure this medicine is working and that it does not cause unwanted effects. Eye examinations should be included.

This medicine increases the sensitivity of your skin and lips to sunlight. Therefore, *exposure to the sun, even through window glass or on a cloudy day, could cause a serious burn.* If you must go out during the daylight hours:

- *Before each treatment, cover your skin for at least 24 hours* by wearing protective clothing, such as long-sleeved shirts, full-length slacks, wide-brimmed hat, and gloves. In addition, *protect your lips with a special sun block lipstick that has a protection factor of at least 15.* Check with your doctor before using sun block products on other parts of your body before a treatment, since sun block products should not be used on the areas of your skin that are to be treated.
- *After each treatment, cover your skin for at least 8 hours* by wearing protective clothing. In addition, use a sun block product that has a protection factor of at least 15 on your lips and on those areas of your body that cannot be covered.

If you have any questions about this, check with your doctor or pharmacist.

Your skin may continue to be sensitive to sunlight for some time after treatment with this medicine. Use extra caution for at least 48 hours following each treatment if you plan to spend any time in the sun. Do not sunbathe during this time.

For 24 hours after you take each dose of trioxsalen, your eyes should be protected during daylight hours with special wraparound sunglasses that totally block or absorb ultraviolet light (ordinary sunglasses are not adequate). This is to prevent cataracts. Your doctor will tell you what kind of sunglasses to use. These glasses should be worn even in indirect light, such as light coming through window glass or on a cloudy day.

Eating certain foods while you are taking trixosalen may increase your skin's sensitivity to sunlight. To help prevent this, avoid eating limes, figs, parsley, parsnips, mustard, carrots, and celery while you are being treated with this medicine.

This medicine may cause your skin to become dry or itchy. *However, check with your doctor before applying anything to your skin to treat this problem.*

Side Effects of This Medicine

Along with its needed effects, a medicine may cause some unwanted effects. Although not all of these side effects may occur, if they do occur they may need medical attention.

Check with your doctor immediately if you think you have taken an overdose or if any of the following side effects occur, since they may indicate a serious burn:

Blistering and peeling of skin; reddened, sore skin; swelling, especially of feet or lower legs

Other side effects may occur that usually do not need medical attention. These side effects may go away during treatment as your body adjusts to the medicine. However, check with your doctor if any of the following side effects continue for more than 48 hours or are bothersome:

More common

Itching of skin; nausea

Less common

Dizziness; headache; mental depression; nervousness; trouble in sleeping

There is an increased risk of developing skin cancer after use of trioxsalen. You should check your body regularly and show your doctor any skin sores that do not heal, new skin growths, and skin growths that have changed in the way they look or feel.

Premature aging of the skin may occur as a result of prolonged trioxsalen therapy. This effect is permanent and is similar to what happens when a person sunbathes for long periods of time.

Other side effects not listed above may also occur in some patients. If you notice any other effects, check with your doctor.

Annual revision: September 1990

TROPICAMIDE Ophthalmic

Some commonly used brand names are:

In the U.S.

I-Picamide	Ocu-Tropic
Mydriacyl	Spectro-Cyl
Mydriafair	Tropicacyl

Generic name product may also be available.

In Canada

Minims Tropicamide	Tropicacyl
Mydriacyl	

Description

Tropicamide (troe-PIK-a-mide) is used to dilate (enlarge) the pupil. It is used before eye examinations. Tropicamide may also be used before and after eye surgery.

This medicine is available only with your doctor's prescription, in the following dosage form:

Ophthalmic

- Ophthalmic solution (eye drops) (U.S. and Canada)

It is very important that you read and understand the following information. If any of it causes you special concern, check with your doctor. Also, *if you have any questions* or if you want more information about this medicine or your medical problem, *ask your doctor, nurse, or pharmacist*.

Before Using This Medicine

In deciding to use a medicine, the risks of taking the medicine must be weighed against the good it will do. This is a decision you and your doctor will make. For tropicamide, the following should be considered:

Allergies—Tell your doctor if you have ever had any unusual or allergic reaction to tropicamide. Also tell your doctor and pharmacist if you are allergic to any other substances, such as preservatives.

Pregnancy—Studies on effects in pregnancy have not been done in either humans or animals.

Breast-feeding—Tropicamide has not been reported to cause problems in nursing babies.

Children—Children may be especially sensitive to the effects of tropicamide. This may increase the chance or severity of some of the side effects during treatment.

Older adults—Many medicines have not been studied specifically in older people. Therefore, it may not be known whether they work exactly the same way they do in younger adults or if they cause different side effects or problems in older people. Although there is no specific information comparing use of tropicamide in the elderly with use in other age groups, this medicine is not expected to cause different side effects or problems in older people than it does in younger adults.

Other medicines—Although certain medicines should not be used together at all, in other cases two different medicines may be used together even if an interaction might occur. In these cases, your doctor may want to change the dose, or other precautions may be necessary. Tell your doctor and pharmacist if you are using any other prescription or nonprescription (over-the-counter [OTC]) medicine.

Other medical problems—The presence of other medical problems may affect the use of tropicamide. Make sure you tell your doctor if you have any other medical problems, especially:

- Brain damage (in children) or
- Down's syndrome (mongolism) or
- Spastic paralysis (in children)—Tropicamide may make the condition worse.

Precautions While Using This Medicine

After this medicine is applied to your eyes:

- Your pupils will become unusually large and you will have blurring of vision, especially for close objects. *Make sure your vision is clear before you drive, use machines, or do anything else that could be dangerous if you are not able to see well.*
- Your eyes will become more sensitive to light than they are normally. When you go out during the daylight hours, even on cloudy days, *wear sunglasses that block ultraviolet (UV) light to protect your eyes from sunlight and other bright lights.* Ordinary sunglasses may not protect your eyes. If you have any questions about the kind of sunglasses to wear, check with your doctor.
- If these effects continue for longer than 24 hours after the medicine is used, check with your doctor.

Side Effects of This Medicine

Along with its needed effects, a medicine may cause some unwanted effects. Although not all of these side effects may occur, if they do occur they may need medical attention.

Check with your doctor as soon as possible if any of the following side effects occur:

Symptoms of too much medicine being absorbed into the body

Clumsiness or unsteadiness; confusion; fast heartbeat; flushing or redness of face; hallucinations (seeing, hearing, or feeling things that are not there); increased thirst or dryness of mouth; skin rash; slurred speech; swollen stomach in infants; unusual behavior, especially in children; unusual drowsiness, tiredness, or weakness

Other side effects may occur that usually do not need medical attention. These side effects may go away during treatment as your body adjusts to the medicine. However, check with your doctor if any of the following side effects continue or are bothersome:

More common

Stinging of the eye when the medicine is applied

Other side effects not listed above may also occur in some patients. If you notice any other effects, check with your doctor.

Annual revision: 11/21/91

TYPHOID VACCINE LIVE ORAL Systemic†

A commonly used brand name in the U.S. is Vivotif Berna.

†Not commercially available in Canada.

Description

Typhoid (TYE-foid) fever is a serious disease that can cause death. It is caused by a germ called *Salmonella typhi*, and is spread most often through infected food or water. Typhoid may also be spread by close person-to-person contact with infected persons (such as occurs with persons living in the same household). Some infected persons do not appear to be sick, but they can still spread the germ to others.

Typhoid fever is very rare in the U.S. and other areas of the world that have good water and sewage (waste) systems. However, it is a problem in parts of the world that do not have such systems. If you are traveling to certain countries or remote (out-of-the-way) areas, typhoid vaccine will help protect you from typhoid fever. The U.S. Centers for Disease Control (CDC) currently recommend caution in the following areas of the world:

- Africa
- Asia
- Latin America

Typhoid vaccine taken by mouth helps prevent typhoid fever, but does not provide 100% protection. Therefore, it is very important to avoid infected persons and food and water that may be infected, even if you have taken the vaccine.

To get the best possible protection against typhoid, you should complete the vaccine dosing schedule (all 4 doses of the vaccine) at least 1 week before travel to areas where you may be exposed to typhoid.

If you will be traveling regularly to parts of the world where typhoid is a problem, you should get a booster (repeat) dose of the vaccine every 5 years.

Typhoid vaccine is available only from a health care provider, in the following dosage form:

Oral

- Enteric-coated capsules (U.S.)

It is very important that you read and understand the following information. If any of it causes you special concern, check with your doctor. Also, *if you have any questions* or if you want more information about this medicine or your medical problem, *ask your doctor, nurse, or pharmacist.*

Before Using This Vaccine

In deciding to use a medicine, the risks of taking the medicine must be weighed against the good it will do. This is a decision you and your doctor will make. For typhoid vaccine, the following should be considered:

Allergies—Tell your doctor if you have ever had any unusual or allergic reaction to typhoid vaccine. Also tell your doctor and pharmacist if you are allergic to any other substances, such as foods, preservatives, or dyes. This vaccine contains sucrose and lactose, and the vaccine bacteria are grown in a mixture containing beef.

Pregnancy—Studies on effects in pregnancy have not been done in either humans or animals. Before taking this medicine, make sure your doctor knows if you are pregnant or if you may become pregnant.

Breast-feeding—It is not known whether typhoid vaccine passes into the breast milk. However, this vaccine has not been reported to cause problems in nursing babies.

Children—Typhoid vaccine is not recommended for infants and children up to 6 years of age. Although there is no specific information comparing use of typhoid vaccine in children 6 years of age and over with use in other age groups, this vaccine is not expected to cause different side effects or problems in these children than it does in adults.

Older adults—Many medicines have not been studied specifically in older people. Therefore, it may not be known whether they work exactly the same way they do in younger adults. Although there is no specific information comparing use of typhoid vaccine in the elderly with use in other age groups, this vaccine is not expected to cause different side effects or problems in older people than it does in younger adults.

Other medicines—Although certain medicines should not be used together at all, in other cases two different medicines may be used together even if an interaction might occur. In these cases, your doctor may want to change the dose, or other precautions may be necessary. When you are taking typhoid vaccine, it is especially important that your doctor and pharmacist know if you are taking any of the following:

- Anti-infectives by mouth or by injection (medicine for infection) or
- Antimalarials (medicine for malaria)—These medicines may reduce the useful effect of the typhoid vaccine
- Treatment with x-rays, cancer medicines, or high doses of steroids—Treatment may increase the action of the vaccine, causing an increase in vaccine side effects, or treatment may block the useful effect of the vaccine

Other medical problems—The presence of other medical problems may affect the use of typhoid vaccine. Make sure you tell your doctor if you have any other medical problems, especially:

- Diarrhea or
- Fever or
- Other illness (severe) or
- Stomach or intestinal illness (severe) or
- Vomiting—The condition may reduce the useful effect of the vaccine
- Immune deficiency condition, including HIV or AIDS—The condition may increase the chance of side effects of the vaccine

Before you begin using any new medicine (prescription or nonprescription) or if you develop any new medical problem while you are using this vaccine, check with your doctor, nurse, or pharmacist.

Proper Use of This Vaccine

It is important that all 4 doses of the vaccine be taken exactly as directed. If all the doses are not taken or if doses are not taken at the correct times, the vaccine may not work properly.

The vaccine capsules are meant to dissolve in the intestines. Therefore, they should be inspected to make sure that they are not broken or cracked when you take them. If any are broken or cracked, you will need to replace them.

Typhoid vaccine must be stored in the refrigerator at a temperature between 2 and 8 °C (35.6 and 46.4 °F) at all times. If the vaccine is left at room temperature, it will lose its effectiveness. Therefore, remember to replace unused vaccine in the refrigerator between doses.

Each dose of the vaccine should be taken approximately 1 hour before a meal. Take with a cold or lukewarm drink that has a temperature that does not exceed body temperature, e.g., 37 °C (98.6 °F).

Swallow the capsule whole. Do not chew it before swallowing. Also swallow the capsule as soon as possible after you place it in your mouth.

Dosing—*Follow your doctor's orders or the directions on the label.* The following information includes only the average dose of typhoid vaccine. *If your dose is different, do not change it* unless your doctor tells you to do so:

- Take 1 capsule by mouth every other day for a total of 4 doses.

Missed dose—If you miss a dose of this medicine and you remember it on the day it should be taken, take it as directed. However, if you do not remember the missed dose until the next day, take the missed dose at that time and reschedule your every-other-day doses from then. *It is important that this vaccine be taken exactly as directed so it can give you the most protection against typhoid fever.*

Storage—To store this medicine:

- Keep out of the reach of children.
- *Store in the refrigerator at all times.* However, keep the medicine from freezing.
- Do not keep outdated medicine or medicine no longer needed. Be sure that any discarded medicine is out of the reach of children.

Precautions While Using This Medicine

Tell your doctor that you have taken this vaccine:

- If you are to receive any other live vaccines within 1 month after taking this vaccine.

Side Effects of This Vaccine

Along with its needed effects, a medicine may cause some unwanted effects. Although not all of these side effects may occur, if they do occur they may need medical attention.

Get emergency help immediately if any of the following side effects occur:

Symptoms of allergic reaction

Difficulty in breathing or swallowing; hives; itching, especially of feet or hands; reddening of skin, especially around ears; swelling of eyes, face, or inside of nose; unusual tiredness or weakness (sudden and severe)

Other side effects may occur that usually do not need medical attention. These side effects may go away during treatment as your body adjusts to the medicine. However, check with your doctor if any of the following side effects continue or are bothersome:

Less common or rare

Diarrhea; fever; hives; nausea; skin rash; stomach cramps or pain; vomiting

Other side effects not listed above may also occur in some patients. If you notice any other effects, check with your doctor.

Annual revision: 07/22/92

UNDECYLENIC ACID, COMPOUND Topical

Some commonly used brand names are:

In the U.S.

- Caldesene Medicated Powder
- Cruex Antifungal Cream
- Cruex Antifungal Powder
- Cruex Antifungal Spray Powder
- Decylenes Powder
- Desenex Antifungal Cream
- Desenex Antifungal Liquid
- Desenex Antifungal Ointment
- Desenex Antifungal Penetrating Foam
- Desenex Antifungal Powder
- Desenex Antifungal Spray Powder
- Gordochom Solution

In Canada

- Cruex Aerosol Powder
- Cruex Cream
- Cruex Powder
- Desenex Aerosol Powder
- Desenex Foam
- Desenex Ointment
- Desenex Powder
- Desenex Solution

Description

Compound undecylenic acid (un-de-sill-ENN-ik AS-id) belongs to the group of medicines called antifungals. It is used to treat some types of fungus infections.

Compound undecylenic acid is available without a prescription; however, your doctor may have special instructions on the proper use of this medicine for your medical condition.

Compound undecylenic acid is available in the following dosage forms:

Topical

- Aerosol foam (U.S. and Canada)
- Aerosol powder (U.S. and Canada)
- Cream (U.S. and Canada)
- Ointment (U.S. and Canada)
- Powder (U.S. and Canada)
- Solution (U.S. and Canada)

It is very important that you read and understand the following information. If any of it causes you special concern, check with your doctor or pharmacist. Also, *if you have any questions* or if you want more information about this medicine or your medical problem, *ask your doctor, nurse, or pharmacist.*

Before Using This Medicine

If you are taking this medicine without a prescription, carefully read and follow any precautions on the label. For compound undecylenic acid, the following should be considered:

Allergies—Tell your doctor if you have ever had any unusual or allergic reaction to compound undecylenic acid. Also tell your doctor and pharmacist if you are allergic to any other substances, such as preservatives or dyes.

Pregnancy—Compound undecylenic acid topical preparations have not been shown to cause birth defects or other problems in humans.

Breast-feeding—Compound undecylenic acid topical preparations have not been reported to cause problems in nursing babies.

Children—Compound undecylenic acid should not be used on children up to 2 years of age, unless otherwise directed by your doctor. Although there is no specific information comparing use of compound undecylenic acid topical preparations in children 2 years of age and older with use in other age groups, this medicine is not expected to cause different side effects or problems in children 2 years of age and older than it does in adults.

Older adults—Many medicines have not been studied specifically in older people. Therefore, it may not be known whether they work exactly the same way they do in younger adults or if they cause different side effects or problems in older people. There is no specific information comparing use of compound undecylenic acid in the elderly with use in other age groups.

Other medicines—Although certain medicines should not be used together at all, in other cases two different medicines may be used together even if an interaction might occur. In these cases, your doctor may want to change the dose, or other precautions may be necessary. Tell your doctor and pharmacist if you are using any other topical prescription or nonprescription (over-the-counter [OTC]) medicine that is to be applied to the same area of the skin.

Before you begin using any new medicine (prescription or nonprescription) or if you develop any new medical problem while you are using this medicine, check with your doctor, nurse, or pharmacist.

Proper Use of This Medicine

Before applying compound undecylenic acid, wash the affected and surrounding areas, and dry thoroughly. Then apply enough medicine to cover these areas.

Keep this medicine away from the eyes.

For patients using the *cream form* of this medicine:

- Apply cream generously to affected and surrounding areas. Rub in well.
- Do not use on pus-containing sores or on badly broken skin.

For patients using the *powder form* of this medicine:

- If the powder is used on the feet, sprinkle it between toes, on feet, and in socks and shoes.

For patients using the *aerosol powder or aerosol foam form* of this medicine:

- From a distance of 4 to 6 inches, spray the affected and surrounding areas. If the medicine is used on the feet, spray it between the toes also. The powder may also be sprayed on socks and shoes.

- Do not use this medicine around the eyes, nose, or mouth.
- Do not inhale the aerosol.
- Do not use near heat, near open flame, or while smoking.

To help clear up your infection completely, *keep using this medicine for 2 weeks after burning, itching, or other symptoms have disappeared,* unless otherwise directed by your doctor. *Do not miss any doses.*

Missed dose—If you do miss a dose of this medicine, apply it as soon as possible. Then go back to your regular dosing schedule.

Storage—To store this medicine:
- Keep out of the reach of children.
- Store away from heat and direct light.
- Do not store the powder form of this medicine in the bathroom, near the kitchen sink, or in other damp places. Heat or moisture may cause the medicine to break down.
- Keep the aerosol foam, aerosol powder, cream, ointment, and solution forms of this medicine from freezing.
- Do not puncture, break, or burn the aerosol foam or powder container.
- Do not keep outdated medicine or medicine no longer needed. Be sure that any discarded medicine is out of the reach of children.

Precautions While Using This Medicine

If your skin problem does not improve within 4 weeks, or if it becomes worse, check with your doctor or pharmacist.

To help prevent reinfection after the period of treatment with this medicine, the powder or spray powder form of this medicine may be used each day after bathing and careful drying.

Side Effects of This Medicine

Along with its needed effects, a medicine may cause some unwanted effects. Although not all of these side effects may occur, if they do occur they may need medical attention.

Check with your doctor or pharmacist as soon as possible if the following side effect occurs:

Skin irritation not present before use of this medicine

Other side effects not listed above may also occur in some patients. If you notice any other effects, check with your doctor or pharmacist.

Annual revision: 11/05/91

URACIL MUSTARD Systemic†

Generic name product available in the U.S.

†Not commercially available in Canada.

Description

Uracil (YOOR-a-sill) mustard belongs to the group of medicines known as alkylating agents. It is used to treat some kinds of cancer as well as some noncancerous conditions.

Uracil mustard interferes with the growth of cancer cells, which are eventually destroyed. Since the growth of normal body cells may also be affected by uracil mustard, other effects will also occur. Some of these may be serious and must be reported to your doctor. Other effects, such as hair loss, may not be serious but may cause concern. Some effects may not occur for months or years after the medicine is used.

Before you begin treatment with uracil mustard, you and your doctor should talk about the good this medicine will do as well as the risks of using it.

Uracil mustard is available only with your doctor's prescription, in the following dosage form:

Oral
- Capsules (U.S.)

It is very important that you read and understand the following information. If any of it causes you special concern, check with your doctor or pharmacist. Also, *if you have any questions* or if you want more information about this dietary supplement or your medical problem, *ask your doctor, nurse, pharmacist, or dietitian.*

Before Using This Medicine

In deciding to use a medicine, the risks of taking the medicine must be weighed against the good it will do.

This is a decision you and your doctor will make. For uracil mustard, the following should be considered:

Allergies—Tell your doctor if you have ever had any unusual or allergic reaction to uracil mustard.

Pregnancy—Tell your doctor if you are pregnant or if you intend to have children. This medicine may cause birth defects if either the male or female is taking it at the time of conception or if it is taken during pregnancy. In addition, many cancer medicines may cause sterility which could be permanent. Although sterility has not been reported with this medicine, the possibility should be kept in mind.

Be sure that you have discussed this with your doctor before taking this medicine. It is best to use some kind of birth control while you are taking uracil mustard. Tell your doctor right away if you think you have become pregnant while taking uracil mustard.

Breast-feeding—Tell your doctor if you are breast-feeding or if you intend to breast-feed during treatment with this medicine. Because uracil mustard may cause serious side effects, breast-feeding is generally not recommended while you are receiving it.

Children—Although there is no specific information about the use of uracil mustard in children, it is not expected to cause different side effects or problems in children than it does in adults.

Older adults—Many medicines have not been tested in older people. Therefore, it may not be known whether they work exactly the same way they do in younger adults or if they cause different side effects or problems in older people. There is no specific information about the use of uracil mustard in the elderly.

Other medicines—Although certain medicines should not be used together at all, in other cases two different medicines may be used together even if an interaction might occur. In these cases, your doctor may want to change the dose, or other precautions may be necessary. When you are taking uracil mustard, it is especially important that your doctor and pharmacist know if you are taking any of the following:

- Amphotericin B by injection (e.g., Fungizone) or
- Antithyroid agents (medicine for overactive thyroid) or
- Azathioprine (e.g., Imuran) or
- Chloramphenicol (e.g., Chloromycetin) or
- Colchicine or
- Flucytosine (e.g., Ancobon) or
- Interferon (e.g., Intron A, Roferon-A) or
- Plicamycin (e.g., Mithracin) or
- Zidovudine (e.g., Retrovir) or
- If you have ever been treated with x-rays or cancer medicines—Uracil mustard may increase the effects of these medicines or radiation therapy on the blood
- Probenecid (e.g., Benemid) or
- Sulfinpyrazone (e.g., Anturane)—Uracil mustard may increase the concentration of uric acid in the blood, which these medicines are used to lower

Other medical problems—The presence of other medical problems may affect the use of uracil mustard. Make sure you tell your doctor if you have any other medical problems, especially:

- Chickenpox (including recent exposure) or
- Herpes zoster (shingles)—Risk of severe disease affecting other parts of the body
- Gout (history of) or
- Kidney stones (history of)—Uracil mustard may increase levels of uric acid in the body, which can cause gout or kidney stones
- Infection—Uracil mustard can reduce immunity to infection
- Kidney disease
- Liver disease

Before you begin using any new medicine (prescription or nonprescription) or if you develop any new medical problem while you are using this medicine, check with your doctor, nurse, or pharmacist.

Proper Use of This Medicine

Use this medicine only as directed by your doctor. Do not use more or less of it, and do not use it more often than your doctor ordered. The exact amount of medicine you need has been carefully worked out. Taking too much may increase the chance of side effects, while taking too little may not improve your condition.

While you are using this medicine, your doctor may want you to drink extra fluids so that you will pass more urine. This will help prevent kidney problems and keep your kidneys working well.

Uracil mustard often causes nausea and vomiting. Even if you begin to feel ill, *do not stop using this medicine without first checking with your doctor.* Ask your doctor, nurse, or pharmacist for ways to lessen these effects.

If you vomit shortly after taking a dose of uracil mustard, check with your doctor. You will be told whether to take the dose again or to wait until the next scheduled dose.

Missed dose—If you miss a dose of this medicine, skip the missed dose and go back to your regular dosing schedule. Do not double doses.

Storage—To store this medicine:

- Keep out of the reach of children.
- Store away from heat and direct light.
- Do not store in the bathroom, near the kitchen sink, or in other damp places. Heat or moisture may cause the medicine to break down.
- Do not keep outdated medicine or medicine no longer needed. Be sure that any discarded medicine is out of the reach of children.

Precautions While Using This Medicine

It is very important that your doctor check your progress at regular visits to make sure that this medicine is working properly and to check for unwanted effects.

While you are being treated with uracil mustard, and after you stop treatment with it, *do not have any immunizations (vaccinations) without your doctor's approval.* Uracil mustard may lower your body's resistance and there is a chance you might get the infection the immunization is meant to prevent. Other people living in your household should not take or should not have recently taken oral polio vaccine since there is a chance they could pass the polio virus on to you. Also, avoid other persons who have taken oral polio vaccine. Do not get close to them and do not stay in the same room with them for very long. If you cannot take these precautions, you should consider wearing a protective face mask that covers the nose and mouth.

Uracil mustard can lower the number of white blood cells in your blood temporarily, increasing the chance of getting an infection. It can also lower the number of platelets, which are necessary for proper blood clotting. If this occurs, there are certain precautions you can take, especially when your blood count is low, to reduce the risk of infection or bleeding:

- If you can, avoid people with infections. *Check with your doctor immediately* if you think you are getting an infection or if you get a fever or chills, cough or hoarseness, lower back or side pain, or painful or difficult urination.
- *Check with your doctor immediately* if you notice any unusual bleeding or bruising; black, tarry stools; blood in urine or stools; or pinpoint red spots on your skin.
- Be careful when using a regular toothbrush, dental floss, or toothpick. Your medical doctor, dentist, or nurse may recommend other ways to clean your teeth and gums. Check with your medical doctor before having any dental work done.
- Do not touch your eyes or the inside of your nose unless you have just washed your hands and have not touched anything else in the meantime.
- Be careful not to cut yourself when you are using sharp objects such as a safety razor or fingernail or toenail cutters.
- Avoid contact sports or other situations where bruising or injury could occur.

Side Effects of This Medicine

Along with their needed effects medicines like uracil mustard can sometimes cause unwanted effects such as blood problems, loss of hair, and other side effects. These and others are described below. Also, because of the way these medicines act on the body, there is a chance that they might cause other unwanted effects that may not occur until months or years after the medicine is used. These delayed effects may include certain types of cancer, such as leukemia. Discuss these possible effects with your doctor.

Although not all of the side effects may occur, if they do occur they may need medical attention.

Check with your doctor immediately if any of the following side effects occur:

Less common

Black, tarry stools; blood in urine or stools; cough or hoarseness; fever or chills; lower back or side pain; painful or difficult urination; pinpoint red spots on skin; unusual bleeding or bruising

Check with your doctor as soon as possible if any of the following side effects occur:

Less common

Joint pain; swelling of feet or lower legs

Rare

Sores in mouth and on lips; yellow eyes or skin

Other side effects may occur that usually do not need medical attention. These side effects may go away during treatment as your body adjusts to the medicine. Also, your doctor or nurse may be able to tell you about ways to prevent or reduce some of these side effects. Check with your doctor or nurse if any of the following side effects continue or are bothersome or if you have any questions about them:

More common

Diarrhea; nausea or vomiting

Less common

Darkening of the skin; irritability; mental depression; nervousness; skin rash and itching

This medicine may cause a temporary loss of hair in some people. After treatment with uracil mustard has ended, normal hair growth should return.

After you stop taking uracil mustard, it may still produce some side effects that need attention. During this period of time, check with your doctor if you notice any of the following:

Black, tarry stools; blood in urine or stools; cough or hoarseness; fever or chills; lower back or side pain; painful or difficult urination; pinpoint red spots on skin; unusual bleeding or bruising

Other side effects not listed above may also occur in some patients. If you notice any other effects, check with your doctor.

Annual revision: September 1990
Interim revision: 08/11/93

UREA Intra-amniotic

A commonly used brand name in the U.S. is Ureaphil. Another commonly used name is carbamide.

Description

Intra-amniotic urea (yoor-EE-a) is given by injection into the uterus to cause abortion. It is to be administered only by or under the immediate care of your doctor. It is available in the following dosage form:

Parenteral

- Injection (U.S.)

It is very important that you read and understand the following information. If any of it causes you special concern, check with your doctor. Also, *if you have any questions* or if you want more information about this medicine or your medical problem, *ask your doctor, nurse, or pharmacist.*

Before Receiving This Medicine

In deciding to use a medicine, the risks of taking the medicine must be weighed against the good it will do. This is a decision you and your doctor will make. For urea, the following should be considered:

Allergies—Tell your doctor if you have ever had any unusual or allergic reaction to urea. Also tell your doctor and pharmacist if you are allergic to any other substances, such as foods, preservatives, or dyes.

Teenagers—Although there is no specific information comparing use of urea in adolescent females, with use in other age groups, this medicine is not expected to cause different side effects or problems in adolescent females than it does in adults.

Other medicines—Although certain medicines should not be used together at all, in other cases two different medicines may be used together even if an interaction might occur. In these cases, your doctor may want to change the dose, or other precautions may be necessary. Tell your doctor and pharmacist if you are taking any other prescription or nonprescription (over-the-counter [OTC]) medicine.

Other medical problems—The presence of other medical problems may affect the use of urea. Make sure you tell your doctor if you have any other medical problems, especially:

- Diabetes mellitus (sugar diabetes)
- Fibroid tumors of the uterus
- Kidney disease
- Liver disease
- Sickle cell disease

Proper Use of This Medicine

During the abortion procedure, you should drink fluids to help prevent your body from losing too much water.

Side Effects of This Medicine

Along with its needed effects, a medicine may cause some unwanted effects. Although not all of these side effects may occur, if they do occur they may need medical attention.

Check with your doctor or nurse immediately if either of the following side effects occurs during the time that the injection is being given:

Pain in lower abdomen; weakness

Check with your doctor or nurse as soon as possible if any of the following side effects occur:

Rare

Confusion; irregular heartbeat; muscle cramps or pain; numbness, tingling, pain, or weakness in hands or feet; unusual tiredness or weakness; weakness and heaviness of legs

Other side effects may occur that usually do not need medical attention. However, check with your doctor or nurse if any of the following side effects continue or are bothersome:

More common

Nausea or vomiting

Less common or rare

Headache

After the procedure is completed, this procedure may still produce some side effects that need medical attention. Check with your doctor if you notice any of the following side effects:

Chills or shivering; fever; foul-smelling vaginal discharge; increase in bleeding of the uterus; pain in lower abdomen

Other side effects not listed above may also occur in some patients. If you notice any other effects, check with your doctor or nurse.

Annual revision: 08/18/93

URINE GLUCOSE AND KETONE TEST KITS FOR HOME USE

This information applies to the following medicines:

Copper Reduction Urine Glucose Test
Glucose Oxidase Urine Glucose Test
Nitroprusside Urine Ketone Test
Urine Glucose and Ketone (Combined) Test

Some commonly used brand names are:

For Copper Reduction Urine Glucose Test

In the U.S.

Clinitest

In Canada

Clinitest

For Glucose Oxidase Urine Glucose Test

In the U.S.

Biotel/diabetes
Chemstrip uG
Clinistix
Diastix
Tes-tape

In Canada

Clinistix
Diastix
Tes-tape

For Nitroprusside Urine Ketone Test

In the U.S.

Acetest
Chemstrip K
KetoStix

In Canada

Acetest
KetoStix

For Urine Glucose and Ketone (Combined) Test

In the U.S.

Chemstrip uGK
Keto-diastix

In Canada

Chemstrip uGK
Keto-diastix

Description

Diabetes mellitus (sugar diabetes) is a condition that causes problems in controlling the amount of sugar (glucose) in the blood. This is because the pancreas gland does not work properly to make enough insulin to allow the body to handle glucose the right way. Normally, insulin helps glucose enter body cells so it can be used for energy. It also helps the body store extra nutrients and release them for energy when needed. If there is not enough insulin, the unused glucose builds up in the blood. Some of this extra glucose will be passed into the urine. Having extra glucose in the blood for many years causes damage to blood vessels and nerves. Eventually, the body organs (especially the eyes, heart, kidneys, and lower limbs) are damaged. People with diabetes who carefully control their condition may be less likely to develop these problems.

When body cells are not able to use glucose because of the shortage of insulin, they use stored fats instead. Abnormally fast use of fats causes a buildup of their breakdown product, ketones, in the blood. The ketones make the blood more acid, resulting in a condition called ketoacidosis. The combined ketone and acid condition is poisonous to the brain, causing the patient to become confused and drowsy. Coma and death may follow if the problem is not corrected.

Patients with diabetes are taught to test their urine or blood for glucose and ketones as part of a program to manage their diabetes. Blood tests for glucose are considered by most doctors to be the best way to monitor diabetes. Urine tests are mostly used by patients who do not need insulin to control their diabetes and patients whose disease is stable, or those who are not able to take blood samples. These tests may also be used in addition to blood tests when monitoring must be done often, such as on sick days.

Testing for ketones is important when blood or urine tests are high for glucose, or when a patient is sick or cannot eat. Ketone testing is especially important during pregnancy, because insulin needs change rapidly and ketones are damaging to the fetus. Some products test for glucose and ketones on the same strip.

Before Using This Test Kit

It is important to get the best results possible from these urine tests. Therefore, the following should be considered by you and your diabetes care provider before choosing which urine test is the best for you or what adjustments may be needed when you are testing your urine:

Diet—Foods that color the urine may make the test colors harder to read. Check the urine sample for unusual color when test results are not what you expect.

Medicines—Certain medicines may affect the results of your testing. When a new medicine is prescribed for you, ask your diabetes care provider about possible problems with the test you usually use. Also, make sure you tell your diabetes care provider about any medicines you may use.

Medicines that color the urine may make the test colors harder to read. Check the urine sample for unusual color when your urine test results are not what you expect.

Many medicines (including nonprescription products such as vitamins, aspirin, and iron) may cause false test results, especially with certain tablet products.

Other medical problems—The presence of certain medical problems may affect the results of your testing. Check with your diabetes care provider if you have any other medical conditions, including:.

- Vision problems—If you are color-blind or have poor vision, you will need someone to help you in reading your test results

Proper Use of This Test

Usually your diabetes care provider (doctor, nurse, or diabetes educator) will help you choose and learn to use a test product. Some tests are more sensitive, easier to use, or more likely to be affected by other medicines and conditions. The test product should be matched to your needs.

Once the choice of a urine test is made by the diabetes care provider or teacher, you should use it at the planned times, as often as instructed. This may be 4 or more times a day for some patients. Doing the test often allows for better control of your diabetes.

Buy only the product recommended by your doctor or diabetes specialist or center. Do not switch products without the advice of one of these professionals. The printed instructions on the proper use of these urine test kits are different for each product. You could get confusing results with a different product until you learn its proper use.

To use:

- Wash and dry your hands.
- Collect a urine sample in a clean, dry container according to the written package instructions or your diabetes specialist's instructions. Do not refrigerate the urine or let it stand for more than one-half hour (30 minutes) before testing it.
- Choose a well-lighted area with normal room temperature and humidity, with a clean, dry working surface to perform the test. You will also need a watch, timer, or clock that can measure in seconds and a cold water faucet nearby.
- Wash and dry your hands before handling the test materials. Be careful not to touch the testing areas. Skin oils or perspiration may affect the test chemicals and cause a false result. It is also important that you use clean, dry test kit materials. Traces of old test chemicals or soaps can cause false test results. Reused containers or droppers should be rinsed with distilled water and allowed to dry between uses.
- Read and follow the test kit instructions carefully. Soon after you take out a test strip, tablet, or piece of tape, close the container.
- For test strips, dip the strip in the urine for one second and tap it on the edge of the container to remove the extra urine. You may also hold the strip directly in your urine stream to wet the test areas.
- Compare the color of the test strip to the color chart on the package at the end of the timing period. You may hold the strip right next to the color chart. The color should be the same on all of the wet area.
- When you are using tests that require drops of urine to be put into a test tube, hold the dropper straight up and down. Carefully count the water and urine drops as you drop them in the test tube. Place the test tube in its holder and wait for any boiling to stop. (After the boiling stops, the test tube will still be hot, so be careful not to burn your fingers.)
- 15 seconds after boiling has stopped, read the test results by matching the color of the urine in the test tube with the proper color chart. You may want to hold the color chart right next to the test tube. If your test kit has more than one method, make sure to use the correct color chart, based on the number of drops you use.
- For *Acetest*, allow each drop to soak into the tablet and read the test at 15 seconds.
- Do the test control, if one is recommended in the package instructions.
- Record your test results.

Storage—To store these products:

- Keep out of the reach of children. Test kit chemicals can be poisonous if swallowed.
- Store these test kits in their original containers. Keep the container tightly closed. Recap the test product container immediately after use.
- Keep in a cool, dry place, away from heat, humidity (such as the bathroom or shower area), and direct sunlight. Heat-exposed test kits will not work properly.
- Do not put test kits in the refrigerator. Keep the product from freezing.
- Check the expiration date printed on the package before purchasing. Do not use an outdated test kit. Outdated test kits will not work correctly.
- Do not use tablets or strips that have changed color or are falling apart. This is a sign that they are no longer good and will not give correct results.
- Unused liquids may be poured down the drain. Any urine or tests with urine in them should be flushed in the toilet. Be sure that any discarded test kit is out of the reach of children.

About Your Test Results

After you have your urine test results, you should write them in a log book or diary, along with any other problems you may be having. Your diabetes care providers can then give you any advice you will need to help you best control your diabetes.

Use the guidelines (rules) that your doctor has given you on what to do when your results show that your diabetes is not under the proper control. Usually these rules involve adjustments in your diet, medicines, or exercise. Depending upon your diabetes control program, you may be able to make some of these adjustments or handle some problems by yourself or at home with telephone advice from your doctor's office. However, some problems are serious enough that you will need to see your doctor to get your diabetes under control again.

Notify your doctor, nurse, or diabetes educator if you are not sure of your test results for any reason. Your control of your diabetes depends on your understanding of diabetes and its treatment as well as the decisions you make every day.

Having high levels of glucose in your urine (or blood) and finding ketones in your urine may indicate a hidden illness or infection. Prompt notification of your doctor is important to get additional treatment to regain control of your condition, and to avoid complications.

If you have any other questions about your results or the use of diabetic urine test kits, ask your diabetes care provider or pharmacist. Also, most kits have a toll-free number advice to call for advice.

Annual revision: 10/26/92

URINARY TRACT INFECTION TEST KITS FOR HOME USE†

A commonly used brand name in the U.S. is Biotel/uti.

†Not commercialy available in Canada.

Description

Urinary tract infection test kits are designed to help detect infections of the urinary tract. Urinary tract infections (UTIs) may also be called bladder infections, cystitis, kidney infections, or pyelonephritis, depending on the part of the urinary system where the infection is found. Most infections begin in the bladder and, if untreated, may move up the ureters to the kidneys. Although a patient may not feel ill or know that he or she has an infection, the infection may cause damage to the kidneys if it is not treated.

Certain people are more likely to get these infections. Women, some diabetics, patients who have had UTIs before, persons who use urinary catheters, or persons with spinal cord injuries may have these infections more often. Pregnant women who get bladder infections may develop kidney infections more easily, and their UTIs may cause serious problems with the pregnancy.

Patients who are likely to get infections without feeling any symptoms may check for infection by using a home test kit. The UTI test detects nitrite, a chemical in the urine. Bacteria that commonly infect the urinary tract make nitrite from the nitrates that are normally present in one's diet. The patient checks for infection by dipping the test strip with a chemically treated pad in the urine and watching for the pad to change color. If nitrites are present, the test pad turns pink. The patient should notify his or her physician that the test is positive so that further testing or antibiotic treatment can be started, if necessary.

Some doctors may also have a patient use the UTI test kit after finishing his or her treatment for a urinary tract infection to see if the infection has cleared.

It is very important that you read and understand the following information. If any of it causes you special concern, check with your doctor. Also, *if you have any questions* or if you want more information about this test or your medical problem, *ask your doctor, nurse, or pharmacist.* Most kits also provide a toll-free number for advice on using the kits.

Before Using This Test Kit

To get the best results possible from urinary tract infection test kits, the following should be considered before you use these test kits:

Diet—For 10 hours before using the test, avoid eating foods that are high in vitamin C (for example, citrus fruits, tomatoes, strawberries, cantaloupes, raw peppers). The vitamin C may block the test reaction.

For 1 day before using the test, avoid eating foods that make the urine more basic (alkaline). Foods that make the urine alkaline include citrus fruits and juices, milk and other dairy products, and peanuts.

Medicines—Certain medicines may affect the results of the urinary tract infection test. Check with your doctor if you are taking any medicines, especially:

- Acetazolamide (e.g., Diamox) or
- Antacids—These medicines make the urine more basic (alkaline); avoid taking these medicines for 1 day before using the test
- Antibiotics—Some antibiotics may react with the test materials used in this kit.
- Phenazopyridine (e.g., Pyridium)—Do not use the test if you are taking phenazopyridine or other medicines that turn the urine red. Such medicines may appear to cause a positive test reaction even if an infection is not present.
- Vitamin C—Avoid taking large amounts (more than 250 mg) of vitamin C for 10 hours before using the test. The vitamin C may block the test reaction

Proper Use of This Test

Check the expiration date printed on the package before buying the test kit. Do not use outdated strips. Outdated test kits will not work properly.

Read test instructions carefully. Use the test only after you understand the instructions. Most test kits include a toll-free number for consumer questions, or you may ask questions of your doctor, nurse, or pharmacist.

Have someone help you to read the test if you are color-blind or if you cannot see well.

Have a watch or clock with a second hand available, to time the test carefully.

To make sure that the results of your test are not affected:

- Avoid touching the test pads, because skin oils or perspiration may affect the reactions.
- Test the first morning urine, or urine that has been held in the bladder for more than 4 hours.
- Use a clean, dry container to catch the urine sample, or pass the test strip through the stream of urine.
- Test fresh urine. Do not refrigerate the urine or let it stand for more than one-half hour before testing.
- If you have collected the urine in a container, dip the strip in the urine sample for 1 second and tap it on the edge of the container to remove the excess.
- In 30 or 40 seconds, depending on the product used and the directions given, look at the test strip for any trace of pink color. Any color should be uniform, not just appearing in spots or around the edges. You may hold the test strip next to the color chart on the container for comparison.

Do the "test control" if there is one in the package.

Recap the test strip container immediately after use.

Do the test for 3 mornings in a row or as directed by your doctor. It is more likely that you will be able to tell if you have an infection if testing is done more than 1 day.

Record results and report them to your medical doctor.

Storage—To store this product:

- Keep out of the reach of children.
- Do not store in warm, humid conditions or in direct sunlight.

About Your Test Results

If any of your tests show any trace of pink, notify your doctor so that more testing can be done or treatment can be started.

If testing is negative, but you have symptoms of a urinary tract infection, check with your doctor. These symptoms may include:

- Bloody or cloudy urine;
- Burning or pain when you urinate;
- Fever and chills; and
- Frequent and/or sudden urge to urinate;
- General ill feeling;
- Lower abdominal or back pain.

Some infections may be caused by bacteria that do not make nitrites and so are not detected by this test. Your doctor can use other tests to determine if you have such an infection.

It is important to get medical treatment for a urinary tract infection. Untreated infections can cause damage to your kidneys or other health problems. Treatment is usually by an antibiotic that can be taken by mouth.

Annual revision: 07/16/92

UROFOLLITROPIN Systemic

A commonly used brand name in the U.S. and Canada is Metrodin. Other commonly used names are follicle-stimulating hormone and FSH.

Description

Urofollitropin (YOO-roe-fall-ee-troe-pin) is a fertility drug that is identical to the hormone called follicle-stimulating hormone (FSH) that is produced naturally by the pituitary gland.

FSH is primarily responsible for stimulating growth of the ovarian follicle, which includes the developing egg, the cells surrounding the egg that produce the hormones needed to support a pregnancy, and the fluid around the egg. As the ovarian follicle grows, an increasing amount of the hormone estrogen (ESS-troe-jen) is produced by the cells in the follicle and released into the bloodstream. Estrogen causes the endometrium (lining of the uterus) to thicken before ovulation occurs. The higher blood levels of estrogen will also provide a cue to the hypothalamus and pituitary gland to slow the production and release of FSH.

Another pituitary hormone, luteinizing hormone (LH), also helps to increase the amount of estrogen produced by the follicle cells. However, the main function of LH is to cause ovulation. The sharp rise in the blood level of LH that triggers ovulation is sometimes called the LH surge. After ovulation, the group of hormone-producing follicle cells become what is called the corpus luteum and will produce estrogen and large amounts of another hormone, progesterone (proe-JESS-ter-one). Progesterone causes the endometrium to mature so that it can support the egg after it is fertilized. If implantation of a fertilized egg does not occur, the levels of estrogen and progesterone decrease and the endometrium sloughs off (e.g., menstruation occurs).

Urofollitropin is usually given in combination with human chorionic gonadotropin (hCG). The actions of hCG are almost identical to those of LH. It is given to simulate the natural LH surge. This results in predictable ovulation.

Urofollitropin is often used in women who have low levels of FSH and too-high levels of LH. Women with polycystic ovary syndrome usually have hormone levels such as this and are treated with urofollitropin to make up for the low amounts of FSH. Many women being treated with urofollitropin have already tried clomiphene (e.g., Serophene) and have not been able to conceive yet. Urofollitropin may also be used to cause the ovary to produce several follicles, which can then be harvested for use in gamete intrafallopian transfer (GIFT) or in vitro fertilization (IVF).

Urofollitropin is to be given only by or under the supervision of your doctor. It is available in the following dosage form:

Parenteral

- Injection (U.S. and Canada)

It is very important that you read and understand the following information. If any of it causes you special concern, check with your doctor. Also, *if you have any questions* or if you want more information about this medicine or your medical problem, *ask your doctor, nurse, or pharmacist.*

Before Receiving This Medicine

In deciding to use a medicine, the risks of taking the medicine must be weighed against the good it will do. This is a decision you and your doctor will make. For urofollitropin, the following should be considered:

Allergies—Tell your doctor if you have ever had any unusual or allergic reaction to urofollitropin. Also tell your doctor and pharmacist if you are allergic to any other substances, such as foods, preservatives, or dyes.

Pregnancy—If you become pregnant as a result of using this medicine, there is an increased chance of a multiple pregnancy.

Other medicines—Although certain medicines should not be used together at all, in other cases two different medicines may be used together even if an interaction might occur. In these cases, your doctor may want to change the dose, or other precautions may be necessary. Tell your doctor or pharmacist if you are taking any other prescription or nonprescription (over-the-counter [OTC]) medicine.

Other medical problems—The presence of other medical problems may affect the use of urofollitropin. Make sure you tell your doctor if you have any other medical problems, especially:

- Cyst on ovary—Urofollitropin can cause further growth of cysts on the ovary
- Unusual vaginal bleeding—Some irregular vaginal bleeding is a sign that the endometrium is growing too rapidly, possibly of endometrial cancer, or some hormone imbalances; the increases in estrogen production caused by urofollitropin can make these problems worse. If a hormonal imbalance is present, it should be treated before the beginning of menotropins therapy

Before you begin using any new medicine (prescription or nonprescription) or if you develop any new medical problem while you are using this medicine, check with your doctor, nurse, or pharmacist.

Precautions While Receiving This Medicine

It is very important that your doctor check your progress at regular visits to make sure that the medicine is working properly and to check for unwanted effects. Your doctor will likely want to monitor the development of the ovarian follicle(s) by measuring the amount of estrogen in your bloodstream and by checking the size of the follicle(s) with ultrasound examinations.

If your doctor has asked you to record your basal body temperature (BBT) daily, make sure that you do this every day. It is important that intercourse take place around the time of ovulation to give you the best chance of becoming pregnant.

Side Effects of This Medicine

Along with its needed effects, a medicine may cause some unwanted effects. Although not all of these side effects may occur, if they do occur they may need medical attention.

Check with your doctor as soon as possible if any of the following side effects occur:

More common

Abdominal or pelvic pain; bloating (mild); redness, pain, or swelling at the injection site

Less common or rare

Abdominal or stomach pain (severe); bloating (moderate to severe); decreased amount of urine; feeling of indigestion; fever and chills; nausea, vomiting, or diarrhea (continuing or severe); pelvic pain (severe); shortness of breath; skin rash or hives; swelling of lower legs; weight gain (rapid)

Other side effects may occur that usually do not need medical attention. These side effects may go away during treatment as your body adjusts to the medicine. However, check with your doctor if any of the following side effects continue or are bothersome:

Less common or rare

Breast tenderness; diarrhea (mild); nausea; vomiting

After you stop using this medicine, your body may need time to adjust. The length of time this takes depends on the amount of medicine you were using and how long you used it. During this period of time check with your doctor if you notice any of the following side effects:

Abdominal or stomach pain (severe); bloating (moderate to severe); decreased amount of urine; feeling of indigestion; nausea, vomiting, or diarrhea (continuing or severe); pelvic pain (severe); shortness of breath; swelling of lower legs; weight gain (rapid)

Other side effects not listed above may also occur in some patients. If you notice any other effects, check with your doctor.

Annual revision: 07/08/92

URSODIOL Systemic†

A commonly used brand name in the U.S. is Actigall.

Another commonly used name is ursodeoxycholic acid.

†Not commercially available in Canada.

Description

Ursodiol (ur-so-DYE-ole) is used in the treatment of gallstone disease. It is taken by mouth to dissolve the gallstones.

Ursodiol is used in patients who do not need to have their gallbladder removed or in those in whom surgery is best avoided because of other medical problems. However, ursodiol works only in those patients whose gallstones are made of cholesterol and works best when these stones are small and of the "floating" type.

Ursodiol is available only with your doctor's prescription, in the following dosage form:

Oral

- Capsules (U.S.)

It is very important that you read and understand the following information. If any of it causes you special concern, check with your doctor. Also, *if you have any questions* or if you want more information about this medicine or your medical problem, *ask your doctor, nurse, or pharmacist.*

Before Using This Medicine

In deciding to use a medicine, the risks of taking the medicine must be weighed against the good it will do. This is a decision you and your doctor will make. For ursodiol, the following should be considered:

Allergies—Tell your doctor if you have ever had any unusual or allergic reaction to ursodiol or other products containing bile acids.

Diet—It is thought that body weight and the kind of diet the patient follows may affect how fast the stones dissolve and whether new stones will form. However, check with your doctor before going on any diet.

Pregnancy—Studies have not been done in humans. However, ursodiol has not been shown to cause birth defects or other problems in animal studies.

Breast-feeding—It is not known whether ursodiol passes into the breast milk. However, this medicine has not been reported to cause problems in nursing babies.

Children—Although there is no specific information comparing use of ursodiol in children with use in other age groups, this medicine is not expected to cause different side effects or problems in children than it does in adults.

Older adults—Many medicines have not been studied specifically in older people. Therefore, it may not be known whether they work exactly the same way they do in younger adults. Although there is no specific information comparing use of ursodiol in the elderly with use in other age groups, this medicine is not expected to cause different side effects or problems in older people than it does in younger adults.

Other medicines—Although certain medicines should not be used together at all, in other cases 2 different medicines may be used together even if an interaction might occur. In these cases, your doctor may want to change the dose, or other precautions may be necessary. Tell your doctor and pharmacist if you are taking any other prescription or nonprescription (over-the-counter [OTC]) medicine.

Other medical problems—The presence of other medical problems may affect the use of ursodiol. Make sure you tell your doctor if you have any other medical problems, especially:

- Biliary tract problems or
- Pancreatitis (inflammation of pancreas)—These conditions may make it necessary to have surgery since treatment with ursodiol would take too long

Before you begin using any new medicine (prescription or nonprescription) or if you develop any new medical problem while you are using this medicine, check with your doctor, nurse, or pharmacist.

Proper Use of This Medicine

Take ursodiol with meals for best results, unless otherwise directed by your doctor.

Take ursodiol for the full time of treatment, even if you begin to feel better. If you stop taking this medicine too soon, the gallstones may not dissolve as fast or may not dissolve at all.

Missed dose—If you miss a dose of this medicine, take it as soon as possible or double your next dose.

Storage—To store this medicine:

- Keep out of the reach of children.
- Store away from heat and direct light.
- Do not store in the bathroom, near the kitchen sink, or in other damp places. Heat or moisture may cause the medicine to break down.
- Do not keep outdated medicine or medicine no longer needed. Be sure that any discarded medicine is out of the reach of children.

Precautions While Using This Medicine

It is important that your doctor check your progress at regular visits. Laboratory tests will have to be done every few months while you are taking this medicine to make sure that the gallstones are dissolving and your liver is working properly.

Do not take aluminum-containing antacids (e.g., ALternaGEL, Maalox) while taking ursodiol. To do so may keep ursodiol from working properly. Before using an antacid, check with your doctor, nurse, or pharmacist.

Check with your doctor immediately if severe abdominal or stomach pain, especially toward the upper right side, and severe nausea and vomiting occur. These symptoms may mean that you have other medical problems or that your gallstone condition needs your doctor's attention.

Side Effects of This Medicine

Along with its needed effects, a medicine may cause some unwanted effects. The following side effect may go away during treatment as your body adjusts to the medicine. However, check with your doctor if it continues or is bothersome:

Less common or rare

Diarrhea

Other side effects not listed above may also occur in some patients. If you notice any other effects, check with your doctor.

Additional Information

Once a medicine has been approved for marketing for a certain use, experience may show that it is also useful for other medical problems. Although these uses are not included in product labeling, ursodiol is used in certain patients with the following medical conditions:

- Chronic liver disease
- Risk of gallstones (in patients who are in a weight-reduction program)
- Liver transplant (to help reduce the risk of rejection)

There is no additional information relating to proper use, precautions, or side effects for these uses.

Annual revision: 11/11/91

VALPROIC ACID Systemic

This information applies to the following medicines:
Divalproex (dye-VAL-pro-ex)
Valproic Acid (val-PRO-ic acid)

Some commonly used brand names are:

For Divalproex
In the U.S.
Depakote
Depakote Sprinkle
In Canada
Epival

For Valproic Acid
In the U.S.
Depakene
Myproic Acid
Generic name product may also be available.
In Canada
Depakene

Description

Valproic acid and divalproex belong to the group of medicines called anticonvulsants. They are used to control certain types of seizures in the treatment of epilepsy. Valproic acid and divalproex may be used alone or with other seizure medicine.

Divalproex forms valproic acid in the body. Therefore, the following information applies to both medicines.

This medicine is available only with your doctor's prescription, in the following dosage forms:

Oral

Divalproex
- Delayed-release capsules (U.S.)
- Delayed-release tablets (U.S. and Canada)

Valproic Acid
- Capsules (U.S. and Canada)
- Syrup (U.S. and Canada)

It is very important that you read and understand the following information. If any of it causes you special concern, check with your doctor. Also, *if you have any questions* or if you want more information about this medicine or your medical problem, *ask your doctor, nurse, or pharmacist.*

Before Using This Medicine

In deciding to use a medicine, the risks of taking the medicine must be weighed against the good it will do. This is a decision you and your doctor will make. For valproic acid and divalproex, the following should be considered:

Allergies—Tell your doctor if you have ever had any unusual or allergic reaction to divalproex or valproic acid. Also tell your doctor and pharmacist if you are allergic to any other substances, such as foods or dyes.

Pregnancy—Valproic acid and divalproex have been reported to cause birth defects when taken by the mother during the first 3 months of pregnancy. Also, animal studies have shown that valproic acid causes birth defects when taken in doses several times greater than doses used in humans. However, these medicines may be necessary to control seizures in some pregnant patients. Be sure you have discussed this with your doctor.

Breast-feeding—Valproic acid and divalproex pass into the breast milk, but their effect on the nursing baby is not known. It may be necessary for you to take another medicine or to stop breast-feeding during treatment with valproic acid or divalproex. Be sure you have discussed the risks and benefits of this medicine with your doctor.

Children—Abdominal or stomach cramps, nausea or vomiting, tiredness or weakness, and yellow eyes or skin may be especially likely to occur in children, who are usually more sensitive to the effects of valproic acid and divalproex. Children up to 2 years of age and those taking more than 1 medicine for seizure control may be more likely to develop serious side effects.

Older adults—Elderly people are especially sensitive to the effects of valproic acid or divalproex. This may increase the chance of side effects during treatment.

Other medicines—Although certain medicines should not be used together at all, in other cases 2 different medicines may be used together even if an interaction might occur. In these cases, your doctor may want to change the dose, or other precautions may be necessary. When you are taking valproic acid or divalproex, it is especially important that your doctor and pharmacist know if you are taking any of the following:

- Acetaminophen (e.g., Tylenol) (with long-term, high-dose use) or
- Amiodarone (e.g., Cordarone) or
- Anabolic steroids (nandrolone [e.g., Anabolin], oxandrolone [e.g., Anavar], oxymetholone [e.g., Anadrol], stanozolol [e.g., Winstrol]) or
- Androgens (male hormones) or
- Anti-infectives by mouth or injection (medicine for infection) or
- Antithyroid agents (medicine for overactive thyroid) or
- Barbiturates or
- Carbamazepine (e.g., Tegretol) or
- Carmustine (e.g., BiCNU) or
- Chloroquine (e.g., Aralen) or
- Dantrolene (e.g., Dantrium) or
- Daunorubicin (e.g., Cerubidine) or
- Disulfiram (e.g., Antabuse) or
- Estrogens (female hormones) or
- Etretinate (e.g., Tegison) or
- Gold salts (medicine for arthritis) or
- Hydroxychloroquine (e.g., Plaquenil) or
- Mercaptopurine (e.g., Purinethol) or
- Methotrexate (e.g., Mexate) or

- Methyldopa (e.g., Aldomet) or
- Naltrexone (e.g., Trexan) (with long-term, high-dose use) or
- Oral contraceptives (birth control pills) containing estrogen or
- Phenothiazines (acetophenazine [e.g., Tindal], chlorpromazine [e.g., Thorazine], fluphenazine [e.g., Prolixin], mesoridazine [e.g., Serentil], perphenazine [e.g., Trilafon], prochlorperazine [e.g., Compazine], promazine [e.g., Sparine], promethazine [e.g., Phenergan], thioridazine [e.g., Mellaril], trifluoperazine [e.g., Stelazine], triflupromazine [e.g., Vesprin], trimeprazine [e.g., Temaril]) or
- Plicamycin (e.g., Mithracin)—There is an increased risk of serious side effects to the liver
- Central nervous system (CNS) depressants (medicine that causes drowsiness) or
- Tricyclic antidepressants (medicine for depression)—Valproic acid and divalproex may increase CNS depressant effects
- Carbenicillin by injection (e.g., Geopen)
- Dipyridamole (e.g., Persantine) or
- Inflammation or pain medicine, except narcotics, or
- Pentoxifylline (e.g., Trental) or
- Sulfinpyrazone (e.g., Anturane) or
- Ticarcillin (e.g., Ticar)—Valproic acid or divalproex may increase the chance of bleeding because of decreased blood clotting ability; the potential of aspirin, medicine for inflammation or pain, or sulfinpyrazone to cause stomach ulcer and bleeding may also increase the chance of bleeding in patients taking valproic acid or divalproex
- Heparin—There is an increased risk of side effects that may cause bleeding
- Mefloquine—The amount of valproic acid or divalproex that you need to take may change
- Other anticonvulsants (medicine for seizures)—There is an increased risk of seizures

Other medical problems—The presence of other medical problems may affect the use of valproic acid or divalproex. Make sure you tell your doctor if you have any other medical problems, especially:

- Blood disease or
- Brain disease or
- Kidney disease—There is an increased risk of serious side effects
- Liver disease—Valproic acid or divalproex may make the condition worse

Before you begin using any new medicine (prescription or nonprescription) or if you develop any new medical problem while you are using this medicine, check with your doctor, nurse, or pharmacist.

Proper Use of This Medicine

For patients taking *the capsule form* of valproic acid:

- Swallow the capsule whole without chewing or breaking. This is to prevent irritation of the mouth or throat.

For patients taking *the delayed-release capsule form* of divalproex:

- Swallow the capsule whole, or sprinkle the contents on a small amount of soft food such as applesauce or pudding and swallow without chewing.

For patients taking *the delayed-release tablet form* of this medicine:

- Take the tablet with water, not milk, and swallow it whole without chewing, breaking, or crushing. This is to prevent damage to the special coating that helps lessen irritation of the stomach.

For patients taking *the syrup form* of this medicine:

- The syrup may be mixed with any liquid or added to food for a better taste.

This medicine may be taken with meals or snacks to reduce stomach upset.

This medicine must be taken exactly as directed by your doctor to prevent seizures and lessen the possibility of side effects.

Dosing—The dose of valproic acid or divalproex will be different for different patients. *Follow your doctor's orders or the directions on the label.* The following information includes only the average doses of valproic acid or divalproex. *If your dose is different, do not change it* unless your doctor tells you to do so.

- The number of capsules or tablets or teaspoonfuls of syrup that you take depends on the strength of the medicine. Also, *the number of doses you take each day, the time allowed between doses, and the length of time you take the medicine depend on the medical problem for which you are using valproic acid or divalproex.*
- If valproic acid or divalproex is the only medicine you are taking for seizures:

  —Adults and adolescents: Dose is based on body weight. The usual dose is 5 to 15 milligrams per kilogram (2.3 to 6.9 milligrams per pound) to start. Your doctor may increase your dose gradually every week by 5 to 10 milligrams per kilogram of body weight if needed. However, the dose is usually not more than 60 milligrams per kilogram of body weight a day. If the total dose a day is greater than 250 milligrams, it is usually divided into smaller doses and taken two or more times during the day.

  —Children 1 to 12 years of age: Dose is based on body weight. The usual dose is 15 to 45 milligrams per kilogram (6.9 to 20.7 milligrams per pound) to start. The doctor may increase the dose gradually every week by 5 to 10 milligrams per kilogram of body weight if needed.
- If you are taking more than one medicine for seizures:

  —Adults and adolescents: Dose is based on body weight. The usual dose is 10 to 30 milligrams per kilogram (4.6 to 13.8 milligrams per pound) to start. Your doctor may increase your dose gradually every week by 5 to 10 milligrams per kilogram of body weight if needed. If the total dose a day is greater than 250 milligrams, it is usually divided into smaller doses and taken two or more times during the day.

—Children 1 to 12 years of age: Dose is based on body weight. The usual dose is 30 to 100 milligrams per kilogram (13.8 to 45.5 milligrams per pound).

Missed dose—If you miss a dose of this medicine, and your dosing schedule is:

- One dose a day—Take the missed dose as soon as possible. However, if you do not remember until the next day, skip the missed dose and go back to your regular dosing schedule. Do not double doses.
- Two or more doses a day—If you remember within 6 hours of the missed dose, take it right away. Then take the rest of the doses for that day at equally spaced times. Do not double doses.

If you have any questions about this, check with your doctor.

Storage—To store this medicine:

- Keep out of the reach of children.
- Store away from heat and direct light.
- Do not store the capsule or tablet form of this medicine in the bathroom, near the kitchen sink, or in other damp places. Heat or moisture may cause the medicine to break down.
- Keep the syrup form of this medicine from freezing.
- Do not keep outdated medicine or medicine no longer needed. Be sure that any discarded medicine is out of the reach of children.

Precautions While Using This Medicine

Your doctor should check your progress at regular visits, especially for the first few months you take this medicine. This is necessary to allow dose adjustments and to reduce any unwanted effects.

Do not stop taking valproic acid or divalproex without first checking with your doctor. Your doctor may want you to gradually reduce the amount you are taking before stopping completely. Stopping the medicine suddenly may cause you to have seizures again.

Before you have any medical tests, tell the doctor in charge that you are taking this medicine. The results of the metyrapone and thyroid function tests may be affected by this medicine.

Before having any kind of surgery, dental treatment, or emergency treatment, tell the medical doctor or dentist in charge that you are taking this medicine. Valproic acid or divalproex may change the time it takes your blood to clot, which may increase the chance of bleeding. Also, taking valproic acid or divalproex together with medicines that are used during surgery or dental or emergency treatments may increase the CNS depressant effects.

Valproic acid and divalproex will add to the effects of alcohol and other CNS depressants (medicines that slow down the nervous system, possibly causing drowsiness). Some examples of CNS depressants are antihistamines or medicine for hay fever, other allergies, or colds; sedatives, tranquilizers, or sleeping medicine; prescription pain medicine or narcotics; barbiturates; medicine for seizures; muscle relaxants; or anesthetics, including some dental anesthetics. *Check with your doctor before taking any of the above while you are using this medicine.*

For diabetic patients:

- This medicine may interfere with urine tests for ketones and give false-positive results.

Your doctor may want you to carry a medical identification card or bracelet stating that you are taking this medicine.

This medicine may cause some people to become drowsy or less alert than they are normally. *Make sure you know how you react to this medicine before you drive, use machines, or do anything else that could be dangerous if you are not alert.*

Side Effects of This Medicine

Along with its needed effects, a medicine may cause some unwanted effects. Although not all of these side effects may occur, if they do occur they may need medical attention.

Check with your doctor as soon as possible if any of the following side effects occur:

Less common

Abdominal or stomach cramps (severe); behavioral, mood, or mental changes; continuous, uncontrolled back-and-forth and/or rolling eye movements; double vision; increase in seizures; loss of appetite; nausea or vomiting (continuing); spots before eyes; swelling of face; tiredness and weakness; unusual bleeding or bruising; yellow eyes or skin

Other side effects may occur that usually do not need medical attention. These side effects may go away during treatment as your body adjusts to the medicine. However, check with your doctor if any of the following side effects continue or are bothersome:

More common

Abdominal or stomach cramps (mild); change in menstrual periods; diarrhea; hair loss; indigestion; loss of appetite; nausea and vomiting; trembling of hands and arms; unusual weight loss or gain

Less common or rare
Clumsiness or unsteadiness; constipation; dizziness; drowsiness; headache; skin rash; unusual excitement, restlessness, or irritability

Other side effects not listed above may also occur in some patients. If you notice any other effects, check with your doctor.

Additional Information

Once a medicine has been approved for marketing for a certain use, experience may show that it is also useful for other medical problems. Although these uses are not included in product labeling, valproic acid and divalproex are used in certain patients with the following medical condition:

- Bipolar disorder (manic-depressive illness)

Other than the above information, there is no additional information relating to proper use, precautions, or side effects for these uses.

Annual revision: 03/09/93

VANCOMYCIN Oral

A commonly used brand name in the U.S. and Canada is Vancocin.

Description

Vancomycin (van-koe-MYE-sin) belongs to the family of medicines called antibiotics. Antibiotics are medicines used in the treatment of infections caused by bacteria. They work by killing bacteria or preventing their growth. Vancomycin will not work for colds, flu, or other virus infections.

When oral vancomycin is taken by mouth, it is not absorbed very much and works inside the intestinal tract to treat certain types of colitis (an inflammation of the small or large intestine). Vancomycin may also be used for other conditions as determined by your doctor.

Vancomycin is available only with your doctor's prescription, in the following dosage forms:

Oral
- Capsules (U.S. and Canada)
- Oral solution (U.S.)

It is very important that you read and understand the following information. If any of it causes you special concern, check with your doctor. Also, *if you have any questions* or if you want more information about this medicine or your medical problem, *ask your doctor, nurse, or pharmacist.*

Before Using This Medicine

In deciding to use a medicine, the risks of taking the medicine must be weighed against the good it will do. This is a decision you and your doctor will make. For oral vancomycin, the following should be considered:

Allergies—Tell your doctor if you have ever had any unusual or allergic reaction to oral vancomycin. Also tell your doctor and pharmacist if you are allergic to any other substances, such as foods, preservatives, or dyes.

Pregnancy—Studies with oral vancomycin have not been done in either humans or animals.

Breast-feeding—Vancomycin passes into the breast milk. However, when taken by mouth, only small amounts of vancomycin are absorbed into the mother's body. In addition, vancomycin is not absorbed very much from the digestive tract (stomach and intestines) of the nursing infant.

Children—Although there is no specific information comparing use of oral vancomycin in children with use in other age groups, this medicine is not expected to cause different side effects or problems in children than it does in adults.

Older adults—Elderly people may be more sensitive to the effects of oral vancomycin. This may increase the chance of a loss of hearing and ringing or buzzing or a feeling of fullness in the ears.

Other medicines—Although certain medicines should not be used together at all, in other cases two different medicines may be used together even if an interaction might occur. In these cases, your doctor may want to change the dose, or other precautions may be necessary. When you are taking oral vancomycin, it is especially important that your doctor and pharmacist know if you are taking any of the following:

- Cholestyramine (e.g., Questran) or
- Colestipol (e.g., Colestid)—Use of these medicines with oral vancomycin may decrease the effects of oral vancomycin

Other medical problems—The presence of other medical problems may affect the use of oral vancomycin. Make sure you tell your doctor if you have any other medical problems, especially:

- Kidney disease, severe, or
- Loss of hearing, or deafness, history of, or
- Other inflammatory bowel disorders—Patients with these medical problems may have an increased chance of side effects

Before you begin using any new medicine (prescription or nonprescription) or if you develop any new medical problem while you are using this medicine, check with your doctor, nurse, or pharmacist.

Proper Use of This Medicine

For patients taking the *oral liquid form* of vancomycin:

- Use a specially marked measuring spoon or other device to measure each dose accurately. The average household teaspoon may not hold the right amount of liquid.
- Do not use after the expiration date on the label. The medicine may not work properly after that date. Check with your pharmacist if you have any questions about this.

To help clear up your colitis completely, *keep taking this medicine for the full time of treatment,* even if you begin to feel better after a few days. If you stop taking this medicine too soon, your symptoms may return. *Do not miss any doses.*

Dosing—The dose of oral vancomycin will be different for different patients. *Follow your doctor's orders or the directions on the label.* The following information includes only the average doses of oral vancomycin. *If your dose is different, do not change it* unless your doctor tells you to do so.

- The number of capsules or teaspoonfuls of solution that you take depends on the strength of the medicine. Also, *the number of doses you take each day, the time allowed between doses, and the length of time you take the medicine depend on the medical problem for which you are taking oral vancomycin.*
- For *oral* dosage forms (capsules, oral solution):
  —Adults and adolescents: 125 to 500 milligrams every 6 hours for 5 to 10 days.
  —Children: Dose is based on body weight and must be determined by the doctor. The usual dose is 10 milligrams per kilogram of body weight (22 milligrams per pound). This dose is taken every 6 hours for 5 to 10 days.

Missed dose—If you miss a dose of this medicine, take it as soon as possible. However, if it is almost time for your next dose, skip the missed dose and go back to your regular dosing schedule. Do not double doses.

Storage—To store this medicine:

- Keep out of the reach of children.
- Store away from heat and direct light.
- Do not store the capsule form of this medicine in the bathroom, near the kitchen sink, or in other damp places. Heat or moisture may cause the medicine to break down.
- Store the oral liquid form of vancomycin in the refrigerator because heat will cause this medicine to break down. However, keep the medicine from freezing. Follow the directions on the label.
- Do not keep outdated medicine or medicine no longer needed. Be sure that any discarded medicine is out of the reach of children.

Precautions While Using This Medicine

It is important that your doctor check your progress during and after treatment. This is to make sure that the colitis is cleared up completely.

If the symptoms of your colitis do not improve within a few days, or if they become worse, check with your doctor.

If your doctor orders cholestyramine or colestipol for your colitis, do not take vancomycin by mouth within 3 to 4 hours of taking either of these medicines. To do so may keep vancomycin from working properly.

If you are taking this medicine for diarrhea caused by other antibiotics, do not take any other diarrhea medicine without first checking with your doctor or pharmacist. These medicines may make your diarrhea worse or make it last longer.

Side Effects of This Medicine

Along with its needed effects, a medicine may cause some unwanted effects. Although not all of these side effects may occur, if they do occur they may need medical attention.

Check with your doctor immediately if any of the following side effects occur:

Rare

Loss of hearing; ringing or buzzing or a feeling of fullness in the ears

Note: The above side effects may also occur up to several weeks after you stop taking this medicine.

Other side effects may occur that usually do not need medical attention. These side effects may go away during treatment as your body adjusts to the medicine. However,

check with your doctor if any of the following side effects continue or are bothersome:

More common

Bitter or unpleasant taste; nausea or vomiting

Other side effects not listed above may also occur in some patients. If you notice any other effects, check with your doctor.

Annual revision: 02/23/93

VANCOMYCIN Systemic

Some commonly used brand names are:

In the U.S.

Lyphocin
Vancoled
Vancocin

Generic name product may also be available.

In Canada

Vancocin

Description

Vancomycin (van-koe-MYE-sin) belongs to the family of medicines called antibiotics. Antibiotics are medicines used in the treatment of infections caused by bacteria. They work by killing bacteria or preventing their growth. Vancomycin will not work for colds, flu, or other virus infections.

Vancomycin is used to treat infections in many different parts of the body. It is sometimes given with other antibiotics. Vancomycin is also used in patients with heart valve disease (e.g., rheumatic fever) or prosthetic (artificial) heart valves who are allergic to penicillin. This medicine is used to prevent endocarditis (inflammation of the lining of the heart) in these patients who are having dental work or surgery done on the upper respiratory tract (for example, nose or throat). Vancomycin may also be used for other conditions as determined by your doctor.

Vancomycin given by injection is usually used for serious infections in which other medicines may not work. However, this medicine may also cause some serious side effects, including damage to your hearing and kidneys. These side effects may be more likely to occur in elderly patients. You and your doctor should talk about the good this medicine will do as well as the risks of receiving it.

Vancomycin is available only with your doctor's prescription, in the following dosage form:

Parenteral

- Injection (U.S. and Canada)

It is very important that you read and understand the following information. If any of it causes you special concern, check with your doctor. Also, *if you have any questions* or if you want more information about this medicine or your medical problem, *ask your doctor, nurse, or pharmacist.*

Before Receiving This Medicine

In deciding to use a medicine, the risks of taking the medicine must be weighed against the good it will do. This is a decision you and your doctor will make. For vancomycin, the following should be considered:

Allergies—Tell your doctor if you have ever had any unusual or allergic reaction to vancomycin. Also tell your doctor and pharmacist if you are allergic to any other substances, such as foods, preservatives, or dyes.

Pregnancy—Vancomycin has not been reported to cause hearing loss or kidney damage in the infants of women given vancomycin during their second or third trimesters of pregnancy. It has also not been reported to cause birth defects in animal studies.

Breast-feeding—Vancomycin passes into breast milk. However, this medicine has not been reported to cause problems in nursing babies.

Children—Vancomycin can cause serious side effects in any patient. Therefore, it is especially important that you discuss with the child's doctor the good that this medicine will do as well as the risks of using it.

Older adults—Elderly people may be especially sensitive to the effects of vancomycin. This may increase the chance of hearing or kidney damage.

Other medicines—Although certain medicines should not be used together at all, in other cases two different medicines may be used together even if an interaction might occur. In these cases, your doctor may want to change the dose, or other precautions may be necessary. When you are receiving vancomycin, it is especially important that your doctor and pharmacist know if you are taking any of the following:

- Aminoglycosides by injection (amikacin [e.g., Amikin], gentamicin [e.g., Garamycin], kanamycin [e.g., Kantrex], neomycin [e.g., Mycifradin], netilmicin [e.g., Netromycin], streptomycin, tobramycin [e.g., Nebcin]) or
- Amphotericin B by injection (e.g., Fungizone) or
- Bacitracin by injection or
- Bumetanide by injection (e.g., Bumex) or
- Capreomycin (e.g., Capastat) or
- Cisplatin (e.g., Platinol) or
- Cyclosporine (e.g., Sandimmune) or
- Ethacrynic acid by injection (e.g., Edecrin) or
- Furosemide by injection (e.g., Lasix) or

- Paromomycin (e.g., Humatin) or
- Polymyxins, especially colistimethate (e.g., Coly-Mycin M) and polymyxin B (e.g., Aerosporin) or
- Streptozocin (e.g., Zanosar)—Use of these medicines with vancomycin may increase the chance of side effects

Other medical problems—The presence of other medical problems may affect the use of vancomycin. Make sure you tell your doctor if you have any other medical problems, especially:

- Kidney disease or
- Loss of hearing, or deafness, history of—Patients with kidney disease or a history of hearing loss or deafness may have an increased chance of side effects

Before you begin using any new medicine (prescription or nonprescription) or if you develop any new medical problem while you are using this medicine, check with your doctor, nurse, or pharmacist.

Proper Use of This Medicine

Some medicines given by injection may sometimes be given at home to patients who do not need to be in the hospital for the full time of treatment. If you are receiving this medicine at home, *make sure you clearly understand and carefully follow your doctor's instructions.*

To help clear up your infection completely, *vancomycin must be given for the full time of treatment,* even if you begin to feel better after a few days. Also, this medicine works best when there is a constant amount in the blood or stool. To help keep the amount constant, vancomycin must be given on a regular schedule.

Side Effects of This Medicine

Along with its needed effects, a medicine may cause some unwanted effects. Although not all of these side effects may occur, if they do occur they may need medical attention.

Check with your doctor or nurse immediately if any of the following side effects occur:

Less common

Change in the frequency of urination or amount of urine; difficulty in breathing; drowsiness; increased thirst; loss of appetite; nausea or vomiting; weakness

Rare

Loss of hearing; ringing or buzzing or a feeling of fullness in the ears

Note: The above side effects may also occur up to several weeks after you stop receiving this medicine.

Symptoms of "red-neck syndrome"—Rare

Chills or fever; fainting; fast heartbeat; itching; nausea or vomiting; rash or redness of the face, base of neck, upper body, back, and arms; tingling; unpleasant taste

Note: Symptoms of the "red-neck syndrome" are more common when vancomycin is given by direct or rapid injection.

The above side effects, except the "red-neck syndrome," are more likely to occur in the elderly, who are usually more sensitive to the effects of vancomycin.

Other side effects not listed above may also occur in some patients. If you notice any other effects, check with your doctor.

Annual revision: 09/20/92

VASOPRESSIN Systemic

Some commonly used brand names are:

In the U.S.
Pitressin
Generic name product may also be available.

In Canada
Pitressin
Pressyn

Description

Vasopressin (vay-soe-PRESS-in) is a hormone naturally produced by your body. It is necessary to maintain good health. Lack of vasopressin causes your body to lose too much water.

Vasopressin is used to control the frequent urination, increased thirst, and loss of water associated with diabetes insipidus (water diabetes).

Vasopressin also may be used for other conditions as determined by your doctor.

This medicine is available only with your doctor's prescription, in the following dosage form:

Parenteral

- Injection (U.S. and Canada)

It is very important that you read and understand the following information. If any of it causes you special concern, check with your doctor. Also, *if you have any questions* or if you want more information about this medicine or your medical problem, *ask your doctor, nurse, or pharmacist.*

Before Receiving This Medicine

In deciding to use a medicine, the risks of taking the medicine must be weighed against the good it will do. This is a decision you and your doctor will make. For vasopressin, the following should be considered:

Allergies—Tell your doctor if you have ever had any unusual or allergic reaction to vasopressin. Also tell your doctor and pharmacist if you are allergic to any other substances, such as foods, preservatives, or dyes.

Pregnancy—Vasopressin has not been shown to cause birth defects or other problems in humans.

Breast-feeding—Vasopressin has not been reported to cause problems in nursing babies.

Children—Children may be especially sensitive to the effects of vasopressin. This may increase the chance of side effects during treatment.

Older adults—Many medicines have not been studied specifically in older people. Therefore, it may not be known whether they work exactly the same way they do in younger adults or if they cause different side effects or problems in older people. Although there is no specific information comparing the use of vasopressin in the elderly with use in other age groups, the elderly may be more sensitive to its effects.

Other medicines—Although certain medicines should not be used together at all, in other cases two different medicines may be used together even if an interaction might occur. In these cases, your doctor may want to change the dose, or other precautions may be necessary. Tell your doctor and pharmacist if you are taking any other prescription or nonprescription (over-the-counter [OTC]) medicine.

Other medical problems—The presence of other medical problems may affect the use of vasopressin. Make sure you tell your doctor if you have any other medical problems, especially:

- Asthma or
- Epilepsy or
- Heart disease or
- Kidney disease or
- Migraine headaches—If fluid retention (keeping more body water) caused by vasopressin occurs too fast, these conditions may be worsened
- Heart or blood vessel disease—Vasopressin can cause chest pain or a heart attack; it can also increase blood pressure

Before you begin using any new medicine (prescription or nonprescription) or if you develop any new medical problem while you are using this medicine, check with your doctor, nurse, or pharmacist.

Proper Use of This Medicine

Use this medicine only as directed. Do not use more of it and do not use it more often than your doctor ordered. To do so may increase the chance of side effects.

Missed dose—If you miss a dose of this medicine, use it as soon as possible. However, if it is almost time for your next dose, skip the missed dose and go back to your regular dosing schedule. Do not double doses.

Storage—To store this medicine:

- Keep out of the reach of children.
- Store away from heat and direct light.
- Keep from freezing.
- Do not keep outdated medicine or medicine no longer needed. Be sure that any discarded medicine is out of the reach of children.

Side Effects of This Medicine

Along with its needed effects, a medicine may cause some unwanted effects. Although not all of these effects may occur, if they do occur they may need medical attention.

Check with your doctor immediately if any of the following side effects occur since they may be signs or symptoms of an allergic reaction or overdose:

Rare

Chest pain; coma; confusion; convulsions (seizures); drowsiness; fever; headache (continuing); problems with urination; redness of skin; skin rash, hives, or itching; swelling of face, feet, hands, or mouth; weight gain; wheezing or troubled breathing

Other side effects may occur that usually do not need medical attention. These side effects may go away during treatment as your body adjusts to the medicine. However, check with your doctor if any of the following side effects continue or are bothersome:

Less common

Abdominal or stomach cramps; belching; diarrhea; dizziness or lightheadedness; increased sweating; increased urge for bowel movement; nausea or vomiting; pale skin; passage of gas; "pounding" in head; trembling; white-colored area around mouth

Other side effects not listed above may also occur in some patients. If you notice any other effects, check with your doctor.

Annual revision: 08/26/93

VIDARABINE Ophthalmic

A commonly used brand name in the U.S. and Canada is Vira-A. Other commonly used names are arabinoside and ara-A.

Description

Vidarabine (vye-DARE-a-been) ophthalmic preparations are used to treat virus infections of the eye.

Vidarabine is available only with your doctor's prescription, in the following dosage form:

Ophthalmic

- Ophthalmic ointment (U.S. and Canada)

It is very important that you read and understand the following information. If any of it causes you special concern, check with your doctor. Also, *if you have any questions* or if you want more information about this medicine or your medical problem, *ask your doctor, nurse, or pharmacist.*

Before Using This Medicine

In deciding to use a medicine, the risks of using the medicine must be weighed against the good it will do. This is a decision you and your doctor will make. For vidarabine, the following should be considered:

Allergies—Tell your doctor if you have ever had any unusual or allergic reaction to vidarabine. Also tell your doctor and pharmacist if you are allergic to any other substances, such as preservatives.

Pregnancy—Studies have not been done in humans. Studies in rats and rabbits have shown that vidarabine, given by injection, causes birth defects. In addition, studies in rabbits have shown that vidarabine, applied as a 10% ointment to the skin, may cause birth defects or other problems. However, these doses are much higher than those used in the eyes of humans. Therefore, the chance that vidarabine ophthalmic ointment would cause birth defects or other problems in humans is very small.

Breast-feeding—It is not known whether vidarabine, applied to the eyes, is absorbed into the body and passes into the breast milk. Although most medicines pass into breast milk in small amounts, many of them may be used safely while breast-feeding. Mothers who are taking this medicine and who wish to breast-feed should discuss this with their doctor.

Children—Although there is no specific information comparing use of vidarabine in children with use in other age groups, it is not expected to cause different side effects or problems in children than it does in adults.

Older adults—Many medicines have not been studied specifically in older people. Therefore, it may not be known whether they work exactly the same way they do in younger adults or if they cause different side effects or problems in older people. There is no specific information comparing use of vidarabine in the elderly with use in other age groups.

Other medicines—Although certain medicines should not be used together at all, in other cases two different medicines may be used together even if an interaction might occur. In these cases, your doctor may want to change the dose, or other precautions may be necessary. Tell your doctor and pharmacist if you are using any other prescription or nonprescription (over-the-counter [OTC]) medicine in your eyes.

Before you begin using any new medicine (prescription or nonprescription) or if you develop any new medical problem while you are using this medicine, check with your doctor, nurse, or pharmacist.

Proper Use of This Medicine

To use:

- First, wash your hands. Then pull the lower eyelid away from the eye to form a pouch. Squeeze a thin strip of ointment into the pouch. A 1.25-cm (approximately ½-inch) strip of ointment is usually enough unless otherwise directed by your doctor. Gently close the eyes and keep them closed for 1 or 2 minutes to allow the medicine to come into contact with the infection.
- To keep the medicine as germ-free as possible, do not touch the applicator tip to any surface (including the eye). After using vidarabine eye ointment, wipe the tip of the ointment tube with a clean tissue and keep the tube tightly closed.

Do not use this medicine more often or for a longer time than your doctor ordered. To do so may cause problems in the eyes. If you have any questions about this, check with your doctor.

To help clear up your infection completely, *keep using this medicine for the full time of treatment,* even if your symptoms have disappeared. *Do not miss any doses.*

Dosing—The dose of ophthalmic vidarabine will be different for different patients. *Follow your doctor's orders or the directions on the label.* The following information includes only the average doses of ophthalmic vidarabine. *If your dose is different, do not change it* unless your doctor tells you to do so.

The number of doses you use each day, the time allowed between doses, and the length of time you use the medicine depend on the medical problem for which you are using ophthalmic vidarabine.

- For *ophthalmic ointment* dosage forms:
  —For virus eye infection:
    - Adults and children—Use in each eye every three hours (five times a day). After healing has occurred, the dose may be reduced to two times a day for seven days more.

Missed dose—If you miss a dose of this medicine, apply it as soon as possible. However, if it is almost time for your next dose, skip the missed dose and go back to your regular dosing schedule.

Storage—To store this medicine:
- Keep out of the reach of children.
- Store away from heat and direct light.
- Keep the medicine from freezing.
- Do not keep outdated medicine or medicine no longer needed. Be sure that any discarded medicine is out of the reach of children.

Precautions While Using This Medicine

After application, eye ointments usually cause your vision to blur for a few minutes.

It is very important that you keep your appointments with your doctor. If your symptoms become worse, check with your doctor sooner.

This medicine may cause your eyes to become more sensitive to light than they are normally. Wearing sunglasses and avoiding too much exposure to bright light may help lessen the discomfort.

Side Effects of This Medicine

Along with its needed effects, a medicine may cause some unwanted effects. Although not all of these side effects may occur, if they do occur they may need medical attention.

Check with your doctor as soon as possible if any of the following side effects occur:

Increased sensitivity of eyes to light; itching, redness, swelling, pain, burning, or other sign of irritation not present before use of this medicine

Other side effects may occur that usually do not need medical attention. These side effects may go away during treatment as your body adjusts to the medicine. However, check with your doctor if either of the following side effects continues or is bothersome:

Excess flow of tears; feeling of something in the eye

Other side effects not listed above may also occur in some patients. If you notice any other effects, check with your doctor.

Annual revision: 07/01/93

VINBLASTINE Systemic

Some commonly used brand names are:

In the U.S.
Velban
Velsar
Generic name product may also be available.

In Canada
Velbe

Description

Vinblastine (vin-BLAS-teen) belongs to the group of medicines known as antineoplastic agents. It is used to treat some kinds of cancer as well as some noncancerous conditions.

Vinblastine interferes with the growth of cancer cells, which are eventually destroyed. Since the growth of normal body cells may also be affected by vinblastine, other effects will also occur. Some of these may be serious and must be reported to your doctor. Other effects, such as hair loss, may not be serious but may cause concern. Some effects do not occur for months or years after the medicine is used.

Before you begin treatment with vinblastine, you and your doctor should talk about the good this medicine will do as well as the risks of using it.

Vinblastine is to be administered only by or under the immediate supervision of your doctor. It is available in the following dosage form:

Parenteral
- Injection (U.S. and Canada)

It is very important that you read and understand the following information. If any of it causes you special concern, check with your doctor. Also, *if you have any questions* or if you want more information about this medicine or your medical problem, *ask your doctor, nurse, or pharmacist.*

Before Using This Medicine

In deciding to use a medicine, the risks of taking the medicine must be weighed against the good it will do. This is a decision you and your doctor will make. For vinblastine, the following should be considered:

Allergies—Tell your doctor if you have ever had any unusual or allergic reaction to vinblastine.

Pregnancy—Tell your doctor if you are pregnant or if you intend to have children. This medicine may cause birth defects if either the male or female is taking it at the time of conception or if it is taken during pregnancy. In addition, many cancer medicines may cause sterility which could be permanent. Although sterility has not been reported with this medicine, vinblastine may interfere with production of sperm and the possibility should be kept in mind.

Be sure that you have discussed this with your doctor before receiving this medicine. It is best to use some kind of birth control while you are receiving vinblastine. Tell your doctor right away if you think you have become pregnant while receiving vinblastine.

Breast-feeding—Tell your doctor if you are breast-feeding or if you intend to breast-feed during treatment with this medicine. Because vinblastine may cause serious side effects, breast-feeding is generally not recommended while you are receiving it.

Children—This medicine has been tested in children and has not been shown to cause different side effects or problems than it does in adults.

Older adults—Many medicines have not been tested in older people. Therefore, it may not be known whether they work exactly the same way they do in younger adults or if they cause different side effects or problems in older people. There is no specific information about the use of vinblastine in the elderly.

Other medicines—Although certain medicines should not be used together at all, in other cases two different medicines may be used together even if an interaction might occur. In these cases, your doctor may want to change the dose, or other precautions may be necessary. When you are receiving vinblastine, it is especially important that your doctor and pharmacist know if you are taking any of the following:

- Amphotericin B by injection (e.g., Fungizone) or
- Antithyroid agents (medicine for overactive thyroid) or
- Azathioprine (e.g., Imuran) or
- Chloramphenicol (e.g., Chloromycetin) or
- Colchicine or
- Flucytosine (e.g., Ancobon) or
- Interferon (e.g., Intron A, Roferon-A) or
- Plicamycin (e.g., Mithracin) or
- Zidovudine (e.g., Retrovir) or
- If you have ever been treated with x-rays or cancer medicines—Vinblastine may increase the effects of these medicines or radiation therapy on the blood
- Probenecid (e.g., Benemid) or
- Sulfinpyrazone (e.g., Anturane)—Vinblastine may increase the concentration of uric acid in the blood, which these medicines are used to lower

Other medical problems—The presence of other medical problems may affect the use of vinblastine. Make sure you tell your doctor if you have any other medical problems, especially:

- Chickenpox (including recent exposure) or
- Herpes zoster (shingles)—Risk of severe disease affecting other parts of the body
- Gout (history of) or
- Kidney stones (history of)—Vinblastine may increase levels of uric acid in the body, which can cause gout or kidney stones
- Infection—Vinblastine can reduce immunity to infection
- Liver disease—Effects may be increased because of slower removal of vinblastine from the body

Before you begin using any new medicine (prescription or nonprescription) or if you develop any new medical problem while you are using this medicine, check with your doctor, nurse, or pharmacist.

Proper Use of This Medicine

Vinblastine is sometimes given together with certain other medicines. If you are using a combination of medicines, it is important that you receive each one at the proper time. If you are taking some of these medicines by mouth, ask your doctor, nurse, or pharmacist to help you plan a way to take them at the right times.

While you are using this medicine, your doctor may want you to drink extra fluids so that you will pass more urine. This will help prevent kidney problems and keep your kidneys working well.

Vinblastine sometimes causes nausea and vomiting. However, it is very important that you continue to receive the medicine, even if you begin to feel ill. Ask your doctor, nurse, or pharmacist for ways to lessen these effects.

Precautions While Using This Medicine

It is very important that your doctor check your progress at regular visits to make sure that this medicine is working properly and to check for unwanted effects.

While you are being treated with vinblastine, and after you stop treatment with it, *do not have any immunizations (vaccinations) without your doctor's approval.* Vinblastine may lower your body's resistance and there is a chance you might get the infection the immunization is meant to prevent. Other people living in your household should not take oral polio vaccine since there is a chance they could pass the polio virus on to you. Also, avoid persons who have taken oral polio vaccine. Do not get close to them, and do not stay in the same room with them for very long. If you cannot take these precautions, you should consider wearing a protective face mask that covers the nose and mouth.

Vinblastine can temporarily lower the number of white blood cells in your blood, increasing the chance of getting an infection. It can also lower the number of platelets, which are necessary for proper blood clotting. If this occurs, there are certain precautions you can take, especially when your blood count is low, to reduce the risk of infection or bleeding:

- If you can, avoid people with infections. *Check with your doctor immediately* if you think you are getting an infection or if you get a fever or chills, cough or hoarseness, lower back or side pain, or painful or difficult urination.
- *Check with your doctor immediately* if you notice any unusual bleeding or bruising; black, tarry stools; blood in urine or stools; or pinpoint red spots on your skin.
- Be careful when using a regular toothbrush, dental floss, or toothpick. Your medical doctor, dentist, or nurse may recommend other ways to clean your teeth and gums. Check with your medical doctor before having any dental work done.
- Do not touch your eyes or the inside of your nose unless you have just washed your hands and have not touched anything else in the meantime.
- Be careful not to cut yourself when you are using sharp objects such as a safety razor or fingernail or toenail cutters.
- Avoid contact sports or other situations where bruising or injury could occur.

If vinblastine accidentally seeps out of the vein into which it is injected, it may damage the skin and cause some scarring. *Tell the doctor or nurse right away if you notice redness, pain, or swelling at the place of injection.*

Side Effects of This Medicine

Along with their needed effects medicines like vinblastine can sometimes cause unwanted effects such as blood problems, loss of hair, and other side effects. These and others are described below. Also, because of the way these medicines act on the body, there is a chance that they might cause other unwanted effects that may not occur until months or years after the medicine is used. These delayed effects may include certain types of cancer, such as leukemia. Discuss these possible effects with your doctor.

Although not all of these side effects may occur, if they do occur they may need medical attention.

Check with your doctor or nurse immediately if any of the following side effects occur:

Less common

Cough or hoarseness; fever or chills; lower back or side pain; painful or difficult urination; pain or redness at place of injection

Rare

Black, tarry stools; blood in urine or stools; pinpoint red spots on skin; unusual bleeding or bruising

Check with your doctor or nurse as soon as possible if any of the following side effects occur:

Less common

Joint pain; sores in mouth and on lips; swelling of feet or lower legs

Rare

Difficulty in walking; dizziness; double vision; drooping eyelids; headache; jaw pain; mental depression; numbness or tingling in fingers and toes; pain in fingers and toes; pain in testicles; weakness

Other side effects may occur that usually do not need medical attention. These side effects may go away during treatment as your body adjusts to the medicine. Also, your doctor or nurse may be able to tell you about ways to prevent or reduce some of these side effects. Check with your doctor or nurse if any of the following side effects continue or are bothersome or if you have any questions about them:

Less common

Muscle pain; nausea and vomiting

This medicine often causes a temporary loss of hair. After treatment with vinblastine has ended, or sometimes even during treatment, normal hair growth should return.

Other side effects not listed above may also occur in some patients. If you notice any other effects, check with your doctor.

Annual revision: September 1990
Interim revision: 08/02/93

VINCRISTINE Systemic

Some commonly used brand names are:

In the U.S.
- Oncovin
- Vincasar PFS
- Vincrex

Generic name product may also be available.

In Canada
- Oncovin

Description

Vincristine (vin-KRIS-teen) belongs to the group of medicines known as antineoplastic agents. It is used to treat some kinds of cancer as well as some noncancerous conditions.

Vincristine interferes with the growth of cancer cells, which are eventually destroyed. Since the growth of normal body cells may also be affected by vincristine, other effects will also occur. Some of these may be serious and must be reported to your doctor. Other effects, such as hair loss, may not be serious but may cause concern. Some effects may not occur for months or years after the medicine is used.

Before you begin treatment with vincristine, you and your doctor should talk about the good this medicine will do as well as the risks of using it.

Vincristine is to be administered only by or under the immediate supervision of your doctor. It is available in the following dosage form:

Parenteral
- Injection (U.S. and Canada)

It is very important that you read and understand the following information. If any of it causes you special concern, check with your doctor. Also, *if you have any questions* or if you want more information about this medicine or your medical problem, *ask your doctor, nurse, or pharmacist.*

Before Using This Medicine

In deciding to use a medicine, the risks of taking the medicine must be weighed against the good it will do. This is a decision you and your doctor will make. For vincristine, the following should be considered:

Allergies—Tell your doctor if you have ever had any unusual or allergic reaction to vincristine.

Pregnancy—Tell your doctor if you are pregnant or if you intend to have children. There is a chance that this medicine may cause birth defects if either the male or female is taking it at the time of conception or if it is taken during pregnancy. Vincristine causes birth defects and death of the fetus in animals. In addition, many cancer medicines may cause sterility, which could be permanent. Although sterility has not been reported with this medicine, the possibility should be kept in mind.

Be sure that you have discussed this with your doctor before receiving this medicine. It is best to use some kind of birth control while you are receiving vincristine. Tell your doctor right away if you think you have become pregnant while receiving vincristine.

Breast-feeding—Tell your doctor if you are breast-feeding or if you intend to breast-feed during treatment with this medicine. Because vincristine may cause serious side effects, breast-feeding is generally not recommended while you are receiving it.

Children—This medicine has been tested in children and has not been shown to cause different side effects or problems than it does in adults.

Older adults—Nervous system effects may be more likely to occur in the elderly, who are usually more sensitive to the effects of vincristine.

Other medicines—Although certain medicines should not be used together at all, in other cases two different medicines may be used together even if an interaction might occur. In these cases, your doctor may want to change the dose, or other precautions may be necessary. When you are receiving vincristine, it is especially important that your doctor and pharmacist know if you are taking any of the following:

- Probenecid (e.g., Benemid) or
- Sulfinpyrazone (e.g., Anturane)—Vincristine may increase the concentration of uric acid in the blood, which these medicines are used to lower
- If you have ever been treated with x-rays or cancer medicines—Vincristine may increase the effects of these medicines or radiation therapy on the blood

Other medical problems—The presence of other medical problems may affect the use of vincristine. Make sure you tell your doctor if you have any other medical problems, especially:

- Chickenpox (including recent exposure) or
- Herpes zoster (shingles)—Risk of severe disease affecting other parts of the body
- Gout (history of) or
- Kidney stones (history of)—Vincristine may increase levels of uric acid in the body, which can cause gout or kidney stones
- Infection—Vincristine can reduce immunity to infection
- Liver disease—Effects may be increased because of slower removal of vincristine from the body
- Nerve or muscle disease—May be worsened

Before you begin using any new medicine (prescription or nonprescription) or if you develop any new medical problem while you are using this medicine, check with your doctor, nurse, or pharmacist.

Proper Use of This Medicine

Vincristine is often given together with certain other medicines. If you are using a combination of medicines, it is important that you receive each one at the proper time. If you are taking some of these medicines by mouth, ask your doctor, nurse, or pharmacist to help you plan a way to take them at the right times.

While you are using this medicine, it may be necessary to drink extra fluids so that you will pass more urine. This will help prevent kidney problems and keep your kidneys working well. Ask your doctor if this is necessary for you.

This medicine sometimes causes nausea and vomiting. However, it is very important that you continue to receive the medicine, even if you begin to feel ill. Ask your doctor, nurse, or pharmacist for ways to lessen these effects.

Vincristine frequently causes constipation and stomach cramps. Your doctor may want you to take a laxative. However, do not decide to take these medicines on your own without first checking with your doctor.

Precautions While Using This Medicine

It is very important that your doctor check your progress at regular visits to make sure that vincristine is working properly and to check for unwanted effects.

While you are being treated with vincristine, and after you stop treatment with it, *do not have any immunizations (vaccinations) without your doctor's approval.* Vincristine may lower your body's resistance and there is a chance you might get the infection the immunization is meant to prevent. Other people living in your household should not take or should not have recently taken oral polio vaccine since there is a chance they could pass the polio virus on to you. Also, avoid other persons who have taken oral polio vaccine. Do not get close to them, and do not stay in the same room with them for very long. If you cannot take these precautions, you should consider wearing a protective face mask that covers the nose and mouth.

If vincristine accidentally seeps out of the vein into which it is injected, it may damage some tissues and cause scarring. *Tell the doctor or nurse right away if you notice redness, pain, or swelling at the place of injection.*

Side Effects of This Medicine

Along with their needed effects, medicines like vincristine can sometimes cause unwanted effects such as blood problems, nervous system problems, loss of hair, and other side effects. These and others are described below. Also, because of the way these medicines act on the body, there is a chance that they might cause other unwanted effects that may not occur until months or years after the medicine is used. These delayed effects may include certain types of cancer, such as leukemia. Discuss these possible effects with your doctor.

Although not all of these side effects may occur, if they do occur they may need medical attention.

Check with your doctor or nurse immediately if the following side effects occur:

Less common

Pain or redness at place of injection

Rare

Black, tarry stools; blood in urine or stools; cough or hoarseness; fever or chills; pinpoint red spots on skin; unusual bleeding or bruising

Check with your doctor or nurse as soon as possible if any of the following side effects occur:

More common

Blurred or double vision; constipation; difficulty in walking; drooping eyelids; headache; jaw pain; joint pain; lower back or side pain; numbness or tingling in fingers and toes; pain in fingers and toes; pain in testicles; stomach cramps; swelling of feet or lower legs; weakness

Less common

Agitation; bed-wetting; confusion; convulsions (seizures); decrease or increase in urination; dizziness or lightheadedness when getting up from a lying or sitting position; hallucinations (seeing, hearing, or feeling things that are not there); lack of sweating; loss of appetite; mental depression; painful or difficult urination; trouble in sleeping; unconsciousness

Rare

Sores in mouth and on lips

Other side effects may occur that usually do not need medical attention. These side effects may go away during treatment as your body adjusts to the medicine. Also, your doctor or nurse may be able to tell you about ways to prevent or reduce some of these side effects. Check with your doctor or nurse if any of the following side effects continue or are bothersome or if you have any questions about them:

Less common

Bloating; diarrhea; loss of weight; nausea and vomiting; skin rash

This medicine often causes a temporary loss of hair. After treatment with vincristine has ended, or sometimes even during treatment, normal hair growth should return.

Other side effects not listed above may also occur in some patients. If you notice any other effects, check with your doctor.

Annual revision: September 1990
Interim revision: 08/11/93

VITAMIN A Systemic

A commonly used brand name in the U.S. and Canada is Aquasol A.
Another commonly used name is retinol.
Generic name product may also be available in the U.S. and Canada.

Description

Vitamins (VYE-ta-mins) are compounds that you *must* have for growth and health. They are needed in small amounts only and are usually available in the foods that you eat. Vitamin A is necessary for normal growth and health and for healthy eyes and skin.

Lack of vitamin A may lead to a rare condition called night blindness (problems seeing in the dark), as well as dry eyes, eye infections, skin problems, and slowed growth. Your doctor may treat these problems by prescribing vitamin A for you.

Patients with the following conditions may be more likely to have a deficiency of vitamin A:

- Intestine diseases
- Infections (continuing or chronic)
- Pancreas disease
- Stomach removal
- Stress (continuing)

In addition, infants receiving unfortified formula may need vitamin A supplements.

Vitamin A absorption will be impaired in any condition in which fat malabsorption occurs.

If any of the above apply to you, you should take vitamin A supplements only on the advice of your physician after need has been established.

Claims that vitamin A is effective for treatment of conditions such as acne or lung diseases, or for treatment of eye problems, wounds, or dry or wrinkled skin not caused by lack of vitamin A have not been proven. Although vitamin A is being used to prevent certain types of cancer, there is not enough information to show that this is effective.

Some strengths of vitamin A are available without a prescription. However, it may be a good idea to check with your doctor before taking vitamin A on your own. *Taking large amounts over long periods may cause serious unwanted effects.*

Vitamin A is available in the following dosage forms:

Oral

- Capsules (U.S. and Canada)
- Solution (U.S.)
- Tablets (U.S.)

Parenteral

- Injection (U.S.)

It is very important that you read and understand the following information. If any of it causes you special concern, check with your doctor or pharmacist. Also, *if you have any questions* or if you want more information about this dietary supplement or your medical problem, *ask your doctor, nurse, pharmacist, or dietitian.*

Importance of Diet

Vitamin supplements should be taken only if you cannot get enough vitamins in your diet; however, some diets may not contain all of the vitamins you need. This may occur with rapid weight loss, unusual diets (such as some reducing diets in which choice of foods is very limited), prolonged intravenous feeding, or malnutrition. In order to get enough vitamins and minerals in your diet, it is important that you eat a balanced and varied diet. Follow carefully any diet program your doctor may recommend. For your specific vitamin and/or mineral needs, ask your doctor or dietitian for a list of appropriate foods.

Vitamin A activity is found in various foods including yellow-orange fruits and vegetables; dark green, leafy vegetables; whole milk; fortified skim milk; liver; and margarine. Vitamin A comes in different forms. Retinols are a kind of vitamin A found in foods that come from animals (meat, milk, eggs). The form of vitamin A found in plants is called beta-carotene. Food processing may destroy some of the vitamins. For example, freezing may reduce the amount of vitamin A in foods.

Vitamins alone will not take the place of a good diet and will not provide energy. Your body needs other substances found in food, such as protein, minerals, carbohydrates, and fat. Vitamins themselves often cannot work without the presence of other foods. For example, fat is needed so that vitamin A can be absorbed into the body.

In some cases, it may not be possible for you to get enough food to supply you with the proper vitamins. In other cases, the amount of vitamins you need may be increased above normal. Therefore, a vitamin supplement may be needed.

Experts have developed a list of recommended dietary allowances (RDA) for most of the vitamins. The RDA are not an exact number but a general idea of how much you need. They do not cover amounts needed for problems caused by a serious lack of vitamins.

In the past, the RDA for vitamin A have been expressed in Units (U). This term Units has been replaced by retinol equivalents (RE) or micrograms (mcg) of retinol, with 1 RE equal to 1 mcg of retinol. One RE of vitamin A is equal to 3.33 Units of vitamin A.

The RDA for vitamin A are:

- Infants and children—
  - Birth to 1 year of age: 375 mcg or RE per day.
  - 1 to 3 years of age: 400 mcg or RE per day.
  - 4 to 6 years of age: 500 mcg or RE per day.
  - 7 to 10 years of age: 700 mcg or RE per day.
- Adolescent and adult males—
  - 11 years of age and over: 1000 mcg or RE per day.
- Adolescent and adult females—
  - 11 years of age and over: 800 mcg or RE per day.
- Pregnant females—800 mcg or RE per day.
- Breast-feeding females—
  - First 6 months: 1300 mcg or RE per day.
  - Second 6 months: 1200 mcg or RE per day.

Remember:

- The total amount of each vitamin that you get every day includes what you get from the foods that you eat *and* what you may take as a supplement.
- Your total amount should not be greater than the RDA, unless ordered by your doctor. *Taking too much vitamin A over a period of time may cause harmful effects.*

Before Using This Dietary Supplement

If you are taking this dietary supplement without a prescription, carefully read and follow any precautions on the label. For vitamin A, the following should be considered:

Allergies—Tell your doctor if you have ever had any unusual or allergic reaction to vitamin A. Also tell your doctor and pharmacist if you are allergic to any other substances, such as foods, preservatives, or dyes.

Pregnancy—It is especially important that you are receiving enough vitamins when you become pregnant and that you continue to receive the right amount of vitamins throughout your pregnancy. The healthy growth and development of the fetus depend on a steady supply of nutrients from the mother.

However, taking too much vitamin A during pregnancy can also cause harmful effects such as birth defects or slow or reduced growth in the child.

Breast-feeding—It is especially important that you receive the right amounts of vitamins so that your baby will also get the vitamins needed to grow properly. However, taking large amounts of a dietary supplement while breast-feeding may be harmful to the mother and/or baby and should be avoided.

Children—Normal daily requirements vary according to age. It is especially important that children receive enough vitamins in their diet for healthy growth and development. Side effects are more likely to occur in young children who are more sensitive than adults to the effects of vitamin A, especially with high doses.

Older adults—Some studies have shown that the elderly may be at risk of high blood levels of vitamin A with long-term use.

Medicines or other dietary supplements—Although certain medicines or dietary supplements should not be used together at all, in other cases they may be used together even if an interaction might occur. In these cases, your doctor may want to change the dose, or other precautions may be necessary. When you are taking vitamin A, it is especially important that your doctor and pharmacist know if you are taking any of the following:

- Isotretinoin (e.g., Accutane)—Use with vitamin A may cause high blood levels of vitamin A, which may increase the chance of side effects

Other medical problems—The presence of other medical problems may affect the use of vitamin A. Make sure you tell your doctor if you have any other medical problems, especially:

- Alcoholism, chronic, or
- Liver disease—Vitamin A use may make liver problems worse
- Kidney disease—May cause high blood levels of vitamin A which may increase the chance of side effects

Proper Use of This Dietary Supplement

Do not take more than the recommended daily amount. Vitamin A is stored in the body and *taking too much over a period of time can cause poisoning and even death.* Some people believe that taking very large doses of vitamins (called megadoses or megavitamin therapy) is useful for treating certain medical problems. Studies have not proven this. Large doses should be taken only under the direction of your doctor after need has been identified.

For patients taking the *oral liquid form* of vitamin A:

- This preparation is to be taken by mouth even though it comes in a dropper bottle.
- This dietary supplement may be dropped directly into the mouth or mixed with cereal, fruit juice, or other food.

Missed dose—If you miss taking a vitamin for one or more days there is no cause for concern, since it takes some time for your body to become seriously low in vitamins. However, if your doctor has recommended that you take this vitamin, try to remember to take it as directed every day.

Storage—To store this dietary supplement:

- Keep out of the reach of children.
- Store away from heat and direct light.
- Do not store in the bathroom, near the kitchen sink or in other damp places. Heat or moisture may cause the dietary supplement to break down.
- Keep the oral liquid form of this dietary supplement from freezing.
- Do not keep outdated dietary supplements or those no longer needed. Be sure that any discarded dietary supplement is out of the reach of children.

Side Effects of This Dietary Supplement

Along with its needed effects, a dietary supplement may cause some unwanted effects. Vitamin A does not usually cause any side effects at normal recommended doses. *However, taking large amounts of vitamin A over a period of time may cause some unwanted effects that can be serious. Check with your doctor immediately* if any of the following side effects occur, since they may be signs of sudden overdose:

Bleeding from gums or sore mouth; bulging soft spot on head (in babies); confusion or unusual excitement; diarrhea; dizziness or drowsiness; double vision; headache (severe); irritability (severe); peeling of skin, especially on lips and palms; vomiting (severe)

Check with your doctor as soon as possible if any of the following side effects occur, since they may also be signs of gradual overdose:

Bone or joint pain; convulsions (seizures); drying or cracking of skin or lips; fever; general feeling of discomfort or illness or weakness; headache; increased sensitivity of skin to sunlight; increase in frequency of urination, especially at night, or in amount of urine; irritability; loss of appetite; loss of hair; stomach pain; unusual tiredness; vomiting; yellow-orange patches on soles of feet, palms of hands, or skin around nose and lips

Other side effects not listed above may also occur in some patients. If you notice any other effects, check with your doctor or pharmacist.

Annual revision: 02/18/92
Interim revision: 08/21/92

VITAMIN B_{12} Systemic

This information applies to the following medicines:

Cyanocobalamin (sye-an-oh-koe-BAL-a-min)
Hydroxocobalamin (hye-drox-oh-koe-BAL-a-min)

Some commonly used brand names are:

For Cyanocobalamin

In the U.S.

Cobex
Crystamine
Crysti-12
Cyanoject
Cyomin
Rubesol-1000
Rubramin PC

Generic name product may also be available.

In Canada

Anacobin
Bedoz
Rubion
Rubramin

Generic name product may also be available.

For Hydroxocobalamin†

In the U.S.

Alphamine
Hydrobexan
Hydro-Cobex
Hydro-Crysti-12
LA-12

Generic name product may also be available.

†Not commercially available in Canada.

Description

Vitamins (VYE-ta-mins) are compounds that you *must* have for growth and health. They are needed in small amounts only and are usually available in the foods that you eat. Vitamin B_{12} is necessary for healthy blood. Cyanocobalamin and hydroxocobalamin are man-made forms of vitamin B_{12}.

Some people have a medical problem called pernicious anemia in which vitamin B_{12} is not absorbed from the intestine. Others may have a badly diseased intestine or have had a large part of their stomach or intestine removed, so that vitamin B_{12} cannot be absorbed. These people need to receive vitamin B_{12} by injection.

Patients with the following conditions also may be more likely to have a deficiency of vitamin B_{12}:

- Alcoholism
- Anemia, hemolytic
- Fever (continuing)
- Genetic disorders such as homocystinuria and/or methylmalonic aciduria

- Intestine diseases
- Infections (continuing or chronic)
- Kidney disease
- Liver disease
- Pancreas disease
- Stomach disease
- Stress (continuing)
- Worm infections

If any of these conditions apply to you, you should take vitamin B_{12} supplements only on the advice of your doctor after need has been established.

Lack of vitamin B_{12} may lead to anemia (weak blood), stomach problems, and nerve damage. Your doctor may treat this by prescribing vitamin B_{12} for you.

Claims that vitamin B_{12} is effective for treatment of various conditions such as aging, allergies, eye problems, slow growth, poor appetite or malnutrition, skin problems, tiredness, mental problems, sterility, thyroid disease, and nerve diseases have not been proven. Many of these treatments involve large and expensive amounts of vitamins.

Some strengths of the B vitamins are available only with your doctor's prescription. Others are available without a prescription. However, it may be a good idea to check with your doctor before taking vitamin B_{12} on your own.

Vitamin B_{12} is available in the following dosage forms:

Oral

Cyanocobalamin
- Tablets (U.S. and Canada)

Parenteral

Cyanocobalamin
- Injection (U.S. and Canada)

Hydroxocobalamin
- Injection (U.S.)

It is very important that you read and understand the following information. If any of it causes you special concern, check with your doctor or pharmacist. Also, *if you have any questions* or if you want more information about this medicine or your medical problem, *ask your doctor, nurse, pharmacist, or dietitian.*

Importance of Diet

Vitamin supplements should be taken only if you cannot get enough vitamins in your diet; however, some diets may not contain all of the vitamins you need. This may occur with rapid weight loss, unusual diets such as some reducing diets in which choice of foods is very limited, or strict vegetarian (vegan-vegetarian) or macrobiotic diets, prolonged intravenous feeding, or malnutrition. A balanced diet should provide all the vitamins you normally need.

In order to get enough vitamins and minerals in your diet, it is important that you eat a balanced and varied diet. Follow carefully any diet program your doctor may recommend. For your specific vitamin and/or mineral needs, ask your doctor or dietitian for a list of appropriate foods.

Vitamin B_{12} is found in various foods, including fish, egg yolk, milk, and fermented cheeses. It is *not* found in any vegetables. Ordinary cooking probably does not destroy the vitamin B_{12} in food.

Vitamins alone will not take the place of a good diet and will not provide energy. Your body also needs other substances found in food, such as protein, minerals, carbohydrates, and fat. Vitamins themselves often cannot work without the presence of other foods.

In some cases, it may not be possible for you to get enough food to supply you with the proper vitamins. In other cases, the amount of vitamins you need may be increased above normal. Therefore, a vitamin supplement may be needed.

Experts have developed a list of recommended dietary allowances (RDA) for most of the vitamins. The RDA are not an exact number but a general idea of how much you need. They do not cover amounts needed for problems caused by a serious lack of vitamins.

The RDA for vitamin B_{12} are:

- Infants and children—
  - Birth to 6 months of age: 0.3 micrograms (mcg) per day.
  - 6 months to 1 year of age: 0.5 mcg per day.
  - 1 to 3 years of age: 0.7 mcg per day.
  - 4 to 6 years of age: 1 mcg per day.
  - 7 to 10 years of age: 1.4 mcg per day.
- Adolescent and adult males—11 years of age and over: 2 mcg per day.
- Adolescent and adult females—11 years of age and over: 2 mcg per day.
- Pregnant females—2.2 mcg per day.
- Breast-feeding females—2.6 mcg per day.

Remember:

- The total amount of each vitamin that you get every day includes what you get from the foods that you eat *and* what you may take as a supplement.
- Your total amount should not be greater than the RDA, unless ordered by your doctor.

Before Using This Dietary Supplement

If you are taking this medicine without a prescription, carefully read and follow any precautions on the label. For vitamin B_{12}, the following should be considered:

Allergies—Tell your doctor if you have ever had any unusual or allergic reaction to vitamin B_{12}. Also, tell your doctor or pharmacist if you are allergic to any other substances, such as foods, preservatives, or dyes.

Pregnancy—It is especially important that you are receiving enough vitamins when you become pregnant and that you continue to receive the right amount of vitamins throughout your pregnancy. Healthy fetal growth and development depend on a steady supply of nutrients from mother to fetus. However, taking large amounts of a dietary supplement in pregnancy may be harmful to the mother and/or fetus and should be avoided.

You may need vitamin B_{12} supplements if you are a strict vegetarian (vegan-vegetarian). Too little vitamin B_{12} can cause harmful effects such as anemia or nervous system injury.

Breast-feeding—It is especially important that you receive the right amounts of vitamins so that your baby will also get the vitamins needed to grow properly. If you are a strict vegetarian, your baby may not be getting the vitamin B_{12} needed. However, taking large amounts of a dietary supplement while breast-feeding may be harmful to the mother and/or baby and should be avoided.

Children—Normal daily requirements vary according to age. It is especially important that children receive enough vitamins in their diet for healthy growth and development.

Older adults—It is important that older people continue to receive enough vitamins in their diet for good health.

Medicines or other dietary supplements—Although certain medicines or dietary supplement should not be used together at all, in other cases they may be used together even if an interaction might occur. In these cases, your doctor may want to change the dose, or other precautions may be necessary. Tell your doctor and pharmacist if you are taking any other dietary supplement or any prescription or nonprescription (over-the-counter [OTC]) medicine.

Other medical problems—The presence of other medical problems may affect the use of vitamin B_{12}. Make sure you tell your doctor if you have any other medical problems, especially:

- Leber's disease (an eye disease)—Vitamin B_{12} may make this condition worse

Proper Use of This Dietary Supplement

Some people believe that taking very large doses of vitamins (called megadoses or megavitamin therapy) is useful for treating certain medical problems. Studies have not proven this. Large doses should be taken only under the direction of your doctor after need has been identified.

For patients receiving vitamin B_{12} by injection for pernicious anemia or if part of the stomach or intestine has been removed:

- You will have to receive treatment for the rest of your life. You must continue to receive this medicine even if you feel well, in order to prevent future problems.

Missed dose—If you miss taking a vitamin for one or more days there is no cause for concern, since it takes some time for your body to become seriously low in vitamins. However, if your doctor has recommended that you take this vitamin, try to remember to take it as directed.

Storage—To store this dietary supplement:

- Keep out of the reach of children.
- Store away from heat and direct light.
- Do not store in the bathroom, near the kitchen sink, or in other damp places. Heat or moisture may cause the dietary supplement to break down.
- Do not keep outdated dietary supplement or those no longer needed. Be sure that any discarded dietary supplement is out of the reach of children.

Side Effects of This Dietary Supplement

Along with its needed effects, a dietary supplement may cause some unwanted effects. Cyanocobalamin or hydroxocobalamin do not usually cause any side effects. *However, check with your doctor immediately* if any of the following side effects occur:

Rare—soon after receiving injection only

Skin rash or itching; wheezing

Check with your doctor as soon as possible if either of the following side effects continues or is bothersome:

Less common

Diarrhea; itching of skin

Other side effects not listed above may also occur in some patients. If you notice any other effects, check with your doctor or pharmacist.

Annual revision: 01/29/92
Interim revision: 06/02/92

VITAMIN D and Related Compounds Systemic

This information applies to the following medicines:

Alfacalcidol (al-fa-KAL-si-dol)
Calcifediol (kal-si-fe-DYE-ole)
Calcitriol (kal-si-TRYE-ole)
Dihydrotachysterol (dye-hye-droh-tak-ISS-ter-ole)
Ergocalciferol (er-goe-kal-SIF-e-role)

Some commonly used brand names are:

For Alfacalcidol*
In Canada
One-Alpha

For Calcifediol†
In the U.S.
Calderol

For Calcitriol
In the U.S.
Calcijex
Rocaltrol
In Canada
Rocaltrol

For Dihydrotachysterol
In the U.S.
DHT
DHT Intensol
Hytakerol
In Canada
Hytakerol

For Ergocalciferol
In the U.S.
Calciferol
Drisdol
Deltalin
Generic name product may also be available.
In Canada
Calciferol
Drisdol
Ostoforte
Radiostol Forte

*Not commercially available in the U.S.
†Not commercially available in Canada.

Description

Vitamins (VYE-ta-mins) are compounds that you *must* have for growth and health. They are needed in small amounts only and are available in the foods that you eat. Vitamin D is necessary for strong bones and teeth.

Lack of vitamin D may lead to a condition called rickets, especially in children, in which bones and teeth are weak. In adults it may cause a condition called osteomalacia, in which calcium is lost from bones so that they become weak. Your doctor may treat these problems by prescribing vitamin D for you. Vitamin D is also sometimes used to treat other diseases in which calcium is not used properly by the body.

Ergocalciferol is the form of vitamin D used in vitamin supplements.

Patients with the following conditions may be more likely to have a deficiency of vitamin D:

Alcoholism
Intestine diseases
Kidney disease
Liver disease
Pancreas disease
Surgical removal of stomach

In addition, individuals and breast-fed infants who lack exposure to sunlight, as well as dark-skinned individuals, may be more likely to have a vitamin D deficiency.

If any of the above apply to you, you should take vitamin D supplements only on the advice of your doctor after need has been established.

Alfacalcidol, calcifediol, calcitriol, and dihydrotachysterol are forms of vitamin D used to treat hypocalcemia (not enough calcium in the blood). Alfacalcidol, calcifediol, and calcitriol are also used to treat certain types of bone disease that may occur with kidney disease in patients who are undergoing kidney dialysis.

Claims that vitamin D is effective for treatment of arthritis and prevention of nearsightedness or nerve problems have not been proven. Some psoriasis patients may benefit from vitamin D supplements; however, controlled studies have not been performed.

Some strengths of ergocalciferol and all strengths of alfacalcidol, calcifediol, calcitriol, and dihydrotachysterol are available only with your doctor's prescription. Other strengths of ergocalciferol are available without a prescription. However, it may be a good idea to check with your doctor before taking vitamin D on your own. *Taking large amounts over long periods may cause serious unwanted effects.*

Vitamin D and related compounds are available in the following dosage forms:

Oral

Alfacalcidol
- Capsules (Canada)
- Oral solution (Canada)

Calcifediol
- Capsules (U.S.)

Calcitriol
- Capsules (U.S. and Canada)

Dihydrotachysterol
- Capsules (U.S. and Canada)
- Oral solution (U.S.)
- Tablets (U.S.)

Ergocalciferol
- Capsules (U.S. and Canada)
- Oral solution (U.S. and Canada)
- Tablets (U.S. and Canada)

Parenteral

Calcitriol
- Injection (U.S. and Canada)

Ergocalciferol
- Injection (U.S. and Canada)

It is very important that you read and understand the following information. If any of it causes you special concern, check with your doctor or pharmacist. Also, *if you have any questions* or if you want more information about this dietary supplement or your medical problem, *ask your doctor, nurse, pharmacist, or dietitian.*

Importance of Diet

For dietary supplement use only:

- Dietary supplements should be taken only if you cannot get enough vitamins in your diet; however, some diets may not contain all of the vitamins you need. This may occur with rapid weight loss, unusual diets (such as strict vegetarian or macrobiotic diets that do not include milk or reducing diets in which choice of foods is very limited), prolonged intravenous feeding, or malnutrition. A balanced diet should provide all the vitamins you normally need.

In order to get enough vitamins and minerals in your diet, it is important that you eat a balanced and varied diet. Follow carefully any diet program your doctor may recommend. For your specific vitamin and/or mineral needs, ask your doctor or dietitian for a list of appropriate foods.

Vitamin D is found naturally only in fish and fish-liver oils. However, it is also found in milk (vitamin D–fortified). Cooking does not affect the vitamin D in foods. Vitamin D is sometimes called the "sunshine vitamin" since it is made in your skin when you are exposed to sunlight. If you eat a balanced diet and get outside in the sunshine at least 1.5 to 2 hours a week, you should be getting all the vitamin D you need.

Vitamins alone will not take the place of a good diet and will not provide energy. Your body also needs other substances found in food such as protein, minerals, carbohydrates, and fat. Vitamins themselves often cannot work without the presence of other foods. For example, fat is needed so that vitamin D can be absorbed into the body.

In some cases, it may not be possible for you to get enough food to supply you with the proper vitamins. In other cases, the amount of vitamins you need may be increased above normal. Therefore, a vitamin supplement may be needed.

Experts have developed a list of recommended dietary allowances (RDA) for most of the vitamins. The RDA are not an exact number but a general idea of how much you need. They do not cover amounts needed for problems caused by a serious lack of vitamins.

In the past, the RDA for vitamin D have been expressed in Units (U). This term has been replaced by micrograms (mcg) of vitamin D.

The RDA for vitamin D are:

- Infants and children—
  - Birth to 6 months of age: 7.5 micrograms (mcg) (300 Units) per day.
  - 6 months to 10 years of age: 10 mcg (400 Units) per day.
- Adolescent and adult males—
  - 11 to 25 years of age: 10 mcg (400 Units) per day.
  - 25 years of age and over: 5 mcg (200 Units) per day.
- Adolescent and adult females—
  - 11 to 25 years of age: 10 mcg (400 Units) per day.
  - 25 years of age and over: 5 mcg (200 Units) per day.
- Pregnant females—10 mcg (400 Units) per day.
- Breast-feeding females—10 mcg (400 Units) per day.

Remember:

- The total amount of each vitamin that you get every day includes what you get from the foods that you eat *and* what you may take as a supplement.
- Your total amount should not be greater than the RDA, unless ordered by your doctor. *Taking too much vitamin D over a period of time may cause harmful effects.*

Before Using This Dietary Supplement

If you are taking this dietary supplement without a prescription, carefully read and follow any precautions on the label. For vitamin D and related compounds, the following should be considered:

Allergies—Tell your doctor if you have ever had any unusual or allergic reaction to alfacalcidol, calcifediol, calcitriol, dihydrotachysterol, or ergocalciferol. Also, tell your doctor and pharmacist if you are allergic to any other substances, such as foods, preservatives, or dyes.

Pregnancy—It is especially important that you are receiving enough vitamin D when you become pregnant and that you continue to receive the right amounts of vitamins throughout your pregnancy. The healthy growth and development of the fetus depend on a steady supply of nutrients from the mother.

You may need vitamin D supplements if you are a strict vegetarian (vegan-vegetarian) and/or have little exposure to sunlight and do not drink vitamin D-fortified milk.

Taking too much alfacalcidol, calcifediol, calcitriol, dihydrotachysterol, or ergocalciferol can also be harmful to the fetus. Taking more than your doctor has recommended can cause your baby to be more sensitive than usual to its effects, can cause problems with a gland called the parathyroid, and can cause a defect in the baby's heart.

Breast-feeding—It is especially important that you receive the right amounts of vitamins so that your baby will also get the vitamins needed to grow properly. Infants who are totally breast-fed and have little exposure to the sun may require vitamin D supplementation. However, taking large amounts of a dietary supplement while breast-feeding may be harmful to the mother and/or baby and should be avoided.

Only small amounts of alfacalcidol, calcifediol, calcitriol, or dihydrotachysterol pass into breast milk and these amounts have not been reported to cause problems in nursing babies.

Children—Normal daily requirements vary according to age. It is especially important that children receive enough vitamins in their diet for healthy growth and development. Some studies have shown that infants who are totally breast-fed, especially with dark-skinned mothers, and have little exposure to sunlight may be at risk of vitamin D deficiency. Your doctor may prescribe a vitamin/mineral supplement that contains vitamin D. Some infants may be sensitive to even small amounts of alfacalcidol, calcifediol, calcitriol, dihydrotachysterol, or ergocalciferol. Also, children may show slowed growth when receiving large doses of alfacalcidol, calcifediol, calcitriol, dihydrotachysterol, or ergocalciferol for a long time.

Older adults—It is important that older people continue to receive enough vitamins in their diet for good health. Studies have shown that older adults may have lower blood levels of vitamin D than younger adults, especially those who have little exposure to sunlight. Your doctor may recommend that you take a vitamin supplement that contains vitamin D.

Medicines or other dietary supplements—Although certain medicines or dietary supplements should not be used together at all, in other cases they may be used together even if an interaction might occur. In these cases, your doctor may want to change the dose, or other precautions may be necessary. When you are taking vitamin D and related compounds it is especially important that your doctor and pharmacist know if you are taking any of the following:

- Antacids containing magnesium—Use of these products with any vitamin D–related compound may result in high blood levels of magnesium, especially in patients with kidney disease
- Calcium-containing preparations or
- Thiazide diuretics (water pills)—Use of these medicines with vitamin D may cause high blood levels of calcium and increase the chance of side effects
- Vitamin D and related compounds, other—Use of vitamin D with a related compound may cause high blood levels of vitamin D and increase the chance of side effects.

Other medical problems—The presence of other medical problems may affect the use of vitamin D and related compounds. Make sure you tell your doctor if you have any other medical problems, especially:

- Heart or blood vessel disease—Alfacalcidol, calcifediol, calcitriol, or dihydrotachysterol may cause hypercalcemia (high blood levels of calcium), which may make these conditions worse
- Kidney disease—High blood levels of alfacalcidol, calcifediol, calcitriol, dihydrotachysterol, or ergocalciferol may result, which may increase the chance of side effects
- Sarcoidosis—May increase sensitivity to alfacalcidol, calcifediol, calcitriol, dihydrotachysterol, or ergocalciferol and increase the chance of side effects

Proper Use of This Dietary Supplement

For use as a dietary supplement:

- *Do not take more than the recommended daily amount.* Vitamin D is stored in the body, and taking too much over a period of time can cause poisoning and even death. Some people believe that taking very large doses of vitamins (called megadoses or megavitamin therapy) is useful for treating certain medical problems. Studies have not proven this. Large doses should be taken only under the direction of your doctor after need has been identified.

If you have any questions about this, check with your doctor or pharmacist.

For patients taking the *oral liquid form* of this dietary supplement:

- This preparation should be taken by mouth even though it comes in a dropper bottle.
- This dietary supplement may be dropped directly into the mouth or mixed with cereal, fruit juice, or other food.

While you are taking alfacalcidol, calcifediol, calcitriol, or dihydrotachysterol, your doctor may want you to follow a special diet or take a calcium supplement. Be sure to follow instructions carefully. If you are already taking a calcium supplement or any medicine containing calcium, make sure your doctor knows.

Missed dose—

- *For use as a dietary supplement:* If you miss taking a dietary supplement for one or more days there is no cause for concern, since it takes some time for your body to become seriously low in vitamins. However, if your doctor has recommended that you take this dietary supplement, try to remember to take it as directed every day.
- If you are taking this medicine for a reason other than as a dietary supplement and you miss a dose and your dosing schedule is:

  —One dose every other day: Take the missed dose as soon as possible if you remember it on the day it should be taken. However, if you do not remember the missed dose until the next day, take it at that time. Then skip a day and start your dosing schedule again. Do not double doses.

—One dose a day: Take the missed dose as soon as possible. Then go back to your regular dosing schedule. However, if you do not remember the missed dose until the next day, skip the missed dose and go back to your regular dosing schedule. Do not double doses.

—More than one dose a day: Take the missed dose as soon as possible. Then go back to your regular dosing schedule. However, if it is almost time for your next dose, skip the missed dose and go back to your regular dosing schedule. Do not double doses.

If you have any questions about this, check with your doctor.

Storage—To store this dietary supplement:
- Keep out of the reach of children.
- Store away from heat and direct light.
- Do not store in the bathroom, near the kitchen sink, or in other damp places. Heat or moisture may cause the dietary supplement to break down.
- Keep the oral liquid form of the dietary supplement from freezing.
- Do not keep outdated dietary supplements or those no longer needed. Be sure that any discarded dietary supplement is out of the reach of children.

Precautions While Using This Dietary Supplement

If you are taking this medicine for a reason other than as a dietary supplement, *your doctor should check your progress at regular visits* to make sure that it does not cause unwanted effects.

Do not take any nonprescription (over-the-counter [OTC]) medicine or dietary supplement that contains calcium, phosphorus, or vitamin D while you are taking any of these dietary supplements unless you have been told to do so by your doctor. The extra calcium, phosphorus, or vitamin D may increase the chance of side effects.

Do not take antacids or other medicines containing magnesium while you are taking any of these medicines. Taking these medicines together may cause unwanted effects.

Side Effects of This Dietary Supplement

Along with its needed effects, a dietary supplement may cause some unwanted effects. Alfacalcidol, calcifediol, calcitriol, dihydrotachysterol, and ergocalciferol do not usually cause any side effects when taken as directed. However, *taking large amounts over a period of time may cause some unwanted effects that can be serious.*

Check with your doctor immediately if any of the following effects occur:

Late symptoms of severe overdose

High blood pressure; irregular heartbeat; stomach pain (severe)

Check with your doctor as soon as possible if any of the following effects occur:

Early symptoms of overdose

Constipation (especially in children or adolescents); diarrhea; dryness of mouth; headache (continuing); increased thirst; increase in frequency of urination, especially at night, or in amount of urine; loss of appetite; metallic taste; nausea or vomiting (especially in children or adolescents); unusual tiredness or weakness

Late symptoms of overdose

Bone pain; cloudy urine; drowsiness; increased sensitivity of eyes to light or irritation of eyes; itching of skin; mood or mental changes; muscle pain; nausea or vomiting; weight loss

Other side effects not listed above may also occur in some patients. If you notice any other effects, check with your doctor.

Annual revision: 08/03/92
Interim revision: 08/18/92

VITAMIN E Systemic

Some commonly used brand names are:

In the U.S.

Aquasol E
E-Vitamin Succinate
Liqui-E
Pheryl-E
Vita Plus E

Generic name product may also be available.

In Canada

Aquasol E
Webber Vitamin E

Generic name product may also be available.

Another commonly used name is alpha tocopherol.

Description

Vitamins (VYE-ta-mins) are compounds that you *must* have for growth and health. They are needed in only small amounts and are available in the foods that you eat. Vitamin E prevents a chemical reaction called oxidation, which can sometimes result in harmful effects in your body. It is also important for the proper function of nerves and muscles.

Patients with the following conditions may be more likely to have a deficiency of vitamin E:
- Intestine disease
- Liver disease
- Pancreas disease
- Surgical removal of stomach

If any of the above apply to you, you should take vitamin E supplements only on the advice of your doctor after need has been established.

Infants who are receiving a formula that is not fortified with vitamin E may be likely to have a vitamin E deficiency. Also, diets high in polyunsaturated fatty acids may increase your need for vitamin E.

Claims that vitamin E is effective for treatment of cancer and for prevention or treatment of acne, aging, loss of hair, bee stings, liver spots on the hands, bursitis, diaper rash, frostbite, stomach ulcer, heart attacks, labor pains, certain blood diseases, miscarriage, muscular dystrophy, poor posture, sexual impotence, sterility, infertility, menopause, sunburn, and lung damage from air pollution have not been proven. Although vitamin E is being used to prevent certain types of cancer, there is not enough information to show that this is effective.

Vitamin E is available without a prescription. However, it may be a good idea to check with your doctor before taking vitamin E on your own. Lack of vitamin E is extremely rare, except in people who have a disease in which it is not absorbed into the body.

If you are using vitamin E for reasons other than as a vitamin supplement, most of the following information will not apply to you.

Vitamin E is available in the following dosage forms:

Oral
- Capsules (U.S. and Canada)
- Oral solution (U.S. and Canada)
- Tablets (U.S.)
- Chewable tablets (U.S.)

It is very important that you read and understand the following information. If any of it causes you special concern, check with your doctor or pharmacist. Also, *if you have any questions* or if you want more information about this dietary supplement or your medical problem, *ask your doctor, nurse, pharmacist, or dietitian.*

Importance of Diet

Vitamin supplements should be taken only if you cannot get enough vitamins in your diet; however, intravenous feeding solutions may not contain enough vitamin E and may cause your body to become low in vitamin E if they are used for a long time.

In order to get enough vitamins and minerals in your diet, it is important that you eat a balanced and varied diet. Follow carefully any diet program your doctor may recommend. For your specific vitamin and/or mineral needs, ask your doctor or dietitian for a list of appropriate foods.

Vitamin E is found in various foods including vegetable oils (corn, cottonseed, soybean, safflower), wheat germ, whole-grain cereals, and green leafy vegetables. Cooking and storage may destroy some of the vitamin E in foods.

Vitamin supplements alone will not take the place of a good diet and will not provide energy. Your body also needs other substances found in food such as protein, minerals, carbohydrates, and fat. Vitamins themselves often cannot work without the presence of other foods. For example, small amounts of fat are needed so that vitamin E can be absorbed into the body.

In some cases, it may not be possible for you to get enough food to supply you with the proper vitamins. In other cases, the amount of vitamins you need may be increased above normal. Therefore, a vitamin supplement may be needed. However, lack of vitamin E is very rare.

Experts have developed Recommended Dietary Allowances (RDA) for vitamins and other nutrients based on the amount you need for good health. RDA cover the needs of most healthy people. They do not cover the needs of those who require extra vitamins or nutrients because of disease or serious lack of good nutrition. RDA should not be thought of as the amount of vitamins or other nutrients you need every day. Instead, they are the amounts you should eat on an average over time.

Vitamin E is available in various forms, including *d-* or *dl*-alpha tocopheryl acetate, *d-* or *dl*-alpha tocopherol, and *d-* or *dl*-alpha tocopheryl acid succinate. In the past, the RDA for vitamin E have been expressed in Units. This term has been replaced by alpha tocopherol equivalents (alpha-TE) or milligrams (mg) of *d*-alpha tocopherol. One Unit is equivalent to 1 mg of *dl*-alpha tocopherol acetate or 0.6 mg *d*-alpha tocopherol. Most products available in stores continue to be labeled in Units.

The RDAs for vitamin E are:
- Infants and children—
  - Birth to 6 months of age: 3 mg alpha-TE (5 Units) per day.
  - 6 months to 1 year of age: 4 mg alpha-TE (6.7 Units) per day.
  - 1 to 3 years of age: 6 mg alpha-TE (10 Units) per day.
  - 4 to 10 years of age: 7 mg alpha-TE (11.7 Units) per day.
- Adolescent and adult males—11 years of age and over: 10 mg alpha-TE (16.7 Units) per day.
- Adolescent and adult females—11 years of age and over: 8 mg alpha-TE (13 Units) per day.
- Pregnant females—10 mg alpha-TE (16.7 Units) per day.

- Breast-feeding females—
  First 6 months: 12 mg alpha-TE (20 Units) per day.
  Second 6 months: 11 mg alpha-TE (18 Units) per day.

Remember:

- The total amount of each vitamin that you get every day includes what you get from the foods that you eat *and* what you may take as a supplement.
- The total amount you get, averaged over several days, should not be greater than twice the RDA, unless ordered by your doctor. Taking more than 400 Units of vitamin E a day over a period of time may cause nausea, stomach cramps, or muscle weakness.

Before Using This Dietary Supplement

If you are taking this dietary supplement without a prescription, carefully read and follow any precautions on the label. For vitamin E, the following should be considered:

Allergies—Tell your doctor if you have ever had any unusual or allergic reaction to vitamin E. Also, tell your doctor and pharmacist if you are allergic to any other substances, such as foods, preservatives, or dyes.

Pregnancy—It is especially important that you are receiving enough vitamins when you become pregnant and that you continue to receive the right amount of vitamins throughout your pregnancy. The healthy growth and development of the fetus depend on a steady supply of nutrients from the mother. However, taking large amounts of a dietary supplement during pregnancy may be harmful and should be avoided.

Breast-feeding—It is especially important that you receive the right amounts of vitamins so that your baby will also get the vitamins needed to grow properly. You should also check with your doctor if you are giving your baby an unfortified formula. In that case, the baby must get the vitamins needed some other way. However, taking large amounts of a dietary supplement while breast-feeding may be harmful to the mother and/or baby and should be avoided.

Children—Normal daily requirements vary according to age. It is especially important that children receive enough vitamins in their diet for healthy growth and development. You should check with your doctor if you are giving your baby an unfortified formula. In that case, the baby must get the vitamins needed some other way. Some studies have shown that premature infants may have low levels of vitamin E. Your doctor may recommend a vitamin E supplement.

Older adults—It is important that older people continue to receive enough vitamins in their diet for good health. Although there is no specific information about the use of vitamin E in older people in doses higher than the normal daily requirements, it is not expected to cause different side effects or problems in older people than in younger adults.

Medicines or other dietary supplements—Although certain medicines or dietary supplements should not be used together at all, in other cases they may be used together even if an interaction might occur. In these cases, your doctor may want to change the dose, or other precautions may be necessary. Tell your doctor and pharmacist if you are taking any other prescription or nonprescription (over-the-counter [OTC]) medicine.

Other medical problems—The presence of other medical problems may affect the use of vitamin E. Make sure you tell your doctor if you have any other medical problems, especially:

- Bleeding problems—Vitamin E may make this condition worse

Proper Use of This Dietary Supplement

Do not take more than the recommended daily amount. Vitamin E is stored in the body, and taking more than 400 Units a day over a period of time may cause harmful effects. Some of these effects are described below. Some people believe that taking very large doses of vitamins (called megadoses or megavitamin therapy) is useful for treating certain medical problems. Studies have not proven this. Large doses should be taken only under the direction of your doctor after need has been identified.

For patients taking the *oral liquid form of this dietary supplement:*

- This preparation should be taken by mouth even though it comes in a dropper bottle.
- This dietary supplement may be dropped directly into the mouth or mixed with cereal, fruit juice, or other food.

Missed dose—If you miss taking a vitamin for one or more days there is no cause for concern, since it takes some time for your body to become seriously low in vitamins. However, if your doctor has recommended that you take this vitamin, try to remember to take it as directed every day.

Storage—To store this dietary supplement:

- Keep out of the reach of children.
- Store away from heat and direct light.
- Do not store in the bathroom, near the kitchen sink, or in other damp places. Heat or moisture may cause the dietary supplement to break down.
- Keep the oral liquid form of this dietary supplement from freezing.

- Do not keep outdated dietary supplements or those no longer needed. Be sure that any discarded dietary supplement is out of the reach of children.

Side Effects of This Dietary Supplement

Along with its needed effects, a dietary supplement may cause some unwanted effects. When used for short periods of time at recommended doses, vitamin E usually does not cause any side effects. However, check with your doctor as soon as possible if any of the following side effects occur:

With doses greater than 400 Units a day and long-term use

Blurred vision; diarrhea; dizziness; headache; nausea or stomach cramps; unusual tiredness or weakness

Other side effects not listed above may also occur in some patients. If you notice any other effects, check with your doctor.

Annual revision: 06/22/93

VITAMIN K Systemic

This information applies to the following medicines:

Menadiol (men-a-DYE-ole)
Phytonadione (fye-toe-na-DYE-one)

Some commonly used brand names are:

For Menadiol

In the U.S.
Synkayvite

In Canada
Synkayvite

For Phytonadione

In the U.S.
AquaMEPHYTON
Mephyton
Konakion

In Canada
Konakion

Generic name product may also be available.

Another commonly used name is phytomenadione.

Description

Vitamins (VYE-ta-mins) are compounds that you *must* have for growth and health. They are needed in only small amounts and are usually available in the foods that you eat. Vitamin K is necessary for normal clotting of the blood.

Vitamin K is found in various foods including green leafy vegetables, meat, and dairy products. If you eat a balanced diet containing these foods, you should be getting all the vitamin K you need. Little vitamin K is lost from foods with ordinary cooking.

Lack of vitamin K is rare but may lead to problems with blood clotting and increased bleeding. Your doctor may treat this by prescribing vitamin K for you.

Vitamin K is routinely given to newborn infants to prevent bleeding problems.

This medicine is available only with your doctor's prescription, in the following dosage forms:

Oral

Menadiol
- Tablets (U.S. and Canada)

Phytonadione
- Tablets (U.S.)

Parenteral

Menadiol
- Injection (U.S.)

Phytonadione
- Injection (U.S. and Canada)

It is very important that you read and understand the following information. If any of it causes you special concern, check with your doctor. Also, *if you have any questions* or if you want more information about this medicine or your medical problem, *ask your doctor, nurse, or pharmacist.*

Before Using This Medicine

In deciding to use a medicine, the risks of taking the medicine must be weighed against the good it will do. This is a decision you and your doctor will make. For Vitamin K, the following should be considered:

Allergies—Tell your doctor if you have ever had any unusual or allergic reaction to vitamin K. Also tell your doctor and pharmacist if you are allergic to any other substances, such as foods, preservatives, or dyes.

Pregnancy—Vitamin K has not been reported to cause birth defects or other problems in humans.

Breast-feeding—Vitamin K taken by the mother has not been reported to cause problems in nursing babies. You should also check with your doctor if you are giving your baby an unfortified formula. In that case, the baby must get the vitamins needed some other way.

Children—Children may be especially sensitive to the effects of vitamin K, especially menadiol. This may increase the chance of side effects during treatment.

Older adults—Many medicines have not been tested in older people. Therefore, it may not be known whether they work exactly the same way they do in younger adults or if they cause different side effects or problems in older people. There is no specific information about the use of vitamin K in the elderly.

Other medicines—Although certain medicines should not be used together at all, in other cases two different medicines may be used together even if an interaction might occur. In these cases, your doctor may want to change the dose, or other precautions may be necessary. When you are taking vitamin K, it is especially important that your doctor and pharmacist know if you are taking any of the following:

- Acetohydroxamic acid (e.g., Lithostat) or
- Antidiabetics, oral (diabetes medicine you take by mouth) or
- Dapsone or
- Furazolidone (e.g., Furoxone) or
- Methyldopa (e.g., Aldomet) or
- Nitrofurantoin (e.g., Furadantin) or
- Primaquine or
- Procainamide (e.g., Pronestyl) or
- Quinidine (e.g., Quinidex) or
- Quinine (e.g., Quinamm) or
- Sulfonamides (sulfa medicine) or
- Sulfoxone (e.g., Diasone)—The chance of a serious side effect may be increased, especially with menadiol
- Anticoagulants (blood thinners)—Vitamin K decreases the effects of these medicines and is sometimes used to treat bleeding caused by anticoagulants; however, anyone receiving an anticoagulant should not take any supplement that contains vitamin K (alone or in combination with other vitamins or nutrients) unless it has been ordered by their doctor

Other medical problems—The presence of other medical problems may affect the use of vitamin K. Make sure you tell your doctor if you have any other medical problems, especially:

- Cystic fibrosis or
- Diarrhea (prolonged) or
- Intestinal problems—These conditions may interfere with absorption of vitamin K into the body when it is taken by mouth; higher doses may be needed, or the medicine may have to be injected
- Glucose-6-phosphate dehydrogenase (G6PD) deficiency or
- Liver disease—The chance of unwanted effects may be increased

Before you begin using any new medicine (prescription or nonprescription) or if you develop any new medical problem while you are using this medicine, check with your doctor, nurse, or pharmacist.

Proper Use of This Medicine

Take this medicine only as directed by your doctor. Do not take more or less of it, do not take it more often, and do not take it for a longer time than your doctor ordered. To do so may cause serious unwanted effects such as blood clotting problems.

Your doctor should check your progress at regular visits. A blood test must be taken regularly to see how fast your blood is clotting. This will help your doctor decide how much medicine you need.

Missed dose—If you miss a dose of this medicine, take it as soon as possible. However, if it is almost time for your next dose, skip the missed dose and go back to your regular dosing schedule. Do not double doses. *Tell your doctor about any doses you miss.*

Storage—To store this medicine:

- Keep out of the reach of children.
- Store away from heat and direct light.
- Do not store in the bathroom, near the kitchen sink, or in other damp places. Heat or moisture may cause the medicine to break down.
- Do not keep outdated medicine or medicine no longer needed. Be sure that any discarded medicine is out of the reach of children.

Precautions While Using This Medicine

Tell all medical doctors and dentists you go to that you are taking this medicine.

Always check with your doctor, nurse, or pharmacist before you start or stop taking any other medicine. This includes any nonprescription (over-the-counter [OTC]) medicine, even aspirin. Other medicines may change the way this medicine affects your body.

Side Effects of This Medicine

Along with its needed effects, a medicine may cause some unwanted effects. Although vitamin K does not usually cause side effects that need medical attention, check with your doctor if any of the following side effects continue or are bothersome:

Less common

Flushing of face; redness, pain, or swelling at place of injection; unusual taste

Other side effects not listed above may also occur in some patients. If you notice any other effects, check with your doctor.

Annual revision: August 1990

VITAMINS AND FLUORIDE Systemic

This information applies to the following medicines:

Multiple Vitamins and Fluoride
Vitamins A, D, and C and Fluoride

Some commonly used brand names are:

For Multiple Vitamins and Fluoride

In the U.S.

Adeflor
Mulvidren-F
Poly-Vi-Flor
Vi-Daylin/F

In Canada

Adeflor
Poly-Vi-Flor

For Vitamins A, D, and C and Fluoride

In the U.S.

Cari-Tab
Tri-Vi-Flor

In Canada

Tri-Vi-Flor

Description

This medicine is a combination of vitamins and fluoride. Vitamins are used when the daily diet does not include enough of the vitamins needed for good health.

Fluoride has been found to be helpful in reducing the number of cavities in the teeth. It is usually present naturally in drinking water. However, some areas of the country do not have a high enough level of fluoride in the water. To make up for this, extra fluorides may be added to the diet. Some children may require both dietary fluorides and fluoride treatments by the dentist. Use of a fluoride toothpaste or rinse may be helpful, as well.

Taking fluorides does not replace good dental habits. These include eating a good diet, brushing and flossing teeth frequently, and having regular dental checkups.

This medicine is available only with your medical doctor's or dentist's prescription, in the following dosage forms:

Oral

- Oral solution (U.S. and Canada)
- Chewable Tablets (U.S. and Canada)

It is very important that you read and understand the following information. If any of it causes you special concern, check with your doctor or dentist. Also, *if you have any questions* or if you want more information about this dietary supplement or your medical problem, *ask your doctor, dentist, nurse, pharmacist, or dietitian.*

Before Using This Dietary Supplement

In deciding to use a dietary supplement, the risks of taking the dietary supplement must be weighed against the good it will do. This is a decision you and your medical doctor or dentist will make. For multiple vitamins and fluoride, the following should be considered:

Allergies—Tell your medical doctor or dentist if you have ever had any unusual or allergic reactions to fluoride. Also, tell your medical doctor, dentist, and pharmacist if you are allergic to any other substances, such as foods, preservatives, or dyes.

Pregnancy—Fluoride occurs naturally in water and has not been shown to cause problems in infants of mothers who drank fluoridated water or took recommended doses of supplements.

Breast-feeding—Small amounts of fluoride pass into breast milk; however, problems have not been documented with normal intake.

Children—Doses of fluoride that are too large or are taken for a long time may cause bone problems and teeth discoloration in children.

Older adults—This dietary supplement has not been shown to cause different side effects or problems in older people than it does in younger adults.

Medicines or other dietary supplements—Although certain medicines or dietary supplements should not be used together at all, in other cases they may be used together even if an interaction might occur. In these cases, your medical doctor or dentist may want to change the dose, or other precautions may be necessary. When you are taking multiple vitamins and fluoride it is especially important that your medical doctor or dentist, and pharmacist know if you are taking any of the following:

- Anticoagulants, coumarin- or indandione-derivative (blood thinners)—Use with vitamin K (in the multiple vitamins and fluoride preparations) may prevent the anticoagulant from working properly
- Iron supplements—Use with vitamin E (in the multiple vitamins and fluoride preparation) may prevent the iron supplement from working properly
- Vitamin D and related compounds—Use with vitamin D (in the multiple vitamins and fluoride preparations) may cause high blood levels of vitamin D, which may increase the chance of side effects

Other medical problems—The presence of other medical problems may affect the use of multiple vitamins and fluoride. Make sure you tell your medical doctor or dentist if you have any other medical problems, especially:

- Dental fluorosis (teeth discoloration)—Fluorides may make this condition worse

Proper Use of This Dietary Supplement

Take this dietary supplement only as directed by your medical doctor or dentist. Do not take more of it and do not take it more often than ordered. Taking too much fluoride and some vitamins (especially vitamins A and D) over a period of time may cause unwanted effects.

Do not take multiple vitamins and fluoride products at the same time as taking foods that contain calcium. It is best to space them 1 to 2 hours apart, to get the full benefit from the medicine.

For patients taking the *chewable tablet form* of this dietary supplement:

- Tablets should be chewed or crushed before they are swallowed.
- This dietary supplement works best if it is taken at bedtime, after the teeth have been thoroughly brushed.

For patients taking the *oral liquid form of* this dietary supplement:

- This dietary supplement is to be taken by mouth even though it comes in a dropper bottle. The amount to be taken is to be measured with the specially marked dropper.
- *Always store this dietary supplement in the original plastic container.* It has been designed to give you the correct dose. Also, fluoride will interact with glass and should not be stored in glass containers.
- This dietary supplement may be dropped directly into the mouth or mixed with cereal, fruit juice, or other food.

Missed dose—If you miss a dose of this dietary supplement, take it as soon as you remember. However, if it is almost time for the next dose, skip the missed dose and go back to your regular dosing schedule. Do not double doses.

Storage—To store this dietary supplement:

- Keep this dietary supplement out of the reach of children, since overdose is especially dangerous in children.
- Store away from heat and direct light.
- Do not store in the bathroom, near the kitchen sink, or in other damp places. Heat or moisture may cause the dietary supplement to break down.
- Protect the oral solution from freezing.
- Do not keep outdated dietary supplements or those no longer needed. Be sure that any discarded dietary supplement is out of the reach of children.

Precautions While Using This Dietary Supplement

The level of fluoride present in the water is different in different parts of the country. If you move to another area, check with a medical doctor or dentist in the new area as soon as possible to see if this medicine is still needed or if the dose needs to be changed. Also, check with your medical doctor or dentist if you change infant feeding habits (e.g., breast-feeding to infant formula), drinking water (e.g., city water to nonfluoridated bottled water), or filtering systems (e.g., tap water to filtered tap water).

Inform your medical doctor or dentist as soon as possible if you notice white, brown, or black spots on the teeth. These are signs of too much fluoride.

Side Effects of This Dietary Supplement

Along with its needed effects, a dietary supplement may cause some unwanted effects. Although not all of these side effects may occur, if they do occur they may need medical attention.

When the correct amount of this dietary supplement is used, side effects usually are rare. However, *taking an overdose of fluoride may cause serious problems.*

Stop taking this dietary supplement and check with your medical doctor immediately if any of the following side effects occur, as they may be signs of severe fluoride overdose:

Black, tarry stools; bloody vomit; diarrhea; drowsiness; faintness; increased watering of mouth; nausea or vomiting; shallow breathing; stomach cramps or pain; tremors; unusual excitement; watery eyes; weakness

Check with your medical doctor or dentist as soon as possible if the following side effects occur, as some may be early signs of possible chronic fluoride overdose:

Pain and aching of bones; skin rash; sores in the mouth and on the lips; stiffness; white, brown, or black discoloration of teeth

Other side effects not listed above may also occur in some patients. If you notice any other effects, check with your medical doctor or dentist.

Annual revision: September 1990
Interim revision: 08/21/92

XYLOMETAZOLINE Nasal

Some commonly used brand names are:

In the U.S.

Chlorohist-LA	Otrivin Nasal Drops
Neo-Synephrine II Long Acting Nasal Spray Adult Strength	Otrivin Nasal Spray
Neo-Synephrine II Long Acting Nose Drops Adult Strength	Otrivin Pediatric Nasal Drops

Generic name product may also be available.

In Canada

Otrivin Decongestant Nose Drops	Otrivin Pediatric Nasal Spray
Otrivin Nasal Spray	Otrivin With M-D Pump
Otrivin Pediatric Decongestant Nose Drops	

Description

Xylometazoline (zye-loe-met-AZ-oh-leen) is used for the temporary relief of congestion or stuffiness in the nose caused by hay fever or other allergies, colds, or sinus trouble.

This medicine may also be used for other conditions as determined by your doctor.

This medicine is available without a prescription; however, your doctor may have special instructions on the proper use or dose for your medical condition.

Xylometazoline is available in the following dosage forms:

Nasal
- Nasal drops (U.S. and Canada)
- Nasal spray (U.S. and Canada)

It is very important that you read and understand the following information. If any of it causes you special concern, check with your doctor or pharmacist. Also, *if you have any questions* or if you want more information about this medicine or your medical problem, *ask your doctor, nurse, or pharmacist.*

Before Using This Medicine

If you are using this medicine without a prescription, carefully read and follow any precautions on the label. For xylometazoline, the following should be considered:

Allergies—Tell your doctor if you have ever had any unusual or allergic reaction to xylometazoline or to any of the other nasal decongestants. Also tell your doctor and pharmacist if you are allergic to any other substances, such as foods, preservatives, or dyes.

Pregnancy—Xylometazoline may be absorbed into the body. However, xylometazoline has not been shown to cause birth defects or other problems in humans.

Breast-feeding—Xylometazoline may be absorbed into the body. However, xylometazoline has not been reported to cause problems in nursing babies.

Children—Children may be especially sensitive to the effects of xylometazoline. This may increase the chance of side effects during treatment.

Older adults—Many medicines have not been tested in older people. Therefore, it may not be known whether they work exactly the same way they do in younger adults or if they cause different side effects or problems in older people. There is no specific information about the use of xylometazoline in the elderly.

Other medicines—Although certain medicines should not be used together at all, in other cases two different medicines may be used together even if an interaction might occur. In these cases, your doctor may want to change the dose, or other precautions may be necessary. When you are using xylometazoline, it is especially important that your doctor and pharmacist know if you are taking any other prescription or nonprescription (over-the-counter [OTC]) medicine.

Other medical problems—The presence of other medical problems may affect the use of xylometazoline. Make sure you tell your doctor if you have any other medical problems, especially:

- Diabetes mellitus (sugar diabetes)
- Heart or blood vessel disease or
- High blood pressure—Xylometazoline may make the condition worse
- Overactive thyroid

Before you begin using any new medicine (prescription or nonprescription) or if you develop any new medical problem while you are using this medicine, check with your doctor, nurse, or pharmacist.

Proper Use of This Medicine

To use the *nose drops*:
- Blow your nose gently. Tilt the head back while standing or sitting up, or lie down on a bed and hang head over the side. Place the drops into each nostril and keep the head tilted back for a few minutes to allow the medicine to spread throughout the nose.
- Rinse the dropper with hot water and dry with a clean tissue. Replace the cap right after use.

To use the *nose spray*:
- Blow your nose gently. With the head upright, spray the medicine into each nostril. Sniff briskly while squeezing the bottle quickly and firmly. For best results, spray once into each nostril, wait 3 to 5 minutes to allow the medicine to work, then blow your

nose gently and thoroughly. Repeat until the complete dose is used.

- Rinse the tip of the spray bottle with hot water taking care not to suck water into the bottle, and dry with a clean tissue. Replace the cap right after use.

To avoid spreading the infection, do not use the container for more than one person.

Use this medicine only as directed. Do not use more of it, do not use it more often, and do not use it for longer than 3 days, unless otherwise directed by your doctor. To do so may make your runny or stuffy nose worse and may also increase the chance of side effects.

Missed dose—If you miss a dose of this medicine and you remember within an hour or so of the missed dose, use it right away. However, if you do not remember until later, skip the missed dose and go back to your regular dosing schedule. Do not double doses.

Storage—To store this medicine:

- Keep out of the reach of children.
- Store away from heat and direct light.
- Keep the medicine from freezing.
- Do not keep outdated medicine or medicine no longer needed. Be sure that any discarded medicine is out of the reach of children.

Side Effects of This Medicine

Along with its needed effects, a medicine may cause some unwanted effects. Although not all of these side effects may occur, if they do occur they may need medical attention.

When this medicine is used for short periods of time at low doses, side effects usually are rare. However, check with your doctor as soon as possible if any of the following occur:

Increase in runny or stuffy nose

Symptoms of too much medicine being absorbed into the body

Blurred vision; headache or lightheadedness; nervousness; pounding, irregular, or fast heartbeat; trouble in sleeping

Other side effects may occur that usually do not need medical attention. These side effects may go away during treatment as your body adjusts to the medicine. However, check with your doctor or pharmacist if any of the following side effects continue or are bothersome:

Burning, dryness, or stinging of inside of nose; sneezing

Other side effects not listed above may also occur in some patients. If you notice any other effects, check with your doctor or pharmacist.

Annual revision: October 1990

YOHIMBINE Systemic

Some commonly used brand names are:

In the U.S.

Actibine	Yocon
Aphrodyne	Yohimex

Generic name product may also be available.

In Canada

Yocon
Yohimide

Generic name product may also be available.

Description

Yohimbine (yo-HIM-been) is used to treat men who are impotent (not able to have sex). It is taken by mouth to help produce erections.

The way yohimbine works is not known for sure. It is thought, however, to work by increasing the body's production of certain chemicals that help produce erections. It does not work in all men who are impotent.

Yohimbine is available only with your doctor's prescription, in the following dosage form:

Oral

- Tablets (U.S. and Canada)

It is very important that you read and understand the following information. If any of it causes you special concern, check with your doctor. Also, *if you have any questions* or if you want more information about this medicine or your medical problem, *ask your doctor, nurse, or pharmacist.*

Before Using This Medicine

In deciding to use a medicine, the risks of taking the medicine must be weighed against the good it will do. This is a decision you and your doctor will make. For yohimbine, the following should be considered:

Allergies—Tell your doctor if you have ever had any unusual or allergic reaction to yohimbine or any of the rauwolfia alkaloids, such as deserpidine (e.g, Harmonyl), rauwolfia serpentina (e.g., Raudixin), or reserpine (e.g., Serpalan). Also tell your doctor and pharmacist if you are allergic to any other substances, such as foods, preservatives, or dyes.

Older adults—Many medicines have not been studied specifically in older people. Therefore, it may not be known whether they work exactly the same way they do in younger adults. Although there is no specific information comparing use of yohimbine in the elderly with use in other age groups, this medicine has been used in some elderly patients and has not been shown to cause different side effects or problems in older people than it does in younger adults.

Other medicines—Although certain medicines should not be used together at all, in other cases two different medicines may be used together even if an interaction might occur. In these cases, your doctor may want to change the dose, or other precautions may be necessary. Tell your doctor and pharmacist if you are taking any other prescription or nonprescription (over-the-counter [OTC]) medicine.

Other medical problems—The presence of other medical problems may affect the use of yohimbine. Make sure you tell your doctor if you have any other medical problems, especially:

- Angina pectoris or
- Depression or
- Other psychiatric illness or
- Heart disease or
- High blood pressure or
- Kidney disease—Yohimbine may make these conditions worse
- Liver disease—Effects of yohimbine may be increased because of slower removal from the body

Before you begin using any new medicine (prescription or nonprescription) or if you develop any new medical problem while you are using this medicine, check with your doctor, nurse, or pharmacist.

Proper Use of This Medicine

This medicine usually begins to work about 2 to 3 weeks after you begin to take it.

Dosing—The dose of yohimbine will be different for different patients. *Follow your doctor's orders or the directions on the label.* The following information includes only the average doses of yohimbine. *If your dose is different, do not change it* unless your doctor tells you to do so:

- The number of tablets that you take depends on the strength of the medicine.
- For *oral* dosage forms (tablets):
  —Adults: 5.4 to 6 milligrams three times a day.

Missed dose—If you miss a dose of this medicine, take it as soon as possible. However, if it is almost time for your next dose, skip the missed dose and go back to your regular dosing schedule. Do not double doses.

Storage—To store this medicine:

- Keep out of the reach of children.
- Store away from heat and direct light.
- Do not store in the bathroom, near the kitchen sink, or in other damp places. Heat or moisture may cause the medicine to break down.
- Keep the medicine from freezing. Do not refrigerate.

- Do not keep outdated medicine or medicine no longer needed. Be sure that any discarded medicine is out of the reach of children.

Precautions While Using This Medicine

It is important that your doctor check your progress at regular visits to make sure that this medicine is working properly.

Use yohimbine exactly as directed by your doctor. Do not use more of it and do not use it more often than ordered. If too much is used, the risk of side effects such as fast heartbeat and high blood pressure is increased.

Side Effects of This Medicine

Along with its needed effects, a medicine may cause some unwanted effects. Although not all of these side effects may occur, if they do occur they may need medical attention.

Check with your doctor as soon as possible if any of the following side effects occur:

Less common

Fast heartbeat; increased blood pressure

Other side effects may occur that usually do not need medical attention. These side effects may go away during treatment as your body adjusts to the medicine. However, check with your doctor if any of the following side effects continue or are bothersome:

Less common

Dizziness; headache; irritability; nervousness or restlessness

Rare

Nausea and vomiting; skin flushing; sweating; tremor

Other side effects not listed above may also occur in some patients. If you notice any other effects, check with your doctor.

Annual revision: 10/24/92

ZALCITABINE Systemic

A commonly used brand name in the U.S. and Canada is HIVID. Another commonly used name is ddC.

Description

Zalcitabine (zal-SITE-a-been) (also known as ddC) is used in the treatment of the infection caused by the human immunodeficiency virus (HIV). HIV is the virus that causes acquired immune deficiency syndrome (AIDS).

Zalcitabine (ddC) will not cure or prevent HIV infection or AIDS; however, it helps inhibit HIV from reproducing and appears to slow down the destruction of the immune system. This may help delay the development of problems usually related to AIDS or HIV disease. Zalcitabine will not keep you from spreading HIV to other people. People who receive this medicine may continue to have other problems usually related to AIDS or HIV disease.

Zalcitabine may cause some serious side effects, including peripheral neuropathy, a problem involving the nerves. Symptoms of peripheral neuropathy include tingling, burning, numbness, or pain in the hands or feet. Zalcitabine may also cause pancreatitis (inflammation of the pancreas). Symptoms of pancreatitis include stomach pain, and nausea and vomiting. *Check with your doctor if any new health problems or symptoms occur while you are taking zalcitabine.*

Zalcitabine is available only with your doctor's prescription, in the following dosage form:

Oral

- Tablets (U.S. and Canada)

It is very important that you read and understand the following information. If any of it causes you special concern, check with your doctor. Also, *if you have any questions* or if you want more information about this medicine or your medical problem, *ask your doctor, nurse, or pharmacist.*

Before Using This Medicine

In deciding to use a medicine, the risks of taking the medicine must be weighed against the good it will do. This is a decision you and your doctor will make. For zalcitabine, the following should be considered:

Allergies—Tell your doctor if you have ever had any unusual or allergic reaction to zalcitabine. Also tell your doctor and pharmacist if you are allergic to any other substances, such as foods, preservatives, or dyes.

Pregnancy—Zalcitabine has not been studied in pregnant women. However, studies in animals have shown that zalcitabine causes birth defects when given in very high doses. Before taking this medicine, make sure your doctor knows if you are pregnant or if you may become pregnant.

Breast-feeding—It is not known whether zalcitabine passes into the breast milk. However, if your baby does not already have the AIDS virus, there is a chance that you could pass it to your baby by breast-feeding. Talk to your doctor first if you are thinking about breast-feeding your baby.

Children—Zalcitabine can cause serious side effects in any patient. Therefore, it is especially important that you discuss with your child's doctor the good that this medicine may do as well as the risks of using it. Your child must be seen frequently and your child's progress carefully followed by the doctor while the child is taking zalcitabine.

Older adults—Zalcitabine has not been studied specifically in older people. Therefore, it is not known whether it causes different side effects or problems in the elderly than it does in younger adults.

Other medicines—Although certain medicines should not be used together at all, in other cases two different medicines may be used together even if an interaction might occur. In these cases, your doctor may want to change the dose, or other precautions may be necessary. When you are taking zalcitabine, it is especially important that your doctor and pharmacist know if you are taking any of the following:

- Alcohol or
- Asparaginase (e.g., Elspar) or
- Azathioprine (e.g., Imuran) or
- Estrogens (female hormones) or
- Furosemide (e.g., Lasix) or
- Methyldopa (e.g., Aldomet) or
- Nitrofurantoin (e.g., Furadantin, Macrodantin) or
- Pentamidine by injection (e.g., Pentam, Pentacarinat) or
- Sulfonamides (e.g., Bactrim, Septra) or
- Sulindac (e.g., Clinoril) or
- Tetracyclines or
- Thiazide diuretics (water pills) (e.g., Diuril, Hydrodiuril) or
- Valproic acid (e.g., Depakote)—Use of these medicines with zalcitabine may increase the chance of pancreatitis (inflammation of the pancreas)
- Aminoglycosides by injection (amikacin [e.g., Amikin], gentamicin [e.g., Garamycin], kanamycin [e.g., Kantrex], neomycin [e.g., Mycifradin], netilmicin [e.g., Netromycin], streptomycin, tobramycin [e.g., Nebcin]) or
- Amphotericin B (e.g., Fungizone) or
- Foscarnet (e.g., Foscavir)—Use of these medicines with zalcitabine may increase the chance of side effects
- Chloramphenicol (e.g., Chloromycetin) or
- Cisplatin (e.g., Platinol) or
- Dapsone (e.g., Avlosulfon) or
- Ethambutol (e.g., Myambutol) or
- Ethionamide (e.g., Trecator-SC) or
- Hydralazine (e.g., Apresoline) or

- Isoniazid (e.g., Nydrazid) or
- Lithium (e.g., Eskalith, Lithobid) or
- Metronidazole (e.g., Flagyl) or
- Nitrofurantoin (e.g., Furadantin, Macrodantin) or
- Nitrous oxide or
- Phenytoin (e.g., Dilantin) or
- Vincristine (e.g., Oncovin)—Use of these medicines with zalcitabine may increase the chance of peripheral neuropathy (tingling, burning, numbness, or pain in your hands or feet)

Other medical problems—The presence of other medical problems may affect the use of zalcitabine. Make sure you tell your doctor if you have any other medical problems, especially:

- Alcohol abuse or
- Increased blood triglycerides (or a history of) or
- Pancreatitis (or a history of)—Patients with these medical problems may be at increased risk of pancreatitis (inflammation of the pancreas)
- Liver disease—Zalcitabine may make liver disease worse in patients with liver disease or a history of alcohol abuse
- Kidney disease—Patients with kidney disease may have an increased chance of side effects
- Peripheral neuropathy—Zalcitabine may make this condition worse

Before you begin using any new medicine (prescription or nonprescription) or if you develop any new medical problem while you are using this medicine, check with your doctor, nurse, or pharmacist.

Proper Use of This Medicine

Take this medicine exactly as directed by your doctor. Do not take more of it, do not take it more often, and do not take it for a longer time than your doctor ordered. Also, do not stop taking this medicine without checking with your doctor first.

Keep taking zalcitabine for the full time of treatment, even if you begin to feel better.

This medicine works best when there is a constant amount in the blood. *To help keep the amount constant, do not miss any doses.* If you need help in planning the best times to take your medicine, check with your doctor, nurse, or pharmacist.

Only take medicine that your doctor has prescribed specifically for you. Do not share your medicine with others.

Dosing—The dose of zalcitabine will be different for different patients. *Follow your doctor's orders or the directions on the label.* The following information includes only the average doses of zalcitabine. Your dose may be different if you have kidney disease. *If your dose is different, do not change it* unless your doctor tells you to do so:

- Adults and children 13 years of age and older: 0.75 mg, together with 200 mg of zidovudine, every eight hours.
- Children up to 12 years of age: Use and dose is based on body weight and must be determined by your doctor.

Missed dose—If you miss a dose of this medicine, take it as soon as possible. However, if it is almost time for your next dose, skip the missed dose and go back to your regular dosing schedule. Do not double doses.

Storage—To store this medicine:

- Keep out of the reach of children.
- Store away from heat and direct light.
- Do not store in the bathroom, near the kitchen sink, or in other damp places. Heat or moisture may cause the medicine to break down.
- Do not keep outdated medicine or medicine no longer needed. Be sure that any discarded medicine is out of the reach of children.

Precautions While Using This Medicine

It is very important that your doctor check your progress at regular visits.

Do not take any other medicines without checking with your doctor first. To do so may increase the chance of side effects from zalcitabine.

HIV may be acquired from or spread to other people through infected body fluids, including blood, vaginal fluid, or semen. *If you are infected, it is best to avoid any sexual activity involving an exchange of body fluids with other people. If you do have sex, always wear (or have your partner wear) a condom ("rubber").* Only use condoms made of latex, and *use them every time you have vaginal, anal, or oral sex.* The use of a spermicide (such as nonoxynol-9) may also help prevent transmission of HIV if it is not irritating to the vagina, rectum, or mouth. Spermicides have been shown to kill HIV in lab tests. Do not use oil-based jelly, cold cream, baby oil, or shortening as a lubricant—these products can cause the rubber to break. Lubricants without oil, such as *K-Y Jelly*, are recommended. Women may wish to carry their own condoms. Birth control pills and diaphragms will help protect against pregnancy, but they will not prevent someone from giving or getting the AIDS virus. *If you inject drugs*, get help to stop. *Do not share needles or equipment with anyone.* In some cities, more than half of the drug users are infected, and sharing even 1 needle or syringe can spread the virus. If you have any questions about this, check with your doctor, nurse, or pharmacist.

Side Effects of This Medicine

Along with its needed effects, a medicine may cause some unwanted effects. Although not all of these side effects

may occur, if they do occur they may need medical attention.

Check with your doctor immediately if any of the following side effects occur:

More common

Tingling, burning, numbness, or pain in the hands, arms, feet, or legs

Less common

Fever; joint pain; muscle pain; skin rash; ulcers in the mouth and throat

Rare

Fever and sore throat; nausea and vomiting; stomach pain

Other side effects may occur that usually do not need medical attention. These side effects may go away during treatment as your body adjusts to the medicine. However, check with your doctor if any of the following side effects continue or are bothersome:

Less common

Diarrhea; headache

Other side effects not listed above may also occur in some patients. If you notice any other effects, check with your doctor.

Annual revision: 03/03/93

ZIDOVUDINE Systemic

Some commonly used brand names are:

In the U.S.

Retrovir

In Canada

Apo-Zidovudine

Retrovir

Novo-AZT

Another commonly used name is AZT.

Description

Zidovudine (zye-DOE-vue-deen) (also known as AZT) is used in the treatment of the infection caused by the human immunodeficiency virus (HIV). HIV is the virus responsible for acquired immune deficiency syndrome (AIDS). Zidovudine is also used to slow the progression of disease in patients infected with HIV who have early symptoms or no symptoms at all.

Zidovudine will not cure or prevent HIV infection or AIDS. It appears to slow down the destruction of the immune system caused by HIV. This may help delay the development of symptoms related to advanced HIV disease. However, it will not keep you from spreading the virus to other people. People who receive this medicine may continue to have the problems usually related to AIDS or HIV disease.

HIV infection can result in a very serious, usually fatal, disease. An estimated 1 to 1.5 million persons in the United States are currently infected with HIV. It has become one of the leading causes of death in men and women under the age of 45 and in children between 1 and 5 years of age.

HIV primarily attacks certain white blood cells in the body and slowly, over several years, breaks down the body's immune system. When this happens, the person may get other serious infections as well. These include serious fungus infections, *Pneumocystis* (noo-moe-SISS-tis) *carinii* pneumonia (PCP), and cytomegalovirus (CMV) infections, which can affect the retina of the eyes, the lungs, and the stomach and intestines. The person may also develop certain kinds of cancer, such as non-Hodgkin's lymphoma or Kaposi's sarcoma, a form of cancer usually involving purplish tumors of the skin or mouth. AZT may be given with other medicines to treat these problems.

Although most cases of HIV infection in the U.S. have occurred in homosexual and bisexual men, HIV infection has increased most rapidly in people exposed to the virus through heterosexual contact. Other people at risk of contracting HIV are intravenous drug users, their sexual partners and people who received transfusions with blood or blood products contaminated with the AIDS virus and their sexual partners. Children born to mothers infected with HIV are also at risk of getting the virus.

This virus is spread from person to person by infected body fluids, such as blood, semen, vaginal fluids (including menstrual blood), and breast milk. HIV is almost always spread by the intimate exchange of these fluids that occurs during unprotected sex (vaginal, anal, and possibly oral) with someone who is infected with the virus, and/or by sharing contaminated needles and syringes when injecting drugs. HIV is also spread from an infected mother to her fetus during pregnancy or childbirth, and, rarely, through breast-feeding. It is not spread by casual contact, such as touching, shaking hands, coughing, sneezing, or routine everyday contact, such as working in the same office, going to the same school, or eating in the same restaurant.

HIV can infect people of any age, sex, race, or sexual orientation. Because symptoms may take months, or more often years, to appear, an infected person may look and feel fine. During this time a person may spread the infection to others without knowing it.

The early symptoms of HIV infection may include fever; night sweats; swollen glands in the neck, armpit, and/or groin; unexplained weight loss; profound tiredness; yeast infections in the mouth; diarrhea; continuing cough; weakness; loss of appetite; or in women, vaginal yeast infections.

Zidovudine may cause some serious side effects, including bone marrow problems. Symptoms of bone marrow problems include fever, chills, or sore throat; pale skin; and unusual tiredness or weakness. These problems may require blood transfusions or temporarily stopping treatment with zidovudine. *Check with your doctor if any new health problems or symptoms occur while you are taking zidovudine.*

Zidovudine is available only with your doctor's prescription, in the following dosage forms:

Oral

- Capsules (U.S. and Canada)
- Syrup (U.S. and Canada)

Parenteral

- Injection (U.S. and Canada)

It is very important that you read and understand the following information. If any of it causes you special concern, check with your doctor. Also, *if you have any questions* or if you want more information about this medicine or your medical problem, *ask your doctor, nurse, or pharmacist.*

Before Using This Medicine

In deciding to use a medicine, the risks of taking the medicine must be weighed against the good it will do. This is a decision you and your doctor will make. For zidovudine, the following should be considered:

Allergies—Tell your doctor if you have ever had any unusual or allergic reaction to zidovudine. Also tell your doctor and pharmacist if you are allergic to any other substances, such as foods, preservatives, or dyes.

Pregnancy—Zidovudine crosses the placenta. Studies in pregnant women have not been completed. However, zidovudine has not been shown to cause birth defects in studies in rats and rabbits given this medicine by mouth in doses many times larger than the human dose.

Breast-feeding—It is not known whether zidovudine passes into the breast milk. However, if your baby does not have the AIDS virus, there is a chance that you could pass it to your baby by breast-feeding. Talk to your doctor first if you are thinking about breast-feeding your baby.

Children—Zidovudine can cause serious side effects in any patient. Therefore, it is especially important that you discuss with your child's doctor the good that this medicine may do as well as the risks of using it. Your child must be carefully followed, and frequently seen, by the doctor while he or she is taking zidovudine.

Older adults—Zidovudine has not been studied specifically in older people. Therefore, it is not known whether it causes different side effects or problems in the elderly than it does in younger adults.

Other medicines—Although certain medicines should not be used together at all, in other cases 2 different medicines may be used together even if an interaction might occur. In these cases, your doctor may want to change the dose, or other precautions may be necessary. When you are taking zidovudine, it is especially important that your doctor and pharmacist know if you are taking any of the following:

- Amphotericin B by injection (e.g., Fungizone) or
- Antineoplastics (cancer medicine) or
- Antithyroid agents (medicine for overactive thyroid) or
- Azathioprine (e.g., Imuran) or
- Chloramphenicol (e.g., Chloromycetin) or
- Colchicine or
- Cyclophosphamide (e.g., Cytoxan) or
- Flucytosine (e.g., Ancobon) or
- Ganciclovir (e.g., Cytovene) or
- Interferon (e.g., Intron A, Roferon-A) or
- Mercaptopurine (e.g., Purinethol) or
- Methotrexate (e.g., Mexate) or
- Plicamycin (e.g., Mithracin)—Caution should be used if these medicines and zidovudine are used together; taking zidovudine while you are using or receiving these medicines may make anemia and other blood problems worse
- Clarithromycin (e.g., Biaxin)—Clarithromycin may decrease the amount of zidovudine in the blood
- Probenecid (e.g., Benemid)—Probenecid may increase the blood levels of zidovudine, increasing the chance of side effects

Other medical problems—The presence of other medical problems may affect the use of zidovudine. Make sure you tell your doctor if you have any other medical problems, especially:

- Anemia or other blood problems—Zidovudine may make these conditions worse
- Liver disease—Patients with liver disease may have an increase in side effects from zidovudine
- Low amounts of folic acid or vitamin B_{12} in the blood—Zidovudine may worsen anemia caused by a decrease of folic acid or vitamin B_{12}

Before you begin using any new medicine (prescription or nonprescription) or if you develop any new medical problem while you are using this medicine, check with your doctor, nurse, or pharmacist.

Proper Use of This Medicine

Patient information sheets about zidovudine are available. Read this information carefully.

Take this medicine exactly as directed by your doctor. Do not take more of it, do not take it more often, and do not take it for a longer time than your doctor ordered. Also, do not stop taking this medicine without checking with your doctor first.

Keep taking zidovudine for the full time of treatment, even if you begin to feel better.

For patients using *zidovudine syrup:*

- Use a specially marked measuring spoon or other device to measure each dose accurately. The average household teaspoon may not hold the right amount of liquid.

This medicine works best when there is a constant amount in the blood. *To help keep the amount constant, do not miss any doses.* If you need help in planning the best times to take your medicine, check with your doctor, nurse, or pharmacist.

Missed dose—If you do miss a dose of this medicine, take it as soon as possible. However, if it is almost time for your next dose, skip the missed dose and go back to your regular dosing schedule. Do not double doses.

Storage—To store this medicine:

- Keep out of the reach of children.
- Store away from heat and direct light.
- Do not store in the bathroom, near the kitchen sink, or in other damp places. Heat or moisture may cause the medicine to break down.
- Do not keep outdated medicine or medicine no longer needed. Be sure that any discarded medicine is out of the reach of children.

Precautions While Using This Medicine

It is very important that your doctor check your progress at regular visits. This medicine may cause blood problems.

Do not take any other medicines without checking with your doctor first. To do so may increase the chance of side effects from zidovudine.

Zidovudine may cause blood problems. These problems may result in a greater chance of certain infections and slow healing. Therefore, you should be careful when using regular toothbrushes, dental floss, and toothpicks not to damage your gums. Check with your medical doctor or dentist if you have any questions about proper oral hygiene (mouth care) during treatment.

HIV may be acquired from or spread to other people through infected body fluids, including blood, vaginal fluid, or semen. *If you are infected, it is best to avoid any sexual activity involving an exchange of body fluids with other people. If you do have sex, always wear (or have your partner wear) a condom ("rubber").* Only use condoms made of latex, and *use them every time you have vaginal, anal, or oral sex.* The use of a spermicide (such as nonoxynol-9) may also help prevent transmission of HIV if it is not irritating to the vagina, rectum, or mouth. Spermicides have been shown to kill HIV in lab tests. Do not use oil-based jelly, cold cream, baby oil, or shortening as a lubricant—these products can cause the rubber to break. Lubricants without oil, such as *K-Y Jelly*, are recommended. Women may wish to carry their own condoms. Birth control pills and diaphragms will help protect against pregnancy, but they will not prevent someone from giving or getting the AIDS virus. *If you inject drugs,* get help to stop. *Do not share needles with anyone.* In some cities, more than half of the drug users are infected and sharing even 1 needle can spread the virus. If you have any questions about this, check with your doctor, nurse, or pharmacist.

Side Effects of This Medicine

Along with its needed effects, a medicine may cause some unwanted effects. Although not all of these side effects may occur, if they do occur they may need medical attention.

Check with your doctor immediately if any of the following side effects occur:

More common

Fever, chills, or sore throat; pale skin; unusual tiredness or weakness

Note: The above side effects may also occur up to weeks or months after you stop taking this medicine.

Rare

Abdominal discomfort; confusion; convulsions (seizures); general feeling of discomfort; loss of appetite; mania; muscle tenderness and weakness; nausea

Other side effects may occur that usually do not need medical attention. These side effects may go away during treatment as your body adjusts to the medicine. However, check with your doctor if any of the following side effects continue or are bothersome:

More common

Headache (severe); muscle soreness; nausea; trouble in sleeping

Less common

Bluish-brown colored bands on nails

Other side effects not listed above may also occur in some patients. If you notice any other effects, check with your doctor.

Additional Information

Once a medicine has been approved for marketing for a certain use, experience may show that it is also useful

for other medical problems. Although this use is not included in product labeling, zidovudine is used in certain patients with the following medical condition:

- Human immunodeficiency virus (HIV) infection due to occupational exposure (possible prevention of)

Other than the above information, there is no additional information relating to proper use, precautions, or side effects for this use.

Annual revision: 11/11/92

ZINC SUPPLEMENTS Systemic

This information applies to the following medicines:

Zinc Chloride (zink KLOR-ide)
Zinc Gluconate (GLOO-coh-nate)
Zinc Sulfate (SUL-fate)

Some commonly used brand names are:

For Zinc Chloride†
In the U.S.
Generic name product may be available.

For Zinc Gluconate
In the U.S.
Generic name product may be available.
In Canada
Generic name product may be available.

For Zinc Sulfate
In the U.S.
Orazinc
Verazinc
Zinc-220
Zincate
Zinkaps-220
Generic name product may also be available.
In Canada
PMS Egozinc
Generic name product may also be available.

†Not commercially available in Canada.

Description

Zinc supplements are used to prevent or treat zinc deficiency.

The body needs zinc for normal growth and health. For patients who are unable to get enough zinc in their regular diet or who have a need for more zinc, zinc supplements may be necessary. They are generally taken by mouth but some patients may have to receive them by injection.

Zinc supplements may be used for other conditions as determined by your doctor.

Lack of zinc may lead to poor night vision and wound-healing, a decrease in sense of taste and smell, a reduced ability to fight infections, and poor development of reproductive organs.

Patients with the following conditions may be more likely to have a deficiency of zinc:

- Acrodermatitis enteropathica (a lack of absorption of zinc from the intestine)
- Alcoholism
- Burns
- Diabetes mellitus (sugar diabetes)
- Down's syndrome
- Eating disorders
- Intestine diseases
- Infections (continuing or chronic)
- Kidney disease
- Liver disease
- Pancreas disease
- Sickle cell disease
- Skin disorders
- Stomach removal
- Stress (continuing)
- Thalassemia
- Trauma (prolonged)

In addition, premature infants may need additional zinc.

If any of the above apply to you, you should take zinc supplements only on the advice of your doctor after need has been established.

Claims that zinc is effective in preventing vision loss in the elderly have not been proven. Zinc has not been proven effective in the treatment of porphyria.

Some zinc preparations are available only with your doctor's prescription. Others are available without a prescription; however, your doctor may have special instructions on the proper use and dose for your condition.

Zinc supplements are available in the following dosage forms:

Oral
Zinc Gluconate
- Tablets (U.S. and Canada)

Zinc Sulfate
- Capsules (U.S. and Canada)
- Tablets (U.S.)

Parenteral
Zinc Chloride
- Injection (U.S.)

Zinc Sulfate
- Injection (U.S. and Canada)

It is very important that you read and understand the following information. If any of it causes you special concern, check with your doctor or pharmacist. Also, *if you have any questions* or if you want more information about this dietary supplement or your medical problem, *ask your doctor, nurse, pharmacist, or dietitian.*

Importance of Diet

Many nutritionists recommend that, if possible, people should get all the zinc they need from foods. However, some people do not get enough zinc from their diet. For example, people on weight-loss diets may consume too little food to provide enough zinc. Others may need more zinc than normal. For such people, a zinc supplement is important.

In order to get enough vitamins and minerals in your regular diet, it is important that you eat a balanced and varied diet. Follow carefully any diet program your doctor or dietitian may recommend. For your specific vitamin and/or mineral needs, ask your doctor for a list of appropriate foods.

Zinc is found in various foods, including lean red meats, seafoods (especially herring and oysters), peas, and beans. Zinc is also found in whole grains; however, large amounts of whole-grains have been found to decrease the amount of zinc that is absorbed. Additional zinc may be added to the diet through treated (galvanized) cookware. Foods stored in uncoated tin cans may cause less zinc to be available for absorption from food.

Experts have developed a list of Recommended Dietary Allowances (RDA) of zinc. The RDA is not an exact number but a general idea of how much you need every day. The RDAs do not cover amounts needed for problems caused by a serious lack of zinc.

The RDA for zinc are:

- Infants and children—
  Birth to 1 year of age: 5 mg per day.
  1 to 10 years of age: 10 mg per day.
- Adolescent and adult males—11 years of age and over: 15 mg per day.
- Adolescent and adult females—11 years of age and over: 12 mg per day.
- Pregnant females—15 mg per day.
- Breast-feeding females—
  First 6 months: 19 mg per day.
  Second 6 months: 16 mg per day.

Remember:

- The total amount of zinc that you get every day includes what you get from the foods that you eat *and* what you may take as a supplement.
- This total amount should not be greater than the RDA, unless ordered by your doctor.

Before Using This Dietary Supplement

If you are taking this dietary supplement without a prescription, carefully read and follow any precautions on the label. For zinc supplements, the following should be considered:

Allergies—Tell your doctor and pharmacist if you are allergic to any substances, such as foods, preservatives, or dyes.

Pregnancy—It is especially important that you are receiving enough vitamins and minerals when you become pregnant and that you continue to receive the right amount of vitamins and minerals throughout your pregnancy. The healthy growth and development of the fetus depend on a steady supply of nutrients from the mother. There is evidence that low blood levels of zinc may lead to problems in pregnancy or defects in the baby. However, taking large amounts of a dietary supplement in pregnancy may be harmful to the mother and/or fetus and should be avoided.

Breast-feeding—It is important that you receive the right amounts of vitamins and minerals so that your baby will also get the vitamins and minerals needed to grow properly. However, taking large amounts of a dietary supplement while breast-feeding may be harmful to the mother and/or baby and should be avoided.

Children—It is especially important that children receive enough zinc in their diet for healthy growth and development. Although there is no specific information comparing use of zinc in children with use in other age groups, this medicine is not expected to cause different side effects or problems in children than it does in adults.

Older adults—It is important that older people continue to receive enough zinc in their daily diets. There is some evidence that the elderly may be at risk of becoming deficient in zinc due to poor food selection, decreased absorption of zinc by the body, or medicines that decrease absorption of zinc or increase loss of zinc from the body.

Medicines or other dietary supplements—Although certain medicines or dietary supplements should not be used together at all, in other cases they may be used together even if an interaction might occur. In these cases, your doctor may want to change the dose, or other precautions may be necessary. When you are taking zinc supplements, it is especially important that your doctor and pharmacist know if you are taking any of the following:

- Copper supplements or
- Penicillamine and other medicines that bind with metals or
- Tetracycline (medicine for infection)—Use with zinc supplements may cause these medicines to be less effective; zinc supplements should be given at least 2 hours after copper supplements, penicillamine, or tetracycline

- Iron supplements—Use with zinc supplements may cause the zinc to be less effective; zinc supplements should be given at least 2 hours after iron supplements

Other medical problems—The presence of other medical problems may affect the use of zinc supplements. Make sure you tell your doctor if you have any other medical problems, especially:

- Copper deficiency—Zinc supplements may make this condition worse

Proper Use of This Dietary Supplement

Zinc supplements are most effective if they are taken at least 1 hour before or 2 hours after meals. However, if zinc supplements cause stomach upset, they may be taken with a meal. You should tell your doctor if you are taking your zinc supplement with meals.

Some people believe that taking very large doses of a vitamin or mineral (called megadoses) is useful for treating certain medical problems. Studies have not proven this. Large doses should be taken only under the direction of your doctor after need has been identified.

If you miss taking zinc supplements for one or more days there is no cause for concern, since it takes some time for your body to become seriously low in zinc. However, if your doctor has recommended that you take zinc, try to remember to take it as directed every day.

Storage—To store this dietary supplement:

- Keep out of the reach of children.
- Store away from heat and direct light.
- Do not store in the bathroom, near the kitchen sink, or in other damp places. Heat or moisture may cause the dietary supplement to break down.
- Keep the dietary supplement from freezing. Do not refrigerate.
- Do not keep outdated dietary supplements or those no longer needed. Be sure that any discarded dietary supplement is out of the reach of children.

Precautions While Using This Dietary Supplement

When zinc combines with certain foods it may not be absorbed into your body and it will do you no good. If you are taking zinc, the following foods should be avoided or taken 2 hours after you take zinc:

- Bran
- Fiber-containing foods
- Phosphorus-containing foods such as milk or poultry
- Whole-grain breads and cereals

Do not take zinc supplements and copper, iron, or phosphorus supplements at the same time. It is best to space doses of these products 2 hours apart, to get the full benefit from each dietary supplement.

Side Effects of This Dietary Supplement

Along with its needed effects, a dietary supplement may cause some unwanted effects. Although not all of these side effects may occur, if they do occur they may need medical attention.

Check with your doctor as soon as possible if any of the following side effects occur:

Rare—With large doses

Chills; continuing ulcers or sores in mouth or throat; fever; heartburn; indigestion; nausea; sore throat; unusual tiredness or weakness

Symptoms of overdose

Chest pain; dizziness; fainting; shortness of breath; vomiting; yellow eyes or skin

Other side effects not listed above may also occur in some patients. If you notice any other effects, check with your doctor.

Additional Information

Once a medicine or dietary supplement has been approved for marketing for a certain use, experience may show that it is also useful for other medical problems. Although this use is not included in product labeling, zinc supplements are used in certain patients with the following medical condition:

- Wilson's disease (a disease of too much copper in the body)

Other than the above information, there is no additional information relating to proper use, precautions, or side effects for this use.

Annual revision: 02/03/92
Interim revision: 08/21/92

Glossary

Abdomen—The internal body area between the chest and pelvis.

Abortifacient—Medicine that causes abortion.

Abrade—Scrape or rub away the outer cover or layer of a part.

Absorption—Passing into the body; incorporation of substances into or across tissues of the body, for example, digested food into the blood from the small intestine, or poisons through the skin.

Achlorhydria—Absence of acid that normally would be found in the stomach.

Acidifier, urinary—Medicine that makes the urine more acidic.

Acidosis—Build-up of too much acid in the body fluids and tissues.

Acromegaly—Enlargement of the face, hands, and feet because of too much growth hormone.

Acute—Sharp or intense; describes a condition that begins suddenly, has severe symptoms, and usually lasts a short length of time.

Addison's disease—Disease caused by not enough secretion of hormones by the adrenal glands.

Adhesion—The union by connective tissue of two parts that are normally separate (such as parts of a joint).

Adjunct—An additional or secondary treatment that is helpful but is not necessary to treatment of a particular condition; not effective for that condition if used alone.

Adjuvant—1. A substance added to or used with another substance to assist its action. 2. Something that assists or enhances the effectiveness of medical treatment.

Adrenal cortex—Outer layer of tissue of the adrenal gland, which produces hormones.

Adrenal glands—Two triangle-shaped organs located next to the kidneys. They produce the hormones epinephrine and norepinephrine and other hormones related to metabolism and sexual development and functioning.

Adrenaline—See epinephrine.

Adrenal medulla—Inner part of the adrenal gland, which produces epinephrine and norepinephrine.

Adrenocorticoids—See corticosteroids.

Aerosol—Suspension of very small liquid or solid particles in compressed gas; drugs in aerosol form are dispensed in the form of a mist by releasing the gas.

African sleeping sickness—See Trypanosomiasis, African.

Agoraphobia—Fear of public places or open spaces.

Agranulocytosis—Disorder in which there is a severe decrease in the number of granulocytes in the blood.

AIDS (acquired immunodeficiency syndrome)—Disease caused by human immunodeficiency virus (HIV). The disease results in a breakdown of the body's immune system, which makes a person more likely to get other infections and some forms of cancer.

Alcohol-abuse deterrent—Medicine used to help alcoholics avoid the use of alcohol.

Alkaline—Having a pH of more than 7. Opposite of acidic.

Alkalizer, urinary—Medicine used to make the urine more alkaline.

Alkalosis—Build-up of too much alkalinity in the body fluids and tissues.

Alopecia—Loss or absence of hair from areas where it normally is present; baldness.

Altitude sickness agent—Medicine used to prevent or lessen some of the effects of high altitude on the body.

Alzheimer's disease—Progressive disorder of thinking and other mental processes, usually beginning in late middle age.

Aminoglycosides—A class of chemically related antibiotics used to treat some serious types of bacterial infections.

Anabolic steroids—Synthetic forms of androgens.

Analgesic—Medicine that relieves pain without causing unconsciousness.

Anaphylaxis—Sudden, severe allergic reaction.

Androgens—Male hormones, such as testosterone.

Anemia—Symptom of various diseases that exists because of too little hemoglobin in the blood.

Anesthesiologist—A physician who is qualified to give an anesthetic and other medicines to a patient before and during surgery.

Anesthetic—Medicine that causes a loss of sensation, sometimes through loss of consciousness.

Aneurysm—Dilatation or saclike swelling and weakening of the wall of an artery, vein, or the heart.

Angina—Pain, tightness, or feeling of heaviness in the chest, due mostly to lack of oxygen to the heart muscle. The pain may be felt in the left shoulder and arm instead of or in addition to the chest. Symptoms often occur during exercise.

Angioedema—Allergic condition marked by continuing swelling and severe itching of areas of the skin.

Anorexia—Loss of appetite for food.

Anoxia—Absence of oxygen. The term is sometimes incorrectly used for hypoxia, which means an abnormally low amount of oxygen in the body.

Antacid—Medicine used to neutralize excess acid in the stomach.

Antagonist—Drug or other substance that blocks or works against the action of another.

Anthelmintic—Medicine used to treat infections caused by worms.

Antiacne agent—Medicine used to treat acne.

Antiadrenal—Medicine used to prevent an overactive adrenal gland (adrenal cortex) from producing too much cortisone-like hormone.

Antianemic—Agent that prevents or corrects anemia.

Antianginal—Medicine used to prevent or treat angina attacks.

Antianxiety agent—Medicine used to treat nervousness, tension, or anxiety.

Antiarrhythmic—Medicine used to treat irregular heartbeats.

Antiasthmatic—Medicine used to treat asthma.

Antibacterial—Medicine that kills bacteria or stops their growth.

Antibiotic—Medicine used to treat infections.

Antibody—Special kind of blood protein that helps the body fight infection.

Antibulimic—Medicine used to treat bulimia.

Anticholelithic—Medicine that dissolves gallstones.

Anticoagulant—Medicine that prevents blood clots from being formed in the blood vessels.

Anticonvulsant—Medicine used to prevent or treat convulsions (seizures).

Antidepressant—Medicine used to treat mental depression.

Antidiabetic agent—Medicine used to control blood sugar levels in patients with diabetes mellitus (sugar diabetes).

Antidiarrheal—Medicine used to treat diarrhea.

Antidiuretic—Medicine used to help hold water in the body (for example, in patients with diabetes insipidus [water diabetes]).

Antidote—Medicine used to prevent or treat harmful effects of another medicine or a poison.

Antidyskinetic—Medicine used to help treat the loss of muscle control caused by certain diseases or some other medicines.

Antidysmenorrheal—Medicine used to treat menstrual cramps.

Antiemetic—Medicine used to prevent or treat nausea and vomiting.

Antiendometriotic—Medicine used to treat endometriosis.

Antienuretic—Medicine used to help prevent bedwetting.

Antifibrotic—Medicine used to treat fibrosis.

Antiflatulent—Medicine used to help relieve excess gas in the stomach or intestines.

Antifungal—Medicine used to treat infections caused by a fungus.

Antiglaucoma agent—Medicine used to treat glaucoma.

Antigout agent—Medicine used to prevent or relieve gout attacks.

Antihemorrhagic—Medicine used to prevent or help stop serious bleeding.

Antihistamine—Medicine used to prevent or relieve the symptoms of allergies (such as hay fever).

Antihypercalcemic—Medicine used to help lower the amount of calcium in the blood.

Antihyperlipidemic—Medicine used to help lower the amount of cholesterol or other fat-like substances in the blood.

Antihyperphosphatemic—Medicine used to help lower the amount of phosphate in the blood.

Antihypertensive—Medicine used to treat high blood pressure.

Antihyperuricemic—Medicine used to prevent or treat gout or other medical problems caused by too much uric acid in the blood.

Antihypocalcemic—Medicine used to increase calcium blood levels in patients with too little calcium.

Antihypoglycemic—Medicine used to increase blood sugar levels in patients with low blood sugar.

Antihypokalemic—Medicine used to increase potassium blood levels in patients with too little potassium.

Antihypoparathyroid—Medicine used to treat the effects of an underactive parathyroid gland.

Anti-infective—Medicine used to treat infection.

Anti-inflammatory—Medicine used to relieve pain, swelling, and other symptoms caused by inflammation.

Anti-inflammatory, nonsteroidal—An anti-inflammatory medicine that is not a cortisone-like medicine.

Anti-inflammatory, steroidal—A cortisone-like anti-inflammatory medicine.

Antimanic—Medicine used to treat manic-depressive mental illness.

Antimetabolite—Medicine that interferes with the normal processes within cells, preventing their growth.

Antimuscarinic—Medicine used to block the effects of a certain chemical in the body; often used to reduce smooth muscle spasms, especially abdominal or stomach cramps or spasms.

Antimyasthenic—Medicine used to treat myasthenia gravis.

Antimyotonic—Medicine used to prevent or relieve nighttime leg cramps or muscle spasms.

Antineoplastic—Medicine used to treat cancer.

Antineuralgic—Medicine used to treat neuralgia.

Antiprotozoal—Medicine used to treat infections caused by protozoa (tiny, one-celled animals).

Antipsoriatic—Medicine used to treat psoriasis.

Antipsychotic—Medicine used to treat certain nervous, mental, and emotional conditions.

Antipyretic—Medicine used to reduce high fever.

Antirheumatic—Medicine used to treat arthritis (rheumatism).

Antirosacea—Medicine used to treat rosacea.

Antiseborrheic—Medicine used to treat dandruff and seborrhea.

Antiseptic—Medicine that stops the growth of germs. Used on the surface of the skin to prevent the development of infections in cuts, scrapes, and wounds.

Antispasmodic—Medicine used to reduce smooth muscle spasms (for example, stomach, intestinal, or urinary tract spasms).

Antispastic—Medicine used to treat muscle spasms.

Antithyroid agent—Medicine used to treat an overactive thyroid gland.

Antitremor agent—Medicine used to treat tremors (trembling or shaking).

Antitubercular—Medicine used to treat tuberculosis (TB).

Antitussive—Medicine used to relieve cough.

Antiulcer agent—Medicine used to treat stomach and duodenal ulcers.

Antivertigo agent—Medicine used to prevent dizziness.

Antiviral—Medicine used to treat infections caused by a virus.

Anxiety—An emotional state in which there is apprehension, worry, or tension in reaction to imagined danger or dread of a situation; may include sweating, increased pulse, trembling, weakness, and fatigue.

Apnea—Temporary state of not breathing.

Apoplexy—See Stroke.

Appendicitis—Inflammation of the appendix.

Appetite stimulant—Medicine used to help increase the desire for food.

Appetite suppressant—Medicine used in weight control programs to help decrease the desire for food.

Arrhythmia—Loss of the normal rhythm of the heartbeat.

Arteritis, temporal—Inflammatory disease of the blood vessels, usually of the head; occurs in older people.

Arthralgia—Pain in a joint.

Arthritis, rheumatoid—Chronic disease of the joints, marked by pain and swelling at the sites.

Ascites—Accumulation of fluid in the abdominal cavity.

Asthma—Disease marked by inflammation of the bronchial tubes (air passages). During an attack, air passages become constricted, causing wheezing and difficult breathing. Attacks may be brought on by allergens, virus infection, cold air, or exercise.

Atherosclerosis—Common disease of the arteries in which fat deposits thicken and harden the artery walls.

Avoid—To keep away from deliberately.

Bacteremia—Presence of bacteria in the blood.

Bacterium—Tiny, one-celled organism. Many types of bacteria are responsible for a number of diseases and infections.

Bancroft's filariasis—Disease transmitted by mosquitos in which an infection with the filarial worm occurs. Affects the lymph system, producing inflammation.

Beriberi—Disorder caused by too little vitamin B_1 (thiamine), marked by an accumulation of fluid in the body, extreme weight loss, inflammation of nerves, or paralysis.

Bile—Thick fluid produced by the liver and stored in the gallbladder. Bile helps in the digestion of food.

Bile duct—Tubular passage through which bile passes from the liver to the gallbladder.

Bilharziasis—See Manson's schistosomiasis.

Biliary—Relating to bile, the bile duct, or the gallbladder.

Bipolar disorder—Also called "manic-depressive illness." Severe mental illness marked by repeated episodes of depression and mania.

Bisexual—One whose sexual attraction is toward persons of both sexes.

Black fever—See Leishmaniasis, visceral.

Blackwater fever—Condition, marked by dark urine, rarely seen as a complication of malaria.

Blood fluke—See Manson's schistosomiasis.

Bone marrow—Soft material contained within the cavities of bones. One form produces red blood cells.

Bone marrow depression—Condition in which the production of blood cells and platelets by the red bone marrow is decreased.

Bone resorption inhibitor—Medicine used to prevent or treat certain types of bone disorders, such as Paget's disease of the bone.

Bowel disease, inflammatory, suppressant—Medicine used to treat certain intestinal disorders, such as colitis.

Bradycardia—Slow heart rate, usually less than 60 beats per minute.

Bronchitis—Inflammation of the bronchial tubes (air passages) of the lungs.

Bronchodilator—Medicine used to open up the bronchial tubes (air passages) of the lungs to increase the flow of air through them.

Buccal—Relating to the cheek. A buccal medicine is taken by placing it in the cheek pocket and letting it slowly dissolve.

Bulimia—Disturbance in eating behavior marked by bouts of excessive eating followed by self-induced vomiting and diarrhea, hard exercise, or fasting.

Bursa—Small fluid-filled sac present where body parts move over one another (such as a joint) to help reduce friction.

Bursitis—Inflammation of a bursa.

Candidiasis of the mouth—Also called "thrush" or "white mouth." Overgrowth of the yeast *Candida* in the mouth marked by white patches on the tongue or inside the mouth.

Candidiasis of the vagina—Yeast infection of the vagina caused by the yeast *Candida;* associated with itching, burning, and a cheesy or curd-like white discharge.

Cardiac—Relating to the heart.

Cardiac arrhythmia—Irregularity or loss of the normal rhythm of the heartbeat.

Cardiac load-reducing agent—Medicine used to ease the workload of the heart by allowing the blood to flow through the blood vessels more easily.

Cardiotonic—Medicine used to improve the strength and efficiency of the heart.

Caries, dental—Also called "cavities." Tooth decay, sometimes causing pain, and leading to the crumbling of the tooth.

Cataract—An opacity (cloudiness) in the eye lens that impairs vision or causes blindness.

Catheter—Tube inserted into a small opening in the body so that fluids can be put in or taken out.

Caustic—Burning or corrosive agent; irritating and destructive to living tissue.

Cavities—See Caries, dental.

Central nervous system—Part of the nervous system that is composed of the brain and spinal cord.

Cerebral palsy—Brain condition resulting in weakness and poor coordination of the limbs.

Cervix—Lower end or necklike part of the uterus.

Chemotherapy—Treatment of illness or disease by chemical agents. The term most commonly refers to the use of drugs to treat cancer.

Chickenpox—See Varicella.

Chlamydia—A family of microorganisms that cause a variety of diseases in humans. One form is transmitted by sexual contact.

Cholesterol—Fat-like substance found in the blood and most tissues. Too much cholesterol is associated with several potential health risks, especially atherosclerosis (hardening of the arteries).

Chronic—Describes a condition of long duration, which is often of gradual onset and may involve very slow changes. Note that the term "chronic" has nothing to do with how serious the condition is.

Cirrhosis—Liver disease marked by abnormal cell growth, which may in turn lead to other serious conditions.

Clitoris—Small, elongated, erectile organ that is the female counterpart of the penis.

CNS—See Central nervous system.

Cold sores—See Herpes simplex.

Colic—Waves of sudden severe abdominal pain, which are usually separated by relatively pain-free intervals.

Colitis—Inflammation of the colon (bowel).

Colostomy—Operation in which part of the colon (bowel) is brought through the abdominal wall to create an artificial opening. The contents of the intestine are discharged through the opening, bypassing the rest of the intestines.

Coma—State of unconsciousness from which the patient cannot be aroused.

Coma, hepatic—Disturbances in mental function and the nervous system caused by severe liver disease.

Condom—Thin sheath or cover worn over the penis during sexual intercourse to prevent pregnancy or infection.

Congestive heart failure—Condition resulting from inability of the heart to pump strongly enough to maintain adequate blood flow; characterized by breathlessness and edema.

Conjunctiva—Delicate mucous membrane covering the front of the eye and the inside of the eyelid.

Conjunctivitis—Inflammation of the conjunctiva.

Constriction—Squeezing together and becoming narrower or smaller, such as constriction of blood vessels or eye pupils.

Contagious disease—Disease that can be transmitted from one person to another.

Contamination—To make impure or unclean, especially by introducing germs or unclean material into or on normally sterile substances or objects.

Contraceptive—Medicine or device used to prevent pregnancy.

Corticosteroids—Group of cortisone-like hormones that are secreted by the adrenal cortex and are critical to the body. The two major groups of corticosteroids are glucocorticoids, which affect fat and body metabolism, and mineralocorticoids, which regulate salt/water balance. Also known as adrenocorticoids.

Cortisol—Natural hormone produced by the adrenal cortex, important for carbohydrate, protein, and fat metabolism and for the normal response to stress; synthetic cortisol (hydrocortisone) is used to treat inflammations, allergies, collagen diseases, rheumatic disorders, and adrenal failure.

Cot death—See Sudden infant death syndrome (SIDS).

Cowpox—See Vaccinia.

Creutzfeldt-Jakob disease—Rare disease, probably caused by a slow-acting virus that affects the brain and nervous system.

Crib death—See Sudden infant death syndrome (SIDS).

Crohn's disease—Condition in which parts of the digestive tract become thick and inflamed.

Croup—Inflammation and blockage of the larynx (voice box) in young children.

Crystalluria—Presence of crystals in the urine.

Cushing's syndrome—Condition in which the adrenal gland produces too much cortisone-like hormone, leading to weight gain, round face, and high blood pressure.

Cycloplegia—Paralysis of certain eye muscles, which can be useful in resting the muscles; useful in certain eye examinations.

Cycloplegic—Medicine used to induce cycloplegia.

Cyst—Abnormal sac or closed cavity filled with liquid or semisolid matter.

Cystic—Marked by cysts.

Cystic fibrosis—Hereditary disease of infants, children, and young adults in which exocrine glands do not function normally; excess mucus production causes serious lung disease.

Cystine—An amino acid found in most proteins; it is produced by the digestion of the protein.

Cystitis, interstitial—Inflammation of the bladder, predominantly in women, with frequent urge to urinate and painful urination.

Cytomegalovirus—One of a group of viruses. One form is sexually transmitted and can cause blindness and be fatal in patients with weakened immune systems.

Cytoplasm—Material that surrounds the nucleus of a cell.

Cytotoxic agent—Chemical that kills cells or stops cell division; used to treat cancer.

Decongestant, nasal—Medicine used to help relieve nasal congestion (stuffy nose).

Decongestant, ophthalmic—Medicine used in the eye to relieve redness, burning, itching, or other irritation.

Decubitus—Act of lying down or the position taken in lying down.

Decubitus ulcer—Bedsore; damage to the skin and underlying tissues caused by constant pressure.

Dental—Related to the teeth or gums.

Depression, mental—Condition marked by deep sadness; associated with lack of any pleasurable interest in life. Other symptoms include disturbances in sleep, appetite, and concentration, and difficulty in performing day-to-day tasks.

Dermatitis herpetiformis—Skin disease marked by sores and itching.

Dermatitis, seborrheic—Type of eczema found on the scalp and face.

Dermatomyositis—Inflammatory disorder of the skin and underlying tissues, including breakdown of muscle fibers.

Diabetes insipidus—Disorder in which the patient produces large amounts of urine and is constantly thirsty. Also called "water diabetes."

Diabetes mellitus—Disorder in which the body cannot process sugars to produce energy; either the body does not produce enough insulin or the body tissues are unable to use the insulin present. This leads to too much sugar in the blood (hyperglycemia). Also called "sugar diabetes."

Diagnose—Find out the cause or nature of a disorder by an examination or laboratory tests.

Diagnostic procedure—A process carried out to determine the cause or nature of a condition, disease, or disorder.

Dialysis, renal—Artificial technique for removing waste materials or poisons from the blood when the kidneys are not working properly.

Digestant—Medicine used to help the stomach digest food.

Diplopia—Awareness of two images of a single object at one time; double vision.

Diuretic—Also called "water pill." Medicine that increases the amount of urine produced by helping the kidneys get rid of water and salt.

Diverticulitis—Inflammation of a diverticulum in the intestinal tract.

Diverticulum—Sac or pouch opening from a canal or cavity.

Down's syndrome—Also called "mongolism." Mental retardation caused by a defect in the genes. Patients with Down's syndrome are marked physically by a round head, flat nose, slightly slanted eyes, and short stature.

DNA—Deoxyribonucleic acid; the genetic material in cells that controls heredity.

Duct—Tube or channel, especially one that serves to carry secretions from a gland.

Dumdum fever—See Leishmaniasis, visceral.

Duodenal ulcer—Open sore in that part of the small intestine closest to the stomach.

Duodenum—First of the three parts of the small intestine.

Dyskinesia—Refers to abnormal, involuntary movement or a defect in voluntary movement.

Dyspnea—Labored or difficult breathing or respiration.

Eczema—Inflammation of the skin, marked by itching and rash.

Edema—Swelling of body tissue due to accumulation of fluids, usually first noticed in the feet or lower legs.

Eighth-cranial-nerve disease—Disease of the eighth cranial (brain) nerve, resulting in dizziness, loss of balance, loss of hearing, nausea, or vomiting.

Electrolyte—Substance that can, when in solution, conduct an electric current. In medical use, these substances are needed for normal functioning of the body. Body electrolytes include bicarbonate, chloride, sodium, potassium, etc.

Embolism—Sudden blocking of an artery by a blood clot or other foreign substances carried to the place of obstruction by the blood.

Embryo—In humans, a developing fertilized egg within the uterus (womb) from about two to eight weeks after fertilization.

Emergency—Extremely serious unexpected or sudden happening or situation that calls for immediate action.

Emollient—Substance that soothes and softens an irritated surface, such as the skin.

Emphysema—Lung condition in which too much air accumulates in lung tissue because of blockage or narrowing of the bronchial tubes (air passages), leading to troubled breathing and heart problems.

Encephalitis—Inflammation of the brain.

Encephalopathy—Any degenerative disease of the brain; caused by many different medical conditions.

Endocarditis—Inflammation of the lining of the heart, leading to fever, heart murmurs, and heart failure.

Endometriosis—Condition in which material similar to the lining of the uterus (womb) appears at other sites within the pelvic cavity, causing pain and bleeding.

Enteric coating—Coating on tablets which allows them to pass through the stomach unchanged before being broken up in the intestine and being absorbed. Used to protect the stomach from the medicine and/or the medicine from the stomach's acid.

Enteritis—Inflammation of the small intestine, usually causing diarrhea.

Enuresis—Urinating while asleep (bedwetting).

Enzyme—Type of protein produced by living cells that is important for normal chemical reactions in the body.

Eosinophil—Variety of leukocyte or other granulocyte readily stained by the dye eosin.

Eosinophilia—Condition in which the number of eosinophils in the blood is abnormally high.

Epidural space—Area in the spinal column into which medicines (usually for pain) can be administered.

Epilepsy—Any of a group of brain disorders featuring sudden attacks of seizures and other symptoms.

Epinephrine—Hormone secreted by the adrenal medulla. It stimulates the heart, constricts blood vessels, and relaxes muscles. Also known as adrenaline.

EPO—See erythropoietin.

Ergot alkaloids—Medicines that cause narrowing of blood vessels; used to treat migraine headaches, and to reduce bleeding in childbirth.

Erythropoietin—Hormone secreted by the kidney. It controls the production of red blood cells by the bone marrow; also available as a synthetic drug (EPO).

Esophagus—The muscular tube extending from the pharynx to the stomach.

Estrogen—Female hormone necessary for the normal sexual development of the female and for the regulation of the menstrual cycle during the childbearing years.

Exocrine gland—Any gland that discharges its secretion through a duct.

Exophthalmos—Thrusting forward of the eyeballs in their sockets giving the appearance of the eyes sticking out too far.

Expectorant—Medicine used to help remove mucus or phlegm in the lungs by coughing or spitting it up.

Extrapyramidal symptoms—Movement disorders occurring with certain diseases or with use of certain drugs, including trembling and shaking of hands and fingers, twisting movements of the body, shuffling walk, and stiffness of arms or legs.

Familial Mediterranean fever—Also called polyserositis. Inherited condition involving inflammation of the lining of the chest, abdomen, and joints.

Fasciculation—Small, spontaneous contraction of a few muscle fibers, which is visible through the skin; muscular twitching.

Favism—Inherited condition resulting from sensitivity to broad (fava) beans; marked by fever, vomiting, diarrhea, and acute destruction of red blood cells.

Fertility—Capacity to bring about the start of pregnancy.

Fetus—In humans, a developing baby within the uterus (womb) from about the beginning of the third month of pregnancy until birth.

Fibrocystic—Having benign (noncancerous) tumors of connective tissue.

Fibroid tumor—A noncancerous tumor of the uterus formed of fibrous or fully developed connective tissue.

Fibrosis—Condition in which the skin and underlying tissues tighten and become less flexible.

Fistula—Abnormal tubelike passage connecting two internal organs or one that leads from an abscess or internal organ to the body surface.

Flatulence—Excessive amount of air or gas in the stomach or intestine.

Flu—See Influenza.

Flushing—Temporary redness of the face and/or neck.

Fungus—Any of a group of simple plants that live off of other living matter; includes molds and yeasts.

Fungus infection—Infection caused by a fungus. Some common fungus infections are tinea pedis (athlete's foot), tinea capitis (ringworm of the scalp), tinea cruris (ringworm of the groin or jock itch), and mouth or vaginal candidiasis (yeast infections).

Gait—Manner of walk.

Gamma globulin—Type of protein found in the blood that is important in the body's immunity to infection.

Gastric—Relating to the stomach.

Gastric acid secretion inhibitor—Medicine used to decrease the amount of acid produced by the stomach.

Gastroenteritis—Inflammation of the stomach and intestine.

Gastroesophageal reflux—Backward flow into the esophagus of the contents of the stomach and duodenum. The condition is often characterized by "heartburn."

Gastroparesis, diabetic—Condition brought on by diabetes in which the stomach does not function as it should.

Generic—General in nature; relating to an entire group or class. In relation to medicines, the general name of a drug substance; not owned by one specific group as would be true for a trademark or brand name.

Genital—1. Relating to the organs concerned with reproduction; the sexual organs. 2. Relating to reproduction.

Genital warts—Small growths found on the genitals or around the anus; caused by a virus. The disease may be transmitted by sexual contact.

Gilles de la Tourette syndrome—See Tourette's disorder.

Gingiva—Gums.

Gingival hyperplasia—Enlargement of the gums.

Gingivitis—Inflammation of the gums.

Glandular fever—See Mononucleosis.

Glaucoma—Condition of abnormally high pressure in the eye; may lead to loss of vision if not treated.

Glomeruli—Clusters of capillaries in the nephron of the kidney that act as a filter of the blood.

Glomerulonephritis—Inflammation of the glomeruli of the kidney not caused by infection.

Glucose-6-phosphate dehydrogenase (G6PD) deficiency—Lack of or reduced amounts of an enzyme (glucose-6-phosphate dehydrogenase) that breaks down certain sugar compounds in the body.

Gluten—Type of protein found primarily in wheat and rye.

Goiter—Enlargement of the thyroid gland that causes the neck to swell. Condition usually results from a lack of iodine or overactivity of the thyroid gland.

Gonadotropin—Hormone that stimulates the actions of the sex organs.

Gonorrhea—An infectious disease, usually transmitted by sexual contact. It causes infection in the genital mucous membranes in both men and women.

Gout—Disease in which too much uric acid builds up in the blood and joints, leading to painful swelling.

Granulation—Small, fleshy outgrowths on the healing surface of a wound or ulcer; a normal stage in healing.

Granulocyte—Any cell, especially a white blood cell, containing granules in its cytoplasm.

Granulocytopenia—Abnormal reduction of the number of granulocytes in the blood; agranulocytosis.

Granuloma—A growth or mass of granulation tissue produced in response to chronic infection, inflammation, a foreign body, or to unknown causes.

Graves' disease—Disorder in which too much thyroid hormone is present in the blood.

Groin—The area between the abdomen and thigh.

Guillain-Barré syndrome—Nerve disease marked by sudden numbness and weakness in the limbs that may progress to complete paralysis.

Gynecomastia—Excessive development of the breasts in the male.

Hair follicle—Sheath of tissue surrounding a hair root.

Hansen's disease—See Leprosy.

Hartnup disease—Hereditary disease in which the body has trouble processing certain chemicals, leading to mental retardation, rough skin, and problems with muscle coordination.

Heart attack—See Myocardial infarction.

Hematuria—Presence of blood or blood cells in the urine.

Hemoglobin—Iron-containing substance found in red blood cells that transports oxygen from the lungs to the tissues of the body.

Hemolytic anemia—Type of anemia caused by destruction of red blood cells.

Hemophilia—Hereditary blood disease in males in which blood clotting is delayed, leading to excessive and uncontrolled bleeding even after minor injuries.

Hemorrhoids—Also called "piles." Enlarged veins in the walls of the anus.

Hepatic—Relating to the liver.

Hepatitis—Inflammation of the liver.

Hernia, hiatal—Condition in which the stomach passes partly into the chest through the opening for the esophagus in the diaphragm.

Herpes simplex—The virus that causes "cold sores." These are an inflammation of the skin resulting in small, painful blisters. Infection may occur either around the mouth or, in the case of genital herpes, around the genitals (sex organs).

Herpes zoster—Also called "shingles," an infectious disease usually marked by pain and blisters along one nerve, often on the face, chest, stomach, or back. The infection is caused by the virus that also causes chickenpox.

Heterosexual—One whose sexual attraction is toward persons of the opposite sex.

High blood pressure—See Hypertension.

Hirsutism—Adult male pattern of hair growth in women.

HIV (human immunodeficiency virus)—Virus that causes AIDS.

Hodgkin's disease—Malignant condition marked by swelling of the lymph nodes, with weight loss and fever.

Homosexual—One whose sexual attraction is toward persons of the same sex.

Hormone—Substance produced in one part of the body (such as a gland), which then passes into the bloodstream and travels to other organs or tissues, where it carries out its effect.

Hot flashes—Sensations of heat of the face, neck, and upper body, often accompanied by sweating and flushing.

Hydrocortisone—See cortisol.

Hyperactivity—Abnormally increased activity.

Hyperammonemia—Elevated concentration of ammonia or its compounds in the blood.

Hypercalcemia—Too much calcium in the blood.

Hypercalciuria—Too much calcium in the urine.

Hypercholesterolemia—Excessive amount of cholesterol in the blood.

Hyperglycemia—High blood sugar.

Hyperkalemia—Abnormally high amount of potassium in the blood.

Hyperkeratosis—Overgrowth or thickening of the outer horny layer of the skin.

Hyperlipidemia—General term for too high a level of any or all of the lipids in the blood plasma.

Hyperphosphatemia—Too much phosphate in the blood.

Hypersensitivity—Excessive response by the body's immune system to a foreign substance.

Hypertension—Also called "high blood pressure." Blood pressure in the arteries (blood vessels) that is higher than normal for the patient's age group. Hypertension often shows no outward signs or symptoms but may lead to a number of serious health problems.

Hyperthermia—Very high body temperature.

Hyperthyroidism—1. Overactivity of the thyroid gland. 2. Condition caused by excessive secretion of the thyroid gland, which results in an increase in metabolism.

Hypocalcemia—Too little calcium in the blood.

Hypoglycemia—Low blood sugar.

Hypokalemia—Abnormally low amount of potassium in the blood.

Hypotension, orthostatic—Fall in blood pressure that occurs upon standing up.

Hypothalamus—Area of the brain that controls a number of body functions, including temperature, thirst, hunger, sexual and emotional activity, and sleep.

Hypothermia—Very low body temperature.

Hypoxia—Broad term meaning intake of oxygen or its use by the body is inadequate.

Ileostomy—Operation in which the ileum is brought through the abdominal wall to create an artificial opening. The contents of the intestine are discharged through the opening, bypassing the colon (bowel).

Ileum—Lowest of the three portions of the small intestine.

Immune deficiency condition—Lack of immune response to protect against infectious disease.

Immune system—Complex network of the body that defends against foreign substances or organisms that may harm the body.

Immunizing agent, active—Agent that causes the body to produce its own antibodies for protection against certain infections.

Immunocompromised—Having natural immunity decreased because of irradiation, certain medicine or diseases, and other conditions.

Immunosuppressant—Medicine that reduces the body's natural immunity.

Impetigo—Contagious bacterial skin infection common in babies and children in which skin redness develops into blisters that break and form a thick crust.

Implant—1. Special form of medicine, often a small pellet or rod, that is inserted into the body or beneath the skin so that the medicine will be released continuously over a period of time. 2. To insert or graft material or an object into a body site. 3. Material or an object inserted into a body site, such as a lens implant or a breast implant. 4. Action of a fertilized ovum becoming attached or embedded in the uterus.

Impotence—Difficulty or inability of the male to have or maintain an erection of the penis.

Incontinence—Inability to control natural passage of urine or of bowel movements.

Infertility—Medical condition which results in the difficulty or inability of a woman to become pregnant or of a man to cause pregnancy.

Inflammation—Pain, redness, swelling, and heat in a part of the body, usually in response to injury or illness.

Influenza—Also called "flu." Highly contagious virus infection of the respiratory tract, marked by coughing, headache, chills, fever, muscle pain, and general weakness.

Ingredient—One of the parts or substances that make up a mixture or compound.

Inhalation—Medicine used by being breathed (inhaled) into the lungs. Some inhalations work locally in the lungs, while others produce their effects elsewhere in the body.

Inhibitor—Substance that prevents a process or reaction.

Inner ear—Inner portion of the ear; a liquid filled system of cavities and ducts that make up the organs of hearing and balance.

Insomnia—Inability to sleep or remain asleep.

Insulin—Hormone that enables the body to use sugar. Used in the treatment and control of diabetes mellitus (sugar diabetes).

Interstitial plasma cell pneumonia—See Pneumocystis pneumonia.

Intra-amniotic—Within the sac that contains the fetus and amniotic fluid.

Intra-arterial—Into an artery.

Intracavernosal—Into the corpus cavernosa (cavities in the penis that, when filled with blood, produce an erection).

Intracavitary—Into a body cavity (for example, the chest cavity or bladder).

Intramuscular—Into a muscle.

Intrauterine device (IUD)—Small plastic or metal device placed in the uterus (womb) to prevent pregnancy.

Intravenous—Into a vein.

Irrigation—Washing out a body cavity or wound with a solution of a medicine.

Ischemia—Condition caused by inadequate blood flow to a part of the body; caused by constriction or blocking of blood vessels that supply the part of the body affected.

Jaundice—Yellowing of the eyes and skin due to too much of a certain pigment in the bile.

Jock itch—Ringworm of the groin.

Kala-azar—See Leishmaniasis, visceral.

Kaposi's sarcoma—Malignant skin tumor. One form occurs in immunocompromised patients, for example, transplant recipients and AIDS patients.

Keratolytic—Medicine used to soften hardened areas of the skin (e.g., warts).

Ketoacidosis—Type of acidosis associated with diabetes.

Lactation—Secretion of breast milk.

Larvae—Young or immature insects.

Larynx—Organ that serves as a passage for air from the pharynx to the lungs; it contains the vocal cords.

Laxative—Medicine taken to encourage bowel movements.

Laxative, bulk-forming—Laxative that acts by absorbing liquid in the intestines and swelling to form a soft, bulky stool. The bowel is then stimulated normally by the presence of the bulky mass.

Laxative, hyperosmotic—Laxative that acts by drawing water into the bowel from surrounding body tissues. This provides a soft stool mass and increased bowel action.

Laxative, lubricant—Laxative that acts by coating the bowel and the stool mass with a waterproof film. This keeps moisture in the stool. The stool remains soft and its passage is made easier.

Laxative, stimulant—Also called contact laxative. Laxative that acts directly on the intestinal wall. The direct stimulation increases the muscle contractions that move the stool mass along.

Laxative, stool softener—Also called emollient laxative. Laxative that acts by helping liquids mix into the stool and prevent dry, hard stool masses. The stool remains soft and its passage is made easier.

Legionnaires' disease—Lung infection caused by a certain bacterium.

Leishmaniasis, visceral—Also called "black fever," "Dumdum fever," or "kala-azar." Tropical disease, transmitted by sandfly bites, which causes liver and spleen enlargement, anemia, weight loss, and fever.

Lennox-Gastaut syndrome—Type of childhood epilepsy.

Leprosy—Also called "Hansen's disease." Chronic disease affecting the skin, mucous membranes, and nerves. Symptoms include skin patches and loss of feeling and paralysis in the hands and feet leading to disfigurement and deformity.

Leukemia—Disease of the blood and bone marrow in which too many white blood cells are produced, resulting in anemia, bleeding, and low resistance to infections.

Leukocyte—White blood cell; any blood cell that contains a nucleus.

Leukoderma—See Vitiligo.

Leukopenia—Abnormal reduction in the total number of leukocytes in the blood.

Local effect—Affecting only the area to which something is being applied.

Loiasis—The state of being infected by a roundworm.

Lugol's solution—Transparent, deep brown liquid containing iodine and potassium iodide, which may be given before a radiopharmaceutical medicine.

Lupus—See Lupus erythematosus, systemic.

Lupus erythematosus, systemic—Also called "lupus" or "SLE" (systemic lupus erythematosus). Chronic inflammatory disease affecting the skin and various internal organs.

Lymph—Fluid that bathes the tissues. It is formed in tissue spaces all over the body and circulated by the lymphatic system.

Lymphatic system—Network of vessels that conveys lymph from the tissue fluids to the bloodstream.

Lymph node—Small, rounded body found at intervals along the lymphatic system. The nodes act as filters for the lymph by keeping bacteria and other foreign particles from entering the bloodstream. They also produce lymphocytes.

Lymphocyte—Any of a number of white blood cells found in the blood, lymph, and lymphatic tissues. They are involved in immunity.

Lymphoma—Malignant tumor of lymph nodes or tissue.

Lyse—To cause breakdown. In cells, damage or rupture of the membrane results in destruction of the cell.

Macrobiotic—Vegetarian diet consisting mostly of whole grains.

Malignant—Describing a condition that becomes continually worse if untreated; also used to mean cancerous.

Malnutrition—Condition caused by unbalanced or insufficient diet.

Mammogram—X-ray picture of the breast, usually taken to check for abnormal growths.

Mania—Mental state in which fast talking and excited feelings or actions are out of control.

Manson's schistosomiasis—Also called "blood fluke" or "bilharziasis." Tropical infection in which worms enter the body from contaminated water and settle in the intestines, causing anemia and inflammation.

Mast cells—Special cells in the body that release substances, such as histamine, that cause allergic reactions.

Mastocytosis—Accumulation of too many mast cells in tissues.

Megavitamin therapy—Taking very large doses of vitamins to prevent or treat certain medical problems.

Melanoma—Highly malignant cancer tumor, usually occurring on the skin.

Meniere's disease—Disease affecting the inner ear that is characterized by a group of symptoms including ringing in the ears, hearing loss, and dizziness.

Meningitis—Inflammation of the tissues that surround the brain and spinal cord.

Menopause—The time in a woman's life when the ovaries no longer produce an egg cell at regular times and menstruation stops.

Methemoglobin—Substance formed from hemoglobin in which iron has been oxidized and does not function as an oxygen carrier.

Methemoglobinemia—Presence of methemoglobin in the blood.

Middle ear—Chamber of the ear lying behind the eardrum and containing the structures that conduct sound.

Migraine—Throbbing headache thought to be caused by enlarged blood vessels, usually affecting one side of the head.

Miotic—Medicine used in the eye that causes the pupil to constrict (become smaller).

Mongolism—See Down's syndrome.

Mono—See Mononucleosis.

Monoclonal—Derived from a single cell; related to production of drugs by genetic engineering (e.g., monoclonal antibodies).

Mononucleosis—Also called "mono" or "glandular fever." Infectious viral disease occurring mostly in adolescents and young adults, marked by fever, sore throat, swelling of the lymph nodes in the neck and armpits, and by severe fatigue.

Motility—Ability to move without outside aid, force, or cause.

Mucolytic—Medicine that breaks down or dissolves mucus.

Mucosal—Relating to the mucous membrane.

Mucous membrane—Moist layer of tissue surrounding or lining many body structures and cavities, including the mouth, lips, inside of nose, anus, and vagina.

Mucus—Thick fluid produced by the body as a protective barrier, as a lubricant, and as a carrier of enzymes.

Multiple sclerosis (MS)—Chronic, progressive nerve disease marked by unsteadiness, shakiness, and problems in speech.

Myasthenia gravis—Chronic disease marked by abnormal weakness, and sometimes paralysis, of certain muscles.

Mydriatic—Medicine used in the eye that causes the pupil to dilate (become larger).

Myelogram—X-ray picture of the spinal cord.

Myeloma, multiple—Cancerous bone marrow disease that affects the body's ability to fight infections.

Myocardial infarction—Also called "heart attack." Interruption of blood supply to the heart, leading to sudden, severe chest pain, and damage to the heart muscle.

Myocardial reinfarction prophylactic—Medicine used to help prevent additional heart attacks in patients who have already had one attack.

Myotonia congenita—Hereditary muscle disorder marked by difficulty in relaxing a muscle or releasing a grip after any strong effort.

Narcolepsy—Extreme tendency to fall asleep suddenly.

Nasal—Relating to the nose.

Nasogastric (NG) tube—Tube that is inserted through the nose, down the throat, and into the stomach, so that medicine, food, or nutrients may be administered to patients who cannot swallow.

Nebulizer—Instrument that administers liquid in the form of a fine spray.

Necrosis—Death of tissue, cells, or a part of a structure or organ, surrounded by healthy parts.

Neoplasm—Also called tumor. New and abnormal growth of tissue in or on a part of the body, in which the multiplication of cells is uncontrolled and progressive.

Nephron—Unit of the kidney that acts as a filter of the blood; formation of urine is a result.

Neuralgia—Pain along the course of one or more nerves, occurring suddenly and intensely.

Neuralgia, trigeminal—Also called "tic douloureux." Severe burning or stabbing pain along the nerves in the face.

Neuritis, optic—Disease of the nerves in the eye.

Neuritis, peripheral—Inflammation of terminal nerves or the nerve endings.

Neutropenia—Abnormal reduction of neutrophils in the blood.

Nicotinamide adenine dinucleotide (NADH) methemoglobin reductase deficiency—Reduced ability of the blood to carry oxygen caused by the lack of or reduced amount of a specific enzyme.

Nodule—Small, rounded mass, lump, or swelling.

Nonsuppurative—Not discharging pus.

NSAIDs (nonsteroidal anti-inflammatory drugs)—Refers to a group of medicines used to treat inflammation and pain.

Nucleus—Part of the cell that contains DNA.

Nystagmus—Rapid, involuntary movements of the eyeball that may be from side to side, up and down, around, or in a mixed direction.

Obesity—Excess accumulation of fat in the body along with an increase in body weight that exceeds the healthy range for the body's frame.

Obstetrics—Field of medicine concerned with the care of women during pregnancy and childbirth.

Occlusive dressing—Dressing (such as plastic kitchen wrap) that completely cuts off air to the skin.

Occult—Concealed, hidden, or of unknown cause; cannot be seen by the human eye; detectable only by microscope or chemical testing, as for occult blood in the stools or feces.

Ophthalmic—Relating to the eye.

Opioid—1. Any synthetic narcotic with opium-like actions; not derived from opium. 2. Natural chemicals that produce opium-like effects by acting at the same cell sites where opium exerts action.

Oral—Relating to the mouth.

Orchitis—Inflammation of the testis.

Osteitis deformans—See Paget's disease.

Osteomalacia—Softening of the bones due to lack of vitamin D.

Osteoporosis—Loss of calcium from bone tissue, resulting in bones that are brittle and easily fractured.

OTC (over the counter)—Refers to medicine or devices available without a prescription.

Otic—Relating to the ear.

Otitis media—Inflammation of the middle ear.

Ototoxicity—Having a harmful effect on the organs or nerves of the ear concerned with hearing and balance.

Ovary—Female reproductive organ that produces egg cells and sex hormones. There are two ovaries, one on each side of the uterus.

Overactive thyroid—Condition in which the thyroid gland produces extra thyroid hormones; may cause fast heartbeat, tremors, nervousness, and increased sweating.

Ovulation—Process by which an ovum is released from the ovary. In human menstruating females, this usually occurs once a month.

Ovum—Mature female reproductive cell, or egg cell. It is capable of developing into a new organism if fertilized.

Paget's disease—Also called "osteitis deformans." Chronic bone disease, marked by thickening of the bones and severe pain.

Pancreatitis—Inflammation of the pancreas.

Pancytopenia—Reduction in the number of red cells, all types of white cells, and platelets in the blood.

Paralysis agitans—See Parkinson's disease.

Parathyroid glands—Two pairs of small bodies situated beside the thyroid gland; secrete parathyroid hormone that regulates the distribution of calcium and phosphorus in the body.

Parenteral—Injecting a medicine into the body using a needle and syringe.

Parkinsonism—See Parkinson's disease.

Parkinson's disease—Also called "Parkinsonism," "paralysis agitans," or "shaking palsy." Brain disease marked by tremor (shaking), stiffness, and difficulty in moving.

Patent ductus arteriosus (PDA)—Condition in newborn babies in which an important blood vessel in the heart fails to close as it should, resulting in faulty circulation and serious health problems.

Pediculicide—Medicine that kills lice.

Pediculosis—Infestation of the body or scalp with lice.

Pellagra—Disease caused by too little niacin, which results in scaly skin, diarrhea, and mental depression.

Pemphigus—Skin disease marked by successive outbreaks of blisters.

Peptic ulcer—Open sore in esophagus, stomach, or duodenum, caused by acidic gastric juice.

Peritoneum—Closed sac, formed by a membrane that lines the walls of the abdomen and covers the liver, stomach, spleen, gallbladder, and intestines.

Peritonitis—Inflammation of the peritoneum.

Peyronie's disease—Dense, fiber-like growth in the penis, which can be felt as an irregular hard lump, and which usually causes bending and pain when the penis is erect.

Pharynx—Space just behind the mouth that serves as a passageway for food from the mouth to the esophagus and for air from the nose and mouth to the larynx.

Phenol—Substance used as a preservative for injections.

Pheochromocytoma (PCC)—Tumor of the adrenal gland.

Phlebitis—Inflammation of a vein.

Phlegm—Thick mucus produced in the respiratory passages.

Piles—See Hemorrhoids.

Pituitary gland—Pea-sized body located at the base of the skull. It produces a number of hormones that are essential to normal body growth and functioning.

Placebo—Also called "sugar pill." Medicine that has no active medicinal substance but may help to relieve a condition because the patient believes it will.

Plaque, dental—Mixture of saliva, bacteria, and carbohydrates that forms on the teeth, leading to caries (cavities) and gum disease.

Platelet—Disc-shaped structure in the blood that performs several functions relating to blood clotting.

Platelet aggregation inhibitor—Medicine used to help prevent the platelets in the blood from clumping together. This effect reduces the chance of heart attack or stroke in certain patients.

Pleura—Membrane covering the lungs.

Pneumococcal—Relating to certain bacteria that cause pneumonia.

Pneumocystis pneumonia—A very serious type of pneumonia usually affecting persons with weakened immune systems, such as occurs in AIDS.

Polymorphous light eruption—A skin problem in certain people, which results from exposure to sunlight.

Polymyalgia rheumatica—Rheumatic disease, most common in elderly patients, which causes aching and stiffness in the shoulders and hips.

Polyp—Swollen or tumorous tissue that may or may not be cancerous.

Porphyria—Rare, inherited blood disease in which there is a disturbance of porphyrin metabolism.

Prevent—To stop or to keep from happening.

Priapism—Prolonged abnormal, painful erection of the penis.

Proctitis—Inflammation of the rectum.

Progestin—Female hormone necessary during the child-bearing years for the development of the milk-producing glands, and for the proper regulation of the menstrual cycle.

Prolactin—Hormone secreted by cells of the anterior pituitary gland that stimulates and maintains milk flow in women following childbirth.

Prolactinoma—A type of pituitary tumor often associated with galactorrhea and menstrual irregularity.

Prophylactic—1. Agent or medicine used to prevent the occurrence of a specific condition. 2. Condom.

Prostate—Gland surrounding the neck of the male urethra just below the base of the bladder. It secretes a fluid that constitutes a major portion of the semen.

Prosthesis—Any artificial substitute for a missing body part.

Protozoa—Tiny, one-celled animals; some cause diseases in humans.

Psoralen—Chemical found in plants and used in certain perfumes and medicines. Exposure to a psoralen and then to sunlight may increase the risk of severe burning.

Psoriasis—Chronic skin disease marked by itchy, scaly, red patches.

Psychosis—Severe mental illness marked by loss of contact with reality, often involving delusions, hallucinations, and disordered thinking.

Purpura—Condition marked by bleeding into the skin; skin rash or spots are first red, darken to purple, then fade to brownish-yellow.

PUVA—The combination of a psoralen, such as methoxsalen or trioxsalen, and ultraviolet light A; used to treat psoriasis and some other skin conditions.

Rachischisis—See Spina bifida.

Radiopaque agent—Substance that makes it easier to see an area of the body with x-rays. Radiopaque agents are used to help diagnose a variety of medical problems.

Radiopharmaceutical—Radioactive agent used to diagnose certain medical problems or treat certain diseases.

Raynaud's syndrome—Condition marked by paleness, numbness, and discomfort in the fingers when they are exposed to cold.

Rectal—Relating to the rectum.

Renal—Relating to the kidneys.

Reye's syndrome—Serious disease affecting the liver and brain that sometimes occurs after a virus infection, such as influenza or chickenpox. It occurs most often in young children and teenagers. The first sign of Reye's syndrome is usually severe, prolonged vomiting.

Rheumatic heart disease—Heart disease marked by scarring and chronic inflammation of the heart and its valves, occurring after rheumatic fever.

Rhinitis—Inflammation of the mucous membrane inside the nose.

Rickets—Bone disease caused by too little vitamin D, resulting in soft and malformed bones.

Ringworm—See Tinea.

Risk—The possibility of injury or of suffering harm.

River blindness—Disease in which one is infected with worms of the Onchocera type. The condition can progress to different eye nerve conditions or blindness. Also called Roble's disease, blinding filarial disease, and craw-craw.

Rosacea—Skin disease of the face, usually in middle-aged and older persons. Also called adult acne.

Sarcoidosis—Chronic disorder in which the lymph nodes in many parts of the body are enlarged, and small fleshy swellings develop in the lungs, liver, and spleen.

Scabicide—Medicine used to treat scabies (itch mite) infection.

Scabies—Contagious dermatitis caused by a mite burrowing under the skin that results in severe itching and redness.

Schizophrenia—Severe mental disorder in which thinking, mood, and behavior are disturbed.

Scintigram—Image obtained by detecting radiation emitted from a radiopharmaceutical introduced into the body.

Scleroderma—Persistent hardening and shrinking of the skin.

Scotoma—Area of decreased vision or total loss of vision in a part of the visual field.

Scrotum—Sac that holds the testes (male sex glands).

Scurvy—Disease caused by a deficiency of vitamin C (ascorbic acid), marked by bleeding gums, bleeding beneath the skin, and body weakness.

Seborrhea—Skin condition caused by the excess release of a thick, semi-fluid substance from the sebaceous glands.

Secretion—1. Process in which a gland releases a substance into the body for use. 2. The substance released by the gland.

Sedative-hypnotic—Medicine used to treat nervousness, restlessness, or insomnia.

Sedation—A relaxed or calmed state.

Seizure—Sudden, unnatural involuntary contraction or series of contractions of the muscles.

Semen—Fluid released from the penis at sexual climax. It is made up of sperm suspended in secretions from the reproductive tract.

Severe—Of a great degree, such as very serious pain or distress.

Shaking palsy—See Parkinson's disease.

Shingles—See Herpes zoster.

Shock—Severe disruption of cellular metabolism associated with reduced blood volume and blood pressure too low to supply adequate blood to the tissues.

Shunt—Surgical tube used to transfer blood or other fluid from one part of the body to another.

SIADH (secretion of inappropriate antidiuretic hormone) syndrome—Disease in which the body retains (keeps) more fluid and loses more sodium than normal.

Sickle cell anemia—Hereditary blood disease that predominantly affects blacks; name comes from the sickle-shaped red blood cells found in the blood of patients.

Sinusitis—Inflammation of a sinus.

Sjögren's syndrome—Condition marked by dry eyes, dry mouth, and arthritis.

Skeletal muscle relaxant—Medicine used to relax certain muscles and help relieve the pain and discomfort caused by strains, sprains, or other injury to the muscles.

SLE—See Lupus erythematosus, systemic.

Spastic paralysis—Weakness of a limb because of too much reflex response.

Spermicide—Substance that kills sperm.

Spina bifida—Also called "rachischisis." Birth defect in which the infant's spinal cord is partially exposed through a hole in the backbone.

Stenosis—Abnormal narrowing of a passage or duct of the body.

Sterility—1. Inability to produce offspring. 2. The state of being free of living microorganisms.

Stimulant, respiratory—Medicine used to stimulate breathing.

Stomatitis—Inflammation of the mucous membrane of the mouth.

Streptokinase—Enzyme that dissolves blood clots.

Stroke—Also called "apoplexy." Sudden weakness or paralysis, usually affecting one side of the body. Stroke occurs when the flow of blood to an area of the brain is interrupted.

Stye—Infection of one or more sebaceous glands of the eyelid, marked by swelling.

Subcutaneous—Under the skin.

Sublingual—Under the tongue. A sublingual medicine is taken by placing it under the tongue and letting it slowly dissolve.

Sudden infant death syndrome (SIDS)—Also called "crib death" or "cot death." Death of an infant, usually while asleep, from an unknown cause.

Sugar diabetes—See Diabetes mellitus.

Sugar pill—See Placebo.

Sulfite—Type of preservative; causes allergic reactions, such as asthma, in sensitive patients.

Sulfone—Medicine that acts against the bacteria that cause leprosy.

Sunscreen—Substance, usually a cream or lotion, that blocks the sun and ultraviolet light and helps prevent sunburn when applied to the skin.

Suppository—Mass of medicated material shaped for insertion into the rectum, vagina, or urethra. Suppository is solid at room temperature but melts at body temperature.

Suppressant—Medicine that stops an action or condition.

Suspension—A liquid in which the drug is not dissolved. When left standing for a period of time, particles settle at the bottom of the liquid and the top portion turns clear. When shaken it is ready for use.

Syncope—Sudden loss of consciousness due to inadequate blood flow to the brain; fainting.

Syphilis—An infectious disease, usually transmitted by sexual contact. The three stages of the disease may be separated by months or years.

Syringe—Device used to inject liquids into the body, remove material from a part of the body, or wash out a body cavity.

Systemic—For general effects throughout the body; applies to most medicines when taken by mouth or given by injection.

Tachycardia—Abnormal rapid beating of the heart, usually applied to a heart rate over 100 beats per minute in adults.

Temporomandibular joint (TMJ)—Hinge that connects the lower jaw to the skull.

Tendinitis—Inflammation of a tendon.

Teratogenic—Causing abnormal development in an embryo or fetus resulting in birth defects.

Testosterone—Principal male sex hormone.

Tetany—Condition marked by spasm and twitching of the muscles, particularly those of the hands, feet and face; caused by a decrease in the calcium concentration in the blood.

Therapeutic—Relating to the treatment of a specific condition.

Thimerosal—Chemical used as a preservative in some medicines, and as an antiseptic and disinfectant.

Thrombolytic agent—Substance that dissolves blood clots.

Thrombophlebitis—Inflammation of a vein associated with the formation of a thrombus.

Thrombus—Blood clot that obstructs a blood vessel or a cavity of the heart.

Thrush—See Candidiasis of the mouth.

Thyroid gland—Large gland in the base of the neck. It releases thyroid hormone, which controls body metabolism.

Thyrotoxicosis—Condition resulting from excessive amounts of thyroid hormones in the blood.

Tic—Repeated involuntary movement or spasm of a muscle.

Tic douloureux—See Neuralgia, trigeminal.

Tinea—Also called "ringworm." Fungus infection of the surface of the skin, particularly the scalp, feet, and nails.

Topical—For local effects when applied directly to the skin.

Tourette's disorder—Also called "Gilles de la Tourette syndrome." Condition usually marked with motor (jerking movements) and vocal (grunts, sniffs) tics.

Toxemia—Blood poisoning caused by bacteria growth at the site of infection.

Toxemia of pregnancy—Disease occurring in pregnant women in which there are metabolic disturbances that may result in hypertension, edema, excess protein in the urine, convulsions, and coma.

Toxic—Poisonous; potentially deadly.

Toxoplasmosis—Disease caused by a blood protozoan, usually transmitted to humans from cats or by eating raw meat; generally the symptoms are mild and self-limited.

Tracheostomy—A surgical opening through the throat into the trachea (windpipe) to permit a patient to breathe easily.

Tranquilizer—Medicine that produces a calming effect. It is used to relieve mental anxiety and tension.

Transdermal disk—Patch applied to the skin as a means of administering medicine; medicine contained in the patch is absorbed into the body through the skin.

Trichomoniasis—Infection of the vagina resulting in inflammation of genital tissues and discharge. It can be passed on to males.

Triglyceride—Fatty substance present in food or formed in the body from carbohydrates; stored in adipose tissue as fat.

Trypanosome fever—See Trypanosomiasis, African.

Trypanosomiasis, African—Also called "African sleeping sickness." Tropical disease, transmitted by tsetse fly bites, which causes fever, headache, and chills, followed by enlarged lymph nodes and anemia. Months or even years later, the disease affects the central nervous system, causing drowsiness and lethargy, coma, and death.

Tuberculosis (TB)—Infectious disease, usually of the lungs, marked by fever, night sweats, weight loss, and coughing up blood. TB can occur in almost any organ of the body or other body tissue.

Tumor—Abnormal growth or enlargement in or on a part of the body.

Tyramine—Chemical present in many foods and beverages. Its structure and action in the body are similar to epinephrine.

Ulcer—Open sore or break in the skin or mucous membrane; often fails to heal and is accompanied by inflammation.

Ulcerative colitis—Chronic, recurrent inflammation and ulceration of the colon.

Ulceration—1. Formation or development of an ulcer. 2. Condition of an area marked with ulcers loosely associated with one another.

Underactive thyroid—Condition occurring when the thyroid does not produce enough hormone, thus causing cell metabolism to slow down.

Ureter—Tube through which urine passes from the kidney to the bladder.

Urethra—Tube through which urine passes from the bladder to the outside of the body.

Urticaria—Hives; an eruption of itching wheals on the skin.

Vaccine—Medicine given by mouth or by injection to produce immunity to a certain infection.

Vaccinia—Also called "cowpox." Mild virus infection causing symptoms similar to smallpox.

Vaginal—Relating to the vagina.

Varicella—Also called "chickenpox." Very infectious virus disease marked by fever and itchy rash that develops into blisters and then scabs.

Vascular—Relating to the blood vessels.

Vasodilator—Medicine that dilates the blood vessels, permitting increased blood flow.

Ventricular fibrillation—Life-threatening condition of fine, quivering, irregular movements of many individual muscle fibers of the ventricular muscle; replaces the normal heart beat and interrupts pumping function.

Ventricle—A small cavity, such as one of the two lower chambers of the heart or one of the several cavities of the brain.

Vertigo—Sensation of whirling motion, either of oneself or of one's surroundings.

Veterinary—Relating to the medical care of animals.

Virus—Any of a group of simple microbes that are too small to be seen by a light microscope. They can grow and reproduce only in living cells. Many cause serious diseases in humans.

Vitiligo—Also called "leukoderma." Condition in which some areas of skin lose their color and turn white.

von Willebrand's disease—Hereditary blood disease in which blood clotting is delayed, leading to excessive and uncontrolled bleeding even after minor injuries.

Water diabetes—See Diabetes insipidus.

Water pill—See Diuretic.

Wheal—Temporary, small, raised area of the skin, usually accompanied by itching or burning; welt.

Wheezing—A whistling sound made when there is difficulty in breathing.

White mouth—See Candidiasis of the mouth.

Wilson's disease—Inborn defect in the body's ability to process copper. Too much copper may lead to jaundice, cirrhosis, mental retardation, or symptoms like those of Parkinson's disease.

Zollinger-Ellison syndrome—Disorder in which the stomach produces too much acid, leading to ulcers.

Appendix I

COMBINATION CHEMOTHERAPY

ABVD Systemic

This information applies to the following medicines:

Doxorubicin (dox-oh-ROO-bi-sin) (by injection)
Bleomycin (blee-oh-MYE-sin) (by injection)
Vinblastine (vin-BLAS-teen) (by injection)
Dacarbazine (da-KAR-ba-zeen) (by injection)

Some commonly used brand names are:

For Doxorubicin

In the U.S.

Adriamycin PFS
Adriamycin RDF
Rubex

Generic name product may also be available.

In Canada

Adriamycin PFS
Adriamycin RDF

For Bleomycin

In the U.S. and Canada

Blenoxane

For Vinblastine

In the U.S.

Velban
Velsar

Generic name product may also be available.

In Canada

Velbe

For Dacarbazine

In the U.S.

DTIC-Dome

Generic name product may also be available.

In Canada

DTIC

About Your Medicine

This combination therapy consists of four cancer medicines. They are used together to treat Hodgkin's disease and some other kinds of cancer.

If any of the information causes you special concern or if you want additional information about your medicine and its use, check with your doctor, nurse, or pharmacist.

Before Using This Medicine

Discuss with your doctor the possible side effects that may be caused by this medicine. Some of them may be serious and/or long term.

Tell your doctor, nurse, and pharmacist if you. . .

- are allergic to any medicine, either prescription or nonprescription (OTC);
- are pregnant or intend to have children;
- are breast-feeding an infant;
- are taking *any* other prescription or nonprescription (OTC) medicine;
- have *any* other medical problems;
- have ever been treated with x-rays or cancer medicines;
- smoke.

Proper Use of This Medicine

While you are using this combination of medicines, your doctor may want you to drink extra fluids so that you will pass more urine. This will help prevent kidney problems and keep your kidneys working well.

Precautions

It is very important that your doctor check your progress at regular visits to make sure that this medicine is working properly and to check for unwanted effects.

While you are being treated with these medicines, and after you stop treatment with them, *do not have any immunizations (vaccinations) without your doctor's approval*. Also, try to avoid people with infections.

If doxorubicin or vinblastine accidentally seeps out of the vein into which it is injected, it may damage some tissues and cause scarring. *Tell the doctor or nurse right away if you notice redness, pain, or swelling at the place of injection.*

Possible Side Effects

Side effects that should be reported *immediately*:

Black, tarry stools
Blood in urine or stools
Confusion

- Cough or hoarseness
- Faintness
- Fast or irregular heartbeat
- Fever or chills
- Lower back or side pain
- Painful or difficult urination
- Pain or redness at place of injection
- Pinpoint red spots on skin
- Shortness of breath
- Swelling of feet and lower legs
- Unusual bleeding or bruising
- Wheezing

Side effects that should be reported as soon as possible:

- Darkening or redness of skin (after x-ray treatment)
- Difficulty in walking
- Dizziness
- Double vision
- Drooping eyelids
- Headache
- Jaw pain
- Joint pain
- Mental depression
- Numbness, tingling, or pain in fingers and toes
- Pain in testicles
- Red streaks along injected vein
- Skin rash or itching
- Sores in mouth and on lips
- Stomach pain
- Weakness

Side effects that usually do not need medical attention (however, check with your doctor or nurse if they continue or are bothersome):

- Changes in fingernails or toenails
- Darkening of soles, palms, or nails
- Diarrhea
- Flushing or numbness of face
- Loss of hair
- Muscle pain
- Nausea and vomiting
- Reddish urine
- Swelling of fingers

After you stop receiving these medicines, they may still produce some side effects that need attention. During this period of time, *check with your doctor or nurse immediately* if you notice:

- Cough
- Fast or irregular heartbeat
- Shortness of breath
- Swelling of feet and lower legs

Also, check with your doctor or nurse if you notice:

- Black, tarry stools
- Blood in urine or stools
- Fever or chills
- Lower back or side pain
- Painful or difficult urination
- Pinpoint red spots on skin
- Unusual bleeding or bruising

Other side effects not listed above may also occur in some patients. If you notice any other effects, check with your doctor or nurse.

Annual revision: 05/22/91

BACOP Systemic

This information applies to the following medicines:

- Bleomycin (blee-oh-MYE-sin) (by injection)
- Doxorubicin (dox-oh-ROO-bi-sin) (by injection)
- Cyclophosphamide (sye-kloe-FOSS-fa-mide) (by injection)
- Vincristine (vin-KRIS-teen) (by injection)
- Prednisone (PRED-ni-sone) (by mouth)

Some commonly used brand names are:

For Bleomycin

In the U.S. and Canada

Blenoxane

For Doxorubicin

In the U.S.

Adriamycin PFS
Adriamycin RDF
Rubex

Generic name product may also be available.

In Canada

Adriamycin PFS
Adriamycin RDF

For Cyclophosphamide

In the U.S.

Cytoxan
Neosar

Generic name product may also be available.

In Canada

Cytoxan
Procytox

For Vincristine

In the U.S.

Oncovin
Vincasar PFS
Vincrex

Generic name product may also be available.

In Canada

Oncovin

For Prednisone

In the U.S.

Deltasone
Liquid Pred
Meticorten
Orasone
Prednicen-M
Prednisone Intensol
Sterapred
Sterapred DS

Generic name product may also be available.

In Canada

Apo-Prednisone
Deltasone
Winpred

Generic name product may also be available.

About Your Medicine

This combination therapy consists of four cancer medicines (bleomycin, doxorubicin, cyclophosphamide, vincristine) and an adrenocorticoid (prednisone). They are used together to treat some kinds of cancer.

If any of the information causes you special concern or if you want additional information about your medicine and its use, check with your doctor, nurse, or pharmacist.

Before Using This Medicine

Discuss with your doctor the possible side effects that may be caused by this medicine. Some of them may be serious and/or long term.

Tell your doctor, nurse, and pharmacist if you. . .

- are allergic to any medicine, either prescription or nonprescription (OTC);
- are pregnant or intend to have children;
- are breast-feeding an infant;
- are taking *any* other prescription or nonprescription (OTC) medicine;
- have *any* other medical problems;
- have ever been treated with x-rays or cancer medicines;
- smoke.

Proper Use of This Medicine

Use each of these medicines exactly as directed by your doctor. The exact amount of each medicine that you need and the best times to take each one have been carefully worked out. Ask your doctor, nurse, or pharmacist to help you plan a way to take each of your medicines at the right times.

Take prednisone with food to help prevent stomach upset. If stomach upset, burning, or pain continues, check with your doctor.

While you are receiving these medicines, especially cyclophosphamide, it is important that you drink extra fluids so that you will pass more urine. Also, empty your bladder frequently, including at least once during the night. This will help prevent kidney and bladder problems and keep your kidneys working well. Some patients may have to drink up to 7 to 12 cups (3 quarts) of fluid a day. If you have any questions about this, check with your doctor.

If you miss a dose of prednisone and you remember it within a few hours, take it as soon as you remember it. However, if several hours have passed or if it is almost time for the next dose, *check with your doctor*. Do not double doses.

Precautions

It is very important that your doctor check your progress at regular visits to make sure that this medicine is working properly and to check for unwanted effects.

While you are being treated with these medicines, and after you stop treatment with them, *do not have any immunizations (vaccinations) without your doctor's approval*. Also, try to avoid people with infections.

If doxorubicin or vincristine accidentally seeps out of the vein into which it is injected, it may damage some tissues and cause scarring. *Tell the doctor or nurse right away if you notice redness, pain, or swelling at the place of injection.*

Possible Side Effects

Side effects that should be reported *immediately:*

Black, tarry stools
Blood in urine or stools
Confusion
Cough or hoarseness
Faintness
Fast or irregular heartbeat
Fever or chills
Lower back or side pain
Pain at place of injection
Painful or difficult urination
Pinpoint red spots on skin
Shortness of breath
Sweating
Swelling of feet and lower legs
Unusual bleeding or bruising
Wheezing

Side effects that should be reported as soon as possible:

Agitation
Bed-wetting
Blurred or double vision
Constipation
Convulsions (seizures)
Darkening or redness of skin (after x-ray treatment)
Difficulty in walking
Dizziness
Drooping eyelids
Frequent urination
Hallucinations (seeing, hearing, or feeling things that are not there)
Headache
Jaw pain
Joint pain
Lack of sweating
Mental depression
Missing menstrual periods
Numbness, tingling, or pain in fingers and toes

Pain in testicles
Red streaks along injected vein
Sores in mouth and on lips
Stomach cramps
Unusual thirst
Unusual tiredness or weakness
Yellow eyes or skin

Side effects that usually do not need medical attention (however, check with your doctor or nurse if they continue or are bothersome):

Bloating
Darkening of soles, palms, or nails
Diarrhea
Flushing or redness of face
Itching of skin
Loss of appetite
Loss of hair
Nausea or vomiting
Reddish urine
Skin rash or colored bumps on fingertips, elbows, or palms
Skin redness or tenderness
Swelling of fingers

After you stop receiving these medicines, they may still produce some side effects that need attention. During this period of time, *check with your doctor or nurse immediately* if you notice:

Blood in urine
Cough
Fast or irregular heartbeat
Shortness of breath
Swelling of feet and lower legs

Other side effects not listed above may also occur in some patients. If you notice any other effects, check with your doctor or nurse.

Annual revision: 05/22/91

BCVPP Systemic

This information applies to the following medicines:

Carmustine (kar-MUS-teen) (by injection)
Cyclophosphamide (sye-kloe-FOSS-fa-mide) (by injection)
Vinblastine (vin-BLAS-teen) (by injection)
Procarbazine (pro-KAR-ba-zeen) (by mouth)
Prednisone (PRED-ni-sone) (by mouth)

Some commonly used brand names are:

For Carmustine

In the U.S. and Canada
BiCNU

Another commonly used name is BCNU.

For Cyclophosphamide

In the U.S.
Cytoxan
Neosar

Generic name product may also be available.

In Canada
Cytoxan
Procytox

For Vinblastine

In the U.S.
Velban
Velsar

Generic name product may also be available.

In Canada
Velbe

For Procarbazine

In the U.S.
Matulane

In Canada
Natulan

For Prednisone

In the U.S.
Deltasone
Liquid Pred
Meticorten
Orasone
Prednicen-M
Prednisone Intensol
Sterapred
Sterapred DS

Generic name product may also be available.

In Canada
Apo-Prednisone
Deltasone
Winpred

Generic name product may also be available.

About Your Medicine

This combination therapy consists of four cancer medicines (carmustine, cyclophosphamide, vinblastine, procarbazine) and an adrenocorticoid (prednisone). They are used together to treat Hodgkin's disease and some other kinds of cancer.

If any of the information causes you special concern or if you want additional information about your medicine and its use, check with your doctor, nurse, or pharmacist.

Before Using This Medicine

Discuss with your doctor the possible side effects that may be caused by this medicine. Some of them may be serious and/or long term.

Tell your doctor, nurse, and pharmacist if you. . .

- are allergic to any medicine, either prescription or nonprescription (OTC);
- are pregnant or intend to have children;
- are breast-feeding an infant;
- are taking *any* other prescription or nonprescription (OTC) medicine;
- have *any* other medical problems;

- have ever been treated with x-rays or cancer medicines;
- smoke.

Proper Use of This Medicine

Use each of these medicines exactly as directed by your doctor. The exact amount of each medicine that you need and the best times to take each one have been carefully worked out. Ask your doctor, nurse, or pharmacist to help you plan a way to take each of your medicines at the right times.

Take prednisone with food to help prevent stomach upset. If stomach upset, burning, or pain continues, check with your doctor.

While you are using these medicines, especially cyclophosphamide, it is important that you drink extra fluids so that you will pass more urine. Also, empty your bladder frequently, including at least once during the night. This will help prevent kidney and bladder problems and keep your kidneys working well. Some patients may have to drink up to 7 to 12 cups (3 quarts) of fluid a day. If you have any questions about this, check with your doctor.

If you miss a dose of prednisone or procarbazine and you remember it within a few hours, take it as soon as you remember it. However, if several hours have passed or if it is almost time for the next dose, *check with your doctor*. Do not double doses.

Precautions

It is very important that your doctor check your progress at regular visits.

When taken with certain foods, drinks, or other medicines, *procarbazine* can cause very dangerous reactions. *To avoid such reactions:*

- Do not eat foods that have a high tyramine content (most common in foods that are aged or fermented to increase their flavor).
- Do not drink alcoholic beverages or alcohol-free or reduced-alcohol beer and wine.
- Do not eat or drink large amounts of caffeine-containing food or beverages.
- Do not take any other medicine unless prescribed by your doctor, including OTC or nonprescription medicines.

After you stop using procarbazine you must continue to obey the above rules of caution for at least 2 weeks.

Procarbazine may cause some people to become drowsy or less alert than they are normally. *Make sure you know how you react to this medicine before you drive, use machines, or do anything else that could be dangerous if you are not alert.*

While you are receiving these medicines, and for several weeks after you stop treatment:

- *Do not have any immunizations (vaccinations) without your doctor's approval.* Also, try to avoid people with infections.
- If you are going to have surgery or emergency treatment, *tell the medical doctor or dentist in charge that you have been taking this medicine.*

Possible Side Effects

Side effects that should be reported *immediately*:

Black, tarry stools
Blood in urine or stools
Chest pain
Cough or hoarseness
Enlarged pupils of eyes
Fast or slow or irregular heartbeat
Fever or chills
Headache (severe)
Increased sensitivity of eyes to light
Increased sweating (possibly with fever or cold, clammy skin)
Lower back or side pain
Painful or difficult urination
Pain or redness at place of injection
Pinpoint red spots on skin
Shortness of breath (sudden)
Stiff or sore neck
Unusual bleeding or bruising

Side effects that should be reported as soon as possible:

Bloody vomit
Diarrhea
Dizziness, confusion, or agitation
Double vision
Drooping eyelids
Fainting
Flushing of face
Hallucinations (seeing, hearing, or feeling things that are not there)
Increase or decrease in urination
Jaw pain
Joint pain
Mental depression
Missing menstrual periods
Numbness, tingling, or pain in fingers or toes
Pain in testicles
Shortness of breath
Sores in mouth and on lips
Swelling of feet or lower legs
Thickening of bronchial secretions
Unsteadiness or awkwardness
Unusual thirst
Unusual tiredness or weakness
Yellow eyes or skin

Side effects that usually do not need medical attention (however, check with your doctor or nurse if they continue or are bothersome):

- Constipation
- Darkening of skin and fingernails
- Difficulty in swallowing
- Discoloration of skin along vein of injection
- Dry mouth
- Loss of appetite
- Loss of hair
- Muscle pain or twitching
- Nausea or vomiting
- Nightmares
- Skin rash, hives, or itching
- Sleeplessness
- Stomach pain
- Swollen lips

After you stop receiving these medicines, they may still produce some side effects that need attention. During this period of time, *check with your doctor or nurse immediately* if you notice:

- Blood in urine

Also, check with your doctor or nurse if you notice:

- Black, tarry stools
- Blood in urine or stools
- Cough or hoarseness
- Fever or chills
- Lower back or side pain
- Painful or difficult urination
- Pinpoint red spots on skin
- Shortness of breath
- Unusual bleeding or bruising

Other side effects not listed above may also occur in some patients. If you notice any other effects, check with your doctor or nurse.

Annual revision: 05/22/91

BEP Systemic

This information applies to the following medicines:

- Bleomycin (blee-oh-MYE-sin) (by injection)
- Etoposide (e-TOE-poe-side) (by injection)
- Cisplatin (sis-PLA-tin) (by injection)

Some commonly used brand names are:

For Bleomycin
In the U.S. and Canada
Blenoxane

For Etoposide
In the U.S. and Canada
VePesid

Another commonly used name is VP-16.

For Cisplatin
In the U.S.
Platinol
Platinol-AQ
In Canada
Platinol
Platinol-AQ

Generic name product may also be available.

About Your Medicine

This combination therapy consists of three cancer medicines. They are used together to treat some kinds of cancer.

If any of the information causes you special concern or if you want additional information about your medicine and its use, check with your doctor, nurse, or pharmacist.

Before Using This Medicine

Discuss with your doctor the possible side effects that may be caused by this medicine. Some of them may be serious and/or long term.

Tell your doctor, nurse, and pharmacist if you. . .

- are allergic to any medicine, either prescription or nonprescription (OTC);
- are pregnant or intend to have children;
- are breast-feeding an infant;
- are taking *any* other prescription or nonprescription (OTC) medicine;
- have *any* other medical problems;
- have ever been treated with x-rays or cancer medicines;
- smoke.

Proper Use of This Medicine

While you are receiving these medicines, your doctor may want you to drink extra fluids so that you will pass more urine. This will help prevent kidney problems and keep your kidneys working well.

These medicines often cause nausea, vomiting, and loss of appetite, which may be severe. However, it is very important that you continue to receive the medicines, even if you begin to feel ill. Ask your doctor, nurse, or pharmacist for ways to lessen these effects.

Precautions

It is very important that your doctor check your progress at regular visits to make sure that these medicines are working properly and to check for unwanted effects.

While you are being treated with these medicines, and after you stop treatment with them, *do not have any immunizations (vaccinations) without your doctor's approval.* Also, try to avoid people with infections.

Possible Side Effects

Side effects that should be reported *immediately:*

Black, tarry stools
Blood in urine or stools
Confusion
Cough or hoarseness
Faintness
Fast heartbeat
Fever or chills
Lower back or side pain
Painful or difficult urination
Pinpoint red spots on skin
Redness, pain, or swelling at place of injection
Shortness of breath or wheezing
Sweating
Swelling of face
Unusual bleeding or bruising

Side effects that should be reported as soon as possible:

Agitation or confusion
Blurred vision or change in ability to see colors (especially blue or yellow)
Convulsions (seizures)
Joint pain
Loss of balance
Loss of reflexes
Loss of taste
Numbness or tingling in fingers, toes, or face
Ringing in ears
Sores in mouth or on lips
Swelling of feet or lower legs
Trouble in hearing
Trouble in walking
Unusual tiredness or weakness

Side effects that usually do not need medical attention (however, check with your doctor or nurse if they continue or are bothersome):

Darkening or thickening of skin
Diarrhea
Itching of skin
Loss of appetite
Loss of hair
Nausea and vomiting
Skin rash or colored bumps on fingertips, elbows, or palms
Skin redness or tenderness
Swelling of fingers

After you stop receiving these medicines, they may still produce some side effects that need attention. During this period of time, *check with your doctor or nurse as soon as possible* if you notice:

Black, tarry stools
Blood in urine or stools
Cough or hoarseness
Decrease in urination
Fever or chills
Loss of balance
Lower back or side pain
Painful or difficult urination
Pinpoint red spots on skin
Ringing in ears
Shortness of breath
Swelling of feet or lower legs
Trouble in hearing
Unusual bleeding or bruising

Other side effects not listed above may also occur in some patients. If you notice any other effects, check with your doctor or nurse.

Annual revision: 07/07/92

CAE Systemic

This information applies to the following medicines:

Cyclophosphamide (sye-kloe-FOSS-fa-mide) (by injection)
Doxorubicin (dox-oh-ROO-bi-sin) (by injection)
Etoposide (e-TOE-poe-side) (by injection)

Some commonly used brand names are:

For Cyclophosphamide

In the U.S.

Cytoxan
Neosar

Generic name product may also be available.

In Canada

Cytoxan
Procytox

For Doxorubicin

In the U.S.

Adriamycin PFS
Adriamycin RDF
Rubex

Generic name product may also be available.

In Canada

Adriamycin PFS
Adriamycin RDF

For Etoposide
In the U.S. and Canada
VePesid
Another commonly used name is VP-16.

About Your Medicine

This combination therapy consists of three cancer medicines. They are used together to treat some kinds of cancer.

If any of the information causes you special concern or if you want additional information about your medicine and its use, check with your doctor, nurse, or pharmacist.

Before Using This Medicine

Discuss with your doctor the possible side effects that may be caused by this medicine. Some of them may be serious and/or long term.

Tell your doctor, nurse, and pharmacist if you. . .

- are allergic to any medicine, either prescription or nonprescription (OTC);
- are pregnant or intend to have children;
- are breast-feeding an infant;
- are taking *any* other prescription or nonprescription (OTC) medicine;
- have *any* other medical problems;
- have ever been treated with x-rays or cancer medicines.

Proper Use of This Medicine

While you are receiving these medicines, especially cyclophosphamide, it is important that you drink extra fluids so that you will pass more urine. Also, empty your bladder frequently, including at least once during the night. This will help prevent kidney and bladder problems and keep your kidneys working well. Some patients may have to drink up to 7 to 12 cups (3 quarts) of fluid a day. If you have any questions about this, check with your doctor.

Precautions

It is very important that your doctor check your progress at regular visits to make sure that this medicine is working properly and to check for unwanted effects.

While you are being treated with these medicines, and after you stop treatment with them, *do not have any immunizations (vaccinations) without your doctor's approval.* Also, try to avoid people with infections.

If doxorubicin accidentally seeps out of the vein into which it is injected, it may damage some tissues and cause scarring. *Tell the doctor or nurse right away if you notice redness, pain, or swelling at the place of injection.*

Possible Side Effects

Side effects that should be reported *immediately:*

Black, tarry stools
Blood in urine or stools
Cough or hoarseness
Fast or irregular heartbeat
Fever or chills
Lower back or side pain
Painful or difficult urination
Pinpoint red spots on skin
Shortness of breath
Swelling of feet and lower legs
Unusual bleeding or bruising
Wheezing

Side effects that should be reported as soon as possible:

Darkening or redness of skin (after x-ray treatment)
Decrease or increase in urination
Difficulty in walking
Dizziness, confusion, or agitation
Joint pain
Missing menstrual periods
Numbness or tingling in fingers and toes
Red streaks along injected vein
Sores in mouth and on lips
Unusual tiredness or weakness
Yellow eyes or skin

Side effects that usually do not need medical attention (however, check with your doctor or nurse if they continue or are bothersome):

Darkening of soles, palms, or nails
Diarrhea or stomach pain
Flushing or redness of face
Headache
Increased sweating
Loss of appetite
Loss of hair
Nausea or vomiting
Reddish urine
Skin rash, hives, or itching
Swollen lips

After you stop receiving these medicines, they may still produce some side effects that need attention. During this period of time, *check with your doctor or nurse immediately* if you notice:

Blood in urine
Fast or irregular heartbeat
Shortness of breath
Swelling of feet and lower legs

Other side effects not listed above may also occur in some patients. If you notice any other effects, check with your doctor or nurse.

Annual revision: 05/22/91

CAF Systemic

This information applies to the following medicines:
Cyclophosphamide (sye-kloe-FOSS-fa-mide) (by mouth)
Doxorubicin (dox-oh-ROO-bi-sin) (by injection)
Fluorouracil (flure-oh-YOOR-a-sill) (by injection)

Some commonly used brand names are:

For Cyclophosphamide
In the U.S.
Cytoxan
In Canada
Cytoxan
Procytox

For Doxorubicin
In the U.S.
Adriamycin PFS
Adriamycin RDF
Rubex
Generic name product may also be available.
In Canada
Adriamycin PFS
Adriamycin RDF

For Fluorouracil
In the U.S. and Canada
Adrucil
Generic name product may also be available.

Another commonly used name is 5-FU.

About Your Medicine

This combination therapy consists of three cancer medicines. They are used together to treat breast cancer and some other kinds of cancer.

If any of the information causes you special concern or if you want additional information about your medicine and its use, check with your doctor, nurse, or pharmacist.

Before Using This Medicine

Discuss with your doctor the possible side effects that may be caused by this medicine. Some of them may be serious and/or long term.

Tell your doctor, nurse, and pharmacist if you. . .

- are allergic to any medicine, either prescription or nonprescription (OTC);
- are pregnant or intend to have children;
- are breast-feeding an infant;
- are taking *any* other prescription or nonprescription (OTC) medicine;
- have *any* other medical problems;
- have ever been treated with x-rays or cancer medicines.

Proper Use of This Medicine

Use each of these medicines exactly as directed by your doctor. The exact amount of each medicine that you need and the best times to take each one have been carefully worked out. Ask your doctor, nurse, or pharmacist to help you plan a way to take each of your medicines at the right times.

While you are using these medicines, especially cyclophosphamide, it is important that you drink extra fluids so that you will pass more urine. Also, empty your bladder frequently, including at least once during the night. This will help prevent kidney and bladder problems and keep your kidneys working well. Some patients may have to drink up to 7 to 12 cups (3 quarts) of fluid a day. If you have any questions about this, check with your doctor.

If you vomit shortly after taking a dose of cyclophosphamide, check with your doctor. You will be told whether to take the dose again or to wait until the next scheduled dose.

If you miss a dose of cyclophosphamide, do not take the missed dose at all and do not double the next one. Instead, go back to your regular dosing schedule and check with your doctor.

Precautions

It is very important that your doctor check your progress at regular visits to make sure that these medicines are working properly and to check for unwanted effects.

While you are being treated with these medicines, and after you stop treatment with them, *do not have any immunizations (vaccinations) without your doctor's approval*. Also, try to avoid people with infections.

If doxorubicin accidentally seeps out of the vein into which it is injected, it may damage some tissues and cause scarring. *Tell the doctor or nurse right away if you notice redness, pain, or swelling at the place of injection.*

Possible Side Effects

Side effects that should be reported *immediately*:
Black, tarry stools
Blood in urine or stools
Cough or hoarseness
Diarrhea
Fast or irregular heartbeat
Fever or chills
Heartburn
Lower back or side pain
Nausea and vomiting (severe)
Pain at place of injection
Painful or difficult urination
Pinpoint red spots on skin

Shortness of breath
Sores in mouth and on lips
Stomach cramps
Swelling of feet and lower legs
Unusual bleeding or bruising
Wheezing

Side effects that should be reported as soon as possible:

Chest pain
Darkening or redness of skin (after x-ray treatment)
Dizziness, confusion, or agitation
Frequent urination
Joint pain
Missing menstrual periods
Red streaks along injected vein
Tingling of hands and feet, followed by pain, redness, and swelling
Trouble with balance
Unusual thirst
Unusual tiredness or weakness
Yellow eyes or skin

Side effects that usually do not need medical attention (however, check with your doctor or nurse if they continue or are bothersome):

Darkening of soles, palms, or nails
Flushing or redness of face
Headache
Increased sweating
Loss of appetite
Loss of hair
Nausea and vomiting
Reddish urine
Skin rash, hives, or itching
Swollen lips

After you stop receiving these medicines, they may still produce some side effects that need attention. During this period of time, *check with your doctor or nurse immediately* if you notice:

Black, tarry stools
Blood in urine or stools
Cough or hoarseness
Fast or irregular heartbeat
Fever or chills
Lower back or side pain
Painful or difficult urination
Pinpoint red spots on skin
Shortness of breath
Swelling of feet and lower legs
Unusual bleeding or bruising

Other side effects not listed above may also occur in some patients. If you notice any other effects, check with your doctor or nurse.

Annual revision: 07/07/92

CAMP Systemic

This information applies to the following medicines:

Cyclophosphamide (sye-kloe-FOSS-fa-mide) (by injection)
Doxorubicin (dox-oh-ROO-bi-sin) (by injection)
Methotrexate (meth-o-TREX-ate) (by injection)
Procarbazine (pro-KAR-ba-zeen) (by mouth)

Some commonly used brand names are:

For Cyclophosphamide

In the U.S.

Cytoxan
Neosar

Generic name product may also be available.

In Canada

Cytoxan
Procytox

For Doxorubicin

In the U.S.

Adriamycin PFS
Adriamycin RDF
Rubex

Generic name product may also be available.

In Canada

Adriamycin PFS
Adriamycin RDF

For Methotrexate

In the U.S.

Folex
Folex PFS
Mexate
Mexate-AQ

Generic name product may also be available.

In Canada

Generic name product available.

For Procarbazine

In the U.S.

Matulane

In Canada

Natulan

About Your Medicine

This combination therapy consists of four cancer medicines. They are used together to treat lung cancer and some other kinds of cancer.

If any of the information causes you special concern or if you want additional information about your medicine and its use, check with your doctor, nurse, or pharmacist.

Before Using This Medicine

Discuss with your doctor the possible side effects that may be caused by this medicine. Some of them may be serious and/or long term.

Tell your doctor, nurse, and pharmacist if you. . .

- are allergic to any medicine, either prescription or nonprescription (OTC);
- are pregnant or intend to have children;
- are breast-feeding an infant;
- are taking *any* other prescription or nonprescription (OTC) medicine;
- have *any* other medical problems;
- have ever been treated with x-rays or cancer medicines.

Proper Use of This Medicine

Take procarbazine exactly as directed by your doctor. The exact amount that you need and the best times to take it have been carefully worked out.

While you are receiving these medicines, especially cyclophosphamide, it is important that you drink extra fluids so that you will pass more urine. Also, empty your bladder frequently, including at least once during the night. This will help prevent kidney and bladder problems and keep your kidneys working well. Some patients may have to drink up to 7 to 12 cups (3 quarts) of fluid a day. If you have any questions about this, check with your doctor.

If you vomit shortly after taking a dose of procarbazine, check with your doctor. You will be told whether to take the dose again or to wait until the next scheduled dose.

If you miss a dose of procarbazine and you remember it within a few hours, take it as soon as you remember it. However, if several hours have passed or if it is almost time for the next dose, *check with your doctor*. Do not double doses.

Precautions

It is very important that your doctor check your progress at regular visits.

When taken with certain foods, drinks, or other medicines, procarbazine can cause very dangerous reactions. *To avoid such reactions:*

- Do not eat foods that have a high tyramine content (most common in foods that are aged or fermented to increase their flavor).
- Do not drink alcoholic beverages or alcohol-free or reduced-alcohol beer and wine.
- Do not eat or drink large amounts of caffeine-containing foods or beverages.
- Do not take any other medicine unless prescribed by your doctor, including OTC or nonprescription medicines.

After you stop using procarbazine you must continue to obey the above rules of caution for at least 2 weeks.

Do not drink alcohol while using methotrexate. Alcohol can increase the chance of liver problems.

Do not take medicine for inflammation or pain without first checking with your doctor. These medicines may increase the effects of methotrexate, which could be harmful.

While you are being treated with these medicines, and after you stop treatment with them, *do not have any immunizations (vaccinations) without your doctor's approval.* Also, try to avoid people with infections.

If doxorubicin accidentally seeps out of the vein into which it is injected, it may damage some tissues and cause scarring. *Tell the doctor or nurse right away if you notice redness, pain, or swelling at the place of injection.*

Procarbazine may cause some people to become drowsy or less alert than they are normally. *Make sure you know how you react to this medicine before you drive, use machines, or do anything else that could be dangerous if you are not alert.*

If you are going to have surgery or emergency treatment, *tell the medical doctor or dentist in charge that you have been taking procarbazine.*

Possible Side Effects

Side effects that should be reported *immediately*:

Black, tarry stools
Blood in urine or stools
Bloody vomit
Blurred vision
Chest pain
Confusion
Convulsions (seizures)
Cough or hoarseness
Diarrhea
Enlarged pupils of eyes
Fast or slow or irregular heartbeat
Fever or chills
Headache (severe)
Increased sensitivity of eyes to light
Increased sweating (possibly with fever or cold, clammy skin)
Lower back or side pain
Pain at place of injection
Painful or difficult urination
Pinpoint red spots on skin
Reddening of skin
Shortness of breath
Sores in mouth and on lips
Stiff or sore neck
Stomach cramps
Swelling of feet and lower legs
Unusual bleeding or bruising
Wheezing

Side effects that should be reported as soon as possible:

- Agitation
- Back pain
- Darkening or redness of skin (after x-ray treatment)
- Difficulty in walking
- Dizziness
- Frequent urination
- Hallucinations (seeing, hearing, or feeling things that are not there)
- Joint pain
- Missing menstrual periods
- Numbness or tingling in fingers and toes
- Pain in testicles
- Red streaks along injected vein
- Unsteadiness or awkwardness
- Unusual thirst
- Unusual tiredness or weakness
- Yellow eyes or skin

Side effects that usually do not need medical attention (however, check with your doctor or nurse if they continue or are bothersome):

- Acne
- Boils
- Constipation
- Darkening of soles, palms, or nails
- Drowsiness
- Flushing or redness of face
- Loss of appetite
- Loss of hair
- Mental depression
- Nausea or vomiting
- Nervousness or restlessness
- Pale skin
- Reddish urine
- Skin rash, hives, or itching
- Skin redness or tenderness
- Trouble in sleeping

After you stop receiving these medicines, they may still produce some side effects that need attention. During this period of time, *check with your doctor or nurse immediately* if you notice:

- Blood in urine
- Fast or irregular heartbeat
- Shortness of breath
- Swelling of feet or lower legs

Other side effects not listed above may also occur in some patients. If you notice any other effects, check with your doctor or nurse.

Annual revision: 05/22/91

CAP Systemic

This information applies to the following medicines:

- Cyclophosphamide (sye-kloe-FOSS-fa-mide) (by injection)
- Doxorubicin (dox-oh-ROO-bi-sin) (by injection)
- Cisplatin (sis-PLA-tin) (by injection)

Some commonly used brand names are:

For Cyclophosphamide

In the U.S.

Cytoxan
Neosar

Generic name product may also be available.

In Canada

Cytoxan
Procytox

For Doxorubicin

In the U.S.

Adriamycin PFS
Adriamycin RDF
Rubex

Generic name product may also be available.

In Canada

Adriamycin PFS
Adriamycin RDF

For Cisplatin

In the U.S.

Platinol
Platinol-AQ

In Canada

Platinol
Platinol-AQ

Generic name product may also be available.

About Your Medicine

This combination therapy consists of three cancer medicines. They are used together to treat cancer of the ovaries and some other kinds of cancer.

If any of the information causes you special concern or if you want additional information about your medicine and its use, check with your doctor, nurse, or pharmacist.

Before Using This Medicine

Discuss with your doctor the possible side effects that may be caused by this medicine. Some of them may be serious and/or long term.

Tell your doctor, nurse, and pharmacist if you. . .

- are allergic to any medicine, either prescription or nonprescription (OTC);
- are pregnant or intend to have children;
- are breast-feeding an infant;
- are taking *any* other prescription or nonprescription (OTC) medicine;
- have *any* other medical problems;

- have ever been treated with x-rays or cancer medicines.

Proper Use of This Medicine

While you are receiving these medicines, especially cyclophosphamide, it is important that you drink extra fluids so that you will pass more urine. Also, empty your bladder frequently, including at least once during the night. This will help prevent kidney and bladder problems and keep your kidneys working well. Some patients may have to drink up to 7 to 12 cups (3 quarts) of fluid a day. If you have any questions about this, check with your doctor.

Precautions

It is very important that your doctor check your progress at regular visits to make sure that this medicine is working properly and to check for unwanted effects.

While you are being treated with these medicines, and after you stop treatment with them, *do not have any immunizations (vaccinations) without your doctor's approval.* Also, try to avoid people with infections.

If doxorubicin or cisplatin accidentally seeps out of the vein into which it is injected, it may damage some tissues and cause scarring. *Tell the doctor or nurse right away if you notice redness, pain, or swelling at the place of injection.*

Possible Side Effects

Side effects that should be reported *immediately*:

Black, tarry stools
Blood in urine or stools
Cough or hoarseness
Dizziness or faintness (shortly after a dose)
Fast or irregular heartbeat
Fever or chills
Lower back or side pain
Painful or difficult urination
Pinpoint red spots on skin
Shortness of breath
Swelling of face
Swelling of feet and lower legs
Unusual bleeding or bruising
Wheezing

Side effects that should be reported as soon as possible:

Blurred or double vision
Change in ability to see colors (especially blue or yellow)
Convulsions (seizures)
Darkening or redness of skin (after x-ray treatment)
Decrease or increase in urination
Dizziness, confusion, or agitation
Joint pain
Loss of balance
Loss of reflexes
Missing menstrual periods
Numbness, tingling, or pain in fingers and toes
Red streaks along injected vein
Ringing in ears
Sores in mouth and on lips
Trouble in hearing
Trouble in walking
Unusual tiredness or weakness
Yellow eyes or skin

Side effects that usually do not need medical attention (however, check with your doctor or nurse if they continue or are bothersome):

Darkening of soles, palms, or nails
Diarrhea or stomach pain
Flushing or redness of face
Headache
Loss of appetite
Loss of hair
Nausea or vomiting
Reddish urine
Skin rash, hives, or itching
Swollen lips
Unusual increase in sweating

After you stop receiving these medicines, they may still produce some side effects that need attention. During this period of time, *check with your doctor or nurse immediately* if you notice:

Black, tarry stools
Blood in urine or stools
Cough or hoarseness
Decrease in urination
Fast or irregular heartbeat
Fever or chills
Loss of balance
Lower back or side pain
Painful or difficult urination
Pinpoint red spots on skin
Ringing in ears
Shortness of breath
Swelling of feet and lower legs
Trouble in hearing
Unusual bleeding or bruising

Other side effects not listed above may also occur in some patients. If you notice any other effects, check with your doctor or nurse.

Annual revision: 07/07/92

CAV Systemic

This information applies to the following medicines:

Cyclophosphamide (sye-kloe-FOSS-fa-mide) (by injection)
Doxorubicin (dox-oh-ROO-bi-sin) (by injection)
Vincristine (vin-KRIS-teen) (by injection)

Some commonly used brand names are:

For Cyclophosphamide

In the U.S.

Cytoxan
Neosar

Generic name product may also be available.

In Canada

Cytoxan
Procytox

For Doxorubicin

In the U.S.

Adriamycin PFS
Adriamycin RDF
Rubex

Generic name product may also be available.

In Canada

Adriamycin PFS
Adriamycin RDF

For Vincristine

In the U.S.

Oncovin
Vincasar PFS
Vincrex

Generic name product may also be available.

In Canada

Oncovin

About Your Medicine

This combination therapy consists of three cancer medicines. They are used together to treat lung cancer and some other kinds of cancer.

If any of the information causes you special concern or if you want additional information about your medicine and its use, check with your doctor, nurse, or pharmacist.

Before Using This Medicine

Discuss with your doctor the possible side effects that may be caused by this medicine. Some of them may be serious and/or long term.

Tell your doctor, nurse, and pharmacist if you. . .

- are allergic to any medicine, either prescription or nonprescription (OTC);
- are pregnant or intend to have children;
- are breast-feeding an infant;
- are taking *any* other prescription or nonprescription (OTC) medicine;
- have *any* other medical problems;
- have ever been treated with x-rays or cancer medicines.

Proper Use of This Medicine

While you are receiving these medicines, especially cyclophosphamide, it is important that you drink extra fluids so that you will pass more urine. Also, empty your bladder frequently, including at least once during the night. This will help prevent kidney and bladder problems and keep your kidneys working well. Some patients may have to drink up to 7 to 12 cups (3 quarts) of fluid a day. If you have any questions about this, check with your doctor.

Precautions

It is very important that your doctor check your progress at regular visits to make sure that this medicine is working properly and to check for unwanted effects.

While you are being treated with these medicines, and after you stop treatment with them, *do not have any immunizations (vaccinations) without your doctor's approval.* Also, try to avoid people with infections.

If doxorubicin or vincristine accidentally seeps out of the vein into which it is injected, it may damage some tissues and cause scarring. *Tell the doctor or nurse right away if you notice redness, pain, or swelling at the place of injection.*

Possible Side Effects

Side effects that should be reported *immediately*:

Black, tarry stools
Blood in urine or stools
Cough or hoarseness
Fast or irregular heartbeat
Fever or chills
Lower back or side pain
Painful or difficult urination
Pinpoint red spots on skin
Shortness of breath
Swelling of feet and lower legs
Unusual bleeding or bruising
Wheezing

Side effects that should be reported as soon as possible:

Bed-wetting
Blurred or double vision
Constipation
Convulsions (seizures)
Darkening or redness of skin (after x-ray treatment)
Decrease or increase in urination
Difficulty in walking
Dizziness, confusion, or agitation
Drooping eyelids
Hallucinations (seeing, hearing, or feeling things that are not there)

Headache
Jaw pain
Joint pain
Lack of sweating
Mental depression
Missing menstrual periods
Numbness, tingling, or pain in fingers and toes
Pain in testicles
Red streaks along injected vein
Sores in mouth and on lips
Stomach cramps
Trouble in sleeping
Unusual tiredness or weakness
Yellow eyes or skin

Side effects that usually do not need medical attention (however, check with your doctor or nurse if they continue or are bothersome):

Bloating
Darkening of soles, palms, or nails
Diarrhea
Flushing or redness of face
Increased sweating
Loss of appetite
Loss of hair
Nausea or vomiting
Reddish urine
Skin rash, hives, or itching
Swollen lips

After you stop receiving these medicines, they may still produce some side effects that need attention. During this period of time, *check with your doctor or nurse immediately* if you notice:

Blood in urine
Fast or irregular heartbeat
Shortness of breath
Swelling of feet and lower legs

Other side effects not listed above may also occur in some patients. If you notice any other effects, check with your doctor or nurse.

Annual revision: 05/22/91

CEP Systemic

This information applies to the following medicines:

Cyclophosphamide (sye-kloe-FOSS-fa-mide) (by injection)
Etoposide (e-TOE-poe-side) (by injection)
Cisplatin (sis-PLA-tin) (by injection)

Some commonly used brand names are:

For Cyclophosphamide

In the U.S.

Cytoxan
Neosar

Generic name product may also be available.

In Canada

Cytoxan
Procytox

For Etoposide

In the U.S. and Canada

VePesid

Another commonly used name is VP-16.

For Cisplatin

In the U.S.

Platinol
Platinol-AQ

In Canada

Platinol
Platinol-AQ

Generic name product may also be available.

About Your Medicine

This combination therapy consists of three cancer medicines. They are used together to treat some kinds of cancer.

If any of the information causes you special concern or if you want additional information about your medicine and its use, check with your doctor, nurse, or pharmacist.

Before Using This Medicine

Discuss with your doctor the possible side effects that may be caused by this medicine. Some of them may be serious and/or long term.

Tell your doctor, nurse, and pharmacist if you. . .

- are allergic to any medicine, either prescription or nonprescription (OTC);
- are pregnant or intend to have children;
- are breast-feeding an infant;
- are taking *any* other prescription or nonprescription (OTC) medicine;
- have *any* other medical problems;
- have ever been treated with x-rays or cancer medicines.

Proper Use of This Medicine

While you are receiving these medicines, especially cyclophosphamide, it is important that you drink extra fluids so that you will pass more urine. Also, empty your bladder frequently, including at least once during the night. This will help prevent kidney and bladder problems and keep your kidneys working well. Some patients may have to drink up to 7 to 12 cups (3 quarts) of fluid a day. If you have any questions about this, check with your doctor.

These medicines often cause nausea, vomiting, and loss of appetite, which may be severe. However, it is very important that you continue to receive the medicines, even if you begin to feel ill. Ask your doctor, nurse, or pharmacist for ways to lessen these effects.

Precautions

It is very important that your doctor check your progress at regular visits to make sure that this medicine is working properly and to check for unwanted effects.

While you are being treated with these medicines, and after you stop treatment with them, *do not have any immunizations (vaccinations) without your doctor's approval.* Also, try to avoid people with infections.

If cisplatin accidentally seeps out of the vein into which it is injected, it may damage some tissues and cause scarring. *Tell the doctor or nurse right away if you notice redness, pain, or swelling at the place of injection.*

Possible Side Effects

Side effects that should be reported *immediately*:

Black, tarry stools
Blood in urine or stools
Cough or hoarseness
Dizziness or faintness (shortly after a dose)
Fast or irregular heartbeat
Fever or chills
Lower back or side pain
Pain at place of injection
Painful or difficult urination
Pinpoint red spots on skin
Swelling of face
Unusual bleeding or bruising
Wheezing

Side effects that should be reported as soon as possible:

Blurred or double vision
Change in ability to see colors (especially blue or yellow)
Convulsions (seizures)
Decrease or increase in urination
Dizziness, confusion, or agitation
Loss of balance
Loss of reflexes
Missing menstrual periods
Numbness, tingling, or pain in fingers and toes
Ringing in ears
Shortness of breath
Sores in mouth and on lips
Swelling of feet or lower legs
Trouble in hearing
Trouble in walking
Unusual tiredness or weakness
Yellow eyes or skin

Side effects that usually do not need medical attention (however, check with your doctor or nurse if they continue or are bothersome):

Darkening of skin and fingernails
Diarrhea or stomach pain
Flushing or redness of face
Increased sweating
Loss of appetite
Loss of hair
Nausea or vomiting
Skin rash, hives, or itching
Swollen lips

After you stop receiving these medicines, they may still produce some side effects that need attention. During this period of time, *check with your doctor or nurse immediately* if you notice:

Black, tarry stools
Blood in urine or stools
Cough or hoarseness
Decrease in urination
Fever or chills
Loss of balance
Lower back or side pain
Painful or difficult urination
Pinpoint red spots on skin
Ringing in ears
Swelling of feet or lower legs
Trouble in hearing
Unusual bleeding or bruising

Other side effects not listed above may also occur in some patients. If you notice any other effects, check with your doctor or nurse.

Annual revision: 07/07/92

CHOP Systemic

This information applies to the following medicines:

Cyclophosphamide (sye-kloe-FOSS-fa-mide) (by injection)
Doxorubicin (dox-oh-ROO-bi-sin) (by injection)
Vincristine (vin-KRIS-teen) (by injection)
Prednisone (PRED-ni-sone) (by mouth)

Some commonly used brand names are:

For Cyclophosphamide

In the U.S.

Cytoxan
Neosar

Generic name product may also be available.

In Canada

Cytoxan
Procytox

For Doxorubicin

In the U.S.

Adriamycin PFS
Adriamycin RDF
Rubex

Generic name product may also be available.

In Canada

Adriamycin PFS
Adriamycin RDF

For Vincristine

In the U.S.

Oncovin
Vincasar PFS
Vincrex

Generic name product may also be available.

In Canada

Oncovin

For Prednisone

In the U.S.

Deltasone
Liquid Pred
Meticorten
Orasone
Prednicen-M
Prednisone Intensol
Sterapred
Sterapred DS

Generic name product may also be available.

In Canada

Apo-Prednisone
Deltasone
Winpred

Generic name product may also be available.

About Your Medicine

This combination therapy consists of three cancer medicines (cyclophosphamide, doxorubicin, vincristine) and an adrenocorticoid (prednisone). They are used together to treat some lymphomas and some other kinds of cancer.

If any of the information causes you special concern or if you want additional information about your medicine and its use, check with your doctor, nurse, or pharmacist.

Before Using This Medicine

Discuss with your doctor the possible side effects that may be caused by this medicine. Some of them may be serious and/or long term.

Tell your doctor, nurse, and pharmacist if you. . .

- are allergic to any medicine, either prescription or nonprescription (OTC);
- are pregnant or intend to have children;
- are breast-feeding an infant;
- are taking *any* other prescription or nonprescription (OTC) medicine;
- have *any* other medical problems;
- have ever been treated with x-rays or cancer medicines.

Proper Use of This Medicine

Use each of these medicines exactly as directed by your doctor. The exact amount of each medicine that you need and the best times to take each one have been carefully worked out. Ask your doctor, nurse, or pharmacist to help you plan a way to take each of your medicines at the right times.

Take prednisone with food to help prevent stomach upset. If stomach upset, burning, or pain continues, check with your doctor.

While you are receiving these medicines, especially cyclophosphamide, it is important that you drink extra fluids so that you will pass more urine. Also, empty your bladder frequently, including at least once during the night. This will help prevent kidney and bladder problems and keep your kidneys working well. Some patients may have to drink up to 7 to 12 cups (3 quarts) of fluid a day. If you have any questions about this, check with your doctor.

If you miss a dose of prednisone and you remember it within a few hours, take it as soon as you remember it. However, if several hours have passed or if it is almost time for the next dose, *check with your doctor*. Do not double doses.

Precautions

It is very important that your doctor check your progress at regular visits to make sure that this medicine is working properly and to check for unwanted effects.

While you are being treated with these medicines, and after you stop treatment with them, *do not have any immunizations (vaccinations) without your doctor's approval.* Also, try to avoid people with infections.

If doxorubicin or vincristine accidentally seeps out of the vein into which it is injected, it may damage some tissues and cause scarring. *Tell the doctor or nurse right away if you notice redness, pain, or swelling at the place of injection.*

Possible Side Effects

Side effects that should be reported *immediately:*

- Black, tarry stools
- Blood in urine or stools
- Cough or hoarseness
- Fast or irregular heartbeat
- Fever or chills
- Lower back or side pain
- Pain at place of injection
- Painful or difficult urination
- Pinpoint red spots on skin
- Shortness of breath
- Swelling of feet and lower legs
- Unusual bleeding or bruising
- Wheezing

Side effects that should be reported as soon as possible:

- Bed-wetting
- Blurred or double vision
- Constipation
- Convulsions (seizures)
- Darkening or redness of skin (after x-ray treatment)
- Decrease or increase in urination
- Difficulty in walking
- Dizziness, confusion, or agitation
- Drooping eyelids
- Hallucinations (seeing, hearing, or feeling things that are not there)
- Headache
- Jaw pain
- Joint pain
- Lack of sweating
- Mental depression
- Missing menstrual periods
- Numbness, tingling, or pain in fingers and toes
- Pain in testicles
- Red streaks along injected vein
- Sores in mouth and on lips
- Stomach cramps
- Trouble in sleeping
- Unusual thirst
- Unusual tiredness or weakness
- Yellow eyes or skin

Side effects that usually do not need medical attention (however, check with your doctor or nurse if they continue or are bothersome):

- Bloating
- Diarrhea
- Flushing or redness of face
- Increased sweating
- Loss of appetite
- Loss of hair
- Nausea or vomiting
- Reddish urine
- Skin rash, hives, or itching
- Swollen lips

After you stop receiving these medicines, they may still produce some side effects that need attention. During this period of time, *check with your doctor or nurse immediately* if you notice:

- Blood in urine
- Fast or irregular heartbeat
- Shortness of breath
- Swelling of feet and lower legs

Other side effects not listed above may also occur in some patients. If you notice any other effects, check with your doctor or nurse.

Annual revision: 05/22/91

CISPLATIN AND CYCLOPHOSPHAMIDE Systemic

This information applies to the following medicines:

Cisplatin (sis-PLA-tin) (by injection)
Cyclophosphamide (sye-kloe-FOSS-fa-mide) (by injection)

Some commonly used brand names are:

For Cisplatin

In the U.S.
Platinol
Platinol-AQ

In Canada
Platinol
Platinol-AQ

Generic name product may also be available.

For Cyclophosphamide

In the U.S.
Cytoxan
Neosar

Generic name product may also be available.

In Canada
Cytoxan
Procytox

About Your Medicine

This combination therapy consists of two cancer medicines. They are used together to treat some kinds of cancer.

If any of the information causes you special concern or if you want additional information about your medicine and its use, check with your doctor, nurse, or pharmacist.

Before Using This Medicine

Discuss with your doctor the possible side effects that may be caused by this medicine. Some of them may be serious and/or long term.

Tell your doctor, nurse, and pharmacist if you. . .

- are allergic to any medicine, either prescription or nonprescription (OTC);
- are pregnant or intend to have children;
- are breast-feeding an infant;
- are taking *any* other prescription or nonprescription (OTC) medicine;
- have *any* other medical problems;
- have ever been treated with x-rays or cancer medicines.

Proper Use of This Medicine

While you are receiving these medicines, especially cyclophosphamide, it is important that you drink extra fluids so that you will pass more urine. Also, empty your bladder frequently, including at least once during the night. This will help prevent kidney and bladder problems and keep your kidneys working well. Some patients may have to drink up to 7 to 12 cups (3 quarts) of fluid a day. If you have any questions about this, check with your doctor.

Precautions

It is very important that your doctor check your progress at regular visits to make sure that this medicine is working properly and to check for unwanted effects.

While you are being treated with these medicines, and after you stop treatment with them, *do not have any immunizations (vaccinations) without your doctor's approval.* Also, try to avoid people with infections.

If cisplatin accidentally seeps out of the vein into which it is injected, it may damage some tissues and cause scarring. *Tell the doctor or nurse right away if you notice redness, pain, or swelling at the place of injection.*

Possible Side Effects

Side effects that should be reported *immediately*:

Black, tarry stools
Blood in urine or stools
Cough or hoarseness
Dizziness or faintness (shortly after a dose)
Fast or irregular heartbeat
Fever or chills
Lower back or side pain
Painful or difficult urination
Pinpoint red spots on skin
Swelling of face
Unusual bleeding or bruising
Wheezing

Side effects that should be reported as soon as possible:

Blurred or double vision
Change in ability to see colors (especially blue or yellow)
Convulsions (seizures)
Decrease or increase in urination
Dizziness, confusion, or agitation
Loss of balance
Loss of reflexes
Missing menstrual periods
Numbness, tingling, or pain in fingers and toes
Ringing in ears
Shortness of breath
Sores in mouth and on lips
Swelling of feet or lower legs
Trouble in hearing
Trouble in walking
Unusual tiredness or weakness
Yellow eyes or skin

Side effects that usually do not need medical attention (however, check with your doctor or nurse if they continue or are bothersome):

Darkening of skin and fingernails
Diarrhea or stomach pain
Flushing or redness of face
Increased sweating
Loss of appetite
Loss of hair
Nausea or vomiting
Skin rash, hives, or itching
Swollen lips

After you stop receiving these medicines, they may still produce some side effects that need attention. During this period of time, *check with your doctor or nurse immediately* if you notice:

Black, tarry stools
Blood in urine or stools
Cough or hoarseness
Decrease in urination
Fever or chills
Loss of balance
Lower back or side pain
Painful or difficult urination
Pinpoint red spots on skin
Ringing in ears
Swelling of feet or lower legs
Trouble in hearing
Unusual bleeding or bruising

Other side effects not listed above may also occur in some patients. If you notice any other effects, check with your doctor or nurse.

Annual revision: 07/07/92

CISPLATIN, FLUOROURACIL, AND LEUCOVORIN Systemic

This information applies to the following medicines:
Cisplatin (sis-PLA-tin) (by injection)
Fluorouracil (flure-oh-YOOR-a-sill) (by injection)
Leucovorin (loo-koe-VOR-in) (by injection)

Some commonly used brand names are:

For Cisplatin
In the U.S.
Platinol
Platinol-AQ
In Canada
Platinol
Platinol-AQ
Generic name product may also be available.

For Fluorouracil
In the U.S. and Canada
Adrucil
Generic name product may also be available.
Another commonly used name is 5-FU.

For Leucovorin
In the U.S.
Wellcovorin
Generic name product may also be available.
In Canada
Generic name product available.
Other commonly used names are citrovorum factor and folinic acid.

About Your Medicine

This combination therapy consists of two cancer medicines plus leucovorin. They are given together to treat some kinds of cancer.

If any of the information causes you special concern or if you want additional information about your medicine and its use, check with your doctor, nurse, or pharmacist.

Before Using This Medicine

Discuss with your doctor the possible side effects that may be caused by this medicine. Some of them may be serious and/or long term.

Tell your doctor, nurse, and pharmacist if you. . .

- are allergic to any medicine, either prescription or nonprescription (OTC);
- are pregnant or intend to have children;
- are breast-feeding an infant;
- are taking *any* other prescription or nonprescription (OTC) medicine;
- have *any* other medical problems;
- have ever been treated with x-rays or cancer medicines.

Proper Use of This Medicine

While you are receiving these medicines, your doctor may want you to drink extra fluids so that you will pass more urine. This will help prevent kidney problems and keep your kidneys working well.

These medicines often cause nausea and vomiting. However, it is very important that you continue to receive the medicines, even if you begin to feel ill. Ask your doctor, nurse, or pharmacist for ways to lessen these effects.

Precautions

It is very important that your doctor check your progress at regular visits to make sure that this medicine is working properly and to check for unwanted effects.

While you are being treated with these medicines, and after you stop treatment with them, *do not have any immunizations (vaccinations) without your doctor's approval.* Also, try to avoid people with infections.

If cisplatin accidentally seeps out of the vein into which it is injected, it may damage some tissues and cause scarring. *Tell the doctor or nurse right away if you notice redness, pain, or swelling at the place of injection.*

Possible Side Effects

Side effects that should be reported *immediately*:

Black, tarry stools
Blood in urine or stools
Cough or hoarseness
Diarrhea
Dizziness or faintness (shortly after a dose)
Fast heartbeat
Fever or chills
Heartburn
Lower back or side pain
Nausea and vomiting (severe)
Painful or difficult urination
Pinpoint red spots on skin
Skin rash, hives, or itching
Sores in mouth and on lips
Stomach cramps
Swelling of face
Unusual bleeding or bruising
Wheezing

Side effects that should be reported as soon as possible:

Agitation or confusion
Blurred vision
Change in ability to see colors (especially blue or yellow)
Chest pain
Convulsions (seizures)
Joint pain
Loss of balance
Loss of reflexes
Loss of taste
Numbness or tingling in fingers, toes, or face

Shortness of breath
Swelling of feet or lower legs
Tingling of hands and feet, followed by pain, redness, and swelling
Trouble in hearing or ringing in ears
Trouble in walking
Unusual tiredness or weakness

Side effects that usually do not need medical attention (however, check with your doctor or nurse if they continue or are bothersome):

Loss of appetite
Loss of hair
Nausea and vomiting

After you stop receiving these medicines, they may still produce some side effects that need attention. During this period of time, *check with your doctor or nurse immediately* if you notice:

Black, tarry stools
Blood in urine or stools
Cough or hoarseness
Decrease in urination
Fever or chills
Loss of balance
Lower back or side pain
Painful or difficult urination
Pinpoint red spots on skin
Ringing in ears
Swelling of feet or lower legs
Trouble in hearing
Unusual bleeding or bruising

Other side effects not listed above may also occur in some patients. If you notice any other effects, check with your doctor or nurse.

Annual revision: 07/07/92

CISPLATIN, VINBLASTINE, AND FLUOROURACIL Systemic

This information applies to the following medicines:

Cisplatin (sis-PLA-tin) (by injection)
Vinblastine (vin-BLAS-teen) (by injection)
Fluorouracil (flure-oh-YOOR-a-sill) (by injection)

Some commonly used brand names are:

For Cisplatin

In the U.S.
Platinol
Platinol-AQ

In Canada
Platinol
Platinol-AQ

Generic name product may also be available.

For Vinblastine

In the U.S.
Velban
Velsar

Generic name product may also be available.

In Canada
Velbe

For Fluorouracil

In the U.S. and Canada
Adrucil

Generic name product may also be available.

Another commonly used name is 5-FU.

About Your Medicine

This combination therapy consists of three cancer medicines. They are used together to treat some kinds of cancer.

If any of the information causes you special concern or if you want additional information about your medicine and its use, check with your doctor, nurse, or pharmacist.

Before Using This Medicine

Discuss with your doctor the possible side effects that may be caused by this medicine. Some of them may be serious and/or long term.

Tell your doctor, nurse, and pharmacist if you. . .

- are allergic to any medicine, either prescription or nonprescription (OTC);
- are pregnant or intend to have children;
- are breast-feeding an infant;
- are taking *any* other prescription or nonprescription (OTC) medicine;
- have *any* other medical problems;
- have ever been treated with x-rays or cancer medicines.

Proper Use of This Medicine

While you are receiving these medicines, your doctor may want you to drink extra fluids so that you will pass more urine. This will help prevent kidney problems and keep your kidneys working well.

These medicines often cause nausea and vomiting. However, it is very important that you continue to receive the medicines, even if you begin to feel ill. Ask your doctor, nurse, or pharmacist for ways to lessen these effects.

Precautions

It is very important that your doctor check your progress at regular visits to make sure that this medicine is working properly and to check for unwanted effects.

While you are being treated with these medicines, and after you stop treatment with them, *do not have any immunizations (vaccinations) without your doctor's approval.* Also, try to avoid people with infections.

If cisplatin or vinblastine accidentally seeps out of the vein into which it is injected, it may damage some tissues and cause scarring. *Tell the doctor or nurse right away if you notice redness, pain, or swelling at the place of injection.*

Possible Side Effects

Side effects that should be reported *immediately*:

- Black, tarry stools
- Blood in urine or stools
- Cough or hoarseness
- Diarrhea
- Dizziness or faintness (shortly after a dose)
- Fast heartbeat
- Fever or chills
- Heartburn
- Lower back or side pain
- Nausea and vomiting (severe)
- Painful or difficult urination
- Pinpoint red spots on skin
- Sores in mouth and on lips
- Stomach cramps
- Swelling of face
- Unusual bleeding or bruising
- Wheezing

Side effects that should be reported as soon as possible:

- Agitation or confusion
- Blurred or double vision
- Change in ability to see colors (especially blue or yellow)
- Chest pain
- Convulsions (seizures)
- Dizziness
- Drooping eyelids
- Headache or jaw pain
- Joint pain
- Loss of balance
- Loss of reflexes
- Loss of taste
- Mental depression
- Numbness or tingling in fingers, toes, or face
- Pain in fingers and toes
- Pain in testicles
- Shortness of breath
- Swelling of feet or lower legs
- Tingling of hands and feet, followed by pain, redness, and swelling
- Trouble in hearing or ringing in ears
- Trouble in walking
- Unusual tiredness or weakness

Side effects that usually do not need medical attention (however, check with your doctor or nurse if they continue or are bothersome):

- Loss of appetite
- Loss of hair
- Muscle pain
- Nausea and vomiting
- Skin rash and itching

After you stop receiving these medicines, they may still produce some side effects that need attention. During this period of time, *check with your doctor or nurse immediately* if you notice:

- Black, tarry stools
- Blood in urine or stools
- Cough or hoarseness
- Decrease in urination
- Difficulty in hearing
- Fever or chills
- Loss of balance
- Lower back or side pain
- Painful or difficult urination
- Pinpoint red spots on skin
- Ringing in ears
- Swelling of feet or lower legs
- Unusual bleeding or bruising

Other side effects not listed above may also occur in some patients. If you notice any other effects, check with your doctor or nurse.

Annual revision: 07/07/92

CMF Systemic

This information applies to the following medicines:

- Cyclophosphamide (sye-kloe-FOSS-fa-mide) (by mouth)
- Methotrexate (meth-o-TREX-ate) (by injection)
- Fluorouracil (flure-oh-YOOR-a-sill) (by injection)

Some commonly used brand names are:

For Cyclophosphamide

In the U.S.

Cytoxan

In Canada

Cytoxan

Procytox

For Methotrexate

In the U.S.

Folex
Folex PFS
Mexate
Mexate-AQ

Generic name product may also be available.

In Canada

Generic name product available.

For Fluorouracil

In the U.S. and Canada

Adrucil

Generic name product may also be available.

Another commonly used name is 5-FU.

About Your Medicine

This combination therapy consists of three cancer medicines. They are used together to treat breast cancer and some other kinds of cancer.

If any of the information causes you special concern or if you want additional information about your medicine and its use, check with your doctor, nurse, or pharmacist.

Before Using This Medicine

Discuss with your doctor the possible side effects that may be caused by this medicine. Some of them may be serious and/or long term.

Tell your doctor, nurse, and pharmacist if you...

- are allergic to any medicine, either prescription or nonprescription (OTC);
- are pregnant or intend to have children;
- are breast-feeding an infant;
- are taking *any* other prescription or nonprescription (OTC) medicine;
- have *any* other medical problems;
- have ever been treated with x-rays or cancer medicines.

Proper Use of This Medicine

Use each of these medicines exactly as directed by your doctor. The exact amount of each medicine that you need and the best times to take each one have been carefully worked out. Ask your doctor, nurse, or pharmacist to help you plan a way to take each of your medicines at the right times.

While you are receiving these medicines, especially cyclophosphamide, it is important that you drink extra fluids so that you will pass more urine. Also, empty your bladder frequently, including at least once during the night. This will help prevent kidney and bladder problems and keep your kidneys working well. Some patients may have to drink up to 7 to 12 cups (3 quarts) of fluid a day. If you have any questions about this, check with your doctor.

If you vomit shortly after taking a dose of cyclophosphamide, check with your doctor. You will be told whether to take the dose again or to wait until the next scheduled dose.

If you miss a dose of cyclophosphamide, do not take the missed dose at all and do not double the next one. Instead, go back to your regular dosing schedule and check with your doctor.

Precautions

It is very important that your doctor check your progress at regular visits to make sure that these medicines are working properly and to check for unwanted effects.

Do not drink alcohol while using methotrexate. Alcohol can increase the chance of liver problems.

Do not take medicine for inflammation or pain without first checking with your doctor. These medicines may increase the effects of methotrexate, which could be harmful.

While you are being treated with these medicines, and after you stop treatment with them, *do not have any immunizations (vaccinations) without your doctor's approval.* Also, try to avoid people with infections.

Possible Side Effects

Side effects that should be reported *immediately*:

Black, tarry stools
Blood in urine or stools
Bloody vomit
Blurred vision
Convulsions (seizures)
Cough or hoarseness
Diarrhea
Fever or chills
Lower back or side pain
Nausea and vomiting (severe)
Painful or difficult urination
Pinpoint red spots on skin
Reddening of skin
Shortness of breath
Sores in mouth and on lips
Stomach pain
Swelling of feet or lower legs
Unusual bleeding or bruising

Side effects that should be reported as soon as possible:

Back pain
Chest pain
Dark urine
Dizziness, confusion, or agitation
Drowsiness

Fast heartbeat
Frequent urination
Headache
Joint pain
Missing menstrual periods
Redness, swelling, or pain at place of injection
Tingling of hands and feet, followed by pain, redness, and swelling
Trouble with balance
Unusual thirst
Unusual tiredness or weakness
Yellow eyes or skin

Side effects that usually do not need medical attention (however, check with your doctor or nurse if they continue or are bothersome):

Acne
Boils
Darkening of skin and fingernails
Flushing or redness of face
Increased sweating
Loss of appetite
Loss of hair
Nausea or vomiting
Pale skin
Skin rash, hives, or itching
Swollen lips

After you stop receiving these medicines, they may still produce some side effects that need attention. During this period of time, *check with your doctor or nurse immediately* if you notice:

Black, tarry stools
Blood in urine or stools
Cough or hoarseness
Fever or chills
Lower back or side pain
Painful or difficult urination
Pinpoint red spots on skin
Unusual bleeding or bruising

Other side effects not listed above may also occur in some patients. If you notice any other effects, check with your doctor or nurse.

Annual revision: 07/07/92

CMFP Systemic

This information applies to the following medicines:

Cyclophosphamide (sye-kloe-FOSS-fa-mide) (by mouth)
Methotrexate (meth-o-TREX-ate) (by injection)
Fluorouracil (flure-oh-YOOR-a-sill) (by injection)
Prednisone (PRED-ni-sone) (by mouth)

Some commonly used brand names are:

For Cyclophosphamide

In the U.S.
Cytoxan

In Canada
Cytoxan
Procytox

For Methotrexate

In the U.S.
Folex
Folex PFS
Mexate
Mexate-AQ
Generic name product may also be available.

In Canada
Generic name product available.

For Fluorouracil

In the U.S. and Canada
Adrucil
Generic name product may also be available.

Another commonly used name is 5-FU.

For Prednisone

In the U.S.
Deltasone
Liquid Pred
Meticorten
Orasone
Prednicen-M
Prednisone Intensol
Sterapred
Sterapred DS
Generic name product may also be available.

In Canada
Apo-Prednisone
Deltasone
Winpred
Generic name product may also be available.

About Your Medicine

This combination therapy consists of three cancer medicines (cyclophosphamide, methotrexate, fluorouracil) and an adrenocorticoid (prednisone). They are used together to treat some other kinds of cancer.

If any of the information causes you special concern or if you want additional information about your medicine and its use, check with your doctor, nurse, or pharmacist.

Before Using This Medicine

Discuss with your doctor the possible side effects that may be caused by this medicine. Some of them may be serious and/or long term.

Tell your doctor, nurse, and pharmacist if you. . .

- are allergic to any medicine, either prescription or nonprescription (OTC);
- are pregnant or intend to have children;
- are breast-feeding an infant;
- are taking *any* other prescription or nonprescription (OTC) medicine;

- have *any* other medical problems;
- have ever been treated with x-rays or cancer medicines.

Proper Use of This Medicine

Use each of these medicines exactly as directed by your doctor. The exact amount of each medicine that you need and the best times to take each one have been carefully worked out. Ask your doctor, nurse, or pharmacist to help you plan a way to take each of your medicines at the right times.

Take prednisone with food to help prevent stomach upset. If stomach upset, burning, or pain continues, check with your doctor.

While you are using these medicines, especially cyclophosphamide, it is important that you drink extra fluids so that you will pass more urine. Also, empty your bladder frequently, including at least once during the night. This will help prevent kidney and bladder problems and keep your kidneys working well. Some patients may have to drink up to 7 to 12 cups (3 quarts) of fluid a day. If you have any questions about this, check with your doctor.

If you vomit shortly after taking a dose of cyclophosphamide, check with your doctor. You will be told whether to take the dose again or to wait until the next scheduled dose.

If you miss a dose of cyclophosphamide, do not take the missed dose at all and do not double the next one. Instead, go back to your regular dosing schedule and check with your doctor.

If you miss a dose of prednisone and you remember it within a few hours, take it as soon as you remember it. However, if several hours have passed or if it is almost time for the next dose, *check with your doctor.* Do not double doses.

Precautions

It is very important that your doctor check your progress at regular visits to make sure that these medicines are working properly and to check for unwanted effects.

Do not drink alcohol while using methotrexate. Alcohol can increase the chance of liver problems.

Do not take medicine for inflammation or pain without first checking with your doctor. These medicines may increase the effects of methotrexate, which could be harmful.

While you are being treated with these medicines, and after you stop treatment with them, *do not have any immunizations (vaccinations) without your doctor's approval.* Also, try to avoid people with infections.

Possible Side Effects

Side effects that should be reported *immediately:*

Black, tarry stools
Blood in urine or stools
Bloody vomit
Blurred vision
Confusion
Convulsions (seizures)
Cough or hoarseness
Diarrhea
Fever or chills
Lower back or side pain
Nausea and vomiting (severe)
Painful or difficult urination
Pinpoint red spots on skin
Reddening of skin
Shortness of breath
Sores in mouth and on lips
Stomach pain
Swelling of feet or lower legs
Unusual bleeding or bruising

Side effects that should be reported as soon as possible:

Back pain
Chest pain
Dark urine
Dizziness, confusion, or agitation
Drowsiness
Fast heartbeat
Frequent urination
Headache
Joint pain
Missing menstrual periods
Redness, swelling, or pain at place of injection
Tingling of hands and feet, followed by pain, redness, and swelling
Trouble with balance
Unusual thirst
Unusual tiredness or weakness
Yellow eyes or skin

Side effects that usually do not need medical attention (however, check with your doctor or nurse if they continue or are bothersome):

Acne
Boils
Darkening of skin and fingernails
Flushing or redness of face
Increased sweating
Loss of appetite
Loss of hair
Nausea or vomiting
Pale skin
Skin rash, hives, or itching
Swollen lips

After you stop receiving these medicines, they may still produce some side effects that need attention. During this period of time, *check with your doctor or nurse immediately* if you notice:

Black, tarry stools
Blood in urine or stools
Cough or hoarseness
Fever or chills
Lower back or side pain
Painful or difficult urination
Pinpoint red spots on skin
Unusual bleeding or bruising

Other side effects not listed above may also occur in some patients. If you notice any other effects, check with your doctor or nurse.

Annual revision: 07/07/92

COMLA Systemic

This information applies to the following medicines:

Cyclophosphamide (sye-kloe-FOSS-fa-mide) (by injection)
Vincristine (vin-KRIS-teen) (by injection)
Methotrexate (meth-o-TREX-ate) (by injection)
Leucovorin (loo-koe-VOR-in) (by mouth or injection)
Cytarabine (sye-TARE-a-been) (by injection)

Some commonly used brand names are:

For Cyclophosphamide

In the U.S.

Cytoxan
Neosar

Generic name product may also be available.

In Canada

Cytoxan
Procytox

For Vincristine

In the U.S.

Oncovin
Vincasar PFS
Vincrex

Generic name product may also be available.

In Canada

Oncovin

For Methotrexate

In the U.S

Folex
Folex PFS
Mexate
Mexate-AQ

Generic name product may also be available.

In Canada

Generic name product available.

For Leucovorin

In the U.S.

Wellcovorin

Generic name product may also be available.

In Canada

Generic name product available.

Other commonly used names are citrovorum factor and folinic acid.

For Cytarabine

In the U.S.

Cytosar-U

In Canada

Cytosar

Other commonly used names are ara-C and cytosine arabinoside.

About Your Medicine

This combination therapy consists of four cancer medicines. They are used together to treat some kinds of cancer.

To prevent too much damage by methotrexate to normal cells, leucovorin is also given by mouth or injection as an antidote.

If any of the information causes you special concern or if you want additional information about your medicine and its use, check with your doctor, nurse, or pharmacist.

Before Using This Medicine

Discuss with your doctor the possible side effects that may be caused by this medicine. Some of them may be serious and/or long term.

Tell your doctor, nurse, and pharmacist if you. . .

- are allergic to any medicine, either prescription or nonprescription (OTC);
- are pregnant or intend to have children;
- are breast-feeding an infant;
- are taking *any* other prescription or nonprescription (OTC) medicine;
- have *any* other medical problems;
- have ever been treated with x-rays or cancer medicines.

Proper Use of This Medicine

Use each of these medicines exactly as directed by your doctor. The exact amount of each medicine that you need and the best times to take each one have been carefully worked out. Ask your doctor, nurse, or pharmacist to help you plan a way to take each of your medicines at the right times.

While you are receiving these medicines, especially cyclophosphamide, it is important that you drink extra fluids so that you will pass more urine. Also, empty your bladder frequently, including at least once during the night. This will help prevent kidney and bladder problems and keep your kidneys working well. Some patients may have to drink up to 7 to 12 cups (3 quarts) of fluid a day. If you have any questions about this, check with your doctor.

For patients taking leucovorin by mouth:

- Leucovorin works best when there is a constant amount in the blood. *To help keep this amount constant, do not miss any doses. Also, it is best to take each dose at evenly spaced times day and night.* If this interferes with your sleep or other daily activities, or if you need help in planning the best times to take your medicine, check with your doctor, nurse, or pharmacist.
- If you vomit shortly after taking a dose of leucovorin, check with your doctor. You will be told whether to take the dose again or to wait until the next scheduled dose.
- If you miss a dose of leucovorin, *check with your doctor right away.* Your doctor may want you to take extra leucovorin to make up for what you missed. Do not take more medicine on your own, however, since it is very important that you receive the right dose at the right time.

Precautions

It is very important that your doctor check your progress at regular visits to make sure that these medicines are working properly and to check for unwanted effects.

Do not drink alcohol while using methotrexate. Alcohol can increase the chance of liver problems.

Do not take medicine for inflammation or pain without first checking with your doctor. These medicines may increase the effects of methotrexate, which could be harmful.

While you are being treated with these medicines, and after you stop treatment with them, *do not have any immunizations (vaccinations) without your doctor's approval.* Also, try to avoid people with infections.

If vincristine accidentally seeps out of the vein into which it is injected, it may damage some tissues and cause scarring. *Tell the doctor or nurse right away if you notice redness, pain, or swelling at the place of injection.*

Possible Side Effects

Side effects that should be reported *immediately:*

Black, tarry stools
Blood in urine or stools
Bloody vomit
Blurred vision
Confusion
Convulsions (seizures)
Cough or hoarseness
Diarrhea
Fever or chills
Lower back or side pain
Painful or difficult urination
Pinpoint red spots on skin
Reddening of skin
Shortness of breath
Sores in mouth and on lips
Stomach pain
Swelling of feet and lower legs
Unusual bleeding or bruising

Side effects that should be reported as soon as possible:

Back pain
Bed-wetting
Bone or muscle pain
Chest pain
Constipation
Dark urine
Decrease or increase in urination
Difficulty in swallowing
Difficulty in walking
Dizziness, confusion, or agitation
Double vision
Drooping eyelids
Drowsiness
Fast or irregular heartbeat
Hallucinations (seeing, hearing, or feeling things that are not there)
Headache
Jaw pain
Joint pain
Lack of sweating
Mental depression
Missing menstrual periods
Numbness, tingling, or pain in fingers and toes
Pain in testicles
Trouble in sleeping
Unusual thirst
Unusual tiredness or weakness
Yellow eyes or skin

Side effects that usually do not need medical attention (however, check with your doctor or nurse if they continue or are bothersome):

Bloating
Darkening of soles, palms, or nails
Flushing or redness of face
Increased sweating
Loss of appetite
Loss of hair
Nausea or vomiting
Skin rash, hives, or itching
Swollen lips

After you stop receiving these medicines, they may still produce some side effects that need attention. During this period of time, *check with your doctor or nurse immediately* if you notice:

- Black, tarry stools
- Blood in urine or stools
- Cough or hoarseness
- Fever or chills
- Lower back or side pain
- Painful or difficult urination
- Pinpoint red spots on skin
- Unusual bleeding or bruising

Other side effects not listed above may also occur in some patients. If you notice any other effects, check with your doctor or nurse.

Annual revision: 05/22/91

COPA Systemic

This information applies to the following medicines:

- Cyclophosphamide (sye-kloe-FOSS-fa-mide) (by injection)
- Vincristine (vin-KRIS-teen) (by injection)
- Prednisone (PRED-ni-sone) (by mouth)
- Doxorubicin (dox-oh-ROO-bi-sin) (by injection)

Some commonly used brand names are:

For Cyclophosphamide

In the U.S.

Cytoxan
Neosar

Generic name product may also be available.

In Canada

Cytoxan
Procytox

For Vincristine

In the U.S.

Oncovin
Vincasar PFS
Vincrex

Generic name product may also be available.

In Canada

Oncovin

For Prednisone

In the U.S.

Deltasone
Liquid Pred
Meticorten
Orasone
Prednicen-M
Prednisone Intensol
Sterapred
Sterapred DS

Generic name product may also be available.

In Canada

Apo-Prednisone
Deltasone
Winpred

Generic name product may also be available.

For Doxorubicin

In the U.S.

Adriamycin PFS
Adriamycin RDF
Rubex

Generic name product may also be available.

In Canada

Adriamycin PFS
Adriamycin RDF

About Your Medicine

This combination therapy consists of three cancer medicines (cyclophosphamide, doxorubicin, vincristine) and an adrenocorticoid (prednisone). They are used together to treat some lymphomas and some other kinds of cancer.

If any of the information causes you special concern or if you want additional information about your medicine and its use, check with your doctor, nurse, or pharmacist.

Before Using This Medicine

Discuss with your doctor the possible side effects that may be caused by this medicine. Some of them may be serious and/or long term.

Tell your doctor, nurse, and pharmacist if you. . .

- are allergic to any medicine, either prescription or nonprescription (OTC);
- are pregnant or intend to have children;
- are breast-feeding an infant;
- are taking *any* other prescription or nonprescription (OTC) medicine;
- have *any* other medical problems;
- have ever been treated with x-rays or cancer medicines.

Proper Use of This Medicine

Use each of these medicines exactly as directed by your doctor. The exact amount of each medicine that you need and the best times to take each one have been carefully worked out. Ask your doctor, nurse, or pharmacist to help you plan a way to take each of your medicines at the right times.

Take prednisone with food to help prevent stomach upset. If stomach upset, burning, or pain continues, check with your doctor.

While you are receiving these medicines, especially cyclophosphamide, it is important that you drink extra fluids so that you will pass more urine. Also, empty your bladder frequently, including at least once during the night. This will help prevent kidney and bladder problems and keep your kidneys working well. Some patients may have to drink up to 7 to 12 cups (3 quarts) of fluid a day. If you have any questions about this, check with your doctor.

If you miss a dose of prednisone and you remember it within a few hours, take it as soon as you remember it. However, if several hours have passed or if it is almost time for the next dose, *check with your doctor*. Do not double doses.

Precautions

It is very important that your doctor check your progress at regular visits to make sure that this medicine is working properly and to check for unwanted effects.

While you are being treated with these medicines, and after you stop treatment with them, *do not have any immunizations (vaccinations) without your doctor's approval*. Also, try to avoid people with infections.

If doxorubicin or vincristine accidentally seeps out of the vein into which it is injected, it may damage some tissues and cause scarring. *Tell the doctor or nurse right away if you notice redness, pain, or swelling at the place of injection.*

Possible Side Effects

Side effects that should be reported *immediately*:

- Black, tarry stools
- Blood in urine or stools
- Cough or hoarseness
- Fast or irregular heartbeat
- Fever or chills
- Lower back or side pain
- Pain at place of injection
- Painful or difficult urination
- Pinpoint red spots on skin
- Shortness of breath
- Swelling of feet and lower legs
- Unusual bleeding or bruising
- Wheezing

Side effects that should be reported as soon as possible:

- Bed-wetting
- Blurred or double vision
- Constipation
- Convulsions (seizures)
- Darkening or redness of skin (after x-ray treatment)
- Decrease or increase in urination
- Difficulty in walking
- Dizziness, confusion, or agitation
- Drooping eyelids
- Hallucinations (seeing, hearing, or feeling things that are not there)
- Headache
- Jaw pain
- Joint pain
- Lack of sweating
- Mental depression
- Missing menstrual periods
- Numbness, tingling, or pain in fingers and toes
- Pain in testicles
- Red streaks along injected vein
- Sores in mouth and on lips
- Stomach cramps
- Trouble in sleeping
- Unusual thirst
- Unusual tiredness or weakness
- Yellow eyes or skin

Side effects that usually do not need medical attention (however, check with your doctor or nurse if they continue or are bothersome):

- Bloating
- Diarrhea
- Flushing or redness of face
- Increased sweating
- Loss of appetite
- Loss of hair
- Nausea or vomiting
- Reddish urine
- Skin rash, hives, or itching
- Swollen lips

After you stop receiving these medicines, they may still produce some side effects that need attention. During this period of time, *check with your doctor or nurse immediately* if you notice:

- Blood in urine
- Fast or irregular heartbeat
- Shortness of breath
- Swelling of feet and lower legs

Other side effects not listed above may also occur in some patients. If you notice any other effects, check with your doctor or nurse.

Annual revision: 05/22/91

COP-BLAM Systemic

This information applies to the following medicines:

- Cyclophosphamide (sye-kloe-FOSS-fa-mide) (by injection)
- Vincristine (vin-KRIS-teen) (by injection)
- Prednisone (PRED-ni-sone) (by mouth)
- Bleomycin (blee-oh-MYE-sin) (by injection)
- Doxorubicin (dox-oh-ROO-bi-sin) (by injection)
- Procarbazine (pro-KAR-ba-zeen) (by mouth)

Some commonly used brand names are:

For Cyclophosphamide

In the U.S.

Cytoxan
Neosar

Generic name product may also be available.

In Canada

Cytoxan
Procytox

For Vincristine

In the U.S.

Oncovin
Vincasar PFS
Vincrex

Generic name product may also be available.

In Canada

Oncovin

For Prednisone

In the U.S.

Deltasone
Liquid Pred
Meticorten
Orasone
Prednicen-M
Prednisone Intensol
Sterapred
Sterapred DS

Generic name product may also be available.

In Canada

Apo-Prednisone
Deltasone
Winpred

Generic name product may also be available.

For Bleomycin

In the U.S. and Canada

Blenoxane

For Doxorubicin

In the U.S.

Adriamycin PFS
Adriamycin RDF
Rubex

Generic name product may also be available.

In Canada

Adriamycin PFS
Adriamycin RDF

For Procarbazine

In the U.S.

Matulane

In Canada

Natulan

About Your Medicine

This combination therapy consists of five cancer medicines (cyclophosphamide, vincristine, bleomycin, doxorubicin, procarbazine) and an adrenocorticoid (prednisone). They are used together to treat some kinds of cancer.

If any of the information causes you special concern or if you want additional information about your medicine and its use, check with your doctor, nurse, or pharmacist.

Before Using This Medicine

Discuss with your doctor the possible side effects that may be caused by this medicine. Some of them may be serious and/or long term.

Tell your doctor, nurse, and pharmacist if you. . .

- are allergic to any medicine, either prescription or nonprescription (OTC);
- are pregnant or intend to have children;
- are breast-feeding an infant;
- are taking *any* other prescription or nonprescription (OTC) medicine;
- have *any* other medical problems;
- have ever been treated with x-rays or cancer medicines;
- smoke.

Proper Use of This Medicine

Use each of these medicines exactly as directed by your doctor. The exact amount of each medicine that you need and the best times to take each one have been carefully worked out. Ask your doctor, nurse, or pharmacist to help you plan a way to take each of your medicines at the right times.

Take prednisone with food to help prevent stomach upset. If stomach upset, burning, or pain continues, check with your doctor.

While you are receiving these medicines, especially cyclophosphamide, it is important that you drink extra fluids so that you will pass more urine. Also, empty your bladder frequently, including at least once during the night. This will help prevent kidney and bladder problems and keep your kidneys working well. Some patients may have to drink up to 7 to 12 cups (3 quarts) of fluid a day. If you have any questions about this, check with your doctor.

If you miss a dose of prednisone or procarbazine and you remember it within a few hours, take it as soon as you remember it. However, if several hours have passed or if it is almost time for the next dose, *check with your doctor.* Do not double doses.

Precautions

It is very important that your doctor check your progress at regular visits to make sure that this medicine is working properly and to check for unwanted effects.

When taken with certain foods, drinks, or other medicines, *procarbazine* can cause very dangerous reactions. *To avoid such reactions:*

- Do not eat foods that have a high tyramine content (most common in foods that are aged or fermented to increase their flavor).
- Do not drink alcoholic beverages or alcohol-free or reduced-alcohol beer and wine.

- Do not eat or drink large amounts of caffeine-containing food or beverages.
- Do not take any other medicine unless prescribed by your doctor, including OTC or nonprescription medicines.

After you stop using procarbazine you must continue to obey the above rules of caution for at least 2 weeks.

Procarbazine may cause blurred vision or make some people drowsy or less alert than they are normally. *Make sure you know how you react to this medicine before you drive, use machines, or do anything else that could be dangerous if you are unable to see well or are not alert.*

While you are being treated with these medicines, and for several weeks after you stop treatment with them:

- *Do not have any immunizations (vaccinations) without your doctor's approval.* Also, try to avoid people with infections.
- If you are going to have surgery or emergency treatment, *tell the medical doctor or dentist in charge that you have been taking this medicine.*

If doxorubicin or vincristine accidentally seeps out of the vein into which it is injected, it may damage some tissues and cause scarring. *Tell the doctor or nurse right away if you notice redness, pain, or swelling at the place of injection.*

Possible Side Effects

Side effects that should be reported *immediately:*

Black, tarry stools
Blood in urine or stools
Bloody vomit
Chest pain (severe)
Confusion
Cough or hoarseness
Enlarged pupils of eyes
Faintness
Fast, slow, or irregular heartbeat
Fever or chills
Headache (severe)
Increased sensitivity of eyes to light
Increased sweating (possibly with fever or cold, clammy skin)
Lower back or side pain
Pain at place of injection
Painful or difficult urination
Pinpoint red spots on skin
Shortness of breath
Stiff or sore neck
Swelling of feet and lower legs
Unusual bleeding or bruising
Wheezing

Side effects that should be reported as soon as possible:

Agitation
Bed-wetting
Blurred or double vision
Constipation
Convulsions (seizures)
Darkening or redness of skin (after x-ray treatment)
Diarrhea
Difficulty in walking
Dizziness
Drooping eyelids
Fainting
Frequent urination
Hallucinations (seeing, hearing, or feeling things that are not there)
Jaw pain
Joint pain
Lack of sweating
Mental depression
Missing menstrual periods
Numbness, tingling, or pain in fingers and toes
Pain in testicles
Red streaks along injected vein
Skin rash, hives, or itching
Sores in mouth and on lips
Stomach cramps
Thickening of bronchial secretions
Unsteadiness or awkwardness
Unusual thirst
Unusual tiredness or weakness
Yellow eyes or skin

Side effects that usually do not need medical attention (however, check with your doctor or nurse if they continue or are bothersome):

Bloating
Blurred vision
Colored bumps on fingertips, elbows, or palms
Darkening of soles, palms, or nails
Drowsiness
Dry mouth
Flushing or redness of face
Itching of skin
Loss of appetite
Loss of hair
Muscle pain or twitching
Nausea or vomiting
Nightmares
Reddish urine
Skin redness or tenderness
Swelling of fingers
Trouble in sleeping

After you stop receiving these medicines, they may still produce some side effects that need attention. During this period of time, *check with your doctor or nurse immediately* if you notice:

Blood in urine
Cough
Fast or irregular heartbeat
Shortness of breath
Swelling of feet and lower legs

Other side effects not listed above may also occur in some patients. If you notice any other effects, check with your doctor or nurse.

Annual revision: 05/22/91

CVP Systemic

This information applies to the following medicines:

Cyclophosphamide (sye-kloe-FOSS-fa-mide) (by injection)
Vincristine (vin-KRIS-teen) (by injection)
Prednisone (PRED-ni-sone) (by mouth)

Some commonly used brand names are:

For Cyclophosphamide

In the U.S.

Cytoxan
Neosar

Generic name product may also be available.

In Canada

Cytoxan
Procytox

For Vincristine

In the U.S.

Oncovin
Vincasar PFS
Vincrex

Generic name product may also be available.

In Canada

Oncovin

For Prednisone

In the U.S.

Deltasone
Liquid Pred
Meticorten
Orasone
Prednicen-M
Prednisone Intensol
Sterapred
Sterapred DS

Generic name product may also be available.

In Canada

Apo-Prednisone
Deltasone
Winpred

Generic name product may also be available.

About Your Medicine

This combination therapy consists of two cancer medicines (cyclophosphamide, vincristine) and an adrenocorticoid (prednisone). They are used together to treat some lymphomas and some other kinds of cancer.

If any of the information causes you special concern or if you want additional information about your medicine and its use, check with your doctor, nurse, or pharmacist.

Before Using This Medicine

Discuss with your doctor the possible side effects that may be caused by this medicine. Some of them may be serious and/or long term.

Tell your doctor, nurse, and pharmacist if you. . .

- are allergic to any medicine, either prescription or nonprescription (OTC);
- are pregnant or intend to have children;
- are breast-feeding an infant;
- are taking *any* other prescription or nonprescription (OTC) medicine;
- have *any* other medical problems;
- have ever been treated with x-rays or cancer medicines.

Proper Use of This Medicine

Use each of these medicines exactly as directed by your doctor. The exact amount of each medicine that you need and the best times to take each one have been carefully worked out. Ask your doctor, nurse, or pharmacist to help you plan a way to take each of your medicines at the right times.

Take prednisone with food to help prevent stomach upset. If stomach upset, burning, or pain continues, check with your doctor.

While you are receiving these medicines, especially cyclophosphamide, it is important that you drink extra fluids so that you will pass more urine. Also, empty your bladder frequently, including at least once during the night. This will help prevent kidney and bladder problems and keep your kidneys working well. Some patients may have to drink up to 7 to 12 cups (3 quarts) of fluid a day. If you have any questions about this, check with your doctor.

If you miss a dose of prednisone and you remember it within a few hours, take it as soon as you remember it. However, if several hours have passed or if it is almost time for the next dose, *check with your doctor*. Do not double doses.

Precautions

It is very important that your doctor check your progress at regular visits to make sure that these medicines are working properly and to check for unwanted effects.

While you are being treated with these medicines, and after you stop treatment with them, *do not have any immunizations (vaccinations) without your doctor's approval*. Also, try to avoid people with infections.

If vincristine accidentally seeps out of the vein into which it is injected, it may damage some tissues and cause scarring. *Tell the doctor or nurse right away if you notice redness, pain, or swelling at the place of injection.*

Possible Side Effects

Side effects that should be reported *immediately:*

Black, tarry stools
Blood in urine or stools
Cough or hoarseness

- Fever or chills
- Lower back or side pain
- Pain at place of injection
- Painful or difficult urination
- Pinpint red spots on skin
- Shortness of breath (sudden)
- Unusual bleeding or bruising

Side effects that should be reported as soon as possible:

- Bed-wetting
- Blurred or double vision
- Constipation
- Convulsions (seizures)
- Decrease or increase in urination
- Difficulty in walking
- Dizziness, confusion, or agitation
- Drooping eyelids
- Fast or irregular heartbeat
- Hallucinations (seeing, hearing, or feeling things that are not there)
- Headache
- Jaw pain
- Joint pain
- Lack of sweating
- Mental depression
- Missing menstrual periods
- Numbness, tingling, or pain in fingers and toes
- Pain in testicles
- Shortness of breath
- Sores in mouth and on lips
- Stomach cramps
- Swelling of feet and lower legs
- Trouble in sleeping
- Unusual thirst
- Unusual tiredness or weakness
- Yellow eyes or skin

Side effects that usually do not need medical attention (however, check with your doctor or nurse if they continue or are bothersome):

- Bloating
- Darkening of soles, palms, or nails
- Diarrhea
- Flushing or redness of face
- Increased sweating
- Loss of appetite
- Loss of hair
- Nausea or vomiting
- Skin rash, hives, or itching
- Swollen lips

After you stop receiving these medicines, they may still produce some side effects that need attention. During this period of time, *check with your doctor or nurse immediately* if you notice:

- Blood in urine

Other side effects not listed above may also occur in some patients. If you notice any other effects, check with your doctor or nurse.

Annual revision: 05/22/91

CVPP Systemic

This information applies to the following medicines:

- Cyclophosphamide (sye-kloe-FOSS-fa-mide) (by injection)
- Vincristine (vin-KRIS-teen) (by injection)
- Procarbazine (pro-KAR-ba-zeen) (by mouth)
- Prednisone (PRED-ni-sone) (by mouth)

Some commonly used brand names are:

For Cyclophosphamide

In the U.S.

Cytoxan
Neosar

Generic name product may also be available.

In Canada

Cytoxan
Procytox

For Vincristine

In the U.S.

Oncovin
Vincrex
Vincasar PFS

Generic name product may also be available.

In Canada

Oncovin

For Procarbazine

In the U.S.

Matulane

In Canada

Natulan

For Prednisone

In the U.S.

Deltasone
Prednicen-M
Liquid Pred
Prednisone Intensol
Meticorten
Sterapred
Orasone
Sterapred DS

Generic name product may also be available.

In Canada

Apo-Prednisone
Winpred
Deltasone

Generic name product may also be available.

About Your Medicine

This combination therapy consists of three cancer medicines (cyclophosphamide, vincristine, procarbazine) and an adrenocorticoid (prednisone). They are used together to treat some lymphomas and some other kinds of cancer.

If any of the information causes you special concern or if you want additional information about your medicine and its use, check with your doctor, nurse, or pharmacist.

Before Using This Medicine

Discuss with your doctor the possible side effects that may be caused by this medicine. Some of them may be serious and/or long term.

Tell your doctor, nurse, and pharmacist if you. . .

- are allergic to any medicine, either prescription or nonprescription (OTC);
- are pregnant or intend to have children;
- are breast-feeding an infant;
- are taking *any* other prescription or nonprescription (OTC) medicine;
- have *any* other medical problems;
- have ever been treated with x-rays or cancer medicines.

Proper Use of This Medicine

Use each of these medicines exactly as directed by your doctor. The exact amount of each medicine that you need and the best times to take each one have been carefully worked out. Ask your doctor, nurse, or pharmacist to help you plan a way to take each of your medicines at the right times.

Take prednisone with food to help prevent stomach upset. If stomach upset, burning, or pain continues, check with your doctor.

While you are receiving these medicines, especially cyclophosphamide, it is important that you drink extra fluids so that you will pass more urine. Also, empty your bladder frequently, including at least once during the night. This will help prevent kidney and bladder problems and keep your kidneys working well. Some patients may have to drink up to 7 to 12 cups (3 quarts) of fluid a day. If you have any questions about this, check with your doctor.

If you miss a dose of prednisone or procarbazine and you remember it within a few hours, take it as soon as you remember it. However, if several hours have passed or if it is almost time for the next dose, *check with your doctor.* Do not double doses.

Precautions

It is very important that your doctor check your progress at regular visits to make sure that these medicines are working properly and to check for unwanted effects.

When taken with certain foods, drinks, or other medicines, *procarbazine* can cause very dangerous reactions. *To avoid such reactions:*

- Do not eat foods that have a high tyramine content (most common in foods that are aged or fermented to increase their flavor).
- Do not drink alcoholic beverages or alcohol-free or reduced-alcohol beer and wine.
- Do not eat or drink large amounts of caffeine-containing food or beverages.
- Do not take any other medicine unless prescribed by your doctor, including OTC or nonprescription medicines.

After you stop using procarbazine you must continue to obey the above rules of caution for at least 2 weeks.

Procarbazine may cause some people to become drowsy or less alert than they are normally. *Make sure you know how you react to this medicine before you drive, use machines, or do anything else that could be dangerous if you are not alert.*

While you are being treated with these medicines, and after you stop treatment with them, *do not have any immunizations (vaccinations) without your doctor's approval.* Also, try to avoid people with infections.

If you are going to have surgery or emergency treatment, *tell the medical doctor or dentist in charge that you have been taking this medicine.*

If vincristine accidentally seeps out of the vein into which it is injected, it may damage some tissues and cause scarring. *Tell the doctor or nurse right away if you notice redness, pain, or swelling at the place of injection.*

Possible Side Effects

Side effects that should be reported *immediately*:

Black, tarry stools
Blood in urine or stools
Chest pain
Cough or hoarseness
Enlarged pupils of eyes
Fast or slow or irregular heartbeat
Fever or chills
Headache (severe)
Increased sensitivity of eyes to light
Increased sweating (possibly with fever or cold, clammy skin)
Lower back or side pain
Pain at place of injection
Painful or difficult urination
Pinpoint red spots on skin
Shortness of breath (sudden)
Stiff or sore neck
Unusual bleeding or bruising

Side effects that should be reported as soon as possible:

Bed-wetting
Bloody vomit
Blurred or double vision
Constipation
Convulsions (seizures)
Decrease or increase in urination
Diarrhea
Dizziness, confusion, or agitation
Drooping eyelids
Fainting
Hallucinations (seeing, hearing, or feeling things that are not there)
Jaw pain
Joint pain
Lack of sweating
Mental depression
Missing menstrual periods
Numbness, tingling, or pain in fingers and toes
Pain in testicles
Shortness of breath
Sores in mouth and on lips
Stomach cramps
Swelling of feet and lower legs
Thickening of bronchial secretions
Trouble in sleeping
Trouble in walking
Unsteadiness or awkwardness
Unusual thirst
Unusual tiredness or weakness
Yellow eyes or skin

Side effects that usually do not need medical attention (however, check with your doctor or nurse if they continue or are bothersome):

Bloating
Darkening of soles, palms, or nails
Difficulty in swallowing
Dry mouth
Flushing or redness of face
Loss of appetite
Loss of hair
Muscle pain or twitching
Nausea or vomiting
Nightmares
Skin rash, hives, or itching
Swollen lips

After you stop receiving these medicines, they may still produce some side effects that need attention. During this period of time, *check with your doctor or nurse immediately* if you notice:

Blood in urine

Other side effects not listed above may also occur in some patients. If you notice any other effects, check with your doctor or nurse.

Annual revision: 05/22/91

CYCLOPHOSPHAMIDE, VINCRISTINE, AND METHOTREXATE Systemic

This information applies to the following medicines:

Cyclophosphamide (sye-kloe-FOSS-fa-mide) (by injection)
Vincristine (vin-KRIS-teen) (by injection)
Methotrexate (meth-o-TREX-ate) (by injection)

Some commonly used brand names are:

For Cyclophosphamide

In the U.S.

Cytoxan
Neosar

Generic name product may also be available.

In Canada

Cytoxan
Procytox

For Vincristine

In the U.S.

Oncovin
Vincasar PFS
Vincrex

Generic name product may also be available.

In Canada

Oncovin

For Methotrexate

In the U.S.

Folex
Folex PFS
Mexate
Mexate-AQ

Generic name product may also be available.

In Canada

Generic name product available.

About Your Medicine

This combination therapy consists of three cancer medicines. They are used together to treat some kinds of cancer.

If any of the information causes you special concern or if you want additional information about your medicine and its use, check with your doctor, nurse, or pharmacist.

Before Using This Medicine

Discuss with your doctor the possible side effects that may be caused by this medicine. Some of them may be serious and/or long term.

Tell your doctor, nurse, and pharmacist if you. . .

- are allergic to any medicine, either prescription or nonprescription (OTC);
- are pregnant or intend to have children;

- are breast-feeding an infant;
- are taking *any* other prescription or nonprescription (OTC) medicine;
- have *any* other medical problems;
- have ever been treated with x-rays or cancer medicines.

Proper Use of This Medicine

While you are receiving these medicines, especially cyclophosphamide, it is important that you drink extra fluids so that you will pass more urine. Also, empty your bladder frequently, including at least once during the night. This will help prevent kidney and bladder problems and keep your kidneys working well. Some patients may have to drink up to 7 to 12 cups (3 quarts) of fluid a day. If you have any questions about this, check with your doctor.

Precautions

It is very important that your doctor check your progress at regular visits to make sure that these medicines are working properly and to check for unwanted effects.

Do not drink alcohol while using methotrexate. Alcohol can increase the chance of liver problems.

Do not take medicine for inflammation or pain without first checking with your doctor. These medicines may increase the effects of methotrexate, which could be harmful.

While you are being treated with these medicines, and after you stop treatment with them, *do not have any immunizations (vaccinations) without your doctor's approval.* Also, try to avoid people with infections.

If vincristine accidentally seeps out of the vein into which it is injected, it may damage some tissues and cause scarring. *Tell the doctor or nurse right away if you notice redness, pain, or swelling at the place of injection.*

Possible Side Effects

Side effects that should be reported *immediately:*

Black, tarry stools
Blood in urine or stools
Bloody vomit
Blurred or double vision
Confusion
Convulsions (seizures)
Cough or hoarseness
Diarrhea
Fever or chills
Lower back or side pain
Pain at place of injection
Painful or difficult urination
Pinpoint red spots on skin
Reddening of skin
Shortness of breath
Sores in mouth and on lips
Stomach pain
Swelling of feet and lower legs
Unusual bleeding or bruising

Side effects that should be reported as soon as possible:

Back pain
Bed-wetting
Constipation
Dark urine
Decrease or increase in urination
Difficulty in walking
Dizziness or agitation
Drooping eyelids
Drowsiness
Fast or irregular heartbeat
Hallucinations (seeing, hearing, or feeling things that are not there)
Headache
Jaw pain
Joint pain
Lack of sweating
Mental depression
Missing menstrual periods
Numbness, tingling, or pain in fingers and toes
Pain in testicles
Trouble in sleeping
Unusual thirst
Unusual tiredness or weakness
Yellow eyes or skin

Side effects that usually do not need medical attention (however, check with your doctor or nurse if they continue or are bothersome):

Acne
Bloating
Boils
Darkening of soles, palms, or nails
Flushing or redness of face
Increased sweating
Loss of appetite
Loss of hair
Nausea or vomiting
Pale skin
Skin rash, hives, or itching
Swollen lips

After you stop receiving these medicines, they may still produce some side effects that need attention. During this period of time, *check with your doctor or nurse immediately* if you notice:

Blood in urine

Other side effects not listed above may also occur in some patients. If you notice any other effects, check with your doctor or nurse.

Annual revision: 05/22/91

DOXORUBICIN AND CISPLATIN Systemic

This information applies to the following medicines:

Doxorubicin (dox-oh-ROO-bi-sin) (by injection)
Cisplatin (sis-PLA-tin) (by injection)

Some commonly used brand names are:

For Doxorubicin

In the U.S.

Adriamycin PFS
Adriamycin RDF
Rubex

Generic name product may also be available.

In Canada

Adriamycin PFS
Adriamycin RDF

For Cisplatin

In the U.S.

Platinol
Platinol-AQ

In Canada

Platinol
Platinol-AQ

Generic name product may also be available.

About Your Medicine

This combination therapy consists of two cancer medicines. They are used together to treat some kinds of cancer.

If any of the information causes you special concern or if you want additional information about your medicine and its use, check with your doctor, nurse, or pharmacist.

Before Using This Medicine

Discuss with your doctor the possible side effects that may be caused by this medicine. Some of them may be serious and/or long term.

Tell your doctor, nurse, and pharmacist if you. . .

- are allergic to any medicine, either prescription or nonprescription (OTC);
- are pregnant or intend to have children;
- are breast-feeding an infant;
- are taking *any* other prescription or nonprescription (OTC) medicine;
- have *any* other medical problems;
- have ever been treated with x-rays or cancer medicines.

Proper Use of This Medicine

While you are receiving these medicines, your doctor may want you to drink extra fluids so that you will pass more urine. This will help prevent kidney problems and keep your kidneys working well.

Precautions

It is very important that your doctor check your progress at regular visits to make sure that this medicine is working properly and to check for unwanted effects.

While you are being treated with these medicines, and after you stop treatment with them, *do not have any immunizations (vaccinations) without your doctor's approval.* Also, try to avoid people with infections.

If doxorubicin or cisplatin accidentally seeps out of the vein into which it is injected, it may damage some tissues and cause scarring. *Tell the doctor or nurse right away if you notice redness, pain, or swelling at the place of injection.*

Possible Side Effects

Side effects that should be reported *immediately*:

Black, tarry stools
Blood in urine or stools
Cough or hoarseness
Dizziness or faintness (shortly after a dose)
Fast or irregular heartbeat
Fever or chills
Lower back or side pain
Painful or difficult urination
Pinpoint red spots on skin
Shortness of breath
Swelling of face
Swelling of feet and lower legs
Unusual bleeding or bruising
Wheezing

Side effects that should be reported as soon as possible:

Agitation or confusion
Blurred or double vision
Change in ability to see colors (especially blue or yellow)
Convulsions (seizures)
Darkening or redness of skin (after x-ray treatment)
Decrease in urination
Joint pain
Loss of balance
Loss of reflexes
Loss of taste
Numbness, tingling, or pain in fingers and toes
Red streaks along injected vein
Ringing in ears
Skin rash or itching
Sores in mouth and on lips
Trouble in hearing
Trouble in walking
Unusual tiredness or weakness

Side effects that usually do not need medical attention (however, check with your doctor or nurse if they continue or are bothersome):

Darkening of soles, palms, or nails
Diarrhea

Loss of appetite
Loss of hair
Nausea or vomiting
Reddish urine

After you stop receiving these medicines, they may still produce some side effects that need attention. During this period of time, *check with your doctor or nurse immediately* if you notice:

Black, tarry stools
Blood in urine or stools
Cough or hoarseness
Decrease in urination
Fast or irregular heartbeat
Fever or chills
Loss of balance
Lower back or side pain
Painful or difficult urination
Pinpoint red spots on skin
Ringing in ears
Shortness of breath
Swelling of feet and lower legs
Trouble in hearing
Unusual bleeding or bruising

Other side effects not listed above may also occur in some patients. If you notice any other effects, check with your doctor or nurse.

Annual revision: 07/07/92

DOXORUBICIN and CYCLOPHOSPHAMIDE Systemic

This information applies to the following medicines:

Doxorubicin (dox-oh-ROO-bi-sin) (by injection)
Cyclophosphamide (sye-kloe-FOSS-fa-mide) (by injection or by mouth)

Some commonly used brand names are:

For Doxorubicin

In the U.S.

Adriamycin PFS
Adriamycin RDF
Rubex

Generic name product may also be available.

In Canada

Adriamycin PFS
Adriamycin RDF

For Cyclophosphamide

In the U.S.

Cytoxan
Neosar

Generic name product may also be available.

In Canada

Cytoxan
Procytox

About Your Medicine

This combination therapy consists of two cancer medicines. They are used together to treat some kinds of cancer, including breast cancer.

If any of the information causes you special concern or if you want additional information about your medicine and its use, check with your doctor, nurse, or pharmacist.

Before Using This Medicine

Discuss with your doctor the possible side effects that may be caused by this medicine. Some of them may be serious and/or long term.

Tell your doctor, nurse, and pharmacist if you. . .

- are allergic to any medicine, either prescription or nonprescription (OTC);
- are pregnant or intend to have children;
- are breast-feeding an infant;
- are taking *any* other prescription or nonprescription (OTC) medicine;
- have *any* other medical problems;
- have ever been treated with x-rays or cancer medicines.

Proper Use of This Medicine

While you are using these medicines, especially cyclophosphamide, it is important that you drink extra fluids so that you will pass more urine. Also, empty your bladder frequently, including at least once during the night. This will help prevent kidney and bladder problems and keep your kidneys working well. Some patients may have to drink up to 7 to 12 cups (3 quarts) of fluid a day. If you have any questions about this, check with your doctor.

If you are taking *cyclophosphamide by mouth:*

- If you vomit shortly after taking a dose of cyclophosphamide, check with your doctor. You will be told whether to take the dose again or to wait until the next scheduled dose.
- If you miss a dose of this medicine, do not take the missed dose at all and do not double the next one. Instead, go back to your regular dosing schedule and check with your doctor.

Precautions

It is very important that your doctor check your progress at regular visits to make sure that this medicine is working properly and to check for unwanted effects.

While you are being treated with these medicines, and after you stop treatment with them, *do not have any immunizations (vaccinations) without your doctor's approval.* Also, try to avoid people with infections.

If doxorubicin accidentally seeps out of the vein into which it is injected, it may damage some tissues and cause scarring. *Tell the doctor or nurse right away if you notice redness, pain, or swelling at the place of injection.*

Possible Side Effects

Side effects that should be reported *immediately*:

- Blood in urine
- Fast or irregular heartbeat
- Fever or chills
- Painful urination
- Shortness of breath
- Swelling of feet and lower legs
- Unusual bleeding or bruising
- Wheezing

Side effects that should be reported as soon as possible:

- Black, tarry stools
- Cough
- Darkening or redness of skin (after x-ray treatment)
- Decrease or increase in urination
- Dizziness, confusion, or agitation
- Joint pain
- Lower back, side, or stomach pain
- Missing menstrual periods
- Sores in mouth and on lips
- Unusual tiredness or weakness

Side effects that usually do not need medical attention (however, check with your doctor or nurse if they continue or are bothersome):

- Darkening of soles, palms, or nails
- Diarrhea
- Flushing or redness of face
- Headache
- Increased sweating
- Loss of appetite
- Loss of hair
- Nausea or vomiting
- Reddish urine
- Skin rash, hives, or itching
- Swollen lips

After you stop receiving these medicines, they may still produce some side effects that need attention. During this period of time, *check with your doctor or nurse immediately* if you notice:

- Blood in urine
- Fast or irregular heartbeat
- Shortness of breath
- Swelling of feet and lower legs

Other side effects not listed above may also occur in some patients. If you notice any other effects, check with your doctor or nurse.

Annual revision: 05/22/91

ETOPOSIDE AND CISPLATIN Systemic

This information applies to the following medicines:

Etoposide (e-TOE-poe-side) (by injection)
Cisplatin (sis-PLA-tin) (by injection)

Some commonly used brand names are:

For Etoposide

In the U.S. and Canada
VePesid

Another commonly used name is VP-16.

For Cisplatin

In the U.S.
Platinol
Platinol-AQ

In Canada
Platinol
Platinol-AQ

Generic name product may also be available.

About Your Medicine

This combination therapy consists of two cancer medicines. They are used together to treat some kinds of cancer.

If any of the information causes you special concern or if you want additional information about your medicine and its use, check with your doctor, nurse, or pharmacist.

Before Using This Medicine

Discuss with your doctor the possible side effects that may be caused by this medicine. Some of them may be serious and/or long term.

Tell your doctor, nurse, and pharmacist if you. . .

- are allergic to any medicine, either prescription or nonprescription (OTC);
- are pregnant or intend to have children;
- are breast-feeding an infant;
- are taking *any* other prescription or nonprescription (OTC) medicine;
- have *any* other medical problems;

- have ever been treated with x-rays or cancer medicines.

Proper Use of This Medicine

While you are receiving these medicines, your doctor may want you to drink extra fluids so that you will pass more urine. This will help prevent kidney problems and keep your kidneys working well.

These medicines often cause nausea, vomiting, and loss of appetite, which may be severe. However, it is very important that you continue to receive the medicines, even if you begin to feel ill. Ask your doctor, nurse, or pharmacist for ways to lessen these effects.

Precautions

It is very important that your doctor check your progress at regular visits to make sure that these medicines are working properly and to check for unwanted effects.

While you are being treated with these medicines, and after you stop treatment with them, *do not have any immunizations (vaccinations) without your doctor's approval.* Also, try to avoid people with infections.

Possible Side Effects

Side effects that should be reported *immediately*:

Black, tarry stools
Blood in urine or stools
Cough or hoarseness
Dizziness or faintness (shortly after a dose)
Fast heartbeat
Fever or chills
Lower back or side pain
Painful or difficult urination
Pinpoint red spots on skin
Redness, pain, or swelling at place of injection
Shortness of breath or wheezing
Swelling of face
Unusual bleeding or bruising

Side effects that should be reported as soon as possible:

Agitation or confusion
Blurred vision or change in ability to see colors (especially blue or yellow)
Convulsions (seizures)
Joint pain
Loss of balance
Loss of reflexes
Loss of taste
Numbness or tingling in fingers, toes, or face
Ringing in ears
Sores in mouth or on lips
Swelling of feet or lower legs
Trouble in hearing
Trouble in walking
Unusual tiredness or weakness

Side effects that usually do not need medical attention (however, check with your doctor or nurse if they continue or are bothersome):

Diarrhea
Loss of appetite
Loss of hair
Nausea and vomiting

After you stop receiving these medicines, they may still produce some side effects that need attention. During this period of time, *check with your doctor or nurse as soon as possible* if you notice:

Black, tarry stools
Blood in urine or stools
Cough or hoarseness
Decrease in urination
Fever or chills
Loss of balance
Lower back or side pain
Painful or difficult urination
Pinpoint red spots on skin
Ringing in ears
Swelling of feet or lower legs
Trouble in hearing
Unusual bleeding or bruising

Other side effects not listed above may also occur in some patients. If you notice any other effects, check with your doctor or nurse.

Annual revision: 07/07/92

FAC Systemic

This information applies to the following medicines:

Fluorouracil (flure-oh-YOOR-a-sill) (by injection)
Doxorubicin (dox-oh-ROO-bi-sin) (by injection)
Cyclophosphamide (sye-kloe-FOSS-fa-mide) (by injection)

Some commonly used brand names are:

For Fluorouracil

In the U.S. and Canada

Adrucil

Generic name product may also be available.

Another commonly used name is 5-FU.

For Doxorubicin

In the U.S.

Adriamycin PFS
Adriamycin RDF
Rubex

Generic name product may also be available.

In Canada

Adriamycin PFS
Adriamycin RDF

For Cyclophosphamide

In the U.S.

Cytoxan
Neosar

In Canada

Cytoxan
Procytox

About Your Medicine

This combination therapy consists of three cancer medicines. They are used together to treat breast cancer and some other kinds of cancer.

If any of the information causes you special concern or if you want additional information about your medicine and its use, check with your doctor, nurse, or pharmacist.

Before Using This Medicine

Discuss with your doctor the possible side effects that may be caused by this medicine. Some of them may be serious and/or long term.

Tell your doctor, nurse, and pharmacist if you. . .

- are allergic to any medicine, either prescription or nonprescription (OTC);
- are pregnant or intend to have children;
- are breast-feeding an infant;
- are taking *any* other prescription or nonprescription (OTC) medicine;
- have *any* other medical problems;
- have ever been treated with x-rays or cancer medicines.

Proper Use of This Medicine

While you are using these medicines, especially cyclophosphamide, it is important that you drink extra fluids so that you will pass more urine. Also, empty your bladder frequently, including at least once during the night. This will help prevent kidney and bladder problems and keep your kidneys working well. Some patients may have to drink up to 7 to 12 cups (3 quarts) of fluid a day. If you have any questions about this, check with your doctor.

Precautions

It is very important that your doctor check your progress at regular visits to make sure that these medicines are working properly and to check for unwanted effects.

While you are being treated with these medicines, and after you stop treatment with them, *do not have any immunizations (vaccinations) without your doctor's approval.* Also, try to avoid people with infections.

If doxorubicin accidentally seeps out of the vein into which it is injected, it may damage some tissues and cause scarring. *Tell the doctor or nurse right away if you notice redness, pain, or swelling at the place of injection.*

Possible Side Effects

Side effects that should be reported *immediately*:

Black, tarry stools
Blood in urine or stools
Cough or hoarseness
Diarrhea
Fast or irregular heartbeat
Fever or chills
Heartburn
Lower back or side pain
Nausea and vomiting (severe)
Pain at place of injection
Painful or difficult urination
Pinpoint red spots on skin
Shortness of breath
Sores in mouth and on lips
Stomach cramps
Swelling of feet and lower legs
Unusual bleeding or bruising
Wheezing

Side effects that should be reported as soon as possible:

Chest pain
Darkening or redness of skin (after x-ray treatment)
Dizziness, confusion, or agitation
Frequent urination
Joint pain
Missing menstrual periods
Red streaks along injected vein
Tingling of hands and feet, followed by pain, redness, and swelling

Trouble with balance
Unusual thirst
Unusual tiredness or weakness
Yellow eyes or skin

Side effects that usually do not need medical attention (however, check with your doctor or nurse if they continue or are bothersome):

Darkening of soles, palms, or nails
Flushing or redness of face
Headache
Increased sweating
Loss of appetite
Loss of hair
Nausea and vomiting
Reddish urine
Skin rash, hives, or itching
Swollen lips

After you stop receiving these medicines, they may still produce some side effects that need attention. During this period of time, *check with your doctor or nurse immediately* if you notice:

Black, tarry stools
Blood in urine or stools
Cough or hoarseness
Fast or irregular heartbeat
Fever or chills
Lower back or side pain
Painful or difficult urination
Pinpoint red spots on skin
Shortness of breath
Swelling of feet and lower legs
Unusual bleeding or bruising

Other side effects not listed above may also occur in some patients. If you notice any other effects, check with your doctor or nurse.

Annual revision: 07/07/92

FAM Systemic

This information applies to the following medicines:

Fluorouracil (flure-oh-YOOR-a-sill) (by injection)
Doxorubicin (dox-oh-ROO-bi-sin) (by injection)
Mitomycin (mye-toe-MYE-sin) (by injection)

Some commonly used brand names are:

For Fluorouracil

In the U.S. and Canada

Adrucil

Generic product may also be available.

Another commonly used name is 5-FU.

For Doxorubicin

In the U.S.

Adriamycin PFS
Adriamycin RDF
Rubex

Generic name product may also be available.

In Canada

Adriamycin PFS
Adriamycin RDF

For Mitomycin

In the U.S. and Canada

Mutamycin

About Your Medicine

This combination therapy consists of three cancer medicines. They are used together to treat stomach and pancreas cancer and some other kinds of cancer.

If any of the information causes you special concern or if you want additional information about your medicine and its use, check with your doctor, nurse, or pharmacist.

Before Using This Medicine

Discuss with your doctor the possible side effects that may be caused by this medicine. Some of them may be serious and/or long term.

Tell your doctor, nurse, and pharmacist if you. . .

- are allergic to any medicine, either prescription or nonprescription (OTC);
- are pregnant or intend to have children;
- are breast-feeding an infant;
- are taking *any* other prescription or nonprescription (OTC) medicine;
- have *any* other medical problems;
- have ever been treated with x-rays or cancer medicines.

Proper Use of This Medicine

While you are receiving these medicines, your doctor may want you to drink extra fluids so that you will pass more urine. This will help prevent kidney problems and keep your kidneys working well.

Precautions

It is very important that your doctor check your progress at regular visits to make sure that these medicines are working properly and to check for unwanted effects.

While you are being treated with these medicines, and after you stop treatment with them, *do not have any immunizations (vaccinations) without your doctor's approval.* Also, try to avoid people with infections.

If doxorubicin or mitomycin accidentally seeps out of the vein into which it is injected, it may damage some tissues and cause scarring. *Tell the doctor or nurse right away if you notice redness, pain, or swelling at the place of injection.*

Possible Side Effects

Side effects that should be reported *immediately*:

Black, tarry stools
Blood in urine or stools
Cough or hoarseness
Diarrhea
Fast or irregular heartbeat
Fever or chills
Heartburn
Lower back or side pain
Nausea and vomiting (severe)
Painful or difficult urination
Pain or redness at place of injection
Pinpoint red spots on skin
Shortness of breath
Stomach cramps
Swelling of feet and lower legs
Sores in mouth and on lips
Unusual bleeding or bruising
Wheezing

Side effects that should be reported as soon as possible:

Bloody vomit
Chest pain
Darkening or redness of skin (after x-ray treatment)
Decreased urination
Joint pain
Red streaks along injected vein
Tingling of hands and feet, followed by pain, redness, and swelling
Trouble with balance

Side effects that usually do not need medical attention (however, check with your doctor or nurse if they continue or are bothersome):

Darkening of soles, palms, or nails
Loss of appetite
Loss of hair
Nausea and vomiting
Numbness or tingling in fingers or toes
Reddish urine
Skin rash or itching
Unusual tiredness or weakness

After you stop receiving these medicines, they may still produce some side effects that need attention. During this period of time, *check with your doctor or nurse immediately* if you notice:

Black, tarry stools
Blood in urine or stools
Cough or hoarseness
Decreased urination
Fast or irregular heartbeat
Fever or chills
Lower back or side pain
Painful or difficult urination
Pinpoint red spots on skin
Shortness of breath
Swelling of feet and lower legs
Unusual bleeding or bruising

Other side effects not listed above may also occur in some patients. If you notice any other effects, check with your doctor or nurse.

Annual revision: 07/07/92

FLUOROURACIL AND CISPLATIN Systemic

This information applies to the following medicines:

Fluorouracil (flure-oh-YOOR-a-sill) (by injection)
Cisplatin (sis-PLA-tin) (by injection)

Some commonly used brand names are:

For Fluorouracil
In the U.S. and Canada
Adrucil
Generic name product may also be available.
Another commonly used name is 5-FU.

For Cisplatin
In the U.S.
Platinol
Platinol-AQ
In Canada
Platinol
Platinol-AQ
Generic name product may also be available.

About Your Medicine

This combination therapy consists of two cancer medicines. They are used together to treat some kinds of cancer.

If any of the information causes you special concern or if you want additional information about your medicine and its use, check with your doctor, nurse, or pharmacist.

Before Using This Medicine

Discuss with your doctor the possible side effects that may be caused by this medicine. Some of them may be serious and/or long term.

Tell your doctor, nurse, and pharmacist if you...

- are allergic to any medicine, either prescription or nonprescription (OTC);
- are pregnant or intend to have children;
- are breast-feeding an infant;
- are taking *any* other prescription or nonprescription (OTC) medicine;
- have *any* other medical problems;
- have ever been treated with x-rays or cancer medicines.

Proper Use of This Medicine

While you are receiving these medicines, your doctor may want you to drink extra fluids so that you will pass more urine. This will help prevent kidney problems and keep your kidneys working well.

These medicines often cause nausea and vomiting. However, it is very important that you continue to receive the medicines, even if you begin to feel ill. Ask your doctor, nurse, or pharmacist for ways to lessen these effects.

Precautions

It is very important that your doctor check your progress at regular visits to make sure that this medicine is working properly and to check for unwanted effects.

While you are being treated with these medicines, and after you stop treatment with them, *do not have any immunizations (vaccinations) without your doctor's approval.* Also, try to avoid people with infections.

If cisplatin accidentally seeps out of the vein into which it is injected, it may damage some tissues and cause scarring. *Tell the doctor or nurse right away if you notice redness, pain, or swelling at the place of injection.*

Possible Side Effects

Side effects that should be reported *immediately*:

Black, tarry stools
Blood in urine or stools
Cough or hoarseness
Diarrhea
Dizziness or faintness (shortly after a dose)
Fast heartbeat
Fever or chills
Heartburn
Lower back or side pain
Nausea and vomiting (severe)
Painful or difficult urination
Pinpoint red spots on skin
Sores in mouth and on lips
Stomach cramps
Swelling of face
Unusual bleeding or bruising
Wheezing

Side effects that should be reported as soon as possible:

Agitation or confusion
Blurred vision
Change in ability to see colors (especially blue or yellow)
Chest pain
Convulsions (seizures)
Joint pain
Loss of balance
Loss of reflexes
Loss of taste
Numbness or tingling in fingers, toes, or face
Shortness of breath
Swelling of feet or lower legs
Tingling of hands and feet, followed by pain, redness, and swelling
Trouble in hearing or ringing in ears
Trouble in walking
Unusual tiredness or weakness

Side effects that usually do not need medical attention (however, check with your doctor or nurse if they continue or are bothersome):

Loss of appetite
Loss of hair
Nausea and vomiting
Skin rash and itching

After you stop receiving these medicines, they may still produce some side effects that need attention. During this period of time, *check with your doctor or nurse immediately* if you notice:

Black, tarry stools
Blood in urine or stools
Cough or hoarseness
Decrease in urination
Fever or chills
Loss of balance
Lower back or side pain
Painful or difficult urination
Pinpoint red spots on skin
Ringing in ears
Swelling of feet or lower legs
Trouble in hearing
Unusual bleeding or bruising

Other side effects not listed above may also occur in some patients. If you notice any other effects, check with your doctor or nurse.

Annual revision: 07/07/92

FLUOROURACIL AND LEUCOVORIN Systemic

This information applies to the following medicines:

Fluorouracil (flure-oh-YOOR-a-sill) (by injection)
Leucovorin (loo-koe-VOR-in) (by injection)

Some commonly used brand names are:

For Fluorouracil

In the U.S. and Canada

Adrucil

Generic name product may also be available.

Another commonly used name is 5-FU.

For Leucovorin

In the U.S.

Wellcovorin

Generic name product may also be available.

In Canada

Generic name product available.

Other commonly used names are citrovorum factor and folinic acid.

About Your Medicine

This combination therapy consists of a cancer medicine plus leucovorin. They are given together to treat some kinds of cancer.

If any of the information causes you special concern or if you want additional information about your medicine and its use, check with your doctor, nurse, or pharmacist.

Before Using This Medicine

Discuss with your doctor the possible side effects that may be caused by this medicine. Some of them may be serious and/or long term.

Tell your doctor, nurse, and pharmacist if you...

- are allergic to any medicine, either prescription or nonprescription (OTC);
- are pregnant or intend to have children;
- are breast-feeding an infant;
- are taking *any* other prescription or nonprescription (OTC) medicine;
- have *any* other medical problems;
- have ever been treated with x-rays or cancer medicines.

Proper Use of This Medicine

Fluorouracil often causes nausea and vomiting. However, it is very important that you continue to receive the medicine, even if you begin to feel ill. Ask your doctor, nurse, or pharmacist for ways to lessen these effects.

Precautions

It is very important that your doctor check your progress at regular visits to make sure that this medicine is working properly and to check for unwanted effects.

While you are being treated with these medicines, and after you stop treatment with them, *do not have any immunizations (vaccinations) without your doctor's approval*. Also, try to avoid people with infections.

Possible Side Effects

Side effects that should be reported *immediately*:

Black, tarry stools
Blood in urine or stools
Cough or hoarseness
Diarrhea
Fever or chills
Heartburn
Lower back or side pain
Nausea and vomiting (severe)
Painful or difficult urination
Pinpoint red spots on skin
Skin rash, hives, or itching
Sores in mouth and on lips
Stomach cramps
Unusual bleeding or bruising
Wheezing

Side effects that should be reported as soon as possible:

Chest pain
Shortness of breath
Tingling of hands and feet, followed by pain, redness, and swelling
Trouble with balance

Side effects that usually do not need medical attention (however, check with your doctor or nurse if they continue or are bothersome):

Dry or cracked skin
Loss of appetite
Nausea and vomiting

After you stop receiving these medicines, they may still produce some side effects that need attention. During this period of time, *check with your doctor or nurse immediately* if you notice:

Black, tarry stools
Blood in urine or stools
Cough or hoarseness
Decrease in urination
Fever or chills
Loss of balance
Lower back or side pain

Painful or difficult urination
Pinpoint red spots on skin
Ringing in ears
Swelling of feet or lower legs
Trouble in hearing
Unusual bleeding or bruising

Other side effects not listed above may also occur in some patients. If you notice any other effects, check with your doctor or nurse.

Annual revision: 07/07/92

MACC Systemic

This information applies to the following medicines:
Methotrexate (meth-o-TREX-ate) (by injection)
Doxorubicin (dox-oh-ROO-bi-sin) (by injection)
Cyclophosphamide (sye-kloe-FOSS-fa-mide) (by injection)
Lomustine (loe-MUS-teen) (by mouth)

Some commonly used brand names are:

For Methotrexate
In the U.S.
Folex
Folex PFS
Mexate
Mexate-AQ
Generic name product may also be available.
In Canada
Generic name product available.

For Doxorubicin
In the U.S.
Adriamycin PFS
Adriamycin RDF
Rubex
Generic name product may also be available.
In Canada
Adriamycin PFS
Adriamycin RDF

For Cyclophosphamide
In the U.S.
Cytoxan
Neosar
Generic name product may also be available.
In Canada
Cytoxan
Procytox

For Lomustine
In the U.S. and Canada
CeeNU

Another commonly used name is CCNU.

About Your Medicine

This combination therapy consists of four cancer medicines. They are used together to treat some kinds of cancer.

If any of the information causes you special concern or if you want additional information about your medicine and its use, check with your doctor, nurse, or pharmacist.

Before Using This Medicine

Discuss with your doctor the possible side effects that may be caused by this medicine. Some of them may be serious and/or long term.

Tell your doctor, nurse, and pharmacist if you. . .

- are allergic to any medicine, either prescription or nonprescription (OTC);
- are pregnant or intend to have children;
- are breast-feeding an infant;
- are taking *any* other prescription or nonprescription (OTC) medicine;
- have *any* other medical problems;
- have ever been treated with x-rays or cancer medicines;
- smoke.

Proper Use of This Medicine

Use each of these medicines exactly as directed by your doctor. The exact amount of each medicine that you need and the best times to take each one have been carefully worked out. Ask your doctor, nurse, or pharmacist to help you plan a way to take each of your medicines at the right times.

In order that you receive the proper dose of lomustine, there may be two or more different types of capsules in the container. This is not an error. It is important that you take all of the capsules in the container as one dose so that you receive the right dose of the medicine.

While you are receiving these medicines, especially cyclophosphamide, it is important that you drink extra fluids so that you will pass more urine. Also, empty your bladder frequently, including at least once during the night. This will help prevent kidney and bladder problems and keep your kidneys working well. Some patients may have to drink up to 7 to 12 cups (3 quarts) of fluid a day. If you have any questions about this, check with your doctor.

If you vomit shortly after taking a dose of lomustine, check with your doctor. You may be told to take the dose again.

Precautions

It is very important that your doctor check your progress at regular visits to make sure that this medicine is working properly and to check for unwanted effects.

Do not drink alcohol while using methotrexate. Alcohol can increase the chance of liver problems.

Do not take medicine for inflammation or pain without first checking with your doctor. These medicines may increase the effects of methotrexate, which could be harmful.

While you are being treated with these medicines, and after you stop treatment with them, *do not have any immunizations (vaccinations) without your doctor's approval.* Also, try to avoid people with infections.

If doxorubicin accidentally seeps out of the vein into which it is injected, it may damage some tissues and cause scarring. *Tell the doctor or nurse right away if you notice redness, pain, or swelling at the place of injection.*

Possible Side Effects

Side effects that should be reported *immediately:*

- Black, tarry stools
- Blood in urine or stools
- Bloody vomit
- Blurred or double vision
- Confusion
- Convulsions (seizures)
- Cough or hoarseness
- Diarrhea
- Fast or irregular heartbeat
- Fever or chills
- Lower back or side pain
- Pain at place of injection
- Painful or difficult urination
- Pinpoint red spots on skin
- Reddening of skin
- Shortness of breath
- Sores in mouth and on lips
- Stomach pain
- Swelling of feet and lower legs
- Unusual bleeding or bruising
- Wheezing

Side effects that should be reported as soon as possible:

- Agitation
- Awkwardness
- Back pain
- Darkening or redness of skin (after x-ray treatment)
- Dark urine
- Dizziness
- Drowsiness
- Frequent urination
- Headache
- Jaw pain
- Joint pain
- Missing menstrual periods
- Red streaks along injected vein
- Slurred speech
- Unusual thirst
- Unusual tiredness or weakness
- Yellow eyes or skin

Side effects that usually do not need medical attention (however, check with your doctor or nurse if they continue or are bothersome):

- Acne
- Bloating
- Boils
- Darkening of soles, palms, or nails
- Flushing or redness of face
- Itching of skin
- Loss of appetite
- Loss of hair
- Nausea or vomiting
- Pale skin
- Reddish urine
- Skin rash or colored bumps on fingertips, elbows, or palms
- Sweating

After you stop receiving these medicines, they may still produce some side effects that need attention. During this period of time, *check with your doctor or nurse immediately* if you notice:

- Blood in urine
- Cough
- Fast or irregular heartbeat
- Shortness of breath
- Swelling of feet and lower legs

Other side effects not listed above may also occur in some patients. If you notice any other effects, check with your doctor or nurse.

Annual revision: 07/07/92

MACOP-B Systemic

This information applies to the following medicines:

- Methotrexate (meth-o-TREX-ate) (by injection)
- Leucovorin (loo-koe-VOR-in) (by mouth or injection)
- Doxorubicin (dox-oh-ROO-bi-sin) (by injection)
- Cyclophosphamide (sye-kloe-FOSS-fa-mide) (by injection)
- Vincristine (vin-KRIS-teen) (by injection)
- Prednisone (PRED-ni-sone) (by mouth)
- Bleomycin (blee-oh-MYE-sin) (by injection)

Some commonly used brand names are:

For Methotrexate

In the U.S.

Folex — Mexate
Folex PFS — Mexate-AQ

Generic name product may also be available.

In Canada

Generic name product available.

For Leucovorin
In the U.S.
Wellcovorin
Generic name product may also be available.
In Canada
Generic name product available.
Other commonly used names are citrovorum factor and folinic acid.

For Doxorubicin
In the U.S.
Adriamycin PFS
Adriamycin RDF
Rubex
Generic name product may also be available.
In Canada
Adriamycin PFS
Adriamycin RDF

For Cyclophosphamide
In the U.S.
Cytoxan
Neosar
Generic name product may also be available.
In Canada
Cytoxan
Procytox

For Vincristine
In the U.S.
Oncovin
Vincasar PFS
Vincrex
Generic name product may also be available.
In Canada
Oncovin

For Prednisone
In the U.S.
Deltasone
Liquid Pred
Meticorten
Orasone
Prednicen-M
Prednisone Intensol
Sterapred
Sterapred DS
Generic name product may also be available.
In Canada
Apo-Prednisone
Deltasone
Winpred
Generic name product may also be available.

For Bleomycin
In the U.S. and Canada
Blenoxane

About Your Medicine

This combination therapy consists of five cancer medicines (methotrexate, doxorubicin, cyclophosphamide, vincristine, bleomycin) and an adrenocorticoid (prednisone). They are used together to treat some lymphomas and some other kinds of cancer.

To prevent too much damage by methotrexate to normal cells, leucovorin is also given by mouth or injection as an antidote.

If any of the information causes you special concern or if you want additional information about your medicine and its use, check with your doctor, nurse, or pharmacist.

Before Using This Medicine

Discuss with your doctor the possible side effects that may be caused by this medicine. Some of them may be serious and/or long term.

Tell your doctor, nurse, and pharmacist if you. . .

- are allergic to any medicine, either prescription or nonprescription (OTC);
- are pregnant or intend to have children;
- are breast-feeding an infant;
- are taking *any* other prescription or nonprescription (OTC) medicine;
- have *any* other medical problems;
- have ever been treated with x-rays or cancer medicines;
- smoke.

Proper Use of This Medicine

Use each of these medicines exactly as directed by your doctor. The exact amount of each medicine that you need and the best times to take each one have been carefully worked out. Ask your doctor, nurse, or pharmacist to help you plan a way to take each of your medicines at the right times.

For patients *taking prednisone:*

- *Take prednisone with food* to help prevent stomach upset. If stomach upset, burning, or pain continues, check with your doctor.
- If you miss a dose of prednisone and you remember it within a few hours, take it as soon as you remember it. However, if several hours have passed or if it is almost time for the next dose, *check with your doctor*. Do not double doses.

For patients *taking leucovorin by mouth:*

- Leucovorin works best when there is a constant amount in the blood. *To help keep this amount constant, do not miss any doses. Also, it is best to take each dose at evenly spaced times day and night*. If this interferes with your sleep or other daily activities, or if you need help in planning the best times to take your medicine, check with your doctor, nurse, or pharmacist.
- If you vomit shortly after taking a dose of leucovorin, check with your doctor. You will be told whether to take the dose again or to wait until the next scheduled dose.

- If you miss a dose of leucovorin, *check with your doctor right away*. Your doctor may want you to take extra leucovorin to make up for what you missed. Do not take more medicine on your own, however, since it is very important that you receive the right dose at the right time.

While you are receiving these medicines, especially cyclophosphamide, it is important that you drink extra fluids so that you will pass more urine. Also, empty your bladder frequently, including at least once during the night. This will help prevent kidney and bladder problems and keep your kidneys working well. Some patients may have to drink up to 7 to 12 cups (3 quarts) of fluid a day. If you have any questions about this, check with your doctor.

Precautions

It is very important that your doctor check your progress at regular visits to make sure that this medicine is working properly and to check for unwanted effects.

Do not drink alcohol while using methotrexate. Alcohol can increase the chance of liver problems.

Do not take medicine for inflammation or pain without first checking with your doctor. These medicines may increase the effects of methotrexate, which could be harmful.

While you are being treated with these medicines, and after you stop treatment with them, *do not have any immunizations (vaccinations) without your doctor's approval.* Also, try to avoid people with infections.

If doxorubicin or vincristine accidentally seeps out of the vein into which it is injected, it may damage some tissues and cause scarring. *Tell the doctor or nurse right away if you notice redness, pain, or swelling at the place of injection.*

Possible Side Effects

Side effects that should be reported *immediately*:

Black, tarry stools
Blood in urine or stools
Bloody vomit
Blurred vision
Confusion
Convulsions (seizures)
Cough or hoarseness
Diarrhea
Faintness
Fast or irregular heartbeat
Fever or chills
Lower back or side pain
Pain at place of injection
Painful or difficult urination
Pinpoint red spots on skin
Reddening of skin
Shortness of breath
Sores in mouth and on lips
Stomach pain
Sweating
Swelling of feet and lower legs
Unusual bleeding or bruising
Wheezing

Side effects that should be reported as soon as possible:

Agitation
Back pain
Bed-wetting
Constipation
Darkening or redness of skin (after x-ray treatment)
Dark urine
Difficulty in walking
Dizziness
Double vision
Drooping eyelids
Drowsiness
Frequent urination
Hallucinations (seeing, hearing, or feeling things that are not there)
Headache
Jaw pain
Joint pain
Lack of sweating
Mental depression
Missing menstrual periods
Numbness, tingling, or pain in fingers and toes
Pain in testicles
Red streaks along injected vein
Unusual thirst
Unusual tiredness or weakness
Yellow eyes or skin

Side effects that usually do not need medical attention (however, check with your doctor or nurse if they continue or are bothersome):

Acne
Bloating
Boils
Darkening of soles, palms, or nails
Flushing or redness of face
Itching of skin
Loss of appetite
Loss of hair
Nausea or vomiting
Pale skin
Reddish urine
Skin rash or colored bumps on fingertips, elbows, or palms
Skin redness or tenderness
Swelling of fingers

After you stop receiving these medicines, they may still produce some side effects that need attention. During this period of time, *check with your doctor or nurse immediately* if you notice:

Blood in urine
Cough
Fast or irregular heartbeat
Shortness of breath
Swelling of feet and lower legs

Other side effects not listed above may also occur in some patients. If you notice any other effects, check with your doctor or nurse.

Annual revision: 05/22/91

M-BACOD Systemic

This information applies to the following medicines:

Methotrexate (meth-o-TREX-ate) (by injection)
Bleomycin (blee-oh-MYE-sin) (by injection)
Doxorubicin (dox-oh-ROO-bi-sin) (by injection)
Cyclophosphamide (sye-kloe-FOSS-fa-mide) (by injection)
Vincristine (vin-KRIS-teen) (by injection)
Dexamethasone (dex-a-METH-a-sone) (by mouth)

Some commonly used brand names are:

For Methotrexate

In the U.S.

Folex
Folex PFS
Mexate
Mexate-AQ

Generic name product may also be available.

In Canada

Generic name product available.

For Bleomycin

In the U.S. and Canada

Blenoxane

For Doxorubicin

In the U.S.

Adriamycin PFS
Adriamycin RDF
Rubex

Generic name product may also be available.

In Canada

Adriamycin PFS
Adriamycin RDF

For Cyclophosphamide

In the U.S.

Cytoxan
Neosar

Generic name product may also be available.

In Canada

Cytoxan
Procytox

For Vincristine

In the U.S.

Oncovin
Vincasar PFS
Vincrex

Generic name product may also be available.

In Canada

Oncovin

For Dexamethasone

In the U.S.

Decadron
Dexamethasone Intensol
Dexone
Hexadrol
Mymethasone

Generic name product may also be available.

In Canada

Deronil
Dexasone
Hexadrol
Oradexon

Generic name product may also be available.

About Your Medicine

This combination therapy consists of five cancer medicines (methotrexate, bleomycin, doxorubicin, cyclophosphamide, vincristine) and an adrenocorticoid (dexamethasone). They are used together to treat some lymphomas and some other kinds of cancer.

If any of the information causes you special concern or if you want additional information about your medicine and its use, check with your doctor, nurse, or pharmacist.

Before Using This Medicine

Discuss with your doctor the possible side effects that may be caused by this medicine. Some of them may be serious and/or long term.

Tell your doctor, nurse, and pharmacist if you...

- are allergic to any medicine, either prescription or nonprescription (OTC);
- are pregnant or intend to have children;
- are breast-feeding an infant;
- are taking *any* other prescription or nonprescription (OTC) medicine;
- have *any* other medical problems;
- have ever been treated with x-rays or cancer medicines;
- smoke.

Proper Use of This Medicine

Use each of these medicines exactly as directed by your doctor. The exact amount of each medicine that you need and the best times to take each one have been carefully worked out. Ask your doctor, nurse, or pharmacist to help you plan a way to take each of your medicines at the right times.

Take dexamethasone with food to help prevent stomach upset. If stomach upset, burning, or pain continues, check with your doctor.

While you are receiving these medicines, especially cyclophosphamide, it is important that you drink extra fluids so that you will pass more urine. Also, empty your bladder frequently, including at least once during the night. This will help prevent kidney and bladder problems and keep your kidneys working well. Some patients may have to drink up to 7 to 12 cups (3 quarts) of fluid a day. If you have any questions about this, check with your doctor.

If you miss a dose of dexamethasone and you remember it within a few hours, take it as soon as you remember it. However, if several hours have passed or if it is almost time for the next dose, *check with your doctor.* Do not double doses.

Precautions

It is very important that your doctor check your progress at regular visits to make sure that this medicine is working properly and to check for unwanted effects.

Do not drink alcohol while using methotrexate. Alcohol can increase the chance of liver problems.

Do not take medicine for inflammation or pain without first checking with your doctor. These medicines may increase the effects of methotrexate, which could be harmful.

While you are being treated with these medicines, and after you stop treatment with them, *do not have any immunizations (vaccinations) without your doctor's approval.* Also, try to avoid people with infections.

If doxorubicin or vincristine accidentally seeps out of the vein into which it is injected, it may damage some tissues and cause scarring. *Tell the doctor or nurse right away if you notice redness, pain, or swelling at the place of injection.*

Possible Side Effects

Side effects that should be reported *immediately*:

- Black, tarry stools
- Blood in urine or stools
- Bloody vomit
- Blurred vision
- Confusion
- Convulsions (seizures)
- Cough or hoarseness
- Diarrhea
- Faintness
- Fast or irregular heartbeat
- Fever or chills
- Lower back or side pain
- Pain at place of injection
- Painful or difficult urination
- Pinpoint red spots on skin
- Reddening of skin
- Shortness of breath
- Sores in mouth and on lips
- Stomach pain
- Sweating
- Swelling of feet and lower legs
- Unusual bleeding or bruising
- Wheezing

Side effects that should be reported as soon as possible:

- Agitation
- Back pain
- Bed-wetting
- Constipation
- Darkening or redness of skin (after x-ray treatment)
- Dark urine
- Difficulty in walking
- Dizziness
- Double vision
- Drooping eyelids
- Drowsiness
- Frequent urination
- Hallucinations (seeing, hearing, or feeling things that are not there)
- Headache
- Jaw pain
- Joint pain
- Lack of sweating
- Mental depression
- Missing menstrual periods
- Numbness, tingling, or pain in fingers and toes
- Pain in testicles
- Red streaks along injected vein
- Unusual thirst
- Unusual tiredness or weakness
- Yellow eyes or skin

Side effects that usually do not need medical attention (however, check with your doctor or nurse if they continue or are bothersome):

- Acne
- Bloating
- Boils
- Darkening of soles, palms, or nails
- Flushing or redness of face
- Itching of skin
- Loss of appetite
- Loss of hair
- Nausea or vomiting
- Pale skin
- Reddish urine
- Skin rash or colored bumps on fingertips, elbows, or palms
- Skin redness or tenderness
- Swelling of fingers

After you stop receiving these medicines, they may still produce some side effects that need attention. During this period of time, *check with your doctor or nurse immediately* if you notice:

Blood in urine
Cough
Fast or irregular heartbeat
Shortness of breath
Swelling of feet and lower legs

Other side effects not listed above may also occur in some patients. If you notice any other effects, check with your doctor or nurse.

Annual revision: 05/22/91

M-BACOP Systemic

This information applies to the following medicines:
- Methotrexate (meth-o-TREX-ate) (by injection)
- Leucovorin (loo-koe-VOR-in) (by mouth or injection)
- Bleomycin (blee-oh-MYE-sin) (by injection)
- Doxorubicin (dox-oh-ROO-bi-sin) (by injection)
- Cyclophosphamide (sye-kloe-FOSS-fa-mide) (by injection)
- Vincristine (vin-KRIS-teen) (by injection)
- Prednisone (PRED-ni-sone) (by mouth)

Some commonly used brand names are:

For Methotrexate

In the U.S.

Folex
Folex PFS
Mexate
Mexate-AQ

Generic name product may also be available.

In Canada

Generic name product available.

For Leucovorin

In the U.S.

Wellcovorin

Generic name product may also be available.

In Canada

Generic name product available.

Other commonly used names are citrovorum factor and folinic acid.

For Bleomycin

In the U.S. and Canada

Blenoxane

For Doxorubicin

In the U.S.

Adriamycin PFS
Adriamycin RDF
Rubex

Generic name product may also be available.

In Canada

Adriamycin PFS
Adriamycin RDF

For Cyclophosphamide

In the U.S.

Cytoxan
Neosar

Generic name product may also be available.

In Canada

Cytoxan
Procytox

For Vincristine

In the U.S.

Oncovin
Vincasar PFS
Vincrex

Generic name product may also be available.

In Canada

Oncovin

For Prednisone

In the U.S.

Deltasone
Liquid Pred
Meticorten
Orasone
Prednicen-M
Prednisone Intensol
Sterapred
Sterapred DS

Generic name product may also be available.

In Canada

Apo-Prednisone
Deltasone
Winpred

Generic name product may also be available.

About Your Medicine

This combination therapy consists of five cancer medicines (methotrexate, bleomycin, doxorubicin, cyclophosphamide, vincristine) and an adrenocorticoid (prednisone). They are used together to treat some kinds of cancer.

To prevent too much damage by methotrexate to normal cells, leucovorin is also given by mouth or injection as an antidote.

If any of the information causes you special concern or if you want additional information about your medicine and its use, check with your doctor, nurse, or pharmacist.

Before Using This Medicine

Discuss with your doctor the possible side effects that may be caused by this medicine. Some of them may be serious and/or long term.

Tell your doctor, nurse, and pharmacist if you. . .
- are allergic to any medicine, either prescription or nonprescription (OTC);
- are pregnant or intend to have children;
- are breast-feeding an infant;
- are taking *any* other prescription or nonprescription (OTC) medicine;
- have *any* other medical problems;
- have ever been treated with x-rays or cancer medicines;
- smoke.

Proper Use of This Medicine

Use each of these medicines exactly as directed by your doctor. The exact amount of each medicine that you need and the best times to take each one have been carefully worked out. Ask your doctor, nurse, or pharmacist to help you plan a way to take each of your medicines at the right times.

For patients *taking prednisone:*

- *Take prednisone with food* to help prevent stomach upset. If stomach upset, burning, or pain continues, check with your doctor.
- If you miss a dose of prednisone and you remember it within a few hours, take it as soon as you remember it. However, if several hours have passed or if it is almost time for the next dose, *check with your doctor.* Do not double doses.

For patients *taking leucovorin by mouth:*

- Leucovorin works best when there is a constant amount in the blood. *To help keep this amount constant, do not miss any doses. Also, it is best to take each dose at evenly spaced times day and night.* If this interferes with your sleep or other daily activities, or if you need help in planning the best times to take your medicine, check with your doctor, nurse, or pharmacist.
- If you vomit shortly after taking a dose of leucovorin, check with your doctor. You will be told whether to take the dose again or to wait until the next scheduled dose.
- If you miss a dose of leucovorin, *check with your doctor right away.* Your doctor may want you to take extra leucovorin to make up for what you missed. Do not take more medicine on your own, however, since it is very important that you receive the right dose at the right time.

While you are receiving these medicines, especially cyclophosphamide, it is important that you drink extra fluids so that you will pass more urine. Also, empty your bladder frequently, including at least once during the night. This will help prevent kidney and bladder problems and keep your kidneys working well. Some patients may have to drink up to 7 to 12 cups (3 quarts) of fluid a day. If you have any questions about this, check with your doctor.

Precautions

It is very important that your doctor check your progress at regular visits to make sure that this medicine is working properly and to check for unwanted effects.

Do not drink alcohol while using methotrexate. Alcohol can increase the chance of liver problems.

Do not take medicine for inflammation or pain without first checking with your doctor. These medicines may increase the effects of methotrexate, which could be harmful.

While you are being treated with these medicines, and after you stop treatment with them, *do not have any immunizations (vaccinations) without your doctor's approval.* Also, try to avoid people with infections.

If doxorubicin or vincristine accidentally seeps out of the vein into which it is injected, it may damage some tissues and cause scarring. *Tell the doctor or nurse right away if you notice redness, pain, or swelling at the place of injection.*

Possible Side Effects

Side effects that should be reported *immediately:*

Black, tarry stools
Blood in urine or stools
Bloody vomit
Blurred or double vision
Confusion
Convulsions (seizures)
Cough or hoarseness
Diarrhea
Faintness
Fast or irregular heartbeat
Fever or chills
Lower back or side pain
Pain at place of injection
Painful or difficult urination
Pinpoint red spots on skin
Reddening of skin
Shortness of breath
Sores in mouth and on lips
Stomach pain
Sweating
Swelling of feet and lower legs
Unusual bleeding or bruising
Wheezing

Side effects that should be reported as soon as possible:

Agitation
Back pain
Bed-wetting
Constipation
Dark urine
Difficulty in walking
Darkening or redness of skin (after x-ray treatment)
Dizziness
Drooping eyelids
Drowsiness
Frequent urination
Hallucinations (seeing, hearing, or feeling things that are not there)
Headache
Jaw pain
Joint pain
Lack of sweating
Mental depression

- Missing menstrual periods
- Numbness, tingling, or pain in fingers and toes
- Pain in testicles
- Red streaks along injected vein
- Unusual thirst
- Unusual tiredness or weakness
- Yellow eyes or skin

Side effects that usually do not need medical attention (however, check with your doctor or nurse if they continue or are bothersome):

- Acne
- Bloating
- Boils
- Darkening of soles, palms, or nails
- Flushing or redness of face
- Itching of skin
- Loss of appetite
- Loss of hair
- Nausea or vomiting
- Pale skin
- Reddish urine
- Skin rash or colored bumps on fingertips, elbows, or palms
- Skin redness or tenderness
- Swelling of fingers

After you stop receiving these medicines, they may still produce some side effects that need attention. During this period of time, *check with your doctor or nurse immediately* if you notice:

- Blood in urine
- Cough
- Fast or irregular heartbeat
- Shortness of breath
- Swelling of feet and lower legs

Other side effects not listed above may also occur in some patients. If you notice any other effects, check with your doctor or nurse.

Annual revision: 05/22/91

METHOTREXATE, High-dose, with LEUCOVORIN Rescue Systemic

This information applies to the following medicines:

Methotrexate (meth-o-TREX-ate) (by injection)
Leucovorin (loo-koe-VOR-in) (by mouth or injection)

Some commonly used brand names are:

For Methotrexate

In the U.S.

Folex — Mexate
Folex PFS — Mexate-AQ

Generic name product may also be available.

In Canada

Generic name product available.

For Leucovorin

In the U.S.

Wellcovorin

Generic name product may also be available.

In Canada

Generic name product available.

Other commonly used names are citrovorum factor and folinic acid.

About Your Medicine

Methotrexate belongs to the group of medicines known as antimetabolites. It is given in high doses by injection to treat some kinds of cancer.

To prevent too much damage by methotrexate to normal cells, leucovorin is also given by mouth or injection as an antidote.

If any of the information causes you special concern or if you want additional information about your medicine and its use, check with your doctor, nurse, or pharmacist.

Before Using This Medicine

Discuss with your doctor the possible side effects that may be caused by this medicine. Some of them may be serious and/or long term.

Tell your doctor, nurse, and pharmacist if you. . .

- are allergic to any medicine, either prescription or nonprescription (OTC);
- are pregnant or intend to have children;
- are breast-feeding an infant;
- are taking *any* other prescription or nonprescription (OTC) medicine;
- have *any* other medical problems;
- have ever been treated with x-rays or cancer medicines;
- drink alcohol.

Proper Use of This Medicine

For patients *taking leucovorin by mouth:*

- Leucovorin works best when there is a constant amount in the blood. *To help keep this amount constant, do not miss any doses. Also, it is best to take each dose at evenly spaced times day and night.* If this interferes with your sleep or other daily activities, or if you need help in planning the best times to take your medicine, check with your doctor, nurse, or pharmacist.

- If you vomit shortly after taking a dose of leucovorin, check with your doctor. You will be told whether to take the dose again or to wait until the next scheduled dose.
- If you miss a dose of leucovorin, *check with your doctor right away*. Your doctor may want you to take extra leucovorin to make up for what you missed. Do not take more medicine on your own, however, since it is very important that you receive the right dose at the right time.

Precautions

Do not drink alcohol while using methotrexate. Alcohol can increase the chance of liver problems.

Do not take medicine for inflammation or pain without first checking with your doctor. These medicines may increase the effects of methotrexate, which could be harmful.

While you are being treated with methotrexate, and after you stop treatment with it, *do not have any immunizations (vaccinations) without your doctor's approval*. Also, try to avoid people with infections.

Possible Side Effects

Side effects that should be reported *immediately*:

Black, tarry stools
Blood in urine or stools
Bloody vomit
Blurred vision
Confusion
Convulsions (seizures)
Cough or hoarseness
Diarrhea
Fever or chills
Lower back or side pain
Painful or difficult urination
Pinpoint red spots on skin
Reddening of skin
Shortness of breath
Sores in mouth and on lips
Stomach pain
Swelling of feet or lower legs
Unusual bleeding or bruising

Side effects that should be reported as soon as possible:

Back pain
Dark urine
Dizziness
Drowsiness
Headache
Joint pain
Unusual tiredness or weakness
Yellow eyes or skin

Side effects that usually do not need medical attention (however, check with your doctor or nurse if they continue or are bothersome):

Acne
Boils
Loss of appetite
Loss of hair
Nausea or vomiting
Pale skin
Skin rash or itching

After you stop using methotrexate, it may still produce some side effects that need attention. During this period of time, check with your doctor or nurse as soon as possible if you notice:

Back pain
Blurred vision
Confusion
Convulsions (seizures)
Dizziness
Drowsiness
Fever
Headache
Unusual tiredness or weakness

Other side effects not listed above may also occur in some patients. If you notice any other effects, check with your doctor or nurse.

Annual revision: 05/22/91

MOPP Systemic

This information applies to the following medicines:

Mechlorethamine (me-klor-ETH-a-meen) (by injection)
Vincristine (vin-KRIS-teen) (by injection)
Procarbazine (pro-KAR-ba-zeen) (by mouth)
Prednisone (PRED-ni-sone) (by mouth)

Some commonly used brand names are:

For Mechlorethamine
In the U.S. and Canada
Mustargen
Another commonly used name is nitrogen mustard.

For Vincristine
In the U.S.
Oncovin
Vincrex
Vincasar PFS
Generic name product may also be available.
In Canada
Oncovin

For Procarbazine
In the U.S.
Matulane
In Canada
Natulan

For Prednisone
In the U.S.

Deltasone	Prednicen-M
Liquid Pred	Prednisone Intensol
Meticorten	Sterapred
Orasone	Sterapred DS

Generic name product may also be available.

In Canada

Apo-Prednisone	Winpred
Deltasone	

Generic name product may also be available.

About Your Medicine

This combination therapy consists of three cancer medicines (mechlorethamine, procarbazine, vincristine) and an adrenocorticoid (prednisone). They are used together to treat Hodgkin's disease and some other kinds of cancer.

If any of the information causes you special concern or if you want additional information about your medicine and its use, check with your doctor, nurse, or pharmacist.

Before Using This Medicine

Discuss with your doctor the possible side effects that may be caused by this medicine. Some of them may be serious and/or long term.

Tell your doctor, nurse, and pharmacist if you. . .

- are allergic to any medicine, either prescription or nonprescription (OTC);
- are pregnant or intend to have children;
- are breast-feeding an infant;
- are taking *any* other prescription or nonprescription (OTC) medicine;
- have *any* other medical problems;
- have ever been treated with x-rays or cancer medicines;
- have recently had a heart attack or stroke.

Proper Use of This Medicine

Use each of these medicines exactly as directed by your doctor. The exact amount of each medicine that you need and the best times to take each one have been carefully worked out. Ask your doctor, nurse, or pharmacist to help you plan a way to take each of your medicines at the right times.

Take prednisone with food to help prevent stomach upset. If stomach upset, burning, or pain continues, check with your doctor.

While you are using this combination of medicines, it may be necessary to drink extra fluids so that you will pass more urine. This will help prevent kidney problems and keep your kidneys working well. Ask your doctor if this is necessary for you.

This combination of medicines commonly causes nausea and vomiting. Even if you begin to feel ill, *do not stop using these medicines without first checking with your doctor.* Ask your doctor, nurse, or pharmacist for ways to lessen these effects.

If you vomit shortly after taking a dose of prednisone or procarbazine, check with your doctor. You will be told whether to take the dose again or to wait until the next scheduled dose.

If you miss a dose of prednisone or procarbazine and you remember it within a few hours, take it as soon as you remember it. However, if several hours have passed or if it is almost time for the next dose, *check with your doctor.* Do not double doses.

Precautions

It is very important that your doctor check your progress at regular visits.

When taken with certain foods, drinks, or other medicines, procarbazine can cause very dangerous reactions. *To avoid such reactions:*

- Do not eat foods that have a high tyramine content (most common in foods that are aged or fermented to increase their flavor).
- Do not drink alcoholic beverages or alcohol-free or reduced-alcohol beer and wine.
- Do not eat or drink large amounts of caffeine-containing foods or beverages.
- Do not take any other medicine unless prescribed by your doctor, including OTC or nonprescription medicines.

After you stop using procarbazine you must continue to obey the above rules of caution for at least 2 weeks.

Procarbazine may cause some people to become drowsy or less alert than they are normally. *Make sure you know how you react to this medicine before you drive, use machines, or do anything else that could be dangerous if you are not alert.*

While you are receiving these medicines, and for several weeks after you stop treatment:

- *Do not have any immunizations (vaccinations) without your doctor's approval.* Also, try to avoid people with infections.
- If you are going to have surgery or emergency treatment, *tell the medical doctor or dentist in charge that you have been taking this medicine.*

Possible Side Effects

Side effects that should be reported *immediately*:

Black, tarry stools
Blood in urine or stools
Chest pain
Cough or hoarseness
Enlarged pupils of eyes
Fast or slow or irregular heartbeat
Fever or chills
Headache (severe)
Increased sensitivity of eyes to light
Increased sweating (possibly with fever or cold, clammy skin)
Lower back or side pain
Painful or difficult urination
Pain or redness at place of injection
Pinpoint red spots on skin
Stiff or sore neck
Unusual bleeding or bruising
Wheezing

Side effects that should be reported as soon as possible:

Confusion
Constipation
Convulsions (seizures)
Hallucinations (seeing, hearing, or feeling things that are not there)
Jaw pain
Missing menstrual periods
Numbness, tingling, or burning of fingers, toes, or face
Shortness of breath
Skin rash, hives, or itching
Sores in mouth and on lips
Stomach cramps
Unsteadiness or awkwardness
Weakness
Yellow eyes or skin

Side effects that usually do not need medical attention (however, check with your doctor or nurse if they continue or are bothersome):

Drowsiness
Increase in appetite
Indigestion
Loss of hair
Nausea and vomiting
Nervousness or restlessness
Trouble in sleeping

Other side effects not listed above may also occur in some patients. If you notice any other effects, check with your doctor or nurse.

Annual revision: 05/22/91

MVAC Systemic

This information applies to the following medicines:

Methotrexate (meth-o-TREX-ate) (by injection)
Vinblastine (vin-BLAS-teen) (by injection)
Doxorubicin (dox-oh-ROO-bi-sin) (by injection)
Cisplatin (sis-PLA-tin) (by injection)

Some commonly used brand names are:

For Methotrexate
In the U.S.
Folex
Folex PFS
Mexate
Mexate-AQ
Generic name product may also be available.
In Canada
Generic name product available.

For Vinblastine
In the U.S.
Velban
Velsar
Generic name product may also be available.
In Canada
Velbe

For Doxorubicin
In the U.S.
Adriamycin PFS
Adriamycin RDF
Rubex
Generic name product may also be available.
In Canada
Adriamycin PFS
Adriamycin RDF

For Cisplatin
In the U.S.
Platinol
Platinol-AQ
In Canada
Platinol
Platinol-AQ
Generic name product may also be available.

About Your Medicine

This combination therapy consists of four cancer medicines. They are used together to treat breast cancer and some other kinds of cancer.

If any of the information causes you special concern or if you want additional information about your medicine and its use, check with your doctor, nurse, or pharmacist.

Before Using This Medicine

Discuss with your doctor the possible side effects that may be caused by this medicine. Some of them may be serious and/or long term.

Tell your doctor, nurse, and pharmacist if you. . .

- are allergic to any medicine, either prescription or nonprescription (OTC);
- are pregnant or intend to have children;
- are breast-feeding an infant;
- are taking *any* other prescription or nonprescription (OTC) medicine;
- have *any* other medical problems;
- have ever been treated with x-rays or cancer medicines.

Proper Use of This Medicine

While you are receiving this combination of medicines, your doctor may want you to drink extra fluids so that you will pass more urine. This will help prevent kidney problems and keep your kidneys working well.

Precautions

It is very important that your doctor check your progress at regular visits to make sure that these medicines are working properly and to check for unwanted effects.

Do not drink alcohol while using methotrexate. Alcohol can increase the chance of liver problems.

Do not take medicine for inflammation or pain without first checking with your doctor. These medicines may increase the effects of methotrexate, which could be harmful.

While you are being treated with these medicines, and after you stop treatment with them, *do not have any immunizations (vaccinations) without your doctor's approval.* Also, try to avoid people with infections.

If doxorubicin or cisplatin accidentally seeps out of the vein into which it is injected, it may damage some tissues and cause scarring. *Tell the doctor or nurse right away if you notice redness, pain, or swelling at the place of injection.*

Possible Side Effects

Side effects that should be reported *immediately:*

Black, tarry stools
Blood in urine or stools
Bloody vomit
Blurred vision
Confusion
Convulsions (seizures)
Cough or hoarseness
Diarrhea
Dizziness or faintness (shortly after a dose)
Fast or irregular heartbeat
Fever or chills
Painful or difficult urination
Pain or redness at place of injection
Pinpoint red spots on skin
Reddening of skin
Shortness of breath or wheezing
Sores in mouth and on lips
Stomach pain
Swelling of face
Swelling of feet and lower legs
Unusual bleeding or bruising

Side effects that should be reported as soon as possible:

Back pain
Change in ability to see colors (especially blue or yellow)
Darkening or redness of skin (after x-ray treatment)
Dark urine
Dizziness or drowsiness
Double vision
Drooping eyelids
Headache
Jaw pain
Joint pain
Loss of balance
Loss of reflexes
Mental depression
Numbness or tingling in fingers, toes, or face
Pain in fingers and toes
Pain in testicles
Red streaks along injected vein
Ringing in ears
Trouble in hearing
Trouble in walking
Unusual tiredness or weakness
Yellow eyes or skin

Side effects that usually do not need medical attention (however, check with your doctor or nurse if they continue or are bothersome):

Loss of appetite
Loss of hair
Nausea and vomiting
Reddish urine

After you stop receiving these medicines, they may still produce some side effects that need attention. During this period of time, *check with your doctor or nurse immediately* if you notice:

Fast or irregular heartbeat
Shortness of breath
Swelling of feet and lower legs

Also, check with your doctor or nurse if you notice:

Black, tarry stools
Blood in urine or stools
Cough or hoarseness
Decrease in urination
Fever or chills
Loss of balance
Lower back or side pain

Painful or difficult urination
Pinpoint red spots on skin
Ringing in ears
Trouble in hearing
Unusual bleeding or bruising

Other side effects not listed above may also occur in some patients. If you notice any other effects, check with your doctor or nurse.

Annual revision: 07/07/92

MVCF Systemic

This information applies to the following medicines:

Mitomycin (mye-toe-MYE-sin) (by injection)
Vincristine (vin-KRIS-teen) (by injection)
Cisplatin (sis-PLA-tin) (by injection)
Fluorouracil (flure-oh-YOOR-a-sill) (by injection)

Some commonly used brand names are:

For Mitomycin
In the U.S. and Canada
Mutamycin

For Vincristine
In the U.S
Oncovin
Vincasar PFS
Vincrex
Generic name product may also be available.
In Canada
Oncovin

For Cisplatin
In the U.S.
Platinol
Platinol-AQ
In Canada
Platinol
Platinol-AQ
Generic name product may also be available.

For Fluorouracil
In the U.S. and Canada
Adrucil
Generic name product may also be available.

Another commonly used name is 5-FU.

About Your Medicine

This combination therapy consists of four cancer medicines. They are used together to treat some kinds of cancer.

If any of the information causes you special concern or if you want additional information about your medicine and its use, check with your doctor, nurse, or pharmacist.

Before Using This Medicine

Discuss with your doctor the possible side effects that may be caused by this medicine. Some of them may be serious and/or long term.

Tell your doctor, nurse, and pharmacist if you. . .

- are allergic to any medicine, either prescription or nonprescription (OTC);
- are pregnant or intend to have children;
- are breast-feeding an infant;
- are taking *any* other prescription or nonprescription (OTC) medicine;
- have *any* other medical problems;
- have ever been treated with x-rays or cancer medicines.

Proper Use of This Medicine

While you are receiving these medicines, your doctor may want you to drink extra fluids so that you will pass more urine. This will help prevent kidney problems and keep your kidneys working well.

These medicines often cause nausea and vomiting. However, it is very important that you continue to receive the medicines, even if you begin to feel ill. Ask your doctor, nurse, or pharmacist for ways to lessen these effects.

Precautions

It is very important that your doctor check your progress at regular visits to make sure that this medicine is working properly and to check for unwanted effects.

While you are being treated with these medicines, and after you stop treatment with them, *do not have any immunizations (vaccinations) without your doctor's approval.* Also, try to avoid people with infections.

If mitomycin, vincristine, or cisplatin accidentally seeps out of the vein into which it is injected, it may damage some tissues and cause scarring. *Tell the doctor or nurse right away if you notice redness, pain, or swelling at the place of injection.*

Possible Side Effects

Side effects that should be reported *immediately:*

Black, tarry stools
Blood in urine or stools
Cough or hoarseness
Diarrhea

- Dizziness or faintness (shortly after a dose of cisplatin)
- Fast heartbeat
- Fever or chills
- Heartburn
- Lower back or side pain
- Nausea and vomiting (severe)
- Painful or difficult urination
- Pinpoint red spots on skin
- Sores in mouth and on lips
- Stomach cramps
- Swelling of face
- Unusual bleeding or bruising
- Wheezing

Side effects that should be reported as soon as possible:

- Agitation or confusion
- Bed-wetting
- Blurred or double vision
- Change in ability to see colors (especially blue or yellow)
- Chest pain
- Constipation
- Convulsions (seizures)
- Decrease or increase in urination
- Dizziness
- Drooping eyelids
- Headache or jaw pain
- Joint pain
- Loss of appetite or taste
- Loss of balance
- Loss of reflexes
- Mental depression
- Numbness or tingling in fingers, toes, or face
- Pain in fingers and toes
- Pain in testicles
- Shortness of breath
- Swelling of feet or lower legs
- Tingling of hands and feet, followed by pain, redness, and swelling
- Trouble in hearing or ringing in ears
- Trouble in sleeping
- Trouble in walking
- Unusual tiredness or weakness

Side effects that usually do not need medical attention (however, check with your doctor or nurse if they continue or are bothersome):

- Bloating
- Loss of hair
- Loss of weight
- Nausea and vomiting
- Purple-colored bands on nails
- Skin rash and itching

After you stop receiving these medicines, they may still produce some side effects that need attention. During this period of time, *check with your doctor or nurse immediately* if you notice:

- Black, tarry stools
- Blood in urine or stools
- Cough or hoarseness
- Decrease in urination
- Fever or chills
- Loss of balance
- Lower back or side pain
- Painful or difficult urination
- Pinpoint red spots on skin
- Ringing in ears
- Shortness of breath
- Swelling of feet or lower legs
- Trouble in hearing
- Unusual bleeding or bruising

Other side effects not listed above may also occur in some patients. If you notice any other effects, check with your doctor or nurse.

Annual revision: 07/07/92

PEB Systemic

This information applies to the following medicines:

- Cisplatin (sis-PLA-tin) (by injection)
- Etoposide (e-TOE-poe-side) (by injection)
- Bleomycin (blee-oh-MYE-sin) (by injection)

Some commonly used brand names are:

For Cisplatin

In the U.S.
Platinol
Platinol-AQ

In Canada
Platinol
Platinol-AQ

Generic name product may also be available.

For Etoposide

In the U.S. and Canada
VePesid

Another commonly used name is VP-16.

For Bleomycin

In the U.S. and Canada
Blenoxane

About Your Medicine

This combination therapy consists of three cancer medicines. They are used together to treat some kinds of cancer.

If any of the information causes you special concern or if you want additional information about your medicine and its use, check with your doctor, nurse, or pharmacist.

Before Using This Medicine

Discuss with your doctor the possible side effects that may be caused by this medicine. Some of them may be serious and/or long term.

Tell your doctor, nurse, and pharmacist if you. . .

- are allergic to any medicine, either prescription or nonprescription (OTC);
- are pregnant or intend to have children;
- are breast-feeding an infant;
- are taking *any* other prescription or nonprescription (OTC) medicine;
- have *any* other medical problems;
- have ever been treated with x-rays or cancer medicines;
- smoke.

Proper Use of This Medicine

While you are receiving these medicines, your doctor may want you to drink extra fluids so that you will pass more urine. This will help prevent kidney problems and keep your kidneys working well.

These medicines often cause nausea, vomiting, and loss of appetite, which may be severe. However, it is very important that you continue to receive the medicines, even if you begin to feel ill. Ask your doctor, nurse, or pharmacist for ways to lessen these effects.

Precautions

It is very important that your doctor check your progress at regular visits to make sure that these medicines are working properly and to check for unwanted effects.

While you are being treated with these medicines, and after you stop treatment with them, *do not have any immunizations (vaccinations) without your doctor's approval.* Also, try to avoid people with infections.

Possible Side Effects

Side effects that should be reported *immediately:*

Black, tarry stools
Blood in urine or stools
Confusion
Cough or hoarseness
Faintness
Fast heartbeat
Fever or chills
Lower back or side pain
Painful or difficult urination
Pinpoint red spots on skin
Redness, pain, or swelling at place of injection
Shortness of breath or wheezing
Sweating
Swelling of face
Unusual bleeding or bruising

Side effects that should be reported as soon as possible:

Agitation or confusion
Blurred vision or change in ability to see colors (especially blue or yellow)
Convulsions (seizures)
Joint pain
Loss of balance
Loss of reflexes
Loss of taste
Numbness or tingling in fingers, toes, or face
Ringing in ears
Sores in mouth or on lips
Swelling of feet or lower legs
Trouble in hearing
Trouble in walking
Unusual tiredness or weakness

Side effects that usually do not need medical attention (however, check with your doctor or nurse if they continue or are bothersome):

Darkening or thickening of skin
Diarrhea
Itching of skin
Loss of appetite
Loss of hair
Nausea and vomiting
Skin rash or colored bumps on fingertips, elbows, or palms
Skin redness or tenderness
Swelling of fingers

After you stop receiving these medicines, they may still produce some side effects that need attention. During this period of time, *check with your doctor or nurse as soon as possible* if you notice:

Black, tarry stools
Blood in urine or stools
Cough or hoarseness
Decrease in urination
Fever or chills
Loss of balance
Lower back or side pain
Painful or difficult urination
Pinpoint red spots on skin
Ringing in ears
Shortness of breath
Swelling of feet or lower legs
Trouble in hearing
Unusual bleeding or bruising

Other side effects not listed above may also occur in some patients. If you notice any other effects, check with your doctor or nurse.

Annual revision: 07/07/92

ProMACE and CytaBOM Systemic

This information applies to the following medicines:

Prednisone (PRED-ni-sone) (by mouth)
Methotrexate (meth-o-TREX-ate) (by injection)
Leucovorin (loo-koe-VOR-in) (by mouth or injection)
Doxorubicin (dox-oh-ROO-bi-sin) (by injection)
Cyclophosphamide (sye-kloe-FOSS-fa-mide) (by injection)
Etoposide (e-TOE-po-side) (by injection)
Vincristine (vin-KRIS-teen) (by injection)
Bleomycin (blee-oh-MYE-sin) (by injection)

Some commonly used brand names are:

For Prednisone

In the U.S.

Deltasone
Liquid Pred
Meticorten
Orasone
Prednicen-M
Prednisone Intensol
Sterapred
Sterapred DS

Generic name product may also be available.

In Canada

Apo-Prednisone
Deltasone
Winpred

Generic name product may also be available.

For Methotrexate

In the U.S.

Folex
Folex PFS
Mexate
Mexate-AQ

Generic name product may also be available.

In Canada

Generic name product available.

For Leucovorin

In the U.S.

Wellcovorin

Generic name product may also be available.

In Canada

Generic name product available.

Other commonly used names are citrovorum factor and folinic acid.

For Doxorubicin

In the U.S.

Adriamycin PFS
Adriamycin RDF
Rubex

Generic name product may also be available.

In Canada

Adriamycin PFS
Adriamycin RDF

For Cyclophosphamide

In the U.S.

Cytoxan
Neosar

Generic name product may also be available.

In Canada

Cytoxan
Procytox

For Etoposide

In the U.S. and Canada

VePesid

For Vincristine

In the U.S.

Oncovin
Vincasar PFS
Vincrex

Generic name product may also be available.

In Canada

Oncovin

For Bleomycin

In the U.S. and Canada

Blenoxane

About Your Medicine

This combination therapy consists of six cancer medicines (methotrexate, doxorubicin, cyclophosphamide, etoposide, vincristine, bleomycin) and an adrenocorticoid (prednisone). They are used together to treat some lymphomas and some other kinds of cancer.

To prevent too much damage by methotrexate to normal cells, leucovorin is also given by mouth or injection as an antidote.

If any of the information causes you special concern or if you want additional information about your medicine and its use, check with your doctor, nurse, or pharmacist.

Before Using This Medicine

Discuss with your doctor the possible side effects that may be caused by this medicine. Some of them may be serious and/or long term.

Tell your doctor, nurse, and pharmacist if you. . .

- are allergic to any medicine, either prescription or nonprescription (OTC);
- are pregnant or intend to have children;
- are breast-feeding an infant;
- are taking *any* other prescription or nonprescription (OTC) medicine;
- have *any* other medical problems;
- have ever been treated with x-rays or cancer medicines;
- smoke.

Proper Use of This Medicine

Use each of these medicines exactly as directed by your doctor. The exact amount of each medicine that you need and the best times to take each one have been carefully worked out. Ask your doctor, nurse, or pharmacist to help you plan a way to take each of your medicines at the right times.

For patients *taking prednisone:*

- *Take prednisone with food* to help prevent stomach upset. If stomach upset, burning, or pain continues, check with your doctor.
- If you miss a dose of prednisone and you remember it within a few hours, take it as soon as you remember it. However, if several hours have passed or if it is

almost time for the next dose, *check with your doctor.* Do not double doses.

For patients *taking leucovorin by mouth:*

- Leucovorin works best when there is a constant amount in the blood. *To help keep this amount constant, do not miss any doses. Also, it is best to take each dose at evenly spaced times day and night.* If this interferes with your sleep or other daily activities, or if you need help in planning the best times to take your medicine, check with your doctor, nurse, or pharmacist.
- If you vomit shortly after taking a dose of leucovorin, check with your doctor. You will be told whether to take the dose again or to wait until the next scheduled dose.
- If you miss a dose of leucovorin, *check with your doctor right away.* Your doctor may want you to take extra leucovorin to make up for what you missed. Do not take more medicine on your own, however, since it is very important that you receive the right dose at the right time.

While you are receiving these medicines, especially cyclophosphamide, it is important that you drink extra fluids so that you will pass more urine. Also, empty your bladder frequently, including at least once during the night. This will help prevent kidney and bladder problems and keep your kidneys working well. Some patients may have to drink up to 7 to 12 cups (3 quarts) of fluid a day. If you have any questions about this, check with your doctor.

Precautions

It is very important that your doctor check your progress at regular visits to make sure that this medicine is working properly and to check for unwanted effects.

Do not drink alcohol while using methotrexate. Alcohol can increase the chance of liver problems.

Do not take medicine for inflammation or pain without first checking with your doctor. These medicines may increase the effects of methotrexate, which could be harmful.

While you are being treated with these medicines, and after you stop treatment with them, *do not have any immunizations (vaccinations) without your doctor's approval.* Also, try to avoid people with infections.

If doxorubicin or vincristine accidentally seeps out of the vein into which it is injected, it may damage some tissues and cause scarring. *Tell the doctor or nurse right away if you notice redness, pain, or swelling at the place of injection.*

Possible Side Effects

Side effects that should be reported *immediately*:

Black, tarry stools
Blood in urine or stools
Bloody vomit
Blurred vision
Confusion
Convulsions (seizures)
Cough or hoarseness
Diarrhea
Faintness
Fast or irregular heartbeat
Fever or chills
Lower back or side pain
Pain at place of injection
Painful or difficult urination
Pinpoint red spots on skin
Reddening of skin
Shortness of breath
Sores in mouth and on lips
Stomach pain
Sweating
Swelling of feet and lower legs
Unusual bleeding or bruising
Wheezing

Side effects that should be reported as soon as possible:

Agitation
Back pain
Bed-wetting
Constipation
Darkening or redness of skin (after x-ray treatment)
Dark urine
Difficulty in walking
Dizziness
Double vision
Drooping eyelids
Drowsiness
Frequent urination
Hallucinations (seeing, hearing, or feeling things that are not there)
Headache
Jaw pain
Joint pain
Lack of sweating
Mental depression
Missing menstrual periods
Numbness, tingling, or pain in fingers and toes
Pain in testicles
Red streaks along injected vein
Unusual thirst
Unusual tiredness or weakness
Yellow eyes or skin

Side effects that usually do not need medical attention (however, check with your doctor or nurse if they continue or are bothersome):

Acne
Bloating
Boils
Darkening of soles, palms, or nails

Flushing or redness of face
Itching of skin
Loss of appetite
Loss of hair
Nausea or vomiting
Pale skin
Reddish urine
Skin rash or colored bumps on fingertips, elbows, or palms
Skin redness or tenderness
Swelling of fingers

After you stop receiving these medicines, they may still produce some side effects that need attention. During this period of time, *check with your doctor or nurse immediately* if you notice:

Blood in urine
Cough
Fast or irregular heartbeat
Shortness of breath
Swelling of feet and lower legs

Other side effects not listed above may also occur in some patients. If you notice any other effects, check with your doctor or nurse.

Annual revision: 05/22/91

PVB Systemic

This information applies to the following medicines:

Cisplatin (sis-PLA-tin) (by injection)
Vinblastine (vin-BLAS-teen) (by injection)
Bleomycin (blee-oh-MYE-sin) (by injection)

Some commonly used brand names are:

For Cisplatin
In the U.S.
Platinol
Platinol-AQ
In Canada
Platinol
Platinol-AQ
Generic name product may also be available.

For Vinblastine
In the U.S.
Velban
Velsar
Generic name product may also be available.
In Canada
Velbe

For Bleomycin
In the U.S. and Canada
Blenoxane

About Your Medicine

This combination therapy consists of three cancer medicines. They are used to treat some kinds of cancer.

If any of the information causes you special concern or if you want additional information about your medicine and its use, check with your doctor, nurse, or pharmacist.

Before Using This Medicine

Discuss with your doctor the possible side effects that may be caused by this medicine. Some of them may be serious and/or long term.

Tell your doctor, nurse, and pharmacist if you. . .

- are allergic to any medicine, either prescription or nonprescription (OTC);
- are pregnant or intend to have children;
- are breast-feeding an infant;
- are taking *any* other prescription or nonprescription (OTC) medicine;
- have *any* other medical problems;
- have ever been treated with x-rays or cancer medicines;
- smoke.

Proper Use of This Medicine

While you are receiving this medicine, your doctor may want you to drink extra fluids so that you will pass more urine. This will help prevent kidney problems and keep your kidneys working well.

These medicines often cause nausea and vomiting. However, it is very important that you continue to receive the medicines, even if you begin to feel ill. Ask your doctor, nurse, or pharmacist for ways to lessen these effects.

Precautions

It is very important that your doctor check your progress at regular visits to make sure that this medicine is working properly and to check for unwanted effects.

While you are being treated with these medicines, and for several weeks after you stop treatment with them, *do not have any immunizations (vaccinations) without your doctor's approval.* Also, try to avoid people with infections.

If cisplatin or vinblastine accidentally seeps out of the vein into which it is injected, it may damage some tissues and cause scarring. *Tell the doctor or nurse right away if you notice redness, pain, or swelling at the place of injection.*

Possible Side Effects

Side effects that should be reported *immediately:*

Black, tarry stools
Blood in urine or stools
Confusion
Cough or hoarseness
Dizziness or faintness (shortly after a dose of cisplatin)
Faintness
Fast heartbeat
Fever or chills
Lower back or side pain
Painful or difficult urination
Pinpoint red spots on skin
Sweating
Swelling of face
Unusual bleeding or bruising
Wheezing

Side effects that should be reported as soon as possible:

Blurred or double vision
Change in ability to see colors
Chest pain
Convulsions (seizures)
Dizziness
Drooping eyelids
Headache or jaw pain
Joint pain
Loss of balance
Loss of reflexes
Loss of taste
Mental depression
Numbness or tingling in fingers, toes, or face
Pain in fingers and toes
Pain in testicles
Shortness of breath
Sores in mouth and on lips
Swelling of feet or lower legs
Trouble in hearing or ringing in ears
Trouble in walking
Unusual tiredness or weakness

Side effects that usually do not need medical attention (however, check with your doctor or nurse if they continue or are bothersome):

Darkening or thickening of skin
Itching of skin
Loss of appetite
Loss of hair
Muscle pain
Nausea and vomiting
Skin rash or colored bumps on fingertips, elbows, or palms
Skin redness or tenderness
Swelling of fingers

After you stop receiving these medicines, they may still produce some side effects that need attention. During this period of time, *check with your doctor or nurse immediately* if you notice:

Black, tarry stools
Blood in urine or stools
Cough or hoarseness
Decrease in urination
Fever or chills
Loss of balance
Lower back or side pain
Painful or difficult urination
Pinpoint red spots on skin
Ringing in ears
Shortness of breath
Swelling of feet or lower legs
Trouble in hearing
Unusual bleeding or bruising

Other side effects not listed above may also occur in some patients. If you notice any other effects, check with your doctor or nurse.

Annual revision: 07/07/92

TMF Systemic

This information applies to the following medicines:

Thiotepa (thye-oh-TEP-a) (by injection)
Methotrexate (meth-o-TREX-ate) (by injection)
Fluorouracil (flure-oh-YOOR-a-sill) (by injection)

Some commonly used brand names are:

For Thiotepa

In the U.S. and Canada

Generic name product available.

For Methotrexate

In the U.S.

Folex
Folex PFS
Mexate
Mexate-AQ

Generic name product may also be available.

In Canada

Generic name product available.

For Fluorouracil
In the U.S. and Canada
Adrucil
Generic name product may also be available.
Another commonly used name is 5-FU.

About Your Medicine

This combination therapy consists of three cancer medicines. They are used together to treat breast cancer and some other kinds of cancer.

If any of the information causes you special concern or if you want additional information about your medicine and its use, check with your doctor, nurse, or pharmacist.

Before Using This Medicine

Discuss with your doctor the possible side effects that may be caused by this medicine. Some of them may be serious and/or long term.

Tell your doctor, nurse, and pharmacist if you. . .

- are allergic to any medicine, either prescription or nonprescription (OTC);
- are pregnant or intend to have children;
- are breast-feeding an infant;
- are taking *any* other prescription or nonprescription (OTC) medicine;
- have *any* other medical problems;
- have ever been treated with x-rays or cancer medicines.

Proper Use of This Medicine

While you are using these medicines, it may be necessary that you drink extra fluids so that you will pass more urine. This will help prevent kidney problems and keep your kidneys working well. If you have any questions about this, check with your doctor.

Precautions

It is very important that your doctor check your progress at regular visits to make sure that these medicines are working properly and to check for unwanted effects.

Do not drink alcohol while using methotrexate. Alcohol can increase the chance of liver problems.

Do not take medicine for inflammation or pain without first checking with your doctor. These medicines may increase the effects of methotrexate, which could be harmful.

While you are being treated with these medicines, and after you stop treatment with them, *do not have any immunizations (vaccinations) without your doctor's approval.* Also, try to avoid people with infections.

Possible Side Effects

Side effects that should be reported *immediately:*

Black, tarry stools
Blood in urine or stools
Bloody vomit
Blurred vision
Confusion
Convulsions (seizures)
Cough or hoarseness
Diarrhea
Fever or chills
Lower back or side pain
Nausea and vomiting (severe)
Painful or difficult urination
Pinpoint red spots on skin
Reddening of skin
Shortness of breath
Skin rash
Sores in mouth and on lips
Stomach pain
Swelling of feet or lower legs
Tightness of throat
Unusual bleeding or bruising
Wheezing

Side effects that should be reported as soon as possible:

Back pain
Dark urine
Dizziness, confusion, or agitation
Drowsiness
Headache
Joint pain
Redness, swelling, or pain at place of injection
Tingling of hands and feet, followed by pain, redness, and swelling
Trouble with balance
Unusual tiredness or weakness
Yellow eyes or skin

Side effects that usually do not need medical attention (however, check with your doctor or nurse if they continue or are bothersome):

Acne
Boils
Loss of appetite
Loss of hair
Nausea or vomiting
Pale skin

After you stop receiving these medicines, they may still produce some side effects that need attention. During this period of time, *check with your doctor or nurse immediately* if you notice:

Black, tarry stools
Blood in urine or stools
Cough or hoarseness

Fever or chills
Lower back or side pain
Painful or difficult urination
Pinpoint red spots on skin
Unusual bleeding or bruising

Other side effects not listed above may also occur in some patients. If you notice any other effects, check with your doctor or nurse.

Annual revision: 07/07/92

VAC Systemic

This information applies to the following medicines:

Dactinomycin (dak-ti-noe-MYE-sin) (by injection)
Cyclophosphamide (sye-kloe-FOSS-fa-mide) (by mouth)
Vincristine (vin-KRIS-teen) (by injection)

Some commonly used brand names are:

For Vincristine

In the U.S.

Oncovin
Vincasar PFS
Vincrex

Generic name product may also be available.

In Canada

Oncovin

For Dactinomycin

In the U.S. and Canada

Cosmegen

Another commonly used name is actinomycin-D.

For Cyclophosphamide

In the U.S.

Cytoxan

In Canada

Cytoxan
Procytox

About Your Medicine

This combination therapy consists of three cancer medicines. They are used together to treat some kinds of cancer.

If any of the information causes you special concern or if you want additional information about your medicine and its use, check with your doctor, nurse, or pharmacist.

Before Using This Medicine

Discuss with your doctor the possible side effects that may be caused by this medicine. Some of them may be serious and/or long term.

Tell your doctor, nurse, and pharmacist if you. . .

- are allergic to any medicine, either prescription or nonprescription (OTC);
- are pregnant or intend to have children;
- are breast-feeding an infant;
- are taking *any* other prescription or nonprescription (OTC) medicine;
- have *any* other medical problems;
- have ever been treated with x-rays or cancer medicines.

Proper Use of This Medicine

While you are receiving these medicines, especially cyclophosphamide, it is important that you drink extra fluids so that you will pass more urine. Also, empty your bladder frequently, including at least once during the night. This will help prevent kidney and bladder problems and keep your kidneys working well. Some patients may have to drink up to 7 to 12 cups (3 quarts) of fluid a day. If you have any questions about this, check with your doctor.

Precautions

It is very important that your doctor check your progress at regular visits to make sure that these medicines are working properly and to check for unwanted effects.

While you are being treated with these medicines, and after you stop treatment with them, *do not have any immunizations (vaccinations) without your doctor's approval.* Also, try to avoid people with infections.

If vincristine or dactinomycin accidentally seeps out of the vein into which it is injected, it may damage some tissues and cause scarring. *Tell the doctor or nurse right away if you notice redness, pain, or swelling at the place of injection.*

Possible Side Effects

Side effects that should be reported *immediately:*

Black, tarry stools
Blood in urine or stools
Cough or hoarseness
Fever or chills
Lower back or side pain
Pain at place of injection
Painful or difficult urination
Pinpoint red spots on skin
Shortness of breath (sudden)

- Unusual bleeding or bruising
- Wheezing

Side effects that should be reported as soon as possible:

- Bed-wetting
- Blurred or double vision
- Constipation
- Convulsions (seizures)
- Decrease or increase in urination
- Diarrhea (continuing)
- Difficulty in swallowing
- Difficulty in walking
- Dizziness, confusion, or agitation
- Drooping eyelids
- Fast or irregular heartbeat
- Hallucinations (seeing, hearing, or feeling things that are not there)
- Headache
- Heartburn
- Jaw pain
- Joint pain
- Lack of sweating
- Mental depression
- Missing menstrual periods
- Numbness, tingling, or pain in fingers and toes
- Pain in testicles
- Shortness of breath
- Sores in mouth and on lips
- Stomach cramps
- Swelling of feet and lower legs
- Trouble in sleeping
- Unusual thirst
- Unusual tiredness or weakness
- Yellow eyes or skin

Side effects that usually do not need medical attention (however, check with your doctor or nurse if they continue or are bothersome):

- Acne
- Bloating
- Darkening of soles, palms, or nails
- Flushing or redness of skin
- Increased sweating
- Loss of appetite
- Loss of hair
- Nausea or vomiting
- Skin rash, hives, or itching
- Swollen lips

After you stop receiving these medicines, they may still produce some side effects that need attention. During this period of time, *check with your doctor or nurse immediately* if you notice:

- Blood in urine

Also, check with your doctor if you notice:

- Black, tarry stools
- Blood in urine or stools
- Cough or hoarseness
- Diarrhea
- Fever or chills
- Lower back or side pain
- Painful or difficult urination
- Pinpoint red spots on skin
- Sores in mouth and on lips
- Stomach pain
- Unusual bleeding or bruising
- Yellow eyes or skin

Other side effects not listed above may also occur in some patients. If you notice any other effects, check with your doctor or nurse.

Annual revision: 05/22/91

VAD Systemic

This information applies to the following medicines:

- Vincristine (vin-KRIS-teen) (by injection)
- Doxorubicin (dox-oh-ROO-bi-sin) (by injection)
- Dexamethasone (dex-a-METH-a-zone) (by mouth)

Some commonly used brand names are:

For Vincristine

In the U.S.

- Oncovin
- Vincrex
- Vincasar PFS

Generic name product may also be available.

In Canada

- Oncovin

For Doxorubicin

In the U.S.

- Adriamycin PFS
- Rubex
- Adriamycin RDF

Generic name product may also be available.

In Canada

- Adriamycin PFS
- Adriamycin RDF

For Dexamethasone

In the U.S.

- Decadron
- Hexadrol
- Dexamethasone Intensol
- Mymethasone
- Dexone

Generic name product may also be available.

In Canada

- Deronil
- Hexadrol
- Dexasone
- Oradexon

Generic name product may also be available.

About Your Medicine

This combination therapy consists of two cancer medicines (vincristine and doxorubicin) and an adrenocorticoid (dexamethasone). They are used together to treat some lymphomas and some other kinds of cancer.

If any of the information causes you special concern or if you want additional information about your medicine and its use, check with your doctor, nurse, or pharmacist.

Before Using This Medicine

Discuss with your doctor the possible side effects that may be caused by this medicine. Some of them may be serious and/or long term.

Tell your doctor, nurse, and pharmacist if you. . .

- are allergic to any medicine, either prescription or nonprescription (OTC);
- are pregnant or intend to have children;
- are breast-feeding an infant;
- are taking *any* other prescription or nonprescription (OTC) medicine;
- have *any* other medical problems;
- have ever been treated with x-rays or cancer medicines.

Proper Use of This Medicine

Use each of these medicines exactly as directed by your doctor. The exact amount of each medicine that you need and the best times to take each one have been carefully worked out. Ask your doctor, nurse, or pharmacist to help you plan a way to take each of your medicines at the right times.

Take dexamethasone with food to help prevent stomach upset. If stomach upset, burning, or pain continues, check with your doctor.

While you are receiving these medicines, your doctor may want you to drink extra fluids so that you will pass more urine. This will help prevent kidney problems and keep your kidneys working well.

If you miss a dose of dexamethasone and you remember it within a few hours, take it as soon as you remember it. However, if several hours have passed or if it is almost time for the next dose, *check with your doctor.* Do not double doses.

Precautions

It is very important that your doctor check your progress at regular visits to make sure that this medicine is working properly and to check for unwanted effects.

While you are being treated with these medicines, and after you stop treatment with them, *do not have any immunizations (vaccinations) without your doctor's approval.* Also, try to avoid people with infections.

If doxorubicin or vincristine accidentally seeps out of the vein into which it is injected, it may damage some tissues and cause scarring. *Tell the doctor or nurse right away if you notice redness, pain, or swelling at the place of injection.*

Possible Side Effects

Side effects that should be reported *immediately:*

Black, tarry stools
Blood in urine or stools
Cough or hoarseness
Fast or irregular heartbeat
Fever or chills
Lower back or side pain
Pain at place of injection
Painful or difficult urination
Pinpoint red spots on skin
Shortness of breath
Swelling of feet and lower legs
Unusual bleeding or bruising

Side effects that should be reported as soon as possible:

Bed-wetting
Blurred or double vision
Constipation
Convulsions (seizures)
Darkening or redness of skin (after x-ray treatment)
Decrease or increase in urination
Difficulty in walking
Dizziness, confusion, or agitation
Drooping eyelids
Hallucinations (seeing, hearing, or feeling things that are not there)
Headache
Jaw pain
Joint pain
Lack of sweating
Mental depression
Numbness, tingling, or pain in fingers and toes
Pain in testicles
Red streaks along injected vein
Skin rash or itching
Sores in mouth and on lips
Stomach cramps
Trouble in sleeping
Weakness

Side effects that usually do not need medical attention (however, check with your doctor or nurse if they continue or are bothersome):

Bloating
Diarrhea
Loss of hair
Nausea or vomiting
Reddish urine

After you stop receiving these medicines, they may still produce some side effects that need attention. During this period of time, *check with your doctor or nurse immediately* if you notice:

Fast or irregular heartbeat
Shortness of breath
Swelling of feet and lower legs

Other side effects not listed above may also occur in some patients. If you notice any other effects, check with your doctor or nurse.

Annual revision: 05/22/91

VBMCP Systemic

This information applies to the following medicines:

Vincristine (vin-KRIS-teen) (by injection)
Carmustine (kar-MUS-teen) (by injection)
Melphalan (MEL-fa-lan) (by mouth)
Cyclophosphamide (sye-kloe-FOSS-fa-mide) (by injection)
Prednisone (PRED-ni-sone) (by mouth)

Some commonly used brand names are:

For Vincristine

In the U.S.

Oncovin
Vincasar PFS
Vincrex

Generic name product may also be available.

In Canada

Oncovin

For Carmustine

In the U.S. and Canada

BiCNU

Another commonly used name is BCNU.

For Melphalan

In the U.S. and Canada

Alkeran

For Cyclophosphamide

In the U.S.

Cytoxan
Neosar

Generic name product may also be available.

In Canada

Cytoxan
Procytox

For Prednisone

In the U.S.

Deltasone
Liquid Pred
Meticorten
Orasone
Prednicen-M
Prednisone Intensol
Sterapred
Sterapred DS

Generic name product may also be available.

In Canada

Apo-Prednisone
Deltasone
Winpred

Generic name product may also be available.

About Your Medicine

This combination therapy consists of four cancer medicines (vincristine, carmustine, melphalan, cyclophosphamide) and an adrenocorticoid (prednisone). They are used together to treat multiple myeloma and some other kinds of cancer.

If any of the information causes you special concern or if you want additional information about your medicine and its use, check with your doctor, nurse, or pharmacist.

Before Using This Medicine

Discuss with your doctor the possible side effects that may be caused by this medicine. Some of them may be serious and/or long term.

Tell your doctor, nurse, and pharmacist if you. . .

- are allergic to any medicine, either prescription or nonprescription (OTC);
- are pregnant or intend to have children;
- are breast-feeding an infant;
- are taking *any* other prescription or nonprescription (OTC) medicine;
- have *any* other medical problems;
- have ever been treated with x-rays or cancer medicines;
- smoke.

Proper Use of This Medicine

Use each of these medicines exactly as directed by your doctor. The exact amount of each medicine that you need and the best times to take each one have been carefully worked out. Ask your doctor, nurse, or pharmacist to help you plan a way to take each of your medicines at the right times.

Take prednisone with food to help prevent stomach upset. If stomach upset, burning, or pain continues, check with your doctor.

While you are receiving these medicines, especially cyclophosphamide, it is important that you drink extra fluids so that you will pass more urine. Also, empty your bladder frequently, including at least once during the night. This will help prevent kidney and bladder problems and keep your kidneys working well. Some patients may have to drink up to 7 to 12 cups (3 quarts) of fluid a day.

If you have any questions about this, check with your doctor.

If you miss a dose of prednisone or melphalan and you remember it within a few hours, take it as soon as you remember it. However, if several hours have passed or if it is almost time for the next dose, *check with your doctor*. Do not double doses.

Precautions

It is very important that your doctor check your progress at regular visits to make sure that this medicine is working properly and to check for unwanted effects.

While you are being treated with these medicines, and after you stop treatment with them, *do not have any immunizations (vaccinations) without your doctor's approval*. Also, try to avoid people with infections.

If carmustine or vincristine accidentally seeps out of the vein into which it is injected, it may damage some tissues and cause scarring. *Tell the doctor or nurse right away if you notice redness, pain, or swelling at the place of injection.*

Possible Side Effects

Side effects that should be reported *immediately:*

- Black, tarry stools
- Blood in urine or stools
- Confusion
- Convulsions (seizures)
- Cough or hoarseness
- Diarrhea
- Fever or chills
- Lower back or side pain
- Pain at place of injection
- Painful or difficult urination
- Pinpoint red spots on skin
- Reddening of skin
- Shortness of breath
- Skin rash or itching (sudden)
- Stomach pain
- Swelling of feet and lower legs
- Unusual bleeding or bruising

Side effects that should be reported as soon as possible:

- Back pain
- Bed-wetting
- Constipation
- Dark urine
- Decrease or increase in urination
- Difficulty in walking
- Dizziness, confusion, or agitation
- Double vision
- Drooping eyelids
- Drowsiness
- Flushing or redness of face
- Hallucinations (seeing, hearing, or feeling things that are not there)
- Headache
- Jaw pain
- Joint pain
- Lack of sweating
- Mental depression
- Missing menstrual periods
- Numbness, tingling, or pain in fingers and toes
- Pain in testicles
- Sores in mouth and on lips
- Trouble in sleeping
- Unusual thirst
- Unusual tiredness or weakness
- Yellow eyes or skin

Side effects that usually do not need medical attention (however, check with your doctor or nurse if they continue or are bothersome):

- Bloating
- Difficulty in swallowing
- Increased sweating
- Loss of appetite
- Loss of hair
- Nausea or vomiting
- Swollen lips

After you stop receiving these medicines, they may still produce some side effects that need attention. During this period of time, *check with your doctor or nurse immediately* if you notice:

- Black, tarry stools
- Blood in urine or stools
- Cough or hoarseness
- Fever or chills
- Lower back or side pain
- Painful or difficult urination
- Pinpoint red spots on skin
- Shortness of breath
- Unusual bleeding or bruising

Other side effects not listed above may also occur in some patients. If you notice any other effects, check with your doctor or nurse.

Annual revision: 05/22/91

VINCRISTINE, PREDNISONE, AND ASPARAGINASE Systemic

This information applies to the following medicines:
- Vincristine (vin-KRIS-teen) (by injection)
- Prednisone (PRED-ni-sone) (by mouth)
- Asparaginase (a-SPARE-a-gin-ase) (by injection)

Some commonly used brand names are:

For Vincristine

In the U.S.

Oncovin
Vincrex
Vincasar PFS

Generic name product may also be available.

In Canada

Oncovin

For Prednisone

In the U.S.

Deltasone
Prednicen-M
Liquid Pred
Prednisone Intensol
Meticorten
Sterapred
Orasone
Sterapred DS

Generic name product may also be available.

In Canada

Apo-Prednisone
Winpred
Deltasone

Generic name product may also be available.

For Asparaginase

In the U.S.

Elspar

In Canada

Kidrolase

Another commonly used name is colaspase.

About Your Medicine

This combination therapy consists of two cancer medicines (vincristine, asparaginase) and an adrenocorticoid (prednisone). They are used together to treat some kinds of cancer.

If any of the information causes you special concern or if you want additional information about your medicine and its use, check with your doctor, nurse, or pharmacist.

Before Using This Medicine

Discuss with your doctor the possible side effects that may be caused by this medicine. Some of them may be serious and/or long term.

Tell your doctor, nurse, and pharmacist if you. . .
- are allergic to any medicine, either prescription or nonprescription (OTC);
- are pregnant or intend to have children;
- are breast-feeding an infant;
- are taking *any* other prescription or nonprescription (OTC) medicine;
- have *any* other medical problems;
- have ever been treated with x-rays or cancer medicines.

Proper Use of This Medicine

Use each of these medicines exactly as directed by your doctor. The exact amount of each medicine that you need and the best times to take each one have been carefully worked out. Ask your doctor, nurse, or pharmacist to help you plan a way to take each of your medicines at the right times.

Take prednisone with food to help prevent stomach upset. If stomach upset, burning, or pain continues, check with your doctor.

While you are receiving these medicines, your doctor may want you to drink extra fluids so that you will pass more urine. This will help prevent kidney problems and keep your kidneys working well.

If you miss a dose of prednisone and you remember it within a few hours, take it as soon as you remember it. However, if several hours have passed or if it is almost time for the next dose, *check with your doctor*. Do not double doses.

Precautions

It is very important that your doctor check your progress at regular visits to make sure that these medicines are working properly and to check for unwanted effects.

While you are being treated with these medicines, and after you stop treatment with them, *do not have any immunizations (vaccinations) without your doctor's approval.* Also, try to avoid people with infections.

If vincristine accidentally seeps out of the vein into which it is injected, it may damage some tissues and cause scarring. *Tell the doctor or nurse right away if you notice redness, pain, or swelling at the place of injection.*

Possible Side Effects

Side effects that should be reported *immediately:*

Black, tarry stools
Blood in urine or stools
Cough or hoarseness
Difficulty in breathing
Fever or chills
Joint pain
Lower back or side pain
Pain at place of injection
Painful or difficult urination
Pinpoint red spots on skin
Puffy face
Skin rash or itching

Stomach pain (severe) with nausea and vomiting
Unusual bleeding or bruising

Side effects that should be reported as soon as possible:

Bed-wetting
Blurred or double vision
Confusion
Constipation
Convulsions (seizures)
Decrease or increase in urination
Difficulty in walking
Dizziness or lightheadedness
Drooping eyelids
Drowsiness
Hallucinations (seeing, hearing, or feeling things that are not there)
Headache
Inability to move arm or leg
Jaw pain
Lack of sweating
Mental depression
Missing menstrual periods
Nervousness
Numbness, tingling, or pain in fingers and toes
Pain in testicles
Sores in mouth and on lips
Stomach cramps
Swelling of feet and lower legs
Trouble in sleeping
Unusual thirst
Unusual tiredness or weakness
Yellow eyes or skin

Side effects that usually do not need medical attention (however, check with your doctor or nurse if they continue or are bothersome):

Bloating
Diarrhea
Loss of appetite
Loss of hair
Nausea or vomiting

After you stop receiving these medicines, they may still produce some side effects that need attention. During this period of time, *check with your doctor or nurse immediately* if you notice:

Stomach pain (severe) with nausea and vomiting

Other side effects not listed above may also occur in some patients. If you notice any other effects, check with your doctor or nurse.

Annual revision: 05/22/91

Stomach pain (severe) with nausea and vomiting
Unusual bleeding or bruising

Side effects that should be reported as soon as possible:

Bed-wetting
Blurred or double vision
Confusion
Constipation
Convulsions (seizures)
Decrease or increase in urination
Difficulty in walking
Drooping eyelids
Drowsiness
Hallucinations (seeing, hearing, or feeling things that are not there)
Headache
Inability to move arms or legs
Jaw pain
Lack of sweating
Mental depression
Missing menstrual periods
Nervousness
Numbness, tingling, or pain in fingers and toes
Pain in testicles
Sores in mouth and on lips
Stomach cramps
Swelling of feet and lower legs
Sudden weakness
Unusual tiredness
Unusual tiredness or weakness
Yellow eyes or skin

Side effects that usually do not need medical attention (however, check with your doctor or nurse if they continue or are bothersome):

Bloating
Diarrhea
Loss of appetite
Loss of hair
Nausea or vomiting

After you stop receiving these medicines, they may still produce some side effects that need attention. During this period of time, check with your doctor or nurse immediately if you notice:

Stomach pain (severe) with nausea and vomiting

Other side effects not listed above may also occur in some patients. If you notice any other effects, check with your doctor or nurse.

Annual revision: 07/22/94

II

Appendix II

ADDITIONAL MONOGRAPHS

The following monographs were finalized too late to be included in the regular alphabetic pagination of this volume.

ALBENDAZOLE Systemic*†

Some commonly used brand names are Eskazole and Zentel.

*Not commercially available in the U.S.
†Not commercially available in Canada.

Description

Albendazole (al-BEN-da-zole) is used to treat worm infections. Albendazole works by keeping the worm from absorbing sugar (glucose), so that the worm loses energy and dies.

Albendazole is used to treat:

- Common roundworms (ascariasis);
- Hookworms (ancylostomiasis and necatoriasis);
- Hydatid disease (echinococcosis);
- Pinworms (enterobiasis or oxyuriasis);
- Tapeworms (taeniasis);
- Threadworms (strongyloidiasis);
- Whipworms (trichuriasis).

This medicine may also be used for other worm infections as determined by your doctor.

Albendazole is available only with your doctor's prescription, in the following dosage forms:

Oral

- Oral suspension (United Kingdom)
- Tablets (United Kingdom)

It is very important that you read and understand the following information. If any of it causes you special concern, check with your doctor. Also, *if you have any questions* or if you want more information about this medicine or your medical problem, *ask your doctor, nurse, or pharmacist.*

Before Using This Medicine

In deciding to use a medicine, the risks of taking the medicine must be weighed against the good it will do. This is a decision you and your doctor will make. For albendazole, the following should be considered:

Allergies—Tell your doctor if you have ever had any unusual or allergic reaction to albendazole. Also tell your doctor and pharmacist if you are allergic to any other substances, such as foods, preservatives, or dyes.

Pregnancy—Albendazole has not been studied in pregnant women. However, studies in animals have shown that albendazole can cause birth defects or other problems. Before taking this medicine, make sure your doctor knows if you are pregnant or if you may become pregnant.

Women of childbearing age (15 to 40 years) should take the medicine within 7 days of the start of their period (menstrual cycle). Birth control must be used during treatment and for one month after stopping treatment with albendazole.

Breast-feeding—It is not known whether albendazole passes into human breast milk. Although most medicines pass into breast milk in small amounts, many of them may be used safely while breast-feeding. Mothers who are taking this medicine and who wish to breast-feed should discuss this with their doctor.

Children—Although there is no specific information comparing use of albendazole in children with use in other age groups, this medicine is not expected to cause different side effects or problems in children than it does in adults.

Older adults—Many medicines have not been studied specifically in older people. Therefore, it may not be known whether they work exactly the same way they do in younger adults or if they cause different side effects or problems in older people. There is no specific information comparing use of albendazole in the elderly with use in other age groups.

II

Other medical problems—The presence of other medical problems may affect the use of albendazole. Make sure you tell your doctor if you have any other medical problems, especially:

- Liver disease—Patients with liver disease may have an increased chance of side effects

Before you begin using any new medicine (prescription or nonprescription) or if you develop any new medical problem while you are using this medicine, check with your doctor, nurse, or pharmacist.

Proper Use of This Medicine

No special preparations (fasting, laxatives, or enemas) are necessary before, during, or immediately after treatment with albendazole.

Albendazole is best taken with meals, especially with food containing fat, to help your body absorb the medicine better.

For patients taking the *tablet form* of albendazole:

- Tablets may be chewed, swallowed whole with a small amount of liquid, or crushed and mixed with food.

To help clear up your infection completely, *take this medicine exactly as directed by your doctor for the full time of treatment.* In some infections, a second treatment in 2 to 3 weeks with this medicine may be needed to clear up the infection completely. *Do not miss any doses.*

Pinworms may be easily passed from one person to another, especially among persons in the same household. Therefore, all household members may have to be treated at the same time to prevent their infection or reinfection.

Dosing—The dose of albendazole will be different for different patients. *Follow your doctor's orders or the directions on the label.* The following information includes only the average doses of albendazole. *If your dose is different, do not change it* unless your doctor tells you to do so.

The number of tablets or teaspoonfuls of suspension that you take depends on the strength of the medicine. Also, *the number of doses you take each day, the time allowed between doses, and the length of time you take the medicine depend on the medical problem for which you are taking albendazole* .

- For *oral* dosage forms (oral suspension and tablets):
  —For common roundworms, hookworms, pinworms, and whipworms:
    - Adults and children over 2 years of age—400 milligrams (mg) once a day for one day. Treatment may need to be repeated in 3 weeks.
    - Children up to 2 years of age—200 mg once a day for one day. Treatment may need to be repeated in 3 weeks.

  —For tapeworms and threadworms:
    - Adults and children over 2 years of age—400 mg once a day for three days in a row. Treatment may need to be repeated in 3 weeks.
    - Children up to 2 years of age—200 mg once a day for three days in a row. Treatment may need to be repeated in 3 weeks.

  —For hydatid disease:
    - Adults—800 mg per day for twenty-eight days. Treatment may be repeated when necessary or in 2 weeks.
    - Children up to 6 years of age—Dosage has not been established.
    - Children 6 years of age and over—Dose is based on body weight and must be determined by your doctor. However, the usual dose is 12 mg of albendazole per kilogram (5.5 milligrams per pound) of body weight per day for 28 days. Treatment may be repeated when necessary.

Missed dose—If you miss a dose of this medicine, take it as soon as possible. However, if it is almost time for your next dose, skip the missed dose and go back to your regular dosing schedule. Do not double doses.

Storage—To store this medicine:

- Keep out of the reach of children.
- Store away from heat and direct light.
- Do not store in the bathroom, near the kitchen sink, or in other damp places. Heat or moisture may cause the medicine to break down.
- Keep the suspension form of this medicine from freezing.
- Do not keep outdated medicine or medicine no longer needed. Be sure that any discarded medicine is out of the reach of children.

Precautions While Using This Medicine

It is important that your doctor check your progress after treatment. This is to make sure that the infection is cleared up completely, and to allow your doctor to check for any unwanted effects.

If your symptoms do not improve after you have taken this medicine for the full course of treatment, or if they become worse, check with your doctor.

While you are taking albendazole, it is important that you use birth control, since this medicine can cause birth defects or other problems.

For patients taking albendazole for *hookworms*:

- In hookworm infections, anemia may occur. Therefore, your doctor may want you to take iron supplements. If so, it is important to take iron every day while you are being treated for hookworm infection.

Do not miss any doses. Your doctor may also want you to keep taking iron supplements for at least 3 to 6 months after you stop taking albendazole. If you have any questions about this, check with your doctor.

For patients taking albendazole for *hydatid disease*:

- Avoid contacts with infected dogs; animal waste should be burned or buried to prevent reinfection of dogs.

For patients taking albendazole for *pinworms*:

- In some patients, pinworms may return after treatment with albendazole. Wear pajamas and underwear to sleep, take a bath every day, and wash (not shake) all bedding and nightclothes (pajamas) after treatment to help prevent reinfection. Treatment may be repeated after 3 weeks.
- Pinworms may be easily passed from one person to another, especially among persons in the same household. Therefore, all household members may have to be treated at the same time to prevent their infection or reinfection.

For patients taking albendazole for *roundworms* and *whipworms*:

- Good health habits, such as proper disposal of waste, are required to help prevent reinfection.

For patients taking albendazole for *tapeworms*:

- Check or inspect the meat carefully.
- Cook all pork and beef thoroughly before eating. You may also freeze, or refrigerate and salt, the meat for a long period of time. All of these measures will destroy or kill the worm that may be present in the meat and will help prevent reinfection.

For patients taking albendazole for *threadworms*:

- Cook vegetables thoroughly before eating. This will destroy or kill the worm that may be present in the vegetables and will help prevent reinfection.

Side Effects of This Medicine

Along with its needed effects, a medicine may cause some unwanted effects. Although not all of these side effects may occur, if they do occur they may need medical attention.

Check with your doctor as soon as possible if any of the following side effects occur:

Rare

Fever; skin rash or itching; sore throat; unusual tiredness and weakness

Other side effects may occur that usually do not need medical attention. These side effects may go away during treatment as your body adjusts to the medicine. However, check with your doctor if any of the following side effects continue or are bothersome:

Less common

Abdominal or stomach upset or pain; diarrhea; dizziness; headache; nausea; vomiting

Rare

Thinning or loss of hair

Other side effects not listed above may also occur in some patients. If you notice any other effects, check with your doctor.

Additional Information

Once a medicine has been approved for marketing for a certain use, experience may show that it is also useful for other medical problems. Although these uses are not included in product labeling, albendazole is used in certain patients with the following infections:

- Capillariasis
- Clonorchiasis
- Giardiasis
- Neurocysticercosis
- Trichinosis
- Trichostrongyliasis

For patients taking this medicine for *giardiasis*:

- Household contacts and sexual partners of infected patients should be seen by the doctor to prevent spread of infection to others. After treatment, it is important that your doctor check to see whether or not the infection in your body has been cleared up completely.

Other than the above information, there is no additional information relating to proper use, precautions, or side effects for these uses.

Annual revision: 08/18/93

ALDESLEUKIN Systemic†

A commonly used brand name in the U.S. is Proleukin.
Other commonly used names are interleukin-2 and IL-2.

†Not commercially available in Canada.

Description

Aldesleukin (al-des-LOO-kin) is a synthetic (man-made) version of a substance called interleukin-2. Interleukins are produced naturally by cells in the body to help white blood cells work. Aldesleukin is used to treat cancer of the kidney.

Aldesleukin causes some other very serious effects in addition to its helpful effects. Some effects can be fatal. For that reason, aldesleukin is given only in the hospital. If severe side effects occur, which is common, treatment in an intensive care unit (ICU) may be necessary. Other effects may not be serious but may cause concern. Before you begin treatment with aldesleukin, you and your doctor should talk about the good this medicine will do as well as the risks of using it.

Aldesleukin is to be administered only by or under the immediate supervision of your doctor. It is available in the following dosage form:

Parenteral

- Injection (U.S.)

It is very important that you read and understand the following information. If any of it causes you special concern, check with your doctor. Also, *if you have any questions* or if you want more information about this medicine or your medical problem, *ask your doctor, nurse, or pharmacist.*

Before Using This Medicine

In deciding to use a medicine, the risks of taking the medicine must be weighed against the good it will do. This is a decision you and your doctor will make. For aldesleukin, the following should be considered:

Allergies—Tell your doctor if you have ever had any unusual or allergic reaction to aldesleukin.

Pregnancy—Aldesleukin has not been studied in humans or in animals. However, because this medicine may cause serious side effects, use during pregnancy is usually not recommended.

Be sure that you have discussed this with your doctor before receiving this medicine.

Breast-feeding—It is not known whether aldesleukin passes into breast milk.

Children—There is no specific information comparing use of aldesleukin in children with use in other age groups.

Older adults—Many medicines have not been studied specifically in older people. Therefore, it may not be known whether they work exactly the same way they do in younger adults. There is no specific information comparing use of aldesleukin in the elderly with use in other age groups.

Other medicines—Although certain medicines should not be used together at all, in other cases two different medicines may be used together even if an interaction might occur. In these cases, your doctor may want to change the dose, or other precautions may be necessary. Tell your doctor and pharmacist if you are taking *any* other medicine.

Other medical problems—The presence of other medical problems may affect the use of aldesleukin. Make sure you tell your doctor if you have any other medical problems, especially:

- Chickenpox (including recent exposure) or
- Herpes zoster (shingles)—Risk of severe disease affecting other parts of the body
- Heart disease or
- Immune system problems or
- Liver disease or
- Lung disease or
- Psoriasis or
- Underactive thyroid—May be worsened by aldesleukin
- Infection—Aldesleukin may decrease your body's ability to fight infection
- Kidney disease—Effects of aldesleukin may be increased because of slower removal from the body
- Mental problems—Aldesleukin may make them worse
- Seizures (history of)—Aldesleukin can cause seizures

Before you begin using any new medicine (prescription or nonprescription) or if you develop any new medical problem while you are using this medicine, check with your doctor, nurse, or pharmacist.

Precautions While Using This Medicine

Aldesleukin can temporarily affect the white blood cells in your blood, increasing the chance of getting an infection. It can also lower the number of platelets, which are necessary for proper blood clotting. If this occurs, there are certain precautions you can take, especially when your blood count is low, to reduce the risk of infection or bleeding:

- If you can, avoid people with infections. *Check with your doctor immediately* if you think you are getting an infection or if you get a fever or chills, cough or hoarseness, lower back or side pain, or painful or difficult urination.

- *Check with your doctor immediately* if you notice any unusual bleeding or bruising; black, tarry stools; blood in urine or stools; or pinpoint red spots on your skin.
- Be careful when using a regular toothbrush, dental floss, or toothpick. Your medical doctor, dentist, or nurse may recommend other ways to clean your teeth and gums. Check with your medical doctor before having any dental work done.
- Do not touch your eyes or the inside of your nose unless you have just washed your hands and have not touched anything else in the meantime.
- Be careful not to cut yourself when you are using sharp objects such as a safety razor or fingernail or toenail cutters.
- Avoid contact sports or other situations where bruising or injury could occur.

Side Effects of This Medicine

Along with its needed effects, a medicine may cause some unwanted effects. Some side effects will have signs or symptoms that you can see or feel. Your doctor may watch for others by doing certain tests.

Check with your doctor or nurse immediately if any of the following side effects occur:

More common

Fever or chills; shortness of breath

Less common

Black, tarry stools; blisters on skin; blood in urine; bloody vomit; chest pain; cough or hoarseness; lower back or side pain; painful or difficult urination; pinpoint red spots on skin; stomach pain (severe); unusual bleeding or bruising

Check with your doctor or nurse as soon as possible if any of the following side effects occur:

More common

Agitation; confusion; diarrhea; dizziness; drowsiness; mental depression; nausea and vomiting; sores in mouth and on lips; tingling of hands or feet; unusual decrease in urination; unusual tiredness; weight gain of 5 to 10 pounds or more

Less common

Bloating and stomach pain; blurred or double vision; faintness; fast or irregular heartbeat; loss of taste; rapid breathing; redness, swelling, and soreness of tongue; trouble in speaking; yellow eyes and skin

Rare

Changes in menstrual periods; clumsiness; coldness; convulsions (seizures); listlessness; muscle aches; pain or redness at site of injection; sudden inability to move; swelling in the front of the neck; swelling of feet or lower legs; weakness

This medicine may also cause the following side effects that your doctor will watch for:

More common

Anemia; heart problems; kidney problems; liver problems; low blood pressure; low platelet counts in blood; low white blood cell counts; other blood problems; underactive thyroid

Other side effects may occur that usually do not need medical attention. These side effects may go away during treatment as your body adjusts to the medicine. Also, your doctor or nurse may be able to tell you about ways to prevent or reduce some of these side effects. Check with your doctor or nurse if any of the following side effects continue or are bothersome or if you have any questions about them:

More common

Dry skin; loss of appetite; skin rash or redness with burning or itching, followed by peeling; unusual feeling of discomfort or illness

Less common

Constipation; headache; joint pain; muscle pain

Other side effects not listed above may also occur in some patients. If you notice any other effects, check with your doctor.

Annual revision: 09/15/93

AMLODIPINE Systemic†

A commonly used brand name in the U.S. is Norvasc.

†Not commercially available in Canada.

Description

Amlodipine (am-LOE-di-peen) is a calcium channel blocker used to treat angina (chest pain) and high blood pressure. Amlodipine affects the movement of calcium into the cells of the heart and blood vessels. As a result, amlodipine relaxes blood vessels and increases the supply of blood and oxygen to the heart while reducing its workload.

High blood pressure adds to the workload of the heart and arteries. If it continues for a long time, the heart and arteries may not function properly. This can damage the blood vessels of the brain, heart, and kidneys, resulting in a stroke, heart failure, or kidney failure. High blood pressure may also increase the risk of heart attacks. These problems may be less likely to occur if blood pressure is controlled.

This medicine is available only with your doctor's prescription, in the following dosage form:

Oral

- Tablets (U.S.)

It is very important that you read and understand the following information. If any of it causes you special concern, check with your doctor. Also, *if you have any questions* or if you want more information about this medicine or your medical problem, *ask your doctor, nurse, or pharmacist.*

Before Using This Medicine

In deciding to use a medicine, the risks of taking the medicine must be weighed against the good it will do. This is a decision you and your doctor will make. For amlodipine, the following should be considered:

Allergies—Tell your doctor if you have ever had any unusual or allergic reaction to amlodipine. Also tell your doctor and pharmacist if you are allergic to any other substances, such as foods, preservatives, or dyes.

Pregnancy—Amlodipine has not been studied in pregnant women. However, studies in animals have shown that, at very high doses, amlodipine may cause fetal death. Before taking this medicine, make sure your doctor knows if you are pregnant or if you may become pregnant.

Breast-feeding—It is not known whether amlodipine passes into breast milk. Although most medicines pass into breast milk in small amounts, many of them may be used safely while breast-feeding. Mothers who are taking this medicine and who wish to breast-feed should discuss this with their doctor.

Children—Studies on this medicine have been done only in adult patients, and there is no specific information comparing use of amlodipine in children with use in other age groups.

Older adults—Elderly people may be especially sensitive to the effects of amlodipine. This may increase the chance of side effects during treatment.

Other medicines—Although certain medicines should not be used together at all, in other cases two different medicines may be used together even if an interaction might occur. In these cases, your doctor may want to change the dose, or other precautions may be necessary. Tell your doctor and pharmacist if you are using any other prescription or nonprescription (over-the-counter [OTC]) medicine.

Other medical problems—The presence of other medical problems may affect the use of amlodipine. Make sure you tell your doctor if you have any other medical problems, especially:

- Congestive heart failure—There is a small chance that amlodipine may make this condition worse
- Liver disease—Higher blood levels of amlodipine may result and a smaller dose may be needed
- Very low blood pressure—Amlodipine may make this condition worse

Before you begin using any new medicine (prescription or nonprescription) or if you develop any new medical problem while you are using this medicine, check with your doctor, nurse, or pharmacist.

Proper Use of This Medicine

Take this medicine exactly as directed even if you feel well and do not notice any chest pain. Do not take more of this medicine and do not take it more often than your doctor ordered. Do not miss any doses.

For patients taking this medicine *for high blood pressure:*

- In addition to the use of the medicine your doctor has prescribed, treatment for your high blood pressure may include weight control and care in the types of food you eat, especially foods high in sodium (salt). Your doctor will tell you which of these are most important for you. You should check with your doctor before changing your diet.
- Many patients who have high blood pressure will not notice any signs of the problem. In fact, many may feel normal. It is very important that you *take your medicine exactly as directed* and that you keep your appointments with your doctor even if you feel well.
- Remember that this medicine will not cure your high blood pressure but it does help control it. Therefore, you must continue to take it as directed if you expect to lower your blood pressure and keep it down. *You may have to take high blood pressure medicine for the rest of your life.* If high blood pressure is not treated, it can cause serious problems such as heart failure, blood vessel disease, stroke, or kidney disease.

Dosing—The dose of amlodipine will be different for different patients. *Follow your doctor's orders or the directions on the label.* The following information includes only the average doses of amlodipine. *If your dose is different, do not change it* unless your doctor tells you to do so.

The number of tablets that you take depends on the strength of the medicine.

- For *oral* dosage form (tablets):
  - —For angina (chest pain):
    - Adults—5 to 10 milligrams (mg) once a day.
    - Children—Use must be determined by your doctor.
  - —For high blood pressure:
    - Adults—2.5 to 10 mg once a day.
    - Children—Use must be determined by your doctor.

Missed dose—If you miss a dose of this medicine, take it as soon as possible. However, if it is almost time for your next dose, skip the missed dose and go back to your regular dosing schedule. Do not double doses.

Storage—To store this medicine:

- Keep out of the reach of children.
- Store away from heat and direct light.
- Do not store in the bathroom, near the kitchen sink, or in other damp places. Heat or moisture may cause the medicine to break down.
- Keep the medicine from freezing. Do not refrigerate.
- Do not keep outdated medicine or medicine no longer needed. Be sure that any discarded medicine is out of the reach of children.

Precautions While Using This Medicine

It is important that your doctor check your progress at regular visits. This will allow your doctor to make sure the medicine is working properly and to change the dosage if needed.

If you have been using this medicine regularly for several weeks, do not suddenly stop using it. Stopping suddenly may cause your chest pain or high blood pressure to come back or get worse. Check with your doctor for the best way to reduce gradually the amount you are taking before stopping completely.

Chest pain resulting from exercise or physical exertion usually is reduced or prevented by this medicine. This may tempt you to be too active. *Make sure you discuss with your doctor a safe amount of exercise for your medical problem.*

After taking a dose of this medicine you may get a headache that lasts for a short time. This should become less noticeable after you have taken this medicine for a while. If this effect continues, or if the headaches are severe, check with your doctor.

In some patients, tenderness, swelling, or bleeding of the gums may appear soon after treatment with this medicine is started. Brushing and flossing your teeth carefully and regularly and massaging your gums may help prevent this. *See your dentist regularly* to have your teeth cleaned. Check with your medical doctor or dentist if you have any questions about how to take care of your teeth and gums, or if you notice any tenderness, swelling, or bleeding of your gums.

For patients taking this medicine *for high blood pressure:*

- *Do not take other medicines unless they have been discussed with your doctor.* This especially includes over-the-counter (nonprescription) medicines for appetite control, asthma, colds, cough, hay fever, or sinus problems, since they may tend to increase your blood pressure.

Side Effects of This Medicine

Along with its needed effects, a medicine may cause some unwanted effects. Although not all of these side effects may occur, if they do occur they may need medical attention.

Check with your doctor as soon as possible if any of the following side effects occur:

More common

Swelling of ankles or feet

Less common

Dizziness; pounding heartbeat

Rare

Chest pain; dizziness or lightheadedness when getting up from a lying or sitting position; slow heartbeat

Other side effects may occur that usually do not need medical attention. These side effects may go away during treatment as your body adjusts to the medicine. However, check with your doctor if any of the following side effects continue or are bothersome:

More common

Flushing; headache

Less common

Nausea; unusual tiredness or weakness

Other side effects not listed above may also occur in some patients. If you notice any other effects, check with your doctor.

Annual revision: 08/12/93

ANTIHEMOPHILIC FACTOR Systemic

Some commonly used brand names are:

In the U.S.

Hemofil M	MelATE
Humate-P	Monoclate-P
Hyate:C	Profilate OSD
Koate-HP	Recombinate
Kogenate	

Generic name product may also be available.

In Canada

Koate-HP
Recombinate

Other commonly used names are AHF and factor VIII.

Description

Antihemophilic (an-tee-hee-moe-FIL-ik) factor (AHF) is a protein produced naturally in the body. It helps the blood form clots to stop bleeding.

Hemophilia A, also called classical hemophilia, is a condition in which the body does not make enough AHF. If you do not have enough AHF and you become injured, your blood will not form clots as it should, and you may bleed into and damage your muscles and joints. One type of AHF is used to treat another condition called von Willebrand disease, in which there is a risk of bleeding. AHF also may be used for other conditions as determined by your doctor.

The AHF that your doctor will give you is obtained naturally from human or pig blood, or artificially by a man-made process.

AHF obtained from human blood has been treated. It is not likely to contain harmful viruses such as hepatitis B virus; non-A, non-B hepatitis; or human immunodeficiency virus (HIV), the virus that causes acquired immunodeficiency syndrome (AIDS). The man-made and pork AHF products do not contain these viruses.

AHF is available only with your doctor's prescription, in the following dosage form:

Parenteral

- Injection (U.S. and Canada)

It is very important that you read and understand the following information. If any of it causes you special concern, check with your doctor. Also, *if you have any questions* or if you want more information about this medicine or your medical problem, *ask your doctor, nurse, or pharmacist.*

Before Using This Medicine

In deciding to use a medicine, the risks of taking the medicine must be weighed against the good it will do. This is a decision you and your doctor will make. For antihemophilic factor (AHF), the following should be considered:

Allergies—Tell your doctor if you have ever had any unusual or allergic reaction to AHF. Also tell your doctor and pharmacist if you are allergic to any other substances, such as foods, preservatives, or dyes.

Pregnancy—Studies on effects in pregnancy have not been done in either humans or animals.

Breast-feeding—It is not known whether AHF passes into breast milk. Although most medicines pass into breast milk in small amounts, many of them may be used safely while breast-feeding. Mothers who are using this medicine and who wish to breast-feed should discuss this with their doctor.

Children—This medicine has been tested in children and, in effective doses, has not been shown to cause different side effects or problems than it does in adults.

Older adults—This medicine has been tested and has not been shown to cause different side effects or problems in older people than it does in younger adults.

Other medicines—Although certain medicines should not be used together at all, in other cases two different medicines may be used together even if an interaction might occur. In these cases, your doctor may want to change the dose, or other precautions may be necessary. Tell your doctor and pharmacist if you are using any other prescription or nonprescription (over-the-counter [OTC]) medicine.

Other medical problems—The presence of other medical problems may affect the use of AHF. Make sure you tell your doctor if you have any other medical problems.

Before you begin using any new medicine (prescription or nonprescription) or if you develop any new medical problem while you are using this medicine, check with your doctor, nurse, or pharmacist.

Proper Use of This Medicine

Some medicines given by injection may sometimes be given at home to patients who do not need to be in the hospital. If you are using this medicine at home, your doctor or nurse will teach you how to prepare and inject the medicine. You will have a chance to practice preparing and injecting it. *Be certain that you understand exactly how the medicine is to be prepared and injected.* To prepare this medicine:

- Take the dry medicine and the liquid (diluent) out of the refrigerator or freezer and bring them to room temperature, as directed by your doctor.

- When injecting the liquid (diluent) into the dry medicine, *aim the stream of liquid (diluent) against the wall of the container of dry medicine* to prevent foaming.
- *Swirl the container gently to dissolve the medicine. Do not shake the container.*

Use this medicine right away. It should not be kept longer than 1 or 3 hours after it has been prepared, as directed on the package or by your doctor.

A plastic disposable syringe and filter needle must be used with this medicine. The medicine may stick to the inside of a glass syringe, and you may not receive a full dose.

Do not reuse syringes and needles. Put used syringes and needles in a puncture-resistant disposable container, or dispose of them as directed by your doctor, nurse, or pharmacist.

Dosing—The dose of antihemophilic factor (AHF) will be different for different patients. The dose you receive will be based on:

- Your body weight.
- The amount of AHF your body is able to make.
- How much, how often, and where in your body you are bleeding.
- Whether or not your body has built up a defense (antibody) against this medicine.

Your dose of this medicine may even be different at different times. It is important that you *follow your doctor's orders.*

Missed dose—If you miss a dose of this medicine, check with your doctor as soon as possible for instructions. If you cannot reach your doctor, use your usual dose as soon as you remember.

Storage—To store this medicine:

- Keep out of the reach of children.
- Some AHF products must be stored in the refrigerator and some in the freezer. However, some of them may be kept at room temperature for short periods of time. Store this medicine as directed by your doctor or by the manufacturer.
- Do not keep outdated medicine or medicine no longer needed. Be sure that any discarded medicine is out of the reach of children.

Precautions While Using This Medicine

If you were recently diagnosed with hemophilia A, you should receive hepatitis B vaccine to reduce even further your risk of getting hepatitis B from antihemophilic factor.

It is recommended that you carry identification stating that you have hemophilia A, and what medicine you are using. If you have any questions about what kind of identification to carry, check with your doctor, nurse, or pharmacist.

After a while, your body may build up a defense (antibody) against this medicine. *Tell your doctor if this medicine seems to be less effective than usual.*

Side Effects of This Medicine

Along with its needed effects, a medicine may cause some unwanted effects. Some side effects will have signs or symptoms that you can see or feel. Your doctor may watch for others by doing certain tests.

Check with your doctor immediately if any of the following side effects occur, because they may mean that you are having a serious allergic reaction to the medicine:

Less common or rare

Changes in facial skin color; fast or irregular breathing; puffiness or swelling of the eyelids or around the eyes; shortness of breath, troubled breathing, tightness in chest, and/or wheezing; skin rash, hives, and/or itching

Also, check with your doctor as soon as possible if any of the following occur:

Less common or rare

Chills; fever; nausea; tenderness, pain, swelling, warmth, skin discoloration, and noticeable veins over affected area; unusual bleeding or bruising; unusual tiredness or weakness

Other side effects may occur that usually do not need medical attention. These side effects may go away during treatment as your body adjusts to the medicine. However, check with your doctor if any of the following side effects continue or are bothersome:

Less common

Burning, stinging, or swelling at place of injection; dizziness or lightheadedness; dry mouth or bad taste in mouth; headache; nosebleed; redness of face; vomiting

Other side effects not listed above may also occur in some patients. If you notice any other effects, check with your doctor.

Annual revision: 07/30/93

CIPROFLOXACIN Ophthalmic

A commonly used brand name in the U.S. and Canada is Ciloxan.

Description

Ophthalmic ciprofloxacin (sip-roe-FLOX-a-sin) is used in the eye to treat bacterial infections of the eye and corneal ulcers of the eye. Ophthalmic ciprofloxacin works by killing bacteria.

Ciprofloxacin ophthalmic preparation is available only with your doctor's prescription, in the following dosage form:

Ophthalmic

- Ophthalmic solution (eye drops) (U.S. and Canada)

It is very important that you read and understand the following information. If any of it causes you special concern, check with your doctor. Also, *if you have any questions* or if you want more information about this medicine or your medical problem, *ask your doctor, nurse, or pharmacist.*

Before Using This Medicine

In deciding to use a medicine, the risks of using the medicine must be weighed against the good it will do. This is a decision you and your doctor will make. For ophthalmic ciprofloxacin, the following should be considered:

Allergies—Tell your doctor if you have ever had any unusual or allergic reaction to ophthalmic or systemic ciprofloxacin (e.g., Cipro) or any related medicines, such as cinoxacin (e.g., Cinobac), norfloxacin (e.g., Chibroxin or Noroxin), ofloxacin (e.g., Floxin), or nalidixic acid (e.g., NegGram). Also tell your doctor and pharmacist if you are allergic to any other substances, such as foods, preservatives, or dyes.

Pregnancy—Ciprofloxacin has not been studied in pregnant women. However, studies in animals have not shown that ciprofloxacin causes birth defects.

Breast-feeding—It is not known whether ophthalmic ciprofloxin passes into breast milk. However, ciprofloxacin given by mouth does pass into breast milk. Although most medicines pass into breast milk in small amounts, many of them may be used safely while breast-feeding. Mothers who are using this medicine and who wish to breast-feed should discuss this with their doctor.

Children—Use is not recommended in infants and children up to 12 years of age. In children 12 years of age and older, this medicine is not expected to cause different side effects or problems than it does in adults.

Older adults—Many medicines have not been studied specifically in older people. Therefore, it may not be known whether they work exactly the same way they do in younger adults or if they cause different side effects or problems in older people. There is no specific information comparing use of ophthalmic ciprofloxacin in the elderly with use in other age groups.

Other medicines—Although certain medicines should not be used together at all, in other cases two different medicines may be used together even if an interaction might occur. In these cases, your doctor may want to change the dose, or other precautions may be necessary. Tell your doctor and pharmacist if you using any other prescription or nonprescription (over-the-counter [OTC]) medicine that is to be used in the eye.

Before you begin using any new medicine (prescription or nonprescription) or if you develop any new medical problem while you are using this medicine, check with your doctor, nurse, or pharmacist.

Proper Use of This Medicine

To use:

- First, wash your hands. Then tilt the head back and pull the lower eyelid away from the eye to form a pouch. Drop the medicine into the pouch and gently close the eyes. Do not blink. Keep the eyes closed for 1 or 2 minutes to allow the medicine to come into contact with the infection.
- If you think you did not get the drop of medicine into your eyes properly, use another drop.
- To keep the medicine as germ-free as possible, do not touch the applicator tip to any surface (including the eye). Also, keep the container tightly closed.

To help clear up your eye infection completely, *keep using ophthalmic ciprofloxacin for the full time of treatment*, even if your symptoms have disappeared. *Do not miss any doses.*

Dosing—The dose of ophthalmic ciprofloxacin will be different for different patients. *Follow your doctor's orders or the directions on the label.* The following information includes only the average doses of ophthalmic ciprofloxacin. *If your dose is different, do not change it* unless your doctor tells you to do so.

The number of doses you use each day, the time allowed between doses, and the length of time you use the medicine depend on the medical problem for which you are using ophthalmic ciprofloxacin.

- For *ophthalmic solution* dosage form:
  —For bacterial conjunctivitis:
    - Adults and children 12 years of age and older—Use 1 drop in each eye every two hours, while you are awake, for two days. Then use 1 drop in

each eye every four hours, while you are awake, for the next five days.

• Infants and children up to 12 years of age—Use and dose must be determined by your doctor.

—For corneal ulcers:

• Adults and children 12 years of age and older—On day one, use 1 drop in the affected eye every fifteen minutes for six hours, then 1 drop every thirty minutes for the rest of the day, while you are awake. On day two, use 1 drop every hour, while you are awake. On days three through fourteen, use 1 drop every four hours, while you are awake.

• Infants and children up to 12 years of age—Use and dose must be determined by your doctor.

Missed dose—If you miss a dose of this medicine, use it as soon as possible. However, if it is almost time for your next dose, skip the missed dose and go back to your regular dosing schedule.

Storage—To store this medicine:

- Keep out of the reach of children.
- Store away from heat and direct light.
- Keep the medicine from freezing. Do not refrigerate.
- Do not keep outdated medicine or medicine no longer needed. Be sure that any discarded medicine is out of the reach of children.

Precautions While Using This Medicine

If your eye infection does not improve within a few days, or if it becomes worse, check with your doctor.

This medicine may cause your eyes to become more sensitive to light than they are normally. Wearing sunglasses and avoiding too much exposure to bright light may help lessen the discomfort.

Side Effects of This Medicine

Along with its needed effects, a medicine may cause some unwanted effects. Although not all of these side effects may occur, if they do occur they may need medical attention.

Check with your doctor as soon as possible if any of the following side effects occur:

Rare

Blurred vision or other change in vision; irritation (severe) or redness of eye; nausea; skin rash

Other side effects may occur that usually do not need medical attention. These side effects may go away during treatment as your body adjusts to the medicine. However, check with your doctor if any of the following side effects continue or are bothersome:

More common

Burning or other discomfort of eye; crusting or crystals in corner of eye

Less common

Bad taste following use in the eye; feeling of something in eye; itching of eye; redness of the lining of the eyelids

Rare

Increased sensitivity of eyes to light; swelling of eyelid; tearing of eye

Other side effects not listed above may also occur in some patients. If you notice any other effects, check with your doctor.

Annual revision: 07/29/93

CISAPRIDE Systemic

A commonly used brand name in the U.S. and Canada is Prepulsid.

Description

Cisapride (SIS-a-pride) is a medicine that increases the movements or contractions of the stomach and intestines. It is used to treat symptoms such as heartburn caused by a backward flow of stomach acid into the esophagus.

Cisapride is available only with your doctor's prescription. It is available in the following dosage forms:

Oral

- Oral suspension (Canada)
- Tablets (U.S. and Canada)

It is very important that you read and understand the following information. If any of it causes you special concern, check with your doctor. Also, *if you have any questions* or if you want more information about this medicine or your medical problem, *ask your doctor, nurse, or pharmacist.*

Before Using This Medicine

In deciding to use a medicine, the risks of taking the medicine must be weighed against the good it will do.

This is a decision you and your doctor will make. For cisapride, the following should be considered:

Allergies—Tell your doctor if you have ever had any unusual or allergic reaction to cisapride. Also tell your doctor and pharmacist if you are allergic to any other substances, such as foods, preservatives, or dyes.

Pregnancy—Cisapride has not been studied in pregnant women. However, studies in animals have shown that cisapride causes harm to the fetus. Before taking this medicine, make sure your doctor knows if you are pregnant or if you may become pregnant.

Breast-feeding—Although cisapride passes into the breast milk, it has not been shown to cause problems in nursing babies.

Children—This medicine has been tested in a limited number of children. In effective doses, the medicine has not been shown to cause different side effects or problems than it does in adults.

Older adults—Elderly people are especially sensitive to the effects of cisapride. Cisapride stays in the body longer so the dose may be different than in younger people.

Other medicines—Although certain medicines should not be used together at all, in other cases two different medicines may be used together even if an interaction might occur. In these cases, your doctor may want to change the dose, or other precautions may be necessary. When you are taking cisapride, it is especially important that your doctor and pharmacist know if you are taking any of the following:

- Amantadine (e.g., Symmetrel) or
- Anticholinergics (medicine for abdominal or stomach spasms or cramps) or
- Antidepressants (medicine for depression) or
- Antidyskinetics (medicine for Parkinson's disease or other conditions affecting control of muscles) or
- Antihistamines or
- Antipsychotics (medicine for mental illness) or
- Buclizine (e.g., Bucladin) or
- Carbamazepine (e.g., Tegretol) or
- Cyclizine (e.g., Marezine) or
- Cyclobenzaprine (e.g., Flexeril) or
- Disopyramide (e.g., Norpace) or
- Flavoxate (e.g., Urispas) or
- Ipratropium (e.g., Atrovent) or
- Meclizine (e.g., Antivert) or
- Methylphenidate (e.g., Ritalin) or
- Orphenadrine (e.g., Norflex) or
- Oxybutynin (e.g., Ditropen) or
- Procainamide (e.g., Pronestyl) or
- Promethazine (e.g., Phenergan) or
- Quinidine (e.g., Quinidex) or
- Trimeprazine (e.g., Temaril)—Cisapride may decrease the absorption of these medicines and cause them to be less effective

Other medical problems—The presence of other medical problems may affect the use of cisapride. Make sure you tell your doctor if you have any other medical problems, especially:

- Abdominal or stomach bleeding or
- Intestinal blockage—Cisapride may make these conditions worse
- Epilepsy or history of seizures—Cisapride has been reported to cause seizures in patients with a history of seizures
- Kidney disease or
- Liver disease—Higher blood levels of cisapride may result and a smaller dose may be needed

Before you begin using any new medicine (prescription or nonprescription) or if you develop any new medical problem while you are using this medicine, check with your doctor, nurse, or pharmacist.

Proper Use of This Medicine

Take this medicine 15 minutes before meals and at bedtime with a beverage, unless otherwise directed by your doctor.

Dosing—The dose of cisapride will be different for different patients. *Follow your doctor's orders or the directions on the label.* The following information includes only the average doses of cisapride. *If your dose is different, do not change it* unless your doctor tells you to do so.

- For *oral* dosage form (tablets and solution):
  —For heartburn caused by gastroesophageal reflux:
    - Adults and children 12 years of age and older: 5 to 20 milligrams (mg) of cisapride two to four times a day. Cisapride should be taken fifteen minutes before meals and at bedtime.
    - Children up to 12 years of age: Dose is based on body weight. The dose is usually 0.15 to 0.3 mg of cisapride per kilogram (0.07 to 0.14 mg per pound) of body weight three to four times a day, fifteen minutes before meals.

Missed dose—If you miss a dose of this medicine, take it as soon as possible. However, if it is almost time for your next dose, skip the missed dose and go back to your regular dosing schedule. Do not double doses.

Storage—To store this medicine:

- Keep out of the reach of children.
- Store away from heat and direct light.
- Do not store in the bathroom, near the kitchen sink, or in other damp places. Heat or moisture may cause the medicine to break down.
- Keep the medicine from freezing. Do not refrigerate.
- Do not keep outdated medicine or medicine no longer needed. Be sure that any discarded medicine is out of the reach of children.

Precautions While Using This Medicine

This medicine may cause your body to absorb alcohol more quickly than you normally would. Therefore, you may notice the effects sooner. *Check with your doctor before drinking alcohol while you are using this medicine.*

This medicine may cause some people to become drowsy or less alert than they are normally. *Make sure you know how you react to this medicine before you drive, use machines, or do anything else that could be dangerous if you are dizzy or are not alert.*

Side Effects of This Medicine

Along with its needed effects, a medicine may cause some unwanted effects. Although not all of these side effects may occur, if they do occur they may need medical attention.

Check with your doctor immediately if the following side effect occurs:

Rare

Seizures

Note: Seizures have occurred only in patients with a history of seizures.

Other side effects may occur that usually do not need medical attention. These side effects may go away during treatment as your body adjusts to the medicine. However, check with your doctor if any of the following side effects continue or are bothersome:

Less common

Abdominal cramping, constipation, diarrhea, drowsiness, headache, nausea, unusual tiredness or weakness

Other side effects not listed above may also occur in some patients. If you notice any other effects, check with your doctor.

Additional Information

Once a medicine has been approved for marketing for a certain use, experience may show that it is also useful for other medical problems. Although this use is not included in product labeling, cisapride is used in certain patients with the following medical condition:

- Gastroparesis (stomach condition)

Other than the above information, there is no additional information relating to proper use, precautions, or side effects for this use.

Annual revision: 08/27/93

ENTERAL NUTRITION FORMULAS Systemic

This information applies to the following enteral nutrition formulas:

Enteral nutrition, blenderized
Enteral nutrition, disease-specific
Enteral nutrition, fiber-containing
Enteral nutrition, milk-based
Enteral nutrition, modular
Enteral nutrition, monomeric (elemental)
Enteral nutrition, polymeric

Some commonly used brand names are:

For Blenderized Enteral Nutrition

In the U.S.

Compleat Modified
Compleat Regular
Vitaneed

In Canada

Compleat Modified

For Disease-specific Enteral Nutrition

In the U.S.

Amin-aid
Glucerna
Hepatic-Aid II
Immun-Aid
Impact
Impact with Fiber
Lipisorb
Nepro
NutriHep
NutriVent
Perative
Protain XL
Pulmocare
Stresstein
Suplena
TraumaCal
Traum-Aid HBC
Travasorb Hepatic Diet
Travasorb Renal Diet

In Canada

Citrotein
Glucerna
Impact
Nepro
Pulmocare
Suplena

For Fiber-containing Enteral Nutrition

In the U.S.

Ensure with Fiber
Fiberlan
Fibersource
Fibersource HN
Impact with Fiber
Jevity
Nutren 1.0 with Fiber
NutriSource
NutriSource HN
Pediasure with Fiber
Profiber
Replete with Fiber
Sustacal with Fiber
Ultracal

In Canada

Ensure with Fiber
Jevity
NutriSource
NutriSource HN

For Milk-based Enteral Nutrition

In the U.S.

Carnation Instant Breakfast
Carnation Instant Breakfast No Sugar Added
Great Shake
Lonalac
Menu Magic Instant Breakfast
Menu Magic Milk Shake
Meritene
Sustagen
Tasty Shake

In Canada
Meritene
Sustagen

For Modular Enteral Nutrition

In the U.S.
Casec
Elementra
MCT Oil
Microlipid
Moducal
Polycose
ProMod
Propac
Sumacal

In Canada
MCT Oil
Polycose
ProMod

For Monomeric (Elemental) Enteral Nutrition

In the U.S.
Accupep HPF
Alitraq
Criticare HN
Peptamen
Reabilan
Reabilan HN
Tolerex
Travasorb HN
Travasorb STD
Vital High Nitrogen
Vivonex T.E.N.

In Canada
Tolerex
Vital High Nitrogen
Vivonex T.E.N.

For Polymeric Enteral Nutrition

In the U.S.
Attain
CitriSource
Citrotein
Comply
Ensure
Ensure HN
Ensure Plus
Ensure Plus HN
Entrition Half-Strength
Entrition HN
Introlan
Introlite
Isocal
Isocal HCN
Isocal HN
Isolan
Isosource
Isosource HN
Isotein HN
Magnacal
Nutren 1.0
Nutren 1.5
Nutren 2.0
Nutrilan Flavored Supplements
Osmolite
Osmolite HN
Pediasure
Pre-Attain
Precision HN
Precision Isotonic Diet
Precision Low Residue
Promote
Replete
Resource
Resource Plus
Sustacal
Sustacal 8.8
Sustacal HC
TwoCal HN
Ultralan

In Canada
CitriSource
Enercal
Ensure
Ensure High Protein
Ensure Plus
Isosource
Isosource HN
Osmolite HN
Pediasure
Resource
Resource Plus

Description

Enteral nutrition formulas are used as nutritional replacements for patients who are unable to get enough nutrients in their diet. These formulas are taken by mouth or through a feeding tube and are used by the body for energy and to form substances needed for normal body functions.

Patients with the following conditions may be more likely to need enteral feedings:

- Acquired immunodeficiency syndrome (AIDS)
- Burns
- Cancer
- Infections, prolonged
- Kidney problems
- Liver problems
- Lung problems
- Pancreas problems
- Stomach problems
- Surgery
- Trauma
- Vomiting, prolonged

Enteral nutrition formulas are available without a prescription. However, they should only be used under medical supervision.

The benefits of enteral formulas in healthy people have not been proven.

Enteral nutrition formulas are available in the following dosage forms:

Oral

Blenderized Enteral Nutrition
- Oral solution (U.S. and Canada)

Disease-specific Enteral Nutrition
- Oral solution (U.S. and Canada)
- Powder for solution (U.S. and Canada)

Fiber-containing Enteral Nutrition
- Oral solution (U.S. and Canada)

Milk-based Enteral Nutrition
- Oral solution (U.S.)
- Powder for solution (U.S. and Canada)

Modular Enteral Nutrition
- Oil (U.S. and Canada)
- Oral solution (U.S. and Canada)
- Oral powder (U.S. and Canada)

Monomeric Enteral Nutrition
- Oral solution (U.S. and Canada)
- Powder for solution (U.S.)

Polymeric Enteral Nutrition
- Oral solution (U.S. and Canada)
- Powder for solution (U.S.)

It is very important that you read and understand the following information. If any of it causes you special concern, check with your doctor or pharmacist. Also, *if you have any questions* or if you want more information about this enteral nutrition formula or your medical problem, *ask your doctor, nurse, pharmacist, or dietitian.*

Before Using This Enteral Nutrition Formula

If you are taking any of these enteral nutrition formulas without a prescription, carefully read and follow any precautions on the label. For enteral nutrition formulas, the following should be considered:

Allergies—Tell your doctor if you have ever had any unusual or allergic reaction to any of the ingredients listed for your enteral nutrition formula. Also tell your doctor and pharmacist if you are allergic to any other substances, such as foods, preservatives, or dyes.

Pregnancy—Studies on effects in pregnancy have not been done in either humans or animals.

Breast-feeding—This enteral nutrition formula has not been reported to cause problems in nursing babies.

Children—Caution should be used when giving enteral feedings to children less than one year of age. Very young children may not be able to eliminate the feeding from the body. Although there is no specific information about the use of enteral feedings in older children, it is not expected to cause different side effects or problems in these children than it does in adults.

Older adults—Older adults may be at risk of developing problems related to the use of a nasogastric tube (tube going through the nose into the stomach), such as aspiration (sucking fluid into the lungs) or removing the nasogastric tube. The enteral feeding itself has not been shown to cause different side effects or problems in older people than it does in younger adults.

Medicines—Although certain medications and enteral nutrition formulas should not be used together at all, in other cases they may be used together even if an interaction might occur. In these cases, your doctor may want to change the dose, or other precautions may be necessary. Tell your doctor and pharmacist if you are taking any prescription or nonprescription (over-the-counter [OTC]) medicine.

Other medical problems—The presence of other medical problems may affect the use of enteral feedings. Make sure you tell your doctor if you have any other medical problems, especially:

- Breathing problems or
- Dehydration or
- Diabetes mellitus (sugar diabetes) or
- Diarrhea or
- Heart problems or
- Hyperglycemia (high levels of sugar in the blood) or
- Hyperlipidemia or
- Lactose intolerance or
- Liver problems or
- Pancreas problems—Enteral feedings may make these conditions worse; your doctor may recommend a special formula for your condition
- Intestine problems or
- Stomach problems—These problems may prevent enteral formulas from being absorbed properly
- Kidney problems—Higher blood levels of certain ingredients of the enteral feeding may result, and a smaller amount of enteral feeding may be needed.
- Malnutrition, severe—Heart and nerve problems have been reported when feeding a patient who is severely malnourished; enteral formula may need to be used in smaller amounts

Proper Use of This Enteral Nutrition Formula

Your enteral feeding may be given by mouth or by a feeding tube. Use the amount recommended by your doctor.

For patients taking the *oral liquid* form of enteral nutrition:

- This preparation is in ready-to-use form. No dilution is needed unless directed by your physician.
- Shake the preparation well before opening. Refrigerate after opening, out of the reach of children. Most formulas can be kept in the refrigerator for 1 to 2 days. Check the label of your product.

For patients using the *powder* form of this preparation:

- For mixing or other use, follow carefully the instructions on the package.
- Any unused solution should be kept in the refrigerator, out of the reach of children. Most formulas can be kept in the refrigerator for 1 to 2 days. Check the label of your product.

Storage—To store the unopened container:

- Keep out of the reach of children.
- Store away from heat and direct light.
- Do not store in the bathroom, near the kitchen sink, or in other damp places. Heat or moisture may cause the enteral nutrition formula to break down.
- Keep the enteral nutrition formula from freezing. Do not refrigerate, unless the product has been opened or mixed.
- Do not keep outdated enteral nutrition formulas or those no longer needed. Be sure that any discarded enteral nutrition formula is out of the reach of children.

Precautions While Using This Enteral Nutrition Formula

Enteral feedings must be handled properly to protect them from bacteria. Enteral feedings should be used for no more than 12 hours at room temperature and then should be discarded.

If you are taking your enteral feeding through a tube, enteral formulas that are too thick may clog the feeding tube. If this happens, check with your doctor, nurse, dietitian, or pharmacist.

Side Effects of This Enteral Nutrition Formula

Some problems may result from improper use of an enteral formula or use of the incorrect formula in your condition. Check with your doctor if any of the following problems occur:

More common

Confusion; convulsions (seizures); decrease in urine volume; dryness of mouth; frequent urination; increased thirst; irregular heartbeat; mood or mental changes; muscle cramps or pain; numbness or tingling in hands, feet, or lips; respiratory distress, shortness of breath or difficulty breathing; unexplained nervousness; unusual tiredness or weakness; weakness or heaviness of legs; weak pulse

Other problems may occur that usually do not need medical attention. They may go away during treatment as your body adjusts to the enteral nutrition formula. However, check with your doctor if any of the following side effects continue or are bothersome:

More common

Constipation; diarrhea; nausea or vomiting

Other side effects not listed above may also occur in some patients. If you notice any other effects, check with your doctor.

Annual revision: 08/31/93

FACTOR IX Systemic

Some commonly used brand names are:

In the U.S.

- AlphaNine
- AlphaNine SD
- Bebulin VH
- Konȳne 80
- Mononine
- Profilnine Heat-Treated
- Proplex T

In Canada

- AlphaNine
- Bebulin VH

Other commonly used names are Christmas factor, plasma thromboplastin component (PTC), and prothrombin complex concentrate (PCC).

Description

Factor IX is a protein produced naturally in the body. It helps the blood form clots to stop bleeding. Injections of factor IX are used to treat hemophilia B, which is sometimes called Christmas disease. This is a condition in which the body does not make enough factor IX. If you do not have enough factor IX and you become injured, your blood will not form clots as it should, and you may bleed into and damage your muscles and joints.

Injections of one form of factor IX, called factor IX complex, also are used to treat certain people with hemophilia A. In hemophilia A, sometimes called classical hemophilia, the body does not make enough factor VIII, and, just as in hemophilia B, the blood cannot form clots as it should. Injections of factor IX complex may be used in patients in whom the medicine used to treat hemophilia A is no longer effective. Injections of factor IX complex also may be used for other conditions as determined by your doctor.

The factor IX product that your doctor will give you is obtained naturally from human blood. It has been treated and is not likely to contain harmful viruses such as hepatitis B virus, hepatitis C (non-A, non-B) virus, or human immunodeficiency virus (HIV), the virus that causes acquired immunodeficiency syndrome (AIDS).

Factor IX is available only with your doctor's prescription, in the following dosage form:

Parenteral

- Injection (U.S. and Canada)

It is very important that you read and understand the following information. If any of it causes you special concern, check with your doctor. Also, *if you have any questions* or if you want more information about this medicine or your medical problem, *ask your doctor, nurse, or pharmacist.*

Before Using This Medicine

In deciding to use a medicine, the risks of using the medicine must be weighed against the good it will do. This is a decision you and your doctor will make. For factor IX, the following should be considered:

Allergies—Tell your doctor if you have ever had any unusual or allergic reaction to injections of factor IX or mouse protein. Also tell your doctor and pharmacist if you are allergic to any other substances, such as foods, preservatives, or dyes.

Pregnancy—Studies on effects in pregnancy have not been done in either humans or animals.

Breast-feeding—It is not known whether the ingredients in factor IX products pass into breast milk. Although most medicines pass into breast milk in small amounts, many of them may be used safely while breast-feeding. Mothers who are using this medicine and who wish to breast-feed should discuss this with their doctor.

Children—Blood clots may be especially likely to occur in premature and newborn babies, who are usually more sensitive than adults to the effects of injections of factor IX.

Older adults—This medicine has been tested and has not been shown to cause different side effects or problems in older people than it does in younger adults.

Other medicines—Although certain medicines should not be used together at all, in other cases two different medicines may be used together even if an interaction might occur. In these cases, your doctor may want to change the dose, or other precautions may be necessary. Tell your doctor and pharmacist if you are using any other prescription or nonprescription (over-the-counter [OTC]) medicine.

Other medical problems—The presence of other medical problems may affect the use of factor IX products. Make sure you tell your doctor if you have any other medical problems, especially:

- Liver disease—Risk of bleeding or developing blood clots may be increased

Before you begin using any new medicine (prescription or nonprescription) or if you develop any new medical problem while you are using this medicine, check with your doctor, nurse, or pharmacist.

Proper Use of This Medicine

Some medicines given by injection may sometimes be given at home to patients who do not need to be in the hospital. If you are using this medicine at home, your doctor or nurse will teach you how to prepare and inject the medicine. You will have a chance to practice preparing and injecting it. *Be sure that you understand exactly how the medicine is to be prepared and injected.*

To prepare this medicine:

- Take the dry medicine and the liquid (diluent) out of the refrigerator and *bring them to room temperature*, as directed by your doctor.
- When injecting the liquid (diluent) into the dry medicine, *aim the stream of liquid (diluent) against the wall of the container of dry medicine* to prevent foaming.
- *Swirl the container gently to dissolve the medicine. Do not shake the container.*

Use this medicine right away. It should not be kept longer than 3 hours after it has been prepared.

A plastic disposable syringe and filter needle must be used with this medicine. The medicine may stick to the inside of a glass syringe, and you may not receive a full dose.

Do not reuse syringes and needles. Put used syringes and needles in a puncture-resistant disposable container, or dispose of them as directed by your doctor, nurse, or pharmacist.

Dosing—The dose of factor IX will be different for different patients. The dose you receive will be based on:

- The condition for which you are using this medicine.
- Your body weight.
- The amount of factor IX your body is able to make.
- How much, how often, and where in your body you are bleeding.
- Whether or not your body has built up a defense (antibody) against this medicine.

Your dose of this medicine may even be different at different times. It is important that you *follow your doctor's orders.*

Missed dose—If you miss a dose of this medicine, check with your doctor as soon as possible for instructions.

Storage—To store this medicine:

- Keep out of the reach of children.
- Some factor IX products must be stored in the refrigerator, and some may be kept at room temperature for short periods of time. Store this medicine as directed by your doctor or the manufacturer.
- Do not keep outdated medicine or medicine no longer needed. Be sure that any discarded medicine is out of the reach of children.

Precautions While Using This Medicine

If you were recently diagnosed with hemophilia B, you should receive a hepatitis B vaccine to reduce even further your risk of getting hepatitis B from factor IX products.

After a while, your body may build up a defense (antibody) against this medicine. *Tell your doctor if this medicine seems to be less effective than usual.*

It is recommended that you carry identification stating that you have hemophilia A or hemophilia B. If you have any questions about what kind of identification to carry, check with your doctor, nurse, or pharmacist.

Side Effects of This Medicine

Along with its needed effects, a medicine may cause some unwanted effects. Although not all of these side effects may occur, if they do occur they may need medical attention.

Check with your doctor immediately if any of the following side effects occur, because they may mean that you are having a serious allergic reaction to the medicine:

Less common or rare

Changes in facial skin color; fast or irregular breathing; puffiness or swelling of the eyelids or around the eyes; shortness of breath, troubled breathing, tightness in chest, and/or wheezing; skin rash, hives, and/or itching

Also, check with your doctor immediately if any of the following side effects occur, because they may mean that you are developing a problem with blood clotting:

More common

Bluish coloring (especially of the hands and feet); convulsions; dizziness or lightheadedness when getting up from a lying or sitting position; increased heart rate; large blue or purplish patches in the skin (at places of injection); nausea or vomiting; pains in chest, groin, or legs (especially calves); persistent bleeding from puncture sites, gums, inner linings of the nose and/or mouth, or blood in the stool or urine; severe pain or pressure in the chest and/or the neck, back, or left arm; severe, sudden headache; shortness of breath or fast breathing; sudden loss of coordination; sudden and unexplained slurred speech, vision changes, and/or weakness or numbness in arm or leg

Also, check with your doctor immediately if any of the following side effects occur, because they may mean that your medicine is being given too fast:

Less common

Burning or stinging at place of injection; changes in blood pressure or pulse rate; chills; drowsiness; fever; headache; nausea or vomiting; redness of face; shortness of breath

Other side effects not listed above may also occur in some patients. If you notice any other effects, check with your doctor.

Annual revision: 08/27/93

GADODIAMIDE Diagnostic†

A commonly used brand name in the U.S. is Omniscan.

†Not commercially available in Canada.

Description

Gadodiamide (gad-oh-DYE-a-mide) is a paramagnetic agent. Paramagnetic agents are used to help provide a clear picture during magnetic resonance imaging (MRI), a special kind of diagnostic procedure. MRI uses magnets and computers to create images or "pictures" of certain areas inside the body. Unlike x-rays, it does not involve radiation.

Gadodiamide is given by injection before MRI to help diagnose problems or diseases of the brain or the spine.

Gadodiamide is to be used only by or under the supervision of a doctor. It is available in the following dosage form:

Parenteral

- Injection (U.S.)

It is very important that you read and understand the following information. If any of it causes you special concern, check with your doctor. Also, *if you have any questions* or if you want more information about this test or your medical problem, *ask your doctor, nurse, or pharmacist.*

Before Having This Test

In deciding to use a diagnostic test, any risks of the test must be weighed against the good it will do. This is a decision you and your doctor will make. Also, test results may be affected by other things. For gadodiamide, the following should be considered:

Allergies—Tell your doctor if you have ever had any unusual or allergic reaction to contrast agents like gadodiamide. Also, tell your doctor if you are allergic to any other substances, such as foods, preservatives, or dyes.

Pregnancy—Studies have not been done in humans. However, studies in animals at doses higher than human doses have shown that gadodiamide increases the risk of birth defects in the offspring. Also, it is not known yet what effect the magnetic field used in MRI might have on the development of the human fetus. Be sure you have discussed this with your doctor.

Breast-feeding—It is not known whether gadodiamide passes into breast milk. However, your doctor may want you to stop breast-feeding for some time after receiving gadodiamide. Be sure you have discussed this with your doctor.

Children—Although there is no specific information comparing use of gadodiamide in children with use in other age groups, this agent is not expected to cause different side effects or problems in children than it does in adults.

Older adults—Gadodiamide has been used in older people and has not been shown to cause different side effects or problems in older people than it does in younger adults.

Other medical problems—The presence of other medical problems may affect the use of gadodiamide. Make sure you tell your doctor if you have any other medical problems, especially:

- Allergies or asthma (history of)—If you have a history of these conditions, the risk of having a reaction, such as an allergic reaction, to the gadodiamide is greater
- Hemolytic anemia—Gadodiamide may make this condition worse
- Kidney disease (severe)—Gadodiamide may accumulate in the body, which may increase the chance of side effects
- Sickle cell disease—There may be a greater risk of blood vessel problems in patients with this condition

Preparation for This Test

Your doctor may have special instructions for you in preparation for your test, depending on the type of test you are having. If you do not understand the instructions you receive or if you have not received any instructions, check with your doctor in advance.

Side Effects of This Medicine

Along with its needed effects, contrast agents like gadodiamide may cause some unwanted effects. Although not all of these side effects may occur, if they do occur they may need medical attention.

Less common or rare

Itching, watery eyes; skin rash or hives; swelling of face; thickening of tongue; wheezing, tightness in chest, or troubled breathing

Other side effects may occur that usually do not need medical attention. These side effects may go away as your body adjusts to this agent. However, check with your doctor if any of the following side effects continue or are bothersome:

More common

Dizziness; headache; nausea

Less common or rare

Anxiety; changes in taste; chest pains; confusion; convulsions (seizures); diarrhea; dryness of mouth; pain at injection site; unusual warmth and flushing of skin

Other side effects not listed above may also occur in some patients. If you notice any other effects, check with your doctor.

Annual revision: 08/17/93

GADOTERIDOL Diagnostic†

A commonly used brand name in the U.S. is ProHance.

†Not commercially available in Canada.

Description

Gadoteridol (gad-oh-TER-i-dol) is a paramagnetic agent. Paramagnetic agents are used to help provide a clear picture during magnetic resonance imaging (MRI). MRI is a special kind of diagnostic procedure. It uses magnets and computers to create images or "pictures" of certain areas inside the body. Unlike x-rays, it does not involve radiation.

Gadoteridol is given by injection before MRI to help diagnose problems or diseases of the brain or the spine.

Gadoteridol is to be used only by or under the supervision of a doctor. It is available in the following dosage form:

Parenteral

- Injection (U.S.)

It is very important that you read and understand the following information. If any of it causes you special concern, check with your doctor. Also, *if you have any questions* or if you want more information about this test or your medical problem, *ask your doctor, nurse, or pharmacist.*

Before Having This Test

In deciding to use a diagnostic test, any risks of the test must be weighed against the good it will do. This is a decision you and your doctor will make. Also, test results may be affected by other things. For gadoteridol, the following should be considered:

Allergies—Tell your doctor if you have ever had any unusual or allergic reaction to contrast agents like gadoteridol. Also, tell your doctor if you are allergic to any other substances, such as foods, preservatives, or dyes.

Pregnancy—Studies have not been done in humans. However, studies in animals given doses many times higher than human doses have shown that gadoteridol increased the risk of losing the fetus or caused side effects in the offspring. Also, it is not known yet what effect the magnetic field used in MRI might have on the development of the human fetus. Be sure you have discussed this with your doctor.

Breast-feeding—It is not known if gadoteridol passes into the breast milk. However, your doctor may want you to stop breast-feeding for some time after receiving gadoteridol. Be sure you have discussed this with your doctor.

Children—Gadoteridol has been used in a limited number of children. In effective doses, it has not been shown to cause different side effects or problems than it does in adults.

Older adults—Gadoteridol has been used in older people and has not been shown to cause different side effects or problems in older people than it does in younger adults.

Other medical problems—The presence of other medical problems may affect the use of gadoteridol. Make sure you tell your doctor if you have any other medical problems, especially:

- Allergies or asthma (history of)—If you have a history of these conditions, the risk of having a reaction, such as an allergic reaction to the gadoteridol, is greater
- Anemia—This condition may get worse with the use of gadoteridol
- Kidney disease (severe)—Gadoteridol may accumulate in the body, which may increase the chance of side effects
- Sickle cell disease—There may be a greater risk of blood vessel problems in patients with this condition.

Preparation for This Test

Your doctor may have special instructions for you in preparation for your test, depending on the type of test. If you do not understand the instructions you receive or if you have not received any instructions, check with your doctor in advance.

Side Effects of This Medicine

Along with its needed effects, contrast agents like gadoteridol may cause some unwanted effects. Although not all of these side effects may occur, if they do occur they may need medical attention.

Less common or rare

Fast or irregular heartbeat; itching, watery eyes; low blood pressure; skin rash or hives; swelling of face; thickening of tongue; wheezing, tightness in chest, or troubled breathing

Other side effects may occur that usually do not need medical attention. These side effects may go away as your body adjusts to this agent. However, check with your doctor if any of the following side effects continue or are bothersome:

More common

Changes in taste; nausea or vomiting

Less common or rare

Anxiety; confusion; diarrhea; dizziness; headache; pain at injection site; unusual warmth and flushing of skin

Other side effects not listed above may also occur in some patients. If you notice any other effects, check with your doctor.

Annual revision: 08/17/93

HALOFANTRINE Systemic*†

A commonly used brand name is Halfan.

*Not commercially available in the U.S.
†Not commercially available in Canada.

Description

Halofantrine (ha-loe-FAN-trin) is used to treat certain types of malaria infection. It works by killing the malaria parasites (tiny one-celled animals).

Halofantrine is available only with your doctor's prescription, in the following dosage forms:

Oral

- Oral suspension (United Kingdom)
- Tablets (United Kingdom)

It is very important that you read and understand the following information. If any of it causes you special concern, check with your doctor. Also, *if you have any questions* or if you want more information about this medicine or your medical problem, *ask your doctor, nurse, or pharmacist.*

Before Using This Medicine

In deciding to use a medicine, the risks of taking the medicine must be weighed against the good it will do. This is a decision you and your doctor will make. For halofantrine, the following should be considered:

Allergies—Tell your doctor if you have ever had any unusual or allergic reaction to halofantrine. Also tell your doctor and pharmacist if you are allergic to any other substances, such as foods, preservatives, or dyes.

Pregnancy—Halofantrine has not been studied in pregnant women. However, it has been found to cause unwanted effects, including death of the fetus, in animals. Before taking this medicine, make sure your doctor knows if you are pregnant or if you may become pregnant.

Breast-feeding—Halofantrine may pass into breast milk and cause unwanted effects in nursing babies. It may be necessary for you to take another medicine or to stop breast-feeding while taking halofantrine. Be sure you have discussed the risks and benefits of the medicine with your doctor.

Children—Although there is no specific information comparing use of halofantrine in children with use in other age groups, this medicine is not expected to cause different side effects or problems in children than it does in adults.

Older adults—Many medicines have not been studied specifically in older people. Therefore, it may not be known whether they work exactly the same way they do in younger adults or if they cause different side effects or problems in older people. There is no specific information comparing use of halofantrine in the elderly with use in other age groups.

Other medicines—Although certain medicines should not be used together at all, in other cases two different medicines may be used together even if an interaction might occur. In these cases, your doctor may want to change the dose, or other precautions may be necessary. When you are taking halofantrine, it is especially important that your doctor and pharmacist know if you are taking any of the following:

- Mefloquine (e.g., Lariam)—Recent use of mefloquine or use of mefloquine with halofantrine may cause fast and irregular heartbeat

Other medical problems—The presence of other medical problems may affect the use of halofantrine. Make sure you tell your doctor if you have any other medical problems, especially:

- Heart problems especially abnormal heartbeat or
- Thiamine deficiency or
- Unexplained sudden fainting—These conditions increase the chance of side effects affecting the heart, including fast irregular heartbeat

Before you begin using any new medicine (prescription or nonprescription) or if you develop any new medical problem while you are using this medicine, check with your doctor, nurse, or pharmacist.

Proper Use of This Medicine

Halofantrine is best taken on an empty stomach to decrease the chance of side effects.

To help clear up your infection completely, *take this medicine exactly as directed by your doctor for the full time of treatment.* Your symptoms may come back if you stop your treatment too early. Your doctor may also instruct you to take a second course of treatment after one week.

Dosing—The dose of halofantrine will be different for different patients. *Follow your doctor's orders or the directions on the label.* The following information includes only the average doses of halofantrine. *If your dose is different, do not change it* unless your doctor tells you to do so.

The number of tablets or teaspoonfuls of suspension that you take depends on the strength of the medicine. Also, *the number of doses you take each day, the time allowed between doses, and the length of time you take the medicine depend on the medical problem for which you are taking halofantrine.*

- For malaria:
  - —For *oral* dosage form (oral suspension):
    - Adults and children over 12 years of age—500 milligrams (mg), taken on an empty stomach every six hours three times a day for one day. Treatment may need to be repeated after one week.
    - Children—Dose is based on age and/or body weight. Treatment may need to be repeated after one week.
      - —1 to 2 years of age: 100 mg, taken on an empty stomach every six hours three times a day for one day.
      - —2 to 5 years of age: 150 mg, taken on an empty stomach every six hours three times a day for one day.
      - —5 to 8 years of age: 200 mg, taken on an empty stomach every six hours three times a day for one day.
      - —8 to 10 years of age: 250 mg, taken on an empty stomach every six hours three times a day for one day.
      - —10 to 12 years of age: 300 mg, taken on an empty stomach every six hours three times a day for one day.
  - —For *oral* dosage form (tablets):
    - Adults and children over 37 kilograms (81.4 pounds) of body weight—500 mg, taken on an empty stomach every six hours three times a day for one day. Treatment may need to be repeated after one week.
    - Children—Dose is based on body weight and must be determined by your doctor. Treatment may need to be repeated after one week.
      - —Up to 23 kilograms (50.6 pounds) of body weight: Dosage has not been established.
      - —23 to 31 kilograms (50.6 to 68.2 pounds) of body weight: 250 mg, taken on an empty

stomach every six hours three times a day for one day.

—32 to 37 kilograms (70.4 to 81.4 pounds) of body weight: 375 mg, taken on an empty stomach every six hours three times a day for one day.

Missed dose—If you miss a dose of this medicine, take it as soon as possible. However, if it is almost time for your next dose, skip the missed dose and go back to your regular dosing schedule. Do not double doses.

Storage—To store this medicine:

- Keep out of the reach of children.
- Store away from heat and direct light.
- Do not store in the bathroom, near the kitchen sink, or in other damp places. Heat or moisture may cause the medicine to break down.
- Keep the liquid form of this medicine from freezing.
- Do not keep outdated medicine or medicine no longer needed. Be sure that any discarded medicine is out of the reach of children.

Precautions While Using This Medicine

It is important that your doctor check your progress after treatment. This is to make sure that the infection is cleared up completely, and to allow your doctor to check for any unwanted effects.

If your symptoms do not improve after you have taken this medicine for the full course of treatment, or if they become worse, check with your doctor.

Malaria is spread by the bites of certain kinds of infected female mosquitoes. If you are living in, or will be traveling to, an area where there is a chance of getting malaria, the following mosquito-control measures will help to prevent infection:

- If possible, avoid going out between dusk and dawn because it is at these times when mosquitoes most commonly bite.
- Wear long-sleeved shirts and long trousers to protect your arms and legs, especially from dusk through dawn when mosquitoes are out.
- Apply insect repellant, preferably one containing DEET, to uncovered areas of the skin from dusk through dawn when mosquitoes are out.
- If possible, sleep in a screened or air-conditioned room or under mosquito netting sprayed with insecticide to avoid being bitten by malaria-carrying mosquitoes.
- Use mosquito coils or sprays to kill mosquitoes in living and sleeping quarters during evening and nighttime hours.

Side Effects of This Medicine

Along with its needed effects, a medicine may cause some unwanted effects. Although not all of these side effects may occur, if they do occur they may need medical attention.

Check with your doctor immediately if any of the following side effects occur:

Rare

Anxiety; black or decreased amount of urine; chest or lower back pain; fast and irregular heartbeat; feeling restless; flushing of the whole body; rapid breathing

Other side effects may occur that usually do not need medical attention. These side effects may go away during treatment as your body adjusts to the medicine. However, check with your doctor if any of the following side effects continue or are bothersome:

Less common

Abdominal or stomach pain; diarrhea; nausea; skin itching or rash; vomiting

Other side effects not listed above may also occur in some patients. If you notice any other effects, check with your doctor.

Annual revision: 08/31/93

INFANT FORMULAS Systemic

Some commonly used brand names are:

For Infant Formulas, Hypoallergenic

In the U.S.

Alimentum	Pregestimil
Nutramigen	

In Canada

Alimentum	Pregestimil
Nutramigen	

For Infant Formulas, Milk-based

In the U.S.

Carnation Follow-Up Formula	Similac 27
Carnation Good Start	Similac with Iron 20
Enfamil	Similac with Iron 24
Enfamil Human Milk Fortifier	Similac Natural Care Human Milk Fortifier
Enfamil with Iron	Similac PM 60/40
Enfamil Premature Formula	Similac Special Care 20
Enfamil Premature Formula with Iron	Similac Special Care 24
Gerber Baby Formula	Similac Special Care with Iron 24
Lactofree	SMA 13
Preemie SMA 20	SMA 20
Preemie SMA 24	SMA 24
Similac 13	SMA 27
Similac 20	SMA Lo-Iron 13
Similac 24	SMA Lo-Iron 20
	SMA Lo-Iron 24

In Canada

Preemie SMA 20	Similac Special Care 24
Preemie SMA 24	SMA 13
Similac 13	SMA 20
Similac 20	SMA 24
Similac 24	SMA 27
Similac 27	SMA Lo-Iron 13
Similac PM 60/40	SMA Lo-Iron 20
Similac Special Care 20	SMA Lo-Iron 24

For Infant Formulas, Soy-based

In the U.S.

Gerber Soy Formula	Nursoy
Isomil	ProSobee
Isomil SF	RCF
I-Soyalac	Soyalac

In Canada

Isomil	ProSobee
Nursoy	RCF

Description

Infant formulas are used to supply all or part of the nutrients infants need for growth and development. These formulas are used by the body for energy and to form substances for normal body functions.

The amount and type of nutrients contained in infant formulas are regulated by the Food and Drug Administration (FDA). The FDA also regulates the manufacturing process, labeling, and recall procedure for infant formulas.

Infant formulas are available without a prescription. However, they should only be used under medical supervision. They are available in the following forms:

Oral

Infant Formulas, Hypoallergenic (for infants allergic to milk)
- Oral concentrate (U.S. and Canada)
- Oral solution (U.S. and Canada)
- Powder for oral solution (U.S. and Canada)

Infant Formulas, Milk-based (for infants not allergic to milk)
- Oral concentrate (U.S.)
- Oral powder (U.S.)
- Oral solution (U.S. and Canada)
- Powder for oral solution (U.S. and Canada)

Infant Formulas, Soy-based (for infants allergic to milk but not to soy)
- Oral concentrate (U.S. and Canada)
- Oral solution (U.S. and Canada)
- Powder for oral solution (U.S. and Canada)

It is very important that you read and understand the following information. If any of it causes you special concern, check with your infant's doctor or dietitian. Also, *if you have any questions* or if you want more information about this infant formula, *ask your doctor, nurse, pharmacist, or dietitian.*

Before Using This Infant Formula

If you are giving your infant this infant formula, carefully read and follow any precautions on the label. For infant formulas, the following should be considered:

Allergies—Tell your doctor if your infant has ever had any unusual or allergic reaction to infant formulas. Also tell your doctor and pharmacist if your infant is allergic to any other substances, such as foods, preservatives, or dyes.

Children—Problems may occur if the infant formula is not mixed properly or is not used under medical care.

Medicines, dietary supplements, or infant formulas—Although certain medicines, dietary supplements, or infant formulas should not be used together at all, in other cases they may be used together even if an interaction might occur. In these cases, your doctor may want to change the feeding schedule, or other precautions may be necessary. When you are giving your infant an infant formula, it is especially important that your doctor and pharmacist know if you are giving your infant any dietary supplements or any prescription or nonprescription (over-the-counter [OTC]) medicine.

Other medical problems—The presence of other medical problems may affect the use of infant formulas. Make sure you tell your doctor if your infant has any medical problems, especially:

- Breathing problems or
- Dehydration or
- Diabetes mellitus (sugar diabetes) or
- Diarrhea or
- Heart problems or
- Hyperglycemia (high levels of sugar in the blood) or
- Liver problems or
- Pancreas problems—Infant formulas may make these conditions worse
- Intestine problems or
- Stomach problems—These problems may prevent infant formulas from being absorbed properly
- Kidney problems—Higher blood levels of certain ingredients of the infant formula may result, and a smaller amount of infant formula may be needed
- Phenylketonuria—Infant formulas contain phenylalanine, which may make the condition worse

Proper Use of This Infant Formula

Infant formulas may be given by mouth or, in some cases, by a tube feeding. Use the amount of infant formula and the feeding schedule recommended by your doctor.

For infants receiving the *concentrate or powder for oral solution* form of this preparation:

- For mixing or other use, follow carefully the instructions on the package.
- Any unused solution should be kept in the refrigerator. Most formulas can be kept in the refrigerator for 1 to 2 days. Check the label of your product.

For infants receiving the *oral liquid* form of this preparation:

- This preparation is in ready-to-use form. No dilution is needed unless directed by your doctor.
- Shake the preparation well before opening. Refrigerate after opening. Most formulas can be kept in the refrigerator for 1 to 2 days. Check the label of your product.

For infants receiving *Enfamil Human Milk Fortifier*:

- This powder should be added to mother's breast milk. For mixing or other use, follow carefully the instructions on the package.
- Any unused solution should be kept in the refrigerator for up to 1 day.

For infants receiving *Similac Natural Care*:

- This liquid should be added to the mother's breast milk. It may also be fed alternating with breast milk to low-birth-weight infants as directed by the infant's doctor. For mixing or other use, follow carefully the instructions on the package.
- Any unused solution should be kept in the refrigerator for up to 1 day.

Feeding—The amount of an infant formula to be given will be different for different infants. *Follow your doctor's orders.*

Storage—To store the unopened container:

- Keep out of the reach of children.
- Store away from heat and direct light.
- Do not store in the bathroom, near the kitchen sink, or in other damp places. Heat or moisture may cause the infant formula to break down.
- Keep the infant formula from freezing. Do not refrigerate until after the product has been opened or mixed.
- Do not keep outdated infant formulas or those no longer needed. Be sure that any discarded infant formula is out of the reach of children.

Side Effects of This Infant Formula

Along with its needed effects, an infant formula may cause some unwanted effects. Although not all of these side effects may occur, if they do occur they may need medical attention.

More common

Diarrhea; unusual thirst; unusual tiredness or weakness

Note: Diarrhea can lead to severe fluid loss in your infant very quickly. Diarrhea can be caused by improper infant formula preparation. Make sure that you are following the directions for mixing on the container of your product.

Less common

Signs of milk allergy (hives, wheezing); signs of milk intolerance (abdominal bloating, diarrhea, stomach cramps, vomiting)

Annual revision: 09/23/93

ITRACONAZOLE Systemic†

A commonly used brand name in the U.S. is Sporanox.

†Not commercially available in Canada.

Description

Itraconazole (i-tra-KOE-na-zole) is used to help overcome serious fungus infections that may occur in different parts of the body. This medicine may also be used for other problems as determined by your doctor.

Itraconazole is available only with your doctor's prescription, in the following dosage form:

Oral

- Capsules (U.S.)

It is very important that you read and understand the following information. If any of it causes you special concern, check with your doctor. Also, *if you have any questions* or if you want more information about this medicine or your medical problem, *ask your doctor, nurse, or pharmacist.*

Before Using This Medicine

In deciding to use a medicine, the risks of taking the medicine must be weighed against the good it will do. This is a decision you and your doctor will make. For itraconazole, the following should be considered:

Allergies—Tell your doctor if you have ever had any unusual or allergic reaction to itraconazole or other related medicines, such as fluconazole, ketoconazole, or miconazole. Also tell your doctor and pharmacist if you are allergic to any other substances, such as foods, preservatives, or dyes.

Pregnancy—Itraconazole has not been studied in pregnant women. However, studies in some animals have shown that itraconazole, taken in high doses, may cause harm to the mother and the fetus. It has caused birth defects in animals. Before taking this medicine, make sure your doctor knows if you are pregnant or if you may become pregnant.

Breast-feeding—Itraconazole passes into breast milk. Be sure you have discussed the risks and benefits of this medicine with your doctor.

Children—A small number of children have been safely treated with itraconazole. Be sure to discuss with your child's doctor the use of this medicine in children.

Older adults—Many medicines have not been studied specifically in older people. Therefore, it may not be known whether they work exactly the same way they do in younger adults or if they cause different side effects or problems in older people. There is no specific information comparing use of itraconazole in the elderly with use in other age groups.

Other medicines—Although certain medicines should not be used together at all, in other cases 2 different medicines may be used together even if an interaction might occur. In these cases, your doctor may want to change the dose, or other precautions may be necessary. When you are taking itraconazole, it is especially important that your doctor and pharmacist know if you are taking any of the following:

- Antacids or
- Cimetidine (e.g., Tagamet) or
- Didanosine (e.g., Videx, ddI) or
- Famotidine (e.g., Pepcid) or
- Nizatidine (e.g., Axid) or
- Ranitidine (e.g., Zantac)—Use of these medicines may decrease the effects of itraconazole. Didanosine must not be taken at the same time as itraconazole. These other medicines should be taken at least 2 hours after itraconazole
- Astemizole (e.g., Hismanal) or
- Terfenadine (e.g., Seldane)—Itraconazole may increase the chance of serious side effects of astemizole or terfenadine. These medicines should not be taken with itraconazole
- Carbamazepine (e.g., Tegretol) or
- Phenytoin (e.g., Dilantin) or
- Rifampin (e.g., Rifadin)—These medicines may decrease the effects of itraconazole
- Cyclosporine (e.g., Sandimmune) or
- Digoxin (e.g., Lanoxin) or
- Warfarin (e.g., Coumadin)—Itraconazole may increase the effects of these medicines, which may increase the chance of side effects

Other medical problems—The presence of other medical problems may affect the use of itraconazole. Make sure you tell your doctor if you have any other medical problems, especially:

- Achlorhydria (absence of stomach acid) or
- Hypochlorhydria (decreased amount of stomach acid)—Itraconazole may not be absorbed from the stomach as well in patients who have low or no stomach acid
- Liver disease—Liver disease may increase the chance of side effects caused by itraconazole

Before you begin using any new medicine (prescription or nonprescription) or if you develop any new medical problem while you are using this medicine, check with your doctor, nurse, or pharmacist.

Proper Use of This Medicine

Itraconazole should be taken with a meal or snack so that the medicine is fully absorbed into the body.

To help clear up your infection completely, *keep taking your medicine for the full time of treatment,* even if you begin to feel better after a few days. Since fungus infections may be very slow to clear up, you may have to continue taking this medicine every day for as long as 6 months to a year or more. Some fungus infections never clear up completely and need continuous treatment. If you stop taking this medicine too soon, your symptoms may return.

This medicine works best when there is a constant amount in the blood or urine. *To help keep the amount constant, do not miss any doses. Also, it is best to take each dose at the same time every day.* If you need help in planning the best time to take your medicine, check with your doctor, nurse, or pharmacist.

Dosing—The dose of itraconazole may be different for different patients. *Follow your doctor's orders or the directions on the label.* The following information includes only the average doses of itraconazole. *If your dose is different, do not change it* unless your doctor tells you to do so.

The number of capsules that you take depends on the strength of the medicine. Also, *the number of doses you take each day, the time allowed between doses, and the length of time you take the medicine depend on the medical problem for which you are taking itraconazole.*

- For the *oral* dosage form (capsules):
  - —For treatment of blastomycosis or histoplasmosis:
    - Adults and teenagers—200 milligrams (mg) taken with food once a day. The dose may be increased if necessary, up to a total daily dose of 400 mg. Doses above 200 mg per day should be given in two divided doses.
    - Children—Use and dose must be determined by your doctor.

Missed dose—If you miss a dose of this medicine, take it as soon as possible. This will help to keep a constant amount of medicine in the blood. However, if it is almost time for your next dose, skip the missed dose and go back to your regular dosing schedule. Do not double doses.

Storage—To store this medicine:

- Keep out of the reach of children.
- Store away from heat and direct light.
- Do not store in the bathroom, near the kitchen sink, or in other damp places. Heat or moisture may cause the medicine to break down.
- Do not keep outdated medicine or medicine no longer needed. Be sure that any discarded medicine is out of the reach of children.

Precautions While Using This Medicine

It is important that your doctor check your progress at regular visits. This will allow your doctor to check for any unwanted effects.

If your symptoms do not improve within a few weeks (or months for some infections), or if they become worse, check with your doctor.

If you are taking antacids, cimetidine (e.g., Tagamet), famotidine (e.g., Pepcid), nizatidine (e.g., Axid), or ranitidine (e.g., Zantac) while you are taking itraconazole, take the other medicine at least 2 hours after you take itraconazole. If you take these medicines at the same time that you take itraconazole, they will keep itraconazole from working properly.

Side Effects of This Medicine

Along with its needed effects, a medicine may cause some unwanted effects. Although not all of these effects may occur, if they do occur they may need medical attention.

Check with your doctor immediately if any of the following side effects occur:

Less common

Skin rash

Rare

Dark or amber urine; loss of appetite; pale stools; stomach pain; unusual tiredness or weakness; yellow eyes or skin

Other side effects may occur that usually do not need medical attention. These side effects may go away during treatment as your body adjusts to the medicine. However, check with your doctor if any of the following side effects continue or are bothersome:

Less common

Constipation; diarrhea; headache; loss of appetite; nausea or vomiting

Other side effects not listed above may also occur in some patients. If you notice any other effects, check with your doctor.

Additional Information

Once a medicine has been approved for marketing for a certain use, experience may show that it is also useful for other medical problems. Although these uses are not included in product labeling, itraconazole is used in certain patients with the following medical conditions:

- Aspergillosis
- Candidal infections of the mouth, throat, or vagina
- Coccidioidomycosis
- Cryptococcal meningitis

- Cryptococcosis
- Histoplasmosis (suppression)
- Onychomycosis
- Tinea corporis (ringworm of the body)
- Tinea cruris (ringworm of the groin; jock itch)
- Tinea manuum (ringworm of the hand)
- Tinea pedis (ringworm of the foot; athlete's foot)

Other than the above information, there is no additional information relating to proper use, precautions, or side effects for these uses.

Annual revision: 08/03/93

JAPANESE ENCEPHALITIS VIRUS VACCINE Systemic†

A commonly used brand name in the U.S. is Je-Vax.

†Not commercially available in Canada.

Description

Japanese encephalitis (in-cef-a-LY-tis) virus vaccine is an immunizing agent used to help prevent infection by the Japanese encephalitis virus. Japanese encephalitis is caused by the bite of a mosquito that lives in certain parts of Asia. The vaccine works by causing your body to produce its own protection (antibodies) against the virus.

This vaccine is available only from your doctor or other authorized health care provider, in the following dosage form:

Parenteral

- Injection (U.S.)

It is very important that you read and understand the following information. If any of it causes you special concern, check with your doctor. Also, *if you have any questions* or if you want more information about this medicine or your medical problem, *ask your doctor, nurse, or pharmacist.*

Before Receiving This Vaccine

In deciding to use a medicine, the risks of receiving the medicine must be weighed against the good it will do. This is a decision you and your doctor will make. For Japanese encephalitis virus vaccine, the following should be considered:

Allergies—Tell your doctor if you have ever had any unusual or allergic reaction to thimerosal, formaldehyde, gelatin, or rodent protein or brain products. Also tell your doctor and pharmacist if you are allergic to any other substances, such as foods, preservatives, or dyes.

Pregnancy—Studies on effects in pregnancy have not been done in either humans or animals.

Breast-feeding—It is not known whether this vaccine passes into breast milk. Although most medicines pass into breast milk in small amounts, many of them may be used safely while breast-feeding. Mothers who are receiving this vaccine and who wish to breast-feed should discuss this with their doctor.

Children—Studies on this vaccine have been done only in adults and children 1 year of age and older. There is no specific information comparing use of this vaccine in infants under 1 year of age with use in other age groups.

Older adults—Many medicines have not been studied specifically in older people. Therefore, it may not be known whether they work exactly the same way they do in younger adults. Although there is no specific information comparing use of Japanese encephalitis virus vaccine in the elderly with use in other age groups, this vaccine is not expected to cause different side effects or problems in older people than it does in younger adults. In addition, immunization may be especially useful for the elderly, since older persons may have a higher risk of illness following infection with the Japanese encephalitis virus.

Other medical problems—The presence of other medical problems may affect the use of this vaccine. Make sure you tell your doctor if you have any other medical problems, especially:

- Hives (history of)—May increase the chance of side effects of the vaccine

Before you begin using any new medicine (prescription or nonprescription) or if you develop any new medical problem while you are receiving this vaccine, check with your doctor, nurse, or pharmacist.

Proper Use of This Vaccine

It is important that you receive 3 doses of the vaccine. If there is not enough time for you to get all 3 doses, you may get 2 doses of the vaccine. However, *2 doses of the vaccine will not protect you as well as 3 doses.*

It is important that you receive all 3 doses of the vaccine at least 10 days before you plan on traveling out of the country. There is a chance of side effects that do not show up right away, and, if they do occur, they may need medical attention. In addition, the 10 days will give your body time to produce antibodies against the Japanese encephalitis virus.

Dosing—The number of doses you receive and the time allowed between doses of Japanese encephalitis virus vaccine will be different for different patients.

- For help preventing Japanese encephalitis:
  - —For *injection* dosage form:
    - Adults and children 1 year of age and older—One dose injected under the skin on days zero, seven, and thirty, for a total of three doses.
    - Children up to 1 year of age—Use and dose must be determined by your doctor.

Precautions After Receiving This Vaccine

Since the vaccine may not protect everyone completely, *it is very important that you still use precautions to reduce your chance of mosquito bites.* These include using insect repellents and mosquito netting, wearing protective clothing, and staying indoors during twilight and after dark.

Side Effects of This Vaccine

Along with its needed effects, a medicine may cause some unwanted effects. Although not all of these side effects may occur, if they do occur they may need medical attention. *It is very important that you tell your doctor about any side effect that occurs after a dose of the vaccine,* even if the side effect goes away without treatment. Some types of side effects may mean that you should not receive any more doses of the vaccine.

Get emergency help immediately if the following side effect occurs:

Rare

Swelling of face, lips, eyelids, throat, tongue, hands, or feet

Check with your doctor immediately if any of the following side effects occur:

Rare

Hives; tiredness or weakness (severe or unusual); wheezing or troubled breathing

Although the following side effects usually do not need medical attention and may go away on their own, *their presence may also mean that more serious side effects are about to occur.* Therefore, check with your doctor as soon as possible if any of the following side effects occur:

More common

Tenderness, soreness, redness, or swelling at place of injection

Less common

Abdominal pain; aches or pains in muscles; chills or fever; dizziness; general feeling of discomfort or illness; headache; itching or skin rash; nausea or vomiting

Rare

Joint swelling

Other side effects not listed above may also occur in some patients. If you notice any other effects, check with your doctor.

Annual revision: 06/21/93

LIDOCAINE AND PRILOCAINE Topical

A commonly used brand name in the U.S. and Canada is EMLA.

Another commonly used name for lidocaine is lignocaine.

Description

This medicine contains a mixture of 2 local anesthetics (an-ess-THET-iks), lidocaine (LYE-doe-kane) and prilocaine (PRIL-oh-kane). It is used to produce numbness or loss of feeling before certain painful procedures, such as injections, drawing blood from a vein, or removing small growths (warts, for example) from the skin.

This medicine deadens the nerve endings in the skin. It does not cause unconsciousness as general anesthetics used for surgery do.

In the U.S., this medicine is available only with your doctor's prescription. In Canada, it is available without a prescription. However, your doctor may have special instructions on the proper use and dose, depending on the reason you are using this medicine.

Topical

- Cream (U.S. and Canada)

It is very important that you read and understand the following information. If any of it causes you special concern, check with your doctor or pharmacist. Also, *if you have any questions* or if you want more information about this medicine or your medical problem, *ask your doctor, nurse, or pharmacist.*

Before Using This Medicine

In deciding to use a medicine, the risks of using the medicine must be weighed against the good it will do.

This is a decision you and your doctor will make. For this medicine, the following should be considered:

Allergies—Tell your doctor if you have ever had any unusual or allergic reaction to lidocaine, prilocaine, or other local anesthetics given by injection or applied to any part of the body as a liquid, cream, ointment, or spray. Also tell your doctor and pharmacist if you are allergic to any other substances, such as foods, preservatives, or dyes.

Pregnancy—This mixture of lidocaine and prilocaine has not been studied in pregnant women. However, lidocaine and prilocaine (separately) have been given to pregnant women and have not been reported to cause birth defects or other problems.

Breast-feeding—Small amounts of lidocaine, and probably of prilocaine also, pass into breast milk. Many medicines that pass into breast milk in small amounts may be used safely while breast-feeding. Mothers who are breast-feeding and who wish to use this medicine should discuss this with their doctor.

Children—This medicine has been tested in children. Very young children (less than 1 year of age) may be especially sensitive to the effects of lidocaine and prilocaine. This may increase the chance of side effects. However, in effective doses, this medicine has not been shown to cause different side effects or problems in children older than 1 year of age than it does in adults.

Young children are often frightened when they receive injections or have other painful procedures done. This medicine helps prevent pain, but it will not calm a frightened child. Parents can help by staying calm and by comforting and reassuring the child.

Older adults—This medicine has not been studied specifically in older people. However, it is possible that the chance of some side effects may be increased in elderly people. Experience with local anesthetics given by injection or applied to other areas of the body (for example, the throat or the inside of the mouth) has shown that elderly people are usually more sensitive than younger adults to the effects of local anesthetics.

Other medicines—Although certain medicines should not be used together at all, in other cases two different medicines may be used together even if an interaction might occur. In these cases, your doctor may want to change the dose, or other precautions may be necessary. Before using this medicine, tell your doctor, nurse, or pharmacist if you are taking any other prescription or nonprescription (over-the-counter [OTC]) medicine, especially:

- Sulfonamides (sulfa medicine)—The chance of a side effect (methemoglobinemia) may be increased, especially in infants.

Other medical problems—The presence of other medical problems may affect the use of this medicine. Make sure you tell your doctor if you have any other medical problems, especially:

- Broken or inflamed skin, burns, or open wounds at place of application or
- Atopic dermatitis or
- Eczema—More of this medicine can be absorbed into the body quickly, which increases the chance of side effects
- Glucose-6-phosphate dehydrogenase (G6PD) deficiency—A possible side effect of this medicine (methemoglobinemia) may be more likely to occur
- Liver disease (severe)—The chance of side effects may be increased if large amounts of this medicine are absorbed into the body quickly
- Methemoglobinemia—This medicine may make your condition worse

Proper Use of This Medicine

For safe and effective use of this medicine:

- Use this medicine only when directed to do so by your doctor or nurse. *Do not use it for any other reason without first checking with your doctor.* This medicine may be more likely than other topical anesthetics to cause unwanted effects if it is used too much, because more of it is absorbed into the body through the skin.
- Unless otherwise directed by your doctor or nurse, *do not apply this medicine to open wounds, burns, or broken or inflamed skin.*
- *Be careful not to get any of this medicine in your eyes,* because it can cause severe eye irritation. If any of the medicine does get into your eye, *do not rub or wipe the eye, even if it hurts. Instead, check with your doctor right away.*
- Be careful not to get any of this medicine on your lips or in your mouth.
- *Follow carefully any directions given to you by your doctor or nurse about how this medicine should be used.* If you have not received other instructions about how to apply this medicine, *follow the patient directions that come with the medicine.*
- *Check with your doctor or nurse if you have any questions* about how to apply this medicine, where to apply it, or what time to apply it.

To use:

- Apply a thick layer of medicine to the area or areas where local anesthesia (numbness or loss of feeling) is needed. *Do not spread out the medicine.*
- This medicine is used together with a special bandage (called an occlusive dressing). *Check with your doctor, nurse, or pharmacist if you did not receive any bandages with the medicine.* Cover the medicine with the bandage. *Seal the edges of the bandage tightly, making sure that none of the medicine leaks out.* Do not lift the bandage or otherwise disturb it.

Keeping the medicine tightly covered helps it work properly.

- If your doctor or nurse has directed you to remove the bandage and wipe off the medicine after a certain amount of time, follow the directions carefully. Then clean the area with the antiseptic solution recommended by your doctor or nurse. *If your doctor or nurse has not directed you to remove the bandage and the medicine, keep them in place until your doctor or nurse removes them.*

Dosing—The dose of this medicine will be different for different patients. *Follow your doctor's orders or the directions that come with the medicine.* The following information includes only the average doses of this medicine. *If your dose is different, do not change it* unless your doctor tells you to do so.

- For *topical* dosage form (cream):
  - —For preventing pain caused by injections or drawing blood from a vein:
    - Adults and children—Apply 2.5 grams of cream (one-half of the amount in a 5-gram tube) in a thick layer to an area about two inches by two inches (twenty to twenty-five square centimeters) in size. Your doctor or nurse may direct you to apply the medicine in two places. The medicine should remain in place, covered by the bandage that comes with it, for at least one hour.
  - —For preventing pain caused by certain procedures:
    - Adults—The size of the area to be covered by a thick layer of this medicine and the amount of time that the medicine must be kept in place depend on the procedure that is being done. The medicine sometimes needs to be kept in place, covered with the bandage, for two hours or more.
    - Children—The size of the area to be covered by a thick layer of this medicine and the amount of time that the medicine must be kept in place depend on the procedure being done. However, the largest area that may be covered by this medicine depends on the child's weight and must be determined by your doctor. The medicine sometimes needs to be kept in place, covered with the bandage, for two hours or more.

Storage—To store this medicine:

- Keep out of the reach of children.
- Store away from heat and direct light.
- Keep the medicine from freezing.
- Do not keep outdated medicine or medicine no longer needed. Be sure that any discarded medicine is out of the reach of children.

Precautions After Using This Medicine

After applying this medicine to the skin of a child, *watch the child carefully to make sure that he or she does not loosen or remove the bandage. Also, keep the child from getting any of the medicine into his or her mouth.* This medicine can cause serious side effects, especially in children, if any of it gets into the mouth or is swallowed.

During the time that the area to which the medicine was applied feels numb, serious injury can occur without your knowing about it. *Be especially careful to avoid injury until the anesthetic wears off or feeling returns to the area.* For example, do not scratch or rub the area or allow very hot or very cold objects to touch it.

Side Effects of This Medicine

Along with its needed effects, a medicine may cause some unwanted effects. Although not all of these side effects may occur, if they do occur they may need medical attention.

The following side effects may mean that a serious allergic reaction is occurring. Check with your doctor or get emergency help immediately if they occur, especially if several of them occur at the same time.

Rare

Coughing, shortness of breath, troubled breathing, tightness in chest, or wheezing; difficulty in swallowing; large, hive-like swellings on eyelids, face, lips, or tongue; severe dizziness or feeling faint; skin rash, itching, or hives; stuffy nose

Also check with your doctor or nurse, or get emergency help right away, if any of the following side effects occur:

Signs of too much medicine being absorbed into the body

Blue or blue-purple color of lips, fingernails, or skin; blurred or double vision; dark urine; dizziness or drowsiness; feeling hot, cold, or numb; headache; irregular or fast heartbeat; muscle twitching or trembling; nausea or vomiting; ringing or buzzing in the ears; shortness of breath or troubled breathing; unusual excitement, nervousness, or restlessness; unusual tiredness or weakness

Note: The above side effects are not likely to occur when usual amounts of this medicine are used properly. However, they may occur if the medicine is used too often, applied to broken skin (for example, cuts or scrapes), applied to very large areas, or kept on the skin too long.

Other side effects may occur that usually do not need medical attention. However, check with your doctor if any of the following side effects continue or are bothersome:

More common

Burning feeling, swelling, itching, or skin rash at place of application (without other signs of an allergic reaction listed above); white or red skin at place of application

Other side effects not listed above may also occur in some patients. If you notice any other effects, check with your doctor.

Additional Information

Once a medicine has been approved for marketing for a certain use, experience may show that it is also useful for other uses. Although this use is not included in product labeling, this medicine is used to produce loss of feeling in the genital area of adults before certain kinds of procedures are done. When used for this purpose, the medicine will be applied and removed by your doctor.

Other than the above information, there is no additional information relating to precautions or side effects for this use.

Annual revision: 08/18/93

LORACARBEF Systemic†

A commonly used brand name in the U.S. is Lorabid.

†Not commercially available in Canada.

Description

Loracarbef (loe-ra-KAR-bef) is used to treat bacterial infections in many different parts of the body. It works by killing bacteria or preventing their growth. This medicine will not work for colds, flu, or other virus infections.

Loracarbef is available only with your doctor's prescription, in the following dosage forms:

Oral

- Capsules (U.S.)
- Oral suspension (U.S.)

It is very important that you read and understand the following information. If any of it causes you special concern, check with your doctor. Also, *if you have any questions* or if you want more information about this medicine or your medical problem, *ask your doctor, nurse, or pharmacist.*

Before Using This Medicine

In deciding to use a medicine, the risks of taking the medicine must be weighed against the good it will do. This is a decision you and your doctor will make. For loracarbef, the following should be considered:

Allergies—Tell your doctor if you have ever had any unusual or allergic reaction to loracarbef or to any related medicines such as penicillins or cephalosporins. Also tell your doctor and pharmacist if you are allergic to any other substances, such as foods, preservatives, or dyes.

Pregnancy—Loracarbef has not been studied in pregnant women. However, loracarbef has not been shown to cause birth defects or other problems in animal studies.

Breast-feeding—It is not known whether loracarbef passes into breast milk.

Children—This medicine has been tested in a limited number of children 6 months of age and older. In effective doses, the medicine has not been shown to cause different side effects or problems than it does in adults.

Older adults—This medicine has been tested in a limited number of elderly patients and has not been shown to cause different side effects or problems in older people than it does in younger adults.

Other medicines—Although certain medicines should not be used together at all, in other cases two different medicines may be used together even if an interaction might occur. In these cases, your doctor may want to change the dose, or other precautions may be necessary. When you are taking loracarbef, it is especially important that your doctor and pharmacist know if you are taking any of the following:

- Probenecid (e.g., Benemid)—Probenecid increases the blood level of loracarbef, increasing the chance of side effects

Other medical problems—The presence of other medical problems may affect the use of loracarbef. Make sure you tell your doctor if you have any other medical problems, especially:

- Kidney disease—Kidney disease may increase the blood level of loracarbef, increasing the chance of side effects

Before you begin using any new medicine (prescription or nonprescription) or if you develop any new medical problem while you are using this medicine, check with your doctor, nurse, or pharmacist.

Proper Use of This Medicine

Loracarbef should be taken at least 1 hour before or at least 2 hours after meals.

To help clear up your infection completely, *keep taking loracarbef for the full time of treatment,* even if you begin to feel better after a few days. *If you have a "strep" infection, you should keep taking this medicine for at least 10 days. This is especially important in "strep" infections. Serious heart problems could develop later* if your infection is not cleared up completely. Also, if you stop taking this medicine too soon, your symptoms may return.

This medicine works best when there is a constant amount in the blood or urine. *To help keep the amount constant, do not miss any doses. Also, it is best to take the doses at evenly spaced times, day and night.* If this interferes with your sleep or other daily activities, or if you need help in planning the best times to take your medicine, check with your doctor, nurse, or pharmacist.

Dosing—The dose of loracarbef will be different for different patients. *Follow your doctor's orders or the directions on the label.* The following information includes only the average doses of loracarbef. Your dose may be different if you have kidney disease. *If your dose is different, do not change it* unless your doctor tells you to do so.

The number of capsules or teaspoonfuls of suspension that you take depends on the strength of the medicine. Also, *the number of doses you take each day, the time allowed between doses, and the length of time you take the medicine depend on the medical problem for which you are taking loracarbef.*

- For *oral* dosage forms (capsules or oral suspension):
  - —For bronchitis:
    - Adults and children 13 years of age and older—200 to 400 milligrams (mg) every twelve hours for seven days.
    - Children 6 months to 12 years of age—Use and dose to be determined by your doctor.
  - —For otitis media (ear infection):
    - Children 6 months to 12 years of age—Dose is based on body weight and must be determined by your doctor.
  - —For pneumonia:
    - Adults and children 13 years of age and older—400 mg every twelve hours for fourteen days.
    - Children 6 months to 12 years of age—Use and dose to be determined by your doctor.
  - —For sinusitis:
    - Adults and children 13 years of age and older—400 mg every twelve hours for ten days.
    - Children 6 months to 12 years of age—Use and dose to be determined by your doctor.
  - —For skin and soft tissue infections:
    - Adults and children 13 years of age and older—200 mg every twelve hours for seven days.
    - Children 6 months to 12 years of age—Dose is based on body weight and must be determined by your doctor.
  - —For streptococcal pharyngitis ("strep throat"):
    - Adults and children 13 years of age and older—200 mg every twelve hours for ten days.
    - Children 6 months to 12 years of age—Dose is based on body weight and must be determined by your doctor.
  - —For urinary tract infections:
    - Adults and children 13 years of age and older—200 to 400 mg every twelve to twenty-four hours for seven to fourteen days.
    - Children 6 months to 12 years of age—Use and dose to be determined by your doctor.

Missed dose—If you do miss a dose of this medicine, take it as soon as possible. This will help to keep a constant amount of medicine in the blood or urine. However, if it is almost time for your next dose, skip the missed dose and go back to your regular dosing schedule. Do not double doses.

Storage—To store this medicine:

- Keep out of the reach of children.
- Store away from heat and direct light.
- Do not store the capsule form of this medicine in the bathroom, near the kitchen sink, or in other damp places. Heat or moisture may cause the medicine to break down.
- Do not keep outdated medicine or medicine no longer needed. Be sure that any discarded medicine is out of the reach of children.

Precautions While Using This Medicine

If your symptoms do not improve within a few days, or if they become worse, check with your doctor.

In some patients, loracarbef may cause diarrhea.

- Severe diarrhea may be a sign of a serious side effect. *Do not take any diarrhea medicine without first checking with your doctor.* Diarrhea medicines may make your diarrhea worse or last longer.
- For mild diarrhea, diarrhea medicine containing kaolin or attapulgite (e.g., Kaopectate tablets, Diasorb) may be taken. However, other kinds of diarrhea medicine should not be taken. They may make your diarrhea worse or last longer.
- If you have any questions about this or if mild diarrhea continues or gets worse, check with your doctor or pharmacist.

Side Effects of This Medicine

Along with its needed effects, a medicine may cause some unwanted effects. Although not all of these side effects may occur, if they do occur they may need medical attention.

Check with your doctor as soon as possible if any of the following side effects occur:

More common

Itching; skin rash

Other side effects may occur that usually do not need medical attention. These side effects may go away during treatment as your body adjusts to the medicine. However, check with your doctor if any of the following side effects continue or are bothersome:

More common

Diarrhea; loss of appetite; nausea and vomiting; stomach pain

Rare

Dizziness; drowsiness; headache; itching or discharge from the vagina; nervousness; trouble in sleeping

Other side effects not listed above may also occur in some patients. If you notice any other effects, check with your doctor.

Annual revision: 08/18/93

NEDOCROMIL Inhalation

A commonly used brand name in the U.S. and Canada is Tilade.

Description

Nedocromil (ne-DOK-roe-mil) is used to prevent the symptoms of asthma. When it is used regularly, nedocromil lessens the number and severity of asthma attacks by reducing inflammation in the lungs. Nedocromil is also used just before exposure to substances (for example, allergens, chemicals, cold air, or air pollutants) that cause reactions, to prevent bronchospasm (wheezing or difficulty in breathing). In addition, nedocromil is used to prevent bronchospasm caused by exercise. This medicine will not help an asthma or bronchospasm attack that has already started.

When nedocromil is used to prevent symptoms of asthma, it may be used with other asthma medicines, such as bronchodilators (medicines that open up narrowed breathing passages) and corticosteroids (cortisone-like medicine).

Nedocromil works by acting on certain inflammatory cells in the lungs to prevent them from releasing substances that cause asthma or bronchospasm.

This medicine is available only with your doctor's prescription, in the following dosage form:

Inhalation

- Inhalation aerosol (U.S. and Canada)

It is very important that you read and understand the following information. If any of it causes you special concern, check with your doctor. Also, *if you have any questions* or if you want more information about this medicine or your medical problem, *ask your doctor, nurse, or pharmacist.*

Before Using This Medicine

In deciding to use a medicine, the risks of using the medicine must be weighed against the good it will do. This is a decision you and your doctor will make. For nedocromil, the following should be considered:

Allergies—Tell your doctor if you have ever had any unusual or allergic reaction to nedocromil or to any other inhalation aerosol medicine.

Pregnancy—Nedocromil has not been studied in pregnant women. However, nedocromil has not been shown to cause birth defects or other problems in animal studies.

Breast-feeding—It is not known whether nedocromil passes into breast milk. Although most medicines pass into breast milk in small amounts, many of them may be used safely while breast-feeding. Mothers who are using this medicine and who wish to breast-feed should discuss this with their doctor.

Children—Nedocromil has been tested in a limited number of children 6 years of age and older. In effective doses, it is not expected to cause different side effects or problems in children than it does in adults.

Older adults—Many medicines have not been studied specifically in older people. Therefore, it may not be known whether they work the same way they do in younger adults. Although there is no specific information comparing the use of nedocromil in the elderly with use in other age groups, it is not expected to cause different side effects or problems in older people than it does in younger adults.

Before you begin using any new medicine (prescription or nonprescription) or if you develop any new medical problem while you are using this medicine, check with your doctor, nurse, or pharmacist.

Proper Use of This Medicine

Nedocromil is used to help prevent symptoms of asthma or bronchospasm (wheezing or difficulty in breathing). When this medicine is used regularly, it decreases the number and severity of asthma attacks. Nedocromil will not relieve an asthma or bronchospasm attack that has already started.

Nedocromil inhalation aerosol usually comes with patient directions. Read them carefully before using this medicine.

The nedocromil aerosol canister provides about 56 or 112 inhalations, depending on the size of the canister your doctor ordered. You should keep a record of the number of inhalations you use so you will know when the canister is almost empty. This canister, unlike other aerosol canisters, cannot be floated in water to test its fullness.

This medicine is used with a metered dose inhaler. If you do not understand the directions or you are not sure how to use the inhaler, ask your doctor, nurse, or pharmacist to show you what to do. Also, ask your doctor, nurse, or pharmacist to check often your method of using the inhaler.

When you use the inhaler for the first time, or if you have not used it for a while, the inhaler may not deliver the right amount of medicine with the first puff. Therefore, before using the inhaler, you should test it to make sure it works properly.

To test the inhaler before using the first time or if not used for a while:

- Insert the metal canister firmly into the clean mouthpiece according to the manufacturer's instructions. Check to make sure the canister is placed properly into the mouthpiece.
- Take the cover off the mouthpiece and shake the inhaler well.
- Hold the canister against a light background and press the top of the canister, spraying the medicine into the air. If you see a fine mist of medicine, you will know the inhaler is working properly and that you will get the right amount of medicine when you use it.

To use the inhaler:

- Hold the inhaler upright, using your thumb and forefinger, with the mouthpiece end down and pointing toward you.
- Gently shake the inhaler and canister well.
- Hold the mouthpiece away from your mouth and breathe out slowly to the end of a normal breath.
- Use the inhalation method recommended by your doctor.
  —One method is to place the mouthpiece about 1 to 2 inches (2 fingerwidths) in front of your widely opened mouth. Make sure the inhaler is aimed properly into your mouth.
  —Another method is to place the mouthpiece in your mouth between your teeth and over your tongue with your lips closed around it.
  —Also, your doctor may want you to use a spacer device with the inhaler. A spacer is attached to the end of the inhaler to help deliver the medicine to the lungs. Use the spacer according to the manufacturer's instructions.
- Tilt your head back a little. Start to breathe in slowly and deeply through your mouth and, at the same time, press the top of the canister once to get one puff of medicine. Continue to breathe in slowly until you have taken a full breath. It is important to press down on the canister and breathe in at the same time so you will get the correct amount of medicine deep into your lungs. This step may be difficult at first and can be practiced in front of a mirror. If you are using the closed-mouth method and you see a fine mist of medicine coming from your mouth or nose, you are not using your inhaler correctly.
- Hold your breath for several seconds. This allows more of the medicine to enter your lungs.
- Take the mouthpiece away from your mouth and breathe out slowly.
- If your doctor has told you to inhale more than one puff of medicine at each dose, take the second puff following exactly the same steps you used for the first puff.
- If your doctor told you to use an inhaled bronchodilator before using nedocromil, you should wait at least 2 minutes after using the bronchodilator before using nedocromil. This allows the nedocromil to get deeper into your lungs.
- When you are finished, replace the cover of the mouthpiece to keep it clean.

To clean the inhaler:

- Clean the inhaler often to prevent build-up of medicine and blocking of the mouthpiece. The mouthpiece can be washed every day and should be washed at least twice a week.
- Remove the metal canister from the inhaler and set aside. Do not get the canister wet.
- Wash the mouthpiece in hot water.
- Shake off the excess water and let the mouthpiece air dry completely before replacing the metal canister and cover.

For patients using nedocromil regularly (for example, every day):

- *In order for nedocromil to work properly, it must be inhaled every day in regularly spaced doses as ordered by your doctor.*
- Usually about 2 weeks may pass before you begin to feel the full effects of this medicine.

Missed dose—If you are using nodocromil regularly and you miss a dose of this medicine, take it as soon as possible. Then take any remaining doses for that day at regularly spaced intervals.

Dosing—The dose of nedocromil will be different for different patients. *Follow your doctor's orders or the directions on the label.* The following information includes only the average doses of nedocromil. *If your dose is different, do not change it* unless your doctor tells you to do so:

- For *inhalation* dosage form (inhalation aerosol):
  —For prevention of asthma symptoms:
    - Adults and children 12 years of age or older—3.5 or 4 milligrams (mg) (2 puffs) two to four times a day at regular intervals.
    - Children up to 12 years of age—Use and dose must be determined by the doctor.

  —For prevention of bronchospasm caused by exercise or a substance:
    - Adults and children 12 years of age or older—3.5 or 4 milligrams (mg) (2 puffs) as a single dose up to thirty minutes before exercise or exposure to any substance that may cause an attack.
    - Children up to 12 years of age—Use and dose must be determined by the doctor.

Storage—To store this medicine:

- Keep out of the reach of children.
- Store away from heat and direct sunlight.
- Keep the medicine from freezing.
- Do not puncture, break, or burn the aerosol container, even if it is empty.
- Do not keep outdated medicine or medicine no longer needed. Be sure that any discarded medicine is out of the reach of children.
- Always keep the dust cover on the mouthpiece when the inhaler is not in use.

Precautions While Using This Medicine

If your symptoms do not improve or if your condition becomes worse, check with your doctor.

You may also be taking a corticosteroid or a bronchodilator for asthma along with this medicine. *Do not stop taking the corticosteroid or bronchodilator even if your asthma seems better, unless told to do so by your doctor.*

Throat irritation and/or an unpleasant taste may occur after you use this medicine. Gargling and rinsing the mouth after each dose may help prevent these effects.

Side Effects of This Medicine

Along with its needed effects, a medicine may cause some unwanted effects. Although not all of these side effects may occur, if they do occur they may need medical attention.

Check with your doctor as soon as possible if any of the following side effects occur:

Less common

Increased wheezing, tightness in chest, or difficulty in breathing

Other side effects may occur that usually do not need medical attention. These side effects may go away during treatment as your body adjusts to the medicine. However, check with your doctor if any of the following side effects continue or are bothersome:

Less common

Cough; headache; nausea; throat irritation

After you use the nedocromil inhalation aerosol, you may notice an unpleasant taste. This may be expected and will go away when you stop using the medicine.

Other side effects not listed above may also occur in some patients. If you notice any other effects, check with your doctor.

Annual revision: 09/23/93

PACLITAXEL Systemic

A commonly used brand name in the U.S. and Canada is Taxol.

Description

Paclitaxel (pak-li-TAX-el) belongs to the group of medicines called antineoplastics. It is used to treat cancer of the ovary.

Paclitaxel interferes with the growth of cancer cells, which are eventually destroyed. Since the growth of normal body cells may also be affected by paclitaxel, other effects will also occur. Some of these may be serious and must be reported to your doctor. Other effects may not be serious but may cause concern. Some effects may not occur for months or years after the medicine is used.

Paclitaxel may also be used to treat other conditions as determined by your doctor.

Before you begin treatment with paclitaxel, you and your doctor should talk about the good this medicine will do as well as the risks of using it.

Paclitaxel is to be administered only by or under the immediate supervision of your doctor. It is available in the following dosage form:

Parenteral

- Injection (U.S. and Canada)

It is very important that you read and understand the following information. If any of it causes you special concern, check with your doctor. Also, *if you have any questions* or if you want more information about this medicine or your medical problem, *ask your doctor, nurse, or pharmacist.*

Before Using This Medicine

In deciding to use a medicine, the risks of taking the medicine must be weighed against the good it will do. This is a decision you and your doctor will make. For paclitaxel, the following should be considered:

Allergies—Tell your doctor if you have ever had any unusual or allergic reaction to paclitaxel.

Pregnancy—Tell your doctor if you are pregnant or if you intend to become pregnant. Studies in rats and rabbits have shown that paclitaxel causes miscarriages and deaths of the fetus, as well as problems in the mother.

Be sure that you have discussed this with your doctor before taking this medicine. It is best to use some kind of birth control while you are receiving paclitaxel. Tell your doctor right away if you think you have become pregnant while receiving paclitaxel.

Breast-feeding—It is not known whether paclitaxel passes into breast milk. However, because this medicine may cause serious side effects, breast-feeding is generally not recommended while you are receiving it.

Children—There is no specific information comparing use of paclitaxel in children with use in other age groups.

Older adults—This medicine has been tested in a limited number of patients and has not been shown to cause different side effects or problems in older people than it does in younger adults.

Other medicines—Although certain medicines should not be used together at all, in other cases two different medicines may be used together even if an interaction might occur. In these cases, your doctor may want to change the dose, or other precautions may be necessary. When you are receiving paclitaxel, it is especially important that your doctor and pharmacist know if you are taking any of the following:

- Amphotericin B by injection (e.g., Fungizone) or
- Antithyroid agents (medicine for overactive thyroid) or
- Azathioprine (e.g., Imuran) or
- Chloramphenicol (e.g., Chloromycetin) or
- Colchicine or
- Flucytosine (e.g., Ancobon) or
- Ganciclovir (e.g., Cytovene) or
- Interferon (e.g., Intron A, Roferon-A) or
- Plicamycin (e.g., Mithracin) or
- Zidovudine (e.g., AZT, Retrovir) or
- If you have ever been treated with x-rays or cancer medicines—Paclitaxel may increase the effects of these medicines or radiation therapy on the blood

Other medical problems—The presence of other medical problems may affect the use of paclitaxel. Make sure you tell your doctor if you have any other medical problems, especially:

- Chickenpox (including recent exposure) or
- Herpes zoster (shingles)—Risk of severe disease affecting other parts of the body
- Heart rhythm problems—May be made worse by paclitaxel
- Infection—Paclitaxel may decrease your body's ability to fight infection

Before you begin using any new medicine (prescription or nonprescription) or if you develop any new medical problem while you are using this medicine, check with your doctor, nurse, or pharmacist.

Proper Use of This Medicine

This medicine often causes nausea and vomiting, which is usually mild. However, it is very important that you continue to receive the medicine even if you begin to feel ill. Ask your doctor, nurse, or pharmacist for ways to lessen these effects.

Precautions While Using This Medicine

It is very important that your doctor check your progress at regular visits to make sure that this medicine is working properly and to check for unwanted effects.

While you are being treated with paclitaxel, and after you stop treatment with it, *do not have any immunizations (vaccinations) without your doctor's approval.* Paclitaxel may lower your body's resistance and there is a chance you might get the infection the immunization is meant to prevent. In addition, other persons living in your household should not take oral polio vaccine since there is a chance they could pass the polio virus on to you. Also, avoid persons who have taken oral polio vaccine. Do not get close to them and do not stay in the same room with them for very long. If you cannot take these precautions, you should consider wearing a protective face mask that covers the nose and mouth.

Paclitaxel can temporarily lower the number of white blood cells in your blood, increasing the chance of getting an infection. It can also lower the number of platelets, which are necessary for proper blood clotting. If this occurs, there are certain precautions you can take, especially when your blood count is low, to reduce the risk of infection or bleeding:

- If you can, avoid people with infections. *Check with your doctor immediately* if you think you are getting an infection or if you get a fever or chills, cough or hoarseness, lower back or side pain, or painful or difficult urination.
- *Check with your doctor immediately* if you notice any unusual bleeding or bruising; black, tarry stools; blood in urine or stools; or pinpoint red spots on your skin.
- Be careful when using a regular toothbrush, dental floss, or toothpick. Your medical doctor, dentist, or nurse may recommend other ways to clean your teeth and gums. Check with your medical doctor before having any dental work done.
- Do not touch your eyes or the inside of your nose unless you have just washed your hands and have not touched anything else in the meantime.
- Be careful not to cut yourself when you are using sharp objects such as a safety razor or fingernail or toenail cutters.
- Avoid contact sports or other situations where bruising or injury could occur.

Side Effects of This Medicine

Along with its needed effects, a medicine may cause some unwanted effects. Some side effects will have signs or symptoms that you can see or feel. Your doctor may watch for others by doing certain tests.

Also, because of the way these medicines act on the body, there is a chance that they might cause other unwanted effects that may not occur until months or years after the medicine is used. These delayed effects may include certain types of cancer. Discuss these possible effects with your doctor.

Check with your doctor immediately if any of the following side effects occur:

More common

Cough or hoarseness; fever or chills; lower back or side pain; painful or difficult urination

Less common

Black, tarry stools; blood in urine or stools; pinpoint red spots on skin; unusual bleeding or bruising

Rare

Shortness of breath (severe); skin reaction (severe)

Check with your doctor as soon as possible if any of the following side effects occur:

More common

Flushing of face; shortness of breath; skin rash or itching

Rare

Pain or redness at place of injection; sores in mouth and on lips (usually get better within 7 days after treatment)

This medicine may also cause the following side effects that your doctor will watch out for:

More common

Anemia; low white blood cell count; low platelet count in blood

Less common

Low blood pressure; slow heartbeat; effects on liver

Other side effects may occur that usually do not need medical attention. These side effects may go away during treatment as your body adjusts to the medicine. Also, your doctor or nurse may be able to tell you about ways to prevent or reduce some of these side effects. Check with your doctor or nurse if any of the following side effects continue or are bothersome or if you have any questions about them:

More common

Diarrhea; nausea and vomiting; numbness, burning, or tingling in hands or feet; pain in joints or muscles, especially in arms or legs (begins 2 to 3 days after treatment and may last up to 5 days)

This medicine usually causes a temporary and total loss of hair (including eyebrows, eyelashes, and pubic hair) about 2 to 3 weeks after treatment begins. After treatment with paclitaxel has ended, normal hair growth should return.

Other side effects not listed above may also occur in some patients. If you notice any other effects, check with your doctor.

Annual revision: 09/15/93

PIPERAZINE Systemic

A commonly used brand name in Canada is Entacyl.
Generic name product may also be available in the U.S.

Description

Piperazine (PI-per-a-zeen) belongs to the family of medicines called anthelmintics (ant-hel-MIN-tiks). Anthelmintics are used in the treatment of worm infections.

Piperazine is used to treat:

- common roundworms (ascariasis) and
- pinworms (enterobiasis; oxyuriasis).

Piperazine works by paralyzing the worms. They are then passed in the stool.

Piperazine is available only with your doctor's prescription, in the following dosage forms:

Oral

- Granules for oral solution (Canada)
- Oral suspension (Canada)
- Tablets (U.S.)

It is very important that you read and understand the following information. If any of it causes you special concern, check with your doctor. Also, *if you have any questions* or if you want more information about this medicine or your medical problem, *ask your doctor, nurse, or pharmacist.*

Before Using This Medicine

In deciding to use a medicine, the risks of taking the medicine must be weighed against the good it will do. This is a decision you and your doctor will make. For piperazine, the following should be considered:

Allergies—Tell your doctor if you have ever had any unusual or allergic reaction to piperazine or ethylenediamine. Also tell your doctor and pharmacist if you are allergic to any other substances, such as foods, preservatives, or dyes.

Pregnancy—Piperazine has not been studied in pregnant women. Piperazine has not been shown to cause birth defects or other problems in animal studies. However, piperazine, taken by mouth, may be changed within the body into a substance that may cause cancer. Before taking piperazine, make sure your doctor knows if you are pregnant or if you may become pregnant.

Breast-feeding—Although it is not known whether piperazine passes into the breast milk, piperazine has not been reported to cause problems in nursing babies.

Children—Children may be especially sensitive to the effects of piperazine. This may increase the chance of side effects during treatment.

Older adults—Many medicines have not been studied specifically in older people. Therefore, it may not be known whether they work exactly the same way they do in younger adults or if they cause different side effects or problems in older people. There is no specific information comparing use of piperazine in the elderly with use in other age groups.

Other medicines—Although certain medicines should not be used together at all, in other cases two different medicines may be used together even if an interaction might occur. In these cases, your doctor may want to change the dose, or other precautions may be necessary. When you are taking piperazine, it is especially important that your doctor and pharmacist know if you are taking any of the following:

- Phenothiazines (acetophenazine [e.g., Tindal], chlorpromazine [e.g., Thorazine], fluphenazine [e.g., Prolixin], mesoridazine [e.g., Serentil], perphenazine[e.g., Trilafon], prochlorperazine [e.g., Compazine], promazine [e.g., Sparine], promethazine [e.g., Phenergan], thioridazine [e.g., Mellaril], trifluoperazine [e.g., Stelazine], triflupromazine [e.g., Vesprin], trimeprazine [e.g., Temaril])—Taking piperazine and a phenothiazine together may increase the risk of convulsions
- Pyrantel (e.g., Antiminth)—Taking piperazine and pyrantel together may decrease the effects of piperazine

Other medical problems—The presence of other medical problems may affect the use of piperazine. Make sure you tell your doctor if you have any other medical problems, especially:

- Kidney disease or
- Liver disease—Patients with kidney or liver disease may have an increased chance of side effects
- Seizure disorder, especially a history of epilepsy—Piperazine may make the condition worse

Before you begin using any new medicine (prescription or nonprescription) or if you develop any new medical problem while you are using this medicine, check with your doctor, nurse, or pharmacist.

Proper Use of This Medicine

No special preparation (for example, special diet, fasting, other medicines, laxatives, or enemas) are necessary before, during, or immediately after you take piperazine.

Piperazine may be taken with or without food or on a full or empty stomach. However, if your doctor tells you to take the medicine a certain way, take it exactly as directed.

For patients taking the *granules for oral solution form* of piperazine:

- Dissolve the contents of 1 packet of granules in 57 mL (about 2 ounces) of water, milk, or fruit juice.

- Be sure to drink all of the liquid to get the full dose of medicine.

Take this medicine only as directed. Do not take more of it and do not take it more often than your doctor ordered. To do so may increase the chance of serious side effects.

To help clear up your infection completely, *take this medicine in regularly spaced doses as ordered by your doctor.* In some infections a second treatment with this medicine may be required to clear up the infection completely. *Do not miss any doses.*

For patients taking piperazine for *pinworms*:

- Pinworms may be easily passed from one person to another, especially among persons in the same household. Therefore, all household members may have to be treated at the same time to prevent their infection or reinfection.

Dosing—The dose of piperazine will be different for different patients. *Follow your doctor's orders or the directions on the label.* The following information includes only the average doses of piperazine. *If your dose is different, do not change it* unless your doctor tells you to do so.

The number of tablets or teaspoonfuls of solution or suspension of the medicine that you take depends on the strength of the medicine. Also, *the number of doses you take each day, the time allowed between doses, and the length of time you take the medicine depend on the medical problem for which you are taking piperazine.*

- For *oral suspension* or *granules for oral solution* dosage form:
  - —For common roundworms or pinworms:
    - Adults and children over 14 years of age—1.8 grams of oral suspension or 2 grams of granules for oral solution three times a day for one day. Treatment may need to be repeated in two weeks.
    - Children—Dose is based on age and/or body weight. Treatment may need to be repeated in two weeks.
      - —Up to 2 years of age: 600 milligrams (mg) of oral suspension three times a day for one day.
      - —2 to 8 years of age: 1.2 grams of oral suspension two times a day or 2 grams of granules for oral solution once a day, for one day.
      - —8 to 14 years of age: 1.2 grams of oral suspension three times a day or 2 grams of granules for oral solution two times a day, for one day.
- For *tablet* dosage form:
  - —For common roundworms:
    - Adults—3.5 grams (piperazine hexahydrate) per day for two days in a row. Treatment may need to be repeated in one week.
    - Children—Dose is based on body weight and must be determined by your doctor. However, the usual dose is 75 mg (piperazine hexahydrate) per kilogram (34 mg per pound) of body weight per day for two days in a row. Treatment may need to be repeated in one week.
  - —For pinworms:
    - Adults and children—Dose is based on body weight and must be determined by your doctor. However, the usual dose is 65 mg (piperazine hexahydrate) per kilogram (29.5 mg per pound) of body weight per day for seven days in a row. Treatment may need to be repeated in one week.

Missed dose—If you miss a dose of this medicine, take it as soon as possible. However, if it is almost time for your next dose, skip the missed dose and go back to your regular dosing schedule. Do not double doses.

Storage—To store this medicine:

- Keep out of the reach of children. Overdose of piperazine is very dangerous in young children.
- Store away from heat and direct light.
- Do not store in the bathroom, near the kitchen sink, or in other damp places. Heat or moisture may cause the medicine to break down.
- Keep the liquid form of this medicine from freezing.
- Do not keep outdated medicine or medicine no longer needed. Be sure that any discarded medicine is out of the reach of children.

Precautions While Using This Medicine

It is important that your doctor check your progress after treatment. This is to make sure that the infection is cleared up completely, and to allow your doctor to check for any unwanted effects.

If your symptoms do not improve after you have taken this medicine for the full course of treatment, or if they become worse, check with your doctor.

For patients taking piperazine for *pinworms*:

- In some patients, pinworms may return after treatment with piperazine. Washing (not shaking) all bedding and nightclothes (pajamas) after treatment may help to prevent this.

Side Effects of This Medicine

Along with its needed effects, a medicine may cause some unwanted effects. Although not all of these side effects may occur, if they do occur they may need medical attention.

Check with your doctor immediately if any of the following side effects occur:

Rare

Fever, joint pain, skin rash, or itching

Symptoms of overdose

Convulsions (seizures); difficulty in breathing; muscle weakness

Other side effects may occur that usually do not need medical attention. These side effects may go away during treatment as your body adjusts to the medicine. However, check with your doctor if any of the following side effects continue or are bothersome:

Less common

Abdominal or stomach cramps or pain; diarrhea; dizziness; drowsiness; headache; muscle weakness; nausea or vomiting; tremors

Other side effects not listed above may also occur in some patients. If you notice any other effects, check with your doctor.

Annual revision: 08/02/93

RIFABUTIN Systemic

A commonly used brand name in the U.S. and Canada is Mycobutin.

Description

Rifabutin (rif-a-BUE-tin) is used to help prevent *Mycobacterium avium* complex (MAC) disease from causing disease throughout the body in patients with advanced human immunodeficiency virus (HIV) infection. MAC is an infection caused by two similar bacteria, *Mycobacterium avium* and *Mycobacterium intracellulare. Mycobacterium avium* is more common in patients with HIV infection. MAC may also occur in other patients whose immune system is not working properly. Symptoms of MAC in people with AIDS (acquired immunodeficiency syndrome) include fever, night sweats, chills, weight loss, and weakness. Rifabutin will not work for colds, flu, or most other infections.

Rifabutin is available only with your doctor's prescription, in the following dosage form:

Oral

- Capsules (U.S. and Canada)

It is very important that you read and understand the following information. If any of it causes you special concern, check with your doctor. Also, *if you have any questions* or if you want more information about this medicine or your medical problem, *ask your doctor, nurse, or pharmacist.*

Before Using This Medicine

In deciding to use a medicine, the risks of taking the medicine must be weighed against the good it will do. This is a decision you and your doctor will make. For rifabutin, the following should be considered:

Allergies—Tell your doctor if you have ever had any unusual or allergic reaction to rifabutin or rifampin. Also tell your doctor and pharmacist if you are allergic to any other substances, such as foods, preservatives, or dyes.

Pregnancy—Rifabutin has not been studied in pregnant women. However, studies in animals have shown that rifabutin causes birth defects. Before you take this medicine, make sure your doctor knows if you are pregnant or if you may become pregnant.

Breast-feeding—It is not known whether rifabutin passes into the breast milk. However, if your baby does not have the AIDS virus, there is a chance that you could pass the virus to your baby by breast-feeding. Talk to your doctor first if you are thinking about breast-feeding your baby.

Children—Studies on this medicine have only been done in adult patients, and there is no specific information comparing use of rifabutin in children with use in other age groups. However, studies are being done to determine the best dose for children.

Older adults—Many medicines have not been studied specifically in older people. Therefore, it may not be known whether they work exactly the same way they do in younger adults. Although there is no specific information comparing use of rifabutin in the elderly with use in other age groups, this medicine is not expected to cause different side effects or problems in older people than it does in younger adults.

Other medicines—Although certain medicines should not be used together at all, in other cases two different medicines may be used together even if an interaction might occur. In these cases, your doctor may want to change the dose, or other precautions may be necessary. When you are taking rifabutin, it is especially important that your doctor and pharmacist know if you are taking any of the following:

- Zidovudine (e.g., AZT, Retrovir)—Use of rifabutin with zidovudine may lower the amount of zidovudine in the blood

Other medical problems—The presence of other medical problems may affect the use of rifabutin. Make sure you tell your doctor if you have any other medical problems, especially:

- Active tuberculosis—Patients with active tuberculosis should not receive rifabutin alone to prevent MAC. Rifabutin may be used with other medicines when treating tuberculosis. However, when rifabutin is used alone, it will not cure tuberculosis. Tuberculosis germs may develop a resistance to rifabutin and other similar medicines. This may make future treatment of tuberculosis more difficult

Before you begin using any new medicine (prescription or nonprescription) or if you develop any new medical problem while you are using this medicine, check with your doctor, nurse, or pharmacist.

Proper Use of This Medicine

Rifabutin may be taken on an empty stomach (either 1 hour before or 2 hours after a meal). However, if this medicine upsets your stomach, you may want to take it with food.

For *patients unable to swallow capsules:*

- The contents of the capsules may be mixed with applesauce. Be sure to take all the food to get the full dose of medicine.

To help prevent MAC disease, *it is very important that you keep taking this medicine for the full time of treatment.* You may have to take it every day for many months. *It is important that you do not miss any doses.*

Dosing—The dose of rifabutin may be different for different patients. *Follow your doctor's orders or the directions on the label.* The following information includes only the average doses of rifabutin. *If your dose is different, do not change it* unless your doctor tells you to do so.

- For *oral* dosage forms (capsules):
  - —For the prevention of *Mycobacterium avium* complex:
    - Adults and teenagers—300 milligrams (mg) once a day, or 150 mg two times a day. The medicine may be taken with food if this medicine upsets your stomach.
    - Children—Use and dose must be determined by your doctor.

Missed dose—If you miss a dose of this medicine, take it as soon as possible. However, if it is almost time for your next dose, skip the missed dose and go back to your regular dosing schedule. Do not double doses. *If this medicine is taken on an irregular schedule, side effects may occur more often and may be more serious than usual.* If you have any questions about this, check with your doctor or pharmacist.

Storage—To store this medicine:

- Keep out of the reach of children.
- Store away from heat and direct light.
- Do not store in the bathroom, near the kitchen sink, or in other damp places. Heat or moisture may cause the medicine to break down.
- Do not keep outdated medicine or medicine no longer needed. Be sure that any discarded medicine is out of the reach of children.

Precautions While Using This Medicine

It is very important that your doctor check your progress at regular visits.

Rifabutin will cause your urine, stool, saliva, sputum, sweat, and tears to turn reddish orange to reddish brown. This is to be expected while you are taking this medicine. This effect may cause soft contact lenses to become permanently discolored. Standard cleaning solutions may not take out all the discoloration. Therefore, *it is best not to wear soft contact lenses while taking this medicine.* Hard contact lenses are not discolored by rifabutin. If you have any questions about this, check with your doctor.

Side Effects of This Medicine

Along with its needed effects, a medicine may cause some unwanted effects. Although not all of these side effects may occur, if they do occur they may need medical attention.

Check with your doctor immediately if any of the following side effects occur:

More common

Skin rash

Rare

Eye pain; joint pain; loss of vision

Other side effects may occur that usually do not need medical attention. These side effects may go away during treatment as your body adjusts to the medicine. However, check with your doctor if any of the following side effects continue or are bothersome:

More common

Nausea; vomiting

This medicine commonly causes reddish orange to reddish brown discoloration of urine, stools, saliva, sputum, sweat, and tears. This side effect does not usually need medical attention. However, tears that have been discolored by this medicine may also discolor soft contact lenses (see *Precautions While Using This Medicine*).

Other side effects not listed above may also occur in some patients. If you notice any other effects, check with your doctor.

Annual revision: 08/18/93

Appendix III

ADDITIONAL PRODUCTS AND USES

The following information is new information not included in the text of this book. It has not gone through the USP DI review process. Refer to the Glossary for definitions of medical and technical terms.

GENERIC NAME (*Brand name*)	DOSAGE FORM(S)	USE	COMMENTS
Acenocoumarol (*Sintrom* [Canada])	Tablets	Anticoagulant	For general information that may apply to all coumarin-derivative anticoagulants, see *Anticoagulants (Systemic)*
Acetaminophen		Analgesic; Antipyretic	
(*Aspirin Free Anacin Maximum Strength Caplets,* Robins [U.S.]; *Aspirin Free Anacin Maximum Strength Gel Caplets,* Robins [U.S.]; *Aspirin Free Anacin Maximum Strength Tablets,* Robins [U.S.])	Tablets		Additional brand name products
(*Actimol* [Canada])	Chewable Tablets Oral Suspension Tablets		Additional Canadian brand name products
Acetaminophen and Caffeine (*Aspirin Free Bayer Select Maximum Strength Headache Pain Relief Caplets* [U.S.])	Tablets	Analgesic	Additional brand name product
Acetaminophen and Calcium Carbonate (*Extra Strength Tylenol Headache Plus Caplets* [U.S.])	Tablets	Analgesic-antacid, for pain accompanied by heartburn, acid indigestion, and/or upset stomach	Additional combination product
Acetaminophen, Calcium Carbonate, Magnesium Carbonate, and Magnesium Oxide (*Aspirin Free Excedrin Dual Caplets* [U.S.])	Tablets	Analgesic-antacid, for pain accompanied by heartburn, acid indigestion, and/or upset stomach	Additional combination product
Acetazolamide (*Storzolamide* [U.S.])	Tablets	Antiglaucoma agent; Anticonvulsant, in epilepsy	Additional brand name product
Amdinocillin Pivoxil Hydrochloride (*Selexid* [Canada])	Tablets	Antibacterial (systemic), for urinary tract infections	Canadian drug product For general information that may apply to all penicillins, see *Penicillins (Systemic)*
Amsacrine (*Amsa P-D* [Canada])	Injection	Antineoplastic, for leukemia	Canadian drug product
Anileridine (*Leritine* [Canada])	Tablets Injection	Analgesic, for moderate to severe pain	An opioid analgesic For general information that may apply to all opioid analgesics, see *Narcotic Analgesics—For Pain Relief (Systemic)*
Aspirin (*Bayer Enteric* [U.S.])	Delayed-release Tablets	Analgesic; Antirheumatic; Antipyretic	Additional brand name product

Additional Products and Uses *(continued)*

GENERIC NAME (*Brand name*)	DOSAGE FORM(S)	USE	COMMENTS
Atenolol and Chlorthalidone (Generic [U.S.])	Tablets	Antihypertensive	Available generically
Beclomethasone Dipropionate (*Beclodisk* [Canada])	Powder for Inhalation	Adrenocorticoid (inhalation-local); Antiasthmatic, for chronic asthma	Dosage form available in Canada Intended for use only with *Beclodisk Diskhaler*
Benzydamine Hydrochloride (*Tantum* [Canada])	Oral Topical Solution	Analgesic (oral-local), for mouth and throat pain	Canadian drug product
Betamethasone Dipropionate (*Occlucort* [Canada])	Lotion	Corticosteroid (topical); Anti-inflammatory, steroidal (topical), for skin disorders	Canadian brand name product
Betamethasone Disodium Phosphate (*Betnesol* [Canada])	Dental Pellets	Corticosteroid (topical); Anti-inflammatory (steroidal), for mouth ulcers	Dosage form available in Canada; for use in mouth For general information that may apply to this medication see *Corticosteroids—Medium to Very High Potency (Topical)*
Betaxolol Hydrochloride and Chlorthalidone (*Kerledex* [U.S.])	Tablets	Antihypertensive	Additional combination product For general information that may apply to this medication, see *Beta-adrenergic Blocking Agents and Thiazide Diuretics (Systemic)*
Brompheniramine Maleate and Phenylpropanolamine Hydrochloride		Antihistamine-decongestant, for cough and cold symptoms and other upper respiratory problems	Additional dosage forms; OTC
(*Dimetapp Cold and Allergy* [U.S.])	Chewable Tablets		
(*Dimetapp Maximum Strength Liquigels* [U.S.])	Capsules		
Brompheniramine Maleate and Pseudoephedrine Hydrochloride (*Touro A&H* [U.S.])	Extended-release Capsules	Antihistamine-decongestant, for cough and cold symptoms and other upper respiratory problems	Additional brand name product
Budesonide (*Pulmicort; Pulmicort Spacer* [Canada])	Inhalation Aerosol	Adrenocorticoid (inhalation-local); Antiasthmatic, for chronic asthma	*Pulmicort Spacer* contains a spacer device For general information that may apply to this medication, see *Corticosteroids (Inhalation)*
Bufexamac (*Norfemac* [Canada]; *Parfenac* [Canada])	Cream Ointment	Anti-inflammatory (nonsteroidal), for skin or rectal inflammation	Canadian drug products
Butorphanol Tartrate (*Stadol NS* [U.S.])	Nasal Solution	Analgesic	Additional dosage form

Additional Products and Uses *(continued)*

GENERIC NAME (*Brand name*)	DOSAGE FORM(S)	USE	COMMENTS
Calcium Acetate (Generic [U.S.])	Tablets	Antihyperphosphatemic, for lowering blood phosphate levels	Available generically
Calcium Polycarbophil (*FiberNorm* [U.S.])	Tablets	Laxative; Antidiarrheal	Additional brand name product; OTC
Captopril (*Apo-Capto* [Canada]; *Novo-Captoril* [Canada]; *Syn-Captopril* [Canada])	Tablets	Antihypertensive; Vasodilator, for congestive heart failure	Canadian brand name products
Carboxymethylcellulose (*Cellufresh* [U.S.]; *Celluvisc* [U.S.])	Ophthalmic Solution	Protectant (ophthalmic); Artificial tears	Additional brand name products; OTC
Chlorpheniramine Maleate and Phenylephrine Hydrochloride (*EDA-HIST* [U.S.])	Oral Solution	Antihistamine-decongestant, for cough and cold symptoms and other upper respiratory problems	Additional brand name product; contains 5% alcohol
Chlorpheniramine Maleate, Phenylephrine Hydrochloride, and Acetaminophen (*Dristan Cold* [U.S.])	Tablets	Antihistamine-decongestant-analgesic for cough and cold symptoms and other upper respiratory problems	Additional brand name product; OTC
Chlorpheniramine Maleate, Phenylephrine Hydrochloride, Codeine Phosphate, and Ammonium Chloride (*Statuss Expectorant* [U.S.])	Oral Solution	Antihistamine-decongestant-antitussive-expectorant for cough and cold symptoms and other upper respiratory problems	Additional combination product; contains 5% alcohol; Schedule V For general information that may apply to this medication, see *Cough/Cold Combinations (Systemic)*
Chlorpheniramine Maleate, Phenylephrine Hydrochloride, and Hydrocodone Bitartrate (*Endal-HD Plus* [U.S.])	Oral Solution	Antihistamine-decongestant-antitussive-for cough and cold symptoms and other upper respiratory problems	Additional brand name product; alcohol free; Schedule III
Chlorpheniramine Maleate and Phenylpropanolamine Hydrochloride (*Tripalgen Cold* [U.S.])	Syrup	Antihistamine-decongestant, for cough and cold symptoms and other upper respiratory problems	Additional brand name product; OTC
Chlorpheniramine Maleate, Phenylpropanolamine Hydrochloride, and Aspirin (*BC Cold Powder* [U.S.])	for Oral Solution	Antihistamine-decongestant-analgesic, for cough and cold symptoms and other upper respiratory problems	Additional brand name product; OTC
Chlorpheniramine Maleate, Phenyltoloxamine Citrate, Phenylephrine Hydrochloride, and Phenylpropanolamine Hydrochloride (*Par Decon* [U.S.])	Extended-release Tablets	Antihistamine-decongestant, for cough and cold symptoms and other upper respiratory problems	Additional brand name product
Chlorpheniramine Maleate and Pseudoephedrine Hydrochloride (*Children's NyQuil* [U.S.])	Oral Solution	Antihistamine-decongestant, for cough and cold symptoms and other upper respiratory problems	Additional brand name product; OTC
Chlorpheniramine Maleate, Pseudoephedrine Hydrochloride, and Acetaminophen (*Tylenol Allergy Sinus Gelcaps* [U.S.])	Tablets	Antihistamine-decongestant-analgesic, for cough and cold symptoms and other upper respiratory problems	Additional brand name product; OTC

Additional Products and Uses *(continued)*

GENERIC NAME (*Brand name*)	DOSAGE FORM(S)	USE	COMMENTS
Chlorpheniramine Maleate, Pseudoephedrine Hydrochloride, Dextromethorphan Hydrobromide, and Acetaminophen (*Comtrex Hot Flu Relief* [U.S.]; *Comtrex Multi-Symptom Hot Flu Relief* [U.S.]; *Dristan Cold and Flu* [U.S.]; *TheraFlu Nighttime Maximum Strength* [U.S.])	for Oral Solution	Antihistamine-decongestant-antitussive-analgesic, for cough and cold symptoms and other upper respiratory problems	Additional brand name products; OTC
Chlorpheniramine Tannate, Pyrilamine Tannate, and Phenylephrine Tannate (*Tritann Pediatric* [U.S.])	Oral Suspension	Antihistamine-decongestant, for cough and cold symptoms and other upper respiratory problems	Additional brand name product
Choline Salicylate and Cetyl-dimethyl-benzyl-ammonium Chloride (*Teejel* [Canada])	Gel	Analgesic (oral-local), for teething or mouth pain	Contains 39% alcohol Should not be used by patients who cannot take other salicylates
Cladribine (*Leustatin* [U.S.])	Injection	Antineoplastic, for leukemia	U.S. drug product
Clarithromycin (*Biaxin* [Canada])	Tablets	Antibacterial (systemic), for infections in many different parts of the body	Now available in Canada
Clemastine Fumarate (*Tavist-1* [U.S.]) (Generic [U.S.])	Tablets	Antihistamine	Now available OTC Available generically
Clemastine Fumarate and Phenylpropanolamine Hydrochloride (*Tavist-D* [U.S.])	Extended-release Tablets	Antihistamine-decongestant, for cough and cold symptoms and other upper respiratory problems	Now available OTC
Clindamycin Phosphate (*Cleocin* [U.S.])	Vaginal Cream	Anti-infective, for vaginal infections	Additional dosage form
Clioquinol and Flumethasone Pivalate (*Locacorten Vioform* [Canada])	Cream Ointment	Antibacterial-antifungal-corticosteroid (topical), for skin inflammation, infection, and itching	Canadian combination products For general information that may apply to this combination, see *Clioquinol and Hydrocortisone (Topical)*
Clioquinol and Flumethasone Pivalate (*Locacorten Vioform* [Canada])	Otic Solution	Antibacterial-antifungal-corticosteroid (otic), for ear infections	Canadian combination product For general information that may apply to all otic corticosteroids, see *Corticosteroids (Otic)*
Clobazam (*Frisium* [Canada])	Tablets	Anticonvulsant	Canadian drug product
Clotrimazole (*FemCare* [U.S.]; *Mycelex-7* [U.S.])	Vaginal Cream Vaginal Tablets	Antifungal (vaginal), for fungus infections of the vagina	Additional brand name products; OTC
Cyproterone Acetate (*Androcur* [Canada])	Tablets Injection	Antineoplastic, for prostate cancer	Canadian drug product
Debrisoquine Sulfate (*Declinax* [Canada])	Tablets	Antihypertensive	Canadian drug product

Additional Products and Uses *(continued)*

GENERIC NAME (*Brand name*)	DOSAGE FORM(S)	USE	COMMENTS
Desogestrel and Ethinyl Estradiol (*Desogen 28* [U.S.])	Tablets	Estrogen-Progestin; Contraceptive (systemic)	Additional combination product For general information that may apply to this combination, see *Estrogens and Progestins (Oral Contraceptives) (Systemic)*
Dexbrompheniramine Maleate and Pseudoephedrine Sulfate (*Cheracol Sinus* [U.S.])	Extended-release Tablets	Antihistamine-decongestant, for cough and cold symptoms and other upper respiratory problems	Additional brand name product; OTC
Dextromethorphan Hydrobromide		Antitussive	Additional brand name products; OTC
(*Creo-Terpin* [U.S.])	Oral Solution		Contains 25% alcohol
(*Robitussin Maximum Strength Cough* [U.S.])	Syrup		Contains 1.4% alcohol
Dextromethorphan Hydrobromide and Acetaminophen (*Tylenol Cough* [U.S.])	Oral Solution	Antitussive-analgesic, for cough and cold symptoms and other upper respiratory problems	Additional combination product; contains 10% alcohol; OTC For general information that may apply to this combination, see *Cough/Cold Combinations (Systemic)*
Dextromethorphan Hydrobromide and Guaifenesin (*Safe Tussin 30* [U.S.])	Oral Solution	Antitussive-expectorant, for cough and cold symptoms and other upper respiratory problems	Additional brand name product; OTC; contains no sugar, no alcohol, and no dyes
Diclofenac (*Apo-Diclo* [Canada]; *Novo-Difenac* [Canada]; *Nu-Diclo* [Canada])	Delayed-release Tablets	Antirheumatic (nonsteroidal anti-inflammatory)	Canadian brand name products
Diethylamine Salicylate (*Algesal* [Canada])	Cream	Analgesic (topical), for muscle and joint pain	Caution required in patients who cannot take other salicylates
Diflunisal (Generic [U.S.])	Tablets	Antirheumatic (nonsteroidal anti-inflammatory); Analgesic, for migraine headache	Available generically
Dimenhydrinate (*Children's Dramamine* [U.S.])	Elixir	Antiemetic; Antivertigo	Additional brand name product; OTC; contains 5% alcohol
Diphenhydramine Hydrochloride		Antihistamine; Antidyskinetic; Antiemetic; Antivertigo agent; Sedative-hypnotic	Additional brand name products; OTC
(*Dormin* [U.S.])	Capsules		
(*Silphen* [U.S.])	Syrup		Also used for coughs of colds or allergy
Diphenhydramine Hydrochloride, Pseudoephedrine Hydrochloride, and Acetaminophen (*Benadryl Allergy/Sinus Headache Caplets* [U.S.])	Tablets	Antihistamine-decongestant-analgesic, for cough and cold symptoms and other upper respiratory problems	Additional brand name product; OTC

Additional Products and Uses *(continued)*

GENERIC NAME (*Brand name*)	DOSAGE FORM(S)	USE	COMMENTS
Diphenhydramine Hydrochloride, Pseudoephedrine Hydrochloride, Dextromethorphan Hydrobromide, and Acetaminophen (*Contac Night Caplets* [U.S.])	Tablets	Antihistamine-decongestant-antitussive-analgesic, for cough and cold symptoms and other upper respiratory problems	Additional brand name product; available in a dual package that also contains *Contac Day Caplets*; OTC
Dipyridamole and Aspirin (*Asasantine* [Canada])	Capsules	Platelet aggregation inhibitor	For general information that may apply to this combination, see *Dipyridamole (Therapeutic)* and *Salicylates (Systemic)*
Domperidone (*Motilium* [Canada])	Tablets	Stomach and intestine stimulant; Antiemetic, drug-related	Canadian drug product
Enalapril Maleate and Hydrochlorothiazide (*Vaseretic* [Canada])	Tablets	Antihypertensive	Canadian brand name product
Epinephrine (*Ana-Guard Epinephrine* [U.S.])	Injection	Antiallergic (systemic)	Additional brand name product
Epirubicin Hydrochloride (*Pharmorubicin* [Canada])	for Injection	Antineoplastic, for breast cancer	Canadian drug product
Erythromycin	Topical	Antiacne agent (topical)	
(*E/Gel* [U.S.]; *Emgel* [U.S.])	Gel		Additional brand name products
(*Theramycin Z* [U.S.])	Solution		
(Generic [U.S.])	Gel		Available generically
Estrogens, Conjugated (*Mannest* [U.S.])	Tablets	Estrogen replacement therapy; Antineoplastic, for breast or prostate cancer; Osteoporosis prophylactic	Additional brand name product
Felbamate (*Felbatol* [U.S.])	Tablets Oral Suspension	Anticonvulsant, for some types of epilepsy, including Lennox-Gastaut syndrome in children	U.S. drug product
Fentanyl (*Duragesic* [U.S.])	Transdermal System	Analgesic, for chronic pain	First opioid analgesic available in a transdermal system Controlled substance—Schedule II
Flucloxacillin Sodium (*Fluclox* [Canada])	Capsules for Oral Solution	Antibacterial (systemic), for infections in many different parts of the body	Canadian drug products For general information that may apply to all penicillins, see *Penicillins (Systemic)*
Fluocinonide (Generic [U.S.])	Ointment	Corticosteroid (topical); Anti-inflammatory, steroidal (topical), for skin disorders	Available generically
Fluocinonide, Procinonide, and Ciprocinonide (*Trisyn* [Canada])	Cream	Corticosteroid (topical); Anti-inflammatory (steroidal), for skin disorders	For general information that may apply to all topical corticosteroids, see *Corticosteroids—Medium to Very High Potency (Topical)*
Fluoxetine (*Prozac* [Canada])	Capsules	Antibulimic	Additional use in Canada

Additional Products and Uses *(continued)*

GENERIC NAME (*Brand name*)	DOSAGE FORM(S)	USE	COMMENTS
Fluphenazine Hydrochloride (Generic [U.S.])	Elixir	Antipsychotic	Available generically
Flurbiprofen		Antirheumatic	
(*Apo-Flurbiprofen* [Canada])	Tablets		Canadian brand name product
(*Froben SR* [Canada])	Extended-release Capsules		Capsules are to be swallowed whole
Fluspirilene (*Imap* [Canada]; *Imap Forte* [Canada])	Injection	Antipsychotic	Canadian drug products
Framycetin Sulfate (*Soframycin* [Canada])	Ophthalmic Ointment Ophthalmic Solution	Antibacterial (ophthalmic), for eye infections	Canadian drug products Belongs to the group of *Streptomyces*-derived antibiotics (including neomycin, paromomycin, kanamycin)
Framycetin Sulfate (*Sofra-Tulle* [Canada])	Impregnated Gauze	Antibacterial (topical), for skin or burn infections	Canadian drug product Belongs to the group of *Streptomyces*-derived antibiotics (including neomycin, paromomycin, kanamycin)
Framycetin Sulfate and Gramicidin (*Soframycin* [Canada])	Ointment	Antibacterial (topical), for skin or burn infections	Canadian combination product
Framycetin Sulfate, Gramicidin, and Dexamethasone (*Sofracort Eye-Ear Drops* and *Sofracort Eye-Ear Ointment* [Canada])	Ophthalmic Ointment Ophthalmic Solution	Antibacterial-adrenocorticoid (ophthalmic), for eye infections	Canadian combination products
Framycetin Sulfate, Gramicidin, and Dexamethasone (*Sofracort Eye-Ear Drops* and *Sofracort Eye-Ear Ointment* [Canada])	Otic Ointment Otic Solution	Antibacterial-corticosteroid (otic), for ear infections	Canadian combination products
Fusidic Acid (*Fucidin* [Canada])	for Injection Oral Suspension Tablets	Antibacterial (systemic), for infections in many different parts of the body	Canadian drug products
Fusidic Acid (*Fucidin* [Canada])	Cream Impregnated Gauze Ointment	Antibacterial (topical), for skin or burn infections	Canadian drug products
Gonadorelin Acetate (*Lutrepulse* [U.S.])	for Injection	Hormone, for treatment of infertility	Additional FDA-approved use Intended for use only with *Lutrepulse* pump
Guaifenesin (*Touro Ex* [U.S.])	Extended-release Capsules	Expectorant	Additional brand name product
Hydrocortisone (*Anusol-HC 2.5%* [U.S.]; *Prevex HC* [Canada])	Cream	Corticosteroid (topical); Anti-inflammatory, steroidal (topical), for skin disorders	U.S. and Canadian brand name products
Hydrocortisone Acetate (*Gynecort 10* [U.S.]; *Lanacort 10* [U.S.])	Cream	Corticosteroid (topical); Anti-inflammatory, steroidal (topical), for skin disorders	Additional brand name products; OTC

Additional Products and Uses *(continued)*

GENERIC NAME (*Brand name*)	DOSAGE FORM(S)	USE	COMMENTS
Hydrocortisone and Urea (*Sential* [Canada])	Cream	Corticosteroid (topical); Anti-inflammatory, steroidal (topical), for skin disorders	Canadian brand name product For general information that may apply to this medication, see *Corticosteroids—Low Potency (Topical)*
Ibuprofen		Antirheumatic (nonsteroidal anti-inflammatory); Analgesic; Antipyretic; Antidysmenorrheal	
(*Bayer Select Pain Relief Formula Caplets* [U.S.]; *Cramp End,* [U.S.]; *Excedrin-IB Caplets* [U.S.]; *Excedrin-IB Tablets* [U.S.]; *Ibu* [U.S.]; *Ibu 200* [U.S.]; *Ibu-4* [U.S.]; *Ibu-6* [U.S.]; *Ibu-8* [U.S.]; *Ibifon-600 Caplets* [U.S.]; *Saleto-200 Saleto-400* [U.S.]; *Saleto-600* [U.S.]; *Saleto-800* [U.S.])	Tablets		Additional brand name products
(*Motrin, Children's* [U.S.])	Oral Suspension		Brand name change—formerly *PediaProfen*
(*Midol-IB* [U.S.])	Tablets		Brand name change—formerly *Midol-200*
Indomethacin (*Nu-Indo* [Canada])	Capsules	Antirheumatic (nonsteroidal anti-inflammatory); Antigout agent	Canadian brand name product
Iodinated Glycerol (*Par Glycerol* [U.S.])	Elixir	Mucolytic	Additional brand name product
Ipratropium Bromide (*Atrovent* [Canada])	Nasal Inhalation	Antiallergic (nasal), for hay fever or other allergies	Dosage form available in Canada
Isosorbide Dinitrate (*Coradur* [Canada])	Extended-release Tablets	Antianginal	Canadian brand name product
Isotretinoin (*Isotrex* [Canada])	Gel	Antiacne agent (topical)	Canadian brand name product
Ketoprofen		Antirheumatic (nonsteroidal anti-inflammatory)	
(*Apo-Keto* [Canada])	Capsules		Canadian brand name products
(*Apo-Keto-E* [Canada])	Delayed-release Capsules		
(*Apo-Keto-E* [Canada]; *Novo-Keto-EC* [Canada])	Delayed-release Tablets		
(*Oruvail* [Canada])	Extended-release Capsules		
(*Rhodis-EC* [Canada])			Brand name change—formerly *Rhodis-E*
Ketorolac Tromethamine (*Acular* [U.S.])	Ophthalmic Solution	Anti-inflammatory, nonsteroidal (ophthalmic), for itching of eyes caused by allergies	Additional brand name product For general information that may apply to all ophthalmic nonsteroidal anti-inflammatory agents, see *Anti-inflammatory Agents, Nonsteroidal (Ophthalmic)*

Additional Products and Uses *(continued)*

GENERIC NAME (*Brand name*)	DOSAGE FORM(S)	USE	COMMENTS
Ketotifen Fumarate (*Zaditen* [Canada])	Syrup Tablets	Antiallergic (systemic); Asthma prophylactic in children	Canadian drug product
Leuprolide Acetate		Hormone-like agent for treatment of premature puberty	Additional FDA-approved use; additional brand name products
(*Lupron Depot-Ped* [U.S.])	for Injection		
(*Lupron for Pediatric Use* [U.S.])	Injection		
Levodopa and Benserazide (*Prolopa* [Canada])	Capsules	Antidyskinetic, for symptoms of Parkinson's disease	Canadian drug product
Levonorgestrel (*Norplant* [U.S.])	Implants	Progestin; Contraceptive (systemic)	Additional dosage form
Liothyronine Sodium (*Triostat* [U.S.])	Injection	Thyroid hormone	Additional dosage form
Loperamide Hydrochloride		Antidiarrheal	Additional brand name products; OTC
(*Kaopectate II Caplets* [U.S.])	Tablets		
(*Pepto Diarrhea Control* [U.S.])	Oral Solution		Contains 5.25% alcohol
(Generic [U.S.])	Capsules		Available generically
Meclofenamate Sodium (*Meclomen* [U.S.])	Capsules	Antidysmenorrheal	Additional FDA-approved use
Medroxyprogesterone Acetate (*Depo-Provera* [U.S.])	Sterile Suspension	Progestin; Contraceptive (systemic)	Additional FDA-approved use
Melphalan Hydrochloride (*Alkeran* [U.S.])	for Injection	Antineoplastic, for multiple myeloma	Additional dosage form
Mesalamine (*Asacol* [U.S. and Canada])	Delayed-release Tablets	Inflammatory bowel disease suppressant	Additional dosage form in the U.S. Enteric-coated tablets Another name is aminosalicylic acid
Metaproterenol Sulfate (*Prometa* [U.S.])	Syrup	Bronchodilator	Additional brand name product
Metformin Hydrochloride (*Glucophage* [Canada])	Tablets	Antidiabetic	Canadian drug product Metformin should be taken with food or meals to minimize gastric upset
Methyldopa (*Nu-Medopa* [Canada])	Tablets	Antihypertensive	Canadian brand name product
Metoprolol Tartrate (*Nu-Metop* [Canada])	Tablets	Antianginal; Antihypertensive; Myocardial reinfarction prophylactic	Canadian brand name product
Metronidazole			
(*Flagyl* [Canada])	Vaginal Cream Vaginal Suppositories	Antiprotozoal (vaginal), for trichomoniasis	Additional dosage forms in Canada
(*MetroGel-Vaginal* [U.S.]	Vaginal Gel	Anti-infective (vaginal) for vaginal infections	Additional dosage form in the U.S.
Metronidazole (*MetroGel* [Canada])	Topical Gel	Antirosacea	Now available in Canada

Additional Products and Uses *(continued)*

GENERIC NAME (*Brand name*)	DOSAGE FORM(S)	USE	COMMENTS
Metronidazole and Nystatin (*Flagystatin* [Canada])	Vaginal Cream Vaginal Suppositories Vaginal Tablets	Antiprotozoal-antifungal (vaginal), for yeast infections or trichomoniasis	Canadian combination products
Morphine Sulfate (*Oramorph SR* [U.S.])	Extended-release Tablets	Analgesic, for chronic pain	Additional brand name product
Nafarelin Acetate (*Synarel* [U.S.])	Nasal Solution	Hormone-like agent for treatment of premature puberty	Additional FDA-approved use
Naftifine (*Naftin* [U.S.])	Gel	Antifungal (topical), for ringworm of the body, jock itch, or athlete's foot	Additional dosage form
Naproxen		Antirheumatic (nonsteroidal anti-inflammatory); Analgesic; Antidysmenorrheal	
(*Naprosyn-E* [Canada])	Delayed-release Tablets		Additional dosage form in Canada
(*Nu-Naprox* [Canada])	Tablets		Canadian brand name product
Nicotinamide (*Papulex* [Canada])	Gel	Antiacne agent (topical)	Canadian drug product
Nifedipine (*Adalat CC* [U.S.])	Extended-release Tablets	Antihypertensive	Additional brand name product; should be taken on an empty stomach; do not chew, divide, or crush tablets
Nilutamide (*Anandron* [Canada])	Tablets	Antineoplastic, for prostate cancer	Canadian drug product
Nitrofurantoin (*Macrobid* [U.S.])	Extended-release Capsules	Antibacterial (systemic), for urinary tract infections	Additional dosage form
Nitroglycerin (*Nitro-Dur* [Canada])	Transdermal Systems	Antianginal	Canadian brand name product
Norethindrone and Ethinyl Estradiol (*Jenest-28* [U.S.])	Tablets	Estrogen-Progestin; Contraceptive (systemic)	Additional brand name product
Norgestimate and Ethinyl Estradiol (*Ortho-Cyclen 21* [U.S.]; *Ortho-Cyclen 28* [U.S.]; *Ortho Tri-Cyclen 21* [U.S.]; *Ortho Tri-Cyclen 28* [U.S.])	Tablets	Estrogen-Progestin; Contraceptive (systemic)	Additional combination products For general information that may apply to this combination, see *Estrogens and Progestins (Oral Contraceptives) (Systemic)*
Ondansetron			
(*Zofran* [U.S.])	Tablets	Antiemetic, following cancer chemotherapy	Additional dosage form
(*Zofran* [Canada])	Injection Tablets	Antiemetic, following cancer chemotherapy or radiation therapy	Now available in Canada
Paroxetine (*Paxil* [U.S.])	Tablets	Antidepressant	U.S. drug product

Additional Products and Uses *(continued)*

GENERIC NAME (*Brand name*)	DOSAGE FORM(S)	USE	COMMENTS
Permethrin			Additional brand name products
(*Elimite* [U.S.]; *Nix Dermal Cream* [Canada])	Cream	Scabicide, for scabies	
(*Nix Creme Rinse* [U.S. and Canada])	Lotion	Pediculicide, for head lice	OTC in U.S.; formerly Rx Now available in Canada Note—Permethrin 0.5% is used also as a repellant in the form of a contact spray for clothing (not skin) to prevent the bites of ixodid ticks. The bites of ixodid ticks infected with *Borrelia burgdorferi* cause Lyme disease
Pheniramine Maleate, Pyrilamine Maleate, Phenylephrine Hydrochloride, Phenylpropanolamine Hydrochloride, and Hydrocodone Bitartrate (*Statuss Green* [U.S.])	Oral Solution	Antihistamine-decongestant-antitussive, for cough and cold symptoms and other upper respiratory problems	Additional brand name product; contains 5% alcohol; Schedule III
Phenylbutazone (*Cotylbutazone* [U.S.])	Capsules	Antirheumatic (nonsteriodal anti-inflammatory); Antigout agent	Additional brand name product
Phenylephrine Hydrochloride, Phenylpropanolamine Hydrochloride, and Guaifenesin (*Despec* [U.S.])	Oral Solution	Decongestant-expectorant, for cough and cold symptoms and other upper respiratory problems	Additional brand name product
Phenylpropanolamine Hydrochloride and Guaifenesin		Decongestant-expectorant, for cough and cold symptoms and other upper respiratory problems	Additional brand name products
(*Despec* [U.S.])	Extended-release Capsules		
(*Stamoist LA* [U.S.]; *ULR-LA* [U.S.])	Extended-release Tablets		
Piroxicam	Capsules	Antirheumatic (nonsteroidal anti-inflammatory)	
(*Nu-Pirox* [Canada])			Canadian brand name product
(Generic [U.S.])			Available generically
Pivampicillin (*Pondocillin* [Canada])	for Oral Suspension Tablets	Antibacterial (systemic), for infections in many different parts of the body	Canadian drug product For general information that may apply to all penicillins, see *Penicillins (Systemic)*
Pizotyline Hydrogen Maleate (*Sandomigran* [Canada]; *Sandomigran DS* [Canada])	Tablets	Migraine headache preventive	Dosage should be decreased gradually over a 2-week period prior to discontinuation, to prevent rebound headache
Podofilox (*Condylox* [U.S.])	Topical solution	Cytotoxic (topical), for venereal warts	U.S. drug product
Progesterone (*Progestasert* [U.S.])	Intrauterine System	Contraceptive (intrauterine-local)	Patient informed consent forms must be completed before insertion of the system

Additional Products and Uses *(continued)*

GENERIC NAME (*Brand name*)	DOSAGE FORM(S)	USE	COMMENTS
Propoxyphene Hydrochloride and Acetaminophen (*Proxy 65* [U.S.])	Tablets	Analgesic	Additional brand name product
Pseudoephedrine Hydrochloride and Acetaminophen (*Bayer Select Maximum Strength Sinus Pain Relief Caplets* [U.S.]; *Tylenol Sinus Maximum Strength Gel-caps* [U.S.])	Tablets	Decongestant-analgesic, for congestion and headache caused by sinusitis, colds, or allergies	Additional brand name products; OTC
Pseudoephedrine Hydrochloride and Dextromethorphan Hydrobromide (*Robitussin Maximum Strength Cough and Cold* [U.S.])	Oral Solution	Decongestant-antitussive, for cough and cold symptoms and other upper respiratory problems	Additional dosage form; OTC
Pseudoephedrine Hydrochloride, Dextromethorphan Hydrobromide, and Acetaminophen		Decongestant-antitussive-analgesic, for cough and cold symptoms and other upper respiratory problems	OTC
(*Contac Day Caplets* [U.S.])	Tablets		Additional brand name product; available in a dual package that also contains *Contac Night Caplets*
(*Dristan Juice Mix-in Cold, Flu, and Cough* [U.S.])	for Oral Solution		Additional dosage form
(*Tylenol Cold No Drowsiness Formula Gelcaps* [U.S.])	Tablets		Additional brand name product
(*Tylenol Cough with Decongestant* [U.S.])	Oral Solution		Additional dosage form; contains 10% alcohol
Pseudoephedrine Hydrochloride, Dextromethorphan Hydrobromide, Guaifenesin, and Acetaminophen		Decongestant-antitussive-expectorant-analgesic, for cough and cold symptoms and other upper respiratory problems	OTC
(*DayQuil Liquicaps* [U.S.])	Capsules		Additional dosage form
(*DayQuil Non-Drowsy Cold/Flu* [U.S.])	Oral Solution		Additional brand name product
Pseudoephedrine Hydrochloride and Guaifenesin (*Stamoist E* [U.S.]); *GuaiMAX-D* [U.S.])	Extended-release Tablets	Decongestant-expectorant, for cough and cold symptoms and other upper respiratory problems	Additional brand name products
Pseudoephedrine Hydrochloride and Ibuprofen (*Dimetapp Sinus Caplets* [U.S.])	Tablets	Decongestant-analgesic, for congestion and headache caused by sinusitis, colds, or allergies	Additional brand name product; OTC
Pyrethrins and Piperonyl Butoxide (*Lice-Enz Foam and Comb Lice Killing Shampoo Kit* [U.S.])	Solution Shampoo	Pediculicide, for head lice	Additional brand name product; OTC
Pyrilamine Maleate, Pseudoephedrine Hydrochloride, Dextromethorphan Hydrobromide, and Acetaminophen (*Robitussin Night Relief* [U.S.])	Oral Solution	Antihistamine-decongestant-antitussive-analgesic, for cough and cold symptoms and other upper respiratory problems	Reformulated product; pseudoephedrine hydrochloride replaces phenylephrine hydrochloride; OTC

Additional Products and Uses *(continued)*

GENERIC NAME (*Brand name*)	DOSAGE FORM(S)	USE	COMMENTS
Pyrithione (*Theraplex Z* [U.S.])	Lotion Shampoo	Antiseborrheic (topical), for dandruff and other scalp disorders	Additional brand name product
Remoxipride Hydrochloride Monohydrate (*Roxiam* [Canada])	Capsules Injection	Antipsychotic	Canadian drug product
Risperidone (*Risperdal* [Canada])	Tablets	Antipsychotic	Canadian drug product
Salicylic Acid and Sulfur (*Diasporal Cream* [U.S.])	Cream	Antiacne agent (topical)	Additional brand name product; additional dosage form; OTC
Sulconazole Nitrate (*Exelderm* [U.S.])	Cream Topical Solution	Antifungal (topical), for treatment of ringworm of the body, jock itch, athlete's foot, or sun fungus	Treatment of athlete's foot is an additional FDA-approved use for the cream dosage form only
Sulfadiazine and Trimethoprim (*Coptin* [Canada])	Tablets Oral Suspension	Antibacterial (systemic), for urinary tract infections	Canadian combination products For general information that may apply to this combination, see *Sulfamethoxazole and Trimethoprim (Systemic)*
Teniposide (*Vumon* [Canada])	Injection	Antineoplastic	Canadian drug product
Tenoxicam (*Mobiflex* [Canada])	Tablets	Antirheumatic (nonsteroidal anti-inflammatory); Anti-inflammatory (nonsteroidal), for bursitis, tendinitis, or shoulder or hip inflammation	Canadian drug product For general information that may apply to all anti-inflammatory analgesics, see *Anti-inflammatory Analgesics (Systemic)*
Testosterone (*Testopel* [U.S.])	Pellets	Androgen, for treatment of androgen deficiency and delayed puberty in boys	Additional dosage form
Theophylline (*Theo-Sav* [U.S.]; *Theox* [U.S.])	Extended-release Tablets	Bronchodilator; Asthma prophylactic	Additional brand name products
Theophylline, Ephedrine Hydrochloride, and Phenobarbital (*T.E.P.* [U.S.])	Tablets	Bronchodilator	Additional brand name product; OTC
Tiaprofenic Acid		Antirheumatic (nonsteroidal anti-inflammatory)	
(*Albert Tiafen* [Canada])	Tablets		Canadian brand name product
(*Surgam SR* [Canada])	Extended-release Capsules		Additional dosage form in Canada
Tioconazole (*Trosyd Dermal Cream* [Canada])	Cream	Antifungal (topical), for treatment of ringworm of the body, jock itch, athlete's foot, sun fungus, or other skin fungus infections	Canadian drug product
Tolmetin Sodium (Generic [U.S.])	Capsules Tablets	Antirheumatic (nonsteroidal anti-inflammatory)	Available generically
Triamcinolone Acetonide (*Nasacort* [U.S.])	Nasal Aerosol	Adrenocorticoid (nasal); Anti-inflammatory, steroidal (nasal), for hay fever or other allergies	Additional dosage form For general information that may apply to all nasal adrenocorticoids, see *Corticosteroids (Nasal)*

Additional Products and Uses *(continued)*

GENERIC NAME (*Brand name*)	DOSAGE FORM(S)	USE	COMMENTS
Triethanolamine Salicylate (*Myoflex* [Canada]; *Royflex* [Canada])	Cream	Analgesic (topical), for muscle and joint pain	Should not be used by patients who cannot take other salicylates
Triprolidine Hydrochloride and Pseudoephedrine Hydrochloride (*Atrofed* [U.S.])	Tablets	Antihistamine-decongestant, for upper respiratory problems caused by colds or allergies	Additional brand name product; OTC
Vindesine Sulfate (*Eldisine* [Canada])	for Injection	Antineoplastic, for leukemia	Canadian drug product
Zolpidem (*Ambien* [U.S.])	Tablets	Sedative-hypnotic, for insomnia	U.S. drug product

IV

Appendix IV

PICTOGRAMS

The pictograms included in this appendix represent selected commonly used directions for appropriate drug use or identify information that patients should share with their health care provider. They are intended to be used in a fashion that will reinforce other printed or oral instructions and as a reminder to patients as to the proper way to take or store their medication. It is possible that an individual reacting to the pictograms will have a different interpretation than what is intended. Because of this potential for misinterpretation, the pictograms should *not* be used as the sole means of transferring information to the patient.

In general, three different geometric shapes are used for the pictograms. A circle with a diagonal line through it represents a "do not" instruction; a triangle indicates a precaution; and a rectangle provides basic information on how to use the medication. If the pictogram transmits a message relating to how the patient should or should not take a medication, the inset image will be that of a person with his/her hand to the mouth in the act of taking a medication. If the pictogram message relates to the physical handling of the medication itself, the inset depicts a medication container with an Rx on it.

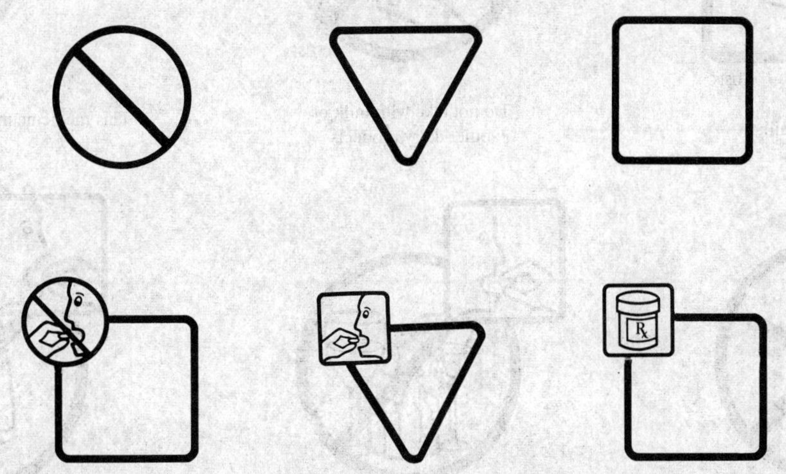

If you have any comments on these pictograms, especially ideas generated from actual patient use, or if you have ideas for additional pictograms, please contact:

Drug Information Division
USPC
12601 Twinbrook Parkway
Rockville, MD 20852

NOTE: The health care professional using the pictograms for a patient must decide which pictograms apply to the specific medication the patient is using. If photocopies of the pages that follow are used for patient education purposes, the provider should cross out pictograms that do not apply to a specific medication or otherwise indicate those symbols which are or are not applicable to that patient.

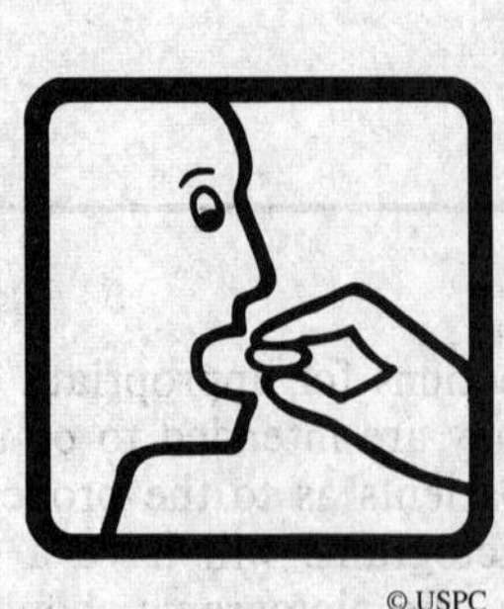
© USPC

Take by mouth

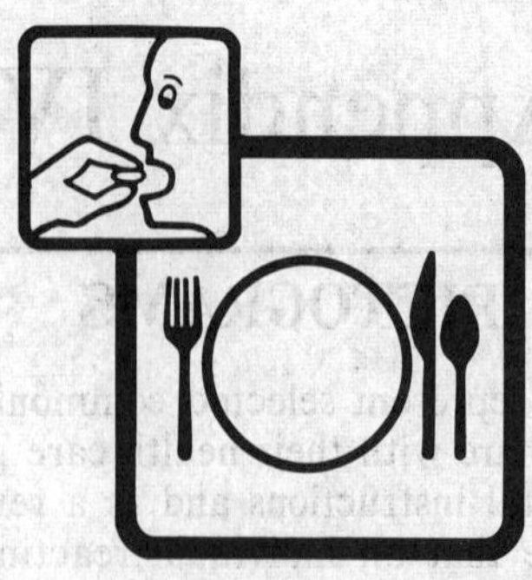
© USPC

Take with meals

© USPC

Do not take with meals

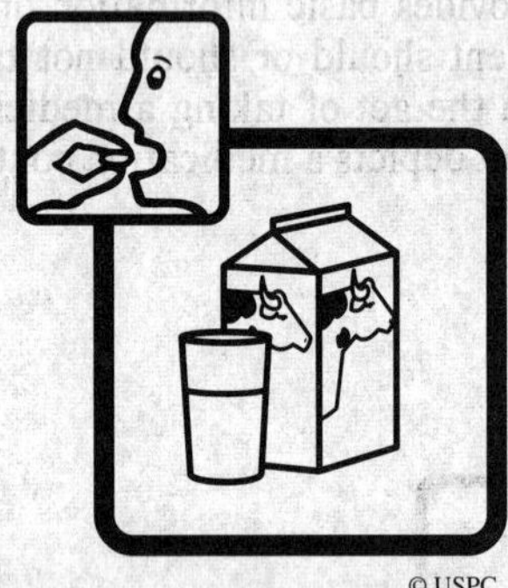
© USPC

Take with milk

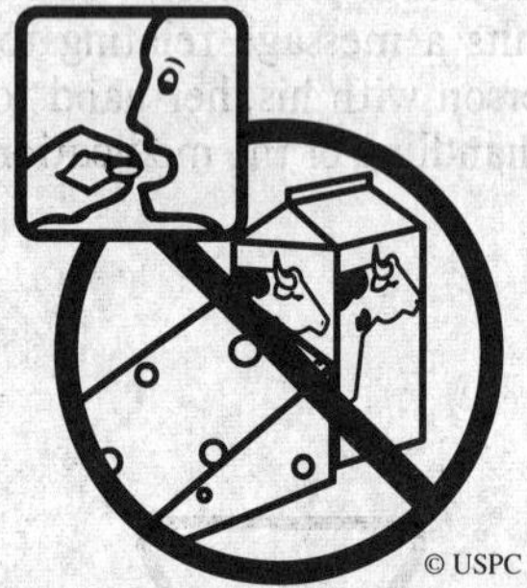
© USPC

Do not take with milk or other dairy products

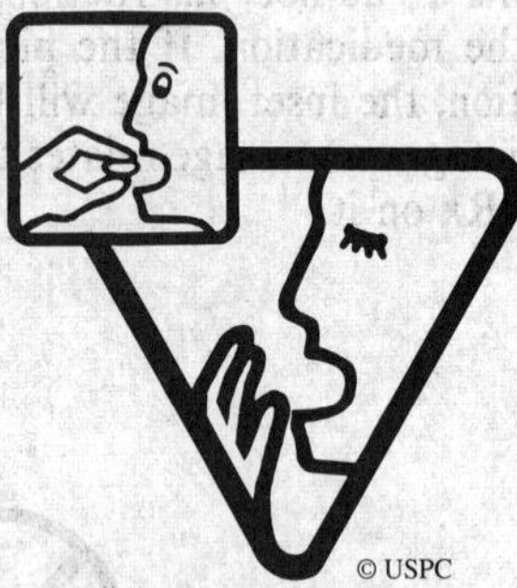
© USPC

This medicine may make you drowsy

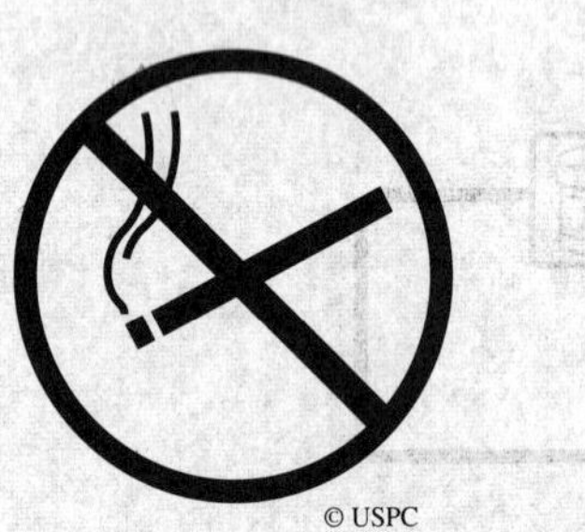
© USPC

Do not smoke

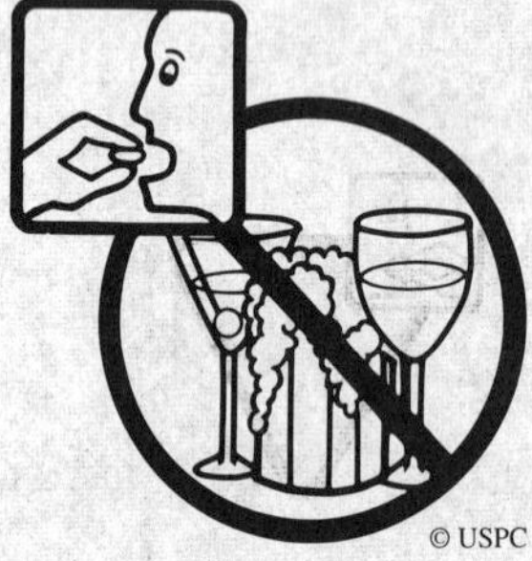
© USPC

Do not drink alcohol when taking this medicine

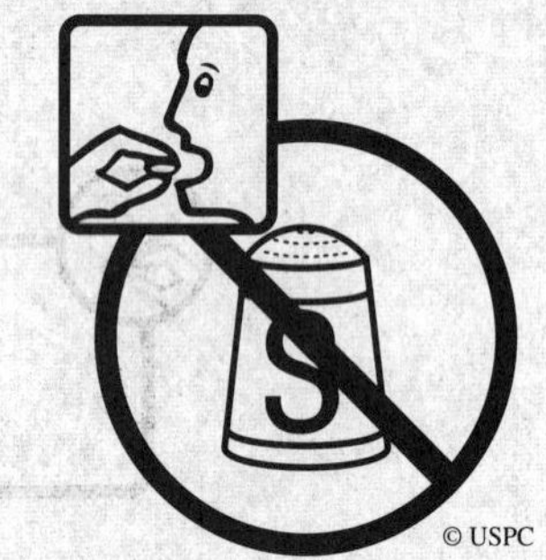

© USPC

Do not use additional salt

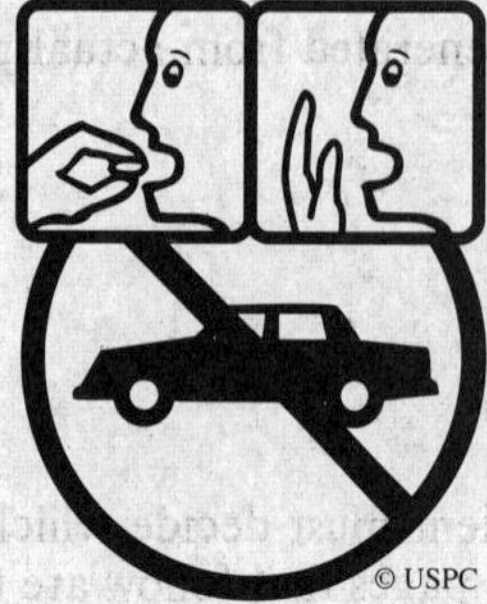
© USPC

Do not drive if this medicine makes you sleepy

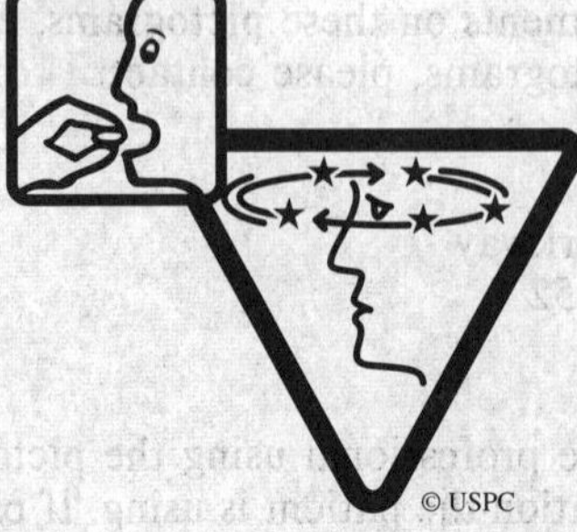
© USPC

This medicine may make you dizzy

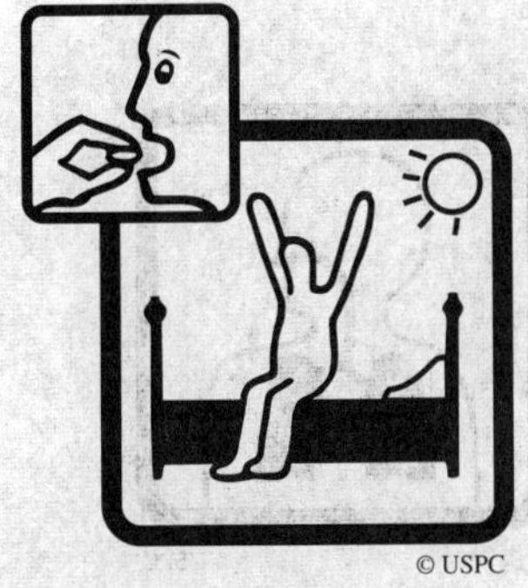

Take in the morning

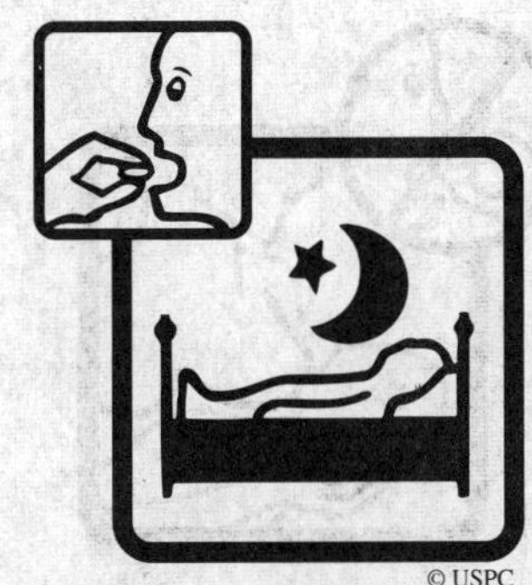

Take at bedtime

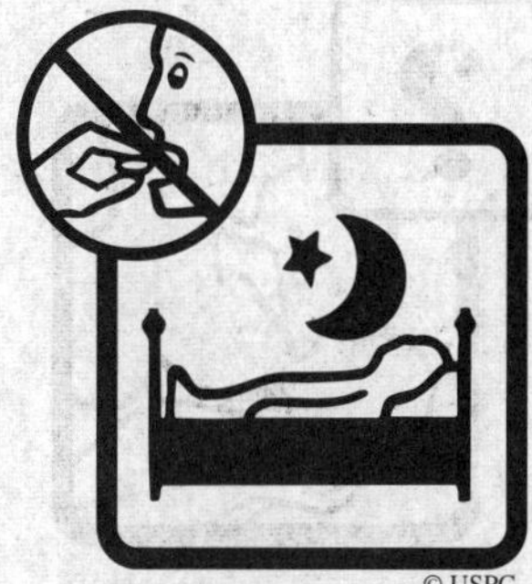

Do not take at bedtime

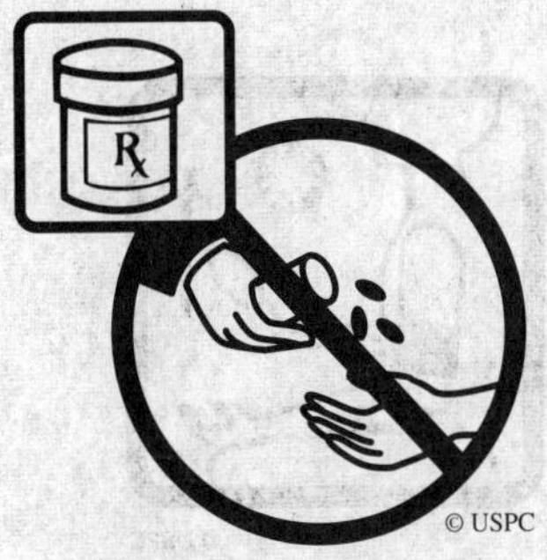

Do not share your medicine with others

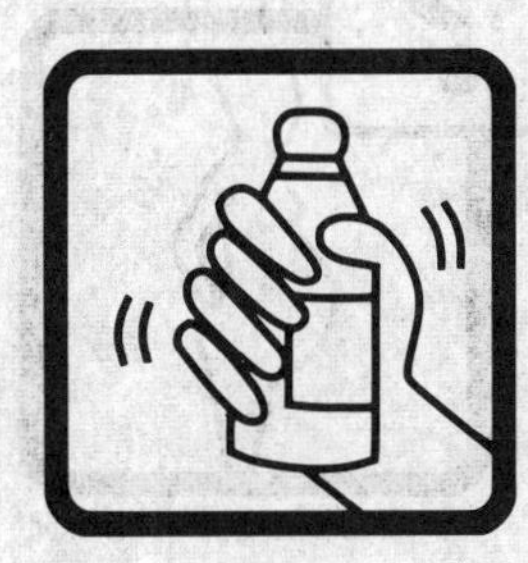

Shake well

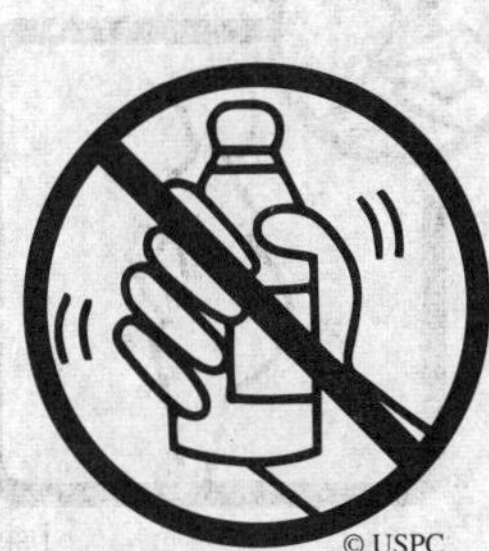

Do not shake

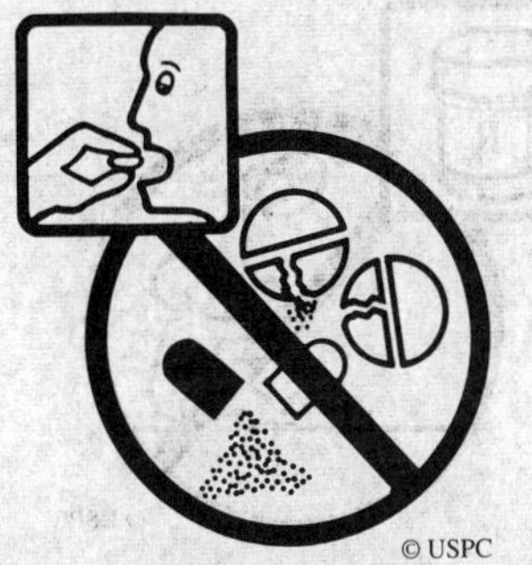

Do not break or crush tablets or open capsules

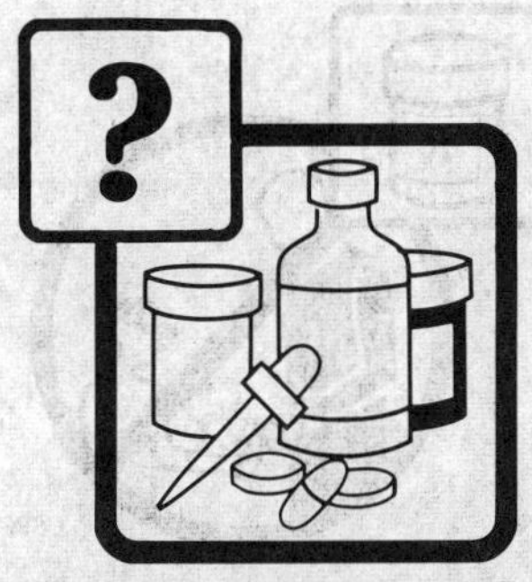

Are you taking any other medicines?

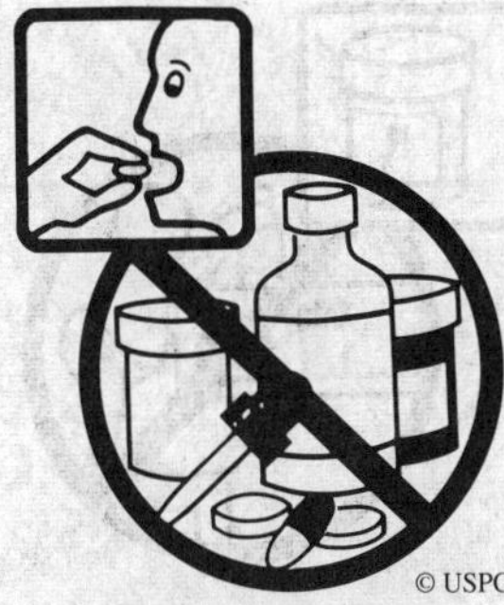

Do not take other medicines with this medicine

Do not store near heat or in sunlight

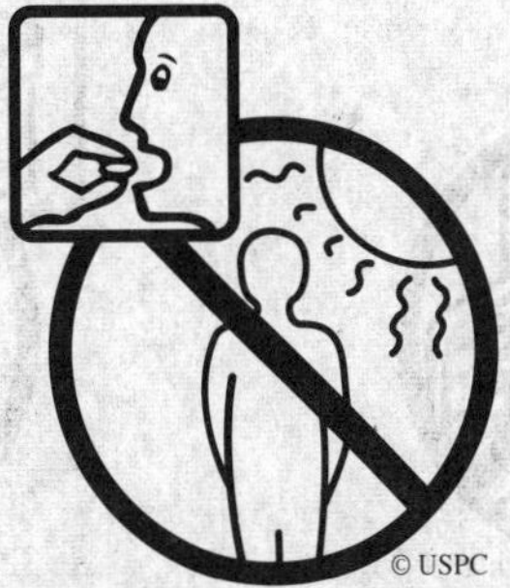

Avoid too much sun or use of sunlamp

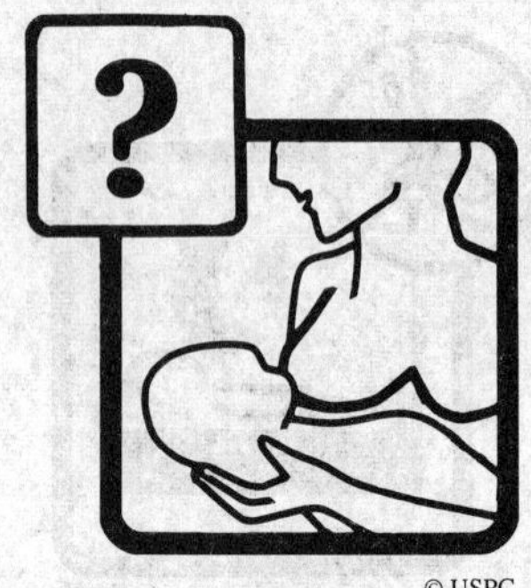

Are you breast-feeding?

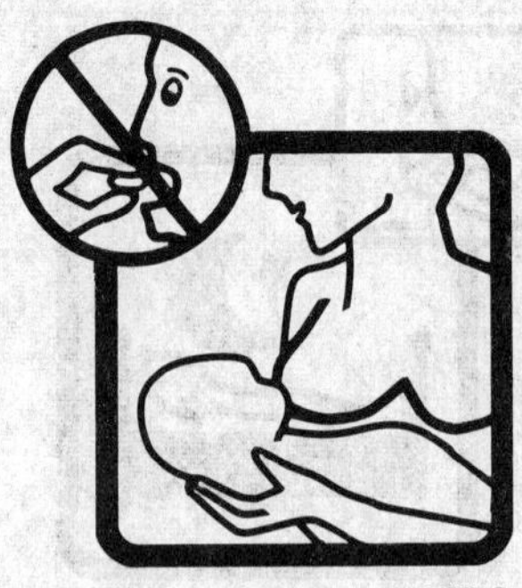

Do not take if breast-feeding

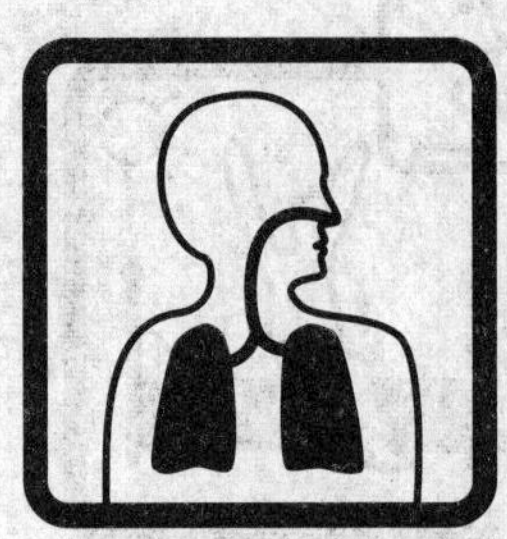

For lungs/respiratory problems

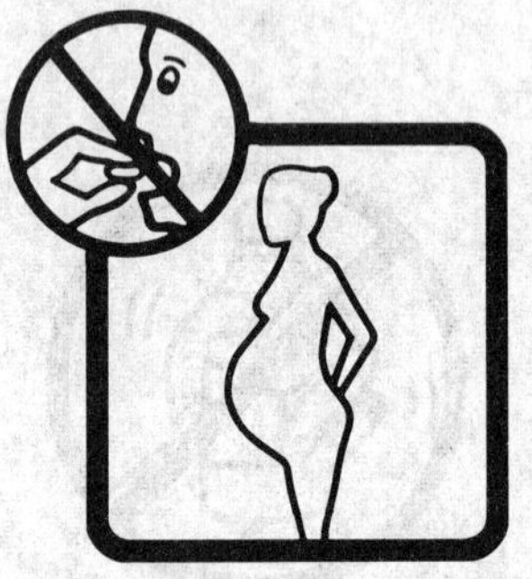

Do not take if pregnant

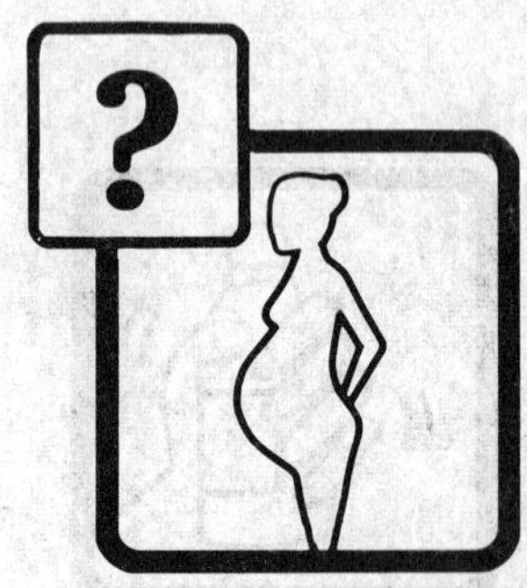

Are you pregnant or do you intend to become pregnant?

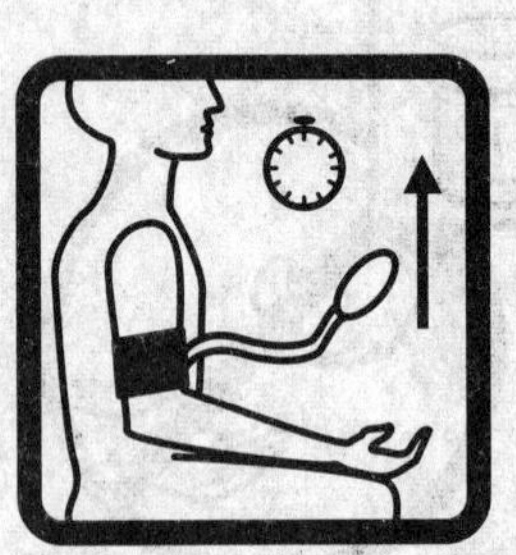

For hypertension (high blood pressure)

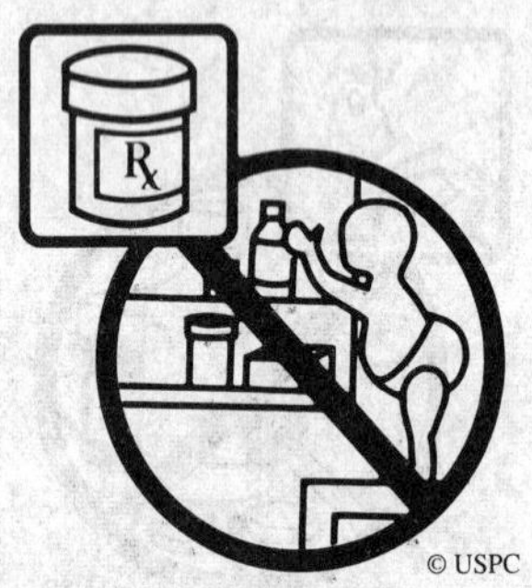

Store medicine out of reach of children

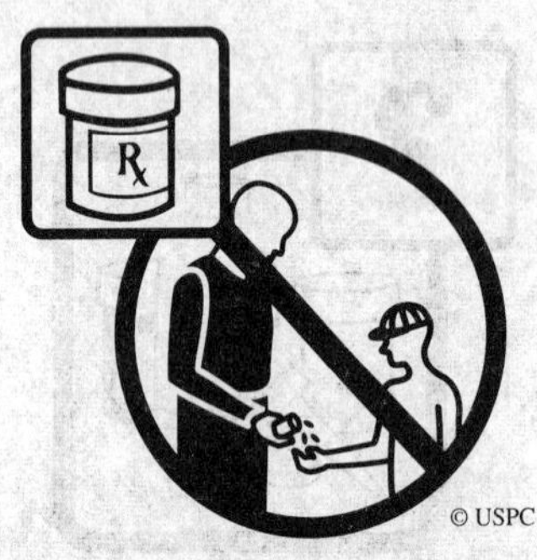

Do not give medicine to children

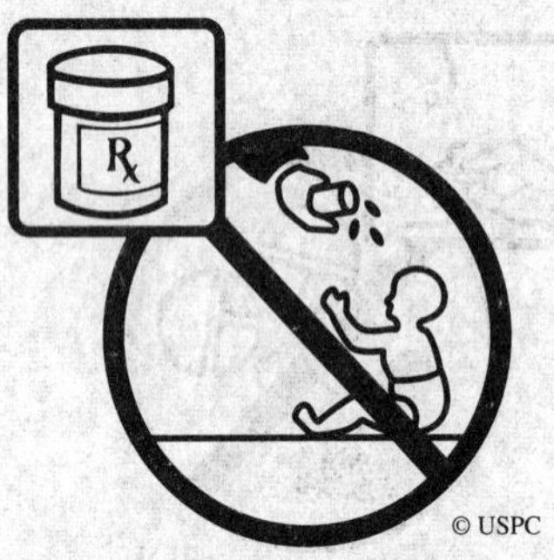

Do not give medicine to babies

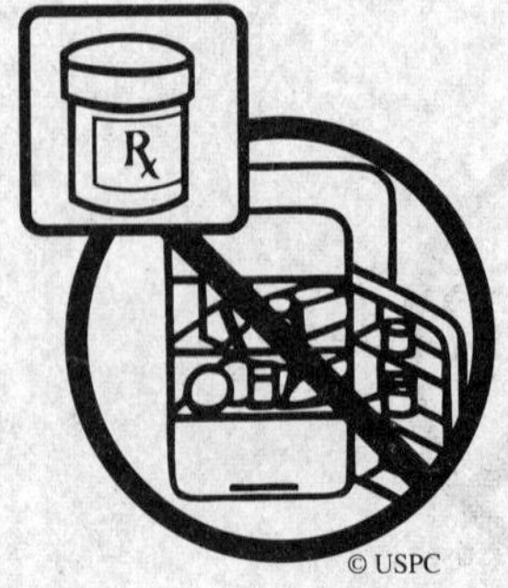

Do not refrigerate

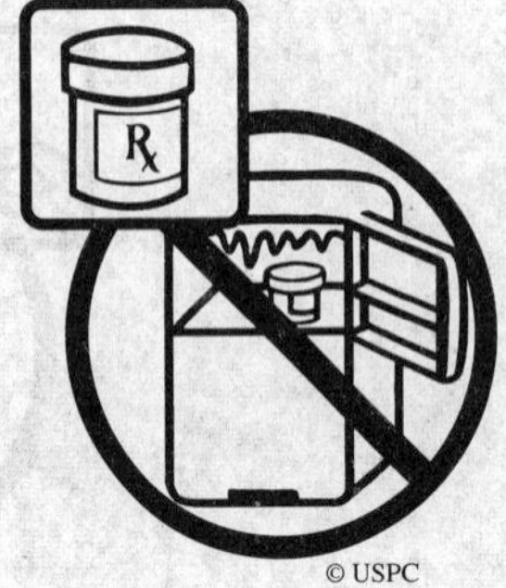

Do not freeze

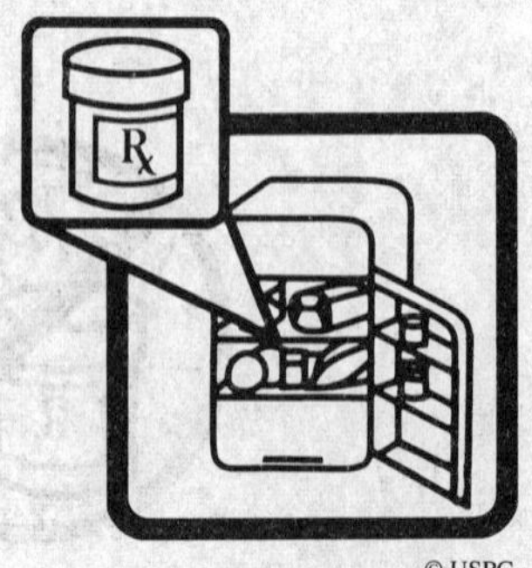

Store in refrigerator

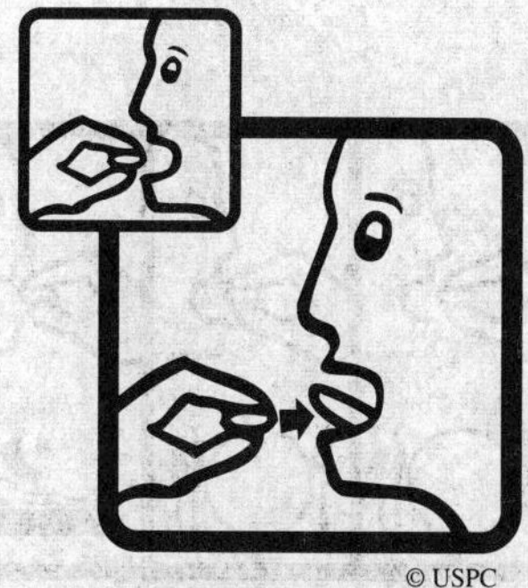

Dissolve under the tongue

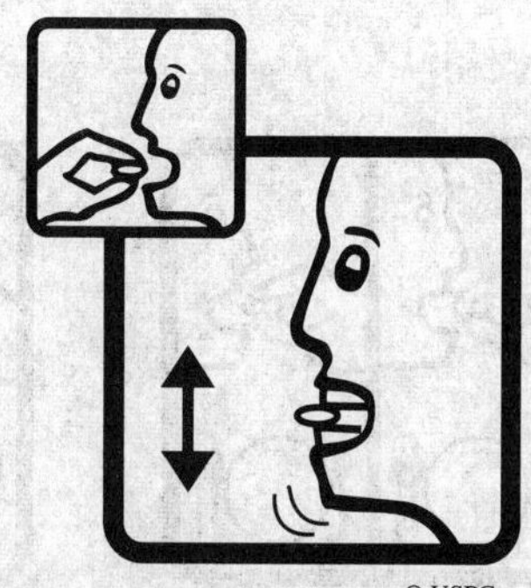

Chew

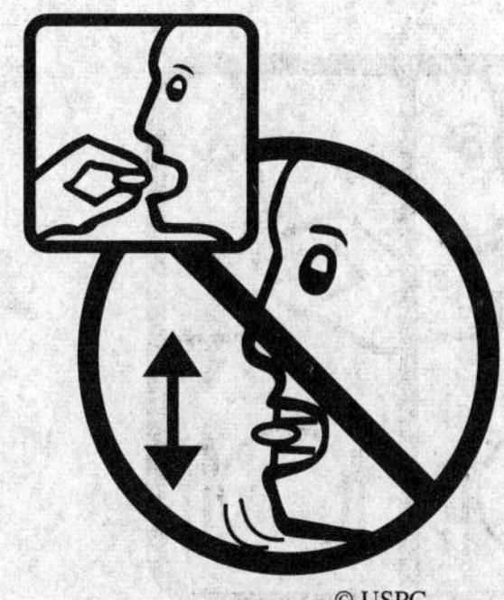

Do not chew

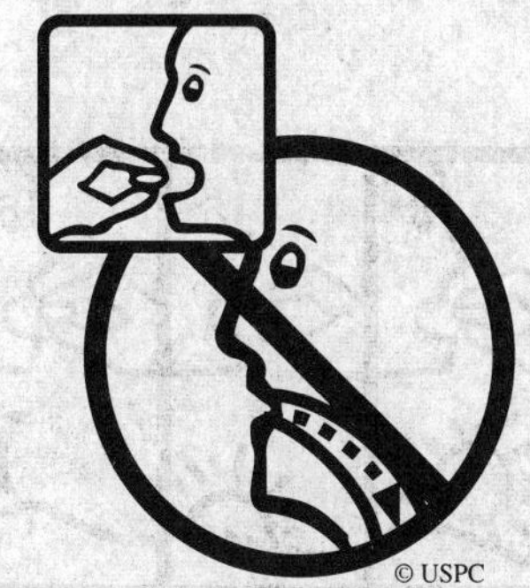

Do not swallow

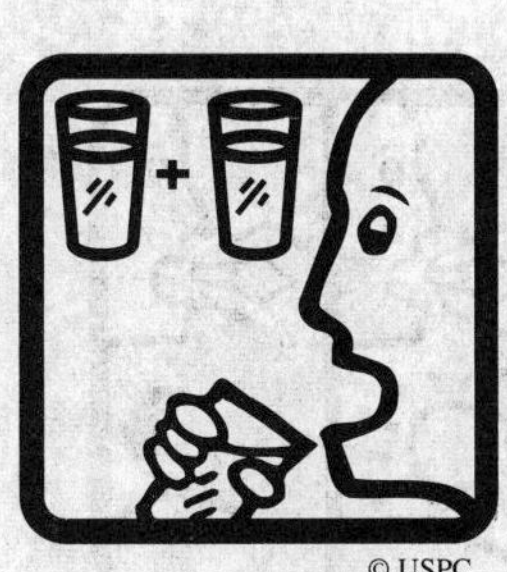

Drink additional water

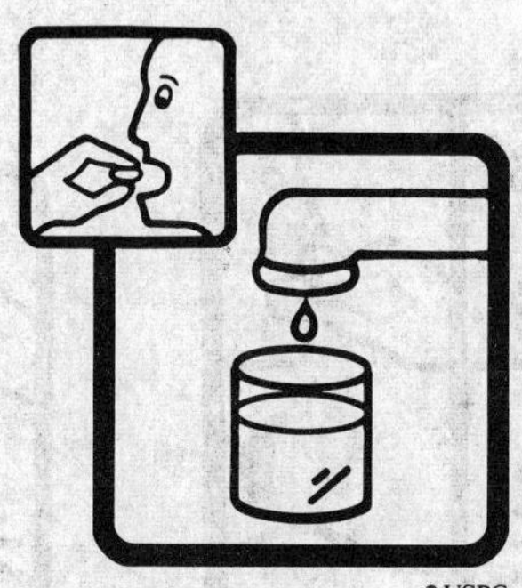

Take with glass of water

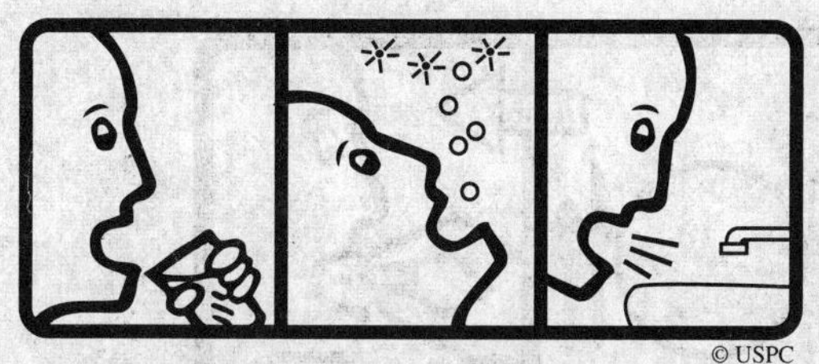

Use this medicine as a gargle

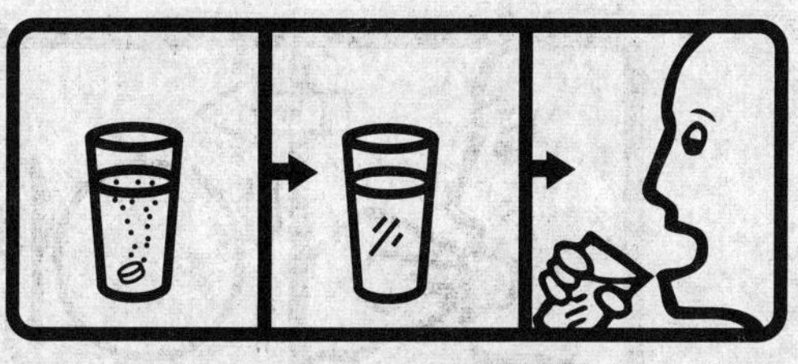

Dissolve in water

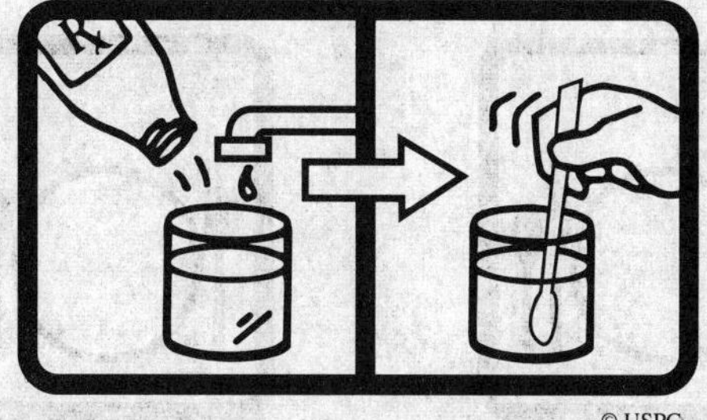

Dilute with water

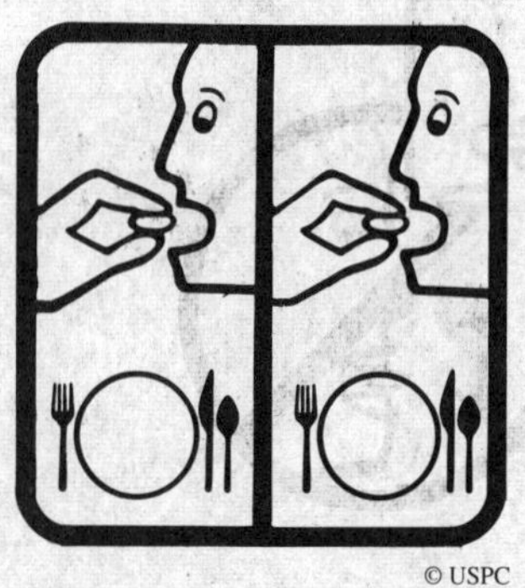
© USPC

Take 2 times a day with meals

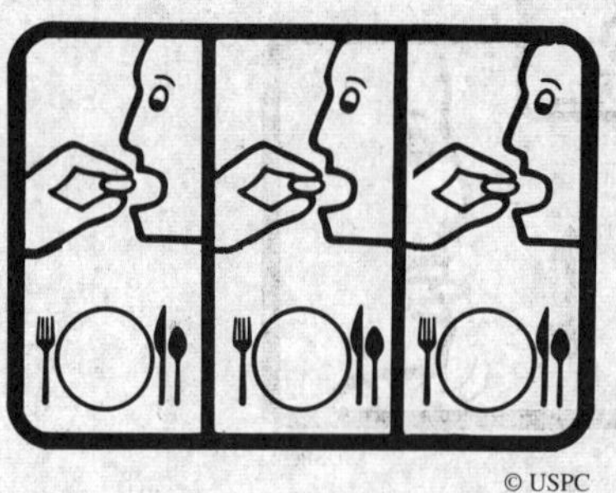
© USPC

Take 3 times a day with meals

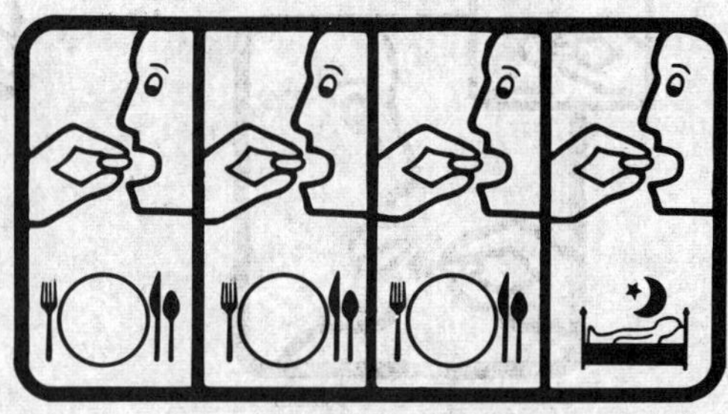
© USPC

Take 4 times a day, with meals and at bedtime

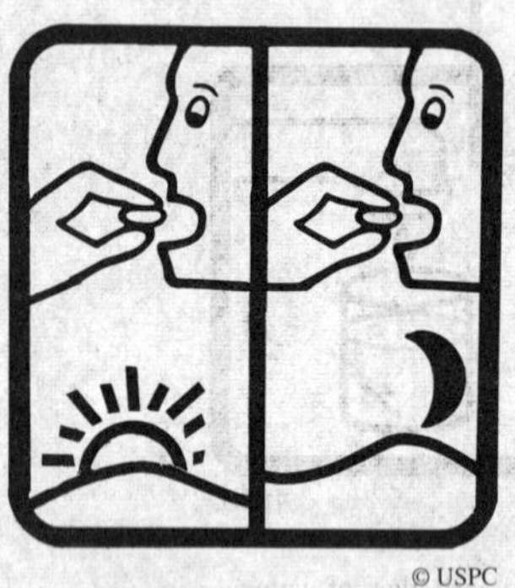
© USPC

Take 2 times a day

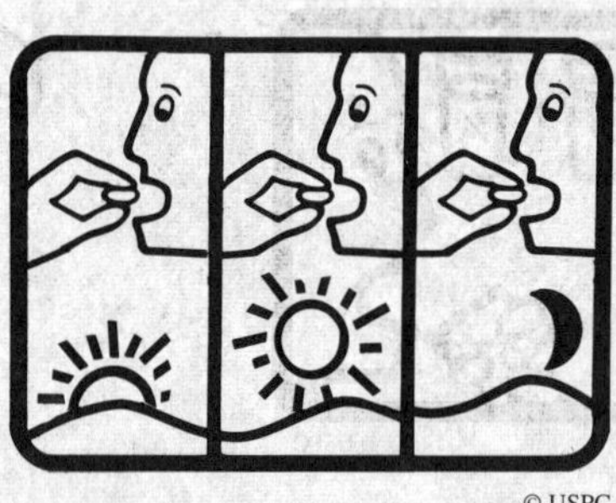
© USPC

Take 3 times a day

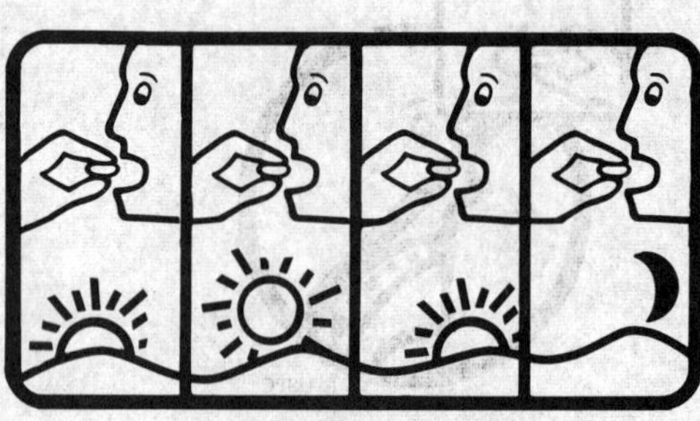
© USPC

Take 4 times a day

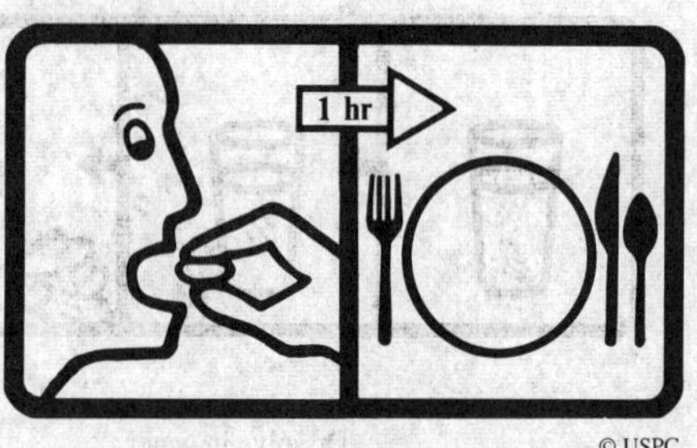

© USPC

Take 1 hour before meals

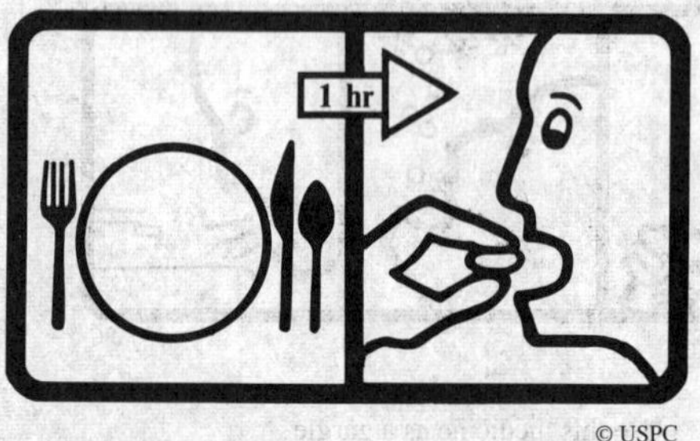

© USPC

Take 1 hour after meals

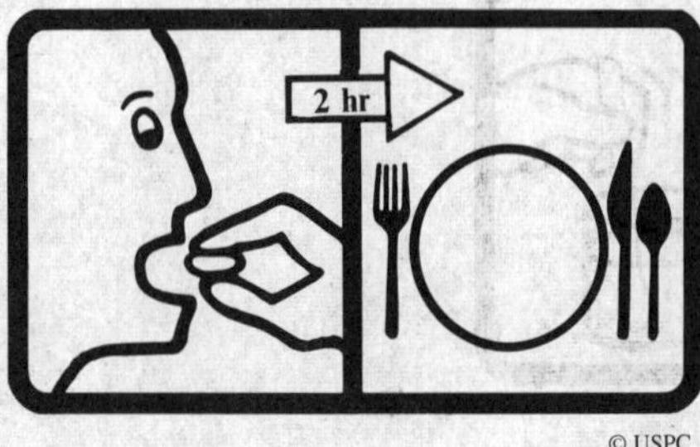

© USPC

Take 2 hours before meals

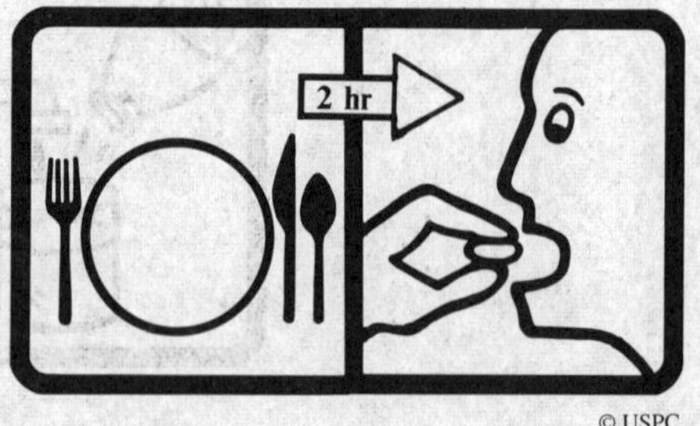

© USPC

Take 2 hours after meals

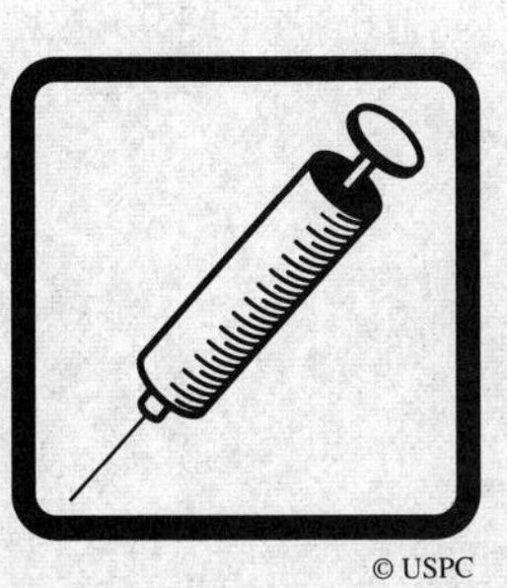

Injection

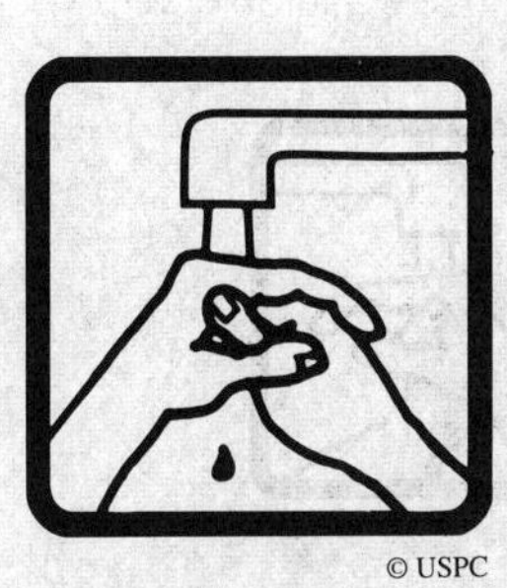

Wash hands

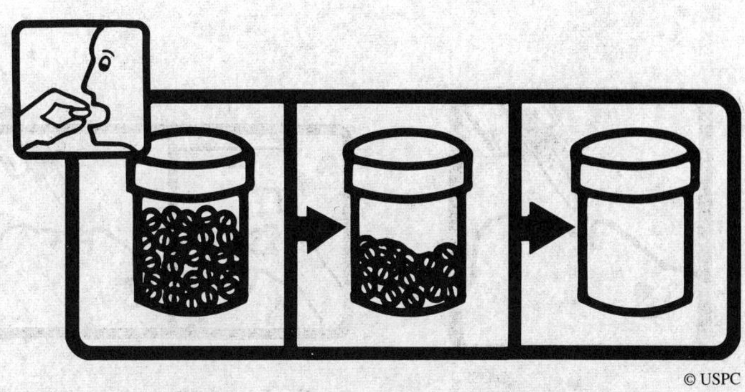

Take until gone

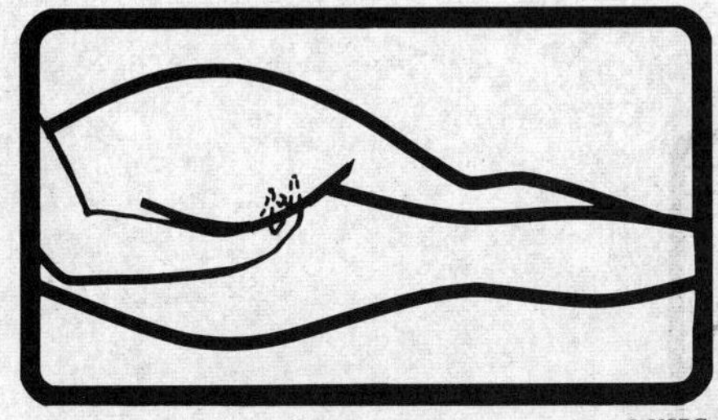

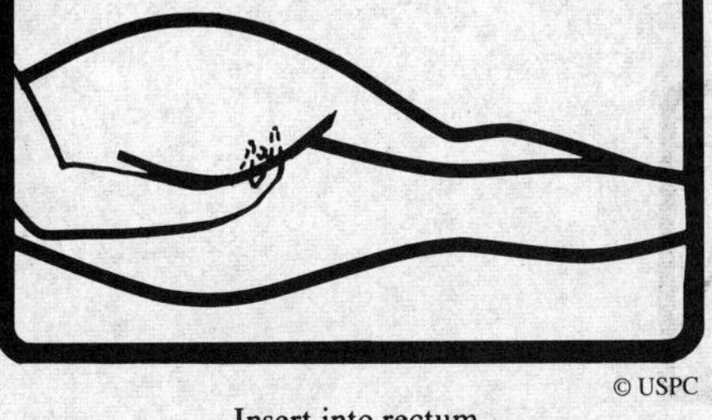

Insert into rectum

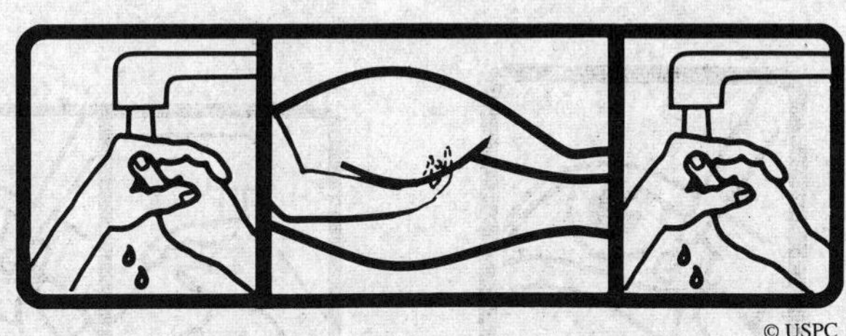

Wash hands/Insert into rectum/Wash hands again

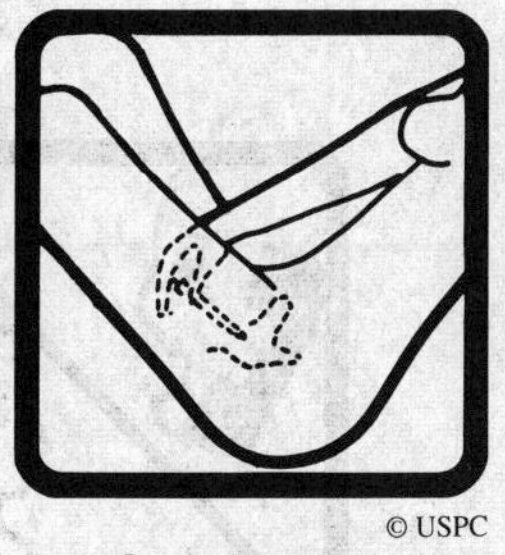

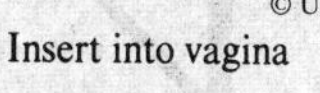

Insert into vagina

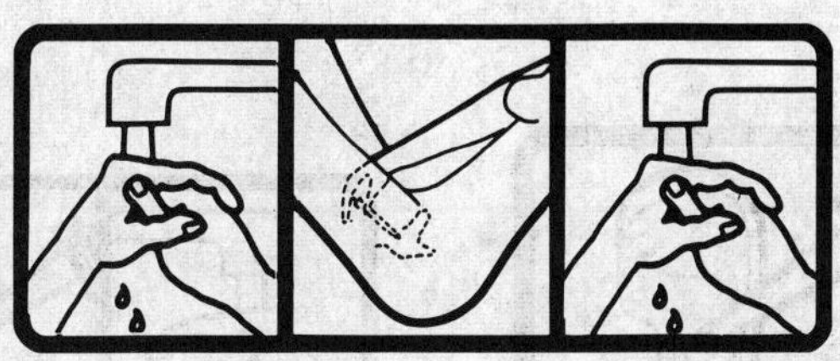

Wash hands/Insert into vagina/Wash hands again

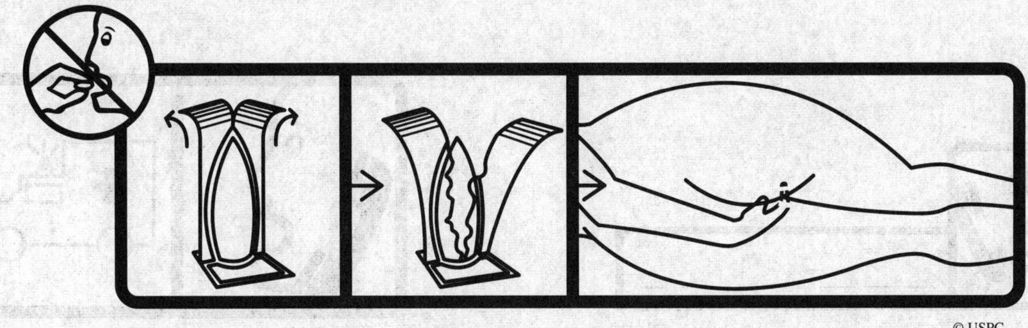

Remove foil from suppository before inserting into rectum

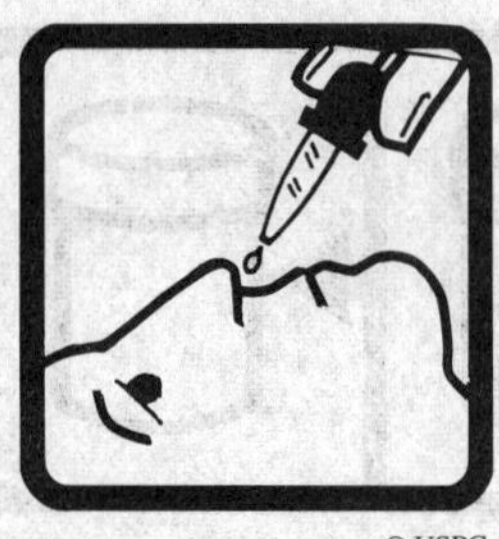

© USPC

Place drops in nose

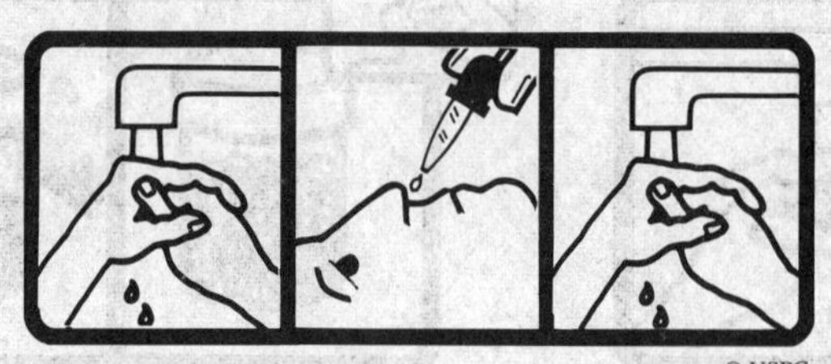

© USPC

Wash hands/Place drops in nose/Wash hands again

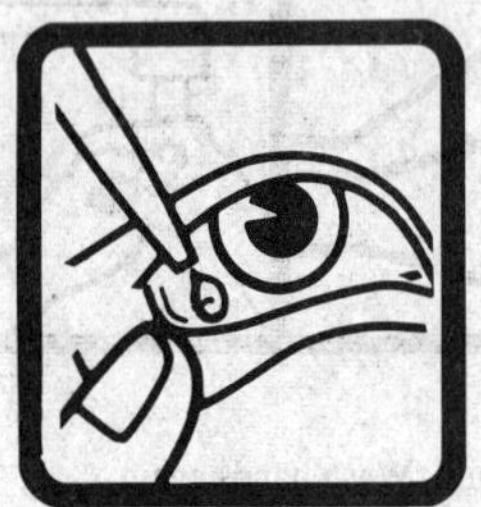

© USPC

Place drops in lower eyelid

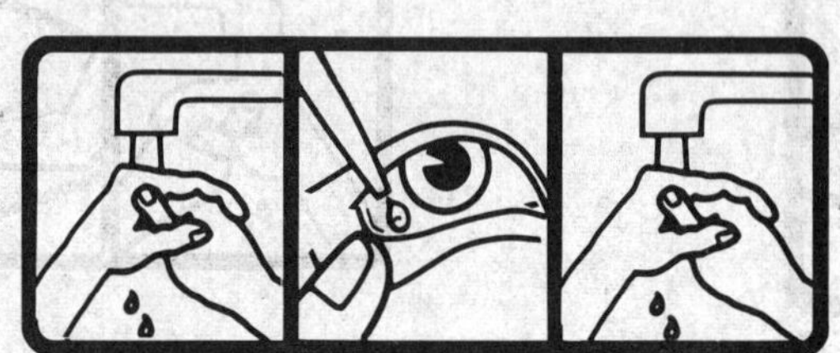

© USPC

Wash hands/Place drops in lower eyelid/Wash hands again

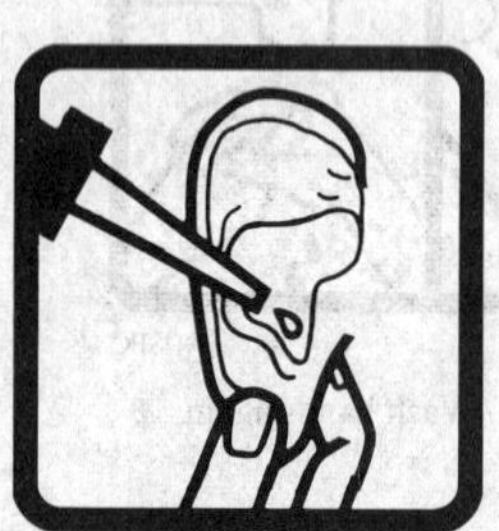

© USPC

Place drops in ear

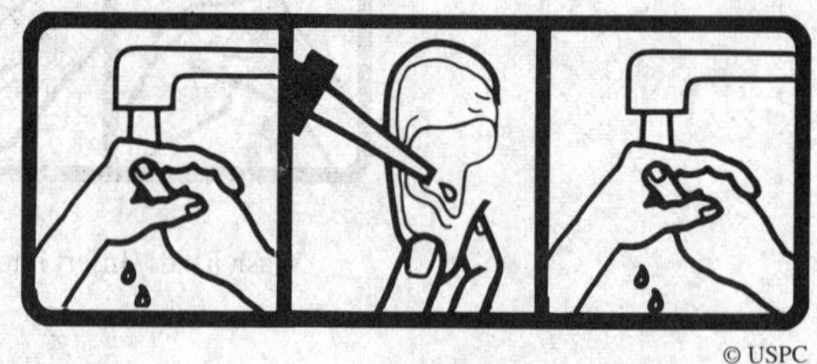

© USPC

Wash hands/Place drops in ear/Wash hands again

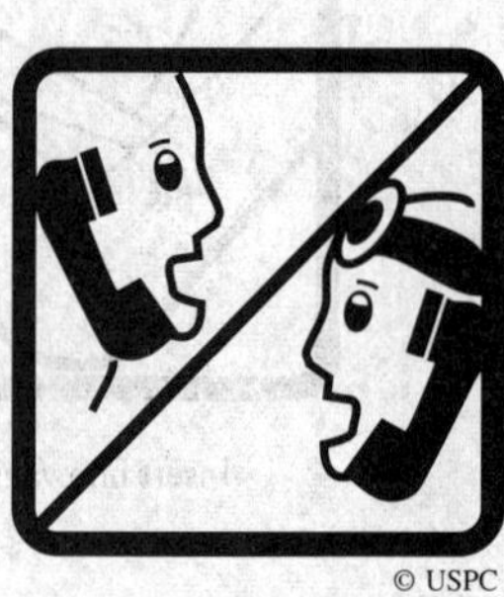

© USPC

Call your doctor

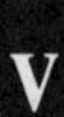

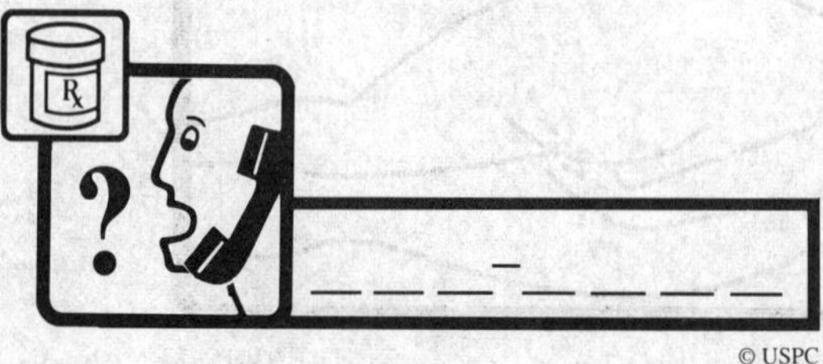

© USPC

If you have questions, call this number

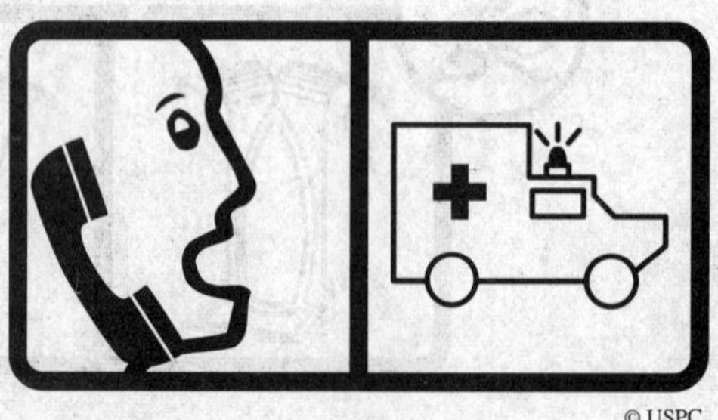

© USPC

Get emergency help

Appendix V

CATEGORIES OF USE

The following categories of use and the specific drugs listed under each entry are intended only as a useful reference for the consumer and should not be used to make decisions concerning the appropriateness of therapy in a particular instance. The drugs included under each entry should not be considered interchangeable for any given patient. In many instances, the drugs differ significantly with regard to effectiveness, seriousness of side effects, and other critical considerations.

You can find specific information for each drug in the individual monographs; look in the index for the appropriate page number. A glossary of terms can be found on page 1447. Should you desire additional information or if you have any questions as to how this information may relate to you in particular, ask your doctor, nurse, pharmacist, or other health care provider.

The information for this listing has been extracted from the USP DI data base. The category terminology used is intentionally broad in scope, and each entry may cover a wide range of specific indications. These specific indications may not be readily apparent to the reader. In addition, certain uses for some of the drugs listed may not have been specifically included in the manufacturer's product information, but they may be considered appropriate therapy in selected patients as defined by current medical practice.

Readers are reminded that the information in this text is selected and not considered to be complete. Absence of a drug from a category of use listing is not meant to imply that it is inappropriate for such use. On the other hand, presence of a drug in a category of use listing does not necessarily mean that the drug is appropriate for use in a particular patient.

A

Abortifacient
- Carboprost (Systemic)
- Dinoprost (Intra-amniotic)
- Dinoprostone (Cervical/Vaginal)
- Sodium Chloride (Intra-amniotic)
- Urea (Intra-amniotic)

Acidifier, urinary
- Potassium Phosphates (Systemic)
- Potassium and Sodium Phosphates (Systemic)

Adrenocorticoid
- Betamethasone—Glucocorticoid Effects (Systemic)
- Cortisone—Glucocorticoid Effects (Systemic)
- Dexamethasone—Glucocorticoid Effects (Systemic)
- Hydrocortisone—Glucocorticoid Effects (Systemic)
- Methylprednisolone—Glucocorticoid Effects (Systemic)
- Paramethasone—Glucocorticoid Effects (Systemic)
- Prednisolone—Glucocorticoid Effects (Systemic)
- Prednisone—Glucocorticoid Effects (Systemic)
- Triamcinolone—Glucocorticoid Effects (Systemic)

Adrenocorticoid-antiseptic, otic
- Desonide and Acetic Acid (Otic)
- Hydrocortisone and Acetic Acid (Otic)

Adrenocorticoid, inhalation
- Beclomethasone (Inhalation)
- Budesonide (Inhalation)
- Dexamethasone (Inhalation)
- Flunisolide (Inhalation)
- Triamcinolone (Inhalation)

Adrenocorticoid, mineralocorticoid
- Fludrocortisone (Systemic)

Adrenocorticoid, nasal
- Beclomethasone (Nasal)
- Dexamethasone (Nasal)
- Flunisolide (Nasal)
- Triamcinolone (Nasal)

Adrenocorticoid, ophthalmic
- Betamethasone (Ophthalmic)
- Dexamethasone (Ophthalmic)
- Fluorometholone (Ophthalmic)
- Hydrocortisone (Ophthalmic)
- Medrysone (Ophthalmic)
- Prednisolone (Ophthalmic)

Adrenocorticoid, otic
- Betamethasone (Otic)
- Dexamethasone (Otic)
- Hydrocortisone (Otic)

Adrenocorticotropic hormone
- Corticotropin—Glucocorticoid Effects (Systemic)

Alcohol-abuse deterrent
- Disulfiram (Systemic)

Aldosterone antagonist
- Spironolactone (Systemic)

Alkalizer, systemic
- Potassium Citrate and Citric Acid (Systemic)
- Sodium Bicarbonate (Systemic)
- Sodium Citrate and Citric Acid (Systemic)
- Tricitrates (Systemic)

Alkalizer, urinary
- Potassium Citrate (Systemic)
- Potassium Citrate and Citric Acid (Systemic)
- Potassium Citrate and Sodium Citrate (Systemic)
- Sodium Bicarbonate (Systemic)
- Sodium Citrate and Citric Acid (Systemic)
- Tricitrates (Systemic)

Alpha$_1$-antitrypsin replenisher
- Alpha$_1$-proteinase Inhibitor, Human (Systemic)

5-Alpha-reductase inhibitor
- Finasteride (Systemic)

Altitude sickness, acute, agent
- Acetazolamide (Systemic)

Amnestic
- Diazepam (Systemic)
- Lorazepam (Systemic)

Amyloidosis suppressant
- Colchicine (Systemic)

Anabolic steroid
- Nandrolone (Systemic)
- Oxandrolone (Systemic)
- Oxymetholone (Systemic)
- Stanozolol (Systemic)

Analgesia adjunct
- Caffeine (Systemic)

Analgesic
- Acetaminophen (Systemic)
- Acetaminophen and Aspirin (Systemic)
- Acetaminophen, Aspirin, and Caffeine (Systemic)
- Acetaminophen, Aspirin, and Caffeine, Buffered (Systemic)
- Acetaminophen, Aspirin, and Salicylamide, Buffered (Systemic)
- Acetaminophen, Aspirin, Salicylamide, and Caffeine (Systemic)
- Acetaminophen, Aspirin, Salicylamide, Codeine, and Caffeine (Systemic)
- Acetaminophen and Caffeine (Systemic)
- Acetaminophen and Codeine (Systemic)
- Acetaminophen, Codeine, and Caffeine (Systemic)
- Acetaminophen and Salicylamide (Systemic)
- Acetaminophen, Salicylamide, and Caffeine (Systemic)
- Anileridine (Systemic)
- Aspirin (Systemic)
- Aspirin, Buffered (Systemic)
- Aspirin and Caffeine (Systemic)
- Aspirin and Caffeine, Buffered (Systemic)
- Aspirin, Caffeine, and Dihydrocodeine (Systemic)
- Aspirin and Codeine (Systemic)
- Aspirin, Codeine, and Caffeine (Systemic)
- Aspirin, Codeine, and Caffeine, Buffered (Systemic)
- Buprenorphine (Systemic)
- Butalbital and Acetaminophen (Systemic)
- Butalbital, Acetaminophen, and Caffeine (Systemic)
- Butalbital and Aspirin (Systemic)
- Butalbital, Aspirin, and Caffeine (Systemic)
- Butalbital, Aspirin, Codeine, and Caffeine (Systemic)
- Butorphanol (Systemic)
- Choline Salicylate (Systemic)
- Choline and Magnesium Salicylates (Systemic)
- Codeine (Systemic)
- Dezocine (Systemic)
- Diflunisal (Systemic)

V

Analgesic *(continued)*
- Dihydrocodeine, Acetaminophen, and Caffeine (Systemic)
- Etodolac (Systemic)
- Fenoprofen (Systemic)
- Fentanyl (Systemic)
- Floctafenine (Systemic)
- Hydrocodone (Systemic)
- Hydrocodone and Acetaminophen (Systemic)
- Hydrocodone and Aspirin (Systemic)
- Hydrocodone, Aspirin, and Caffeine (Systemic)
- Hydromorphone (Systemic)
- Ibuprofen (Systemic)
- Ketoprofen (Systemic)
- Ketorolac (Systemic)
- Levorphanol (Systemic)
- Magnesium Salicylate (Systemic)
- Meclofenamate (Systemic)
- Mefenamic Acid (Systemic)
- Meperidine (Systemic)
- Meperidine and Acetaminophen (Systemic)
- Meprobamate and Aspirin (Systemic)
- Methadone (Systemic)
- Methotrimeprazine (Systemic)
- Morphine (Systemic)
- Nalbuphine (Systemic)
- Naproxen (Systemic)
- Opium (Systemic)
- Oxycodone (Systemic)
- Oxycodone and Acetaminophen (Systemic)
- Oxycodone and Aspirin (Systemic)
- Oxymorphone (Systemic)
- Pentazocine (Systemic)
- Pentazocine and Acetaminophen (Systemic)
- Pentazocine and Aspirin (Systemic)
- Pentazocine and Naloxone (Systemic)
- Phenobarbital, Aspirin, and Codeine (Systemic)
- Propoxyphene (Systemic)
- Propoxyphene and Acetaminophen (Systemic)
- Propoxyphene and Aspirin (Systemic)
- Propoxyphene, Aspirin, and Caffeine (Systemic)
- Salsalate (Systemic)
- Sodium Salicylate (Systemic)

Analgesic-anesthetic, otic
- Antipyrine and Benzocaine (Otic)

Analgesic-antacid
- Acetaminophen, Calcium Carbonate, Potassium and Sodium Bicarbonates, and Citric Acid (Systemic)
- Acetaminophen, Sodium Bicarbonate, and Citric Acid (Systemic)
- Aspirin, Sodium Bicarbonate, and Citric Acid (Systemic)

Analgesic, oral-local
- Benzydamine (Oral)
- Choline Salicylate and Cetyl-dimethyl-benzyl-ammonium Chloride (Oral)

Analgesic–skeletal muscle relaxant
- Chlorzoxazone and Acetaminophen (Systemic)
- Orphenadrine and Aspirin (Systemic)

Analgesic, specific pain syndromes, topical
- Capsaicin (Topical)

Analgesic, topical
- Diethylamine Salicylate (Topical)
- Triethanolamine Salicylate (Topical)

Analgesic, in trigeminal neuralgia
- Baclofen (Systemic)

Analgesic, urinary
- Phenazopyridine (Systemic)

Androgen
- Fluoxymesterone (Systemic)
- Methyltestosterone (Systemic)
- Testosterone (Systemic)

Androgen-estrogen
- Diethylstilbestrol and Methyltestosterone (Systemic)
- Estrogens, Conjugated, and Methyltestosterone (Systemic)
- Estrogens, Esterified, and Methyltestosterone (Systemic)
- Fluoxymesterone and Ethinyl Estradiol (Systemic)
- Testosterone and Estradiol (Systemic)

Anesthesia adjunct
- Buprenorphine (Systemic)
- Etomidate (Systemic)
- Propofol (Systemic)
- Scopolamine (Systemic)

Anesthesia adjunct, opioid analgesic
- Alfentanil (Systemic)
- Butorphanol (Systemic)
- Fentanyl (Systemic)
- Hydromorphone (Systemic)
- Levorphanol (Systemic)
- Meperidine (Systemic)
- Morphine (Systemic)
- Nalbuphine (Systemic)
- Oxymorphone (Systemic)
- Pentazocine (Systemic)
- Sufentanil (Systemic)

Anesthetic, general
- Enflurane (Systemic)
- Etomidate (Systemic)
- Halothane (Systemic)
- Isoflurane (Systemic)
- Ketamine (Systemic)
- Methohexital (Systemic)
- Methoxyflurane (Systemic)
- Nitrous Oxide (Systemic)
- Propofol (Systemic)
- Thiamylal (Systemic)
- Thiopental (Systemic)

Anesthetic, general, adjunct
- Midazolam (Systemic)

Anesthetic, local
- Bupivacaine (Parenteral-Local)
- Chloroprocaine (Parenteral-Local)
- Etidocaine (Parenteral-Local)
- Lidocaine (Parenteral-Local)
- Lidocaine and Prilocaine (Topical)
- Mepivacaine (Parenteral-Local)
- Prilocaine (Parenteral-Local)
- Procaine (Parenteral-Local)
- Propoxycaine and Procaine (Parenteral-Local)
- Tetracaine (Parenteral-Local)

Anesthetic, local, adjunct
- Epinephrine (Oral/Injection)
- Midazolam (Systemic)

Anesthetic, local, dental
- Benzocaine (Dental)
- Butacaine (Dental)
- Dyclonine (Dental)
- Lidocaine (Dental)
- Tetracaine (Dental)

Anesthetic, local, ophthalmic
- Proparacaine (Ophthalmic)
- Tetracaine (Ophthalmic)

Anesthetic, local, rectal
- Benzocaine (Rectal)
- Dibucaine (Rectal)
- Pramoxine (Rectal)
- Tetracaine (Rectal)
- Tetracaine and Menthol (Rectal)

Anesthetic, local, topical
- Benzocaine (Topical)
- Benzocaine and Menthol (Topical)
- Butamben (Topical)
- Dibucaine (Topical)
- Lidocaine (Topical)
- Pramoxine (Topical)
- Pramoxine and Menthol (Topical)
- Tetracaine (Topical)
- Tetracaine and Menthol (Topical)

Anesthetic-vasoconstrictor, mucosal-local
- Cocaine (Mucosal-Local)

Angioedema, hereditary, prophylactic
- Danazol (Systemic)

Antacid
- Alumina and Magnesia (Oral)
- Alumina, Magnesia, and Calcium Carbonate (Oral)
- Alumina, Magnesia, and Simethicone (Oral)
- Alumina and Magnesium Carbonate (Oral)
- Alumina and Magnesium Trisilicate (Oral)
- Alumina, Magnesium Trisilicate, and Sodium Bicarbonate (Oral)
- Aluminum Carbonate, Basic (Oral)
- Aluminum Hydroxide (Oral)
- Bismuth Subsalicylate (Oral)
- Calcium Carbonate (Oral)
- Calcium Carbonate (Systemic)
- Calcium Carbonate and Magnesia (Oral)
- Calcium Carbonate, Magnesia, and Simethicone (Oral)
- Calcium and Magnesium Carbonates (Oral)
- Calcium and Magnesium Carbonates and Magnesium Oxide (Oral)
- Calcium Carbonate and Simethicone (Oral)
- Dihydroxyaluminum Aminoacetate (Oral)
- Dihydroxyaluminum Sodium Carbonate (Oral)
- Magaldrate (Oral)
- Magaldrate and Simethicone (Oral)
- Magnesium Carbonate and Sodium Bicarbonate (Oral)
- Magnesium Hydroxide (Oral)
- Magnesium Oxide (Oral)
- Magnesium Trisilicate, Alumina, and Magnesia (Oral)
- Simethicone, Alumina, Calcium Carbonate, and Magnesia (Oral)
- Simethicone, Alumina, Magnesium Carbonate, and Magnesia (Oral)
- Sodium Bicarbonate (Systemic)

Anthelmintic, oral-local
- Niclosamide (Oral)
- Pyrantel (Oral)
- Pyrvinium (Oral)

Anthelmintic, systemic
- Albendazole (Systemic)
- Diethylcarbamazine (Systemic)
- Ivermectin (Systemic)
- Mebendazole (Systemic)
- Metronidazole (Systemic)
- Oxamniquine (Systemic)
- Piperazine (Systemic)
- Praziquantel (Systemic)
- Thiabendazole (Systemic)

Anthelmintic, topical
- Thiabendazole (Topical)

Antiacne agent, systemic
- Erythromycin (Systemic)
- Isotretinoin (Systemic)
- Minocycline (Systemic)
- Tetracycline (Systemic)

Antiacne agent, topical
- Alcohol and Acetone (Topical)
- Alcohol and Sulfur (Topical)
- Benzoyl Peroxide (Topical)
- Clindamycin (Topical)
- Erythromycin (Topical)
- Erythromycin and Benzoyl Peroxide (Topical)
- Isotretinoin (Topical)
- Meclocycline (Topical)
- Nicotinamide (Topical)
- Resorcinol and Sulfur (Topical)
- Salicylic Acid (Topical)
- Salicylic Acid and Sulfur (Topical)
- Sulfur (Topical)
- Sulfurated Lime (Topical)
- Tetracycline (Topical)
- Tretinoin (Topical)

Antiadrenal
- Aminoglutethimide (Systemic)
- Ketoconazole (Systemic)
- Metyrapone (Systemic)
- Mitotane (Systemic)
- Trilostane (Systemic)

Antiadrenergic
- Acebutolol (Systemic)
- Atenolol (Systemic)
- Betaxolol (Systemic)
- Carteolol (Systemic)
- Labetalol (Systemic)
- Metoprolol (Systemic)
- Nadolol (Systemic)
- Oxprenolol (Systemic)
- Penbutolol (Systemic)
- Pindolol (Systemic)
- Propranolol (Systemic)
- Sotalol (Systemic)
- Timolol (Systemic)

Antiallergic, inhalation
- Cromolyn (Inhalation)
- Nedocromil (Inhalation)

Antiallergic, nasal
- Cromolyn (Nasal)
- Ipratropium (Nasal)

Antiallergic, ophthalmic
- Cromolyn (Ophthalmic)

Antiallergic, systemic
- Cromolyn (Oral)
- Epinephrine (Oral/Injection)
- Ketotifen (Systemic)

Antianemic
- Cyanocobalamin (Systemic)
- Epoetin (Systemic)
- Ferrous Fumarate (Systemic)
- Ferrous Gluconate (Systemic)
- Ferrous Sulfate (Systemic)
- Fluoxymesterone (Systemic)
- Hydroxocobalamin (Systemic)
- Iron Dextran (Systemic)
- Iron-Polysaccharide (Systemic)
- Iron Sorbitol (Systemic)
- Leucovorin (Systemic)
- Nandrolone (Systemic)
- Oxymetholone (Systemic)
- Stanozolol (Systemic)
- Testosterone (Systemic)

Antianginal
- Acebutolol (Systemic)
- Amlodipine (Systemic)
- Amyl Nitrite (Systemic)
- Atenolol (Systemic)
- Bepridil (Systemic)
- Carteolol (Systemic)
- Diltiazem (Systemic)
- Erythrityl Tetranitrate—Oral (Systemic)
- Erythrityl Tetranitrate—Sublingual, Chewable, or Buccal (Systemic)

Antianginal *(continued)*
- Felodipine (Systemic)
- Isosorbide Dinitrate—Oral (Systemic)
- Isosorbide Dinitrate—Sublingual, Chewable, or Buccal (Systemic)
- Isradipine (Systemic)
- Labetalol (Systemic)
- Metoprolol (Systemic)
- Nadolol (Systemic)
- Nicardipine (Systemic)
- Nifedipine (Systemic)
- Nitroglycerin—Lingual Aerosol (Systemic)
- Nitroglycerin—Oral (Systemic)
- Nitroglycerin—Sublingual, Chewable, or Buccal (Systemic)
- Nitroglycerin—Topical (Systemic)
- Oxprenolol (Systemic)
- Penbutolol (Systemic)
- Pentaerythritol Tetranitrate—Oral (Systemic)
- Pindolol (Systemic)
- Propranolol (Systemic)
- Sotalol (Systemic)
- Timolol (Systemic)
- Verapamil (Systemic)

Antiangioedema, hereditary, agent
- Oxymetholone (Systemic)
- Stanozolol (Systemic)

Antianxiety agent
- Alprazolam (Systemic)
- Bromazepam (Systemic)
- Buspirone (Systemic)
- Chlordiazepoxide (Systemic)
- Chlormezanone (Systemic)
- Clorazepate (Systemic)
- Diazepam (Systemic)
- Halazepam (Systemic)
- Hydroxyzine (Systemic)
- Ketazolam (Systemic)
- Lorazepam (Systemic)
- Meprobamate (Systemic)
- Oxazepam (Systemic)
- Prazepam (Systemic)

Antianxiety agent–antidepressant
- Chlordiazepoxide and Amitriptyline (Systemic)
- Loxapine (Systemic)

Antianxiety therapy adjunct
- Acebutolol (Systemic)
- Metoprolol (Systemic)
- Oxprenolol (Systemic)
- Propranolol (Systemic)
- Sotalol (Systemic)
- Timolol (Systemic)

Antiarrhythmic
- Acebutolol (Systemic)
- Amiodarone (Systemic)
- Atenolol (Systemic)
- Atropine (Systemic)
- Digitoxin (Systemic)
- Digoxin (Systemic)
- Diltiazem (Systemic)
- Disopyramide (Systemic)
- Encainide (Systemic)
- Flecainide (Systemic)
- Glycopyrrolate (Systemic)
- Hyoscyamine (Systemic)
- Lidocaine—For Self-Injection (Systemic)
- Metoprolol (Systemic)
- Mexiletine (Systemic)
- Moricizine (Systemic)
- Nadolol (Systemic)
- Oxprenolol (Systemic)
- Phenytoin (Systemic)
- Procainamide (Systemic)
- Propafenone (Systemic)
- Propranolol (Systemic)

Antiarrhythmic *(continued)*
- Quinidine (Systemic)
- Scopolamine (Systemic)
- Sotalol (Systemic)
- Timolol (Systemic)
- Tocainide (Systemic)
- Verapamil (Systemic)

Antiasthmatic
- Astemizole (Systemic)
- Beclomethasone (Inhalation)
- Budesonide (Inhalation)
- Dexamethasone (Inhalation)
- Flunisolide (Inhalation)
- Loratadine (Systemic)
- Terfenadine (Systemic)
- Triamcinolone (Inhalation)

Antibacterial-adrenocorticoid, ophthalmic
- Framycetin, Gramicidin, and Dexamethasone (Ophthalmic)

Antibacterial-adrenocorticoid, otic
- Colistin, Neomycin, and Hydrocortisone (Otic)
- Neomycin, Polymyxin B, and Hydrocortisone (Otic)

Antibacterial-analgesic, urinary tract
- Sulfamethoxazole and Phenazopyridine (Systemic)
- Sulfisoxazole and Phenazopyridine (Systemic)

Antibacterial-antifungal-corticosteroid, otic
- Clioquinol and Flumethasone (Otic)

Antibacterial-antifungal-corticosteroid, topical
- Clioquinol and Flumethasone (Topical)
- Clioquinol and Hydrocortisone (Topical)

Antibacterial, antileprosy agent
- Dapsone (Systemic)
- Ethionamide (Systemic)
- Rifampin (Systemic)

Antibacterial, antimycobacterial
- Aminosalicylate Sodium (Systemic)
- Capreomycin (Systemic)
- Clofazimine (Systemic)
- Cycloserine (Systemic)
- Ethambutol (Systemic)
- Ethionamide (Systemic)
- Isoniazid (Systemic)
- Pyrazinamide (Systemic)
- Rifabutin (Systemic)
- Rifampin (Systemic)
- Rifampin and Isoniazid (Systemic)
- Streptomycin (Systemic)

Antibacterial-corticosteroid, ophthalmic
- Neomycin, Polymyxin B, and Hydrocortisone (Ophthalmic)

Antibacterial-corticosteroid, otic
- Framycetin, Gramicidin, and Dexamethasone (Otic)

Antibacterial, dental
- Chlorhexidine (Dental)

Antibacterial, ophthalmic
- Chloramphenicol (Ophthalmic)
- Chlortetracycline (Ophthalmic)
- Ciprofloxacin (Ophthalmic)
- Erythromycin (Ophthalmic)
- Framycetin (Ophthalmic)
- Gentamicin (Ophthalmic)
- Neomycin (Ophthalmic)
- Neomycin, Polymyxin B, and Bacitracin (Ophthalmic)
- Neomycin, Polymyxin B, and Gramicidin (Ophthalmic)
- Norfloxacin (Ophthalmic)
- Sulfacetamide (Ophthalmic)
- Sulfisoxazole (Ophthalmic)
- Tetracycline (Ophthalmic)
- Tobramycin (Ophthalmic)

Antibacterial, oral-local
- Furazolidone (Oral)
- Vancomycin (Oral)

Antibacterial, otic
- Chloramphenicol (Otic)
- Gentamicin (Otic)

Antibacterial, systemic
- Amdinocillin (Systemic)
- Amikacin (Systemic)
- Amoxicillin (Systemic)
- Amoxicillin and Clavulanate (Systemic)
- Ampicillin (Systemic)
- Ampicillin and Sulbactam (Systemic)
- Azithromycin (Systemic)
- Azlocillin (Systemic)
- Aztreonam (Systemic)
- Bacampicillin (Systemic)
- Carbenicillin (Systemic)
- Cefaclor (Systemic)
- Cefadroxil (Systemic)
- Cefamandole (Systemic)
- Cefazolin (Systemic)
- Cefixime (Systemic)
- Cefmetazole (Systemic)
- Cefonicid (Systemic)
- Cefoperazone (Systemic)
- Ceforanide (Systemic)
- Cefotaxime (Systemic)
- Cefotetan (Systemic)
- Cefoxitin (Systemic)
- Ceftazidime (Systemic)
- Ceftizoxime (Systemic)
- Ceftriaxone (Systemic)
- Cefuroxime (Systemic)
- Cephalexin (Systemic)
- Cephalothin (Systemic)
- Cephapirin (Systemic)
- Cephradine (Systemic)
- Chloramphenicol (Systemic)
- Cinoxacin (Systemic)
- Ciprofloxacin (Systemic)
- Clarithromycin (Systemic)
- Clindamycin (Systemic)
- Cloxacillin (Systemic)
- Cyclacillin (Systemic)
- Cycloserine (Systemic)
- Demeclocycline (Systemic)
- Dicloxacillin (Systemic)
- Doxycycline (Systemic)
- Enoxacin (Systemic)
- Erythromycin (Systemic)
- Erythromycin and Sulfisoxazole (Systemic)
- Flucloxacillin (Systemic)
- Fusidic Acid (Systemic)
- Gentamicin (Systemic)
- Imipenem and Cilastatin (Systemic)
- Immune Globulin Intravenous (Human) (Systemic)
- Kanamycin (Systemic)
- Lincomycin (Systemic)
- Lomefloxacin (Systemic)
- Loracarbef (Systemic)
- Methacycline (Systemic)
- Methenamine (Systemic)
- Methicillin (Systemic)
- Metronidazole (Systemic)
- Mezlocillin (Systemic)
- Minocycline (Systemic)
- Moxalactam (Systemic)
- Nafcillin (Systemic)
- Nalidixic Acid (Systemic)
- Netilmicin (Systemic)
- Nitrofurantoin (Systemic)
- Norfloxacin (Systemic)
- Ofloxacin (Systemic)
- Oxacillin (Systemic)
- Oxytetracycline (Systemic)

Antibacterial, systemic *(continued)*
- Penicillin G (Systemic)
- Penicillin V (Systemic)
- Piperacillin (Systemic)
- Pivampicillin (Systemic)
- Rifampin (Systemic)
- Spectinomycin (Systemic)
- Streptomycin (Systemic)
- Sulfacytine (Systemic)
- Sulfadiazine (Systemic)
- Sulfadiazine and Trimethoprim (Systemic)
- Sulfamethoxazole (Systemic)
- Sulfamethoxazole and Trimethoprim (Systemic)
- Sulfisoxazole (Systemic)
- Tetracycline (Systemic)
- Ticarcillin (Systemic)
- Ticarcillin and Clavulanate (Systemic)
- Tobramycin (Systemic)
- Trimethoprim (Systemic)
- Vancomycin (Systemic)

Antibacterial, topical
- Chloramphenicol (Topical)
- Chlortetracycline (Topical)
- Clindamycin (Topical)
- Clioquinol (Topical)
- Erythromycin (Topical)
- Framycetin (Topical)
- Framycetin and Gramicidin (Topical)
- Fusidic Acid (Topical)
- Gentamicin (Topical)
- Mafenide (Topical)
- Mupirocin (Topical)
- Neomycin (Topical)
- Neomycin and Polymyxin B (Topical)
- Neomycin, Polymyxin B, and Bacitracin (Topical)
- Silver Sulfadiazine (Topical)
- Tetracycline (Topical)

Antibacterial, urinary
- Sulfamethizole (Systemic)

Antibiotic therapy adjunct
- Probenecid (Systemic)

Antibulimic
- Amitriptyline (Systemic)
- Clomipramine (Systemic)
- Desipramine (Systemic)
- Fluoxetine (Systemic)
- Imipramine (Systemic)

Anticataplectic
- Clomipramine (Systemic)
- Desipramine (Systemic)
- Imipramine (Systemic)
- Protriptyline (Systemic)

Anticholelithic
- Chenodiol (Systemic)
- Ursodiol (Systemic)

Anticholinergic
- Anisotropine (Systemic)
- Atropine (Systemic)
- Belladonna (Systemic)
- Clidinium (Systemic)
- Dicyclomine (Systemic)
- Glycopyrrolate (Systemic)
- Homatropine (Systemic)
- Hyoscyamine (Systemic)
- Isopropamide (Systemic)
- Mepenzolate (Systemic)
- Methantheline (Systemic)
- Methscopolamine (Systemic)
- Oxyphencyclimine (Systemic)
- Pirenzepine (Systemic)
- Propantheline (Systemic)
- Scopolamine (Systemic)
- Tridihexethyl (Systemic)

Anticholinergic-antibacterial-analgesic, urinary tract
- Atropine, Hyoscyamine, Methenamine, Methylene Blue, Phenyl Salicylate, and Benzoic Acid (Systemic)

Anticholinergic-sedative
- Atropine, Hyoscyamine, Scopolamine, and Phenobarbital (Systemic)
- Atropine and Phenobarbital (Systemic)
- Belladonna and Butabarbital (Systemic)
- Belladonna and Phenobarbital (Systemic)
- Chlordiazepoxide and Clidinium (Systemic)
- Hyoscyamine and Phenobarbital (Systemic)

Anticoagulant
- Acenocoumarol (Systemic)
- Anisindione (Systemic)
- Dicumarol (Systemic)
- Heparin (Systemic)
- Warfarin (Systemic)

Anticonvulsant
- Acetazolamide (Systemic)
- Amobarbital (Systemic)
- Carbamazepine (Systemic)
- Clobazam (Systemic)
- Clonazepam (Systemic)
- Clorazepate (Systemic)
- Diazepam (Systemic)
- Divalproex (Systemic)
- Ethosuximide (Systemic)
- Ethotoin (Systemic)
- Felbamate (Systemic)
- Lorazepam (Systemic)
- Mephenytoin (Systemic)
- Mephobarbital (Systemic)
- Metharbital (Systemic)
- Methsuximide (Systemic)
- Nitrazepam (Systemic)
- Paraldehyde (Systemic)
- Paramethadione (Systemic)
- Pentobarbital (Systemic)
- Phenacemide (Systemic)
- Phenobarbital (Systemic)
- Phensuximide (Systemic)
- Phenytoin (Systemic)
- Primidone (Systemic)
- Secobarbital (Systemic)
- Trimethadione (Systemic)
- Valproic Acid (Systemic)

Anticonvulsant, specific in infantile myoclonic seizures
- Corticotropin—Glucocorticoid Effects (Systemic)

Antidepressant
- Amitriptyline (Systemic)
- Amoxapine (Systemic)
- Bupropion (Systemic)
- Clomipramine (Systemic)
- Desipramine (Systemic)
- Doxepin (Systemic)
- Fluoxetine (Systemic)
- Imipramine (Systemic)
- Isocarboxazid (Systemic)
- Maprotiline (Systemic)
- Nortriptyline (Systemic)
- Paroxetine (Systemic)
- Phenelzine (Systemic)
- Protriptyline (Systemic)
- Sertraline (Systemic)
- Tranylcypromine (Systemic)
- Trazodone (Systemic)
- Trimipramine (Systemic)

Antidepressant therapy adjunct
- Lithium (Systemic)

Antidiabetic
Acetohexamide (Systemic)
Chlorpropamide (Systemic)
Glipizide (Systemic)
Glyburide (Systemic)
Insulin (Systemic)
Metformin (Systemic)
Tolazamide (Systemic)
Tolbutamide (Systemic)
Antidiarrheal
Calcium Polycarbophil (Oral)
Codeine (Systemic)
Glycopyrrolate (Systemic)
Morphine (Systemic)
Opium Tincture (Systemic)
Polycarbophil (Oral)
Psyllium Hydrophilic Mucilloid (Oral)
Antidiarrheal, acquired immunodeficiency syndrome (AIDS)
Octreotide (Systemic)
Antidiarrheal, adsorbent
Attapulgite (Oral)
Charcoal, Activated (Oral)
Kaolin and Pectin (Oral)
Kaolin, Pectin, Belladonna Alkaloids, and Opium (Systemic)
Kaolin, Pectin, and Paregoric (Systemic)
Antidiarrheal, antiperistaltic
Difenoxin and Atropine (Systemic)
Diphenoxylate and Atropine (Systemic)
Loperamide (Oral)
Antidiarrheal, antisecretory
Bismuth Subsalicylate (Oral)
Antidiarrheal, gastrointestinal tumor
Octreotide (Systemic)
Antidiarrheal, postoperative colonic bile acids
Cholestyramine (Oral)
Colestipol (Oral)
Antidiuretic
Carbamazepine (Systemic)
Chlorpropamide (Systemic)
Antidiuretic, central diabetes insipidus
Clofibrate (Systemic)
Desmopressin (Systemic)
Lypressin (Systemic)
Vasopressin (Systemic)
Antidiuretic, central and nephrogenic diabetes insipidus
Bendroflumethiazide (Systemic)
Benzthiazide (Systemic)
Chlorothiazide (Systemic)
Chlorthalidone (Systemic)
Cyclothiazide (Systemic)
Hydrochlorothiazide (Systemic)
Hydroflumethiazide (Systemic)
Methyclothiazide (Systemic)
Metolazone (Systemic)
Polythiazide (Systemic)
Quinethazone (Systemic)
Trichlormethiazide (Systemic)
Antidiuretic, primary nocturnal enuresis
Desmopressin (Systemic)
Antidote, adsorbent-laxative
Charcoal, Activated (Oral)
Antidote, anion-exchange resin
Cholestyramine (Oral)
Antidote, to beta-adrenergic blocking agents
Glucagon (Systemic)
Antidote, to calcium channel blocking agents
Glucagon (Systemic)
Antidote, to cholinesterase inhibitors
Atropine (Systemic)
Hyoscyamine (Systemic)
Antidote, to cyanide poisoning
Amyl Nitrite (Systemic)
Antidote, to cycloserine poisoning
Pyridoxine (Vitamin B_6) (Systemic)

Antidote, to drug-induced hypoprothrombinemia
Menadiol (Systemic)
Phytonadione (Systemic)
Antidote, to ergot alkaloid poisoning
Prazosin (Systemic)
Antidote, to folic acid antagonists
Leucovorin (Systemic)
Antidote, to heavy metals
Penicillamine (Systemic)
Antidote, to isoniazid poisoning
Pyridoxine (Vitamin B_6) (Systemic)
Antidote, to muscarine
Atropine (Systemic)
Hyoscyamine (Systemic)
Antidote, to nondepolarizing neuromuscular block
Neostigmine (Systemic)
Pyridostigmine (Systemic)
Antidote, to organophosphate pesticides
Atropine (Systemic)
Antidyskinetic
Amantadine (Systemic)
Benztropine (Systemic)
Biperiden (Systemic)
Bromocriptine (Systemic)
Carbidopa and Levodopa (Systemic)
Diphenhydramine (Systemic)
Ethopropazine (Systemic)
Levodopa (Systemic)
Levodopa and Benserazide (Systemic)
Procyclidine (Systemic)
Selegiline (Systemic)
Trihexyphenidyl (Systemic)
Antidyskinetic, dopamine agonist
Pergolide (Systemic)
Antidyskinetic, Gilles de la Tourette's syndrome
Haloperidol (Systemic)
Pimozide (Systemic)
Antidyskinetic, Huntington's chorea
Chlorpromazine (Systemic)
Haloperidol (Systemic)
Thioridazine (Systemic)
Antidysmenorrheal
Belladonna (Systemic)
Clonidine (Systemic)
Diclofenac (Systemic)
Etodolac (Systemic)
Flurbiprofen (Systemic)
Ibuprofen (Systemic)
Indomethacin (Systemic)
Isoxsuprine (Systemic)
Ketoprofen (Systemic)
Meclofenamate (Systemic)
Mefenamic Acid (Systemic)
Naproxen (Systemic)
Scopolamine (Systemic)
Antiemetic
Buclizine (Systemic)
Chlorpromazine (Systemic)
Cyclizine (Systemic)
Dimenhydrinate (Systemic)
Diphenhydramine (Systemic)
Diphenidol (Systemic)
Dronabinol (Systemic)
Fructose, Dextrose, and Phosphoric Acid (Oral)
Haloperidol (Systemic)
Hydroxyzine (Systemic)
Meclizine (Systemic)
Metoclopramide (Systemic)
Nabilone (Systemic)
Ondansetron (Systemic)
Perphenazine (Systemic)
Prochlorperazine (Systemic)
Promethazine (Systemic)
Scopolamine (Systemic)
Thiethylperazine (Systemic)

Antiemetic *(continued)*
Triflupromazine (Systemic)
Trimethobenzamide (Systemic)
Antiemetic, in cancer chemotherapy
Corticotropin—Glucocorticoid Effects (Systemic)
Dexamethasone—Glucocorticoid Effects (Systemic)
Hydrocortisone—Glucocorticoid Effects (Systemic)
Lorazepam (Systemic)
Prednisone—Glucocorticoid Effects (Systemic)
Antiemetic, drug-related
Domperidone (Systemic)
Antiendometriotic agent
Nafarelin (Systemic)
Antienuretic
Amitriptyline (Systemic)
Imipramine (Systemic)
Antifatigue, specifically in multiple sclerosis
Amantadine (Systemic)
Antifibrinolytic
Aminocaproic Acid (Systemic)
Tranexamic Acid (Systemic)
Antifibrotic
Aminobenzoate Potassium (Systemic)
Antiflatulent
Charcoal, Activated (Oral)
Simethicone (Oral)
Antifungal
Dapsone (Systemic)
Antifungal-adrenocorticoid, topical
Clotrimazole and Betamethasone (Topical)
Nystatin and Triamcinolone (Topical)
Antifungal, ophthalmic
Natamycin (Ophthalmic)
Antifungal, oral-local
Clotrimazole (Oral)
Nystatin (Oral)
Antifungal, systemic
Amphotericin B (Systemic)
Fluconazole (Systemic)
Flucytosine (Systemic)
Griseofulvin (Systemic)
Itraconazole (Systemic)
Ketoconazole (Systemic)
Miconazole (Systemic)
Potassium Iodide (Systemic)
Antifungal, topical
Carbol-Fuchsin (Topical)
Ciclopirox (Topical)
Clioquinol (Topical)
Clotrimazole (Topical)
Econazole (Topical)
Haloprogin (Topical)
Ketoconazole (Topical)
Mafenide (Topical)
Miconazole (Topical)
Naftifine (Topical)
Nystatin (Topical)
Oxiconazole (Topical)
Silver Sulfadiazine (Topical)
Sulconazole (Topical)
Terbinafine (Topical)
Tioconazole (Topical)
Tolnaftate (Topical)
Antifungal, vaginal
Butoconazole (Vaginal)
Clotrimazole (Vaginal)
Econazole (Vaginal)
Gentian Violet (Vaginal)
Miconazole (Vaginal)
Nystatin (Vaginal)
Terconazole (Vaginal)
Tioconazole (Vaginal)

Antiglaucoma agent, ophthalmic
- Betaxolol (Ophthalmic)
- Carbachol (Ophthalmic)
- Carteolol (Ophthalmic)
- Demecarium (Ophthalmic)
- Dipivefrin (Ophthalmic)
- Echothiophate (Ophthalmic)
- Epinephrine (Ophthalmic)
- Isoflurophate (Ophthalmic)
- Levobunolol (Ophthalmic)
- Metipranolol (Ophthalmic)
- Physostigmine (Ophthalmic)
- Pilocarpine (Ophthalmic)
- Timolol (Ophthalmic)

Antiglaucoma agent, systemic
- Acetazolamide (Systemic)
- Dichlorphenamide (Systemic)
- Glycerin (Systemic)
- Methazolamide (Systemic)
- Timolol (Systemic)

Antigout agent
- Allopurinol (Systemic)
- Colchicine (Systemic)
- Etodolac (Systemic)
- Fenoprofen (Systemic)
- Ibuprofen (Systemic)
- Indomethacin (Systemic)
- Ketoprofen (Systemic)
- Naproxen (Systemic)
- Phenylbutazone (Systemic)
- Piroxicam (Systemic)
- Probenecid (Systemic)
- Probenecid and Colchicine (Systemic)
- Sulfinpyrazone (Systemic)
- Sulindac (Systemic)

Antihemorrhagic
- Aminocaproic Acid (Systemic)
- Antihemophilic Factor (Systemic)
- Desmopressin (Systemic)
- Factor IX (Systemic)
- Phytonadione (Systemic)
- Tranexamic Acid (Systemic)

Antihemorrhagic, postabortion uterine bleeding
- Carboprost (Systemic)
- Dinoprostone (Cervical/Vaginal)
- Methylergonovine (Systemic)
- Oxytocin (Systemic)

Antihemorrhagic, postpartum uterine bleeding
- Carboprost (Systemic)
- Dinoprostone (Cervical/Vaginal)
- Methylergonovine (Systemic)
- Oxytocin (Systemic)

Antihemorrhagic, topical
- Epinephrine (Oral/Injection)

Antihistaminic, H_1-receptor
- Astemizole (Systemic)
- Azatadine (Systemic)
- Bromodiphenhydramine (Systemic)
- Brompheniramine (Systemic)
- Carbinoxamine (Systemic)
- Cetirizine (Systemic)
- Chlorpheniramine (Systemic)
- Clemastine (Systemic)
- Cyproheptadine (Systemic)
- Dexchlorpheniramine (Systemic)
- Dimenhydrinate (Systemic)
- Diphenhydramine (Systemic)
- Diphenylpyraline (Systemic)
- Doxylamine (Systemic)
- Hydroxyzine (Systemic)
- Loratadine (Systemic)
- Methdilazine (Systemic)
- Phenindamine (Systemic)
- Promethazine (Systemic)
- Pyrilamine (Systemic)
- Terfenadine (Systemic)
- Trimeprazine (Systemic)

Antihistaminic, H_1-receptor *(continued)*
- Tripelennamine (Systemic)
- Triprolidine (Systemic)

Antihistaminic (H_1-receptor)-antitussive
- Bromodiphenhydramine and Codeine (Systemic)
- Chlorpheniramine and Dextromethorphan (Systemic)
- Phenyltoloxamine and Hydrocodone (Systemic)
- Promethazine and Codeine (Systemic)
- Promethazine and Dextromethorphan (Systemic)

Antihistaminic (H_1-receptor)-antitussive-analgesic
- Chlorpheniramine, Codeine, Aspirin, and Caffeine (Systemic)
- Chlorpheniramine, Dextromethorphan, and Acetaminophen (Systemic)

Antihistaminic (H_1-receptor)-antitussive-expectorant
- Bromodiphenhydramine, Diphenhydramine, Codeine, Ammonium Chloride, and Potassium Guaiacolsulfonate (Systemic)
- Chlorpheniramine, Codeine, and Guaifenesin (Systemic)
- Diphenhydramine, Codeine, and Ammonium Chloride (Systemic)
- Diphenhydramine, Dextromethorphan, and Ammonium Chloride (Systemic)
- Phenindamine, Hydrocodone, and Guaifenesin (Systemic)
- Pheniramine, Codeine, and Guaifenesin (Systemic)
- Pheniramine, Pyrilamine, Hydrocodone, Potassium Citrate, and Ascorbic Acid (Systemic)

Antihistaminic (H_1-receptor)-decongestant
- Azatadine and Pseudoephedrine (Systemic)
- Brompheniramine and Phenylephrine (Systemic)
- Brompheniramine, Phenylephrine, and Phenylpropanolamine (Systemic)
- Brompheniramine and Phenylpropanolamine (Systemic)
- Brompheniramine, Phenyltoloxamine, and Phenylephrine (Systemic)
- Brompheniramine and Pseudoephedrine (Systemic)
- Carbinoxamine and Pseudoephedrine (Systemic)
- Chlorpheniramine, Phenindamine, and Phenylpropanolamine (Systemic)
- Chlorpheniramine and Phenylephrine (Systemic)
- Chlorpheniramine, Phenylephrine, and Phenylpropanolamine (Systemic)
- Chlorpheniramine and Phenylpropanolamine (Systemic)
- Chlorpheniramine, Phenyltoloxamine, and Phenylephrine (Systemic)
- Chlorpheniramine, Phenyltoloxamine, Phenylephrine, and Phenylpropanolamine (Systemic)
- Chlorpheniramine and Pseudoephedrine (Systemic)
- Chlorpheniramine, Pyrilamine, and Phenylephrine (Systemic)
- Chlorpheniramine, Pyrilamine, Phenylephrine, and Phenylpropanolamine (Systemic)
- Clemastine and Phenylpropanolamine (Systemic)
- Dexbrompheniramine and Pseudoephedrine (Systemic)
- Diphenhydramine and Pseudoephedrine (Systemic)

Antihistaminic (H_1-receptor)-decongestant *(continued)*
- Pheniramine, Phenyltoloxamine, Pyrilamine, and Phenylpropanolamine (Systemic)
- Pheniramine, Pyrilamine, and Phenylpropanolamine (Systemic)
- Promethazine and Phenylephrine (Systemic)
- Promethazine and Pseudoephedrine (Systemic)
- Terfenadine and Pseudoephedrine (Systemic)
- Triprolidine and Pseudoephedrine (Systemic)

Antihistaminic (H_1-receptor)-decongestant-analgesic
- Brompheniramine, Phenylephrine, Phenylpropanolamine, and Acetaminophen (Systemic)
- Brompheniramine, Phenylpropanolamine, and Acetaminophen (Systemic)
- Brompheniramine, Phenylpropanolamine, and Aspirin (Systemic)
- Chlorpheniramine, Phenylephrine, and Acetaminophen (Systemic)
- Chlorpheniramine, Phenylephrine, Acetaminophen, and Caffeine (Systemic)
- Chlorpheniramine, Phenylephrine, Acetaminophen, and Salicylamide (Systemic)
- Chlorpheniramine, Phenylephrine, Acetaminophen, Salicylamide, and Caffeine (Systemic)
- Chlorpheniramine, Phenylpropanolamine, and Acetaminophen (Systemic)
- Chlorpheniramine, Phenylpropanolamine, Acetaminophen, and Caffeine (Systemic)
- Chlorpheniramine, Phenylpropanolamine, and Aspirin (Systemic)
- Chlorpheniramine, Phenylpropanolamine, Aspirin, and Caffeine (Systemic)
- Chlorpheniramine, Phenyltoloxamine, Phenylpropanolamine, and Acetaminophen (Systemic)
- Chlorpheniramine, Pseudoephedrine, and Acetaminophen (Systemic)
- Chlorpheniramine, Pyrilamine, Phenylephrine, and Acetaminophen (Systemic)
- Chlorpheniramine, Pyrilamine, Phenylephrine, Phenylpropanolamine, and Acetaminophen (Systemic)
- Dexbrompheniramine, Pseudoephedrine, and Acetaminophen (Systemic)
- Diphenhydramine, Phenylpropanolamine, and Aspirin (Systemic)
- Diphenhydramine, Pseudoephedrine, and Acetaminophen (Systemic)
- Pheniramine, Phenylephrine, Sodium Salicylate, and Caffeine (Systemic)
- Pheniramine, Pyrilamine, Phenylpropanolamine, and Aspirin (Systemic)
- Phenyltoloxamine, Phenylpropanolamine, and Acetaminophen (Systemic)
- Pyrilamine, Phenylephrine, Aspirin, and Caffeine (Systemic)
- Pyrilamine, Phenylpropanolamine, Acetaminophen, and Caffeine (Systemic)
- Triprolidine, Pseudoephedrine, and Acetaminophen (Systemic)

Antihistaminic (H_1-receptor)-decongestant-anticholinergic
- Brompheniramine, Phenyltoloxamine, Pseudoephedrine, and Atropine (Systemic)
- Chlorpheniramine, Phenylephrine, and Methscopolamine (Systemic)

Antihistaminic (H_1-receptor)-decongestant-anticholinergic *(continued)*
- Chlorpheniramine, Phenylephrine, Phenylpropanolamine, Atropine, Hyoscyamine, and Scopolamine (Systemic)
- Chlorpheniramine, Phenylpropanolamine, and Methscopolamine (Systemic)

Antihistaminic (H_1-receptor)-decongestant-antitussive
- Brompheniramine, Phenylephrine, Phenylpropanolamine, and Codeine (Systemic)
- Brompheniramine, Phenylephrine, Phenylpropanolamine, and Dextromethorphan (Systemic)
- Brompheniramine, Phenylpropanolamine, and Codeine (Systemic)
- Brompheniramine, Phenylpropanolamine, and Dextromethorphan (Systemic)
- Brompheniramine, Pseudoephedrine, and Dextromethorphan (Systemic)
- Carbinoxamine, Pseudoephedrine, and Dextromethorphan (Systemic)
- Chlorpheniramine, Ephedrine, Phenylephrine, and Carbetapentane (Systemic)
- Chlorpheniramine, Phenylephrine, and Dextromethorphan (Systemic)
- Chlorpheniramine, Phenylephrine, and Hydrocodone (Systemic)
- Chlorpheniramine, Phenylephrine, Phenylpropanolamine, and Codeine (Systemic)
- Chlorpheniramine, Phenylephrine, Phenylpropanolamine, and Dextromethorphan (Systemic)
- Chlorpheniramine, Phenylephrine, Phenylpropanolamine, and Dihydrocodeine (Systemic)
- Chlorpheniramine, Phenylpropanolamine, and Caramiphen (Systemic)
- Chlorpheniramine, Phenylpropanolamine, and Dextromethorphan (Systemic)
- Chlorpheniramine, Pseudoephedrine, and Codeine (Systemic)
- Chlorpheniramine, Pseudoephedrine, and Dextromethorphan (Systemic)
- Chlorpheniramine, Pseudoephedrine, and Hydrocodone (Systemic)
- Diphenylpyraline, Phenylephrine, and Codeine (Systemic)
- Diphenylpyraline, Phenylephrine, and Dextromethorphan (Systemic)
- Diphenylpyraline, Phenylephrine, and Hydrocodone (Systemic)
- Pheniramine, Pyrilamine, Phenylephrine, Phenylpropanolamine, and Hydrocodone (Systemic)
- Pheniramine, Pyrilamine, Phenylpropanolamine, and Codeine (Systemic)
- Pheniramine, Pyrilamine, Phenylpropanolamine, and Dextromethorphan (Systemic)
- Pheniramine, Pyrilamine, Phenylpropanolamine, and Hydrocodone (Systemic)
- Promethazine, Phenylephrine, and Codeine (Systemic)
- Pyrilamine, Phenylephrine, and Codeine (Systemic)
- Pyrilamine, Phenylephrine, and Dextromethorphan (Systemic)
- Pyrilamine, Phenylephrine, and Hydrocodone (Systemic)
- Triprolidine, Pseudoephedrine, and Codeine (Systemic)
- Triprolidine, Pseudoephedrine, and Dextromethorphan (Systemic)

Antihistaminic (H_1-receptor)-decongestant-antitussive-analgesic
- Chlorpheniramine, Phenindamine, Phenylephrine, Dextromethorphan, Acetaminophen, Salicylamide, Caffeine, and Ascorbic Acid (Systemic)
- Chlorpheniramine, Pheniramine, Pyrilamine, Phenylephrine, Hydrocodone, Salicylamide, Caffeine, and Ascorbic Acid (Systemic)
- Chlorpheniramine, Phenylephrine, Dextromethorphan, Acetaminophen, and Salicylamide (Systemic)
- Chlorpheniramine, Phenylephrine, Hydrocodone, Acetaminophen, and Caffeine (Systemic)
- Chlorpheniramine, Phenylpropanolamine, Dextromethorphan, and Acetaminophen (Systemic)
- Chlorpheniramine, Phenylpropanolamine, Dextromethorphan, Acetaminophen, and Caffeine (Systemic)
- Chlorpheniramine, Pseudoephedrine, Dextromethorphan, and Acetaminophen (Systemic)
- Diphenhydramine, Pseudoephedrine, Dextromethorphan, and Acetaminophen (Systemic)
- Doxylamine, Pseudoephedrine, Dextromethorphan, and Acetaminophen (Systemic)
- Pheniramine, Pyrilamine, Phenylpropanolamine, Codeine, Acetaminophen, and Caffeine (Systemic)
- Pyrilamine, Phenylephrine, Dextromethorphan, and Acetaminophen (Systemic)
- Pyrilamine, Phenylpropanolamine, Dextromethorphan, and Sodium Salicylate (Systemic)
- Pyrilamine, Pseudoephrine, Dextromethorphan, and Acetaminophen (Systemic)

Antihistaminic (H_1-receptor)-decongestant-antitussive-expectorant
- Brompheniramine, Phenylephrine, Phenylpropanolamine, Codeine, and Guaifenesin (Systemic)
- Brompheniramine, Phenylephrine, Phenylpropanolamine, Hydrocodone, and Guaifenesin (Systemic)
- Chlorpheniramine, Ephedrine, Phenylephrine, Dextromethorphan, Ammonium Chloride, and Ipecac (Systemic)
- Chlorpheniramine, Phenindamine, Pyrilamine, Phenylephrine, Hydrocodone, and Ammonium Chloride (Systemic)
- Chlorpheniramine, Phenylephrine, Codeine, and Ammonium Chloride (Systemic)
- Chlorpheniramine, Phenylephrine, Codeine, Ammonium Chloride, Potassium Guaiacolsulfonate, and Sodium Citrate (Systemic)
- Chlorpheniramine, Phenylephrine, Codeine, and Potassium Iodide (Systemic)
- Chlorpheniramine, Phenylephrine, Dextromethorphan, and Guaifenesin (Systemic)
- Chlorpheniramine, Phenylephrine, Dextromethorphan, Guaifenesin, and Ammonium Chloride (Systemic)
- Chlorpheniramine, Phenylephrine, Phenylpropanolamine, Carbetapentane, and Potassium Guaiacolsulfonate (Systemic)
- Chlorpheniramine, Phenylpropanolamine, Dextromethorphan, and Ammonium Chloride (Systemic)
- Chlorpheniramine, Phenyltoloxamine, Ephedrine, Codeine, and Guaiacol Carbonate (Systemic)

Antihistaminic (H_1-receptor)-decongestant-antitussive-expectorant *(continued)*
- Chlorpheniramine, Phenyltoloxamine, Phenylpropanolamine, Dextromethorphan, and Guaifenesin (Systemic)
- Diphenylpyraline, Phenylephrine, Hydrocodone, and Guaifenesin (Systemic)
- Pheniramine, Pyrilamine, Phenylpropanolamine, Dextromethorphan, and Ammonium Chloride (Systemic)
- Pheniramine, Pyrilamine, Phenylpropanolamine, Dextromethorphan, and Guaifenesin (Systemic)
- Pheniramine, Pyrilamine, Phenylpropanolamine, Hydrocodone, and Guaifenesin (Systemic)
- Pyrilamine, Phenylephrine, Hydrocodone, and Ammonium Chloride (Systemic)
- Pyrilamine, Phenylpropanolamine, Dextromethorphan, Guaifenesin, Potassium Citrate, and Citric Acid (Systemic)
- Triprolidine, Pseudoephedrine, Codeine, and Guaifenesin (Systemic)

Antihistaminic (H_1-receptor)-decongestant-antitussive-expectorant-analgesic
- Chlorpheniramine, Phenylephrine, Phenylpropanolamine, Dextromethorphan, Guaifenesin, and Acetaminophen (Systemic)
- Chlorpheniramine, Phenylpropanolamine, Codeine, Guaifenesin, and Acetaminophen (Systemic)
- Chlorpheniramine, Phenylpropanolamine, Hydrocodone, Guaifenesin, and Salicylamide (Systemic)
- Chlorpheniramine, Pseudoephedrine, Dextromethorphan, Guaifenesin, and Aspirin (Systemic)
- Pheniramine, Phenylephrine, Codeine, Sodium Citrate, Sodium Salicylate, and Caffeine (Systemic)

Antihistaminic (H_1-receptor)-decongestant-expectorant
- Brompheniramine, Phenylephrine, Phenylpropanolamine, and Guaifenesin (Systemic)
- Carbinoxamine, Pseudoephedrine, and Guaifenesin (Systemic)
- Chlorpheniramine, Ephedrine, and Guaifenesin (Systemic)
- Chlorpheniramine, Phenylephrine, and Guaifenesin (Systemic)
- Chlorpheniramine, Phenylpropanolamine, and Guaifenesin (Systemic)
- Chlorpheniramine, Phenylpropanolamine, Guaifenesin, Sodium Citrate, and Citric Acid (Systemic)
- Chlorpheniramine, Pseudoephedrine, and Guaifenesin (Systemic)
- Dexchlorpheniramine, Pseudoephedrine, and Guaifenesin (Systemic)
- Pheniramine, Pyrilamine, Phenylpropanolamine, and Guaifenesin (Systemic)

Antihyperammonemic
- Lactulose (Oral)
- Sodium Benzoate and Sodium Phenylacetate (Systemic)

Antihyperbilirubinemic
- Phenobarbital (Systemic)

Antihypercalcemic
- Bumetanide (Systemic)
- Chloroquine (Systemic)
- Ethacrynic Acid (Systemic)
- Etidronate (Systemic)

Antihypercalcemic *(continued)*
Furosemide (Systemic)
Gallium Nitrate (Systemic)
Hydroxychloroquine (Systemic)
Pamidronate (Systemic)
Plicamycin (Systemic)
Antihypercalcemic therapy adjunct
Calcitonin-Human (Systemic)
Calcitonin-Salmon (Systemic)
Antihypercalciuric
Plicamycin (Systemic)
Antihyperkalemic
Calcium Chloride (Systemic)
Calcium Glubionate (Systemic)
Calcium Gluconate (Systemic)
Antihyperlipidemic
Cholestyramine (Oral)
Clofibrate (Systemic)
Colestipol (Oral)
Dextrothyroxine (Systemic)
Gemfibrozil (Systemic)
Lovastatin (Systemic)
Niacin (Systemic)
Pravastatin (Systemic)
Probucol (Systemic)
Psyllium Hydrophilic Mucilloid (Oral)
Simvastatin (Systemic)
Antihypermagnesemic
Calcium Chloride (Systemic)
Calcium Glubionate (Systemic)
Calcium Gluceptate (Systemic)
Calcium Gluconate (Systemic)
Antihyperoxaluric
Cholestyramine (Oral)
Antihyperphosphatemic
Aluminum Carbonate (Oral)
Aluminum Hydroxide (Oral)
Calcium Acetate (Systemic)
Calcium Carbonate (Oral)
Calcium Carbonate (Systemic)
Calcium Citrate (Systemic)
Antihyperprolactinemic
Bromocriptine (Systemic)
Antihypertensive
Acebutolol (Systemic)
Amiloride (Systemic)
Amiloride and Hydrochlorothiazide (Systemic)
Amlodipine (Systemic)
Atenolol (Systemic)
Atenolol and Chlorthalidone (Systemic)
Benazepril (Systemic)
Bendroflumethiazide (Systemic)
Benzthiazide (Systemic)
Betaxolol (Systemic)
Betaxolol and Chlorthalidone (Systemic)
Bisoprolol (Systemic)
Bumetanide (Systemic)
Captopril (Systemic)
Captopril and Hydrochlorothiazide (Systemic)
Carteolol (Systemic)
Chlorothiazide (Systemic)
Chlorthalidone (Systemic)
Clonidine (Systemic)
Clonidine and Chlorthalidone (Systemic)
Cyclothiazide (Systemic)
Debrisoquine (Systemic)
Deserpidine (Systemic)
Deserpidine and Hydrochlorothiazide (Systemic)
Deserpidine and Methyclothiazide (Systemic)
Diltiazem (Systemic)
Doxazosin (Systemic)
Enalapril (Systemic)

Antihypertensive *(continued)*
Enalapril and Hydrochlorothiazide (Systemic)
Ethacrynic Acid (Systemic)
Felodipine (Systemic)
Fosinopril (Systemic)
Furosemide (Systemic)
Guanabenz (Systemic)
Guanadrel (Systemic)
Guanethidine (Systemic)
Guanethidine and Hydrochlorothiazide (Systemic)
Guanfacine (Systemic)
Hydralazine (Systemic)
Hydralazine and Hydrochlorothiazide (Systemic)
Hydrochlorothiazide (Systemic)
Hydroflumethiazide (Systemic)
Indapamide (Systemic)
Isradipine (Systemic)
Labetalol (Systemic)
Labetalol and Hydrochlorothiazide (Systemic)
Lisinopril (Systemic)
Lisinopril and Hydrochlorothiazide (Systemic)
Mecamylamine (Systemic)
Methyclothiazide (Systemic)
Methyldopa (Systemic)
Methyldopa and Chlorothiazide (Systemic)
Methyldopa and Hydrochlorothiazide (Systemic)
Metolazone (Systemic)
Metoprolol (Systemic)
Metoprolol and Hydrochlorothiazide (Systemic)
Minoxidil (Systemic)
Nadolol (Systemic)
Nadolol and Bendroflumethiazide (Systemic)
Nicardipine (Systemic)
Nifedipine (Systemic)
Oxprenolol (Systemic)
Penbutolol (Systemic)
Pindolol (Systemic)
Pindolol and Hydrochlorothiazide (Systemic)
Polythiazide (Systemic)
Prazosin (Systemic)
Prazosin and Polythiazide (Systemic)
Propranolol (Systemic)
Propranolol and Hydrochlorothiazide (Systemic)
Quinapril (Systemic)
Quinethazone (Systemic)
Ramipril (Systemic)
Rauwolfia Serpentina (Systemic)
Rauwolfia Serpentina and Bendroflumethiazide (Systemic)
Reserpine (Systemic)
Reserpine and Chlorothiazide (Systemic)
Reserpine and Chlorthalidone (Systemic)
Reserpine, Hydralazine, and Hydrochlorothiazide (Systemic)
Reserpine and Hydrochlorothiazide (Systemic)
Reserpine and Hydroflumethiazide (Systemic)
Reserpine and Methyclothiazide (Systemic)
Reserpine and Polythiazide (Systemic)
Reserpine and Trichlormethiazide (Systemic)
Sotalol (Systemic)
Spironolactone (Systemic)
Spironolactone and Hydrochlorothiazide (Systemic)
Terazosin (Systemic)

Antihypertensive *(continued)*
Timolol (Systemic)
Timolol and Hydrochlorothiazide (Systemic)
Triamterene (Systemic)
Triamterene and Hydrochlorothiazide (Systemic)
Trichlormethiazide (Systemic)
Verapamil (Systemic)
Antihypertensive, ocular
Apraclonidine (Ophthalmic)
Antihypertensive, pheochromocytoma
Metyrosine (Systemic)
Phenoxybenzamine (Systemic)
Antihyperthyroid agent
Iodine, Strong (Systemic)
Ipodate (Diagnostic)
Methimazole (Systemic)
Potassium Iodide (Systemic)
Propylthiouracil (Systemic)
Sodium Iodide (Systemic)
Sodium Iodide I 131 (Diagnostic)
Sodium Iodide I 131 (Therapeutic)
Antihyperuricemic
Allopurinol (Systemic)
Probenecid (Systemic)
Sulfinpyrazone (Systemic)
Antihypocalcemic
Alfacalcidol (Systemic)
Calcifediol (Systemic)
Calcitriol (Systemic)
Calcium Carbonate (Oral)
Calcium Carbonate (Systemic)
Calcium Chloride (Systemic)
Calcium Citrate (Systemic)
Calcium Glubionate (Systemic)
Calcium Gluceptate (Systemic)
Calcium Gluconate (Systemic)
Calcium Glycerophosphate and Calcium Lactate (Systemic)
Calcium Lactate (Systemic)
Calcium Lactate-Gluconate and Calcium Carbonate (Systemic)
Calcium Phosphate, Dibasic (Systemic)
Calcium Phosphate, Tribasic (Systemic)
Dihydrotachysterol (Systemic)
Ergocalciferol (Systemic)
Antihypoglycemic
Diazoxide (Oral)
Glucagon (Systemic)
Antihypoglycemic, pancreatic tumor
Octreotide (Systemic)
Antihypokalemic
Amiloride (Systemic)
Amiloride and Hydrochlorothiazide (Systemic)
Potassium Acetate (Systemic)
Potassium Bicarbonate (Systemic)
Potassium Bicarbonate and Potassium Chloride (Systemic)
Potassium Bicarbonate and Potassium Citrate (Systemic)
Potassium Chloride (Systemic)
Potassium Chloride, Potassium Bicarbonate, and Potassium Citrate (Systemic)
Potassium Gluconate (Systemic)
Potassium Gluconate and Potassium Chloride (Systemic)
Potassium Gluconate and Potassium Citrate (Systemic)
Spironolactone (Systemic)
Spironolactone and Hydrochlorothiazide (Systemic)
Triamterene (Systemic)
Triamterene and Hydrochlorothiazide (Systemic)
Trikates (Systemic)

Antihypomagnesemic
- Magnesium Chloride (Systemic)
- Magnesium Citrate (Systemic)
- Magnesium Gluceptate (Systemic)
- Magnesium Gluconate (Systemic)
- Magnesium Hydroxide (Systemic)
- Magnesium Lactate (Systemic)
- Magnesium Oxide (Systemic)
- Magnesium Pidolate (Systemic)
- Magnesium Sulfate (Systemic)

Antihypoparathyroid
- Calcitriol (Systemic)
- Dihydrotachysterol (Systemic)
- Ergocalciferol (Systemic)

Antihypotensive
- Dihydroergotamine (Systemic)

Antihypotensive, carcinoid crisis
- Octreotide (Systemic)

Antihypotensive, idiopathic orthostatic
- Fludrocortisone (Systemic)

Anti-infective, vaginal
- Clindamycin (Vaginal)
- Metronidazole (Vaginal)

Anti-inflammatory, inhalation
- Nedocromil (Inhalation)

Anti-inflammatory, local, interstitial cystitis
- Dimethyl Sulfoxide (Mucosal)

Anti-inflammatory, nonsteroidal
- Aspirin (Systemic)
- Aspirin, Buffered (Systemic)
- Aspirin and Caffeine (Systemic)
- Aspirin and Caffeine, Buffered (Systemic)
- Choline Salicylate (Systemic)
- Choline and Magnesium Salicylates (Systemic)
- Etodolac (Systemic)
- Indomethacin (Systemic)
- Magnesium Salicylate (Systemic)
- Naproxen (Systemic)
- Salsalate (Systemic)
- Sodium Salicylate (Systemic)
- Sulindac (Systemic)
- Tenoxicam (Systemic)

Anti-inflammatory, nonsteroidal, ophthalmic
- Diclofenac (Ophthalmic)
- Flurbiprofen (Ophthalmic)
- Indomethacin (Ophthalmic)
- Ketorolac (Ophthalmic)

Anti-inflammatory, nonsteroidal, topical
- Bufexamac (Topical)

Anti-inflammatory, steroidal
- Betamethasone—Glucocorticoid Effects (Systemic)
- Cortisone—Glucocorticoid Effects (Systemic)
- Dexamethasone—Glucocorticoid Effects (Systemic)
- Hydrocortisone—Glucocorticoid Effects (Systemic)
- Methylprednisolone—Glucocorticoid Effects (Systemic)
- Paramethasone—Glucocorticoid Effects (Systemic)
- Prednisolone—Glucocorticoid Effects (Systemic)
- Prednisone—Glucocorticoid Effects (Systemic)
- Triamcinolone—Glucocorticoid Effects (Systemic)

Anti-inflammatory, steroidal, nasal
- Beclomethasone (Nasal)
- Dexamethasone (Nasal)
- Flunisolide (Nasal)
- Triamcinolone (Nasal)

Anti-inflammatory, steroidal, ophthalmic
- Betamethasone (Ophthalmic)
- Dexamethasone (Ophthalmic)
- Fluorometholone (Ophthalmic)
- Hydrocortisone (Ophthalmic)
- Medrysone (Ophthalmic)
- Prednisolone (Ophthalmic)

Anti-inflammatory, steroidal, otic
- Betamethasone (Otic)
- Desonide and Acetic Acid (Otic)
- Dexamethasone (Otic)
- Hydrocortisone (Otic)
- Hydrocortisone and Acetic Acid (Otic)

Anti-inflammatory, steroidal, topical
- Alclometasone (Topical)
- Amcinonide (Topical)
- Beclomethasone (Topical)
- Betamethasone (Dental)
- Betamethasone (Topical)
- Clobetasol (Topical)
- Clobetasone (Topical)
- Clocortolone (Topical)
- Desonide (Topical)
- Desoximetasone (Topical)
- Dexamethasone (Topical)
- Diflorasone (Topical)
- Diflucortolone (Topical)
- Flumethasone (Topical)
- Fluocinolone (Topical)
- Fluocinonide (Topical)
- Fluocinonide, Procinonide, and Ciprocinonide (Topical)
- Flurandrenolide (Topical)
- Fluticasone (Topical)
- Halcinonide (Topical)
- Halobetasol (Topical)
- Hydrocortisone (Dental)
- Hydrocortisone (Rectal)
- Hydrocortisone (Topical)
- Hydrocortisone Acetate (Topical)
- Hydrocortisone Butyrate (Topical)
- Hydrocortisone and Urea (Topical)
- Hydrocortisone Valerate (Topical)
- Mometasone (Topical)
- Triamcinolone (Dental)
- Triamcinolone (Topical)

Anti-Kawasaki disease, systemic
- Immune Globulin Intravenous (Human) (Systemic)

Antimalarial
- Halofantrine (Systemic)
- Mefloquine (Systemic)

Antimanic
- Carbamazepine (Systemic)
- Lithium (Systemic)

Antimigraine agent
- Sumatriptan (Systemic)

Antimyasthenic
- Ambenonium (Systemic)
- Neostigmine (Systemic)
- Pyridostigmine (Systemic)

Antimydriatic
- Dapiprazole (Ophthalmic)

Antimyotonic
- Quinine (Systemic)

Antinarcolepsy adjunct
- Imipramine (Systemic)
- Protriptyline (Systemic)

Antineoplastic
- Aldesleukin (Systemic)
- Altretamine (Systemic)
- Aminoglutethimide (Systemic)
- Amsacrine (Systemic)
- Asparaginase (Systemic)
- Bacillus Calmette-Guérin (BCG) Live (Mucosal-Local)
- Bleomycin (Systemic)

Antineoplastic *(continued)*
- Buserelin (Systemic)
- Busulfan (Systemic)
- Carboplatin (Systemic)
- Carmustine (Systemic)
- Chlorambucil (Systemic)
- Chlorotrianisene (Systemic)
- Chromic Phosphate P 32 (Therapeutic)
- Cisplatin (Systemic)
- Cladribine (Systemic)
- Cyclophosphamide (Systemic)
- Cyproterone (Systemic)
- Cytarabine (Systemic)
- Dacarbazine (Systemic)
- Dactinomycin (Systemic)
- Daunorubicin (Systemic)
- Diethylstilbestrol (Systemic)
- Doxorubicin (Systemic)
- Epirubicin (Systemic)
- Estradiol (Systemic)
- Estramustine (Systemic)
- Estrogens, Conjugated (Systemic)
- Estrogens, Esterified (Systemic)
- Estrone (Systemic)
- Ethinyl Estradiol (Systemic)
- Etoposide (Systemic)
- Floxuridine (Systemic)
- Fludarabine (Systemic)
- Fluorouracil (Systemic)
- Fluoxymesterone (Systemic)
- Flutamide (Systemic)
- Goserelin (Systemic)
- Hydroxyprogesterone (Systemic)
- Hydroxyurea (Systemic)
- Idarubicin (Systemic)
- Ifosfamide (Systemic)
- Interferon Alfa-2a, Recombinant (Systemic)
- Interferon Alfa-2b, Recombinant (Systemic)
- Interferon Alfa-n1 (lns) (Systemic)
- Interferon Alfa-n3 (Systemic)
- Iobenguane, Radioiodinated (Therapeutic)
- Ketoconazole (Systemic)
- Leuprolide (Systemic)
- Levothyroxine (Systemic)
- Liothyronine (Systemic)
- Liotrix (Systemic)
- Lomustine (Systemic)
- Mechlorethamine (Systemic)
- Medroxyprogesterone (Systemic)
- Megestrol (Systemic)
- Melphalan (Systemic)
- Mercaptopurine (Systemic)
- Methotrexate—For Cancer (Systemic)
- Methoxsalen (Systemic)
- Methyltestosterone (Systemic)
- Mitomycin (Systemic)
- Mitotane (Systemic)
- Mitoxantrone (Systemic)
- Nandrolone (Systemic)
- Nilutamide (Systemic)
- Paclitaxel (Systemic)
- Pentostatin (Systemic)
- Plicamycin (Systemic)
- Procarbazine (Systemic)
- Sodium Iodide I 131 (Therapeutic)
- Sodium Phosphate P 32 (Therapeutic)
- Streptozocin (Systemic)
- Tamoxifen (Systemic)
- Teniposide (Systemic)
- Testolactone (Systemic)
- Testosterone (Systemic)
- Thioguanine (Systemic)
- Thiotepa (Systemic)
- Thyroglobulin (Systemic)
- Thyroid (Systemic)

Antineoplastic *(continued)*
- Thyrotropin (Systemic)
- Uracil Mustard (Systemic)
- Vinblastine (Systemic)
- Vincristine (Systemic)
- Vindesine (Systemic)

Antineoplastic adjunct
- Leucovorin (Systemic)
- Levamisole (Systemic)

Antineoplastic, topical
- Fluorouracil (Topical)
- Mechlorethamine (Topical)

Antineuralgia adjunct
- Fluphenazine (Systemic)

Antineuralgic
- Amitriptyline (Systemic)
- Clomipramine (Systemic)
- Desipramine (Systemic)
- Doxepin (Systemic)
- Imipramine (Systemic)
- Maprotiline (Systemic)
- Nortriptyline (Systemic)
- Trazodone (Systemic)
- Trimipramine (Systemic)

Antineuralgic, specific pain syndromes
- Carbamazepine (Systemic)

Antineuralgic, specific pain syndromes, topical
- Capsaicin (Topical)

Antineuralgic, trigeminal neuralgia
- Phenytoin (Systemic)

Antineutropenic
- Filgrastim (Systemic)
- Sargramostim (Systemic)

Antiobsessional agent
- Fluoxetine (Systemic)

Antiobsessive-compulsive agent
- Clomipramine (Systemic)

Antiosteolytic
- Colchicine (Systemic)

Antipanic agent
- Alprazolam (Systemic)
- Chlordiazepoxide (Systemic)
- Clomipramine (Systemic)
- Clonazepam (Systemic)
- Desipramine (Systemic)
- Diazepam (Systemic)
- Doxepin (Systemic)
- Imipramine (Systemic)
- Lorazepam (Systemic)
- Nortriptyline (Systemic)
- Phenelzine (Systemic)
- Tranylcypromine (Systemic)

Antiparalytic, familial periodic paralysis
- Acetazolamide (Systemic)

Antipolyneuropathy agent
- Immune Globulin Intravenous (Human) (Systemic)

Antiprotozoal
- Amphotericin B (Systemic)
- Atovaquone (Systemic)
- Chloroquine (Systemic)
- Clindamycin (Systemic)
- Dapsone (Systemic)
- Demeclocycline (Systemic)
- Doxycycline (Systemic)
- Furazolidone (Oral)
- Hydroxychloroquine (Systemic)
- Iodoquinol (Oral)
- Methacycline (Systemic)
- Metronidazole (Systemic)
- Minocycline (Systemic)
- Oxytetracycline (Systemic)
- Pentamidine (Inhalation)
- Pentamidine (Systemic)
- Primaquine (Systemic)
- Pyrimethamine (Systemic)
- Quinacrine (Systemic)

Antiprotozoal *(continued)*
- Quinine (Systemic)
- Sulfadoxine and Pyrimethamine (Systemic)
- Sulfamethoxazole (Systemic)
- Sulfamethoxazole and Trimethoprim (Systemic)
- Sulfisoxazole (Systemic)
- Tetracycline (Systemic)

Antiprotozoal-antifungal, vaginal
- Metronidazole and Nystatin (Vaginal)

Antiprotozoal, systemic
- Albendazole (Systemic)
- Eflornithine (Systemic)

Antiprotozoal, vaginal
- Metronidazole (Vaginal)

Antipruritic
- Doxepin (Systemic)

Antipruritic, cholestasis
- Cholestyramine (Oral)
- Colestipol (Oral)

Antipsoriatic, systemic
- Etretinate (Systemic)
- Methotrexate—For Noncancerous Conditions (Systemic)
- Methoxsalen (Systemic)
- Trioxsalen (Systemic)

Antipsoriatic, topical
- Anthralin (Topical)
- Coal Tar (Topical)
- Methoxsalen (Topical)
- Salicylic Acid (Topical)
- Salicylic Acid, Sulfur, and Coal Tar (Topical)

Antipsychotic
- Acetophenazine (Systemic)
- Carbamazepine (Systemic)
- Chlorpromazine (Systemic)
- Chlorprothixene (Systemic)
- Clozapine (Systemic)
- Flupenthixol (Systemic)
- Fluphenazine (Systemic)
- Fluspirilene (Systemic)
- Haloperidol (Systemic)
- Loxapine (Systemic)
- Mesoridazine (Systemic)
- Methotrimeprazine (Systemic)
- Molindone (Systemic)
- Pericyazine (Systemic)
- Perphenazine (Systemic)
- Pimozide (Systemic)
- Pipotiazine (Systemic)
- Prochlorperazine (Systemic)
- Promazine (Systemic)
- Remoxipride (Systemic)
- Risperidone (Systemic)
- Thiopropazate (Systemic)
- Thioproperazine (Systemic)
- Thioridazine (Systemic)
- Thiothixene (Systemic)
- Trifluoperazine (Systemic)
- Triflupromazine (Systemic)

Antipsychotic-antidepressant
- Perphenazine and Amitriptyline (Systemic)

Antipyretic
- Acetaminophen (Systemic)
- Acetaminophen and Aspirin (Systemic)
- Acetaminophen, Aspirin, and Caffeine (Systemic)
- Acetaminophen, Aspirin, and Caffeine, Buffered (Systemic)
- Acetaminophen, Aspirin, and Salicylamide, Buffered (Systemic)
- Acetaminophen, Aspirin, Salicylamide, and Caffeine (Systemic)
- Acetaminophen and Caffeine (Systemic)
- Acetaminophen and Salicylamide (Systemic)

Antipyretic *(continued)*
- Acetaminophen, Salicylamide, and Caffeine (Systemic)
- Aspirin (Systemic)
- Aspirin, Buffered (Systemic)
- Aspirin and Caffeine (Systemic)
- Aspirin and Caffeine, Buffered (Systemic)
- Choline Salicylate (Systemic)
- Choline and Magnesium Salicylates (Systemic)
- Ibuprofen (Systemic)
- Indomethacin (Systemic)
- Magnesium Salicylate (Systemic)
- Salsalate (Systemic)
- Sodium Salicylate (Systemic)

Antirheumatic
- Aspirin (Systemic)
- Flurbiprofen (Systemic)

Antirheumatic, disease-modifying
- Auranofin (Systemic)
- Aurothioglucose (Systemic)
- Azathioprine (Systemic)
- Chloroquine (Systemic)
- Gold Sodium Thiomalate (Systemic)
- Hydroxychloroquine (Systemic)
- Methotrexate—For Noncancerous Conditions (Systemic)
- Penicillamine (Systemic)
- Sulfasalazine (Systemic)

Antirheumatic, nonsteroidal anti-inflammatory
- Aspirin (Systemic)
- Aspirin, Buffered (Systemic)
- Aspirin and Caffeine (Systemic)
- Aspirin and Caffeine, Buffered (Systemic)
- Choline Salicylate (Systemic)
- Choline and Magnesium Salicylates (Systemic)
- Diclofenac (Systemic)
- Diflunisal (Systemic)
- Etodolac (Systemic)
- Fenoprofen (Systemic)
- Flurbiprofen (Systemic)
- Ibuprofen (Systemic)
- Indomethacin (Systemic)
- Ketoprofen (Systemic)
- Magnesium Salicylate (Systemic)
- Meclofenamate (Systemic)
- Nabumetone (Systemic)
- Naproxen (Systemic)
- Oxaprozin (Systemic)
- Phenylbutazone (Systemic)
- Piroxicam (Systemic)
- Salsalate (Systemic)
- Sodium Salicylate (Systemic)
- Sulindac (Systemic)
- Tenoxicam (Systemic)
- Tiaprofenic Acid (Systemic)
- Tolmetin (Systemic)

Antirosacea agent, systemic
- Isotretinoin (Systemic)

Antirosacea agent, topical
- Metronidazole (Topical)
- Sulfur (Topical)

Antiseborrheic
- Chloroxine (Topical)
- Coal Tar (Topical)
- Pyrithione (Topical)
- Salicylic Acid (Topical)
- Salicylic Acid and Sulfur (Topical)
- Salicylic Acid, Sulfur, and Coal Tar (Topical)
- Selenium Sulfide (Topical)
- Sulfur (Topical)

Antispasmodic
- Glucagon (Systemic)

Antispasmodic, gastrointestinal
Dicyclomine (Systemic)
Oxyphencyclimine (Systemic)
Scopolamine (Systemic)
Antispasmodic, urinary tract
Atropine (Systemic)
Flavoxate (Systemic)
Oxybutynin (Systemic)
Scopolamine (Systemic)
Antispastic
Baclofen (Systemic)
Dantrolene (Systemic)
Antithrombotic
Aspirin (Systemic)
Aspirin, Buffered (Systemic)
Aspirin and Caffeine (Systemic)
Aspirin and Caffeine, Buffered (Systemic)
Ticlopidine (Systemic)
Antithrombotic adjunct
Dipyridamole (Systemic)
Antitremor agent
Acebutolol (Systemic)
Atenolol (Systemic)
Chlordiazepoxide (Systemic)
Diazepam (Systemic)
Lorazepam (Systemic)
Metoprolol (Systemic)
Nadolol (Systemic)
Oxprenolol (Systemic)
Pindolol (Systemic)
Propranolol (Systemic)
Sotalol (Systemic)
Timolol (Systemic)
Antitussive
Benzonatate (Systemic)
Chlophedianol (Systemic)
Codeine (Systemic)
Dextromethorphan (Systemic)
Diphenhydramine (Systemic)
Hydrocodone (Systemic)
Hydromorphone (Systemic)
Methadone (Systemic)
Morphine (Systemic)
Antitussive-analgesic
Dextromethorphan and Acetaminophen (Systemic)
Antitussive-anticholinergic
Hydrocodone and Homatropine (Systemic)
Antitussive-expectorant
Codeine and Calcium Iodide (Systemic)
Codeine and Guaifenesin (Systemic)
Codeine and Iodinated Glycerol (Systemic)
Dextromethorphan and Guaifenesin (Systemic)
Dextromethorphan, Guaifenesin, Potassium Citrate, and Citric Acid (Systemic)
Dextromethorphan and Iodinated Glycerol (Systemic)
Hydrocodone and Guaifenesin (Systemic)
Hydrocodone and Potassium Guaiacolsulfonate (Systemic)
Hydromorphone and Guaifenesin (Systemic)
Antiulcer agent
Amitriptyline (Systemic)
Bismuth Subsalicylate (Oral)
Cimetidine (Systemic)
Doxepin (Systemic)
Famotidine (Systemic)
Misoprostol (Systemic)
Nizatidine (Systemic)
Omeprazole (Systemic)
Ranitidine (Systemic)
Sucralfate (Oral)
Trimipramine (Systemic)

Antiurolithic, calcium calculi
Bendroflumethiazide (Systemic)
Benzthiazide (Systemic)
Cellulose Sodium Phosphate (Systemic)
Chlorothiazide (Systemic)
Chlorthalidone (Systemic)
Cyclothiazide (Systemic)
Hydrochlorothiazide (Systemic)
Hydroflumethiazide (Systemic)
Magnesium Hydroxide (Oral)
Methyclothiazide (Systemic)
Metolazone (Systemic)
Polythiazide (Systemic)
Potassium Phosphates (Systemic)
Potassium and Sodium Phosphates (Systemic)
Quinethazone (Systemic)
Trichlormethiazide (Systemic)
Antiurolithic, calcium oxalate calculi
Allopurinol (Systemic)
Potassium Citrate (Systemic)
Potassium Citrate and Citric Acid (Systemic)
Antiurolithic, calcium phosphate calculi
Potassium Citrate (Systemic)
Potassium Citrate and Citric Acid (Systemic)
Antiurolithic, cystine calculi
Acetazolamide (Systemic)
Penicillamine (Systemic)
Potassium Citrate (Systemic)
Potassium Citrate and Citric Acid (Systemic)
Potassium Citrate and Sodium Citrate (Systemic)
Sodium Citrate and Citric Acid (Systemic)
Tiopronin (Systemic)
Tricitrates (Systemic)
Antiurolithic, phosphate calculi
Aluminum Carbonate (Oral)
Aluminum Hydroxide (Oral)
Antiurolithic, struvite calculi
Acetohydroxamic Acid (Systemic)
Antiurolithic, uric acid calculi
Acetazolamide (Systemic)
Allopurinol (Systemic)
Potassium Citrate (Systemic)
Potassium Citrate and Citric Acid (Systemic)
Potassium Citrate and Sodium Citrate (Systemic)
Sodium Citrate and Citric Acid (Systemic)
Tricitrates (Systemic)
Antivertigo agent
Belladonna (Systemic)
Dimenhydrinate (Systemic)
Diphenhydramine (Systemic)
Diphenidol (Systemic)
Meclizine (Systemic)
Promethazine (Systemic)
Scopolamine (Systemic)
Antiviral, ophthalmic
Idoxuridine (Ophthalmic)
Trifluridine (Ophthalmic)
Vidarabine (Ophthalmic)
Antiviral, systemic
Acyclovir (Systemic)
Amantadine (Systemic)
Didanosine (Systemic)
Foscarnet (Systemic)
Ganciclovir (Systemic)
Immune Globulin Intravenous (Human) (Systemic)
Ribavirin (Systemic)
Zalcitabine (Systemic)
Zidovudine (Systemic)

Antiviral, topical
Acyclovir (Topical)
Appetite stimulant
Cyproheptadine (Systemic)
Dronabinol (Systemic)
Appetite suppressant
Benzphetamine (Systemic)
Diethylpropion (Systemic)
Fenfluramine (Systemic)
Mazindol (Systemic)
Phendimetrazine (Systemic)
Phentermine (Systemic)
Phenylpropanolamine (Systemic)
Asthma prophylactic
Albuterol (Inhalation)
Aminophylline (Systemic)
Bitolterol (Inhalation)
Cromolyn (Inhalation)
Epinephrine (Inhalation)
Isoetharine (Inhalation)
Ketotifen (Systemic)
Metaproterenol (Inhalation)
Nedocromil (Inhalation)
Oxtriphylline (Systemic)
Pirbuterol (Inhalation)
Procaterol (Inhalation)
Terbutaline (Inhalation)
Theophylline (Systemic)

B–C

Benign prostatic hypertrophy therapy
Phenoxybenzamine (Systemic)
Biological response modifier
Aldesleukin (Systemic)
Interferon Alfa-2a, Recombinant (Systemic)
Interferon Alfa-2b, Recombinant (Systemic)
Interferon Alfa-n1 (lns) (Systemic)
Interferon Alfa-n3 (Systemic)
Interferon, Gamma (Systemic)
Levamisole (Systemic)
Blood viscosity–reducing agent
Pentoxifylline (Systemic)
Bone resorption inhibitor
Calcitonin-Human (Systemic)
Calcitonin-Salmon (Systemic)
Etidronate (Systemic)
Pamidronate (Systemic)
Plicamycin (Systemic)
Bowel disease, inflammatory, suppressant
Azathioprine (Systemic)
Mesalamine (Rectal)
Metronidazole (Systemic)
Olsalazine (Oral)
Sulfasalazine (Systemic)
Bowel preparation, preoperative, adjunct
Erythromycin (Systemic)
Kanamycin (Oral)
Neomycin (Oral)
Bronchodilator
Albuterol (Inhalation)
Albuterol (Oral/Injection)
Aminophylline (Systemic)
Bitolterol (Inhalation)
Dyphylline (Systemic)
Ephedrine (Oral/Injection)
Epinephrine (Inhalation)
Epinephrine (Oral/Injection)
Ethylnorepinephrine (Oral/Injection)
Fenoterol (Inhalation)
Fenoterol (Oral/Injection)
Ipratropium (Inhalation)
Isoetharine (Inhalation)
Isoproterenol (Inhalation)
Isoproterenol (Oral/Injection)

Bronchodilator *(continued)*
- Metaproterenol (Inhalation)
- Metaproterenol (Oral/Injection)
- Oxtriphylline (Systemic)
- Oxtriphylline and Guaifenesin (Systemic)
- Pirbuterol (Inhalation)
- Procaterol (Inhalation)
- Terbutaline (Inhalation)
- Terbutaline (Oral/Injection)
- Theophylline (Systemic)
- Theophylline, Ephedrine, and Phenobarbital (Systemic)
- Theophylline and Guaifenesin (Systemic)

Bronchodilator-decongestant
- Isoproterenol and Phenylephrine (Systemic)

Buffer, neutralizing
- Sodium Citrate and Citric Acid (Systemic)
- Tricitrates (Systemic)

Calcium pyrophosphate deposition disease suppressant
- Colchicine (Systemic)

Cardiac stimulant
- Epinephrine (Oral/Injection)
- Isoproterenol (Oral/Injection)

Cardiotonic
- Calcium Chloride (Systemic)
- Calcium Glubionate (Systemic)
- Calcium Gluconate (Systemic)
- Digitoxin (Systemic)
- Digoxin (Systemic)

Caustic
- Salicylic Acid (Topical)

Cerumen removal adjunct
- Antipyrine and Benzocaine (Otic)

Chelating agent
- Deferoxamine (Systemic)
- Penicillamine (Systemic)
- Succimer (Systemic)
- Trientine (Systemic)

Chemonucleolytic, herniated lumbar intervertebral disc therapy
- Chymopapain (Parenteral-Local)

Cholelitholytic
- Monooctanoin (Local)

Cholinergic
- Bethanechol (Systemic)

Cholinergic adjunct, curariform block
- Atropine (Systemic)
- Glycopyrrolate (Systemic)
- Hyoscyamine (Systemic)

Cholinergic, cholinesterase inhibitor
- Ambenonium (Systemic)
- Neostigmine (Systemic)
- Pyridostigmine (Systemic)

Cholinergic enhancer
- Cisapride (Systemic)

Cleansing agent, astringent
- Alcohol and Acetone (Topical)

Cleansing agent, astringent-keratolytic
- Alcohol and Sulfur (Topical)

Cleansing agent, defatting
- Alcohol and Acetone (Topical)

Cleansing agent, defatting-keratolytic
- Alcohol and Sulfur (Topical)

Collagenase synthesis/secretion inhibitor
- Phenytoin (Systemic)

Contraceptive
- Condoms

Contraceptive, intrauterine-local
- Progesterone (Intrauterine)

Contraceptive, postcoital, systemic
- Norgestrel and Ethinyl Estradiol (Systemic)

Contraceptive, systemic
- Desogestrel and Ethinyl Estradiol (Systemic)
- Ethynodiol Diacetate and Ethinyl Estradiol (Systemic)

Contraceptive, systemic *(continued)*
- Levonorgestrel (Systemic)
- Levonorgestrel and Ethinyl Estradiol (Systemic)
- Medroxyprogesterone (Systemic)
- Norethindrone (Systemic)
- Norethindrone Acetate and Ethinyl Estradiol (Systemic)
- Norethindrone and Ethinyl Estradiol (Systemic)
- Norethindrone and Mestranol (Systemic)
- Norgestimate and Ethinyl Estradiol (Systemic)
- Norgestrel (Systemic)
- Norgestrel and Ethinyl Estradiol (Systemic)

Contraceptive, vaginal
- Benzalkonium Chloride (Vaginal)
- Nonoxynol 9 (Vaginal)
- Octoxynol 9 (Vaginal)

Copper absorption inhibitor
- Zinc (Systemic)

Corticosteroid, topical
- Alcometasone (Topical)
- Amcinonide (Topical)
- Beclomethasone (Topical)
- Betamethasone (Dental)
- Betamethasone (Topical)
- Clobetasol (Topical)
- Clobetasone (Topical)
- Clocortolone (Topical)
- Desonide (Topical)
- Desoximetasone (Topical)
- Dexamethasone (Topical)
- Diflorasone (Topical)
- Diflucortolone (Topical)
- Flumethasone (Topical)
- Fluocinolone (Topical)
- Fluocinonide (Topical)
- Fluocinonide, Procinonide, and Ciprocinonide (Topical)
- Flurandrenolide (Topical)
- Fluticasone (Topical)
- Halcinonide (Topical)
- Halobetasol (Topical)
- Hydrocortisone (Dental)
- Hydrocortisone (Rectal)
- Hydrocortisone (Topical)
- Hydrocortisone Acetate (Topical)
- Hydrocortisone Butyrate (Topical)
- Hydrocortisone and Urea (Topical)
- Hydrocortisone Valerate (Topical)
- Mometasone (Topical)
- Triamcinolone (Dental)
- Triamcinolone (Topical)

Cryptorchidism therapy adjunct
- Chorionic Gonadotropin (Systemic)

Cycloplegic
- Atropine (Ophthalmic)
- Cyclopentolate (Ophthalmic)
- Homatropine (Ophthalmic)
- Scopolamine (Ophthalmic)
- Tropicamide (Ophthalmic)

Cyclostimulant, accommodative esotropia
- Demecarium (Ophthalmic)
- Echothiophate (Ophthalmic)
- Isoflurophate (Ophthalmic)

Cytotoxic, topical
- Podofilox (Topical)
- Podophyllum (Topical)

D

Decongestant-analgesic
- Phenylephrine and Acetaminophen (Systemic)
- Phenylpropanolamine and Acetaminophen (Systemic)

Decongestant-analgesic *(continued)*
- Phenylpropanolamine, Acetaminophen, and Aspirin (Systemic)
- Phenylpropanolamine, Acetaminophen, Aspirin, and Caffeine (Systemic)
- Phenylpropanolamine, Acetaminophen, Salicylamide, and Caffeine (Systemic)
- Phenylpropanolamine and Aspirin (Systemic)
- Pseudoephedrine and Acetaminophen (Systemic)
- Pseudoephedrine, Acetaminophen, and Caffeine (Systemic)
- Pseudoephedrine and Aspirin (Systemic)
- Pseudoephedrine, Aspirin, and Caffeine (Systemic)
- Pseudoephedrine and Ibuprofen (Systemic)

Decongestant-antitussive
- Phenylephrine and Dextromethorphan (Systemic)
- Phenylpropanolamine and Caramiphen (Systemic)
- Phenylpropanolamine and Dextromethorphan (Systemic)
- Phenylpropanolamine and Hydrocodone (Systemic)
- Pseudoephedrine and Codeine (Systemic)
- Pseudoephedrine and Dextromethorphan (Systemic)
- Pseudoephedrine and Hydrocodone (Systemic)

Decongestant-antitussive-analgesic
- Phenylpropanolamine, Dextromethorphan, and Acetaminophen (Systemic)
- Pseudoephedrine, Dextromethorphan, and Acetaminophen (Systemic)

Decongestant-antitussive-expectorant
- Phenylephrine, Dextromethorphan, and Guaifenesin (Systemic)
- Phenylephrine, Hydrocodone, and Guaifenesin (Systemic)
- Phenylpropanolamine, Codeine, and Guaifenesin (Systemic)
- Phenylpropanolamine, Dextromethorphan, and Guaifenesin (Systemic)
- Pseudoephedrine, Codeine, and Guaifenesin (Systemic)
- Pseudoephedrine, Dextromethorphan, and Guaifenesin (Systemic)
- Pseudoephedrine, Hydrocodone, and Guaifenesin (Systemic)

Decongestant-antitussive-expectorant-analgesic
- Phenylephrine, Dextromethorphan, Guaifenesin, and Acetaminophen (Systemic)
- Pseudoephedrine, Dextromethorphan, Guaifenesin, and Acetaminophen (Systemic)

Decongestant-expectorant
- Ephedrine and Guaifenesin (Systemic)
- Ephedrine and Potassium Iodide (Systemic)
- Phenylephrine, Phenylpropanolamine, and Guaifenesin (Systemic)
- Phenylpropanolamine and Guaifenesin (Systemic)
- Pseudoephedrine and Guaifenesin (Systemic)

Decongestant-expectorant-analgesic
- Phenylephrine, Guaifenesin, Acetaminophen, Salicylamide, and Caffeine (Systemic)

Decongestant, nasal, systemic
- Ephedrine (Oral/Injection)
- Phenylpropanolamine (Systemic)
- Pseudoephedrine (Systemic)

Decongestant, ophthalmic
- Naphazoline (Ophthalmic)
- Oxymetazoline (Ophthalmic)
- Phenylephrine (Ophthalmic)

Decongestant, topical
Oxymetazoline (Nasal)
Phenylephrine (Nasal)
Xylometazoline (Nasal)
Deferoxamine adjunct, chronic iron overdose
Ascorbic Acid (Systemic)
Dementia symptoms treatment adjunct
Ergoloid Mesylates (Systemic)
Dental caries prophylactic
Sodium Fluoride (Systemic)
Dermatitis herpetiformis suppressant
Colchicine (Systemic)
Dapsone (Systemic)
Sulfapyridine (Systemic)
Diagnostic aid, accommodative esotropia
Demecarium (Ophthalmic)
Echothiophate (Ophthalmic)
Isoflurophate (Ophthalmic)
Diagnostic aid adjunct, antispasmodic
Glucagon (Systemic)
Diagnostic aid adjunct, ischemic heart disease
Dipyridamole (Systemic)
Diagnostic aid adjunct, red blood cell disease
Ascorbic Acid (Systemic)
Diagnostic aid adjunct, renal disease
Furosemide (Systemic)
Diagnostic aid, adrenocortical function
Corticotropin—Glucocorticoid Effects (Systemic)
Diagnostic aid, angiography
Dinoprost (Intra-amniotic)
Diagnostic aid, bronchial airway hyperreactivity
Methacholine (Inhalation)
Diagnostic aid, bronchial studies
Acetylcysteine (Inhalation)
Diagnostic aid, cardiac function
Amyl Nitrite (Systemic)
Diagnostic aid, contact lens procedures
Hydroxypropyl Methylcellulose (Ophthalmic)
Diagnostic aid, coronary vasospasm
Ergonovine (Systemic)
Diagnostic aid, Cushing's syndrome
Dexamethasone—Glucocorticoid Effects (Systemic)
Diagnostic aid, cycloplegic
Tropicamide (Ophthalmic)
Diagnostic aid, diabetes insipidus
Vasopressin (Systemic)
Diagnostic aid, endogenous depression
Dexamethasone—Glucocorticoid Effects (Systemic)
Diagnostic aid, folate deficiency
Folic Acid (Vitamin B_9) (Systemic)
Diagnostic aid, gastric function
Histamine (Diagnostic)
Pentagastrin (Diagnostic)
Diagnostic aid, gastrointestinal bleeding
Sodium Chromate Cr 51 (Diagnostic)
Sodium Pertechnetate Tc 99m (Diagnostic)
Technetium Tc 99m Sulfur Colloid (Diagnostic)
Diagnostic aid, gastroscopy
Simethicone (Oral)
Diagnostic aid, glycosuria
Urine Test Kit for Glucose and Ketone Testing
Urine Test Kit for Glucose Testing
Diagnostic aid, gonioscopy
Hydroxypropyl Methylcellulose (Ophthalmic)
Diagnostic aid, hypogonadism
Chorionic Gonadotropin (Systemic)
Diagnostic aid, hypoparathyroidism vs. pseudohypoparathyroidism
Teriparatide (Systemic)

Diagnostic aid, hypothalamic-pituitary-gonadal axis function
Clomiphene (Systemic)
Gonadorelin (Systemic)
Diagnostic aid, hypothalamic-pituitary-thyroid axis function
Protirelin (Diagnostic)
Diagnostic aid, iron absorption
Ferrous Citrate Fe 59 (Diagnostic)
Diagnostic aid, iron metabolism
Ferrous Citrate Fe 59 (Diagnostic)
Diagnostic aid, ketonuria
Urine Test Kit for Glucose and Ketone Testing
Urine Test Kit for Ketone Testing
Diagnostic aid, myasthenia gravis
Neostigmine (Systemic)
Diagnostic aid, mydriatic
Phenylephrine (Ophthalmic)
Tropicamide (Ophthalmic)
Diagnostic aid, occult bleeding
Fecal Occult Blood Test Kits
Diagnostic aid, ovarian function
Clomiphene (Systemic)
Diagnostic aid, ovulation
Ovulation Prediction Test Kits for Home Use
Diagnostic aid, pancreatic function
Bentiromide (Diagnostic)
Pancrelipase (Systemic)
Diagnostic aid, paramagnetic, brain disorders
Gadodiamide (Diagnostic)
Gadopentetate (Diagnostic)
Gadoteridol (Diagnostic)
Diagnostic aid, paramagnetic, spine disorders
Gadodiamide (Diagnostic)
Gadopentetate (Diagnostic)
Gadoteridol (Diagnostic)
Diagnostic aid, parkinsonism
Apomorphine (Systemic)
Diagnostic aid, pituitary function
Metyrapone (Systemic)
Diagnostic aid, placental reserve
Oxytocin (Systemic)
Diagnostic aid, platelet survival
Sodium Chromate Cr 51 (Diagnostic)
Diagnostic aid, pregnancy
Pregnancy Test Kits for Home Use
Diagnostic aid, primary hyperaldosteronism
Spironolactone (Systemic)
Diagnostic aid, radioactive, adrenomedullary disorders
Iobenguane, Radioiodinated (Diagnostic)
Diagnostic aid, radioactive, blood loss
Radioiodinated Albumin (Diagnostic)
Diagnostic aid, radioactive, bone disease
Technetium Tc 99m Medronate (Diagnostic)
Technetium Tc 99m Oxidronate (Diagnostic)
Technetium Tc 99m Pyrophosphate (Diagnostic)
Technetium Tc 99m (Pyro- and trimeta-) Phosphates (Diagnostic)
Diagnostic aid, radioactive, brain disorders
Fludeoxyglucose F 18 (Diagnostic)
Iofetamine I 123 (Diagnostic)
Sodium Pertechnetate Tc 99m (Diagnostic)
Technetium Tc 99m Exametazime (Diagnostic)
Diagnostic aid, radioactive, cardiac disease
Ammonia N 13 (Diagnostic)
Fludeoxyglucose F 18 (Diagnostic)
Rubidium Rb 82 (Diagnostic)
Technetium Tc 99m Albumin (Diagnostic)
Technetium Tc 99m Pyrophosphate (Diagnostic)

Diagnostic aid, radioactive, cardiac disease *(continued)*
Technetium Tc 99m (Pyro- and trimeta-) Phosphates (Diagnostic)
Technetium Tc 99m Sestamibi (Diagnostic)
Technetium Tc 99m Teboroxime (Diagnostic)
Diagnostic aid, radioactive, cardiac disorders
Sodium Pertechnetate Tc 99m (Diagnostic)
Diagnostic aid, radioactive, cerebral disorders
Technetium Tc 99m Gluceptate (Diagnostic)
Diagnostic aid, radioactive, cerebrospinal fluid flow disorders
Indium In 111 Pentetate (Diagnostic)
Technetium Tc 99m Pentetate (Diagnostic)
Diagnostic aid, radioactive, cerebrovascular disease
Ammonia N 13 (Diagnostic)
Iofetamine I 123 (Diagnostic)
Technetium Tc 99m Exametazime (Diagnostic)
Xenon Xe 133 (Diagnostic)
Diagnostic aid, radioactive, cyanocobalamin malabsorption syndromes
Cyanocobalamin Co 57 (Diagnostic)
Diagnostic aid, radioactive, extrahepatic malignant disease
Indium In 111 Satumomab Pendetide (Diagnostic)
Diagnostic aid, radioactive, focal inflammatory lesions
Gallium Citrate Ga 67 (Diagnostic)
Diagnostic aid, radioactive, gastroesophageal disorders
Technetium Tc 99m Sulfur Colloid (Diagnostic)
Diagnostic aid, radioactive, gastrointestinal bleeding
Technetium Tc 99m (Pyro- and trimeta-) Phosphates (Diagnostic)
Diagnostic aid, radioactive, gastrointestinal disorders
Sodium Pertechnetate Tc 99m (Diagnostic)
Technetium Tc 99m Sulfur Colloid (Diagnostic)
Diagnostic aid, radioactive, hepatic disease
Ammonia N 13 (Diagnostic)
Fludeoxyglucose F 18 (Diagnostic)
Technetium Tc 99m Sulfur Colloid (Diagnostic)
Diagnostic aid, radioactive, hepatobiliary disorders
Technetium Tc 99m Disofenin (Diagnostic)
Technetium Tc 99m Lidofenin (Diagnostic)
Technetium Tc 99m Mebrofenin (Diagnostic)
Diagnostic aid, radioactive, inflammatory lesions
Indium In 111 Oxyquinoline (Diagnostic)
Technetium Tc 99m Exametazime (Diagnostic)
Diagnostic aid, radioactive, intracranial lesions
Technetium Tc 99m Gluceptate (Diagnostic)
Technetium Tc 99m Pentetate (Diagnostic)
Diagnostic aid, radioactive, ischemic heart disease
Thallous Chloride Tl 201 (Diagnostic)
Diagnostic aid, radioactive, myocardial infarction
Thallous Chloride Tl 201 (Diagnostic)
Diagnostic aid, radioactive, nasolacrimal disorders
Sodium Pertechnetate Tc 99m (Diagnostic)
Diagnostic aid, radioactive, neoplastic disease
Fludeoxyglucose F 18 (Diagnostic)
Gallium Citrate Ga 67 (Diagnostic)

Diagnostic aid, radioactive, neuroendocrine tumors
Iobenguane, Radioiodinated (Diagnostic)
Diagnostic aid, radioactive, parathyroid disorders
Technetium Tc 99m Sestamibi (Diagnostic)
Thallous Chloride Tl 201 (Diagnostic)
Diagnostic aid, radioactive, pulmonary disease
Krypton Kr 81m (Diagnostic)
Technetium Tc 99m Albumin Aggregated (Diagnostic)
Technetium Tc 99m Pentetate (Diagnostic)
Xenon Xe 127 (Diagnostic)
Xenon Xe 133 (Diagnostic)
Diagnostic aid, radioactive, pulmonary emboli
Krypton Kr 81m (Diagnostic)
Diagnostic aid, radioactive, red blood cell disease
Sodium Chromate Cr 51 (Diagnostic)
Diagnostic aid, radioactive, renal disorders
Iodohippurate Sodium I 123 (Diagnostic)
Iodohippurate Sodium I 131 (Diagnostic)
Iothalamate Sodium I 125 (Diagnostic)
Technetium Tc 99m Gluceptate (Diagnostic)
Technetium Tc 99m Mertiatide (Diagnostic)
Technetium Tc 99m Pentetate (Diagnostic)
Technetium Tc 99m Succimer (Diagnostic)
Diagnostic aid, radioactive, salivary gland disorders
Sodium Pertechnetate Tc 99m (Diagnostic)
Diagnostic aid, radioactive, spleen disease
Sodium Chromate Cr 51(Diagnostic)
Technetium Tc 99m Sulfur Colloid (Diagnostic)
Diagnostic aid, radioactive, thrombosis
Indium In 111 Oxyquinoline (Diagnostic)
Diagnostic aid, radioactive, thyroid disorders
Fludeoxyglucose F 18 (Diagnostic)
Sodium Iodide I 123 (Diagnostic)
Sodium Iodide I 131 (Diagnostic)
Sodium Iodide I 131 (Therapeutic)
Sodium Pertechnetate Tc 99m (Diagnostic)
Technetium Tc 99m Sestamibi (Diagnostic)
Diagnostic aid, radioactive, urinary bladder disorders
Sodium Pertechnetate Tc 99m (Diagnostic)
Diagnostic aid, radioactive, urinary tract obstructions
Iodohippurate Sodium I 123 (Diagnostic)
Iodohippurate Sodium I 131 (Diagnostic)
Diagnostic aid, radioactive, vascular disorders
Sodium Pertechnetate Tc 99m (Diagnostic)
Diagnostic aid, radiography of the bowel
Simethicone (Oral)
Diagnostic aid, radiopaque, biliary tract disorders
Diatrizoates (Diagnostic)
Iodipamide (Diagnostic)
xol (Diagnostic)
Iopamidol (Diagnostic)
Iothalamate (Diagnostic)
Ioversol (Diagnostic)
Diagnostic aid, radiopaque, brain disorders
Diatrizoates (Diagnostic)
Iopamidol (Diagnostic)
Iothalamate (Diagnostic)
Ioxaglate (Diagnostic)
Metrizamide (Diagnostic)
Diagnostic aid, radiopaque, breast disease
Diatrizoates (Diagnostic)
Diagnostic aid, radiopaque, cardiac disease
Diatrizoates (Diagnostic)
Iohexol (Diagnostic)
Iopamidol (Diagnostic)
Iothalamate (Diagnostic)
Ioversol (Diagnostic)
Ioxaglate (Diagnostic)
Metrizamide (Diagnostic)
Diagnostic aid, radiopaque, central nervous system disorders
Iohexol (Diagnostic)
Iopamidol (Diagnostic)
Metrizamide (Diagnostic)
Diagnostic aid, radiopaque, cerebrospinal fluid disorders
Iohexol (Diagnostic)
Iopamidol (Diagnostic)
Metrizamide (Diagnostic)
Diagnostic aid, radiopaque contrast enhancer adjunct in computed tomography
Diatrizoates (Diagnostic)
Iohexol (Diagnostic)
Diagnostic aid, radiopaque contrast enhancer in computed tomography
Diatrizoates (Diagnostic)
Iohexol (Diagnostic)
Iopamidol (Diagnostic)
Iothalamate (Diagnostic)
Ioversol (Diagnostic)
Ioxaglate (Diagnostic)
Diagnostic aid, radiopaque, disk disease
Diatrizoates (Diagnostic)
Diagnostic aid, radiopaque, gallbladder disorders
Iocetamic Acid (Diagnostic)
Iodipamide (Diagnostic)
Iopanoic Acid (Diagnostic)
Ipodate (Diagnostic)
Tyropanoate (Diagnostic)
Diagnostic aid, radiopaque, gastrointestinal disorders
Barium Sulfate (Diagnostic)
Diatrizoates (Diagnostic)
Diagnostic aid, radiopaque, gastrointestinal tract disorders
Iohexol (Diagnostic)
Diagnostic aid, radiopaque, joint disease
Diatrizoates (Diagnostic)
Iohexol (Diagnostic)
Iopamidol (Diagnostic)
Iothalamate (Diagnostic)
Ioversol (Diagnostic)
Ioxaglate (Diagnostic)
Metrizamide (Diagnostic)
Diagnostic aid, radiopaque, pancreas disease
Iothalamate (Diagnostic)
Diagnostic aid, radiopaque, peritoneal disorders
Iohexol (Diagnostic)
Iopamidol (Diagnostic)
Ioversol (Diagnostic)
Diagnostic aid, radiopaque, pregnancy disorders
Diatrizoates (Diagnostic)
Diagnostic aid, radiopaque, sexual anomalies
Diatrizoate and Iodipamide (Diagnostic, Mucosal)
Diagnostic aid, radiopaque, spinal disease
Metrizamide (Diagnostic)
Diagnostic aid, radiopaque, splenic and portal vein disorders
Diatrizoates (Diagnostic)
Diagnostic aid, radiopaque, urinary tract disorders
Diatrizoates (Diagnostic)
Diatrizoates (Diagnostic, Mucosal)
Iohexol (Diagnostic)
Iohexol (Diagnostic, Mucosal)
Iopamidol (Diagnostic)
Iothalamate (Diagnostic)
Iothalamate (Diagnostic, Mucosal)
Ioversol (Diagnostic)
Ioxaglate (Diagnostic)
Metrizamide (Diagnostic)
Diagnostic aid, radiopaque, uterus and fallopian tube disorders
Diatrizoate and Iodipamide (Diagnostic, Mucosal)
Diatrizoates (Diagnostic, Mucosal)
Iohexol (Diagnostic, Mucosal)
Ioxaglate (Diagnostic, Mucosal)
Diagnostic aid, radiopaque, vascular disease
Diatrizoates (Diagnostic)
Iohexol (Diagnostic)
Iopamidol (Diagnostic)
Iothalamate (Diagnostic)
Ioversol (Diagnostic)
Ioxaglate (Diagnostic)
Metrizamide (Diagnostic)
Diagnostic aid, renal function
Inulin (Diagnostic)
Phenolsulfonphthalein (Diagnostic)
Diagnostic aid, renal tubular acidosis
Fludrocortisone (Systemic)
Diagnostic aid, residual bladder urine
Phenolsulfonphthalein (Diagnostic)
Diagnostic aid, thyroid function
Levothyroxine (Systemic)
Liothyronine (Systemic)
Thyrotropin (Systemic)
Diagnostic aid, urinary tract infection
Urinary Tract Infection Test Kits for Home Use
Diagnostic aid, utero-placental insufficiency
Oxytocin (Systemic)
Diagnostic aid, vitamin deficiency
Cyanocobalamin (Systemic)
Hydroxocobalamin (Systemic)
Dietary supplement
Magnesium Chloride (Systemic)
Magnesium Citrate (Systemic)
Magnesium Gluceptate (Systemic)
Magnesium Gluconate (Systemic)
Magnesium Hydroxide (Systemic)
Magnesium Lactate (Systemic)
Magnesium Oxide (Systemic)
Magnesium Pidolate (Systemic)
Magnesium Sulfate (Systemic)
Digestant
Pancrelipase (Systemic)
Digestant-anticholinergic-sedative
Pancreatin, Pepsin, Bile Salts, Hyoscyamine, Atropine, Scopolamine, and Phenobarbital (Systemic)
Diuretic
Amiloride (Systemic)
Amiloride and Hydrochlorothiazide (Systemic)
Bendroflumethiazide (Systemic)
Benzthiazide (Systemic)
Bumetanide (Systemic)
Chlorothiazide (Systemic)
Chlorthalidone (Systemic)
Cyclothiazide (Systemic)
Ethacrynic Acid (Systemic)
Furosemide (Systemic)
Glycerin (Systemic)
Hydrochlorothiazide (Systemic)
Hydroflumethiazide (Systemic)
Indapamide (Systemic)
Methyclothiazide (Systemic)
Metolazone (Systemic)
Polythiazide (Systemic)
Quinethazone (Systemic)
Spironolactone (Systemic)
Spironolactone and Hydrochlorothiazide (Systemic)
Triamterene (Systemic)
Triamterene and Hydrochlorothiazide (Systemic)
Trichlormethiazide (Systemic)

Diuretic, syndrome of inappropriate antidiuretic hormone
 Demeclocycline (Systemic)
Diuretic, urinary alkalinizing
 Acetazolamide (Systemic)
Dopamine agonist
 Bromocriptine (Systemic)
Dopaminergic blocking agent
 Metoclopramide (Systemic)
Drying agent, topical
 Carbol-Fuchsin (Topical)
Duchenne muscular dystrophy therapy adjunct
 Dantrolene (Systemic)

E–L

Electrolyte replenisher
 Calcium Chloride (Systemic)
 Calcium Glubionate (Systemic)
 Calcium Gluceptate (Systemic)
 Calcium Gluconate (Systemic)
 Dextrose and Electrolytes (Systemic)
 Magnesium Chloride (Systemic)
 Magnesium Sulfate (Systemic)
 Oral Rehydration Salts (Systemic)
 Potassium Acetate (Systemic)
 Potassium Bicarbonate (Systemic)
 Potassium Bicarbonate and Potassium Chloride (Systemic)
 Potassium Bicarbonate and Potassium Citrate (Systemic)
 Potassium Chloride (Systemic)
 Potassium Chloride, Potassium Bicarbonate, and Potassium Citrate (Systemic)
 Potassium Gluconate (Systemic)
 Potassium Gluconate and Potassium Chloride (Systemic)
 Potassium Gluconate and Potassium Citrate (Systemic)
 Potassium Phosphates (Systemic)
 Potassium and Sodium Phosphates (Systemic)
 Rice Syrup Solids and Electrolytes (Systemic)
 Sodium Bicarbonate (Systemic)
 Sodium Phosphates (Systemic)
 Trikates (Systemic)
Emetic
 Apomorphine (Systemic)
 Ipecac (Oral)
Enzyme, adenosine deaminase, replenisher
 Pegademase (Systemic)
Enzyme, glucocerebrosidase, replenisher
 Alglucerase (Systemic)
Enzyme, pancreatic, replenisher
 Pancrelipase (Systemic)
Estrogen-progestin
 Desogestrel and Ethinyl Estradiol (Systemic)
 Ethynodiol Diacetate and Ethinyl Estradiol (Systemic)
 Levonorgestrel and Ethinyl Estradiol (Systemic)
 Norethindrone Acetate and Ethinyl Estradiol (Systemic)
 Norethindrone and Ethinyl Estradiol (Systemic)
 Norethindrone and Mestranol (Systemic)
 Norgestimate and Ethinyl Estradiol (Systemic)
 Norgestrel and Ethinyl Estradiol (Systemic)
Estrogen, systemic
 Chlorotrianisene (Systemic)
 Diethylstilbestrol (Systemic)
 Estradiol (Systemic)
 Estrogens, Conjugated (Systemic)
 Estrogens, Esterified (Systemic)
Estrogen, systemic *(continued)*
 Estrone (Systemic)
 Estropipate (Systemic)
 Ethinyl Estradiol (Systemic)
 Quinestrol (Systemic)
Estrogen, vaginal
 Dienestrol (Vaginal)
 Estradiol (Vaginal)
 Estrogens, Conjugated (Vaginal)
 Estrone (Vaginal)
 Estropipate (Vaginal)
Evacuant, bowel
 Polyethylene Glycol and Electrolytes (Local)
Expectorant
 Guaifenesin (Systemic)
Familial Mediterranean fever suppressant
 Colchicine (Systemic)
Gastric acid pump inhibitor
 Omeprazole (Systemic)
Gastric acid secretion inhibitor
 Cimetidine (Systemic)
 Famotidine (Systemic)
 Nizatidine (Systemic)
 Ranitidine (Systemic)
Gastric mucosa protectant
 Misoprostol (Systemic)
 Sucralfate (Oral)
Gastrointestinal emptying, delayed, adjunct
 Cisapride (Systemic)
 Metoclopramide (Systemic)
Gonadotropic principle
 Clomiphene (Systemic)
Gonadotropin
 Chorionic Gonadotropin (Systemic)
 Menotropins (Systemic)
 Urofollitropin (Systemic)
Gonadotropin inhibitor
 Danazol (Systemic)
 Nafarelin (Systemic)
Gonadotropin-releasing hormone (GnRH) agonist
 Leuprolide (Systemic)
Gonadotropin-releasing hormone (GnRH) analog
 Nafarelin (Systemic)
Gonad-stimulating principle
 Gonadorelin (Systemic)
Granulopoietic
 Lithium (Systemic)
Growth hormone
 Somatrem (Systemic)
 Somatropin (Systemic)
Growth hormone suppressant, acromegaly
 Bromocriptine (Systemic)
 Octreotide (Systemic)
Hair growth stimulant, alopecia androgenetica, topical
 Minoxidil (Topical)
Hair growth stimulant, alopecia areata, systemic
 Methoxsalen (Systemic)
Hair growth stimulant, alopecia areata, topical
 Anthralin (Topical)
 Methoxsalen (Topical)
Headache, tension, prophylactic
 Isocarboxazid (Systemic)
 Phenelzine (Systemic)
 Tranylcypromine (Systemic)
Headache, vascular, prophylactic
 Isocarboxazid (Systemic)
 Phenelzine (Systemic)
 Tranylcypromine (Systemic)
Hematopoietic stimulant
 Filgrastim (Systemic)
 Sargramostim (Systemic)
Hemorrhagic cystitis prophylactic
 Mesna (Systemic)
Hepatic encephalopathy therapy adjunct
 Kanamycin (Oral)
 Neomycin (Oral)
Histamine H_2-receptor antagonist
 Cimetidine (Systemic)
 Famotidine (Systemic)
 Nizatidine (Systemic)
 Ranitidine (Systemic)
HMG-CoA reductase inhibitor
 Lovastatin (Systemic)
 Pravastatin (Systemic)
 Simvastatin (Systemic)
Hormone-like agent for treatment of premature puberty
 Leuprolide (Systemic)
 Nafarelin (Systemic)
Hormone, for treatment in infertility
 Gonadorelin (Systemic)
Hydrocholeretic
 Dehydrocholic Acid (Oral)
Hypertrophic cardiomyopathy therapy adjunct
 Acebutolol (Systemic)
 Atenolol (Systemic)
 Metoprolol (Systemic)
 Nadolol (Systemic)
 Oxprenolol (Systemic)
 Pindolol (Systemic)
 Propranolol (Systemic)
 Sotalol (Systemic)
 Timolol (Systemic)
 Verapamil (Systemic)
Immunizing agent, active
 Diphtheria and Tetanus Toxoids and Pertussis Vaccine Adsorbed (Systemic)
 Haemophilus b Conjugate Vaccine (Systemic)
 Haemophilus b Polysaccharide Vaccine (Systemic)
 Hepatitis B Vaccine Recombinant (Systemic)
 Influenza Virus Vaccine (Systemic)
 Japanese Encephalitis Virus Vaccine (Systemic)
 Measles Virus Vaccine Live (Systemic)
 Meningococcal Polysaccharide Vaccine (Systemic)
 Mumps Virus Vaccine Live (Systemic)
 Pneumococcal Vaccine Polyvalent (Systemic)
 Poliovirus Vaccine (Systemic)
 Rubella Virus Vaccine Live (Systemic)
 Tetanus Toxoid (Systemic)
 Typhoid Vaccine Live Oral (Systemic)
Immunizing agent, passive
 Immune Globulin Intravenous (Human) (Systemic)
Immunomodulator
 Interferon, Gamma (Systemic)
Immunosuppressant
 Azathioprine (Systemic)
 Betamethasone—Glucocorticoid Effects (Systemic)
 Chlorambucil (Systemic)
 Corticotropin—Glucocorticoid Effects (Systemic)
 Cortisone—Glucocorticoid Effects (Systemic)
 Cyclophosphamide (Systemic)
 Cyclosporine (Systemic)
 Dexamethasone—Glucocorticoid Effects (Systemic)
 Hydrocortisone—Glucocorticoid Effects (Systemic)
 Mercaptopurine (Systemic)
 Methylprednisolone—Glucocorticoid Effects (Systemic)
 Muromonab-CD3 (Systemic)

Immunosuppressant *(continued)*
Paramethasone—Glucocorticoid Effects (Systemic)
Prednisolone—Glucocorticoid Effects (Systemic)
Prednisone—Glucocorticoid Effects (Systemic)
Triamcinolone—Glucocorticoid Effects (Systemic)
Impotence therapy
Alprostadil (Intracavernosal)
Papaverine (Intracavernosal)
Impotence therapy adjunct
Phentolamine and Papaverine (Intracavernosal)
Impotence therapy agent
Yohimbine (Systemic)
Infertility therapy adjunct
Bromocriptine (Systemic)
Chorionic Gonadotropin (Systemic)
Clomiphene (Systemic)
Menotropins (Systemic)
Urofollitropin (Systemic)
Inflammatory bowel disease suppressant
Mesalamine (Rectal)
Iodine replenisher
Iodine, Strong (Systemic)
Potassium Iodide (Systemic)
Keratinization stabilizer
Isotretinoin (Systemic)
Keratolytic, topical
Benzoyl Peroxide (Topical)
Coal Tar (Topical)
Resorcinol (Topical)
Resorcinol and Sulfur (Topical)
Salicylic Acid (Topical)
Salicylic Acid and Sulfur (Topical)
Salicylic Acid, Sulfur, and Coal Tar (Topical)
Sulfur (Topical)
Sulfurated Lime (Topical)
Tretinoin (Topical)
Labor, premature, inhibitor
Isoxsuprine (Systemic)
Terbutaline (Oral/Injection)
Lactation inhibitor
Bromocriptine (Systemic)
Lactation stimulant
Oxytocin (Systemic)
Laxative, bulk-forming
Calcium Polycarbophil (Oral)
Malt Soup Extract (Oral)
Malt Soup Extract and Psyllium (Oral)
Methylcellulose (Oral)
Polycarbophil (Oral)
Psyllium (Oral)
Psyllium Hydrophilic Mucilloid (Oral)
Psyllium Hydrophilic Mucilloid and Carboxymethylcellulose (Oral)
Laxative, bulk-forming and stimulant
Psyllium Hydrophilic Mucilloid and Senna (Oral)
Psyllium Hydrophilic Mucilloid and Sennosides (Oral)
Psyllium and Senna (Oral)
Laxative, bulk-forming, stimulant, and stool softener (emollient)
Carboxymethylcellulose, Casanthranol, and Docusate (Oral)
Laxative, bulk-forming and stool softener (emollient)
Carboxymethylcellulose and Docusate (Oral)
Laxative, carbon dioxide–releasing
Potassium Bitartrate and Sodium Bicarbonate (Rectal)
Laxative, hyperosmotic
Glycerin (Rectal)
Sodium Phosphates (Rectal)
Laxative, hyperosmotic, lactulose
Lactulose (Oral)
Laxative, hyperosmotic and lubricant
Milk of Magnesia and Mineral Oil (Oral)
Milk of Magnesia, Mineral Oil, and Glycerin (Oral)
Laxative, hyperosmotic, lubricant, and stimulant
Mineral Oil, Glycerin, and Phenolphthalein (Oral)
Laxative, hyperosmotic, saline
Magnesium Citrate (Oral)
Magnesium Hydroxide (Oral)
Magnesium Oxide (Oral)
Magnesium Sulfate (Oral)
Sodium Phosphate (Oral)
Laxative, lubricant
Mineral Oil (Oral)
Mineral Oil (Rectal)
Laxative, lubricant and stimulant
Mineral Oil and Cascara Sagrada (Oral)
Mineral Oil and Phenolphthalein (Oral)
Laxative, stimulant
Bisacodyl (Rectal)
Senna (Rectal)
Laxative, stimulant or contact
Bisacodyl (Oral)
Casanthranol (Oral)
Cascara Sagrada (Oral)
Cascara Sagrada and Aloe (Oral)
Cascara Sagrada and Phenolphthalein (Oral)
Castor Oil (Oral)
Dehydrocholic Acid (Oral)
Phenolphthalein (Oral)
Senna (Oral)
Sennosides (Oral)
Laxative, stimulant and stool softener (emollient)
Bisacodyl and Docusate (Oral)
Casanthranol and Docusate (Oral)
Danthron and Docusate (Oral)
Dehydrocholic Acid and Docusate (Oral)
Dehydrocholic Acid, Docusate, and Phenolphthalein (Oral)
Docusate and Phenolphthalein (Oral)
Senna and Docusate (Oral)
Laxative, stool softener (emollient)
Docusate (Oral)
Docusate (Rectal)
Poloxamer 188 (Oral)
Lubricant, ophthalmic
Hydroxypropyl Methylcellulose (Ophthalmic)
Lupus erythematosus suppressant
Azathioprine (Systemic)
Chloroquine (Systemic)
Hydroxychloroquine (Systemic)

M–S

Malignant hyperthermia therapy adjunct
Dantrolene (Systemic)
Mast cell stabilizer
Cromolyn (Inhalation)
Cromolyn (Oral)
Mast cell stabilizer, nasal
Cromolyn (Nasal)
Mast cell stabilizer, ophthalmic
Cromolyn (Ophthalmic)
Menopausal syndrome therapy adjunct
Clonidine (Systemic)
Methemoglobinemia (idiopathic) therapy adjunct
Ascorbic Acid (Systemic)
Migraine headache preventive
Pizotyline (Systemic)
Miosis inhibitor, in ophthalmic surgery
Diclofenac (Ophthalmic)
Flurbiprofen (Ophthalmic)
Indomethacin (Ophthalmic)
Suprofen (Ophthalmic)
Miotic
Carbachol (Ophthalmic)
Physostigmine (Ophthalmic)
Pilocarpine (Ophthalmic)
Monoclonal antibody
Muromonab-CD3 (Systemic)
Mucolytic
Acetylcysteine (Inhalation)
Iodinated Glycerol (Systemic)
Muscle phosphorylase deficiency therapy adjunct
Dantrolene (Systemic)
Mydriatic
Atropine (Ophthalmic)
Cyclopentolate (Ophthalmic)
Homatropine (Ophthalmic)
Phenylephrine (Ophthalmic)
Scopolamine (Ophthalmic)
Tropicamide (Ophthalmic)
Myocardial infarction prophylactic
Acebutolol (Systemic)
Aspirin (Systemic)
Aspirin, Buffered (Systemic)
Aspirin and Caffeine (Systemic)
Aspirin and Caffeine, Buffered (Systemic)
Atenolol (Systemic)
Metoprolol (Systemic)
Nadolol (Systemic)
Oxprenolol (Systemic)
Propranolol (Systemic)
Sotalol (Systemic)
Timolol (Systemic)
Myocardial infarction therapy
Acebutolol (Systemic)
Atenolol (Systemic)
Metoprolol (Systemic)
Nadolol (Systemic)
Oxprenolol (Systemic)
Propranolol (Systemic)
Sotalol (Systemic)
Timolol (Systemic)
Myocardial reinfarction prophylactic
Aspirin (Systemic)
Aspirin, Buffered (Systemic)
Aspirin and Caffeine (Systemic)
Aspirin and Caffeine, Buffered (Systemic)
Metoprolol (Systemic)
Myocardial reinfarction prophylactic adjunct
Dipyridamole (Systemic)
Neuroleptic-induced akathisia therapy
Betaxolol (Systemic)
Metoprolol (Systemic)
Nadolol (Systemic)
Propranolol (Systemic)
Neuroleptic malignant syndrome therapy
Bromocriptine (Systemic)
Neuroleptic malignant syndrome therapy adjunct
Dantrolene (Systemic)
Neuromuscular blocking agent
Atracurium (Systemic)
Gallamine (Systemic)
Metocurine (Systemic)
Pancuronium (Systemic)
Succinylcholine (Systemic)
Tubocurarine (Systemic)
Vecuronium (Systemic)
Neuromuscular blocking agent, ophthalmic
Botulinum Toxin Type A (Parenteral-Local)

Nutritional replacement
  Enteral Nutrition Formulas (Systemic)
  Infant Formulas (Systemic)
Nutritional supplement
  Levocarnitine (Systemic)
  Sodium Fluoride (Systemic)
Nutritional supplement, fatty acid
  Fat Emulsions (Systemic)
Nutritional supplement, mineral
  Ammonium Molybdate (Systemic)
  Calcium Carbonate (Systemic)
  Calcium Citrate (Systemic)
  Calcium Glubionate (Systemic)
  Calcium Gluceptate and Calcium Gluconate (Systemic)
  Calcium Gluconate (Systemic)
  Calcium Lactate (Systemic)
  Calcium Lactate-Gluconate and Calcium Carbonate (Systemic)
  Calcium Phosphate, Dibasic (Systemic)
  Calcium Phosphate, Tribasic (Systemic)
  Chromic Chloride (Systemic)
  Chromium (Systemic)
  Copper Gluconate (Systemic)
  Copper Sulfate (Systemic)
  Manganese Gluconate (Systemic)
  Manganese Sulfate (Systemic)
  Selenious Acid (Systemic)
  Selenium (Systemic)
  Sodium Iodide (Systemic)
  Zinc (Systemic)
Nutritional supplement, vitamin
  Ascorbic Acid (Systemic)
  Beta-carotene (Systemic)
  Biotin (Systemic)
  Calcifediol (Systemic)
  Calcitriol (Systemic)
  Calcium Pantothenate (Systemic)
  Cyanocobalamin (Systemic)
  Ergocalciferol (Systemic)
  Folic Acid (Vitamin B_9) (Systemic)
  Hydroxocobalamin (Systemic)
  Niacin (Vitamin B_3) (Systemic)
  Niacinamide (Systemic)
  Pantothenic Acid (Vitamin B_5) (Systemic)
  Pyridoxine (Vitamin B_6) (Systemic)
  Riboflavin (Vitamin B_2) (Systemic)
  Thiamine (Vitamin B_1) (Systemic)
  Vitamin A (Systemic)
  Vitamin E (Systemic)
Nutritional supplement, vitamin, prothrombogenic
  Menadiol (Systemic)
  Phytonadione (Systemic)
Opioid (narcotic) abuse therapy adjunct
  Naltrexone (Systemic)
Opioid (narcotic) antagonist
  Naltrexone (Systemic)
Opioid withdrawal syndrome suppressant
  Clonidine (Systemic)
Osmotic agent, meconium ileus
  Diatrizoates (Diagnostic)
Osteoporosis prophylactic
  Diethylstilbestrol (Systemic)
  Estradiol (Systemic)
  Estrogens, Conjugated (Systemic)
  Estrogens, Esterified (Systemic)
  Estropipate (Systemic)
  Ethinyl Estradiol (Systemic)
Osteoporosis therapy adjunct
  Calcitonin-Human (Systemic)
  Calcitonin-Salmon (Systemic)
Oxytocic
  Carboprost (Systemic)
  Dinoprostone (Cervical/Vaginal)
  Oxytocin (Systemic)

Parkinsonism therapy adjunct
  Orphenadrine (Systemic)
Pediculicide
  Lindane (Topical)
  Malathion (Topical)
  Permethrin (Topical)
  Pyrethrins and Piperonyl Butoxide (Topical)
Peristaltic stimulant
  Metoclopramide (Systemic)
Pheochromocytoma therapy adjunct
  Acebutolol (Systemic)
  Atenolol (Systemic)
  Labetalol (Systemic)
  Metoprolol (Systemic)
  Nadolol (Systemic)
  Oxprenolol (Systemic)
  Propranolol (Systemic)
  Sotalol (Systemic)
  Timolol (Systemic)
Photosensitivity suppressant, erythropoietic protoporphyria
  Beta-carotene—For Photosensitivity (Systemic)
Pituitary, anterior, hormone
  Corticotropin—Glucocorticoid Effects (Systemic)
Pituitary, posterior, hormone
  Vasopressin (Systemic)
Platelet aggregation inhibitor
  Aspirin (Systemic)
  Aspirin, Buffered (Systemic)
  Aspirin and Caffeine (Systemic)
  Aspirin and Caffeine, Buffered (Systemic)
  Aspirin, Sodium Bicarbonate, and Citric Acid (Systemic)
  Dipyridamole (Systemic)
  Dipyridamole and Aspirin (Systemic)
  Ticlopidine (Systemic)
Platelet count stimulator, systemic
  Immune Globulin Intravenous (Human) (Systemic)
Polymorphous light eruption suppressant
  Beta-carotene—For Photosensitivity (Systemic)
  Chloroquine (Systemic)
  Hydroxychloroquine (Systemic)
Porphyria cutanea tarda suppressant
  Chloroquine (Systemic)
  Hydroxychloroquine (Systemic)
Priapism reversal agent
  Epinephrine (Oral/Injection)
Progestin
  Hydroxyprogesterone (Systemic)
  Levonorgestrel (Systemic)
  Medroxyprogesterone (Systemic)
  Norethindrone (Systemic)
  Norgestrel (Systemic)
  Progesterone (Systemic)
Prostaglandin
  Dinoprostone (Cervical/Vaginal)
Prostaglandin synthesis inhibitor
  Diclofenac (Ophthalmic)
  Flurbiprofen (Ophthalmic)
  Indomethacin (Ophthalmic)
  Suprofen (Ophthalmic)
Prostaglandin synthesis inhibitor, renal (Bartter's syndrome)
  Indomethacin (Systemic)
Protectant, ophthalmic
  Carboxymethylcellulose (Ophthalmic)
  Hydroxypropyl Cellulose (Ophthalmic)
  Hydroxypropyl Methylcellulose (Ophthalmic)
Pulmonary edema therapy adjunct
  Morphine (Systemic)

Radiation protectant, thyroid gland
  Iodine, Strong (Systemic)
  Potassium Iodide (Systemic)
Repigmenting agent, systemic
  Methoxsalen (Systemic)
  Trioxsalen (Systemic)
Repigmenting agent, topical
  Methoxsalen (Topical)
Respiratory stimulant adjunct
  Caffeine (Systemic)
  Caffeine, Citrated (Systemic)
Scabicide
  Crotamiton (Topical)
  Lindane (Topical)
  Permethrin (Topical)
  Sulfur (Topical)
  Sulfurated Lime (Topical)
Sedative-hypnotic
  Alprazolam (Systemic)
  Amobarbital (Systemic)
  Aprobarbital (Systemic)
  Bromazepam (Systemic)
  Butabarbital (Systemic)
  Chloral Hydrate (Systemic)
  Chlordiazepoxide (Systemic)
  Clorazepate (Systemic)
  Diazepam (Systemic)
  Diphenhydramine (Systemic)
  Doxylamine (Systemic)
  Estazolam (Systemic)
  Ethchlorvynol (Systemic)
  Ethinamate (Systemic)
  Flurazepam (Systemic)
  Glutethimide (Systemic)
  Halazepam (Systemic)
  Ketazolam (Systemic)
  Lorazepam (Systemic)
  Methyprylon (Systemic)
  Midazolam (Systemic)
  Nitrazepam (Systemic)
  Oxazepam (Systemic)
  Pentobarbital (Systemic)
  Phenobarbital (Systemic)
  Prazepam (Systemic)
  Promethazine (Systemic)
  Propiomazine (Systemic)
  Propofol (Systemic)
  Quazepam (Systemic)
  Secobarbital (Systemic)
  Temazepam (Systemic)
  Triazolam (Systemic)
  Trimeprazine (Systemic)
  Zolpidem (Systemic)
Sedative, preoperative
  Methotrimeprazine (Systemic)
Senility symptoms treatment adjunct
  Isoxsuprine (Systemic)
Sexually transmitted disease prophylactic
  Condoms
Skeletal muscle relaxant
  Carisoprodol (Systemic)
  Chlorphenesin (Systemic)
  Chlorzoxazone (Systemic)
  Cyclobenzaprine (Systemic)
  Metaxalone (Systemic)
  Methocarbamol (Systemic)
  Orphenadrine (Systemic)
  Phenytoin (Systemic)
Skeletal muscle relaxant adjunct
  Diazepam (Systemic)
  Lorazepam (Systemic)
Smoking cessation adjunct
  Nicotine (Systemic)
Solubilizing agent, cholesterol
  Monooctanoin (Local)

Stimulant, central nervous system
- Amphetamine (Systemic)
- Amphetamine and Dextroamphetamine Resin Complex (Systemic)
- Caffeine (Systemic)
- Caffeine, Citrated (Systemic)
- Dextroamphetamine (Systemic)
- Ephedrine (Oral/Injection)
- Methamphetamine (Systemic)
- Methylphenidate (Systemic)
- Pemoline (Systemic)

Stimulant, respiratory
- Aminophylline (Systemic)
- Theophylline (Systemic)

Stomach and intestine stimulant
- Domperidone (Systemic)

Subarachnoid hemorrhage therapy
- Flunarizine (Systemic)
- Nicardipine (Systemic)
- Nimodipine (Systemic)

Suppressant, narcotic abstinence syndrome
- Methadone (Systemic)
- Opium Tincture (Systemic)

Surgical aid
- Epinephrine (Ophthalmic)

Surgical aid, antihemorrhagic
- Epinephrine (Oral/Injection)

Surgical aid, decongestant
- Epinephrine (Oral/Injection)

Surgical aid, mydriatic
- Epinephrine (Oral/Injection)

Sympathomimetic (adrenergic) agent
- Phenylpropanolamine (Systemic)

T–Z

Tears, artificial
- Carboxymethylcellulose (Ophthalmic)
- Hydroxypropyl Cellulose (Ophthalmic)
- Hydroxypropyl Methylcellulose (Ophthalmic)

Thrombolytic
- Alteplase, Recombinant (Systemic)
- Anistreplase (Systemic)
- Streptokinase (Systemic)
- Urokinase (Systemic)

Thrombosis prophylaxis adjunct
- Dihydroergotamine (Systemic)

Thyroid hormone
- Levothyroxine (Systemic)
- Liothyronine (Systemic)
- Liotrix (Systemic)
- Thyroglobulin (Systemic)
- Thyroid (Systemic)

Thyroid inhibitor
- Potassium Iodide (Systemic)

Thyrotoxicosis therapy adjunct
- Acebutolol (Systemic)
- Atenolol (Systemic)
- Metoprolol (Systemic)
- Nadolol (Systemic)
- Oxprenolol (Systemic)
- Propranolol (Systemic)
- Sotalol (Systemic)
- Timolol (Systemic)

Thyrotropic hormone
- Thyrotropin (Systemic)

Tocolytic
- Ritodrine (Systemic)

Urinary tract infection treatment adjunct
- Acetohydroxamic Acid (Systemic)

Urticaria therapy adjunct
- Cimetidine (Systemic)
- Ephedrine (Oral/Injection)

Uterine stimulant
- Dinoprost (Intra-amniotic)
- Dinoprostone (Cervical/Vaginal)
- Ergonovine (Systemic)
- Methylergonovine (Systemic)

Vascular headache prophylactic
- Atenolol (Systemic)
- Clonidine (Systemic)
- Ergotamine, Belladonna Alkaloids, and Phenobarbital (Systemic)
- Fenoprofen (Systemic)
- Flunarizine (Systemic)
- Ibuprofen (Systemic)
- Indomethacin (Systemic)
- Lithium (Systemic)
- Mefenamic Acid (Systemic)
- Methysergide (Systemic)
- Metoprolol (Systemic)
- Nadolol (Systemic)
- Naproxen (Systemic)
- Propranolol (Systemic)
- Timolol (Systemic)
- Verapamil (Systemic)

Vascular headache suppressant
- Cyproheptadine (Systemic)
- Diflunisal (Systemic)
- Dihydroergotamine (Systemic)
- Ergotamine (Systemic)
- Ergotamine and Caffeine (Systemic)
- Ergotamine, Caffeine, and Belladonna Alkaloids (Systemic)
- Ergotamine, Caffeine, Belladonna Alkaloids, and Pentobarbital (Systemic)
- Ergotamine, Caffeine, and Cyclizine (Systemic)
- Ergotamine, Caffeine, and Dimenhydrinate (Systemic)
- Ergotamine, Caffeine, and Diphenhydramine (Systemic)

Vascular headache suppressant *(continued)*
- Etodolac (Systemic)
- Fenoprofen (Systemic)
- Floctafenine (Systemic)
- Ibuprofen (Systemic)
- Indomethacin (Systemic)
- Ketoprofen (Systemic)
- Meclofenamate (Systemic)
- Mefenamic Acid (Systemic)
- Naproxen (Systemic)

Vascular headache suppressant, migraine
- Isometheptene, Dichloralphenazone, and Acetaminophen (Systemic)

Vasodilator
- Papaverine (Systemic)

Vasodilator, congestive heart failure
- Benazepril (Systemic)
- Captopril (Systemic)
- Captopril and Hydrochlorothiazide (Systemic)
- Enalapril (Systemic)
- Enalapril and Hydrochlorothiazide (Systemic)
- Erythrityl Tetranitrate—Oral (Systemic)
- Erythrityl Tetranitrate—Sublingual, Chewable, or Buccal (Systemic)
- Hydralazine (Systemic)
- Isosorbide Dinitrate—Oral (Systemic)
- Isosorbide Dinitrate—Sublingual, Chewable, or Buccal (Systemic)
- Lisinopril (Systemic)
- Lisinopril and Hydrochlorothiazide (Systemic)
- Nitroglycerin—Lingual Aerosol (Systemic)
- Nitroglycerin—Oral (Systemic)
- Nitroglycerin—Sublingual, Chewable, or Buccal (Systemic)
- Nitroglycerin—Topical (Systemic)
- Pentaerythritol Tetranitrate—Oral (Systemic)
- Prazosin (Systemic)
- Quinapril (Systemic)
- Ramipril (Systemic)

Vasopressor
- Ephedrine (Oral/Injection)
- Epinephrine (Oral/Injection)

Vasospastic therapy adjunct
- Deserpidine (Systemic)
- Isoxsuprine (Systemic)
- Nicotinyl Alcohol (Systemic)
- Nylidrin (Systemic)
- Prazosin (Systemic)
- Rauwolfia Serpentina (Systemic)
- Reserpine (Systemic)

Vitamin replenisher–dental caries prophylactic
- Vitamins and Fluoride (Systemic)

VI

Appendix VI

THE MEDICINE CHART

The Medicine Chart presents photographs of the most frequently prescribed medicines in the United States. In general, commonly used brand name products and a representative sampling of generic products have been included. The pictorial listing is not intended to be inclusive and does not represent all products on the market. Only selected solid oral dosage forms (capsules and tablets) have been included. The inclusion of a product does not mean the USPC has any particular knowledge that the product included has properties different from other products, nor should it be interpreted as an endorsement by USPC. Similarly, the fact that a particular product has not been included does not indicate that the product has been judged by the USPC to be unsatisfactory or unacceptable.

The drug products in *The Medicine Chart* are listed alphabetically by generic name of active ingredient(s). To quickly locate a particular medicine, check the product listing index that follows. This listing provides brand and generic names and directs the user to the appropriate page and chart location. In addition, any identifying code found on the surface of a capsule or tablet that might be useful in making a correct identification is included in the parentheses that follow the product's index entry. Please note that these codes may change as manufacturers reformulate or redesign their products. In addition, some companies may not manufacture all of their own products. In some of these cases, the imprinting on the tablet or capsule may be that of the actual manufacturer and not of the company marketing the product.

An inverted cross-index has also been included to help identify products by their identifying codes. These codes may not be unique to a given product; they are intended for use in initial identification only. In this cross-index, the codes are listed first in alpha-numeric order, accompanied by their generic or brand names and page and chart location.

Brand names are in *italics*. An asterisk next to the generic name of the active ingredient(s) indicates that the solid oral dosage forms containing the ingredient(s) are available only from a single source with no generic equivalents currently available in the U.S. Where multiple source products are shown, it must be kept in mind that other products may also be available.

The size and color of the products shown are intended to match the actual product as closely as possible; however, there may be some differences due to variations caused by the photographic process. Also, manufacturers may occasionally change the color, imprinting, or shape of their products, and for a period of time both the "old" and the newly changed dosage form may be on the market. Such changes may not occur uniformly thoughout the different dosages of the product. These types of changes will be incorporated in subsequent versions of the chart as they are brought to our attention.

Use of this chart is limited to serving as an initial guide in identifying drug products. The identity of a product should be verified further before any action is taken.

*In thousands of units of lipase/amylase/protease, respectively.

INVERTED CROSS-INDEX

DAN 5682—Schein/Danbury Triamterene and Hydrochlorothiazide Tablets 75/50 mg........... MC-24, A2
DAN 5693—Schein/Danbury Prazosin Capsules 5 mg.. MC-19, B6
DAN 5696—Schein/Danbury Prazosin Capsules 2 mg.. MC-19, B6
DAN 5697—Schein/Danbury Prazosin Capsules 1 mg.. MC-19, B6
DAN 5708—Schein/Danbury Clindamycin Capsules 150 mg...................................... MC-5, C6
DAN 5730—Schein/Danbury Baclofen Tablets 10 mg... MC-2, D7
DAN 5731—Schein/Danbury Baclofen Tablets 20 mg... MC-2, D7
DAN 5782—Schein/Danbury Atenolol and Chlorthalidone Tablets 50/25 mg.................. MC-2, C3
DAN 5783—Schein/Danbury Atenolol and Chlorthalidone Tablets 100/25 mg.................MC-2, C3
DF—*Hytrin* Tablets 1 mg.............................. MC-22, A3
DH—*Hytrin* Tablets 2 mg.............................. MC-22, A3
DI—*Hytrin* Tablets 10 mg............................. MC-22, A3
DJ—*Hytrin* Tablets 5 mg.............................. MC-22, A3
dp 25—*Levoxine* Tablets 0.025 mg.................... MC-13, B2
dp 50—*Levoxine* Tablets 0.05 mg..................... MC-13, B2
dp 75—*Levoxine* Tablets 0.075 mg.................... MC-13, B2
dp 88—*Levoxine* Tablets 0.088 mg.................... MC-13, B2
dp 100—*Levoxine* Tablets 0.1 mg..................... MC-13, B2
dp 112—*Levoxine* Tablets 0.112 mg................... MC-13, B3
dp 125—*Levoxine* Tablets 0.125 mg................... MC-13, B3
dp 150—*Levoxine* Tablets 0.15 mg.................... MC-13, B3
dp 175—*Levoxine* Tablets 0.175 mg................... MC-13, B3
dp 200—*Levoxine* Tablets 0.2 mg..................... MC-13, B3
dp 300—*Levoxine* Tablets 0.3 mg..................... MC-13, B3
DS—*Anaprox* Tablets 500 mg.......................... MC-16, A4
DS 02C—*Septra* Tablets 800/160 mg................... MC-21, C3
D 03—*Danocrine* Capsules 50 mg...................... MC-6, C1
D 04—*Danocrine* Capsules 100 mg..................... MC-6, C1
D 05—*Danocrine* Capsules 200 mg..................... MC-6, C1
D 35—*Demerol* Tablets 50 mg......................... MC-14, B3
D 37—*Demerol* Tablets 100 mg........................ MC-14, B3
EA—Abbott Erythromycin Tablets 500 mg................ MC-9, A5
EB—Abbott Erythromycin Tablets 250 mg................ MC-9, A5
EC—*Ery-Tab* Delayed-release Tablets 250 mg.......... MC-9, A6
ED—*Ery-Tab* Delayed-release Tablets 500 mg.......... MC-9, A6
EE—*E.E.S.* Tablets 400 mg........................... MC-9, B6
EH—*Ery-Tab* Delayed-release Tablets 333 mg.......... MC-9, A6
EK—*PCE* Delayed-release Tablets 500 mg.............. MC-9, A7
ER—Abbott Erythromycin Delayed-release Capsules 250 mg.. MC-9, A4
ES—*Erythrocin* Tablets 250 mg....................... MC-9, C2
ET—*Erythrocin* Tablets 500 mg....................... MC-9, C2
GG 27—Geneva Hydrochlorothiazide Tablets 50 mg.... MC-11, B7
GG 28—Geneva Hydrochlorothiazide Tablets 25 mg.... MC-11, B7
GG 35—Geneva Thioridazine Tablets 150 mg........... MC-22, D6
GG 36—Geneva Thioridazine Tablets 200 mg........... MC-22, D6
GG 45—Geneva Dipyridamole Tablets 50 mg............ MC-7, D6
GG 49—Geneva Dipyridamole Tablets 25 mg............ MC-7, D6
GG 51—Geneva Trifluoperazine Tablets 1 mg.......... MC-24, A5
GG 53—Geneva Trifluoperazine Tablets 2 mg.......... MC-24, A5
GG 55—Geneva Trifluoperazine Tablets 5 mg.......... MC-24, A5
GG 56—Geneva Disopyramide Capsules 100 mg.......... MC-8, A2
GG 57—Geneva Disopyramide Capsules 150 mg.......... MC-8, A2
GG 58—Geneva Trifluoperazine Tablets 10 mg......... MC-24, A5
GG 61—Geneva Chlorpropamide Tablets 100 mg......... MC-5, A4
GG 71—Geneva Propranolol Tablets 10 mg............. MC-20, B2
GG 72—Geneva Propranolol Tablets 20 mg............. MC-20, B2
GG 73—Geneva Propranolol Tablets 40 mg............. MC-20, B2
GG 74—Geneva Propranolol Tablets 60 mg............. MC-20, B2
GG 75—Geneva Propranolol Tablets 80 mg............. MC-20, B2
GG 81—Geneva Clonidine Tablets 0.1 mg.............. MC-5, D3
GG 82—Geneva Clonidine Tablets 0.2 mg.............. MC-5, D3
GG 83—Geneva Clonidine Tablets 0.3 mg.............. MC-5, D3
GG 85—Geneva Spironolactone Tablets 25 mg......... MC-21, B3
GG 95—Geneva Spironolactone and Hydrochlorothiazide Tablets 25/25 mg.................. MC-21, B6
GG 101—Geneva Methocarbamol Tablets 750 mg........ MC-14, B6
GG 103—Geneva Metronidazole Tablets 250 mg........ MC-15, B6
GG 104—Geneva Methyldopa Tablets 125 mg........... MC-14, C4
GG 111—Geneva Methyldopa Tablets 250 mg........... MC-14, C4
GG 118—Geneva Chlorpheniramine, Phenylpropanolamine, Phenylephrine, and Phenyltoloxamine Extended-release Tablets 40/10/15/5 mg............ MC-4, D6
GG 119—Geneva Butalbital, Aspirin, and Caffeine Tablets 50/325/40 mg.................................... MC-3, B7
GG 124—Geneva Haloperidol Tablets 2 mg........... MC-11, A4
GG 125—Geneva Haloperidol Tablets 5 mg........... MC-11, A4
GG 126—Geneva Haloperidol Tablets 10 mg.......... MC-11, A4
GG 132—Geneva Verapamil Tablets 80 mg............ MC-24, C2
GG 133—Geneva Verapamil Tablets 120 mg........... MC-24, C2
GG 134—Geneva Haloperidol Tablets 20 mg.......... MC-11, A4
GG 141—Geneva Meclizine Tablets 12.5 mg.......... MC-14, A3
GG 144—Geneva Chlorpropamide Tablets 250 mg...... MC-5, A4
GG 167—Geneva Desipramine Tablets 100 mg......... MC-6, C3
GG 168—Geneva Desipramine Tablets 150 mg......... MC-6, C3
GG 172—Geneva Triamterene and Hydrochlorothiazide Tablets 75/50 mg............... MC-23, D7
GG 190—Geneva Methocarbamol Tablets 500 mg....... MC-14, B6
GG 195—Geneva Metronidazole Tablets 500 mg....... MC-15, B6
GG 219—Geneva Methyldopa and Hydrochlorothiazide Tablets 250/15 mg.............. MC-14, D2
GG 242—Geneva Methyclothiazide Tablets 5 mg...... MC-14, C3
GG 243—Geneva Methyldopa and Hydrochlorothiazide Tablets 500/30 mg.............. MC-14, D3
GG 244—Geneva Methyclothiazide Tablets 2.5 mg.... MC-14, C3
GG 254—Geneva Fenoprofen Tablets 600 mg.......... MC-10, A3
GG 261—Geneva Meclizine Tablets 25 mg............ MC-14, A3
GG 263—Geneva Atenolol Tablets 50 mg............. MC-2, B3
GG 264—Geneva Atenolol Tablets 100 mg............ MC-2, B3
GG 265—Geneva Methyldopa and Hydrochlorothiazide Tablets 250/25 mg.............. MC-14, D2
GG 270—Geneva Tolazamide Tablets 100 mg.......... MC-23, B7
GG 271—Geneva Tolazamide Tablets 250 mg.......... MC-23, B7
GG 272—Geneva Tolazamide Tablets 500 mg.......... MC-23, B7
GG 289—Geneva Methyldopa and Hydrochlorothiazide Tablets 500/50 mg.............. MC-14, D3
GG 437—Geneva Chlorpromazine Tablets 100 mg...... MC-5, A1
GG 457—Geneva Chlorpromazine Tablets 200 mg...... MC-5, A1
GG 464—Geneva Dipyridamole Tablets 75 mg......... MC-7, D6
GG 471—Geneva Methyldopa Tablets 500 mg.......... MC-14, C4
GG 472—Geneva Procainamide Extended-release Tablets 250 mg.................................... MC-19, C6
GG 473—Geneva Procainamide Extended-release Tablets 500 mg.................................... MC-19, C6
GG 474—Geneva Procainamide Extended-release Tablets 750 mg.................................... MC-19, C6
GG 501—Geneva Nitroglycerin Extended-release Capsules 6.5 mg.................................. MC-16, C6
GG 511—Geneva Nitroglycerin Extended-release Capsules 2.5 mg.................................. MC-16, C6
GG 512—Geneva Nitroglycerin Extended-release Capsules 9 mg.................................... MC-16, C6
GG 517—Geneva Indomethacin Capsules 25 mg........ MC-12, B5
GG 518—Geneva Indomethacin Capsules 50 mg........ MC-12, B5
GG 533—Geneva Diphenhydramine Capsules 25 mg..... MC-7, C6
GG 541—Geneva Diphenhydramine Capsules 50 mg..... MC-7, C6
GG 551—Geneva Procainamide Capsules 250 mg....... MC-19, C5
GG 552—Geneva Procainamide Capsules 375 mg....... MC-19, C5
GG 553—Geneva Procainamide Capsules 500 mg....... MC-19, C5
GG 558—Geneva Fenoprofen Capsules 200 mg......... MC-10, A2
GG 559—Geneva Fenoprofen Capsules 300 mg......... MC-10, A2
GG 572—Geneva Doxepin Capsules 25 mg............. MC-8, B1
GG 573—Geneva Doxepin Capsules 50 mg............. MC-8, B2
GG 574—Geneva Doxepin Capsules 75 mg............. MC-8, B2
GG 576—Geneva Doxepin Capsules 10 mg............. MC-8, B1
GG 577—Geneva Doxepin Capsules 100 mg............ MC-8, B2
GG 589—Geneva Thiothixene Capsules 1 mg.......... MC-23, A5
GG 596—Geneva Thiothixene Capsules 2 mg.......... MC-23, A5
GG 597—Geneva Thiothixene Capsules 5 mg.......... MC-23, A5
GG 598—Geneva Thiothixene Capsules 10 mg......... MC-23, A5
H09—*Ilosone* Capsules 250 mg..................... MC-9, B4
H11—Lederle Hydralazine Tablets 25 mg............ MC-11, B2
H12—Lederle Hydralazine Tablets 50 mg............ MC-11, B2
H69—*Keflex* Capsules 250 mg...................... MC-4, C1
H71—*Keflex* Capsules 500 mg...................... MC-4, C1
H76—*Nalfon* Capsules 200 mg...................... MC-9, D7
H77—*Nalfon* Capsules 300 mg...................... MC-9, D7

H 203—Schein Tetracycline Capsules 500 mg MC-22, B4
H 214—Schein Tetracycline Capsules 250 mg Blue/Yellow MC-22, B4
IBU 400—Boots Laboratories Ibuprofen Tablets 400 mg MC-11, D7
IBU 600—Boots Laboratories Ibuprofen Tablets 600 mg MC-11, D7
IBU 800—Boots Laboratories Ibuprofen Tablets 800 mg MC-11, D7
J10—*Eskalith CR* Extended-release Tablets 450 mg MC-13, C6
KL—*Biaxin* Tablets 500 mg MC-5, C3
KT—*Biaxin* Tablets 250 mg MC-5, C3
K2—*Dilaudid* Tablets 2 mg MC-11, C6
K4—*Dilaudid* Tablets 4 mg MC-11, C6
LL 200—*Suprax* Tablets 200 mg MC-4, B2
LU—*Ogen* Tablets 0.625 mg MC-9, C7
LV—*Ogen* Tablets 1.25 mg MC-9, C7
LX—*Ogen* Tablets 2.5 mg MC-9, C7
L 9—*Ledercillin VK* Tablets 500 mg MC-18, B4
L 10—*Ledercillin VK* Tablets 250 mg MC-18, B4
MJ 5—*BuSpar* Tablets 5 mg MC-3, B5
MJ 10—*BuSpar* Tablets 10 mg MC-3, B5
MJ 10 mEq 770—*Klotrix* Extended-release Tablets 750 mg MC-19, A4
MJ 755—*Estrace* Tablets 1 mg MC-9, C4
MJ 756—*Estrace* Tablets 2 mg MC-9, C4
MJ 775—*Desyrel* Tablets 50 mg MC-23, D2
MJ 776—*Desyrel* Tablets 100 mg MC-23, D2
MJ 778—*Desyrel* Tablets 150 mg Dividose MC-23, D2
MJ 784—*Duricef* Capsules 500 mg MC-4, A7
MJ 785—*Duricef* Tablets 1 gram MC-4, B1
MO—*Toprol XL* Extended-release Tablets 50 mg MC-15, B3
MP 44—Mutual Benztropine Tablets 1 mg MC-3, A5
MP 47—Mutual Albuterol Tablets 2 mg MC-1, B2
MP 50—Mutual Tolmetin Tablets 200 mg MC-23, C6
MP 71—Purepac Allopurinol Tablets 100 mg MC-1, B7
MP 74—Mutual Chlorzoxazone Tablets 500 mg MC-5, B5
MP 80—Mutual Allopurinol Tablets 300 mg MC-1, B7
MP 88—Mutual Albuterol Tablets 4 mg MC-1, B2
MP 108—Mutual Quinidine Sulfate Tablets 200 mg MC-20, D6
MP 112—Mutual Sulindac Tablets 150 mg MC-21, D2
MP 114—Mutual Trazodone Tablets 100 mg MC-23, D3
MP 116—Mutual Sulindac Tablets 200 mg MC-21, D2
MP 118—Mutual Trazodone Tablets 50 mg MC-23, D3
MP 124—Mutual Quinidine Sulfate Tablets 300 mg MC-20, D6
MP 142—Mutual Benztropine Tablets 2 mg MC-3, A5
MP 146—Mutual Atenolol Tablets 50 mg MC-2, B6
MP 147—Mutual Atenolol Tablets 100 mg MC-2, B6
MP 152—Mutual Atenolol and Chlorthalidone Tablets 100/25 mg MC-2, C2
MP 153—Mutual Atenolol and Chlorthalidone Tablets 50/25 mg MC-2, C2
MS—*Toprol XL* Extended-release Tablets 100 mg MC-15, B3
MSD 14—*Vasotec* Tablets 2.5 mg MC-8, D4
MSD 19—*Prinivil* Tablets 5 mg MC-13, B5
MSD 20—*Decadron* Tablets 0.25 mg MC-6, C6
MSD 21—*Cogentin* Tablets 0.5 mg MC-3, A4
MSD 23—*Elavil* Tablets 10 mg MC-1, D2
MSD 25—*Indocin* Capsules 25 mg MC-12, B6
MSD 41—*Decadron* Tablets 0.5 mg MC-6, C6
MSD 42—*HydroDIURIL* Tablets 25 mg MC-11, C1
MSD 45—*Elavil* Tablets 25 mg MC-1, D2
MSD 50—*Indocin* Capsules 50 mg MC-12, B6
MSD 59—*Blocadren* Tablets 5 mg MC-23, B3
MSD 60—*Cogentin* Tablets 2 mg MC-3, A4
MSD 63—*Decadron* Tablets 0.75 mg MC-6, C6
MSD 72—*Proscar* Tablets 5 mg MC-10, A7
MSD 95—*Decadron* Tablets 1.5 mg MC-6, C7
MSD 97—*Decadron* Tablets 4 mg MC-6, C7
MSD 102—*Elavil* Tablets 50 mg MC-1, D2
MSD 105—*HydroDIURIL* Tablets 50 mg MC-11, C1
MSD 106—*Prinivil* Tablets 10 mg MC-13, B5
MSD 135—*Aldomet* Tablets 125 mg MC-14, C5
MSD 136—*Blocadren* Tablets 10 mg MC-23, B3
MSD 140—*Prinzide* Tablets 20/12.5 mg MC-13, B7
MSD 142—*Prinzide* Tablets 20/25 mg MC-13, B7
MSD 147—*Decadron* Tablets 6 mg MC-6, C7
MSD 207—*Prinivil* Tablets 20 mg MC-13, B5
MSD 237—*Prinivil* Tablets 40 mg MC-13, B5
MSD 401—*Aldomet* Tablets 250 mg MC-14, C5
MSD 410—*HydroDIURIL* Tablets 100 mg MC-11, C1
MSD 423—*Aldoril* Tablets 250/15 mg MC-14, D4
MSD 430—*Elavil* Tablets 75 mg MC-1, D2
MSD 435—*Elavil* Tablets 100 mg MC-1, D2
MSD 437—*Blocadren* Tablets 20 mg MC-23, B3
MSD 451—*Plendil* Tablets 5 mg MC-9, D6
MSD 452—*Plendil* Tablets 10 mg MC-9, D6
MSD 456—*Aldoril* Tablets 250/25 mg MC-14, D4
MSD 516—*Aldomet* Tablets 500 mg MC-14, C5
MSD 517—*Triavil* Tablets 4/50 mg MC-18, C4
MSD 635—*Cogentin* Tablets 1 mg MC-3, A4
MSD 673—*Elavil* Tablets 150 mg MC-1, D3
MSD 675—*Dolobid* Tablets 250 mg MC-7, B3
MSD 693—*Indocin SR* Extended-release Capsules 75 mg MC-12, B7
MSD 694—*Aldoril* Tablets 500/30 mg MC-14, D5
MSD 697—*Dolobid* Tablets 500 mg MC-7, B3
MSD 705—*Noroxin* Tablets 400 mg MC-17, A7
MSD 707—*Tonocard* Tablets 400 mg MC-23, B6
MSD 709—*Tonocard* Tablets 600 mg MC-23, B6
MSD 712—*Vasotec* Tablets 5 mg MC-8, D4
MSD 713—*Vasotec* Tablets 10 mg MC-8, D4
MSD 714—*Vasotec* Tablets 20 mg MC-8, D4
MSD 720—*Vaseretic* Tablets 10/25 mg MC-8, D5
MSD 726—*Zocor* Tablets 5 mg MC-21, B1
MSD 731—*Mevacor* Tablets 20 mg MC-14, A1
MSD 732—*Mevacor* Tablets 40 mg MC-14, A1
MSD 735—*Zocor* Tablets 10 mg MC-21, B1
MSD 742—*Prilosec* Delayed-release Capsules 20 mg ... MC-17, C1
MSD 914—*Triavil* Tablets 2/10 mg MC-18, C3
MSD 917—*Moduretic* Tablets 5/50 mg MC-1, C5
MSD 921—*Triavil* Tablets 2/25 mg MC-18, C3
MSD 931—*Flexeril* Tablets 10 mg MC-6, B4
MSD 934—*Triavil* Tablets 4/10 mg MC-18, C3
MSD 935—*Aldoril* Tablets 500/50 mg MC-14, D5
MSD 941—*Clinoril* Tablets 150 mg MC-21, D1
MSD 942—*Clinoril* Tablets 200 mg MC-21, D1
MSD 946—*Triavil* Tablets 4/25 mg MC-18, C4
MSD 963—*Pepcid* Tablets 20 mg MC-9, D5
MSD 964—*Pepcid* Tablets 40 mg MC-9, D5
MT 4—*Pancrease* Delayed-release Capsules 4/20/25 ... MC-18, A5
MT 10—*Pancrease* Delayed-release Capsules 10/30/30 .... MC-18, A5
MT 16—*Pancrease* Delayed-release Capsules 16/48/48 .... MC-18, A6
MT 25—*Pancrease* Delayed-release Capsules 25/75/75 .... MC-18, A6
MY—*Toprol XL* Extended-release Capsules 200 mg MC-15, B3
M 1—Mylan Clonidine and Chlorthalidone Tablets 0.1/15 mg MC-6, A3
M2—Schein/Danbury Furosemide Tablets 20 mg MC-10, D1
M 3—*Minocin* Tablets 50 mg MC-15, C4
M 5—*Minocin* Tablets 100 mg MC-15, C4
M8—*Maxzide* Tablets 75/50 mg MC-24, A1
M9—*Maxzide* Tablets 37.5/25 mg MC-24, A1
M 27—Mylan Clonidine and Chlorthalidone Tablets 0.2/15 mg MC-6, A3
M 30—Mylan Clorazepate Tablets 3.75 mg MC-6, A6
M 31—Mylan Allopurinol Tablets 100 mg MC-1, C1
M 40—Mylan Clorazepate Tablets 7.5 mg MC-6, A6
M 45—*Minocin* Capsules 50 mg MC-15, C3
M 46—*Minocin* Capsules 100 mg MC-15, C3
M 54—Mylan Thioridazine Tablets 10 mg MC-22, D7
M 55—Mylan Timolol Tablets 5 mg MC-23, B4
M 58—Mylan Thioridazine Tablets 25 mg MC-22, D7
M 59—Mylan Thioridazine Tablets 50 mg MC-22, D7
M 61—Mylan Thioridazine Tablets 100 mg MC-22, D7
M 70—Mylan Clorazepate Tablets 15 mg MC-6, A6
M 71—Mylan Allopurinol Tablets 300 mg MC-1, C1
M 72—Mylan Clonidine and Chlorthalidone Tablets 0.3/15 mg MC-6, A3
M 221—Mylan Timolol Tablets 10 mg MC-23, B4
NE—*Asacol* Extended-release Tablets 400 mg MC-14, B4
NE—*Entex PSE* Tablets 120/600 mg MC-20, D1

NE—*Nicolar* Tablets 500 mg ... MC-16, A7
NR—*Depakote* Delayed-release Tablets 250 mg ... MC-8, A6
NS—*Depakote* Delayed-release Tablets 500 mg ... MC-8, A6
NT—*Depakote* Delayed-release Tablets 125 mg ... MC-8, A6
N 21—*NegGram* Tablets 250 mg ... MC-16, A1
N 22—*NegGram* Tablets 500 mg ... MC-16, A1
N 23—*NegGram* Tablets 1 gram ... MC-16, A2
P—*Demulen 1/35-28* Tablets Inert ... MC-9, D2
P—*Demulen 1/50-28* Tablets Inert ... MC-9, D3
PAA—*Trinalin* Extended-release Tablets 1/120 mg ... MC-2, D3
P-D 007—*Dilantin* Chewable Tablets 50 mg ... MC-18, D4
P-D 180—*Pyridium* Tablets 100 mg ... MC-18, C5
P-D 181—*Pyridium* Tablets 200 mg ... MC-18, C5
P-D 204—*Procan SR* Extended-release Tablets 500 mg ... MC-19, C7
P-D 205—*Procan SR* Extended-release Tablets 750 mg ... MC-19, D1
P-D 207—*Procan SR* Extended-release Tablets 1 gram ... MC-19, D1
P-D 362—*Dilantin* Capsules 100 mg ... MC-18, D5
P-D 365—*Dilantin* Capsules 30 mg ... MC-18, D5
P-D 471—*Benadryl* Capsules 25 mg ... MC-7, C7
P-D 473—*Benadryl* Capsules 50 mg ... MC-7, C7
P-D 552—*Centrax* Capsules 5 mg ... MC-19, B3
P-D 553—*Centrax* Capsules 10 mg ... MC-19, B3
P-D 622—*Loestrin Fe 1/20* Tablets 75 mg ... MC-17, A3
P-D 622—*Loestrin Fe 1.5/30* Tablets 75 mg ... MC-17, A4
P-D 696—*Eryc* Delayed-release Capsules 250 mg ... MC-9, B3
P-D 915—*Loestrin Fe 1/20* Tablets 1/0.02 mg ... MC-17, A3
P-D 915—*Loestrin 21 1/20* Tablets 1/0.02 mg ... MC-17, A1
P-D 916—*Loestrin Fe 1.5/30* Tablets 1.5/0.03 mg ... MC-17, A4
P-D 916—*Loestrin 21 1.5/30* Tablets 1.5/0.03 mg ... MC-17, A2
PPP 207—*Corgard* Tablets 40 mg ... MC-15, D5
PPP 208—*Corgard* Tablets 120 mg ... MC-15, D5
PPP 232—*Corgard* Tablets 20 mg ... MC-15, D5
PPP 241—*Corgard* Tablets 80 mg ... MC-15, D5
PPP 246—*Corgard* Tablets 160 mg ... MC-15, D5
PPP 606—*Naturetin* Tablets 5 mg ... MC-3, A2
PPP 618—*Naturetin* Tablets 10 mg ... MC-3, A2
PPP 775—*Pronestyl-SR* Extended-release Tablets 500 mg ... MC-19, D4
PPP 863—*Prolixin* Tablets 1 mg ... MC-10, B4
PPP 864—*Prolixin* Tablets 2.5 mg ... MC-10, B4
PPP 877—*Prolixin* Tablets 5 mg ... MC-10, B4
PPP 956—*Prolixin* Tablets 10 mg ... MC-10, B4
P7F—*Mepron* Tablets 250 mg ... MC-2, C5
P 44—Lederle Propranolol Tablets 10 mg ... MC-20, B3
P 45—Lederle Propranolol Tablets 20 mg ... MC-20, B3
P 46—Lederle Propranolol Tablets 40 mg ... MC-20, B3
P 47—Lederle Propranolol Tablets 80 mg ... MC-20, B3
P 65—Lederle Propranolol Tablets 60 mg ... MC-20, B3
rPr 351—*Slo-Phyllin* Tablets 100 mg ... MC-22, D1
rPr 352—*Slo-Phyllin* Tablets 200 mg ... MC-22, D1
R021—Purepac Flurazepam Capsules 15 mg ... MC-10, C1
R022—Purepac Flurazepam Capsules 30 mg ... MC-10, C1
R 497—Purepac Nifedipine Capsules 10 mg ... MC-16, B7
R 520—Purepac Tolmetin Capsules 400 mg ... MC-23, C7
R 530—Purepac Nifedipine Capsules 20 mg ... MC-16, B7
SKF—*Dyazide* Capsules 50/25 mg ... MC-24, A3
SKF—*Ornade* Extended-release Capsules 75/12 mg ... MC-23, C2
SKF C44—*Compazine* Extended-release Capsules 10 mg ... MC-19, D7
SKF C46—*Compazine* Extended-release Capsules 15 mg ... MC-19, D7
SKF C66—*Compazine* Tablets 5 mg ... MC-20, A1
SKF C67—*Compazine* Tablets 10 mg ... MC-20, A1
SKF C69—*Compazine* Tablets 25 mg ... MC-20, A1
SR 80—*Calan SR* Extended-release Tablets 180 mg ... MC-24, D3
SR 120—*Calan SR* Extended-release Tablets 120 mg ... MC-24, D2
SR 240—*Calan SR* Extended-release Tablets 240 mg ... MC-24, D3
S04—*Stelazine* Tablets 2 mg ... MC-24, A6
S 5—*Eldepryl* Tablets 5 mg ... MC-21, A6
TL—*Tranxene T-Tab* Tablets 3.75 mg ... MC-6, A5
TM—*Tranxene T-Tab* Tablets 7.5 mg ... MC-6, A5
TN—*Tranxene T-Tab* Tablets 15 mg ... MC-6, A5
TX—*Tranxene SD* Tablets 11.25 mg ... MC-6, A4
TY—*Tranxene SD* Tablets 22.5 mg ... MC-6, A4
T9A—*Lanoxin* Tablets 0.5 mg ... MC-7, B5
T37—*Talacen* Tablets 25/650 mg ... MC-18, B7
T 51—*Talwin Nx* Tablets 50/0.5 mg ... MC-18, C1
T64—*Thorazine* Extended-release Capsules 75 mg ... MC-5, A2
T74—*Thorazine* Tablets 25 mg ... MC-5, A3
UC—ProSom Tablets 1 mg ... MC-9, C3
UD—ProSom Tablets 2 mg ... MC-9, C3
U05—*Ilosone* Chewable Tablets 125 mg ... MC-9, B5
U25—*Ilosone* Chewable Tablets 250 mg ... MC-9, B5
U 121—*Loniten* Tablets 2.5 mg ... MC-15, C7
V7—*Verelan* Extended-release Capsules 180 mg ... MC-24, C3
V8—*Verelan* Extended-release Capsules 120 mg ... MC-24, C3
V9—*Verelan* Extended-resease Capsules 240 mg ... MC-24, C4
WC 242—Warner Chilcott Carbamazepine Chewable Tablets 100 mg ... MC-3, D6
WC 407—Warner Chilcott Tetracycline Capsules 250 mg ... MC-22, B6
WC 445—Warner Chilcott Clonidine Tablets 0.3 mg ... MC-6, A1
WC 607—Warner Chilcott Phenobarbital Tablets 60 mg ... MC-18, C6
WC 615—Warner Chilcott Minocycline Capsules 50 mg ... MC-15, C5
WC 616—Warner Chilcott Minocycline Capsules 100 mg ... MC-15, C5
WC 697—Warner Chilcott Tetracycline Capsules 500 mg ... MC-22, B6
WC 698—Warner Chilcott Phenobarbital Tablets 100 mg ... MC-18, C6
WC 699—Warner Chilcott Phenobarbital Tablets 15 mg ... MC-18, C6
WC 700—Warner Chilcott Phenobarbital Tablets 30 mg ... MC-18, C6
WC 773—Warner Chilcott Sulindac Tablets 150 mg ... MC-21, D4
WC 774—Warner Chilcott Sulindac Tablets 200 mg ... MC-21, D4
WHR 1354—*Slo-Phyllin* Extended-release Capsules 60 mg ... MC-22, C7
WHR 1356—*Slo-Phyllin* Extended-release Capsules 250 mg ... MC-22, C7
X3A—*Lanoxin* Tablets 0.25 mg ... MC-7, B5
Y2B—*Septra* Tablets 400/80 mg ... MC-21, C3
Y3B—*Lanoxin* Tablets 0.125 mg ... MC-7, B5
Y9C 100—*Retrovir* Capsules 100 mg ... MC-24, D6
Z2931—Rugby Methyldopa Tablets 250 mg ... MC-14, C7
Z2932—Rugby Methyldopa Tablets 500 mg ... MC-14, C7
0051—*Lopurin* Tablets 100 mg ... MC-1, B5
0052—*Lopurin* Tablets 300 mg ... MC-1, B5
0.125—*Halcion* Tablets 0.125 mg ... MC-24, A4
0.25—*Halcion* Tablets 0.25 mg ... MC-24, A4
0.25—*Xanax* Tablets 0.25 mg ... MC-1, C3
0.3—*Premarin* Tablets 0.3 mg ... MC-9, C5
0.5—*Bumex* Tablets 0.5 mg ... MC-3, B3
0.5—*Xanax* Tablets 0.5 mg ... MC-1, C3
0.5/35—*Genora 0.5/35-21* Tablets 0.5/0.035 mg ... MC-16, D6
0.625—*Premarin* Tablets 0.625 mg ... MC-9, C5
0.9—*Premarin* Tablets 0.9 mg ... MC-9, C5
051—Purepac Diazepam Tablets 2 mg ... MC-6, D3
052—Purepac Diazepam Tablets 5 mg ... MC-6, D3
053—Purepac Diazepam Tablets 10 mg ... MC-6, D3
058—Barr Diphenhydramine Capsules 25 mg ... MC-7, C5
059—Barr Diphenhydramine Capsules 50 mg ... MC-7, C5
063—Purepac Lorazepam Tablets 2 mg ... MC-13, D5
067—Purepac Oxazepam Capsules 10 mg ... MC-17, C7
069—Purepac Oxazepam Capsules 15 mg ... MC-17, C7
073—Purepac Oxazepam Capsules 30 mg ... MC-17, C7
076—Purepac Temazepam Capsules 15 mg ... MC-22, A1
077—Purepac Temazepam Capsules 30 mg ... MC-22, A1
078—Purepac Clorazepate Tablets 3.75 mg ... MC-6, A7
081—Purepac Clorazepate Tablets 7.5 mg ... MC-6, A7
083—Purepac Clorazepate Tablets 15 mg ... MC-6, A7
085—Purepac Propoxyphene Napsylate and Acetaminophen Tablets 100/650 mg ... MC-20, B1
094—*Vibramycin* Capsules 50 mg ... MC-8, C4
095—*Mycelex Troche* Lozenges 10 mg ... MC-6, B1
095—*Vibramycin* Capsules 100 mg ... MC-8, C4
099—*Vibra-tabs* Tablets 100 mg ... MC-8, C5
09A—*Proloprim* Tablets 100 mg ... MC-24, B1

0115 3875—Rugby Meclizine Chewable Tablets 25 mg ... MC-14, A5
0149 0007—*Macrodantin* Capsules 25 mg ... MC-16, C4
0149 0008—*Macrodantin* Capsules 50 mg ... MC-16, C4
0149 0009—*Macrodantin* Capsules 100 mg ... MC-16, C4
0149 0030—*Dantrium* Capsules 25 mg ... MC-6, C2
0149 0031—*Dantrium* Capsules 50 mg ... MC-6, C2
0149 0033—*Dantrium* Capsules 100 mg ... MC-6, C2
0149 0412—*Entex* Capsules 5/45/200 mg ... MC-18, D1
0149 0436—*Entex LA* Extended-release Tablets 75/400 mg ... MC-18, D3
0230—Rugby Doxycycline Capsules 100 mg ... MC-8, C7
0280—Rugby Doxycycline Capsules 50 mg ... MC-8, C7
0665 4160—Solvay Lithium Capsules ... MC-13, C7
0920—*Dilatrate-SR* Extended-release Capsules 40 mg ... MC-12, C1
½—*Haldol* Tablets 0.5 mg ... MC-11, A5
½—*Mykrox* Tablets 0.5 mg ... MC-15, B1
1—*Bumex* Tablets 1 mg ... MC-3, B3
1—*Haldol* Tablets 1 mg ... MC-11, A5
1—*Tenex* Tablets 1 mg ... MC-11, A1
1—*Tylenol with Codeine* Tablets 300/7.5 mg ... MC-1, A1
1.0—*Xanax* Tablets 1 mg ... MC-1, C3
1.25—*Micronase* Tablets 1.25 mg ... MC-10, D5
1.25—*Premarin* Tablets 1.25 mg ... MC-9, C6
1.25 mg—*Altace* Capsules 1.25 mg ... MC-21, A1
1/35—*Genora 1/35-28* Tablets 1/0.035 mg ... MC-16, D7
1/50—*Genora 1/50-28* Tablets 1/0.05 mg ... MC-17, A6
1A—*Cartrol* Tablets 2.5 mg ... MC-4, A5
1C—*Cartrol* Tablets 5 mg ... MC-4, A5
1 mg—*Cardura* Tablets 1 mg ... MC-8, A7
2—*Bumex* Tablets 2 mg ... MC-3, B4
2—*Coumadin* Tablets 2 mg ... MC-24, D4
2—*Haldol* Tablets 2 mg ... MC-11, A5
2—*Halotestin* Tablets 2 mg ... MC-10, B3
2—*Medrol* Tablets 2 mg ... MC-15, A2
2—*Tenex* Tablets 2 mg ... MC-11, A1
2—*Tylenol with Codeine* Tablets 300/15 mg ... MC-1, A1
2—*Valium* Tablets 2 mg ... MC-6, D5
2—*Ventolin* Tablets 2 mg ... MC-1, B1
2—*Xanax* Tablets 2 mg ... MC-1, C3
2 mg—*Cardura* Tablets 2 mg ... MC-8, A7
.25—*Rocaltrol* Capsules 0.25 mcg ... MC-3, C4
2½—*Coumadin* Tablets 2.5 mg ... MC-24, D4
2½—*Zaroxolyn* Tablets 2.5 mg ... MC-15, B2
2.5—*Deltasone* Tablets 2.5 mg ... MC-19, C3
2.5—*DynaCirc* Capsules 2.5 mg ... MC-12, D5
2.5—*Micronase* Tablets 2.5 mg ... MC-10, D5
2.5—*Norvasc* Tablets 2.5 mg ... MC-1, D4
2.5—*Premarin* Tablets 2.5 mg ... MC-9, C6
2.5—*Provera* Tablets 2.5 mg ... MC-14, B1
2.5 mg—*Altace* Capsules 2.5 mg ... MC-21, A1
3—*Empirin with Codeine* Tablets 325/30 mg ... MC-2, B1
3—*Ritalin* Tablets 10 mg ... MC-14, D7
3—*Tylenol with Codeine* Tablets 300/30 mg ... MC-1, A2
4—*Empirin with Codeine* Tablets 325/60 mg ... MC-2, B1
4—*Medrol* Tablets 4 mg ... MC-15, A2
4—Mylan Fluphenazine Tablets 1 mg ... MC-10, B5
4—*Tylenol with Codeine* Tablets 300/60 mg ... MC-1, A2
4—*Ventolin* Tablets 4 mg ... MC-1, B1
4—*Zofran* Tablets 4 mg ... MC-17, C2
4 mg—*Cardura* Tablets 4 mg ... MC-8, A7
.5—*Rocaltrol* Capsules 0.5 mcg ... MC-3, C4
5—*Accupril* Tablets 5 mg ... MC-20, D3
5—*Cortef* Tablets 5 mg ... MC-11, C5
5—*Coumadin* Tablets 5 mg ... MC-24, D5
5—*Deltasone* Tablets 5 mg ... MC-19, C3
5—*Dyna Circ* Capsules 5 mg ... MC-12, D5
5—*Haldol* Tablets 5 mg ... MC-11, A5
5—*Halotestin* Tablets 5 mg ... MC-10, B3
5—*Isordil* Sublingual Tablets 5 mg ... MC-12, C4
5—*Libritabs* Tablets 5 mg ... MC-4, C7
5—*Librium* Capsules 5 mg ... MC-4, C6
5—*Lotensin* Tablets 5 mg ... MC-3, A1
5—*Micronase* Tablets 5 mg ... MC-10, D5
5—*Norvasc* Tablets 5 mg ... MC-1, D4
5—*Provera* Tablets 5 mg ... MC-14, B1
5—*Reglan* Tablets 5 mg ... MC-15, A5
5—*Valium* Tablets 5 mg ... MC-6, D5
5—*Zaroxolyn* Tablets 5 mg ... MC-15, B2
5 mg—*Altace* Capsules 5 mg ... MC-21, A1
6—*Rufen* Tablets 600 mg ... MC-12, A1
6—*Serax* Capsules 15 mg ... MC-17, D2
7—*Lozol* Tablets 1.25 mg ... MC-12, B4
7—*Ritalin* Tablets 5 mg ... MC-14, D7
7.5—*Doral* Tablets 7.5 mg ... MC-20, D2
7.5 mg—*Restoril* Capsules 7.5 mg ... MC-22, A2
7½—*Coumadin* Tablets 7.5 mg ... MC-24, D5
8—*Dilaudid* Tablets 8 mg ... MC-11, C6
8—*Klor-Con* Extended-release Tablets 600 mg ... MC-19, B1
8—*Lozol* Tablets 2.5 mg ... MC-12, B2
8—*Medrol* Tablets 8 mg ... MC-15, A2
8—*Rufen* Tablets 800 mg ... MC-12, A1
8—*Zofran* Tablets 8 mg ... MC-17, C2
8 mg—*Cardura* Tablets 8 mg ... MC-8, A7
9—Mylan Fluphenazine Tablets 2.5 mg ... MC-10, B6
10—*Accupril* Tablets 10 mg ... MC-20, D3
10—*Accutane* Capsules 10 mg ... MC-12, D4
10—*Atarax* Tablets 10 mg ... MC-11, D3
10—*Bentyl* Capsules 10 mg ... MC-7, A5
10—*Cortef* Tablets 10 mg ... MC-11, C5
10—*Coumadin* Tablets 10 mg ... MC-24, D5
10—*Deltasone* Tablets 10 mg ... MC-19, C3
10—*Haldol* Tablets 10 mg ... MC-11, A5
10—*Halotestin* Tablets 10 mg ... MC-10, B3
10—*Inderal* Tablets 10 mg ... MC-20, C2
10—*Isordil* Sublingual Tablets 10 mg ... MC-12, C4
10—*K-Dur* Extended-release Tablets 750 mg ... MC-19, A3
10—*Kerlone* Tablets 10 mg ... MC-3, A7
10—*Klor-Con* Extended-release Tablets 750 mg ... MC-19, B1
10—*Libritabs* Tablets 10 mg ... MC-4, C7
10—*Librium* Capsules 10 mg ... MC-4, C6
10—*Loniten* Tablets 10 mg ... MC-15, C7
10—*Lotensin* Tablets 10 mg ... MC-3, A1
10—*Norvasc* Tablets 10 mg ... MC-1, D4
10—*Pravachol* Tablets 10 mg ... MC-19, B2
10—*Provera* Tablets 10 mg ... MC-14, B1
10—*Valium* Tablets 10 mg ... MC-6, D5
10—*Zaroxolyn* Tablets 10 mg ... MC-15, B2
10-0364—Schein Nifedipine Capsules 10 mg ... MC-16, C1
10 mg—*Altace* Capsules 10 mg ... MC-21, A1
11—*Tri-Levlen 28* Tablets Inert ... MC-13, A4
15—Biocraft Penicillin V Tablets 250 mg Round ... MC-18, B3
15—*Dalmane* Capsules 15 mg ... MC-10, C2
15—*Doral* Tablets 15 mg ... MC-20, D2
15—*Ionamin* Capsules 15 mg ... MC-18, C7
15—*Valrelease* Extended-release Capsules 15 mg ... MC-6, D4
16—Biocraft Penicillin V Tablets 250 mg Oval ... MC-18, B3
16—*Medrol* Tablets 16 mg ... MC-15, A3
16—*Ritalin-SR* Extended-release Tablets 20 mg ... MC-15, A1
17—Biocraft Penicillin V Tablets 500 mg Round ... MC-18, B3
17 12—*Carafate* Tablets 1 gram ... MC-21, C2
18—*Didrex* Tablets 25 mg ... MC-3, A3
19—*Phenergan* Tablets 12.5 mg ... MC-20, A2
20—*Accupril* Tablets 20 mg ... MC-20, D3
20—*Accutane* Capsules 20 mg ... MC-12, D4
20—*Bentyl* Tablets 20 mg ... MC-7, A6
20—*Cortef* Tablets 20 mg ... MC-11, C5
20—*Deltasone* Tablets 20 mg ... MC-19, C3
20—*Haldol* Tablets 20 mg ... MC-11, A5
20—*Inderal* Tablets 20 mg ... MC-20, C2
20—*ISMO* Tablets 20 mg ... MC-12, D3
20—*K-Dur* Tablets 1500 mg ... MC-19, A3
20—*Kerlone* Tablets 20 mg ... MC-3, A7
20—*Lotensin* Tablets 20 mg ... MC-3, A1
20—*Paxil* Tablets 20 mg ... MC-18, A7
20—*Pravachol* Tablets 20 mg ... MC-19, B2
20—*Tofranil-PM* Capsules 75 mg ... MC-12, B1
20-0364—Schein Nifedipine Capsules 20 mg ... MC-16, C1
20 (R)—*Hygroton* Tablets 50 mg ... MC-5, B2
21—*Hygroton* Tablets 100 mg ... MC-5, B2
21—*Levlen 21 and 28* Tablets 0.15/0.03 mg ... MC-13, A3
22—*Esidrix* Tablets 25 mg ... MC-11, B6
22—*Levatol* Tablets 20 mg ... MC-18, B1

200—*Proloprim* Tablets 200 mg MC-24, B1
200—*Synthroid* Tablets 0.2 mg MC-13, B1
200—*Theo-Dur* Extended-release Tablets 200 mg MC-22, C4
200—*Theo-Dur Sprinkle* Extended-release Capsules 200 mg MC-22, C3
200—*Tolectin* Tablets 200 mg MC-23, C4
200—*Trandate* Tablets 200 mg MC-12, D7
200—*Vascor* Tablets 200 mg MC-3, A6
200—*Zovirax* Capsules 200 mg MC-1, A6
200 mg—*Floxin* Tablets 200 mg MC-17, B7
200 mg—*Lodine* Capsules 200 mg MC-9, D4
200 mg—*Slo-bid* Extended-release Capsules 200 mg MC-22, C6
200 SKF—*Tagamet* Tablets 200 mg MC-5, B6
210—*Antivert* Tablets 12.5 mg MC-14, A4
211—*Antivert* Tablets 25 mg MC-14, A4
211—*Grifulvin V* Tablets 250 mg MC-10, D6
211—Mylan Chlordiazepoxide and Amitriptyline Tablets 5/12.5 mg MC-4, D1
214—*Antivert* Tablets 50 mg MC-14, A4
214—*Grifulvin V* Tablets 500 mg MC-14, D6
214—Mylan Haloperidol Tablets 2 mg MC-11, A6
227—*Phenergan* Tablets 50 mg MC-20, A2
227 227—*Normozide* Tablets 200/25 mg MC-13, A2
235 235—*Normozide* Tablets 100/25 mg MC-13, A2
239—Apothecon Cephalexin Capsules 500 mg MC-4, B6
240 mg—*Betapace* Tablets 240 mg MC-21, B2
240 mg—*Cardizem CD* Capsules 240 mg MC-7, B6
240 mg—*Dilacor XR* Extended-release Capsules 240 mg MC-7, C4
244—*Normodyne* Tablets 100 mg MC-13, A1
250—*Amoxil* Capsules 250 mg MC-1, D6
250—*Amoxil* Chewable Tablets 250 mg MC-1, D7
250—*Ethmozine* Tablets 250 mg MC-15, D2
250—*Keftab* Tablets 250 mg MC-4, C2
250—*Lorelco* Tablets 250 mg MC-19, C4
250—*Naprosyn* Tablets 250 mg MC-16, A3
250—*Orinase* Tablets 250 mg MC-23, C2
250—*Slo-Niacin* Extended-release Tablets 250 mg MC-16, B1
250—*Ticlid* Tablets 250 mg MC-23, B2
250—*Tigan* Capsules 250 mg MC-24, A7
250—*Tolinase* Tablets 250 mg MC-23, C1
250—*V-Cillin K* Tablets 250 mg MC-18, B5
250mg—*E-Mycin* Delayed-release Tablets 250 mg MC-9, B2
250 mg—*Nicobid* Extended-release Capsules 250 mg MC-16, A5
250 mg—*Panmycin* Capsules 250 mg MC-22, B5
250/125—*Augmentin* Tablets 250/125 mg MC-2, A2
252—Barr Dipyridamole Tablets 25 mg MC-7, D4
253—Purepac Methyldopa Tablets 250 mg MC-14, C6
255—Purepac Methyldopa Tablets 500 mg MC-14, C6
257—Mylan Haloperidol Tablets 1 mg MC-11, A6
259—Barr Erythromycin Ethylsuccinate Tablets 400 mg MC-9, C1
260—Barr Thioridazine Tablets 10 mg MC-22, D4
260—*Procardia* Capsules 10 mg MC-16, B5
261—Barr Thioridazine Tablets 25 mg MC-22, D4
261—*Procardia* Capsules 20 mg MC-16, B5
261—Purepac Methyldopa and Hydrochlorothiazide Tablets 250/15 mg MC-14, D6
262—Barr Thioridazine Tablets 50 mg MC-22, D4
263—Barr Thioridazine Tablets 100 mg MC-22, D4
263—Purepac Methyldopa and Hydrochlorothiazide Tablets 250/25 mg MC-14, D6
267—Barr Chlorthalidone Tablets 25 mg MC-5, A7
268—Barr Chlorthalidone Tablets 50 mg MC-5, A7
269—Purepac Metoclopramide Tablets 10 mg MC-15, A4
274—*Anaprox* Tablets 275 mg MC-16, A4
277—Mylan Chlordiazepoxide and Amitriptyline Tablets 10/25 mg MC-4, D1
280—Purepac Haloperidol Tablets 1 mg MC-11, A7
281—Purepac Haloperidol Tablets 2 mg MC-11, A7
282—Purepac Haloperidol Tablets 5 mg MC-11, A7
283—*Corzide* Tablets 40/5 mg MC-15, D7
284—*Corzide* Tablets 80/5 mg MC-15, D7
285—Barr Dipyridamole Tablets 50 mg MC-7, D4
286—Barr Dipyridamole Tablets 75 mg MC-7, D4
286—Purepac Haloperidol Tablets 10 mg MC-11, A7
287—Purepac Haloperidol Tablets 20 mg MC-11, A7
289—Purepac Haloperidol Tablets 0.5 mg MC-11, A7
295—Barr Doxycycline Tablets 100 mg MC-8, C3
296—Barr Doxycycline Capsules 50 mg MC-8, C2
297—Barr Doxycycline Capsules 100 mg MC-8, C2
300—*Ethmozine* Tablets 300 mg MC-15, D3
300—*Rythmol* Tablets 300 mg MC-20, A3
300—*Synthroid* Tablets 0.3 mg MC-13, B1
300—*Theo-Dur* Extended-release Tablets 300 mg MC-22, C4
300—*Trandate* Tablets 300 mg MC-12, D7
300—*Vascor* Tablets 300 mg MC-3, A6
300—*Zantac* Tablets 300 mg MC-21, A2
300—*Zyloprim* Tablets 300 mg MC-1, B6
300mg—*Motrin* Tablets 300 mg MC-12, A6
300 MG—*Actigall* Capsules 300 mg MC-24, B3
300 mg—*Cardizem CD* Capsules 300 mg MC-7, B7
300 mg—*Cleocin* Capsules 300 mg MC-5, C7
300 mg—*Floxin* Tablets 300 mg MC-17, B7
300 mg—*Lodine* Tablets 300 mg MC-9, D4
300 mg—*Slo-bid* Extended-release Capsules 300 mg MC-22, C6
300 SKF—*Tagamet* Tablets 300 mg MC-5, B6
302—Schein/Danbury Furosemide Tablets 80 mg MC-10, D1
305—*Zithromax* Capsules 250 mg MC-2, D5
309—*Omnipen* Capsules 500 mg MC-2, A6
317—Barr Propoxyphene Napsylate and Acetaminophen Tablets 50/325 mg MC-20, A5
317—Purepac Fenoprofen Tablets 600 mg MC-10, A4
317—*Serax* Tablets 15 mg MC-17, D3
318—Barr Propoxyphene Napsylate and Acetaminophen Tablets 100/650 mg White MC-20, A5
321—Purepac Propranolol Tablets 60 mg MC-20, B4
322—*Feldene* Capsules 10 mg MC-19, A1
323—*Feldene* Capsules 20 mg MC-19, A1
327—Barr Thioridazine Tablets 150 mg MC-22, D5
327—Mylan Haloperidol Tablets 5 mg MC-11, A6
328—Barr Thioridazine Tablets 200 mg MC-22, D5
331—Barr Disopyramide Capsules 100 mg MC-8, A1
331—Purepac Propranolol Tablets 40 mg MC-20, B4
332—Barr Disopyramide Capsules 150 mg MC-8, A1
333—Purepac Propranolol Tablets 80 mg MC-20, B4
333mg—*E-Mycin* Delayed-release Tablets 333 mg MC-9, B2
338—*Capozide* Tablets 25/15 mg MC-3, C7
349—*Capozide* Tablets 25/25 mg MC-3, C7
351—Mylan Haloperidol Tablets 0.5 mg MC-11, A6
358—Purepac Propranolol and Hydrochlorothiazide Tablets 40/25 mg MC-20, C3
360—Purepac Propranolol and Hydrochlorothiazide Tablets 80/25 mg MC-20, C3
370—Barr Lorazepam Tablets 0.5 mg MC-13, D4
371—Barr Lorazepam Tablets 1 mg MC-13, D4
372—Barr Lorazepam Tablets 2 mg MC-13, D4
373—Barr Oxazepam Tablets 15 mg MC-17, C6
374—Barr Oxazepam Capsules 10 mg MC-17, C5
375—Barr Oxazepam Capsules 15 mg MC-17, C5
375—*Naprosyn* Tablets 375 mg MC-16, A3
376—Barr Oxazepam Capsules 30 mg MC-17, C5
377—Barr Flurazepam Capsules 15 mg MC-10, B7
378—Barr Flurazepam Capsules 30 mg MC-10, B7
381—Barr Meperidine Tablets 50 mg MC-14, B2
382—Barr Meperidine Tablets 100 mg MC-14, B2
384—*Capozide* Tablets 50/15 mg MC-3, D1
387—*Ceftin* Tablets 250 mg MC-4, B4
388—Purepac Spironolactone Tablets 25 mg MC-21, B4
390—*Capozide* Tablets 50/25 mg MC-3, D1
390—*Pen-Vee K* Tablets 500 mg MC-18, B6
391 391—*Normozide* Tablets 300/25 mg MC-13, A2
393—*Diabinese* Tablets 100 mg MC-5, A5
394—*Ceftin* Tablets 500 mg MC-4, B5
394—*Diabinese* Tablets 250 mg MC-5, A5
395—*Ceftin* Tablets 125 mg MC-4, B4
400—*Maxaquin* Tablets 400 mg MC-13, D1
400—*Rufen* Tablets 400 mg MC-12, A1
400—*Suprax* Tablets 400 mg MC-4, B2
400—*Vascor* Tablets 400 mg MC-3, A6
400 mg—*Floxin* Tablets 400 mg MC-17, B7
400mg—*Motrin* Tablets 400 mg MC-12, A6
400 SKF—*Tagamet* Tablets 400 mg MC-5, B7
404—Purepac Tetracycline Capsules 250 mg MC-22, B3

406—Purepac Tetracycline Capsules 500 mg MC-22, B3
411—*Glucotrol* Tablets 5 mg.......... MC-10, D3
412—*Glucotrol* Tablets 10 mg.......... MC-10, D3
419—Barr Ibuprofen Tablets 400 mg.......... MC-11, D6
420—Barr Ibuprofen Tablets 600 mg.......... MC-11, D6
425—Barr Verapamil Tablets 80 mg.......... MC-24, B5
430—*Minizide* Capsules 1/0.5 mg MC-19, B7
431—*Minipress* Capsules 1 mg MC-19, B4
431—*Pronestyl* Tablets 250 mg.......... MC-19, D3
431—*Proventil* Extended-release Tablets 4 mg MC-1, B4
432—*Minizide* Capsules 2/0.5 mg MC-19, B7
434—*Pronestyl* Tablets 375 mg.......... MC-19, D3
436—*Minizide* Capsules 5/0.5 mg MC-19, B7
437—*Minipress* Capsules 2 mg MC-19, B4
438—*Minipress* Capsules 5 mg MC-19, B4
438—*Normodyne* Tablets 300 mg.......... MC-13, A1
438—*Pronestyl* Tablets 500 mg.......... MC-19, D3
439—Purepac Trazodone Tablets 50 mg MC-23, D4
441—Purepac Trazodone Tablets 100 mg MC-23, D4
443—Warner Chilcott Clonidine Tablets 0.1 mg MC-6, A1
444—Warner Chilcott Clonidine Tablets 0.2 mg MC-6, A1
445—*Ovral-28* Tablets Inert MC-17, B2
450—*Capoten* Tablets 12.5 mg MC-3, C5
452—*Capoten* Tablets 25 mg MC-3, C5
455—Barr Verapamil Tablets 120 mg MC-24, B5
458—*Claritin* Tablets 10 mg MC-13, D3
470—Barr Propoxyphene Napsylate and Acetaminophen Tablets 100/650 mg Pink.......... MC-20, A5
473—Purepac Verapamil Tablets 80 mg MC-24, C5
475—Purepac Verapamil Tablets 120 mg MC-24, C5
477—Barr Haloperidol Tablets 0.5 mg.......... MC-11, A2
478—Barr Haloperidol Tablets 1 mg MC-11, A2
479—Barr Haloperidol Tablets 2 mg MC-11, A2
480—Barr Haloperidol Tablets 5 mg MC-11, A2
481—Barr Haloperidol Tablets 10 mg MC-11, A3
482—Barr Haloperidol Tablets 20 mg MC-11, A3
482—*Capoten* Tablets 50 mg.......... MC-3, C6
485—*Capoten* Tablets 100 mg.......... MC-3, C6
486—*Lo-Ovral-21 and -28* Tablets Inert MC-17, B1
486—*Nordette-28* Tablets Inert.......... MC-13, A5
487—Barr Temazepam Capsules 15 mg.......... MC-21, D6
488—Barr Temazepam Capsules 30 mg.......... MC-21, D6
499—Barr Ibuprofen Tablets 800 mg.......... MC-11, D6
500—*Amoxil* Capsules 500 mg MC-1, D6
500—*Flagyl* Tablets 500 mg MC-15, C2
500—*Keftab* Tablets 500 mg MC-4, C2
500—*Lorelco* Tablets 500 mg MC-19, C4
500—*Naprosyn* Tablets 500 mg.......... MC-16, A3
500—*Nicobid* Extended-release Capsules 500 mg.......... MC-16, A6
500—*Orinase* Tablets 500 mg MC-23, C2
500—Purepac Prazosin Capsules 1 mg.......... MC-19, B5
500—*Relafen* Tablets 500 mg MC-15, D4
500—*Slo-Niacin* Extended-release Tablets 500 mg MC-16, B1
500—*Tolinase* Tablets 500 mg MC-23, C1
500—*V-Cillin K* Tablets 500 mg.......... MC-18, B5
500/125—*Augmentin* Tablets 500/125 mg MC-2, A2
501—Purepac Prazosin Capsules 2 mg.......... MC-19, B5
502—Purepac Prazosin Capsules 5 mg.......... MC-19, B5
512—*Cipro* Tablets 250 mg MC-5, C1
513—*Cipro* Tablets 500 mg MC-5, C2
514—*Cipro* Tablets 750 mg MC-5, C2
515—*Quibron* Capsules 300/180 mg MC-22, D3
516—*Quibron* Capsules 150/90 mg MC-22, D3
521—*Lufyllin* Tablets 200 mg.......... MC-8, D3
521—Mylan Propoxyphene Napsylate and Acetaminophen Tablets 100/65 mg White.......... MC-20, A7
534—*Sinequan* Capsules 10 mg.......... MC-8, B3
535—*Ortho-Novum 7/7/7-21 and -28* Tablets 0.5/0.035 mg.......... MC-16, D5
535—*Sinequan* Capsules 25 mg.......... MC-8, B3
536—*Sinequan* Capsules 50 mg.......... MC-8, B3
537—*Sinequan* Capsules 150 mg.......... MC-8, B4
538—*Sinequan* Capsules 100 mg.......... MC-8, B4
539—*Sinequan* Capsules 75 mg.......... MC-8, B4
541—*Vistaril* Capsules 25 mg MC-11, D2
542—*Vistaril* Capsules 50 mg MC-11, D2
543—*Roxicet* Tablets 5/325 mg MC-18, A1
543—*Vistaril* Capsules 100 mg MC-11, D2
550—Barr Cephradine Capsules 250 mg MC-4, C4
551—Barr Cephradine Capsules 500 mg MC-4, C4
555 19—Barr Hydrochlorothiazide Tablets 25 mg MC-11, B5
555 20—Barr Hydrochlorothiazide Tablets 50 mg MC-11, B5
555 169—Barr Furosemide Tablets 40 mg.......... MC-10, C6
555 192—Barr Hydrochlorothiazide Tablets 100 mg MC-11, B5
555 196—Barr Furosemide Tablets 80 mg.......... MC-10, C6
555 444—Barr Triamterene and Hydrochlorothiazide Tablets 75/50 mg.......... MC-23, D6
555 585—Barr Chlorzoxazone Tablets 500 mg MC-5, B3
559—*Wymox* Capsules 250 mg.......... MC-2, A1
560—*Wymox* Capsules 500 mg.......... MC-2, A1
571—*Navane* Capsules 1 mg MC-23, A6
572—*Navane* Capsules 2 mg MC-23, A6
573—*Navane* Capsules 5 mg MC-23, A6
574—*Navane* Capsules 10 mg MC-23, A7
577—*Navane* Capsules 20 mg MC-23, A7
583—*Ovcon 35-21 and -28* Tablets 0.4/0.035 mg.......... MC-16, D2
584—Barr Erythromycin Delayed-release Capsules 250 mg.......... MC-9, B1
584—*Ovcon 50-21 and -28* Tablets 1/0.05 mg MC-16, D3
600—*Nolvadex* Tablets 10 mg.......... MC-21, D5
600—*Tolectin* Tablets 600 mg.......... MC-23, C4
600mg—*Motrin* Tablets 600 mg MC-12, A7
601—*Pro-Banthine* Tablets 15 mg.......... MC-20, A4
603—*Sumycin* Tablets 500 mg MC-22, B1
609—*Monopril* Tablets 20 mg.......... MC-10, C5
611—*Pro-Banthine* Tablets 7.5 mg MC-20, A4
641—*Triphasil-21 and -28* Tablets 0.05/0.03 mg.......... MC-13, A6
642—*Triphasil-21 and -28* Tablets 0.075/0.04 mg.......... MC-13, A6
643—*Triphasil-21 and -28* Tablets 0.125/0.03 mg.......... MC-13, A6
647—*Sinemet* Tablets 10/100 mg.......... MC-4, A1
648—*Veetids* Tablets 500 mg.......... MC-18, B2
650—*Sinemet* Tablets 25/100 mg.......... MC-4, A1
650—*Triphasil-28* Tablets Inert MC-13, A6
654—*Sinemet* Tablets 25/250 mg.......... MC-4, A1
655—*Sumycin* Capsules 250 mg MC-22, A7
663—*Sumycin* Tablets 250 mg MC-22, B1
684—*Veetids* Tablets 250 mg.......... MC-18, B2
703—*Trinalin* Extended-release Tablets 1/120 mg.......... MC-2, D3
710—Mylan Cyclobenzaprine Tablets 10 mg.......... MC-6, B5
715—Mylan Timolol Tablets 20 mg MC-23, B4
731—*Lufyllin* Tablets 400 mg MC-8, D3
750—*Relafen* Tablets 750 mg MC-15, D4
750—*Robaxin* Tablets 750 mg.......... MC-14, B7
750—*Slo-Niacin* Extended-release Tablets 750 mg MC-16, B1
752—*Normodyne* Tablets 200 mg.......... MC-13, A1
756—*Pronestyl* Capsules 375 mg MC-19, D2
757—*Pronestyl* Capsules 500 mg MC-19, D2
758—*Pronestyl* Capsules 250 mg MC-19, D2
760—*Sorbitrate* Sublingual Tablets 5 mg MC-12, D2
761—*Sorbitrate* Sublingual Tablets 10 mg MC-12, D2
763—*Sumycin* Capsules 500 mg MC-22, A7
770—*Sorbitrate* Tablets 5 mg MC-12, C5
773—*Sorbitrate* Tablets 30 mg MC-12, C6
774—*Sorbitrate* Tablets 40 mg MC-12, C6
780—*Sorbitrate* Tablets 10 mg MC-13, C5
800—*Zovirax* Tablets 800 mg MC-1, A7
800mg—*Motrin* Tablets 800 mg MC-12, A7
800 SKF—*Tagamet* Tablets 800 mg.......... MC-5, B7
810—*Sorbitrate* Chewable Tablets 5 mg MC-12, C7
811—*Adalat* Capsules 10 mg.......... MC-16, B4
815—*Sorbitrate* Chewable Tablets 10 mg MC-12, C7
820—*Sorbitrate* Tablets 20 mg MC-12, C5
821—*Adalat* Capsules 20 mg.......... MC-16, B4
850—*Ovcon 35-28* Tablets Inert MC-16, D2
850—*Ovcon 50-28* Tablets Inert MC-16, D3
853—*Sorbitrate* Sublingual Tablets 2.5 mg.......... MC-12, D2
855—*Nimotop* Capsules 30 mg MC-16, C2
880—*Sorbitrate SA* Extended-release Tablets 40 mg.......... MC-12, D1
901—*Lortab* Tablets 2.5/500 mg MC-11, C4
902—*Lortab* Tablets 5/500 mg MC-11, C4
903—*Lortab* Tablets 7.5/500 mg MC-11, C4
1001—*Aldactone* Tablets 25 mg MC-21, B5
1011—*Aldactazide* Tablets 25/25 mg MC-21, C1
1021—*Aldactazide* Tablets 50/50 mg MC-21, C1

1031—*Aldactone* Tablets 100 mg MC-21, B5
1041—*Aldactone* Tablets 50 mg MC-21, B5
1375—*Ditropan* Tablets 5 mg MC-17, D4
1381—*Daypro* Tablets 600 mg MC-17, C4
1451—*Cytotec* Tablets 0.1 mg MC-15, D1
1461—*Cytotec* Tablets 0.2 mg MC-15, D1
1771—*Cardizem* Tablets 30 mg MC-7, C2
1772—*Cardizem* Tablets 60 mg MC-7, C2
1800—*Ortho-Est* Tablets 1.25 mg MC-9, D1
1801—*Ortho-Est* Tablets 0.625 mg MC-9, D1
1831—*Flagyl* Tablets 250 mg MC-15, C2
2103—*Soma Compound* Tablets 200/325 mg MC-4, A3
2150—Mylan Meclofenamate Capsules 50 mg MC-14, A6
2403—*Soma Compound with Codeine* Tablets 200/325/16 mg MC-4, A4
2437—*Cardene* Capsules 20 mg MC-16, B2
2438—*Cardene* Capsules 30 mg MC-16, B2
2732—*Norpace CR* Extended-release Capsules 100 mg MC-8, A5
2742—*Norpace CR* Extended-release Capsules 150 mg MC-8, A5
2752—*Norpace* Capsules 100 mg MC-8, A3
2762—*Norpace* Capsules 150 mg MC-8, A3
2832—*Theo-24* Extended-release Capsules 100 mg MC-22, D2
2842—*Theo-24* Extended-release Capsules 200 mg MC-22, D2
2852—*Theo-24* Extended-release Capsules 300 mg MC-22, D2
3000—Mylan Meclofenamate Capsules 100 mg MC-14, A6
3061—*Ceclor* Capsules 250 mg MC-4, A6
3062—*Ceclor* Capsules 500 mg MC-4, A6
3071—Rugby Amitriptyline Tablets 10 mg MC-1, C7
3072—Rugby Amitriptyline Tablets 25 mg MC-1, C7
3073—Rugby Amitriptyline Tablets 50 mg MC-1, C7
3074—Rugby Amitriptyline Tablets 75 mg MC-1, C7
3075—Rugby Amitriptyline Tablets 100 mg MC-1, D1
3076—Rugby Amitriptyline Tablets 150 mg MC-1, D1
3105—*Prozac* Capsules 20 mg MC-10, B2
3144—*Axid* Capsules 150 mg MC-16, D1
3145—*Axid* Capsules 300 mg MC-16, D1
3170—*Lorabid* Capsules 200 mg MC-3, D2
3597—*Diphenhist* Tablets 25 mg MC-7, D2
3736—Rugby Doxepin Capsules 10 mg MC-8, B5
3737—Rugby Doxepin Capsules 75 mg MC-8, B6
3738—Rugby Doxepin Capsules 150 mg MC-8, B6
3874—Rugby Hydroxyzine Tablets 10 mg MC-11, D4
3875—Rugby Hydroxyzine Tablets 25 mg MC-11, D4
3876—Rugby Hydroxyzine Tablets 50 mg MC-11, D4
3952—Rugby Levothyroxine Tablets 0.1 mg MC-13, B4
3953—Rugby Levothyroxine Tablets 0.15 mg MC-13, B4
3958—Rugby Levothyroxine Tablets 0.3 mg MC-13, B4
3977—Rugby Ibuprofen Tablets 400 mg MC-12, A2
3978—Rugby Ibuprofen Tablets 600 mg MC-12, A2
3979—Rugby Ibuprofen Tablets 800 mg MC-12, A3
4010—Mylan Temazepam Capsules 15 mg MC-21, D7
4018—Rugby Metronidazole Tablets 250 mg MC-15, B7
4019—Rugby Metronidazole Tablets 500 mg MC-15, B7
4042—Rugby Metoclopramide Tablets 10 mg MC-15, A6
4125—*Isordil* Extended-release Tablets 40 mg MC-12, C3
4132—*Surmontil* Capsules 25 mg MC-24, B2
4133—*Surmontil* Capsules 50 mg MC-24, B2
4152—*Isordil* Tablets 5 mg MC-12, C2
4153—*Isordil* Tablets 10 mg MC-12, C2
4154—*Isordil* Tablets 20 mg MC-12, C2
4158—*Surmontil* Capsules 100 mg MC-24, B2
4159—*Isordil* Tablets 30 mg MC-12, C2
4188—*Cordarone* Tablets 200 mg MC-1, C6
4191—*Synalgos-DC* Capsules 356.4/30/16 mg MC-2, A7
4192—*Isordil* Tablets 40 mg MC-12, C2
4250—*Donnatal* Tablets 0.0194/0.1037/0.0065/16.2 mg MC-2, C7
4309—Rugby Propranolol Tablets 10 mg MC-20, B5
4313—Rugby Propranolol Tablets 20 mg MC-20, B5
4314—Rugby Propranolol Tablets 40 mg MC-20, B5
4315—Rugby Propranolol Tablets 60 mg MC-20, B5
4316—Rugby Propranolol Tablets 80 mg MC-20, B5
4325—Rugby Prednisone Tablets 10 mg MC-19, C2
4326—Rugby Prednisone Tablets 20 mg MC-19, C2
4381—Rugby Levothyroxine Tablets 0.2 mg MC-13, B4
4402—Rugby Propranolol and Hydrochlorothiazide Tablets 40/25 mg MC-20, C4
4403—Rugby Propranolol and Hydrochlorothiazide Tablets 80/25 mg MC-20, C4
4564—Rugby Doxepin Capsules 25 mg MC-8, B5
4565—Rugby Doxepin Capsules 50 mg MC-8, B5
4566—Rugby Doxepin Capsules 100 mg MC-8, B6
4812—Rugby Verapamil Tablets 80 mg MC-24, C6
4932—Rugby Verapamil Tablets 120 mg MC-24, C6
5050—Mylan Temazepam Capsules 30 mg MC-21, D7
5100—*Penetrex* Tablets 200 mg MC-8, D6
5140—*Penetrex* Tablets 400 mg MC-8, D6
5401—*Ambien* Tablets 5 mg MC-24, D7
5421—*Ambien* Tablets 10 mg MC-24, D7
5455—Schein/Danbury Chlorpropamide Tablets 250 mg MC-5, A6
5496—Schein/Danbury Spironolactone and Hydrochlorothiazide Tablets 25/25 mg MC-21, B7
5522—Schein/Danbury Hydroxyzine Tablets 10 mg MC-11, D5
5523—Schein/Danbury Hydroxyzine Tablets 25 mg MC-11, D5
5538—Schein/Danbury Quinidine Gluconate Extended-release Tablets 324 mg MC-20, D5
5540—Schein/Danbury Metronidazole Tablets 250 mg MC-15, C1
5542—Schein/Danbury Thioridazine Tablets 25 mg MC-23, A3
5543—Schein/Danbury Allopurinol Tablets 100 mg MC-1, C2
5544—Schein/Danbury Allopurinol Tablets 300 mg MC-1, C2
5546—Schein/Danbury Sulfamethoxazole and Trimethoprim Tablets 400/80 mg MC-21, C5
5547—Schein/Danbury Sulfamethoxazole and Trimethoprim Tablets 800/160 mg MC-21, C5
5552—Schein/Danbury Metronidazole Tablets 500 mg MC-15, C1
5553—Schein/Danbury Doxycycline Tablets 100 mg MC-8, D2
5562—Schein/Danbury Procainamide Extended-release Tablets 250 mg MC-19, D6
5565—Schein/Danbury Hydroxyzine Tablets 50 mg MC-11, D5
5566—Schein/Danbury Thioridazine Tablets 10 mg MC-23, A3
5568—Schein/Danbury Thioridazine Tablets 50 mg MC-23, A3
5569—Schein/Danbury Thioridazine Tablets 100 mg MC-23, A4
5575—Schein/Danbury Furosemide Tablets 40 mg MC-10, D1
5579—Schein/Danbury Chlorpropamide Tablets 100 mg MC-5, A6
5580—Schein/Danbury Thioridazine Tablets 150 mg MC-23, A4
5581—Schein/Danbury Thioridazine Tablets 200 mg MC-23, A4
5584—Schein/Danbury Ibuprofen Tablets 400 mg MC-12, A4
5585—Schein/Danbury Ibuprofen Tablets 200 mg MC-12, A4
5586—Schein/Danbury Ibuprofen Tablets 600 mg MC-12, A5
5587—Schein/Danbury Methyldopa Tablets 500 mg MC-14, D1
5588—Schein/Danbury Methyldopa Tablets 250 mg MC-14, D1
5589—Schein/Danbury Metoclopramide Tablets 10 mg MC-15, A7
5592—Schein/Danbury Thiothixene Capsules 2 mg MC-23, B1
5593—Schein/Danbury Thiothixene Capsules 1 mg MC-23, B1
5594—Schein/Danbury Thiothixene Capsules 10 mg MC-23, B1
5595—Schein/Danbury Thiothixene Capsules 5 mg MC-23, B1
5599—Schein/Danbury Trazodone Tablets 100 mg MC-23, D5
5600—Schein/Danbury Trazodone Tablets 50 mg MC-23, D5
5601—Schein/Danbury Verapamil Tablets 80 mg MC-24, C7
5602—Schein/Danbury Verapamil Tablets 120 mg MC-24, C7
5644—Schein/Danbury Ibuprofen Tablets 800 mg MC-12, A5
5658—Schein/Danbury Cyclobenzaprine Tablets 10 mg MC-6, B6
5660—Schein/Danbury Sulindac Tablets 200 mg MC-21, D3
5661—Schein/Danbury Sulindac Tablets 150 mg MC-21, D3
5704—Schein/Danbury Fenoprofen Tablets 600 mg MC-10, A5
5710—Schein/Danbury Albuterol Tablets 2 mg MC-1, B3
5711—Schein/Danbury Albuterol Tablets 4 mg MC-1, B3
5736—Schein/Danbury Timolol Tablets 5 mg MC-23, B5
5737—Schein/Danbury Timolol Tablets 10 mg MC-23, B5
5738—Schein/Danbury Timolol Tablets 20 mg MC-23, B5
5777—Schein/Danbury Atenolol Tablets 50 mg MC-2, B7
5778—Schein/Danbury Atenolol Tablets 100 mg MC-2, B7
6251—*Phenaphen with Codeine* Tablets 650/30 mg MC-1, A5
7278—*Polymox* and *Trimox* Capsules 250 mg MC-1, D5
7279—*Polymox* and *Trimox* Capsules 500 mg MC-1, D5
7658—*Dynapen* Capsules 500 mg MC-7, D2
7720—*Cefzil* Tablets 250 mg MC-4, B3
7721—*Cefzil* Tablets 500 mg MC-4, B3

7892—*Dynapen* Capsules 125 mg MC-7, D1
7893—*Dynapen* Capsules 250 mg MC-7, D1
7977—*Prostaphlin* Capsules 250 mg. MC-17, C3
7982—*Prostaphlin* Capsules 500 mg. MC-17, C3
7992—*Principen* Capsules 250 mg MC-2, A4
7993—*Principen* Capsules 500 mg MC-2, A4

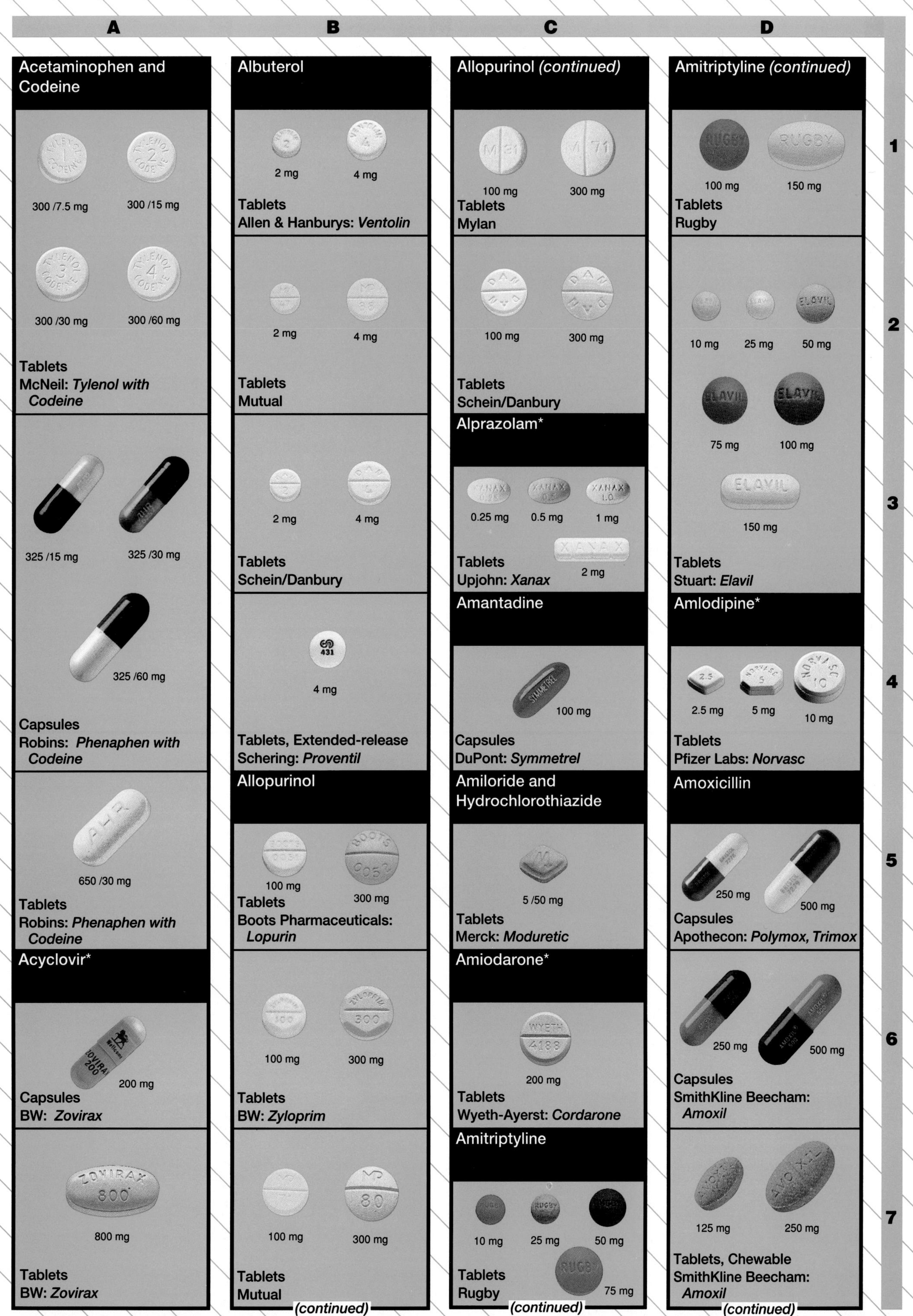

* Single source product for solid oral dosage forms in the U.S.

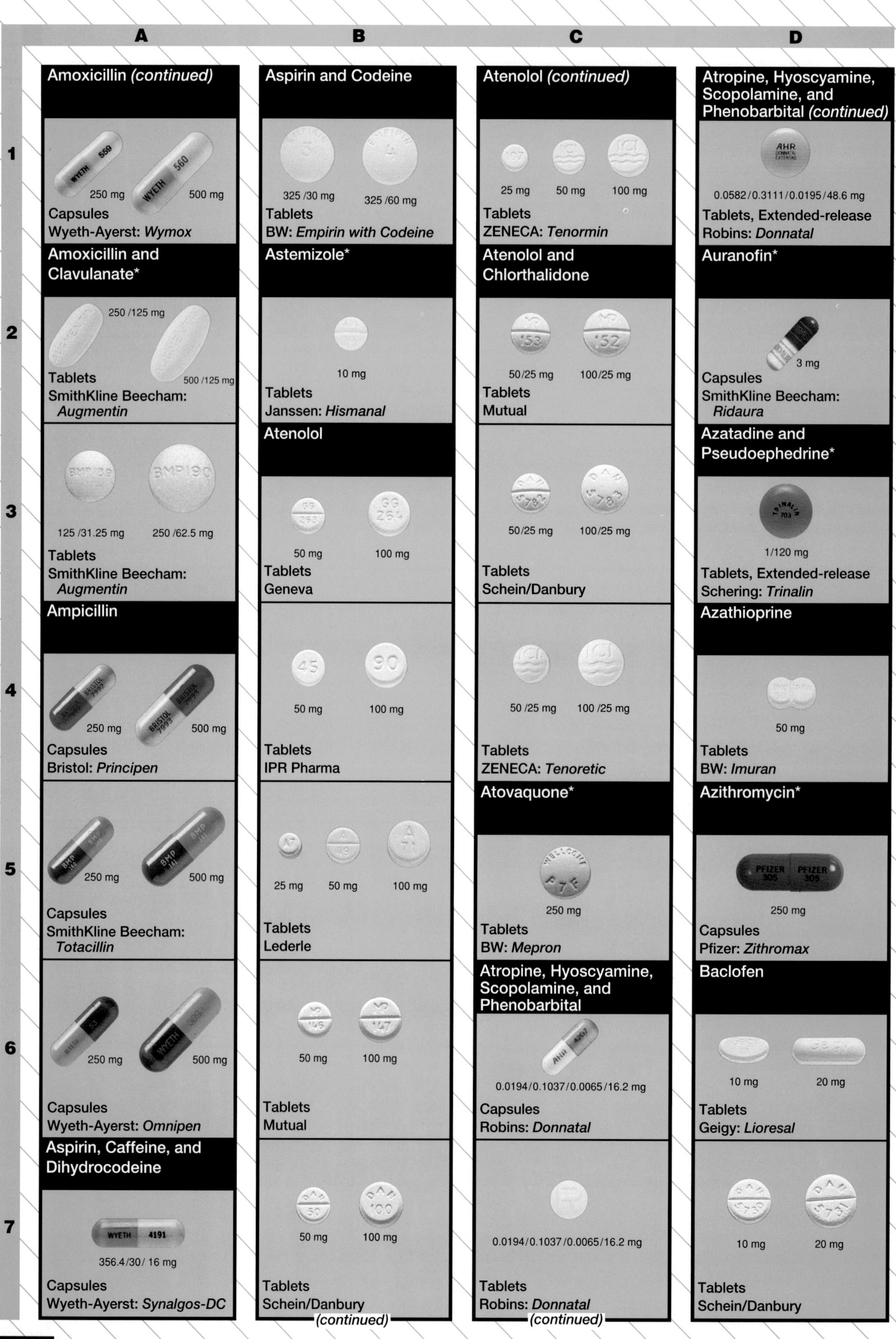

* Single source product for solid oral dosage forms in the U.S.

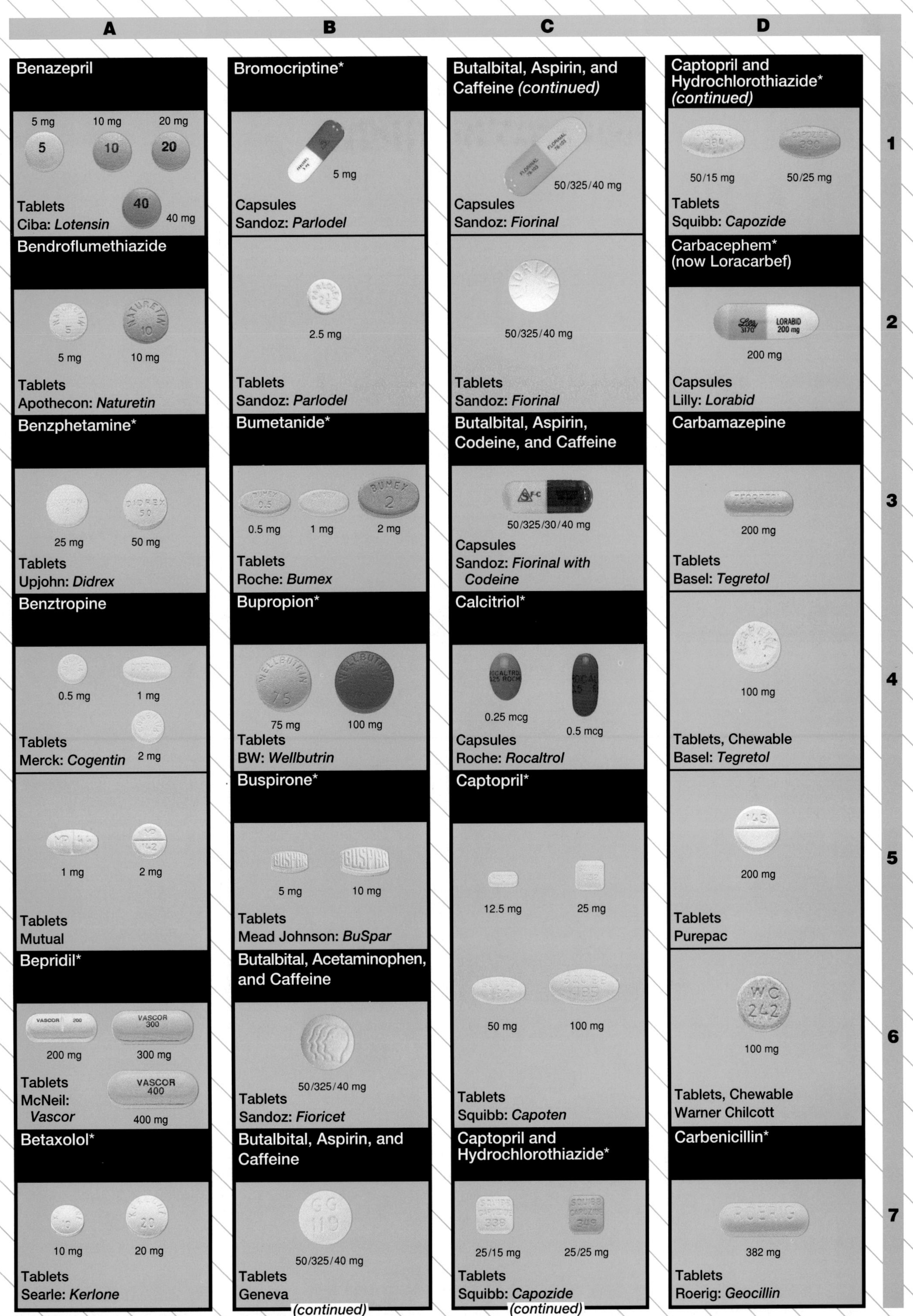

* Single source product for solid oral dosage forms in the U.S.

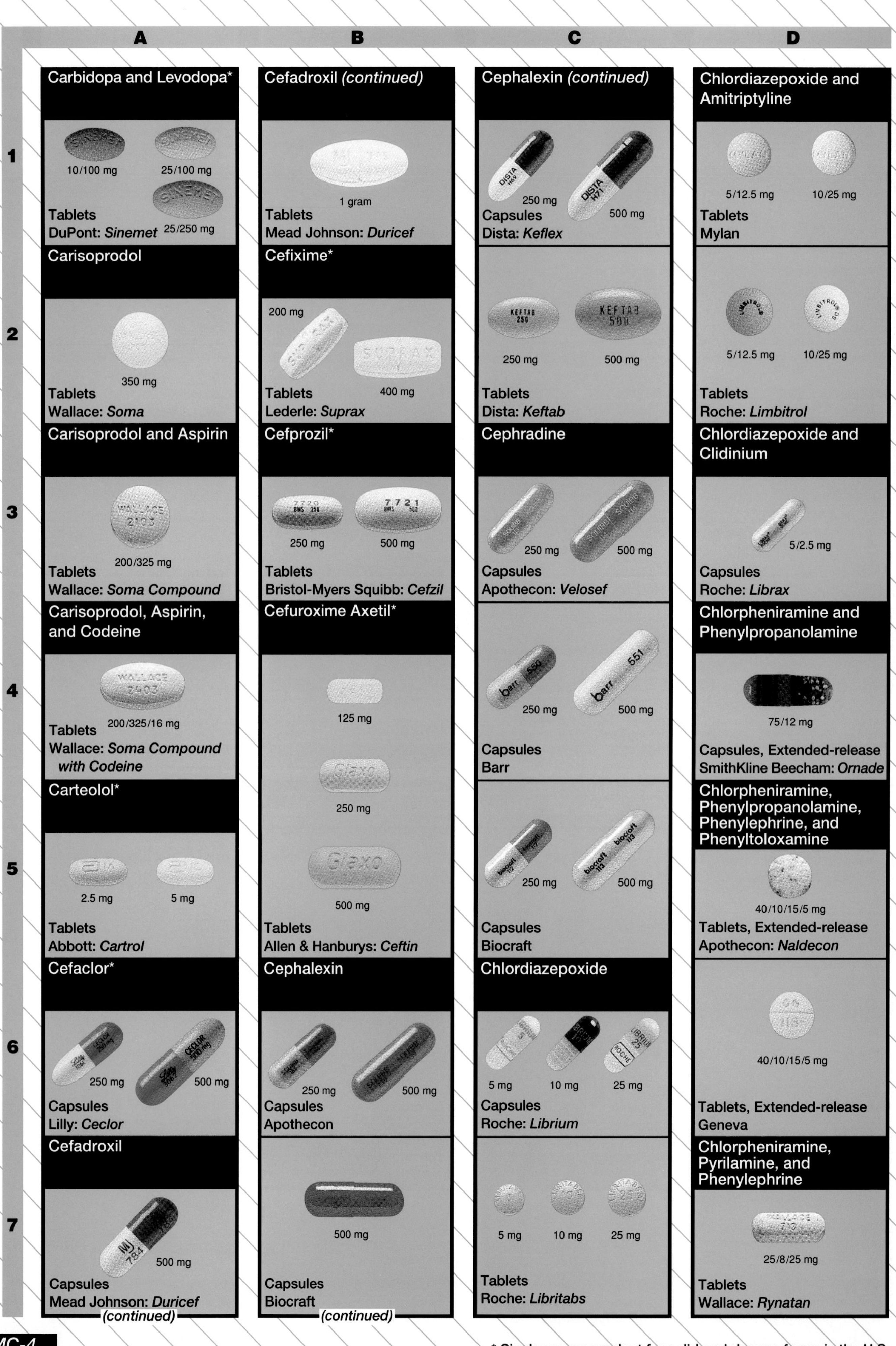

* Single source product for solid oral dosage forms in the U.S.

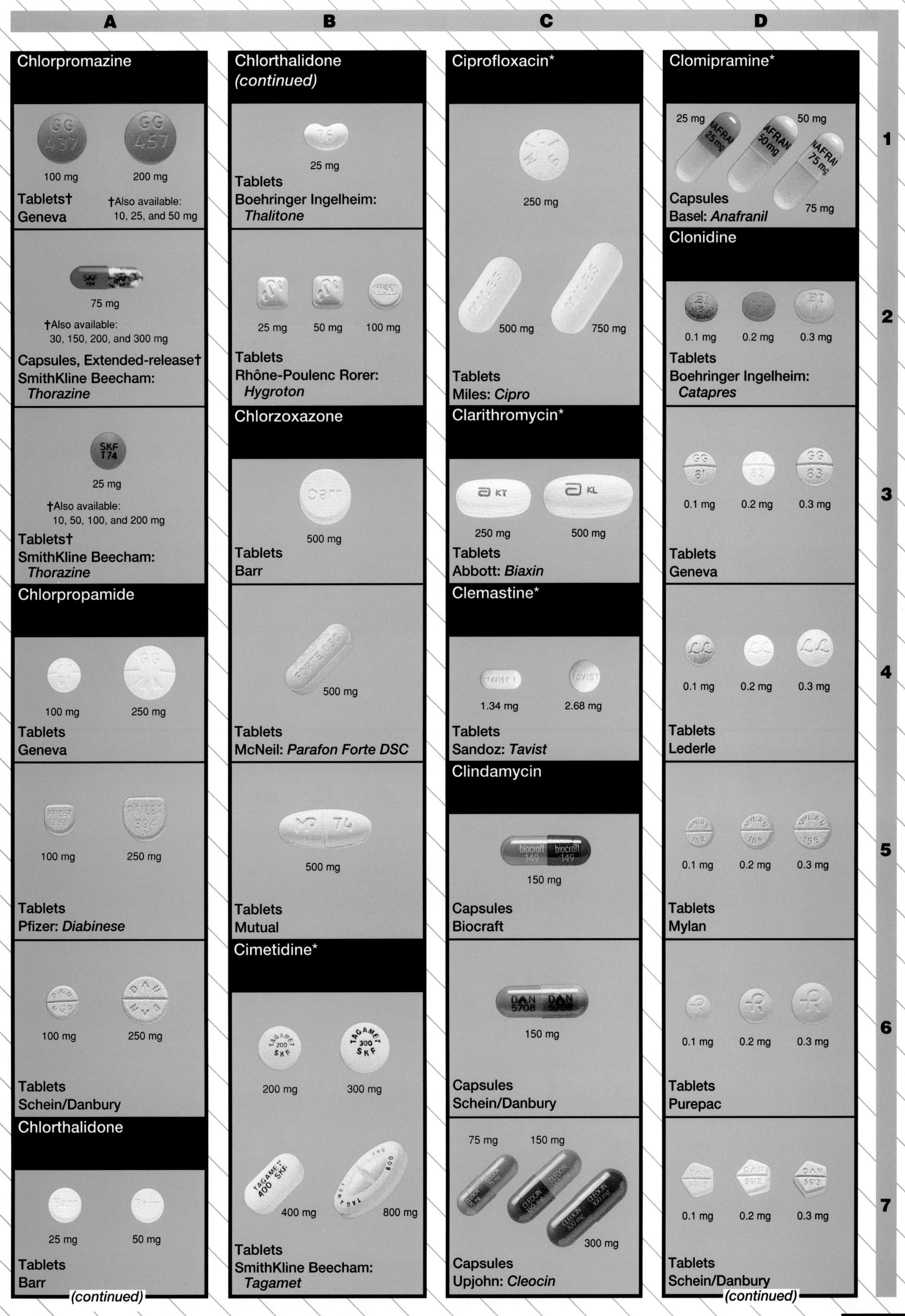

* Single source product for solid oral dosage forms in the U.S.

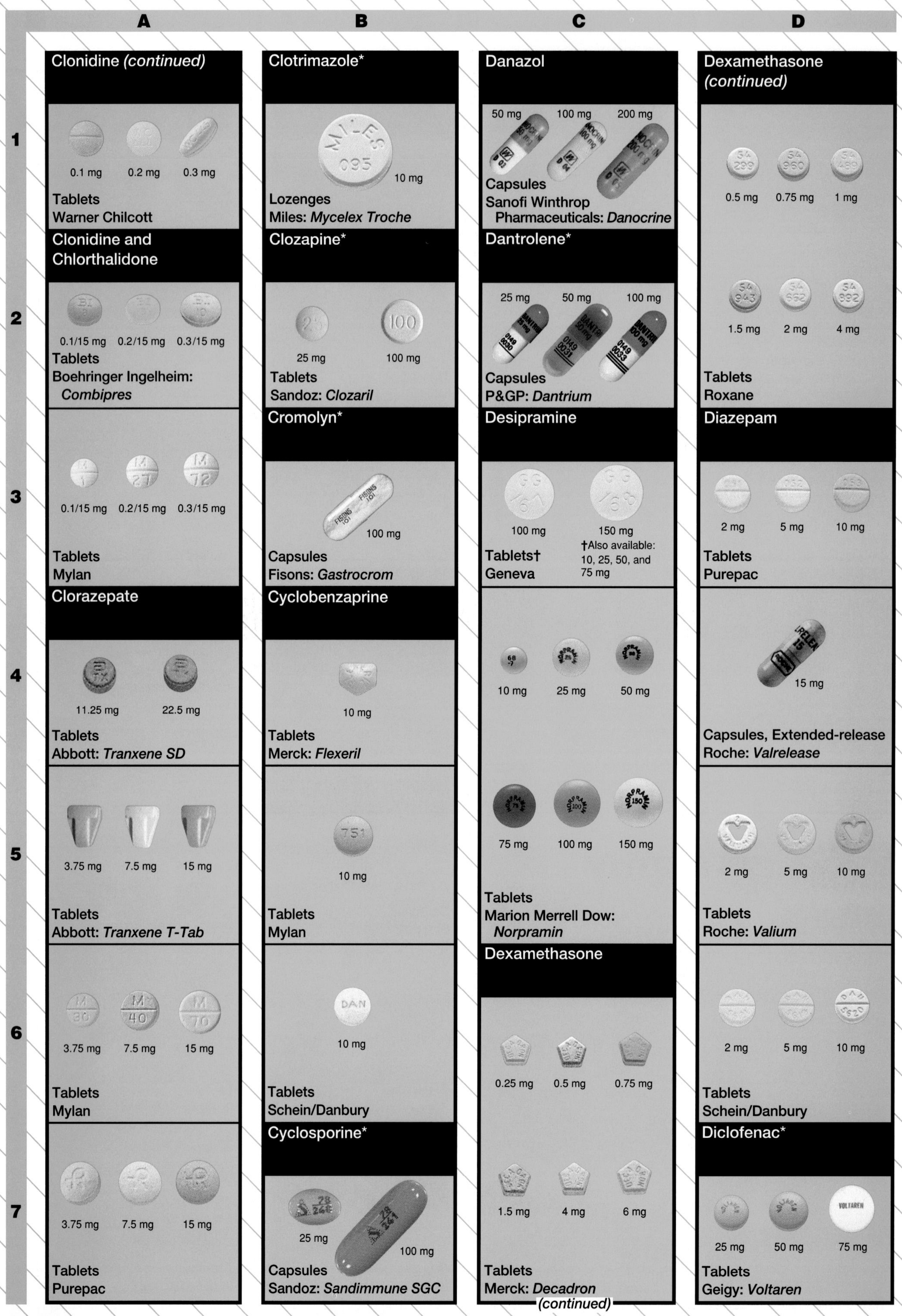

* Single source product for solid oral dosage forms in the U.S.

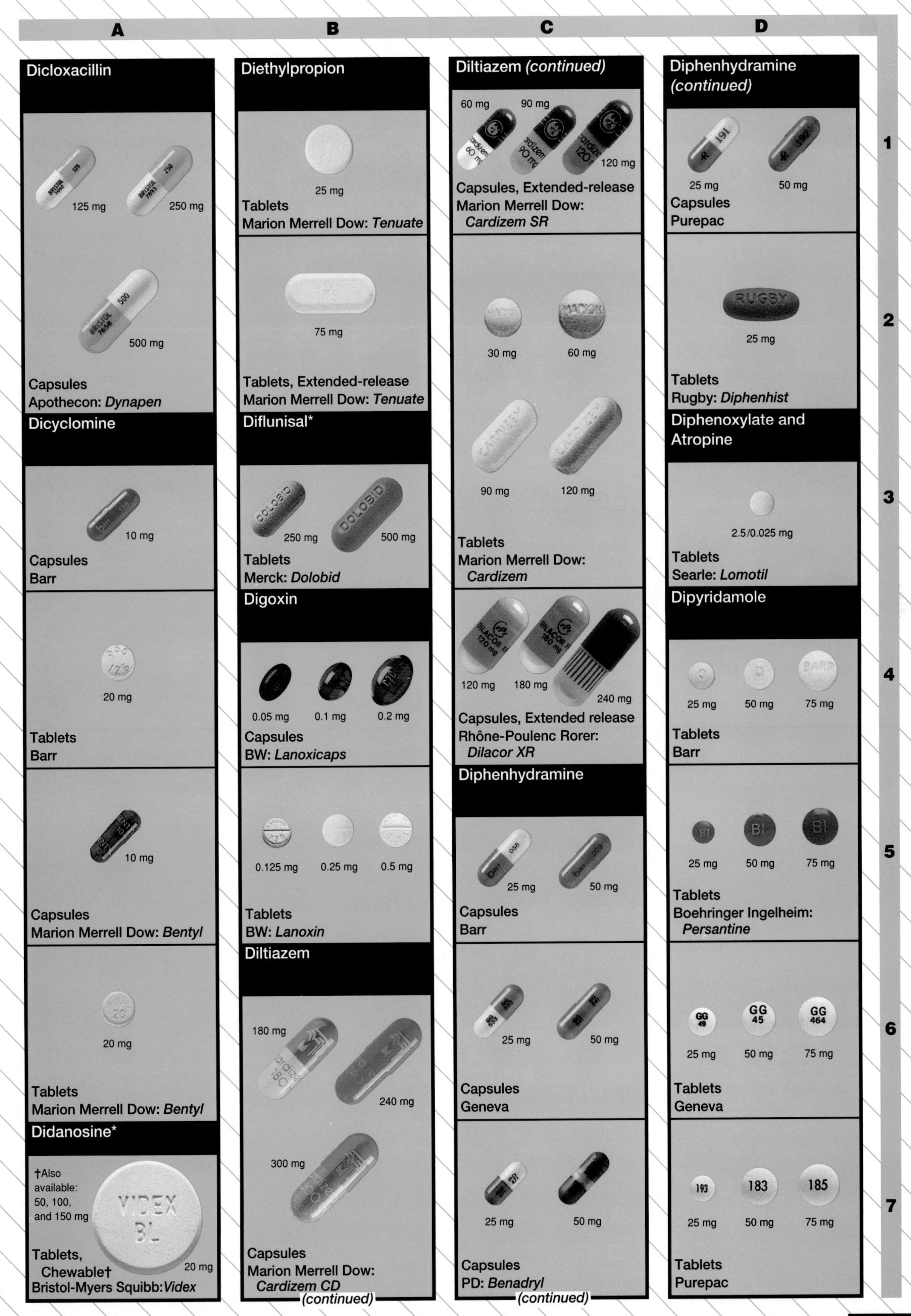

* Single source product for solid oral dosage forms in the U.S.

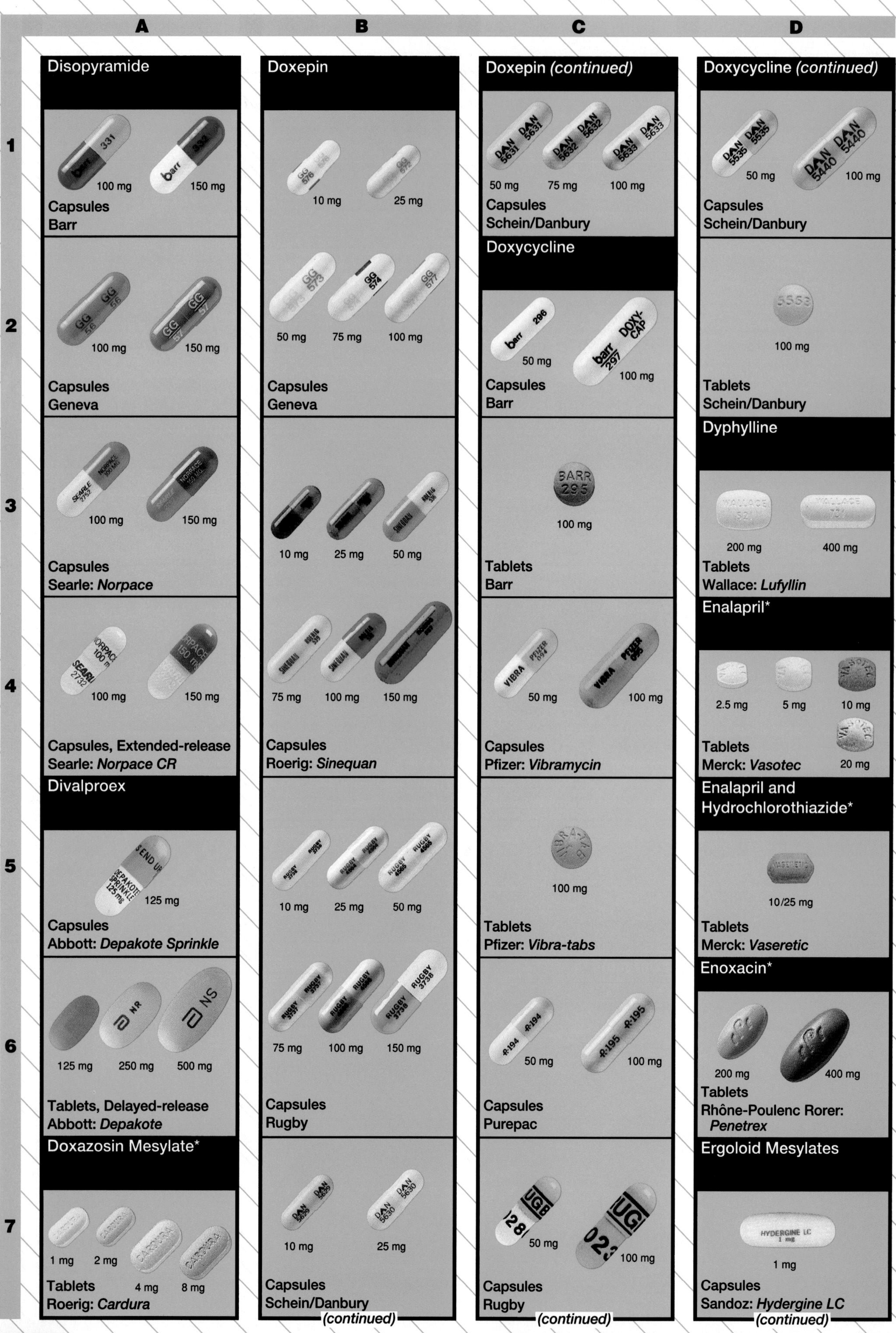

* Single source product for solid oral dosage forms in the U.S.

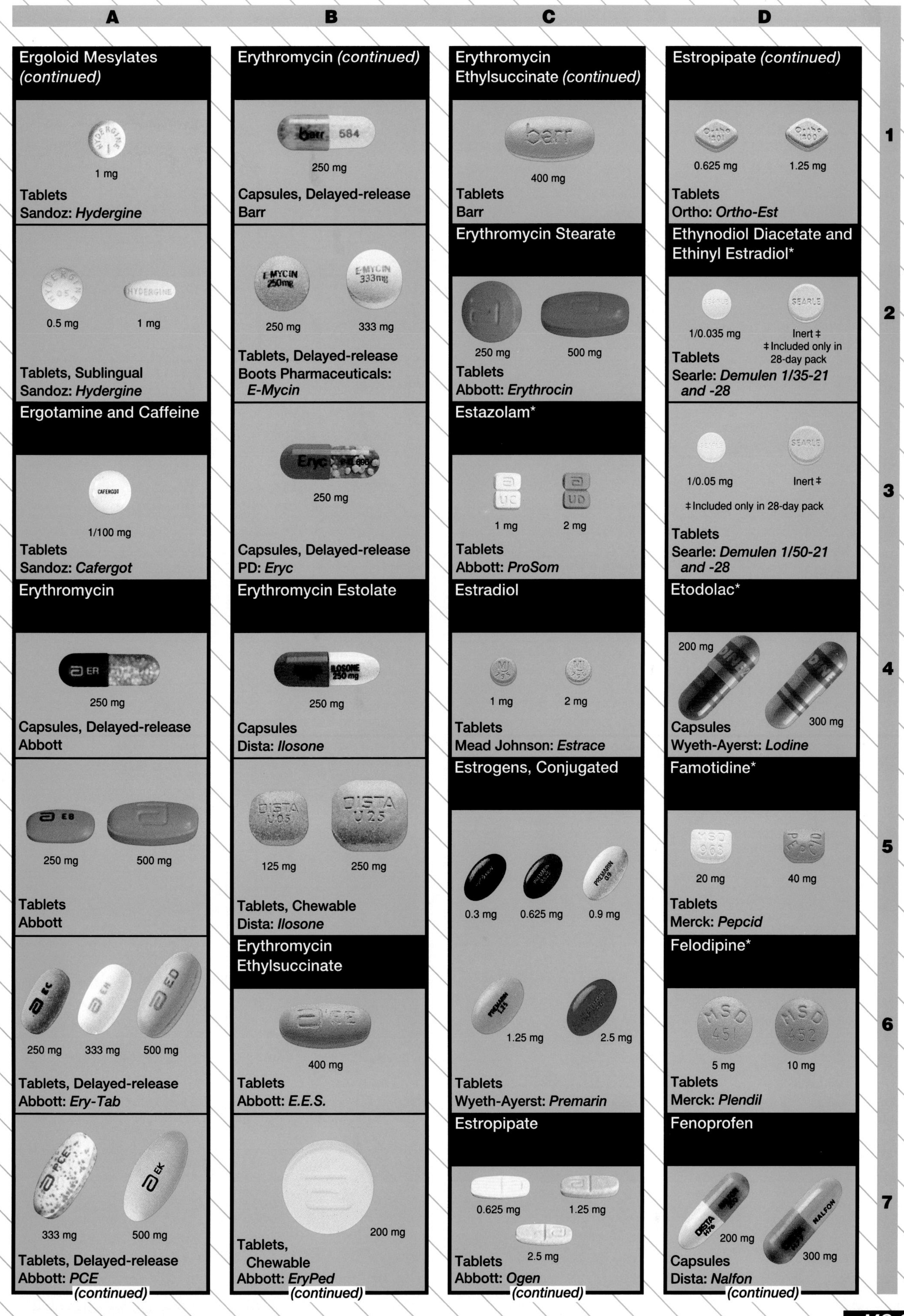

* Single source product for solid oral dosage forms in the U.S.

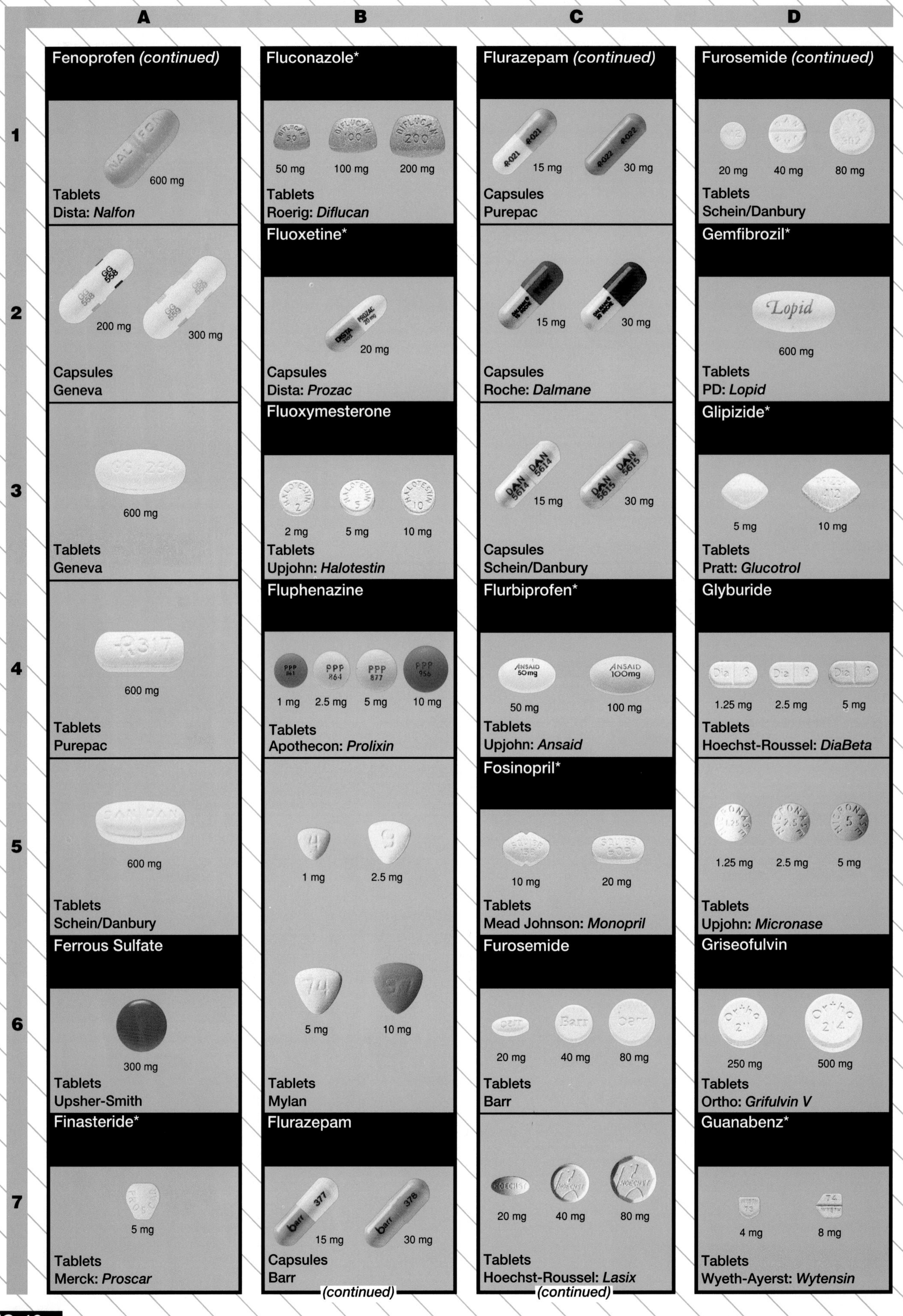

* Single source product for solid oral dosage forms in the U.S.

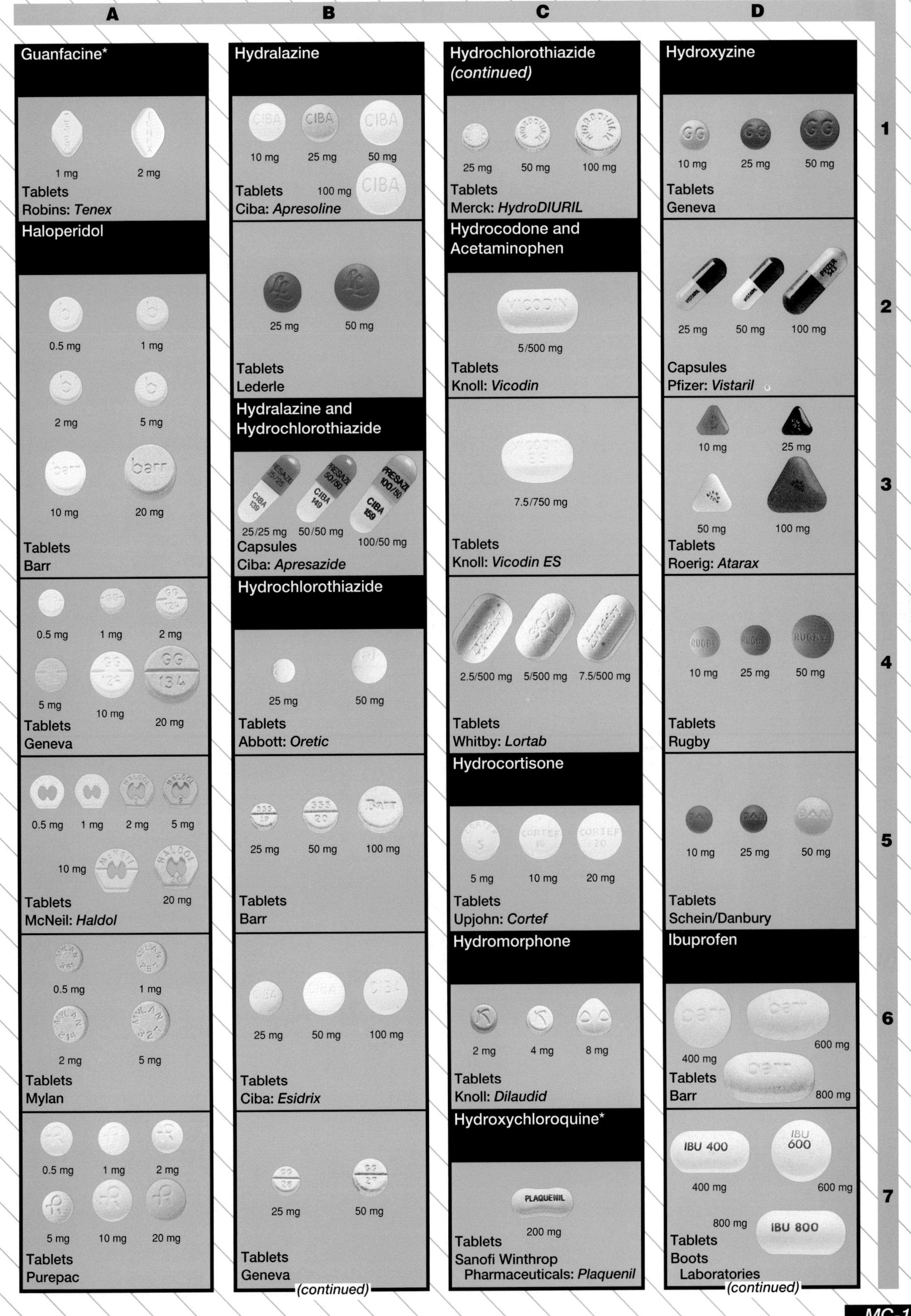

* Single source product for solid oral dosage forms in the U.S.

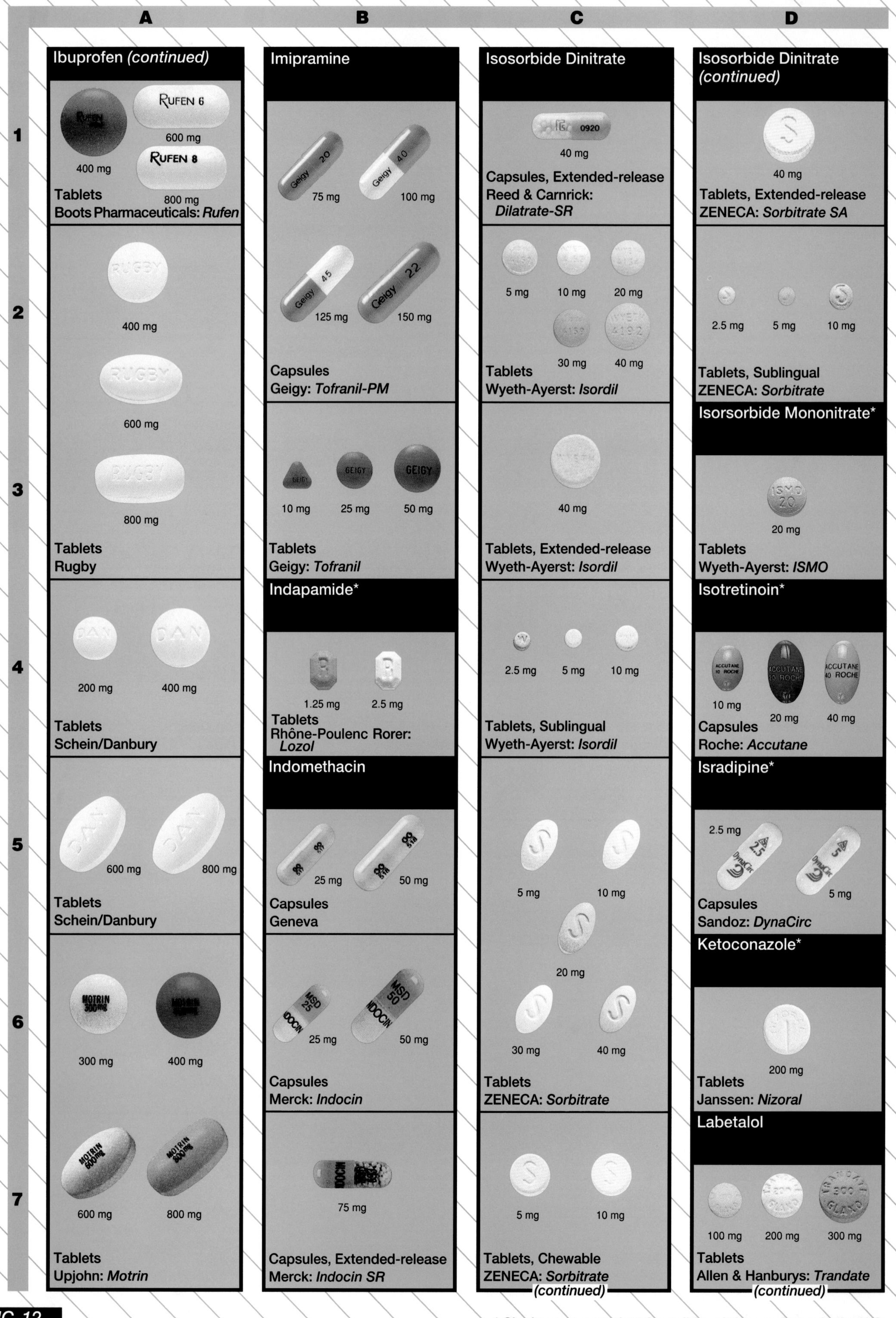
A
B
C
D
1
2
3
4
5
6
7
Ibuprofen (continued)
RUFEN 6
RUFEN 8
400 mg
600 mg
800 mg
Tablets
Boots Pharmaceuticals: Rufen
RUGBY
400 mg
600 mg
800 mg
Tablets
Rugby
DAN
200 mg
400 mg
Tablets
Schein/Danbury
600 mg
800 mg
Tablets
Schein/Danbury
MOTRIN 300mg
300 mg
400 mg
600 mg
800 mg
Tablets
Upjohn: Motrin
Imipramine
Geigy 20
Geigy 40
75 mg
100 mg
Geigy 45
Geigy 22
125 mg
150 mg
Capsules
Geigy: Tofranil-PM
GEIGY
10 mg
25 mg
50 mg
Tablets
Geigy: Tofranil
Indapamide*
1.25 mg
2.5 mg
Tablets
Rhône-Poulenc Rorer: Lozol
Indomethacin
25 mg
50 mg
Capsules
Geneva
MSD 25 INDOCIN
MSD 50 INDOCIN
25 mg
50 mg
Capsules
Merck: Indocin
75 mg
Capsules, Extended-release
Merck: Indocin SR
Isosorbide Dinitrate
0920
40 mg
Capsules, Extended-release
Reed & Carnrick: Dilatrate-SR
5 mg
10 mg
20 mg
30 mg
40 mg
Tablets
Wyeth-Ayerst: Isordil
40 mg
Tablets, Extended-release
Wyeth-Ayerst: Isordil
2.5 mg
5 mg
10 mg
Tablets, Sublingual
Wyeth-Ayerst: Isordil
5 mg
10 mg
20 mg
30 mg
40 mg
Tablets
ZENECA: Sorbitrate
5 mg
10 mg
Tablets, Chewable
ZENECA: Sorbitrate
(continued)
Isosorbide Dinitrate (continued)
40 mg
Tablets, Extended-release
ZENECA: Sorbitrate SA
2.5 mg
5 mg
10 mg
Tablets, Sublingual
ZENECA: Sorbitrate
Isorsorbide Mononitrate*
ISMO 20
20 mg
Tablets
Wyeth-Ayerst: ISMO
Isotretinoin*
ACCUTANE 10 ROCHE
ACCUTANE 20 ROCHE
ACCUTANE 40 ROCHE
10 mg
20 mg
40 mg
Capsules
Roche: Accutane
Isradipine*
2.5 mg
DynaCirc
5 mg
Capsules
Sandoz: DynaCirc
Ketoconazole*
200 mg
Tablets
Janssen: Nizoral
Labetalol
100 mg
200 mg
300 mg
Tablets
Allen & Hanburys: Trandate
(continued)
* Single source product for solid oral dosage forms in the U.S.

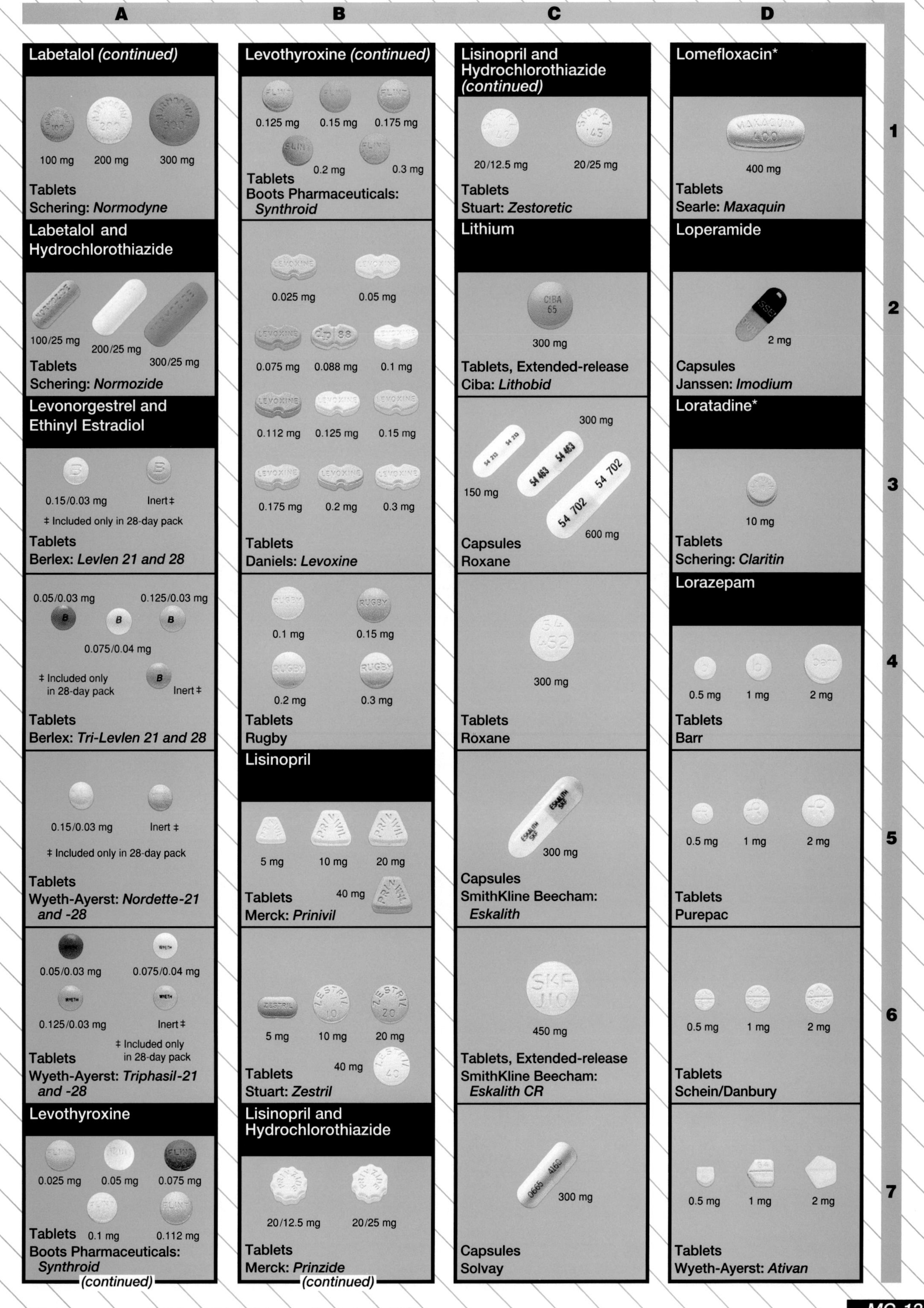

* Single source product for solid oral dosage forms in the U.S.

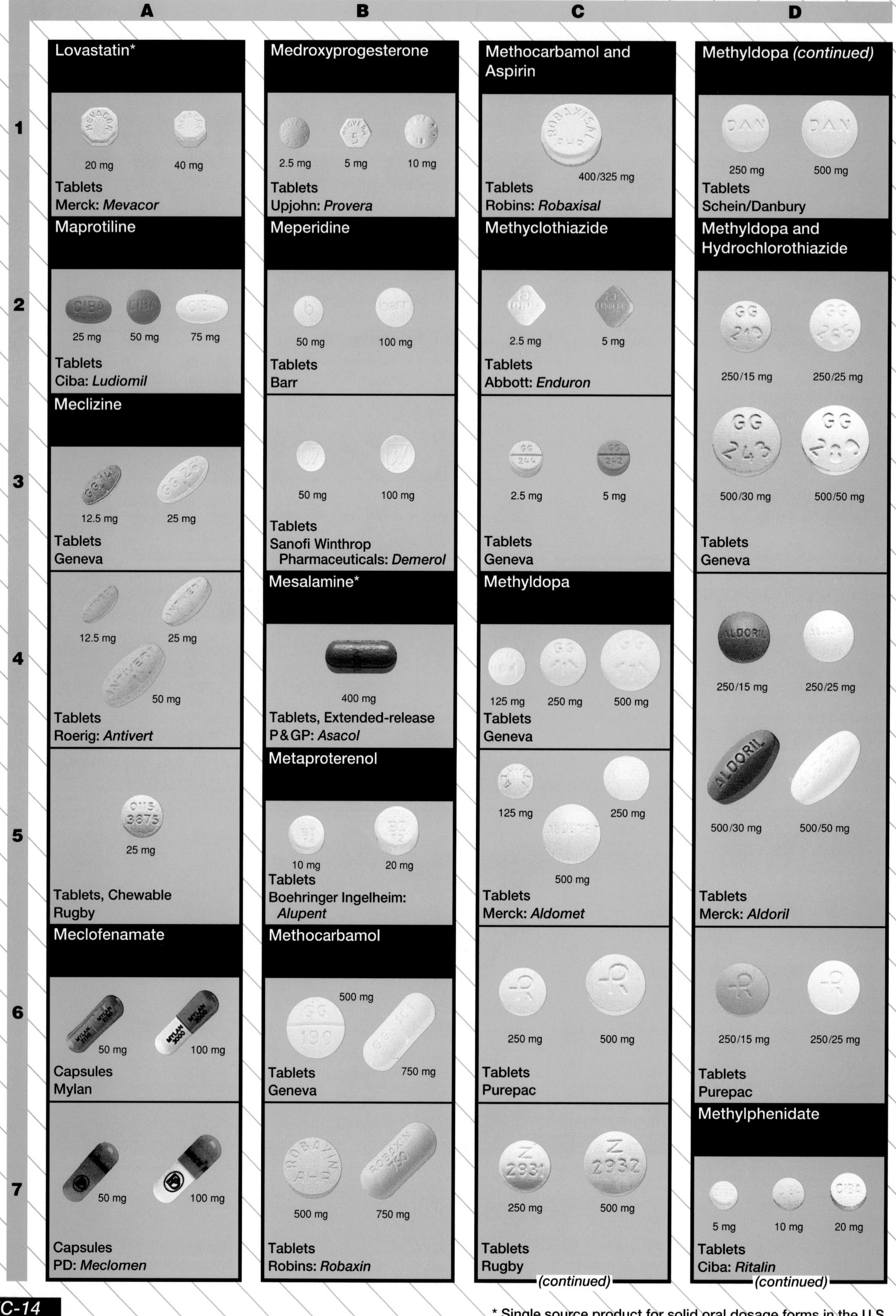
A
B
C
D
1
2
3
4
5
6
7
Lovastatin*
20 mg
40 mg
Tablets
Merck: Mevacor
Maprotiline
25 mg
50 mg
75 mg
Tablets
Ciba: Ludiomil
Meclizine
12.5 mg
25 mg
Tablets
Geneva
12.5 mg
25 mg
50 mg
Tablets
Roerig: Antivert
25 mg
Tablets, Chewable
Rugby
Meclofenamate
50 mg
100 mg
Capsules
Mylan
50 mg
100 mg
Capsules
PD: Meclomen
Medroxyprogesterone
2.5 mg
5 mg
10 mg
Tablets
Upjohn: Provera
Meperidine
50 mg
100 mg
Tablets
Barr
50 mg
100 mg
Tablets
Sanofi Winthrop Pharmaceuticals: Demerol
Mesalamine*
400 mg
Tablets, Extended-release
P&GP: Asacol
Metaproterenol
10 mg
20 mg
Tablets
Boehringer Ingelheim: Alupent
Methocarbamol
500 mg
750 mg
Tablets
Geneva
500 mg
750 mg
Tablets
Robins: Robaxin
Methocarbamol and Aspirin
400/325 mg
Tablets
Robins: Robaxisal
Methyclothiazide
2.5 mg
5 mg
Tablets
Abbott: Enduron
2.5 mg
5 mg
Tablets
Geneva
Methyldopa
125 mg
250 mg
500 mg
Tablets
Geneva
125 mg
250 mg
500 mg
Tablets
Merck: Aldomet
250 mg
500 mg
Tablets
Purepac
250 mg
500 mg
Tablets
Rugby
(continued)
Methyldopa (continued)
250 mg
500 mg
Tablets
Schein/Danbury
Methyldopa and Hydrochlorothiazide
250/15 mg
250/25 mg
500/30 mg
500/50 mg
Tablets
Geneva
250/15 mg
250/25 mg
500/30 mg
500/50 mg
Tablets
Merck: Aldoril
250/15 mg
250/25 mg
Tablets
Purepac
Methylphenidate
5 mg
10 mg
20 mg
Tablets
Ciba: Ritalin
(continued)
* Single source product for solid oral dosage forms in the U.S.

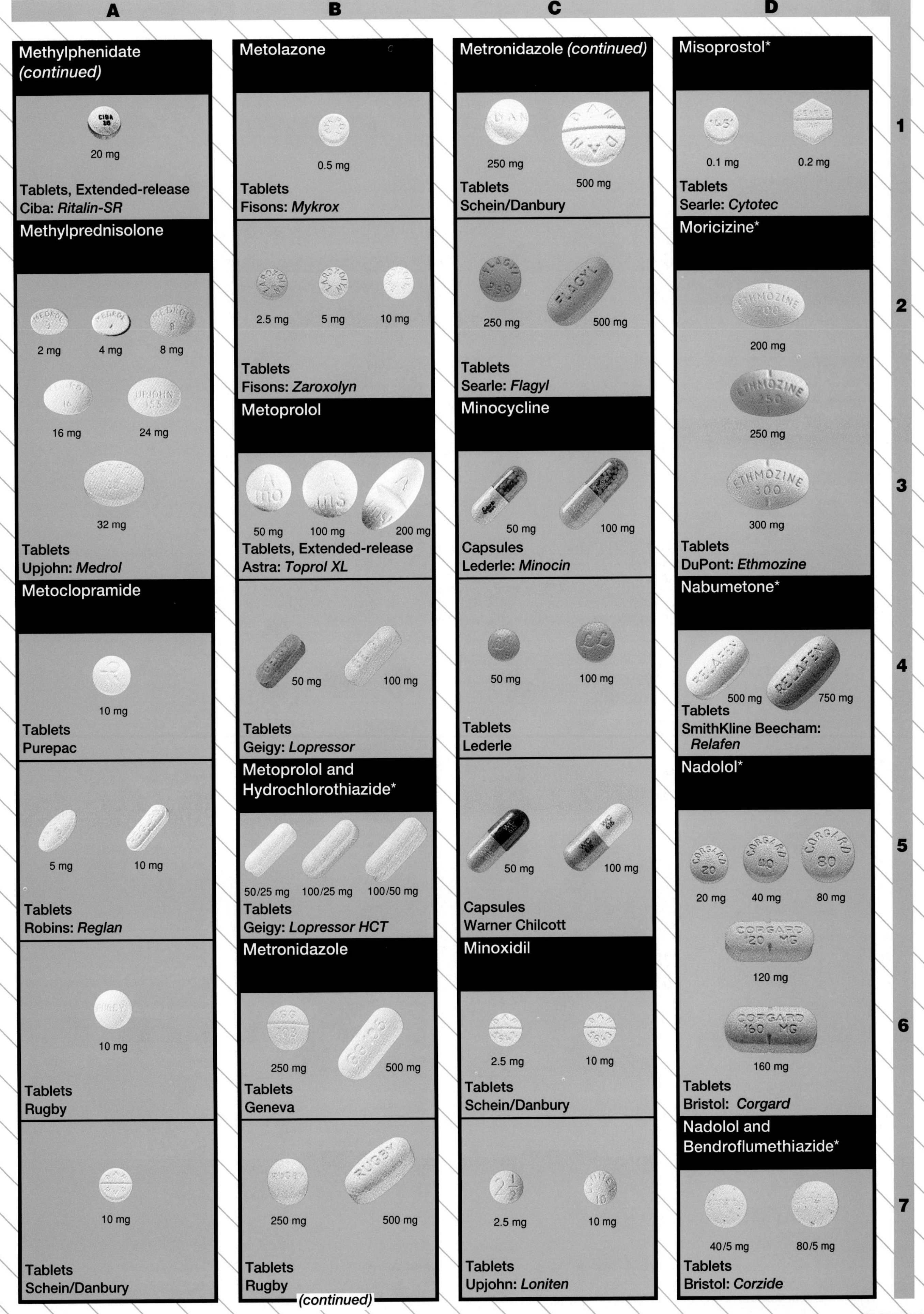

* Single source product for solid oral dosage forms in the U.S.

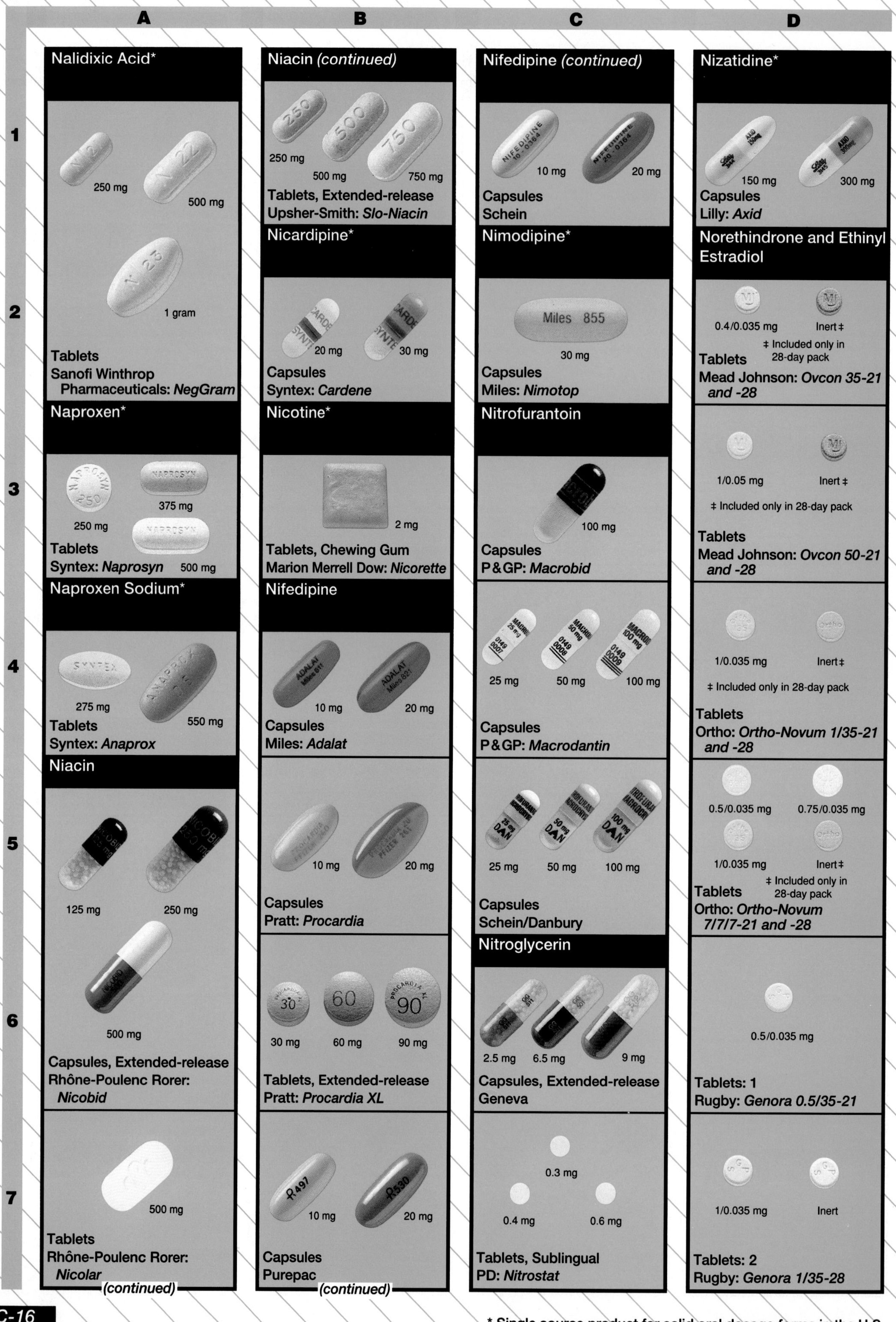

* Single source product for solid oral dosage forms in the U.S.

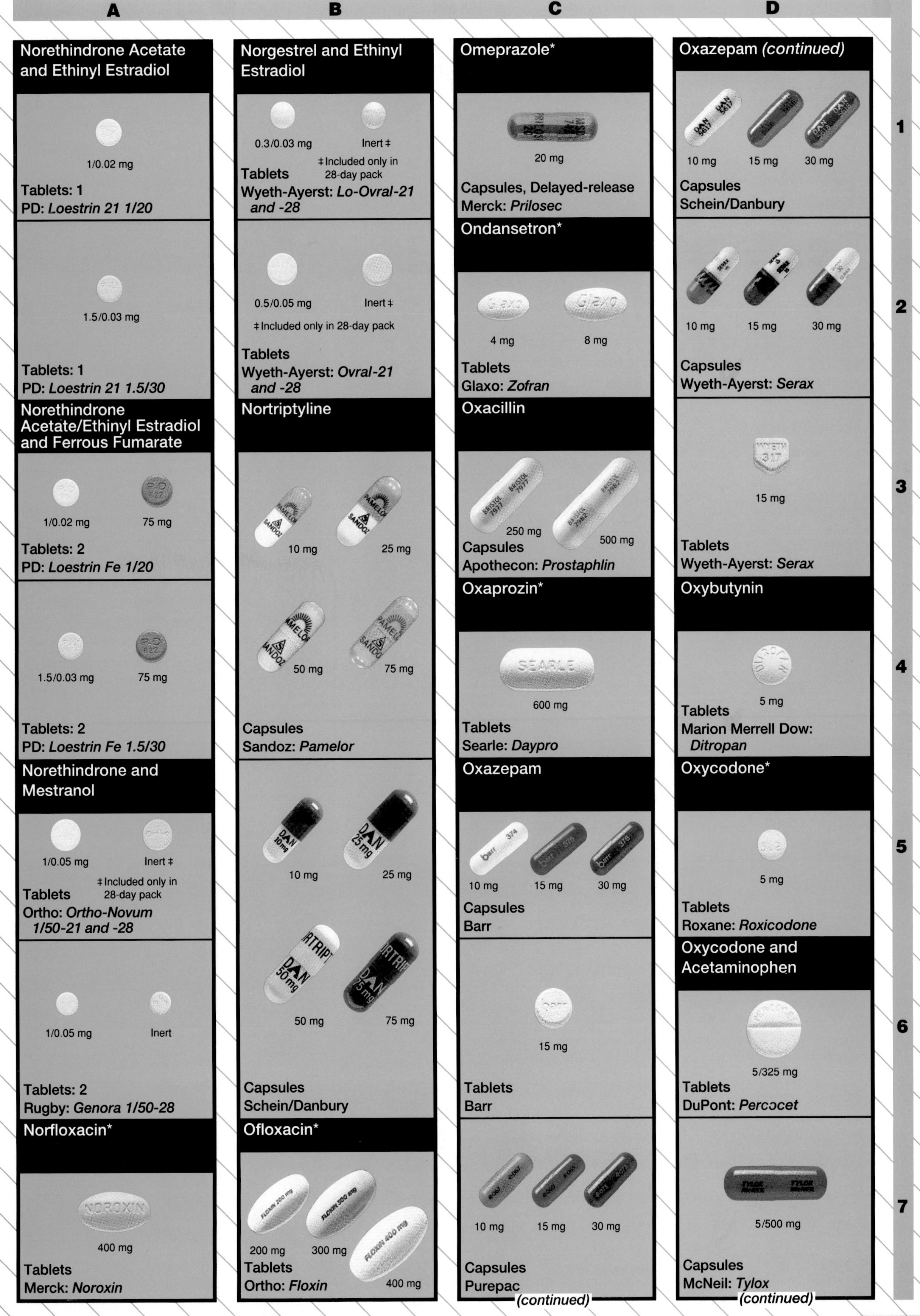

* Single source product for solid oral dosage forms in the U.S.

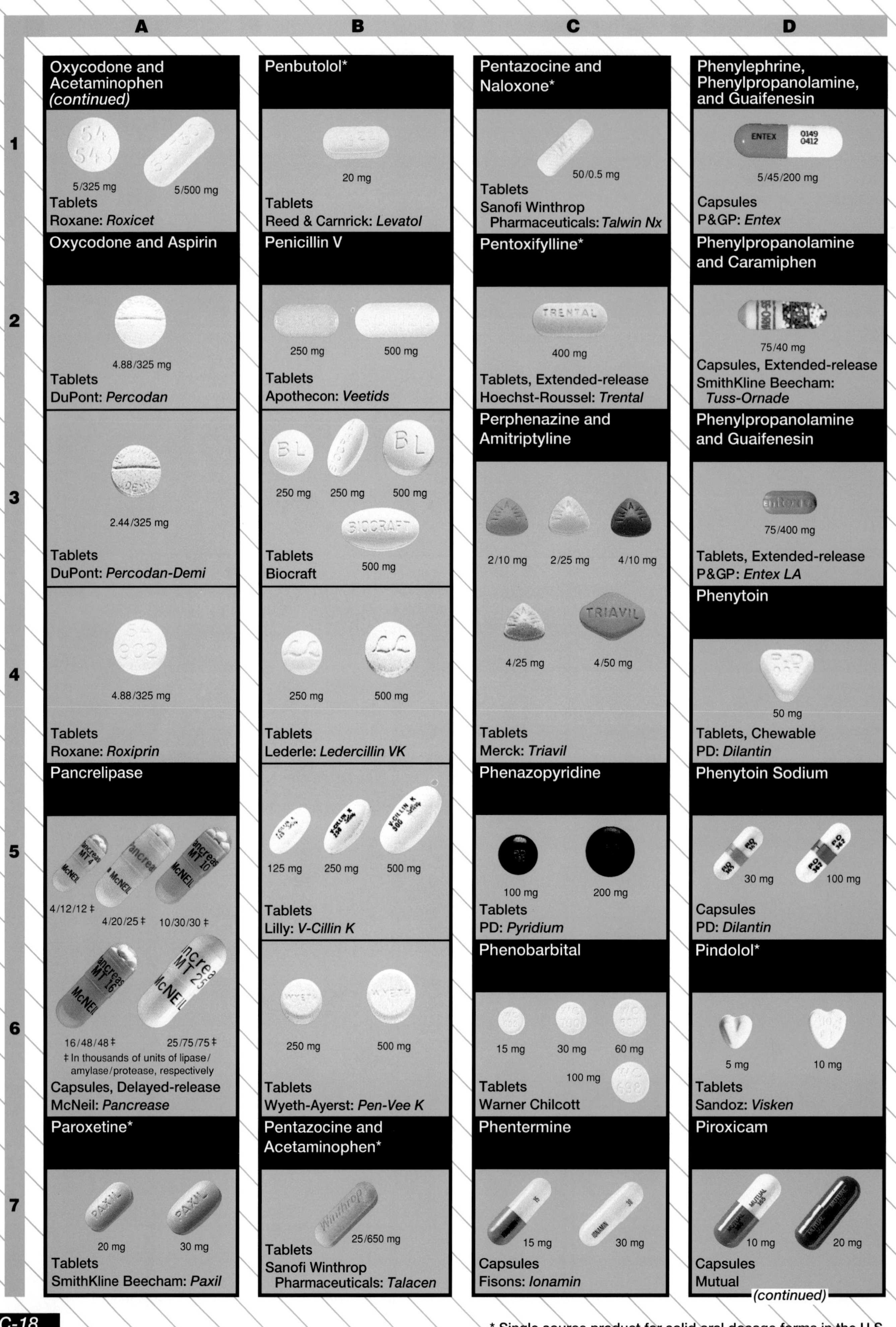
A
B
C
D
1
2
3
4
5
6
7
Oxycodone and Acetaminophen (continued)
5/325 mg
5/500 mg
Tablets
Roxane: Roxicet
Oxycodone and Aspirin
4.88/325 mg
Tablets
DuPont: Percodan
2.44/325 mg
Tablets
DuPont: Percodan-Demi
4.88/325 mg
Tablets
Roxane: Roxiprin
Pancrelipase
4/12/12 ‡
4/20/25 ‡
10/30/30 ‡
16/48/48 ‡
25/75/75 ‡
‡ In thousands of units of lipase/amylase/protease, respectively
Capsules, Delayed-release
McNeil: Pancrease
Paroxetine*
PAXIL
20 mg
30 mg
Tablets
SmithKline Beecham: Paxil
Penbutolol*
20 mg
Tablets
Reed & Carnrick: Levatol
Penicillin V
250 mg
500 mg
Tablets
Apothecon: Veetids
BL
250 mg
250 mg
500 mg
BIOCRAFT
Tablets
Biocraft
500 mg
250 mg
500 mg
Tablets
Lederle: Ledercillin VK
125 mg
250 mg
500 mg
Tablets
Lilly: V-Cillin K
WYETH
250 mg
500 mg
Tablets
Wyeth-Ayerst: Pen-Vee K
Pentazocine and Acetaminophen*
Winthrop
25/650 mg
Tablets
Sanofi Winthrop Pharmaceuticals: Talacen
Pentazocine and Naloxone*
50/0.5 mg
Tablets
Sanofi Winthrop Pharmaceuticals: Talwin Nx
Pentoxifylline*
TRENTAL
400 mg
Tablets, Extended-release
Hoechst-Roussel: Trental
Perphenazine and Amitriptyline
2/10 mg
2/25 mg
4/10 mg
TRIAVIL
4/25 mg
4/50 mg
Tablets
Merck: Triavil
Phenazopyridine
100 mg
200 mg
Tablets
PD: Pyridium
Phenobarbital
15 mg
30 mg
60 mg
100 mg
Tablets
Warner Chilcott
Phentermine
15 mg
30 mg
Capsules
Fisons: Ionamin
Phenylephrine, Phenylpropanolamine, and Guaifenesin
ENTEX 0149 0412
5/45/200 mg
Capsules
P&GP: Entex
Phenylpropanolamine and Caramiphen
75/40 mg
Capsules, Extended-release
SmithKline Beecham: Tuss-Ornade
Phenylpropanolamine and Guaifenesin
75/400 mg
Tablets, Extended-release
P&GP: Entex LA
Phenytoin
50 mg
Tablets, Chewable
PD: Dilantin
Phenytoin Sodium
30 mg
100 mg
Capsules
PD: Dilantin
Pindolol*
5 mg
10 mg
Tablets
Sandoz: Visken
Piroxicam
10 mg
20 mg
Capsules
Mutual
(continued)
* Single source product for solid oral dosage forms in the U.S.

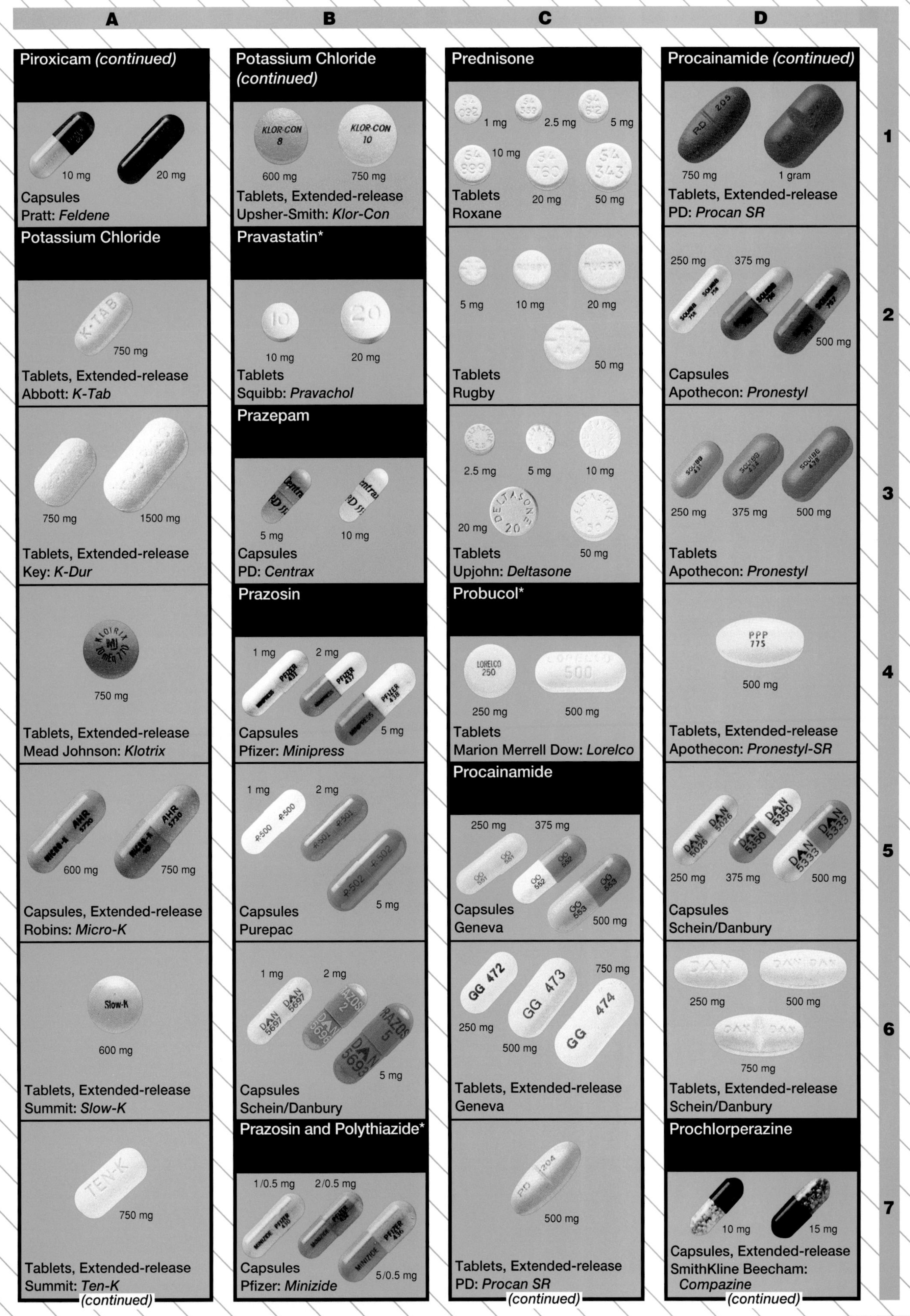

* Single source product for solid oral dosage forms in the U.S.

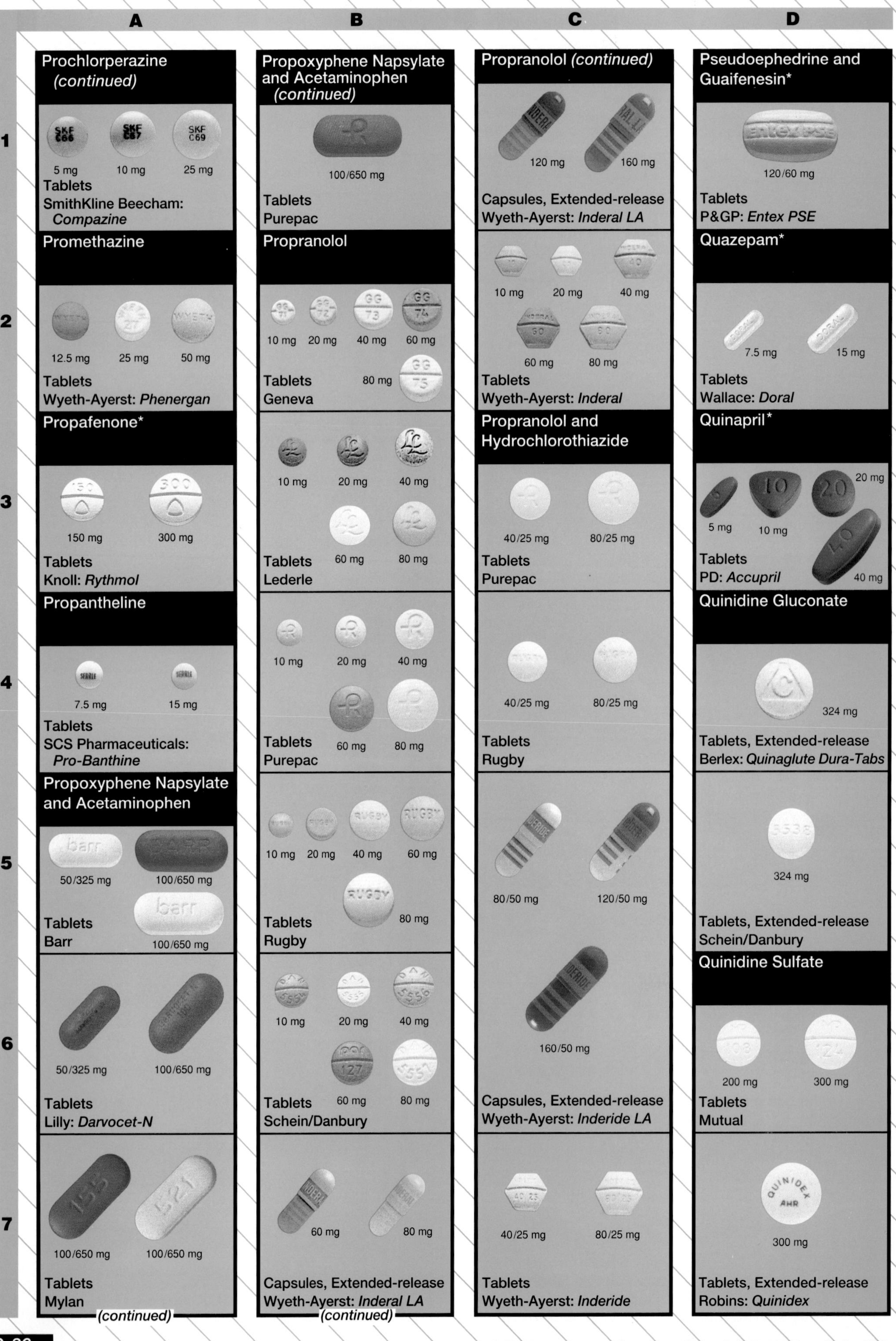

* Single source product for solid oral dosage forms in the U.S.

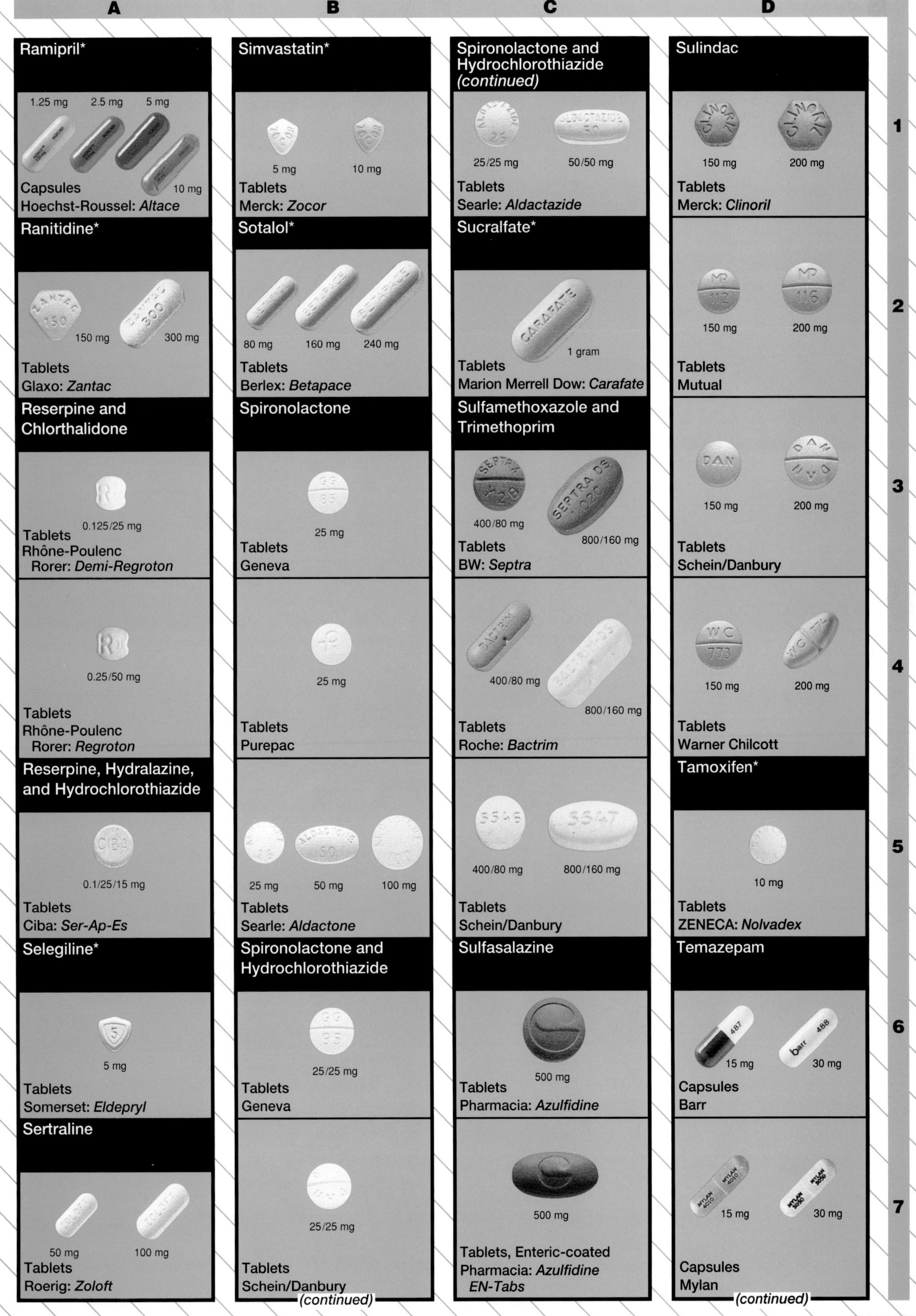

* Single source product for solid oral dosage forms in the U.S.

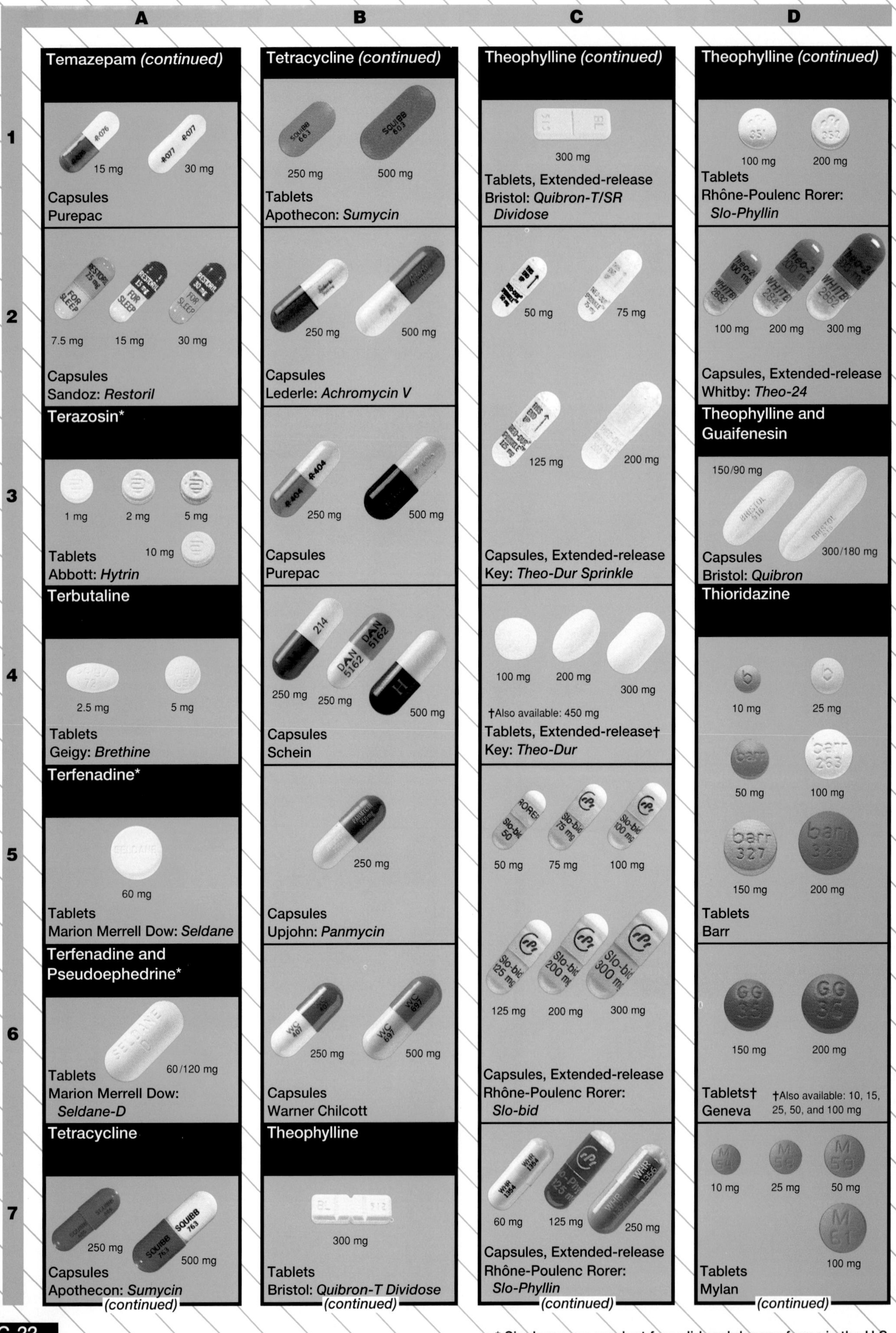

* Single source product for solid oral dosage forms in the U.S.

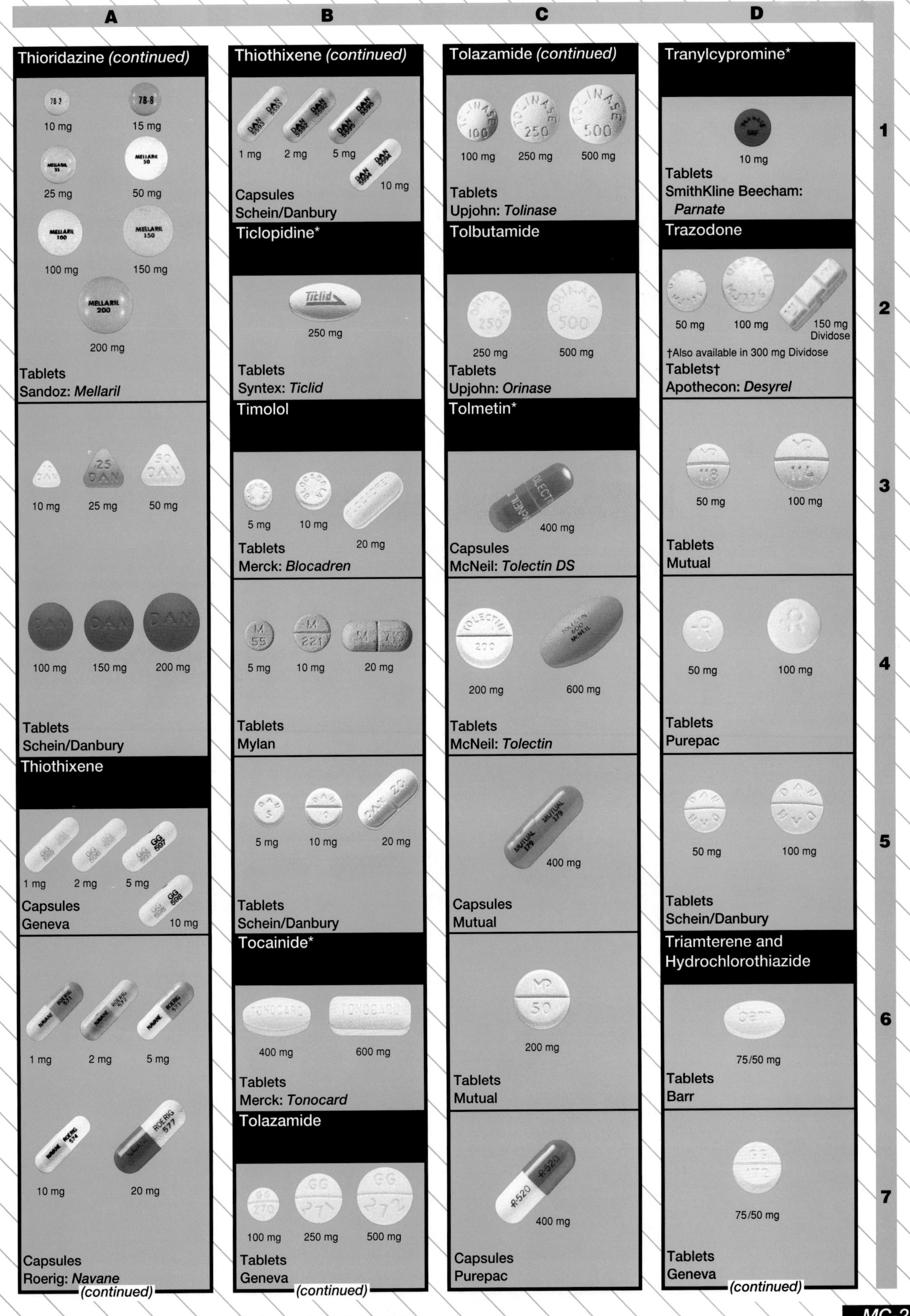

* Single source product for solid oral dosage forms in the U.S.

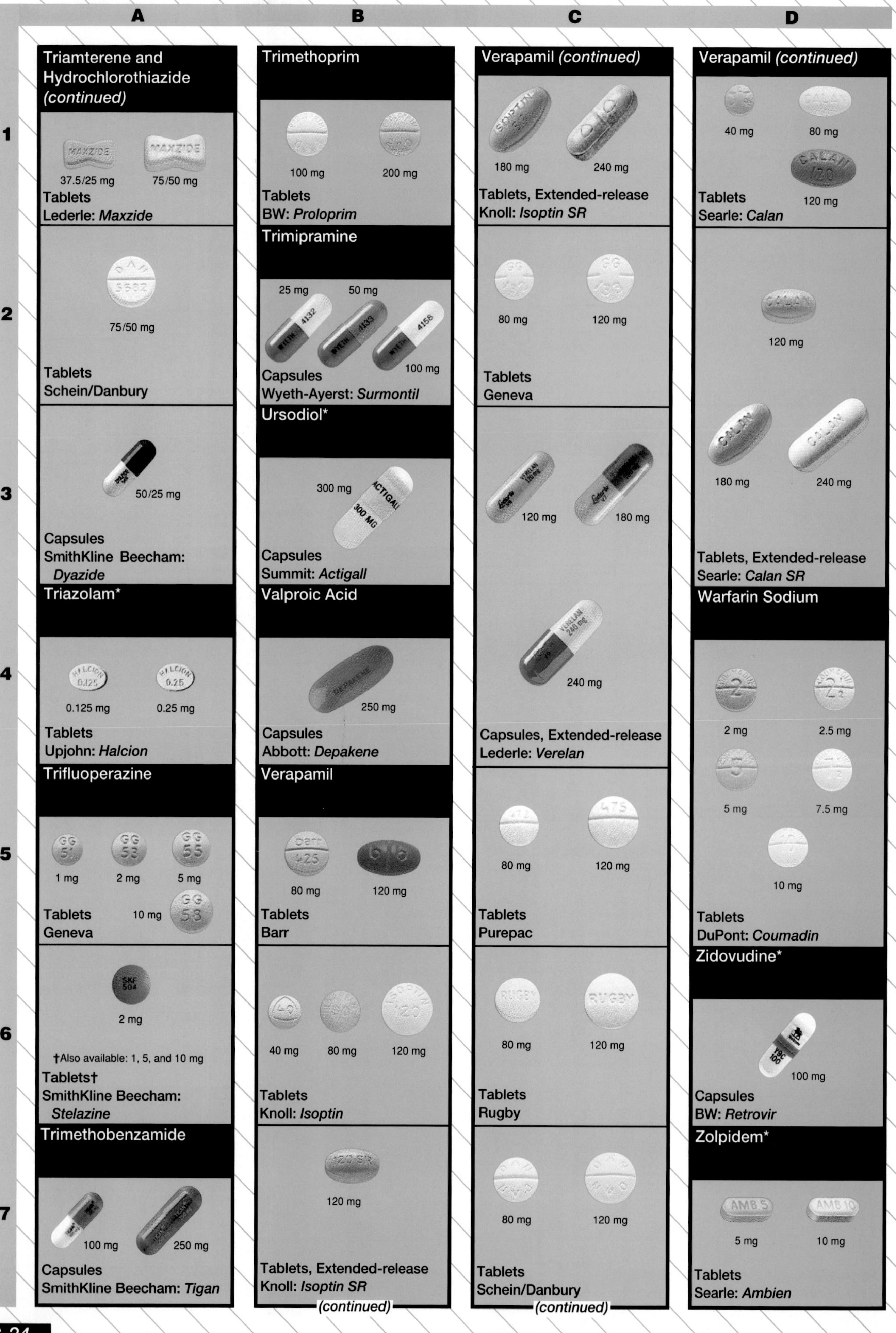

* Single source product for solid oral dosage forms in the U.S.

Appendix VII

PREGNANCY PRECAUTION LISTING

The following medicines, selected from those included in this publication, have specific precautions in regard to use during pregnancy. For specific information, consult the individual monographs; look in the index for the page number.

The use of any medicine during pregnancy must be carefully considered. The physician and the patient must balance the expected benefits against the possible risks.

Absence of a drug from the list is not meant to imply that it is safe for use in pregnant patients. For many drugs, it is not known whether a problem exists; experimentation on pregnant women is generally not done. Knowledge is usually gained only from the accumulated experience over many years in giving a drug to pregnant women who really needed its benefits. Also, well-planned studies in pregnant animals may reveal problems, although the relation of such findings to pregnant humans and their babies may not be known. Problems suggested by animal studies are often included in the warnings in this book.

Readers are reminded that the information in this text is selected and not considered to be complete.

A–D

Acebutolol (Systemic)
Acetaminophen and Aspirin (Systemic)
Acetaminophen, Aspirin, and Caffeine (Systemic)
Acetaminophen, Aspirin, and Caffeine, Buffered (Systemic)
Acetaminophen, Aspirin, and Salicylamide, Buffered (Systemic)
Acetaminophen, Aspirin, Salicylamide, and Caffeine (Systemic)
Acetaminophen, Aspirin, Salicylamide, Codeine, and Caffeine (Systemic)
Acetaminophen, Calcium Carbonate, Potassium and Sodium Bicarbonates, and Citric Acid (Systemic)
Acetaminophen and Codeine (Systemic)
Acetaminophen, Codeine, and Caffeine (Systemic)
Acetaminophen and Salicylamide (Systemic)
Acetaminophen, Salicylamide, and Caffeine (Systemic)
Acetaminophen, Sodium Bicarbonate, and Citric Acid (Systemic)
Acetazolamide (Systemic)
Acetohexamide (Systemic)
Acetohydroxamic Acid (Systemic)
Acetophenazine (Systemic)
Acyclovir (Systemic)
Albendazole (Systemic)
Albuterol (Inhalation)
Albuterol (Oral/Injection)
Alclometasone (Topical)
Aldesleukin (Systemic)
Alfacalcidol (Systemic)
Alfentanil (Systemic)
Allopurinol (Systemic)
Alprazolam (Systemic)
Alteplase, Recombinant (Systemic)
Altretamine (Systemic)
Alumina and Magnesia (Oral)
Alumina, Magnesia, and Calcium Carbonate (Oral)
Alumina, Magnesia, and Simethicone (Oral)
Alumina and Magnesium Carbonate (Oral)
Alumina and Magnesium Trisilicate (Oral)
Alumina, Magnesium Trisilicate, and Sodium Bicarbonate (Oral)
Aluminum Carbonate, Basic (Oral)
Aluminum Hydroxide (Oral)
Amantadine (Systemic)
Ambenonium (Systemic)
Amcinonide (Topical)
Amikacin (Systemic)
Amiloride (Systemic)
Amiloride and Hydrochlorothiazide (Systemic)
Aminocaproic Acid (Systemic)
Aminoglutethimide (Systemic)
Aminophylline (Systemic)
Aminosalicylate Sodium (Systemic)
Amiodarone (Systemic)
Amitriptyline (Systemic)
Amlodipine (Systemic)
Ammonia N 13 (Diagnostic)
Amobarbital (Systemic)
Amoxapine (Systemic)
Amphetamine (Systemic)
Amphetamine and Dextroamphetamine Resin Complex (Systemic)
Amyl Nitrite (Systemic)
Anisindione (Systemic)
Anistreplase (Systemic)
Aprobarbital (Systemic)
Ascorbic Acid (Systemic)
Asparaginase (Systemic)
Aspirin (Systemic)
Aspirin, Buffered (Systemic)
Aspirin and Caffeine (Systemic)
Aspirin, Caffeine, and Dihydrocodeine (Systemic)
Aspirin and Codeine (Systemic)
Aspirin, Codeine, and Caffeine (Systemic)
Aspirin, Codeine, and Caffeine, Buffered (Systemic)
Aspirin, Sodium Bicarbonate, and Citric Acid (Systemic)
Astemizole (Systemic)
Atenolol (Systemic)
Atenolol and Chlorthalidone (Systemic)
Atovaquone (Systemic)
Atropine (Systemic)
Atropine, Hyoscyamine, Scopolamine, and Phenobarbital (Systemic)
Atropine and Phenobarbital (Systemic)
Auranofin (Systemic)
Aurothioglucose (Systemic)
Azatadine and Pseudoephedrine (Systemic)
Azathioprine (Systemic)
Baclofen (Systemic)
Barium Sulfate (Diagnostic)
Beclomethasone (Inhalation)
Beclomethasone (Nasal)
Beclomethasone (Topical)
Belladonna and Butabarbital (Systemic)
Belladonna and Phenobarbital (Systemic)
Benazepril (Systemic)
Bendroflumethiazide (Systemic)
Benzphetamine (Systemic)
Benzthiazide (Systemic)
Bepridil (Systemic)
Beta-carotene (Systemic)
Betamethasone (Ophthalmic)
Betamethasone (Topical)
Betamethasone—Glucocorticoid Effects (Systemic)
Betaxolol (Ophthalmic)
Betaxolol (Systemic)
Bismuth Subsalicylate (Oral)
Bisoprolol (Systemic)
Bitolterol (Inhalation)
Bleomycin (Systemic)
Bromazepam (Systemic)
Bromocriptine (Systemic)
Bromodiphenhydramine and Codeine (Systemic)
Bromodiphenhydramine, Diphenhydramine, Codeine, Ammonium Chloride, and Potassium Guaiacolsulfonate (Systemic)
Brompheniramine and Phenylephrine (Systemic)
Brompheniramine, Phenylephrine, and Phenylpropanolamine (Systemic)
Brompheniramine, Phenylephrine, Phenylpropanolamine, and Acetaminophen (Systemic)
Brompheniramine, Phenylephrine, Phenylpropanolamine, and Codeine (Systemic)
Brompheniramine, Phenylephrine, Phenylpropanolamine, Codeine, and Guaifenesin (Systemic)
Brompheniramine, Phenylephrine, Phenylpropanolamine, Hydrocodone, and Guaifenesin (Systemic)
Brompheniramine and Phenylpropanolamine (Systemic)
Brompheniramine, Phenylpropanolamine, and Acetaminophen (Systemic)
Brompheniramine, Phenylpropanolamine, and Aspirin (Systemic)
Brompheniramine, Phenylpropanolamine, and Codeine (Systemic)
Brompheniramine, Phenyltoloxamine, and Phenylephrine (Systemic)
Brompheniramine, Phenyltoloxamine, Pseudoephedrine, and Atropine (Systemic)
Brompheniramine and Pseudoephedrine (Systemic)

VII

Brompheniramine, Pseudoephedrine, and Dextromethorphan (Systemic)
Buclizine (Systemic)
Bumetanide (Systemic)
Bupivacaine (Parenteral-Local)
Buprenorphine (Systemic)
Bupropion (Systemic)
Busulfan (Systemic)
Butabarbital (Systemic)
Butalbital and Acetaminophen (Systemic)
Butalbital, Acetaminophen, and Caffeine (Systemic)
Butalbital and Aspirin (Systemic)
Butalbital, Aspirin, and Caffeine (Systemic)
Butalbital, Aspirin, Codeine, and Caffeine (Systemic)
Butoconazole (Vaginal)
Butorphanol (Systemic)
Caffeine (Systemic)
Caffeine, Citrated (Systemic)
Calcifediol (Systemic)
Calcitonin-Human (Systemic)
Calcitonin-Salmon (Systemic)
Calcitriol (Systemic)
Calcium Carbonate (Oral)
Calcium Carbonate and Magnesia (Oral)
Calcium Carbonate, Magnesia, and Simethicone (Oral)
Calcium and Magnesium Carbonates (Oral)
Calcium and Magnesium Carbonates and Magnesium Oxide (Oral)
Calcium Carbonate and Simethicone (Oral)
Capreomycin (Systemic)
Captopril (Systemic)
Captopril and Hydrochlorothiazide (Systemic)
Carbamazepine (Systemic)
Carbidopa and Levodopa (Systemic)
Carbinoxamine and Pseudoephedrine (Systemic)
Carbinoxamine, Pseudoephedrine, and Dextromethorphan (Systemic)
Carbinoxamine, Pseudoephedrine, and Guaifenesin (Systemic)
Carboplatin (Systemic)
Carmustine (Systemic)
Carteolol (Ophthalmic)
Carteolol (Systemic)
Castor Oil (Oral)
Cefoxitin (Systemic)
Cellulose Sodium Phosphate (Systemic)
Chenodiol (Systemic)
Chloral Hydrate (Systemic)
Chlorambucil (Systemic)
Chloramphenicol (Systemic)
Chlordiazepoxide (Systemic)
Chlordiazepoxide and Amitriptyline (Systemic)
Chlordiazepoxide and Clidinium (Systemic)
Chloroprocaine (Parenteral-Local)
Chloroquine (Systemic)
Chlorothiazide (Systemic)
Chlorotrianisene (Systemic)
Chlorpheniramine, Codeine, Aspirin, and Caffeine (Systemic)
Chlorpheniramine, Codeine, and Guaifenesin (Systemic)
Chlorpheniramine, Phenindamine, Phenylephrine, Dextromethorphan, Acetaminophen, Salicylamide, Caffeine, and Ascorbic Acid (Systemic)
Chlorpheniramine, Phenindamine, and Phenylpropanolamine (Systemic)
Chlorpheniramine, Phenindamine, Pyrilamine, Phenylephrine, Hydrocodone, and Ammonium Chloride (Systemic)
Chlorpheniramine, Pheniramine, Pyrilamine, Phenylephrine, Hydrocodone, Salicylamide, Caffeine, and Ascorbic Acid (Systemic)
Chlorpheniramine and Phenylephrine (Systemic)
Chlorpheniramine, Phenylephrine, and Acetaminophen (Systemic)
Chlorpheniramine, Phenylephrine, Acetaminophen, and Caffeine (Systemic)
Chlorpheniramine, Phenylephrine, Acetaminophen, and Salicylamide (Systemic)
Chlorpheniramine, Phenylephrine, Acetaminophen, Salicylamide, and Caffeine (Systemic)
Chlorpheniramine, Phenylephrine, Codeine, Ammonium Chloride, Potassium Guaiacolsulfonate, and Sodium Citrate (Systemic)
Chlorpheniramine, Phenylephrine, Codeine, and Potassium Iodide (Systemic)
Chlorpheniramine, Phenylephrine, Dextromethorphan, Acetaminophen, and Salicylamide (Systemic)
Chlorpheniramine, Phenylephrine, and Hydrocodone (Systemic)
Chlorpheniramine, Phenylephrine, Hydrocodone, Acetaminophen, and Caffeine (Systemic)
Chlorpheniramine, Phenylephrine, and Phenylpropanolamine (Systemic)
Chlorpheniramine, Phenylephrine, Phenylpropanolamine, Atropine, Hyoscyamine, and Scopolamine (Systemic)
Chlorpheniramine, Phenylephrine, Phenylpropanolamine, and Codeine (Systemic)
Chlorpheniramine, Phenylephrine, Phenylpropanolamine, and Dihydrocodeine (Systemic)
Chlorpheniramine and Phenylpropanolamine (Systemic)
Chlorpheniramine, Phenylpropanolamine, and Acetaminophen (Systemic)
Chlorpheniramine, Phenylpropanolamine, Acetaminophen, and Caffeine (Systemic)
Chlorpheniramine, Phenylpropanolamine, and Aspirin (Systemic)
Chlorpheniramine, Phenylpropanolamine, Aspirin, and Caffeine (Systemic)
Chlorpheniramine, Phenylpropanolamine, Codeine, Guaifenesin, and Acetaminophen (Systemic)
Chlorpheniramine, Phenylpropanolamine, Dextromethorphan, Acetaminophen, and Caffeine (Systemic)
Chlorpheniramine, Phenylpropanolamine, Hydrocodone, Guaifenesin, and Salicylamide (Systemic)
Chlorpheniramine, Phenylpropanolamine, and Methscopolamine (Systemic)
Chlorpheniramine, Phenyltoloxamine, Ephedrine, Codeine, and Guaiacol Carbonate (Systemic)
Chlorpheniramine, Phenyltoloxamine, and Phenylephrine (Systemic)
Chlorpheniramine, Phenyltoloxamine, Phenylephrine, and Phenylpropanolamine (Systemic)
Chlorpheniramine, Phenyltoloxamine, Phenylpropanolamine, and Acetaminophen (Systemic)
Chlorpheniramine and Pseudoephedrine (Systemic)
Chlorpheniramine, Pseudoephedrine, and Acetaminophen (Systemic)
Chlorpheniramine, Pseudoephedrine, and Codeine (Systemic)
Chlorpheniramine, Pseudoephedrine, and Dextromethorphan (Systemic)
Chlorpheniramine, Pseudoephedrine, Dextromethorphan, and Acetaminophen (Systemic)
Chlorpheniramine, Pseudoephedrine, Dextromethorphan, Guaifenesin, and Aspirin (Systemic)
Chlorpheniramine, Pseudoephedrine, and Guaifenesin (Systemic)
Chlorpheniramine, Pseudoephedrine, and Hydrocodone (Systemic)
Chlorpheniramine, Pyrilamine, and Phenylephrine (Systemic)
Chlorpheniramine, Pyrilamine, Phenylephrine, and Acetaminophen (Systemic)
Chlorpheniramine, Pyrilamine, Phenylephrine, and Phenylpropanolamine (Systemic)
Chlorpheniramine, Pyrilamine, Phenylephrine, Phenylpropanolamine, and Acetaminophen (Systemic)
Chlorpromazine (Systemic)
Chlorpropamide (Systemic)
Chlorprothixene (Systemic)
Chlorthalidone (Systemic)
Chlorzoxazone and Acetaminophen (Systemic)
Cholestyramine (Oral)
Choline Salicylate (Systemic)
Choline and Magnesium Salicylates (Systemic)
Chorionic Gonadotropin (Systemic)
Chromic Phosphate P 32 (Therapeutic)
Cimetidine (Systemic)
Cinoxacin (Systemic)
Ciprofloxacin (Ophthalmic)
Ciprofloxacin (Systemic)
Cisapride (Systemic)
Cisplatin (Systemic)
Clarithromycin (Systemic)
Clemastine and Phenylpropanolamine (Systemic)
Clioquinol and Hydrocortisone (Topical)
Clobetasol (Topical)
Clobetasone (Topical)
Clocortolone (Topical)
Clofazimine (Systemic)
Clofibrate (Systemic)
Clomiphene (Systemic)
Clomipramine (Systemic)
Clonazepam (Systemic)
Clonidine (Systemic)
Clonidine and Chlorthalidone (Systemic)
Clorazepate (Systemic)
Clotrimazole (Oral)
Clotrimazole (Vaginal)
Clotrimazole and Betamethasone (Topical)
Cocaine (Mucosal-Local)
Codeine (Systemic)
Codeine and Calcium Iodide (Systemic)
Codeine and Guaifenesin (Systemic)
Codeine and Iodinated Glycerol (Systemic)
Colchicine (Systemic)
Colestipol (Oral)
Corticotropin—Glucocorticoid Effects (Systemic)
Cortisone—Glucocorticoid Effects (Systemic)
Cromolyn (Inhalation)
Cromolyn (Nasal)
Cromolyn (Ophthalmic)
Cromolyn (Oral)
Cyanocobalamin Co 57 (Diagnostic)
Cyclizine (Systemic)
Cyclophosphamide (Systemic)
Cyclosporine (Systemic)
Cyclothiazide (Systemic)

Cytarabine (Systemic)
Dacarbazine (Systemic)
Dactinomycin (Systemic)
Danazol (Systemic)
Daunorubicin (Systemic)
Deferoxamine (Systemic)
Demecarium (Ophthalmic)
Demeclocycline (Systemic)
Deserpidine (Systemic)
Deserpidine and Hydrochlorothiazide (Systemic)
Deserpidine and Methyclothiazide (Systemic)
Desipramine (Systemic)
Desonide (Topical)
Desoximetasone (Topical)
Dexamethasone (Inhalation)
Dexamethasone (Nasal)
Dexamethasone (Ophthalmic)
Dexamethasone (Topical)
Dexamethasone—Glucocorticoid Effects (Systemic)
Dexbrompheniramine and Pseudoephedrine (Systemic)
Dexbrompheniramine, Pseudoephedrine, and Acetaminophen (Systemic)
Dexchlorpheniramine, Pseudoephedrine, and Guaifenesin (Systemic)
Dextroamphetamine (Systemic)
Dextromethorphan and Iodinated Glycerol (Systemic)
Dezocine (Systemic)
Diatrizoate and Iodipamide (Diagnostic, Mucosal)
Diatrizoates (Diagnostic)
Diatrizoates (Diagnostic, Mucosal)
Diazepam (Systemic)
Diazoxide (Oral)
Dichlorphenamide (Systemic)
Diclofenac (Ophthalmic)
Diclofenac (Systemic)
Dicumarol (Systemic)
Dicyclomine (Systemic)
Dienestrol (Vaginal)
Diethylcarbamazine (Systemic)
Diethylstilbestrol (Systemic)
Diethylstilbestrol and Methyltestosterone (Systemic)
Difenoxin and Atropine (Systemic)
Diflorasone (Topical)
Diflucortolone (Topical)
Diflunisal (Systemic)
Digitoxin (Systemic)
Digoxin (Systemic)
Dihydrocodeine, Acetaminophen, and Caffeine (Systemic)
Dihydroergotamine (Systemic)
Dihydrotachysterol (Systemic)
Dihydroxyaluminum Aminoacetate (Oral)
Dihydroxyaluminum Sodium Carbonate (Oral)
Diltiazem (Systemic)
Dimethyl Sulfoxide (Mucosal)
Dinoprost (Intra-amniotic)
Dinoprostone (Cervical/Vaginal)
Diphenhydramine, Codeine, and Ammonium Chloride (Systemic)
Diphenhydramine, Phenylpropanolamine, and Aspirin (Systemic)
Diphenhydramine and Pseudoephedrine (Systemic)
Diphenhydramine, Pseudoephedrine, and Acetaminophen (Systemic)
Diphenhydramine, Pseudoephedrine, Dextromethorphan, and Acetaminophen (Systemic)
Diphenoxylate and Atropine (Systemic)
Diphenylpyraline, Phenylephrine, and Codeine (Systemic)
Diphenylpyraline, Phenylephrine, and Hydrocodone (Systemic)
Diphenylpyraline, Phenylephrine, Hydrocodone, and Guaifenesin (Systemic)
Disopyramide (Systemic)
Disulfiram (Systemic)
Divalproex (Systemic)
Doxazosin (Systemic)
Doxepin (Systemic)
Doxorubicin (Systemic)
Doxycycline (Systemic)
Doxylamine (Systemic)
Doxylamine, Pseudoephedrine, Dextromethorphan, and Acetaminophen (Systemic)
Dronabinol (Systemic)

E–N

Echothiophate (Ophthalmic)
Econazole (Topical)
Eflornithine (Systemic)
Enalapril (Systemic)
Enalapril and Hydrochlorothiazide (Systemic)
Enflurane (Systemic)
Enoxacin (Systemic)
Ephedrine (Oral/Injection)
Ephedrine and Potassium Iodide (Systemic)
Epinephrine (Inhalation)
Epinephrine (Oral/Injection)
Ergocalciferol (Systemic)
Ergonovine (Systemic)
Ergotamine (Systemic)
Ergotamine, Belladonna Alkaloids, and Phenobarbital (Systemic)
Ergotamine and Caffeine (Systemic)
Ergotamine, Caffeine, and Belladonna Alkaloids (Systemic)
Ergotamine, Caffeine, Belladonna Alkaloids, and Pentobarbital (Systemic)
Ergotamine, Caffeine, and Cyclizine (Systemic)
Ergotamine, Caffeine, and Dimenhydrinate (Systemic)
Ergotamine, Caffeine, and Diphenhydramine (Systemic)
Erythromycin Estolate (Systemic)
Erythromycin and Sulfisoxazole (Systemic)
Estazolam (Systemic)
Estradiol (Systemic)
Estradiol (Vaginal)
Estramustine (Systemic)
Estrogens, Conjugated (Systemic)
Estrogens, Conjugated (Vaginal)
Estrogens, Conjugated, and Methyltestosterone (Systemic)
Estrogens, Esterified (Systemic)
Estrogens, Esterified, and Methyltestosterone (Systemic)
Estrone (Systemic)
Estrone (Vaginal)
Estropipate (Systemic)
Estropipate (Vaginal)
Ethacrynic Acid (Systemic)
Ethambutol (Systemic)
Ethchlorvynol (Systemic)
Ethinyl Estradiol (Systemic)
Ethionamide (Systemic)
Ethosuximide (Systemic)
Ethotoin (Systemic)
Ethynodiol Diacetate and Ethinyl Estradiol (Systemic)
Etidocaine (Parenteral-Local)
Etidronate (Systemic)
Etodolac (Systemic)
Etomidate (Systemic)
Etoposide (Systemic)
Etretinate (Systemic)
Felodipine (Systemic)
Fenfluramine (Systemic)
Fenoprofen (Systemic)
Fentanyl (Systemic)
Ferrous Citrate Fe 59 (Diagnostic)
Filgrastim (Systemic)
Finasteride (Systemic)
Flecainide (Systemic)
Floctafenine (Systemic)
Floxuridine (Systemic)
Fluconazole (Systemic)
Flucytosine (Systemic)
Fludarabine (Systemic)
Fludeoxyglucose F 18 (Diagnostic)
Fludrocortisone (Systemic)
Flumethasone (Topical)
Flunarizine (Systemic)
Flunisolide (Inhalation)
Flunisolide (Nasal)
Fluocinolone (Topical)
Fluocinonide (Topical)
Fluorometholone (Ophthalmic)
Fluorouracil (Systemic)
Fluorouracil (Topical)
Fluoxymesterone (Systemic)
Fluoxymesterone and Ethinyl Estradiol (Systemic)
Flupenthixol (Systemic)
Fluphenazine (Systemic)
Flurandrenolide (Topical)
Flurazepam (Systemic)
Flurbiprofen (Ophthalmic)
Flurbiprofen (Systemic)
Flutamide (Systemic)
Fluticasone (Topical)
Foscarnet (Systemic)
Fosinopril (Systemic)
Furosemide (Systemic)
Gadodiamide (Diagnostic)
Gadopentetate (Diagnostic)
Gadoteridol (Diagnostic)
Gallium Citrate Ga 67 (Diagnostic)
Ganciclovir (Systemic)
Gemfibrozil (Systemic)
Gentamicin (Systemic)
Glipizide (Systemic)
Glutethimide (Systemic)
Glyburide (Systemic)
Glycopyrrolate (Systemic)
Gold Sodium Thiomalate (Systemic)
Gonadorelin (Systemic)
Griseofulvin (Systemic)
Guanabenz (Systemic)
Guanethidine and Hydrochlorothiazide (Systemic)
Guanfacine (Systemic)
Halazepam (Systemic)
Halcinonide (Topical)
Halobetasol (Topical)
Halofantrine (Systemic)
Haloperidol (Systemic)
Halothane (Systemic)
Heparin (Systemic)
Hydralazine (Systemic)

Hydralazine and Hydrochlorothiazide (Systemic)
Hydrochlorothiazide (Systemic)
Hydrocodone (Systemic)
Hydrocodone and Acetaminophen (Systemic)
Hydrocodone and Aspirin (Systemic)
Hydrocodone, Aspirin, and Caffeine (Systemic)
Hydrocodone and Guaifenesin (Systemic)
Hydrocodone and Homatropine (Systemic)
Hydrocodone and Potassium Guaiacolsulfonate (Systemic)
Hydrocortisone (Dental)
Hydrocortisone (Ophthalmic)
Hydrocortisone (Rectal)
Hydrocortisone (Topical)
Hydrocortisone Acetate (Topical)
Hydrocortisone Butyrate (Topical)
Hydrocortisone—Glucocorticoid Effects (Systemic)
Hydrocortisone Valerate (Topical)
Hydroflumethiazide (Systemic)
Hydromorphone (Systemic)
Hydromorphone and Guaifenesin (Systemic)
Hydroxychloroquine (Systemic)
Hydroxyprogesterone (Systemic)
Hydroxyurea (Systemic)
Hydroxyzine (Systemic)
Hyoscyamine (Systemic)
Hyoscyamine and Phenobarbital (Systemic)
Ibuprofen (Systemic)
Idarubicin (Systemic)
Idoxuridine (Ophthalmic)
Ifosfamide (Systemic)
Imipenem and Cilastatin (Systemic)
Imipramine (Systemic)
Indapamide (Systemic)
Indium In 111 Oxyquinoline (Diagnostic)
Indium In 111 Pentetate (Diagnostic)
Indium In 111 Satumomab Pendetide (Diagnostic)
Indomethacin (Ophthalmic)
Indomethacin (Systemic)
Interferon Alfa-2a, Recombinant (Systemic)
Interferon Alfa-2b, Recombinant (Systemic)
Interferon, Gamma (Systemic)
Iobenguane, Radioiodinated (Diagnostic)
Iobenguane, Radioiodinated (Therapeutic)
Iocetamic Acid (Diagnostic)
Iodinated Glycerol (Systemic)
Iodine, Strong (Systemic)
Iodipamide (Diagnostic)
Iodohippurate Sodium I 123 (Diagnostic)
Iodohippurate Sodium I 131 (Diagnostic)
Iofetamine I 123 (Diagnostic)
Iohexol (Diagnostic)
Iohexol (Diagnostic, Mucosal)
Iopamidol (Diagnostic)
Iopanoic Acid (Diagnostic)
Iothalamate (Diagnostic)
Iothalamate (Diagnostic, Mucosal)
Iothalamate Sodium I 125 (Diagnostic)
Ioversol (Diagnostic)
Ioxaglate (Diagnostic)
Ioxaglate (Diagnostic, Mucosal)
Ipodate (Diagnostic)
Ipratropium (Inhalation)
Iron Dextran (Systemic)
Isocarboxazid (Systemic)
Isoflurane (Systemic)
Isoflurophate (Ophthalmic)
Isoniazid (Systemic)
Isoproterenol and Phenylephrine (Systemic)
Isosorbide Dinitrate—Oral (Systemic)
Isosorbide Dinitrate—Sublingual, Chewable, or Buccal (Systemic)
Isotretinoin (Systemic)
Isoxsuprine (Systemic)
Isradipine (Systemic)
Itraconazole (Systemic)
Ivermectin (Systemic)
Japanese Encephalitis Virus Vaccine (Systemic)
Kanamycin (Systemic)
Kaolin, Pectin, Belladonna Alkaloids, and Opium (Systemic)
Kaolin, Pectin, and Paregoric (Systemic)
Ketamine (Systemic)
Ketazolam (Systemic)
Ketoconazole (Systemic)
Ketoconazole (Topical)
Ketoprofen (Systemic)
Ketorolac (Systemic)
Krypton Kr 81m (Diagnostic)
Labetalol (Systemic)
Labetalol and Hydrochlorothiazide (Systemic)
Leuprolide (Systemic)
Levamisole (Systemic)
Levobunolol (Ophthalmic)
Levodopa (Systemic)
Levonorgestrel and Ethinyl Estradiol (Systemic)
Levorphanol (Systemic)
Lidocaine (Parenteral-Local)
Lidocaine—For Self-Injection (Systemic)
Lindane (Topical)
Lisinopril (Systemic)
Lisinopril and Hydrochlorothiazide (Systemic)
Lithium (Systemic)
Lomefloxacin (Systemic)
Lomustine (Systemic)
Loperamide (Oral)
Lorazepam (Systemic)
Lovastatin (Systemic)
Loxapine (Systemic)
Mafenide (Topical)
Magaldrate (Oral)
Magaldrate and Simethicone (Oral)
Magnesium Carbonate and Sodium Bicarbonate (Oral)
Magnesium Citrate (Oral)
Magnesium Hydroxide (Oral)
Magnesium Hydroxide and Mineral Oil (Oral)
Magnesium Hydroxide, Mineral Oil, and Glycerin (Oral)
Magnesium Oxide (Oral)
Magnesium Salicylate (Systemic)
Magnesium Sulfate (Oral)
Magnesium Sulfate (Systemic)
Magnesium Trisilicate, Alumina, and Magnesia (Oral)
Mazindol (Systemic)
Measles Virus Vaccine Live (Systemic)
Mebendazole (Systemic)
Mecamylamine (Systemic)
Mechlorethamine (Systemic)
Mechlorethamine (Topical)
Meclizine (Systemic)
Meclocycline (Topical)
Meclofenamate (Systemic)
Medroxyprogesterone (Systemic)
Medrysone (Ophthalmic)
Mefenamic Acid (Systemic)
Mefloquine (Systemic)
Megestrol (Systemic)
Melphalan (Systemic)
Menadiol (Systemic)
Meningococcal Polysaccharide Vaccine (Systemic)
Menotropins (Systemic)
Meperidine (Systemic)
Meperidine and Acetaminophen (Systemic)
Mephenytoin (Systemic)
Mephobarbital (Systemic)
Mepivacaine (Parenteral-Local)
Meprobamate (Systemic)
Meprobamate and Aspirin (Systemic)
Mercaptopurine (Systemic)
Mesoridazine (Systemic)
Metaproterenol (Inhalation)
Metaproterenol (Oral/Injection)
Methacholine (Inhalation)
Methacycline (Systemic)
Methadone (Systemic)
Methamphetamine (Systemic)
Metharbital (Systemic)
Methazolamide (Systemic)
Methdilazine (Systemic)
Methimazole (Systemic)
Methohexital (Systemic)
Methotrexate—For Cancer (Systemic)
Methotrexate—For Noncancerous Conditions (Systemic)
Methotrimeprazine (Systemic)
Methoxyflurane (Systemic)
Methsuximide (Systemic)
Methyclothiazide (Systemic)
Methyldopa and Chlorothiazide (Systemic)
Methyldopa and Hydrochlorothiazide (Systemic)
Methylergonovine (Systemic)
Methylprednisolone—Glucocorticoid Effects (Systemic)
Methyltestosterone (Systemic)
Metipranolol (Ophthalmic)
Metolazone (Systemic)
Metoprolol (Systemic)
Metoprolol and Hydrochlorothiazide (Systemic)
Metrizamide (Diagnostic)
Metronidazole (Systemic)
Metyrapone (Systemic)
Mexiletine (Systemic)
Miconazole (Vaginal)
Midazolam (Systemic)
Mineral Oil (Oral)
Mineral Oil and Cascara Sagrada (Oral)
Mineral Oil, Glycerin, and Phenolphthalein (Oral)
Mineral Oil and Phenolphthalein (Oral)
Minocycline (Systemic)
Minoxidil (Systemic)
Minoxidil (Topical)
Misoprostol (Systemic)
Mitomycin (Systemic)
Mitotane (Systemic)
Mitoxantrone (Systemic)
Molindone (Systemic)
Mometasone (Topical)
Morphine (Systemic)
Moxalactam (Systemic)
Mumps Virus Vaccine Live (Systemic)
Nabilone (Systemic)
Nabumetone (Systemic)
Nadolol (Systemic)
Nadolol and Bendroflumethiazide (Systemic)
Nafarelin (Systemic)
Nalbuphine (Systemic)
Nalidixic Acid (Systemic)
Naltrexone (Systemic)
Nandrolone (Systemic)
Naproxen (Systemic)

Neomycin (Oral)
Neomycin (Systemic)
Neomycin, Polymyxin B, and Hydrocortisone (Ophthalmic)
Neomycin, Polymyxin B, and Hydrocortisone (Otic)
Neostigmine (Systemic)
Netilmicin (Systemic)
Nicardipine (Systemic)
Nicotine (Systemic)
Nifedipine (Systemic)
Nimodipine (Systemic)
Nitrazepam (Systemic)
Nitrofurantoin (Systemic)
Nitrous Oxide (Systemic)
Nizatidine (Systemic)
Norethindrone (Systemic)
Norethindrone Acetate and Ethinyl Estradiol (Systemic)
Norethindrone and Ethinyl Estradiol (Systemic)
Norethindrone and Mestranol (Systemic)
Norfloxacin (Ophthalmic)
Norfloxacin (Systemic)
Norgestrel (Systemic)
Norgestrel and Ethinyl Estradiol (Systemic)
Nortriptyline (Systemic)
Nystatin and Triamcinolone (Topical)

O–Z

Ofloxacin (Systemic)
Olsalazine (Oral)
Omeprazole (Systemic)
Opium (Systemic)
Opium Tincture (Systemic)
Orphenadrine and Aspirin (Systemic)
Oxamniquine (Systemic)
Oxandrolone (Systemic)
Oxaprozin (Systemic)
Oxazepam (Systemic)
Oxprenolol (Systemic)
Oxtriphylline (Systemic)
Oxtriphylline and Guaifenesin (Systemic)
Oxycodone (Systemic)
Oxycodone and Acetaminophen (Systemic)
Oxycodone and Aspirin (Systemic)
Oxymetholone (Systemic)
Oxymorphone (Systemic)
Oxytetracycline (Systemic)
Oxytocin (Systemic)
Paclitaxel (Systemic)
Pamidronate (Systemic)
Paraldehyde (Systemic)
Paramethadione (Systemic)
Paramethasone—Glucocorticoid Effects (Systemic)
Paregoric (Systemic)
Pemoline (Systemic)
Penbutolol (Systemic)
Penicillamine (Systemic)
Pentamidine (Inhalation)
Pentamidine (Systemic)
Pentazocine (Systemic)
Pentazocine and Acetaminophen (Systemic)
Pentazocine and Aspirin (Systemic)
Pentazocine and Naloxone (Systemic)
Pentobarbital (Systemic)
Pentostatin (Systemic)
Pentoxifylline (Systemic)
Pericyazine (Systemic)
Perphenazine (Systemic)
Perphenazine and Amitriptyline (Systemic)
Phenacemide (Systemic)
Phenelzine (Systemic)
Phenindamine, Hydrocodone, and Guaifenesin (Systemic)
Pheniramine, Codeine, and Guaifenesin (Systemic)
Pheniramine, Phenylephrine, Codeine, Sodium Citrate, Sodium Salicylate, and Caffeine (Systemic)
Pheniramine, Phenylephrine, Sodium Salicylate, and Caffeine (Systemic)
Pheniramine, Phenyltoloxamine, Pyrilamine, and Phenylpropanolamine (Systemic)
Pheniramine, Pyrilamine, Hydrocodone, Potassium Citrate, and Ascorbic Acid (Systemic)
Pheniramine, Pyrilamine, Phenylephrine, Phenylpropanolamine, and Hydrocodone (Systemic)
Pheniramine, Pyrilamine, and Phenylpropanolamine (Systemic)
Pheniramine, Pyrilamine, Phenylpropanolamine, and Aspirin (Systemic)
Pheniramine, Pyrilamine, Phenylpropanolamine, and Codeine (Systemic)
Pheniramine, Pyrilamine, Phenylpropanolamine, Codeine, Acetaminophen, and Caffeine (Systemic)
Pheniramine, Pyrilamine, Phenylpropanolamine, and Hydrocodone (Systemic)
Pheniramine, Pyrilamine, Phenylpropanolamine, Hydrocodone, and Guaifenesin (Systemic)
Phenobarbital (Systemic)
Phenobarbital, Aspirin, and Codeine (Systemic)
Phensuximide (Systemic)
Phenylbutazone (Systemic)
Phenylephrine and Acetaminophen (Systemic)
Phenylephrine, Guaifenesin, Acetaminophen, Salicylamide, and Caffeine (Systemic)
Phenylephrine, Hydrocodone, and Guaifenesin (Systemic)
Phenylpropanolamine (Systemic)
Phenylpropanolamine and Acetaminophen (Systemic)
Phenylpropanolamine, Acetaminophen, and Aspirin (Systemic)
Phenylpropanolamine, Acetaminophen, Aspirin, and Caffeine (Systemic)
Phenylpropanolamine, Acetaminophen, Salicylamide, and Caffeine (Systemic)
Phenylpropanolamine and Aspirin (Systemic)
Phenylpropanolamine, Codeine, and Guaifenesin (Systemic)
Phenylpropanolamine and Hydrocodone (Systemic)
Phenyltoloxamine and Hydrocodone (Systemic)
Phenyltoloxamine, Phenylpropanolamine, and Acetaminophen (Systemic)
Phenytoin (Systemic)
Phytonadione (Systemic)
Pimozide (Systemic)
Pindolol (Systemic)
Pindolol and Hydrochlorothiazide (Systemic)
Piperazine (Systemic)
Pipotiazine (Systemic)
Pirbuterol (Inhalation)
Piroxicam (Systemic)
Plicamycin (Systemic)
Pneumococcal Vaccine Polyvalent (Systemic)
Podophyllum (Topical)
Poliovirus Vaccine (Systemic)
Polythiazide (Systemic)
Potassium Iodide (Systemic)
Pravastatin (Systemic)
Prazepam (Systemic)
Praziquantel (Systemic)
Prazosin and Polythiazide (Systemic)
Prednisolone (Ophthalmic)
Prednisolone—Glucocorticoid Effects (Systemic)
Prednisone—Glucocorticoid Effects (Systemic)
Prilocaine (Parenteral-Local)
Primaquine (Systemic)
Primidone (Systemic)
Probenecid and Colchicine (Systemic)
Procainamide (Systemic)
Procaine (Parenteral-Local)
Procarbazine (Systemic)
Prochlorperazine (Systemic)
Progesterone (Systemic)
Promazine (Systemic)
Promethazine (Systemic)
Promethazine and Codeine (Systemic)
Promethazine and Phenylephrine (Systemic)
Promethazine, Phenylephrine, and Codeine (Systemic)
Promethazine and Pseudoephedrine (Systemic)
Propafenone (Systemic)
Propofol (Systemic)
Propoxycaine and Procaine (Parenteral-Local)
Propoxyphene (Systemic)
Propoxyphene and Acetaminophen (Systemic)
Propoxyphene and Aspirin (Systemic)
Propoxyphene, Aspirin, and Caffeine (Systemic)
Propranolol (Systemic)
Propranolol and Hydrochlorothiazide (Systemic)
Propylthiouracil (Systemic)
Protirelin (Diagnostic)
Protriptyline (Systemic)
Pseudoephedrine (Systemic)
Pseudoephedrine and Acetaminophen (Systemic)
Pseudoephedrine, Acetaminophen, and Caffeine (Systemic)
Pseudoephedrine and Aspirin (Systemic)
Pseudoephedrine, Aspirin, and Caffeine (Systemic)
Pseudoephedrine and Codeine (Systemic)
Pseudoephedrine, Codeine, and Guaifenesin (Systemic)
Pseudoephedrine and Dextromethorphan (Systemic)
Pseudoephedrine, Dextromethorphan, and Acetaminophen (Systemic)
Pseudoephedrine, Dextromethorphan, and Guaifenesin (Systemic)
Pseudoephedrine, Dextromethorphan, Guaifenesin, and Acetaminophen (Systemic)
Pseudoephedrine and Guaifenesin (Systemic)
Pseudoephedrine and Hydrocodone (Systemic)
Pseudoephedrine, Hydrocodone, and Guaifenesin (Systemic)
Pseudoephedrine and Ibuprofen (Systemic)
Pyridostigmine (Systemic)
Pyridoxine (Systemic)
Pyrilamine, Phenylephrine, Aspirin, and Caffeine (Systemic)
Pyrilamine, Phenylephrine, and Codeine (Systemic)
Pyrilamine, Phenylephrine, and Hydrocodone (Systemic)
Pyrilamine, Phenylephrine, Hydrocodone, and Ammonium Chloride (Systemic)
Pyrilamine, Phenylpropanolamine, Acetaminophen, and Caffeine (Systemic)
Pyrilamine, Phenylpropanolamine, Dextromethorphan, and Sodium Salicylate (Systemic)
Pyrimethamine (Systemic)

Quazepam (Systemic)
Quinacrine (Systemic)
Quinapril (Systemic)
Quinestrol (Systemic)
Quinethazone (Systemic)
Quinidine (Systemic)
Quinine (Systemic)
Radioiodinated Albumin (Diagnostic)
Ramipril (Systemic)
Rauwolfia Serpentina (Systemic)
Rauwolfia Serpentina and Bendroflumethiazide (Systemic)
Reserpine (Systemic)
Reserpine and Chlorothiazide (Systemic)
Reserpine and Chlorthalidone (Systemic)
Reserpine, Hydralazine, and Hydrochlorothiazide (Systemic)
Reserpine and Hydrochlorothiazide (Systemic)
Reserpine and Hydroflumethiazide (Systemic)
Reserpine and Methyclothiazide (Systemic)
Reserpine and Polythiazide (Systemic)
Reserpine and Trichlormethiazide (Systemic)
Ribavirin (Systemic)
Rifabutin (Systemic)
Rifampin (Systemic)
Rifampin and Isoniazid (Systemic)
Ritodrine (Systemic)
Rubella Virus Vaccine Live (Systemic)
Rubidium Rb 82 (Diagnostic)
Salicylic Acid (Topical)
Salicylic Acid and Sulfur (Topical)
Salicylic Acid, Sulfur, and Coal Tar (Topical)
Salsalate (Systemic)
Scopolamine (Systemic)
Secobarbital (Systemic)
Secobarbital and Amobarbital (Systemic)
Selenious Acid (Systemic)
Selenium (Systemic)
Selenium Sulfide (Topical)
Sertraline (Systemic)
Silver Sulfadiazine (Topical)
Simethicone, Alumina, Calcium Carbonate, and Magnesia (Oral)
Simethicone, Alumina, Magnesium Carbonate and Magnesia (Oral)
Simvastatin (Systemic)
Sodium Bicarbonate (Systemic)
Sodium Chromate Cr 51 (Diagnostic)
Sodium Iodide (Systemic)
Sodium Iodide I 123 (Diagnostic)
Sodium Iodide I 131 (Diagnostic)
Sodium Iodide I 131 (Therapeutic)
Sodium Pertechnetate Tc 99m (Diagnostic)
Sodium Phosphate (Oral)
Sodium Phosphate P 32 (Therapeutic)
Sodium Phosphates (Oral)
Sodium Salicylate (Systemic)
Sotalol (Systemic)
Spironolactone (Systemic)
Spironolactone and Hydrochlorothiazide (Systemic)
Stanozolol (Systemic)
Streptokinase (Systemic)
Streptomycin (Systemic)
Streptozocin (Systemic)
Succimer (Systemic)
Sufentanil (Systemic)
Sulfadoxine and Pyrimethamine (Systemic)
Sulfamethoxazole (Systemic)
Sulfamethoxazole and Phenazopyridine (Systemic)
Sulfamethoxazole and Trimethoprim (Systemic)
Sulfanilamide (Vaginal)
Sulfanilamide, Aminacrine, and Allantoin (Vaginal)
Sulfapyridine (Systemic)
Sulfasalazine (Systemic)
Sulfisoxazole (Systemic)
Sulfisoxazole and Phenazopyridine (Systemic)
Sulindac (Systemic)
Sumatriptan (Systemic)
Suprofen (Ophthalmic)
Tamoxifen (Systemic)
Technetium Tc 99m Albumin (Diagnostic)
Technetium Tc 99m Albumin Aggregated (Diagnostic)
Technetium Tc 99m Disofenin (Diagnostic)
Technetium Tc 99m Exametazime (Diagnostic)
Technetium Tc 99m Gluceptate (Diagnostic)
Technetium Tc 99m Lidofenin (Diagnostic)
Technetium Tc 99m Mebrofenin (Diagnostic)
Technetium Tc 99m Medronate (Diagnostic)
Technetium Tc 99m Mertiatide (Diagnostic)
Technetium Tc 99m Oxidronate (Diagnostic)
Technetium Tc 99m Pentetate (Diagnostic)
Technetium Tc 99m Pyrophosphate (Diagnostic)
Technetium Tc 99m (Pyro- and trimeta-) Phosphates (Diagnostic)
Technetium Tc 99m Sestamibi (Diagnostic)
Technetium Tc 99m Succimer (Diagnostic)
Technetium Tc 99m Sulfur Colloid (Diagnostic)
Technetium Tc 99m Teboroxime (Diagnostic)
Temazepam (Systemic)
Terazosin (Systemic)
Terbutaline (Inhalation)
Terbutaline (Oral/Injection)
Terconazole (Vaginal)
Terfenadine (Systemic)
Terfenadine and Pseudoephedrine (Systemic)
Testolactone (Systemic)
Testosterone (Systemic)
Testosterone and Estradiol (Systemic)
Tetracaine (Parenteral-Local)
Tetracycline (Systemic)
Thallous Chloride Tl 201 (Diagnostic)
Theophylline (Systemic)
Theophylline, Ephedrine, Guaifenesin, and Butabarbital (Systemic)
Theophylline, Ephedrine, Guaifenesin, and Phenobarbital (Systemic)
Theophylline, Ephedrine, and Hydroxyzine (Systemic)
Theophylline, Ephedrine, and Phenobarbital (Systemic)
Theophylline and Guaifenesin (Systemic)
Thiabendazole (Systemic)
Thiamylal (Systemic)
Thiethylperazine (Systemic)
Thioguanine (Systemic)
Thiopental (Systemic)
Thiopropazate (Systemic)
Thioproperazine (Systemic)
Thioridazine (Systemic)
Thiotepa (Systemic)
Thiothixene (Systemic)
Tiaprofenic Acid (Systemic)
Ticlopidine (Systemic)
Timolol (Ophthalmic)
Timolol (Systemic)
Timolol and Hydrochlorothiazide (Systemic)
Tioconazole (Vaginal)
Tiopronin (Systemic)
Tobramycin (Systemic)
Tocainide (Systemic)
Tolazamide (Systemic)
Tolbutamide (Systemic)
Tolmetin (Systemic)
Tranylcypromine (Systemic)
Trazodone (Systemic)
Tretinoin (Topical)
Triamcinolone (Dental)
Triamcinolone (Inhalation)
Triamcinolone (Topical)
Triamcinolone—Glucocorticoid Effects (Systemic)
Triamterene (Systemic)
Triamterene and Hydrochlorothiazide (Systemic)
Triazolam (Systemic)
Trichlormethiazide (Systemic)
Trientine (Systemic)
Trifluoperazine (Systemic)
Triflupromazine (Systemic)
Trifluridine (Ophthalmic)
Trilostane (Systemic)
Trimeprazine (Systemic)
Trimethadione (Systemic)
Trimethobenzamide (Systemic)
Trimethoprim (Systemic)
Trimipramine (Systemic)
Triple Sulfa (Vaginal)
Triprolidine and Pseudoephedrine (Systemic)
Triprolidine, Pseudoephedrine, and Acetaminophen (Systemic)
Triprolidine, Pseudoephedrine, and Codeine (Systemic)
Triprolidine, Pseudoephedrine, Codeine, and Guaifenesin (Systemic)
Triprolidine, Pseudoephedrine, and Dextromethorphan (Systemic)
Typhoid Vaccine Live Oral (Systemic)
Tyropanoate (Diagnostic)
Uracil Mustard (Systemic)
Urofollitropin (Systemic)
Urokinase (Systemic)
Valproic Acid (Systemic)
Vasopressin (Systemic)
Verapamil (Systemic)
Vinblastine (Systemic)
Vincristine (Systemic)
Vitamin A (Systemic)
Warfarin (Systemic)
Xenon Xe 127 (Diagnostic)
Xenon Xe 133 (Diagnostic)
Zalcitabine (Systemic)
Zidovudine (Systemic)

VIII

Appendix VIII

BREAST-FEEDING PRECAUTION LISTING

The following medicines, selected from those included in this publication, have specific precautions in regard to use while breast-feeding. For specific information, consult the individual monographs; look in the index for the page number.

The use of any medicine while breast-feeding must be carefully considered. The physician and the patient must balance the expected benefits against the possible risks.

Absence of a drug from the list is not meant to imply that it is safe for use while breast-feeding. For many drugs, it is not known whether a problem exists; experimentation on women who are breast-feeding is generally not done. Knowledge is usually gained only from the accumulated experience over many years in giving a drug to breast-feeding women who really needed its benefits. Also, well-planned studies in breast-feeding animals may reveal problems, although the relation of such findings to humans may not be known. Problems suggested by animal studies are often included in the warnings in this book.

Readers are reminded that the information in this text is selected and not considered to be complete.

A–B

Acebutolol (Systemic)
Acetohexamide (Systemic)
Acetohydroxamic Acid (Systemic)
Acetophenazine (Systemic)
Albuterol (Inhalation)
Albuterol (Oral/Injection)
Alclometasone (Topical)
Alprazolam (Systemic)
Altretamine (Systemic)
Amcinonide (Topical)
Aminophylline (Systemic)
Amiodarone (Systemic)
Ammonia N 13 (Diagnostic)
Amobarbital (Systemic)
Amoxicillin (Systemic)
Amoxicillin and Clavulanate (Systemic)
Ampicillin (Systemic)
Ampicillin and Sulbactam (Systemic)
Amyl Nitrite (Systemic)
Anisindione (Systemic)
Anisotropine (Systemic)
Apraclonidine (Ophthalmic)
Aprobarbital (Systemic)
Asparaginase (Systemic)
Aspirin (Systemic)
Aspirin, Buffered (Systemic)
Aspirin and Caffeine (Systemic)
Aspirin, Caffeine, and Dihydrocodeine (Systemic)
Aspirin and Codeine (Systemic)
Aspirin, Codeine, and Caffeine (Systemic)
Aspirin, Codeine, and Caffeine, Buffered (Systemic)
Astemizole (Systemic)
Atenolol (Systemic)
Atenolol and Chlorthalidone (Systemic)
Atropine (Ophthalmic)
Atropine (Systemic)
Atropine, Hyoscyamine, Scopolamine, and Phenobarbital (Systemic)
Atropine and Phenobarbital (Systemic)
Auranofin (Systemic)
Aurothioglucose (Systemic)
Azatadine (Systemic)
Azatadine and Pseudoephedrine (Systemic)
Azathioprine (Systemic)
Azlocillin (Systemic)
Bacampicillin (Systemic)
Beclomethasone (Inhalation)
Beclomethasone (Nasal)
Beclomethasone (Topical)
Belladonna (Systemic)
Belladonna and Butabarbital (Systemic)
Belladonna and Phenobarbital (Systemic)
Bendroflumethiazide (Systemic)
Benzthiazide (Systemic)
Benztropine (Systemic)
Betamethasone (Topical)
Betamethasone—Glucocorticoid Effects (Systemic)
Betaxolol (Ophthalmic)
Betaxolol (Systemic)
Biperiden (Systemic)
Bismuth Subsalicylate (Oral)
Bisoprolol (Systemic)
Bleomycin (Systemic)
Bromazepam (Systemic)
Bromocriptine (Systemic)
Bromodiphenhydramine (Systemic)
Bromodiphenhydramine and Codeine (Systemic)
Bromodiphenhydramine, Diphenhydramine, Codeine, Ammonium Chloride, and Potassium Guaiacolsulfonate (Systemic)
Brompheniramine (Systemic)
Brompheniramine and Phenylephrine (Systemic)
Brompheniramine, Phenylephrine, and Phenylpropanolamine (Systemic)
Brompheniramine, Phenylephrine, Phenylpropanolamine, and Acetaminophen (Systemic)
Brompheniramine, Phenylephrine, Phenylpropanolamine, and Codeine (Systemic)
Brompheniramine, Phenylephrine, Phenylpropanolamine, Codeine, and Guaifenesin (Systemic)
Brompheniramine, Phenylephrine, Phenylpropanolamine, and Dextromethorphan (Systemic)
Brompheniramine, Phenylephrine, Phenylpropanolamine, and Guaifenesin (Systemic)
Brompheniramine, Phenylephrine, Phenylpropanolamine, Hydrocodone, and Guaifenesin (Systemic)
Brompheniramine and Phenylpropanolamine (Systemic)
Brompheniramine, Phenylpropanolamine, and Acetaminophen (Systemic)
Brompheniramine, Phenylpropanolamine, and Aspirin (Systemic)
Brompheniramine, Phenylpropanolamine, and Codeine (Systemic)
Brompheniramine, Phenylpropanolamine, and Dextromethorphan (Systemic)
Brompheniramine, Phenyltoloxamine, and Phenylephrine (Systemic)
Brompheniramine, Phenyltoloxamine, Pseudoephedrine, and Atropine (Systemic)
Brompheniramine and Pseudoephedrine (Systemic)
Brompheniramine, Pseudoephedrine, and Dextromethorphan (Systemic)
Buclizine (Systemic)
Buprenorphine (Systemic)
Bupropion (Systemic)
Busulfan (Systemic)
Butabarbital (Systemic)
Butalbital and Acetaminophen (Systemic)
Butalbital, Acetaminophen, and Caffeine (Systemic)
Butalbital and Aspirin (Systemic)
Butalbital, Aspirin, and Caffeine (Systemic)
Butalbital, Aspirin, Codeine, and Caffeine (Systemic)

C

Caffeine (Systemic)
Caffeine, Citrated (Systemic)
Calcitonin-Human (Systemic)
Calcitonin-Salmon (Systemic)
Carbamazepine (Systemic)
Carbenicillin (Systemic)
Carbidopa and Levodopa (Systemic)
Carbinoxamine (Systemic)

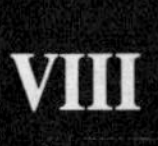

Carbinoxamine and Pseudoephedrine (Systemic)
Carbinoxamine, Pseudoephedrine, and Dextromethorphan (Systemic)
Carbinoxamine, Pseudoephedrine, and Guaifenesin (Systemic)
Carboplatin (Systemic)
Carisoprodol (Systemic)
Carmustine (Systemic)
Carteolol (Systemic)
Cascara Sagrada (Oral)
Cascara Sagrada and Aloe (Oral)
Cascara Sagrada and Phenolphthalein (Oral)
Cetirizine (Systemic)
Chloral Hydrate (Systemic)
Chlorambucil (Systemic)
Chloramphenicol (Systemic)
Chlordiazepoxide (Systemic)
Chlordiazepoxide and Amitriptyline (Systemic)
Chlordiazepoxide and Clidinium (Systemic)
Chloroquine (Systemic)
Chlorothiazide (Systemic)
Chlorotrianisene (Systemic)
Chlorpheniramine (Systemic)
Chlorpheniramine, Codeine, Aspirin, and Caffeine (Systemic)
Chlorpheniramine, Codeine, and Guaifenesin (Systemic)
Chlorpheniramine and Dextromethorphan (Systemic)
Chlorpheniramine, Dextromethorphan, and Acetaminophen (Systemic)
Chlorpheniramine, Ephedrine, and Guaifenesin (Systemic)
Chlorpheniramine, Ephedrine, Phenylephrine, and Carbetapentane (Systemic)
Chlorpheniramine, Ephedrine, Phenylephrine, Dextromethorphan, Ammonium Chloride, and Ipecac (Systemic)
Chlorpheniramine, Phenindamine, Phenylephrine, Dextromethorphan, Acetaminophen, Salicylamide, Caffeine, and Ascorbic Acid (Systemic)
Chlorpheniramine, Phenindamine, and Phenylpropanolamine (Systemic)
Chlorpheniramine, Phenindamine, Pyrilamine, Phenylephrine, Hydrocodone, and Ammonium Chloride (Systemic)
Chlorpheniramine, Pheniramine, Pyrilamine, Phenylephrine, Hydrocodone, Salicylamide, Caffeine, and Ascorbic Acid (Systemic)
Chlorpheniramine and Phenylephrine (Systemic)
Chlorpheniramine, Phenylephrine, and Acetaminophen (Systemic)
Chlorpheniramine, Phenylephrine, Acetaminophen, and Caffeine (Systemic)
Chlorpheniramine, Phenylephrine, Acetaminophen, and Salicylamide (Systemic)
Chlorpheniramine, Phenylephrine, Acetaminophen, Salicylamide, and Caffeine (Systemic)
Chlorpheniramine, Phenylephrine, Codeine, Ammonium Chloride, Potassium Guaiacolsulfonate, and Sodium Citrate (Systemic)
Chlorpheniramine, Phenylephrine, Codeine, and Potassium Iodide (Systemic)
Chlorpheniramine, Phenylephrine, and Dextromethorphan (Systemic)
Chlorpheniramine, Phenylephrine, Dextromethorphan, Acetaminophen, and Salicylamide (Systemic)
Chlorpheniramine, Phenylephrine, Dextromethorphan, and Guaifenesin (Systemic)
Chlorpheniramine, Phenylephrine, Dextromethorphan, Guaifenesin, and Ammonium Chloride (Systemic)
Chlorpheniramine, Phenylephrine, and Guaifenesin (Systemic)
Chlorpheniramine, Phenylephrine, and Hydrocodone (Systemic)
Chlorpheniramine, Phenylephrine, Hydrocodone, Acetaminophen, and Caffeine (Systemic)
Chlorpheniramine, Phenylephrine, and Methscopolamine (Systemic)
Chlorpheniramine, Phenylephrine, and Phenylpropanolamine (Systemic)
Chlorpheniramine, Phenylephrine, Phenylpropanolamine, Atropine, Hyoscyamine, and Scopolamine (Systemic)
Chlorpheniramine, Phenylephrine, Phenylpropanolamine, Carbetapentane, and Potassium Guaiacolsulfonate (Systemic)
Chlorpheniramine, Phenylephrine, Phenylpropanolamine, and Codeine (Systemic)
Chlorpheniramine, Phenylephrine, Phenylpropanolamine, and Dextromethorphan (Systemic)
Chlorpheniramine, Phenylephrine, Phenylpropanolamine, Dextromethorphan, Guaifenesin, and Acetaminophen (Systemic)
Chlorpheniramine, Phenylephrine, Phenylpropanolamine, and Dihydrocodeine (Systemic)
Chlorpheniramine and Phenylpropanolamine (Systemic)
Chlorpheniramine, Phenylpropanolamine, and Acetaminophen (Systemic)
Chlorpheniramine, Phenylpropanolamine, Acetaminophen, and Caffeine (Systemic)
Chlorpheniramine, Phenylpropanolamine, and Aspirin (Systemic)
Chlorpheniramine, Phenylpropanolamine, Aspirin, and Caffeine (Systemic)
Chlorpheniramine, Phenylpropanolamine, and Caramiphen (Systemic)
Chlorpheniramine, Phenylpropanolamine, Codeine, Guaifenesin, and Acetaminophen (Systemic)
Chlorpheniramine, Phenylpropanolamine, and Dextromethorphan (Systemic)
Chlorpheniramine, Phenylpropanolamine, Dextromethorphan, and Acetaminophen (Systemic)
Chlorpheniramine, Phenylpropanolamine, Dextromethorphan, Acetaminophen, and Caffeine (Systemic)
Chlorpheniramine, Phenylpropanolamine, Dextromethorphan, and Ammonium Chloride (Systemic)
Chlorpheniramine, Phenylpropanolamine, and Guaifenesin (Systemic)
Chlorpheniramine, Phenylpropanolamine, Guaifenesin, Sodium Citrate, and Citric Acid (Systemic)
Chlorpheniramine, Phenylpropanolamine, Hydrocodone, Guaifenesin, and Salicylamide (Systemic)
Chlorpheniramine, Phenylpropanolamine, and Methscopolamine (Systemic)
Chlorpheniramine, Phenyltoloxamine, Ephedrine, Codeine, and Guaiacol Carbonate (Systemic)
Chlorpheniramine, Phenyltoloxamine, and Phenylephrine (Systemic)
Chlorpheniramine, Phenyltoloxamine, Phenylephrine, and Phenylpropanolamine (Systemic)
Chlorpheniramine, Phenyltoloxamine, Phenylpropanolamine, and Acetaminophen (Systemic)
Chlorpheniramine, Phenyltoloxamine, Phenylpropanolamine, Dextromethorphan, and Guaifenesin (Systemic)
Chlorpheniramine and Pseudoephedrine (Systemic)
Chlorpheniramine, Pseudoephedrine, and Acetaminophen (Systemic)
Chlorpheniramine, Pseudoephedrine, and Codeine (Systemic)
Chlorpheniramine, Pseudoephedrine, and Dextromethorphan (Systemic)
Chlorpheniramine, Pseudoephedrine, Dextromethorphan, and Acetaminophen (Systemic)
Chlorpheniramine, Pseudoephedrine, Dextromethorphan, Guaifenesin, and Aspirin (Systemic)
Chlorpheniramine, Pseudoephedrine, and Guaifenesin (Systemic)
Chlorpheniramine, Pseudoephedrine, and Hydrocodone (Systemic)
Chlorpheniramine, Pyrilamine, and Phenylephrine (Systemic)
Chlorpheniramine, Pyrilamine, Phenylephrine, and Acetaminophen (Systemic)
Chlorpheniramine, Pyrilamine, Phenylephrine, and Phenylpropanolamine (Systemic)
Chlorpheniramine, Pyrilamine, Phenylephrine, Phenylpropanolamine, and Acetaminophen (Systemic)
Chlorpromazine (Systemic)
Chlorpropamide (Systemic)
Chlorprothixene (Systemic)
Chlorthalidone (Systemic)
Cholestyramine (Oral)
Choline Salicylate (Systemic)
Choline and Magnesium Salicylates (Systemic)
Chromic Phosphate P 32 (Therapeutic)
Cimetidine (Systemic)
Cinoxacin (Systemic)
Ciprofloxacin (Systemic)
Cisplatin (Systemic)
Clemastine (Systemic)
Clemastine and Phenylpropanolamine (Systemic)
Clidinium (Systemic)
Clobetasol (Topical)
Clobetasone (Topical)
Clocortolone (Topical)
Clofazimine (Systemic)
Clofibrate (Systemic)
Clonazepam (Systemic)
Clorazepate (Systemic)
Clotrimazole and Betamethasone (Topical)
Cloxacillin (Systemic)
Clozapine (Systemic)
Cocaine (Mucosal-Local)
Codeine and Calcium Iodide (Systemic)
Codeine and Guaifenesin (Systemic)
Codeine and Iodinated Glycerol (Systemic)

Colchicine (Systemic)
Cortisone—Glucocorticoid Effects (Systemic)
Cyanocobalamin Co 57 (Diagnostic)
Cyclacillin (Systemic)
Cyclizine (Systemic)
Cyclophosphamide (Systemic)
Cyclosporine (Systemic)
Cyclothiazide (Systemic)
Cyproheptadine (Systemic)
Cytarabine (Systemic)

D–F

Dacarbazine (Systemic)
Dactinomycin (Systemic)
Danazol (Systemic)
Danthron and Docusate (Oral)
Dantrolene (Systemic)
Dapsone (Systemic)
Daunorubicin (Systemic)
Demecarium (Ophthalmic)
Demeclocycline (Systemic)
Deserpidine (Systemic)
Deserpidine and Hydrochlorothiazide (Systemic)
Deserpidine and Methyclothiazide (Systemic)
Desonide (Topical)
Desoximetasone (Topical)
Dexamethasone (Inhalation)
Dexamethasone (Nasal)
Dexamethasone (Topical)
Dexamethasone—Glucocorticoid Effects (Systemic)
Dexbrompheniramine and Pseudoephedrine (Systemic)
Dexbrompheniramine, Pseudoephedrine, and Acetaminophen (Systemic)
Dexchlorpheniramine (Systemic)
Dexchlorpheniramine, Pseudoephedrine, and Guaifenesin (Systemic)
Dextromethorphan and Iodinated Glycerol (Systemic)
Diatrizoate and Iodipamide (Diagnostic, Mucosal)
Diatrizoates (Diagnostic)
Diatrizoates (Diagnostic, Mucosal)
Diazepam (Systemic)
Dicloxacillin (Systemic)
Dicumarol (Systemic)
Dicyclomine (Systemic)
Dienestrol (Vaginal)
Diethylstilbestrol (Systemic)
Diethylstilbestrol and Methyltestosterone (Systemic)
Difenoxin and Atropine (Systemic)
Diflorasone (Topical)
Diflucortolone (Topical)
Dihydroergotamine (Systemic)
Dimenhydrinate (Systemic)
Diphenhydramine (Systemic)
Diphenhydramine, Codeine, and Ammonium Chloride (Systemic)
Diphenhydramine, Dextromethorphan, and Ammonium Chloride (Systemic)
Diphenhydramine, Phenylpropanolamine, and Aspirin (Systemic)
Diphenhydramine and Pseudoephedrine (Systemic)
Diphenhydramine, Pseudoephedrine, and Acetaminophen (Systemic)
Diphenhydramine, Pseudoephedrine, Dextromethorphan, and Acetaminophen (Systemic)
Diphenoxylate and Atropine (Systemic)
Diphenylpyraline (Systemic)
Diphenylpyraline, Phenylephrine, and Codeine (Systemic)
Diphenylpyraline, Phenylephrine, and Dextromethorphan (Systemic)
Diphenylpyraline, Phenylephrine, and Hydrocodone (Systemic)
Diphenylpyraline, Phenylephrine, Hydrocodone, and Guaifenesin (Systemic)
Doxepin (Systemic)
Doxorubicin (Systemic)
Doxycycline (Systemic)
Doxylamine (Systemic)
Doxylamine, Pseudoephedrine, Dextromethorphan, and Acetaminophen (Systemic)
Dronabinol (Systemic)
Echothiophate (Ophthalmic)
Econazole (Topical)
Enoxacin (Systemic)
Ephedrine (Oral/Injection)
Ephedrine and Potassium Iodide (Systemic)
Epinephrine (Inhalation)
Epinephrine (Oral/Injection)
Ergonovine (Systemic)
Ergotamine (Systemic)
Ergotamine, Belladonna Alkaloids, and Phenobarbital (Systemic)
Ergotamine and Caffeine (Systemic)
Ergotamine, Caffeine, and Belladonna Alkaloids (Systemic)
Ergotamine, Caffeine, Belladonna Alkaloids, and Pentobarbital (Systemic)
Ergotamine, Caffeine, and Cyclizine (Systemic)
Ergotamine, Caffeine, and Dimenhydrinate (Systemic)
Ergotamine, Caffeine, and Diphenhydramine (Systemic)
Erythromycin and Sulfisoxazole (Systemic)
Estazolam (Systemic)
Estradiol (Systemic)
Estradiol (Vaginal)
Estrogens, Conjugated (Systemic)
Estrogens, Conjugated (Vaginal)
Estrogens, Conjugated, and Methyltestosterone (Systemic)
Estrogens, Esterified (Systemic)
Estrogens, Esterified, and Methyltestosterone (Systemic)
Estrone (Systemic)
Estrone (Vaginal)
Estropipate (Systemic)
Estropipate (Vaginal)
Ethinyl Estradiol (Systemic)
Ethopropazine (Systemic)
Ethotoin (Systemic)
Ethynodiol Diacetate and Ethinyl Estradiol (Systemic)
Etoposide (Systemic)
Etretinate (Systemic)
Famotidine (Systemic)
Ferrous Citrate Fe 59 (Diagnostic)
Floxuridine (Systemic)
Fludarabine (Systemic)
Fludeoxyglucose F 18 (Diagnostic)
Fludrocortisone (Systemic)
Flumethasone (Topical)
Flunisolide (Inhalation)
Flunisolide (Nasal)
Fluocinolone (Topical)
Fluocinonide (Topical)
Fluorouracil (Systemic)
Fluorouracil (Topical)
Fluoxymesterone (Systemic)
Fluoxymesterone and Ethinyl Estradiol (Systemic)
Flupenthixol (Systemic)
Fluphenazine (Systemic)
Flurandrenolide (Topical)
Flurazepam (Systemic)
Fluticasone (Topical)
Furazolidone (Oral)

G–O

Gallium Citrate Ga 67 (Diagnostic)
Gallium Nitrate (Systemic)
Ganciclovir (Systemic)
Gemfibrozil (Systemic)
Glipizide (Systemic)
Glutethimide (Systemic)
Glyburide (Systemic)
Glycopyrrolate (Systemic)
Gold Sodium Thiomalate (Systemic)
Guanethidine (Systemic)
Guanethidine and Hydrochlorothiazide (Systemic)
Halazepam (Systemic)
Halcinonide (Topical)
Halobetasol (Topical)
Halofantrine (Systemic)
Haloperidol (Systemic)
Heparin (Systemic)
Homatropine (Systemic)
Hydralazine and Hydrochlorothiazide (Systemic)
Hydrochlorothiazide (Systemic)
Hydrocodone and Aspirin (Systemic)
Hydrocodone, Aspirin, and Caffeine (Systemic)
Hydrocodone and Guaifenesin (Systemic)
Hydrocodone and Homatropine (Systemic)
Hydrocodone and Potassium Guaiacolsulfonate (Systemic)
Hydrocortisone (Dental)
Hydrocortisone (Rectal)
Hydrocortisone (Topical)
Hydrocortisone Acetate (Topical)
Hydrocortisone Butyrate (Topical)
Hydrocortisone—Glucocorticoid Effects (Systemic)
Hydrocortisone Valerate (Topical)
Hydroflumethiazide (Systemic)
Hydromorphone and Guaifenesin (Systemic)
Hydroxychloroquine (Systemic)
Hydroxyprogesterone (Systemic)
Hydroxyurea (Systemic)
Hydroxyzine (Systemic)
Hyoscyamine (Systemic)
Hyoscyamine and Phenobarbital (Systemic)
Idarubicin (Systemic)
Ifosfamide (Systemic)
Indium In 111 Oxyquinoline (Diagnostic)
Indium In 111 Pentetate (Diagnostic)
Indium In 111 Satumomab Pendetide (Diagnostic)
Indomethacin (Systemic)
Interferon Alfa-2a, Recombinant (Systemic)
Interferon Alfa-2b, Recombinant (Systemic)
Interferon Alfa-n1 (lns) (Systemic)

Interferon Alfa-n3 (Systemic)
Interferon, Gamma (Systemic)
Iobenguane, Radioiodinated (Diagnostic)
Iobenguane, Radioiodinated (Therapeutic)
Iocetamic Acid (Diagnostic)
Iodinated Glycerol (Systemic)
Iodine, Strong (Systemic)
Iodipamide (Diagnostic)
Iodohippurate Sodium I 123 (Diagnostic)
Iodohippurate Sodium I 131 (Diagnostic)
Iofetamine I 123 (Diagnostic)
Iohexol (Diagnostic)
Iohexol (Diagnostic, Mucosal)
Iopamidol (Diagnostic)
Iopanoic Acid (Diagnostic)
Iothalamate (Diagnostic)
Iothalamate (Diagnostic, Mucosal)
Iothalamate Sodium I 125 (Diagnostic)
Ioversol (Diagnostic)
Ioxaglate (Diagnostic)
Ioxaglate (Diagnostic, Mucosal)
Ipodate (Diagnostic)
Isoflurophate (Ophthalmic)
Isoniazid (Systemic)
Isopropamide (Systemic)
Isotretinoin (Systemic)
Kaolin, Pectin, Belladonna Alkaloids, and Opium (Systemic)
Ketazolam (Systemic)
Ketoconazole (Systemic)
Krypton Kr 81m (Diagnostic)
Labetalol (Systemic)
Labetalol and Hydrochlorothiazide (Systemic)
Leuprolide (Systemic)
Levodopa (Systemic)
Levonorgestrel and Ethinyl Estradiol (Systemic)
Lindane (Topical)
Lithium (Systemic)
Lomefloxacin (Systemic)
Lomustine (Systemic)
Loratadine (Systemic)
Lorazepam (Systemic)
Lovastatin (Systemic)
Mafenide (Topical)
Magnesium Salicylate (Systemic)
Mechlorethamine (Systemic)
Mechlorethamine (Topical)
Meclizine (Systemic)
Meclofenamate (Systemic)
Medroxyprogesterone (Systemic)
Mefloquine (Systemic)
Megestrol (Systemic)
Melphalan (Systemic)
Mepenzolate (Systemic)
Mephobarbital (Systemic)
Meprobamate (Systemic)
Meprobamate and Aspirin (Systemic)
Mercaptopurine (Systemic)
Mesoridazine (Systemic)
Methacycline (Systemic)
Methadone (Systemic)
Methantheline (Systemic)
Metharbital (Systemic)
Methdilazine (Systemic)
Methicillin (Systemic)
Methimazole (Systemic)
Methotrexate—For Cancer (Systemic)
Methotrexate—For Noncancerous Conditions (Systemic)
Methotrimeprazine (Systemic)
Methscopolamine (Systemic)
Methyclothiazide (Systemic)
Methyldopa and Chlorothiazide (Systemic)
Methyldopa and Hydrochlorothiazide (Systemic)
Methylergonovine (Systemic)
Methylprednisolone—Glucocorticoid Effects (Systemic)
Methyltestosterone (Systemic)
Methysergide (Systemic)
Metoclopramide (Systemic)
Metolazone (Systemic)
Metoprolol (Systemic)
Metoprolol and Hydrochlorothiazide (Systemic)
Metrizamide (Diagnostic)
Metronidazole (Systemic)
Metyrapone (Systemic)
Mexiletine (Systemic)
Mezlocillin (Systemic)
Mineral Oil and Cascara Sagrada (Oral)
Minocycline (Systemic)
Minoxidil (Topical)
Misoprostol (Systemic)
Mitomycin (Systemic)
Mitoxantrone (Systemic)
Mometasone (Topical)
Muromonab-CD3 (Systemic)
Nabilone (Systemic)
Nadolol (Systemic)
Nadolol and Bendroflumethiazide (Systemic)
Nafcillin (Systemic)
Naftifine (Topical)
Nalidixic Acid (Systemic)
Nicotine (Systemic)
Nitrazepam (Systemic)
Nitrofurantoin (Systemic)
Nizatidine (Systemic)
Norethindrone (Systemic)
Norethindrone Acetate and Ethinyl Estradiol (Systemic)
Norethindrone and Ethinyl Estradiol (Systemic)
Norethindrone and Mestranol (Systemic)
Norfloxacin (Ophthalmic)
Norfloxacin (Systemic)
Norgestrel (Systemic)
Norgestrel and Ethinyl Estradiol (Systemic)
Nystatin and Triamcinolone (Topical)
Ofloxacin (Systemic)
Omeprazole (Systemic)
Orphenadrine and Aspirin (Systemic)
Oxacillin (Systemic)
Oxazepam (Systemic)
Oxprenolol (Systemic)
Oxtriphylline (Systemic)
Oxtriphylline and Guaifenesin (Systemic)
Oxybutynin (Systemic)
Oxycodone and Aspirin (Systemic)
Oxyphencyclimine (Systemic)
Oxytetracycline (Systemic)

P

Paclitaxel (Systemic)
Pancreatin, Pepsin, Bile Salts, Hyoscyamine, Atropine, Scopolamine, and Phenobarbital (Systemic)
Paramethasone—Glucocorticoid Effects (Systemic)
Penbutolol (Systemic)
Penicillin G (Systemic)
Penicillin V (Systemic)
Pentamidine (Systemic)
Pentazocine and Aspirin (Systemic)
Pentobarbital (Systemic)
Pentostatin (Systemic)
Pentoxifylline (Systemic)
Pergolide (Systemic)
Pericyazine (Systemic)
Permethrin (Topical)
Perphenazine (Systemic)
Perphenazine and Amitriptyline (Systemic)
Phenindamine (Systemic)
Phenindamine, Hydrocodone, and Guaifenesin (Systemic)
Pheniramine, Codeine, and Guaifenesin (Systemic)
Pheniramine, Phenylephrine, Codeine, Sodium Citrate, Sodium Salicylate, and Caffeine (Systemic)
Pheniramine, Phenylephrine, Sodium Salicylate, and Caffeine (Systemic)
Pheniramine, Phenyltoloxamine, Pyrilamine, and Phenylpropanolamine (Systemic)
Pheniramine, Pyrilamine, Hydrocodone, Potassium Citrate, and Ascorbic Acid (Systemic)
Pheniramine, Pyrilamine, Phenylephrine, Phenylpropanolamine, and Hydrocodone (Systemic)
Pheniramine, Pyrilamine, and Phenylpropanolamine (Systemic)
Pheniramine, Pyrilamine, Phenylpropanolamine, and Aspirin (Systemic)
Pheniramine, Pyrilamine, Phenylpropanolamine, and Codeine (Systemic)
Pheniramine, Pyrilamine, Phenylpropanolamine, Codeine, Acetaminophen, and Caffeine (Systemic)
Pheniramine, Pyrilamine, Phenylpropanolamine, and Dextromethorphan (Systemic)
Pheniramine, Pyrilamine, Phenylpropanolamine, Dextromethorphan, and Ammonium Chloride (Systemic)
Pheniramine, Pyrilamine, Phenylpropanolamine, Dextromethorphan, and Guaifenesin (Systemic)
Pheniramine, Pyrilamine, Phenylpropanolamine, and Guaifenesin (Systemic)
Pheniramine, Pyrilamine, Phenylpropanolamine, and Hydrocodone (Systemic)
Pheniramine, Pyrilamine, Phenylpropanolamine, Hydrocodone, and Guaifenesin (Systemic)
Phenobarbital (Systemic)
Phenobarbital, Aspirin, and Codeine (Systemic)
Phenylbutazone (Systemic)
Phenylephrine and Acetaminophen (Systemic)
Phenylephrine, Guaifenesin, Acetaminophen, Salicylamide, and Caffeine (Systemic)
Phenylephrine, Hydrocodone, and Guaifenesin (Systemic)
Phenylpropanolamine and Acetaminophen (Systemic)
Phenylpropanolamine, Acetaminophen, and Aspirin (Systemic)
Phenylpropanolamine, Acetaminophen, Aspirin, and Caffeine (Systemic)
Phenylpropanolamine, Acetaminophen, Salicylamide, and Caffeine (Systemic)
Phenylpropanolamine and Aspirin (Systemic)
Phenylpropanolamine, Codeine, and Guaifenesin (Systemic)

Phenylpropanolamine and Hydrocodone (Systemic)
Phenyltoloxamine and Hydrocodone (Systemic)
Phenyltoloxamine, Phenylpropanolamine, and Acetaminophen (Systemic)
Phenytoin (Systemic)
Pimozide (Systemic)
Pindolol (Systemic)
Pindolol and Hydrochlorothiazide (Systemic)
Piperacillin (Systemic)
Pipotiazine (Systemic)
Pirenzepine (Systemic)
Piroxicam (Systemic)
Poliovirus Vaccine (Systemic)
Polythiazide (Systemic)
Potassium Iodide (Systemic)
Pravastatin (Systemic)
Prazepam (Systemic)
Praziquantel (Systemic)
Prednisolone—Glucocorticoid Effects (Systemic)
Prednisone—Glucocorticoid Effects (Systemic)
Primidone (Systemic)
Probenecid and Colchicine (Systemic)
Probucol (Systemic)
Procarbazine (Systemic)
Prochlorperazine (Systemic)
Procyclidine (Systemic)
Progesterone (Systemic)
Promazine (Systemic)
Promethazine (Systemic)
Promethazine and Codeine (Systemic)
Promethazine and Dextromethorphan (Systemic)
Promethazine and Phenylephrine (Systemic)
Promethazine, Phenylephrine, and Codeine (Systemic)
Promethazine and Pseudoephedrine (Systemic)
Propantheline (Systemic)
Propoxyphene and Aspirin (Systemic)
Propoxyphene, Aspirin, and Caffeine (Systemic)
Propranolol (Systemic)
Propranolol and Hydrochlorothiazide (Systemic)
Propylthiouracil (Systemic)
Protirelin (Diagnostic)
Pseudoephedrine (Systemic)
Pseudoephedrine and Acetaminophen (Systemic)
Pseudoephedrine, Acetaminophen, and Caffeine (Systemic)
Pseudoephedrine and Aspirin (Systemic)
Pseudoephedrine, Aspirin, and Caffeine (Systemic)
Pseudoephedrine and Codeine (Systemic)
Pseudoephedrine, Codeine, and Guaifenesin (Systemic)
Pseudoephedrine and Dextromethorphan (Systemic)
Pseudoephedrine, Dextromethorphan, and Acetaminophen (Systemic)
Pseudoephedrine, Dextromethorphan, and Guaifenesin (Systemic)
Pseudoephedrine, Dextromethorphan, Guaifenesin, and Acetaminophen (Systemic)
Pseudoephedrine and Guaifenesin (Systemic)
Pseudoephedrine and Hydrocodone (Systemic)
Pseudoephedrine, Hydrocodone, and Guaifenesin (Systemic)
Pseudoephedrine and Ibuprofen (Systemic)
Pyrilamine (Systemic)
Pyrilamine, Phenylephrine, Aspirin, and Caffeine (Systemic)
Pyrilamine, Phenylephrine, and Codeine (Systemic)
Pyrilamine, Phenylephrine, and Dextromethorphan (Systemic)
Pyrilamine, Phenylephrine, Dextromethorphan, and Acetaminophen (Systemic)
Pyrilamine, Phenylephrine, and Hydrocodone (Systemic)
Pyrilamine, Phenylephrine, Hydrocodone, and Ammonium Chloride (Systemic)
Pyrilamine, Phenylpropanolamine, Acetaminophen, and Caffeine (Systemic)
Pyrilamine, Phenylpropanolamine, Dextromethorphan, Guaifenesin, Potassium Citrate, and Citric Acid (Systemic)
Pyrilamine, Phenylpropanolamine, Dextromethorphan, and Sodium Salicylate (Systemic)
Pyrimethamine (Systemic)

Q–Z

Quazepam (Systemic)
Quinestrol (Systemic)
Quinethazone (Systemic)
Radioiodinated Albumin (Diagnostic)
Ranitidine (Systemic)
Rauwolfia Serpentina (Systemic)
Rauwolfia Serpentina and Bendroflumethiazide (Systemic)
Reserpine (Systemic)
Reserpine and Chlorothiazide (Systemic)
Reserpine and Chlorthalidone (Systemic)
Reserpine, Hydralazine, and Hydrochlorothiazide (Systemic)
Reserpine and Hydrochlorothiazide (Systemic)
Reserpine and Hydroflumethiazide (Systemic)
Reserpine and Methyclothiazide (Systemic)
Reserpine and Polythiazide (Systemic)
Reserpine and Trichlormethiazide (Systemic)
Ribavirin (Systemic)
Rifampin and Isoniazid (Systemic)
Rubidium Rb 82 (Diagnostic)
Salicylic Acid (Topical)
Salicylic Acid and Sulfur (Topical)
Salicylic Acid, Sulfur, and Coal Tar (Topical)
Salsalate (Systemic)
Scopolamine (Systemic)
Secobarbital (Systemic)
Secobarbital and Amobarbital (Systemic)
Silver Sulfadiazine (Topical)
Simvastatin (Systemic)
Sodium Chromate Cr 51 (Diagnostic)
Sodium Iodide (Systemic)
Sodium Iodide I 123 (Diagnostic)
Sodium Iodide I 131 (Diagnostic)
Sodium Iodide I 131 (Therapeutic)
Sodium Pertechnetate Tc 99m (Diagnostic)
Sodium Phosphate P 32 (Therapeutic)
Sodium Salicylate (Systemic)
Sotalol (Systemic)
Streptozocin (Systemic)
Sulfacytine (Systemic)
Sulfadiazine (Systemic)
Sulfadoxine and Pyrimethamine (Systemic)
Sulfamethizole (Systemic)
Sulfamethoxazole (Systemic)
Sulfamethoxazole and Phenazopyridine (Systemic)
Sulfamethoxazole and Trimethoprim (Systemic)
Sulfanilamide (Vaginal)
Sulfanilamide, Aminacrine, and Allantoin (Vaginal)
Sulfapyridine (Systemic)
Sulfasalazine (Systemic)
Sulfisoxazole (Systemic)
Sulfisoxazole and Phenazopyridine (Systemic)
Tamoxifen (Systemic)
Technetium Tc 99m Albumin (Diagnostic)
Technetium Tc 99m Albumin Aggregated (Diagnostic)
Technetium Tc 99m Disofenin (Diagnostic)
Technetium Tc 99m Exametazime (Diagnostic)
Technetium Tc 99m Gluceptate (Diagnostic)
Technetium Tc 99m Lidofenin (Diagnostic)
Technetium Tc 99m Mebrofenin (Diagnostic)
Technetium Tc 99m Medronate (Diagnostic)
Technetium Tc 99m Mertiatide (Diagnostic)
Technetium Tc 99m Oxidronate (Diagnostic)
Technetium Tc 99m Pentetate (Diagnostic)
Technetium Tc 99m Pyrophosphate (Diagnostic)
Technetium Tc 99m (Pyro- and trimeta-) Phosphates (Diagnostic)
Technetium Tc 99m Sestamibi (Diagnostic)
Technetium Tc 99m Succimer (Diagnostic)
Technetium Tc 99m Sulfur Colloid (Diagnostic)
Technetium Tc 99m Teboroxime (Diagnostic)
Temazepam (Systemic)
Terbutaline (Inhalation)
Terbutaline (Oral/Injection)
Terfenadine (Systemic)
Terfenadine and Pseudoephedrine (Systemic)
Teriparatide (Systemic)
Testosterone (Systemic)
Testosterone and Estradiol (Systemic)
Tetracycline (Systemic)
Thallous Chloride Tl 201 (Diagnostic)
Theophylline (Systemic)
Theophylline, Ephedrine, Guaifenesin, and Butabarbital (Systemic)
Theophylline, Ephedrine, Guaifenesin, and Phenobarbital (Systemic)
Theophylline, Ephedrine, and Hydroxyzine (Systemic)
Theophylline, Ephedrine, and Phenobarbital (Systemic)
Theophylline and Guaifenesin (Systemic)
Thiabendazole (Systemic)
Thiethylperazine (Systemic)
Thioguanine (Systemic)
Thiopropazate (Systemic)
Thioproperazine (Systemic)
Thioridazine (Systemic)
Thiotepa (Systemic)
Thiothixene (Systemic)
Ticarcillin (Systemic)
Ticarcillin and Clavulanate (Systemic)
Timolol (Ophthalmic)
Timolol (Systemic)
Timolol and Hydrochlorothiazide (Systemic)
Tiopronin (Systemic)
Tolazamide (Systemic)
Tolbutamide (Systemic)

Triamcinolone (Dental)
Triamcinolone (Inhalation)
Triamcinolone (Topical)
Triamcinolone—Glucocorticoid Effects (Systemic)
Triazolam (Systemic)
Trichlormethiazide (Systemic)
Tridihexethyl (Systemic)
Trifluoperazine (Systemic)
Triflupromazine (Systemic)
Trihexyphenidyl (Systemic)
Trimeprazine (Systemic)
Trimethoprim (Systemic)
Tripelennamine (Systemic)
Triple Sulfa (Vaginal)
Triprolidine (Systemic)
Triprolidine and Pseudoephedrine (Systemic)
Triprolidine, Pseudoephedrine, and Acetaminophen (Systemic)
Triprolidine, Pseudoephedrine, and Codeine (Systemic)
Triprolidine, Pseudoephedrine, Codeine, and Guaifenesin (Systemic)
Triprolidine, Pseudoephedrine, and Dextromethorphan (Systemic)
Tyropanoate (Diagnostic)
Uracil Mustard (Systemic)
Vinblastine (Systemic)
Vincristine (Systemic)
Xenon Xe 127 (Diagnostic)
Xenon Xe 133 (Diagnostic)
Zidovudine (Systemic)

Appendix IX

ATHLETES PRECAUTIONS

Banned Substances and the Athlete

Since the beginning of organized competition, athletes have tried to gain every possible advantage over their competitors. Sometimes this competitive edge is gained fairly by training harder or developing new and improved methods. Recently, however, many athletes have tried to gain an advantage through the use of substances that affect the body in ways that can improve athletic performance. These substances are called ergogenic aids, which may be drugs, herbal products, or substances that are produced by the body. Ergogenic aids can be defined as any natural or man-made substance that can increase strength, endurance, or flexibility. Increasing use of ergogenic aids, and the drug-related deaths of several well-known athletes, have led the National Collegiate Athletic Association (NCAA) and United States Olympic Committee (USOC) to monitor more closely the use of drugs and other ergogenic aids by athletes. The NCAA and USOC have established lists of banned substances, as well as education and testing programs. The use of substances that are on these lists is illegal by NCAA and USOC rules, and can result in an athlete being disqualified from an event and other penalties. In most cases, banned substances are also used in doses that are much higher than those recommended by doctors, and can cause dangerous and even permanent or life-threatening side effects.

The brief descriptions of banned substances that are listed below have been compiled using information in the USP DI database, NCAA and USOC publications, and other sources. The lists that follow these descriptions are unofficial and, due to the sometimes rapid changes in the NCAA and USOC lists, may be incomplete or inaccurate. These lists are meant to be an example of the kinds of substances that may be banned, and should not be used in the place of the USOC or NCAA lists. Before using or advising an athlete to use a substance, always check with the appropriate governing body. The NCAA Drug-Testing/Education Program phone number is 913-339-1906; the USOC Drug Education Program toll-free hotline number is 1-800-233-0393. Both of these lists are constantly updated to address any changes in the drug use patterns of athletes.

What Athletes Should Know About Banned Substances and Use of Medications

Information for the Athlete:

Athletes should always check with the appropriate governing body for their sport before taking **any** medicines or substances. Even medicines that a physician may prescribe for common conditions such as allergies may contain a substance that is banned by the NCAA or USOC. Nonprescription, or over-the-counter (OTC), medicines may also be banned. It is important that athletes check with the appropriate governing body for their sport to be sure that a substance is not banned. A medicine that may work equally well and is not banned can often be substituted for a banned one.

The NCAA and USOC maintain different lists of banned substances, and have different rules regarding procedures, drug testing, and violations. Also, there are different lists of banned substances for some USOC sports or events; and the NCAA riflery list contains some substances that are not included in the rest of the NCAA list. Athletes should always know the different drugs that are banned for their sport or event, and should consult the governing body for their sport before taking any substances that could be banned.

Once it is determined that a drug is not banned, it should be taken exactly as recommended by the physician, nurse, pharmacist, dentist, or other health care provider. Patients should always feel free to ask these professionals any questions that they have about their medicines or treatment. Athletes may also want to ask about any possible effect that taking a medicine can have on their status with the NCAA or USOC, and if any changes should be made in their training or competition schedule. Athletes should always know what medicines they are taking and why they were prescribed, as well as any special warnings or instructions, potential drug interactions, and/or possible side effects that they can cause.

Classes of NCAA and/or USOC Banned Substances

Stimulants:

Central nervous system (CNS) stimulants include a wide range of drugs in many dosage forms. Some stimulants, such as amphetamines, are used to treat children with attention-deficit hyperactivity disorder (ADHD) and people who have narcolepsy. Because stimulants can increase the heart rate and flow of blood and oxygen, they are often used by athletes to quicken reaction times, heighten alertness, and reduce fatigue. However, the abuse of these substances can cause dangerous reactions in the athlete's body. During exercise or competition, some of the athlete's bodily functions (such as heart rate and blood pressure) can be increased to very stressful levels. With stimulant use, these functions can be increased to dangerously high levels that can result in stroke, heartbeat irregularities, and heart attack. When taken in unusually high doses, some common stimulants (caffeine, for example) are considered toxic and can even cause death. When stimulants are taken to relieve fatigue, the body's natural warning signals can be covered up. This can place the athlete at greater risk of injury and dangerous reactions. Heat exhaustion and collapse can also occur. Athletes also take stimulants for the mental effects that they believe these drugs can have, such as increased competitiveness, aggressiveness, and self-confidence. These effects can also place the athlete at a greater risk of injury. Stimulants can also cause depression and thought disorders.

Some banned stimulants can be found in common products, such as cough/cold medications. Some herbal products (teas, some dietary supplements) may also contain banned substances, such as ephedrine. Athletes should always check to be sure that even common products do not contain stimulants that are banned by the NCAA and/or USOC.

Caffeine is one of the most widely used and often abused stimulants in the world. It is found in many common products, including coffee, tea, chocolate, some sodas, and many common medications. Caffeine can be very dangerous when taken at very high doses, and the NCAA and USOC ban certain levels of caffeine use. The NCAA prohibits urinary concentrations of caffeine that exceed 15 micrograms/mL; the USOC limit is 12 micrograms/mL.

The following stimulants may be banned by the NCAA and/or USOC (listed by generic name with examples of commonly used brand names in parentheses):

- Amphetamine
- Amphetamine and Dextroamphetamine Resin Complex (e.g., Biphetamine)
- Benzphetamine (e.g., Didrex)
- Caffeine (e.g., NoDoz)
- Caffeine, Citrated
- Cocaine
- Dextroamphetamine (e.g., Dexedrine)
- Diethylpropion (e.g., Tenuate)
- Ephedrine
- Isoproterenol (e.g., Isuprel)
- Metaproterenol (e.g., Alupent, Metaprel)
- Methamphetamine (e.g., Desoxyn)
- Methylphenidate (e.g., Ritalin)
- Pemoline (e.g., Cylert)
- Phendimetrazine (e.g., Anorex)
- Phentermine (e.g., Fastin)
- Phenylpropanolamine (e.g., Dexatrim)
- Pseudoephedrine (e.g., Sudafed)

Beta-blockers:

Beta-adrenergic blocking agents, commonly called beta-blockers, are used to treat high blood pressure, to treat chest pain, to prevent additional heart attacks in heart attack patients, and for a number of other conditions, such as irregular heartbeat and migraine headaches. Ophthalmic beta-blockers are commonly used to treat glaucoma.

Some forms of beta-blockers are used by athletes in certain sports (mainly the shooting events) because they lower the heart rate, which steadies the nerves (and trigger finger). It has even been suggested that shooters' heart rates can be so slowed by beta-blockers that they are able to shoot between heartbeats. Use of these drugs can give the athlete an unfair advantage, and is banned for all riflery competition by the NCAA. The USOC permits the use of ophthalmic beta-blockers, and tests for beta-blocker abuse in the following events (this list is subject to change): archery, biathlon, bobsled, diving, equestrian, fencing, figure skating, gymnastics, luge, modern pentathlon (shooting), sailing, shooting, and ski jumping.

The following beta-blockers may be banned by the NCAA and/or USOC (listed by generic name):

- Acebutolol (e.g., Sectral)
- Alprenolol (e.g., Aptin)
- Atenolol (e.g., Tenormin)
- Betaxolol* (e.g., Kerlone)
- Atenolol and Chlorthalidone (e.g., Tenoretic)
- Labetolol and Hydrochlorothiazide (e.g., Normozide)
- Metoprolol (e.g., Lopressor)
- Metoprolol and Hydrochlorothiazide (e.g., Lopressor HCT)
- Nadolol (e.g., Corgard)
- Nadolol and Bendroflumethiazide (e.g., Corzide)
- Oxprenolol (e.g., Trasicor)
- Pindolol (e.g., Visken)
- Pindolol and Hydrochlorothiazide (e.g., Viskazide)
- Propranolol (e.g., Inderal)
- Propranolol and Hydrochlorothiazide (e.g., Inderide)
- Sotalol (e.g., Sotacor)
- Timolol* (e.g., Blocadren)
- Timolol and Hydrochlorothiazide (.e.g, Timolide)

*Ophthalmic use of these drugs is allowed by the USOC; any use is banned by the NCAA.

Diuretics:

Diuretics act on the kidneys to increase the flow of urine. They are commonly used to reduce the amount of water in the body. Diuretics are often used to treat high blood pressure, and may be used for other conditions as well. Athletes use diuretics to lose weight rapidly. The rapid flushing of water from the body, however, can result in harmful effects such as dehydration, muscle cramps, and exhaustion, among others. Athletes also take diuretics to reduce the concentrations of other banned substances in their urine. Use of diuretics is banned by both the NCAA and USOC.

The following diuretics may be banned by the NCAA and/or USOC (listed by generic name):

- Acetazolamide (e.g., Diamox)
- Amiloride (e.g., Midamor)
- Bendroflumethiazide (e.g., Naturetin)
- Benzthiazide (e.g., Exna)
- Bumetanide (e.g., Bumex)
- Chlorothiazide (e.g., Diuril)
- Chlorthalidone (e.g., Hygroton)
- Cyclothiazide (e.g., Anhydron)
- Ethacrynic Acid (e.g., Edecrin)
- Furosemide (e.g., Lasix)
- Hydrochlorothiazide (e.g., HydroDIURIL)
- Hydroflumethiazide (e.g., Saluron)
- Indapamide (e.g., Lozol)
- Methyclothiazide (e.g., Aquatensin)
- Metolazone (e.g., Zaroxolyn)
- Polythiazide (e.g., Renese)
- Quinethazone (e.g., Hydromox)
- Spironolactone (e.g., Aldactone)
- Triamterene (e.g., Dyrenium)
- Trichlormethiazide (e.g., Metahydrin)

Blood Doping:

Blood doping is the practice of administering blood or blood-related products to an athlete to enhance his or her performance. Blood doping is usually practiced by endurance athletes, who expect the additional red blood cells (which carry oxygen) to increase their endurance. An unnecessary transfusion can place the athlete at risk of side effects such as allergic reaction, bacterial contamination, and hepatitis. The manipulation of the blood, especially the process of adding red blood cells (or "red blood cell packing") creates serious risks due to the high red blood cell concentration that may result. Because the concentration of red blood cells in endurance athletes can rise due to fluid loss during competition, the added red blood cells can thicken the blood. As the blood thickens the athlete is at increasing risk of blood clotting, stroke, and heart failure. Using additional (unneeded) blood is similar to using any other performance-enhancing aid, and the process of blood doping is banned by both the NCAA and USOC.

Peptide Hormones and Analogs:

Peptide hormones carry messages between organs in the body. Man-made versions of these substances are called analogs. The peptide hormones and analogs most abused by athletes are those that cause the release of growth-related chemicals in the body. When they are produced naturally, these substances act in a positive manner upon the body (stimulating growth and muscle mass, for instance). When these effects are unnecessarily produced by a man-made substance, however, they upset the body's chemical balance, and can cause dangerous and long-term side effects.

Human growth hormone (GH) is produced by the pituitary gland and is needed for growth in children. If a child fails to grow normally because his or her body is not producing enough GH, this substance may be used to stimulate growth. The analogs of GH are called somatrem and somatropin. Athletes use GH and its analogs in the same manner as anabolic steroids. They believe that these substances will increase strength and muscle mass, stimulate growth, and strengthen the tendons and ligaments. Because it acts on the pituitary gland, however, GH stimulates the growth of other tissues and organs as well. This can result in very dangerous side effects. These effects can include the development of diabetes; abnormal growth of the bones and internal organs such as the heart, kidneys, and liver; hardening of the arteries; and high blood pressure. Leukemia has also been reported in several short-stature children who were treated with GH.

GH, and other analogs with similar effects, such as chorionic gonadotropin and corticotropin (ACTH), and growth hormone releasing factor, are banned by the NCAA and USOC.

Erythropoietin (EPO) is produced by the body (mainly in the kidneys) and causes the bone marrow to produce red blood cells. **Epoetin** is a man-made version of erythropoietin, and is used to treat or prevent anemia (a disease caused by a lack of red blood cells). Athletes take epoetin to increase levels of red blood cells in hopes of increasing their endurance. With use of these substances, however, the athlete's red blood cell concentration may rise above acceptable and safe levels. The thickening of the blood that can result may cause blood clotting, stroke, and heart failure. There is also evidence that links the use of epoetin to the heart attack-related deaths of several endurance athletes. Use of epoetin in this manner is equivalent to blood doping, and is banned by both the NCAA and USOC.

Anabolic Steroids:

Anabolic steroids are analogs of **testosterone**, a naturally produced male sex hormone (an androgen) that stimulates the growth of reproductive and body tissue, protein synthesis, and the development of male traits. Accepted medical uses for these drugs include helping patients gain weight following a severe illness, injury, or continuing infection, if they have failed to gain or maintain normal weight, or for patients with AIDS wasting syndrome; as well as treatment of certain types of anemia, certain kinds of breast cancer (in women), and hereditary angioedema.

Athletes take anabolic steroids because they believe that these drugs will increase the growth and development of muscle mass and strength. Whether steroids produce these effects is a subject of debate in the medical and athletic communities, and has yet to be definitely proven or disproven. When used for this purpose, however, steroids are usually taken in dangerously high doses that can exceed recommended doses by ten to one-hundred times.

When taken in very high doses, steroids often have serious and sometimes permanent side effects that include tumors of the liver, liver cancer, and liver disease; as well as premature heart disease. Steroid use in young males may result in stunted growth; enlarged penis; increased frequency of erections; severe acne; unnatural hair growth; and unexplained darkening of the skin. In adult males, side effects can include enlargement of breasts or breast soreness; enlargement of the prostate gland; frequent or continuing erections; frequent urge to urinate; increased and inappropriate aggessiveness and sexual appetite ("roid rage"); kidney dysfunction; premature baldness; and reduction of the testicles. Adult females may be subject to side effects that include abnormal menstrual cycles; enlargement of the clitoris; and the development of masculine traits such as deepening of the voice, unnatural hair growth on the face and body, and/or hair loss.

The following androgens and anabolic steroids are banned by the NCAA and/or USOC (listed by generic name):

- Fluoxymesterone (e.g., Halotestin)
- Methyltestosterone (e.g., Oreton)
- Nandrolone (e.g., Durabolin)
- Oxandrolone (e.g., Anavar)
- Oxymetholone (e.g., Anadrol)
- Stanozolol (e.g., Winstrol)

Other Banned Classes and Substances:

Some recreational drugs, such as **marijuana** and **heroin,** are banned by the NCAA. Because these substances are not believed to improve performance, they are not banned by the USOC (although marijuana is banned by the national governing bodies of some sports). **Cocaine,** which some may consider a recreational drug, is banned as a stimulant and local anesthetic by the NCAA and USOC. Several other drugs, such as **LSD, PCP, mescaline,** and **angel dust,** are not believed to improve performance and are not banned. Both the NCAA and USOC, however, strongly discourage the use of these substances. **Alcohol** is banned for all riflery events by the NCAA, but is not banned by the USOC (it may be banned by national governing bodies of particular sports, such as the rifle events). Use of any **tobacco** product on the field of play is banned in NCAA championship events (baseball dugouts are considered to be in the field of play).

Corticosteroids are anti-inflammatory drugs that may be produced by the body or man-made. Corticosteroids are not banned by the NCAA. However, corticosteroids that you take by mouth or inject into the muscle or vein are banned by the USOC. Use of topical and inhaled corticosteroids is not banned by the USOC. Local or intra-articular injections of these substances for medical purposes is not banned. However, permission to compete while using them in this manner must be requested before the event by a letter from the team doctor, and granted by the USOC or International Olympic Committee (IOC) Medical Commission (whichever is responsible for testing at the particular event).

The following corticosteroids (when taken by mouth or injected) may be banned or require official permission for use by USOC athletes (listed by generic name):

- Betamethasone (e.g., Celestone)
- Corticotropin (e.g., Acthar)

- Cortisone (e.g., Cortone)
- Dexamethasone (e.g., Decadron)
- Hydrocortisone (e.g., Cortef, Solu-Cortef)
- Methylprednisolone (e.g., Depo-Medrol, Medrol)
- Paramethasone (e.g., Haldrone)
- Prednisolone (e.g., Delta-cortef, Hydeltrasol)
- Prednisone (e.g., Meticorten)
- Triamcinolone (e.g., Aristocort)

Certain types of **local anesthetics** may contain other drugs that are banned by the NCAA and USOC. The use of topical local anesthetics is permitted by both bodies, but there are certain restrictions placed upon their use by injection.

The following local anesthetics may be banned by the NCAA and/or USOC (listed by generic name):

- Bupivacaine (e.g., Marcaine)
- Chloroprocaine (e.g., Nesacaine)
- Cocaine
- Etidocaine (e.g., Duranest-MPF)
- Lidocaine (e.g., Xylocaine)
- Mepivacaine (e.g., Carbocaine)
- Prilocaine (e.g., Citanest Plain)
- Procaine (e.g., Novocain)
- Propoxycaine and Procaine (e.g., Ravocaine and Novocain with Neo-Cobefrin)

Note: The lists of drugs that are included above are unofficial and are not meant to be used as a substitute for NCAA and/or USOC banned substance information. The only way to be sure if a substance is banned for a particular sport or event is to consult the appropriate governing body.

Index

Brand names are in *italics*. There are many brands and different manufacturers of drugs and the listing of selected American and Canadian brand names and manufacturers is intended only for ease of reference. There are additional brands and manufacturers that have not been included. The inclusion of a brand name does not mean the USPC has any particular knowledge that the brand listed has properties different from other brands of the same drug, nor should it be interpreted as an endorsement by the USPC. Similarly, the fact that a particular brand has not been included does not indicate that the product has been judged to be unsatisfactory or unacceptable. The page numbers MC-1 to MC-24 refer to the product identification photographs in The Medicine Chart (Appendix VI).

A

B

C

D

E

F

G

I

J

K

L

M

N

O

P

Q

R

S

T

U

V

W

X

Y

Z